2025

ICD-10-CM
FOR PHYSICIANS

Jackie L. Koesterman, CPC
Coding and Reimbursement Specialist
JDK Medical Coding EDU
Grand Forks, North Dakota

BUCK'S

INCLUDES
NETTER'S
ANATOMY
ART

ELSEVIER

Elsevier
3251 Riverport Lane
St. Louis, Missouri 63043

BUCK'S 2025 ICD-10-CM FOR PHYSICIANS   ISBN: 978-0-443-26151-0

Notice

Practitioners and researchers must always rely on their own experience and knowledge in evaluating and using any information, methods, compounds or experiments described herein. Because of rapid advances in the medical sciences, in particular, independent verification of diagnoses and drug dosages should be made. To the fullest extent of the law, no responsibility is assumed by Elsevier, authors, editors or contributors for any injury and/or damage to persons or property as a matter of products liability, negligence or otherwise, or from any use or operation of any methods, products, instructions, or ideas contained in the material herein.

Previous editions copyrighted 2024, 2023, 2022, 2021, 2020, 2019, 2018, 2017, 2016, 2015, 2014, 2013, 2010

International Standard Book Number: 978-0-443-26151-0

Senior Content Strategist: Luke Held
Content Development Manager: Danielle Frazier
Senior Content Development Specialist: Joshua S. Rapplean
Publishing Services Manager: Deepthi Unni
Project Manager: Nayagi Anandan
Senior Book Designer: Maggie Reid

Printed in Canada

Last digit is the print number: 9 8 7 6 5 4 3 2 1

 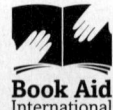

Working together
to grow libraries in
developing countries

www.elsevier.com • www.bookaid.org

DEDICATION

To all who require of themselves the highest level of accuracy, integrity, and professionalism. You enhance our profession and are a tremendous asset to health care. May this manual be of assistance to you.

With Greatest Admiration.

Carol J. Buck, MS

DEVELOPMENT OF THIS EDITION

Lead Technical Collaborator

Jackie L. Koesterman, CPC
Coding and Reimbursement Specialist
JDK Medical Coding EDU
Grand Forks, North Dakota

Query Team

Patricia Cordy Henricksen, MS, CHCA, CPC-I, CPC, CCP-P, ASC-PM
AAPC-Approved Instructor
Auditing, Coding, and Education Specialist
Soterion Medical Services
Lexington, Kentucky

CONTENTS

GUIDE TO USING THE 2025 ICD-10-CM FOR PHYSICIANS

Medical coding has long been a part of the health care profession. Through the years medical coding systems have become more complex and extensive. Today, medical coding is an intricate and immense process that is present in every health care setting. The increased use of electronic submissions for health care services only increases the need for coders who understand the coding process.

2025 ICD-10-CM for Physicians, Professional Edition was developed to help meet the needs of coding professionals at all levels by offering a comprehensive coding text at a reasonable price.

All material strictly adheres to the latest government versions available at the time of publication. Updates from the *Definitions of Medicare Code Edits* (MCE) will be posted to the companion website (www.codingupdates.com) when available.

Illustrations and Items

The ICD-10-CM Tabular List contains illustrations, pictures, and items to assist you in understanding difficult terminology, diseases/conditions, or coding in a specific category. Items are always shaded with ███████ ink so that the added material is not mistaken for official notations or instructions. ████████ shading is used for other annotations in the text. Your ideas on what other descriptions or illustrations should be in future editions of this text are always appreciated.

Instructional Notations

Includes Notes

Includes

The word "Includes" appears immediately under certain categories to further define, or give examples of, the content of the category.

Excludes Notes

The ICD-10-CM has two types of excludes notes. Each note has a different definition for use, but they are both similar in that they indicate that codes excluded from each other are independent of each other.

Excludes1

A type 1 Excludes note is a pure excludes. It means "NOT CODED HERE!" An Excludes1 note indicates that the code excluded should never be used at the same time as the code above the Excludes1 note. An Excludes1 is for use when two conditions cannot occur together, such as a congenital form versus an acquired form of the same condition.

Excludes2

A type 2 Excludes note represents "NOT INCLUDED HERE." An Excludes2 note indicates that the condition excluded is not part of the condition it is excluded from, but a patient may have both conditions at the same time. When an Excludes2 note appears under a code, it is acceptable to use both the code and the excluded code together.

Code First/Use Additional Code notes (etiology/manifestation paired codes)

Certain conditions have both an underlying etiology and multiple body system manifestations due to the underlying etiology. For such conditions the ICD-10-CM has a coding convention that requires the underlying condition be sequenced first, followed by the manifestation. Wherever such a combination exists, there is a "use additional code" note at the etiology code, and a "code first" note at the manifestation code. These instructional notes indicate the proper sequencing order of the codes, etiology followed by manifestation.

In most cases the manifestation codes will have in the code title, "in diseases classified elsewhere." Codes with this title are a component of the etiology/manifestation convention. The code title indicates that it is a manifestation code. "In diseases classified elsewhere" codes are never permitted to be used as first-listed or principal diagnosis codes. They must be used in conjunction with an underlying condition code, and they must be listed following the underlying condition.

Use additional

The words indicate an instructional note that another code may be needed.

Code first

The words indicate an instructional note that directs the coder to sequence the underlying condition before the manifestation.

Code also

A "code also" note instructs that two codes may be required to fully describe a condition, but the sequencing of the two codes is discretionary, depending on the severity of the conditions and the reason for the encounter.

7th characters and placeholder X

For codes less than 6 characters that require a 7th character, a placeholder X should be assigned for all characters less than 6. The 7th character must always be the 7th character of a code.

Annotated

Throughout the manual, revisions, additions, and deleted codes or words are indicated by the following symbols:

⇒ **Revised:** Revisions within the line or code from the previous edition are indicated by the arrow.

▶ **New:** Additions to the previous edition are indicated by the triangle.

~~deleted~~ **Deleted:** Deletions from the previous edition are struck through.

ICD-10-CM Tabular List Symbols

● **Use Additional Character(s):** The red stop sign cautions that the code requires additional character(s) to ensure the greatest specificity.

X For codes less than 6 characters that require a 7th character, a placeholder X should be assigned for all characters less than 6. The 7th character must always be the 7th character of a code.

OGCR The *Official Guidelines for Coding and Reporting* symbol includes the placement of a portion of a guideline as that guideline pertains to the code by which it is located. The complete OGCR are located in Part I.

🔧 The **Hierarchical condition category (HCC)** was initiated in 2004 for the reimbursement for patients with Medicare Advantage plans (Medicare Part C). HCC is based on a list of chronic or severity of illness diagnosis codes that CMS uses to determine reimbursements to Medicare Advantage plans. The HCC risk adjustment factor data is calculated for an entire year for encounters of the patient's care.

▶ **Manifestation Code:** Describes the manifestation of an underlying disease, not the disease itself, and therefore should not be assigned as a principal diagnosis, according to the *Definitions of Medicare Code Edits* (MCE).

Age conflict: The *Definitions of Medicare Code Edits* (MCE) detects inconsistencies between a patient's age and diagnosis. For example, a 5-year-old patient with benign prostatic hypertrophy or a 78-year-old pregnant female.

The diagnosis is clinically and virtually impossible in a patient of the stated age. Therefore, either the diagnosis or the age is presumed to be incorrect. There are four age categories for diagnoses in the *Definitions of Medicare Code Edits* (MCE):

N • Newborn. Age of 0 years; a subset of diagnoses intended only for newborns and neonates (e.g., fetal distress, perinatal jaundice).

P • Pediatric. Age range is 0-17 years inclusive (e.g., Reye's syndrome, routine child health exam).

M • Maternity. Age range is 9-64 years inclusive (e.g., diabetes in pregnancy, antepartum pulmonary complication).

A • Adult. Age range is 15-124 years inclusive (e.g., senile delirium, mature cataract).

♀♂ **Sex conflict:** *Definitions of Medicare Code Edits* (MCE) detects inconsistencies between a patient's sex and any diagnosis or procedure on the patient's record. For example, a male patient with cervical cancer (diagnosis) or a female patient with a prostatectomy (procedure). In both instances, the indicated diagnosis or the procedure conflicts with the stated sex of the patient. Therefore, either the patient's diagnosis, procedure, or sex is presumed to be incorrect.

Key words

Highlight identifies key words within similar code descriptions in a particular category.

Coding Clinic Identifies the year, quarter, and page number that presents information about an ICD-10-CM code in the American Hospital Association's *Coding Clinic*® for ICD-10-CM.

Visit codingupdates.com for the full list of *2025* Present on Admission codes.

SYMBOLS AND CONVENTIONS

ICD-10-CM Tabular

Use Additional Character(s): The red stop sign cautions you that the code requires additional character(s) to ensure greatest specificity.

Volume 1, Tabular List

● **K22** **Other diseases of esophagus**
  Excludes2 esophageal varices (I85.-)

X● **V00.01** **Pedestrian on foot injured in collision with roller-skater**

A02.20 **Localized salmonella infection, unspecified**

Placeholder X: The red X reminds you that for codes less than 6 characters that require a 7th character, a placeholder X should be assigned to all characters less than 6.

Unspecified: These codes are for use when the information in the medical record is insufficient to assign a more specific code. For those categories for which an unspecified code is not provided, the "other specified" code may represent both other and unspecified.

Use additional code: Located at the etiology code and directs you to assign a manifestation code.

A48.3 **Toxic shock syndrome**
  Use additional code to identify the organism (B95, B96)

Code first indicates the etiology code is to be first-listed before the manifestation code.

B39 **Histoplasmosis**
  Code first associated AIDS (B20)

Notes define terms or give coding instructions.

E34.0 **Carcinoid syndrome**
  Note: May be used as an additional code to identify functional activity associated with a carcinoid tumor.

Codes or index entries are for purposes of illustration only and may not be current.

OGCR Section I.C.6.B.5.

Neoplasm Related Pain Code G89.3 is assigned to pain documented as being related, associated or due to cancer, primary or secondary malignancy, or tumor. This code is assigned regardless of whether the pain is acute or chronic.

OGCR: The *Official Guidelines for Coding and Reporting* are placed near the codes to which they refer and are highlighted.

I70.2 **Atherosclerosis of native arteries of the extremities**
Mönckeberg's (medial) sclerosis

Use additional code, if applicable, to identify chronic total occlusion of artery of extremity (I70.92)

code, if applicable, directs the coder to other conditions that may be appropriate to report.

I74 **Arterial embolism and thrombosis**
Includes   embolic infarction
embolic occlusion
thrombotic infarction
thrombotic occlusion

The word "and" should be interpreted to mean either "and" or "or" when it appears in a statement.

Bold typeface is used on all codes and titles.

I83.001 **Varicose veins of unspecified lower extremity with ulcer of thigh**

"with" should be interpreted to mean "associated with" or "due to."

K73.2 **Chronic active hepatitis, not elsewhere classified**

"not elsewhere classified" or **NEC** identifies a code that is assigned only when the information at hand specifies a condition for which no more specific code is available.

"not otherwise specified" or **NOS** is equivalent to unspecified.

W13.9 **Fall from, out of or through building, not otherwise specified**

Codes or index entries are for purposes of illustration only and may not be current.

Excludes1 means "NOT CODED HERE!" An Excludes1 note indicates that the code excluded should never be assigned at the same time as the code above the Excludes1 note.

Includes: This note appears immediately under a three-character code title to further define, or give examples of, the content.

Codes titled "other" or "other specified" are for use when the information in the medical record provides detail for which a specific code does not exist.

Pediatric Age, Ø-17, according to the *Definitions of Medicare Code Edits* (MCE).

Females Only according to the *Definitions of Medicare Code Edits* (MCE).

M19 **Other and unspecified osteoarthritis**
  Excludes1 polyarthritis (M15.-)
  Excludes2 arthrosis of spine (M47.-)
            hallux rigidus (M20.2)
            osteoarthritis of spine (M47.-)

A06 **Amebiasis**
  Includes infection due to Entamoeba histolytica

E26.01 **Conn's syndrome**
       Code also adrenal adenoma (D35.0)

E25.8 **Other adrenogenital disorders**

O00.2 **Ovarian pregnancy** M

P02.20 **Newborn (suspected to be) affected by unspecified morphological and functional abnormalities of placenta** N

L21.0 **Seborrhea capitis** P
       Cradle cap

G30.1 **Alzheimer's disease with late onset** A

B37.3 **Candidiasis of vulva and vagina** ♀

C60.1 **Malignant neoplasm of glans penis** ♂

Excludes2 represents "NOT INCLUDED HERE." An Excludes2 note indicates that the condition excluded is not part of the condition represented by the code, but a patient may have both conditions at the same time and it is acceptable to use both the code and the excluded code together, when appropriate.

Code also instructs that two codes may be required to fully describe a condition, but this note does not provide sequencing direction.

Maternity DX (Diagnosis) for ages 9-64 according to the *Definitions of Medicare Code Edits* (MCE).

Newborn, Age Ø, according to the *Definitions of Medicare Code Edits* (MCE).

Adult Age, 15-124, according to the *Definitions of Medicare Code Edits* (MCE).

Males Only according to the *Definitions of Medicare Code Edits* (MCE).

Codes or index entries are for purposes of illustration only and may not be current.

Manifestation according to the *Definitions of Medicare Code Edits* (MCE).

▶H22 *Disorders of iris and ciliary body in diseases classified elsewhere*

Code first underlying disease, such as:
gout (M1A-, M10.-)

Key Term Highlight identifies key words within similar code descriptions in a particular category.

F10.21   Alcohol dependence, **in remission** ◀

Coding Clinic identifies the year, quarter, and page number that presents information about an ICD-10-PCS code in the American Hospital Association's *Coding Clinic®*.

B96.5   Pseudomonas (aeruginosa) (mallei) (pseudomallei) as the cause of diseases classified elsewhere
▶ Coding Clinic: 2015, Q1, P18

Codes or index entries are for purposes of illustration only and may not be current.

Alphabetic Index

Main terms are in **bold** typeface.

Aberrant (congenital) —*see also* Malposition, congenital
adrenal gland Q89.1

Etiology code first followed by the manifestation code in **brackets**. The code in brackets is always to be sequenced second.

Amyloid heart (disease) E85.4 *[I43]*

Amylophagia —*see* Pica

"**see**" indicates another term should be referenced.

Angiofibroma —*see also* Neoplasm, benign, by site

"**see also**" follows a main term and instructs that there is another main term that may also be referenced.

Appendicitis (pneumococcal) (retrocecal) K37
    with
        perforation NOS K35.32
        peritoneal abscess K35.33

A default code is listed next to the main term and represents that condition most commonly associated with the main term. If a condition is documented in a medical record without any additional information, such as acute or chronic, the default code should be assigned.

Use Additional Character(s): The red stop sign cautions you that the code requires additional character(s) to ensure greatest specificity.

Abrasion T14.8
    ankle S90.51-●

Codes or index entries are for purposes of illustration only and may not be current.

No Change	**CHAPTER 1**	
No Change	**CERTAIN INFECTIOUS AND PARASITIC DISEASES (A00-B99)**	

INTESTINAL INFECTIOUS DISEASES (A00-A09)

No Change	**A04**	Other bacterial intestinal infections
No Change		A04.7 Enterocolitis due to Clostridium difficile
Add		Clostridioides difficile colitis

TUBERCULOSIS (A15-A19)

No Change	**A18**	Tuberculosis of other organs
No Change		A18.4 Tuberculosis of skin and subcutaneous tissue
Revise from		Lupus excedens
		Lupus exedens

INFECTIONS WITH A PREDOMINANTLY SEXUAL MODE OF TRANSMISSION (A50-A64)

No Change	**A50**	Congenital syphilis
No Change		A50.4 Late congenital neurosyphilis [juvenile neurosyphilis]
No Change		A50.45 Juvenile general paresis
Revise from		Juvenile tabetoparetic neurosyphilis
		Juvenile taboparetic neurosyphilis

RICKETTSIOSES (A75-A79)

No Change	**A77**	Spotted fever [tick-borne rickettsioses]
No Change		A77.4 Ehrlichiosis
Revise from		A77.41 Ehrlichiosis chafeensis [E. chafeensis]
		A77.41 Ehrlichiosis chaffeensis [E. chaffeensis]

No Change	**CHAPTER 2**	
No Change	**NEOPLASMS (C00-D49)**	

MALIGNANT NEOPLASMS OF BREAST (C50)

No Change	**C50**	Malignant neoplasm of breast
No Change		Use Additional
Revise from		code to identify estrogen receptor status (Z17.0, Z17.1)
		code to identify estrogen, and other hormones and factors receptor status (Z17.-)

MALIGNANT NEUROENDOCRINE TUMORS (C7A)

No Change	**C7A**	Malignant neuroendocrine tumors
No Change		Use Additional
Revise from		carcinoid syndrome (E34.0)
		carcinoid syndrome (E34.00)

MALIGNANT NEOPLASMS OF LYMPHOID, HEMATOPOIETIC AND RELATED TISSUE (C81-C96)

No Change	**C81**	Hodgkin lymphoma
No Change		C81.0 Nodular lymphocyte predominant Hodgkin lymphoma
Add		C81.0A Nodular lymphocyte predominant Hodgkin lymphoma, in remission
No Change		C81.1 Nodular sclerosis Hodgkin lymphoma
Add		C81.1A Nodular sclerosis Hodgkin lymphoma, in remission
No Change		C81.2 Mixed cellularity Hodgkin lymphoma
Add		C81.2A Mixed cellularity Hodgkin lymphoma, in remission
No Change		C81.3 Lymphocyte depleted Hodgkin lymphoma
Add		C81.3A Lymphocyte depleted Hodgkin lymphoma, in remission
No Change		C81.4 Lymphocyte-rich Hodgkin lymphoma
Add		C81.4A Lymphocyte-rich Hodgkin lymphoma, in remission
No Change		C81.7 Other Hodgkin lymphoma
Add		C81.7A Other Hodgkin lymphoma, in remission
No Change		C81.9 Hodgkin lymphoma, unspecified
Add		C81.9A Hodgkin lymphoma, unspecified, in remission
No Change	**C82**	Follicular lymphoma
No Change		C82.0 Follicular lymphoma grade I
Add		C82.0A Follicular lymphoma grade I, in remission
No Change		C82.1 Follicular lymphoma grade II
Add		C82.1A Follicular lymphoma grade II, in remission
No Change		C82.2 Follicular lymphoma grade III, unspecified
Add		C82.2A Follicular lymphoma grade III, unspecified, in remission
No Change		C82.3 Follicular lymphoma grade IIIa
Add		C82.3A Follicular lymphoma grade IIIa, in remission
No Change		C82.4 Follicular lymphoma grade IIIb
Add		C82.4A Follicular lymphoma grade IIIb, in remission
No Change		C82.5 Diffuse follicle center lymphoma
Add		C82.5A Diffuse follicle center lymphoma, in remission
No Change		C82.6 Cutaneous follicle center lymphoma
Add		C82.6A Cutaneous follicle center lymphoma, in remission
No Change		C82.8 Other types of follicular lymphoma
Add		C82.8A Other types of follicular lymphoma, in remission
No Change		C82.9 Follicular lymphoma, unspecified
Add		C82.9A Follicular lymphoma, unspecified, in remission

No Change	**C83**	**Non-follicular lymphoma**	
No Change		**C83.0**	**Small cell B-cell lymphoma**
No Change		**Excludes1**	
			Waldenström macroglobulinemia (C88.0)
			Waldenström macroglobulinemia (C88.00)
Add		**C83.0A**	**Small cell B-cell lymphoma, in remission**
No Change		**C83.1**	**Mantle cell lymphoma**
Add		**C83.1A**	**Mantle cell lymphoma, in remission**
Add			Centrocytic lymphoma, in remission
No Change		**C83.3**	**Diffuse large B-cell lymphoma**
Add			Diffuse large B-cell lymphoma, subtype not specified
No Change			**C83.39** **Diffuse large B-cell lymphoma, extranodal and solid organ sites**
Add			**C83.390** **Primary central nervous system lymphoma**
Add			PCNSL of brain
Add			PCNSL of meninges
Add			PCNSL of spinal cord
Add			PCNSL NOS
Add			**Excludes1** Primary central nervous system lymphoma, Burkitt (C83.79)
Add			Primary central nervous system lymphoma, lymphoblastic (C83.59)
Add			Primary central nervous system lymphoma, other (C83.89)
Add			Primary central nervous system lymphoma, peripheral T-cell (C84.49)
Add			**C83.398** **Diffuse large B-cell lymphoma of other extranodal and solid organ sites**
Add		**C83.3A**	**Diffuse large B-cell lymphoma, in remission**
No Change		**C83.5**	**Lymphoblastic (diffuse) lymphoma**
		C83.5A	**Lymphoblastic (diffuse) lymphoma, in remission**
No Change		**C83.7**	**Burkitt lymphoma**
		C83.7A	**Burkitt lymphoma, in remission**
No Change		**C83.8**	**Other non-follicular lymphoma**
		C83.8A	**Other non-follicular lymphoma, in remission**
No Change		**C83.9**	**Non-follicular (diffuse) lymphoma, unspecified**
		C83.9A	**Non-follicular (diffuse) lymphoma, unspecified, in remission**
No Change	**C84**	**Mature T/NK-cell lymphomas**	
No Change		**C84.0**	**Mycosis fungoides**
		C84.0A	**Mycosis fungoides, in remission**
No Change		**C84.1**	**Sézary disease**
		C84.1A	**Sézary disease, in remission**
No Change		**C84.4**	**Peripheral T-cell lymphoma, not elsewhere classified**
Add			**C84.4A** **Peripheral T-cell lymphoma, not elsewhere classified, in remission**
No Change		**C84.6**	**Anaplastic large cell lymphoma, ALK-positive**
Add			**C84.6A** **Anaplastic large cell lymphoma, ALK-positive, in remission**
No Change		**C84.7**	**Anaplastic large cell lymphoma, ALK-negative**
Add			**C84.7B** **Anaplastic large cell lymphoma, ALK-negative, in remission**
No Change		**C84.A**	**Cutaneous T-cell lymphoma, unspecified**
Add			**C84.AA** **Cutaneous T-cell lymphoma, unspecified, in remission**
No Change		**C84.Z**	**Other mature T/NK-cell lymphomas**
		Excludes1	
Revise from			angioimmunoblastic T-cell lymphoma (C86.5)
Revise to			angioimmunoblastic T-cell lymphoma (C86.50)
Revise from			blastic NK-cell lymphoma (C86.4)
Revise to			blastic NK-cell lymphoma (C86.40)
Revise from			enteropathy-type T-cell lymphoma (C86.2)
Revise to			enteropathy-type T-cell lymphoma (C86.20)
Revise from			extranodal NK-cell lymphoma, nasal type (C86.0)
Revise to			extranodal NK-cell lymphoma, nasal type (C86.00)
Revise from			hepatosplenic T-cell lymphoma (C86.1)
Revise to			hepatosplenic T-cell lymphoma (C86.10)
Revise from			primary cutaneous CD30-positive T-cell proliferations (C86.6)
Revise to			primary cutaneous CD30-positive T-cell proliferations (C86.60)
Revise from			subcutaneous panniculitis-like T-cell lymphoma (C86.3)
Revise to			subcutaneous panniculitis-like T-cell lymphoma (C86.30)
Add			**C84.ZA** **Other mature T/NK-cell lymphomas, in remission**
No Change		**C84.9**	**Mature T/NK-cell lymphomas, unspecified**
Add			**C84.9A** **Mature T/NK-cell lymphomas, unspecified, in remission**
No Change	**C85**	**Other specified and unspecified types of non-Hodgkin lymphoma**	
No Change		**C85.1**	**Unspecified B-cell lymphoma**
Add			**C85.1A** **Unspecified B-cell lymphoma, in remission**
No Change		**C85.2**	**Mediastinal (thymic) large B-cell lymphoma**
Add			**C85.2A** **Mediastinal (thymic) large B-cell lymphoma, in remission**
No Change		**C85.8**	**Other specified types of non-Hodgkin lymphoma**
Add			**C85.8A** **Other specified types of non-Hodgkin lymphoma, in remission**
No Change		**C85.9**	**Non-Hodgkin lymphoma, unspecified**
Add			**C85.9A** **Non-Hodgkin lymphoma, unspecified, in remission**

No Change	C86	**Other specified types of T/NK-cell lymphoma**
No Change	C86.0	**Extranodal NK/T-cell lymphoma, nasal type**
Add	C86.00	**Extranodal NK/T-cell lymphoma, nasal type not having achieved remission**
Add		Extranodal NK/T-cell lymphoma, nasal type NOS
Add		Extranodal NK/T-cell lymphoma, nasal type with failed remission
Add	C86.01	**Extranodal NK/T-cell lymphoma, nasal type, in remission**
No Change	C86.1	**Hepatosplenic T-cell lymphoma**
Add	C86.10	**Hepatosplenic T-cell lymphoma not having achieved remission**
Add		Hepatosplenic T-cell lymphoma NOS
Add		Hepatosplenic T-cell lymphoma with failed remission
Add	C86.11	**Hepatosplenic T-cell lymphoma, in remission**
No Change	C86.2	**Enteropathy-type (intestinal) T-cell lymphoma**
Add	C86.20	**Enteropathy-type (intestinal) T-cell lymphoma not having achieved remission**
Add		Enteropathy associated T-cell lymphoma NOS
Add		Enteropathy associated T-cell lymphoma not having achieved remission
Add		Enteropathy associated T-cell lymphoma with failed remission
Add		Enteropathy-type (intestinal) T-cell lymphoma NOS
Add		Enteropathy-type (intestinal) T-cell lymphoma with failed remission
Add	C86.21	**Enteropathy-type (intestinal) T-cell lymphoma, in remission**
Add		Enteropathy associated T-cell lymphoma, in remission
No Change	C86.3	**Subcutaneous panniculitis-like T-cell lymphoma**
Add	C86.30	**Subcutaneous panniculitis-like T-cell lymphoma not having achieved remission**
Add		Subcutaneous panniculitis-like T-cell lymphoma NOS
Add		Subcutaneous panniculitis-like T-cell lymphoma with failed remission
	C86.31	**Subcutaneous panniculitis-like T-cell lymphoma, in remission**
No Change	C86.4	**Blastic NK-cell lymphoma**
Add	C86.40	**Blastic NK-cell lymphoma not having achieved remission**
Add		Blastic NK-cell lymphoma NOS
Add		Blastic NK-cell lymphoma with failed remission
Add		Blastic plasmacytoid dendritic cell neoplasm (BPDCN) NOS
Add		Blastic plasmacytoid dendritic cell neoplasm (BPDCN) not having achieved remission
Add		Blastic plasmacytoid dendritic cell neoplasm (BPDCN) with failed remission
Add	C86.41	**Blastic NK-cell lymphoma, in remission**
Add		Blastic plasmacytoid dendritic cell neoplasm (BPDCN), in remission

No Change	C86.5	**Angioimmunoblastic T-cell lymphoma**
Add	C86.50	**Angioimmunoblastic T-cell lymphoma not having achieved remission**
Add		Angioimmunoblastic lymphadenopathy with dysproteinemia (AILD) NOS
Add		Angioimmunoblastic lymphadenopathy with dysproteinemia (AILD) not having achieved remission
Add		Angioimmunoblastic lymphadenopathy with dysproteinemia (AILD) with failed remission
Add		Angioimmunoblastic T-cell lymphoma NOS
Add		Angioimmunoblastic T-cell lymphoma with failed remission
Add	C86.51	**Angioimmunoblastic T-cell lymphoma, in remission**
Add		Angioimmunoblastic lymphadenopathy with dysproteinemia (AILD), in remission
No Change	C86.6	**Primary cutaneous CD30-positive T-cell proliferations**
Add	C86.60	**Primary cutaneous CD30-positive T-cell proliferations not having achieved remission**
Add		Lymphomatoid papulosis NOS
Add		Lymphomatoid papulosis not having achieved remission
Add		Lymphomatoid papulosis with failed remission
Add		Primary cutaneous anaplastic large cell lymphoma NOS
Add		Primary cutaneous anaplastic large cell lymphoma not having achieved remission
Add		Primary cutaneous anaplastic large cell lymphoma with failed remission
Add		Primary cutaneous CD30-positive large T-cell lymphoma NOS
Add		Primary cutaneous CD30-positive large T-cell lymphoma not having achieved remission
Add		Primary cutaneous CD30-positive large T-cell lymphoma with failed remission
Add		Primary cutaneous CD30-positive T-cell proliferations NOS
Add		Primary cutaneous CD30-positive T-cell proliferations with failed remission
Add	C86.61	**Primary cutaneous CD30-positive T-cell proliferations, in remission**
No Change	C88	**Malignant immunoproliferative diseases and certain other B-cell lymphomas**
No Change	C88.0	**Waldenström macroglobulinemia**
Add	C88.00	**Waldenström macroglobulinemia not having achieved remission**
Add		Lymphoplasmacytic lymphoma with IgM-production, NOS
Add		Lymphoplasmacytic lymphoma with IgM-production not having achieved remission
Add		Lymphoplasmacytic lymphoma with IgM-production with failed remission
Add		Macroglobulinemia (idiopathic) (primary) NOS
Add		Macroglobulinemia (idiopathic) (primary) not having achieved remission
Add		Macroglobulinemia (idiopathic) (primary) with failed remission
Add		Waldenström macroglobulinemia NOS
Add		Waldenström macroglobulinemia with failed remission
Add	C88.01	**Waldenström macroglobulinemia, in remission**

No Change		C88.2	Heavy chain disease
Add		C88.20	Heavy chain disease not having achieved remission
Add			Franklin disease NOS
Add			Franklin disease not having achieved remission
Add			Franklin disease with failed remission
Add			Gamma heavy chain disease NOS
Add			Gamma heavy chain disease not having achieved remission
Add			Gamma heavy chain disease with failed remission
Add			Heavy chain disease NOS
			Heavy chain disease with failed remissionMu heavy chain disease not having achieved remission
Add			Mu heavy chain disease NOS
Add			Mu heavy chain disease not having achieved remission
Add			Mu heavy chain disease with failed remission
Add		C88.21	Heavy chain disease, in remission
No Change	C88.3		Immunoproliferative small intestinal disease
Add		C88.30	Immunoproliferative small intestinal disease not having achieved remission
Add			Alpha heavy chain disease NOS
Add			Alpha heavy chain disease not having achieved remission
Add			Alpha heavy chain disease with failed remission
Add			Immunoproliferative small intestinal disease NOS
Add			Immunoproliferative small intestinal disease with failed remission
Add			Mediterranean lymphoma NOS
Add			Mediterranean lymphoma not having achieved remission
Add			Mediterranean lymphoma with failed remission
Add		C88.31	Immunoproliferative small intestinal disease, in remission
No Change	C88.4		Extranodal marginal zone B-cell lymphoma of mucosa-associated lymphoid tissue [MALT-lymphoma]
Add		C88.40	Extranodal marginal zone B-cell lymphoma of mucosa-associated lymphoid tissue [MALT-lymphoma] not having achieved remission
Add			Extranodal marginal zone B-cell lymphoma of mucosa-associated lymphoid tissue [MALT-lymphoma] NOS
Add			Extranodal marginal zone B-cell lymphoma of mucosa-associated lymphoid tissue [MALT-lymphoma] with failed remission
Add			Lymphoma of bronchial-associated lymphoid tissue [BALT-lymphoma] NOS
Add			Lymphoma of bronchial-associated lymphoid tissue [BALT-lymphoma] not having achieved remission
Add			Lymphoma of bronchial-associated lymphoid tissue [BALT-lymphoma] with failed remission
Add			Lymphoma of skin-associated lymphoid tissue [SALT-lymphoma] NOS
Add			Lymphoma of skin-associated lymphoid tissue [SALT-lymphoma] not having achieved remission
Add			Lymphoma of skin-associated lymphoid tissue [SALT-lymphoma] with failed remission

Add		C88.41	Extranodal marginal zone B-cell lymphoma of mucosa-associated lymphoid tissue [MALT-lymphoma], in remission
No Change	C88.8		Other malignant immunoproliferative diseases
Add		C88.80	Other malignant immunoproliferative diseases not having achieved remission
Add			Other malignant immunoproliferative diseases NOS
Add			Other malignant immunoproliferative diseases with failed remission
Add		C88.81	Other malignant immunoproliferative diseases, in remission
No Change	C88.9		Malignant immunoproliferative disease, unspecified
Add		C88.90	Malignant immunoproliferative disease, unspecified not having achieved remission
Add			Immunoproliferative disease NOS
Add			Immunoproliferative disease NOS not having achieved remission
Add			Immunoproliferative disease NOS with failed remission
Add			Malignant immunoproliferative disease, unspecified NOS
Add			Malignant immunoproliferative disease, unspecified with failed remission
Add		C88.91	Malignant immunoproliferative disease, unspecified, in remission

No Change			**IN SITU NEOPLASMS (D00-D09)**
No Change	D05		Carcinoma in situ of breast
Add		Excludes2	malignant neoplasm of breast (C50.-)

No Change			**BENIGN NEUROENDOCRINE TUMORS (D3A)**
No Change	D3A		Benign neuroendocrine tumors
No Change		Use Additional	
Revise from			carcinoid syndrome (E34.0)
Revise to			carcinoid syndrome (E34.00)

No Change **CHAPTER 3**

No Change

DISEASES OF THE BLOOD AND BLOOD-FORMING ORGANS AND CERTAIN DISORDERS INVOLVING THE IMMUNE MECHANISM (D50-D89)

No Change			**APLASTIC AND OTHER ANEMIAS AND OTHER BONE MARROW FAILURE SYNDROMES (D60-D64)**
No Change	D61		Other aplastic anemias and other bone marrow failure syndromes
No Change		D61.0	Constitutional aplastic anemia
Add		D61.03	Fanconi anemia
Add			Fanconi pancytopenia
Add			Fanconi's anemia
Add		Excludes1	Fanconi syndrome (E72.0-)
No Change		D61.09	Other constitutional aplastic anemia
Delete			Fanconi's anemia

No Change			**CERTAIN DISORDERS INVOLVING THE IMMUNE MECHANISM (D80-D89)**
No Change	D89		Other disorders involving the immune mechanism, not elsewhere classified
No Change		D89.8	Other specified disorders involving the immune mechanism, not elsewhere classified
No Change		D89.83	Cytokine release syndrome
Add			Use Additional code for adverse effect, if applicable, to identify immune checkpoint inhibitors and immunostimulant drugs (T45.AX5)

No Change	**CHAPTER 4**
No Change	**ENDOCRINE, NUTRITIONAL AND METABOLIC DISEASES (E00-E89)**

No Change		**DISORDERS OF THYROID GLAND (E00-E07)**
No Change **E07**		Other disorders of thyroid
No Change	**E07.1**	Dyshormogenetic goiter
Add		Dyshormonogenetic goiter
Add		Familial dyshormonogenetic goiter

No Change		**DIABETES MELLITUS (E08-E13)**

No Change **E08** Diabetes mellitus due to underlying condition

Add Use Additional injectable non-insulin antidiabetic drugs (Z79.85)

No Change **E08.6** Diabetes mellitus due to underlying condition with other specified complications

No Change **E08.64** Diabetes mellitus due to underlying condition with hypoglycemia

Add Use Additional code for hypoglycemia level, if applicable (E16.A-)

No Change **E09** Drug or chemical induced diabetes mellitus

Add Use Additional injectable non-insulin antidiabetic drugs (Z79.85)

No Change **E09.6** Drug or chemical induced diabetes mellitus with other specified complications

No Change **E09.64** Drug or chemical induced diabetes mellitus with hypoglycemia

Add Use Additional code for hypoglycemia level, if applicable (E16.A-)

No Change **E10** Type 1 diabetes mellitus

No Change **E10.6** Type 1 diabetes mellitus with other specified complications

No Change **E10.64** Type 1 diabetes mellitus with hypoglycemia

Add Use Additional code for hypoglycemia level, if applicable (E16.A-)

Add **E10.A** Type 1 diabetes mellitus, presymptomatic
Early-stage type 1 diabetes mellitus

Add **E10.A0** Type 1 diabetes mellitus, presymptomatic, unspecified

Add **E10.A1** Type 1 diabetes mellitus, presymptomatic, Stage 1
Multiple confirmed islet autoantibodies with normoglycemia

Add **E10.A2** Type 1 diabetes mellitus, presymptomatic, Stage 2

Add Confirmed islet autoimmunity with dysglycemia

No Change **E11** Type 2 diabetes mellitus

Add Use Additional injectable non-insulin antidiabetic drugs (Z79.85)

No Change **E11.6** Type 2 diabetes mellitus with other specified complications

No Change **E11.64** Type 2 diabetes mellitus with hypoglycemia

Add Use Additional code for hypoglycemia level, if applicable (E16.A-)

No Change **E13** Other specified diabetes mellitus

Add Use Additional injectable non-insulin antidiabetic drugs (Z79.85)

No Change **E13.6** Other specified diabetes mellitus with other specified complications

No Change **E13.64** Other specified diabetes mellitus with hypoglycemia

Add Use Additional code for hypoglycemia level, if applicable (E16.A-)

No Change **OTHER DISORDERS OF GLUCOSE REGULATION AND PANCREATIC INTERNAL SECRETION (E15-E16)**

No Change **E16** Other disorders of pancreatic internal secretion

No Change **E16.0** Drug-induced hypoglycemia without coma

No Change Use Additional

Delete code for adverse effect, if applicable, to identify drug (T36-T50 with fifth or sixth character 5)

Add code for hypoglycemia level, if applicable (E16.A-)

No Change **E16.1** Other hypoglycemia

Add Use Additional code for hypoglycemia level, if applicable (E16.A-)

No Change **E16.2** Hypoglycemia, unspecified

Add Use Additional code for hypoglycemia level, if applicable (E16.A-)

No Change **E16.A** Hypoglycemia level

Add **E16.A1** Hypoglycemia level 1
Add Decreased blood glucose level 1

Add **E16.A2** Hypoglycemia level 2
Add Decreased blood glucose level 2

Add **E16.A3** Hypoglycemia level 3
Add Decreased blood glucose level 3

No Change **DISORDERS OF OTHER ENDOCRINE GLANDS (E20-E35)**

No Change **E34** Other endocrine disorders

No Change **E34.0** Carcinoid syndrome

Delete **Note:** May be used as an Additional code to identify functional activity associated with a carcinoid tumor.

Add Code also the underlying disorder, such as:
Add primary neuroendocrine tumors (C7A.-)
Add secondary neuroendocrine tumors (C7B.-)

Add **E34.00** Carcinoid syndrome, unspecified
Add Carcinoid disease, unspecified

Add **E34.01** Carcinoid heart syndrome
Add Carcinoid heart disease
Add Hedinger syndrome

Add **E34.09** Other carcinoid syndrome
Add Carcinoid disease NEC
Add Carcinoid syndrome NEC
Add Other carcinoid disease

No Change **OVERWEIGHT, OBESITY AND OTHER HYPERALIMENTATION (E65-E68)**

No Change **E66** Overweight and obesity

No Change Use Additional

Revise from code to identify body mass index (BMI), if known (Z68.-)

Revise to code to identify body mass index (BMI), if known, for adults (Z68.1-Z68.45) or pediatrics (Z68.5-)

Delete **Excludes1** adiposogenital dystrophy (E23.6)
Delete lipomatosis NOS (E88.2)
Delete lipomatosis dolorosa [Dercum] (E88.2)
Delete Prader-Willi syndrome (Q87.11)

Add **Excludes2** adiposogenital dystrophy (E23.6)
Add lipomatosis dolorosa [Dercum] (E88.2)
Add lipomatosis NOS (E88.2)
Add Prader-Willi syndrome (Q87.11)

No Change **E66.8** Other obesity

Add **E66.81** Obesity class
Add **E66.811** Obesity, class 1
Add **E66.812** Obesity, class 2
Add **E66.813** Obesity, class 3

Add **E66.89** Other obesity not elsewhere classified

No Change		**METABOLIC DISORDERS (E70-E88)**
No Change **E74**		Other disorders of carbohydrate metabolism
No Change	**E74.8**	Other specified disorders of carbohydrate metabolism
Add		**E74.82** Disorders of citrate metabolism
Add		**E74.820** SLC13A5 Citrate Transporter Disorder
Add		**E74.829** Other disorders of citrate metabolism
No Change **E87**		Other disorders of fluid, electrolyte and acid-base balance
No Change	**E87.0**	Hyperosmolality and hypernatremia
Delete		**Excludes1** diabetes with hyperosmolarity (E08, E09, E11, E13 with final characters .00 or .01)
Add		**Excludes2** diabetes with hyperosmolarity (E08, E09, E11, E13 with final characters .00 or .01)
No Change **E88**		Other and unspecified metabolic disorders
No Change	**E88.0**	Disorders of plasma-protein metabolism, not elsewhere classified
No Change		**Excludes1**
Revise from		Waldenström macroglobulinemia (C88.0)
Revise to		Waldenström macroglobulinemia (C88.00)
No Change	**E88.8**	Other specified metabolic disorders
Add		**E88.82** Obesity due to disruption of MC4R pathway
Add		Use Additional code, if applicable, to identify associated manifestations, such as polyphagia (R63.2)
Add		Use Additional code to identify body mass index (BMI), if known (Z68.-)

No Change **CHAPTER 5**

No Change **MENTAL, BEHAVIORAL AND NEURODEVELOPMENTAL DISORDERS (F01-F99)**

No Change **MENTAL DISORDERS DUE TO KNOWN PHYSIOLOGICAL CONDITIONS (F01-F09)**

No Change **F01**		Vascular dementia
No Change		*Code first*
Delete		the underlying physiological condition or sequelae of cerebrovascular disease.
Add		, if applicable, any causal condition
No Change **F02**		Dementia in other diseases classified elsewhere
No Change		*Code first*
Delete		dementia with Lewy bodies (G31.83)
Delete		dementia with Parkinsonism (G31.83)
Add		neurocognitive disorder with Lewy bodies (G31.83)
Add		other frontotemporal neurocognitive disorder (G31.90)
No Change **F03**		Unspecified dementia
Delete		**Excludes1** senility NOS (R41.81)
No Change		**Excludes2**
Add		dementia with delirium or acute confusional state (F05)
Delete		senile dementia with delirium or acute confusional state (F05)

No Change **F06**		Other mental disorders due to known physiological condition
No Change		**Excludes1**
Revise from		unspecified dementia (F03)
Revise to		unspecified dementia (F03.-)
No Change	**F06.7**	Mild neurocognitive disorder due to known physiological condition
No Change		*Code first*
Delete		frontotemporal neurocognitive disorder (G31.09)
Add		other frontotemporal neurocognitive disorder (G31.09)
No Change		**Excludes1**
Revise from		dementia (F01.-, F02.-, F03)
Revise to		dementia (F01.-, F02.-, F03.-)

No Change **SCHIZOPHRENIA, SCHIZOTYPAL, DELUSIONAL, AND OTHER NON-MOOD PSYCHOTIC DISORDERS (F20-F29)**

No Change **F20**		Schizophrenia
Add		Use Additional code, if applicable, to identify:
Add		other specified cognitive deficit (R41.84-)

No Change **ANXIETY, DISSOCIATIVE, STRESS-RELATED, SOMATOFORM AND OTHER NONPSYCHOTIC MENTAL DISORDERS (F40-F48)**

No Change **F45**		Somatoform disorders
No Change	**F45.2**	Hypochondriacal disorders
No Change		**F45.22** Body dysmorphic disorder
Add		Bigorexia
Add		Muscle dysmorphia

No Change **BEHAVIORAL SYNDROMES ASSOCIATED WITH PHYSIOLOGICAL DISTURBANCES AND PHYSICAL FACTORS (F50-F59)**

No Change **F50**		Eating disorders
No Change	**F50.0**	Anorexia nervosa
No Change		**F50.01** Anorexia nervosa, restricting type
Add		**F50.010** Anorexia nervosa, restricting type, mild
Add		Anorexia nervosa, restricting type, with a body mass index greater than or equal to 17 kg/m2
Add		**F50.011** Anorexia nervosa, restricting type, moderate
Add		Anorexia nervosa, restricting type, with a body mass index of 16.0-16.99 kg/m2
Add		**F50.012** Anorexia nervosa, restricting type, severe
Add		Anorexia nervosa, restricting type, with a body mass index of 15.0-15.99 kg/m2
Add		**F50.013** Anorexia nervosa, restricting type, extreme
Add		Anorexia nervosa, restricting type, with a body mass index of less than 15.0 kg/m2
Add		**F50.014** Anorexia nervosa, restricting type, in remission
Add		Anorexia nervosa, restricting type, in full remission
Add		Anorexia nervosa, restricting type, in partial remission
Add		**F50.019** Anorexia nervosa, restricting type, unspecified

No Change		F50.02 Anorexia nervosa, binge eating/purging type
No Change		**Excludes1**
Revise from		bulimia nervosa (F50.2)
Revise to		bulimia nervosa (F50.2-)
Add		F50.020 **Anorexia nervosa, binge eating/purging type, mild**
Add		Anorexia nervosa, binge eating/purging type, with a body mass index greater than or equal to 17 kg/m2
Add		F50.021 **Anorexia nervosa, binge eating/purging type, moderate**
Add		Anorexia nervosa, binge eating/purging type, with a body mass index of 16.0-16.99 kg/m2
Add		F50.022 **Anorexia nervosa, binge eating/purging type, severe**
Add		Anorexia nervosa, binge eating/purging type, with a body mass index of 15.0-15.99 kg/m2
Add		F50.023 **Anorexia nervosa, binge eating/purging type, extreme**
Add		Anorexia nervosa, binge eating/purging type, with a body mass index of less than 15.0 kg/m2
Add		F50.024 **Anorexia nervosa, binge eating/ purging type, in remission**
Add		Anorexia nervosa, binge eating/purging type, in full remission
Add		Anorexia nervosa, binge eating/purging type, in partial remission
Add		F50.029 **Anorexia nervosa, binge eating/purging type, unspecified**
No Change	F50.2	**Bulimia nervosa**
No Change		**Excludes1**
Revise from		anorexia nervosa, binge eating/ purging type (F50.02)
Revise to		anorexia nervosa, binge eating/ purging type (F50.02-)
Add	F50.20	**Bulimia nervosa, unspecified**
Add	F50.21	**Bulimia nervosa, mild**
Add		Bulimia nervosa with 1-3 episodes of inappropriate compensatory behavior per week
Add	F50.22	**Bulimia nervosa, moderate**
Add		Bulimia nervosa with 4-7 episodes of inappropriate compensatory behavior per week
Add	F50.23	**Bulimia nervosa, severe**
Add		Bulimia nervosa with 8-13 episodes of inappropriate compensatory behavior per week
Add	F50.24	**Bulimia nervosa, extreme**
Add		Bulimia nervosa with 14 or more episodes of inappropriate compensatory behavior per week
Add	F50.25	**Bulimia nervosa, in remission**
Add		Bulimia nervosa, in full remission
Add		Bulimia nervosa, in partial remission

No Change	F50.8	**Other eating disorders**
Delete		**Excludes2** pica of infancy and childhood (F98.3)
No Change	F50.81	**Binge eating disorder**
Add		F50.810 **Binge eating disorder, mild**
Add		Binge eating disorder with 1-3 binge eating episodes per week
Add		F50.811 **Binge eating disorder, moderate**
Add		Binge eating disorder with 4-7 binge eating episodes per week
Add		F50.812 **Binge eating disorder, severe**
Add		Binge eating disorder with 8-13 binge eating episodes per week
Add		F50.813 **Binge eating disorder, extreme**
Add		Binge eating disorder with 14 or more eating episodes per week
Add		F50.814 **Binge eating disorder, in remission**
Add		Binge eating disorder, in full remission
Add		Binge eating disorder, in partial remission
Add		F50.819 **Binge eating disorder, unspecified**
No Change	F50.82	**Avoidant/restrictive food intake disorder**
Add		Avoidant/restrictive food intake disorder, in remission
Add	F50.83	**Pica in adults**
Add		Pica in adults, in remission
Add		**Excludes1** pica in infancy and childhood (F98.3)
Add	F50.84	**Rumination disorder in adults**
Add		Rumination disorder in adults, in remission
Add		**Excludes1** rumination disorder in infancy and childhood (F98.21)
No Change	F50.89	**Other specified eating disorder**
Delete		Pica in adults

BEHAVIORAL AND EMOTIONAL DISORDERS WITH ONSET USUALLY OCCURRING IN CHILDHOOD AND ADOLESCENCE (F90-F98)

No Change

No Change F98		**Other behavioral and emotional disorders with onset usually occurring in childhood and adolescence**
No Change	F98.2	**Other feeding disorders of infancy and childhood**
Revise from	F98.21	**Rumination disorder of infancy**
Revise to	F98.21	**Rumination disorder of infancy and childhood**
Add		Rumination disorder in infancy or childhood, in remission
Add		**Excludes1** rumination disorder in adults (F50.84)
No Change	F98.3	**Pica of infancy and childhood**
Add		Pica in infancy or childhood, in remission
Add		**Excludes1** pica in adults (F50.83)

No Change **CHAPTER 6**

No Change # DISEASES OF THE NERVOUS SYSTEM (G00-G99)

No Change ## EXTRAPYRAMIDAL AND MOVEMENT DISORDERS (G20-G26)

No Change **G21** Secondary parkinsonism
No Change **Excludes1**
Delete   dementia with Parkinsonism (G31.83)
Add   neurocognitive disorder with Lewy bodies (G31.83)

No Change ## OTHER DEGENERATIVE DISEASES OF THE NERVOUS SYSTEM (G30-G32)

No Change **G30** Alzheimer's disease
No Change **Excludes1**
Revise from   senile dementia NOS (F03)
Revise to   senile dementia NOS (F03.-)

No Change **G31** Other degenerative diseases of nervous system, not elsewhere classified
No Change **G31.8** Other specified degenerative diseases of nervous system
No Change **G31.84** Mild cognitive impairment of uncertain or unknown etiology
No Change   **Excludes1**
Revise from   dementia (F01.-, F02.-, F03)
Revise to   dementia (F01.-, F02.-, F03.-)

No Change ## EPISODIC AND PAROXYSMAL DISORDERS (G40-G47)

No Change **G40** Epilepsy and recurrent seizures
No Change **G40.8** Other epilepsy and recurrent seizures
Add **G40.84** KCNQ2-related epilepsy
Add **G40.841** KCNQ2-related epilepsy, not intractable, with status epilepticus
Add **G40.842** KCNQ2-related epilepsy, not intractable, without status epilepticus
     KCNQ2-related epilepsy NOS
Add **G40.843** KCNQ2-related epilepsy, intractable, with status epilepticus
Add **G40.844** KCNQ2-related epilepsy, intractable, without status epilepticus

No Change ## OTHER DISORDERS OF THE NERVOUS SYSTEM (G89-G99)

No Change **G90** Disorders of autonomic nervous system
No Change **G90.8** Other disorders of autonomic nervous system
Add **G90.81** Serotonin syndrome
Add   Serotonin toxicity
Add   *Code first poisoning due to drug or toxin, such as:*
Add   linezolid (T36.8X- with sixth character 1-4)
Add   monoamine oxidase inhibitors (T43.1X with sixth character 1-4)
Add   selective serotonin and norepinephrine reuptake inhibitors [SSNRI] (T43.21 with sixth character 1-4)
Add   selective serotonin reuptake inhibitors [SSRI] (T43.22 with sixth character 1-4)
Add   Use Additional code for adverse effect, if applicable, to identify drug, such as:
Add   linezolid (T36.8X5)
Add   monoamine oxidase inhibitors (T43.1X5)
Add   selective serotonin and norepinephrine reuptake inhibitors [SSNRI] (T43.215)
Add   selective serotonin reuptake inhibitors [SSRI] (T43.225)
Add   Use Additional code, if applicable, to identify:
Add   disseminated intravascular coagulation (D65)
Add   hypertensive crisis (I16.-)
Add   metabolic acidosis (E87.2-)
Add   shock, not elsewhere classified (R57.-)
Add   toxic encephalopathy (G92.-)
Add   ventricular tachycardia (I47.2-)
Add **G90.89** Other disorders of autonomic nervous system

No Change **G93** Other disorders of brain
No Change **G93.4** Other and unspecified encephalopathy
Revise from **G93.42** Megaloencephalic leukoencephalopathy with subcortical cysts
Revise to **G93.42** Megalencephalic leukoencephalopathy with subcortical cysts
Add **G93.45** Developmental and epileptic encephalopathy
Add   Early infantile epileptic encephalopathy
Add   Code also, if applicable, associated disorders such as:
Add   developmental disorders of scholastic skills (F81.-)
Add   developmental disorder of speech and language (F80.-)
Add   epilepsy, by specific type (G40.-)
Add   intellectual disabilities (F70-F79)
Add   other neurodevelopmental disorder (F88)
Add   pervasive developmental disorders (F84.-)

No Change **CHAPTER 7**

No Change **DISEASES OF THE EYE AND ADNEXA (H00-H59)**

No Change **GLAUCOMA (H40-H42)**

No Change **H42** Glaucoma in diseases classified elsewhere
No Change   *Code first*
Revise from   Reiger's anomaly (Q13.81)
Revise to   Rieger anomaly (Q13.81)

No Change **DISORDERS OF VITREOUS BODY AND GLOBE (H43-H44)**

No Change **H44** Disorders of globe
No Change **H44.2** Degenerative myopia
No Change   **H44.2A** Degenerative myopia with choroidal neovascularization
Revise from   **H44.2A3** Degenerative myopia with choroidal neovascularization, bilateral eye
Revise to   **H44.2A3** Degenerative myopia with choroidal neovascularization, bilateral
No Change   **H44.2B** Degenerative myopia with macular hole
Revise from   **H44.2B3** Degenerative myopia with macular hole, bilateral eye
Revise to   **H44.2B3** Degenerative myopia with macular hole, bilateral
No Change   **H44.2C** Degenerative myopia with retinal detachment
Revise from   **H44.2C3** Degenerative myopia with retinal detachment, bilateral eye
Revise to   **H44.2C3** Degenerative myopia with retinal detachment, bilateral
No Change   **H44.2D** Degenerative myopia with foveoschisis
Revise from   **H44.2D3** Degenerative myopia with foveoschisis, bilateral eye
Revise to   **H44.2D3** Degenerative myopia with foveoschisis, bilateral
No Change   **H44.2E** Degenerative myopia with other maculopathy
Revise from   **H44.2E3** Degenerative myopia with other maculopathy, bilateral eye
Revise to   **H44.2E3** Degenerative myopia with other maculopathy, bilateral

No Change **CHAPTER 9**

No Change **DISEASES OF THE CIRCULATORY SYSTEM (I00-I99)**

No Change **CHRONIC RHEUMATIC HEART DISEASES (I05-I09)**

No Change **I08** Multiple valve diseases
Delete   **Excludes1** multiple valve disease specified a nonrheumatic (I34.-, I35.-, I36.-, I37.-, I38.-, Q22.-, Q23.-, Q24.8-)
Add   **Excludes2** multiple valve disease specified as nonrheumatic (I34.-, I35.-, I36.-, I37.-, I38.-, Q22.-, Q23.-, Q24.8-)

No Change **HYPERTENSIVE DISEASES (I10-I1A)**

No Change **I16** Hypertensive crisis
No Change **I16.1** Hypertensive emergency
Add   Use Additional code, if applicable, to identify specific organ dysfunction, such as:
Add   acute kidney injury (N17.-)
Add   acute myocardial infarction (I21.-)
Add   acute pulmonary edema (left and/or right ventricular failure) (J81.0, I50.-)
Add   aortic dissection (I71.0-)
Add   cerebral hemorrhage (I60.-. I61.-, I62.-)
Add   cerebral infarction (I63.-)
Add   eclampsia (O15.-)
Add   hypertensive encephalopathy (I67.4)
Add   seizure (R56.9)

No Change **ISCHEMIC HEART DISEASES (I20-I25)**

No Change **I21** Acute myocardial infarction
No Change **I21.A** Other type of myocardial infarction
No Change   **I21.A1** Myocardial infarction type 2
No Change   *Code first*
Revise from   the underlying cause, such as:
Revise to   , if applicable, the underlying cause, such as:

No Change **PULMONARY HEART DISEASE AND DISEASES OF PULMONARY CIRCULATION (I26-I28)**

No Change **I26** Pulmonary embolism
No Change **I26.0** Pulmonary embolism with acute cor pulmonale
Add   **I26.03** Cement embolism of pulmonary artery with acute cor pulmonale
Add   *Code first* complication of other artery following a procedure (T81.718)
Add   **I26.04** Fat embolism of pulmonary artery with acute cor pulmonale
Add   *Code first,* if applicable:
Add   complication of other artery following a procedure (T81.718)
Add   traumatic fat embolism (T79.1)
No Change   **I26.09** Other pulmonary embolism with acute cor pulmonale
Add   Other thrombotic pulmonary embolism with acute cor pulmonale
No Change **I26.9** Pulmonary embolism without acute cor pulmonale
Revise from   **I26.93** Single subsegmental pulmonary embolism without acute cor pulmonale
Revise to   **I26.93** Single subsegmental thrombotic pulmonary embolism without acute cor pulmonale
Revise from   **I26.94** Multiple subsegmental pulmonary emboli without acute cor pulmonale
Revise to   **I26.94** Multiple subsegmental thrombotic pulmonary emboli without acute cor pulmonale
Add   **I26.95** Cement embolism of pulmonary artery without acute cor pulmonale
Add   *Code first* complication of other artery following a procedure (T81.718)
Add   **I26.96** Fat embolism of pulmonary artery without acute cor pulmonale
Add   *Code first,* if applicable:
complication of other artery following a procedure (T81.718)
Add   traumatic fat embolism (T79.1)
No Change   **I26.99** Other pulmonary embolism without acute cor pulmonale
Add   Other thrombotic pulmonary embolism without acute cor pulmonale

No Change | **OTHER FORMS OF HEART DISEASE (I30-I5A)**

No Change I30 | **Acute pericarditis**
No Change | **Excludes1**
Revise from | viral pericarditis due to Coxsakie virus (B33.23)
Revise to | viral pericarditis due to Coxsackie virus (B33.23)

No Change I35 | **Nonrheumatic aortic valve disorders**
Delete | **Excludes1** aortic valve disorder of unspecified cause but with diseases of mitral and/or tricuspid valve(s) (I08.-)
Delete | aortic valve disorder specified as congenital (Q23.0, Q23.1)
Delete | aortic valve disorder specified as rheumatic (I06.-)
Delete | hypertrophic subaortic stenosis (I42.1)
Add | Code also, if applicable, bicuspid aortic valve (Q23.81)
Add | **Excludes2** aortic valve disorder of unspecified cause but with diseases of mitral and/or tricuspid valve(s) (I08.-)
Add | aortic valve disorder specified as congenital (Q23.0, Q23.1)
Add | aortic valve disorder specified as rheumatic (I06.-)
Add | hypertrophic subaortic stenosis (I42.1)

No Change **CHAPTER 10**

No Change **DISEASES OF THE RESPIRATORY SYSTEM (J00-J99)**

No Change | **INFLUENZA AND PNEUMONIA (J09-J18)**

No Change J13 | **Pneumonia due to Streptococcus pneumoniae**
No Change | *Code first*
Revise from | associated influenza, if applicable (J09.X1, J10.0-, J11.0-)
Revise from | , if applicable, associated influenza (J09.X1, J10.0-, J11.0-)
No Change | Code also
Delete | associated abscess, if applicable (J85.1)
Add | , if applicable, any associated condition such as:
Add | abscess (J85.1)
Add | aspiration pneumonia (J69.-)

No Change J14 | **Pneumonia due to Hemophilus influenzae**
No Change | *Code first*
Revise from | associated influenza, if applicable (J09.X1, J10.0-, J11.0-)
Revise to | , if applicable, associated influenza (J09.X1, J10.0-, J11.0-)
No Change | Code also
Delete | associated abscess, if applicable (J85.1)
Add | , if applicable, any associated condition such as:
Add | abscess (J85.1)
Add | aspiration pneumonia (J69.-)

No Change J15 | **Bacterial pneumonia, not elsewhere classified**
No Change | *Code first*
Revise from | associated influenza, if applicable (J09.X1, J10.0-, J11.0-)
Revise to | , if applicable, associated influenza (J09.X1, J10.0-, J11.0-)
No Change | Code also
Delete | associated abscess, if applicable (J85.1)
Add | , if applicable, any associated condition such as:
Add | abscess (J85.1)
Add | aspiration pneumonia (J69.-)

No Change J16 | **Pneumonia due to other infectious organisms, not elsewhere classified**
No Change | *Code first*
Revise from | associated influenza, if applicable (J09.X1, J10.0-, J11.0-)
Revise to | , if applicable, associated influenza (J09.X1, J10.0-, J11.0-)
No Change | Code also
Delete | associated abscess, if applicable (J85.1)
Add | , if applicable, any associated condition such as:
Add | abscess (J85.1)
Add | aspiration pneumonia (J69.-)

No Change J17 | **Pneumonia in diseases classified elsewhere**
Add | Code also, if applicable, any associated condition such as:
Add | abscess (J85.1)
Add | aspiration pneumonia (J69.-)

No Change J18 | **Pneumonia, unspecified organism**
No Change | *Code first*
Revise from | associated influenza, if applicable (J09.X1, J10.0-, J11.0-)
Revise to | , if applicable, associated influenza (J09.X1, J10.0-, J11.0-)
Add | Code also, if applicable, any associated condition such as:
Add | aspiration pneumonia (J69.-)
Delete | **Excludes1** abscess of lung with pneumonia (J85.1)
Delete | aspiration pneumonia due to anesthesia during labor and delivery (O74.0)
Delete | aspiration pneumonia due to anesthesia during pregnancy (O29)
Delete | aspiration pneumonia due to anesthesia during puerperium (O89.0)
Delete | aspiration pneumonia due to solids and liquids (J69.-)
Delete | aspiration pneumonia NOS (J69.0)
Delete | lipid pneumonia (J69.1)
Delete | pneumonitis due to external agents (J67-J70)
Add | **Excludes2** abscess of lung with pneumonia (J85.1)
Add | aspiration pneumonia due to anesthesia during labor and delivery (O74.0)
Add | aspiration pneumonia due to anesthesia during pregnancy (O29)
Add | aspiration pneumonia due to anesthesia during puerperium (O89.0)
Add | aspiration pneumonia due to solids and liquids (J69.-)
Add | aspiration pneumonia NOS (J69.0)
Add | lipid pneumonia (J69.1)
Add | pneumonitis due to external agents (J67-J70)

No Change | **OTHER ACUTE LOWER RESPIRATORY INFECTIONS (J20-J22)**

No Change J21 | **Acute bronchiolitis**
No Change | J21.9 | **Acute bronchiolitis, unspecified**
No Change | **Excludes1**
Revise from | chronic bronchiolitis (J44.-)
Revise to | chronic bronchiolitis (J44.89)

No Change		**OTHER DISEASES OF UPPER RESPIRATORY TRACT (J30-J39)**
No Change	J34	Other and unspecified disorders of nose and nasal sinuses
No Change	J34.8	Other specified disorders of nose and nasal sinuses
Add	J34.82	Nasal valve collapse
Add		Nasal valve compromise
Add		Nasal valve stenosis
Add		*Code first* underlying cause, such as: deviated nasal septum (J34.2)
Add	J34.820	Internal nasal valve collapse
Add	J34.8200	Internal nasal valve collapse, unspecified
Add	J34.8201	Internal nasal valve collapse, static
Add		Narrowing of the septum, head of the inferior turbinate and the upper lateral cartilage
Add	J34.8202	Internal nasal valve collapse, dynamic
Add		Collapse or falling of the upper, middle sidewall of the nose on inspiration
Add	J34.821	External nasal valve collapse
Add	J34.8210	External nasal valve collapse, unspecified
Add	J34.8211	External nasal valve collapse, static
Add		Fixed narrowing of the caudal septum, lower lateral cartilage, alar rim and nasal sill
Add	J34.8212	External nasal valve collapse, dynamic
Add		Collapse or falling of the lower sidewall or nostril of the nose on inspiration
Add	J34.829	Nasal valve collapse, unspecified
Add		Nasal valve collapse, NOS

LUNG DISEASES DUE TO EXTERNAL AGENTS (J60-J70)

No Change	J69	Pneumonitis due to solids and liquids
Add		Code also, if applicable, other types of pneumonias

OTHER RESPIRATORY DISEASES PRINCIPALLY AFFECTING THE INTERSTITIUM (J80-J84)

No Change	J84	Other interstitial pulmonary diseases
Add		Code also, if applicable, associated condition

SUPPURATIVE AND NECROTIC CONDITIONS OF THE LOWER RESPIRATORY TRACT (J85-J86)

No Change	J86	Pyothorax
No Change	J86.0	Pyothorax with fistula
Add		Code also, if applicable, disruption of internal operation (surgical) wound (T81.32-)

No Change **CHAPTER 11**

No Change
DISEASES OF THE DIGESTIVE SYSTEM (K00-K95)

DISEASES OF ORAL CAVITY AND SALIVARY GLANDS (K00-K14)

No Change	K14	Diseases of tongue
No Change		**Excludes2**
Revise from		leukedema of tongue (K13.29)
Revise to		leukoedema of tongue (K13.29)

DISEASES OF ESOPHAGUS, STOMACH AND DUODENUM (K20-K31)

No Change	K31	Other diseases of stomach and duodenum
No Change	K31.6	Fistula of stomach and duodenum
Add		Code also, if applicable, disruption of internal operation (surgical) wound (T81.32-)

NONINFECTIVE ENTERITIS AND COLITIS (K50-K52)

No Change	K50	Crohn's disease [regional enteritis]
Add		Use Additional code to identify any associated fistulas, if applicable:
Add		anal fistula (K60.3-)
Add		anorectal fistula (K60.5-)
Add		rectal fistula (K60.4-)
No Change	K51	Ulcerative colitis
Add		Use Additional code to identify any associated fistulas, if applicable:
Add		anal fistula (K60.3-)
Add		anorectal fistula (K60.5-)
Add		rectal fistula (K60.4-)

OTHER DISEASES OF INTESTINES (K55-K64)

No Change	K58	Irritable bowel syndrome
Revise from	K58.9	Irritable bowel syndrome without diarrhea
Revise to	K58.9	Irritable bowel syndrome, unspecified
No Change	K60	Fissure and fistula of anal and rectal regions
Add		**Excludes2** abscess or cellulitis of anal and rectal regions (K61.-)
No Change	K60.3	Anal fistula
Add		*Code first*, if applicable:
Add		Crohn's disease (K50.-)
Add		ulcerative colitis (K51.-)
Add		**Excludes1** congenital fistula (Q43.6)
Add	K60.30	Anal fistula, unspecified
Add		Anal fistula NOS
Add	K60.31	Anal fistula, simple
Add		Low intersphincteric anal fistula
Add		Superficial anal fistula
Add	K60.311	Anal fistula, simple, initial
Add		Anal fistula, simple, new
Add	K60.312	Anal fistula, simple, persistent
Add		Anal fistula, simple, chronic
Add	K60.313	Anal fistula, simple, recurrent
Add		Anal fistula simple, occurring following complete healing
Add	K60.319	Anal fistula, simple, unspecified

Add		**K60.32**	**Anal fistula, complex**
Add			Extrasphincteric anal fistula
Add			High intersphincteric anal fistula
Add			Suprasphincteric anal fistula
Add			Transsphincteric anal fistula
Add			Code also, if applicable:
			perianal abscess (K61.0)
			rectovaginal fistula (N82.3)
			stenosis of anus and rectum (K62.4)
Add			**K60.321 Anal fistula, complex, initial**
Add			Anal fistula, complex, new
Add			**K60.322 Anal fistula, complex, persistent**
Add			Anal fistula, complex, chronic
Add			**K60.323 Anal fistula, complex, recurrent**
Add			Anal fistula complex, occurring following complete healing
Add			**K60.329 Anal fistula, complex, unspecified**
No Change	**K60.4**	**Rectal fistula**	
Add		*Code first, if applicable:*	
Add		Crohn's disease (K50.-)	
Add		ulcerative colitis (K51.-)	
Add		**Excludes1** congenital fistula (Q43.6)	
Add		**K60.40**	**Rectal fistula, unspecified**
Add			Rectal fistula NOS
Add		**K60.41**	**Rectal fistula, simple**
Add			Low intersphincteric rectal fistula
Add			Superficial rectal fistula
Add			**K60.411 Rectal fistula, simple, initial**
Add			Rectal, fistula, simple, new
Add			**K60.412 Rectal fistula, simple, persistent**
Add			Rectal fistula, simple, chronic
Add			**K60.413 Rectal fistula, simple, recurrent**
Add			Rectal fistula simple, occurring following complete healing
Add			**K60.419 Rectal fistula, simple, unspecified**
Add		**K60.42**	**Rectal fistula, complex**
Add			Extrasphincteric rectal fistula
Add			High intersphincteric rectal fistula
Add			Suprasphincteric rectal fistula
Add			Transsphincteric rectal fistula
Add			Code also, if applicable:
			perianal abscess (K61.0)
			rectovaginal fistula (N82.3)
			stenosis of anus and rectum (K62.4)
Add			**K60.421 Rectal fistula, complex, initial**
Add			Rectal fistula, complex, new
Add			**K60.422 Rectal fistula, complex, persistent**
Add			Rectal fistula, complex, chronic
Add			**K60.423 Rectal fistula, complex, recurrent**
Add			Rectal fistula complex occurring following complete healing
Add			**K60.429 Rectal fistula, complex, unspecified**
No Change	**K60.5**	**Anorectal fistula**	
Add		*Code first, if applicable:*	
Add		Crohn's disease (K50.-)	
Add		ulcerative colitis (K51.-)	
Add		**Excludes1** congenital fistula (Q43.6)	
Add		**K60.50**	**Anorectal fistula, unspecified**
Add			Anorectal fistula NOS

Add		**K60.51**	**Anorectal fistula, simple**
Add			Low intersphincteric anorectal fistula
Add			Superficial anorectal fistula
Add			**K60.511 Anorectal fistula, simple, initial**
Add			Anorectal fistula, simple, new
Add			**K60.512 Anorectal fistula, simple, persistent**
Add			Anorectal fistula, simple, chronic
Add			**K60.513 Anorectal fistula, simple, recurrent**
Add			Anorectal fistula simple, occurring following complete healing
Add			**K60.519 Anorectal fistula, simple, unspecified**
Add		**K60.52**	**Anorectal fistula, complex**
Add			Extrasphincteric anorectal fistula
Add			High intersphincteric anorectal fistula
Add			Suprasphincteric anorectal fistula
Add			Transsphincteric anorectal fistula
Add			Code also, if applicable:
			perianal abscess (K61.0)
			rectovaginal fistula (N82.3)
			stenosis of anus and rectum (K62.4)
Add			**K60.521 Anorectal fistula, complex, initial**
Add			Anorectal fistula, complex, new
Add			**K60.522 Anorectal fistula, complex, persistent**
Add			Anorectal fistula, complex, chronic
Add			**K60.523 Anorectal fistula, complex, recurrent**
Add			Anorectal fistula complex, occurring following complete healing
Add			**K60.529 Anorectal fistula, complex, unspecified**
No Change	**K63**	**Other diseases of intestine**	
No Change		**K63.2**	**Fistula of intestine**
Add			Code also, if applicable, disruption of internal operation (surgical) wound (T81.32-)

No Change **DISORDERS OF GALLBLADDER, BILIARY TRACT AND PANCREAS (K80-K87)**

No Change	**K82**	**Other diseases of gallbladder**	
No Change		**K82.3**	**Fistula of gallbladder**
Add			Code also, if applicable, disruption of internal operation (surgical) wound (T81.32-)

No Change **CHAPTER 12**

No Change # DISEASES OF THE SKIN AND SUBCUTANEOUS TISSUE (L00-L99)

No Change **DERMATITIS AND ECZEMA (L20-L30)**

No Change	**L29**	**Pruritus**	
No Change		**L29.8**	**Other pruritus**
Add			**L29.81 Cholestatic pruritus**
Add			Code also, if applicable, type of liver disease
Add			Use Additional code for adverse effect, if applicable, to identify drug (T36-T50 with fifth or sixth character 5)
Add			**L29.89 Other pruritus**

No Change	**PAPULOSQUAMOUS DISORDERS (L40-L45)**	

No Change **L43** **Lichen planus**
No Change   **Excludes1**
Revise from   lichen planopilaris (L66.1)
Revise to   lichen planopilaris (L66.1-)

DISORDERS OF SKIN APPENDAGES (L60-L75)

No Change **L66** **Cicatricial alopecia [scarring hair loss]**
No Change   **L66.1** **Lichen planopilaris**
Delete   Follicular lichen planus
Add   **L66.10** **Lichen planopilaris, unspecified**
Add   **L66.11** **Classic lichen planopilaris**
Add   Follicular lichen planus
Add   **L66.12** **Frontal fibrosing alopecia**
Add   FFA
Add   **L66.19** **Other lichen planopilaris**
Add   Lassueur Graham-Little Piccardi syndrome
No Change   **L66.8** **Other cicatricial alopecia**
Add   **L66.81** **Central centrifugal cicatricial alopecia**
Add   CCCA
Add   **L66.89** **Other cicatricial alopecia**

No Change **CHAPTER 13**

No Change **DISEASES OF THE MUSCULOSKELETAL SYSTEM AND CONNECTIVE TISSUE (M00-M99)**

No Change **OTHER DORSOPATHIES (M50-M54)**

No Change **M51** **Thoracic, thoracolumbar, and lumbosacral intervertebral disc disorders**
No Change   **M51.3** **Other thoracic, thoracolumbar and lumbosacral intervertebral disc degeneration**
No Change   **M51.36** **Other intervertebral disc degeneration, lumbar region**
Add   **M51.360** **Other intervertebral disc degeneration, lumbar region with discogenic back pain only**
Add   Other intervertebral disc degeneration, lumbar region with axial back pain only
Add   **M51.361** **Other intervertebral disc degeneration, lumbar region with lower extremity pain only**
Add   Other intervertebral disc degeneration, lumbar region with leg pain only
Add   Other intervertebral disc degeneration, lumbar region with referred sclerotomal pain only
Add   **M51.362** **Other intervertebral disc degeneration, lumbar region with discogenic back pain and lower extremity pain**
Add   Other intervertebral disc degeneration, lumbar region with discogenic back pain and leg pain
Add   Other intervertebral disc degeneration, lumbar region with axial back pain and referred sclerotomal pain

Add   **M51.369** **Other intervertebral disc degeneration, lumbar region without mention of lumbar back pain or lower extremity pain**
Add   Other intervertebral disc degeneration, lumbar region without mention of lumbar back pain or leg pain
Add   Other intervertebral disc degeneration, lumbar region, NOS
No Change   **M51.37** **Other intervertebral disc degeneration, lumbosacral region**
Add   **M51.370** **Other intervertebral disc degeneration, lumbosacral region with discogenic back pain only**
Add   Other intervertebral disc degeneration, lumbosacral region with axial back pain only
Add   **M51.371** **Other intervertebral disc degeneration, lumbosacral region with lower extremity pain only**
Add   Other intervertebral disc degeneration, lumbosacral region with leg pain only
Add   Other intervertebral disc degeneration, lumbosacral region with referred sclerotomal pain only
Add   **M51.372** **Other intervertebral disc degeneration, lumbosacral region with discogenic back pain and lower extremity pain**
Add   Other intervertebral disc degeneration, lumbosacral region with discogenic back pain and leg pain
Add   Other intervertebral disc degeneration, lumbosacral region with axial back pain and referred sclerotomal pain
Add   **M51.379** **Other intervertebral disc degeneration, lumbosacral region without mention of lumbar back pain or lower extremity pain**
Add   Other intervertebral disc degeneration, lumbosacral region without mention of lumbar back pain or leg pain
Add   Other intervertebral disc degeneration, lumbosacral region, NOS

No Change	M54	Dorsalgia	
No Change		M54.3	Sciatica
Add			**Excludes1** intervertebral disc degeneration, lumbar region with lower extremity pain only (M51.361)
Add			intervertebral disc degeneration, lumbosacral region with lower extremity pain only (M51.371)
No Change		M54.4	Lumbago with sciatica
Add			**Excludes1** intervertebral disc degeneration, lumbar region with discogenic back pain and lower extremity pain (M51.362)
Add			intervertebral disc degeneration, lumbosacral region with discogenic back pain and lower extremity pain (M51.372)
No Change		M54.5	Low back pain
Add			**Excludes1** intervertebral disc degeneration, lumbar region with discogenic back pain only (M51.360)
Add			intervertebral disc degeneration, lumbosacral region with discogenic back pain only (M51.370)

No Change   **DISORDERS OF MUSCLES (M60-M63)**

No Change	M62	Other disorders of muscle	
No Change		M62.8	Other specified disorders of muscle
Add			M62.85 Dysfunction of the multifidus muscles, lumbar region

No Change   **DISORDERS OF SYNOVIUM AND TENDON (M65-M67)**

No Change	M65	Synovitis and tenosynovitis		
No Change		M65.9	Synovitis and tenosynovitis, unspecified	
Add			M65.90	Unspecified synovitis and tenosynovitis, unspecified site
Add			M65.91	Unspecified synovitis and tenosynovitis, shoulder
Add				M65.911 Unspecified synovitis and tenosynovitis, right shoulder
Add				M65.912 Unspecified synovitis and tenosynovitis, left shoulder
Add				M65.919 Unspecified synovitis and tenosynovitis, unspecified shoulder
Add			M65.92	Unspecified synovitis and tenosynovitis, upper arm
Add				M65.921 Unspecified synovitis and tenosynovitis, right upper arm
Add				M65.922 Unspecified synovitis and tenosynovitis, left upper arm
Add				M65.929 Unspecified synovitis and tenosynovitis, unspecified upper arm
Add			M65.93	Unspecified synovitis and tenosynovitis, forearm
Add				M65.931 Unspecified synovitis and tenosynovitis, right forearm
Add				M65.932 Unspecified synovitis and tenosynovitis, left forearm
Add				M65.939 Unspecified synovitis and tenosynovitis, unspecified forearm

Add		M65.94	Unspecified synovitis and tenosynovitis, hand
Add			M65.941 Unspecified synovitis and tenosynovitis, right hand
Add			M65.942 Unspecified synovitis and tenosynovitis, left hand
Add			M65.949 Unspecified synovitis and tenosynovitis, unspecified hand
Add		M65.95	Unspecified synovitis and tenosynovitis, thigh
Add			M65.951 Unspecified synovitis and tenosynovitis, right thigh
Add			M65.952 Unspecified synovitis and tenosynovitis, left thigh
Add			M65.959 Unspecified synovitis and tenosynovitis, unspecified thigh
Add		M65.96	Unspecified synovitis and tenosynovitis, lower leg
Add			M65.961 Unspecified synovitis and tenosynovitis, right lower leg
Add			M65.962 Unspecified synovitis and tenosynovitis, left lower leg
Add			M65.969 Unspecified synovitis and tenosynovitis, unspecified lower leg
Add		M65.97	Unspecified synovitis and tenosynovitis, ankle and foot
Add			M65.971 Unspecified synovitis and tenosynovitis, right ankle and foot
Add			M65.972 Unspecified synovitis and tenosynovitis, left ankle and foot
Add			M65.979 Unspecified synovitis and tenosynovitis, unspecified ankle and foot
Add		M65.98	Unspecified synovitis and tenosynovitis, other site
Add		M65.99	Unspecified synovitis and tenosynovitis, multiple sites

No Change   **CHONDROPATHIES (M91-M94)**

No Change	M92	Other juvenile osteochondrosis	
No Change		M92.8	Other specified juvenile osteochondrosis
Delete			Calcaneal apophysitis

No Change **CHAPTER 14**

No Change **DISEASES OF THE GENITOURINARY SYSTEM (N00-N99)**

No Change   **OTHER DISEASES OF THE URINARY SYSTEM (N30-N39)**

No Change	N39	Other disorders of urinary system	
No Change		N39.0	Urinary tract infection, site not specified
Add			**Excludes1** pyonephrosis (N13.6)

No Change **CHAPTER 15**

No Change **PREGNANCY, CHILDBIRTH AND THE PUERPERIUM (O00-O9A)**

No Change **OTHER MATERNAL DISORDERS PREDOMINANTLY RELATED TO PREGNANCY (O20-O29)**

No Change O24   Diabetes mellitus in pregnancy, childbirth, and the puerperium

No Change   O24.1   Pre-existing type 2 diabetes mellitus, in pregnancy, childbirth and the puerperium

Add   Use Additional injectable non-insulin antidiabetic drugs (Z79.85)

No Change   O24.3   Unspecified pre-existing diabetes mellitus in pregnancy, childbirth and the puerperium

Add   Use Additional injectable non-insulin antidiabetic drugs (Z79.85)

No Change   O24.8   Other pre-existing diabetes mellitus in pregnancy, childbirth, and the puerperium

Add   Use Additional injectable non-insulin antidiabetic drugs (Z79.85)

No Change   O24.9   Unspecified diabetes mellitus in pregnancy, childbirth and the puerperium

Add   Use Additional
Revise from   code for long-term (current) use of insulin (Z79.4)
Revise to   code (for):
Add   from categories E08, E09 and E13 to further identify any manifestation
Add   injectable non-insulin antidiabetic drugs (Z79.85)
Add   long-term (current) use of insulin (Z79.4)

No Change **CHAPTER 16**

No Change **CERTAIN CONDITIONS ORIGINATING IN THE PERINATAL PERIOD (P00-P96)**

No Change **TRANSITORY ENDOCRINE AND METABOLIC DISORDERS SPECIFIC TO NEWBORN (P70-P74)**

No Change P72   Other transitory neonatal endocrine disorders

Add   **Excludes1**   dyshormonogenetic goiter (E07.1)

No Change **CHAPTER 17**

No Change **CONGENITAL MALFORMATIONS, DEFORMATIONS AND CHROMOSOMAL ABNORMALITIES (Q00-Q99)**

No Change **CONGENITAL MALFORMATIONS OF EYE, EAR, FACE AND NECK (Q10-Q18)**

No Change Q13   Congenital malformations of anterior segment of eye

No Change   Q13.8   Other congenital malformations of anterior segment of eye

Revise from   Q13.81   Rieger's anomaly
Revise to   Q13.81   Rieger anomaly
Add   Axenfeld-Rieger syndrome
Add   Code also any other associated congenital malformations such as cardiac defects

No Change **CONGENITAL MALFORMATIONS OF THE CIRCULATORY SYSTEM (Q20-Q28)**

No Change Q23   Congenital malformations of aortic and mitral valves

No Change   Q23.1   Congenital insufficiency of aortic valve
Delete   Bicuspid aortic valve

No Change   Q23.8   Other congenital malformations of aortic and mitral valves

Add   Q23.81   Bicuspid aortic valve
Add   Congenital bicuspid aortic valve
Add   Unicuspid (congenital) aortic valve (at birth)

Add   Code also, if applicable, acquired aortic valve disorders, such as:
Add   aortic (valve) insufficiency (nonrheumatic) (I35.1)
Add   aortic (valve) stenosis (nonrheumatic) (I35.0)
Add   aortic (valve) stenosis with insufficiency (nonrheumatic) (I35.2)

Add   Q23.82   Congenital mitral valve cleft leaflet
Add   Cleft mitral valve leaflet at birth

Add   Q23.88   Other congenital malformations of aortic and mitral valves

No Change **OTHER CONGENITAL MALFORMATIONS (Q80-Q89)**

No Change Q87   Other specified congenital malformation syndromes affecting multiple systems

No Change   Q87.8   Other specified congenital malformation syndromes, not elsewhere classified

Add   Q87.86   Kleefstra syndrome

No Change **CHAPTER 18**

No Change **SYMPTOMS, SIGNS AND ABNORMAL CLINICAL AND LABORATORY FINDINGS, NOT ELSEWHERE CLASSIFIED (R00-R99)**

No Change **SYMPTOMS AND SIGNS INVOLVING THE DIGESTIVE SYSTEM AND ABDOMEN (R10-R19)**

No Change R11   Nausea and vomiting
No Change   **Excludes1**
Revise from   vomiting associated with bulimia nervosa (F50.2)
Revise to   vomiting associated with bulimia nervosa (F50.2-)

No Change   R11.1   Vomiting
No Change   R11.15   Cyclical vomiting syndrome unrelated to migraine

No Change   **Excludes2**
Revise from   bulimia nervosa (F50.2)
Revise to   bulimia nervosa (F50.20)

No Change		**SYMPTOMS AND SIGNS INVOLVING COGNITION, PERCEPTION, EMOTIONAL STATE AND BEHAVIOR (R40-R46)**	

No Change	**R41**	Other symptoms and signs involving cognitive functions and awareness	
No Change		**R41.0** Disorientation, unspecified	
Add		**Excludes1** delirium due to known physiological condition (F05)	
No Change		**R41.8** Other symptoms and signs involving cognitive functions and awareness	
No Change			**R41.84** Other specified cognitive deficit
			Code first the underlying condition, if known, such as:
Add			*known, such as:*
Add			schizophrenia (F20.-)
Add			**R41.85** Anosognosia
No Change			**R41.89** Other symptoms and signs involving cognitive functions and awareness
Delete			Anosognosia

No Change		**GENERAL SYMPTOMS AND SIGNS (R50-R69)**	

No Change	**R54**	Age-related physical debility	
No Change		**Excludes1**	
Revise from		senile psychosis (F03)	
Revise to		senile psychosis (F03.-)	
No Change	**R63**	Symptoms and signs concerning food and fluid intake	
No Change		**Excludes1**	
Revise from		bulimia NOS (F50.2)	
Revise to		bulimia NOS (F50.2-)	

No Change		**ABNORMAL FINDINGS ON EXAMINATION OF BLOOD, WITHOUT DIAGNOSIS (R70-R79)**	

No Change	**R73**	Elevated blood glucose level	
No Change		**R73.0** Abnormal glucose	
Add		**Excludes1** type 1 diabetes mellitus, presymptomatic (E10.A-)	

No Change # CHAPTER 19

No Change ## INJURY, POISONING AND CERTAIN OTHER CONSEQUENCES OF EXTERNAL CAUSES (S00-T88)

No Change		**INJURIES TO THE HEAD (S00-S09)**	

No Change	**S06**	Intracranial injury	
No Change		**S06.3** Focal traumatic brain injury	
No Change			**S06.34** Traumatic hemorrhage of right cerebrum
No Change			**S06.341** Traumatic hemorrhage of right cerebrum with loss of consciousness of 30 minutes or less
Revise from			Traumatic hemorrhage of right cerebrum with loss of consciousness
Revise to			Traumatic hemorrhage of right cerebrum with brief loss of consciousness

No Change		**INJURIES TO THE THORAX (S20-S29)**	

No Change	**S22**	Fracture of rib(s), sternum and thoracic spine	
No Change		Code also	
Revise from		, if applicable, any associated:	
Revise from		, if applicable, any associated condition such as:	
Add		traumatic hemopneumothorax (S27.2)	
Add		traumatic hemothorax (S27.1-)	
Add		traumatic pneumothorax (S27.0)	

No Change		**POISONING BY, ADVERSE EFFECTS OF AND UNDERDOSING OF DRUGS, MEDICAMENTS AND BIOLOGICAL SUBSTANCES (T36-T50)**	

No Change	**T45**	Poisoning by, adverse effect of and underdosing of primarily systemic and hematological agents, not elsewhere classified	
No Change		**T45.1** Poisoning by, adverse effect of and underdosing of antineoplastic and immunosuppressive drugs	
Add		**Excludes1** poisoning by, adverse effect of and underdosing of immune checkpoint inhibitors and immunostimulant drugs (T45.A)	
Add		**T45.A** Poisoning by, adverse effect of and underdosing of immune checkpoint inhibitors and immunostimulant drugs	
Add		**Excludes1** poisoning by, adverse effect of and underdosing of antineoplastic and immunosuppressive drug (T45.1)	
Add			**T45.AX** Poisoning by, adverse effect of and underdosing of immune checkpoint inhibitors and immunostimulant drugs
Add			**T45.AX1** Poisoning by immune checkpoint inhibitors and immunostimulant drugs, accidental (unintentional)
Add			Poisoning by immune checkpoint inhibitors and immunosuppressive drugs NOS
Add			**T45.AX2** Poisoning by immune checkpoint inhibitors and immunostimulant drugs, intentional self-harm
Add			**T45.AX3** Poisoning by immune checkpoint inhibitors and immunostimulant drugs, assault
Add			**T45.AX4** Poisoning by immune checkpoint inhibitors and immunostimulant drugs, undetermined
Add			**T45.AX5** Adverse effect of immune checkpoint inhibitors and immunostimulant drugs
Add			**T45.AX6** Underdosing of immune checkpoint inhibitors and immunostimulant drugs

No Change		**TOXIC EFFECTS OF SUBSTANCES CHIEFLY NONMEDICINAL AS TO SOURCE (T51-T65)**	

No Change	**T63**	Toxic effect of contact with venomous animals and plants	
		T63.4 Toxic effect of venom of other arthropods	
Add		Use Additional code, if applicable, for anaphylactic shock (T78.2)	
No Change	**T65**	Toxic effect of other and unspecified substances	
No Change		**T65.3** Toxic effect of nitroderivatives and aminoderivatives of benzene and its homologues	
Revise from		Toxic effect of anilin [benzenamine]	
Revise to		Toxic effect of aniline [benzenamine]	

No Change	**COMPLICATIONS OF SURGICAL AND MEDICAL CARE, NOT ELSEWHERE CLASSIFIED (T80-T88)**	
No Change	**T80**	**Complications following infusion, transfusion and therapeutic injection**
No Change	**T80.8**	**Other complications following infusion, transfusion and therapeutic injection**
No Change	**T80.82**	**Complication of immune effector cellular therapy**
Add	Excludes2	adverse effect of immune checkpoint inhibitors and immunostimulant drugs (T45.AX5)
Add	**T81**	**Complications of procedures, not elsewhere classified**
No Change	**T81.3**	**Disruption of wound, not elsewhere classified**
No Change	**T81.32**	**Disruption of internal operation (surgical) wound, not elsewhere classified**
Delete		Deep disruption or dehiscence of operation wound NOS
Delete		Disruption or dehiscence of closure of internal organ or other internal tissue
Delete		Disruption or dehiscence of closure of muscle or muscle flap
Delete		Disruption or dehiscence of closure of ribs or rib cage
Delete		Disruption or dehiscence of closure of skull or craniotomy
Delete		Disruption or dehiscence of closure of sternum or sternotomy
Delete		Disruption or dehiscence of closure of tendon or ligament
Delete		Disruption or dehiscence of closure of superficial or muscular fascia
Add	**T81.320**	**Disruption or dehiscence of gastrointestinal tract anastomosis, repair, or closure**
Add	**T81.321**	**Disruption or dehiscence of closure of internal operation (surgical) wound of abdominal wall muscle or fascia**
Add	**T81.328**	**Disruption or dehiscence of closure of other specified internal operation (surgical) wound**
Add		Disruption or dehiscence of closure of muscle or muscle flap (other than abdominal wall muscle)
Add		Disruption or dehiscence of closure of ribs or rib cage
Add		Disruption or dehiscence of closure of skull or craniotomy
Add		Disruption or dehiscence of closure of sternum or sternotomy
Add		Disruption or dehiscence of closure of tendon or ligament
Add		Disruption or dehiscence of closure of superficial or muscular fascia (other than abdominal wall fascia)
Add	**T81.329**	**Deep disruption or dehiscence of operation wound, unspecified**
Add		Deep disruption or dehiscence of operation wound NOS

No Change	**T81.4**	**Infection following a procedure**
Add		Code also, if applicable, disruption of internal operation (surgical) wound (T81.32-)
No Change	**T81.8**	**Other complications of procedures, not elsewhere classified**
No Change	**T81.83**	**Persistent postprocedural fistula**
Add		Code also, if applicable, disruption of internal operation (surgical) wound (T81.32-)
No Change		Use Additional
Revise from		anal fistula (K60.3)
Revise to		anal fistula (K60.3-)
Revise from		anorectal fistula (K60.5)
Revise to		anorectal fistula (K60.5-)

No Change **CHAPTER 21**

No Change

FACTORS INFLUENCING HEALTH STATUS AND CONTACT WITH HEALTH SERVICES (Z00-Z99)

No Change   This chapter contains the following blocks:

Revise from	Z17	Estrogen receptor status
Revise to	Z17	Estrogen, and other hormones and factors receptor status

No Change   **GENETIC CARRIER AND GENETIC SUSCEPTIBILITY TO DISEASE (Z14-Z15)**

No Change	**Z15**	**Genetic susceptibility to disease**
Add	**Z15.1**	**Genetic susceptibility to epilepsy and neurodevelopmental disorders**
Add		Code also, if applicable, related disorders such as:
Add		developmental and epileptic encephalopathy (G93.45)
Add		developmental disorder of speech and language (F80.-)
Add		developmental disorders of scholastic skills (F81.-)
Add		epilepsy, by specific type (G40.-)
Add		intellectual disabilities (F70-F79)
Add		other neurodevelopmental disorder (F88)
Add		pervasive developmental disorders (F84.-)
Add	**Z15.2**	**Genetic susceptibility to obesity**
Add		Code also, if applicable, any associated manifestations, such as:
Add		other obesity (E66.8-)
Add		polyphagia (R63.2)
Add		Use Additional code to identify body mass index (BMI), if known (Z68.-)

Revise from		**ESTROGEN RECEPTOR STATUS (Z17)**
Revise to		**ESTROGEN, AND OTHER HORMONES AND FACTORS RECEPTOR STATUS (Z17)**
Revise from	**Z17**	**Estrogen receptor status**
Revise to	**Z17**	**Estrogen, and other hormones and factors receptor status**
Add		Note: Use one code, as available, for each receptor: Z17.0, Z17.1, Z17.2-, Z17.3-
Add		Code first malignant neoplasm, such as: malignant neoplasm of ovary (C56.-)
Add	**Z17.2**	**Progesterone receptor status**
Add	**Z17.21**	**Progesterone receptor positive status** PR+
Add	**Z17.22**	**Progesterone receptor negative status** PR-
Add	**Z17.3**	**Human epidermal growth factor 2 receptor**
Add	**Z17.31**	**Human epidermal growth factor receptor 2 positive status** HER2+

Add	Z17.32	Human epidermal growth factor receptor 2 negative status
Add		HER2-
Add	Z17.4	Combined receptor status
Add		**Note:** Assign a code from subcategory Z17.4- when only a combined receptor status is documented
Add	Z17.41	Hormone receptor positive
Add		HR+
Add		Z17.410	Hormone receptor positive with human epidermal growth factor receptor 2 positive status
Add			HR+ with HER2+
Add		Z17.411	Hormone receptor positive with human epidermal growth factor receptor 2 negative status
Add			HR+ with HER2-
Add	Z17.42	Hormone receptor negative
Add		HR-
Add		Z17.420	Hormone receptor negative with human epidermal growth factor receptor 2 positive status
Add			HR- with HER2+
Add		Z17.421	Hormone receptor negative with human epidermal growth factor receptor 2 negative status
Add			HR- with HER2-
Add			TNBC
Add			Triple negative breast cancer

ENCOUNTERS FOR OTHER SPECIFIC HEALTH CARE (Z40-Z53) *No Change*

No Change Z45	Encounter for adjustment and management of implanted device
No Change	Z45.3	Encounter for adjustment and management of implanted devices of the special senses
No Change		Z45.32	Encounter for adjustment and management of implanted hearing device
No Change		**Excludes1**
Revise from			Encounter for fitting and adjustment of hearing aide (Z46.1)
Revise to			Encounter for fitting and adjustment of hearing aid (Z46.1)
No Change Z51	Encounter for other aftercare and medical care
Add	Z51.A	Encounter for sepsis aftercare

No Change **PERSONS WITH POTENTIAL HEALTH HAZARDS RELATED TO SOCIOECONOMIC AND PSYCHOSOCIAL CIRCUMSTANCES (Z55-Z65)**

No Change Z59	Problems related to housing and economic circumstances
No Change	Z59.7	Insufficient social insurance and welfare support
Add		Insufficient social and welfare insurance
Add		Z59.71	Insufficient health insurance coverage
Add			Inadequate social insurance
Add			Insufficient social insurance
Add			No health insurance coverage
Add		Z59.72	Insufficient welfare support
Add			Inadequate welfare support

BLOOD TYPE (Z67) *No Change*

No Change Z67	Blood type
Add	Z67.A	Duffy phenotype
Add		Z67.A1	Duffy null
Add			Duffy phenotype Fy(a-b-)
Add		Z67.A2	Duffy a positive
Add			Duffy phenotype Fy(a+b-)
Add		Z67.A3	Duffy b positive
Add			Duffy phenotype Fy(a-b+)
Add		Z67.A4	Duffy a and b positive
Add			Duffy phenotype Fy(a+b+)

No Change **BODY MASS INDEX [BMI] (Z68)**

No Change Z68	Body mass index [BMI]
No Change	Z68.5	Body mass index [BMI] pediatric
Revise from		Z68.54	Body mass index [BMI] pediatric, greater than or equal to 95th percentile for age
Revise to		Z68.54	Body mass index [BMI] pediatric, 95th percentile for age to less than 120% of the 95th percentile for age
Add		Z68.55	Body mass index [BMI] pediatric, 120% of the 95th percentile for age to less than 140% of the 95th percentile for age
Add		Z68.56	Body mass index [BMI] pediatric, greater than or equal to 140% of the 95th percentile for age

No Change **PERSONS WITH POTENTIAL HEALTH HAZARDS RELATED TO FAMILY AND PERSONAL HISTORY AND CERTAIN CONDITIONS INFLUENCING HEALTH STATUS (Z77-Z99)**

No Change Z79	Long term (current) drug therapy
No Change	Z79.6	Long term (current) use of immunomodulators and immunosuppressants
No Change		Z79.62	Long term (current) use of immunosuppressant
No Change			Z79.624	Long term (current) use of inhibitors of nucleotide synthesis
Revise from				Long term (current) use omycophenolate
Revise to				Long term (current) use of mycophenolate
No Change Z83	Family history of other specific disorders
No Change	Z83.7	Family history of diseases of the digestive system
Add		Z83.72	Family history of familial adenomatous polyposis
No Change Z86	Personal history of certain other diseases
No Change	Z86.0	Personal history of in-situ and benign neoplasms and neoplasms of uncertain behavior
No Change		Z86.01	Personal history of benign neoplasm
Revise from			Z86.010	Personal history of colonic polyps
Revise to			Z86.010	Personal history of colon polyps
Add				Personal history of colorectal polyps
Add				Personal history of rectal polyps
Add				Z86.0100	Personal history of colon polyps, unspecified
Add					Personal history of colon polyps NOS

Add		Z86.0101	Personal history of adenomatous and serrated colon polyps
			Personal history of tubular adenoma polyps
Add			Personal history of sessile adenomatous colon polyp
Add			Personal history of sessile serrated colon polyp
Add			Personal history of tubulovillous adenoma polyps
Add			Personal history of villous adenoma polyps
Add			Personal history of traditional serrated adenoma polyps
Add		Z86.0102	Personal history of hyperplastic colon polyps
Add		Z86.0109	Personal history of other colon polyps

No Change	Z91		Personal risk factors, not elsewhere classified
No Change		Z91.1	Patient's noncompliance with medical treatment and regimen
No Change		Z91.12	Patient's intentional underdosing of medication regimen
			Excludes1 adverse effect of prescribed drug taken as directed-code to adverse effect
Delete			
Delete			poisoning (overdose)-code to poisoning

No Change		Z91.13	Patient's unintentional underdosing of medication regimen
Delete			**Excludes1** adverse effect of prescribed drug taken as directed-code to adverse effect
Delete			poisoning (overdose)-code to poisoning
No Change		Z91.14	Patient's other noncompliance with medication regimen
Add			*Code first, if applicable, adverse effect of underdosing (T36-T50)*
No Change	Z92		Personal history of medical treatment
No Change		Z92.2	Personal history of drug therapy
No Change		Z92.22	Personal history of monoclonal drug therapy
Add			**Excludes2** personal history of immune checkpoint inhibitor therapy (Z92.26)
Add		Z92.26	Personal history of immune checkpoint inhibitor therapy
Add			Personal history of ICI drug therapy
No Change		Z92.8	Personal history of other medical treatment
No Change		Z92.85	Personal history of cellular therapy
Add			**Excludes2** personal history of immune checkpoint inhibitor therapy (Z92.26)
No Change	Z93		Artificial opening status
No Change		Z93.2	Ileostomy status
Add			Ileal pouch status
Add			Kock pouch status

PART I

Introduction

ICD-10-CM Official Guidelines for Coding and Reporting FY2025
(October 1, 2024 - September 30, 2025)

Narrative changes appear in **bold** text
Items <u>underlined</u> have been moved within the guidelines since the 2024 version
Italics are used to indicate revisions to heading changes

The Centers for Medicare and Medicaid Services (CMS) and the National Center for Health Statistics (NCHS), two departments within the U.S. Federal Government's Department of Health and Human Services (DHHS), provide the following guidelines for coding and reporting using the International Classification of Diseases, 10th Revision, Clinical Modification (ICD-10-CM). These guidelines should be used as a companion document to the official version of the ICD-10-CM as published on the NCHS website. The ICD-10-CM is a morbidity classification published by the United States for classifying diagnoses and reason for visits in all health care settings. The ICD-10-CM is based on the ICD-10, the statistical classification of disease published by the World Health Organization (WHO).

These guidelines have been approved by the four organizations that make up the Cooperating Parties for the ICD-10-CM: the American Hospital Association (AHA), the American Health Information Management Association (AHIMA), CMS, and NCHS.

These guidelines are a set of rules that have been developed to accompany and complement the official conventions and instructions provided within the ICD-10-CM itself. The instructions and conventions of the classification take precedence over guidelines. These guidelines are based on the coding and sequencing instructions in the Tabular List and Alphabetic Index of ICD-10-CM, but provide additional instruction. Adherence to these guidelines when assigning ICD-10-CM diagnosis codes is required under the Health Insurance Portability and Accountability Act (HIPAA). The diagnosis codes (Tabular List and Alphabetic Index)

have been adopted under HIPAA for all health care settings. A joint effort between the health care provider and the coder is essential to achieve complete and accurate documentation, code assignment, and reporting of diagnoses and procedures. These guidelines have been developed to assist both the health care provider and the coder in identifying those diagnoses that are to be reported. The importance of consistent, complete documentation in the medical record cannot be overemphasized. Without such documentation accurate coding cannot be achieved. The entire record should be reviewed to determine the specific reason for the encounter and the conditions treated.

The term "encounter" is used for all settings, including hospital admissions. In the context of these guidelines, the term "provider" is used throughout the guidelines to mean physician or any qualified health care practitioner who is legally accountable for establishing the patient's diagnosis. Only this set of guidelines, approved by the Cooperating Parties, is official.

The guidelines are organized into sections. Section I includes the structure and conventions of the classification and general guidelines that apply to the entire classification, and chapter-specific guidelines that correspond to the chapters as they are arranged in the classification. Section II includes guidelines for selection of principal diagnosis for non-outpatient settings. Section III includes guidelines for reporting additional diagnoses in non-outpatient settings. Section IV is for outpatient coding and reporting. It is necessary to review all sections of the guidelines to fully understand all of the rules and instructions needed to code properly.

ICD-10-CM Official Guidelines for Coding and Reporting

Section I. Conventions, General Coding Guidelines and Chapter Specific Guidelines

A. Conventions for the ICD-10-CM
1. The Alphabetic Index and Tabular List
2. Format and Structure:
3. Use of codes for reporting purposes
4. Placeholder character
5. 7th Characters
6. Abbreviations
   a. Alphabetic Index abbreviations
   b. Tabular List abbreviations
7. Punctuation
8. Use of "and"
9. Other and Unspecified codes
   a. "Other" codes
   b. "Unspecified" codes
10. Includes Notes
11. Inclusion terms
12. Excludes Notes
   a. Excludes1
   b. Excludes2
13. Etiology/manifestation convention ("code first", "use additional code" and "in diseases classified elsewhere" notes)
14. "And"
15. "With"
16. "See" and "See Also"
17. "Code also note"
18. Default codes
19. Code assignment and Clinical Criteria

B. General Coding Guidelines
1. Locating a code in the ICD-10-CM
2. Level of Detail in Coding
3. Code or codes from A00.0 through T88.9, Z00-Z99.8, U00-U85
4. Signs and symptoms
5. Conditions that are an integral part of a disease process
6. Conditions that are not an integral part of a disease process
7. Multiple coding for a single condition
8. Acute and Chronic Conditions
9. Combination Code
10. Sequela (Late Effects)
11. Impending or Threatened Condition
12. Reporting Same Diagnosis Code more than Once
13. Laterality
14. Documentation by Clinicians Other than the Patient's Provider
15. Syndromes
16. Documentation of Complications of Care
17. Borderline Diagnosis
18. Use of Sign/Symptom/Unspecified Codes
19. Coding for Healthcare Encounters in Hurricane Aftermath
   a. Use of External Cause of Morbidity Codes
   b. Sequencing of External Causes of Morbidity Codes
   c. Other External Causes of Morbidity Code Issues
   d. Use of Z codes

C. Chapter-Specific Coding Guidelines
1. Chapter 1: Certain Infectious and Parasitic Diseases (A00-B99, U07.1, U09.9)
   a. Human Immunodeficiency Virus (HIV) Infections
   b. Infectious agents as the cause of diseases classified to other chapters
   c. Infections resistant to antibiotics
   d. Sepsis, Severe Sepsis, and Septic Shock infection resistant to antibiotics
   e. Methicillin Resistant Staphylococcus aureus (MRSA) Conditions
   f. Zika virus infection
   g. Coronavirus infections
2. Chapter 2: Neoplasms (C00-D49)
   a. *Admission/Encounter for treatment of primary site*
   b. *Admission/Encounter for t*reatment of secondary site
   c. Coding and sequencing of complications
   d. Primary malignancy previously excised
   e. Admissions/Encounters involving chemotherapy, immunotherapy and radiation therapy
   f. Admission/encounter to determine extent of malignancy
   g. Symptoms, signs, and abnormal findings listed in Chapter 18 associated with neoplasms
   h. Admission/encounter for pain control/management
   i. Malignancy in two or more noncontiguous sites
   j. Disseminated malignant neoplasm, unspecified
   k. Malignant neoplasm without specification of site
   l. Sequencing of neoplasm codes
   m. Current malignancy versus personal history of malignancy
   n. Leukemia, Multiple Myeloma, and Malignant Plasma Cell Neoplasms in remission versus personal history
   o. Aftercare following surgery for neoplasm
   p. Follow-up care for completed treatment of a malignancy
   q. Prophylactic organ removal for prevention of malignancy
   r. Malignant neoplasm associated with transplanted organ
   s. Breast Implant Associated Anaplastic Large Cell Lymphoma
   t. Secondary malignant neoplasm of lymphoid tissue
3. Chapter 3: Disease of the Blood and Blood-Forming Organs and Certain Disorders Involving the Immune Mechanism (D50-D89)
4. Chapter 4: Endocrine, Nutritional, and Metabolic Diseases (E00-E89)
   a. Diabetes mellitus
5. Chapter 5: Mental, Behavioral, and Neurodevelopmental disorders (F01 – F99)
   a. Pain disorders related to psychological factors
   b. Mental and behavioral disorders due to psychoactive substance use
   c. Factitious Disorder
6. Chapter 6: Diseases of the Nervous System (G00-G99)
   a. Dominant/nondominant side
   b. Pain - Category G89

GUIDELINES (ICD-10-CM)

21. Chapter 21: Factors Influencing Health Status and Contact with Health Services (Z00-Z99)
    a. Use of Z Codes in Any Healthcare Setting
    b. Z Codes Indicate a Reason for an Encounter or Provide Additional Information about a Patient Encounter
    c. Categories of Z Codes
22. Chapter 22: Codes for Special Purposes (U00-U85)

Section II. Selection of Principal Diagnosis

A. Codes for symptoms, signs, and ill-defined conditions
B. Two or more interrelated conditions, each potentially meeting the definition for principal diagnosis
C. Two or more diagnoses that equally meet the definition for principal diagnosis
D. Two or more comparative or contrasting conditions
E. A symptom(s) followed by contrasting/comparative diagnoses
F. Original treatment plan not carried out
G. Complications of surgery and other medical care
H. Uncertain Diagnosis
I. Admission from Observation Unit
    1. Admission Following Medical Observation
    2. Admission Following Post-Operative Observation
J. Admission from Outpatient Surgery
K. Admissions/Encounters for Rehabilitation

Section III. Reporting Additional Diagnoses

A. Previous conditions
B. Abnormal findings
C. Uncertain Diagnosis

Section IV. Diagnostic Coding and Reporting Guidelines for Outpatient Services

A. Selection of first-listed condition
    1. Outpatient Surgery
    2. Observation Stay
B. Codes from A00.0 through T88.9, Z00-Z99, U00-U85
C. Accurate reporting of ICD-10-CM diagnosis codes
D. Codes that describe symptoms and signs
E. Encounters for circumstances other than a disease or injury
F. Level of Detail in Coding
    1. ICD-10-CM codes with 3, 4, 5, 6, or 7 characters
    2. Use of full number of characters required for a code
    3. Highest level of specificity
G. ICD-10-CM code for the diagnosis, condition, problem, or other reason for encounter/visit
H. Uncertain diagnosis
I. Chronic diseases
J. Code all documented conditions that coexist
K. Patients receiving diagnostic services only
L. Patients receiving therapeutic services only
M. Patients receiving preoperative evaluations only
N. Ambulatory surgery
O. Routine outpatient prenatal visits
P. Encounters for general medical examinations with abnormal findings
Q. Encounters for routine health screenings

Appendix I: Present on Admission Reporting Guidelines

Section I. Conventions, General Coding Guidelines, and Chapter Specific Guidelines

The conventions, general guidelines, and chapter-specific guidelines are applicable to all health care settings unless otherwise indicated. The conventions and instructions of the classification take precedence over guidelines.

A. **Conventions for the ICD-10-CM**
   The conventions for the ICD-10-CM are the general rules for use of the classification independent of the guidelines. These conventions are incorporated within the Alphabetic Index and Tabular List of the ICD-10-CM as instructional notes.

   1. **The Alphabetic Index and Tabular List**
      The ICD-10-CM is divided into the Alphabetic Index, an alphabetical list of terms and their corresponding code, and the Tabular List, a structured list of codes divided into chapters based on body system or condition. The Alphabetic Index consists of the following parts: the Index of Diseases and Injury, the Index of External Causes of Injury, the Table of Neoplasms, and the Table of Drugs and Chemicals.
      See Section I.C.2. **Neoplasms**
      See Section I.C.19. Adverse effects, poisoning, underdosing and toxic effects

   2. **Format and Structure:**
      The ICD-10-CM Tabular List contains categories, subcategories and codes. Characters for categories, subcategories and codes may be either a letter or a number. All categories are 3 characters. A 3-character category that has no further subdivision is equivalent to a code. Subcategories are either 4 or 5 characters. Codes may be 3, 4, 5, 6 or 7 characters. That is, each level of subdivision after a category is a subcategory. The final level of subdivision is a code. Codes that have applicable 7th characters are still referred to as codes, not subcategories. A code that has an applicable 7th character is considered invalid without the 7th character.
      The ICD-10-CM uses an indented format for ease in reference

   3. **Use of codes for reporting purposes**
      For reporting purposes only codes are permissible, not categories or subcategories, and any applicable 7th character is required.

   4. **Placeholder character**
      The ICD-10-CM utilizes a placeholder character "X". The "X" is used as a placeholder at certain codes to allow for future expansion. An example of this is at the poisoning, adverse effect and underdosing codes, categories T36-T50. Where a placeholder exists, the X must be used in order for the code to be considered a valid code.

   5. **7th Characters**
      Certain ICD-10-CM categories have applicable 7th characters. The applicable 7th character is required for all codes within the category, or as the notes in the Tabular List instruct. The 7th character must always be the 7th character in the data field. If a

code that requires a 7th character is not 6 characters, a placeholder X must be used to fill in the empty characters.

6. **Abbreviations**

   a. **Alphabetic Index abbreviations**

      NEC "Not elsewhere classifiable"
      This abbreviation in the Alphabetic Index represents "other specified". When a specific code is not available for a condition the Alphabetic Index directs the coder to the "other specified" code in the Tabular List.

      NOS "Not otherwise specified"
      This abbreviation is the equivalent of unspecified.

   b. **Tabular List abbreviations**

      NEC "Not elsewhere classifiable"
      This abbreviation in the Tabular List represents "other specified". When a specific code is not available for a condition, the Tabular List includes an NEC entry under a code to identify the code as the "other specified" code.

      NOS "Not otherwise specified"
      This abbreviation is the equivalent of unspecified.

7. **Punctuation**

   [ ] Brackets are used in the Tabular List to enclose synonyms, alternative wording or explanatory phrases. Brackets are used in the Alphabetic Index to identify manifestation codes.

   ( ) Parentheses are used in both the Alphabetic Index and Tabular List to enclose supplementary words that may be present or absent in the statement of a disease or procedure without affecting the code number to which it is assigned. The terms within the parentheses are referred to as nonessential modifiers. The nonessential modifiers in the Alphabetic Index to Diseases apply to subterms following a main term except when a nonessential modifier and a subentry are mutually exclusive, the subentry takes precedence. For example, in the ICD-10-CM Alphabetic Index under the main term Enteritis, "acute" is a nonessential modifier and "chronic" is a subentry. In this case, the nonessential modifier "acute" does not apply to the subentry "chronic".

   : Colons are used in the Tabular List after an incomplete term which needs one or more of the modifiers following the colon to make it assignable to a given category.

8. **Use of "and".**

   See Section I.A.14. Use of the term "And"

9. **Other and Unspecified codes**

   a. **"Other" codes**
   Codes titled "other" or "other specified" are for use when the information in the medical record provides detail for which a specific code does not exist. Alphabetic Index entries with NEC in the line designate "other" codes in the Tabular List.

These Alphabetic Index entries represent specific disease entities for which no specific code exists so the term is included within an "other" code.

   b. **"Unspecified" codes**
   Codes titled "unspecified" are for use when the information in the medical record is insufficient to assign a more specific code. For those categories for which an unspecified code is not provided, the "other specified" code may represent both other and unspecified.
   See Section I.B.18 Use of signs/symptoms/unspecified codes

10. **Includes Notes**
    This note appears immediately under a 3-character code title to further define, or give examples of, the content of the category.

11. **Inclusion terms**
    List of terms is included under some codes. These terms are the conditions for which that code is to be used. The terms may be synonyms of the code title, or, in the case of "other specified" codes, the terms are a list of the various conditions assigned to that code. The inclusion terms are not necessarily exhaustive. Additional terms found only in the Alphabetic Index may also be assigned to a code.

12. **Excludes Notes**
    The ICD-10-CM has two types of excludes notes. Each type of note has a different definition for use, but they are all similar in that they indicate that codes excluded from each other are independent of each other.

    a. **Excludes1**
    A type 1 Excludes note is a pure excludes note. It means "NOT CODED HERE!" An Excludes1 note indicates that the code excluded should never be used at the same time as the code above the Excludes1 note. An Excludes1 is used when two conditions cannot occur together, such as a congenital form versus an acquired form of the same condition.

    An exception to the Excludes1 definition is the circumstance when the two conditions are unrelated to each other. If it is not clear whether the two conditions involving an Excludes1 note are related or not, query the provider. For example, code F45.8, Other somatoform disorders, has an Excludes1 note for "sleep related teeth grinding (G47.63)" because "teeth grinding" is an inclusion term under F45.8. Only one of these two codes should be assigned for teeth grinding. However, psychogenic dysmenorrhea is also an inclusion term under F45.8, and a patient could have both this condition and sleep-related teeth grinding. In this case, the two conditions are clearly unrelated to each other, and so it would be appropriate to report F45.8 and G47.63 together.

    b. **Excludes2**
    A Type 2 Excludes note represents "Not included here." An excludes2 note indicates that the condition excluded is not part of the condition represented by the code, but a patient may have both conditions at the same time. When

an Excludes2 note appears under a code, it is acceptable to use both the code and the excluded code together, when appropriate.

13. **Etiology/manifestation convention ("code first", "use additional code" and "in diseases classified elsewhere" notes)**

Certain conditions have both an underlying etiology and multiple body system manifestations due to the underlying etiology. For such conditions, the ICD-10-CM has a coding convention that requires the underlying condition be sequenced first, if applicable, followed by the manifestation. Wherever such a combination exists, there is a "use additional code" note at the etiology code, and a "code first" note at the manifestation code. These instructional notes indicate the proper sequencing order of the codes, etiology followed by manifestation.

In most cases the manifestation codes will have in the code title, "in diseases classified elsewhere." Codes with this title are a component of the etiology/manifestation convention. The code title indicates that it is a manifestation code. "In diseases classified elsewhere" codes are never permitted to be used as first-listed or principal diagnosis codes. They must be used in conjunction with an underlying condition code and they must be listed following the underlying condition. See category F02, Dementia in other diseases classified elsewhere, for an example of this convention.

There are manifestation codes that do not have "in diseases classified elsewhere" in the title. For such codes, there is a "use additional code" note at the etiology code and a "code first" note at the manifestation code and the rules for sequencing apply.

In addition to the notes in the Tabular List, these conditions also have a specific Alphabetic Index entry structure. In the Alphabetic Index both conditions are listed together with the etiology code first followed by the manifestation codes in brackets. The code in brackets is always to be sequenced second.

An example of the etiology/manifestation convention is dementia with Parkinson's disease. In the Alphabetic Index, **a** code **from category G20** is listed first, followed by code F02.80 or F02.81 in brackets. A code from category G20- represents the underlying etiology, Parkinson's disease, and must be sequenced first, whereas *codes* F02.80 and F02.81 represent the manifestation of dementia in diseases classified elsewhere, with or without behavioral disturbance.

"Code first" and "Use additional code" notes are also used as sequencing rules in the classification for certain codes that are not part of an etiology/manifestation combination.

See Section I.B.7. Multiple coding for a single condition.

14. **"And"**

The word "and" should be interpreted to mean either "and" or "or" when it appears in a title.

For example, cases of "tuberculosis of bones", "tuberculosis of joints" and "tuberculosis of bones and joints" are classified to subcategory A18.0, Tuberculosis of bones and joints.

15. **"With"**

The word "with" or "in" should be interpreted to mean "associated with" or "due to" when it appears in a code title, the Alphabetic Index, (either under a main term or subterm) or an instructional note in the Tabular List. The classification presumes a causal relationship between the two conditions linked by these terms in the Alphabetic Index or Tabular List. These conditions should be coded as related even in the absence of provider documentation explicitly linking them, unless the documentation clearly states the conditions are unrelated or when another guideline exists that specifically requires a documented linkage between two conditions (e.g., sepsis guideline for "acute organ dysfunction that is not clearly associated with the sepsis").

For conditions not specifically linked by these relational terms in the classification or when a guideline requires that a linkage between two conditions be explicitly documented provider documentation must link the conditions in order to code them as related.

The word "with" in the Alphabetic Index is sequenced immediately following the main term or subterm, not in alphabetical order.

16. **"See" and "See Also"**

The "see" instruction following a main term in the Alphabetic Index indicates that another term should be referenced. It is necessary to go to the main term referenced with the "see" note to locate the correct code.

A "see also" instruction following a main term in the Alphabetic Index instructs that there is another main term that may also be referenced that may provide additional Alphabetic Index entries that may be useful. It is not necessary to follow the "see also" note when the original main term provides the necessary code.

17. **"Code also" note**

A "code also" note instructs that two codes may be required to fully describe a condition, but this note does not provide sequencing direction. The sequencing depends on the circumstances of the encounter.

18. **Default codes**

A code listed next to a main term in the ICD-10-CM Alphabetic Index is referred to as a default code. The default code represents that condition that is most commonly associated with the main term, or is the unspecified code for the condition. If a condition is documented in a medical record (for example, appendicitis) without any additional information, such as acute or chronic, the default code should be assigned.

19. **Code assignment and Clinical Criteria**

The assignment of a diagnosis code is based on the provider's diagnostic statement that the condition exists. The provider's statement that the patient has a particular condition is sufficient. Code assignment is not based on clinical criteria used by the provider to establish the diagnosis. **If there is** conflicting medical record documentation, query the provider.

B. General Coding Guidelines

1. Locating a code in the ICD-10-CM

To select a code in the classification that corresponds to a diagnosis or reason for visit documented in a medical record, first locate the term in the Alphabetic Index, and then verify the code in the Tabular List. Read and be guided by instructional notations that appear in both the Alphabetic Index and the Tabular List.

It is essential to use both the Alphabetic Index and Tabular List when locating and assigning a code. The Alphabetic Index does not always provide the full code. Selection of the full code, including laterality and any applicable 7th character can only be done in the Tabular List. A dash (-) at the end of an Alphabetic Index entry indicates that additional characters are required. Even if a dash is not included at the Alphabetic Index entry, it is necessary to refer to the Tabular List to verify that no 7th character is required.

2. Level of Detail in Coding

Diagnosis codes are to be used and reported at their highest number of characters available and to the highest level of specificity documented in the medical record.

ICD-10-CM diagnosis codes are composed of codes with 3, 4, 5, 6, or 7 characters. Codes with three characters are included in ICD-10-CM as the heading of a category of codes that may be further subdivided by the use of 4th and/or 5th characters and/or 6th characters, which provide greater detail.

A 3-character code is to be used only if it is not further subdivided. A code is invalid if it has not been coded to the full number of characters required for that code, including the 7th character, if applicable.

3. Code or codes from A00.0 through T88.9, Z00-Z99.8, U00-U85

The appropriate code or codes from A00.0 through T88.9, Z00-Z99.8 and U00-U85 must be used to identify diagnoses, symptoms, conditions, problems, complaints or other reason(s) for the encounter/visit.

4. Signs and symptoms

Codes that describe symptoms and signs, as opposed to diagnoses, are acceptable for reporting purposes when a related definitive diagnosis has not been established (confirmed) by the provider. Chapter 18 of ICD-10-CM, Symptoms, Signs, and Abnormal Clinical and Laboratory Findings, Not Elsewhere Classified (codes R00.0 - R99) contains many, but not all codes for symptoms.

See Section I.B.18 Use of signs/symptoms/unspecified codes

5. Conditions that are an integral part of a disease process

Signs and symptoms that are associated routinely with a disease process should not be assigned as additional codes, unless otherwise instructed by the classification.

6. Conditions that are not an integral part of a disease process

Additional signs and symptoms that may not be associated routinely with a disease process should be coded when present.

7. Multiple coding for a single condition

In addition to the etiology/manifestation convention that requires two codes to fully describe a single condition that affects multiple body systems, there are other single conditions that also require more than one code. "Use additional code" notes are found in the Tabular List at codes that are not part of an etiology/manifestation pair where a secondary code is useful to fully describe a condition. The sequencing rule is the same as the etiology/manifestation pair, "use additional code" indicates that a secondary code should be added, if known.

For example, for bacterial infections that are not included in Chapter 1, a secondary code from category B95, Streptococcus, Staphylococcus, and Enterococcus, as the cause of diseases classified elsewhere, or B96, Other bacterial agents as the cause of diseases classified elsewhere, may be required to identify the bacterial organism causing the infection. A "use additional code" note will normally be found at the infectious disease code, indicating a need for the organism code to be added as a secondary code.

"Code first" notes are also under certain codes that are not specifically manifestation codes but may be due to an underlying cause. When there is a "code first" note and an underlying condition is present, the underlying condition should be sequenced first, if known.

"Code, if applicable, any causal condition first," notes indicate that this code may be assigned as a principal diagnosis when the causal condition is unknown or not applicable. If a causal condition is known, then the code for that condition should be sequenced as the principal or first-listed diagnosis.

Multiple codes may be needed for sequela, complication codes and obstetric codes to more fully describe a condition. See the specific guidelines for these conditions for further instruction.

8. Acute and Chronic Conditions

If the same condition is described as both acute (subacute) and chronic, and separate subentries exist in the Alphabetic Index at the same indentation level, code both and sequence the acute (subacute) code first.

9. Combination Code

A combination code is a single code used to classify:
Two diagnoses, or
A diagnosis with an associated secondary process (manifestation)
A diagnosis with an associated complication
Combination codes are identified by referring to subterm entries in the Alphabetic Index and by reading the inclusion and exclusion notes in the Tabular List.

Assign only the combination code when that code fully identifies the diagnostic conditions involved or when the Alphabetic Index so directs. Multiple coding should not be used when the classification provides a combination code that clearly identifies all of the elements documented in the diagnosis. When the combination code lacks necessary specificity in describing the manifestation or complication, an additional code should be used as a secondary code.

10. **Sequela (Late Effects)**
A sequela is the residual effect (condition produced) after the acute phase of an illness or injury has terminated. There is no time limit on when a sequela code can be used. The residual may be apparent early, such as in cerebral infarction, or it may occur months or years later, such as that due to a previous injury. Examples of sequela include: scar formation resulting from a burn, deviated septum due to a nasal fracture, and infertility due to tubal occlusion from old tuberculosis. Coding of sequela generally requires two codes sequenced in the following order: the condition or nature of the sequela is sequenced first. The sequela code is sequenced second.

An exception to the above guidelines are those instances where the code for the sequela is followed by a manifestation code identified in the Tabular List and title, or the sequela code has been expanded (at the 4th, 5th, or 6th character levels) to include the manifestation(s). The code for the acute phase of an illness or injury that led to the sequela is never used with a code for the late effect.

See Section I.C.9. Sequelae of cerebrovascular disease
See Section I.C.15. Sequelae of complication of pregnancy, childbirth and the puerperium
See Section I.C.19. Application of 7th characters for Chapter 19

11. **Impending or Threatened Condition**
Code any condition described at the time of discharge as "impending" or "threatened" as follows:
If it did occur, code as confirmed diagnosis.
If it did not occur, reference the Alphabetic Index to determine if the condition has a subentry term for "impending" or "threatened" and also reference main term entries for "Impending" and for "Threatened."
If the subterms are listed, assign the given code.
If the subterms are not listed, code the existing underlying condition(s) and not the condition described as impending or threatened.

12. **Reporting Same Diagnosis Code More Than Once**
Each unique ICD-10-CM diagnosis code may be reported only once for an encounter. This applies to bilateral conditions when there are no distinct codes identifying laterality or two different conditions classified to the same ICD-10-CM diagnosis code.

13. **Laterality**
Some ICD-10-CM codes indicate laterality, specifying whether the condition occurs on the left, right or is bilateral. If no bilateral code is provided and the condition is bilateral, assign separate codes for both the left and right side. If the side is not identified in the medical record, assign the code for the unspecified side.

When a patient has a bilateral condition and each side is treated during separate encounters, assign the "bilateral" code (as the condition still exists on both sides), including for the encounter to treat the first side. For the second encounter for treatment after one side has previously been treated and the condition no longer exists on that side, assign the appropriate unilateral code for the side where the condition still exists (e.g., cataract surgery performed on each eye in separate encounters). The bilateral code would not be assigned for the subsequent encounter, as the patient no longer has the condition in the previously-treated site. If the treatment on the first side did not completely resolve the condition, then the bilateral code would still be appropriate.

When laterality is not documented by the patient's provider, code assignment for the affected side may be based on medical record documentation from other clinicians. If there is conflicting medical record documentation regarding the affected side, the patient's provider should be queried for clarification. Codes for "unspecified" side should rarely be used, such as when the documentation in the record is insufficient to determine the affected side and it is not possible to obtain clarification.

14. **Documentation by Clinicians Other than the Patient's Provider**
Code assignment is based on the documentation by the patient's provider (i.e., physician or other qualified healthcare practitioner legally accountable for establishing the patient's diagnosis). There are a few exceptions when code assignment may be based on medical record documentation from clinicians who are not the patient's provider (i.e., physician or other qualified healthcare practitioner legally accountable for establishing the patient's diagnosis).

In this context, "clinicians" other than the patient's provider refer to healthcare professionals permitted, based on regulatory or accreditation requirements or internal hospital policies, to document in a patient's official medical record.

These exceptions include codes for:
- Body Mass Index (BMI)
- Depth of non-pressure chronic ulcers
- Pressure ulcer stage
- Coma scale
- NIH stroke scale (NIHSS)
- Social determinants of health (SDOH) **classified to Chapter 21**
- Laterality
- Blood alcohol level

This information is typically, **or may be,** documented by other clinicians involved in the care of the patient (e.g., a dietitian often documents the BMI, a nurse often documents the pressure ulcer stages, and an emergency medical technician often documents the coma scale). However, the associated diagnosis (such as overweight, obesity, acute stroke, pressure ulcer, or a condition classifiable to category F10, Alcohol related disorders) must be documented by the patient's provider. If there is conflicting medical record documentation, either from the same clinician or different clinicians, the patient's provider should be queried for clarification.

The BMI, coma scale, and NIHSS blood alcohol level codes, codes for social determinants of health **and underimmunization status** should only be reported as secondary diagnoses.

See Section I.C.21.c.17 for additional information regarding coding social determinants of health.

15. Syndromes

Follow the Alphabetic Index guidance when coding syndromes. In the absence of Alphabetic Index guidance, assign codes for the documented manifestations of the syndrome. Additional codes for manifestations that are not an integral part of the disease process may also be assigned when the condition does not have a unique code.

16. Documentation of Complications of Care

Code assignment is based on the provider's documentation of the relationship between the condition and the care or procedure, unless otherwise instructed by the classification. The guideline extends to any complications of care, regardless of the chapter the code is located in. It is important to note that not all conditions that occur during or following medical care or surgery are classified as complications. There must be a cause-and-effect relationship between the care provided and the condition, and **the documentation must support that the condition is clinically significant. It is not necessary for the provider to explicitly document the term "complication." For example, if the condition alters the course of the surgery as documented in the operative report, then it is would be appropriate to report a complication code.** Query the provider for clarification **if the documentation is not clear as to the relationship between the condition and the care or procedure.**

17. Borderline Diagnosis

If the provider documents a "borderline" diagnosis at the time of discharge, the diagnosis is coded as confirmed, unless the classification provides a specific entry (e.g., borderline diabetes). If a borderline condition has a specific index entry in ICD-10-CM, it should be coded as such. Since borderline conditions are not uncertain diagnoses, no distinction is made between the care setting (inpatient versus outpatient). Whenever the documentation is unclear regarding a borderline condition, coders are encouraged to query for clarification.

18. Use of Sign/Symptom/Unspecified Codes

Sign/symptom and "unspecified" codes have acceptable, even necessary, uses. While specific diagnosis codes should be reported when they are supported by the available medical record documentation and clinical knowledge of the patient's health condition, there are instances when signs/symptoms or unspecified codes are the best choices for accurately reflecting the healthcare encounter. Each healthcare encounter should be coded to the level of certainty known for that encounter.

As stated in the introductory section of these official coding guidelines, a joint effort between the healthcare provider and the coder is essential to achieve complete and accurate documentation, code assignment, and reporting of diagnoses and procedures. The importance of consistent, complete documentation in the medical record cannot be overemphasized. Without such documentation accurate coding cannot be achieved. The entire record should be reviewed to determine the specific reason for the encounter and the conditions treated.

If a definitive diagnosis has not been established by the end of the encounter, it is appropriate to report codes for sign(s) and/or symptom(s) in lieu of a definitive diagnosis. When sufficient clinical information isn't known or available about a particular health condition to assign a more specific code, it is acceptable to report the appropriate "unspecified" code (e.g., a diagnosis of pneumonia has been determined, but not the specific type). Unspecified codes should be reported when they are the codes that most accurately reflect what is known about the patient's condition at the time of that particular encounter. It would be inappropriate to select a specific code that is not supported by the medical record documentation or conduct medically unnecessary diagnostic testing in order to determine a more specific code.

19. Coding for Healthcare Encounters in Hurricane Aftermath

a. Use of External Cause of Morbidity Codes

An external cause of morbidity code should be assigned to identify the cause of the injury(ies) incurred as a result of the hurricane. The use of external cause of morbidity codes is supplemental to the application of ICD-10-CM codes. External cause of morbidity codes are never to be recorded as a principal diagnosis (first-listed in non-inpatient settings). The appropriate injury code should be sequenced before any external cause codes. The external cause of morbidity codes capture how the injury or health condition happened (cause), the intent (unintentional or accidental; or intentional, such as suicide or assault), the place where the event occurred, the activity of the patient at the time of the event, and the person's status (e.g., civilian, military). They should not be assigned for encounters to treat hurricane victims' medical conditions when no injury, adverse effect or poisoning is involved. External cause of morbidity codes should be assigned for each encounter for care and treatment of the injury. External cause of morbidity codes may be assigned in all health care settings. For the purpose of capturing complete and accurate ICD-10-CM data in the aftermath of the hurricane, a healthcare setting should be considered as any location where medical care is provided by licensed healthcare professionals.

b. Sequencing of External Causes of Morbidity Codes

Codes for cataclysmic events, such as a hurricane, take priority over all other external cause codes except child and adult abuse and terrorism and should be sequenced before other external cause of injury codes. Assign as many external cause of morbidity codes as necessary to fully explain each cause. For example, if an injury occurs as a result of a building collapse during the hurricane, external cause codes for both the hurricane and the building collapse should be assigned, with the external causes code for hurricane being sequenced as the first external cause code. For injuries incurred as a direct result of the hurricane, assign the appropriate code(s) for the injuries, followed by the code X37.0-, Hurricane (with the appropriate 7th character), and any other applicable external cause of injury codes. Code X37.0- also should be assigned when an injury is incurred as a result of flooding caused by a levee breaking related to the hurricane. Code X38.-, Flood (with the appropriate 7th character), should be assigned when an injury is from flooding resulting directly from the storm. Code X36.0.-, Collapse of dam or man-made structure, should not be assigned when the cause of the collapse is due to the hurricane. Use of code X36.0- is limited to collapses of man-made structures due to earth surface movements, not due to storm surges directly from a hurricane.

c. Other External Causes of Morbidity Code Issues

For injuries that are not a direct result of the hurricane, such as an evacuee that has incurred an injury as a result of a motor vehicle accident, assign the appropriate external cause of morbidity code(s) to describe the cause of the injury, but do not assign code X37.0-, Hurricane. If it is not clear whether the injury was a direct result of the hurricane, assume the injury is due to the hurricane and assign code X37.0-, Hurricane, as well as any other applicable external cause of morbidity codes. In addition to code X37.0-, Hurricane, other possible applicable external cause of morbidity codes include:

X30-	Exposure to excessive natural heat
X31-	Exposure to excessive natural cold
X38-	Flood

d. Use of Z codes

Z codes (other reasons for healthcare encounters) may be assigned as appropriate to further explain the reasons for presenting for healthcare services, including transfers between healthcare facilities or provide additional information relevant to a patient encounter. The ICD-10-CM Official Guidelines for Coding and Reporting identify which codes maybe assigned as principal or first-listed diagnosis only, secondary diagnosis only, or principal/first-listed or secondary (depending on the circumstances). Possible applicable Z codes include:

Z59.0-	Homelessness
Z59.1	Inadequate housing
Z59.5	Extreme poverty
Z75.1	Person awaiting admission to adequate facility elsewhere
Z75.3	Unavailability and inaccessibility of health-care facilities
Z75.4	Unavailability and inaccessibility of other helping agencies
Z76.2	Encounter for health supervision and care of other healthy infant and child
Z99.12	Encounter for respirator [ventilator] dependence during power failure

The external cause of morbidity codes and the Z codes listed above are not an all-inclusive list. Other codes may be applicable to the encounter based upon the documentation. Assign as many codes as necessary to fully explain each healthcare encounter. Since patient history information may be very limited, use any available documentation to assign the appropriate external cause of morbidity and Z codes.

C. Chapter-Specific Coding Guidelines

In addition to general coding guidelines, there are guidelines for specific diagnoses and/or conditions in the classification. Unless otherwise indicated, these guidelines apply to all health care settings. Please refer to Section II for guidelines on the selection of principal diagnosis.

1. Chapter 1: Certain Infectious and Parasitic Diseases (A00-B99, U07.1, U09.9)

a. Human Immunodeficiency Virus (HIV) Infections

1) Code only confirmed cases

Code only confirmed cases of HIV infection/illness. This is an exception to the hospital inpatient guideline Section II, H.

In this context, "confirmation" does not require documentation of positive serology or culture for HIV; the provider's diagnostic statement that the patient is HIV positive, or has an HIV-related illness is sufficient.

2) Selection and sequencing of HIV codes

(a) Patient admitted for HIV-related condition

If a patient is admitted for an HIV-related condition, the principal diagnosis should be B20, Human immunodeficiency virus [HIV] disease followed by additional diagnosis codes for all reported HIV-related conditions.

An exception to this guideline is if the reason for admission is hemolytic-uremic syndrome associated with HIV disease. Assign code D59.31, Infection-associated hemolytic-uremic syndrome, followed by code B20, Human immunodeficiency virus [HIV] disease.

ICD-10-CM PHYSICIAN EDITION

GUIDELINES (ICD-10-CM)

(b) Patient with HIV disease admitted for unrelated condition

If a patient with HIV disease is admitted for an unrelated condition (such as a traumatic injury), the code for the unrelated condition (e.g., the nature of injury code) should be the principal diagnosis. Other diagnoses would be B20 followed by additional diagnosis codes for all reported HIV-related conditions.

(c) Whether the patient is newly diagnosed

Whether the patient is newly diagnosed or has had previous admissions/encounters for HIV conditions is irrelevant to the sequencing decision.

(d) Asymptomatic human immunodeficiency virus

Z21, Asymptomatic human immunodeficiency virus [HIV] infection status, is to be applied when the patient without any documentation of symptoms is listed as being "HIV positive," "known HIV," "HIV test positive," or similar terminology. Do not use this code if the term "AIDS" or "HIV disease" is used or if the patient is treated for any HIV-related illness or is described as having any condition(s) resulting from his/her HIV positive status; use B20 in these cases.

(e) Patients with inconclusive HIV serology

Patients with inconclusive HIV serology, but no definitive diagnosis or manifestations of the illness, may be assigned code R75, Inconclusive laboratory evidence of human immunodeficiency virus [HIV].

(f) Previously diagnosed HIV-related illness

Patients with any known prior diagnosis of an HIV-related illness should be coded to B20. Once a patient has developed an HIV-related illness, the patient should always be assigned code B20 on every subsequent admission/encounter. Patients previously diagnosed with any HIV illness (B20) should never be assigned to R75 or Z21, Asymptomatic human immunodeficiency virus [HIV] infection status.

(g) HIV Infection in Pregnancy, Childbirth and the Puerperium

During pregnancy, childbirth or the puerperium, a patient admitted (or presenting for a health care encounter) because of an HIV-related illness should receive a principal diagnosis code of O98.7-, Human immunodeficiency [HIV] disease complicating pregnancy, childbirth and the puerperium, followed by B20 and the code(s) for the HIV-related illness(es). Codes from Chapter 15 always take sequencing priority.

Patients with asymptomatic HIV infection status admitted (or presenting for a health care encounter) during pregnancy, childbirth, or the puerperium should receive codes of O98.7- and Z21.

(h) Encounters for testing for HIV

If a patient is being seen to determine his/her HIV status, use code Z11.4, Encounter for screening for human immunodeficiency virus [HIV]. Use additional codes for any associated high-risk behavior, if applicable.

If a patient with signs or symptoms is being seen for HIV testing, code the signs and symptoms. An additional counseling code Z71.7, Human immunodeficiency virus [HIV] counseling, may be used if counseling is provided during the encounter for the test.

When a patient returns to be informed of his/her HIV test results and the test result is negative, use code Z71.7, Human immunodeficiency virus [HIV] counseling.

If the results are positive, see previous guidelines and assign codes as appropriate.

(i) HIV managed by antiretroviral medication

If a patient with documented HIV disease, HIV-related illness or AIDS is currently managed on antiretroviral medications, assign code B20, Human immunodeficiency virus [HIV] disease. Code Z79.899, Other long term (current) drug therapy, may be assigned as an additional code to identify the long-term (current) use of antiretroviral medications.

(j) Encounter for HIV Prophylaxis Measures

When a patient is seen for administration of pre-exposure prophylaxis medication for HIV, assign code Z29.81, Encounter for HIV pre-exposure prophylaxis. Pre-exposure prophylaxis (PrEP) is intended to prevent infection in people who are at risk for getting HIV through sex or injection drug use. Any risk factors for HIV should also be coded.

b. Infectious agents as the cause of diseases classified to other chapters

Certain infections are classified in chapters other than Chapter 1 and no organism is identified as part of the infection code. In these instances, it is necessary to use an additional code from Chapter 1 to identify the organism. A code from category B95, Streptococcus, Staphylococcus, and Enterococcus as the cause of diseases classified to other chapters, B96, Other bacterial agents as the cause of diseases classified to other chapters, or B97, Viral agents as the cause of diseases classified to other chapters, is to be used as an additional code to identify the organism. An instructional note will be found at the infection code advising that an additional organism code is required.

c. Infections resistant to antibiotics

Many bacterial infections are resistant to current antibiotics. It is necessary to identify all infections documented as antibiotic resistant. Assign a code from category Z16, Resistance to antimicrobial drugs, following the infection code only if the infection code does not identify drug resistance.

d. Sepsis, Severe Sepsis, and Septic Shock
   1) Coding of Sepsis and Severe Sepsis
      (a) Sepsis
For a diagnosis of sepsis, assign the appropriate code for the underlying systemic infection. If the type of infection or causal organism is not further specified, assign code A41.9, Sepsis, unspecified organism.

A code from subcategory R65.2, Severe sepsis, should not be assigned unless severe sepsis or an associated acute organ dysfunction is documented.

   (i) Negative or inconclusive blood cultures and sepsis
   Negative or inconclusive blood cultures do not preclude a diagnosis of sepsis in patients with clinical evidence of the condition, however, the provider should be queried.

   (ii) Urosepsis
   The term urosepsis is a nonspecific term. It is not to be considered synonymous with sepsis. It has no default code in the Alphabetic Index. Should a provider use this term, he/she must be queried for clarification.

   (iii) Sepsis with organ dysfunction
   If a patient has sepsis and associated acute organ dysfunction or multiple organ dysfunction (MOD), follow the instructions for coding severe sepsis.

   (iv) Acute organ dysfunction that is not clearly associated with the sepsis
   If a patient has sepsis and an acute organ dysfunction, but the medical record documentation indicates that the acute organ dysfunction is related to a medical condition other than the sepsis, do not assign a code from subcategory R65.2, Severe sepsis. An acute organ dysfunction must be associated with the sepsis in order to assign the severe sepsis code. If the documentation is not clear as to whether an acute organ dysfunction is related to the sepsis or another medical condition, query the provider.

      (b) Severe sepsis
The coding of severe sepsis requires a minimum of 2 codes: first a code for the underlying systemic infection, followed by a code from subcategory R65.2, Severe sepsis. If the causal organism is not documented, assign code A41.9, Sepsis, unspecified organism, for the infection. Additional code(s) for the associated acute organ dysfunction are also required.

Due to the complex nature of severe sepsis, some cases may require querying the provider prior to assignment of the codes.

   2) Septic shock
      (a) Septic shock generally refers to circulatory failure associated with severe sepsis, and therefore, it represents a type of acute organ dysfunction.
For all cases of septic shock, the code for the systemic infection should be sequenced first, followed by code R65.21, Severe sepsis with septic shock or code T81.12, Postprocedural septic shock. Any additional codes for the other acute organ dysfunctions should also be assigned. As noted in the sequencing instructions in the Tabular List, the code for septic shock cannot be assigned as a principal diagnosis.

   3) Sequencing of severe sepsis
If severe sepsis is present on admission, and meets the definition of principal diagnosis, the underlying systemic infection should be assigned as principal diagnosis followed by the appropriate code from subcategory R65.2 as required by the sequencing rules in the Tabular List. A code from subcategory R65.2 can never be assigned as a principal diagnosis.

When severe sepsis develops during an encounter (it was not present on admission) the underlying systemic infection and the appropriate code from subcategory R65.2 should be assigned as secondary diagnoses.

Severe sepsis may be present on admission but the diagnosis may not be confirmed until sometime after admission. If the documentation is not clear whether severe sepsis was present on admission, the provider should be queried.
For infection-associated hemolytic-uremic syndrome with severe sepsis, see guideline I.C.1.d.9.

   4) Sepsis or severe sepsis with a localized infection
If the reason for admission is sepsis or severe sepsis and a localized infection, such as pneumonia or cellulitis, a code(s) for the underlying systemic infection should be assigned first and the code for the localized infection should be assigned as a secondary diagnosis. If the patient has severe sepsis, a code from subcategory R65.2 should also be assigned as a secondary diagnosis. If the patient is admitted with a localized infection, such as pneumonia, and sepsis/severe sepsis doesn't develop until after admission, the localized infection should be assigned first, followed by the appropriate sepsis/severe sepsis codes.
For hemolytic-uremic syndrome associated with sepsis, see guideline I.C.1.d.9.

   5) Sepsis due to a postprocedural infection
      (a) Documentation of causal relationship
As with all postprocedural complications, code assignment is based on the provider's documentation of the relationship between the infection and the procedure.

      (b) Sepsis due to a postprocedural infection
For **sepsis** following a **postprocedural wound (surgical site) infection**, a code from **T81.41** to T81.43, Infection following a procedure, or a

code from O86.00 to O86.03, Infection of obstetric surgical wound, that identifies the site of the infection should be **sequenced** first, if known. Assign an additional code for sepsis following a procedure (T81.44) or sepsis following an obstetrical procedure (O86.04). Use an additional code to identify the infectious agent. If the patient has severe sepsis the appropriate code from subcategory R65.2 should also be assigned with the additional code(s) for any acute organ dysfunction.

For infections following infusion, transfusion, therapeutic injection, or immunization, a code from subcategory T80.2, Infections following infusion, transfusion, and therapeutic injection, or code T88.0-, Infection following immunization, should be coded first, followed by the code for the specific infection. If the patient has severe sepsis, the appropriate code from subcategory R65.2 should also be assigned, with the additional codes(s) for any acute organ dysfunction.

(c) Postprocedural infection and postprocedural septic shock

If a postprocedural infection has resulted in postprocedural septic shock, assign the codes indicated above for sepsis due to a postprocedural infection, followed by code T81.12-, Postprocedural septic shock. Do not assign code R65.21, Severe sepsis with septic shock. Additional code(s) should be assigned for any acute organ dysfunction.

6) Sepsis and severe sepsis associated with a noninfectious process (condition)

In some cases a noninfectious process (condition), such as trauma, may lead to an infection which can result in sepsis or severe sepsis. If sepsis or severe sepsis is documented as associated with a noninfectious condition, such as a burn or serious injury, and this condition meets the definition for principal diagnosis, the code for the noninfectious condition should be sequenced first, followed by the code for the resulting infection. If severe sepsis is present, a code from subcategory R65.2 should also be assigned with any associated organ dysfunction(s) codes. It is not necessary to assign a code from subcategory R65.1, Systemic inflammatory response syndrome (SIRS) of non-infectious origin, for these cases.

If the infection meets the definition of principal diagnosis it should be sequenced before the non-infectious condition. When both the associated non-infectious condition and the infection meet the definition of principal diagnosis either may be assigned as principal diagnosis.

Only one code from category R65, Symptoms and signs specifically associated with systemic inflammation and infection, should be assigned. Therefore, when a non-infectious condition leads to an infection resulting in severe sepsis, assign the appropriate code from subcategory R65.2, Severe sepsis. Do not additionally assign a code from subcategory R65.1, Systemic inflammatory response syndrome (SIRS) of non-infectious origin.

See Section I.C.18. SIRS due to non-infectious process

7) Sepsis and septic shock complicating abortion, pregnancy, childbirth, and the puerperium

See Section I.C.15. Sepsis and septic shock complicating abortion, pregnancy, childbirth and the puerperium

8) Newborn sepsis

See Section I.C.16. f. Bacterial sepsis of Newborn

9) Hemolytic-uremic syndrome associated with sepsis

If the reason for admission is hemolytic-uremic syndrome that is associated with sepsis, assign code D59.31, Infection-associated hemolytic-uremic syndrome, as the principal diagnosis. Codes for the underlying systemic infection and any other conditions (such as severe sepsis) should be assigned as secondary diagnoses.

e. Methicillin Resistant Staphylococcus aureus (MRSA) Conditions

1) Selection and sequencing of MRSA codes

(a) Combination codes for MRSA infection

When a patient is diagnosed with an infection that is due to methicillin resistant Staphylococcus aureus (MRSA), and that infection has a combination code that includes the causal organism (e.g., sepsis, pneumonia) assign the appropriate combination code for the condition (e.g., code A41.02, Sepsis due to Methicillin resistant Staphylococcus aureus or code J15.212, Pneumonia due to Methicillin resistant Staphylococcus aureus). Do not assign code B95.62, Methicillin resistant Staphylococcus aureus infection as the cause of diseases classified elsewhere, as an additional code because the combination code includes the type of infection and the MRSA organism. Do not assign a code from subcategory Z16.11, Resistance to penicillins, as an additional diagnosis.

See Section C.1. for instructions on coding and sequencing of sepsis and severe sepsis.

(b) Other codes for MRSA infection

When there is documentation of a current infection (e.g., wound infection, stitch abscess, urinary tract infection) due to MRSA, and that infection does not have a combination code that includes the causal organism, assign the appropriate code to identify the condition along with code B95.62, Methicillin resistant Staphylococcus aureus infection as the cause of diseases classified elsewhere for the MRSA infection. Do not assign a code from subcategory Z16.11, Resistance to penicillins.

(c) Methicillin susceptible Staphylococcus aureus (MSSA) and MRSA colonization

The condition or state of being colonized or carrying MSSA or MRSA is called colonization or carriage, while an individual person is described as being colonized or being a carrier. Colonization means that MSSA or MSRA is present on or in the body without necessarily causing illness. A positive MRSA colonization test might be documented by the provider as "MRSA screen positive" or "MRSA nasal swab positive".

13

Assign code Z22.322, Carrier or suspected carrier of Methicillin resistant Staphylococcus aureus, for patients documented as having MRSA colonization. Assign code Z22.321, Carrier or suspected carrier of Methicillin susceptible Staphylococcus aureus, for patients documented as having MSSA colonization. Colonization is not necessarily indicative of a disease process or as the cause of a specific condition the patient may have unless documented as such by the provider.

(d) MRSA colonization and infection
If a patient is documented as having both MRSA colonization and infection during a hospital admission, code Z22.322, Carrier or suspected carrier of Methicillin resistant Staphylococcus aureus, and a code for the MRSA infection may both be assigned.

f. Zika virus infections
1) Code only confirmed cases
Code only a confirmed diagnosis of Zika virus (A92.5, Zika virus disease) as documented by the provider. This is an exception to the hospital inpatient guideline Section II, H.

In this context, "confirmation" does not require documentation of the type of test performed; the provider's diagnostic statement that the condition is confirmed is sufficient. This code should be assigned regardless of the stated mode of transmission.

If the provider documents "suspected", "possible" or "probable" Zika, do not assign code A92.5. Assign a code(s) explaining the reason for encounter (such as fever, rash, or joint pain) or Z20.821, Contact with and (suspected) exposure to Zika virus.

g. Coronavirus infections
1) COVID-19 infection (infection due to SARS-CoV-2)
(a) Code only confirmed cases
Code only a confirmed diagnosis of the 2019 novel coronavirus disease (COVID-19) as documented by the provider, or documentation of a positive COVID-19 test result. For a confirmed diagnosis, assign code U07.1, COVID-19. This is an exception to the hospital inpatient guideline Section II, H. In this context, "confirmation" does not require documentation of a positive test result for COVID-19; the provider's documentation that the individual has COVID-19 is sufficient.

If the provider documents "suspected," "possible," "probable," or "inconclusive" COVID-19, do not assign code U07.1. Instead, code the signs and symptoms reported. *See guideline I.C.1.g.1.g.*
(b) Sequencing of codes
When COVID-19 meets the definition of principal diagnosis, code U07.1, COVID-19, should be sequenced first, followed by the appropriate codes for associated manifestations, except when another guideline requires that certain codes be sequenced first, such as obstetrics, sepsis, or transplant complications.

For a COVID-19 infection that progresses to sepsis, see Section I.C.1.d. Sepsis, Severe Sepsis, and Septic Shock
See Section I.C.15.s. for COVID-19 infection in pregnancy, childbirth, and the puerperium
See Section I.C.16.h. for COVID-19 infection in newborn
For a COVID-19 infection in a lung transplant patient, see Section I.C.19.g.3.a. Transplant complications other than kidney.

(c) Acute respiratory manifestations of COVID-19
When the reason for the encounter/admission is a respiratory manifestation of COVID-19, assign code U07.1, COVID-19, as the principal/first-listed diagnosis and assign code(s) for the respiratory manifestation(s) as additional diagnoses.

The following conditions are examples of common respiratory manifestations of COVID-19.

(i) Pneumonia
For a patient with pneumonia confirmed as due to COVID-19, assign codes U07.1, COVID-19, and J12.89, Other viral pneumonia.
(ii) Acute bronchitis
For a patient with acute bronchitis confirmed as due to COVID-19, assign codes U07.1, and J20.8, Acute bronchitis due to other specified organisms.
Bronchitis not otherwise specified (NOS) due to COVID-19 should be coded using code U07.1 and J40, Bronchitis, not specified as acute or chronic.
(iii) Lower respiratory infection
If the COVID-19 is documented as being associated with a lower respiratory infection, not otherwise specified (NOS), or an acute respiratory infection, NOS, codes U07.1 and J22, Unspecified acute lower respiratory infection, should be assigned.
If the COVID-19 is documented as being associated with a respiratory infection, NOS, codes U07.1 and J98.8, Other specified respiratory disorders, should be assigned.
(iv) Acute respiratory distress syndrome
For acute respiratory distress syndrome (ARDS) due to COVID-19, assign codes U07.1, and J80, Acute respiratory distress syndrome.
(v) Acute respiratory failure
For acute respiratory failure due to COVID-19, assign code U07.1, and code J96.0-, Acute respiratory failure.

(d) Non-respiratory manifestations of COVID-19

When the reason for the encounter/admission is a **nonrespiratory** manifestation (e.g., viral enteritis) of COVID-19, assign code U07.1, COVID-19, as the principal/first-listed diagnosis and assign code(s) for the manifestation(s) as additional diagnoses.

(e) Exposure to COVID-19

For asymptomatic individuals with actual or suspected exposure to COVID-19, assign code Z20.828, Contact with and (suspected) exposure to other viral communicable diseases.

For symptomatic individuals with actual or suspected exposure to COVID-19 and the infection has been ruled out, or test results are inconclusive or unknown, assign code Z20.828, Contact with and (suspected) exposure to other viral communicable diseases. See guideline I.C.21.c.1, Contact/Exposure, for additional guidance regarding the use of category Z20 codes.

If COVID-19 is confirmed, see guideline I.C.1.g.1.a.

(f) Screening for COVID-19

For screening for COVID-19, including preoperative testing, assign code Z11.52, Encounter for screening for COVID-19.

(g) Signs and symptoms without definitive diagnosis of **COVID19**

For patients presenting with any signs/symptoms associated with COVID-19 (such as fever, etc.) but a definitive diagnosis has not been established, assign the appropriate code(s) for each of the presenting signs and symptoms such as:

- R05.1, Acute cough, or R05.9, Cough, unspecified
- R06.02 Shortness of breath
- R50.9 Fever, unspecified

If a patient with signs/symptoms associated with COVID-19 also has an actual or suspected contact with or exposure to COVID-19, assign Z20.828, Contact with and (suspected) exposure to other viral communicable diseases, as an additional code.

(h) Asymptomatic individuals who test positive for COVID-19

For asymptomatic individuals who test positive for COVID-19, see guideline I.C.1.g.1.a. Although the individual is asymptomatic, the individual has tested positive and is considered to have the COVID-19 infection.

(i) Personal history of COVID-19

For patients with a history of COVID-19, assign code Z86.19, Personal history of other infectious and parasitic diseases.

(j) Follow-up visits after COVID-19 infection has resolved

For individuals who previously had COVID-19 without residual symptom(s) or condition(s), and are being seen for follow-up evaluation, and COVID-19 test results are negative, assign codes Z09, Encounter for follow-up examination after completed treatment for conditions other than malignant neoplasm, and Z86.19, Personal history of other infectious and parasitic diseases.

For follow-up visits for individuals with symptom(s) or condition(s) related to a previous COVID-19 infection, see guideline I.C.1.g.1.m.

See Section I.C.21.c.8, Factors influencing health states and contact with health services, Follow-up

(k) Encounter for antibody testing

For an encounter for antibody testing that is not being performed to confirm a current COVID-19 infection, nor is a follow-up test after resolution of COVID-19, assign Z01.84, Encounter for antibody response examination.

Follow the applicable guidelines above if the individual is being tested to confirm a current COVID-19 infection.

For follow-up testing after a COVID-19 infection, see guideline I.C.1.g.1.j.

(l) Multisystem Inflammatory Syndrome

For individuals with multisystem inflammatory syndrome (MIS) and COVID-19, assign code U07.1, COVID-19, as the principal/first-listed diagnosis and assign code M35.81, Multisystem inflammatory syndrome, as an additional diagnosis.

If an individual with a history of COVID-19 develops MIS, assign codes M35.81, Multisystem inflammatory syndrome, and U09.9, Post COVID-19 condition, unspecified.

If an individual with a known or suspected exposure to COVID-19, and no current COVID-19 infection or history of COVID-19, develops MIS, assign codes M35.81, Multisystem inflammatory syndrome, and Z20.822, Contact with and (suspected) exposure to COVID-19.

Additional codes should be assigned for any associated complications of MIS.

(m) Post COVID-19 Condition

For sequela of COVID-19, or associated symptoms or conditions that develop following a previous COVID-19 infection, assign a code(s) for the specific symptom(s) or condition(s) related to the previous COVID-19 infection, if known, and code U09.9, Post COVID-19 condition, unspecified.

Code U09.9 should not be assigned for manifestations of an active (current) COVID-19 infection.

If a patient has a condition(s) associated with a previous COVID-19 infection and develops a new active (current) COVID-19 infection, code U09.9 may be assigned in conjunction with code U07.1, COVID-19, to identify that the patient also has a condition(s) associated with a previous COVID-19 infection. Code(s) for the specific condition(s) associated with the previous COVID-19 infection and code(s) for manifestation(s) of the new active (current) COVID-19 infection should also be assigned.

(n) Underimmunization for COVID-19 Status Code Z28.310, Unvaccinated for COVID-19, may be assigned when the patient has not received a COVID-19 vaccine of any type. Code

Z28.311, Partially vaccinated for COVID-19, may be assigned when the patient has been partially vaccinated for COVID-19 as per the recommendations of the Centers for Disease Control and Prevention (CDC) in place at the time of the encounter. For information, visit the CDC's website

https://www.cdc.gov/coronavirus/2019-ncov/vaccines/.

See Section I.B.14. for underimmunization documentation by clinicians other than patient's provider.

2. Chapter 2: Neoplasms (C00-D49)
General guidelines

Chapter 2 of the ICD-10-CM contains the codes for most benign and all malignant neoplasms. Certain benign neoplasms, such as prostatic adenomas, may be found in the specific body system chapters. To properly code a neoplasm it is necessary to determine from the record if the neoplasm is benign, in-situ, malignant, or of uncertain histologic behavior. If malignant, any secondary (metastatic) sites should also be determined.

Primary malignant neoplasms overlapping site boundaries

A primary malignant neoplasm that overlaps two or more contiguous (next to each other) sites should be classified to the subcategory/code .8 ("overlapping lesion"), unless the combination is specifically indexed elsewhere. For multiple neoplasms of the same site that are not contiguous such as tumors in different quadrants of the same breast, codes for each site should be assigned.

Malignant neoplasm of ectopic tissue

Malignant neoplasms of ectopic tissue are to be coded to the site of origin mentioned (e.g., ectopic pancreatic malignant neoplasms involving the stomach are coded to malignant neoplasm of pancreas, unspecified) (C25.9).

The neoplasm table in the Alphabetic Index should be referenced first. However, if the histological term is documented, that term should be referenced first, rather than going immediately to the Neoplasm Table, in order to determine which column in the Neoplasm Table is appropriate. For example, if the documentation indicates "adenoma," refer to the term in the Alphabetic Index to review the entries under this term and the instructional note to "see also neoplasm, by site, benign." The table provides the proper code based on the type of neoplasm and the site. It is important to select the proper column in the table that corresponds to the type of neoplasm. The Tabular List should then be referenced to verify that the correct code has been selected from the table and that a more specific site code does not exist.

See Section I.C.21. Factors influencing health status and contact with health services, Status, for information regarding Z15.0, codes for genetic susceptibility to cancer.

a. *Admission/Encounter for treatment of primary site*

If the **malignancy is chiefly responsible for occasioning the patient admission/encounter and treatment is directed at the primary site,** designate the **primary** malignancy as the principal /**first-listed** diagnosis.

The only exception to this guideline is if the administration of chemotherapy, immunotherapy or external beam radiation therapy **is chiefly responsible for occasioning the admission/encounter. In that case,** assign the appropriate Z51.— code as the first-listed or principal diagnosis, and the **underlying** diagnosis or problem for which the service is being performed as a secondary diagnosis.

b. *Admission/Encounter for treatment of secondary site*

When a patient is admitted because of a primary neoplasm with metastasis and treatment is directed toward the secondary site only, the secondary neoplasm is designated as the principal diagnosis even though the primary malignancy is still present.

c. Coding and sequencing of complications

Coding and sequencing of complications associated with the malignancies or with the therapy thereof are subject to the following guidelines:

1) Anemia associated with malignancy

When admission/encounter is for management of an anemia associated with the malignancy, and the treatment is only for anemia, the appropriate code for the malignancy is sequenced as the principal or first-listed diagnosis followed by the appropriate code for the anemia (such as code D63.0, Anemia in neoplastic disease).

2) Anemia associated with chemotherapy, immunotherapy and radiation therapy

When the admission/encounter is for management of an anemia associated with an adverse effect of the administration of chemotherapy or immunotherapy and the only treatment is for the anemia, the anemia code is sequenced first followed by the appropriate codes for the neoplasm and the adverse effect (T45.1X5, Adverse effect of antineoplastic and immunosuppressive drugs).

When the admission/encounter is for management of an anemia associated with an adverse effect of radiotherapy, the anemia code should be sequenced first, followed by the appropriate neoplasm code and code Y84.2, Radiological procedure and radiotherapy as the cause of abnormal reaction of the patient, or of later complication, without mention of misadventure at the time of the procedure.

3) Management of dehydration due to the malignancy

When the admission/encounter is for management of dehydration due to the malignancy and only the dehydration is being treated (intravenous rehydration), the dehydration is sequenced first, followed by the code(s) for the malignancy.

4) Treatment of a complication resulting from a surgical procedure

When the admission/encounter is for treatment of a complication resulting from a surgical procedure, designate the complication as the principal or first-listed diagnosis if treatment is directed at resolving the complication.

d. Primary malignancy previously excised

When a primary malignancy has been previously excised or eradicated from its site and there is no further treatment directed to that site and there is no evidence of any existing primary malignancy, at that site a code from category Z85, Personal history of malignant neoplasm, should be used to indicate the former site of the malignancy. Any mention of extension, invasion, or metastasis to another site is coded as a secondary malignant neoplasm to that site. The secondary site may be the principal or first-listed diagnosis with the Z85 code used as a secondary code.

See section I.C.2.t. Secondary malignant neoplasm of lymphoid tissue.

e. Admissions/Encounters involving chemotherapy, immunotherapy and radiation therapy

1) Episode of care involves surgical removal of neoplasm

When an episode of care involves the surgical removal of a neoplasm, primary or secondary site, followed by adjunct chemotherapy or radiation treatment during the same episode of care, the code for the neoplasm should be assigned as principal or first-listed diagnosis.

2) Patient admission/encounter chiefly for administration of chemotherapy, immunotherapy and radiation therapy

If a patient admission/encounter is **chiefly** for the administration of chemotherapy, immunotherapy or external beam radiation therapy assign code Z51.0, Encounter for antineoplastic radiation therapy, or Z51.11, Encounter for antineoplastic chemotherapy, or Z51.12, Encounter for antineoplastic immunotherapy as the first-listed or principal diagnosis. If a patient receives more than one of these therapies during the same admission, more than one of these codes may be assigned, in any sequence.

The malignancy for which the therapy is being administered should be assigned as a secondary diagnosis.

If a patient admission/encounter is for the insertion or implantation of radioactive elements (e.g., brachytherapy) the appropriate code for the malignancy is sequenced as the principal or first-listed diagnosis. Code Z51.0 should not be assigned.

3) Patient admitted for radiation therapy, chemotherapy or immunotherapy and develops complications

When a patient is admitted for the purpose of external beam radiotherapy, immunotherapy or chemotherapy and develops complications such as uncontrolled nausea and vomiting or dehydration, the principal or first-listed diagnosis is Z51.0, Encounter for antineoplastic radiation therapy, or Z51.11, Encounter for antineoplastic chemotherapy, or Z51.12, Encounter for antineoplastic immunotherapy followed by any codes for the complications.

When a patient is admitted for the purpose of insertion or implantation of radioactive elements (e.g., brachytherapy) and develops complications such as uncontrolled nausea and vomiting or dehydration, the principal or first-listed diagnosis is the appropriate code for the malignancy followed by any codes for the complications.

f. Admission/encounter to determine extent of malignancy

When the reason for admission/encounter is to determine the extent of the malignancy, or for a procedure such as paracentesis or thoracentesis, the primary malignancy or appropriate metastatic site is designated as the principal or first-listed diagnosis, even though chemotherapy or radiotherapy is administered.

g. Symptoms, signs, and abnormal findings listed in Chapter 18 associated with neoplasms

Symptoms, signs, and ill-defined conditions listed in Chapter 18 characteristic of, or associated with, an existing primary or secondary site malignancy cannot be used to replace the malignancy as principal or first-listed diagnosis, regardless of the number of admissions or encounters for treatment and care of the neoplasm.

See Section I.C.21. Factors influencing health status and contact with health services, Encounter for prophylactic organ removal.

h. Admission/encounter for pain control/management

See Section I.C.6. for information on coding admission/encounter for pain control/management.

i. Malignancy in two or more noncontiguous sites

A patient may have more than one malignant tumor in the same organ. These tumors may represent different primaries or metastatic disease, depending on the site. Should the documentation be unclear, the provider should be queried as to the status of each tumor so that the correct codes can be assigned.

j. Disseminated malignant neoplasm, unspecified

Code C80.0, Disseminated malignant neoplasm, unspecified, is for use only in those cases where the patient has advanced metastatic disease and no known primary or secondary sites are specified. It should not be used in place of assigning codes for the primary site and all known secondary sites.

k. Malignant neoplasm without specification of site

Code C80.1, Malignant (primary) neoplasm, unspecified, equates to Cancer, unspecified. This code should only be used when no determination can be made as to the primary site of a malignancy. This code should rarely be used in the inpatient setting.

l. Sequencing of neoplasm codes

1) Encounter for treatment of primary malignancy

If the reason for the encounter is for treatment of a primary malignancy, assign the malignancy as the principal/first-listed diagnosis. The primary site is to be sequenced first, followed by any metastatic sites.

2) Encounter for treatment of secondary malignancy

When an encounter is for a primary malignancy with metastasis and treatment is directed toward the metastatic (secondary) site(s) only, the metastatic site(s) is designated as the principal/first-listed diagnosis. The primary malignancy is coded as an additional code.

3) Malignant neoplasm in a pregnant patient

When a pregnant patient has a malignant neoplasm, a code from subcategory O9A.1-, Malignant neoplasm complicating pregnancy, childbirth, and the puerperium, should be sequenced first, followed by the appropriate code from Chapter 2 to indicate the type of neoplasm.

4) Encounter for complication associated with a neoplasm

When an encounter is for management of a complication associated with a neoplasm, such as dehydration, and the treatment is only for the complication, the complication is coded first, followed by the appropriate code(s) for the neoplasm.

The exception to this guideline is anemia. When the admission/encounter is for management of an anemia associated with the malignancy, and the treatment is only for anemia, the appropriate code for the malignancy is sequenced as the principal or first-listed diagnosis followed by code D63.0, Anemia in neoplastic disease.

5) Complication from surgical procedure for treatment of a neoplasm

When an encounter is for treatment of a complication resulting from a surgical procedure performed for the treatment of the neoplasm, designate the complication as the principal/first-listed diagnosis. See the guideline regarding the coding of a current malignancy versus personal history to determine if the code for the neoplasm should also be assigned.

6) Pathologic fracture due to a neoplasm

When an encounter is for a pathological fracture due to a neoplasm, and the focus of treatment is the fracture, a code from subcategory M84.5, Pathological fracture in neoplastic disease, should be sequenced first, followed by the code for the neoplasm.

If the focus of treatment is the neoplasm with an associated pathological fracture, the neoplasm code should be sequenced first, followed by a code from M84.5 for the pathological fracture.

m. Current malignancy versus personal history of malignancy

When a primary malignancy has been excised but further treatment, such as an additional surgery for the malignancy, radiation therapy or chemotherapy is directed to that site, the primary malignancy code should be used until treatment is completed.

When a primary malignancy has been previously excised or eradicated from its site, there is no further treatment (of the malignancy) directed to that site, and there is no evidence of any existing primary malignancy at that site, a code from category Z85, Personal history of malignant neoplasm, should be used to indicate the former site of the malignancy.

Codes from subcategories Z85.0 – Z85.85 should only be assigned for the former site of a primary malignancy, not the site of a secondary malignancy. Code Z85.89, may be assigned for the former site(s) of either a primary or secondary malignancy.

See Section I.C.21. Factors influencing health status and contact with health services, History (of)

n. Leukemia, Multiple Myeloma, and Malignant Plasma Cell Neoplasms in remission versus personal history

The categories for leukemia, and category C90, Multiple myeloma and malignant plasma cell neoplasms, have codes indicating whether or not the leukemia has achieved remission. There are also codes Z85.6, Personal history of leukemia, and Z85.79, Personal history of other malignant neoplasms of lymphoid, hematopoietic and related tissues. If the documentation is unclear, as to whether the leukemia has achieved remission, the provider should be queried.

See Section I.C.21. Factors influencing health status and contact with health services, History (of)

o. Aftercare following surgery for neoplasm

See Section I.C.21. Factors influencing health status and contact with health services, Aftercare

p. Follow-up care for completed treatment of a malignancy

See Section I.C.21. Factors influencing health status and contact with health services, Follow-up

q. Prophylactic organ removal for prevention of malignancy

See Section I.C. 21, Factors influencing health status and contact with health services, Prophylactic organ removal

r. Malignant neoplasm associated with transplanted organ

A malignant neoplasm of a transplanted organ should be coded as a transplant complication. Assign first the appropriate code from category T86.-, Complications of transplanted organs and tissue, followed by code C80.2, Malignant neoplasm associated with transplanted organ. Use an additional code for the specific malignancy.

s. Breast Implant Associated Anaplastic Large Cell Lymphoma

Breast implant associated anaplastic large cell lymphoma (BIA-ALCL) is a type of lymphoma that can develop around breast implants. Assign code C84.7A, Anaplastic large cell lymphoma, ALK-negative, breast, for BIA-ALCL or C84.7B, Anaplastic large cell lymphoma, ALK-negative, in remission, for BIA-ALCL in remission. Do not assign a complication code from chapter 19.

t. Secondary malignant neoplasm of lymphoid tissue

When a malignant neoplasm of lymphoid tissue metastasizes beyond the lymph nodes, a code from categories C81-C85 with a final character identifying "extranodal and solid organ sites" should be assigned rather than a code for the secondary neoplasm of the affected solid organ. For example, for metastasis of diffuse large B-cell lymphoma to the lung, brain and left adrenal gland, assign code C83.398, Diffuse large B-cell lymphoma of other extranodal and solid organ sites.

3. Chapter 3: Disease of the blood and blood-forming organs and certain disorders involving the immune mechanism (D50-D89)
Reserved for future guideline expansion

4. Chapter 4: Endocrine, Nutritional, and Metabolic Diseases (E00-E89)

a. Diabetes mellitus
The diabetes mellitus codes are combination codes that include the type of diabetes mellitus, the body system affected, and the complications affecting that body system. As many codes within a particular category as are necessary to describe all of the complications of the disease may be used. They should be sequenced based on the reason for a particular encounter. Assign as many codes from categories E08 – E13 as needed to identify all of the associated conditions that the patient has.

1) Type of diabetes
The age of a patient is not the sole determining factor, though most type 1 diabetics develop the condition before reaching puberty. For this reason type 1 diabetes mellitus is also referred to as juvenile diabetes.

(a) Presymptomatic Type 1 Diabetes Mellitus Codes E10.A-, Type 1 diabetes mellitus, presymptomatic, are assigned for early-stage type 1 diabetes that predates the onset of symptoms.

2) Type of diabetes mellitus not documented
If the type of diabetes mellitus is not documented in the medical record the default is E11.-, Type 2 diabetes mellitus.

3) Diabetes mellitus and the use of insulin, oral hypoglycemics, and injectable non-insulin drugs
If the documentation in a medical record does not indicate the type of diabetes but does indicate that the patient uses insulin, code E11, Type 2 diabetes mellitus, should be assigned. Additional code(s) should be assigned from category Z79 to identify the long-term (current) use of insulin or oral hypoglycemic drugs, or injectable non-insulin antidiabetic, as follows: If the patient is treated with both oral **hypoglycemic drugs** and insulin, both code Z79.4, Long term (current) use of insulin, and code Z79.84, Long term (current) use of oral hypoglycemic drugs, should be assigned. If the patient is treated with both insulin and an injectable non-insulin antidiabetic drug, assign codes Z79.4, Long-term (current) use of insulin, and **Z79.85, Long-term (current) use of injectable non-insulin antidiabetic drugs.** If the patient is treated with both oral hypoglycemic drugs and an injectable non-insulin antidiabetic drug, assign codes Z79.84, Long-term (current) use of oral hypoglycemic drugs, and **Z79.85, Long-term (current) use of injectable non-insulin antidiabetic drugs.** Code Z79.4 should not be assigned if insulin is given temporarily to bring a type 2 patient's blood sugar under control during an encounter.

4) Diabetes mellitus in pregnancy and gestational diabetes
See Section I.C.15. Diabetes mellitus in pregnancy.
See Section I.C.15. Gestational (pregnancy induced) diabetes

5) Complications due to insulin pump malfunction

(a) Underdose of insulin due to insulin pump failure
An underdose of insulin due to an insulin pump failure should be assigned to a code from subcategory T85.6, Mechanical complication of other specified internal and external prosthetic devices, implants and grafts, that specifies the type of pump malfunction, as the principal or first-listed code, followed by code T38.3X6-, Underdosing of insulin and oral hypoglycemic [antidiabetic] drugs. Additional codes for the type of diabetes mellitus and any associated complications due to the underdosing should also be assigned.

(b) Overdose of insulin due to insulin pump failure
The principal or first-listed code for an encounter due to an insulin pump malfunction resulting in an overdose of insulin, should also be T85.6-, Mechanical complication of other specified internal and external prosthetic devices, implants and grafts, followed by code T38.3X1-, Poisoning by insulin and oral hypoglycemic [antidiabetic] drugs, accidental (unintentional).

6) Secondary diabetes mellitus
Codes under categories E08, Diabetes mellitus due to underlying condition, E09, Drug or chemical induced diabetes mellitus and E13, Other specified diabetes mellitus, identify complications/manifestations associated with secondary diabetes mellitus. Secondary diabetes is always caused by another condition or event (e.g., cystic fibrosis, malignant neoplasm of pancreas, pancreatectomy, adverse effect of drug, or poisoning).

(a) Secondary diabetes mellitus and the use of insulin or hypoglycemic drugs
For patients with secondary diabetes mellitus who routinely use insulin or oral hypoglycemic drugs, or injectable non-insulin drugs, an additional code(s) from category Z79 should be assigned to identify the long-term (current) use of insulin or oral hypoglycemic drugs, or non-injectable non-insulin drugs as follows: If the patient is treated

with both oral **hypoglycemic drugs** and insulin, both code Z79.4, Long term (current) use of insulin, and code Z79.84, Long term (current) use of oral hypoglycemic drugs, should be assigned. If the patient is treated with both insulin and an injectable non-insulin antidiabetic drug, assign codes Z79.4, Long- term (current) use of insulin, and **Z79.85, Long-term (current) use of injectable non-insulin antidiabetic drugs.** If the patient is treated with both oral hypoglycemic drugs and an injectable non-insulin antidiabetic drug, assign codes Z79.84, Long-term (current) use of oral hypoglycemic drugs, and **Z79.85, Long-term (current) use of injectable non-insulin antidiabetic drugs.** Code Z79.4 should not be assigned if insulin is given temporarily to bring a type 2 patient's blood sugar under control during an encounter.

(b) Assigning and sequencing secondary diabetes codes and its causes

The sequencing of the secondary diabetes codes in relationship to codes for the cause of the diabetes is based on the Tabular List instructions for categories E08, E09 and E13.

(i) Secondary diabetes mellitus due to pancreatectomy
For postpancreatectomy diabetes mellitus (lack of insulin due to the surgical removal of all or part of the pancreas), assign code E89.1, Postprocedural hypoinsulinemia. Assign a code from category E13 as the principal or firstlisted diagnosis and a code from subcategory Z90.41-, Acquired absence of pancreas, as additional codes.

(ii) Secondary diabetes due to drugs
Secondary diabetes may be caused by an adverse effect of correctly administered medications, poisoning or sequela of poisoning.

See Section I.C.19.e for coding of adverse effects and poisoning, and Section I.C.20 for external cause code reporting.

5. Chapter 5: Mental, Behavioral and Neurodevelopmental disorders (F01 – F99)

a. Pain disorders related to psychological factors
Assign code F45.41, for pain that is exclusively related to psychological disorders. As indicated by the Excludes1 note under category G89, a code from category G89 should not be assigned with code F45.41

Code F45.42, Pain disorders with related psychological factors, should be used with a code from category G89, Pain, not elsewhere classified, if there is documentation of a psychological component for a patient with acute or chronic pain.

See Section I.C.6. Pain

b. Mental and behavioral disorders due to psychoactive substance use

1) In Remission
Selection of codes **describing** "in remission" for categories F10-F19, Mental and behavioral disorders

due to psychoactive substance use (categories F10-F19 with -11, -.21, **-91**) requires the provider's clinical judgment **and** are assigned only on the basis of provider documentation (as defined in the Official Guidelines for Coding and Reporting), unless otherwise instructed by the classification.

Mild substance use disorders in early or sustained remission are classified to the appropriate codes for substance abuse in remission, and moderate or severe substance use disorders in early or sustained remission are classified to the appropriate codes for substance dependence in remission.

2) Psychoactive Substance Use, Abuse and Dependence
When the provider documentation refers to use, abuse and dependence of the same substance (e.g., alcohol, opioid, cannabis, etc.), only one code should be assigned to identify the pattern of use based on the following hierarchy:
- If both use and abuse are documented, assign only the code for abuse
- If both abuse and dependence are documented, assign only the code for dependence
- If use, abuse and dependence are all documented, assign only the code for dependence
- If both use and dependence are documented, assign only the code for dependence.

3) Psychoactive Substance Use, Unspecified
As with all other unspecified diagnoses, the codes for unspecified psychoactive substance use disorders (F10.9-, F11.9-, F12.9-, F13.9-, F15.9-, F16.9-, F18.9-, F19.9-) should only be assigned based on provider documentation and when they meet the definition of a reportable diagnosis (see Section III, Reporting Additional Diagnoses). These codes are to be used only when the psychoactive substance use is associated 1with a substance related disorder (chapter 5 such as sexual dysfunction and sleep disorder, or a mental or behavioral disorder) or medical condition, and such a relationship is documented by the provider.

4) Medical Conditions Due to Psychoactive Substance Use, Abuse and Dependence
Medical conditions due to substance use, abuse, and dependence are not classified as substance-induced disorders. Assign the diagnosis code for the medical condition as directed by the Alphabetical Index along with the appropriate psychoactive substance use, abuse or dependence code. For example, for alcoholic pancreatitis due to alcohol dependence, assign the appropriate code from subcategory K85.2, Alcohol induced acute pancreatitis, and the appropriate code from subcategory F10.2, such as code F10.20, Alcohol dependence, uncomplicated. It would not be appropriate to assign code F10.288, Alcohol dependence with other alcohol-induced disorder.

5) Blood Alcohol Level

A code from category Y9Ø, Evidence of alcohol involvement determined by blood alcohol level, may be assigned when this information is documented and the patient's provider has documented a condition classifiable to category F1Ø, Alcohol related disorders. The blood alcohol level does not need to be documented by the patient's provider in order for it to be coded.

See Section I.B.14. for blood alcohol level documentation by clinicians other than patient's provider.

c. Factitious Disorder

Factitious disorder imposed on self or Munchausen's syndrome is a disorder in which a person falsely reports or causes his or her own physical or psychological signs or symptoms. For patients with documented factitious disorder on self or Munchausen's syndrome, assign the appropriate code from subcategory F68.1-, Factitious disorder imposed on self.

Munchausen's syndrome by proxy (MSBP) is a disorder in which a caregiver (perpetrator) falsely reports or causes an illness or injury in another person (victim) under his or her care, such as a child, an elderly adult, or a person who has a disability. The condition is also referred to as "factitious disorder imposed on another" or "factitious disorder by proxy." The perpetrator, not the victim, receives this diagnosis. Assign code F68.A, Factitious disorder imposed on another, to the perpetrator's record. For the victim of a patient suffering from MSBP, assign the appropriate code from categories T74, Adult and child abuse, neglect and other maltreatment, confirmed, or T76, Adult and child abuse, neglect and other maltreatment, suspected.

See Section I.C.19.f. Adult and child abuse, neglect and other maltreatment

d. Dementia

The ICD-10-CM classifies dementia (categories FØ1, FØ2, and FØ3) on the basis of the etiology and severity (unspecified, mild, moderate or severe). Selection of the appropriate severity level requires the provider's clinical judgment and codes should be assigned only on the basis of provider documentation (as defined in the *Official Guidelines for Coding and Reporting*), unless otherwise instructed by the classification. If the documentation does not provide information about the severity of the dementia, assign the appropriate code for unspecified severity.

If a patient is admitted to an inpatient acute care hospital or other inpatient facility setting with dementia at one severity level and it progresses to a higher severity level, assign one code for the highest severity level reported during the stay.

6. Chapter 6: Diseases of the Nervous System (GØØ-G99)

a. Dominant/nondominant side

Codes from category G81, Hemiplegia and hemiparesis, and subcategories, G83.1, Monoplegia of lower limb, G83.2, Monoplegia of upper limb, and G83.3, Monoplegia, unspecified, identify whether the dominant or nondominant side is affected. Should the affected side be documented, but not specified as dominant or nondominant, and the classification system does not indicate a default, code selection is as follows:

- For ambidextrous patients, the default should be dominant.
- If the left side is affected, the default is non-dominant.
- If the right side is affected, the default is dominant.

b. Pain - Category G89

1) General coding information

Codes in category G89, Pain, not elsewhere classified, may be used in conjunction with codes from other categories and chapters to provide more detail about acute or chronic pain and neoplasm-related pain, unless otherwise indicated below.

If the pain is not specified as acute or chronic, post-thoracotomy, postprocedural, or neoplasm-related, do not assign codes from category G89.

A code from category G89 should not be assigned if the underlying (definitive) diagnosis is known, unless the reason for the encounter is pain control/management and not management of the underlying condition.

When an admission or encounter is for a procedure aimed at treating the underlying condition (e.g., spinal fusion, kyphoplasty), a code for the underlying condition (e.g., vertebral fracture, spinal stenosis) should be assigned as the principal diagnosis. No code from category G89 should be assigned.

(a) Category G89 Codes as Principal or First-Listed Diagnosis

Category G89 codes are acceptable as principal diagnosis or the first-listed code:

- When pain control or pain management is the reason for the admission/encounter (e.g., a patient with displaced intervertebral disc, nerve impingement and severe back pain presents for injection of steroid into the spinal canal). The underlying cause of the pain should be reported as an additional diagnosis, if known.
- When a patient is admitted for the insertion of a neurostimulator for pain control, assign the appropriate pain code as the principal or first-listed diagnosis. When an admission or encounter is for a procedure aimed at treating the underlying condition and a neurostimulator is inserted for pain control during the same admission/encounter, a code for the underlying condition should be assigned as the principal diagnosis and the appropriate pain code should be assigned as a secondary diagnosis.

(b) Use of Category G89 Codes in Conjunction with Site-Specific Pain Codes

(i) Assigning Category G89 and Site-Specific Pain Codes

Codes from category G89 may be used in conjunction with codes that identify the site of pain (including codes from Chapter 18) if the category G89 code provides additional information. For example, if the code describes the site of the pain, but does not fully describe whether the pain is acute or chronic, then both codes should be assigned.

(ii) Sequencing of Category G89 Codes with Site-Specific Pain Codes

The sequencing of category G89 codes with site-specific pain codes (including Chapter 18 codes), is dependent on the circumstances of the encounter/admission as follows:

- If the encounter is for pain control or pain management, assign the code from category G89 followed by the code identifying the specific site of pain (e.g., encounter for pain management for acute neck pain from trauma is assigned code G89.11, Acute pain due to trauma, followed by code M54.2, Cervicalgia, to identify the site of pain).
- If the encounter is for any other reason except pain control or pain management, and a related definitive diagnosis has not been established (confirmed) by the provider, assign the code for the specific site of pain first, followed by the appropriate code from category G89.

2) Pain due to devices, implants and grafts
See Section I.C.19. Pain due to medical devices

3) Postoperative Pain
The provider's documentation should be used to guide the coding of postoperative pain, as well as Section III. Reporting Additional Diagnoses and Section IV. Diagnostic Coding and Reporting in the Outpatient Setting.

The default for post-thoracotomy and other postoperative pain not specified as acute or chronic is the code for the acute form.

Routine or expected postoperative pain immediately after surgery should not be coded.

(a) Postoperative pain not associated with specific postoperative complication
Postoperative pain not associated with a specific postoperative complication is assigned to the appropriate postoperative pain code in category G89.

(b) Postoperative pain associated with specific postoperative complication
Postoperative pain associated with a specific postoperative complication (such as painful wire sutures) is assigned to the appropriate code(s) found in Chapter 19, Injury, poisoning, and certain other consequences of external causes. If appropriate, use additional code(s) from category G89 to identify acute or chronic pain (G89.18 or G89.28).

4) Chronic pain
Chronic pain is classified to subcategory G89.2. There is no time frame defining when pain becomes chronic pain. The provider's documentation should be used to guide use of these codes.

5) Neoplasm Related Pain
Code G89.3 is assigned to pain documented as being related, associated or due to cancer, primary or secondary malignancy, or tumor. This code is assigned regardless of whether the pain is acute or chronic.

This code may be assigned as the principal or first-listed code when the stated reason for the admission/encounter is documented as pain control/pain management. The underlying neoplasm should be reported as an additional diagnosis.

When the reason for the admission/encounter is management of the neoplasm and the pain associated with the neoplasm is also documented, code G89.3 may be assigned as an additional diagnosis. It is not necessary to assign an additional code for the site of the pain.

See Section I.C.2 for instructions on the sequencing of neoplasms for all other stated reasons for the admission/encounter (except for pain control/pain management).

6) Chronic pain syndrome
Central pain syndrome (G89.0) and chronic pain syndrome (G89.4) are different than the term "chronic pain," and therefore codes should only be used when the provider has specifically documented this condition.

See Section I.C.5. Pain disorders related to psychological factors

7. Chapter 7: Diseases of the Eye and Adnexa (H00-H59)

a. Glaucoma
1) Assigning Glaucoma Codes
Assign as many codes from category H40, Glaucoma, as needed to identify the type of glaucoma, the affected eye, and the glaucoma stage.

2) Bilateral glaucoma with same type and stage
When a patient has bilateral glaucoma and both eyes are documented as being the same type and stage, and there is a code for bilateral glaucoma, report only the code for the type of glaucoma, bilateral, with the seventh character for the stage.

When a patient has bilateral glaucoma and both eyes are documented as being the same type and stage, and the classification does not provide a code for bilateral glaucoma (i.e., subcategories H40.10, H40.11 and H40.20) report only one code for the type of glaucoma with the appropriate seventh character for the stage.

3) Bilateral glaucoma stage with different types or stages
When a patient has bilateral glaucoma and each eye is documented as having a different type or stage, and the classification distinguishes laterality, assign the appropriate code for each eye rather than the code for bilateral glaucoma.

When a patient has bilateral glaucoma and each eye is documented as having a different type, and the classification does not distinguish laterality (i.e., subcategories H40.10, H40.11 and H40.20), assign one code for each type of glaucoma with the appropriate 7th character for the stage.

When a patient has bilateral glaucoma and each eye is documented as having the same type, but different stage, and the classification does not distinguish laterality (i.e., subcategories H40.10, H40.11 and H40.20), assign a code for the type of glaucoma for each eye with the 7th character for the specific glaucoma stage documented for each eye.

4) Patient admitted with glaucoma and stage evolves during the admission

If a patient is admitted with glaucoma and the stage progresses during the admission, assign the code for highest stage documented.

5) Indeterminate stage glaucoma

Assignment of the 7th character "4" for "indeterminate stage" should be based on the clinical documentation. The 7th character "4" is used for glaucomas whose stage cannot be clinically determined. This 7th character should not be confused with the 7th character "0", unspecified, which should be assigned when there is no documentation regarding the stage of the glaucoma.

b. Blindness

If "blindness" or "low vision" of both eyes is documented but the visual impairment category is not documented, assign code H54.3, Unqualified visual loss, both eyes. If "blindness" or "low vision" in one eye is documented but the visual impairment category is not documented, assign a code from H54.6-, Unqualified visual loss, one eye. If "blindness" or "visual loss" is documented without any information about whether one or both eyes are affected, assign code H54.7, Unspecified visual loss.

8. Chapter 8: Diseases of the Ear and Mastoid Process (H60-H95)

Reserved for future guideline expansion

9. Chapter 9: Diseases of the Circulatory System (I00-I99)

a. Hypertension

The classification presumes a causal relationship between hypertension and heart involvement and between hypertension and kidney involvement, as the two conditions are linked by the term "with" in the Alphabetic Index. These conditions should be coded as related even in the absence of provider documentation explicitly linking them, unless the documentation clearly states the conditions are unrelated.

For hypertension and conditions not specifically linked by relational terms such as "with," "associated with" or "due to" in the classification, provider documentation must link the conditions in order to code them as related.

1) Hypertension with Heart Disease

Hypertension with heart conditions classified to I50.- or I51.4-I51.7, I51.89, I51.9, are assigned to, a code from category I11, Hypertensive heart disease. Use additional code(s) from category I50, Heart failure, to identify the type(s) of heart failure in those patients with heart failure.

The same heart conditions (I50.-, I51.4-I51.7, I51.89, I51.9) with hypertension are coded separately if the provider has documented they are unrelated to the hypertension. Sequence according to the circumstances of the admission/encounter.

2) Hypertensive Chronic Kidney Disease

Assign codes from category I12, Hypertensive chronic kidney disease, when both hypertension and a condition classifiable to category N18, Chronic kidney disease (CKD), are present. CKD should not be coded as hypertensive if the provider indicates the CKD is not related to the hypertension.

The appropriate code from category N18 should be used as a secondary code with a code from category I12 to identify the stage of chronic kidney disease.

See Section I.C.14. Chronic kidney disease.

If a patient has hypertensive chronic kidney disease and acute renal failure, the acute renal failure should also be coded. Sequence according to the circumstances of the admission/encounter.

3) Hypertensive Heart and Chronic Kidney Disease

Assign codes from combination category I13, Hypertensive heart and chronic kidney disease, when there is hypertension with both heart and kidney involvement. If heart failure is present, assign an additional code from category I50 to identify the type of heart failure.

The appropriate code from category N18, Chronic kidney disease, should be used as a secondary code with a code from category I13 to identify the stage of chronic kidney disease.

See Section I.C.14. Chronic kidney disease.

The codes in category I13, Hypertensive heart and chronic kidney disease, are combination codes that include hypertension, heart disease and chronic kidney disease. The Includes note at I13 specifies that the conditions included at I11 and I12 are included together in I13. If a patient has hypertension, heart disease and chronic kidney disease then a code from I13 should be used, not individual codes for hypertension, heart disease and chronic kidney disease, or codes from I11 or I12.

For patients with both acute renal failure and chronic kidney disease the acute renal failure should also be coded. Sequence according to the circumstances of the admission/encounter.

4) Hypertensive Cerebrovascular Disease

For hypertensive cerebrovascular disease, first assign the appropriate code from categories I60-I69, followed by the appropriate hypertension code.

5) Hypertensive Retinopathy

Subcategory H35.0, Background retinopathy and retinal vascular changes, should be used with a code from category I10 – I15, Hypertensive disease to include the systemic hypertension. The sequencing is based on the reason for the encounter.

6) Hypertension, Secondary
Secondary hypertension is due to an underlying condition. Two codes are required: one to identify the underlying etiology and one from category I15 to identify the hypertension. Sequencing of codes is determined by the reason for admission/encounter.

7) Hypertension, Transient
Assign code R03.0, Elevated blood pressure reading without diagnosis of hypertension, unless patient has an established diagnosis of hypertension. Assign code O13.-, Gestational [pregnancy-induced] hypertension without significant proteinuria, or O14.-, Pre-eclampsia, for transient hypertension of pregnancy.

8) Hypertension, Controlled
This diagnostic statement usually refers to an existing state of hypertension under control by therapy. Assign the appropriate code from categories I10-I15, Hypertensive diseases.

9) Hypertension, Uncontrolled
Uncontrolled hypertension may refer to untreated hypertension or hypertension not responding to current therapeutic regimen. In either case, assign the appropriate code from categories I10-I15, Hypertensive diseases.

10) Hypertensive Crisis
Assign a code from category I16, Hypertensive crisis, for documented hypertensive urgency, hypertensive emergency or unspecified hypertensive crisis. Code also any identified hypertensive disease (I10-I15). The sequencing is based on the reason for the encounter.

11) Pulmonary Hypertension
Pulmonary hypertension is classified to category I27, Other pulmonary heart diseases. For secondary pulmonary hypertension (I27.1, I27.2-), code also any associated conditions or adverse effects of drugs or toxins. The sequencing is based on the reason for the encounter, except for adverse effects of drugs.
See Section I.C.19.e

12) Hypertension, Resistant
Resistant hypertension refers to blood pressure of a patient with hypertension that remains above goal in spite of the use of antihypertensive medications. Assign code I1A.0, Resistant hypertension, as an additional code when apparent treatment resistant hypertension, treatment resistant hypertension, or true resistant hypertension is documented by the provider. A code for the specific type of existing hypertension is sequenced first, if known.

b. Atherosclerotic Coronary Artery Disease and Angina
ICD-10-CM has combination codes for atherosclerotic heart disease with angina pectoris. The subcategories for these codes are I25.11, Atherosclerotic heart disease of native coronary artery with angina pectoris and I25.7, Atherosclerosis of coronary artery bypass graft(s) and coronary artery of transplanted heart with angina pectoris.

When using one of these combination codes it is not necessary to use an additional code for angina pectoris. A causal relationship can be assumed in a patient with both atherosclerosis and angina pectoris, unless the documentation indicates the angina is due to something other than the atherosclerosis.

If a patient with coronary artery disease is admitted due to an acute myocardial infarction (AMI), the AMI should be sequenced before the coronary artery disease.
See Section I.C.9. Acute myocardial infarction (AMI)

c. Intraoperative and Postprocedural Cerebrovascular Accident
Medical record documentation should clearly specify the cause-and-effect relationship between the medical intervention and the cerebrovascular accident in order to assign a code for intraoperative or postprocedural cerebrovascular accident.

Proper code assignment depends on whether it was an infarction or hemorrhage and whether it occurred intraoperatively or postoperatively. If it was a cerebral hemorrhage, code assignment depends on the type of procedure performed.

d. Sequelae of Cerebrovascular Disease
1) Category I69, Sequelae of Cerebrovascular disease
Category I69 is used to indicate conditions classifiable to categories I60-I67 as the causes of sequela (neurologic deficits), themselves classified elsewhere. These "late effects" include neurologic deficits that persist after initial onset of conditions classifiable to categories I60-I67. The neurologic deficits caused by cerebrovascular disease may be present from the onset or may arise at any time after the onset of the condition classifiable to categories I60-I67.

Codes from category I69, Sequelae of cerebrovascular disease, that specify hemiplegia, hemiparesis and monoplegia identify whether the dominant or nondominant side is affected. Should the affected side be documented, but not specified as dominant or nondominant, and the classification system does not indicate a default, code selection is as follows:
- For ambidextrous patients, the default should be dominant.
- If the left side is affected, the default is nondominant.
- If the right side is affected, the default is dominant.

2) Codes from category I69 with codes from I60-I67
Codes from category I69 may be assigned on a health care record with codes from I60-I67, if the patient has a current cerebrovascular disease and deficits from an old cerebrovascular disease.

3) Codes from category I69 and Personal history of transient ischemic attack (TIA) and cerebral infarction (Z86.73)
Codes from category I69 should not be assigned if the patient does not have neurologic deficits.
See Section I.C.21. 4. History (of) for use of personal history codes

e. Acute myocardial infarction (AMI)

1) Type 1 ST elevation myocardial infarction (STEMI) and non ST elevation myocardial infarction (NSTEMI)

The ICD-10-CM codes for type 1 acute myocardial infarction (AMI) identify the site, such as anterolateral wall or true posterior wall. Subcategories I21.0-I21.2 and code I21.3 are used for type 1 ST elevation myocardial infarction (STEMI). Code I21.4, Non-ST elevation (NSTEMI) myocardial infarction, is used for type 1 non ST elevation myocardial infarction (NSTEMI) and nontransmural MIs.

If a type 1 NSTEMI evolves to STEMI, assign the STEMI code. If a type 1 STEMI converts to NSTEMI due to thrombolytic therapy, it is still coded as STEMI.

For encounters occurring while the myocardial infarction is equal to, or less than, 4 weeks old, including transfers to another acute setting or a postacute setting, and the myocardial infarction meets the definition for "other diagnoses" (see Section III, Reporting Additional Diagnoses), codes from category I21 may continue to be reported. For encounters after the 4 week time frame and the patient is still receiving care related to the myocardial infarction, the appropriate aftercare code should be assigned, rather than a code from category I21. For old or healed myocardial infarctions not requiring further care, code I25.2, Old myocardial infarction, may be assigned.

2) Acute myocardial infarction, unspecified

Code I21.9, Acute myocardial infarction, unspecified, is the default for unspecified acute myocardial infarction or unspecified type. If only type 1 STEMI or transmural MI without the site is documented, assign code I21.3, ST elevation (STEMI) myocardial infarction of unspecified site.

3) AMI documented as nontransmural or subendocardial but site provided

If an AMI is documented as nontransmural or subendocardial, but the site is provided, it is still coded as a subendocardial AMI.

See Section I.C.21.3 for information on coding status post administration of tPA in a different facility within the last 24 hours.

4) Subsequent acute myocardial infarction

A code from category I22, Subsequent ST elevation (STEMI) and non ST elevation (NSTEMI) myocardial infarction, is to be used when a patient who has suffered a type 1 or unspecified AMI has a new AMI within the 4 week time frame of the initial AMI. A code from category I22 must be used in conjunction with a code from category I21. The sequencing of the I22 and I21 codes depends on the circumstances of the encounter.

Do not assign code I22 for subsequent myocardial infarctions other than type 1 or unspecified. For subsequent type 2 AMI assign only code I21.A1. For subsequent type 4 or type 5 AMI, assign only code I21.A9.

If a subsequent myocardial infarction of one type occurs within 4 weeks of a myocardial infarction of a different type, assign the appropriate codes from category I21 to identify each type. Do not assign a code from I22. Codes from category I22 should only be assigned if both the initial and subsequent myocardial infarctions are type 1 or unspecified.

5) Other Types of Myocardial Infarction

The ICD-10-CM provides codes for different types of myocardial infarction. Type 1 myocardial infarctions are assigned to codes I21.0-I21.4.

Type 2 myocardial infarction (myocardial infarction due to demand ischemia or secondary to ischemic imbalance) is assigned to code I21.A1, Myocardial infarction type 2 with the underlying cause coded first, if applicable. Do not assign code I24.8, Other forms of acute ischemic heart disease, for the demand ischemia. If a type 2 AMI is described as NSTEMI or STEMI, only assign code I21.A1. Codes I21.01-I21.4 should only be assigned for type 1 AMIs.

Acute myocardial infarctions type 3, 4a, 4b, 4c, and 5 are assigned to code I21.A9, Other myocardial infarction type.

The "Code also" and "Code first" notes should be followed related to complications, and for coding of postprocedural myocardial infarctions during or following cardiac surgery.

6) Myocardial Infarction with Coronary Microvascular Dysfunction

Coronary microvascular dysfunction (CMD) is a condition that impacts the microvasculature by restricting microvascular flow and increasing microvascular resistance. Code I21.B, Myocardial infarction with coronary microvascular dysfunction, is assigned for myocardial infarction with coronary microvascular disease, myocardial infarction with coronary microvascular dysfunction, and myocardial infarction with non-obstructive coronary arteries (MINOCA) with microvascular disease.

10. Chapter 10: Diseases of the Respiratory System (J00-J99, U07.1)

a. Chronic Obstructive Pulmonary Disease [COPD] and Asthma

1) Acute exacerbation of chronic obstructive bronchitis and asthma

The codes in categories J44 and J45 distinguish between uncomplicated cases and those in acute exacerbation. An acute exacerbation is a worsening or a decompensation of a chronic condition. An acute exacerbation is not equivalent to an infection superimposed on a chronic condition, though an exacerbation may be triggered by an infection.

b. Acute Respiratory Failure

1) Acute respiratory failure as principal diagnosis

A code from subcategory J96.0, Acute respiratory failure, or subcategory J96.2, Acute and chronic respiratory failure, may be assigned as a principal diagnosis when it is the condition established after study to be chiefly responsible for occasioning the admission to the hospital, and the selection is supported by the Alphabetic Index and Tabular List. However, chapter-specific coding guidelines (such as obstetrics, poisoning, HIV, newborn) that provide sequencing direction take precedence.

2) Acute respiratory failure as secondary diagnosis

Respiratory failure may be listed as a secondary diagnosis if it occurs after admission, or if it is present on admission, but does not meet the definition of principal diagnosis.

3) Sequencing of acute respiratory failure and another acute condition

When a patient is admitted with respiratory failure and another acute condition (e.g., myocardial infarction, cerebrovascular accident, aspiration pneumonia), the principal diagnosis will not be the same in every situation. This applies whether the other acute condition is a respiratory or nonrespiratory condition. Selection of the principal diagnosis will be dependent on the circumstances of admission. If both the respiratory failure and the other acute condition are equally responsible for occasioning the admission to the hospital, and there are no chapter-specific sequencing rules, the guideline regarding two or more diagnoses that equally meet the definition for principal diagnosis (Section II, C.) may be applied in these situations.

If the documentation is not clear as to whether acute respiratory failure and another condition are equally responsible for occasioning the admission, query the provider for clarification.

c. Influenza due to certain identified influenza viruses

Code only confirmed cases of influenza due to certain identified influenza viruses (category J09), and due to other identified influenza virus (category J10). This is an exception to the hospital inpatient guideline Section II, H. (Uncertain Diagnosis).

In this context, "confirmation" does not require documentation of positive laboratory testing specific for avian or other novel influenza A or other identified influenza virus. However, coding should be based on the provider's diagnostic statement that the patient has avian influenza, or other novel influenza A, for category J09, or has another particular identified strain of influenza, such as H1N1 or H3N2, but not identified as novel or variant, for category J10.

If the provider records "suspected" or "possible" or "probable" avian influenza, or novel influenza, or other identified influenza, then the appropriate influenza code from category J11, Influenza due to unidentified influenza virus, should be assigned. A code from category J09, Influenza due to certain identified influenza viruses, should not be assigned nor should a code from category J10, Influenza due to other identified influenza virus.

d. Ventilator associated Pneumonia

1) Documentation of Ventilator associated Pneumonia

As with all procedural or postprocedural complications, code assignment is based on the provider's documentation of the relationship between the condition and the procedure.

Code J95.851, Ventilator associated pneumonia, should be assigned only when the provider has documented ventilator associated pneumonia (VAP). An additional code to identify the organism (e.g., Pseudomonas aeruginosa, code B96.5) should also be assigned. Do not assign an additional code from categories J12-J18 to identify the type of pneumonia.

Code J95.851 should not be assigned for cases where the patient has pneumonia and is on a mechanical ventilator and the provider has not specifically stated that the pneumonia is ventilator-associated pneumonia. If the documentation is unclear as to whether the patient has a pneumonia that is a complication attributable to the mechanical ventilator, query the provider.

2) Ventilator associated Pneumonia Develops after Admission

A patient may be admitted with one type of pneumonia (e.g., code J13, Pneumonia due to Streptococcus pneumonia) and subsequently develop VAP. In this instance, the principal diagnosis would be the appropriate code from categories J12-J18 for the pneumonia diagnosed at the time of admission. Code J95.851, Ventilator associated pneumonia, would be assigned as an additional diagnosis when the provider has also documented the presence of ventilator associated pneumonia.

e. Vaping-related disorders

For patients presenting with condition(s) related to vaping, assign code U07.0, Vaping-related disorder, as the principal diagnosis. For lung injury due to vaping, assign only code U07.0. Assign additional codes for other manifestations, such as acute respiratory failure (subcategory J96.0-) or pneumonitis (code J68.0).

Associated respiratory signs and symptoms due to vaping, such as cough, shortness of breath, etc., are not coded separately, when a definitive diagnosis has been established. However, it would be appropriate to code separately any gastrointestinal symptoms, such as diarrhea and abdominal pain.

11. **Chapter 11: Diseases of the Digestive System (K00-K95)**
Reserved for future guideline expansion

12. **Chapter 12: Diseases of the Skin and Subcutaneous Tissue (L00-L99)**

a. Pressure ulcer stage codes

1) Pressure ulcer stages

Codes in category L89, Pressure ulcer, identify the site and stage of the pressure ulcer.

The ICD-10-CM classifies pressure ulcer stages based on severity, which is designated by stages 1-4, deep tissue pressure injury, unspecified stage, and unstageable.

Assign as many codes from category L89 as needed to identify all the pressure ulcers the patient has, if applicable.

See Section I.B.14 for pressure ulcer stage documentation by clinicians other than patient's provider

2) Unstageable pressure ulcers

Assignment of the code for unstageable pressure ulcer (L89.--Ø) should be based on the clinical documentation. These codes are used for pressure ulcers whose stage cannot be clinically determined (e.g., the ulcer is covered by eschar or has been treated with a skin or muscle graft). This code should not be confused with the codes for unspecified stage (L89.--9). When there is no documentation regarding the stage of the pressure ulcer, assign the appropriate code for unspecified stage (L89.9).

If during an encounter, the stage of an unstageable pressure ulcer is revealed after debridement, assign only the code for the stage revealed following debridement.

3) Documented pressure ulcer stage

Assignment of the pressure ulcer stage code should be guided by clinical documentation of the stage or documentation of the terms found in the Alphabetic Index. For clinical terms describing the stage that are not found in the Alphabetic Index, and there is no documentation of the stage, the provider should be queried.

4) Patients admitted with pressure ulcers documented as healed

No code is assigned if the documentation states that the pressure ulcer is completely healed at the time of admission.

5) Pressure ulcers documented as healing

Pressure ulcers described as healing should be assigned the appropriate pressure ulcer stage code based on the documentation in the medical record. If the documentation does not provide information about the stage of the healing pressure ulcer, assign the appropriate code for unspecified stage.

If the documentation is unclear as to whether the patient has a current (new) pressure ulcer or if the patient is being treated for a healing pressure ulcer, query the provider.

For ulcers that were present on admission but healed at the time of discharge, assign the code for the site and stage of the pressure ulcer at the time of admission.

6) Patient admitted with pressure ulcer evolving into another stage during the admission

If a patient is admitted to an inpatient hospital with a pressure ulcer at one stage and it progresses to a higher stage, two separate codes should be assigned: one code for the site and stage of the ulcer on admission and a second code for the same ulcer site and the highest stage reported during the stay.

7) Pressure-induced deep tissue damage

For pressure-induced deep tissue damage or deep tissue pressure injury, assign only the appropriate code for pressure-induced deep tissue damage (L89.--6).

b. Non-Pressure Chronic Ulcers

1) Patients admitted with non-pressure ulcers documented as healed

No code is assigned if the documentation states that the non-pressure ulcer is completely healed at the time of admission.

2) Non-pressure ulcers documented as healing

Non-pressure ulcers described as healing should be assigned the appropriate non-pressure ulcer code based on the documentation in the medical record. If the documentation does not provide information about the severity of the healing non-pressure ulcer, assign the appropriate code for unspecified severity.

If the documentation is unclear as to whether the patient has a current (new) non-pressure ulcer or if the patient is being treated for a healing non-pressure ulcer, query the provider.

For ulcers that were present on admission but healed at the time of discharge, assign the code for the site and severity of the non-pressure ulcer at the time of admission.

3) Patient admitted with non-pressure ulcer that progresses to another severity level during the admission

If a patient is admitted to an inpatient hospital with a non-pressure ulcer at one severity level and it progresses to a higher severity level, two separate codes should be assigned: one code for the site and severity level of the ulcer on admission and a second code for the same ulcer site and the highest severity level reported during the stay.

See Section I.B.14 for pressure ulcer stage documentation by clinicians other than patient's provider

13. Chapter 13: Diseases of the Musculoskeletal System and Connective Tissue (MØØ-M99)

a. Site and laterality

Most of the codes within Chapter 13 have site and laterality designations. The site represents the bone, joint or the muscle involved. For some conditions where more than one bone, joint or muscle is usually involved, such as osteoarthritis, there is a "multiple sites" code available. For categories where no multiple site code is provided and more than one bone, joint or muscle is involved, multiple codes should be used to indicate the different sites involved.

1) Bone versus joint

For certain conditions, the bone may be affected at the upper or lower end (e.g., avascular necrosis of bone, M87, Osteoporosis, M80, M81). Though the portion of the bone affected may be at the joint, the site designation will be the bone, not the joint.

b. Acute traumatic versus chronic or recurrent musculoskeletal conditions

Many musculoskeletal conditions are a result of previous injury or trauma to a site, or are recurrent conditions. Bone, joint or muscle conditions that are the result of a healed injury are usually found in Chapter 13. Recurrent bone, joint or muscle conditions are also usually found in Chapter 13. Any current, acute injury should be coded to the appropriate injury code from Chapter 19. Chronic or recurrent conditions should generally be coded with a code from Chapter 13. If it is difficult to determine from the documentation in the record which code is best to describe a condition, query the provider.

c. Coding of Pathologic Fractures

Seventh character A is for use as long as the patient is receiving active treatment for the fracture. While the patient may be seen by a new or different provider over the course of treatment for a pathological fracture, assignment of the 7th character is based on whether the patient is undergoing active treatment and not whether the provider is seeing the patient for the first time.

Seventh character, D is to be used for encounters after the patient has completed active treatment for the fracture and is receiving routine care for the fracture during the healing or recovery phase. The other 7th characters, listed under each subcategory in the Tabular List, are to be used for subsequent encounters for treatment of problems associated with the healing, such as malunions, nonunions, and sequelae.

Care for complications of surgical treatment for fracture repairs during the healing or recovery phase should be coded with the appropriate complication codes.

See Section I.C.19. Coding of traumatic fractures

d. Osteoporosis

Osteoporosis is a systemic condition, meaning that all bones of the musculoskeletal system are affected. Therefore, site is not a component of the codes under category M81, Osteoporosis without current pathological fracture. The site codes under category M80, Osteoporosis with current pathological fracture, identify the site of the fracture, not the osteoporosis.

1) Osteoporosis without pathological fracture

Category M81, Osteoporosis without current pathological fracture, is for use for patients with osteoporosis who do not currently have a pathologic fracture due to the osteoporosis, even if they have had a fracture in the past. For patients with a history of osteoporosis fractures, status code Z87.310, Personal history of (healed) osteoporosis fracture, should follow the code from M81.

2) Osteoporosis with current pathological fracture

Category M80, Osteoporosis with current pathological fracture, is for patients who have a current pathologic fracture at the time of an encounter. The codes under M80 identify the site of the fracture. A code from category M80, not a traumatic fracture code, should be used for any patient with known osteoporosis who suffers a fracture, even if the patient had a minor fall or trauma, if that fall or trauma would not usually break a normal, healthy bone.

e. Multisystem Inflammatory Syndrome

See Section I.C.1.g.1.l for Multisystem Inflammatory Syndrome

14. Chapter 14: Diseases of Genitourinary System (N00-N99)

a. Chronic kidney disease

1) Stages of chronic kidney disease (CKD)

The ICD-10-CM classifies CKD based on severity. The severity of CKD is designated by stages 1-5. Stage 2, code N18.2, equates to mild CKD; stage 3, codes N18.30-N18.32, equate to moderate CKD;

and stage 4, code N18.4, equates to severe CKD. Code N18.6, End stage renal disease (ESRD), is assigned when the provider has documented end-stage-renal disease (ESRD).

If both a stage of CKD and ESRD are documented, assign code N18.6 only.

2) Chronic kidney disease and kidney transplant status

Patients who have undergone kidney transplant may still have some form of chronic kidney disease (CKD) because the kidney transplant may not fully restore kidney function. Therefore, the presence of CKD alone does not constitute a transplant complication. Assign the appropriate N18 code for the patient's stage of CKD and code Z94.0, Kidney transplant status. If a transplant complication such as failure or rejection or other transplant complication is documented, see Section I.C.19.g for information on coding complications of a kidney transplant. If the documentation is unclear as to whether the patient has a complication of the transplant, query the provider.

3) Chronic kidney disease with other conditions

Patients with CKD may also suffer from other serious conditions, most commonly diabetes mellitus and hypertension. The sequencing of the CKD code in relationship to codes for other contributing conditions is based on the conventions in the Tabular List.

See I.C.9. Hypertensive chronic kidney disease.
See I.C.19. Chronic kidney disease and kidney transplant complications.

15. Chapter 15: Pregnancy, Childbirth, and the Puerperium (O00-O9A)

a. General Rules for Obstetric Cases

1) Codes from chapter 15 and sequencing priority

Obstetric cases require codes from chapter 15, codes in the range O00O9A, Pregnancy, Childbirth, and the Puerperium. Chapter 15 codes have sequencing priority over codes from other chapters. Additional codes from other chapters may be used in conjunction with chapter 15 codes to further specify conditions. Should the provider document that the pregnancy is incidental to the encounter, then code Z33.1, Pregnant state, incidental, should be used in place of any chapter 15 codes. It is the provider's responsibility to state that the condition being treated is not affecting the pregnancy.

2) Chapter 15 codes used only on the maternal record

Chapter 15 codes are to be used only on the maternal record, never on the record of the newborn.

3) Final character for trimester

The majority of codes in Chapter 15 have a final character indicating the trimester of pregnancy. The timeframes for the trimesters are indicated at the beginning of the chapter. If trimester is not a component of a code it is because the condition always occurs in a specific trimester, or the concept of trimester of pregnancy is not applicable. Certain codes have characters for only certain trimesters because the condition does not occur in all trimesters, but it may occur in more than just one.

Assignment of the final character for trimester should be based on the provider's documentation of the trimester (or number of weeks) for the current admission/encounter. This applies to the assignment of trimester for pre-existing conditions as well as those that develop during or are due to the pregnancy. The provider's documentation of the number of weeks may be used to assign the appropriate code identifying the trimester.

Whenever delivery occurs during the current admission, and there is an "in childbirth" option for the obstetric complication being coded, the "in childbirth" code should be assigned.

When the classification does not provide an obstetric code with an "in childbirth" option, it is appropriate to assign a code describing the current trimester.

4) Selection of trimester for inpatient admissions that encompass more than one trimester

In instances when a patient is admitted to a hospital for complications of pregnancy during one trimester and remains in the hospital into a subsequent trimester, the trimester character for the antepartum complication code should be assigned on the basis of the trimester when the complication developed, not the trimester of the discharge. If the condition developed prior to the current admission/encounter or represents a pre-existing condition, the trimester character for the trimester at the time of the admission/encounter should be assigned.

5) Unspecified trimester

Each category that includes codes for trimester has a code for "unspecified trimester." The "unspecified trimester" code should rarely be used, such as when the documentation in the record is insufficient to determine the trimester and it is not possible to obtain clarification.

6) 7th character for fetus identification

Where applicable, a 7th character is to be assigned for certain categories (O31, O32, O33.3 - O33.6, O35, O36, O40, O41, O60.1, O60.2, O64, and O69) to identify the fetus for which the complication code applies.

Assign 7th character "0":
- For single gestations
- When the documentation in the record is insufficient to determine the fetus affected and it is not possible to obtain clarification.
- When it is not possible to clinically determine which fetus is affected.

7) Completed weeks of gestation

In ICD-10-CM, "completed" weeks of gestation refers to full weeks. For example, if the provider documents gestation at 39 weeks and 6 days, the code for 39 weeks of gestation should be assigned, as the patient has not yet reached 40 completed weeks.

b. Selection of OB Principal or First-listed Diagnosis

1) Routine outpatient prenatal visits

For routine outpatient prenatal visits when no complications are present, a code from category Z34, Encounter for supervision of normal pregnancy, should be used as the first-listed diagnosis. These codes should not be used in conjunction with chapter 15 codes.

2) Supervision of High-Risk Pregnancy

Codes from category O09, Supervision of high-risk pregnancy, are intended for use only during the prenatal period. For complications during the labor or delivery episode as a result of a high-risk pregnancy, assign the applicable complication codes from chapter 15. If there are no complications during the labor or delivery episode, assign code O80, Encounter for full-term uncomplicated delivery.

For routine prenatal outpatient visits for patients with high-risk pregnancies, a code from category O09, Supervision of high-risk pregnancy, should be used as the first-listed diagnosis. Secondary Chapter 15 codes may be used in conjunction with these codes if appropriate.

3) Episodes when no delivery occurs

In episodes when no delivery occurs, the principal diagnosis should correspond to the principal complication of the pregnancy which necessitated the encounter. Should more than one complication exist, all of which are treated or monitored, any of the complication codes may be sequenced first.

4) When a delivery occurs

When an obstetric patient is admitted and delivers during that admission, the condition that prompted the admission should be sequenced as the principal diagnosis. If multiple conditions prompted the admission, sequence the one most related to the delivery as the principal diagnosis. A code for any complication of the delivery should be assigned as an additional diagnosis. In cases of cesarean delivery, if the patient was admitted with a condition that resulted in the performance of a cesarean procedure, that condition should be selected as the principal diagnosis. If the reason for the admission was unrelated to the condition resulting in the cesarean delivery, the condition related to the reason for the admission should be selected as the principal diagnosis.

5) Outcome of delivery

A code from category Z37, Outcome of delivery, should be included on every maternal record when a delivery has occurred. These codes are not to be used on subsequent records or on the newborn record.

c. Pre-existing conditions versus conditions due to the pregnancy

Certain categories in Chapter 15 distinguish between conditions of the mother that existed prior to pregnancy (pre-existing) and those that are a direct result of pregnancy. When assigning codes from Chapter 15, it is important to assess if a condition was pre-existing prior to pregnancy or developed during or due to the pregnancy in order to assign the correct code.

Categories that do not distinguish between pre-existing and pregnancy-related conditions may be used for either. It is acceptable to use codes specifically for the puerperium with codes complicating pregnancy and childbirth if a condition arises postpartum during the delivery encounter.

d. Pre-existing hypertension in pregnancy
Category O10, Pre-existing hypertension complicating pregnancy, childbirth and the puerperium, includes codes for hypertensive heart and hypertensive chronic kidney disease. When assigning one of the O10 codes that includes hypertensive heart disease or hypertensive chronic kidney disease, it is necessary to add a secondary code from the appropriate hypertension category to specify the type of heart failure or chronic kidney disease.

See Section I.C.9. Hypertension.

e. Fetal Conditions Affecting the Management of the Mother
1) Codes from categories O35 and O36
Codes from categories O35, Maternal care for known or suspected fetal abnormality and damage, and O36, Maternal care for other fetal problems, are assigned only when the fetal condition is actually responsible for modifying the management of the mother, i.e., by requiring diagnostic studies, additional observation, special care, or termination of pregnancy. The fact that the fetal condition exists does not justify assigning a code from this series to the mother's record.

2) In utero surgery
In cases when surgery is performed on the fetus, a diagnosis code from category O35, Maternal care for known or suspected fetal abnormality and damage, should be assigned identifying the fetal condition. Assign the appropriate procedure code for the procedure performed.

No code from Chapter 16, the perinatal codes, should be used on the mother's record to identify fetal conditions. Surgery performed in utero on a fetus is still to be coded as an obstetric encounter.

f. HIV Infection in Pregnancy, Childbirth and the Puerperium
During pregnancy, childbirth or the puerperium, a patient admitted because of an HIV-related illness should receive a principal diagnosis from subcategory O98.7-, Human immunodeficiency [HIV] disease complicating pregnancy, childbirth and the puerperium, followed by the code(s) for the HIV-related illness(es).

Patients with asymptomatic HIV infection status admitted during pregnancy, childbirth, or the puerperium should receive codes of O98.7- and Z21, Asymptomatic human immunodeficiency virus [HIV] infection status.

g. Diabetes mellitus in pregnancy
Diabetes mellitus is a significant complicating factor in pregnancy. Pregnant patients who are diabetic should be assigned a code from

category O24, Diabetes mellitus in pregnancy, childbirth, and the puerperium, first, followed by the appropriate diabetes code(s) (E08-E13) from Chapter 4.

h. Longterm use of insulin and oral hypoglycemics
See section I.C.4.a.3 for information on the longterm use of insulin and oral hypoglycemics.

i. Gestational (pregnancy induced) diabetes
Gestational (pregnancy induced) diabetes can occur during the second and third trimester of pregnancy in patients who were not diabetic prior to pregnancy. Gestational diabetes can cause complications in the pregnancy similar to those of pre-existing diabetes mellitus. It also puts the patient at greater risk of developing diabetes after the pregnancy. Codes for gestational diabetes are in subcategory O24.4, Gestational diabetes mellitus. No other code from category O24, Diabetes mellitus in pregnancy, childbirth, and the puerperium, should be used with a code from O24.4.

The codes under subcategory O24.4 include diet controlled, insulin controlled, and controlled by oral hypoglycemic drugs. If a patient with gestational diabetes is treated with both diet and insulin, only the code for insulin-controlled is required. If a patient with gestational diabetes is treated with both diet and oral hypoglycemic medications, only the code for "controlled by oral hypoglycemic drugs" is required. Codes Z79.4, Long-term (current) use of insulin, Z79.84, Long-term (current) use of oral hypoglycemic drugs, **and Z79.85, Long-term (current) use of injectable non-insulin antidiabetic drugs,** should not be assigned with codes from subcategory O24.4.

An abnormal glucose tolerance in pregnancy is assigned a code from subcategory O99.81, Abnormal glucose complicating pregnancy, childbirth, and the puerperium.

j. Sepsis and septic shock complicating abortion, pregnancy, childbirth and the puerperium
When assigning a chapter 15 code for sepsis complicating abortion, pregnancy, childbirth, and the puerperium, a code for the specific type of infection should be assigned as an additional diagnosis. If severe sepsis is present, a code from subcategory R65.2, Severe sepsis, and code(s) for associated organ dysfunction(s) should also be assigned as additional diagnoses.

k. Puerperal sepsis
Code O85, Puerperal sepsis, should be assigned with a secondary code to identify the causal organism (e.g., for a bacterial infection, assign a code from category B95-B96, Bacterial infections in conditions classified elsewhere). A code from category A40, Streptococcal sepsis, or A41, Other sepsis, should not be used for puerperal sepsis. If applicable, use additional codes to identify severe sepsis (R65.2-) and any associated acute organ dysfunction.

Code O85 should not be assigned for sepsis following an obstetrical procedure (See Section I.C.1.d.5.b., Sepsis due to a postprocedural infection).

l. Alcohol, tobacco and drug use during pregnancy, childbirth and the puerperium
1) Alcohol use during pregnancy, childbirth and the puerperium
Codes under subcategory O99.31, Alcohol use complicating pregnancy, childbirth, and the puerperium, should be assigned for any pregnancy case when a patient uses alcohol during the pregnancy or postpartum. A secondary code from category F10, Alcohol related disorders, should also be assigned to identify manifestations of the alcohol use.

2) Tobacco use during pregnancy, childbirth and the puerperium
Codes under subcategory O99.33, Smoking (tobacco) complicating pregnancy, childbirth, and the puerperium, should be assigned for any pregnancy case when a patient uses any type of tobacco product during the pregnancy or postpartum. A secondary code from category F17, Nicotine dependence, should also be assigned to identify the type of nicotine dependence.

3) Drug use during pregnancy, childbirth and the puerperium
Codes under subcategory O99.32, Drug use complicating pregnancy, childbirth, and the puerperium, should be assigned for any pregnancy case when a patient uses drugs during the pregnancy or postpartum. This can involve illegal drugs, or inappropriate use or abuse of prescription drugs. Secondary code(s) from categories F11-F16 and F18-F19 should also be assigned to identify manifestations of the drug use.

m. Poisoning, toxic effects, adverse effects and underdosing in a pregnant patient
A code from subcategory O9A.2, Injury, poisoning and certain other consequences of external causes complicating pregnancy, childbirth, and the puerperium, should be sequenced first, followed by the appropriate injury, poisoning, toxic effect, adverse effect or underdosing code, and then the additional code(s) that specifies the condition caused by the poisoning, toxic effect, adverse effect or underdosing.

See Section I.C.19. Adverse effects, poisoning, underdosing and toxic effects.

n. Normal Delivery, Code O80
1) Encounter for full term uncomplicated delivery
Code O80 should be assigned when a patient is admitted for a full-term normal delivery and delivers a single, healthy infant without any complications antepartum, during the delivery, or postpartum during the delivery episode. Code O80 is always a principal diagnosis. It is not to be used if any other code from chapter 15 is needed to describe a current complication of the antenatal, delivery, or postnatal period. Additional codes from other chapters may be used with code O80 if they are not related to or are in any way complicating the pregnancy.

2) Uncomplicated delivery with resolved antepartum complication
Code O80 may be used if the patient had a complication at some point during the pregnancy, but the complication is not present at the time of the admission for delivery.

3) Outcome of delivery for O80
Z37.0, Single live birth, is the only outcome of delivery code appropriate for use with O80.

o. The Peripartum and Postpartum Periods
1) Peripartum and Postpartum periods
The postpartum period begins immediately after delivery and continues for six weeks following delivery. The peripartum period is defined as the last month of pregnancy to five months postpartum.

2) Peripartum and postpartum complication
A postpartum complication is any complication occurring within the six week period.

3) Pregnancy-related complications after 6-week period
Chapter 15 codes may also be used to describe pregnancy-related complications after the peripartum or postpartum period if the provider documents that a condition is pregnancy related.

4) Admission for routine postpartum care following delivery outside hospital
When the mother delivers outside the hospital prior to admission and is admitted for routine postpartum care and no complications are noted, code Z39.0, Encounter for care and examination of mother immediately after delivery, should be assigned as the principal diagnosis.

5) Pregnancy associated cardiomyopathy
Pregnancy associated cardiomyopathy, code O90.3, is unique in that it may be diagnosed in the third trimester of pregnancy but may continue to progress months after delivery. For this reason, it is referred to as peripartum cardiomyopathy. Code O90.3 is only for use when the cardiomyopathy develops as a result of pregnancy in a patient who did not have pre-existing heart disease.

p. Code O94, Sequelae of complication of pregnancy, childbirth, and the puerperium
1) Code O94
Code O94, Sequelae of complication of pregnancy, childbirth, and the puerperium, is for use in those cases when an initial complication of a pregnancy develops a sequela or sequelae requiring care or treatment at a future date.

2) After the initial postpartum period
This code may be used at any time after the initial postpartum period.

3) Sequencing of Code O94
This code, like all sequela codes, is to be sequenced following the code describing the sequelae of the complication.

q. Termination of Pregnancy and Spontaneous abortions

1) Abortion with Liveborn Fetus

When an attempted termination of pregnancy results in a liveborn fetus assign code Z33.2, Encounter for elective termination of pregnancy and a code from category Z37, Outcome of Delivery.

2) Retained Products of Conception following an abortion

Subsequent encounters for retained products of conception following a spontaneous abortion or elective termination of pregnancy, without complications are assigned O03.4, Incomplete spontaneous abortion without complication or code O07.4, Failed attempted termination of pregnancy without complication. This advice is appropriate even when the patient was discharged previously with a discharge diagnosis of complete abortion. If the patient has a specific complication associated with the spontaneous abortion or elective termination of pregnancy in addition to retained products of conception, assign the appropriate complication code (e.g., O03.-, O04.-, O07.-) instead of code O03.4 or O07.4

3) Complications leading to abortion

Codes from chapter 15 may be used as additional codes to identify any documented complications of the pregnancy in conjunction with codes in categories in O04, O07 and O08.

4) Hemorrhage following elective abortion

For hemorrhage post elective abortion, assign code O04.6, Delayed or excessive hemorrhage following (induced) termination of pregnancy. Do not assign code O72.1, Other immediate postpartum hemorrhage, as this code should not be assigned for post abortion conditions.

r. Abuse in a pregnant patient

For suspected or confirmed cases of abuse of a pregnant patient, a code(s) from subcategories O9A.3, Physical abuse complicating pregnancy, childbirth, and the puerperium, O9A.4, Sexual abuse complicating pregnancy, childbirth, and the puerperium, and O9A.5, Psychological abuse complicating pregnancy, childbirth, and the puerperium, should be sequenced first, followed by the appropriate codes (if applicable) to identify any associated current injury due to physical abuse, sexual abuse, and the perpetrator of abuse.

See Section I.C.19. Adult and child abuse, neglect and other maltreatment.

s. COVID-19 infection in pregnancy, childbirth, and the puerperium

During pregnancy, childbirth or the puerperium, when COVID-19 is the reason for admission/encounter, code O98.5-, Other viral diseases complicating pregnancy, childbirth and the puerperium, should be sequenced as the principal/first-listed diagnosis, and code U07.1, COVID-19, and the appropriate codes for associated manifestation(s) should be assigned as additional diagnoses. Codes from Chapter 15 always take sequencing priority.

If the reason for admission/encounter is unrelated to COVID-19 but the patient tests positive for COVID-19 during the admission/encounter, the appropriate code for the reason for admission/encounter should be sequenced as the principal/first-listed diagnosis, and codes O98.5- and U07.1, as well as the appropriate codes for associated COVID-19 manifestations, should be assigned as additional diagnoses.

16. Chapter 16: Certain Conditions Originating in the Perinatal Period (P00-P96)

For coding and reporting purposes the perinatal period is defined as before birth through the 28th day following birth. The following guidelines are provided for reporting purposes

a. General Perinatal Rules

1) Use of Chapter 16 Codes

Codes in this chapter are never for use on the maternal record. Codes from Chapter 15, the obstetric chapter, are never permitted on the newborn record. Chapter 16 codes may be used throughout the life of the patient if the condition is still present.

2) Principal Diagnosis for Birth Record

When coding the birth episode in a newborn record, assign a code from category Z38, Liveborn infants according to place of birth and type of delivery, as the principal diagnosis. A code from category Z38 is assigned only once, to a newborn at the time of birth. If a newborn is transferred to another institution, a code from category Z38 should not be used at the receiving hospital.

A code from category Z38 is used only on the newborn record, not on the mother's record.

3) Use of Codes from other Chapters with Codes from Chapter 16

Codes from other chapters may be used with codes from chapter 16 if the codes from the other chapters provide more specific detail. Codes for signs and symptoms may be assigned when a definitive diagnosis has not been established. If the reason for the encounter is a perinatal condition, the code from chapter 16 should be sequenced first.

4) Use of Chapter 16 Codes after the Perinatal Period

Should a condition originate in the perinatal period, and continue throughout the life of the patient, the perinatal code should continue to be used regardless of the patient's age.

5) Birth process or community acquired conditions

If a newborn has a condition that may be either due to the birth process or community acquired and the documentation does not indicate which it is, the default is due to the birth process and the code from Chapter 16 should be used. If the condition is community-acquired, a code from Chapter 16 should not be assigned.

For COVID-19 infection in a newborn, see guideline I.C.16.h.

6) Code all clinically significant conditions

All clinically significant conditions noted on routine newborn examination should be coded. A condition is clinically significant if it requires:

- clinical evaluation; or
- therapeutic treatment; or
- diagnostic procedures; or
- extended length of hospital stay; or
- increased nursing care and/or monitoring; or
- has implications for future health care needs

Note: The perinatal guidelines listed above are the same as the general coding guidelines for "additional diagnoses," except for the final point regarding implications for future health care needs. Codes should be assigned for conditions that have been specified by the provider as having implications for future health care needs.

b. Observation and Evaluation of Newborns for Suspected Conditions not Found

1) Use of Z05 codes

Assign a code from category Z05, Observation and evaluation of newborn for suspected **diseases and** conditions ruled out, to identify those instances when a healthy newborn is evaluated for a suspected condition/**disease** that is determined after study not to be present. Do not use a code from category Z05 when the patient **is documented to have** signs or symptoms of a suspected problem; in such cases code the sign or symptom.

2) Z05 on other than the birth record

A code from category Z05 may also be assigned as a principal or firstlisted code for readmissions or encounters when the code from category Z38 code no longer applies. Codes from category Z05 are for use only for healthy newborns and infants for which no condition after study is found to be present.

3) Z05 on a birth record

A code from category Z05 is to be used as a secondary code after the code from category Z38, Liveborn infants according to place of birth and type of delivery.

c. Coding Additional Perinatal Diagnoses

1) Assigning codes for conditions that require treatment

Assign codes for conditions that require treatment or further investigation, prolong the length of stay, or require resource utilization.

2) Codes for conditions specified as having implications for future health care needs

Assign codes for conditions that have been specified by the provider as having implications for future health care needs.

Note: This guideline should not be used for adult patients.

d. Prematurity and Fetal Growth Retardation

Providers utilize different criteria in determining prematurity. A code for prematurity should not be assigned unless it is documented. Assignment of codes in categories P05, Disorders of newborn related to slow fetal growth and fetal malnutrition, and P07, Disorders of newborn related to short gestation and low birth weight, not elsewhere classified, should be based on the recorded birth weight and estimated gestational age.

When both birth weight and gestational age are available, two codes from category P07 should be assigned, with the code for birth weight sequenced before the code for gestational age.

e. Low birth weight and immaturity status

Codes from category P07, Disorders of newborn related to short gestation and low birth weight, not elsewhere classified, are for use for a child or adult who was premature or had a low birth weight as a newborn and this is affecting the patient's current health status.

See Section I.C.21. Factors influencing health status and contact with health services, Status.

f. Bacterial Sepsis of Newborn

Category P36, Bacterial sepsis of newborn, includes congenital sepsis. If a perinate is documented as having sepsis without documentation of congenital or community acquired, the default is congenital and a code from category P36 should be assigned. If the P36 code includes the causal organism, an additional code from category B95, Streptococcus, Staphylococcus, and Enterococcus as the cause of diseases classified elsewhere, or B96, Other bacterial agents as the cause of diseases classified elsewhere, should not be assigned. If the P36 code does not include the causal organism, assign an additional code from category B96. If applicable, use additional codes to identify severe sepsis (R65.2-) and any associated acute organ dysfunction.

g. Stillbirth

Code P95, Stillbirth, is only for use in institutions that maintain separate records for stillbirths. No other code should be used with P95. Code P95 should not be used on the mother's record.

h. COVID-19 Infection in Newborn

For a newborn that tests positive for COVID-19, assign code U07.1, COVID-19, and the appropriate codes for associated manifestation(s) in neonates/newborns in the absence of documentation indicating a specific type of transmission. For a newborn that tests positive for COVID-19 and the provider documents the condition was contracted in utero or during the birth process, assign codes P35.8, Other congenital viral diseases, and U07.1, COVID-19. When coding the birth episode in a newborn record, the appropriate code from category Z38, Liveborn infants according to place of birth and type of delivery, should be assigned as the principal diagnosis.

17. Chapter 17: Congenital malformations, deformations, and chromosomal abnormalities (Q00-Q99)

Assign an appropriate code(s) from categories Q00-Q99, Congenital malformations, deformations, and chromosomal abnormalities when a malformation/deformation or chromosomal abnormality is documented. A malformation/deformation/or chromosomal abnormality may be the principal/first-listed diagnosis on a record or a secondary diagnosis.

When a malformation/deformation/or chromosomal abnormality does not have a unique code assignment, assign additional code(s) for any manifestations that may be present.

When the code assignment specifically identifies the malformation/deformation/or chromosomal abnormality, manifestations that are an inherent component of the anomaly should not be coded separately. Additional codes should be assigned for manifestations that are not an inherent component.

Codes from Chapter 17 may be used throughout the life of the patient. If a congenital malformation or deformity has been corrected, a personal history code should be used to identify the history of the malformation or deformity. Although present at birth, a malformation/deformation/or chromosomal abnormality may not be identified until later in life. Whenever the condition is diagnosed by the provider, it is appropriate to assign a code from codes Q00-Q99.

For the birth admission, the appropriate code from category Z38, Liveborn infants, according to place of birth and type of delivery, should be sequenced as the principal diagnosis, followed by any congenital anomaly codes, Q00-Q99.

18. **Chapter 18: Symptoms, signs, and abnormal clinical and laboratory findings, not elsewhere classified (R00-R99)**

Chapter 18 includes symptoms, signs, abnormal results of clinical or other investigative procedures, and ill-defined conditions regarding which no diagnosis classifiable elsewhere is recorded. Signs and symptoms that point to a specific diagnosis have been assigned to a category in other chapters of the classification.

a. Use of symptom codes
Codes that describe symptoms and signs are acceptable for reporting purposes when a related definitive diagnosis has not been established (confirmed) by the provider.

b. Use of a symptom code with a definitive diagnosis code
Codes for signs and symptoms may be reported in addition to a related definitive diagnosis when the sign or symptom is not routinely associated with that diagnosis, such as the various signs and symptoms associated with complex syndromes. The definitive diagnosis code should be sequenced before the symptom code.

Signs or symptoms that are associated routinely with a disease process should not be assigned as additional codes, unless otherwise instructed by the classification.

c. Combination codes that include symptoms
ICD-10-CM contains a number of combination codes that identify both the definitive diagnosis and common symptoms of that diagnosis. When using one of these combination codes, an additional code should not be assigned for the symptom.

d. Repeated falls
Code R29.6, Repeated falls, is for use for encounters when a patient has recently fallen and the reason for the fall is being investigated.

Code Z91.81, History of falling, is for use when a patient has fallen in the past and is at risk for future falls. When appropriate, both codes R29.6 and Z91.81 may be assigned together.

e. Coma
Code R40.20, Unspecified coma, **should** be assigned **when the underlying cause of the coma is not known, or the cause is a traumatic brain injury and the coma scale is not documented in the medical record.**

Do not report codes for unspecified coma, individual or total Glasgow coma scale scores for a patient with a medically induced coma or a sedated patient.

1) Coma Scale
The coma scale codes (R40.21- to R40.24-) can be used in conjunction with traumatic brain injury codes. These codes **cannot be used with code R40.2A, Nontraumatic coma due to underlying condition. They** are primarily for use by trauma registries, but they may be used in any setting where this information is collected. The coma scale codes should be sequenced after the diagnosis code(s).

These codes, one from each subcategory, are needed to complete the scale. The 7th character indicates when the scale was recorded. The 7th character should match for all three codes.

At a minimum, report the initial score documented on presentation at your facility. This may be a score from the emergency medicine technician (EMT) or in the emergency department. If desired, a facility may choose to capture multiple coma scale scores.

Assign code R40.24-, Glasgow coma scale, total score, when only the total score is documented in the medical record and not the individual score(s).

If multiple coma scores are captured within the first 24 hours after hospital admission, assign only the code for the score at the time of admission. ICD-10-CM does not classify coma scores that are reported after admission but less than 24 hours later.

See Section I.B.14. for coma scale documentation by clinicians other than patient's provider

f. Functional quadriplegia
GUIDELINE HAS BEEN DELETED EFFECTIVE OCTOBER 1, 2017

g. SIRS due to Non-Infectious Process
The systemic inflammatory response syndrome (SIRS) can develop as a result of certain non-infectious disease processes, such as trauma, malignant neoplasm, or pancreatitis. When SIRS is documented with a noninfectious condition, and no subsequent infection is documented, the code for the underlying condition, such as an injury, should be assigned, followed by code R65.10, Systemic inflammatory response syndrome (SIRS) of non-infectious origin without acute organ dysfunction, or code R65.11, Systemic inflammatory response syndrome (SIRS) of non-infectious origin with acute organ dysfunction. If an associated acute organ dysfunction is documented, the appropriate code(s) for the specific type of organ dysfunction(s)

should be assigned in addition to code R65.11. If acute organ dysfunction is documented, but it cannot be determined if the acute organ dysfunction is associated with SIRS or due to another condition (e.g., directly due to the trauma), the provider should be queried.

h. Death NOS
Code R99, Ill-defined and unknown cause of mortality, is only for use in the very limited circumstance when a patient who has already died is brought into an emergency department or other healthcare facility and is pronounced dead upon arrival. It does not represent the discharge disposition of death.

i. NIHSS Stroke Scale
The NIH stroke scale (NIHSS) codes (R29.7- -) can be used in conjunction with acute stroke codes **(I60-I63)** to identify the patient's neurological status and the severity of the stroke. The stroke scale codes should be sequenced after the acute stroke diagnosis code(s).

At a minimum, report the initial score documented. If desired, a facility may choose to capture multiple stroke scale scores.

See Section I.B.14 for NIHSS stroke scale documentation by clinicians other than patient's provider

19. **Chapter 19: Injury, poisoning, and certain other consequences of external causes (S00-T88)**

a. Application of 7th Characters in Chapter 19
Most categories in chapter 19 have a 7th character requirement for each applicable code. Most categories in this chapter have three 7th character values (with the exception of fractures): A, initial encounter, D, subsequent encounter and S, sequela. Categories for traumatic fractures have additional 7th character values. While the patient may be seen by a new or different provider over the course of treatment for an injury, assignment of the 7th character is based on whether the patient is undergoing active treatment and not whether the provider is seeing the patient for the first time.

For complication codes, active treatment refers to treatment for the condition described by the code, even though it may be related to an earlier precipitating problem. For example, code T84.50XA, Infection and inflammatory reaction due to unspecified internal joint prosthesis, initial encounter, is used when active treatment is provided for the infection, even though the condition relates to the prosthetic device, implant or graft that was placed at a previous encounter.

7th character "A", initial encounter is used for each encounter where the patient is receiving active treatment for the condition.

7th character "D" subsequent encounter is used for encounters after the patient has completed active treatment of the condition and is receiving routine care for the condition during the healing or recovery phase.

The aftercare Z codes should not be used for aftercare for conditions such as injuries or poisonings, where 7th characters are provided to identify subsequent care. For example, for aftercare of an injury, assign the acute injury code with the 7th character "D" (subsequent encounter).

7th character "S", sequela, is for use for complications or conditions that arise as a direct result of a condition, such as scar formation after a burn. The scars are sequelae of the burn. When using 7th character "S", it is necessary to use both the injury code that precipitated the sequela and the code for the sequela itself. The "S" is added only to the injury code, not the sequela code. The 7th character "S" identifies the injury responsible for the sequela. The specific type of sequela (e.g., scar) is sequenced first, followed by the injury code.

See Section I.B.10. Sequelae, (Late Effects)

b. Coding of Injuries
When coding injuries, assign separate codes for each injury unless a combination code is provided, in which case the combination code is assigned. Codes from category T07, Unspecified multiple injuries should not be assigned in the inpatient setting unless information for a more specific code is not available. Traumatic injury codes (S00-T14.9) are not to be used for normal, healing surgical wounds or to identify complications of surgical wounds.

The code for the most serious injury, as determined by the provider and the focus of treatment, is sequenced first.

1) Superficial injuries
Superficial injuries such as abrasions or contusions are not coded when associated with more severe injuries of the same site.

2) Primary injury with damage to nerves/ blood vessels
When a primary injury results in minor damage to peripheral nerves or blood vessels, the primary injury is sequenced first with additional code(s) for injuries to nerves and spinal cord (such as category S04), and/or injury to blood vessels (such as category S15). When the primary injury is to the blood vessels or nerves, that injury should be sequenced first.

3) Iatrogenic injuries
Injury codes from Chapter 19 should not be assigned for injuries that occur during, or as a result of, a medical intervention. Assign the appropriate complication code(s).

c. Coding of Traumatic Fractures
The principles of multiple coding of injuries should be followed in coding fractures. Fractures of specified sites are coded individually by site in accordance with both the provisions within categories S02, S12, S22, S32, S42, S49, S52, S59, S62, S72, S79, S82, S89, S92 and the level of detail furnished by medical record content.

A fracture not indicated as open or closed should be coded to closed. A fracture not indicated whether displaced or not displaced should be coded to displaced.

More specific guidelines are as follows:

1) Initial vs. subsequent encounter for fractures

Traumatic fractures are coded using the appropriate 7th character for initial encounter (A, B, C) for each encounter where the patient is receiving active treatment for the fracture. The appropriate 7th character for initial encounter should also be assigned for a patient who delayed seeking treatment for the fracture or nonunion.

Fractures are coded using the appropriate 7th character for subsequent care for encounters after the patient has completed active treatment of the fracture and is receiving routine care for the fracture during the healing or recovery phase.

Care for complications of surgical treatment for fracture repairs during the healing or recovery phase should be coded with the appropriate complication codes.

Care of complications of fractures, such as malunion and nonunion, should be reported with the appropriate 7th character for subsequent care with nonunion (K, M, N,) or subsequent care with malunion (P, Q, R).

Malunion/nonunion: The appropriate 7th character for initial encounter should also be assigned for a patient who delayed seeking treatment for the fracture or nonunion.

The open fracture designations in the assignment of the 7th character for fractures of the forearm, femur and lower leg, including ankle are based on the Gustilo open fracture classification. When the Gustilo classification type is not specified for an open fracture, the 7th character for open fracture type I or II should be assigned (B, E, H, M, Q).

A code from category M80, not a traumatic fracture code, should be used for any patient with known osteoporosis who suffers a fracture, even if the patient had a minor fall or trauma, if that fall or trauma would not usually break a normal, healthy bone.

See Section I.C.13. Osteoporosis.

The aftercare Z codes should not be used for aftercare for traumatic fractures. For aftercare of a traumatic fracture, assign the acute fracture code with the appropriate 7th character.

2) Multiple fractures sequencing

Multiple fractures are sequenced in accordance with the severity of the fracture.

3) Physeal fractures

For physeal fractures, assign only the code identifying the type of physeal fracture. Do not assign a separate code to identify the specific bone that is fractured.

d. Coding of Burns and Corrosions

The ICD-10-CM makes a distinction between burns and corrosions. The burn codes are for thermal burns, except sunburns, that come from a heat source, such as a fire or hot appliance. The burn codes are also for burns resulting from electricity and radiation. Corrosions are burns due to chemicals. The guidelines are the same for burns and corrosions.

Current burns (T20-T25) are classified by depth, extent and by agent (X code). Burns are classified by depth as first degree (erythema), second degree (blistering), and third degree (full-thickness involvement). Burns of the eye and internal organs (T26-T28) are classified by site, but not by degree.

1) Sequencing of burn and related condition codes

Sequence first the code that reflects the highest degree of burn when more than one burn is present.

  a. When the reason for the admission or encounter is for treatment of external multiple burns, sequence first the code that reflects the burn of the highest degree.

  b. When a patient has both internal and external burns, the circumstances of admission govern the selection of the principal diagnosis or first-listed diagnosis.

  c. When a patient is admitted for burn injuries and other related conditions such as smoke inhalation and/or respiratory failure, the circumstances of admission govern the selection of the principal or first-listed diagnosis.

2) Burns of the same anatomic site

Classify burns of the same anatomic site and on the same side but of different degrees to the subcategory identifying the highest degree recorded in the diagnosis (e.g., for second and third degree burns of right thigh, assign only code T24.311-).

3) Non-healing burns

Non-healing burns are coded as acute burns.

Necrosis of burned skin should be coded as a non-healed burn.

4) Infected burn

For any documented infected burn site, use an additional code for the infection.

5) Assign separate codes for each burn site

When coding burns, assign separate codes for each burn site. Category T30, Burn and corrosion, body region unspecified is extremely vague and should rarely be used.

Codes for burns of "multiple sites" should only be assigned when the medical record documentation does not specify the individual sites.

6) Burns and corrosions classified according to extent of body surface involved

Assign codes from category T31, Burns classified according to extent of body surface involved, or T32, Corrosions classified according to extent of body surface involved, for acute burns or corrosions when the site of the burn or corrosion is not specified or when there is a need for additional data. It is advisable to use category T31 as additional coding when needed to provide data for evaluating burn mortality, such as that needed by burn units. It is also advisable to use category T31 as an additional code for reporting purposes when there is mention of a thirddegree burn involving 20 percent or more of the body surface. Codes from categories T31 and T32 should not be used for sequelae of burns or corrosions.

Categories T31 and T32 are based on the classic "rule of nines" in estimating body surface involved: head and neck are assigned nine percent, each arm nine percent, each leg 18 percent, the anterior trunk 18 percent, posterior trunk 18 percent, and genitalia one percent. Providers may change these percentage assignments where necessary to accommodate infants and children who have proportionately larger heads than adults, and patients who have large buttocks, thighs, or abdomen that involve burns.

7) Encounters for treatment of sequela of burns

Encounters for the treatment of the late effects of burns or corrosions (i.e., scars or joint contractures) should be coded with a burn or corrosion code with the 7th character "S" for sequela.

8) Sequelae with a late effect code and current burn

When appropriate, both a code for a current burn or corrosion with 7th character "A" or "D" and a burn or corrosion code with 7th character "S" may be assigned on the same record (when both a current burn and sequelae of an old burn exist). Burns and corrosions do not heal at the same rate and a current healing wound may still exist with sequela of a healed burn or corrosion.

See Section I.B.10. Sequela, (Late Effects)

9) Use of an external cause code with burns and corrosions

An external cause code should be used with burns and corrosions to identify the source and intent of the burn, as well as the place where it occurred.

e. Adverse Effects, Poisoning, Underdosing and Toxic Effects

Codes in categories T36-T65 are combination codes that include the substance that was taken as well as the intent. No additional external cause code is required for poisonings, toxic effects, adverse effects and underdosing codes.

1) Do not code directly from the Table of Drugs

Do not code directly from the Table of Drugs and Chemicals. Always refer back to the Tabular List.

2) Use as many codes as necessary to describe

Use as many codes as necessary to describe completely all drugs, medicinal or biological substances.

3) If the same code would describe the causative agent

If the same code would describe the causative agent for more than one adverse reaction, poisoning, toxic effect or underdosing, assign the code only once.

4) If two or more drugs, medicinal or biological substances

If two or more drugs, medicinal or biological substances are taken, code each individually unless a combination code is listed in the Table of Drugs and Chemicals.

If multiple unspecified drugs, medicinal or biological substances were taken, assign the appropriate code from subcategory T50.91, Poisoning by, adverse effect of and underdosing of multiple unspecified drugs, medicaments and biological substances.

5) The occurrence of drug toxicity is classified in ICD-10-CM as follows:

(a) Adverse Effect

When coding an adverse effect of a drug that has been correctly prescribed and properly administered, assign the appropriate code for the nature of the adverse effect followed by the appropriate code for the adverse effect of the drug (T36-T50). The code for the drug should have a 5th or 6th character "5" (for example T36.0X5-) Examples of the nature of an adverse effect are tachycardia, delirium, gastrointestinal hemorrhaging, vomiting, hypokalemia, hepatitis, renal failure, or respiratory failure.

(b) Poisoning

When coding a poisoning or reaction to the improper use of a medication (e.g., overdose, wrong substance given or taken in error, wrong route of administration), first assign the appropriate code from categories T36-T50. The poisoning codes have an associated intent as their 5th or 6th character (accidental, intentional self-harm, assault and undetermined). If the intent of the poisoning is unknown or unspecified, code the intent as accidental intent. The undetermined intent is only for use if the documentation in the record specifies that the intent cannot be determined. Use additional code(s) for all manifestations of poisonings.

If there is also a diagnosis of abuse or dependence of the substance, the abuse or dependence is assigned as an additional code.

Examples of poisoning include:

(i) Error was made in drug prescription Errors made in drug prescription or in the administration of the drug by provider, nurse, patient, or other person.

(ii) Overdose of a drug intentionally taken If an overdose of a drug was intentionally taken or administered and resulted in drug toxicity, it would be coded as a poisoning.

(iii) Nonprescribed drug taken with correctly prescribed and properly administered drug.
If a nonprescribed drug or medicinal agent was taken in combination with a correctly prescribed and properly administered drug, any drug toxicity or other reaction resulting from the interaction of the two drugs would be classified as a poisoning.

(iv) Interaction of drug(s) and alcohol.
When a reaction results from the interaction of a drug(s) and alcohol, this would be classified as poisoning.

See Section I.C.4. if poisoning is the result of insulin pump malfunctions.

For Sequela (Late Effects) see Section I.B.10.

(c) Underdosing

Underdosing refers to taking less of a medication than is prescribed by a provider or a manufacturer's instruction. Discontinuing the use of a prescribed medication on the patient's own initiative (not directed by the patient's provider) is also classified as an underdosing. For underdosing, assign the code from categories T36-T50 (fifth or sixth character "6").

Documentation of a change in the patient's condition is not required in order to assign an underdosing code.

Documentation that the patient is taking less of a medication than is prescribed or discontinued the prescribed medication is sufficient for code assignment.

Codes for underdosing should never be assigned as principal or first-listed codes. If a patient has a relapse or exacerbation of the medical condition for which the drug is prescribed because of the reduction in dose, then the medical condition itself should be coded.

Noncompliance (Z91.12-, Z91.13-, **Z91.14-** and **Z91.A4-**) or complication of care (Y63.6-Y63.9) codes are to be used with an underdosing code to indicate intent, if known.

(d) Toxic Effects

When a harmful substance is ingested or comes in contact with a person, this is classified as a toxic effect. The toxic effect codes are in categories T51-T65. **When coding a toxic effect, assign the toxic effect code first, followed by codes for all associated manifestations of the toxic effect.**

Toxic effect codes have an associated intent: accidental, intentional self-harm, assault and undetermined.

For Sequela (Late Effects) see Section I.B.10. Sequela

f. Adult and child abuse, neglect and other maltreatment

Sequence first the appropriate code from categories T74, Adult and child abuse, neglect and other maltreatment, confirmed, or T76, Adult and child abuse, neglect and other maltreatment, suspected, for abuse, neglect and other maltreatment, followed by any accompanying mental health or injury code(s).

If the documentation in the medical record states abuse or neglect it is coded as confirmed (T74.-). It is coded as suspected if it is documented as suspected (T76.-).

For cases of confirmed abuse or neglect an external cause code from the assault section (X92-Y09) should be added to identify the cause of any physical injuries. A perpetrator code (Y07) should be added when the perpetrator of the abuse is known. For suspected cases of abuse or neglect, do not report external cause or perpetrator code.

If a suspected case of abuse, neglect or mistreatment is ruled out during an encounter code Z04.71, Encounter for examination and observation following alleged physical adult abuse, ruled out,

or code Z04.72, Encounter for examination and observation following alleged child physical abuse, ruled out, should be used, not a code from T76.

If a suspected case of alleged rape or sexual abuse is ruled out during an encounter code Z04.41, Encounter for examination and observation following alleged adult rape or code Z04.42, Encounter for examination and observation following alleged child rape, should be used, not a code from T76.

If a suspected case of forced sexual exploitation or forced labor exploitation is ruled out during an encounter, code Z04.81, Encounter for examination and observation of victim following forced sexual exploitation, or code Z04.82, Encounter for examination and observation of victim following forced labor exploitation, should be used, not a code from T76.

See Section I.C.15. Abuse in a pregnant patient.

g. Complications of care

1) General guidelines for complications of care

(a) Documentation of complications of care

See Section I.B.16. for information on documentation of complications of care.

2) Pain due to medical devices

Pain associated with devices, implants or grafts left in a surgical site (for example painful hip prosthesis) is assigned to the appropriate code(s) found in Chapter 19, Injury, poisoning, and certain other consequences of external causes. Specific codes for pain due to medical devices are found in the T code section of the ICD-10-CM. Use additional code(s) from category G89 to identify acute or chronic pain due to presence of the device, implant or graft (G89.18 or G89.28).

3) Transplant complications

(a) Transplant complications other than kidney

Codes under category T86, Complications of transplanted organs and tissues, are for use for both complications and rejection of transplanted organs. A transplant complication code is only assigned if the complication affects the function of the transplanted organ. Two codes are required to fully describe a transplant complication: the appropriate code from category T86 and a secondary code that identifies the complication.

Pre-existing conditions or conditions that develop after the transplant are not coded as complications unless they affect the function of the transplanted organs.

See Section I.C.21. for transplant organ removal status
See Section I.C.2. for malignant neoplasm associated with transplanted organ.

See I.C.1.d.4. for sequencing of sepsis due to infection in transplanted organ

(b) Kidney transplant complications

Patients who have undergone kidney transplant may still have some form of chronic kidney disease (CKD) because the kidney transplant may not fully restore kidney function. Code T86.1- should be

GUIDELINES (ICD-10-CM)

assigned for documented complications of a kidney transplant, such as transplant failure or rejection or other transplant complication. Code T86.1- should not be assigned for post kidney transplant patients who have chronic kidney (CKD) unless a transplant complication such as transplant failure or rejection is documented. If the documentation is unclear as to whether the patient has a complication of the transplant, query the provider.

Conditions that affect the function of the transplanted kidney, other than CKD, should be assigned a code from subcategory T86.1, Complications of transplanted organ, Kidney, and a secondary code that identifies the complication.

For patients with CKD following a kidney transplant, but who do not have a complication such as failure or rejection, *see Section I.C.14. Chronic kidney disease and kidney transplant status.*

See I.C.1.d.4. for sequencing of sepsis due to infection in transplanted organ

4) Complication codes that include the external cause

As with certain other T codes, some of the complications of care codes have the external cause included in the code. The code includes the nature of the complication as well as the type of procedure that caused the complication. No external cause code indicating the type of procedure is necessary for these codes.

5) Complications of care codes within the body system chapters

Intraoperative and postprocedural complication codes are found within the body system chapters with codes specific to the organs and structures of that body system. These codes should be sequenced first, followed by a code(s) for the specific complication, if applicable.

Complication codes from the body system chapters should be assigned for intraoperative and postprocedural complications (e.g., the appropriate complication code from chapter 9 would be assigned for a vascular intraoperative or postprocedural complication) unless the complication is specifically indexed to a T code in chapter 19.

20. Chapter 20: External Causes of Morbidity (V00-Y99)

The external causes of morbidity codes should never be sequenced as the first-listed or principal diagnosis.

External cause codes are intended to provide data for injury research and evaluation of injury prevention strategies. These codes capture how the injury or health condition happened (cause), the intent (unintentional or accidental; or intentional, such as suicide or assault), the place where the event occurred the activity of the patient at the time of the event, and the person's status (e.g., civilian, military).

There is no national requirement for mandatory ICD-10-CM external cause code reporting. Unless a provider is subject to a state-based external cause code reporting mandate or these codes are required by a particular payer, reporting of ICD-10-CM codes in Chapter 20, External Causes of Morbidity, is not required. In the absence of a mandatory reporting requirement, providers are encouraged to voluntarily report external cause codes, as they provide valuable data for injury research and evaluation of injury prevention strategies.

a. General External Cause Coding Guidelines

1) Used with any code in the range of A00.0-T88.9, Z00-Z99

An external cause code may be used with any code in the range of A00.0-T88.9, Z00-Z99, classification that represents a health condition due to an external cause. Though they are most applicable to injuries, they are also valid for use with such things as infections or diseases due to an external source, and other health conditions, such as a heart attack that occurs during strenuous physical activity.

2) External cause code used for length of treatment

Assign the external cause code, with the appropriate 7th character (initial encounter, subsequent encounter or sequela) for each encounter for which the injury or condition is being treated.

Most categories in Chapter 20 have a 7th character requirement for each applicable code. Most categories in this chapter have three 7th character values: A, initial encounter, D, subsequent encounter and S, sequela. While the patient may be seen by a new or different provider over the course of treatment for an injury or condition, assignment of the 7th character for external cause should match the 7th character of the code assigned for the associated injury or condition for the encounter.

3) Use the full range of external cause codes

Use the full range of external cause codes to completely describe the cause, the intent, the place of occurrence, and if applicable, the activity of the patient at the time of the event, and the patient's status, for all injuries, and other health conditions due to an external cause.

4) Assign as many external cause codes as necessary

Assign as many external cause codes as necessary to fully explain each cause. If only one external code can be recorded, assign the code most related to the principal diagnosis.

5) The selection of the appropriate external cause code

The selection of the appropriate external cause code is guided by the Alphabetic Index of External Causes and by Inclusion and Exclusion notes in the Tabular List.

6) External cause code can never be a principal diagnosis

An external cause code can never be a principal (first-listed) diagnosis.

7) Combination external cause codes

Certain of the external cause codes are combination codes that identify sequential events that result in an injury, such as a fall which results in striking against an object. The injury may be due to either event or both. The combination external cause code used should correspond to the sequence of events regardless of which caused the most serious injury.

8) No external cause code needed in certain circumstances

No external cause code from Chapter 20 is needed if the external cause and intent are included in a code from another chapter (e.g., T36.0X1- Poisoning by penicillins, accidental (unintentional)).

b. Place of Occurrence Guideline

Codes from category Y92, Place of occurrence of the external cause, are secondary codes for use after other external cause codes to identify the location of the patient at the time of injury or other condition.

Generally, a place of occurrence code is assigned only once, at the initial encounter for treatment. However, in the rare instance that a new injury occurs during hospitalization, an additional place of occurrence code may be assigned. No 7th characters are used for Y92.

Do not use place of occurrence code Y92.9 if the place is not stated or is not applicable.

c. Activity Code

Assign a code from category Y93, Activity code, to describe the activity of the patient at the time the injury or other health condition occurred.

An activity code is used only once, at the initial encounter for treatment. Only one code from Y93 should be recorded on a medical record.

The activity codes are not applicable to poisonings, adverse effects, misadventures or sequela.

Do not assign Y93.9, Unspecified activity, if the activity is not stated.

A code from category Y93 is appropriate for use with external cause and intent codes if identifying the activity provides additional information about the event.

d. Place of Occurrence, Activity, and Status Codes Used with other External Cause Code

When applicable, place of occurrence, activity, and external cause status codes are sequenced after the main external cause code(s). Regardless of the number of external cause codes assigned, generally there should be only one place of occurrence code, one activity code, and one external cause status code assigned to an encounter. However, in the rare instance that a new injury occurs during hospitalization, an additional place of occurrence code may be assigned.

e. If the Reporting Format Limits the Number of External Cause Codes

If the reporting format limits the number of external cause codes that can be used in reporting clinical data, report the code for the cause/intent most related to the principal diagnosis. If the format permits capture of additional external cause codes, the cause/intent, including medical misadventures, of the additional events should be reported rather than the codes for place, activity, or external status.

f. Multiple External Cause Coding Guidelines

More than one external cause code is required to fully describe the external cause of an illness or injury. The assignment of external cause codes should be sequenced in the following priority:

If two or more events cause separate injuries, an external cause code should be assigned for each cause. The first-listed external cause code will be selected in the following order:

External codes for child and adult abuse take priority over all other external cause codes.
See Section I.C.19., Child and Adult abuse guidelines.

External cause codes for terrorism events take priority over all other external cause codes except child and adult abuse.

External cause codes for cataclysmic events take priority over all other external cause codes except child and adult abuse and terrorism.

External cause codes for transport accidents take priority over all other external cause codes except cataclysmic events, child and adult abuse and terrorism.

Activity and external cause status codes are assigned following all causal (intent) external cause codes.

The first-listed external cause code should correspond to the cause of the most serious diagnosis due to an assault, accident, or self-harm, following the order of hierarchy listed above.

g. Child and Adult Abuse Guideline

Adult and child abuse, neglect and maltreatment are classified as assault. Any of the assault codes may be used to indicate the external cause of any injury resulting from the confirmed abuse.

For confirmed cases of abuse, neglect and maltreatment, when the perpetrator is known, a code from Y07, Perpetrator of maltreatment and neglect, should accompany any other assault codes.
See Section I.C.19. Adult and child abuse, neglect and other maltreatment

h. Unknown or Undetermined Intent Guideline

If the intent (accident, self-harm, assault) of the cause of an injury or other condition is unknown or unspecified, code the intent as accidental intent. All transport accident categories assume accidental intent.

1) Use of undetermined intent

External cause codes for events of undetermined intent are only for use if the documentation in the record specifies that the intent cannot be determined.

i. Sequelae (Late Effects) of External Cause Guidelines

1) Sequelae external cause codes

Sequela are reported using the external cause code with the 7th character "S" for sequela. These codes should be used with any report of a late effect or sequela resulting from a previous injury.
See Section I.B.10. Sequela (Late Effects)

2) Sequela external cause code with a related current injury

A sequela external cause code should never be used with a related current nature of injury code.

3) Use of sequela external cause codes for subsequent visits

Use a late effect external cause code for subsequent visits when a late effect of the initial injury is being treated. Do not use a late effect external cause code for subsequent visits for follow-up care (e.g., to assess healing, to receive rehabilitative therapy) of the injury when no late effect of the injury has been documented.

j. Terrorism Guidelines

1) Cause of injury identified by the Federal Government (FBI) as terrorism

When the cause of an injury is identified by the Federal Government (FBI) as terrorism, the first-listed external cause code should be a code from category Y38, Terrorism. The definition of terrorism employed by the FBI is found at the inclusion note at the beginning of category Y38. Use additional code for place of occurrence (Y92.-). More than one Y38 code may be assigned if the injury is the result of more than one mechanism of terrorism.

2) Cause of an injury is suspected to be the result of terrorism

When the cause of an injury is suspected to be the result of terrorism a code from category Y38 should not be assigned. Suspected cases should be classified as assault.

3) Code Y38.9, Terrorism, secondary effects

Assign code Y38.9, Terrorism, secondary effects, for conditions occurring subsequent to the terrorist event. This code should not be assigned for conditions that are due to the initial terrorist act.

It is acceptable to assign code Y38.9 with another code from Y38 if there is an injury due to the initial terrorist event and an injury that is a subsequent result of the terrorist event.

k. External Cause Status

A code from category Y99, External cause status, should be assigned whenever any other external cause code is assigned for an encounter, including an Activity code, except for the events noted below. Assign a code from category Y99, External cause status, to indicate the work status of the person at the time the event occurred. The status code indicates whether the event occurred during military activity, whether a non-military person was at work, whether an individual including a student or volunteer was involved in a non-work activity at the time of the causal event.

A code from Y99, External cause status, should be assigned, when applicable, with other external cause codes, such as transport accidents and falls. The external cause status codes are not applicable to poisonings, adverse effects, misadventures or late effects.

Do not assign a code from category Y99 if no other external cause codes (cause, activity) are applicable for the encounter.

An external cause status code is used only once, at the initial encounter for treatment. Only one code from Y99 should be recorded on a medical record.

Do not assign code Y99.9, Unspecified external cause status, if the status is not stated.

21. **Chapter 21: Factors influencing health status and contact with health services (Z00-Z99)**
Note: The chapter-specific guidelines provide additional information about the use of Z codes for specified encounters.

a. Use of Z Codes in Any Healthcare Setting

Z codes are for use in any healthcare setting. Z codes may be used as either a first-listed (principal diagnosis code in the inpatient setting) or secondary code, depending on the circumstances of the encounter. Certain Z codes may only be used as first-listed or principal diagnosis.

b. Z Codes Indicate a Reason for an Encounter *or Provide Additional Information about a Patient Encounter*

Z codes are not procedure codes. A corresponding procedure code must accompany a Z code to describe any procedure performed.

c. Categories of Z Codes

1) Contact/Exposure

Category Z20 indicates contact with, and suspected exposure to, communicable diseases. These codes are for patients who are suspected to have been exposed to a disease by close personal contact with an infected individual or are in an area where a disease is epidemic.

Category Z77, Other contact with and (suspected) exposures hazardous to health, indicates contact with and suspected exposures hazardous to health.

Contact/exposure codes may be used as a first-listed code to explain an encounter for testing, or, more commonly, as a secondary code to identify a potential risk.

2) Inoculations and vaccinations

Code Z23 is for encounters for inoculations and vaccinations. It indicates that a patient is being seen to receive a prophylactic inoculation against a disease. Procedure codes are required to identify the actual administration of the injection and the type(s) of immunizations given. Code Z23 may be used as a secondary code if the inoculation is given as a routine part of preventive health care, such as a well-baby visit.

3) Status

Status codes indicate that a patient is either a carrier of a disease or has the sequelae or residual of a past disease or condition. This includes such things as the presence of prosthetic or mechanical devices resulting from past treatment. A status code is informative, because the status may affect the course of treatment and its outcome. A status code is distinct from a history code. The history code indicates that the patient no longer has the condition.

A status code should not be used with a diagnosis code from one of the body system chapters, if the diagnosis code includes the information provided by the status code. For example, code Z94.1, Heart transplant status, should not be used with a code from subcategory T86.2, Complications of heart transplant. The status code does not provide additional information. The complication code indicates that the patient is a heart transplant patient.

For encounters for weaning from a mechanical ventilator, assign a code from subcategory J96.1, Chronic respiratory failure, followed by code Z99.11, Dependence on respirator [ventilator] status.

The status Z codes/categories are:

Z14   Genetic carrier
Genetic carrier status indicates that a person carries a gene, associated with a particular disease, which may be passed to offspring who may develop that disease. The person does not have the disease and is not at risk of developing the disease.

Z15   Genetic susceptibility to disease Genetic susceptibility indicates that a person has a gene that increases the risk of that person developing the disease.

Codes from category Z15 should not be used as principal or first-listed codes. If the patient has the condition to which he/she is susceptible, and that condition is the reason for the encounter, the code for the current condition should be sequenced first. If the patient is being seen for follow-up after completed treatment for this condition, and the condition no longer exists, a follow-up code should be sequenced first, followed by the appropriate personal history and genetic susceptibility codes. If the purpose of the encounter is genetic counseling associated with procreative management, code Z31.5, Encounter for genetic counseling, should be assigned as the first-listed code, followed by a code from category Z15. Additional codes should be assigned for any applicable family or personal history.

Z16   Resistance to antimicrobial drugs
This code indicates that a patient has a condition that is resistant to antimicrobial drug treatment. Sequence the infection code first.

Z17   Estrogen, and other hormones and factors receptor status

Z18   Retained foreign body fragments

Z19   Hormone sensitivity malignancy status

Z21   Asymptomatic HIV infection status This code indicates that a patient has tested positive for HIV but has manifested no signs or symptoms of the disease.

Z22   Carrier of infectious disease Carrier status indicates that a person harbors the specific organisms of a disease without manifest symptoms and is capable of transmitting the infection.

Z28.3   Underimmunization status

See Section I.B.14. for underimmunization documentation by clinicians other than the patient's provider.

Z33.1   Pregnant state, incidental This code is a secondary code only for use when the pregnancy is in no way complicating the reason for visit. Otherwise, a code from the obstetric chapter is required.

Z66   Do not resuscitate
This code may be used when it is documented by the provider that a patient is on do not resuscitate status at any time during the stay.

Z67   Blood type

Z68   Body mass index (BMI)
BMI codes should only be assigned when there is an associated reportable diagnosis (such as obesity). Do not assign BMI codes during pregnancy.

See Section I.B.14 for BMI documentation by clinicians other than the patient's provider.

Z74.01   Bed confinement status

Z76.82   Awaiting organ transplant status

Z78   Other specified health status
Code Z78.1, Physical restraint status, may be used when it is documented by the provider that a patient has been put in restraints during the current encounter. Please note that this code should not be reported when it is documented by the provider that a patient is temporarily restrained during a procedure.

Z79   Long-term (current) drug therapy
Codes from this category indicate a patient's continuous use of a prescribed drug (including such things as aspirin therapy) for the long-term treatment of a condition or for prophylactic use. It is not for use for patients who have addictions to drugs. This subcategory is not for use of medications for detoxification or maintenance programs to prevent withdrawal symptoms (e.g., methadone maintenance for opiate dependence). Assign the appropriate code for the drug use, abuse, or dependence instead.

Assign a code from Z79 if the patient is receiving a medication for an extended period as a prophylactic measure (such as for the prevention of deep vein thrombosis) or as treatment of a chronic condition (such as arthritis) or a disease requiring a lengthy course of treatment (such as cancer). Do not assign a code from category Z79 for medication being administered for a brief period of time to treat an acute illness or injury (such as a course of antibiotics to treat acute bronchitis).

Z88   Allergy status to drugs, medicaments and biological substances Except: Z88.9, Allergy status to unspecified drugs, medicaments and biological substances status

Z89   Acquired absence of limb

Z90   Acquired absence of organs, not elsewhere classified

Z91.0-   Allergy status, other than to drugs and biological substances

Z92.82   Status post administration of tPA (rtPA) in a different facility within the last 24 hours prior to admission to a current facility Assign code Z92.82, Status post administration of tPA (rtPA) in a different facility within the last 24 hours prior to admission to current facility, as a secondary diagnosis when a patient is received by transfer into a facility and documentation indicates they were administered tissue plasminogen activator (tPA) within the last 24 hours prior to admission to the current facility. This guideline applies even if the patient is still receiving the tPA at the time they are received into the current facility. The appropriate code for the condition for which the tPA was administered (such as cerebrovascular disease or myocardial infarction) should be assigned first. Code Z92.82 is only applicable to the receiving facility record and not to the transferring facility record.

Z93   Artificial opening status
Z94   Transplanted organ and tissue status
Z95   Presence of cardiac and vascular implants and grafts
Z96   Presence of other functional implants
Z97   Presence of other devices
Z98   Other postprocedural states

Assign code Z98.85, Transplanted organ removal status, to indicate that a transplanted organ has been previously removed. This code should not be assigned for the encounter in which the transplanted organ is removed. The complication necessitating removal of the transplant organ should be assigned for that encounter.

See Section I.C.19. for information on the coding of organ transplant complications.

Z99   Dependence on enabling machines and devices, not elsewhere classified

Note: Categories Z89-Z90 and Z93-Z99 are for use only if there are no complications or malfunctions of the organ or tissue replaced, the amputation site or the equipment on which the patient is dependent.

4) History (of)

There are two types of history Z codes, personal and family. Personal history codes explain a patient's past medical condition that no longer exists and is not receiving any treatment, but that has the potential for recurrence, and therefore may require continued monitoring.

Family history codes are for use when a patient has a family member(s) who has had a particular disease that causes the patient to be at higher risk of also contracting the disease.

Personal history codes may be used in conjunction with follow-up codes and family history codes may be used in conjunction with screening codes to explain the need for a test or procedure. History codes are also acceptable on any medical record regardless of the reason for visit. A history of an illness, even if no longer present, is important information that may alter the type of treatment ordered.

The reason for the encounter (for example, screening or counseling) should be sequenced first and the appropriate personal and/or family history code(s) should be assigned as additional diagnos(es).

The history Z code categories are:

Z80   Family history of primary malignant neoplasm
Z81   Family history of mental and behavioral disorders
Z82   Family history of certain disabilities and chronic diseases (leading to disablement)
Z83   Family history of other specific disorders
Z84   Family history of other conditions
Z85   Personal history of malignant neoplasm
Z86   Personal history of certain other diseases
Z87   Personal history of other diseases and conditions
Z91.4-   Personal history of psychological trauma, not elsewhere classified
Z91.5   Personal history of self-harm
Z91.81   History of falling
Z91.82   Personal history of military deployment
Z91.85   Personal history of military service
Z92   Personal history of medical treatment Except: Z92.0, Personal history of contraception Except: Z92.82, Status post administration of tPA (rtPA) in a different facility within the last 24 hours prior to admission to a current facility

5) Screening

Screening is the testing for disease or disease precursors in seemingly well individuals so that early detection and treatment can be provided for those who test positive for the disease (e.g., screening mammogram).

The testing of a person to rule out or confirm a suspected diagnosis because the patient has some sign or symptom is a diagnostic examination, not a screening. In these cases, the sign or symptom is used to explain the reason for the test.

A screening code may be a first-listed code if the reason for the visit is specifically the screening exam. It may also be used as an additional code if the screening is done during an office visit for other health problems. A screening code is not necessary if the screening is inherent to a routine examination, such as a pap smear done during a routine pelvic examination.

Should a condition be discovered during the screening then the code for the condition may be assigned as an additional diagnosis.

The Z code indicates that a screening exam is planned. A procedure code is required to confirm that the screening was performed.

The screening Z codes/categories:

Z11 Encounter for screening for infectious and parasitic diseases

Z12 Encounter for screening for malignant neoplasms

Z13 Encounter for screening for other diseases and disorders Except: Z13.9, Encounter for screening, unspecified

Z36 Encounter for antenatal screening for mother

6) Observation

There are three observation Z code categories. They are for use in very limited circumstances when a person is being observed for a suspected condition that is ruled out. The observation codes are not for use if an injury or illness or any signs or symptoms related to the suspected condition are present. In such cases the diagnosis/symptom code is used with the corresponding external cause code.

The observation codes are primarily to be used as a principal/first-listed diagnosis. An observation code may be assigned as a secondary diagnosis code when the patient is being observed for a condition that is ruled out and is unrelated to the principal/first-listed diagnosis. Also, when the principal diagnosis is required to be a code from category Z38, Liveborn infants according to place of birth and type of delivery, then a code from category Z05, Encounter for observation and evaluation of newborn for suspected diseases and conditions ruled out, is sequenced after the Z38 code. Additional codes may be used in addition to the observation code, but only if they are unrelated to the suspected condition being observed.

Codes from subcategory Z03.7, Encounter for suspected maternal and fetal conditions ruled out, may either be used as a first-listed or as an additional code assignment depending on the case. They are for use in very limited circumstances on a maternal record when an encounter is for a suspected maternal or fetal condition that is ruled out during that encounter (for example, a maternal or fetal condition may be suspected due to an abnormal test result). These codes should not be used when the condition is confirmed. In those cases, the confirmed condition should be coded. In addition, these codes are not for use if an illness or any signs or symptoms related to the suspected condition or problem are present. In such cases the diagnosis/symptom code is used.

Additional codes may be used in addition to the code from subcategory Z03.7, but only if they are unrelated to the suspected condition being evaluated.

Codes from subcategory Z03.7, may not be used for encounters for antenatal screening of mother. *See Section I.C.21. Screening.*

For encounters for suspected fetal condition that are inconclusive following testing and evaluation, assign the appropriate code from category O35, O36, O40 or O41.

The observation Z code categories:

Z03 Encounter for medical observation for suspected diseases and conditions ruled out

Z04 Encounter for examination and observation for other reasons Except: Z04.9, Encounter for examination and observation for unspecified reason

Z05 Encounter for observation and evaluation of newborn for suspected diseases and conditions ruled out

7) Aftercare

Aftercare visit codes cover situations when the initial treatment of a disease has been performed and the patient requires continued care during the healing or recovery phase, or for the long-term consequences of the disease. The aftercare Z code should not be used if treatment is directed at a current, acute disease. The diagnosis code is to be used in these cases.

Exceptions to this rule are codes Z51.0, Encounter for antineoplastic radiation therapy, and codes from subcategory Z51.1, Encounter for antineoplastic chemotherapy and immunotherapy. These codes are to be first-listed, followed by the diagnosis code when a patient's encounter is solely to receive radiation therapy, chemotherapy, or immunotherapy for the treatment of a neoplasm. If the reason for the encounter is more than one type of antineoplastic therapy, code Z51.0 and a code from subcategory Z51.1 may be assigned together, in which case one of these codes would be reported as a secondary diagnosis.

The aftercare Z codes should also not be used for aftercare for injuries. For aftercare of an injury, assign the acute injury code with the appropriate 7th character (for subsequent encounter).

The aftercare codes are generally first-listed to explain the specific reason for the encounter. An aftercare code may be used as an additional code when some type of aftercare is provided in addition to the reason for admission and no diagnosis code is applicable. An example of this would be the closure of a colostomy during an encounter for treatment of another condition.

Aftercare codes should be used in conjunction with other aftercare codes or diagnosis codes to provide better detail on the specifics of an aftercare encounter visit, unless otherwise directed by the classification. The sequencing of multiple aftercare codes depends on the circumstances of the encounter.

Certain aftercare Z code categories need a secondary diagnosis code to describe the resolving condition or sequelae. For others, the condition is included in the code title.

Additional Z code aftercare category terms include fitting and adjustment, and attention to artificial openings.

Status Z codes may be used with aftercare Z codes to indicate the nature of the aftercare. For example code Z95.1, Presence of aortocoronary bypass graft, may be used with code Z48.812, Encounter for surgical aftercare following surgery on the circulatory system, to indicate the surgery for which the aftercare is being performed. A status code should not be used when the aftercare code indicates the type of status, such as using Z43.0, Encounter for attention to tracheostomy, with Z93.0, Tracheostomy status.

The aftercare Z category/codes:

Z42 Encounter for plastic and reconstructive surgery following medical procedure or healed injury
Z43 Encounter for attention to artificial openings
Z44 Encounter for fitting and adjustment of external prosthetic device
Z45 Encounter for adjustment and management of implanted device
Z46 Encounter for fitting and adjustment of other devices
Z47 Orthopedic aftercare
Z48 Encounter for other postprocedural aftercare
Z49 Encounter for care involving renal dialysis
Z51 Encounter for other aftercare and medical care

8) Follow-up

The follow-up codes are used to explain continuing surveillance following completed treatment of a disease, condition, or injury. They imply that the condition has been fully treated and no longer exists. They should not be confused with aftercare codes, or injury codes with a 7th character for subsequent encounter, that explain ongoing care of a healing condition or its sequelae. Follow-up codes may be used in conjunction with history codes to provide the full picture of the healed condition and its treatment. The follow-up code is sequenced first, followed by the history code.

A follow-up code may be used to explain multiple visits. Should a condition be found to have recurred on the follow-up visit, then the diagnosis code for the condition should be assigned in place of the follow-up code.

The follow-up Z **codes/**categories:

Z08 Encounter for follow-up examination after completed treatment for malignant neoplasm
Z09 Encounter for follow-up examination after completed treatment for conditions other than malignant neoplasm
Codes Z08, Encounter for follow-up examination after completed treatment for malignant neoplasm, and Z09, Encounter for follow up examination after completed treatment for conditions other than malignant neoplasm, may be assigned following any type of completed treatment modality (including both medical and surgical treatments).
Z39 Encounter for maternal postpartum care and examination

9) Donor

Codes in category Z52, Donors of organs and tissues, are used for living individuals who are donating blood or other body tissue. These codes are for individuals donating for others, as well as for self-donations. They are not used to identify cadaveric donations.

10) Counseling

Counseling Z codes are used when a patient or family member receives assistance in the aftermath of an illness or injury, or when support is required in coping with family or social problems.

The counseling Z codes/categories:

Z30.0- Encounter for general counseling and advice on contraception
Z31.5 Encounter for procreative genetic counseling
Z31.6- Encounter for general counseling and advice on procreation
Z32.2 Encounter for childbirth instruction
Z32.3 Encounter for childcare instruction
Z69 Encounter for mental health services for victim and perpetrator of abuse
Z70 Counseling related to sexual attitude, behavior and orientation
Z71 Persons encountering health services for other counseling and medical advice, not elsewhere classified
Note: Code Z71.84, Encounter for health counseling related to travel, is to be used for health risk and safety counseling for future travel purposes. Code Z71.85, Encounter for immunization safety counseling, is to be used for counseling of the patient or caregiver regarding the safety of a vaccine. This code should not be used for the provision of general information regarding risks and potential side effects during routine encounters for the administration of vaccines.
Code Z71.87, Encounter for pediatric-to-adult transition counseling, should be assigned when pediatric-to-adult transition counseling is the sole reason for the encounter or when this counseling is provided in addition to other services, such as treatment of a chronic condition. If both transition counseling and treatment of a medical condition are provided during the same encounter, the code(s) for the medical condition(s) treated and code Z71.87 should be assigned, with sequencing depending on the circumstances of the encounter.
Z76.81 Expectant mother prebirth pediatrician visit

11) Encounters for Obstetrical and Reproductive Services

See Section I.C.15. Pregnancy, Childbirth, and the Puerperium, for further instruction on the use of these codes.

Z codes for pregnancy are for use in those circumstances when none of the problems or complications included in the codes from the Obstetrics chapter exist (a routine prenatal visit or postpartum care). Codes in category Z34, Encounter for supervision of normal pregnancy, are always first listed and are not to be used with any other code from the OB chapter.

Codes in category Z3A, Weeks of gestation, may be assigned to provide additional information about the pregnancy. Category Z3A codes should not be assigned for pregnancies with abortive outcomes (categories O00-O08), elective termination of pregnancy (code Z33.2), nor for postpartum conditions, as category Z3A is not applicable to these conditions. The date of the admission should be used to determine weeks of gestation for inpatient admissions that encompass more than one gestational week.

The outcome of delivery, category Z37, should be included on all maternal delivery records. It is always a secondary code. Codes in category Z37 should not be used on the newborn record.

Z codes for family planning (contraceptive) or procreative management and counseling should be included on an obstetric record either during the pregnancy or the postpartum stage, if applicable.

Z codes/categories for obstetrical and reproductive services:

Z30	Encounter for contraceptive management
Z31	Encounter for procreative management
Z32.2	Encounter for childbirth instruction
Z32.3	Encounter for childcare instruction
Z33	Pregnant state
Z34	Encounter for supervision of normal pregnancy
Z36	Encounter for antenatal screening of mother
Z3A	Weeks of gestation
Z37	Outcome of delivery
Z39	Encounter for maternal postpartum care and examination
Z76.81	Expectant mother prebirth pediatrician visit

12) Newborns and Infants
See Section I.C.16. Newborn (Perinatal) Guidelines, for further instruction on the use of these codes.

Newborn Z codes/categories:

Z76.1	Encounter for health supervision and care of foundling
Z00.1-	Encounter for routine child health examination
Z38	Liveborn infants according to place of birth and type of delivery

13) Routine and Administrative Examinations
The Z codes allow for the description of encounters for routine examinations, such as, a general check-up, or, examinations for administrative purposes, such as, a pre-employment physical. The codes are not to be used if the examination is for diagnosis of a suspected condition or for treatment purposes. In such cases the diagnosis code is used. During a routine exam, should a diagnosis or condition be discovered, it should be coded as an additional code. Pre-existing and chronic conditions and history codes may also be included as additional codes as long as the examination is for administrative purposes and not focused on any particular condition.

Some of the codes for routine health examinations distinguish between "with" and "without" abnormal findings. Code assignment depends on the information that is known at the time the encounter is being coded. For example, if no abnormal findings were found during the examination, but the encounter is being coded before test results are back, it is acceptable to assign the code for "without abnormal findings." When assigning a code for "with abnormal findings," additional code(s) should be assigned to identify the specific abnormal finding(s).

Pre-operative examination and pre-procedural laboratory examination Z codes are for use only in those situations when a patient is being cleared for a procedure or surgery and no treatment is given.

The Z codes/categories for routine and administrative examinations:

Z00	Encounter for general examination without complaint, suspected or reported diagnosis
Z01	Encounter for other special examination without complaint, suspected or reported diagnosis
Z02	Encounter for administrative examination Except: Z02.9, Encounter for administrative examinations, unspecified
Z32.0-	Encounter for pregnancy test

14) Miscellaneous Z Codes
The miscellaneous Z codes capture a number of other health care encounters that do not fall into one of the other categories. Some of these codes identify the reason for the encounter; others are for use as additional codes that provide useful information on circumstances that may affect a patient's care and treatment.

Prophylactic Organ Removal
For encounters specifically for prophylactic removal of an organ (such as prophylactic removal of breasts due to a genetic susceptibility to cancer or a family history of cancer), the principal or first-listed code should be a code from category Z40, Encounter for prophylactic surgery, followed by the appropriate codes to identify the associated risk factor (such as genetic susceptibility or family history).

If the patient has a malignancy of one site and is having prophylactic removal at another site to prevent either a new primary malignancy or metastatic disease, a code for the malignancy should also be assigned in addition to a code from subcategory Z40.0, Encounter for prophylactic surgery for risk factors related to malignant neoplasms. A Z40.0 code should not be assigned if the patient is having organ removal for treatment of a malignancy, such as the removal of the testes for the treatment of prostate cancer.

Miscellaneous Z codes/categories:

Z28   Immunization not carried out
      Except: Z28.3, Underimmunization status

Z29   Encounter for other prophylactic measures

Z40   Encounter for prophylactic surgery

Z41   Encounter for procedures for purposes other than remedying health state
      Except: Z41.9, Encounter for procedure for purposes other than remedying health state, unspecified

Z72   Problems related to lifestyle
      Note: These codes should be assigned only when the documentation specifies that the patient has an associated problem

Z73   Problems related to life management difficulty
      Note: These codes should be assigned only when the documentation specifies that the patient has an associated problem.

Z74   Problems related to care provider dependency Except: Z74.01, Bed confinement status

Z75   Problems related to medical facilities and other health care

Z76.0 Encounter for issue of repeat prescription

Z76.3 Healthy person accompanying sick person

Z76.4 Other boarder to healthcare facility

Z76.5 Malingerer [conscious simulation]

Z91.1- Patient's noncompliance with medical treatment and regimen

Z91.A- Caregiver's noncompliance with patient's medical treatment and regimen

Z91.83 Wandering in diseases classified elsewhere

Z91.84- Oral health risk factors

Z91.89 Other specified personal risk factors, not elsewhere classified

See Section I.B.14 for Z55-Z65 Persons with potential health hazards related to socioeconomic and psychosocial circumstances, documentation by clinicians other than the patient's provider

15) Nonspecific Z Codes

Certain Z codes are so non-specific, or potentially redundant with other codes in the classification, that there can be little justification for their use in the inpatient setting. Their use in the outpatient setting should be limited to those instances when there is no further documentation to permit more precise coding. Otherwise, any sign or symptom or any other reason for visit that is captured in another code should be used.

Nonspecific Z codes/categories:

Z02.9 Encounter for administrative examinations, unspecified

Z04.9 Encounter for examination and observation for unspecified reason

Z13.9 Encounter for screening, unspecified

Z41.9 Encounter for procedure for purposes other than remedying health state, unspecified

Z52.9 Donor of unspecified organ or tissue

Z86.59 Personal history of other mental and behavioral disorders

Z88.9 Allergy status to unspecified drugs, medicaments and biological substances status

Z92.0 Personal history of contraception

16) Z Codes That May Only be Principal/First-Listed Diagnosis

The following Z codes/categories may only be reported as the principal/first-listed diagnosis, except when there are multiple encounters on the same day and the medical records for the encounters are combined:

Z00   Encounter for general examination without complaint, suspected or reported diagnosis
      Except: Z00.6

Z01   Encounter for other special examination without complaint, suspected or reported diagnosis

Z02   Encounter for administrative examination

Z04   Encounter for examination and observation for other reasons

Z33.2 Encounter for elective termination of pregnancy

Z31.81 Encounter for male factor infertility in female patient

Z31.83 Encounter for assisted reproductive fertility procedure cycle

Z31.84 Encounter for fertility preservation procedure

Z34   Encounter for supervision of normal pregnancy

Z39   Encounter for maternal postpartum care and examination

Z38   Liveborn infants according to place of birth and type of delivery

Z40   Encounter for prophylactic surgery

Z42   Encounter for plastic and reconstructive surgery following medical procedure or healed injury

Z51.0 Encounter for antineoplastic radiation therapy

Z51.1- Encounter for antineoplastic chemotherapy and immunotherapy

Z52   Donors of organs and tissues Except: Z52.9, Donor of unspecified organ or tissue

Z76.1 Encounter for health supervision and care of foundling

Z76.2 Encounter for health supervision and care of other healthy infant and child

Z99.12 Encounter for respirator [ventilator] dependence during power failure

17) Social Determinants of Health

Social determinants of health (SDOH) codes describing social problems, conditions, or risk factors that influence a patient's health should be assigned when this information is documented in the patient's medical record. Assign as many SDOH codes as are necessary to describe all of the social problems, conditions, or risk factors documented during the current episode of care. For example, a patient who lives alone may suffer an acute injury temporarily impacting their ability to perform routine activities of daily living. When documented as such, this would support assignment of code Z60.2, Problems related to living alone. However, merely living alone, without documentation of a risk or unmet need for assistance at home, would not support assignment of code Z60.2. Documentation by a clinician (or patient-reported information that is signed off by a clinician) that the patient expressed concerns with access and availability of food would support assignment of code Z59.41, Food insecurity. Similarly, medical record documentation indicating the patient is homeless would support assignment of a code from subcategory Z59.0-, Homelessness.

For social determinants of health **classified to chapter 21**, such as information found in categories Z55-Z65, Persons with potential health hazards related to socioeconomic and psychosocial circumstances, code assignment may be based on medical record documentation from clinicians involved in the care of the patient who are not the patient's provider since this information represents social information, rather than medical diagnoses.

For example, coding professionals may utilize documentation of social information from social workers, community health workers, case managers, or nurses, if their documentation is included in the official medical record.

Patient self-reported documentation may be used to assign codes for social determinants of health, as long as the patient self-reported information is signed-off by and incorporated into the medical record by either a clinician or provider.

Social determinants of health codes are located primarily in these Z code categories:

Z55	Problems related to education and literacy
Z56	Problems related to employment and unemployment
Z57	Occupational exposure to risk factors
Z58	Problems related to physical environment
Z59	Problems related to housing and economic circumstances
Z60	Problems related to social environment
Z62	Problems related to upbringing
Z63	Other problems related to primary support group, including family circumstances
Z64	Problems related to certain psychosocial circumstances
Z65	Problems related to other psychosocial circumstances

See Section I.B.14. Documentation by Clinicians Other than the Patient's Provider.

22. **Chapter 22: Codes for Special Purposes (U00-U85)**

U07.0	Vaping-related disorder (see Section I.C.10.e., Vaping-related disorders)
U07.1	COVID-19 (see Section I.C.1.g.1., COVID-19 infection)
U09.9	Post COVID-19 condition, unspecified (see Section I.C.1.g.1.m)

Section II. Selection of Principal Diagnosis

The circumstances of inpatient admission always govern the selection of principal diagnosis. The principal diagnosis is defined in the Uniform Hospital Discharge Data Set (UHDDS) as "that condition established after study to be chiefly responsible for occasioning the admission of the patient to the hospital for care."

The UHDDS definitions are used by hospitals to report inpatient data elements in a standardized manner. These data elements and their definitions can be found in the July 31, 1985, Federal Register (Vol. 50, No, 147), pp. 31038-40.

Since that time, the application of the UHDDS definitions has been expanded to include all nonoutpatient settings (acute care, short term, long-term care and psychiatric hospitals; home health agencies; rehab facilities; nursing homes, etc. . . .). The UHDDS definitions also apply to hospice services (all levels of care).

In determining principal diagnosis, coding conventions in the ICD-10-CM, the Tabular List and Alphabetic Index take precedence over these official coding guidelines.

(See Section I.A., Conventions for the ICD-10-CM)

The importance of consistent, complete documentation in the medical record cannot be overemphasized. Without such documentation the application of all coding guidelines is a difficult, if not impossible, task.

A. **Codes for symptoms, signs, and ill-defined conditions**

Codes for symptoms, signs, and ill-defined conditions from Chapter 18 are not to be used as principal diagnosis when a related definitive diagnosis has been established.

B. **Two or more interrelated conditions, each potentially meeting the definition for principal diagnosis**

When there are two or more interrelated conditions (such as diseases in the same ICD-10-CM chapter or manifestations characteristically associated with a certain disease) potentially meeting the definition of principal diagnosis, either condition may be sequenced first, unless the circumstances of the admission, the therapy provided, the Tabular List, or the Alphabetic Index indicate otherwise.

C. **Two or more diagnoses that equally meet the definition for principal diagnosis**

In the unusual instance when two or more diagnoses equally meet the criteria for principal diagnosis as determined by the circumstances of admission, diagnostic workup and/or therapy provided, and the Alphabetic Index, Tabular List, or another coding guidelines does not provide sequencing direction, any one of the diagnoses may be sequenced first.

D. Two or more comparative or contrasting conditions.

In those rare instances when two or more contrasting or comparative diagnoses are documented as "either/or" (or similar terminology), they are coded as if the diagnoses were confirmed and the diagnoses are sequenced according to the circumstances of the admission. If no further determination can be made as to which diagnosis should be principal, either diagnosis may be sequenced first

E. A symptom(s) followed by contrasting/ comparative diagnoses

GUIDELINE HAS BEEN DELETED EFFECTIVE OCTOBER 1, 2014

F. Original treatment plan not carried out

Sequence as the principal diagnosis the condition, which after study occasioned the admission to the hospital, even though treatment may not have been carried out due to unforeseen circumstances.

G. Complications of surgery and other medical care

When the admission is for treatment of a complication resulting from surgery or other medical care, the complication code is sequenced as the principal diagnosis. If the complication is classified to the T80-T88 series and the code lacks the necessary specificity in describing the complication, an additional code for the specific complication should be assigned.

H. Uncertain Diagnosis

If the diagnosis documented at the time of discharge is qualified as "probable," "suspected," "likely," "questionable," "possible," or "still to be ruled out," "compatible with," "consistent with," or other similar terms indicating uncertainty, code the condition as if it existed or was established. The bases for these guidelines are the diagnostic workup, arrangements for further workup or observation, and initial therapeutic approach that correspond most closely with the established diagnosis.

Note: This guideline is applicable only to inpatient admissions to short-term, acute, long-term care and psychiatric hospitals.

I. Admission from Observation Unit

1. Admission Following Medical Observation

When a patient is admitted to an observation unit for a medical condition, which either worsens or does not improve, and is subsequently admitted as an inpatient of the same hospital for this same medical condition, the principal diagnosis would be the medical condition which led to the hospital admission.

2. Admission Following Post-Operative Observation

When a patient is admitted to an observation unit to monitor a condition (or complication) that develops following outpatient surgery, and then is subsequently admitted as an inpatient of the same hospital, hospitals should apply the Uniform Hospital Discharge Data Set (UHDDS) definition of principal diagnosis as "that condition established after study to be chiefly responsible for occasioning the admission of the patient to the hospital for care."

J. Admission from Outpatient Surgery

When a patient receives surgery in the hospital's outpatient surgery department and is subsequently admitted for continuing inpatient care at the same hospital, the following guidelines should be followed in selecting the principal diagnosis for the inpatient admission:

- If the reason for the inpatient admission is a complication, assign the complication as the principal diagnosis.
- If no complication, or other condition, is documented as the reason for the inpatient admission, assign the reason for the outpatient surgery as the principal diagnosis.
- If the reason for the inpatient admission is another condition unrelated to the surgery, assign the unrelated condition as the principal diagnosis.

K. Admissions/Encounters for Rehabilitation

When the purpose for the admission/encounter is rehabilitation, sequence first the code for the condition for which the service is being performed. For example, for an admission/encounter for rehabilitation for right-sided dominant hemiplegia following a cerebrovascular infarction, report code I69.351, Hemiplegia and hemiparesis following cerebral infarction affecting right dominant side, as the first-listed or principal diagnosis.

If the condition for which the rehabilitation service is being provided is no longer present, report the appropriate aftercare code as the first-listed or principal diagnosis, unless the rehabilitation service is being provided following an injury. For rehabilitation services following active treatment of an injury, assign the injury code with the appropriate seventh character for subsequent encounter as the first-listed or principal diagnosis. For example, if a patient with severe degenerative osteoarthritis of the hip, underwent hip replacement and the current encounter/ admission is for rehabilitation, report code Z47.1, Aftercare following joint replacement surgery, as the first-listed or principal diagnosis. If the patient requires rehabilitation post hip replacement for right intertrochanteric femur fracture, report code S72.141D, Displaced intertrochanteric fracture of right femur, subsequent encounter for closed fracture with routine healing, as the first-listed or principal diagnosis.

See Section I.C.21.c.7., Factors influencing health states and contact with health services, Aftercare.

See Section I.C.19.a., for additional information about the use of 7th characters for injury codes.

Section III. Reporting Additional Diagnoses

GENERAL RULES FOR OTHER (ADDITIONAL) DIAGNOSES

For reporting purposes the definition for "other diagnoses" is interpreted as additional **clinically significant** conditions that affect patient care in terms of requiring:

    clinical evaluation; or

    therapeutic treatment; or

    diagnostic procedures; or

    extended length of hospital stay; or

    increased nursing care and/or monitoring.

The UHDDS item #11-b defines Other Diagnoses as "all conditions that coexist at the time of admission, that develop subsequently, or that affect the treatment received and/or the length of stay. Diagnoses that relate to an earlier episode which have no bearing on the current hospital stay are to be excluded." UHDDS definitions apply to inpatients in acute care, short-term, long term care and psychiatric hospital setting. The UHDDS definitions are used by acute care short-term hospitals to report inpatient data elements in a standardized manner. These data elements and their definitions can be found in the July 31, 1985, Federal Register (Vol. 50, No, 147), pp. 31038-40.

Since that time, the application of the UHDDS definitions has been expanded to include all non-outpatient settings (acute care, short term, long term care and psychiatric hospitals; home health agencies; rehab facilities; nursing homes, etc. . .). The UHDDS definitions also apply to hospice services (all levels of care).

The following guidelines are to be applied in designating "other diagnoses" when neither the Alphabetic Index nor the Tabular List in ICD-10-CM provide direction. The listing of the diagnoses in the patient record is the responsibility of the provider.

A. Previous conditions

If the provider has included a diagnosis in the final diagnostic statement, such as the discharge summary or the face sheet, it should ordinarily be coded. Some providers include in the diagnostic statement resolved conditions or diagnoses and status-post procedures from previous admissions that have no bearing on the current stay. Such conditions are not to be reported and are coded only if required by hospital policy.

However, history codes (categories Z80-Z87) may be used as secondary codes if the historical condition or family history has an impact on current care or influences treatment.

B. Abnormal findings

Abnormal findings (laboratory, x-ray, pathologic, and other diagnostic results) are not coded and reported unless the provider indicates their clinical significance. If the findings are outside the normal range and the provider has ordered other tests to evaluate the condition or prescribed treatment, it is appropriate to ask the provider whether the abnormal finding should be added.

Please note: This differs from the coding practices in the outpatient setting for coding encounters for diagnostic tests that have been interpreted by a provider.

C. Uncertain Diagnosis

If the diagnosis documented at the time of discharge is qualified as "probable," "suspected," "likely," "questionable," "possible," or "still to be ruled out," "compatible with," "consistent with," or other similar terms indicating uncertainty, code the condition as if it existed or was established. The bases for these guidelines are the diagnostic workup, arrangements for further workup or observation, and initial therapeutic approach that correspond most closely with the established diagnosis.

Note: This guideline is applicable only to inpatient admissions to short-term, acute, long-term care and psychiatric hospitals.

Section IV. Diagnostic Coding and Reporting Guidelines for Outpatient Services

These coding guidelines for outpatient diagnoses have been approved for use by hospitals/ providers in coding and reporting hospital-based outpatient services and provider-based office visits. Guidelines in Section I, Conventions, general coding guidelines and chapter-specific guidelines, should also be applied for outpatient services and office visits.

Information about the use of certain abbreviations, punctuation, symbols, and other conventions used in the ICD-10-CM Tabular List (code numbers and titles), can be found in Section IA of these guidelines, under "Conventions Used in the Tabular List." Section I.B. contains general guidelines that apply to the entire classification. Section I.C. contains chapter-specific guidelines that correspond to the chapters as they are arranged in the classification. Information about the correct sequence to use in finding a code is also described in Section I.

The terms encounter and visit are often used interchangeably in describing outpatient service contacts and, therefore, appear together in these guidelines without distinguishing one from the other.

Though the conventions and general guidelines apply to all settings, coding guidelines for outpatient and provider reporting of diagnoses will vary in a number of instances from those for inpatient diagnoses, recognizing that:

The Uniform Hospital Discharge Data Set (UHDDS) definition of principal diagnosis does not apply to hospital-based outpatient services and provider-based office visits.

Coding guidelines for inconclusive diagnoses (probable, suspected, rule out, etc.) were developed for inpatient reporting and do not apply to outpatients.

A. Selection of first-listed condition

In the outpatient setting, the term first-listed diagnosis is used in lieu of principal diagnosis.

In determining the first-listed diagnosis the coding conventions of ICD-10-CM, as well as the general and disease specific guidelines take precedence over the outpatient guidelines.

Diagnoses often are not established at the time of the initial encounter/visit. It may take two or more visits before the diagnosis is confirmed.

The most critical rule involves beginning the search for the correct code assignment through the Alphabetic Index. Never begin searching initially in the Tabular List as this will lead to coding errors.

1. Outpatient Surgery
When a patient presents for outpatient surgery (same day surgery), code the reason for the surgery as the first-listed diagnosis (reason for the encounter), even if the surgery is not performed due to a contraindication.

2. Observation Stay
When a patient is admitted for observation for a medical condition, assign a code for the medical condition as the first-listed diagnosis.

When a patient presents for outpatient surgery and develops complications requiring admission to observation, code the reason for the surgery as the first reported diagnosis (reason for the encounter), followed by codes for the complications as secondary diagnoses.

B. Codes from A00.0 through T88.9, Z00-Z99, U00-U85
The appropriate code(s) from A00.0 through T88.9, Z00-Z99, and U00-U85 must be used to identify diagnoses, symptoms, conditions, problems, complaints, or other reason(s) for the encounter/visit.

C. Accurate reporting of ICD-10-CM diagnosis codes
For accurate reporting of ICD-10-CM diagnosis codes, the documentation should describe the patient's condition, using terminology which includes specific diagnoses as well as symptoms, problems, or reasons for the encounter. There are ICD-10-CM codes to describe all of these.

D. Codes that describe symptoms and signs
Codes that describe symptoms and signs, as opposed to diagnoses, are acceptable for reporting purposes when a diagnosis has not been established (confirmed) by the provider. Chapter 18 of ICD-10-CM, Symptoms, Signs, and Abnormal Clinical and Laboratory Findings Not Elsewhere Classified (codes R00-R99) contains many, but not all codes for symptoms.

E. Encounters for circumstances other than a disease or injury
ICD-10-CM provides codes to deal with encounters for circumstances other than a disease or injury. The Factors Influencing Health Status and Contact with Health Services codes (Z00-Z99) are provided to deal with occasions when circumstances other than a disease or injury are recorded as diagnosis or problems.
See Section I.C.21., Factors influencing health status and contact with health services.

F. Level of Detail in Coding
1. ICD-10-CM codes with 3, 4, 5, 6 or 7 characters
ICD-10-CM is composed of codes with 3, 4, 5, 6 or 7 characters. Codes with three characters are included in ICD-10-CM as the heading of a category of codes that may be further subdivided by the use of fourth, fifth, sixth or seventh characters to provide greater specificity.

2. Use of full number of characters required for a code
A 3-character code is to be used only if it is not further subdivided. A code is invalid if it has not been coded to the full number of characters required for that code, including the 7th character, if applicable.

3. Highest level of specificity
Code to the highest level of specificity when supported by the medical record documentation.

G. ICD-10-CM code for the diagnosis, condition, problem, or other reason for encounter/visit
List first the ICD-10-CM code for the diagnosis, condition, problem, or other reason for encounter/visit shown in the medical record to be chiefly responsible for the services provided. List additional codes that describe any coexisting conditions. In some cases the first-listed diagnosis may be a symptom when a diagnosis has not been established (confirmed) by the provider.

H. Uncertain diagnosis
Do not code diagnoses documented as "probable," "suspected," "questionable," "rule out," "compatible with," "consistent with," or "working diagnosis" or other similar terms indicating uncertainty. Rather, code the condition(s) to the highest degree of certainty for that encounter/visit, such as symptoms, signs, abnormal test results, or other reason for the visit.

Please note: This differs from the coding practices used by short-term, acute care, long-term care and psychiatric hospitals.

I. Chronic diseases
Chronic diseases treated on an ongoing basis may be coded and reported as many times as the patient receives treatment and care for the condition(s)

J. Code all documented conditions that coexist
Code all documented conditions that coexist at the time of the encounter/visit, and that require or affect patient care treatment or management. Do not code conditions that were previously treated and no longer exist. However, history codes (categories Z80-Z87) may be used as secondary codes if the historical condition or family history has an impact on current care or influences treatment.

K. Patients receiving diagnostic services only
For patients receiving diagnostic services only during an encounter/visit, sequence first the diagnosis, condition, problem, or other reason for encounter/visit shown in the medical record to be chiefly responsible for the outpatient services provided during the encounter/visit. Codes for other diagnoses (e.g., chronic conditions) may be sequenced as additional diagnoses.

For encounters for routine laboratory/radiology testing in the absence of any signs, symptoms, or associated diagnosis, assign Z01.89, Encounter for other specified special examinations. If routine testing is performed during the same encounter as a test to evaluate a sign, symptom, or diagnosis, it is appropriate to assign both the Z code and the code describing the reason for the non-routine test.

For outpatient encounters for diagnostic tests that have been interpreted by a physician, and the final report is available at the time of coding, code any confirmed or definitive diagnosis(es) documented in the interpretation. Do not code related signs and symptoms as additional diagnoses.

Please note: This differs from the coding practice in the hospital inpatient setting regarding abnormal findings on test results.

L. Patients receiving therapeutic services only

For patients receiving therapeutic services only during an encounter/visit, sequence first the diagnosis, condition, problem, or other reason for encounter/visit shown in the medical record to be chiefly responsible for the outpatient services provided during the encounter/visit. Codes for other diagnoses (e.g., chronic conditions) may be sequenced as additional diagnoses.

The only exception to this rule is that when the primary reason for the admission/encounter is chemotherapy or radiation therapy, the appropriate Z code for the service is listed first, and the diagnosis or problem for which the service is being performed listed second.

M. Patients receiving preoperative evaluations only

For patients receiving preoperative evaluations only, sequence first a code from subcategory Z01.81, Encounter for pre-procedural examinations, to describe the pre-op consultations. Assign a code for the condition to describe the reason for the surgery as an additional diagnosis. Code also any findings related to the pre-op evaluation.

N. Ambulatory surgery

For ambulatory surgery, code the diagnosis for which the surgery was performed. If the postoperative diagnosis is known to be different from the preoperative diagnosis at the time the diagnosis is confirmed, select the postoperative diagnosis for coding, since it is the most definitive.

O. Routine outpatient prenatal visits

See Section I.C.15., Routine outpatient prenatal visits.

P. Encounters for general medical examinations with abnormal findings

The subcategories for encounters for general medical examinations, Z00.0- and encounter for routine child health examination, Z00.12-, provide codes for with and without abnormal findings. Should a general medical examination result in an abnormal finding, the code for general medical examination with abnormal finding should be assigned as the first-listed diagnosis. An examination with abnormal findings refers to a condition/diagnosis that is newly identified or a change in severity of a chronic condition (such as uncontrolled hypertension, or an acute exacerbation of chronic obstructive pulmonary disease) during a routine physical examination. A secondary code for the abnormal finding should also be coded.

Q. Encounters for routine health screenings

See Section I.C.21., Factors influencing health status and contact with health services, Screening

Appendix I
Present on Admission Reporting Guidelines

Introduction

These guidelines are to be used as a supplement to the ICD-10-CM Official Guidelines for Coding and Reporting to facilitate the assignment of the Present on Admission (POA) indicator for each diagnosis and external cause of injury code reported on claim forms (UB-Ø4 and 837 Institutional).

These guidelines are not intended to replace any guidelines in the main body of the ICD-10-CM Official Guidelines for Coding and Reporting. The POA guidelines are not intended to provide guidance on when a condition should be coded, but rather, how to apply the POA indicator to the final set of diagnosis codes that have been assigned in accordance with Sections I, II, and III of the official coding guidelines. Subsequent to the assignment of the ICD-10-CM codes, the POA indicator should then be assigned to those conditions that have been coded.

As stated in the Introduction to the ICD-10-CM Official Guidelines for Coding and Reporting, a joint effort between the healthcare provider and the coder is essential to achieve complete and accurate documentation, code assignment, and reporting of diagnoses and procedures. The importance of consistent, complete documentation in the medical record cannot be overemphasized. Medical record documentation from any provider involved in the care and treatment of the patient may be used to support the determination of whether a condition was present on admission or not. In the context of the official coding guidelines, the term "provider" means a physician or any qualified healthcare practitioner who is legally accountable for establishing the patient's diagnosis.

These guidelines are not a substitute for the provider's clinical judgment as to the determination of whether a condition was/was not present on admission. The provider should be queried regarding issues related to the linking of signs/symptoms, timing of test results, and the timing of findings.

Please see the CDC website for the detailed list of ICD-10-CM codes that do not require the use of a POA indicator (https://www.cdc.gov/nchs/icd/icd-1Ø-cm/files.html). The codes and categories on this exempt list are for circumstances regarding the healthcare encounter or factors influencing health status that do not represent a current disease or injury or that describe conditions that are always present on admission.

General Reporting Requirements

All claims involving inpatient admissions to general acute care hospitals or other facilities that are subject to a law or regulation mandating collection of present on admission information.

Present on admission is defined as present at the time the order for inpatient admission occurs—conditions that develop during an outpatient encounter, including emergency department, observation, or outpatient surgery, are considered as present on admission.

POA indicator is assigned to principal and secondary diagnoses (as defined in Section II of the Official Guidelines for Coding and Reporting) and the external cause of injury codes.

Issues related to inconsistent, missing, conflicting or unclear documentation must still be resolved by the provider.

If a condition would not be coded and reported based on UHDDS definitions and current official coding guidelines, then the POA indicator would not be reported.

Reporting Options

Y - Yes

N - No

U - Unknown

W - Clinically undetermined

Unreported/Not used - (Exempt from POA reporting)

Reporting Definitions

Y = present at the time of inpatient admission

N = not present at the time of inpatient admission

U = documentation is insufficient to determine if condition is present on admission

W = provider is unable to clinically determine whether condition was present on admission or not

Timeframe for POA Identification and Documentation

There is no required timeframe as to when a provider (per the definition of "provider" used in these guidelines) must identify or document a condition to be present on admission. In some clinical situations, it may not be possible for a provider to make a definitive diagnosis (or a condition may not be recognized or reported by the patient) for a period of time after admission. In some cases it may be several days before the provider arrives at a definitive diagnosis. This does not mean that the condition was not present on admission. Determination of whether the condition was present on admission or not will be based on the applicable POA guideline as identified in this document, or on the provider's best clinical judgment.

If at the time of code assignment the documentation is unclear as to whether a condition was present on admission or not, it is appropriate to query the provider for clarification.

Assigning the POA Indicator

Condition is on the "Exempt from Reporting" list

Leave the "present on admission" field blank if the condition is on the list of ICD-10-CM codes for which this field is not applicable. This is the only circumstance in which the field may be left blank.

POA Explicitly Documented

Assign "Y" for any condition the provider explicitly documents as being present on admission.

Assign "N" for any condition the provider explicitly documents as not present at the time of admission.

Conditions diagnosed prior to inpatient admission

Assign "Y" for conditions that were diagnosed prior to admission (example: hypertension, diabetes mellitus, asthma)

Conditions diagnosed during the admission but clearly present before admission

Assign "Y" for conditions diagnosed during the admission that were clearly present but not diagnosed until after admission occurred.

Diagnoses subsequently confirmed after admission are considered present on admission if at the time of admission they are documented as suspected, possible, rule out, differential diagnosis, or constitute an underlying cause of a symptom that is present at the time of admission.

Condition develops during outpatient encounter prior to inpatient admission

Assign "Y" for any condition that develops during an outpatient encounter prior to a written order for inpatient admission.

Documentation does not indicate whether condition was present on admission

Assign "U" when the medical record documentation is unclear as to whether the condition was present on admission. "U" should not be routinely assigned and used only in very limited circumstances. Coders are encouraged to query the providers when the documentation is unclear.

Documentation states that it cannot be determined whether the condition was or was not present on admission

Assign "W" when the medical record documentation indicates that it cannot be clinically determined whether or not the condition was present on admission.

Chronic condition with acute exacerbation during the admission

If a single code identifies both the chronic condition and the acute exacerbation, see POA guidelines pertaining to codes that contain multiple clinical concepts.

If a single code only identifies the chronic condition and not the acute exacerbation (e.g., acute exacerbation of chronic leukemia), assign "Y."

Conditions documented as possible, probable, suspected, or rule out at the time of discharge

If the final diagnosis contains a possible, probable, suspected, or rule out diagnosis, and this diagnosis was based on signs, symptoms or clinical findings suspected at the time of inpatient admission, assign "Y."

If the final diagnosis contains a possible, probable, suspected, or rule out diagnosis, and this diagnosis was based on signs, symptoms or clinical findings that were not present on admission, assign "N".

Conditions documented as impending or threatened at the time of discharge

If the final diagnosis contains an impending or threatened diagnosis, and this diagnosis is based on symptoms or clinical findings that were present on admission, assign "Y".

If the final diagnosis contains an impending or threatened diagnosis, and this diagnosis is based on symptoms or clinical findings that were not present on admission, assign "N".

Acute and Chronic Conditions

Assign "Y" for acute conditions that are present at time of admission and "N" for acute conditions that are not present at time of admission.

Assign "Y" for chronic conditions, even though the condition may not be diagnosed until after admission.

If a single code identifies both an acute and chronic condition, see the POA guidelines for codes that contain multiple clinical concepts.

Codes That Contain Multiple Clinical Concepts

Assign "N" if at least one of the clinical concepts included in the code was not present on admission (e.g., COPD with acute exacerbation and the exacerbation was not present on admission; gastric ulcer that does not start bleeding until after admission; asthma patient develops status asthmaticus after admission).

Assign "Y" if all of the clinical concepts included in the code were present on admission (e.g., duodenal ulcer that perforates prior to admission).

For infection codes that include the causal organism, assign "Y" if the infection (or signs of the infection) were present on admission, even though the culture results may not be known until after admission (e.g., patient is admitted with pneumonia and the provider documents Pseudomonas as the causal organism a few days later).

Same Diagnosis Code for Two or More Conditions

When the same ICD-10-CM diagnosis code applies to two or more conditions during the same encounter (e.g., two separate conditions classified to the same ICD-10-CM diagnosis code):

Assign "Y" if all conditions represented by the single ICD-10-CM code were present on admission (e.g., bilateral unspecified age-related cataracts).

Assign "N" if any of the conditions represented by the single ICD-10-CM code was not present on admission (e.g., traumatic secondary and recurrent hemorrhage and seroma is assigned to a single code T79.2, but only one of the conditions was present on admission).

Obstetrical conditions

Whether or not the patient delivers during the current hospitalization does not affect assignment of the POA indicator. The determining factor for POA assignment is whether the pregnancy complication or obstetrical condition described by the code was present at the time of admission or not.

If the pregnancy complication or obstetrical condition was present on admission (e.g., patient admitted in preterm labor), assign "Y".

If the pregnancy complication or obstetrical condition was not present on admission (e.g., 2nd degree laceration during delivery, postpartum hemorrhage that occurred during current hospitalization, fetal distress develops after admission), assign "N".

If the obstetrical code includes more than one diagnosis and any of the diagnoses identified by the code were not present on admission assign "N".

(e.g., Category O11, Pre-existing hypertension with pre-eclampsia)

Perinatal conditions

Newborns are not considered to be admitted until after birth. Therefore, any condition present at birth or that developed in utero is considered present at admission and should be assigned "Y". This includes conditions that occur during delivery (e.g., injury during delivery, meconium aspiration, exposure to streptococcus B in the vaginal canal).

Congenital conditions and anomalies

Assign "Y" for congenital conditions and anomalies except for categories Q00-Q99, Congenital anomalies, which are on the exempt list. Congenital conditions are always considered present on admission.

External cause of injury codes

Assign "Y" for any external cause code representing an external cause of morbidity that occurred prior to inpatient admission (e.g., patient fell out of bed at home, patient fell out of bed in emergency room prior to admission).

Assign "N" for any external cause code representing an external cause of morbidity that occurred during inpatient hospitalization (e.g., patient fell out of hospital bed during hospital stay, patient experienced an adverse reaction to a medication administered after inpatient admission).

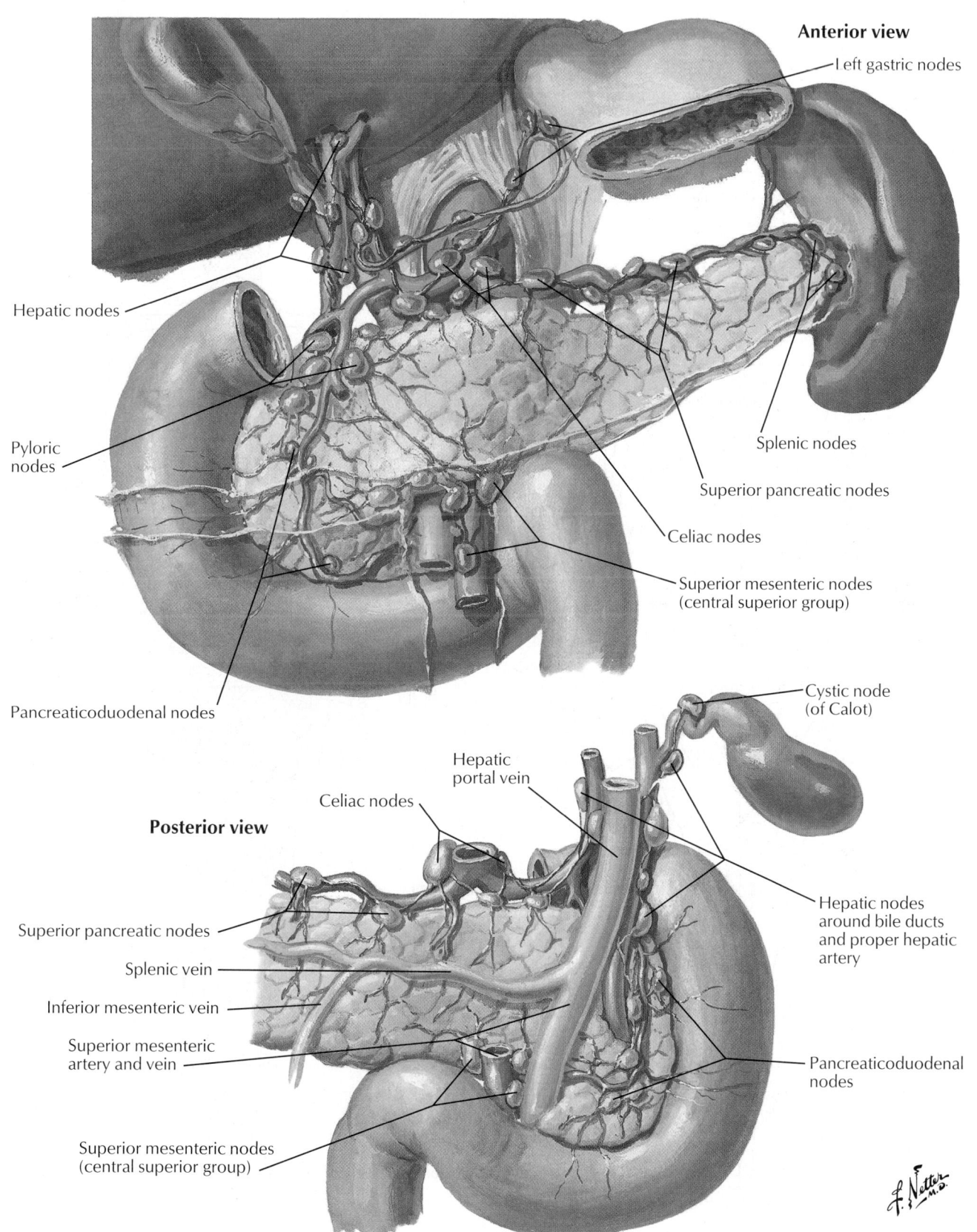

Anterior view

Left gastric nodes

Hepatic nodes

Pyloric nodes

Pancreaticoduodenal nodes

Splenic nodes

Superior pancreatic nodes

Celiac nodes

Superior mesenteric nodes (central superior group)

Posterior view

Cystic node (of Calot)

Hepatic portal vein

Celiac nodes

Hepatic nodes around bile ducts and proper hepatic artery

Superior pancreatic nodes

Splenic vein

Inferior mesenteric vein

Superior mesenteric artery and vein

Pancreaticoduodenal nodes

Superior mesenteric nodes (central superior group)

ANATOMY ILLUSTRATIONS

Levels of principal dermatomes

C5	Clavicles
C5, 6, 7	Lateral parts of upper limbs
C8, T1	Medial sides of upper limbs
C6	Thumb
C6, 7, 8	Hand
C8	Ring and little fingers
T4	Level of nipples
T10	Level of umbilicus
L1	Inguinal or groin regions
L1, 2, 3, 4	Anterior and inner surfaces of lower limbs
L4, 5, S1	Foot
L4	Medial side of great toe
S1, 2, L5	Posterior and other surfaces of lower limbs
S1	Lateral margin of foot and little toe
S2, 3, 4	Perineum

Plate 2 Schematic demarcation of Dermatomes. (Miller MD, Hart JA, MacKnight JM: Essential Orthopaedics, ed 2, Philadelphia, 2020, Elsevier.)

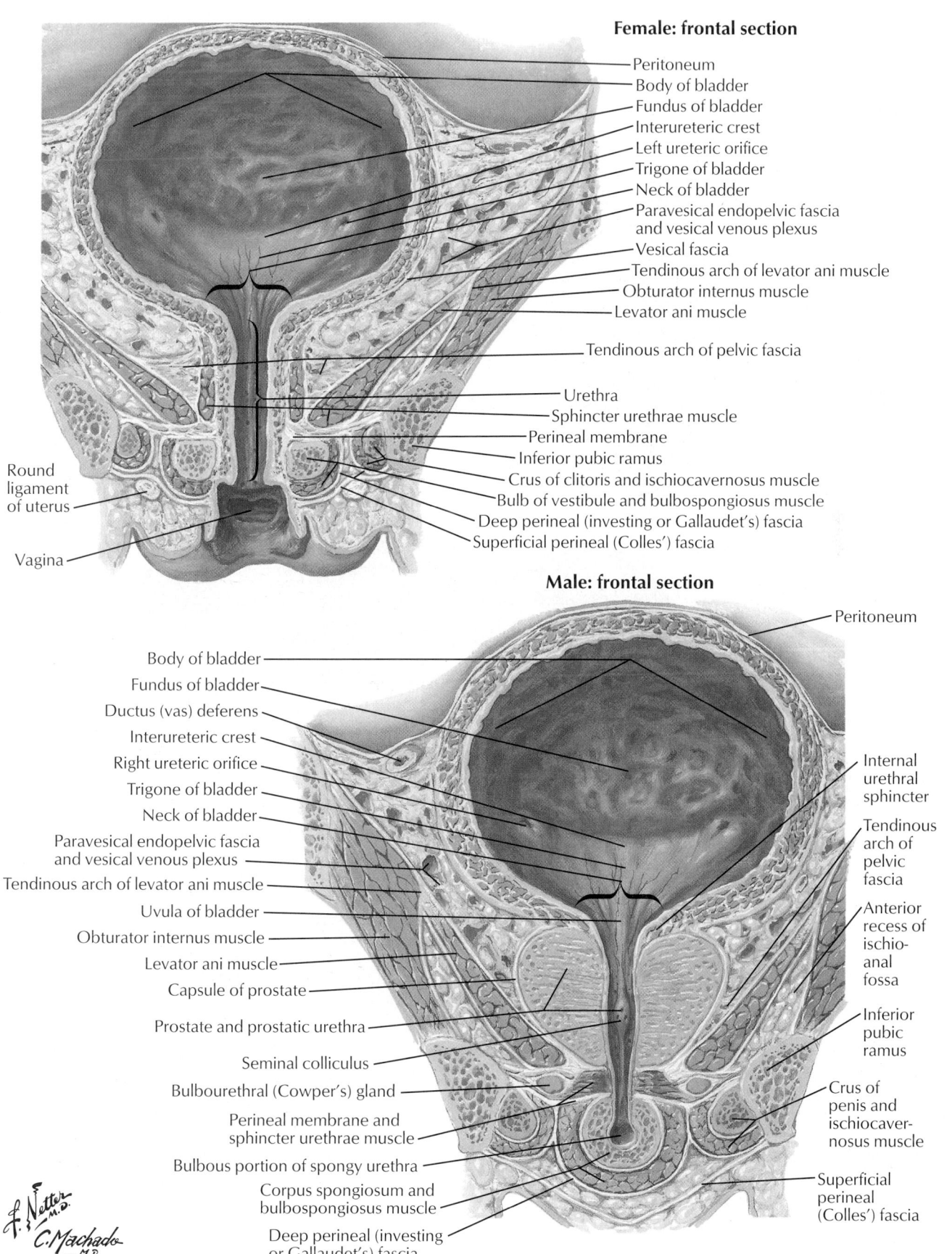

Female: frontal section

- Peritoneum
- Body of bladder
- Fundus of bladder
- Interureteric crest
- Left ureteric orifice
- Trigone of bladder
- Neck of bladder
- Paravesical endopelvic fascia and vesical venous plexus
- Vesical fascia
- Tendinous arch of levator ani muscle
- Obturator internus muscle
- Levator ani muscle
- Tendinous arch of pelvic fascia
- Urethra
- Sphincter urethrae muscle
- Perineal membrane
- Inferior pubic ramus
- Crus of clitoris and ischiocavernosus muscle
- Bulb of vestibule and bulbospongiosus muscle
- Deep perineal (investing or Gallaudet's) fascia
- Superficial perineal (Colles') fascia

- Round ligament of uterus
- Vagina

Male: frontal section

- Peritoneum
- Body of bladder
- Fundus of bladder
- Ductus (vas) deferens
- Interureteric crest
- Right ureteric orifice
- Trigone of bladder
- Neck of bladder
- Paravesical endopelvic fascia and vesical venous plexus
- Tendinous arch of levator ani muscle
- Uvula of bladder
- Obturator internus muscle
- Levator ani muscle
- Capsule of prostate
- Prostate and prostatic urethra
- Seminal colliculus
- Bulbourethral (Cowper's) gland
- Perineal membrane and sphincter urethrae muscle
- Bulbous portion of spongy urethra
- Corpus spongiosum and bulbospongiosus muscle
- Deep perineal (investing or Gallaudet's) fascia

- Internal urethral sphincter
- Tendinous arch of pelvic fascia
- Anterior recess of ischio-anal fossa
- Inferior pubic ramus
- Crus of penis and ischiocavernosus muscle
- Superficial perineal (Colles') fascia

ANATOMY ILLUSTRATIONS

Sites of ectopic implantation

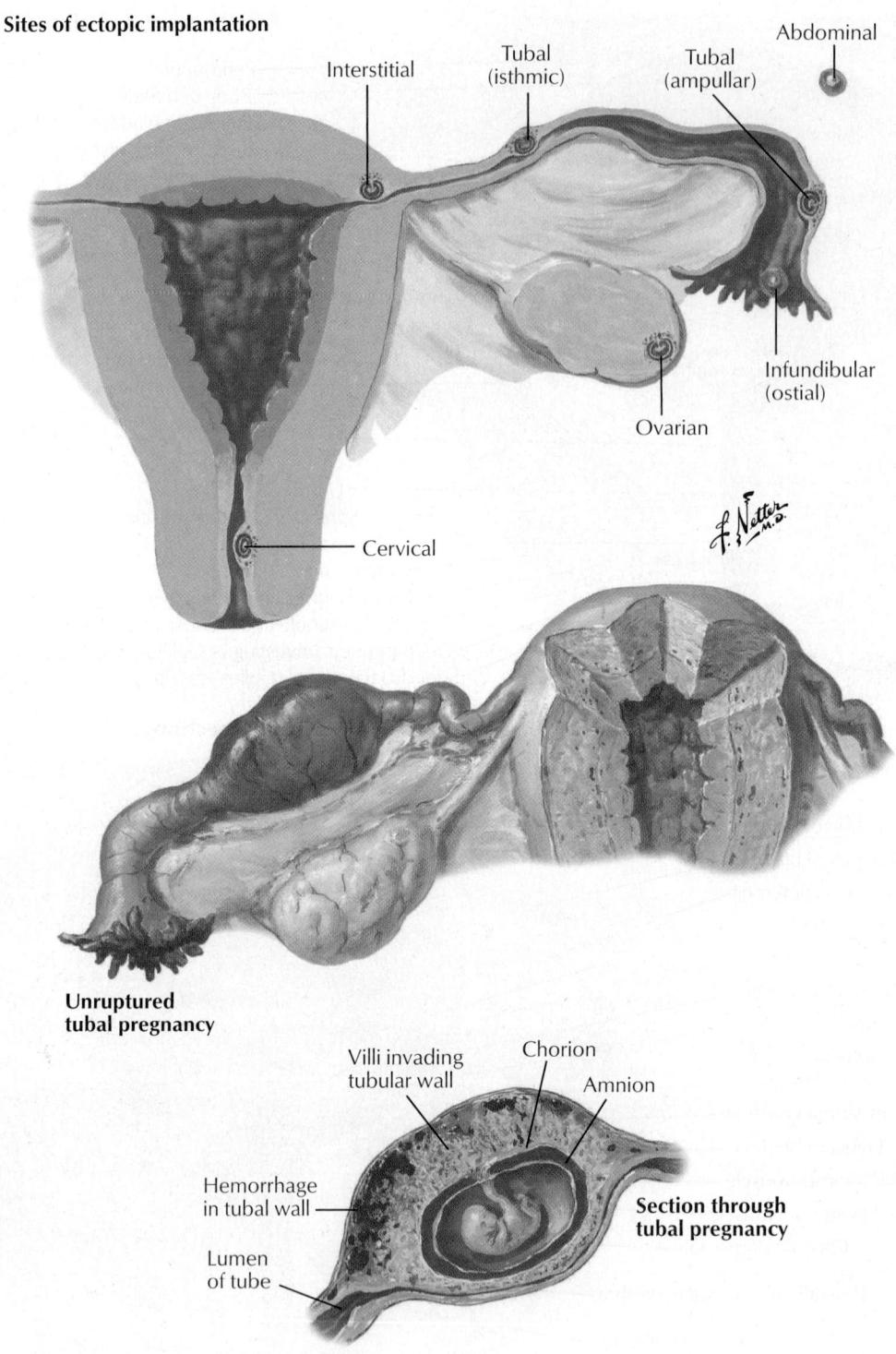

Interstitial

Tubal (isthmic)

Tubal (ampullar)

Abdominal

Infundibular (ostial)

Ovarian

Cervical

Unruptured tubal pregnancy

Villi invading tubular wall

Chorion

Amnion

Hemorrhage in tubal wall

Lumen of tube

Section through tubal pregnancy

Skin of penis

Superficial fascia of penis (Colles' fascia)

Deep (Buck's) fascia of penis

Testicular artery

Ductus deferens

Artery to ductus deferens

Genital branch of genitofemoral nerve

Pampiniform (venous) plexus

Epididymis

Appendix of epididymis

Appendix of testis

Testis (covered by visceral layer of tunica vaginalis)

Parietal layer of tunica vaginalis

Superficial inguinal ring

External spermatic fascia

Cremaster muscle and fascia

Septum of scrotum (formed by dartos fascia)

Superficial (dartos) fascia of scrotum

Skin of scrotum

Superficial (dartos) fascia of scrotum

External spermatic fascia

Cremaster muscle and fascia

Internal spermatic fascia

Parietal layer of tunica vaginalis

Epididymis

Testis (covered by visceral layer of tunica vaginalis)

Skin of scrotum

ANATOMY ILLUSTRATIONS

I Olfactory

III Oculomotor

II Optic

IV Trochlear
VI Abducens

V Trigeminal

VII Facial

VIII Vestibulocochlear

X Vagus

XII Hypoglossal

IX
Glossopharyngeal

XI Accessory

Plate 6 Cranial Nerves (12 pairs) are known by their numbers (Roman numerals) and names. (Herlihy BL: The Human Body in Health and Illness, ed 6, St. Louis, 2018, Elsevier.)

Superior view

Medial branch ⎱ Supraorbital nerve
Lateral branch ⎰

Supratrochlear nerve

Medial rectus muscle

Superior oblique muscle

Infratrochlear nerve

Nasociliary nerve

Trochlear nerve (IV)

Common tendinous ring

Ophthalmic nerve (V₁)

Optic nerve (II)

Internal carotid artery and nerve plexus

Oculomotor nerve (III)

Trochlear nerve (IV)

Abducent nerve (VI)

Tentorium cerebelli

Levator palpebrae superioris muscle

Superior rectus muscle

Lacrimal gland

Lacrimal nerve

Lateral rectus muscle

Frontal nerve

Maxillary nerve (V₂)

Meningeal branch of maxillary nerve

Mandibular nerve (V₃)

Lesser petrosal nerve

Meningeal branch of mandibular nerve

Greater petrosal nerve

Trigeminal (semilunar) ganglion

Tentorial (meningeal) branch of ophthalmic nerve

Superior view:
levator palpebrae superioris, superior rectus, and superior oblique muscles partially cut away

Supratrochlear nerve *(cut)*

Supraorbital nerve branches *(cut)*

Infratrochlear nerve

Anterior ethmoidal nerve

Optic nerve (II)

Posterior ethmoidal nerve

Superior branch of oculomotor nerve (III) *(cut)*

Nasociliary nerve

Internal carotid plexus

Trochlear nerve (IV) *(cut)*

Oculomotor nerve (III)

Abducent nerve (VI)

Long ciliary nerves

Short ciliary nerves

Lacrimal nerve

Ciliary ganglion

Parasympathetic root of ciliary ganglion (from inferior branch of oculomotor nerve)

Sympathetic root of ciliary ganglion (from internal carotid plexus)

Sensory root of ciliary ganglion (from nasociliary nerve)

Branches to inferior and medial rectus muscles

Abducent nerve (VI)

Inferior branch of oculomotor nerve (III)

Lacrimal nerve

Frontal nerve *(cut)*

Ophthalmic nerve (V₁)

ANATOMY ILLUSTRATIONS

Proper palmar digital nerves (median nerve)

Medial two lumbricals innervated by ulnar nerve

Cutaneous innervation of the median nerve in the hand

Cutaneous innervation of the dorsal branch of the ulnar nerve

Cutaneous innervation of the palmar branch of the median nerve

Palmar view

Dorsal view

Lateral two lumbricals innervated by median nerve

Proper palmar digital nerve (ulnar nerve)

Intrinsic muscles innervated by ulnar nerve except the thenar muscles and the two lateral lumbricals

Common palmar digital nerve

Hypothenar muscles innervated by ulnar nerve

Palmaris brevis

Deep branch of the ulnar nerve

Superficial branch of the ulnar nerve

Palmar branch of the ulnar nerve

Ulnar nerve

Ulna

Common palmar digital nerves (median nerve)

Cutaneous innervation of the superficial branch of the ulnar nerve in the hand

Thenar muscles innervated by median nerve

Recurrent branch of median nerve

Cutaneous innervation of the palmar branch of the ulnar nerve

Palmar view

Palmar branch of the median nerve

Median nerve

Radius

Cutaneous innervation of the median nerve in the hand

Innervation of the hand, median and ulnar nerves (palmar view)

Dorsal view

Plate 8 Innervation of the Hand: Median and Ulnar Nerves (From Drake RL, Vogl AW, Mitchell AWM, Tibbitts RM, Richardson PE: Gray's Atlas of Anatomy, ed 2, Philadelphia, 2015, Churchill Livingstone.)

Arteries and nerves of forearm (anterior view)

Biceps brachii

Posterior cutaneous nerve of forearm (cut) (from radial nerve)

Lateral cutaneous nerve of forearm (cut) (from musculocutaneous nerve)

Biceps brachii tendon

Radial artery

Brachioradialis

Ulnar nerve

Medial cutaneous nerve of forearm (from medial cord of brachial plexus)

Median nerve

Brachial artery

Medial epicondyle

Bicipital aponeurosis

Radial artery

Palmaris longus tendon

Median nerve

Thenar muscles

Palmar branch of median nerve

Palmar aponeurosis

Ulnar artery

Brachioradialis tendon (cut)

Palmar branch of ulnar nerve

Hypothenar muscles

Radial nerve

Brachial artery

Lateral epicondyle

Radial recurrent artery

Deep branch radial nerve

Radial artery

Supinator

Superficial branch radial nerve

Common interosseous artery

Posterior interosseous artery

Interosseous membrane

Pronator teres (cut)

Perforating branches of anterior interosseous artery

Median nerve

Recurrent interosseous artery

Ulnar nerve

Humeral head of pronator teres (cut)

Posterior interosseous artery

Anterior ulnar recurrent artery

Humeral head of flexor carpi ulnaris

Posterior ulnar recurrent artery

Ulnar head of pronator teres

Ulnar artery

Anterior interosseous nerve

Anterior interosseous artery

Radial artery

Interosseous membrane

Flexor digitorum superficialis (cut)

Flexor digitorum profundus

Superficial palmar branch of radial artery

Dorsal branch of ulnar nerve

Flexor carpi radialis tendon (cut)

Flexor retinaculum

Superficial palmar branch of radial artery

Palmar branch of median nerve

Flexor carpi ulnaris tendon (cut)

Ulnar nerve

Palmar branch of ulnar nerve

Deep palmar branch of ulnar artery

Deep palmar arch

Superficial palmar arch

Superior ulnar collateral artery

Inferior ulnar collateral artery

Radial collateral artery

Brachial artery

Radial recurrent artery

Anterior ulnar recurrent artery

Posterior ulnar recurrent artery

Common interosseous artery

Anterior interosseous artery

Ulnar artery

Radius

Ulna

Superficial palmar branch of radial artery

Pisiform

Superficial palmar arch

Deep palmar arch

Plate 9 Arteries and Nerves of the Forearm (Anterior View) (From Drake RL, Vogl AW, Mitchell AWM, Tibbitts RM, Richardson PE: Gray's Atlas of Anatomy, ed 2, Philadelphia, 2015, Churchill Livingstone.)

ANATOMY ILLUSTRATIONS

Lateral cutaneous branch of subcostal nerve

Inguinal ligament (Poupart's)

Superficial circumflex iliac vein

Femoral branches of genitofemoral nerve

Lateral femoral cutaneous nerve

Saphenous opening (fossa ovalis)

Fascia lata

Anterior cutaneous branches of femoral nerve

Patellar nerve plexus

Branches of lateral sural cutaneous nerve (from common fibular [peroneal] nerve)

Deep fascia of leg (crural fascia)

Superficial fibular (peroneal) nerve
Medial dorsal cutaneous branch

Intermediate dorsal cutaneous branch

Small saphenous vein and lateral dorsal cutaneous nerve (from sural nerve)

Lateral dorsal digital nerve and vein of 5th toe

Dorsal metatarsal veins

Dorsal digital nerves and veins

Superficial epigastric vein

Ilioinguinal nerve (scrotal branch) (usually passes through superficial inguinal ring)

Genital branch of genitofemoral nerve

Femoral vein

Superficial external pudendal vein

Accessory saphenous vein

Great saphenous vein

Cutaneous branches of obturator nerve

Infrapatellar branch of saphenous nerve

Saphenous nerve (terminal branch of femoral nerve)

Great saphenous vein

Dorsal digital nerves

Dorsal venous arch

Dorsal digital nerve and vein of medial side of great toe

Dorsal digital branch of deep fibular (peroneal) nerve

ANATOMY ILLUSTRATIONS

Plate 10 Superficial Nerves and Veins of Lower Limb: Anterior View. (Copyright 2024 Elsevier Inc. All rights reserved. www.netterimages.com. Image ID: 4846)

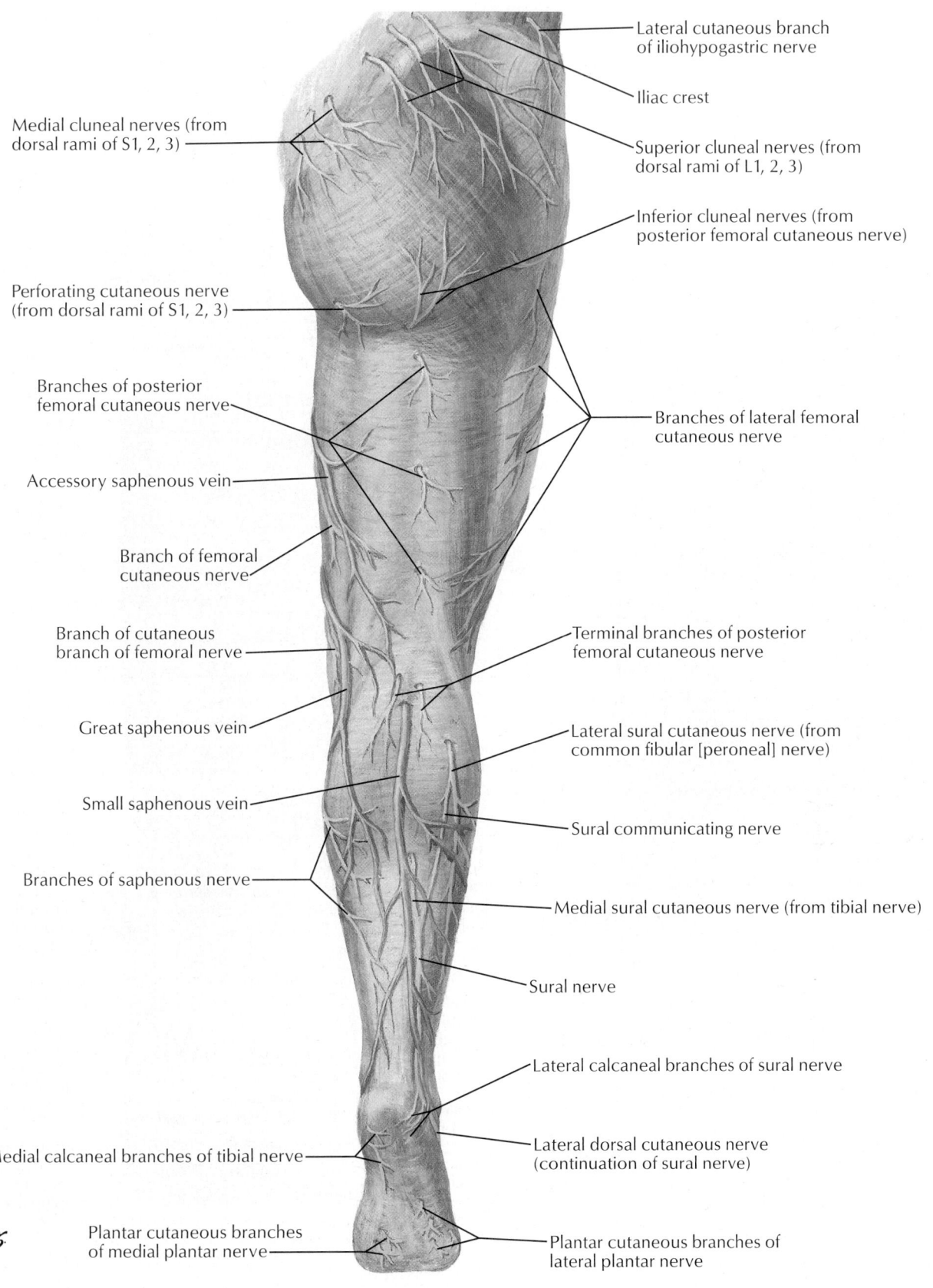

Lateral cutaneous branch of iliohypogastric nerve

Iliac crest

Medial cluneal nerves (from dorsal rami of S1, 2, 3)

Superior cluneal nerves (from dorsal rami of L1, 2, 3)

Inferior cluneal nerves (from posterior femoral cutaneous nerve)

Perforating cutaneous nerve (from dorsal rami of S1, 2, 3)

Branches of posterior femoral cutaneous nerve

Branches of lateral femoral cutaneous nerve

Accessory saphenous vein

Branch of femoral cutaneous nerve

Branch of cutaneous branch of femoral nerve

Terminal branches of posterior femoral cutaneous nerve

Great saphenous vein

Lateral sural cutaneous nerve (from common fibular [peroneal] nerve)

Small saphenous vein

Sural communicating nerve

Branches of saphenous nerve

Medial sural cutaneous nerve (from tibial nerve)

Sural nerve

Lateral calcaneal branches of sural nerve

Medial calcaneal branches of tibial nerve

Lateral dorsal cutaneous nerve (continuation of sural nerve)

Plantar cutaneous branches of medial plantar nerve

Plantar cutaneous branches of lateral plantar nerve

ANATOMY ILLUSTRATIONS

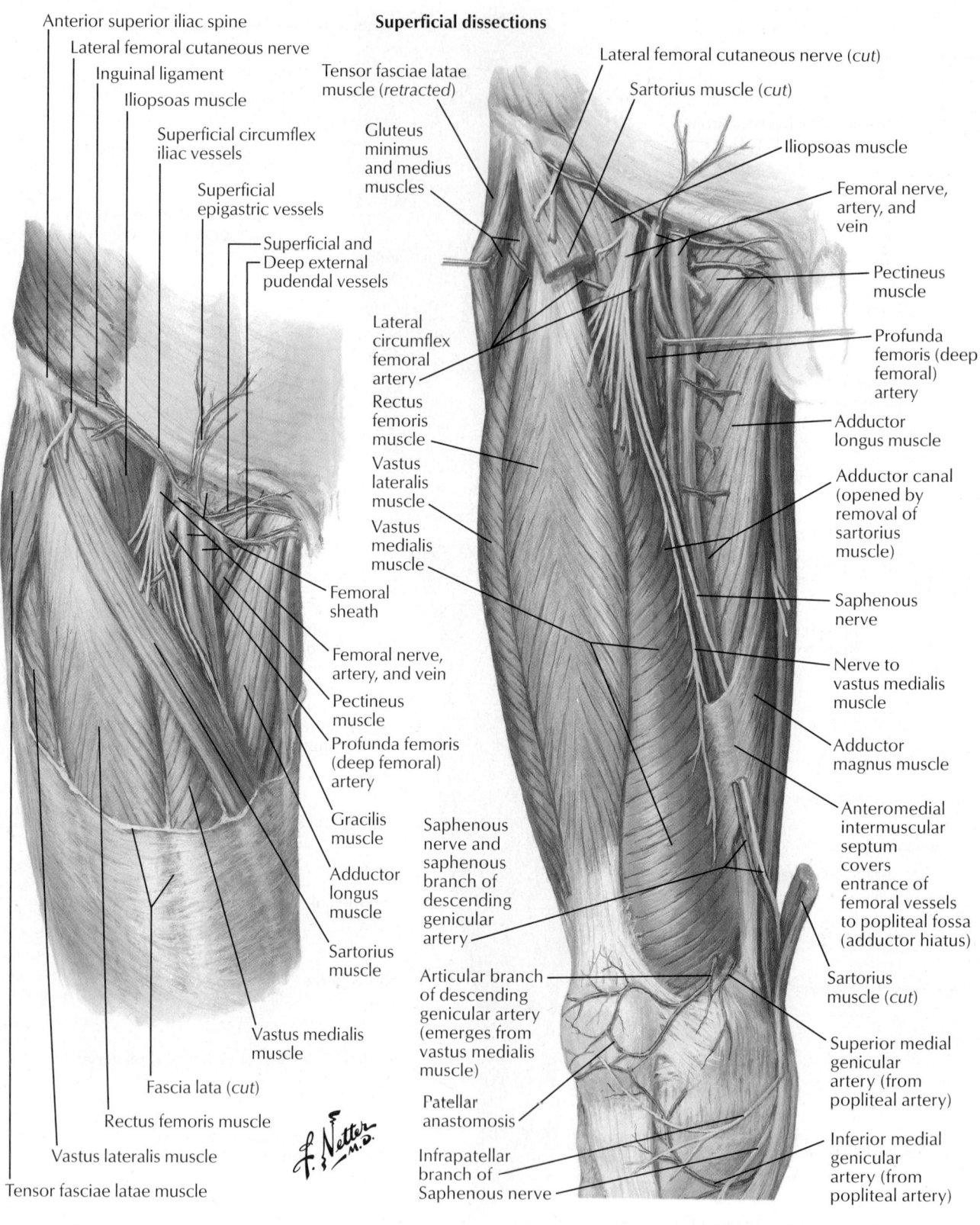

Anterior superior iliac spine
Lateral femoral cutaneous nerve
Inguinal ligament
Iliopsoas muscle
Superficial circumflex iliac vessels
Superficial epigastric vessels
Superficial and Deep external pudendal vessels

Superficial dissections

Tensor fasciae latae muscle (*retracted*)
Gluteus minimus and medius muscles
Lateral circumflex femoral artery
Rectus femoris muscle
Vastus lateralis muscle
Vastus medialis muscle
Femoral sheath
Femoral nerve, artery, and vein
Pectineus muscle
Profunda femoris (deep femoral) artery
Gracilis muscle
Adductor longus muscle
Sartorius muscle
Vastus medialis muscle
Fascia lata (*cut*)
Rectus femoris muscle
Vastus lateralis muscle
Tensor fasciae latae muscle

Lateral femoral cutaneous nerve (*cut*)
Sartorius muscle (*cut*)
Iliopsoas muscle
Femoral nerve, artery, and vein
Pectineus muscle
Profunda femoris (deep femoral) artery
Adductor longus muscle
Adductor canal (opened by removal of sartorius muscle)
Saphenous nerve
Nerve to vastus medialis muscle
Adductor magnus muscle
Anteromedial intermuscular septum covers entrance of femoral vessels to popliteal fossa (adductor hiatus)
Sartorius muscle (*cut*)
Superior medial genicular artery (from popliteal artery)
Inferior medial genicular artery (from popliteal artery)

Saphenous nerve and saphenous branch of descending genicular artery
Articular branch of descending genicular artery (emerges from vastus medialis muscle)
Patellar anastomosis
Infrapatellar branch of Saphenous nerve

F. Netter M.D.

ANATOMY ILLUSTRATIONS

Plate 12 Arteries and Nerves of Thigh: Anterior Views. (Copyright 2024 Elsevier Inc. All rights reserved. www.netterimages.com. Image ID: 4475)

68

Deep dissection

Deep circumflex iliac artery

Lateral femoral cutaneous nerve

Sartorius muscle (*cut*)

Iliopsoas muscle

Tensor fasciae latae muscle (*retracted*)

Gluteus medius and minimus muscles

Femoral nerve

Rectus femoris muscle (*cut*)

Ascending, transverse and descending branches of Lateral circumflex femoral artery

Medial circumflex femoral artery

Pectineus muscle (*cut*)

Profunda femoris (deep femoral) artery

Perforating branches

Adductor longus muscle (*cut*)

Vastus lateralis muscle

Vastus intermedius muscle

Rectus femoris muscle (*cut*)

Saphenous nerve

Anteromedial intermuscular septum (*opened*)

Vastus medialis muscle

Quadriceps femoris tendon

Patella and patellar anastomosis

Medial patellar retinaculum

Patellar ligament

External iliac artery and vein

Inguinal ligament (Poupart's)

Femoral artery and vein (*cut*)

Pectineus muscle (*cut*)

Obturator canal

Obturator externus muscle

Adductor longus muscle (*cut*)

Anterior branch and Posterior branch of obturator nerve

Quadratus femoris muscle

Adductor brevis muscle

Branches of posterior branch of obturator nerve

Adductor magnus muscle

Gracilis muscle

Cutaneous branch of obturator nerve

Femoral artery and vein (*cut*)

Descending genicular artery
Articular branch
Saphenous branch

Adductor hiatus

Sartorius muscle (*cut*)

Adductor magnus tendon

Adductor tubercle on medial epicondyle of femur

Superior medial genicular artery (from popliteal artery)

Infrapatellar branch of Saphenous nerve

Inferior medial genicular artery (from popliteal artery)

ANATOMY ILLUSTRATIONS

Plate 13 Arteries and Nerves of Thigh: Posterior View. (Copyright 2024 Elsevier Inc. All rights reserved. www.netterimages.com. Image ID: 49316)

69

Deep dissection

Superior cluneal nerves

Gluteus maximus muscle (*cut*)

Medial cluneal nerves

Inferior gluteal artery and nerve

Pudendal nerve

Nerve to obturator internus
(and superior gemellus)

Posterior femoral
cutaneous nerve

Sacrotuberous ligament

Ischial tuberosity

Inferior cluneal nerves (*cut*)

Adductor magnus muscle

Gracilis muscle

Sciatic nerve

Muscular branches of sciatic nerve

Semitendinosus muscle (*retracted*)

Semimembranosus muscle

Sciatic nerve

Articular branch

Adductor hiatus

Popliteal vein and artery

Superior medial genicular artery

Medial epicondyle of femur

Tibial nerve

Gastrocnemius muscle (medial head)

Medial sural cutaneous nerve

Small saphenous vein

Iliac crest

Gluteal aponeurosis and
gluteus medius muscle (*cut*)

Superior gluteal artery and nerve

Gluteus minimus muscle

Tensor fasciae latae muscle

Piriformis muscle

Gluteus medius muscle (*cut*)

Superior gemellus muscle

Greater trochanter of femur

Obturator internus muscle

Inferior gemellus muscle

Gluteus maximus muscle (*cut*)

Quadratus femoris muscle

Medial circumflex femoral
artery

Vastus lateralis muscle
and iliotibial tract

Adductor minimus part of
adductor magnus muscle

1st perforating artery (from
profunda femoris artery)

Adductor magnus muscle

2nd and 3rd perforating arteries
(from profunda femoris artery)

4th perforating artery (from
profunda femoris artery)

Long head (*retracted*) ⎫ Biceps femoris
Short head ⎭ muscle

Superior lateral genicular artery

Common fibular (peroneal) nerve

Plantaris muscle

Gastrocnemius muscle (lateral head)

Lateral sural cutaneous nerve

ANATOMY ILLUSTRATIONS

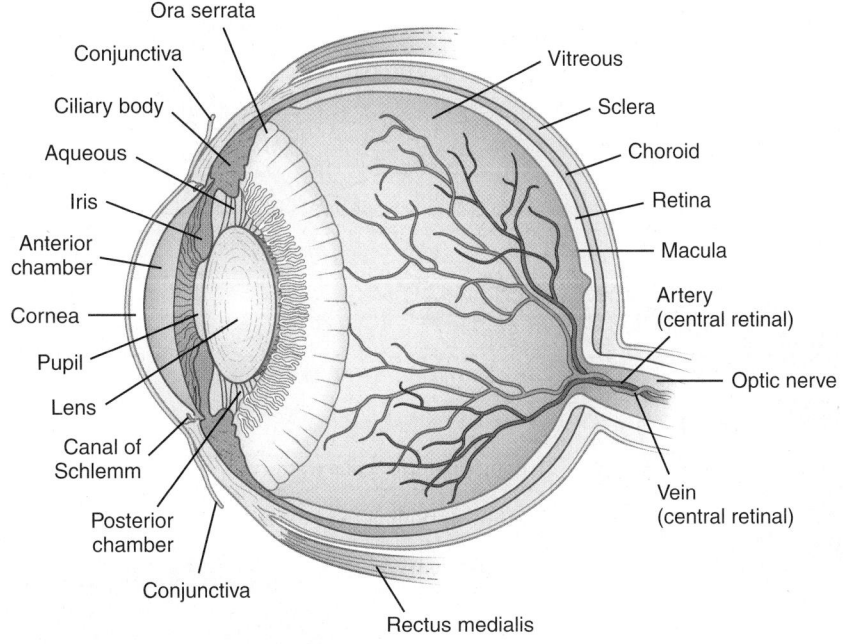

Ora serrata

Conjunctiva

Ciliary body

Aqueous

Iris

Anterior chamber

Cornea

Pupil

Lens

Canal of Schlemm

Posterior chamber

Conjunctiva

Rectus medialis

Vitreous

Sclera

Choroid

Retina

Macula

Artery (central retinal)

Optic nerve

Vein (central retinal)

Plate 15   Anatomy of the eye. (Dehn RW, Asprey DP: Essential Clinical Procedures, ed 3, Philadelphia, 2013, Saunders.)

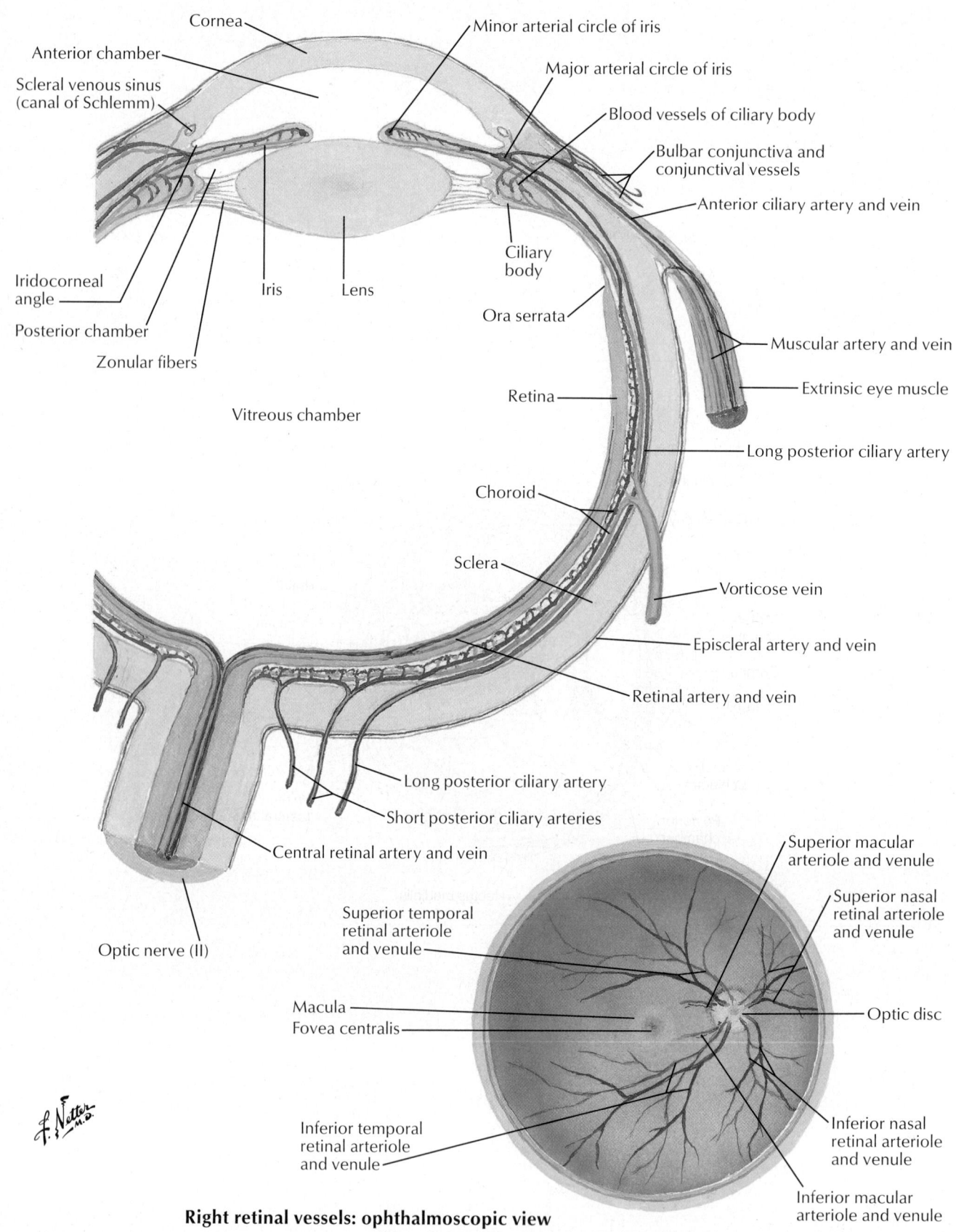

Cornea

Anterior chamber

Scleral venous sinus (canal of Schlemm)

Minor arterial circle of iris

Major arterial circle of iris

Blood vessels of ciliary body

Bulbar conjunctiva and conjunctival vessels

Anterior ciliary artery and vein

Ciliary body

Ora serrata

Iridocorneal angle

Iris

Lens

Posterior chamber

Zonular fibers

Vitreous chamber

Muscular artery and vein

Extrinsic eye muscle

Retina

Long posterior ciliary artery

Choroid

Sclera

Vorticose vein

Episcleral artery and vein

Retinal artery and vein

Long posterior ciliary artery

Short posterior ciliary arteries

Central retinal artery and vein

Optic nerve (II)

Superior macular arteriole and venule

Superior nasal retinal arteriole and venule

Superior temporal retinal arteriole and venule

Macula

Fovea centralis

Optic disc

Inferior nasal retinal arteriole and venule

Inferior temporal retinal arteriole and venule

Inferior macular arteriole and venule

Right retinal vessels: ophthalmoscopic view

Plate 16   Intrinsic Arteries and Veins of Eye. (Copyright 2024 Elsevier Inc. All rights reserved. www.netterimages.com. Image ID: 49107)

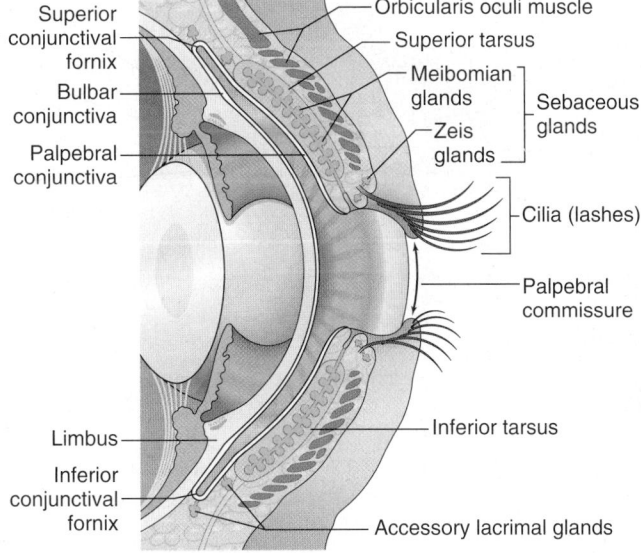

Superior conjunctival fornix

Bulbar conjunctiva

Palpebral conjunctiva

Orbicularis oculi muscle

Superior tarsus

Meibomian glands

Zeis glands

Sebaceous glands

Cilia (lashes)

Palpebral commissure

Limbus

Inferior conjunctival fornix

Inferior tarsus

Accessory lacrimal glands

Plate 17 Anatomy of the conjunctiva and eyelids. (Kumar V, Abbas AK, Aster JC: Robbins and Cotran Pathologic Basis of Disease, ed 9, Philadelphia, 2015, Saunders.)

Superior palpebral conjunctiva: tarsal (meibomian) glands shining through

Seen through cornea { Pupil / Iris

Corneoscleral junction (corneal limbus)

Bulbar conjunctiva over sclera

Inferior conjunctival fornix

Inferior palpebral conjunctiva: tarsal glands shining through

Superior lacrimal papilla and punctum

Plica semilunaris

Lacrimal caruncle in lacrimal lake (lacus lacrimalis)

Inferior lacrimal papilla and punctum

Plate 18　Eyelid.

Orbital part of
lacrimal gland

Palpebral part of
lacrimal gland

Excretory ducts of
lacrimal gland

Plica semilunaris

Lacrimal caruncle

Inferior lacrimal papilla and punctum

Superior lacrimal papilla and punctum

Lacrimal canaliculi

Lacrimal sac

Nasolacrimal duct

Opening of
nasolacrimal duct

Frontal bone (*cut away*)

Orbital part of
lacrimal gland

Palpebral part of
lacrimal gland

Excretory ducts of
lacrimal gland

Plica semilunaris
and lacrimal lake

Lacrimal caruncle

Inferior lacrimal papilla and punctum

Opening of nasolacrimal duct
and site of Hasner's valve

Superior lacrimal papilla and punctum

Lacrimal canaliculi

Lacrimal sac

Nasolacrimal du

Middle nasal
concha

Nasal cavity

Inferior nasal
concha (*cut*)

Inferior nasal meatu

Plate 19   Lacrimal Apparatus. (Copyright 2024 Elsevier Inc. All rights reserved. www.netterimages.com. Image ID: 49103)

Plate 20 Pathway of Sound. (LaFleur Brooks D, LaFleur Brooks M: Basic Medical Language, ed 4, St. Louis, 2013, Mosby.)

Plate 21 Middle ear structures. (©Elsevier Collection.)

RIGHT TYMPANIC MEMBRANE

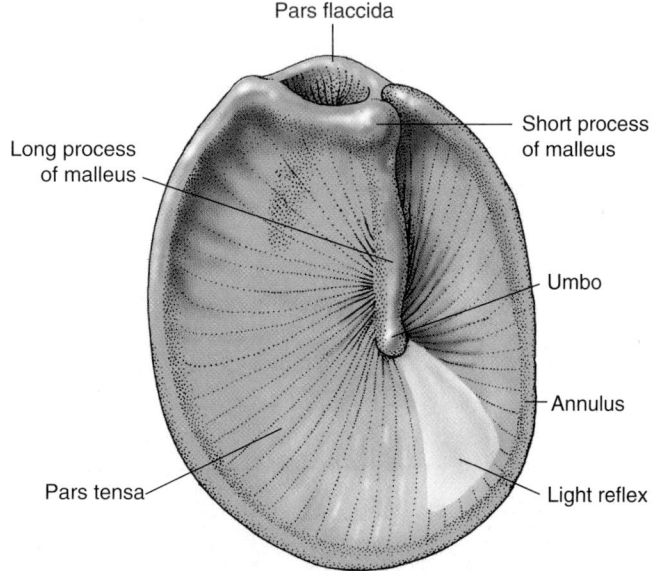

Pars flaccida

Short process
of malleus

Long process
of malleus

Umbo

Annulus

Pars tensa

Light reflex

Plate 22 Structural landmarks of tympanic membrane. (Ignatavicius DD, Workman ML: Medical-Surgical Nursing: Patient-Centered Collaborative Care, ed 7, St. Louis, 2013, Saunders.)

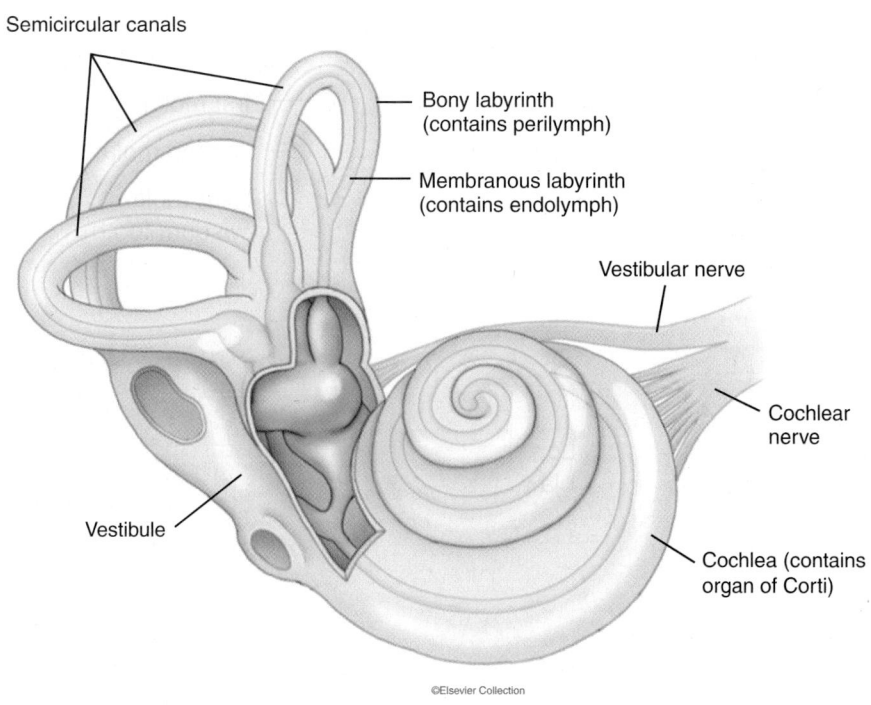

Semicircular canals

Bony labyrinth
(contains perilymph)

Membranous labyrinth
(contains endolymph)

Vestibular nerve

Cochlear
nerve

Vestibule

Cochlea (contains
organ of Corti)

©Elsevier Collection

Plate 23 Inner ear structures. (©Elsevier Collection.)

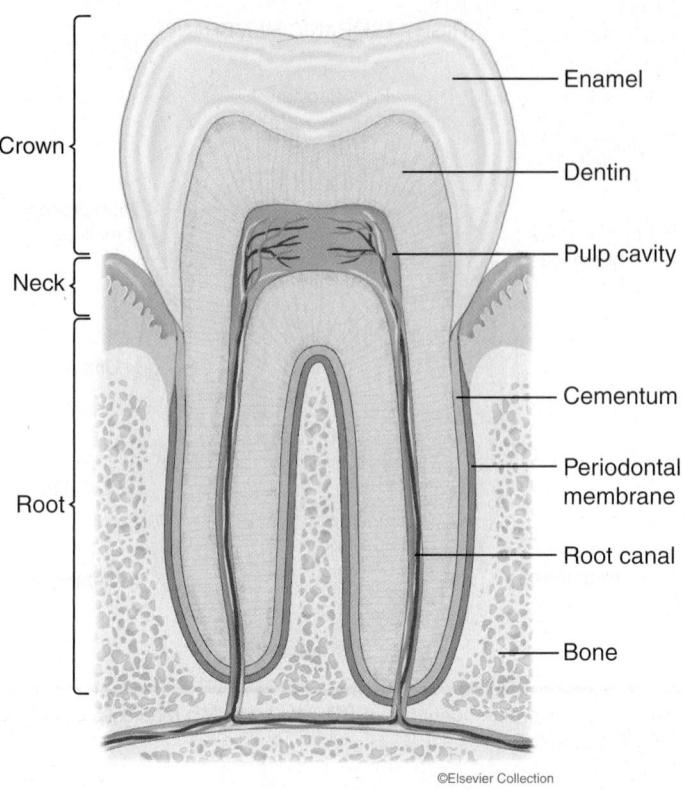

Crown

Neck

Root

Enamel

Dentin

Pulp cavity

Cementum

Periodontal membrane

Root canal

Bone

©Elsevier Collection

Plate 24 The Tooth. (©Elsevier Collection).

Central incisor

Lateral incisor

Canine

First premolar

Second premolar

First molar

Second molar

Third molar
(wisdom tooth)

Upper
jaw

Lower
jaw

©Elsevier Collection

Plate 25 Adult Teeth. (©Elsevier Collection).

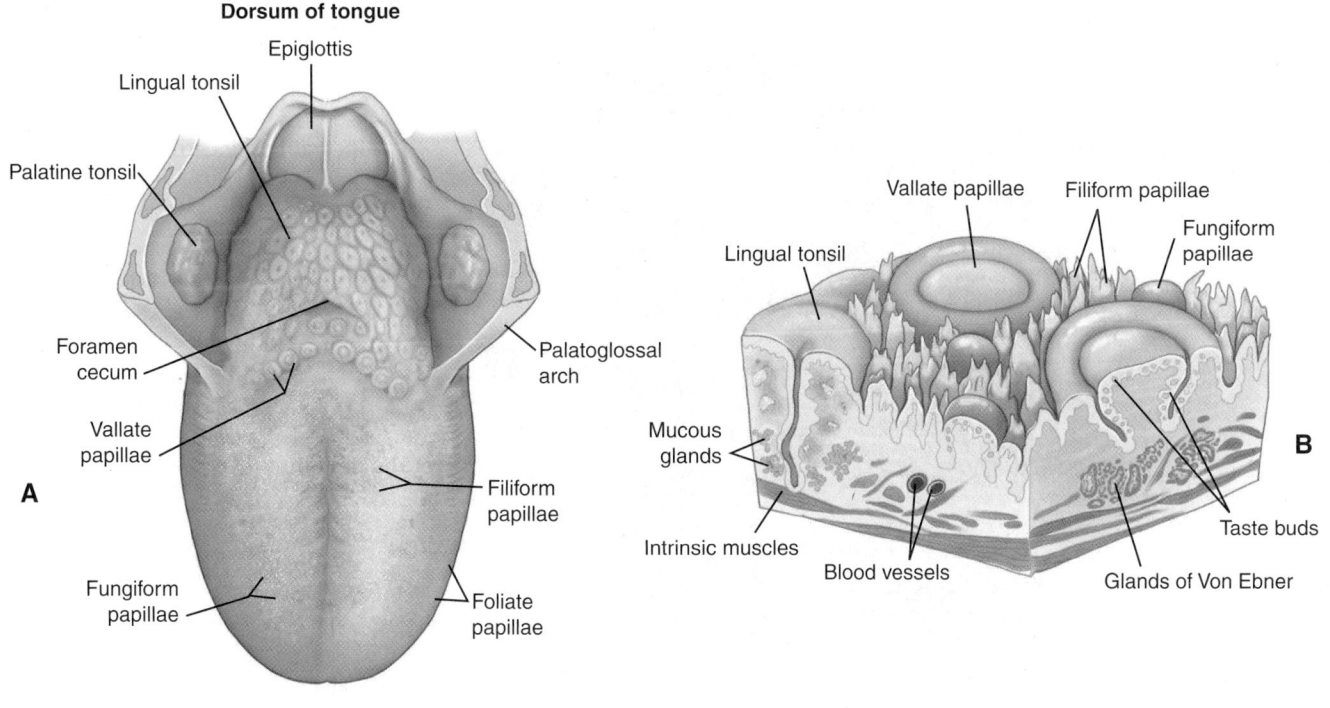

Dorsum of tongue

Epiglottis

Lingual tonsil

Palatine tonsil

Foramen cecum

Vallate papillae

A

Fungiform papillae

Palatoglossal arch

Filiform papillae

Foliate papillae

Vallate papillae

Filiform papillae

Lingual tonsil

Fungiform papillae

Mucous glands

Intrinsic muscles

Blood vessels

Taste buds

Glands of Von Ebner

B

© Elsevier Collection

Plate 26   A, Dorsal view of tongue showing the roughened large lingual tonsils on the posterior of the tongue and the foliate papillae on the side. B, Section of dorsal of the tongue showing a cutaway through lingual papillae and showing von Ebner's glands at the base of the vallate papilla. (Brand RW, Isselhard DE: *Anatomy of Orofacial Structures: A Comprehensive Approach*, ed 8, St. Louis, 2019, Elsevier.)

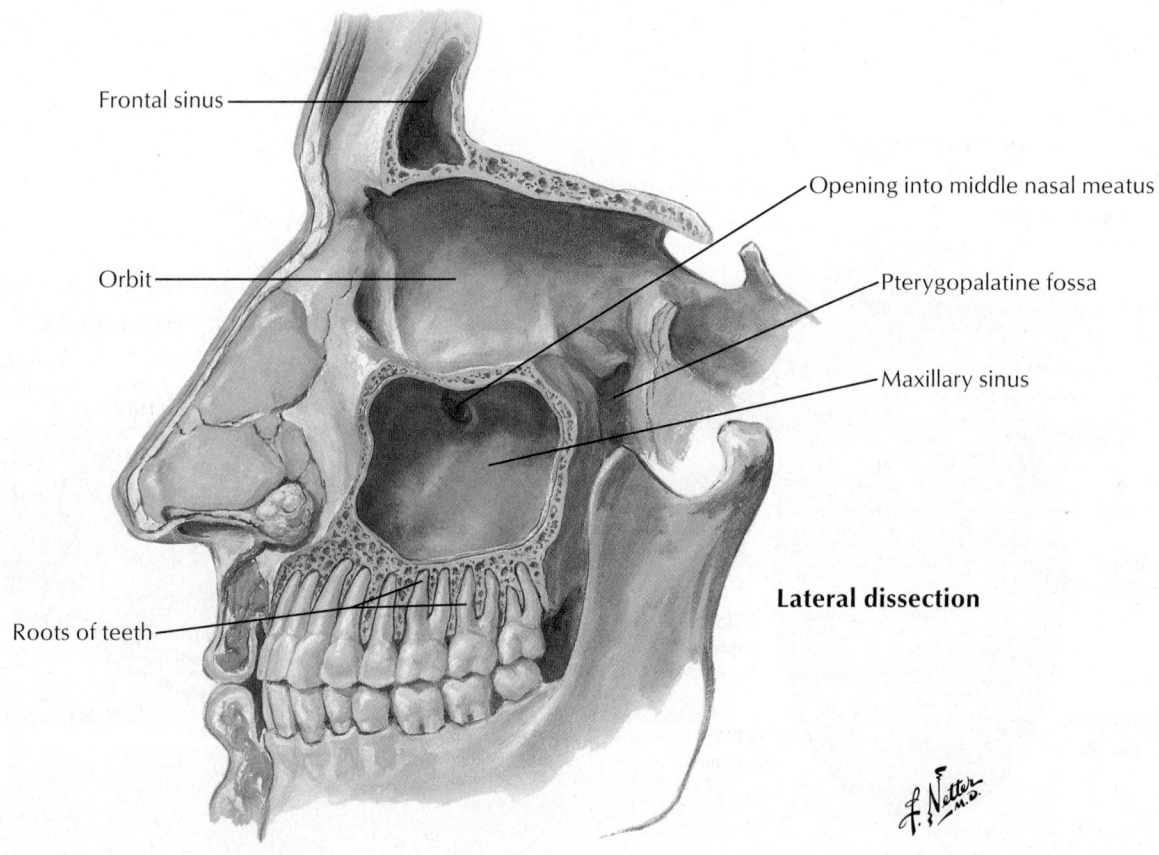

Frontal sinus

Opening into middle nasal meatus

Orbit

Pterygopalatine fossa

Maxillary sinus

Lateral dissection

Roots of teeth

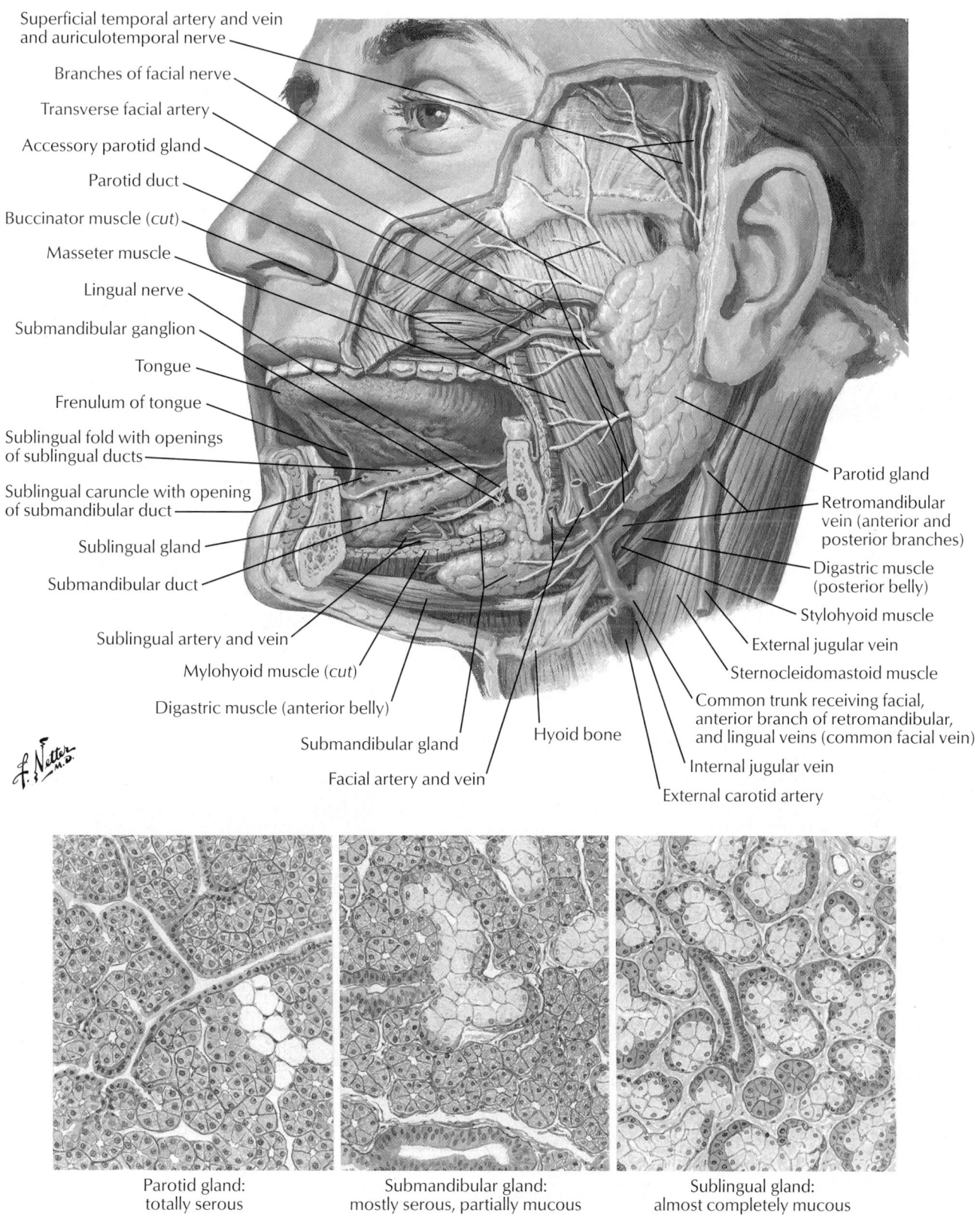

Superficial temporal artery and vein and auriculotemporal nerve

Branches of facial nerve

Transverse facial artery

Accessory parotid gland

Parotid duct

Buccinator muscle (*cut*)

Masseter muscle

Lingual nerve

Submandibular ganglion

Tongue

Frenulum of tongue

Sublingual fold with openings of sublingual ducts

Sublingual caruncle with opening of submandibular duct

Sublingual gland

Submandibular duct

Sublingual artery and vein

Mylohyoid muscle (*cut*)

Digastric muscle (anterior belly)

Submandibular gland

Facial artery and vein

Hyoid bone

Parotid gland

Retromandibular vein (anterior and posterior branches)

Digastric muscle (posterior belly)

Stylohyoid muscle

External jugular vein

Sternocleidomastoid muscle

Common trunk receiving facial, anterior branch of retromandibular, and lingual veins (common facial vein)

Internal jugular vein

External carotid artery

Parotid gland: totally serous

Submandibular gland: mostly serous, partially mucous

Sublingual gland: almost completely mucous

Coronary Arteries: Arteriographic Views

Right coronary artery: left anterior oblique view

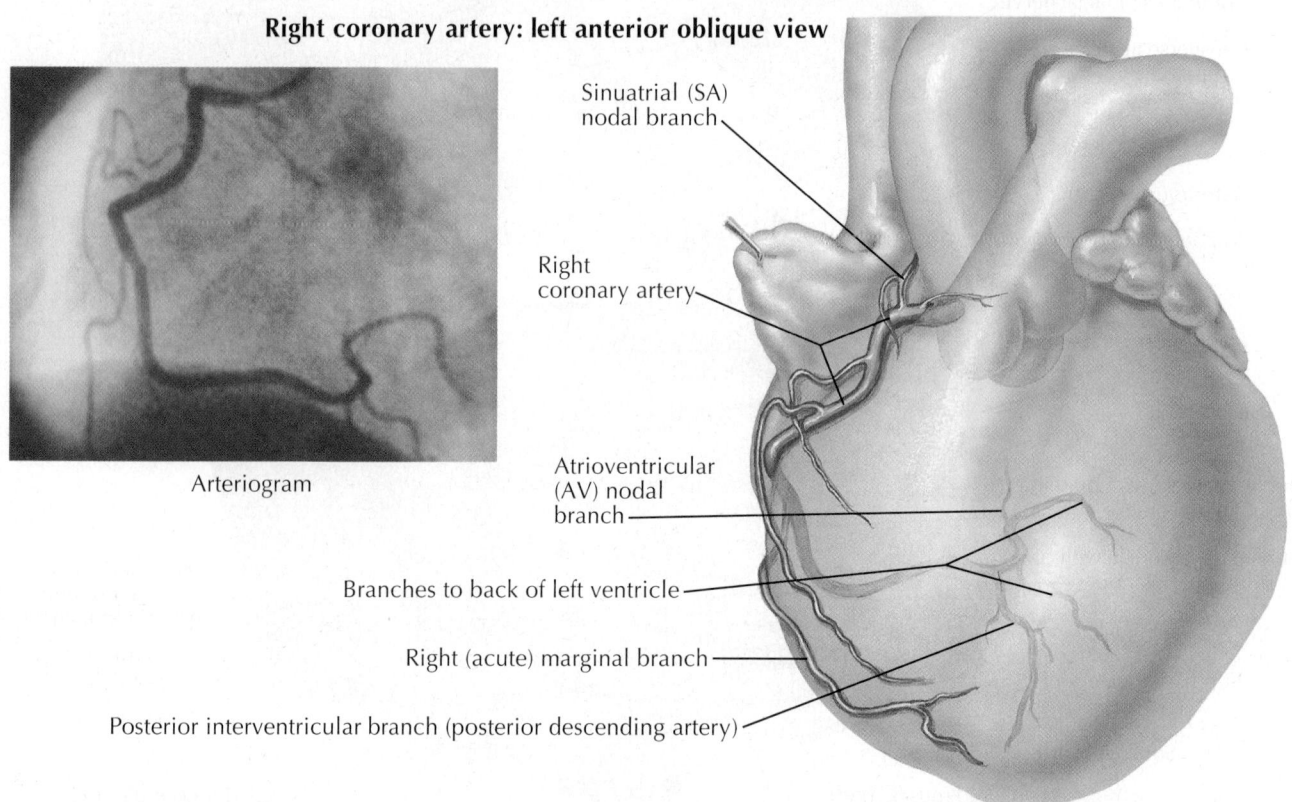

Sinuatrial (SA) nodal branch

Right coronary artery

Atrioventricular (AV) nodal branch

Branches to back of left ventricle

Right (acute) marginal branch

Posterior interventricular branch (posterior descending artery)

Arteriogram

Right coronary artery: right anterior oblique view

Sinuatrial (SA) nodal branch

Conus (arteriosus) branch

Right coronary artery

Right (acute) marginal branch

Arteriogram

Atrioventricular (AV) nodal branch

Right posterolateral branches (to back of left ventricle)

Posterior interventricular branch (posterior descending artery)

ANATOMY ILLUSTRATIONS

Left coronary artery: left anterior oblique view

Left coronary artery

Circumflex branch

Anterior interventricular branch (left anterior descending)

Diagonal branches of anterior interventricular branch

Atrioventricular branch of circumflex branch

Left (obtuse) marginal branch

Posterolateral branches

(Perforating) interventricular septal branches

Arteriogram

Left coronary artery: right anterior oblique view

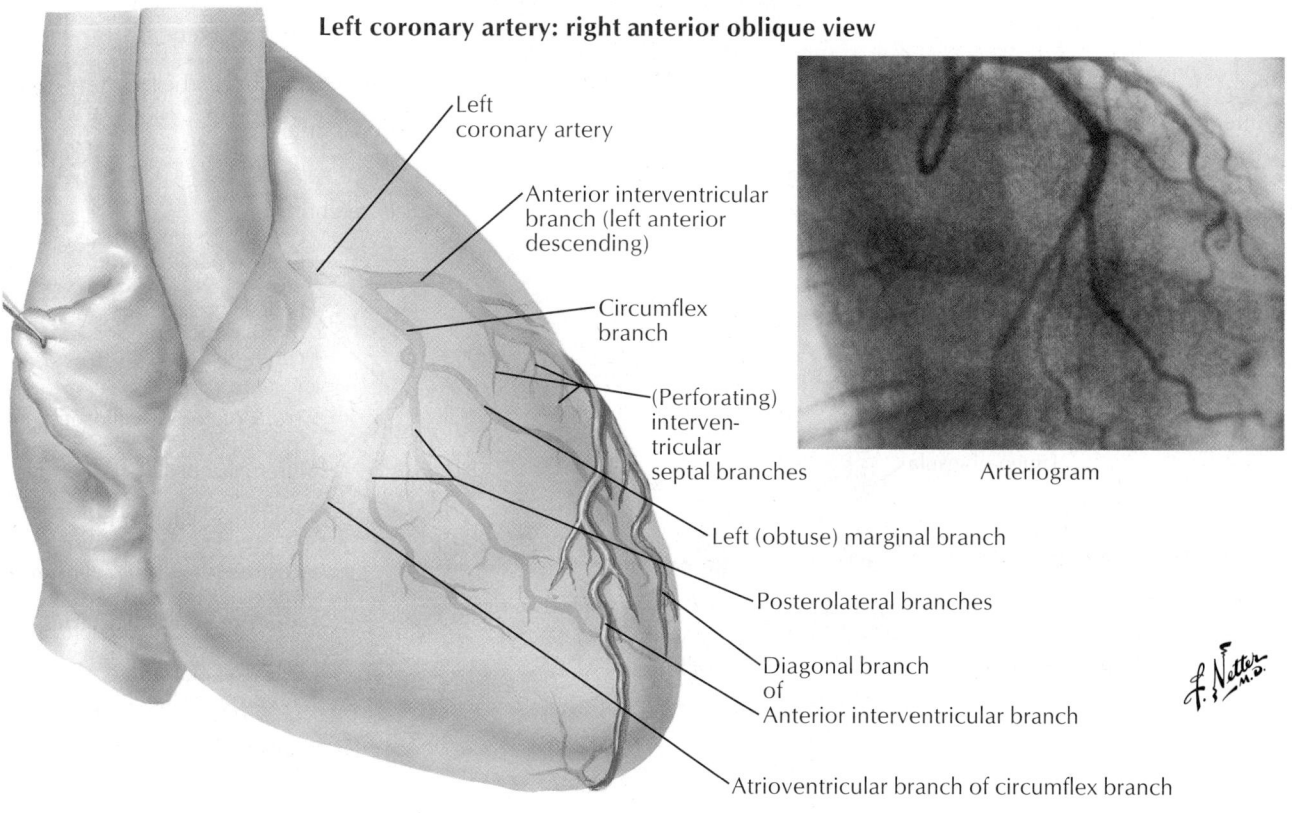

Left coronary artery

Anterior interventricular branch (left anterior descending)

Circumflex branch

(Perforating) interventricular septal branches

Left (obtuse) marginal branch

Posterolateral branches

Diagonal branch of Anterior interventricular branch

Atrioventricular branch of circumflex branch

Arteriogram

ANATOMY ILLUSTRATIONS

Corpus callosum

Anterolateral central (lenticulostriate) arteries

Lateral frontobasal (orbitofrontal) artery

Prefrontal artery

Precentral (pre-Rolandic) and central (Rolandic) sulcal arteries

Anterior parietal (postcentral sulcal) artery

Posterior parietal artery

Branch to angular gyrus

Temporal branches (anterior, middle, and posterior)

Middle cerebral artery and branches (deep in lateral cerebral [Sylvian] sulcus)

Anterior communicating artery

Posterior communicating artery

Anterior inferior cerebellar artery (AICA)

Posterior spinal artery

Paracentral artery

Medial frontal branches

Pericallosal artery

Callosomarginal artery

Polar frontal artery

Anterior cerebral arteries

Medial frontobasal (orbitofrontal) artery

Distal medial striate artery (recurrent artery of Heubner)

Internal carotid artery

Anterior choroidal artery

Posterior cerebral artery

Superior cerebellar artery

Basilar and pontine arteries

Labyrinthine (internal acoustic) artery

Vertebral artery

Posterior inferior cerebellar artery (PICA)

Anterior spinal artery

Corpus striatum (caudate and lentiform nuclei)

Anterolateral central (lenticulostriate) arteries

Insula (island of Reil)

Limen of insula

Precentral (pre-Rolandic), central (Rolandic) sulcal, and parietal arteries

Lateral cerebral (Sylvian) sulcus

Temporal branches of middle cerebral artery

Temporal lobe

Middle cerebral artery

Internal carotid artery

Falx cerebri

Callosomarginal arteries and Pericallosal arteries (branches of anterior cerebral arteries)

Trunk of corpus callosum

Internal capsule

Septum pellucidum

Rostrum of corpus callosum

Anterior cerebral arteries

Distal medial striate artery (recurrent artery of Heubner)

Anterior communicating artery

Optic chiasm

ANATOMY ILLUSTRATIONS

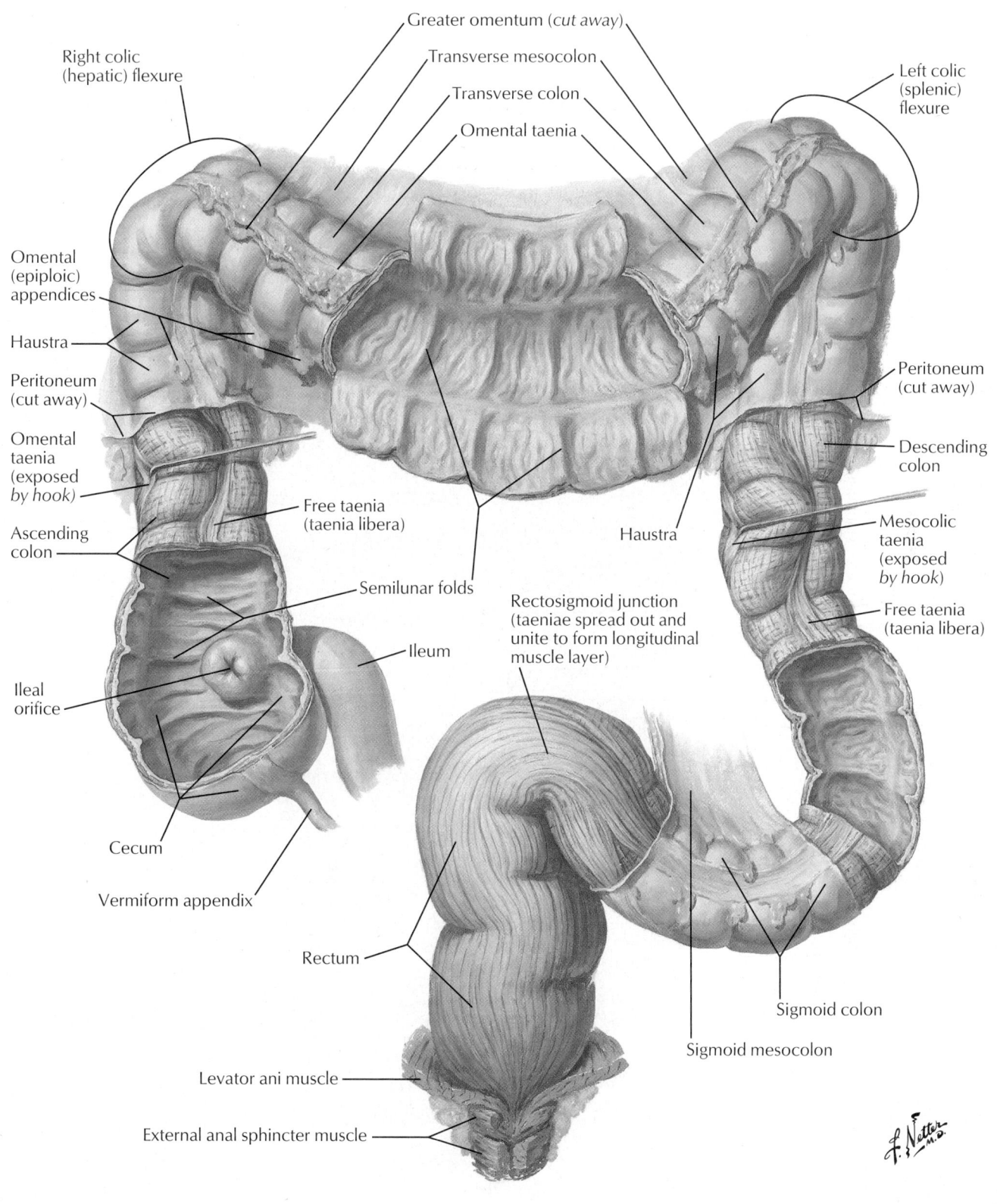

Right colic (hepatic) flexure

Greater omentum (*cut away*)

Transverse mesocolon

Transverse colon

Omental taenia

Left colic (splenic) flexure

Omental (epiploic) appendices

Haustra

Peritoneum (cut away)

Omental taenia (exposed *by hook*)

Ascending colon

Free taenia (taenia libera)

Haustra

Peritoneum (cut away)

Descending colon

Mesocolic taenia (exposed *by hook*)

Semilunar folds

Rectosigmoid junction (taeniae spread out and unite to form longitudinal muscle layer)

Free taenia (taenia libera)

Ileum

Ileal orifice

Cecum

Vermiform appendix

Rectum

Sigmoid colon

Sigmoid mesocolon

Levator ani muscle

External anal sphincter muscle

Plate 32 Mucosa and Musculature of Large Intestine. (Copyright 2024 Elsevier Inc. All rights reserved. www.netterimages.com. Image ID: 4778)

Transverse Section: T3–4 Intervertebral Disc, Manubrium

T3–4

Plate 244

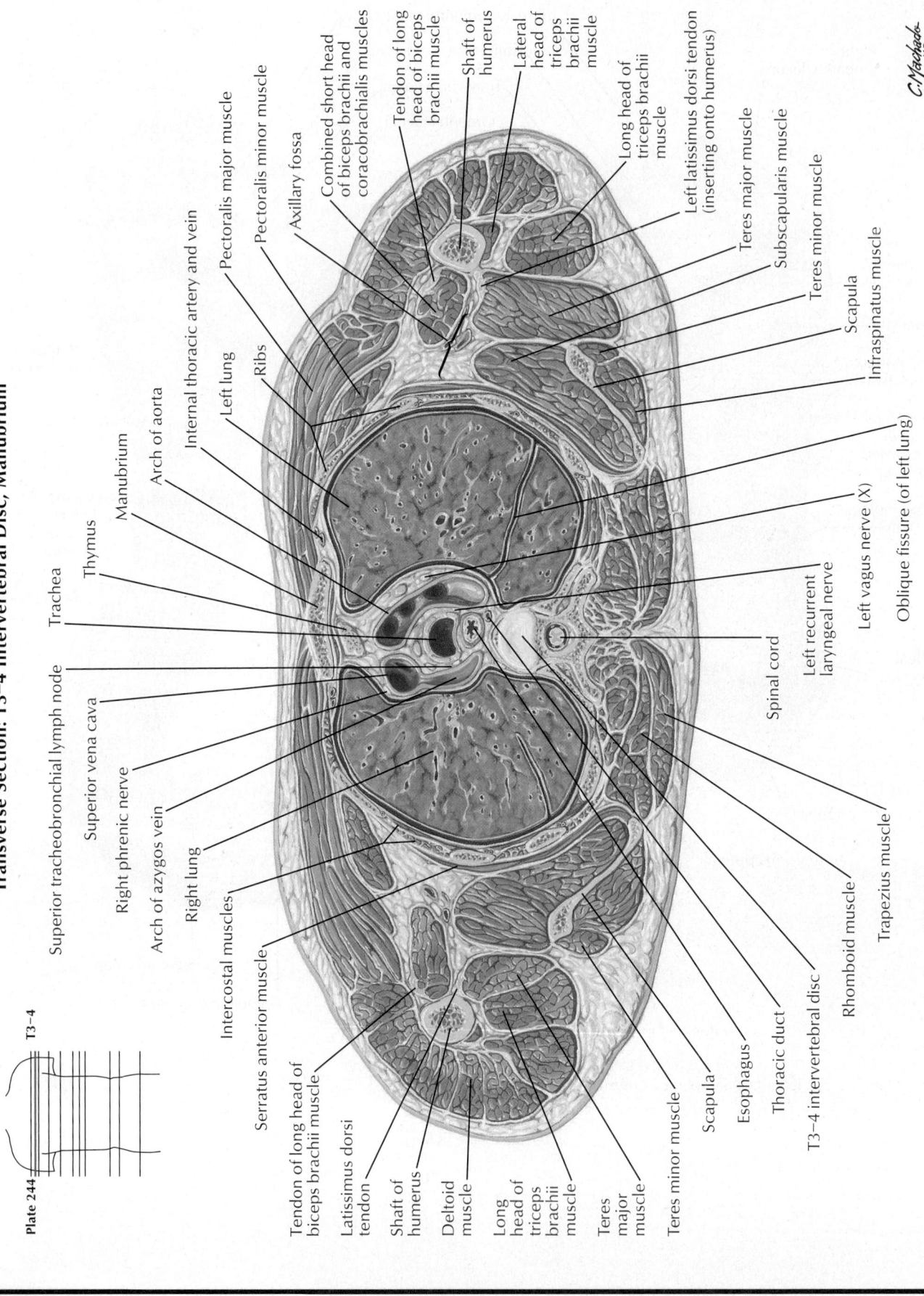

Superior tracheobronchial lymph node

Trachea

Thymus

Manubrium

Arch of aorta

Internal thoracic artery and vein

Pectoralis major muscle

Pectoralis minor muscle

Axillary fossa

Combined short head of biceps brachii and coracobrachialis muscles

Tendon of long head of biceps brachii muscle

Shaft of humerus

Lateral head of triceps brachii muscle

Long head of triceps brachii muscle

Left latissimus dorsi tendon (inserting onto humerus)

Teres major muscle

Subscapularis muscle

Teres minor muscle

Scapula

Infraspinatus muscle

Left lung

Ribs

Oblique fissure (of left lung)

Left vagus nerve (X)

Left recurrent laryngeal nerve

Spinal cord

Trapezius muscle

Rhomboid muscle

T3–4 intervertebral disc

Thoracic duct

Esophagus

Scapula

Teres minor muscle

Teres major muscle

Long head of triceps brachii muscle

Deltoid muscle

Shaft of humerus

Latissimus dorsi tendon

Tendon of long head of biceps brachii muscle

Serratus anterior muscle

Intercostal muscles

Right lung

Arch of azygos vein

Right phrenic nerve

Superior vena cava

Plate 33 Cross Section of Thorax at T3-4 Disc Level. (Copyright 2024 Elsevier Inc. All rights reserved. www.netterimages.com. Image ID: 4880)

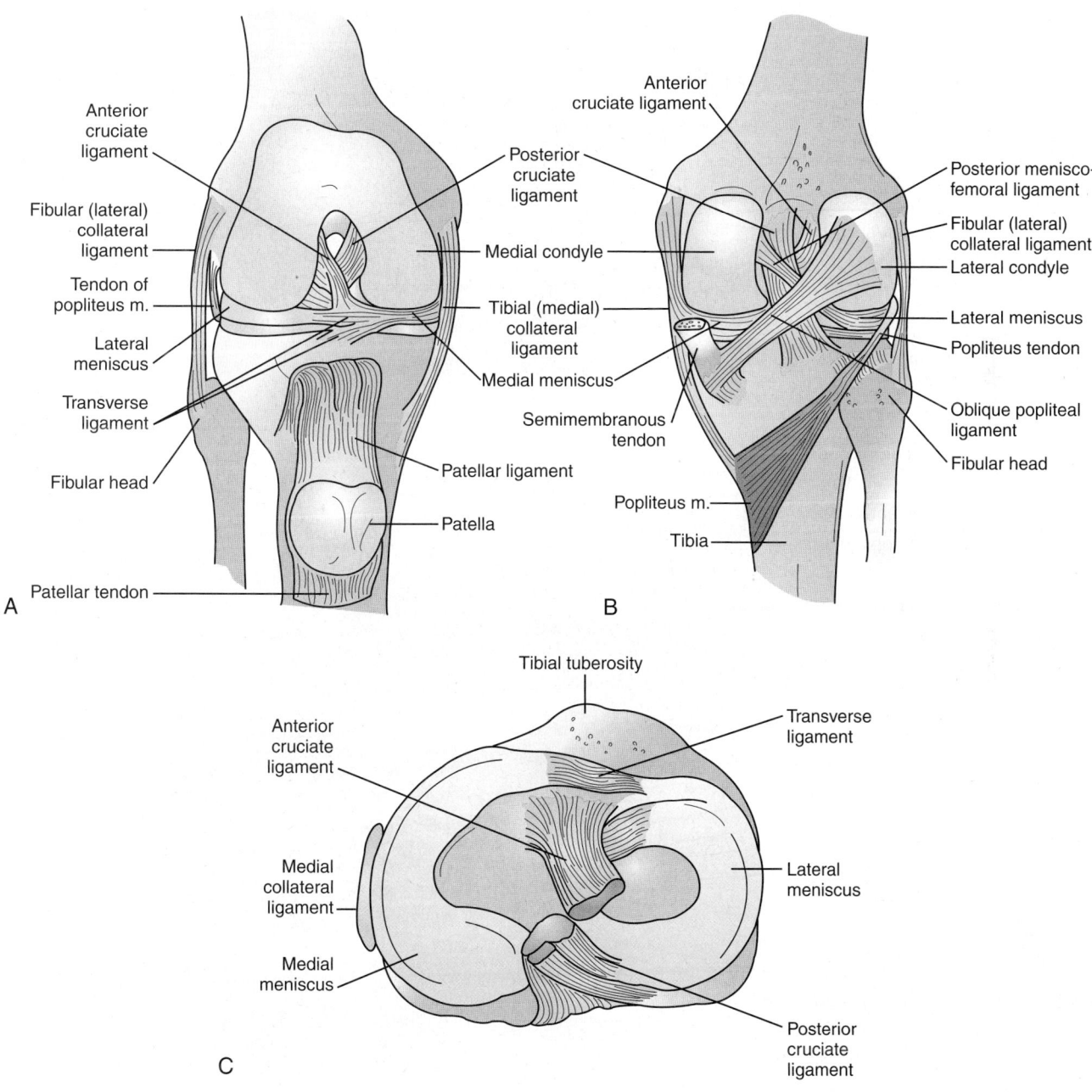

A

Anterior
cruciate
ligament

Fibular (lateral)
collateral
ligament

Tendon of
popliteus m.

Lateral
meniscus

Transverse
ligament

Fibular head

Patellar tendon

Posterior
cruciate
ligament

Medial condyle

Tibial (medial)
collateral
ligament

Medial meniscus

Patellar ligament

Patella

B

Anterior
cruciate ligament

Semimembranous
tendon

Popliteus m.

Tibia

Posterior menisco-
femoral ligament

Fibular (lateral)
collateral ligament

Lateral condyle

Lateral meniscus

Popliteus tendon

Oblique popliteal
ligament

Fibular head

C

Tibial tuberosity

Anterior
cruciate
ligament

Medial
collateral
ligament

Medial
meniscus

Transverse
ligament

Lateral
meniscus

Posterior
cruciate
ligament

Plate 34 Knee joint opened; anterior, posterior, and proximal views. A, Anterior view of the knee joint, opened by folding the patella and patellar ligament inferiorly. On the lateral side is the fibular collateral ligament, separated by the popliteal tendon from the lateral meniscus. On the medial side, the tibial collateral ligament is attached to the medial meniscus. The anterior and posterior cruciate ligaments are seen between the femoral condyles. B, Posterior view of the opened knee joint with a more complete view of the posterior cruciate ligament. C, The femur is removed, showing the proximal (articular) end of the right tibia. On the medial side is the gently curved medial meniscus; on the lateral side is the more tightly curved lateral meniscus. The anterior end of the medial meniscus is anchored to the surface of the tibia by the transverse ligament. The cut ends of the anterior and posterior cruciate ligaments are shown, as well as the meniscofemoral ligament. (Fritz S: Mosby's Essential Sciences for Therapeutic Massage: Anatomy, Physiology, Biomechanics, and Pathology, ed 5, St. Louis, 2017, Elsevier.)

Paramedian (sagittal) dissection

Ureter

Uterine (fallopian) tube

Ovary

Ligament of ovary

Round ligament of uterus

Broad ligament (*cut*)

Superior pubic ramus (*cut*)

Inferior pubic ramus (*cut*)

Ischiocavernosus muscle

Body of clitoris

Labia minora

Labium majus

Rectouterine pouch (of Douglas)

Peritoneum (*cut edge*)

Vesicouterine pouch

Rectum

Ureter

Urinary bladder

Vagina

Pelvic diaphragm (levator ani muscle)

Deep transverse perineal muscle (*cut*)

External anal sphincter muscle

Median (sagittal) section

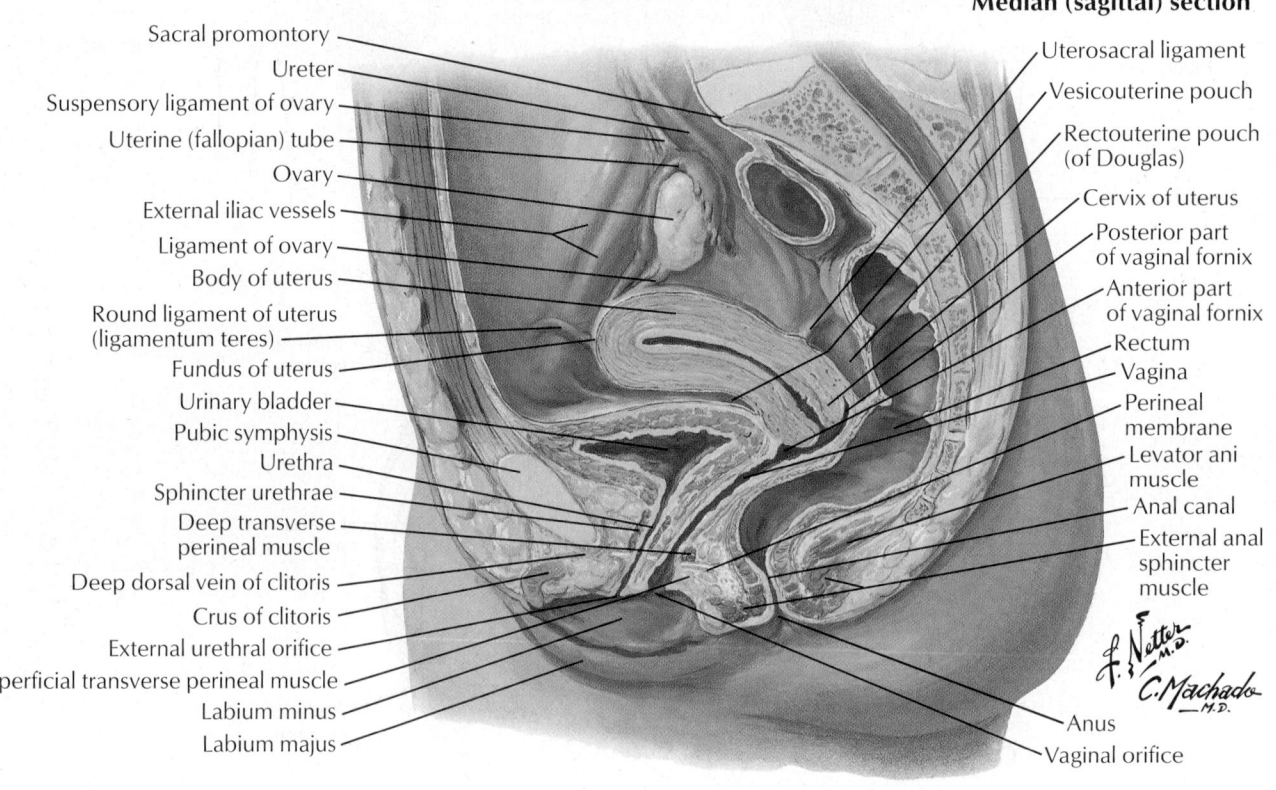

Sacral promontory

Ureter

Suspensory ligament of ovary

Uterine (fallopian) tube

Ovary

External iliac vessels

Ligament of ovary

Body of uterus

Round ligament of uterus (ligamentum teres)

Fundus of uterus

Urinary bladder

Pubic symphysis

Urethra

Sphincter urethrae

Deep transverse perineal muscle

Deep dorsal vein of clitoris

Crus of clitoris

External urethral orifice

Superficial transverse perineal muscle

Labium minus

Labium majus

Uterosacral ligament

Vesicouterine pouch

Rectouterine pouch (of Douglas)

Cervix of uterus

Posterior part of vaginal fornix

Anterior part of vaginal fornix

Rectum

Vagina

Perineal membrane

Levator ani muscle

Anal canal

External anal sphincter muscle

Anus

Vaginal orifice

F. Netter M.D.

C. Machado M.D.

Plate 35 Pelvic Viscera and Perineum: Female. (Copyright 2024 Elsevier Inc. All rights reserved. www.netterimages.com. Image ID: 4463)

PART II

Alphabetic Index

ICD-10-CM INDEX TO DISEASES AND INJURIES

A

Aarskog's syndrome Q87.19
Abandonment —*see* Maltreatment
Abasia (-astasia) (hysterical) F44.4
Abderhalden-Kaufmann-Lignac syndrome
  (cystinosis) E72.04
Abdomen, abdominal —*see also* condition
  acute R10.0
  angina K55.1
  muscle deficiency syndrome Q79.4
Abdominalgia —*see* Pain, abdominal
Abduction contracture, hip or other joint —*see*
  Contraction, joint
Aberrant (congenital) —*see also* Malposition,
  congenital
  adrenal gland Q89.1
  artery (peripheral) Q27.8
    basilar NEC Q28.1
    cerebral Q28.3
    coronary Q24.5
    digestive system Q27.8
    eye Q15.8
    lower limb Q27.8
    precerebral Q28.1
    pulmonary Q25.79
    renal Q27.2
    retina Q14.1
    specified site NEC Q27.8
    subclavian Q27.8
    upper limb Q27.8
    vertebral Q28.1
  breast Q83.8
  endocrine gland NEC Q89.2
  hepatic duct Q44.5
  pancreas Q45.3
  parathyroid gland Q89.2
  pituitary gland Q89.2
  sebaceous glands, mucous membrane, mouth,
    congenital Q38.6
  spleen Q89.09
  subclavian artery Q27.8
  thymus (gland) Q89.2
  thyroid gland Q89.2
  vein (peripheral) NEC Q27.8
    cerebral Q28.3
    digestive system Q27.8
    lower limb Q27.8
    precerebral Q28.1
    specified site NEC Q27.8
    upper limb Q27.8
Aberration
  distantial —*see* Disturbance, visual
  mental F99
Abetalipoproteinemia E78.6
Abiotrophy R68.89
Ablatio, ablation
  retinae —*see* Detachment, retina
Ablepharia, ablepharon Q10.3
Abnormal, abnormality, abnormalities —*see also*
  Anomaly
  acid-base balance (mixed) E87.4
  albumin R77.0
  alphafetoprotein R77.2
  alveolar ridge K08.9
  anatomical relationship Q89.9
  apertures, congenital, diaphragm Q79.1
  atrial septal, specified NEC Q21.19
  auditory perception H93.29-•
    diplacusis —*see* Diplacusis
    hyperacusis —*see* Hyperacusis
    recruitment —*see* Recruitment, auditory
    threshold shift —*see* Shift, auditory threshold
  autosomes Q99.9
    fragile site Q95.5
  basal metabolic rate R94.8
  biosynthesis, testicular androgen E29.1
  bleeding time R79.1
  blood amino-acid level R79.83
  blood level (of)
    cobalt R79.0
    copper R79.0
    iron R79.0
    lithium R78.89
    magnesium R79.0
    mineral NEC R79.0
    zinc R79.0
  blood pressure
    elevated R03.0
    low reading (nonspecific) R03.1

Abnormal, abnormality, abnormalities *(Continued)*
  blood sugar R73.09
  blood-gas level R79.81
  bowel sounds R19.15
    absent R19.11
    hyperactive R19.12
  brain scan R94.02
  breathing R06.9
  caloric test R94.138
  cerebrospinal fluid R83.9
    cytology R83.6
    drug level R83.2
    enzyme level R83.0
    hormones R83.1
    immunology R83.4
    microbiology R83.5
    nonmedicinal level R83.3
    specified type NEC R83.8
  chemistry, blood R79.9
    C-reactive protein R79.82
    drugs —*see* Findings, abnormal, in blood
    gas level R79.81
    minerals R79.0
    pancytopenia D61.818
    PTT R79.1
    specified NEC R79.89
    toxins —*see* Findings, abnormal, in blood
  chest sounds (friction) (rales) R09.89
  chromosome, chromosomal Q99.9
    with more than three X chromosomes, female
      Q97.1
    analysis result R89.8
      bronchial washings R84.8
      cerebrospinal fluid R83.8
      cervix uteri NEC R87.89
      nasal secretions R84.8
      nipple discharge R89.8
      peritoneal fluid R85.89
      pleural fluid R84.8
      prostatic secretions R86.8
      saliva R85.89
      seminal fluid R86.8
      sputum R84.8
      synovial fluid R89.8
      throat scrapings R84.8
      vagina R87.89
      vulva R87.89
      wound secretions R89.8
    dicentric replacement Q93.2
    ring replacement Q93.2
    sex Q99.8
      female phenotype Q97.9
        specified NEC Q97.8
      male phenotype Q98.9
        specified NEC Q98.8
      structural male Q98.6
    specified NEC Q99.8
  clinical findings NEC R68.89
  coagulation D68.9
    newborn, transient P61.6
    profile R79.1
    time R79.1
  communication —*see* Fistula
  conjunctiva, vascular H11.41-•
  coronary artery Q24.5
  cortisol-binding globulin E27.8
  course, eustachian tube Q17.8
  creatinine clearance R94.4
  cytology
    anus R85.619
      atypical squamous cells cannot exclude
        high grade squamous intraepithelial
        lesion (ASC-H) R85.611
      atypical squamous cells of undetermined
        significance (ASC-US) R85.610
      cytologic evidence of malignancy R85.614
      high grade squamous intraepithelial lesion
        (HGSIL) R85.613
      human papillomavirus (HPV) DNA test
        high risk positive R85.81
        low risk positive R85.82
      inadequate smear R85.615
      low grade squamous intraepithelial lesion
        (LGSIL) R85.612
      satisfactory anal smear but lacking
        transformation zone R85.616
      specified NEC R85.618
      unsatisfactory smear R85.615
    female genital organs —*see* Abnormal,
      Papanicolaou (smear)

Abnormal, abnormality, abnormalities *(Continued)*
  dark adaptation curve H53.61
  dentofacial NEC —*see* Anomaly, dentofacial
  development, developmental Q89.9
    central nervous system Q07.9
  diagnostic imaging
    abdomen, abdominal region NEC R93.5
    biliary tract R93.2
    bladder R93.41
    breast R92.8
    central nervous system NEC R90.89
    cerebrovascular NEC R90.89
    coronary circulation R93.1
    digestive tract NEC R93.3
    gastrointestinal (tract) R93.3
    genitourinary organs R93.89
    head R93.0
    heart R93.1
    intrathoracic organ NEC R93.89
    kidney R93.42-•
    limbs R93.6
    liver R93.2
    lung (field) R91.8
    musculoskeletal system NEC R93.7
    renal pelvis R93.41
    retroperitoneum R93.5
    site specified NEC R93.89
    skin and subcutaneous tissue R93.89
    skull R93.0
    testis R93.81-•
    urinary organs specified NEC R93.49
    ureter R93.41
  direction, teeth, fully erupted M26.30
  ear ossicles, acquired NEC H74.39-•
    ankylosis —*see* Ankylosis, ear ossicles
    discontinuity —*see* Discontinuity, ossicles, ear
    partial loss —*see* Loss, ossicles, ear (partial)
  Ebstein Q22.5
  echocardiogram R93.1
  echoencephalogram R90.81
  echogram —*see* Abnormal, diagnostic imaging
  electrocardiogram [ECG] [EKG] R94.31
  electroencephalogram [EEG] R94.01
  electrolyte —*see* Imbalance, electrolyte
  electromyogram [EMG] R94.131
  electro-oculogram [EOG] R94.110
  electrophysiological intracardiac studies R94.39
  electroretinogram [ERG] R94.111
  erythrocytes
    congenital, with perinatal jaundice D58.9
  feces (color) (contents) (mucus) R19.5
  finding —*see* Findings, abnormal, without
    diagnosis
  fluid
    amniotic —*see* Abnormal, specimen, specified
    cerebrospinal —*see* Abnormal, cerebrospinal
      fluid
    peritoneal —*see* Abnormal, specimen,
      digestive organs
    pleural —*see* Abnormal, specimen, respiratory
      organs
    synovial —*see* Abnormal, specimen, specified
    thorax (bronchial washings) (pleural fluid) —
      see Abnormal, specimen, respiratory
      organs
    vaginal —*see* Abnormal, specimen, female
      genital organs
  form
    teeth K00.2
    uterus —*see* Anomaly, uterus
  function studies
    auditory R94.120
    bladder R94.8
    brain R94.09
    cardiovascular R94.30
    ear R94.128
    endocrine NEC R94.7
    eye NEC R94.118
    kidney R94.4
    liver R94.5
    nervous system
      central NEC R94.09
      peripheral NEC R94.138
    pancreas R94.8
    placenta R94.8
    pulmonary R94.2
    special senses NEC R94.128
    spleen R94.8
    thyroid R94.6
    vestibular R94.121

▶ New   ⟹ Revised   ~~deleted~~ Deleted   • Use Additional Character(s)

Abnormal, abnormality, abnormalities (Continued)
 gait —see Gait
  hysterical F44.4
 gastrin secretion E16.4
 globulin R77.1
  cortisol-binding E27.8
  thyroid-binding E07.89
 glomerular, minor —see also N00-N07 with
   fourth character .0 N05.0
 glucagon secretion E16.3
 glucose tolerance (test) (non-fasting) R73.09
 gravitational (G) forces or states (effect of) T75.81
 hair (color) (shaft) L67.9
  specified NEC L67.8
 hard tissue formation in pulp (dental) K04.3
 head movement R25.0
 heart
  rate R00.9
   specified NEC R00.8
  shadow R93.1
  sounds NEC R01.2
 hemoglobin (disease) —see also Disease,
   hemoglobin D58.2
  trait —see Trait, hemoglobin, abnormal
 histology NEC R89.7
 immunological findings R89.4
  in serum R76.9
   specified NEC R76.8
 increase in appetite R63.2
 involuntary movement —see Abnormal,
   movement, involuntary
 jaw closure M26.51
 karyotype R89.8
 kidney function test R94.4
 knee jerk R29.2
 leukocyte (cell) (differential) NEC D72.9
 liver function test (see also Elevated, liver
   function, test) R79.89
 loss of
  height R29.890
  weight R63.4
 mammogram NEC R92.8
  calcification (calculus) R92.1
  microcalcification R92.0
 Mantoux test R76.11
 movement (disorder) —see also Disorder,
   movement
  head R25.0
  involuntary R25.9
   fasciculation R25.3
   of head R25.0
   spasm R25.2
   specified type NEC R25.8
   tremor R25.1
 myoglobin (Aberdeen) (Annapolis) R89.7
 neonatal screening P09.9
  for
   congenital adrenal hyperplasia P09.2
   congenital endocrine disease P09.2
   congenital hematologic disorders P09.3
   critical congenital heart disease P09.5
   cystic fibrosis P09.4
   hemoglobinopathy P09.3
   hypothyroidism P09.2
   inborn errors of metabolism P09.1
   neonatal hearing loss P09.6
   red cell membrane defects P09.3
   sickle cell P09.3
   specified NEC P09.8
 oculomotor study R94.113
 palmar creases Q82.8
 Papanicolaou (smear)
  anus R85.619
   atypical squamous cells cannot exclude
      high grade squamous intraepithelial
      lesion (ASC-H) R85.611
   atypical squamous cells of undetermined
      significance (ASC-US) R85.610
   cytologic evidence of malignancy R85.614
   high grade squamous intraepithelial lesion
      (HGSIL) R85.613
   human papillomavirus (HPV) DNA test
    high risk positive R85.81
    low risk postive R85.82
   inadequate smear R85.615
   low grade squamous intraepithelial lesion
      (LGSIL) R85.612
   satisfactory anal smear but lacking
      transformation zone R85.616
   specified NEC R85.618
   unsatisfactory smear R85.615

Abnormal, abnormality, abnormalities
 — (Continued)
 Papanicolaou (smear) (Continued)
  bronchial washings R84.6
  cerebrospinal fluid R83.6
  cervix R87.619
   atypical squamous cells cannot exclude
      high grade squamous intraepithelial
      lesion (ASC-H) R87.611
   atypical squamous cells of undetermined
      significance (ASC-US) R87.610
   cytologic evidence of malignancy
      R87.614
   high grade squamous intraepithelial lesion
      (HGSIL) R87.613
   inadequate smear R87.615
   low grade squamous intraepithelial lesion
      (LGSIL) R87.612
   non-atypical endometrial cells R87.618
   satisfactory cervical smear but lacking
      transformation zone R87.616
   specified NEC R87.618
   thin preparaton R87.619
   unsatisfactory smear R87.615
  nasal secretions R84.6
  nipple discharge R89.6
  peritoneal fluid R85.69
  pleural fluid R84.6
  prostatic secretions R86.6
  saliva R85.69
  seminal fluid R86.6
  sites NEC R89.6
  sputum R84.6
  synovial fluid R89.6
  throat scrapings R84.6
  vagina R87.629
   atypical squamous cells cannot exclude
      high grade squamous intraepithelial
      lesion (ASC-H) R87.621
   atypical squamous cells of undetermined
      significance (ASC-US) R87.620
   cytologic evidence of malignancy
      R87.624
   high grade squamous intraepithelial lesion
      (HGSIL) R87.623
   inadequate smear R87.625
   low grade squamous intraepithelial lesion
      (LGSIL) R87.622
   specified NEC R87.628
   thin preparation R87.629
   unsatisfactory smear R87.625
  vulva R87.69
  wound secretions R89.6
 partial thromboplastin time (PTT) R79.1
 pelvis (bony) —see Deformity, pelvis
 percussion, chest (tympany) R09.89
 periods (grossly) —see Menstruation
 phonocardiogram R94.39
 plantar reflex R29.2
 plasma
  protein R77.9
   specified NEC R77.8
  viscosity R70.1
 pleural (folds) Q34.0
 posture R29.3
 product of conception O02.9
  specified type NEC O02.89
 prothrombin time (PT) R79.1
 pulmonary
  artery, congenital Q25.79
  function, newborn P28.89
  test results R94.2
 pulsations in neck R00.2
 pupillary H21.56-•
  function (reaction) (reflex) —see Anomaly,
    pupil, function
 radiological examination —see Abnormal,
   diagnostic imaging
 red blood cell(s) (morphology) (volume) R71.8
 reflex —see Reflex
 renal function test R94.4
 response to nerve stimulation R94.130
 retinal correspondence H53.31
 retinal function study R94.111
 rhythm, heart —see also Arrhythmia
 saliva —see Abnormal, specimen, digestive
   organs
 scan
  kidney R94.4
  liver R93.2
  thyroid R94.6

Abnormal, abnormality, abnormalities (Continued)
 secretion
  gastrin E16.4
  glucagon E16.3
 semen, seminal fluid —see Abnormal, specimen,
   male genital organs
 serum level (of)
  acid phosphatase R74.8
  alkaline phosphatase R74.8
  amylase R74.8
  enzymes R74.9
   specified NEC R74.8
  lipase R74.8
  triacylglycerol lipase R74.8
 shape
  gravid uterus —see Anomaly, uterus
 sinus venosus Q21.06
 size, tooth, teeth K00.2
 spacing, tooth, teeth, fully erupted M26.30
 specimen
  digestive organs (peritoneal fluid) (saliva)
    R85.9
   cytology R85.69
   drug level R85.2
   enzyme level R85.0
   histology R85.7
   hormones R85.1
   immunology R85.4
   microbiology R85.5
   nonmedicinal level R85.3
   specified type NEC R85.89
  female genital organs (secretions) (smears)
    R87.9
   cytology R87.69
    cervix R87.619
     human papillomavirus (HPV) DNA
       test
       high risk positive R87.810
       low risk positive R87.820
      inadequate (unsatisfactory) smear
        R87.615
     non-atypical endometrial cells R87.618
     specified NEC R87.618
    vagina R87.629
     human papillomavirus (HPV) DNA
       test
       high risk positive R87.811
       low risk positive R87.821
      inadequate (unsatisfactory) smear
        R87.625
    vulva R87.69
   drug level R87.2
   enzyme level R87.0
   histological R87.7
   hormones R87.1
   immunology R87.4
   microbiology R87.5
   nonmedicinal level R87.3
   specified type NEC R87.89
  male genital organs (prostatic secretions)
    (semen) R86.9
   cytology R86.6
   drug level R86.2
   enzyme level R86.0
   histological R86.7
   hormones R86.1
   immunology R86.4
   microbiology R86.5
   nonmedicinal level R86.3
   specified type NEC R86.8
  nipple discharge —see Abnormal, specimen,
    specified
  respiratory organs (bronchial washings) (nasal
    secretions) (pleural fluid) (sputum) R84.9
   cytology R84.6
   drug level R84.2
   enzyme level R84.0
   histology R84.7
   hormones R84.1
   immunology R84.4
   microbiology R84.5
   nonmedicinal level R84.3
   specified type NEC R84.8
  specified organ, system and tissue NOS R89.9
   cytology R89.6
   drug level R89.2
   enzyme level R89.0
   histology R89.7
   hormones R89.1
   immunology R89.4
   microbiology R89.5

Abnormal, abnormality, abnormalities — *(Continued)*
  specimen *(Continued)*
    specified organ, system and tissue *(Continued)*
      nonmedicinal level R89.3
      specified type NEC R89.8
    synovial fluid —*see* Abnormal, specimen, specified
    thorax (bronchial washings) (pleural fluids) — *see* Abnormal, specimen, respiratory organs
    vagina (secretion) (smear) R87.629
    vulva (secretion) (smear) R87.69
    wound secretion —*see* Abnormal, specimen, specified
   spermatozoa —*see* Abnormal, specimen, male genital organs
  sputum (amount) (color) (odor) R09.3
  stool (color) (contents) (mucus) R19.5
   bloody K92.1
   guaiac positive R19.5
  synchondrosis Q78.8
  thermography —*see also* Abnormal, diagnostic imaging R93.89
  thyroid-binding globulin E07.89
  tooth, teeth (form) (size) K00.2
  toxicology (findings) R78.9
  transport protein E88.09
  tumor marker NEC R97.8
  ultrasound results —*see* Abnormal, diagnostic imaging
  umbilical cord complicating delivery O69.9
  urination NEC R39.198
  urine (constituents) R82.90
   bile R82.2
   cytological examination R82.89
   drugs R82.5
   fat R82.0
   glucose R81
   heavy metals R82.6
   hemoglobin R82.3
   histological examination R82.89
   ketones R82.4
   microbiological examination (culture) R82.79
   myoglobin R82.1
   positive culture R82.79
   protein —*see* Proteinuria
   specified substance NEC R82.998
    chromoabnormality NEC R82.91
   substances nonmedical R82.6
  uterine hemorrhage —*see* Hemorrhage, uterus
  vectorcardiogram R94.39
  visually evoked potential (VEP) R94.112
  white blood cells D72.9
   specified NEC D72.89
  X-ray examination —*see* Abnormal, diagnostic imaging
Abnormity (any organ or part) —*see* Anomaly
Abocclusion M26.29
  hemolytic disease (newborn) P55.1
  incompatibility reaction ABO —*see* Complication(s), transfusion, incompatibility reaction, ABO
Abolition, language R48.8
Aborter, habitual or recurrent —*see* Loss (of), pregnancy, recurrent
Abortion (complete) (spontaneous) O03.9
  with
   retained products of conception —*see* Abortion, incomplete
  attempted (elective) (failed) O07.4
   complicated by O07.30
    afibrinogenemia O07.1
    cardiac arrest O07.36
    chemical damage of pelvic organ(s) O07.34
    circulatory collapse O07.31
    cystitis O07.38
    defibrination syndrome O07.1
    electrolyte imbalance O07.33
    embolism (air) (amniotic fluid) (blood clot) (fat) (pulmonary) (septic) (soap) O07.2
    endometritis O07.0
    genital tract and pelvic infection O07.0
    hemolysis O07.1
    hemorrhage (delayed) (excessive) O07.1
    infection
     genital tract or pelvic O07.0
     urinary tract tract O07.38
    intravascular coagulation O07.1
    laceration of pelvic organ(s) O07.34
    metabolic disorder O07.33

Abortion *(Continued)*
  attempted *(Continued)*
   complicated by *(Continued)*
    oliguria O07.32
    oophoritis O07.0
    parametritis O07.0
    pelvic peritonitis O07.0
    perforation of pelvic organ(s) O07.34
    renal failure or shutdown O07.32
    salpingitis or salpingo-oophoritis O07.0
    sepsis O07.37
    shock O07.31
    specified condition NEC O07.39
    tubular necrosis (renal) O07.32
    uremia O07.32
    urinary tract infection O07.38
    venous complication NEC O07.35
     embolism (air) (amniotic fluid) (blood clot) (fat) (pulmonary) (septic) (soap) O07.2
  complicated (by) (following) O03.80
   afibrinogenemia O03.6
   cardiac arrest O03.86
   chemical damage of pelvic organ(s) O03.84
   circulatory collapse O03.81
   cystitis O03.88
   defibrination syndrome O03.6
   electrolyte imbalance O03.83
   embolism (air) (amniotic fluid) (blood clot) (fat) (pulmonary) (septic) (soap) O03.7
   endometritis O03.5
   genital tract and pelvic infection O03.5
   hemolysis O03.6
   hemorrhage (delayed) (excessive) O03.6
   infection
    genital tract or pelvic O03.5
    urinary tract O03.88
   intravascular coagulation O03.6
   laceration of pelvic organ(s) O03.84
   metabolic disorder O03.83
   oliguria O03.82
   oophoritis O03.5
   parametritis O03.5
   pelvic peritonitis O03.5
   perforation of pelvic organ(s) O03.84
   renal failure or shutdown O03.82
   salpingitis or salpingo-oophoritis O03.5
   sepsis O03.87
   shock O03.81
   specified condition NEC O03.89
   tubular necrosis (renal) O03.82
   uremia O03.82
   urinary tract infection O03.88
   venous complication NEC O03.85
    embolism (air) (amniotic fluid) (blood clot) (fat) (pulmonary) (septic) (soap) O03.7
  failed —*see* Abortion, attempted
  habitual or recurrent N96
   with current abortion —*see* categories O03-O04
   without current pregnancy N96
   care in current pregnancy O26.2-●
  incomplete (spontaneous) O03.4
   complicated (by) (following) O03.30
    afibrinogenemia O03.1
    cardiac arrest O03.36
    chemical damage of pelvic organ(s) O03.34
    circulatory collapse O03.31
    cystitis O03.38
    defibrination syndrome O03.1
    electrolyte imbalance O03.33
    embolism (air) (amniotic fluid) (blood clot) (fat) (pulmonary) (septic) (soap) O03.2
    endometritis O03.0
    genital tract and pelvic infection O03.0
    hemolysis O03.1
    hemorrhage (delayed) (excessive) O03.1
    infection
     genital tract or pelvic O03.0
     urinary tract O03.38
    intravascular coagulation O03.1
    laceration of pelvic organ(s) O03.34
    metabolic disorder O03.33
    oliguria O03.32
    oophoritis O03.0
    parametritis O03.0
    pelvic peritonitis O03.0
    perforation of pelvic organ(s) O03.34
    renal failure or shutdown O03.32
    salpingitis or salpingo-oophoritis O03.0
    sepsis O03.37

Abortion *(Continued)*
  incomplete (spontaneous) *(Continued)*
   complicated *(Continued)*
    shock O03.31
    specified condition NEC O03.39
    tubular necrosis (renal) O03.32
    uremia O03.32
    urinary infection O03.38
    venous complication NEC O03.35
     embolism (air) (amniotic fluid) (blood clot) (fat) (pulmonary) (septic) (soap) O03.2
  induced (encounter for) Z33.2
   complicated by O04.80
    afibrinogenemia O04.6
    cardiac arrest O04.86
    chemical damage of pelvic organ(s) O04.84
    circulatory collapse O04.81
    cystitis O04.88
    defibrination syndrome O04.6
    electrolyte imbalance O04.83
    embolism (air) (amniotic fluid) (blood clot) (fat) (pulmonary) (septic) (soap) O04.7
    endometritis O04.5
    genital tract and pelvic infection O04.5
    hemolysis O04.6
    hemorrhage (delayed) (excessive) O04.6
    infection
     genital tract or pelvic O04.5
     urinary tract O04.88
    intravascular coagulation O04.6
    laceration of pelvic organ(s) O04.84
    metabolic disorder O04.83
    oliguria O04.82
    oophoritis O04.5
    parametritis O04.5
    pelvic peritonitis O04.5
    perforation of pelvic organ(s) O04.84
    renal failure or shutdown O04.82
    salpingitis or salpingo-oophoritis O04.5
    sepsis O04.87
    shock O04.81
    specified condition NEC O04.89
    tubular necrosis (renal) O04.82
    uremia O04.82
    urinary tract infection O04.88
    venous complication NEC O04.85
     embolism (air) (amniotic fluid) (blood clot) (fat) (pulmonary) (septic) (soap) O04.7
  inevitable O03.4
  missed O02.1
  spontaneous —*see* Abortion (complete) (spontaneous)
   threatened O20.0
  threatened (spontaneous) O20.0
  tubal O00.10-●
   with intrauterine pregnancy O00.11-
Abortus fever A23.1
Aboulomania F60.7
Abrami's disease D59.8
Abramov-Fiedler myocarditis (acute isolated myocarditis) I40.1
Abrasion T14.8
  abdomen, abdominal (wall) S30.811
  alveolar process S00.512
  ankle S90.51-●
  antecubital space —*see* Abrasion, elbow
  anus S30.817
  arm (upper) S40.81-●
  auditory canal —*see* Abrasion, ear
  auricle —*see* Abrasion, ear
  axilla —*see* Abrasion, arm
  back, lower S30.810
  breast S20.11-●
  brow S00.81
  buttock S30.810
  calf —*see* Abrasion, leg
  canthus —*see* Abrasion, eyelid
  cheek S00.81
   internal S00.512
  chest wall —*see* Abrasion, thorax
  chin S00.81
  clitoris S30.814
  cornea S05.0-●
  costal region —*see* Abrasion, thorax
  dental K03.1
  digit(s)
   foot —*see* Abrasion, toe
   hand —*see* Abrasion, finger
  ear S00.41-●

▶ New   ⇒ Revised   ~~deleted~~ Deleted   ● Use Additional Character(s)

Abrasion (Continued)
elbow S50.31-●
epididymis S30.813
epigastric region S30.811
epiglottis S10.11
esophagus (thoracic) S27.818
 cervical S10.11
eyebrow —see Abrasion, eyelid
eyelid S00.21-●
face S00.81
finger(s) S60.41-●
 index S60.41-●
 little S60.41-●
 middle S60.41-●
 ring S60.41-●
flank S30.811
foot (except toe(s) alone) S90.81-●
 toe —see Abrasion, toe
forearm S50.81-●
 elbow only —see Abrasion, elbow
forehead S00.81
genital organs, external
 female S30.816
 male S30.815
groin S30.811
gum S00.512
hand S60.51-●
head S00.91
 ear —see Abrasion, ear
 eyelid —see Abrasion, eyelid
 lip S00.511
 nose S00.31
 oral cavity S00.512
 scalp S00.01
 specified site NEC S00.81
heel —see Abrasion, foot
hip S70.21-●
inguinal region S30.811
interscapular region S20.419
jaw S00.81
knee S80.21-●
labium (majus) (minus) S30.814
larynx S10.11
leg (lower) S80.81-●
 knee —see Abrasion, knee
 upper —see Abrasion, thigh
lip S00.511
lower back S30.810
lumbar region S30.810
malar region S00.81
mammary —see Abrasion, breast
mastoid region S00.81
mouth S00.512
nail
 finger —see Abrasion, finger
 toe —see Abrasion, toe
nape S10.81
nasal S00.31
neck S10.91
 specified site NEC S10.81
 throat S10.11
nose S00.31
occipital region S00.01
oral cavity S00.512
orbital region —see Abrasion, eyelid
palate S00.512
palm —see Abrasion, hand
parietal region S00.01
pelvis S30.810
penis S30.812
perineum
 female S30.814
 male S30.810
periocular area —see Abrasion, eyelid
phalanges
 finger —see Abrasion, finger
 toe —see Abrasion, toe
pharynx S10.11
pinna —see Abrasion, ear
popliteal space —see Abrasion, knee
prepuce S30.812
pubic region S30.810
pudendum
 female S30.816
 male S30.815
sacral region S30.810
scalp S00.01
scapular region —see Abrasion, shoulder
scrotum S30.813
shin —see Abrasion, leg
shoulder S40.21-●

Abrasion (Continued)
skin NEC T14.8
sternal region S20.319
submaxillary region S00.81
submental region S00.81
subungual
 finger(s) —see Abrasion, finger
 toe(s) —see Abrasion, toe
supraclavicular fossa S10.81
supraorbital S00.81
temple S00.81
temporal region S00.81
testis S30.813
thigh S70.31-●
thorax, thoracic (wall) S20.91
 back S20.91
 front S20.31-●
throat S10.11
thumb S60.31-●
toe(s) (lesser) S90.416
 great S90.41-●
tongue S00.512
tooth, teeth (dentifrice) (habitual) (hard tissues)
 (occupational) (ritual) (traditional) K03.1
trachea S10.11
tunica vaginalis S30.813
tympanum, tympanic membrane —see Abrasion,
 ear
uvula S00.512
vagina S30.814
vocal cords S10.11
vulva S30.814
wrist S60.81-●
Abrism —see Poisoning, food, noxious, plant
Abruptio placentae O45.9-●
with
 afibrinogenemia O45.01-●
 coagulation defect O45.00-●
  specified NEC O45.09-●
 disseminated intravascular coagulation
  O45.02-●
 hypofibrinogenemia O45.01-●
 specified NEC O45.8-●
Abruption, placenta —see Abruptio placentae
Abscess (connective tissue) (embolic) (fistulous)
 (infective) (metastatic) (multiple) (pernicious)
 (pyogenic) (septic) L02.91
with
 diverticular disease (intestine) K57.80
  with bleeding K57.81
  large intestine K57.20
   with
    bleeding K57.21
    small intestine K57.40
     with bleeding K57.41
  small intestine K57.00
   with
    bleeding K57.01
    large intestine K57.40
     with bleeding K57.41
 lymphangitis - code by site under Abscess
abdomen, abdominal
 cavity K65.1
 wall L02.211
abdominopelvic K65.1
accessory sinus —see Sinusitis
adrenal (capsule) (gland) E27.8
alveolar K04.7
 with sinus K04.6
ambic A06.4
 brain (and liver or lung abscess) A06.6
 genitourinary tract A06.82
 liver (without mention of brain or lung
  abscess) A06.4
 lung (and liver) (without mention of brain
  abscess) A06.5
 specified site NEC A06.89
 spleen A06.89
anaerobic A48.0
ankle —see Abscess, lower limb
anorectal K61.2
antecubital space —see Abscess, upper limb
antrum (chronic) (Highmore) —see Sinusitis,
 maxillary
anus K61.0
apical (tooth) K04.7
 with sinus (alveolar) K04.6
appendix K35.33
areola (acute) (chronic) (nonpuerperal) N61.1
 puerperal, postpartum or gestational —see
  Infection, nipple

Abscess (Continued)
arm (any part) —see Abscess, upper limb
artery (wall) I77.89
atheromatous I77.2
auricle, ear —see Abscess, ear, external
axilla (region) L02.41-●
 lymph gland or node L04.2
back (any part, except buttock) L02.212
Bartholin's gland N75.1
 with
  abortion —see Abortion, by type
   complicated by, sepsis
  ectopic or molar pregnancy O08.0
 following ectopic or molar pregnancy O08.0
Bezold's —see Mastoiditis, acute
bilharziasis B65.1
bladder (wall) —see Cystitis, specified type NEC
bone (subperiosteal) —see also Osteomyelitis,
 specified type NEC
 accessory sinus (chronic) —see Sinusitis
 chronic or old —see Osteomyelitis, chronic
 jaw (lower) (upper) M27.2
 mastoid —see Mastoiditis, acute, subperiosteal
 petrous —see Petrositis
 spinal (tuberculous) A18.01
  nontuberculous —see Osteomyelitis,
   vertebra
bowel K63.0
brain (any part) (cystic) (otogenic) G06.0
 amebic (with abscess of any other site) A06.6
 gonococcal A54.82
 pheomycotic (chromomycotic) B43.1
 tuberculous A17.81
breast (acute) (chronic) (nonpuerperal) N61.1
 newborn P39.0
 puerperal, postpartum, gestational —see
  Mastitis, obstetric, purulent
broad ligament N73.2
 acute N73.0
 chronic N73.1
Brodie's (localized) (chronic) M86.8X-●
bronchi J98.09
buccal cavity K12.2
bulbourethral gland N34.0
bursa M71.00
 ankle M71.07-●
 elbow M71.02-●
 foot M71.07-●
 hand M71.04-●
 hip M71.05-●
 knee M71.06-●
 multiple sites M71.09
 pharyngeal J39.1
 shoulder M71.01-●
 specified site NEC M71.08
 wrist M71.03-●
buttock L02.31
canthus —see Blepharoconjunctivitis
cartilage —see Disorder, cartilage, specified type
 NEC
cecum K35.33
cerebellum, cerebellar G06.0
 sequelae G09
cerebral (embolic) G06.0
 sequelae G09
cervical (meaning neck) L02.11
 lymph gland or node L04.0
cervix (stump) (uteri) —see Cervicitis
cheek (external) L02.01
 inner K12.2
chest J86.9
 with fistula J86.0
 wall L02.213
chin L02.01
choroid —see Inflammation, chorioretinal
circumtonsillar J36
cold (lung) (tuberculous) —see also Tuberculosis,
 abscess, lung
 articular —see Tuberculosis, joint
colon (wall) K63.0
colostomy K94.02
conjunctiva —see Conjunctivitis, acute
cornea H16.31-●
corpus
 cavernosum N48.21
 luteum —see Oophoritis
Cowper's gland N34.0
cranium G06.0
cul-de-sac (Douglas') (posterior) —see Peritonitis,
 pelvic, female
cutaneous —see Abscess, by site

Abscess *(Continued)*
 dental K04.7
  with sinus (alveolar) K04.6
 dentoalveolar K04.7
  with sinus K04.6
 diaphragm, diaphragmatic K65.1
 Douglas' cul-de-sac or pouch —*see* Peritonitis,
   pelvic, female
 Dubois A50.59
 ear (middle) —*see also* Otitis, media, suppurative
  acute —*see* Otitis, media, suppurative, acute
  external H60.0-●
 entamebic —*see* Abscess, amebic
 enterostomy K94.12
 epididymis N45.4
 epidural G06.2
  brain G06.0
  spinal cord G06.1
 epiglottis J38.7
 epiploon, epiploic K65.1
 erysipelatous —*see* Erysipelas
 esophagus K20.80
 ethmoid (bone) (chronic) (sinus) J32.2
 external auditory canal —*see* Abscess, ear,
   external
 extradural G06.2
  brain G06.0
   sequelae G09
  spinal cord G06.1
 extraperitoneal K68.19
 eye —*see* Endophthalmitis, purulent
 eyelid H00.03-●
 face (any part, except ear, eye and nose)
   L02.01
 fallopian tube —*see* Salpingitis
 fascia M72.8
 fauces J39.1
 fecal K63.0
 femoral (region) —*see* Abscess, lower limb
 filaria, filarial —*see* Infestation, filarial
 finger (any) —*see also* Abscess, hand
  nail —*see* Cellulitis, finger
 foot L02.61-●
 forehead L02.01
 frontal sinus (chronic) J32.1
 gallbladder K81.0
 genital organ or tract
  female (external) N76.4
  male N49.9
   multiple sites N49.8
   specified NEC N49.8
 gestational mammary O91.11-●
 gestational subareolar O91.11-●
 gingival
  aggressive K05.20
   generalized K05.229
    moderate K05.222
    severe K05.223
    slight K05.221
   localized K05.219
    moderate K05.212
    severe K05.213
    slight K05.211
 gland, glandular (lymph) (acute) —*see*
   Lymphadenitis, acute
 gluteal (region) L02.31
 gonorrheal —*see* Gonococcus
 groin L02.214
 gum
  aggressive K05.20
   generalized K05.229
    moderate K05.222
    severe K05.223
    slight K05.221
   localized K05.219
    moderate K05.212
    severe K05.213
    slight K05.211
 hand L02.51-●
 head NEC L02.811
  face (any part, except ear, eye and nose)
    L02.01
 heart —*see* Carditis
 heel —*see* Abscess, foot
 helminthic —*see* Infestation, helminth
 hepatic (cholangitic) (hematogenic)
   (lymphogenic) (pylephlebitic) K75.0
  amebic A06.4
 hip (region) —*see* Abscess, lower limb
 horseshoe K61.31
 ileocecal K35.33
 ileostomy (bud) K94.12

Abscess *(Continued)*
 iliac (region) L02.214
  fossa K35.33
 infraclavicular (fossa) —*see* Abscess, upper limb
 inguinal (region) L02.214
  lymph gland or node L04.1
 intersphincteric K61.4
 intestine, intestinal NEC K63.0
  rectal K61.1
 intra-abdominal —*see also* Abscess, peritoneum
   K65.1
  following procedure T81.43
   obstetrical O86.03
  postprocedural T81.43
   retroperitoneal K68.11
 intracranial G06.0
 intramammary —*see* Abscess, breast
 intramuscular, following procedure T81.44
  obstetrical O86.02
 intraorbital —*see* Abscess, orbit
 intraperitoneal K65.1
 intrasphincteric (anus) K61.4
 intraspinal G06.1
 intratonsillar J36
 ischiorectal (fossa) (specified NEC) K61.39
 jaw (bone) (lower) (upper) M27.2
 joint —*see* Arthritis, pyogenic or pyemic
  spine (tuberculous) A18.01
   nontuberculous —*see* Spondylopathy,
     infective
 kidney N15.1
  with calculus N20.0
   with hydronephrosis N13.6
  puerperal (postpartum) O86.21
 knee —*see also* Abscess, lower limb
  joint M00.9
 labium (majus) (minus) N76.4
 lacrimal
  caruncle —*see* Inflammation, lacrimal,
    passages, acute
  gland —*see* Dacryoadenitis
  passages (duct) (sac) —*see* Inflammation,
    lacrimal, passages, acute
 lacunar N34.0
 larynx J38.7
 lateral (alveolar) K04.7
  with sinus K04.6
 leg (any part) —*see* Abscess, lower limb
 lens H27.8
 lingual K14.0
  tonsil J36
 lip K13.0
 Littre's gland N34.0
 liver (cholangitic) (hematogenic) (lymphogenic)
   (pylephlebitic) (pyogenic) K75.0
  amebic (due to Entamoeba histolytica)
    (dysenteric) (tropical) A06.4
   with
    brain abscess (and liver or lung abscess)
      A06.6
    lung abscess A06.5
 loin (region) L02.211
 lower limb L02.41-●
 lumbar (tuberculous) A18.01
  nontuberculous L02.212
 lung (miliary) (putrid) J85.2
  with pneumonia J85.1
   due to specified organism (*see* Pneumonia,
     in (due to))
  amebic (with liver abscess) A06.5
   with
    brain abscess A06.6
    pneumonia A06.5
 lymph, lymphatic, gland or node (acute) —*see*
   also Lymphadenitis, acute
  mesentery I88.0
 malar M27.2
 mammary gland —*see* Abscess, breast
 marginal, anus K61.0
 mastoid —*see* Mastoiditis, acute
 maxilla, maxillary M27.2
  molar (tooth) K04.7
   with sinus K04.6
  premolar K04.7
  sinus (chronic) J32.0
 mediastinum J85.3
 meibomian gland —*see* Hordeolum
 meninges G06.2
 mesentery, mesenteric K65.1
 mesosalpinx —*see* Salpingitis
 mons pubis L02.215
 mouth (floor) K12.2

Abscess *(Continued)*
 muscle —*see* Myositis, infective
 myocardium I40.0
 nabothian (follicle) —*see* Cervicitis
 nasal J32.9
 nasopharyngeal J39.1
 navel L02.216
  newborn P38.9
   with mild hemorrhage P38.1
   without hemorrhage P38.9
 neck (region) L02.11
  lymph gland or node L04.0
 nephritic —*see* Abscess, kidney
 nipple N61.1
  associated with
   lactation —*see* Pregnancy, complicated by
   pregnancy —*see* Pregnancy, complicated by
 nose (external) (fossa) (septum) J34.0
  sinus (chronic) —*see* Sinusitis
 omentum K65.1
 operative wound T81.49
 orbit, orbital —*see* Cellulitis, orbit
 otogenic G06.0
 ovary, ovarian (corpus luteum) —*see* Oophoritis
 oviduct —*see* Oophoritis
 palate (soft) K12.2
  hard M27.2
 palmar (space) —*see* Abscess, hand
 pancreas (duct) —*see* Pancreatitis, acute
 parafrenal N48.21
 parametric, parametrium N73.2
  acute N73.0
  chronic N73.1
 paranephric N15.1
 parapancreatic —*see* Pancreatitis, acute
 parapharyngeal J39.0
 pararectal K61.1
 parasinus —*see* Sinusitis
 parauterine (*see also* Disease, pelvis,
   inflammatory) N73.2
 paravaginal —*see* Vaginitis
 parietal region (scalp) L02.811
 parodontal —*see* Periodontitis, aggressive,
   localized
 parotid (duct) (gland) K11.3
  region K12.2
 pectoral (region) L02.213
 pelvis, pelvic
  female —*see* Disease, pelvis, inflammatory
  male, peritoneal K65.1
 penis N48.21
  gonococcal (accessory gland) (periurethral)
    A54.1
 perianal K61.0
 periapical K04.7
  with sinus (alveolar) K04.6
 periappendicular K35.33
 pericardial I30.1
 pericecal K35.33
 pericemental —*see* Periodontitis, aggressive,
   localized
 pericholecystic —*see* Cholecystitis, acute
 pericoronal —*see* Periodontitis, aggressive,
   localized
 peridental —*see* Periodontitis, aggressive, localized
 perimetric —*see also* Disease, pelvis,
   inflammatory N73.2
 perinephric, perinephritic —*see* Abscess, kidney
 perineum, perineal (superficial) L02.215
  urethra N34.0
 periodontal (parietal) —*see* Periodontitis,
   aggressive, localized
  apical K04.7
 periosteum, periosteal —*see also* Osteomyelitis,
   specified type NEC
  with osteomyelitis —*see also* Osteomyelitis,
    specified type NEC
   acute —*see* Osteomyelitis, acute
   chronic —*see* Osteomyelitis, chronic
 peripharyngeal J39.0
 peripleuritic J86.9
  with fistula J86.0
 periprostatic N41.2
 perirectal K61.1
 perirenal (tissue) —*see* Abscess, kidney
 perisinuous (nose) —*see* Sinusitis
 peritoneum, peritoneal (perforated) (ruptured)
   K65.1
  with appendicitis (*see also* Appendicitis) K35.33
  pelvic
   female —*see* Peritonitis, pelvic, female
   male K65.1

▶ New   ⟹ Revised   ~~deleted~~ Deleted   ● Use Additional Character(s)

Abscess —(Continued)
  peritoneum, peritoneal (Continued)
    postoperative T81.43
    puerperal, postpartum, childbirth O85
    tuberculous A18.31
  peritonsillar J36
  perityphlic K35.33
  periureteral N28.89
  periurethral N34.0
    gonococcal (accessory gland) (periurethral)
        A54.1
  periuterine —see also Disease, pelvis,
      inflammatory N73.2
  perivesical —see Cystitis, specified type NEC
  petrous bone —see Petrositis
  phagedenic NOS L02.91
    chancroid A57
  pharynx, pharyngeal (lateral) J39.1
  pilonidal L05.01
  pituitary (gland) E23.6
  pleura J86.9
    with fistula J86.0
  popliteal —see Abscess, lower limb
  postcecal K35.33
  postlaryngeal J38.7
  postnasal J34.0
  postoperative (any site) (see also Infection,
      postoperative wound) T81.49
    retroperitoneal K68.11
  postpharyngeal J39.0
  posttonsillar J36
  post-typhoid A01.09
  pouch of Douglas —see Peritonitis, pelvic, female
  premammary —see Abscess, breast
  prepatellar —see Abscess, lower limb
  presacral K68.19
  prostate N41.2
    gonococcal (acute) (chronic) A54.22
  psoas muscle K68.12
  puerperal - code by site under Puerperal, abscess
  pulmonary —see Abscess, lung
  pulp, pulpal (dental) K04.01
    irreversible K04.02
    reversible K04.01
  rectovaginal septum K63.0
  rectovesical —see Cystitis, specified type NEC
  rectum K61.1
  renal —see Abscess, kidney
  retina —see Inflammation, chorioretinal
  retrobulbar —see Abscess, orbit
  retrocecal K65.1
  retrolaryngeal J38.7
  retromammary —see Abscess, breast
  retroperitoneal NEC K68.19
    postprocedural K68.11
  retropharyngeal J39.0
  retrouterine —see Peritonitis, pelvic, female
  retrovesical —see Cystitis, specified type NEC
  root, tooth K04.7
    with sinus (alveolar) K04.6
  round ligament —see also Disease, pelvis,
      inflammatory N73.2
  rupture (spontaneous) NOS L02.91
  sacrum (tuberculous)
    nontuberculous M46.28
  salivary (duct) (gland) K11.3
  scalp (any part) L02.811
  scapular —see Osteomyelitis, specified type NEC
  sclera —see Scleritis
  scrofulous (tuberculous) A18.2
  scrotum N49.2
  seminal vesicle N49.0
  septal, dental K04.7
    with sinus (alveolar) K04.6
  serous —see Periostitis
  shoulder (region) —see Abscess, upper limb
  sigmoid K63.0
  sinus (accessory) (chronic) (nasal) —see also
      Sinusitis
    intracranial venous (any) G06.0
  Skene's duct or gland N34.0
  skin —see Abscess, by site
  specified site NEC L02.818
  spermatic cord N49.1
  sphenoidal (sinus) (chronic) J32.3
  spinal cord (any part) (staphylococcal) G06.1
    tuberculous A17.81
  spine (column) (tuberculous) A18.01
    epidural G06.1
    nontuberculous —see Osteomyelitis, vertebra
  spleen D73.3
    amebic A06.89

Abscess (Continued)
  stitch T81.41
    following an obstetrical procedure O86.01
  subarachnoid G06.2
    brain G06.0
    spinal cord G06.1
  subareolar —see Abscess, breast
  subcecal K35.33
  subcutaneous —see also Abscess, by site
    following procedure T81.41
      obstetrical O86.01
    pheomycotic (chromomycotic) B43.2
  subdiaphragmatic K65.1
  subdural G06.2
    brain G06.0
      sequelae G09
    spinal cord G06.1
  sub-fascial, following an obstetrical procedure
      O86.02
  subgaleal L02.811
  subhepatic K65.1
  sublingual K12.2
    gland K11.3
  submammary —see Abscess, breast
  submandibular (region) (space) (triangle) K12.2
    gland K11.3
  submaxillary (region) L02.01
    gland K11.3
  submental L02.01
    gland K11.3
  subperiosteal —see Osteomyelitis, specified type
      NEC
  subphrenic K65.1
    following an obstetrical procedure O86.03
    postoperative T81.43
  suburethral N34.0
  sudoriparous L75.8
  supraclavicular (fossa) —see Abscess, upper limb
  supralevator K61.5
  suprapelvic, acute N73.0
  suprarenal (capsule) (gland) E27.8
  sweat gland L74.8
  tear duct —see Inflammation, lacrimal, passages,
      acute
  temple L02.01
  temporal region L02.01
  temporosphenoidal G06.0
  tendon (sheath) M65.00
    ankle M65.07-●
    foot M65.07-●
    forearm M65.03-●
    hand M65.04-●
    lower leg M65.06-●
    pelvic region M65.05-●
    shoulder region M65.01-●
    specified site NEC M65.08
    thigh M65.05-●
    upper arm M65.02-●
  testis N45.4
  thigh —see Abscess, lower limb
  thorax J86.9
    with fistula J86.0
  throat J39.1
  thumb —see also Abscess, hand
    nail —see Cellulitis, finger
  thymus (gland) E32.1
  thyroid (gland) E06.0
  toe (any) —see also Abscess, foot
    nail —see Cellulitis, toe
  tongue (staphylococcal) K14.0
  tonsil(s) (lingual) J36
  tonsillopharyngeal J36
  tooth, teeth (root) K04.7
    with sinus (alveolar) K04.6
    supporting structures NEC —see Periodontitis,
        aggressive, localized
  trachea J39.8
  trunk L02.219
    abdominal wall L02.211
    back L02.212
    chest wall L02.213
    groin L02.214
    perineum L02.215
    umbilicus L02.216
  tubal —see Salpingitis
  tuberculous —see Tuberculosis, abscess
  tubo-ovarian —see Salpingo-oophoritis
  tunica vaginalis N49.1
  umbilicus L02.216
  upper
    limb L02.41-●
    respiratory J39.8

Abscess (Continued)
  urethral (gland) N34.0
  urinary N34.0
  uterus, uterine (wall) —see also Endometritis
    ligament —see also Disease, pelvis,
        inflammatory N73.2
    neck —see Cervicitis
  uvula K12.2
  vagina (wall) —see Vaginitis
  vaginorectal —see Vaginitis
  vas deferens N49.1
  vermiform appendix K35.33
  vertebra (column) (tuberculous) A18.01
    nontuberculous —see Osteomyelitis, vertebra
  vesical —see Cystitis, specified type NEC
  vesico-uterine pouch —see Peritonitis, pelvic,
      female
  vitreous (humor) —see Endophthalmitis,
      purulent
  vocal cord J38.3
  von Bezold's —see Mastoiditis, acute
  vulva N76.4
  vulvovaginal gland N75.1
  web space —see Abscess, hand
  wound T81.49
  wrist —see Abscess, upper limb
Absence (of) (organ or part) (complete or partial)
  adrenal (gland) (congenital) Q89.1
    acquired E89.6
  albumin in blood E88.09
  alimentary tract (congenital) Q45.8
    upper Q40.8
  alveolar process (acquired) —see Anomaly,
      alveolar
  ankle (acquired) Z89.44-●
  anus (congenital) Q42.3
    with fistula Q42.2
  aorta (congenital) Q25.41
  appendix, congenital Q42.8
  arm (acquired) Z89.20-●
    above elbow Z89.22-●
      congenital (with hand present) —see
          Agenesis, arm, with hand present
          and hand —see Agenesis, forearm, and
              hand
    below elbow Z89.21-●
      congenital (with hand present) —see
          Agenesis, arm, with hand present
          and hand —see Agenesis, forearm, and
              hand
    congenital —see Defect, reduction, upper limb
    shoulder (following explantation of shoulder
        joint prosthesis) (joint) (with or without
        presence of antibiotic-impregnated
        cement spacer) Z89.23-●
      congenital (with hand present) —see
          Agenesis, arm, with hand present
  artery (congenital) (peripheral) Q27.8
    brain Q28.3
    coronary Q24.5
    pulmonary Q25.79
    specified NEC Q27.8
    umbilical Q27.0
  atrial septum (congenital) Q21.19
  auditory canal (congenital) (external) Q16.1
  auricle (ear), congenital Q16.0
  bile, biliary duct, congenital Q44.5
  bladder (acquired) Z90.6
    congenital Q64.5
  bowel sounds R19.11
  brain Q00.0
    part of Q04.3
  breast(s) (and nipple(s)) (acquired) Z90.1-●
    congenital Q83.8
  broad ligament Q50.6
  bronchus (congenital) Q32.4
  canaliculus lacrimalis, congenital Q10.4
  cerebellum (vermis) Q04.3
  cervix (acquired) (with uterus) Z90.710
    with remaining uterus Z90.712
    congenital Q51.5
  chin, congenital Q18.8
  cilia, (congenital) Q10.3
    acquired —see Madarosis
  clitoris (congenital) Q52.6
  coccyx, congenital Q76.49
  cold sense R20.8
  congenital
    lumen —see Atresia
    organ or site NEC —see Agenesis
    septum —see Imperfect, closure
  corpus callosum Q04.0

Absence *(Continued)*
  cricoid cartilage, congenital Q31.8
  diaphragm (with hernia), congenital Q79.1
  digestive organ(s) or tract, congenital Q45.8
    acquired NEC Z90.49
    upper Q40.8
  ductus arteriosus Q28.8
  duodenum (acquired) Z90.49
    congenital Q41.0
  ear, congenital Q16.9
    acquired H93.8-●
    auricle Q16.0
    external Q16.0
    inner Q16.5
    lobe, lobule Q17.8
    middle, except ossicles Q16.4
      ossicles Q16.3
    ossicles Q16.3
  ejaculatory duct (congenital) Q55.4
  endocrine gland (congenital) NEC Q89.2
    acquired E89.89
  epididymis (congenital) Q55.4
    acquired Z90.79
  epiglottis, congenital Q31.8
  esophagus (congenital) Q39.8
    acquired (partial) Z90.49
  eustachian tube (congenital) Q16.2
  extremity (acquired) Z89.9
    congenital Q73.0
    knee (following explanation of knee joint
      prosthesis) (joint) (with or without
      presence of antibiotic-impregnated
      cement spacer) Z89.52-●
    lower (above knee) Z89.619
      below knee Z89.51-●
    upper —*see* Absence, arm
  eye (acquired) Z90.01
    congenital Q11.1
    muscle (congenital) Q10.3
  eyeball (acquired) Z90.01
  eyelid (fold) (congenital) Q10.3
    acquired Z90.01
  face, specified part NEC Q18.8
  fallopian tube(s) (acquired) Z90.79
    congenital Q50.6
  family member (causing problem in home)
    NEC —*see also* Disruption, family
    Z63.32
  femur, congenital —*see* Defect, reduction, lower
    limb, longitudinal, femur
  fibrinogen (congenital) D68.2
    acquired D65
  finger(s) (acquired) Z89.02-●
    congenital —*see* Agenesis, hand
  foot (acquired) Z89.43-●
    congenital —*see* Agenesis, foot
  forearm (acquired) —*see* Absence, arm, below
    elbow
  gallbladder (acquired) Z90.49
    congenital Q44.0
  gamma globulin in blood D80.1
    hereditary D80.0
  genital organs
    acquired (female) (male) Z90.79
    female, congenital Q52.8
      external Q52.71
      internal NEC Q52.8
    male, congenital Q55.8
  genitourinary organs, congenital NEC
    female Q52.8
    male Q55.8
  globe (acquired) Z90.01
    congenital Q11.1
  glottis, congenital Q31.8
  hand and wrist (acquired) Z89.11-●
    congenital —*see* Agenesis, hand
  head, part (acquired) NEC Z90.09
  heat sense R20.8
  hip (following explanation of hip joint
    prosthesis) (joint) (with or without presence
    of antibiotic-impregnated cement spacer)
    Z89.62-●
  hymen (congenital) Q52.4
  ileum (acquired) Z90.49
    congenital Q41.2
  immunoglobulin, isolated NEC D80.3
    IgA D80.2
    IgG D80.3
    IgM D80.4
  incus (acquired) —*see* Loss, ossicles, ear
    congenital Q16.3
  inner ear, congenital Q16.5

Absence *(Continued)*
  intestine (acquired) (small) Z90.49
    congenital Q41.9
      specified NEC Q41.8
    large Z90.49
      congenital Q42.9
        specified NEC Q42.8
  iris, congenital Q13.1
  jejunum (acquired) Z90.49
    congenital Q41.1
  joint
    acquired
      hip (following explanation of hip joint
        prosthesis) (with or without presence
        of antibiotic-impregnated cement
        spacer) Z89.62-●
      knee (following explanation of knee joint
        prosthesis) (with or without presence
        of antibiotic-impregnated cement
        spacer) Z89.52-●
      shoulder (following explanation of
        shoulder joint prosthesis) (with or
        without presence of antibiotic-
        impregnated cement spacer) Z89.23-●
    congenital NEC Q74.8
  kidney(s) (acquired) Z90.5
    congenital Q60.2
      bilateral Q60.1
      unilateral Q60.0
  knee (following explanation of knee joint
    prosthesis) (joint) (with or without presence
    of antibiotic-impregnated cement spacer)
    Z89.52-●
  labyrinth, membranous Q16.5
  larynx (congenital) Q31.8
    acquired Z90.02
  leg (acquired) (above knee) Z89.61-●
    below knee (acquired) Z89.51-●
    congenital —*see* Defect, reduction, lower
      limb
  lens (acquired) —*see also* Aphakia
    congenital Q12.3
    post cataract extraction Z98.4-●
  limb (acquired) —*see* Absence, extremity
  lip Q38.6
  liver (congenital) Q44.79
  lung (fissure) (lobe) (bilateral) (unilateral)
    (congenital) Q33.3
    acquired (any part) Z90.2
  menstruation —*see* Amenorrhea
  muscle (congenital) (pectoral) Q79.8
    ocular Q10.3
  neck, part Q18.8
  neutrophil —*see* Agranulocytosis
  nipple(s) (with breast(s)) (acquired) Z90.1-●
    congenital Q83.2
  nose (congenital) Q30.1
    acquired Z90.09
  organ
    of Corti, congenital Q16.5
    or site, congenital NEC Q89.8
      acquired NEC Z90.89
  osseous meatus (ear) Q16.4
  ovary (acquired)
    bilateral Z90.722
    congenital
      bilateral Q50.02
      unilateral Q50.01
    unilateral Z90.721
  oviduct (acquired)
    bilateral Z90.722
    congenital Q50.6
    unilateral Z90.721
  pancreas (congenital) Q45.0
    acquired Z90.410
      complete Z90.410
      partial Z90.411
      total Z90.410
  parathyroid gland (acquired) E89.2
    congenital Q89.2
  patella, congenital Q74.1
  penis (congenital) Q55.5
    acquired Z90.79
  pericardium (congenital) Q24.8
  pituitary gland (congenital) Q89.2
    acquired E89.3
  prostate (acquired) Z90.79
    congenital Q55.4
  pulmonary valve Q22.0
  punctum lacrimale (congenital) Q10.4
  radius, congenital —*see* Defect, reduction, upper
    limb, longitudinal, radius

Absence *(Continued)*
  rectum (congenital) Q42.1
    with fistula Q42.0
    acquired Z90.49
  respiratory organ NOS Q34.9
  rib (acquired) Z90.89
    congenital Q76.6
  sacrum, congenital Q76.49
  salivary gland(s), congenital Q38.4
  scrotum, congenital Q55.29
  seminal vesicles (congenital) Q55.4
    acquired Z90.79
  septum
    atrial (congenital) Q21.19
    between aorta and pulmonary artery
      Q21.4
    ventricular (congenital) Q20.4
  sex chromosome
    female phenotype Q97.8
    male phenotype Q98.8
  skull bone (congenital) Q75.8
    with
      anencephaly Q00.0
      encephalocele —*see* Encephalocele
      hydrocephalus Q03.9
        with spina bifida —*see* Spina bifida, by
          site, with hydrocephalus
      microcephaly Q02
  spermatic cord, congenital Q55.4
  spine, congenital Q76.49
  spleen (congenital) Q89.01
    acquired Z90.81
  sternum, congenital Q76.7
  stomach (acquired) (partial) Z90.3
    congenital Q40.2
  superior vena cava, congenital Q26.8
  teeth, tooth (congenital) K00.0
    acquired (complete) K08.109
      class I K08.101
      class II K08.102
      class III K08.103
      class IV K08.104
      due to
        caries K08.139
          class I K08.131
          class II K08.132
          class III K08.133
          class IV K08.134
        periodontal disease K08.129
          class I K08.121
          class II K08.122
          class III K08.123
          class IV K08.124
      specified NEC K08.199
        class I K08.191
        class II K08.192
        class III K08.193
        class IV K08.194
      trauma K08.119
        class I K08.111
        class II K08.112
        class III K08.113
        class IV K08.114
    partial K08.409
      class I K08.401
      class II K08.402
      class III K08.403
      class IV K08.404
      due to
        caries K08.439
          class I K08.431
          class II K08.432
          class III K08.433
          class IV K08.434
        periodontal disease K08.429
          class I K08.421
          class II K08.422
          class III K08.423
          class IV K08.424
      specified NEC K08.499
        class I K08.491
        class II K08.492
        class III K08.493
        class IV K08.494
      trauma K08.419
        class I K08.411
        class II K08.412
        class III K08.413
        class IV K08.414
  tendon (congenital) Q79.8
  testis (congenital) Q55.0
    acquired Z90.79

▶ New   ➡ Revised   ~~deleted~~ Deleted   ● Use Additional Character(s)

Absence *(Continued)*
  thumb (acquired) Z89.01-●
    congenital —*see* Agenesis, hand
  thymus gland Q89.2
  thyroid (gland) (acquired) E89.0
    cartilage, congenital Q31.8
    congenital E03.1
  toe(s) (acquired) Z89.42-●
    with foot —*see* Absence, foot and ankle
    congenital —*see* Agenesis, foot
    great Z89.41-●
  tongue, congenital Q38.3
  trachea (cartilage), congenital Q32.1
  transverse aortic arch, congenital Q25.49
  tricuspid valve Q22.4
  umbilical artery, congenital Q27.0
  upper arm and forearm with hand present,
      congenital —*see* Agenesis, arm, with hand
      present
  ureter (congenital) Q62.4
    acquired Z90.6
  urethra, congenital Q64.5
  uterus (acquired) Z90.710
    with cervix Z90.710
    with remaining cervical stump Z90.711
    congenital Q51.0
  uvula, congenital Q38.5
  vagina, congenital Q52.0
  vas deferens (congenital) Q55.4
    acquired Z90.79
  vein (peripheral) congenital NEC Q27.8
    cerebral Q28.3
    digestive system Q27.8
    great Q26.8
    lower limb Q27.8
    portal Q26.5
    precerebral Q28.1
    specified site NEC Q27.8
    upper limb Q27.8
  vena cava (inferior) (superior), congenital
      Q26.8
  ventricular septum Q20.4
  vertebra, congenital Q76.49
  von Willebrand factor, complete (near) (see also
      Disease, von Willebrand) D68.03
  vulva, congenital Q52.71
  wrist (acquired) Z89.12-●
Absorbent system disease I87.8
Absorption
  carbohydrate, disturbance K90.49
  chemical —*see* Table of Drugs and
      Chemicals
    through placenta (newborn) P04.9
      environmental substance P04.6
      nutritional substance P04.5
      obstetric anesthetic or analgesic drug
          P04.0
  drug NEC —*see* Table of Drugs and Chemicals
    addictive
      through placenta (newborn) (*see also*
          Newborn, affected by, maternal,
          use of) P04.40
        cocaine P04.41
        hallucinogens P04.42
        specified drug NEC P04.49
    medicinal
      through placenta (newborn) P04.19
    through placenta (newborn) P04.19
      obstetric anesthetic or analgesic drug
          P04.0
  fat, disturbance K90.49
    pancreatic K90.3
  noxious substance —*see* Table of Drugs and
      Chemicals
  protein, disturbance K90.49
  starch, disturbance K90.49
  toxic substance —*see* Table of Drugs and
      Chemicals
  uremic —*see* Uremia
Abstinence symptoms, syndrome
  alcohol F10.239
    with delirium F10.231
  cocaine F14.23
  neonatal P96.1
  nicotine —*see* Dependence, drug, nicotine, with,
      withdrawal
  opioid F11.93
    with dependence F11.23
  psychoactive NEC F19.939
    with
      delirium F19.931
      dependence F19.239

Abstinence symptoms, syndromec —
    (Continued)
  psychoactive *(Continued)*
    with *(Continued)*
      dependence *(Continued)*
        with
          delirium F19.231
          perceptual disturbance F19.232
        uncomplicated F19.230
      perceptual disturbance F19.932
    uncomplicated F19.930
  sedative F13.939
    with
      delirium F13.931
      dependence F13.239
        with
          delirium F13.231
          perceptual disturbance F13.232
        uncomplicated F13.230
      perceptual disturbance F13.932
    uncomplicated F13.930
  stimulant NEC F15.93
    with dependence F15.23
Abulia R68.89
Abulomania F60.7
Abuse
  adult —*see* Maltreatment, adult
    as reason for
      couple seeking advice (including offender)
          Z63.0
  alcohol (non-dependent) F10.10
    with
      anxiety disorder F10.180
      intoxication F10.129
        with delirium F10.121
        uncomplicated F10.120
      mood disorder F10.14
      other specified disorder F10.188
      psychosis F10.159
        delusions F10.150
        hallucinations F10.151
      sexual dysfunction F10.181
      sleep disorder F10.182
      unspecified disorder F10.19
      withdrawal F10.139
        with
          perceptual disturbance
              F10.132
          delirium F10.131
          uncomplicated F10.130
    counseling and surveillance Z71.41
    in remission (early) (sustained) F10.11
  amphetamine (or related substance) —*see also*
      Abuse, drug, stimulant NEC
    stimulant NEC F15.10
      with
        anxiety disorder F15.180
        intoxication F15.129
          with
            delirium F15.121
            perceptual disturbance
                F15.122
        withdrawal F15.13
  analgesics (non-prescribed) (over the counter)
      F55.8
  antacids F55.0
  antidepressants —*see* Abuse, drug, psychoactive
      NEC
  anxiolytic —*see* Abuse, drug, sedative
  barbiturates —*see* Abuse, drug, sedative
  caffeine —*see* Abuse, drug, stimulant NEC
  cannabis, cannabinoids —*see* Abuse, drug,
      cannabis
  child —*see* Maltreatment, child
  cocaine —*see* Abuse, drug, cocaine
  drug NEC (non-dependent) F19.10
    with sleep disorder F19.182
    amphetamine type —*see* Abuse, drug,
        stimulant NEC
    analgesics (non-prescribed) (over the counter)
        F55.8
    antacids F55.0
    antidepressants —*see* Abuse, drug,
        psychoactive NEC
    anxiolytics —*see* Abuse, drug, sedative
    barbiturates —*see* Abuse, drug, sedative
    caffeine —*see* Abuse, drug, stimulant
        NEC
    cannabis F12.10
      with
        anxiety disorder F12.180
        intoxication F12.129

Abuse *(Continued)*
  drug NEC *(Continued)*
    cannabis *(Continued)*
      with *(Continued)*
        intoxication *(Continued)*
          with
            delirium F12.121
            perceptual disturbance F12.122
          uncomplicated F12.120
        other specified disorder F12.188
        psychosis F12.159
          delusions F12.150
          hallucinations F12.151
        unspecified disorder F12.19
        withdrawal F12.13
      in remission (early) (sustained) F12.11
    cocaine F14.10
      with
        anxiety disorder F14.180
        intoxication F14.129
          with
            delirium F14.121
            perceptual disturbance F14.122
          uncomplicated F14.120
        mood disorder F14.14
        other specified disorder F14.188
        psychosis F14.159
          delusions F14.150
          hallucinations F14.151
        sexual dysfunction F14.181
        sleep disorder F14.182
        unspecified disorder F14.19
        withdrawal F14.13
      in remission (early) (sustained) F14.11
    counseling and surveillance Z71.51
    hallucinogen F16.10
      with
        anxiety disorder F16.180
        flashbacks F16.183
        intoxication F16.129
          with
            delirium F16.121
            perceptual disturbance F16.122
          uncomplicated F16.120
        mood disorder F16.14
        other specified disorder F16.188
        perception disorder, persisting F16.183
        psychosis F16.159
          delusions F16.150
          hallucinations F16.151
        unspecified disorder F16.19
      in remission (early) (sustained) F16.11
    hashish —*see* Abuse, drug, cannabis
    herbal or folk remedies F55.1
    hormones F55.3
    hypnotics —*see* Abuse, drug, sedative
    inhalant F18.10
      with
        anxiety disorder F18.180
        dementia, persisting F18.17
        intoxication F18.129
          with delirium F18.121
          uncomplicated F18.120
        mood disorder F18.14
        other specified disorder F18.188
        psychosis F18.159
          delusions F18.150
          hallucinations F18.151
        unspecified disorder F18.19
      in remission (early) (sustained) F18.11
    in remission (early) (sustained) F19.11
    laxatives F55.2
    LSD —*see* Abuse, drug, hallucinogen
    marihuana —*see* Abuse, drug, cannabis
    morphine type (opioids) —*see* Abuse, drug,
        opioid
    opioid F11.10
      with
        intoxication F11.129
          with
            delirium F11.121
            perceptual disturbance F11.122
          uncomplicated F11.120
        mood disorder F11.14
        opioid-associated amnestic syndrome
            F11.188
        other specified disorder F11.188
        psychosis F11.159
          delusions F11.150
          hallucinations F11.151
        sexual dysfunction F11.181
        sleep disorder F11.182

Abuse *(Continued)*
  drug NEC *(Continued)*
    opioid *(Continued)*
      with *(Continued)*
        unspecified disorder F11.19
        withdrawal F11.13
      in remission (early) (sustained) F11.11
    PCP (phencyclidine) (or related substance) —*see*
      Abuse, drug, hallucinogen
    psychoactive NEC F19.10
      with
        amnestic disorder F19.16
        anxiety disorder F19.180
        dementia F19.17
        intoxication F19.129
          with
            delirium F19.121
            perceptual disturbance
              F19.122
          uncomplicated F19.120
        mood disorder F19.14
        other specified disorder F19.188
        psychosis F19.159
          delusions F19.150
          hallucinations F19.151
        sexual dysfunction F19.181
        sleep disorder F19.182
        unspecified disorder F19.19
        withdrawal F19.139
          with
            perceptual disturbance F19.132
          delirium F19.131
          uncomplicated F19.130
    sedative, hypnotic or anxiolytic F13.10
      with
        anxiety disorder F13.180
        intoxication F13.129
          with delirium F13.121
          uncomplicated F13.120
        mood disorder F13.14
        other specified disorder F13.188
        psychosis F13.159
          delusions F13.150
          hallucinations F13.151
        sexual dysfunction F13.181
        sleep disorder F13.182
        unspecified disorder F13.19
        withdrawal F13.139
          with
            perceptual disturbance F13.132
          delirium F13.131
          uncomplicated F13.130
      in remission (early) (sustained) F13.11
    solvent —*see* Abuse, drug, inhalant
    steroids F55.3
    stimulant NEC F15.10
      with
        anxiety disorder F15.180
        intoxication F15.129
          with
            delirium F15.121
            perceptual disturbance F15.122
          uncomplicated F15.120
        mood disorder F15.14
        other specified disorder F15.188
        psychosis F15.159
          delusions F15.150
          hallucinations F15.151
        sexual dysfunction F15.181
        sleep disorder F15.182
        unspecified disorder F15.19
        withdrawal F15.13
      in remission (early) (sustained) F15.11
    tranquilizers —*see* Abuse, drug, sedative
    vitamins F55.4
    hallucinogens —*see* Abuse, drug, hallucinogen
    hashish —*see* Abuse, drug, cannabis
    herbal or folk remedies F55.1
    hormones F55.3
    hypnotic —*see* Abuse, drug, sedative
    inhalant —*see* Abuse, drug, inhalant
    laxatives F55.2
    LSD —*see* Abuse, drug, hallucinogen
    marihuana —*see* Abuse, drug, cannabis
    morphine type (opioids) —*see* Abuse, drug,
      opioid
    non-psychoactive substance NEC F55.8
      antacids F55.0
      folk remedies F55.1
      herbal remedies F55.1
      hormones F55.3
      laxatives F55.2

Abuse *(Continued)*
  non-psychoactive substance NEC *(Continued)*
    steroids F55.3
    vitamins F55.4
  opioids —*see* Abuse, drug, opioid
  PCP (phencyclidine) (or related substance) —*see*
    Abuse, drug, hallucinogen
  physical (adult) (child) —*see* Maltreatment
  psychoactive substance —*see* Abuse, drug,
    psychoactive NEC
  psychological (adult) (child) —*see* Maltreatment
  sedative —*see* Abuse, drug, sedative
  sexual —*see* Maltreatment
  solvent —*see* Abuse, drug, inhalant
  steroids F55.3
  vitamins F55.4
Acalculia R48.8
  developmental F81.2
Acanthamebiasis (with) B60.10
  conjunctiva B60.12
  keratoconjunctivitis B60.13
  meningoencephalitis B60.11
  other specified B60.19
Acanthocephaliasis B83.8
Acanthocheilonemiasis B74.4
Acanthocytosis E78.6
Acantholysis L11.9
Acanthosis (acquired) (nigricans) L83
  benign Q82.8
  congenital Q82.8
  seborrheic L82.1
    inflamed L82.0
  tongue K14.3
Acapnia E87.3
Acarbia E87.29
Acardia, acardius Q89.8
Acardiacus amorphus Q89.8
Acardiotrophia I51.4
Acariasis B88.0
  scabies B86
Acarodermatitis (urticarioides) B88.0
Acarophobia F40.218
Acatalasemia, acatalasia E80.3
Acathisia (drug induced) G25.71
Accelerated atrioventricular conduction
  I45.6
Accentuation of personality traits (type A)
  Z73.1
Accessory (congenital)
  adrenal gland Q89.1
  anus Q43.4
  appendix Q43.4
  atrioventricular conduction I45.6
  auditory ossicles Q16.3
  auricle (ear) Q17.0
  biliary duct or passage Q44.5
  bladder Q64.79
  blood vessels NEC Q27.9
    coronary Q24.5
  bone NEC Q79.8
  breast tissue, axilla Q83.1
  carpal bones Q74.0
  cecum Q43.4
  chromosome(s) NEC (nonsex) Q92.9
    with complex rearrangements NEC Q92.5
      seen only at prometaphase Q92.8
    13 —*see* Trisomy, 13
    18 —*see* Trisomy, 18
    21 —*see* Trisomy, 21
    partial Q92.9
    sex
      female phenotype Q97.8
  coronary artery Q24.5
  cusp(s), heart valve NEC Q24.8
    pulmonary Q22.3
  cystic duct Q44.5
  digit(s) Q69.9
  ear (auricle) (lobe) Q17.0
  endocrine gland NEC Q89.2
  eye muscle Q10.3
  eyelid Q10.3
  face bone(s) Q75.8
  fallopian tube (fimbria) (ostium) Q50.6
  finger(s) Q69.0
  foreskin N47.8
  frontonasal process Q75.8
  gallbladder Q44.1
  genital organ(s)
    female Q52.8
      external Q52.79
      internal NEC Q52.8
    male Q55.8

Accessory *(Continued)*
  genitourinary organs NEC Q89.8
    female Q52.8
    male Q55.8
  hallux Q69.2
  heart Q24.8
    valve NEC Q24.8
      pulmonary Q22.3
  hepatic ducts Q44.5
  hymen Q52.4
  intestine (large) (small) Q43.4
  kidney Q63.0
  lacrimal canal Q10.6
  leaflet, heart valve NEC Q24.8
  ligament, broad Q50.6
  liver Q44.79
    duct Q44.5
  lobule (ear) Q17.0
  lung (lobe) Q33.1
  muscle Q79.8
  navicular of carpus Q74.0
  nervous system, part NEC Q07.8
  nipple Q83.3
  nose Q30.8
  organ or site not listed —*see* Anomaly, by site
  ovary Q50.31
  oviduct Q50.6
  pancreas Q45.3
  parathyroid gland Q89.2
  parotid gland (and duct) Q38.4
  pituitary gland Q89.2
  preauricular appendage Q17.0
  prepuce N47.8
  renal arteries (multiple) Q27.2
  rib Q76.6
    cervical Q76.5
  roots (teeth) K00.2
  salivary gland Q38.4
  sesamoid bones Q74.8
    foot Q74.2
    hand Q74.0
  skin tags Q82.8
  spleen Q89.09
  sternum Q76.7
  submaxillary gland Q38.4
  tarsal bones Q74.2
  teeth, tooth K00.1
  tendon Q79.8
  thumb Q69.1
  thymus gland Q89.2
  thyroid gland Q89.2
  toes Q69.2
  tongue Q38.3
  tooth, teeth K00.1
  tragus Q17.0
  ureter Q62.5
  urethra Q64.79
  urinary organ or tract NEC Q64.8
  uterus Q51.28
  vagina Q52.10
  valve, heart NEC Q24.8
    pulmonary Q22.3
  vertebra Q76.49
  vocal cords Q31.8
  vulva Q52.79
Accident
  birth —*see* Birth, injury
  cardiac —*see* Infarct, myocardium
  cerebrovascular (ischemic) I63.9
    aborted I63.9
    chronic (old) (remote) (imaging) (without
      sequelae) Z86.73
      with residual defects - see Sequelae,
        disease, cerebrovascular
    embolic I63.-●
    hemorrhagic —*see* Hemorrhage, intracranial,
      intracerebral
    old (without sequelae) Z86.73
      with sequelae (of) —*see* Sequelae,
        infarction, cerebral
    thrombotic I63.-
  coronary —*see* Infarct, myocardium
  craniovascular I63.9
  vascular, brain I63.9
Accidental —*see* condition
Accommodation (disorder) —*see also* condition
  hysterical paralysis of F44.89
  insufficiency of H52.4
  paresis —*see* Paresis, of accommodation
  spasm —*see* Spasm, of accommodation
Accouchement —*see* Delivery
Accreta placenta O43.21-●

▶ New   ⇒ Revised   ~~deleted~~ Deleted   ● Use Additional Character(s)

Accretio cordis (nonrheumatic) I31.0
Accretions, tooth, teeth K03.6
Acculturation difficulty Z60.3
Accumulation secretion, prostate N42.89
Acephalia, acephalism, acephalus, acephaly
    Q00.0
Acephalobrachia monster Q89.8
Acephalochirus monster Q89.8
Acephalogaster Q89.8
Acephalostomus monster Q89.8
Acephalothorax Q89.8
Acerophobia F40.298
Acetonemia R79.89
    in Type 1 diabetes E10.10
        with coma E10.11
Acetonuria R82.4
Achalasia (cardia) (esophagus) K22.0
    congenital Q39.5
    pylorus Q40.0
    sphincteral NEC K59.89
Ache(s) —see Pain
Acheilia Q38.6
Achillobursitis —see Tendinitis, Achilles
Achillodynia —see Tendinitis, Achilles
Achlorhydria, achlorhydric (neurogenic) K31.83
    anemia D50.8
    diarrhea K31.83
    psychogenic F45.8
    secondary to vagotomy K91.1
Achluophobia F40.228
Acholia K82.8
Acholuric jaundice (familial) (splenomegalic) —see
    also Spherocytosis
    acquired D59.8
Achondrogenesis Q77.0
Achondroplasia (osteosclerosis congenita) Q77.4
Achroma, cutis L80
Achromat (ism), achromatopsia (acquired)
    (congenital) H53.51
Achromia, congenital —see Albinism
Achromia parasitica B36.0
Achylia gastrica K31.89
    psychogenic F45.8
Acid
    burn —see Corrosion
    deficiency
        amide nicotinic E52
        ascorbic E54
        folic E53.8
        nicotinic E52
        pantothenic E53.8
    intoxication (see also Acidosis) E87.29
    peptic disease K30
    phosphatase deficiency E83.39
    stomach K30
        psychogenic F45.8
Acidemia (see also Acidosis) E87.20
    argininosuccinic E72.22
    isovaleric E71.110
    metabolic - see also Acidosis, metabolic
    newborn P19.9
        first noted before onset of labor P19.0
        first noted during labor P19.1
        noted at birth P19.2
    methylmalonic E71.120
    pipecolic E72.3
    propionic E71.121
Acidity, gastric (high) K30
    psychogenic F45.8
Acidocytopenia —see Agranulocytosis
Acidocytosis D72.10
Acidopenia —see Agranulocytosis
Acidosis (lactic) E87.20
    in Type 1 diabetes E10.10
        with coma E10.11
    kidney, tubular N25.89
    lactic E87.20
        acute E87.21
        chronic E87.22
    metabolic NEC E87.20
        acute E87.21
        chronic E87.22
        hyperchloremic, of newborn P74.421
        with respiratory acidosis E87.4
        late, of newborn P74.0
    mixed metabolic and respiratory, newborn P84
    newborn P84
    renal (hyperchloremic) (tubular) N25.89
    respiratory E87.29
        acute J96.02
        chronic J96.12
        complicated by

Acidosis (Continued)
    respiratory (Continued)
        complicated by (Continued)
            metabolic
                acidosis E87.4
                alkalosis E87.4
            specified NEC E87.29
Aciduria
    4-hydroxybutyric E72.81
    argininosuccinic E72.22
    gamma-hydroxybutyric E72.81
    glutaric (type I) E72.3
        type II E71.313
        type III E71.5-●
    orotic (congenital) (hereditary) (pyrimidine
        deficiency) E79.89
        anemia D53.0
Acladiosis (skin) B36.0
Aclasis, diaphyseal Q78.6
Acleistocardia Q21.19
Aclusion —see Anomaly, dentofacial, malocclusion
Acne L70.9
    artificialis L70.8
    atrophica L70.2
    cachecticorum (Hebra) L70.8
    conglobata L70.1
    cystic L70.0
    decalvans L66.2
    excoriée (des jeunes filles) L70.5
    frontalis L70.2
    indurata L70.0
    infantile L70.4
    keloid L73.0
    lupoid L70.2
    necrotic, necrotica (miliaris) L70.2
    neonatal L70.4
    nodular L70.0
    occupational L70.8
    picker's L70.5
    pustular L70.0
    rodens L70.2
    rosacea L71.9
    specified NEC L70.8
    tropica L70.3
    varioliformis L70.2
    vulgaris L70.0
Acnitis (primary) A18.4
Acosta's disease T70.29
Acoustic —see condition
Acousticophobia F40.298
ACPO (acute colonic pseudo-obstruction) K59.81
Acquired —see also condition
    immunodeficiency syndrome (AIDS) B20
Acrania Q00.0
Acroangiodermatitis I78.9
Acroasphyxia, chronic I73.89
Acrobystitis N47.7
Acrocephalopolysyndactyly Q87.0
Acrocephalosyndactyly Q87.0
Acrocephaly Q75.009
Acrochondrohyperplasia —see Syndrome, Marfan
Acrocyanosis I73.89
    newborn P28.2
        meaning transient blue hands and feet - omit
            code
Acrodermatitis L30.8
    atrophicans (chronica) L90.4
    continua (Hallopeau) L40.2
    enteropathica (hereditary) E83.2
    Hallopeau's L40.2
    infantile papular L44.4
    perstans L40.2
    pustulosa continua L40.2
    recalcitrant pustular L40.2
Acrodynia —see Poisoning, mercury
Acromegaly, acromegalia E22.0
Acromelalgia I73.81
Acromicria, acromikria Q79.8
Acronyx L60.0
Acropachy, thyroid —see Thyrotoxicosis
Acroparesthesia (simple) (vasomotor) I73.89
Acropathy, thyroid —see Thyrotoxicosis
Acrophobia F40.241
Acroposthitis N47.7
Acroscleriasis, acroscleroderma, acrosclerosis —
    see Sclerosis, systemic
Acrosphacelus I96
Acrospiroma, eccrine —see Neoplasm, skin, benign
Acrostealgia —see Osteochondropathy
Acrotrophodynia —see Immersion
ACTH ectopic syndrome E24.3
Actinic —see condition

Actinobacillosis, actinobacillus A28.8
    mallei A24.0
    muris A25.1
Actinomyces israelii (infection) —see
    Actinomycosis
Actinomycetoma (foot) B47.1
Actinomycosis, actinomycotic A42.9
    with pneumonia A42.0
    abdominal A42.1
    cervicofacial A42.2
    cutaneous A42.89
    gastrointestinal A42.1
    pulmonary A42.0
    sepsis A42.7
    specified site NEC A42.89
Actinoneuritis G62.82
Action, heart
    disorder I49.9
    irregular I49.9
        psychogenic F45.8
Activated protein C resistance D68.51
Activation
    mast cell (disorder) (syndrome) D89.40
        idiopathic D89.42
        monoclonal D89.41
        secondary D89.43
        specified type NEC D89.49
Active —see condition
Acute —see also condition
    abdomen R10.0
    gallbladder —see Cholecystitis, acute
Acyanotic heart disease (congenital) Q24.9
Acystia Q64.5
Adair-Dighton syndrome (brittle bones and blue
    sclera, deafness) Q78.0
Adamantinoblastoma —see Ameloblastoma
Adamantinoma —see also Cyst, calcifying
    odontogenic
    long bones C40.90
        lower limb C40.2-●
        upper limb C40.0-●
    malignant C41.1
        jaw (bone) (lower) C41.1
            upper C41.0
    tibial C40.2-●
Adamantoblastoma —see Ameloblastoma
Adams-Stokes (-Morgagni) disease or syndrome
    I45.9
Adaption reaction —see Disorder, adjustment
Addiction —see also Dependence F19.20
    alcohol, alcoholic (ethyl) (methyl) (wood)
        (without remission) F10.20
        with remission F10.21
    drug —see Dependence, drug
    ethyl alcohol (without remission) F10.20
        with remission F10.21
    heroin —see Dependence, drug, opioid
    methyl alcohol (without remission) F10.20
        with remission F10.21
    methylated spirit (without remission) F10.20
        with remission F10.21
    morphine(-like substances) —see Dependence,
        drug, opioid
    nicotine —see Dependence, drug, nicotine
    opium and opioids —see Dependence, drug,
        opioid
    tobacco —see Dependence, drug, nicotine
Addisonian crisis E27.2
Addison's
    anemia (pernicious) D51.0
    disease (bronze) or syndrome E27.1
        tuberculous A18.7
    keloid L94.0
Addison-Biermer anemia (pernicious) D51.0
Addison-Schilder complex E71.528
Additional —see also Accessory
    chromosome(s) (see also Trisomy) Q99.8
        21 —see Trisomy, 21
        marker —see Extra, marker chromosomes
        sex —see Abnormal, chromosome, sex
Adduction contracture, hip or other joint —see
    Contraction, joint
Adenitis —see also Lymphadenitis
    acute, unspecified site L04.9
    axillary I88.9
        acute L04.2
        chronic or subacute I88.1
    Bartholin's gland N75.8
    bulbourethral gland —see Urethritis
    cervical I88.9
        acute L04.0
        chronic or subacute I88.1

Adenitis *(Continued)*
  chancroid (Hemophilus ducreyi) A57
  chronic, unspecified site I88.1
  Cowper's gland —*see* Urethritis
  due to Pasteurella multocida (P. septica) A28.0
  epidemic, acute B27.09
  gangrenous L04.9
  gonorrheal NEC A54.89
  groin I88.9
    acute L04.1
    chronic or subacute I88.1
  infectious (acute) (epidemic) B27.09
  inguinal I88.9
    acute L04.1
    chronic or subacute I88.1
  lymph gland or node, except mesenteric I88.9
    acute —*see* Lymphadenitis, acute
    chronic or subacute I88.1
  mesenteric (acute) (chronic) (nonspecific)
      (subacute) I88.0
  parotid gland (suppurative) —*see* Sialoadenitis
  salivary gland (any) (suppurative) —*see*
      Sialoadenitis
  scrofulous (tuberculous) A18.2
  Skene's duct or gland —*see* Urethritis
  strumous, tuberculous A18.2
  subacute, unspecified site I88.1
  sublingual gland (suppurative) —*see* Sialoadenitis
  submandibular gland (suppurative) —*see*
      Sialoadenitis
  submaxillary gland (suppurative) —*see*
      Sialoadenitis
  tuberculous —*see* Tuberculosis, lymph gland
  urethral gland —*see* Urethritis
  Wharton's duct (suppurative) —*see* Sialoadenitis
Adenoacanthoma —*see* Neoplasm, malignant, by
    site
Adenoameloblastoma —*see* Cyst, calcifying
    odontogenic
Adenocarcinoid (tumor) —*see* Neoplasm,
    malignant, by site
Adenocarcinoma —*see also* Neoplasm, malignant,
    by site
  acidophil
    specified site —*see* Neoplasm, malignant, by
        site
    unspecified site C75.1
  adrenal cortical C74.0-●
  alveolar —*see* Neoplasm, lung, malignant
  apocrine
    breast —*see* Neoplasm, breast, malignant
    in situ
      breast D05.8-●
      specified site NEC —*see* Neoplasm, skin,
          in situ
      unspecified site D04.9
    specified site NEC —*see* Neoplasm, skin,
        malignant
    unspecified site C44.99
  basal cell
    specified site —*see* Neoplasm, skin, malignant
    unspecified site C08.9
  basophil
    specified site —*see* Neoplasm, malignant, by
        site
    unspecified site C75.1
  bile duct type C22.1
    liver C22.1
    specified site NEC —*see* Neoplasm, malignant,
        by site
    unspecified site C22.1
  bronchiolar —*see* Neoplasm, lung, malignant
  bronchioloalveolar —*see* Neoplasm, lung,
      malignant
  ceruminous C44.29-●
  cervix, in situ (*see also* Carcinoma, cervix uteri, in
      situ) D06.9
  chromophobe
    specified site —*see* Neoplasm, malignant, by
        site
    unspecified site C75.1
  diffuse type
    specified site —*see* Neoplasm, malignant, by
        site
    unspecified site C16.9
  duct
    infiltrating
      with Paget's disease —*see* Neoplasm,
          breast, malignant
      specified site —*see* Neoplasm, malignant,
          by site

Adenocarcinoma *(Continued)*
  duct *(Continued)*
    infiltrating *(Continued)*
      unspecified site (female) C50.91-●
        male C50.92-●
    specified site —*see* Neoplasm, malignant, by
        site
    unspecified site
      female C56.9
      male C61
  eosinophil
    specified site —*see* Neoplasm, malignant, by
        site
    unspecified site C75.1
  follicular
    with papillary C73
    moderately differentiated C73
    specified site —*see* Neoplasm, malignant, by
        site
    trabecular C73
    unspecified site C73
    well differentiated C73
  Hurthle cell C73
  in
    adenomatous
      polyposis coli C18.9
  infiltrating duct
    with Paget's disease —*see* Neoplasm, breast,
        malignant
    specified site —*see* Neoplasm, malignant, by
        site
    unspecified site (female) C50.91-●
      male C50.92-●
  inflammatory
    specified site —*see* Neoplasm, malignant, by
        site
    unspecified site (female) C50.91-●
      male C50.92-●
  intestinal type
    specified site —*see* Neoplasm, malignant, by
        site
    unspecified site C16.9
  intracystic papillary
  intraductal
    breast D05.1-●
    noninfiltrating
      breast D05.1-●
      papillary
        with invasion
          specified site —*see* Neoplasm,
              malignant, by site
          unspecified site (female) C50.91-●
            male C50.92-●
        breast D05.1-●
        specified site NEC —*see* Neoplasm, in
            situ, by site
        unspecified site D05.1-●
      specified site NEC —*see* Neoplasm, in situ,
          by site
      unspecified site D05.1-●
    papillary
      with invasion
        specified site —*see* Neoplasm, malignant,
            by site
        unspecified site (female) C50.91-●
          male C50.92-●
      breast D05.1-●
      specified site —*see* Neoplasm, in situ, by site
      unspecified site D05.1-●
    specified site NEC —*see* Neoplasm, in situ,
        by site
    unspecified site D05.1-●
  islet cell
    with exocrine, mixed
      specified site —*see* Neoplasm, malignant,
          by site
      unspecified site C25.9
    pancreas C25.4
    specified site NEC —*see* Neoplasm, malignant,
        by site
    unspecified site C25.4
  lobular
    in situ
      breast D05.0-●
      specified site NEC —*see* Neoplasm, in situ,
          by site
      unspecified site D05.0-●
    specified site —*see* Neoplasm, malignant, by
        site
    unspecified site (female) C50.91-●
      male C50.92-●

Adenocarcinoma *(Continued)*
  mucoid —*see also* Neoplasm, malignant, by site
    cell
      specified site —*see* Neoplasm, malignant,
          by site
      unspecified site C75.1
  nonencapsulated sclerosing C73
  papillary
    with follicular C73
    follicular variant C73
    intraductal (noninfiltrating)
      with invasion
        specified site —*see* Neoplasm, malignant,
            by site
        unspecified site (female) C50.91-●
          male C50.92-●
      breast D05.1-●
      specified site NEC —*see* Neoplasm, in situ,
          by site
      unspecified site D05.1-●
    serous
      specified site —*see* Neoplasm, malignant,
          by site
      unspecified site C56.9
  papillocystic
    specified site —*see* Neoplasm, malignant, by
        site
    unspecified site C56.9
  pseudomucinous
    specified site —*see* Neoplasm, malignant, by
        site
    unspecified site C56.9
  renal cell C64-●
  sebaceous —*see* Neoplasm, skin, malignant, by
      site
  serous —*see also* Neoplasm, malignant, by site
    papillary
      specified site —*see* Neoplasm, malignant,
          by site
      unspecified site C56.9
  sweat gland —*see* Neoplasm, skin, malignant
  water-clear cell C75.0
Adenocarcinoma-in-situ —*see also* Neoplasm, in
    situ, by site
  breast D05.9-●
Adenofibroma
  clear cell —*see* Neoplasm, benign, by site
  endometrioid D27.9
    borderline malignancy D39.10
    malignant C56-●
  mucinous
    specified site —*see* Neoplasm, benign, by site
    unspecified site D27.9
  papillary
    specified site —*see* Neoplasm, benign, by site
    unspecified site D27.9
  prostate —*see* Enlargement, enlarged, prostate
  serous
    specified site —*see* Neoplasm, benign, by site
    unspecified site D27.9
  specified site —*see* Neoplasm, benign, by site
  unspecified site D27.9
Adenofibrosis
  breast —*see* Fibroadenosis, breast
  endometrioid N80.00
Adenoiditis (chronic) J35.02
  with tonsillitis J35.03
  acute J03.90
    recurrent J03.91
    specified organism NEC J03.80
      recurrent J03.81
    staphylococcal J03.80
      recurrent J03.81
    streptococcal J03.00
      recurrent J03.01
Adenoids —*see* condition
Adenolipoma —*see* Neoplasm, benign, by site
Adenolipomatosis, Launois-Bensaude E88.89
Adenolymphoma
  specified site —*see* Neoplasm, benign, by site
  unspecified site D11.9
Adenoma —*see also* Neoplasm, benign, by site
  acidophil
    specified site —*see* Neoplasm, benign, by site
    unspecified site D35.2
  acidophil-basophil, mixed
    specified site —*see* Neoplasm, benign, by site
    unspecified site D35.2
  adrenal (cortical) D35.00
    clear cell D35.00
    compact cell D35.00

Adenoma *(Continued)*
  adrenal *(Continued)*
    glomerulosa cell D35.00
    heavily pigmented variant D35.00
    mixed cell D35.00
  alpha-cell
    pancreas D13.7
    specified site NEC —*see* Neoplasm, benign,
        by site
    unspecified site D13.7
  alveolar D14.30
  apocrine
    breast D24-●
    specified site NEC —*see* Neoplasm, skin,
        benign, by site
    unspecified site D23.9
  basal cell D11.9
  basophil
    specified site —*see* Neoplasm, benign, by site
    unspecified site D35.2
  basophil-acidophil, mixed
    specified site —*see* Neoplasm, benign, by site
    unspecified site D35.2
  beta-cell
    pancreas D13.7
    specified site NEC —*see* Neoplasm, benign,
        by site
    unspecified site D13.7
  bile duct D13.4
    common D13.5
    extrahepatic D13.5
    intrahepatic D13.4
    specified site NEC —*see* Neoplasm, benign,
        by site
    unspecified site D13.4
  black D35.00
  bronchial D38.1
    cylindroid type —*see* Neoplasm, lung,
        malignant
  ceruminous D23.2-●
  chief cell D35.1
  chromophobe
    specified site —*see* Neoplasm, benign, by
        site
    unspecified site D35.2
  colloid
    specified site —*see* Neoplasm, benign, by site
    unspecified site D34
  eccrine, papillary —*see* Neoplasm, skin, benign
  endocrine, multiple
    single specified site —*see* Neoplasm, uncertain
        behavior, by site
    two or more specified sites D44-●
    unspecified site D44.9
  endometrioid —*see also* Neoplasm, benign
    borderline malignancy —*see* Neoplasm,
        uncertain behavior, by site
  eosinophil
    specified site —*see* Neoplasm, malignant, by
        site
    unspecified site D35.2
  fetal
    specified site —*see* Neoplasm, benign, by site
    unspecified site D34
  follicular
    specified site —*see* Neoplasm, benign, by site
    unspecified site D34
  hepatocellular D13.4
  Hurthle cell D34
  islet cell
    pancreas D13.7
    specified site NEC —*see* Neoplasm, benign,
        by site
    unspecified site D13.7
  liver cell D13.4
  macrofollicular
    specified site —*see* Neoplasm, benign, by site
    unspecified site D34
  malignant, malignum —*see* Neoplasm,
        malignant, by site
  microcystic
    pancreas D13.6
    specified site NEC —*see* Neoplasm, benign,
        by site
    unspecified site D13.6
  microfollicular
    specified site —*see* Neoplasm, benign, by site
    unspecified site D34
  mucoid cell
    specified site —*see* Neoplasm, benign, by site
    unspecified site D35.2

Adenoma *(Continued)*
  multiple endocrine
    single specified site —*see* Neoplasm, uncertain
        behavior, by site
    two or more specified sites D44-●
    unspecified site D44.9
  nipple D24-●
  papillary —*see also* Neoplasm, benign, by site
    eccrine —*see* Neoplasm, skin, benign, by site
  Pick's tubular
    specified site —*see* Neoplasm, benign, by
        site
    unspecified site
      female D27.9
      male D29.20
  pleomorphic
    carcinoma in —*see* Neoplasm, salivary gland,
        malignant
      specified site —*see* Neoplasm, malignant,
          by site
      unspecified site C08.9
  polypoid —*see also* Neoplasm, benign
    adenocarcinoma in —*see* Neoplasm,
        malignant, by site
    adenocarcinoma in situ —*see* Neoplasm, in
        situ, by site
➡ prostate —*see* Neoplasm, prostate, benign
  rete cell D29.20
  sebaceous —*see* Neoplasm, skin, benign
  Sertoli cell
    specified site —*see* Neoplasm, benign, by site
    unspecified site
      female D27.9
      male D29.20
  skin appendage —*see* Neoplasm, skin, benign
  sudoriferous gland —*see* Neoplasm, skin, benign
  sweat gland —*see* Neoplasm, skin, benign
  testicular
    specified site —*see* Neoplasm, benign, by site
    unspecified site
      female D27.9
      male D29.20
  tubular —*see also* Neoplasm, benign, by site
    adenocarcinoma in —*see* Neoplasm,
        malignant, by site
    adenocarcinoma in situ —*see* Neoplasm, in
        situ, by site
    Pick's
      specified site —*see* Neoplasm, benign
      unspecified site
        female D27.9
        male D29.20
  tubulovillous —*see also* Neoplasm, benign, by
      site
    adenocarcinoma in —*see* Neoplasm,
        malignant, by site
    adenocarcinoma in situ —*see* Neoplasm, in
        situ, by site
  villous —*see* Neoplasm, uncertain behavior, by site
    adenocarcinoma in —*see* Neoplasm,
        malignant, by site
    adenocarcinoma in situ —*see* Neoplasm, in
        situ, by site
  water-clear cell D35.1
Adenomatosis
  endocrine (multiple) E31.20
    single specified site —*see* Neoplasm, uncertain
        behavior, by site
  erosive of nipple D24-●
  pluriendocrine —*see* Adenomatosis, endocrine
  pulmonary D38.1
    malignant —*see* Neoplasm, lung, malignant
    specified site —*see* Neoplasm, benign, by site
    unspecified site D12.6
Adenomatous
  goiter (nontoxic) E04.9
    with hyperthyroidism —*see* Hyperthyroidism,
        with, goiter, nodular
    toxic —*see* Hyperthyroidism, with, goiter,
        nodular
Adenomyoma —*see also* Neoplasm, benign, by site
  prostate —*see* Enlarged, prostate
Adenomyometritis N80.00
Adenomyosis (uterus) N80.03
Adenopathy (lymph gland) R59.9
  generalized R59.1
  inguinal R59.0
  localized R59.0
  mediastinal R59.0
  mesentery R59.0
  syphilitic (secondary) A51.49

Adenopathy *(Continued)*
  tracheobronchial R59.0
    tuberculous A15.4
      primary (progressive) A15.7
  tuberculous —*see also* Tuberculosis, lymph gland
    tracheobronchial A15.4
      primary (progressive) A15.7
Adenosalpingitis —*see* Salpingitis
Adenosarcoma —*see* Neoplasm, malignant, by site
Adenosclerosis I88.8
Adenosis (sclerosing) breast —*see* Fibroadenosis,
    breast
Adenovirus, as cause of disease classified
    elsewhere B97.0
Adentia (complete) (partial) —*see* Absence, teeth
Adherent —*see also* Adhesions
  labia (minora) N90.89
  pericardium (nonrheumatic) I31.0
    rheumatic I09.2
  placenta (with hemorrhage) O72.0
    without hemorrhage O73.0
  prepuce, newborn N47.0
  scar (skin) L90.5
  tendon in scar L90.5
Adhesions, adhesive (postinfective) K66.0
  with intestinal obstruction K56.50
    complete K56.52
    incomplete K56.51
    partial K56.51
  abdominal (wall) —*see* Adhesions, peritoneum
  appendix K38.8
  bile duct (common) (hepatic) K83.8
  bladder (sphincter) N32.89
  bowel —*see* Adhesions, peritoneum
  cardiac I31.0
    rheumatic I09.2
  cecum —*see* Adhesions, peritoneum
  cervicovaginal N88.1
    congenital Q52.8
    postpartal O90.89
    old N88.1
  cervix N88.1
  ciliary body NEC —*see* Adhesions, iris
  clitoris N90.89
  colon —*see* Adhesions, peritoneum
  common duct K83.8
  congenital —*see also* Anomaly, by site
    fingers —*see* Syndactylism, complex, fingers
    omental, anomalous Q43.3
    peritoneal Q43.3
    tongue (to gum or roof of mouth) Q38.3
  conjunctiva (acquired) H11.21-●
    congenital Q15.8
  cystic duct K82.8
  diaphragm —*see* Adhesions, peritoneum
  due to foreign body —*see* Foreign body
  duodenum —*see* Adhesions, peritoneum
  ear
    middle H74.1-●
  epididymis N50.89
  epidural —*see* Adhesions, meninges
  epiglottis J38.7
  eyelid H02.59
  female pelvis N73.6
  gallbladder K82.8
  globe H44.89
  heart I31.0
    rheumatic I09.2
  ileocecal (coil) —*see* Adhesions, peritoneum
  ileum —*see* Adhesions, peritoneum
  intestine —*see also* Adhesions, peritoneum
    with obstruction K56.50
      complete K56.52
      incomplete K56.51
      partial K56.51
  intra-abdominal —*see* Adhesions, peritoneum
  iris H21.50-●
    anterior H21.51-●
    goniosynechiae H21.52-●
    posterior H21.54-●
    to corneal graft T85.898
  joint —*see* Ankylosis
    knee M23.8X
    temporomandibular M26.61-●
  labium (majus) (minus), congenital Q52.5
  liver —*see* Adhesions, peritoneum
  lung J98.4
  mediastinum J98.59
  meninges (cerebral) (spinal) G96.12
    congenital Q07.8
    tuberculous (cerebral) (spinal) A17.0

Adhesions, adhesive *(Continued)*
  mesenteric —*see* Adhesions, peritoneum
  nasal (septum) (to turbinates) J34.89
  ocular muscle —*see* Strabismus, mechanical
  omentum —*see* Adhesions, peritoneum
  ovary N73.6
    congenital (to cecum, kidney or omentum) Q50.39
  paraovarian N73.6
  pelvic (peritoneal)
    female N73.6
      postprocedural N99.4
    male —*see* Adhesions, peritoneum
    postpartal (old) N73.6
    tuberculous A18.17
  penis to scrotum (congenital) Q55.8
  periappendiceal —*see also* Adhesions, peritoneum
  pericardium (nonrheumatic) I31.0
    focal I31.8
    rheumatic I09.2
    tuberculous A18.84
  pericholecystic K82.8
  perigastric —*see* Adhesions, peritoneum
  periovarian N73.6
  periprostatic N42.89
  perirectal —*see* Adhesions, peritoneum
  perirenal N28.89
  peritoneum, peritoneal (postinfective) K66.0
    with obstruction (intestinal) K56.50
      complete K56.52
      incomplete K56.51
      partial K56.51
    congenital Q43.3
    pelvic, female N73.6
      postprocedural N99.4
    postpartal, pelvic N73.6
    postprocedural K66.0
    to uterus N73.6
  peritubal N73.6
  periureteral N28.89
  periuterine N73.6
  perivesical N32.89
  perivesicular (seminal vesicle) N50.89
  pleura, pleuritic J94.8
    tuberculous NEC A15.6
  pleuropericardial J94.8
  postoperative (gastrointestinal tract) K66.0
    with obstruction —*see also* Obstruction, intestine, postoperative K91.30
    due to foreign body accidentally left in wound —*see* Foreign body, accidentally left during a procedure
    pelvic peritoneal N99.4
    urethra —*see* Stricture, urethra, postprocedural
    vagina N99.2
  postpartal, old (vulva or perineum) N90.89
  preputial, prepuce N47.5
  pulmonary J98.4
  pylorus —*see* Adhesions, peritoneum
  sciatic nerve —*see* Lesion, nerve, sciatic
  seminal vesicle N50.89
  shoulder (joint) —*see* Capsulitis, adhesive
  sigmoid flexure —*see* Adhesions, peritoneum
  spermatic cord (acquired) N50.89
    congenital Q55.4
  spinal canal G96.12
  stomach —*see* Adhesions, peritoneum
  subscapular —*see* Capsulitis, adhesive
  temporomandibular M26.61-●
  tendinitis —*see also* Tenosynovitis, specified type NEC
    shoulder —*see* Capsulitis, adhesive
  testis N44.8
  tongue, congenital (to gum or roof of mouth) Q38.3
    acquired K14.8
  trachea J39.8
  tubo-ovarian N73.6
  tunica vaginalis N44.8
  uterus N73.6
    internal N85.6
    to abdominal wall N73.6
  vagina (chronic) N89.5
    postoperative N99.2
  vitreomacular H43.82-●
  vitreous H43.89
  vulva N90.89
Adiaspiromycosis B48.8
Adie (-Holmes) pupil or syndrome —*see* Anomaly, pupil, function, tonic pupil

Adiponecrosis neonatorum P83.88
Adiposis —*see also* Obesity
  cerebralis E23.6
  dolorosa E88.2
Adiposity —*see also* Obesity
  heart —*see* Degeneration, myocardial
  localized E65
Adiposogenital dystrophy E23.6
Adjustment
  disorder —*see* Disorder, adjustment
  implanted device —*see* Encounter (for), adjustment (of)
  prosthesis, external —*see* Fitting
  reaction —*see* Disorder, adjustment
Administration of tPA (rtPA) in a different facility within the last 24 hours prior to admission to current facility Z92.82
Admission (for) —*see also* Encounter (for)
  adjustment (of)
    artificial
      arm Z44.00-●
        complete Z44.01-●
        partial Z44.02-●
      eye Z44.2
      leg Z44.10-●
        complete Z44.11-●
        partial Z44.12-●
    brain neuropacemaker Z46.2
      implanted Z45.42
    breast
      implant Z45.81
      prosthesis (external) Z44.3
    colostomy belt Z46.89
    contact lenses Z46.0
    cystostomy device Z46.6
    dental prosthesis Z46.3
    device NEC
      abdominal Z46.89
      implanted Z45.89
        cardiac Z45.09
          defibrillator (with synchronous cardiac pacemaker) Z45.02
          pacemaker (cardiac resynchronization therapy (CRT-P)) Z45.018
          pulse generator Z45.010
          resynchronization therapy defibrillator (CRT-D) Z45.02
        hearing device Z45.328
          bone conduction Z45.320
          cochlear Z45.321
        infusion pump Z45.1
        nervous system Z45.49
          CSF drainage Z45.41
          hearing device —*see* Admission, adjustment, device, implanted, hearing device
          neuropacemaker Z45.42
          visual substitution Z45.31
        specified NEC Z45.89
        vascular access Z45.2
        visual substitution Z45.31
      nervous system Z46.2
        implanted —*see* Admission, adjustment, device, implanted, nervous system
    orthodontic Z46.4
    prosthetic Z44.9
      arm —*see* Admission, adjustment, artificial, arm
      breast Z44.3
      dental Z46.3
      eye Z44.2
      leg —*see* Admission, adjustment, artificial, leg
      specified type NEC Z44.8
    substitution
      auditory Z46.2
        implanted —*see* Admission, adjustment, device, implanted, hearing device
      nervous system Z46.2
        implanted —*see* Admission, adjustment, device, implanted, nervous system
      visual Z46.2
        implanted Z45.31
    urinary Z46.6
    hearing aid Z46.1
      implanted —*see* Admission, adjustment, device, implanted, hearing device
    ileostomy device Z46.89
    intestinal appliance or device NEC Z46.89

Admission *(Continued)*
  adjustment *(Continued)*
    neuropacemaker (brain) (peripheral nerve) (spinal cord) Z46.2
      implanted Z45.42
    orthodontic device Z46.4
    orthopedic (brace) (cast) (device) (shoes) Z46.89
    pacemaker (cardiac resynchronization therapy (CRT-P))
      cardiac Z45.018
        pulse generator Z45.010
      nervous system Z46.2
        implanted Z45.42
    portacath (port-a-cath) Z45.2
    prosthesis Z44.9
      arm —*see* Admission, adjustment, artificial, arm
      breast Z44.3
      dental Z46.3
      eye Z44.2
      leg —*see* Admission, adjustment, artificial, leg
      specified NEC Z44.8
    spectacles Z46.0
  aftercare (*see also* Aftercare) Z51.89
    postpartum
      immediately after delivery Z39.0
      routine follow-up Z39.2
    radiation therapy (antineoplastic) Z51.0
  ► sepsis Z51.A
  attention to artificial opening (of) Z43.9
    artificial vagina Z43.7
    colostomy Z43.3
    cystostomy Z43.5
    enterostomy Z43.4
    gastrostomy Z43.1
    ileostomy Z43.2
    jejunostomy Z43.4
    nephrostomy Z43.6
    specified site NEC Z43.8
      intestinal tract Z43.4
      urinary tract Z43.6
    tracheostomy Z43.0
    ureterostomy Z43.6
    urethrostomy Z43.6
  breast augmentation or reduction Z41.1
  breast reconstruction following mastectomy Z42.1
  change of
    dressing (nonsurgical) Z48.00
    neuropacemaker device (brain) (peripheral nerve) (spinal cord) Z46.2
      implanted Z45.42
    surgical dressing Z48.01
  circumcision, ritual or routine (in absence of diagnosis) Z41.2
  clinical research investigation (control) (normal comparison) (participant) Z00.6
  contraceptive management Z30.9
  cosmetic surgery NEC Z41.1
  counseling (*see also* Counseling)
    dietary Z71.3
    gestational carrier Z31.7
    HIV Z71.7
    human immunodeficiency virus Z71.7
    nonattending third party Z71.0
    procreative management NEC Z31.69
  delivery, full-term, uncomplicated O80
    cesarean, without indication O82
  desensitization to allergens Z51.6
  dietary surveillance and counseling Z71.3
  ear piercing Z41.3
  examination at health care facility (adult) —*see also* Examination Z00.00
    with abnormal findings Z00.01
    clinical research investigation (control) (normal comparison) (participant) Z00.6
    dental Z01.20
      with abnormal findings Z01.21
    donor (potential) Z00.5
    ear Z01.10
      with abnormal findings NEC Z01.118
        following failed vision screening Z01.020
          with abnormal findings Z01.021
    eye Z01.00
      with abnormal findings Z01.01
    general, specified reason NEC Z00.8
    hearing Z01.10
      with abnormal findings NEC Z01.118
    infant or child (over 28 days old) Z00.129
      with abnormal findings Z00.121

Admission *(Continued)*
  examination at health care facility *(Continued)*
    postpartum checkup Z39.2
    psychiatric (general) Z00.8
      requested by authority Z04.6
    vision Z01.00
      with abnormal findings Z01.01
        following failed vision screening Z01.020
          with abnormal findings Z01.021
      infant or child (over 28 days old) Z00.129
        with abnormal findings Z00.121
  fitting (of)
    artificial
      arm —*see* Admission, adjustment, artificial,
        arm
      eye Z44.2
      leg —*see* Admission, adjustment, artificial, leg
    brain neuropacemaker Z46.2
      implanted Z45.42
    breast prosthesis (external) Z44.3
    colostomy belt Z46.89
    contact lenses Z46.0
    cystostomy device Z46.6
    dental prosthesis Z46.3
    dentures Z46.3
    device NEC
      abdominal Z46.89
      nervous system Z46.2
        implanted —*see* Admission, adjustment,
          device, implanted, nervous system
      orthodontic Z46.4
      prosthetic Z44.9
        breast Z44.3
        dental Z46.3
        eye Z44.2
      substitution
        auditory Z46.2
          implanted —*see* Admission,
            adjustment, device, implanted,
            hearing device
        nervous system Z46.2
          implanted —*see* Admission,
            adjustment, device, implanted,
            nervous system
        visual Z46.2
          implanted Z45.31
    hearing aid Z46.1
    ileostomy device Z46.89
    intestinal appliance or device NEC Z46.89
    neuropacemaker (brain) (peripheral nerve)
      (spinal cord) Z46.2
      implanted Z45.42
    orthodontic device Z46.4
    orthopedic device (brace) (cast) (shoes) Z46.89
    prosthesis Z44.9
      arm —*see* Admission, adjustment, artificial,
        arm
      breast Z44.3
      dental Z46.3
      eye Z44.2
      leg —*see* Admission, adjustment, artificial, leg
      specified type NEC Z44.8
    spectacles Z46.0
  follow-up examination Z09
  intrauterine device management Z30.431
    initial prescription Z30.014
  mental health evaluation Z00.8
    requested by authority Z04.6
  observation —*see* Observation
  Papanicolaou smear, cervix Z12.4
    for suspected malignant neoplasm Z12.4
  plastic and reconstructive surgery following
    medical procedure or healed injury NEC
    Z42.8
  plastic surgery, cosmetic NEC Z41.1
  postpartum observation
    immediately after delivery Z39.0
    routine follow-up Z39.2
  poststerilization (for restoration) Z31.0
    aftercare Z31.42
  procreative management Z31.9
  prophylactic (measure) —*see also* Encounter,
    prophylactic measures
    organ removal Z40.00
      breast Z40.01
      fallopian tube(s) Z40.03
        with ovary(s) Z40.02
      ovary(s) Z40.02
      specified organ NEC Z40.09
      testes Z40.09
  vaccination Z23

Admission *(Continued)*
  psychiatric examination (general) Z00.8
    requested by authority Z04.6
  radiation therapy (antineoplastic) Z51.0
  reconstructive surgery following medical
    procedure or healed injury NEC Z42.8
  removal of
    cystostomy catheter Z43.5
    drains Z48.03
    dressing (nonsurgical) Z48.00
    implantable subdermal contraceptive Z30.46
    intrauterine contraceptive device Z30.432
    neuropacemaker (brain) (peripheral nerve)
      (spinal cord) Z46.2
      implanted Z45.42
    staples Z48.02
    surgical dressing Z48.01
    sutures Z48.02
    ureteral stent Z46.6
  respirator [ventilator] use during power failure
    Z99.12
  restoration of organ continuity (poststerilization)
    Z31.0
    aftercare Z31.42
  sensitivity test —*see also* Test, skin
    allergy NEC Z01.82
    Mantoux Z11.1
  tuboplasty following previous sterilization Z31.0
    aftercare Z31.42
  vasoplasty following previous sterilization Z31.0
    aftercare Z31.42
  vision examination Z01.00
    with abnormal findings Z01.01
      following failed vision screening Z01.020
        with abnormal findings Z01.021
    infant or child (over 28 days old) Z00.129
      with abnormal findings Z00.121
  waiting period for admission to other facility
    Z75.1
Adnexitis (suppurative) —*see* Salpingo-oophoritis
Adolescent X-linked adrenoleukodystrophy
    E71.521
Adrenal (gland) —*see* condition
Adrenalism, tuberculous A18.7
Adrenalitis, adrenitis E27.8
  autoimmune E27.1
  meningococcal, hemorrhagic A39.1
Adrenarche, premature E27.0
Adrenocortical syndrome —*see* Cushing's,
    syndrome
Adrenogenital syndrome E25.9
  acquired E25.8
  congenital E25.0
  salt loss E25.0
Adrenogenitalism, congenital E25.0
Adrenoleukodystrophy E71.529
  neonatal E71.511
  X-linked E71.529
    Addison only phenotype E71.528
    Addison-Schilder E71.528
    adolescent E71.521
    adrenomyeloneuropathy E71.522
    childhood cerebral E71.520
    other specified E71.528
Adrenomyeloneuropathy E71.522
Adventitious bursa —*see* Bursopathy, specified
    type NEC
Adverse effect —*see* Table of Drugs and Chemicals,
    categories T36-T50, with 6th character 5
Advice —*see* Counseling
Adynamia (episodica) (hereditary) (periodic) G72.3
Aeration lung imperfect, newborn —*see*
    Atelectasis
Aerobullosis T70.3
Aerocele —*see* Embolism, air
Aerodermectasia
  subcutaneous (traumatic) T79.7
Aerodontalgia T70.29
Aeroembolism T70.3
Aerogenes capsulatus infection A48.0
Aero-otitis media T70.0
Aerophagy, aerophagia (psychogenic) F45.8
Aerophobia F40.228
Aerosinusitis T70.1
Aerotitis T70.0
Affection —*see* Disease
Afibrinogenemia —*see also* Defect, coagulation
    D68.8
  acquired D65
  congenital D68.2
  following ectopic or molar pregnancy O08.1

Afibrinogenemia *(Continued)*
  in abortion —*see* Abortion, by type, complicated
    by, afibrinogenemia
  puerperal O72.3
African
  sleeping sickness B56.9
  tick fever A68.1
  trypanosomiasis B56.9
    gambian B56.0
    rhodesian B56.1
Aftercare —*see also* Care Z51.89
  following surgery (for) (on)
    amputation Z47.81
    attention to
      drains Z48.03
      dressings (nonsurgical) Z48.00
        surgical Z48.01
      sutures Z48.02
    circulatory system Z48.812
    delayed (planned) wound closure Z48.1
    digestive system Z48.815
    explantation of joint prosthesis (staged
      procedure)
      hip Z47.32
      knee Z47.33
      shoulder Z47.31
    genitourinary system Z48.816
    joint replacement Z47.1
    neoplasm Z48.3
    nervous system Z48.811
    oral cavity Z48.814
    organ transplant
      bone marrow Z48.290
      heart Z48.21
      heart-lung Z48.280
      kidney Z48.22
      liver Z48.23
      lung Z48.24
      multiple organs NEC Z48.288
      specified NEC Z48.298
    orthopedic NEC Z47.89
    planned wound closure Z48.1
    removal of internal fixation device Z47.2
    respiratory system Z48.813
    scoliosis Z47.82
    sense organs Z48.810
    skin and subcutaneous tissue Z48.817
    specified body system
      circulatory Z48.812
      digestive Z48.815
      genitourinary Z48.816
      nervous Z48.811
      oral cavity Z48.814
      respiratory Z48.813
      sense organs Z48.810
      skin and subcutaneous tissue Z48.817
      teeth Z48.814
    specified NEC Z48.89
    spinal Z47.89
    teeth Z48.814
  fracture — code to fracture with seventh
    character D
  involving
    removal of
      drains Z48.03
      dressings (nonsurgical) Z48.00
      staples Z48.02
      surgical dressings Z48.01
      sutures Z48.02
    neuropacemaker (brain) (peripheral nerve)
      (spinal cord) Z46.2
      implanted Z45.42
    orthopedic NEC Z47.89
  postprocedural —*see* Aftercare, following surgery
After-cataract —*see* Cataract, secondary
Agalactia (primary) O92.3
  elective, secondary or therapeutic O92.5
Agammaglobulinemia (acquired (secondary))
    (nonfamilial) D80.1
  with
    immunoglobulin-bearing B-lymphocytes D80.1
    lymphopenia D81.9
  autosomal recessive (Swiss type) D80.0
  Bruton's X-linked D80.0
  common variable (CVAgamma) D80.1
  congenital sex-linked D80.0
  hereditary D80.0
  lymphopenic D81.9
  Swiss type (autosomal recessive) D80.0
  X-linked (with growth hormone deficiency)
    (Bruton) D80.0

Aganglionosis (bowel) (colon) Q43.1
Age (old) —*see* Senility
Agenesis
  adrenal (gland) Q89.1
  alimentary tract (complete) (partial) NEC Q45.8
    upper Q40.8
  anus, anal (canal) Q42.3
    with fistula Q42.2
  aorta Q25.41
  appendix Q42.8
  arm (complete) Q71.0-●
    with hand present Q71.1-●
  artery (peripheral) Q27.9
    brain Q28.3
    coronary Q24.5
    pulmonary Q25.79
    specified NEC Q27.8
    umbilical Q27.0
  auditory (canal) (external) Q16.1
  auricle (ear) Q16.0
  bile duct or passage Q44.5
  bladder Q64.5
  bone Q79.9
  brain Q00.0
    part of Q04.3
  breast (with nipple present) Q83.8
    with absent nipple Q83.0
  bronchus Q32.4
  canaliculus lacrimalis Q10.4
  carpus —*see* Agenesis, hand
  cartilage Q79.9
  cecum Q42.8
  cerebellum Q04.3
  cervix Q51.5
  chin Q18.8
  cilia Q10.3
  circulatory system, part NOS Q28.9
  clavicle Q74.0
  clitoris Q52.6
  coccyx Q76.49
  colon Q42.9
    specified NEC Q42.8
  corpus callosum Q04.0
  cricoid cartilage Q31.8
  diaphragm (with hernia) Q79.1
  digestive organ(s) or tract (complete) (partial)
    NEC Q45.8
    upper Q40.8
  ductus arteriosus Q28.8
  duodenum Q41.0
  ear Q16.9
    auricle Q16.0
    lobe Q17.8
  ejaculatory duct Q55.4
  endocrine (gland) NEC Q89.2
  epiglottis Q31.8
  esophagus Q39.8
  eustachian tube Q16.2
  eye Q11.1
    adnexa Q15.8
  eyelid (fold) Q10.3
  face
    bones NEC Q75.8
    specified part NEC Q18.8
  fallopian tube Q50.6
  femur —*see* Defect, reduction, lower limb,
    longitudinal, femur
  fibula —*see* Defect, reduction, lower limb,
    longitudinal, fibula
  finger (complete) (partial) —*see* Agenesis, hand
  foot (and toes) (complete) (partial) Q72.3-●
  forearm (with hand present) —*see* Agenesis, arm,
    with hand present
    and hand Q71.2-●
  gallbladder Q44.0
  gastric Q40.2
  genitalia, genital (organ(s))
    female Q52.8
      external Q52.71
      internal NEC Q52.8
    male Q55.8
  glottis Q31.8
  hair Q84.0
  hand (and fingers) (complete) (partial) Q71.3-●
  heart Q24.8
    valve NEC Q24.8
      pulmonary Q22.0
  hepatic Q44.79
  humerus —*see* Defect, reduction, upper limb
  hymen Q52.4
  ileum Q41.2

Agenesis (*Continued*)
  incus Q16.3
  intestine (small) Q41.9
    large Q42.9
      specified NEC Q42.8
  iris (dilator fibers) Q13.1
  jaw M26.09
  jejunum Q41.1
  kidney(s) (partial) Q60.2
    bilateral Q60.1
    unilateral Q60.0
  labium (majus) (minus) Q52.71
  labyrinth, membranous Q16.5
  lacrimal apparatus Q10.4
  larynx Q31.8
  leg (complete) Q72.0-●
    with foot present Q72.1-●
    lower leg (with foot present) —*see* Agenesis,
      leg, with foot present
    and foot Q72.2-●
  lens Q12.3
  limb (complete) Q73.0
    lower —*see* Agenesis, leg
    upper —*see* Agenesis, arm
  lip Q38.0
  liver Q44.79
  lung (fissure) (lobe) (bilateral) (unilateral) Q33.3
  mandible, maxilla M26.09
  metacarpus —*see* Agenesis, hand
  metatarsus —*see* Agenesis, foot
  muscle Q79.8
    eyelid Q10.3
    ocular Q15.8
  musculoskeletal system NEC Q79.8
  nail(s) Q84.3
  neck, part Q18.8
  nerve Q07.8
  nervous system, part NEC Q07.8
  nipple Q83.2
  nose Q30.1
  nuclear Q07.8
  organ
    of Corti Q16.5
    or site not listed —*see* Anomaly, by site
  osseous meatus (ear) Q16.1
  ovary
    bilateral Q50.02
    unilateral Q50.01
  oviduct Q50.6
  pancreas Q45.0
  parathyroid (gland) Q89.2
  parotid gland(s) Q38.4
  patella Q74.1
  pelvic girdle (complete) (partial) Q74.2
  penis Q55.5
  pericardium Q24.8
  pituitary (gland) Q89.2
  prostate Q55.4
  punctum lacrimale Q10.4
  radioulnar —*see* Defect, reduction, upper limb
  radius —*see* Defect, reduction, upper limb,
    longitudinal, radius
  rectum Q42.1
    with fistula Q42.0
  renal Q60.2
    bilateral Q60.1
    unilateral Q60.0
  respiratory organ NEC Q34.8
  rib Q76.6
  roof of orbit Q75.8
  round ligament Q52.8
  sacrum Q76.49
  salivary gland Q38.4
  scapula Q74.0
  scrotum Q55.29
  seminal vesicles Q55.4
  septum
    atrial Q21.19
    between aorta and pulmonary artery Q21.4
    ventricular Q20.4
  shoulder girdle (complete) (partial) Q74.0
  skull (bone) Q75.8
    with
      anencephaly Q00.0
      encephalocele —*see* Encephalocele
      hydrocephalus Q03.9
        with spina bifida —*see* Spina bifida, by
          site, with hydrocephalus
      microcephaly Q02
  spermatic cord Q55.4
  spinal cord Q06.0

Agenesis (*Continued*)
  spine Q76.49
  spleen Q89.01
  sternum Q76.7
  stomach Q40.2
  submaxillary gland(s) (congenital) Q38.4
  tarsus —*see* Agenesis, foot
  tendon Q79.8
  testicle Q55.0
  thymus (gland) Q89.2
  thyroid (gland) E03.1
    cartilage Q31.8
  tibia —*see* Defect, reduction, lower limb,
    longitudinal, tibia
  tibiofibular —*see* Defect, reduction, lower limb,
    specified type NEC
  toe (and foot) (complete) (partial) —*see* Agenesis,
    foot
  tongue Q38.3
  trachea (cartilage) Q32.1
  ulna —*see* Defect, reduction, upper limb,
    longitudinal, ulna
  upper limb —*see* Agenesis, arm
  ureter Q62.4
  urethra Q64.5
  urinary tract NEC Q64.8
  uterus Q51.0
  uvula Q38.5
  vagina Q52.0
  vas deferens Q55.4
  vein(s) (peripheral) Q27.9
    brain Q28.3
    great NEC Q26.8
    portal Q26.5
  vena cava (inferior) (superior) Q26.8
  vermis of cerebellum Q04.3
  vertebra Q76.49
  vulva Q52.71
Ageusia R43.2
Agitated —*see* condition
Agitation R45.1
Aglossia (congenital) Q38.3
Aglossia-adactylia syndrome Q87.0
Aglycogenosis E74.00
Agnosia (body image) (other senses) (tactile)
  R48.1
  developmental F88
  verbal R48.1
    auditory R48.1
      developmental F80.2
    developmental F80.2
  visual (object) R48.3
Agoraphobia F40.00
  with panic disorder F40.01
  without panic disorder F40.02
Agrammatism R48.8
Agranulocytopenia —*see* Agranulocytosis
Agranulocytosis (chronic) (cyclical) (genetic)
  (infantile) (periodic) (pernicious) (*see also*
  Neutropenia) D70.9
  congenital D70.0
  cytoreductive cancer chemotherapy sequela
    D70.1
  drug-induced D70.2
    due to cytoreductive cancer chemotherapy
      D70.1
  due to infection D70.3
  secondary D70.4
    drug-induced D70.2
      due to cytoreductive cancer chemotherapy
        D70.1
Agraphia (absolute) R48.8
  with alexia R48.0
  developmental F81.81
Ague (dumb) —*see* Malaria
Agyria Q04.3
Ahumada-del Castillo syndrome E23.0
Aichomophobia F40.298
AIDS (related complex) B20
Ailment heart —*see* Disease, heart
Ailurophobia F40.218
Ainhum (disease) L94.6
AIN —*see* Neoplasia, intraepithelial, anal
AIPHI (acute idiopathic pulmonary hemorrhage in
  infants (over 28 days old)) R04.81
Air
  anterior mediastinum J98.2
  compressed, disease T70.3
  conditioner lung or pneumonitis J67.7
  embolism (artery) (cerebral) (any site) T79.0
    with ectopic or molar pregnancy O08.2

▶ New   ⇒ Revised   ~~deleted~~ Deleted   ● Use Additional Character(s)

Allergy, allergic *(Continued)*
nasal, seasonal due to pollen J30.1
pneumonia J82.89
pollen (any) (hay fever) J30.1
  asthma —*see* Asthma, allergic extrinsic
primrose J30.1
primula J30.1
proctocolitis K52.29
purpura D69.0
ragweed (hay fever) (pollen) J30.1
  asthma —*see* Asthma, allergic extrinsic
rose (pollen) J30.1
seasonal NEC J30.2
Senecio jacobae (pollen) J30.1
serum —*see also* Reaction, serum T80.69
  anaphylactic shock T80.59
shock (anaphylactic) T78.2
  due to
    administration of blood and blood products T80.51
    adverse effect of correct medicinal substance properly administered T88.6
    immunization T80.52
    serum NEC T80.59
    vaccination T80.52
  specific NEC T78.49
tree (any) (hay fever) (pollen) J30.1
  asthma —*see* Asthma, allergic extrinsic
upper respiratory J30.9
urticaria L50.0
vaccine —*see* Allergy, serum
wheat —*see* Allergy, food
Allescheriasis B48.2
Alligator skin disease Q80.9
Allocheiria, allochiria R20.8
Almeida's disease —*see* Paracoccidioidomycosis
Alopecia (hereditaria) (seborrheica) L65.9
androgenic L64.9
  drug-induced L64.0
  specified NEC L64.8
areata L63.9
  ophiasis L63.2
  specified NEC L63.8
  totalis L63.0
  universalis L63.1
cicatricial L66.9
  ▶central centrifugal L66.81
  ▶specified NEC L66.89
circumscripta L63.9
congenital, congenitalis Q84.0
due to cytotoxic drugs NEC L65.8
▶frontal fibrosing L66.12
mucinosa L65.2
postinfective NEC L65.8
postpartum L65.0
premature L64.8
specific (syphilitic) A51.32
specified NEC L65.8
syphilitic (secondary) A51.32
totalis (capitis) L63.0
universalis (entire body) L63.1
X-ray L58.1
Alpers' disease G31.81
Alpine sickness T70.29
Alport syndrome Q87.81
ALTE (apparent life threatening event) in newborn and infant R68.13
Alteration (of), **Altered**
awareness
  transient R40.4
  unintended under general anesthesia, during procedure T88.53
mental status R41.82
pattern of family relationships affecting child Z62.898
sensation
  following
    cerebrovascular disease I69.998
      cerebral infarction I69.398
      intracerebral hemorrhage I69.198
      nontraumatic intracranial hemorrhage NEC I69.298
      specified disease NEC I69.898
      subarachnoid hemorrhage I69.098
Alternating —*see* condition
Altitude, high (effects) —*see* Effect, adverse, high altitude
Aluminosis (of lung) J63.0
Alveolitis
allergic (extrinsic) —*see* Pneumonitis, hypersensitivity

Alveolitis *(Continued)*
due to
  Aspergillus clavatus J67.4
  Cryptostroma corticale J67.6
fibrosing (cryptogenic) (idiopathic) J84.112
jaw M27.3
sicca dolorosa M27.3
Alveolus, alveolar —*see* condition
Alymphocytosis D72.810
thymic (with immunodeficiency) D82.1
Alymphoplasia, thymic D82.1
Alzheimer's disease or sclerosis —*see* Disease, Alzheimer's
Amastia (with nipple present) Q83.8
with absent nipple Q83.0
Amathophobia F40.228
Amaurosis (acquired) (congenital) —*see also* Blindness
fugax G45.3
hysterical F44.6
Leber's congenital H35.50
uremic —*see* Uremia
Amaurotic idiocy (infantile) (juvenile) (late) E75.4
Amaxophobia F40.248
Ambiguous genitalia Q56.4
Amblyopia (congenital) (ex anopsia) (partial) (suppression) H53.00-●
anisometropic —*see* Amblyopia, refractive
deprivation H53.01-●
hysterical F44.6
nocturnal —*see also* Blindness, night
  vitamin A deficiency E50.5
refractive H53.02-●
strabismic H53.03-●
suspect H53.04-●
tobacco H53.8
toxic NEC H53.8
uremic —*see* Uremia
Ameba, amebic (histolytica) —*see also* Amebiasis
abscess (liver) A06.4
Amebiasis A06.9
with abscess —*see* Abscess, amebic
acute A06.0
chronic (intestine) A06.1
  with abscess —*see* Abscess, amebic
cutaneous A06.7
cutis A06.7
cystitis A06.81
genitourinary tract NEC A06.82
hepatic —*see* Abscess, liver, amebic
intestine A06.0
nondysenteric colitis A06.2
skin A06.7
specified site NEC A06.89
Ameboma (of intestine) A06.3
Amelia Q73.0
lower limb —*see* Agenesis, leg
upper limb —*see* Agenesis, arm
Ameloblastoma —*see also* Cyst, calcifying odontogenic
long bones C40.9-●
  lower limb C40.2-●
  upper limb C40.0-●
malignant C41.1
  jaw (bone) (lower) C41.1
    upper C41.0
tibial C40.2-●
Amelogenesis imperfecta K00.5
nonhereditaria (segmentalis) K00.4
Amenorrhea N91.2
hyperhormonal E28.8
primary N91.0
secondary N91.1
Amentia —*see* Disability, intellectual
Meynert's (nonalcoholic) F04
American
leishmaniasis B55.2
mountain tick fever A93.2
Ametropia —*see* Disorder, refraction
AMH (asymptomatic microscopic hematuria) R31.21
Amianthosis J61
Amimia R48.8
Amino-acid disorder E72.9
anemia D53.0
Aminoacidopathy E72.9
Aminoaciduria E72.9
Amnes (t)ic syndrome (post-traumatic) F04
induced by
  alcohol F10.96
    with dependence F10.26

Amnes (t)ic syndrome *(Continued)*
induced by *(Continued)*
  psychoactive NEC F19.96
    with
      abuse F19.16
      dependence F19.26
  sedative F13.96
    with dependence F13.26
Amnesia R41.3
anterograde R41.1
auditory R48.8
dissociative F44.0
  with dissociative fugue F44.1
hysterical F44.0
postictal in epilepsy —*see* Epilepsy
psychogenic F44.0
retrograde R41.2
transient global G45.4
Amnion, amniotic —*see* condition
Amnionitis —*see* Pregnancy, complicated by
Amok F68.8
Amoral traits F60.89
Amphetamine (or other stimulant) —induced
anxiety disorder F15.980
bipolar and related disorder F15.94
delirium F15.921
depressive disorder F15.94
obsessive-compulsive and related disorder F15.988
psychotic disorder F15.959
sexual dysfunction F15.981
sleep disorder F15.982
stimulant withdrawal F15.23
Ampulla
lower esophagus K22.89
phrenic K22.89
Amputation —*see also* Absence, by site, acquired
neuroma (postoperative) (traumatic) —*see* Complications, amputation stump, neuroma
stump (surgical)
  abnormal, painful, or with complication (late) —*see* Complications, amputation stump
  healed or old NOS Z89.9
traumatic (complete) (partial)
  arm (upper) (complete) S48.91-●
    at
      elbow S58.01-●
        partial S58.02-●
      shoulder joint (complete) S48.01-●
        partial S48.02-●
    between
      elbow and wrist (complete) S58.11-●
        partial S58.12-●
      shoulder and elbow (complete) S48.11-●
        partial S48.12-●
    partial S48.92-●
  breast (complete) S28.21-●
    partial S28.22-●
  clitoris (complete) S38.211
    partial S38.212
  ear (complete) S08.11-●
    partial S08.12-●
  finger (complete) (metacarpophalangeal) S68.11-●
    index S68.11-●
    little S68.11-●
    middle S68.11-●
    partial S68.12-●
      index S68.12-●
      little S68.12-●
      middle S68.12-●
      ring S68.12-●
    ring S68.11-●
    thumb —*see* Amputation, traumatic, thumb
    transphalangeal (complete) S68.61-●
      index S68.61-●
      little S68.61-●
      middle S68.61-●
      partial S68.62-●
        index S68.62-●
        little S68.62-●
        middle S68.62-●
        ring S68.62-●
      ring S68.61-●
  foot (complete) S98.91-●
    at ankle level S98.01-●
      partial S98.02-●

▶ New ⟹ Revised ~~deleted~~ Deleted ● Use Additional Character(s)

Amputation *(Continued)*
  traumatic *(Continued)*
    foot *(Continued)*
      midfoot S98.31-●
        partial S98.32-●
      partial S98.92-●
    forearm (complete) S58.91-●
      at elbow level (complete) S58.01-●
        partial S58.02-●
      between elbow and wrist (complete)
          S58.11-●
        partial S58.12-●
      partial S58.92-●
    genital organ(s) (external)
      female (complete) S38.211
        partial S38.212
      male
        penis (complete) S38.221
          partial S38.222
        scrotum (complete) S38.231
          partial S38.232
        testes (complete) S38.231
          partial S38.232
    hand (complete) (wrist level) S68.41-●
      finger(s) alone —*see* Amputation, traumatic,
          finger
      partial S68.42-●
      thumb alone —*see* Amputation, traumatic,
          thumb
      transmetacarpal (complete) S68.71-●
        partial S68.72-●
    head
      ear —*see* Amputation, traumatic, ear
      nose (partial) S08.812
        complete S08.811
      part S08.89
        scalp S08.0
    hip (and thigh) (complete) S78.91-●
      at hip joint (complete) S78.01-●
        partial S78.02-●
      between hip and knee (complete)
          S78.11-●
        partial S78.12-●
      partial S78.92-●
    labium (majus) (minus) (complete) S38.21-●
      partial S38.21-●
    leg (lower) S88.91-●
      at knee level S88.01-●
        partial S88.02-●
      between knee and ankle S88.11-●
        partial S88.12-●
      partial S88.92-●
    nose (partial) S08.812
      complete S08.811
    penis (complete) S38.221
      partial S38.222
    scrotum (complete) S38.231
      partial S38.232
    shoulder —*see* Amputation, traumatic, arm
      at shoulder joint —*see* Amputation,
          traumatic, arm, at shoulder joint
    testes (complete) S38.231
      partial S38.232
    thigh —*see* Amputation, traumatic, hip
    thorax, part of S28.1
      breast —*see* Amputation, traumatic, breast
    thumb (complete) (metacarpophalangeal)
        S68.01-●
      partial S68.02-●
      transphalangeal (complete) S68.51-●
        partial S68.52-●
    toe (lesser) S98.13-●
      great S98.11-●
        partial S98.12-●
      more than one S98.21-●
        partial S98.22-●
      partial S98.14-●
    vulva (complete) S38.211
      partial S38.212
Amputee (bilateral) (old) Z89.9
Amsterdam dwarfism Q87.19
Amusia R48.8
  developmental F80.89
Amyelencephalus, amyelencephaly Q00.0
Amyelia Q06.0
Amygdalitis —*see* Tonsillitis
Amygdalolith J35.8
Amyloid heart (disease) E85.4 *[I43]*
Amyloidosis (generalized) (primary) E85.9
  with lung involvement E85.4 *[J99]*
  familial E85.2

Amyloidosis *(Continued)*
  genetic E85.2
  heart E85.4 *[I43]*
  hemodialysis-associated E85.3
  light chain (AL) E85.81
  liver E85.4 *[K77]*
  localized E85.4
  neuropathic heredofamilial E85.1
  non-neuropathic heredofamilial E85.0
  organ limited E85.4
  Portuguese E85.1
  pulmonary E85.4 *[J99]*
  secondary systemic E85.3
  senile systemic (SSA) E85.82
  skin (lichen) (macular) E85.4 *[L99]*
  specified NEC E85.89
  subglottic E85.4 *[J99]*
  wild-type transthyretin-related (ATTR)
      E85.82
Amylopectinosis (brancher enzyme deficiency)
    E74.03
Amylophagia —*see* Pica
Amyoplasia congenita Q79.8
Amyotonia M62.89
  congenita G70.2
Amyotrophia, amyotrophy, amyotrophic
    G71.8
  congenita Q79.8
  diabetic —*see* Diabetes, amyotrophy
  lateral sclerosis G12.21
  neuralgic G54.5
  spinal progressive G12.25
Anacidity, gastric K31.83
  psychogenic F45.8
Anaerosis of newborn P28.89
Analbuminemia E88.09
Analgesia —*see* Anesthesia
Analphalipoproteinemia E78.6
Anaphylactic
  purpura D69.0
  shock or reaction —*see* Shock, anaphylactic
Anaphylactoid shock or reaction —*see* Shock,
    anaphylactic
Anaphylactoid syndrome of pregnancy O88.01-●
Anaphylaxis —*see* Shock, anaphylactic
Anaplasia cervix —*see also* Dysplasia, cervix
    N87.9
Anaplasmosis [A. phagocytophilum] (transfusion
    transmitted) A79.82
  human A77.49
Anarthria R47.1
Anasarca R60.1
  cardiac —*see* Failure, heart, congestive
  lung J18.2
  newborn P83.2
  nutritional E43
  pulmonary J18.2
  renal N04.9
Anastomosis
  aneurysmal —*see* Aneurysm
  arteriovenous ruptured brain I60.8
  intestinal K63.89
    complicated NEC K91.89
      involving urinary tract N99.89
  intracerebral I61.8
  intraparenchymal I61.8
  intraventricular I61.5
  retinal and choroidal vessels (congenital) Q14.8
  subarachnoid I60.8
Anatomical narrow angle H40.03-●
Ancylostoma, ancylostomiasis (braziliense)
    (caninum) (ceylanicum) (duodenale) B76.0
  Necator americanus B76.1
Andersen's disease (glycogen storage) E74.09
Anderson-Fabry disease E75.21
Andes disease T70.29
Andrews' disease (bacterid) L08.89
Androblastoma
  benign
    specified site —*see* Neoplasm, benign, by site
    unspecified site
      female D27.9
      male D29.20
  malignant
    specified site —*see* Neoplasm, malignant, by
        site
    unspecified site
      female C56.9
      male C62.90
  specified site —*see* Neoplasm, uncertain
      behavior, by site

Androblastoma *(Continued)*
  tubular
    with lipid storage
      specified site —*see* Neoplasm, benign, by
          site
      unspecified site
        female D27.9
        male D29.20
    specified site —*see* Neoplasm, benign, by site
    unspecified site
      female D27.9
      male D29.20
  unspecified site
    female D39.10
    male D40.10
Androgen insensitivity syndrome —*see also*
    Syndrome, androgen insensitivity
    E34.50
Androgen resistance syndrome —*see also*
    Syndrome, androgen insensitivity E34.50
Android pelvis Q74.2
  with disproportion (fetopelvic) O33.3
    causing obstructed labor O65.3
Androphobia F40.290
Anectasis, pulmonary (newborn) —*see* Atelectasis
Anemia (essential) (general) (hemoglobin
    deficiency) (infantile) (primary) (profound)
    D64.9
  with (due to) (in)
    disorder of
      anaerobic glycolysis D55.29
      pentose phosphate pathway D55.1
    koilonychia D50.9
  achlorhydric D50.8
  achrestic D53.1
  Addison (-Biermer) (pernicious) D51.0
  agranulocytic —*see* Agranulocytosis
  amino-acid-deficiency D53.0
  aplastic D61.9
    congenital D61.09
    drug-induced D61.1
    due to
      drugs D61.1
      external agents NEC D61.2
      infection D61.2
      radiation D61.2
    idiopathic D61.3
    red cell (pure) D60.9
      chronic D60.0
      congenital D61.01
      specified type NEC D60.8
      transient D60.1
    specified type NEC D61.89
    toxic D61.2
  aregenerative
    congenital D61.09
  asiderotic D50.9
  atypical (primary) D64.9
  Baghdad spring D55.0
  Balantidium coli A07.0
  Biermer's (pernicious) D51.0
  blood loss (chronic) D50.0
    acute D62
  bothriocephalus B70.0 *[D63.8]*
  brickmaker's B76.9 *[D63.8]*
  cerebral I67.89
  childhood D58.9
  chloritic D50.8
  chronic
    blood loss D50.0
    hemolytic D58.9
      idiopathic D59.9
    simple D53.9
  chronica congenita aregenerativa D61.09
  combined system disease NEC D51.0 *[G32.0]*
    due to dietary vitamin B12 deficiency D51.3
        [G32.0]
  complicating pregnancy, childbirth or
      puerperium —*see* Pregnancy, complicated
      by (management affected by), anemia
  congenital P61.4
    aplastic D61.09
    due to isoimmunization NOS P55.9
    dyserythropoietic, dyshematopoietic D64.4
    following fetal blood loss P61.3
    Heinz body D58.2
    hereditary hemolytic NOS D58.9
    pernicious D51.0
    spherocytic D58.0
  Cooley's (erythroblastic) D56.1
  cytogenic D51.0

Anemia *(Continued)*
  deficiency D53.9
    2, 3 diphosphoglycurate mutase D55.29
    2, 3 PG D55.29
    6 phosphogluconate dehydrogenase D55.1
    6-PGD D55.1
    amino-acid D53.0
    combined B12 and folate D53.1
    enzyme D55.9
      drug-induced (hemolytic) D59.2
      glucose-6-phosphate dehydrogenase
        (G6PD) D55.0
      glycolytic D55.29
      nucleotide metabolism D55.3
      related to hexose monophosphate (HMP)
        shunt pathway NEC D55.1
      specified type NEC D55.8
    erythrocytic glutathione D55.1
    folate D52.9
      dietary D52.0
      drug-induced D52.1
    folic acid D52.9
      dietary D52.0
      drug-induced D52.1
    G SH D55.1
    G6PD D55.0
    GGS-R D55.1
    glucose-6-phosphate dehydrogenase D55.0
    glutathione reductase D55.1
    glyceraldehyde phosphate dehydrogenase
      D55.29
    hexokinase D55.29
    iron D50.9
      secondary to blood loss (chronic) D50.0
    nutritional D53.9
      with
        poor iron absorption D50.8
        specified deficiency NEC D53.8
    phosphofructo-aldolase D55.29
    phosphoglycerate kinase D55.29
    PK D55.21
    protein D53.0
    pyruvate kinase D55.21
    transcobalamin II D55.22
    triose-phosphate isomerase D55.29
    vitamin B12 NOS D51.9
      dietary D51.3
      due to
        intrinsic factor deficiency D51.0
        selective vitamin B12 malabsorption with
          proteinuria D51.1
      pernicious D51.0
      specified type NEC D51.8
  Diamond-Blackfan (congenital hypoplastic)
    D61.01
  dibothriocephalus B70.0 *[D63.8]*
  dimorphic D53.1
  diphasic D53.1
  Diphyllobothrium (Dibothriocephalus) B70.0
    [D63.8]
  due to (in) (with)
    antineoplastic chemotherapy D64.81
    blood loss (chronic) D50.0
      acute D62
    chemotherapy, antineoplastic D64.81
    chronic disease classified elsewhere NEC
      D63.8
    chronic kidney disease D63.1
    deficiency
      amino acid D53.0
      copper D53.8
      folate (folic acid) D52.9
        dietary D52.0
        drug-induced D52.1
      molybdenum D53.8
      protein D53.0
      zinc D53.8
    dietary vitamin B12 deficiency D51.3
    disorder of
      glutathione metabolism D55.1
      nucleotide metabolism D55.3
    drug —*see also* Anemia, by type —*see also* Table of
      Drugs and Chemicals
    end stage renal disease D63.1
    enzyme disorder D55.9
    fetal blood loss P61.3
    fish tapeworm (D latum) infestation B70.0
      [D63.8]
    hemorrhage (chronic) D50.0
      acute D62
    impaired absorption D50.9

Anemia *(Continued)*
  due to *(Continued)*
    loss of blood (chronic) D50.0
      acute D62
    myxedema E03.9 *[D63.8]*
    Necator americanus B76.1 *[D63.8]*
    prematurity P61.2
    selective vitamin B12 malabsorption with
      proteinuria D51.1
    transcobalamin II deficiency D51.2
  Dyke-Young type (secondary) (symptomatic)
    D59.19
  dyserythropoietic (congenital) D64.4
  dyshematopoietic (congenital) D64.4
  Egyptian B76.9 *[D63.8]*
  elliptocytosis —*see* Elliptocytosis
  enzyme-deficiency, drug-induced D59.2
  epidemic —*see also* Ancylostomiasis B76.9 *[D63.8]*
  erythroblastic
    familial D56.1
    newborn —*see also* Disease, hemolytic P55.9
    of childhood D56.1
  erythrocytic glutathione deficiency D55.1
  erythropoietin-resistant anemia (EPO resistant
    anemia) D63.1
  Faber's (achlorhydric anemia) D50.9
  factitious (self-induced blood letting) D50.0
  familial erythroblastic D56.1
  ~~Fanconi's (congenital pancytopenia) D61.09~~
  ▶ Fanconi ('s) D61.03
  favism D55.0
  fish tapeworm (D. latum) infestation B70.0
    [D63.8]
  folate (folic acid) deficiency D52.9
  glucose-6-phosphate dehydrogenase (G6PD)
    deficiency D55.0
  glutathione-reductase deficiency D55.1
  goat's milk D52.0
  granulocytic —*see* Agranulocytosis
  Heinz body, congenital D58.2
  hemolytic D58.9
    acquired D59.9
      with hemoglobinuria NEC D59.6
      autoimmune NEC D59.19
      infectious D59.4
      specified type NEC D59.8
      toxic D59.4
    acute D59.9
      due to enzyme deficiency specified type
        NEC D55.8
      Lederer's D59.19
    autoimmune D59.10
      cold D59.12
      drug-induced D59.0
      mixed D59.13
      warm D59.11
    chronic D58.9
      idiopathic D59.9
    cold type (secondary) (symptomatic) D59.12
    congenital (spherocytic) —*see* Spherocytosis
    due to
      cardiac conditions D59.4
      drugs (nonautoimmune) D59.2
        autoimmune D59.0
      enzyme disorder D55.9
        drug-induced D59.2
      presence of shunt or other internal
        prosthetic device D59.4
    familial D58.9
    hereditary D58.9
      due to enzyme disorder D55.9
        specified type NEC D55.8
      specified type NEC D58.8
    idiopathic (chronic) D59.9
    mechanical D59.4
    microangiopathic D59.4
    mixed type (primary) (secondary)
      (symptomatic) D59.13
    nonautoimmune D59.4
      drug-induced D59.2
    nonspherocytic
      congenital or hereditary NEC D55.8
        glucose-6-phosphate dehydrogenase
          deficiency D55.0
        pyruvate kinase deficiency D55.21
        type
          I D55.1
          II D55.29
      type
        I D55.1
        II D55.29

Anemia *(Continued)*
  hemolytic *(Continued)*
    primary
      autoimmune
        cold type D59.12
        mixed type D59.13
        warm type D59.11
    secondary D59.4
      autoimmune
        cold type D59.12
        mixed type D59.13
        warm type D59.11
    specified (hereditary) type NEC D58.8
    Stransky-Regala type —*see also*
      Hemoglobinopathy D58.8
    symptomatic D59.4
      autoimmune
        cold type D59.12
        mixed type D59.13
        warm type D59.11
    toxic D59.4
    warm type (primary) (secondary)
      (symptomatic) D59.11
  hemorrhagic (chronic) D50.0
    acute D62
  Herrick's D57.1
  hexokinase deficiency D55.29
  hookworm B76.9 *[D63.8]*
  hypochromic (idiopathic) (microcytic)
    (normoblastic) D50.9
    due to blood loss (chronic) D50.0
      acute D62
    familial sex-linked D64.0
    pyridoxine-responsive D64.3
    sideroblastic, sex-linked D64.0
  hypoplasia, red blood cells D61.9
    congenital or familial D61.01
  hypoplastic (idiopathic) D61.9
    congenital or familial (of childhood) D61.01
  hypoproliferative (refractive) D61.9
  idiopathic D64.9
    aplastic D61.3
    hemolytic, chronic D59.9
  in (due to) (with)
    chronic kidney disease D63.1
    end stage renal disease D63.1
    failure, kidney (renal) D63.1
    neoplastic disease —*see also* Neoplasm
      D63.0
  intertropical —*see also* Ancylostomiasis
    D63.8
  iron deficiency D50.9
    secondary to blood loss (chronic) D50.0
      acute D62
    specified type NEC D50.8
  Joseph-Diamond-Blackfan (congenital
    hypoplastic) D61.01
  Lederer's (hemolytic) D59.19
  leukoerythroblastic D61.82
  macrocytic D53.9
    nutritional D52.0
    tropical D52.8
  malarial (*see also* Malaria) B54 *[D63.8]*
  malignant (progressive) D51.0
  malnutrition D53.9
  marsh (*see also* Malaria) B54 *[D63.8]*
  Mediterranean (with other hemoglobinopathy)
    D56.9
  megaloblastic D53.1
    combined B12 and folate deficiency
      D53.1
    hereditary D51.1
    nutritional D52.0
    orotic aciduria D53.0
    refractory D53.1
    specified type NEC D53.1
  megalocytic D53.1
  microcytic (hypochromic) D50.9
    due to blood loss (chronic) D50.0
      acute D62
    familial D56.8
  microdrepanocytosis D57.40
  microelliptopoikilocytic (Rietti-Greppi-Micheli)
    D56.9
  miner's B76.9 *[D63.8]*
  myelodysplastic D46.9
  myelofibrosis D75.81
  myelogenous D64.89
  myelopathic D64.89
  myelophthisic D61.82
  myeloproliferative D47.Z9

▶ New   ⇒ Revised   ~~deleted~~ Deleted   ● Use Additional Character(s)

Anemia *(Continued)*
  newborn P61.4
    due to
      ABO (antibodies, isoimmunization,
        maternal/fetal incompatibility) P55.1
      Rh (antibodies, isoimmunization,
        maternal/fetal incompatibility) P55.0
    following fetal blood loss P61.3
    posthemorrhagic (fetal) P61.3
  nonspherocytic hemolytic —*see* Anemia,
    hemolytic, nonspherocytic
  normocytic (infectional) D64.9
    due to blood loss (chronic) D50.0
      acute D62
    myelophthisic D61.82
  nutritional (deficiency) D53.9
    with
      poor iron absorption D50.8
      specified deficiency NEC D53.8
    megaloblastic D52.0
  of prematurity P61.2
  orotaciduric (congenital) (hereditary) D53.0
  osteosclerotic D64.89
  ovalocytosis (hereditary) —*see* Elliptocytosis
  paludal —*see also* Malaria B54 *[D63.8]*
  pernicious (congenital) (malignant) (progressive)
    D51.0
  pleochromic D64.89
    of sprue D52.8
  posthemorrhagic (chronic) D50.0
    acute D62
    newborn P61.3
  postoperative (postprocedural)
    due to (acute) blood loss D62
      chronic blood loss D50.0
    specified NEC D64.89
  postpartum O90.81
  pressure D64.89
  progressive D64.9
    malignant D51.0
    pernicious D51.0
  protein-deficiency D53.0
  pseudoleukemica infantum D64.89
  pure red cell D60.9
    congenital D61.01
  pyridoxine-responsive D64.3
  pyruvate kinase deficiency D55.21
  refractory D46.4
    with
      excess of blasts D46.20
        1 (RAEB 1) D46.21
        2 (RAEB 2) D46.22
        in transformation (RAEB T) —*see*
          Leukemia, acute myeloblastic
      hemochromatosis D46.1
      sideroblasts (ring) (RARS) D46.1
    without ring sideroblasts, so stated D46.0
    without sideroblasts without excess of blasts
      D46.0
    megaloblastic D53.1
    sideroblastic D46.1
    sideropenic D50.9
  Rietti-Greppi-Micheli D56.9
  scorbutic D53.2
  secondary to
    blood loss (chronic) D50.0
      acute D62
    hemorrhage (chronic) D50.0
      acute D62
  semiplastic D61.89
  sickle-cell —*see* Disease, sickle-cell
  sideroblastic D64.3
    hereditary D64.0
    hypochromic, sex-linked D64.0
    pyridoxine-responsive NEC D64.3
    refractory D46.1
    secondary (due to)
      disease D64.1
      drugs and toxins D64.2
    specified type NEC D64.3
  sideropenic (refractory) D50.9
    due to blood loss (chronic) D50.0
      acute D62
  simple chronic D53.9
  specified type NEC D64.89
  spherocytic (hereditary) —*see* Spherocytosis
  splenic D64.89
  splenomegalic D64.89
  stomatocytosis D58.8
  syphilitic (acquired) (late) A52.79 *[D63.8]*
  target cell D64.89

Anemia *(Continued)*
  thalassemia D56.9
  thrombocytopenic —*see* Thrombocytopenia
  toxic D61.2
  tropical B76.9 *[D63.8]*
    macrocytic D52.8
  tuberculous A18.89 *[D63.8]*
  vegan D51.3
  vitamin
    B6-responsive D64.3
    B12 deficiency (dietary) pernicious D51.0
  von Jaksch's D64.89
  Witts' (achlorhydric anemia) D50.8
Anemophobia F40.228
Anencephalus, anencephaly Q00.0
Anergasia —*see* Psychosis, organic
Anesthesia, anesthetic R20.0
  complication or reaction NEC —*see also*
    Complications, anesthesia T88.59
    due to
      correct substance properly administered —
        see Table of Drugs and Chemicals, by
        drug, adverse effect
      overdose or wrong substance given —*see*
        Table of Drugs and Chemicals, by
        drug, poisoning
      unintended awareness under general
        anesthesia during procedure T88.53
      personal history of Z92.84
  cornea H18.81-●
  dissociative F44.6
  functional (hysterical) F44.6
  hyperesthetic, thalamic G89.0
  hysterical F44.6
  local skin lesion R20.0
  sexual (psychogenic) F52.1
  shock (due to) T88.2
  skin R20.0
  testicular N50.9
Anetoderma (maculosum) (of) L90.8
  Jadassohn-Pellizzari L90.2
  ~~Schweninger-Buzzi L90.1~~
  ▶ Schweninger-Buzzi L90.1
Aneurin deficiency E51.9
Aneurysm (anastomotic) (artery) (cirsoid) (diffuse)
  (false) (fusiform) (multiple) (saccular) I72.9
  abdominal (aorta) I71.40
    infrarenal I71.43
      ruptured I71.33
    juxtarenal I71.42
      ruptured I71.32
    pararenal I71.41
      ruptured I71.31
    ruptured I71.30
    syphilitic A52.01
  aorta, aortic (nonsyphilitic) I71.9
    abdominal I71.40
      dissecting —*see* Dissection, aorta, abdominal
      ruptured I71.30
    arch I71.22
      ruptured I71.12
    arteriosclerotic I71.9
      ruptured I71.8
    ascending I71.21
      ruptured I71.11
    congenital Q25.43
    descending I71.9
      abdominal I71.40
        ruptured I71.30
      ruptured I71.8
      thoracic I71.23
        ruptured I71.13
    dissecting —*see* Dissection, aorta
    root Q25.43
    ruptured I71.8
    sinus, congenital Q25.43
    syphilitic A52.01
    thoracic I71.20
      ruptured I71.10
    thoracoabdominal I71.60
      paravisceral I71.62
        ruptured I71.52
      ruptured I71.50
      supraceliac I71.61
        ruptured I71.51
    thorax, thoracic I71.20
      arch I71.22
        ruptured I71.12
      ascending I71.21
        ruptured I71.11
      descending I71.23
        ruptured I71.13

Aneurysm *(Continued)*
  aorta, aortic *(Continued)*
    thorax, thoracic *(Continued)*
      ruptured I71.10
        arch I71.12
        ascending I71.11
        descending I71.13
      transverse I71.22
        ruptured I71.12
    valve (heart) —*see also* Endocarditis, aortic
      I35.8
  arteriosclerotic I72.9
    cerebral I67.1
      ruptured —*see* Hemorrhage, intracranial,
        subarachnoid
  arteriovenous (congenital) —*see also*
    Malformation, arteriovenous
    acquired I77.0
      brain I67.1
        ruptured —*see* Aneurysm,
          arteriorvenous, brain, ruptured
      coronary I25.41
      pulmonary I28.0
    brain Q28.2
      ruptured I60.8
        intracerebral I61.8
        intraparenchymal I61.8
        intraventricular I61.5
        subarachnoid I60.8
    peripheral —*see* Malformation, arteriovenous,
      peripheral
    precerebral vessels Q28.0
    specified site NEC —*see also* Malformation,
      arteriovenous
      acquired I77.0
  basal —*see* Aneurysm, brain
  basilar (trunk) I72.5
  berry (congenital) (nonruptured) I67.1
    ruptured I60.7
  brain I67.1
    arteriosclerotic I67.1
      ruptured —*see* Hemorrhage, intracranial,
        subarachnoid
    arteriovenous (congenital) (nonruptured)
      Q28.2
      acquired I67.1
      ➡ruptured —*see* Aneurysm,
        arteriorvenous, brain, ruptured
      ➡ruptured —*see* Aneurysm, arteriorvenous,
        brain, ruptured
    berry (congenital) (nonruptured) I67.1
      ruptured —*see also* Hemorrhage,
        intracranial, subarachnoid I60.7
    congenital Q28.3
      aorta (root) (sinus) Q25.43
      ruptured I60.7
    meninges I67.1
      ruptured I60.8
    miliary (congenital) (nonruptured) I67.1
      ruptured —*see also* Hemorrhage,
        intracranial, subarachnoid I60.7
    mycotic I67.1
      with endocarditis - *see also* Endocarditis
      ruptured —*see* Hemorrhage, intracranial,
        subarachnoid
    syphilitic (hemorrhage) A52.05
  cardiac (false) —*see also* Aneurysm,
    heart I25.3
  carotid artery (common) (external) I72.0
    internal (intracranial) I67.1
      extracranial portion I72.0
      ruptured into brain I60.0-●
    syphilitic A52.09
      intracranial A52.05
  cavernous sinus I67.1
    arteriovenous (congenital) (nonruptured) Q28.3
      ruptured I60.8
  celiac I72.8
  central nervous system, syphilitic A52.05
  cerebral —*see* Aneurysm, brain
  chest —*see* Aneurysm, thorax
  circle of Willis I67.1
    congenital Q28.3
      ruptured I60.6
    ruptured I60.6
  common iliac artery I72.3
  congenital (peripheral) Q27.8
    aorta (root) (sinus) Q25.43
    brain Q28.3
      ruptured I60.7
    coronary Q24.5

Aneurysm *(Continued)*
  congenital *(Continued)*
    digestive system Q27.8
    lower limb Q27.8
    pulmonary Q25.79
    retina Q14.1
    specified site NEC Q27.8
    upper limb Q27.8
  conjunctiva —*see* Abnormality, conjunctiva, vascular
  conus arteriosus —*see* Aneurysm, heart
  coronary (arteriosclerotic) (artery) I25.41
    arteriovenous, congenital Q24.5
    congenital Q24.5
    ruptured —*see* Infarct, myocardium
    syphilitic A52.06
    vein I25.89
  cylindroid (aorta) I71.9
    ruptured I71.8
    syphilitic A52.01
  ductus arteriosus Q25.0
  endocardial, infective (any valve) I33.0
  femoral (artery) (ruptured) I72.4
  gastroduodenal I72.8
  gastroepiploic I72.8
  heart (wall) (chronic or with a stated duration of over 4 weeks) I25.3
    valve —*see* Endocarditis
  hepatic I72.8
  iliac (common) (artery) (ruptured) I72.3
  infective I72.9
    endocardial (any valve) I33.0
  innominate (nonsyphilitic) I72.8
    syphilitic A52.09
  interauricular septum —*see* Aneurysm, heart
  interventricular septum —*see* Aneurysm, heart
  intrathoracic (nonsyphilitic) (*see also* Aneurysm, aorta, thorax) I71.20
    ruptured (*see also* Aneurysm, aorta, thorax, ruptured) I71.10
    syphilitic A52.01
  lower limb I72.4
  lung (pulmonary artery) I28.1
  mediastinal (nonsyphilitic) I72.8
    syphilitic A52.09
  miliary (congenital) I67.1
    ruptured —*see* Hemorrhage, intracerebral, subarachnoid, intracranial
  mitral (heart) (valve) I34.89
  mural —*see* Aneurysm, heart
  mycotic I72.9
    endocardial (any valve) I33.0
    ruptured, brain —*see* Hemorrhage, intracerebral, subarachnoid
  myocardium —*see* Aneurysm, heart
  neck I72.0
  pancreaticoduodenal I72.8
  patent ductus arteriosus Q25.0
  peripheral NEC I72.8
    congenital Q27.8
      digestive system Q27.8
      lower limb Q27.8
      specified site NEC Q27.8
      upper limb Q27.8
  popliteal (artery) (ruptured) I72.4
  precerebral
    congenital (nonruptured) Q28.1
    specified site, NEC I72.5
  pulmonary I28.1
    arteriovenous Q25.72
      acquired I28.0
    syphilitic A52.09
    valve (heart) —*see* Endocarditis, pulmonary
  racemose (peripheral) I72.9
    congenital —*see* Aneurysm, congenital
  radial I72.1
  Rasmussen NEC A15.0
  renal (artery) I72.2
  retina —*see also* Disorder, retina, microaneurysms
    congenital Q14.1
    diabetic —*see* E08-E13 with .3-●
  sinus of Valsalva Q25.43
  specified NEC I72.8
  spinal (cord) I72.8
    syphilitic (hemorrhage) A52.09
  splenic I72.8
  subclavian (artery) (ruptured) I72.8
    syphilitic A52.09
  superior mesenteric I72.8

Aneurysm *(Continued)*
  syphilitic (aorta) A52.01
    central nervous system A52.05
    congenital (late) A50.54 *[I79.0]*
    spine, spinal A52.09
  thoracoabdominal (aorta) I71.60
    ruptured I71.50
    syphilitic A52.01
  thorax, thoracic (aorta) (arch) (nonsyphilitic) —*see* Aneurysm, aorta, thorax
    ruptured —*see* Aneurysm, aorta, thorax, ruptured
    syphilitic A52.01
  traumatic (complication) (early), specified site —*see* Injury, blood vessel
  tricuspid (heart) (valve) I07.8
  ulnar I72.1
  upper limb (ruptured) I72.1
  valve, valvular —*see* Endocarditis
  visceral NEC I72.8
  venous —*see also* Varix I86.8
    congenital Q27.8
      digestive system Q27.8
      lower limb Q27.8
      specified site NEC Q27.8
      upper limb Q27.8
  ventricle —*see* Aneurysm, heart
  vertebral artery I72.6
  visceral NEC I72.8
Angelman syndrome Q93.51
Anger R45.4
Angiectasis, angiectopia I99.8
Angiitis I77.6
  allergic granulomatous M30.1
  hypersensitivity M31.0
  necrotizing M31.9
    specified NEC M31.8
  nervous system, granulomatous I67.7
Angina (attack) (cardiac) (chest) (heart) (pectoris) (syndrome) (vasomotor) I20.9
  with
    atherosclerotic heart disease —*see* Arteriosclerosis, coronary (artery)
    coronary microvascular disease I20.81
    coronary microvascular dysfunction I20.81
    documented spasm I20.1
  abdominal K55.1
  accelerated —*see* Angina, unstable
  agranulocytic —*see* Agranulocytosis
  angiospastic —*see* Angina, with documented spasm
  aphthous B08.5
  crescendo —*see* Angina, unstable
  croupous J05.0
  cruris I73.9
  de novo effort —*see* Angina, unstable
  diphtheritic, membranous A36.0
  equivalent I20.89
  exudative, chronic J37.0
  following acute myocardial infarction I23.7
  gangrenous diphtheritic A36.0
  intestinal K55.1
  Ludovici K12.2
  Ludwig's K12.2
  malignant diphtheritic A36.0
  membranous J05.0
    diphtheritic A36.0
    Vincent's A69.1
  mesenteric K55.1
  monocytic —*see* Mononucleosis, infectious
  of effort —*see* Angina, specified NEC
  phlegmonous J36
    diphtheritic A36.0
  post-infarctional I23.7
  pre-infarctional —*see* Angina, unstable
  Prinzmetal —*see* Angina, with documented spasm
  progressive —*see* Angina, unstable
  pseudomembranous A69.1
  pultaceous, diphtheritic A36.0
  refractory I20.2
  spasm-induced —*see* Angina, with documented spasm
  specified NEC I20.89
  stable I20.89
  stenocardia —*see* Angina, specified NEC
  stridulous, diphtheritic A36.2
  tonsil J36
  trachealis J05.0
  unstable I20.0
  variant —*see* Angina, with documented spasm

Angina *(Continued)*
  Vincent's A69.1
  worsening effort —*see* Angina, unstable
Angioblastoma —*see* Neoplasm, connective tissue, uncertain behavior
Angiocholecystitis —*see* Cholecystitis, acute
Angiocholitis —*see also* Cholecystitis, acute K83.09
Angiodysgenesis spinalis G95.19
Angiodysplasia (cecum) (colon) K55.20
  with bleeding K55.21
  duodenum (and stomach) K31.819
    with bleeding K31.811
  stomach (and duodenum) K31.819
    with bleeding K31.811
Angioedema (allergic) (any site) (with urticaria) T78.3
  episodic, with eosinophilia D72.118
  hereditary D84.1
Angioendothelioma —*see* Neoplasm, uncertain behavior, by site
  benign D18.00
    intra-abdominal D18.03
    intracranial D18.02
    skin D18.01
    specified site NEC D18.09
  bone —*see* Neoplasm, bone, malignant
  Ewing's —*see* Neoplasm, bone, malignant
Angioendotheliomatosis C85.8-●
Angiofibroma —*see also* Neoplasm, benign, by site
  juvenile
    specified site —*see* Neoplasm, benign, by site
    unspecified site D10.6
Angiohemophilia (A) (B) —*see* Disease, von Willebrand
Angioid streaks (choroid) (macula) (retina) H35.33
Angiokeratoma —*see* Neoplasm, skin, benign
  corporis diffusum E75.21
Angioleiomyoma —*see* Neoplasm, connective tissue, benign
Angiolipoma —*see also* Lipoma
  infiltrating —*see* Lipoma
Angioma —*see also* Hemangioma, by site
  capillary I78.1
  hemorrhagicum hereditaria I78.0
  intra-abdominal D18.03
  intracranial D18.02
  malignant —*see* Neoplasm, connective tissue, malignant
  plexiform D18.00
    intra-abdominal D18.03
    intracranial D18.02
    skin D18.01
    specified site NEC D18.09
  senile I78.1
  serpiginosum L81.7
  skin D18.01
  specified site NEC D18.09
  spider I78.1
  stellate I78.1
  venous Q28.3
Angiomatosis Q82.8
  bacillary A79.89
  encephalotrigeminal Q85.89
  hemorrhagic familial I78.0
  hereditary familial I78.0
  liver K76.4
Angiomyolipoma —*see* Lipoma
Angiomyoliposarcoma —*see* Neoplasm, connective tissue, malignant
Angiomyoma —*see* Neoplasm, connective tissue, benign
Angiomyosarcoma —*see* Neoplasm, connective tissue, malignant
Angiomyxoma —*see* Neoplasm, connective tissue, uncertain behavior
Angioneurosis F45.8
Angioneurotic edema (allergic) (any site) (with urticaria) T78.3
  hereditary D84.1
Angiopathia, angiopathy I99.9
  cerebral I67.9
    amyloid E85.4 *[I68.0]*
  diabetic (peripheral) —*see* Diabetes, angiopathy
  peripheral I73.9
    diabetic —*see* Diabetes, angiopathy
    specified type NEC I73.89
  retinae syphilitica A52.05
  retinalis (juvenilis)
    diabetic —*see* Diabetes, retinopathy
    proliferative —*see* Retinopathy, proliferative

Angiosarcoma —*see also* Neoplasm, connective
   tissue, malignant
   liver C22.3
Angiosclerosis —*see* Arteriosclerosis
Angiospasm (peripheral) (traumatic) (vessel) (see
   also Vasospasm) I73.9
   brachial plexus G54.0
   cerebral G45.9
   cervical plexus G54.2
   nerve
      arm —*see* Mononeuropathy, upper limb
         axillary G54.0
         median —*see* Lesion, nerve, median
         ulnar —*see* Lesion, nerve, ulnar
      axillary G54.0
      leg —*see* Mononeuropathy, lower limb
         median —*see* Lesion, nerve, median
         plantar —*see* Lesion, nerve, plantar
         ulnar —*see* Lesion, nerve, ulnar
Angiospastic disease or edema I73.9
Angiostrongyliasis
   due to
      Parastrongylus
         cantonensis B83.2
         costaricensis B81.3
      intestinal B81.3
Anguillulosis —*see* Strongyloidiasis
Angulation
   cecum —*see* Obstruction, intestine
   coccyx (acquired) —*see also* subcategory M43.8
      congenital NEC Q76.49
   femur (acquired) —*see also* Deformity, limb,
      specified type NEC, thigh
      congenital Q74.2
   intestine (large) (small) —*see* Obstruction,
      intestine
   sacrum (acquired) —*see also* subcategory M43.8
      congenital NEC Q76.49
   sigmoid (flexure) —*see* Obstruction, intestine
   spine —*see* Dorsopathy, deforming, specified NEC
   tibia (acquired) —*see also* Deformity, limb,
      specified type NEC, lower leg
      congenital Q74.2
   ureter N13.5
      with infection N13.6
   wrist (acquired) —*see also* Deformity, limb,
      specified type NEC, forearm
      congenital Q74.0
Angulus infectiosus (lips) K13.0
Anhedonia R45.84
   sexual F52.0
Anhidrosis L74.4
Anhydration E86.0
Anhydremia E86.0
Anidrosis L74.4
Aniridia (congenital) Q13.1
Anisakiasis (infection) (infestation) B81.0
Anisakis larvae infestation B81.0
Aniseikonia H52.32
Anisocoria (pupil) H57.02
   congenital Q13.2
Anisocytosis R71.8
Anisometropia (congenital) H52.31
Ankle —*see* condition
Ankyloblepharon (eyelid) (acquired) —*see also*
   Blepharophimosis
   filiforme (adnatum) (congenital) Q10.3
   total Q10.3
Ankyloglossia Q38.1
Ankylosis (fibrous) (osseous) (joint) M24.60
   ankle M24.67-●
   arthrodesis status Z98.1
   cricoarytenoid (cartilage) (joint) (larynx) J38.7
   dental K03.5
   ear ossicles H74.31-●
   elbow M24.62-●
   foot M24.67-●
   hand M24.64-●
   hip M24.65-●
   incostapedial joint (infectional) —*see* Ankylosis,
      ear ossicles
   jaw (temporomandibular) M26.61-●
   knee M24.66-●
   lumbosacral (joint) M43.27
   postoperative (status) Z98.1
   produced by surgical fusion, status Z98.1
   sacro-iliac (joint) M43.28
   shoulder M24.61-●
   specified site NEC M24.69
   spine (joint) —*see also* Fusion, spine
      spondylitic —*see* Spondylitis, ankylosing

Ankylosis *(Continued)*
   surgical Z98.1
   temporomandibular M26.61-●
   tooth, teeth (hard tissues) K03.5
   wrist M24.63-●
Ankylostoma —*see* Ancylostoma
Ankylostomiasis —*see* Ancylostomiasis
Ankylurethria —*see* Stricture, urethra
Annular —*see also* condition
   detachment, cervix N88.8
   organ or site, congenital NEC —*see* Distortion
   pancreas (congenital) Q45.1
Anoctaminopathy G71.035
Anodontia (complete) (partial) (vera) K00.0
   acquired K08.10
Anomaly, anomalous (congenital) (unspecified
   type) Q89.9
   abdominal wall NEC Q79.59
   acoustic nerve Q07.8
   adrenal (gland) Q89.1
   Alder (-Reilly) (leukocyte granulation)
      D72.0
   alimentary tract Q45.9
      upper Q40.9
   alveolar M26.70
      hyperplasia M26.79
         mandibular M26.72
         maxillary M26.71
      hypoplasia M26.79
         mandibular M26.74
         maxillary M26.73
      ridge (process) M26.79
      specified NEC M26.79
   ankle (joint) Q74.2
   anus Q43.9
   aorta (arch) NEC Q25.40
      coarctation (preductal) (postductal) Q25.1
   aortic cusp or valve Q23.9
   appendix Q43.8
   apple peel syndrome Q41.1
   aqueduct of Sylvius Q03.0
      with spina bifida —*see* Spina bifida, with
         hydrocephalus
   arm Q74.0
   arteriovenous NEC
      coronary Q24.5
      gastrointestinal Q27.33
         acquired —*see* Angiodysplasia
   artery (peripheral) Q27.9
      basilar NEC Q28.1
      cerebral Q28.3
      coronary Q24.5
      digestive system Q27.8
      eye Q15.8
      great Q25.9
         specified NEC Q25.8
      lower limb Q27.8
      peripheral Q27.9
         specified NEC Q27.8
      pulmonary NEC Q25.79
      renal Q27.2
      retina Q14.1
      specified site NEC Q27.8
      subclavian Q27.8
         origin Q25.48
      umbilical Q27.0
      upper limb Q27.8
      vertebral NEC Q28.1
   aryteno-epiglottic folds Q31.8
   atrial
      bands or folds Q20.8
      septa Q21.10
   atrioventricular
      excitation I45.6
      septum Q21.0
   auditory canal Q17.8
   auricle
      ear Q17.8
         causing impairment of hearing Q16.9
      heart Q20.8
   Axenfeld's Q15.0
   back Q89.9
   band
      atrial Q20.8
      heart Q24.8
      ventricular Q24.8
   Bartholin's duct Q38.4
   biliary duct or passage Q44.5
   bladder Q64.70
      absence Q64.5
      diverticulum Q64.6

Anomaly, anomalous *(Continued)*
   bladder *(Continued)*
      exstrophy Q64.10
         cloacal Q64.12
         extroversion Q64.19
         specified type NEC Q64.19
         supravesical fissure Q64.11
      neck obstruction Q64.31
      specified type NEC Q64.79
   bone Q79.9
      arm Q74.0
      face Q75.9
      leg Q74.2
      pelvic girdle Q74.2
      shoulder girdle Q74.0
      skull Q75.9
        with
           anencephaly Q00.0
           encephalocele —*see* Encephalocele
           hydrocephalus Q03.9
              with spina bifida —*see* Spina bifida, by
                 site, with hydrocephalus
           microcephaly Q02
   brain (multiple) Q04.9
      vessel Q28.3
   breast Q83.9
   broad ligament Q50.6
   bronchus Q32.4
   bulbus cordis Q21.9
   bursa Q79.9
   canal of Nuck Q52.4
   canthus Q10.3
   capillary Q27.9
   cardiac Q24.9
      chambers Q20.9
         specified NEC Q20.8
      septal closure Q21.9
         specified NEC Q21.8
      valve NEC Q24.8
         pulmonary Q22.3
   cardiovascular system Q28.8
   carpus Q74.0
   caruncle, lacrimal Q10.6
   cascade stomach Q40.2
   cauda equina Q06.3
   cecum Q43.9
   cerebral Q04.9
      vessels Q28.3
   cervix Q51.9
   Chédiak-Higashi(-Steinbrinck) (congenital
      gigantism of peroxidase granules) E70.330
   cheek Q18.9
   chest wall Q67.8
      bones Q76.9
   chin Q18.9
   chordae tendineae Q24.8
   choroid Q14.3
      plexus Q07.8
   chromosomes, chromosomal Q99.9
      D (1) —*see* condition, chromosome 13
      E (3) —*see* condition, chromosome 18
      G —*see* condition, chromosome 21
      sex
         female phenotype Q97.8
         gonadal dysgenesis (pure) Q99.1
         Klinefelter's Q98.4
         male phenotype Q98.9
         Turner's Q96.9
      specified NEC Q99.8
   cilia Q10.3
   circulatory system Q28.9
   clavicle Q74.0
   clitoris Q52.6
   coccyx Q76.49
   colon Q43.9
   common duct Q44.5
   communication
      coronary artery Q24.5
      left ventricle with right atrium Q21.0
   concha (ear) Q17.3
   connection
      portal vein Q26.5
      pulmonary venous Q26.4
         partial Q26.3
         total Q26.2
      renal artery with kidney Q27.2
   cornea (shape) Q13.4
   coronary artery or vein Q24.5
   cranium —*see* Anomaly, skull
   cricoid cartilage Q31.8
   cystic duct Q44.5

Anomaly, anomalous (Continued)
dental
  alveolar —see Anomaly, alveolar
  arch relationship M26.20
    specified NEC M26.29
dentofacial M26.9
  alveolar —see Anomaly, alveolar
  dental arch relationship M26.20
    specified NEC M26.29
  functional M26.50
    specified NEC M26.59
  jaw-cranial base relationship M26.10
    asymmetry M26.12
      maxillary M26.11
    specified type NEC M26.19
  jaw size M26.00
    macrogenia M26.05
    mandibular
      hyperplasia M26.03
      hypoplasia M26.04
    maxillary
      hyperplasia M26.01
      hypoplasia M26.02
    microgenia M26.06
    specified type NEC M26.09
  malocclusion M26.4
    dental arch relationship NEC M26.29
    jaw-cranial base relationship —see
      Anomaly, dentofacial, jaw-cranial base
      relationship
    jaw size —see Anomaly, dentofacial, jaw
      size
  specified type NEC M26.89
  temporomandibular joint M26.60-●
    adhesions M26.61-●
    ankylosis M26.61-●
    arthralgia M26.62-●
    articular disc M26.63-●
    specified type NEC M26.69
  tooth position, fully erupted M26.30
    specified NEC M26.39
dermatoglyphic Q82.8
diaphragm (apertures) NEC Q79.1
digestive organ(s) or tract Q45.9
  lower Q43.9
  upper Q40.9
distance, interarch (excessive) (inadequate)
  M26.25
distribution, coronary artery Q24.5
ductus
  arteriosus Q25.0
  botalli Q25.0
duodenum Q43.9
dura (brain) Q04.9
  spinal cord Q06.9
ear (external) Q17.9
  causing impairment of hearing Q16.9
  inner Q16.5
  middle (causing impairment of hearing) Q16.4
    ossicles Q16.3
Ebstein's (heart) (tricuspid valve) Q22.5
ectodermal Q82.9
Eisenmenger's (ventricular septal defect) Q21.8
ejaculatory duct Q55.4
elbow Q74.0
endocrine gland NEC Q89.2
epididymis Q55.4
epiglottis Q31.8
esophagus Q39.9
eustachian tube Q17.8
eye Q15.9
  anterior segment Q13.9
    specified NEC Q13.89
  posterior segment Q14.9
    specified NEC Q14.8
  ptosis (eyelid) Q10.0
  specified NEC Q15.8
eyebrow Q18.8
eyelid Q10.3
  ptosis Q10.0
face Q18.9
  bone(s) Q75.9
fallopian tube Q50.6
fascia Q79.9
femur NEC Q74.2
fibula NEC Q74.2
finger Q74.0
fixation, intestine Q43.3
flexion (joint) NOS Q74.9
  hip or thigh Q65.89
foot NEC Q74.2
  varus (congenital) Q66.3-●

Anomaly, anomalous (Continued)
foramen
  Botalli Q21.12
  ovale Q21.12
forearm Q74.0
forehead Q75.8
form, teeth K00.2
fovea centralis Q14.1
frontal bone —see Anomaly, skull
gallbladder (position) (shape) (size) Q44.1
Gartner's duct Q52.4
gastrointestinal tract Q45.9
genitalia, genital organ(s) or system
  female Q52.9
    external Q52.70
    internal NOS Q52.9
  male Q55.9
    hydrocele P83.5
    specified NEC Q55.8
genitourinary NEC
  female Q52.9
  male Q55.9
Gerbode Q21.0
glottis Q31.8
granulation or granulocyte, genetic
  (constitutional) (leukocyte) D72.0
gum Q38.6
gyri Q07.9
hair Q84.2
hand Q74.0
hard tissue formation in pulp K04.3
head —see Anomaly, skull
heart Q24.9
  auricle Q20.8
  bands or folds Q24.8
  fibroelastosis cordis I42.4
  obstructive NEC Q22.6
  patent ductus arteriosus (Botalli) Q25.0
  septum Q21.9
    auricular Q21.19
    interatrial Q21.19
    interventricular Q21.0
      with pulmonary stenosis or atresia,
        dextraposition of aorta and
        hypertrophy of right ventricle Q21.3
    specified NEC Q21.8
    ventricular Q21.0
      with pulmonary stenosis or atresia,
        dextraposition of aorta and
        hypertrophy of right ventricle
        Q21.3
  tetralogy of Fallot Q21.3
  valve NEC Q24.8
    aortic
      bicuspid valve Q23.81
        functional, with stenosis - see Stenosis,
        aortic (valve)
      insufficiency Q23.1
      stenosis Q23.0
        subaortic Q24.4
    mitral
      insufficiency Q23.3
      stenosis Q23.2
    pulmonary Q22.3
      atresia Q22.0
      insufficiency Q22.2
      stenosis Q22.1
        infundibular Q24.3
        subvalvular Q24.3
    tricuspid
      atresia Q22.4
      stenosis Q22.4
  ventricle Q20.8
heel NEC Q74.2
Hegglin's D72.0
hemianencephaly Q00.0
hemicephaly Q00.0
hemicrania Q00.0
hepatic duct Q44.5
hip NEC Q74.2
hourglass stomach Q40.2
humerus Q74.0
hydatid of Morgagni
  female Q50.5
  male (epididymal) Q55.4
    testicular Q55.29
hymen Q52.4
hypersegmentation of neutrophils, hereditary
  D72.0
hypophyseal Q89.2
ileocecal (coil) (valve) Q43.9
ileum Q43.9

Anomaly, anomalous (Continued)
ilium NEC Q74.2
integument Q84.9
  specified NEC Q84.8
interarch distance (excessive) (inadequate) M26.25
intervertebral cartilage or disc Q76.49
intestine (large) (small) Q43.9
  with anomalous adhesions, fixation or
    malrotation Q43.3
iris Q13.2
ischium NEC Q74.2
jaw —see Anomaly, dentofacial
  alveolar —see Anomaly, alveolar
  jaw-cranial base relationship —see Anomaly,
    dentofacial, jaw-cranial base relationship
jejunum Q43.8
joint Q74.9
  specified NEC Q74.8
Jordan's D72.0
kidney(s) (calyx) (pelvis) Q63.9
  artery Q27.2
  specified NEC Q63.8
Klippel-Feil (brevicollis) Q76.1
knee Q74.1
labium (majus) (minus) Q52.70
labyrinth, membranous Q16.5
lacrimal apparatus or duct Q10.6
larynx, laryngeal (muscle) Q31.9
  web (bed) Q31.0
lens Q12.9
leukocytes, genetic D72.0
  granulation (constitutional) D72.0
lid (fold) Q10.3
ligament Q79.9
  broad Q50.6
  round Q52.8
limb Q74.9
  lower NEC Q74.2
    reduction deformity —see Defect, reduction,
      lower limb
  upper Q74.0
lip Q38.0
liver Q44.79
  duct Q44.5
lower limb NEC Q74.2
lumbosacral (joint) (region) Q76.49
  kyphosis —see Kyphosis, congenital
  lordosis —see Lordosis, congenital
lung (fissure) (lobe) Q33.9
mandible —see Anomaly, dentofacial
maxilla —see Anomaly, dentofacial
May (-Hegglin) D72.0
meatus urinarius NEC Q64.79
meningeal bands or folds Q07.9
  constriction of Q07.8
  spinal Q06.9
meninges Q07.9
  cerebral Q04.8
  spinal Q06.9
meningocele Q05.9
mesentery Q45.9
metacarpus Q74.0
metatarsus NEC Q74.2
middle ear Q16.4
  ossicles Q16.3
mitral (leaflets) (valve) Q23.9
  Cleft Q23.82
  insufficiency Q23.3
  specified NEC Q23.88
  stenosis Q23.2
mouth Q38.6
Müllerian —see also Anomaly, by site
  uterus NEC Q51.818
multiple NEC Q89.7
muscle Q79.9
  eyelid Q10.3
musculoskeletal system, except limbs Q79.9
myocardium Q24.8
nail Q84.6
narrowness, eyelid Q10.3
nasal sinus (wall) Q30.8
neck (any part) Q18.9
nerve Q07.9
  acoustic Q07.8
  optic Q07.8
nervous system (central) Q07.9
nipple Q83.9
nose, nasal (bones) (cartilage) (septum) (sinus)
  Q30.9
  specified NEC Q30.8
ocular muscle Q15.8
omphalomesenteric duct Q43.0

A

▶ New   ⇒ Revised   ~~deleted~~ Deleted   ● Use Additional Character(s)

Anomaly, anomalous *(Continued)*
  opening, pulmonary veins Q26.4
  optic
    disc Q14.2
    nerve Q07.8
  opticociliary vessels Q13.2
  orbit (eye) Q10.7
  organ Q89.9
    of Corti Q16.5
  origin
    artery
      innominate Q25.8
      pulmonary Q25.79
      renal Q27.2
      subclavian Q25.48
  osseous meatus (ear) Q16.1
  ovary Q50.39
  oviduct Q50.6
  palate (hard) (soft) NEC Q38.5
  pancreas or pancreatic duct Q45.3
  papillary muscles Q24.8
  parathyroid gland Q89.2
  paraurethral ducts Q64.79
  parotid (gland) Q38.4
  patella Q74.1
  Pelger-Huët (hereditary hyposegmentation) D72.0
  pelvic girdle NEC Q74.2
  pelvis (bony) NEC Q74.2
    rachitic E64.3
  penis (glans) Q55.69
  pericardium Q24.8
  peripheral vascular system Q27.9
  Peter's Q13.4
  pharynx Q38.8
  pigmentation L81.9
    congenital Q82.8
  pituitary (gland) Q89.2
  pleural (folds) Q34.0
  portal vein Q26.5
    connection Q26.5
  position, tooth, teeth, fully erupted M26.30
    specified NEC M26.39
  precerebral vessel Q28.1
  prepuce Q55.69
  prostate Q55.4
  pulmonary Q33.9
    artery NEC Q25.79
    valve Q22.3
      atresia Q22.0
      insufficiency Q22.2
      specified type NEC Q22.3
      stenosis Q22.1
        infundibular Q24.3
        subvalvular Q24.3
    venous connection Q26.4
      partial Q26.3
      total Q26.2
  pupil Q13.2
    function H57.00
      anisocoria H57.02
      Argyll Robertson pupil H57.01
      miosis H57.03
      mydriasis H57.04
      specified type NEC H57.09
      tonic pupil H57.05-●
  pylorus Q40.3
  radius Q74.0
  rectum Q43.9
  reduction (extremity) (limb)
    femur (longitudinal) —*see* Defect, reduction, lower limb, longitudinal, femur
    fibula (longitudinal) —*see* Defect, reduction, lower limb, longitudinal, fibula
    lower limb —*see* Defect, reduction, lower limb
    radius (longitudinal) —*see* Defect, reduction, upper limb, longitudinal, radius
    tibia (longitudinal) —*see* Defect, reduction, lower limb, longitudinal, tibia
    ulna (longitudinal) —*see* Defect, reduction, upper limb, longitudinal, ulna
    upper limb —*see* Defect, reduction, upper limb
  refraction —*see* Disorder, refraction
  renal Q63.9
    artery Q27.2
    pelvis Q63.9
      specified NEC Q63.8
  respiratory system Q34.9
    specified NEC Q34.8
  retina Q14.1

Anomaly, anomalous *(Continued)*
  rib Q76.6
    cervical Q76.5
    ~~Rieger's Q13.81~~
  ▶ Rieger Q13.81
  rotation —*see* Malrotation
    hip or thigh Q65.89
  round ligament Q52.8
  sacroiliac (joint) NEC Q74.2
  sacrum NEC Q76.49
    kyphosis —*see* Kyphosis, congenital
    lordosis —*see* Lordosis, congenital
  saddle nose, syphilitic A50.57
  salivary duct or gland Q38.4
  scapula Q74.0
  scrotum —*see* Malformation, testis and scrotum
  sebaceous gland Q82.9
  seminal vesicles Q55.4
  sense organs NEC Q07.8
  sex chromosomes NEC —*see also* Anomaly, chromosomes
    female phenotype Q97.8
    male phenotype Q98.9
  shoulder (girdle) (joint) Q74.0
  sigmoid (flexure) Q43.9
  simian crease Q82.8
  sinus of Valsalva Q25.49
  skeleton generalized Q78.9
  skin (appendage) Q82.9
  skull Q75.9
    with
      anencephaly Q00.0
      encephalocele —*see* Encephalocele
      hydrocephalus Q03.9
        with spina bifida —*see* Spina bifida, by site, with hydrocephalus
      microcephaly Q02
  specified organ or site NEC Q89.8
  spermatic cord Q55.4
  spine, spinal NEC Q76.49
    column NEC Q76.49
      kyphosis —*see* Kyphosis, congenital
      lordosis —*see* Lordosis, congenital
    cord Q06.9
    nerve root Q07.8
  spleen Q89.09
    agenesis Q89.01
  stenonian duct Q38.4
  sternum NEC Q76.7
  stomach Q40.3
  submaxillary gland Q38.4
  tarsus NEC Q74.2
  tendon Q79.9
  testis —*see* Malformation, testis and scrotum
  thigh NEC Q74.2
  thorax (wall) Q67.8
    bony Q76.9
  throat Q38.8
  thumb Q74.0
  thymus gland Q89.2
  thyroid (gland) Q89.2
    cartilage Q31.8
  tibia NEC Q74.2
    saber A50.56
  toe Q74.2
  tongue Q38.3
  tooth, teeth K00.9
    eruption K00.6
    position, fully erupted M26.30
    spacing, fully erupted M26.30
  trachea (cartilage) Q32.1
  tragus Q17.9
  tricuspid (leaflet) (valve) Q22.9
    atresia or stenosis Q22.4
    Ebstein's Q22.5
  Uhl's (hypoplasia of myocardium, right ventricle) Q24.8
  ulna Q74.0
  umbilical artery Q27.0
  union
    cricoid cartilage and thyroid cartilage Q31.8
    thyroid cartilage and hyoid bone Q31.8
    trachea with larynx Q31.8
  upper limb Q74.0
  urachus Q64.4
  ureter Q62.8
    obstructive NEC Q62.39
      cecoureterocele Q62.32
      orthotopic ureterocele Q62.31
  urethra Q64.70
    absence Q64.5
    double Q64.74

Anomaly, anomalous *(Continued)*
  urethra *(Continued)*
    fistula to rectum Q64.73
    obstructive Q64.39
      stricture Q64.32
    prolapse Q64.71
    specified type NEC Q64.79
  urinary tract Q64.9
  uterus Q51.9
    with only one functioning horn Q51.4
  uvula Q38.5
  vagina Q52.4
  valleculae Q31.8
  valve (heart) NEC Q24.8
    coronary sinus Q24.5
    inferior vena cava Q24.8
    pulmonary Q22.3
    sinus coronario Q24.5
    venae cavae inferioris Q24.8
  vas deferens Q55.4
  vascular Q27.9
    brain Q28.3
    ring Q25.45
  vein(s) (peripheral) Q27.9
    brain Q28.3
    cerebral Q28.3
    coronary Q24.5
    developmental Q28.3
    great Q26.9
      specified NEC Q26.8
  vena cava (inferior) (superior) Q26.9
  venous —*see* Anomaly, vein(s)
  venous return Q26.8
  ventricular
    bands or folds Q24.8
    septa Q21.0
  vertebra Q76.49
    kyphosis —*see* Kyphosis, congenital
    lordosis —*see* Lordosis, congenital
  vesicourethral orifice Q64.79
  vessel(s) Q27.9
    optic papilla Q14.2
    precerebral Q28.1
  vitelline duct Q43.0
  vitreous body or humor Q14.0
  vulva Q52.70
  wrist (joint) Q74.0
Anomia R48.8
Anonychia (congenital) Q84.3
  acquired L60.8
Anophthalmos, anophthalmus (congenital) (globe) Q11.1
  acquired Z90.01
Anopia, anopsia H53.46-●
  quadrant H53.46-●
Anorchia, anorchism, anorchidism Q55.0
Anorexia R63.0
  hysterical F44.89
  nervosa F50.00
    atypical F50.9
    ▶ binge-eating type F50.2-●
    ▶ with purging F50.02-●
    ▶ restricting type F50.01-●
Anorgasmy, psychogenic (female) F52.31
  male F52.32
Anosmia R43.0
  hysterical F44.6
  postinfectional J39.8
▶ Anosognosia R41.85
Anosteoplasia Q78.9
Anovulatory cycle N97.0
Anoxemia R09.02
  newborn P84
Anoxia (pathological) R09.02
  altitude T70.29
  cerebral G93.1
    complicating
      anesthesia (general) (local) or other sedation T88.59
        in labor and delivery O74.3
        in pregnancy O29.21-●
        postpartum, puerperal O89.2
      delivery (cesarean) (instrumental) O75.4
    during a procedure G97.81
    newborn P84
    resulting from a procedure G97.82
  due to
    drowning T75.1
    high altitude T70.29
  heart —*see* Insufficiency, coronary
  intrauterine P84

Anoxia *(Continued)*
  myocardial —*see* Insufficiency, coronary
  newborn P84
  spinal cord G95.11
  systemic (by suffocation) (low content in
      atmosphere) —*see* Asphyxia, traumatic
Anteflexion —*see* Anteversion
Antenatal
  care (normal pregnancy) Z34.90
  screening (encounter for) of mother —*see also*
      Encounter, antenatal screening
      Z36.9
Antepartum —*see* condition
Anterior —*see* condition
Antero-occlusion M26.220
Anteversion
  cervix —*see* Anteversion, uterus
  femur (neck), congenital Q65.89
  uterus, uterine (cervix) (postinfectional)
      (postpartal, old) N85.4
    congenital Q51.818
    in pregnancy or childbirth —*see* Pregnancy,
        complicated by
Anthophobia F40.228
Anthracosilicosis J60
Anthracosis (lung) (occupational) J60
  lingua K14.3
Anthrax A22.9
  with pneumonia A22.1
  cerebral A22.8
  colitis A22.2
  cutaneous A22.0
  gastrointestinal A22.2
  inhalation A22.1
  intestinal A22.2
  meningitis A22.8
  pulmonary A22.1
  respiratory A22.1
  sepsis A22.7
  specified manifestation NEC A22.8
Anthropoid pelvis Q74.2
  with disproportion (fetopelvic) O33.0
Anthropophobia F40.10
  generalized F40.11
Antibodies, maternal (blood group) —*see*
      Isoimmunization, affecting management of
      pregnancy
  anti-D —*see* Isoimmunization, affecting
      management of pregnancy, Rh
      newborn P55.0
Antibody
  anticardiolipin R76.0
    with
      hemorrhagic disorder D68.312
      hypercoagulable state D68.61
  antiphosphatidylglycerol R76.0
    with
      hemorrhagic disorder D68.312
      hypercoagulable state D68.61
  antiphosphatidylinositol R76.0
    with
      hemorrhagic disorder D68.312
      hypercoagulable state D68.61
  antiphosphatidylserine R76.0
    with
      hemorrhagic disorder D68.312
      hypercoagulable state D68.61
  antiphospholipid R76.0
    with
      hemorrhagic disorder D68.312
      hypercoagulable state D68.61
Anticardiolipin syndrome D68.61
Anticoagulant, circulating (intrinsic) —*see also* -
      Disorder, hemorrhagic D68.318
  drug-induced (extrinsic) —*see also* - Disorder,
      hemorrhagic D68.32
  iatrogenic D68.32
Antidiuretic hormone syndrome E22.2
Antimonial cholera —*see* Poisoning, antimony
Antiphospholipid
  antibody
    with hemorrhagic disorder D68.312
  syndrome D68.61
Antisocial personality F60.2
Antithrombinemia —*see* Circulating
      anticoagulants
Antithromboplastinemia D68.318
Antithromboplastinogenemia D68.318
Antitoxin complication or reaction —*see*
      Complications, vaccination
Antlophobia F40.228

Antritis J32.0
  maxilla J32.0
    acute J01.00
      recurrent J01.01
  stomach K29.50
    with bleeding K29.51
Antrum, antral —*see* condition
Anuria R34
  calculous (impacted) (recurrent) —*see also*
      Calculus, urinary N20.9
  following
    abortion —*see* Abortion by type complicated
        by, renal failure
    ectopic or molar pregnancy O08.4
  newborn P96.0
  postprocedural N99.0
  postrenal N13.8
  puerperal O90.49
  traumatic (following crushing) T79.5
Anus, anal —*see* condition
Anusitis K62.89
Anxiety F41.9
  depression F41.8
  episodic paroxysmal F41.0
  generalized F41.1
  hysteria F41.8
  neurosis F41.1
  panic type F41.0
  reaction F41.1
  separation, abnormal (of childhood) F93.0
  specified NEC F41.8
  state F41.1
Aorta, aortic —*see* condition
Aortectasia —*see* Ectasia, aorta
  with aneurysm —*see* Aneurysm, aorta
Aortitis (nonsyphilitic) (calcific) I77.6
  arteriosclerotic I70.0
  Doehle-Heller A52.02
  luetic A52.02
  rheumatic —*see* Endocarditis, acute, rheumatic
  specific (syphilitic) A52.02
  syphilitic A52.02
    congenital A50.54 *[I79.1]*
Apathetic thyroid storm —*see* Thyrotoxicosis
Apathy R45.3
Apeirophobia F40.228
Apepsia K30
  psychogenic F45.8
Aperistalsis, esophagus K22.0
Apertognathia M26.29
Apert's syndrome Q87.0
Aphagia R13.0
  psychogenic F50.9
Aphakia (acquired) (postoperative) H27.0-●
  congenital Q12.3
Aphasia (amnestic) (global) (nominal) (semantic)
      (syntactic) R47.01
  acquired, with epilepsy (Landau-Kleffner
      syndrome) —*see* Epilepsy, specified NEC
  auditory (developmental) F80.2
  developmental (receptive type) F80.2
    expressive type F80.1
    Wernicke's F80.2
  following
    cerebrovascular disease I69.920
      cerebral infarction I69.320
      intracerebral hemorrhage I69.120
      nontraumatic intracranial hemorrhage NEC
          I69.220
      specified disease NEC I69.820
      subarachnoid hemorrhage I69.020
  primary progressive (*see also* Dementia, in,
      diseases specified elsewhere) G31.01
      [F02.80]
    with behavioral disturbance (*see also*
        Dementia, in, diseases specified
        elsewhere) G31.01 *[F02.81-●]*
  progressive isolated (*see also* Dementia, in,
      diseases specified elsewhere) G31.01 *[F02.80]*
    with behavioral disturbance (*see also*
        Dementia, in, diseases specified
        elsewhere) G31.01 *[F02.81-●]*
  sensory F80.2
  syphilis, tertiary A52.19
  Wernicke's (developmental) F80.2
Aphonia (organic) R49.1
  hysterical F44.4
  psychogenic F44.4
Aphthae, aphthous —*see also* condition
  Bednar's K12.0
  cachectic K14.0

Aphthae, aphthous *(Continued)*
  epizootic B08.8
  fever B08.8
  oral (recurrent) K12.0
  stomatitis (major) (minor) K12.0
  thrush B37.0
  ulcer (oral) (recurrent) K12.0
    genital organ(s) NEC
      female N76.6
      male N50.89
    larynx J38.7
Apical —*see* condition
Apiphobia F40.218
Aplasia —*see also* Agenesis
  abdominal muscle syndrome Q79.4
  alveolar process (acquired) —*see* Anomaly, alveolar
    congenital Q38.6
  aorta (congenital) Q25.41
  axialis extracorticalis (congenita) E75.29
  bone marrow (myeloid) D61.9
    congenital D61.01
  brain Q00.0
    part of Q04.3
  bronchus Q32.4
  cementum K00.4
  cerebellum Q04.3
  cervix (congenital) Q51.5
  congenital pure red cell D61.01
  corpus callosum Q04.0
  cutis congenita Q84.8
  erythrocyte congenital D61.01
  extracortical axial E75.29
  eye Q11.1
  fovea centralis (congenital) Q14.1
  gallbladder, congenital Q44.0
  iris Q13.1
  labyrinth, membranous Q16.5
  limb (congenital) Q73.8
    lower —*see* Defect, reduction, lower limb
    upper —*see* Agenesis, arm
  lung, congenital (bilateral) (unilateral) Q33.3
  pancreas Q45.0
  parathyroid-thymic D82.1
  Pelizaeus-Merzbacher E75.27
  penis Q55.5
  prostate Q55.4
  red cell (with thymoma) D60.9
    acquired D60.9
      due to drugs D60.9
    adult D60.9
    chronic D60.0
    congenital D61.01
    constitutional D61.01
    due to drugs D60.9
    hereditary D61.01
    of infants D61.01
    primary D61.01
    pure D61.01
      due to drugs D60.9
    specified type NEC D60.8
    transient D60.1
  round ligament Q52.8
  skin Q84.8
  spermatic cord Q55.4
  spleen Q89.01
  testicle Q55.0
  thymic, with immunodeficiency D82.1
  thyroid (congenital) (with myxedema) E03.1
  uterus Q51.0
  ventral horn cell Q06.1
Apnea, apneic (of) (spells) R06.81
  newborn P28.40
    central P28.41
    mixed P28.43
    obstructive P28.42
    sleep
      primary P28.30
        central P28.31
        mixed P28.33
        obstructive P28.32
        specified NEC P28.39
    specified NEC P28.49
  prematurity P28.49
  sleep G47.30
    central (primary) G47.31
      idiopathic G47.31
      in conditions classified elsewhere G47.37
    obstructive (adult) (pediatric) G47.33
      hypopnea G47.33
    primary central G47.31
    specified NEC G47.39

▶ New   ⇒ Revised   ~~deleted~~ Deleted   ● Use Additional Character(s)

Apneumatosis, newborn P28.0
Apocrine metaplasia (breast) —*see* Dysplasia, mammary, specified type NEC
Apophysitis (bone) —*see also* Osteochondropathy
▥calcaneus M92.6
juvenile M92.9
Apoplectiform convulsions (cerebral ischemia) I67.82
Apoplexia, apoplexy, apoplectic
adrenal A39.1
heart (auricle) (ventricle) —*see* Infarct, myocardium
heat T67.01
hemorrhagic (stroke) —*see* Hemorrhage, intracranial
meninges, hemorrhagic —*see* Hemorrhage, intracranial, subarachnoid
uremic N18.9 *[168.8]*
Appearance
bizarre R46.1
specified NEC R46.89
very low level of personal hygiene R46.0
Appendage
epididymal (organ of Morgagni) Q55.4
intestine (epiploic) Q43.8
preauricular Q17.0
testicular (organ of Morgagni) Q55.29
Appendicitis (pneumococcal) (retrocecal) K37
with
gangrene K35.891
with localized peritonitis K35.31
perforation NOS K35.32
peritoneal abscess K35.33
peritonitis NEC K35.33
generalized K35.209
with
abscess K35.219
with perforation or rupture K35.211
following rupture or perforation of appendix NOS K35.211
without perforation or rupture K35.210
perforation or rupture K35.201
following rupture or perforation of appendix NOS K35.201
without rupture or perforation of appendix K35.200
localized K35.30
with
gangrene K35.32
perforation K35.32
and abscess K35.33
ruptured NOS (with localized peritonitis) K35.32
acute (catarrhal) (fulminating) (obstructive) (retrocecal) (suppurative) K35.80
with
gangrene K35.891
peritoneal abscess K35.33
peritonitis NEC K35.33
generalized K35.209
with
abscess K35.219
with perforation or rupture K35.211
following rupture or perforation of appendix NOS K35.211
without perforation or rupture K35.210
perforation or rupture K35.201
following rupture or perforation of appendix NOS K35.201
without rupture or perforation of appendix K35.200
localized K35.30
with
gangrene K35.32
perforation K35.32
and abscess K35.33
specified NEC K35.890
with gangrene K35.891
with localized peritonitis K35.31
amebic A06.89
chronic (recurrent) K36
exacerbation —*see* Appendicitis, with, gangrene
gangrenous —*see* Appendicitis, acute
healed (obliterative) K36
interval K36
neurogenic K36
obstructive K36
recurrent K36

Appendicitis *(Continued)*
relapsing K36
ruptured NOS (with localized peritonitis) K35.32
subacute (adhesive) K36
subsiding K36
suppurative —*see* Appendicitis, acute
tuberculous A18.32
Appendicopathia oxyurica B80
Appendix, appendicular —*see also* condition
epididymis Q55.4
Morgagni
female Q50.5
male (epididymal) Q55.4
testicular Q55.29
testis Q55.29
Appetite
depraved —*see* Pica
excessive R63.2
lack or loss —*see also* Anorexia R63.0
nonorganic origin F50.89
psychogenic F50.89
perverted (hysterical) —*see* Pica
Apple peel syndrome Q41.1
Apprehension state F41.1
Apprehensiveness, abnormal F41.9
Approximal wear K03.0
Apraxia (classic) (ideational) (ideokinetic) (ideomotor) (motor) (verbal) R48.2
following
cerebrovascular disease I69.990
cerebral infarction I69.390
intracerebral hemorrhage I69.190
nontraumatic intracranial hemorrhage NEC I69.290
specified disease NEC I69.890
subarachnoid hemorrhage I69.090
oculomotor, congenital H51.8
Aptyalism K11.7
Apudoma —*see* Neoplasm, uncertain behavior, by site
Aqueous misdirection H40.83-●
Arabicum elephantiasis —*see* Infestation, filarial
Arachnitis —*see* Meningitis
Arachnodactyly —*see* Syndrome, Marfan
Arachnoiditis (acute) (adhesive) (basal) (brain) (cerebrospinal) —*see* Meningitis
Arachnophobia F40.210
Arboencephalitis, Australian A83.4
Arborization block (heart) I45.5
ARC (AIDS-related complex) B20
Arch
aortic Q25.49
bovine Q25.49
Arches —*see* condition
Arcuate uterus Q51.810
Arcuatus uterus Q51.810
Arcus (cornea) senilis —*see* Degeneration, cornea, senile
Arc-welder's lung J63.4
Areflexia R29.2
Areola —*see* condition
Argentaffinoma —*see also* Neoplasm, uncertain behavior, by site
malignant —*see* Neoplasm, malignant, by site
▥syndrome E34.09
Argininemia E72.21
Arginosuccinic aciduria E72.22
Argyll Robertson phenomenon, pupil or syndrome (syphilitic) A52.19
atypical H57.09
nonsyphilitic H57.09
Argyria, argyriasis
conjunctival H11.13-●
from drug or medicament —*see* Table of Drugs and Chemicals, by substance
Argyrosis, conjunctival H11.13-●
Arhinencephaly Q04.1
Ariboflavinosis E53.0
Arm —*see* condition
Arnold-Chiari disease, obstruction or syndrome (type II) Q07.00
with
hydrocephalus Q07.02
with spina bifida Q07.03
spina bifida Q07.01
with hydrocephalus Q07.03
type III —*see* Encephalocele
type IV Q04.8
Aromatic amino-acid metabolism disorder E70.9
specified NEC E70.89

Arousals, confusional G47.51
Arrest, arrested
cardiac I46.9
complicating
abortion —*see* Abortion, by type, complicated by, cardiac arrest
anesthesia (general) (local) or other sedation —*see* Table of Drugs and Chemicals, by drug
in labor and delivery O74.2
in pregnancy O29.11-●
postpartum, puerperal O89.1
delivery (cesarean) (instrumental) O75.4
due to
cardiac condition I46.2
specified condition NEC I46.8
intraoperative I97.71-●
newborn P29.81
personal history, successfully resuscitated Z86.74
postprocedural I97.12-●
obstetric procedure O75.4
cardiorespiratory —*see* Arrest, cardiac
circulatory —*see* Arrest, cardiac
deep transverse O64.0
development or growth
bone —*see* Disorder, bone, development or growth
child R62.50
tracheal rings Q32.1
epiphyseal
complete
femur M89.15-●
humerus M89.12-●
tibia M89.16-●
ulna M89.13-●
forearm M89.13-●
specified NEC M89.13-●
ulna —*see* Arrest, epiphyseal, by type, ulna
lower leg M89.16-●
specified NEC M89.168
tibia —*see* Arrest, epiphyseal, by type, tibia
partial
femur M89.15-●
humerus M89.12-●
tibia M89.16-●
ulna M89.13-●
specified NEC M89.18
granulopoiesis —*see* Agranulocytosis
growth plate —*see* Arrest, epiphyseal
heart —*see* Arrest, cardiac
legal, anxiety concerning Z65.3
physeal —*see* Arrest, epiphyseal
respiratory R09.2
newborn P28.81
sinus I45.5
spermatogenesis (complete) —*see* Azoospermia
incomplete —*see* Oligospermia
transverse (deep) O64.0
Arrhenoblastoma
benign
specified site —*see* Neoplasm, benign, by site
unspecified site
female D27.9
male D29.20
malignant
specified site —*see* Neoplasm, malignant, by site
unspecified site
female C56.9
male C62.90
specified site —*see* Neoplasm, uncertain behavior, by site
unspecified site
female D39.10
male D40.10
Arrhythmia (auricle)(cardiac) (juvenile)(nodal) (reflex)(supraventricular)(transitory) (ventricle) I49.9
block I45.9
extrasystolic I49.49
newborn
bradycardia P29.12
occurring before birth P03.819
before onset of labor P03.810
during labor P03.811
tachycardia P29.11
psychogenic F45.8
sinus I49.8
specified NEC I49.8
vagal R55
ventricular re-entry I47.0

Arrillaga-Ayerza syndrome (pulmonary sclerosis
  with pulmonary hypertension) I27.0
Arsenical pigmentation L81.8
  from drug or medicament —*see* Table of Drugs
    and Chemicals
Arsenism —*see* Poisoning, arsenic
Arterial —*see* condition
Arteriofibrosis —*see* Arteriosclerosis
Arteriolar sclerosis —*see* Arteriosclerosis
Arteriolith —*see* Arteriosclerosis
Arteriolitis I77.6
  necrotizing, kidney I77.5
  renal —*see* Hypertension, kidney
Arteriolosclerosis —*see* Arteriosclerosis
Arterionephrosclerosis —*see* Hypertension, kidney
Arteriopathy I77.9
  cerebral autosomal dominant, with subcortical
    infarcts and leukoencephalopathy
    (CADASIL) I67.850
Arteriosclerosis, arteriosclerotic (diffuse)
    (obliterans) (of) (senile) (with calcification)
    I70.90
  with
    chronic limb-threatening ischemia —*see*
      Arteriosclerosis, with critical limb
      ischemia
    critical limb ischemia
      bypass graft I70.329
        autologous vein graft I70.429
          leg I70.429
            with
              gangrene (and intermittent
                claudication, rest pain, and
                ulcer) I70.469
              rest pain (and intermittent
                claudication) I70.429
            bilateral I70.423
              with
                gangrene (and intermittent
                  claudication, rest pain,
                  and ulcer) I70.463
                rest pain (and intermittent
                  claudication) I70.423
            left I70.422
              with
                gangrene (and intermittent
                  claudication, rest pain,
                  and ulcer) I70.462
                rest pain (and intermittent
                  claudication) I70.422
                ulceration (and intermittent
                  claudication and rest
                  pain) I70.449
                ankle I70.443
                calf I70.442
                foot site NEC I70.445
                heel I70.444
                lower leg NEC I70.448
                mid foot I70.444
                thigh I70.441
            right I70.421
              with
                gangrene (and intermittent
                  claudication, rest pain,
                  and ulcer) I70.461
                rest pain (and intermittent
                  claudication) I70.421
                ulceration (and intermittent
                  claudication and rest
                  pain) I70.439
                ankle I70.433
                calf I70.432
                foot site NEC I70.435
                heel I70.434
                lower leg NEC I70.438
                midfoot I70.434
                thigh I70.431
        leg I70.329
          with
            gangrene (and intermittent
              claudication, rest pain, and
              ulcer) I70.369
            rest pain (and intermittent
              claudication) I70.329
          bilateral I70.323
            with
              gangrene (and intermittent
                claudication, rest pain, and
                ulcer) I70.363
              rest pain (and intermittent
                claudication) I70.323

Arteriosclerosis, arteriosclerotic (*Continued*)
  with (*Continued*)
    critical limb ischemia (*Continued*)
      bypass graft (*Continued*)
        leg (*Continued*)
          left I70.322
            with
              rest pain (and intermittent
                claudication) I70.322
              ulceration (and intermittent
                claudication and rest pain)
                I70.349
              ankle I70.343
              calf I70.342
              foot site NEC I70.345
              heel I70.344
              lower leg NEC I70.348
              midfoot I70.344
              thigh I70.341
          right I70.321
            with
              gangrene (and intermittent
                claudication, rest pain, and
                ulcer) I70.361
              rest pain (and intermittent
                claudication) I70.321
              ulceration (and intermittent
                claudication and rest pain)
                I70.339
              ankle I70.333
              calf I70.332
              foot site NEC I70.335
              heel I70.334
              lower leg NEC I70.338
              midfoot I70.334
              thigh I70.331
        nonautologous biological graft I70.529
          leg I70.529
            with
              gangrene (and intermittent
                claudication, rest pain, and
                ulcer) I70.569
              rest pain (and intermittent
                claudication) I70.529
            bilateral I70.523
              with
                gangrene (and intermittent
                  claudication, rest pain,
                  and ulcer) I70.563
                rest pain (and intermittent
                  claudication) I70.523
            left I70.522
              with
                gangrene (and intermittent
                  claudication, rest pain,
                  and ulcer) I70.562
                rest pain (and intermittent
                  claudication) I70.522
                ulceration (and intermittent
                  claudication and rest
                  pain) I70.549
                ankle I70.543
                calf I70.542
                foot site NEC I70.545
                heel I70.544
                lower leg NEC I70.548
                midfoot I70.544
                thigh I70.541
            right I70.521
              with
                gangrene (and intermittent
                  claudication, rest pain,
                  and ulcer) I70.561
                rest pain (and intermittent
                  claudication) I70.521
                ulceration (and intermittent
                  claudication and rest
                  pain) I70.539
                ankle I70.533
                calf I70.532
                foot site NEC I70.535
                heel I70.534
                lower leg NEC I70.538
                midfoot I70.534
                thigh I70.531
        nonbiological graft I70.629
          leg I70.629
            with
              gangrene (and intermittent
                claudication, rest pain, and
                ulcer) I70.669

Arteriosclerosis, arteriosclerotic (*Continued*)
  with (*Continued*)
    critical limb ischemia (*Continued*)
      bypass graft (*Continued*)
        nonbiological graf (*Continued*)
          leg (*Continued*)
            with (*Continued*)
              rest pain (and intermittent
                claudication) I70.629
            bilateral I70.623
              with
                gangrene (and intermittent
                  claudication, rest pain,
                  and ulcer) I70.663
                rest pain (and intermittent
                  claudication) I70.623
            left I70.622
              with
                gangrene (and intermittent
                  claudication, rest pain,
                  and ulcer) I70.662
                rest pain (and intermittent
                  claudication) I70.622
                ulceration (and intermittent
                  claudication and rest
                  pain) I70.649
                ankle I70.643
                calf I70.642
                foot site NEC I70.645
                heel I70.644
                lower leg NEC I70.648
                midfoot I70.644
                thigh I70.641
            right I70.621
              with
                gangrene (and intermittent
                  claudication, rest pain,
                  and ulcer) I70.661
                rest pain (and intermittent
                  claudication) I70.621
                ulceration (and intermittent
                  claudication and rest
                  pain) I70.639
                ankle I70.633
                calf I70.632
                foot site NEC I70.635
                heel I70.634
                lower leg NEC I70.638
                midfoot I70.634
                thigh I70.631
        specified graft NEC I70.729
          leg I70.729
            with
              gangrene (and intermittent
                claudication, rest pain, and
                ulcer) I70.769
              rest pain (and intermittent
                claudication) I70.729
            bilateral I70.723
              with
                gangrene (and intermittent
                  claudication, rest pain,
                  and ulcer) I70.763
                rest pain (and intermittent
                  claudication)
                  I70.723
            left I70.722
              with
                gangrene (and intermittent
                  claudication, rest pain,
                  and ulcer) I70.762
                rest pain (and intermittent
                  claudication)
                  I70.722
                ulceration (and intermittent
                  claudication and rest
                  pain) I70.749
                ankle I70.743
                calf I70.742
                foot site NEC I70.745
                heel I70.744
                lower leg NEC I70.748
                midfoot I70.744
                thigh I70.741
            right I70.721
              with
                gangrene (and intermittent
                  claudication, rest pain,
                  and ulcer) I70.761
                rest pain (and intermittent
                  claudication) I70.721

Arteriosclerosis, arteriosclerotic *(Continued)*
 with *(Continued)*
  critical limb ischemia *(Continued)*
   bypass graft *(Continued)*
    specified graft NEC *(Continued)*
     leg *(Continued)*
      right *(Continued)*
       with *(Continued)*
        ulceration (and intermittent
          claudication and rest
          pain) I70.739
         ankle I70.733
         calf I70.732
         foot site NEC I70.735
         heel I70.734
         lower leg NEC I70.738
         midfoot I70.734
         thigh I70.731
   leg I70.229
    with
     gangrene (and intermittent
       claudication, rest pain, and ulcer)
       I70.269
     rest pain (and intermittent
       claudication) I70.229
    bilateral I70.223
     with
      gangrene (and intermittent
        claudication, rest pain, and
        ulcer) I70.263
      rest pain (and intermittent
        claudication) I70.223
    left I70.222
     with
      gangrene (and intermittent
        claudication, rest pain, and
        ulcer) I70.262
      rest pain (and intermittent
        claudication) I70.222
      ulceration (and intermittent
        claudication and rest pain)
        I70.249
       ankle I70.243
       calf I70.242
       foot site NEC I70.245
       heel I70.244
       lower leg NEC I70.248
       midfoot I70.244
       thigh I70.241
    right I70.221
     with
      gangrene (and intermittent
        claudication, rest pain, and
        ulcer) I70.261
      rest pain (and intermittent
        claudication) I70.221
      ulceration (and intermittent
        claudication and rest pain)
        I70.239
       ankle I70.233
       calf I70.232
       foot site NEC I70.235
       heel I70.234
       lower leg NEC I70.238
       midfoot I70.234
       thigh I70.231
 aorta I70.0
 arteries of extremities —*see* Arteriosclerosis,
   extremities
 with
  chronic limb-threatening ischemia —*see*
    Arteriosclerosis, with critical limb
    ischemia
  critical limb ischemia —*see* Arteriosclerosis,
    with critical limb ischemia
 brain I67.2
  with infarction —*see* Occlusion, artery, brain
    or cerebral, with infarction
 bypass graft
  with
   chronic limb-threatening ischemia —*see*
     Arteriosclerosis, with critical limb
     ischemia
   critical limb ischemia —*see* Arteriosclerosis,
     with critical limb ischemia
  coronary —*see* Arteriosclerosis, coronary,
    bypass graft
  extremities —*see* Arteriosclerosis, extremities,
    bypass graft
 cardiac —*see* Disease, heart, ischemic,
   atherosclerotic

Arteriosclerosis, arteriosclerotic *(Continued)*
 cardiopathy —*see* Disease, heart, ischemic,
   atherosclerotic
 cardiorenal —*see* Hypertension, cardiorenal
 cardiovascular —*see* Disease, heart, ischemic,
   atherosclerotic
 carotid —*see also* Occlusion, artery, carotid
   I65.2-●
 central nervous system I67.2
  with infarction —*see* Occlusion, artery,
    cerebral or precerebral, with infarction
 cerebral I67.2
  with infarction —*see* Occlusion, artery, brain
    or cerebral, with infarction
 cerebrovascular I67.2
  with infarction —*see* Occlusion, artery, brain
    or cerebral, with infarction
 coronary (artery) I25.10
  bypass graft I25.810
   with
    angina pectoris I25.709
     with documented spasm I25.701
     refractory I25.702
     specified type NEC I25.708
     unstable I25.700
    ischemic chest pain I25.709
   autologous artery I25.810
    with
     angina pectoris I25.729
      with documented spasm I25.721
      refractory I25.722
      specified type I25.728
      unstable I25.720
     ischemic chest pain I25.729
   autologous vein I25.810
    with
     angina pectoris I25.719
      with documented spasm I25.711
      refractory I25.712
      specified type I25.718
      unstable I25.710
     ischemic chest pain I25.719
  bypass graft I25.810
   nonautologous biological I25.810
    with
     angina pectoris I25.739
      with documented spasm I25.731
      refractory I25.732
      specified type I25.738
      unstable I25.730
     ischemic chest pain I25.739
   specified type NEC I25.810
    with
     angina pectoris I25.799
      with documented spasm
        I25.791
      refractory I25.792
      specified type I25.798
      unstable I25.790
     ischemic chest pain I25.799
  due to
   calcified coronary lesion (severely)
     I25.84
   lipid rich plaque I25.83
  native vessel
   with
    angina pectoris I25.119
     with documented spasm I25.111
     refractory I25.112
     specified type NEC I25.118
     unstable I25.110
    ischemic chest pain I25.119
  transplanted heart I25.811
   bypass graft I25.812
    with
     angina pectoris I25.769
      with documented spasm
        I25.761
      refractory I25.762
      specified type I25.768
      unstable I25.760
     ischemic chest pain I25.769
   native coronary artery I25.811
    with
     angina pectoris I25.759
      with documented spasm
        I25.751
      refractory I25.752
      specified type I25.758
      unstable I25.750
     ischemic chest pain I25.759

Arteriosclerosis, arteriosclerotic *(Continued)*
 extremities (native arteries) I70.209
  with
   chronic limb-threatening ischemia —*see*
     Arteriosclerosis, with critical limb
     ischemia
   critical limb ischemia —*see* Arteriosclerosis,
     with critical limb ischemia
  bypass graft I70.309
   with
    chronic limb-threatening ischemia —*see*
      Arteriosclerosis, with critical limb
      ischemia
    critical limb ischemia —*see*
      Arteriosclerosis, with critical limb
      ischemia
   autologous vein graft I70.409
    leg I70.409
     with
      gangrene (and intermittent
        claudication, rest pain and
        ulcer) I70.469
      intermittent claudication
        I70.419
      rest pain (and intermittent
        claudication) I70.429
     bilateral I70.403
      with
       gangrene (and intermittent
         claudication, rest pain and
         ulcer) I70.463
       intermittent claudication
         I70.413
       rest pain (and intermittent
         claudication) I70.423
      specified type NEC I70.493
     left I70.402
      with
       gangrene (and intermittent
         claudication, rest pain and
         ulcer) I70.462
       intermittent claudication
         I70.412
       rest pain (and intermittent
         claudication) I70.422
       ulceration (and intermittent
         claudication and rest pain)
         I70.449
        ankle I70.443
        calf I70.442
        foot site NEC I70.445
        heel I70.444
        lower leg NEC I70.448
        midfoot I70.444
        thigh I70.441
      specified type NEC I70.492
     right I70.401
      with
       gangrene (and intermittent
         claudication, rest pain and
         ulcer) I70.461
       intermittent claudication
         I70.411
       with
        rest pain (and intermittent
          claudication) I70.421
        ulceration (and intermittent
          claudication and rest pain)
          I70.439
         ankle I70.433
         calf I70.432
         foot site NEC I70.435
         heel I70.434
         lower leg NEC I70.438
         midfoot I70.434
         thigh I70.431
      specified type NEC I70.491
     specified type NEC I70.499
    specified NEC I70.408
     with
      gangrene (and intermittent
        claudication, rest pain and
        ulcer) I70.468
      intermittent claudication
        I70.418
      rest pain (and intermittent
        claudication) I70.428
      ulceration (and intermittent
        claudication and rest pain)
        I70.45
     specified type NEC I70.498

Arteriosclerosis, arteriosclerotic (Continued)
  coronary (artery) (Continued)
    bypass graft (Continued)
      leg I70.309
        with
          gangrene (and intermittent
            claudication, rest pain and ulcer)
            I70.369
          intermittent claudication I70.319
          rest pain (and intermittent
            claudication) I70.329
      bilateral I70.303
        with
          gangrene (and intermittent
            claudication, rest pain and
            ulcer) I70.363
          intermittent claudication I70.313
          rest pain (and intermittent
            claudication) I70.323
        specified type NEC I70.393
      left I70.302
        with
          gangrene (and intermittent
            claudication, rest pain and
            ulcer) I70.362
          intermittent claudication I70.312
          rest pain (and intermittent
            claudication) I70.322
          ulceration (and intermittent
            claudication and rest pain)
            I70.349
            ankle I70.343
            calf I70.342
            foot site NEC I70.345
            heel I70.344
            lower leg NEC I70.348
            midfoot I70.344
            thigh I70.341
        specified type NEC I70.392
      right I70.301
        with
          gangrene (and intermittent
            claudication, rest pain and
            ulcer) I70.361
          intermittent claudication I70.311
          rest pain (and intermittent
            claudication) I70.321
          ulceration (and intermittent
            claudication and rest pain)
            I70.339
            ankle I70.333
            calf I70.332
            foot site NEC I70.335
            heel I70.334
            lower leg NEC I70.338
            midfoot I70.334
            thigh I70.331
        specified type NEC I70.391
      specified type NEC I70.399
    nonautologous biological graft I70.509
      leg I70.509
        with
          gangrene (and intermittent
            claudication, rest pain and
            ulcer) I70.569
          intermittent claudication I70.519
          rest pain (and intermittent
            claudication) I70.529
      bilateral I70.503
        with
          gangrene (and intermittent
            claudication, rest pain and
            ulcer) I70.563
          intermittent claudication I70.513
          rest pain (and intermittent
            claudication) I70.523
        specified type NEC I70.593
      left I70.502
        with
          gangrene (and intermittent
            claudication, rest pain and
            ulcer) I70.562
          intermittent claudication I70.512
          rest pain (and intermittent
            claudication) I70.522
          ulceration (and intermittent
            claudication and rest pain)
            I70.549
            ankle I70.543
            calf I70.542
            foot site NEC I70.545

Arteriosclerosis, arteriosclerotic (Continued)
  coronary (artery) (Continued)
    bypass graft (Continued)
      nonautologous biological graft (Continued)
        leg (Continued)
          left (Continued)
            with (Continued)
              ulceration (Continued)
                heel I70.544
                lower leg NEC I70.548
                midfoot I70.544
                thigh I70.541
            specified type NEC I70.592
          right I70.501
            with
              gangrene (and intermittent
                claudication, rest pain and
                ulcer) I70.561
              intermittent claudication I70.511
              rest pain (and intermittent
                claudication) I70.521
              ulceration (and intermittent
                claudication and rest pain)
                I70.539
                ankle I70.533
                calf I70.532
                foot site NEC I70.535
                heel I70.534
                lower leg NEC I70.538
                midfoot I70.534
                thigh I70.531
            specified type NEC I70.591
          specified type NEC I70.599
        specified NEC I70.508
          with
            gangrene (and intermittent
              claudication, rest pain and
              ulcer) I70.568
            intermittent claudication I70.518
            rest pain (and intermittent
              claudication) I70.528
            ulceration (and intermittent
              claudication and rest pain)
              I70.55
          specified type NEC I70.598
    nonbiological graft I70.609
      leg I70.609
        with
          gangrene (and intermittent
            claudication, rest pain and
            ulcer) I70.669
          intermittent claudication I70.619
          rest pain (and intermittent
            claudication) I70.629
      bilateral I70.603
        with
          gangrene (and intermittent
            claudication, rest pain and
            ulcer) I70.663
          intermittent claudication I70.613
          rest pain (and intermittent
            claudication) I70.623
        specified type NEC I70.693
      left I70.602
        with
          gangrene (and intermittent
            claudication, rest pain and
            ulcer) I70.662
          intermittent claudication
            I70.612
          rest pain (and intermittent
            claudication) I70.622
          ulceration (and intermittent
            claudication and rest pain)
            I70.649
            ankle I70.643
            calf I70.642
            foot site NEC I70.645
            heel I70.644
            lower leg NEC I70.648
            midfoot I70.644
            thigh I70.641
        specified type NEC I70.692
      right I70.601
        with
          gangrene (and intermittent
            claudication, rest pain and
            ulcer) I70.661
          intermittent claudication I70.611
          rest pain (and intermittent
            claudication) I70.621

Arteriosclerosis, arteriosclerotic (Continued)
  coronary (artery) (Continued)
    bypass graft (Continued)
      nonbiological graft (Continued)
        leg (Continued)
          right (Continued)
            with (Continued)
              ulceration (and intermittent
                claudication and rest pain)
                I70.639
                ankle I70.633
                calf I70.632
                foot site NEC I70.635
                heel I70.634
                lower leg NEC I70.638
                midfoot I70.634
                thigh I70.631
            specified type NEC I70.691
          specified type NEC I70.699
        specified NEC I70.608
          with
            gangrene (and intermittent
              claudication, rest pain and
              ulcer) I70.668
            intermittent claudication I70.618
            rest pain (and intermittent
              claudication) I70.628
            ulceration (and intermittent
              claudication and rest pain)
              I70.65
          specified type NEC I70.698
      specified graft NEC I70.709
        leg I70.709
          with
            gangrene (and intermittent
              claudication, rest pain and
              ulcer) I70.769
            intermittent claudication I70.719
            rest pain (and intermittent
              claudication) I70.729
        bilateral I70.703
          with
            gangrene (and intermittent
              claudication, rest pain and
              ulcer) I70.763
            intermittent claudication
              I70.713
            rest pain (and intermittent
              claudication) I70.723
          specified type NEC I70.793
        left I70.702
          with
            gangrene (and intermittent
              claudication, rest pain and
              ulcer) I70.762
            intermittent claudication
              I70.712
            rest pain (and intermittent
              claudication) I70.722
            ulceration (and intermittent
              claudication and rest pain)
              I70.749
              ankle I70.743
              calf I70.742
              foot site NEC I70.745
              heel I70.744
              lower leg NEC I70.748
              midfoot I70.744
              thigh I70.741
          specified type NEC I70.792
        right I70.701
          with
            gangrene (and intermittent
              claudication, rest pain and
              ulcer) I70.761
            intermittent claudication I70.711
            rest pain (and intermittent
              claudication) I70.721
            ulceration (and intermittent
              claudication and rest pain)
              I70.739
              ankle I70.733
              calf I70.732
              foot site NEC I70.735
              heel I70.734
              lower leg NEC I70.738
              midfoot I70.734
              thigh I70.731
          specified type NEC I70.791
        specified type NEC I70.799
      specified NEC I70.708

▶ New　　⟹ Revised　　~~deleted~~ Deleted　　● Use Additional Character(s)

Arteriosclerosis, arteriosclerotic (Continued)
  coronary (artery) (Continued)
    bypass graft (Continued)
      specified graft NEC (Continued)
        specified NEC (Continued)
          with
            gangrene (and intermittent
              claudication, rest pain and
              ulcer) I70.768
            intermittent claudication
              I70.718
            rest pain (and intermittent
              claudication) I70.728
            ulceration (and intermittent
              claudication and rest pain)
              I70.75
          specified type NEC I70.798
      specified NEC I70.308
        with
          gangrene (and intermittent
            claudication, rest pain and ulcer)
            I70.368
          intermittent claudication I70.318
          rest pain (and intermittent
            claudication) I70.328
          ulceration (and intermittent
            claudication and rest pain)
            I70.35
        specified type NEC I70.398
  leg I70.209
    with
      gangrene (and intermittent claudication,
        rest pain and ulcer) I70.269
      intermittent claudication I70.219
      rest pain (and intermittent claudication)
        I70.229
    bilateral I70.203
      with
        gangrene (and intermittent
          claudication, rest pain and ulcer)
          I70.263
        intermittent claudication I70.213
        rest pain (and intermittent
          claudication) I70.223
      specified type NEC I70.293
    left I70.202
      with
        gangrene (and intermittent
          claudication, rest pain and ulcer)
          I70.262
        intermittent claudication I70.212
        rest pain (and intermittent
          claudication) I70.222
        ulceration (and intermittent
          claudication and rest pain)
          I70.249
          ankle I70.243
          calf I70.242
          foot site NEC I70.245
          heel I70.244
          lower leg NEC I70.248
          midfoot I70.244
          thigh I70.241
      specified type NEC I70.292
    right I70.201
      with
        gangrene (and intermittent
          claudication, rest pain and ulcer)
          I70.261
        intermittent claudication I70.211
        rest pain (and intermittent
          claudication) I70.221
        ulceration (and intermittent
          claudication and rest pain)
          I70.239
          ankle I70.233
          calf I70.232
          foot site NEC I70.235
          heel I70.234
          lower leg NEC I70.238
          midfoot I70.234
          thigh I70.231
      specified type NEC I70.291
    specified type NEC I70.299
  specified site NEC I70.208
    with
      gangrene (and intermittent claudication,
        rest pain and ulcer) I70.268
      intermittent claudication I70.218
      rest pain (and intermittent claudication)
        I70.228

rteriosclerosis, arteriosclerotic (Continued)
  coronary (artery) (Continued)
    specified site NEC (Continued)
      with (Continued)
        ulceration (and intermittent claudication
          and rest pain) I70.25
      specified type NEC I70.298
  generalized I70.91
  heart (disease) —see Arteriosclerosis, coronary
    (artery)
  kidney —see Hypertension, kidney
  medial —see Arteriosclerosis, extremities
  mesenteric (artery) K55.1
  Mönckeberg's —see Arteriosclerosis, extremities
  myocarditis I51.4
  peripheral (of extremities) —see Arteriosclerosis,
    extremities
  pulmonary (idiopathic) I27.0
  renal (arterioles) —see also Hypertension, kidney
    artery I70.1
  retina (vascular) I70.8 [H35.0-●]
  specified artery NEC I70.8
  spinal (cord) G95.19
  vertebral (artery) I67.2
    with infarction - see Occlusion, artery,
      vertebral, with infarction
Arteriospasm I73.9
Arteriovenous —see condition
Arteritis I77.6
  allergic M31.0
  aorta (nonsyphilitic) I77.6
    syphilitic A52.02
  aortic arch M31.4
  brachiocephalic M31.4
  brain I67.7
    syphilitic A52.04
  cerebral I67.7
    in
      diseases classified elsewhere I68.2
      systemic lupus erythematosus M32.19
    listerial A32.89
    syphilitic A52.04
    tuberculous A18.89
  coronary (artery) I25.89
    rheumatic I01.8
      chronic I09.89
    syphilitic A52.06
  cranial (left) (right), giant cell M31.6
  deformans —see Arteriosclerosis
  giant cell NEC M31.6
    with polymyalgia rheumatica M31.5
  necrosing or necrotizing M31.9
    specified NEC M31.8
  nodosa M30.0
  obliterans —see Arteriosclerosis
  pulmonary I28.8
  rheumatic —see Fever, rheumatic
  senile —see Arteriosclerosis
  suppurative I77.2
  syphilitic (general) A52.09
    brain A52.04
    coronary A52.06
    spinal A52.09
  temporal, giant cell M31.6
  young female aortic arch syndrome M31.4
Artery, arterial —see also condition
  abscess I77.89
  single umbilical Q27.0
Arthralgia (allergic) —see also Pain, joint
  in caisson disease T70.3
  temporomandibular M26.62
Arthritis, arthritic (acute) (chronic) (nonpyogenic)
  (subacute) M19.90
  allergic —see Arthritis, specified form NEC
  ankylosing (crippling) (spine) —see also
    Spondylitis, ankylosing
    sites other than spine —see Arthritis, specified
      form NEC
  atrophic —see Osteoarthritis
    spine —see Spondylitis, ankylosing
  back —see Spondylopathy, inflammatory
  blennorrhagic (gonococcal) A54.42
  Charcot's —see Arthropathy, neuropathic
    diabetic —see Diabetes, arthropathy,
      neuropathic
    syringomyelic G95.0
  chylous (filarial) —see also category M01 B74.9
  climacteric (any site) NEC —see Arthritis,
    specified form NEC
  crystal (-induced) —see Arthritis, in, crystals
  deformans —see Osteoarthritis

Arthritis, arthritic (Continued)
  degenerative —see Osteoarthritis
  due to or associated with
    acromegaly E22.0
    brucellosis —see Brucellosis
    caisson disease T70.3
    diabetes —see Diabetes, arthropathy
    dracontiasis —see also category M01 B72
    enteritis NEC
      regional —see Enteritis, regional
    erysipelas —see also category M01 A46
    erythema
      epidemic A25.1
      nodosum L52
    filariasis NOS B74.9
    glanders A24.0
    helminthiasis —see also category M01 B83.9
    hemophilia D66 [M36.2]
    Henoch-(Schönlein) purpura D69.0 [M36.4]
    human parvovirus —see also category M01
      B97.6
    infectious disease NEC —see category M01
    leprosy (see also category M01) —see also
      Leprosy A30.9
    Lyme disease A69.23
    mycobacteria —see also category M01 A31.8
    parasitic disease NEC —see also category M01
      B89
    paratyphoid fever (see also category M01)—see
      also Fever, paratyphoid A01.4
    rat bite fever —see also category M01 A25.1
    regional enteritis —see Enteritis, regional
    respiratory disorder NOS J98.9
    serum sickness —see also Reaction, serum
      T80.69
    syringomyelia G95.0
    typhoid fever A01.04
  epidemic erythema A25.1
  facet joint (see also Spondylosis) M47.819
  febrile —see Fever, rheumatic
  gonococcal A54.42
  gouty (acute) —see Gout
  in (due to)
    acromegaly —see also subcategory M14.8-
      ● E22.0
    amyloidosis —see also subcategory M14.8-
      ● E85.4
    bacterial disease —see also subcategory M01
      A49.9
    Behçet's syndrome M35.2
    caisson disease —see also subcategory M14.8-●
      T70.3
    coliform bacilli (Escherichia coli) —see
      Arthritis, in, pyogenic organism NEC
    crystals M11.9
      dicalcium phosphate —see Arthritis, in,
        crystals, specified type NEC
      hydroxyapatite M11.0-●
      pyrophosphate —see Arthritis, in, crystals,
        specified type NEC
      specified type NEC M11.80
        ankle M11.87-●
        elbow M11.82-●
        foot joint M11.87-●
        hand joint M11.84-●
        hip M11.85-●
        knee M11.86-●
        multiple sites M11.8-●
        shoulder M11.81-●
        vertebrae M11.88
        wrist M11.83-●
    dermatoarthritis, lipoid E78.81
    dracontiasis (dracunculiasis) —see also
      category M01 B72
    endocrine disorder NEC —see also
      subcategory M14.8-● E34.9
    enteritis, infectious NEC —see also category
      M01 A09
      specified organism NEC —see also category
        M01 A08.8
    erythema
      multiforme —see also subcategory M14.8-●
        L51.9
      nodosum —see also subcategory M14.8-●
        L52
    gout —see Gout
    helminthiasis NEC —see also category M01
      B83.9
    hemochromatosis —see also subcategory
      M14.8-● E83.118
    hemoglobinopathy NEC D58.2 [M36.3]

Arthritis, arthritic *(Continued)*
  in *(Continued)*
    hemophilia NEC D66 *[M36.2]*
    Hemophilus influenzae M00.8-● *[B96.3]*
    Henoch(-Schönlein) purpura D69.0 *[M36.4]*
    hyperparathyroidism NEC —*see also*
      subcategory M14.8-● E21.3
    hypersensitivity reaction NEC T78.49 *[M36.4]*
    hypogammaglobulinemia —*see also*
      subcategory M14.8-● D80.1
    hypothyroidism NEC —*see also* subcategory
      M14.8-● E03.9
    infection —*see* Arthritis, pyogenic or pyemic
      spine —*see* Spondylopathy, infective
    infectious disease NEC —*see* category M01
    leprosy —*see also* category M01 A30.9
    leukemia NEC C95.9-● *[M36.1]*
    lipoid dermatoarthritis E78.81
    Lyme disease A69.23
    Mediterranean fever, familial —*see also*
      subcategory M14.8-● M04.1
    Meningococcus A39.83
    metabolic disorder NEC —*see also* subcategory
      M14.8-● E88.9
    multiple myelomatosis C90.0-● *[M36.1]*
    mumps B26.85
    mycosis NEC —*see also* category M01 B49
    myelomatosis (multiple) C90.0-● *[M36.1]*
    neurological disorder NEC G98.0
    ochronosis —*see also* subcategory M14.8-●
      E70.29
    O'nyong-nyong —*see also* category M01 A92.1
    parasitic disease NEC —*see also* category M01
      B89
    paratyphoid fever —*see also* category M01
      A01.4
    Pseudomonas —*see* Arthritis, pyogenic,
      bacterial NEC
    psoriasis L40.50
    pyogenic organism NEC —*see* Arthritis,
      pyogenic, bacterial NEC
    Reiter's disease —*see* Reiter's disease
    respiratory disorder NEC —*see also*
      subcategory M14.8-● J98.9
    reticulosis, malignant —*see also* subcategory
      M14.8-● C86.0-●
    rubella B06.82
    Salmonella (arizonae) (cholerae-suis)
      (enteritidis) (typhimurium) A02.23
    sarcoidosis D86.86
    specified bacteria NEC —*see* Arthritis,
      pyogenic, bacterial NEC
    sporotrichosis B42.82
    syringomyelia G95.0
    thalassemia NEC D56.9 *[M36.3]*
    tuberculosis —*see* Tuberculosis, arthritis
    typhoid fever A01.04
    urethritis, Reiter's —*see* Reiter's disease
    viral disease NEC —*see also* category M01 B34.9
  infectious or infective —*see also* Arthritis,
    pyogenic or pyemic
    spine —*see* Spondylopathy, infective
  juvenile M08.90
    with systemic onset —*see* Still's disease
    ankle M08.97-●
    elbow M08.92-●
    foot joint M08.97-●
    hand joint M08.94-●
    hip M08.95-●
    knee M08.96 ●
    multiple site M08.99
    pauciarticular M08.40
      ankle M08.47-●
      elbow M08.42-●
      foot joint M08.47-●
      hand joint M08.44-●
      hip M08.45-●
      knee M08.46-●
      shoulder M08.41-●
      specified site NEC M08.4A
      vertebrae M08.48
      wrist M08.43-●
    psoriatic L40.54
    rheumatoid —*see* Arthritis, rheumatoid,
      juvenile
    shoulder M08.91-●
    specified site NEC M08.9A
    specified type NEC M08.80
      ankle M08.87-●
      elbow M08.82-●
      foot joint M08.87-●

Arthritis, arthritic *(Continued)*
  juvenile *(Continued)*
    specified type NEC *(Continued)*
      hand joint M08.84-●
      hip M08.85-●
      knee M08.86-●
      multiple site M08.89
      shoulder M08.81-●
      specified joint NEC M08.88
      vertebrae M08.88
      wrist M08.83-●
    vertebra M08.98
    wrist M08.93-●
  meaning osteoarthritis —*see* Osteoarthritis
  meningococcal A39.83
  menopausal (any site) NEC —*see* Arthritis,
    specified form NEC
  mutilans (psoriatic) L40.52
  mycotic NEC —*see also* category M01 B49
  neuropathic (Charcot) —*see* Arthropathy,
    neuropathic
    diabetic —*see* Diabetes, arthropathy, neuropathic
    nonsyphilitic NEC G98.0
    syringomyelic G95.0
  ochronotic —*see also* subcategory M14.8-● E70.29
  palindromic (any site) —*see* Rheumatism,
    palindromic
  pneumococcal M00.10
    ankle M00.17-●
    elbow M00.12-●
    foot joint —*see* Arthritis, pneumococcal, ankle
    hand joint M00.14-●
    hip M00.15-●
    knee M00.16-●
    multiple site M00.19
    shoulder M00.11-●
    vertebra M00.18
    wrist M00.13-●
  postdysenteric —*see* Arthropathy, postdysenteric
  postmeningococcal A39.84
  postrheumatic, chronic —*see* Arthropathy,
    postrheumatic, chronic
  primary progressive —*see also* Arthritis, specified
    form NEC
    spine —*see* Spondylitis, ankylosing
  psoriatic L40.50
  purulent (any site except spine) —*see* Arthritis,
    pyogenic or pyemic
    spine —*see* Spondylopathy, infective
  pyogenic or pyemic (any site except spine) M00.9
    bacterial NEC M00.80
      ankle M00.87-●
      elbow M00.82-●
      foot joint —*see* Arthritis, pyogenic, bacterial
        NEC, ankle
      hand joint M00.84-●
      hip M00.85-●
      knee M00.86-●
      multiple site M00.89
      shoulder M00.81-●
      vertebra M00.88
      wrist M00.83-●
    pneumococcal —*see* Arthritis, pneumococcal
    spine —*see* Spondylopathy, infective
    staphylococcal —*see* Arthritis, staphylococcal
    streptococcal —*see* Arthritis, streptococcal NEC
      pneumococcal —*see* Arthritis,
        pneumococcal
  reactive —*see* Reiter's disease
  rheumatic —*see also* Arthritis, rheumatoid
    acute or subacute —*see* Fever, rheumatic
  rheumatoid M06.9
    with
      carditis —*see* Rheumatoid, carditis
      endocarditis —*see* Rheumatoid, carditis
      heart involvement NEC —*see* Rheumatoid,
        carditis
      lung involvement —*see* Rheumatoid, lung
      myocarditis —*see* Rheumatoid, carditis
      myopathy —*see* Rheumatoid, myopathy
      pericarditis —*see* Rheumatoid, carditis
      polyneuropathy —*see* Rheumatoid,
        polyneuropathy
      rheumatoid factor —*see* Arthritis,
        rheumatoid, seropositive
      splenoadenomegaly and leukopenia —*see*
        Felty's syndrome
      vasculitis —*see* Rheumatoid, vasculitis
      visceral involvement NEC —*see*
        Rheumatoid, arthritis, with
        involvement of organs NEC

Arthritis, arthritic *(Continued)*
  rheumatoid *(Continued)*
    juvenile (with or without rheumatoid factor)
      M08.00
      with systemic onset —*see* Still's disease
      ankle M08.07-●
      elbow M08.02-●
      foot joint M08.07-●
      hand joint M08.04-●
      hip M08.05-●
      knee M08.06-●
      multiple site M08.09
      shoulder M08.01-●
      specified site NEC M08.0A
      vertebra M08.08
      wrist M08.03-●
    seronegative M06.00
      ankle M06.07-●
      elbow M06.02-●
      foot joint M06.07-●
      hand joint M06.04-●
      hip M06.05-●
      knee M06.06-●
      multiple sites M06.09
      shoulder M06.01-●
      specified site NEC M06.0A
      vertebra M06.08
      wrist M06.03-●
    seropositive M05.9
      without organ involvement M05.70
        ankle M05.77-●
        elbow M05.72-●
        foot joint M05.77-●
        hand joint M05.74-●
        hip M05.75-●
        knee M05.76-●
        multiple sites M05.79
        shoulder M05.71-●
        specified site NEC M05.7A
        vertebra —*see* Spondylitis, ankylosing
        wrist M05.73-●
      specified NEC M05.80
        ankle M05.87-●
        elbow M05.82-●
        foot joint M05.87-●
        hand joint M05.84-●
        hip M05.85-●
        knee M05.86-●
        multiple sites M05.89
        specified site NEC M05.8A
        shoulder M05.81-●
        vertebra —*see* Spondylitis, ankylosing
        wrist M05.83-●
    specified type NEC M06.80
      ankle M06.87-●
      elbow M06.82-●
      foot joint M06.87-●
      hand joint M06.84-●
      hip M06.85-●
      knee M06.86-●
      multiple site M06.89
      shoulder M06.81-●
      specified site NEC M06.8A
      vertebra M06.88
      wrist M06.83-●
    spine —*see* Spondylitis, ankylosing
  rubella B06.82
  scorbutic —*see also* subcategory M14.8-● E54
  senile or senescent —*see* Osteoarthritis
  septic (any site except spine) —*see* Arthritis,
    pyogenic or pyemic
    spine —*see* Spondylopathy, infective
  serum (nontherapeutic) (therapeutic) —*see*
    Arthropathy, postimmunization
  specified form NEC M13.80
    ankle M13.87-●
    elbow M13.82-●
    foot joint M13.87-●
    hand joint M13.84-●
    hip M13.85-●
    knee M13.86-●
    multiple site M13.89
    shoulder M13.81-●
    specified joint NEC M13.88
    wrist M13.83-●
  spine —*see also* Spondylosis
    infectious or infective NEC —*see*
      Spondylopathy, infective
    Marie-Strümpell —*see* Spondylitis, ankylosing
    pyogenic —*see* Spondylopathy, infective
    rheumatoid —*see* Spondylitis, ankylosing

▶ New   ➠ Revised   ~~deleted~~ Deleted   ● Use Additional Character(s)

Arthritis, arthritic *(Continued)*
  spine *(Continued)*
    traumatic (old) —*see* Spondylopathy,
      traumatic
    tuberculous A18.01
  staphylococcal M00.00
    ankle M00.07-●
    elbow M00.02-●
    foot joint —*see* Arthritis, staphylococcal, ankle
    hand joint M00.04-●
    hip M00.05-●
    knee M00.06-●
    multiple site M00.09
    shoulder M00.01-●
    vertebra M00.08
    wrist M00.03-●
  streptococcal NEC M00.20
    ankle M00.27-●
    elbow M00.22-●
    foot joint —*see* Arthritis, streptococcal, ankle
    hand joint M00.24-●
    hip M00.25-●
    knee M00.26-●
    multiple site M00.29
    shoulder M00.21-●
    vertebra M00.28
    wrist M00.23-●
  suppurative —*see* Arthritis, pyogenic or pyemic
  syphilitic (late) A52.16
    congenital A50.55 *[M12.80]*
  syphilitica deformans (Charcot) A52.16
  temporomandibular joint M26.65-●
  toxic of menopause (any site) —*see* Arthritis,
    specified form NEC
  transient —*see* Arthropathy, specified form NEC
  traumatic (chronic) —*see* Arthropathy, traumatic
  tuberculous A18.02
    spine A18.01
  uratic —*see* Gout
  urethritica (Reiter's) —*see* Reiter's disease
  vertebral —*see* Spondylopathy, inflammatory
  villous (any site) —*see* Arthropathy, specified
    form NEC
Arthrocele —*see* Effusion, joint
Arthrodesis status Z98.1
Arthrodynia —*see also* Pain, joint
Arthrodysplasia Q74.9
Arthrofibrosis, joint —*see* Ankylosis
Arthrogryposis (congenital) Q68.8
  multiplex congenita Q74.3
Arthrokatadysis M24.7
Arthropathy (*see also* Arthritis) M12.9
  Charcot's —*see* Arthropathy, neuropathic
    diabetic —*see* Diabetes, arthropathy,
      neuropathic
    syringomyelic G95.0
  cricoarytenoid J38.7
  crystal(-induced) —*see* Arthritis, in, crystals
  diabetic NEC —*see* Diabetes, arthropathy
  distal interphalangeal, psoriatic L40.51
  enteropathic M07.60
    ankle M07.67-●
    elbow M07.62-●
    foot joint M07.67-●
    hand joint M07.64-●
    hip M07.65-●
    knee M07.66-●
    multiple site M07.69
    shoulder M07.61-●
    vertebra M07.68
    wrist M07.63-●
  facet joint (*see also* Spondylosis) M47.819
  following intestinal bypass M02.00
    ankle M02.07-●
    elbow M02.02-●
    foot joint M02.07-●
    hand joint M02.04-●
    hip M02.05-●
    knee M02.06-●
    multiple site M02.09
    shoulder M02.01-●
    vertebra M02.08
    wrist M02.03-●
  gouty —*see also* Gout
    in (due to)
      Lesch-Nyhan syndrome E79.1 *[M14.8-●]*
      sickle-cell disorders D57-● *[M14.8-●]*
  hemophilic NEC D66 *[M36.2]*
    in (due to)
      hyperparathyroidism NEC E21.3 *[M14.8-●]*
      metabolic disease NOS E88.9 *[M14.8-●]*

Arthropathy *(Continued)*
  hemophilic NEC *(Continued)*
    acromegaly E22.0 *[M14.8-●]*
    amyloidosis E85.4 *[M14.8-●]*
    blood disorder NOS D75.9 *[M36.3]*
    diabetes —*see* Diabetes, arthropathy
    endocrine disease NOS E34.9 *[M14.8-●]*
    erythema
      multiforme L51.9 *[M14.8-●]*
      nodosum L52 *[M14.8-●]*
    hemochromatosis E83.118 *[M14.8-●]*
    hemoglobinopathy NEC D58.2 *[M36.3]*
    hemophilia NEC D66 *[M36.2]*
    Henoch-Schönlein purpura D69.0 *[M36.4]*
    hyperthyroidism E05.90 *[M14.8-●]*
    hypothyroidism E03.9 *[M14.8-●]*
    infective endocarditis I33.0 *[M12.80]*
    leukemia NEC C95.9-● *[M36.1]*
    malignant histiocytosis C96.A *[M36.1]*
    metabolic disease NOS E88.9 *[M14.8-●]*
    multiple myeloma C90.0-● *[M36.1]*
    neoplastic disease NOS (*see also* Neoplasm)
      D49.9 *[M36.1]*
    nutritional deficiency —*see also* subcategory
      M14.8-● E63.9
    psoriasis NOS L40.50
    sarcoidosis D86.86
    syphilis (late) A52.77
      congenital A50.55 *[M12.80]*
    thyrotoxicosis —*see also* subcategory M14.8-●
      E05.90
    ulcerative colitis K51.90 *[M07.60]*
    viral hepatitis (postinfectious) NEC B19.9
      [M12.80]
    Whipple's disease —*see also* subcategory
      M14.8-● K90.81
  Jaccoud —*see* Arthropathy, postrheumatic,
    chronic
  juvenile —*see* Arthritis, juvenile
    psoriatic L40.54
  mutilans (psoriatic) L40.52
  neuropathic (Charcot) M14.60
    ankle M14.67-●
    diabetic —*see* Diabetes, arthropathy,
      neuropathic
    elbow M14.62-●
    foot joint M14.67-●
    hand joint M14.64-●
    hip M14.65-●
    knee M14.66-●
    multiple site M14.69
    nonsyphilitic NEC G98.0
    shoulder M14.61-●
    syringomyelic G95.0
    vertebra M14.68
    wrist M14.63-●
  osteopulmonary —*see* Osteoarthropathy,
    hypertrophic, specified NEC
  postdysenteric M02.10
    ankle M02.17-●
    elbow M02.12-●
    foot joint M02.17-●
    hand joint M02.14-●
    hip M02.15-●
    knee M02.16-●
    multiple site M02.19
    shoulder M02.11-●
    vertebra M02.18
    wrist M02.13-●
  postimmunization M02.20
    ankle M02.27-●
    elbow M02.22-●
    foot joint M02.27-●
    hand joint M02.24-●
    hip M02.25-●
    knee M02.26-●
    multiple site M02.29
    shoulder M02.21-●
    vertebra M02.28
    wrist M02.23-●
  postinfectious NEC B99 *[M12.80]*
    in (due to)
      enteritis due to Yersinia enterocolitica A04.6
        [M12.80]
      syphilis A52.77
      viral hepatitis NEC B19.9 *[M12.80]*
  postrheumatic, chronic (Jaccoud) M12.00
    ankle M12.07-●
    elbow M12.02-●
    foot joint M12.07-●
    hand joint M12.04-●

Arthropathy *(Continued)*
  postrheumatic, chronic *(Continued)*
    hip M12.05-●
    knee M12.06-●
    multiple site M12.09
    shoulder M12.01-●
    specified joint NEC M12.08
    vertebrae M12.08
    wrist M12.03-●
  psoriatic NEC L40.59
    interphalangeal, distal L40.51
  reactive M02.9
    in (due to)
      infective endocarditis I33.0 *[M02.9]*
    specified type NEC M02.80
      ankle M02.87-●
      elbow M02.82-●
      foot joint M02.87-●
      hand joint M02.84-●
      hip M02.85-●
      knee M02.86-●
      multiple site M02.89
      shoulder M02.81-●
      vertebra M02.88
      wrist M02.83-●
  specified form NEC M12.80
    ankle M12.87-●
    elbow M12.82-●
    foot joint M12.87-●
    hand joint M12.84-●
    hip M12.85-●
    knee M12.86-●
    multiple site M12.89
    shoulder M12.81-●
    specified joint NEC M12.88
    vertebrae M12.88
    wrist M12.83-●
  syringomyelic G95.0
  tabes dorsalis A52.16
  tabetic A52.16
  temporomandibular joint M26.65-●
  transient —*see* Arthropathy, specified form NEC
  traumatic M12.50
    ankle M12.57-●
    elbow M12.52-●
    foot joint M12.57-●
    hand joint M12.54-●
    hip M12.55-●
    knee M12.56-●
    multiple site M12.59
    shoulder M12.51-●
    specified joint NEC M12.58
    vertebrae M12.58
    wrist M12.53-●
Arthropyosis —*see* Arthritis, pyogenic or pyemic
Arthrosis (deformans) (degenerative) (localized) —
  see also Osteoarthritis M19.90
  spine —*see* Spondylosis
Arthus' phenomenon or reaction T78.41
  due to
    drug —*see* Table of Drugs and Chemicals, by
      drug
Articular —*see* condition
Articulation, reverse (teeth) M26.24
Artificial
  insemination complication —*see* Complications,
    artificial, fertilization
  opening status (functioning) (without
    complication) Z93.9
    anus (colostomy) Z93.3
    colostomy Z93.3
    cystostomy Z93.50
      appendico-vesicostomy Z93.52
      cutaneous Z93.51
      specified NEC Z93.59
    enterostomy Z93.4
    gastrostomy Z93.1
    ileostomy (ileal pouch) (Kock pouch) Z93.2
    intestinal tract NEC Z93.4
    jejunostomy Z93.4
    nephrostomy Z93.6
    specified site NEC Z93.8
    tracheostomy Z93.0
    ureterostomy Z93.6
    urethrostomy Z93.6
    urinary tract NEC Z93.6
    vagina Z93.8
  vagina status Z93.8
Arytenoid —*see* condition
Asadollahi-Rauch syndrome Q87.85
Asbestosis (occupational) J61

ASC-H (atypical squamous cells cannot exclude high grade squamous intraepithelial lesion on cytologic smear)
  anus R85.611
  cervix R87.611
  vagina R87.621
ASC-US (atypical squamous cells of undetermined significance on cytologic smear)
  anus R85.610
  cervix R87.610
  vagina R87.620
Ascariasis B77.9
  with
    complications NEC B77.89
    intestinal complications B77.0
    pneumonia, pneumonitis B77.81
Ascaridosis, ascaridiasis —see Ascariasis
Ascaris (infection) (infestation) (lumbricoides) —see Ascariasis
Ascending —see condition
Aschoff's bodies —see Myocarditis, rheumatic
Ascites (abdominal) R18.8
  cardiac —see also Failure, heart, right I50.810
  chylous (nonfilarial) I89.8
    filarial —see Infestation, filarial
  due to
    cirrhosis, alcoholic K70.31
    hepatitis
      alcoholic K70.11
      chronic active K71.51
    S. japonicum B65.2
  heart —see also Failure, heart, right I50.810
  malignant R18.0
  pseudochylous R18.8
  syphilitic A52.74
  tuberculous A18.31
Aseptic —see condition
Asherman's syndrome N85.6
Asialia K11.7
Asiatic cholera —see Cholera
Asimultagnosia (simultanagnosia) R48.3
Askin's tumor —see Neoplasm, connective tissue, malignant
Asocial personality F60.2
Asomatognosia R41.4
Aspartylglucosaminuria E77.1
Asperger's disease or syndrome F84.5
Aspergilloma —see Aspergillosis
Aspergillosis (with pneumonia) B44.9
  bronchopulmonary, allergic B44.81
  disseminated B44.7
  generalized B44.7
  pulmonary NEC B44.1
    allergic B44.81
    invasive B44.0
  specified NEC B44.89
  tonsillar B44.2
Aspergillus (flavus) (fumigatus) (infection) (terreus) —see Aspergillosis
Aspermatogenesis —see Azoospermia
Aspermia (testis) —see Azoospermia
Asphyxia, asphyxiation (by) R09.01
  antenatal P84
  birth P84
  bunny bag —see Asphyxia, due to, mechanical threat to breathing, trapped in bed clothes
  crushing S28.0
  drowning T75.1
  gas, fumes, or vapor —see Table of Drugs and Chemicals
  inhalation —see Inhalation
  intrauterine P84
  local I73.00
    with gangrene I73.01
  mucus —see also Foreign body, respiratory tract, causing asphyxiation
  newborn P84
  pathological R09.01
  postnatal P84
    mechanical —see Asphyxia, due to, mechanical threat to breathing
  prenatal P84
  reticularis R23.1
  strangulation —see Asphyxia, due to, mechanical threat to breathing
  submersion T75.1
  traumatic T71.9
    due to
      crushed chest S28.0
      foreign body (in) —see Foreign body, respiratory tract, causing asphyxia

Asphyxia, asphyxiation (Continued)
  traumatic (Continued)
    due to (Continued)
      low oxygen content of ambient air T71.20
        due to
          being trapped in
            low oxygen environment T71.29
            in car trunk T71.221
              circumstances undetermined T71.224
              done with intent to harm by another person T71.223
                self T71.222
            in refrigerator T71.231
              circumstances undetermined T71.234
              done with intent to harm by another person T71.233
                self T71.232
      cave-in T71.21
      mechanical threat to breathing (accidental) T71.191
        circumstances undetermined T71.194
        done with intent to harm by another person T71.193
          self T71.192
        hanging T71.161
          circumstances undetermined T71.164
          done with intent to harm by another person T71.163
            self T71.162
        plastic bag T71.121
          circumstances undetermined T71.124
          done with intent to harm by another person T71.123
            self T71.122
        smothering
          in furniture T71.151
            circumstances undetermined T71.154
            done with intent to harm by another person T71.153
              self T71.152
          under
            another person's body T71.141
              circumstances undetermined T71.144
              done with intent to harm T71.143
            pillow T71.111
              circumstances undetermined T71.114
              done with intent to harm by another person T71.113
                self T71.112
      trapped in bed clothes T71.131
        circumstances undetermined T71.134
        done with intent to harm by another person T71.133
          self T71.132
  vomiting, vomitus —see Foreign body, respiratory tract, causing asphyxia
Aspiration
  amniotic (clear) fluid (newborn) P24.10
    with
      pneumonia (pneumonitis) P24.11
      respiratory symptoms P24.11
  blood
    newborn (without respiratory symptoms) P24.20
    with
      pneumonia (pneumonitis) P24.21
      respiratory symptoms P24.21
    specified age NEC —see Foreign body, respiratory tract
  bronchitis J69.0
  food or foreign body —see Foreign body, by site
  liquor (amnii) (newborn) P24.10
    with
      pneumonia (pneumonitis) P24.11
      respiratory symptoms P24.11
  meconium (newborn) (without respiratory symptoms) P24.00
    with
      pneumonitis (pneumonitis) P24.01
      respiratory symptoms P24.01
  milk (newborn) (without respiratory symptoms) P24.30
    with
      pneumonia (pneumonitis) P24.31
      respiratory symptoms P24.31
  specified age NEC —see Foreign body, respiratory tract

Aspiration (Continued)
  mucus —see also Foreign body, by site, causing asphyxia
    newborn P24.10
      with
        pneumonia (pneumonitis) P24.11
        respiratory symptoms P24.11
    neonatal P24.9
      specific NEC (without respiratory symptoms) P24.80
      with
        pneumonia (pneumonitis) P24.81
        respiratory symptoms P24.81
    newborn P24.9
      specific NEC (without respiratory symptoms) P24.80
      with
        pneumonia (pneumonitis) P24.81
        respiratory symptoms P24.81
  pneumonia J69.0
  pneumonitis J69.0
  syndrome of newborn —see Aspiration, by substance, with pneumonia
  vernix caseosa (newborn) P24.80
    with
      pneumonia (pneumonitis) P24.81
      respiratory symptoms P24.81
  vomitus —see also Foreign body, respiratory tract
    newborn (without respiratory symptoms) P24.30
    with
      pneumonia (pneumonitis) P24.31
      respiratory symptoms P24.31
Asplenia (congenital) Q89.01
▶functional D73.0
  postsurgical Z90.81
Assam fever B55.0
Assault, sexual —see Maltreatment
Assmann's focus NEC A15.0
Astasia (-abasia) (hysterical) F44.4
Asteatosis cutis L85.3
Astereognosia, astereognosis R48.1
Asterixis R27.8
  in liver disease K71.3
Asteroid hyalitis —see Deposit, crystalline
Asthenia, asthenic R53.1
  cardiac —see also Failure, heart I50.9
    psychogenic F45.8
  cardiovascular —see also Failure, heart I50.9
    psychogenic F45.8
  heart —see also Failure, heart I50.9
    psychogenic F45.8
  hysterical F44.4
  myocardial —see also Failure, heart I50.9
    psychogenic F45.8
  nervous F48.8
  neurocirculatory F45.8
  neurotic F48.8
  psychogenic F48.8
  psychoneurotic F48.8
  psychophysiologic F48.8
  reaction (psychophysiologic) F48.8
  senile R54
Asthenopia —see also Discomfort, visual
  hysterical F44.6
  psychogenic F44.6
Asthenospermia —see Abnormal, specimen, male genital organs
Asthma, asthmatic (bronchial) (catarrh) (spasmodic) J45.909
  with
    chronic obstructive bronchitis J44.89
      with
        acute lower respiratory infection J44.0
        exacerbation (acute) J44.1
    chronic obstructive pulmonary disease J44.89
      with
        acute lower respiratory infection J44.0
        exacerbation (acute) J44.1
    exacerbation (acute) J45.901
    hay fever —see Asthma, allergic extrinsic
    rhinitis, allergic —see Asthma, allergic extrinsic
    status asthmaticus J45.902
  allergic extrinsic J45.909
    with
      exacerbation (acute) J45.901
      status asthmaticus J45.902
  atopic —see Asthma, allergic extrinsic
  cardiac —see Failure, ventricular, left
  cardiobronchial I50.1

Asthma, asthmatic *(Continued)*
childhood J45.909
  with
    exacerbation (acute) J45.901
    status asthmaticus J45.902
chronic obstructive J44.89
  with
    acute lower respiratory infection J44.0
    exacerbation (acute) J44.1
collier's J60
cough variant J45.991
detergent J69.8
due to
  detergent J69.8
  inhalation of fumes J68.3
eosinophilic J82.83
extrinsic, allergic —*see* Asthma, allergic extrinsic
grinder's J62.8
hay —*see* Asthma, allergic extrinsic
heart I50.1
idiosyncratic —*see* Asthma, nonallergic
intermittent (mild) J45.20
  with
    exacerbation (acute) J45.21
    status asthmaticus J45.22
intrinsic, nonallergic —*see* Asthma, nonallergic
Kopp's E32.8
late-onset J45.909
  with
    exacerbation (acute) J45.901
    status asthmaticus J45.902
mild intermittent J45.20
  with
    exacerbation (acute) J45.21
    status asthmaticus J45.22
mild persistent J45.30
  with
    exacerbation (acute) J45.31
    status asthmaticus J45.32
Millar's (laryngismus stridulus) J38.5
miner's J60
mixed J45.909
  with
    exacerbation (acute) J45.901
    status asthmaticus J45.902
moderate persistent J45.40
  with
    exacerbation (acute) J45.41
    status asthmaticus J45.42
nervous —*see* Asthma, nonallergic
nonallergic (intrinsic) J45.909
  with
    exacerbation (acute) J45.901
    status asthmaticus J45.902
persistent
  mild J45.30
    with
      exacerbation (acute) J45.31
      status asthmaticus J45.32
  moderate J45.40
    with
      exacerbation (acute) J45.41
      status asthmaticus J45.42
  severe J45.50
    with
      exacerbation (acute) J45.51
      status asthmaticus J45.52
platinum J45.998
pneumoconiotic NEC J64
potter's J62.8
predominantly allergic J45.909
psychogenic F54
pulmonary eosinophilic J82.83
red cedar J67.8
Rostan's I50.1
sandblaster's J62.8
sequoiosis J67.8
severe persistent J45.50
  with
    exacerbation (acute) J45.51
    status asthmaticus J45.52
specified NEC J45.998
stonemason's J62.8
thymic E32.8
tuberculous —*see* Tuberculosis, pulmonary
Wichmann's (laryngismus stridulus) J38.5
wood J67.8
Astigmatism (compound) (congenital) H52.20-●
irregular H52.21-●
regular H52.22-●
Astraphobia F40.220

Astroblastoma
specified site —*see* Neoplasm, malignant, by site
unspecified site C71.9
Astrocytoma (cystic)
anaplastic
  specified site —*see* Neoplasm, malignant, by site
  unspecified site C71.9
fibrillary
  specified site —*see* Neoplasm, malignant, by site
  unspecified site C71.9
fibrous
  specified site —*see* Neoplasm, malignant, by site
  unspecified site C71.9
gemistocytic
  specified site —*see* Neoplasm, malignant, by site
  unspecified site C71.9
juvenile
  specified site —*see* Neoplasm, malignant, by site
  unspecified site C71.9
pilocytic
  specified site —*see* Neoplasm, malignant, by site
  unspecified site C71.9
piloid
  specified site —*see* Neoplasm, malignant, by site
  unspecified site C71.9
protoplasmic
  specified site —*see* Neoplasm, malignant, by site
  unspecified site C71.9
specified site NEC —*see* Neoplasm, malignant, by site
subependymal D43.2
  giant cell
    specified site —*see* Neoplasm, uncertain behavior, by site
    unspecified site D43.2
  specified site —*see* Neoplasm, uncertain behavior, by site
  unspecified site D43.2
unspecified site C71.9
Astroglioma
specified site —*see* Neoplasm, malignant, by site
unspecified site C71.9
Asymbolia R48.8
Asymmetry —*see also* Distortion
between native and reconstructed breast N65.1
face Q67.0
jaw (lower) —*see* Anomaly, dentofacial, jaw-cranial base relationship, asymmetry
Asynergia, asynergy R27.8
ventricular I51.89
Asystole (heart) —*see* Arrest, cardiac
At risk
for
  dental caries Z91.849
    high Z91.843
    low Z91.841
    moderate Z91.842
  falling Z91.81
  feeling loneliness Z65.8
  social isolation Z91.89
Ataxia, ataxy, ataxic R27.0
acute R27.8
autosomal recessive Friedreich G11.11
brain (hereditary) G11.9
cerebellar (hereditary) G11.9
  with defective DNA repair G11.3
  alcoholic G31.2
  early-onset G11.10
    with
      essential tremor G11.19
      myoclonus [Hunt's ataxia] G11.19
      retained tendon reflexes G11.19
    in
      alcoholism G31.2
      myxedema E03.9 *[G13.2]*
      neoplastic disease —*see also* Neoplasm D49.9 *[G32.81]*
      specified disease NEC G32.81
  late-onset (Marie's) G11.2
cerebral (hereditary) G11.9
congenital nonprogressive G11.0
family, familial —*see* Ataxia, hereditary

Ataxia, ataxy, ataxic *(Continued)*
following
  cerebrovascular disease I69.993
    cerebral infarction I69.393
    intracerebral hemorrhage I69.193
    nontraumatic intracranial hemorrhage NEC I69.293
    specified disease NEC I69.893
    subarachnoid hemorrhage I69.093
Friedreich's (heredofamilial) (cerebellar) (spinal) G11.11
gait R26.0
  hysterical F44.4
general R27.8
gluten M35.9 *[G32.81]*
  with celiac disease K90.0 *[G32.81]*
hereditary G11.9
  with neuropathy G60.2
  cerebellar —*see* Ataxia, cerebellar
  spastic G11.4
  specified NEC G11.8
  spinal (Friedreich's) G11.11
heredofamilial —*see* Ataxia, hereditary
Hunt's G11.19
hysterical F44.4
locomotor (progressive) (syphilitic) (partial) (spastic) A52.11
  diabetic —*see* Diabetes, ataxia
Marie's (cerebellar) (heredofamilial) (late-onset) G11.2
nonorganic origin F44.4
nonprogressive, congenital G11.0
psychogenic F44.4
Roussy-Lévy G60.0
Sanger-Brown's (hereditary) G11.2
spastic hereditary G11.4
spinal
  hereditary (Friedreich's) G11.11
  progressive (syphilitic) A52.11
spinocerebellar, X-linked recessive G11.19
telangiectasia (Louis-Bar) G11.3
Ataxia-telangiectasia (Louis-Bar) G11.3
Atelectasis (massive) (partial) (pressure) (pulmonary) J98.11
newborn P28.10
  due to resorption P28.11
  partial P28.19
  primary P28.0
  secondary P28.19
primary (newborn) P28.0
tuberculous —*see* Tuberculosis, pulmonary
Atelocardia Q24.9
Atelomyelia Q06.1
Atheroembolism
of
  extremities
    lower I75.02-●
    upper I75.01-●
  kidney I75.81
  specified NEC I75.89
Atheroma, atheromatous —*see also* Arteriosclerosis I70.90
aorta, aortic I70.0
  valve —*see also* Endocarditis, aortic I35.8
aorto-iliac I70.0
artery —*see* Arteriosclerosis
basilar (artery) I67.2
carotid (artery) (common) (internal) I67.2
cerebral (arteries) I67.2
coronary (artery) I25.10
  with angina pectoris —*see* Arteriosclerosis, coronary (artery)
degeneration —*see* Arteriosclerosis
heart, cardiac —*see* Disease, heart, ischemic, atherosclerotic
mitral (valve) I34.89
myocardium, myocardial —*see* Disease, heart, ischemic, atherosclerotic
pulmonary valve (heart) —*see also* Endocarditis, pulmonary I37.8
tricuspid (heart) (valve) I36.8
valve, valvular —*see* Endocarditis
vertebral (artery) I67.2
Atheromatosis —*see* Arteriosclerosis
Atherosclerosis —*see also* Arteriosclerosis
coronary
  artery I25.10
    with angina pectoris —*see* Arteriosclerosis, coronary (artery),

Atherosclerosis (Continued)
  coronary (Continued)
    artery (Continued)
      due to
        calcified coronary lesion (severely) I25.84
        lipid rich plaque I25.83
      transplanted heart I25.811
        bypass graft I25.812
          with angina pectoris —see Arteriosclerosis, coronary (artery)
        native coronary artery I25.811
          with angina pectoris —see Arteriosclerosis, coronary (artery)
Athetosis (acquired) R25.8
  bilateral (congenital) G80.3
  congenital (bilateral) (double) G80.3
  double (congenital) G80.3
  unilateral R25.8
Athlete's
  foot B35.3
  heart I51.7
Athrepsia E41
Athyrea (acquired) —see also Hypothyroidism
  congenital E03.1
Atonia, atony, atonic
  bladder (sphincter) (neurogenic) N31.2
  capillary I78.8
  cecum K59.89
    psychogenic F45.8
  colon —see Atony, intestine
  congenital P94.2
  esophagus K22.89
  intestine K59.89
    psychogenic F45.8
  stomach K31.89
    neurotic or psychogenic F45.8
  uterus (during labor) O62.2
    with hemorrhage (postpartum) O72.1
    postpartum (with hemorrhage) O72.1
      without hemorrhage O75.89
Atopy —see History, allergy
Atransferrinemia, congenital E88.09
Atresia, atretic
  alimentary organ or tract NEC Q45.8
    upper Q40.8
  ani, anus, anal (canal) Q42.3
    with fistula Q42.2
  aorta (ring) Q25.29
  aortic (orifice) (valve) Q23.0
    arch Q25.21
    congenital with hypoplasia of ascending aorta and defective development of left ventricle (with mitral stenosis) Q23.4
    in hypoplastic left heart syndrome Q23.4
  aqueduct of Sylvius Q03.0
    with spina bifida —see Spina bifida, with hydrocephalus
  artery NEC Q27.8
    cerebral Q28.3
    coronary Q24.5
    digestive system Q27.8
    eye Q15.8
    lower limb Q27.8
    pulmonary Q25.5
    specified site NEC Q27.8
    umbilical Q27.0
    upper limb Q27.8
  auditory canal (external) Q16.1
  bile duct (common) (congenital) (hepatic) Q44.2
    acquired —see Obstruction, bile duct
  bladder (neck) Q64.39
    obstruction Q64.31
  bronchus Q32.4
  cecum Q42.8
  cervix (acquired) N88.2
    congenital Q51.828
    in pregnancy or childbirth —see Anomaly, cervix, in pregnancy or childbirth
      causing obstructed labor O65.5
  choana Q30.0
  colon Q42.9
    specified NEC Q42.8
  common duct Q44.2
  cricoid cartilage Q31.8
  cystic duct Q44.2
    acquired K82.8
      with obstruction K82.0
  digestive organs NEC Q45.8
  duodenum Q41.0
  ear canal Q16.1
  ejaculatory duct Q55.4

Atresia, atretic (Continued)
  epiglottis Q31.8
  esophagus Q39.0
    with tracheoesophageal fistula Q39.1
  eustachian tube Q17.8
  fallopian tube (congenital) Q50.6
    acquired N97.1
  follicular cyst N83.0-●
  foramen of
    Luschka Q03.1
      with spina bifida —see Spina bifida, with hydrocephalus
    Magendie Q03.1
      with spina bifida —see Spina bifida, with hydrocephalus
  gallbladder Q44.1
  genital organ
    external
      female Q52.79
      male Q55.8
    internal
      female Q52.8
      male Q55.8
  glottis Q31.8
  gullet Q39.0
    with tracheoesophageal fistula Q39.1
  heart valve NEC Q24.8
    pulmonary Q22.0
    tricuspid Q22.4
  hymen Q52.3
    acquired (postinfective) N89.6
  ileum Q41.2
  intestine (small) Q41.9
    large Q42.9
      specified NEC Q42.8
  iris, filtration angle Q15.0
  jejunum Q41.1
  lacrimal apparatus Q10.4
  larynx Q31.8
  meatus urinarius Q64.33
  mitral valve Q23.2
    in hypoplastic left heart syndrome Q23.4
  nares (anterior) (posterior) Q30.0
  nasopharynx Q34.8
  nose, nostril Q30.0
    acquired J34.89
  organ or site NEC Q89.8
  osseous meatus (ear) Q16.1
  oviduct (congenital) Q50.6
    acquired N97.1
  parotid duct Q38.4
    acquired K11.8
  pulmonary (artery) Q25.5
    valve Q22.0
  pulmonic Q22.0
  pupil Q13.2
  rectum Q42.1
    with fistula Q42.0
  salivary duct Q38.4
    acquired K11.8
  sublingual duct Q38.4
    acquired K11.8
  submandibular duct Q38.4
    acquired K11.8
  submaxillary duct Q38.4
    acquired K11.8
  thyroid cartilage Q31.8
  trachea Q32.1
  tricuspid valve Q22.4
  ureter Q62.10
    pelvic junction Q62.11
    vesical orifice Q62.12
  ureteropelvic junction Q62.11
  ureterovesical orifice Q62.12
  urethra (valvular) Q64.39
    stricture Q64.32
  urinary tract NEC Q64.8
  uterus Q51.818
    acquired N85.8
  vagina (congenital) Q52.4
    acquired (postinfectional) (senile) N89.5
  vas deferens Q55.3
  vascular NEC Q27.8
    cerebral Q28.3
    digestive system Q27.8
    lower limb Q27.8
    specified site NEC Q27.8
    upper limb Q27.8
  vein NEC Q27.8
    digestive system Q27.8
    great Q26.8

Atresia, atretic (Continued)
  vein NEC (Continued)
    lower limb Q27.8
    portal Q26.5
    pulmonary Q26.4
      partial Q26.3
      total Q26.2
    specified site NEC Q27.8
    upper limb Q27.8
  vena cava (inferior) (superior) Q26.8
  vesicourethral orifice Q64.31
  vulva Q52.79
    acquired N90.5
Atrichia, atrichosis —see Alopecia
Atrophia —see also Atrophy
  cutis senilis L90.8
    due to radiation L57.8
  gyrata of choroid and retina H31.23
  senilis R54
    dermatological L90.8
      due to radiation (nonionizing) (solar) L57.8
  unguium L60.3
    congenita Q84.6
Atrophie blanche (en plaque) (de Milian) L95.0
Atrophoderma, atrophodermia (of) L90.9
  diffusum (idiopathic) L90.4
  maculatum L90.8
    et striatum L90.8
      due to syphilis A52.79
    syphilitic A51.39
  neuriticum L90.8
  Pasini and Pierini L90.3
  pigmentosum Q82.1
  reticulatum symmetricum faciei L66.4
  senile L90.8
    due to radiation (nonionizing) (solar) L57.8
  vermiculata (cheeks) L66.4
Atrophy, atrophic (of)
  adrenal (capsule) (gland) E27.49
    primary (autoimmune) E27.1
  alveolar process or ridge (edentulous) K08.20
  anal sphincter (disuse) N81.84
  appendix K38.8
  arteriosclerotic —see Arteriosclerosis
  bile duct (common) (hepatic) K83.8
  bladder N32.89
    neurogenic N31.8
  blanche (en plaque) (of Milian) L95.0
  bone (senile) NEC —see also Disorder, bone, specified type NEC
    due to
      tabes dorsalis (neurogenic) A52.11
  brain (cortex) (progressive) G31.9
    frontotemporal circumscribed (see also Dementia, in, diseases specified elsewhere) G31.01 [F02.80]
      with behavioral disturbance (see also Dementia, in, diseases specified elsewhere) G31.01 [F02.81-●]
    senile NEC G31.1
  breast N64.2
    obstetric —see Disorder, breast, specified type NEC
  buccal cavity K13.79
  cardiac —see Degeneration, myocardial
  cartilage (infectional) (joint) —see Disorder, cartilage, specified NEC
  cerebellar —see Atrophy, brain
  cerebral —see Atrophy, brain
  cervix (mucosa) (senile) (uteri) N88.8
    menopausal N95.8
  Charcot-Marie-Tooth G60.0
  choroid (central) (macular) (myopic) (retina) H31.10-●
    diffuse secondary H31.12-●
    gyrate H31.23
    senile H31.11-●
  ciliary body —see Atrophy, iris
  conjunctiva (senile) H11.89
  corpus cavernosum N48.89
  cortical —see Atrophy, brain
  cystic duct K82.8
  Déjérine-Thomas G23.8
  disuse NEC —see Atrophy, muscle
  Duchenne-Aran G12.21
  ear H93.8-●
  edentulous alveolar ridge K08.20
  endometrium (senile) N85.8
    cervix N88.8
  enteric K63.89
  epididymis N50.89

▶ New   ⇒ Revised   ~~deleted~~ Deleted   ● Use Additional Character(s)

Atrophy, atrophic *(Continued)*
eyeball —*see* Disorder, globe, degenerated
   condition, atrophy
eyelid (senile) —*see* Disorder, eyelid,
   degenerative
facial (skin) L90.9
fallopian tube (senile) N83.32-●
   with ovary N83.33-●
fascioscapulohumeral (Landouzy-Déjérine)
   G71.02
fatty, thymus (gland) E32.8
gallbladder K82.8
gastric K29.40
   with bleeding K29.41
gastrointestinal K63.89
glandular I89.8
globe H44.52-●
gum —*see* Recession, gingival
hair L67.8
heart (brown) —*see* Degeneration, myocardial
hemifacial Q67.4
   Romberg G51.8
infantile E41
   paralysis, acute —*see* Poliomyelitis, paralytic
intestine K63.89
iris (essential) (progressive) H21.26-●
   specified NEC H21.29
kidney (senile) (terminal) —*see also* Sclerosis,
   renal N26.1
   congenital or infantile Q60.5
     bilateral Q60.4
     unilateral Q60.3
   hydronephrotic —*see* Hydronephrosis
lacrimal gland (primary) H04.14-●
   secondary H04.15-●
Landouzy-Déjérine G71.02
laryngitis, infective J37.0
larynx J38.7
Leber's optic (hereditary) H47.22
lip K13.0
liver (yellow) K72.90
   with coma K72.91
   acute, subacute K72.00
     with coma K72.01
   chronic K72.10
     with coma K72.11
lung (senile) J98.4
macular (dermatological) L90.8
   syphilitic, skin A51.39
     striated A52.79
mandible (edentulous) K08.20
   minimal K08.21
   moderate K08.22
   severe K08.23
maxilla K08.20
   minimal K08.24
   moderate K08.25
   severe K08.26
muscle, muscular (diffuse) (general) (idiopathic)
   (primary) M62.50
   ankle M62.57-●
   back M62.5A9
     cervical M62.5A0
     lumbosacral M62.5A2
     thoracic M62.5A1
   Duchenne-Aran G12.21
   foot M62.57-●
   forearm M62.53-●
   hand M62.54-●
   infantile spinal G12.0
   lower leg M62.56-●
   multiple sites M62.59
   myelopathic —*see* Atrophy, muscle, spinal
   myotonic G71.11
   neuritic G58.9
   neuropathic (peroneal) (progressive) G60.0
   pelvic (disuse) N81.84
   peroneal G60.0
   progressive (bulbar) G12.21
     adult G12.1
     infantile (spinal) G12.0
     spinal G12.25
       adult G12.1
       infantile G12.0
   pseudohypertrophic G71.02
   shoulder region M62.51-●
   specified site NEC M62.58
   spinal G12.9
     adult form G12.1
     Aran-Duchenne G12.21
     childhood form, type II G12.1

Atrophy, atrophic *(Continued)*
muscle, muscular *(Continued)*
   spinal *(Continued)*
     distal G12.1
     hereditary NFC G12.1
     infantile, type I (Werdnig-Hoffmann) G12.0
     juvenile form, type III (Kugelberg-
       Welander) G12.1
     progressive G12.25
     scapuloperoneal form G12.1
     specified NEC G12.8
   syphilitic A52.78
   thigh M62.55-●
   upper arm M62.52-●
myocardium —*see* Degeneration, myocardial
myometrium (senile) N85.8
   cervix N88.8
myopathic NEC —*see* Atrophy, muscle
myotonia G71.11
nail L60.3
nasopharynx J31.1
nerve —*see also* Disorder, nerve
   abducens —*see* Strabismus, paralytic, sixth
     nerve
   accessory G52.8
   acoustic or auditory —*see* subcategory H93.3
   cranial G52.9
     eighth (auditory) —*see* subcategory H93.3
     eleventh (accessory) G52.8
     fifth (trigeminal) G52.8
     first (olfactory) G52.0
     fourth (trochlear) —*see* Strabismus,
       paralytic, fourth nerve
     second (optic) H47.20
     sixth (abducens) —*see* Strabismus,
       paralytic, sixth nerve
     tenth (pneumogastric) (vagus) G52.2
     third (oculomotor) —*see* Strabismus,
       paralytic, third nerve
     twelfth (hypoglossal) G52.3
   hypoglossal G52.3
   oculomotor —*see* Strabismus, paralytic, third
     nerve
   olfactory G52.0
   optic (papillomacular bundle)
     syphilitic (late) A52.15
       congenital A50.44
   pneumogastric G52.2
   trigeminal G50.8
   trochlear —*see* Strabismus, paralytic, fourth
     nerve
   vagus (pneumogastric) G52.2
neurogenic, bone, tabetic A52.11
nutritional E43
   with marasmus E41
old age R54
olivopontocerebellar G23.8
optic (nerve) H47.20
   glaucomatous H47.23-●
   hereditary H47.22
   primary H47.21-●
   specified type NEC H47.29-●
   syphilitic (late) A52.15
     congenital A50.44
orbit H05.31-●
ovary (senile) N83.31-●
   with fallopian tube N83.33-●
oviduct (senile) —*see* Atrophy, fallopian tube
palsy, diffuse (progressive) G12.22
pancreas (duct) (senile) K86.89
parotid gland K11.0
pelvic muscle N81.84
penis N48.89
pharynx J39.2
pluriglandular E31.8
   autoimmune E31.0
polyarthritis M15.9
prostate N42.89
pseudohypertrophic (muscle) G71.02
renal —*see also* Sclerosis, renal N26.1
retina, retinal (postinfectional) H35.89
rhinitis J31.0
salivary gland K11.0
scar L90.5
sclerosis, lobar (of brain) (*see also* Dementia,
   in, diseases specified elsewhere) G31.09
   [F02.80]
   with behavioral disturbance (*see also* Dementia,
     in, diseases specified elsewhere) G31.09
     [F02.81-●]
scrotum N50.89

Atrophy, atrophic *(Continued)*
seminal vesicle N50.89
senile R54
   due to radiation (nonionizing) (solar) L57.8
skin (patches) (spots) L90.9
   degenerative (senile) L90.8
   due to radiation (nonionizing) (solar) L57.8
   senile L90.8
spermatic cord N50.89
spinal (acute) (cord) G95.89
   muscular —*see* Atrophy, muscle, spinal
   paralysis G12.20
     acute —*see* Poliomyelitis, paralytic
     meaning progressive muscular atrophy
       G12.25
   spine (column) —*see* Spondylopathy, specified
     NEC
spleen (senile) D73.0
stomach K29.40
   with bleeding K29.41
striate (skin) L90.6
   syphilitic A52.79
subcutaneous L90.9
sublingual gland K11.0
submandibular gland K11.0
submaxillary gland K11.0
Sudeck's —*see* Algoneurodystrophy
suprarenal (capsule) (gland) E27.49
   primary E27.1
systemic affecting central nervous system
   in
     myxedema E03.9 *[G13.2]*
     neoplastic disease —*see also* Neoplasm
       D49.9 *[G13.1]*
     specified disease NEC G13.8
tarso-orbital fascia, congenital Q10.3
testis N50.0
thenar, partial —*see* Syndrome, carpal tunnel
thymus (fatty) E32.8
thyroid (gland) (acquired) E03.4
   with cretinism E03.1
   congenital (with myxedema) E03.1
tongue (senile) K14.8
   papillae K14.4
trachea J39.8
tunica vaginalis N50.89
turbinate J34.89
tympanic membrane (nonflaccid) H73.82-●
   flaccid H73.81-●
upper respiratory tract J39.8
uterus, uterine (senile) N85.8
   cervix N88.8
   due to radiation (intended effect) N85.8
     adverse effect or misadventure N99.89
vagina (senile) N95.2
vas deferens N50.89
vascular I99.8
vertebra (senile) —*see* Spondylopathy, specified
   NEC
vulva (senile) N90.5
Werdnig-Hoffmann G12.0
yellow —*see* Failure, hepatic
Attack, attacks
   with alteration of consciousness (with
     automatisms) —*see* Epilepsy, localization-
     related, symptomatic, with complex partial
     seizures
   without alteration of consciousness —*see*
     Epilepsy, localization-related, symptomatic,
     with simple partial seizures
   Adams-Stokes I45.9
   akinetic —*see* Epilepsy, generalized, specified
     NEC
   angina —*see* Angina
   atonic —*see* Epilepsy, generalized, specified
     NEC
   benign shuddering G25.83
   cataleptic —*see* Catalepsy
   coronary —*see* Infarct, myocardium
   cyanotic, newborn P28.2
   drop NEC R55
   epileptic —*see* Epilepsy
   heart —*see* infarct, myocardium
   hysterical F44.9
   jacksonian —*see* Epilepsy, localization-related,
     symptomatic, with simple partial seizures
   myocardium, myocardial —*see* Infarct,
     myocardium
   myoclonic —*see* Epilepsy, generalized, specified
     NEC
   panic F41.0

Attack, attacks *(Continued)*
  psychomotor —*see* Epilepsy, localization-related,
      symptomatic, with complex partial seizures
  salaam —*see* Epilepsy, spasms
  schizophreniform, brief F23
  shuddering, benign G25.83
  Stokes-Adams I45.9
  syncope R55
  transient ischemic (TIA) G45.9
      specified NEC G45.8
  unconsciousness R55
      hysterical F44.89
  vasomotor R55
  vasovagal (paroxysmal) (idiopathic) R55
Attention (to)
  artificial
      opening (of) Z43.9
          digestive tract NEC Z43.4
              colon Z43.3
              ilium Z43.2
              stomach Z43.1
          specified NEC Z43.8
          trachea Z43.0
          urinary tract NEC Z43.6
              cystostomy Z43.5
              nephrostomy Z43.6
              ureterostomy Z43.6
              urethrostomy Z43.6
      vagina Z43.7
  colostomy Z43.3
  cystostomy Z43.5
  deficit disorder or syndrome F98.8
      with hyperactivity —*see* Disorder, attention-
          deficit hyperactivity
  gastrostomy Z43.1
  ileostomy Z43.2
  jejunostomy Z43.4
  nephrostomy Z43.6
  surgical dressings Z48.01
  sutures Z48.02
  tracheostomy Z43.0
  ureterostomy Z43.6
  urethrostomy Z43.6
Attrition
  gum —*see* Recession, gingival
  tooth, teeth (excessive) (hard tissues) K03.0
Atypical, atypism —*see also* condition
  cells (on cytolgocial smear) (endocervical)
      (endometrial) (glandular)
          cervix R87.619
          vagina R87.629
  cervical N87.9
  endometrium N85.9
      hyperplasia N85.00
  parenting situation Z62.9
Auditory —*see* condition
Aujeszky's disease B33.8
Aurantiasis, cutis E67.1
Auricle, auricular —*see also* condition
  cervical Q18.2
Auriculotemporal syndrome G50.8
Austin Flint murmur (aortic insufficiency) I35.1
Australian
  Q fever A78
  X disease A83.4
Autism, autistic (childhood) (infantile) F84.0
  atypical F84.9
  spectrum disorder F84.0
▶ Autoantibodies, multiple confirmed islet, with
      normoglycemia E10.A1
Autodigestion R68.89
Autoerythrocyte sensitization (syndrome) D69.2
Autographism L50.3
Autoimmune
  disease (systemic) M35.9
  inhibitors to clotting factors D68.311
  lymphoproliferative syndrome [ALPS] D89.82
  thyroiditis E06.3
▶ Autoimmunity, confirmed islet, with dysglycemia
      E10.A2
Autointoxication R68.89
Automatism G93.89
  with temporal sclerosis G93.81
  epileptic —*see* Epilepsy, localization- related,
      symptomatic, with complex partial seizures
  paroxysmal, idiopathic —*see* Epilepsy,
      localization-related, symptomatic, with
      complex partial seizures
Autonomic, autonomous
  bladder (neurogenic) N31.2
  hysteria seizure F44.5

Autosensitivity, erythrocyte D69.2
Autosensitization, cutaneous L30.2
Autosome —*see* condition by chromosome
  involved
Autotopagnosia R48.1
Autotoxemia R68.89
Autumn —*see* condition
Avellis' syndrome G46.8
Aversion
  oral R63.39
      newborn P92.-●
      nonorganic origin F98.2
  sexual F52.1
Aviator's
  disease or sickness —*see* Effect, adverse, high
      altitude
  ear T70.0
Avitaminosis (multiple) —*see also* Deficiency,
      vitamin E56.9
  B E53.9
      with
          beriberi E51.11
          pellagra E52
  B2 E53.0
  B6 E53.1
  B12 E53.8
  D E55.9
      with rickets E55.0
  G E53.0
  K E56.1
  nicotinic acid E52
AVNRT (atrioventricular nodal re-entrant
      tachycardia) I47.19
AVRT (atrioventricular nodal re-entrant
      tachycardia) I47.19
Avulsion (traumatic)
  blood vessel —*see* Injury, blood vessel
  bone —*see* Fracture, by site
  cartilage —*see also* Dislocation, by site
      symphyseal (inner), complicating delivery
          O71.6
  external site other than limb —*see* Wound, open,
      by site
  eye S05.7-●
  head (intracranial)
      external site NEC S08.89
      scalp S08.0
  internal organ or site —*see* Injury, by site
  joint —*see also* Dislocation, by site
      capsule —*see* Sprain, by site
  kidney S37.06-●
  ligament —*see* Sprain, by site
  limb —*see also* Amputation, traumatic, by site
      skin and subcutaneous tissue —*see* Wound,
          open, by site
  muscle —*see* Injury, muscle
  nerve (root) —*see* Injury, nerve
  scalp S08.0
  skin and subcutaneous tissue —*see* Wound,
      open, by site
  spleen S36.032
  symphyseal cartilage (inner), complicating
      delivery O71.6
  tendon —*see* Injury, muscle
  tooth S03.2
Awareness of heart beat R00.2
Axenfeld's
  anomaly or syndrome Q15.0
  degeneration (calcareous) Q13.4
Axilla, axillary —*see also* condition
  breast Q83.1
Axonotmesls —*see* Injury, nerve
Ayerza's disease or syndrome (pulmonary artery
      sclerosis with pulmonary hypertension) I27.0
Azoospermia (organic) N46.01
  due to
      drug therapy N46.021
      efferent duct obstruction N46.023
      infection N46.022
      radiation N46.024
      specified cause NEC N46.029
      systemic disease N46.025
Azotemia R79.89
  meaning uremia N19
Aztec ear Q17.3
Azygos
  continuation inferior vena cava Q26.8
  lobe (lung) Q33.1

—————— **B** ——————

Baastrup's disease —*see* Kissing spine
Babesiosis B60.00
  due to
      Babesia
          divergens B60.03
          duncani B60.02
          KO-1 B60.09
          microti B60.01
          MO-1 B60.03
          species
              unspecified B60.00
          venatorum B60.09
      specified NEC B60.09
Babington's disease (familial hemorrhagic
      telangiectasia) I78.0
Babinski's syndrome A52.79
Baby
  crying constantly R68.11
  floppy (syndrome) P94.2
Bacillary —*see* condition
Bacilluria R82.71
Bacillus —*see also* Infection, bacillus
  abortus infection A23.1
  anthracis infection A22.9
  coli infection —*see also* Escherichia coli
      B96.20
  Flexner's A03.1
  mallei infection A24.0
  Shiga's A03.0
  suipestifer infection —*see* Infection, salmonella
Back —*see* condition
Backache (postural) M54.9
  sacroiliac M53.3
  specified NEC M54.89
Backflow —*see* Reflux
Backward reading (dyslexia) F81.0
Bacteremia R78.81
  with sepsis —*see* Sepsis
Bactericholia —*see* Cholecystitis, acute
Bacterid, bacteride (pustular) L40.3
Bacterium, bacteria, bacterial
  agent NEC, as cause of disease classified
      elsewhere B96.89
  in blood —*see* Bacteremia
  in urine —*see* Bacteriuria
➡Bacteriuria, bacteruria (asymptomatic) R82.71
  ~~asymptomatic R82.71~~
Bacteroides
  fragilis, as cause of disease classified elsewhere
      B96.6
Bad
  heart —*see* Disease, heart
  trip
      due to drug abuse —*see* Abuse, drug,
          hallucinogen
      due to drug dependence —*see* Dependence,
          drug, hallucinogen
Baelz's disease (cheilitis glandularis apostematosa)
      K13.0
Baerensprung's disease (eczema marginatum)
      B35.6
Bagasse disease or pneumonitis J67.1
Bagassosis J67.1
Baker's cyst —*see* Cyst, Baker's
Bakwin-Krida syndrome (metaphyseal dysplasia)
      Q78.5
Balancing side interference M26.56
Balanitis (circinata) (erosiva) (gangrenosa)
      (phagedenic) (vulgaris) N48.1
  amebic A06.82
  candidal B37.42
  due to Haemophilus ducreyi A57
  gonococcal (acute) (chronic) A54.23
  xerotica obliterans N48.0
Balanoposthitis N47.6
  gonococcal (acute) (chronic) A54.23
  ulcerative (specific) A63.8
Balanorrhagia —*see* Balanitis
Balantidiasis, balantidiosis A07.0
Bald tongue K14.4
Baldness —*see also* Alopecia
  male-pattern —*see* Alopecia, androgenic
Balkan grippe A78
Balloon disease —*see* Effect, adverse, high
      altitude
Balo's disease (concentric sclerosis) G37.5
Bamberger-Marie disease —*see* Osteoarthropathy,
      hypertrophic, specified type NEC
Bancroft's filariasis B74.0

▶ New ⇒ Revised ~~deleted~~ Deleted ● Use Additional Character(s)

Band(s)
adhesive —see Adhesions, peritoneum
anomalous or congenital —see also Anomaly, by site
   heart (atrial) (ventricular) Q24.8
   intestine Q43.3
   omentum Q43.3
cervix N88.1
constricting, congenital Q79.8
gallbladder (congenital) Q44.1
intestinal (adhesive) —see Adhesions, peritoneum
obstructive
   intestine K56.50
     complete K56.52
     incomplete K56.51
     partial K56.51
   peritoneum K56.50
     complete K56.52
     incomplete K56.51
     partial K56.51
periappendiceal, congenital Q43.3
peritoneal (adhesive) —see Adhesions, peritoneum
uterus N73.6
   internal N85.6
vagina N89.5
Bandemia D72.825
Bandl's ring (contraction), complicating delivery O62.4
Bangkok hemorrhagic fever A91
Bang's disease (brucella abortus) A23.1
Bankruptcy (anxiety concerning) Z59.86
Bannister's disease T78.3
hereditary D84.1
Banti's disease or syndrome (with cirrhosis) (with portal hypertension) K76.6
Bar, median, prostate —see Enlargement, enlarged, prostate
Barcoo disease or rot —see Ulcer, skin
Barlow's disease E54
Barodontalgia T70.29
Baron Münchausen syndrome —see Disorder, factitious
Barosinusitis T70.1
Barotitis T70.0
Barotrauma T70.29
odontalgia T70.29
otitic T70.0
sinus T70.1
Barraquer (-Simons) disease or syndrome (progressive lipodystrophy) E88.1
Barré-Guillain disease or syndrome G61.0
Barré-Liéou syndrome (posterior cervical sympathetic) M53.0
Barrel chest M95.4
Barrett's
disease —see Barrett's, esophagus
esophagus K22.70
   with dysplasia K22.719
     high grade K22.711
     low grade K22.710
   without dysplasia K22.70
syndrome —see Barrett's, esophagus
ulcer K22.10
   with bleeding K22.11
   without bleeding K22.10
Barth syndrome E78.71
Bársony (-Polgár) (-Teschendorf) syndrome (corkscrew esophagus) K22.4
Bartholinitis (suppurating) N75.8
gonococcal (acute) (chronic) (with abscess) A54.1
Bartonellosis A44.9
cutaneous A44.1
mucocutaneous A44.1
specified NEC A44.8
systemic A44.0
Barton's fracture S52.56- •
Bartter's syndrome E26.81
Basal —see condition
Basan's (hidrotic) ectodermal dysplasia Q82.4
Baseball finger —see Dislocation, finger
Basedow's disease (exophthalmic goiter) —see Hyperthyroidism, with, goiter
Basic —see condition
Basilar —see condition
Bason's (hidrotic) ectodermal dysplasia Q82.4
Basopenia —see Agranulocytosis
Basophilia D72.824
Basophilism (cortico-adrenal) (Cushing's) (pituitary) E24.0

Bassen-Kornzweig disease or syndrome E78.6
Bat ear Q17.5
Bateman's
disease B08.1
purpura (senile) D69.2
Bathing cramp T75.1
Bathophobia F40.248
Batten (-Mayou) disease E75.4
retina E75.4 [H36.89]
Batten-Steinert syndrome G71.11
Battered —see Maltreatment
Battey Mycobacterium infection A31.0
Battle exhaustion F43.0
Battledore placenta O43.19- •
Baumgarten-Cruveilhier cirrhosis, disease or syndrome K74.69
Bauxite fibrosis (of lung) J63.1
Bayle's disease (general paresis) A52.17
Bazin's disease (primary) (tuberculous) A18.4
Beach ear —see Swimmer's, ear
Beaded hair (congenital) Q84.1
Béal conjunctivitis or syndrome B30.2
Beard's disease (neurasthenia) F48.8
Beat(s)
atrial, premature I49.1
ectopic I49.49
elbow —see Bursitis, elbow
escaped, heart I49.49
hand —see Bursitis, hand
knee —see Bursitis, knee
premature I49.40
   atrial I49.1
   auricular I49.1
   supraventricular I49.1
Beau's
disease or syndrome —see Degeneration, myocardial
lines (transverse furrows on fingernails) L60.4
Bechterev's syndrome —see Spondylitis, ankylosing
Beck's syndrome (anterior spinal artery occlusion) I65.8
Becker's
cardiomyopathy I42.8
disease
   idiopathic mural endomyocardial disease I42.3
   myotonia congenita, recessive form G71.12
dystrophy G71.01
pigmented hairy nevus D22.5
Beckwith-Wiedemann syndrome Q87.3
Bed confinement status Z74.01
Bed-sharing, infant Z72.823
Bed sore —see Ulcer, pressure, by site
Bedbug bite(s) —see Bite(s), by site, superficial, insect
Bedclothes, asphyxiation or suffocation by —see Asphyxia, traumatic, due to, mechanical, trapped
Bednar's
aphthae K12.0
tumor —see Neoplasm, malignant, by site
Bedridden Z74.01
Bedsore —see Ulcer, pressure, by site
Bedwetting —see Enuresis
Bee sting (with allergic or anaphylactic shock) T63.44- •
Beer drinker's heart (disease) I42.6
Begbie's disease (exophthalmic goiter) —see Hyperthyroidism, with, goiter
Behavior
antisocial
   adult Z72.811
   child or adolescent Z72.810
disorder, disturbance —see Disorder, conduct
disruptive —see Disorder, conduct
drug seeking Z76.5
inexplicable R46.2
marked evasiveness R46.5
obsessive-compulsive R46.81
overactivity R46.3
poor responsiveness R46.4
self-damaging (life-style) Z72.89
sleep-incompatible Z72.821
slowness R46.4
specified NEC R46.89
strange (and inexplicable) R46.2
suspiciousness R46.5
type A pattern Z73.1
undue concern or preoccupation with stressful events R46.6
verbosity and circumstantial detail obscuring reason for contact R46.7

Behcet's disease or syndrome M35.2
Behr's disease —see Degeneration, macula
Beigel's disease or morbus (white piedra) B36.2
Bejel A65
Bekhterev's syndrome —see Spondylitis, ankylosing
Belching —see Eructation
Bell's
mania F30.8
palsy, paralysis G51.0
   infant or newborn P11.3
spasm G51.3- •
Bence Jones albuminuria or proteinuria NEC R80.3
Bends T70.3
Benedikt's paralysis or syndrome G46.3
Benign (see also condition)
prostatic hyperplasia —see Hyperplasia, prostate
Bennett's fracture (displaced) S62.21- •
Benson's disease —see Deposit, crystalline
Bent
back (hysterical) F44.4
nose M95.0
   congenital Q67.4
Bereavement (uncomplicated) Z63.4
Bergeron's disease (hysterical chorea) F44.4
Berger's disease —see Nephropathy, IgA
Beriberi (dry) E51.11
heart (disease) E51.12
polyneuropathy E51.11
wet E51.12
   involving circulatory system E51.11
Berlin's disease or edema (traumatic) S05.8X- •
Berlock (berloque) dermatitis L56.2
Bernard-Horner syndrome G90.2
Bernard-Soulier disease or thrombopathia D69.1
Bernhardt (-Roth) disease —see Mononeuropathy, lower limb, meralgia paresthetica
Bernheim's syndrome —see Failure, heart, right
Bertielliasis B71.8
Berylliosis (lung) J63.2
Besnier-Boeck (-Schaumann) disease —see Sarcoidosis
Besnier's
lupus pernio D86.3
prurigo L20.0
Bestiality F65.89
Best's disease H35.50
Beta-mercaptolactate-cysteine disulfiduria E72.09
Betalipoproteinemia, broad or floating E78.2
Betting and gambling Z72.6
pathological (compulsive) F63.0
Bezoar T18.9
intestine T18.3
stomach T18.2
Bezold's abscess —see Mastoiditis, acute
Bianchi's syndrome R48.8
Bicornate or bicornis uterus Q51.3
in pregnancy or childbirth O34.00
   causing obstructed labor O65.5
Bicuspid aortic valve Q23.81
▶ functional, with stenosis —see Stenosis, aortic (valve)
Biedl-Bardet syndrome Q87.83
Bielschowsky (-Jansky) disease E75.4
Biermer's (pernicious) anemia or disease D51.0
Biett's disease L93.0
Bifid (congenital)
apex, heart Q24.8
clitoris Q52.6
kidney Q63.8
nose Q30.2
patella Q74.1
scrotum Q55.29
toe NEC Q74.2
tongue Q38.3
ureter Q62.8
uterus Q51.3
uvula Q35.7
Biforis uterus (suprasimplex) Q51.3
Bifurcation (congenital)
gallbladder Q44.1
kidney pelvis Q63.8
renal pelvis Q63.8
rib Q76.6
tongue, congenital Q38.3
trachea Q32.1
ureter Q62.8
urethra Q64.74
vertebra Q76.49
Big spleen syndrome D73.1

Bigeminal pulse R00.8
▶ Bigorexia F45.22
Bilateral —*see* condition
Bile
  duct —*see* condition
  pigments in urine R82.2
Bilharziasis —*see also* Schistosomiasis
  chyluria B65.0
  cutaneous B65.3
  galacturia B65.0
  hematochyluria B65.0
  intestinal B65.1
  lipemia B65.9
  lipuria B65.0
  oriental B65.2
  piarhemia B65.9
  pulmonary NOS B65.9 *[J99]*
    pneumonia B65.9 *[J17]*
  tropical hematuria B65.0
  vesical B65.0
Biliary —*see* condition
Bilirubin metabolism disorder E80.7
  specified NEC E80.6
Bilirubinemia, familial nonhemolytic E80.4
Bilirubinuria R82.2
Biliuria R82.2
Bilocular stomach K31.2
Binswanger's disease I67.3
Biparta, bipartite
  carpal scaphoid Q74.0
  patella Q74.1
  vagina Q52.10
BI-RADS —*see* Breast, Imaging Reporting and
  Data System
Bird
  face Q75.8
  fancier's disease or lung J67.2
Birt-Hogg-Dube syndrome Q87.89
Birth
  complications in mother —*see* Delivery,
    complicated
  compression during NOS P15.9
  defect —*see* Anomaly
  immature (less than 37 completed weeks) —*see*
    Preterm, newborn
    extremely (less than 28 completed weeks) —
      see Immaturity, extreme
  inattention, at or after —*see* Maltreatment, child,
    neglect
  injury NOS P15.9
    basal ganglia P11.1
    brachial plexus NEC P14.3
    brain (compression) (pressure) P11.2
    central nervous system NOS P11.9
    cerebellum P11.1
    cerebral hemorrhage P10.1
    external genitalia P15.5
    eye P15.3
    face P15.4
    fracture
      bone P13.9
        specified NEC P13.8
      clavicle P13.4
      femur P13.2
      humerus P13.3
      long bone, except femur P13.3
      radius and ulna P13.3
      skull P13.0
      spine P11.5
      tibia and fibula P13.3
    intracranial P11.2
      laceration or hemorrhage P10.9
        specified NEC P10.8
    intraventricular hemorrhage P10.2
    laceration
      brain P10.1
      by scalpel P15.8
      peripheral nerve P14.9
    liver P15.0
    meninges
      brain P11.1
      spinal cord P11.5
    nerve
      brachial plexus P14.3
      cranial NEC (except facial) P11.4
      facial P11.3
      peripheral P14.9
      phrenic (paralysis) P14.2
    paralysis
      facial nerve P11.3
      spinal P11.5

Birth (*Continued*)
  injury (*Continued*)
    penis P15.5
    rupture
      spinal cord P11.5
    scalp P12.9
    scalpel wound P15.8
    scrotum P15.5
    skull NEC P13.1
      fracture P13.0
    specified type NEC P15.8
    spinal cord P11.5
    spine P11.5
    spleen P15.1
    sternomastoid (hematoma) P15.2
    subarachnoid hemorrhage P10.3
    subcutaneous fat necrosis P15.6
    subdural hemorrhage P10.0
    tentorial tear P10.4
    testes P15.5
    vulva P15.5
  lack of care, at or after —*see* Maltreatment, child,
    neglect
  neglect, at or after —*see* Maltreatment, child,
    neglect
  palsy or paralysis, newborn, NOS (birth injury)
    P14.9
  premature (infant) —*see* Preterm,
    newborn
  shock, newborn P96.89
  trauma —*see* Birth, injury
  weight
    4000 grams to 4499 grams P08.1
    4500 grams or more P08.0
    low (2499 grams or less) —*see* Low,
      birthweight
    extremely (999 grams or less) —*see* Low,
      birthweight, extreme
Birthmark Q82.5
Bisalbuminemia E88.09
Biskra's button B55.1
Bite(s) (animal) (human)
  abdomen, abdominal
    wall S31.159
      with penetration into peritoneal cavity
        S31.659
      epigastric region S31.152
        with penetration into peritoneal cavity
          S31.652
      left
        lower quadrant S31.154
          with penetration into peritoneal cavity
            S31.654
        upper quadrant S31.151
          with penetration into peritoneal cavity
            S31.651
      periumbilic region S31.155
        with penetration into peritoneal cavity
          S31.655
      right
        lower quadrant S31.153
          with penetration into peritoneal cavity
            S31.653
        upper quadrant S31.150
          with penetration into peritoneal cavity
            S31.650
      superficial NEC S30.871
        insect S30.861
  alveolar (process) —*see* Bite, oral
    cavity
  amphibian (venomous) —*see* Venom, bite,
    amphibian
  animal —*see also* Bite, by site
    venomous —*see* Venom
  ankle S91.05-●
    superficial NEC S90.57-●
      insect S90.56-●
  antecubital space —*see* Bite, elbow
  anus S31.835
    superficial NEC S30.877
      insect S30.867
  arm (upper) S41.15-●
    lower —*see* Bite, forearm
    superficial NEC S40.87-●
      insect S40.86-●
  arthropod NEC —*see* Venom, bite,
    arthropod
  auditory canal (external) (meatus) —*see* Bite,
    ear
  auricle, ear —*see* Bite, ear
  axilla —*see* Bite, arm

Bite (*Continued*)
  back —*see also* Bite, thorax, back
    lower S31.050
      with penetration into retroperitoneal space
        S31.051
      superficial NEC S30.870
        insect S30.860
  bedbug —*see* Bite(s), by site, superficial,
    insect
  breast S21.05-●
    superficial NEC S20.17-●
      insect S20.16-●
  brow —*see* Bite, head, specified site NEC
  buttock S31.805
    left S31.825
    right S31.815
    superficial NEC S30.870
      insect S30.860
  calf —*see* Bite, leg
  canaliculus lacrimalis —*see* Bite, eyelid
  canthus, eye —*see* Bite, eyelid
  centipede —*see* Toxicity, venom, arthropod,
    centipede
  cheek (external) S01.45-●
    internal —*see* Bite, oral cavity
    superficial NEC S00.87
      insect S00.86
  chest wall —*see* Bite, thorax
  chigger B88.0
  chin —*see* Bite, head, specified site NEC
  clitoris —*see* Bite, vulva
  costal region —*see* Bite, thorax
  digit(s)
    hand —*see* Bite, finger
    toe —*see* Bite, toe
  ear (canal) (external) S01.35-●
    superficial NEC S00.47-●
      insect S00.46-●
  elbow S51.05-●
    superficial NEC S50.37-●
      insect S50.36-●
  epididymis —*see* Bite, testis
  epigastric region —*see* Bite, abdomen
  epiglottis —*see* Bite, neck, specified site NEC
  esophagus, cervical S11.25
    superficial NEC S10.17
      insect S10.16
  eyebrow —*see* Bite, eyelid
  eyelid S01.15-●
    superficial NEC S00.27-●
      insect S00.26-●
  face NEC —*see* Bite, head, specified site NEC
  finger(s) S61.259
    with
      damage to nail S61.359
    index S61.258
      with
        damage to nail S61.358
      left S61.251
        with
          damage to nail S61.351
      right S61.250
        with
          damage to nail S61.350
      superficial NEC S60.478
        insect S60.46-●
    little S61.25-●
      with
        damage to nail S61.35-●
      superficial NEC S60.47-●
        insect S60.46-●
    middle S61.25-●
      with
        damage to nail S61.35-●
      superficial NEC S60.47-●
        insect S60.46-●
    ring S61.25-●
      with
        damage to nail S61.35-●
      superficial NEC S60.47-●
        insect S60.46-●
    superficial NEC S60.479
      insect S60.469
    thumb —*see* Bite, thumb
  flank —*see* Bite, abdomen, wall
  flea —*see* Bite, by site, superficial,
    insect
  foot (except toe(s) alone) S91.35-●
    superficial NEC S90.87-●
      insect S90.86-●
    toe —*see* Bite, toe

▶ New   ⇒ Revised   ~~deleted~~ Deleted   ● Use Additional Character(s)

Bite *(Continued)*
  forearm S51.85-●
    elbow only —*see* Bite, elbow
    superficial NEC S50.87-●
      insect S50.86-●
  forehead —*see* Bite, head, specified site
    NEC
  genital organs, external
    female S31.552
      superficial NEC S30.876
        insect S30.866
      vagina and vulva —*see* Bite, vulva
    male S31.551
      penis —*see* Bite, penis
      scrotum —*see* Bite, scrotum
      superficial NEC S30.875
        insect S30.865
      testes —*see* Bite, testis
  groin —*see* Bite, abdomen, wall
  gum —*see* Bite, oral cavity
  hand S61.45-●
    finger —*see* Bite, finger
    superficial NEC S60.57-●
      insect S60.56-●
    thumb —*see* Bite, thumb
  head S01.95
    cheek —*see* Bite, cheek
    ear —*see* Bite, ear
    eyelid —*see* Bite, eyelid
    lip —*see* Bite, lip
    nose —*see* Bite, nose
    oral cavity —*see* Bite, oral cavity
    scalp —*see* Bite, scalp
    specified site NEC S01.85
      superficial NEC S00.87
        insect S00.86
    superficial NEC S00.97
      insect S00.96
    temporomandibular area —*see* Bite, cheek
  heel —*see* Bite, foot
  hip S71.05-●
    superficial NEC S70.27-●
      insect S70.26-●
  hymen S31.45
  hypochondrium —*see* Bite, abdomen, wall
  hypogastric region —*see* Bite, abdomen, wall
  inguinal region —*see* Bite, abdomen, wall
  insect —*see* Bite, by site, superficial, insect
  instep —*see* Bite, foot
  interscapular region —*see* Bite, thorax, back
  jaw —*see* Bite, head, specified site NEC
  knee S81.05-●
    superficial NEC S80.27-●
      insect S80.26-●
  labium (majus) (minus) —*see* Bite, vulva
  lacrimal duct —*see* Bite, eyelid
  larynx S11.015
    superficial NEC S10.17
      insect S10.16
  leg (lower) S81.85-●
    ankle —*see* Bite, ankle
    foot —*see* Bite, foot
    knee —*see* Bite, knee
    superficial NEC S80.87-●
      insect S80.86-●
    toe —*see* Bite, toe
    upper —*see* Bite, thigh
  lip S01.551
    superficial NEC S00.571
      insect S00.561
  lizard (venomous) —*see* Venom, bite, reptile
  loin —*see* Bite, abdomen, wall
  lower back —*see* Bite, back, lower
  lumbar region —*see* Bite, back, lower
  malar region —*see* Bite, head, specified site NEC
  mammary —*see* Bite, breast
  marine animals (venomous) —*see* Toxicity,
    venom, marine animal
  mastoid region —*see* Bite, head, specified site NEC
  mouth —*see* Bite, oral cavity
  nail
    finger —*see* Bite, finger
    toe —*see* Bite, toe
  nape —*see* Bite, neck, specified site NEC
  nasal (septum) (sinus) —*see* Bite, nose
  nasopharynx —*see* Bite, head, specified site NEC
  neck S11.95
    involving
      cervical esophagus —*see* Bite, esophagus,
        cervical
      larynx —*see* Bite, larynx

Bite *(Continued)*
  neck *(Continued)*
    involving *(Continued)*
      pharynx —*see* Bite, pharynx
      thyroid gland S11.15
      trachea —*see* Bite, trachea
    specified site NEC S11.85
      superficial NEC S10.87
        insect S10.86
    superficial NEC S10.97
      insect S10.96
    throat S11.85
      superficial NEC S10.17
        insect S10.16
  nose (septum) (sinus) S01.25
    superficial NEC S00.37
      insect S00.36
  occipital region —*see* Bite, scalp
  oral cavity S01.552
    superficial NEC S00.572
      insect S00.562
  orbital region —*see* Bite, eyelid
  palate —*see* Bite, oral cavity
  palm —*see* Bite, hand
  parietal region —*see* Bite, scalp
  pelvis S31.050
    with penetration into retroperitoneal space
      S31.051
    superficial NEC S30.870
      insect S30.860
  penis S31.25
    superficial NEC S30.872
      insect S30.862
  perineum
    female —*see* Bite, vulva
    male —*see* Bite, pelvis
  periocular area (with or without lacrimal
    passages) —*see* Bite, eyelid
  phalanges
    finger —*see* Bite, finger
    toe —*see* Bite, toe
  pharynx S11.25
    superficial NEC S10.17
      insect S10.16
  pinna —*see* Bite, ear
  poisonous —*see* Venom
  popliteal space —*see* Bite, knee
  prepuce —*see* Bite, penis
  pubic region —*see* Bite, abdomen, wall
  rectovaginal septum —*see* Bite, vulva
  red bug B88.0
  reptile NEC —*see also* Venom, bite,
    reptile
    nonvenomous —*see* Bite, by site
    snake —*see* Venom, bite, snake
  sacral region —*see* Bite, back, lower
  sacroiliac region —*see* Bite, back, lower
  salivary gland —*see* Bite, oral cavity
  scalp S01.05
    superficial NEC S00.07
      insect S00.06
  scapular region —*see* Bite, shoulder
  scrotum S31.35
    superficial NEC S30.873
      insect S30.863
  sea-snake (venomous) —*see* Toxicity, venom,
    snake, sea snake
  shin —*see* Bite, leg
  shoulder S41.05-●
    superficial NEC S40.27-●
      insect S40.26-●
  snake —*see also* Venom, bite, snake
    nonvenomous —*see* Bite, by site
  spermatic cord —*see* Bite, testis
  spider (venomous) —*see* Toxicity, venom, spider
    nonvenomous —*see* Bite, by site, superficial,
      insect
  sternal region —*see* Bite, thorax, front
  submaxillary region —*see* Bite, head, specified
    site NEC
  submental region —*see* Bite, head, specified site
    NEC
  subungual
    finger(s) —*see* Bite, finger
    toe —*see* Bite, toe
  superficial —*see* Bite, by site, superficial
  supraclavicular fossa S11.85
  supraorbital —*see* Bite, head, specified site
    NEC
  temple, temporal region —*see* Bite, head,
    specified site NEC

Bite *(Continued)*
  temporomandibular area —*see* Bite, cheek
  testis S31.35
    superficial NEC S30.873
      insect S30.863
  thigh S71.15-●
    superficial NEC S70.37-●
      insect S70.36-●
  thorax, thoracic (wall) S21.95
    back S21.25-●
      with penetration into thoracic cavity
        S21.45-●
    breast —*see* Bite, breast
    front S21.15-●
      with penetration into thoracic cavity
        S21.35-●
    superficial NEC S20.97
      back S20.47-●
      front S20.37-●
      insect S20.96
        back S20.46-●
        front S20.36-●
  throat —*see* Bite, neck, throat
  thumb S61.05-●
    with
      damage to nail S61.15-●
    superficial NEC S60.37-●
      insect S60.36-●
  thyroid S11.15
    superficial NEC S10.87
      insect S10.86
  toe(s) S91.15-●
    with
      damage to nail S91.25-●
    great S91.15-●
      with
        damage to nail S91.25-●
    lesser S91.15-●
      with
        damage to nail S91.25-●
    superficial NEC S90.47-●
      great S90.47-●
      insect S90.46-●
        great S90.46-●
  tongue S01.552
  trachea S11.025
    superficial NEC S10.17
      insect S10.16
  tunica vaginalis —*see* Bite, testis
  tympanum, tympanic membrane —*see* Bite, ear
  umbilical region S31.155
  uvula —*see* Bite, oral cavity
  vagina —*see* Bite, vulva
  venomous —*see* Venom
  vocal cords S11.035
    superficial NEC S10.17
      insect S10.16
  vulva S31.45
    superficial NEC S30.874
      insect S30.864
  wrist S61.55-●
    superficial NEC S60.87-●
      insect S60.86-●
Biting, cheek or lip K13.1
Biventricular failure (heart) I50.82
Björck (-Thorson) syndrome (malignant carcinoid)
  E34.09
Black
  death A20.9
  eye S00.1-●
  hairy tongue K14.3
  heel (foot) S90.3-●
  lung (disease) J60
  palm (hand) S60.22-●
Blackfan-Diamond anemia or syndrome
  (congenital hypoplastic anemia) D61.01
Blackhead L70.0
Blackout R55
Bladder —*see* condition
Blast (air) (hydraulic) (immersion) (underwater)
  blindness S05.8X-●
  injury
    abdomen or thorax —*see* Injury, by site
    ear (acoustic nerve trauma) —*see* Injury, nerve,
      acoustic, specified type NEC
    syndrome NEC T70.8
Blastoma —*see* Neoplasm, malignant, by site
  pulmonary —*see* Neoplasm, lung, malignant
Blastomycosis, blastomycotic B40.9
  Brazilian —*see* Paracoccidioidomycosis
  cutaneous B40.3

Blastomycosis, blastomycotic (Continued)
  disseminated B40.7
  European —see Cryptococcosis
  generalized B40.7
  keloidal B48.0
  North American B40.9
  primary pulmonary B40.0
  pulmonary B40.2
    acute B40.0
    chronic B40.1
  skin B40.3
  South American —see Paracoccidioidomycosis
  specified NEC B40.89
Bleb(s) R23.8
  emphysematous (lung) (solitary) J43.9
  endophthalmitis H59.43
  filtering (vitreous), after glaucoma surgery
    Z98.83
  inflammed (infected), postprocedural H59.40
    stage 1 H59.41
    stage 2 H59.42
    stage 3 H59.43
  lung (ruptured) J43.9
    congenital —see Atelectasis
    newborn P25.8
  subpleural (emphysematous) J43.9
Blebitis, postprocedural H59.40
  stage 1 H59.41
  stage 2 H59.42
  stage 3 H59.43
Bleeder (familial) (hereditary) —see Hemophilia
Bleeding —see also Hemorrhage
  anal K62.5
  anovulatory N97.0
  atonic, following delivery O72.1
  capillary I78.8
    puerperal O72.2
  contact (postcoital) N93.0
  due to uterine subinvolution N85.3
  ear —see Otorrhagia
  excessive, associated with menopausal onset
    N92.4
  familial —see Defect, coagulation
  following intercourse N93.0
  gastrointestinal K92.2
  hemorrhoids —see Hemorrhoids
  intermenstrual (regular) N92.3
    irregular N92.1
  intraoperative —see Complication,
    intraoperative, hemorrhage
  irregular N92.6
  menopausal N92.4
  newborn, intraventricular —see Newborn,
    affected by, hemorrhage, intraventricular
  nipple N64.59
  nose R04.0
  ovulation N92.3
  perimenopausal N92.4
  postclimacteric N95.0
  postcoital N93.0
  postmenopausal N95.0
  postoperative —see Complication,
    postprocedural, hemorrhage
  preclimacteric N92.4
  pre-pubertal vaginal N93.1
  puberty (excessive, with onset of menstrual
    periods) N92.2
  rectum, rectal K62.5
    newborn P54.2
  tendencies —see Defect, coagulation
  throat R04.1
  tooth socket (post-extraction) K91.840
  umbilical stump P51.9
  uterus, uterine NEC N93.9
    climacteric N92.4
    dysfunctional or functional N93.8
    menopausal N92.4
    preclimacteric or premenopausal N92.4
    unrelated to menstrual cycle N93.9
  vagina, vaginal (abnormal) N93.9
    dysfunctional or functional N93.8
    newborn P54.6
    pre-pubertal N93.1
  vicarious N94.89
Blennorrhagia, blennorrhagic —see Gonorrhea
Blennorrhea (acute) (chronic) —see also Gonorrhea
  inclusion (neonatal) (newborn) P39.1
  lower genitourinary tract (gonococcal)
    A54.00
  neonatorum (gonococcal ophthalmia) A54.31
Blepharelosis —see Entropion

Blepharitis (angularis) (ciliaris) (eyelid) (marginal)
  (nonulcerative) H01.009
  herpes zoster B02.39
  left H01.006
    lower H01.005
    upper H01.004
    upper and lower H01.00B
  right H01.003
    lower H01.002
    upper H01.001
    upper and lower H01.00A
  squamous H01.029
    left H01.026
      lower H01.025
      upper H01.024
      upper and lower H01.02B
    right H01.023
      lower H01.022
      upper H01.021
      upper and lower H01.02A
  ulcerative H01.019
    left H01.016
      lower H01.015
      upper H01.014
      upper and lower H01.01B
    right H01.013
      lower H01.012
      upper H01.011
      upper and lower H01.01B
Blepharochalasis H02.30
  congenital Q10.0
  left H02.36
    lower H02.35
    upper H02.34
  right H02.33
    lower H02.32
    upper H02.31
Blepharoclonus H02.59
Blepharoconjunctivitis H10.50-●
  angular H10.52-●
  contact H10.53-●
  ligneous H10.51-●
Blepharophimosis (eyelid) H02.529
  congenital Q10.3
  left H02.526
    lower H02.525
    upper H02.524
  right H02.523
    lower H02.522
    upper H02.521
Blepharoptosis H02.40-●
  congenital Q10.0
  mechanical H02.41-●
  myogenic H02.42-●
  neurogenic H02.43-●
  paralytic H02.43-●
Blepharopyorrhea, gonococcal A54.39
Blepharospasm G24.5
  drug induced G24.01
Blighted ovum O02.0
Blind —see also Blindness
  bronchus (congenital) Q32.4
  loop syndrome K90.2
    congenital Q43.8
  sac, fallopian tube (congenital) Q50.6
  spot, enlarged —see Defect, visual field,
    localized, scotoma, blind spot area
  tract or tube, congenital NEC —see Atresia, by
    site
Blindness (acquired) (congenital) (both eyes)
  H54.0X-●
  blast S05.8X-●
  color —see Deficiency, color vision
  concussion S05.8X-●
  cortical H47.619
    left brain H47.612
    right brain H47.611
  day H53.11
  due to injury (current episode) S05.9-●
    sequelae — code to injury with seventh
      character S
  eclipse (total) —see Retinopathy, solar
  emotional (hysterical) F44.6
  face H53.16
  hysterical F44.6
  legal (both eyes) (USA definition) H54.8
  mind R48.8
  night H53.60
    abnormal dark adaptation curve H53.61
    acquired H53.62
    congenital H53.63

Blindness (Continued)
  night (Continued)
    specified type NEC H53.69
    vitamin A deficiency E50.5
  one eye (other eye normal) H54.40
    left (normal vision on right) H54.42-●
      low vision on right H54.12-●
    low vision, other eye H54.10
    right (normal vision on left) H54.41-●
      low vision on left H54.11-●
  psychic R48.8
  river B73.01
  snow —see Photokeratitis
  sun, solar —see Retinopathy, solar
  transient —see Disturbance, vision, subjective,
    loss, transient
  traumatic (current episode) S05.9-●
  word (developmental) F81.0
    acquired R48.0
    secondary to organic lesion R48.0
Blister (nonthermal)
  abdominal wall S30.821
  alveolar process S00.522
  ankle S90.52-●
  antecubital space —see Blister, elbow
  anus S30.827
  arm (upper) S40.82-●
  auditory canal —see Blister, ear
  auricle —see Blister, ear
  axilla —see Blister, arm
  back, lower S30.820
  beetle dermatitis L24.89
  breast S20.12-●
  brow S00.82
  calf —see Blister, leg
  canthus —see Blister, eyelid
  cheek S00.82
    internal S00.522
  chest wall —see Blister, thorax
  chin S00.82
  costal region —see Blister, thorax
  digit(s)
    foot —see Blister, toe
    hand —see Blister, finger
  due to burn —see Burn, by site, second
    degree
  ear S00.42-●
  elbow S50.32-●
  epiglottis S10.12
  esophagus, cervical S10.12
  eyebrow —see Blister, eyelid
  eyelid S00.22-●
  face S00.82
  fever B00.1
  finger(s) S60.429
    index S60.42-●
    little S60.42-●
    middle S60.42-●
    ring S60.42-●
  foot (except toe(s) alone) S90.82-●
    toe —see Blister, toe
  forearm S50.82-●
    elbow only —see Blister, elbow
  forehead S00.82
  fracture - omit code
  genital organ
    female S30.826
    male S30.825
  gum S00.522
  hand S60.52-●
  head S00.92
    ear —see Blister, ear
    eyelid —see Blister, eyelid
    lip S00.521
    nose S00.32
    oral cavity S00.522
    scalp S00.02
    specified site NEC S00.82
  heel —see Blister, foot
  hip S70.22-●
  interscapular region S20.429
  jaw S00.82
  knee S80.22-●
  larynx S10.12
  leg (lower) S80.82-●
    knee —see Blister, knee
    upper —see Blister, thigh
  lip S00.521
  malar region S00.82
  mammary —see Blister, breast
  mastoid region S00.82

▶ New   ⇒ Revised   ~~deleted~~ Deleted   ● Use Additional Character(s)

Blister (*Continued*)
mouth S00.522
multiple, skin, nontraumatic R23.8
nail
finger —*see* Blister, finger
toe —*see* Blister, toe
nasal S00.32
neck S10.92
specified site NEC S10.82
throat S10.12
nose S00.32
occipital region S00.02
oral cavity S00.522
orbital region —*see* Blister, eyelid
palate S00.522
palm —*see* Blister, hand
parietal region S00.02
pelvis S30.820
penis S30.822
periocular area —*see* Blister, eyelid
phalanges
finger —*see* Blister, finger
toe —*see* Blister, toe
pharynx S10.12
pinna —*see* Blister, ear
popliteal space —*see* Blister, knee
scalp S00.02
scapular region —*see* Blister, shoulder
scrotum S30.823
shin —*see* Blister, leg
shoulder S40.22-●
sternal region S20.329
submaxillary region S00.82
submental region S00.82
subungual
finger(s) —*see* Blister, finger
toe(s) —*see* Blister, toe
supraclavicular fossa S10.82
supraorbital S00.82
temple S00.82
temporal region S00.82
testis S30.823
thermal —*see* Burn, by site, second
degree
thigh S70.32-●
thorax, thoracic (wall) S20.92
back S20.42-●
front S20.32-●
throat S10.12
thumb S60.32-●
toe(s) S90.42-●
great S90.42-●
tongue S00.522
trachea S10.12
tympanum, tympanic membrane —*see* Blister,
ear
upper arm —*see* Blister, arm (upper)
uvula S00.522
vagina S30.824
vocal cords S10.12
vulva S30.824
wrist S60.82-●
Bloating R14.0
Bloch-Sulzberger disease or syndrome Q82.3
Block, blocked
alveolocapillary J84.10
arborization (heart) I45.5
arrhythmic I45.9
atrioventricular (incomplete) (partial)
I44.30
with atrioventricular dissociation I44.2
complete I44.2
congenital Q24.6
congenital Q24.6
first degree I44.0
second degree (types I and II) I44.1
specified NEC I44.39
third degree I44.2
types I and II I44.1
auriculoventricular —*see* Block, atrioventricular
bifascicular (cardiac) I45.2
bundle-branch (complete) (false) (incomplete)
I45.4
bilateral I45.2
left I44.7
with right bundle branch block I45.2
hemiblock I44.60
anterior I44.4
posterior I44.5
incomplete I44.7
with right bundle branch block I45.2

Block, blocked (*Continued*)
bundle-branc (*Continued*)
right I45.10
with
left bundle branch block I45.2
left fascicular block I45.2
specified NEC I45.19
Wilson's type I45.19
cardiac I45.9
conduction I45.9
complete I44.2
fascicular (left) I44.60
anterior I44.4
posterior I44.5
right I45.0
specified NEC I44.69
foramen Magendie (acquired) G91.1
congenital Q03.1
with spina bifida —*see* Spina bifida, by site,
with hydrocephalus
heart I45.9
bundle branch I45.4
bilateral I45.2
complete (atrioventricular) I44.2
congenital Q24.6
first degree (atrioventricular) I44.0
second degree (atrioventricular) I44.1
specified type NEC I45.5
third degree (atrioventricular) I44.2
hepatic vein I82.0
intraventricular (nonspecific) I45.4
bundle branch
bilateral I45.2
kidney N28.9
postcystoscopic or postprocedural N99.0
Mobitz (types I and II) I44.1
myocardial —*see* Block, heart
nodal I45.5
organ or site, congenital NEC —*see* Atresia, by
site
portal (vein) I81
second degree (types I and II) I44.1
sinoatrial I45.5
sinoauricular I45.5
third degree I44.2
trifascicular I45.3
tubal N97.1
vein NOS I82.90
Wenckebach (types I and II) I44.1
Blockage —*see* Obstruction
Blocq's disease F44.4
Blood
constituents, abnormal R78.9
disease D75.9
donor —*see* Donor, blood
dyscrasia D75.9
with
abortion —*see* Abortion, by type,
complicated by, hemorrhage
ectopic pregnancy O08.1
molar pregnancy O08.1
following ectopic or molar pregnancy O08.1
newborn P61.9
puerperal, postpartum O72.3
flukes NEC —*see* Schistosomiasis
in
feces K92.1
occult R19.5
urine —*see* Hematuria
mole O02.0
occult in feces R19.5
pressure
decreased, due to shock following injury T79.4
examination only Z01.30
fluctuating I99.8
high —*see* Hypertension
borderline R03.0
incidental reading, without diagnosis of
hypertension R03.0
low —*see also* Hypotension
incidental reading, without diagnosis of
hypotension R03.1
spitting —*see* Hemoptysis
staining cornea —*see* Pigmentation, cornea,
stromal
transfusion
reaction or complication —*see* Complications,
transfusion
type
A (Rh positive) Z67.10
Rh negative Z67.11

Blood (*Continued*)
type (*Continued*)
AB (Rh positive) Z67.30
Rh negative Z67.31
B (Rh positive) Z67.20
Rh negative Z67.21
O (Rh positive) Z67.40
Rh negative Z67.41
Rh (positive) Z67.90
negative Z67.91
vessel rupture —*see* Hemorrhage
vomiting —*see* Hematemesis
Blood-forming organs, disease D75.9
Bloodgood's disease —*see* Mastopathy, cystic
Bloom (-Machacek)(-Torre) syndrome Q82.8
Blount disease or osteochondrosis
M92.51-●
Blue
baby Q24.9
diaper syndrome E72.09
dome cyst (breast) —*see* Cyst, breast
dot cataract Q12.0
nevus D22.9
sclera Q13.5
with fragility of bone and deafness Q78.0
toe syndrome I75.02-●
Blueness —*see* Cyanosis
Blues, postpartal O90.6
baby O90.6
Blurring, visual H53.8
Blushing (abnormal) (excessive) R23.2
BMI —*see* Body, mass index
Boarder, hospital NEC Z76.4
accompanying sick person Z76.3
healthy infant or child Z76.2
foundling Z76.1
Bockhart's impetigo L01.02
**Bodechtel-Guttman disease (subacute sclerosing
panencephalitis)** A81.1
Boder-Sedgwick syndrome (ataxia- telangiectasia)
G11.3
Body, bodies
Aschoff's —*see* Myocarditis, rheumatic
asteroid, vitreous —*see* Deposit, crystalline
cytoid (retina) —*see* Occlusion, artery, retina
drusen (degenerative) (macula) (retinal) —*see
also* Degeneration, macula, drusen
optic disc —*see* Drusen, optic disc
foreign —*see* Foreign body
loose
joint, except knee —*see* Loose, body, joint
knee M23.4-●
sheath, tendon —*see* Disorder, tendon,
specified type NEC
mass index (BMI)
adult
19.9 or less Z68.1
20.0-20.9 Z68.20
21.0-21.9 Z68.21
22.0-22.9 Z68.22
23.0-23.9 Z68.23
24.0-24.9 Z68.24
25.0-25.9 Z68.25
26.0-26.9 Z68.26
27.0-27.9 Z68.27
28.0-28.9 Z68.28
29.0-29.9 Z68.29
30.0-30.9 Z68.30
31.0-31.9 Z68.31
32.0-32.9 Z68.32
33.0-33.9 Z68.33
34.0-34.9 Z68.34
35.0-35.9 Z68.35
36.0-36.9 Z68.36
37.0-37.9 Z68.37
38.0-38.9 Z68.38
39.0-39.9 Z68.39
40.0-44.9 Z68.41
45.0-49.9 Z68.42
50.0-59.9 Z68.43
60.0-69.9 Z68.44
70 and over Z68.45
pediatric
5th percentile to less than 85th percentile
for age Z68.52
85th percentile to less than 95th percentile
for age Z68.53
~~greater than or equal to ninety-fifth
percentile for age Z68.54~~
▶ 95th percentile for age to less than 120% of
the 95th percentile for age Z68.54

Body, bodies (Continued)
mass index (BMI) (Continued)
pediatric (Continued)
▶ 120% of the 95th percentile for age to less than 140% of the 95th percentile for age Z68.55
▶ greater than or equal to 140% of the 95th percentile for age Z68.56
less than fifth percentile for age Z68.51
Mooser's A75.2
rice —see also Loose, body, joint
knee M23.4-●
rocking F98.4
Boeck's
disease or sarcoid —see Sarcoidosis
lupoid (miliary) D86.3
Boerhaave's syndrome (spontaneous esophageal rupture) K22.3
Boggy
cervix N88.8
uterus N85.8
Boil —see also Furuncle, by site
Aleppo B55.1
Baghdad B55.1
Delhi B55.1
lacrimal
gland —see Dacryoadenitis
passages (duct) (sac) —see Inflammation, lacrimal, passages, acute
Natal B55.1
orbit, orbital —see Abscess, orbit
tropical B55.1
Bold hives —see Urticaria
Bombé, iris —see Membrane, pupillary
Bone —see condition
Bonnevie-Ullrich syndrome —see also Turner's syndrome Q87.19
Bonnier's syndrome —see subcategory H81.8
Bonvale dam fever T73.3
Bony block of joint —see Ankylosis
BOOP (bronchiolitis obliterans organized pneumonia) J84.89
Borderline
diabetes mellitus R73.03
hypertension R03.0
osteopenia M85.8-●
pelvis, with obstruction during labor O65.1
personality F60.3
Borna disease A83.9
Bornholm disease B33.0
Boston exanthem A88.0
Botalli, ductus (patent) (persistent) Q25.0
Bothriocephalus latus infestation B70.0
Botulism (foodborne intoxication) A05.1
infant A48.51
non-foodborne A48.52
wound A48.52
Bouba —see Yaws
Bouchard's nodes (with arthropathy) M15.2
Bouffée délirante F23
Bouillaud's disease or syndrome (rheumatic heart disease) I01.9
Bourneville's disease Q85.1
Boutonniere deformity (finger) —see Deformity, finger, boutonniere
Bouveret (-Hoffmann) syndrome (paroxysmal tachycardia) I47.9
Bovine heart —see Hypertrophy, cardiac
Bowel —see condition
Bowen's
dermatosis (precancerous) —see Neoplasm, skin, in situ
disease —see Neoplasm, skin, in situ
epithelioma —see Neoplasm, skin, in situ
type
epidermoid carcinoma-in-situ —see Neoplasm, skin, in situ
intraepidermal squamous cell carcinoma —see Neoplasm, skin, in situ
Bowing
femur —see also Deformity, limb, specified type NEC, thigh
congenital Q68.3
fibula —see also Deformity, limb, specified type NEC, lower leg
congenital Q68.4
forearm —see Deformity, limb, specified type NEC, forearm
leg(s), long bones, congenital Q68.5
radius —see Deformity, limb, specified type NEC, forearm

Bowing (Continued)
tibia —see also Deformity, limb, specified type NEC, lower leg
congenital Q68.4
Bowleg(s) (acquired) M21.16-●
congenital Q68.5
rachitic E64.3
Boyd's dysentery A03.2
Brachial —see condition
Brachycardia R00.1
Brachycephaly, non-deformational Q75.022
Bradley's disease A08.19
Bradyarrhythmia, cardiac I49.8
Bradycardia (sinoatrial) (sinus) (vagal) R00.1
neonatal P29.12
reflex G90.09
tachycardia syndrome I49.5
Bradykinesia R25.8
Bradypnea R06.89
Bradytachycardia I49.5
Brailsford's disease or osteochondrosis —see Osteochondrosis, juvenile, radius
Brain —see also condition
death G93.82
syndrome —see Syndrome, brain
Branched-chain amino-acid disorder E71.2
Branchial —see condition
cartilage, congenital Q18.2
Branchiogenic remnant (in neck) Q18.0
Brandt's syndrome (acrodermatitis enteropathica) E83.2
Brash (water) R12
Bravais-Jacksonian epilepsy —see Epilepsy, localization-related, symptomatic, with simple partial seizures
Braxton Hicks contractions —see False, labor
Brazilian leishmaniasis B55.2
BRBPR K62.5
Break, retina (without detachment) H33.30-●
with retinal detachment —see Detachment, retina
horseshoe tear H33.31-●
multiple H33.33-●
round hole H33.32-●
Breakdown
device, graft or implant —see also Complications, by site and type, mechanical T85.618
arterial graft NEC —see Complication, cardiovascular device, mechanical, vascular
breast (implant) T85.41
catheter NEC T85.618
cystostomy T83.010
dialysis (renal) T82.41
intraperitoneal T85.611
Hopkins T83.018
ileostomy T83.018
infusion NEC T82.514
cranial T85.610
epidural T85.610
intrathecal T85.610
spinal T85.610
subarachnoid T85.610
subdural T85.610
nephrostomy T83.012
urethral indwelling T83.011
urinary NEC T83.018
urostomy T83.018
electronic (electrode) (pulse generator) (stimulator)
bone T84.310
cardiac T82.119
electrode T82.110
pulse generator T82.111
specified type NEC T82.118
nervous system —see Complication, prosthetic device, mechanical, electronic nervous system stimulator
urinary —see Complication, genitourinary, device, urinary, mechanical
fixation, internal (orthopedic) NEC — see Complication, fixation device, mechanical
gastrointestinal —see Complications, prosthetic device, mechanical, gastrointestinal device
genital NEC T83.418
intrauterine contraceptive device T83.31
penile prosthesis (cylinder) (implanted) (pump) (reservoir) T83.410
testicular prosthesis T83.411

Breakdown (Continued)
device, graft or implant (Continued)
heart NEC —see Complication, cardiovascular device, mechanical
intrathecal infusion pump T85.615
joint prosthesis —see Complications..., joint prosthesis, internal, mechanical, by site
nervous system, specified device NEC T85.615
ocular NEC —see Complications, prosthetic device, mechanical, ocular device
orthopedic NEC —see Complication, orthopedic, device, mechanical
specified NEC T85.618
subcutaneous device pocket
nervous system prosthetic device, implant, or graft T85.890
other internal prosthetic device, implant, or graft T85.898
sutures, permanent T85.612
used in bone repair —see Complications, fixation device, internal (orthopedic), mechanical
urinary NEC T83.118
graft T83.21
sphincter, implanted T83.111
stent (ileal conduit) (nephroureteral) T83.113
ureteral indwelling T83.112
vascular NEC —see Complication, cardiovascular device, mechanical
ventricular intracranial shunt T85.01
nervous F48.8
perineum O90.1
respirator J95.850
specified NEC J95.859
ventilator J95.850
specified NEC J95.859
Breast —see also condition
buds E30.1
in newborn P96.89
dense R92.3-
Imaging Reporting and Data System (BI-RADS) : A R92.31-●
Imaging Reporting and Data System (BI-RADS) : B R92.32-●
Imaging Reporting and Data System (BI-RADS) : C R92.33-●
Imaging Reporting and Data System (BI-RADS) : D R92.34-●
Imaging Reporting and Data System (BI-RADS) : 1 R92.31-●
Imaging Reporting and Data System (BI-RADS) : 2 R92.32-●
Imaging Reporting and Data System (BI-RADS) : 3 R92.33-●
Imaging Reporting and Data System (BI-RADS) : 4 R92.34-●
nodule —see also Lump, breast N63.0
Breath
foul R19.6
holder, child R06.89
holding spell R06.89
shortness R06.02
Breathing
labored —see Hyperventilation
mouth R06.5
causing malocclusion M26.5
periodic R06.3
high altitude G47.32
Breathlessness R06.81
Breda's disease —see Yaws
Breech presentation (mother) O32.1
causing obstructed labor O64.1
footling O32.8
causing obstructed labor O64.8
incomplete O32.8
causing obstructed labor O64.8
Breisky's disease N90.4
Brennemann's syndrome I88.0
Brenner
tumor (benign) D27.9
borderline malignancy D39.1-●
malignant C56
proliferating D39.1
Bretonneau's disease or angina A36.0
Breus' mole O02.0
Brevicollis Q76.49
Brickmakers' anemia B76.9 [D63.8]
Bridge, myocardial Q24.5
Bright red blood per rectum (BRBPR) K62.5

Bright's disease —*see also* Nephritis
arteriosclerotic —*see* Hypertension, kidney
Brill (-Zinsser) disease (recrudescent typhus) A75.1
Brill-Symmers' disease C82.90
▸Brion-Kayser disease —*see* Fever, paratyphoid
Briquet's disorder or syndrome F45.0
Brissaud's
infantilism or dwarfism E23.0
motor-verbal tic F95.2
Brittle
bones disease Q78.0
nails L60.3
congenital Q84.6
Broad —*see also* condition
beta disease E78.2
ligament laceration syndrome N83.8
Broad- or floating-betalipoproteinemia E78.2
Brock's syndrome (atelectasis due to enlarged lymph nodes) J98.19
Brocq-Duhring disease (dermatitis herpetiformis) L13.0
Brodie's abscess or disease M86.8X-●
Broken
arches —*see also* Deformity, limb, flat foot
arm (meaning upper limb) —*see* Fracture, arm
back —*see* Fracture, vertebra
bone —*see* Fracture
implant or internal device —*see* Complications, by site and type, mechanical
leg (meaning lower limb) —*see* Fracture, leg
nose S02.2
tooth, teeth —*see* Fracture, tooth
Bromhidrosis, bromidrosis L75.0
Bromidism, bromism G92.8
chronic (dependence) F13.20
due to
correct substance properly administered —*see* Table of Drugs and Chemicals, by drug, adverse effect
overdose or wrong substance given or taken —*see* Table of Drugs and Chemicals, by drug, poisoning
Bromidrosiphobia F40.298
Bronchi, bronchial —*see* condition
Bronchiectasis (cylindrical) (diffuse) (fusiform) (localized) (saccular) J47.9
with
acute
bronchitis J47.0
lower respiratory infection J47.0
exacerbation (acute) J47.1
congenital Q33.4
tuberculous NEC —*see* Tuberculosis, pulmonary
Bronchiolectasis —*see* Bronchiectasis
Bronchiolitis (acute) (infective) (subacute) J21.9
with
bronchospasm or obstruction J21.9
influenza, flu or grippe —*see* Influenza, with, respiratory manifestations NEC
chemical (chronic) J68.4
acute J68.0
chronic (fibrosing) J44.89
obliterative J44.81
due to
external agent —*see* Bronchitis, acute, due to
human metapneumovirus J21.1
respiratory syncytial virus (RSV) J21.0
specified organism NEC J21.8
fibrosa obliterans J44.81
influenzal —*see* Influenza, with, respiratory manifestations NEC
obliterans (*see also* Bronchiolitis, obliterative) J44.81
with organizing pneumonia (BOOP) J84.89
syndrome J44.81
obliterative (chronic) (subacute) (*see also* Bronchiolitis, obliterans) J44.81
due to chemicals, gases, fumes or vapors (inhalation) (*see also* Disease, respiratory, chronic, due to chemicals, gases, fumes or vapors) J44.81
due to fumes or vapors (*see also* Disease, respiratory, chronic, due to chemicals, gases, fumes or vapors) J44.81
respiratory, interstitial lung disease J84.115
Bronchitis (diffuse) (fibrinous) (hypostatic) (infective) (membranous) J40
with
influenza, flu or grippe —*see* Influenza, with, respiratory manifestations NEC

Bronchitis *(Continued)*
with *(Continued)*
obstruction (airway) (lung) J44.89
tracheitis (15 years of age and above) J40
acute or subacute J20.9
chronic J42
under 15 years of age J20.9
acute or subacute (with bronchospasm or obstruction) J20.9
with
bronchiectasis J47.0
chronic obstructive pulmonary disease J44.0
chemical (due to gases, fumes or vapors) J68.0
due to
fumes or vapors J68.0
Haemophilus influenzae J20.1
Mycoplasma pneumoniae J20.0
radiation J70.0
specified organism NEC J20.8
Streptococcus J20.2
virus
coxsackie J20.3
echovirus J20.7
parainfluenzae J20.4
respiratory syncytial (RSV) J20.5
rhinovirus J20.6
viral NEC J20.8
allergic (acute) J45.909
with
exacerbation (acute) J45.901
status asthmaticus J45.902
arachidic T17.528
aspiration (due to food and vomit) J69.0
asthmatic J45.9
chronic J44.89
with
acute lower respiratory infection J44.0
exacerbation (acute) J44.1
capillary —*see* Pneumonia, broncho
caseous (tuberculous) A15.5
Castellani's A69.8
catarrhal (15 years of age and above) J40
acute —*see* Bronchitis, acute
chronic J41.0
under 15 years of age J20.9
chemical (acute) (subacute) J68.0
chronic (*see also* Disease, respiratory, chronic, due to chemicals, gases, fumes or vapors) J42
due to fumes or vapors (*see also* Disease, respiratory, chronic, due to chemicals, gases, fumes or vapors) J42
chronic J68.4
chronic J42
with
airways obstruction J44.89
tracheitis (chronic) J42
asthmatic (obstructive) J44.89
catarrhal J41.0
chemical (due to fumes or vapors) (*see also* Disease, respiratory, chronic, due to chemicals, gases, fumes or vapors) J42
due to
chemicals, gases, fumes or vapors (inhalation) (*see also* Disease, respiratory, chronic, due to chemicals, gases, fumes or vapors) J42
radiation J70.1
tobacco smoking J41.0
emphysematous J44.89
mucopurulent J41.1
non-obstructive J41.0
obliterans —*see* Bronchiolitis, obliterans
obstructive J44.89
purulent J41.1
simple J41.0
croupous —*see* Bronchitis, acute
due to gases, fumes or vapors (chemical) J68.0
emphysematous (obstructive) J44.89
exudative —*see* Bronchitis, acute
fetid J41.1
grippal —*see* Influenza, with, respiratory manifestations NEC
in those under 15 years age —*see* Bronchitis, acute
chronic —*see* Bronchitis, chronic
influenzal —*see* Influenza, with, respiratory manifestations NEC
mixed simple and mucopurulent J41.8
moulder's J62.8

Bronchitis *(Continued)*
mucopurulent (chronic) (recurrent) J41.1
acute or subacute J20.9
simple (mixed) J41.8
obliterans (chronic) —*see* Bronchiolitis, obliterans
obstructive (chronic) (diffuse) J44.89
pituitous J41.1
pneumococcal, acute or subacute J20.2
pseudomembranous, acute or subacute —*see* Bronchitis, acute
purulent (chronic) (recurrent) J41.1
acute or subacute —*see* Bronchitis, acute
putrid J41.1
senile (chronic) J42
simple and mucopurulent (mixed) J41.8
smokers' J41.0
spirochetal NEC A69.8
subacute —*see* Bronchitis, acute
suppurative (chronic) J41.1
acute or subacute —*see* Bronchitis, acute
tuberculous A15.5
under 15 years of age —*see* Bronchitis, acute
chronic —*see* Bronchitis, chronic
viral NEC, acute or subacute —*see also* Bronchitis, acute J20.8
Bronchoalveolitis J18.0
Bronchoaspergillosis B44.1
Bronchocele meaning goiter E04.0
Broncholithiasis J98.09
tuberculous NEC A15.5
Bronchomalacia J98.09
congenital Q32.2
Bronchomycosis NOS B49 *[J99]*
candidal B37.1
Bronchopleuropneumonia —*see* Pneumonia, broncho
Bronchopneumonia —*see* Pneumonia, broncho
Bronchopneumonitis —*see* Pneumonia, broncho
Bronchopulmonary —*see* condition
Bronchopulmonitis —*see* Pneumonia, broncho
Bronchorrhagia (*see* Hemoptysis)
Bronchorrhea J98.09
acute J20.9
chronic (infective) (purulent) J42
Bronchospasm (acute) J98.01
with
bronchiolitis, acute J21.9
bronchitis, acute (conditions in J20) —*see* Bronchitis, acute
due to external agent —*see* condition, respiratory, acute, due to
exercise induced J45.990
Bronchospirochetosis A69.8
Castellani A69.8
Bronchostenosis J98.09
Bronchus —*see* condition
Brontophobia F40.220
Bronze baby syndrome P83.88
Brooke's tumor —*see* Neoplasm, skin, benign
Brown enamel of teeth (hereditary) K00.5
Brown's sheath syndrome H50.61-●
Brown-Séquard disease, paralysis or syndrome G83.81
Bruce sepsis A23.0
Brucellosis (infection) A23.9
abortus A23.1
canis A23.3
dermatitis A23.9
melitensis A23.0
mixed A23.8
sepsis A23.9
melitensis A23.0
specified NEC A23.8
suis A23.2
Bruck-de Lange disease Q87.19
Bruck's disease —*see* Deformity, limb
BRUE (brief resolved unexplained event) R68.13
Brugsch's syndrome Q82.8
Bruise (skin surface intact) —*see also* Contusion
with
open wound —*see* Wound, open
internal organ —*see* Injury, by site
newborn P54.5
scalp, due to birth injury, newborn P12.3
umbilical cord O69.5
Bruit (arterial) R09.89
cardiac R01.1
Brush burn —*see* Abrasion, by site
Bruton's X-linked agammaglobulinemia D80.0

Bruxism
  psychogenic F45.8
  sleep related G47.63
Bubbly lung syndrome P27.0
Bubo I88.8
  blennorrhagic (gonococcal) A54.89
  chancroidal A57
  climatic A55
  due to Haemophilus ducreyi A57
  gonococcal A54.89
  indolent (nonspecific) I88.8
  inguinal (nonspecific) I88.8
    chancroidal A57
    climatic A55
    due to H. ducreyi A57
    infective I88.8
  scrofulous (tuberculous) A18.2
  soft chancre A57
  suppurating —see Lymphadenitis, acute
  syphilitic (primary) A51.0
    congenital A50.07
  tropical A55
  virulent (chancroidal) A57
Bubonic plague A20.0
Bubonocele —see Hernia, inguinal
Buccal —see condition
Buchanan's disease or osteochondrosis
    M91.0
Buchem's syndrome (hyperostosis corticalis) M85.2
Bucket-handle fracture or tear (semilunar
    cartilage) —see Tear, meniscus
Budd-Chiari syndrome (hepatic vein thrombosis)
    I82.0
Budgerigar fancier's disease or lung J67.2
Buds
  breast E30.1
    in newborn P96.89
Buerger's disease (thromboangiitis obliterans) I73.1
Bulbar —see condition
Bulbus cordis (left ventricle) (persistent)
    Q21.8
▶Bulimia (nervosa) F50.2-●
  atypical F50.9
  normal weight F50.9
Bulky
  stools R19.5
  uterus N85.2
Bulla (e) R23.8
  lung (emphysematous) (solitary) J43.9
    newborn P25.8
Bullet wound —see also Puncture
  fracture - code as Fracture, by site
  internal organ —see Injury, by site
Bundle
  branch block (complete) (false) (incomplete) —
      see Block, bundle-branch
  of His —see condition
Bunion M21.61-●
  tailor's M21.62-●
Bunionette M21.62-●
Buphthalmia, buphthalmos (congenital)
    Q15.0
Burdwan fever B55.0
Bürger-Grütz disease or syndrome E78.3
Buried
  penis (congenital) Q55.64
    acquired N48.83
  roots K08.3
Burke's syndrome K86.89
Burkholderia
  cepacia A49.8
  mallei A24.0
  pseudomallei —see Melioidosis
Burkitt
  cell leukemia C91.0-●
  lymphoma (malignant) C83.7-●
    small noncleaved, diffuse C83.7-●
    spleen C83.77
    undifferentiated C83.7-●
  tumor C83.7-●
  type
    acute lymphoblastic leukemia C91.0-●
    undifferentiated C83.7-●
Burn (electricity) (flame) (hot gas, liquid or hot
    object) (radiation) (steam) (thermal)
    T30.0
  abdomen, abdominal (muscle) (wall)
      T21.02
    first degree T21.12
    second degree T21.22
    third degree T21.32

Burn (Continued)
  above elbow T22.039
    first degree T22.139
    left T22.032
      first degree T22.132
      second degree T22.232
      third degree T22.332
    right T22.031
      first degree T22.131
      second degree T22.231
      third degree T22.331
    second degree T22.239
    third degree T22.339
  acid (caustic) (external) (internal) —see
      Corrosion, by site
  alimentary tract NEC T28.2
    esophagus T28.1
    mouth T28.0
    pharynx T28.0
  alkaline (caustic) (external) (internal) —see
      Corrosion, by site
  ankle T25.019
    first degree T25.119
    left T25.012
      first degree T25.112
      second degree T25.212
      third degree T25.312
    multiple with foot —see Burn, lower, limb,
        multiple, ankle and foot
    right T25.011
      first degree T25.111
      second degree T25.211
      third degree T25.311
    second degree T25.219
    third degree T25.319
  anus —see Burn, buttock
  arm (lower) (upper) —see Burn, upper,
      limb
  axilla T22.049
    first degree T22.149
    left T22.042
      first degree T22.142
      second degree T22.242
      third degree T22.342
    right T22.041
      first degree T22.141
      second degree T22.241
      third degree T22.341
    second degree T22.249
    third degree T22.349
  back (lower) T21.04
    first degree T21.14
    second degree T21.24
    third degree T21.34
    upper T21.03
      first degree T21.13
      second degree T21.23
      third degree T21.33
  blisters - code as Burn, second degree, by
      site
  breast(s) —see Burn, chest wall
  buttock(s) T21.05
    first degree T21.15
    second degree T21.25
    third degree T21.35
  calf T24.039
    first degree T24.139
    left T24.032
      first degree T24.132
      second degree T24.232
      third degree T24.332
    right T24.031
      first degree T24.131
      second degree T24.231
      third degree T24.331
    second degree T24.239
    third degree T24.339
  canthus (eye) —see Burn, eyelid
  caustic acid or alkaline —see Corrosion, by
      site
  cervix T28.3
  cheek T20.06
    first degree T20.16
    second degree T20.26
    third degree T20.36
  chemical (acids) (alkalines) (caustics) (external)
      (internal) —see Corrosion, by site
  chest wall T21.01
    first degree T21.11
    second degree T21.21
    third degree T21.31

Burn (Continued)
  chin T20.03
    first degree T20.13
    second degree T20.23
    third degree T20.33
  colon T28.2
  conjunctiva (and cornea) —see Burn, cornea
  cornea (and conjunctiva) T26.1-●
    chemical —see Corrosion, cornea
  corrosion (external) (internal) —see Corrosion,
      by site
  deep necrosis of underlying tissue - code as
      Burn, third degree, by site
  dorsum of hand T23.069
    first degree T23.169
    left T23.062
      first degree T23.162
      second degree T23.262
      third degree T23.362
    right T23.061
      first degree T23.161
      second degree T23.261
      third degree T23.361
    second degree T23.269
    third degree T23.369
  due to ingested chemical agent —see Corrosion,
      by site
  ear (auricle) (external) (canal) T20.01
    first degree T20.11
    second degree T20.21
    third degree T20.31
  elbow T22.029
    first degree T22.129
    left T22.022
      first degree T22.122
      second degree T22.222
      third degree T22.322
    right T22.021
      first degree T22.121
      second degree T22.221
      third degree T22.321
    second degree T22.229
    third degree T22.329
  epidermal loss - code as Burn, second degree,
      by site
  erythema, erythematous - code as Burn, first
      degree, by site
  esophagus T28.1
  extent (percentage of body surface)
    less than 10 percent T31.0
    10-19 percent T31.10
      with 0-9 percent third degree burns T31.10
      with 10-19 percent third degree burns
          T31.11
    20-29 percent T31.20
      with 0-9 percent third degree burns T31.20
      with 10-19 percent third degree burns
          T31.21
      with 20-29 percent third degree burns
          T31.22
    30-39 percent T31.30
      with 0-9 percent third degree burns
          T31.30
      with 10-19 percent third degree burns
          T31.31
      with 20-29 percent third degree burns
          T31.32
      with 30-39 percent third degree burns
          T31.33
    40-49 percent T31.40
      with 0-9 percent third degree burns
          T31.40
      with 10-19 percent third degree burns
          T31.41
      with 20-29 percent third degree burns
          T31.42
      with 30-39 percent third degree burns
          T31.43
      with 40-49 percent third degree burns
          T31.44
    50-59 percent T31.50
      with 0-9 percent third degree burns T31.50
      with 10-19 percent third degree burns T31.51
      with 20-29 percent third degree burns T31.52
      with 30-39 percent third degree burns T31.53
      with 40-49 percent third degree burns T31.54
      with 50-59 percent third degree burns T31.55
    60-69 percent T31.60
      with 0-9 percent third degree burns T31.60
      with 10-19 percent third degree burns T31.61
      with 20-29 percent third degree burns T31.62

▶ New   ⟹ Revised   ~~deleted~~ Deleted   ● Use Additional Character(s)

▶ New   ⇨ Revised   ~~deleted~~ Deleted   ● Use Additional Character(s)

Burn (*Continued*)
  upper limb (*Continued*)
    multiple sites (*Continued*)
      right T22.091
        first degree T22.191
          second degree T22.291
          third degree T22.391
        second degree T22.299
        third degree T22.399
    scapular region —*see* Burn, scapular region
    second degree T22.20
    shoulder —*see* Burn, shoulder
    third degree T22.30
    wrist —*see* Burn, wrist
  uterus T28.3
  vagina T28.3
  vulva —*see* Burn, genital organs, external, female
  wrist T23.079
    first degree T23.179
    left T23.072
      first degree T23.172
      second degree T23.272
      third degree T23.372
    multiple sites with hand T23.099
      first degree T23.199
      left T23.092
        first degree T23.192
        second degree T23.292
        third degree T23.392
      right T23.091
        first degree T23.191
        second degree T23.291
        third degree T23.391
      second degree T23.299
      third degree T23.399
    right T23.071
      first degree T23.171
      second degree T23.271
      third degree T23.371
    second degree T23.279
    third degree T23.379
Burnett's syndrome E83.52
Burning
  feet syndrome E53.9
  sensation R20.8
  tongue K14.6
Burn-out (state) Z73.0
Burns' disease or osteochondrosis —*see* Osteochondrosis, juvenile, ulna
Bursa —*see* condition
Bursitis M71.9
  Achilles —*see* Tendinitis, Achilles
  adhesive —*see* Bursitis, specified NEC
  ankle —*see* Enthesopathy, ankle and tarsus
  calcaneal —*see* Enthesopathy, foot, specified type NEC
  collateral ligament, tibial —*see* Bursitis, tibial collateral
  due to use, overuse, pressure —*see also* Disorder, soft tissue, due to use, specified type NEC
    specified NEC —*see* Disorder, soft tissue, due to use, specified NEC
  Duplay's M75.0
  elbow NEC M70.3-●
    olecranon M70.2-●
  finger —*see* Disorder, soft tissue, due to use, specified type NEC, hand
  foot —*see* Enthesopathy, foot, specified type NEC
  gonococcal A54.49
  gouty —*see* Gout
  hand M70.1-●
  hip NEC M70.7-●
    trochanteric M70.6-●
  infective NEC M71.10
    abscess —*see* Abscess, bursa
    ankle M71.17-●
    elbow M71.12-●
    foot M71.17-●
    hand M71.14-●
    hip M71.15-●
    knee M71.16-●
    multiple sites M71.19
    shoulder M71.11-●
    specified site NEC M71.18
    wrist M71.13-●
  ischial —*see* Bursitis, hip
  knee NEC M70.5-●
    prepatellar M70.4-●
  occupational NEC —*see also* Disorder, soft tissue, due to, use

Bursitis (*Continued*)
  olecranon —*see* Bursitis, elbow, olecranon
  pharyngeal J39.1
  popliteal —*see* Bursitis, knee
  prepatellar M70.4-●
  radiohumeral M70.3-●
  rheumatoid M06.20
    ankle M06.27-●
    elbow M06.22-●
    foot joint M06.27-●
    hand joint M06.24-●
    hip M06.25-●
    knee M06.26-●
    multiple site M06.29
    shoulder M06.21-●
    vertebra M06.28
    wrist M06.23-●
  scapulohumeral —*see* Bursitis, shoulder
  semimembranous muscle (knee) —*see* Bursitis, knee
  shoulder M75.5-●
    adhesive —*see* Capsulitis, adhesive
  specified NEC M71.50
    ankle M71.57-●
    due to use, overuse or pressure —*see* Disorder, soft tissue, due to, use
    elbow M71.52-●
    foot M71.57-●
    hand M71.54-●
    hip M71.55-●
    knee M71.56-●
    shoulder —*see* Bursitis, shoulder
    specified site NEC M71.58
    tibial collateral M76.4-●
    wrist M71.53-●
  subacromial —*see* Bursitis, shoulder
  subcoracoid —*see* Bursitis, shoulder
  subdeltoid —*see* Bursitis, shoulder
  syphilitic A52.78
  Thornwaldt, Tornwaldt J39.2
  tibial collateral M76.4-●
  toe —*see* Enthesopathy, foot, specified type NEC
  trochanteric (area) —*see* Bursitis, hip, trochanteric
  wrist —*see* Bursitis, hand
Bursopathy M71.9
  specified type NEC M71.80
    ankle M71.87-●
    elbow M71.82-●
    foot M71.87-●
    hand M71.84-●
    hip M71.85-●
    knee M71.86-●
    multiple sites M71.89
    shoulder M71.81-●
    specified site NEC M71.88
    wrist M71.83-●
Burst stitches or sutures (complication of surgery) T81.31
  external operation wound T81.31
  internal operation wound (*see also* Dehiscence, closure) T81.328
    abdominal wall muscle or fascia T81.321
    specified NEC T81.328
Buruli ulcer A31.1
Bury's disease L95.1
Buschke's
  disease —*see* Cryptococcosis by site
  scleredema —*see* Sclerosis, systemic
Busse-Buschke disease —*see* Cryptococcosis by site
Buttock —*see* condition
Button
  Biskra B55.1
  Delhi B55.1
  oriental B55.1
Buttonhole deformity (finger) —*see* Deformity, finger, boutonniere
Bwamba fever A92.8
Byssinosis J66.0
Bywaters' syndrome T79.5

<hr>C<hr>

Cachexia E43
  cancerous R64
  cardiac —*see* Disease, heart
  dehydration E86.0
  due to
    malnutrition R64
    underlying condition E88.A
  exophthalmic —*see* Hyperthyroidism
  heart —*see* Disease, heart
  hypophyseal E23.0
  hypopituitary E23.0
  lead —*see* Poisoning, lead
  malignant R64
  marsh —*see* Malaria
  nervous F48.8
  old age R54
  paludal —*see* Malaria
  pituitary E23.0
  pulmonary R64
  renal N28.9
  saturnine —*see* Poisoning, lead
  senile R54
  Simmonds' E23.0
  splenica D73.0
  strumipriva E03.4
  tuberculous NEC —*see* Tuberculosis
CADASIL (cerebral autosomal dominant arteriopathy with subcortical infarcts and leukoencephalopathy) I67.850
Café au lait spots L81.3
Caffeine-induced
  anxiety disorder F15.980
  sleep disorder F15.982
Caffey's syndrome Q78.8
Caisson disease T70.3
Cake kidney Q63.1
Caked breast (puerperal, postpartum) O92.79
Calabar swelling B74.3
Calcaneal spur —*see* Spur, bone, calcaneal
Calcaneo-apophysitis M92.6
Calcareous —*see* condition
Calcicosis J62.8
Calciferol (vitamin D) deficiency E55.9
  with rickets E55.0
Calcification
  adrenal (capsule) (gland) E27.49
    tuberculous E35 [B90.8]
  aorta I70.0
  artery (annular) —*see* Arteriosclerosis
  auricle (ear) —*see* Disorder, pinna, specified type NEC
  basal ganglia G23.8
  bladder N32.89
    due to Schistosoma hematobium B65.0
  brain (cortex) —*see* Calcification, cerebral
  bronchus J98.09
  bursa M71.40
    ankle M71.47-●
    elbow M71.42-●
    foot M71.47-●
    hand M71.44-●
    hip M71.45-●
    knee M71.46-●
    multiple sites M71.49
    shoulder M75.3-●
    specified site NEC M71.48
    wrist M71.43-●
  cardiac —*see* Degeneration, myocardial
  cerebral (cortex) G93.89
    artery I67.2
  cervix (uteri) N88.8
  choroid plexus G93.89
  conjunctiva —*see* Concretion, conjunctiva
  corpora cavernosa (penis) N48.89
  cortex (brain) —*see* Calcification, cerebral
  dental pulp (nodular) K04.2
  dentinal papilla K00.4
  fallopian tube N83.8
  falx cerebri G96.198
  gallbladder K82.8
  general E83.59
  heart —*see also* Degeneration, myocardial
    valve —*see also* Endocarditis
    mitral —*see* Calcification, mitral
  idiopathic infantile arterial (IIAC) Q28.8
  intervertebral cartilage or disc (postinfective) —*see* Disorder, disc, specified NEC
  intracranial —*see* Calcification, cerebral
  joint —*see* Disorder, joint, specified type NEC

Calcification (Continued)
kidney N28.89
  tuberculous N29 [B90.1]
larynx (senile) J38.7
lens —see Cataract, specified NEC
lung (active) (postinfectional) J98.4
  tuberculous B90.9
lymph gland or node (postinfectional)
    I89.8
  tuberculous —see also Tuberculosis, lymph
      gland B90.8
mammographic R92.1
massive (paraplegic) —see Myositis, ossificans,
    in, quadriplegia
medial —see Arteriosclerosis, extremities
meninges (cerebral) (spinal) G96.198
metastatic E83.59
mitral (valve)
  annular I34.81
    nonrheumatic I34.81
    rheumatic I05.8
  annulus I34.81
    nonrheumatic I34.81
    rheumatic I05.8
Mönckeberg's —see Arteriosclerosis,
    extremities
muscle M61.9
  due to burns —see Myositis, ossificans, in,
      burns
  paralytic —see Myositis, ossificans, in,
      quadriplegia
  specified type NEC M61.40
    ankle M61.47-●
    foot M61.47-●
    forearm M61.43-●
    hand M61.44-●
    lower leg M61.46-●
    multiple sites M61.49
    pelvic region M61.45-●
    shoulder region M61.41-●
    specified site NEC M61.48
    thigh M61.45-●
    upper arm M61.42-●
myocardium, myocardial —see Degeneration,
    myocardial
ovary N83.8
pancreas K86.89
penis N48.89
periarticular —see Disorder, joint, specified type
    NEC
pericardium —see also Pericarditis I31.1
pineal gland E34.8
pleura J94.8
  postinfectional J94.8
  tuberculous NEC B90.9
pulpal (dental) (nodular) K04.2
sclera H15.89
spleen D73.89
subcutaneous L94.2
suprarenal (capsule) (gland) E27.49
tendon (sheath) —see also Tenosynovitis,
    specified type NEC
  with bursitis, synovitis or tenosynovitis —see
      Tendinitis, calcific
trachea J39.8
ureter N28.89
vitreous —see Deposit, crystalline
Calcified —see Calcification
Calcinosis (interstitial) (tumoral) (universalis)
    E83.59
  with Raynaud's phenomenon, esophageal
      dysfunction, sclerodactyly, telangiectasia
      (CREST syndrome) M34.1
  circumscripta (skin) L94.2
  cutis L94.2
Calciphylaxis —see also Calcification, by site
    E83.59
Calcium
  deposits —see Calcification, by site
  metabolism disorder E83.50
  salts or soaps in vitreous —see Deposit,
      crystalline
Calciuria R82.994
Calculi —see Calculus
Calculosis, intrahepatic —see Calculus, bile
    duct
Calculus, calculi, calculous
  ampulla of Vater —see Calculus, bile duct
  anuria (impacted) (recurrent) —see also Calculus,
      urinary N20.9
  appendix K38.1

Calculus, calculi, calculous (Continued)
bile duct (common) (hepatic) K80.50
  with
    calculus of gallbladder —see Calculus,
        gallbladder and bile duct
    cholangitis K80.30
      with
        cholecystitis —see Calculus, bile duct,
            with cholecystitis
        obstruction K80.31
      acute K80.32
        with
          chronic cholangitis K80.36
            with obstruction K80.37
          obstruction K80.33
      chronic K80.34
        with
          acute cholangitis K80.36
            with obstruction K80.37
          obstruction K80.35
    cholecystitis (with cholangitis) K80.40
      with obstruction K80.41
      acute K80.42
        with
          chronic cholecystitis K80.46
            with obstruction K80.47
          obstruction K80.43
      chronic K80.44
        with
          acute cholecystitis K80.46
            with obstruction K80.47
          obstruction K80.45
    obstruction K80.51
biliary —see also Calculus, gallbladder
  with bile duct involvement - see also Calculus,
      bile duct
  specified NEC K80.80
    with obstruction K80.81
bilirubin, multiple —see Calculus, gallbladder
bladder (encysted) (impacted) (urinary)
    (diverticulum) N21.0
bronchus J98.09
calyx (kidney) (renal) —see Calculus, kidney
cholesterol (pure) (solitary) —see Calculus,
    gallbladder
common duct (bile) —see Calculus, bile duct
conjunctiva —see Concretion, conjunctiva
cystic N21.0
  duct —see Calculus, gallbladder
dental (subgingival) (supragingival) K03.6
diverticulum
  bladder N21.0
  kidney N20.0
epididymis N50.89
gallbladder K80.20
  with
    bile duct calculus —see Calculus,
        gallbladder and bile duct
    cholecystitis K80.10
      with obstruction K80.11
      acute K80.00
        with
          chronic cholecystitis K80.12
            with obstruction K80.13
          obstruction K80.01
      chronic K80.10
        with
          acute cholecystitis K80.12
            with obstruction K80.13
          obstruction K80.11
      specified NEC K80.18
        with obstruction K80.19
    obstruction K80.21
gallbladder and bile duct K80.70
  with
    cholecystitis K80.60
      with obstruction K80.61
      acute K80.62
        with
          chronic cholecystitis K80.66
            with obstruction K80.67
          obstruction K80.63
      chronic K80.64
        with
          acute cholecystitis K80.66
            with obstruction K80.67
          obstruction K80.65
    obstruction K80.71
hepatic (duct) —see Calculus, bile duct
hepatobiliary K80.80
  with obstruction K80.81

Calculus, calculi, calculous (Continued)
ileal conduit N21.8
intestinal (impaction) (obstruction) K56.49
kidney (impacted) (multiple) (pelvis) (recurrent)
    (staghorn) N20.0
  with calculus, ureter N20.2
  with hydronephrosis N13.2
    with infection N13.6
  congenital Q63.8
  with hydronephrosis N13.2
    with infection N13.6
lacrimal passages —see Dacryolith
liver (impacted) —see Calculus, bile duct
lung J98.4
mammographic R92.1
nephritic (impacted) (recurrent) —see Calculus,
    kidney
nose J34.89
pancreas (duct) K86.89
parotid duct or gland K11.5
pelvis, encysted —see Calculus, kidney
prostate N42.0
pulmonary J98.4
pyelitis (impacted) (recurrent) N20.0
  with hydronephrosis N13.6
pyelonephritis (impacted) (recurrent) —see
    category N20
  with hydronephrosis N13.6
renal (impacted) (recurrent) —see Calculus,
    kidney
salivary (duct) (gland) K11.5
seminal vesicle N50.89
staghorn —see Calculus, kidney
Stensen's duct K11.5
stomach K31.89
sublingual duct or gland K11.5
  congenital Q38.4
submandibular duct, gland or region K11.5
submaxillary duct, gland or region K11.5
suburethral N21.8
tonsil J35.8
tooth, teeth (subgingival) (supragingival) K03.6
tunica vaginalis N50.89
ureter (impacted) (recurrent) N20.1
  with calculus, kidney N20.2
    with hydronephrosis N13.2
      with infection N13.6
  with hydronephrosis N13.2
    with infection N13.6
ureteropelvic junction N20.1
urethra (impacted) N21.1
urinary (duct) (impacted) (passage) (tract) N20.9
  with hydronephrosis N13.2
    with infection N13.6
  in (due to)
    lower N21.9
      specified NEC N21.8
vagina N89.8
vesical (impacted) N21.0
Wharton's duct K11.5
xanthine E79.82 [N22]
Caliectasis N28.89
Caliectasis N28.89
California
  disease B38.9
  encephalitis A83.5
Caligo cornea —see Opacity, cornea, central
Callositas, callosity (infected) L84
Callus (infected) L84
  bone —see Osteophyte
  excessive, following fracture - code as
      Sequelae of fracture
CALME (childhood asymmetric labium majus
    enlargement) N90.61
Calorie deficiency or malnutrition —see also
    Malnutrition E46
Calpainopathy (primary) G71.032
  autosomal dominant G71.031
  autosomal recessive G71.032
Calvé-Perthes disease —see Legg-Calve-Perthes
    disease
Calvé's disease —see Osteochondrosis, juvenile,
    spine
Calvities —see Alopecia, androgenic
Cameroon fever —see Malaria
Camptocormia (hysterical) F44.4
Camurati-Engelmann syndrome Q78.3
Canal —see also condition
  atrioventricular Q21.20
    common Q21.23
    incomplete Q21.21

▶ New   ⇒ Revised   ~~deleted~~ Deleted   ● Use Additional Character(s)

Canal *(Continued)*
  atrioventricular *(Continued)*
    intermediate Q21.22
    partial Q21.21
    transitional Q21.22
Canaliculitis (lacrimal) (acute) (subacute)
  H04.33-●
  Actinomyces A42.89
  chronic H04.42-●
Canavan disease E75.28
Canceled procedure (surgical) Z53.9
  because of
    contraindication Z53.09
      smoking Z53.01
    left against medical advice (AMA) Z53.29
    patient's decision Z53.20
      for reasons of belief or group pressure Z53.1
      specified reason NEC Z53.29
    specified reason NEC Z53.8
Cancer —*see also* Neoplasm, by site, malignant
  bile duct type, liver C22.1
  blood —*see* Leukemia
  breast —*see also* Neoplasm, breast, malignant
    C50.91-●
  hepatocellular C22.0
  lung —*see also* Neoplasm, lung, malignant
    C34.90-●
  ovarian —*see also* Neoplasm, ovary, malignant
    C56.9-●
  unspecified site (primary) C80.1
Cancer (o)phobia F45.29
Cancerous —*see* Neoplasm, malignant, by site
Cancrum oris A69.0
Candidiasis, candidal B37.9
  balanitis B37.42
  bronchitis B37.1
  cheilitis B37.83
  congenital P37.5
  cystitis B37.41
  disseminated B37.7
  endocarditis B37.6
  enteritis B37.82
  esophagitis B37.81
  intertrigo B37.2
  lung B37.1
  meningitis B37.5
  mouth B37.0
  nails B37.2
  neonatal P37.5
  onychia B37.2
  oral B37.0
  osteomyelitis B37.89
  otitis externa B37.84
  paronychia B37.2
  perionyxis B37.2
  pneumonia B37.1
  proctitis B37.82
  pulmonary B37.1
  pyelonephritis B37.49
  sepsis B37.7
  skin B37.2
  specified site NEC B37.89
  stomatitis B37.0
  systemic B37.7
  urethritis B37.41
  urogenital site NEC B37.49
  vagina (acute) B37.31
    chronic (recurrent) B37.32
  vulva (acute) B37.31
    chronic (recurrent) B37.32
  vulvovaginitis (acute) B37.31
    chronic (recurrent) B37.32
Candidid L30.2
Candidosis —*see* Candidiasis
Candiru infection or infestation B88.8
Canities (premature) L67.1
  congenital Q84.2
Canker (mouth) (sore) K12.0
  rash A38.9
Cannabinosis J66.2
Cannabis induced
  anxiety disorder F12.980
  psychotic disorder F12.959
  sleep disorder F12.988
Canton fever A75.9
Cantrell's syndrome Q87.89
Capillariasis (intestinal) B81.1
  hepatic B83.8
Capillary —*see* condition
Caplan's syndrome —*see* Rheumatoid, lung
Capsule —*see* condition

Capsulitis (joint) —*see also* Enthesopathy
  adhesive (shoulder) M75.0-●
  hepatic K65.8
  labyrinthine —*see* Otosclerosis, specified NEC
  thyroid E06.9
Caput
  crepitus Q75.8
  medusae I86.8
  succedaneum P12.81
Car sickness T75.3
Carapata (disease) A68.0
Carate —*see* Pinta
Carbon lung J60
Carbuncle L02.93
  abdominal wall L02.231
  anus K61.0
  auditory canal, external —*see* Abscess, ear, external
  auricle ear —*see* Abscess, ear, external
  axilla L02.43-●
  back (any part) L02.232
  breast N61.1
  buttock L02.33
  cheek (external) L02.03
  chest wall L02.233
  chin L02.03
  corpus cavernosum N48.21
  ear (any part) (external) (middle) —*see* Abscess, ear, external
  external auditory canal —*see* Abscess, ear, external
  eyelid —*see* Abscess, eyelid
  face NEC L02.03
  femoral (region) —*see* Carbuncle, lower limb
  finger —*see* Carbuncle, hand
  flank L02.231
  foot L02.63-●
  forehead L02.03
  genital —*see* Abscess, genital
  gluteal (region) L02.33
  groin L02.234
  hand L02.53-●
  head NEC L02.831
  heel —*see* Carbuncle, foot
  hip —*see* Carbuncle, lower limb
  kidney —*see* Abscess, kidney
  knee —*see* Carbuncle, lower limb
  labium (majus) (minus) N76.4
  lacrimal
    gland —*see* Dacryoadenitis
    passages (duct) (sac) —*see* Inflammation, lacrimal, passages, acute
  leg —*see* Carbuncle, lower limb
  lower limb L02.43-●
  malignant A22.0
  navel L02.236
  neck L02.13
  nose (external) (septum) J34.0
  orbit, orbital —*see* Abscess, orbit
  palmar (space) —*see* Carbuncle, hand
  partes posteriores L02.33
  pectoral region L02.233
  penis N48.21
  perineum L02.235
  pinna —*see* Abscess, ear, external
  popliteal —*see* Carbuncle, lower limb
  scalp L02.831
  seminal vesicle N49.0
  shoulder —*see* Carbuncle, upper limb
  specified site NEC L02.838
  temple (region) L02.03
  thumb —*see* Carbuncle, hand
  toe —*see* Carbuncle, foot
  trunk L02.239
    abdominal wall L02.231
    back L02.232
    chest wall L02.233
    groin L02.234
    perineum L02.235
    umbilicus L02.236
  umbilicus L02.236
  upper limb L02.43-●
  urethra N34.0
  vulva N76.4
Carbunculus —*see* Carbuncle
Carcinoid (tumor) —*see* Tumor, carcinoid
Carcinoidosis E34.00
  heart E34.01
Carcinoma (malignant) —*see also* Neoplasm, by site, malignant
  acidophil
    specified site —*see* Neoplasm, malignant, by site
    unspecified site C75.1

Carcinoma *(Continued)*
  acidophil-basophil, mixed
    specified site —*see* Neoplasm, malignant, by site
    unspecified site C75.1
  adnexal (skin) —*see* Neoplasm, skin, malignant
  adrenal cortical C74.0-●
  alveolar —*see* Neoplasm, lung, malignant
    cell —*see* Neoplasm, lung, malignant
  ameloblastic C41.1
    upper jaw (bone) C41.0
  apocrine
    breast —*see* Neoplasm, breast, malignant
    specified site NEC —*see* Neoplasm, skin, malignant
    unspecified site C44.99
  basal cell (pigmented) *(see also* Neoplasm, skin, malignant) C44.91
    fibro-epithelial —*see* Neoplasm, skin, malignant
    morphea —*see* Neoplasm, skin, malignant
    multicentric —*see* Neoplasm, skin, malignant
  basaloid
  basal-squamous cell, mixed —*see* Neoplasm, skin, malignant
  basophil
    specified site —*see* Neoplasm, malignant, by site
    unspecified site C75.1
  basophil-acidophil, mixed
    specified site —*see* Neoplasm, malignant, by site
    unspecified site C75.1
  basosquamous —*see* Neoplasm, skin, malignant
  bile duct
    with hepatocellular, mixed C22.0
    liver C22.1
    specified site NEC —*see* Neoplasm, malignant, by site
    unspecified site C22.1
  branchial or branchiogenic C10.4
  bronchial or bronchogenic —*see* Neoplasm, lung, malignant
  bronchiolar —*see* Neoplasm, lung, malignant
  bronchioloalveolar —*see* Neoplasm, lung, malignant
  C cell
    specified site —*see* Neoplasm, malignant, by site
    unspecified site C73
  ceruminous C44.29-●
  cervix uteri
    in situ D06.9
      endocervix D06.0
      exocervix D06.1
      specified site NEC D06.7
  chorionic
    specified site —*see* Neoplasm, malignant, by site
    unspecified site
      female C58
      male C62.90
  chromophobe
    specified site —*see* Neoplasm, malignant, by site
    unspecified site C75.1
  cloacogenic
    specified site —*see* Neoplasm, malignant, by site
    unspecified site C21.2
  diffuse type
    specified site —*see* Neoplasm, malignant, by site
    unspecified site C16.9
  duct (cell)
    with Paget's disease —*see* Neoplasm, breast, malignant
    infiltrating
      with lobular carcinoma (in situ)
        specified site —*see* Neoplasm, malignant, by site
        unspecified site (female) C50.91-●
          male C50.92-●
      specified site —*see* Neoplasm, malignant, by site
      unspecified site (female) C50.91-●
        male C50.92-●
  ductal
    with lobular
      specified site —*see* Neoplasm, malignant, by site
      unspecified site (female) C50.91-●
        male C50.92-●

Carcinoma (Continued)
  ductular, infiltrating
    specified site —see Neoplasm, malignant, by
        site
    unspecified site (female) C50.91-●
        male C50.92-●
  embryonal
    liver C22.7
  endometrioid
    specified site —see Neoplasm, malignant, by
        site
    unspecified site
        female C56.9
        male C61
  eosinophil
    specified site —see Neoplasm, malignant, by
        site
    unspecified site C75.1
  epidermoid —see also Neoplasm, skin malignant
    in situ, Bowen's type —see Neoplasm, skin,
        in situ
  fibroepithelial, basal cell —see Neoplasm, skin,
        malignant
  follicular
    with papillary (mixed) C73
    moderately differentiated C73
    pure follicle C73
    specified site —see Neoplasm, malignant, by
        site
    trabecular C73
    unspecified site C73
    well differentiated C73
  generalized, with unspecified primary site
        C80.0
  glycogen-rich —see Neoplasm, breast,
        malignant
  granulosa cell C56-●
  hepatic cell C22.0
  hepatocellular C22.0
    with bile duct, mixed C22.0
    fibrolamellar C22.0
  hepatocholangiolitic C22.0
  Hurthle cell C73
  in
    adenomatous
        polyposis coli C18.9
    ⟹pleomorphic adenoma —see Neoplasm,
        salivary gland or duct,
        malignant
    situ —see Carcinoma-in-situ
  infiltrating
    duct
        with lobular
            specified site —see Neoplasm, malignant,
                by site
            unspecified site (female) C50.91-●
                male C50.92-●
        with Paget's disease —see Neoplasm,
            breast, malignant
        specified site —see Neoplasm, malignant
        unspecified site (female) C50.91-●
            male C50.92-●
    ductular
        specified site —see Neoplasm, malignant
        unspecified site (female) C50.91-●
            male C50.92-●
    lobular
        specified site —see Neoplasm, malignant
        unspecified site (female) C50.91-●
            male C50.92-●
  inflammatory
    specified site —see Neoplasm, malignant
    unspecified site (female) C50.91-●
        male C50.92-●
  intestinal type
    specified site —see Neoplasm, malignant, by
        site
    unspecified site C16.9
  intracystic
    noninfiltrating —see Neoplasm, in situ, by site
  intraductal (noninfiltrating)
    with Paget's disease —see Neoplasm, breast,
        malignant
    breast D05.1-●
    papillary
        with invasion
            specified site —see Neoplasm, malignant,
                by site
            unspecified site (female) C50.91-●
                male C50.92-●
        breast D05.1-●

Carcinoma (Continued)
  intraductal (Continued)
    papillary (Continued)
        specified site NEC —see Neoplasm,
            in situ, by site
        unspecified site (female) D05.1-●
    specified site NEC —see Neoplasm,
        in situ, by site
    unspecified site (female) D05.1-●
  intraepidermal —see Neoplasm, in situ
    squamous cell, Bowen's type —see Neoplasm,
        skin, in situ
  intraepithelial —see Neoplasm, in situ, by site
    squamous cell —see Neoplasm, in situ, by
        site
  intraosseous C41.1
    upper jaw (bone) C41.0
  islet cell
    with exocrine, mixed
        specified site —see Neoplasm, malignant,
            by site
        unspecified site C25.9
    pancreas C25.4
    specified site NEC —see Neoplasm, malignant,
        by site
    unspecified site C25.4
  juvenile, breast —see Neoplasm, breast,
        malignant
  large cell
    small cell
        specified site —see Neoplasm, malignant,
            by site
        unspecified site C34.90
  Leydig cell (testis)
    specified site —see Neoplasm, malignant, by
        site
    unspecified site
        female C56.9
        male C62.90
  lipid-rich (female) C50.91-●
        male C50.92-●
  liver cell C22.0
  liver NEC C22.7
  lobular (infiltrating)
    with intraductal
        specified site —see Neoplasm, malignant,
            by site
        unspecified site (female) C50.91-●
            male C50.92-●
    noninfiltrating
        breast D05.0-●
        specified site NEC —see Neoplasm, in situ,
            by site
        unspecified site D05.0-●
    specified site —see Neoplasm, malignant, by
        site
    unspecified site (female) C50.91-●
        male C50.92-●
  medullary
    with
        amyloid stroma
            specified site —see Neoplasm, malignant,
                by site
            unspecified site C73
        lymphoid stroma
            specified site —see Neoplasm, malignant,
                by site
            unspecified site (female) C50.91-●
                male C50.92-●
  Merkel cell C4A.9
    anal margin C4A.51
    anal skin C4A.51
    canthus C4A.1-●
    ear and external auricular canal C4A.2-●
    external auricular canal C4A.2-●
    eyelid, including canthus C4A.1-●
    face C4A.30
        specified NEC C4A.39
    hip C4A.7-●
    lip C4A.0
    lower limb, including hip C4A.7-●
    neck C4A.4
    nodal presentation C7B.1
    nose C4A.31
    overlapping sites C4A.8
    perianal skin C4A.51
    scalp C4A.4
    secondary C7B.1
    shoulder C4A.6-●
    skin of breast C4A.52
    trunk NEC C4A.59

Carcinoma (Continued)
  Merkel cell (Continued)
    upper limb, including shoulder C4A.6-●
    visceral metastatic C7B.1
  metastatic —see Neoplasm, secondary
  metatypical —see Neoplasm, skin,
        malignant
  morphea, basal cell —see Neoplasm, skin,
        malignant
  mucoid
    cell
        specified site —see Neoplasm, malignant,
            by site
        unspecified site C75.1
  neuroendocrine —see also Tumor,
        neuroendocrine
    high grade, any site C7A.1
    poorly differentiated, any site C7A.1
  nonencapsulated sclerosing C73
  noninfiltrating
    intracystic —see Neoplasm, in situ, by
        site
    intraductal
        breast D05.1-●
        papillary
            breast D05.1-●
            specified site NEC —see Neoplasm, in
                situ, by site
            unspecified site D05.1-●
        specified site —see Neoplasm, in situ, by
            site
        unspecified site D05.1-●
    lobular
        breast D05.0-●
        specified site NEC —see Neoplasm, in situ,
            by site
        unspecified site (female) D05.0-●
  oat cell
    specified site —see Neoplasm, malignant, by
        site
    unspecified site C34.90
  odontogenic C41.1
    upper jaw (bone) C41.0
  papillary
    with follicular (mixed) C73
    follicular variant C73
    intraductal (noninfiltrating)
        with invasion
            specified site —see Neoplasm, malignant,
                by site
            unspecified site (female) C50.91-●
                male C50.92-●
        breast D05.1-●
        specified site NEC —see Neoplasm, in situ,
            by site
        unspecified site D05.1-●
    serous
        specified site —see Neoplasm, malignant,
            by site
    surface
        specified site —see Neoplasm, malignant,
            by site
        unspecified site C56.9
    unspecified site C56.9
  papillocystic
    specified site —see Neoplasm, malignant, by
        site
    unspecified site C56.9
  parafollicular cell
    specified site —see Neoplasm, malignant, by
        site
    unspecified site C73
  pilomatrix —see Neoplasm, skin, malignant
  pseudomucinous
    specified site —see Neoplasm, malignant, by
        site
    unspecified site C56.9
  renal cell C64-●
  Schmincke —see Neoplasm, nasopharynx,
        malignant
  Schneiderian
    specified site —see Neoplasm, malignant, by
        site
    unspecified site C30.0
  sebaceous —see Neoplasm, skin,
        malignant
  secondary —see also Neoplasm, secondary, by
        site
    Merkel cell C7B.1
  secretory, breast —see Neoplasm, breast,
        malignant

▶ New   ⟹ Revised   ~~deleted~~ Deleted   ● Use Additional Character(s)

Carcinoma *(Continued)*
 serous
  papillary
   specified site —*see* Neoplasm, malignant,
     by site
   unspecified site C56.9
  surface, papillary
   specified site —*see* Neoplasm, malignant,
     by site
   unspecified site C56.9
 Sertoli cell
  specified site —*see* Neoplasm, malignant, by
    site
  unspecified site C62.90
   female C56.9
   male C62.90
 skin appendage —*see* Neoplasm, skin,
   malignant
 small cell
  fusiform cell
   specified site —*see* Neoplasm, malignant,
     by site
   unspecified site C34.90
  intermediate cell
   specified site —*see* Neoplasm, malignant,
     by site
   unspecified site C34.90
  large cell
   specified site —*see* Neoplasm, malignant,
     by site
   unspecified site C34.90
 solid
  with amyloid stroma
   specified site —*see* Neoplasm, malignant,
     by site
   unspecified site C73
  microinvasive
   specified site —*see* Neoplasm, malignant,
     by site
   unspecified site C53.9
 sweat gland —*see* Neoplasm, skin, malignant
 theca cell C56.-●
 thymic C37
 unspecified site (primary) C80.1
 water-clear cell C75.0
Carcinoma-in-situ —*see also* Neoplasm, in situ,
   by site
 breast NOS D05.9-●
  specified type NEC D05.8-●
 epidermoid —*see also* Neoplasm, in situ, by site
  with questionable stromal invasion
   cervix D06.9
  specified site NEC —*see* Neoplasm, in situ,
    by site
  unspecified site D06.9
 Bowen's type —*see* Neoplasm, skin, in situ
 intraductal
  breast D05.1-●
  specified site NEC —*see* Neoplasm, in situ,
    by site
  unspecified site D05.1-●
 lobular
  with
   infiltrating duct
    breast (female) C50.91-●
     male C50.92-●
    specified site NEC —*see* Neoplasm,
      malignant
    unspecified site (female) C50.91-●
     male C50.92-●
   intraductal
    breast D05.8-●
    specified site NEC —*see* Neoplasm, in
      situ, by site
    unspecified site (female) D05.8-●
  breast D05.0-●
  specified site NEC —*see* Neoplasm, in situ,
    by site
  unspecified site D05.0-●
 squamous cell —*see also* Neoplasm, in situ, by
   site
  with questionable stromal invasion
   cervix D06.9
  specified site NEC —*see* Neoplasm, in situ,
    by site
  unspecified site D06.9
Carcinomaphobia F45.29
Carcinomatosis C80.0
 peritonei C78.6
 unspecified site (primary) (secondary)
   C80.0

Carcinosarcoma —*see* Neoplasm, malignant, by site
 embryonal —*see* Neoplasm, malignant, by site
Cardia, cardial —*see* condition
Cardiac —*see also* condition
 death, sudden —*see* Arrest, cardiac
 pacemaker
  in situ Z95.0
  management or adjustment Z45.018
 tamponade I31.4
Cardialgia —*see* Pain, precordial
Cardiectasis —*see* Hypertrophy, cardiac
Cardiochalasia K21.9
Cardiomalacia I51.5
Cardiomegalia glycogenica diffusa E74.02 *[143]*
Cardiomegaly —*see also* Hypertrophy, cardiac
 congenital Q24.8
 glycogen E74.02 *[143]*
 idiopathic I51.7
Cardiomyoliposis I51.5
Cardiomyopathy (familial) (idiopathic) I42.9
 alcoholic I42.6
 amyloid E85.4 *[143]*
  transthyretin-related (ATTR) familial E85.4
    [143]
 arteriosclerotic —*see* Disease, heart, ischemic,
   atherosclerotic
 beriberi E51.12
 cobalt-beer I42.6
 congenital I42.4
 congestive I42.0
 constrictive NOS I42.5
 dilated I42.0
 due to
  alcohol I42.6
  beriberi E51.12
  cardiac glycogenosis E74.02 *[143]*
  drugs I42.7
  external agents NEC I42.7
  Friedreich's ataxia G11.11
  myotonia atrophica G71.11 *[143]*
  progressive muscular dystrophy *(see also*
    Dystrophy, muscular, by type) G71.09
    [143]
 glycogen storage E74.02 *[143]*
 hypertensive —*see* Hypertension, heart
 hypertrophic (nonobstructive) I42.2
  obstructive I42.1
   congenital Q24.8
 in
  Chagas' disease (chronic) B57.2
   acute B57.0
  sarcoidosis D86.85
 ischemic I25.5
 metabolic E88.9 *[143]*
  thyrotoxic E05.90 *[143]*
   with thyroid storm E05.91 *[143]*
 newborn I42.8
  congenital I42.4
 non-ischemic *(see also* by cause) I42.8
 nutritional E63.9 *[143]*
  beriberi E51.12
 obscure of Africa I42.8
 peripartum O90.3
 postpartum O90.3
 restrictive NEC I42.5
 rheumatic I09.0
 secondary I42.9
 specified NEC I42.8
 stress induced I51.81
 takotsubo I51.81
 thyrotoxic E05.90 *[143]*
  with thyroid storm E05.91 *[143]*
 toxic NEC I42.7
 transthyretin-related (ATTR) familial amyloid
   E85.4
 tuberculous A18.84
 viral B33.24
Cardionephritis —*see* Hypertension, cardiorenal
Cardionephropathy —*see* Hypertension,
   cardiorenal
Cardionephrosis —*see* Hypertension, cardiorenal
Cardiopathia nigra I27.0
Cardiopathy —*see also* Disease, heart I51.9
 idiopathic I42.9
 mucopolysaccharidosis E76.3 *[152]*
Cardiopericarditis —*see* Pericarditis
Cardiophobia F45.29
Cardiorenal —*see* condition
Cardiorrhexis —*see* Infarct, myocardium
Cardiosclerosis —*see* Disease, heart, ischemic,
   atherosclerotic

Cardiosis —*see* Disease, heart
Cardiospasm (esophagus) (reflex) (stomach) K22.0
 congenital Q39.5
  with megaesophagus Q39.5
Cardiostenosis —*see* Disease, heart
Cardiosymphysis I31.0
Cardiovascular —*see* condition
Carditis (acute) (bacterial) (chronic) (subacute) I51.89
 meningococcal A39.50
 rheumatic —*see* Disease, heart, rheumatic
 rheumatoid —*see* Rheumatoid, carditis
 viral B33.20
Care (of) (for) (following)
 child (routine) Z76.2
 family member (handicapped) (sick)
  creating problem for family Z63.6
  provided away from home for holiday relief
    Z75.5
  unavailable, due to
   absence (person rendering care) (sufferer)
     Z74.2
   inability (any reason) of person rendering
     care Z74.2
 foundling Z76.1
 holiday relief Z75.5
 improper —*see* Maltreatment
 lack of (at or after birth) (infant) —*see*
   Maltreatment, child, neglect
 lactating mother Z39.1
 palliative Z51.5
 postpartum
  immediately after delivery Z39.0
  routine follow-up Z39.2
 respite Z75.5
 unavailable, due to
  absence of person rendering care
    Z74.2
  inability (any reason) of person rendering
    care Z74.2
 well-baby Z76.2
Caries
 bone NEC A18.03
 dental (dentino enamel junction)
   (early childhood) (of dentine)
   (pre-eruptive) (recurrent) (to the pulp)
   K02.9
  arrested (coronal) (root) K02.3
  chewing surface
   limited to enamel K02.51
   penetrating into dentin K02.52
   penetrating into pulp K02.53
  coronal surface
   chewing surface
    limited to enamel K02.51
    penetrating into dentin K02.52
    penetrating into pulp K02.53
   pit and fissure surface
    limited to enamel K02.51
    penetrating into dentin K02.52
    penetrating into pulp K02.53
   smooth surface
    limited to enamel K02.61
    penetrating into dentin K02.62
    penetrating into pulp K02.63
  pit and fissure surface
   limited to enamel K02.51
   penetrating into dentin K02.52
   penetrating into pulp K02.53
  primary, cervical origin K02.52
  root K02.7
  smooth surface
   limited to enamel K02.61
   penetrating into dentin K02.62
   penetrating into pulp K02.63
 external meatus —*see* Disorder, ear, external,
   specified type NEC
 hip (tuberculous) A18.02
 initial (tooth)
  chewing surface K02.51
  pit and fissure surface K02.51
  smooth surface K02.61
 knee (tuberculous) A18.02
 labyrinth —*see* subcategory H83.8
 limb NEC (tuberculous) A18.03
 mastoid process (chronic) —*see* Mastoiditis,
   chronic
  tuberculous A18.03
 middle ear —*see* subcategory H74.8
 nose (tuberculous) A18.03
 orbit (tuberculous) A18.03
 ossicles, ear —*see* Abnormal, ear ossicles

Caries *(Continued)*
  petrous bone —*see* Petrositis
  root (dental) (tooth) K02.7
  sacrum (tuberculous) A18.01
  spine, spinal (column) (tuberculous)
    A18.01
    syphilitic A52.77
      congenital (early) A50.02 *[M90.80]*
  tooth, teeth —*see* Caries, dental
  tuberculous A18.03
  vertebra (column) (tuberculous) A18.01
Carious teeth —*see* Caries, dental
Carneous mole O02.0
Carnitine insufficiency E71.40
Carotenemia (dietary) E67.1
Carotenosis (cutis) (skin) E67.1
Carotid body or sinus syndrome G90.01
Carotidynia G90.01
Carpal tunnel syndrome —*see* Syndrome, carpal
  tunnel
Carpenter's syndrome Q87.0
Carpopedal spasm —*see* Tetany
Carr-Barr-Plunkett syndrome Q97.1
Carrier (suspected) of
  Acinetobacter baumannii Z22.349
    carbapenem-resistant Z22.340
    carbapenem-sensitive Z22.341
  amebiasis Z22.1
  bacterial disease NEC Z22.39
    diphtheria Z22.2
    intestinal infectious NEC Z22.1
      typhoid Z22.0
    meningococcal Z22.31
    sexually transmitted Z22.4
    specified NEC Z22.39
    staphylococcal (Methicillin susceptible) Z22.321
      Methicillin resistant Z22.322
    streptococcal Z22.338
      group B Z22.330
        complicating pregnancy or delivery
          O99.82-●
    typhoid Z22.0
  cholera Z22.1
  diphtheria Z22.2
  E. coli (Escherichia coli) Z22.35-
  Enterobacterales Z22.359
    carbapenem-resistant Z22.350
    carbapenem-sensitive Z22.358
    Enterobacterales, specified type NEC Z22.358
    ESBL-producing Z22.358
    extended-spectrum beta-lactamase producing
      Z22.358
  gastrointestinal pathogens NEC Z22.1
  genetic Z14.8
    cystic fibrosis Z14.1
    hemophilia A (asymptomatic) Z14.01
      symptomatic Z14.02
  gestational, pregnant Z33.1
  gonorrhea Z22.4
  HAA (hepatitis Australian-antigen) B18.8
  HB (c)(s)-AG B18.1
  hepatitis (viral) B18.9
    Australia-antigen (HAA) B18.8
    B surface antigen (HBsAg) B18.1
      with acute delta- (super)infection B17.0
    C B18.2
    specified NEC B18.8
  human T-cell lymphotropic virus type-1 (HTLV-
    1) infection Z22.6
  infectious organism Z22.9
    specified NEC Z22.8
  K. pneumoniae (Klebsiella pneumoniae) Z22.35-
  meningococci Z22.31
  Salmonella typhosa Z22.0
  serum hepatitis —*see* Carrier, hepatitis
  staphylococci (Methicillin susceptible) Z22.321
    Methicillin resistant Z22.322
  streptococci Z22.338
    group B Z22.330
      complicating pregnancy or delivery
        O99.82-●
  syphilis Z22.4
  typhoid Z22.0
  venereal disease NEC Z22.4
Carrion's disease A44.0
Carter's relapsing fever (Asiatic) A68.1
Cartilage —*see* condition
Caruncle (inflamed)
  conjunctiva (acute) —*see* Conjunctivitis, acute
  labium (majus) (minus) N90.89
  lacrimal —*see* Inflammation, lacrimal, passages

Caruncle *(Continued)*
  myrtiform N89.8
  urethral (benign) N36.2
Cascade stomach K31.2
Caseation lymphatic gland (tuberculous)
  A18.2
Cassidy (-Scholte) syndrome (malignant carcinoid)
  E34.09
Castellani's disease A69.8
Castration, traumatic, male S38.231
Casts in urine R82.998
Cat
  cry syndrome Q93.4
  ear Q17.3
  eye syndrome Q92.8
Catabolism, senile R54
Catalepsy (hysterical) F44.2
  schizophrenic F20.2
Cataplexy (idiopathic) —*see* Narcolepsy
Cataract (cortical) (immature) (incipient) H26.9
  with
    neovascularization —*see* Cataract,
      complicated
  age-related —*see* Cataract, senile
  anterior
    and posterior axial embryonal
      Q12.0
    pyramidal Q12.0
  associated with
    galactosemia E74.21 *[H28]*
    myotonic disorders G71.19 *[H28]*
  blue Q12.0
  central Q12.0
  cerulean Q12.0
  complicated H26.20
    with
      neovascularization H26.21-●
      ocular disorder H26.22-●
      glaucomatous flecks H26.23-●
  congenital Q12.0
  coraliform Q12.0
  coronary Q12.0
  crystalline Q12.0
  diabetic —*see* Diabetes, cataract
  drug-induced H26.3-●
  due to
    ocular disorder —*see* Cataract, complicated
    radiation H26.8
  electric H26.8
  extraction status Z98.4-●
  glass-blower's H26.8
  heat ray H26.8
  heterochromic —*see* Cataract, complicated
  hypermature —*see* Cataract, senile, morgagnian
    type
  in (due to)
    chronic iridocyclitis —*see* Cataract,
      complicated
    diabetes —*see* Diabetes, cataract
    endocrine disease E34.9 *[H28]*
    eye disease —*see* Cataract, complicated
    hypoparathyroidism E20.9 *[H28]*
    malnutrition-dehydration E46 *[H28]*
    metabolic disease E88.9 *[H28]*
    myotonic disorders G71.19 *[H28]*
    nutritional disease E63.9 *[H28]*
  infantile —*see* Cataract, presenile
  irradiational —*see* Cataract, specified NEC
  juvenile —*see* Cataract, presenile
  malnutrition-dehydration E46 *[H28]*
  morgagnian —*see* Cataract, senile, morgagnian
    type
  myotonic G71.19 *[H28]*
  myxedema E03.9 *[H28]*
  nuclear
    embryonal Q12.0
    sclerosis —*see* Cataract, senile, nuclear
  presenile H26.00-●
    combined forms H26.06-●
    cortical H26.01-●
    lamellar —*see* Cataract, presenile,
      cortical
    nuclear H26.03-●
    specified NEC H26.09
    subcapsular polar (anterior) H26.04-●
      posterior H26.05-●
    zonular —*see* Cataract, presenile, cortical
  secondary H26.40
    Soemmering's ring H26.41-●
    specified NEC H26.49-●
    to eye disease —*see* Cataract, complicated

Cataract *(Continued)*
  senile H25.9
    brunescens —*see* Cataract, senile, nuclear
    combined forms H25.81-●
    coronary —*see* Cataract, senile, incipient
    cortical H25.01-●
    hypermature —*see* Cataract, senile,
      morgagnian type
    incipient (mature) (total) H25.09-●
      cortical —*see* Cataract, senile, cortical
      subcapsular —*see* Cataract, senile,
        subcapsular
    morgagnian type (hypermature) H25.2-●
    nuclear (sclerosis) H25.1-●
    polar subcapsular (anterior) (posterior) —*see*
      Cataract, senile, incipient
    punctate —*see* Cataract, senile, incipient
    specified NEC H25.89
    subcapsular polar (anterior) H25.03-●
      posterior H25.04-●
  snowflake —*see* Diabetes, cataract
  specified NEC H26.8
  toxic —*see* Cataract, drug-induced
  traumatic H26.10-●
    localized H26.11-●
    partially resolved H26.12-●
    total H26.13-●
  zonular (perinuclear) Q12.0
Cataracta —*see also* Cataract
  brunescens —*see* Cataract, senile, nuclear
  centralis pulverulenta Q12.0
  cerulea Q12.0
  complicata —*see* Cataract, complicated
  congenita Q12.0
  coralliformis Q12.0
  coronaria Q12.0
  diabetic —*see* Diabetes, cataract
  membranacea
    accreta —*see* Cataract, secondary
    congenita Q12.0
  nigra —*see* Cataract, senile, nuclear
  sunflower —*see* Cataract, complicated
Catarrh, catarrhal (acute) (febrile) (infectious)
  (inflammation) *(see also* condition) J00
  bronchial —*see* Bronchitis
  chest —*see* Bronchitis
  chronic J31.0
  due to congenital syphilis A50.03
  enteric —*see* Enteritis
  eustachian H68.009
  fauces —*see* Pharyngitis
  gastrointestinal —*see* Enteritis
  gingivitis K05.00
    nonplaque induced K05.01
    plaque induced K05.00
  hay —*see* Fever, hay
  intestinal —*see* Enteritis
  larynx, chronic J37.0
  liver B15.9
    with hepatic coma B15.0
  lung —*see* Bronchitis
  middle ear, chronic —*see* Otitis, media,
    nonsuppurative, chronic, serous
  mouth K12.1
  nasal (chronic) —*see* Rhinitis
  nasobronchial J31.1
  nasopharyngeal (chronic) J31.1
    acute J00
  pulmonary —*see* Bronchitis
  spring (eye) (vernal) —*see* Conjunctivitis, acute,
    atopic
  summer (hay) —*see* Fever, hay
  throat J31.2
  tubotympanal —*see also* Otitis, media,
    nonsuppurative
    chronic —*see* Otitis, media, nonsuppurative,
      chronic, serous
Catatonia (schizophrenic) F20.2
Catatonic
  disorder due to known physiologic condition
    F06.1
  schizophrenia F20.2
  stupor R40.1
Cat-scratch —*see also* Abrasion
  disease or fever A28.1
Cauda equina —*see* condition
Cauliflower ear M95.1-●
Causalgia (upper limb) G56.4-●
  lower limb G57.7-●
Cause
  external, general effects T75.89

▶ New   ⇒ Revised   ~~deleted~~ Deleted   ● Use Additional Character(s)

Caustic burn —*see* Corrosion, by site
Cavare's disease (familial periodic paralysis) G72.3
Cave-in, injury
　crushing (severe) —*see* Crush
　suffocation —*see* Asphyxia, traumatic, due to
　　low oxygen, due to cave-in
Cavernitis (penis) N48.29
Cavernositis N48.29
Cavernous —*see* condition
Cavitation of lung —*see also* Tuberculosis,
　　pulmonary
　nontuberculous J98.4
Cavities, dental —*see* Caries, dental
Cavity
　lung —*see* Cavitation of lung
　optic papilla Q14.2
　pulmonary —*see* Cavitation of lung
Cavovarus foot, congenital Q66.1-●
Cavus foot (congenital) Q66.7-●
　acquired —*see* Deformity, limb, foot, specified
　　NEC
Cazenave's disease L10.2
CCCA (central centrifugal cicatricial alopecia)
　　L66.81
CDKL5 (Cyclin-Dependent Kinase-Like 5
　　Deficiency Disorder) G40.42
Cecitis K52.9
　with perforation, peritonitis, or rupture K65.8
Cecoureterocele Q62.32
Cecum —*see* condition
Celiac
　artery compression syndrome I77.4
　disease (with steatorrhea) K90.0
　infantilism K90.0
Cell(s), cellular —*see also* condition
　in urine R82.998
Cellulitis (diffuse) (phlegmonous) (septic)
　　(suppurative) L03.90
　abdominal wall L03.311
　anaerobic A48.0
　ankle —*see* Cellulitis, lower limb
　anus K61.0
　arm —*see* Cellulitis, upper limb
　auricle (ear) —*see* Cellulitis, ear
　axilla L03.11-●
　back (any part) L03.312
　breast (acute) (nonpuerperal) (subacute) N61.0
　　nipple N61.0
　broad ligament
　　acute N73.0
　buttock L03.317
　cervical (meaning neck) L03.221
　cervix (uteri) —*see* Cervicitis
　cheek (external) L03.211
　　internal K12.2
　chest wall L03.313
　chronic L03.90
　clostridial A48.0
　corpus cavernosum N48.22
　digit
　　finger —*see* Cellulitis, finger
　　toe —*see* Cellulitis, toe
　Douglas' cul-de-sac or pouch
　　acute N73.0
　drainage site (following operation) T81.49
　ear (external) H60.1-●
　eosinophilic (granulomatous) L98.3
　erysipelatous —*see* Erysipelas
　external auditory canal —*see* Cellulitis, ear
　eyelid —*see* Abscess, eyelid
　face NEC L03.211
　finger (intrathecal) (periosteal) (subcutaneous)
　　(subcuticular) L03.01-●
　foot —*see* Cellulitis, lower limb
　gangrenous —*see* Gangrene
　genital organ NEC
　　female (external) N76.4
　　male N49.9
　　　multiple sites N49.8
　　　specified NEC N49.8
　gluteal (region) L03.317
　gonococcal A54.89
　groin L03.314
　hand —*see* Cellulitis, upper limb
　head NEC L03.811
　　face (any part, except ear, eye and nose)
　　　L03.211
　heel —*see* Cellulitis, lower limb
　hip —*see* Cellulitis, lower limb
　jaw (region) L03.211
　knee —*see* Cellulitis, lower limb

Cellulitis *(Continued)*
　labium (majus) (minus) —*see* Vulvitis
　lacrimal passages —*see* Inflammation, lacrimal,
　　passages
　larynx J38.7
　leg —*see* Cellulitis, lower limb
　lip K13.0
　lower limb L03.11-●
　　toe —*see* Cellulitis, toe
　mouth (floor) K12.2
　multiple sites, so stated L03.90
　nasopharynx J39.1
　navel L03.316
　　newborn P38.9
　　　with mild hemorrhage P38.1
　　　without hemorrhage P38.9
　neck (region) L03.221
　nipple (acute) (nonpuerperal) (subacute)
　　N61.0
　nose (septum) (external) J34.0
　orbit, orbital H05.01-●
　palate (soft) K12.2
　pectoral (region) L03.313
　pelvis, pelvic (chronic)
　　female —*see also* Disease, pelvis, inflammatory
　　　N73.2
　　　acute N73.0
　　following ectopic or molar pregnancy O08.0
　　male K65.0
　penis N48.22
　perineal, perineum L03.315
　periorbital L03.213
　perirectal K61.1
　peritonsillar J36
　periurethral N34.0
　periuterine —*see also* Disease, pelvis,
　　inflammatory N73.2
　　acute N73.0
　pharynx J39.1
　preseptal L03.213
　rectum K61.1
　retroperitoneal K68.9
　round ligament
　　acute N73.0
　scalp (any part) L03.811
　scrotum N49.2
　seminal vesicle N49.0
　shoulder —*see* Cellulitis, upper limb
　specified site NEC L03.818
　submandibular (region) (space) (triangle) K12.2
　　gland K11.3
　submaxillary (region) K12.2
　　gland K11.3
　thigh —*see* Cellulitis, lower limb
　thumb (intrathecal) (periosteal) (subcutaneous)
　　(subcuticular) —*see* Cellulitis, finger
　toe (intrathecal) (periosteal) (subcutaneous)
　　(subcuticular) L03.03-●
　tonsil J36
　trunk L03.319
　　abdominal wall L03.311
　　back (any part) L03.312
　　buttock L03.317
　　chest wall L03.313
　　groin L03.314
　　perineal, perineum L03.315
　　umbilicus L03.316
　tuberculous (primary) A18.4
　umbilicus L03.316
　upper limb L03.11-●
　　axilla —*see* Cellulitis, axilla
　　finger —*see* Cellulitis, finger
　　thumb —*see* Cellulitis, finger
　vaccinal T88.0
　vocal cord J38.3
　vulva —*see* Vulvitis
　wrist —*see* Cellulitis, upper limb
Cementoblastoma, benign —*see* Cyst, calcifying
　　odontogenic
Cementoma —*see* Cyst, calcifying odontogenic
Cementoperiostitis —*see* Periodontitis
Cementosis K03.4
Central auditory processing disorder H93.25
Central pain syndrome G89.0
Cephalematocele, cephal (o)hematocele
　newborn P52.8
　　birth injury P10.8
　traumatic —*see* Hematoma, brain
Cephalematoma, cephalhematoma (calcified)
　newborn (birth injury) P12.0
　traumatic —*see* Hematoma, brain

Cephalgia, cephalalgia —*see also* Headache
　histamine G44.009
　　intractable G44.001
　　not intractable G44.009
　trigeminal autonomic (TAC) NEC G44.099
　　intractable G44.091
　　not intractable G44.099
Cephalic —*see* condition
Cephalitis —*see* Encephalitis
Cephalocele —*see* Encephalocele
Cephalomenia N94.89
Cephalopelvic —*see* condition
Cerclage (with cervical incompetence) in
　pregnancy —*see* Incompetence, cervix, in
　pregnancy
Cerebellitis —*see* Encephalitis
Cerebellum, cerebellar —*see* condition
Cerebral —*see* condition
Cerebritis —*see* Encephalitis
Cerebro-hepato-renal syndrome Q87.89
Cerebromalacia —*see* Softening, brain
　sequelae of cerebrovascular disease I69.398
Cerebroside lipidosis E75.22
Cerebrospasticity (congenital) G80.1
Cerebrospinal —*see* condition
Cerebrum —*see* condition
Ceroid-lipofuscinosis, neuronal E75.4
Cerumen (accumulation) (impacted) H61.2-●
Cervical —*see also* condition
　auricle Q18.2
　dysplasia in pregnancy —*see* Abnormal, cervix,
　　in pregnancy or childbirth
　erosion in pregnancy —*see* Abnormal, cervix, in
　　pregnancy or childbirth
　fibrosis in pregnancy —*see* Abnormal, cervix, in
　　pregnancy or childbirth
　fusion syndrome Q76.1
　rib Q76.5
　shortening (complicating pregnancy) O26.87-●
Cervicalgia M54.2
Cervicitis (acute) (atrophic) (chronic) (nonvenereal)
　　(senile) (subacute) (with ulceration) N72
　with
　　abortion —*see* Abortion, by type complicated by
　　　genital tract and pelvic infection
　　ectopic pregnancy O08.0
　　molar pregnancy O08.0
　chlamydial A56.09
　gonococcal A54.03
　herpesviral A60.03
　puerperal (postpartum) O86.11
　syphilitic A52.76
　trichomonal A59.09
　tuberculous A18.16
Cervicocolpitis (emphysematosa) (*see also*
　　Cervicitis) N72
Cervix —*see* condition
Cesarean delivery, previous, affecting
　　management of pregnancy O34.219
　classical (vertical) scar O34.212
　isthmocele (non-pregnant state) N85.A
　maternal care for O34.22
　low transverse scar O34.211
　mid-transverse T incision O34.218
　scar
　　defect (non-pregnant state) N85.A
　　maternal care for O34.22
　　specified type NEC O34.218
Céstan (-Chenais) paralysis or syndrome G46.3
Céstan-Raymond syndrome I65.8
Cestode infestation B71.9
　specified type NEC B71.8
Cestodiasis B71.9
Chabert's disease A22.9
Chacaleh E53.8
Chafing L30.4
Chagas' (-Mazza) disease (chronic) B57.2
　with
　　cardiovascular involvement NEC B57.2
　　digestive system involvement B57.30
　　　megacolon B57.32
　　　megaesophagus B57.31
　　　other specified B57.39
　　megacolon B57.32
　　megaesophagus B57.31
　　myocarditis B57.2
　　nervous system involvement B57.40
　　　meningitis B57.41
　　　meningoencephalitis B57.42
　　　other specified B57.49
　　specified organ involvement NEC B57.5

Chagas' disease *(Continued)*
  acute (with) B57.1
    cardiovascular NEC B57.0
    myocarditis B57.0
Chagres fever B50.9
Chairridden Z74.09
Chalasia (cardiac sphincter) K21.9
Chalazion H00.19
  left H00.16
    lower H00.15
    upper H00.14
  right H00.13
    lower H00.12
    upper H00.11
Chalcosis —*see also* Disorder, globe, degenerative,
    chalcosis
  cornea —*see* Deposit, cornea
  crystalline lens —*see* Cataract, complicated
  retina H35.89
Chalicosis (pulmonum) J62.8
Chancre (any genital site) (hard) (hunterian)
    (mixed) (primary) (seronegative)
    (seropositive) (syphilitic) A51.0
  congenital A50.07
  conjunctiva NEC A51.2
▶ ducreyi A57
  Ducrey's A57
  extragenital A51.2
  eyelid A51.2
  lip A51.2
  nipple A51.2
  Nisbet's A57
  of
    carate A67.0
    pinta A67.0
    yaws A66.0
  palate, soft A51.2
  phagedenic A57
  simple A57
  soft A57
    bubo A57
    palate A51.2
  urethra A51.0
  yaws A66.0
Chancroid (anus) (genital) (penis) (perineum)
    (rectum) (urethra) (vulva) A57
Chandler's disease (osteochondritis dissecans,
    hip) —*see* Osteochondritis, dissecans, hip
Change(s) (in) (of) —*see also* Removal
  arteriosclerotic —*see* Arteriosclerosis
  bone —*see also* Disorder, bone
    diabetic —*see* Diabetes, bone change
  bowel habit R19.4
  cardiorenal (vascular) —*see* Hypertension,
    cardiorenal
  cardiovascular —*see* Disease, cardiovascular
  circulatory I99.9
  cognitive (mild) (organic) R41.89
  color, tooth, teeth
    during formation K00.8
    posteruptive K03.7
  contraceptive device Z30.433
  corneal membrane H18.30
    Bowman's membrane fold or rupture H18.31-●
    Descemet's membrane
      fold H18.32-●
      rupture H18.33-●
  coronary —*see* Disease, heart, ischemic
  degenerative, spine or vertebra —*see*
    Spondylosis
  dental pulp, regressive K04.2
  dressing (nonsurgical) Z48.00
    surgical Z48.01
  heart —*see* Disease, heart
  hip joint —*see* Derangement, joint, hip
  hyperplastic larynx J38.7
  hypertrophic
    nasal sinus J34.89
    turbinate, nasal J34.3
    upper respiratory tract J39.8
  indwelling catheter Z46.6
  inflammatory —*see also* Inflammation
    sacroiliac M46.1
  job, anxiety concerning Z56.1
  joint —*see* Derangement, joint
  life —*see* Menopause
  mental status R41.82
  minimal (glomerular) —*see also* N00-N07 with
    fourth character .0 N05.0
  myocardium, myocardial —*see* Degeneration,
    myocardial - of life —*see* Menopause

Change *(Continued)*
  pacemaker Z45.018
    pulse generator Z45.010
  personality (enduring) F68.8
    due to (secondary to)
      general medical condition F07.0
    secondary (nonspecific) F60.89
  regressive, dental pulp K04.2
  renal —*see* Disease, renal
  retina H35.9
    myopic —*see also* Myopia, degenerative H44.2-●
  sacroiliac joint M53.3
  senile —*see also* condition R54
  sensory R20.8
  skin R23.9
    acute, due to ultraviolet radiation L56.9
      specified NEC L56.8
    chronic, due to nonionizing radiation L57.9
      specified NEC L57.8
    cyanosis R23.0
    flushing R23.2
    pallor R23.1
    petechiae R23.3
    specified change NEC R23.8
    swelling —*see* Mass, localized
    texture R23.4
  trophic
    arm —*see* Mononeuropathy, upper limb
    leg —*see* Mononeuropathy, lower limb
  vascular I99.9
  vasomotor I73.9
  voice R49.9
    psychogenic F44.4
    specified NEC R49.8
Changing sleep-work schedule, affecting sleep
    G47.26
Changuinola fever A93.1
Chapping skin T69.8
Charcot-Marie-Tooth disease, paralysis or
    syndrome G60.0
Charcot's
  arthropathy —*see* Arthropathy, neuropathic
  cirrhosis K74.3
  disease (tabetic arthropathy) A52.16
  joint (disease) (tabetic) A52.16
    diabetic —*see* Diabetes, with, arthropathy
    syringomyelic G95.0
  syndrome (intermittent claudication) I73.9
CHARGE association Q89.8
Charley-horse (quadriceps) M62.831
  traumatic (quadriceps) S76.11-●
Charlouis' disease —*see* Yaws
Cheadle's disease E54
Checking (of)
  cardiac pacemaker (battery) (electrode(s))
    Z45.018
    pulse generator Z45.010
  implantable subdermal contraceptive Z30.46
  intrauterine contraceptive device Z30.431
  wound Z48.0-●
    due to injury - code to Injury, by site, using
      appropriate seventh character for
      subsequent encounter
    postoperative - see Aftercare
Check-up —*see* Examination
Chédiak-Higashi (-Steinbrinck) syndrome
    (congenital gigantism of peroxidase granules)
    E70.330
Cheek —*see* condition
Cheese itch B88.0
Cheese-washer's lung J67.8
Cheese-worker's lung J67.8
Cheilitis (acute) (angular) (catarrhal) (chronic)
    (exfoliative) (gangrenous) (glandular)
    (infectional) (suppurative) (ulcerative)
    (vesicular) K13.0
  actinic (due to sun) L56.8
    other than from sun L59.8
  candidal B37.83
Cheilodynia K13.0
Cheiloschisis —*see* Cleft, lip
Cheilosis (angular) K13.0
  with pellagra E52
  due to
    vitamin B2 (riboflavin) deficiency E53.0
Cheiromegaly M79.89
Cheiropompholyx L30.1
Cheloid —*see* Keloid
Chemical burn —*see* Corrosion, by site
Chemodectoma —*see* Paraganglioma,
  nonchromaffin

Chemosis, conjunctiva —*see* Edema, conjunctiva
Chemotherapy (session) (for)
  cancer Z51.11
  neoplasm Z51.11
Cherubism M27.8
Chest —*see* condition
Cheyne-Stokes breathing (respiration) R06.3
Chiari's
  disease or syndrome (hepatic vein thrombosis)
    I82.0
  malformation
    type I G93.5
    type II —*see* Spina bifida
  net Q24.8
Chicago disease B40.9
Chickenpox —*see* Varicella
Chiclero ulcer or sore B55.1
Chigger (infestation) B88.0
Chignon (disease) B36.8
  newborn (from vacuum extraction) (birth injury)
    P12.1
Chilaiditi's syndrome (subphrenic displacement,
    colon) Q43.3
Chilblain(s) (lupus) T69.1
▥ Child —*see also* Problem, child
  custody dispute Z65.3
Childbirth —*see* Delivery
Childhood
  cerebral X-linked adrenoleukodystrophy
    E71.520
  period of rapid growth Z00.2
Chill(s) R68.83
  with fever R50.9
  without fever R68.83
  congestive in malarial regions B54
Chilomastigiasis A07.8
Chimera 46,XX/46,XY Q99.0
Chin —*see* condition
Chinese dysentery A03.9
Chionophobia F40.228
Chitral fever A93.1
Chlamydia, chlamydial A74.9
  cervicitis A56.09
  conjunctivitis A74.0
  cystitis A56.01
  endometritis A56.11
  epididymitis A56.19
  female
    pelvic inflammatory disease A56.11
    pelviperitonitis A56.11
  orchitis A56.19
  peritonitis A74.81
  pharyngitis A56.4
  proctitis A56.3
  psittaci (infection) A70
  salpingitis A56.11
  sexually-transmitted infection NEC A56.8
  specified NEC A74.89
  urethritis A56.01
  vulvovaginitis A56.02
Chlamydiosis —*see* Chlamydia
Chloasma (skin) (idiopathic) (symptomatic) L81.1
  eyelid H02.719
    hyperthyroid E05.90 *[H02.719]*
      with thyroid storm E05.91 *[H02.719]*
    left H02.716
      lower H02.715
      upper H02.714
    right H02.713
      lower H02.712
      upper H02.711
Chloroma C92.3-●
Chlorosis D50.9
  Egyptian B76.9 *[D63.8]*
  miner's B76.9 *[D63.8]*
Chlorotic anemia D50.8
Chocolate cyst (ovary) N80.10-●
Choked
  disc or disk —*see* Papilledema
  on food, phlegm, or vomitus NOS —*see* Foreign
    body, by site
  while vomiting NOS —*see* Foreign body, by site
Chokes (resulting from bends) T70.3
Choking sensation R09.89
Cholangiectasis K83.8
Cholangiocarcinoma
  with hepatocellular carcinoma, combined C22.0
  liver C22.1
  specified site NEC —*see* Neoplasm, malignant,
    by site
  unspecified site C22.1

▶ New   ➡ Revised   ~~deleted~~ Deleted   ● Use Additional Character(s)

Cholangiohepatitis K83.8
  due to fluke infestation B66.1
Cholangiohepatoma C22.0
Cholangiolitis (acute) (chronic) (extrahepatic)
  (gangrenous) (intrahepatic) K83.09
  paratyphoidal —see Fever, paratyphoid
  typhoidal A01.09
Cholangioma D13.4
  malignant —see Cholangiocarcinoma
Cholangitis (ascending) (primary) (recurrent)
  (sclerosing) (secondary) (stenosing)
  (suppurative) K83.09
  with calculus, bile duct —see Calculus, bile duct,
    with cholangitis
  chronic nonsuppurative destructive K74.3
  primary K83.09
    sclerosing K83.01
  sclerosing K83.09
Cholecystectasia K82.8
Cholecystitis K81.9
  with
    calculus, stones in
      bile duct (common) (hepatic) —see
        Calculus, bile duct, with cholecystitis
      cystic duct —see Calculus, gallbladder, with
        cholecystitis
      gallbladder —see Calculus, gallbladder,
        with cholecystitis
      choledocholithiasis —see Calculus, bile duct,
        with cholecystitis
      cholelithiasis —see Calculus, gallbladder, with
        cholecystitis
    gangrene of gallbladder K82.A1
    perforation of gallbladder K82.A2
  acute (emphysematous) (gangrenous)
    (suppurative) K81.0
    with
      calculus, stones in
        cystic duct —see Calculus, gallbladder,
          with cholecystitis, acute
        gallbladder —see Calculus, gallbladder,
          with cholecystitis, acute
        choledocholithiasis —see Calculus, bile
          duct, with cholecystitis, acute
        cholelithiasis —see Calculus, gallbladder,
          with cholecystitis, acute
      chronic cholecystitis K81.2
        with gallbladder calculus K80.12
          with obstruction K80.13
  chronic K81.1
    with acute cholecystitis K81.2
      with gallbladder calculus K80.12
        with obstruction K80.13
  emphysematous (acute) —see Cholecystitis,
    acute
  gangrenous —see Cholecystitis, acute
  paratyphoidal, current A01.4
  suppurative —see Cholecystitis, acute
  typhoidal A01.09
Cholecystolithiasis —see Calculus, gallbladder
Choledochitis (suppurative) K83.09
Choledocholith —see Calculus, bile duct
Choledocholithiasis (common duct) (hepatic
  duct) —see Calculus, bile duct
  cystic —see Calculus, gallbladder
  typhoidal A01.09
Cholelithiasis (cystic duct) (gallbladder)
  (impacted) (multiple) —see Calculus,
    gallbladder
  bile duct (common) (hepatic) —see Calculus,
    bile duct
  hepatic duct —see Calculus, bile duct
  specified NEC K80.80
    with obstruction K80.81
Cholemia —see also Jaundice
  familial (simple) (congenital) E80.4
  Gilbert's E80.4
Choleperitoneum, choleperitonitis K65.3
Cholera (Asiatic) (epidemic) (malignant) A00.9
  antimonial —see Poisoning, antimony
  classical A00.0
  due to Vibrio cholerae 01 A00.9
    biovar cholerae A00.0
    biovar eltor A00.1
    el tor A00.1
  el tor A00.1
Cholerine —see Cholera
Cholestasis NEC K83.1
  with hepatocyte injury K71.0
  due to total parenteral nutrition (TPN) K76.89
  pure K71.0

Cholesteatoma (ear) (middle) (with reaction)
  H71.9-●
  attic H71.0-●
  external ear (canal) H60.4-●
  mastoid H71.2-●
  postmastoidectomy cavity (recurrent) —see
    Complications, postmastoidectomy,
    recurrent cholesteatoma
  recurrent (postmastoidectomy) —see
    Complications, postmastoidectomy,
    recurrent cholesteatoma
  tympanum H71.1-●
Cholesteatosis, diffuse H71.3-●
Cholesteremia E78.00
Cholesterin in vitreous —see Deposit, crystalline
Cholesterol
  deposit
    retina H35.89
    vitreous —see Deposit, crystalline
  elevated (high) E78.00
    with elevated (high) triglycerides E78.2
    screening for Z13.220
  imbibition of gallbladder K82.4
Cholesterolemia (essential) (pure) E78.00
  familial E78.01
  hereditary E78.01
Cholesterolosis, cholesterosis (gallbladder) K82.4
  cerebrotendinous E75.5
Cholocolic fistula K82.3
Choluria R82.2
Chondritis M94.8X9
  aural H61.03-●
  costal (Tietze's) M94.0
  external ear H61.03-●
  patella, posttraumatic —see Chondromalacia,
    patella
  pinna H61.03-●
  purulent M94.8X-●
  tuberculous NEC A18.02
    intervertebral A18.01
Chondroblastoma —see also Neoplasm, bone,
  benign
  malignant —see Neoplasm, bone, malignant
Chondrocalcinosis M11.20
  ankle M11.27-●
  elbow M11.22-●
  familial M11.10
    ankle M11.17-●
    elbow M11.12-●
    foot joint M11.17-●
    hand joint M11.14-●
    hip M11.15-●
    knee M11.16-●
    multiple site M11.19
    shoulder M11.11-●
    vertebrae M11.18
    wrist M11.13-●
  foot joint M11.27-●
  hand joint M11.24-●
  hip M11.25-●
  knee M11.26-●
  multiple site M11.29
  shoulder M11.21-●
  specified type NEC M11.20
    ankle M11.27-●
    elbow M11.22-●
    foot joint M11.27-●
    hand joint M11.24-●
    hip M11.25-●
    knee M11.26-●
    multiple site M11.29
    shoulder M11.21-●
    vertebrae M11.28
    wrist M11.23-●
  vertebrae M11.28
  wrist M11.23-●
Chondrodermatitis nodularis helicis or
  anthelicis —see Perichondritis, ear
Chondrodysplasia Q78.9
  with hemangioma Q78.4
  calcificans congenita Q77.3
  fetalis Q77.4
  metaphyseal (Jansen's) (McKusick's) (Schmid's)
    Q78.8
  punctata Q77.3
Chondrodystrophy, chondrodystrophia (familial)
  (fetalis) (hypoplastic) Q78.9
  calcificans congenita Q77.3
  myotonic (congenital) G71.13
  punctata Q77.3
Chondroectodermal dysplasia Q77.6

Chondrogenesis imperfecta Q77.4
Chondrolysis M94.35-●
Chondroma —see also Neoplasm, cartilage, benign
  juxtacortical —see Neoplasm, bone, benign
  periosteal —see Neoplasm, bone, benign
Chondromalacia (systemic) M94.20
  acromioclavicular joint M94.21-●
  ankle M94.27-●
  elbow M94.22-●
  foot joint M94.27-●
  glenohumeral joint M94.21-●
  hand joint M94.24-●
  hip M94.25-●
  knee M94.26-●
    patella M22.4-●
  multiple sites M94.29
  patella M22.4-●
  rib M94.28
  sacroiliac joint M94.259
  shoulder M94.21-●
  sternoclavicular joint M94.21-●
  vertebral joint M94.28
  wrist M94.23-●
Chondromatosis —see also Neoplasm, cartilage,
  uncertain behavior
  internal Q78.4
Chondromyxosarcoma —see Neoplasm, cartilage,
  malignant
Chondro-osteodysplasia (Morquio-Brailsford type)
  E76.219
Chondro-osteodystrophy E76.29
Chondro-osteoma —see Neoplasm, bone, benign
Chondropathia tuberosa M94.0
Chondrosarcoma —see Neoplasm, cartilage,
  malignant
  juxtacortical —see Neoplasm, bone, malignant
  mesenchymal —see Neoplasm, connective tissue,
    malignant
  myxoid —see Neoplasm, cartilage, malignant
Chordee (nonvenereal) N48.89
  congenital Q54.4
  gonococcal A54.09
Chorditis (fibrinous) (nodosa) (tuberosa) J38.2
Chordoma —see Neoplasm, vertebral (column),
  malignant
Chorea (chronic) (gravis) (posthemiplegic) (senile)
  (spasmodic) G25.5
  with
    heart involvement I02.0
      active or acute (conditions in I01-●) I02.0
      rheumatic I02.9
        with valvular disorder I02.0
      rheumatic heart disease (chronic) (inactive)
        (quiescent) — code to rheumatic heart
        condition involved
  drug-induced G25.4
  habit F95.8
  hereditary G10
  Huntington's G10
  hysterical F44.4
  minor I02.9
    with heart involvement I02.0
  progressive G25.5
    hereditary G10
  rheumatic (chronic) I02.9
    with heart involvement I02.0
  Sydenham's I02.9
    with heart involvement —see Chorea, with
      rheumatic heart disease
    nonrheumatic G25.5
Choreoathetosis (paroxysmal) G25.5
Chorioadenoma (destruens) D39.2
Chorioamnionitis O41.12-●
Chorioangioma D26.7
Choriocarcinoma —see Neoplasm, malignant, by
  site
  combined with
    embryonal carcinoma —see Neoplasm,
      malignant, by site
    other germ cell elements —see Neoplasm,
      malignant, by site
    teratoma —see Neoplasm, malignant, by site
  specified site —see Neoplasm, malignant, by site
  unspecified site
    female C58
    male C62.90
Chorioencephalitis (acute) (lymphocytic) (serous)
  A87.2
Chorioepithelioma —see Choriocarcinoma
Choriomeningitis (acute) (lymphocytic) (serous)
  A87.2

Chorionepithelioma —*see* Choriocarcinoma
Chorioretinitis —*see also* Inflammation,
   chorioretinal
  disseminated —*see also* Inflammation,
    chorioretinal, disseminated
   in neurosyphilis A52.19
  Egyptian B76.9 [D63.8]
  focal —*see also* Inflammation, chorioretinal,
    focal
  histoplasmic B39.9 [H32]
  in (due to)
   histoplasmosis B39.9 [H32]
   syphilis (secondary) A51.43
    late A52.71
   toxoplasmosis (acquired) B58.01
    congenital (active) P37.1 [H32]
   tuberculosis A18.53
  juxtapapillary, juxtapapillaris —*see*
    Inflammation, chorioretinal, focal,
    juxtapapillary
  leprous A30.9 [H32]
  miner's B76.9 [D63.8]
  progressive myopia (degeneration) —*see also*
    Myopia, degenerative H44.2-●
  syphilitic (secondary) A51.43
   congenital (early) A50.01 [H32]
    late A50.32
   late A52.71
  tuberculous A18.53
Chorioretinopathy, central serous H35.71-●
Choroid —*see* condition
Choroideremia H31.21
Choroiditis —*see* Chorioretinitis
Choroidopathy —*see* Disorder, choroid
Choroidoretinitis —*see* Chorioretinitis
Choroidoretinopathy, central serous —*see*
   Chorioretinopathy, central serous
Christian-Weber disease M35.6
Christmas disease D67
Chromaffinoma —*see also* Neoplasm, benign, by
   site
  malignant —*see* Neoplasm, malignant, by site
Chromatopsia —*see* Deficiency, color vision
Chromhidrosis, chromidrosis L75.1
Chromoblastomycosis —*see* Chromomycosis
Chromoconversion R82.91
Chromomycosis B43.9
  brain abscess B43.1
  cerebral B43.1
  cutaneous B43.0
  skin B43.0
  specified NEC B43.8
  subcutaneous abscess or cyst B43.2
Chromophytosis B36.0
Chromosome —*see* condition by chromosome
   involved
  D (1) —*see* condition, chromosome 13
  E (3) —*see* condition, chromosome 18
  G —*see* condition, chromosome 21
Chromotrichomycosis B36.8
Chronic —*see* condition
  fracture —*see* Fracture, pathological
Churg-Strauss syndrome M30.1
Chyle cyst, mesentery I89.8
Chylocele (nonfilarial) I89.8
  filarial —*see also* Infestation, filarial B74.9 [N51]
  tunica vaginalis N50.89
   filarial —*see also* Infestation, filarial B74.9
    [N51]
Chylomicronemia (fasting) (with
   hyperprebetalipoproteinemia) E78.3
Chylopericardium I31.39
  acute I30.9
Chylothorax (nonfilarial) J94.0
  filarial —*see also* Infestation, filarial B74.9 [J91.8]
Chylous —*see* condition
Chyluria (nonfilarial) R82.0
  due to
   bilharziasis B65.0
   Brugia (malayi) B74.1
    timori B74.2
   schistosomiasis (bilharziasis) B65.0
   Wuchereria (bancrofti) B74.0
  filarial —*see* Infestation, filarial
Cicatricial (deformity) —*see* Cicatrix
Cicatrix (adherent) (contracted) (painful)
   (vicious) —*see also* Scar L90.5
  adenoid (and tonsil) J35.8
  alveolar process M26.79
  anus K62.89
  auricle —*see* Disorder, pinna, specified type NEC

Cicatrix (Continued)
  bile duct (common) (hepatic) K83.8
  bladder N32.89
  bone —*see* Disorder, bone, specified type NEC
  brain G93.89
  cervix (postoperative) (postpartal) N88.1
  common duct K83.8
  cornea H17.9
   tuberculous A18.59
  duodenum (bulb), obstructive K31.5
  esophagus K22.2
  eyelid —*see* Disorder, eyelid function
  hypopharynx J39.2
  lacrimal passages —*see* Obstruction, lacrimal
  larynx J38.7
  lung J98.4
  middle ear —*see* subcategory H74.8
  mouth K13.79
  muscle M62.89
   with contracture —*see* Contraction, muscle
    NEC
  nasopharynx J39.2
  palate (soft) K13.79
  penis N48.89
  pharynx J39.2
  prostate N42.89
  rectum K62.89
  retina —*see* Scar, chorioretinal
  semilunar cartilage —*see* Derangement,
    meniscus
  seminal vesicle N50.89
  skin L90.5
   infected L08.89
   postinfective L90.5
   tuberculous B90.8
  specified site NEC L90.5
  throat J39.2
  tongue K14.8
  tonsil (and adenoid) J35.8
  trachea J39.8
  tuberculous NEC B90.9
  urethra N36.8
  uterus N85.8
  vagina N89.8
   postoperative N99.2
  vocal cord J38.3
  wrist, constricting (annular) L90.5
CIDP (chronic inflammatory demyelinating
   polyneuropathy) G61.81
CIN —*see* Neoplasia, intraepithelial, cervix
CINCA (chronic infantile neurological, cutaneous
   and articular syndrome)
   M04.2
Cinchonism —*see* Deafness, ototoxic
  correct substance properly administered —*see*
    Table of Drugs and Chemicals, by drug,
    adverse effect
  overdose or wrong substance given or taken —
    see Table of Drugs and Chemicals, by drug,
    poisoning
Circle of Willis —*see* condition
Circular —*see* condition
Circulating anticoagulants —*see also* - Disorder,
   hemorrhagic D68.318
  due to drugs —*see also* - Disorder, hemorrhagic
    D68.32
  following childbirth O72.3
Circulation
  collateral, any site I99.8
  defective (lower extremity) I99.9
   congenital Q28.9
  embryonic Q28.9
  failure (peripheral) R57.9
   newborn P29.89
  fetal, persistent P29.38
  heart, incomplete Q28.9
Circulatory system —*see* condition
Circulus senilis (cornea) —*see* Degeneration,
   cornea, senile
Circumcision (in absence of medical indication)
   (ritual) (routine) Z41.2
Circumscribed —*see* condition
Circumvallate placenta O43.11-●
Cirrhosis, cirrhotic (hepatic) (liver) K74.60
  alcoholic K70.30
   with ascites K70.31
  atrophic —*see* Cirrhosis, liver
  Baumgarten-Cruveilhier K74.69
  biliary (cholangiolitic) (cholangitic)
    (hypertrophic) (obstructive)
    (pericholangiolitic) K74.5

Cirrhosis, cirrhotic (Continued)
  biliary (Continued)
   due to
    Clonorchiasis B66.1
    flukes B66.3
   primary K74.3
   secondary K74.4
  cardiac (of liver) K76.1
  Charcot's K74.3
  cholangiolitic, cholangitic, cholostatic (primary)
    K74.3
  congestive K76.1
  Cruveilhier-Baumgarten K74.69
  cryptogenic (liver) K74.69
  due to
   hepatolenticular degeneration E83.01
   Wilson's disease E83.01
   xanthomatosis E78.2
  fatty K76.0
   alcoholic K70.0
  Hanot's (hypertrophic) K74.3
  hepatic —*see* Cirrhosis, liver
  hypertrophic K74.3
  Indian childhood K74.69
  kidney —*see* Sclerosis, renal
  Laennec's K70.30
   with ascites K70.31
   alcoholic K70.30
    with ascites K70.31
   nonalcoholic K74.69
  liver K74.60
   alcoholic K70.30
    with ascites K70.31
   fatty K70.0
   congenital P78.81
   syphilitic A52.74
  lung (chronic) J84.10
  macronodular K74.69
   alcoholic K70.30
    with ascites K70.31
  micronodular K74.69
   alcoholic K70.30
    with ascites K70.31
  mixed type K74.69
  monolobular K74.3
  nephritis —*see* Sclerosis, renal
  nutritional K74.69
   alcoholic K70.30
    with ascites K70.31
  obstructive —*see* Cirrhosis, biliary
  ovarian N83.8
  pancreas (duct) K86.89
  pigmentary E83.110
  portal K74.69
   alcoholic K70.30
    with ascites K70.31
  postnecrotic K74.69
   alcoholic K70.30
    with ascites K70.31
  pulmonary J84.10
  renal —*see* Sclerosis, renal
  spleen D73.2
  stasis K76.1
  Todd's K74.3
  unilobar K74.3
  xanthomatous (biliary) K74.5
   due to xanthomatosis (familial) (metabolic)
    (primary) E78.2
Cistern, subarachnoid R93.0
Citrullinemia E72.23
Citrullinuria E72.23
Civatte's disease or poikiloderma L57.3
CLAD —*see* Dysfunction, chronic, lung allograft
Clam digger's itch B65.3
Clammy skin R23.1
Clap —*see* Gonorrhea
Clarke-Hadfield syndrome (pancreatic infantilism)
   K86.89
Clark's paralysis G80.9
Clastothrix L67.8
Claude Bernard-Horner syndrome G90.2
  traumatic —*see* Injury, nerve, cervical
    sympathetic
Claude's disease or syndrome G46.3
Claudicatio venosa intermittens I87.8
Claudication (intermittent) I73.9
  cerebral (artery) G45.9
  spinal cord (arteriosclerotic) G95.19
   syphilitic A52.09
  venous (axillary) I87.8
Claustrophobia F40.240

▶ New   ➡ Revised   ~~deleted~~ Deleted   ● Use Additional Character(s)

Clavus (infected) L84
Clawfoot (congenital) Q66.89
　acquired —see Deformity, limb, clawfoot
Clawhand (acquired) —see also Deformity, limb,
　　clawhand
　congenital Q68.1
Clawtoe (congenital) Q66.89
　acquired —see Deformity, toe, specified NEC
Clay eating —see Pica
Cleansing of artificial opening —see Attention to,
　　artificial, opening
Cleft (congenital) —see also Imperfect, closure
　alveolar process M26.79
　branchial (persistent) Q18.2
　cyst Q18.0
　　fistula Q18.0
　　sinus Q18.0
　cricoid cartilage, posterior Q31.8
　foot Q72.7
　hand Q71.6
　lip (unilateral) Q36.9
　　with cleft palate Q37.9
　　　hard Q37.1
　　　　with soft Q37.5
　　　soft Q37.3
　　　　with hard Q37.5
　　bilateral Q36.0
　　　with cleft palate Q37.8
　　　　hard Q37.0
　　　　　with soft Q37.4
　　　　soft Q37.2
　　　　　with hard Q37.4
　　median Q36.1
▶ mitral valve leaflet (at birth) (congenital) Q23.82
　nose Q30.2
　palate Q35.9
　　with cleft lip (unilateral) Q37.9
　　　bilateral Q37.8
　　hard Q35.1
　　　with
　　　　cleft lip (unilateral) Q37.1
　　　　　bilateral Q37.0
　　　　soft Q35.5
　　　　　with cleft lip (unilateral) Q37.5
　　　　　　bilateral Q37.4
　　medial Q35.5
　　soft Q35.3
　　　with
　　　　cleft lip (unilateral) Q37.3
　　　　　bilateral Q37.2
　　　　hard Q35.5
　　　　　with cleft lip (unilateral) Q37.5
　　　　　　bilateral Q37.4
　penis Q55.69
　scrotum Q55.29
　thyroid cartilage Q31.8
　uvula Q35.7
Cleidocranial dysostosis Q74.0
Cleptomania F63.2
Clicking hip (newborn) R29.4
Climacteric (female) —see also Menopause
　arthritis (any site) NEC —see Arthritis, specified
　　　form NEC
　depression (single episode) F32.89
　　recurrent episode F33.8
　male (symptoms) (syndrome) NEC N50.89
　melancholia (single episode) F32.89
　　recurrent episode F33.8
　paranoid state F22
　polyarthritis NEC —see Arthritis, specified form
　　　NEC
　symptoms (female) N95.1
Clinical research investigation (clinical trial)
　　(control subject) (normal comparison)
　　(participant) Z00.6
Clitoris —see condition Cloaca (persistent) Q43.7
Clonorchiasis, clonorchis infection (liver) B66.1
Clonus R25.8
Closed bite M26.29
Clostridium (C.) perfringens, as cause of disease
　　classified elsewhere B96.7
Closure
　congenital, nose Q30.0
　cranial sutures, premature Q75.009
　defective or imperfect NEC —see Imperfect,
　　　closure
　fistula, delayed —see Fistula
　foramen ovale, imperfect Q21.12
　hymen N89.6
　interauricular septum, defective Q21.19
　interventricular septum, defective Q21.0

Closure (Continued)
　lacrimal duct —see also Stenosis, lacrimal, duct
　　congenital Q10.5
　nose (congenital) Q30.0
　　acquired M95.0
　of artificial opening —see Attention to, artificial,
　　　opening
　primary angle, without glaucoma damage
　　　H40.06-●
　vagina N89.5
　valve —see Endocarditis
　vulva N90.5
Clot (blood) —see also Embolism
　artery (obstruction) (occlusion) —see Embolism
　bladder N32.89
　brain (intradural or extradural) —see Occlusion,
　　　artery, cerebral
　circulation I74.9
　heart —see also Infarct, myocardium
　　not resulting in infarction I51.3
　vein —see Thrombosis
Clouded state R40.1
　epileptic —see Epilepsy, specified NEC
　paroxysmal —see Epilepsy, specified NEC
Cloudy antrum, antra J32.0
Clouston's (hidrotic) ectodermal dysplasia Q82.4
Cloverleaf skull Q75.051
Clubbed nail pachydermoperiostosis M89.40 [L62]
Clubbing of finger(s) (nails) R68.3
Clubfinger R68.3
　congenital Q68.1
Clubfoot (congenital) Q66.89
　acquired —see Deformity, limb, clubfoot
　equinovarus Q66.0-●
　paralytic —see Deformity, limb, clubfoot
Clubhand (congenital) (radial) Q71.4-●
　acquired —see Deformity, limb, clubhand
Clubnail R68.3
　congenital Q84.6
Clump, kidney Q63.1
Clumsiness, clumsy child syndrome F82
Cluttering F98.81
Clutton's joints A50.51 [M12.80]
Coagulation, intravascular (diffuse)
　　(disseminated) —see also Defibrination
　　syndrome
　complicating abortion —see Abortion, by type,
　　　complicated by, intravascular coagulation
　COVID-19 associated (see also COVID-19) D65
　following ectopic or molar pregnancy O08.1
Coagulopathy —see also Defect, coagulation
　consumption D65
　intravascular D65
　　newborn P60
Coalition
　calcaneo-scaphoid Q66.89
　tarsal Q66.89
Coalminer's
　elbow —see Bursitis, elbow, olecranon
　lung or pneumoconiosis J60
Coalworker's lung or pneumoconiosis J60
Coarctation
　aorta (preductal) (postductal) Q25.1
　pulmonary artery Q25.71
Coated tongue K14.3
Coats' disease (exudative retinopathy) —see
　　Retinopathy, exudative
Cocaine-induced
　anxiety disorder F14.980
　bipolar and related disorder F14.94
　depressive disorder F14.94
　obsessive-compulsive and related disorder F14.988
　psychotic disorder F14.959
　sleep disorder F14.982
　sexual dysfunction F14.981
Cocainism —see Disorder, cocaine use
Coccidioidomycosis B38.9
　cutaneous B38.3
　disseminated B38.7
　generalized B38.7
　meninges B38.4
　prostate B38.81
　pulmonary B38.2
　　acute B38.0
　　chronic B38.1
　skin B38.3
　specified NEC B38.89
Coccidioidosis —see Coccidioidomycosis
Coccidiosis (intestinal) A07.3
Coccydynia, coccygodynia M53.3
Coccyx —see condition

Cochin-China diarrhea K90.1
Cockayne's syndrome Q87.19
Cocked up toe —see Deformity, toe, specified NEC
Cock's peculiar tumor L72.3
Codman's tumor —see Neoplasm, bone, benign
Coenurosis B71.8
Coffee-worker's lung J67.8
Cogan's syndrome H16.32-●
　oculomotor apraxia H51.8
Coitus, painful (female) N94.10
　male N53.12
　psychogenic F52.6
Cold J00
　with influenza, flu, or grippe —see Influenza,
　　　with, respiratory manifestations NEC
　agglutinin disease or hemoglobinuria (chronic)
　　　D59.12
　bronchial —see Bronchitis
　chest —see Bronchitis
　common (head) J00
　effects of T69.9
　　specified effect NEC T69.8
　excessive, effects of T69.9
　　specified effect NEC T69.8
　exhaustion from T69.8
　exposure to T69.9
　　specified effect NEC T69.8
　head J00
　injury syndrome (newborn) P80.0
　on lung —see Bronchitis
　rose J30.1
　sensitivity, auto-immune D59.12
　symptoms J00
　virus J00
Coldsore B00.1
Colibacillosis A49.8
　as the cause of other disease (see also Escherichia
　　　coli) B96.20
　generalized (see also Sepsis, Escherichia coli) A41.50
Colic (bilious) (infantile) (intestinal) (recurrent)
　　(spasmodic) R10.83
　abdomen R10.83
　　psychogenic F45.8
　appendix, appendicular K38.8
　bile duct —see Calculus, bile duct
　biliary —see Calculus, bile duct
　common duct —see Calculus, bile duct
　cystic duct —see Calculus, gallbladder
　Devonshire NEC —see Poisoning, lead
　gallbladder —see Calculus, gallbladder
　gallstone —see Calculus, gallbladder
　　gallbladder or cystic duct —see Calculus,
　　　gallbladder
　hepatic (duct) —see Calculus, bile duct
　hysterical F45.8
　kidney N23
　lead NEC —see Poisoning, lead
　mucous K58.9
　　with diarrhea K58.0
　　psychogenic F54
　nephritic N23
　painter's NEC —see Poisoning, lead
　pancreas K86.89
　psychogenic F45.8
　renal N23
　saturnine NEC —see Poisoning, lead
　ureter N23
　urethral N36.8
　　due to calculus N21.1
　uterus NEC N94.89
　　menstrual —see Dysmenorrhea
　worm NOS B83.9
Colicystitis —see Cystitis
Colitis (acute) (catarrhal) (chronic) (noninfective)
　　(hemorrhagic) (see also Enteritis) K52.9
　allergic K52.29
　　with
　　　food protein-induced enterocolitis
　　　　syndrome K52.21
　　　proctocolitis K52.29
　amebic (acute) —see also Amebiasis A06.0
　　nondysenteric A06.2
　anthrax A22.2
　bacillary —see Infection, Shigella
　balantidial A07.0
▶ Clostridioides difficile
　▶ not specified as recurrent A04.72
　▶ recurrent A04.71
　Clostridium difficile
　　not specified as recurrent A04.72
　　recurrent A04.71

Colitis *(Continued)*
  coccidial A07.3
  collagenous K52.831
  cystica superficialis K52.89
  dietary counseling and surveillance (for) Z71.3
  dietetic —*see also* Colitis, allergic K52.29
  drug-induced K52.1
  due to radiation K52.0
  eosinophilic K52.82
  food hypersensitivity —*see also* Colitis, allergic K52.29
  giardial A07.1
  granulomatous —*see* Enteritis, regional, large intestine
  infectious —*see* Enteritis, infectious
  indeterminate, so stated K52.3
  ischemic K55.9
    acute (subacute) —*see also* Ischemia, intestine, acute K55.039
    chronic K55.1
    due to mesenteric artery insufficiency K55.1
    fulminant (acute) —*see also* Ischemia, intestine, acute K55.039
  left sided K51.50
    with
      abscess K51.514
      complication K51.519
        specified NEC K51.518
      fistula K51.513
      obstruction K51.512
      rectal bleeding K51.511
  lymphocytic K52.832
  membranous
    psychogenic F54
  microscopic K52.839
    specified NEC K52.838
  mucous —*see* Syndrome, irritable, bowel
    psychogenic F54
  noninfective K52.9
    specified NEC K52.89
  polyposa —*see* Polyp, colon, inflammatory
  protozoal A07.9
  pseudomembranous
    not specified as recurrent A04.72
    recurrent A04.71
  pseudomucinous —*see* Syndrome, irritable, bowel
  regional —*see* Enteritis, regional, large intestine
    infectious A09
  segmental —*see* Enteritis, regional, large intestine
  septic —*see* Enteritis, infectious
  spastic K58.9
    with diarrhea K58.0
    psychogenic F54
  staphylococcal A04.8
    foodborne A05.0
  subacute ischemic —*see also* Ischemia, intestine, acute K55.039
  thromboulcerative —*see also* Ischemia, intestine, acute K55.039
  toxic NEC K52.1
    ~~due to Clostridium difficile~~
      ~~not specified as recurrent A04.72~~
      ~~recurrent A04.71~~
    ▶due to
      ▶Clostridioides difficile
        ▶not specified as recurrent A04.72
        ▶recurrent A04.71
      ▶Clostridium difficile
        ▶not specified as recurrent A04.72
        ▶recurrent A04.71
  transmural —*see* Enteritis, regional, large intestine
  trichomonal A07.8
  tuberculous (ulcerative) A18.32
  ulcerative (chronic) K51.90
    with
      complication K51.919
        abscess K51.914
        fistula K51.913
        obstruction K51.912
        rectal bleeding K51.911
        specified complication NEC K51.918
    enterocolitis —*see* Enterocolitis, ulcerative
    ileocolitis —*see* Ileocolitis, ulcerative
    mucosal proctocolitis —*see* Proctocolitis, mucosal

Colitis *(Continued)*
  ulcerative (chronic) *(Continued)*
    proctitis —*see* Proctitis, ulcerative
    pseudopolyposis —*see* Polyp, colon, inflammatory
    psychogenic F54
    rectosigmoiditis —*see* Rectosigmoiditis, ulcerative
    specified type NEC K51.80
      with
        complication K51.819
          abscess K51.814
          fistula K51.813
          obstruction K51.812
          rectal bleeding K51.811
          specified complication NEC K51.818
Collagenosis, collagen disease (nonvascular) (vascular) M35.9
  cardiovascular I42.8
  reactive perforating L87.1
  specified NEC M35.89
Collapse R55
  adrenal E27.2
  cardiorespiratory R57.0
  cardiovascular R57.0
    newborn P29.89
  circulatory (peripheral) R57.9
    during or after labor and delivery O75.1
    following ectopic or molar pregnancy O08.3
    newborn P29.89
  during or
    after labor and delivery O75.1
    resulting from a procedure, not elsewhere classified T81.10
  external ear canal —*see* Stenosis, external ear canal
  general R55
  heart —*see* Disease, heart
  heat T67.1
  hysterical F44.89
  labyrinth, membranous (congenital) Q16.5
  lung (massive) —*see also* Atelectasis J98.19
    pressure due to anesthesia (general) (local) or other sedation T88.2
      during labor and delivery O74.1
      in pregnancy O29.02-●
      postpartum, puerperal O89.09
  myocardial —*see* Disease, heart
▶nasal valve J34.829
  ▶external J34.8210
    ▶dynamic J34.8212
    ▶static J34.8211
  ▶internal J34.8200
    ▶dynamic J34.8202
    ▶static J34.8201
  nervous F48.8
  neurocirculatory F45.8
  nose M95.0
  ▶lower sidewall or nostril, on inspiration J34.8212
  ▶upper, middle sidewall, on inspiration J34.8202
  postoperative T81.10
  pulmonary —*see also* Atelectasis J98.19
    newborn —*see* Atelectasis
  trachea J39.8
  tracheobronchial J98.09
  valvular —*see* Endocarditis
  vascular (peripheral) R57.9
    during or after labor and delivery O75.1
    following ectopic or molar pregnancy O08.3
    newborn P29.89
      vertebra M48.50-●
    cervical region M48.52-●
    cervicothoracic region M48.53-●
    in (due to)
      neoplasm (metastasis) M84.58-●
      osteoporosis —*see also* Osteoporosis M80.88
        cervical region M80.88
        cervicothoracic region M80.88
        lumbar region M80.88
        lumbosacral region M80.88
        multiple sites M80.88
        occipito-atlanto-axial region M80.88
        sacrococcygeal region M80.88
        thoracic region M80.88
        thoracolumbar region M80.88
      specified disease NEC M48.50-●
        cervical region M48.52-●
        cervicothoracic region M48.53-●
        lumbar region M48.56-●

Collapse *(Continued)*
  vascular *(Continued)*
    in (due to) *(Continued)*
      specified disease *(Continued)*
        lumbosacral region M48.57-●
        occipito-atlanto-axial region M48.51-●
        sacrococcygeal region M48.58-●
        thoracic region M48.54-●
        thoracolumbar region M48.55-●
      lumbar region M48.56-●
      lumbosacral region M48.57-●
      occipito-atlanto-axial region M48.51-●
      sacrococcygeal region M48.58-●
      thoracic region M48.54-●
      thoracolumbar region M48.55-●
Collateral —*see also* condition
  circulation (venous) I87.8
  dilation, veins I87.8
Colles' fracture S52.53-
Collet (-Sicard) syndrome G52.7
Collier's asthma or lung J60
Collodion baby Q80.2
Colloid nodule (of thyroid) (cystic) E04.1
Coloboma (iris) Q13.0
  eyelid Q10.3
  fundus Q14.8
  lens Q12.2
  optic disc (congenital) Q14.2
    acquired H47.31-●
Coloenteritis —*see* Enteritis
Colon —*see* condition
Colonization
  MRSA (Methicillin resistant Staphylococcus aureus) Z22.322
  MSSA (Methicillin susceptible Staphylococcus aureus) Z22.321
  status —*see* Carrier (suspected) of
Coloptosis K63.4
Color blindness —*see* Deficiency, color vision
Colostomy
  attention to Z43.3
  fitting or adjustment Z46.89
  malfunctioning K94.03
  status Z93.3
Colpitis (acute) —*see* Vaginitis
Colpocele N81.5
Colpocystitis —*see* Vaginitis
Colpospasm N94.2
Column, spinal, vertebral —*see* condition
Coma R40.20
  with
    motor response (none) R40.231
      abnormal R40.233
      abnormal extensor posturing to pain or noxious stimuli (<2 years of age) R40.232
      abnormal flexure posturing to pain or noxious stimuli (0-5 years of age) R40.233
      extension R40.232
      extensor posturing to pain or noxious stimuli (2-5 years of age) R40.232
      flexion/decorticate posturing (<2 years of age) R40.233
      flexion withdrawal R40.234
      localizes pain (2-5 years of age) R40.235
      normal or spontaneous movement (<2 years of age) R40.236
      obeys commands (2-5 years of age) R40.236
      score of
        1 R40.231
        2 R40.232
        3 R40.233
        4 R40.234
        5 R40.235
        6 R40.236
      withdraws from pain or noxious stimuli (0-5 years of age) R40.234
      withdraws to touch (<2 years of age) R40.235
    opening of eyes (never) R40.211
      in response to
        pain R40.212
        sound R40.213
      score of
        1 R40.211
        2 R40.212
        3 R40.213
        4 R40.214
      spontaneous R40.214

Coma *(Continued)*
  with *(Continued)*
    verbal response (none) R40.221
      confused conversation R40.224
      cooing or babbling or crying appropriately
        (<2 years of age) R40.225
      inappropriate crying or screaming
        (<2 years of age) R40.223
      inappropriate words R40.223
      inappropriate words (2-5 years of age)
        R40.224
      incomprehensible sounds (2-5 years of age)
        R40.222
      incomprehensible words R40.222
      irritable cries (<2 years of age) R40.224
      moans/grunts to pain; restless
        (<2 years old) R40.222
      oriented R40.225
      score of
        1 R40.221
        2 R40.222
        3 R40.223
        4 R40.224
        5 R40.225
      screaming (2-5 years of age) R40.223
      uses appropriate words (2-5 years of age)
        R40.225
  eclamptic —*see* Eclampsia
  epileptic —*see* Epilepsy
  Glasgow, scale score —*see* Glasgow coma scale
  hepatic —*see* Failure, hepatic, by type, with coma
  hyperglycemic (diabetic) —*see* Diabetes, by type,
    with hyperosmolarity, with coma
  hyperosmolar (diabetic) —*see* Diabetes, by type,
    with hyperosmolarity, with coma
  hypoglycemic (diabetic) —*see* Diabetes, by type,
    with hypoglycemia, with coma
    nondiabetic E15
  in diabetes —*see* Diabetes, coma
  insulin-induced —*see* Coma, hypoglycemic
  ketoacidotic (diabetic) —*see* Diabetes, by type,
    with ketoacidosis, with coma
  myxedematous E03.5
  newborn P91.5
  nontraumatic, due to underlying condition R40.2A
  persistent vegetative state R40.3
  secondary R40.2A
  specified NEC, without documented Glasgow
    coma scale score, or with partial Glasgow
    coma scale score reported R40.244
Comatose —*see* Coma
Combat fatigue F43.0
Combined —*see* condition
Comedo, comedones (giant) L70.0
Comedocarcinoma —*see also* Neoplasm, breast,
    malignant
  noninfiltrating
    breast D05.8-●
    specified site —*see* Neoplasm, in situ, by site
    unspecified site D05.8-●
Comedomastitis —*see* Ectasia, mammary duct
Comminuted fracture - code as Fracture, closed
Common
  arterial trunk Q20.0
  atrioventricular canal Q21.23
  atrium Q21.19
  cold (head) J00
  truncus (arteriosus) Q20.0
  variable immunodeficiency —*see*
    Immunodeficiency, common variable
  ventricle Q20.4
Commotio, commotion (current)
  brain —*see* Injury, intracranial, concussion
  cerebri —*see* Injury, intracranial, concussion
  retinae S05.8X-●
  spinal cord —*see* Injury, spinal cord, by region
  spinalis —*see* Injury, spinal cord, by region
Communication
  between
    base of aorta and pulmonary artery Q21.4
    left ventricle and right atrium Q20.5
    pericardial sac and pleural sac Q34.8
    pulmonary artery and pulmonary vein,
      congenital Q25.72
  congenital between uterus and digestive or
    urinary tract Q51.7
Compartment syndrome (deep) (posterior)
    (traumatic) T79.A0
  abdomen T79.A3
  lower extremity (hip, buttock, thigh, leg, foot,
    toes) T79.A2

Compartment syndrome *(Continued)*
  nontraumatic
    abdomen M79.A3
    lower extremity (hip, buttock, thigh, leg, foot,
      toes) M79.A2-●
    specified site NEC M79.A9
    upper extremity (shoulder, arm, forearm,
      wrist, hand, fingers) M79.A1-●
  specified site NEC T79.A9
  upper extremity (shoulder, arm, forearm, wrist,
    hand, fingers) T79.A1
Compensation
  failure —*see* Disease, heart
  neurosis, psychoneurosis —*see* Disorder,
    factitious
Complaint —*see also* Disease
  bowel, functional K59.9
    psychogenic F45.8
  intestine, functional K59.9
    psychogenic F45.8
  kidney —*see* Disease, renal
  miners' J60
Complete —*see* condition
Complex
  Addison-Schilder E71.528
  cardiorenal —*see* Hypertension,
    cardiorenal
  Costen's M26.69
  disseminated mycobacterium avium-
    intracellulare (DMAC) A31.2
  Eisenmenger's (ventricular septal defect)
    I27.83
  hypersexual F52.8
  jumped process, spine —*see* Dislocation,
    vertebra
  primary, tuberculous A15.7
  Schilder-Addison E71.528
  subluxation (vertebral) M99.19
    abdomen M99.19
    acromioclavicular M99.17
    cervical region M99.11
    cervicothoracic M99.11
    costochondral M99.18
    costovertebral M99.18
    head region M99.10
    hip M99.15
    lower extremity M99.16
    lumbar region M99.13
    lumbosacral M99.13
    occipitocervical M99.10
    pelvic region M99.15
    pubic M99.15
    rib cage M99.18
    sacral region M99.14
    sacrococcygeal M99.14
    sacroiliac M99.14
    specified NEC M99.19
    sternochondral M99.18
    sternoclavicular M99.17
    thoracic region M99.12
    thoracolumbar M99.12
    upper extremity M99.17
  Taussig-Bing (transposition, aorta and
    overriding pulmonary artery) Q20.1
Complication(s) (from) (of)
  accidental puncture or laceration during a
    procedure (of) —*see* Complications,
    intraoperative (intraprocedural), puncture
    or laceration
  amputation stump (surgical) (late) NEC T87.9
    dehiscence T87.81
    infection or inflammation T87.40
      lower limb T87.4-●
      upper limb T87.4-●
    necrosis T87.50
      lower limb T87.5-●
      upper limb T87.5-●
    neuroma T87.30
      lower limb T87.3-●
      upper limb T87.3-●
    specified type NEC T87.89
  anastomosis (and bypass) —*see also*
    Complications, prosthetic device or implant
    intestinal (internal) NEC K91.89
      involving urinary tract N99.89
    urinary tract (involving intestinal tract) N99.89
    vascular —*see* Complications, cardiovascular
      device or implant
  anesthesia, anesthetic —*see also* Anesthesia,
    complication T88.59
    brain, postpartum, puerperal O89.2

Complication *(Continued)*
  anesthesia, anesthetic *(Continued)*
    cardiac
      in
        labor and delivery O74.2
        pregnancy O29.19-●
      postpartum, puerperal O89.1
    central nervous system
      in
        labor and delivery O74.3
        pregnancy O29.29-●
      postpartum, puerperal O89.2
    difficult or failed intubation T88.4
      in pregnancy O29.6-●
    failed sedation (conscious) (moderate) during
      procedure T88.52
    general, unintended awareness during
      procedure T88.53
    hyperthermia, malignant T88.3
    hypothermia T88.51
    intubation failure T88.4
    malignant hyperthermia T88.3
    pulmonary
      in
        labor and delivery O74.1
        pregnancy NEC O29.09-●
      postpartum, puerperal O89.09
    shock T88.2
    spinal and epidural
      in
        labor and delivery NEC O74.6
          headache O74.5
        pregnancy NEC O29.5X-●
      postpartum, puerperal NEC O89.5
        headache O89.4
    unintended awareness under general
      anesthesia during procedure T88.53
  anti-reflux device —*see* Complications,
    esophageal anti-reflux device
  aortic (bifurcation) graft —*see* Complications,
    graft, vascular
  aortocoronary (bypass) graft —*see*
    Complications, coronary artery (bypass)
    graft
  aortofemoral (bypass) graft —*see* Complications,
    extremity artery (bypass) graft
  arteriovenous
    fistula, surgically created T82.9
      embolism T82.818
      fibrosis T82.828
      hemorrhage T82.838
      infection or inflammation T82.7
      mechanical
        breakdown T82.510
        displacement T82.520
        leakage T82.530
        malposition T82.520
        obstruction T82.590
        perforation T82.590
        protrusion T82.590
      pain T82.848
      specified type NEC T82.898
      stenosis T82.858
      thrombosis T82.868
    shunt, surgically created T82.9
      embolism T82.818
      fibrosis T82.828
      hemorrhage T82.838
      infection or inflammation T82.7
      mechanical
        breakdown T82.511
        displacement T82.521
        leakage T82.531
        malposition T82.521
        obstruction T82.591
        perforation T82.591
        protrusion T82.591
      pain T82.848
      specified type NEC T82.898
      stenosis T82.858
      thrombosis T82.868
  arthroplasty —*see* Complications, joint prosthesis
  artificial
    fertilization or insemination N98.9
      attempted introduction (of)
        embryo in embryo transfer N98.3
        ovum following in vitro fertilization
          N98.2
      hyperstimulation of ovaries N98.1
      infection N98.0
      specified NEC N98.8

Complication *(Continued)*
  artificial *(Continued)*
    heart T82.9
      embolism T82.817
      fibrosis T82.827
      hemorrhage T82.837
      infection or inflammation T82.7
      mechanical
        breakdown T82.512
        displacement T82.522
        leakage T82.532
        malposition T82.522
        obstruction T82.592
        perforation T82.592
        protrusion T82.592
      pain T82.847
      specified type NEC T82.897
      stenosis T82.857
      thrombosis T82.867
    opening
      cecostomy —*see* Complications, colostomy
      colostomy —*see* Complications, colostomy
      cystostomy —*see* Complications, cystostomy
      enterostomy —*see* Complications, enterostomy
      gastrostomy —*see* Complications, gastrostomy
      ileostomy —*see* Complications, enterostomy
      jejunostomy —*see* Complications, enterostomy
      nephrostomy —*see* Complications, stoma, urinary tract
      tracheostomy —*see* Complications, tracheostomy
      ureterostomy —*see* Complications, stoma, urinary tract
      urethrostomy —*see* Complications, stoma, urinary tract
  balloon implant or device
    gastrointestinal T85.9
      embolism T85.818
      fibrosis T85.828
      hemorrhage T85.838
      infection and inflammation T85.79
      pain T85.848
      specified type NEC T85.898
      stenosis T85.858
      thrombosis T85.868
    vascular (counterpulsation) T82.9
      embolism T82.818
      fibrosis T82.828
      hemorrhage T82.838
      infection or inflammation T82.7
      mechanical
        breakdown T82.513
        displacement T82.523
        leakage T82.533
        malposition T82.523
        obstruction T82.593
        perforation T82.593
        protrusion T82.593
      pain T82.848
      specified type NEC T82.898
      stenosis T82.858
      thrombosis T82.868
  bariatric procedure
    gastric band procedure K95.09
      infection K95.01
    specified procedure NEC K95.89
      infection K95.81
  bile duct implant (prosthetic) T85.9
    embolism T85.818
    fibrosis T85.828
    hemorrhage T85.838
    infection and inflammation T85.79
    mechanical
      breakdown T85.510
      displacement T85.520
      malfunction T85.510
      malposition T85.520
      obstruction T85.590
      perforation T85.590
      protrusion T85.590
      specified NEC T85.590
    pain T85.848
    specified type NEC T85.898
    stenosis T85.858
    thrombosis T85.868
  bladder device (auxiliary) —*see* Complications, genitourinary, device or implant, urinary system

Complication *(Continued)*
  bleeding (postoperative) —*see* Complication, postoperative, hemorrhage
    intraoperative —*see* Complication, intraoperative, hemorrhage
  blood vessel graft —*see* Complications, graft, vascular
  bone
    device NEC T84.9
      embolism T84.81
      fibrosis T84.82
      hemorrhage T84.83
      infection or inflammation T84.7
      mechanical
        breakdown T84.318
        displacement T84.328
        malposition T84.328
        obstruction T84.398
        perforation T84.398
        protrusion T84.398
      pain T84.84
      specified type NEC T84.89
      stenosis T84.85
      thrombosis T84.86
    graft —*see* Complications, graft, bone
    growth stimulator (electrode) —*see* Complications, electronic stimulator device, bone
    marrow transplant —*see* Complications, transplant, bone, marrow
  brain neurostimulator (electrode) —*see* Complications, electronic stimulator device, brain
  breast implant (prosthetic) T85.9
    capsular contracture T85.44
    embolism T85.818
    fibrosis T85.828
    hemorrhage T85.838
    infection and inflammation T85.79
    mechanical
      breakdown T85.41
      displacement T85.42
      leakage T85.43
      malposition T85.42
      obstruction T85.49
      perforation T85.49
      protrusion T85.49
      specified NEC T85.49
    pain T85.848
    specified type NEC T85.898
    stenosis T85.858
    thrombosis T85.868
  bypass —*see also* Complications, prosthetic device or implant
    aortocoronary —*see* Complications, coronary artery (bypass) graft
    arterial —*see also* Complications, graft, vascular
      extremity —*see* Complications, extremity artery (bypass) graft
  cardiac —*see also* Disease, heart
    device, implant or graft T82.9
      embolism T82.817
      fibrosis T82.827
      hemorrhage T82.837
      infection or inflammation T82.7
        valve prosthesis T82.6
      mechanical
        breakdown T82.519
          specified device NEC T82.518
        displacement T82.529
          specified device NEC T82.528
        leakage T82.539
          specified device NEC T82.538
        malposition T82.529
          specified device NEC T82.528
        obstruction T82.599
          specified device NEC T82.598
        perforation T82.599
          specified device NEC T82.598
        protrusion T82.599
          specified device NEC T82.598
      pain T82.847
      specified type NEC T82.897
      stenosis T82.857
      thrombosis T82.867
  cardiovascular device, graft or implant T82.9
    aortic graft —*see* Complications, graft, vascular
    arteriovenous
      fistula, artificial —*see* Complication, arteriovenous, fistula, surgically created

Complication *(Continued)*
  cardiovascular device *(Continued)*
    arteriovenous *(Continued)*
      shunt —*see* Complication, arteriovenous, shunt, surgically created
    artificial heart —*see* Complication, artificial, heart
    balloon (counterpulsation) device —*see* Complication, balloon implant, vascular
    carotid artery graft —*see* Complications, graft, vascular
    coronary bypass graft —*see* Complication, coronary artery (bypass) graft
    dialysis catheter (vascular) —*see* Complication, catheter, dialysis
    electronic T82.9
      electrode T82.9
        embolism T82.817
        fibrosis T82.827
        hemorrhage T82.837
        infection T82.7
        mechanical
          breakdown T82.110
          displacement T82.120
          leakage T82.190
          obstruction T82.190
          perforation T82.190
          protrusion T82.190
          specified type NEC T82.190
        pain T82.847
        specified NEC T82.897
        stenosis T82.857
        thrombosis T82.867
      embolism T82.817
      fibrosis T82.827
      hemorrhage T82.837
      infection T82.7
      mechanical
        breakdown T82.119
        displacement T82.129
        leakage T82.199
        obstruction T82.199
        perforation T82.199
        protrusion T82.199
        specified type NEC T82.199
      pain T82.847
      pulse generator T82.9
        embolism T82.817
        fibrosis T82.827
        hemorrhage T82.837
        infection T82.7
        mechanical
          breakdown T82.111
          displacement T82.121
          leakage T82.191
          obstruction T82.191
          perforation T82.191
          protrusion T82.191
          specified type NEC T82.191
        pain T82.847
        specified NEC T82.897
        stenosis T82.857
        thrombosis T82.867
      specified condition NEC T82.897
      specified device NEC T82.9
        embolism T82.817
        fibrosis T82.827
        hemorrhage T82.837
        infection T82.7
        mechanical
          breakdown T82.118
          displacement T82.128
          leakage T82.198
          obstruction T82.198
          perforation T82.198
          protrusion T82.198
          specified type NEC T82.198
        pain T82.847
        specified NEC T82.897
        stenosis T82.857
        thrombosis T82.867
      stenosis T82.857
      thrombosis T82.867
    extremity artery graft —*see* Complication, extremity artery (bypass) graft
    femoral artery graft —*see* Complication, extremity artery (bypass) graft
  heart
    transplant —*see* Complication, transplant, heart

Complication *(Continued)*
    cystostomy (stoma) N99.518
        catheter —*see* Complications, catheter,
            cystostomy
        hemorrhage N99.510
        infection N99.511
        malfunction N99.512
        specified type NEC N99.518
    delivery —*see also* Complications, obstetric O75.9
        procedure (instrumental) (manual) (surgical)
            O75.4
        specified NEC O75.89
    dialysis (peritoneal) (renal) —*see also*
            Complications, infusion
        catheter (vascular) —*see* Complication,
            catheter, dialysis
            peritoneal, intraperitoneal —*see*
                Complications, catheter,
                intraperitoneal
    dorsal column (spinal) neurostimulator —*see*
            Complications, electronic stimulator device,
            spinal cord
    drug NEC T88.7
    ear procedure —*see also* Disorder, ear
        intraoperative H95.88-•
            hematoma —*see* Complications,
                intraoperative, hematoma (of), ear
            hemorrhage —*see* Complications,
                intraoperative, hemorrhage (of), ear
            laceration —*see* Complications,
                intraoperative, puncture or
                laceration..., ear
            seroma —*see* Complications,
                postprocedural, seroma (of), mastoid
                process
            specified NEC H95.88-•
        postoperative H95.89-•
            external ear canal stenosis H95.81-•
            hematoma —*see* Complications,
                postprocedural, hemorrhage
                (hematoma) (of), ear
            hemorrhage —*see* Complications,
                postprocedural, hemorrhage
                (hematoma) (of), ear
            postmastoidectomy —*see* Complications,
                postmastoidectomy
            specified NEC H95.89-•
    ectopic pregnancy O08.9
        damage to pelvic organs O08.6
        embolism O08.2
        genital infection O08.0
        hemorrhage (delayed) (excessive) O08.1
        metabolic disorder O08.5
        renal failure O08.4
        shock O08.3
        specified type NEC O08.0
        venous complication NEC O08.7
    electronic stimulator device
        bladder (urinary) —*see* Complications,
            electronic stimulator device, urinary
        bone T84.9
            breakdown T84.310
            displacement T84.320
            embolism T84.81
            fibrosis T84.82
            hemorrhage T84.83
            infection or inflammation T84.7
            malfunction T84.310
            malposition T84.320
            mechanical NEC T84.390
            obstruction T84.390
            pain T84.84
            perforation T84.390
            protrusion T84.390
            specified type NEC T84.89
            stenosis T84.85
            thrombosis T84.86
        brain T85.9
            embolism T85.810
            fibrosis T85.820
            hemorrhage T85.830
            infection and inflammation T85.731
            mechanical
                breakdown T85.110
                displacement T85.120
                leakage T85.190
                malposition T85.120
                obstruction T85.190
                perforation T85.190
                protrusion T85.190
                specified NEC T85.190

Complication *(Continued)*
    electronic stimulator device *(Continued)*
        brain *(Continued)*
            pain T85.840
            specified type NEC T85.890
            stenosis T85.850
            thrombosis T85.860
        cardiac (defibrillator) (pacemaker) —*see*
                Complications, cardiovascular device or
                implant, electronic
        generator (brain) (gastric) (peripheral) (sacral)
                (spinal)
            breakdown T85.113
            displacement T85.123
            leakage T85.193
            malposition T85.123
            obstruction T85.193
            perforation T85.193
            protrusion T85.193
            specified NEC T85.193
        muscle T84.9
            breakdown T84.418
            displacement T84.428
            embolism T84.81
            fibrosis T84.82
            hemorrhage T84.83
            infection or inflammation T84.7
            mechanical NEC T84.498
            pain T84.84
            specified type NEC T84.89
            stenosis T84.85
            thrombosis T84.86
        nervous system T85.9
            brain —*see* Complications, electronic
                stimulator device, brain
            cranial nerve —*see* Complications,
                electronic stimulator device,
                peripheral nerve
            embolism T85.810
            fibrosis T85.820
            gastric nerve —*see* Complications,
                electronic stimulator device,
                peripheral nerve
            hemorrhage T85.830
            infection and inflammation T85.738
            mechanical
                breakdown T85.118
                displacement T85.128
                leakage T85.199
                malposition T85.128
                obstruction T85.199
                perforation T85.199
                protrusion T85.199
                specified NEC T85.199
            pain T85.840
            peripheral nerve —*see* Complications,
                electronic stimulator device,
                peripheral nerve
            sacral nerve —*see* Complications, electronic
                stimulator device, peripheral
                nerve
            specified type NEC T85.890
            spinal cord —*see* Complications, electronic
                stimulator device, spinal cord
            stenosis T85.850
            thrombosis T85.860
            vagal nerve —*see* Complications, electronic
                stimulator device, peripheral nerve
        peripheral nerve T85.9
            embolism T85.810
            fibrosis T85.820
            hemorrhage T85.830
            infection and inflammation T85.732
            mechanical
                breakdown T85.111
                displacement T85.121
                leakage T85.191
                malposition T85.121
                obstruction T85.191
                perforation T85.191
                protrusion T85.191
                specified NEC T85.191
            pain T85.840
            specified type NEC T85.890
            stenosis T85.850
            thrombosis T85.860
        spinal cord T85.9
            embolism T85.810
            fibrosis T85.820
            hemorrhage T85.830
            infection and inflammation T85.733

Complication *(Continued)*
    electronic stimulator device *(Continued)*
        spinal cord *(Continued)*
            mechanical
                breakdown T85.112
                displacement T85.122
                leakage T85.192
                malposition T85.122
                obstruction T85.192
                perforation T85.192
                protrusion T85.192
                specified NEC T85.192
            pain T85.840
            specified type NEC T85.890
            stenosis T85.850
            thrombosis T85.860
        urinary T83.9
            embolism T83.81
            fibrosis T83.82
            hemorrhage T83.83
            infection and inflammation T83.598
            mechanical
                breakdown T83.110
                displacement T83.120
                malposition T83.120
                perforation T83.190
                protrusion T83.190
                specified NEC T83.190
            pain T83.84
            specified type NEC T83.89
            stenosis T83.85
            thrombosis T83.86
    electroshock therapy T88.9
        specified NEC T88.8
    endocrine E34.9
        postprocedural
            adrenal hypofunction E89.6
            hypoinsulinemia E89.1
            hypoparathyroidism E89.2
            hypopituitarism E89.3
            hypothyroidism E89.0
            ovarian failure E89.40
                asymptomatic E89.40
                symptomatic E89.41
            specified NEC E89.89
            testicular hypofunction E89.5
    endodontic treatment NEC M27.59
    enterostomy (stoma) K94.10
        hemorrhage K94.11
        infection K94.12
        malfunction K94.13
        mechanical K94.13
        specified complication NEC K94.19
    episiotomy, disruption O90.1
    esophageal anti-reflux device T85.9
        embolism T85.818
        fibrosis T85.828
        hemorrhage T85.838
        infection and inflammation T85.79
        mechanical
            breakdown T85.511
            displacement T85.521
            malfunction T85.511
            malposition T85.521
            obstruction T85.591
            perforation T85.591
            protrusion T85.591
            specified NEC T85.591
        pain T85.848
        specified type NEC T85.898
        stenosis T85.858
        thrombosis T85.868
    esophagostomy K94.30
        hemorrhage K94.31
        infection K94.32
        malfunction K94.33
        mechanical K94.33
        specified complication NEC K94.39
    extracorporeal circulation T80.90
    extremity artery (bypass) graft T82.9
        arteriosclerosis —*see* Arteriosclerosis,
            extremities, bypass graft
        embolism T82.818
        fibrosis T82.828
        hemorrhage T82.838
        infection and inflammation T82.7
        mechanical
            breakdown T82.318
                femoral artery T82.312
            displacement T82.328
                femoral artery T82.322

▶ New   ⇒ Revised   ~~deleted~~ Deleted   • Use Additional Character(s)

Complication *(Continued)*
  extremity arter *(Continued)*
    mechanical *(Continued)*
      leakage T82.338
        femoral artery T82.332
      malposition T82.328
        femoral artery T82.322
      obstruction T82.398
        femoral artery T82.392
      perforation T82.398
        femoral artery T82.392
      protrusion T82.398
        femoral artery T82.392
    pain T82.848
    specified type NEC T82.898
    stenosis T82.858
    thrombosis T82.868
  eye H57.9
    corneal graft —*see* Complications, graft,
      cornea
    implant (prosthetic) T85.9
      embolism T85.818
      fibrosis T85.828
      hemorrhage T85.838
      infection and inflammation
        T85.79
      mechanical
        breakdown T85.318
        displacement T85.328
        leakage T85.398
        malposition T85.328
        obstruction T85.398
        perforation T85.398
        protrusion T85.398
        specified NEC T85.398
      pain T85.848
      specified type NEC T85.898
      stenosis T85.858
      thrombosis T85.868
    intraocular lens —*see* Complications,
      intraocular lens
    orbital prosthesis —*see* Complications, orbital
      prosthesis
  female genital N94.9
    device, implant or graft NEC —*see*
      Complications, genitourinary, device or
      implant, genital tract
  femoral artery (bypass) graft —*see* Complication,
    extremity artery (bypass) graft
  fixation device, internal (orthopedic)
    T84.9
    infection and inflammation T84.60
      arm T84.61-●
        humerus T84.61-●
        radius T84.61-●
        ulna T84.61-●
      leg T84.629
        femur T84.62-●
        fibula T84.62-●
        tibia T84.62-●
      specified site NEC T84.69
      spine T84.63
    mechanical
      breakdown
        limb T84.119
          carpal T84.210
          femur T84.11-●
          fibula T84.11-●
          humerus T84.11-●
          metacarpal T84.210
          metatarsal T84.213
          phalanx
            foot T84.213
            hand T84.210
          radius T84.11-●
          tarsal T84.213
          tibia T84.11-●
          ulna T84.11-●
        specified bone NEC T84.218
        spine T84.216
      displacement
        limb T84.129
          carpal T84.220
          femur T84.12-●
          fibula T84.12-●
          humerus T84.12-●
          metacarpal T84.220
          metatarsal T84.223
          phalanx
            foot T84.223
            hand T84.220

Complication *(Continued)*
  fixation device, internal *(Continued)*
    mechanical *(Continued)*
      displacement *(Continued)*
        limb *(Continued)*
          radius T84.12-●
          tarsal T84.223
          tibia T84.12-●
          ulna T84.12-●
        specified bone NEC T84.228
        spine T84.226
      malposition —*see* Complications, fixation
        device, internal, mechanical,
        displacement
      obstruction —*see* Complications, fixation
        device, internal, mechanical, specified
        type NEC
      perforation —*see* Complications, fixation
        device, internal, mechanical, specified
        type NEC
      protrusion —*see* Complications, fixation
        device, internal, mechanical, specified
        type NEC
      specified type NEC
        limb T84.199
          carpal T84.290
          femur T84.19-●
          fibula T84.19-●
          humerus T84.19-●
          metacarpal T84.290
          metatarsal T84.293
          phalanx
            foot T84.293
            hand T84.290
          radius T84.19-●
          tarsal T84.293
          tibia T84.19-●
          ulna T84.19-●
        specified bone NEC T84.298
        vertebra T84.296
    specified type NEC T84.89
      embolism T84.81
      fibrosis T84.82
      hemorrhage T84.83
      pain T84.84
      specified complication NEC T84.89
      stenosis T84.85
      thrombosis T84.86
  following
    acute myocardial infarction NEC
      I23.8
      aneurysm (false) (of cardiac wall) (of heart
        wall) (ruptured) I23.3
      angina I23.7
      atrial
        septal defect I23.1
        thrombosis I23.6
      cardiac wall rupture I23.3
      chordae tendinae rupture I23.4
      defect
        septal
          atrial (heart) I23.1
          ventricular (heart) I23.2
      hemopericardium I23.0
      papillary muscle rupture I23.5
      rupture
        cardiac wall I23.3
          with hemopericardium I23.0
        chordae tendineae I23.4
        papillary muscle I23.5
      specified NEC I23.8
      thrombosis
        atrium I23.6
        auricular appendage I23.6
        ventricle (heart) I23.6
      ventricular
        septal defect I23.2
        thrombosis I23.6
    ectopic or molar pregnancy O08.9
      cardiac arrest O08.81
      sepsis O08.82
      specified type NEC O08.89
      urinary tract infection O08.83
    termination of pregnancy —*see*
      Abortion
  gastrointestinal K92.9
    bile duct prosthesis —*see* Complications, bile
      duct implant
    esophageal anti-reflux device —*see*
      Complications, esophageal anti-reflux
      device

Complication *(Continued)*
  gastrointestinal *(Continued)*
    postoperative
      colostomy —*see* Complications, colostomy
      dumping syndrome K91.1
      enterostomy —*see* Complications,
        enterostomy
      gastrostomy —*see* Complications,
        gastrostomy
      malabsorption NEC K91.2
      obstruction —*see also* Obstruction, intestine,
        postoperative K91.30
      postcholecystectomy syndrome K91.5
      specified NEC K91.89
      vomiting after GI surgery K91.0
    prosthetic device or implant
      bile duct prosthesis —*see* Complications,
        bile duct implant
      esophageal anti-reflux device —*see*
        Complications, esophageal
        anti-reflux device
      specified type NEC
        embolism T85.818
        fibrosis T85.828
        hemorrhage T85.838
        mechanical
          breakdown T85.518
          displacement T85.528
          malfunction T85.518
          malposition T85.528
          obstruction T85.598
          perforation T85.598
          protrusion T85.598
          specified NEC T85.598
        pain T85.848
        specified complication NEC T85.898
        stenosis T85.858
        thrombosis T85.868
  gastrostomy (stoma) K94.20
    hemorrhage K94.21
    infection K94.22
    malfunction K94.23
    mechanical K94.23
    specified complication NEC K94.29
  genitourinary
    device or implant T83.9
      genital tract T83.9
        infection or inflammation T83.69
        intrauterine contraceptive device —*see*
          Complications, intrauterine,
          contraceptive device
        mechanical —*see* Complications, by
          device, mechanical
        mesh —*see* Complications, prosthetic
          device or implant, mesh
        penile prosthesis —*see* Complications,
          prosthetic device, penile
        specified type NEC T83.89
          embolism T83.81
          fibrosis T83.82
          hemorrhage T83.83
          pain T83.84
          specified complication NEC T83.89
          stenosis T83.85
          thrombosis T83.86
        vaginal mesh —*see* Complications,
          prosthetic device or implant, mesh
      urinary system T83.9
        cystostomy catheter —*see* Complication,
          catheter, cystostomy
        electronic stimulator —*see*
          Complications, electronic stimulator
          device, urinary
        indwelling urethral catheter —*see*
          Complications, catheter, urethral,
          indwelling
        infection or inflammation T83.598
          indwelling urethral catheter T83.511
        kidney transplant —*see* Complication,
          transplant, kidney
        organ graft —*see* Complication, graft,
          urinary organ
        specified type NEC T83.89
          embolism T83.81
          fibrosis T83.82
          hemorrhage T83.83
          mechanical T83.198
            breakdown T83.118
            displacement T83.128
            malfunction T83.118
            malposition T83.128

Complication *(Continued)*
  genitourinary *(Continued)*
    device or implant *(Continued)*
      urinary system *(Continued)*
        specified type *(Continued)*
          mechanical *(Continued)*
            obstruction T83.198
            perforation T83.198
            protrusion T83.198
            specified NEC T83.198
          sphincter, implanted T83.191
          stent (ileal conduit) (nephroureteral)
            T83.193
          ureteral indwelling T83.192
          pain T83.84
          specified complication NEC T83.89
          stenosis T83.85
          thrombosis T83.86
        sphincter implant —*see* Complications,
          implant, urinary sphincter
    postprocedural
      pelvic peritoneal adhesions N99.4
      renal failure N99.0
      specified NEC N99.89
      stoma —*see* Complications, stoma, urinary
        tract
      urethral stricture —*see* Stricture, urethra,
        postprocedural
      vaginal
        adhesions N99.2
        vault prolapse N99.3
  graft (bypass) (patch) —*see also* Complications,
      prosthetic device or implant
    aorta —*see* Complications, graft, vascular
    arterial —*see* Complication, graft, vascular
    bone T86.839
      failure T86.831
      infection T86.832
      mechanical T84.318
        breakdown T84.318
        displacement T84.328
        protrusion T84.398
        specified type NEC T84.398
      rejection T86.830
      specified type NEC T86.838
    carotid artery —*see* Complications, graft,
        vascular
    cornea T86.849-
      failure T86.841-
      infection T86.842-
      mechanical T85.398
        breakdown T85.318
        displacement T85.328
        protrusion T85.398
        specified type NEC T85.398
      rejection T86.840-
      retroprosthetic membrane T85.398
      specified type NEC T86.848-
    femoral artery (bypass) —*see* Complication,
        extremity artery (bypass) graft
    genital organ or tract —*see* Complications,
        genitourinary, device or implant, genital
        tract
    muscle T84.9
      breakdown T84.410
      displacement T84.420
      embolism T84.81
      fibrosis T84.82
      hemorrhage T84.83
      infection and inflammation T84.7
      mechanical NEC T84.490
      pain T84.84
      specified type NEC T84.89
      stenosis T84.85
      thrombosis T84.86
    nerve —*see* Complication, prosthetic device or
        implant, specified NEC
    skin —*see* Complications, prosthetic device or
        implant, skin graft
    tendon T84.9
      breakdown T84.410
      displacement T84.420
      embolism T84.81
      fibrosis T84.82
      hemorrhage T84.83
      infection and inflammation T84.7
      mechanical NEC T84.490
      pain T84.84
      specified type NEC T84.89
      stenosis T84.85
      thrombosis T84.86

Complication *(Continued)*
  graft *(Continued)*
    urinary organ T83.9
      embolism T83.81
      fibrosis T83.82
      hemorrhage T83.83
      infection and inflammation T83.598
        indwelling urethral catheter T83.511
      mechanical
        breakdown T83.21
        displacement T83.22
        erosion T83.24
        exposure T83.25
        leakage T83.23
        malposition T83.22
        obstruction T83.29
        perforation T83.29
        protrusion T83.29
        specified NEC T83.29
      pain T83.84
      specified type NEC T83.89
      stenosis T83.85
      thrombosis T83.86
    vascular T82.9
      embolism T82.818
      femoral artery —*see* Complication,
        extremity artery (bypass) graft
      fibrosis T82.828
      hemorrhage T82.838
      mechanical
        breakdown T82.319
          aorta (bifurcation) T82.310
          carotid artery T82.311
          specified vessel NEC T82.318
        displacement T82.329
          aorta (bifurcation) T82.320
          carotid artery T82.321
          specified vessel NEC T82.328
        leakage T82.339
          aorta (bifurcation) T82.330
          carotid artery T82.331
          specified vessel NEC T82.338
        malposition T82.329
          aorta (bifurcation) T82.320
          carotid artery T82.321
          specified vessel NEC T82.328
        obstruction T82.399
          aorta (bifurcation) T82.390
          carotid artery T82.391
          specified vessel NEC T82.398
        perforation T82.399
          aorta (bifurcation) T82.390
          carotid artery T82.391
          specified vessel NEC T82.398
        protrusion T82.399
          aorta (bifurcation) T82.390
          carotid artery T82.391
          specified vessel NEC T82.398
      pain T82.848
      specified complication NEC T82.898
      stenosis T82.858
      thrombosis T82.868
  heart I51.9
    assist device
      infection and inflammation T82.7
    following acute myocardial infarction —
      see Complications, following, acute
      myocardial infarction
    postoperative —*see* Complications, circulatory
      system
    transplant —*see* Complication, transplant, heart
      and lung(s) —*see* Complications, transplant,
        heart, with lung
    valve
      graft (biological) T82.9
        embolism T82.817
        fibrosis T82.827
        hemorrhage T82.837
        infection and inflammation T82.7
        mechanical T82.228
          breakdown T82.221
          displacement T82.222
          leakage T82.223
          malposition T82.222
          obstruction T82.228
          perforation T82.228
          protrusion T82.228
        pain T82.847
        specified type NEC T82.897
        stenosis T82.857
        thrombosis T82.867

Complication *(Continued)*
  heart *(Continued)*
    valve *(Continued)*
      prosthesis T82.9
        embolism T82.817
        fibrosis T82.827
        hemorrhage T82.837
        infection or inflammation T82.6
        mechanical T82.09
          breakdown T82.01
          displacement T82.02
          leakage T82.03
          malposition T82.02
          obstruction T82.09
          perforation T82.09
          protrusion T82.09
        pain T82.847
        specified type NEC T82.897
          mechanical T82.09
        stenosis T82.857
        thrombosis T82.867
  hematoma
    intraoperative —*see* Complication,
      intraoperative, hemorrhage
    postprocedural —*see* Complication,
      postprocedural, hematoma
  hemodialysis —*see* Complications, dialysis
  hemorrhage
    intraoperative —*see* Complication,
      intraoperative, hemorrhage
    postprocedural —*see* Complication,
      postprocedural, hemorrhage
  IEC (immune effector cellular) therapy T80.82
  ileostomy (stoma) —*see* Complications,
    enterostomy
  immune effector cellular (IEC) therapy T80.82
  immunization (procedure) —*see* Complications,
    vaccination
  implant —*see also* Complications, by site and type
    urinary sphincter T83.9
      embolism T83.81
      fibrosis T83.82
      hemorrhage T83.83
      infection and inflammation T83.591
      mechanical
        breakdown T83.111
        displacement T83.121
        leakage T83.191
        malposition T83.121
        obstruction T83.191
        perforation T83.191
        protrusion T83.191
        specified NEC T83.191
      pain T83.84
      specified type NEC T83.89
      stenosis T83.85
      thrombosis T83.86
  infusion (procedure) T80.90
    air embolism T80.0
    blood —*see* Complications, transfusion
    catheter —*see* Complications, catheter
    infection T80.29
    pump —*see* Complications, cardiovascular,
      device or implant
    sepsis T80.29
    serum reaction —*see also* Reaction, serum T80.69
      anaphylactic shock —*see also* Shock,
        anaphylactic T80.59
    specified type NEC T80.89
  inhalation therapy NEC T81.81
  injection (procedure) T80.90
    drug reaction —*see* Reaction, drug
    infection T80.29
    sepsis T80.29
    serum (prophylactic) (therapeutic) —*see*
      Complications, vaccination
    specified type NEC T80.89
    vaccine (any) —*see* Complications, vaccination
  inoculation (any) —*see* Complications,
    vaccination
  insulin pump
    infection and inflammation T85.72
    mechanical
      breakdown T85.614
      displacement T85.624
      leakage T85.633
      malposition T85.624
      obstruction T85.694
      perforation T85.694
      protrusion T85.694
      specified NEC T85.694

Complication *(Continued)*
  intestinal pouch NEC K91.858
  intraocular lens (prosthetic) T85.9
    embolism T85.818
    fibrosis T85.828
    hemorrhage T85.838
    infection and inflammation T85.79
    mechanical
      breakdown T85.21
      displacement T85.22
      malposition T85.22
      obstruction T85.29
      perforation T85.29
      protrusion T85.29
      specified NEC T85.29
    pain T85.848
    specified type NEC T85.898
    stenosis T85.858
    thrombosis T85.868
  intraoperative (intraprocedural)
    cardiac arrest —*see also* Infarct, myocardium, associated with revascularization procedure
      during cardiac surgery I97.710
      during other surgery I97.711
    cardiac functional disturbance NEC —*see also* Infarct, myocardium, associated with revascularization procedure
      during cardiac surgery I97.790
      during other surgery I97.791
    hemorrhage (hematoma) (of)
      circulatory system organ or structure
        during cardiac bypass I97.411
        during cardiac catheterization I97.410
        during other circulatory system procedure I97.418
        during other procedure I97.42
      digestive system organ
        during procedure on digestive system K91.61
        during procedure on other organ K91.62
      ear
        during procedure on ear and mastoid process H95.21
        during procedure on other organ H95.22
      endocrine system organ or structure
        during procedure on endocrine system organ or structure E36.01
        during procedure on other organ E36.02
      eye and adnexa
        during ophthalmic procedure H59.11-●
        during other procedure H59.12-●
      genitourinary organ or structure
        during procedure on genitourinary organ or structure N99.61
        during procedure on other organ N99.62
      mastoid process
        during procedure on ear and mastoid process H95.21
        during procedure on other organ H95.22
      musculoskeletal structure
        during musculoskeletal surgery M96.810
        during non-orthopedic surgery M96.811
        during orthopedic surgery M96.810
      nervous system
        during a nervous system procedure G97.31
        during other procedure G97.32
      respiratory system
        during other procedure J95.62
        during procedure on respiratory system organ or structure J95.61
      skin and subcutaneous tissue
        during a dermatologic procedure L76.01
        during a procedure on other organ L76.02
      spleen
        during a procedure on other organ D78.02
        during a procedure on the spleen D78.01
    puncture or laceration (accidental) (unintentional) (of)
      brain
        during a nervous system procedure G97.48
        during other procedure G97.49
      circulatory system organ or structure
        during circulatory system procedure I97.51
        during other procedure I97.52

Complication *(Continued)*
  intraoperative *(Continued)*
    puncture or laceration *(Continued)*
      digestive system
        during procedure on digestive system K91.71
        during procedure on other organ K91.72
      ear
        during procedure on ear and mastoid process H95.31
        during procedure on other organ H95.32
      endocrine system organ or structure
        during procedure on endocrine system organ or structure E36.11
        during procedure on other organ E36.12
      eye and adnexa
        during ophthalmic procedure H59.21-●
        during other procedure H59.22-●
      genitourinary organ or structure
        during procedure on genitourinary organ or structure N99.71
        during procedure on other organ N99.72
      mastoid process
        during procedure on ear and mastoid process H95.31
        during procedure on other organ H95.32
      musculoskeletal structure
        during musculoskeletal surgery M96.820
        during non-orthopedic surgery M96.821
        during orthopedic surgery M96.820
      nervous system
        during a nervous system procedure G97.48
        during other procedure G97.49
      respiratory system
        during other procedure J95.72
        during procedure on respiratory system organ or structure J95.71
      skin and subcutaneous tissue
        during a dermatologic procedure L76.11
        during a procedure on other organ L76.12
      spleen
        during a procedure on other organ D78.12
        during a procedure on the spleen D78.11
    specified NEC
      circulatory system I97.88
      digestive system K91.81
      ear H95.88
      endocrine system E36.8
      eye and adnexa H59.88
      genitourinary system N99.81
      mastoid process H95.88
      musculoskeletal structure M96.89
      nervous system G97.81
      respiratory system J95.88
      skin and subcutaneous tissue L76.81
      spleen D78.81
  intraperitoneal catheter (dialysis) (infusion) —*see* Complication(s), catheter, intraperitoneal dialysis
  intrathecal infusion pump
    infection and inflammation T85.738
    mechanical
      breakdown T85.615
      displacement T85.625
      leakage T85.635
      malfunction T85.695
      malposition T85.625
      obstruction T85.695
      perforation T85.695
      protrusion T85.695
      specified NEC T85.695
  intrauterine
    contraceptive device
      embolism T83.81
      fibrosis T83.82
      hemorrhage T83.83
      infection and inflammation T83.69
      mechanical
        breakdown T83.31
        displacement T83.32
        malposition T83.32
        obstruction T83.39
        perforation T83.39
        protrusion T83.39
        specified NEC T83.39
      pain T83.84
      specified type NEC T83.89
      stenosis T83.85
      thrombosis T83.86
    procedure (fetal), to newborn P96.5

Complication *(Continued)*
  jejunostomy (stoma) —*see* Complications, enterostomy
  joint prosthesis, internal T84.9
    breakage (fracture) T84.01-●
    dislocation T84.02-●
    displacement T84.02-●
    fracture T84.01-●
    infection or inflammation T84.50
      hip T84.5-●
      knee T84.5-●
      specified joint NEC T84.59
    instability T84.02-●
    malposition —*see* Complications, joint prosthesis, mechanical, displacement
    mechanical
      breakage, broken T84.01-●
      dislocation T84.02-●
      fracture T84.01-●
      instability T84.02-●
      leakage —*see* Complications, joint prosthesis, mechanical, specified NEC
      loosening T84.039
        hip T84.03-●
        knee T84.03-●
        specified joint NEC T84.038
      obstruction —*see* Complications, joint prosthesis, mechanical, specified NEC
      ▶osteolysis T84.059
      ▶hip T84.05-●
      ▶knee T84.05-●
      perforation —*see* Complications, joint prosthesis, mechanical, specified NEC
      osteolysis T84.059
        ~~hip T84.05-●~~
        ~~knee T84.05-●~~
        other specified joint T84.058
      periprosthetic osteolysis, by site T84.05-●
      protrusion —*see* Complications, joint prosthesis, mechanical, specified NEC
      specified complication NEC T84.099
        hip T84.09-●
        knee T84.09-●
        other specified joint T84.098
      subluxation T84.02-●
      wear of articular bearing surface T84.069
        hip T84.06-●
        knee T84.06-●
        other specified joint T84.068
    specified joint NEC T84.89
      embolism T84.81
      fibrosis T84.82
      hemorrhage T84.83
      pain T84.84
      specified complication NEC T84.89
      stenosis T84.85
      thrombosis T84.86
    subluxation T84.02-●
  kidney transplant —*see* Complications, transplant, kidney
  labor O75.9
    specified NEC O75.89
  liver transplant (immune or nonimmune) —*see* Complications, transplant, liver
  lumbar puncture G97.1
    cerebrospinal fluid leak G97.0
    headache or reaction G97.1
  lung transplant —*see* Complications, transplant, lung
    and heart —*see* Complications, transplant, lung, with heart
  male genital N50.9
    device, implant or graft —*see* Complications, genitourinary, device or implant, genital tract
    postprocedural or postoperative —*see* Complications, genitourinary, postprocedural
    specified NEC N99.89
  mastoid (process) procedure
    intraoperative H95.88-●
      hematoma —*see* Complications, intraoperative, hemorrhage (hematoma) (of), mastoid process
      hemorrhage —*see* Complications, intraoperative, hemorrhage (hematoma) (of), mastoid process
      laceration —*see* Complications, intraoperative, puncture or laceration..., mastoid process
    specified NEC H95.88-●

Complication *(Continued)*
  mastoid (process) procedure *(Continued)*
    postmastoidectomy —*see* Complications,
        postmastoidectomy
    postoperative H95.89-●
      external ear canal stenosis H95.81-●
      hematoma —*see* Complications...,
          postprocedural, hematoma (of),
          mastoid process
      hemorrhage —*see* Complications...,
          postprocedural, hemorrhage (of),
          mastoid process
      postmastoidectomy —*see* Complications,
          postmastoidectomy
      seroma —*see* Complications,
          postprocedural, seroma (of), mastoid
          process
      specified NEC H95.89-●
  mastoidectomy cavity —*see* Complications,
      postmastoidectomy
  mechanical —*see* Complications, by site and
      type, mechanical
  medical procedures (*see also* Complication(s),
      intraoperative) T88.9
  metabolic E88.9
    postoperative E89.89
    specified NEC E89.89
  molar pregnancy NOS O08.9
    damage to pelvic organs O08.6
    embolism O08.2
    genital infection O08.0
    hemorrhage (delayed) (excessive) O08.1
    metabolic disorder O08.5
    renal failure O08.4
    shock O08.3
    specified type NEC O08.0
    venous complication NEC O08.7
  musculoskeletal system —*see also* Complication,
      intraoperative (intraprocedural), by site
    device, implant or graft NEC —*see*
        Complications, orthopedic, device or
        implant
    internal fixation (nail) (plate) (rod) —*see*
        Complications, fixation device,
        internal
    joint prosthesis —*see* Complications, joint
        prosthesis
    postoperative (postprocedural) M96.89
      with osteoporosis —*see* Osteoporosis
      fracture following insertion of device —
          see Fracture, following insertion of
          orthopedic implant, joint prosthesis or
          bone plate
      joint instability after prosthesis removal
          M96.89
      lordosis M96.4
      postlaminectomy syndrome NEC M96.1
        kyphosis M96.2
      pseudarthrosis M96.0
      specified complication NEC M96.89
    post radiation M96.89
      kyphosis M96.3
      scoliosis M96.5
      specified complication NEC M96.89
  nephrostomy (stoma) —*see* Complications,
      stoma, urinary tract, external NEC
  nervous system G98.8
    central G96.9
      device, implant or graft —*see also*
          Complication, prosthetic device or
          implant, specified NEC
      electronic stimulator (electrode(s)) —*see*
          Complications, electronic stimulator
          device
      specified NEC
        infection and inflammation T85.738
        mechanical T85.695
          breakdown T85.615
          displacement T85.625
          leakage T85.635
          malfunction T85.695
          malposition T85.625
          obstruction T85.695
          perforation T85.695
          protrusion T85.695
          specified NEC T85.695
      ventricular shunt —*see* Complications,
          ventricular shunt
      electronic stimulator (electrode(s)) —*see*
          Complications, electronic stimulator
          device

Complication *(Continued)*
  nervous system *(Continued)*
    postprocedural G97.82
      intracranial hypotension G97.2
      specified NEC G97.82
      spinal fluid leak G97.0
    newborn, due to intrauterine (fetal) procedure
        P96.5
  nonabsorbable (permanent) sutures —*see*
      Complication, sutures, permanent
  obstetric O75.9
    procedure (instrumental) (manual) (surgical)
        specified NEC O75.4
    specified NEC O75.89
    surgical wound NEC O90.89
      hematoma O90.2
      infection O86.00
  ocular lens implant —*see* Complications,
      intraocular lens
  ophthalmologic
    postprocedural bleb —*see* Blebitis
  orbital prosthesis T85.9
    embolism T85.818
    fibrosis T85.828
    hemorrhage T85.838
    infection and inflammation T85.79
    mechanical
      breakdown T85.31-●
      displacement T85.32-●
      malposition T85.32-●
      obstruction T85.39-●
      perforation T85.39-●
      protrusion T85.39-●
      specified NEC T85.39-●
    pain T85.848
    specified type NEC T85.898
    stenosis T85.858
    thrombosis T85.868
  organ or tissue transplant (partial) (total) —*see*
      Complications, transplant
  orthopedic —*see also* Disorder, soft tissue
    device or implant T84.9
      bone
        device or implant —*see* Complication,
            bone, device NEC
        graft —*see* Complication, graft, bone
      breakdown T84.418
      displacement T84.428
      electronic bone stimulator —*see*
          Complications, electronic stimulator
          device, bone
      embolism T84.81
      fibrosis T84.82
      fixation device —*see* Complication, fixation
          device, internal
      hemorrhage T84.83
      infection or inflammation T84.7
      joint prosthesis —*see* Complication, joint
          prosthesis, internal
      malfunction T84.418
      malposition T84.428
      mechanical NEC T84.498
      muscle graft —*see* Complications, graft,
          muscle
      obstruction T84.498
      pain T84.84
      perforation T84.498
      protrusion T84.498
      specified complication NEC T84.89
      stenosis T84.85
      tendon graft —*see* Complications, graft,
          tendon
      thrombosis T84.86
    fracture (following insertion of device) —
        see Fracture, following insertion of
        orthopedic implant, joint prosthesis or
        bone plate
    postprocedural M96.89
      fracture —*see* Fracture, following insertion
          of orthopedic implant, joint prosthesis
          or bone plate
      postlaminectomy syndrome NEC M96.1
        kyphosis M96.3
        lordosis M96.4
      postradiation
        kyphosis M96.2
        scoliosis M96.5
      pseudarthrosis post-fusion M96.0
      specified type NEC M96.89
  pacemaker (cardiac) —*see* Complications,
      cardiovascular device or implant, electronic

Complication *(Continued)*
  pancreas transplant —*see* Complications,
      transplant, pancreas
  penile prosthesis (implant) —*see* Complications,
      prosthetic device, penile
  perfusion NEC T80.90
  perineal repair (obstetrical) NEC O90.89
    disruption O90.1
    hematoma O90.2
    infection (following delivery) O86.09
  phototherapy T88.9
    specified NEC T88.8
  postmastoidectomy NEC H95.19-●
    cyst, mucosal H95.13-●
    granulation H95.12-●
    inflammation, chronic H95.11-●
    recurrent cholesteatoma H95.0-●
  postoperative —*see* Complications,
      postprocedural
    circulatory —*see* Complications, circulatory
        system
    ear —*see* Complications, ear
    endocrine —*see* Complications, endocrine
    eye —*see* Complications, eye
    lumbar puncture G97.1
      cerebrospinal fluid leak G97.0
    nervous system (central) (peripheral) —*see*
        Complications, nervous system
    respiratory system —*see* Complications,
        respiratory system
  postprocedural —*see also* Complications, surgical
      procedure
    cardiac arrest —*see also* Infarct, myocardium,
        associated with revascularization
        procedure
      following cardiac surgery I97.120
      following other surgery I97.121
    cardiac functional disturbance NEC —*see also*
        Infarct, myocardium, associated with
        revascularization procedure
      following cardiac surgery I97.190
      following other surgery I97.191
    cardiac insufficiency
      following cardiac surgery I97.110
      following other surgery I97.111
    chorioretinal scars following retinal surgery
        H59.81-●
    following cataract surgery
      cataract (lens) fragments H59.02-●
      cystoid macular edema H59.03-●
      specified NEC H59.09-●
      vitreous (touch) syndrome H59.01-●
    heart failure
      following cardiac surgery I97.130
      following other surgery I97.131
    hematoma (of)
      circulatory system organ or structure
        following cardiac bypass I97.631
        following cardiac catheterization I97.630
        following other circulatory system
            procedure I97.638
        following other procedure I97.621
      digestive system
        following procedure on digestive system
            K91.870
        following procedure on other organ
            K91.871
      ear
        following other procedure H95.52
        following procedure on ear and mastoid
            process H95.51
      endocrine system
        following endocrine system procedure
            E89.820
        following other procedure E89.821
      eye and adnexa
        following ophthalmic procedure
            H59.33-●
        following other procedure H59.34-●
      genitourinary organ or structure
        following procedure on genitourinary
            organ or structure N99.840
        following procedure on other organ
            N99.841
      mastoid process
        following other procedure H95.52
        following procedure on ear and mastoid
            process H95.51
      musculoskeletal structure
        following musculoskeletal surgery
            M96.840

▶ New   ⇒ Revised   ~~deleted~~ Deleted   ● Use Additional Character(s)

Complication *(Continued)*
  postprocedural *(Continued)*
    hematoma *(Continued)*
      musculoskeletal structure *(Continued)*
        following non-orthopedic surgery M96.841
        following orthopedic surgery M96.840
      nervous system
        following nervous system procedure G97.61
        following other procedure G97.62
      respiratory system
        following other procedure J95.861
        following procedure on respiratory system organ or structure J95.860
      skin and subcutaneous tissue
        following dermatologic procedure L76.31
        following procedure on other organ L76.32
      spleen
        following procedure on other organ D78.32
        following procedure on the spleen D78.31
    hemorrhage (of)
      circulatory system organ or structure
        following cardiac bypass I97.611
        following cardiac catheterization I97.610
        following other circulatory system procedure I97.618
        following other procedure I97.620
      digestive system
        following procedure on digestive system K91.840
        following procedure on other organ K91.841
      ear
        following other procedure H95.42
        following procedure on ear and mastoid process H95.41
      endocrine system
        following endocrine system procedure E89.810
        following other procedure E89.811
      eye and adnexa
        following ophthalmic procedure H59.31-●
        following other procedure H59.32-●
      genitourinary organ or structure
        following procedure on genitourinary organ or structure N99.820
        following procedure on other organ N99.821
      mastoid process
        following other procedure H95.42
        following procedure on ear and mastoid process H95.41
      musculoskeletal structure
        following musculoskeletal surgery M96.830
        following non-orthopedic surgery M96.831
        following orthopedic surgery M96.830
      nervous system
        following nervous system procedure G97.51
        following other procedure G97.52
      respiratory system
        following other procedure J95.831
        following procedure on respiratory system organ or structure J95.830
      skin and subcutaneous tissue
        following dermatologic procedure L76.21
        following a procedure on other organ L76.22
      spleen
        following procedure on other organ D78.22
        following procedure on the spleen D78.21
    seroma (of)
      circulatory system organ or structure
        following cardiac bypass I97.641
        following cardiac catheterization I97.640
        following other circulatory system procedure I97.648
        following other procedure I97.622
      digestive system
        following procedure on digestive system K91.872
        following procedure on other organ K91.873

Complication *(Continued)*
  postprocedural *(Continued)*
    seroma *(Continued)*
      ear
        following other procedure H95.54
        following procedure on ear and mastoid process H95.53
      endocrine system
        following endocrine system procedure E89.822
        following other procedure E89.823
      eye and adnexa
        following ophthalmic procedure H59.35-●
        following other procedure H59.36-●
      genitourinary organ or structure
        following procedure on genitourinary organ or structure N99.842
        following procedure on other organ N99.843
      mastoid process
        following other procedure H95.54
        following procedure on ear and mastoid process H95.53
      musculoskeletal structure
        following musculoskeletal surgery M96.842
        following non-orthopedic surgery M96.843
        following orthopedic surgery M96.842
      nervous system
        following nervous system procedure G97.63
        following other procedure G97.64
      respiratory system
        following other procedure J95.863
        following procedure on respiratory system organ or structure J95.862
      skin and subcutaneous tissue
        following dermatologic procedure L76.33
        following procedure on other organ L76.34
      spleen
        following procedure on other organ D78.34
        following procedure on the spleen D78.33
    specified NEC
      circulatory system I97.89
      digestive K91.89
      ear H95.89
      endocrine E89.89
      eye and adnexa H59.89
      genitourinary N99.89
      mastoid process H95.89
      metabolic E89.89
      musculoskeletal structure M96.89
      nervous system G97.82
      respiratory system J95.89
      skin and subcutaneous tissue L76.82
      spleen D78.89
  pregnancy NEC —*see* Pregnancy, complicated by
  prosthetic device or implant T85.9
    bile duct —*see* Complications, bile duct implant
    breast —*see* Complications, breast implant
    bulking agent
      ureteral
        erosion T83.714
        exposure T83.724
      urethral
        erosion T83.713
        exposure T83.723
    cardiac and vascular NEC —*see* Complications, cardiovascular device or implant
    corneal transplant —*see* Complications, graft, cornea
    electronic nervous system stimulator —*see* Complications, electronic stimulator device
    epidural infusion catheter —*see* Complications, catheter, epidural
    esophageal anti-reflux device —*see* Complications, esophageal anti-reflux device
    genital organ or tract —*see* Complications, genitourinary, device or implant, genital tract
      specified NEC T83.79
    heart valve —*see* Complications, heart, valve, prosthesis

Complication *(Continued)*
  postprocedural *(Continued)*
    prosthetic device or implant *(Continued)*
      infection or inflammation T85.79
        intestine transplant T86.852
        liver transplant T86.43
        lung transplant T86.812
        pancreas transplant T86.892
        skin graft T86.822
      intraocular lens —*see* Complications, intraocular lens
      intraperitoneal (dialysis) catheter —*see* Complication(s), catheter, intraperitoneal dialysis
      joint —*see* Complications, joint prosthesis, internal
      mechanical NEC T85.698
        dialysis catheter (vascular) —*see also* Complication, catheter, dialysis, mechanical
        peritoneal —*see* Complication(s), catheter, intraperitoneal dialysis
        gastrointestinal device T85.598
        ocular device T85.398
        subdural (infusion) catheter T85.690
        suture, permanent T85.692
          that for bone repair —*see* Complications, fixation device, internal (orthopedic), mechanical
        ventricular shunt
          breakdown T85.01
          displacement T85.02
          leakage T85.03
          malposition T85.02
          obstruction T85.09
          perforation T85.09
          protrusion T85.09
          specified NEC T85.09
      mesh
        erosion (to surrounding organ or tissue) T83.718
          urethral (into pelvic floor muscles) T83.712
          vaginal (into pelvic floor muscles) T83.711
        exposure (into surrounding organ or tissue) T83.728
          urethral (through urethral wall) T83.722
          vaginal (into vagina) (through vaginal wall) T83.721
      orbital —*see* Complications, orbital prosthesis
      penile T83.9
        embolism T83.81
        fibrosis T83.82
        hemorrhage T83.83
        infection and inflammation T83.61
        mechanical
          breakdown T83.410
          displacement T83.420
          leakage T83.490
          malposition T83.420
          obstruction T83.490
          perforation T83.490
          protrusion T83.490
          specified NEC T83.490
        pain T83.84
        specified type NEC T83.89
        stenosis T83.85
        thrombosis T83.86
      prosthetic materials NEC
        erosion (to surrounding organ or tissue) T83.718
        exposure (into surrounding organ or tissue) T83.728
      skin graft T86.829
        artificial skin or decellularized allodermis
          embolism T85.818
          fibrosis T85.828
          hemorrhage T85.838
          infection and inflammation T85.79
          mechanical
            breakdown T85.613
            displacement T85.623
            malfunction T85.613
            malposition T85.623
            obstruction T85.693
            perforation T85.693
            protrusion T85.693
            specified NEC T85.693
          pain T85.848
          specified type NEC T85.898
          stenosis T85.858
          thrombosis T85.868

Complication *(Continued)*
  prosthetic device or implant *(Continued)*
    skin graft *(Continued)*
      failure T86.821
      infection T86.822
      rejection T86.820
      specified NEC T86.828
    sling
      urethral (female) (male)
        erosion T83.712
        exposure T83.722
    specified NEC T85.9
      embolism T85.818
      fibrosis T85.828
      hemorrhage T85.838
      infection and inflammation T85.79
      mechanical
        breakdown T85.618
        displacement T85.628
        leakage T85.638
        malfunction T85.618
        malposition T85.628
        obstruction T85.698
        perforation T85.698
        protrusion T85.698
        specified NEC T85.698
      pain T85.848
      specified type NEC T85.898
      stenosis T85.858
      thrombosis T85.868
    subdural infusion catheter *—see*
      Complications, catheter, subdural
    sutures *—see* Complications, sutures
    urinary organ or tract NEC *—see*
      Complications, genitourinary, device or
      implant, urinary system
    vascular *—see* Complications, cardiovascular
      device, graft or implant
    ventricular shunt *—see* Complications,
      ventricular shunt (device)
  puerperium *—see* Puerperal
  puncture, spinal G97.1
    cerebrospinal fluid leak G97.0
    headache or reaction G97.1
  pyelogram N99.89
  radiation
    kyphosis M96.2
    scoliosis M96.5
  reattached
    extremity (infection) (rejection)
      lower T87.1X-●
      upper T87.0X-●
    specified body part NEC T87.2
  reconstructed breast
    asymmetry between native and reconstructed
      breast N65.1
    deformity N65.0
    disproportion between native and
      reconstructed breast N65.1
    excess tissue N65.0
    misshappen N65.0
  reimplant NEC *—see also* Complications,
    prosthetic device or implant
    limb (infection) (rejection) *—see*
      Complications, reattached, extremity
    organ (partial) (total) *—see* Complications,
      transplant
    prosthetic device NEC *—see* Complications,
      prosthetic device
  renal N28.9
    allograft *—see* Complications, transplant, kidney
    dialysis *—see* Complications, dialysis
  respirator
    mechanical J95.850
      specified NEC J95.859
  respiratory system J98.9
    device, implant or graft *—see* Complication,
      prosthetic device or implant, specified
      NEC
    lung transplant *—see* Complications,
      prosthetic device or implant, lung
      transplant
    postoperative J95.89
      air leak J95.812
      Mendelson's syndrome (chemical
        pneumonitis) J95.4
      pneumothorax J95.811
      pulmonary insufficiency (acute) (after
        nonthoracic surgery) J95.2
        chronic J95.3
        following thoracic surgery J95.1

Complication *(Continued)*
  respiratory system *(Continued)*
    postoperative *(Continued)*
      respiratory failure (acute) J95.821
        acute and chronic J95.822
      specified NEC J95.89
      subglottic stenosis J95.5
      tracheostomy complication *—see*
        Complications, tracheostomy
    therapy T81.89
  sedation during labor and delivery O74.9
    cardiac O74.2
    central nervous system O74.3
    pulmonary NEC O74.1
  shunt *—see also* Complications, prosthetic device
    or implant
    arteriovenous *—see* Complications,
      arteriovenous, shunt
    ventricular (communicating) *—see*
      Complications, ventricular shunt
  skin
    graft T86.829
      failure T86.821
      infection T86.822
      rejection T86.820
      specified type NEC T86.828
  spinal
    anesthesia *—see* Complications, anesthesia,
      spinal
    catheter (epidural) (subdural) *—see*
      Complications, catheter
    puncture or tap G97.1
      cerebrospinal fluid leak G97.0
      headache or reaction G97.1
  stent
    bile duct *—see* Complications, bile duct
      prosthesis
    ureteral indwelling
      breakdown T83.112
      displacement T83.122
      leakage T83.192
      malposition T83.122
      obstruction T83.192
      perforation T83.192
      protrusion T83.192
      specified NEC T83.192
    urinary (ileal conduit) (nephroureteral) T83.193
      embolism T83.81
      fibrosis T83.82
      hemorrhage T83.83
      infection and inflammation T83.593
      mechanical
        breakdown T83.113
        displacement T83.123
        leakage T83.193
        malposition T83.123
        obstruction T83.193
        perforation T83.193
        protrusion T83.193
        specified NEC T83.193
      pain T83.84
      specified type NEC T83.89
      stenosis T83.85
      thrombosis T83.86
    vascular
      end stent stenosis *—see* Restenosis, stent
      in stent stenosis *—see* Restenosis, stent
  stoma
    digestive tract
      colostomy *—see* Complications, colostomy
      enterostomy *—see* Complications,
        enterostomy
      esophagostomy *—see* Complications,
        esophagostomy
      gastrostomy *—see* Complications,
        gastrostomy
    urinary tract N99.528
      continent N99.538
        hemorrhage N99.530
        herniation N99.533
        infection N99.531
        malfunction N99.532
        specified type NEC N99.538
        stenosis N99.534
      cystostomy *—see* Complications, cystostomy
      external NOS N99.528
      hemorrhage N99.520
      herniation N99.523
      incontinent N99.528
        hemorrhage N99.520
        herniation N99.523

Complication *(Continued)*
  stoma *(Continued)*
    urinary tracte *(Continued)*
      incontinent *(Continued)*
        infection N99.521
        malfunction N99.522
        specified type NEC N99.528
        stenosis N99.524
      infection N99.521
      malfunction N99.522
      specified type NEC N99.528
      stenosis N99.524
  stomach banding *—see* Complication(s), bariatric
    procedure
  stomach stapling *—see* Complication(s), bariatric
    procedure
  surgical material, nonabsorbable *—see*
    Complication, suture, permanent
  surgical procedure (on) T81.9
    amputation stump (late) *—see* Complications,
      amputation stump
    cardiac *—see* Complications, circulatory
      system
    cholesteatoma, recurrent *—see* Complications,
      postmastoidectomy, recurrent
      cholesteatoma
    circulatory (early) *—see* Complications,
      circulatory system
    digestive system *—see* Complications,
      gastrointestinal
    dumping syndrome (postgastrectomy)
      K91.1
    ear *—see* Complications, ear
    elephantiasis or lymphedema I97.89
      postmastectomy I97.2
    emphysema (surgical) T81.82
    endocrine *—see* Complications, endocrine
    eye *—see* Complications, eye
    fistula (persistent postoperative) T81.83
    foreign body inadvertently left in wound
      (sponge) (suture) (swab) *—see* Foreign
      body, accidentally left during a
      procedure
    gastrointestinal *—see* Complications,
      gastrointestinal
    genitourinary NEC N99.89
    hematoma
      intraoperative *—see* Complication,
        intraoperative, hemorrhage
      postprocedural *—see* Complication,
        postprocedural, hematoma
    hemorrhage
      intraoperative *—see* Complication,
        intraoperative, hemorrhage
      postprocedural *—see* Complication,
        postprocedural, hemorrhage
    hepatic failure K91.82
    hyperglycemia (postpancreatectomy) E89.1
    hypoinsulinemia (postpancreatectomy)
      E89.1
    hypoparathyroidism (postparathyroidectomy)
      E89.2
    hypopituitarism (posthypophysectomy)
      E89.3
    hypothyroidism (post-thyroidectomy)
      E89.0
    intestinal obstruction *—see also* Obstruction,
      intestine, postoperative K91.30
    intracranial hypotension following ventricular
      shunting (ventriculostomy) G97.2
    lymphedema I97.89
      postmastectomy I97.2
    malabsorption (postsurgical) NEC K91.2
      osteoporosis *—see* Osteoporosis,
        postsurgical malabsorption
    mastoidectomy cavity NEC *—see*
      Complications, postmastoidectomy
    metabolic E89.89
      specified NEC E89.89
    musculoskeletal *—see* Complications,
      musculoskeletal system
    nervous system (central) (peripheral) *—see*
      Complications, nervous system
    ovarian failure E89.40
      asymptomatic E89.40
      symptomatic E89.41
    peripheral vascular *—see* Complications,
      surgical procedure, vascular
    postcardiotomy syndrome I97.0
    postcholecystectomy syndrome K91.5
    postcommissurotomy syndrome I97.0

▶ New   ⇒ Revised   ~~deleted~~ Deleted   ● Use Additional Character(s)

Complication *(Continued)*
  vascular *(Continued)*
    device or implant *(Continued)*
      mechanical *(Continued)*
        perforation T82.599
          specified device NEC T82.598
        protrusion T82.599
          specified device NEC T82.598
      pain T82.848
      specified type NEC T82.898
      stenosis T82.858
      thrombosis T82.868
    dialysis catheter —*see* Complication, catheter,
      dialysis
    following infusion, therapeutic injection or
      transfusion T80.1
    graft T82.9
      embolism T82.818
      fibrosis T82.828
      hemorrhage T82.838
      mechanical
        breakdown T82.319
          aorta (bifurcation) T82.310
          carotid artery T82.311
          specified vessel NEC T82.318
        displacement T82.329
          aorta (bifurcation) T82.320
          carotid artery T82.321
          specified vessel NEC T82.328
        leakage T82.339
          aorta (bifurcation) T82.330
          carotid artery T82.331
          femoral artery T82.332
          specified vessel NEC T82.338
        malposition T82.329
          aorta (bifurcation) T82.320
          carotid artery T82.321
          specified vessel NEC T82.328
        obstruction T82.399
          aorta (bifurcation) T82.390
          carotid artery T82.391
          specified vessel NEC T82.398
        perforation T82.399
          aorta (bifurcation) T82.390
          carotid artery T82.391
          specified vessel NEC T82.398
        protrusion T82.399
          aorta (bifurcation) T82.390
          carotid artery T82.391
          specified vessel NEC T82.398
      pain T82.848
      specified complication NEC T82.898
      stenosis T82.858
      thrombosis T82.868
    postoperative —*see* Complications,
      postoperative, circulatory
    vena cava device (filter) (sieve) (umbrella) —*see*
      Complications, umbrella device,
      vascular
  ventilation therapy NEC T81.81
  ventilator
    mechanical J95.850
      specified NEC J95.859
  ventricular (communicating) shunt (device)
    T85.9
    embolism T85.810
    fibrosis T85.820
    hemorrhage T85.830
    infection and inflammation T85.730
    mechanical
      breakdown T85.01
      displacement T85.02
      leakage T85.03
      malposition T85.02
      obstruction T85.09
      perforation T85.09
      protrusion T85.09
      specified NEC T85.09
    pain T85.840
    specified type NEC T85.890
    stenosis T85.850
    thrombosis T85.860
  wire suture, permanent (implanted) —*see*
    Complications, suture, permanent
Compressed air disease T70.3
Compression
  with injury - code by Nature of injury
  artery I77.1
    celiac, syndrome I77.4
  brachial plexus G54.0

Compression *(Continued)*
  brain (stem) G93.5
    due to
      contusion (diffuse) (*see also* Injury,
        intracranial, diffuse) S06.A0
        with herniation S06.A1
      focal (*see also* Injury, intracranial, focal)
        S06.A0
        with herniation S06.A1
      injury NEC (*see also* Injury, intracranial,
        diffuse) S06.A0
    nontraumatic G93.5
    traumatic (*see also* Injury, intracranial, diffuse)
      S06.A0
      with herniation S06.A1
  bronchus J98.09
  cauda equina G83.4
  celiac (artery) (axis) I77.4
  cerebral —*see* Compression, brain
  cervical plexus G54.2
  cord
    spinal —*see* Compression, spinal
    umbilical —*see* Compression, umbilical
      cord
  cranial nerve G52.9
    eighth —*see* subcategory H93.3
    eleventh G52.8
    fifth G50.8
    first G52.0
    fourth —*see* Strabismus, paralytic, fourth
      nerve
    ninth G52.1
    second —*see* Disorder, nerve, optic
    seventh G51.8
    sixth —*see* Strabismus, paralytic, sixth
      nerve
    tenth G52.2
    third —*see* Strabismus, paralytic, third
      nerve
    twelfth G52.3
  diver's squeeze T70.3
  during birth (newborn) P15.9
  esophagus K22.2
  eustachian tube —*see* Obstruction, eustachian
    tube, cartilagenous
  facies Q67.1
  fracture
    nontraumatic NOS —*see* Collapse, vertebra
    pathological —*see* Fracture, pathological
    traumatic —*see* Fracture, traumatic
  heart —*see* Disease, heart
  intestine —*see* Obstruction, intestine
  laryngeal nerve, recurrent G52.2
    with paralysis of vocal cords and larynx J38.00
      bilateral J38.02
      unilateral J38.01
  lumbosacral plexus G54.1
  lung J98.4
  lymphatic vessel I89.0
  medulla —*see* Compression, brain
  nerve —*see also* Disorder, nerve G58.9
    arm NEC —*see* Mononeuropathy, upper limb
    axillary G54.0
    cranial —*see* Compression, cranial nerve
    leg NEC —*see* Mononeuropathy, lower limb
    median (in carpal tunnel) —*see* Syndrome,
      carpal tunnel
    optic —*see* Disorder, nerve, optic
    plantar —*see* Lesion, nerve, plantar
    posterior tibial (in tarsal tunnel) —*see*
      Syndrome, tarsal tunnel
    root or plexus NOS (in) G54.9
      intervertebral disc disorder NEC —
        see Disorder, disc, with, radiculopathy
      with myelopathy —*see* Disorder, disc,
        with, myelopathy
      neoplastic disease —*see also* Neoplasm
        D49.9 [G55]
      spondylosis —*see* Spondylosis, with
        radiculopathy
    sciatic (acute) —*see* Lesion, nerve, sciatic
    sympathetic G90.89
    traumatic —*see* Injury, nerve
    ulnar —*see* Lesion, nerve, ulnar
    upper extremity NEC —*see* Mononeuropathy,
      upper limb
  spinal (cord) G95.20
    by displacement of intervertebral disc NEC —
      see also Disorder, disc, with,
      myelopathy

Compression *(Continued)*
  spinal *(Continued)*
    nerve root NOS G54.9
      due to displacement of intervertebral
        disc NEC —*see* Disorder, disc, with,
        radiculopathy
      with myelopathy —*see* Disorder, disc,
        with, myelopathy
    specified NEC G95.29
    spondylogenic (cervical) (lumbar,
      lumbosacral) (thoracic) —*see*
      Spondylosis, with myelopathy NEC
    anterior —*see* Syndrome, anterior, spinal
      artery, compression
    traumatic —*see* Injury, spinal cord, by region
  subcostal nerve (syndrome) —*see*
    Mononeuropathy, upper limb, specified
    NEC
  sympathetic nerve NEC G90.89
  syndrome T79.5
  trachea J39.8
  ulnar nerve (by scar tissue) —*see* Lesion, nerve,
    ulnar
  umbilical cord
    complicating delivery O69.2
      cord around neck O69.1
      prolapse O69.0
      specified NEC O69.2
  ureter N13.5
  vein I87.1
  vena cava (inferior) (superior) I87.1
Compulsion, compulsive
  gambling F63.0
  neurosis F42.8
  personality F60.5
  states F42.8
  swearing F42.8
    in Gilles de la Tourette's syndrome F95.2
  tics and spasms F95.9
Concato's disease (pericardial polyserositis) A19.9
  nontubercular I31.1
  pleural —*see* Pleurisy, with effusion
Concavity chest wall M95.4
Concealed penis Q55.64
Concern (normal) about sick person in family
  Z63.6
Concrescence (teeth) K00.2
Concretio cordis I31.1
  rheumatic I09.2
  appendicular K38.1
  canaliculus —*see* Dacryolith
  clitoris N90.89
  conjunctiva H11.12-●
  eyelid —*see* Disorder, eyelid, specified type NEC
  lacrimal passages —*see* Dacryolith
  prepuce (male) N47.8
  salivary gland (any) K11.5
  seminal vesicle N50.89
  tonsil J35.8
Concussion (brain) (cerebral) (current) S06.0X9
  with
    loss of consciousness
      30 minutes or less S06.0X1
        brief S06.0X1
      status unknown S06.0XA
      unspecified duration S06.0X9
    no loss of consciousness S06.0X0
  blast (air) (hydraulic) (immersion) (underwater)
    abdomen or thorax —*see* Injury, blast, by site
    ear with acoustic nerve injury —*see* Injury,
      nerve, acoustic, specified type NEC
  cauda equina S34.3
  conus medullaris S34.02
  ocular S05.8X-●
  spinal (cord)
    cervical S14.0
    lumbar S34.01
    sacral S34.02
    thoracic S24.0
  syndrome F07.81
  without loss of consciousness S06.0X0
Condition —*see also* Disease
  post COVID-19 U09.9
Conditions arising in the perinatal period —*see*
  Newborn, affected by
Conduct disorder —*see* Disorder, conduct
Condyloma A63.0
  acuminatum A63.0
  gonorrheal A54.09
  latum A51.31

▶ New   ⇒ Revised   ~~deleted~~ Deleted   ● Use Additional Character(s)

Condyloma *(Continued)*
  syphilitic A51.31
    congenital A50.07
  venereal, syphilitic A51.31
Conflagration —*see also* Burn
  asphyxia (by inhalation of gases, fumes or
    vapors) —*see also* Table of Drugs and
    Chemicals T59.9-●
Conflict (with) —*see also* Discord
  family Z73.9
  grandparent-child Z62.831
  group home staff-child Z62.833
  kinship-care child Z62.831
  marital Z63.0
    involving divorce or estrangement
      Z63.5
  non-parental relative legal guardian-child
    Z62.831
  non-parental relative-child Z62.831
  non-relative guardian-child Z62.832
  other relative-child Z62.831
  parent-child Z62.820
    parent-adopted child Z62.821
    parent-biological child Z62.820
    parent-foster child Z62.822
  parent-step child Z62.823
  social role NEC Z73.5
Confluent —*see* condition
Confusion, confused R41.0
  epileptic F05
  mental state (psychogenic) F44.89
  psychogenic F44.89
  reactive (from emotional stress, psychological
    trauma) F44.89
Confusional arousals G47.51
Congelation T69.9
Congenital —*see also* condition
  aortic septum Q25.49
  intrinsic factor deficiency D51.0
  malformation —*see* Anomaly
Congestion, congestive
  bladder N32.89
  bowel K63.89
  brain G93.89
  breast N64.59
  bronchial J98.09
  catarrhal J31.0
  chest R09.89
  chill, malarial —*see* Malaria
  circulatory NEC I99.8
  duodenum K31.89
  eye —*see* Hyperemia, conjunctiva
  facial, due to birth injury P15.4
  general R68.89
  glottis J37.0
  heart —*see* Failure, heart, congestive
  hepatic K76.1
  hypostatic (lung) —*see* Edema, lung
  intestine K63.89
  kidney N28.89
  labyrinth —*see* subcategory H83.8
  larynx J37.0
  liver K76.1
  lung R09.89
    active or acute —*see* Pneumonia
  malaria, malarial —*see* Malaria
  nasal R09.81
  nose R09.81
  orbit, orbital —*see also* Exophthalmos
    inflammatory (chronic) —*see* Inflammation,
      orbit
  ovary N83.8
  pancreas K86.89
  pelvic, female N94.89
  pleural J94.8
  prostate (active) N42.1
  pulmonary —*see* Congestion, lung
  renal N28.89
  retina H35.81
  seminal vesicle N50.1
  spinal cord G95.19
  spleen (chronic) D73.2
  stomach K31.89
  trachea —*see* Tracheitis
  urethra N36.8
  uterus N85.8
    with subinvolution N85.3
  venous (passive) I87.8
  viscera R68.89
Congestive —*see* Congestion

Conical
  cervix (hypertrophic elongation) N88.4
  cornea —*see* Keratoconus
  teeth K00.2
Conjoined twins Q89.4
Conjugal maladjustment Z63.0
  involving divorce or estrangement Z63.5
Conjunctiva —*see* condition
Conjunctivitis (staphylococcal) (streptococcal)
    NOS H10.9
  Acanthamoeba B60.12
  acute H10.3-●
    atopic H10.1-●
    chemical —*see also* Corrosion, cornea
      H10.21-●
    mucopurulent H10.02-●
      follicular H10.01-●
    pseudomembranous H10.22-●
    serous except viral H10.23-●
      viral —*see* Conjunctivitis, viral
    toxic H10.21-●
  adenoviral (acute) (follicular) B30.1
  allergic (acute) —*see* Conjunctivitis, acute,
      atopic
    chronic H10.45
    vernal H10.44
  anaphylactic —*see* Conjunctivitis, acute, atopic
  Apollo B30.3
  atopic (acute) —*see* Conjunctivitis, acute, atopic
  Béal's B30.2
  blennorrhagic (gonococcal) (neonatorum)
      A54.31
  chemical (acute) —*see also* Corrosion, cornea
      H10.21-●
  chlamydial A74.0
    due to trachoma A71.1
    neonatal P39.1
  chronic (nodosa) (petrificans) (phlyctenular)
      H10.40-●
    allergic H10.45
      vernal H10.44
    follicular H10.43-●
    giant papillary H10.41-●
    simple H10.42-●
    vernal H10.44
  coxsackievirus 24 B30.3
  diphtheritic A36.86
  due to
    dust —*see* Conjunctivitis, acute, atopic
    filariasis B74.9
    mucocutaneous leishmaniasis B55.2
  enterovirus type 70 (hemorrhagic) B30.3
  epidemic (viral) B30.9
    hemorrhagic B30.3
  gonococcal (neonatorum) A54.31
  granular (trachomatous) A71.1
    sequelae (late effect) B94.0
  hemorrhagic (acute) (epidemic) B30.3
  herpes zoster B02.31
  in (due to)
    Acanthamoeba B60.12
    adenovirus (acute) (follicular) B30.1
    Chlamydia A74.0
    coxsackievirus 24 B30.3
    diphtheria A36.86
    enterovirus type 70 (hemorrhagic) B30.3
    filariasis B74.9
    gonococci A54.31
    herpes (simplex) virus B00.53
      zoster B02.31
    infectious disease NEC B99
    meningococci A39.89
    mucocutaneous leishmaniasis B55.2
    rosacea H10.82-●
    syphilis (late) A52.71
    zoster B02.31
  inclusion A74.0
  infantile P39.1
    gonococcal A54.31
  Koch-Weeks' —*see* Conjunctivitis, acute,
      mucopurulent
  light —*see* Conjunctivitis, acute, atopic
  ligneous —*see* Blepharoconjunctivitis, ligneous
  meningococcal A39.89
  mucopurulent —*see* Conjunctivitis, acute,
      mucopurulent
  neonatal P39.1
    gonococcal A54.31
  Newcastle B30.8
  of Béal B30.2

Conjunctivitis *(Continued)*
  parasitic
    filariasis B74.9
    mucocutaneous leishmaniasis B55.2
  Parinaud's H10.89
  petrificans H10.89
  rosacea H10.82-●
  specified NEC H10.89
  swimming-pool B30.1
  trachomatous A71.1
    acute A71.0
    sequelae (late effect) B94.0
  traumatic NEC H10.89
  tuberculous A18.59
  tularemic A21.1
  tularensis A21.1
  viral B30.9
    due to
      adenovirus B30.1
      enterovirus B30.3
    specified NEC B30.8
Conjunctivochalasis H11.82-●
Connective tissue —*see* condition
Conn's syndrome E26.01
Conradi (-Hunermann) disease Q77.3
Consanguinity Z84.3
  counseling Z71.89
Conscious simulation (of illness) Z76.5
Consecutive —*see* condition
Consolidation lung (base) —*see* Pneumonia,
    lobar
Constipation (atonic) (neurogenic) (simple)
    (spastic) K59.00
  chronic K59.09
    idiopathic K59.04
  drug-induced K59.03
  functional K59.04
  outlet dysfunction K59.02
  psychogenic F45.8
  slow transit K59.01
  specified NEC K59.09
Constitutional —*see also* condition
  substandard F60.7
Constitutionally substandard F60.7
Constriction —*see also* Stricture
  auditory canal —*see* Stenosis, external ear canal
  bronchial J98.09
  duodenum K31.5
  esophagus K22.2
  external
    abdomen, abdominal (wall) S30.841
    alveolar process S00.542
    ankle S90.54-●
    antecubital space —*see* Constriction, external,
      forearm
    arm (upper) S40.84-●
    auricle —*see* Constriction, external, ear
    axilla —*see* Constriction, external, arm
    back, lower S30.840
    breast S20.14-●
    brow S00.84
    buttock S30.840
    calf —*see* Constriction, external, leg
    canthus —*see* Constriction, external, eyelid
    cheek S00.84
      internal S00.542
    chest wall —*see* Constriction, external, thorax
    chin S00.84
    clitoris S30.844
    costal region —*see* Constriction, external,
      thorax
    digit(s)
      foot —*see* Constriction, external, toe
      hand —*see* Constriction, external, finger
    ear S00.44-●
    elbow S50.34-●
    epididymis S30.843
    epigastric region S30.841
    esophagus, cervical S10.14
    eyebrow —*see* Constriction, external, eyelid
    eyelid S00.24-●
    face S00.84
    finger(s) S60.44-●
      index S60.44-●
      little S60.44-●
      middle S60.44-●
      ring S60.44-●
    flank S30.841
    foot (except toe(s) alone) S90.84-●
      toe —*see* Constriction, external, toe

Constriction *(Continued)*
  external *(Continued)*
    forearm S50.84-●
      elbow only —*see* Constriction, external, elbow
    forehead S00.84
    genital organs, external
      female S30.846
      male S30.845
    groin S30.841
    gum S00.542
    hand S60.54-●
    head S00.94
      ear —*see* Constriction, external, ear
      eyelid —*see* Constriction, external, eyelid
      lip S00.541
      nose S00.34
      oral cavity S00.542
      scalp S00.04
      specified site NEC S00.84
    heel —*see* Constriction, external, foot
    hip S70.24-●
    inguinal region S30.841
    interscapular region S20.449
    jaw S00.84
    knee S80.24-●
      knee —*see* Constriction, external, knee
      upper —*see* Constriction, external, thigh
    lip S00.541
    lower back S30.840
    lumbar region S30.840
    malar region S00.84
    mammary —*see* Constriction, external, breast
    mastoid region S00.84
    mouth S00.542
    nail
      finger —*see* Constriction, external, finger
      toe —*see* Constriction, external, toe
    nasal S00.34
    neck S10.94
      specified site NEC S10.84
      throat S10.14
    nose S00.34
    occipital region S00.04
    oral cavity S00.542
    orbital region —*see* Constriction, external, eyelid
    palate S00.542
    palm —*see* Constriction, external, hand
    parietal region S00.04
    pelvis S30.840
    penis S30.842
    perineum
      female S30.844
      male S30.840
    periocular area —*see* Constriction, external, eyelid
    phalanges
      finger —*see* Constriction, external, finger
      toe —*see* Constriction, external, toe
    pharynx S10.14
    pinna —*see* Constriction, external, ear
    popliteal space —*see* Constriction, external, knee
    prepuce S30.842
    pubic region S30.840
    pudendum
      female S30.846
      male S30.845
    sacral region S30.840
    scalp S00.04
    scapular region —*see* Constriction, external, shoulder
    scrotum S30.843
    shin —*see* Constriction, external, leg
    shoulder S40.24-●
    sternal region S20.349
    submaxillary region S00.84
    submental region S00.84
    subungual
      finger(s) —*see* Constriction, external, finger
      toe(s) —*see* Constriction, external, toe
    supraclavicular fossa S10.84
    supraorbital S00.84
    temple S00.84
    temporal region S00.84
    testis S30.843
    thigh S70.34-●

Constriction *(Continued)*
  external *(Continued)*
    thorax, thoracic (wall) S20.94
      back S20.44-●
      front S20.34-●
    throat S10.14
    thumb S60.34-●
    toe(s) (lesser) S90.44-●
      great S90.44-●
    tongue S00.542
    trachea S10.14
    tunica vaginalis S30.843
    uvula S00.542
    vagina S30.844
    vulva S30.844
    wrist S60.84-●
  gallbladder —*see* Obstruction, gallbladder
  intestine —*see* Obstruction, intestine
  larynx J38.6
    congenital Q31.8
      specified NEC Q31.8
      subglottic Q31.1
  organ or site, congenital NEC —*see* Atresia, by site
  prepuce (acquired) (congenital) N47.1
  pylorus (adult hypertrophic) K31.1
    congenital or infantile Q40.0
    newborn Q40.0
  ring dystocia (uterus) O62.4
  spastic —*see also* Spasm
    ureter N13.5
  ureter N13.5
    with infection N13.6
  urethra —*see* Stricture, urethra
  visual field (peripheral) (functional) —*see* Defect, visual field
Constrictive —*see* condition
Consultation
  without complaint or sickness Z71.9
    feared complaint unfounded Z71.1
    specified reason NEC Z71.89
  medical —*see* Counseling, medical
  religious Z71.81
  specified reason NEC Z71.89
  spiritual Z71.81
Consumption —*see* Tuberculosis
Contact (with) —*see also* Exposure (to)
  acariasis Z20.7
  AIDS virus Z20.6
  air pollution Z77.110
  algae and algae toxins Z77.121
  algae bloom Z77.121
  anthrax Z20.810
  aromatic (hazardous) compounds NEC Z77.028
  aromatic amines Z77.020
  aromatic dyes NOS Z77.028
  arsenic Z77.010
  asbestos Z77.090
  bacterial disease NEC Z20.818
  benzene Z77.021
  blue-green algae bloom Z77.121
  body fluids (potentially hazardous) Z77.21
  brown tide Z77.121
  chemicals (chiefly nonmedicinal) (hazardous) NEC Z77.098
  cholera Z20.09
  chromium compounds Z77.018
  communicable disease Z20.9
    bacterial NEC Z20.818
    specified NEC Z20.89
    viral NEC Z20.828
    Zika virus Z20.821
  coronavirus (disease) (novel) 2019 Z20.822
  COVID-19 Z20.822
  cyanobacteria bloom Z77.121
  dyes Z77.098
  Escherichia coli (E. coli) Z20.01
  fiberglass —*see* Table of Drugs and Chemicals, fiberglass
  German measles Z20.4
  gonorrhea Z20.2
  hazardous metals NEC Z77.018
  hazardous substances NEC Z77.29
  hazards in the physical environment NEC Z77.128
  hazards to health NEC Z77.9
  HIV Z20.6
  HTLV-III/LAV Z20.6
  human immunodeficiency virus (HIV) Z20.6
  infection Z20.9
    specified NEC Z20.89
  infestation (parasitic) NEC Z20.7

Contact *(Continued)*
  intestinal infectious disease NEC Z20.09
    Escherichia coli (E. coli) Z20.01
  lead Z77.011
  meningococcus Z20.811
  mold (toxic) Z77.120
  nickel dust Z77.018
  noise Z77.122
  parasitic disease Z20.7
  pediculosis Z20.7
  pfiesteria piscicida Z77.121
  poliomyelitis Z20.89
  pollution
    air Z77.110
    environmental NEC Z77.118
    soil Z77.112
    water Z77.111
  polycyclic aromatic hydrocarbons Z77.028
  positive maternal group B streptococcus P00.82
  rabies Z20.3
  radiation, naturally occurring NEC Z77.123
  radon Z77.123
  red tide (Florida) Z77.121
  rubella Z20.4
  SARS-CoV-2 Z20.822
  sexually-transmitted disease Z20.2
  smallpox (laboratory) Z20.89
  syphilis Z20.2
  tuberculosis Z20.1
  uranium Z77.012
  varicella Z20.820
  venereal disease Z20.2
  viral disease NEC Z20.828
  viral hepatitis Z20.5
  water pollution Z77.111
  Zika virus Z20.821
Contamination, food —*see* Intoxication, foodborne
Contraception, contraceptive
  advice Z30.09
  counseling Z30.09
  device (intrauterine) (in situ) Z97.5
    causing menorrhagia T83.83
    checking Z30.431
    complications —*see* Complications, intrauterine, contraceptive device
    in place Z97.5
    initial prescription Z30.014
    reinsertion Z30.433
    removal Z30.432
    replacement Z30.433
  emergency (postcoital) Z30.012
  initial prescription Z30.019
    barrier Z30.018
    diaphragm Z30.018
    injectable Z30.013
    intrauterine device Z30.014
    pills Z30.011
    postcoital (emergency) Z30.012
    specified type NEC Z30.018
    subdermal implantable Z30.017
    transdermal patch hormonal Z30.016
    vaginal ring hormonal Z30.015
  maintenance Z30.40
    barrier Z30.49
    diaphragm Z30.49
    examination Z30.8
    injectable Z30.42
    intrauterine device Z30.431
    pills Z30.41
    specified type NEC Z30.49
    subdermal implantable Z30.46
    transdermal patch hormonal Z30.45
    vaginal ring hormonal Z30.44
  management Z30.9
    specified NEC Z30.8
  postcoital (emergency) Z30.012
  prescription Z30.019
    repeat Z30.40
  sterilization Z30.2
  surveillance (drug) —*see* Contraception, maintenance
Contraction(s), contracture, contracted
  Achilles tendon —*see also* Short, tendon, Achilles
    congenital Q66.89
  amputation stump (surgical) (flexion) (late) next proximal joint T87.89
  anus K59.89
  bile duct (common) (hepatic) K83.8
  bladder N32.89
    neck or sphincter N32.0

▶ New   ⇒ Revised   ~~deleted~~ Deleted   ● Use Additional Character(s)

Contusion *(Continued)*
  intra-abdominal organ S36.92
    colon —*see* Injury, intestine, large, contusion
    liver S36.112
    pancreas —*see* Contusion, pancreas
    rectum S36.62
    small intestine —*see* Injury, intestine, small,
      contusion
    specified organ NEC S36.892
    spleen —*see* Contusion, spleen
    stomach S36.32
  iris (eye) —*see* Contusion, eyeball
  jaw S00.83
  jejunum S36.428
  kidney S37.01-●
    major (greater than 2 cm) S37.02-●
    minor (less than 2 cm) S37.01-●
  knee S80.0-●
  labium (majus) (minus) S30.23
  lacrimal apparatus, gland or sac S05.8X-●
  larynx S10.0
  leg (lower) S80.1-●
    knee —*see* Contusion, knee
  lens —*see* Contusion, eyeball
  lip S00.531
  liver S36.112
  lower back S30.0
  lumbar region S30.0
  lung S27.329
    bilateral S27.322
    unilateral S27.321
  malar region S00.83
  mastoid region S00.83
  membrane, brain —*see* Injury, intracranial,
    diffuse
    focal —*see* Injury, intracranial, focal
  mesentery S36.892
  mesosalpinx S37.892
  mouth S00.532
  muscle —*see* Contusion, by site
  nail
    finger —*see* Contusion, finger, with damage
      to nail
    toe —*see* Contusion, toe, with damage to nail
  nasal S00.33
  neck S10.93
    specified site NEC S10.83
    throat S10.0
  nerve —*see* Injury, nerve
  newborn P54.5
  nose S00.33
  occipital
    lobe (brain) —*see* Injury, intracranial, diffuse
      focal —*see* Injury, intracranial,
        focal
    region (scalp) S00.03
  orbit (region) (tissues) S05.1-●
  ovary S37.429
    bilateral S37.422
    unilateral S37.421
  palate S00.532
  pancreas S36.229
    body S36.221
    head S36.220
    tail S36.222
  parietal
    lobe (brain) —*see* Injury, intracranial, diffuse
      focal —*see* Injury, intracranial, focal
    region (scalp) S00.03
  pelvic organ S37.92
    adrenal gland S37.812
    bladder S37.22
    fallopian tube —*see* Contusion, fallopian tube
    kidney —*see* Contusion, kidney
    ovary —*see* Contusion, ovary
    prostate S37.822
    specified organ NEC S37.892
    ureter S37.12
    urethra S37.32
    uterus S37.62
  pelvis S30.0
  penis S30.21
  perineum
    female S30.23
    male S30.0
  periocular area S00.1-●
  peritoneum S36.81
  periurethral tissue —*see* Contusion,
    urethra
  pharynx S10.0
  pinna —*see* Contusion, ear

Contusion *(Continued)*
  popliteal space —*see* Contusion, knee
  prepuce S30.21
  prostate S37.822
  pubic region S30.1
  pudendum
    female S30.202
    male S30.201
  quadriceps femoris —*see* Contusion, thigh
  rectum S36.62
  retroperitoneum S36.892
  round ligament S37.892
  sacral region S30.0
  scalp S00.03
    due to birth injury P12.3
  scapular region —*see* Contusion, shoulder
  sclera —*see* Contusion, eyeball
  scrotum S30.22
  seminal vesicle S37.892
  shoulder S40.01-●
  skin NEC T14.8
  small intestine —*see* Injury, intestine, small,
    contusion
  spermatic cord S30.22
  spinal cord —*see* Injury, spinal cord,
    by region
    cauda equina S34.3
    conus medullaris S34.139
  spleen S36.029
    major S36.021
    minor S36.020
  sternal region S20.219
  stomach S36.32
  subconjunctival S05.1-●
  subcutaneous NEC T14.8
  submaxillary region S00.83
  submental region S00.83
  subperiosteal NEC T14.8
  subungual
    finger —*see* Contusion, finger, with damage
      to nail
    toe —*see* Contusion, toe, with damage to nail
  supraclavicular fossa S10.83
  supraorbital S00.83
  suprarenal gland S37.812
  temple (region) S00.83
  temporal
    lobe (brain) —*see* Injury, intracranial, diffuse
      focal —*see* Injury, intracranial, focal
    region S00.83
  testis S30.22
  thigh S70.1-●
  thorax (wall) S20.20
    back S20.22-●
    front S20.21-●
  throat S10.0
  thumb S60.01-●
    with damage to nail S60.11-●
  toe(s) (lesser) S90.12-●
    with damage to nail S90.22-●
    great S90.11-●
      with damage to nail S90.21-●
  tongue S00.532
  trachea (cervical) S10.0
    thoracic S27.52
  tunica vaginalis S30.22
  tympanum, tympanic membrane —*see*
    Contusion, ear
  ureter S37.12
  urethra S37.32
  urinary organ NEC S37.892
  uterus S37.62
  uvula S00.532
  vagina S30.23
  vas deferens S37.892
  vesical S37.22
  vocal cord(s) S10.0
  vulva S30.23
  wrist S60.21-●
Conus (congenital) (any type) Q14.8
  cornea —*see* Keratoconus
  medullaris syndrome G95.81
Conversion hysteria, neurosis or reaction
  F44.9
Converter, tuberculosis (test reaction) R76.11
Conviction (legal), anxiety concerning
  Z65.0
  with imprisonment Z65.1
Convulsions (idiopathic) —*see also* Seizure(s) R56.9
  apoplectiform (cerebral ischemia) I67.82
  dissociative F44.5

Convulsions *(Continued)*
  epileptic —*see* Epilepsy
  epileptiform, epileptoid —*see* Epilepsy
  ether (anesthetic) —*see* Table of Drugs and
    Chemicals, by drug
  febrile R56.00
    with status epilepticus G40.901
    complex R56.01
      with status epilepticus G40.901
    simple R56.00
  hysterical F44.5
  infantile P90
    epilepsy —*see* Epilepsy
  jacksonian —*see* Epilepsy, localization-related,
    symptomatic, with simple partial seizures
  myoclonic G25.3
  newborn P90
  obstetrical (nephritic) (uremic) —*see* Eclampsia
  paretic A52.17
  post traumatic R56.1
  psychomotor —*see* Epilepsy, localization-related,
    symptomatic, with complex partial
    seizures
  recurrent R56.9
  reflex R25.8
  scarlatinal A38.8
  tetanus, tetanic —*see* Tetanus
  thymic E32.8
Convulsive —*see also* Convulsions
Cooley's anemia D56.1
Coolie itch B76.9
Cooper's
  disease —*see* Mastopathy, cystic
  hernia —*see* Hernia, abdomen, specified site
    NEC
Copra itch B88.0
Coprophagy F50.89
Coprophobia F40.298
Coproporphyria, hereditary E80.29
Cor
  biloculare Q20.8
  bovis, bovinum —*see* Hypertrophy, cardiac
  pulmonale I27.81
    acute I26.09
      without pulmonary embolism I27.81
    chronic I27.81
      with chronic pulmonary embolism I27.82
  triatriatum, triatrium Q24.2
  triloculare Q20.8
    biatrium Q20.4
    biventriculare Q21.19
Corbus' disease (gangrenous balanitis) N48.1
Cord —*see also* condition
  around neck
    complicating delivery O69.81
      with compression O69.1
  bladder G95.89
    tabetic A52.19
Cordis ectopia Q24.8
Corditis (spermatic) N49.1
Corectopia Q13.2
Cori's disease (glycogen storage) E74.03
Corkhandler's disease or lung J67.3
Corkscrew esophagus K22.4
Corkworker's disease or lung J67.3
Corn (infected) L84
Cornea —*see also* condition
  donor Z52.5
  plana Q13.4
Cornelia de Lange syndrome Q87.19
Cornu cutaneum L85.8
Cornual gestation or pregnancy O00.80
  with intrauterine pregnancy O00.81
Coronary (artery) —*see* condition
Coronavirus (infection)
  as cause of disease classified elsewhere B97.29
  coronavirus-19 U07.1
  COVID-19 U07.1
  SARS-associated B97.21
Corpora —*see also* condition
  amylacea, prostate N42.89
  cavernosa —*see* condition
Corpulence —*see* Obesity
Corpus —*see* condition
Corrected transposition Q20.5
Corrosion (injury) (acid) (caustic) (chemical) (lime)
  (external) (internal) T30.4
  abdomen, abdominal (muscle) (wall) T21.42
    first degree T21.52
    second degree T21.62
    third degree T21.72

Corrosion *(Continued)*
  forehead T20.46
    first degree T20.56
    second degree T20.66
    third degree T20.76
  fourth degree - code as Corrosion, third degree,
      by site
  full thickness skin loss - code as Corrosion, third
      degree, by site
  gastrointestinal tract NEC T28.7
  genital organs
    external
      female T21.47
        first degree T21.57
        second degree T21.67
        third degree T21.77
      male T21.46
        first degree T21.56
        second degree T21.66
        third degree T21.76
    internal T28.8
  groin —*see* Corrosion, abdominal wall
  hand(s) T23.409
    back —*see* Corrosion, dorsum of hand
    finger —*see* Corrosion, finger
    first degree T23.509
    left T23.402
      first degree T23.502
      second degree T23.602
      third degree T23.702
    multiple sites with wrist T23.499
      first degree T23.599
      left T23.492
        first degree T23.592
        second degree T23.692
        third degree T23.792
      right T23.491
        first degree T23.591
        second degree T23.691
        third degree T23.791
      second degree T23.699
      third degree T23.799
    palm —*see* Corrosion, palm
    right T23.401
      first degree T23.501
      second degree T23.601
      third degree T23.701
    second degree T23.609
    third degree T23.709
    thumb —*see* Corrosion, thumb
  head (and face) (and neck) T20.40
    cheek —*see* Corrosion, cheek
    chin —*see* Corrosion, chin
    ear —*see* Corrosion, ear
    eye(s) only —*see* Corrosion, eye
    first degree T20.50
    forehead —*see* Corrosion, forehead
    lip —*see* Corrosion, lip
    multiple sites T20.49
      first degree T20.59
      second degree T20.69
      third degree T20.79
    neck —*see* Corrosion, neck
    nose —*see* Corrosion, nose
    scalp —*see* Corrosion, scalp
    second degree T20.60
    third degree T20.70
  hip(s) —*see* Corrosion, lower, limb
  inhalation —*see* Corrosion, respiratory tract
  internal organ(s) *(see also* Corrosion, by site) T28.90
    alimentary tract T28.7
      esophagus T28.6
    esophagus T28.6
    genitourinary T28.8
    mouth T28.5
    pharynx T28.5
    specified organ NEC T28.99
  interscapular region —*see* Corrosion, back, upper
  intestine (large) (small) T28.7
  knee T24.429
    first degree T24.529
    left T24.422
      first degree T24.522
      second degree T24.622
      third degree T24.722
    right T24.421
      first degree T24.521
      second degree T24.621
      third degree T24.721
    second degree T24.629
    third degree T24.729

Corrosion *(Continued)*
  labium (majus) (minus) —*see* Corrosion, genital
      organs, external, female
  lacrimal apparatus, duct, gland or sac —
      see Corrosion, eye, specified site
      NEC
  larynx T27.4
    with lung T27.5
  leg(s) (meaning lower limb(s)) —*see* Corrosion,
      lower limb
  limb(s)
    lower —*see* Corrosion, lower, limb
    upper —*see* Corrosion, upper limb
  lip(s) T20.42
    first degree T20.52
    second degree T20.62
    third degree T20.72
  lower
    back —*see* Corrosion, back
    limb T24.409
      ankle —*see* Corrosion, ankle
      calf —*see* Corrosion, calf
      first degree T24.509
      foot —*see* Corrosion, foot
      hip —*see* Corrosion, thigh
      knee —*see* Corrosion, knee
      left T24.402
        first degree T24.502
        second degree T24.602
        third degree T24.702
      multiple sites, except ankle and foot
          T24.499
        ankle and foot T25.499
          first degree T25.599
          left T25.492
            first degree T25.592
            second degree T25.692
            third degree T25.792
          right T25.491
            first degree T25.591
            second degree T25.691
            third degree T25.791
          second degree T25.699
          third degree T25.799
        first degree T24.599
        left T24.492
          first degree T24.592
          second degree T24.692
          third degree T24.792
        right T24.491
          first degree T24.591
          second degree T24.691
          third degree T24.791
        second degree T24.699
        third degree T24.799
      right T24.401
        first degree T24.501
        second degree T24.601
        third degree T24.701
      second degree T24.609
      thigh —*see* Corrosion, thigh
      third degree T24.709
  lung (with larynx and trachea) T27.5
  mouth T28.5
  neck T20.47
    first degree T20.57
    second degree T20.67
    third degree T20.77
  nose (septum) T20.44
    first degree T20.54
    second degree T20.64
    third degree T20.74
  ocular adnexa —*see* Corrosion, eye
  orbit region —*see* Corrosion, eyelid
  palm T23.459
    first degree T23.559
    left T23.452
      first degree T23.552
      second degree T23.652
      third degree T23.752
    right T23.451
      first degree T23.551
      second degree T23.651
      third degree T23.751
    second degree T23.659
    third degree T23.759
  partial thickness - code as Corrosion, unspecified
      degree, by site
  pelvis —*see* Corrosion, trunk
  penis —*see* Corrosion, genital organs, external,
      male

Corrosion *(Continued)*
  perineum
    female —*see* Corrosion, genital organs,
        external, female
    male —*see* Corrosion, genital organs, external,
        male
  periocular area —*see* Corrosion, eyelid
  pharynx T28.5
  rectum T28.7
  respiratory tract T27.7
    larynx —*see* Corrosion, larynx
    specified part NEC T27.6
    trachea —*see* Corrosion, larynx
  sac, lacrimal —*see* Corrosion, eye, specified site
      NEC
  scalp T20.45
    first degree T20.55
    second degree T20.65
    third degree T20.75
  scapular region T22.469
    first degree T22.569
    left T22.462
      first degree T22.562
      second degree T22.662
      third degree T22.762
    right T22.461
      first degree T22.561
      second degree T22.661
      third degree T22.761
    second degree T22.669
    third degree T22.769
  sclera —*see* Corrosion, eye, specified site
      NEC
  scrotum —*see* Corrosion, genital organs,
      external, male
  shoulder T22.459
    first degree T22.559
    left T22.452
      first degree T22.552
      second degree T22.652
      third degree T22.752
    right T22.451
      first degree T22.551
      second degree T22.651
      third degree T22.751
    second degree T22.659
    third degree T22.759
  stomach T28.7
  temple —*see* Corrosion, head
  testis —*see* Corrosion, genital organs, external,
      male
  thigh T24.419
    first degree T24.519
    left T24.412
      first degree T24.512
      second degree T24.612
      third degree T24.712
    right T24.411
      first degree T24.511
      second degree T24.611
      third degree T24.711
    second degree T24.619
    third degree T24.719
  thorax (external) —*see* Corrosion,
      trunk
  throat (meaning pharynx) T28.5
  thumb(s) T23.419
    first degree T23.519
    left T23.412
      first degree T23.512
      second degree T23.612
      third degree T23.712
    multiple sites with fingers
        T23.449
      first degree T23.549
      left T23.442
        first degree T23.542
        second degree T23.642
        third degree T23.742
      right T23.441
        first degree T23.541
        second degree T23.641
        third degree T23.741
      second degree T23.649
      third degree T23.749
    right T23.411
      first degree T23.511
      second degree T23.611
      third degree T23.711
    second degree T23.619
    third degree T23.719

▶ New   ⇒ Revised   ~~deleted~~ Deleted   ● Use Additional Character(s)

Corrosion (Continued)
toe T25.439
first degree T25.539
left T25.432
first degree T25.532
second degree T25.632
third degree T25.732
right T25.431
first degree T25.531
second degree T25.631
third degree T25.731
second degree T25.639
third degree T25.739
tongue T28.5
tonsil(s) T28.5
total body —see Corrosion, multiple body
regions
trachea T27.4
with lung T27.5
trunk T21.40
abdominal wall —see Corrosion, abdominal
wall
anus —see Corrosion, buttock
axilla —see Corrosion, upper limb
back —see Corrosion, back
breast —see Corrosion, chest wall
buttock —see Corrosion, buttock
chest wall —see Corrosion, chest wall
first degree T21.50
flank —see Corrosion, abdominal wall
genital
female —see Corrosion, genital organs,
external, female
male —see Corrosion, genital organs,
external, male
groin —see Corrosion, abdominal wall
interscapular region —see Corrosion, back,
upper
labia —see Corrosion, genital organs, external,
female
lower back —see Corrosion, back
penis —see Corrosion, genital organs, external,
male
perineum
female —see Corrosion, genital organs,
external, female
male —see Corrosion, genital organs,
external, male
scapular region —see Corrosion, upper limb
scrotum —see Corrosion, genital organs,
external, male
second degree T21.60
shoulder —see Corrosion, upper limb
specified site NEC T21.49
first degree T21.59
second degree T21.69
third degree T21.79
testes —see Corrosion, genital organs,
external, male
third degree T21.70
upper back —see Corrosion, back, upper
vagina T28.8
vulva —see Corrosion, genital organs,
external, female
unspecified site with extent of body surface
involved specified
less than 10 percent T32.0
10-19 percent (0-9 percent third degree) T32.10
with 10-19 percent third degree T32.11
20-29 percent (0-9 percent third degree) T32.20
with
10-19 percent third degree T32.21
20-29 percent third degree T32.22
30-39 percent (0-9 percent third degree) T32.30
with
10-19 percent third degree T32.31
20-29 percent third degree T32.32
30-39 percent third degree T32.33
40-49 percent (0-9 percent third degree) T32.40
with
10-19 percent third degree T32.41
20-29 percent third degree T32.42
30-39 percent third degree T32.43
40-49 percent third degree T32.44
50-59 percent (0-9 percent third degree) T32.50
with
10-19 percent third degree T32.51
20-29 percent third degree T32.52
30-39 percent third degree T32.53
40-49 percent third degree T32.54
50-59 percent third degree T32.55

Corrosion (Continued)
unspecified site with extent of body surface
involved specified (Continued)
60-69 percent (0-9 percent third degree) T32.60
with
10-19 percent third degree T32.61
20-29 percent third degree T32.62
30-39 percent third degree T32.63
40-49 percent third degree T32.64
50-59 percent third degree T32.65
60-69 percent third degree T32.66
70-79 percent (0-9 percent third degree) T32.70
with
10-19 percent third degree T32.71
20-29 percent third degree T32.72
30-39 percent third degree T32.73
40-49 percent third degree T32.74
50-59 percent third degree T32.75
60-69 percent third degree T32.76
70-79 percent third degree T32.77
80-89 percent (0-9 percent third degree) T32.80
with
10-19 percent third degree T32.81
20-29 percent third degree T32.82
30-39 percent third degree T32.83
40-49 percent third degree T32.84
50-59 percent third degree T32.85
60-69 percent third degree T32.86
70-79 percent third degree T32.87
80-89 percent third degree T32.88
90 percent or more (0-9 percent third degree)
T32.90
with
10-19 percent third degree T32.91
20-29 percent third degree T32.92
30-39 percent third degree T32.93
40-49 percent third degree T32.94
50-59 percent third degree T32.95
60-69 percent third degree T32.96
70-79 percent third degree T32.97
80-89 percent third degree T32.98
90-99 percent third degree T32.99
upper limb (axilla) (scapular region) T22.40
above elbow —see Corrosion, above elbow
axilla —see Corrosion, axilla
elbow —see Corrosion, elbow
first degree T22.50
forearm —see Corrosion, forearm
hand —see Corrosion, hand
interscapular region —see Corrosion, back,
upper
multiple sites T22.499
first degree T22.599
left T22.492
first degree T22.592
second degree T22.692
third degree T22.792
right T22.491
first degree T22.591
second degree T22.691
third degree T22.791
second degree T22.699
third degree T22.799
scapular region —see Corrosion, scapular
region
second degree T22.60
shoulder —see Corrosion, shoulder
third degree T22.70
wrist —see Corrosion, hand
uterus T28.8
vagina T28.8
vulva —see Corrosion, genital organs, external,
female
wrist T23.479
first degree T23.579
left T23.472
first degree T23.572
second degree T23.672
third degree T23.772
multiple sites with hand T23.499
first degree T23.599
left T23.492
first degree T23.592
second degree T23.692
third degree T23.792
right T23.491
first degree T23.591
second degree T23.691
third degree T23.791
second degree T23.699
third degree T23.799

Corrosion (Continued)
wrist (Continued)
right T23.471
first degree T23.571
second degree T23.671
third degree T23.771
second degree T23.679
third degree T23.779
Corrosive burn —see Corrosion
Corsican fever —see Malaria
Cortical —see condition
Cortico-adrenal —see condition
Coryza (acute) J00
with grippe or influenza —see Influenza, with,
respiratory manifestations NEC
syphilitic
congenital (chronic) A50.05
Co-sleeping, child-caregiver Z72.823
Costen's syndrome or complex M26.69
Costiveness —see Constipation
Costochondritis M94.0
Cot death R99
Cotard's syndrome F22
Cotia virus B08.8
Cotton wool spots (retinal) H35.81
~~Cotungo's disease — see Sciatica~~
▶ **Cotugno disease** —see Sciatica
Cough (affected) (epidemic) (nervous) R05.9
with hemorrhage —see Hemoptysis
acute R05.1
bronchial R05.8
with grippe or influenza —see Influenza, with,
respiratory manifestations NEC
chronic R05.3
functional F45.8
hysterical F45.8
laryngeal, spasmodic R05.8
paroxysmal, due to Bordetella pertussis (without
pneumonia) A37.00
with pneumonia A37.01
persistent R05.3
refractory R05.3
psychogenic F45.8
smokers' J41.0
specified NEC R05.8
subacute R05.2
syncope R05.4
tea taster's B49
unexplained R05.3
Counseling (for) Z71.9
abuse NEC
perpetrator Z69.82
victim Z69.81
alcohol abuser Z71.41
family Z71.42
child abuse
nonparental
perpetrator Z69.021
victim Z69.020
parental
perpetrator Z69.011
victim Z69.010
consanguinity Z71.89
contraceptive Z30.09
dietary Z71.3
drug abuser Z71.51
family member Z71.52
exercise Z71.82
family Z71.89
fertility preservation (prior to cancer therapy)
(prior to removal of gonads) Z31.62
for non-attending third party Z71.0
related to sexual behavior or orientation Z70.2
genetic
nonprocreative Z71.83
procreative NEC Z31.5
gestational carrier Z31.7
health (advice) (education) (instruction) —see
Counseling, medical
risk for travel (international) Z71.84
human immunodeficiency virus (HIV) Z71.7
immunization safety Z71.85
impotence Z70.1
insulin pump use Z46.81
medical (for) Z71.9
boarding school resident Z59.3
consanguinity Z71.89
feared complaint and no disease found
Z71.1
human immunodeficiency virus (HIV) Z
71.7

Counseling (*Continued*)
  medical (*Continued*)
    institutional resident Z59.3
    on behalf of another Z71.0
      related to sexual behavior or orientation Z70.2
    person living alone (*see also* Consultation, specified reason NEC) Z60.2
    specified reason NEC Z71.89
  natural family planning
    procreative Z31.61
    to avoid pregnancy Z30.02
  pediatric-to-adult transition Z71.87
  perpetrator (of)
    abuse NEC Z69.82
    child abuse
      non-parental Z69.021
      parental Z69.011
    rape NEC Z69.82
    spousal abuse Z69.12
  procreative NEC Z31.69
    fertility preservation (prior to cancer therapy) (prior to removal of gonads) Z31.62
    using natural family planning Z31.61
  promiscuity Z70.1
  rape victim Z69.81
  religious Z71.81
  safety for travel (international) Z71.84
  sex, sexual (related to) Z70.9
    attitude(s) Z70.0
    behavior or orientation Z70.1
    combined concerns Z70.3
    non-responsiveness Z70.1
    on behalf of third party Z70.2
    specified reason NEC Z70.8
  socioeconomic factors Z71.88
  specified reason NEC Z71.89
  spiritual Z71.81
  spousal abuse (perpetrator) Z69.12
    victim Z69.11
  substance abuse Z71.89
    alcohol Z71.41
    drug Z71.51
    tobacco Z71.6
  travel (international) Z71.84
  tobacco use Z71.6
  use (of)
    insulin pump Z46.81
  vaccine product safety Z71.85
  victim (of)
    abuse Z69.81
    child abuse
      by parent Z69.010
      non-parental Z69.020
    rape NEC Z69.81
Coupled rhythm R00.8
Couvelaire syndrome or uterus (complicating delivery) O45.8X-●
COVID-19 U07.1
  condition post U09.9
  contact (with) Z20.822
  exposure (to) Z20.822
  history of (personal) Z86.16
  long (haul) U09.9
  pneumonia J12.82
  screening Z11.52
  sequelae (post acute) U09.9
Cowperitis —*see* Urethritis
Cowper's gland —*see* condition
Cowpox B08.010
  due to vaccination T88.1
Coxa
  magna M91.4-●
  plana M91.2-●
  valga (acquired) —*see also* Deformity, limb, specified type NEC, thigh
    congenital Q65.81
    sequelae (late effect) of rickets E64.3
  vara (acquired) —*see also* Deformity, limb, specified type NEC, thigh
    congenital Q65.82
    sequelae (late effect) of rickets E64.3
Coxalgia, coxalgic (nontuberculous) —*see also* Pain, joint, hip
  tuberculous A18.02
Coxitis —*see* Monoarthritis, hip
Coxsackie (virus) (infection) B34.1
  as cause of disease classified elsewhere B97.11
  carditis B33.20
  central nervous system NEC A88.8
  endocarditis B33.21

Coxsackie (*Continued*)
  enteritis A08.39
  meningitis (aseptic) A87.0
  myocarditis B33.22
  pericarditis B33.23
  pharyngitis B08.5
  pleurodynia B33.0
  specific disease NEC B33.8
Crabs, meaning pubic lice B85.3
Crack baby P04.41
Cracked nipple N64.0
  associated with
    lactation O92.13
    pregnancy O92.11-●
    puerperium O92.12
Cracked tooth K03.81
Cradle cap L21.0
Craft neurosis F48.8
Cramp(s) R25.2
  abdominal —*see* Pain, abdominal
  bathing T75.1
  colic R10.83
    psychogenic F45.8
  due to immersion T75.1
  fireman T67.2
  heat T67.2
  immersion T75.1
  intestinal —*see* Pain, abdominal
    psychogenic F45.8
  leg, sleep related G47.62
  limb (lower) (upper) NEC R25.2
    sleep related G47.62
  linotypist's F48.8
    organic G25.89
  muscle (limb) (general) R25.2
    due to immersion T75.1
    psychogenic F45.8
  occupational (hand) F48.8
    organic G25.89
  salt-depletion E87.1
  sleep related, leg G47.62
  stoker's T67.2
  swimmer's T75.1
  telegrapher's F48.8
    organic G25.89
  typist's F48.8
    organic G25.89
  uterus N94.89
    menstrual —*see* Dysmenorrhea
  writer's F48.8
    organic G25.89
Cranial —*see* condition
Craniocleidodysostosis Q74.0
Craniofenestria (skull) Q75.8
Craniolacunia (skull) Q75.8
Craniopagus Q89.4
Craniopathy, metabolic M85.2
Craniopharyngeal —*see* condition
Craniopharyngioma D44.4
Craniorachischisis (totalis) Q00.1
Cranioschisis Q75.8
Craniostenosis Q75.009
Craniosynostosis Q75.009
  bilateral Q75.002
  coronal Q75.029
    bilateral Q75.022
    unilateral Q75.021
  lambdoid Q75.049
    bilateral Q75.042
    unilateral Q75.041
  metopic Q75.03
  multi-suture, specified NEC Q75.058
  sagittal Q75.01
  single-suture, specified NEC Q75.08
  unilateral Q75.001
Craniotabes (cause unknown) M83.8
  neonatal P96.3
  rachitic E64.3
  syphilitic A50.56
Cranium —*see* condition
Craw-craw —*see* Onchocerciasis
Creaking joint —*see* Derangement, joint, specified type NEC
Creeping
  eruption B76.9
  palsy or paralysis G12.22
Crenated tongue K14.8
Creotoxism A05.9
Crepitus
  caput Q75.8
  joint —*see* Derangement, joint, specified type NEC

Crescent or conus choroid, congenital Q14.3
CREST syndrome M34.1
Cretin, cretinism (congenital) (endemic) (nongoitrous) (sporadic) E00.9
  pelvis
    with disproportion (fetopelvic) O33.0
      causing obstructed labor O65.0
  type
    hypothyroid E00.1
    mixed E00.2
    myxedematous E00.1
    neurological E00.0
Creutzfeldt-Jakob disease or syndrome (with dementia) A81.00
  familial A81.09
  iatrogenic A81.09
  specified NEC A81.09
  sporadic A81.09
  variant (vCJD) A81.01
Crib death R99
Cribriform hymen Q52.3
Cri-du-chat syndrome Q93.4
Crigler-Najjar disease or syndrome E80.5
Crime, victim of Z65.4
Crimean hemorrhagic fever A98.0
Criminalism F60.2
Crisis
  abdomen R10.0
  acute reaction F43.0
  addisonian E27.2
  adrenal (cortical) E27.2
  celiac K90.0
  Dietl's N13.8
  emotional —*see also* Disorder, adjustment
    acute reaction to stress F43.0
    specific to childhood and adolescence F93.8
  glaucomatocyclitic —*see* Glaucoma, secondary, inflammation
  heart —*see* Failure, heart
  nitritoid I95.2
    correct substance properly administered —*see* Table of Drugs and Chemicals, by drug, adverse effect
    overdose or wrong substance given or taken —*see* Table of Drugs and Chemicals, by drug, poisoning
  oculogyric H51.8
    psychogenic F45.8
  Pel's (tabetic) A52.11
  psychosexual identity F64.2
  renal N28.0
  sickle-cell (*see also* Disease, sickle-cell, by type, with crisis) D57.00
    with
      acute chest syndrome D57.01
      cerebral vascular involvement D57.03
      complication specified NEC D57.09
      pain (vaso-occlusive) D57.00
      splenic sequestration D57.02
  state (acute reaction) F43.0
  tabetic A52.11
  thyroid —*see* Thyrotoxicosis with thyroid storm
  thyrotoxic —*see* Thyrotoxicosis with thyroid storm
Crocq's disease (acrocyanosis) I73.89
Crohn's disease —*see* Enteritis, regional
Crooked septum, nasal J34.2
Cross syndrome E70.328
Crossbite (anterior) (posterior) M26.24
Cross-eye —*see* Strabismus, convergent concomitant
Croup, croupous (catarrhal) (infectious) (inflammatory) (nondiphtheritic) J05.0
  bronchial J20.9
  diphtheritic A36.2
  false J38.5
  spasmodic J38.5
    diphtheritic A36.2
  stridulous J38.5
    diphtheritic A36.2
Crouzon's disease Q75.1
Crowding, tooth, teeth, fully erupted M26.31
CRST syndrome M34.1
Cruchet's disease A85.8
Cruelty in children —*see also* Disorder, conduct
Crural ulcer —*see* Ulcer, lower limb
Crush, crushed, crushing T14.8
  abdomen S38.1
  ankle S97.0-●
  arm (upper) (and shoulder) S47.-●
  axilla —*see* Crush, arm

▶ New   ⇒ Revised   ~~deleted~~ Deleted   ● Use Additional Character(s)

Crush, crushed, crushing (Continued)
  back, lower S38.1
  buttock S38.1
  cheek S07.0
  chest S28.0
  cranium S07.1
  ear S07.0
  elbow S57.0-●
  extremity
    lower
      ankle —see Crush, ankle
      below knee —see Crush, leg
      foot —see Crush, foot
      hip —see Crush, hip
      knee —see Crush, knee
      thigh —see Crush, thigh
      toe —see Crush, toe
    upper
      below elbow S67.9-●
      elbow —see Crush, elbow
      finger —see Crush, finger
      forearm —see Crush, forearm
      hand —see Crush, hand
      thumb —see Crush, thumb
      upper arm —see Crush, arm
      wrist —see Crush, wrist
  face S07.0
  finger(s) S67.1-●
    with hand (and wrist) —see Crush, hand,
      specified site NEC
    index S67.19-●
    little S67.19-●
    middle S67.19-●
    ring S67.19-●
    thumb —see Crush, thumb
  foot S97.8-●
    toe —see Crush, toe
  forearm S57.8-●
  genitalia, external
    female S38.002
      vagina S38.03
      vulva S38.03
    male S38.001
      penis S38.01
      scrotum S38.02
      testis S38.02
  hand (except fingers alone) S67.2-●
    with wrist S67.4-●
  head S07.9
    specified NEC S07.8
  heel —see Crush, foot
  hip S77.0-●
    with thigh S77.2-●
  internal organ (abdomen, chest, or pelvis) NEC
    T14.8
  knee S87.0-●
  labium (majus) (minus) S38.03
  larynx S17.0
  leg (lower) S87.8-●
    knee —see Crush, knee
  lip S07.0
  lower
    back S38.1
    leg —see Crush, leg
  neck S17.9
  nerve —see Injury, nerve
  nose S07.0
  pelvis S38.1
  penis S38.01
  scalp S07.8
  scapular region —see Crush, arm
  scrotum S38.02
  severe, unspecified site T14.8
  shoulder (and upper arm) —see Crush, arm
  skull S07.1
  syndrome (complication of trauma) T79.5
  testis S38.02
  thigh S77.1-●
    with hip S77.2-●
  throat S17.8
  thumb S67.0-●
    with hand (and wrist) —see Crush, hand,
      specified site NEC
  toe(s) S97.10-●
    great S97.11-●
    lesser S97.12-●
  trachea S17.0
  vagina S38.03
  vulva S38.03
  wrist S67.3-●
    with hand S67.4-●

Crusta lactea L21.0
Crusts R23.4
Crutch paralysis —see Injury, brachial plexus
Cruveilhier-Baumgarten cirrhosis, disease or
  syndrome K74.69
Cruveilhier's atrophy or disease G12.8
Crying (constant) (continuous) (excessive)
  child, adolescent, or adult R45.83
  infant (baby) (newborn) R68.11
Cryofibrinogenemia D89.2
Cryoglobulinemia (essential) (idiopathic) (mixed)
  (primary) (purpura) (secondary) (vasculitis)
  D89.1
  with lung involvement D89.1 [J99]
Cryptitis (anal) (rectal) K62.89
Cryptococcosis, cryptococcus (infection)
  (neoformans) B45.9
  bone B45.3
  cerebral B45.1
  cutaneous B45.2
  disseminated B45.7
  generalized B45.7
  meningitis B45.1
  meningocerebralis B45.1
  osseous B45.3
  pulmonary B45.0
  skin B45.2
  specified NEC B45.8
Cryptopapillitis (anus) K62.89
Cryptophthalmos Q11.2
  syndrome Q87.0
Cryptorchid, cryptorchism, cryptorchidism Q53.9
  bilateral Q53.20
    abdominal Q53.211
    perineal Q53.22
  unilateral Q53.10
    abdominal Q53.111
    perineal Q53.12
Cryptosporidiosis A07.2
  hepatobiliary B88.8
  respiratory B88.8
Cryptostromosis J67.6
Crystalluria R82.998
Cubitus
  congenital Q68.8
  valgus (acquired) M21.0-●
    congenital Q68.8
    sequelae (late effect) of rickets E64.3
  varus (acquired) M21.1-●
    congenital Q68.8
    sequelae (late effect) of rickets E64.3
Cultural deprivation or shock Z60.3
Curling esophagus K22.4
Curling's ulcer —see Ulcer, peptic, acute
Curschmann (-Batten) (-Steinert) disease or
  syndrome G71.11
Curse, Ondine's —see Apnea, sleep
Curvature
  organ or site, congenital NEC —see Distortion
  penis (lateral) Q55.61
  Pott's (spinal) A18.01
  radius, idiopathic, progressive (congenital)
    Q74.0
  spine (acquired) (angular) (idiopathic) (incorrect)
    (postural) —see Dorsopathy, deforming
    congenital Q67.5
    due to or associated with
      Charcot-Marie-Tooth disease —see also
        subcategory M49.8 G60.0
      osteitis
        deformans M88.88
        fibrosa cystica —see also subcategory
          M49.8 E21.0
      tuberculosis (Pott's curvature) A18.01
    sequelae (late effect) of rickets E64.3
    tuberculous A18.01
Cushingoid due to steroid therapy E24.2
  correct substance properly administered —see
    Table of Drugs and Chemicals, by drug,
    adverse effect
  overdose or wrong substance given or taken —
    see Table of Drugs and Chemicals, by drug,
    poisoning
Cushing's
  syndrome or disease E24.9
    drug-induced E24.2
    iatrogenic E24.2
    pituitary-dependent E24.0
    specified NEC E24.8
  ulcer —see Ulcer, peptic, acute
Cusp, Carabelli - omit code

Cut (external) —see also Laceration
  muscle —see Injury, muscle
Cutaneous —see also condition
  hemorrhage R23.3
  larva migrans B76.9
Cutis —see also condition
  hyperelastica Q82.8
    acquired L57.4
  laxa (hyperelastica) —see Dermatolysis
  marmorata R23.8
  osteosis L94.2
  pendula —see Dermatolysis
  rhomboidalis nuchae L57.2
  verticis gyrata Q82.8
    acquired L91.8
Cyanosis R23.0
  due to
    patent foramen botalli Q21.12
    persistent foramen ovale Q21.12
  enterogenous D74.8
  paroxysmal digital —see Raynaud's disease
    with gangrene I73.01
  retina, retinal H35.89
Cyanotic heart disease I24.9
  congenital Q24.9
Cycle
  anovulatory N97.0
  menstrual, irregular N92.6
Cyclencephaly Q04.9
Cyclical vomiting, in migraine (see also Vomiting,
    cyclical) G43.A0
  psychogenic F50.89
Cyclitis —see also Iridocyclitis H20.9
  chronic —see Iridocyclitis, chronic
  Fuchs' heterochromic H20.81-●
  granulomatous —see Iridocyclitis, chronic
  lens-induced —see Iridocyclitis, lens-induced
  posterior H30.2-●
Cycloid personality F34.0
Cyclophoria H50.54
Cyclopia, cyclops Q87.0
Cyclopism Q87.0
Cyclosporiasis A07.4
Cyclothymia F34.0
Cyclothymic personality F34.0
Cyclotropia H50.41-●
Cylindroma —see also Neoplasm, malignant, by
    site
  eccrine dermal —see Neoplasm, skin, benign
  skin —see Neoplasm, skin, benign
Cylindruria R82.998
Cynanche
  diphtheritic A36.2
  tonsillaris J36
Cynophobia F40.218
Cynorexia R63.2
Cyphosis —see Kyphosis
Cyprus fever —see Brucellosis
Cyst (colloid) (mucous) (simple) (retention)
  adenoid (infected) J35.8
  adrenal gland E27.8
    congenital Q89.1
  air, lung J98.4
  allantoic Q64.4
  alveolar process (jaw bone) M27.40
  amnion, amniotic O41.8X-●
  aneurysmal M27.49
  anterior
    chamber (eye) —see Cyst, iris
    nasopalatine K09.1
  antrum J34.1
  anus K62.89
  apical (tooth) (periodontal) K04.8
  appendix K38.8
  arachnoid, brain (acquired) G93.0
    congenital Q04.6
  arytenoid J38.7
  Baker's M71.2-●
    ruptured M66.0
    tuberculous A18.02
  Bartholin's gland N75.0
  bile duct (common) (hepatic) K83.5
  bladder (multiple) (trigone) N32.89
  blue dome (breast) —see Cyst, breast
  bone (local) NEC M85.60
    aneurysmal M85.50
      ankle M85.57-●
      foot M85.57-●
      forearm M85.53-●
      hand M85.54-●
      jaw M27.49

▶ New   ⟹ Revised   ~~deleted~~ Deleted   ● Use Additional Character(s)

Cyst (Continued)
jaw (bone) (Continued)
  hemorrhagic M27.49
  traumatic M27.49
joint NEC —see Disorder, joint, specified type NEC
kidney N28.1
  acquired N28.1
  calyceal —see Hydronephrosis
  congenital Q61.00
    more than one (multiple) Q61.02
      specified as polycystic Q61.3
        adult type (autosomal dominant) Q61.2
        infantile type (autosomal recessive) NEC Q61.19
          collecting duct dilation Q61.11
  pyelogenic —see Hydronephrosis
  simple N28.1
  solitary (single) N28.1
    acquired N28.1
congenital Q61.01
labium (majus) (minus) N90.7
  sebaceous N90.7
lacrimal —see also Disorder, lacrimal system, specified NEC
  gland H04.13-●
  passages or sac —see Disorder, lacrimal system, specified NEC
larynx J38.7
lateral periodontal K09.0
lens H27.8
  congenital Q12.8
lip (gland) K13.0
liver (idiopathic) (simple) K76.89
  congenital Q44.6
  hydatid B67.8
    granulosus B67.0
    multilocularis B67.5
lung J98.4
  congenital Q33.0
  giant bullous J43.9
lutein N83.1-●
lymphangiomatous D18.1
lymphoepithelial, oral soft tissue K09.8
macula —see Degeneration, macula, hole
malignant —see Neoplasm, malignant, by site
mammary gland —see Cyst, breast
mandible M27.40
  dentigerous K09.0
  radicular K04.8
maxilla M27.40
  dentigerous K09.0
  radicular K04.8
medial, face and neck Q18.8
median
  anterior maxillary K09.1
  palatal K09.1
mediastinum, congenital Q34.1
meibomian (gland) —see Chalazion
  infected —see Hordeolum
membrane, brain G93.0
meninges (cerebral) G93.0
  spinal G96.198
meniscus, knee —see Derangement, knee, meniscus, cystic
mesentery, mesenteric K66.8
  chyle I89.8
mesonephric duct
  female Q50.5
  male Q55.4
milk N64.89
Morgagni (hydatid)
  female Q50.5
  male (epididymal) Q55.4
    testicular Q55.29
mouth K09.8
Müllerian duct Q50.4
  appendix testis Q55.29
  cervix Q51.6
  fallopian tube Q50.4
  female Q50.4
  male Q55.29
  prostatic utricle Q55.4
  vagina (embryonal) Q52.4
multilocular (ovary) D39.10
  benign —see Neoplasm, benign, by site
myometrium N85.8
nabothian (follicle) (ruptured) N88.8
nasoalveolar K09.1
nasolabial K09.1
nasopalatine (anterior) (duct) K09.1

Cyst (Continued)
nasopharynx J39.2
neoplastic —see Neoplasm, uncertain behavior, by site
  benign —see Neoplasm, benign, by site
nerve root
  cervical G96.191
  lumbar G96.191
  sacral G96.191
  thoracic G96.191
nervous system NEC G96.89
neuroenteric (congenital) Q06.8
nipple —see Cyst, breast
nose (turbinates) J34.1
  sinus J34.1
odontogenic, developmental K09.0
omentum (lesser) K66.8
  congenital Q45.8
ora serrata —see Cyst, retina, ora serrata
oral
  region K09.9
    developmental (nonodontogenic) K09.1
    specified NEC K09.8
  soft tissue K09.9
    specified NEC K09.8
orbit H05.81-●
ovary, ovarian (twisted) N83.20-●
  adherent N83.20-●
  chocolate N80.10-●
  corpus
    albicans N83.29-●
    luteum (hemorrhagic) N83.1-●
  dermoid D27.9
  developmental Q50.1
  due to failure of involution NEC N83.20-●
  endometrial N80.10-●
  follicular (graafian) (hemorrhagic) N83.0-●
  hemorrhagic N83.20-●
  in pregnancy or childbirth O34.8-●
    with obstructed labor O65.5
  multilocular D39.10
  pseudomucinous D27.9
  retention N83.29-●
  serous N83.20-●
  specified NEC N83.29-●
  theca lutein (hemorrhagic) N83.1-●
  tuberculous A18.18
oviduct N83.8
palate (median) (fissural) K09.1
palatine papilla (jaw) K09.1
pancreas, pancreatic (hemorrhagic) (true) K86.2
  congenital Q45.2
  false K86.3
paralabral
  hip M24.85-●
  shoulder S43.43-●
paramesonephric duct Q50.4
  female Q50.4
  male Q55.29
paranephric N28.1
paraphysis, cerebri, congenital Q04.6
parasitic B89
parathyroid (gland) E21.4
paratubal N83.8
paraurethral duct N36.8
paroophoron Q50.5
parotid gland K11.6
parovarian Q50.5
pelvis, female N94.89
  in pregnancy or childbirth O34.8-●
    causing obstructed labor O65.5
penis (sebaceous) N48.89
periapical K04.8
pericardial (congenital) Q24.8
  acquired (secondary) I31.8
pericoronal K09.0
perineural G96.191
periodontal K04.8
  lateral K09.0
peripelvic (lymphatic) N28.1
peritoneum K66.8
  chylous I89.8
periventricular, acquired, newborn P91.1
pharynx (wall) J39.2
pilar L72.11
pilonidal (infected) (rectum) L05.91
  with abscess L05.01
  malignant C44.59-●
pituitary (duct) (gland) E23.6
placenta O43.19-●
pleura J94.8

Cyst (Continued)
popliteal —see Cyst, Baker's
porencephalic Q04.6
  acquired G93.0
postanal (infected) —see Cyst, pilonidal
postmastoidectomy cavity (mucosal) —see Complications, postmastoidectomy, cyst
preauricular Q18.1
prepuce N47.4
  congenital Q55.69
primordial (jaw) K09.0
prostate N42.83
pseudomucinous (ovary) D27.9
pupillary, miotic H21.27-●
radicular (residual) K04.8
radiculodental K04.8
ranular K11.8
Rathke's pouch E23.6
rectum (epithelium) (mucous) K62.89
renal —see Cyst, kidney
residual (radicular) K04.8
retention (ovary) N83.29-●
  salivary gland K11.6
retina H33.19-●
  ora serrata H33.11-●
  parasitic H33.12-●
retroperitoneal K68.9
sacrococcygeal (dermoid) —see Cyst, pilonidal
salivary gland or duct (mucous extravasation or retention) K11.6
Sampson's N80.10-●
sclera H15.89
scrotum L72.9
  sebaceous L72.3
sebaceous (duct) (gland) L72.3
  breast —see Dysplasia, mammary, specified type NEC
  eyelid —see Cyst, eyelid
  genital organ NEC
    female N94.89
    male N50.89
  scrotum L72.3
semilunar cartilage (knee) (multiple) —see Derangement, knee, meniscus, cystic
seminal vesicle N50.89
serous (ovary) N83.20-●
sinus (accessory) (nasal) J34.1
Skene's gland N36.8
skin L72.9
  breast —see Dysplasia, mammary, specified type NEC
  epidermal, epidermoid L72.0
  epithelial L72.0
  eyelid —see Cyst, eyelid
  genital organ NEC
    female N90.7
    male N50.89
  inclusion L72.0
  scrotum L72.9
  sebaceous L72.3
  sweat gland or duct L74.8
solitary
  bone —see Cyst, bone, solitary
  jaw M27.40
  kidney N28.1
spermatic cord N50.89
sphenoid sinus J34.1
spinal meninges G96.198
spleen NEC D73.4
  congenital Q89.09
  hydatid —see also Echinococcus B67.99 [D77]
Stafne's M27.0
subarachnoid intrasellar R93.0
subcutaneous, pheomycotic (chromomycotic) B43.2
subdural (cerebral) G93.0
  spinal cord G96.198
sublingual gland K11.6
submandibular gland K11.6
submaxillary gland K11.6
suburethral N36.8
suprarenal gland E27.8
suprasellar —see Cyst, brain
sweat gland or duct L74.8
synovial —see also Cyst, bursa
  ruptured —see Rupture, synovium
Tarlov G96.191
tarsal —see Chalazion
tendon (sheath) —see Disorder, tendon, specified type NEC

Cyst *(Continued)*
  testis N44.2
    tunica albuginea N44.1
  theca lutein (ovary) N83.1-●
  Thornwaldt's J39.2
  thymus (gland) E32.8
  thyroglossal duct (infected) (persistent) Q89.2
  thyroid (gland) E04.1
  thyrolingual duct (infected) (persistent) Q89.2
  tongue K14.8
  tonsil J35.8
  tooth —*see* Cyst, dental
  Tornwaldt's J39.2
  trichilemmal (proliferating) L72.12
  trichodermal L72.12
  tubal (fallopian) N83.8
    inflammatory —*see* Salpingitis, chronic
  tubo-ovarian N83.8
    inflammatory N70.13
  tunica
    albuginea testis N44.1
    vaginalis N50.89
  turbinate (nose) J34.1
  Tyson's gland N48.89
  urachus, congenital Q64.4
  ureter N28.89
  ureterovesical orifice N28.89
  urethra, urethral (gland) N36.8
  uterine ligament N83.8
  uterus (body) (corpus) (recurrent) N85.8
    embryonic Q51.818
      cervix Q51.6
  vagina, vaginal (implantation) (inclusion)
    (squamous cell) (wall) N89.8
    embryonic Q52.4
  vallecula, vallecular (epiglottis) J38.7
  vesical (orifice) N32.89
  vitreous body H43.89
  vulva (implantation) (inclusion) N90.7
    congenital Q52.79
    sebaceous gland N90.7
  vulvovaginal gland N90.7
  wolffian
    female Q50.5
    male Q55.4
Cystadenocarcinoma —*see* Neoplasm, malignant,
  by site
  bile duct C22.1
  endometrioid —*see* Neoplasm, malignant, by site
    specified site —*see* Neoplasm, malignant, by
      site
    unspecified site
      female C56.9
      male C61
  mucinous
    papillary
      specified site —*see* Neoplasm, malignant,
        by site
      unspecified site C56.9
    specified site —*see* Neoplasm, malignant, by
      site
    unspecified site C56.9
  papillary
    mucinous
      specified site —*see* Neoplasm, malignant,
        by site
      unspecified site C56.9
    pseudomucinous
      specified site —*see* Neoplasm, malignant,
        by site
      unspecified site C56.9
    serous
      specified site —*see* Neoplasm, malignant,
        by site
      unspecified site C56.9
    specified site —*see* Neoplasm, malignant, by
      site
    unspecified site C56.9
  pseudomucinous
    papillary
      specified site —*see* Neoplasm, malignant,
        by site
      unspecified site C56.9
    specified site —*see* Neoplasm, malignant, by
      site
    unspecified site C56.9
  serous
    papillary
      specified site —*see* Neoplasm, malignant,
        by site
      unspecified site C56.9

Cystadenocarcinoma *(Continued)*
  serous *(Continued)*
    specified site —*see* Neoplasm, malignant, by
      site
    unspecified site C56.9
Cystadenofibroma
  clear cell —*see* Neoplasm, benign, by site
  endometrioid D27.9
    borderline malignancy D39.1-●
    malignant C56.-●
  mucinous
    specified site —*see* Neoplasm, benign, by site
    unspecified site D27.9
  serous
    specified site —*see* Neoplasm, benign, by site
    unspecified site D27.9
  specified site —*see* Neoplasm, benign, by site
  unspecified site D27.9
Cystadenoma —*see also* Neoplasm, benign, by site
  bile duct D13.4
  endometrioid —*see* Neoplasm, benign, by site
    borderline malignancy —*see* Neoplasm,
      uncertain behavior, by site
  malignant —*see* Neoplasm, malignant, by site
  mucinous
    borderline malignancy
      ovary C56.-●
      specified site NEC —*see* Neoplasm,
        uncertain behavior, by site
      unspecified site C56.9
    papillary
      borderline malignancy
        ovary C56.-●
        specified site NEC —*see* Neoplasm,
          uncertain behavior, by site
        unspecified site C56.9
      specified site —*see* Neoplasm, benign, by site
      unspecified site D27.9
    specified site —*see* Neoplasm, benign, by site
    unspecified site D27.9
  papillary
    borderline malignancy
      ovary C56-●
      specified site NEC —*see* Neoplasm,
        uncertain behavior, by site
      unspecified site C56.9
    lymphomatosum
      specified site —*see* Neoplasm, benign, by
        site
      unspecified site D11.9
    mucinous
      borderline malignancy
        ovary C56.-●
        specified site NEC —*see* Neoplasm,
          uncertain behavior, by site
        unspecified site C56.9
      specified site —*see* Neoplasm, benign, by
        site
      unspecified site D27.9
    pseudomucinous
      borderline malignancy
        ovary C56.-●
        specified site NEC —*see* Neoplasm,
          uncertain behavior, by site
        unspecified site C56.9
      specified site —*see* Neoplasm, benign, by
        site
      unspecified site D27.9
    serous
      borderline malignancy
        ovary C56.-●
        specified site NEC —*see* Neoplasm,
          uncertain behavior, by site
        unspecified site C56.9
      specified site —*see* Neoplasm, benign, by
        site
      unspecified site D27.9
    specified site —*see* Neoplasm, benign, by site
    unspecified site D27.9
  pseudomucinous
    borderline malignancy
      ovary C56.-●
      specified site NEC —*see* Neoplasm,
        uncertain behavior, by site
      unspecified site C56.9
    papillary
      borderline malignancy
        ovary C56.-●
        specified site NEC —*see* Neoplasm,
          uncertain behavior, by site
        unspecified site C56.9

Cystadenoma *(Continued)*
  pseudomucinous *(Continued)*
    papillary *(Continued)*
      specified site —*see* Neoplasm, benign, by
        site
      unspecified site D27.9
    specified site —*see* Neoplasm, benign, by site
    unspecified site D27.9
  serous
    borderline malignancy
      ovary C56.-●
      specified site NEC —*see* Neoplasm,
        uncertain behavior, by site
      unspecified site C56.9
    papillary
      borderline malignancy
        ovary C56.-●
        specified site NEC —*see* Neoplasm,
          uncertain behavior, by site
        unspecified site C56.9
      specified site —*see* Neoplasm, benign, by
        site
      unspecified site D27.9
    specified site —*see* Neoplasm, benign, by site
    unspecified site D27.9
Cystathionine synthase deficiency E72.11
Cystathioninemia E72.19
Cystathioninuria E72.19
Cystic —*see also* condition
  breast (chronic) —*see* Mastopathy, cystic
  corpora lutea (hemorrhagic) N83.1-●
  duct —*see* condition
  eyeball (congenital) Q11.0
  fibrosis —*see* Fibrosis, cystic
  kidney (congenital) Q61.9
    adult type Q61.2
    infantile type NEC Q61.19
      collecting duct dilatation Q61.11
    medullary Q61.5
  liver, congenital Q44.6
  lung disease J98.4
    congenital Q33.0
  mastitis, chronic —*see* Mastopathy, cystic
  medullary, kidney Q61.5
  meniscus —*see* Derangement, knee, meniscus,
    cystic
  ovary N83.20-●
Cysticercosis, cysticerciasis B69.9
  with
    epileptiform fits B69.0
    myositis B69.81
  brain B69.0
  central nervous system B69.0
  cerebral B69.0
  ocular B69.1
  specified NEC B69.89
Cysticercus cellulose infestation —*see*
  Cysticercosis
Cystinosis (malignant) E72.04
Cystinuria E72.01
Cystitis (exudative) (hemorrhagic) (septic)
  (suppurative) N30.90
  with
    fibrosis —*see* Cystitis, chronic, interstitial
    hematuria N30.91
    leukoplakia —*see* Cystitis, chronic, interstitial
    malakoplakia —*see* Cystitis, chronic,
      interstitial
    metaplasia —*see* Cystitis, chronic, interstitial
    prostatitis N41.3
  acute N30.00
    with hematuria N30.01
    of trigone N30.30
      with hematuria N30.31
  allergic —*see* Cystitis, specified type NEC
  amebic A06.81
  bilharzial B65.9 *[N33]*
  blennorrhagic (gonococcal) A54.01
  bullous —*see* Cystitis, specified type NEC
  calculous N21.0
  chlamydial A56.01
  chronic N30.20
    with hematuria N30.21
    interstitial N30.10
      with hematuria N30.11
    of trigone N30.30
      with hematuria N30.31
    specified NEC N30.20
      with hematuria N30.21
  cystic (a) —*see* Cystitis, specified type NEC
  diphtheritic A36.85

▶ New   ⇒ Revised   ~~deleted~~ Deleted   ● Use Additional Character(s)

Cystitis *(Continued)*
  echinococcal
    granulosus B67.39
    multilocularis B67.69
  emphysematous —*see* Cystitis, specified type
    NEC
  encysted —*see* Cystitis, specified type NEC
  eosinophilic —*see* Cystitis, specified type NEC
  follicular —*see* Cystitis, of trigone
  gangrenous —*see* Cystitis, specified type NEC
  glandularis —*see* Cystitis, specified type NEC
  gonococcal A54.01
  incrusted —*see* Cystitis, specified type NEC
  interstitial (chronic) —*see* Cystitis, chronic,
    interstitial
  irradiation N30.40
    with hematuria N30.41
  irritation —*see* Cystitis, specified type NEC
  malignant —*see* Cystitis, specified type NEC
  of trigone N30.30
    with hematuria N30.31
  panmural —*see* Cystitis, chronic, interstitial
  polyposa —*see* Cystitis, specified type NEC
  prostatic N41.3
  puerperal (postpartum) O86.22
  radiation —*see* Cystitis, irradiation
  specified type NEC N30.80
    with hematuria N30.81
  subacute —*see* Cystitis, chronic
  submucous —*see* Cystitis, chronic, interstitial
  syphilitic (late) A52.76
  trichomonal A59.03
  tuberculous A18.12
  ulcerative —*see* Cystitis, chronic, interstitial
Cystocele (-urethrocele)
  female N81.10
    with prolapse of uterus —*see* Prolapse, uterus
    lateral N81.12
    midline N81.11
    paravaginal N81.12
  in pregnancy or childbirth O34.8-●
    causing obstructed labor O65.5
  male N32.89
Cystolithiasis N21.0
Cystoma —*see also* Neoplasm, benign, by site
  endometrial, ovary N80.10-●
  mucinous
    specified site —*see* Neoplasm, benign, by site
    unspecified site D27.9
  serous
    specified site —*see* Neoplasm, benign, by site
    unspecified site D27.9
  simple (ovary) N83.29-●
Cystoplegia N31.2
Cystoptosis N32.89
Cystopyelitis —*see* Pyelonephritis
Cystorrhagia N32.89
Cystosarcoma phyllodes D48.6-●
  benign D24-●
  malignant —*see* Neoplasm, breast, malignant
Cystostomy
  attention to Z43.5
  complication —*see* Complications, cystostomy
  status Z93.50
    appendico-vesicostomy Z93.52
    cutaneous Z93.51
    specified NEC Z93.59
Cystourethritis —*see* Urethritis
Cystourethrocele —*see also* Cystocele
  female N81.10
    with uterine prolapse —*see* Prolapse, uterus
    lateral N81.12
    midline N81.11
    paravaginal N81.12
  male N32.89
Cytomegalic inclusion disease
  congenital P35.1
Cytomegalovirus infection B25.9
Cytomycosis (reticuloendothelial) B39.4
Cytopenia D75.9
  refractory
    with multilineage dysplasia D46.A
    and ring sideroblasts (RCMD RS) D46.B
Czerny's disease (periodic hydrarthrosis of the
  knee) —*see* Effusion, joint, knee

D

Daae (-Finsen) disease (epidemic pleurodynia)
  B33.0
Dabney's grip B33.0
Da Costa's syndrome F45.8
Dacryoadenitis, dacryadenitis H04.00-●
  acute H04.01-●
  chronic H04.02-●
Dacryocystitis H04.30-●
  acute H04.32-●
  chronic H04.41-●
  neonatal P39.1
  phlegmonous H04.31-●
  syphilitic A52.71
    congenital (early) A50.01
  trachomatous, active A71.1
    sequelae (late effect) B94.0
~~Dacryocystoblennorrhea —see Inflammation,~~
  ~~lacrimal, passages, chronic~~
▶Dacryocystoblennorrhea —*see* see Inflammation,
  lacrimal, passages, chronic
Dacryocystocele —*see* Disorder, lacrimal system,
  changes
Dacryolith, dacryolithiasis H04.51-●
Dacryoma —*see* Disorder, lacrimal system,
  changes
Dacryopericystitis —*see* Dacryocystitis
Dacryops H04.11-●
Dacryostenosis —*see also* Stenosis, lacrimal
  congenital Q10.5
Dactylitis
  bone —*see* Osteomyelitis
  sickle-cell D57.00
    Hb C D57.219
    Hb SS D57.00
    specified NEC D57.819
  skin L08.9
  syphilitic A52.77
  tuberculous A18.03
Dactylolysis spontanea (ainhum) L94.6
Dactylosymphysis Q70.9
  fingers —*see* Syndactylism, complex, fingers
  toes —*see* Syndactylism, complex, toes
Damage
  arteriosclerotic —*see* Arteriosclerosis
  brain (nontraumatic) G93.9
    anoxic, hypoxic G93.1
      resulting from a procedure G97.82
    child NEC G80.9
    due to birth injury P11.2
  cardiorenal (vascular) —*see* Hypertension,
    cardiorenal
  cerebral NEC —*see* Damage, brain
  coccyx, complicating delivery O71.6
  coronary —*see* Disease, heart, ischemic
  deep tissue, pressure-induced —*see also* L89 with
    final character .6
  eye, birth injury P15.3
  liver (nontraumatic) K76.9
    alcoholic K70.9
    due to drugs —*see* Disease, liver, toxic
    toxic —*see* Disease, liver, toxic
  lung
    dabbing (related) U07.0
    electronic cigarette (related) U07.0
    vaping (associated) (device) (product) (use)
      U07.0
  medication T88.7
  organ
    dabbing (related) U07.0
    electronic cigarette (related) U07.0
    vaping (associated) (device) (product) (use)
      U07.0
  pelvic
    joint or ligament, during delivery O71.6
    organ NEC
      during delivery O71.5
      following ectopic or molar pregnancy O08.6
  renal —*see* Disease, renal
  subendocardium, subendocardial —*see*
    Degeneration, myocardial
  vascular I99.9
Dana-Putnam syndrome (subacute combined
  sclerosis with pernicious anemia) —*see*
  Degeneration, combined
Danbolt (-Cross) syndrome (acrodermatitis
  enteropathica) E83.2
Dandruff L21.0
Dandy-Walker syndrome Q03.1
  with spina bifida —*see* Spina bifida

Danlos' syndrome (*see also* Syndrome, Ehler-
  Danlos) Q79.60
Darier (-White) disease (congenital) Q82.8
  meaning erythema annulare centrifugum L53.1
Darier-Roussy sarcoid D86.3
Darling's disease or histoplasmosis B39.4
Darwin's tubercle Q17.8
Dawson's (inclusion body) encephalitis A81.1
De Beurmann (-Gougerot) disease B42.1
De la Tourette's syndrome F95.2
De Lange's syndrome Q87.19
De Morgan's spots (senile angiomas) I78.1
De Quervain's
  disease (tendon sheath) M65.4
  syndrome E34.51
  thyroiditis (subacute granulomatous thyroiditis)
    E06.1
De Toni-Fanconi (-Debré) syndrome E72.09
  with cystinosis E72.04
Dead
  fetus, retained (mother) O36.4
    early pregnancy O02.1
  labyrinth —*see* subcategory H83.2
  ovum, retained O02.0
Deaf nonspeaking NEC H91.3
Deafmutism (acquired) (congenital) NEC H91.3
  hysterical F44.6
  syphilitic, congenital —*see also* subcategory
    H94.8 A50.09
Deafness (acquired) (complete) (hereditary)
    (partial) H91.9-●
  with blue sclera and fragility of bone Q78.0
  auditory fatigue —*see* Deafness, specified type NEC
  aviation T70.0
    nerve injury —*see* Injury, nerve, acoustic,
      specified type NEC
  boilermaker's —*see* subcategory H83.3
  central —*see* Deafness, sensorineural
  conductive H90.2
    and sensorineural
      mixed H90.8
        bilateral H90.6
      bilateral H90.0
      unilateral H90.1-●
        with restricted hearing on the contralateral
          side H90.A-●
  congenital H90.5
    with blue sclera and fragility of bone Q78.0
  due to toxic agents —*see* Deafness, ototoxic
  emotional (hysterical) F44.6
  functional (hysterical) F44.6
  high frequency H91.9-●
  hysterical F44.6
  low frequency H91.9-●
  mental R48.8
  mixed conductive and sensorineural H90.8
    bilateral H90.6
    unilateral H90.7-●
  nerve —*see* Deafness, sensorineural
  neural —*see* Deafness, sensorineural
  noise-induced —*see also* subcategory H83.3
    nerve injury —*see* Injury, nerve, acoustic,
      specified type NEC
  nonspeaking H91.3
  ototoxic —*see* subcategory H91.0
  perceptive —*see* Deafness, sensorineural
  psychogenic (hysterical) F44.6
  sensorineural H90.5
    and conductive
      mixed H90.8
        bilateral H90.6
      bilateral H90.3
      unilateral H90.4-●
        with restricted hearing on the contralateral
          side H90.A-●
  sensory —*see* Deafness, sensorineural
  specified type NEC —*see* subcategory H91.8
  sudden (idiopathic) H91.2-●
  syphilitic A52.15
  transient ischemic H93.01-●
  traumatic —*see* Injury, nerve, acoustic, specified
    type NEC
  word (developmental) H93.25
Death (cause unknown) (of) (unexplained)
    (unspecified cause) R99
  brain G93.82
  cardiac (sudden) (with successful
    resuscitation) —*see* Arrest, cardiac
    family history of Z82.41
    personal history of Z86.74
  family member (assumed) Z63.4

Debt, burdensome Z59.86
Debility (chronic) (general) (nervous) R53.81
  congenital or neonatal NOS P96.9
  nervous R53.81
  old age R54
  senile R54
Débove's disease (splenomegaly) R16.1
Decalcification
  bone —see Osteoporosis
  teeth K03.89
Decapsulation, kidney N28.89
Decay
  dental —see Caries, dental
  senile R54
  tooth, teeth —see Caries, dental
Deciduitis (acute)
  following ectopic or molar pregnancy O08.0
Decline (general) —see Debility
  cognitive, age-associated R41.81
Decompensation
  cardiac (acute) (chronic) —see Disease, heart
  cardiovascular —see Disease, cardiovascular
  heart —see Disease, heart
  hepatic —see Failure, hepatic
  myocardial (acute) (chronic) —see Disease,
    heart
  respiratory J98.8
Decompression sickness T70.3
Decrease (d)
  absolute neutrophile count —see Neutropenia
  blood
  ▶glucose
    ▶level 1 E16.A1
    ▶level 2 E16.A2
    ▶level 3 E16.A3
    platelets —see Thrombocytopenia
    pressure R03.1
      due to shock following
        injury T79.4
        operation T81.19
  estrogen E28.39
    postablative E89.40
      asymptomatic E89.40
      symptomatic E89.41
  fragility of erythrocytes D58.8
  function
    lipase (pancreatic) K90.3
    ovary in hypopituitarism E23.0
    parenchyma of pancreas K86.89
    pituitary (gland) (anterior) (lobe) E23.0
      posterior (lobe) E23.0
  functional activity R68.89
  glucose R73.09
  hematocrit R71.0
  hemoglobin R71.0
  leukocytes D72.819
    specified NEC D72.818
  libido R68.82
  lymphocytes D72.810
  platelets D69.6
  respiration, due to shock following injury T79.4
  sexual desire R68.82
  tear secretion NEC —see Syndrome, dry eye
  tolerance
    fat K90.49
    glucose R73.09
    pancreatic K90.3
    salt and water E87.8
  vision NEC H54.7
  white blood cell count D72.819
    specified NEC D72.818
Decubitus (ulcer) —see Ulcer, pressure, by site
  cervix N86
Deepening acetabulum —see Derangement, joint,
    specified type NEC, hip
Defect, defective Q89.9
  3-beta-hydroxysteroid dehydrogenase E25.0
  11-hydroxylase E25.0
  21-hydroxylase E25.0
  abdominal wall, congenital Q79.59
  antibody immunodeficiency D80.9
  aorticopulmonary septum Q21.4
  atrial septal Q21.1
    coronary sinus Q21.13
    following acute myocardial infarction (current
      complication) I23.1
    ostium primum type (type I) Q21.20
      with
        common atrioventricular valves and
          moderate or larger inlet VSD
          Q21.23

Defect, defective (Continued)
  atrial septal (Continued)
    ostium primum type (Continued)
      with (Continued)
        separate atrioventricular valves
          Q21.21
        and small or restrictive inlet VSD
          Q21.22
    ostium secundum type (patent persistent)
      (type II) Q21.11
    sinus venosus Q21.16
      inferior Q21.15
      superior Q21.14
    specified NEC Q21.19
    vena cava type
      inferior Q21.15
      superior Q21.14
  atrioventricular
    canal Q21.20
    septal
      common Q21.23
      complete Q21.23
      incomplete Q21.21
      intermediate Q21.22
      partial Q21.21
      transitional Q21.22
      unspecified as to partial or complete
        Q21.20
    septum Q21.20
  auricular septal Q21.10
  bilirubin excretion NEC E80.6
  biosynthesis, androgen (testicular) E29.1
  bulbar septum Q21.0
  catalase E80.3
  cell membrane receptor complex (CR3) D71
  circulation I99.9
    congenital Q28.9
    newborn Q28.9
  coagulation (factor) —see also Deficiency, factor
    D68.9
    with
      ectopic pregnancy O08.1
      molar pregnancy O08.1
    acquired D68.4
    antepartum with hemorrhage —see
      Hemorrhage, antepartum, with
      coagulation defect
  COVID-19 associated coagulopathy D68.8
    due to
      liver disease D68.4
      vitamin K deficiency D68.4
    hereditary NEC D68.2
    intrapartum O67.0
    newborn, transient P61.6
    postpartum O99.13
      with hemorrhage O72.3
    specified type NEC D68.8
  complement system D84.1
  conduction (heart) I45.9
    bone —see Deafness, conductive
  congenital, organ or site not listed —see
    Anomaly, by site
  coronary sinus Q21.13
  cushion, endocardial Q21.20
    common Q21.23
    incomplete Q21.21
    intermediate Q21.22
    transitional Q21.22
  degradation, glycoprotein E77.1
  dental bridge, crown, fillings —see Defect, dental
    restoration
  dental restoration K08.50
    specified NEC K08.59
  dentin (hereditary) K00.5
  Descemet's membrane, congenital Q13.89
  developmental —see also Anomaly
    cauda equina Q06.3
  diaphragm
    with elevation, eventration or hernia —see
      Hernia, diaphragm
    congenital Q79.1
      with hernia Q79.0
      gross (with hernia) Q79.0
  ectodermal, congenital Q82.9
  Eisenmenger's Q21.8
  enzyme
    catalase E80.3
    peroxidase E80.3
  esophagus, congenital Q39.9
  extensor retinaculum M62.89
  fibrin polymerization D68.2

Defect, defective (Continued)
  filling
    bladder R93.41
    kidney R93.42-●
    renal pelvis R93.41
    stomach R93.3
    ureter R93.41
    urinary organs, specified NEC R93.49
  GABA (gamma aminobutyric acid) metabolic
    E72.81
  Gerbode Q21.0
  glucose transport, blood-brain barrier E74.810
  glycoprotein degradation E77.1
  Hageman (factor) D68.2
  hearing —see Deafness
  high grade F70
  home, technical, preventing adequate care
    Z59.19
  interatrial septal Q21.19
  interauricular septal Q21.19
  interventricular septal Q21.0
    with dextroposition of aorta, pulmonary
      stenosis and hypertrophy of right
      ventricle Q21.3
    in tetralogy of Fallot Q21.3
  intervertebral annular fibrosis (see also Disease,
    intervertebral disc, by site) M51.9
    lumbar M51.A0
      large M51.A2
      small M51.A1
    lumbosacral M51.A3
      large M51.A5
      small M51.A4
  learning (specific) —see Disorder, learning
  lymphocyte function antigen-1 (LFA-1) D84.0
  lysosomal enzyme, post-translational
    modification E77.0
  major osseous M89.70
    ankle M89.77-●
    carpus M89.74-●
    clavicle M89.71-●
    femur M89.75-●
    fibula M89.76-●
    fingers M89.74-●
    foot M89.77-●
    forearm M89.73-●
    hand M89.74-●
    humerus M89.72-●
    lower leg M89.76-●
    metacarpus M89.74-●
    metatarsus M89.77-●
    multiple sites M89.79
    pelvic region M89.75-●
    pelvis M89.75-●
    radius M89.73-●
    scapula M89.71-●
    shoulder region M89.71-●
    specified NEC M89.78
    tarsus M89.77-●
    thigh M89.75-●
    tibia M89.76-●
    toes M89.77-●
    ulna M89.73-●
  mental —see Disability, intellectual
  modification, lysosomal enzymes, post-
    translational E77.0
  obstructive, congenital
    renal pelvis Q62.39
    ureter Q62.39
      atresia —see Atresia, ureter
      cecoureterocele Q62.32
      megaureter Q62.2
      orthotopic ureterocele Q62.31
  osseous, major M89.70
    ankle M89.77-●
    carpus M89.74-●
    clavicle M89.71-●
    femur M89.75-●
    fibula M89.76-●
    fingers M89.74-●
    foot M89.77-●
    forearm M89.73-●
    hand M89.74-●
    humerus M89.72-●
    lower leg M89.76-●
    metacarpus M89.74-●
    metatarsus M89.77-●
    multiple sites M89.9
    pelvic region M89.75-●
    pelvis M89.75-●
    radius M89.73-●

Defect, defective (Continued)

osseous, major (Continued)

scapula M89.71-●

shoulder region M89.71-●

specified NEC M89.78

tarsus M89.77-●

thigh M89.75-●

tibia M89.76-●

toes M89.77-●

ulna M89.73-●

osteochondral NEC —see also Deformity M95.8-●

ostium

primum Q21.20

secundum Q21.11

peroxidase E80.3

placental blood supply —see Insufficiency, placental

platelets, qualitative D69.1

constitutional —see Disease, von Willebrand

postural NEC, spine —see Dorsopathy, deforming

qualitative, of von Willebrand factor

with

decreased platelet adhesion and selective deficiency of high-molecular-weight multimers (see also Disease, von Willebrand) D68.020

defective platelet adhesion with a normal size distribution of von Willebrand factor multimers (see also Disease, von Willebrand) D68.022

defective von Willebrand factor to factor VIII binding (see also Disease, von Willebrand) D68.023

high-molecular-weight von Willebrand factor loss (see also Disease, von Willebrand) D68.021

hyper-adhesive forms (see also Disease, von Willebrand) D68.021

increased affinity for platelet glycoprotein Ib (see also Disease, von Willebrand) D68.021

markedly decreased affinity for factor VIII (see also Disease, von Willebrand) D68.023

in von Willebrand factor function, with no further subtyping (see also Disease, von Willebrand) D68.029

reduction

limb Q73.8

lower Q72.9-●

absence —see Agenesis, leg

foot —see Agenesis, foot

longitudinal

femur Q72.4-●

fibula Q72.6-●

tibia Q72.5-●

specified type NEC Q72.89-●

split foot Q72.7-●

specified type NEC Q73.8

upper Q71.9-●

absence —see Agenesis, arm

forearm —see Agenesis, forearm

hand —see Agenesis, hand

lobster-claw hand Q71.6-●

longitudinal

radius Q71.4-●

ulna Q71.5-●

specified type NEC Q71.89-●

renal pelvis Q63.8

obstructive Q62.39

respiratory system, congenital Q34.9

restoration, dental K08.50

specified NEC K08.59

retinal nerve bundle fibers H35.89

septal (heart) NOS Q21.9

acquired (atrial) (auricular) (ventricular) (old) I51.0

atrial (see also Defect, atrial septal) Q21.10

concurrent with acute myocardial infarction —see Infarct, myocardium

following acute myocardial infarction (current complication) I23.1

ventricular —see also Defect, ventricular septal Q21.0

sinus venosus (see also Defect, atrial septal, sinus venosus) Q21.16

speech —see Disorder, speech

developmental F80.9

specified NEC R47.89

Defect, defective (Continued)

Taussig-Bing (aortic transposition and overriding pulmonary artery) Q20.1

teeth, wedge K03.1

vascular (local) I99.9

congenital Q27.9

ventricular septal Q21.0

concurrent with acute myocardial infarction —see Infarct, myocardium

following acute myocardial infarction (current complication) I23.2

in tetralogy of Fallot Q21.3

vision NEC H54.7

visual field H53.40

bilateral

heteronymous H53.47

homonymous H53.46-●

generalized contraction H53.48-●

localized

arcuate H53.43-●

scotoma (central area) H53.41-●

blind spot area H53.42-●

sector H53.43-●

specified type NEC H53.45-●

voice R49.9

specified NEC R49.8

wedge, tooth, teeth (abrasion) K03.1

Deferentitis N49.1

gonorrheal (acute) (chronic) A54.23

Defibrination (syndrome) D65

antepartum —see Hemorrhage, antepartum, with coagulation defect, disseminated intravascular coagulation

following ectopic or molar pregnancy O08.1

intrapartum O67.0

newborn P60

postpartum O72.3

Deficiency, deficient

3-beta hydroxysteroid dehydrogenase E25.0

11-hydroxylase E25.0

21-hydroxylase E25.0

5-alpha reductase (with male pseudohermaphroditism) E29.1

AADC (aromatic L-amino acid decarboxylase) E70.81

abdominal muscle syndrome Q79.4

AC globulin (congenital) (hereditary) D68.2

acquired D68.4

accelerator globulin (Ac G) (blood) D68.2

acid phosphatase E83.39

acid sphingomyelinase (ASMD) E75.249

type

A E75.240

A/B E75.244

B E75.241

activating factor (blood) D68.2

ADA2 (adenosine deaminase 2) D81.32

adenosine deaminase (ADA) D81.30

with severe combined immunodeficiency (SCID) D81.31

partial (type 1) D81.39

specified NEC D81.39

type 1 (without SCID) (without severe combined immunodeficiency) D81.39

type 2 D81.32

aldolase (hereditary) E74.19

alpha-1-antitrypsin E88.01

amino-acids E72.9

anemia —see Anemia

aneurin E51.9

antibody with

hyperimmunoglobulinemia D80.6

near-normal immunoglobins D80.6

antidiuretic hormone E23.2

anti-hemophilic

factor (A) D66

B D67

C D68.1

globulin (AHG) NEC D66

antithrombin (antithrombin III) D68.59

aromatic L-amino acid decarboxylase (AADC) E70.81

ascorbic acid E54

attention (disorder) (syndrome) F98.8

with hyperactivity —see Disorder, attention-deficit hyperactivity

autoprothrombin

I D68.2

II D67

C D68.2

beta-glucuronidase E76.29

Deficiency, deficient (Continued)

biotin E53.8

biotin-dependent carboxylase D81.819

biotinidase D81.810

brancher enzyme (amylopectinosis) E74.03

C1 esterase inhibitor (C1-INH) D84.1

calciferol E55.9

with

adult osteomalacia M83.8

rickets —see Rickets

calcium (dietary) E58

calorie, severe E43

with marasmus E41

and kwashiorkor E42

cardiac —see Insufficiency, myocardial

carnitine E71.40

due to

hemodialysis E71.43

inborn errors of metabolism E71.42

Valproic acid therapy E71.43

iatrogenic E71.43

muscle palmityltransferase E71.314

primary E71.41

secondary E71.448

carotene E50.9

central nervous system G96.89

ceruloplasmin (Wilson) E83.01

choline E53.8

Christmas factor D67

chromium E61.4

chronic neurovisceral acid sphingomyelinase E75.244

chronic visceral acid sphingomyelinase E75.241

clotting (blood) —see also Deficiency, coagulation factor D68.9

clotting factor NEC (hereditary) —see also Deficiency, factor D68.2

coagulation NOS D68.9

with

ectopic pregnancy O08.1

molar pregnancy O08.1

acquired (any) D68.4

antepartum hemorrhage —see Hemorrhage, antepartum, with coagulation defect

clotting factor NEC —see also Deficiency, factor D68.2

due to

hyperprothrombinemia D68.4

liver disease D68.4

vitamin K deficiency D68.4

newborn, transient P61.6

postpartum O72.3

specified NEC D68.8

cognitive F09

color vision H53.50

achromatopsia H53.51

acquired H53.52

deuteranomaly H53.53

protanomaly H53.54

specified type NEC H53.59

tritanomaly H53.55

combined glucocorticoid and mineralocorticoid E27.49

contact factor D68.2

copper (nutritional) E61.0

corticoadrenal E27.40

primary E27.1

craniofacial axis Q75.009

cyanocobalamin E53.8

debrancher enzyme (limit dextrinosis) E74.03

dehydrogenase

long chain/very long chain acyl CoA E71.310

medium chain acyl CoA E71.311

short chain acyl CoA E71.312

diet E63.9

dihydropyrimidine dehydrogenase (DPD) E88.89

disaccharidase E73.9

edema —see Malnutrition, severe

endocrine E34.9

energy-supply —see Malnutrition

enzymes, circulating NEC E88.09

ergosterol E55.9

with

adult osteomalacia M83.8

rickets —see Rickets

essential fatty acid (EFA) E63.0

eye movements

saccadic H55.81

smooth pursuit H55.82

Deficiency, deficient *(Continued)*
  factor —*see also* Deficiency, coagulation
    Hageman D68.2
    I (congenital) (hereditary) D68.2
    II (congenital) (hereditary) D68.2
    IX (congenital) (functional) (hereditary) (with functional defect) D67
    multiple (congenital) D68.8
      acquired D68.4
    V (congenital) (hereditary) D68.2
    Hageman D68.2
    VII (congenital) (hereditary) D68.2
    VIII (congenital) (functional) (hereditary) (with functional defect) D66
      with vascular defect —*see* Disease, von Willebrand
    X (congenital) (hereditary) D68.2
    XI (congenital) (hereditary) D68.1
    XII (congenital) (hereditary) D68.2
    XIII (congenital) (hereditary) D68.2
  femoral, proximal focal (congenital) —*see* Defect, reduction, lower limb, longitudinal, femur
  fibrin-stabilizing factor (congenital) (hereditary) D68.2
    acquired D68.4
  fibrinase D68.2
  fibrinogen (congenital) (hereditary) D68.2
    acquired D65
  folate E53.8
  folic acid E53.8
  foreskin N47.3
  fructokinase E74.11
  fructose 1,6-diphosphatase E74.19
  fructose-1-phosphate aldolase E74.19
  GABA (gamma aminobutyric acid) transaminase E72.81
  GABA-T (gamma aminobutyric acid transaminase) E72.81
  galactokinase E74.29
  galactose-1-phosphate uridyl transferase E74.29
  gammaglobulin in blood D80.1
    hereditary D80.0
  glass factor D68.2
  glucocorticoid E27.49
    mineralocorticoid E27.49
  glucose-6-phosphatase E74.01
  glucose-6-phosphate dehydrogenase anemia
    anemia D55.0
    without anemia D75.A
  glucose transporter protein type 1 E74.810
  glucuronyl transferase E80.5
  Glut1 E74.810
  glycogen synthetase E74.09
  gonadotropin (isolated) E23.0
  growth hormone (idiopathic) (isolated) E23.0
  Hageman factor D68.2
  hemoglobin D64.9
  hepatophosphorylase E74.09
  homogentisate 1,2-dioxygenase E70.29
  hormone
    anterior pituitary (partial) NEC E23.0
      growth E23.0
    growth (isolated) E23.0
    pituitary E23.0
    testicular E29.1
  hypoxanthine-(guanine)-phosphoribosyltransferase (HG-PRT) (total HG-PRT) E79.1
  immunity D84.9
    cell-mediated D84.89
      with thrombocytopenia and eczema D82.0
    combined D81.9
    humoral D80.9
    IgA (secretory) D80.2
    IgG D80.3
    IgM D80.4
  immuno —*see* Immunodeficiency
  immunoglobulin, selective
    A (IgA) D80.2
    G (IgG) (subclasses) D80.3
    M (IgM) D80.4
  infantile neurovisceral acid sphingomyelinase E75.240
  inositol (B complex) E53.8
  intrinsic
    factor (congenital) D51.0
    sphincter N36.42
      with urethral hypermobility N36.43
  iodine E61.8
    congenital syndrome —*see* Syndrome, iodine-deficiency, congenital

Deficiency, deficient *(Continued)*
  iron E61.1
    anemia D50.9
  kalium E87.6
  kappa-light chain D80.8
  labile factor (congenital) (hereditary) D68.2
    acquired D68.4
  lacrimal fluid (acquired) —*see also* Syndrome, dry eye
    congenital Q10.6
  lactase
    congenital E73.0
    secondary E73.1
  Laki-Lorand factor D68.2
  LCAD (long chain acyl CoA dehydrogenase deficiency) E71.310
  lecithin cholesterol acyltransferase E78.6
  lipocaic K86.89
  lipoprotein (familial) (high density) E78.6
  liver phosphorylase E74.09
  lysosomal alpha-1, 4 glucosidase E74.02
  lysosome-associated membrane protein 2 [LAMP2] E74.05
  magnesium E61.2
  major histocompatibility complex
    class I D81.6
    class II D81.7
  manganese E61.3
  MCAD (medium chain acyl CoA dehydrogenase deficiency) E71.311
  menadione (vitamin K) E56.1
    newborn P53
  mental (familial) (hereditary) —*see* Disability, intellectual
  methylenetetrahydrofolate reductase (MTHFR) E72.12
  mevalonate kinase M04.1
  mineral NEC E61.8
  mineralocorticoid E27.49
    with glucocorticoid E27.49
  molybdenum (nutritional) E61.5
  moral F60.2
  multiple nutrient elements E61.7
  multiple sulfatase (MSD) E75.26
  muscle
    carnitine (palmityltransferase) E71.314
    phosphofructokinase E74.09
  myoadenylate deaminase E79.2
  myocardial —*see* Insufficiency, myocardial
  myophosphorylase E74.04
  NADH diaphorase or reductase (congenital) D74.0
  NADH-methemoglobin reductase (congenital) D74.0
  natrium E87.1
  niacin (amide) (-tryptophan) E52
  nicotinamide E52
  nicotinic acid E52
  number of teeth —*see* Anodontia
  nutrient element E61.9
    multiple E61.7
    specified NEC E61.8
  nutrition, nutritional (*see also* Nutrition deficient) E63.9
    sequelae —*see* Sequelae, nutritional deficiency
    specified NEC E63.8
  of interleukin 1 receptor antagonist [DIRA] M04.8
  ornithine transcarbamylase E72.4
  ovarian E28.39
  oxygen —*see* Anoxia
  pantothenic acid E53.8
  parathyroid (gland) E20.9
  perineum (female) N81.89
  phenylalanine hydroxylase E70.1
  phosphoenolpyruvate carboxykinase E74.4
  phosphofructokinase E74.19
  ~~phosphomannomutase E74.818~~
  ▶ phosphomannomutase E74.818
  phosphomannose isomerase E74.818
  phosphomannosyl mutase E74.818
  phosphorylase kinase, liver E74.09
  pituitary hormone (isolated) E23.0
  plasma thromboplastin
    antecedent (PTA) D68.1
    component (PTC) D67
  plasminogen (type 1) (type 2) E88.02
  platelet NEC D69.1
    constitutional —*see* Disease, von Willebrand
  polyglandular E31.8
    autoimmune E31.0

Deficiency, deficient *(Continued)*
  potassium (K) E87.6
  prepuce N47.3
  proaccelerin (congenital) (hereditary) D68.2
    acquired D68.4
  proconvertin factor (congenital) (hereditary) D68.2
    acquired D68.4
  protein —*see also* Malnutrition E46
    anemia D53.0
    C D68.59
    S D68.59
  prothrombin (congenital) (hereditary) D68.2
    acquired D68.4
  Prower factor D68.2
  pseudocholinesterase E88.09
  PTA (plasma thromboplastin antecedent) D68.1
  PTC (plasma thromboplastin component) D67
  purine nucleoside phosphorylase (PNP) D81.5
  pyracin (alpha) (beta) E53.1
  pyridoxal E53.1
  pyridoxamine E53.1
  pyridoxine (derivatives) E53.1
  pyruvate
    carboxylase E74.4
    dehydrogenase E74.4
  riboflavin (vitamin B2) E53.0
  salt E87.1
  SCAD (short chain acyl CoA dehydrogenase deficiency) E71.312
  secretion
    ovary E28.39
    salivary gland (any) K11.7
    urine R34
  selenium (dietary) E59
  serum antitrypsin, familial E88.01
  short stature homeobox gene (SHOX)
    with
      dyschondrosteosis Q78.8
      short stature (idiopathic) E34.328
      Turner's syndrome Q96.9
  sodium (Na) E87.1
  SPCA (factor VII) D68.2
  sphincter, intrinsic N36.42
    with urethral hypermobility N36.43
  stable factor (congenital) (hereditary) D68.2
    acquired D68.4
  Stuart-Prower (factor X) D68.2
  succinic semialdehyde dehydrogenase E72.81
  sucrase E74.39
  sulfatase E75.26
  sulfite oxidase E72.19
  thiamin, thiaminic (chloride) E51.9
    beriberi (dry) E51.11
      wet E51.12
  thrombokinase D68.2
    newborn P53
  thyroid (gland) —*see* Hypothyroidism
  tocopherol E56.0
  tooth bud K00.0
  transcobalamine II (anemia) D51.2
  vanadium E61.6
  vascular I99.9
  vasopressin E23.2
  vertical ridge K06.8
  viosterol —*see* Deficiency, calciferol
  vitamin (multiple) NOS E56.9
    A E50.9
      with
        Bitot's spot (corneal) E50.1
        follicular keratosis E50.8
        keratomalacia E50.4
        manifestations NEC E50.8
        night blindness E50.5
        scar of cornea, xerophthalmic E50.6
        xeroderma E50.8
        xerophthalmia E50.7
        xerosis
          conjunctival E50.0
            and Bitot's spot E50.1
          cornea E50.2
            and ulceration E50.3
      sequelae E64.1
    B (complex) NOS E53.9
      with
        beriberi (dry) E51.11
          wet E51.12
        pellagra E52

▶ New   ⇒ Revised   ~~deleted~~ Deleted   ● Use Additional Character(s)

Deficiency, deficient *(Continued)*
vitamin (multiple) *(Continued)*
B1 NOS E51.9
beriberi (dry) E51.11
with circulatory system manifestations E51.11
wet E51.12
B12 E53.8
B2 (riboflavin) E53.0
B6 E53.1
C E54
sequelae E64.2
D E55.9
with
adult osteomalacia M83.8
rickets —*see* Rickets
25-hydroxylase E83.32
E E56.0
folic acid E53.8
G E53.0
group B E53.9
specified NEC E53.8
H (biotin) E53.8
K E56.1
of newborn P53
nicotinic E52
P E56.8
PP (pellagra-preventing) E52
specified NEC E56.8
thiamin E51.9
beriberi —*see* Beriberi
VLCAD (very long chain acyl CoA dehydrogenase deficiency) E71.310
von Willebrand factor
partial quantitative (*see also* Disease, von Willebrand) D68.01
total quantitative (*see also* Disease, von Willebrand) D68.03
zinc, dietary E60
Deficit —*see also* Deficiency
attention and concentration R41.840
following
cerebral infarction I69.310
cerebrovascular disease I69.910
specified disease NEC I69.810
nontraumatic
intracerebral hemorrhage I69.110
specified intracranial hemorrhage NEC I69.210
subarachnoid hemorrhage I69.010
disorder —*see* Attention, deficit
cognitive
communication R41.841
emotional
following
cerebral infarction I69.315
cerebrovascular disease I69.915
specified disease NEC I69.815
nontraumatic
intracerebral hemorrhage I69.115
specified intracranial hemorrhage NEC I69.215
subarachnoid hemorrhage I69.015
following
cerebral infarction I69.319
cerebrovascular disease I69.919
specified disease NEC I69.819
nontraumatic
intracerebral hemorrhage I69.119
specified intracranial hemorrhage NEC I69.219
subarachnoid hemorrhage I69.019
social
following
cerebral infarction I69.315
cerebrovascular disease I69.915
specified disease NEC I69.815
nontraumatic
intracerebral hemorrhage I69.115
specified intracranial hemorrhage NEC I69.215
subarachnoid hemorrhage I69.015
cognitive NEC R41.89
following
cerebral infarction I69.318
cerebrovascular disease I69.918
specified disease NEC I69.818

Deficit *(Continued)*
cognitive *(Continued)*
following *(Continued)*
nontraumatic
intracerebral hemorrhage I69.118
specified intracranial hemorrhage NEC I69.218
subarachnoid hemorrhage I69.018
concentration R41.840
executive function R41.844
following
cerebral infarction I69.314
cerebrovascular disease I69.914
specified disease NEC I69.814
nontraumatic
intracerebral hemorrhage I69.114
specified intracranial hemorrhage NEC I69.214
subarachnoid hemorrhage I69.014
frontal lobe R41.844
following
cerebral infarction I69.314
cerebrovascular disease I69.914
specified disease NEC I69.814
nontraumatic
intracerebral hemorrhage I69.114
specified intracranial hemorrhage NEC I69.214
subarachnoid hemorrhage I69.014
memory
following
cerebral infarction I69.311
cerebrovascular disease I69.911
specified disease NEC I69.811
nontraumatic
intracerebral hemorrhage I69.111
specified intracranial hemorrhage NEC I69.211
subarachnoid hemorrhage I69.011
neurologic NEC R29.818
ischemic
reversible (RIND) I63.9
prolonged (PRIND) I63.9
oxygen R09.02
prolonged reversible ischemic neurologic (PRIND) I63.9
psychomotor R41.843
following
cerebral infarction I69.313
cerebrovascular disease I69.913
specified disease NEC I69.813
nontraumatic
intracerebral hemorrhage I69.113
specified intracranial hemorrhage NEC I69.213
subarachnoid hemorrhage I69.013
visuospatial R41.842
following
cerebral infarction I69.312
cerebrovascular disease I69.912
specified disease NEC I69.812
nontraumatic
intracerebral hemorrhage I69.112
specified intracranial hemorrhage NEC I69.212
subarachnoid hemorrhage I69.012
Deflection
radius —*see* Deformity, limb, specified type NEC, forearm
septum (acquired) (nasal) (nose) J34.2
spine —*see* Curvature, spine
turbinate (nose) J34.2
Defluvium
capillorum —*see* Alopecia
ciliorum —*see* Madarosis
unguium L60.8
Deformity Q89.9
abdomen, congenital Q89.9
abdominal wall
acquired M95.8
congenital Q79.59
acquired (unspecified site) M95.9
adrenal gland Q89.1
alimentary tract, congenital Q45.9
upper Q40.9
ankle (joint) (acquired) —*see also* Deformity, limb, lower leg
abduction —*see* Contraction, joint, ankle
congenital Q68.8

Deformity *(Continued)*
ankle *(Continued)*
contraction —*see* Contraction, joint, ankle
specified type NEC —*see* Deformity, limb, foot, specified NEC
anus (acquired) K62.89
congenital Q43.9
aorta (arch) (congenital) Q25.40
acquired I77.89
aortic
arch, acquired I77.89
cusp or valve (congenital) Q23.88
acquired —*see also* Endocarditis, aortic I35.8
arm (acquired) (upper) —*see also* Deformity, limb, upper arm
congenital Q68.8
forearm —*see* Deformity, limb, forearm
artery (congenital) (peripheral) NOS Q27.9
acquired I77.89
coronary (acquired) I25.9
congenital Q24.5
umbilical Q27.0
atrial septal (*see also* Defect, atrial septal) Q21.10
auditory canal (external) (congenital) —*see also* Malformation, ear, external
acquired —*see* Disorder, ear, external, specified type NEC
auricle
ear (congenital) —*see also* Malformation, ear, external
acquired —*see* Disorder, pinna, deformity
back —*see* Dorsopathy, deforming
bile duct (common) (congenital) (hepatic) Q44.5
acquired K83.8
biliary duct or passage (congenital) Q44.5
acquired K83.8
bladder (neck) (trigone) (sphincter) (acquired) N32.89
congenital Q64.79
bone (acquired) NOS M95.9
congenital Q79.9
turbinate M95.0
brain (congenital) Q04.9
acquired G93.89
reduction Q04.3
breast (acquired) N64.89
congenital Q83.9
reconstructed N65.0
bronchus (congenital) Q32.4
acquired NEC J98.09
bursa, congenital Q79.9
canaliculi (lacrimalis) (acquired) —*see also* Disorder, lacrimal system, changes
congenital Q10.6
canthus, acquired —*see* Disorder, eyelid, specified type NEC
capillary (acquired) I78.8
cardiovascular system, congenital Q28.9
caruncle, lacrimal (acquired) —*see also* Disorder, lacrimal system, changes
congenital Q10.6
cascade, stomach K31.2
cecum (congenital) Q43.9
acquired K63.89
cerebral, acquired G93.89
congenital Q04.9
cervix (uterus) (acquired) NEC N88.8
congenital Q51.9
cheek (acquired) M95.2
congenital Q18.9
chest (acquired) (wall) M95.4
congenital Q67.8
sequelae (late effect) of rickets E64.3
chin (acquired) M95.2
congenital Q18.9
choroid (congenital) Q14.3
acquired H31.8
plexus Q07.8
acquired G96.198
cicatricial —*see* Cicatrix
cilia, acquired —*see* Disorder, eyelid, specified type NEC
clavicle (acquired) M95.8
congenital Q68.8
clitoris (congenital) Q52.6
acquired N90.89
clubfoot —*see* Clubfoot
coccyx (acquired) —*see* subcategory M43.8
colon (congenital) Q43.9
acquired K63.89

Deformity (*Continued*)
concha (ear), congenital —*see also* Malformation, ear, external
  acquired —*see* Disorder, pinna, deformity
cornea (acquired) H18.70
  congenital Q13.4
  descemetocele —*see* Descemetocele
  ectasia —*see* Ectasia, cornea
  specified NEC H18.79-●
  staphyloma —*see* Staphyloma, cornea
coronary artery (acquired) I25.9
  congenital Q24.5
cranium (acquired) —*see* Deformity, skull
cricoid cartilage (congenital) Q31.8
  acquired J38.7
cystic duct (congenital) Q44.5
  acquired K82.8
Dandy-Walker Q03.1
  with spina bifida —*see* Spina bifida
diaphragm (congenital) Q79.1
  acquired J98.6
digestive organ NOS Q45.9
ductus arteriosus Q25.0
duodenal bulb K31.89
duodenum (congenital) Q43.9
  acquired K31.89
dura —*see* Deformity, meninges
ear (acquired) —*see also* Disorder, pinna, deformity
  congenital (external) Q17.9
    internal Q16.5
    middle Q16.4
      ossicles Q16.3
    ossicles Q16.3
ectodermal (congenital) NEC Q84.9
ejaculatory duct (congenital) Q55.4
  acquired N50.89
elbow (joint) (acquired) —*see also* Deformity, limb, upper arm
  congenital Q68.8
  contraction —*see* Contraction, joint, elbow
endocrine gland NEC Q89.2
epididymis (congenital) Q55.4
  acquired N50.89
epiglottis (congenital) Q31.8
  acquired J38.7
esophagus (congenital) Q39.9
  acquired K22.89
eustachian tube (congenital) NEC Q17.8
eye, congenital Q15.9
eyebrow (congenital) Q18.8
eyelid (acquired) —*see also* Disorder, eyelid, specified type NEC
  congenital Q10.3
face (acquired) M95.2
  congenital Q18.9
fallopian tube, acquired N83.8
femur (acquired) —*see* Deformity, limb, specified type NEC, thigh
fetal
  with fetopelvic disproportion O33.7
  causing obstructed labor O66.3
finger (acquired) M20.00-●
  boutonniere M20.02-●
  congenital Q68.1
  flexion contracture —*see* Contraction, joint, hand
  mallet finger M20.01-●
  specified NEC M20.09-●
  swan-neck M20.03-●
flexion (joint) (acquired) —*see also* Deformity, limb, flexion M21.20
  congenital NOS Q74.9
    hip Q65.89
foot (acquired) —*see also* Deformity, limb, lower leg
  cavovarus (congenital) Q66.1-●
  congenital NOS Q66.9-●
    specified type NEC Q66.89
  specified type NEC —*see* Deformity, limb, foot, specified NEC
  valgus (congenital) Q66.6
    acquired —*see* Deformity, valgus, ankle
  varus (congenital) NEC Q66.3-●
    acquired —*see* Deformity, varus, ankle
forearm (acquired) —*see also* Deformity, limb, forearm
  congenital Q68.8
forehead (acquired) M95.2
  congenital Q75.8
frontal bone (acquired) M95.2
  congenital Q75.8

Deformity (*Continued*)
gallbladder (acquired) Q44.1
  acquired K82.8
gastrointestinal tract (congenital) NOS Q45.9
  acquired K63.89
genitalia, genital organ(s) or system NEC
  female (congenital) Q52.9
    acquired N94.89
    external Q52.70
  male (congenital) Q55.9
    acquired N50.89
globe (eye) (congenital) Q15.8
  acquired H44.89
gum, acquired NEC K06.8
hand (acquired) —*see* Deformity, limb, hand
  congenital Q68.1
head (acquired) M95.2
  congenital Q75.8
heart (congenital) Q24.9
  septum Q21.9
    auricular (*see also* Defect, atrial septal) Q21.10
    ventricular Q21.0
  valve (congenital) NEC Q24.8
    acquired —*see* Endocarditis
heel (acquired) —*see* Deformity, foot
hepatic duct (congenital) Q44.5
  acquired K83.8
hip (joint) (acquired) —*see also* Deformity, limb, thigh
  congenital Q65.9
  due to (previous) juvenile osteochondrosis —*see* Coxa, plana
  flexion —*see* Contraction, joint, hip
hourglass —*see* Contraction, hourglass
humerus (acquired) M21.82-●
  congenital Q74.0
hypophyseal (congenital) Q89.2
ileocecal (coil) (valve) (acquired) K63.89
  congenital Q43.9
ileum (congenital) Q43.9
  acquired K63.89
ilium (acquired) M95.5
  congenital Q74.2
integument (congenital) Q84.9
intervertebral cartilage or disc (acquired) —*see* Disorder, disc, specified NEC
intestine (large) (small) (congenital) NOS Q43.9
  acquired K63.89
intrinsic minus or plus (hand) —*see* Deformity, limb, specified type NEC, forearm
iris (acquired) H21.89
  congenital Q13.2
ischium (acquired) M95.5
  congenital Q74.2
jaw (acquired) (congenital) M26.9
joint (acquired) NEC M21.90
  congenital Q68.8
  elbow M21.92-●
  hand M21.94-●
  hip M21.95-●
  knee M21.96-●
  shoulder M21.92-●
  wrist M21.93-●
kidney(s) (calyx) (pelvis) (congenital) Q63.9
  acquired N28.89
  artery (congenital) Q27.2
    acquired I77.89
Klippel-Feil (brevicollis) Q76.1
knee (acquired) NEC —*see also* Deformity, limb, lower leg
  congenital Q68.2
labium (majus) (minus) (congenital) Q52.79
  acquired N90.89
lacrimal passages or duct (congenital) NEC Q10.6
  acquired —*see* Disorder, lacrimal system, changes
larynx (muscle) (congenital) Q31.8
  acquired J38.7
  web (glottic) Q31.0
leg (upper) (acquired) NEC —*see also* Deformity, limb, thigh
  congenital Q68.8
  lower leg —*see* Deformity, limb, lower leg
lens (acquired) H27.8
  congenital Q12.9
lid (fold) (acquired) —*see also* Disorder, eyelid, specified type NEC
  congenital Q10.3

Deformity (*Continued*)
ligament (acquired) —*see* Disorder, ligament
  congenital Q79.9
limb (acquired) M21.90
  clawfoot M21.53-●
  clawhand M21.51-●
    congenital Q68.1
  clubfoot M21.54-●
  clubhand M21.52-●
  congenital, except reduction deformity Q74.9
  flat foot M21.4-●
  flexion M21.20
    ankle M21.27-●
    elbow M21.22-●
    finger M21.24-●
    hip M21.25-●
    knee M21.26-●
    shoulder M21.21-●
    toe M21.27-●
    wrist M21.23-●
  foot
    claw —*see* Deformity, limb, clawfoot
    club —*see* Deformity, limb, clubfoot
    drop M21.37-●
    flat —*see* Deformity, limb, flat foot
    specified NEC M21.6X-●
  forearm M21.93-●
  hand M21.94-●
  lower leg M21.96-●
  specified type NEC M21.80
    forearm M21.83-●
    lower leg M21.86-●
    thigh M21.85-●
    upper arm M21.82-●
  thigh M21.95-●
  unequal length M21.70
    short site is
      femur M21.75-●
      fibula M21.76-●
      humerus M21.72-●
      radius M21.73-●
      tibia M21.76-●
      ulna M21.73-●
  upper arm M21.92-●
  valgus —*see* Deformity, valgus
  varus —*see* Deformity, varus
  wrist drop M21.33-●
lip (acquired) NEC K13.0
  congenital Q38.0
liver (congenital) Q44.70
  acquired K76.89
lumbosacral (congenital) (joint) (region) Q76.49
  acquired —*see* subcategory M43.8
  kyphosis —*see* Kyphosis, congenital
  lordosis —*see* Lordosis, congenital
lung (congenital) Q33.9
  acquired J98.4
lymphatic system, congenital Q89.9
Madelung's (radius) Q74.0
mandible (acquired) (congenital) M26.9
maxilla (acquired) (congenital) M26.9
meninges or membrane (congenital) Q07.9
  cerebral Q04.8
    acquired G96.198
  spinal cord (congenital) Q06.-●
    acquired G96.198
metacarpus (acquired) —*see* Deformity, limb, forearm
  congenital Q74.0
metatarsus (acquired) —*see* Deformity, foot
  congenital Q66.9-●
middle ear (congenital) Q16.4
  ossicles Q16.3
mitral (leaflets) (valve) I05.8
  parachute Q23.2
  stenosis, congenital Q23.2
mouth (acquired) K13.79
  congenital Q38.6
multiple, congenital NEC Q89.7
muscle (acquired) M62.89
  congenital Q79.9
    sternocleidomastoid Q68.0
musculoskeletal system (acquired) M95.9
  congenital Q79.9
  specified NEC M95.8
nail (acquired) L60.8
  congenital Q84.6
nasal —*see* Deformity, nose
neck (acquired) M95.3
  congenital Q18.9
    sternocleidomastoid Q68.0

▶ New   ⟹ Revised   ~~deleted~~ Deleted   ● Use Additional Character(s)

Deformity (Continued)
nervous system (congenital) Q07.9
nipple (congenital) Q83.9
  acquired N64.89
nose (acquired) (cartilage) M95.0
  bone (turbinate) M95.0
  congenital Q30.9
    bent or squashed Q67.4
  saddle M95.0
    syphilitic A50.57
  septum (acquired) J34.2
    congenital Q30.8
  sinus (wall) (congenital) Q30.8
    acquired M95.0
  syphilitic (congenital) A50.57
    late A52.73
ocular muscle (congenital) Q10.3
  acquired —see Strabismus, mechanical
opticociliary vessels (congenital) Q13.2
orbit (eye) (acquired) H05.30
  atrophy —see Atrophy, orbit
  congenital Q10.7
  due to
    bone disease NEC H05.32-●
    trauma or surgery H05.33-●
  enlargement —see Enlargement, orbit
  exostosis —see Exostosis, orbit
organ of Corti (congenital) Q16.5
ovary (congenital) Q50.39
  acquired N83.8
oviduct, acquired N83.8
palate (congenital) Q38.5
  acquired M27.8
  cleft (congenital) —see Cleft, palate
pancreas (congenital) Q45.3
  acquired K86.89
parathyroid (gland) Q89.2
parotid (gland) (congenital) Q38.4
  acquired K11.8
patella (acquired) —see Disorder, patella,
    specified NEC
pelvis, pelvic (acquired) (bony) M95.5
  with disproportion (fetopelvic) O33.0
    causing obstructed labor O65.0
  congenital Q74.2
  rachitic sequelae (late effect) E64.3
penis (glans) (congenital) Q55.69
  acquired N48.89
pericardium (congenital) Q24.8
  acquired —see Pericarditis
pharynx (congenital) Q38.8
  acquired J39.2
pinna, acquired —see also Disorder, pinna,
    deformity
  congenital Q17.9
pituitary (congenital) Q89.2
posture —see Dorsopathy, deforming
prepuce (congenital) Q55.69
  acquired N47.8
prostate (congenital) Q55.4
  acquired N42.89
pupil (congenital) Q13.2
  acquired —see Abnormality, pupillary
pylorus (congenital) Q40.3
  acquired K31.89
rachitic (acquired), old or healed E64.3
radius (acquired) —see also Deformity, limb,
    forearm
  congenital Q68.8
rectum (congenital) Q43.9
  acquired K62.89
reduction (extremity) (limb), congenital (see also
    condition and site) Q73.8
  brain Q04.3
  lower —see Defect, reduction, lower limb
  upper —see Defect, reduction, upper limb
renal —see Deformity, kidney
respiratory system (congenital) Q34.9
rib (acquired) M95.4
  congenital Q76.6
    cervical Q76.5
rotation (joint) (acquired) —see Deformity, limb,
    specified site NEC
  congenital Q74.9
  hip —see Deformity, limb, specified type NEC,
    thigh
    congenital Q65.89
sacroiliac joint (congenital) Q74.2
  acquired —see subcategory M43.8
sacrum (acquired) —see subcategory
    M43.8

Deformity (Continued)
saddle
  back —see Lordosis
  nose M95.0
    syphilitic A50.57
salivary gland or duct (congenital) Q38.4
  acquired K11.8
scapula (acquired) M95.8
  congenital Q68.8
scrotum (congenital) —see also Malformation,
    testis and scrotum
  acquired N50.89
seminal vesicles (congenital) Q55.4
  acquired N50.89
septum, nasal (acquired) J34.2
shoulder (joint) (acquired) —see Deformity, limb,
    upper arm
  congenital Q74.0
  contraction —see Contraction, joint, shoulder
sigmoid (flexure) (congenital) Q43.9
  acquired K63.89
skin (congenital) Q82.9
skull (acquired) M95.2
  congenital Q75.8
    with
      anencephaly Q00.0
      encephalocele —see Encephalocele
      hydrocephalus Q03.9
        with spina bifida —see Spina bifida, by
          site, with hydrocephalus
      microcephaly Q02
soft parts, organs or tissues (of pelvis)
  in pregnancy or childbirth NEC O34.8-●
    causing obstructed labor O65.5
spermatic cord (congenital) Q55.4
  acquired N50.89
  torsion —see Torsion, spermatic cord
spinal —see Dorsopathy, deforming
  column (acquired) —see Dorsopathy,
    deforming
  congenital Q67.5
  cord (congenital) Q06.9
    acquired G95.89
  nerve root (congenital) Q07.9
spine (acquired) —see also Dorsopathy,
    deforming
  congenital Q67.5
  rachitic E64.3
  specified NEC —see Dorsopathy, deforming,
    specified NEC
spleen
  acquired D73.89
  congenital Q89.09
Sprengel's (congenital) Q74.0
sternocleidomastoid (muscle), congenital Q68.0
sternum (acquired) M95.4
  congenital NEC Q76.7
stomach (congenital) Q40.3
  acquired K31.89
submandibular gland (congenital) Q38.4
submaxillary gland (congenital) Q38.4
  acquired K11.8
talipes —see Talipes
testis (congenital) —see also Malformation, testis
    and scrotum
  acquired N44.8
  torsion —see Torsion, testis
thigh (acquired) —see also Deformity, limb, thigh
  congenital NEC Q68.8
thorax (acquired) (wall) M95.4
  congenital Q67.8
  sequelae of rickets E64.3
thumb (acquired) —see also Deformity, finger
  congenital NEC Q68.1
thymus (tissue) (congenital) Q89.2
thyroid (gland) (congenital) Q89.2
  cartilage Q31.8
    acquired J38.7
tibia (acquired) —see also Deformity, limb,
    specified type NEC, lower leg
  congenital NEC Q68.8
  saber (syphilitic) A50.56
toe (acquired) M20.6-●
  congenital Q66.9-●
  hallux rigidus M20.2-●
  hallux valgus M20.1-●
  hallux varus M20.3-●
  hammer toe M20.4-●
  specified NEC M20.5X-●
tongue (congenital) Q38.3
  acquired K14.8

Deformity (Continued)
tooth, teeth K00.2
trachea (rings) (congenital) Q32.1
  acquired J39.8
transverse aortic arch (congenital) Q25.49
tricuspid (leaflets) (valve) I07.8
  atresia or stenosis Q22.4
  Ebstein's Q22.5
trunk (acquired) M95.8
  congenital Q89.9
ulna (acquired) —see also Deformity, limb, forearm
  congenital NEC Q68.8
urachus, congenital Q64.4
ureter (opening) (congenital) Q62.8
  acquired N28.89
urethra (congenital) Q64.79
  acquired N36.8
urinary tract (congenital) Q64.9
  urachus Q64.4
uterus (congenital) Q51.9
  acquired N85.8
uvula (congenital) Q38.5
vagina (acquired) N89.8
  congenital Q52.4
valgus NEC M21.00
  ankle M21.07-●
  elbow M21.02-●
  hip M21.05-●
  knee M21.06-●
valve, valvular (congenital) (heart) Q24.8
  acquired —see Endocarditis
varus NEC M21.10
  ankle M21.17-●
  elbow M21.12-●
  hip M21.15
  knee M21.16-●
  tibia —see Osteochondrosis, juvenile, tibia
vas deferens (congenital) Q55.4
  acquired N50.89
vein (congenital) Q27.9
  great Q26.9
vertebra —see Dorsopathy, deforming
vertical talus (congenital) Q66.80
  left foot Q66.82
  right foot Q66.81
vesicourethral orifice (acquired) N32.89
  congenital NEC Q64.79
vessels of optic papilla (congenital) Q14.2
visual field (contraction) —see Defect, visual field
vitreous body, acquired H43.89
vulva (congenital) Q52.79
  acquired N90.89
wrist (joint) (acquired) —see also Deformity, limb,
    forearm
  congenital Q68.8
  contraction —see Contraction, joint, wrist
Degeneration, degenerative
  adrenal (capsule) (fatty) (gland) (hyaline)
    (infectional) E27.8
  amyloid —see also Amyloidosis E85.9
  anterior cornua, spinal cord G12.29
  anterior labral S43.49-●
  aorta, aortic I70.0
    fatty I77.89
  aortic valve (heart) —see Endocarditis, aortic
  arteriovascular —see Arteriosclerosis
  artery, arterial (atheromatous) (calcareous) —see
    also Arteriosclerosis
    cerebral, amyloid E85.4 [I68.0]
    medial —see Arteriosclerosis, extremities
  articular cartilage NEC —see Derangement, joint,
    articular cartilage, by site
  atheromatous —see Arteriosclerosis
  basal nuclei or ganglia G23.9
    specified NEC G23.8
  bone NEC —see Disorder, bone, specified type
    NEC
  brachial plexus G54.0
  brain (cortical) (progressive) G31.9
    alcoholic G31.2
    arteriosclerotic I67.2
    childhood G31.9
      specified NEC G31.89
    cystic G31.89
      congenital Q04.6
    in
      alcoholism G31.2
      beriberi E51.2
      cerebrovascular disease I67.9
      congenital hydrocephalus Q03.9
        with spina bifida —see also Spina bifida

Degeneration, degenerative *(Continued)*
  brain *(Continued)*
    in *(Continued)*
      Fabry-Anderson disease E75.21
      Gaucher's disease E75.22
      Hunter's syndrome E76.1
      lipidosis
        cerebral E75.4
        generalized E75.6
      mucopolysaccharidosis —*see*
          Mucopolysaccharidosis
      myxedema E03.9 *[G32.89]*
      neoplastic disease —*see also* Neoplasm
          D49.6 *[G32.89]*
      Niemann-Pick disease E75.249 *[G32.89]*
      sphingolipidosis E75.3 *[G32.89]*
      vitamin B12 deficiency E53.8 *[G32.89]*
    senile NEC G31.1
  breast N64.89
  Bruch's membrane —*see* Degeneration, choroid
  capillaries (fatty) I78.8
    amyloid E85.89 *[I79.8]*
  cardiac —*see also* Degeneration, myocardial
    valve, valvular —*see* Endocarditis
  cardiorenal —*see* Hypertension, cardiorenal
  cardiovascular —*see also* Disease, cardiovascular
    renal —*see* Hypertension, cardiorenal
  cerebellar NOS G31.9
    alcoholic G31.2
    primary (hereditary) (sporadic) G11.9
  cerebral —*see* Degeneration, brain
  cerebrovascular I67.9
    due to hypertension I67.4
  cervical plexus G54.2
  cervix N88.8
    due to radiation (intended effect) N88.8
      adverse effect or misadventure N99.89
  chamber angle H21.21-●
  changes, spine or vertebra —*see* Spondylosis
  chorioretinal —*see also* Degeneration, choroid
    hereditary H31.20
  choroid (colloid) (drusen) H31.10-●
    atrophy —*see* Atrophy, choroidal
    hereditary —*see* Dystrophy, choroidal,
        hereditary
  ciliary body H21.22-●
  cochlear —*see* subcategory H83.8
  combined (spinal cord) (subacute) E53.8 *[G32.0]*
    with anemia (pernicious) D51.0 *[G32.0]*
      due to dietary vitamin B12 deficiency D51.3
          [G32.0]
    in (due to)
      vitamin B12 deficiency E53.8 *[G32.0]*
      anemia D51.9 *[G32.0]*
  conjunctiva H11.10
    concretions —*see* Concretion, conjunctiva
    deposits —*see* Deposit, conjunctiva
    pigmentations —*see* Pigmentation,
        conjunctiva
    pinguecula —*see* Pinguecula
    xerosis —*see* Xerosis, conjunctiva
  cornea H18.40
    calcerous H18.43
      band keratopathy H18.42-●
    familial, hereditary —*see* Dystrophy, cornea
    hyaline (of old scars) H18.49
    keratomalacia —*see* Keratomalacia
    nodular H18.45-●
    peripheral H18.46-●
    senile H18.41-●
    specified type NEC H18.49
  cortical (cerebellar) (parenchymatous) G31.89
    alcoholic G31.2
    diffuse, due to arteriopathy I67.2
  corticobasal G31.85
  cutis L98.8
    amyloid E85.4 *[L99]*
  dental pulp K04.2
  disc disease —*see* Degeneration, intervertebral
      disc, by site
  dorsolateral (spinal cord) —*see* Degeneration,
      combined
  extrapyramidal G25.9
  eye, macular —*see also* Degeneration, macula
    congenital or hereditary —*see* Dystrophy,
        retina
  facet joints —*see* Spondylosis
  fatty
    liver NEC K76.0
      alcoholic K70.0
  grey matter (brain) (Alpers') G31.81

Degeneration, degenerative *(Continued)*
  heart —*see also* Degeneration, myocardial
    amyloid E85.4 *[I43]*
    atheromatous —*see* Disease, heart, ischemic,
        atherosclerotic
    ischemic —*see* Disease, heart, ischemic
  hepatolenticular (Wilson's) E83.01
  hepatorenal K76.7
  hyaline (diffuse) (generalized)
    localized —*see* Degeneration, by site
  infrapatellar fat pad M79.4
  intervertebral disc
    with
      myelopathy —*see* Disorder, disc, with,
          myelopathy
      radiculitis or radiculopathy —*see* Disorder,
          disc, with, radiculopathy
    cervical, cervicothoracic —*see* Disorder, disc,
        cervical, degeneration
      with
        myelopathy —*see* Disorder, disc, cervical,
            with myelopathy
        neuritis, radiculitis or radiculopathy —
            see Disorder, disc, cervical, with
            neuritis
    lumbar region M51.36-●
      with
        myelopathy M51.06
        neuritis, radiculitis, radiculopathy or
            sciatica M51.16
    lumbosacral region M51.37-●
      with
        neuritis, radiculitis, radiculopathy or
            sciatica M51.17
    sacrococcygeal region M53.3
    thoracic region M51.34
      with
        myelopathy M51.04
        neuritis, radiculitis, radiculopathy
            M51.14
    thoracolumbar region M51.35
      with
        myelopathy M51.05
        neuritis, radiculitis, radiculopathy
            M51.15
  intestine, amyloid E85.4
  iris (pigmentary) H21.23-●
  ischemic —*see* Ischemia
  joint disease —*see* Osteoarthritis
  kidney N28.89
    amyloid E85.4 *[N29]*
    cystic, congenital Q61.9
    fatty N28.89
    polycystic Q61.3
      adult type (autosomal dominant) Q61.2
      infantile type (autosomal recessive) NEC
          Q61.19
      collecting duct dilatation Q61.11
  Kuhnt-Junius —*see also* Degeneration, macula
      H35.32-●
  lens —*see* Cataract
  lenticular (familial) (progressive) (Wilson's)
      (with cirrhosis of liver) E83.01
  liver (diffuse) NEC K76.89
    amyloid E85.4 *[K77]*
    cystic K76.89
      congenital Q44.6
    fatty NEC K76.0
      alcoholic K70.0
    hypertrophic K76.89
    parenchymatous, acute or subacute K72.00
      with coma K72.01
    pigmentary K76.89
    toxic (acute) K71.9
  lung J98.4
  lymph gland I89.8
    hyaline I89.8
  macula, macular (acquired) (age-related) (senile)
      H35.30
    angioid streaks H35.33
    atrophic age-related H35.31-●
    congenital or hereditary —*see* Dystrophy, retina
    cystoid H35.35-●
    drusen H35.36-●
    dry age-related H35.31-●
    exudative H35.32-●
    hole H35.34-●
    nonexudative H35.31-●
    puckering H35.37-●
    toxic H35.38-●
    wet age-related H35.32-●

Degeneration, degenerative *(Continued)*
  membranous labyrinth, congenital (causing
      impairment of hearing) Q16.5
  meniscus —*see* Derangement, meniscus
  mitral —*see* Insufficiency, mitral
  Mönckeberg's —*see* Arteriosclerosis, extremities
  motor centers, senile G31.1
  multi-system G90.3
  mural —*see* Degeneration, myocardial
  muscle (fatty) (fibrous) (hyaline) (progressive)
      M62.89
    heart —*see* Degeneration, myocardial
  myelin, central nervous system G37.9
  myocardial, myocardium (fatty) (hyaline)
      (senile) I51.5
    with rheumatic fever (conditions in I00) I09.0
      active, acute or subacute I01.2
        with chorea I02.0
      inactive or quiescent (with chorea) I09.0
    hypertensive —*see* Hypertension, heart
    rheumatic —*see* Degeneration, myocardial,
        with rheumatic fever
    syphilitic A52.06
  nasal sinus (mucosa) J32.9
    frontal J32.1
    maxillary J32.0
  nerve —*see* Disorder, nerve
  nervous system G31.9
    alcoholic G31.2
    amyloid E85.4 *[G99.8]*
    autonomic G90.9
    fatty G31.89
    specified NEC G31.89
  nipple N64.89
  olivopontocerebellar (hereditary) (familial) G23.8
  osseous labyrinth —*see* subcategory H83.8
  ovary N83.8
    cystic N83.20-●
    microcystic N83.20-●
  pallidal pigmentary (progressive) G23.0
  pancreas K86.89
    tuberculous A18.83
  penis N48.89
  pigmentary (diffuse) (general)
    localized —*see* Degeneration, by site
    pallidal (progressive) G23.0
  pineal gland E34.8
  pituitary (gland) E23.6
  popliteal fat pad M79.4
  posterolateral (spinal cord) —*see* Degeneration,
      combined
  pulmonary valve (heart) I37.8
  pulp (tooth) K04.2
  pupillary margin H21.24-●
  renal —*see* Degeneration, kidney
  retina H35.9
    hereditary (cerebroretinal) (congenital)
        (juvenile) (macula) (peripheral)
        (pigmentary) —*see* Dystrophy,
        retina
    Kuhnt-Junius —*see also* Degeneration, macula
        H35.32-●
    macula (cystic) (exudative) (hole)
        (nonexudative) (pseudohole) (senile)
        (toxic) —*see* Degeneration, macula
    peripheral H35.40
      lattice H35.41-●
      microcystoid H35.42-●
      paving stone H35.43-●
      secondary
        pigmentary H35.45-●
        vitreoretinal H35.46-●
      senile reticular H35.44-●
    pigmentary (primary) —*see also* Dystrophy,
        retina
    secondary —*see* Degeneration, retina,
        peripheral, secondary
    posterior pole —*see* Degeneration, macula
  saccule, congenital (causing impairment of
      hearing) Q16.5
  senile R54
    brain G31.1
    cardiac, heart or myocardium —*see*
        Degeneration, myocardial
    motor centers G31.1
    vascular —*see* Arteriosclerosis
  sinus (cystic) —*see also* Sinusitis
    polypoid J33.1
  skin L98.8
    amyloid E85.4 *[L99]*
    colloid L98.8

▶ New   ⇒ Revised   ~~deleted~~ Deleted   ● Use Additional Character(s)

Degeneration, degenerative (Continued)
spinal (cord) G31.89
  amyloid E85.4 [G32.89]
  combined (subacute) —see Degeneration,
    combined
  dorsolateral —see Degeneration, combined
  familial NEC G31.89
  fatty G31.89
  funicular —see Degeneration, combined
  posterolateral —see Degeneration,
    combined
  subacute combined —see Degeneration,
    combined
  tuberculous A17.81
spleen D73.0
  amyloid E85.4 [D77]
stomach K31.89
striatonigral G23.2
suprarenal (capsule) (gland) E27.8
synovial membrane (pulpy) —see Disorder,
    synovium, specified type NEC
tapetoretinal —see Dystrophy, retina
thymus (gland) E32.8
  fatty E32.8
thyroid (gland) E07.89
tricuspid (heart) (valve) I07.9
tuberculous NEC —see Tuberculosis
turbinate J34.89
uterus (cystic) N85.8
vascular (senile) —see Arteriosclerosis
  hypertensive —see Hypertension
vitreoretinal, secondary —see Degeneration,
    retina, peripheral, secondary, vitreoretinal
vitreous (body) H43.81-●
Wallerian —see Disorder, nerve
Wilson's hepatolenticular E83.01
Deglutition
paralysis R13.0
  hysterical F44.4
pneumonia J69.0
Degos' disease I77.89
Dehiscence (of)
amputation stump T87.81
cesarean wound O90.0
closure of
  ▶abdominal wall muscle or fascia T81.321
  cornea T81.31
  ⫸craniotomy T81.328
  ⫸fascia (muscular) (superficial) T81.328
  ▶gastrointestinal tract anastomosis, repair, or
    closure T81.320
  ⫸internal organ or tissue T81.328
  laceration (external) (internal) T81.33
  ⫸ligament T81.328
  mucosa T81.31
  ⫸muscle or muscle flap T81.328
  ▶ribs or rib cage T81.328
  skin and subcutaneous tissue (full-thickness)
    (superficial) T81.31
  ⫸skull T81.328
  ⫸sternum (sternotomy) T81.328
  ⫸tendon T81.328
  traumatic laceration (external) (internal)
    T81.33
episiotomy O90.1
operation wound NEC T81.31
  ▶deep T81.329
  external operation wound (superficial)
    T81.31
  ⫸internal operation wound (deep) T81.329
    ▶abdominal wall muscle or fascia
      T81.321
    ▶specified NEC T81.328
perineal wound (postpartum) O90.1
traumatic injury wound repair T81.33
wound T81.30
  traumatic repair T81.33
Dehydration E86.0
newborn P74.1
Déjérine-Roussy syndrome G93.89
Déjérine-Sottas disease or neuropathy
  (hypertrophic) G60.0
Déjérine-Thomas atrophy G23.8
Delay, delayed
any plane in pelvis
  complicating delivery O66.9
birth or delivery NOS O63.9
closure, ductus arteriosus (Botalli) P29.38
coagulation —see Defect, coagulation
conduction (cardiac) (ventricular) I45.9
delivery, second twin, triplet, etc O63.2

Delay, delayed (Continued)
development R62.50
  global F88
  intellectual (specific) F81.9
  language F80.9
    due to hearing loss F80.4
  learning F81.9
  milestone R62.0
  pervasive F84.9
  physiological R62.50
    specified stage NEC R62.0
  reading F81.0
  sexual E30.0
  speech F80.9
    due to hearing loss F80.4
  spelling F81.81
ejaculation F52.32
gastric emptying K30
menarche E30.0
menstruation (cause unknown) N91.0
milestone R62.0
passage of meconium (newborn) P76.0
primary respiration P28.9
puberty (constitutional) E30.0
separation of umbilical cord P96.82
sexual maturation, female E30.0
sleep phase syndrome G47.21
union, fracture —see Fracture, by site
vaccination Z28.9
Deletion(s)
autosome Q93.9
  identified by fluorescence in situ
    hybridization (FISH) Q93.89
  identified by in situ hybridization (ISH)
    Q93.89
chromosome
  with complex rearrangements NEC Q93.7
  part of NEC Q93.59
  seen only at prometaphase Q93.89
  short arm
    4 Q93.3
    5p Q93.4
    22q11.2 Q93.81
  specified NEC Q93.89
long arm chromosome 18 or 21 Q93.89
  with complex rearrangements NEC Q93.7
microdeletions NEC Q93.88
Delhi boil or button B55.1
Delinquency (juvenile) (neurotic) F91.8
group Z72.810
Delinquent immunization status Z28.3
⫸**Delirium, delirious** (acute or subacute)
  (not alcohol or drug-induced) R41.0
  with
    ▶dementia (see also Dementia) F05
  alcoholic (acute) (tremens) (withdrawal)
    F10.921
    with intoxication F10.921
      in
        abuse F10.121
        dependence F10.221
    due to (secondary to)
      alcohol
        intoxication F10.921
          in
            abuse F10.121
            dependence F10.221
        withdrawal F10.231
      amphetamine intoxication F15.921
        in
          abuse F15.121
          dependence F15.221
      anxiolytic
        intoxication F13.921
          in
            abuse F13.121
            dependence F13.221
        withdrawal F13.231
      cannabis intoxication (acute) F12.921
        in
          abuse F12.121
          dependence F12.221
      cocaine intoxication (acute) F14.921
        in
          abuse F14.121
          dependence F14.221
      general medical condition F05
      hallucinogen intoxication F16.921
        in
          abuse F16.121
          dependence F16.221

Delirium, delirious (Continued)
due to (Continued)
  hypnotic
    intoxication F13.921
      in
        abuse F13.121
        dependence F13.221
    withdrawal F13.231
  inhalant intoxication (acute) F18.921
    in
      abuse F18.121
      dependence F18.221
  multiple etiologies F05
  opioid intoxication (acute) F11.921
    in
      abuse F11.121
      dependence F11.221
  other (or unknown) substance F19.921
  phencyclidine intoxication (acute) F16.921
    in
      abuse F16.121
      dependence F16.221
  psychoactive substance NEC intoxication
    (acute) F19.921
    in
      abuse F19.121
      dependence F19.221
  sedative
    intoxication F13.921
      in
        abuse F13.121
        dependence F13.221
    withdrawal F13.231
  unknown etiology R41.0
exhaustion F43.0
hysterical F44.89
postprocedural (postoperative) F05
puerperal F05
thyroid —see Thyrotoxicosis with thyroid storm
traumatic —see Injury, intracranial
tremens (alcohol-induced) F10.231
  sedative-induced F13.231
Delivery (childbirth) (labor)
arrested active phase O62.1
cesarean (for)
  without indication O82
  abnormal
    pelvis (bony) (deformity) (major) NEC with
      disproportion (fetopelvic) O33.0
      with obstructed labor O65.0
    presentation or position O32.9
  abruptio placentae —see also Abruptio
    placentae 045.9-●
  acromion presentation O32.2
  atony, uterus O62.2
  breech presentation O32.1
    incomplete O32.8
  brow presentation O32.3
  cephalopelvic disproportion O33.9
  cerclage O34.3-●
  chin presentation O32.3
  cicatrix of cervix O34.4-●
  contracted pelvis (general)
    inlet O33.2
    outlet O33.3
  cord presentation or prolapse O69.0
  cystocele O34.8-●
  deformity (acquired) (congenital)
    pelvic organs or tissues NEC O34.8-●
    pelvis (bony) NEC O33.0
  disproportion NOS O33.9
  eclampsia —see Eclampsia
  face presentation O32.3
  failed
    forceps O66.5
    induction of labor O61.9
      instrumental O61.1
      mechanical O61.1
      medical O61.0
      specified NEC O61.8
      surgical O61.1
    trial of labor NOS O66.40
      following previous cesarean delivery
        O66.41
    vacuum extraction O66.5
    ventouse O66.5
  fetal-maternal hemorrhage O43.01-●
  hemorrhage (intrapartum) O67.9
    with coagulation defect O67.0
    specified cause NEC O67.8
  high head at term O32.4

Delivery *(Continued)*
  cesarean *(Continued)*
    hydrocephalic fetus O33.6
    incarceration of uterus O34.51-●
    incoordinate uterine action O62.4
    increased size, fetus O33.5
    inertia, uterus O62.2
      primary O62.0
      secondary O62.1
    isthmocele O34.22
    lateroversion, uterus O34.59-●
    mal lie O32.9
    malposition
      fetus O32.9
      pelvic organs or tissues NEC O34.8-●
      uterus NEC O34.59-●
    malpresentation NOS O32.9
    oblique presentation O32.2
    occurring after 37 completed weeks of
        gestation but before 39 completed weeks
        gestation due to (spontaneous) onset of
        labor O75.82
    oversize fetus O33.5
    pelvic tumor NEC O34.8-●
    placenta previa O44.0-●
      complete O44.0-●
        with hemorrhage O44.1-●
    placental insufficiency O36.51-●
    planned, occurring after 37 completed weeks
        of gestation but before 39 completed
        weeks gestation due to (spontaneous)
        onset of labor O75.82
    polyp, cervix O34.4-●
      causing obstructed labor O65.5
    poor dilatation, cervix O62.0
    pre-eclampsia O14.94
      mild O14.04
      moderate O14.04
      severe O14.14
        with hemolysis, elevated liver enzymes
            and low platelet count (HELLP)
            O14.24
    previous
      cesarean delivery O34.219
        classical (vertical) scar O34.212
        isthmocele O34.22
        low transverse scar O34.211
        mid-transverse T incision O34.218
      scar
        defect (isthmocele) O34.22
        specified type NEC O34.218
      surgery (to)
        cervix O34.4-●
        gynecological NEC O34.8-●
        rectum O34.7-●
        uterus O34.29
        vagina O34.6-●
    prolapse
      arm or hand O32.2
      uterus O34.52-●
    prolonged labor NOS O63.9
    rectocele O34.8-●
    retroversion
      uterus O34.53-●
    rigid
      cervix O34.4-●
      pelvic floor O34.8-●
      perineum O34.7-●
      vagina O34.6-●
      vulva O34.7-●
    sacculation, pregnant uterus O34.59-●
    scar(s)
      cervix O34.4-●
      cesarean delivery O34.219
        classical (vertical) O34.212
        isthmocele O34.22
        low transverse O34.211
        mid-transverse T incision O34.218
        scar
          defect (isthmocele) O34.22
          specified type NEC O34.218
      defect (isthmocele) O34.22
      transmural uterine O34.29
      uterus O34.29
    Shirodkar suture in situ O34.3-●
    shoulder presentation O32.2
    stenosis or stricture, cervix O34.4-●
    streptococcus group B (GBS) carrier state
        O99.824
    transmural uterine scar O34.29
    transverse presentation or lie O32.2

Delivery *(Continued)*
  cesarean *(Continued)*
    tumor, pelvic organs or tissues NEC O34.8-●
      cervix O34.4-●
    umbilical cord presentation or prolapse O69.0
  completely normal case O80
  complicated O75.9
    by
      abnormal, abnormality (of)
        forces of labor O62.9
          specified type NEC O62.8
        glucose O99.814
        uterine contractions NOS O62.9
      abruptio placentae —*see also* Abruptio
          placentae O45.9-●
      abuse
        physical O9A.32
        psychological O9A.52
        sexual O9A.42
      adherent placenta O72.0
        without hemorrhage O73.0
      alcohol use O99.314
      anemia (pre-existing) O99.02
      anesthetic death O74.8
      annular detachment of cervix O71.3
      atony, uterus O62.2
      attempted vacuum extraction and forceps
          O66.5
      Bandl's ring O62.4
      bariatric surgery status O99.844
      biliary tract disorder O26.62
      bleeding —*see* Delivery, complicated by,
          hemorrhage
      blood disorder NEC O99.12
      cervical dystocia (hypotonic) O62.2
        primary O62.0
        secondary O62.1
      circulatory system disorder O99.42
      compression of cord (umbilical) NEC O69.2
      condition NEC O99.892
      contraction, contracted ring O62.4
      cord (umbilical)
        around neck
          with compression O69.1
          without compression O69.81
        bruising O69.5
        complication O69.9
          specified NEC O69.89
        compression NEC O69.2
        entanglement O69.2
          without compression O69.82
        hematoma O69.5
        presentation O69.0
        prolapse O69.0
        short O69.3
        thrombosis (vessels) O69.5
        vascular lesion O69.5
      Couvelaire uterus O45.8X-●
      damage to (injury to) NEC
        perineum O71.82
        periurethral tissue O71.82
        vulva O71.82
      delay following rupture of membranes
          (spontaneous) —*see* Pregnancy,
          complicated by, premature rupture of
          membranes
      depressed fetal heart tones O76
      diabetes O24.92
        gestational O24.429
          diet controlled O24.420
          insulin controlled O24.424
          oral drug controlled (antidiabetic)
              (hypoglycemic) O24.425
        pre-existing O24.32
          specified NEC O24.82
          type 1 O24.02
          type 2 O24.12
      diastasis recti (abdominis) O71.89
      dilatation
        bladder O66.8
        cervix incomplete, poor or slow O62.0
      disease NEC O99.892
      disruptio uteri —*see* Delivery, complicated
          by, rupture, uterus
      drug use O99.324
      dysfunction, uterus NOS O62.9
        hypertonic O62.4
        hypotonic O62.2
          primary O62.0
          secondary O62.1
        incoordinate O62.4

Delivery *(Continued)*
  complicated *(Continued)*
    by *(Continued)*
      eclampsia O15.1
      embolism (pulmonary) —*see* Embolism,
          obstetric
      endocrine, nutritional or metabolic disease
          NEC O99.284
      failed
        attempted vaginal birth after previous
            cesarean delivery O66.41
        induction of labor O61.9
          instrumental O61.1
          mechanical O61.1
          medical O61.0
          specified NEC O61.8
          surgical O61.1
        trial of labor O66.40
      female genital mutilation O65.5
      fetal
        abnormal acid-base balance O68
        acidemia O68
        acidosis O68
        alkalosis O68
        death, early O02.1
        deformity O66.3
        heart rate or rhythm (abnormal) (non-
            reassuring) O76
        hypoxia O77.8
        stress O77.9
          due to drug administration O77.1
          electrocardiographic evidence of O77.8
          specified NEC O77.8
          ultrasound evidence of O77.8
      fever during labor O75.2
      gastric banding status O99.844
      gastric bypass status O99.844
      gastrointestinal disease NEC O99.62
      gestational
        diabetes O24.429
          diet controlled O24.420
          insulin (and diet) controlled
              O24.424
          oral drug controlled (antidiabetic)
              (hypoglycemic) O24.425
        edema O12.04
          with proteinuria O12.24
        proteinuria O12.14
      gonorrhea O98.22
      hematoma O71.7
        ischial spine O71.7
        pelvic O71.7
        vagina O71.7
        vulva or perineum O71.7
      hemorrhage (uterine) O67.9
        associated with
          afibrinogenemia O67.0
          coagulation defect O67.0
          hyperfibrinolysis O67.0
          hypofibrinogenemia O67.0
        due to
          low implantation of placenta O44.5-●
          low-lying placenta O44.5-●
          placenta previa O44.1-●
            marginal O44.3-●
            partial O44.3-●
          premature separation of placenta
              (normally implanted) (*see also*
              Abruptio placentae) O45.9-●
          retained placenta O72.0
          uterine leiomyoma O67.8
        placenta NEC O67.8
        postpartum NEC (atonic) (immediate)
            O72.1
          with retained or trapped placenta
              O72.0
          delayed O72.2
          secondary O72.2
          third stage O72.0
      hourglass contraction, uterus O62.4
      hypertension, hypertensive (pre-
          existing) —*see* Hypertension,
          complicated by, childbirth (labor)
      hypotension O26.5-●
      incomplete dilatation (cervix) O62.0
      incoordinate uterus contractions
          O62.4
      inertia, uterus O62.2
        during latent phase of labor O62.0
        primary O62.0
        secondary O62.1

▶ New   ⇒ Revised   ~~deleted~~ Deleted   ● Use Additional Character(s)

Delivery *(Continued)*
  complicated *(Continued)*
    by *(Continued)*
      infection (maternal) O98.92
        carrier state NEC O99.834
        gonorrhea O98.22
        human immunodeficiency virus (HIV) O98.72
        sexually transmitted NEC O98.32
        specified NEC O98.82
        syphilis O98.12
        tuberculosis O98.02
        viral hepatitis O98.42
        viral NEC O98.52
      injury (to mother) *(see also* Delivery, complicated, by, damage to) O71.9
        nonobstetric O9A.22
        caused by abuse *—see* Delivery, complicated by, abuse
      intrauterine fetal death, early O02.1
      inversion, uterus O71.2
      laceration (perineal) O70.9
        anus (sphincter) O70.4
          with third degree laceration *—see also* Delivery, complicated, by, laceration, perineum, third degree O70.20
            with mucosa O70.3
          without third degree laceration O70.4
        bladder (urinary) O71.5
        bowel O71.5
        cervix (uteri) O71.3
        fourchette O70.0
        hymen O70.0
        labia O70.0
        pelvic
          floor O70.1
          organ NEC O71.5
        perineum, perineal O70.9
          first degree O70.0
          fourth degree O70.3
          muscles O70.1
          second degree O70.1
          skin O70.0
          slight O70.0
          third degree O70.20
            with
              both external anal sphincter (EAS) and internal anal sphincter (IAS) torn (IIIc) O70.23
              less than 50% of external anal sphincter (EAS) thickness torn (IIIa) O70.21
              more than 50% external anal sphincter (EAS) thickness torn (IIIb) O70.22
              IIIa O70.21
              IIIb O70.22
              IIIc O70.23
        peritoneum (pelvic) O71.5
        rectovaginal (septum) (without perineal laceration) O71.4
          with perineum *—see also* Delivery, complicated, by, laceration, perineum, third degree O70.20
            with anal or rectal mucosa O70.3
        specified NEC O71.89
        sphincter ani *—see* Delivery, complicated, by, laceration, anus (sphincter)
        urethra O71.5
        uterus O71.81
          before labor O71.81
        vagina, vaginal (deep) (high) (without perineal laceration) O71.4
          with perineum O70.0
          muscles, with perineum O70.1
        vulva O70.0
      liver disorder O26.62
      malignancy O9A.12
      malnutrition O25.2
      malposition, malpresentation
        without obstruction O32.9 *—see also* Delivery, complicated by, obstruction
          breech O32.1
          compound O32.6
          face (brow) (chin) O32.3
          footling O38.8
          high head O32.4

Delivery *(Continued)*
  complicated *(Continued)*
    by *(Continued)*
      malposition, malpresentation *(Continued)*
        without obstruction *(Continued)*
          oblique O32.2
          specified NEC O32.8
          transverse O32.2
          unstable lie O32.0
        placenta O44.0-●
          with hemorrhage O44.1-●
        uterus or cervix O65.5
      meconium in amniotic fluid O77.0
      mental disorder NEC O99.344
      metrorrhexis *—see* Delivery, complicated by, rupture, uterus
      nervous system disorder O99.354
      obesity (pre-existing) O99.214
      obesity surgery status O99.844
      obstetric trauma O71.9
        specified NEC O71.89
      obstructed labor
        due to
          breech (complete) (frank) presentation O64.1
            incomplete O64.8
          brow presentation O64.3
          buttock presentation O64.1
          chin presentation O64.2
          compound presentation O64.5
          contracted pelvis O65.1
          deep transverse arrest O64.0
          deformed pelvis O65.5
          dystocia (fetal) O66.9
            due to
              conjoined twins O66.3
              fetal
                abnormality NEC O66.3
                ascites O66.3
                hydrops O66.3
                meningomyelocele O66.3
                sacral teratoma O66.3
                tumor O66.3
             hydrocephalic fetus O66.3
            shoulder O66.0
          face presentation O64.2
          fetopelvic disproportion O65.4
          footling presentation O64.8
          impacted shoulders O66.0
          incomplete rotation of fetal head O64.0
          large fetus O66.2
          locked twins O66.1
          malposition O64.9
            specified NEC O64.8
          malpresentation O64.9
            specified NEC O64.8
          multiple fetuses NEC O66.6
          pelvic
            abnormality (maternal) O65.9
              organ O65.5
              specified NEC O65.8
            contraction
              inlet O65.2
              mid-cavity O65.3
              outlet O65.3
          persistent (position)
            occipitoiliac O64.0
            occipitoposterior O64.0
            occipitosacral O64.0
            occipitotransverse O64.0
          prolapsed arm O64.4
          shoulder presentation O64.4
        specified NEC O66.8
      pathological retraction ring, uterus O62.4
      penetration, pregnant uterus by instrument O71.1
      perforation *—see* Delivery, complicated by, laceration
      placenta, placental
        ablatio *—see also* Abruptio placentae O45.9-●
        abnormality O43.9-●
          specified NEC O43.89-●
        abruptio *—see also* Abruptio placentae O45.9-●
        accreta O43.21-●
        adherent (with hemorrhage) O72.0
          without hemorrhage O73.0
        detachment (premature) *—see also* Abruptio placentae O45.9-●

Delivery *(Continued)*
  complicated *(Continued)*
    by *(Continued)*
      malposition, malpresentation *(Continued)*
        disorder O43.9-●
          specified NEC O43.89-●
        hemorrhage NEC O67.8
        increta O43.22-●
        low (implantation) (lying) O44.4-●
          with hemorrhage O44.5-●
        malformation O43.10-●
        malposition O44.0-●
          without hemorrhage O44.1-●
        percreta O43.23-●
        previa (central) (complete) (lateral) (total) O44.0-●
          with hemorrhage O44.1-●
            marginal O44.2-●
              with hemorrhage O44.3-●
            partial O44.2-●
              with hemorrhage O44.3-●
        retained (with hemorrhage) O72.0
          without hemorrhage O73.0
        separation (premature) O45.9-●
          specified NEC O45.8X-●
        vicious insertion O44.1-●
      precipitate labor O62.3
      premature rupture, membranes *(see also* Pregnancy, complicated by, premature rupture of membranes) O42.90
      prolapse
        arm or hand O32.2
        cord (umbilical) O69.0
        foot or leg O32.8
        uterus O34.52-●
      prolonged labor O63.9
        first stage O63.0
        second stage O63.1
      protozoal disease (maternal) O98.62
      respiratory disease NEC O99.52
      retained membranes or portions of placenta O72.2
        without hemorrhage O73.1
      retarded birth O63.9
      retention of secundines (with hemorrhage) O72.0
        without hemorrhage O73.0
        partial O72.2
          without hemorrhage O73.1
      rupture
        bladder (urinary) O71.5
        cervix O71.3
        pelvic organ NEC O71.5
        urethra O71.5
        uterus (during or after labor) O71.1
          before labor O71.0-●
      separation, pubic bone (symphysis pubis) O71.6
      shock O75.1
      shoulder presentation O64.4
      skin disorder NEC O99.72
      spasm, cervix O62.4
      stenosis or stricture, cervix O65.5
      streptococcus group B (GBS) carrier state O99.824
      subluxation of symphysis (pubis) O26.72
      syphilis (maternal) O98.12
      tear (obstetric) *—see* Delivery, complicated by, laceration
      tetanic uterus O62.4
      trauma (obstetrical) *—see also* Delivery, complicated, by, damage to O71.9
        non-obstetric O9A.22
        periurethral O71.82
        specified NEC O71.89
      tuberculosis (maternal) O98.02
      tumor, pelvic organs or tissues NEC O65.5
      umbilical cord around neck
        with compression O69.1
        without compression O69.81
      uterine inertia O62.2
        during latent phase of labor O62.0
        primary O62.0
        secondary O62.1
      vasa previa O69.4
      velamentous insertion of cord O43.12-●
    specified complication NEC O75.89
  delayed NOS O63.9
    following rupture of membranes
      artificial O75.5
    second twin, triplet, etc. O63.2

Delivery *(Continued)*
  forceps, low following failed vacuum extraction
      O66.5
  missed (at or near term) O36.4
  normal O80
  obstructed —*see* Delivery, complicated by,
      obstructed labor
  precipitate O62.3
  preterm —*see also* Pregnancy, complicated by,
      preterm labor O60.10
  spontaneous O80
  term pregnancy NOS O80
  uncomplicated O80
  vaginal, following previous cesarean delivery
      O34.219
    classical (vertical) scar O34.212
    low transverse scar O34.211
    mid-transverse T incision O34.218
    scar
      defect (isthmocele) O34.22
      specified type NEC O34.218]
Delusions (paranoid) —*see* Disorder, delusional
Dementia (degenerative (primary)) (persisting)
    (unspecified severity) (without behavioral
    disturbance, psychotic disturbance, mood
    disturbance, and anxiety) F03.90
  with
    aberrant motor behavior (exit-seeking)
        (pacing) (restlessness) (rocking) F03.911
  ▶acute confusional state F05
    agitation F03.911
    anxiety F03.94
    behavioral disturbances (sexual disinhibition)
        (sleep disturbance) (social disinhibition)
        F03.918
      specified NEC F03.918
    Lewy bodies (*see also* Dementia, in, diseases
        specified elsewhere) G31.83 [F02.80]
      with behavioral disturbance (*see also*
          Dementia, in, diseases specified
          elsewhere) G31.83 [F02.81-●]
    mood disturbance (anhedonia) (apathy)
        (depression) F03.93
  ▶old age (senile) F03
    ▶Alzheimer's type —*see* Disease,
        Alzheimer's, late onset
    Parkinson's disease (*see also* Dementia, in,
        diseases specified elsewhere) G20.A1
        [F02.80]
      with behavioral disturbance G20.A1
          [F02.81-●]
    Parkinsonism (*see also* Dementia, in, diseases
        specified elsewhere) G20.C [F02.80]
      with behavioral disturbance (*see also*
          Dementia, in, diseases specified
          elsewhere) G20.C [F02.81-●]
    psychotic disturbance (delusional
        state) (hallucinations) (paranoia)
        (suspiciousness) F03.92
    verbal or physical behaviors (anger)
        (aggression) (combativeness) (profanity)
        (shouting) (threatening)(violence) F03.911
  alcoholic F10.97
    with dependence F10.27
  Alzheimer's type —*see* Disease, Alzheimer's
  arteriosclerotic —*see* Dementia, vascular
  atypical, Alzheimer's type —*see* Disease,
      Alzheimer's, specified NEC
  congenital —*see* Disability, intellectual
  frontal (lobe) (*see also* Dementia, in, diseases
      specified elsewhere) G31.09 [F02.80]
    with behavioral disturbance (*see also*
        Dementia, in, diseases specified
        elsewhere) G31.09 [F02.81-●]
  frontotemporal (*see also* Dementia, in, diseases
      specified elsewhere) G31.09 [F02.80]
    with behavioral disturbance (*see also*
        Dementia, in, diseases specified
        elsewhere) G31.09 [F02.81-●]
    specified NEC (*see also* Dementia, in, diseases
        specified elsewhere) G31.09 [F02.80]
      with behavioral disturbance (*see also*
          Dementia, in, diseases specified
          elsewhere) G31.09 [F02.81-●]
  in (due to)
    alcohol F10.97
      with dependence F10.27
    Alzheimer's disease —*see* Disease,
        Alzheimer's
    arteriosclerotic brain disease —*see* Dementia,
        vascular

Dementia *(Continued)*
  in (due to) *(Continued)*
    cerebral lipidoses (*see also* Dementia, in,
        diseases specified elsewhere) E75.-
        ● [F02.80]
      with behavioral disturbance (*see also*
          Dementia, in, diseases specified
          elsewhere) E75.-● [F02.81-●]
    Creutzfeldt-Jakob disease —*see also*
        Creutzfeldt-Jakob disease or syndrome
        (with dementia) A81.00
    diseases specified elsewhere (unspecified
        severity) (without behavioral
        disturbance, psychotic disturbance,
        mood disturbance, and anxiety)
        F02.80
      with
        aberrant motor behavior (exit-seeking)
            (pacing) (restlessness) (rocking)
            F02.811
        agitation F02.811
        anxiety F02.84
        behavioral disturbances (sexual
            disinhibition) (sleep disturbance)
            (social disinhibition) F02.818
          specified NEC F02.818
        mood disturbance (anhedonia) (apathy)
            (depression) F02.83
        psychotic disturbance (delusional
            state) (hallucinations) (paranoia)
            (suspiciousness) F02.82
        verbal or physical behaviors (anger)
            (aggression) (combativeness)
            (profanity) (shouting) (threatening)
            (violence) F02.811
      mild F02.A0
        with
          aberrant motor behavior (exit-seeking)
              (pacing) (restlessness) (rocking)
              F02.A11
          agitation F02.A11
          anxiety F02.A4
          behavioral disturbances (sexual
              disinhibition) (sleep disturbance)
              (social disinhibition) F02.A18
            specified NEC F02.A18
          mood disturbance (anhedonia)
              (apathy) (depression) F02.A3
          psychotic disturbance (delusional
              state) (hallucinations) (paranoia)
              (suspiciousness) F02.A2
          verbal or physical behaviors (anger)
              (aggression) (combativeness)
              (profanity) (shouting)
              (threatening)(violence) F02.A11
      moderate F02.B0
        with
          aberrant motor behavior (exit-seeking)
              (pacing) (restlessness) (rocking)
              F02.B11
          agitation F02.B11
          anxiety F02.B4
          behavioral disturbances (sexual
              disinhibition) (sleep disturbance)
              (social disinhibition) F02.B18
            specified NEC F02.B18
          mood disturbance (anhedonia)
              (apathy) (depression) F02.B3
          psychotic disturbance (delusional
              state) (hallucinations) (paranoia)
              (suspiciousness) F02.B2
          verbal or physical behaviors (anger)
              (aggression) (combativeness)
              (profanity) (shouting)
              (threatening)(violence) F02.B11
      severe F02.C0
        with
          aberrant motor behavior (exit-seeking)
              (pacing) (restlessness) (rocking)
              F02.C11
          agitation F02.C11
          anxiety F02.C4
          behavioral disturbances (sexual
              disinhibition) (sleep disturbance)
              (social disinhibition) F02.C18
            specified NEC F02.C18
          mood disturbance (anhedonia)
              (apathy) (depression) F02.C3
          psychotic disturbance (delusional
              state) (hallucinations) (paranoia)
              (suspiciousness) F02.C2

Dementia *(Continued)*
  in (due to) *(Continued)*
    diseases specified elsewhere *(Continued)*
      severe *(Continued)*
        with *(Continued)*
          verbal or physical behaviors (anger)
              (aggression) (combativeness)
              (profanity) (shouting)
              (threatening)(violence)
              F02.C11
    epilepsy (*see also* Dementia, in, diseases
        specified elsewhere) G40.-● [F02.80]
      with behavioral disturbance (*see also*
          Dementia, in, diseases specified
          elsewhere) G40.-● [F02.81-●]
    hepatolenticular degeneration (*see also*
        Dementia, in, diseases specified
        elsewhere) E83.01 [F02.80]
      with behavioral disturbance (*see also*
          Dementia, in, diseases specified
          elsewhere) E83.01 [F02.81-●]
    human immunodeficiency virus (HIV) disease
        (*see also* Dementia, in, diseases specified
        elsewhere) B20 [F02.80]
      with behavioral disturbance (*see also*
          Dementia, in, diseases specified
          elsewhere) B20 [F02.81-●]
    Huntington's disease or chorea (*see also*
        Dementia, in, diseases specified
        elsewhere) G10 [F02.80]
      with behavioral disturbance (*see also*
          Dementia, in, diseases specified
          elsewhere) G10 [F02.81-●]
    hypercalcemia (*see also* Dementia, in, diseases
        specified elsewhere) E83.52 [F02.80]
      with behavioral disturbance (*see also*
          Dementia, in, diseases specified
          elsewhere) E83.52 [F02.81-●]
    hypothyroidism, acquired (*see also* Dementia,
        in, diseases specified elsewhere) E03.9
        [F02.80]
      with behavioral disturbance (*see also*
          Dementia, in, diseases specified
          elsewhere) E03.9 [F02.81-●]
      due to iodine deficiency (*see also* Dementia,
          in, diseases specified elsewhere) E01.8
          [F02.80]
        with behavioral disturbance (*see also*
            Dementia, in, diseases specified
            elsewhere) E01.8 [F02.81-●]
    inhalants F18.97
      with dependence F18.27
    multiple
      etiologies F03
      sclerosis (*see also* Dementia, in, diseases
          specified elsewhere) G35
          [F02.80]
        with behavioral disturbance (*see also*
            Dementia, in, diseases specified
            elsewhere) G35 [F02.81-●]
    neurosyphilis (*see also* Dementia, in, diseases
        specified elsewhere) A52.17
        [F02.80]
      with behavioral disturbance (*see also*
          Dementia, in, diseases specified
          elsewhere) A52.17 [F02.81-●]
      juvenile (*see also* Dementia, in, diseases
          specified elsewhere) A50.49 [F02.80]
        with behavioral disturbance (*see also*
            Dementia, in, diseases specified
            elsewhere) A50.49 [F02.81-●]
    niacin deficiency (*see also* Dementia, in,
        diseases specified elsewhere) E52
        [F02.80]
      with behavioral disturbance (*see also*
          Dementia, in, diseases specified
          elsewhere) E52 [F02.81-●]
    paralysis agitans (*see also* Dementia, in,
        diseases specified elsewhere) G20.C
        [F02.80]
      with behavioral disturbance (*see also*
          Dementia, in, diseases specified
          elsewhere) G20.C [F02.81-●]
    Parkinson's disease (*see also* Dementia, in,
        diseases specified elsewhere) G20.A1
        [F02.80]
    pellagra (*see also* Dementia, in, diseases
        specified elsewhere) E52 [F02.80]
      with behavioral disturbance (*see also*
          Dementia, in, diseases specified
          elsewhere) E52 [F02.81-●]

▶ New   ⇒ Revised   ~~deleted~~ Deleted   ● Use Additional Character(s)

Dementia *(Continued)*
  in (due to) *(Continued)*
    Pick's G31.01 *(see also* Dementia, in, diseases
      specified elsewhere) [F02.80]
      with behavioral disturbance *(see also*
        Dementia, in, diseases specified
        elsewhere) G31.01 *[F02.81-●]*
    polyarteritis nodosa *(see also* Dementia, in,
      diseases specified elsewhere) M30.0
      [F02.80]
      with behavioral disturbance *(see also*
        Dementia, in, diseases specified
        elsewhere) M30.0 *[F02.81-●]*
    psychoactive drug F19.97
      with dependence F19.27
      inhalants F18.97
        with dependence F18.27
      sedatives, hypnotics or anxiolytics F13.97
        with dependence F13.27
    sedatives, hypnotics or anxiolytics F13.97
      with dependence F13.27
    systemic lupus erythematosus *(see also*
      Dementia, in, diseases specified
      elsewhere) M32.-● *[F02.80]*
      with behavioral disturbance *(see also*
        Dementia, in, diseases specified
        elsewhere) M32.-● *[F02.81-●]*
    trypanosomiasis
      African *(see also* Dementia, in, diseases
        specified elsewhere) B56.9
        [F02.80]
        with behavioral disturbance *(see also*
          Dementia, in, diseases specified
          elsewhere) B56.9 *[F02.81-●]*
    unknown etiology *(see also* Dementia, in,
      diseases specified elsewhere) F03.-●
    vitamin B12 deficiency *(see also* Dementia,
      in, diseases specified elsewhere) E53.8
      [F02.80]
      with behavioral disturbance *(see also*
        Dementia, in, diseases specified
        elsewhere) E53.8 *[F02.81-●]*
    volatile solvents F18.97
      with dependence F18.27
  infantile, infantilis F84.3
  Lewy body *(see also* Dementia, in, diseases
    specified elsewhere) G31.83 *[F02.80]*
    with behavioral disturbance *(see also*
      Dementia, in, diseases specified
      elsewhere) G31.83 *[F02.81-●]*
  mild F02.A0
    with
      aberrant motor behavior (exit-seeking)
        (pacing) (restlessness) (rocking) F02.
        A11
      agitation F02.A11
      anxiety F02.A4
      behavioral disturbances (sexual
        disinhibition) (sleep disturbance)
        (social disinhibition) F02.A18
        specified NEC F02.A18
      mood disturbance (anhedonia) (apathy)
        (depression) F02.A3
      psychotic disturbance (delusional
        state) (hallucinations) (paranoia)
        (suspiciousness) F02.A2
      verbal or physical behaviors (anger)
        (aggression) (combativeness)
        (profanity) (shouting) (threatening)
        (violence) F02.A11
  moderate F02.B0
    with
      aberrant motor behavior (exit-seeking)
        (pacing) (restlessness) (rocking)
        F02.B11
      agitation F02.B11
      anxiety F02.B4
      behavioral disturbances (sexual
        disinhibition) (sleep disturbance)
        (social disinhibition) F02.B18
        specified NEC F02.B18
      mood disturbance (anhedonia) (apathy)
        (depression) F02.B3
      psychotic disturbance (delusional
        state) (hallucinations) (paranoia)
        (suspiciousness) F02.B2
      verbal or physical behaviors (anger)
        (aggression) (combativeness)
        (profanity) (shouting) (threatening)
        (violence)
        F02.B11

Dementia *(Continued)*
  multi-infarct —*see* Dementia, vascular
  paralytica, paralytic (syphilitic) *(see also*
    Dementia, in, diseases specified elsewhere)
    A52.17 *[F02.80]*
    with behavioral disturbance *(see also*
      Dementia, in, diseases specified
      elsewhere) A52.17 *[F02.81-●]*
    juvenilis A50.45
  paretic A52.17
  praecox —*see* Schizophrenia
  presenile F03
    Alzheimer's type —*see* Disease, Alzheimer's,
      early onset
  primary degenerative F03
  progressive, syphilitic A52.17
  senile F03
    with acute confusional state F05
    Alzheimer's type —*see* Disease, Alzheimer's,
      late onset
    depressed or paranoid type F03
  severe F02.C0
    with
      aberrant motor behavior (exit-seeking)
        (pacing) (restlessness) (rocking) F02.
        C11
      agitation F02.C11
      anxiety F02.C4
      behavioral disturbances (sexual
        disinhibition) (sleep disturbance)
        (social disinhibition) F02.C18
        specified NEC F02.C18
      mood disturbance (anhedonia) (apathy)
        (depression) F02.C3
      psychotic disturbance (delusional
        state) (hallucinations) (paranoia)
        (suspiciousness) F02.C2
      verbal or physical behaviors (anger)
        (aggression) (combativeness)
        (profanity) (shouting) (threatening)
        (violence) F02.C11
  vascular (acute onset) (mixed) (multi-infarct)
    (subcortical) (unspecified severity)
    (without behavioral disturbance, psychotic
    disturbance, mood disturbance, and
    anxiety) F01.50
    with
      aberrant motor behavior (exit-seeking)
        (pacing) (restlessness) (rocking)
        F01.511
      agitation F01.511
      anxiety F01.54
      behavioral disturbances (sleep disturbance)
        (sexual disinhibition) (social
        disinhibition) F01.518
        specified NEC F01.518
      mood disturbance (anhedonia) (apathy)
        (depression) F01.53
      psychotic disturbance (delusional
        state) (hallucinations) (paranoia)
        (suspiciousness) F01.52
      verbal or physical behaviors (anger)
        (aggression) (combativeness)
        (profanity) (shouting) (threatening)
        (violence) F01.511
    mild F01.A0
      with
        aberrant motor behavior (exit-seeking)
          (pacing) (restlessness) (rocking)
          F01.A11
        agitation F01.A11
        anxiety F01.A4
        behavioral disturbances (sleep
          disturbance) (sexual disinhibition)
          (social disinhibition) F01.A18
          specified NEC F01.A18
        mood disturbance (anhedonia) (apathy)
          (depression) F01.A3
        psychotic disturbance (delusional
          state) (hallucinations) (paranoia)
          (suspiciousness) F01.A2
        verbal or physical behaviors (anger)
          (aggression) (combativeness)
          (profanity) (shouting) (threatening)
          (violence) F01.A11
    moderate F01.B0
      with
        aberrant motor behavior (exit-seeking)
          (pacing) (restlessness) (rocking)
          F01.B11
        agitation F01.B11

Dementia *(Continued)*
  vascular *(Continued)*
    moderate *(Continued)*
      with *(Continued)*
        anxiety F01.B4
        behavioral disturbances (sleep
          disturbance) (sexual disinhibition)
          (social disinhibition) F01.B18
          specified NEC F01.B18
        mood disturbance (anhedonia) (apathy)
          (depression) F01.B3
        psychotic disturbance (delusional
          state) (hallucinations) (paranoia)
          (suspiciousness) F01.B2
        verbal or physical behaviors (anger)
          (aggression) (combativeness)
          (profanity) (shouting) (threatening)
          (violence) F01.B11
    severe F01.C0
      with
        aberrant motor behavior (exit-seeking)
          (pacing) (restlessness) (rocking)
          F01.C11
        agitation F01.C11
        anxiety F01.C4
        behavioral disturbances (sleep
          disturbance) (sexual disinhibition)
          (social disinhibition) F01.C18
          specified NEC F01.C18
        mood disturbance (anhedonia) (apathy)
          (depression) F01.C3
        psychotic disturbance (delusional
          state) (hallucinations) (paranoia)
          (suspiciousness) F01.C2
        verbal or physical behaviors (anger)
          (aggression) (combativeness)
          (profanity) (shouting) (threatening)
          (violence) F01.C11
Demineralization, bone —*see* Osteoporosis
Demodex folliculorum (infestation) B88.0
Demophobia F40.248
Demoralization R45.3
Demyelination, demyelinization
  central nervous system G37.9
    specified NEC G37.89
  corpus callosum (central) G37.1
  disseminated, acute G36.9
    specified NEC G36.8
  global G35
  in optic neuritis G36.0
Dengue (classical) (fever) A90
  hemorrhagic A91
  sandfly A93.1
Dennie-Marfan syphilitic syndrome A50.45
Dens evaginatus, in dente or invaginatus K00.2
Dense breasts *(see also* Density, breast) R92.30●
Density
  breast R92.30●
    mammographic●
      extreme R92.34-●
      fatty tissue R92.31-●
      fibroglandular R92.32-●
      heterogeneous R92.33-●
  increased, bone (disseminated) (generalized)
    (spotted) —*see* Disorder, bone, density and
    structure, specified type NEC
  low R92.30●
  lung (nodular) J98.4
Dental —*see also* condition
  examination Z01.20
    with abnormal findings Z01.21
  restoration
    aesthetically inadequate or displeasing K08.56
    defective K08.50
      specified NEC K08.59
    failure of marginal integrity K08.51
    failure of periodontal anatomical integrity
      K08.54
Dentia praecox K00.6
Denticles (pulp) K04.2
Dentigerous cyst K09.0
Dentin
  irregular (in pulp) K04.3
  opalescent K00.5
  secondary (in pulp) K04.3
  sensitive K03.89
Dentinogenesis imperfecta K00.5
Dentinoma —*see* Cyst, calcifying odontogenic
Dentition (syndrome) K00.7
  delayed K00.6
  difficult K00.7

Dentition *(Continued)*
  precocious K00.6
  premature K00.6
  retarded K00.6
Dependence (on) (syndrome) F19.20
  with remission F19.21
  alcohol (ethyl) (methyl) (without remission)
    F10.20
    with
      amnestic disorder, persisting F10.26
      anxiety disorder F10.280
      dementia, persisting F10.27
      intoxication F10.229
        with delirium F10.221
        uncomplicated F10.220
      mood disorder F10.24
      psychotic disorder F10.259
        with
          delusions F10.250
          hallucinations F10.251
      remission F10.21
      sexual dysfunction F10.281
      sleep disorder F10.282
      specified disorder NEC F10.288
      withdrawal F10.239
        with
          delirium F10.231
          perceptual disturbance F10.232
        uncomplicated F10.230
    counseling and surveillance Z71.41
    in remission F10.21
  amobarbital —*see* Dependence, drug, sedative
  amphetamine(s) (type) —*see* Dependence, drug,
    stimulant NEC
  amytal (sodium) —*see* Dependence, drug,
    sedative
  analgesic NEC F55.8
  anesthetic (agent) (gas) (general) (local) NEC —
    see Dependence, drug, psychoactive NEC
  anxiolytic NEC —*see* Dependence, drug, sedative
  barbital(s) —*see* Dependence, drug, sedative
  barbiturate(s) (compounds) (drugs classifiable to
    T42) —*see* Dependence, drug, sedative
  benzedrine —*see* Dependence, drug, stimulant
    NEC
  bhang —*see* Dependence, drug, cannabis
  bromide(s) NEC —*see* Dependence, drug,
    sedative
  caffeine —*see* Dependence, drug, stimulant NEC
  cannabis (sativa) (indica) (resin) (derivatives)
    (type) —*see* Dependence, drug, cannabis
  chloral (betaine) (hydrate) —*see* Dependence,
    drug, sedative
  chlordiazepoxide —*see* Dependence, drug,
    sedative
  coca (leaf) (derivatives) —*see* Dependence, drug,
    cocaine
  cocaine —*see* Dependence, drug, cocaine
  codeine —*see* Dependence, drug, opioid
  combinations of drugs F19.20
  dagga —*see* Dependence, drug, cannabis
  demerol —*see* Dependence, drug, opioid
  dexamphetamine —*see* Dependence, drug,
    stimulant NEC
  dexedrine —*see* Dependence, drug, stimulant
    NEC
  dextromethorphan —*see* Dependence, drug,
    opioid
  dextromoramide —*see* Dependence, drug, opioid
  dextro-nor-pseudo-ephedrine —*see* Dependence,
    drug, stimulant NEC
  dextrorphan —*see* Dependence, drug, opioid
  diazepam —*see* Dependence, drug,
  sedative
  dilaudid —*see* Dependence, drug, opioid
  D-lysergic acid diethylamide —*see* Dependence,
    drug, hallucinogen
  drug NEC F19.20
    with sleep disorder F19.282
    cannabis F12.20
      with
        anxiety disorder F12.280
        intoxication F12.229
          with
            delirium F12.221
            perceptual disturbance F12.222
          uncomplicated F12.220
        other specified disorder F12.288
        psychosis F12.259
          delusions F12.250
          hallucinations F12.251

Dependence *(Continued)*
  drug *(Continued)*
    cannabis *(Continued)*
      with *(Continued)*
        unspecified disorder F12.29
        withdrawal F12.23
      in remission F12.21
    cocaine F14.20
      with
        anxiety disorder F14.280
        intoxication F14.229
          with
            delirium F14.221
            perceptual disturbance F14.222
          uncomplicated F14.220
        mood disorder F14.24
        other specified disorder F14.288
        psychosis F14.259
          delusions F14.250
          hallucinations F14.251
        sexual dysfunction F14.281
        sleep disorder F14.282
        unspecified disorder F14.29
        withdrawal F14.23
      in remission F14.21
      withdrawal symptoms in newborn P96.1
    counseling and surveillance Z71.51
    hallucinogen F16.20
      with
        anxiety disorder F16.280
        flashbacks F16.283
        intoxication F16.229
          with delirium F16.221
          uncomplicated F16.220
        mood disorder F16.24
        other specified disorder F16.288
        perception disorder, persisting F16.283
        psychosis F16.259
          delusions F16.250
          hallucinations F16.251
        unspecified disorder F16.29
      in remission F16.21
    in remission F19.21
    inhalant F18.20
      with
        anxiety disorder F18.280
        dementia, persisting F18.27
        intoxication F18.229
          with delirium F18.221
          uncomplicated F18.220
        mood disorder F18.24
        other specified disorder F18.288
        psychosis F18.259
          delusions F18.250
          hallucinations F18.251
        unspecified disorder F18.29
      in remission F18.21
    nicotine F17.200
      with disorder F17.209
        in remission F17.201
        specified disorder NEC F17.208
        withdrawal F17.203
      chewing tobacco F17.220
        with disorder F17.229
          in remission F17.221
          specified disorder NEC F17.228
          withdrawal F17.223
      cigarettes F17.210
        with disorder F17.219
          in remission F17.211
          specified disorder NEC F17.218
          withdrawal F17.213
      specified product NEC F17.290
        with disorder F17.299
          remission F17.291
          specified disorder NEC F17.298
          withdrawal F17.293
    opioid F11.20
      with
        intoxication F11.229
          with
            delirium F11.221
            perceptual disturbance F11.222
          uncomplicated F11.220
        mood disorder F11.24
        opioid-associated amnestic syndrome
          F11.288
        other specified disorder F11.288
        psychosis F11.259
          delusions F11.250
          hallucinations F11.251

Dependence *(Continued)*
  drug *(Continued)*
    opioid *(Continued)*
      with *(Continued)*
        sexual dysfunction F11.281
        sleep disorder F11.282
        unspecified disorder F11.29
        withdrawal F11.23
      in remission F11.21
    psychoactive NEC F19.20
      with
        amnestic disorder F19.26
        anxiety disorder F19.280
        dementia F19.27
        intoxication F19.229
          with
            delirium F19.221
            perceptual disturbance F19.222
          uncomplicated F19.220
        mood disorder F19.24
        other specified disorder F19.288
        psychosis F19.259
          delusions F19.250
          hallucinations F19.251
        sexual dysfunction F19.281
        sleep disorder F19.282
        unspecified disorder F19.29
        withdrawal F19.239
          with
            delirium F19.231
            perceptual disturbance F19.232
          uncomplicated F19.230
    in remission F19.21
    sedative, hypnotic or anxiolytic F13.20
      with
        amnestic disorder F13.26
        anxiety disorder F13.280
        dementia, persisting F13.27
        intoxication F13.229
          with delirium F13.221
          uncomplicated F13.220
        mood disorder F13.24
        other specified disorder F13.288
        psychosis F13.259
          delusions F13.250
          hallucinations F13.251
        sexual dysfunction F13.281
        sleep disorder F13.282
        unspecified disorder F13.29
        withdrawal F13.239
          with
            delirium F13.231
            perceptual disturbance F13.232
          uncomplicated F13.230
      in remission F13.21
    stimulant NEC F15.20
      with
        anxiety disorder F15.280
        intoxication F15.229
          with
            delirium F15.221
            perceptual disturbance F15.222
          uncomplicated F15.220
        mood disorder F15.24
        other specified disorder F15.288
        psychosis F15.259
          delusions F15.250
          hallucinations F15.251
        sexual dysfunction F15.281
        sleep disorder F15.282
        unspecified disorder F15.29
        withdrawal F15.23
      in remission F15.21
  ethyl
    alcohol (without remission) F10.20
      with remission F10.21
    bromide —*see* Dependence, drug, sedative
    carbamate F19.20
    chloride F19.20
    morphine —*see* Dependence, drug, opioid
  ganja —*see* Dependence, drug, cannabis
  glue (airplane) (sniffing) —*see* Dependence,
    drug, inhalant
  glutethimide —*see* Dependence, drug, sedative
  hallucinogenics —*see* Dependence, drug,
    hallucinogen
  hashish —*see* Dependence, drug, cannabis
  hemp —*see* Dependence, drug, cannabis
  heroin (salt) (any) —*see* Dependence, drug,
    opioid
  hypnotic NEC —*see* Dependence, drug, sedative

▶ New   ⇒ Revised   ~~deleted~~ Deleted   ● Use Additional Character(s)

Derangement *(Continued)*
- joint (internal) *(Continued)*
  - specified type *(Continued)*
    - hip M24.85-●
    - shoulder M24.81-●
    - specified site NEC M24.89
    - wrist M24.83-●
  - temporomandibular M26.69
  - knee (recurrent) M23.9-●
    - ligament disruption, spontaneous M23.60-●
      - anterior cruciate M23.61-●
      - capsular M23.67-●
      - instability, chronic M23.5-●
      - lateral collateral M23.64-●
      - medial collateral M23.63-●
      - posterior cruciate M23.62-●
    - loose body M23.4-●
    - meniscus M23.30-●
      - cystic M23.00-●
        - lateral M23.002
          - anterior horn M23.04-●
          - posterior horn M23.05-●
          - specified NEC M23.06-●
        - medial M23.005
          - anterior horn M23.01-●
          - posterior horn M23.02-●
          - specified NEC M23.03-●
      - degenerate —*see* Derangement, knee, meniscus, specified NEC
      - detached —*see* Derangement, knee, meniscus, specified NEC
      - due to old tear or injury M23.20-●
        - lateral M23.20-●
          - anterior horn M23.24-●
          - posterior horn M23.25-●
          - specified NEC M23.26-●
        - medial M23.20-●
          - anterior horn M23.21-●
          - posterior horn M23.22-●
          - specified NEC M23.23-●
      - retained —*see* Derangement, knee, meniscus, specified NEC
      - specified NEC M23.30-●
        - lateral M23.30-●
          - anterior horn M23.34-●
          - posterior horn M23.35-●
          - specified NEC M23.36-●
        - medial M23.30-●
          - anterior horn M23.31-●
          - posterior horn M23.32-●
          - specified NEC M23.33-●
    - old M23.8X-●
    - specified NEC —*see* subcategory M23.8
  - low back NEC —*see* Dorsopathy, specified NEC
  - meniscus —*see* Derangement, knee, meniscus
  - mental —*see* Psychosis
  - patella, specified NEC —*see* Disorder, patella, derangement NEC
  - semilunar cartilage (knee) —*see* Derangement, knee, meniscus, specified NEC
  - shoulder (internal) —*see* Derangement, joint, shoulder
- **Dercum's disease** E88.2
- **Derealization** (neurotic) F48.1
- **Dermal** —*see* condition
- **Dermaphytid** —*see* Dermatophytosis
- **Dermatitis** (eczematous) L30.9
  - ab igne L59.0
  - acarine B88.0
  - actinic (due to sun) L57.8
    - other than from sun L59.8
  - allergic —*see* Dermatitis, contact, allergic
  - ambustionis, due to burn or scald —*see* Burn
  - amebic A06.7
  - ammonia L22
  - arsenical (ingested) L27.8
  - artefacta L98.1
    - psychogenic F54
  - atopic L20.9
    - psychogenic F54
    - specified NEC L20.89
  - autoimmune progesterone L30.8
  - berlock, berloque L56.2
  - blastomycotic B40.3
  - blister beetle L24.89
  - bullous, bullosa L13.9
    - mucosynechial, atrophic L12.1
    - seasonal L30.8
    - specified NEC L13.8
  - calorica L59.0
    - due to burn or scald —*see* Burn

Dermatitis *(Continued)*
- caterpillar L24.89
- cercarial B65.3
- combustionis L59.0
  - due to burn or scald —*see* Burn
- congelationis T69.1
- contact (occupational) L25.9
  - allergic L23.9
    - due to
      - adhesives L23.1
      - cement L23.5
      - chemical products NEC L23.5
      - chromium L23.0
      - cosmetics L23.2
      - dander (cat) (dog) L23.81
      - drugs in contact with skin L23.3
      - dyes L23.4
      - food in contact with skin L23.6
      - hair (cat) (dog) L23.81
      - insecticide L23.5
      - metals L23.0
      - nickel L23.0
      - plants, non-food L23.7
      - plastic L23.5
      - rubber L23.5
      - specified agent NEC L23.89
  - due to
    - cement L25.3
    - chemical products NEC L25.3
    - cosmetics L25.0
    - dander (cat) (dog) L23.81
    - drugs in contact with skin L25.1
    - dyes L25.2
    - food in contact with skin L25.4
    - hair (cat) (dog) L23.81
    - plants, non-food L25.5
    - specified agent NEC L25.8
  - irritant L24.9
    - due to
      - body fluids L24.A0
        - feces L24.A2
        - incontinence (dual) (fecal) (urinary) 24.A2
        - saliva L24.A1
        - specified NEC L24.A9
        - urine L24.A2
        - wound exudate L24.A9
      - cement L24.5
      - chemical products NEC L24.5
      - cosmetics L24.3
      - detergents L24.0
      - drugs in contact with skin L24.4
      - exudate L24.A9
      - food in contact with skin L24.6
      - friction L24.A0
      - oils and greases L24.1
      - plants, non-food L24.7
    - related to
      - colostomy L24.B3
      - endotracheal tube L24.A9
      - enterocutaneous fistula L24.B3
      - gastrostomy L24.B1
      - ileostomy L24.B3
      - jejunostomy L24.B1
      - saliva or spit fistula L24.B1
      - stoma or fistula L24.B0
        - digestive L24.B1
        - fecal or urinary L24.B3
        - respiratory L24.B2
        - tracheostomy L24.B2
      - solvents L24.2
    - specified agent NEC L24.89
- contusiformis L52
- desquamative L30.8
- diabetic —*see* E08-E13 with .620
- diaper L22
- diphtheritica A36.3
- dry skin L85.3
- due to
  - acetone (contact) (irritant) L24.2
  - acids (contact) (irritant) L24.5
  - adhesive(s) (allergic) (contact) (plaster) L23.1
    - irritant L24.5
  - alcohol (irritant) (skin contact) (substances in category T51) L24.2
    - taken internally L27.8
  - alkalis (contact) (irritant) L24.5
  - arsenic (ingested) L27.8
  - carbon disulfide (contact) (irritant) L24.2
  - caustics (contact) (irritant) L24.5

Dermatitis *(Continued)*
- due to *(Continued)*
  - cement (contact) L25.3
  - cereal (ingested) L27.2
  - chemical(s) NEC L25.3
    - taken internally L27.8
  - chlorocompounds L24.2
  - chromium (contact) (irritant) L24.81
  - coffee (ingested) L27.2
  - cold weather L30.8
  - cosmetics (contact) L25.0
    - allergic L23.2
    - irritant L24.3
  - cyclohexanes L24.2
  - dander (cat) (dog) L23.81
  - Demodex species B88.0
  - Dermanyssus gallinae B88.0
  - detergents (contact) (irritant) L24.0
  - dichromate L24.81
  - drugs and medicaments (generalized) (internal use) L27.0
    - external —*see* Dermatitis, due to, drugs, in contact with skin
    - in contact with skin L25.1
      - allergic L23.3
      - irritant L24.4
    - localized skin eruption L27.1
    - specified substance —*see* Table of Drugs and Chemicals
  - dyes (contact) L25.2
    - allergic L23.4
    - irritant L24.89
  - epidermophytosis —*see* Dermatophytosis
  - esters L24.2
  - external irritant NEC L24.9
  - exudate L24.A9
  - fish (ingested) L27.2
  - flour (ingested) L27.2
  - food (ingested) L27.2
    - in contact with skin L25.4
  - fruit (ingested) L27.2
  - furs (allergic) (contact) L23.81
  - glues —*see* Dermatitis, due to, adhesives
  - glycols L24.2
  - greases NEC (contact) (irritant) L24.1
  - hair (cat) (dog) L23.81
  - hot
    - objects and materials —*see* Burn
    - weather or places L59.0
  - hydrocarbons L24.2
  - infrared rays L59.8
  - ingestion, ingested substance L27.9
    - chemical NEC L27.8
    - drugs and medicaments —*see* Dermatitis, due to, drugs
    - food L27.2
    - specified NEC L27.8
  - insecticide in contact with skin L24.5
  - internal agent L27.9
    - drugs and medicaments (generalized) —*see* Dermatitis, due to, drugs
    - food L27.2
  - irradiation —*see* Dermatitis, due to, radioactive substance
  - ketones L24.2
  - lacquer tree (allergic) (contact) L23.7
  - light (sun) NEC L57.8
    - acute L56.8
    - other L59.8
  - Liponyssoides sanguineus B88.0
  - low temperature L30.8
  - meat (ingested) L27.2
  - metals, metal salts (contact) (irritant) L24.81
  - milk (ingested) L27.2
  - nickel (contact) (irritant) L24.81
  - nylon (contact) (irritant) L24.5
  - oils NEC (contact) (irritant) L24.1
  - paint solvent (contact) (irritant) L24.2
  - petroleum products (contact) (irritant) (substances in T52) L24.2
  - plants NEC (contact) L25.5
    - allergic L23.7
    - irritant L24.7
  - plasters (adhesive) (any) (allergic) (contact) L23.1
    - irritant L24.5
  - plastic (contact) L25.3
  - preservatives (contact) —*see* Dermatitis, due to, chemical, in contact with skin
  - primrose (allergic) (contact) L23.7
  - primula (allergic) (contact) L23.7

▶ New   ➡ Revised   ~~deleted~~ Deleted   ● Use Additional Character(s)

Dermatitis *(Continued)*
  due to *(Continued)*
    radiation L59.8
      nonionizing (chronic exposure) L57.8
        sun NEC L57.8
          acute L56.8
    radioactive substance L58.9
      acute L58.0
      chronic L58.1
    radium L58.9
      acute L58.0
      chronic L58.1
    ragweed (allergic) (contact) L23.7
    Rhus (allergic) (contact) (diversiloba)
        (radicans) (toxicodendron) (venenata)
        (verniciflua) L23.7
    rubber (contact) L24.5
    Senecio jacobaea (allergic) (contact)
        L23.7
    solvents (contact) (irritant) (substances in
        categories T52) L24.2
    specified agent NEC (contact) L25.8
      allergic L23.89
      irritant L24.89
    sunshine NEC L57.8
      acute L56.8
    tetrachlorethylene (contact) (irritant)
        L24.2
    toluene (contact) (irritant) L24.2
    turpentine (contact) L24.2
    ultraviolet rays (sun NEC) (chronic exposure)
        L57.8
      acute L56.8
    vaccine or vaccination L27.0
      specified substance —*see* Table of Drugs
          and Chemicals
    varicose veins —*see* Varix, leg, with,
        inflammation
    X-rays L58.9
      acute L58.0
      chronic L58.1
  dyshydrotic L30.1
  dysmenorrheica N94.6
  escharotica —*see* Burn
  exfoliative, exfoliativa (generalized) L26
    neonatorum L00
  eyelid —*(see also* Dermatosis, eyelid)
      H01.9
    allergic H01.119
      left H01.116
        lower H01.115
        upper H01.114
      right H01.113
        lower H01.112
        upper H01.111
    contact —*see* Dermatitis, eyelid, allergic
    due to
      Demodex species B88.0
      herpes (zoster) B02.39
        simplex B00.59
      eczematous H01.139
        left H01.136
          lower H01.135
          upper H01.134
        right H01.133
          lower H01.132
          upper H01.131
      specified NEC H01.149
  facta, factitia, factitial L98.1
    psychogenic F54
  flexural NEC L20.82
  friction L30.4
  fungus B36.9
    specified type NEC B36.8
  gangrenosa, gangrenous infantum
      L08.0
  harvest mite B88.0
  heat L59.0
  herpesviral, vesicular (ear) (lip) B00.1
  herpetiformis (bullous) (erythematous)
      (pustular) (vesicular) L13.0
    juvenile L12.2
    senile L12.0
  hiemalis L30.8
  hypostatic, hypostatica —*see* Varix, leg, with,
      inflammation
  infectious eczematoid L30.3
  infective L30.3
  irritant —*see* Dermatitis, contact, irritant
  Jacquet's (diaper dermatitis) L22
  Leptus B88.0

Dermatitis *(Continued)*
  lichenified NEC L28.0
  medicamentosa (generalized) (internal use) —*see*
      Dermatitis, due to drugs
  mite B88.0
  multiformis L13.0
    juvenile L12.2
  napkin L22
  neurotica L13.0
  nummular L30.0
  papillaris capillitii L73.0
  pellagrous E52
  perioral L71.0
  photocontact L56.2
  polymorpha dolorosa L13.0
  pruriginosa L13.0
  pruritic NEC L30.8
  psychogenic F54
  purulent L08.0
  pustular
    contagious B08.02
    subcorneal L13.1
  pyococcal L08.0
  pyogenica L08.0
  repens L40.2
  Ritter's (exfoliativa) L00
  Schamberg's L81.7
  schistosome B65.3
  seasonal bullous L30.8
  seborrheic L21.9
    infantile L21.1
    specified NEC L21.8
  sensitization NOS L23.9
  septic L08.0
  solare L57.8
  specified NEC L30.8
  stasis I87.2
    with
      varicose ulcer —*see* Varix, leg, with ulcer,
          with inflammation
      varicose veins —*see* Varix, leg, with,
          inflammation
    due to postthrombotic syndrome —*see*
        Syndrome, postthrombotic
  suppurative L08.0
  traumatic NEC L30.4
  trophoneurotica L13.0
  ultraviolet (sun) (chronic exposure) L57.8
    acute L56.8
  varicose —*see* Varix, leg, with, inflammation
  vegetans L10.1
  verrucosa B43.0
  vesicular, herpesviral B00.1
Dermatoarthritis, lipoid E78.81
Dermatochalasis, eyelid H02.839
  left H02.836
    lower H02.835
    upper H02.834
  right H02.833
    lower H02.832
    upper H02.831
Dermatofibroma (lenticulare) —*see* Neoplasm,
    skin, benign
  protuberans —*see* Neoplasm, skin, uncertain
      behavior
Dermatofibrosarcoma (pigmented) (protuberans)
    —*see* Neoplasm, skin, malignant
Dermatographia L50.3
Dermatolysis (exfoliativa) (congenital)
    Q82.8
  acquired L57.4
  eyelids —*see* Blepharochalasis
  palpebrarum —*see* Blepharochalasis
  senile L57.4
Dermatomegaly NEC Q82.8
Dermatomucosomyositis *(see also*
    Dermatomyositis) M33.10
  with
    myopathy M33.12
    respiratory involvement M33.11
    specified organ involvement NEC
        M33.19
Dermatomycosis B36.9
  furfuracea B36.0
  specified type NEC B36.8
Dermatomyositis (acute) (chronic) —*see also*
    Dermatopolymyositis
  adult —*see also* Dermatomyositis, specified NEC
      M33.10
  in (due to) neoplastic disease —*see also*
      Neoplasm D49.9 *[M36.0]*

Dermatomyositis *(Continued)*
  juvenile M33.00
    with
      myopathy M33.02
      respiratory involvement M33.01
      specified organ involvement NEC M33.09
        amyopathic M33.03
      without myopathy M33.03
  specified NEC M33.10
    with
      myopathy M33.12
      respiratory involvement M33.11
      specified organ involvement NEC M33.19
        amyopathic M33.13
      without myopathy M33.13
Dermatoneuritis of children —*see* Poisoning,
    mercury
Dermatophilosis A48.8
Dermatophytid L30.2
Dermatophytide —*see* Dermatophytosis
Dermatophytosis (epidermophyton) (infection)
    (Microsporum) (tinea) (Trichophyton)
    B35.9
  beard B35.0
  body B35.4
  capitis B35.0
  corporis B35.4
  deep-seated B35.8
  disseminated B35.8
  foot B35.3
  granulomatous B35.8
  groin B35.6
  hand B35.2
  nail B35.1
  perianal (area) B35.6
  scalp B35.0
  specified NEC B35.8
Dermatopolymyositis M33.90
  with
    myopathy M33.92
    respiratory involvement M33.91
    specified organ involvement NEC M33.99
      amyopathic M33.93
  in neoplastic disease —*see also* Neoplasm D49.9
      [M36.0]
  juvenile M33.00
    with
      myopathy M33.02
      respiratory involvement M33.01
      specified organ involvement NEC
          M33.09
        amyopathic M33.03
        without myopathy M33.03
  specified NEC M33.10
    myopathy M33.12
    respiratory involvement M33.11
    specified organ involvement NEC M33.19
      amyopathic M33.13
      without myopathy M33.13
  without myopathy M33.93
Dermatopolyneuritis —*see* Poisoning, mercury
Dermatorrhexis *(see also* Syndrome, Ehlers-Danlos)
    Q79.60
  acquired L57.4
Dermatosclerosis —*see also* Scleroderma
  localized L94.0
Dermatosis L98.9
  Andrews' L08.89
  Bowen's —*see* Neoplasm, skin, in situ
  bullous L13.9
    specified NEC L13.8
  exfoliativa L26
  eyelid (noninfectious) *(see also* Dermatitis, eyelid)
      H01.9
    discoid lupus erythematosus —*see* Lupus,
        erythematosus, eyelid
    xeroderma —*see* Xeroderma, acquired,
        eyelid
  factitial L98.1
  febrile neutrophilic L98.2
  gonococcal A54.89
  herpetiformis L13.0
    juvenile L12.2
  linear IgA L13.8
  menstrual NEC L98.8
  neutrophilic, febrile L98.2
  occupational —*see* Dermatitis, contact
  papulosa nigra L82.1
  pigmentary L81.9
    progressive L81.7
    Schamberg's L81.7

Dermatosis *(Continued)*
  psychogenic F54
  purpuric, pigmented L81.7
  pustular, subcorneal L13.1
  transient acantholytic L11.1
Dermographia, dermographism L50.3
Dermoid (cyst) —*see also* Neoplasm, benign, by site
  with malignant transformation C56-●
  due to radiation (nonionizing) L57.8
Dermopathy
  infiltrative with thyrotoxicosis —*see*
    Thyrotoxicosis
  nephrogenic fibrosing L90.8
Dermophytosis —*see* Dermatophytosis
Descemetocele H18.73-●
Descemet's membrane —*see* condition
Descending —*see* condition
Descensus uteri —*see* Prolapse, uterus
Desert
  rheumatism B38.0
  sore —*see* Ulcer, skin
Desertion (newborn) —*see* Maltreatment
Desmoid (extra-abdominal) (tumor) —*see*
    Neoplasm, connective tissue, uncertain
    behavior
  abdominal wall D48.113
  back D48.117
  buttock D48.116
  chest wall D48.111
  extremity
    lower D48.116
    upper D48.115
  head and neck D48.110
  intraabdominal D48.114
  intrathoracic D48.112
  pelvic cavity D48.114
  pelvic girdle D48.116
  peritoneal D48.114
  retroperitoneal D48.114
  shoulder girdle D48.115
  site unspecified D48.119
  specified site NEC D48.118
Despondency F32.A
Desquamation, skin R23.4
Destruction, destructive —*see also* Damage
  articular facet —*see also* Derangement, joint,
      specified type NEC
    knee M23.8X-●
    vertebra —*see* Spondylosis
  bone —*see also* Disorder, bone, specified type NEC
    syphilitic A52.77
  joint —*see also* Derangement, joint, specified
      type NEC
    sacroiliac M53.3
  rectal sphincter K62.89
  septum (nasal) J34.89
  tuberculous NEC —*see* Tuberculosis
  tympanum, tympanic membrane
      (nontraumatic) —*see* Disorder, tympanic
      membrane, specified NEC
  vertebral disc —*see* Degeneration, intervertebral
      disc
Destructiveness —*see also* Disorder, conduct
  adjustment reaction —*see* Disorder, adjustment
Desultory labor O62.2
Detachment
  cartilage —*see* Sprain
  cervix, annular N88.8
    complicating delivery O71.3
  choroid (old) (postinfectional) (simple)
      (spontaneous) H31.40-●
    hemorrhagic H31.41-●
    serous H31.42-●
  ligament —*see* Sprain
  meniscus (knee) —*see also* Derangement, knee,
      meniscus, specified NEC
    current injury —*see* Tear, meniscus
    due to old tear or injury —*see* Derangement,
        knee, meniscus, due to old tear
  retina (without retinal break) (serous) H33.2-●
    with retinal:
      break H33.00-●
        giant H33.03-●
        multiple H33.02-●
        single H33.01-●
      dialysis H33.04-●
    pigment epithelium —*see* Degeneration,
        retina, separation of layers, pigment
        epithelium detachment
    rhegmatogenous —*see* Detachment, retina,
        with retinal, break

Detachment *(Continued)*
  retina *(Continued)*
    specified NEC H33.8
    total H33.05-●
      traction H33.4-●
  vitreous (body) H43.81
Detergent asthma J69.8
Deterioration
  epileptic F06.8
  general physical R53.81
  heart, cardiac —*see* Degeneration, myocardial
  mental —*see* Psychosis
  myocardial, myocardium —*see* Degeneration,
      myocardial
  senile (simple) R54
Deuteranomaly (anomalous trichromat) H53.53
Deuteranopia (complete) (incomplete) H53.53
Development
  abnormal, bone Q79.9
  arrested R62.50
    bone —*see* Arrest, development or growth,
        bone
    child R62.50
    due to malnutrition E45
  defective, congenital —*see also* Anomaly, by site
    cauda equina Q06.3
    left ventricle Q24.8
      in hypoplastic left heart syndrome Q23.4
    valve Q24.8
      pulmonary Q22.3
  delayed (*see also* Delay, development) R62.50
    arithmetical skills F81.2
    language (skills) (expressive) F80.1
    learning skill F81.9
    mixed skills F88
    motor coordination F82
    reading F81.0
    specified learning skill NEC F81.89
    speech F80.9
    spelling F81.81
    written expression F81.81
  imperfect, congenital —*see also* Anomaly, by site
    heart Q24.9
    lungs Q33.6
  incomplete
    bronchial tree Q32.4
    organ or site not listed —*see* Hypoplasia, by site
    respiratory system Q34.9
  sexual, precocious NEC E30.1
  tardy, mental (*see also* Disability, intellectual) F79
Developmental —*see* condition
  testing, infant or child —*see* Examination, child
Devergie's disease (pityriasis rubra pilaris) L44.0
Deviation (in)
  conjugate palsy (eye) (spastic) H51.0
  esophagus (acquired) K22.89
  eye, skew H51.8
  midline (jaw) (teeth) (dental arch) M26.29
    specified site NEC —*see* Malposition
  nasal septum J34.2
    congenital Q67.4
  opening and closing of the mandible M26.53
  organ or site, congenital NEC —*see* Malposition,
      congenital
  septum (nasal) (acquired) J34.2
    congenital Q67.4
  sexual F65.9
    bestiality F65.89
    erotomania F52.8
    exhibitionism F65.2
    fetishism, fetishistic F65.0
      transvestism F65.1
    frotteurism F65.81
    masochism F65.51
    multiple F65.89
    necrophilia F65.89
    nymphomania F52.8
    pederosis F65.4
    pedophilia F65.4
    sadism, sadomasochism F65.52
    satyriasis F52.8
    specified type NEC F65.89
    transvestism F64.1
    voyeurism F65.3
  teeth, midline M26.29
  trachea J39.8
  ureter, congenital Q62.61
Device
  cerebral ventricle (communicating) in situ Z98.2
  contraceptive —*see* Contraceptive, device
  drainage, cerebrospinal fluid, in situ Z98.2

Devic's disease G36.0
Devil's
  grip B33.0
  pinches (purpura simplex) D69.2
Devitalized tooth K04.99
Devonshire colic —*see* Poisoning, lead
Dextraposition, aorta Q20.3
  in tetralogy of Fallot Q21.3
Dextrinosis, limit (debrancher enzyme deficiency)
    E74.03
Dextrocardia (true) Q24.0
  with
    complete transposition of viscera
        Q89.3
    situs inversus Q89.3
Dextrotransposition, aorta Q20.3
d-glycericacidemia E72.59
Dhat syndrome F48.8
Dhobi itch B35.6
Di George's syndrome D82.1
Di Guglielmo's disease C94.0-●
Diabetes, diabetic (mellitus) (sugar) E11.9
  with
    amyotrophy E11.44
    arthropathy NEC E11.618
    autonomic (poly)neuropathy E11.43
    cataract E11.36
    Charcot's joints E11.610
    chronic kidney disease E11.22
    circulatory complication NEC E11.59
    coma due to
      hyperosmolarity E11.01
      hypoglycemia E11.641
      ketoacidosis E11.11
    complication E11.8
      specified NEC E11.69
    dermatitis E11.620
    foot ulcer E11.621
    gangrene E11.52
    gastroparalysis E11.43
    gastroparesis E11.43
    glomerulonephrosis, intracapillary
        E11.21
    glomerulosclerosis, intercapillary E11.21
    hyperglycemia E11.65
    hyperosmolarity E11.00
      with coma E11.01
    hypoglycemia E11.649
      with coma E11.641
    ketoacidosis E11.10
      with coma E11.11
    kidney complications NEC E11.29
    Kimmelstiel-Wilson disease E11.21
    loss of protective sensation (LOPS) —*see*
        Diabetes, by type, with neuropathy
    mononeuropathy E11.41
    myasthenia E11.44
    necrobiosis lipoidica E11.620
    nephropathy E11.21
    neuralgia E11.42
    neurologic complication NEC E11.49
    neuropathic arthropathy E11.610
    neuropathy E11.40
    ophthalmic complication NEC E11.39
    oral complication NEC E11.638
    osteomyelitis E11.69
    periodontal disease E11.630
    peripheral angiopathy E11.51
      with gangrene E11.52
    polyneuropathy E11.42
    renal complication NEC E11.29
    renal tubular degeneration E11.29
    retinopathy E11.319
      with macular edema E11.311
        resolved following treatment E11.37
      nonproliferative E11.329
        with macular edema E11.321
        mild E11.329
          with macular edema E11.321
        moderate E11.339
          with macular edema E11.331
        severe E11.349
          with macular edema E11.341
      proliferative E11.359
        with
          combined traction retinal detachment
              and rhegmatogenous retinal
              detachment E11.354
          macular edema E11.351
          stable proliferative diabetic
              retinopathy E11.355

▶ New   ⇒ Revised   ~~deleted~~ Deleted   ● Use Additional Character(s)

Diabetes, diabetic *(Continued)*
  with *(Continued)*
    retinopathy *(Continued)*
      proliferative *(Continued)*
        with *(Continued)*
          traction retinal detachment involving the macula E11.352
          traction retinal detachment not involving the macula E11.353
    skin complication NEC E11.628
    skin ulcer NEC E11.622
  brittle —*see* Diabetes, type 1
  bronzed E83.110
  complicating pregnancy —*see* Pregnancy, complicated by, diabetes
  dietary counseling and surveillance Z71.3
  due to
    autoimmune process —*see* Diabetes, type 1
    immune mediated pancreatic islet beta-cell destruction —*see* Diabetes, type 1
  due to drug or chemical E09.9
    with
      amyotrophy E09.44
      arthropathy NEC E09.618
      autonomic (poly)neuropathy E09.43
      cataract E09.36
      Charcot's joints E09.610
      chronic kidney disease E09.22
      circulatory complication NEC E09.59
      complication E09.8
        specified NEC E09.69
      dermatitis E09.620
      foot ulcer E09.621
      gangrene E09.52
      gastroparalysis E09.43
      gastroparesis E09.43
      glomerulonephrosis, intracapillary E09.21
      glomerulosclerosis, intercapillary E09.21
      hyperglycemia E09.65
      hyperosmolarity E09.00
        with coma E09.01
      hypoglycemia E09.649
        with coma E09.641
      ketoacidosis E09.10
        with coma E09.11
      kidney complications NEC E09.29
      Kimmelstiel-Wilson disease E09.21
      mononeuropathy E09.41
      myasthenia E09.44
      necrobiosis lipoidica E09.620
      nephropathy E09.21
      neuralgia E09.42
      neurologic complication NEC E09.49
      neuropathic arthropathy E09.610
      neuropathy E09.40
      ophthalmic complication NEC E09.39
      oral complication NEC E09.638
      periodontal disease E09.630
      peripheral angiopathy E09.51
        with gangrene E09.52
      polyneuropathy E09.42
      renal complication NEC E09.29
      renal tubular degeneration E09.29
      retinopathy E09.319
        with macular edema E09.311
          resolved following treatment E09.37
        nonproliferative E09.329
          with macular edema E09.321
          mild E09.329
            with macular edema E09.321
          moderate E09.339
            with macular edema E09.331
          severe E09.349
            with macular edema E09.341
        proliferative E09.359
          with
            combined traction retinal detachment and rhegmatogenous retinal detachment E09.354
            macular edema E09.351
            stable proliferative diabetic retinopathy E09.355
            traction retinal detachment involving the macula E09.352
            traction retinal detachment not involving the macula E09.353
    skin complication NEC E09.628
    skin ulcer NEC E09.622

  due to underlying condition E08.9
    with
      amyotrophy E08.44
      arthropathy NEC E08.618
      autonomic (poly)neuropathy E08.43
      cataract E08.36
      Charcot's joints E08.610
      chronic kidney disease E08.22
      circulatory complication NEC E08.59
      complication E08.8
        specified NEC E08.69
      dermatitis E08.620
      foot ulcer E08.621
      gangrene E08.52
      gastroparalysis E08.43
      gastroparesis E08.43
      glomerulonephrosis, intracapillary E08.21
      glomerulosclerosis, intercapillary E08.21
      hyperglycemia E08.69
      hyperosmolarity E08.00
        with coma E08.01
      hypoglycemia E08.649
        with coma E08.641
      ketoacidosis E08.10
        with coma E08.11
      kidney complications NEC E08.29
      Kimmelstiel-Wilson disease E08.21
      mononeuropathy E08.41
      myasthenia E08.44
      necrobiosis lipoidica E08.620
      nephropathy E08.21
      neuralgia E08.42
      neurologic complication NEC E08.49
      neuropathic arthropathy E08.610
      neuropathy E08.40
      ophthalmic complication NEC E08.39
      oral complication NEC E08.638
      periodontal disease E08.630
      peripheral angiopathy E08.51
        with gangrene E08.52
      polyneuropathy E08.42
      renal complication NEC E08.29
      renal tubular degeneration E08.29
      retinopathy E08.319
        with macular edema E08.311
          resolved following treatment E08.37
        nonproliferative E08.329
          with macular edema E08.321
          mild E08.329
            with macular edema E08.321
          moderate E08.339
            with macular edema E08.331
          severe E08.349
            with macular edema E08.341
        proliferative E08.359
          with
            combined traction retinal detachment and rhegmatogenous retinal detachment E08.354
            macular edema E08.351
            stable proliferative diabetic retinopathy E08.355
            traction retinal detachment involving the macula E08.352
            traction retinal detachment not involving the macula E08.353
    skin complication NEC E08.628
    skin ulcer NEC E08.622
  gestational (in pregnancy) O24.419
    affecting newborn P70.0
    diet-controlled O24.410
    in childbirth O24.429
      diet-controlled O24.420
      insulin (and diet) controlled O24.424
      oral drug controlled (antidiabetic) (hypoglycemic) O24.425
    insulin (and diet) controlled O24.414
    oral drug controlled (antidiabetic) (hypoglycemic) O24.415
    puerperal O24.439
      diet-controlled O24.430
      insulin (and diet) controlled O24.434
      oral drug controlled (antidiabetic) (hypoglycemic) O24.435
  hepatogenous E13.9
  idiopathic —*see* Diabetes, type 1
  inadequately controlled —*see* Diabetes, by type, with hyperglycemia

  insipidus E23.2
    nephrogenic N25.1
    pituitary E23.2
    vasopressin resistant N25.1
  insulin dependent — code to type of diabetes
  juvenile-onset —*see* Diabetes, type 1
  ketosis-prone —*see* Diabetes, type 1
  latent R73.03
  neonatal (transient) P70.2
  non-insulin dependent — code to type of diabetes
  out of control —*see* Diabetes, by type, with hyperglycemia
  phosphate E83.39
  poorly controlled —*see* Diabetes, by type, with hyperglycemia
  postpancreatectomy —*see* Diabetes, specified type NEC
  postprocedural —*see* Diabetes, specified type NEC
  retina, hemorrhage E13.39
  secondary diabetes mellitus NEC —*see* Diabetes, specified type NEC
  specified type NEC E13.9
    with
      amyotrophy E13.44
      arthropathy NEC E13.618
      autonomic (poly)neuropathy E13.43
      cataract E13.36
      Charcot's joints E13.610
      chronic kidney disease E13.22
      circulatory complication NEC E13.59
      complication E13.8
        specified NEC E13.69
      dermatitis E13.620
      foot ulcer E13.621
      gangrene E13.52
      gastroparalysis E13.43
      gastroparesis E13.43
      glomerulonephrosis, intracapillary E13.21
      glomerulosclerosis, intercapillary E13.21
      hyperglycemia E13.65
      hyperosmolarity E13.00
        with coma E13.01
      hypoglycemia E13.649
        with coma E13.641
      ketoacidosis E13.10
        with coma E13.11
      kidney complications NEC E13.29
      Kimmelstiel-Wilson disease E13.21
      mononeuropathy E13.41
      myasthenia E13.44
      necrobiosis lipoidica E13.620
      nephropathy E13.21
      neuralgia E13.42
      neurologic complication NEC E13.49
      neuropathic arthropathy E13.610
      neuropathy E13.40
      ophthalmic complication NEC E13.39
      oral complication NEC E13.638
      periodontal disease E13.630
      peripheral angiopathy E13.51
        with gangrene E13.52
      polyneuropathy E13.42
      renal complication NEC E13.29
      renal tubular degeneration E13.29
      retinopathy E13.319
        with macular edema E13.311
          resolved following treatment E13.37
        nonproliferative E13.329
          with macular edema E13.321
          mild E13.329
            with macular edema E13.321
          moderate E13.339
            with macular edema E13.331
          severe E13.349
            with macular edema E13.341
        proliferative E13.359
          with
            combined traction retinal detachment and rhegmatogenous retinal detachment E13.354
            macular edema E13.351
            stable proliferative diabetic retinopathy E13.355
            traction retinal detachment involving the macula E13.352
            traction retinal detachment not involving the macula E13.353

Diabetes, diabetic (Continued)
    specified type (Continued)
        with (Continued)
            skin complication NEC E13.628
            skin ulcer NEC E13.622
    steroid-induced —see Diabetes, due to, drug or
        chemical
    type 1 E10.9
        with
            amyotrophy E10.44
            arthropathy NEC E10.618
            autonomic (poly)neuropathy E10.43
            cataract E10.36
            Charcot's joints E10.610
            chronic kidney disease E10.22
            circulatory complication NEC E10.59
            coma due to
                hypoglycemia E11.641
                ketoacidosis E11.11
            complication E10.8
                specified NEC E10.69
            dermatitis E10.620
            foot ulcer E10.621
            gangrene E10.52
            gastroparalysis E10.43
            gastroparesis E10.43
            glomerulonephrosis, intracapillary E10.21
            glomerulosclerosis, intercapillary E10.21
            hyperglycemia E10.65
            hypoglycemia E10.649
                with coma E10.641
            ketoacidosis E10.10
                with coma E10.11
            kidney complications NEC E10.29
            Kimmelstiel-Wilson disease E10.21
            mononeuropathy E10.41
            myasthenia E10.44
            necrobiosis lipoidica E10.620
            nephropathy E10.21
            neuralgia E10.42
            neurologic complication NEC E10.49
            neuropathic arthropathy E10.610
            neuropathy E10.40
            ophthalmic complication NEC E10.39
            oral complication NEC E10.638
            osteomyelitis E10.69
            periodontal disease E10.630
            peripheral angiopathy E10.51
                with gangrene E10.52
            polyneuropathy E10.42
            renal complication NEC E10.29
            renal tubular degeneration E10.29
            retinopathy E10.319
                with macular edema E10.311
                    resolved following treatment E10.37
                nonproliferative E10.329
                    with macular edema E10.321
                    mild E10.329
                        with macular edema E10.321
                    moderate E10.339
                        with macular edema E10.331
                    severe E10.349
                        with macular edema E10.341
                proliferative E10.359
                    with
                        combined traction retinal
                            detachment and
                            rhegmatogenous retinal
                            detachment E13.354
                        macular edema E13.351
                        stable proliferative diabetic
                            retinopathy E13.355
                        traction retinal detachment
                            involving the macula E13.352
                        traction retinal detachment not
                            involving the macula E13.353
            skin complication NEC E10.628
            skin ulcer NEC E10.622
    ► early-stage E10.A-●
    ► presymptomatic E10.A0
        ► Stage 1 E10.A1
        ► Stage 2 E10.A2
    type 2 E11.9
        with
            amyotrophy E11.44
            arthropathy NEC E11.618
            autonomic (poly)neuropathy E11.43
            cataract E11.36
            Charcot's joints E11.610
            chronic kidney disease E11.22
            circulatory complication NEC E11.59

Diabetes, diabetic (Continued)
    type 2 (Continued)
        with (Continued)
            coma due to
                hyperosmolarity E11.01
                hypoglycemia E11.641
                ketoacidosis E11.1-●
            complication E11.8
                specified NEC E11.69
            dermatitis E11.620
            foot ulcer E11.621
            gangrene E11.52
            gastroparalysis E11.43
            gastroparesis E11.43
            glomerulonephrosis, intracapillary E11.21
            glomerulosclerosis, intercapillary E11.21
            hyperglycemia E11.65
            hyperosmolarity E11.00
                with coma E11.01
            hypoglycemia E11.649
                with coma E11.641
            ketoacidosis E11.10
                with coma E11.11
            kidney complications NEC E11.29
            Kimmelstiel-Wilson disease E11.21
            mononeuropathy E11.41
            myasthenia E11.44
            necrobiosis lipoidica E11.620
            nephropathy E11.21
            neuralgia E11.42
            neurologic complication NEC E11.49
            neuropathic arthropathy E11.610
            neuropathy E11.40
            ophthalmic complication NEC E11.39
            oral complication NEC E11.638
            osteomyelitis E11.69
            periodontal disease E11.630
            peripheral angiopathy E11.51
                with gangrene E11.52
            polyneuropathy E11.42
            renal complication NEC E11.29
            renal tubular degeneration E11.29
            retinopathy E11.319
                with macular edema E11.311
                    resolved following treatment E11.37
                nonproliferative E11.329
                    with macular edema E11.321
                    mild E11.329
                        with macular edema E11.321
                    moderate E11.339
                        with macular edema E11.331
                    severe E11.349
                        with macular edema E11.341
                proliferative E11.359
                    with
                        combined traction retinal
                            detachment and
                            rhegmatogenous retinal
                            detachment E11.354
                        macular edema E11.351
                        stable proliferative diabetic
                            retinopathy E11.355
                        traction retinal detachment
                            involving the macula E11.352
                        traction retinal detachment not
                            involving the macula E11.353
            skin complication NEC E11.628
            skin ulcer NEC E11.622
    uncontrolled
    meaning
        hyperglycemia —see Diabetes, by type,
            with, hyperglycemia
        hypoglycemia —see Diabetes, by type, with,
            hypoglycemia
Diacyclothrombopathia D69.1
Diagnosis deferred R69
Dialysis (intermittent) (treatment)
    noncompliance (with) Z91.158
        due to financial hardship Z91.151
    renal (hemodialysis) (peritoneal), status Z99.2
    retina, retinal —see Detachment, retina, with
        retinal, dialysis
Diamond-Blackfan anemia (congenital
    hypoplastic) D61.01
Diamond-Gardener syndrome (autoerythrocyte
    sensitization) D69.2
Diaper rash L22
Diaphoresis (excessive) R61
Diaphragm —see condition
Diaphragmalgia R07.1
Diaphragmatitis, diaphragmitis J98.6

Diaphysial aclasis Q78.6
Diaphysitis —see Osteomyelitis, specified type
    NEC
Diarrhea, diarrheal (disease) (infantile)
    (inflammatory) R19.7
    achlorhydric K31.83
    allergic K52.29
        due to
            colitis —see Colitis, allergic
            enteritis —see Enteritis, allergic
    amebic —see also Amebiasis A06.0
        with abscess —see Abscess, amebic
        acute A06.0
        chronic A06.1
        nondysenteric A06.2
    bacillary —see Dysentery, bacillary
    balantidial A07.0
    cachectic NEC K52.89
    Chilomastix A07.8
    choleriformis A00.1
    chronic (noninfectious) K52.9
    coccidial A07.3
    Cochin-China K90.1
        strongyloidiasis B78.0
    Dientamoeba A07.8
    dietetic —see also Diarrhea, allergic
        K52.29
    drug-induced K52.1
    due to
        bacteria A04.9
            specified NEC A04.8
        Campylobacter A04.5
        Capillaria philippinensis B81.1
        Clostridium difficile
            not specified as recurrent A04.72
            recurrent A04.71
        Clostridium perfringens (C) (F) A04.8
        Cryptosporidium A07.2
        drugs K52.1
        Escherichia coli A04.4
            enteroaggregative A04.4
            enterohemorrhagic A04.3
            enteroinvasive A04.2
            enteropathogenic A04.0
            enterotoxigenic A04.1
            specified NEC A04.4
        food hypersensitivity —see also Diarrhea,
            allergic K52.29
        Necator americanus B76.1
        S. japonicum B65.2
        specified organism NEC A08.8
            bacterial A04.8
            viral A08.39
        Staphylococcus A04.8
        Trichuris trichiuria B79
        virus —see Enteritis, viral
        Yersinia enterocolitica A04.6
    dysenteric A09
    endemic A09
    epidemic A09
    flagellate A07.9
    Flexner's (ulcerative) A03.1
    functional K59.1
        following gastrointestinal surgery
            K91.89
        psychogenic F45.8
    Giardia lamblia A07.1
    giardial A07.1
    hill K90.1
    infectious A09
    malarial —see Malaria
    mite B88.0
    mycotic NEC B49
    neonatal (noninfectious) P78.3
    nervous F45.8
    neurogenic K59.1
    noninfectious K52.9
    postgastrectomy K91.1
    postvagotomy K91.1
    protozoal A07.9
        specified NEC A07.8
    psychogenic F45.8
    specified
        bacterium NEC A04.8
        virus NEC A08.39
    strongyloidiasis B78.0
    toxic K52.1
    trichomonal A07.8
    tropical K90.1
    tuberculous A18.32
    viral —see Enteritis, viral

► New   ⇒ Revised   ~~deleted~~ Deleted   ● Use Additional Character(s)

Diastasis
    cranial bones M84.88
        congenital NEC Q75.8
    joint (traumatic) —see Dislocation
    muscle M62.00
        ankle M62.07-●
        congenital Q79.8
        foot M62.07-●
        forearm M62.03-●
        hand M62.04-●
        lower leg M62.06-●
        pelvic region M62.05-●
        shoulder region M62.01-●
        specified site NEC M62.08
        thigh M62.05-●
        upper arm M62.02-●
    recti (abdomen)
        complicating delivery O71.89
        congenital Q79.59
Diastema, tooth, teeth, fully erupted M26.32
Diastematomyelia Q06.2
Diataxia, cerebral G80.4
Diathesis
    allergic —see History, allergy
    bleeding (familial) D69.9
    cystine (familial) E72.00
    gouty —see Gout
    hemorrhagic (familial) D69.9
        newborn NEC P53
    spasmophilic R29.0
Diaz's disease or osteochondrosis (juvenile)
        (talus) —see Osteochondrosis, juvenile, tarsus
Dibothriocephalus, dibothriocephaliasis (latus)
        (infection) (infestation) B70.0
    larval B70.1
Dicephalus, dicephaly Q89.4
Dichotomy, teeth K00.2
Dichromat, dichromatopsia (congenital) —see
        Deficiency, color vision
Dichuchwa A65
Dicroceliasis B66.2
Didelphia, didelphys —see Double uterus
Didymitis N45.1
    with orchitis N45.3
Dietary
    inadequacy or deficiency E63.9
    surveillance and counseling Z71.3
Dietl's crisis N13.8
Dieulafoy lesion (hemorrhagic)
    duodenum K31.82
    esophagus K22.89
    intestine (colon) K63.81
    stomach K31.82
Difficult, difficulty (in)
    acculturation Z60.3
    feeding R63.30
        elderly R63.39
        infant NOS R63.39
        newborn P92.9
            breast P92.5
            specified NEC P92.8
        nonorganic (infant or child) F98.29
        specified NEC R63.39
    intubation, in anesthesia T88.4
    mechanical, gastroduodenal stoma K91.89
        causing obstruction —see also Obstruction,
            intestine, postoperative K91.30
    micturition
        need to immediately re-void R39.191
        position dependent R39.192
        specified NEC R39.198
    reading (developmental) F81.0
        secondary to emotional disorders F93.9
    spelling (specific) F81.81
        with reading disorder F81.89
        due to inadequate teaching Z55.8
    swallowing —see Dysphagia
    understanding
        health related information Z55.6
        medication instructions Z55.6
    walking R26.2
    work
        conditions NEC Z56.5
        schedule Z56.3
Diffuse —see condition
DiGeorge's syndrome (thymic hypoplasia) D82.1
Digestive —see condition
Dihydropyrimidine dehydrogenase disease
        (DPD) E88.89
Diktyoma —see Neoplasm, malignant, by site
Dilaceration, tooth K00.4

Dilatation
    anus K59.89
        venule —see Hemorrhoids
    aorta (focal) (general) —see Ectasia, aorta
        with aneurysm —see Aneurysm, aorta
        congenital Q25.44
    artery —see Aneurysm
    bladder (sphincter) N32.89
        congenital Q64.79
    blood vessel I99.8
    bronchial J47.9
        with
            exacerbation (acute) J47.1
            lower respiratory infection J47.0
    calyx N28.89
        due to obstruction —see Hydronephosis
    capillaries I78.8
    cardiac (acute) (chronic) —see also Hypertrophy,
            cardiac
        congenital Q24.8
            valve NEC Q24.8
                pulmonary Q22.3
        valve —see Endocarditis
    cavum septi pellucidi Q06.8
    cervix (uteri) —see also Incompetency, cervix
        incomplete, poor, slow complicating delivery
            O62.0
    colon K59.39
        congenital Q43.1
        psychogenic F45.8
        toxic K59.31
    common duct (acquired) K83.8
        congenital Q44.5
    cystic duct (acquired) K82.8
        congenital Q44.5
    duct, mammary —see Ectasia, mammary duct
    duodenum K59.89
    esophagus K22.89
        congenital Q39.5
        due to achalasia K22.0
    eustachian tube, congenital Q17.8
    gallbladder K82.8
    gastric —see Dilatation, stomach
    heart (acute) (chronic) —see also Hypertrophy,
            cardiac
        congenital Q24.8
        valve —see Endocarditis
    ileum K59.89
        psychogenic F45.8
    jejunum K59.89
        psychogenic F45.8
    kidney (calyx) (collecting structures) (cystic)
            (parenchyma) (pelvis) (idiopathic) N28.89
        due to obstruction —see Hydronephrosis
    lacrimal passages or duct —see Disorder,
            lacrimal system, changes
    lymphatic vessel I89.0
    mammary duct —see Ectasia, mammary
            duct
    Meckel's diverticulum (congenital) Q43.0
        malignant —see Table of Neoplasms, small
            intestine, malignant
    myocardium (acute) (chronic) —see
            Hypertrophy, cardiac organ or site,
            congenital NEC —see Distortion
    pancreatic duct K86.89
    pericardium —see Pericarditis
    pharynx J39.2
    prostate N42.89
    pulmonary
        artery (idiopathic) I28.8
        valve, congenital Q22.3
    pupil H57.04
    rectum K59.39
    saccule, congenital Q16.5
    salivary gland (duct) K11.8
    sphincter ani K62.89
    stomach K31.89
        acute K31.0
        psychogenic F45.8
    submaxillary duct K11.8
    trachea, congenital Q32.1
    ureter (idiopathic) N28.82
        congenital Q62.2
        due to obstruction N13.4
    urethra (acquired) N36.8
    vasomotor I73.9
    vein I86.8
    ventricular, ventricle (acute) (chronic) —see also
            Hypertrophy, cardiac
        cerebral, congenital Q04.8

Dilatation (Continued)
    venule NEC I86.8
    vesical orifice N32.89
Dilated, dilation —see Dilatation
Diminished, diminution
    hearing (acuity) —see Deafness
    sense or sensation (cold) (heat) (tactile)
            (vibratory) R20.8
    vision NEC H54.7
    vital capacity R94.2
Diminuta taenia B71.0
Dimitri-Sturge-Weber disease Q85.89
Dimple
    congenital sacral Q82.6
    parasacral Q82.6
    pilonidal or postanal —see Cyst, pilonidal
Dioctophyme renalis (infection) (infestation) B83.8
Dipetalonemiasis B74.4
Diphallus Q55.69
Diphtheria, diphtheritic (gangrenous)
        (hemorrhagic) A36.9
    carrier (suspected) Z22.2
    cutaneous A36.3
    faucial A36.0
    infection of wound A36.3
    laryngeal A36.2
    myocarditis A36.81
    nasal, anterior A36.89
    nasopharyngeal A36.1
    neurological complication A36.89
    pharyngeal A36.0
    specified site NEC A36.89
    tonsillar A36.0
Diphyllobothriasis (intestine) B70.0
    larval B70.1
Diplacusis H93.22-●
Diplegia (upper limbs) G83.0
    congenital (cerebral) G80.8
    facial G51.0
    lower limbs G82.20
    spastic G80.1
Diplococcus, diplococcal —see condition
Diplopia H53.2
Dipsomania F10.20
    with
        psychosis —see Psychosis, alcoholic
        remission F10.21
Dipylidiasis B71.1
DIRA (deficiency of interleukin 1 receptor
        antagonist) M04.8
Direction, teeth, abnormal, fully erupted M26.30
Dirofilariasis B74.8
Dirt-eating child F98.3
Disability, disabilities
    heart —see Disease, heart
    intellectual F79
        with
            autistic features F84.9
                pathogenic CHAMP1 (genetic) (variant)
                    F78.A9
                pathogenic HNRNPH2 (genetic)
                    (variant) F78.A9
                pathogenic SATB2 (genetic) (variant)
                    F78.A9
                pathogenic SETBP1 (genetic) (variant)
                    F78.A9
                pathogenic STXBP1 (genetic) (variant)
                    F78.A9
                pathogenic SYNGAP1 (genetic) (variant)
                    F78.A1
            autosomal dominant F78.A9
            autosomal recessive F78.A9
            genetic related F78.A9
                with
                    pathogenic CHAMP1 (variant)
                        F78.A9
                    pathogenic HNRNPH2 (variant) F78.
                        A9
                    pathogenic SATB2 (variant) F78.A9
                    pathogenic SETBP1 (variant) F78.A9
                    pathogenic STXBP1 (variant) F78.A9
                    pathogenic SYNGAP1 (variant) F78.
                        A1
                specified NEC F78.A9
                SYNGAP1-related F78.A1
        in
            autosomal dominant mental retardation
                F78.A9
            autosomal recessive mental retardation
                F78.A9
            SATB2-associated syndrome F78.A9

Disability, disabilities (Continued)
  intellectual (Continued)
    with (Continued)
      in (Continued)
        SETBP1 disorder F78.A9
        STXBP1 encephalopathy with epilepsy
          (see also Encephalopathy; and see
          also Epilepsy) F78.A9
        X-linked mental retardation (syndromic)
          (Bain type) F78.A9
      mild (I.Q. 50-69) F70
      moderate (I.Q. 35-49) F71
      profound (I.Q. under 20) F73
      severe (I.Q. 20-34) F72
      specified level NEC F78.A9
      SYNGAP1-related F78.A1
      X-linked (syndromic) (Bain type) F78.A9
  knowledge acquisition F81.9
  learning F81.9
  limiting activities Z73.6
  spelling, specific F81.81
Disappearance of family member Z63.4
Disarticulation —see Amputation
  meaning traumatic amputation —see
    Amputation, traumatic
Discharge (from)
  abnormal finding in —see Abnormal, specimen
  breast (female) (male) N64.52
  diencephalic autonomic idiopathic —
    see Epilepsy, specified NEC
  ear —see also Otorrhea
    blood —see Otorrhagia
  excessive urine R35.89
  nipple N64.52
  penile R36.9
  postnasal R09.82
  prison, anxiety concerning Z65.2
  urethral R36.9
    without blood R36.0
    hematospermia R36.1
  vaginal N89.8
Discitis, diskitis M46.40
  cervical region M46.42
  cervicothoracic region M46.43
  lumbar region M46.46
  lumbosacral region M46.47
  multiple sites M46.49
  occipito-atlanto-axial region M46.41
  pyogenic —see Infection, intervertebral
    disc, pyogenic
  sacrococcygeal region M46.48
  thoracic region M46.44
  thoracolumbar region M46.45
Discoid
  meniscus (congenital) Q68.6
  semilunar cartilage (congenital) —see
    Derangement, knee, meniscus,
    specified NEC
Discoloration
  nails L60.8
  teeth (posteruptive) K03.7
    during formation K00.8
Discomfort
  chest R07.89
  visual H53.14-●
Discontinuity, ossicles, ear H74.2-●
Discord (with)
  boss Z56.4
  classmates Z55.4
  counselor Z64.4
  employer Z56.4
  family Z63.8
  fellow employees Z56.4
  in-laws Z63.1
  landlord Z59.2
  lodgers Z59.2
  neighbors Z59.2
  probation officer Z64.4
  social worker Z64.4
  teachers Z55.4
  workmates Z56.4
Discordant connection
  atrioventricular (congenital) Q20.5
  ventriculoarterial Q20.3
Discrepancy
  centric occlusion maximum intercuspation
    M26.55
  leg length (acquired) —see Deformity, limb,
    unequal length
    congenital —see Defect, reduction, lower limb
  uterine size date O26.84-●

Discrimination
  ethnic Z60.5
  political Z60.5
  racial Z60.5
  religious Z60.5
  sex Z60.5
Disease, diseased —see also Syndrome
  absorbent system I87.8
  acid-peptic K30
  Acosta's T70.29
  Adams-Stokes (-Morgagni) (syncope with heart
    block) I45.9
  Addison's anemia (pernicious) D51.0
  adenoids (and tonsils) J35.9
  adrenal (capsule) (cortex) (gland) (medullary)
    E27.9
    hyperfunction E27.0
    specified NEC E27.8
  ainhum L94.6
  airway
    obstructive, chronic J44.9
      due to
        cotton dust J66.0
        specific organic dusts NEC J66.8
    reactive —see Asthma
  akamushi (scrub typhus) A75.3
  Albers-Schönberg (marble bones) Q78.2
  Albert's —see Tendinitis, Achilles
  Alexander G31.86
  alimentary canal K63.9
  alligator-skin Q80.9
    acquired L85.0
  alpha heavy chain C88.3-●
  alpine T70.29
  altitude T70.20
  alveolar ridge
    edentulous K06.9
      specified NEC K06.8
  alveoli, teeth K08.9
  Alzheimer's (see also Dementia, in, diseases
    specified elsewhere) G30.9 [F02.80]
    with behavioral disturbance (see also
      Dementia, in, diseases specified
      elsewhere) G30.9 [F02.81-●]
    early onset (see also Dementia, in, diseases
      specified elsewhere) G30.0 [F02.80]
      with behavioral disturbance (see also
        Dementia, in, diseases specified
        elsewhere) G30.0 [F02.81-●]
    late onset (see also Dementia, in, diseases
      specified elsewhere) G30.1 [F02.80]
      with behavioral disturbance (see also
        Dementia, in, diseases specified
        elsewhere) G30.1 [F02.81-●]
    specified NEC (see also Dementia, in,
      diseases specified elsewhere) G30.8
      [F02.80]
      with behavioral disturbance (see also
        Dementia, in, diseases specified
        elsewhere) G30.8 [F02.81-●]
  amyloid —see Amyloidosis
  Andersen's (glycogenosis IV) E74.09
  Andes T70.29
  Andrews' (bacterid) L08.89
  angiospastic I73.9
    cerebral G45.9
    vein I87.8
  anterior
    chamber H21.9
    horn cell G12.29
  antiglomerular basement membrane (anti-GBM)
    antibody M31.0
    tubulo-interstitial nephritis N12
  Antopol E74.05
  antral —see Sinusitis, maxillary
  anus K62.9
    specified NEC K62.89
  aorta (nonsyphilitic) I77.9
    syphilitic NEC A52.02
  aortic (heart) (valve) I35.9
    rheumatic I06.9
  Apollo B30.3
  aponeuroses —see Enthesopathy
  appendix K38.9
    specified NEC K38.8
  aqueous (chamber) H21.9
  Arnold-Chiari —see Arnold-Chiari disease
  arterial (see also Disease, artery) I77.9
    occlusive (see also Occlusion, by site
      due to stricture or stenosis I77.1
    peripheral I73.9

Disease, diseased (Continued)
  arteriocardiorenal —see Hypertension,
    cardiorenal
  arteriolar (generalized) (obliterative) I77.9
  arteriorenal —see Hypertension, kidney
  arteriosclerotic —see also Arteriosclerosis
    cardiovascular —see Disease, heart, ischemic,
      atherosclerotic
    coronary (artery) —see Disease, heart,
      ischemic, atherosclerotic
    heart —see Disease, heart, ischemic,
      atherosclerotic
  artery (see also Disease, arterial) I77.9
    cerebral I67.9
    coronary I25.10
      with angina pectoris —see Arteriosclerosis,
        coronary (artery)
    peripheral I73.9
  arthropod-borne NOS (viral) A94
    specified type NEC A93.8
  atticoantral, chronic H66.20
    left H66.22
      with right H66.23
    right H66.21
      with left H66.23
  auditory canal —see Disorder, ear, external
  auricle, ear NEC —see Disorder, pinna
  Australian X A83.4
  autoimmune (systemic) NOS M35.9
    hemolytic D59.10
      cold type (primary) (secondary)
        (symptomatic) D59.12
      drug-induced D59.0
      mixed type (primary) (secondary)
        (symptomatic) D59.13
      warm type (primary) (secondary)
        (symptomatic) D59.11
    thyroid E06.3
  autoinflammatory M04.9
    NOD2-associated M04.8
    specified type NEC M04.8
  aviator's —see Effect, adverse, high altitude
  Ayerza's (pulmonary artery sclerosis with
    pulmonary hypertension) I27.0
  Babington's (familial hemorrhagic telangiectasia)
    I78.0
  bacterial A49.9
    specified NEC A48.8
    zoonotic A28.9
      specified type NEC A28.8
  Baelz's (cheilitis glandularis apostematosa)
    K13.0
  bagasse J67.1
  balloon —see Effect, adverse, high altitude
  Bang's (brucella abortus) A23.1
  Bannister's T78.3
  barometer makers' —see Poisoning, mercury
  Barraquer (-Simons') (progressive
    lipodystrophy) E88.1
  Barrett's —see Barrett's, esophagus
  Bartholin's gland N75.9
  basal ganglia G25.9
    degenerative G23.9
      specified NEC G23.8
    specified NEC G25.89
  Basedow's (exophthalmic goiter) —see
    Hyperthyroidism, with, goiter (diffuse)
  Bateman's B08.1
  Batten-Steinert G71.11
  Battey A31.0
  Beard's (neurasthenia) F48.8
  Becker
    idiopathic mural endomyocardial I42.3
    myotonia congenita G71.12
  Begbie's (exophthalmic goiter) —see
    Hyperthyroidism, with, goiter (diffuse)
  behavioral, organic F07.9
  Beigel's (white piedra) B36.2
  Benson's —see Deposit, crystalline
  Bernard-Soulier (thrombopathy) D69.1
  Bernhardt (-Roth) —see Mononeuropathy, lower
    limb, meralgia paresthetica
  Biermer's (pernicious anemia) D51.0
  bile duct (common) (hepatic) K83.9
    with calculus, stones —see Calculus, bile duct
    specified NEC K83.8
  biliary (tract) K83.9
    specified NEC K83.8
  Billroth's —see Spina bifida
  bird fancier's J67.2
  black lung J60

▶ New   ⇒ Revised   ~~deleted~~ Deleted   ● Use Additional Character(s)

Disease, diseased *(Continued)*
bladder N32.9
  in (due to)
    schistosomiasis (bilharziasis) B65.0 *[N33]*
    specified NEC N32.89
bleeder's D66
blood D75.9
  forming organs D75.9
  vessel I99.9
Bloodgood's —*see* Mastopathy, cystic
Blount M92.51-●
Bodechtel-Guttmann (subacute sclerosing
    panencephalitis) A81.1
bone —*see also* Disorder, bone
  aluminum M83.4
  fibrocystic NEC
    jaw M27.49
bone-marrow D75.9
Borna A83.9
Bornholm (epidemic pleurodynia) B33.0
Bouchard's (myopathic dilatation of the
    stomach) K31.0
Bouillaud's (rheumatic heart disease) I01.9
Bourneville (-Brissaud) (tuberous sclerosis)
    Q85.1
Bouveret (-Hoffmann) (paroxysmal tachycardia)
    I47.9
bowel K63.9
  functional K59.9
    psychogenic F45.8
brain G93.9
  arterial, artery I67.9
  arteriosclerotic I67.2
  congenital Q04.9
  degenerative —*see* Degeneration, brain
  inflammatory —*see* Encephalitis
  organic G93.9
    arteriosclerotic I67.2
  parasitic NEC B71.9 *[G94]*
  senile NEC G31.1
  specified NEC G93.89
breast (*see also* Disorder, breast) N64.9
  cystic (chronic) —*see* Mastopathy, cystic
  fibrocystic —*see* Mastopathy, cystic
  Paget's
    female, unspecified side C50.91-●
    male, unspecified side C50.92-●
  specified NEC N64.89
Breda's —*see* Yaws
Bretonneau's (diphtheritic malignant angina)
    A36.0
Bright's —*see* Nephritis
  arteriosclerotic —*see* Hypertension,
    kidney
Brill's (recrudescent typhus) A75.1
Brill-Zinsser (recrudescent typhus) A75.1
Brion-Kayser —*see* Fever, paratyphoid
broad
  beta E78.2
  ligament (noninflammatory) N83.9
    inflammatory —*see* Disease, pelvis,
      inflammatory
    specified NEC N83.8
Brocq-Duhring (dermatitis herpetiformis) L13.0
Brocq's
  meaning
    dermatitis herpetiformis L13.0
    prurigo L28.2
bronchopulmonary J98.4
bronchus NEC J98.09
bronze Addison's E27.1
  tuberculous A18.7
budgerigar fancier's J67.2
Buerger's (thromboangiitis obliterans) I73.1
bullous L13.9
  chronic of childhood L12.2
  specified NEC L13.8
Bürger-Grütz (essential familial hyperlipemia)
    E78.3
bursa —*see* Bursopathy
caisson T70.3
California —*see* Coccidioidomycosis
Canavan E75.28
capillaries I78.9
  specified NEC I78.8
Carapata A68.0
▶carcinoid E34.00
  ▶heart E34.01
  ▶specified NEC E34.09
cardiac —*see* Disease, heart
cardiopulmonary, chronic I27.9

Disease, diseased *(Continued)*
cardiorenal (hepatic) (hypertensive) (vascular) —
    see Hypertension, cardiorenal
cardiovascular (atherosclerotic) I25.10
  with angina pectoris —*see* Arteriosclerosis,
    coronary (artery),
  congenital Q28.9
  hypertensive —*see* Hypertension, heart
  newborn P29.9
    specified NEC P29.89
  renal (hypertensive) —*see* Hypertension,
    cardiorenal
  syphilitic (asymptomatic) A52.00
cartilage —*see* Disorder, cartilage
Castellani's A69.8
Castleman (unicentric) (multicentric) D47.Z2
  HHV-8-associated —*see also* Herpesvirus,
    human, 8 D47.Z2
cat-scratch A28.1
Cavare's (familial periodic paralysis) G72.3
cecum K63.9
celiac (adult) (infantile) (with steatorrhea) K90.0
cellular tissue L98.9
central core G71.29
cerebellar, cerebellum —*see* Disease, brain
cerebral —*see also* Disease, brain
  degenerative —*see* Degeneration, brain
cerebrospinal G96.9
cerebrovascular I67.9
  acute I67.89
    embolic I63.4-●
    thrombotic I63.3-●
  arteriosclerotic I67.2
  hereditary NEC I67.858
  specified NEC I67.89
cervix (uteri) (noninflammatory) N88.9
  inflammatory —*see* Cervicitis
  specified NEC N88.8
Chabert's A22.9
Chandler's (osteochondritis dissecans, hip) —*see*
    Osteochondritis, dissecans, hip
Charlouis —*see* Yaws
Chédiak-Steinbrinck (-Higashi) (congenital
    gigantism of peroxidase granules) E70.330
chest J98.9
Chiari's (hepatic vein thrombosis) I82.0
Chicago B40.9
Chignon B36.8
chigo, chigoe B88.1
childhood granulomatous D71
Chinese liver fluke B66.1
chlamydial A74.9
  specified NEC A74.89
cholecystic K82.9
choroid H31.9
  specified NEC H31.8
Christmas D67
chronic bullous of childhood L12.2
chylomicron retention E78.3
ciliary body H21.9
  specified NEC H21.89
circulatory (system) NEC I99.8
  newborn P29.9
  syphilitic A52.00
    congenital A50.54
coagulation factor deficiency (congenital) —*see*
    Defect, coagulation
coccidioidal —*see* Coccidioidomycosis
cold
  agglutinin or hemoglobinuria D59.12
    paroxysmal D59.6
  hemagglutinin (chronic) D59.12
collagen NOS (nonvascular) (vascular) M35.9
  specified NEC M35.89
colon K63.9
  functional K59.9
    congenital Q43.2
  ischemic —*see also* Ischemia, intestine, acute
    K55.039
colonic inflammatory bowel, unclassified (IBDU)
    K52.3
combined system —*see* Degeneration, combined
compressed air T70.3
Concato's (pericardial polyserositis) A19.9
  nontubercular I31.1
  pleural —*see* Pleurisy, with effusion
conjunctiva H11.9
  chlamydial A74.0
  specified NEC H11.89
  viral B30.9
    specified NEC B30.8

Disease, diseased *(Continued)*
connective tissue, systemic (diffuse) M35.9
  in (due to)
    hypogammaglobulinemia D80.1 *[M36.8]*
    ochronosis E70.29 *[M36.8]*
    specified NEC M35.89
Conor and Bruch's (boutonneuse fever) A77.1
Cooper's —*see* Mastopathy, cystic
Cori's (glycogenosis III) E74.03
corkhandler's or corkworker's J67.3
cornea H18.9
  specified NEC H18.89-●
coronary (artery) —*see* Disease, heart, ischemic,
    atherosclerotic
  congenital Q24.5
  microvascular
    with
      angina pectoris I20.81
      myocardial infarction I21.B
    acute I24.81
    chronic I25.85
  ostial, syphilitic (aortic) (mitral) (pulmonary)
    A52.03
corpus cavernosum N48.9
  specified NEC N48.89
~~Cotugno's —see Sciatica~~
▶Cotugno —*see* Sciatica
COVID-19 U07.1
coxsackie (virus) NEC B34.1
cranial nerve NOS G52.9
Creutzfeldt-Jakob —*see* Creutzfeldt-Jakob
    disease or syndrome
Crocq's (acrocyanosis) I73.89
Crohn's —*see* Enteritis, regional
Curschmann G71.11
cystic
  breast (chronic) —*see* Mastopathy, cystic
  kidney, congenital Q61.9
  liver, congenital Q44.6
  lung J98.4
    congenital Q33.0
cytomegalic inclusion (generalized) B25.9
  with pneumonia B25.0
  congenital P35.1
cytomegaloviral B25.9
  specified NEC B25.8
Czerny's (periodic hydrarthrosis of the knee) —
    see Effusion, joint, knee
Daae (-Finsen) (epidemic pleurodynia) B33.0
Danon E74.05
Darling's —*see* Histoplasmosis capsulati
Débove's (splenomegaly) R16.1
deer fly —*see* Tularemia
Degos' I77.8
demyelinating, demyelinizating (nervous
    system) G37.9
  multiple sclerosis G35
  specified NEC G37.89
dense deposit —*see also* N00-N07 with fourth
    character .6 N05.6
deposition, hydroxyapatite —*see* Disease,
    hydroxyapatite deposition
de Quervain's (tendon sheath) M65.4
  thyroid (subacute granulomatous thyroiditis)
    E06.1
Devergie's (pityriasis rubra pilaris) L44.0
Devic's G36.0
diaphorase deficiency D74.0
diaphragm J98.6
diarrheal, infectious NEC A09
digestive system K92.9
  specified NEC K92.89
disc, degenerative —*see* Degeneration,
    intervertebral disc
discogenic —*see also* Displacement, intervertebral
    disc NEC
  with myelopathy —*see* Disorder, disc, with,
    myelopathy
diverticular —*see* Diverticula
Dubois (thymus) A50.59 *[E35]*
Duchenne-Griesinger G71.01
Duchenne's
  muscular dystrophy G71.01
  pseudohypertrophy, muscles G71.01
ductless glands E34.9
Duhring's (dermatitis herpetiformis) L13.0
duodenum K31.9
  specified NEC K31.89
Dupré's (meningism) R29.1
Dupuytren's (muscle contracture) M72.0
Durand-Nicholas-Favre (climatic bubo) A55

Disease, diseased *(Continued)*
  Duroziez's (congenital mitral stenosis) Q23.2
  ear —*see* Disorder, ear
  Eberth's —*see* Fever, typhoid
  Ebola (virus) A98.4
  Ebstein's heart Q22.5
  Echinococcus —*see* Echinococcus
  echovirus NEC B34.1
  Eddowes' (brittle bones and blue sclera) Q78.0
  edentulous (alveolar) ridge K06.9
    specified NEC K06.8
  Edsall's T67.2
  Eichstedt's (pityriasis versicolor) B36.0
  Eisenmenger's (irreversible) I27.83
  Ellis-van Creveld (chondroectodermal dysplasia)
    Q77.6
  end stage renal (ESRD) N18.6
    due to hypertension I12.0
  endocrine glands or system NEC E34.9
  endomyocardial (eosinophilic) I42.3
  English (rickets) E55.0
  enteroviral, enterovirus NEC B34.1
    central nervous system NEC A88.8
  epidemic B99.9
    specified NEC B99.8
  epididymis N50.9
  Erb (-Landouzy) G71.02
  Erdheim-Chester (ECD) E88.89
  esophagus K22.9
    functional K22.4
    psychogenic F45.8
    specified NEC K22.89
  Eulenburg's (congenital paramyotonia) G71.19
  eustachian tube —*see* Disorder, eustachian tube
  external
    auditory canal —*see* Disorder, ear, external
    ear —*see* Disorder, ear, external
  extrapyramidal G25.9
    specified NEC G25.89
  eye H57.9
    anterior chamber H21.9
    inflammatory NEC H57.89
    muscle (external) —*see* Strabismus
    specified NEC H57.89
    syphilitic —*see* Oculopathy, syphilitic
  eyeball H44.9
    specified NEC H44.89
  eyelid —*see* Disorder, eyelid
    specified NEC —*see* Disorder, eyelid, specified
      type NEC
  eyeworm of Africa B74.3
  facial nerve (seventh) G51.9
    newborn (birth injury) P11.3
  Fahr (of brain) G23.8
  Fahr Volhard (of kidney) I12.-●
  fallopian tube (noninflammatory) N83.9
    inflammatory —*see* Salpingo-oophoritis
    specified NEC N83.8
  familial periodic paralysis G72.3
  ~~Fanconi's (congenital pancytopenia) D61.09~~
▶ Fanconi ('s) D61.03
  fascia NEC —*see also* Disorder, muscle
    inflammatory —*see* Myositis
    specified NEC M62.89
  Fauchard's (periodontitis) —*see* Periodontitis
  Favre-Durand-Nicolas (climatic bubo) A55
  Fede's K14.0
  Feer's —*see* Poisoning, mercury
  female pelvic inflammatory —*see also* Disease,
    pelvis, inflammatory N73.9
    syphilitic (secondary) A51.42
    tuberculous A18.17
  Fernels' (aortic aneurysm) I71.9
  fibrocaseous of lung —*see* Tuberculosis,
    pulmonary
  fibrocystic —*see* Fibrocystic disease
  Fiedler's (leptospiral jaundice) A27.0
  fifth B08.3
  file-cutter's —*see* Poisoning, lead
  fish-skin Q80.9
    acquired L85.0
  Flajani (-Basedow) (exophthalmic goiter) —*see*
    Hyperthyroidism, with, goiter (diffuse)
  flax-dresser's J66.1
  fluke —*see* Infestation, fluke
  foot and mouth B08.8
  foot process N04.9
  Forbes' (glycogenosis III) E74.03
  Fordyce-Fox (apocrine miliaria) L75.2
  Fordyce's (ectopic sebaceous glands) (mouth)
    Q38.6

Disease, diseased *(Continued)*
  Forestier's (rhizomelic pseudopolyarthritis)
    M35.3
    meaning ankylosing hyperostosis —*see*
      Hyperostosis, ankylosing
  Fothergill's
    neuralgia —*see* Neuralgia, trigeminal
    scarlatina anginosa A38.9
  Fournier (gangrene) N49.3
    female N76.82
      vagina and vulva N76.82
  fourth B08.8
  Fox (-Fordyce) (apocrine miliaria) L75.2
  Francis' —*see* Tularemia
▶ Franklin C88.2-●
  Frei's (climatic bubo) A55
  Friedreich's
    combined systemic or ataxia G11.11
    myoclonia G25.3
  frontal sinus —*see* Sinusitis, frontal
  fungus NEC B49
  Gaisböck's (polycythemia hypertonica) D75.1
  gallbladder K82.9
    calculus —*see* Calculus, gallbladder
    cholecystitis —*see* Cholecystitis
    cholesterolosis K82.4
    fistula —*see* Fistula, gallbladder
    hydrops K82.1
    obstruction —*see* Obstruction, gallbladder
    perforation K82.2
    specified NEC K82.8
▶ gamma heavy chain C88.2-●
  Gamna's (siderotic splenomegaly) D73.2
  Gamstorp's (adynamia episodica hereditaria)
    G72.3
  Gandy-Nanta (siderotic splenomegaly) D73.2
  ganister J62.8
  gastric —*see* Disease, stomach
  gastroesophageal reflux (GERD) K21.9
    with esophagitis (without bleeding) K21.00
    with bleeding K21.01
  gastrointestinal (tract) K92.9
    amyloid E85.4
    functional K59.9
      psychogenic F45.8
    specified NEC K92.89
  Gee (-Herter) (-Heubner) (-Thaysen) (nontropical
    sprue) K90.0
  genital organs
    female N94.9
    male N50.9
  Gerhardt's (erythromelalgia) I73.81
  Gibert's (pityriasis rosea) L42
  Gierke's (glycogenosis I) E74.01
  Gilles de la Tourette's (motor-verbal tic) F95.2
  gingiva K06.9
    plaque induced K05.00
    specified NEC K06.8
  gland (lymph) I89.9
  Glanzmann's (hereditary hemorrhagic
    thrombasthenia) D69.1
  glass-blower's (cataract) —*see* Cataract, specified
    NEC
    salivary gland hypertrophy K11.1
  Glisson's —*see* Rickets
  globe H44.9
    specified NEC H44.89
  glomerular —*see also* Glomerulonephritis
    with edema —*see* Nephrosis
    acute —*see* Nephritis, acute
    chronic —*see* Nephritis, chronic
    minimal change N05.0
    rapidly progressive N01.9
  glycogen storage E74.00
    Andersen's E74.09
    Cori's E74.03
    Forbes' E74.03
    generalized E74.00
    glucose-6-phosphatase deficiency E74.01
    heart E74.02 *[143]*
    hepatorenal E74.09
    Hers' E74.09
    liver and kidney E74.09
    lysosomal E74.02
      with acid maltase deficiency E74.02
      without acid maltase deficiency E74.05
    McArdle's E74.04
    muscle phosphofructokinase E74.09
    myocardium E74.02 *[143]*
    Pompe's E74.02
    Tauri's E74.09

Disease, diseased *(Continued)*
  glycogen storage *(Continued)*
    type IIB E74.05
    type 0 E74.09
    type I E74.01
    type II E74.02
    type III E74.03
    type IV E74.09
    type V E74.04
    type VI-XI E74.09
    Von Gierke's E74.01
  Goldstein's (familial hemorrhagic telangiectasia)
    I78.0
  gonococcal NOS A54.9
  graft-versus-host (GVH) D89.813
    acute D89.810
    acute on chronic D89.812
    chronic D89.811
  grainhandler's J67.8
  granulomatous (childhood) (chronic) D71
  Graves' (exophthalmic goiter) —*see*
    Hyperthyroidism, with, goiter (diffuse)
  Griesinger's —*see* Ancylostomiasis
  Grisel's M43.6
  Gruby's (tinea tonsurans) B35.0
  Guillain-Barré G61.0
  Guinon's (motor-verbal tic) F95.2
  gum K06.9
  gynecological N94.9
  H (Hartnup's) E72.02
  Haff —*see* Poisoning, mercury
  Hageman (congenital factor XII deficiency) D68.2
  hair (color) (shaft) L67.9
    follicles L73.9
      specified NEC L73.8
  Hamman's (spontaneous mediastinal
    emphysema) J98.2
  hand, foot and mouth B08.4
  Hansen's —*see* Leprosy
  Hantavirus, with pulmonary manifestations
    B33.4
    with renal manifestations A98.5
  Harada's H30.81-●
  Hartnup (pellagra-cerebellar ataxia-renal
    aminoaciduria) E72.02
  Hart's (pellagra-cerebellar ataxia-renal
    aminoaciduria) E72.02
  Hashimoto's (struma lymphomatosa) E06.3
  Hb —*see* Disease, hemoglobin
  heart (organic) I51.9
    with
      pulmonary edema (acute) —*see also* Failure,
        ventricular, left I50.1
      rheumatic fever (conditions in I00)
        active I01.9
          with chorea I02.0
          specified NEC I01.8
        inactive or quiescent (with chorea) I09.9
          specified NEC I09.89
    amyloid E85.4 *[143]*
    aortic (valve) I35.9
    arteriosclerotic or sclerotic (senile) —*see*
      Disease, heart, ischemic, atherosclerotic
    artery, arterial —*see* Disease, heart, ischemic,
      atherosclerotic
    beer drinkers' I42.6
    beriberi (wet) E51.12
    black I27.0
    congenital Q24.9
      cyanotic Q24.9
      specified NEC Q24.8
    coronary —*see* Disease, heart, ischemic
    cryptogenic I51.9
    fibroid —*see* Myocarditis
    functional I51.89
      psychogenic F45.8
    glycogen storage E74.02 *[143]*
    gonococcal A54.83
    hypertensive —*see* Hypertension, heart
    hyperthyroid —*see also* Hyperthyroidism
      E05.90 *[143]*
      with thyroid storm E05.91 *[143]*
    ischemic (chronic or with a stated duration of
      over 4 weeks) I25.9
      atherosclerotic (of) I25.10
        with angina pectoris —*see*
          Arteriosclerosis, coronary
          (artery)
        coronary artery bypass graft —*see*
          Arteriosclerosis, coronary (artery),
          cardiomyopathy I25.5

▶ New   ⇒ Revised   ~~deleted~~ Deleted   ● Use Additional Character(s)

Disease, diseased *(Continued)*
  heart *(Continued)*
    ischemic *(Continued)*
      diagnosed on ECG or other special
        investigation, but currently presenting
        no symptoms I25.6
      silent I25.6
      specified form NEC
        acute I24.89
        chronic I25.89
    kyphoscoliotic I27.1
    meningococcal A39.50
      endocarditis A39.51
      myocarditis A39.52
      pericarditis A39.53
    mitral I05.9
      specified NEC I05.8
    muscular —*see* Degeneration, myocardial
    psychogenic (functional) F45.8
    pulmonary (chronic) I27.9
      in schistosomiasis B65.9 *[152]*
      specified NEC I27.89
    rheumatic (chronic) (inactive) (old) (quiescent)
      (with chorea) I09.9
      active or acute I01.9
        with chorea (acute) (rheumatic)
          (Sydenham's) I02.0
      specified NEC I09.89
    senile —*see* Myocarditis
    syphilitic A52.06
      aortic A52.03
        aneurysm A52.01
      congenital A50.54 *[152]*
    thyrotoxic —*see also* Thyrotoxicosis E05.90 *[143]*
      with thyroid storm E05.91 *[143]*
    valve, valvular (obstructive) (regurgitant) —
      see also Endocarditis
      congenital NEC Q24.8
        pulmonary Q22.3
    vascular —*see* Disease, cardiovascular
  heavy chain NEC C88.2-●
    alpha C88.3-●
    gamma C88.2-●
    mu C88.2-●
  Hebra's
    pityriasis
      maculata et circinata L42
      rubra pilaris L44.0
    prurigo L28.2
  hematopoietic organs D75.9
  hemoglobin or Hb
    abnormal (mixed) NEC D58.2
      with thalassemia D56.9
    AS genotype D57.3
    Bart's D56.0
    C (Hb-C) D58.2
      with other abnormal hemoglobin NEC
        D58.2
      elliptocytosis D58.1
      Hb-S D57.2-●
      sickle-cell D57.2-●
      thalassemia D56.8
    Constant Spring D58.2
    D (Hb-D) D58.2
    E (Hb-E) D58.2
    E-beta thalassemia D56.5
    elliptocytosis D58.1
    H (Hb-H) (thalassemia) D56.0
      with other abnormal hemoglobin NEC
        D56.9
      Constant Spring D56.0
    I thalassemia D56.9
    M D74.0
    S or SS D57.1
      with
        acute chest syndrome D57.01
        cerebral vascular involvement D57.03
        crisis (painful) D57.00
          with complication specified NEC D57.09
        pain (vaso-occlusive) D57.00
        splenic sequestration D57.02
      beta plus D57.44
        with
          acute chest syndrome D57.451
          cerebral vascular involvement D57.453
          crisis D57.459
            with specified complication NEC
              D57.458
          pain (vaso-occlusive) D57.459
          splenic sequestration D57.452
        without crisis D57.44

Disease, diseased *(Continued)*
  hemoglobin or Hb *(Continued)*
    S or SS *(Continued)*
      beta zero D57.42
        with
          acute chest syndrome D57.431
          cerebral vascular involvement D57.433
          crisis D57.439
            with specified complication NEC
              D57.438
          pain (vaso-occlusive) D57.439
          splenic sequestration D57.432
        without crisis D57.42
    SC D57.2-●
    SD D57.8-●
    SE D57.8-●
    spherocytosis D58.0
    unstable, hemolytic D58.2
  hemolytic (newborn) P55.9
    autoimmune D59.10
      cold type (primary) (secondary)
        (symptomatic) D59.12
      mixed type (primary) (secondary)
        (symptomatic) D59.13
      warm type (primary) (secondary)
        (symptomatic) D59.11
    drug-induced D59.0
    due to or with
      incompatibility
        ABO (blood group) P55.1
        blood (group) (Duffy) (K) (Kell) (Kidd)
          (Lewis) (M) (S) NEC P55.8
        Rh (blood group) (factor) P55.0
      Rh negative mother P55.0
    specified type NEC P55.8
    unstable hemoglobin D58.2
  hemorrhagic D69.9
    newborn P53
  Henoch (-Schönlein) (purpura nervosa) D69.0
  hepatic —*see* Disease, liver
  hepatobiliary K83.9
    toxic K71.9
  hepatolenticular E83.01
  heredodegenerative NEC
    spinal cord G95.89
  herpesviral, disseminated B00.7
  Hers' (glycogenosis VI) E74.09
  Herter (-Gee) (-Heubner) (nontropical sprue) K90.0
  Heubner-Herter (nontropical sprue) K90.0
  high fetal gene or hemoglobin thalassemia D56.9
  Hildenbrand's —*see* Typhus
  hip (joint) M25.9
    congenital Q65.89
    suppurative M00.9
    tuberculous A18.02
  His (-Werner) (trench fever) A79.0
  Hodgson's (*see also* Aneurysm, aorta, thorax)
    I71.20
    ruptured (*see also* Aneurysm, aorta, thorax,
      ruptured) I71.10
  Holla —*see* Spherocytosis
  hookworm B76.9
    specified NEC B76.8
  host-versus-graft D89.813
    acute D89.810
    acute on chronic D89.812
    chronic D89.811
  human immunodeficiency virus (HIV) B20
  Huntington's G10
    with dementia (*see also* Dementia, in, diseases
      specified elsewhere) G10 *[F02.80]*
  Hunt's (herpetic geniculate ganglionitis)
    (neuralgia) B02.21
    dyssynergia cerebellaris myoclonica G11.19
  Hutchinson's (cheiropompholyx) —*see*
    Hutchinson's disease
  hyaline (diffuse) (generalized)
    membrane (lung) (newborn) P22.0
      adult J80
  hydatid —*see* Echinococcus
  hydroxyapatite deposition M11.00
    ankle M11.07-●
    elbow M11.02-●
    foot joint M11.07-●
    hand joint M11.04-●
    hip M11.05-●
    knee M11.06-●
    multiple site M11.09
    shoulder M11.01-●
    vertebra M11.08
    wrist M11.03-●

Disease, diseased *(Continued)*
  hyperkinetic —*see* Hyperkinesia
  hypertensive —*see* Hypertension
  hypophysis E23.7
  Iceland G93.39
  I-cell E77.0
  IgG4-related D89.84
  immune D89.9
  immunoglobulin G4-related D89.84
  immunoproliferative (malignant) C88.9-●
    small intestinal C88.3-●
    specified NEC C88.8-●
  inclusion B25.9
    salivary gland B25.9
  infectious, infective B99.9
    congenital P37.9
      specified NEC P37.8
      viral P35.9
        specified type NEC P35.8
    specified NEC B99.8
  inflammatory
    penis N48.29
      abscess N48.21
      cellulitis N48.22
    prepuce N47.7
      balanoposthitis N47.6
    tubo-ovarian —*see* Salpingo-oophoritis
  intervertebral disc —*see also* Disorder, disc
    with myelopathy —*see* Disorder, disc, with,
      myelopathy
    cervical, cervicothoracic —*see* Disorder, disc,
      cervical
      with
        myelopathy —*see* Disorder, disc, cervical,
          with myelopathy
        neuritis, radiculitis or radiculopathy —
          see Disorder, disc, cervical, with
          neuritis
        specified NEC —*see* Disorder, disc,
          cervical, specified type NEC
    lumbar (with)
      myelopathy M51.06
      neuritis, radiculitis, radiculopathy or
        sciatica M51.16
      specified NEC M51.86
    lumbosacral (with)
      neuritis, radiculitis, radiculopathy or
        sciatica M51.17
      specified NEC M51.87
    specified NEC —*see* Disorder, disc, specified
      NEC
    thoracic (with)
      myelopathy M51.04
      neuritis, radiculitis or radiculopathy M51.14
      specified NEC M51.84
    thoracolumbar (with)
      myelopathy M51.05
      neuritis, radiculitis or radiculopathy M51.15
      specified NEC M51.85
  intestine K63.9
    functional K59.9
      psychogenic F45.8
      specified NEC K59.89
    organic K63.9
    protozoal A07.9
    specified NEC K63.89
  iris H21.9
    specified NEC H21.89
  iron metabolism or storage E83.10
  island (scrub typhus) A75.3
  itai-itai —*see* Poisoning, cadmium
  Jakob-Creutzfeldt —*see* Creutzfeldt-Jakob
    disease or syndrome
  jaw M27.9
    fibrocystic M27.49
    specified NEC M27.8
  jigger B88.1
  joint —*see also* Disorder, joint
    Charcot's —*see* Arthropathy, neuropathic
      (Charcot)
    degenerative —*see* Osteoarthritis
      multiple M15.9
      spine —*see* Spondylosis
    facet joint (*see also* Spondylosis) M47.819
    hypertrophic —*see* Osteoarthritis
    sacroiliac M53.3
    specified NEC —*see* Disorder, joint, specified
      type NEC
    spine NEC —*see* Dorsopathy
    suppurative —*see* Arthritis, pyogenic or
      pyemic

Disease, diseased *(Continued)*
    Jourdain's (acute gingivitis) K05.00
        nonplaque induced K05.01
        plaque induced K05.00
    Kaschin-Beck (endemic polyarthritis) M12.10
        ankle M12.17-●
        elbow M12.12-●
        foot joint M12.17-●
        hand joint M12.14-●
        hip M12.15-●
        knee M12.16-●
        multiple site M12.19
        shoulder M12.11-●
        vertebra M12.18
        wrist M12.13-●
    Katayama B65.2
    Kedani (scrub typhus) A75.3
    Keshan E59
    kidney (functional) (pelvis) N28.9
        chronic N18.9
            hypertensive —*see* Hypertension, kidney
            stage 1 N18.1
            stage 2 (mild) N18.2
            stage 3 (moderate) N18.30
                stage 3a N18.31
                stage 3b N18.32
            stage 4 (severe) N18.4
            stage 5 N18.5
        complicating pregnancy —*see* Pregnancy,
            complicated by, renal disease
        cystic (congenital) Q61.9
        diabetic —*see* E08-E13 with .22
        fibrocystic (congenital) Q61.8
        hypertensive —*see* Hypertension, kidney
        in (due to)
            schistosomiasis (bilharziasis) B65.9 *[N29]*
        multicystic Q61.4
        polycystic Q61.3
            adult type Q61.2
            childhood type NEC Q61.19
                collecting duct dilatation Q61.11
    Kimmelstiel (-Wilson) (intercapillary polycystic
        (congenital) glomerulosclerosis) —*see*
        E08-E13 with .21
    Kimura D21.9
        specified site (*see* Neoplasm, connective tissue
            benign)
    Kinnier Wilson's (hepatolenticular degeneration)
        E83.01
    kissing —*see* Mononucleosis, infectious
    Klebs' —*see also* Glomerulonephritis N05.-●
    Klippel-Feil (brevicollis) Q76.1
    Köhler-Pellegrini-Stieda (calcification, knee
        joint) —*see* Bursitis, tibial collateral
    Kok Q89.8
    König's (osteochondritis dissecans) —*see*
        Osteochondritis, dissecans
    Korsakoff's (nonalcoholic) F04
        alcoholic F10.96
            with dependence F10.26
    Kostmann's (infantile genetic agranulocytosis)
        D70.0
    kuru A81.81
    Kyasanur Forest A98.2
    labyrinth, ear —*see* Disorder, ear, inner
    lacrimal system —*see* Disorder, lacrimal system
    Lafora body (*see also* Epilepsy, progressive,
        Lafora) G40.C09
    Lancereaux-Mathieu (leptospiral jaundice) A27.0
    Landry's G61.0
    Larrey-Weil (leptospiral jaundice) A27.0
    larynx J38.7
    legionnaires' A48.1
        nonpneumonic A48.2
    Lenegre's I44.2
    lens H27.9
        specified NEC H27.8
    Lev's (acquired complete heart block) I44.2
    Lewy body (dementia) (*see also* Dementia,
        in, diseases specified elsewhere) G31.83
        [F02.80]
        with behavioral disturbance (*see also*
            Dementia, in, diseases specified
            elsewhere) G31.83 *[F02.81-●]*
    Lichtheim's (subacute combined sclerosis with
        pernicious anemia) D51.0
    Lightwood's (renal tubular acidosis) N25.89
    Lignac's (cystinosis) E72.04
    lip K13.0
    lipid-storage E75.6
        specified NEC E75.5

Disease, diseased *(Continued)*
    Lipschütz's N76.6
    liver (chronic) (organic) K76.9
        alcoholic (chronic) K70.9
            acute —*see* Disease, liver, alcoholic,
                hepatitis
            cirrhosis K70.30
                with ascites K70.31
            failure K70.40
                with coma K70.41
            fatty liver K70.0
            fibrosis K70.2
            hepatitis K70.10
                with ascites K70.11
            sclerosis K70.2
        cystic, congenital Q44.6
        drug-induced (idiosyncratic) (toxic)
            (predictable) (unpredictable) —*see*
            Disease, liver, toxic
        end stage K72.1-●
            due to hepatitis —*see* Hepatitis
            with coma K72.11
        fatty, nonalcoholic (NAFLD) K76.0
            alcoholic K70.0
        fibrocystic (congenital) Q44.6
        fluke
            Chinese B66.1
            oriental B66.1
            sheep B66.3
        gestational alloimmune (GALD) P78.84
        glycogen storage E74.09 *[K77]*
        in (due to)
            schistosomiasis (bilharziasis) B65.9 *[K77]*
        inflammatory K75.9
            alcoholic K70.1
            specified NEC K75.89
        polycystic (congenital) Q44.6
        toxic K71.9
            with
                cholestasis K71.0
                cirrhosis (liver) K71.7
                fibrosis (liver) K71.7
                focal nodular hyperplasia K71.8
                hepatic granuloma K71.8
                hepatic necrosis K71.10
                    with coma K71.11
                hepatitis NEC K71.6
                    acute K71.2
                    chronic
                        active K71.50
                            with ascites K71.51
                        lobular K71.4
                        persistent K71.3
                lupoid K71.50
                    with ascites K71.51
                peliosis hepatis K71.8
                veno-occlusive disease (VOD) of liver
                  K71.8
        veno-occlusive K76.5
    Lobo's (keloid blastomycosis) B48.0
    Lobstein's (brittle bones and blue sclera) Q78.0
    Ludwig's (submaxillary cellulitis) K12.2
    lumbosacral region M53.87
    lung J98.4
        black J60
        congenital Q33.9
        cystic J98.4
            congenital Q33.0
        dabbing (related) U07.0
        electronic cigarette (related) U07.0
        fibroid (chronic) —*see* Fibrosis, lung
        fluke B66.4
            oriental B66.4
        in
            amyloidosis E85.4 *[J99]*
            sarcoidosis D86.0
            Sjögren's syndrome M35.02
            systemic
                lupus erythematosus M32.13
                sclerosis M34.81
        interstitial J84.9
            drug-induced —*see* Disorder, lung,
                interstitial, drug-induced
            of childhood, specified NEC J84.848
                drug-induced —*see* Disorder, lung,
                    interstitial, drug-induced
            respiratory bronchiolitis J84.115
            specified NEC J84.89
            with progressive fibrotic phenotype, in
                diseases classified elsewhere
                J84.170

Disease, diseased *(Continued)*
    lung *(Continued)*
        obstructive (chronic) J44.9
            with
                acute
                    bronchitis J44.0
                    exacerbation NEC J44.1
                    lower respiratory infection J44.0
                alveolitis, allergic J67.9
▶   asthma J44.89
                bronchiectasis J47.9
                  with
                    exacerbation (acute) J47.1
                    lower respiratory infection J47.0
                bronchitis J44.89
                  with
                    exacerbation (acute) J44.1
                    lower respiratory infection J44.0
                emphysema J43.9
                hypersensitivity pneumonitis J67.9
            decompensated J44.1
                with
                  exacerbation (acute) J44.1
        polycystic J98.4
            congenital Q33.0
        rheumatoid (diffuse) (interstitial) —*see*
            Rheumatoid, lung
        vaping (associated) (device) (product) (use)
            U07.0
    Lutembacher's (atrial septal defect with mitral
        stenosis) Q21.19
    Lyme A69.20
    lymphatic (gland) (system) (channel) (vessel)
        I89.9
    lymphoproliferative D47.9
        specified NEC D47.Z9
        T-gamma D47.Z9
        X-linked D82.3
    Magitot's M27.2
    malarial —*see* Malaria
    malignant —*see also* Neoplasm, malignant, by
        site
    Manson's B65.1
    maple bark J67.6
    maple-syrup-urine E71.0
    Marburg (virus) A98.3
    Marion's (bladder neck obstruction) N32.0
    Marsh's (exophthalmic goiter) —*see*
        Hyperthyroidism, with, goiter (diffuse)
    mastoid (process) —*see* Disorder, ear, middle
    Mathieu's (leptospiral jaundice) A27.0
    Maxcy's A75.2
    McArdle (-Schmid-Pearson) (glycogenosis V)
        E74.04
    mediastinum J98.59
    medullary center (idiopathic) (respiratory)
        G93.89
    Meige's (chronic hereditary edema) Q82.0
    meningococcal —*see* Infection, meningococcal
    mental F99
        organic F09
    mesenchymal M35.9
    mesenteric embolic —*see also* Ischemia, intestine,
        acute K55.039
    metabolic, metabolism E88.9
        bilirubin E80.7
    metal-polisher's J62.8
    metastatic —*see also* Neoplasm, secondary, by
        site C79.9
    microvascular — code to condition
    microvillus
        atrophy Q43.8
        inclusion (MVD) Q43.8
    middle ear —*see* Disorder, ear, middle
    Mikulicz' (dryness of mouth, absent or
        decreased lacrimation) K11.8
    Milroy's (chronic hereditary edema) Q82.0
    Minamata —*see* Poisoning, mercury
    minicore G71.29
    Minor's G95.19
    Minot's (hemorrhagic disease, newborn)P53
    Minot-von Willebrand-Jürgens
        (angiohemophilia) —*see* Disease, von
        Willebrand
    Mitchell's (erythromelalgia) I73.81
    mitral (valve) I05.9
        nonrheumatic I34.9
    mixed connective tissue M35.1
    MOG antibody G37.81
    moldy hay J67.0
    Monge's T70.29

▶ New   ➡ Revised   ~~deleted~~ Deleted   ● Use Additional Character(s)

Disease, diseased *(Continued)*
  Morgagni-Adams-Stokes (syncope with heart block) I45.9
  Morgagni's (syndrome) (hyperostosis frontalis interna) M85.2
  Morton's (with metatarsalgia) —*see* Lesion, nerve, plantar
  Morvan's G60.8
  motor neuron (bulbar) (mixed type) (spinal) G12.20
    amyotrophic lateral sclerosis G12.21
    familial G12.24
    progressive bulbar palsy G12.22
    specified NEC G12.29
  moyamoya I67.5
  multicore G71.29
  multiminicore G71.29
  mu heavy chain disease C88.2-●
  muscle —*see also* Disorder, muscle
    inflammatory —*see* Myositis
    ocular (external) —*see* Strabismus
  musculoskeletal system, soft tissue —*see also* Disorder, soft tissue
    specified NEC —*see* Disorder, soft tissue, specified type NEC
  mushroom workers' J67.5
  mycotic B49
  myelin oligodendrocyte glycoprotein antibody G37.81
  myelodysplastic (*see also* Syndrome, myelodysplastic) C94.6
  myelodysplastic/myeloproliferative neoplasm, unclassifiable C94.6
  myeloproliferative D47.1
    chronic D47.1
    not classified C94.6
    specified NEC C94.6
    unclassifiable C94.6
  myocardium, myocardial —*see also* Degeneration, myocardial I51.5
    primary (idiopathic) I42.9
  myoneural G70.9
  Naegeli's D69.1
  nails L60.9
    specified NEC L60.8
  Nairobi (sheep virus) A93.8
  nasal J34.9
  nemaline body G71.21
  nerve —*see* Disorder, nerve
  nervous system G98.8
    autonomic G90.9
    central G96.9
      specified NEC G96.89
    congenital Q07.9
    parasympathetic G90.9
    specified NEC G98.8
    sympathetic G90.9
    vegetative G90.9
  neuromuscular system G70.9
  Newcastle B30.8
  Nicolas (-Durand)-Favre (climatic bubo) A55
  nipple N64.9
    Paget's C50.01-●
      female C50.01-●
      male C50.02-●
  Nishimoto (-Takeuchi) I67.5
  nonarthropod-borne NOS (viral) B34.9
    enterovirus NEC B34.1
  nonautoimmune hemolytic D59.4
    drug-induced D59.2
  Nonne-Milroy-Meige (chronic hereditary edema) Q82.0
  nose J34.9
  nucleus pulposus —*see* Disorder, disc
  nutritional E63.9
  oast-house-urine E72.19
    ocular
      herpesviral B00.50
      zoster B02.30
  obliterative vascular I77.1
  Ohara's —*see* Tularemia
  Opitz's (congestive splenomegaly) D73.2
  Oppenheim-Urbach (necrobiosis lipoidica diabeticorum) —*see* E08-E13 with .620
  optic nerve NEC —*see* Disorder, nerve, optic
    orbit —*see* Disorder, orbit
  organ
    dabbing (related) U07.0
    electronic cigarette (related) U07.0
    vaping (associated) (device) (product) (use) U07.0
  Oriental liver fluke B66.1

Disease, diseased *(Continued)*
  Oriental lung fluke B66.4
  Ormond's N13.5
  Oropouche virus A93.0
  Osler-Rendu (familial hemorrhagic telangiectasia) I78.0
  osteofibrocystic E21.0
  Otto's M24.7
  outer ear —*see* Disorder, ear, external
  ovary (noninflammatory) N83.9
    cystic N83.20-●
    inflammatory —*see* Salpingo-oophoritis
    polycystic E28.2
    specified NEC N83.8
  Owren's (congenital) —*see* Defect, coagulation
  p110d-activating mutation causing senescent T cells, lymphadenopathy, and immunodeficiency [PASLI] D81.82
  pancreas K86.9
    cystic K86.2
    fibrocystic E84.9
    specified NEC K86.89
  panvalvular I08.9
    specified NEC I08.8
  parametrium (noninflammatory) N83.9
  parasitic B89
    cerebral NEC B71.9 *[G94]*
    intestinal NOS B82.9
    mouth B37.0
    skin NOS B88.9
    specified type —*see* Infestation
    tongue B37.0
  parathyroid (gland) E21.5
    specified NEC E21.4
  Parkinson's G20.A1
    with dyskinesia
      with
        fluctuations G20.B2
        OFF episodes G20.B2
      without mention of
        fluctuations G20.B1
        OFF episodes G20.B1
    without dyskinesia
      with
        fluctuations G20.A2
        OFF episodes G20.A2
      without mention of
        fluctuations G20.A1
        OFF episodes G20.A1
  parodontal K05.6
  Parrot's (syphilitic osteochondritis) A50.02
  Parry's (exophthalmic goiter) —*see* Hyperthyroidism, with, goiter (diffuse)
  Parson's (exophthalmic goiter) —*see* Hyperthyroidism, with, goiter (diffuse)
  Paxton's (white piedra) B36.2
  pearl-worker's —*see* Osteomyelitis, specified type NEC
  Pellegrini-Stieda (calcification, knee joint) —*see* Bursitis, tibial collateral
  pelvis, pelvic
    female NOS N94.9
      specified NEC N94.89
    gonococcal (acute) (chronic) A54.24
    inflammatory (female) N73.9
      acute N73.0
      chlamydial A56.11
      chronic N73.1
      specified NEC N73.8
      syphilitic (secondary) A51.42
        late A52.76
      tuberculous A18.17
    organ, female N94.9
    peritoneum, female NEC N94.89
  penis N48.9
    inflammatory N48.29
      abscess N48.21
      cellulitis N48.22
    specified NEC N48.89
  periapical tissues NOS K04.90
  periodontal K05.6
    specified NEC K05.5
  periosteum —*see* Disorder, bone, specified type NEC
  peripheral
    arterial I73.9
    autonomic nervous system G90.9
    nerves —*see* Polyneuropathy
    vascular NOS I73.9
      in diabetes mellitus —*see* Diabetes, by type, with peripheral angiopathy

Disease, diseased *(Continued)*
  peritoneum K66.9
    pelvic, female NEC N94.89
    specified NEC K66.8
  persistent mucosal (middle ear) H66.20
    left H66.22
      with right H66.23
    right H66.21
      with left H66.23
  Petit's —*see* Hernia, abdomen, specified site NEC
  pharynx J39.2
    specified NEC J39.2
  Phocas' —*see* Mastopathy, cystic
  photochromogenic (acid-fast bacilli) (pulmonary) A31.0
    nonpulmonary A31.9
  Pick's (*see also* Dementia, in, diseases specified elsewhere) G31.01 *[F02.80]*
    with behavioral disturbance (*see also* Dementia, in, diseases specified elsewhere) G31.01 *[F02.81-●]*
    brain (*see also* Dementia, in, diseases specified elsewhere) G31.01 *[F02.80]*
      with behavioral disturbance (*see also* Dementia, in, diseases specified elsewhere) G31.01 *[F02.81-●]*
    of pericardium (pericardial pseudocirrhosis of liver) I31.1
  pigeon fancier's J67.2
  pineal gland E34.8
  pink —*see* Poisoning, mercury
  Pinkus' (lichen nitidus) L44.1
  pinworm B80
  Piry virus A93.8
  pituitary (gland) E23.7
  pituitary-snuff-taker's J67.8
  pleura (cavity) J94.9
    specified NEC J94.8
  pneumatic drill (hammer) T75.21
  Pollitzer's (hidradenitis suppurativa) L73.2
  polycystic
    kidney or renal Q61.3
      adult type Q61.2
      childhood type NEC Q61.19
        collecting duct dilatation Q61.11
    liver or hepatic Q44.6
    lung or pulmonary J98.4
      congenital Q33.0
    ovary, ovaries E28.2
    spleen Q89.09
  polyethylene T84.05-●
  Pompe's (glycogenosis II) E74.02
  Posadas-Wernicke B38.9
  Potain's (pulmonary edema) —*see* Edema, lung
  prepuce N47.8
    inflammatory N47.7
      balanoposthitis N47.6
  Pringle's (tuberous sclerosis) Q85.1
  prion, central nervous system A81.9
    specified NEC A81.89
  prostate N42.9
    specified NEC N42.89
  protozoal B64
    acanthamebiasis —*see* Acanthamebiasis
    African trypanosomiasis —*see* African trypanosomiasis
    babesiosis —(*see also* Babesiosis) B60.00
    Chagas disease —*see* Chagas disease
    intestine, intestinal A07.9
    leishmaniasis —*see* Leishmaniasis
    malaria —*see* Malaria
    naegleriasis B60.2
    pneumocystosis B59
    specified organism NEC B60.8
    toxoplasmosis —*see* Toxoplasmosis
  pseudo-Hurler's E77.0
  psychiatric F99
  psychotic —*see* Psychosis
  Puente's (simple glandular cheilitis) K13.0
  puerperal —*see also* Puerperal O90.89
  pulmonary —*see also* Disease, lung
    artery I28.9
    chronic obstructive J44.9
      with
        acute bronchitis J44.0
          exacerbation (acute) J44.1
        lower respiratory infection (acute) J44.0
      decompensated J44.1
        with
          exacerbation (acute) J44.1

Disease, diseased *(Continued)*
  pulmonary *(Continued)*
    heart I27.9
      specified NEC I27.89
    hypertensive (vascular) —*see also*
      Hypertension, pulmonary I27.20
      primary (idiopathic) I27.0
    valve I37.9
      rheumatic I09.89
  pulp (dental) NOS K04.90
  pulseless M31.4
  Putnam's (subacute combined sclerosis with
    pernicious anemia) D51.0
  Pyle (-Cohn) (metaphyseal dysplasia) Q78.5
  ragpicker's or ragsorter's A22.1
  Raynaud's —*see* Raynaud's disease
  reactive airway —*see* Asthma
  Reclus' (cystic) —*see* Mastopathy, cystic
  rectum K62.9
    specified NEC K62.89
  Refsum's (heredopathia atactica
    polyneuritiformis) G60.1
  renal (functional) (pelvis) —*see also* Disease,
    kidney N28.9
    with
      edema —*see* Nephrosis
      glomerular lesion —*see* Glomerulonephritis
        with edema —*see* Nephrosis
      interstitial nephritis N12
    acute N28.9
    chronic —*see also* Disease, kidney, chronic
      N18.9
    cystic, congenital Q61.9
    diabetic —*see* E08-E13 with .22
    end-stage (failure) N18.6
      due to hypertension I12.0
    fibrocystic (congenital) Q61.8
    hypertensive —*see* Hypertension, kidney
    lupus M32.14
    phosphate-losing (tubular) N25.0
    polycystic (congenital) Q61.3
      adult type Q61.2
      childhood type NEC Q61.19
        collecting duct dilatation Q61.11
    rapidly progressive N01.9
    subacute N01.9
  Rendu-Osler-Weber (familial hemorrhagic
    telangiectasia) I78.0
  renovascular (arteriosclerotic) —*see*
    Hypertension, kidney
  respiratory (tract) J98.9
    acute or subacute NOS J06.9
      due to
        chemicals, gases, fumes or vapors
          (inhalation) J68.3
        external agent J70.9
          specified NEC J70.8
        radiation J70.0
        smoke inhalation J70.5
      noninfectious J39.8
    chronic NOS J98.9
      due to
        chemicals, gases, fumes or vapors J68.4
        external agent J70.9
          specified NEC J70.8
        radiation J70.1
      newborn P27.9
        specified NEC P27.8
    due to
      chemicals, gases, fumes or vapors J68.9
        acute or subacute NEC J68.3
        chronic J68.4
      external agent J70.9
        specified NEC J70.8
    newborn P28.9
      specified type NEC P28.89
    upper J39.9
      acute or subacute J06.9
      noninfectious NEC J39.8
      specified NEC J39.8
      streptococcal J06.9
  retina, retinal H35.9
    Batten's or Batten-Mayou E75.4 *[H36.89]*
    specified NEC H35.89
  rheumatoid —*see* Arthritis, rheumatoid
  rickettsial NOS A79.9
    specified type NEC A79.89
  Riga (-Fede) (cachectic aphthae) K14.0
  Riggs' (compound periodontitis) —*see*
    Periodontitis
  Ritter's L00

Disease, diseased *(Continued)*
  Rivalta's (cervicofacial actinomycosis) A42.2
  rod body G71.21
  Robles' (onchocerciasis) B73.01
  Roger's (congenital interventricular septal
    defect) Q21.0
  Rosenthal's (factor XI deficiency) D68.1
  Ross River B33.1
  Rossbach's (hyperchlorhydria) K31.89
    psychogenic F45.8
  Rotes Quérol —*see* Hyperostosis, ankylosing
  Roth (-Bernhardt) —*see* Mononeuropathy, lower
    limb, meralgia paresthetica
  Runeberg's (progressive pernicious anemia)
    D51.0
  sacroiliac NEC M53.3
  salivary gland or duct K11.9
    inclusion B25.9
    specified NEC K11.8
    virus B25.9
  sandworm B76.9
  Schimmelbusch's —*see* Mastopathy, cystic
  Schmorl's —*see* Schmorl's disease or nodes
  Schönlein (-Henoch) (purpura rheumatica) D69.0
  Schottmüller's —*see* Fever, paratyphoid
  Schultz's (agranulocytosis) —*see*
    Agranulocytosis
  Schwalbe-Ziehen-Oppenheim G24.1
  Schwartz-Jampel G71.13
  sclera H15.9
    specified NEC H15.89
  scrofulous (tuberculous) A18.2
  scrotum N50.9
  sebaceous glands L73.9
  semilunar cartilage, cystic —*see also*
    Derangement, knee, meniscus, cystic
  seminal vesicle N50.9
  serum NEC —*see also* Reaction, serum T80.69
  sexually transmitted A64
    anogenital
      herpesviral infection —*see* Herpes, anogenital
      warts A63.0
    chancroid A57
    chlamydial infection —*see* Chlamydia
    gonorrhea —*see* Gonorrhea
    granuloma inguinale A58
    specified organism NEC A63.8
    syphilis —*see* Syphilis
    trichomoniasis —*see* Trichomoniasis
  Sézary C84.1-●
  shimamushi (scrub typhus) A75.3
  shipyard B30.0
  sickle-cell D57.1
    with
      acute chest syndrome D57.01
      cerebral vascular involvement D57.03
      crisis (painful) D57.00
        with
          complication specified NEC D57.09
          dactylitis D57.04
      dactylitis D57.04
      pain (vaso-occlusive) D57.00
      priapism D57.09
      splenic sequestration D57.02
    elliptocytosis D57.8-●
    Hb-C D57.20
      with
        acute chest syndrome D57.211
        cerebral vascular involvement D57.213
        crisis (painful) D57.219
          with
            dactylitis D57.214
            specified complication NEC
              D57.218
        dactylitis D57.214
        pain (vaso-occlusive) D57.219
        priapism D57.218
        splenic sequestration D57.212
      without crisis D57.20
    Hb-SD D57.80
      with
        acute chest syndrome D57.811
        cerebral vascular involvement D57.813
        crisis (painful) D57.819
          with
            complication specified NEC D57.818
            dactylitis D57.814
        dactylitis D57.814
        pain (vaso-occlusive) D57.819
        splenic sequestration D57.812
      without crisis D57.80

Disease, diseased *(Continued)*
  sickle-cell *(Continued)*
    Hb-SE D57.80
      with
        acute chest syndrome D57.811
        cerebral vascular involvement D57.813
        crisis (painful) D57.819
          with
            complication specified NEC
              D57.818
            dactylitis D57.814
        dactylitis D57.814
        pain (vaso-occlusive) D57.819
        splenic sequestration D57.812
      without crisis D57.80
    specified NEC D57.80
      with
        acute chest syndrome D57.811
        cerebral vascular involvement D57.813
        crisis (painful) D57.819
          with
            complication specified NEC
              D57.818
            dactylitis D57.814
        dactylitis D57.814
        pain (vaso-occlusive) D57.819
        splenic sequestration D57.812
      without crisis D57.80
    spherocytosis D57.80
      with
        acute chest syndrome D57.811
        cerebral vascular involvement D57.813
        crisis (painful) D57.819
          with complication specified NEC
            D57.818
        pain (vaso-occlusive) D57.819
        splenic sequestration D57.812
      without crisis D57.80
    thalassemia D57.40
      with
        acute chest syndrome D57.411
          with dactylitis D57.414
          with specified complication NEC
            D57.418
        cerebral vascular involvement D57.413
        crisis (painful) D57.419
          with specified complication NEC
            D57.418
        dactylitis D57.414
        pain (vaso-occlusive) D57.419
        splenic sequestration D57.412
      beta plus D57.44
        with
          acute chest syndrome D57.451
            with dactylitis D57.454
          cerebral vascular involvement D57.453
          crisis D57.459
            with specified complication NEC
              D57.458
          dactylitis D57.454
          pain (vaso-occlusive) D57.459
          splenic sequestration D57.452
        without crisis D57.44
      beta zero D57.42
        with
          acute chest syndrome D57.431
            with dactylitis D57.434
          cerebral vascular involvement D57.433
          crisis D57.439
            with specified complication NEC
              D57.438
          dactylitis D57.434
          pain (vaso-occlusive) D57.439
          splenic sequestration D57.432
        without crisis D57.42
  silo-filler's J68.8
    bronchitis J68.0
    pneumonitis J68.0
    pulmonary edema J68.1
  simian B B00.4
  Simons' (progressive lipodystrophy) E88.1
  sin nombre virus B33.4
  sinus —*see* Sinusitis
  Sirkari's B55.0
  sixth B08.20
    due to human herpesvirus 6 B08.21
    due to human herpesvirus 7 B08.22
  skin L98.9
    due to metabolic disorder NEC E88.9 *[L99]*
    specified NEC L98.8
  slim (HIV) B20

Disease, diseased (Continued)
small vessel I73.9
Sneddon-Wilkinson (subcorneal pustular
    dermatosis) L13.1
South African creeping B88.0
spinal (cord) G95.9
    congenital Q06.9
    specified NEC G95.89
spine —see also Spondylopathy
    joint —see Dorsopathy
    tuberculous A18.01
spinocerebellar (hereditary) G11.9
    specified NEC G11.8
spleen D73.9
    amyloid E85.4 [D77]
    organic D73.9
    polycystic Q89.09
    postinfectional D73.89
sponge-diver's —see Toxicity, venom, marine
    animal, sea anemone
Startle Q89.8
Steinert's G71.11
Sticker's (erythema infectiosum) B08.3
Stieda's (calcification, knee joint) —see Bursitis,
    tibial collateral
Stokes' (exophthalmic goiter) —see
    Hyperthyroidism, with, goiter (diffuse)
Stokes-Adams (syncope with heart block) I45.9
stomach K31.9
    functional, psychogenic F45.8
    specified NEC K31.89
stonemason's J62.8
storage
    glycogen —see Disease, glycogen storage
    mucopolysaccharide —see
        Mucopolysaccharidosis
striatopallidal system NEC G25.89
Stuart-Prower (congenital factor X deficiency)
    D68.2
Stuart's (congenital factor X deficiency) D68.2
subcutaneous tissue —see Disease, skin
supporting structures of teeth K08.9
    specified NEC K08.89
suprarenal (capsule) (gland) E27.9
    hyperfunction E27.0
    specified NEC E27.8
sweat glands L74.9
    specified NEC L74.8
Sweeley-Klionsky E75.21
Swift (-Feer) —see Poisoning, mercury
swimming-pool granuloma A31.1
Sylvest's (epidemic pleurodynia) B33.0
sympathetic nervous system G90.9
synovium —see Disorder, synovium
syphilitic —see Syphilis
systemic tissue mast cell D47.02
tanapox (virus) B08.71
Tangier E78.6
Tarral-Besnier (pityriasis rubra pilaris) L44.0
Tauri's E74.09
tear duct —see Disorder, lacrimal system
tendon, tendinous —see also Disorder, tendon
    nodular —see Trigger finger
terminal vessel I73.9
testis N50.9
thalassemia Hb-S —see Disease, sickle-cell,
    thalassemia
Thaysen-Gee (nontropical sprue) K90.0
Thomsen G71.12
throat J39.2
    septic J02.0
thromboembolic —see Embolism
thymus (gland) E32.9
    specified NEC E32.8
thyroid (gland) E07.9
    heart —see also Hyperthyroidism E05.90 [I43]
        with thyroid storm E05.91 [I43]
    specified NEC E07.8
Tietze's M94.0
tongue K14.9
    specified NEC K14.89
tonsils, tonsillar (and adenoids) J35.9
tooth, teeth K08.9
    hard tissues K03.9
        specified NEC K03.89
    pulp NEC K04.99
    specified NEC K08.89
Tourette's F95.2
trachea NEC J39.8
tricuspid I07.9
    nonrheumatic I36.9

Disease, diseased (Continued)
triglyceride-storage E75.5
trophoblastic —see Mole, hydatidiform
tsutsugamushi A75.3
tube (fallopian) (noninflammatory) N83.9
    inflammatory —see Salpingitis
    specified NEC N83.8
tuberculous NEC —see Tuberculosis
tubo-ovarian (noninflammatory) N83.9
    inflammatory —see Salpingo-oophoritis
    specified NEC N83.8
tubotympanic, chronic —see Otitis, media,
    suppurative, chronic, tubotympanic
tubulo-interstitial N15.9
    specified NEC N15.8
tympanum —see Disorder, tympanic membrane
Uhl's Q24.8
Underwood's (sclerema neonatorum) P83.0
Unverricht (-Lundborg) —see Epilepsy,
    generalized, idiopathic
Urbach-Oppenheim (necrobiosis lipoidica
    diabeticorum) —see E08-E13 with .620
ureter N28.9
    in (due to)
        schistosomiasis (bilharziasis) B65.0 [N29]
urethra N36.9
    specified NEC N36.8
urinary (tract) N39.9
    bladder N32.9
        specified NEC N32.89
    specified NEC N39.8
uterus (noninflammatory) N85.9
    infective —see Endometritis
    inflammatory —see Endometritis
    specified NEC N85.8
uveal tract (anterior) H21.9
    posterior H31.9
vagabond's B85.1
vagina, vaginal (noninflammatory) N89.9
    inflammatory NEC N76.89
    specified NEC N89.8
valve, valvular I38
    multiple I08.9
        specified NEC I08.8
van Creveld-von Gierke (glycogenosis I) E74.01
vas deferens N50.9
    arteriosclerotic —see Arteriosclerosis
    ciliary body NEC —see Disorder, iris, vascular
    hypertensive —see Hypertension
    iris NEC —see Disorder, iris, vascular
    obliterative I77.1
        peripheral I73.9
    occlusive I99.8
    peripheral (occlusive) I73.9
        in diabetes mellitus —see E08-E13 with .51
vasomotor I73.9
vasospastic I73.9
vein I87.9
venereal —see also Disease, sexually transmitted
    A64
    chlamydial NEC A56.8
        anus A56.3
        genitourinary NOS A56.2
        pharynx A56.4
        rectum A56.3
    fifth A55
    sixth A55
    specified nature or type NEC A63.8
vertebra, vertebral —see also Spondylopathy
    disc —see Disorder, disc
vibration —see Vibration, adverse effects
viral, virus —see also Disease, by type of virus
    B34.9
    arbovirus NOS A94
    arthropod-borne NOS A94
    congenital P35.9
        specified NEC P35.8
    Hanta (with renal manifestations) (Dobrava)
        (Puumala) (Seoul) A98.5
        with pulmonary manifestations (Andes)
            (Bayou) (Bermejo) (Black Creek Canal)
            (Choclo) (Juquitiba) (Laguna negra)
            (Lechiguanas) (New York) (Oran) (Sin
            nombre) B33.4
    Hantaan (Korean hemorrhagic fever)
        A98.5
    human immunodeficiency (HIV) B20
    Kunjin A83.4
    nonarthropod-borne NOS B34.9
    Powassan A84.81
    Rocio (encephalitis) A83.6

Disease, diseased (Continued)
viral, virus (Continued)
    Sin nombre (Hantavirus) (cardio)- pulmonary
        syndrome B33.4
    Tahyna B33.8
    vesicular stomatitis A93.8
vitreous H43.9
    specified NEC H43.89
vocal cord J38.3
Volkmann's, acquired T79.6
von Eulenburg's (congenital paramyotonia)
    G71.19
von Gierke's (glycogenosis I) E74.01
von Graefe's —see Strabismus, paralytic,
    ophthalmoplegia, progressive
von Willebrand (-Jürgens) (angiohemophilia)
    D68.00
    acquired D68.04
    platelet-type D68.09
    pseudo D68.09
    specified NEC D68.09
    type 1 D68.01
    type 1C D68.01
    type 2 D68.029
        type 2A D68.020
        type 2B D68.021
        type 2M D68.022
        type 2N D68.023
    type 3 D68.03
Vrolik's (osteogenesis imperfecta) Q78.0
vulva (noninflammatory) N90.9
    inflammatory NEC N76.89
    specified NEC N90.89
Wallgren's (obstruction of splenic vein with
    collateral circulation) I87.8
Wassilieff's (leptospiral jaundice) A27.0
wasting NEC E88.A
    due to
        malnutrition E43
            with marasmus E41
        underlying condition E88.A
Waterhouse-Friderichsen A39.1
Wegner's (syphilitic osteochondritis) A50.02
Weil's (leptospiral jaundice of lung) A27.0
Weir Mitchell's (erythromelalgia) I73.81
Werdnig-Hoffmann G12.0
Wermer's E31.21
Werner-His (trench fever) A79.0
Werner-Schultz (neutropenic splenomegaly)
    D73.81
Wernicke-Posadas B38.9
whipworm B79
white blood cells D72.9
    specified NEC D72.89
white matter R90.82
white-spot, meaning lichen sclerosus et
    atrophicus L90.0
    penis N48.0
    vulva N90.4
Wilkie's K55.1
Wilkinson-Sneddon (subcorneal pustular
    dermatosis) L13.1
Willis' —see Diabetes
Wilson's (hepatolenticular degeneration) E83.01
woolsorter's A22.1
yaba monkey tumor B08.72
yaba pox (virus) B08.72
Zika virus A92.5
zoonotic, bacterial A28.9
    congenital P35.4
    specified type NEC A28.8
Disfigurement (due to scar) L90.5
Disgerminoma —see Dysgerminoma
DISH (diffuse idiopathic skeletal hyperostosis) —see
    Hyperostosis, ankylosing
Disinsertion, retina —see Detachment, retina
Dislocatable hip, congenital Q65.6
Dislocation (articular)
    with fracture —see Fracture
    acromioclavicular (joint) S43.10-●
        with displacement
            100%-200% S43.12-●
            more than 200% S43.13-●
        inferior S43.14-●
        posterior S43.15-●
    ankle S93.0-●
    astragalus —see Dislocation, ankle
    atlantoaxial S13.121
    atlantooccipital S13.111
    atloidooccipital S13.111
    breast bone S23.29

Dislocation (*Continued*)
- capsule, joint code by site under Dislocation
- carpal (bone) —*see* Dislocation, wrist
- carpometacarpal (joint) NEC S63.05-●
  - thumb S63.04-●
- cartilage (joint) - code by site under Dislocation
- cervical spine (vertebra) —*see* Dislocation, vertebra, cervical
- chronic —*see* Dislocation, recurrent
- clavicle —*see* Dislocation, acromioclavicular joint
- coccyx S33.2
- congenital NEC Q68.8
- coracoid —*see* Dislocation, shoulder
- costal cartilage S23.29
- costochondral S23.29
- cricoarytenoid articulation S13.29
- cricothyroid articulation S13.29
- dorsal vertebra —*see* Dislocation, vertebra, thoracic
- ear ossicle —*see* Discontinuity, ossicles, ear
- elbow S53.10-●
  - congenital Q68.8
  - pathological —*see* Dislocation, pathological NEC, elbow
  - radial head alone —*see* Dislocation, radial head
  - recurrent —*see* Dislocation, recurrent, elbow
  - traumatic S53.10-●
    - anterior S53.11-●
    - lateral S53.14-●
    - medial S53.13-●
    - posterior S53.12-●
    - specified type NEC S53.19-●
- eye, nontraumatic —*see* Luxation, globe
- eyeball, nontraumatic —*see* Luxation, globe
- femur
  - distal end —*see* Dislocation, knee
  - proximal end —*see* Dislocation, hip
- fibula
  - distal end —*see* Dislocation, ankle
  - proximal end —*see* Dislocation, knee
- finger S63.25-●
  - index S63.25-●
  - interphalangeal S63.27-●
    - distal S63.29-●
      - index S63.29-●
      - little S63.29-●
      - middle S63.29-●
      - ring S63.29-●
    - index S63.27-●
    - little S63.27-●
    - middle S63.27-●
    - proximal S63.28-●
      - index S63.28-●
      - little S63.28-●
      - middle S63.28-●
      - ring S63.28-●
    - ring S63.27-●
  - little S63.25-●
  - metacarpophalangeal S63.26-●
    - index S63.26-●
    - little S63.26-●
    - middle S63.26-●
    - ring S63.26-●
  - middle S63.25-●
  - recurrent —*see* Dislocation, recurrent, finger
  - ring S63.25-●
  - thumb —*see* Dislocation, thumb
- foot S93.30-●
  - recurrent —*see* Dislocation, recurrent, foot
  - specified site NEC S93.33-●
  - tarsal joint S93.31-●
  - tarsometatarsal joint S93.32-●
  - toe —*see* Dislocation, toe
- fracture —*see* Fracture
- glenohumeral (joint) —*see* Dislocation, shoulder
- glenoid —*see* Dislocation, shoulder
- habitual —*see* Dislocation, recurrent
- hip S73.00-●
  - anterior S73.03-●
    - obturator S73.02-●
  - central S73.04-●
  - congenital (total) Q65.2
    - bilateral Q65.1
    - partial Q65.5
      - bilateral Q65.4
      - unilateral Q65.3-●
    - unilateral Q65.0-●
  - developmental M24.85-●
  - pathological —*see* Dislocation, pathological NEC, hip

Dislocation (*Continued*)
- hip (*Continued*)
  - posterior S73.01-●
  - recurrent —*see* Dislocation, recurrent, hip
- humerus, proximal end —*see* Dislocation, shoulder
- incomplete —*see* Subluxation, by site
- incus —*see* Discontinuity, ossicles, ear
- infracoracoid —*see* Dislocation, shoulder
- innominate (pubic junction) (sacral junction) S33.39
  - acetabulum —*see* Dislocation, hip
- interphalangeal (joint(s))
  - finger S63.279
    - distal S63.29-●
      - index S63.29-●
      - little S63.29-●
      - middle S63.29-●
      - ring S63.29-●
    - index S63.27-●
    - little S63.27-●
    - middle S63.27-●
    - proximal S63.28-●
      - index S63.28-●
      - little S63.28-●
      - middle S63.28-●
      - ring S63.28-●
    - ring S63.27-●
  - foot or toe —*see* Dislocation, toe
  - thumb S63.12-●
- jaw (cartilage) (meniscus) S03.0-●
- joint prosthesis —*see* Complications, joint prosthesis, mechanical, displacement, by site
- knee S83.106
  - cap —*see* Dislocation, patella
  - congenital Q68.2
  - old M23.8X-●
  - patella —*see* Dislocation, patella
  - pathological —*see* Dislocation, pathological NEC, knee
  - proximal tibia
    - anteriorly S83.11-●
    - laterally S83.14-●
    - medially S83.13-●
    - posteriorly S83.12-●
  - recurrent —*see also* Derangement, knee, specified NEC
  - specified type NEC S83.19-●
- lacrimal gland H04.16-●
- lens (complete) H27.10-●
  - anterior H27.12-●
  - congenital Q12.1
  - ocular implant —*see* Complications, intraocular lens
  - partial H27.11-●
  - posterior H27.13-●
  - traumatic S05.8X-●
- ligament code by site under Dislocation
- lumbar (vertebra) —*see* Dislocation, vertebra, lumbar
- lumbosacral (vertebra) —*see also* Dislocation, vertebra, lumbar
  - congenital Q76.49
- mandible S03.0-●
- meniscus (knee) —*see* Tear, meniscus
  - other sites code by site under Dislocation
- metacarpal (bone)
  - distal end —*see* Dislocation, finger
  - proximal end S63.06-●
- metacarpophalangeal (joint)
  - finger S63.26-●
    - index S63.26-●
    - little S63.26-●
    - middle S63.26-●
    - ring S63.26-●
  - thumb S63.11-●
- metatarsal (bone) —*see* Dislocation, foot
- metatarsophalangeal (joint(s)) —*see* Dislocation, toe
- midcarpal (joint) S63.03-●
- midtarsal (joint) —*see* Dislocation, foot
- neck S13.20
  - specified site NEC S13.29
  - vertebra —*see* Dislocation, vertebra, cervical
- nose (septal cartilage) S03.1
- occipitoatloid S13.111
- old —*see* Derangement, joint, specified type NEC
- ossicles, ear —*see* Discontinuity, ossicles, ear
- partial —*see* Subluxation, by site

Dislocation (*Continued*)
- patella S83.006
  - congenital Q74.1
  - lateral S83.01-●
  - recurrent (nontraumatic) M22.0-●
    - incomplete M22.1-●
  - specified type NEC S83.09-●
- pathological NEC M24.30
  - ankle M24.37-●
  - elbow M24.32-●
  - foot joint M24.37-●
  - hand joint M24.34-●
  - hip M24.35-●
  - knee M24.36-●
  - lumbosacral joint —*see* subcategory M53.2
  - pelvic region —*see* Dislocation, pathological, hip
  - sacroiliac —*see* subcategory M53.2
  - shoulder M24.31-●
  - specified site NEC M24.39
  - wrist M24.33-●
- pelvis NEC S33.30
  - specified NEC S33.39
- phalanx
  - finger or hand —*see* Dislocation, finger
  - foot or toe —*see* Dislocation, toe
- prosthesis, internal —*see* Complications, prosthetic device, by site, mechanical
- radial head S53.006
  - anterior S53.01-●
  - posterior S53.02-●
  - specified type NEC S53.09-●
- radiocarpal (joint) S63.02-●
- radiohumeral (joint) —*see* Dislocation, radial head
- radioulnar (joint)
  - distal S63.01-●
  - proximal —*see* Dislocation, elbow
- radius
  - distal end —*see* Dislocation, wrist
  - proximal end —*see* Dislocation, radial head
- recurrent M24.40
  - ankle M24.47-●
  - elbow M24.42-●
  - finger M24.44-●
  - foot joint M24.47-●
  - hand joint M24.44-●
  - hip M24.45-●
  - knee M24.46-●
    - patella —*see* Dislocation, patella, recurrent
  - patella —*see* Dislocation, patella, recurrent
  - sacroiliac —*see* subcategory M53.2
  - shoulder M24.41-●
  - specified site NEC M24.49
  - toe M24.47-●
  - vertebra —*see also* subcategory M43.5
    - atlantoaxial M43.4
      - with myelopathy M43.3
  - wrist M24.43-●
- rib (cartilage) S23.29
- sacrococcygeal S33.2
- sacroiliac (joint) (ligament) S33.2
  - congenital Q74.2
  - recurrent —*see* subcategory M53.2
- sacrum S33.2
- scaphoid (bone) (hand) (wrist) —*see* Dislocation, wrist
  - foot —*see* Dislocation, foot
- scapula —*see* Dislocation, shoulder, girdle, scapula
- semilunar cartilage, knee —*see* Tear, meniscus
- septal cartilage (nose) S03.1
- septum (nasal) (old) J34.2
- sesamoid bone code by site under Dislocation
- shoulder (blade) (ligament) (joint) (traumatic) S43.006
  - acromioclavicular —*see* Dislocation, acromioclavicular
  - chronic —*see* Dislocation, recurrent, shoulder
  - congenital Q68.8
  - girdle S43.30-●
    - scapula S43.31-●
    - specified site NEC S43.39-●
  - humerus S43.00-●
    - anterior S43.01-●
    - inferior S43.03-●
    - posterior S43.02-●
  - pathological —*see* Dislocation, pathological NEC, shoulder
  - recurrent —*see* Dislocation, recurrent, shoulder
  - specified type NEC S43.08-●

▶ New　　➡ Revised　　~~deleted~~ Deleted　　● Use Additional Character(s)

Dislocation (Continued)

spine
  cervical —see Dislocation, vertebra, cervical
  congenital Q76.49
  due to birth trauma P11.5
  lumbar —see Dislocation, vertebra, lumbar
  thoracic —see Dislocation, vertebra,
    thoracic
spontaneous —see Dislocation, pathological
sternoclavicular (joint) S43.206
  anterior S43.21-●
  posterior S43.22-●
sternum S23.29
subglenoid —see Dislocation, shoulder
symphysis pubis S33.4
talus —see Dislocation, ankle
tarsal (bone(s)) (joint(s)) —see Dislocation, foot
tarsometatarsal (joint(s)) —see Dislocation, foot
temporomandibular (joint) S03.0-●
thigh, proximal end —see Dislocation, hip
thorax S23.20
  specified site NEC S23.29
  vertebra —see Dislocation, vertebra
thumb S63.10-●
  interphalangeal joint —see Dislocation,
    interphalangeal (joint), thumb
  metacarpophalangeal joint —see Dislocation,
    metacarpophalangeal (joint), thumb
thyroid cartilage S13.29
tibia
  distal end —see Dislocation, ankle
  proximal end —see Dislocation, knee
tibiofibular (joint)
  distal —see Dislocation, ankle
  superior —see Dislocation, knee
toe(s) S93.106
  great S93.10-●
    interphalangeal joint S93.11-●
    metatarsophalangeal joint S93.12-●
  interphalangeal joint S93.119
  lesser S93.106
    interphalangeal joint S93.11-●
    metatarsophalangeal joint S93.12-●
  metatarsophalangeal joint S93.12-●
tooth S03.2
trachea S23.29
ulna
  distal end S63.07-●
  proximal end —see Dislocation, elbow
ulnohumeral (joint) —see Dislocation, elbow
vertebra (articular process) (body)
  (traumatic)
  cervical S13.101
    atlantoaxial joint S13.121
    atlantooccipital joint S13.111
    atloidooccipital joint S13.111
    joint between
      C0 and C1 S13.111
      C1 and C2 S13.121
      C2 and C3 S13.131
      C3 and C4 S13.141
      C4 and C5 S13.151
      C5 and C6 S13.161
      C6 and C7 S13.171
      C7 and T1 S13.181
    occipitoatloid joint S13.111
  congenital Q76.49
  lumbar S33.101
    joint between
      L1 and L2 S33.111
      L2 and L3 S33.121
      L3 and L4 S33.131
      L4 and L5 S33.141
  nontraumatic —see Displacement,
    intervertebral disc
  partial —see Subluxation, by site
  recurrent NEC —see subcategory M43.5
  thoracic S23.101
    joint between
      T1 and T2 S23.111
      T2 and T3 S23.121
      T3 and T4 S23.123
      T4 and T5 S23.131
      T5 and T6 S23.133
      T6 and T7 S23.141
      T7 and T8 S23.143
      T8 and T9 S23.151
      T9 and T10 S23.153
      T10 and T11 S23.161
      T11 and T12 S23.163
      T12 and L1 S23.171

Dislocation (Continued)

wrist (carpal bone) S63.006
  carpometacarpal joint —see Dislocation,
    carpometacarpal (joint)
  distal radioulnar joint —see Dislocation,
    radioulnar (joint), distal
  metacarpal bone, proximal —see Dislocation,
    metacarpal (bone), proximal end
  midcarpal —see Dislocation, midcarpal (joint)
  radiocarpal joint —see Dislocation, radiocarpal
    (joint)
  recurrent —see Dislocation, recurrent, wrist
  specified site NEC S63.09-●
  ulna —see Dislocation, ulna, distal end
xiphoid cartilage S23.29
Disorder (of) —see also Disease
acantholytic L11.9
  specified NEC L11.8
acute
  psychotic —see Psychosis, acute
  stress F43.0
adjustment (grief) F43.20
  with
    anxiety F43.22
      with depressed mood F43.23
    conduct disturbance F43.24
      with emotional disturbance F43.25
    depressed mood F43.21
      with anxiety F43.23
    other specified symptom F43.29
adrenal (capsule) (gland) (medullary) E27.9
  specified NEC E27.8
adrenogenital (see also Adrenogenital syndrome)
  E25.9
  drug-induced E25.8
  iatrogenic E25.8
  idiopathic E25.8
adult personality (and behavior) F69
  specified NEC F68.8
affective (mood) —see Disorder, mood
aggressive, unsocialized F91.1
alcohol-related F10.99
  with
    amnestic disorder, persisting F10.96
    anxiety disorder F10.980
    dementia, persisting F10.97
    intoxication F10.929
      with delirium F10.921
      uncomplicated F10.920
    mood disorder F10.94
    other specified F10.988
    psychotic disorder F10.959
      with
        delusions F10.950
        hallucinations F10.951
    sexual dysfunction F10.981
    sleep disorder F10.982
alcohol use
  mild F10.10
    with
      alcohol-induced
        anxiety disorder F10.180
        bipolar and related disorder F10.14
        depressive disorder F10.14
        psychotic disorder F10.159
        sexual dysfunction F10.181
        sleep disorder F10.182
      alcohol intoxication F10.129
        delirium F10.121
    in remission (early) (sustained) F10.11
  moderate or severe F10.20
    with
      alcohol-induced
        anxiety disorder F10.280
        bipolar and related disorder F10.24
        depressive disorder F10.24
        major neurocognitive disorder,
          amnestic-confabulatory type
          F10.26
        major neurocognitive disorder,
          nonamnestic-confabulatory type
          F10.27
        mild neurocognitive disorder F10.288
        psychotic disorder F10.259
        sexual dysfunction F10.281
        sleep disorder F10.282
      alcohol intoxication F10.229
        delirium F10.221
    in remission (early) (sustained) F10.21
allergic —see Allergy
alveolar NEC J84.09

Disorder (Continued)

amino-acid
  cystathioninuria E72.19
  cystinosis E72.04
  cystinuria E72.01
  glycinuria E72.09
  homocystinuria E72.11
  metabolism —see Disturbance,
    metabolism, amino-acid
  specified NEC E72.89
  neonatal, transitory P74.8
  renal transport NEC E72.09
  transport NEC E72.09
amnesic, amnestic
  alcohol-induced F10.96
    with dependence F10.26
  due to (secondary to) general medical
    condition F04
  psychoactive NEC-induced F19.96
    with
      abuse F19.16
      dependence F19.26
  sedative, hypnotic or anxiolytic-●
    induced F13.96
    with dependence F13.26
amphetamine-type substance use
  mild F15.10
    in remission (early) (sustained) F15.11
  moderate F15.20
    in remission (early) (sustained) F15.21
  severe F15.20
    in remission (early) (sustained) F15.21
amphetamine (or other stimulant) use
  mild
    with
      amphetamine (or other stimulant)
        -induced
        anxiety disorder F15.180
        bipolar and related disorder F15.14
        depressive disorder F15.14
        obsessive-compulsive and related
          disorder F15.188
        psychotic disorder F15.159
        sexual dysfunction F15.181
      amphetamine, cocaine, or other
        stimulant intoxication
        with perceptual disturbances F15.122
        without perceptual disturbances
          F15.129
      intoxication delirium F15.121
  moderate or severe
    with
      amphetamine (or other stimulant)
        -induced
        anxiety disorder F15.280
        obsessive-compulsive and related
          disorder F15.288
        sexual dysfunction F15.281
        bipolar and related disorder F15.24
        depressive disorder F15.24
        psychotic disorder F15.259
      amphetamine, cocaine, or other
        stimulant intoxication
        with perceptual disturbances
          F15.222
        without perceptual disturbances
          F15.229
      intoxication delirium F15.221
anaerobic glycolysis with anemia D55.29
anxiety F41.9
  due to (secondary to)
    alcohol F10.980
      in
        abuse F10.180
        dependence F10.280
    amphetamine F15.980
      in
        abuse F15.180
        dependence F15.280
    anxiolytic F13.980
      in
        abuse F13.180
        dependence F13.280
    caffeine F15.980
      in
        abuse F15.180
        dependence F15.280
    cannabis F12.980
      in
        abuse F12.180
        dependence F12.280

Disorder *(Continued)*
  anxiety *(Continued)*
    due to *(Continued)*
      cocaine F14.980
        in
          abuse F14.180
          dependence F14.180
      general medical condition F06.4
      hallucinogen F16.980
        in
          abuse F16.180
          dependence F16.280
      hypnotic F13.980
        in
          abuse F13.180
          dependence F13.280
      inhalant F18.980
        in
          abuse F18.180
          dependence F18.280
      phencyclidine F16.980
        in
          abuse F16.180
          dependence F16.280
      psychoactive substance NEC F19.980
        in
          abuse F19.180
          dependence F19.280
      sedative F13.980
        in
          abuse F13.180
          dependence F13.280
      volatile solvents F18.980
        in
          abuse F18.180
          dependence F18.280
    generalized F41.1
    illness F45.21
    mixed
      with depression (mild) F41.8
      specified NEC F41.3
    organic F06.4
    phobic F40.9
      of childhood F40.8
    specified NEC F41.8
  aortic valve —*see* Endocarditis, aortic
  aromatic amino-acid metabolism E70.9
    specified NEC E70.89
  arteriole NEC I77.89
  artery NEC I77.89
  articulation —*see* Disorder, joint
  attachment (childhood)
    disinhibited F94.2
    reactive F94.1
  attention-deficit hyperactivity (adolescent)
      (adult) (child) F98.8
    combined
      presentation F90.2
      type F90.2
    hyperactive
      impulsive presentation F90.1
      type F90.1
    inattentive
      presentation F90.0
      type F90.0
    specified type NEC F90.8
  attention-deficit without hyperactivity
      (adolescent) (adult) (child) F90.0
  auditory processing (central) H93.25
  autism spectrum F84.0
  autistic F84.0
  autoimmune D89.89
  autonomic nervous system G90.9
    ⇒specified NEC G90.89
  avoidant
    child or adolescent F40.10
    restrictive food intake F50.82
  balance
    acid-base E87.8
      mixed E87.4
    electrolyte E87.8
    fluid NEC E87.8
  behavioral (disruptive) —*see* Disorder, conduct
  bereavement, persistent complex F43.81
  beta-amino-acid metabolism E72.89
  bile acid and cholesterol metabolism E78.70
    Barth syndrome E78.71
    other specified E78.79
    Smith-Lemli-Opitz syndrome E78.72
  bilirubin excretion E80.6
  ⇒binge eating F50.81-●

Disorder *(Continued)*
  binocular
    movement H51.9
      convergence
        excess H51.12
        insufficiency H51.11
      internuclear ophthalmoplegia —*see*
        Ophthalmoplegia, internuclear
      palsy of conjugate gaze H51.0
      specified type NEC H51.8
    vision NEC —*see* Disorder, vision, binocular
  bipolar (I) (seasonal) (type 1) F31.9
    and related due to a known physiological
        condition
      with
        manic features F06.33
        manic- or hypomanic-like episodes
            F06.33
        mixed features F06.34
    current (or most recent) episode
      depressed F31.9
        with psychotic features F31.5
        without psychotic features F31.30
          mild F31.31
          moderate F31.32
          severe (without psychotic features)
              F31.4
            with psychotic features F31.5
      hypomanic F31.0
      manic F31.9
        with psychotic features F31.2
        without psychotic features F31.10
          mild F31.11
          moderate F31.12
          severe (without psychotic features)
              F31.13
            with psychotic features F31.2
      mixed F31.60
        mild F31.61
        moderate F31.62
        severe (without psychotic features)
            F31.63
          with psychotic features F31.64
        severe depression (without psychotic
            features) F31.4
          with psychotic features F31.5
    II (type 2) F31.81
    in remission (currently) F31.70
      in full remission
        most recent episode
          depressed F31.76
          hypomanic F31.72
          manic F31.74
          mixed F31.78
      in partial remission
        most recent episode
          depressed F31.75
          hypomanic F31.71
          manic F31.73
          mixed F31.77
    organic F06.30
    single manic episode F30.9
      mild F30.11
      moderate F30.12
      hhsevere (without psychotic symptoms)
          F30.13
        with psychotic symptoms F30.2
    specified NEC F31.89
  bladder N32.9
    functional NEC N31.9
    in schistosomiasis B65.0 *[N33]*
    specified NEC N32.89
  bleeding D68.9
  blood D75.9
    in congenital early syphilis A50.09 *[D77]*
  body dysmorphic F45.22
  bone M89.9
    continuity M84.9
      specified type NEC M84.80
        ankle M84.87-●
        fibula M84.86-●
        foot M84.87-●
        hand M84.84-●
        humerus M84.82-●
        neck M84.88
        pelvis M84.859
        radius M84.83-●
        rib M84.88
        shoulder M84.81-●
        skull M84.88
        thigh M84.85-●

Disorder *(Continued)*
  bone *(Continued)*
    continuity *(Continued)*
      specified type *(Continued)*
        tibia M84.86-●
        ulna M84.83-●
        vertebra M84.88
    density and structure M85.9
      cyst —*see also* Cyst, bone, specified type
          NEC
        aneurysmal —*see* Cyst, bone,
            aneurysmal
        solitary —*see* Cyst, bone, solitary
      diffuse idiopathic skeletal hyperostosis —
          see Hyperostosis, ankylosing
      fibrous dysplasia (monostotic) —*see*
          Dysplasia, fibrous, bone
      fluorosis —*see* Fluorosis, skeletal
      hyperostosis of skull M85.2
      osteitis condensans —*see* Osteitis,
          condensans
      specified type NEC M85.8-●
        ankle M85.87-●
        foot M85.87-●
        forearm M85.83-●
        hand M85.84-●
        lower leg M85.86-●
        multiple sites M85.89
        neck M85.88
        rib M85.88
        shoulder M85.81-●
        skull M85.88
        thigh M85.85-●
        upper arm M85.82-●
        vertebra M85.88
    development and growth NEC M89.20
      carpus M89.24-●
      clavicle M89.21-●
      femur M89.25-●
      fibula M89.26-●
      finger M89.24-●
      humerus M89.22-●
      ilium M89.28
      ischium M89.28
      metacarpus M89.24-●
      metatarsus M89.27-●
      multiple sites M89.29
      neck M89.28
      radius M89.23-●
      rib M89.28
      scapula M89.21-●
      skull M89.28
      tarsus M89.27-●
      tibia M89.26-●
      toe M89.27-●
      ulna M89.23-●
      vertebra M89.28
    specified type NEC M89.8X-●
  brachial plexus G54.0
  branched-chain amino-acid metabolism E71.2
    specified NEC E71.19
  breast N64.9
    agalactia —*see* Agalactia
    associated with
      lactation O92.70
        specified NEC O92.79
      pregnancy O92.20
        specified NEC O92.29
      puerperium O92.20
        specified NEC O92.29
    cracked nipple —*see* Cracked nipple
    galactorrhea —*see* Galactorrhea
    hypogalactia O92.4
    lactation disorder NEC O92.79
    mastitis —*see* Mastitis
    nipple infection —*see* Infection, nipple
    retracted nipple —*see* Retraction, nipple
    specified type NEC N64.89
  Briquet's F45.0
  bullous, in diseases classified elsewhere L14
  caffeine use
    mild
      with
        caffeine-induced
          anxiety disorder F15.180
          sleep disorder F15.182
    moderate or severe
      with
        caffeine-induced
          anxiety disorder F15.280
          sleep disorder F15.282

▶ New   ⇒ Revised   ~~deleted~~ Deleted   ● Use Additional Character(s)

Disorder (Continued)
  cannabis use
    mild F12.10
      with
        cannabis-induced
          anxiety disorder F12.180
          psychotic disorder F12.159
          sleep disorder F12.188
        cannabis intoxication delirium F12.121
          with perceptual disturbances F12.122
          without perceptual disturbances
            F12.129
      in remission (early) (sustained) F12.11
    moderate or severe F12.20
      with
        cannabis-induced
          anxiety disorder F12.280
          psychotic disorder F12.259
          sleep disorder F12.288
        cannabis intoxication
          with perceptual disturbances F12.222
          without perceptual disturbances
            F12.229
          delirium F12.221
      in remission (early) (sustained) F12.21
  carbohydrate
    absorption, intestinal NEC E74.39
    metabolism (congenital) E74.9
      specified NEC E74.89
  cardiac, functional I51.89
  carnitine metabolism E71.40
  cartilage M94.9
    articular NEC —see Derangement, joint,
      articular cartilage
    chondrocalcinosis —see Chondrocalcinosis
    specified type NEC M94.8X-●
      articular —see Derangement, joint, articular
        cartilage
      multiple sites M94.8X0
  catatonia (due to known physiological condition)
    (with another mental disorder) F06.1
  catatonic
    due to (secondary to) known physiological
      condition F06.1
    organic F06.1
  ▶catatonic NOS F06.1
    ▶due to (secondary to) known physiological
      condition F06.1
    ▶organic NOS F06.1
  central auditory processing H93.25
  cervical
    region NEC M53.82
    root (nerve) NEC G54.2
  character NOS F60.9
  childhood disintegrative NEC F84.3
  cholesterol and bile acid metabolism E78.70
    Barth syndrome E78.71
    other specified E78.79
    Smith-Lemli-Opitz syndrome E78.72
  choroid H31.9
    atrophy —see Atrophy, choroid
    degeneration —see Degeneration, choroid
    detachment —see Detachment, choroid
    dystrophy —see Dystrophy, choroid
    hemorrhage —see Hemorrhage, choroid
    rupture —see Rupture, choroid
    scar —see Scar, chorioretinal
    solar retinopathy —see Retinopathy, solar
    specified type NEC H31.8
  ciliary body —see Disorder, iris
    degeneration —see Degeneration, ciliary body
  ▶citrate metabolism NEC E74.829
  ▶citrate transporter, SLC13A5 E74.820
  coagulation (factor) (see also Defect, coagulation)
    D68.9
    newborn, transient P61.6
  cocaine use
    mild F14.10
      with
        amphetamine, cocaine, or other
          stimulant intoxication
          with perceptual disturbances F14.122
          without perceptual disturbances
            F14.129
        cocaine-induced
          anxiety disorder F14.180
          bipolar and related disorder F14.14
          depressive disorder F14.14
          obsessive-compulsive and related
            disorder F14.188
          psychotic disorder F14.159

Disorder (Continued)
  cocaine use (Continued)
    mild (Continued)
      with (Continued)
        cocaine-induced (Continued)
          sexual dysfunction F14.181
          sleep disorder F14.182
        cocaine intoxication delirium F14.121
      in remission (early) (sustained) F14.11
    moderate or severe F14.20
      with
        amphetamine, cocaine, or other
          stimulant intoxication
          with perceptual disturbances F14.222
          without perceptual disturbances F14.229
        cocaine-induced
          anxiety disorder F14.280
          bipolar and related disorder F14.24
          depressive disorder F14.24
          obsessive-compulsive and related
            disorder F14.288
          psychotic disorder F14.259
          sexual dysfunction F14.281
          sleep disorder F14.282
        cocaine intoxication delirium F14.221
      in remission (early) (sustained) F14.21
  coccyx NEC M53.3
  cognitive F09
    due to (secondary to) general medical
      condition F09
    persisting R41.89
      due to
        alcohol F10.97
          with dependence F10.27
        anxiolytics F13.97
          with dependence F13.27
        hypnotics F13.97
          with dependence F13.27
        sedatives F13.97
          with dependence F13.27
        specified substance NEC F19.97
          with
            abuse F19.17
            dependence F19.27
  communication F80.9
    social pragmatic F80.82
  conduct (childhood) F91.9
    adjustment reaction —see Disorder,
      adjustment
    adolescent onset type F91.2
    childhood onset type F91.1
    compulsive F63.9
    confined to family context F91.0
    depressive F91.8
    group type F91.2
    hyperkinetic —see Disorder, attention-deficit
      hyperactivity
    oppositional defiance F91.3
    socialized F91.2
    solitary aggressive type F91.1
    specified NEC F91.8
    unsocialized (aggressive) F91.1
  conduction, heart I45.9
  congenital glycosylation (CDG) E74.89
  conjunctiva H11.9
    infection —see Conjunctivitis
  connective tissue, localized L94.9
    specified NEC L94.8
  conversion (functional neurological symptom
    disorder)
    with
      abnormal movement F44.4
      anesthesia or sensory loss F44.6
      attacks or seizures F44.5
      mixed symptoms F44.7
      special sensory symptoms F44.6
      speech symptoms F44.4
      swallowing symptoms F44.4
      weakness or paralysis F44.4
  convulsive (secondary) —see Convulsions
  cornea H18.9
    deformity —see Deformity, cornea
    degeneration —see Degeneration, cornea
    deposits —see Deposit, cornea
    due to contact lens H18.82-●
      specified as edema —see Edema, cornea
    edema —see Edema, cornea
    keratitis —see Keratitis
    keratoconjunctivitis —see Keratoconjunctivitis
    membrane change —see Change, corneal
      membrane

Disorder (Continued)
  cornea (Continued)
    neovascularization —see Neovascularization,
      cornea
    scar —see Opacity, cornea
    specified type NEC H18.89-●
    ulcer —see Ulcer, cornea
  corpus cavernosum N48.9
  cranial nerve —see Disorder, nerve, cranial
  Cyclin-Dependent Kinase-Like 5 Deficiency
    (CDKL5) G40.42
  cyclothymic F34.0
  defiant oppositional F91.3
  delusional (persistent) (systematized) F22
    induced F24
  depersonalization F48.1
  depressive F32.A
    due to known physiological condition
      with
        depressive features F06.31
        major depressive-like episode F06.32
        mixed features F06.34
    major F32.9
      with psychotic symptoms F32.3
      in remission (full) F32.5
        partial F32.4
      recurrent F33.9
        with psychotic features F33.3
      single episode F32.9
        mild F32.0
        moderate F32.1
        severe (without psychotic symptoms)
          F32.2
          with psychotic symptoms F32.3
    organic F06.31
    persistent F34.1
    recurrent F33.9
      current episode
        mild F33.0
        moderate F33.1
        severe (without psychotic symptoms)
          F33.2
          with psychotic symptoms F33.3
      in remission F33.40
        full F33.42
        partial F33.41
      specified NEC F33.8
    single episode —see Episode, depressive
    specified NEC F32.89
  developmental F89
    arithmetical skills F81.2
    coordination (motor) F82
    expressive writing F81.81
    language F80.9
      expressive F80.1
      mixed receptive and expressive F80.2
      receptive type F80.2
      specified NEC F80.89
    learning F81.9
      arithmetical F81.2
      reading F81.0
    mixed F88
    motor coordination or function F82
    pervasive F84.9
      specified NEC F84.8
    phonological F80.0
    reading F81.0
    scholastic skills —see also Disorder,
      learning
      mixed F81.89
    specified NEC F88
    speech F80.9
      articulation F80.0
      specified NEC F80.89
    written expression F81.81
  diaphragm J98.6
  digestive (system) K92.9
    newborn P78.9
      specified NEC P78.89
    postprocedural —see Complication,
      gastrointestinal
    psychogenic F45.8
  disc (intervertebral) M51.9
    with
      myelopathy
        cervical region M50.00
        cervicothoracic region M50.03
        high cervical region M50.01
        lumbar region M51.06
        mid-cervical region M50.020
        sacrococcygeal region M53.3

Disorder *(Continued)*
  disc (intervertebral) *(Continued)*
    with *(Continued)*
      myelopathy *(Continued)*
        thoracic region M51.04
        thoracolumbar region M51.05
      radiculopathy
        cervical region M50.10
        cervicothoracic region M50.13
        high cervical region M50.11
        lumbar region M51.16
        lumbosacral region M51.17
        mid-cervical region M50.120
        sacrococcygeal region M53.3
        thoracic region M51.14
        thoracolumbar region M51.15
  cervical M50.90
    with
      myelopathy M50.00
        C2-C3 M50.01
        C3-C4 M50.01
        C4-C5 M50.021
        C5-C6 M50.022
        C6-C7 M50.023
        C7-T1 M50.03
        cervicothoracic region M50.03
        high cervical region M50.01
        mid-cervical region M50.020
      neuritis, radiculitis or radiculopathy M50.10
        C2-C3 M50.11
        C3-C4 M50.11
        C4-C5 M50.121
        C5-C6 M50.122
        C6-C7 M50.123
        C7-T1 M50.13
        cervicothoracic region M50.13
        high cervical region M50.11
        mid-cervical region M50.120
    C2-C3 M50.91
    C3-C4 M50.91
    C4-C5 M50.921
    C5-C6 M50.922
    C6-C7 M50.923
    C7-T1 M50.93
    cervicothoracic region M50.93
    degeneration M50.30
      C2-C3 M50.31
      C3-C4 M50.31
      C4-C5 M50.321
      C5-C6 M50.322
      C6-C7 M50.323
      C7-T1 M50.33
      cervicothoracic region M50.33
      high cervical region M50.31
      mid-cervical region M50.320
    displacement M50.20
      C2-C3 M50.21
      C3-C4 M50.21
      C4-C5 M50.221
      C5-C6 M50.222
      C6-C7 M50.223
      C7-T1 M50.23
      cervicothoracic region M50.23
      high cervical region M50.21
      mid-cervical region M50.220
    high cervical region M50.91
    mid-cervical region M50.920
    specified type NEC M50.80
      C2-C3 M50.81
      C3-C4 M50.81
      C4-C5 M50.821
      C5-C6 M50.822
      C6-C7 M50.823
      C7-T1 M50.83
      cervicothoracic region M50.83
      high cervical region M50.81
      mid-cervical region M50.820
  specified NEC
    lumbar region M51.86
    lumbosacral region M51.87
    sacrococcygeal region M53.3
    thoracic region M51.84
    thoracolumbar region M51.85
  disinhibited attachment (childhood) F94.2
  disintegrative, childhood NEC F84.3
  disruptive F91.9
    mood dysregulation F34.81
    specified NEC F91.8
  disruptive behavior —*see* Disorder, conduct
  dissocial personality F60.2

Disorder *(Continued)*
  dissociative F44.9
    affecting
      motor function F44.4
        and sensation F44.7
      sensation F44.6
        and motor function F44.7
    brief reactive F43.0
    due to (secondary to) general medical condition F06.8
    mixed F44.7
    organic F06.8
    other specified NEC F44.89
  double heterozygous sickling —*see* Disease, sickle-cell
  dream anxiety F51.5
  drug induced hemorrhagic D68.32
  drug related F19.99
    abuse —*see* Abuse, drug
    dependence —*see* Dependence, drug
  dysmorphic body F45.22
  dysthymic F34.1
  ear H93.9-●
    bleeding —*see* Otorrhagia
    deafness —*see* Deafness
    degenerative H93.09-●
    discharge —*see* Otorrhea
    external H61.9-●
      auditory canal stenosis —*see* Stenosis, external ear canal
      exostosis —*see* Exostosis, external ear canal
      impacted cerumen —*see* Impaction, cerumen
      otitis —*see* Otitis, externa
      perichondritis —*see* Perichondritis, ear
      pinna —*see* Disorder, pinna
      specified type NEC H61.89-●
        in diseases classified elsewhere H62.8X-●
    inner H83.9-●
      vestibular dysfunction —*see* Disorder, vestibular function
    middle H74.9-●
      adhesive H74.1-●
      ossicle —*see* Abnormal, ear ossicles
      polyp —*see* Polyp, ear (middle)
      specified NEC, in diseases classified elsewhere H75.8-●
    postprocedural —*see* Complications, ear, procedure
    specified NEC, in diseases classified elsewhere H94.8-●
  eating (adult) (psychogenic) F50.9
    anorexia —*see* Anorexia
    binge F50.81-●
    bulimia F50.2-●
    child F98.29
      pica (in remission) F98.3
      rumination disorder (in remission) F98.21
    pica F50.89
      adult (in remission)
      childhood (in remission) F98.3
      specified NEC F50.89
    rumination (see also Rumination) R11.10
      adult (in remission) F50.84
      infancy or childhood (in remission) F98.21
  electrolyte (balance) NEC E87.8
    with
      abortion —*see* Abortion by type
        complicated by specified condition NEC
      ectopic pregnancy O08.5
      molar pregnancy O08.5
    acidosis (metabolic) (respiratory) E87.2
    alkalosis (lactic) (metabolic) E87.20
      acute E87.21
      chronic E87.22
      respiratory E87.29
      specified NEC E87.29
  elimination, transepidermal L87.9
    specified NEC L87.8
  emotional (persistent) F34.9
    of childhood F93.9
      specified NEC F93.8
  endocrine E34.9
    postprocedural E89.89
      specified NEC E89.89
  erectile (male) (organic) —*see also* Dysfunction, sexual, male, erectile N52.9
    nonorganic F52.21
  erythematous —*see* Erythema

Disorder *(Continued)*
  esophagus K22.9
    functional K22.4
    psychogenic F45.8
  eustachian tube H69.9-●
    infection —*see* Salpingitis, eustachian
    obstruction —*see* Obstruction, eustachian tube
    patulous —*see* Patulous, eustachian tube
    specified NEC H69.8-●
  exhibitionistic F65.2
  extrapyramidal G25.9
    in diseases classified elsewhere —*see* category G26
    specified type NEC G25.89
  eye H57.9
    postprocedural —*see* Complication, postprocedural, eye
  eyelid H02.9
    cyst —*see* Cyst, eyelid
    degenerative H02.70
      chloasma —*see* Chloasma, eyelid
      madarosis —*see* Madarosis
      specified type NEC H02.79
      vitiligo —*see* Vitiligo, eyelid
      xanthelasma —*see* Xanthelasma
    dermatochalasis —*see* Dermato-chalasis
    edema —*see* Edema, eyelid
    elephantiasis —*see* Elephantiasis, eyelid
    foreign body, retained —*see* Foreign body, retained, eyelid
    function H02.59
      abnormal innervation syndrome — *see* Syndrome, abnormal innervation
      blepharochalasis —*see* Blepharochalasis
      blepharoclonus —*see* Blepharoclonus
      blepharophimosis —*see* Blepharophimosis
      blepharoptosis —*see* Blepharoptosis
      lagophthalmos —*see* Lagophthalmos
      lid retraction —*see* Retraction, lid
    hypertrichosis —*see* Hypertrichosis, eyelid
    specified type NEC H02.89
    vascular H02.879
      left H02.876
        lower H02.875
        upper H02.874
      right H02.873
        lower H02.872
        upper H02.871
  factitious
    by proxy F68.A
    imposed on another F68.A
    imposed on self F68.10
      with predominantly
        psychological symptoms F68.11
          with physical symptoms F68.13
        physical symptoms F68.12
          with psychological symptoms F68.13
  factor, coagulation —*see* Defect, coagulation
  fatty acid
    metabolism E71.30
      specified NEC E71.39
    oxidation
      LCAD E71.310
      MCAD E71.311
      SCAD E71.312
      specified deficiency NEC E71.318
  feeding (infant or child) —*see also* Disorder, eating R63.30
    or eating disorder F50.9
    pediatric
      acute R63.31
      chronic R63.32
    specified NEC F50.9
  feigned (with obvious motivation) Z76.5
    without obvious motivation — *see* Disorder, factitious
  female
    hypoactive sexual desire F52.0
    orgasmic F52.31
    sexual interest/arousal F52.22
  fetishistic F65.0
  fibroblastic M72.9
    specified NEC M72.8
  fluency
    adult onset F98.5
    childhood onset F80.81
    following
      cerebral infarction I69.323
      cerebrovascular disease I69.923
        specified disease NEC I69.823
      intracerebral hemorrhage I69.123

▶ New   ⇒ Revised   ~~deleted~~ Deleted   ● Use Additional Character(s)

Disorder *(Continued)*
  fluency *(Continued)*
    following *(Continued)*
      nontraumatic intracranial hemorrhage NEC
        I69.223
      subarachnoid hemorrhage I69.023
    in conditions classified elsewhere R47.82
  fluid balance E87.8
  follicular (skin) L73.9
    specified NEC L73.8
  frotteuristic F65.81
  fructose metabolism E74.10
    essential fructosuria E74.11
    fructokinase deficiency E74.11
    fructose-1, 6-diphosphatase deficiency E74.19
    hereditary fructose intolerance E74.12
    other specified E74.19
  functional polymorphonuclear neutrophils D71
  gallbladder, biliary tract and pancreas in diseases
    classified elsewhere K87
  gambling F63.0
  gamma aminobutyric acid (GABA) metabolism
    E72.81
  gamma-glutamyl cycle E72.89
  gastric (functional) K31.9
    motility K30
    psychogenic F45.8
    secretion K30
  gastrointestinal (functional) NOS K92.9
    newborn P78.9
    psychogenic F45.8
  gender-identity or -role F64.9
    childhood F64.2
    effect on relationship F66
    of adolescence or adulthood F64.0
      nontranssexual F64.8
    specified NEC F64.8
    uncertainty F66
  gender incongruence F64.9
    in adolescents and adults F64.0
    of childhood F64.2
  genito-pelvic pain penetration F52.6
  genitourinary system
    female N94.9
    male N50.9
    psychogenic F45.8
  globe H44.9
    degenerated condition H44.50
      absolute glaucoma H44.51-●
      atrophy H44.52-●
      leucocoria H44.53-●
    degenerative H44.30
      chalcosis H44.31-●
      myopia —*see also* Myopia, degenerative
        H44.2-●
      siderosis H44.32-●
      specified type NEC H44.39-●
    endophthalmitis —*see* Endophthalmitis
    foreign body, retained —*see* Foreign body,
      intraocular, old, retained
    hemophthalmos —*see* Hemophthalmos
    hypotony H44.40
      due to
        ocular fistula H44.42-●
        specified disorder NEC H44.43-●
      flat anterior chamber H44.41-●
      primary H44.44-●
    luxation —*see* Luxation, globe
    specified type NEC H44.89
  glomerular (in) N05.9
    amyloidosis E85.4 *[N08]*
    cryoglobulinemia D89.1 *[N08]*
    disseminated intravascular coagulation D65
      [N08]
    Fabry's disease E75.21 *[N08]*
    familial lecithin cholesterol acyltransferase
      deficiency E78.6 *[N08]*
    Goodpasture's syndrome M31.0
    hemolytic-uremic syndrome —*see* Syndrome,
      hemolytic-uremic
    Henoch (-Schönlein) purpura D69.0 *[N08]*
    malariae malaria B52.0
    microscopic polyangiitis M31.7 *[N08]*
    multiple myeloma C90.0-● *[N08]*
    mumps B26.83
    schistosomiasis B65.9 *[N08]*
    sepsis NEC A41.-● *[N08]*
      streptococcal A40.-● *[N08]*
    sickle-cell disorders D57.-● *[N08]*
    strongyloidiasis B78.9 *[N08]*
    subacute bacterial endocarditis I33.0 *[N08]*

Disorder *(Continued)*
  glomerular *(Continued)*
    syphilis A52.75
    systemic lupus erythematosus M32.14
    thrombotic thrombocytopenic purpura
      M31.19 *[N08]*
    ⮕Waldenström macroglobulinemia C88.0-●
      [N08]
    Wegener's granulomatosis M31.31
  gluconeogenesis E74.4
  glucosaminoglycan metabolism —*see* Disorder,
    metabolism, glucosaminoglycan
  glucose transport E74.819
    specified NEC E74.818
  glycine metabolism E72.50
    d-glycericacidemia E72.59
    hyperhydroxyprolinemia E72.59
    hyperoxaluria R82.992
      primary E72.53
    hyperprolinemia E72.59
    non-ketotic hyperglycinemia E72.51
    oxalosis E72.53
    oxaluria E72.53
    sarcosinemia E72.59
    trimethylaminuria E72.52
  glycoprotein metabolism E77.9
    specified NEC E77.8
  grief
    complicated F43.81
    prolonged F43.81
  habit (and impulse) F63.9
    involving sexual behavior NEC F65.9
    specified NEC F63.89
  hallucinogen use
    mild F16.10
      with
        hallucinogen-induced
          anxiety disorder F16.180
          bipolar and related disorder F16.14
          depressive disorder F16.14
          psychotic disorder F16.159
        hallucinogen intoxication delirium
          F16.121
        other hallucinogen intoxication F16.129
      in remission (early) (sustained) F16.11
    moderate or severe F16.20
      with
        hallucinogen-induced
          anxiety disorder F16.280
          bipolar and related disorder F16.24
          depressive disorder F16.24
          psychotic disorder F16.259
        hallucinogen intoxication delirium
          F16.221
        other hallucinogen intoxication
          F16.229
      in remission (early) (sustained) F16.21
  heart action I49.9
  hematological D75.9
    newborn (transient) P61.9
      specified NEC P61.8
  hematopoietic organs D75.9
  hemorrhagic NEC D69.9
    drug-induced D68.32
    due to
      extrinsic circulating anticoagulants D68.32
      increase in
        anti-IIa D68.32
        anti-Xa D68.32
      intrinsic
        circulating anticoagulants D68.318
        increase in
          antithrombin D68.318
          anti-VIIIa D68.318
          anti-IXa D68.318
          anti-XIa D68.318
    following childbirth O72.3
  hemostasis —*see* Defect, coagulation
  histidine metabolism E70.40
    histidinemia E70.41
    other specified E70.49
  hoarding F42.3
  hyperkinetic —*see* Disorder, attention-deficit
    hyperactivity
  hyperleucine-isoleucinemia E71.19
  hypervalinemia E71.19
  hypoactive sexual desire F52.0
  hypochondriacal F45.20
    body dysmorphic F45.22
    neurosis F45.21
    other specified F45.29

Disorder *(Continued)*
  identity
    dissociative F44.81
    illness anxiety F45.21
    of childhood F93.8
  immune mechanism (immunity) D89.9
    specified type NEC D89.89
  impaired renal tubular function N25.9
    specified NEC N25.89
  impulse (control) F63.9
  inflammatory
    pelvic, in diseases classified elsewhere —*see*
      category N74
    penis N48.29
      abscess N48.21
      cellulitis N48.22
  inhalant use
    mild F18.10
      with
        inhalant-induced
          anxiety disorder F18.180
          depressive disorder F18.14
          major neurocognitive disorder F18.17
          mild neurocognitive disorder F18.188
          psychotic disorder F18.159
        inhalant intoxication F18.129
        inhalant intoxication delirium F18.121
      in remission (early) (sustained) F18.11
    moderate or severe F18.20
      with
        inhalant-induced
          anxiety disorder F18.280
          depressive disorder F18.24
          major neurocognitive disorder F18.27
          mild neurocognitive disorder F18.288
          psychotic disorder F18.259
        inhalant intoxication F18.229
        inhalant intoxication delirium F18.221
      in remission (early) (sustained) F18.21
  integument, newborn P83.9
    specified NEC P83.88
  intermittent explosive F63.81
  internal secretion pancreas —*see* Increased,
    secretion, pancreas, endocrine
  intestine, intestinal
    carbohydrate absorption NEC E74.39
      postoperative K91.2
    functional NEC K59.9
      postoperative K91.89
      psychogenic F45.8
    vascular K55.9
      chronic K55.1
      specified NEC K55.8
  intraoperative (intraprocedural) —*see*
    Complications, intraoperative
  involuntary emotional expression (IEED) F48.2
  iris H21.9
    adhesions —*see* Adhesions, iris
    atrophy —*see* Atrophy, iris
    chamber angle recession —*see* Recession,
      chamber angle
    cyst —*see* Cyst, iris
    degeneration —*see* Degeneration, iris
    in diseases classified elsewhere H22
    iridodialysis —*see* Iridodialysis
    iridoschisis —*see* Iridoschisis
    miotic pupillary cyst —*see* Cyst, pupillary
    pupillary
      abnormality —*see* Abnormality, pupillary
      membrane —*see* Membrane, pupillary
    specified type NEC H21.89
    vascular NEC H21.1X-●
  iron metabolism E83.10
    specified NEC E83.19
  isovaleric acidemia E71.110
  jaw, developmental M27.0
    temporomandibular —*see also* Anomaly,
      dentofacial, temporomandibular joint
      M26.60-●
  joint M25.9
    derangement —*see* Derangement, joint
    effusion —*see* Effusion, joint
    fistula —*see* Fistula, joint
    hemarthrosis —*see* Hemarthrosis
    instability —*see* Instability, joint
    osteophyte —*see* Osteophyte
    pain —*see* Pain, joint
    psychogenic F45.8
    specified type NEC M25.80
      ankle M25.87-●
      elbow M25.82-●

Disorder *(Continued)*
 joint *(Continued)*
  specified type *(Continued)*
   foot joint M25.87-●
   hand joint M25.84-●
   hip M25.85-●
   knee M25.86-●
   shoulder M25.81-●
   wrist M25.83-●
  stiffness —*see* Stiffness, joint
 ketone metabolism E71.32
 kidney N28.9
  functional (tubular) N25.9
  in
   schistosomiasis B65.9 *[N29]*
  tubular function N25.9
   specified NEC N25.89
 lacrimal system H04.9
  changes H04.69
   fistula —*see* Fistula, lacrimal
  gland H04.19
   atrophy —*see* Atrophy, lacrimal gland
   cyst —*see* Cyst, lacrimal, gland
   dacryops —*see* Dacryops
   dislocation —*see* Dislocation, lacrimal gland
   dry eye syndrome —*see* Syndrome, dry eye
   infection —*see* Dacryoadenitis
   granuloma —*see* Granuloma, lacrimal
   inflammation —*see* Inflammation, lacrimal
   obstruction —*see* Obstruction, lacrimal
   specified NEC H04.89
 lactation NEC O92.79
 language (developmental) F80.9
  expressive F80.1
  mixed receptive and expressive F80.2
  receptive F80.2
 late luteal phase dysphoric N94.89
 learning (specific) F81.9
  acalculia R48.8
  alexia R48.0
  mathematics F81.2
  reading F81.0
  specified
   with impairment in
    mathematics F81.2
    reading F81.0
    written expression F81.81
  specified NEC F81.89
  spelling F81.81
  written expression F81.81
 lens H27.9
  aphakia —*see* Aphakia
  cataract —*see* Cataract
  dislocation —*see* Dislocation, lens
  specified type NEC H27.8
 ligament M24.20
  ankle M24.27-●
  attachment, spine —*see* Enthesopathy, spinal
  elbow M24.22-●
  foot joint M24.27-●
  hand joint M24.24-●
  hip M24.25-●
  knee —*see* Derangement, knee, specified NEC
  shoulder M24.21-●
  specified site NEC M24.29
  vertebra M24.28
  wrist M24.23-●
 ligamentous attachments —*see also* Enthesopathy
  spine —*see* Enthesopathy, spinal
 lipid
  metabolism, congenital E78.9
  storage E75.6
   specified NEC E75.5
 lipoprotein
  deficiency (familial) E78.6
  metabolism E78.9
   specified NEC E78.89
 liver K76.9
  malarial B54 *[K77]*
 low back —*see also* Dorsopathy, specified NEC
 lumbosacral
  plexus G54.1
  root (nerve) NEC G54.4
 lung, interstitial, drug-induced J70.4
  acute J70.2
  chronic J70.3
  dabbing (related) U07.0
  e-cigarette (related) U07.0
  electronic cigarette (related) U07.0
  vaping (associated) (device) (product)
   (related) (use) U07.0

Disorder *(Continued)*
 lymphoproliferative, post-transplant (PTLD)
  D47.Z1
 lysine and hydroxylysine metabolism E72.3
 major neurocognitive *(see also* Dementia, in (due
  to)) F03-●
 male
  erectile (organic) —*see also* Dysfunction,
   sexual, male, erectile N52.9
   nonorganic F52.21
  hypoactive sexual desire F52.0
  orgasmic F52.32
 manic F30.9
  organic F06.33
 mast cell activation —*see* Activation, mast cell
 mastoid —*see also* Disorder, ear, middle
  postprocedural —*see* Complications, ear,
   procedure
 meninges, specified type NEC G96.198
 meniscus —*see* Derangement, knee,
  meniscus
 menopausal N95.9
  specified NEC N95.8
 menstrual N92.6
  psychogenic F45.8
  specified NEC N92.5
 mental (or behavioral) (nonpsychotic) F99
  due to (secondary to)
   amphetamine
    due to drug abuse —*see* Abuse, drug,
     stimulant
    due to drug dependence —*see*
     Dependence, drug, stimulant
   brain disease, damage and dysfunction F09
   caffeine use
    due to drug abuse —*see* Abuse, drug,
     stimulant
    due to drug dependence —*see*
     Dependence, drug, stimulant
   cannabis use
    due to drug abuse —*see* Abuse, drug,
     cannabis
    due to drug dependence —*see*
     Dependence, drug, cannabis
   general medical condition F09
   sedative or hypnotic use
    due to drug abuse —*see* Abuse, drug,
     sedative
    due to drug dependence —*see*
     Dependence, drug, sedative
   tobacco (nicotine) use —*see* Dependence,
    drug, nicotine
  following organic brain damage F07.9
   frontal lobe syndrome F07.0
   personality change F07.0
   postconcussional syndrome F07.81
   specified NEC F07.89
  infancy, childhood or adolescence F98.9
  neurotic —*see* Neurosis
  organic or symptomatic F09
  presenile, psychotic F03
  problem NEC
  psychoneurotic —*see* Neurosis
  psychotic —*see* Psychosis
  puerperal F53.0
  senile, psychotic NEC F03
 metabolic, amino acid, transitory, newborn P74.8
 metabolism NOS E88.9
  amino-acid E72.9
   aromatic E70.9
    albinism —*see* Albinism
    histidine E70.40
     histidinemia E70.41
     other specified E70.49
    hyperphenylalaninemia E70.1
     classical phenylketonuria E70.0
    other specified E70.89
    tryptophan E70.5
    tyrosine E70.20
     hypertyrosinemia E70.21
     other specified E70.29
   branched chain E71.2
    3-methylglutaconic aciduria
     E71.111
    hyperleucine-isoleucinemia E71.19
    hypervalinemia E71.19
    isovaleric acidemia E71.110
    maple syrup urine disease E71.0
    methylmalonic acidemia E71.120
    organic aciduria NEC E71.118
    other specified E71.19

Disorder *(Continued)*
 metabolism *(Continued)*
  amino-acid *(Continued)*
   branched chain *(Continued)*
    ~~propionate NEC E71.128~~
    ~~propionic acidemia E71.121~~
    ▶propionate NEC E71.128
    ▶propionic acidemia E71.121
   glycine E72.50
    d-glycericacidemia E72.59
    hyperhydroxyprolinemia E72.59
    hyperoxaluria R82.992
     primary E72.53
    hyperprolinemia E72.59
    non-ketotic hyperglycinemia E72.51
    other specified E72.59
    sarcosinemia E72.59
    trimethylaminuria E72.52
   hydroxylysine E72.3
   lysine E72.3
   ornithine E72.4
   other specified E72.89
    beta-amino acid E72.89
    gamma-glutamyl cycle E72.89
   straight-chain E72.89
   sulfur-bearing E72.10
    homocystinuria E72.11
    methylenetetrahydrofolate reductase
     deficiency E72.12
    other specified E72.19
  bile acid and cholesterol metabolism
   E78.70
  bilirubin E80.7
   specified NEC E80.6
  calcium E83.50
   hypercalcemia E83.52
   hypocalcemia E83.51
   other specified E83.59
  carbohydrate E74.9
   specified NEC E74.89
  cholesterol and bile acid metabolism E78.70
  ▶citrate NEC E74.829
  congenital E88.9
  copper E83.00
   specified type NEC E83.09
   Wilson's disease E83.01
  cystinuria E72.01
  fructose E74.10
  galactose E74.20
  glucosaminoglycan E76.9
   mucopolysaccharidosis —*see*
    Mucopolysaccharidosis
   specified NEC E76.8
  glutamine E72.89
  glycine E72.50
  glycogen storage (hepatorenal) E74.09
  glycoprotein E77.9
   specified NEC E77.8
  glycosaminoglycan E76.9
   specified NEC E76.8
  in labor and delivery O75.89
  iron E83.10
  isoleucine E71.19
  leucine E71.19
  lipoid E78.9
  lipoprotein E78.9
   specified NEC E78.89
  magnesium E83.40
   hypermagnesemia E83.41
   hypomagnesemia E83.42
   other specified E83.49
  mineral E83.9
   specified NEC E83.89
  mitochondrial E88.40
   MELAS syndrome E88.41
   MERRF syndrome (myoclonic epilepsy
    associated with ragged-red fibers)
    E88.42
   other specified E88.49
   tRNA synthetases E88.43
  ornithine E72.4
  phosphatases E83.30
  phosphorus E83.30
   acid phosphatase deficiency E83.39
   hypophosphatasia E83.39
   hypophosphatemia E83.39
    familial E83.31
   other specified E83.39
   pseudovitamin D deficiency E83.32
  plasma protein NEC E88.09
  porphyrin —*see* Porphyria

Disorder *(Continued)*
  metabolism *(Continued)*
    postprocedural E89.89
      specified NEC E89.89
    purine E79.9
      specified NEC E79.89
    pyrimidine E79.9
      specified NEC E79.89
    pyruvate E74.4
    serine E72.89
    sodium E87.8
    specified NEC E88.89
    threonine E72.89
    valine E71.19
    zinc E83.2
  methylmalonic acidemia E71.120
  micturition NEC —*see also* Difficulty, micturition
    R39.198
    feeling of incomplete emptying R39.14
    hesitancy R39.11
    poor stream R39.12
    psychogenic F45.8
    split stream R39.13
    straining R39.16
    urgency R39.15
  mild neurocognitive G31.84
    due to known physiological condition
      (without behavioral disturbance) F06.70
    with behavioral disturbance F06.71
  mitochondrial metabolism E88.40
  mitral (valve) —*see* Endocarditis, mitral
  mixed
    anxiety and depressive F41.8
    of scholastic skills (developmental) F81.89
    receptive expressive language F80.2
  mood F39
    bipolar —*see* Disorder, bipolar
    depressive —*see* Disorder, depressive
    due to (secondary to)
      alcohol F10.94
      amphetamine F15.94
        in
          abuse F15.14
          dependence F15.24
      anxiolytic F13.94
        in
          abuse F13.14
          dependence F13.24
      cocaine F14.94
        in
          abuse F14.14
          dependence F14.24
      general medical condition F06.30
      hallucinogen F16.94
        in
          abuse F16.14
          dependence F16.24
      hypnotic F13.94
        in
          abuse F13.14
          dependence F13.24
      inhalant F18.94
        in
          abuse F18.14
          dependence F18.24
      opioid F11.94
        in
          abuse F11.14
          dependence F11.24
      phencyclidine (PCP) F16.94
        in
          abuse F16.14
          dependence F16.24
      physiological condition F06.30
        with
          depressive features F06.31
          major depressive-like episode F06.32
          manic features F06.33
          mixed features F06.34
      psychoactive substance NEC F19.94
        in
          abuse F19.14
          dependence F19.24
      sedative F13.94
        in
          abuse F13.14
          dependence F13.24
      volatile solvents F18.94
        in
          abuse F18.14
          dependence F18.24

Disorder *(Continued)*
  mood *(Continued)*
    manic episode F30.9
      with psychotic symptoms F30.2
      without psychotic symptoms F30.10
        mild F30.11
        moderate F30.12
        severe F30.13
      in remission (full) F30.4
        partial F30.3
      specified type NEC F30.8
    organic F06.30
      right hemisphere F07.89
    persistent F34.9
      cyclothymia F34.0
      dysthymia F34.1
      specified type NEC F34.89
    recurrent F39
    right hemisphere organic F07.89
  movement G25.9
    drug-induced G25.70
      akathisia G25.71
      specified NEC G25.79
    hysterical F44.4
    in diseases classified elsewhere —*see* category
      G26
    periodic limb G47.61
      sleep related G47.61
    sleep related NEC G47.69
    specified NEC G25.89
    stereotyped F98.4
    treatment-induced G25.9
  multiple personality F44.81
  muscle M62.9
    attachment, spine —*see* Enthesopathy, spinal
    in trichinellosis —*see* Trichinellosis, with
      muscle disorder
    psychogenic F45.8
    specified type NEC M62.89
    tone, newborn P94.9
      specified NEC P94.8
  muscular
    attachments —*see also* Enthesopathy
      spine —*see* Enthesopathy, spinal
    urethra N36.44
  musculoskeletal system, soft tissue —*see*
    Disorder, soft tissue
    postprocedural M96.89
    psychogenic F45.8
  myoneural G70.9
    due to lead G70.1
    specified NEC G70.89
    toxic G70.1
  myotonic NEC G71.19
  nail, in diseases classified elsewhere L62
  neck region NEC —*see* Dorsopathy, specified
    NEC
  neonatal onset multisystemic inflammatory
    (NOMID) M04.2
  nerve G58.9
    abducent NEC —*see* Strabismus, paralytic,
      sixth nerve
    accessory G52.8
    acoustic —*see* subcategory H93.3
    auditory —*see* subcategory H93.3
    auriculotemporal G50.8
    axillary G54.0
    cerebral —*see* Disorder, nerve, cranial
    cranial G52.9
      eighth —*see* subcategory H93.3
      eleventh G52.8
      fifth G50.9
      first G52.0
      fourth NEC —*see* Strabismus, paralytic,
        fourth nerve
      multiple G52.7
      ninth G52.1
      second NEC —*see* Disorder, nerve, optic
      seventh NEC G51.8
      sixth NEC —*see* Strabismus, paralytic, sixth
        nerve
      specified NEC G52.8
      tenth G52.2
      third NEC —*see* Strabismus, paralytic, third
        nerve
      twelfth G52.3
    entrapment —*see* Neuropathy, entrapment
    facial G51.9
      specified NEC G51.8
    femoral —*see* Lesion, nerve, femoral
    glossopharyngeal NEC G52.1

Disorder *(Continued)*
  nerve *(Continued)*
    hypoglossal G52.3
    intercostal G58.0
    lateral
      cutaneous of thigh —*see* Mononeuropathy,
        lower limb, meralgia paresthetica
      popliteal —*see* Lesion, nerve, popliteal
    lower limb —*see* Mononeuropathy, lower limb
    medial popliteal —*see* Lesion, nerve, popliteal,
      medial
    median NEC —*see* Lesion, nerve, median
    multiple G58.7
    oculomotor NEC —*see* Strabismus, paralytic,
      third nerve
    olfactory G52.0
    optic NEC H47.09-●
      hemorrhage into sheath —*see* Hemorrhage,
        optic nerve
      ischemic H47.01-●
    peroneal —*see* Lesion, nerve, popliteal
    phrenic G58.8
    plantar —*see* Lesion, nerve, plantar
    pneumogastric G52.2
    posterior tibial —*see* Syndrome, tarsal tunnel
    radial —*see* Lesion, nerve, radial
    recurrent laryngeal G52.2
    root G54.9
      cervical G54.2
      lumbosacral G54.1
      specified NEC G54.8
      thoracic G54.3
    sciatic NEC —*see* Lesion, nerve, sciatic
    specified NEC G58.8
      lower limb —*see* Mononeuropathy, lower
        limb, specified NEC
      upper limb —*see* Mononeuropathy, upper
        limb, specified NEC
    sympathetic G90.9
    tibial —*see* Lesion, nerve, popliteal, medial
    trigeminal G50.9
      specified NEC G50.8
    trochlear NEC —*see* Strabismus, paralytic,
      fourth nerve
    ulnar —*see* Lesion, nerve, ulnar
    upper limb —*see* Mononeuropathy, upper limb
    vagus G52.2
  nervous system G98.8
    autonomic (peripheral) G90.9
      specified NEC G90.89
    central G96.9
      specified NEC G96.89
    parasympathetic G90.9
    specified NEC G98.8
    sympathetic G90.9
    vegetative G90.9
  neurocognitive R41.9
    with Lewy bodies (*see also* Dementia, in,
      diseases specified elsewhere) G31.83
      [F02.-]
    frontotemporal, specified NEC (*see also*
      Dementia, in, diseases specified
      elsewhere) G31.09 [F02.-●]
    major (*see also* Dementia) F03.-●
      due to vascular disease —*see* Dementia,
        vascular
      mild —*see* Dementia, vascular, mild
      moderate —*see* Dementia, vascular,
        moderate
      severe —*see* Dementia, vascular, severe
    in (due to) (other diseases classified
      elsewhere) —*see also* Dementia, in
      (due to) F02.80
      with
        aggressive behavior (*see also* Dementia,
          in (due to)) F02.81-●
        combative behavior (*see also* Dementia,
          in (due to)) F02.81-●
        violent behavior (*see also* Dementia, in
          (due to)) F02.81-●
    mild (of uncertain or unknown etiology)
      (*see also* Disorder, mild neurocognitive)
      G31.84
  neurodevelopmental F89
    specified NEC F88
  neurohypophysis NEC E23.3
  neurological NEC R29.818
  neuromuscular G70.9
    hereditary NEC G71.9
    specified NEC G70.89
    toxic G70.1

Disorder *(Continued)*
  neurotic F48.9
    specified NEC F48.8
  neutrophil, polymorphonuclear D71
  nicotine use —*see* Dependence, drug, nicotine
  nightmare F51.5
  non-rapid eye movement sleep arousal
    sleep terror type F51.4
    sleepwalking type F51.3
  nose J34.9
    specified NEC J34.89
  obsessive-compulsive F42.9
    and related disorder due to a known
      physiological condition F06.8
  odontogenesis NOS K00.9
  opioid use
    with
      opioid-induced psychotic disorder F11.959
        with
          delusions F11.950
          hallucinations F11.951
    due to drug abuse —*see* Abuse, drug, opioid
    due to drug dependence —*see* Dependence,
      drug, opioid
    mild F11.10
      with
        opioid-induced
          anxiety disorder F11.188
          depressive disorder F11.14
          sexual dysfunction F11.181
        opioid intoxication
          with perceptual disturbances F11.122
          delirium F11.121
          without perceptual disturbances
            F11.129
      in remission (early) (sustained) F11.11
    moderate or severe F11.20
      with
        opioid-induced
          anxiety disorder F11.288
          anxiety disorder F11.988
          depressive disorder F11.24
          depressive disorder F11.94
          sexual dysfunction F11.281
          sexual dysfunction F11.981
        opioid intoxication
          with perceptual disturbances F11.222
          delirium F11.221
          without perceptual disturbances
            F11.229
      in remission (early) (sustained) F11.21
  oppositional defiant F91.3
  optic
    chiasm H47.49
      due to
        inflammatory disorder H47.41
        neoplasm H47.42
        vascular disorder H47.43
    disc H47.39-●
      coloboma —*see* Coloboma, optic disc
      drusen —*see* Drusen, optic disc
      pseudopapilledema —*see*
        Pseudopapilledema
    radiations —*see* Disorder, visual, pathway
    tracts —*see* Disorder, visual, pathway
  orbit H05.9
    cyst —*see* Cyst, orbit
    deformity —*see* Deformity, orbit
    edema —*see* Edema, orbit
    enophthalmos —*see* Enophthalmos
    exophthalmos —*see* Exophthalmos
    hemorrhage —*see* Hemorrhage, orbit
    inflammation —*see* Inflammation, orbit
    myopathy —*see* Myopathy, extraocular muscles
    retained foreign body —*see* Foreign body,
      orbit, old
    specified type NEC H05.89
  organic
    anxiety F06.4
    ~~catatonic F06.1~~
    ▶catatonic NOS F06.1
    delusional F06.2
    dissociative F06.8
    emotionally labile (asthenic) F06.8
    mood (affective) F06.30
    schizophrenia-like F06.2
  orgasmic (female) F52.31
    male F52.32
  ornithine metabolism E72.4
  overanxious F41.1
    of childhood F93.8

Disorder *(Continued)*
  pain
    with related psychological factors
      F45.42
    exclusively related to psychological factors
      F45.41
    genito-pelvic penetration disorder F52.6
  pancreatic internal secretion E16.9
    specified NEC E16.8
  panic F41.0
    with agoraphobia F40.01
  papulosquamous L44.9
    in diseases classified elsewhere L45
    specified NEC L44.8
  paranoid F22
    induced F24
    shared F24
  paraphilic F65.9
    specified NEC F65.89
  parathyroid (gland) E21.5
    specified NEC E21.4
  parietoalveolar NEC J84.09
  paroxysmal, mixed R56.9
  patella M22.9-●
    chondromalacia —*see* Chondromalacia,
      patella
    derangement NEC M22.3X-●
    recurrent
      dislocation —*see* Dislocation, patella,
        recurrent
      subluxation —*see* Dislocation, patella,
        recurrent, incomplete
    specified NEC M22.8X-●
  patellofemoral M22.2X-●
  pedophilic F65.4
  pentose phosphate pathway with anemia D55.1
  perception, due to hallucinogens F16.983
    in
      abuse F16.183
      dependence F16.283
  peripheral nervous system NEC G64
  peroxisomal E71.50
    biogenesis
      neonatal adrenoleukodystrophy E71.511
      specified disorder NEC E71.518
      Zellweger syndrome E71.510
    rhizomelic chondrodysplasia punctata E71.540
    specified form NEC E71.548
      group 1 E71.518
      group 2 E71.53
      group 3 E71.542
    X-linked adrenoleukodystrophy E71.529
      adolescent E71.521
      adrenomyeloneuropathy E71.522
      childhood E71.520
      specified form NEC E71.528
    Zellweger-like syndrome E71.541
  persistent
    (somatoform) pain F45.41
    affective (mood) F34.9
  personality —*see also* Personality F60.9
    affective F34.0
    aggressive F60.3
    amoral F60.2
    anankastic F60.5
    antisocial F60.2
    anxious F60.6
    asocial F60.2
    asthenic F60.7
    avoidant F60.6
    borderline F60.3
    change (secondary) due to general medical
      condition F07.0
    compulsive F60.5
    cyclothymic F34.0
    dependent (passive) F60.7
    depressive F34.1
    dissocial F60.2
    emotional instability F60.3
    expansive paranoid F60.0
    explosive F60.3
    following organic brain damage F07.9
    histrionic F60.4
    hyperthymic F34.0
    hypothymic F34.1
    hysterical F60.4
    immature F60.89
    inadequate F60.7
    labile F60.3
    mixed (nonspecific) F60.89
    moral deficiency F60.2

Disorder *(Continued)*
  personality *(Continued)*
    narcissistic F60.81
    negativistic F60.89
    obsessional F60.5
    obsessive (-compulsive) F60.5
    organic F07.9
    overconscientious F60.5
    paranoid F60.0
    passive (-dependent) F60.7
    passive-aggressive F60.89
    pathological NEC F60.9
    pseudosocial F60.2
    psychopathic F60.2
    schizoid F60.1
    schizotypal F21
    self-defeating F60.7
    specified NEC F60.89
    type A F60.5
    unstable (emotional) F60.3
  pervasive, developmental F84.9
  phencyclidine use
    mild F16.10
      with
        phencyclidine-induced
          anxiety disorder F16.180
          bipolar and related disorder F16.14
          depressive disorder F16.14
          psychotic disorder F16.159
        phencyclidine intoxication F16.129
        phencyclidine intoxication delirium
          F16.121
      in remission (early) (sustained) F16.11
    moderate or severe F16.20
      with
        phencyclidine-induced
          anxiety disorder F16.280
          bipolar and related disorder F16.24
          depressive disorder F16.24
          psychotic disorder F16.259
        phencyclidine intoxication F16.229
        phencyclidine intoxication delirium
          F16.221
      in remission (early) (sustained) F16.21
  phobic anxiety, childhood F40.8
  phosphate-losing tubular N25.0
  pigmentation L81.9
    choroid, congenital Q14.3
    diminished melanin formation L81.6
    iron L81.8
    specified NEC L81.8
  pinna (noninfective) H61.10-●
    deformity, acquired H61.11-●
    hematoma H61.12-●
    perichondritis —*see* Perichondritis, ear
    specified type NEC H61.19-●
  pituitary gland E23.7
    iatrogenic (postprocedural) E89.3
    specified NEC E23.6
  platelet-activating anti-PF4, specified NEC
    D75.84
  platelets D69.1
  plexus G54.9
    specified NEC G54.8
  polymorphonuclear neutrophils D71
  porphyrin metabolism —*see* Porphyria
  postconcussional F07.81
  posthallucinogen perception F16.983
    in
      abuse F16.183
      dependence F16.283
  postmenopausal N95.9
    specified NEC N95.8
  postprocedural (postoperative) —*see*
    Complications, postprocedural
  post-transplant lymphoproliferative D47.z1
  post-traumatic stress (PTSD) F43.10
    acute F43.11
    chronic F43.12
  premenstrual dysphoric (PMDD) F32.81
  prepuce N47.8
  propionic acidemia E71.121
  prostate N42.9
    specified NEC N42.89
  psychogenic NOS —*see also* condition F45.9
    anxiety F41.8
    appetite F50.9
    asthenic F48.8
    cardiovascular (system) F45.8
    compulsive F42.8
    cutaneous F54

▶ New   ⇒ Revised   ~~deleted~~ Deleted   ● Use Additional Character(s)

Disorder *(Continued)*
  psychogenic *(Continued)*
    depressive F32.9
    digestive (system) F45.8
    dysmenorrheic F45.8
    dyspneic F45.8
    endocrine (system) F54
    eye NEC F45.8
    feeding —*see* Disorder, eating
    functional NEC F45.8
    gastric F45.8
    gastrointestinal (system) F45.8
    genitourinary (system) F45.8
    heart (function) (rhythm) F45.8
    hyperventilatory F45.8
    hypochondriacal —*see* Disorder,
      hypochondriacal
    intestinal F45.8
    joint F45.8
    learning F81.9
    limb F45.8
    lymphatic (system) F45.8
    menstrual F45.8
    micturition F45.8
    monoplegic NEC F44.4
    motor F44.4
    muscle F45.8
    musculoskeletal F45.8
    neurocirculatory F45.8
    obsessive F42.8
    occupational F48.8
    organ or part of body NEC F45.8
    paralytic NEC F44.4
    phobic F40.9
    physical NEC F45.8
    rectal F45.8
    respiratory (system) F45.8
    rheumatic F45.8
    sexual (function) F52.9
    skin (allergic) (eczematous) F54
    sleep F51.9
    specified part of body NEC F45.8
    stomach F45.8
  psychological F99
    associated with
      disease classified elsewhere F54
      sexual
        development F66
        relationship F66
      uncertainty about gender identity F64.9
  psychomotor NEC F44.4
    hysterical F44.4
  psychoneurotic —*see also* Neurosis
    mixed NEC F48.8
  psychophysiologic —*see* Disorder, somatoform
  psychosexual F65.9
    development F66
    identity of childhood F64.2
  psychosomatic NOS —*see* Disorder, somatoform
    multiple F45.0
    undifferentiated F45.1
  psychotic —*see* Psychosis
    transient (acute) F23
  puberty E30.9
    specified NEC E30.8
  pulmonary (valve) —*see* Endocarditis, pulmonary
  purine metabolism E79.9
  pyrimidine metabolism E79.9
  pyruvate metabolism E74.4
  reactive attachment (childhood) F94.1
  reading R48.0
    developmental (specific) F81.0
  receptive language F80.2
  receptor, hormonal, peripheral —*see also*
    Syndrome, androgen insensitivity E34.50
  recurrent brief depressive F33.8
  reflex R29.2
  refraction H52.7
    aniseikonia H52.32
    anisometropia H52.31
    astigmatism —*see* Astigmatism
    hypermetropia —*see* Hypermetropia
    myopia —*see* Myopia
    presbyopia H52.4
    specified NEC H52.6
  relationship F68.8
    due to sexual orientation F66
  REM sleep behavior G47.52
  renal function, impaired (tubular) N25.9
  resonance R49.9
    specified NEC R49.8

Disorder *(Continued)*
  respiratory function, impaired —*see also* Failure,
    respiration
    postprocedural —*see* Complication,
      postoperative, respiratory system
    psychogenic F45.8
  retina H35.9
    angioid streaks H35.33
    changes in vascular appearance H35.01-●
    degeneration —*see* Degeneration, retina
    dystrophy (hereditary) —*see* Dystrophy, retina
    edema H35.81
    hemorrhage —*see* Hemorrhage, retina
    ischemia H35.82
    macular degeneration —*see* Degeneration,
      macula
    microaneurysms H35.04-●
    microvascular abnormality NEC H35.09
    neovascularization —*see* Neovascularization,
      retina
    retinopathy —*see* Retinopathy
    separation of layers H35.70
      central serous chorioretinopathy H35.71-●
      pigment epithelium detachment (serous)
        H35.72-●
        hemorrhagic H35.73-●
    specified type NEC H35.89
    telangiectasis —*see* Telangiectasis, retina
    vasculitis —*see* Vasculitis, retina
  retroperitoneal K68.9
  right hemisphere organic affective F07.89
  rumination (infant or child) (in remission) F98.21
  ▶adult (in remission)
  sacrum, sacrococcygeal NEC M53.3
  schizoaffective F25.9
    bipolar type F25.0
    depressive type F25.1
    manic type F25.0
    mixed type F25.0
    specified NEC F25.8
  schizoid of childhood F84.5
  schizophrenia spectrum and other psychotic
    disorder F29
    specified NEC F28
  schizophreniform F20.81
    brief F23
  schizotypal (personality) F21
  seasonal affective, recurrent episodes F33.-●
  secretion, thyrocalcitonin E07.0
  sedative, hypnotic, or anxiolytic use
    mild F13.10
      with
        sedative, hypnotic, or anxiolytic-induced
          anxiety disorder F13.180
          bipolar and related disorder F13.14
          depressive disorder F13.14
          psychotic disorder F13.159
          sexual dysfunction F13.181
        sedative, hypnotic, or anxiolytic
          intoxication F13.129
        sedative, hypnotic, or anxiolytic
          intoxication delirium F13.121
      in remission (early) (sustained) F13.11
    moderate or severe F13.20
      with
        sedative, hypnotic, or anxiolytic-induced
          anxiety disorder F13.280
          bipolar and related disorder F13.24
          anxiety disorder depressive disorder
            F13.24
          major neurocognitive disorder F13.27
          mild neurocognitive disorder F13.288
          psychotic disorder F13.259
          sexual dysfunction F13.281
        sedative, hypnotic, or anxiolytic
          intoxication F13.229
        sedative, hypnotic, or anxiolytic
          intoxication delirium F13.221
      in remission (early) (sustained) F13.21
  seizure —*see also* Epilepsy G40.909
    intractable G40.919
      with status epilepticus G40.911
  semantic pragmatic F80.89
    with autism F84.0
  sense of smell R43.1
    psychogenic F45.8
  separation anxiety, of childhood F93.0
  sexual
    arousal, female F52.22
    aversion F52.1
    function, psychogenic F52.9

Disorder *(Continued)*
  sexual *(Continued)*
    interest/arousal, female F52.22
    masochism F65.51
    maturation F66
    nonorganic F52.9
    preference —*see also* Deviation, sexual F65.9
      fetishistic transvestism F65.1
    relationship F66
    sadism F65.52
  shyness, of childhood and adolescence
    F40.10
  sibling rivalry F93.8
  sickle-cell (sickling) (homozygous) —*see* Disease,
    sickle-cell
    heterozygous D57.3
    specified type NEC D57.8-●
    trait D57.3
  sinus (nasal) J34.9
    specified NEC J34.89
  skin L98.9
    atrophic L90.9
      specified NEC L90.8
    granulomatous L92.9
      specified NEC L92.8
    hypertrophic L91.9
      specified NEC L91.8
    infiltrative NEC L98.6
    newborn P83.9
      specified NEC P83.88
    picking F42.4
    psychogenic (allergic) (eczematous) F54
  ▶SLC13A5 Citrate Transporter Disorder E74.820
  sleep G47.9
    breathing-related —*see* Apnea, sleep
    circadian rhythm G47.20
      advance sleep phase type G47.22
      delayed sleep phase type G47.21
      due to
        alcohol
          abuse F10.182
          dependence F10.282
          use F10.982
        amphetamines
          abuse F15.182
          dependence F15.282
          use F15.982
        caffeine
          abuse F15.182
          dependence F15.282
          use F15.982
        cocaine
          abuse F14.182
          dependence F14.282
          use F14.982
        drug NEC
          abuse F19.182
          dependence F19.282
          use F19.982
        opioid
          abuse F11.182
          dependence F11.282
          use F11.982
        psychoactive substance NEC
          abuse F19.182
          dependence F19.282
          use F19.982
        sedative, hypnotic, or anxiolytic
          abuse F13.182
          dependence F13.282
          use F13.982
        stimulant NEC
          abuse F15.182
          dependence F15.282
          use F15.982
      free running type G47.24
      in conditions classified elsewhere G47.27
      irregular sleep wake type G47.23
      jet lag type G47.25
      non-24-hour sleep-wake type G47.24
      shift work type G47.26
      specified NEC G47.29
      due to
        alcohol
          abuse F10.182
          dependence F10.282
          use F10.982
        amphetamine
          abuse F15.182
          dependence F15.282
          use F15.982

Disorder *(Continued)*
 sleep *(Continued)*
  due to *(Continued)*
   anxiolytic
    abuse F13.182
    dependence F13.282
    use F13.982
   caffeine
    abuse F15.182
    dependence F15.282
    use F15.982
   cocaine
    abuse F14.182
    dependence F14.282
    use F14.982
   drug NEC
    abuse F19.182
    dependence F19.282
    use F19.982
   hypnotic
    abuse F13.182
    dependence F13.282
    use F13.982
   opioid
    abuse F11.182
    dependence F11.282
    use F11.982
   psychoactive substance NEC
    abuse F19.182
    dependence F19.282
    use F19.982
   sedative
    abuse F13.182
    dependence F13.282
    use F13.982
   stimulant NEC
    abuse F15.182
    dependence F15.282
    use F15.982
  emotional F51.9
  excessive somnolence —*see* Hypersomnia
  hypersomnia type —*see* Hypersomnia
  initiating or maintaining —*see* Insomnia
  nightmares F51.5
  nonorganic F51.9
   specified NEC F51.8
  parasomnia type G47.50
  specified NEC G47.8
  terrors F51.4
  walking F51.3
 sleep-wake pattern or schedule —*see also*
   Disorder, sleep, circadian rhythm G47.9
  specified NEC G47.8
 social
  anxiety (of childhood) F40.10
   generalized F40.11
  functioning in childhood F94.9
   specified NEC F94.8
  pragmatic F80.82
 soft tissue M79.9
  ankle M79.9
  due to use, overuse and pressure M70.90
   ankle M70.97-●
   bursitis —*see* Bursitis
   foot M70.97-●
   forearm M70.93-●
   hand M70.94-●
   lower leg M70.96-●
   multiple sites M70.99
   pelvic region M70.95-●
   shoulder region M70.91-●
   specified site NEC M70.98
   specified type NEC M70.80
    ankle M70.87-●
    foot M70.87-●
    forearm M70.83-●
    hand M70.84-●
    lower leg M70.86-●
    multiple sites M70.89
    pelvic region M70.85-●
    shoulder region M70.81-●
    specified site NEC M70.88
    thigh M70.85-●
    upper arm M70.82-●
   thigh M70.95-●
   upper arm M70.92-●
  foot M79.9
  forearm M79.9
  hand M79.9
  lower leg M79.9
  multiple sites M79.9

Disorder *(Continued)*
 soft tissue *(Continued)*
  occupational —*see* Disorder, soft tissue, due to
    use, overuse and pressure
  pelvic region M79.9
  shoulder region M79.9
  specified type NEC M79.89
  thigh M79.9
  upper arm M79.9
 somatic symptom F45.1
 somatization F45.0
 somatoform F45.9
  pain (persistent) F45.41
  somatization (multiple) (long-lasting) F45.0
  specified NEC F45.8
  undifferentiated F45.1
 somnolence, excessive —*see* Hypersomnia
 specific
  arithmetical F81.2
  developmental, of motor F82
  reading F81.0
  speech and language F80.9
  spelling F81.81
  written expression F81.81
 speech R47.9
  articulation (functional) (specific) F80.0
  developmental F80.9
  specified NEC R47.89
 speech-sound F80.0
 spelling (specific) F81.81
 spine —*see also* Dorsopathy
  ligamentous or muscular attachments,
    peripheral —*see* Enthesopathy, spinal
  specified NEC —*see* Dorsopathy, specified
    NEC
 stereotyped, habit or movement F98.4
 stimulant use (other) (unspecified)
  mild F15.10
   in remission (early) (sustained) F15.11
  moderate or severe F15.20
   in remission (early) (sustained) F15.21
 stomach (functional) —*see* Disorder, gastric
 stress F43.9
  acute F43.0
  post-traumatic F43.10
   acute F43.11
   chronic F43.12
 substance use (other) (unknown)
  mild F19.10
   with substance-induced
    anxiety disorder F19.180
    bipolar and related disorder F19.14
    depressive disorder F19.14
    major neurocognitive disorder
      F19.17
    mild neurocognitive disorder F19.188
    obsessive-compulsive and related
      disorder F19.188
    sexual dysfunction F19.181
   substance intoxication F19.129
   substance intoxication delirium F19.121
  moderate or severe F19.20
   with substance-induced
    anxiety disorder F19.280
    bipolar and related disorder F19.24
    depressive disorder F19.24
    major neurocognitive disorder
      F19.27
    mild neurocognitive disorder F19.288
    obsessive-compulsive and related
      disorder F19.288
    sexual dysfunction F19.281
   in remission (early) (sustained) F19.21
   substance intoxication F19.229
   substance intoxication delirium F19.221
 sulfur-bearing amino-acid metabolism
   E72.10
 sweat gland (eccrine) L74.9
  apocrine L75.9
   specified NEC L75.8
  specified NEC L74.8
 synovium M67.90
  acromioclavicular M67.91-●
  ankle M67.97-●
  elbow M67.92-●
  foot M67.97-●
  forearm M67.93-●
  hand M67.94-●
  hip M67.95-●
  knee M67.96-●
  multiple sites M67.99

Disorder *(Continued)*
 synovium *(Continued)*
  rupture —*see* Rupture, synovium
  shoulder M67.91-●
  specified type NEC M67.80
   acromioclavicular M67.81-●
   ankle M67.87-●
   elbow M67.82-●
   foot M67.87-●
   hand M67.84-●
   hip M67.85-●
   knee M67.86-●
   multiple sites M67.89
   wrist M67.83-●
  synovitis —*see* Synovitis
  upper arm M67.92-●
  wrist M67.93-●
 temperature regulation, newborn P81.9
  specified NEC P81.8
 temporomandibular joint M26.60-●
 tendon M67.90
  acromioclavicular M67.91-●
  ankle M67.97-●
  contracture —*see* Contracture, tendon
  elbow M67.92-●
  foot M67.97-●
  forearm M67.93-●
  hand M67.94-●
  hip M67.95-●
  knee M67.96-●
  multiple sites M67.99
  rupture —*see* Rupture, tendon
  shoulder M67.91-●
  specified type NEC M67.80
   acromioclavicular M67.81-●
   ankle M67.87-●
   elbow M67.82-●
   foot M67.87-●
   hand M67.84-●
   hip M67.85-●
   knee M67.86-●
   multiple sites M67.89
   trunk M67.88
   wrist M67.83-●
  synovitis —*see* Synovitis
  tendinitis —*see* Tendinitis
  tenosynovitis —*see* Tenosynovitis
  trunk M67.98
  upper arm M67.92-●
  wrist M67.93-●
 thoracic root (nerve) NEC G54.3
 thyrocalcitonin hypersecretion E07.0
 thyroid (gland) E07.9
  function NEC, neonatal, transitory P72.2
  iodine-deficiency related E01.8
  specified NEC E07.89
 tic —*see* Tic
 tobacco use
  chewing tobacco (mild) (moderate)
    (severe)
   in remission (early) (sustained) F17.221
  cigarettes (mild) (moderate) (severe)
   in remission (early) (sustained) F17.211
  mild F17.200
   in remission (early) (sustained) F17.201
  moderate F17.200
   in remission (early) (sustained) F17.201
  severe F17.200
   in remission (early) (sustained) F17.201
  specified product NEC (mild) (moderate)
    (severe)
   in remission (early) (sustained) F17.291
 tooth K08.9
  development K00.9
   specified NEC K00.8
  eruption K00.6
 Tourette's F95.2
 trance and possession F44.89
 transvestic F65.1
 trauma and stressor-related NOS F43.9
  other specified F43.89
  unspecified F43.9
 tricuspid (valve) —*see* Endocarditis, tricuspid
 tryptophan metabolism E70.5
 tubular, phosphate-losing N25.0
 tubulo-interstitial (in)
  brucellosis A23.9 *[N16]*
  cystinosis E72.04
  diphtheria A36.84
  glycogen storage disease E74.00 *[N16]*
  leukemia NEC C95.9-● *[N16]*

▶ New   ⟹ Revised   ~~deleted~~ Deleted   ● Use Additional Character(s)

Disruption (of)
  ciliary body NEC H21.89
  closure of
    ▶abdominal wall muscle or fascia T81.321
      cornea T81.31
    ▷craniotomy T81.328
    ▷fascia (muscular) (superficial) T81.328
    ▷gastrointestinal tract anastomosis, repair, or
        closure T81.32Ø
    ▷internal organ or tissue T81.328
      laceration (external) (internal) T81.33
    ▷ligament T81.328
      mucosa T81.31
    ▷muscle or muscle flap T81.328
    ▷ribs or rib cage T81.328
      skin and subcutaneous tissue (full-thickness)
        (superficial) T81.31
    ▷skull T81.328
    ▷sternum (sternotomy) T81.328
    ▷tendon T81.328
      traumatic laceration (external) (internal)
        T81.33
  family Z63.8
    due to
      absence of family member due to military
        deployment Z63.31
      absence of family member NEC
        Z63.32
      alcoholism and drug addiction in
        family Z63.72
      bereavement Z63.4
      death (assumed) or disappearance of family
        member Z63.4
      divorce or separation Z63.5
      drug addiction in family Z63.72
      return of family member from military
        deployment (current or past conflict)
        Z63.71
      stressful life events NEC Z63.79
  iris NEC H21.89
  ligament(s) —see also Sprain
    knee
      current injury —see Dislocation, knee
      old (chronic) —see Derangement, knee,
        ligament, instability, chronic
      spontaneous NEC —see Derangement,
        knee, disruption ligament
  ossicular chain —see Discontinuity, ossicles, ear
  pelvic ring (stable) S32.81Ø
    unstable S32.811
  traumatic injury wound repair T81.33
  wound T81.3Ø
    episiotomy O9Ø.1
    operation T81.31
      cesarean O9Ø.Ø
    ▶deep T81.329
      external operation wound (superficial)
        T81.31
    ▷internal operation wound (deep)
        T81.329
      ▶abdominal wall muscle or fascia
        T81.321
      ▶specified NEC T81.328
    perineal (obstetric) O9Ø.1
  traumatic injury repair T81.33
Dissatisfaction with
  employment Z56.9
  school environment Z55.4
Dissecting —see condition
Dissection
  aorta I71.ØØ
    abdominal I71.Ø2
    thoracic I71.Ø19
      aortic arch I71.Ø11
      ascending aorta I71.Ø1Ø
      descending thoracic aorta I71.Ø12
    thoracoabdominal I71.Ø3
  artery I77.7Ø
    basilar (trunk) I77.75
    carotid I77.71
    cerebral (nonruptured) I67.Ø
      ruptured —see Hemorrhage, intracranial,
        subarachnoid
    coronary I25.42
    extremity
      lower I77.77
      upper I77.76
    iliac I77.72
    precerebral
      congenital (nonruptured) Q28.1
      specified site NEC I77.75

Dissection (Continued)
  artery (Continued)
    renal I77.73
    specified NEC I77.79
    vertebral I77.74
  precerebral artery, congenital (nonruptured)
    Q28.1
    Heartland A93.8
  traumatic —see Wound, open, by site
  vascular I99.8
  wound —see Wound, open
Disseminated —see condition
Dissociation
  auriculoventricular or atrioventricular (AV) (any
    degree) (isorhythmic) I45.89
    with heart block I44.2
  interference I45.89
Dissociative reaction, state F44.9
Dissolution, vertebra —see Osteoporosis
Distension, distention
  abdomen R14.Ø
  bladder N32.89
  cecum K63.89
  colon K63.89
  gallbladder K82.8
  intestine K63.89
  kidney N28.89
  liver K76.89
  seminal vesicle N5Ø.89
  stomach K31.89
    acute K31.Ø
    psychogenic F45.8
  ureter —see Dilatation, ureter
  uterus N85.8
Distoma hepaticum infestation B66.3
Distomiasis B66.9
  bile passages B66.3
  hemic B65.9
  hepatic B66.3
    due to Clonorchis sinensis B66.1
  intestinal B66.5
  liver B66.3
    due to Clonorchis sinensis B66.1
  lung B66.4
  pulmonary B66.4
Distomolar (fourth molar) KØØ.1
Disto-occlusion (Division I) (Division II) M26.212
Distortion(s) (congenital)
  adrenal (gland) Q89.1
  arm NEC Q68.8
  bile duct or passage Q44.5
  bladder Q64.79
  brain QØ4.9
  cervix (uteri) Q51.9
  chest (wall) Q67.8
    bones Q76.8
  clavicle Q74.Ø
  clitoris Q52.6
  coccyx Q76.49
  common duct Q44.5
  coronary Q24.5
  cystic duct Q44.5
  ear (auricle) (external) Q17.3
    inner Q16.5
    middle Q16.4
      ossicles Q16.3
  endocrine NEC Q89.2
  eustachian tube Q17.8
  eye (adnexa) Q15.8
  face bone(s) NEC Q75.8
  fallopian tube Q50.6
  femur NEC Q68.8
  fibula NEC Q68.8
  finger(s) Q68.1
  foot Q66.9-●
  genitalia, genital organ(s)
    female Q52.8
      external Q52.79
      internal NEC Q52.8
  gyri QØ4.8
  hand bone(s) Q68.1
  heart (auricle) (ventricle) Q24.8
    valve (cusp) Q24.8
  hepatic duct Q44.5
  humerus NEC Q68.8
  hymen Q52.4
  intrafamilial communications Z63.8
  jaw NEC M26.89
  labium (majus) (minus) Q52.79
  leg NEC Q68.8
  lens Q12.8

Distortion(s) (Continued)
  liver Q44.79
  lumbar spine Q76.49
    with disproportion O33.8
      causing obstructed labor O65.Ø
  lumbosacral (joint) (region) Q76.49
    kyphosis —see Kyphosis, congenital
    lordosis —see Lordosis, congenital
  nerve QØ7.8
  nose Q3Ø.8
  organ
    of Corti Q16.5
    or site not listed —see Anomaly, by site
      ossicles, ear Q16.3
  oviduct Q5Ø.6
  pancreas Q45.3
  parathyroid (gland) Q89.2
  pituitary (gland) Q89.2
  radius NEC Q68.8
  sacroiliac joint Q74.2
  sacrum Q76.49
  scapula Q74.Ø
  shoulder girdle Q74.Ø
  skull bone(s) NEC Q75.8
    with
      anencephalus QØØ.Ø
      encephalocele —see Encephalocele
      hydrocephalus QØ3.9
        with spina bifida —see Spina bifida, with
          hydrocephalus
      microcephaly QØ2
  spinal cord QØ6.8
  spine Q76.49
    kyphosis —see Kyphosis, congenital
    lordosis —see Lordosis, congenital
  spleen Q89.Ø9
  sternum NEC Q76.7
  thorax (wall) Q67.8
    bony Q76.8
  thymus (gland) Q89.2
  thyroid (gland) Q89.2
  tibia NEC Q68.8
  toe(s) Q66.9-●
  tongue Q38.3
  trachea (cartilage) Q32.1
  ulna NEC Q68.8
  ureter Q62.8
  urethra Q64.79
    causing obstruction Q64.39
  uterus Q51.9
  vagina Q52.4
  vertebra Q76.49
    kyphosis —see Kyphosis, congenital
    lordosis —see Lordosis, congenital
  visual —see also Disturbance, vision
    shape and size H53.15
  vulva Q52.79
  wrist (bones) (joint) Q68.8
Distress
  abdomen —see Pain, abdominal
  acute respiratory RØ6.Ø3
    syndrome (adult) (child) J8Ø
  epigastric R1Ø.13
  fetal P84
    complicating pregnancy —see Stress, fetal
  gastrointestinal (functional) K3Ø
    psychogenic F45.8
  intestinal (functional) NOS K59.9
    psychogenic F45.8
  maternal, during labor and delivery O75.Ø
  relationship, with spouse or intimate partner Z63.Ø
  respiratory (adult) (child) RØ6.Ø3
    newborn P22.9
      specified NEC P22.8
    orthopnea RØ6.Ø1
    psychogenic F45.8
    shortness of breath RØ6.Ø2
    specified type NEC RØ6.Ø9
Distribution vessel, atypical Q27.9
  coronary artery Q24.5
  precerebral Q28.1
Districhiasis L68.8
Disturbance(s) —see also Disease
  absorption K9Ø.9
    calcium E58
    carbohydrate K9Ø.49
    fat K9Ø.49
      pancreatic K9Ø.3
    protein K9Ø.49
    starch K9Ø.49
    vitamin —see Deficiency, vitamin

Disturbance(s) *(Continued)*
  acid-base equilibrium E87.8
    mixed E87.4
  activity and attention (with hyperkinesis) —*see*
    Disorder, attention-deficit hyperactivity
  amino acid transport E72.00
  assimilation, food K90.9
  auditory nerve, except deafness —*see*
    subcategory H93.3
  behavior —*see* Disorder, conduct
  blood clotting (mechanism) —*see also* Defect,
    coagulation D68.9
  cerebral
    nerve —*see* Disorder, nerve, cranial
    status, newborn P91.9
      specified NEC P91.88
  circulatory I99.9
  conduct —*see also* Disorder, conduct F91.9
    adjustment reaction —*see* Disorder,
      adjustment
    compulsive F63.9
    disruptive F91.9
    hyperkinetic —*see* Disorder, attention-deficit
      hyperactivity
    socialized F91.2
    specified NEC F91.8
    unsocialized F91.1
  coordination R27.8
  cranial nerve —*see* Disorder, nerve, cranial
  deep sensibility —*see* Disturbance, sensation
  digestive K30
    psychogenic F45.8
  electrolyte —*see also* Imbalance, electrolyte
    newborn, transitory P74.49
      hyperammonemia P74.6
      hyperchloremia P74.421
      hyperchloremic metabolic acidosis P74.421
      hypochloremia P74.422
      potassium balance
        hyperkalemia P74.31
        hypokalemia P74.32
      sodium balance
        hypernatremia P74.21
        hyponatremia P74.22
      specified type NEC P74.49
  emotions specific to childhood and adolescence
    F93.9
    with
      anxiety and fearfulness NEC F93.8
      elective mutism F94.0
      oppositional disorder F91.3
      sensitivity (withdrawal) F40.10
      shyness F40.10
      social withdrawal F40.10
    involving relationship problems F93.8
    mixed F93.8
    specified NEC F93.8
  endocrine (gland) E34.9
    neonatal, transitory P72.9
      specified NEC P72.8
  equilibrium R42
  fructose metabolism E74.10
  gait —*see* Gait
    hysterical F44.4
    psychogenic F44.4
  gastrointestinal (functional) K30
    psychogenic F45.8
  habit, child F98.9
  hearing, except deafness and tinnitus —*see*
    Abnormal, auditory perception
  heart, functional (conditions in I44-I50)
    due to presence of (cardiac) prosthesis
      I97.19-●
    postoperative I97.89
      cardiac surgery —*see also* Infarct,
        myocardium, associated with
        revascularization procedure I97.19-●
  hormones E34.9
  innervation uterus (parasympathetic)
    (sympathetic) N85.8
  keratinization NEC
    gingiva K05.10
      nonplaque induced K05.11
      plaque induced K05.10
    lip K13.0
    oral (mucosa) (soft tissue) K13.29
    tongue K13.29
  learning (specific) —*see* Disorder, learning
  memory —*see* Amnesia
    mild, following organic brain damage
      F06.8

Disturbance(s) *(Continued)*
  mental F99
    associated with diseases classified elsewhere
      F54
  metabolism E88.9
    with
      abortion —*see* Abortion, by type with other
        specified complication
      ectopic pregnancy O08.5
      molar pregnancy O08.5
    amino-acid E72.9
      aromatic E70.9
      branched-chain E71.2
      straight-chain E72.89
      sulfur-bearing E72.10
    ammonia E72.20
    arginine E72.21
    arginosuccinic acid E72.22
    carbohydrate E74.9
    cholesterol E78.9
    citrulline E72.23
    cystathionine E72.19
    general E88.9
    glutamine E72.89
    histidine E70.40
    homocystine E72.19
    hydroxylysine E72.3
    in labor or delivery O75.89
    iron E83.10
    lipoid E78.9
    lysine E72.3
    methionine E72.19
    neonatal, transitory P74.9
      calcium and magnesium P71.9
        specified type NEC P71.8
      carbohydrate metabolism P70.9
        specified type NEC P70.8
      specified NEC P74.8
    ornithine E72.4
    phosphate E83.39
    sodium NEC E87.8
    threonine E72.89
    tryptophan E70.5
    tyrosine E70.20
    urea cycle E72.20
  motor R29.2
  nervous, functional R45.0
  neuromuscular mechanism (eye), due to syphilis
    A52.15
  nutritional E63.9
    nail L60.3
  ocular motion H51.9
    psychogenic F45.8
  oculogyric H51.8
    psychogenic F45.8
  oculomotor H51.9
    psychogenic F45.8
  olfactory nerve R43.1
  optic nerve NEC —*see* Disorder, nerve,
    optic
  oral epithelium, including tongue NEC K13.29
  perceptual due to
    alcohol withdrawal F10.232
    amphetamine intoxication F15.922
      in
        abuse F15.122
        dependence F15.222
    anxiolytic withdrawal F13.232
    cannabis intoxication (acute) F12.922
      in
        abuse F12.122
        dependence F12.222
    cocaine intoxication (acute) F14.922
      in
        abuse F14.122
        dependence F14.222
    hypnotic withdrawal F13.232
    opioid intoxication (acute) F11.922
      in
        abuse F11.122
        dependence F11.222
    phencyclidine intoxication (acute) F16.122
    sedative withdrawal F13.232
  personality (pattern) (trait) —*see also* Disorder,
    personality F60.9
    following organic brain damage F07.9
  polyglandular E31.9
    specified NEC E31.8
  potassium balance, newborn
    hyperkalemia P74.31
    hypokalemia P74.32

Disturbance(s) *(Continued)*
  psychogenic F45.9
  psychomotor F44.4
  psychophysical visual H53.16
  pupillary —*see* Anomaly, pupil, function
  reflex R29.2
  rhythm, heart I49.9
  salivary secretion K11.7
  sensation (cold) (heat) (localization) (tactile
    discrimination) (texture) (vibratory) NEC
    R20.9
    hysterical F44.6
    skin R20.9
      anesthesia R20.0
      hyperesthesia R20.3
      hypoesthesia R20.1
      paresthesia R20.2
      specified type NEC R20.8
    smell R43.9
      and taste (mixed) R43.8
      anosmia R43.0
      parosmia R43.1
      specified NEC R43.8
    taste R43.9
      and smell (mixed) R43.8
      parageusia R43.2
      specified NEC R43.8
  sensory —*see* Disturbance, sensation
  situational (transient) —*see also* Disorder,
    adjustment
    acute F43.0
  sleep G47.9
    nonorganic origin F51.9
  smell —*see* Disturbance, sensation, smell
  sociopathic F60.2
  sodium balance, newborn
    hypernatremia P74.21
    hyponatremia P74.22
  speech R47.9
    developmental F80.9
    specified NEC R47.89
  stomach (functional) K31.9
  sympathetic (nerve) G90.9
  taste —*see* Disturbance, sensation, taste
  temperature
    regulation, newborn P81.9
      specified NEC P81.8
    sense R20.8
      hysterical F44.6
  tooth
    eruption K00.6
    formation K00.4
    structure, hereditary NEC K00.5
  touch —*see* Disturbance, sensation
  vascular I99.9
    arteriosclerotic —*see* Arteriosclerosis
  vasomotor I73.9
  vasospastic I73.9
  vision, visual H53.9
    following
      cerebral infarction I69.398
      cerebrovascular disease I69.998
        specified NEC I69.898
      intracerebral hemorrhage I69.198
      nontraumatic intracranial hemorrhage NEC
        I69.298
      specified disease NEC I69.898
      subarachnoid hemorrhage I69.098
    psychophysical H53.16
    specified NEC H53.8
    subjective H53.10
      day blindness H53.11
      discomfort H53.14-●
      distortions of shape and size H53.15
      loss
        sudden H53.13-●
        transient H53.12-●
      specified type NEC H53.19
  voice R49.9
    psychogenic F44.4
    specified NEC R49.8
Diuresis R35.89
Diver's palsy, paralysis or squeeze T70.3
Diverticulitis (acute) K57.92
  bladder —*see* Cystitis
  ileum —*see* Diverticulitis, intestine, small
  intestine K57.92
    with
      abscess, perforation K57.80
        with bleeding K57.81
      bleeding K57.93

Dropsy, dropsical *(Continued)*
  lung —*see* Edema, lung
  newborn due to isoimmunization P56.0
  pericardium —*see* Pericarditis
Drowned, drowning (near) T75.1
Drowsiness R40.0
Drug
  abuse counseling and surveillance Z71.51
  addiction —*see* Dependence
  dependence —*see* Dependence
  habit —*see* Dependence
  harmful use —*see* Abuse, drug
  induced fever R50.2
  overdose —*see* Table of Drugs and Chemicals, by
    drug, poisoning
  poisoning —*see* Table of Drugs and Chemicals,
    by drug, poisoning
  resistant organism infection —*see also* Resistant,
    organism, to, drug Z16.30
  therapy
    long term (current) (prophylactic) —*see*
      Therapy, drug long-term (current)
      (prophylactic)
    short term - omit code
  wrong substance given or taken in error —*see*
    Table of Drugs and Chemicals, by drug,
    poisoning
Drunkenness (without dependence) F10.129
  acute in alcoholism F10.229
  chronic (without remission) F10.20
    with remission F10.21
  pathological (without dependence) F10.129
    with dependence F10.229
  sleep F51.9
Drusen
  macula (degenerative) (retina) —*see*
    Degeneration, macula, drusen
  optic disc H47.32-●
Dry, dryness —*see also* condition
  larynx J38.7
  mouth R68.2
    due to dehydration E86.0
  nose J34.89
  socket (teeth) M27.3
  throat J39.2
DSAP L56.5
Duane's syndrome H50.81-●
Dubin-Johnson disease or syndrome E80.6
Dubois' disease (thymus gland) A50.59 *[E35]*
Dubowitz' syndrome Q87.19
Duchenne-Aran muscular atrophy G12.21
Duchenne-Griesinger disease G71.01
Duchenne's
  disease or syndrome
    motor neuron disease G12.22
    muscular dystrophy G71.01
  locomotor ataxia (syphilitic) A52.11
  paralysis
    birth injury P14.0
    due to or associated with
      motor neuron disease G12.22
      muscular dystrophy G71.01
Ducreyi chancre A57
Ducrey's chancre A57
Duct, ductus —*see* condition
Duffy phenotype —*see* Phenotype, Duffy
Duhring's disease (dermatitis herpetiformis) L13.0
Dullness, cardiac (decreased) (increased) R01.2
Dumb ague —*see* Malaria
Dumbness —*see* Aphasia
Dumdum fever B55.0
Dumping syndrome (postgastrectomy) K91.1
Duodenitis (nonspecific) (peptic) K29.80
  erosive —*see* Ulcer, duodenum
  with bleeding K29.81
Duodenocholangitis —*see* Cholangitis
Duodenum, duodenal —*see* condition
Duplay's bursitis or periarthritis M75.0
Duplication, duplex —*see also* Accessory
  alimentary tract Q45.8
  anus Q43.4
  appendix (and cecum) Q43.4
  biliary duct (any) Q44.5
  bladder Q64.79
  cecum (and appendix) Q43.4
  cervix Q51.820
  chromosome NEC —*see also* Trisomy
    with complex rearrangements NEC Q92.5
    seen only at prometaphase Q92.8
  cystic duct Q44.5
  digestive organs Q45.8

Duplication, duplex *(Continued)*
  esophagus Q39.8
  frontonasal process Q75.8
  intestine (large) (small) Q43.4
  kidney Q63.0
  liver Q44.79
  pancreas Q45.3
  penis Q55.69
  respiratory organs NEC Q34.8
  salivary duct Q38.4
  spinal cord (incomplete) Q06.2
  stomach Q40.2
Dupré's disease (meningism) R29.1
Dupuytren's contraction or disease M72.0
Durand-Nicolas-Favre disease A55
Durotomy (inadvertent) (incidental) G97.41
Duroziez's disease (congenital mitral stenosis)
  Q23.2
Dutton's relapsing fever (West African) A68.1
Dwarfism (*see also* Short, stature) E34.328
  achondroplastic Q77.4
  congenital (*see also* Short, stature) E34.328
  constitutional E34.31
  hypochondroplastic Q77.4
  hypophyseal E23.0
  infantile (*see also* Short, stature) E34.328
  Laron-type (*see also* Short, stature) E34.321
  Lorain (-Levi) type E23.0
  metatropic Q77.8
  nephrotic-glycosuric (with hypophosphatemic
    rickets) E72.09
  nutritional E45
  pancreatic K86.89
  pituitary E23.0
  renal N25.0
  thanatophoric Q77.1
Dyke-Young anemia (secondary) (symptomatic)
  D59.19
Dysacusis —*see* Abnormal, auditory
  perception
Dysadrenocortism E27.9
  hyperfunction E27.0
Dysarthria R47.1
  following
    cerebral infarction I69.322
    cerebrovascular disease I69.922
      specified disease NEC I69.822
    intracerebral hemorrhage I69.122
    nontraumatic intracranial hemorrhage NEC
      I69.222
    subarachnoid hemorrhage I69.022
Dysautonomia (familial) G90.1
Dysbarism T70.3
Dysbasia R26.2
  angiosclerotica intermittens I73.9
  hysterical F44.4
  lordotica (progressiva) G24.1
  nonorganic origin F44.4
  psychogenic F44.4
Dysbetalipoproteinemia (familial) E78.2
Dyscalculia R48.8
  developmental F81.2
Dyschezia K59.00
Dyschondroplasia (with hemangiomata) Q78.4
Dyschromia (skin) L81.9
Dyscollagenosis M35.9
Dyscranio-pygo-phalangy Q87.0
Dyscrasia
  blood (with) D75.9
    antepartum hemorrhage —*see* Hemorrhage,
      antepartum, with coagulation defect
    intrapartum hemorrhage O67.0
    newborn P61.9
      specified type NEC P61.8
    puerperal, postpartum O72.3
  polyglandular, pluriglandular E31.9
Dysendocrinism E34.9
Dysentery, dysenteric (catarrhal) (diarrhea)
  (epidemic) (hemorrhagic) (infectious)
  (sporadic) (tropical) A09
  abscess, liver A06.4
  amebic —*see also* Amebiasis A06.0
    with abscess —*see* Abscess, amebic
    acute A06.0
    chronic A06.1
  arthritis —*see also* category M01 A09
    bacillary —*see also* category M01 A03.9
  bacillary A03.9
    arthritis —*see also* category M01 A03.9
    Boyd A03.2
    Flexner A03.1

Dysentery, dysenteric *(Continued)*
  bacillary *(Continued)*
    Schmitz (-Stutzer) A03.0
    Shiga (-Kruse) A03.0
    Shigella A03.9
      boydii A03.2
      dysenteriae A03.0
      flexneri A03.1
      group A A03.0
      group B A03.1
      group C A03.2
      group D A03.3
      sonnei A03.3
      specified type NEC A03.8
    Sonne A03.3
    specified type NEC A03.8
  balantidial A07.0
  Balantidium coli A07.0
  Boyd's A03.2
  candidal B37.82
  Chilomastix A07.8
  Chinese A03.9
  coccidial A07.3
  Dientamoeba (fragilis) A07.8
  Embadomonas A07.8
  Entamoeba, entamebic —*see* Dysentery, amebic
  Flexner-Boyd A03.2
  Flexner's A03.1
  Giardia lamblia A07.1
  Hiss-Russell A03.1
  Lamblia A07.1
  leishmanial B55.0
  malarial —*see* Malaria
  metazoal B82.0
  monilial B37.82
  protozoal A07.9
  Salmonella A02.0
  schistosomal B65.1
  Schmitz (-Stutzer) A03.0
  Shiga (-Kruse) A03.0
  Shigella NOS —*see* Dysentery, bacillary
  Sonne A03.3
  strongyloidiasis B78.0
  trichomonal A07.8
  viral —*see also* Enteritis, viral A08.4
Dysequilibrium R42
Dysesthesia R20.8
  hysterical F44.6
Dysferlinopathy G71.033
Dysfibrinogenemia (congenital) D68.2
Dysfunction
  adrenal E27.9
    hyperfunction E27.0
  autonomic
    due to alcohol G31.2
    somatoform F45.8
  bladder N31.9
    neurogenic NOS —*see* Dysfunction, bladder,
      neuromuscular
    neuromuscular NOS N31.9
      atonic (motor) (sensory) N31.2
      autonomous N31.2
      flaccid N31.2
      nonreflex N31.2
      reflex N31.1
      specified NEC N31.8
      uninhibited N31.0
  bleeding, uterus N93.8
  cerebral G93.89
  chronic
    coronary microvascular I25.85
    lung allograft J4A.9
      mixed J4A.0
      specified NEC J4A.8
  colon K59.9
    psychogenic F45.8
  colostomy K94.03
  coronary microvascular I25.85
    with
      angina pectoris I20.81
      myocardial infarction I21.B
    acute I24.81
    chronic I25.85
  cystic duct K82.8
  cystostomy (stoma) —*see* Complications,
    cystostomy
  ejaculatory N53.19
    anejaculatory orgasm N53.13
    painful N53.12
    premature F52.4
    retarded N53.11

Dysfunction (Continued)
  endocrine NOS E34.9
  endometrium N85.8
  enterostomy K94.13
  erectile —see Dysfunction, sexual, male, erectile
  feeding, pediatric
    acute R63.31
    chronic R63.32
  gallbladder K82.8
  gastrostomy (stoma) K94.23
  gland, glandular NOS E34.9
    meibomian, of eyelid —see Dysfunction,
        meibomian gland
  heart I51.89
  hemoglobin D75.89
  hepatic K76.89
  hypophysis E23.7
  hypothalamic NEC E23.3
  ileostomy (stoma) K94.13
  jejunostomy (stoma) K94.13
  kidney —see Disease, renal
  labyrinthine —see subcategory H83.2
  left ventricular, following sudden emotional
      stress I51.81
  liver K76.89
  male —see Dysfunction, sexual, male
  meibomian gland, of eyelid H02.889
    left H02.886
      lower H02.885
      upper H02.884
      upper and lower eyelids H02.88B
    right H02.883
      lower H02.882
      upper H02.881
      upper and lower eyelids H02.88A
▶ multifidus muscles, lumbar region M62.85
  orgasmic (female) F52.31
    male F52.32
  ovary E28.9
    specified NEC E28.8
  papillary muscle I51.89
  parathyroid E21.4
  physiological NEC R68.89
    psychogenic F59
  pineal gland E34.8
  pituitary (gland) E23.3
  platelets D69.1
  polyglandular E31.9
    specified NEC E31.8
  psychophysiologic F59
  psychosexual F52.9
    with
      dyspareunia F52.6
      premature ejaculation F52.4
      vaginismus F52.5
  pylorus K31.9
  rectum K59.9
    psychogenic F45.8
  reflex (sympathetic) —see Syndrome, pain,
      complex regional I
  segmental —see Dysfunction, somatic
  senile R54
  sexual (due to) R37
    alcohol F10.981
    amphetamine F15.981
      in
        abuse F15.181
        dependence F15.281
    anxiolytic F13.981
      in
        abuse F13.181
        dependence F13.281
    cocaine F14.981
      in
        abuse F14.181
        dependence F14.281
    excessive sexual drive F52.8
    failure of genital response (male) F52.21
      female F52.22
    female N94.9
      aversion F52.1
      dyspareunia N94.10
        psychogenic F52.6
      frigidity F52.22
      nymphomania F52.8
      orgasmic F52.31
      psychogenic F52.9
        aversion F52.1
        dyspareunia F52.6
        frigidity F52.22
        nymphomania F52.8

Dysfunction (Continued)
  sexual (due to) (Continued)
    female (Continued)
      psychogenic (Continued)
        orgasmic F52.31
        vaginismus F52.5
      vaginismus N94.2
        psychogenic F52.5
    hypnotic F13.981
      in
        abuse F13.181
        dependence F13.281
    inhibited orgasm (female) F52.31
      male F52.32
    lack
      of sexual enjoyment F52.1
      or loss of sexual desire F52.0
    male N53.9
      anejaculatory orgasm N53.13
      ejaculatory N53.19
        painful N53.12
        premature F52.4
        retarded N53.11
      erectile N52.9
        drug induced N52.2
        due to
          disease classified elsewhere N52.1
          drug N52.2
        postoperative (postprocedural) N52.39
          following
            cryotherapy N52.37
            interstitial seed therapy N52.36
            prostate ablative therapy N52.37
            prostatectomy N52.34
              radical N52.31
            radiation therapy N52.35
            radical cystectomy N52.32
            ultrasound ablative therapy N52.37
            urethral surgery N52.33
        psychogenic F52.21
        specified cause NEC N52.8
        vasculogenic
          arterial insufficiency N52.01
            with corporo-venous occlusive
                N52.03
          corporo-venous occlusive N52.02
            with arterial insufficiency N52.03
      impotence —see Dysfunction, sexual, male,
          erectile
      psychogenic F52.9
        aversion F52.1
        erectile F52.21
        orgasmic F52.32
        premature ejaculation F52.4
        satyriasis F52.8
        specified type NEC F52.8
      specified type NEC N53.8
    nonorganic F52.9
      specified NEC F52.8
    opioid F11.981
      in
        abuse F11.181
        dependence F11.281
    orgasmic dysfunction (female) F52.31
      male F52.32
    premature ejaculation F52.4
    psychoactive substances NEC F19.981
      in
        abuse F19.181
        dependence F19.281
    psychogenic F52.9
    sedative F13.981
      in
        abuse F13.181
        dependence F13.281
    sexual aversion F52.1
    vaginismus (nonorganic) (psychogenic) F52.5
  sinoatrial node I49.5
  somatic M99.09
    abdomen M99.09
    acromioclavicular M99.07
    cervical region M99.01
    cervicothoracic M99.01
    costochondral M99.08
    costovertebral M99.08
    head region M99.00
    hip M99.05
    lower extremity M99.06
    lumbar region M99.03
    lumbosacral M99.03
    occipitocervical M99.00

Dysfunction (Continued)
  somatic (Continued)
    pelvic region M99.05
    pubic M99.05
    rib cage M99.08
    sacral region M99.04
    sacrococcygeal M99.04
    sacroiliac M99.04
    specified NEC M99.09
    sternochondral M99.08
    sternoclavicular M99.07
    thoracic region M99.02
    thoracolumbar M99.02
    upper extremity M99.07
  somatoform autonomic F45.8
  stomach K31.89
    psychogenic F45.8
  suprarenal E27.9
    hyperfunction E27.0
  symbolic R48.9
    specified type NEC R48.8
  temporomandibular (joint) M26.69
    joint-pain syndrome M26.62-●
  testicular (endocrine) E29.9
    specified NEC E29.8
  thymus E32.9
  thyroid E07.9
  ureterostomy (stoma) —see Complications,
      stoma, urinary tract
  urethrostomy (stoma) —see Complications,
      stoma, urinary tract
  uterus, complicating delivery O62.9
    hypertonic O62.4
    hypotonic O62.2
      primary O62.0
      secondary O62.1
  ventricular I51.9
    with congestive heart failure —see also Failure,
        heart I50.9
    left, reversible, following sudden emotional
        stress I51.81
Dysgenesis
  gonadal (due to chromosomal anomaly)
      Q96.9
    pure Q99.1
  renal Q60.5
    bilateral Q60.4
    unilateral Q60.3
  reticular D72.0
  tidal platelet D69.3
Dysgerminoma
  specified site —see Neoplasm, malignant,
      by site
  unspecified site
    female C56.9
    male C62.90
Dysgeusia R43.2
Dysgraphia R27.8
Dyshidrosis, dysidrosis L30.1
Dyskaryotic cervical smear R87.619
Dyskeratosis L85.8
  cervix —see Dysplasia, cervix
  congenital Q82.8
  uterus NEC N85.8
Dyskinesia G24.9
  biliary (cystic duct or gallbladder) K82.8
  drug induced
    orofacial G24.01
  esophagus K22.4
  hysterical F44.4
  intestinal K59.89
  nonorganic origin F44.4
  orofacial (idiopathic) G24.4
    drug induced G24.01
  psychogenic F44.4
  subacute, drug induced G24.01
  tardive G24.01
    neuroleptic induced G24.01
  trachea J39.8
  tracheobronchial J98.09
Dyslalia (developmental) F80.0
Dyslexia R48.0
  developmental F81.0
Dyslipidemia E78.5
  depressed HDL cholesterol E78.6
  elevated fasting triglycerides E78.1
Dysmaturity —see also Light for dates
  pulmonary (newborn) (Wilson-Mikity) P27.0
Dysmenorrhea (essential) (exfoliative) N94.6
  congestive (syndrome) N94.6
  primary N94.4

▶ New   ⇒ Revised   ~~deleted~~ Deleted   ● Use Additional Character(s)

Dysmenorrhea *(Continued)*
  psychogenic F45.8
  secondary N94.5
Dysmetabolic syndrome X E88.810
Dysmetria R27.8
Dysmorphia
▶ muscle F45.22
Dysmorphism (due to)
  alcohol Q86.0
  exogenous cause NEC Q86.8
  hydantoin Q86.1
  warfarin Q86.2
Dysmorphophobia (nondelusional) F45.22
  delusional F22
Dysnomia R47.01
Dysorexia R63.0
  psychogenic F50.89
Dysostosis
  cleidocranial, cleidocranialis Q74.0
  craniofacial Q75.1
  Fairbank's (idiopathic familial generalized
      osteophytosis) Q78.9
  mandibulofacial (incomplete) Q75.4
  multiplex E76.01
  oculomandibular Q75.5
Dyspareunia (female) N94.10
  deep N94.12
  male N53.12
  nonorganic F52.6
  psychogenic F52.6
  secondary N94.19
  specified NEC N94.19
  superficial (introital) N94.11
Dyspepsia R10.13
  atonic K30
  functional (allergic) (congenital)
      (gastrointestinal) (occupational) (reflex)
      K30
  intestinal K59.89
  nervous F45.8
  neurotic F45.8
  psychogenic F45.8
Dysphagia R13.10
  cervical R13.19
  following
      cerebral infarction I69.391
      cerebrovascular disease I69.991
          specified NEC I69.891
      intracerebral hemorrhage I69.191
      nontraumatic intracranial hemorrhage NEC
          I69.291
      specified disease NEC I69.891
      subarachnoid hemorrhage I69.091
  functional (hysterical) F45.8
  hysterical F45.8
  nervous (hysterical) F45.8
  neurogenic R13.19
  oral phase R13.11
  oropharyngeal phase R13.12
  pharyngeal phase R13.13
  pharyngoesophageal phase R13.14
  psychogenic F45.8
  sideropenic D50.1
  spastica K22.4
  specified NEC R13.19
Dysphagocytosis, congenital D71
Dysphasia R47.02
  developmental
      expressive type F80.1
      receptive type F80.2
  following
      cerebrovascular disease I69.921
          cerebral infarction I69.321
          intracerebral hemorrhage I69.121
      nontraumatic intracranial hemorrhage NEC
          I69.221
          specified disease NEC I69.821
          subarachnoid hemorrhage I69.021
Dysphonia R49.0
  functional F44.4
  hysterical F44.4
  psychogenic F44.4
  spastica J38.3
Dysphoria
  gender F64.9
      in
          adolescence and adulthood F64.0
          children F64.2
      specified NEC F64.8
      postpartal O90.6
Dyspituitarism E23.3

Dysplasia —*see also* Anomaly
  acetabular, congenital Q65.89
  alveolar capillary, with vein misalignment
      J84.843
  anus (histologically confirmed) (mild)
      (moderate) K62.82
      severe D01.3
  arrhythmogenic right ventricular I42.8
  arterial, fibromuscular I77.3
  asphyxiating thoracic (congenital) Q77.2
  brain Q07.9
  bronchopulmonary, perinatal P27.1
  cervix (uteri) N87.9
      mild N87.0
      moderate N87.1
      severe D06.9
  chondroectodermal Q77.6
  colon D12.6
  craniometaphyseal Q78.58
  dentinal K00.5
  diaphyseal, progressive Q78.3
  dystrophic Q77.5
  ectodermal (anhidrotic) (congenital) (hereditary)
      Q82.4
      hydrotic Q82.8
  epithelial, uterine cervix —*see* Dysplasia,
      cervix
  eye (congenital) Q11.2
  fibrous
      bone NEC (monostotic) M85.00
          ankle M85.07-●
          foot M85.07-●
          forearm M85.03-●
          hand M85.04-●
          lower leg M85.06-●
          multiple site M85.09
          neck M85.08
          rib M85.08
          shoulder M85.01-●
          skull M85.08
          specified site NEC M85.08
          thigh M85.05-●
          toe M85.07-●
          upper arm M85.02-●
          vertebra M85.08
      diaphyseal, progressive Q78.3
      jaw M27.8
      polyostotic Q78.1
  florid osseous —*see also* Cyst, calcifying
      odontogenic
  high grade, focal D12.6
  hip, congenital Q65.89
  joint, congenital Q74.8
  kidney Q61.4
      multicystic Q61.4
  leg Q74.2
  lung, congenital (not associated with short
      gestation) Q33.6
  mammary (gland) (benign) N60.9-●
      cyst (solitary) —*see* Cyst, breast
      cystic —*see* Mastopathy, cystic
      duct ectasia —*see* Ectasia, mammary
          duct
      fibroadenosis —*see* Fibroadenosis, breast
      fibrosclerosis —*see* Fibrosclerosis, breast
      specified type NEC N60.8-●
  metaphyseal Q78.5
  muscle Q79.8
  oculodentodigital Q87.0
  periapical (cemental) (cemento-osseous) —*see*
      Cyst, calcifying odontogenic
  periosteum —*see* Disorder, bone, specified type
      NEC
  polyostotic fibrous Q78.1
  prostate —*see also* Neoplasia, intraepithelial,
      prostate N42.30
      severe D07.5
      specified NEC N42.39
  renal Q61.4
      multicystic Q61.4
  retinal, congenital Q14.1
  right ventricular, arrhythmogenic I42.8
  septo-optic Q04.4
  skin L98.8
  spinal cord Q06.1
  spondyloepiphyseal Q77.7
  thymic, with immunodeficiency D82.1
  vagina N89.3
      mild N89.0
      moderate N89.1
      severe NEC D07.2

Dysplasia *(Continued)*
  vulva N90.3
      mild N90.0
      moderate N90.1
      severe NEC D07.1
Dysplasminogenemia E88.02
Dyspnea (nocturnal) (paroxysmal) R06.00
  asthmatic (bronchial) J45.909
      with
          bronchitis J45.909
              with
                  exacerbation (acute) J45.901
                  status asthmaticus J45.902
              chronic J44.89
          exacerbation (acute) J45.901
          status asthmaticus J45.902
  cardiac —*see* Failure, ventricular, left
  cardiac —*see* Failure, ventricular, left
  functional F45.8
  hyperventilation R06.4
  hysterical F45.8
  newborn P28.89
  psychogenic F45.8
  shortness of breath R06.02
  specified type NEC R06.09
  transfusion-associated [TAD] J95.87
Dyspraxia R27.8
  developmental (syndrome) F82
Dysproteinemia E88.09
Dysreflexia, autonomic G90.4
Dysrhythmia
  cardiac I49.9
      newborn
          bradycardia P29.12
          occurring before birth P03.819
              before onset of labor P03.810
              during labor P03.811
          tachycardia P29.11
      postoperative I97.89
  cerebral or cortical —*see* Epilepsy
Dyssomnia —*see* Disorder, sleep
Dyssynergia
  biliary K83.8
  bladder sphincter N36.44
  cerebellaris myoclonica (Hunt's ataxia) G11.19
Dysthymia F34.1
Dysthyroidism E07.9
Dystocia O66.9
  affecting newborn P03.1
  cervical (hypotonic) O62.2
      affecting newborn P03.6
      primary O62.0
      secondary O62.1
  contraction ring O62.4
  fetal O66.9
      abnormality NEC O66.3
      conjoined twins O66.3
      oversize O66.2
  maternal O66.9
  positional O64.9
  shoulder (girdle) O66.0
      causing obstructed labor O66.0
  uterine NEC O62.4
Dystonia G24.9
  cervical G24.3
  deformans progressiva G24.1
  drug induced NEC G24.09
      acute G24.02
      specified NEC G24.09
  familial G24.1
  idiopathic G24.1
      familial G24.1
      nonfamilial G24.2
      orofacial G24.4
  lenticularis G24.8
  musculorum deformans G24.1
  neuroleptic induced (acute) G24.02
  orofacial (idiopathic) G24.4
  oromandibular G24.4
      due to drug G24.01
  specified NEC G24.8
  torsion (familial) (idiopathic) G24.1
      acquired G24.8
      genetic G24.1
      symptomatic (nonfamilial) G24.2
Dystonic movements R25.8
Dystrophy, dystrophia
  adiposogenital E23.6
  autosomal recessive, childhood type, muscular
      dystrophy resembling Duchenne or Becker
      G71.01

— E —

▶ New   ⇒ Revised   ~~deleted~~ Deleted   ● Use Additional Character(s)

▶ New   ⇒ Revised   ~~deleted~~ Deleted   ● Use Additional Character(s)

Effect, adverse *(Continued)*
  anesthesia —*see also* Anesthesia T88.59
    in labor and delivery O74.9
    local, toxic
      in labor and delivery O74.4-●
      in pregnancy NEC O29.3-●
      postpartum, puerperal O89.3
    postpartum, puerperal O89.9
    specified NEC T88.59
      in labor and delivery O74.8
      postpartum, puerperal O89.8
    spinal and epidural T88.59
      headache T88.59
        in labor and delivery O74.5
        postpartum, puerperal O89.4
      specified NEC
        in labor and delivery O74.6
        postpartum, puerperal O89.5
  antitoxin —*see* Complications, vaccination
  atmospheric pressure T70.9
    due to explosion T70.8
    high T70.3
    low —*see* Effect, adverse, high altitude
    specified effect NEC T70.8
  biological, correct substance properly
      administered —*see* Effect, adverse, drug
  blood (derivatives) (serum) (transfusion) —*see*
      Complications, transfusion
  chemical substance —*see* Table of Drugs and
      Chemicals
  cold (temperature) (weather) T69.9
    chilblains T69.1
    frostbite —*see* Frostbite
    specified effect NEC T69.8
  drugs and medicaments T88.7
    specified drug —*see* Table of Drugs and
        Chemicals, by drug, adverse effect
    specified effect — code to condition
  electric current, electricity (shock) T75.4
    burn —*see* Burn
  exertion (excessive) T73.3
  exposure —*see* Exposure
  external cause NEC T75.89
  foodstuffs T78.1
    allergic reaction —*see* Allergy, food
      causing anaphylaxis —*see* Shock,
          anaphylactic, due to food
    noxious —*see* Poisoning, food, noxious
  gases, fumes, or vapors T59.9-●
    specified agent —*see* Table of Drugs and
        Chemicals
  glue (airplane) sniffing
    due to drug abuse —*see* Abuse, drug, inhalant
    due to drug dependence —*see* Dependence,
        drug, inhalant
  heat —*see* Heat
  high altitude NEC T70.29
    anoxia T70.29
    on
      ears T70.0
      sinuses T70.1
    polycythemia D75.1
  high pressure fluids T70.4
  hot weather —*see* Heat
  hunger T73.0
  immersion, foot —*see* Immersion
  immunization —*see* Complications, vaccination
  immunological agents —*see* Complications,
      vaccination
  infrared (radiation) (rays) NOS T66
    dermatitis or eczema L59.8
  infusion —*see* Complications, infusion
  lack of care of infants —*see* Maltreatment, child
  lightning —*see* Lightning
  medical care T88.9
    specified NEC T88.8
  medicinal substance, correct, properly
      administered —*see* Effect, adverse, drug
  motion T75.3
  noise, on inner ear —*see* subcategory H83.3
  overheated places —*see* Heat
  psychosocial, of work environment Z56.5
  radiation (diagnostic) (infrared) (natural source)
      (therapeutic) (ultraviolet) (X-ray) NOS T66
    dermatitis or eczema —*see* Dermatitis, due to,
        radiation
    fibrosis of lung J70.1
    pneumonitis J70.0
    pulmonary manifestations
      acute J70.0
      chronic J70.1
    skin L59.9

Effect, adverse *(Continued)*
  radioactive substance NOS
    dermatitis or eczema —*see* Radiodermatitis
  reduced temperature T69.9
    immersion foot or hand —*see* Immersion
    specified effect NEC T69.8
  serum NEC *(see also* Reaction, serum) T80.69
    specified NEC T78.8
      external cause NEC T75.89
  strangulation —*see* Asphyxia, traumatic
  submersion T75.1
  thirst T73.1
  toxic —*see* Toxicity
  transfusion —*see* Complications, transfusion
  ultraviolet (radiation) (rays) NOS T66
    burn —*see* Burn
    dermatitis or eczema —*see* Dermatitis, due to,
        ultraviolet rays
      acute L56.8
  vaccine (any) —*see* Complications, vaccination
  vibration —*see* Vibration, adverse effects
  water pressure NEC T70.9
    specified NEC T70.8
  weightlessness T75.82
  whole blood —*see* Complications, transfusion
  work environment Z56.5
Effect(s) (of) (from) —*see* Effect, adverse NEC
Effects, late —*see* Sequelae
Effluvium
  anagen L65.1
  telogen L65.0
Effort syndrome (psychogenic) F45.8
Effusion
  amniotic fluid —*see* Pregnancy, complicated by,
      premature rupture of membranes
  brain (serous) G93.6
  bronchial —*see* Bronchitis
  cerebral G93.6
  cerebrospinal —*see also* Meningitis
    vessel G93.6
  chest —*see* Effusion, pleura
  chylous, chyliform (pleura) J94.0
  intracranial G93.6
  joint M25.40
    ankle M25.47-●
    elbow M25.42-●
    foot joint M25.47-●
    hand joint M25.44-●
    hip M25.45-●
    knee M25.46-●
    shoulder M25.41-●
    specified joint NEC M25.48
    wrist M25.43-●
  malignant pleural J91.0
  meninges —*see* Meningitis
  pericardium, pericardial (noninflammatory) I31.39
    acute —*see* Pericarditis, acute
    malignant, in disease classified elsewhere
        I31.31
    specified type, NEC I31.39
  peritoneal (chronic) R18.8
  pleura, pleurisy, pleuritic, pleuropericardial J90
    chylous, chyliform J94.0
    due to systemic lupus erythematosis M32.13
    in conditions classified elsewhere J91.8
    influenzal —*see* Influenza, with, respiratory
        manifestations NEC
    malignant J91.0
    newborn P28.89
    tuberculous NEC A15.6
      primary (progressive) A15.7
  spinal —*see* Meningitis
  thorax, thoracic —*see* Effusion, pleura
Egg shell nails L60.3
  congenital Q84.6
EGPA (eosinophilic granulomatosis with
    polyangiitis) M30.1
Egyptian splenomegaly B65.1
Ehlers-Danlos syndrome *(see also* Syndrome,
    Ehlers-Danlos) Q79.60
Ehrlichiosis A77.40
  due to
    ~~E. chafeensis A77.41~~
    ▶E. chaffeensis A77.41
    E. ewingii A77.49
    E. muris euclairensis A77.49
    E. sennetsu A79.81
    specified organism NEC A77.49
Eichstedt's disease B36.0
Eisenmenger's
  complex or syndrome I27.83
  defect Q21.8

Ejaculation
  delayed F52.32
  painful N53.12
  premature F52.4
  retarded N53.11
  retrograde N53.14
  semen, painful N53.12
    psychogenic F52.6
Ekbom's syndrome (restless legs) G25.81
Ekman's syndrome (brittle bones and blue sclera)
    Q78.0
Elastic skin Q82.8
  acquired L57.4
Elastofibroma —*see* Neoplasm, connective tissue,
    benign
Elastoma (juvenile) Q82.8
  Miescher's L87.2
Elastomyofibrosis I42.4
Elastosis
  actinic, solar L57.8
  atrophicans (senile) L57.4
  perforans serpiginosa L87.2
  senilis L57.4
Elbow —*see* condition
Electric current, electricity, effects (concussion)
    (fatal) (nonfatal) (shock) T75.4
  burn —*see* Burn
Electric feet syndrome E53.8
Electrocution T75.4
  from electroshock gun (taser) T75.4
Electrolyte imbalance E87.8
  with
    abortion —*see* Abortion by type, complicated
        by, electrolyte imbalance
    ectopic pregnancy O08.5
    molar pregnancy O08.5
Elephantiasis (nonfilarial) I89.0
  arabicum —*see* Infestation, filarial
  bancroftian B74.0
  congenital (any site) (hereditary) Q82.0
  due to
    Brugia (malayi) B74.1
      timori B74.2
    mastectomy I97.2
    Wuchereria (bancrofti) B74.0
  eyelid H02.859
    left H02.856
      lower H02.855
      upper H02.854
    right H02.853
      lower H02.852
      upper H02.851
  filarial, filariensis —*see* Infestation,
      filarial
  glandular I89.0
  graecorum A30.9
  lymphangiectatic I89.0
  lymphatic vessel I89.0
    due to mastectomy I97.2
  scrotum (nonfilarial) I89.0
  streptococcal I89.0
  surgical I97.89
    postmastectomy I97.2
  telangiectodes I89.0
  vulva (nonfilarial) N90.89
Elevated, elevation
  alanine transaminase (ALT) R74.01
  ALT (alanine transaminase) R74.01
  antibody titer R76.0
  aspartate transaminase (AST) R74.01
  AST (aspartate transaminase) R74.01
  basal metabolic rate R94.8
  blood pressure —*see also* Hypertension
    reading (incidental) (isolated) (nonspecific),
        no diagnosis of hypertension
        R03.0
  blood sugar R73.9
  body temperature (of unknown origin)
      R50.9
  C-reactive protein (CRP) R79.82
  cancer antigen 125 [CA 125] R97.1
  carcinoembryonic antigen [CEA] R97.0
  cholesterol E78.00
    with high triglycerides E78.2
  conjugate, eye H51.0
  diaphragm, congenital Q79.1
  erythrocyte sedimentation rate R70.0
  fasting glucose R73.01
  fasting triglycerides E78.1
  finding on laboratory examination —*see*
      Findings, abnormal, inconclusive, without
      diagnosis, by type of exam

Embolism *(Continued)*
  portal (vein) I81
  postoperative, postprocedural
    artery T81.719
      mesenteric T81.710
      renal T81.711
      specified NEC T81.718
    vein T81.72
  precerebral artery —*see* Occlusion, artery,
      precerebral
  puerperal —*see* Embolism, obstetric
  pulmonary (acute) (artery) (vein) I26.99
    with acute cor pulmonale I26.09
  ▶cement I26.95
    ▶with acute cor pulmonale I26.03
    chronic I27.82
  ▶fat I26.96
    ▶with acute cor pulmonale I26.04
    following
      abortion —*see* Abortion by type
          complicated by embolism
      ectopic or molar pregnancy O08.2
    healed or old Z86.711
    in pregnancy, childbirth or puerperium —*see*
        Embolism, obstetric
    multiple subsegmental without acute cor
        pulmonale I26.94
    personal history of Z86.711
    saddle I26.92
      with acute cor pulmonale I26.02
    septic I26.90
      with acute cor pulmonale I26.01
    single subsegmental without acute cor
        pulmonale I26.93
    subsegmental NOS I26.93
  pyemic (multiple) I76
    following
      abortion —*see* Abortion by type
          complicated by embolism
      ectopic or molar pregnancy O08.2
    Hemophilus influenzae A41.3
    pneumococcal A40.3
      with pneumonia J13
    puerperal, postpartum, childbirth (any
        organism) —*see* Embolism, obstetric
    specified organism NEC A41.89
    staphylococcal A41.2
    streptococcal A40.9
  renal (artery) N28.0
    vein I82.3
  retina, retinal —*see* Occlusion, artery,
      retina
  saddle
    abdominal aorta I74.01
    pulmonary artery I26.92
      with acute cor pulmonale I26.02
  septic (arterial) I76
    complicating abortion —*see* Abortion, by type,
        complicated by, embolism
  sinus —*see* Embolism, intracranial, venous
      sinus
  soap complicating abortion —*see* Abortion, by
      type, complicated by, embolism
  spinal cord G95.19
    pyogenic origin G06.1
  spleen, splenic (artery) I74.8
  ▶thrombotic
    ▶specified NEC I26.99
      ▶with acute cor pulmonale I26.09
  upper extremity I74.2
  vein (acute) I82.90
    antecubital I82.61-●
      chronic I82.71-●
    axillary I82.A1-●
      chronic I82.A2-●
    basilic I82.61-●
      chronic I82.71-●
    brachial I82.62-●
      chronic I82.72-●
    brachiocephalic (innominate) I82.290
      chronic I82.291
    calf, muscle I82.46-●
      chronic I82.56-●
    cephalic I82.61-●
      chronic I82.71-●
    chronic I82.91
    deep (DVT) I82.40-●
      calf I82.4Z-●
        chronic I82.5Z-●
      lower leg I82.4Z-●
        chronic I82.5Z-●

Embolism *(Continued)*
  vein *(Continued)*
    deep (DVT) *(Continued)*
      thigh I82.4Y-●
        chronic I82.5Y-●
      upper leg I82.4Y
        chronic I82.5y-●
    femoral I82.41-●
      chronic I82.51-●
    gastrocnemial I82.46-●
      chronic I82.56-●
    iliac (iliofemoral) I82.42-●
      chronic I82.52-●
    innominate I82.290
      chronic I82.291
    internal jugular I82.C1-●
      chronic I82.C2-●
    lower extremity
      deep I82.40-●
        chronic I82.50-●
        specified NEC I82.49-●
          chronic NEC I82.59-●
      distal
        deep I82.4Z-●
      proximal
        deep I82.4Y-●
          chronic I82.5Y-●
      superficial I82.81-●
    peroneal I82.45-●
      chronic I82.55-●
    popliteal I82.43-●
      chronic I82.53-●
    radial I82.62-●
      chronic I82.72-●
    renal I82.3
    saphenous (greater) (lesser) I82.81-●
    soleal I82.46-●
      chronic I82.56-●
    specified NEC I82.890
      chronic NEC I82.891
    subclavian I82.B1-●
      chronic I82.B2-●
    thoracic NEC I82.290
      chronic I82.291
    tibial I82.44-●
      chronic I82.54-●
    ulnar I82.62-●
      chronic I82.72-●
    upper extremity I82.60-●
      chronic I82.70-●
      deep I82.62-●
        chronic I82.72-●
      superficial I82.61-●
        chronic I82.71-●
  vena cava
    inferior (acute) I82.220
      chronic I82.221
    superior (acute) I82.210
      chronic I82.211
  venous sinus G08
  vessels of brain —*see* Occlusion, artery, cerebral
Embolus —*see* Embolism
Embryoma —*see also* Neoplasm, uncertain
    behavior, by site
  benign —*see* Neoplasm, benign, by site
  kidney C64.-●
  liver C22.0
  malignant —*see also* Neoplasm, malignant, by site
    kidney C64.-●
    liver C22.0
    testis C62.9-●
      descended (scrotal) C62.1-●
      undescended C62.0-●
  testis C62.9-●
    descended (scrotal) C62.1-●
    undescended C62.0-●
Embryonic
  circulation Q28.9
  heart Q28.9
  vas deferens Q55.4
Embryopathia NOS Q89.9
Embryotoxon Q13.4
Emesis —*see* Vomiting
Emotional lability R45.86
Emotionality, pathological F60.3
Emotogenic disease —*see* Disorder, psychogenic
Emphysema (atrophic) (bullous) (chronic)
    (interlobular) (lung) (obstructive) (pulmonary)
    (senile) (vesicular) J43.9
  cellular tissue (traumatic) T79.7
    surgical T81.82

Emphysema *(Continued)*
  centrilobular J43.2
  compensatory J98.3
  congenital (interstitial) P25.0
  conjunctiva H11.89
  connective tissue (traumatic) T79.7
    surgical T81.82
  due to chemicals, gases, fumes or vapors (see also
      Disease, respiratory, chronic, due to
      chemicals, gases, fumes or vapors) J43.-●
  eyelid(s) —*see* Disorder, eyelid, specified type NEC
    surgical T81.82
    traumatic T79.7
  interstitial J98.2
    congenital P25.0
    perinatal period P25.0
  laminated tissue T79.7
    surgical T81.82
  mediastinal J98.2
    newborn P25.2
  orbit, orbital —*see* Disorder, orbit, specified type
      NEC
  panacinar J43.1
  panlobular J43.1
  specified NEC J43.8
  subcutaneous (traumatic) T79.7
    nontraumatic J98.2
    postprocedural T81.82
    surgical T81.82
  surgical T81.82
  thymus (gland) (congenital) E32.8
  traumatic (subcutaneous) T79.7
  unilateral J43.0
Empty nest syndrome Z60.0
Empyema (acute) (chest) (double) (pleura)
    (supradiaphragmatic) (thorax) J86.9
  with fistula J86.0
  accessory sinus (chronic) —*see* Sinusitis
  antrum (chronic) —*see* Sinusitis, maxillary
  brain (any part) —*see* Abscess, brain
  ethmoidal (chronic) (sinus) —*see* Sinusitis,
      ethmoidal
  extradural —*see* Abscess, extradural
  frontal (chronic) (sinus) —*see* Sinusitis, frontal
  gallbladder K81.0
  mastoid (process) (acute) —*see* Mastoiditis, acute
  maxilla, maxillary M27.2
    sinus (chronic) —*see* Sinusitis, maxillary
  nasal sinus (chronic) —*see* Sinusitis
  sinus (accessory) (chronic) (nasal) —*see* Sinusitis
  sphenoidal (sinus) (chronic) —*see* Sinusitis,
      sphenoidal
  subarachnoid —*see* Abscess, extradural
  subdural —*see* Abscess, subdural
  tuberculous A15.6
  ureter —*see* Ureteritis
  ventricular —*see* Abscess, brain
En coup de sabre lesion L94.1
Enamel pearls K00.2
Enameloma K00.2
Enanthema, viral B09
Encephalitis (chronic) (hemorrhagic) (idiopathic)
    (nonepidemic) (spurious) (subacute) G04.90
  acute —*see also* Encephalitis, viral A86
    disseminated G04.00
      infectious G04.01
      noninfectious G04.81
      postimmunization (postvaccination) G04.02
      postinfectious G04.01
    inclusion body A85.8
    necrotizing hemorrhagic G04.30
      postimmunization G04.32
      postinfectious G04.31
      specified NEC G04.39
  arboviral, arbovirus NEC A85.2
  arthropod-borne NEC (viral) A85.2
  Australian A83.4
  California (virus) A83.5
  Central European (tick-borne) A84.1
  Czechoslovakian A84.1
  Dawson's (inclusion body) A81.1
  diffuse sclerosing A81.1
  disseminated, acute G04.00
  due to
    cat scratch disease A28.1
    human immunodeficiency virus (HIV) disease
        B20 [G05.3]
    malaria —*see* Malaria
    rickettsiosis —*see* Rickettsiosis
    smallpox inoculation G04.02
    typhus —*see* Typhus

E

▶ New   ⇒ Revised   ~~deleted~~ Deleted   ● Use Additional Character(s)

Encounter (Continued)
  antenatal screening Z36.9
    cervical length Z36.86
    chromosomal anomalies Z36.0
    congenital cardiac abnormalities Z36.83
    elevated maternal serum alphafetoprotein
      level Z36.1
    fetal growth retardation Z36.4
    fetal lung maturity Z36.84
    fetal macrosomia Z36.88
    hydrops fetalis Z36.81
    intrauterine growth restriction (IUGR)/small-
      for-dates Z36.4
    isoimmunization Z36.5
    large-for-dates Z36.88
    malformations Z36.3
    non-visualized anatomy on a previous scan
      Z36.2
    nuchal translucency Z36.82
    raised alphafetoprotein level Z36.1
    risk of pre-term labor Z36.86
    specified type NEC Z36.89
    specified follow-up NEC Z36.2
    specified genetic defects NEC Z36.8A
    Streptococcus B Z36.85
    suspected anomaly Z36.3
    uncertain dates Z36.87
  assisted reproductive fertility procedure cycle
    Z31.83
  blood typing Z01.83
    Rh typing Z01.83
  breast augmentation or reduction Z41.1
  breast implant exchange (different material)
    (different size) Z45.81
  breast reconstruction following mastectomy
    Z42.1
  check-up —see Examination
  chemotherapy for neoplasm Z51.11
  child welfare screening exam Z02.84
  colonoscopy, screening Z12.11
  counseling —see Counseling
  delivery, full-term, uncomplicated O80
    cesarean, without indication O82
  desensitization to allergens Z51.6
  ear piercing Z41.3
  examination —see Examination
  expectant parent(s) (adoptive) pre-birth
    pediatrician visit Z76.81
  fertility preservation procedure (prior to cancer
    therapy) (prior to removal of gonads)
    Z31.84
  fitting (of) —see Fitting (and adjustment) (of)
  genetic
    counseling
      nonprocreative Z71.83
      procreative Z31.5
    testing —see Test, genetic
  hearing conservation and treatment
    Z01.12
  HIV
    pre-exposure prophylaxis Z29.81
    PrEP Z29.81
  immunotherapy for neoplasm Z51.12
  in vitro fertilization cycle Z31.83
  instruction (in)
    child care (postpartal) (prenatal)
      Z32.3
    childbirth Z32.2
    natural family planning
      procreative Z31.61
      to avoid pregnancy Z30.02
  insulin pump titration Z46.81
  joint prosthesis insertion following prior
    explantation of joint prosthesis (staged
    procedure)
    hip Z47.32
    knee Z47.33
    shoulder Z47.31
  laboratory (as part of a general medical
    examination) Z00.00
    with abnormal findings Z00.01
  mental health services (for)
    abuse NEC
      perpetrator Z69.82
      victim Z69.81
    child abuse
      nonparental
        perpetrator Z69.021
        victim Z69.020
      parental
        perpetrator Z69.011
        victim Z69.010

Encounter (Continued)
  mental health services (Continued)
    child neglect
      nonparental
        perpetrator Z69.021
        victim Z69.020
      parental
        perpetrator Z69.011
        victim Z69.010
    child psychological abuse
      nonparental
        perpetrator Z69.021
        victim Z69.020
      parental
        perpetrator Z69.011
        victim Z69.010
    child sexual abuse
      nonparental
        perpetrator Z69.021
        victim Z69.020
      parental
        perpetrator Z69.011
        victim Z69.010
    non-spousal adult abuse
      perpetrator Z69.82
      victim Z69.81
    spousal or partner
      abuse
        perpetrator Z69.12
        victim Z69.11
      neglect
        perpetrator Z69.12
        victim Z69.11
      psychological abuse
        perpetrator Z69.12
        victim Z69.11
      violence
        perpetrator (physical) (sexual)
          Z69.12
        victim (physical) Z69.11
          sexual Z69.81
  observation (for) (ruled out)
    alarm, without findings
      apnea Z03.83
      bradycardia Z03.83
      oximeter Z03.83
    condition suspected related to home
      physiologic monitoring device
      Z03.83
      newborn Z05.81
        apnea alarm Z05.81
        bradycardia alarm Z05.81
        malfunction of home cardiorespiratory
          monitor Z05.81
        non-specific findings home physiologic
          monitoring device Z05.81
        pulse oximeter alarm without findings
          Z05.81
    exposure to (suspected)
      anthrax Z03.810
      biological agent NEC Z03.818
    malfunction of home cardiorespiratory
      monitor Z03.83
    non-specific findings home physiologic
      monitoring device Z03.83
▶ palliative care Z51.5
  pediatrician visit, by expectant parent(s)
    (adoptive) Z76.81
  placental sample (taken vaginally) see
    also Encounter, antenatal screening
    Z36.9
  plastic and reconstructive surgery following
    medical procedure or healed injury NEC
    Z42.8
  postoperative —see Aftercare
  pregnancy
    supervision of —see Pregnancy, supervision of
    test Z32.00
      result negative Z32.02
      result positive Z32.01
  procreative management and counseling for
    gestational carrier Z31.7
  prophylactic measures Z29.9
    antivenin Z29.12
    fluoride administration Z29.3
    HIV pre-exposure Z29.81
    immunotherapy for respiratory syncytial
      virus (RSV) Z29.11
    rabies immune globin Z29.14
    Rho (D) immune globulin Z29.13
    specified NEC Z29.89
  radiation therapy (antineoplastic) Z51.0

Encounter (Continued)
  radiological (as part of a general medical
    examination) Z00.00
    with abnormal findings Z00.01
  reconstructive surgery following medical
    procedure or healed injury NEC Z42.8
  removal (of) —see also Removal
    artificial
      arm Z44.00-●
        complete Z44.01-●
        partial Z44.02-●
      eye Z44.2-●
      leg Z44.10-●
        complete Z44.11-●
        partial Z44.12-●
    breast implant Z45.81
      tissue expander (with or without
        synchronous insertion of permanent
        implant) Z45.81
    device Z46.9
      specified NEC Z46.89
    external
      fixation device — code to fracture with
        seventh character D
      prosthesis, prosthetic device Z44.9
        breast Z44.3-●
        specified NEC Z44.8
    implanted device NEC Z45.89
    insulin pump Z46.81
    internal fixation device Z47.2
    myringotomy device (stent) (tube) Z45.82
    nervous system device NEC Z46.2
      brain neuropacemaker Z46.2
      visual substitution device Z46.2
        implanted Z45.31
    non-vascular catheter Z46.82
    orthodontic device Z46.4
    stent
      ureteral Z46.6
    urinary device Z46.6
  repeat cervical smear to confirm findings of
    recent normal smear following initial
    abnormal smear Z01.42
  respirator [ventilator] use during power failure
    (Z99.12)
  Rh typing Z01.83
  screening —see Screening
  specified NEC Z76.89
  sterilization Z30.2
  suspected condition, ruled out
    amniotic cavity and membrane Z03.71
    cervical shortening Z03.75
    fetal anomaly Z03.73
    fetal growth Z03.74
    maternal and fetal conditions NEC Z03.79
    oligohydramnios Z03.71
    placental problem Z03.72
    polyhydramnios Z03.71
  suspected exposure (to), ruled out
    anthrax Z03.810
    biological agents NEC Z03.818
  termination of pregnancy, elective Z33.2
  testing —see Test
  therapeutic drug level monitoring Z51.81
  titration, insulin pump Z46.81
  to determine fetal viability of pregnancy O36.80
  training
    insulin pump Z46.81
  X ray of chest (as part of a general medical
    examination Z00.00)
    with abnormal findings Z00.01
Encysting —see Cyst
Endarteritis (bacterial, subacute) (infective) I77.6
  brain I67.7
  cerebral or cerebrospinal I67.7
  deformans —see Arteriosclerosis
  embolic —see Embolism
  obliterans —see also Arteriosclerosis
    pulmonary I28.8
  pulmonary I28.8
  retina —see Vasculitis, retina
  senile —see Arteriosclerosis
  syphilitic A52.09
    brain or cerebral A52.04
    congenital A50.54 [I79.8]
  tuberculous A18.89
Endemic —see condition
Endocarditis (chronic) (marantic) (nonbacterial)
    (thrombotic) (valvular) I38
  with rheumatic fever (conditions in I00)
    active —see Endocarditis, acute, rheumatic
    inactive or quiescent (with chorea) I09.1

▶ New   ⇒ Revised   ~~deleted~~ Deleted   ● Use Additional Character(s)

Endocarditis *(Continued)*
  acute or subacute I33.9
    infective I33.0
    rheumatic (aortic) (mitral) (pulmonary)
        (tricuspid) I01.1
      with chorea (acute) (rheumatic)
          (Sydenham's) I02.0
  aortic (heart) (nonrheumatic) (valve) I35.8
    with
      mitral disease I08.0
        with tricuspid (valve) disease I08.3
          active or acute I01.1
            with chorea (acute) (rheumatic)
                (Sydenham's) I02.0
        rheumatic fever (conditions in I00)
          active —*see* Endocarditis, acute, rheumatic
          inactive or quiescent (with chorea) I06.9
      tricuspid (valve) disease I08.2
        with mitral (valve) disease I08.3
    acute or subacute I33.9
    arteriosclerotic I35.8
    rheumatic I06.9
      with mitral disease I08.0
        with tricuspid (valve) disease I08.3
          active or acute I01.1
            with chorea (acute) (rheumatic)
                (Sydenham's) I02.0
        active or acute I01.1
          with chorea (acute) (rheumatic)
              (Sydenham's) I02.0
        specified NEC I06.8
    specified cause NEC I35.8
    syphilitic A52.03
  arteriosclerotic I38
  atypical verrucous (Libman-Sacks) M32.11
  bacterial (acute) (any valve) (subacute) I33.0
  candidal B37.6
  congenital Q24.8
  constrictive I33.0
  Coxiella burnetii A78 *[139]*
  Coxsackie B33.21
  due to
    prosthetic cardiac valve T82.6
    Q fever A78 *[139]*
    Serratia marcescens I33.0
    typhoid (fever) A01.02
  gonococcal A54.83
  infectious or infective (acute) (any valve)
      (subacute) I33.0
  lenta (acute) (any valve) (subacute) I33.0
  Libman-Sacks M32.11
  listerial A32.82
  Löffler's I42.3
  malignant (acute) (any valve) (subacute) I33.0
  meningococcal A39.51
  mitral (chronic) (double) (fibroid) (heart)
      (inactive) (valve) (with chorea) I05.9
    with
      aortic (valve) disease I08.0
        with tricuspid (valve) disease I08.3
          active or acute I01.1
            with chorea (acute) (rheumatic)
                (Sydenham's) I02.0
        rheumatic fever (conditions in I00)
          active —*see* Endocarditis, acute,
              rheumatic
          inactive or quiescent (with chorea) I05.9
      tricuspid (valve) disease I08.1
        with aortic (valve) disease I08.3
    active or acute I01.1
      with chorea (acute) (rheumatic)
          (Sydenham's) I02.0
      bacterial I33.0
    arteriosclerotic I34.89
    nonrheumatic I34.89
      acute or subacute I33.9
    specified NEC I05.8
  monilial B37.6
  multiple valves I08.9
    specified disorders I08.8
  mycotic (acute) (any valve) (subacute) I33.0
  pneumococcal (acute) (any valve) (subacute) I33.0
  pulmonary (chronic) (heart) (valve) I37.8
    with rheumatic fever (conditions in I00)
      active —*see* Endocarditis, acute, rheumatic
      inactive or quiescent (with chorea) I09.89
        with aortic, mitral or tricuspid disease
            I08.8
    acute or subacute I33.9
      rheumatic I01.1
        with chorea (acute) (rheumatic)
            (Sydenham's) I02.0

Endocarditis *(Continued)*
  pulmonary *(Continued)*
    arteriosclerotic I37.8
    congenital Q22.2
    rheumatic (chronic) (inactive) (with chorea)
        I09.89
      active or acute I01.1
        with chorea (acute) (rheumatic)
            (Sydenham's) I02.0
    syphilitic A52.03
  purulent (acute) (any valve) (subacute) I33.0
  Q fever A78 *[139]*
  rheumatic (chronic) (inactive) (with chorea) I09.1
    active or acute (aortic) (mitral) (pulmonary)
        (tricuspid) I01.1
      with chorea (acute) (rheumatic)
          (Sydenham's) I02.0
  rheumatoid —*see* Rheumatoid, carditis
  septic (acute) (any valve) (subacute) I33.0
  streptococcal (acute) (any valve) (subacute)
      I33.0
  subacute —*see* Endocarditis, acute
  suppurative (acute) (any valve) (subacute) I33.0
  syphilitic A52.03
  toxic I33.9
  tricuspid (chronic) (heart) (inactive) (rheumatic)
      (valve) (with chorea) I07.9
    with
      aortic (valve) disease I08.2
        mitral (valve) disease I08.3
      mitral (valve) disease I08.1
        aortic (valve) disease I08.3
      rheumatic fever (conditions in I00)
        active —*see* Endocarditis, acute,
            rheumatic
        inactive or quiescent (with chorea) I07.8
    active or acute I01.1
      with chorea (acute) (rheumatic)
          (Sydenham's) I02.0
    arteriosclerotic I36.8
    nonrheumatic I36.8
      acute or subacute I33.9
    specified cause, except rheumatic I36.8
  tuberculous —*see* Tuberculosis, endocarditis
  typhoid A01.02
  ulcerative (acute) (any valve) (subacute) I33.0
  vegetative (acute) (any valve) (subacute) I33.0
  verrucous (atypical) (nonbacterial)
      (nonrheumatic) M32.11
Endocardium, endocardial —*see also* condition
  cushion defect Q21.20
Endocervicitis —*see also* Cervicitis
  due to intrauterine (contraceptive) device T83.69

  hyperplastic N72
Endocrine —*see* condition
Endocrinopathy, pluriglandular E31.9
Endodontic
  overfill M27.52
  underfill M27.53
Endodontitis K04.01
  irreversible K04.02
  reversible K04.01
Endomastoiditis —*see* Mastoiditis
Endometrioma N80.12-●
Endometriosis N80.9
  abdomen, abdominal N80.C0
    specified site, NEC N80.C9
    wall N80.C19
      fascia and muscular layers N80.C11
      subcutaneous tissue N80.C10
      unspecified depth N80.C19
  appendix N80.549
    deep N80.542
    superficial N80.541
  bladder (unspecified depth) N80.A0
    deep N80.A2
    superficial N80.A1
  bowel N80.50
  broad ligament N80.3C
  cardiothoracic space N80.B6
  cecum N80.539
    N80.532
    superficial N80.531
  cervix N80.0-●
  colon N80.559
    descending N80.559
      deep N80.552
      superficial N80.551
    sigmoid N80.529
      deep N80.522
      superficial N80.521

Endometriosis *(Continued)*
  colon *(Continued)*
    transverse N80.559
      deep N80.552
      superficial N80.551
  cul-de-sac (Douglas')
    anterior (unspecified depth) N80.319
      deep N80.312
      superficial N80.311
    posterior (unspecified depth) N80.329
      deep N80.322
      superficial N80.321
  deep
    involving muscular wall of fallopian tube
        N80.22
    retrocervical N80.02
  diaphragm N80.B39
    deep N80.B32
    superficial N80.B31
    unspecified depth N80.B39
  exocervix N80.01
  extra-pelvic abdominal peritoneum
      N80.C4
  fallopian tube (unspecified depth) N80.20-●
    deep N80.22-●
    superficial N80.21-●
  female genital organ NEC N80.8
  gallbladder N80.8
  inguinal canal N80.C3
  in scar of skin N80.6
  internal N80.02
  intestine N80.50
    small N80.569
      deep (multifocal) N80.562
      superficial N80.561
  lung N80.B2
  mediastinal space N80.B5
  myometrium N80.03
  nerve
    femoral N80.D6
    obturator N80.D3
    pelvic N80.D0
      splanchnic N80.D1
    pudendal N80.D5
    retroperitoneum, NEC N80.D9
    sacral splanchnic N80.D1
    sciatic N80.D4
    specified, NEC N80.D9
  ovary (unspecified depth) N80.10-●
    deep N80.12-●
    superficial N80.11-●
  parametrium N80.399
  pelvic
    brim N80.38-●
      deep N80.37-●
      superficial N80.36-●
    peritoneum N80.30
      specified sites, NEC N80.399
        deep N80.392
        superficial N80.391
    sidewall N80.35-●
      deep N80.34-●
      superficial N80.33-●
  pericardial space N80.B4
  peritoneal (pelvic) N80.30
  pleura N80.B1
  rectovaginal septum N80.40
    with involvement of vagina N80.42
    without involvement of vagina N80.41
  rectum N80.519
    deep (multifocal) N80.512
    superficial N80.511
  retroperitoneum N80.30
  round ligament N80.3C9
  sacral nerve roots N80.D2
  skin (scar) N80.6
  specified site NEC N80.8
  stromal D39.0
  thorax N80.B-●
  umbilicus N80.C2
  ureter N80.A69
    deep N80.A5-●
    extrinsic N80.A4-●
    intrinsic N80.A5-●
    unspecified depth N80.A6-●
  uterosacral ligament(s) N80.3C-●
    deep N80.3B-●
    superficial N80.3A-●
  uterus N80.00
    deep N80.02
    internal N80.02
    superficial N80.01

Endometriosis *(Continued)*
  vagina N80.42
  vulva N80.8
Endometritis (decidual) (nonspecific) (purulent)
      (senile (atrophic) (suppurative) N71.9
  with ectopic pregnancy O08.0
  acute N71.0
  ~~blennorrhagic (gonococcal) (acute) (chronic)~~
      ~~A54.24~~
  ▶blennorrhagic (gonococcal) (acute) (chronic)
      A54.24
  cervix, cervical (with erosion or ectropion) —*see*
      also Cervicitis
      hyperplastic N72
  chlamydial A56.11
  chronic N71.1
  following
      abortion —*see* Abortion by type complicated
          by genital infection
      ectopic or molar pregnancy O08.0
  gonococcal, gonorrheal (acute) (chronic) A54.24
  hyperplastic —*see also* Hyperplasia, endometrial
      N85.00-●
      cervix N72
  puerperal, postpartum, childbirth O86.12
  subacute N71.0
  tuberculous A18.17
Endometrium —*see* condition
Endomyocardiopathy, South African I42.3
Endomyocarditis —*see* Endocarditis
Endomyofibrosis I42.3
Endomyometritis —*see* Endometritis
Endopericarditis —*see* Endocarditis
Endoperineuritis —*see* Disorder, nerve
Endophlebitis —*see* Phlebitis
Endophthalmia —*see* Endophthalmitis, purulent
Endophthalmitis (acute) (infective) (metastatic)
      (subacute) H44.009
  bleb associated H59.4 —*see also* Bleb, inflamed
      (infected), postprocedural
  gonorrheal A54.39
  in (due to)
      cysticercosis B69.1
      onchocerciasis B73.01
      toxocariasis B83.0
  panuveitis —*see* Panuveitis
  parasitic H44.12-●
  purulent H44.00-●
      panophthalmitis —*see* Panophthalmitis
      vitreous abscess H44.02-●
  specified NEC H44.19
  sympathetic —*see* Uveitis, sympathetic
Endosalpingioma D28.2
Endosalpingiosis N94.89
Endosteitis —*see* Osteomyelitis
Endothelioma, bone —*see* Neoplasm, bone,
      malignant
Endotheliosis (hemorrhagic infectional) D69.8
Endotoxemia — code to condition
Endotrachelitis —*see* Cervicitis
Engelmann (-Camurati) syndrome Q78.3
English disease —*see* Rickets
Engman's disease L30.3
Engorgement
  breast N64.59
      newborn P83.4
      puerperal, postpartum O92.79
  lung (passive) —*see* Edema, lung
  pulmonary (passive) —*see* Edema, lung
  stomach K31.89
  venous, retina —*see* Occlusion, retina, vein,
      engorgement
Enlargement, enlarged —*see also* Hypertrophy
  adenoids J35.2
      with tonsils J35.3
  alveolar ridge K08.89
      congenital —*see* Anomaly, alveolar
  apertures of diaphragm (congenital) Q79.1
  gingival K06.1
  heart, cardiac —*see* Hypertrophy, cardiac
  labium majus, childhood asymmetric (CALME)
      N90.61
  lacrimal gland, chronic H04.03-●
  liver —*see* Hypertrophy, liver
  lymph gland or node R59.9
      generalized R59.1
      localized R59.0
  orbit H05.34-●
  organ or site, congenital NEC —*see* Anomaly,
      by site
  parathyroid (gland) E21.0

Enlargement, enlarged *(Continued)*
  pituitary fossa R93.0
  prostate N40.0
      with lower urinary tract symptoms (LUTS)
          N40.1
      nodular N40.3
      nodular N40.2
          with lower urinary tract symptoms
              (LUTS) N40.3
      without lower urinary tract symptoms (LUTS)
          N40.0
      nodular N40.2
  sella turcica R93.0
  spleen —*see* Splenomegaly
  thymus (gland) (congenital) E32.0
  thyroid (gland) —*see* Goiter
  tongue K14.8
  tonsils J35.1
      with adenoids J35.3
  uterus N85.2
  vestibular aqueduct Q16.5
Enophthalmos H05.40-●
  due to
      orbital tissue atrophy H05.41-●
      trauma or surgery H05.42-●
Enostosis M27.8
Entamebic, entamebiasis —*see* Amebiasis
Entanglement
  umbilical cord(s) O69.82
      with compression O69.2
      around neck
          with compression O69.1
          without compression O69.81
      of twins in monoamniotic sac O69.2
      other, with compression O69.2
      other, without compression O69.82
      without compression O69.82
Enteralgia —*see* Pain, abdominal
Enteric —*see* condition
Enteritis (acute) (diarrheal) (hemorrhagic)
      (noninfective) K52.9
  adenovirus A08.2
  aertrycke infection A02.0
  allergic K52.29
      with
          eosinophilic gastritis or gastroenteritis
              K52.81
          food protein-induced enterocolitis
              syndrome K52.21
          food protein-induced enteropathy
              K52.22
          FPIES K52.21
  amebic (acute) A06.0
      with abscess —*see* Abscess, amebic
      chronic A06.1
          with abscess —*see* Abscess, amebic
          nondysenteric A06.2
      nondysenteric A06.2
  astrovirus A08.32
  bacillary NOS A03.9
  bacterial A04.9
      specified NEC A04.8
  calicivirus A08.31
  candidal B37.82
  Chilomastix A07.8
  choleriformis A00.1
  chronic (noninfectious) K52.9
      ulcerative —*see* Colitis, ulcerative
  cicatrizing (chronic) —*see* Enteritis, regional,
      small intestine
  ▶Clostridioides difficile
      ▶not specified as recurrent A04.72
      ▶recurrent A04.71
  Clostridium
      botulinum (food poisoning) A05.1
      difficile
          not specified as recurrent A04.72
          recurrent A04.71
  coccidial A07.3
  coxsackie virus A08.39
  dietetic —*see also* Enteritis, allergic K52.29
  drug-induced K52.1
  due to
      astrovirus A08.32
      calicivirus A08.31
      coxsackie virus A08.39
      drugs K52.1
      echovirus A08.39
      enterovirus NEC A08.39
      food hypersensitivity —*see also* Enteritis,
          allergic K52.29

Enteritis *(Continued)*
  due to *(Continued)*
      infectious organism (bacterial) (viral) —*see*
          Enteritis, infectious
      torovirus A08.39
      Yersinia enterocolitica A04.6
  echovirus A08.39
  eltor A00.1
  enterovirus NEC A08.39
  eosinophilic K52.81
  epidemic (infectious) A09
  fulminant —*see also* Ischemia, intestine, acute
      K55.019
  gangrenous —*see* Enteritis, infectious
  giardial A07.1
  infectious NOS A09
      due to
          adenovirus A08.2
          Aerobacter aerogenes A04.8
          Arizona (bacillus) A02.0
          bacteria NOS A04.9
              specified NEC A04.8
          Campylobacter A04.5
          ▶Clostridioides difficile
              ▶not specified as recurrent A04.72
              ▶recurrent A04.71
          Clostridium difficile
              not specified as recurrent A04.72
              recurrent A04.71
          Clostridium perfringens A04.8
          Enterobacter aerogenes A04.8
          enterovirus A08.39
          Escherichia coli A04.4
              enteroaggregative A04.4
              enterohemorrhagic A04.3
              enteroinvasive A04.2
              enteropathogenic A04.0
              enterotoxigenic A04.1
              specified NEC A04.4
          specified
              bacteria NEC A04.8
              virus NEC A08.39
          Staphylococcus A04.8
          virus NEC A08.4
              specified type NEC A08.39
          Yersinia enterocolitica A04.6
      specified organism NEC A08.8
  influenzal —*see* Influenza, with, digestive
      manifestations
  ischemic K55.9
      acute —*see also* Ischemia, intestine, acute
          K55.019
      chronic K55.1
  microsporidial A07.8
  mucomembranous, myxomembranous —*see*
      Syndrome, irritable bowel
  mucous —*see* Syndrome, irritable bowel
  necroticans A05.2
  necrotizing of newborn —*see* Enterocolitis,
      necrotizing, in newborn
  neurogenic —*see* Syndrome, irritable bowel
  newborn necrotizing —*see* Enterocolitis,
      necrotizing, in newborn
  noninfectious K52.9
  norovirus A08.11
  parasitic NEC B82.9
  paratyphoid (fever) —*see* Fever, paratyphoid
  protozoal A07.9
      specified NEC A07.8
  radiation K52.0
  regional (of) K50.90
      with
          complication K50.919
              abscess K50.914
              fistula K50.913
              intestinal obstruction K50.912
              rectal bleeding K50.911
              specified complication NEC K50.918
      colon —*see* Enteritis, regional, large intestine
      duodenum —*see* Enteritis, regional, small
          intestine
      ileum —*see* Enteritis, regional, small intestine
      jejunum —*see* Enteritis, regional, small
          intestine
      large bowel —*see* Enteritis, regional, large
          intestine
      large intestine (colon) (rectum) K50.10
          with
              complication K50.119
                  abscess K50.114
                  fistula K50.113

▶ New   ⇒ Revised   ~~deleted~~ Deleted   ● Use Additional Character(s)

Enteritis *(Continued)*
  regional *(Continued)*
    large intestine *(Continued)*
      with *(Continued)*
        complication *(Continued)*
          intestinal obstruction K50.112
          rectal bleeding K50.111
          small intestine (duodenum) (ileum)
            (jejunum) involvement K50.80
            with
              complication K50.819
                abscess K50.814
                fistula K50.813
                intestinal obstruction K50.812
                rectal bleeding K50.811
                specified complication NEC
                  K50.818
          specified complication NEC K50.118
      rectum —*see* Enteritis, regional, large intestine
    small intestine (duodenum) (ileum) (jejunum)
      K50.00
      with
        complication K50.019
          abscess K50.014
          fistula K50.013
          intestinal obstruction K50.012
          large intestine (colon) (rectum)
            involvement K50.80
            with
              complication K50.819
                abscess K50.814
                fistula K50.813
                intestinal obstruction
                  K50.812
                rectal bleeding K50.811
                specified complication NEC
                  K50.818
        rectal bleeding K50.011
        specified complication NEC K50.018
rotaviral A08.0
Salmonella, salmonellosis (arizonae) (cholerae-
  suis) (enteritidis) (typhimurium) A02.0
segmental —*see* Enteritis, regional
septic A09
Shigella —*see* Infection, Shigella
small round structured NEC A08.19
spasmodic, spastic —*see* Syndrome, irritable
  bowel
staphylococcal A04.8
  due to food A05.0
torovirus A08.39
toxic NEC K52.1
  ~~due to Clostridium difficile~~
    ~~not specified as recurrent A04.72~~
    ~~recurrent A04.71~~
  ▶ due to
    ▶ Clostridioides difficile
      ▶ not specified as recurrent A04.72
      ▶ recurrent A04.71
    ▶ Clostridium difficile
      ▶ not specified as recurrent A04.72
      ▶ recurrent A04.71
trichomonal A07.8
tuberculous A18.32
typhosa A01.00
ulcerative (chronic) —*see* Colitis, ulcerative
viral A08.4
  adenovirus A08.2
  enterovirus A08.39
  Rotavirus A08.0
  small round structured NEC A08.19
  specified NEC A08.39
  virus specified NEC A08.39
Enterobiasis B80
Enterobius vermicularis (infection) (infestation)
  B80
Enterocele —*see also* Hernia, abdomen
  pelvic, pelvis (acquired) (congenital) N81.5
  vagina, vaginal (acquired) (congenital)
    NEC N81.5
Enterocolitis —*see also* Enteritis K52.9
  ~~due to Clostridium difficile~~
    ~~not specified as recurrent A04.72~~
    ~~recurrent A04.71~~
  ▶ due to
    ▶ Clostridioides difficile
      ▶ not specified as recurrent A04.72
      ▶ recurrent A04.71
    ▶ Clostridium difficile
      ▶ not specified as recurrent A04.72
      ▶ recurrent A04.71

Enterocolitis *(Continued)*
  fulminant ischemic —*see also* Ischemia, intestine,
    acute K55.059
  granulomatous —*see* Enteritis, regional
  hemorrhagic (acute) —*see also* Ischemia,
    intestine, acute K55.059
    chronic K55.1
  infectious NEC A09
  ischemic K55.9
  necrotizing K55.30
    with
      perforation K55.33
      pneumatosis K55.32
      and perforation K55.33
    ~~due to Clostridium difficile~~
      ~~not specified as recurrent A04.72~~
      ~~recurrent A04.71~~
    ▶ due to
      ▶ Clostridioides difficile
        ▶ not specified as recurrent A04.72
        ▶ recurrent A04.71
      ▶ Clostridium difficile
        ▶ not specified as recurrent A04.72
        ▶ recurrent A04.71
    in non-newborn K55.30
      stage 1 (without pneumatosis, without
        perforation) K55.31
      stage 2 (with pneumatosis, without
        perforation) K55.32
      stage 3 (with pneumatosis, with
        perforation) K55.33
    in newborn P77.9
      stage 1 (without pneumatosis, without
        perforation) P77.1
      stage 2 (with pneumatosis, without
        perforation) P77.2
      stage 3 (with pneumatosis, with
        perforation) P77.3
    without pneumatosis or perforation K55.31
  noninfectious K52.9
  newborn —*see* Enterocolitis, necrotizing, in
    newborn
  pseudomembranous (newborn)
    not specified as recurrent A04.72
    recurrent A04.71
  radiation K52.0
    newborn —*see* Enterocolitis, necrotizing, in
      newborn
  ulcerative (chronic) —*see* Pancolitis, ulcerative
    (chronic)
Enterogastritis —*see* Enteritis
Enteropathy K63.9
  celiac-gluten-sensitive K90.0
    non-celiac K90.41
  food protein-induced K52.22
  hemorrhagic, terminal —*see also* Ischemia,
    intestine, acute K55.059
  protein-losing K90.49
Enteroperitonitis —*see* Peritonitis
Enteroptosis K63.4
Enterorrhagia K92.2
Enterospasm —*see also* Syndrome, irritable, bowel
  psychogenic F45.8
Enterostenosis —*see also* Obstruction, intestine,
  specified NEC K56.699
Enterostomy
  complication —*see* Complication, enterostomy
  status Z93.4
Enterovirus, as cause of disease classified
  elsewhere B97.10
  coxsackievirus B97.11
  echovirus B97.12
  other specified B97.19
Enthesopathy (peripheral) M77.5-●
  Achilles tendinitis —*see* Tendinitis, Achilles
  ankle and tarsus M77.9
    specified type NEC —*see* Enthesopathy, foot,
      specified type NEC
  anterior tibial syndrome M76.81-●
  calcaneal spur —*see* Spur, bone, calcaneal
  elbow region M77.8
    lateral epicondylitis —*see* Epicondylitis, lateral
    medial epicondylitis —*see* Epicondylitis, medial
  foot NEC M77.8
    metatarsalgia —*see* Metatarsalgia
    specified type NEC M77.5-●
  forearm M77.8
  gluteal tendinitis —*see* Tendinitis, gluteal
  hand M77.8
  hip —*see* Enthesopathy, lower limb, specified
    type NEC

Enthesopathy *(Continued)*
  iliac crest spur —*see* Spur, bone, iliac crest
  iliotibial band syndrome —*see* Syndrome,
    iliotibial band
  knee —*see* Enthesopathy, lower limb, lower leg,
    specified type NEC
  lateral epicondylitis —*see* Epicondylitis, lateral
  lower limb (excluding foot) M76.9
    Achilles tendinitis —*see* Tendinitis, Achilles
    ankle and tarsus M77.5-
      specified type NEC - *see* Enthesopathy, foot,
        specified type NEC
    anterior tibial syndrome M76.81-●
    gluteal tendinitis —*see* Tendinitis, gluteal
    iliac crest spur —*see* Spur, bone, iliac crest
    iliotibial band syndrome —*see* Syndrome,
      iliotibial band
    patellar tendinitis —*see* Tendinitis, patellar
    pelvic region —*see* Enthesopathy, lower limb,
      specified type NEC
    peroneal tendinitis —*see* Tendinitis, peroneal
    posterior tibial syndrome M76.82-●
    psoas tendinitis —*see* Tendinitis, psoas
    specified type NEC M76.89-●
    tibial collateral bursitis —*see* Bursitis, tibial
      collateral
  medial epicondylitis —*see* Epicondylitis, medial
  multiple sites M77.8
  patellar tendinitis —*see* Tendinitis, patellar
  pelvis M77.8
  periarthritis of wrist —*see* Periarthritis, wrist
  peroneal tendinitis —*see* Tendinitis, peroneal
  posterior tibial syndrome M76.82-●
  psoas tendinitis —*see* Tendinitis, psoas
  shoulder M77.8
  shoulder region —*see* Lesion, shoulder
  specified type NEC M77.8
  spinal M46.00
    cervical region M46.02
    cervicothoracic region M46.03
    lumbar region M46.06
    lumbosacral region M46.07
    multiple sites M46.09
    occipito-atlanto-axial region M46.01
    sacrococcygeal region M46.08
    thoracic region M46.04
    thoracolumbar region M46.05
  tibial collateral bursitis —*see* Bursitis, tibial
    collateral
  upper arm M77.8
  wrist and carpus NEC M77.8
    calcaneal spur —*see* Spur, bone, calcaneal
    periarthritis of wrist —*see* Periarthritis, wrist
Entomophobia F40.218
Entomophthoromycosis B46.8
Entrance, air into vein —*see* Embolism, air
Entrapment, nerve —*see also* Neuropathy,
  entrapment
  muscle
    eye
      extraocular H50.68-●
      oblique
        inferior H50.62-●
        superior H50.66-●
      rectus
        inferior H50.63-●
        lateral H50.64-●
        medial H50.65-●
        superior H50.67-●
Entropion (eyelid) (paralytic) H02.009
  cicatricial H02.019
    left H02.016
      lower H02.015
      upper H02.014
    right H02.013
      lower H02.012
      upper H02.011
  congenital Q10.2
  left H02.006
    lower H02.005
    upper H02.004
  mechanical H02.029
    left H02.026
      lower H02.025
      upper H02.024
    right H02.023
      lower H02.022
      upper H02.021
  right H02.003
    lower H02.002
    upper H02.001

Entropion *(Continued)*
  senile H02.039
    left H02.036
      lower H02.035
      upper H02.034
    right H02.033
      lower H02.032
      upper H02.031
  spastic H02.049
    left H02.046
      lower H02.045
      upper H02.044
    right H02.043
      lower H02.042
      upper H02.041
Enucleated eye (traumatic, current) S05.7-●
Enuresis R32
  functional F98.0
  habit disturbance F98.0
  nocturnal N39.44
    psychogenic F98.0
  nonorganic origin F98.0
  psychogenic F98.0
Eosinopenia —*see* Agranulocytosis
Eosinophilia (allergic) (idiopathic) (secondary)
    D72.10
  with
    angiolymphoid hyperplasia (ALHE) D18.01
  familial D72.19
  hereditary D72.19
  in disease classified elsewhere D72.18
  infiltrative —*see* Eosinophilia, pulmonary
  Löffler's J82.89
  peritoneal —*see* Peritonitis, eosinophilic
  pulmonary NEC J82.89
    acute J82.82
    asthmatic J82.83
    chronic J82.81
  specified NEC D72.19
  tropical (pulmonary) J82.89
Eosinophilia-myalgia syndrome M35.89
Ependymitis (acute) (cerebral) (chronic)
    (granular) —*see* Encephalomyelitis
Ependymoblastoma
  specified site —*see* Neoplasm, malignant, by
    site
  unspecified site C71.9
Ependymoma (epithelial) (malignant)
  anaplastic
    specified site —*see* Neoplasm, malignant, by
      site
    unspecified site C71.9
  benign
    specified site —*see* Neoplasm, benign, by site
    unspecified site D33.2
  myxopapillary D43.2
    specified site —*see* Neoplasm, uncertain
      behavior, by site
    unspecified site D43.2
  papillary D43.2
    specified site —*see* Neoplasm, uncertain
      behavior, by site
    unspecified site D43.2
  specified site —*see* Neoplasm, malignant, by site
  unspecified site C71.9
Ependymopathy G93.89
Ephelis, ephelides L81.2
Epiblepharon (congenital) Q10.3
Epicanthus, epicanthic fold (eyelid) (congenital)
    Q10.3
Epicondylitis (elbow)
  lateral M77.1-●
  medial M77.0-●
Epicystitis —*see* Cystitis
Epidemic —*see* condition
Epidermidalization, cervix —*see* Dysplasia, cervix
Epidermis, epidermal —*see* condition
Epidermodysplasia verruciformis B07.8
Epidermolysis
  bullosa (congenital) Q81.9
    acquired L12.30
      drug-induced L12.31
      specified cause NEC L12.35
    dystrophica Q81.2
    letalis Q81.1
    simplex Q81.0
    specified NEC Q81.8
  necroticans combustiformis L51.2
    due to drug —*see* Table of Drugs and
      Chemicals, by drug
Epidermophytid —*see* Dermatophytosis

Epidermophytosis (infected) —*see*
    Dermatophytosis
Epididymis —*see* condition
Epididymitis (acute) (nonvenereal) (recurrent)
    (residual) N45.1
  with orchitis N45.3
  blennorrhagic (gonococcal) A54.23
  caseous (tuberculous) A18.15
  chlamydial A56.19
  filarial —*see also* Infestation, filarial B74.9 *[N51]*
  gonococcal A54.23
  syphilitic A52.76
  tuberculous A18.15
Epididymo-orchitis —*see also* Epididymitis N45.3
Epidural —*see* condition
Epigastrium, epigastric —*see* condition
Epigastrocele —*see* Hernia, ventral
Epiglottis —*see* condition
Epiglottitis, epiglottiditis (acute) J05.10
  with obstruction J05.11
  chronic J37.0
Epignathus Q89.4
Epilepsia partialis continua —*see also*
    Kozhevnikof's epilepsy G40.1-●
Epilepsy, epileptic, epilepsia (attack) (cerebral)
    (convulsion) (fit) (seizure) G40.909

> Note: the following terms are to be considered
> equivalent to intractable: pharmacoresistant
> (pharmacologically resistant), treatment
> resistant, refractory (medically) and poorly
> controlled

  with
    complex partial seizures —*see* Epilepsy,
      localization-related, symptomatic, with
      complex partial seizures
    grand mal seizures on awakening —
      see Epilepsy, generalized, specified NEC
    myoclonic absences —*see* Epilepsy,
      generalized, specified NEC
    myoclonic-astatic seizures —*see* Epilepsy,
      generalized, specified NEC
    simple partial seizures —*see* Epilepsy,
      localization-related, symptomatic, with
      simple partial seizures
  akinetic —*see* Epilepsy, generalized, specified
    NEC
  benign childhood with centrotemporal EEG
    spikes —*see* Epilepsy, localization-related,
      idiopathic
  benign myoclonic in infancy G40.80-●
  Bravais-jacksonian —*see* Epilepsy, localization-
    related, symptomatic,
    with simple partial seizures
  childhood
    with occipital EEG paroxysms —*see* Epilepsy,
      localization-related, idiopathic
    absence G40.A09
      intractable G40.A19
        with status epilepticus G40.A11
        without status epilepticus G40.A19
      not intractable G40.A09
        with status epilepticus G40.A01
        without status epilepticus G40.A09
  climacteric —*see* Epilepsy, specified NEC
  cysticercosis B69.0
  deterioration (mental) F06.8
  due to syphilis A52.19
  focal —*see* Epilepsy, localization-related,
    symptomatic, with simple partial
    seizures
  generalized
    idiopathic G40.309
      intractable G40.319
        with status epilepticus G40.311
        without status epilepticus G40.319
      not intractable G40.309
        with status epilepticus G40.301
        without status epilepticus G40.309
    specified NEC G40.409
      intractable G40.419
        with status epilepticus G40.411
        without status epilepticus G40.419
      not intractable G40.409
        with status epilepticus G40.401
        without status epilepticus G40.409
  impulsive petit mal —*see* Epilepsy, juvenile
    myoclonic

Epilepsy, epileptic, epilepsia *(Continued)*
  intractable G40.919
    with status epilepticus G40.911
    without status epilepticus G40.919
  juvenile absence G40.A09
    intractable G40.A19
      with status epilepticus G40.A11
      without status epilepticus G40.A19
    not intractable G40.A09
      with status epilepticus G40.A01
      without status epilepticus G40.A09
  juvenile myoclonic G40.B11
    intractable G40.B19
      with status epilepticus G40.B11
      without status epilepticus G40.B19
    not intractable G40.B09
      with status epilepticus G40.B01
      without status epilepticus G40.B09
  ▶ KCNQ2-related G40.842
    ▶ intractable G40.844
      ▶ with status epilepticus G40.843
      ▶ without status epilepticus G40.844
    ▶ not intractable G40.842
      ▶ with status epilepticus G40.841
      ▶ without status epilepticus G40.842
  Lafora progressive myoclonus (*see also* Epilepsy,
    progressive, Lafora) G40.C09
  localization-related (focal) (partial)
    idiopathic G40.009
      with seizures of localized onset G40.009
        intractable G40.019
          with status epilepticus G40.011
          without status epilepticus G40.019
        not intractable G40.009
          with status epilepticus G40.001
          without status epilepticus G40.009
    symptomatic
      with complex partial seizures G40.209
        intractable G40.219
          with status epilepticus G40.211
          without status epilepticus G40.219
        not intractable G40.209
          with status epilepticus G40.201
          without status epilepticus G40.209
      with simple partial seizures G40.109
        intractable G40.119
          with status epilepticus G40.111
          without status epilepticus G40.119
        not intractable G40.109
          with status epilepticus G40.101
          without status epilepticus G40.109
  myoclonus, myoclonic —*see also* Epilepsy,
    generalized, specified NEC
    progressive —*see also* Epilepsy, generalized,
      idiopathic
    Lafora G40.C09
      intractable G40.C19
        with status epilepticus G40.C11
        without status epilepticus G40.C19
      not intractable G40.C09
        with status epilepticus G40.C01
        without status epilepticus G40.C09
    type 1 - see Epilepsy, generalized,
      idiopathic
    type 2 - see Epilepsy, myoclonus,
      progressive, Lafora
    severe, in infancy (SMEI) G40.83-●
  not intractable G40.909
    with status epilepticus G40.901
    without status epilepticus G40.909
  on awakening —*see* Epilepsy, generalized,
    specified NEC
  parasitic NOS B71.9 *[G94]*
  partial —*see* Epilepsy, localization-related,
    symptomatic, with simple partial seizures
  partialis continua —*see also* Kozhevnikof's
    epilepsy G40.1-●
  peripheral —*see* Epilepsy, specified NEC
  polymorphic, in infancy (PMEI) G40.83-●
  procursiva —*see* Epilepsy, localization-related,
    symptomatic, with simple partial seizures
  progressive (familial) myoclonic —*see* Epilepsy,
    myoclonus, progressive
  Lafora (*see also* Epilepsy, progressive, Lafora)
    G40.C09
  reflex —*see* Epilepsy, specified NEC
  related to
    alcohol G40.509
      not intractable G40.509
        with status epilepticus G40.501
        without status epliepticus G40.509

▶ New   ⇒ Revised   ~~deleted~~ Deleted   ● Use Additional Character(s)

Eruption *(Continued)*
 skin (nonspecific) R21
  creeping (meaning hookworm) B76.9
  due to inoculation/vaccination
    (generalized) —*see also* Dermatitis, due
    to, vaccine L27.0
   localized L27.1
  erysipeloid A26.0
  feigned L98.1
  Kaposi's varicelliform B00.0
  lichenoid L28.0
  meaning dermatitis —*see* Dermatitis
  toxic NEC L53.0
 tooth, teeth, abnormal (incomplete) (late)
   (premature) (sequence) K00.6
 vesicular R23.8
Erysipelas (gangrenous) (infantile) (newborn)
  (phlegmonous) (suppurative) A46
 external ear A46 [H62.40]
 puerperal, postpartum O86.89
Erysipeloid A26.9
 cutaneous (Rosenbach's) A26.0
 disseminated A26.8
 sepsis A26.7
 specified NEC A26.8
Erythema, erythematous (infectional)
  (inflammation) L53.9
 ab igne L59.0
 annulare (centrifugum) (rheumaticum) L53.1
 arthriticum epidemicum A25.1
 brucellum —*see* Brucellosis
 chronic figurate NEC L53.3
 chronicum migrans (Borrelia burgdorferi) A69.20
 diaper L22
 due to
  chemical NEC L53.0
   in contact with skin L24.5
  drug (internal use) —*see* Dermatitis, due to,
    drugs
 elevatum diutinum L95.1
 endemic E52
 epidemic, arthritic A25.1
 figuratum perstans L53.3
 gluteal L22
 heat - code by site under Burn, first degree
 ichthyosiforme congenitum bullous Q80.3
 in diseases classified elsewhere L54
 induratum (nontuberculous) L52
  tuberculous A18.4
 infectiosum B08.3
 intertrigo L30.4
 iris L51.9
 marginatum L53.2
  in (due to) acute rheumatic fever I00
 medicamentosum —*see* Dermatitis, due to, drugs
 migrans A26.0
  chronicum A69.20
  tongue K14.1
 multiforme (major) (minor) L51.9
  bullous, bullosum L51.1
  conjunctiva L51.1
  nonbullous L51.0
  pemphigoides L12.0
  specified NEC L51.8
 napkin L22
 neonatorum P83.88
  toxic P83.1
 nodosum L52
  tuberculous A18.4
 palmar L53.8
 pernio T69.1
 rash, newborn P83.88
 scarlatiniform (recurrent) (exfoliative)
   L53.8
 solare L55.0
 specified NEC L53.8
 toxic, toxicum NEC L53.0
  newborn P83.1
 tuberculous (primary) A18.4
Erythematous, erythematosus —*see* condition
Erythermalgia (primary) I73.81
Erythralgia I73.81
Erythrasma L08.1
Erythredema (polyneuropathy) —*see* Poisoning,
  mercury
Erythremia (acute) C94.0-•
 chronic D45
 secondary D75.1
Erythroblastopenia —*see also* Aplasia, red cell
  D60.9
 congenital D61.01

Erythroblastophthisis D61.09
Erythroblastosis (fetalis) (newborn) P55.9
 due to
  ABO (antibodies) (incompatibility)
    (isoimmunization) P55.1
  Rh (antibodies) (incompatibility)
    (isoimmunization) P55.0
Erythrocyanosis (crurum) I73.89
Erythrocythemia —*see* Erythremia
Erythrocytosis (megalosplenic) (secondary) D75.1
 familial D75.0
 oval, hereditary —*see* Elliptocytosis
 secondary D75.1
 stress D75.1
Erythroderma (secondary) —*see also* Erythema L53.9
 bullous ichthyosiform, congenital Q80.3
 desquamativum L21.1
 ichthyosiform, congenital (bullous) Q80.3
 neonatorum P83.88
 psoriaticum L40.8
Erythrodysesthesia, palmar plantar (PPE) L27.1
Erythrogenesis imperfecta D61.09
Erythroleukemia C94.0-•
Erythromelalgia I73.81
Erythrophagocytosis D75.89
Erythrophobia F40.298
Erythroplakia, oral epithelium, and tongue K13.29
Erythroplasia (Queyrat) D07.4
 specified site —*see* Neoplasm, skin, in situ
 unspecified site D07.4
Escherichia coli (E. coli), as cause of disease
   classified elsewhere B96.20
 non-O157 Shiga toxin-producing (with known O
   group) B96.22
 non-Shiga toxin-producing B96.29
 O157 with confirmation of Shiga toxin when H
   antigen is unknown, or is not H7 B96.21
 O157:H- (nonmotile) with confirmation of Shiga
   toxin B96.21
 Shiga toxin-producing (with unspecified O
   group) (STEC) B96.23
 O157 B96.21
 O157:H7 with or without confirmation of Shiga
   toxin-production B96.21
 specified NEC B96.29
Esophagismus K22.4
Esophagitis (acute) (alkaline) (chemical) (chronic)
   (infectional) (necrotic) (peptic) (postoperative)
   (without bleeding) K20.90
 with bleeding K20.91
 candidal B37.81
 due to gastrointestinal reflux disease (without
   bleeding) K21.00
  with bleeding K21.01
 eosinophilic K20.0
 reflux K21.00
  with bleeding K21.01
 specified NEC (without bleeding) K20.80
  with bleeding K20.81
 tuberculous A18.83
 ulcerative K22.10
  with bleeding K22.11
Esophagocele K22.5
Esophagomalacia K22.89
Esophagospasm K22.4
Esophagostenosis K22.2
Esophagostomiasis B81.8
Esophagotracheal —*see* condition
Esophagus —*see* condition
Esophoria H50.51
 convergence, excess H51.12
 divergence, insufficiency H51.8
Esotropia —*see* Strabismus, convergent concomitant
Espundia B55.2
Essential —*see* condition
Esthesioneuroblastoma C30.0
Esthesioneurocytoma C30.0
Esthesioneuroepithelioma C30.0
Esthiomene A55
Estivo-autumnal malaria (fever) B50.9
Estrangement (marital) Z63.5
 parent-child NEC Z62.890
Estriasis —*see* Myiasis
Ethanolism —*see* Alcoholism
Etherism —*see* Dependence, drug, inhalant
Ethmoid, ethmoidal —*see* condition
Ethmoiditis (chronic) (nonpurulent) (purulent) —
   see also Sinusitis, ethmoidal
 influenzal —*see* Influenza, with, respiratory
   manifestations NEC
Woakes' J33.1

Ethylism —*see* Alcoholism
Eulenburg's disease (congenital paramyotonia)
  G71.19
Eumycetoma B47.0
Eunuchoidism E29.1
 hypogonadotropic E23.0
European blastomycosis —*see* Cryptococcosis
Eustachian —*see* condition
Evaluation (for) (of)
 development state
  adolescent Z00.3
  period of
   delayed growth in childhood Z00.70
    with abnormal findings Z00.71
   rapid growth in childhood Z00.2
  puberty Z00.3
 growth and developmental state (period of rapid
   growth) Z00.2
  delayed growth Z00.70
   with abnormal findings Z00.71
 mental health (status) Z00.8
  requested by authority Z04.6
 period of
  delayed growth in childhood Z00.70
   with abnormal findings Z00.71
  rapid growth in childhood Z00.2
 suspected condition —*see* Observation
Evans syndrome D69.41
Event
 apparent life threatening in newborn and infant
   (ALTE) R68.13
 brief resolved unexplained event (BRUE) R68.13
Eventration —*see also* Hernia, ventral
 colon into chest —*see* Hernia, diaphragm
 diaphragm (congenital) Q79.1
Eversion
 bladder N32.89
 cervix (uteri) N86
  with cervicitis N72
 foot NEC —*see also* Deformity, valgus, ankle
  congenital Q66.6
 punctum lacrimale (postinfectional) (senile)
   H04.52-•
 ureter (meatus) N28.89
 urethra (meatus) N36.8
 uterus N81.4
Evidence
 cytologic
  of malignancy on anal smear R85.614
  of malignancy on cervical smear R87.614
  of malignancy on vaginal smear R87.624
Evisceration
 birth injury P15.8
 traumatic NEC
  eye —*see* Enucleated eye
Evulsion —*see* Avulsion
Ewing's sarcoma or tumor —*see* Neoplasm, bone,
  malignant
Examination (for) (following) (general) (of)
   (routine) Z00.00
 with abnormal findings Z00.01
 abuse, physical (alleged), ruled out
  adult Z04.71
  child Z04.72
 adolescent (development state) Z00.3
 alleged rape or sexual assault (victim), ruled out
  adult Z04.41
  child Z04.42
 allergy Z01.82
 annual (adult) (periodic) (physical) Z00.00
  with abnormal findings Z00.01
  gynecological Z01.419
   with abnormal findings Z01.411
 antibody response Z01.84
 blood —*see* Examination, laboratory
 blood pressure Z01.30
  with abnormal findings Z01.31
 cancer staging —*see* Neoplasm, malignant, by
   site
 cervical Papanicolaou smear Z12.4
  as part of routine gynecological examination
    Z01.419
   with abnormal findings Z01.411
 child (over 28 days old) Z00.129
  with abnormal findings Z00.121
  under 28 days old —*see* Newborn,
    examination
 clinical research control or normal comparison
   (control) (participant) Z00.6
 contraceptive (drug) maintenance (routine) Z30.8
  device (intrauterine) Z30.431

▶ New   ⇒ Revised   ~~deleted~~ Deleted   • Use Additional Character(s)

Examination *(Continued)*
dental Z01.20
  with abnormal findings Z01.21
developmental —*see* Examination, child
donor (potential) Z00.5
ear Z01.10
  with abnormal findings NEC Z01.118
eye Z01.00
  with abnormal findings Z01.01
  following failed vision screening Z01.020
    with abnormal findings Z01.021
following
  accident NEC Z04.3
    transport Z04.1
    work Z04.2
  assault, alleged, ruled out
    adult Z04.71
    child Z04.72
  motor vehicle accident Z04.1
  treatment (for) Z09
    combined NEC Z09
      fracture Z09
      malignant neoplasm Z08
    malignant neoplasm Z08
    mental disorder Z09
    specified condition NEC Z09
follow-up (routine) (following) Z09
  chemotherapy NEC Z09
    malignant neoplasm Z08
  fracture Z09
  malignant neoplasm Z08
  postpartum Z39.2
  psychotherapy Z09
  radiotherapy NEC Z09
    malignant neoplasm Z08
  surgery NEC Z09
    malignant neoplasm Z08
forced sexual exploitation Z04.81
forced labor exploitation Z04.82
gynecological Z01.419
  with abnormal findings Z01.411
  for contraceptive maintenance Z30.8
health —*see* Examination, medical
hearing Z01.10
  with abnormal findings NEC Z01.118
  infant or child (over 28 days old)
    Z00.129
    with abnormal findings Z00.121
  following failed hearing screening
    Z01.110
immunity status testing Z01.84
laboratory (as part of a general medical
  examination) Z00.00
  with abnormal findings Z00.01
  preprocedural Z01.812
lactating mother Z39.1
medical (adult) (for) (of) Z00.00
  with abnormal findings Z00.01
  administrative purpose only Z02.9
    specified NEC Z02.89
  admission to
    armed forces Z02.3
    old age home Z02.2
    prison Z02.89
    residential institution Z02.2
    school Z02.0
      following illness or medical treatment
        Z02.0
    summer camp Z02.89
  adoption Z02.82
  blood alcohol or drug level Z02.83
  camp (summer) Z02.89
  clinical research, normal subject (control)
    (participant) Z00.6
  control subject in clinical research (normal
    comparison) (participant) Z00.6
  donor (potential) Z00.5
  driving license Z02.4
  general (adult) Z00.00
    with abnormal findings Z00.01
  immigration Z02.89
  insurance purposes Z02.6
  marriage Z02.89
  medicolegal reasons NEC Z04.89
  naturalization Z02.89
  participation in sport Z02.5
  paternity testing Z02.81
  population survey Z00.8
  pre-employment Z02.1
  pre-operative —*see* Examination,
    pre-procedural

Examination *(Continued)*
medical *(Continued)*
  pre-procedural
    cardiovascular Z01.810
    respiratory Z01.811
    specified NEC Z01.818
  preschool children
    for admission to school Z02.0
  prisoners
    for entrance into prison Z02.89
  recruitment for armed forces Z02.3
  specified NEC Z00.8
  sport competition Z02.5
medicolegal reason NEC Z04.89
  forced sexual exploitation Z04.81
  forced labor exploitation Z04.82
newborn —*see* Newborn, examination
pelvic (annual) (periodic) Z01.419
  with abnormal findings Z01.411
period of rapid growth in childhood Z00.2
periodic (adult) (annual) (routine) Z00.00
  with abnormal findings Z00.01
physical (adult) —*see also* Examination, medical
  Z00.00
  sports Z02.5
postpartum
  immediately after delivery Z39.0
  routine follow-up Z39.2
pre-chemotherapy (antineoplastic) Z01.818
prenatal (normal pregnancy) —*see also*
  Pregnancy, normal Z34.9-●
pre-procedural (pre-operative)
  cardiovascular Z01.810
  laboratory Z01.812
  respiratory Z01.811
  specified NEC Z01.818
  prior to chemotherapy (antineoplastic) Z01.818
psychiatric NEC Z00.8
  follow-up not needing further care Z09
  requested by authority Z04.6
radiological (as part of a general medical
  examination) Z00.00
  with abnormal findings Z00.01
repeat cervical smear to confirm findings of
  recent normal smear following initial
  abnormal smear Z01.42
skin (hypersensitivity) Z01.82
special —*see also* Examination, by type Z01.89
  specified type NEC Z01.89
specified type or reason NEC Z04.89
teeth Z01.20
  with abnormal findings Z01.21
urine —*see* Examination, laboratory
vision Z01.00
  with abnormal findings Z01.01
  following failed vision screening Z01.020
    with abnormal findings Z01.021
  infant or child (over 28 days old) Z00.129
    with abnormal findings Z00.121
Exanthem, exanthema —*see also* Rash
with enteroviral vesicular stomatitis B08.4
Boston A88.0
epidemic with meningitis A88.0 [G02]
subitum B08.20
  due to human herpesvirus 6 B08.21
  due to human herpesvirus 7 B08.22
viral, virus B09
  specified type NEC B08.8
Excess, excessive, excessively
alcohol level in blood R78.0
androgen (ovarian) E28.1
attrition, tooth, teeth K03.0
carotene, carotin (dietary) E67.1
cold, effects of T69.9
  specified effect NEC T69.8
convergence H51.12
crying
  in child, adolescent, or adult R45.83
  in infant R68.11
development, breast N62
divergence H51.8
drinking (alcohol) NEC (without dependence)
  F10.10
  habitual (continual) (without remission)
    F10.20
eating R63.2
estrogen E28.0
fat —*see also* Obesity
  in heart —*see* Degeneration, myocardial
  localized E65
foreskin N47.8

Excess, excessive, excessively *(Continued)*
gas R14.0
glucagon E16.3
heat —*see* Heat
intermaxillary vertical dimension of fully
  erupted teeth M26.37
interocclusal distance of fully erupted teeth
  M26.37
kalium E87.5
large
  colon K59.39
    congenital Q43.8
  infant P08.0
  organ or site, congenital NEC —*see* Anomaly,
    by site
long
  organ or site, congenital NEC —*see* Anomaly,
    by site
menstruation (with regular cycle) N92.0
  with irregular cycle N92.1
napping Z72.821
natrium E87.0
number of teeth K00.1
nutrient (dietary) NEC R63.2
potassium (K) E87.5
salivation K11.7
secretion —*see also* Hypersecretion
  milk O92.6
  sputum R09.3
  sweat R61
sexual drive F52.8
short
  organ or site, congenital NEC —*see* Anomaly,
    by site
  umbilical cord in labor or delivery O69.3
skin L98.7
  and subcutaneous tissue L98.7
  eyelid (acquired) —*see* Blepharochalasis
    congenital Q10.3
sodium (Na) E87.0
spacing of fully erupted teeth M26.32
sputum R09.3
sweating R61
thirst R63.1
  due to deprivation of water T73.1
transportation time Z59.82
tuberosity of jaw M26.07
vitamin
  A (dietary) E67.0
    administered as drug (prolonged intake) —
      see Table of Drugs and Chemicals,
      vitamins, adverse effect
    overdose or wrong substance given or
      taken —*see* Table of Drugs and
      Chemicals, vitamins, poisoning
  D (dietary) E67.3
    administered as drug (prolonged intake) —
      see Table of Drugs and Chemicals,
      vitamins, adverse
      effect
    overdose or wrong substance given or
      taken —*see* Table of Drugs and
      Chemicals, vitamins, poisoning
weight
  gain R63.5
  loss R63.4
Excitability, abnormal, under minor stress
  (personality disorder) F60.3
Excitation
anomalous atrioventricular I45.6
psychogenic F30.8
reactive (from emotional stress, psychological
  trauma) F30.8
Excitement
hypomanic F30.8
manic F30.9
mental, reactive (from emotional stress,
  psychological trauma) F30.8
state, reactive (from emotional stress,
  psychological trauma) F30.8
Excoriation (traumatic) —*see also* Abrasion
neurotic L98.1
skin picking disorder F42.4
Exfoliation
due to erythematous conditions according to
  extent of body surface involved L49.0
  10-19 percent of body surface L49.1
  20-29 percent of body surface L49.2
  30-39 percent of body surface L49.3
  40-49 percent of body surface L49.4
  50-59 percent of body surface L49.5

Exfoliation *(Continued)*
  due to erythematous conditions
      according to extent of body surface
      involved — *(Continued)*
      60-69 percent of body surface L49.6
      70-79 percent of body surface L49.7
      80-89 percent of body surface L49.8
      90-99 percent of body surface L49.9
      less than 10 percent of body surface L49.0
    teeth, due to systemic causes K08.0
Exfoliative —*see* condition
Exhaustion, exhaustive (physical NEC) R53.83
  battle F43.0
  cardiac —*see* Failure, heart
  delirium F43.0
  due to
    cold T69.8
    excessive exertion T73.3
    exposure T73.2
    neurasthenia F48.8
  heart —*see* Failure, heart
  heat —*see also* Heat, exhaustion T67.5
    due to
      salt depletion T67.4
      water depletion T67.3
  maternal, complicating delivery O75.81
  mental F48.8
  myocardium, myocardial —*see* Failure, heart
  nervous F48.8
  old age R54
  psychogenic F48.8
  psychosis F43.0
  senile R54
  vital NEC Z73.0
Exhibitionism F65.2
Exocervicitis —*see* Cervicitis
Exomphalos Q79.2
  meaning hernia —*see* Hernia, umbilicus
Exophoria H50.52
  convergence, insufficiency H51.11
  divergence, excess H51.8
Exophthalmos H05.2-●
  congenital Q15.8
  constant NEC H05.24-●
  displacement, globe —*see* Displacement, globe
  due to thyrotoxicosis (hyperthyroidism) —*see*
      Hyperthyroidism, with, goiter (diffuse)
  dysthyroid —*see* Hyperthyroidism, with, goiter
      (diffuse)
  goiter —*see* Hyperthyroidism, with, goiter (diffuse)
  intermittent NEC H05.25-●
  malignant —*see* Hyperthyroidism, with, goiter
      (diffuse)
  orbital
    edema —*see* Edema, orbit
    hemorrhage —*see* Hemorrhage, orbit
  pulsating NEC H05.26-●
  thyrotoxic, thyrotropic —*see* Hyperthyroidism,
      with, goiter (diffuse)
Exostosis —*see also* Disorder, bone
  cartilaginous —*see* Neoplasm, bone, benign
  congenital (multiple) Q78.6
  external ear canal H61.81-●
  gonococcal A54.49
  jaw (bone) M27.8
  multiple, congenital Q78.6
  orbit H05.35-●
  osteocartilaginous —*see* Neoplasm, bone, benign
  syphilitic A52.77
Exotropia —*see* Strabismus, divergent concomitant
Explanation of
  investigation finding Z71.2
  medication Z71.89
Exploitation
  labor
    confirmed
      adult forced T74.61
      child forced T74.62
    suspected
      adult forced T76.61
      child forced T76.62
  sexual
    confirmed
      adult forced T74.51
      child T74.52
    suspected
      adult forced T76.51
      child T76.52
Exposure (to) —*see also* Contact, with T75.89
  acariasis Z20.7
  AIDS virus Z20.6

Exposure *(Continued)*
  air pollution Z77.110
  algae and algae toxins Z77.121
  algae bloom Z77.121
  anthrax Z20.810
  aromatic amines Z77.020
  aromatic (hazardous) compounds NEC Z77.028
  aromatic dyes NOS Z77.028
  arsenic Z77.010
  asbestos Z77.090
  bacterial disease NEC Z20.818
  benzene Z77.021
  blue-green algae bloom Z77.121
  body fluids (potentially hazardous) Z77.21
  brown tide Z77.121
  chemicals (chiefly nonmedicinal) (hazardous)
      NEC Z77.098
  cholera Z20.09
  chromium compounds Z77.018
  cold, effects of T69.9
    specified effect NEC T69.8
  communicable disease Z20.9
    bacterial NEC Z20.818
    specified NEC Z20.89
    viral NEC Z20.828
    Zika virus Z20.821
    coronavirus (disease) (novel) 2019
        Z20.822
  cyanobacteria bloom Z77.121
  disaster Z65.5
  discrimination Z60.5
  dyes Z77.098
  effects of T73.9
  environmental tobacco smoke (acute) (chronic)
      Z77.22
  Escherichia coli (E. coli) Z20.01
  exhaustion due to T73.2
  fiberglass —*see* Table of Drugs and Chemicals,
      fiberglass
  German measles Z20.4
  gonorrhea Z20.2
  hazardous metals NEC Z77.018
  hazardous substances NEC Z77.29
  hazards in the physical environment NEC
      Z77.128
  hazards to health NEC Z77.9
  human immunodeficiency virus (HIV)
      Z20.6
  human T-lymphotropic virus type-1 (HTLV-1)
      Z20.89
  implanted
    mesh —*see* Complications, prosthetic device
        or implant, mesh
    prosthetic materials NEC —*see* Complications,
        prosthetic materials NEC
  infestation (parasitic) NEC Z20.7
  intestinal infectious disease NEC Z20.09
    Escherichia coli (E. coli) Z20.01
  lead Z77.011
  meningococcus Z20.811
  mold (toxic) Z77.120
  nickel dust Z77.018
  noise Z77.122
  occupational
    air contaminants NEC Z57.39
    dust Z57.2
    environmental tobacco smoke Z57.31
    extreme temperature Z57.6
    noise Z57.0
    radiation Z57.1
    risk factors Z57.9
      specified NEC Z57.8
    toxic agents (gases) (liquids) (solids) (vapors)
        in agriculture Z57.4
    toxic agents (gases) (liquids) (solids) (vapors)
        in industry NEC Z57.5
    vibration Z57.7
  parasitic disease NEC Z20.7
  pediculosis Z20.7
  persecution Z60.5
  pfiesteria piscicida Z77.121
  poliomyelitis Z20.89
  pollution
    air Z77.110
    environmental NEC Z77.118
    soil Z77.112
    water Z77.111
  polycyclic aromatic hydrocarbons Z77.028
  prenatal (drugs) (toxic chemicals) —*see*
      Newborn, affected by, noxious substances
      transmitted via placenta or breast milk

Exposure *(Continued)*
  rabies Z20.3
  radiation, naturally occurring NEC Z77.123
  radon Z77.123
  red tide (Florida) Z77.121
  rubella Z20.4
  second hand tobacco smoke (acute) (chronic)
      Z77.22
    in the perinatal period P96.81
  sexually-transmitted disease Z20.2
  smallpox (laboratory) Z20.89
  syphilis Z20.2
  terrorism Z65.4
  torture Z65.4
  tuberculosis Z20.1
  uranium Z77.012
  varicella Z20.820
  venereal disease Z20.2
  viral disease NEC Z20.828
  war Z65.5
  water pollution Z77.111
    Zika virus Z20.821
Exsanguination —*see* Hemorrhage
Exstrophy
  abdominal contents Q45.8
  bladder Q64.10
    cloacal Q64.12
    specified type NEC Q64.19
    supravesical fissure Q64.11
Extensive —*see* condition
Extra —*see also* Accessory
  marker chromosomes (normal individual)
      Q92.61
    in abnormal individual Q92.62
  rib Q76.6
    cervical Q76.5
Extrasystoles (supraventricular) I49.49
  atrial I49.1
  auricular I49.1
  junctional I49.2
  ventricular I49.3
Extrauterine gestation or pregnancy —*see*
    Pregnancy, by site
Extravasation
  blood R58
  chyle into mesentery I89.8
  pelvicalyceal N13.8
  pyelosinus N13.8
  urine (from ureter) R39.0
  vesicant agent
    antineoplastic chemotherapy T80.810
    other agent NEC T80.818
Extremity —*see* condition, limb
Extrophy —*see* Exstrophy
Extroversion
  bladder Q64.19
  uterus N81.4
    complicating delivery O71.2
    postpartal (old) N81.4
Extruded tooth (teeth) M26.34
Extrusion
  breast implant (prosthetic) T85.42
  eye implant (globe) (ball) T85.328
  intervertebral disc —*see* Displacement,
      intervertebral disc
  ocular lens implant (prosthetic) —*see*
      Complications, intraocular lens
  vitreous —*see* Prolapse, vitreous
Exudate
  causing irritant dermatitis L24.A9
  pleural —*see* Effusion, pleura
  retina H35.89
  wound fluids causing irritant dermatitis L24.A9
Exudative —*see* condition
Eye, eyeball, eyelid —*see* condition
Eyestrain —*see* Disturbance, vision, subjective
Eyeworm disease of Africa B74.3

F

Faber's syndrome (achlorhydric anemia) D50.9
Fabry (-Anderson) disease E75.21
Facet syndrome M47.89-●
Faciocephalalgia, autonomic —*see also*
    Neuropathy, peripheral, autonomic G90.09
Factor(s)
  psychic, associated with diseases classified
      elsewhere F54

Note: heart failure stages A, B, C, and D are
based on the American College of Cardiology
and American Heart Association stages of heart
failure, which complement and should not be
confused with the New York Heart Association
Classification of Heart Failure, into Class I,
Class II, Class III, and Class IV

Failure, failed (Continued)
  renal N19
    with
      tubular necrosis (acute) N17.0
    acute N17.9
      with
        cortical necrosis N17.1
        medullary necrosis N17.2
        tubular necrosis N17.0
      specified NEC N17.8
    chronic N18.9
      hypertensive —see Hypertension, kidney
    congenital P96.0
    end stage (chronic) N18.6
      due to hypertension I12.0
    following
      abortion —see Abortion by type
        complicated by specified
          condition NEC
      crushing T79.5
      ectopic or molar pregnancy O08.4
      labor and delivery (acute) O90.49
    hypertensive —see Hypertension, kidney
    postprocedural N99.0
  respiration, respiratory J96.90
    with
      hypercapnia J96.92
      hypercarbia J96.02
      hypoxia J96.91
    acute J96.00
      with
        hypercapnia J96.02
        hypercarbia J96.92
        hypoxia J96.01
    acute and (on) chronic J96.20
      with
        hypercapnia J96.22
        hypercarbia J96.22
        hypoxia J96.21
    center G93.89
    chronic J96.10
      with
        hypercapnia J96.12
        hypercarbia J96.12
        hypoxia J96.11
    newborn P28.5
    postprocedural (acute) J95.821
      acute and chronic J95.822
  rotation
    cecum Q43.3
    colon Q43.3
    intestine Q43.3
    kidney Q63.2
  sedation (conscious) (moderate) during
    procedure T88.52
    history of Z92.83
  segmentation —see also Fusion
    fingers —see Syndactylism, complex, fingers
    vertebra Q76.49
      with scoliosis Q76.3
  seminiferous tubule, adult E29.1
  senile (general) R54
  sexual arousal (male) F52.21
    female F52.22
  testicular endocrine function E29.1
  to thrive (child over 28 days old) R62.51
    adult R62.7
    newborn P92.6
  transplant T86.92
    bone T86.831
      marrow T86.02
    cornea T86.841-●
    heart T86.22
      with lung(s) T86.32
    intestine T86.851
    kidney T86.12
    liver T86.42
    lung(s) T86.811
      with heart T86.32
    pancreas T86.891
    skin (allograft) (autograft) T86.821
    specified organ or tissue NEC T86.891
    stem cell (peripheral blood) (umbilical cord)
      T86.5
  trial of labor (with subsequent cesarean delivery)
    O66.40
    following previous cesarean delivery O66.41
  tubal ligation N99.89
  urinary —see Disease, kidney, chronic
  vacuum extraction NOS (with subsequent
    cesarean delivery) O66.5

Failure, failed (Continued)
  vasectomy N99.89
  ventouse NOS (with subsequent cesarean
    delivery) O66.5
  ventricular —see also Failure, heart I50.9
    left —see also Failure, heart, left I50.1
      with rheumatic fever (conditions
        in I00)
        active I01.8
          with chorea I02.0
        inactive or quiescent (with chorea) I09.81
      rheumatic (chronic) (inactive) (with chorea)
        I09.81
        active or acute I01.8
          with chorea I02.0
    right —see Failure, heart, right
  vital centers, newborn P91.88
Fainting (fit) R55
Fallen arches —see Deformity, limb, flat foot
Falling, falls (repeated) R29.6
  any organ or part —see Prolapse
Fallopian
  insufflation Z31.41
  tube —see condition
Fallot's
  pentalogy Q21.8
  tetrad or tetralogy Q21.3
  triad or trilogy Q22.3
False —see also condition
  croup J38.5
  joint —see Nonunion, fracture
  labor (pains) O47.9
    at or after 37 completed weeks of gestation
      O47.1
    before 37 completed weeks of gestation
      O47.0-●
  passage, urethra (prostatic) N36.5
  pregnancy F45.8
Family, familial —see also condition
  disruption Z63.8
    involving divorce or separation
      Z63.5
  Li-Fraumeni (syndrome) Z15.01
  planning advice Z30.09
  problem Z63.9
    specified NEC Z63.8
  retinoblastoma C69.2-●
Famine (effects of) T73.0
  edema —see Malnutrition, severe
Fanconi (-de Toni)(-Debré) syndrome
  E72.09
  with cystinosis E72.04
Fanconi's anemia (congenital pancytopenia) D61.09
Fanconi('s) anemia D61.03
Fanconi hypoplastic anemia D61.03
Fanconi panmyelopathy D61.03
Farber's disease or syndrome E75.29
Farcy A24.0
Farmer's
  lung J67.0
  skin L57.8
Farsightedness —see Hypermetropia
Fascia —see condition
Fasciculation R25.3
Fasciitis M72.9
  diffuse (eosinophilic) M35.4
  infective M72.8
    necrotizing M72.6
  necrotizing M72.6
  nodular M72.4
  perirenal (with ureteral obstruction)
    N13.5
    with infection N13.6
  plantar M72.2
  specified NEC M72.8
  traumatic (old) M72.8
    current - code by site under Sprain
Fascioliasis B66.3
Fasciolopsis, fasciolopsiasis (intestinal)
  B66.5
Fascioscapulohumeral myopathy G71.02
Fast pulse R00.0
Fat
  embolism —see Embolism, fat
  excessive —see also Obesity
    in heart —see Degeneration, myocardial
  in stool R19.5
  localized (pad) E65
    heart —see Degeneration, myocardial
    knee M79.4
    retropatellar M79.4

Fat (Continued)
  necrosis
    breast N64.1
    mesentery K65.4
    omentum K65.4
  pad E65
    knee M79.4
Fatigue R53.83
  auditory deafness —see Deafness
  chronic R53.82
  combat F43.0
  general R53.83
    psychogenic F48.8
  heat (transient) T67.6
  muscle M62.89
  myocardium —see Failure, heart
  neoplasm-related R53.0
  nervous, neurosis F48.8
  operational F48.8
  psychogenic (general) F48.8
  senile R54
  voice R49.8
Fatness —see Obesity
Fatty —see also condition
  apron E65
  degeneration —see Degeneration, fatty
  heart (enlarged) —see Degeneration, myocardial
  liver NEC K76.0

    alcoholic K70.0
    nonalcoholic K76.0
  necrosis —see Degeneration, fatty
Fauces —see condition
Fauchard's disease (periodontitis) —see
    Periodontitis
Faucitis J02.9
Favism (anemia) D55.0
Favus —see Dermatophytosis
Fazio-Londe disease or syndrome
  G12.1
Fear complex or reaction F40.9
Fear of —see Phobia
Feared complaint unfounded Z71.1
Febris, febrile —see also Fever
  flava —see also Fever, yellow A95.9
  melitensis A23.0
  pestis —see Plague
  recurrens —see Fever, relapsing
  rubra A38.9
Fecal
  incontinence R15.9
  smearing R15.1
  soiling R15.1
  urgency R15.2
Fecalith (impaction) K56.41
  appendix K38.1
  congenital P76.8
Fede's disease K14.0
Feeble rapid pulse due to shock following injury
  T79.4
Feeble-minded F70
Feeding
  difficulties R63.30
  problem (elderly) (infant) R63.39
    newborn P92.9
      specified NEC P92.8
    nonorganic (adult) —see Disorder,
      eating
Feeling (of)
  foreign body in throat R09.A2
Feer's disease —see Poisoning, mercury
Feet —see condition
Feigned illness Z76.5
Feil-Klippel syndrome (brevicollis) Q76.1
Feinmesser's (hidrotic) ectodermal dysplasia
  Q82.4
Felinophobia F40.218
Felon —see also Cellulitis, digit
  with lymphangitis —see Lymphangitis,
    acute, digit
Felty's syndrome M05.00
  ankle M05.07-●
  elbow M05.02-●
  foot joint M05.07-●
  hand joint M05.04-●
  hip M05.05-●
  knee M05.06-●
  multiple site M05.09
  shoulder M05.01-●
  vertebra —see Spondylitis, ankylosing
  wrist M05.03-●

Female genital cutting status —*see* Female genital
    mutilation status (FGM)
Female genital mutilation status (FGM) N90.810
    specified NEC N90.818
    type I (clitorectomy status) N90.811
    type II (clitorectomy with excision of labia
        minora status) N90.812
    type III (infibulation status) N90.813
    type IV N90.818
Femur, femoral —*see* condition
Fenestration, fenestrated —*see also* Imperfect,
    closure
    aortico-pulmonary Q21.4
    atrial septum Q21.11
    cusps, heart valve NEC Q24.8
        pulmonary Q22.3
    pulmonic cusps Q22.3
Fernell's disease (aortic aneurysm) I71.9
Fertile eunuch syndrome E23.0
Fetid
    breath R19.6
    sweat L75.0
Fetishism F65.0
    transvestic F65.1
Fetus, fetal —*see also* condition
    alcohol syndrome (dysmorphic) Q86.0
    compressus O31.0-●
    hydantoin syndrome Q86.1
    lung tissue P28.0
    papyraceous O31.0-●
Fever (inanition) (of unknown origin) (persistent)
    (with chills) (with rigor) R50.9
    abortus A23.1
    Aden (dengue) A90
    African tick bite A77.8
    African tick-borne A68.1
    American
        mountain (tick) A93.2
        spotted A77.0
    aphthous B08.8
    arbovirus, arboviral A94
        hemorrhagic A94
        specified NEC A93.8
    Argentinian hemorrhagic A96.0
    Assam B55.0
    Australian Q A78
    Bangkok hemorrhagic A91
    Barmah forest A92.8
    Bartonella A44.0
    bilious, hemoglobinuric B50.8
    blackwater B50.8
    blister B00.1
    Bolivian hemorrhagic A96.1
    Bonvale dam T73.3
    boutonneuse A77.1
    brain —*see* Encephalitis
    Brazilian purpuric A48.4
    breakbone A90
    Bullis A77.0
    Bunyamwera A92.8
    Burdwan B55.0
    Bwamba A92.8
    Cameroon —*see* Malaria
    Canton A75.9
    catarrhal (acute) J00
        chronic J31.0
    cat-scratch A28.1
    Central Asian hemorrhagic A98.0
    cerebral —*see* Encephalitis
    cerebrospinal meningococcal A39.0
    Chagres B50.9
    Chandipura A92.8
    Changuinola A93.1
    Charcot's (biliary) (hepatic) (intermittent) —*see*
        Calculus, bile duct
    Chikungunya (viral) (hemorrhagic) A92.0
    Chitral A93.1
    Colombo —*see* Fever, paratyphoid
    Colorado tick (virus) A93.2
    congestive (remittent) —*see* Malaria
    Congo virus A98.0
    continued malarial B50.9
    Corsican —*see* Malaria
    Crimean-Congo hemorrhagic A98.0
    Cyprus —*see* Brucellosis
    dandy A90
    deer fly —*see* Tularemia
    dengue (virus) A90
        hemorrhagic A91
        sandfly A93.1
    desert B38.0

Fever *(Continued)*
    drug induced R50.2
    due to
        conditions classified elsewhere R50.81
        heat T67.01
    enteric A01.00
    enteroviral exanthematous (Boston exanthem)
        A88.0
    ephemeral (of unknown origin) R50.9
    epidemic hemorrhagic A98.5
    erysipelatous —*see* Erysipelas
    estivo-autumnal (malarial) B50.9
    famine A75.0
    five day A79.0
    following delivery O86.4
    Fort Bragg A27.89
    gastroenteric A01.00
    gastromalarial —*see* Malaria
    Gibraltar —*see* Brucellosis
    glandular —*see* Mononucleosis, infectious
    Guama (viral) A92.8
    Haverhill A25.1
    hay (allergic) J30.1
        with asthma (bronchial) J45.909
            with
                exacerbation (acute) J45.901
                status asthmaticus J45.902
        due to
            allergen other than pollen J30.89
            pollen, any plant or tree J30.1
    heat (effects) T67.01
    hematuric, bilious B50.8
    hemoglobinuric (malarial) (bilious) B50.8
    hemorrhagic (arthropod-borne) NOS A94
        with renal syndrome A98.5
        arenaviral A96.9
            specified NEC A96.8
        Argentinian A96.0
        Bangkok A91
        Bolivian A96.1
        Central Asian A98.0
        Chikungunya A92.0
        Crimean-Congo A98.0
        dengue (virus) A91
        epidemic A98.5
        Junin (virus) A96.0
        Korean A98.5
        Kyasanur forest A98.2
        Machupo (virus) A96.1
        mite-borne A93.8
        mosquito-borne A92.8
        Omsk A98.1
        Philippine A91
        Russian A98.5
        Singapore A91
        Southeast Asia A91
        Thailand A91
        tick-borne NEC A93.8
        viral A99
            specified NEC A98.8
    hepatic —*see* Cholecystitis
    herpetic —*see* Herpes
    icterohemorrhagic A27.0
    Indiana A93.8
    infective B99.9
        specified NEC B99.8
    intermittent (bilious) —*see also* Malaria
        of unknown origin R50.9
        pernicious B50.9
    iodide R50.2
    Japanese river A75.3
    jungle —*see also* Malaria
        yellow A95.0
    Junin (virus) hemorrhagic A96.0
    Katayama B65.2
    kedani A75.3
    Kenya (tick) A77.1
    Kew Garden A79.1
    Korean hemorrhagic A98.5
    Lassa A96.2
    Lone Star A77.0
    Machupo (virus) hemorrhagic A96.1
    malaria, malarial —*see* Malaria
    Malta A23.9
    Marseilles A77.1
    marsh —*see* Malaria
    Mayaro (viral) A92.8
    Mediterranean —*see also* Brucellosis A23.9
        familial M04.1
        tick A77.1
    meningeal —*see* Meningitis

Fever *(Continued)*
    Meuse A79.0
    Mexican A75.2
    mianeh A68.1
    miasmatic —*see* Malaria
    mosquito-borne (viral) A92.9
        hemorrhagic A92.8
    mountain —*see also* Brucellosis
        meaning Rocky Mountain spotted fever A77.0
        tick (American) (Colorado) (viral) A93.2
    Mucambo (viral) A92.8
    mud A27.9
    Neapolitan —*see* Brucellosis
    neutropenic D70.9
    newborn P81.9
        environmental P81.0
    Nine-Mile A78
    non-exanthematous tick A93.2
    North Asian tick-borne A77.2
    Omsk hemorrhagic A98.1
    O'nyong-nyong (viral) A92.1
    Oropouche (viral) A93.0
    Oroya A44.0
    pacific coast tick A77.8
    paludal —*see* Malaria
    Panama (malarial) B50.9
    Pappataci A93.1
    paratyphoid A01.4
        A A01.1
        B A01.2
        C A01.3
    parrot A70
    periodic (Mediterranean) M04.1
    persistent (of unknown origin) R50.9
    petechial A39.0
    pharyngoconjunctival B30.2
    Philippine hemorrhagic A91
    phlebotomus A93.1
    Piry (virus) A93.8
    Pixuna (viral) A92.8
    Plasmodium ovale B53.0
    polioviral (nonparalytic) A80.4
    Pontiac A48.2
    postimmunization R50.83
    postoperative R50.82
        due to infection T81.40
    posttransfusion R50.84
    postvaccination R50.83
    presenting with conditions classified elsewhere
        R50.81
    pretibial A27.89
    puerperal O86.4
    Q A78
    quadrilateral A78
    quartan (malaria) B52.9
    Queensland (coastal) (tick) A77.3
    quintan A79.0
    rabbit —*see* Tularemia
    rat-bite A25.9
        due to
            Spirillum A25.0
            Streptobacillus moniliformis A25.1
    recurrent —*see* Fever, relapsing
    relapsing (Borrelia) A68.9
        Carter's (Asiatic) A68.1
        Dutton's (West African) A68.1
        Koch's A68.9
        louse-borne A68.0
        Novy's
            louse-borne A68.0
            tick-borne A68.1
        Obermeyer's (European) A68.0
        tick-borne A68.1
    remittent (bilious) (congestive) (gastric) —*see*
        Malaria
    rheumatic (active) (acute) (chronic) (subacute)
        I00
        with central nervous system involvement
            I02.9
        active with heart involvement —*see* category
            I01
        inactive or quiescent with
            cardiac hypertrophy I09.89
            carditis I09.9
            endocarditis I09.1
                aortic (valve) I06.9
                    with mitral (valve) disease I08.0
                mitral (valve) I05.9
                    with aortic (valve) disease I08.0
                pulmonary (valve) I09.89
                tricuspid (valve) I07.8

Fever *(Continued)*
  rheumatic *(Continued)*
    inactive or quiescent with *(Continued)*
      heart disease NEC I09.89
      heart failure (congestive) (conditions in
        category I50.) I09.81
      left ventricular failure (conditions in
        I50.1-I50.4-) I09.81
      myocarditis, myocardial degeneration
        (conditions in I51.4) I09.0
      pancarditis I09.9
      pericarditis I09.2
  Rift Valley (viral) A92.4
  Rocky Mountain spotted A77.0
  rose J30.1
  Ross River B33.1
  Russian hemorrhagic A98.5
  San Joaquin (Valley) B38.0
  sandfly A93.1
  Sao Paulo A77.0
  scarlet A38.9
  seven day (leptospirosis) (autumnal) (Japanese)
    A27.89
    dengue A90
  shin-bone A79.0
  Singapore hemorrhagic A91
  solar A90
  Songo A98.5
  sore B00.1
  South African tick-bite A68.1
  Southeast Asia hemorrhagic A91
  spinal —*see* Meningitis
  spirillary A25.0
  splenic —*see* Anthrax
  spotted A77.9
    American A77.0
    Brazilian A77.0
    cerebrospinal meningitis A39.0
    Colombian A77.0
    due to Rickettsia
      africae (African tick bite fever) A77.8
      australis A77.3
      conorii A77.1
      parkeri A77.8
      rickettsii A77.0
      sibirica A77.2
      specified type NEC A77.8
    Ehrlichiosis A77.40
      due to
        ~~E. chaffeensis A77.41~~
        ▶ E. chaffeensis A77.41
        specified organism NEC A77.49
    Rocky Mountain A77.0
  steroid R50.2
  streptobacillary A25.1
  subtertian B50.9
  Sumatran mite A75.3
  sun A90
  swamp A27.9
  swine A02.8
  sylvatic, yellow A95.0
  Tahyna B33.8
  tertian —*see* Malaria, tertian
  Thailand hemorrhagic A91
  thermic T67.01
  three-day A93.1
  tick
    American mountain A93.2
    Colorado A93.2
    Kemerovo A93.8
    Mediterranean A77.1
    mountain A93.2
    nonxanthematous A93.2
    Quaranfil A93.8
  tick-bite NEC A93.8
  tick-borne (hemorrhagic) NEC A93.8
  trench A79.0
  tsutsugamushi A75.3
  typhogastric A01.00
  typhoid (abortive) (hemorrhagic) (intermittent)
    (malignant) A01.00
    complicated by
      arthritis A01.04
      heart involvement A01.02
      meningitis A01.01
      osteomyelitis A01.05
      pneumonia A01.03
      specified NEC A01.09
  typhomalarial —*see* Malaria
  typhus —*see* Typhus (fever)
  undulant —*see* Brucellosis

Fever *(Continued)*
  unknown origin R50.9
  uveoparotid D86.89
  valley B38.0
  Venezuelan equine A92.2
  vesicular stomatitis A93.8
  viral hemorrhagic —*see* Fever, hemorrhagic, by
    type of virus
  Volhynian A79.0
  Wesselsbron (viral) A92.8
  West
    African B50.8
    Nile (viral) A92.30
      with
        complications NEC A92.39
        cranial nerve disorders A92.32
        encephalitis A92.31
        encephalomyelitis A92.31
        neurologic manifestation NEC
          A92.32
        optic neuritis A92.32
        polyradiculitis A92.32
  Whitmore's —*see* Melioidosis
  Wolhynian A79.0
  worm B83.9
  yellow A95.9
    jungle A95.0
    sylvatic A95.0
    urban A95.1
  Zika virus A92.5
▶FFA (frontal fibrosing alopecia) L66.12
Fibrillation
  atrial or auricular (established) I48.91
    chronic I48.20
      persistent I48.19
    paroxysmal I48.0
    permanent I48.21
    persistent (chronic) (NOS) (other) I48.19
      longstanding I48.11
  cardiac I49.8
  heart I49.8
  muscular M62.89
  ventricular I49.01
Fibrin
  ball or bodies, pleural (sac) J94.1
  chamber, anterior (eye) (gelatinous exudate) —
    see Iridocyclitis, acute
Fibrinogenolysis —*see* Fibrinolysis
Fibrinogenopenia D68.8
  acquired D65
  congenital D68.2
Fibrinolysis (hemorrhagic) (acquired) D65
  antepartum hemorrhage —*see* Hemorrhage,
    antepartum, with coagulation defect
  following
    abortion —*see* Abortion by type complicated
      by hemorrhage
    ectopic or molar pregnancy O08.1
  intrapartum O67.0
  newborn, transient P60
  postpartum O72.3
Fibrinopenia (hereditary) D68.2
  acquired D68.4
Fibrinopurulent —*see* condition
Fibrinous —*see* condition
Fibroadenoma
  cellular intracanalicular D24-●
  giant D24-●
  intracanalicular
    cellular D24-●
    giant D24-●
    specified site —*see* Neoplasm, benign, by
      site
    unspecified site D24-●
  juvenile D24-●
  pericanalicular
    specified site —*see* Neoplasm, benign, by site
    unspecified site D24-●
  phyllodes D24-●
  prostate D29.1
  specified site NEC —*see* Neoplasm, benign, by
    site
  unspecified site D24-●
Fibroadenosis, breast (chronic) (cystic) (diffuse)
  (periodic) (segmental) N60.2-●
Fibroangioma —*see also* Neoplasm, benign, by site
  juvenile
    specified site —*see* Neoplasm, benign, by site
    unspecified site D10.6
Fibrochondrosarcoma —*see* Neoplasm, cartilage,
  malignant

Fibrocystic
  disease —*see also* Fibrosis, cystic
    breast —*see* Mastopathy, cystic
    jaw M27.49
    kidney (congenital) Q61.8
    liver Q44.6
    pancreas E84.9
  kidney (congenital) Q61.8
Fibrodysplasia ossificans progressiva —*see*
  Myositis, ossificans, progressiva
Fibroelastosis (cordis) (endocardial)
  (endomyocardial) I42.4
Fibroid (tumor) —*see also* Neoplasm, connective
  tissue, benign
  disease, lung (chronic) —*see* Fibrosis, lung
  heart (disease) —*see* Myocarditis
  in pregnancy or childbirth O34.1-●
    causing obstructed labor O65.5
  induration, lung (chronic) —*see* Fibrosis, lung
  lung —*see* Fibrosis, lung
  pneumonia (chronic) —*see* Fibrosis, lung
  uterus —*see also* Leiomyoma, uterus D25.9
Fibrolipoma —*see* Lipoma
Fibroliposarcoma —*see* Neoplasm, connective
  tissue, malignant
Fibroma —*see also* Neoplasm, connective tissue,
  benign
  ameloblastic —*see* Cyst, calcifying odontogenic
  bone (nonossifying) —*see* Disorder, bone,
    specified type NEC
    ossifying —*see* Neoplasm, bone, benign
  cementifying —*see* Neoplasm, bone, benign
  chondromyxoid —*see* Neoplasm, bone,
    benign
  desmoplastic —*see* Neoplasm, connective tissue,
    uncertain behavior
  durum —*see* Neoplasm, connective tissue,
    benign
  fascial —*see* Neoplasm, connective tissue, benign
  invasive —*see* Neoplasm, connective tissue,
    uncertain behavior
  molle —*see* Lipoma
  myxoid —*see* Neoplasm, connective tissue,
    benign
  nasopharynx, nasopharyngeal (juvenile) D10.6
  nonosteogenic (nonossifying) —*see* Dysplasia,
    fibrous
  odontogenic (central) —*see* Cyst, calcifying
    odontogenic
  ossifying —*see* Neoplasm, bone, benign
  periosteal —*see* Neoplasm, bone, benign
  soft —*see* Lipoma
Fibromatosis M72.9
  abdominal —*see* Neoplasm, connective tissue,
    uncertain behavior
  aggressive —*see* Neoplasm, connective tissue,
    uncertain behavior
  congenital generalized —*see* Neoplasm,
    connective tissue, uncertain behavior
  Dupuytren's M72.0
  gingival K06.1
  palmar (fascial) M72.0
  plantar (fascial) M72.2
  pseudosarcomatous (proliferative)
    (subcutaneous) M72.4
  retroperitoneal D48.3
  specified NEC M72.8
Fibromyalgia M79.7
Fibromyoma —*see also* Neoplasm, connective
  tissue, benign
  uterus (corpus) —*see also* Leiomyoma, uterus
    in pregnancy or childbirth —*see* Fibroid, in
      pregnancy or childbirth
    causing obstructed labor O65.5
Fibromyositis M79.7
Fibromyxolipoma D17.9
Fibromyxoma —*see* Neoplasm, connective tissue,
  benign
Fibromyxosarcoma —*see* Neoplasm, connective
  tissue, malignant
Fibro-odontoma, ameloblastic —*see* Cyst,
  calcifying odontogenic
Fibro-osteoma —*see* Neoplasm, bone, benign
Fibroplasia, retrolental H35.17
Fibropurulent —*see* condition
Fibrosarcoma —*see also* Neoplasm, connective
  tissue, malignant
  ameloblastic C41.1
    upper jaw (bone) C41.0
  congenital —*see* Neoplasm, connective tissue,
    malignant

Fibrosarcoma *(Continued)*
fascial —*see* Neoplasm, connective tissue,
    malignant
infantile —*see* Neoplasm, connective tissue,
    malignant
odontogenic C41.1
    upper jaw (bone) C41.0
periosteal —*see* Neoplasm, bone, malignant
Fibrosclerosis
breast N60.3-●
multifocal M35.5
penis (corpora cavernosa) N48.6
Fibrosis, fibrotic
adrenal (gland) E27.8
amnion O41.8X-●
anal papillae K62.89
arteriocapillary —*see* Arteriosclerosis
bladder N32.89
    interstitial —*see* Cystitis, chronic,
        interstitial
    localized submucosal —*see* Cystitis, chronic,
        interstitial
    panmural —*see* Cystitis, chronic, interstitial
breast —*see* Fibrosclerosis, breast
capillary —*see also* Arteriosclerosis I70.90
    lung (chronic) —*see* Fibrosis, lung
cardiac —*see* Myocarditis
cervix N88.8
chorion O41.8X-●
corpus cavernosum (sclerosing) N48.6
cystic (of pancreas) E84.9
    with
        distal intestinal obstruction syndrome
            E84.19
        fecal impaction E84.19
        intestinal manifestations NEC E84.19
        pulmonary manifestations E84.0
        specified manifestations NEC E84.8
due to device, implant or graft —*see also*
        Complications, by site and type, specified
        NEC T85.828
    arterial graft NEC T82.828
    breast (implant) T85.828
    catheter NEC T85.828
        dialysis (renal) T82.828
            intraperitoneal T85.828
        infusion NEC T82.828
            spinal (epidural) (subdural)
                T85.820
        urinary (indwelling) T83.82
    electronic (electrode) (pulse generator)
            (stimulator)
        bone T84.82
        cardiac T82.827
        nervous system (brain) (peripheral nerve)
            (spinal) T85.820
        urinary T83.82
    fixation, internal (orthopedic) NEC
            T84.82
    gastrointestinal (bile duct) (esophagus)
            T85.828
    genital NEC T83.82
    heart NEC T82.827
    joint prosthesis T84.82
    ocular (corneal graft) (orbital implant) NEC
            T85.828
    orthopedic NEC T84.82
    specified NEC T85.828
    urinary NEC T83.82
    vascular NEC T82.828
    ventricular intracranial shunt T85.820
ejaculatory duct N50.89
endocardium —*see* Endocarditis
endomyocardial (tropical) I42.3
epididymis N50.89
eye muscle —*see* Strabismus, mechanical
heart —*see* Myocarditis
hepatic —*see* Fibrosis, liver
hepatolienal (portal hypertension) K76.6
hepatosplenic (portal hypertension) K76.6
infrapatellar fat pad M79.4
intrascrotal N50.89
kidney N26.9
liver K74.00
    with sclerosis K74.2
    advanced K74.02
    alcoholic K70.2
    early K74.01
    stage
        F1 or F2 K74.01
        F3 K74.02

Fibrosis, fibrotic *(Continued)*
lung (atrophic) (chronic) (confluent) (massive)
        (perialveolar) (peribronchial) J84.10
    with
        anthracosilicosis J60
        anthracosis J60
        asbestosis J61
        bagassosis J67.1
        bauxite J63.1
        berylliosis J63.2
        byssinosis J66.0
        calcicosis J62.8
        chalicosis J62.8
        dust reticulation J64
        farmer's lung J67.0
        ganister disease J62.8
        graphite J63.3
        pneumoconiosis NOS J64
        siderosis J63.4
        silicosis J62.8
    capillary J84.10
    congenital P27.8
    diffuse (idiopathic) J84.10
        chemicals, gases, fumes or vapors
            (inhalation) (*see also* Disease,
            respiratory, chronic, due to chemicals,
            gases, fumes or vapors) J84.10
        interstitial J84.10
            acute J84.114
        talc J62.0
    following radiation J70.1
    idiopathic J84.112
    postinflammatory J84.10
    silicotic J62.8
    tuberculous —*see* Tuberculosis,
        pulmonary
lymphatic gland I89.8
median bar —*see* Hyperplasia, prostate
mediastinum (idiopathic) J98.59
meninges G96.198
myocardium, myocardial —*see* Myocarditis
ovary N83.8
oviduct N83.8
pancreas K86.89
penis NEC N48.6
pericardium I31.0
perineum, in pregnancy or childbirth O34.7-●
    causing obstructed labor O65.5
pleura J94.1
popliteal fat pad M79.4
prostate (chronic) —*see* Hyperplasia, prostate
pulmonary —*see also* Fibrosis, lung J84.10
    congenital P27.8
    idiopathic J84.112
rectal sphincter K62.89
retroperitoneal K68.3
    with infection N13.6
    idiopathic (with ureteral obstruction) N13.5
sclerosing mesenteric (idiopathic) K65.4
scrotum N50.89
seminal vesicle N50.89
senile R54
skin L90.5
spermatic cord N50.89
spleen D73.89
    in schistosomiasis (bilharziasis) B65.9 *[D77]*
subepidermal nodular —*see* Neoplasm, skin,
    benign
submucous (oral) (tongue) K13.5
testis N44.8
    chronic, due to syphilis A52.76
thymus (gland) E32.8
tongue, submucous K13.5
tunica vaginalis N50.89
uterus (non-neoplastic) N85.8
vagina N89.8
valve, heart —*see* Endocarditis
vas deferens N50.89
vein I87.8
Fibrositis (periarticular) M79.7
nodular, chronic (Jaccoud's) (rheumatoid) —*see*
        Arthropathy, postrheumatic, chronic
Fibrothorax J94.1
Fibrotic —*see* Fibrosis
Fibrous —*see* condition
Fibroxanthoma —*see also* Neoplasm, connective
        tissue, benign
atypical —*see* Neoplasm, connective tissue,
    uncertain behavior
malignant —*see* Neoplasm, connective tissue,
    malignant

Fibroxanthosarcoma —*see* Neoplasm, connective
        tissue, malignant
Fiedler's
disease (icterohemorrhagic leptospirosis) A27.0
myocarditis (acute) I40.1
Fifth disease B08.3
venereal A55
Filaria, filarial, filariasis —*see* Infestation, filarial
Filatov's disease —*see* Mononucleosis, infectious
File-cutter's disease —*see* Poisoning, lead
Filling defect
biliary tract R93.2
bladder R93.41
duodenum R93.3
gallbladder R93.2
gastrointestinal tract R93.3
intestine R93.3
kidney R93.42-●
stomach R93.3
ureter R93.41
urinary organs, specified NEC R93.49
Fimbrial cyst Q50.4
Financial problem affecting care NOS Z59.9
bankruptcy Z59.89
foreclosure on loan Z59.89
home loan Z59.81-●
strain Z59.86
**Findings, abnormal, inconclusive, without
        diagnosis** —*see also* Abnormal
17-ketosteroids, elevated R82.5
acetonuria R82.4
alcohol in blood R78.0
anisocytosis R71.8
antenatal screening of mother O28.9
    biochemical O28.1
    chromosomal O28.5
    cytological O28.2
    genetic O28.5
    hematological O28.0
    radiological O28.4
    specified NEC O28.8
    ultrasonic O28.3
antibody titer, elevated R76.0
anticardiolipin antibody R76.0
antiphosphatidylglycerol antibody R76.0
antiphosphatidylinositol antibody R76.0
antiphosphatidylserine antibody R76.0
antiphospholipid antibody R76.0
bacteriuria R82.71
bicarbonate E87.8
bile in urine R82.2
blood sugar R73.09
    high R73.9
    low (transient) E16.2
body fluid or substance, specified NEC R88.8
casts, urine R82.998
catecholamines R82.5
cells, urine R82.998
chloride E87.8
cholesterol E78.9
    high E78.00
        with high triglycerides E78.2
chyluria R82.0
cloudy
    dialysis effluent R88.0
    urine R82.90
creatinine clearance R94.4
crystals, urine R82.998
culture
    blood R78.81
    positive —*see* Positive, culture
echocardiogram R93.1
electrolyte level, urinary R82.998
function study NEC R94.8
    bladder R94.8
    endocrine NEC R94.7
        thyroid R94.6
    kidney R94.4
    liver R94.5
    pancreas R94.8
    placenta R94.8
    pulmonary R94.2
    spleen R94.8
gallbladder, nonvisualization R93.2
glucose (tolerance test) (non-fasting) R73.09
glycosuria R81
heart
    shadow R93.1
    sounds R01.2
hematuria R82.3
hematocrit drop (precipitous) R71.0

Findings, abnormal, inconclusive, without
     diagnosis —(Continued)
  hemoglobinuria R82.3
  human papillomavirus (HPV) DNA test
       positive
     cervix
       high risk R87.810
       low risk R87.820
     vagina
       high risk R87.811
       low risk R87.821
  in blood (of substance not normally found in
       blood) R78.9
     addictive drug NEC R78.4
     alcohol (excessive level) R78.0
     cocaine R78.2
     hallucinogen R78.3
     heavy metals (abnormal level)
          R78.79
     lead R78.71
     lithium (abnormal level) R78.89
     opiate drug R78.1
     psychotropic drug R78.5
     specified substance NEC R78.89
     steroid agent R78.6
  indoleacetic acid, elevated R82.5
  ketonuria R82.4
  lactic acid dehydrogenase (LDH) R74.02
  liver function test (see also Elevated, liver
       function, test) R79.89
  mammogram NEC R92.8
     calcification (calculus) R92.1
     inconclusive result R92.2
     microcalcification R92.0
  mediastinal shift R93.89
  melanin, urine R82.998
  myoglobinuria R82.1
  neonatal screening —see Abnormal, neonatal
       screening
  newborn screens, state mandated —see
       Abnormal, neonatal screening
  nonvisualization of gallbladder R93.2
  odor of urine NOS R82.90
  Papanicolaou cervix R87.619
     non-atypical endometrial cells R87.618
  pneumoencephalogram R93.0
  poikilocytosis R71.8
  potassium (deficiency) E87.6
     excess E87.5
  PPD R76.11
  radiologic (X-ray) R93.89
     abdomen R93.5
     biliary tract R93.2
     breast R92.8
     gastrointestinal tract R93.3
     genitourinary organs R93.89
     head R93.0
     inconclusive due to excess body fat of patient
          R93.9
     intrathoracic organs NEC R93.1
     musculoskeletal
       limbs R93.6
       other than limb R93.7
     placenta R93.89
     retroperitoneum R93.5
     skin R93.89
     skull R93.0
     subcutaneous tissue R93.89
     testis R93.81-●
  red blood cell (count) (morphology) (sickling)
       (volume) R71.8
  scan NEC R94.8
     bladder R94.8
     bone R94.8
     kidney R94.4
     liver R93.2
     lung R94.2
     pancreas R94.8
     placental R94.8
     spleen R94.8
     thyroid R94.6
  sedimentation rate, elevated R70.0
  SGOT R74.01
  SGPT R74.01
  sodium (deficiency) E87.1
     excess E87.0
  specified body fluid NEC R88.8
  stress test R94.39
  thyroid (function) (metabolic rate) (scan)
       (uptake) R94.6
  transaminase (level) R74.01

Findings, abnormal, inconclusive, without
     diagnosis —(Continued)
  triglycerides E78.9
     high E78.1
       with high cholesterol E78.2
  tuberculin skin test (without active tuberculosis)
       R76.11
  urine R82.90
     acetone R82.4
     bacteria R82.71
     bile R82.2
     casts or cells R82.998
     chyle R82.0
     culture positive R82.79
     glucose R81
     hemoglobin R82.3
     ketone R82.4
     sugar R81
  vanillylmandelic acid (VMA), elevated R82.5
  vectorcardiogram (VCG) R94.39
  ventriculogram R93.0
  white blood cell (count) (differential)
       (morphology) D72.9
  xerography R92.8
Finger —see condition
Fire, Saint Anthony's —see Erysipelas
Fire-setting
  pathological (compulsive) F63.1
Fish hook stomach K31.89
Fishmeal-worker's lung J67.8
Fissure, fissured
  anus, anal K60.2
     acute K60.0
     chronic K60.1
     congenital Q43.8
  ear, lobule, congenital Q17.8
  epiglottis (congenital) Q31.8
  larynx J38.7
     congenital Q31.8
  lip K13.0
     congenital —see Cleft, lip
  nipple N64.0
     associated with
       lactation O92.13
       pregnancy O92.11-●
       puerperium O92.12
  nose Q30.2
  palate (congenital) —see Cleft, palate
  skin R23.4
  spine (congenital) —see also Spina bifida
     with hydrocephalus —see Spina bifida, by site,
          with hydrocephalus
  tongue (acquired) K14.5
     congenital Q38.3
Fistula (cutaneous) L98.8
  abdomen (wall) K63.2
     bladder N32.2
     intestine NEC K63.2
     ureter N28.89
     uterus N82.5
  abdominorectal K63.2
  abdominosigmoidal K63.2
  abdominothoracic J86.0
  abdominouterine N82.5
     congenital Q51.7
  abdominovesical N32.2
  accessory sinuses —see Sinusitis
  actinomycotic —see Actinomycosis
  alveolar antrum —see Sinusitis, maxillary
  alveolar process K04.6
  ▶anorectal (infectional) K60.50
     ►complex K60.529
       ►chronic K60.522
       ►initial K60.521
       ►new K60.521
       ►occurring following complete healing
            K60.523
       ►persistent K60.522
       ►recurrent K60.523
     ►extrasphincteric K60.52-●
     ►high intersphincteric K60.52-●
     ►low intersphincteric K60.51-●
     ►simple K60.519
       ►chronic K60.512
       ►initial K60.511
       ►new K60.511
       ►occurring following complete healing
            K60.513
       ►persistent K60.512
       ►recurrent K60.513
     ►superficial K60.51-●

Fistula (Continued)
  anorectal —(Continued)
     ►suprasphincteric K60.52-●
     ►transsphincteric K60.52-●
  antrobuccal —see Sinusitis, maxillary
  antrum —see Sinusitis, maxillary
  ▶anus, anal (recurrent) (infectional) K60.30
     ►complex K60.329
       ►chronic K60.322
       ►initial K60.321
       ►new K60.321
       ►occurring following complete healing
            K60.323
       ►persistent K60.322
       ►recurrent K60.323
     ►extrasphincteric K60.32-●
     ►high intersphincteric K60.32-●
     ►low intersphincteric K60.31-●
     ►simple K60.319
       ►chronic K60.312
       ►initial K60.311
       ►new K60.311
       ►occurring following complete healing
            K60.313
       ►persistent K60.312
       ►recurrent K60.313
     ►superficial K60.31-●
     ►suprasphincteric K60.32-●
     ►transsphincteric K60.32-●
     congenital Q43.6
       with absence, atresia and stenosis
            Q42.2
     tuberculous A18.32
  aorta-duodenal I77.2
  appendix, appendicular K38.3
  arteriovenous (acquired) (nonruptured) I77.0
     brain I67.1
       congenital Q28.2
          ruptured —see Fistula, arteriovenous,
               brain, ruptured
       ruptured I60.8
          intracerebral I61.8
          intraparenchymal I61.8
          intraventricular I61.5
          subarachnoid I60.8
     cerebral —see Fistula, arteriovenous, brain
     congenital (peripheral) —see also
          Malformation, arteriovenous
       brain Q28.2
          ruptured —see Fistula, arteriovenous,
               brain, ruptured
       coronary Q24.5
       pulmonary Q25.72
     coronary I25.41
       congenital Q24.5
     pulmonary I28.0
       congenital Q25.72
     surgically created (for dialysis) Z99.2
       complication —see Complication,
            arteriovenous, fistula, surgically
            created
     traumatic —see Injury, blood vessel
  artery I77.2
  aural (mastoid) —see Mastoiditis, chronic
  auricle —see also Disorder, pinna, specified type
       NEC
     congenital Q18.1
  Bartholin's gland N82.8
  bile duct (common) (hepatic) K83.3
     with calculus, stones —see also Calculus, bile
          duct K83.3
  biliary (tract) —see Fistula, bile duct
  bladder (sphincter) NEC —see also Fistula,
       vesico- N32.2
     into seminal vesicle N32.2
  bone —see also Disorder, bone, specified type
       NEC
     with osteomyelitis, chronic —see
          Osteomyelitis, chronic, with draining
          sinus
  brain G93.89
     arteriovenous (acquired) (see Fistula,
          arteriovenous, brain) I67.1
       congenital Q28.2
  branchial (cleft) Q18.0
  branchiogenous Q18.0
  breast N61.0
     puerperal, postpartum or gestational, due
          to mastitis (purulent) —see Mastitis,
          obstetric, purulent
  bronchial J86.0

▶ New   ⇨ Revised   ~~deleted~~ Deleted   ● Use Additional Character(s)

Fistula *(Continued)*
  bronchocutaneous, bronchomediastinal,
    bronchopleural, bronchopleuromediastinal
    (infective) J86.0
    tuberculous NEC A15.5
  bronchoesophageal J86.0
    congenital Q39.2
      with atresia of esophagus Q39.1
  bronchovisceral J86.0
  buccal cavity (infective) K12.2
  cecosigmoidal K63.2
  cecum K63.2
  cerebrospinal (fluid) G96.08
  cervical, lateral Q18.1
  cervicoaural Q18.1
  cervicosigmoidal N82.4
  cervicovesical N82.1
  cervix N82.8
  chest (wall) J86.0
  cholecystenteric —*see* Fistula, gallbladder
  cholecystocolic —*see* Fistula, gallbladder
  cholecystocolonic —*see* Fistula, gallbladder
  cholecystoduodenal —*see* Fistula, gallbladder
  cholecystogastric —*see* Fistula, gallbladder
  cholecystointestinal —*see* Fistula, gallbladder
  choledochoduodenal —*see* Fistula, bile duct
  cholocolic K82.3
  coccyx —*see* Sinus, pilonidal
  colon K63.2
  colostomy K94.09
  colovesical N32.1
  common duct —*see* Fistula, bile duct
  congenital, site not listed —*see* Anomaly, by site
  coronary, arteriovenous I25.41
    congenital Q24.5
  costal region J86.0
  cul-de-sac, Douglas' N82.8
  cystic duct —*see also* Fistula, gallbladder
    congenital Q44.5
  dental K04.6
  diaphragm J86.0
  duodenum K31.6
  ear (external) (canal) —*see* Disorder, ear, external,
    specified type NEC
  enterocolic K63.2
  enterocutaneous K63.2
  enterouterine N82.4
    congenital Q51.7
  enterovaginal N82.4
    congenital Q52.2
    large intestine N82.3
    small intestine N82.2
  enterovesical N32.1
  epididymis N50.89
    tuberculous A18.15
  esophagobronchial J86.0
    congenital Q39.2
      with atresia of esophagus Q39.1
  esophagocutaneous K22.89
  esophagopleural-cutaneous J86.0
  esophagotracheal J86.0
    congenital Q39.2
      with atresia of esophagus Q39.1
  esophagus K22.89
    congenital Q39.2
      with atresia of esophagus Q39.1
  ethmoid —*see* Sinusitis, ethmoidal
  eyeball (cornea) (sclera) —*see* Disorder, globe,
    hypotony
  eyelid H01.8
  fallopian tube, external N82.5
  fecal K63.2
    congenital Q43.6
  from periapical abscess K04.6
  frontal sinus —*see* Sinusitis, frontal
  gallbladder K82.3
    with calculus, cholelithiasis, stones —*see*
      Calculus, gallbladder
  gastric K31.6
  gastrocolic K31.6
    congenital Q40.2
    tuberculous A18.32
  gastroenterocolic K31.6
  gastroesophageal K31.6
  gastrojejunal K31.6
  gastrojejunocolic K31.6
  genital tract (female) N82.9
    specified NEC N82.8
    to intestine NEC N82.4
    to skin N82.5
  hepatic artery-portal vein, congenital Q26.6

Fistula *(Continued)*
  hepatopleural J86.0
  hepatopulmonary J86.0
  ileorectal or ileosigmoidal K63.2
  ileovaginal N82.2
  ileovesical N32.1
  ileum K63.2
  in ano K60.30
    tuberculous A18.32
  inner ear (labyrinth) —*see* subcategory
    H83.1
  intestine NEC K63.2
  intestinocolic (abdominal) K63.2
  intestinoureteral N28.89
  intestinouterine N82.4
  intestinovaginal N82.4
    large intestine N82.3
    small intestine N82.2
  intestinovesical N32.1
  ischiorectal (fossa) K61.39
  jejunum K63.2
  joint M25.10
    ankle M25.17-●
    elbow M25.12-●
    foot joint M25.17-●
    hand joint M25.14-●
    hip M25.15-●
    knee M25.16-●
    shoulder M25.11-●
    specified joint NEC M25.18
    tuberculous —*see* Tuberculosis, joint
    vertebrae M25.18
    wrist M25.13-●
  kidney N28.89
  labium (majus) (minus) N82.8
  labyrinth —*see* subcategory H83.1
  lacrimal (gland) (sac) H04.61-●
  lacrimonasal duct —*see* Fistula, lacrimal
  laryngotracheal, congenital Q34.8
  larynx J38.7
  lip K13.0
    congenital Q38.0
  lumbar, tuberculous A18.01
  lung J86.0
  lymphatic I89.8
  mammary (gland) N61.0
  mastoid (process) (region) —*see* Mastoiditis,
    chronic
  maxillary J32.0
  medial, face and neck Q18.8
  mediastinal J86.0
  mediastinobronchial J86.0
  mediastinocutaneous J86.0
  middle ear —*see* subcategory H74.8
  mouth K12.2
  nasal J34.89
    sinus —*see* Sinusitis
  nasopharynx J39.2
  nipple N64.0
  nose J34.89
  oral (cutaneous) K12.2
    maxillary J32.0
    nasal (with cleft palate) —*see* Cleft,
      palate
  orbit, orbital —*see* Disorder, orbit, specified type
    NEC
  oroantral J32.0
  oviduct, external N82.5
  palate (hard) M27.8
  pancreatic K86.89
  pancreaticoduodenal K86.89
  parotid (gland) K11.4
    region K12.2
  penis N48.89
  perianal K60.30
  pericardium (pleura) (sac) —*see* Pericarditis
  pericecal K63.2
  perineorectal K60.40
  perineosigmoidal K63.2
  perineum, perineal (with urethral involvement)
    NEC N36.0
    tuberculous A18.13
    ureter N28.89
  perirectal K60.40
    tuberculous A18.32
  peritoneum K65.9
  pharyngoesophageal J39.2
  pharynx J39.2
    branchial cleft (congenital) Q18.0
  pilonidal (infected) (rectum) —*see* Sinus,
    pilonidal

Fistula *(Continued)*
  pleura, pleural, pleurocutaneous,
    pleuroperitoneal J86.0
    tuberculous NEC A15.6
  pleuropericardial I31.8
  portal vein-hepatic artery, congenital Q26.6
  postauricular H70.81-●
  postoperative, persistent T81.83
    specified site —*see* Fistula, by site
  preauricular (congenital) Q18.1
  prostate N42.89
  pulmonary J86.0
    arteriovenous I28.0
      congenital Q25.72
    tuberculous —*see* Tuberculosis, pulmonary
  pulmonoperitoneal J86.0
  ▶rectal (infectional) K60.40
    ▶complex K60.429
      ▶chronic K60.422
      ▶initial K60.421
      ▶new K60.421
      ▶occurring following complete healing
        K60.423
      ▶persistent K60.422
      ▶recurrent K60.423
    ▶extrasphincteric K60.42-●
    ▶high intersphincteric K60.42-●
    ▶low intersphincteric K60.41-●
    ▶simple K60.419
      ▶chronic K60.412
      ▶initial K60.411
      ▶new K60.411
      ▶occurring following complete healing
        K60.413
      ▶persistent K60.412
      ▶recurrent K60.413
    ▶superficial K60.41-●
    ▶suprasphincteric K60.42-●
    ▶transsphincteric K60.42-●
  rectolabial N82.4
  rectosigmoid (intercommunicating) K63.2
  rectoureteral N28.89
  rectourethral N36.0
    congenital Q64.73
  rectouterine N82.4
    congenital Q51.7
  rectovaginal N82.3
    congenital Q52.2
    tuberculous A18.18
  rectovesical N32.1
    congenital Q64.79
  rectovesicovaginal N82.3
  rectovulval N82.4
    congenital Q52.79
  rectum (to skin) K60.40
    congenital Q43.6
      with absence, atresia and stenosis
        Q42.0
    tuberculous A18.32
  renal N28.89
  retroauricular —*see* Fistula, postauricular
  salivary duct or gland (any) K11.4
    congenital Q38.4
  scrotum (urinary) N50.89
    tuberculous A18.15
  semicircular canals —*see* subcategory H83.1
  sigmoid K63.2
    to bladder N32.1
  sinus —*see* Sinusitis
  skin L98.8
    to genital tract (female) N82.5
  splenocolic D73.89
  stercoral K63.2
  stomach K31.6
  sublingual gland K11.4
  submandibular gland K11.4
  submaxillary (gland) K11.4
    region K12.2
  thoracic J86.0
    duct I89.8
  thoracoabdominal J86.0
  thoracogastric J86.0
  thoracointestinal J86.0
  thorax J86.0
  thyroglossal duct Q89.2
  thyroid E07.89
  trachea, congenital (external) (internal) Q32.1
  tracheoesophageal J86.0
    congenital Q39.2
      with atresia of esophagus Q39.1
    following tracheostomy J95.04

Fistula (Continued)
  traumatic arteriovenous —see Injury, blood
      vessel, by site
  tuberculous - code by site under Tuberculosis
  typhoid A01.09
  umbilicourinary Q64.8
  urachus, congenital Q64.4
  ureter (persistent) N28.89
  ureteroabdominal N28.89
  ureterorectal N28.89
  ureterosigmoido-abdominal N28.89
  ureterovaginal N82.1
  ureterovesical N32.2
  urethra N36.0
      congenital Q64.79
      tuberculous A18.13
  urethroperineal N36.0
  urethroperineovesical N32.2
  urethrorectal N36.0
      congenital Q64.73
  urethroscrotal N50.89
  urethrovaginal N82.1
  urethrovesical N32.2
  urinary (tract) (persistent) (recurrent) N36.0
  uteroabdominal N82.5
      congenital Q51.7
  uteroenteric, uterointestinal N82.4
      congenital Q51.7
  uterorectal N82.4
      congenital Q51.7
  uteroureteric N82.1
  uterourethral Q51.7
  uterovaginal N82.8
  uterovesical N82.1
      congenital Q51.7
  uterus N82.8
  vagina (postpartal) (wall) N82.8
  vaginocutaneous (postpartal) N82.5
  vaginointestinal NEC N82.4
      large intestine N82.3
      small intestine N82.2
  vaginoperineal N82.5
  vasocutaneous, congenital Q55.7
  vesical NEC N32.2
  vesicoabdominal N32.2
  vesicocervicovaginal N82.1
  vesicocolic N32.1
  vesicocutaneous N32.2
  vesicoenteric N32.1
  vesicointestinal N32.1
  vesicometrorectal N82.4
  vesicoperineal N32.2
  vesicorectal N32.1
      congenital Q64.79
  vesicosigmoidal N32.1
  vesicosigmoidovaginal N82.3
  vesicoureteral N32.2
  vesicoureterovaginal N82.1
  vesicourethral N32.2
  vesicourethrorectal N32.1
  vesicouterine N82.1
      congenital Q51.7
  vesicovaginal N82.0
  vulvorectal N82.4
      congenital Q52.79
Fit R56.9
  epileptic —see Epilepsy
  fainting R55
  hysterical F44.5
  newborn P90
Fitting (and adjustment) (of)
  artificial
      arm —see Admission, adjustment, artificial, arm
      breast Z44.3
      eye Z44.2
      leg —see Admission, adjustment, artificial, leg
  automatic implantable cardiac defibrillator (with
      synchronous cardiac pacemaker) Z45.02
  brain neuropacemaker Z46.2
      implanted Z45.42
  cardiac defibrillator —see Fitting (and
      adjustment) (of), automatic implantable
      cardiac defibrillator
  catheter, non-vascular Z46.82
  colostomy belt Z46.89
  contact lenses Z46.0
  CRT-D (resynchronization therapy defibrillator)
      Z45.02
  CRT-P (cardiac resynchronization therapy
      pacemaker) Z45.018
      pulse generator Z45.010

Fitting (Continued)
  cystostomy device Z46.6
  defibrillator, cardiac —see Fitting (and
      adjustment) (of), automatic implantable
      cardiac defibrillator
  dentures Z46.3
  device NOS Z46.9
      abdominal Z46.89
      gastrointestinal NEC Z46.59
      implanted NEC Z45.89
      nervous system Z46.2
          implanted —see Admission, adjustment,
              device, implanted, nervous system
      orthodontic Z46.4
      orthoptic Z46.0
      orthotic Z46.89
      prosthetic (external) Z44.9
          breast Z44.3
          dental Z46.3
          eye Z44.2
          specified NEC Z44.8
      specified NEC Z46.89
      substitution
          auditory Z46.2
              implanted —see Admission, adjustment,
                  device, implanted, hearing device
          nervous system Z46.2
              implanted —see Admission, adjustment,
                  device, implanted, nervous system
          visual Z46.2
              implanted Z45.31
      urinary Z46.6
  gastric lap band Z46.51
  gastrointestinal appliance NEC Z46.59
  glasses (reading) Z46.0
  hearing aid Z46.1
  ileostomy device Z46.89
  insulin pump Z46.81
  intestinal appliance NEC Z46.89
  myringotomy device (stent) (tube) Z45.82
  neuropacemaker Z46.2
      implanted Z45.42
  non-vascular catheter Z46.82
  orthodontic device Z46.4
  orthopedic device (brace) (cast) (corset) (shoes)
      Z46.89
  pacemaker (cardiac) (cardiac resynchronization
      therapy (CRT-P)) Z45.018
      nervous system (brain) (peripheral nerve)
          (spinal cord) Z46.2
          implanted Z45.42
      pulse generator Z45.010
  portacath (port-a-cath) Z45.2
  prosthesis (external) Z44.9
      arm —see Admission, adjustment, artificial,
          arm
      breast Z44.3
      dental Z46.3
      eye Z44.2
      leg —see Admission, adjustment, artificial, leg
      specified NEC Z44.8
  spectacles Z46.0
  wheelchair Z46.89
Fitzhugh-Curtis syndrome
  due to
      Chlamydia trachomatis A74.81
      ~~Neisseria gonorrhea (gonococcal peritonitis)
          A54.85~~
      ▶Neisseria gonorrhea (gonococcal peritonitis)
          A54.85
Fitz's syndrome (acute hemorrhagic
      pancreatitis) —see also Pancreatitis,
      acute K85.80
Fixation
  joint —see Ankylosis
  larynx J38.7
  stapes —see Ankylosis, ear ossicles
      deafness —see Deafness, conductive
  uterus (acquired) —see Malposition, uterus
  vocal cord J38.3
Flabby ridge K06.8
Flaccid —see also condition
  palate, congenital Q38.5
Flail
  chest S22.5-●
      associated with chest compression and
          cardiopulmonary resuscitation M96.A4
      newborn (birth injury) P13.8
  joint (paralytic) M25.20
      ankle M25.27-●
      elbow M25.22-●

Flail (Continued)
  joint (Continued)
      foot joint M25.27-●
      hand joint M25.24-●
      hip M25.25-●
      knee M25.26-●
      shoulder M25.21-●
      specified joint NEC M25.28
      wrist M25.23-●
Flajani's disease —see Hyperthyroidism, with,
      goiter (diffuse)
Flap, liver K71.3
Flashbacks (residual to hallucinogen use) F16.283
Flat
  affect R45.89
  chamber (eye) —see Disorder, globe, hypotony,
      flat anterior chamber
  chest, congenital Q67.8
  foot (acquired) (fixed type) (painful)
      (postural) —see also Deformity, limb, flat
      foot
      congenital (rigid) (spastic (everted)) Q66.5-●
      rachitic sequelae (late effect) E64.3
  organ or site, congenital NEC —see Anomaly,
      by site
  pelvis M95.5
      with disproportion (fetopelvic) O33.0
          causing obstructed labor O65.0
      congenital Q74.2
Flatau-Schilder disease G37.0
Flatback syndrome M40.30
  lumbar region M40.36
  lumbosacral region M40.37
  thoracolumbar region M40.35
Flattening
  head, femur M89.8X5
  hip —see Coxa, plana
  lip (congenital) Q18.8
  nose (congenital) Q67.4
      acquired M95.0
Flatulence R14.3
  psychogenic F45.8
Flatus R14.3
  vaginalis N89.8
Flax-dresser's disease J66.1
Flea bite —see Injury, bite, by site, superficial, insect
Flecks, glaucomatous (subcapsular) —see Cataract,
      complicated
Fleischer (-Kayser) ring (cornea) H18.04-●
Fleshy mole O02.0
Flexibilitas cerea —see Catalepsy
Flexion
  amputation stump (surgical) T87.89
  cervix —see Malposition, uterus
  contracture, joint —see Contraction, joint
  deformity, joint —see also Deformity, limb,
      flexion M21.20
      hip, congenital Q65.89
  uterus —see also Malposition, uterus
      lateral —see Lateroversion, uterus
Flexner-Boyd dysentery A03.2
Flexner's dysentery A03.1
Flexure —see Flexion
Flint murmur (aortic insufficiency) I35.1
Floater, vitreous —see Opacity, vitreous
Floating
  cartilage (joint) —see also Loose, body, joint
      knee —see Derangement, knee, loose body
  gallbladder, congenital Q44.1
  kidney N28.89
      congenital Q63.8
  spleen D73.89
Flooding N92.0
Floor —see condition
Floppy
  baby syndrome (nonspecific) P94.2
  iris syndrome (intraoperative) (IFIS) H21.81
  nonrheumatic mitral valve syndrome I34.1
Flu —see also Influenza
  avian —see also Influenza, due to, identified
      novel influenza A virus J09.X2
  bird —see also Influenza, due to, identified novel
      influenza A virus J09.X2
  intestinal NEC A08.4
  swine (viruses that normally cause infections in
      pigs) —see also Influenza, due to, identified
      novel influenza A virus J09.X2
Fluctuating blood pressure I99.8
Fluid
  abdomen R18.8
  chest J94.8

▶ New   ⇒ Revised   ~~deleted~~ Deleted   ● Use Additional Character(s)

Fluid *(Continued)*
  heart —*see* Failure, heart, congestive
  joint —*see* Effusion, joint
  loss (acute) E86.9
  lung —*see* Edema, lung
  overload E87.70
    specified NEC E87.79
  peritoneal cavity R18.8
  pleural cavity J94.8
  retention R60.9
Flukes NEC —*see also* Infestation, fluke
  blood NEC —*see* Schistosomiasis
  liver B66.3
Fluor (vaginalis) N89.8
  trichomonal or due to Trichomonas (vaginalis) A59.00
Fluorosis
  dental K00.3
  skeletal M85.10
    ankle M85.17-●
    foot M85.17-●
    forearm M85.13-●
    hand M85.14-●
    lower leg M85.16-●
    multiple site M85.19
    neck M85.18
    rib M85.18
    shoulder M85.11-●
    skull M85.18
    specified site NEC M85.18
    thigh M85.15-●
    toe M85.17-●
    upper arm M85.12-●
    vertebra M85.18
Flush syndrome E34.09
Flushing R23.2
  menopausal N95.1
Flutter
  atrial or auricular I48.92
    atypical I48.4
    type I I48.3
    type II I48.4
    typical I48.3
  heart I49.8
    atrial or auricular I48.92
      atypical I48.4
      type I I48.3
      type II I48.4
      typical I48.3
    ventricular I49.02
    ventricular I49.02
FNHTR (febrile nonhemolytic transfusion reaction) R50.84
Fochier's abscess - code by site under Abscess
Focus, Assmann's —*see* Tuberculosis, pulmonary
Fogo selvagem L10.3
Foix-Alajouanine syndrome G95.19
Fold, folds (anomalous) —*see also* Anomaly, by site
  Descemet's membrane —*see* Change, corneal membrane, Descemet's, fold
  epicanthic Q10.3
  heart Q24.8
Folie à deux F24
Follicle
  cervix (nabothian) (ruptured) N88.8
  graafian, ruptured, with hemorrhage N83.0-●
  nabothian N88.8
Follicular —*see* condition
Folliculitis (superficial) L73.9
  abscedens et suffodiens L66.3
  cyst N83.0-●
  decalvans L66.2
  deep —*see* Furuncle, by site
  gonococcal (acute) (chronic) A54.01
  keloid, keloidalis L73.0
  pustular L01.02
  ulerythematosa reticulata L66.4
Folliculome lipidique
  specified site —*see* Neoplasm, benign, by site
  unspecified site
    female D27.9
    male D29.20
Følling's disease E70.0
Follow-up —*see* Examination, follow-up
Fong's syndrome (hereditary osteo-onychodysplasia) Q87.2
Food
  allergy L27.2
  asphyxia (from aspiration or inhalation) —*see* Foreign body, by site
  choked on —*see* Foreign body, by site

Food *(Continued)*
  deprivation T73.0
    specified kind of food NEC E63.8
  insecurity Z59.41
  intoxication —*see* Poisoning, food
  lack of T73.0
  poisoning —*see* Poisoning, food
  rejection NEC —*see* Disorder, eating
  strangulation or suffocation —*see* Foreign body, by site
  toxemia —*see* Poisoning, food
Foot —*see* condition
Foramen ovale (nonclosure) (patent) (persistent) Q21.12
Forbes' glycogen storage disease E74.03
Fordyce-Fox disease L75.2
Fordyce's disease (mouth) Q38.6
Forearm —*see* condition
Foreclosure on loan Z59.89
Foreign body
  with
    laceration —*see* Laceration, by site, with foreign body
    puncture wound —*see* Puncture, by site, with foreign body
  accidentally left following a procedure T81.509
    aspiration T81.506
      resulting in
        adhesions T81.516
        obstruction T81.526
        perforation T81.536
        specified complication NEC T81.596
    cardiac catheterization T81.505
      resulting in
        acute reaction T81.60
          aseptic peritonitis T81.61
          specified NEC T81.69
        adhesions T81.515
        obstruction T81.525
        perforation T81.535
        specified complication NEC T81.595
    causing
      acute reaction T81.60
        aseptic peritonitis T81.61
        specified complication NEC T81.69
      adhesions T81.519
      aseptic peritonitis T81.61
      obstruction T81.529
      perforation T81.539
      specified complication NEC T81.599
    endoscopy T81.504
      resulting in
        adhesions T81.514
        obstruction T81.524
        perforation T81.534
        specified complication NEC T81.594
    immunization T81.503
      resulting in
        adhesions T81.513
        obstruction T81.523
        perforation T81.533
        specified complication NEC T81.593
    infusion T81.501
      resulting in
        adhesions T81.511
        obstruction T81.521
        perforation T81.531
        specified complication NEC T81.591
    injection T81.503
      resulting in
        adhesions T81.513
        obstruction T81.523
        perforation T81.533
        specified complication NEC T81.593
    kidney dialysis T81.502
      resulting in
        adhesions T81.512
        obstruction T81.522
        perforation T81.532
        specified complication NEC T81.592
    packing removal T81.507
      resulting in
        acute reaction T81.60
          aseptic peritonitis T81.61
          specified NEC T81.69
        adhesions T81.517
        obstruction T81.527
        perforation T81.537
        specified complication NEC T81.597

Foreign body *(Continued)*
  accidentally left following a procedure — *(Continued)*
    puncture T81.506
      resulting in
        adhesions T81.516
        obstruction T81.526
        perforation T81.536
        specified complication NEC T81.596
    specified procedure NEC T81.508
      resulting in
        acute reaction T81.60
          aseptic peritonitis T81.61
          specified NEC T81.69
        adhesions T81.518
        obstruction T81.528
        perforation T81.538
        specified complication NEC T81.598
    surgical operation T81.500
      resulting in
        acute reaction T81.60
          aseptic peritonitis T81.61
          specified NEC T81.69
        adhesions T81.510
        obstruction T81.520
        perforation T81.530
        specified complication NEC T81.590
    transfusion T81.501
      resulting in
        adhesions T81.511
        obstruction T81.521
        perforation T81.531
        specified complication NEC T81.591
  alimentary tract T18.9
    anus T18.5
    colon T18.4
    esophagus —*see* Foreign body, esophagus
    mouth T18.0
    multiple sites T18.8
    rectosigmoid (junction) T18.5
    rectum T18.5
    small intestine T18.3
    specified site NEC T18.8
    stomach T18.2
  anterior chamber (eye) S05.5-●
  auditory canal —*see* Foreign body, entering through orifice, ear
  bronchus T17.508
    causing
      asphyxiation T17.500
        food (bone) (seed) T17.520
        gastric contents (vomitus) T17.510
        specified type NEC T17.590
      injury NEC T17.508
        food (bone) (seed) T17.528
        gastric contents (vomitus) T17.518
        specified type NEC T17.598
  canthus —*see* Foreign body, conjunctival sac
  ciliary body (eye) S05.5-●
  conjunctival sac T15.1-●
  cornea T15.0-●
  entering through orifice
    accessory sinus T17.0
    alimentary canal T18.9
      multiple parts T18.8
      specified part NEC T18.8
    alveolar process T18.0
    antrum (Highmore's) T17.0
    anus T18.5
    appendix T18.4
    auditory canal —*see* Foreign body, entering through orifice, ear
    auricle —*see* Foreign body, entering through orifice, ear
    bladder T19.1
    bronchioles —*see* Foreign body, respiratory tract, specified site NEC
    bronchus (main) —*see* Foreign body, bronchus
    buccal cavity T18.0
    canthus (inner) —*see* Foreign body, conjunctival sac
    cecum T18.4
    cervix (canal) (uteri) T19.3
    colon T18.4
    conjunctival sac —*see* Foreign body, conjunctival sac
    cornea —*see* Foreign body, cornea
    digestive organ or tract NOS T18.9
      multiple parts T18.8
      specified part NEC T18.8
    duodenum T18.3

Foreign body *(Continued)*
  entering through orifice *(Continued)*
    ear (external) T16.-●
    esophagus —*see* Foreign body, esophagus
    eye (external) NOS T15.9-●
      conjunctival sac —*see* Foreign body,
        conjunctival sac
      cornea —*see* Foreign body, cornea
      specified part NEC T15.8-●
    eyeball —*see also* Foreign body, entering
      through orifice, eye, specified part
      NEC
      with penetrating wound —*see* Puncture,
        eyeball
    eyelid —*see also* Foreign body, conjunctival sac
      with
        laceration —*see* Laceration, eyelid, with
          foreign body
        puncture —*see* Puncture, eyelid, with
          foreign body
        superficial injury —*see* Foreign body,
          superficial, eyelid
  gastrointestinal tract T18.9
    multiple parts T18.8
    specified part NEC T18.8
  genitourinary tract T19.9
    multiple parts T19.8
    specified part NEC T19.8
  globe —*see* Foreign body, entering through
    orifice, eyeball
  gum T18.0
  Highmore's antrum T17.0
  hypopharynx —*see* Foreign body,
    pharynx
  ileum T18.3
  intestine (small) T18.3
    large T18.4
  lacrimal apparatus (punctum) —*see* Foreign
    body, entering through orifice, eye,
    specified part NEC
  large intestine T18.4
  larynx —*see* Foreign body, larynx
  lung —*see* Foreign body, respiratory tract,
    specified site NEC
  maxillary sinus T17.0
  mouth T18.0
  nasal sinus T17.0
  nasopharynx —*see* Foreign body, pharynx
  nose (passage) T17.1
  nostril T17.1
  oral cavity T18.0
  palate T18.0
  penis T19.4
  pharynx —*see* Foreign body, pharynx
  piriform sinus —*see* Foreign body, pharynx
  rectosigmoid (junction) T18.5
  rectum T18.5
  respiratory tract —*see* Foreign body,
    respiratory tract
  sinus (accessory) (frontal) (maxillary) (nasal)
    T17.0
    piriform —*see* Foreign body, pharynx
  small intestine T18.3
  stomach T18.2
  suffocation by —*see* Foreign body, by site
  tear ducts or glands —*see* Foreign body,
    entering through orifice, eye, specified
    part NEC
  throat —*see* Foreign body, pharynx
  tongue T18.0
  tonsil, tonsillar (fossa) —*see* Foreign body,
    pharynx
  trachea —*see* Foreign body, trachea
  ureter T19.8
  urethra T19.0
  uterus (any part) T19.3
  vagina T19.2
  vulva T19.2
  esophagus T18.108
    causing
      injury NEC T18.108
        food (bone) (seed) T18.128
        gastric contents (vomitus) T18.118
        specified type NEC T18.198
      tracheal compression T18.100
        food (bone) (seed) T18.120
        gastric contents (vomitus) T18.110
        specified type NEC T18.190
  feeling of, in throat R09.89
  fragment —*see* Retained, foreign body fragments
    (type of)

Foreign body *(Continued)*
  genitourinary tract T19.9
    bladder T19.1
    multiple parts T19.8
    penis T19.4
    specified site NEC T19.8
    urethra T19.0
    uterus T19.3
      IUD Z97.5
    vagina T19.2
      contraceptive device Z97.5
    vulva T19.2
  granuloma (old) (soft tissue) —*see also*
    Granuloma, foreign body
    skin L92.3
  in
    laceration —*see* Laceration, by site, with
      foreign body
    puncture wound —*see* Puncture, by site, with
      foreign body
    soft tissue (residual) M79.5
  inadvertently left in operation wound —*see*
    Foreign body, accidentally left during a
    procedure
  ingestion, ingested NOS T18.9
  inhalation or inspiration —*see* Foreign body, by
    site
  internal organ, not entering through a natural
    orifice - code as specific injury with foreign
    body
  intraocular S05.5-●
    old, retained (nonmagnetic) H44.70-●
      anterior chamber H44.71-●
      ciliary body H44.72-●
      iris H44.72-●
      lens H44.73-●
      magnetic H44.60-●
        anterior chamber H44.61-●
        ciliary body H44.62-●
        iris H44.62-●
        lens H44.63-●
        posterior wall H44.64-●
        specified site NEC H44.69-●
        vitreous body H44.65-●
      posterior wall H44.74-●
      specified site NEC H44.79-●
      vitreous body H44.75-●
  iris —*see* Foreign body, intraocular
  lacrimal punctum —*see* Foreign body, entering
    through orifice, eye, specified part
    NEC
  larynx T17.308
    causing
      asphyxiation T17.300
        food (bone) (seed) T17.320
        gastric contents (vomitus) T17.310
        specified type NEC T17.390
      injury NEC T17.308
        food (bone) (seed) T17.328
        gastric contents (vomitus) T17.318
        specified type NEC T17.398
  lens —*see* Foreign body, intraocular
  ocular muscle S05.4-●
    old, retained —*see* Foreign body, orbit, old
  old or residual
    soft tissue (residual) M79.5
  operation wound, left accidentally —*see* Foreign
    body, accidentally left during a procedure
  orbit S05.4-●
    old, retained H05.5-●
  pharynx T17.208
    causing
      asphyxiation T17.200
        food (bone) (seed) T17.220
        gastric contents (vomitus)
          T17.210
        specified type NEC T17.290
      injury NEC T17.208
        food (bone) (seed) T17.228
        gastric contents (vomitus)
          T17.218
        specified type NEC T17.298
  respiratory tract T17.908
    bronchioles —*see* Foreign body, respiratory
      tract, specified site NEC
    bronchus —*see* Foreign body, bronchus
    causing
      asphyxiation T17.900
        food (bone) (seed) T17.920
        gastric contents (vomitus) T17.910
        specified type NEC T17.990

Foreign body *(Continued)*
  respiratory tract *(Continued)*
    causing *(Continued)*
      injury NEC T17.908
        food (bone) (seed) T17.928
        gastric contents (vomitus) T17.918
        specified type NEC T17.998
    larynx —*see* Foreign body, larynx
    lung —*see* Foreign body, respiratory tract,
      specified site NEC
    multiple parts —*see* Foreign body, respiratory
      tract, specified site NEC
    nasal sinus T17.0
    nasopharynx —*see* Foreign body, pharynx
    nose T17.1
    nostril T17.1
    pharynx —*see* Foreign body, pharynx
    specified site NEC T17.808
      causing
        asphyxiation T17.800
          food (bone) (seed) T17.820
          gastric contents (vomitus) T17.810
          specified type NEC T17.890
        injury NEC T17.808
          food (bone) (seed) T17.828
          gastric contents (vomitus) T17.818
          specified type NEC T17.898
    throat —*see* Foreign body, pharynx
    trachea —*see* Foreign body, trachea
  retained (old) (nonmagnetic) (in)
    anterior chamber (eye) —*see* Foreign body,
      intraocular, old, retained, anterior
      chamber
      magnetic —*see* Foreign body, intraocular,
        old, retained, magnetic, anterior
        chamber
    ciliary body —*see* Foreign body, intraocular,
      old, retained, ciliary body
      magnetic —*see* Foreign body, intraocular,
        old, retained, magnetic, ciliary body
    eyelid H02.819
      left H02.816
        lower H02.815
        upper H02.814
      right H02.813
        lower H02.812
        upper H02.811
    fragments —*see* Retained, foreign body
      fragments (type of)
    globe —*see* Foreign body, intraocular, old,
      retained
      magnetic —*see* Foreign body, intraocular,
        old, retained, magnetic
    intraocular —*see* Foreign body, intraocular,
      old, retained
      magnetic —*see* Foreign body, intraocular,
        old, retained, magnetic
    iris —*see* Foreign body, intraocular, old,
      retained, iris
      magnetic —*see* Foreign body, intraocular,
        old, retained, magnetic, iris
    lens —*see* Foreign body, intraocular, old,
      retained, lens
      magnetic —*see* Foreign body, intraocular,
        old, retained, magnetic, lens
    muscle —*see* Foreign body, retained, soft
      tissue
    orbit —*see* Foreign body, orbit, old
    posterior wall of globe —*see* Foreign body,
      intraocular, old, retained, posterior wall
      magnetic —*see* Foreign body, intraocular,
        old, retained, magnetic, posterior wall
    retrobulbar —*see* Foreign body, orbit, old,
      retrobulbar
    soft tissue M79.5
    vitreous —*see* Foreign body, intraocular, old,
      retained, vitreous body
      magnetic —*see* Foreign body, intraocular,
        old, retained, magnetic, vitreous body
  retina S05.5-●
  sensation - *see* Sensation, foreign body
  superficial, without open wound
    abdomen, abdominal (wall) S30.851
    alveolar process S00.552
    ankle S90.55-●
    antecubital space —*see* Foreign body,
      superficial, forearm
    anus S30.857
    arm (upper) S40.85-●
    auditory canal —*see* Foreign body, superficial,
      ear

▶ New   ➡ Revised   ~~deleted~~ Deleted   ● Use Additional Character(s)

▶ New   ⇒ Revised   ~~deleted~~ Deleted   ● Use Additional Character(s)

Fracture, traumatic (*Continued*)
femur, femora (*Continued*)
shaft (lower third) (middle third) (upper
third) S72.30-●
comminuted (displaced) S72.35-●
nondisplaced S72.35-●
oblique (displaced) S72.33-●
nondisplaced S72.33-●
segmental (displaced) S72.36-●
nondisplaced S72.36-●
specified NEC S72.39-●
spiral (displaced) S72.34-●
nondisplaced S72.34-●
transverse (displaced) S72.32-●
nondisplaced S72.32-●
specified site NEC —*see* subcategory
S72.8
subcapital (displaced) S72.01-●
subtrochanteric (region) (section) (displaced)
S72.2-●
nondisplaced S72.2-●
transcervical —*see* Fracture, femur,
midcervical
transtrochanteric —*see* Fracture, femur,
trochanteric
trochanteric S72.10-●
apophyseal (displaced) S72.13-●
nondisplaced S72.13-●
greater trochanter (displaced) S72.11-●
nondisplaced S72.11-●
intertrochanteric (displaced) S72.14-●
nondisplaced S72.14-●
lesser trochanter (displaced) S72.12-●
nondisplaced S72.12-●
upper end S72.00-●
apophyseal (displaced) S72.13-●
nondisplaced S72.13-●
cervicotrochanteric —*see* Fracture, femur,
upper end, neck, base
epiphysis (displaced) S72.02-●
nondisplaced S72.02-●
head S72.05-●
articular (displaced) S72.06-●
nondisplaced S72.06-●
specified NEC S72.09-●
intertrochanteric (displaced)
S72.14-●
nondisplaced S72.14-●
intracapsular S72.01-●
midcervical (displaced) S72.03-●
nondisplaced S72.03-●
neck S72.00-●
base (displaced) S72.04-●
nondisplaced S72.04-●
specified NEC S72.09-●
pertrochanteric —*see* Fracture, femur, upper
end, trochanteric
physeal S79.00-●
Salter-Harris type I S79.01-●
specified NEC S79.09-●
subcapital (displaced) S72.01-●
subtrochanteric (displaced) S72.2-●
nondisplaced S72.2-●
transcervical —*see* Fracture, femur, upper
end, midcervical
trochanteric S72.10-●
greater (displaced) S72.11-●
nondisplaced S72.11-●
lesser (displaced) S72.12-●
nondisplaced S72.12-●
fibula (shaft) (styloid) S82.40-●
comminuted (displaced) S82.45-●
nondisplaced S82.45-●
following insertion of implant, prosthesis or
plate M96.67-●
involving ankle or malleolus —*see* Fracture,
fibula, lateral malleolus
lateral malleolus (displaced) S82.6-●
nondisplaced S82.6-●
lower end
physeal S89.30-●
Salter-Harris
Type I S89.31-●
Type II S89.32-●
specified NEC S89.39-●
specified NEC S82.83-●
torus S82.82-●
oblique (displaced) S82.43-●
nondisplaced S82.43-●
segmental (displaced) S82.46-●
nondisplaced S82.46-●
specified NEC S82.49-●

Fracture, traumatic (*Continued*)
fibula (*Continued*)
spiral (displaced) S82.44-●
nondisplaced S82.44-●
transverse (displaced) S82.42-●
nondisplaced S82.42-●
upper end
physeal S89.20-●
Salter-Harris
Type I S89.21-●
Type II S89.22-●
specified NEC S89.29-●
specified NEC S82.83-●
torus S82.81-●
finger (except thumb) (displaced) S62.60-●
distal phalanx (displaced) S62.63-●
nondisplaced S62.66-●
index S62.60-●
distal phalanx (displaced) S62.63-●
nondisplaced S62.66-●
middle phalanx (displaced) S62.62-●
nondisplaced S62.65-●
proximal phalanx (displaced) S62.61-●
nondisplaced S62.64-●
little S62.60-●
distal phalanx (displaced) S62.63-●
nondisplaced S62.66-●
middle phalanx (displaced) S62.62-●
nondisplaced S62.65-●
proximal phalanx (displaced) S62.61-●
nondisplaced S62.64-●
middle phalanx (displaced) S62.62-●
nondisplaced S62.65-●
middle S62.60-●
distal phalanx (displaced) S62.63-●
nondisplaced S62.66-●
middle phalanx (displaced) S62.62-●
nondisplaced S62.65-●
proximal phalanx (displaced) S62.61-●
nondisplaced S62.64-●
proximal phalanx (displaced) S62.61-●
nondisplaced S62.64-●
ring S62.60-●
distal phalanx (displaced) S62.63-●
nondisplaced S62.66-●
middle phalanx (displaced) S62.62-●
nondisplaced S62.65-●
proximal phalanx (displaced) S62.61-●
nondisplaced S62.64-●
thumb —*see* Fracture, thumb
following insertion (intraoperative)
(postoperative) of orthopedic implant, joint
prosthesis or bone plate M96.69
femur M96.66-●
fibula M96.67-●
humerus M96.62-●
pelvis M96.65
radius M96.63-●
specified bone NEC M96.69
tibia M96.67-●
ulna M96.63-●
foot S92.90-●
astragalus —*see* Fracture, tarsal, talus
calcaneus —*see* Fracture, tarsal, calcaneus
cuboid —*see* Fracture, tarsal, cuboid
cuneiform —*see* Fracture, tarsal, cuneiform
metatarsal —*see* Fracture, metatarsal
navicular —*see* Fracture, tarsal, navicular
sesamoid S92.81-●
specified NEC S92.81-●
talus —*see* Fracture, tarsal, talus
tarsal —*see* Fracture, tarsal
toe —*see* Fracture, toe
forearm S52.9-●
radius —*see* Fracture, radius
ulna —*see* Fracture, ulna
fossa (anterior) (middle) (posterior) S02.19
fragility —*see* Fracture, pathological, due to
osteoporosis
frontal (bone) (skull) S02.0
sinus S02.19
glenoid (cavity) (scapula) —*see* Fracture, scapula,
glenoid cavity
greenstick —*see* Fracture, by site
hallux —*see* Fracture, toe, great
hand S62.9-●
carpal —*see* Fracture, carpal bone
finger (except thumb) —*see* Fracture, finger
metacarpal —*see* Fracture, metacarpal
navicular (scaphoid) (hand) —*see* Fracture,
carpal bone, navicular
thumb —*see* Fracture, thumb

Fracture, traumatic (*Continued*)
healed or old
with complications - code by Nature of the
complication
heel bone —*see* Fracture, tarsal, calcaneus
Hill-Sachs S42.29-●
hip —*see* Fracture, femur, neck
humerus S42.30-●
anatomical neck —*see* Fracture, humerus,
upper end
articular process —*see* Fracture, humerus,
lower end
capitellum —*see* Fracture, humerus, lower
end, condyle, lateral
distal end —*see* Fracture, humerus, lower end
epiphysis
lower —*see* Fracture, humerus, lower end,
physeal
upper —*see* Fracture, humerus, upper end,
physeal
external condyle —*see* Fracture, humerus,
lower end, condyle, lateral
following insertion of implant, prosthesis or
plate M96.62-●
great tuberosity —*see* Fracture, humerus,
upper end, greater tuberosity
intercondylar —*see* Fracture, humerus, lower
end
internal epicondyle —*see* Fracture, humerus,
lower end, epicondyle, medial
lesser tuberosity —*see* Fracture, humerus,
upper end, lesser tuberosity
lower end S42.40-●
condyle
lateral (displaced) S42.45-●
nondisplaced S42.45-●
medial (displaced) S42.46-●
nondisplaced S42.46-●
epicondyle
lateral (displaced) S42.43-●
nondisplaced S42.43-●
medial (displaced) S42.44-●
incarcerated S42.44-●
nondisplaced S42.44-●
physeal S49.10-●
Salter-Harris
Type I S49.11-●
Type II S49.12-●
Type III S49.13-●
Type IV S49.14-●
specified NEC S49.19-●
specified NEC (displaced)
S42.49-●
nondisplaced S42.49-●
supracondylar (simple) (displaced)
S42.41-●
with intercondylar fracture —*see*
Fracture, humerus, lower end
comminuted (displaced) S42.42-●
nondisplaced S42.42-●
nondisplaced S42.41-●
torus S42.48-●
transcondylar (displaced) S42.47-●
nondisplaced S42.47-●
proximal end —*see* Fracture, humerus, upper
end
shaft S42.30-●
comminuted (displaced) S42.35-●
nondisplaced S42.35-●
greenstick S42.31-●
oblique (displaced) S42.33-●
nondisplaced S42.33-●
segmental (displaced) S42.36-●
nondisplaced S42.36-●
specified NEC S42.39-●
spiral (displaced) S42.34-●
nondisplaced S42.34-●
transverse (displaced) S42.32-●
nondisplaced S42.32-●
supracondylar —*see* Fracture, humerus, lower
end
surgical neck —*see* Fracture, humerus, upper
end, surgical neck
trochlea —*see* Fracture, humerus, lower end,
condyle, medial
tuberosity —*see* Fracture, humerus, upper
end
upper end S42.20-●
anatomical neck —*see* Fracture, humerus,
upper end, specified NEC
articular head —*see* Fracture, humerus,
upper end, specified NEC

Fracture, traumatic *(Continued)*
  humerus *(Continued)*
    upper end *(Continued)*
      epiphysis —*see* Fracture, humerus, upper
        end, physeal
      greater tuberosity (displaced) S42.25-●
        nondisplaced S42.25-●
      lesser tuberosity (displaced) S42.26-●
        nondisplaced S42.26-●
      physeal S49.00-●
        Salter-Harris
          Type I S49.01-●
          Type II S49.02-●
          Type III S49.03-●
          Type IV S49.04-●
        specified NEC (displaced) S49.09-●
      specified NEC (displaced) S42.29-●
        nondisplaced S42.29-●
      surgical neck (displaced) S42.21-●
        four-part S42.24-●
        nondisplaced S42.21-●
        three-part S42.23-●
        two-part (displaced) S42.22-●
          nondisplaced S42.22-●
      torus S42.27-●
      transepiphyseal —*see* Fracture, humerus,
        upper end, physeal
  hyoid bone S12.8
  ilium S32.30-●
    with disruption of pelvic ring —*see*
      Disruption, pelvic ring
    avulsion (displaced) S32.31-●
      nondisplaced S32.31-●
    specified NEC S32.39-●
  impaction, impacted - code as Fracture, by site
  innominate bone —*see* Fracture, ilium
  instep —*see* Fracture, foot
  ischium S32.60-●
    with disruption of pelvic ring —*see*
      Disruption, pelvic ring
    avulsion (displaced) S32.61-●
      nondisplaced S32.61-●
    specified NEC S32.69-●
  jaw (bone) (lower) —*see* Fracture, mandible
    upper —*see* Fracture, maxilla
  joint prosthesis —*see* Complications, joint
    prosthesis, mechanical, breakdown, by site
    periprosthetic —*see* Fracture, traumatic,
      periprosthetic
  knee cap —*see* Fracture, patella
  larynx S12.8
  late effects —*see* Sequelae, fracture
  leg (lower) S82.9-●
    ankle —*see* Fracture, ankle
    femur —*see* Fracture, femur
    fibula —*see* Fracture, fibula
    malleolus —*see* Fracture, ankle
    patella —*see* Fracture, patella
    specified site NEC S82.89-●
    tibia —*see* Fracture, tibia
  lumbar spine —*see* Fracture, vertebra, lumbar
  lumbosacral spine S32.9
  Maisonneuve's (displaced) S82.86-●
    nondisplaced S82.86-●
  malar bone —*see also* Fracture, maxilla S02.400
    left side S02.40B
    right side S02.40A
  malleolus —*see* Fracture, ankle
  malunion —*see* Fracture, by site
  mandible (lower jawbone) S02.609
    alveolus S02.67-●
    angle (of jaw) S02.65-●
    body, unspecified S02.600-●
      left side S02.602
      right side S02.601
    condylar process S02.61-●
    coronoid process S02.63-●
    ramus, unspecified S02.64-●
    specified site NEC S02.69
    subcondylar process S02.62-●
    symphysis S02.66
  manubrium (sterni) S22.21
    dissociation from sternum S22.23
  march —*see* Fracture, traumatic, stress, by site
  maxilla, maxillary (bone) (sinus) (superior)
    (upper jaw) S02.401
    alveolus S02.42
    inferior —*see* Fracture, mandible
    LeFort I S02.411
    LeFort II S02.412
    LeFort III S02.413

Fracture, traumatic *(Continued)*
  maxilla, maxillary *(Continued)*
    left side S02.40D
    right side S02.40C
  metacarpal S62.309
    base (displaced) S62.319
      nondisplaced S62.349
    fifth S62.30-●
      base (displaced) S62.31-●
        nondisplaced S62.34-●
      neck (displaced) S62.33-●
        nondisplaced S62.36-●
      shaft (displaced) S62.32-●
        nondisplaced S62.35-●
      specified NEC S62.398
    first S62.20-●
      base NEC (displaced) S62.23-●
        nondisplaced S62.23-●
      Bennett's —*see* Bennett's fracture
      neck (displaced) S62.25-●
        nondisplaced S62.25-●
      shaft (displaced) S62.24-●
        nondisplaced S62.24-●
      specified NEC S62.29-●
    fourth S62.30-●
      base (displaced) S62.31-●
        nondisplaced S62.34-●
      neck (displaced) S62.33-●
        nondisplaced S62.36-●
      shaft (displaced) S62.32-●
        nondisplaced S62.35-●
      specified NEC S62.39-●
    neck (displaced) S62.33-●
      nondisplaced S62.36-●
    Rolando's —*see* Rolando's fracture
    second S62.30-●
      base (displaced) S62.31-●
        nondisplaced S62.34-●
      neck (displaced) S62.33-●
        nondisplaced S62.36-●
      shaft (displaced) S62.32-●
        nondisplaced S62.35-●
      specified NEC S62.39-●
    shaft (displaced) S62.32-●
      nondisplaced S62.35-●
    specified NEC S62.399
    third S62.30-●
      base (displaced) S62.31-●
        nondisplaced S62.34-●
      neck (displaced) S62.33-●
        nondisplaced S62.36-●
      shaft (displaced) S62.32-●
        nondisplaced S62.35-●
      specified NEC S62.39-●
  metaphyseal —*see* Fracture, traumatic, by site,
    shaft
  metastatic —*see* Fracture, pathological, due to,
    neoplastic disease —*see also* Neoplasm
  metatarsal bone S92.30-●
    fifth (displaced) S92.35-●
      nondisplaced S92.35-●
    first (displaced) S92.31-●
      nondisplaced S92.31-●
    fourth (displaced) S92.34-●
      nondisplaced S92.34-●
    physeal S99.10-●
      Salter-Harris
        Type I S99.11-●
        Type II S99.12-●
        Type III S99.13-●
        Type IV S99.14-●
      specified NEC S99.19-●
    second (displaced) S92.32-●
      nondisplaced S92.32-●
    third (displaced) S92.33-●
      nondisplaced S92.33-●
  Monteggia's —*see* Monteggia's fracture
  multiple
    hand (and wrist) NEC —*see* Fracture, by
      site
    ribs —*see* Fracture, rib, multiple
  nasal (bone(s)) S02.2
  navicular (scaphoid) (foot) —*see also* Fracture,
    tarsal, navicular
    hand —*see* Fracture, carpal, navicular
  neck S12.9
    cervical vertebra S12.9
      fifth (displaced) S12.400
        nondisplaced S12.401
        specified type NEC (displaced) S12.490
          nondisplaced S12.491

Fracture, traumatic *(Continued)*
  neck *(Continued)*
    cervical vertebra *(Continued)*
      first (displaced) S12.000
        burst (stable) S12.01
          unstable S12.02
        lateral mass (displaced)
          S12.040
          nondisplaced S12.041
        nondisplaced S12.001
        posterior arch (displaced)
          S12.030
          nondisplaced S12.031
        specified type NEC (displaced) S12.090
          nondisplaced S12.091
      fourth (displaced) S12.300
        nondisplaced S12.301
        specified type NEC (displaced) S12.390
          nondisplaced S12.391
      second (displaced) S12.100
        dens (anterior) (displaced) (type II)
          S12.110
          nondisplaced S12.112
          posterior S12.111
          specified type NEC (displaced)
            S12.120
            nondisplaced S12.121
        nondisplaced S12.101
        specified type NEC (displaced) S12.190
          nondisplaced S12.191
      seventh (displaced) S12.600
        nondisplaced S12.601
        specified type NEC (displaced) S12.690
          nondisplaced S12.691
      sixth (displaced) S12.500
        nondisplaced S12.501
        specified type NEC (displaced) S12.590
          nondisplaced S12.591
      third (displaced) S12.200
        nondisplaced S12.201
        specified type NEC (displaced) S12.290
          nondisplaced S12.291
    hyoid bone S12.8
    larynx S12.8
    specified site NEC S12.8
    thyroid cartilage S12.8
    trachea S12.8
  neoplastic NEC —*see* Fracture, pathological, due
    to, neoplastic disease
  neural arch —*see* Fracture, vertebra
  newborn —*see* Birth, injury, fracture
  nontraumatic —*see* Fracture, pathological
  nonunion —*see* Nonunion, fracture
  nose, nasal (bone) (septum) S02.2
  occiput —*see* Fracture, skull, base,
    occiput
  odontoid process —*see* Fracture, neck, cervical
    vertebra, second
  olecranon (process) (ulna) —*see* Fracture, ulna,
    upper end, olecranon process
  orbit, orbital (bone) (region) S02.85
    floor (blow-out) S02.3-●
    roof S02.12-●
    wall S02.85
      lateral S02.84-●
      medial S02.83-●
  os
    calcis —*see* Fracture, tarsal,
      calcaneus
    magnum —*see* Fracture, carpal,
      capitate
    pubis —*see* Fracture, pubis
  palate S02.8-●
  parietal bone (skull) S02.0
  patella S82.00-●
    comminuted (displaced) S82.04-●
      nondisplaced S82.04-●
    longitudinal (displaced) S82.02-●
      nondisplaced S82.02-●
    osteochondral (displaced) S82.01-●
      nondisplaced S82.01-●
    specified NEC S82.09-●
    transverse (displaced) S82.03-●
      nondisplaced S82.03-●
  pedicle (of vertebral arch) —*see* Fracture,
    vertebra
  pelvis, pelvic (bone) S32.9
    acetabulum —*see* Fracture, acetabulum
    circle —*see* Disruption, pelvic ring
    following insertion of implant, prosthesis or
      plate M96.65

▶ New   ⇒ Revised   ~~deleted~~ Deleted   ● Use Additional Character(s)

Fracture, traumatic *(Continued)*
  pelvis, pelvic *(Continued)*
    ilium —*see* Fracture, ilium
    ischium —*see* Fracture, ischium
    multiple
      with disruption of pelvic ring (circle) —*see*
        Disruption, pelvic ring
      without disruption of pelvic ring (circle)
        S32.82
    pubis —*see* Fracture, pubis
    sacrum —*see* Fracture, sacrum
    specified site NEC S32.89
  periprosthetic, around internal prosthetic joint
    M97.9
    ankle M97.2-•
    elbow M97.4-•
    finger M97.8
    hip M97.0-•
    knee M97.1-•
    shoulder M97.3-•
    specified joint NEC M97.8
    spine M97.8
    toe M97.8
    wrist M97.8
  phalanx
    foot —*see* Fracture, toe
    hand —*see* Fracture, finger
  pisiform —*see* Fracture, carpal, pisiform
  pond —*see* Fracture, skull
  prosthetic device, internal —*see* Complications,
    prosthetic device, by site, mechanical
  pubis S32.50-•
    with disruption of pelvic ring —*see*
      Disruption, pelvic ring
    specified site NEC S32.59-•
    superior rim S32.59-•
  radius S52.9-•
    distal end —*see* Fracture, radius, lower
      end
    following insertion of implant, prosthesis or
      plate M96.63-•
    head —*see* Fracture, radius, upper end, head
    lower end S52.50-•
      Barton's —*see* Barton's fracture
      Colles' —*see* Colles' fracture
      extraarticular NEC S52.55-•
      intraarticular NEC S52.57-•
      physeal S59.20-•
        Salter-Harris
          Type I S59.21-•
          Type II S59.22-•
          Type III S59.23-•
          Type IV S59.24-•
          specified NEC S59.29-•
      Smith's —*see* Smith's fracture
      specified NEC S52.59-•
      styloid process (displaced) S52.51-•
        nondisplaced S52.51-•
      torus S52.52-•
    neck —*see* Fracture, radius, upper end
    proximal end —*see* Fracture, radius, upper
      end
    shaft S52.30-•
      bent bone S52.38-•
      comminuted (displaced) S52.35-•
        nondisplaced S52.35-•
      Galeazzi's —*see* Galeazzi's fracture
      greenstick S52.31-•
      oblique (displaced) S52.33-•
        nondisplaced S52.33-•
      segmental (displaced) S52.36-•
        nondisplaced S52.36-•
      specified NEC S52.39-•
      spiral (displaced) S52.34-•
        nondisplaced S52.34-•
      transverse (displaced) S52.32-•
        nondisplaced S52.32-•
    upper end S52.10-•
      head (displaced) S52.12-•
        nondisplaced S52.12-•
      neck (displaced) S52.13-•
        nondisplaced S52.13-•
      physeal S59.10-•
        Salter-Harris
          Type I S59.11-•
          Type II S59.12-•
          Type III S59.13-•
          Type IV S59.14-•
          specified NEC S59.19-•
      specified NEC S52.18-•
      torus S52.11-•

Fracture, traumatic *(Continued)*
  ramus
    inferior or superior, pubis —*see* Fracture,
      pubis
    mandible —*see* Fracture, mandible
  restorative material (dental)
    K08.539
    with loss of material K08.531
    without loss of material K08.530
  rib S22.3-•
    with flail chest —*see* Flail, chest
      associated with chest compression and
        cardiopulmonary resuscitation M96.
        A2
    multiple S22.4-•
      with flail chest —*see* Flail, chest
        associated with chest compression and
          cardiopulmonary resuscitation
          M96.A3
  root, tooth —*see* Fracture, tooth
  sacrum S32.10
    specified NEC S32.19
    Type
      1 S32.14
      2 S32.15
      3 S32.16
      4 S32.17
    Zone
      I S32.119
        displaced (minimally) S32.111
          severely S32.112
        nondisplaced S32.110
      II S32.129
        displaced (minimally) S32.121
          severely S32.122
        nondisplaced S32.120
      III S32.139
        displaced (minimally) S32.131
          severely S32.132
        nondisplaced S32.130
  scaphoid (hand) —*see also* Fracture, carpal,
    navicular
    foot —*see* Fracture, tarsal, navicular
  scapula S42.10-•
    acromial process (displaced) S42.12-•
      nondisplaced S42.12-•
    body (displaced) S42.11-•
      nondisplaced S42.11-•
    coracoid process (displaced) S42.13-•
      nondisplaced S42.13-•
    glenoid cavity (displaced) S42.14-•
      nondisplaced S42.14-•
    neck (displaced) S42.15-•
      nondisplaced S42.15-•
    specified NEC S42.19-•
  semilunar bone, wrist —*see* Fracture, carpal,
    lunate
  sequelae —*see* Sequelae, fracture
  sesamoid bone
    foot S92.81-•
    hand —*see* Fracture, carpal
    other —*see* Fracture, traumatic, by site
  shepherd's —*see* Fracture, tarsal, talus
  shoulder (girdle) S42.9-•
    blade —*see* Fracture, scapula
  sinus (ethmoid) (frontal) S02.19
  skull S02.91
    base S02.10-•
      occiput S02.119
        condyle S02.113
          type I S02.110
            left side S02.11B
            right side S02.11A
          type II S02.111
            left side S02.11D
            right side S02.11C
          type III S02.112
            left side S02.11F
            right side S02.11E
          specified NEC S02.118
            left side S02.11H
            right side S02.11G
        specified NEC S02.19-•
    birth injury P13.0
    frontal bone S02.0
    parietal bone S02.0
    specified site NEC S02.8
    temporal bone S02.19
    vault S02.0
  Smith's —*see* Smith's fracture
  sphenoid (bone) (sinus) S02.19

Fracture, traumatic *(Continued)*
  spine —*see* Fracture, vertebra
  spinous process —*see* Fracture, vertebra
  spontaneous (cause unknown) —*see* Fracture,
    pathological
  stave (of thumb) —*see* Fracture, metacarpal, first
  sternum S22.20
    with flail chest —*see* Flail, chest
      associated with chest compression and
        cardiopulmonary resuscitation M96.
        A1
    body S22.22
    manubrium S22.21
    xiphoid (process) S22.24
      associated with chest compression and
        cardiopulmonary resuscitation
        M96.A1
  stress M84.30
    ankle M84.37-•
    carpus M84.34-•
    clavicle M84.31-•
    femoral neck M84.359
    femur M84.35-•
    fibula M84.36-•
    finger M84.34-•
    hip M84.35-•
    humerus M84.32-•
    ilium M84.350
    ischium M84.350
    metacarpus M84.34-•
    metatarsus M84.37-•
    neck —*see* Fracture, fatigue, vertebra
    pelvis M84.350
    radius M84.33-•
    rib M84.38
    scapula M84.31-•
    skull M84.38
    tarsus M84.37-•
    tibia M84.36-•
    toe M84.37-•
    ulna M84.33-•
    vertebra —*see* Fracture, fatigue, vertebra
  supracondylar, elbow —*see* Fracture, humerus,
    lower end, supracondylar
  symphysis pubis —*see* Fracture, pubis
  talus (ankle bone) —*see* Fracture, tarsal, talus
  tarsal bone(s) S92.20-•
    astragalus —*see* Fracture, tarsal, talus
    calcaneus S92.00-•
      anterior process (displaced) S92.02-•
        nondisplaced S92.02-•
      body (displaced) S92.01-•
        nondisplaced S92.01-•
      extraarticular NEC (displaced) S92.05-•
        nondisplaced S92.05-•
      intraarticular (displaced) S92.06-•
        nondisplaced S92.06-•
      physeal S99.00-•
        Salter-Harris
          Type I S99.01-•
          Type II S99.02-•
          Type III S99.03-•
          Type IV S99.04-•
          specified NEC S99.09-•
      tuberosity (displaced) S92.04-•
        avulsion (displaced) S92.03-•
          nondisplaced S92.03-•
        nondisplaced S92.04-•
    cuboid (displaced) S92.21-•
      nondisplaced S92.21-•
    cuneiform
      intermediate (displaced) S92.23-•
        nondisplaced S92.23-•
      lateral (displaced) S92.22-•
        nondisplaced S92.22-•
      medial (displaced) S92.24-•
        nondisplaced S92.24-•
    navicular (displaced) S92.25-•
      nondisplaced S92.25-•
    scaphoid —*see* Fracture, tarsal, navicular
    talus S92.10-•
      avulsion (displaced) S92.15-•
        nondisplaced S92.15-•
      body (displaced) S92.12-•
        nondisplaced S92.12-•
      dome (displaced) S92.14-•
        nondisplaced S92.14-•
      head (displaced) S92.12-•
        nondisplaced S92.12-•
      lateral process (displaced) S92.14-•
        nondisplaced S92.14-•

Fracture, traumatic *(Continued)*
  tarsal bone(s) *(Continued)*
    talus *(Continued)*
      neck (displaced) S92.11-●
        nondisplaced S92.11-●
      posterior process (displaced) S92.13-●
        nondisplaced S92.13-●
      specified NEC S92.19-●
  temporal bone (styloid) S02.19
  thorax (bony) S22.9
    with flail chest —*see* Flail, chest
    rib S22.3-●
      multiple S22.4-●
        with flail chest —*see* Flail, chest
    sternum S22.20
      body S22.22
      manubrium S22.21
      xiphoid process S22.24
        associated with chest compression and
          cardiopulmonary resuscitation
          M96.A1
    vertebra (displaced) S22.009
      burst (stable) S22.001
        unstable S22.002
      eighth S22.069
        burst (stable) S22.061
          unstable S22.062
        specified type NEC S22.068
        wedge compression S22.060
      eleventh S22.089
        burst (stable) S22.081
          unstable S22.082
        specified type NEC S22.088
        wedge compression S22.080
      fifth S22.059
        burst (stable) S22.051
          unstable S22.052
        specified type NEC S22.058
        wedge compression S22.050
      first S22.019
        burst (stable) S22.011
          unstable S22.012
        specified type NEC S22.018
        wedge compression S22.010
      fourth S22.049
        burst (stable) S22.041
          unstable S22.042
        specified type NEC S22.048
        wedge compression S22.040
      ninth S22.079
        burst (stable) S22.071
          unstable S22.072
        specified type NEC S22.078
        wedge compression S22.070
      nondisplaced S22.001
      second S22.029
        burst (stable) S22.021
          unstable S22.022
        specified type NEC S22.028
        wedge compression S22.020
      seventh S22.069
        burst (stable) S22.061
          unstable S22.062
        specified type NEC S22.068
        wedge compression S22.060
      sixth S22.059
        burst (stable) S22.051
          unstable S22.052
        specified type NEC S22.058
        wedge compression S22.050
      specified type NEC S22.008
      tenth S22.079
        burst (stable) S22.071
          unstable S22.072
        specified type NEC S22.078
        wedge compression S22.070
      third S22.039
        burst (stable) S22.031
          unstable S22.032
        specified type NEC S22.038
        wedge compression S22.030
      twelfth S22.089
        burst (stable) S22.081
          unstable S22.082
        specified type NEC S22.088
        wedge compression S22.080
      wedge compression S22.000
  thumb S62.50-●
    distal phalanx (displaced) S62.52-●
      nondisplaced S62.52-●
    proximal phalanx (displaced) S62.51-●
      nondisplaced S62.51-●

Fracture, traumatic *(Continued)*
  thyroid cartilage S12.8
  tibia (shaft) S82.20-●
    comminuted (displaced) S82.25-●
      nondisplaced S82.25-●
    condyles —*see* Fracture, tibia, upper end
    distal end —*see* Fracture, tibia, lower end
    epiphysis
      lower —*see* Fracture, tibia, lower end
      upper —*see* Fracture, tibia, upper end
    following insertion of implant, prosthesis or
      plate M96.67-●
    head (involving knee joint) —*see* Fracture,
      tibia, upper end
    intercondyloid eminence —*see* Fracture, tibia,
      upper end
    involving ankle or malleolus —*see* Fracture,
      ankle, medial malleolus
    lower end S82.30-●
      physeal S89.10-●
        Salter-Harris
          Type I S89.11-●
          Type II S89.12-●
          Type III S89.13-●
          Type IV S89.14-●
          specified NEC S89.19-●
      pilon (displaced) S82.87-●
        nondisplaced S82.87-●
      specified NEC S82.39-●
      torus S82.31-●
    malleolus —*see* Fracture, ankle, medial malleolus
    oblique (displaced) S82.23-●
      nondisplaced S82.23-●
    pilon —*see* Fracture, tibia, lower end, pilon
    proximal end —*see* Fracture, tibia, upper end
    segmental (displaced) S82.26-●
      nondisplaced S82.26-●
    specified NEC S82.29-●
    spine —*see* Fracture, tibia, upper end, spine
    spiral (displaced) S82.24-●
      nondisplaced S82.24-●
    transverse (displaced) S82.22-●
      nondisplaced S82.22-●
    tuberosity —*see* Fracture, tibia, upper end,
      tuberosity
    upper end S82.10-●
      bicondylar (displaced) S82.14-●
        nondisplaced S82.14-●
      lateral condyle (displaced) S82.12-●
        nondisplaced S82.12-●
      medial condyle (displaced) S82.13-●
        nondisplaced S82.13-●
      physeal S89.00-●
        Salter-Harris
          Type I S89.01-●
          Type II S89.02-●
          Type III S89.03-●
          Type IV S89.04-●
          specified NEC S89.09-●
      plateau —*see* Fracture, tibia, upper end,
        bicondylar
      specified NEC S82.19-●
      spine (displaced) S82.11-●
        nondisplaced S82.11-●
      torus S82.16-●
      tuberosity (displaced) S82.15-●
        nondisplaced S82.15-●
  toe S92.91-●
    great (displaced) S92.40-●
      distal phalanx (displaced) S92.42-●
        nondisplaced S92.42-●
      nondisplaced S92.40-●
      proximal phalanx (displaced) S92.41-●
        nondisplaced S92.41-●
      specified NEC S92.49-●
    lesser (displaced) S92.50-●
      distal phalanx (displaced) S92.53-●
        nondisplaced S92.53-●
      middle phalanx (displaced) S92.52-●
        nondisplaced S92.52-●
      nondisplaced S92.50-●
      proximal phalanx (displaced) S92.51-●
        nondisplaced S92.51-●
      specified NEC S92.59-●
    physeal
      phalanx S99.20-●
        Salter-Harris
          Type I S99.21-●
          Type II S99.22-●
          Type III S99.23-●
          Type IV S99.24-●
          specified NEC S99.29-●

Fracture, traumatic *(Continued)*
  tooth (root) S02.5
  trachea (cartilage) S12.8
  transverse process —*see* Fracture, vertebra
  trapezium or trapezoid bone —*see* Fracture,
    carpal
  trimalleolar —*see* Fracture, ankle, trimalleolar
  triquetrum (cuneiform of carpus) —*see* Fracture,
    carpal, triquetrum
  trochanter —*see* Fracture, femur, trochanteric
  tuberosity (external) —*see* Fracture, traumatic,
    by site
  ulna (shaft) S52.20-●
    bent bone S52.28-●
    coronoid process —*see* Fracture, ulna, upper
      end, coronoid process
    distal end —*see* Fracture, ulna, lower end
    following insertion of implant, prosthesis or
      plate M96.63-●
    head S52.60-●
    lower end S52.60-●
      physeal S59.00-●
        Salter-Harris
          Type I S59.01-●
          Type II S59.02-●
          Type III S59.03-●
          Type IV S59.04-●
          specified NEC S59.09-●
      specified NEC S52.69-●
      styloid process (displaced) S52.61-●
        nondisplaced S52.61-●
      torus S52.62-●
    proximal end —*see* Fracture, ulna, upper end
    shaft S52.20-●
      comminuted (displaced) S52.25-●
        nondisplaced S52.25-●
      greenstick S52.21-●
      Monteggia's —*see* Monteggia's fracture
      oblique (displaced) S52.23-●
        nondisplaced S52.23-●
      segmental (displaced) S52.26-●
        nondisplaced S52.26-●
      specified NEC S52.29-●
      spiral (displaced) S52.24-●
        nondisplaced S52.24-●
      transverse (displaced) S52.22-●
        nondisplaced S52.22-●
    upper end S52.00-●
      coronoid process (displaced) S52.04-●
        nondisplaced S52.04-●
      olecranon process (displaced) S52.02-●
        with intraarticular extension S52.03-●
        nondisplaced S52.02-●
          with intraarticular extension S52.03-●
      specified NEC S52.09-●
      torus S52.01-●
  unciform —*see* Fracture, carpal, hamate
  vault of skull S02.0
  vertebra, vertebral (arch) (body) (column)
    (neural arch) (pedicle) (spinous process)
    (transverse process)
    atlas —*see* Fracture, neck, cervical vertebra, first
    axis —*see* Fracture, neck, cervical vertebra,
      second
    cervical (teardrop) S12.9
      axis —*see* Fracture, neck, cervical vertebra,
        second
      first (atlas) —*see* Fracture, neck, cervical
        vertebra, first
      second (axis) —*see* Fracture, neck, cervical
        vertebra, second
    chronic M84.48
    coccyx S32.2
    dorsal —*see* Fracture, thorax, vertebra
    lumbar S32.009
      burst (stable) S32.001
        unstable S32.002
      fifth S32.059
        burst (stable) S32.051
          unstable S32.052
        specified type NEC S32.058
        wedge compression S32.050
      first S32.019
        burst (stable) S32.011
          unstable S32.012
        specified type NEC S32.018
        wedge compression S32.010
      fourth S32.049
        burst (stable) S32.041
          unstable S32.042
        specified type NEC S32.048
        wedge compression S32.040

▶ New   ⇒ Revised   ~~deleted~~ Deleted   ● Use Additional Character(s)

Fracture, traumatic *(Continued)*
  vertebra, vertebral *(Continued)*
    lumbar *(Continued)*
      second S32.029
        burst (stable) S32.021
          unstable S32.022
        specified type NEC S32.028
        wedge compression S32.020
      specified type NEC S32.008
      third S32.039
        burst (stable) S32.031
          unstable S32.032
        specified type NEC S32.038
        wedge compression S32.030
      wedge compression S32.000
    metastatic —*see* Collapse, vertebra, in,
      specified disease NEC —*see also*
      Neoplasm
    newborn (birth injury) P11.5
    sacrum S32.10
      specified NEC S32.19
      Type
        1 S32.14
        2 S32.15
        3 S32.16
        4 S32.17
      Zone
        I S32.119
          displaced (minimally) S32.111
            severely S32.112
          nondisplaced S32.110
        II S32.129
          displaced (minimally) S32.121
            severely S32.122
          nondisplaced S32.120
        III S32.139
          displaced (minimally) S32.131
            severely S32.132
          nondisplaced S32.130
    thoracic —*see* Fracture, thorax, vertebra
  vertex S02.0
  vomer (bone) S02.2
  wrist S62.10-●
    carpal —*see* Fracture, carpal bone
    navicular (scaphoid) (hand) —*see* Fracture,
      carpal, navicular
  xiphisternum, xiphoid (process) S22.24
    associated with chest compression and
      cardiopulmonary resuscitation
      M96.A1
  zygoma S02.442
    left side S02.40F
    right side S02.40E
Fragile, fragility
  autosomal site Q95.5
  bone, congenital (with blue sclera) Q78.0
  capillary (hereditary) D69.8
  hair L67.8
  nails L60.3
  non-sex chromosome site Q95.5
  X chromosome Q99.2
Fragilitas
  crinium L67.8
  ossium (with blue sclerae) (hereditary)
    Q78.0
  unguium L60.3
    congenital Q84.6
Fragments, cataract (lens), following cataract
  surgery H59.02-●
  retained foreign body —*see* Retained, foreign
    body fragments (type of)
Frailty (frail) R54
  mental R41.81
Frambesia, frambesial (tropica) —*see also*
  Yaws
  initial lesion or ulcer A66.0
  primary A66.0
Frambeside
  gummatous A66.4
  of early yaws A66.2
Frambesioma A66.1
Franceschetti-Klein (-Wildervanck) disease or
  syndrome Q75.4
Francis' disease —*see* Tularemia
Franklin disease C88.2-●
Frank's essential thrombocytopenia D69.3
Fraser's syndrome Q87.0
Freckle(s) L81.2
  malignant melanoma in —*see* Melanoma
  melanotic (Hutchinson's) —*see* Melanoma, in
    situ
  retinal D49.81

Frederickson's hyperlipoproteinemia, type
  I and V E78.3
  IIA E78.00
  IIB and III E78.2
  IV E78.1
Freeman Sheldon syndrome Q87.0
Freezing —*see also* Effect, adverse, cold T69.9
Freiberg's disease (infraction of metatarsal head
  or osteochondrosis) —*see* Osteochondrosis,
  juvenile, metatarsus
Frei's disease A55
Fremitus, friction, cardiac R01.2
Frenum, frenulum
  external os Q51.828
  tongue (shortening) (congenital) Q38.1
Frequency micturition (nocturnal) R35.0
  psychogenic F45.8
Frey's syndrome
  auriculotemporal G50.8
  hyperhidrosis L74.52
Friction
  burn —*see* Burn, by site
  fremitus, cardiac R01.2
  precordial R01.2
  sounds, chest R09.89
Friderichsen-Waterhouse syndrome or disease
  A39.1
Friedländer's B (bacillus) NEC —*see also* condition
  A49.8
Friedreich's
  ataxia G11.11
  combined systemic disease G11.11
  facial hemihypertrophy Q67.4
  sclerosis (cerebellum) (spinal cord) G11.11
Frigidity F52.22
Fröhlich's syndrome E23.6
Frontal —*see also* condition
  lobe syndrome F07.0
Frostbite (superficial) T33.90
  with
    partial thickness skin loss —*see* Frostbite
      (superficial), by site
    tissue necrosis T34.90
  abdominal wall T33.3
    with tissue necrosis T34.3
  ankle T33.81-●
    with tissue necrosis T34.81-●
  arm T33.4-●
  with tissue necrosis T34.4-●
    finger(s) —*see* Frostbite, finger
    hand —*see* Frostbite, hand
    wrist —*see* Frostbite, wrist
  ear T33.01-●
    with tissue necrosis T34.01-●
  face T33.09
    with tissue necrosis T34.09
  finger T33.53-●
    with tissue necrosis T34.53-●
  foot T33.82-●
    with tissue necrosis T34.82-●
  hand T33.52-●
    with tissue necrosis T34.52-●
  head T33.09
    with tissue necrosis T34.09
    ear —*see* Frostbite, ear
    nose —*see* Frostbite, nose
  hip (and thigh) T33.6-●
    with tissue necrosis T34.6-●
  knee T33.7-●
    with tissue necrosis T34.7-●
  leg T33.9-●
    with tissue necrosis T34.9-●
    ankle —*see* Frostbite, ankle
    foot —*see* Frostbite, foot
    knee —*see* Frostbite, knee
    lower T33.7-●
      with tissue necrosis T34.7-●
    thigh —*see* Frostbite, hip
    toe —*see* Frostbite, toe
  limb
    lower T33.99
      with tissue necrosis T34.99
    upper —*see* Frostbite, arm
  neck T33.1
    with tissue necrosis T34.1
  nose T33.02
    with tissue necrosis T34.02
  pelvis T33.3
    with tissue necrosis T34.3
  specified site NEC T33.99
    with tissue necrosis T34.99
  thigh —*see* Frostbite, hip

Frostbite *(Continued)*
  thorax T33.2
    with tissue necrosis T34.2
  toes T33.83-●
    with tissue necrosis T34.83-●
  trunk T33.99
    with tissue necrosis T34.99
  wrist T33.51-●
    with tissue necrosis T34.51-●
Frotteurism F65.81
Frozen —*see also* Effect, adverse, cold T69.9
  pelvis (female) N94.89
    male K66.8
  shoulder —*see* Capsulitis, adhesive
Fructokinase deficiency E74.11
Fructose 1,6 diphosphatase deficiency E74.19
Fructosemia (benign) (essential) E74.12
Fructosuria (benign) (essential) E74.11
Fuchs'
  black spot (myopic) —*see also* Myopia,
    degenerative H44.2-●
  dystrophy (corneal endothelium) H18.51-●
  heterochromic cyclitis —*see* Cyclitis, Fuchs'
    heterochromic
Fucosidosis E77.1
Fugue R68.89
  dissociative F44.1
  hysterical (dissociative) F44.1
  postictal in epilepsy —*see* Epilepsy
  reaction to exceptional stress (transient)
    F43.0
Fulminant, fulminating —*see* condition
Functional —*see also* condition
  bleeding (uterus) N93.8
Functioning, intellectual, borderline R41.83
Fundus —*see* condition
Fungemia NOS B49
Fungus, fungous
  cerebral G93.89
  disease NOS B49
  infection —*see* Infection, fungus
Funiculitis (acute) (chronic) (endemic)
  N49.1
  gonococcal (acute) (chronic) A54.23
  tuberculous A18.15
Funnel
  breast (acquired) M95.4
    congenital Q67.6
    sequelae (late effect) of rickets E64.3
  chest (acquired) M95.4
    congenital Q67.6
    sequelae (late effect) of rickets E64.3
  pelvis (acquired) M95.5
    with disproportion (fetopelvic) O33.3
      causing obstructed labor O65.3
    congenital Q74.2
FUO (fever of unknown origin) R50.9
Furfur L21.0
  microsporon B36.0
Furrier's lung J67.8
Furrowed K14.5
  nail(s) (transverse) L60.4
    congenital Q84.6
  tongue K14.5
    congenital Q38.3
Furuncle L02.92
  abdominal wall L02.221
  ankle —*see* Furuncle, lower limb
  antecubital space —*see* Furuncle, upper
    limb
  anus K61.0
  arm —*see* Furuncle, upper limb
  auditory canal, external —*see* Abscess, ear,
    external
  auricle (ear) —*see* Abscess, ear, external
  axilla (region) L02.42-●
  back (any part) L02.222
  breast N61.1
  buttock L02.32
  cheek (external) L02.02
  chest wall L02.223
  chin L02.02
  corpus cavernosum N48.21
  ear, external —*see* Abscess, ear, external
  external auditory canal —*see* Abscess, ear,
    external
  eyelid —*see* Abscess, eyelid
  face L02.02
  femoral (region) —*see* Furuncle, lower
    limb
  finger —*see* Furuncle, hand
  flank L02.221

Furuncle *(Continued)*
  foot L02.62-●
  forehead L02.02
  gluteal (region) L02.32
  groin L02.224
  hand L02.52-●
  head L02.821
    face L02.02
  hip —*see* Furuncle, lower limb
  kidney —*see* Abscess, kidney
  knee —*see* Furuncle, lower limb
  labium (majus) (minus) N76.4
  lacrimal
    gland —*see* Dacryoadenitis
    passages (duct) (sac) —*see* Inflammation,
      lacrimal, passages, acute
  leg (any part) —*see* Furuncle, lower limb
  lower limb L02.42-●
  malignant A22.0
  mouth K12.2
  navel L02.226
  neck L02.12
  nose J34.0
  orbit, orbital —*see* Abscess, orbit
  palmar (space) —*see* Furuncle, hand
  partes posteriores L02.32
  pectoral region L02.223
  penis N48.21
  perineum L02.225
  pinna —*see* Abscess, ear, external
  popliteal —*see* Furuncle, lower limb
  prepatellar —*see* Furuncle, lower limb
  scalp L02.821
  seminal vesicle N49.0
  shoulder —*see* Furuncle, upper limb
  specified site NEC L02.828
  submandibular K12.2
  temple (region) L02.02
  thumb —*see* Furuncle, hand
  toe —*see* Furuncle, foot
  trunk L02.229
    abdominal wall L02.221
    back L02.222
    chest wall L02.223
    groin L02.224
    perineum L02.225
    umbilicus L02.226
  umbilicus L02.226
  upper limb L02.42-●
  vulva N76.4
Furunculosis —*see* Furuncle
Fused —*see* Fusion, fused
Fusion, fused (congenital)
  astragaloscaphoid Q74.2
  atria Q21.19
  auditory canal Q16.1
  auricles, heart Q21.19
  binocular with defective stereopsis H53.32
  bone Q79.8
  cervical spine M43.22
  choanal Q30.0
  commissure, mitral valve Q23.2
  cusps, heart valve NEC Q24.8
    mitral Q23.2
    pulmonary Q22.1
    tricuspid Q22.4
  ear ossicles Q16.3
  fingers Q70.0-●
  hymen Q52.3
  joint (acquired) —*see also* Ankylosis
    congenital Q74.8
  kidneys (incomplete) Q63.1
  labium (majus) (minus) Q52.5
  larynx and trachea Q34.8
  limb, congenital Q74.8
    lower Q74.2
    upper Q74.0
  lobes, lung Q33.8
  lumbosacral (acquired) M43.27
    arthrodesis status Z98.1
    congenital Q76.49
    postprocedural status Z98.1
  nares, nose, nasal, nostril(s) Q30.0
  organ or site not listed —*see* Anomaly, by site
  ossicles Q79.9
    auditory Q16.3
  pulmonic cusps Q22.1
  ribs Q76.6
  sacroiliac (joint) (acquired) M43.28
    arthrodesis status Z98.1
    congenital Q74.2
    postprocedural status Z98.1

Fusion, fused *(Continued)*
  spine (acquired) NEC M43.20
    arthrodesis status Z98.1
    cervical region M43.22
    cervicothoracic region M43.23
    congenital Q76.49
    lumbar M43.26
    lumbosacral region M43.27
    occipito-atlanto-axial region M43.21
    postoperative status Z98.1
    sacrococcygeal region M43.28
    thoracic region M43.24
    thoracolumbar region M43.25
  sublingual duct with submaxillary duct at
    opening in mouth Q38.4
  testes Q55.1
  toes Q70.2
  tooth, teeth K00.2
  trachea and esophagus Q39.8
  twins Q89.4
  vagina Q52.4
  ventricles, heart Q21.0
  vertebra (arch) —*see* Fusion, spine
  vulva Q52.5
Fusospirillosis (mouth) (tongue) (tonsil) A69.1
Fussy baby R68.12

G

Gain in weight (abnormal) (excessive) —*see also*
  Weight, gain
Gaisböck's disease (polycythemia hypertonica)
  D75.1
Gait abnormality R26.9
  ataxic R26.0
  falling R29.6
  hysterical (ataxic) (staggering) F44.4
  paralytic R26.1
  spastic R26.1
  specified type NEC R26.89
  staggering R26.0
  unsteadiness R26.81
  walking difficulty NEC R26.2
Galactocele (breast) N64.89
  puerperal, postpartum O92.79
Galactophoritis N61.0
  gestational, puerperal, postpartum O91.2-●
Galactorrhea O92.6
  not associated with childbirth N64.3
Galactosemia (classic) (congenital) E74.21
Galactosuria E74.29
Galacturia R82.0
  schistosomiasis (bilharziasis) B65.0
GALD (gestational alloimmune liver disease)
  P78.84
Galeazzi's fracture S52.37-●
Galen's vein —*see* condition
Galeophobia F40.218
Gall duct —*see* condition
Gallbladder —*see also* condition
  acute K81.0
Gallop rhythm R00.8
Gallstone (colic) (cystic duct) (gallbladder)
  (impacted) (multiple) —*see also* Calculus,
  gallbladder
  with
    cholecystitis —*see* Calculus, gallbladder, with
      cholecystitis
  bile duct (common) (hepatic) —*see* Calculus,
    bile duct
  causing intestinal obstruction K56.3
  specified NEC K80.80
    with obstruction K80.81
Gambling Z72.6
  pathological (compulsive) F63.0
Gammopathy (of undetermined significance
  [MGUS]) D47.2
  associated with lymphoplasmacytic dyscrasia
    D47.2
  monoclonal D47.2
  polyclonal D89.0
Gamna's disease (siderotic splenomegaly) D73.1
Gamophobia F40.298
Gampsodactylia (congenital) Q66.7-●
Gamstorp's disease (adynamia episodica
  hereditaria) G72.3
Gandy-Nanta disease (siderotic splenomegaly)
  D73.1

Gang
  membership offenses Z72.810
Gangliocytoma D36.10
Ganglioglioma —*see* Neoplasm, uncertain
  behavior, by site
Ganglion (compound) (diffuse) (joint) (tendon
  (sheath)) M67.40
  ankle M67.47-●
  foot M67.47-●
  forearm M67.43-●
  hand M67.44-●
  lower leg M67.46-●
  multiple sites M67.49
  of yaws (early) (late) A66.6
  pelvic region M67.45-●
  periosteal —*see* Periostitis
  shoulder region M67.41-●
  specified site NEC M67.48
  thigh region M67.45-●
  tuberculous A18.09
  upper arm M67.42-●
  wrist M67.43-●
Ganglioneuroblastoma —*see* Neoplasm, nerve,
  malignant
Ganglioneuroma D36.10
  malignant —*see* Neoplasm, nerve, malignant
Ganglioneuromatosis D36.10
Ganglionitis
  fifth nerve —*see* Neuralgia, trigeminal
  gasserian (postherpetic) (postzoster) B02.21
  geniculate G51.1
    newborn (birth injury) P11.3
    postherpetic, postzoster B02.21
  herpes zoster B02.21
  postherpetic geniculate B02.21
Gangliosidosis E75.10
  GM1 E75.19
  GM2 E75.00
    other specified E75.09
    Sandhoff disease E75.01
    Tay-Sachs disease E75.02
  GM3 E75.19
  mucolipidosis IV E75.11
Gangosa A66.5
Gangrene, gangrenous (connective tissue)
  (dropsical) (dry) (moist) (skin) (ulcer) —*see
  also* Necrosis I96
  with diabetes (mellitus) —*see* Diabetes, with
    gangrene
  abdomen (wall) I96
  alveolar M27.3
  appendix K35.80
    with
      peritonitis, localized (*see also* Appendicitis)
        K35.31
  arteriosclerotic (general) (senile) —*see*
    Arteriosclerosis, extremities, with, gangrene
  auricle I96
  Bacillus welchii A48.0
  bladder (infectious) —*see* Cystitis, specified type
    NEC
  bowel, cecum, or colon —*see* Gangrene, intestine
  Clostridium perfringens or welchii A48.0
  cornea H18.89-●
  corpora cavernosa N48.29
    noninfective N48.89
  cutaneous, spreading I96
  decubital —*see* Ulcer, pressure, by site
  diabetic (any site) —*see* Diabetes, with gangrene
  emphysematous —*see* Gangrene, gas
  epidemic —*see* Poisoning, food, noxious, plant
  epididymis (infectional) N45.1
  erysipelas —*see* Erysipelas
  extremity (lower) (upper) I96
  Fournier N49.3
    female N76.82
    vagina and vulva N76.82
  fusospirochetal A69.0
  gallbladder —*see* Cholecystitis, acute
  gas (bacillus) A48.0
    following
      abortion —*see* Abortion by type
        complicated by infection
      ectopic or molar pregnancy O08.0
  glossitis K14.0
  hernia —*see* Hernia, by site, with gangrene
  intestine, intestinal (hemorrhagic) (massive) —
    see also Infarct, intestine K55.069
    with
      mesenteric embolism —*see also* Infarct,
        intestine K55.069
      obstruction —*see* Obstruction, intestine

▶ New   ⇒ Revised   ~~deleted~~ Deleted   ● Use Additional Character(s)

Gangrene, gangrenous *(Continued)*
  laryngitis J04.0
  limb (lower) (upper) I96
  lung J85.0
    spirochetal A69.8
  lymphangitis I89.1
  Meleney's (synergistic) —*see* Ulcer, skin
  mesentery —*see also* Infarct, intestine
      K55.069
    with
        embolism —*see also* Infarct, intestine
            K55.069
        intestinal obstruction —*see* Obstruction,
            intestine
  mouth A69.0
  ovary —*see* Oophoritis
  pancreas —*see* Pancreatitis, acute
  penis N48.29
    noninfective N48.89
  perineum I96
  pharynx —*see also* Pharyngitis
    Vincent's A69.1
  presenile I73.1
  progressive synergistic —*see* Ulcer, skin
  pulmonary J85.0
  pulpal (dental) K04.1
  quinsy J36
  Raynaud's (symmetric gangrene) I73.01
  retropharyngeal J39.2
  scrotum N49.3
    noninfective N50.89
  senile (atherosclerotic) —*see* Arteriosclerosis,
      extremities, with, gangrene
  spermatic cord N49.1
    noninfective N50.89
  spine I96
  spirochetal NEC A69.8
  spreading cutaneous I96
  stomatitis A69.0
  symmetrical I73.01
  testis (infectional) N45.2
    noninfective N44.8
  throat —*see also* Pharyngitis
    diphtheritic A36.0
    Vincent's A69.1
  thyroid (gland) E07.89
  tooth (pulp) K04.1
  tuberculous NEC —*see* Tuberculosis
  tunica vaginalis N49.1
    noninfective N50.89
  umbilicus I96
  uterus —*see* Endometritis
  uvulitis K12.2
  vas deferens N49.1
    noninfective N50.89
  vulva N76.82
Ganister disease J62.8
Ganser's syndrome (hysterical) F44.89
Gardner-Diamond syndrome (autoerythrocyte
    sensitization) D69.2
Gargoylism E76.01
Garré's disease, osteitis (sclerosing),
    osteomyelitis —*see* Osteomyelitis, specified
    type NEC
Garrod's pad, knuckle M72.1
Gartner's duct
  cyst Q52.4
  persistent Q50.6
Gas R14.3
  asphyxiation, inhalation, poisoning, suffocation
      NEC —*see* Table of Drugs and Chemicals
  excessive R14.0
  gangrene A48.0
    following
        abortion —*see* Abortion by type
            complicated by infection
        ectopic or molar pregnancy O08.0
  on stomach R14.0
  pains R14.1
Gastralgia —*see also* Pain, abdominal
Gastrectasis K31.0
  psychogenic F45.8
Gastric —*see* condition
Gastrinoma
  malignant
    pancreas C25.4
    specified site NEC —*see* Neoplasm, malignant,
        by site
    unspecified site C25.4
  specified site —*see* Neoplasm, uncertain
      behavior
  unspecified site D37.9

Gastritis (simple) K29.70
  with bleeding K29.71
  acute (erosive) K29.00
    with bleeding K29.01
  alcoholic K29.20
    with bleeding K29.21
  allergic K29.60
    with bleeding K29.61
  atrophic (chronic) K29.40
    with bleeding K29.41
  chronic (antral) (fundal) K29.50
    with bleeding K29.51
    atrophic K29.40
      with bleeding K29.41
    superficial K29.30
      with bleeding K29.31
  dietary counseling and surveillance Z71.3
  due to diet deficiency E63.9
  eosinophilic K52.81
  giant hypertrophic K29.60
    with bleeding K29.61
  granulomatous K29.60
    with bleeding K29.61
  hypertrophic (mucosa) K29.60
    with bleeding K29.61
  nervous F54
  spastic K29.60
    with bleeding K29.61
  specified NEC K29.60
    with bleeding K29.61
  superficial chronic K29.30
    with bleeding K29.31
  tuberculous A18.83
  viral NEC A08.4
Gastrocarcinoma —*see* Neoplasm, malignant,
    stomach
Gastrocolic —*see* condition
Gastrodisciasis, gastrodiscoidiasis B66.8
Gastroduodenitis K29.90
  with bleeding K29.91
  virus, viral A08.4
    specified type NEC A08.39
Gastrodynia —*see* Pain, abdominal
Gastroenteritis (acute) (chronic) (noninfectious)
    (*see also* Enteritis) K52.9
  allergic K52.29
  with
      eosinophilic gastritis or gastroenteritis K52.81

      food protein-induced enterocolitis syndrome
          K52.21
      food protein-induced enteropathy K52.22
  dietetic —*see also* Gastroenteritis, allergic K52.29

  drug-induced K52.1
  due to
      Cryptosporidium A07.2
      drugs K52.1
      food poisoning —*see* Intoxication,
          foodborne
      radiation K52.0
  eosinophilic K52.81
  epidemic (infectious) A09
  food hypersensitivity —*see also* Gastroenteritis,
      allergic K52.29
  infectious —*see* Enteritis, infectious
  influenzal —*see* Influenza, with gastroenteritis
  noninfectious K52.9
    specified NEC K52.89
  rotaviral A08.0
  Salmonella A02.0
  toxic K52.1
  viral NEC A08.4
    acute infectious A08.39
        type Norwalk A08.11
    infantile (acute) A08.39
    Norwalk agent A08.11
    rotaviral A08.0
    severe of infants A08.39
    specified type NEC A08.39
Gastroenteropathy —*see also* Gastroenteritis K52.9
  acute, due to Norovirus A08.11
  acute, due to Norwalk agent A08.11
  infectious A09
Gastroenteroptosis K63.4
Gastroesophageal laceration-hemorrhage
    syndrome K22.6
Gastrointestinal —*see* condition
Gastrojejunal —*see* condition
Gastrojejunitis —*see also* Enteritis K52.9
Gastrojejunocolic —*see* condition
Gastroliths K31.89

Gastromalacia K31.89
Gastroparalysis K31.84
  diabetic —*see* Diabetes, gastroparalysis
Gastroparesis K31.84
  diabetic —*see* Diabetes, by type, with
      gastroparesis
Gastropathy K31.9
  congestive portal (*see also*, Hypertension, portal)
      K31.89
  erythematous K29.70
  exudative K90.89
  portal hypertensive (*see also*, Hypertension,
      portal) K31.89
  specified NEC K31.89
Gastroptosis K31.89
Gastrorrhagia K92.2
  psychogenic F45.8
Gastroschisis (congenital) Q79.3
Gastrospasm (neurogenic) (reflex) K31.89
  neurotic F45.8
  psychogenic F45.8
Gastrostaxis —*see* Gastritis, with bleeding
Gastrostenosis K31.89
Gastrostomy
  attention to Z43.1
  status Z93.1
Gastrosuccorrhea (continuous) (intermittent)
    K31.89
  neurotic F45.8
  psychogenic F45.8
Gatophobia F40.218
Gaucher's disease or splenomegaly (adult)
    (infantile) E75.22
Gee (-Herter)(-Thaysen) disease (nontropical
    sprue) K90.0
Gélineau's syndrome G47.419
  with cataplexy G47.411
Gemination, tooth, teeth K00.2
Gemistocytoma
  specified site —*see* Neoplasm, malignant, by
      site
  unspecified site C71.9
General, generalized —*see* condition
Genetic
  carrier (status)
    cystic fibrosis Z14.1
    hemophilia A (asymptomatic) Z14.01
        symptomatic Z14.02
    specified NEC Z14.8
  susceptibility to disease NEC Z15.89
    ▶epilepsy Z15.1
    malignant neoplasm Z15.09
        breast Z15.01
        endometrium Z15.04
        ovary Z15.02
        prostate Z15.03
        specified NEC Z15.09
    multiple endocrine neoplasia Z15.81
    ▶neurodevelopmental disorders Z15.1
    ▶obesity Z15.2
Genital —*see* condition
Genito-anorectal syndrome A55
Genitourinary system —*see* condition
Genu
  congenital Q74.1
  extrorsum (acquired) —*see also* Deformity, varus,
      knee
    congenital Q74.1
    sequelae (late effect) of rickets E64.3
  introrsum (acquired) —*see also* Deformity,
      valgus, knee
    congenital Q74.1
    sequelae (late effect) of rickets E64.3
  rachitic (old) E64.3
  recurvatum (acquired) —*see also* Deformity, limb,
      specified type NEC, lower leg
    congenital Q68.2
    sequelae (late effect) of rickets E64.3
  valgum (acquired) (knock-knee) M21.06-●
    congenital Q74.1
    sequelae (late effect) of rickets E64.3
  varum (acquired) (bowleg) M21.16-●
    congenital Q74.1
    sequelae (late effect) of rickets E64.3
Geographic tongue K14.1
Geophagia —*see* Pica
Geotrichosis B48.3
  stomatitis B48.3
Gephyrophobia F40.242
Gerbode defect Q21.0
GERD (gastroesophageal reflux disease)
    K21.9

Gerhardt's
　disease (erythromelalgia) I73.81
　syndrome (vocal cord paralysis) J38.00
　　bilateral J38.02
　　unilateral J38.01
German measles —see also Rubella
　exposure to Z20.4
Germinoblastoma (diffuse) C85.9-●
　follicular C82.9-●
Germinoma —see Neoplasm, malignant, by site
Gerontoxon —see Degeneration, cornea, senile
Gerstmann-Sträussler-Scheinker syndrome (GSS)
　A81.82
Gerstmann's syndrome R48.8
　developmental F81.2
Gestation (period) —see also Pregnancy
　ectopic —see Pregnancy, by site
　multiple O30.9-●
　　greater than quadruplets —see Pregnancy,
　　　multiple (gestation), specified NEC
　　specified NEC —see Pregnancy, multiple
　　　(gestation), specified NEC
Gestational
　mammary abscess O91.11-●
　purulent mastitis O91.11-●
　subareolar abscess O91.11-●
Ghon tubercle, primary infection A15.7
Ghost
　teeth K00.4
　vessels (cornea) H16.41-●
Ghoul hand A66.3
Gianotti-Crosti disease L44.4
Giant
　cell
　　epulis K06.8
　　peripheral granuloma K06.8
　esophagus, congenital Q39.5
　kidney, congenital Q63.3
　urticaria T78.3
　　hereditary D84.1
Giardiasis A07.1
Gibert's disease or pityriasis L42
Giddiness R42
　hysterical F44.89
　psychogenic F45.8
Gierke's disease (glycogenosis I) E74.01
Gigantism (cerebral) (hypophyseal) (pituitary)
　E22.0
　constitutional E34.4
Gilbert's disease or syndrome E80.4
Gilchrist's disease B40.9
Gilford-Hutchinson disease E34.8
Gilles de la Tourette's disease or syndrome
　(motor-verbal tic) F95.2
Gingivitis K05.10
　acute (catarrhal) K05.00
　　necrotizing A69.1
　　nonplaque induced K05.01
　　plaque induced K05.00
　chronic (desquamative) (hyperplastic) (simple
　　marginal) (pregnancy associated)
　　(ulcerative) K05.10
　　nonplaque induced K05.11
　　plaque induced K05.10
　expulsiva —see Periodontitis
　necrotizing ulcerative (acute) A69.1
　pellagrous E52
　　acute necrotizing A69.1
　Vincent's A69.1
Gingivoglossitis K14.0
Gingivopericementitis —see Periodontitis
Gingivosis —see Gingivitis, chronic
Gingivostomatitis K05.10
　herpesviral B00.2
　necrotizing ulcerative (acute) A69.1
Gland, glandular —see condition
Glanders A24.0
Glanzmann (-Naegeli) disease or thrombasthenia
　D69.1
Glasgow coma scale
　total score
　　3-8 R40.243
　　9-12 R40.242
　　13-15 R40.241
Glass-blower's disease (cataract) —see Cataract,
　specified NEC
Glaucoma H40.9
　with
　　increased episcleral venous pressure H40.81-●
　　pseudoexfoliation of lens —see Glaucoma,
　　　open angle, primary, capsular

Glaucoma (Continued)
　absolute H44.51-●
　angle-closure (primary) H40.20-●
　　acute (attack) (crisis) H40.21-●
　　chronic H40.22-●
　　intermittent H40.23-●
　　residual stage H40.24-●
　borderline H40.00-●
　capsular (with pseudoexfoliation of lens) —see
　　Glaucoma, open angle, primary, capsular
　childhood Q15.0
　closed angle —see Glaucoma, angle-closure
　congenital Q15.0
　corticosteroid-induced —see Glaucoma,
　　secondary, drugs
　hypersecretion H40.82-●
　in (due to)
　　amyloidosis E85.4 [H42]
　　aniridia Q13.1 [H42]
　　concussion of globe —see Glaucoma,
　　　secondary, trauma
　　dislocation of lens —see Glaucoma,
　　　secondary
　　disorder of lens NEC —see Glaucoma,
　　　secondary
　　drugs —see Glaucoma, secondary, drugs
　　endocrine disease NOS E34.9 [H42]
　　eye
　　　inflammation —see Glaucoma, secondary,
　　　　inflammation
　　　trauma —see Glaucoma, secondary,
　　　　trauma
　　hypermature cataract —see Glaucoma,
　　　secondary
　　iridocyclitis —see Glaucoma, secondary,
　　　inflammation
　　lens disorder —see Glaucoma, secondary,
　　　Lowe's syndrome E72.03 [H42]
　　metabolic disease NOS E88.9 [H42]
　　ocular disorders NEC —see Glaucoma,
　　　secondary
　　onchocerciasis B73.02
　　pupillary block —see Glaucoma, secondary
　　retinal vein occlusion —see Glaucoma,
　　　secondary
　　Rieger's anomaly Q13.81 [H42]
▶　　Rieger anomaly Q13.81 [H42]
　　rubeosis of iris —see Glaucoma, secondary
　　tumor of globe —see Glaucoma, secondary
　infantile Q15.0
　low tension —see Glaucoma, open angle,
　　primary, low-tension
　malignant H40.83-●
　narrow angle —see Glaucoma, angle-closure
　newborn Q15.0
　noncongestive (chronic) —see Glaucoma, open
　　angle
　nonobstructive —see Glaucoma, open angle
　obstructive —see also Glaucoma, angle-closure
　　due to lens changes —see Glaucoma,
　　　secondary
　open angle H40.10-●
　　primary H40.11-●
　　　capsular (with pseudoexfoliation of lens)
　　　　H40.14-●
　　　low-tension H40.12-●
　　　pigmentary H40.13-●
　　　residual stage H40.15-●
　phacolytic —see Glaucoma, secondary
　pigmentary —see Glaucoma, open angle,
　　primary, pigmentary
　postinfectious —see Glaucoma, secondary,
　　inflammation
　secondary (to) H40.5-●
　　drugs H40.6-●
　　inflammation H40.4-●
　　trauma H40.3-●
　simple (chronic) H40.11-●
　simplex H40.11-●
　specified type NEC H40.89
　suspect H40.00-●
　syphilitic A52.71
　traumatic —see also Glaucoma, secondary,
　　trauma
　　newborn (birth injury) P15.3
　tuberculous A18.59
Glaucomatous flecks (subcapsular) —see Cataract,
　complicated
Glazed tongue K14.4
Gleet (gonococcal) A54.01
Glénard's disease K63.4

Glioblastoma (multiforme)
　with sarcomatous component
　　specified site —see Neoplasm, malignant, by
　　　site
　　unspecified site C71.9
　giant cell
　　specified site —see Neoplasm, malignant, by
　　　site
　　unspecified site C71.9
　specified site —see Neoplasm, malignant, by site
　unspecified site C71.9
Glioma (malignant)
　astrocytic
　　specified site —see Neoplasm, malignant, by
　　　site
　　unspecified site C71.9
　mixed
　　specified site —see Neoplasm, malignant, by
　　　site
　　unspecified site C71.9
　nose Q30.8
　specified site NEC —see Neoplasm, malignant,
　　by site
　subependymal D43.2
　　specified site —see Neoplasm, uncertain
　　　behavior, by site
　　unspecified site D43.2
　unspecified site C71.9
Gliomatosis cerebri C71.0
Glioneuroma —see Neoplasm, uncertain behavior,
　by site
Gliosarcoma
　specified site —see Neoplasm, malignant, by site
　unspecified site C71.9
Gliosis (cerebral) G93.89
　spinal G95.89
Glisson's disease —see Rickets
Globinuria R82.3
Globus (hystericus) F45.8
Glomangioma D18.00
　intra-abdominal D18.03
　intracranial D18.02
　skin D18.01
　specified site NEC D18.09
Glomangiomyoma D18.00
　intra-abdominal D18.03
　intracranial D18.02
　skin D18.01
　specified site NEC D18.09
Glomangiosarcoma —see Neoplasm, connective
　tissue, malignant
Glomerular
　disease in syphilis A52.75
　nephritis —see Glomerulonephritis
Glomerulitis —see Glomerulonephritis
Glomerulonephritis —see also Nephritis N05.9
　with
　　C3
　　　glomerulonephritis N05.A
　　　glomerulopathy N05.A
　　　　with dense deposit disease N05.6
　　edema —see Nephrosis
　　minimal change N05.0
　　minor glomerular abnormality N05.0
　acute N00.9
　chronic N03.9
　crescentic (diffuse) NEC —see also N00-N07 with
　　fourth character .7 N05.7
　dense deposit —see also N00-N07 with fourth
　　character .6 N05.6
　diffuse
　　crescentic —see also N00-N07 with fourth
　　　character .7 N05.7
　　endocapillary proliferative —see also N00N07
　　　with fourth character .4 N05.4
　　membranous —see also N00-N07 with fourth
　　　character .2 N05.2
　　mesangial proliferative —see also N00-N07
　　　with fourth character .3 N05.3
　　mesangiocapillary —see also N00-N07 with
　　　fourth character .5 N05.5
　　sclerosing N18.9
　endocapillary proliferative (diffuse) NEC —see
　　also N00-N07 with fourth character .4 N05.4
　extracapillary NEC —see also N00-N07 with
　　fourth character .7 N05.7
　focal (and segmental) —see also N00-N07 with
　　fourth character .1 N05.1
　hypocomplementemic —see Glomerulonephritis,
　　membranoproliferative
　IgA —see Nephropathy, IgA

Glomerulonephritis (Continued)
immune complex (circulating) NEC N05.8
in (due to)
amyloidosis E85.4 [N08]
bilharziasis B65.9 [N08]
cryoglobulinemia D89.1 [N08]
defibrination syndrome D65 [N08]
diabetes mellitus —see Diabetes, glomerulosclerosis
disseminated intravascular coagulation D65 [N08]
Fabry (-Anderson) disease E75.21 [N08]
Goodpasture's syndrome M31.0
hemolytic-uremic syndrome —see Syndrome, hemolytic-uremic
Henoch (-Schönlein) purpura D69.0 [N08]
lecithin cholesterol acyltransferase deficiency E78.6 [N08]
microscopic polyangiitis M31.7 [N08]
multiple myeloma C90.0-● [N08]
Plasmodium malariae B52.0
schistosomiasis B65.9 [N08]
sepsis A41.9-● [N08]
streptococcal A40-● [N08]
sickle-cell disorders D57.-● [N08]
strongyloidiasis B78.9 [N08]
subacute bacterial endocarditis I33.0 [N08]
syphilis (late) congenital A50.59 [N08]
systemic lupus erythematosus M32.14
thrombotic thrombocytopenic purpura M31.19 [N08]
typhoid fever A01.09
Waldenström macroglobulinemia C88.0-● [N08]
Wegener's granulomatosis M31.31
latent or quiescent N03.9
lobular, lobulonodular —see Glomerulonephritis, membranoproliferative
membranoproliferative (diffuse) (type 1 or 3) — see also N00-N07 with fourth character .5 N05.5
dense deposit (type 2) NEC —see also N00-N07 with fourth character .6 N05.6
membranous (diffuse) NEC —see also N00-N07 with fourth character .2 N05.2
mesangial
IgA/IgG —see Nephropathy, IgA
proliferative (diffuse) NEC —see also N00-N07 with fourth character .3 N05.3
mesangiocapillary (diffuse) NEC —see also N00-N07 with fourth character .5 N05.5
necrotic, necrotizing NEC —see also N00-N07 with fourth character .8 N05.8
nodular —see Glomerulonephritis, membranoproliferative
poststreptococcal NEC N05.9
acute N00.9
chronic N03.9
rapidly progressive N01.9
proliferative NEC —see also N00-N07 with fourth character .8 N05.8
diffuse (lupus) M32.14
rapidly progressive N01.9
sclerosing, diffuse N18.9
specified pathology NEC —see also N00-N07 with fourth character .8 N05.8
subacute N01.9
Glomerulopathy —see Glomerulonephritis
Glomerulosclerosis —see also Sclerosis, renal
intercapillary (nodular) (with diabetes) —see Diabetes, glomerulosclerosis
intracapillary —see Diabetes, glomerulosclerosis
Glossagra K14.6
Glossalgia K14.6
Glossitis (chronic superficial) (gangrenous) (Moeller's) K14.0
areata exfoliativa K14.1
atrophic K14.4
benign migratory K14.1
cortical superficial, sclerotic K14.0
Hunter's D51.0
interstitial, sclerous K14.0
median rhomboid K14.2
pellagrous E52
superficial, chronic K14.0
Glossocele K14.8
Glossodynia K14.6
exfoliativa K14.4
Glossoncus K14.8
Glossopathy K14.9

Glossophytia K14.3
Glossoplegia K14.8
Glossoptosis K14.8
Glossopyrosis K14.6
Glossotrichia K14.3
Glossy skin L90.8
Glottis —see condition
Glottitis —see also Laryngitis J04.0
Glucagonoma
pancreas
benign D13.7
malignant C25.4
uncertain behavior D37.8
specified site NEC
benign —see Neoplasm, benign, by site
malignant —see Neoplasm, malignant, by site
uncertain behavior —see Neoplasm, uncertain behavior, by site
unspecified site
benign D13.7
malignant C25.4
uncertain behavior D37.8
Glucoglycinuria E72.51
Glucose-galactose malabsorption E74.39
Glue
ear —see Otitis, media, nonsuppurative, chronic, mucoid
sniffing (airplane) —see Abuse, drug, inhalant
dependence —see Dependence, drug, inhalant
GLUT1 deficiency syndrome 1, infantile onset E74.810
GLUT1 deficiency syndrome 2, childhood onset E74.810
Glutaric aciduria E72.3
Glycinemia E72.51
Glycinuria (renal) (with ketosis) E72.09
Glycogen
infiltration —see Disease, glycogen storage
storage disease —see Disease, glycogen storage
Glycogenosis (diffuse) (generalized) —see also Disease, glycogen storage
cardiac E74.02 [I43]
diabetic, secondary —see Diabetes, glycogenosis, secondary
pulmonary interstitial J84.842
Glycopenia E16.2
Glycosuria R81
renal (familial) E74.818
Gnathostoma spinigerum (infection) (infestation), gnathostomiasis (wandering swelling) B83.1
Goiter (plunging) (substernal) E04.9
with
hyperthyroidism (recurrent) —see Hyperthyroidism, with, goiter
thyrotoxicosis —see Hyperthyroidism, with, goiter
adenomatous —see Goiter, nodular
cancerous C73
congenital (nontoxic) E03.0
diffuse E03.0
parenchymatous E03.0
transitory, with normal functioning P72.0
cystic E04.2
due to iodine-deficiency E01.1
due to
enzyme defect in synthesis of thyroid hormone E07.1
iodine-deficiency (endemic) E01.2
dyshormonogenetic (familial) E07.1
endemic (iodine-deficiency) E01.2
diffuse E01.0
multinodular E01.1
exophthalmic —see Hyperthyroidism, with, goiter
iodine-deficiency (endemic) E01.2
diffuse E01.0
multinodular E01.1
nodular E01.1
lingual Q89.2
lymphadenoid E06.3
malignant C73
multinodular (cystic) (nontoxic) E04.2
toxic or with hyperthyroidism E05.20
with thyroid storm E05.21
neonatal NEC P72.0
nodular (nontoxic) (due to) E04.9
with
hyperthyroidism E05.20
with thyroid storm E05.21
thyrotoxicosis E05.20
with thyroid storm E05.21

Goiter (Continued)
nodular (Continued)
endemic E01.1
iodine-deficiency E01.1
sporadic E04.9
toxic E05.20
with thyroid storm E05.21
nontoxic E04.9
diffuse (colloid) E04.0
multinodular E04.2
simple E04.0
specified NEC E04.8
uninodular E04.1
simple E04.0
toxic —see Hyperthyroidism, with, goiter
uninodular (nontoxic) E04.1
toxic or with hyperthyroidism E05.10
with thyroid storm E05.11
Goiter-deafness syndrome E07.1
Goldberg syndrome Q89.8
Goldberg-Maxwell syndrome E34.51
Goldblatt's hypertension or kidney I70.1
Goldenhar (-Gorlin) syndrome Q87.0
Goldflam-Erb disease or syndrome G70.00
with exacerbation (acute) G70.01
in crisis G70.01
Goldscheider's disease Q81.8
Goldstein's disease (familial hemorrhagic telangiectasia) I78.0
Golfer's elbow —see Epicondylitis, medial
Gonadoblastoma
specified site —see Neoplasm, uncertain behavior, by site
unspecified site
female D39.10
male D40.10
Gonecystitis —see Vesiculitis
Gongylonemiasis B83.8
Goniosynechiae —see Adhesions, iris, goniosynechiae
Gonococcemia A54.86
Gonococcus, gonococcal (disease) (infection) —see also condition A54.9
anus A54.6
bursa, bursitis A54.49
conjunctiva, conjunctivitis (neonatorum) A54.31
endocardium A54.83
eye A54.30
conjunctivitis A54.31
iridocyclitis A54.32
keratitis A54.33
newborn A54.31
other specified A54.39
fallopian tubes (acute) (chronic) A54.24
genitourinary (organ) (system) (tract) (acute)
lower A54.00
with abscess (accessory gland) (periurethral) A54.1
upper —see also condition A54.29
heart A54.83
iridocyclitis A54.32
joint A54.42
lymphatic (gland) (node) A54.89
meninges, meningitis A54.81
musculoskeletal A54.40
arthritis A54.42
osteomyelitis A54.43
other specified A54.49
spondylopathy A54.41
pelviperitonitis A54.24
pelvis (acute) (chronic) A54.24
pharynx A54.5
proctitis A54.6
pyosalpinx (acute) (chronic) A54.24
rectum A54.6
skin A54.89
specified site NEC A54.89
tendon sheath A54.49
throat A54.5
urethra (acute) (chronic) A54.01
with abscess (accessory gland) (periurethral) A54.1
vulva (acute) (chronic) A54.02
Gonocytoma
specified site —see Neoplasm, uncertain behavior, by site
unspecified site
female D39.10
male D40.10

Gonorrhea (acute) (chronic) A54.9
  Bartholin's gland (acute) (chronic) (purulent) A54.02
    with abscess (accessory gland) (periurethral) A54.1
  bladder A54.01
  cervix A54.03
  conjunctiva, conjunctivitis (neonatorum) A54.31
  contact Z20.2
  Cowper's gland (with abscess) A54.1
  exposure to Z20.2
  fallopian tube (acute) (chronic) A54.24
  kidney (acute) (chronic) A54.21
  lower genitourinary tract A54.00
    with abscess (accessory gland) (periurethral) A54.1
  ovary (acute) (chronic) A54.24
  pelvis (acute) (chronic) A54.24
    female pelvic inflammatory disease A54.24
  penis A54.09
  prostate (acute) (chronic) A54.22
  seminal vesicle (acute) (chronic) A54.23
  specified site not listed —see also Gonococcus A54.89
  spermatic cord (acute) (chronic) A54.23
  urethra A54.01
    with abscess (accessory gland) (periurethral) A54.1
  vagina A54.02
  vas deferens (acute) (chronic) A54.23
  vulva A54.02
Goodall's disease A08.19
Goodpasture's syndrome M31.0
Gopalan's syndrome (burning feet) E53.0
Gorlin-Chaudry-Moss syndrome Q87.0
Gottron's papules L94.4
Gougerot's syndrome (trisymptomatic) L81.7
Gougerot-Blum syndrome (pigmented purpuric lichenoid dermatitis) L81.7
Gougerot-Carteaud disease or syndrome (confluent reticulate papillomatosis) L83
Gouley's syndrome (constrictive pericarditis) I31.1
Goundou A66.6
Gout, chronic (see also Gout, gouty) M1A.9-●
  drug-induced M1A.20
    ankle M1A.27-●
    elbow M1A.22-●
    foot joint M1A.27-●
    hand joint M1A.24-●
    hip M1A.25-●
    knee M1A.26-●
    multiple site M1A.29-●
    shoulder M1A.21-●
    vertebrae M1A.28
    wrist M1A.23-●
  idiopathic M1A.00
    ankle M1A.07-●
    elbow M1A.02-●
    foot joint M1A.07-●
    hand joint M1A.04-●
    hip M1A.05-●
    knee M1A.06-●
    multiple site M1A.09
    shoulder M1A.01-●
    vertebrae M1A.08
    wrist M1A.03-●
  in (due to) renal impairment M1A.30
    ankle M1A.37-●
    elbow M1A.32-●
    foot joint M1A.37-●
    hand joint M1A.34-●
    hip M1A.35-●
    knee M1A.36-●
    multiple site M1A.39
    shoulder M1A.31-●
    vertebrae M1A.38
    wrist M1A.33-●
  lead-induced M1A.10
    ankle M1A.17-●
    elbow M1A.12-●
    foot joint M1A.17-●
    hand joint M1A.14-●
    hip M1A.15-●
    knee M1A.16-●
    multiple site M1A.19
    shoulder M1A.11-●
    vertebrae M1A.18
    wrist M1A.13-●
  primary —see Gout, chronic, idiopathic
  saturnine —see Gout, chronic, lead-induced

Gout, chronic (Continued)
  secondary NEC M1A.40
    ankle M1A.47-●
    elbow M1A.42-●
    foot joint M1A.47-●
    hand joint M1A.44-●
    hip M1A.45-●
    knee M1A.46-●
    multiple site M1A.49
    shoulder M1A.41-●
    vertebrae M1A.48
    wrist M1A.43-●
  syphilitic —see also subcategory M14.8-● A52.77
  tophi M1A.9
Gout, gouty (acute) (attack) (flare) —see also Gout, chronic M10.9-●
  drug-induced M10.20
    ankle M10.27-●
    elbow M10.22-●
    foot joint M10.27-●
    hand joint M10.24-●
    hip M10.25-●
    knee M10.26-●
    multiple site M10.29
    shoulder M10.21-●
    vertebrae M10.28
    wrist M10.23-●
  idiopathic M10.00
    ankle M10.07-●
    elbow M10.02-●
    foot joint M10.07-●
    hand joint M10.04-●
    hip M10.05-●
    knee M10.06-●
    multiple site M10.09
    shoulder M10.01-●
    vertebrae M10.08
    wrist M10.03-●
  in (due to) renal impairment M10.30
    ankle M10.37-●
    elbow M10.32-●
    foot joint M10.37-●
    hand joint M10.34-●
    hip M10.35-●
    knee M10.36-●
    multiple site M10.39
    shoulder M10.31-●
    vertebrae M10.38
    wrist M10.33-●
  lead-induced M10.10
    ankle M10.17-●
    elbow M10.12-●
    foot joint M10.17-●
    hand joint M10.14-●
    hip M10.15-●
    knee M10.16-●
    multiple site M10.19
    shoulder M10.11-●
    vertebrae M10.18
    wrist M10.13-●
  primary —see Gout, idiopathic
  saturnine —see Gout, lead-induced
  secondary NEC M10.40
    ankle M10.47-●
    elbow M10.42-●
    foot joint M10.47-●
    hand joint M10.44-●
    hip M10.45-●
    knee M10.46-●
    multiple site M10.49
    shoulder M10.41-●
    vertebrae M10.48
    wrist M10.43-●
  syphilitic —see also subcategory M14.8-● A52.77
  tophi NEC —see Gout, chronic
Gower's
  muscular dystrophy G71.01
  syndrome (vasovagal attack) R55
Gradenigo's syndrome —see Otitis, media, suppurative, acute
Graefe's disease —see Strabismus, paralytic, ophthalmoplegia, progressive
Graft-versus-host disease D89.813
  acute D89.810
  acute on chronic D89.812
  chronic D89.811
Grain mite (itch) B88.0
Grainhandler's disease or lung J67.8
Grand mal —see Epilepsy, generalized, specified NEC

Grand multipara status only (not pregnant) Z64.1
  pregnant —see Pregnancy, complicated by, grand multiparity
Granite worker's lung J62.8
Granular —see also condition
  inflammation, pharynx J31.2
  kidney (contracting) —see Sclerosis, renal
  liver K74.69
Granulation tissue (abnormal) (excessive) L92.9
  postmastoidectomy cavity —see Complications, postmastoidectomy, granulation
Granulocytopenia (primary) (malignant) —see Agranulocytosis
Granuloma L92.9
  abdomen K66.8
    from residual foreign body L92.3
    pyogenicum L98.0
  actinic L57.5
  annulare (perforating) L92.0
  apical K04.5
  aural —see Otitis, externa, specified NEC
  beryllium (skin) L92.3
  bone
    eosinophilic C96.6
    from residual foreign body —see Osteomyelitis, specified type NEC
    lung C96.6
  brain (any site) G06.0
    schistosomiasis B65.9 [G07]
  canaliculus lacrimalis —see Granuloma, lacrimal
  candidal (cutaneous) B37.2
  cerebral (any site) G06.0
  coccidioidal (primary) (progressive) B38.7
    lung B38.1
    meninges B38.4
  colon K63.89
  conjunctiva H11.22-●
  dental K04.5
  ear, middle —see Cholesteatoma
  eosinophilic C96.6
    bone C96.6
    lung C96.6
    oral mucosa K13.4
    skin L92.2
  eyelid H01.8
  facial (e) L92.2
  foreign body (in soft tissue) NEC M60.20
    ankle M60.27-●
    foot M60.27-●
    forearm M60.23-●
    hand M60.24-●
    in operation wound —see Foreign body, accidentally left during a procedure
    lower leg M60.26-●
    pelvic region M60.25-●
    shoulder region M60.21-●
    skin L92.3
    specified site NEC M60.28
    subcutaneous tissue L92.3
    thigh M60.25-●
    upper arm M60.22-●
  gangraenescens M31.2
  genito-inguinale A58
  giant cell (central) (reparative) (jaw) M27.1
    gingiva (peripheral) K06.8
  gland (lymph) I88.8
  hepatic NEC K75.3
    in (due to)
      berylliosis J63.2 [K77]
      sarcoidosis D86.89
  Hodgkin C81.9-●
  ileum K63.89
  infectious B99.9
    specified NEC B99.8
  inguinale (Donovan) (venereal) A58
  intestine NEC K63.89
  intracranial (any site) G06.0
  intraspinal (any part) G06.1
  iridocyclitis —see Iridocyclitis, chronic
  jaw (bone) (central) M27.1
    reparative giant cell M27.1
  kidney —see also Infection, kidney N15.8
  lacrimal H04.81-●
  larynx J38.7
  lethal midline (faciale) (e) M31.2
  liver NEC —see Granuloma, hepatic
  lung (infectious) —see also Fibrosis, lung
    coccidioidal B38.1
    eosinophilic C96.6
  Majocchi's B35.8
  malignant (facial) (e) M31.2

▶ New   ⇒ Revised   ~~deleted~~ Deleted   ● Use Additional Character(s)

Granuloma (Continued)
  mandible (central) M27.1
  midline (lethal) M31.2
  monilial (cutaneous) B37.2
  nasal sinus —see Sinusitis
  operation wound T81.89
    foreign body —see Foreign body, accidentally
        left during a procedure
    stitch T81.89
    talc —see Foreign body, accidentally left
        during a procedure
  oral mucosa K13.4
  orbit, orbital H05.11-•
  paracoccidioidal B41.8
  penis, venereal A58
  periapical K04.5
  peritoneum K66.8
    due to ova of helminths NOS —see also
        Helminthiasis B83.9 [K67]
  postmastoidectomy cavity —see Complications,
      postmastoidectomy, recurrent
      cholesteatoma
  prostate N42.89
  pudendi (ulcerating) A58
  pulp, internal (tooth) K03.3
  pyogenic, pyogenicum (of) (skin) L98.0
    gingiva K06.8
    maxillary alveolar ridge K04.5
    oral mucosa K13.4
  rectum K62.89
  reticulohistiocytic D76.3
  rubrum nasi L74.8
  Schistosoma —see Schistosomiasis
  septic (skin) L98.0
  silica (skin) L92.3
  sinus (accessory) (infective) (nasal) —see
      Sinusitis
  skin L92.9
    from residual foreign body L92.3
    pyogenicum L98.0
  spine
    syphilitic (epidural) A52.19
    tuberculous A18.01
  stitch (postoperative) T81.89
  suppurative (skin) L98.0
  swimming pool A31.1
  talc —see also Granuloma, foreign body
    in operation wound —see Foreign body,
        accidentally left during a procedure
  telangiectaticum (skin) L98.0
  tracheostomy J95.09
  trichophyticum B35.8
  tropicum A66.4
  umbilical P83.81
  umbilicus P83.81
  urethra N36.8
  uveitis —see Iridocyclitis, chronic
  vagina A58
  venereum A58
  vocal cord J38.3
Granulomatosis L92.9
  with polyangiitis M31.3-•
  eosinophilic, with polyangiitis [EGPA] M30.1
  lymphoid C83.8-•
  miliary (listerial) A32.89
  necrotizing, respiratory M31.30
  progressive septic D71
  specified NEC L92.8
  Wegener's M31.30
    with renal involvement M31.31
Granulomatous tissue (abnormal) (excessive)
    L92.9
Granulosis rubra nasi L74.8
Graphite fibrosis (of lung) J63.3
Graphospasm F48.8
  organic G25.89
Grating scapula M89.8X1
Gravel (urinary) —see Calculus, urinary
Graves' disease —see Hyperthyroidism, with,
    goiter
Gravis —see condition
Grawitz tumor C64.-•
Gray syndrome (newborn) P93.0
Grayness, hair (premature) L67.1
  congenital Q84.2
Green sickness D50.8
Greenfield's disease
  meaning
    concentric sclerosis (encephalitis periaxialis
        concentrica) G37.5
    metachromatic leukodystrophy E75.25

Greenstick fracture - code as Fracture, by site
Grey syndrome (newborn) P93.0
Grief F43.21
  complicated F43.81
  prolonged F43.81
  reaction —see also Disorder, adjustment
      F43.20
Griesinger's disease B76.0
Grinder's lung or pneumoconiosis J62.8
Grinding, teeth
  psychogenic F45.8
  sleep related G47.63
Grip
  Dabney's B33.0
  devil's B33.0
Grippe, grippal —see also Influenza
  Balkan A78
  summer, of Italy A93.1
Grisel's disease M43.6
Groin —see condition
Grooved tongue K14.5
Ground itch B76.9
Grover's disease or syndrome L11.1
Growing pains, children R29.898
Growth (fungoid) (neoplastic) (new) —see also
    Neoplasm
  adenoid (vegetative) J35.8
  benign —see Neoplasm, benign, by site
  malignant —see Neoplasm, malignant, by site
  rapid, childhood Z00.2
  secondary —see Neoplasm, secondary, by site
Gruby's disease B35.0
Guardianship by non-parental relative Z62.23
Gubler-Millard paralysis or syndrome G46.3
Guerin-Stern syndrome Q74.3
Guidance, insufficient anterior (occlusal)
    M26.54
Guillain-Barré disease or syndrome G61.0
  sequelae G65.0
Guinea worms (infection) (infestation) B72
Guinon's disease (motor-verbal tic) F95.2
Gull's disease E03.4
Gum —see condition
Gumboil K04.7
  with sinus K04.6
Gumma (syphilitic) A52.79
  artery A52.09
    cerebral A52.04
  bone A52.77
    of yaws (late) A66.6
  brain A52.19
  cauda equina A52.19
  central nervous system A52.3
  ciliary body A52.71
  congenital A50.59
  eyelid A52.71
  heart A52.06
  intracranial A52.19
  iris A52.71
  kidney A52.75
  larynx A52.73
  leptomeninges A52.19
  liver A52.74
  meninges A52.19
  myocardium A52.06
  nasopharynx A52.73
  neurosyphilitic A52.3
  nose A52.73
  orbit A52.71
  palate (soft) A52.79
  penis A52.76
  pericardium A52.06
  pharynx A52.73
  pituitary A52.79
  scrofulous (tuberculous) A18.4
  skin A52.79
  specified site NEC A52.79
  spinal cord A52.19
  tongue A52.79
  tonsil A52.73
  trachea A52.73
  tuberculous A18.4
  ulcerative due to yaws A66.4
  ureter A52.75
  yaws A66.4
    bone A66.6
Gunn's syndrome Q07.8
Gunshot wound —see also Puncture, open
  fracture - code as Fracture, by site
  internal organs —see Injury, by site
Gynandrism Q56.0

Gynandroblastoma
  specified site —see Neoplasm, uncertain
      behavior, by site
  unspecified site
    female D39.10
    male D40.10
Gynecological examination (periodic) (routine)
    Z01.419
  with abnormal findings Z01.411
Gynecomastia N62
Gynephobia F40.291
Gyrate scalp Q82.8

H

H (Hartnup's) disease E72.02
Haas' disease or osteochondrosis (juvenile) (head
    of humerus) —see Osteochondrosis, juvenile,
    humerus
H-ABC (hypomyelination with atrophy of the
    basal ganglia and cerebellum) G23.3
Habit, habituation
  bad sleep Z72.821
  chorea F95.8
  disturbance, child F98.9
  drug —see Dependence, drug
  irregular sleep Z72.821
  laxative F55.2
  spasm —see Tic
  tic —see Tic
Haemophilus (H.) influenzae, as cause of disease
    classified elsewhere B96.3
Haff disease —see Poisoning, mercury
Hageman's factor defect, deficiency or disease
    D68.2
Haglund's disease or osteochondrosis (juvenile)
    (os tibiale externum) —see Osteochondrosis,
    juvenile, tarsus
Hailey-Hailey disease Q82.8
Hair —see also condition
  plucking F63.3
    in stereotyped movement disorder F98.4
  tourniquet syndrome —see also Constriction,
      external, by site
    finger S60.44-•
    penis S30.842
    thumb S60.34-•
    toe S90.44-•
Hairball in stomach T18.2
Hair-pulling, pathological (compulsive) F63.3
Hairy black tongue K14.3
Half vertebra Q76.49
Halitosis R19.6
Hallerman-Streiff syndrome Q87.0
Hallervorden-Spatz disease G23.0
Hallopeau's acrodermatitis or disease L40.2
Hallucination R44.3
  auditory R44.0
  gustatory R44.2
  olfactory R44.2
  specified NEC R44.2
  tactile R44.2
  visual R44.1
Hallucinosis (chronic) F28
  alcoholic (acute) F10.951
    in
      abuse F10.151
      dependence F10.251
  drug-induced F19.951
    cannabis F12.951
    cocaine F14.951
    hallucinogen F16.151
    in
      abuse F19.151
        cannabis F12.151
        cocaine F14.151
        hallucinogen F16.151
        inhalant F18.151
        opioid F11.151
        sedative, anxiolytic or hypnotic
            F13.151
        stimulant NEC F15.151
      dependence F19.251
        cannabis F12.251
        cocaine F14.251
        hallucinogen F16.251
        inhalant F18.251
        opioid F11.251

Hallucinosis (Continued)
  drug-induced (Continued)
    in (Continued)
      dependence (Continued)
        sedative, anxiolytic or hypnotic F13.251
        stimulant NEC F15.251
      inhalant F18.951
      opioid F11.951
      sedative, anxiolytic or hypnotic F13.951
      stimulant NEC F15.951
    organic F06.0
Hallux
  deformity (acquired) NEC M20.5X-●
  limitus M20.5X-●
  malleus (acquired) NEC M20.3-●
  rigidus (acquired) M20.2-●
    congenital Q74.2
    sequelae (late effect) of rickets E64.3
  valgus (acquired) M20.1-●
    congenital Q66.6
  varus (acquired) M20.3-●
    congenital Q66.3-●
Halo, visual H53.19
Hamartoma, hamartoblastoma Q85.9
  epithelial (gingival), odontogenic, central
    or peripheral —see Cyst, calcifying
    odontogenic
Hamartosis Q85.9
Hamman-Rich syndrome J84.114
Hammer toe (acquired) NEC —see also Deformity,
    toe, hammer toe
  congenital Q66.89
  sequelae (late effect) of rickets E64.3
Hand —see condition
Hand-foot syndrome L27.1
Handicap, handicapped
  educational Z55.9
    specified NEC Z55.8
Hand-Schüller-Christian disease or syndrome
    C96.5
Hanging (asphyxia) (strangulation) (suffocation) —
    see Asphyxia, traumatic, due to mechanical
    threat
Hangnail —see also Cellulitis, digit
  with lymphangitis —see Lymphangitis, acute,
    digit
Hangover (alcohol) F10.129
Hanhart's syndrome Q87.0
Hanot-Chauffard (-Troisier) **syndrome** E83.19
Hanot's cirrhosis or disease K74.3
Hansen's disease —see Leprosy
Hantaan virus disease (Korean hemorrhagic fever)
    A98.5
Hantavirus disease (with renal manifestations)
    (Dobrava) (Puumala) (Seoul) A98.5
  with pulmonary manifestations (Andes) (Bayou)
    (Bermejo) (Black Creek Canal) (Choclo)
    (Juquitiba) (Laguna negra) (Lechiguanas)
    (New York) (Oran) (Sin nombre) B33.4
Happy puppet syndrome Q93.59
Harada's disease or syndrome H30.81-●
Hardening
  artery —see Arteriosclerosis
  brain G93.89
Harelip (complete) (incomplete) —see Cleft, lip
Harlequin (newborn) Q80.4
Harley's disease D59.6
Harmful use (of)
  alcohol F10.10
  anxiolytics —see Abuse, drug, sedative
  cannabinoids —see Abuse, drug, cannabis
  cocaine —see Abuse, drug, cocaine
  drug —see Abuse, drug
  hallucinogens —see Abuse, drug, hallucinogen
  hypnotics —see Abuse, drug, sedative
  opioids —see Abuse, drug, opioid
  PCP (phencyclidine) —see Abuse, drug,
    hallucinogen
  sedatives —see Abuse, drug, sedative
  stimulants NEC —see Abuse, drug, stimulant
Harris' lines —see Arrest, epiphyseal
Hardship, material, due to limited financial
    resources, specified NEC Z59.87
Hartnup's disease E72.02
Harvester's lung J67.0
Harvesting ovum for in vitro fertilization Z31.83
Hashimoto's disease or thyroiditis E06.3
Hashitoxicosis (transient) E06.3
Hassal-Henle bodies or warts (cornea) H18.49
Haut mal —see Epilepsy, generalized, specified
    NEC

Haverhill fever A25.1
Hay fever —see also Fever, hay J30.1
Hayem-Widal syndrome D59.8
Haygarth's nodes M15.8
Haymaker's lung J67.0
Hb (abnormal)
  Bart's disease D56.0
  disease —see Disease, hemoglobin
  trait —see Trait
Head —see condition
Headache R51.9
  with
    orthostatic component NEC R51.0
    positional component NEC R51.0
  allergic NEC G44.89
  associated with sexual activity G44.82
  cervicogenic G44.86
  chronic daily R51.9
  cluster G44.009
    chronic G44.029
      intractable G44.021
      not intractable G44.029
    episodic G44.019
      intractable G44.011
      not intractable G44.019
    intractable G44.001
    not intractable G44.009
  cough (primary) G44.83
  daily chronic R51.9
  drug-induced NEC G44.40
    intractable G44.41
    not intractable G44.40
  exertional (primary) G44.84
  histamine G44.009
    intractable G44.001
    not intractable G44.009
  hypnic G44.81
  lumbar puncture G97.1
  medication overuse G44.40
    intractable G44.41
    not intractable G44.40
  menstrual —see Migraine, menstrual
  migraine (type) —see also Migraine
    G43.909
  nasal septum R51.9
  neuralgiform, short lasting unilateral, with
    conjunctival injection and tearing (SUNCT)
    G44.059
    intractable G44.051
    not intractable G44.059
  new daily persistent (NDPH) G44.52
  orgasmic G44.82
  periodic syndromes in adults and children
    G43.C0
    with refractory migraine G43.C1
    intractable G43.C1
    not intractable G43.C0
    without refractory migraine G43.C0
  postspinal puncture G97.1
  post-traumatic G44.309
    acute G44.319
      intractable G44.311
      not intractable G44.319
    chronic G44.329
      intractable G44.321
      not intractable G44.329
    intractable G44.301
    not intractable G44.309
  pre-menstrual —see Migraine, menstrual
  preorgasmic G44.82
  primary
    cough G44.83
    exertional G44.84
    stabbing G44.85
    thunderclap G44.53
  rebound G44.40
    intractable G44.41
    not intractable G44.40
  short lasting unilateral neuralgiform, with
    conjunctival injection and tearing (SUNCT)
    G44.059
    intractable G44.051
    not intractable G44.059
  specified syndrome NEC G44.89
  spinal and epidural anesthesia - induced
    T88.59
    in labor and delivery O74.5
    in pregnancy O29.4-●
    postpartum, puerperal O89.4
  spinal fluid loss (from puncture) G97.1
  stabbing (primary) G44.85

Headache (Continued)
  tension (-type) G44.209
    chronic G44.229
      intractable G44.221
      not intractable G44.229
    episodic G44.219
      intractable G44.211
      not intractable G44.219
    intractable G44.201
    not intractable G44.209
  thunderclap (primary) G44.53
  vascular NEC G44.1
Healthy
  infant
    accompanying sick mother Z76.3
    receiving care Z76.2
  person accompanying sick person Z76.3
Hearing examination Z01.10
  with abnormal findings NEC Z01.118
  infant or child (over 28 days old) Z00.129
    with abnormal findings Z00.121
  following failed hearing screening Z01.110
  for hearing conservation and treatment Z01.12
Heart —see condition
▶carcinoid - see Syndrome, carcinoid, heart
Heart beat
  abnormality R00.9
    specified NEC R00.8
  awareness R00.2
  rapid R00.0
  slow R00.1
Heartburn R12
  psychogenic F45.8
Heartland virus disease A93.8
Heat (effects) T67.9
  apoplexy T67.01
  burn —see also Burn L55.9
  collapse T67.1
  cramps T67.2
  dermatitis or eczema L59.0
  edema T67.7
  erythema - code by site under Burn, first degree
  excessive T67.9
    specified effect NEC T67.8
  exhaustion T67.5
    anhydrotic T67.3
    due to
      salt (and water) depletion T67.4
      water depletion T67.3
        with salt depletion T67.4
  fatigue (transient) T67.6
  fever T67.01
  hyperpyrexia T67.01
  prickly L74.0
  prostration —see Heat, exhaustion
  pyrexia T67.01
  rash L74.0
  specified effect NEC T67.8
  stroke T67.01
    exertional T67.02
    specified NEC T67.09
  sunburn —see Sunburn
  syncope T67.1
Heavy-for-dates NEC (infant) (4000g to 4499g) P08.1
  exceptionally (4500g or more) P08.0
Hebephrenia, hebephrenic (schizophrenia) F20.1
Heberden's disease or nodes (with arthropathy)
    M15.1
Hebra's
  pityriasis L26
  prurigo L28.2
Heel —see condition
Heerfordt's disease D86.89
Hegglin's anomaly or syndrome D72.0
Heilmeyer-Schoner disease D45
Heine-Medin disease A80.9
Heinz body anemia, congenital D58.2
Heliophobia F40.228
Heller's disease or syndrome F84.3
HELLP syndrome (hemolysis, elevated liver
    enzymes and low platelet count) O14.2-●
  complicating
    childbirth O14.24
    puerperium O14.25
Helminthiasis —see also Infestation, helminth
  Ancylostoma B76.0
  intestinal B82.0
    mixed types (types classifiable to more than
      one of the titles B65.0-B81.3 and B81.8)
      B81.4
    specified type NEC B81.8

▶ New   ⇒ Revised   ~~deleted~~ Deleted   ● Use Additional Character(s)

Helminthiasis *(Continued)*
mixed types (intestinal) (types classifiable to more than one of the titles B65.0-B81.3 and B81.8) B81.4
Necator (americanus) B76.1
specified type NEC B83.8
Heloma L84
Hemangioblastoma —*see* Neoplasm, connective tissue, uncertain behavior
malignant —*see* Neoplasm, connective tissue, malignant
Hemangioendothelioma —*see also* Neoplasm, uncertain behavior, by site
benign D18.00
intra-abdominal D18.03
intracranial D18.02
skin D18.01
specified site NEC D18.09
bone (diffuse) —*see* Neoplasm, bone, malignant
epithelioid —*see also* Neoplasm, uncertain behavior, by site
malignant —*see* Neoplasm, malignant, by site
malignant —*see* Neoplasm, connective tissue, malignant
Hemangiofibroma —*see* Neoplasm, benign, by site
Hemangiolipoma —*see* Lipoma
Hemangioma D18.00
arteriovenous D18.00
intra-abdominal D18.03
intracranial D18.02
skin D18.01
specified site NEC D18.09
capillary I78.1
intra-abdominal D18.03
intracranial D18.02
skin D18.01
specified site NEC D18.09
cavernous D18.00
intra-abdominal D18.03
intracranial D18.02
skin D18.01
specified site NEC D18.09
epithelioid D18.00
intra-abdominal D18.03
intracranial D18.02
skin D18.01
specified site NEC D18.09
histiocytoid D18.00
intra-abdominal D18.03
intracranial D18.02
skin D18.01
specified site NEC D18.09
infantile D18.00
intra-abdominal D18.03
intracranial D18.02
skin D18.01
specified site NEC D18.09
intra-abdominal D18.03
intracranial D18.02
intramuscular D18.00
intra-abdominal D18.03
intracranial D18.02
skin D18.01
specified site NEC D18.09
intrathoracic structures D18.09
juvenile D18.00
malignant —*see* Neoplasm, connective tissue, malignant
plexiform D18.00
intra-abdominal D18.03
intracranial D18.02
skin D18.01
specified site NEC D18.09
racemose D18.00
intra-abdominal D18.03
intracranial D18.02
skin D18.01
specified site NEC D18.09
sclerosing —*see* Neoplasm, skin, benign
simplex D18.00
intra-abdominal D18.03
intracranial D18.02
skin D18.01
specified site NEC D18.09
skin D18.01
specified site NEC D18.09
venous D18.00
intra-abdominal D18.03
intracranial D18.02
skin D18.01
specified site NEC D18.09

Hemangioma *(Continued)*
verrucous keratotic D18.00
intra-abdominal D18.03
intracranial D18.02
skin D18.01
specified site NEC D18.09
Hemangiomatosis (systemic) I78.8
involving single site —*see* Hemangioma
Hemangiopericytoma —*see also* Neoplasm, connective tissue, uncertain behavior
benign —*see* Neoplasm, connective tissue, benign
malignant —*see* Neoplasm, connective tissue, malignant
Hemangiosarcoma —*see* Neoplasm, connective tissue, malignant
Hemarthrosis (nontraumatic) M25.00
ankle M25.07-●
elbow M25.02-●
foot joint M25.07-●
hand joint M25.04-●
hip M25.05-●
in hemophilic arthropathy —*see* Arthropathy, hemophilic
knee M25.06-●
shoulder M25.01-●
specified joint NEC M25.08
traumatic —*see* Sprain, by site
vertebrae M25.08
wrist M25.03-●
Hematemesis K92.0
with ulcer - code by site under Ulcer, with hemorrhage K27.4
newborn, neonatal P54.0
due to swallowed maternal blood P78.2
Hematidrosis L74.8
Hematinuria —*see also* Hemoglobinuria
malarial B50.8
Hematobilia K83.8
Hematocele
female NEC N94.89
with ectopic pregnancy O00.90
with intrauterine pregnancy O00.91
ovary N83.8
male N50.1
Hematochezia —*see also* Melena K92.1
Hematochyluria —*see also* Infestation, filarial
schistosomiasis (bilharziasis) B65.0
Hematocolpos (with hematometra or hematosalpinx) N89.7
Hematocornea —*see* Pigmentation, cornea, stromal
Hematogenous —*see* condition
Hematoma (traumatic) (skin surface intact) —*see also* Contusion
with
injury of internal organs —*see* Injury, by site
open wound —*see* Wound, open
amputation stump (surgical) (late) T87.89
aorta, dissecting I71.00
abdominal I71.02
thoracic (*see also* Dissection, aorta, thoracic) I71.019
thoracoabdominal I71.03
aortic intramural —*see* Dissection, aorta
arterial (complicating trauma) —*see* Injury, blood vessel, by site
auricle —*see* Contusion, ear
nontraumatic —*see* Disorder, pinna, hematoma
birth injury NEC P15.8
brain (traumatic)
with
cerebral laceration or contusion (diffuse) —*see* Injury, intracranial, diffuse
focal —*see* Injury, intracranial, focal
cerebellar, traumatic S06.37-●
intracerebral, traumatic —*see* Injury, intracranial, intracerebral hemorrhage
newborn NEC P52.4
birth injury P10.1
nontraumatic —*see* Hemorrhage, intracranial
subarachnoid, arachnoid, traumatic —*see* Injury, intracranial, subarachnoid hemorrhage
subdural, traumatic —*see* Injury, intracranial, subdural hemorrhage
breast (nontraumatic) N64.89
broad ligament (nontraumatic) N83.7
traumatic S37.892
cerebellar, traumatic S06.37-●

Hematoma *(Continued)*
cerebral —*see* Hematoma, brain
cerebrum S06.36-●
left S06.35-●
right S06.34-●
cesarean delivery wound O90.2
complicating delivery (perineal) (pelvic) (vagina) (vulva) O71.7
corpus cavernosum (nontraumatic) N48.89
epididymis (nontraumatic) N50.1
epidural (traumatic) —*see* Injury, intracranial, epidural hemorrhage
spinal —*see* Injury, spinal cord, by region
episiotomy O90.2
face, birth injury P15.4
genital organ NEC (nontraumatic)
female (nonobstetric) N94.89
traumatic S30.202
male N50.1
traumatic S30.201
internal organs —*see* Injury, by site
intracerebral, traumatic —*see* Injury, intracranial, intracerebral hemorrhage
intraoperative —*see* Complications, intraoperative, hemorrhage
labia (nontraumatic) (nonobstetric) N90.8
liver (subcapsular) (nontraumatic) K76.89
birth injury P15.0
mediastinum —*see* Injury, intrathoracic
mesosalpinx (nontraumatic) N83.7
traumatic S37.898
muscle - code by site under Contusion
nontraumatic
muscle M79.81
soft tissue M79.81
obstetrical surgical wound O90.2
orbit, orbital (nontraumatic) —*see also* Hemorrhage, orbit
traumatic —*see* Contusion, orbit
pelvis (female) (nontraumatic) (nonobstetric) N94.89
obstetric O71.7
traumatic —*see* Injury, by site
penis (nontraumatic) N48.89
birth injury P15.5
perianal (nontraumatic) K64.5
perineal S30.23
complicating delivery O71.7
perirenal —*see* Injury, kidney
peritoneal K66.1
pinna —*see* Contusion, ear
nontraumatic —*see* Disorder, pinna, hematoma
placenta O43.89-●
postoperative (postprocedural) —*see* Complication, postprocedural, hematoma
retroperitoneal (nontraumatic) K68.3
traumatic S36.892
scrotum, superficial S30.22
birth injury P15.5
seminal vesicle (nontraumatic) N50.1
traumatic S37.892
spermatic cord (traumatic) S37.892
nontraumatic N50.1
spinal (cord) (meninges) —*see also* Injury, spinal cord, by region
newborn (birth injury) P11.5
spleen D73.5
intraoperative —*see* Complications, intraoperative, hemorrhage, spleen
postprocedural (postoperative) —*see* Complications, postprocedural, hemorrhage, spleen
sternocleidomastoid, birth injury P15.2
sternomastoid, birth injury P15.2
subarachnoid (traumatic) —*see* Injury, intracranial, subarachnoid hemorrhage
newborn (nontraumatic) P52.5
due to birth injury P10.3
nontraumatic —*see* Hemorrhage, intracranial, subarachnoid
subdural (traumatic) —*see* Injury, intracranial, subdural hemorrhage
newborn (localized) P52.8
birth injury P10.0
nontraumatic —*see* Hemorrhage, intracranial, subdural
superficial, newborn P54.5
testis (nontraumatic) N50.1
birth injury P15.5
tunica vaginalis (nontraumatic) N50.1

Hematoma (Continued)
  umbilical cord, complicating delivery O69.5
  uterine ligament (broad) (nontraumatic) N83.7
    traumatic S37.892
  vagina (ruptured) (nontraumatic) N89.8
    complicating delivery O71.7
  vas deferens (nontraumatic) N50.1
    traumatic S37.892
  vitreous —see Hemorrhage, vitreous
  vulva (nontraumatic) (nonobstetric) N90.89
    complicating delivery O71.7
    newborn (birth injury) P15.5
Hematometra N85.7
  with hematocolpos N89.7
Hematomyelia (central) G95.19
  newborn (birth injury) P11.5
  traumatic T14.8
Hematomyelitis G04.90
Hematoperitoneum —see Hemoperitoneum
Hematophobia F40.230
Hematopneumothorax (see Hemothorax)
Hematopoiesis, cyclic D70.4
Hematoporphyria —see Porphyria
Hematorachis, hematorrhachis G95.19
  newborn (birth injury) P11.5
Hematosalpinx N83.6
  with
    hematocolpos N89.7
    hematometra N85.7
      with hematocolpos N89.7
  infectional —see Salpingitis
Hematospermia R36.1
Hematothorax (see Hemothorax)
Hematuria R31.9
  benign (familial) (of childhood) —see also
    Hematuria, idiopathic
    essential microscopic R31.1
  due to sulphonamide, sulfonamide —see Table of
    Drugs and Chemicals, by drug
  endemic —see also Schistosomiasis B65.0
  gross R31.0
  idiopathic N02.9
    with glomerular lesion
      C3
        glomerulonephritis N02.A
        glomerulopathy N02.A
          with dense deposit disease N02.6
      crescentic (diffuse) glomerulonephritis
        N02.7
      dense deposit disease N02.6
      endocapillary proliferative
        glomerulonephritis N02.4
      focal and segmental hyalinosis or sclerosis
        N02.1
      membranoproliferative (diffuse) N02.5
      membranous (diffuse) N02.2
      mesangial proliferative (diffuse) N02.3
      mesangiocapillary (diffuse) N02.5
      minor abnormality N02.0
      proliferative NEC N02.8
      specified pathology NEC N02.8
  intermittent —see Hematuria, idiopathic
  malarial B50.8
  microscopic NEC (with symptoms) R31.29
    asymptomatic R31.21
    benign essential R31.1
  paroxysmal —see also Hematuria, idiopathic
    nocturnal D59.5
  persistent —see Hematuria, idiopathic
  recurrent —see Hematuria, idiopathic
  tropical —see also Schistosomiasis B65.0
  tuberculous A18.13
Hemeralopia (day blindness) H53.11
  vitamin A deficiency E50.5
Hemi-akinesia R41.4
Hemianalgesia R20.0
Hemianencephaly Q00.0
Hemianesthesia R20.0
Hemianopia, hemianopsia (heteronymous)
  H53.47
  homonymous H53.46-●
  syphilitic A52.71
Hemiathetosis R25.8
Hemiatrophy R68.89
  cerebellar G31.9
  face, facial, progressive (Romberg) G51.8
  tongue K14.8
Hemiballism (us) G25.5
Hemicardia Q24.8
Hemicephalus, hemicephaly Q00.0
Hemichorea G25.5
Hemicolitis, left —see Colitis, left sided

Hemicrania
  congenital malformation Q00.0
  continua G44.51
  meaning migraine —see also Migraine G43.909
  paroxysmal G44.039
    chronic G44.049
      intractable G44.041
      not intractable G44.049
    episodic G44.039
      intractable G44.031
      not intractable G44.039
    intractable G44.031
    not intractable G44.039
Hemidystrophy —see Hemiatrophy
Hemiectromelia Q73.8
Hemihypalgesia R20.8
Hemihypesthesia R20.1
Hemi-inattention R41.4
Hemimegalencephaly Q04.5
Hemimelia Q73.8
  lower limb —see Defect, reduction, lower limb
    specified type NEC
  upper limb —see Defect, reduction, upper limb,
    specified type NEC
Hemiparalysis —see Hemiplegia
Hemiparesis —see Hemiplegia
Hemiparesthesia R20.2
Hemiparkinsonism G20.C
Hemiplegia G81.9-●
  alternans facialis G83.89
  ascending NEC G81.90
    spinal G95.89
  congenital (cerebral) G80.8
    spastic G80.2
  embolic (current episode) I63.4-●
  flaccid G81.0-●
  following
    cerebrovascular disease I69.959
      cerebral infarction I69.35-●
      intracerebral hemorrhage I69.15-●
      nontraumatic intracranial hemorrhage NEC
        I69.25-●
      specified disease NEC I69.85-●
      stroke NOS I69.35-●
      subarachnoid hemorrhage I69.05-●
  hysterical F44.4
  newborn NEC P91.88
    birth injury P11.9
  spastic G81.1-●
    congenital G80.2
  thrombotic (current episode) I63.3-●
Hemisection, spinal cord —see Injury, spinal cord,
  by region
Hemispasm (facial) R25.2
Hemisporosis B48.8
Hemitremor R25.1
Hemivertebra Q76.49
  failure of segmentation with scoliosis Q76.3
  fusion with scoliosis Q76.3
Hemochromatosis E83.119
  with refractory anemia D46.1
  due to repeated red blood cell transfusion E83.111
  hereditary (primary) E83.110
  neonatal P78.84
  primary E83.110
  specified NEC E83.118
Hemoglobin —see also condition
  abnormal (disease) —see Disease, hemoglobin
  AS genotype D57.3
  Constant Spring D58.2
  E-beta thalassemia D56.5
  fetal, hereditary persistence (HPFH) D56.4
  H Constant Spring D56.0
  low NOS D64.9
  S (Hb S), heterozygous D57.3
Hemoglobinemia D59.9
  due to blood transfusion T80.89
  paroxysmal D59.6
    nocturnal D59.5
Hemoglobinopathy (mixed) D58.2
  with thalassemia D56.8
  sickle-cell D57.1
    with thalassemia D57.40
      with
        acute chest syndrome D57.411
        cerebral vascular involvement D57.413
        crisis (painful) D57.419
          with specified complication NEC
            D57.418
        pain (vaso-occlusive) D57.419
        splenic sequestration D57.412
      without crisis D57.40

Hemoglobinuria R82.3
  with anemia, hemolytic, acquired (chronic) NEC
    D59.6
  cold (paroxysmal) (with Raynaud's syndrome)
    D59.6
    agglutinin D59.12
  due to exertion or hemolysis NEC D59.6
  intermittent D59.6
  malarial B50.8
  march D59.6
  nocturnal (paroxysmal) D59.5
  paroxysmal (cold) D59.6
    nocturnal D59.5
Hemolymphangioma D18.1
Hemolysis
  intravascular
    with
      abortion —see Abortion, by type,
        complicated by, hemorrhage
      ectopic or molar pregnancy O08.1
      hemorrhage
        antepartum —see Hemorrhage,
          antepartum, with coagulation
          defect
        intrapartum —see also Hemorrhage,
          complicating, delivery O67.0
      postpartum O72.3
  neonatal (excessive) P58.9
    specified NEC P58.8
Hemolytic —see condition
Hemopericardium I31.2
  following acute myocardial infarction (current
    complication) I23.0
  newborn P54.8
  traumatic —see Injury, heart, with
    hemopericardium
Hemoperitoneum K66.1
  infectional K65.9
  traumatic S36.899
    with open wound —see Wound, open, with,
      abdominal, wall, by site if known,
      penetration into peritoneal cavity
Hemophilia (classical) (familial) (hereditary) D66
  A D66
  B D67
  C D68.1
  acquired D68.311
  autoimmune D68.311
  calcipriva —see also Defect, coagulation D68.4
  nonfamilial —see also Defect, coagulation D68.4
  secondary D68.311
  vascular —see Disease, von Willebrand
Hemophthalmos H44.81-●
Hemopneumothorax —see also Hemothorax
  traumatic S27.2
Hemoptysis R04.2
  newborn P26.9
  tuberculous —see Tuberculosis, pulmonary
Hemorrhage, hemorrhagic (concealed) R58
  abdomen R58
  accidental antepartum —see Hemorrhage,
    antepartum
  acute idiopathic pulmonary, in infants R04.81
  adenoid J35.8
  adrenal (capsule) (gland) E27.49
    medulla E27.8
    newborn P54.4
  after delivery —see Hemorrhage, postpartum
  alveolar
    lung, newborn P26.8
    process K08.89
  alveolus K08.89
  amputation stump (surgical) T87.89
  anemia (chronic) D50.0
    acute D62
  antepartum (with) O46.90
    with coagulation defect O46.00-●
      afibrinogenemia O46.01-●
      disseminated intravascular coagulation
        O46.02-●
      hypofibrinogenemia O46.01-●
      specified defect NEC O46.09-●
    before 20 weeks gestation O20.9
      specified type NEC O20.8
      threatened abortion O20.0
    due to
      abruptio placenta —see also Abruptio
        placentae O45.9-●
      leiomyoma, uterus —see Hemorrhage,
        antepartum, specified cause NEC
      placenta previa O44.1-●
      specified cause NEC —see subcategory O46.8X-●

▶ New   ⇒ Revised   ~~deleted~~ Deleted   ● Use Additional Character(s)

Hemorrhage, hemorrhagic (Continued)
anus (sphincter) K62.5
apoplexy (stroke) —see Hemorrhage,
   intracranial, intracerebral
arachnoid —see Hemorrhage, intracranial,
   subarachnoid
artery R58
  brain —see Hemorrhage, intracranial,
    intracerebral
basilar (ganglion) I61.0
bladder N32.89
bowel K92.2
  newborn P54.3
brain (miliary) (nontraumatic) —see
   Hemorrhage, intracranial, intracerebral
  due to
    birth injury P10.1
    syphilis A52.05
  epidural or extradural (traumatic) —see Injury,
    intracranial, epidural hemorrhage
  newborn P52.4
    birth injury P10.1
  subarachnoid —see Hemorrhage, intracranial,
    subarachnoid
  subdural —see Hemorrhage, intracranial,
    subdural
brainstem (nontraumatic) I61.3
  traumatic S06.38-●
breast N64.59
bronchial tube —see Hemorrhage, lung
bronchopulmonary —see Hemorrhage,
   lung
bronchus —see Hemorrhage, lung
bulbar I61.5
capillary I78.8
  primary D69.8
cecum K92.2
cerebellar, cerebellum (nontraumatic)
   I61.4
  newborn P52.6
  traumatic S06.37-●
cerebral, cerebrum —see also Hemorrhage,
   intracranial, intracerebral
  lobe I61.1
  newborn (anoxic) P52.4
    birth injury P10.1
cerebromeningeal I61.8
cerebrospinal —see Hemorrhage, intracranial,
   intracerebral
cervix (uteri) (stump) NEC N88.8
chamber, anterior (eye) —see Hyphema
childbirth —see Hemorrhage, complicating,
   delivery
choroid H31.30-●
  expulsive H31.31-●
ciliary body —see Hyphema
cochlea —see subcategory H83.8
colon K92.2
complicating
  abortion —see Abortion, by type, complicated
    by, hemorrhage
  delivery O67.9
    associated with coagulation defect
      (afibrinogenemia) (DIC)
      (hyperfibrinolysis) O67.0
    specified cause NEC O67.8
  surgical procedure —see Hemorrhage,
    intraoperative
conjunctiva H11.3-●
  newborn P54.8
cord, newborn (stump) P51.9
corpus luteum (ruptured) cyst N83.1-●
cortical (brain) I61.1
cranial —see Hemorrhage, intracranial
cutaneous R23.3
  due to autosensitivity, erythrocyte D69.2
  newborn P54.5
delayed
  following ectopic or molar pregnancy
    O08.1
  postpartum O72.2
diathesis (familial) D69.9
disease D69.9
  newborn P53
  specified type NEC D69.8
due to or associated with
  afibrinogenemia or other coagulation defect
    (conditions in categories D65-D69)
    antepartum —see Hemorrhage, antepartum,
      with coagulation defect
      intrapartum O67.0
  dental implant M27.61

Hemorrhage, hemorrhagic (Continued)
due to or associated with (Continued)
  device, implant or graft —see also
    Complications, by site and type,
    specified NEC T85.838
    arterial graft NEC T82.838
    breast T85.838
    catheter NEC T85.838
      dialysis (renal) T82.838
        intraperitoneal T85.838
      infusion NEC T82.838
        spinal (epidural) (subdural)
          T85.830
      urinary (indwelling) T83.83
    electronic (electrode) (pulse generator)
      (stimulator)
      bone T84.83
      cardiac T82.837
      nervous system (brain) (peripheral
        nerve) (spinal) T85.830
      urinary T83.83
    fixation, internal (orthopedic) NEC T84.83
    gastrointestinal (bile duct) (esophagus)
      T85.838
    genital NEC T83.83
    heart NEC T82.837
    joint prosthesis T84.83
    ocular (corneal graft) (orbital implant) NEC
      T85.838
    orthopedic NEC T84.83
      bone graft T86.838
    specified NEC T85.838
    urinary NEC T83.83
    vascular NEC T82.838
    ventricular intracranial shunt T85.838
duodenum, duodenal K92.2
  ulcer —see Ulcer, duodenum, with
    hemorrhage
dura mater —see Hemorrhage, intracranial,
   subdural
endotracheal —see Hemorrhage, lung
epicranial subaponeurotic (massive), birth injury
   P12.2
epidural (traumatic) —see also Injury,
   intracranial, epidural hemorrhage
  nontraumatic I62.1
esophagus K22.89
  varix I85.01
    secondary I85.11
excessive, following ectopic gestation
   (subsequent episode) O08.1
extradural (traumatic) —see Injury, intracranial,
   epidural hemorrhage
  birth injury P10.8
  newborn (anoxic) (nontraumatic) P52.8
  nontraumatic I62.1
eye NEC H57.89
  fundus —see Hemorrhage, retina
  lid —see Disorder, eyelid, specified type NEC
fallopian tube N83.6
fibrinogenolysis —see Fibrinolysis
fibrinolytic (acquired) —see Fibrinolysis
from
  ear (nontraumatic) —see Otorrhagia
  tracheostomy stoma J95.01
fundus, eye —see Hemorrhage, retina
funis —see Hemorrhage, umbilicus, cord
gastric —see Hemorrhage, stomach
gastroenteric K92.2
  newborn P54.3
gastrointestinal (tract) K92.2
  newborn P54.3
genital organ, male N50.1
genitourinary (tract) NOS R31.9
gingiva K06.8
globe (eye) —see Hemophthalmos
graafian follicle cyst (ruptured) N83.0-●
gum K06.8
heart I51.89
hypopharyngeal (throat) R04.1
intermenstrual (regular) N92.3
  irregular N92.1
internal (organs) NEC R58
  capsule I61.0
  ear —see subcategory H83.8
  newborn P54.8
intestine K92.2
  newborn P54.3
intra-abdominal R58
intra-alveolar (lung), newborn P26.8
intracerebral (nontraumatic) —see Hemorrhage,
   intracranial, intracerebral

Hemorrhage, hemorrhagic (Continued)
intracranial (nontraumatic) I62.9
  birth injury P10.9
  epidural, nontraumatic I62.1
  extradural, nontraumatic I62.1
  intracerebral (nontraumatic) (in) I61.9
    brain stem I61.3
    cerebellum I61.4
    hemisphere I61.2
      cortical (superficial) I61.1
      subcortical (deep) I61.0
    intraoperative
      during a nervous system procedure
        G97.31
      during other procedure G97.32
    intraventricular I61.5
    multiple localized I61.6
    newborn P52.4
      birth injury P10.1
    postprocedural
      following a nervous system procedure
        G97.51
      following other procedure
        G97.52
    specified NEC I61.8
    superficial I61.1
    traumatic —see Injury, intracranial,
      intracerebral hemorrhage,
      traumatic
      focal —see Injury, intracranial, focal
  newborn P52.9
    specified NEC P52.8
  subarachnoid (nontraumatic) (from) I60.9
    intracranial (cerebral) artery I60.7
      anterior communicating I60.2
      basilar I60.4
      carotid siphon and bifurcation
        I60.0-●
      communicating I60.7
        anterior I60.2
        posterior I60.3-●
      middle cerebral I60.1-●
      posterior communicating I60.3-●
      specified artery NEC I60.6
      vertebral I60.5-●
    newborn P52.5
      birth injury P10.3
    specified NEC I60.8
    traumatic S06.6X-●
  subdural (nontraumatic) I62.00
    acute I62.01
    birth injury P10.0
    chronic I62.03
    newborn (anoxic) (hypoxic) P52.8
      birth injury P10.0
    spinal G95.19
    subacute I62.02
    traumatic —see Injury, intracranial,
      subdural hemorrhage
  traumatic —see Injury, intracranial, focal brain
    injury
intramedullary NEC G95.19
intraocular —see Hemophthalmos
intraoperative, intraprocedural —see
   Complication, hemorrhage (hematoma),
   intraoperative (intraprocedural), by site
intrapartum —see Hemorrhage, complicating,
   delivery
intrapelvic
  female N94.89
  male K66.1
intraperitoneal K66.1
intrapontine I61.3
intraprocedural —see Complication,
   hemorrhage (hematoma), intraoperative
   (intraprocedural), by site
intrauterine N85.7
  complicating delivery —see also Hemorrhage,
    complicating, delivery O67.9
  postpartum —see Hemorrhage, postpartum
intraventricular I61.5
  newborn (nontraumatic) —see also Newborn,
    affected by, hemorrhage P52.3
    due to birth injury P10.2
    grade
      1 P52.0
      2 P52.1
      3 P52.21
      4 P52.22
intravesical N32.89
iris (postinfectional) (postinflammatory)
   (toxic) —see Hyphema

Hemorrhage, hemorrhagic (Continued)
joint (nontraumatic) —see Hemarthrosis
kidney N28.89
knee (joint) (nontraumatic) —see Hemarthrosis, knee
labyrinth —see subcategory H83.8
lenticular striate artery I61.0
ligature, vessel —see Hemorrhage, postoperative
liver K76.89
lung R04.89
newborn P26.9
massive P26.1
specified NEC P26.8
tuberculous —see Tuberculosis, pulmonary
massive umbilical, newborn P51.0
mediastinum —see Hemorrhage, lung
medulla I61.3
membrane (brain) I60.8
spinal cord —see Hemorrhage, spinal cord
meninges, meningeal (brain) (middle) I60.8
spinal cord —see Hemorrhage, spinal cord
mesentery K66.1
metritis —see Endometritis
mouth K13.79
mucous membrane NEC R58
newborn P54.8
muscle M62.89
nail (subungual) L60.8
nasal turbinate R04.0
newborn P54.8
navel, newborn P51.9
newborn P54.9
specified NEC P54.8
nipple N64.59
nose R04.0
newborn P54.8
omentum K66.1
optic nerve (sheath) H47.02-•
orbit, orbital H05.23-•
ovary NEC N83.8
oviduct N83.6
pancreas K86.89
parathyroid (gland) (spontaneous) E21.4
parturition —see Hemorrhage, complicating, delivery
penis N48.89
pericardium, pericarditis I31.2
peritoneum, peritoneal K66.1
peritonsillar tissue J35.8
due to infection J36
petechial R23.3
due to autosensitivity, erythrocyte D69.2
pituitary (gland) E23.6
pleura —see Hemorrhage, lung
polioencephalitis, superior E51.2
polymyositis —see Polymyositis
pons, pontine I61.3
posterior fossa (nontraumatic) I61.8
newborn P52.6
postmenopausal N95.0
postnasal R04.0
postoperative —see Complications, postprocedural, hemorrhage, by site
postpartum NEC (following delivery of placenta) O72.1
delayed or secondary O72.2
retained placenta O72.0
third stage O72.0
pregnancy —see Hemorrhage, antepartum
preretinal —see Hemorrhage, retina
prostate N42.1
puerperal —see Hemorrhage, postpartum
delayed or secondary O72.2
pulmonary R04.89
newborn P26.9
massive P26.1
specified NEC P26.8
tuberculous —see Tuberculosis, pulmonary
purpura (primary) D69.3
rectum (sphincter) K62.5
newborn P54.2
recurring, following initial hemorrhage at time of injury T79.2
renal N28.89
respiratory passage or tract R04.9
specified NEC R04.89
retina, retinal (vessels) H35.6-•
diabetic —see Microaneurysm, retinal, diabetic
retroperitoneal K68.3
scalp R58
scrotum N50.1

Hemorrhage, hemorrhagic (Continued)
secondary (nontraumatic) R58
following initial hemorrhage at time of injury T79.2
seminal vesicle N50.1
skin R23.3
newborn P54.5
slipped umbilical ligature P51.8
spermatic cord N50.1
spinal (cord) G95.19
newborn (birth injury) P11.5
spleen D73.5
intraoperative —see Complications, intraoperative, hemorrhage, spleen
postprocedural —see Complications, postprocedural, hemorrhage, spleen
stomach K92.2
newborn P54.3
ulcer —see Ulcer, stomach, with hemorrhage
subarachnoid (nontraumatic) —see Hemorrhage, intracranial, subarachnoid
subconjunctival —see also Hemorrhage, conjunctiva
birth injury P15.3
subcortical (brain) I61.0
subcutaneous R23.3
subdiaphragmatic R58
subdural (acute) (nontraumatic) —see Hemorrhage, intracranial, subdural
subependymal
newborn P52.0
with intraventricular extension P52.1
and intracerebral extension P52.22
subgaleal P12.2
subhyaloid —see Hemorrhage, retina
subperiosteal —see Disorder, bone, specified type NEC
subretinal —see Hemorrhage, retina
subtentorial —see Hemorrhage, intracranial, subdural
subungual L60.8
suprarenal (capsule) (gland) E27.49
newborn P54.4
tentorium (traumatic) NEC —see Hemorrhage, brain
newborn (birth injury) P10.4
testis N50.1
third stage (postpartum) O72.0
thorax —see Hemorrhage, lung
throat R04.1
thymus (gland) E32.8
thyroid (cyst) (gland) E07.89
tongue K14.8
tonsil J35.8
trachea —see Hemorrhage, lung
tracheobronchial R04.89
newborn P26.0
traumatic — code to specific injury
cerebellar —see Hemorrhage, brain
intracranial —see Hemorrhage, brain
recurring or secondary (following initial hemorrhage at time of injury) T79.2
tuberculous NEC —see also Tuberculosis, pulmonary A15.0
tunica vaginalis N50.1
ulcer - code by site under Ulcer, with hemorrhage K27.4
umbilicus, umbilical
cord
after birth, newborn P51.9
complicating delivery O69.5
newborn P51.9
massive P51.0
slipped ligature P51.8
stump P51.9
urethra (idiopathic) N36.8
uterus, uterine (abnormal) N93.9
climacteric N92.4
complicating delivery —see Hemorrhage, complicating, delivery
dysfunctional or functional N93.8
intermenstrual (regular) N92.3
irregular N92.1
postmenopausal N95.0
postpartum —see Hemorrhage, postpartum
preclimacteric or premenopausal N92.4
prepubertal N93.8
pubertal N92.2
vagina (abnormal) N93.9
newborn P54.6
vas deferens N50.1
vasa previa O69.4

Hemorrhage, hemorrhagic (Continued)
ventricular I61.5
vesical N32.89
viscera NEC R58
newborn P54.8
vitreous (humor) (intraocular) H43.1-•
vulva N90.89
Hemorrhoids (bleeding) (without mention of degree) K64.9
1st degree (grade/stage I) (without prolapse outside of anal canal) K64.0
2nd degree (grade/stage II) (that prolapse with straining but retract spontaneously) K64.1
3rd degree (grade/stage III) (that prolapse with straining and require manual replacement back inside anal canal) K64.2
4th degree (grade/stage IV) (with prolapsed tissue that cannot be manually replaced) K64.3
complicating
pregnancy O22.4
puerperium O87.2
external K64.4
with
thrombosis K64.5
internal (without mention of degree) K64.8
prolapsed K64.8
skin tags
anus K64.4
residual K64.4
specified NEC K64.8
strangulated —see also Hemorrhoids, by degree K64.8
thrombosed —see also Hemorrhoids, by degree K64.5
ulcerated —see also Hemorrhoids, by degree K64.8
Hemosalpinx N83.6
with
hematocolpos N89.7
hematometra N85.7
with hematocolpos N89.7
Hemosiderosis (dietary) E83.19
pulmonary, idiopathic E83.1 [J84.03]
transfusion T80.89
Hemothorax (bacterial) (nontuberculous) J94.2
newborn P54.8
traumatic S27.1
with pneumothorax S27.2
tuberculous NEC A15.6
Henoch (-Schönlein) disease or syndrome (purpura) D69.0
Henpue, henpuye A66.6
Hepar lobatum (syphilitic) A52.74
Hepatalgia K76.89
Hepatitis K75.9
▶A —see Hepatitis, viral, type, A
acute B17.9
with coma K72.01
with hepatic failure —see Failure, hepatic
alcoholic —see Hepatitis, alcoholic
infectious B15.9
non-viral K72.0
▦viral (see also, Hepatitis, viral) B17.9
alcoholic (acute) (chronic) K70.10
with ascites K70.11
amebic —see Abscess, liver, amebic
anicteric (viral) —see Hepatitis, viral
antigen-associated (HAA) —see Hepatitis, B
Australia-antigen (positive) —see Hepatitis, B
autoimmune K75.4
B B19.10
~~with hepatic coma B19.11~~
▶with
▶delta (agent) —see Hepatitis, D
▶hepatic coma B19.11
acute B16.9
with
delta-agent (coinfection) (without hepatic coma) B16.1
with hepatic coma B16.0
hepatic coma (without delta-agent coinfection) B16.2
chronic B18.1
with delta-agent B18.0
bacterial NEC K75.89
C (viral) B19.20
with hepatic coma B19.21
acute B17.10
with hepatic coma B17.11
chronic B18.2
catarrhal (acute) B15.9
with hepatic coma B15.0

Hepatitis *(Continued)*
cholangiolitic K75.89
cholestatic K75.89
chronic K73.9
  active NEC K73.2
  ▶toxic —*see* Disease, liver, toxic, with, hepatitis, chronic, active
  lobular NEC K73.1
  persistent NEC K73.0
  specified NEC K73.8
  ▶toxic —*see* Disease, liver, toxic, with, hepatitis, chronic
  ▶viral —*see* Hepatitis, viral, chronic
cytomegaloviral B25.1
▶D B16.1
  ▶acute B16.1
    ▶with hepatic coma B16.0
    ▶in hepatitis B carrier B17.0
  ▶chronic B18.0
▶delta (agent) —*see* Hepatitis, D
due to ethanol (acute) (chronic) —*see* Hepatitis, alcoholic
epidemic B15.9
  with hepatic coma B15.0
fulminant NEC (viral) —*see* Hepatitis, viral
granulomatous NEC K75.3
herpesviral B00.81
history of
  B Z86.19
  C Z86.19
homologous serum —*see* Hepatitis, viral, type B
in (due to)
  mumps B26.81
  toxoplasmosis (acquired) B58.1
    congenital (active) P37.1 *[K77]*
infectious, infective B15.9
  acute (subacute) B17.9
  chronic B18.9
inoculation —*see* Hepatitis, viral, type B
interstitial (chronic) K74.69
ischemia, ischemic K72.00
lupoid NEC K75.2
malignant NEC (with hepatic failure) K72.90
  with coma K72.91
neonatal giant cell P59.29
neonatal (idiopathic) (toxic) P59.29
newborn P59.29
postimmunization —*see* Hepatitis, viral, type B
post-transfusion —*see* Hepatitis, viral, type B
reactive, nonspecific K75.2
serum —*see* Hepatitis, viral, type B
shock K72.00
specified type NEC
  with hepatic failure —*see* Failure, hepatic
syphilitic (late) A52.74
  congenital (early) A50.08 *[K77]*
    late A50.59 *[K77]*
  secondary A51.45
toxic —*see also* Disease, liver, toxic K71.6
tuberculous A18.83
viral, virus B19.9
  with hepatic coma B19.0
  acute B17.9
  chronic B18.9
    specified NEC B18.8
    type
      B B18.1
        with delta-agent B18.0
      C B18.2
      ▶D B18.0
  congenital P35.3
  coxsackie B33.8 *[K77]*
  cytomegalic inclusion B25.1
  in remission, any type — code to Hepatitis, chronic, by type
  non-A, non-B B17.8
  specified type NEC (with or without coma) B17.8
  type
    A B15.9
      with hepatic coma B15.0
    B B19.10
      with hepatic coma B19.11
      acute B16.9
        with
          delta-agent (coinfection) (without hepatic coma) B16.1
            with hepatic coma B16.0
          hepatic coma (without delta-agent coinfection) B16.2
      chronic B18.1
        with delta-agent B18.0

Hepatitis *(Continued)*
viral, virus *(Continued)*
  type *(Continued)*
    C B19.20
      with hepatic coma B19.21
      acute B17.10
        with hepatic coma B17.11
      chronic B18.2
    ▶D B16.1
      ▶acute B16.1
        ▶with hepatic coma B16.0
        ▶in hepatitis B carrier B17.0
      ▶chronic B18.0
    ▶delta (agent) —*see* Hepatitis, viral, type, D
    E B17.2
    non-A, non-B B17.8
Hepatization lung (acute) —*see* Pneumonia, lobar
Hepatoblastoma C22.2
Hepatocarcinoma C22.0
Hepatocholangiocarcinoma C22.0
Hepatocholangioma, benign D13.4
Hepatocholangitis K75.89
Hepatolenticular degeneration E83.01
Hepatoma (malignant) C22.0
  benign D13.4
  embryonal C22.0
Hepatomegaly —*see also* Hypertrophy, liver
  with splenomegaly R16.2
  congenital Q44.79
  in mononucleosis
    gammaherpesviral B27.09
    infectious specified NEC B27.89
Hepatoptosis K76.89
Hepatorenal syndrome following labor and delivery O90.41
Hepatosis K76.89
Hepatosplenomegaly R16.2
  hyperlipemic (Bürger-Grütz type) E78.3 *[K77]*
Hereditary —*see* condition
Hereditary alpha tryptasemia (syndrome) D89.44
Heredodegeneration, macular —*see* Dystrophy, retina
Heredopathia atactica polyneuritiformis G60.1
Heredosyphilis —*see* Syphilis, congenital
Herlitz' syndrome Q81.1
Hermansky-Pudlak syndrome E70.331
Hermaphrodite, hermaphroditism (true) Q56.0
  46,XX with streak gonads Q99.1
  46,XX/46,XY Q99.0
  46,XY with streak gonads Q99.1
  chimera 46,XX/46,XY Q99.0
Hernia, hernial (acquired) (recurrent) K46.9
  with
    gangrene —*see* Hernia, by site, with, gangrene
    incarceration —*see* Hernia, by site, with, obstruction
    irreducible —*see* Hernia, by site, with, obstruction
    obstruction —*see* Hernia, by site, with, obstruction
    strangulation —*see* Hernia, by site, with, obstruction
  abdomen, abdominal K46.9
    with
      gangrene (and obstruction) K46.1
      obstruction K46.0
    femoral —*see* Hernia, femoral
    incisional —*see* Hernia, incisional
    inguinal —*see* Hernia, inguinal
    specified site NEC K45.8
      with
        gangrene (and obstruction) K45.1
        obstruction K45.0
    umbilical —*see* Hernia, umbilical
    wall —*see* Hernia, ventral
  appendix —*see* Hernia, abdomen
  bladder (mucosa) (sphincter)
    congenital (female) (male) Q79.51
    female —*see* Cystocele
    male N32.89
  brain, congenital —*see* Encephalocele
  cartilage, vertebra —*see* Displacement, intervertebral disc
  cerebral, congenital —*see also* Encephalocele endaural Q01.8
  ciliary body (traumatic) S05.2-●
  colon —*see* Hernia, abdomen
  Cooper's —*see* Hernia, abdomen, specified site NEC
  crural —*see* Hernia, femoral

Hernia, hernial *(Continued)*
diaphragm, diaphragmatic K44.9
  with
    gangrene (and obstruction) K44.1
    obstruction K44.0
  congenital Q79.0
direct (inguinal) —*see* Hernia, inguinal
diverticulum, intestine —*see* Hernia, abdomen
double (inguinal) —*see* Hernia, inguinal, bilateral
due to adhesions (with obstruction) K56.50
epigastric —*see also* Hernia, ventral K43.9
esophageal hiatus —*see* Hernia, hiatal
external (inguinal) —*see* Hernia, inguinal
fallopian tube N83.4-●
fascia M62.89
femoral K41.90
  with
    gangrene (and obstruction) K41.40
      not specified as recurrent K41.40
      recurrent K41.41
    obstruction K41.30
      not specified as recurrent K41.30
      recurrent K41.31
  bilateral K41.20
    with
      gangrene (and obstruction) K41.10
        not specified as recurrent K41.10
        recurrent K41.11
      obstruction K41.00
        not specified as recurrent K41.00
        recurrent K41.01
    not specified as recurrent K41.20
    recurrent K41.21
  not specified as recurrent K41.90
  recurrent K41.91
  unilateral K41.90
    with
      gangrene (and obstruction) K41.40
        not specified as recurrent K41.40
        recurrent K41.41
      obstruction K41.30
        not specified as recurrent K41.30
        recurrent K41.31
    not specified as recurrent K41.90
    recurrent K41.91
foramen magnum G93.5
  congenital Q01.8
funicular (umbilical) —*see also* Hernia, umbilicus
  spermatic (cord) —*see* Hernia, inguinal
gastrointestinal tract —*see* Hernia, abdomen
Hesselbach's —*see* Hernia, femoral, specified site NEC
hiatal (esophageal) (sliding) K44.9
  with
    gangrene (and obstruction) K44.1
    obstruction K44.0
  congenital Q40.1
hypogastric —*see* Hernia, ventral
incarcerated —*see also* Hernia, by site, with obstruction
  with gangrene —*see* Hernia, by site, with gangrene
incisional K43.2
  with
    gangrene (and obstruction) K43.1
    obstruction K43.0
indirect (inguinal) —*see* Hernia, inguinal
inguinal (direct) (external) (funicular) (indirect) (internal) (oblique) (scrotal) (sliding) K40.90
  with
    gangrene (and obstruction) K40.40
      not specified as recurrent K40.40
      recurrent K40.41
    obstruction K40.30
      not specified as recurrent K40.30
      recurrent K40.31
  bilateral K40.20
    with
      gangrene (and obstruction) K40.10
        not specified as recurrent K40.10
        recurrent K40.11
      obstruction K40.00
        not specified as recurrent K40.00
        recurrent K40.01
    not specified as recurrent K40.20
    recurrent K40.21
  not specified as recurrent K40.90
  recurrent K40.91

Hernia, hernial (Continued)
 inguinal (Continued)
  unilateral K40.90
   with
    gangrene (and obstruction) K40.40
     not specified as recurrent K40.40
     recurrent K40.41
    obstruction K40.30
     not specified as recurrent K40.30
     recurrent K40.31
    not specified as recurrent K40.90
    recurrent K40.91
 internal —see also Hernia, abdomen
  inguinal —see Hernia, inguinal
 interstitial —see Hernia, abdomen
 intervertebral cartilage or disc —see
  Displacement, intervertebral disc
 intestine, intestinal —see Hernia, by site
 intra-abdominal —see Hernia, abdomen
 iris (traumatic) S05.2-•
 irreducible —see also Hernia, by site, with
  obstruction
  with gangrene —see Hernia, by site, with
   gangrene
 ischiatic —see Hernia, abdomen, specified site
  NEC
 ischiorectal —see Hernia, abdomen, specified
  site NEC
 lens (traumatic) S05.2-•
 linea (alba) (semilunaris) —see Hernia, ventral
 Littre's —see Hernia, abdomen
 lumbar —see Hernia, abdomen, specified site
  NEC
 lung (subcutaneous) J98.4
 mediastinum J98.59
 mesenteric (internal) —see Hernia, abdomen
 midline —see Hernia, ventral
 muscle (sheath) M62.89
 nucleus pulposus —see Displacement,
  intervertebral disc
 oblique (inguinal) —see Hernia, inguinal
 obstructive —see also Hernia, by site, with
  obstruction
  with gangrene —see Hernia, by site, with
   gangrene
 obturator —see Hernia, abdomen, specified site
  NEC
 omental —see Hernia, abdomen
 ovary N83.4-•
 oviduct N83.4-•
 paraesophageal —see also Hernia, diaphragm
  congenital Q40.1
 parastomal K43.5
  with
   gangrene (and obstruction) K43.4
   obstruction K43.3
 paraumbilical —see Hernia, umbilicus
 perineal —see Hernia, abdomen, specified site
  NEC
 Petit's —see Hernia, abdomen, specified site NEC
 postoperative —see Hernia, incisional
 pregnant uterus —see Abnormal, uterus in
  pregnancy or childbirth
 prevesical N32.89
 properitoneal —see Hernia, abdomen, specified
  site NEC
 pudendal —see Hernia, abdomen, specified site
  NEC
 rectovaginal N81.6
 retroperitoneal —see Hernia, abdomen, specified
  site NEC
 Richter's —see Hernia, abdomen, with
  obstruction
 Rieux's, Riex's —see Hernia, abdomen, specified
  site NEC
 sac condition (adhesion) (dropsy) (inflammation)
  (laceration) (suppuration) - code by site
  under Hernia
 sciatic —see Hernia, abdomen, specified site
  NEC
 scrotum, scrotal —see Hernia, inguinal
 sliding (inguinal) —see also Hernia, inguinal
  hiatus —see Hernia, hiatal
 spigelian —see Hernia, ventral
 spinal —see Spina bifida
 strangulated —see also Hernia, by site, with
  obstruction
  with gangrene —see Hernia, by site, with
   gangrene
 subxiphoid —see Hernia, ventral

Hernia, hernial (Continued)
 supra-umbilicus —see Hernia, ventral
 tendon —see Disorder, tendon, specified type
  NEC
 Treitz's (fossa) —see Hernia, abdomen, specified
  site NEC
 tunica vaginalis Q55.29
 umbilicus, umbilical K42.9
  with
   gangrene (and obstruction) K42.1
   obstruction K42.0
 ureter N28.89
 urethra, congenital Q64.79
 urinary meatus, congenital Q64.79
 uterus N81.4
  pregnant —see Abnormal, uterus in pregnancy
   or childbirth
 vaginal (anterior) (wall) —see Cystocele
 Velpeau's —see Hernia, femoral
 ventral K43.9
  with
   gangrene (and obstruction) K43.7
   obstruction K43.6
  incisional K43.2
   with
    gangrene (and obstruction) K43.1
    obstruction K43.0
  recurrent —see Hernia, incisional
  specified NEC K43.9
   with
    gangrene (and obstruction) K43.7
    obstruction K43.6
 vesical
  congenital (female) (male) Q79.51
  female —see Cystocele
  male N32.89
 vitreous (into wound) S05.2-•
  into anterior chamber —see Prolapse,
   vitreous
Herniation —see also Hernia
 brain (stem) G93.5
  nontraumatic G93.5
  traumatic S06.A1
   cerebellar S06.A1
   subfalcine (cingulate) S06.A1
   tonsillar S06.A1
   transtentorial (central) (upward cerebellar)
    S06.A1
   uncal S06.A1
 cerebral G93.5
  nontraumatic G93.5
  traumatic S06.A1
 mediastinum J98.59
 nucleus pulposus —see Displacement,
  intervertebral disc
Herpangina B08.5
Herpes, herpesvirus, herpetic B00.9
 anogenital A60.9
  perianal skin A60.1
  rectum A60.1
  urogenital tract A60.00
   cervix A60.03
   male genital organ NEC A60.02
   penis A60.01
   specified site NEC A60.09
   vagina A60.04
   vulva A60.04
 blepharitis (zoster) B02.39
  simplex B00.59
 circinatus B35.4
  bullosus L12.0
 conjunctivitis (simplex) B00.53
  zoster B02.31
 cornea B02.33
 encephalitis B00.4
  due to herpesvirus 6 B10.01
  due to herpesvirus 7 B10.09
  specified NEC B10.09
 eye (zoster) B02.30
  simplex B00.50
 eyelid (zoster) B02.39
  simplex B00.59
 facialis B00.1
 febrilis B00.1
 geniculate ganglionitis B02.21
 genital, genitalis A60.00
  female A60.09
  male A60.02
 gestational, gestationis O26.4-•
 gingivostomatitis B00.2

Herpes, herpesvirus, herpetic (Continued)
 human B00.9
  1 —see Herpes, simplex
  2 —see Herpes, simplex
  3 —see Varicella
  4 —see Mononucleosis, Epstein-Barr (virus)
  5 —see Disease, cytomegalic inclusion
   (generalized)
  6
   encephalitis B10.01
   specified NEC B10.81
  7
   encephalitis B10.09
   specified NEC B10.82
  8 B10.89
 infection NEC B10.89
  Kaposi's sarcoma associated B10.89
 iridocyclitis (simplex) B00.51
  zoster B02.32
 iris (vesicular erythema multiforme) L51.9
 iritis (simplex) B00.51
  Kaposi's sarcoma associated B10.89
 keratitis (simplex) (dendritic) (disciform)
  (interstitial) B00.52
  zoster (interstitial) B02.33
 keratoconjunctivitis (simplex) B00.52
  zoster B02.33
 labialis B00.1
 lip B00.1
 meningitis (simplex) B00.3
  zoster B02.1
 ophthalmicus (zoster) NEC B02.30
  simplex B00.50
 penis A60.01
 perianal skin A60.1
 pharyngitis, pharyngotonsillitis B00.2
 rectum A60.1
 scrotum A60.02
 sepsis B00.7
 simplex B00.9
  complicated NEC B00.89
  congenital P35.2
  conjunctivitis B00.53
  external ear B00.1
  eyelid B00.59
  hepatitis B00.81
  keratitis (interstitial) B00.52
  ~~myelitis B00.82~~
  ▶myelitis B00.82
  specified complication NEC B00.89
  visceral B00.89
 stomatitis B00.2
 tonsurans B35.0
 visceral B00.89
 vulva A60.04
 whitlow B00.89
 zoster —see also condition B02.9
  auricularis B02.21
  complicated NEC B02.8
  conjunctivitis B02.31
  disseminated B02.7
  encephalitis B02.0
  eye(lid) B02.39
  geniculate ganglionitis B02.21
  keratitis (interstitial) B02.33
  meningitis B02.1
  myelitis B02.24
  neuritis, neuralgia B02.29
  ophthalmicus NEC B02.30
  oticus B02.21
  polyneuropathy B02.23
  specified complication NEC B02.8
  trigeminal neuralgia B02.22
Herpesvirus (human) —see Herpes
Herpetophobia F40.218
Herrick's anemia —see Disease, sickle-cell
Hers' disease E74.09
Herter-Gee syndrome K90.0
Herxheimer's reaction R68.89
Hesitancy
 of micturition R39.11
 urinary R39.11
Hesselbach's hernia —see Hernia, femoral,
 specified site NEC
Heterochromia (congenital) Q13.2
 cataract —see Cataract, complicated
 cyclitis (Fuchs) —see Cyclitis, Fuchs'
  heterochromic
 hair L67.1
 iritis —see Cyclitis, Fuchs' heterochromic

▶ New   ➡ Revised   ~~deleted~~ Deleted   • Use Additional Character(s)

Heterochromia *(Continued)*
  retained metallic foreign body (nonmagnetic) —
      see Foreign body, intraocular, old,
      retained
    magnetic —*see* Foreign body, intraocular, old,
        retained, magnetic
  uveitis —*see* Cyclitis, Fuchs' heterochromic
Heterophoria —*see* Strabismus, heterophoria
Heterophyes, heterophyiasis (small intestine)
    B66.8
Heterotopia, heterotopic —*see also* Malposition,
    congenital
  cerebralis Q04.8
Heterotropia —*see* Strabismus
Heubner-Herter disease K90.0
Hexadactylism Q69.9
HGSIL (cytology finding) (high grade squamous
    intraepithelial lesion on cytologic smear) (Pap
    smear finding)
  anus R85.613
  cervix R87.613
    biopsy (histology) finding — *see* Neoplasia,
        intraepithelial, cervix, grade II or grade
        III
  vagina R87.623
    biopsy (histology) finding — *see* Neoplasia,
        intraepithelial, vagina, grade II or grade
        III
Hibernoma —*see* Lipoma
Hiccup, hiccough R06.6
  epidemic B33.0
  psychogenic F45.8
Hidden penis (congenital) Q55.64
  acquired N48.83
Hidradenitis (axillaris) (suppurative)
    L73.2
Hidradenoma (nodular) —*see also* Neoplasm, skin,
    benign
  clear cell —*see* Neoplasm, skin, benign
  papillary —*see* Neoplasm, skin, benign
Hidrocystoma —*see* Neoplasm, skin,
    benign
High
  altitude effects T70.20
    anoxia T70.29
    on
        ears T70.0
        sinuses T70.1
    polycythemia D75.1
  arch
    foot Q66.7-●
    palate, congenital Q38.5
  arterial tension —*see* Hypertension
  basal metabolic rate R94.8
  blood pressure —*see also* Hypertension
    borderline R03.0
    reading (incidental) (isolated) (nonspecific),
        without diagnosis of hypertension
        R03.0
  cholesterol E78.00
    with high triglycerides E78.2
  diaphragm (congenital) Q79.1
  expressed emotional level within family Z63.8
  head at term O32.4
  palate, congenital Q38.5
  risk
    infant NEC Z76.2
    sexual behavior (heterosexual) Z72.51
        bisexual Z72.53
        homosexual Z72.52
  scrotal testis, testes
    bilateral Q53.23
    unilateral Q53.13
  temperature (of unknown origin) R50.9
  thoracic rib Q76.6
  triglycerides E78.1
    with high cholesterol E78.2
Hildenbrand's disease A75.0
Hilum —*see* condition
Hip —*see* condition
Hippel's disease Q85.83
Hippophobia F40.218
Hippus H57.09
Hirschsprung's disease or megacolon Q43.1
Hirsutism, hirsuties L68.0
Hirudiniasis
  external B88.3
  internal B83.4
Hiss-Russell dysentery A03.1
Histidinemia, histidinuria E70.41

Histiocytoma —*see also* Neoplasm, skin, benign
  fibrous —*see also* Neoplasm, skin, benign
    atypical —*see* Neoplasm, connective tissue,
        uncertain behavior
    malignant —*see* Neoplasm, connective tissue,
        malignant
Histiocytosis D76.3
  acute differentiated progressive C96.0
  Langerhans' cell NEC C96.6
    multifocal X
        multisystemic (disseminated) C96.0
        unisystemic C96.5
    pulmonary, adult (adult PLCH) J84.82
    unifocal (X) C96.6
  lipid, lipoid D76.3
    essential E75.29
  malignant C96.A
  mononuclear phagocytes NEC D76.1
    Langerhans' cells C96.6
  non-Langerhans cell D76.3
  polyostotic sclerosing D76.3
  sinus, with massive lymphadenopathy D76.3
  syndrome NEC D76.3
  X NEC C96.6
    acute (progressive) C96.0
    chronic C96.6
    multifocal C96.5
    multisystemic C96.0
    unifocal C96.6
Histoplasmosis B39.9
  with pneumonia NEC B39.2
  African B39.5
  American —*see* Histoplasmosis, capsulati
  capsulati B39.4
    disseminated B39.3
    generalized B39.3
    pulmonary B39.2
        acute B39.0
        chronic B39.1
  Darling's B39.4
  duboisii B39.5
  lung NEC B39.2
History
  family (of) —*see also* History, personal (of)
  ▶adenomatous polyposis Z83.72
    alcohol abuse Z81.1
    allergy NEC Z84.89
    anemia Z83.2
    arthritis Z82.61
    asthma Z82.5
    blindness Z82.1
    cardiac death (sudden) Z82.41
    carrier of genetic disease Z84.81
    chromosomal anomaly Z82.79
    chronic
        disabling disease NEC Z82.8
        lower respiratory disease Z82.5
    colonic polyps Z83.719
        adenomatous and serrated Z83.710
        hyperplastic Z83.711
        inflammatory Z83.718
        specified, NEC Z83.718
        tubular adenoma Z83.710
        tubulovillous adenoma Z83.710
        villous adenoma Z83.710
    congenital malformations and deformations
        Z82.79
        polycystic kidney Z82.71
    consanguinity Z84.3
    deafness Z82.2
    diabetes mellitus Z83.3
    disability NEC Z82.8
    disease or disorder (of)
        allergic NEC Z84.89
        behavioral NEC Z81.8
        blood and blood-forming organs Z83.2
        cardiovascular NEC Z82.49
        chronic disabling NEC Z82.8
        digestive Z83.79
        ear NEC Z83.52
        elevated lipoprotein (a) (Lp(a)) Z83.430
        endocrine NEC Z83.49
        eye NEC Z83.518
            glaucoma Z83.511
        familial hypercholesterolemia Z83.42
        genitourinary NEC Z84.2
        glaucoma Z83.511
        hematological Z83.2
        immune mechanism Z83.2
        infectious NEC Z83.1

History *(Continued)*
  family *(Continued)*
    disease or disorder *(Continued)*
        ischemic heart Z82.49
        kidney Z84.1
        lipoprotein metabolism Z83.438
        mental NEC Z81.8
        metabolic Z83.49
        musculoskeletal NEC Z82.69
        neurological NEC Z82.0
        nutritional Z83.49
        parasitic NEC Z83.1
        psychiatric NEC Z81.8
        respiratory NEC Z83.6
        skin and subcutaneous tissue NEC
            Z84.0
        specified NEC Z84.89
    drug abuse NEC Z81.3
    elevated lipoprotein(a) (Lp (a)) Z83.430
    epilepsy Z82.0
    familial hypercholesterolemia Z83.42
    genetic disease carrier Z84.81
    glaucoma Z83.511
    hearing loss Z82.2
    human immunodeficiency virus (HIV)
        infection Z83.0
    Huntington's chorea Z82.0
    hyperlipidemia, familial combined
        Z83.438
    intellectual disability Z81.0
    leukemia Z80.6
    lipidemia NEC Z83.438
    malignant neoplasm (of) NOS Z80.9
        bladder Z80.52
        breast Z80.3
        bronchus Z80.1
        digestive organ Z80.0
        gastrointestinal tract Z80.0
        genital organ Z80.49
            ovary Z80.41
            prostate Z80.42
            specified organ NEC Z80.49
            testis Z80.43
        hematopoietic NEC Z80.7
        intrathoracic organ NEC Z80.2
        kidney Z80.51
        lung Z80.1
        lymphatic NEC Z80.7
        ovary Z80.41
        prostate Z80.42
        respiratory organ NEC Z80.2
        specified site NEC Z80.8
        testis Z80.43
        trachea Z80.1
        urinary organ or tract Z80.59
            bladder Z80.52
            kidney Z80.51
    mental
        disorder NEC Z81.8
    multiple endocrine neoplasia (MEN)
        syndrome Z83.41
    osteoporosis Z82.62
    polycystic kidney Z82.71
  ▶polyposis, adenomatous Z83.72
    polyps (colon) (*see also* History, family, colonic
        polyps) Z83.719
    psychiatric disorder Z81.8
    psychoactive substance abuse NEC
        Z81.3
    respiratory condition NEC Z83.6
        asthma and other lower respiratory
            conditions Z82.5
    self-harmful behavior Z81.8
    SIDS (sudden infant death syndrome)
        Z84.82
    skin condition Z84.0
    specified condition NEC Z84.89
    stroke (cerebrovascular) Z82.3
    substance abuse NEC Z81.4
        alcohol Z81.1
        drug NEC Z81.3
        psychoactive NEC Z81.3
        tobacco Z81.2
    sudden
        cardiac death Z82.41
        infant death syndrome (SIDS)
            Z84.82
    tobacco abuse Z81.2
    violence, violent behavior Z81.8
    visual loss Z82.1

History *(Continued)*
  personal (of) —*see also* History, family (of)
    abuse
      adult Z91.419
        financial Z91.413
        forced labor or sexual exploitation Z91.42
        intimate partner Z91.414
        physical and sexual Z91.410
        psychological Z91.411
      childhood Z62.819
        financial Z62.814
        forced labor or sexual exploitation in childhood Z62.813
        intimate partner Z62.815
        physical Z62.810
        psychological Z62.811
        sexual Z62.810
          in adolescence —*see* History, personal, abuse, childhood
    alcohol dependence F10.21
    allergy (to) Z88.9
      analgesic agent NEC Z88.6
      anesthetic Z88.4
      antibiotic agent NEC Z88.1
      anti-infective agent NEC Z88.3
      contrast media Z91.041
      drugs, medicaments and biological substances Z88.9
        specified NEC Z88.8
      food Z91.018
        additives Z91.02
        beef Z91.014
        eggs Z91.012
        lamb Z91.014
        mammalian meats Z91.014
        milk products Z91.011
        peanuts Z91.010
        pork Z91.014
        red meats Z91.014
        seafood Z91.013
        specified food NEC Z91.018
      insect Z91.038
        bee Z91.030
      latex Z91.040
      medicinal agents Z88.9
        specified NEC Z88.8
      narcotic agent NEC Z88.5
      nonmedicinal agents Z91.048
      penicillin Z88.0
      serum Z88.7
      specified NEC Z91.09
      sulfonamides Z88.2
      vaccine Z88.7
    anaphylactic shock Z87.892
    anaphylaxis Z87.892
    behavioral disorders Z86.59
    benign carcinoid tumor Z86.012
    benign neoplasm Z86.018
      brain Z86.011
      carcinoid Z86.012
    ▶ colonic polyps —*see* History, personal, neoplasm, benign, colon polyp
    brain injury (traumatic) Z87.820
    breast implant removal Z98.86
    calculi, renal Z87.442
    cancer —*see* History, personal (of), malignant neoplasm (of)
    cardiac arrest (death), successfully resuscitated Z86.74
    CAR-T (Chimeric Antigen Receptor T-cell) therapy Z92.850
    cellular therapy Z92.859
      specified NEC Z92.858
    cerebral infarction without residual deficit Z86.73
    certain (corrected) conditions arising in the perinatal period, specified NEC Z87.68
    cervical dysplasia Z87.410
    chemotherapy for neoplastic condition Z92.21
    childhood abuse —*see* History, personal (of), abuse
    Chimeric Antigen Receptor T-cell (CAR-T) therapy Z92.850
    cleft lip (corrected) Z87.730
    cleft palate (corrected) Z87.730
    cloaca, persistent Z87.732
    cloacal malformations Z87.732
    collapsed vertebra (healed) Z87.311
      due to osteoporosis Z87.310
    combat and operational stress reaction Z86.51

History *(Continued)*
  personal *(Continued)*
    congenital malformation (corrected) Z87.798
      circulatory system (corrected) Z87.74
      diaphragmatic hernia Z87.760
      digestive system (corrected) NEC Z87.738
      ear (corrected) Z87.721
      eye (corrected) Z87.720
      face and neck (corrected) Z87.790
      gastroschisis Z87.761
      genitourinary system (corrected) NEC Z87.718
      heart (corrected) Z87.74
      integument (corrected) Z87.768
      limb(s) (corrected) Z87.768
        malformations
          abdominal wall Z87.763
          diaphragm NEC Z87.760
          integument Z87.768
          limbs Z87.768
          musculoskeletal system Z87.768
          prune belly Z87.762
      musculoskeletal system (corrected) Z87.768
      neck (corrected) Z87.790
      necrotizing enterocolitis of newborn (corrected) Z87.61
      nervous system (corrected) NEC Z87.728
      respiratory system (corrected) Z87.75
      sense organs (corrected) NEC Z87.728
      specified NEC Z87.798
      tracheoesophageal
        atresia Z87.731
        fistula Z87.731
    contraception Z92.0
    coronavirus (disease) (novel) 2019 Z86.16
    COVID-19 Z86.16
    deployment (military) Z91.82
    diabetic foot ulcer Z86.31
    disease or disorder (of) Z87.898
      blood and blood-forming organs Z86.2
      circulatory system Z86.79
        specified condition NEC Z86.79
      connective tissue NEC Z87.39
      digestive system Z87.19
        ▶ colonic polyp —*see* History, personal, neoplasm, benign, colon polyp
        peptic ulcer disease Z87.11
        specified condition NEC Z87.19
      ear Z86.69
      endocrine Z86.39
        diabetic foot ulcer Z86.31
        gestational diabetes Z86.32
        specified type NEC Z86.39
      eye Z86.69
      genital (track) system NEC
        female Z87.42
        male Z87.438
      hematological Z86.2
      Hodgkin Z85.71
      immune mechanism Z86.2
      infectious Z86.19
        coronavirus (disease) (novel) 2019 Z86.16
        COVID-19 Z86.16
        malaria Z86.13
        Methicillin resistant Staphylococcus aureus (MRSA) Z86.14
        poliomyelitis Z86.12
        SARS-CoV-2 Z86.16
        specified NEC Z86.19
        tuberculosis Z86.11
      mental NEC Z86.59
      metabolic Z86.39
        diabetic foot ulcer Z86.31
        gestational diabetes Z86.32
        specified type NEC Z86.39
      musculoskeletal NEC Z87.39
      nervous system Z86.69
      nutritional Z86.39
      parasitic Z86.19
      respiratory system NEC Z87.09
      sense organs Z86.69
      skin Z87.2
      specified site or type NEC Z87.898
      subcutaneous tissue Z87.2
      trophoblastic Z87.59
      urinary system NEC Z87.448
    drug dependence —*see* Dependence, drug, by type, in remission

History *(Continued)*
  personal *(Continued)*
    drug therapy
      antineoplastic chemotherapy Z92.21
      estrogen Z92.23
      ▶ ICI (immune checkpoint inhibitor) drug therapy Z92.26
      immunosuppression Z92.25
      inhaled steroids Z92.240
      monoclonal drug Z92.22
      specified NEC Z92.29
      steroid Z92.241
      systemic steroids Z92.241
    dysplasia
      cervical (mild) (moderate) Z87.410
        severe (grade III) Z86.001
      prostatic Z87.430
      vaginal (mild) (moderate) Z87.411
        severe (grade III) Z86.002
      vulvar (mild) (moderate) Z87.412
        severe (grade III) Z86.002
    embolism (venous) Z86.718
      pulmonary Z86.711
    encephalitis Z86.61
    estrogen therapy Z92.23
    extracorporeal membrane oxygenation (ECMO) Z92.81
    failed conscious sedation Z92.83
    failed moderate sedation Z92.83
    fall, falling Z91.81
    forced labor or sexual exploitation Z91.42
      in childhood Z62.813
    fracture (healed)
      fatigue Z87.312
      fragility Z87.310
      osteoporosis Z87.310
      pathological NEC Z87.311
      stress Z87.312
      traumatic Z87.81
    gene therapy Z92.86
    gestational diabetes Z86.32
    hepatitis
      B Z86.19
      C Z86.19
    Hodgkin disease Z85.71
    hyperthermia, malignant Z88.4
    hypospadias (corrected) Z87.710
    hysterectomy Z90.710
    ▶ ICI (immune checkpoint inhibitor) drug therapy Z92.26
    ▶ immune checkpoint inhibitor (ICI) therapy Z92.26
    immunosuppression therapy Z92.25
    in situ neoplasm
      breast Z86.000
      cervix uteri Z86.001
      digestive organs, specified NEC Z86.004
      esophagus Z86.003
      genital organs, specified NEC Z86.002
      melanoma Z86.006
      middle ear Z86.005
      oral cavity Z86.003
      respiratory system Z86.005
      skin Z86.007
      specified NEC Z86.008
      stomach Z86.003
    infection NEC Z86.19
      central nervous system Z86.61
      coronavirus (disease) (novel) 2019 Z86.16
      COVID-19 Z86.16
      latent tuberculosis Z86.15
      Methicillin resistant Staphylococcus aureus (MRSA) Z86.14
      SARS-CoV-2 Z86.16
      urinary (recurrent) (tract) Z87.41
    injury NEC Z87.828
    in utero procedure during pregnancy Z98.870
    in utero procedure while a fetus Z98.871
    irradiation Z92.3
    kidney stones Z87.442
    latent tuberculosis Z86.15
    leukemia Z85.6
    lymphoma (non-Hodgkin) Z85.72
    malignant melanoma (skin) Z85.820
    malignant neoplasm (of) Z85.9
      accessory sinuses Z85.22
      anus NEC Z85.048
        carcinoid Z85.040
      bladder Z85.51
      bone Z85.830
      brain Z85.841

▶ New   ➡ Revised   ~~deleted~~ Deleted   • Use Additional Character(s)

History *(Continued)*
  personal *(Continued)*
    malignant neoplasm *(Continued)*
      breast Z85.3
      bronchus NEC Z85.118
        carcinoid Z85.110
      carcinoid —*see* History, personal (of), malignant neoplasm, by site, carcinoid
      cervix Z85.41
      colon NEC Z85.038
        carcinoid Z85.030
      digestive organ Z85.00
        specified NEC Z85.09
      endocrine gland NEC Z85.858
      epididymis Z85.48
      esophagus Z85.01
      eye Z85.840
      gastrointestinal tract —*see* History, malignant neoplasm, digestive organ
      genital organ
        female Z85.40
          specified NEC Z85.44
        male Z85.45
          specified NEC Z85.49
      hematopoietic NEC Z85.79
      intrathoracic organ Z85.20-●
      kidney NEC Z85.528
        carcinoid Z85.520
      large intestine NEC Z85.038
        carcinoid Z85.030
      larynx Z85.21
      liver Z85.05
      lung NEC Z85.118
        carcinoid Z85.110
      mediastinum Z85.29
      Merkel cell Z85.821
      middle ear Z85.22
      nasal cavities Z85.22
      nervous system NEC Z85.848
        oral cavity Z85.819
        specified site NEC Z85.818
      ovary Z85.43
      pancreas Z85.07
      pelvis Z85.53
      pharynx Z85.819
        specified site NEC Z85.818
      pleura Z85.29
      prostate Z85.46
      rectosigmoid junction NEC Z85.048
        carcinoid Z85.040
      rectum NEC Z85.048
        carcinoid Z85.040
      respiratory organ Z85.20
      sinuses, accessory Z85.22
      skin NEC Z85.828
        melanoma Z85.820
        Merkel cell Z85.821
      small intestine NEC Z85.068
        carcinoid Z85.060
      soft tissue Z85.831
      specified site NEC Z85.89
      stomach NEC Z85.028
        carcinoid Z85.020
      testis Z85.47
      thymus NEC Z85.238
        carcinoid Z85.230
      thyroid Z85.850
      tongue Z85.810
      trachea Z85.12
      ureter Z85.54
      urinary organ or tract Z85.50
        specified NEC Z85.59
      uterus Z85.42
    maltreatment Z91.89
    medical treatment NEC Z92.89
    melanoma Z85.820
      in situ Z86.06
      malignant (skin) Z85.820
    meningitis Z86.61
    mental disorder Z86.59
    Merkel cell carcinoma (skin) Z85.821
    Methicillin resistant Staphylococcus aureus (MRSA) Z86.14
    military deployment Z91.82
    military service Z91.85
    military war, peacekeeping and humanitarian deployment (current or past conflict) Z91.82
    myocardial infarction (old) I25.2

History *(Continued)*
  personal *(Continued)*
    neglect (in)
      adult Z91.412
      childhood Z62.812
    neoplasia
      anal intraepithelial, III [AIN III] Z86.004
      high-grade prostatic intraepithelial, III [HGPIN III] Z86.002
      vaginal intraepithelial, III [VAIN III] Z86.002
      vulvar intraepithelial, III [VIN III] Z86.002
    neoplasm
      benign Z86.018
        brain Z86.011
        colon polyp Z86.0100
          adenomatous (sessile) Z86.0101
          hyperplastic Z86.0102
          serrated (sessile) Z86.0101
          specified NEC Z86.0109
          traditional serrated adenoma Z86.0101
          tubular adenoma Z86.0101
          tubulovillous adenoma Z86.0101
          villous adenoma Z86.0101
      in situ
        breast Z86.000
        cervix uteri Z86.001
        digestive organs, specified NEC Z86.004
        esophagus Z86.003
        genital organs, specified NEC Z86.002
        melanoma Z86.006
        middle ear Z86.005
        oral cavity Z86.003
        respiratory system Z86.005
        skin Z86.007
        specified NEC Z86.008
        stomach Z86.003
      malignant —*see* History of, malignant neoplasm
      uncertain behavior Z86.03
    nephrotic syndrome Z87.441
    nicotine dependence Z87.891
    noncompliance with medical treatment or regimen —*see* Noncompliance
    nutritional deficiency Z86.39
    obstetric complications Z87.59
      childbirth Z87.59
      pregnancy Z87.59
      pre-term labor Z87.51
      puerperium Z87.59
    osteoporosis fractures Z87.31
    parasuicide (attempt) Z91.51
    physical trauma NEC Z87.828
      self-harm or suicide attempt Z91.51
    pneumonia (recurrent) Z87.01
    poisoning NEC Z91.89
      self-harm or suicide attempt Z91.51
    poor personal hygiene Z91.89
    preterm labor Z87.51
    procedure during pregnancy Z98.870
    procedure while a fetus Z98.871
    prolonged reversible ischemic neurologic deficit (PRINO) Z86.73
    prostatic dysplasia Z87.430
    psychiatric disorder NEC Z87.89
    psychological
      abuse
        adult Z91.411
        child Z62.811
      trauma, specified NEC Z91.49
    radiation therapy Z92.3
    removal
      implant
        breast Z98.86
    renal calculi Z87.442
    respiratory condition NEC Z87.09
    retained foreign body fully removed Z87.821
    risk factors NEC Z91.89
    SARS-CoV-2 infection Z86.16
    self-harm
      nonsuicidal Z91.52
      suicidal Z91.51
    self-inflicted injury without suicidal intent Z91.52
    self-injury
      nonsuicidal Z91.52
    self-mutilation Z91.52
    self-poisoning attempt Z91.51
      suicidal behavior Z91.51
    sex reassignment Z87.890
    sleep-wake cycle problem Z72.821

History *(Continued)*
  personal *(Continued)*
    specified NEC Z87.898
    steroid therapy (systemic) Z92.241
      inhaled Z92.240
    stroke without residual deficits Z86.73
    substance abuse NEC F10-F19
    sudden cardiac arrest Z86.74
    sudden cardiac death successfully resuscitated Z86.74
    suicide attempt Z91.51
    surgery NEC Z98.890
      with uterine scar Z98.891
      sex reassignment Z87.890
      transplant —*see* Transplant
    thrombophlebitis Z86.72
    thrombosis (venous) Z86.718
      pulmonary Z86.711
    tobacco dependence Z87.891
    transient ischemic attack (TIA) without residual deficits Z86.73
    trauma (physical) NEC Z87.828
      psychological NEC Z91.49
      self-harm Z91.51
    traumatic brain injury Z87.820
    tuberculosis, latent infection Z86.15
    unhealthy sleep-wake cycle Z72.821
    unintended awareness under general anesthesia Z92.84
    urinary (recurrent) (tract) infection(s) Z87.440
    urinary calculi Z87.42
    uterine scar from previous surgery Z98.891
    vaginal dysplasia Z87.411
    venous thrombosis or embolism Z86.718
      pulmonary Z86.711
    vulvar dysplasia Z87.412
His-Werner disease A79.0
HIV —*see also* Human, immunodeficiency virus B20
  laboratory evidence (nonconclusive) R75
  nonconclusive test (in infants) R75
  positive, seropositive Z21
Hives (bold) —*see* Urticaria
Hoarseness R49.0
Hobo Z59.00
Hodgkin disease —*see* Lymphoma, Hodgkin
Hodgson's (*see also* Aneurysm, aorta, thorax) I71.20
  ruptured (*see also* Aneurysm, aorta, thorax, ruptured) I71.10
Hoffa-Kastert disease E88.89
Hoffa's disease E88.89
Hoffmann-Bouveret syndrome I47.9
Hoffmann's syndrome E03.9 [G73.7]
Hole (round)
  macula H35.34-●
  retina (without detachment) —*see* Break, retina, round hole
    with detachment —*see* Detachment, retina, with retinal, break
Holiday relief care Z75.5
Hollenhorst's plaque —*see* Occlusion, artery, retina
Hollow foot (congenital) Q66.7-●
  acquired —*see* Deformity, limb, foot, specified NEC
Holoprosencephaly Q04.2
Holt-Oram syndrome Q87.2
Homelessness Z59.00
  sheltered Z59.01
  unsheltered Z59.02
Homesickness —*see* Disorder, adjustment
Homocysteinemia R79.83
Homocystinemia R79.83
Homocystinuria E72.11
Homogentisate 1,2-dioxygenase deficiency E70.29
Homologous serum hepatitis (prophylactic) (therapeutic) —*see* Hepatitis, viral, type B
Honeycomb lung J98.4
  congenital Q33.0
Hooded
  clitoris Q52.6
  penis Q55.69
Hookworm (disease) (infection) (infestation) B76.9
  with anemia B76.9 [D63.8]
  specified NEC B76.8
Hordeolum (eyelid) (externum) (recurrent) H00.019
  internum H00.029
    left H00.026
      lower H00.025
      upper H00.024

Hordeolum *(Continued)*
  internum *(Continued)*
    right H00.023
      lower H00.022
      upper H00.021
    left H00.016
      lower H00.015
      upper H00.014
    right H00.013
      lower H00.012
      upper H00.011
Horn
  cutaneous L85.8
  nail L60.2
    congenital Q84.6
Horner (-Claude Bernard) syndrome G90.2
  traumatic —*see* Injury, nerve, cervical sympathetic
Horseshoe kidney (congenital) Q63.1
Horton's headache or neuralgia G44.099
  intractable G44.091
  not intractable G44.099
Hospital hopper syndrome —*see* Disorder,
    factitious
Hospitalism in children —*see* Disorder, adjustment
Hostility R45.5
  towards child Z62.3
Hot flashes
  menopausal N95.1
Hourglass (contracture) —*see also* Contraction,
    hourglass
  stomach K31.89
    congenital Q40.2
    stricture K31.2
Household, housing circumstance affecting care
    Z59.9
  specified NEC Z59.89
Housemaid's knee —*see* Bursitis, prepatellar
HSCT-TMA (hematopoietic stem cell
    transplantation-associated thrombotic
    microangiopathy) M31.11
Hudson (-Stähli) line (cornea) —*see* Pigmentation,
    cornea, anterior
Human
  bite (open wound) —*see also* Bite
    intact skin surface —*see* Bite, superficial
  herpesvirus —*see* Herpes
  immunodeficiency virus (HIV) disease
      (infection) B20
    asymptomatic status Z21
    contact Z20.6
    counseling Z71.7
    dementia (*see also* Dementia, in, diseases
        specified elsewhere) B20 *[F02.80]*
      with behavioral disturbance (*see also*
          Dementia, in, diseases specified
          elsewhere) B20 *[F02.81-●]*
    exposure to Z20.6
    laboratory evidence R75
    type-2 (HIV 2) as cause of disease classified
        elsewhere B97.35
  papillomavirus (HPV)
    DNA test positive
      high risk
        cervix R87.810
        vagina R87.811
      low risk
        cervix R87.820
        vagina R87.821
    screening for Z11.51
  T-cell lymphotropic virus
    type-1 (HTLV-I) infection B33.3
      as cause of disease classified elsewhere B97.33
      carrier Z22.6
    type-2 (HTLV-II) as cause of disease classified
        elsewhere B97.34
Humidifier lung or pneumonitis J67.7
Humiliation (experience) in childhood Z62.898
Humpback (acquired) —*see* Kyphosis
Hunchback (acquired) —*see* Kyphosis
Hunger T73.0
  air, psychogenic F45.8
Hungry bone syndrome E83.81
Hunner's ulcer —*see* Cystitis, chronic, interstitial
Hunter's
  glossitis D51.0
  syndrome E76.1
Huntington's disease or chorea G10
  with dementia (*see also* Dementia, in, diseases
      specified elsewhere) G10 *[F02.80]*
    with behavioral disturbance (*see also*
        Dementia, in, diseases specified
        elsewhere) G10 *[F02.81-●]*

Hunt's
  disease or syndrome (herpetic geniculate
      ganglionitis) B02.21
    dyssynergia cerebellaris myoclonica G11.19
  neuralgia B02.21
Hurler (-Scheie) disease or syndrome E76.02
Hurst's disease G36.1
Hurthle cell
  adenocarcinoma C73
  adenoma D34
  carcinoma C73
  tumor D34
Hutchinson-Boeck disease or syndrome —*see*
    Sarcoidosis
Hutchinson-Gilford disease or syndrome E34.8
Hutchinson's
  disease, meaning
    angioma serpiginosum L81.7
    pompholyx (cheiropompholyx) L30.1
    prurigo estivalis L56.4
    summer eruption or summer prurigo L56.4
  melanotic freckle —*see* Melanoma, in situ
    malignant melanoma in —*see* Melanoma
  teeth or incisors (congenital syphilis) A50.52
  triad (congenital syphilis) A50.53
Hyalin plaque, sclera, senile H15.89
Hyaline membrane (disease) (lung) (pulmonary)
    (newborn) P22.0
Hyalinosis
  cutis (et mucosae) E78.89
  focal and segmental (glomerular) —*see also*
      N00-N07 with fourth character .1 N05.1
Hyalitis, hyalosis, asteroid —*see also* Deposit,
    crystalline
  syphilitic (late) A52.71
Hydatid
  cyst or tumor —*see* Echinococcus
  mole —*see* Hydatidiform mole
  Morgagni
    female Q50.5
    male (epididymal) Q55.4
      testicular Q55.29
Hydatidiform mole (benign) (complicating
    pregnancy) (delivered) (undelivered) O01.9
  classical O01.0
  complete O01.0
  incomplete O01.1
  invasive D39.2
  malignant D39.2
  partial O01.1
Hydatidosis —*see* Echinococcus
Hydradenitis (axillaris) (suppurative) L73.2
Hydradenoma —*see* Hidradenoma
Hydramnios O40.-●
Hydramphaly, hydranencephaly Q04.3
  with spina bifida —*see* Spina bifida, with
      hydrocephalus
Hydrargyrism NEC —*see* Poisoning, mercury
Hydrarthrosis —*see also* Effusion, joint
  gonococcal A54.42
  intermittent M12.40
    ankle M12.47-●
    elbow M12.42-●
    foot joint M12.47-●
    hand joint M12.44-●
    hip M12.45-●
    knee M12.46-●
    multiple site M12.49
    shoulder M12.41-●
    specified joint NEC M12.48
    wrist M12.43-●
  of yaws (early) (late) —*see also* subcategory
      M14.8-● A66.6
  syphilitic (late) A52.77
    congenital A50.55 *[M12.80]*
Hydremia D64.89
Hydrencephalocele (congenital) —*see*
    Encephalocele
Hydrencephalomeningocele (congenital) —*see*
    Encephalocele
Hydroa R23.8
  aestivale L56.4
  vacciniforme L56.4
Hydroadenitis (axillaris) (suppurative) L73.2
Hydrocalycosis —*see* Hydronephrosis
Hydrocele (spermatic cord) (testis) (tunica
    vaginalis) N43.3
  canal of Nuck N94.89
  communicating N43.2
  congenital P83.5
  encysted N43.0

Hydrocele *(Continued)*
  female NEC N94.89
  infected N43.1
  newborn P83.5
  round ligament N94.89
  specified NEC N43.2
  spinalis —*see* Spina bifida
  vulva N90.89
Hydrocephalus (acquired) (external) (internal)
    (malignant) (recurrent) G91.9
  aqueduct Sylvius stricture Q03.0
  causing disproportion O33.6
    with obstructed labor O66.3
  communicating G91.0
  congenital (external) (internal) Q03.9
    with spina bifida Q05.4
      cervical Q05.0
      dorsal Q05.1
      lumbar Q05.2
      lumbosacral Q05.2
      sacral Q05.3
      thoracic Q05.1
      thoracolumbar Q05.1
    specified NEC Q03.8
  due to toxoplasmosis (congenital) P37.1
  foramen Magendie block (acquired) G91.1
    congenital —*see also* Hydrocephalus,
        congenital Q03.1
  in (due to)
    infectious disease NEC B89 *[G91.4]*
    neoplastic disease NEC (*see also* Neoplasm)
        G91.4
    parasitic disease B89 *[G91.4]*
  newborn Q03.9
    with spina bifida —*see* Spina bifida, with
        hydrocephalus
  noncommunicating G91.1
  normal pressure G91.2
    secondary G91.0
  obstructive G91.1
  otitic G93.2
  post-traumatic NEC G91.3
  secondary G91.4
    post-traumatic G91.3
  specified NEC G91.8
  syphilitic, congenital A50.49
Hydrocolpos (congenital) N89.8
Hydrocystoma —*see* Neoplasm, skin, benign
Hydroencephalocele (congenital) —*see*
    Encephalocele
Hydroencephalomeningocele (congenital) —*see*
    Encephalocele
Hydrohematopneumothorax —*see* Hemothorax
Hydromeningitis —*see* Meningitis
Hydromeningocele (spinal) —*see also* Spina bifida
  cranial —*see* Encephalocele
Hydrometra N85.8
Hydrometrocolpos N89.8
Hydromicrocephaly Q02
Hydromphalos (since birth) Q45.8
Hydromyelia Q06.4
Hydromyelocele —*see* Spina bifida
Hydronephrosis (atrophic) (early) (functionless)
    (intermittent) (primary) (secondary) NEC
    N13.30
  with
    infection N13.6
    obstruction (by) (of)
      renal calculus N13.2
        with infection N13.6
      ureteral NEC N13.1
        with infection N13.6
        calculus N13.2
          with infection N13.6
      ureteropelvic junction (congenital)
          Q62.11
        acquired N13.0
          with infection N13.6
    ureteral stricture NEC N13.1
      with infection N13.6
  congenital Q62.0
    due to acquired occlusion of ureteropelvic
        junction N13.0
  specified type NEC N13.39
  tuberculous A18.11
Hydropericarditis —*see* Pericarditis
Hydropericardium —*see* Pericarditis
Hydroperitoneum R18.8
Hydrophobia —*see* Rabies
Hydrophthalmos Q15.0
Hydropneumohemothorax —*see* Hemothorax
Hydropneumopericarditis —*see* Pericarditis

Hydropneumopericardium —*see* Pericarditis
Hydropneumothorax J94.8
  traumatic —*see* Injury, intrathoracic, lung
  tuberculous NEC A15.6
Hydrops R60.9
  abdominis R18.8
  articulorum intermittens —*see* Hydrarthrosis,
      intermittent
  cardiac —*see* Failure, heart, congestive
  causing obstructed labor (mother) O66.3
  endolymphatic H81.0-●
  fetal —*see* Pregnancy, complicated by, hydrops,
      fetalis
  fetalis P83.2
    due to
      ABO isoimmunization P56.0
      alpha thalassemia D56.0
      hemolytic disease P56.90
        specified NEC P56.99
      isoimmunization (ABO) (Rh) P56.0
      other specified nonhemolytic disease NEC
          P83.2
      Rh incompatibility P56.0
    during pregnancy —*see* Pregnancy,
        complicated by, hydrops, fetalis
  gallbladder K82.1
  joint —*see* Effusion, joint
  labyrinth H81.0
  newborn (idiopathic) P83.2
    due to
      ABO isoimmunization P56.0
      alpha thalassemia D56.0
      hemolytic disease P56.90
        specified NEC P56.99
      isoimmunization (ABO) (Rh) P56.0
      Rh incompatibility P56.0
  nutritional —*see* Malnutrition, severe
  pericardium —*see* Pericarditis
  pleura —*see* Hydrothorax
  spermatic cord —*see* Hydrocele
Hydropyonephrosis N13.6
Hydrorachis Q06.4
Hydrorrhea (nasal) J34.89
  pregnancy —*see* Rupture, membranes,
      premature
Hydrosadenitis (axillaris) (suppurative) L73.2
Hydrosalpinx (fallopian tube) (follicularis)
      N70.11
Hydrothorax (double) (pleura) J94.8
  chylous (nonfilarial) I89.8
    filarial —*see also* Infestation, filarial B74.9
        [J91.8]
  traumatic —*see* Injury, intrathoracic
  tuberculous NEC (non primary) A15.6
Hydroureter —*see also* Hydronephrosis
      N13.4
  with infection N13.6
  congenital Q62.39
Hydroureteronephrosis —*see* Hydronephrosis
Hydrourethra N36.8
Hydroxykynureninuria E70.89
Hydroxylysinemia E72.3
Hydroxyprolinemia E72.59
Hygiene, sleep
  abuse Z72.821
  inadequate Z72.821
  poor Z72.821
Hygroma (congenital) (cystic) D18.1
  praepatellare, prepatellar —*see* Bursitis,
      prepatellar
  subdural —*see* Leak, cerebrospinal fluid
Hymen —*see* condition
Hymenolepis, hymenolepiasis (diminuta)
      (infection) (infestation) (nana) B71.0
Hypalgesia R20.8
Hyperacidity (gastric) K31.89
  psychogenic F45.8
Hyperactive, hyperactivity F90.9
  basal cell, uterine cervix —*see* Dysplasia, cervix
  bowel sounds R19.12
  cervix epithelial (basal) —*see* Dysplasia, cervix
  child F90.9
    attention deficit —*see* Disorder, attention-
        deficit hyperactivity
  detrusor muscle N32.81
  gastrointestinal K31.89
    psychogenic F45.8
  nasal mucous membrane J34.3
  stomach K31.89
  thyroid (gland) —*see* Hyperthyroidism
Hyperacusis H93.23-●
Hyperadrenalism E27.5

Hyperadrenocorticism E24.9
  congenital E25.0
  iatrogenic E24.2
    correct substance properly administered —*see*
        Table of Drugs and Chemicals, by drug,
        adverse effect
    overdose or wrong substance given or
        taken —*see* Table of Drugs and
        Chemicals, by drug, poisoning
  not associated with Cushing's syndrome E27.0
  pituitary-dependent E24.0
Hyperaldosteronism E26.9
  familial (type I) E26.02
  glucocorticoid-remediable E26.02
  primary (due to (bilateral) adrenal hyperplasia)
      E26.09
  primary NEC E26.09
  secondary E26.1
  specified NEC E26.89
Hyperalgesia R20.8
Hyperalimentation R63.2
  carotene, carotin E67.1
  specified NEC E67.8
  vitamin
    A E67.0
    D E67.3
Hyperaminoaciduria
  arginine E72.21
  cystine E72.01
  lysine E72.3
  ornithine E72.4
Hyperammonemia (congenital) E72.20
Hyperazotemia —*see* Uremia
Hyperbetalipoproteinemia (familial) E78.00
  with prebetalipoproteinemia E78.2
Hyperbilirubinemia
  constitutional E80.6
  familial conjugated E80.6
  neonatal (transient) —*see* Jaundice, newborn
Hypercalcemia, hypocalciuric, familial E83.52
Hypercalciuria, idiopathic R82.994
Hypercapnia R06.89
  newborn P84
Hypercarotenemia (dietary) E67.1
Hypercementosis K03.4
Hyperchloremia E87.8
Hyperchlorhydria K31.89
  neurotic F45.8
  psychogenic F45.8
Hypercholesterinemia —*see* Hypercholesterolemia
Hypercholesterolemia (essential) (primary) (pure)
      E78.00
  with hyperglyceridemia, endogenous E78.2
  dietary counseling and surveillance Z71.3
  familial E78.01
  hereditary E78.01
Hyperchylia gastrica, psychogenic F45.8
Hyperchylomicronemia (familial) (primary) E78.3
  with hyperbetalipoproteinemia E78.3
Hypercoagulable (state) D68.59
  activated protein C resistance D68.51
  antithrombin (III) deficiency D68.59
  factor V Leiden mutation D68.51
  primary NEC D68.59
  protein C deficiency D68.59
  protein S deficiency D68.59
  prothrombin gene mutation D68.52
  secondary D68.69
  specified NEC D68.69
Hypercoagulation (state) D68.59
Hypercorticalism, pituitary-dependent
      E24.0
Hypercorticosolism —*see* Cushing's, syndrome
Hypercorticosteronism E24.2
  correct substance properly administered —*see*
      Table of Drugs and Chemicals, by drug,
      adverse effect
  overdose or wrong substance given or taken —
      see Table of Drugs and Chemicals, by drug,
      poisoning
Hypercortisonism E24.2
  correct substance properly administered —*see*
      Table of Drugs and Chemicals, by drug,
      adverse effect
  overdose or wrong substance given or taken —
      see Table of Drugs and Chemicals, by drug,
      poisoning
Hyperekplexia Q89.8
Hyperelectrolytemia E87.8
Hyperemesis R11.10
  with nausea R11.2
  gravidarum (mild) O21.0

Hyperemesis (Continued)
  gravidarum (Continued)
    with
      carbohydrate depletion O21.1
      dehydration O21.1
      electrolyte imbalance O21.1
      metabolic disturbance O21.1
    severe (with metabolic disturbance) O21.1
  projectile R11.12
  psychogenic F45.8
Hyperemia (acute) (passive) R68.89
  anal mucosa K62.89
  bladder N32.89
  cerebral I67.89
  conjunctiva H11.43-●
  ear internal, acute —*see* subcategory H83.0
  enteric K59.89
  eye —*see* Hyperemia, conjunctiva
  eyelid (active) (passive) —*see* Disorder, eyelid,
      specified type NEC
  intestine K59.89
  iris —*see* Disorder, iris, vascular
  kidney N28.89
  labyrinth —*see* subcategory H83.0
  liver (active) K76.89
  lung (passive) —*see* Edema, lung
  pulmonary (passive) —*see* Edema, lung
  renal N28.89
  retina H35.89
  stomach K31.89
Hyperesthesia (body surface) R20.3
  larynx (reflex) J38.7
    hysterical F44.89
  pharynx (reflex) J39.2
    hysterical F44.89
Hyperestrogenism (drug-induced) (iatrogenic)
      E28.0
Hyperexplexia Q89.8
Hyperfibrinolysis —*see* Fibrinolysis
Hyperfructosemia E74.19
Hyperfunction
  adrenal cortex, not associated with Cushing's
      syndrome E27.0
    medulla E27.5
      adrenomedullary E27.5
    virilism E25.9
      congenital E25.0
  ovarian E28.8
  pancreas K86.89
  parathyroid (gland) E21.3
  pituitary (gland) (anterior) E22.9
    specified NEC E22.8
  polyglandular E31.1
  testicular E29.0
Hypergammaglobulinemia D89.2
  polyclonal D89.0
  Waldenström D89.0
Hypergastrinemia E16.4
Hyperglobulinemia R77.1
Hyperglycemia, hyperglycemic (transient) R73.9
  coma —*see* Diabetes, by type, with coma
  postpancreatectomy E89.1
Hyperglyceridemia (endogenous) (essential)
      (familial) (hereditary) (pure) E78.1
  mixed E78.3
Hyperglycinemia (non-ketotic) E72.51
Hypergonadism
  ovarian E28.8
  testicular (primary) (infantile) E29.0
Hyperheparinemia D68.32
Hyperhidrosis, hyperidrosis R61
  focal
    primary L74.519
      axilla L74.510
      face L74.511
      palms L74.512
      soles L74.513
    secondary L74.52
  generalized R61
  localized
    primary L74.519
      axilla L74.510
      face L74.511
      palms L74.512
      soles L74.513
    secondary L74.52
  psychogenic F45.8
  secondary R61
    focal L74.52
Hyperhistidinemia E70.41
Hyperhomocysteinemia E72.11
Hyperhydroxyprolinemia E72.59

Hyperinsulinism (functional) E16.1
  with
    coma (hypoglycemic) E15
    encephalopathy E16.1 [G94]
  ectopic E16.1
  therapeutic misadventure (from administration of
    insulin) —see subcategory T38.3
Hyperkalemia E87.5
Hyperkeratosis —see also Keratosis L85.9
  cervix N88.0
  due to yaws (early) (late) (palmar or plantar)
    A66.3
  follicularis Q82.8
    penetrans (in cutem) L87.0
  palmoplantaris climacterica L85.1
  pinta A67.1
  senile (with pruritus) L57.0
  universalis congenita Q80.8
  vocal cord J38.3
  vulva N90.4
Hyperkinesia, hyperkinetic (disease) (reaction)
    (syndrome) (childhood) (adolescence) —see
    also Disorder, attention-deficit hyperactivity
  heart I51.89
Hyperleucine-isoleucinemia E71.19
Hyperlipemia, hyperlipidemia E78.5
  combined E78.2
    familial E78.49
  group
    A E78.00
    B E78.1
    C E78.2
    D E78.3
  mixed E78.2
  specified NEC E78.49
Hyperlipidosis E75.6
  hereditary NEC E75.5
Hyperlipoproteinemia E78.5
  Fredrickson's type
    I E78.3
    IIa E78.00
    IIb E78.2
    III E78.2
    IV E78.1
    V E78.3
  low-density-lipoprotein-type (LDL) E78.00
  very-low-density-lipoprotein-type (VLDL) E78.1
Hyperlucent lung, unilateral J43.0
Hyperlysinemia E72.3
Hypermagnesemia E83.41
  neonatal P71.8
Hypermenorrhea N92.0
Hypermethioninemia E72.19
Hypermetropia (congenital) H52.0-●
Hypermobility, hypermotility
  cecum —see Syndrome, irritable bowel
  coccyx —see subcategory M53.2
  colon —see Syndrome, irritable bowel
    psychogenic F45.8
  ileum K58.9
  intestine —see also Syndrome, irritable bowel
    K58.9
    psychogenic F45.8
  meniscus (knee) —see Derangement, knee,
    meniscus
  scapula —see Instability, joint, shoulder
  stomach K31.89
    psychogenic F45.8
  syndrome M35.7
  urethra N36.41
    with intrinsic sphincter deficiency N36.43
Hypernasality R49.21
Hypernatremia E87.0
Hypernephroma C64.-●
Hyperopia —see Hypermetropia
Hyperorexia nervosa F50.2-●
Hyperornithinemia E72.4
Hyperosmia R43.1
Hyperosmolality (see also, Diabetes, by type, with
    hyperosmolarity) E87.0
Hyperostosis (monomelic) —see also Disorder,
    bone, density and structure, specified NEC
  ankylosing (spine) M48.10
    cervical region M48.12
    cervicothoracic region M48.13
    lumbar region M48.16
    lumbosacral region M48.17
    multiple sites M48.19
    occipito-atlanto-axial region M48.11
    sacrococcygeal region M48.18
    thoracic region M48.14
    thoracolumbar region M48.15

Hyperostosis (Continued)
  cortical (skull) M85.2
    infantile M89.8X-●
  frontal, internal of skull M85.2
  interna frontalis M85.2
  skeletal, diffuse idiopathic —see Hyperostosis,
    ankylosing
  skull M85.2
    congenital Q75.8
  vertebral, ankylosing —see Hyperostosis,
    ankylosing
Hyperovarism E28.8
Hyperoxaluria (primary) R82.992
Hyperparathyroidism E21.3
  primary E21.0
  secondary (renal) N25.81
    non-renal E21.1
  specified NEC E21.2
  tertiary E21.2
Hyperpathia R20.8
Hyperperistalsis R19.2
  psychogenic F45.8
Hyperpermeability, capillary I78.8
Hyperphagia R63.2
Hyperphenylalaninemia NEC E70.1
Hyperphoria (alternating) H50.53
Hyperphosphatemia E83.39
Hyperpiesis, hyperpiesia —see Hypertension
Hyperpigmentation —see also Pigmentation
  melanin NEC L81.4
  postinflammatory L81.0
Hyperpinealism E34.8
Hyperpituitarism E22.9
Hyperplasia, hyperplastic
  adenoids J35.2
  adrenal (capsule) (cortex) (gland) E27.8
    with
      sexual precocity (male) E25.9
        congenital E25.0
      virilism, adrenal E25.9
        congenital E25.0
      virilization (female) E25.9
        congenital E25.0
    congenital E25.0
    salt-losing E25.0
  adrenomedullary E27.5
  angiolymphoid, eosinophilia (ALHE)
    D18.01
  appendix (lymphoid) K38.0
  artery, fibromuscular I77.3
  bone —see also Hypertrophy, bone
    marrow D75.89
  breast —see also Hypertrophy, breast
    atypical, atypia N60.9-●
      ductal N60.9-●
      lobular N60.9-●
  C-cell, thyroid E07.0
  cementation (tooth) (teeth) K03.4
  cervical gland R59.0
  cervix (uteri) (basal cell) (endometrium)
    (polypoid) —see also Dysplasia, cervix
    congenital Q51.828
  clitoris, congenital Q52.6
  denture K06.2
  endocervicitis N72
  endometrium, endometrial (adenomatous)
    (cystic) (glandular) (glandular-cystic)
    (polypoid) N85.00
    with atypia N85.02
    benign N85.01
    cervix —see Dysplasia, cervix
    complex (without atypia) N85.01
    simple (without atypia) N85.01
  epithelial L85.9
    focal, oral, including tongue
      K13.29
    nipple N62
    skin L85.9
    tongue K13.29
    vaginal wall N89.3
  erythroid D75.89
  fibromuscular of artery (carotid) (renal)
    I77.3
  genital
    female NEC N94.89
    male N50.89
  gingiva K06.1
  glandularis cystica uteri (interstitialis) —see also
    Hyperplasia, endometrial N85.00-●
  gum K06.1
  hymen, congenital Q52.4
  irritative, edentulous (alveolar) K06.2

Hyperplasia, hyperplastic (Continued)
  jaw M26.09
    alveolar M26.79
      lower M26.03
        alveolar M26.72
      upper M26.01
        alveolar M26.71
  kidney (congenital) Q63.3
  labia N90.69
    epithelial N90.3
  liver (congenital) Q44.79
    nodular, focal K76.89
  lymph gland or node R59.9
  mandible, mandibular M26.03
    alveolar M26.72
    unilateral condylar M27.8
  maxilla, maxillary M26.01
    alveolar M26.71
  myometrium, myometrial N85.2
  neuroendocrine cell, of infancy J84.841
  nose
    lymphoid J34.89
    polypoid J33.9
  oral mucosa (irritative) K13.6
  organ or site, congenital NEC —see Anomaly,
    by site
  ovary N83.8
  palate, papillary (irritative) K13.6
  pancreatic islet cells E16.9
    alpha E16.8
      with excess
        gastrin E16.4
        glucagon E16.3
    beta E16.1
  parathyroid (gland) E21.0
  pharynx (lymphoid) J39.2
  prostate (adenofibromatous) N40.0
    with lower urinary tract symptoms (LUTS)
      N40.1
    nodular N40.3
    nodular N40.2
      with lower urinary tract symptoms
        (LUTS) N40.3
    without lower urinary tract symptoms (LUTS)
      N40.0
    nodular N40.2
  renal artery I77.89
  reticulo-endothelial (cell) D75.89
  salivary gland (any) K11.1
  Schimmelbusch's —see Mastopathy, cystic
  suprarenal capsule (gland) E27.8
  thymus (gland) (persistent) E32.0
  thyroid (gland) —see Goiter
  tonsils (faucial) (infective) (lingual) (lymphoid)
    J35.1
    with adenoids J35.3
  unilateral condylar M27.8
  uterus, uterine N85.2
    endometrium (glandular) —see also
      Hyperplasia, endometrial N85.00-●
  vulva N90.69
    epithelial N90.3
Hyperpnea —see Hyperventilation
Hyperpotassemia E87.5
Hyperprebetalipoproteinemia (familial)
  E78.1
Hyperprolactinemia E22.1
Hyperprolinemia (type I) (type II) E72.59
Hyperproteinemia E88.09
Hyperprothrombinemia, causing coagulation
  factor deficiency D68.4
Hyperpyrexia R50.9
  heat (effects) T67.01
  malignant, due to anesthetic T88.3
  rheumatic —see Fever, rheumatic
  unknown origin R50.9
Hyper-reflexia R29.2
Hypersalivation K11.7
Hypersecretion
  ACTH (not associated with Cushing's
    syndrome) E27.0
    pituitary E24.0
  adrenaline E27.5
  adrenomedullary E27.5
  androgen (testicular) E29.0
    ovarian (drug-induced) (iatrogenic) E28.1
  calcitonin E07.0
  catecholamine E27.5
  corticoadrenal E24.9
  cortisol E24.9
  epinephrine E27.5
  estrogen E28.0

▶ New   ⇒ Revised   deleted Deleted   ● Use Additional Character(s)

Hypersecretion *(Continued)*
  gastric K31.89
    psychogenic F45.8
  gastrin E16.4
  glucagon E16.3
  hormone(s)
    ACTH (not associated with Cushing's
      syndrome) E27.0
      pituitary E24.0
    antidiuretic E22.2
    growth E22.0
    intestinal NEC E34.1
    ovarian androgen E28.1
    pituitary E22.9
    testicular E29.0
    thyroid stimulating E05.80
      with thyroid storm E05.81
  insulin —*see* Hyperinsulinism
  lacrimal glands —*see* Epiphora
  medulloadrenal E27.5
  milk O92.6
  ovarian androgens E28.1
  salivary gland (any) K11.7
  thyrocalcitonin E07.0
  upper respiratory J39.8
Hypersegmentation, leukocytic, hereditary
    D72.0
Hypersensitive, hypersensitiveness,
    hypersensitivity —*see also* Allergy
  carotid sinus G90.01
  colon —*see* Irritable, colon
  drug T88.7
  gastrointestinal K52.29
    immediate K52.29
    psychogenic F45.8
  labyrinth —*see* subcategory H83.2
  pain R20.8
  pneumonitis —*see* Pneumonitis, allergic
  reaction T78.40
    upper respiratory tract NEC J39.3
Hypersomnia (organic) G47.10
  due to
    alcohol
      abuse F10.182
      dependence F10.282
      use F10.982
    amphetamines
      abuse F15.182
      dependence F15.282
      use F15.982
    caffeine
      abuse F15.182
      dependence F15.282
      use F15.982
    cocaine
      abuse F14.182
      dependence F14.282
      use F14.982
    drug NEC
      abuse F19.182
      dependence F19.282
      use F19.982
    medical condition G47.14
    mental disorder F51.13
    opioid
      abuse F11.182
      dependence F11.282
      use F11.982
    psychoactive substance NEC
      abuse F19.182
      dependence F19.282
      use F19.982
    sedative, hypnotic, or anxiolytic
      abuse F13.182
      dependence F13.282
      use F13.982
    stimulant NEC
      abuse F15.182
      dependence F15.282
      use F15.982
  idiopathic G47.11
    with long sleep time G47.11
    without long sleep time G47.12
  menstrual related G47.13
  nonorganic origin F51.11
    specified NEC F51.19
  not due to a substance or known physiological
    condition F51.11
    specified NEC F51.19
  primary F51.11
  recurrent G47.13
  specified NEC G47.19

Hypersplenia, hypersplenism D73.1
Hyperstimulation, ovaries (associated with
    induced ovulation) N98.1
Hypersusceptibility —*see* Allergy
Hypertelorism (ocular) (orbital) Q75.2
Hypertension, hypertensive (accelerated) (benign)
    (essential) (idiopathic)
    (malignant) (systemic) I10
  with
    heart failure (congestive) I11.0
    heart involvement (conditions in I50.- or
      I51.4-I51.7, I51.89, I51.9, due to
      hypertension) —*see* Hypertension, heart
    kidney involvement —*see* Hypertension,
      kidney
  benign, intracranial G93.2
  borderline R03.0
  cardiorenal (disease) I13.10
    with heart failure I13.0
      with stage 1 through stage 4 chronic kidney
        disease I13.0
      with stage 5 or end stage renal disease I13.2
    without heart failure I13.10
      with stage 1 through stage 4 chronic kidney
        disease I13.10
      with stage 5 or end stage renal disease
        I13.11
  cardiovascular
    disease (arteriosclerotic) (sclerotic) —*see*
      Hypertension, heart
    renal (disease) —*see* Hypertension, cardiorenal
  chronic venous —*see* Hypertension, venous
    (chronic)
  complicating
    childbirth (labor) O16.4
      pre-existing O10.92
        with
          heart disease O10.12
            with renal disease O10.32
          pre-eclampsia O11.4
          renal disease O10.22
            with heart disease O10.32
          essential O10.02
      secondary O10.42
    pregnancy O16.-●
      with edema —*see also* Pre-eclampsia
        O14.9-●
      gestational (pregnancy induced) (without
        proteinuria) O13.-●
        with proteinuria O14.9-●
          mild pre-eclampsia O14.0-●
          moderate pre-eclampsia O14.0-●
          severe pre-eclampsia O14.1-●
            with hemolysis, elevated liver
              enzymes and low platelet
              count (HELLP) O14.2-●
      pre-existing O10.91-●
        with
          heart disease O10.11-●
            with renal disease O10.31-●
          pre-eclampsia —*see* category O11
          renal disease O10.21-●
            with heart disease O10.31-●
          essential O10.01-●
          secondary O10.41-●
      transient O13.-●
    puerperium pre-existing O16.5
      pre-existing
        with
          heart disease O10.13
            with renal disease O10.33
          pre-eclampsia O11.5
          renal disease O10.23
            with heart disease O10.33
          essential O10.03
      pregnancy-induced O13.9
      secondary O10.43
  crisis I16.9
  due to
    endocrine disorders I15.2
    pheochromocytoma (*see also*
      Pheochromocytoma, by type) I15.2
    renal disorders NEC I15.1
      arterial I15.0
    renovascular disorders I15.0
    specified disease NEC I15.8
  emergency I16.1
  encephalopathy I67.4
  gestational (without significant proteinuria)
    (pregnancy-induced) (transient) O13.-●
    with significant proteinuria —*see*
      Pre-eclampsia

Hypertension, hypertensive *(Continued)*
  gestational *(Continued)*
    complicating
      delivery O13.4
      puerperium O13.5
  Goldblatt's I70.1
  heart (disease) (conditions in I51.4-I51.9 due to
    hypertension) I11.9
    with
      heart failure (congestive) I11.0
      kidney disease (chronic) —*see*
        Hypertension, cardiorenal
  intracranial, benign G93.2
  kidney I12.9
    with
      heart disease —*see* Hypertension, cardiorenal
      stage 1 through stage 4 chronic kidney
        disease I12.9
      stage 5 chronic kidney disease (CKD) or
        end stage renal disease (ESRD) I12.0
  lesser circulation I27.0
    maternal O16.-●
  newborn P29.2
    pulmonary (persistent) P29.30
  ocular H40.05-●
  pancreatic duct — code to underlying condition
    with chronic pancreatitis K86.1
  portal (due to chronic liver disease) (idiopathic)
    K76.6
    gastropathy K31.89
    in (due to) schistosomiasis (bilharziasis) B65.9
      [K77]
  postoperative I97.3
  psychogenic F45.8
  pulmonary NEC I27.20
    with
      cor pulmonale (chronic) I27.29
        acute I26.09
      right heart ventricular strain/failure I27.29
        acute I26.09
      right to left shunt related to congenital
        heart disease I27.83
      unclear multifactorial mechanisms I27.29
    arterial (associated) (drug-induced) (toxin-
      induced) I27.21
    chronic thromboembolic I27.24
    due to
      hematologic disorders I27.29
      kyphoscoliotic heart disease I27.1
      left heart disease I27.22
      lung diseases and hypoxia I27.23
      metabolic disorders I27.29
      specified systemic disorders NEC I27.29
    group 1 (associated) (drug-induced) (toxin-
      induced) I27.21
    group 2 I27.22
    group 3 I27.23
    group 4 I27.24
    group 5 I27.29
    of newborn (persistent) P29.30
    secondary
      arterial I27.21
      specified NEC I27.29
    primary (idiopathic) I27.0
  renal —*see* Hypertension, kidney
  renovascular I15.0
  resistant (apparent treatment) (treatment) (true)
    I1A.0
  secondary NEC I15.9
    due to
      endocrine disorders I15.2
      pheochromocytoma (*see also*
        Pheochromocytoma, by type) I15.2
      renal disorders NEC I15.1
        arterial I15.0
      renovascular disorders I15.0
    specified NEC I15.8
  transient R03.0
    of pregnancy O13.●
  urgency I16.0
  venous (chronic)
    due to
      deep vein thrombosis —*see* Syndrome,
        postthrombotic
    idiopathic I87.309
      with
        inflammation I87.32-●
          with ulcer I87.33-●
        specified complication NEC I87.39-●
        ulcer I87.31-●
          with inflammation I87.33-●
      asymptomatic I87.30-●

Hypertensive urgency —*see* Hypertension
Hyperthecosis ovary E28.8
Hyperthermia (of unknown origin) —*see also*
    Hyperpyrexia
malignant, due to anesthesia T88.3
newborn P81.9
    environmental P81.0
Hyperthyroid (recurrent) —*see* Hyperthyroidism
Hyperthyroidism (latent) (pre-adult) (recurrent)
    E05.90
with
    goiter (diffuse) E05.00
      with thyroid storm E05.01
      nodular (multinodular) E05.20
        with thyroid storm E05.21
        uninodular E05.10
          with thyroid storm E05.11
    storm E05.91
due to ectopic thyroid tissue E05.30
    with thyroid storm E05.31
neonatal, transitory P72.1
specified NEC E05.80
    with thyroid storm E05.81
Hypertony, hypertonia, hypertonicity
bladder N31.8
congenital P94.1
stomach K31.89
    psychogenic F45.8
uterus, uterine (contractions) (complicating
    delivery) O62.4
Hypertrichosis L68.9
congenital Q84.2
eyelid H02.869
    left H02.866
      lower H02.865
      upper H02.864
    right H02.863
      lower H02.862
      upper H02.861
lanuginosa Q84.2
    acquired L68.1
localized L68.2
specified NEC L68.8
Hypertriglyceridemia, essential E78.1
Hypertrophy, hypertrophic
adenofibromatous, prostate —*see* Enlargement,
    enlarged, prostate
adenoids (infective) J35.2
    with tonsils J35.3
adrenal cortex E27.8
alveolar process or ridge —*see* Anomaly, alveolar
anal papillae K62.89
artery I77.89
    congenital NEC Q27.8
      digestive system Q27.8
      lower limb Q27.8
      specified site NEC Q27.8
      upper limb Q27.8
auricular —*see* Hypertrophy, cardiac
Bartholin's gland N75.8
bile duct (common) (hepatic) K83.8
bladder (sphincter) (trigone) N32.89
bone M89.30
    carpus M89.34-•
    clavicle M89.31-•
    femur M89.35-•
    fibula M89.36-•
    finger M89.34-•
    humerus M89.32-•
    ilium M89.38
    ischium M89.38
    metacarpus M89.34-•
    metatarsus M89.37-•
    multiple sites M89.39
    neck M89.38
    pubic ramus M89.38
    radius M89.33-•
    rib M89.38
    scapula M89.31-•
    skull M89.38
    tarsus M89.37-•
    tibia M89.36-•
    toe M89.37-•
    ulna M89.33-•
    vertebra M89.38
brain G93.89
breast N62
    cystic —*see* Mastopathy, cystic
    newborn P83.4
    pubertal, massive N62

Hypertrophy, hypertrophic *(Continued)*
breast *(Continued)*
    puerperal, postpartum —*see* Disorder, breast,
      specified type NEC
    senile (parenchymatous) N62
cardiac (chronic) (idiopathic) I51.7
    with rheumatic fever (conditions in I00)
      active I01.8
      inactive or quiescent (with chorea) I09.89
    congenital NEC Q24.8
    fatty —*see* Degeneration, myocardial
    hypertensive —*see* Hypertension, heart
    rheumatic (with chorea) I09.89
      active or acute I01.8
        with chorea I02.0
    valve —*see* Endocarditis
cartilage —*see* Disorder, cartilage, specified type
    NEC
cecum —*see* Megacolon
cervix (uteri) N88.8
    congenital Q51.828
    elongation N88.4
clitoris (cirrhotic) N90.89
    congenital Q52.6
colon —*see also* Megacolon
    congenital Q43.2
conjunctiva, lymphoid H11.89
corpora cavernosa N48.89
cystic duct K82.8
duodenum K31.89
endometrium (glandular) —*see also* Hyperplasia,
    endometrial N85.00-•
    cervix N88.8
epididymis N50.89
esophageal hiatus (congenital) Q79.1
    with hernia —*see* Hernia, hiatal
eyelid —*see* Disorder, eyelid, specified type
    NEC
facet joint (see also Spondylosis) M47.819
fat pad E65
    knee (infrapatellar) (popliteal) (prepatellar)
      (retropatellar) M79.4
foot (congenital) Q74.2
frenulum, frenum (tongue) K14.8
    lip K13.0
gallbladder K82.8
gastric mucosa K29.60
    with bleeding K29.61
gland, glandular R59.9
    generalized R59.1
    localized R59.0
gum (mucous membrane) K06.1
heart (idiopathic) —*see also* Hypertrophy, cardiac
    valve —*see also* Endocarditis I38
hemifacial Q67.4
hepatic —*see* Hypertrophy, liver
hiatus (esophageal) Q79.1
hilus gland R59.0
hymen, congenital Q52.4
ileum K63.89
intestine NEC K63.89
jejunum K63.89
kidney (compensatory) N28.81
    congenital Q63.3
labium (majus) (minus) N90.60
ligament —*see* Disorder, ligament
lingual tonsil (infective) J35.1
    with adenoids J35.3
lip K13.0
    congenital Q18.6
liver R16.0
    acute K76.89
    cirrhotic —*see* Cirrhosis, liver
    congenital Q44.79
    fatty —*see* Fatty, liver
lymph, lymphatic gland R59.9
    generalized R59.1
    localized R59.0
    tuberculous —*see* Tuberculosis, lymph
      gland
mammary gland —*see* Hypertrophy, breast
Meckel's diverticulum (congenital) Q43.0
    malignant —*see* Table of Neoplasms, small
      intestine, malignant
median bar —*see* Hyperplasia, prostate
meibomian gland —*see* Chalazion
meniscus, knee, congenital Q74.1
metatarsal head —*see* Hypertrophy, bone,
    metatarsus
metatarsus —*see* Hypertrophy, bone, metatarsus

Hypertrophy, hypertrophic *(Continued)*
mucous membrane
    alveolar ridge K06.2
    gum K06.1
    nose (turbinate) J34.3
muscle M62.89
muscular coat, artery I77.89
myocardium —*see also* Hypertrophy, cardiac
    idiopathic I42.2
myometrium N85.2
nail L60.2
    congenital Q84.5
nasal J34.89
    alae J34.89
    bone J34.89
    cartilage J34.89
    mucous membrane (septum) J34.3
    sinus J34.89
    turbinate J34.3
nasopharynx, lymphoid (infectional) (tissue)
    (wall) J35.2
nipple N62
organ or site, congenital NEC —*see* Anomaly, by
    site - ovary N83.8
palate (hard) M27.8
    soft K13.79
pancreas, congenital Q45.3
parathyroid (gland) E21.0
parotid gland K11.1
penis N48.89
pharyngeal tonsil J35.2
pharynx J39.2
    lymphoid (infectional) (tissue) (wall)
      J35.2
pituitary (anterior) (fossa) (gland) E23.6
prepuce (congenital) N47.8
    female N90.89
prostate —*see* Enlargement, enlarged, prostate
    congenital Q55.4
pseudomuscular (see also Dystrophy, muscular,
    by type, if applicable)
pylorus (adult) (muscle) (sphincter) K31.1
    congenital or infantile Q40.0
rectal, rectum (sphincter) K62.89
rhinitis (turbinate) J31.0
salivary gland (any) K11.1
    congenital Q38.4
scaphoid (tarsal) —*see* Hypertrophy, bone, tarsus
scar L91.0
scrotum N50.89
seminal vesicle N50.89
sigmoid —*see* Megacolon
skin L91.9
    specified NEC L91.8
spermatic cord N50.89
spleen —*see* Splenomegaly
spondylitis —*see* Spondylosis
stomach K31.89
sublingual gland K11.1
submandibular gland K11.1
suprarenal cortex (gland) E27.8
synovial NEC M67.20
    acromioclavicular M67.21-•
    ankle M67.27-•
    elbow M67.22-•
    foot M67.27-•
    hand M67.24-•
    hip M67.25-•
    knee M67.26-•
    multiple sites M67.29
    specified site NEC M67.28
    wrist M67.23-•
tendon —*see* Disorder, tendon, specified type
    NEC
testis N44.8
    congenital Q55.29
thymic, thymus (gland) (congenital)
    E32.0
thyroid (gland) —*see* Goiter
toe (congenital) Q74.2
    acquired —*see also* Deformity, toe, specified
      NEC
    congenital Q38.2
    papillae (foliate) K14.3
tonsils (faucial) (infective) (lingual) (lymphoid)
    J35.1
    with adenoids J35.3
tunica vaginalis N50.89
ureter N28.89
urethra N36.8

Hypertrophy, hypertrophic *(Continued)*
  uterus N85.2
    neck (with elongation) N88.4
    puerperal O90.89
  uvula K13.79
  vagina N89.8
  vas deferens N50.89
  vein I87.8
  ventricle, ventricular (heart) —*see also*
    Hypertrophy, cardiac
    congenital Q24.8
    in tetralogy of Fallot Q21.3
  verumontanum N36.8
  vocal cord J38.3
  vulva N90.60
    stasis (nonfilarial) N90.69
Hypertropia H50.2-●
Hypertyrosinemia E70.21
Hyperuricemia (asymptomatic) E79.0
Hyperuricosuria R82.993
Hypervalinemia E71.19
Hyperventilation (tetany) R06.4
  hysterical F45.8
  psychogenic F45.8
  syndrome F45.8
Hypervitaminosis (dietary) NEC E67.8
  A E67.0
    administered as drug (prolonged intake) —*see*
      Table of Drugs and Chemicals, vitamins,
      adverse effect
    overdose or wrong substance given or
      taken —*see* Table of Drugs and
      Chemicals, vitamins, poisoning
  B6 E67.2
  D E67.3
    administered as drug (prolonged intake) —*see*
      Table of Drugs and Chemicals, vitamins,
      adverse effect
    overdose or wrong substance given or
      taken —*see* Table of Drugs and
      Chemicals, vitamins, poisoning
  K E67.8
    administered as drug (prolonged intake) —*see*
      Table of Drugs and Chemicals, vitamins,
      adverse effect
    overdose or wrong substance given or
      taken —*see* Table of Drugs and
      Chemicals, vitamins, poisoning
Hypervolemia E87.70
  specified NEC E87.79
Hypesthesia R20.1
  cornea —*see* Anesthesia, cornea
Hyphema H21.0-●
  traumatic S05.1-●
Hypoacidity, gastric K31.89
  psychogenic F45.8
Hypoadrenalism, hypoadrenia E27.40
  primary E27.1
  tuberculous A18.7
Hypoadrenocorticism E27.40
  pituitary E23.0
  primary E27.1
Hypoalbuminemia E88.09
Hypoaldosteronism E27.40
Hypoalphalipoproteinemia E78.6
Hypobarism T70.29
Hypobaropathy T70.29
Hypobetalipoproteinemia (familial) E78.6
Hypocalcemia E83.51
  autosomal dominant E20.810
    type 1 (ADH1) E20.810
    type 2 (ADH2) E20.810
  dietary E58
  neonatal P71.1
    due to cow's milk P71.0
  phosphate-loading (newborn) P71.1
Hypochloremia E87.8
Hypochlorhydria K31.89
  neurotic F45.8
  psychogenic F45.8
Hypochondria, hypochondriac, hypochondriasis
  (reaction) F45.21
  sleep F51.03
Hypochondrogenesis Q77.0
Hypochondroplasia Q77.4
Hypochromasia, blood cells D50.8
Hypodontia —*see* Anodontia
Hypocitraturia R82.991
Hypoeosinophilia D72.89
Hypoesthesia R20.1

Hypofibrinogenemia D68.8
  acquired D65
  congenital (hereditary) D68.2
Hypofunction
  adrenocortical E27.40
    drug-induced E27.3
    postprocedural E89.6
    primary E27.1
  adrenomedullary, postprocedural E89.6
  cerebral R29.818
  corticoadrenal NEC E27.40
  intestinal K59.89
  labyrinth —*see* subcategory H83.2
  ovary E28.39
  pituitary (gland) (anterior) E23.0
  testicular E29.1
    postprocedural (postsurgical) (postirradiation)
      (iatrogenic) E89.5
Hypogalactia O92.4
Hypogammaglobulinemia —*see also*
  Agammaglobulinemia D80.1
  hereditary D80.0
  nonfamilial D80.1
  transient, of infancy D80.7
Hypogenitalism (congenital) —*see* Hypogonadism
Hypoglossia Q38.3
Hypoglycemia (spontaneous) E16.2
  coma E15
    diabetic —*see* Diabetes, by type, with
      hypoglycemia, with coma
  diabetic —*see* Diabetes, hypoglycemia
  dietary counseling and surveillance Z71.3
  drug-induced E16.0
    with coma (nondiabetic) E15
  due to insulin E16.0
    with coma (nondiabetic) E15
    therapeutic misadventure —*see* subcategory
      T38.3
  functional, nonhyperinsulinemic E16.1
  iatrogenic E16.0
    with coma (nondiabetic) E15
  in infant of diabetic mother P70.1
    gestational diabetes P70.0
  infantile E16.1
  leucine-induced E71.19
▶ level
▶   1 E16.A1
▶   2 E16.A2
▶   3 E16.A3
  neonatal (transitory) P70.4
    iatrogenic P70.3
  reactive (not drug-induced) E16.1
  transitory neonatal P70.4
Hypogonadism
  female E28.39
  hypogonadotropic E23.0
  male E29.1
  ovarian (primary) E28.39
  pituitary E23.0
  testicular (primary) E29.1
Hypohidrosis, hypoidrosis L74.4
Hypoinsulinemia, postprocedural E89.1
Hypokalemia E87.6
Hypoleukocytosis —*see* Agranulocytosis
Hypolipoproteinemia (alpha) (beta) E78.6
Hypomagnesemia E83.42
  neonatal P71.2
Hypomania, hypomanic reaction F30.8
Hypomenorrhea —*see* Oligomenorrhea
Hypometabolism R63.8
Hypomotility
  gastrointestinal (tract) K31.89
    psychogenic F45.8
  intestine K59.89
    psychogenic F45.8
  stomach K31.89
    psychogenic F45.8
Hypomyelination - hypogonadotropic
  hypogonadism - hypodontia G11.5
Hypomyelination with atrophy of the basal
  ganglia and cerebellum (H-ABC) G23.3
Hyponasality R49.22
Hyponatremia E87.1
Hypo-osmolality E87.1
Hypo-ovarianism, hypo-ovarism E28.39
Hypoparathyroidism E20.9
  autoimmune E20.812
  due to impaired parathyroid hormone secretion,
    unspecified E20.819
  familial E20.89

Hypoparathyroidism *(Continued)*
  idiopathic E20.0
  isolated E20.818
  neonatal, transitory P71.4
  postprocedural E89.2
  secondary, in diseases classified elsewhere
    E20.811
  specified NEC E20.89
    due to impaired parathyroid hormone
      secretion E20.818
Hypoperfusion (in)
  newborn P96.89
Hypopharyngitis —*see* Laryngopharyngitis
Hypophoria H50.53
Hypophosphatemia, hypophosphatasia (acquired)
  (congenital) (renal) E83.39
  familial E83.31
Hypophyseal, hypophysis —*see also* condition
  dwarfism E23.0
  gigantism E22.0
Hypopiesis —*see* Hypotension
Hypopinealism E34.8
Hypopituitarism (juvenile) E23.0
  drug-induced E23.1
  due to
    hypophysectomy E89.3
    radiotherapy E89.3
  iatrogenic NEC E23.1
  postirradiation E89.3
  postpartum O99.285
  postprocedural E89.3
Hypoplasia, hypoplastic
  adrenal (gland), congenital Q89.1
  alimentary tract, congenital Q45.8
    upper Q40.8
  anus, anal (canal) Q42.3
    with fistula Q42.2
  aorta, aortic Q25.42
    ascending, in hypoplastic left heart syndrome
      Q23.4
    valve Q23.1
      in hypoplastic left heart syndrome Q23.4
  areola, congenital Q83.8
  arm (congenital) —*see* Defect, reduction, upper
    limb
  artery (peripheral) Q27.8
    brain (congenital) Q28.3
    coronary Q24.5
    digestive system Q27.8
    lower limb Q27.8
    pulmonary Q25.79
      functional, unilateral J43.0
    retinal (congenital) Q14.1
    specified site NEC Q27.8
    umbilical Q27.0
    upper limb Q27.8
  auditory canal Q17.8
    causing impairment of hearing Q16.9
  biliary duct or passage Q44.5
  bone NOS Q79.9
    face Q75.8
    marrow D61.9
      megakaryocytic D69.49
    skull —*see* Hypoplasia, skull
  brain Q02
    gyri Q04.3
    part of Q04.3
  breast (areola) N64.82
  bronchus Q32.4
  cardiac Q24.8
  carpus —*see* Defect, reduction, upper limb,
    specified type NEC
  cartilage hair Q78.8
  cecum Q42.8
  cementum K00.4
  cephalic Q02
  cerebellum Q04.3
  cervix (uteri), congenital Q51.821
  clavicle (congenital) Q74.0
  coccyx Q76.49
  colon Q42.9
    specified NEC Q42.8
  corpus callosum Q04.0
  cricoid cartilage Q31.2
  digestive organ(s) or tract NEC Q45.8
    upper (congenital) Q40.8
  ear (auricle) (lobe) Q17.2
    middle Q16.4
  enamel of teeth (neonatal) (postnatal) (prenatal)
    K00.4

Hypoplasia, hypoplastic *(Continued)*
  endocrine (gland) NEC Q89.2
  endometrium N85.8
  epididymis (congenital) Q55.4
  epiglottis Q31.2
  erythroid, congenital D61.01
  esophagus (congenital) Q39.8
  eustachian tube Q17.8
  eye Q11.2
  eyelid (congenital) Q10.3
  face Q18.8
    bone(s) Q75.8
  femur (congenital) —*see* Defect, reduction, lower
      limb, specified type NEC
  fibula (congenital) —*see* Defect, reduction, lower
      limb, specified type NEC
  finger (congenital) —*see* Defect, reduction, upper
      limb, specified type NEC
  focal dermal Q82.8
  foot —*see* Defect, reduction, lower limb,
      specified type NEC
  gallbladder Q44.0
  genitalia, genital organ(s)
    female, congenital Q52.8
      external Q52.79
      internal NEC Q52.8
    in adiposogenital dystrophy E23.6
  glottis Q31.2
  hair Q84.2
  hand (congenital) —*see* Defect, reduction, upper
      limb, specified type NEC
  heart Q24.8
  humerus (congenital) —*see* Defect, reduction,
      upper limb, specified type NEC
  intestine (small) Q41.9
    large Q42.9
      specified NEC Q42.8
  jaw M26.09
    alveolar M26.79
    lower M26.04
      alveolar M26.74
    upper M26.02
      alveolar M26.73
  kidney(s) Q60.5
    bilateral Q60.4
    unilateral Q60.3
  labium (majus) (minus), congenital Q52.79
  larynx Q31.2
  left heart syndrome Q23.4
  leg (congenital) —*see* Defect, reduction, lower
      limb
  limb Q73.8
    lower (congenital) —*see* Defect, reduction,
        lower limb
    upper (congenital) —*see* Defect, reduction,
        upper limb
  liver Q44.79
  lung (lobe) (not associated with short gestation)
      Q33.6
    associated with immaturity, low birth weight,
        prematurity, or short gestation P28.0
  mammary (areola), congenital Q83.8
  mandible, mandibular M26.04
    alveolar M26.74
    unilateral condylar M27.8
  maxillary M26.02
    alveolar M26.73
  medullary D61.9
  megakaryocytic D69.49
  metacarpus —*see* Defect, reduction, upper limb,
      specified type NEC
  metatarsus —*see* Defect, reduction, lower limb,
      specified type NEC
  muscle Q79.8
  nail(s) Q84.6
  nose, nasal Q30.1
  optic nerve H47.03-●
  osseous meatus (ear) Q17.8
  ovary, congenital Q50.39
  pancreas Q45.0
  parathyroid (gland) Q89.2
  parotid gland Q38.4
  patella Q74.1
  pelvis, pelvic girdle Q74.2
  penis (congenital) Q55.62
  peripheral vascular system Q27.8
    digestive system Q27.8
    lower limb Q27.8
    specified site NEC Q27.8
    upper limb Q27.8
  pituitary (gland) (congenital) Q89.2

Hypoplasia, hypoplastic *(Continued)*
  pulmonary (not associated with short gestation)
      Q33.6
    artery, functional J43.0
    associated with short gestation P28.0
  radioulnar —*see* Defect, reduction, upper limb,
      specified type NEC
  radius —*see* Defect, reduction, upper limb
  rectum Q42.1
    with fistula Q42.0
  respiratory system NEC Q34.8
  rib Q76.6
  right heart syndrome Q22.6
  sacrum Q76.49
  scapula Q74.0
  scrotum Q55.1
  shoulder girdle Q74.0
  skin Q82.8
  skull (bone) Q75.8
    with
      anencephaly Q00.0
      encephalocele —*see* Encephalocele
      hydrocephalus Q03.9
        with spina bifida —*see* Spina bifida, by
            site, with hydrocephalus
      microcephaly Q02
  spinal (cord) (ventral horn cell) Q06.1
  spine Q76.49
  sternum Q76.7
  tarsus —*see* Defect, reduction, lower limb,
      specified type NEC
  testis Q55.1
  thymic, with immunodeficiency D82.1
  thymus (gland) Q89.2
    with immunodeficiency D82.1
  thyroid (gland) E03.1
    cartilage Q31.2
  tibiofibular (congenital) —*see* Defect, reduction,
      lower limb, specified type NEC
  toe —*see* Defect, reduction, lower limb, specified
      type NEC
  tongue Q38.3
  Turner's K00.4
  ulna (congenital) —*see* Defect, reduction, upper
      limb
  umbilical artery Q27.0
  unilateral condylar M27.8
  ureter Q62.8
  uterus, congenital Q51.811
  vagina Q52.4
  vascular NEC peripheral Q27.8
    brain Q28.3
    digestive system Q27.8
    lower limb Q27.8
    specified site NEC Q27.8
    upper limb Q27.8
  vein(s) (peripheral) Q27.8
    brain Q28.3
    digestive system Q27.8
    great Q26.8
    lower limb Q27.8
    specified site NEC Q27.8
    upper limb Q27.8
  vena cava (inferior) (superior) Q26.8
  vertebra Q76.49
  vulva, congenital Q52.79
  zonule (ciliary) Q12.8
Hypoplasminogenemia E88.02
Hypopnea, obstructive sleep apnea G47.33
Hypopotassemia E87.6
Hypoproconvertinemia, congenital (hereditary)
    D68.2
Hypoproteinemia E77.8
Hypoprothrombinemia (congenital) (hereditary)
    (idiopathic) D68.2
  acquired D68.4
  newborn, transient P61.6
Hypoptyalism K11.7
Hypopyon (eye) (anterior chamber) —*see*
    Iridocyclitis, acute, hypopyon
Hypopyrexia R68.0
Hyporeflexia R29.2
Hyposecretion
  ACTH E23.0
  antidiuretic hormone E23.2
  ovary E28.39
  salivary gland (any) K11.7
  vasopressin E23.2
Hyposegmentation, leukocytic, hereditary
    D72.0
Hyposiderinemia D50.9

Hypospadias Q54.9
  balanic Q54.0
  coronal Q54.0
  glandular Q54.0
  penile Q54.1
  penoscrotal Q54.2
  perineal Q54.3
  specified NEC Q54.8
Hypospermatogenesis —*see* Oligospermia
Hyposplenism D73.0
Hypostasis pulmonary, passive —*see* Edema, lung
Hypostatic —*see* condition
Hyposthenuria N28.89
Hypotension (arterial) (constitutional) I95.9
  chronic I95.89
  drug-induced I95.2
  due to (of) hemodialysis I95.3
  iatrogenic I95.89
  idiopathic (permanent) I95.0
  intracranial G96.810
    following
      lumbar cerebrospinal fluid shunting G97.83
      specified procedure NEC G97.84
      ventricular shunting (ventriculostomy)
          G97.2
    specified NEC G96.819
    spontaneous G96.811
Hypothermia (accidental) T68
  intra-dialytic I95.3
  maternal, syndrome (following labor and
      delivery) O26.5-●
  neurogenic, orthostatic G90.3
  orthostatic (chronic) I95.1
    due to drugs I95.2
    neurogenic G90.3
  postoperative I95.81
  postural I95.1
  specified NEC I95.89
    due to anesthesia, anesthetic T88.51
  low environmental temperature T68
  neonatal P80.9
    environmental (mild) NEC P80.8
    mild P80.8
    severe (chronic) (cold injury syndrome) P80.0
    specified NEC P80.8
  not associated with low environmental
      temperature R68.0
Hypothyroidism (acquired) E03.9
  autoimmune —*see* Thyroiditis, autoimmune
  congenital (without goiter) E03.1
    with goiter (diffuse) E03.0
  due to
    exogenous substance NEC E03.2
    iodine-deficiency, acquired E01.8
      subclinical E02
    irradiation therapy E89.0
    medicament NEC E03.2
    P-aminosalicylic acid (PAS) E03.2
    phenylbutazone E03.2
    resorcinol E03.2
    sulfonamide E03.2
    surgery E89.0
    thiourea group drugs E03.2
  iatrogenic NEC E03.2
  iodine-deficiency (acquired) E01.8
    congenital —*see* Syndrome, iodine-deficiency,
        congenital
    subclinical E02
  neonatal, transitory P72.2
  postinfectious E03.3
  postirradiation E89.0
  postprocedural E89.0
  postsurgical E89.0
  specified NEC E03.8
  subclinical, iodine-deficiency
      related E02
Hypotonia, hypotonicity, hypotony
  bladder N31.2
  congenital (benign) P94.2
  eye —*see* Disorder, globe, hypotony
Hypotrichosis —*see* Alopecia
Hypotropia H50.2-●
Hypoventilation R06.89
  congenital central alveolar G47.35
  sleep related
    idiopathic nonobstructive alveolar G47.34
    in conditions classified elsewhere G47.36
Hypovitaminosis —*see* Deficiency, vitamin
Hypovolemia E86.1
  surgical shock T81.19
  traumatic (shock) T79.4

Hypoxemia R09.02
  newborn P84
  sleep related, in conditions classified elsewhere G47.36
Hypoxia —see also Anoxia R09.02
  cerebral, during a procedure NEC G97.81
    postprocedural NEC G97.82
  intrauterine P84
  myocardial —see Insufficiency, coronary
  newborn P84
  sleep-related G47.34
Hypsarhythmia —see Epilepsy, generalized, specified NEC
▶Hypsarrhythmia —see Epilepsy, generalized, specified NEC
Hysteralgia, pregnant uterus O26.89- ●
Hysteria, hysterical (conversion) (dissociative state) F44.9
  anxiety F41.8
  convulsions F44.5
  psychosis, acute F44.9
Hysteroepilepsy F44.5

I

IBDU (colonic inflammatory bowel dissease unclassified) K52.3
ICANS (immune effector cell-associated neurotoxicity syndrome) —see Syndrome, immune effector cell-associated neurotoxicity
Ichthyoparasitism due to Vandellia cirrhosa B88.8
Ichthyosis (congenital) Q80.9
  acquired L85.0
  fetalis Q80.4
  hystrix Q80.8
  lamellar Q80.2
  lingual K13.29
  palmaris and plantaris Q82.8
  simplex Q80.0
  vera Q80.8
  vulgaris Q80.0
  X-linked Q80.1
Ichthyotoxism —see Poisoning, fish
  bacterial —see Intoxication, foodborne
Icteroanemia, hemolytic (acquired) D59.9
  congenital —see Spherocytosis
Icterus —see also Jaundice
  conjunctiva R17
  gravis, newborn P55.0
  hematogenous (acquired) D59.9
  hemolytic (acquired) D59.9
    congenital —see Spherocytosis
  hemorrhagic (acute) (leptospiral) (spirochetal) A27.0
    newborn P53
  infectious B15.9
    with hepatic coma B15.0
    leptospiral A27.0
    spirochetal A27.0
  neonatorum —see Jaundice, newborn
  newborn P59.9
  spirochetal A27.0
Ictus solaris, solis T67.01
Ideation
  homicidal R45.850
  suicidal R45.851
Identity disorder (child) F64.9
  gender role F64.2
  psychosexual F64.2
Idioglossia F80.0
Idiopathic —see condition
Idiot, idiocy (congenital) F73
  amaurotic (Bielschowsky(-Jansky)) (family) (infantile (late)) (juvenile (late)) (Vogt-Spielmeyer) E75.4
  microcephalic Q02
Id reaction (due to bacteria) L30.2
IgE asthma J45.909

IIAC (idiopathic infantile arterial calcification) Q28.8
Ileitis (chronic) (noninfectious) —see also Enteritis K52.9
  backwash —see Pancolitis, ulcerative (chronic)
  infectious A09
  regional (ulcerative) —see Enteritis, regional, small intestine
  segmental —see Enteritis, regional
  terminal (ulcerative) —see Enteritis, regional, small intestine
Ileocolitis —see also Enteritis K52.9
  infectious A09
  regional —see Enteritis, regional
  ulcerative K51.0- ●
Ileostomy
  attention to Z43.2
  malfunctioning K94.13
  status (ileal pouch) (Kock pouch) Z93.2
    with complication —see Complications, enterostomy
Ileotyphus —see Typhoid
Ileum —see condition
Ileus (bowel) (colon) (inhibitory) (intestine) K56.7
  adynamic K56.0
  due to gallstone (in intestine) K56.3
  duodenal (chronic) K31.5
  gallstone K56.3
  mechanical NEC —see also Obstruction, intestine, specified K56.699
  meconium P76.0
    in cystic fibrosis E84.11
    meaning meconium plug (without cystic fibrosis) P76.0
  myxedema K59.89
  neurogenic K56.0
    Hirschsprung's disease or megacolon Q43.1
  newborn
    due to meconium P76.0
      in cystic fibrosis E84.11
      meaning meconium plug (without cystic fibrosis) P76.0
    transitory P76.1
  obstructive —see also Obstruction, intestine, specified K56.699
  paralytic K56.0
  postoperative K91.89
Iliac —see condition
Iliotibial band syndrome M76.3- ●
Illiteracy Z55.0
  health Z55.6
Illness —see also Disease R69
  manic-depressive —see Disorder, bipolar
Imbalance R26.89
  autonomic G90.89
  constituents of food intake E63.1
  electrolyte E87.8
    with
      abortion —see Abortion by type, complicated by, electrolyte imbalance
      molar pregnancy O08.5
    due to hyperemesis gravidarum O21.1
    following ectopic or molar pregnancy O08.5
    neonatal, transitory NEC P74.49
      potassium
        hyperkalemia P74.31
        hypokalemia P74.32
      sodium
        hypernatremia P74.21
        hyponatremia P74.22
  endocrine E34.9
  eye muscle NOS H50.9
  hormone E34.9
  hysterical F44.4
  labyrinth —see subcategory H83.2
  posture R29.3
  protein-energy —see Malnutrition
  sympathetic G90.89
Imbecile, imbecility (I.Q. 35-49) F71
Imbedding, intrauterine device T83.39
Imbibition, cholesterol (gallbladder) K82.4

Imbrication, teeth, fully erupted M26.30
Imerslund (-Gräsbeck) syndrome D51.1
Immature —see also Immaturity
  birth (less than 37 completed weeks) —see Preterm, newborn
    extremely (less than 28 completed weeks) —see Immaturity, extreme
  personality F60.89
Immaturity (less than 37 completed weeks) —see also Preterm, newborn
  extreme of newborn (less than 28 completed weeks of gestation) (less than 196 completed days of gestation) (unspecified weeks of gestation) P07.20
    gestational age
      23 completed weeks (23 weeks, 0 days through 23 weeks, 6 days) P07.22
      24 completed weeks (24 weeks, 0 days through 24 weeks, 6 days) P07.23
      25 completed weeks (25 weeks, 0 days through 25 weeks, 6 days) P07.24
      26 completed weeks (26 weeks, 0 days through 26 weeks, 6 days) P07.25
      27 completed weeks (27 weeks, 0 days through 27 weeks, 6 days) P07.26
    less than 23 completed weeks P07.21
  fetus or infant light-for-dates —see Light-for-dates
  lung, newborn P28.0
  organ or site NEC —see Hypoplasia
  pulmonary, newborn P28.0
  reaction F60.89
  sexual (female) (male), after puberty E30.0
Immersion T75.1
  foot T69.02- ●
  hand T69.01- ●
Immobile, immobility
  complete, due to severe physical disability or frailty R53.2
  intestine K59.89
  syndrome (paraplegic) M62.3
Immune reconstitution (inflammatory) syndrome [IRIS] D89.3
Immunization —see also Vaccination
  ABO —see Incompatibility, ABO
    in newborn P55.1
  appropriate for age
    child (over 28 days old) Z00.129
      with abnormal findings Z00.121
  complication —see Complications, vaccination
  encounter for Z23
  not done (not carried out) Z28.9
    because (of)
      acute illness of patient Z28.01
      allergy to vaccine (or component) Z28.04
      caregiver refusal Z28.82
      chronic illness of patient Z28.02
      contraindication NEC Z28.09
      delay in delivery of vaccine Z28.83
      group pressure Z28.1
      guardian refusal Z28.82
      immune compromised state of patient Z28.03
      lack of availability of vaccine Z28.83
      manufacturer delay of vaccine Z28.83
      parent refusal Z28.82
      patient's belief Z28.1
      patient had disease being vaccinated against Z28.81
      patient refusal Z28.21
      religious beliefs of patient Z28.1
      specified reason NEC Z28.89
        of patient Z28.29
      unavailability of vaccine Z28.83
      unspecified patient reason Z28.20
  Rh factor
    affecting management of pregnancy NEC O36.09- ●
      anti-D antibody O36.01- ●
    from transfusion —see Complication(s), transfusion, incompatibility reaction, Rh (factor)
Immunocompromised NOS D84.9
Immunocytoma C83.0- ●

Immunodeficiency D84.9
  with
    adenosine-deaminase deficiency (see also
      Deficiency, adenosine deaminase) D81.30
    antibody defects D80.9
      specified type NEC D80.8
    hyperimmunoglobulinemia D80.6
    increased immunoglobulin M (IgM)
      D80.5
    major defect D82.9
      specified type NEC D82.8
    partial albinism D82.8
    short-limbed stature D82.2
    thrombocytopenia and eczema D82.0
  antibody with
    hyperimmunoglobulinemia D80.6
    near-normal immunoglobulins D80.6
  autosomal recessive, Swiss type D80.0
  combined D81.9
    biotin-dependent carboxylase D81.819
      biotinidase D81.810
      holocarboxylase synthetase D81.818
      specified type NEC D81.818
    severe (SCID) D81.9
      with
        low or normal B-cell numbers D81.2
        low T- and B-cell numbers D81.1
        reticular dysgenesis D81.0
    specified type NEC D81.89
  common variable D83.9
    with
      abnormalities of B-cell numbers and
        function D83.0
      autoantibodies to B- or T-cells D83.2
      immunoregulatory T-cell disorders D83.1
    specified type NEC D83.8
  due to
    conditions classified elsewhere D84.81
    drugs D84.821
    external causes D84.822
    medication (current or past) D84.821
  following hereditary defective response to
    Epstein-Barr virus (EBV) D82.3
  selective, immunoglobulin
    A (IgA) D80.2
    G (IgG) (subclasses) D80.3
    M (IgM) D80.4
  severe combined (SCID) D81.9
    due to adenosine deaminase deficiency
      D81.31
  specified type NEC D84.89
  X-linked, with increased IgM D80.5
Immunodeficient NOS D84.9
Immunosuppressed NOS D84.9
Immunotherapy (encounter for)
  antineoplastic Z51.12
Impaction, impacted
  bowel, colon, rectum —see also Impaction, fecal
    K56.49
    by gallstone K56.3
  calculus —see Calculus
  cerumen (ear) (external) H61.2-•
  cuspid —see Impaction, tooth
  dental (same or adjacent tooth) K01.1
  fecal, feces K56.41
  fracture —see Fracture, by site
  gallbladder —see Calculus, gallbladder
  gallstone(s) —see Calculus, gallbladder
    bile duct (common) (hepatic) —see Calculus,
      bile duct
    cystic duct —see Calculus, gallbladder
    in intestine, with obstruction (any part)
      K56.3
  intestine (calculous) NEC —see also Impaction,
    fecal K56.49
    gallstone, with ileus K56.3
  intrauterine device (IUD) T83.39
  molar —see Impaction, tooth
  shoulder, causing obstructed labor O66.0
  tooth, teeth K01.1
  turbinate J34.89
Impaired, impairment (function)
  auditory discrimination —see Abnormal,
    auditory perception
  cognitive, mild, of uncertain or unknown
    etiology G31.84
  dual sensory Z73.82
  fasting glucose R73.01
  glucose tolerance (oral) R73.02
  hearing —see Deafness
  heart —see Disease, heart

Impaired, impairment (Continued)
  kidney N28.9
    disorder resulting from N25.9
      specified NEC N25.89
  liver K72.90
    with coma K72.91
  mastication K08.89
  mild cognitive G31.84
    of uncertain or unknown etiology
      G31.84
  mild neurocognitive
    due to known physiological condition
      (without behavioral disturbance)
      F06.70
    with behavioral disturbance F06.71
  mobility
    ear ossicles —see Ankylosis, ear ossicles
    requiring care provider Z74.09
  myocardium, myocardial —see Insufficiency,
    myocardial
  rectal sphincter R19.8
  renal (acute) (chronic) N28.9
    disorder resulting from N25.9
      specified NEC N25.89
  vision NEC H54.7
    both eyes H54.3
Impediment, speech (see also Disorder, speech)
  R47.9
  psychogenic (childhood) F98.8
  slurring R47.81
  specified NEC R47.89
Impending
  coronary syndrome I20.0
  delirium tremens F10.239
  myocardial infarction I20.0
Imperception auditory (acquired) —see also
  Deafness
  congenital H93.25
Imperfect
  aeration, lung (newborn) NEC —see Atelectasis
  closure (congenital)
    alimentary tract NEC Q45.8
      lower Q43.8
      upper Q40.8
    atrioventricular ostium Q21.20
    atrium (secundum) Q21.11
    branchial cleft NOS Q18.2
      cyst Q18.0
      fistula Q18.0
      sinus Q18.0
    choroid Q14.3
    cricoid cartilage Q31.8
    cusps, heart valve NEC Q24.8
      pulmonary Q22.3
    ductus
      arteriosus Q25.0
      Botalli Q25.0
    ear drum (causing impairment of hearing)
      Q16.4
    esophagus with communication to bronchus
      or trachea Q39.1
    eyelid Q10.3
    foramen
      botalli Q21.12
      ovale Q21.12
    genitalia, genital organ(s) or system
      female Q52.8
        external Q52.79
        internal NEC Q52.8
      male Q55.8
    glottic Q31.8
    interatrial ostium or septum Q21.19
    interauricular ostium or septum Q21.19
    interventricular ostium or septum Q21.0
    larynx Q31.8
    lip —see Cleft, lip
    nasal septum Q30.3
    nose Q30.2
    omphalomesenteric duct Q43.0
    optic nerve entry Q14.2
    organ or site not listed —see Anomaly, by
      site
    ostium
      interatrial Q21.19
      interauricular Q21.19
      interventricular Q21.0
    palate —see Cleft, palate
    preauricular sinus Q18.1
    retina Q14.1
    roof of orbit Q75.8
    sclera Q13.5

Imperfect (Continued)
  closure (Continued)
    septum
      aorticopulmonary Q21.4
      atrial (secundum) Q21.19
      between aorta and pulmonary artery Q21.4
      heart Q21.9
      interatrial (secundum) Q21.19
      interauricular (secundum) Q21.19
      interventricular Q21.0
        in tetralogy of Fallot Q21.3
      nasal Q30.3
      ventricular Q21.0
        with pulmonary stenosis or atresia,
          dextraposition of aorta, and
          hypertrophy of right ventricle Q21.3
        in tetralogy of Fallot Q21.3
    skull Q75.009
      with
        anencephaly Q00.0
        encephalocele —see Encephalocele
        hydrocephalus Q03.9
          with spina bifida —see Spina bifida, by
            site, with hydrocephalus
        microcephaly Q02
    spine (with meningocele) —see Spina bifida
    trachea Q32.1
    tympanic membrane (causing impairment of
      hearing) Q16.4
    uterus Q51.818
    vitelline duct Q43.0
  erection —see Dysfunction, sexual, male, erectile
  fusion —see Imperfect, closure
  inflation, lung (newborn) —see Atelectasis
  posture R29.3
  rotation, intestine Q43.3
  septum, ventricular Q21.0
Imperfectly descended testis —see Cryptorchid
Imperforate (congenital) —see also Atresia
  anus Q42.3
    with fistula Q42.2
  cervix (uteri) Q51.828
  esophagus Q39.0
    with tracheoesophageal fistula Q39.1
  hymen Q52.3
  jejunum Q41.1
  pharynx Q38.8
  rectum Q42.1
    with fistula Q42.0
  urethra Q64.39
  vagina Q52.4
Impervious (congenital) —see also Atresia
  anus Q42.3
    with fistula Q42.2
  bile duct Q44.2
  esophagus Q39.0
    with tracheoesophageal fistula Q39.1
  intestine (small) Q41.9
    large Q42.9
      specified NEC Q42.8
  rectum Q42.1
    with fistula Q42.0
  ureter —see Atresia, ureter
  urethra Q64.39
Impetiginization of dermatoses L01.1
Impetigo (any organism) (any site) (circinate)
  (contagiosa) (simplex) (vulgaris)
  L01.00
  Bockhart's L01.02
  bullous, bullosa L01.03
  external ear L01.00 [H62.40]
  follicularis L01.02
  furfuracea L30.5
  herpetiformis L40.1
    nonobstetrical L40.1
  neonatorum L01.03
  nonbullous L01.01
  specified type NEC L01.09
  ulcerative L01.09
Impingement (on teeth)
  joint —see Disorder, joint, specified type NEC
  soft tissue
    anterior M26.81
    posterior M26.82
Implant, endometrial N80.9
Implantation
  anomalous —see Anomaly, by site
    ureter Q62.63
  cyst
    external area or site (skin) NEC L72.0
    iris —see Cyst, iris, implantation

Implantation *(Continued)*
  cyst *(Continued)*
    vagina N89.8
    vulva N90.7
  dermoid (cyst) —*see* Implantation, cyst
Impotence (sexual) N52.9
  counseling Z70.1
  organic origin —*see also* Dysfunction, sexual, male, erectile N52.9
  psychogenic F52.21
Impression, basilar Q75.8
Imprisonment, anxiety concerning Z65.1
Improper care (child) (newborn) —*see* Maltreatment
Improperly tied umbilical cord (causing hemorrhage) P51.8
Impulsiveness (impulsive) R45.87
Inability to
  comply with dietary regimen Z91.118
  swallow - see Aphagia
Inaccessible, inaccessibility
  health care NEC Z75.3
    due to
      waiting period Z75.2
        for admission to facility elsewhere Z75.1
  other helping agencies Z75.4
  transportation Z59.82
Inactive —*see* condition
Inadequate, inadequacy
  aesthetics of dental restoration K08.56
  biologic, constitutional, functional, or social F60.7
  development
    child R62.50
    genitalia
      after puberty NEC E30.0
      congenital
        female Q52.8
          external Q52.79
          internal Q52.8
        male Q55.8
    lungs Q33.6
      associated with short gestation P28.0
    organ or site not listed —*see* Anomaly, by site
  diet (causing nutritional deficiency) E63.9
  drinking-water supply Z58.6
  eating habits Z72.4
  environment, household Z59.11
  family support Z63.8
  food (supply) NEC Z59.48
    hunger effects T73.0
  functional F60.7
  household care, due to
    family member
      handicapped or ill Z74.2
      on vacation Z75.5
      temporarily away from home Z74.2
    technical defects in home Z59.19
    temporary absence from home of person rendering care Z74.2
  housing Z59.10
    environmental temperature Z59.11
    heating Z59.11
    space Z59.19
    specified NEC Z59.19
    utilities Z59.12
  income (financial) Z59.6
  intrafamilial communication Z63.8
  material resources due to limited financial resources, specified NEC Z59.87
  mental —*see* Disability, intellectual
  parental supervision or control of child Z62.0
  personality F60.7
  pulmonary
    function R06.89
      newborn P28.5
    ventilation, newborn P28.5
  sample of cytologic smear
    anus R85.615
    cervix R87.615
    vagina R87.625
  social F60.7
    insurance Z59.71
    skills NEC Z73.4
  social support Z60.8
  supervision of child by parent Z62.0
  teaching affecting education Z55.8
  transportation Z59.82
  welfare support Z59.72

Inanition R64
  with edema —*see* Malnutrition, severe
  due to
    deprivation of food T73.0
    malnutrition —*see* Malnutrition
  fever R50.9
Inappropriate
  change in quantitative human chorionic gonadotropin (hCG) in early pregnancy O02.81
  diet or eating habits Z72.4
  level of quantitative human chorionic gonadotropin (hCG) for gestational age in early pregnancy O02.81
  secretion
    antidiuretic hormone (ADH) (excessive) E22.2
      deficiency E23.2
    pituitary (posterior) E22.2
  sinus tachycardia, so stated (IST) I47.11
Inattention at or after birth —*see* Neglect
Incarceration, incarcerated
  enterocele K46.0
    gangrenous K46.1
  epiplocele K46.0
    gangrenous K46.1
  exomphalos K42.0
    gangrenous K42.1
  hernia —*see also* Hernia, by site, with obstruction
    with gangrene —*see* Hernia, by site, with gangrene
  iris, in wound —*see* Injury, eye, laceration, with prolapse
  lens, in wound —*see* Injury, eye, laceration, with prolapse
  omphalocele K42.0
  prison, anxiety concerning Z65.1
  rupture —*see* Hernia, by site
  sarcoepiplocele K46.0
    gangrenous K46.1
  sarcoepiplomphalocele K42.0
    with gangrene K42.1
  uterus N85.8
    gravid O34.51-●
      causing obstructed labor O65.5
Incised wound
  external —*see* Laceration
  internal organs —*see* Injury, by site
Incision, incisional
  hernia K43.2
    with
      gangrene (and obstruction) K43.1
      obstruction K43.0
  surgical, complication —*see* Complications, surgical procedure
  traumatic
    external —*see* Laceration
    internal organs —*see* Injury, by site
Inclusion
  azurophilic leukocytic D72.0
  blennorrhea (neonatal) (newborn) P39.1
  gallbladder in liver (congenital) Q44.1
Incompatibility
  ABO
    affecting management of pregnancy O36.11-●
      anti-A sensitization O36.11-●
      anti-B sensitization O36.19-●
      specified NEC O36.19-●
    infusion or transfusion reaction —*see* Complication(s), transfusion, incompatibility reaction, ABO
    newborn P55.1
  blood (group) (Duffy) (K) (Kell) (Kidd) (Lewis) (M) (S) NEC
    affecting management of pregnancy O36.11-●
      anti-A sensitization O36.11-●
      anti-B sensitization O36.19-●
    infusion or transfusion reaction T80.89
    newborn P55.8
  divorce or estrangement Z63.5
  Rh (blood group) (factor) Z31.82
    affecting management of pregnancy NEC O36.09-●
      anti-D antibody O36.01-●
    infusion or transfusion reaction —*see* Complication(s), transfusion, incompatibility reaction, Rh (factor)
    newborn P55.0
  rhesus —*see* Incompatibility, Rh

Incompetency, incompetent, incompetence
  annular
    aortic (valve) —*see* Insufficiency, aortic
    mitral (valve) I34.0
    pulmonary valve (heart) I37.1
  aortic (valve) —*see* Insufficiency, aortic
  cardiac valve —*see* Endocarditis
  cervix, cervical (os) N88.3
    in pregnancy O34.3-●
  chronotropic I45.89
    with
      autonomic dysfunction G90.89
      ischemic heart disease I25.89
      left ventricular dysfunction I51.89
      sinus node dysfunction I49.8
  esophagogastric (junction) (sphincter) K22.0
  mitral (valve) —*see* Insufficiency, mitral
  pelvic fundus N81.89
  pubocervical tissue N81.82
  pulmonary valve (heart) I37.1
    congenital Q22.3
  rectovaginal tissue N81.83
  tricuspid (annular) (valve) —*see* Insufficiency, tricuspid
  valvular —*see* Endocarditis
    congenital Q24.8
  vein, venous (saphenous) (varicose) —*see* Varix, leg
Incomplete —*see also* condition
  atrioventricular
    canal Q21.21
    septal defect Q21.21
  bladder, emptying R33.9
  defecation R15.0
  endocardial cushion defect Q21.21
  expansion lungs (newborn) NEC —*see* Atelectasis
  rotation, intestine Q43.3
Inconclusive
  diagnostic imaging due to excess body fat of patient R93.9
  findings on diagnostic imaging of breast NEC R92.8
  mammogram R92.2
Incontinence R32
  anal sphincter R15.9
  coital N39.491
  feces R15.9
    nonorganic origin F98.1
  insensible (urinary) N39.42
  overflow N39.490
  postural (urinary) N39.492
  psychogenic F45.8
  rectal R15.9
  reflex N39.498
  stress (female) (male) N39.3
    and urge N39.46
  urethral sphincter R32
  urge N39.41
    and stress (female) (male) N39.46
  urine (urinary) R32
    continuous N39.45
    due to cognitive impairment, or severe physical disability or immobility R39.81
    functional R39.81
    insensible N39.42
    mixed (stress and urge) N39.46
    nocturnal N39.44
    nonorganic origin F98.0
    overflow N39.490
    post dribbling N39.43
    postural N39.492
    reflex N39.498
    specified NEC N39.498
    stress (female) (male) N39.3
      and urge N39.46
    total N39.498
    unaware N39.42
    urge N39.41
      and stress (female) (male) N39.46
Incontinentia pigmenti Q82.3
Incoordinate, incoordination
  esophageal-pharyngeal (newborn) —*see* Dysphagia
  muscular R27.8
  uterus (action) (contractions) (complicating delivery) O62.4
Increase, increased
  abnormal, in development R63.8
  androgens (ovarian) E28.1

Increase, increased *(Continued)*
 anticoagulants (antithrombin) (anti-VIIIa) (anti-IXa) (anti-Xa) (anti-XIa) —*see* Circulating anticoagulants
 cold sense R20.8
 estrogen E28.0
 function
  adrenal
   cortex —*see* Cushing's, syndrome
   medulla E27.5
  pituitary (gland) (anterior) (lobe) E22.9
   posterior E22.2
 heat sense R20.8
 intracranial pressure (benign) G93.2
 permeability, capillaries I78.8
 pressure, intracranial G93.2
 secretion
  gastrin E16.4
  glucagon E16.3
  pancreas, endocrine E16.9
   growth hormone-releasing hormone E16.8
   pancreatic polypeptide E16.8
   somatostatin E16.8
   vasoactive-intestinal polypeptide E16.8
 sphericity, lens Q12.4
 splenic activity D73.1
 venous pressure I87.8
  portal K76.6
Increta placenta O43.22-●
Incrustation, cornea, foreign body (lead) (zinc) — *see* Foreign body, cornea
Incyclophoria H50.54
Incyclotropia —*see* Cyclotropia
Indeterminate sex Q56.4
India rubber skin Q82.8
Indigestion (acid) (bilious) (functional) K30
 catarrhal K31.89
 due to decomposed food NOS A05.9
 nervous F45.8
 psychogenic F45.8
Indirect —*see* condition
Induratio penis plastica N48.6
Induration, indurated
 brain G93.89
 breast (fibrous) N64.51
  puerperal, postpartum O92.29
 broad ligament N83.8
 chancre
  anus A51.1
  congenital A50.07
  extragenital NEC A51.2
 corpora cavernosa (penis) (plastic) N48.6
 liver (chronic) K76.89
 lung (black) (chronic) (fibroid) —*see also* Fibrosis, lung J84.10
  essential brown J84.03
 penile (plastic) N48.6
 phlebitic —*see* Phlebitis
 skin R23.4
Inebriety (without dependence) —*see* Alcohol, intoxication
Inefficiency, kidney N28.9
Inelasticity, skin R23.4
Inequality, leg (length) (acquired) —*see also* Deformity, limb, unequal length
 congenital —*see* Defect, reduction, lower limb
 lower leg —*see* Deformity, limb, unequal length
Inertia
 bladder (neurogenic) N31.2
 stomach K31.89
  psychogenic F45.8
 uterus, uterine during labor O62.2
  during latent phase of labor O62.0
  primary O62.0
  secondary O62.1
 vesical (neurogenic) N31.2
Infancy, infantile, infantilism —*see also* condition
 celiac K90.0
 genitalia, genitals (after puberty) E30.0
 Herter's (nontropical sprue) K90.0
 intestinal K90.0
 Lorain E23.0
 pancreatic K86.89
 pelvis M95.5
  with disproportion (fetopelvic) O33.1
   causing obstructed labor O65.1
 pituitary E23.0
 renal N25.0
 uterus —*see* Infantile, genitalia

Infant(s) —*see also* Infancy
 excessive crying R68.11
 irritable child R68.12
 lack of care —*see* Neglect
 liveborn (singleton) Z38.2
  born in hospital Z38.00
   by cesarean Z38.01
  born outside hospital Z38.1
  multiple NEC Z38.8
   born in hospital Z38.68
    by cesarean Z38.69
   born outside hospital Z38.7
  quadruplet Z38.8
   born in hospital Z38.63
    by cesarean Z38.64
   born outside hospital Z38.7
  quintuplet Z38.8
   born in hospital Z38.65
    by cesarean Z38.66
   born outside hospital Z38.7
  triplet Z38.8
   born in hospital Z38.61
    by cesarean Z38.62
   born outside hospital Z38.7
  twin Z38.5
   born in hospital Z38.30
    by cesarean Z38.31
   born outside hospital Z38.4
 of diabetic mother (syndrome of) P70.1
  gestational diabetes P70.0
Infantile —*see also* condition
 genitalia, genitals E30.0
 os, uterine E30.0
 penis E30.0
 testis E29.1
 uterus E30.0
Infantilism —*see* Infancy
Infarct, infarction
 adrenal (capsule) (gland) E27.49
 appendices epiploicae —*see also* Infarct, intestine K55.069
 bowel —*see also* Infarct, intestine K55.069
 brain (stem) —*see* Infarct, cerebral
 breast N64.89
 brewer's (kidney) N28.0
 cardiac —*see* Infarct, myocardium
 cerebellar —*see* Infarct, cerebral
 cerebral (acute) (*see also* Occlusion, artery cerebral or precerebral, with infarction) I63.9-●
  aborted I63.9
  chronic (imaging) (old) (remote) (without sequelae) Z86.73
   with residual defects - see Sequelae, disease, cerebrovascular
  cortical I63.9
  due to
   cerebral venous thrombosis, nonpyogenic I63.6
   embolism
    cerebral arteries I63.4-●
    precerebral arteries I63.1-●
   occlusion NEC
    cerebral arteries I63.5-●
    precerebral arteries I63.2-●
    small artery I63.81
   stenosis NEC
    cerebral arteries I63.5-●
    precerebral arteries I63.2-●
    small artery I63.81
   thrombosis
    cerebral artery I63.3-●
    precerebral artery I63.0-●
  intraoperative
   during cardiac surgery I97.810
   during other surgery I97.811
  neonatal P91.82-●
  perinatal (arterial ischemic) P91.82-●
  postprocedural
   following cardiac surgery I97.820
   following other surgery I97.821
  specified NEC I63.89
 colon (acute) (agnogenic) (embolic) (hemorrhagic) (nonocclusive) (nonthrombotic) (occlusive) (segmental) (thrombotic) (with gangrene) —*see also* Infarct, intestine K55.049
 coronary artery —*see* Infarct, myocardium
 embolic —*see* Embolism
 fallopian tube N83.8
 gallbladder K82.8

Infarct, infarction *(Continued)*
 heart —*see* Infarct, myocardium
 hepatic K76.3
 hypophysis (anterior lobe) E23.6
 impending (myocardium) I20.0
 intestine (acute) (agnogenic) (embolic) (hemorrhagic) (nonocclusive) (nonthrombotic) (occlusive) (thrombotic) (with gangrene) K55.069
  diffuse K55.062
  focal K55.061
  large K55.049
   diffuse K55.042
   focal K55.041
  small K55.029
   diffuse K55.022
   focal K55.021
 kidney N28.0
 lacunar I63.81
 liver K76.3
 lung (embolic) (thrombotic) —*see* Embolism, pulmonary
 lymph node I89.8
 mesentery, mesenteric (embolic) (thrombotic) (with gangrene) —*see also* Infarct, intestine K55.069
 muscle (ischemic) M62.20
  ankle M62.27-●
  foot M62.27-●
  forearm M62.23-●
  hand M62.24-●
  lower leg M62.26-●
  pelvic region M62.25-●
  shoulder region M62.21-●
  specified site NEC M62.28
  thigh M62.25-●
  upper arm M62.22-●
 myocardium, myocardial (acute) (with stated duration of 4 weeks or less) I21.9
  with
   coronary microvascular disease I21.B
   coronary microvascular dysfunction I21.B
   nonobstructive coronary arteries [MINOCA] with microvascular disease I21.B
  associated with revascularization procedure I21.A9
  diagnosed on ECG, but presenting no symptoms I25.2
  due to
   demand ischemia I21.A1
   ischemic imbalance I21.A1
  healed or old I25.2
  intraoperative —*see also* Infarct, myocardium, associated with revascularization procedure
   during cardiac surgery I97.790
   during other surgery I97.791
  non-Q wave I21.4
  non-ST elevation (NSTEMI) I21.4
   subsequent I22.2
  nontransmural I21.4
  past (diagnosed on ECG or other investigation, but currently presenting no symptoms) I25.2
  postprocedural —*see also* Infarct, myocardium, associated with revascularization procedure
   following cardiac surgery —*see also* Infarct, myocardium, type 4 or type 5 I97.190
   following other surgery I97.191
  Q wave —*see also* Infarct, myocardium, ST elevation, by site I21.3
  secondary to
   demand ischemia I21.A1
   ischemic imbalance I21.A1
  ST elevation (STEMI) I21.3
   anterior (anteroapical) (anterolateral) (anteroseptal) (Q wave) (wall) I21.09
    subsequent I22.0
   inferior (diaphragmatic) (inferolateral) (inferoposterior) (wall) NEC I21.19
    subsequent I22.1
   inferoposterior transmural (Q wave) I21.11
   involving
    coronary artery of anterior wall NEC I21.09
    coronary artery of inferior wall NEC I21.19
    diagonal coronary artery I21.02

▶ New ⇒ Revised ~~deleted~~ Deleted ● Use Additional Character(s)

Infarct, infarction *(Continued)*
myocardium, myocardial *(Continued)*
ST elevation *(Continued)*
involving *(Continued)*
left anterior descending coronary artery I21.02
left circumflex coronary artery I21.21
left main coronary artery I21.01
oblique marginal coronary artery I21.21
right coronary artery I21.11
lateral (apical-lateral) (basal-lateral) (high) I21.29
subsequent I22.8
posterior (posterobasal) (posterolateral) (posteroseptal) (true) I21.29
subsequent I22.8
septal I21.29
subsequent I22.8
specified NEC I21.29
subsequent I22.8
subsequent I22.9
subsequent (recurrent) (reinfarction) I22.9
anterior (anteroapical) (anterolateral) (anteroseptal) (wall) I22.0
diaphragmatic (wall) I22.1
inferior (diaphragmatic) (inferolateral) (inferoposterior) (wall) I22.1
lateral (apical-lateral) (basal-lateral) (high) I22.8
non-ST elevation (NSTEMI) I22.2
posterior (posterobasal) (posterolateral) (posteroseptal) (true) I22.8
septal I22.8
specified NEC I22.8
ST elevation I22.9
anterior (anteroapical) (anterolateral) (anteroseptal) (wall) I22.0
inferior (diaphragmatic) (inferolateral) (inferoposterior) (wall) I22.1
specified NEC I22.8
subendocardial I22.2
transmural I22.9
anterior (anteroapical) (anterolateral) (anteroseptal) (wall) I22.0
diaphragmatic (wall) I22.1
inferior (diaphragmatic) (inferolateral) (inferoposterior) (wall) I22.1
lateral (apical-lateral) (basal-lateral) (high) I22.8
posterior (posterobasal) (posterolateral) (posteroseptal) (true) I22.8
specified NEC I22.8
type 1 —*see also* Infarction, myocardial, subsequent, by site, or by ST elevation or non-ST elevation I22.9
type 2 I21.A1
type 3 I21.A9
type 4 I21.A9
type 5 I21.A9
syphilitic A52.06
transmural *(see also,* Infarct, myocardium, ST elevation, by site) I21.3
anterior (anteroapical) (anterolateral) (anteroseptal) (Q wave) (wall) NEC I21.09
inferior (diaphragmatic) (inferolateral) (inferoposterior) (Q wave) (wall) NEC I21.19
inferoposterior (Q wave) I21.11
lateral (apical-lateral) (basal-lateral) (high) NEC I21.29
posterior (posterobasal) (posterolateral) (posteroseptal) (true) NEC I21.29
septal NEC I21.29
specified NEC I21.29
type 1 —*see also* Infarction, myocardial, by site, or by ST elevation or non-ST elevation I21.9
type 2 I21.A1
type 3 I21.A9
type 4 (a) (b) (c) I21.A9
type 5 I21.A9
nontransmural I21.4
omentum —*see also* Infarct, intestine K55.069
ovary N83.8
pancreas K86.89
papillary muscle —*see* Infarct, myocardium
parathyroid gland E21.4
pituitary (gland) E23.6
placenta O43.81-●
prostate N42.89

Infarct, infarction *(Continued)*
pulmonary (artery) (vein) (hemorrhagic) —*see* Embolism, pulmonary
renal (embolic) (thrombotic) N28.0
retina, retinal (artery) —*see* Occlusion, artery, retina
spinal (cord) (acute) (embolic) (nonembolic) G95.11
spleen D73.5
embolic or thrombotic I74.8
subendocardial (acute) (nontransmural) I21.4
suprarenal (capsule) (gland) E27.49
testis N50.1
thrombotic —*see also* Thrombosis
artery, arterial —*see* Embolism
thyroid (gland) E07.89
ventricle (heart) —*see* Infarct, myocardium
Infecting —*see* condition
Infection, infected, infective (opportunistic) B99.9
with
drug resistant organism —*see* Resistance (to), drug —*see also* specific organism
lymphangitis —*see* Lymphangitis
organ dysfunction (acute) R65.20
with septic shock R65.21
abscess (skin) - code by site under Abscess
Absidia —*see* Mucormycosis
Acanthamoeba —*see* Acanthamebiasis
Acanthocheilonema (perstans) (streptocerca) B74.4
accessory sinus (chronic) —*see* Sinusitis
achorion —*see* Dermatophytosis
Acinetobacter baumannii, as cause of disease classified elsewhere B96.83
Acremonium falciforme B47.0
acromioclavicular M00.9
Actinobacillus (actinomycetem-comitans) A28.8
mallei A24.0
muris A25.1
Actinomadura B47.1
Actinomyces (israelii) —*see also* Actinomycosis A42.9
Actinomycetales —*see* Actinomycosis
actinomycotic NOS —*see* Actinomycosis
adenoid (and tonsil) J03.90
chronic J35.02
adenovirus NEC
as cause of disease classified elsewhere B97.0
unspecified nature or site B34.0
aerogenes capsulatus A48.0
aertrycke —*see* Infection, salmonella
alimentary canal NOS —*see* Enteritis, infectious
Allescheria boydii B48.2
Alternaria B48.8
alveolus, alveolar (process) K04.7
Ameba, amebic (histolytica) —*see* Amebiasis
amniotic fluid, sac or cavity O41.10-●
chorioamnionitis O41.12-●
placentitis O41.14-●
amputation stump (surgical) —*see* Complication, amputation stump, infection
Ancylostoma (duodenalis) B76.0
Anisakiasis, Anisakis larvae B81.0
anthrax —*see* Anthrax
antrum (chronic) —*see* Sinusitis, maxillary
anus, anal (papillae) (sphincter) K62.89
arbovirus (arbor virus) A94
specified type NEC A93.8
artificial insemination N98.0
Ascaris lumbricoides —*see* Ascariasis
Ascomycetes B47.0
Aspergillus (flavus) (fumigatus) (terreus) —*see* Aspergillosis
atypical
acid-fast (bacilli) —*see* Mycobacterium, atypical
mycobacteria —*see* Mycobacterium, atypical
virus A81.9
specified type NEC A81.89
auditory meatus (external) —*see* Otitis, externa, infective
auricle (ear) —*see* Otitis, externa, infective
axillary gland (lymph) L04.2
Bacillus A49.9
abortus A23.1
anthracis —*see* Anthrax
Ducrey's (any location) A57
▶ducreyi (any location) A57
Flexner's A03.1
Friedländer's NEC A49.8
gas (gangrene) A48.0

Infection, infected, infective *(Continued)*
Bacillus *(Continued)*
mallei A24.0
melitensis A23.0
paratyphoid, paratyphosus A01.4
A A01.1
B A01.2
C A01.3
Shiga (-Kruse) A03.0
suipestifer —*see* Infection, salmonella
swimming pool A31.1
typhosa A01.00
welchii —*see* Gangrene, gas
bacterial NOS A49.9
as cause of disease classified elsewhere B96.89
Acinetobacter baumannii B96.83
Bacteroides fragilis [B. fragilis] B96.6
Clostridium perfringens [C. perfringens] B96.7
Cronobacter (sakazakii) B96.89
Enterobacter sakazakii B96.89
Enterococcus B95.2
Escherichia coli [E. coli] (see also Escherichia coli) B96.20
Helicobacter pylori [H.pylori] B96.81
Hemophilus influenzae [H. influenzae] B96.3
Klebsiella pneumoniae [K. pneumoniae] B96.1
Mycoplasma pneumoniae [M. pneumoniae] B96.0
Proteus (mirabilis) (morganii) B96.4
Pseudomonas (aeruginosa) (mallei) (pseudomallei) B96.5
Staphylococcus B95.8
aureus (methicillin susceptible) (MSSA) B95.61
methicillin resistant (MRSA) B95.62
specified NEC B95.7
Streptococcus B95.5
group A B95.0
group B B95.1
pneumoniae B95.3
specified NEC B95.4
Vibrio vulnificus B96.82
specified NEC A48.8
Bacterium
paratyphosum A01.4
A A01.1
B A01.2
C A01.3
typhosum A01.00
Bacteroides NEC A49.8
fragilis, as cause of disease classified elsewhere B96.6
Balantidium coli A07.0
Bartholin's gland N75.8
Basidiobolus B46.8
bile duct (common) (hepatic) —*see* Cholangitis
bladder —*see* Cystitis
Blastomyces, blastomycotic —*see also* Blastomycosis
brasiliensis —*see* Paracoccidioidomycosis
dermatitidis —*see* Blastomycosis
European —*see* Cryptococcosis
Loboi B48.0
North American B40.9
South American —*see* Paracoccidioidomycosis
bleb, postprocedure —*see* Blebitis
bone —*see* Osteomyelitis
Bordetella —*see* Whooping cough
Borrelia bergdorfi A69.20
brain —*see also* Encephalitis G04.90
membranes —*see* Meningitis
septic G06.0
meninges —*see* Meningitis, bacterial
branchial cyst Q18.0
breast —*see* Mastitis
bronchus —*see* Bronchitis
Brucella A23.9
abortus A23.1
canis A23.3
melitensis A23.0
mixed A23.8
specified NEC A23.8
suis A23.2
Brugia (malayi) B74.1
timori B74.2
bursa —*see* Bursitis, infective
buttocks (skin) L08.9

Infection, infected, infective *(Continued)*
  Campylobacter, intestinal A04.5
    as cause of disease classified elsewhere
      B96.81
  Candida (albicans) (tropicalis) —*see* Candidiasis
  candiru B88.8
  Capillaria (intestinal) B81.1
    hepatica B83.8
    philippinensis B81.1
  cartilage —*see* Disorder, cartilage, specified type
    NEC
  catheter-related bloodstream (CRBSI) T80.211
  cat liver fluke B66.0
  cellulitis - code by site under Cellulitis
  central line-associated T80.219
    bloodstream (CLABSI) T80.211
    specified NEC T80.218
  Cephalosporium falciforme B47.0
  cerebrospinal —*see* Meningitis
  cervical gland (lymph) L04.0
  cervix —*see* Cervicitis
  cesarean delivery wound (puerperal) O86.00
  cestodes —*see* Infestation, cestodes
  chest J22
  Chilomastix (intestinal) A07.8
  Chlamydia, chlamydial A74.9
    anus A56.3
    genitourinary tract A56.2
      lower A56.00
      specified NEC A56.19
    lymphogranuloma A55
    pharynx A56.4
    psittaci A70
    rectum A56.3
    sexually transmitted NEC A56.8
  cholera —*see* Cholera
  Cladosporium
    bantianum (brain abscess) B43.1
    carrionii B43.0
    castellanii B36.1
    trichoides (brain abscess) B43.1
    werneckii B36.1
  Clonorchis (sinensis) (liver) B66.1
  ▶Clostridioides
    ▶difficile
      ▶as cause of disease classified elsewhere
        B96.89
      ▶foodborne (disease)
        ▶not specified as recurrent A04.72
        ▶recurrent A04.71
      ▶gas gangrene A48.0
      ▶necrotizing enterocolitis
        ▶not specified as recurrent A04.72
        ▶recurrent A04.71
      ▶sepsis A41.4
  Clostridium NEC
    bifermentans A48.0
    botulinum (food poisoning) A05.1
      infant A48.51
      wound A48.52
    difficile
      as cause of disease classified elsewhere
        B96.89
      foodborne (disease)
        not specified as recurrent A04.72
        recurrent A04.71
      gas gangrene A48.0
      necrotizing enterocolitis
        not specified as recurrent A04.72
        recurrent A04.71
      sepsis A41.4
    gas-forming NEC A48.0
    histolyticum A48.0
    novyi, causing gas gangrene A48.0
    oedematiens A48.0
    perfringens
      as cause of disease classified elsewhere
        B96.7
      due to food A05.2
      foodborne (disease) A05.2
      gas gangrene A48.0
      sepsis A41.4
    septicum, causing gas gangrene A48.0
    sordellii, causing gas gangrene A48.0
    welchii
      as cause of disease classified elsewhere
        B96.7
      foodborne (disease) A05.2
      gas gangrene A48.0
      necrotizing enteritis A05.2
      sepsis A41.4

Infection, infected, infective *(Continued)*
  Coccidioides (immitis) —*see* Coccidioidomycosis
  colon —*see* Enteritis, infectious
  colostomy K94.02
  common duct —*see* Cholangitis
  congenital P39.9
    Candida (albicans) P37.5
    cytomegalovirus P35.1
    hepatitis, viral P35.3
    herpes simplex P35.2
    infectious or parasitic disease P37.9
      specified NEC P37.8
    listeriosis (disseminated) P37.2
    malaria NEC P37.4
      falciparum P37.3
    Plasmodium falciparum P37.3
    poliomyelitis P35.8
    rubella P35.0
    skin P39.4
    toxoplasmosis (acute) (subacute) (chronic)
      P37.1
    tuberculosis P37.0
    urinary (tract) P39.3
    vaccinia P35.8
    virus P35.9
      specified type NEC P35.8
  Conidiobolus B46.8
  coronavirus-2019 U07.1
  coronavirus NEC B34.2
    as cause of disease classified elsewhere
      B97.29
    severe acute respiratory syndrome (SARS
      associated) B97.21
  corpus luteum —*see* Salpingo-oophoritis
  Corynebacterium diphtheriae —*see* Diphtheria
  cotia virus B08.8
  COVID-19 U07.1
  Coxiella burnetii A78
  coxsackie —*see* Coxsackie
  Cronobacter (sakazakii) B96.89
    as cause of disease classified elsewhere B96.89
    generalized A41.59
  Cryptococcus neoformans —*see* Cryptococcosis
  Cryptosporidium A07.2
  Cunninghamella —*see* Mucormycosis
  cyst —*see* Cyst
  cystic duct —*see also* Cholecystitis K81.9
  Cysticercus cellulosae —*see* Cysticercosis
  cytomegalovirus, cytomegaloviral B25.9
    congenital P35.1
    maternal, maternal care for (suspected)
      damage to fetus O35.3
    mononucleosis B27.10
      with
        complication NEC B27.19
        meningitis B27.12
        polyneuropathy B27.11
  delta-agent (acute), in hepatitis B carrier B17.0
  dental (pulpal origin) K04.7
  Deuteromycetes B47.0
  Dicrocoelium dendriticum B66.2
  Dipetalonema (perstans) (streptocerca) B74.4
  diphtherial —*see* Diphtheria
  Diphyllobothrium (adult) (latum) (pacificum)
    B70.0
    larval B70.1
  Diplogonoporus (grandis) B71.8
  Dipylidium caninum B67.4
  Dirofilaria B74.8
  Dracunculus medinensis B72
  Drechslera (hawaiiensis) B43.8
  ~~Ducrey Haemophilus (any location) A57~~
  ▶ducreyi Haemophilus (any location) A57
  due to or resulting from
    artificial insemination N98.0
    Babesia
      divergens (-like) strain B60.03
      duncani (-type) species B60.02
      microti B60.01
      species
        specified NEC B60.09
    central venous catheter T80.219
      bloodstream T80.211
      exit or insertion site T80.212
      localized T80.212
      port or reservoir T80.212
      specified NEC T80.218
      tunnel T80.212
    device, implant or graft —*see also*
      Complications, by site and type,
      infection or inflammation T85.79

Infection, infected, infective *(Continued)*
  due to or resulting from *(Continued)*
    device, implant or graft *(Continued)*
      arterial graft NEC T82.7
      breast (implant) T85.79
      catheter NEC T85.79
        dialysis (renal) T82.7
          central line T80.211
          intraperitoneal T85.71
        infusion NEC T82.7
          cranial T85.735
          intrathecal T85.735
          spinal (epidural) (subdural)
            T85.735
          subarachnoid T85.735
        urinary T83.518
          cystostomy T83.510
          Hopkins T83.518
          ileostomy T83.518
          nephrostomy T83.512
          specified NEC T83.518
          urethral indwelling T83.511
          urostomy T83.518
      electronic (electrode) (pulse generator)
        (stimulator)
        bone T84.7
        cardiac T82.7
        nervous system T85.738
          brain T85.731
          cranial nerve T85.732
          gastric nerve T85.732
          generator pocket T85.734
          neurostimulator generator T85.734
          peripheral nerve T85.732
          sacral nerve T85.732
          spinal cord T85.733
          vagal nerve T85.732
        urinary T83.590
      fixation, internal (orthopedic) NEC —*see*
        Complication, fixation device,
        infection
      gastrointestinal (bile duct) (esophagus)
        T85.79
        neurostimulator electrode (lead) T85.732
      genital NEC T83.69
      heart NEC T82.7
        valve (prosthesis) T82.6
          graft T82.7
      joint prosthesis —*see* Complication, joint
        prosthesis, infection
      ocular (corneal graft) (orbital implant) NEC
        T85.79
      orthopedic NEC T84.7
      ➡penile (cylinder) (pump) (reservoir)
        T83.61
      specified NEC T85.79
      testicular T83.62
      urinary NEC T83.598
        ileal conduit stent T83.593
        implanted neurostimulation T83.590
        implanted sphincter T83.591
        indwelling ureteral stent T83.592
        nephroureteral stent T83.593
        specified stent NEC T83.593
      vascular NEC T82.7
      ventricular intracranial (communicating)
        shunt T85.730
    Hickman catheter T80.219
      bloodstream T80.211
      localized T80.212
      specified NEC T80.218
    immunization or vaccination T88.0
    infusion, injection or transfusion NEC T80.29
      acute T80.22
    injury NEC - code by site under Wound,
      open
    peripherally inserted central catheter (PICC)
      T80.219
      bloodstream T80.211
      localized T80.212
      specified NEC T80.218
    portacath (port-a-cath) T80.219
      bloodstream T80.211
      localized T80.212
      specified NEC T80.218
    protozoa of the order Piroplasmida NEC
      B60.09
    pulmonary artery catheter —*see* Infection,
      due to or resulting from, central venous
      catheter
    surgery T81.40

▶ New   ➡ Revised   ~~deleted~~ Deleted   ● Use Additional Character(s)

Infection, infected, infective *(Continued)*
  due to or resulting from *(Continued)*
    Swan Ganz catheter —*see* Infection, due to or
        resulting from, central venous catheter
    triple lumen catheter T80.219
      bloodstream T80.211
      localized T80.212
      specified NEC T80.218
    umbilical venous catheter T80.219
      bloodstream T80.211
      localized T80.212
      specified NEC T80.218
  during labor NEC O75.3
  ear (middle) —*see also* Otitis media
    external —*see* Otitis, externa, infective
    inner —*see* subcategory H83.0
  Eberthella typhosa A01.00
  Echinococcus —*see* Echinococcus
  echovirus
    as cause of disease classified elsewhere B97.12
    unspecified nature or site B34.1
  endocardium I33.0
  endocervix —*see* Cervicitis
  Entamoeba —*see* Amebiasis
  enteric —*see* Enteritis, infectious
  Enterobacter sakazakii B96.89
  Enterobius vermicularis B80
  enterostomy K94.12
  enterovirus B34.1
    as cause of disease classified elsewhere B97.10
      coxsackievirus B97.11
      echovirus B97.12
      specified NEC B97.19
  Entomophthora B46.8
  Epidermophyton —*see* Dermatophytosis
  epididymis —*see* Epididymitis
  episiotomy (puerperal) O86.09
  Erysipelothrix (insidiosa) (rhusiopathiae) —*see*
      Erysipeloid
  erythema infectiosum B08.3
  Escherichia (E.) coli NEC A49.8
    as cause of disease classified elsewhere —*see
        also* Escherichia coli B96.20
    congenital P39.8
      sepsis P36.4
    generalized A41.51
    intestinal —*see* Enteritis, infectious, due to,
        Escherichia coli
  ethmoidal (chronic) (sinus) —*see* Sinusitis,
      ethmoidal
  eustachian tube (ear) —*see* Salpingitis,
      eustachian
  external auditory canal (meatus) NEC —*see*
      Otitis, externa, infective
  eye (purulent) —*see* Endophthalmitis, purulent
  eyelid —*see* Inflammation, eyelid
  fallopian tube —*see* Salpingo-oophoritis
  Fasciola (gigantica) (hepatica) (indica) B66.3
  Fasciolopsis (buski) B66.5
  filarial —*see* Infestation, filarial
  finger (skin) L08.9
    nail L03.01-●
      fungus B35.1
  fish tapeworm B70.0
    larval B70.1
  flagellate, intestinal A07.9
  fluke —*see* Infestation, fluke
  focal
    teeth (pulpal origin) K04.7
    tonsils J35.01
  Fonsecaea (compactum) (pedrosoi) B43.0
  food —*see* Intoxication, foodborne
  foot (skin) L08.9
    dermatophytic fungus B35.3
  Francisella tularensis —*see* Tularemia
  frontal (sinus) (chronic) —*see* Sinusitis, frontal
  fungus NOS B49
    beard B35.0
    dermatophytic —*see* Dermatophytosis
    foot B35.3
    groin B35.6
    hand B35.2
    nail B35.1
    pathogenic to compromised host only B48.8
    perianal (area) B35.6
    scalp B35.0
    skin B36.9
      foot B35.3
      hand B35.2
      toenails B35.1
  Fusarium B48.8

Infection, infected, infective *(Continued)*
  gallbladder —*see* Cholecystitis
  gas bacillus —*see* Gangrene, gas
  gastrointestinal —*see* Enteritis, infectious
  generalized NEC —*see* Sepsis
  generator pocket, implanted electronic
      neurostimulator T85.734
  genital organ or tract
    female —*see* Disease, pelvis, inflammatory
    male N49.9
      multiple sites N49.8
      specified NEC N49.8
  Ghon tubercle, primary A15.7
  Giardia lamblia A07.1
  gingiva (chronic) K05.10
    acute K05.00
      nonplaque induced K05.01
      plaque induced K05.00
    nonplaque induced K05.11
    plaque induced K05.10
  glanders A24.0
  glenosporopsis B48.0
  Gnathostoma (spinigerum) B83.1
  Gongylonema B83.8
  gonococcal —*see* Gonococcus
  gram-negative bacilli NOS A49.9
  guinea worm B72
  gum (chronic) K05.10
    acute K05.00
      nonplaque induced K05.01
      plaque induced K05.00
    nonplaque induced K05.11
    plaque induced K05.10
  Haemophilus —*see* Infection, Hemophilus
  heart —*see* Carditis
  Helicobacter pylori A04.8
    as cause of disease classified elsewhere B96.81
  helminths B83.9
    intestinal B82.0
      mixed (types classifiable to more than one
          of the titles B65.0-B81.3 and B81.8)
          B81.4
      specified type NEC B81.8
    specified type NEC B83.8
  Hemophilus
    aegyptius, systemic A48.4
    ~~ducrey (any location) A57~~
    ▶ducreyi (any location) A57
    generalized A41.3
    influenzae NEC A49.2
      as cause of disease classified elsewhere
          B96.3
  herpes (simplex) —*see also* Herpes
    congenital P35.2
    disseminated B00.7
    zoster B02.9
  herpesvirus, herpesviral —*see* Herpes
  Heterophyes (heterophyes) B66.8
  hip (joint) NEC M00.9
    due to internal joint prosthesis
      left T84.52
      right T84.51
    skin NEC L08.9
  Histoplasma —*see* Histoplasmosis
    American B39.4
    capsulatum B39.4
  hookworm B76.9
  human
    papilloma virus A63.0
    T-cell lymphotropic virus type-1 (HTLV-1)
        B33.3
  hydrocele N43.0
  Hymenolepis B71.0
  hypopharynx —*see* Pharyngitis
  inguinal (lymph) glands L04.1
    due to soft chancre A57
  intervertebral disc, pyogenic M46.30
    cervical region M46.32
    cervicothoracic region M46.33
    lumbar region M46.36
    lumbosacral region M46.37
    multiple sites M46.39
    occipito-atlanto-axial region M46.31
    sacrococcygeal region M46.38
    thoracic region M46.34
    thoracolumbar region M46.35
  intestine, intestinal —*see* Enteritis, infectious
    specified NEC A08.8
  intra-amniotic affecting newborn NEC P39.2
  intrauterine inflammation O41.12-●
  Isospora belli or hominis A07.3

Infection, infected, infective *(Continued)*
  Japanese B encephalitis A83.0
  jaw (bone) (lower) (upper) M27.2
  joint NEC M00.9
    due to internal joint prosthesis T84.50
  kidney (cortex) (hematogenous) N15.9
    with calculus N20.0
      with hydronephrosis N13.6
    following ectopic gestation O08.83
    pelvis and ureter (cystic) N28.85
    puerperal (postpartum) O86.21
    specified NEC N15.8
  Klebsiella (K.) pneumoniae NEC A49.8
    as cause of disease classified elsewhere B96.1
  knee (joint) NEC M00.9
    due to internal joint prosthesis
      left T84.54
      right T84.53
    joint M00.9
    skin L08.9
  Koch's —*see* Tuberculosis
  labia (majora) (minora) (acute) —*see* Vulvitis
  lacrimal
    gland —*see* Dacryoadenitis
    passages (duct) (sac) —*see* Inflammation,
        lacrimal, passages
  lancet fluke B66.2
  larynx NEC J38.7
  leg (skin) NOS L08.9
  Legionella pneumophila A48.1
    nonpneumonic A48.2
  Leishmania —*see also* Leishmaniasis
    aethiopica B55.1
    braziliensis B55.2
    chagasi B55.0
    donovani B55.0
    infantum B55.0
    major B55.1
    mexicana B55.1
    tropica B55.1
  lentivirus, as cause of disease classified
      elsewhere B97.31
  Leptosphaeria senegalensis B47.0
  Leptospira interrogans A27.9
    autumnalis A27.89
    canicola A27.89
    hebdomadis A27.89
    icterohaemorrhagiae A27.0
    pomona A27.89
    specified type NEC A27.89
  leptospirochetal NEC —*see* Leptospirosis
  Listeria monocytogenes —*see also* Listeriosis
    congenital P37.2
  Loa loa B74.3
    with conjunctival infestation B74.3
    eyelid B74.3
  Loboa loboi B48.0
  local, skin (staphylococcal) (streptococcal) L08.9
    abscess - code by site under Abscess
    cellulitis - code by site under Cellulitis
    specified NEC L08.89
    ulcer —*see* Ulcer, skin
  Loefflerella mallei A24.0
  lung —*see also* Pneumonia J18.9
    atypical Mycobacterium A31.0
    spirochetal A69.8
    tuberculous —*see* Tuberculosis, pulmonary
    virus —*see* Pneumonia, viral
  lymph gland —*see also* Lymphadenitis, acute
    mesenteric I88.0
  lymphoid tissue, base of tongue or posterior
      pharynx, NEC (chronic) J35.03
  Madurella (grisea) (mycetomii) B47.0
  major
    following ectopic or molar pregnancy
        O08.3
    puerperal, postpartum, childbirth O85
  Malassezia furfur B36.0
  Malleomyces
    mallei A24.0
    pseudomallei (whitmori) —*see* Melioidosis
  mammary gland N61.0
  Mansonella (ozzardi) (perstans) (streptocerca)
      B74.4
  mastoid —*see* Mastoiditis
  maxilla, maxillary M27.2
    sinus (chronic) —*see* Sinusitis, maxillary
  mediastinum J98.51
  Medina (worm) B72
  meibomian cyst or gland —*see* Hordeolum
  meninges —*see* Meningitis, bacterial

Infection, infected, infective *(Continued)*
  meningococcal —*see also* condition A39.9
    adrenals A39.1
    brain A39.81
    cerebrospinal A39.0
    conjunctiva A39.89
    endocardium A39.51
    heart A39.50
      endocardium A39.51
      myocardium A39.52
      pericardium A39.53
    joint A39.83
    meninges A39.0
    meningococcemia A39.4
      acute A39.2
      chronic A39.3
    myocardium A39.52
    pericardium A39.53
    retrobulbar neuritis A39.82
    specified site NEC A39.89
  mesenteric lymph nodes or glands NEC
    I88.0
  Metagonimus B66.8
  metatarsophalangeal M00.9
  methicillin
    resistant Staphylococcus aureus (MRSA)
      A49.02
    susceptible Staphylococcus aureus (MSSA)
      A49.01
  Microsporum, microsporic —*see*
    Dermatophytosis
  mixed flora (bacterial) NEC A49.8
  Monilia —*see* Candidiasis
  Monosporium apiospermum B48.2
  mouth, parasitic B37.0
  Mucor —*see* Mucormycosis
  muscle NEC —*see* Myositis, infective
  mycelium NOS B49
  mycetoma B47.9
    actinomycotic NEC B47.1
    mycotic NEC B47.0
  Mycobacterium, mycobacterial —*see*
    Mycobacterium
  Mycoplasma NEC A49.3
    pneumoniae, as cause of disease classified
      elsewhere B96.0
  mycotic NOS B49
    pathogenic to compromised host only B48.8
    skin NOS B36.9
  myocardium NEC I40.0
  nail (chronic)
    with lymphangitis —*see* Lymphangitis, acute,
      digit
    finger L03.01-●
      fungus B35.1
    ingrowing L60.0
    toe L03.03-●
      fungus B35.1
  nasal sinus (chronic) —*see* Sinusitis
  nasopharynx —*see* Nasopharyngitis
  navel L08.82
  Necator americanus B76.1
  Neisseria —*see* Gonococcus
  Neotestudina rosatii B47.0
  newborn P39.9
    intra-amniotic NEC P39.2
    skin P39.4
    specified type NEC P39.8
  nipple N61.0
    associated with
      lactation O91.03
      pregnancy O91.01-●
      puerperium O91.02
  Nocardia —*see* Nocardiosis
  obstetrical surgical wound (puerperal)
    O86.00
    incisional site
      deep O86.02
      superficial O86.01
    organ and space site O86.03
    surgical site specified NEC O86.09
  Oesophagostomum (apiostomum)
    B81.8
  Oestrus ovis —*see* Myiasis
  Oidium albicans B37.9
  Onchocerca (volvulus) —*see* Onchocerciasis -
    oncovirus, as cause of disease classified
      elsewhere B97.32
  operation wound T81.49
  Opisthorchis (felineus) (viverrini) B66.0
  orbit, orbital —*see* Inflammation, orbit

Infection, infected, infective *(Continued)*
  orthopoxvirus NEC B08.09
  ovary —*see* Salpingo-oophoritis
  Oxyuris vermicularis B80
  pancreas (acute) —*see* Pancreatitis, acute
    abscess —*see* Pancreatitis, acute
    specified NEC —*see also* Pancreatitis, acute
      K85.80
  papillomavirus, as cause of disease classified
    elsewhere B97.7
  papovavirus NEC B34.4
  Paracoccidioides brasiliensis —*see*
    Paracoccidioidomycosis
  Paragonimus (westermani) B66.4
  parainfluenza virus B34.8
  parameningococcus NOS A39.9
  parapoxvirus B08.60
    specified NEC B08.69
  parasitic B89
  Parastrongylus
    cantonensis B83.2
    costaricensis B81.3
    paratyphoid A01.4
      Type A A01.1
      Type B A01.2
      Type C A01.3
  paraurethral ducts N34.2
  parotid gland —*see* Sialoadenitis
  parvovirus NEC B34.3
    as cause of disease classified elsewhere B97.6
  Pasteurella NEC A28.0
    multocida A28.0
    pestis —*see* Plague
    pseudotuberculosis A28.0
    septica (cat bite) (dog bite) A28.0
    tularensis —*see* Tularemia
  pelvic, female —*see* Disease, pelvis,
    inflammatory
  Penicillium (marneffei) B48.4
  penis (glans) (retention) NEC N48.29
  periapical K04.5
  peridental, periodontal K05.20
    generalized —*see* Periodontitis, aggressive,
      generalized
    localized —*see* Periodontitis, aggressive,
      localized
  perinatal period P39.9
    specified type NEC P39.8
  perineal repair (puerperal) O86.09
  periorbital —*see* Inflammation, orbit
  perirectal K62.89
  perirenal —*see* Infection, kidney
  peritoneal —*see* Peritonitis
  periureteral N28.89
  Petriellidium boydii B48.2
  pharynx —*see also* Pharyngitis
    coxsackievirus B08.5
    posterior, lymphoid (chronic) J35.03
  Phialophora
    gougerotii (subcutaneous abscess or cyst)
      B43.2
    jeanselmei (subcutaneous abscess or cyst)
      B43.2
    verrucosa (skin) B43.0
  Piedraia hortae B36.3
  pinta A67.9
    intermediate A67.1
    late A67.2
    mixed A67.3
    primary A67.0
  pinworm B80
  pityrosporum furfur B36.0
  pleuro-pneumonia-like organism (PPLO) NEC
    A49.3
    as cause of disease classified elsewhere B96.0
  pneumococcus, pneumococcal NEC A49.1
    as cause of disease classified elsewhere B95.3
    generalized (purulent) A40.3
      with pneumonia J13
  Pneumocystis carinii (pneumonia) B59
  Pneumocystis jiroveci (pneumonia) B59
  port or reservoir T80.212
  postoperative T81.40
  postoperative wound T81.49
  postprocedural T81.40
    surgical site
      deep incisional T81.42
      organ and space T81.43
      specified NEC T81.49
      superficial incisional T81.41
  postvaccinal T88.0

Infection, infected, infective *(Continued)*
  prepuce NEC N47.7
    with penile inflammation N47.6
  prion —*see* Disease, prion, central nervous
    system
  prostate (capsule) —*see* Prostatitis
  Proteus (mirabilis) (morganii) (vulgaris) NEC
    A49.8
    as cause of disease classified elsewhere B96.4
  protozoal NEC B64
    intestinal A07.9
      specified NEC A07.8
    specified NEC B60.8
  Pseudoallescheria boydii B48.2
  Pseudomonas NEC A49.8
    as cause of disease classified elsewhere B96.5
    generalized A41.52
    mallei A24.0
    pneumonia J15.1
    pseudomallei —*see* Melioidosis
  puerperal O86.4
    genitourinary tract NEC O86.89
    major or generalized O85
    minor O86.4
    specified NEC O86.89
  pulmonary —*see* Infection, lung
  purulent —*see* Abscess
  Pyrenochaeta romeroi B47.0
  Q fever A78
  rectum (sphincter) K62.89
  renal —*see also* Infection, kidney
    pelvis and ureter (cystic) N28.85
  reovirus, as cause of disease classified elsewhere
    B97.5
  respiratory (tract) NEC J98.8
    acute J22
    chronic J98.8
    influenzal (upper) (acute) —*see* Influenza,
      with, respiratory manifestations NEC
    lower (acute) J22
      chronic —*see* Bronchitis, chronic
    rhinovirus J00
    syncytial virus (RSV) —*see* Infection, virus,
      respiratory syncytial (RSV)
    upper (acute) NOS J06.9
      chronic J39.8
      streptococcal J06.9
      viral NOS J06.9
        due to respiratory syncytial virus (RSV)
          J06.9 [B97.1]
  resulting from
    presence of internal prosthesis, implant,
      graft —*see* Complications, by site and
      type, infection
  retortamoniasis A07.8
  retroperitoneal NEC K68.9
  retrovirus B33.3
    as cause of disease classified elsewhere B97.30
    human
      immunodeficiency, type 2 (HIV 2) B97.35
      T-cell lymphotropic
        type I (HTLV-I) B97.33
        type II (HTLV-II) B97.34
    lentivirus B97.31
    oncovirus B97.32
    specified NEC B97.39
  Rhinosporidium (seeberi) B48.1
  rhinovirus
    as cause of disease classified elsewhere B97.89
    unspecified nature or site B34.8
  Rhizopus —*see* Mucormycosis
  rickettsial NOS A79.9
  roundworm (large) NEC B82.0
    Ascariasis —*see also* Ascariasis B77.9
  rubella —*see* Rubella
  Saccharomyces —*see* Candidiasis
  salivary duct or gland (any) —*see* Sialoadenitis
  Salmonella (aertrycke) (arizonae) (cholerae-suis)
    (enteritidis) (gallinarum) (suipestifer)
    (typhimurium) A02.9
    with
      (gastro) enteritis A02.0
      sepsis A02.1
      specified manifestation NEC A02.8
    due to food (poisoning) A02.9
    hirschfeldii A01.3
    localized A02.20
      arthritis A02.23
      meningitis A02.21
      osteomyelitis A02.24
      pneumonia A02.22

▶ New   ⇒ Revised   ~~deleted~~ Deleted   ● Use Additional Character(s)

Infection, infected, infective *(Continued)*
  Salmonella *(Continued)*
    localized *(Continued)*
      pyelonephritis A02.25
      specified NEC A02.29
    paratyphi A01.4
      A A01.1
      B A01.2
      C A01.3
    schottmuelleri A01.2
    typhi, typhosa —*see* Typhoid
  Sarcocystis A07.8
  scabies B86
  Schistosoma —*see* Infestation, Schistosoma
  scrotum (acute) NEC N49.2
  seminal vesicle —*see* Vesiculitis
  septic
    localized, skin —*see* Abscess
  Serratia NEC A49.8
    as cause of disease classified elsewhere B96.89
    generalized A41.53
  sheep liver fluke B66.3
  Shigella A03.9
    boydii A03.2
    dysenteriae A03.0
    flexneri A03.1
    group
      A A03.0
      B A03.1
      C A03.2
      D A03.3
    Schmitz (-Stutzer) A03.0
    schmitzii A03.0
    shigae A03.0
    sonnei A03.3
    specified NEC A03.8
  shoulder (joint) NEC M00.9
    due to internal joint prosthesis T84.59
    skin NEC L08.9
  sinus (accessory) (chronic) (nasal) —*see also*
      Sinusitis
    pilonidal —*see* Sinus, pilonidal
    skin NEC L08.89
  Skene's duct or gland —*see* Urethritis
  skin (local) (staphylococcal) (streptococcal) L08.9
    abscess - code by site under Abscess
    cellulitis - code by site under Cellulitis
    due to fungus B36.9
      specified type NEC B36.8
    mycotic B36.9
      specified type NEC B36.8
    newborn P39.4
    ulcer —*see* Ulcer, skin
  slow virus A81.9
    specified NEC A81.89
  Sparganum (mansoni) (proliferum) (baxteri)
      B70.1
  specific —*see also* Syphilis
    to perinatal period —*see* Infection, congenital
  specified NEC B99.8
  spermatic cord NEC N49.1
  sphenoidal (sinus) —*see* Sinusitis,
      sphenoidal
  spinal cord NOS —*see also* Myelitis G04.91
    abscess G06.1
    meninges —*see* Meningitis
    streptococcal G04.89
  Spirillum A25.0
  spirochetal NOS A69.9
    lung A69.8
    specified NEC A69.8
  Spirometra larvae B70.1
  spleen D73.89
  Sporotrichum, Sporothrix (schenckii) —*see*
      Sporotrichosis
  staphylococcal, unspecified site
    aureus (methicillin susceptible) (MSSA)
        A49.01
      methicillin resistant (MRSA) A49.02
    as cause of disease classified elsewhere
        B95.8
      aureus (methicillin susceptible) (MSSA)
          B95.61
        methicillin resistant (MRSA)
            B95.62
      specified NEC B95.7
    food poisoning A05.0
    generalized (purulent) A41.2
    pneumonia —*see* Pneumonia, staphylococcal
  Stellantchasmus falcatus B66.8
  streptobacillus moniliformis A25.1

Infection, infected, infective *(Continued)*
  streptococcal NEC A49.1
    as cause of disease classified elsewhere B95.5
    B genitourinary complicating
      childbirth O98.82
        pregnancy O98.81- •
        puerperium O98.83
    congenital
      sepsis P36.10
        group B P36.0
        specified NEC P36.19
    generalized (purulent) A40.9
  Streptomyces B47.1
  Strongyloides (stercoralis) —*see* Strongyloidiasis
  stump (amputation) (surgical) —*see*
      Complication, amputation stump,
      infection
  subcutaneous tissue, local L08.9
  suipestifer —*see* Infection, salmonella
  swimming pool bacillus A31.1
  Taenia —*see* Infestation, Taenia
  Taeniarhynchus saginatus B68.1
  tapeworm —*see* Infestation,
      tapeworm
  tendon (sheath) —*see* Tenosynovitis, infective
      NEC
  Ternidens diminutus B81.8
  testis —*see* Orchitis
  threadworm B80
  throat —*see* Pharyngitis
  thyroglossal duct K14.8
  toe (skin) L08.9
    cellulitis L03.03- •
      fungus B35.1
    nail L03.03- •
      fungus B35.1
  tongue NEC K14.0
    parasitic B37.0
  tonsil (and adenoid) (faucial) (lingual)
      (pharyngeal) —*see* Tonsillitis
  tooth, teeth K04.7
    irreversible K04.02
    periapical K04.7
  Iperidental, periodontal K05.20
    generalized —*see* Periodontitis, aggressive,
        generalized
    localized —*see* Periodontitis, aggressive,
        localized
    pulp K04.01
      irreversible K04.02
      reversible K04.01
  TORCH —*see* Infection, congenital
    without active infection P00.2
  Torula histolytica —*see* Cryptococcosis
  Toxocara (canis) (cati) (felis) B83.0
  Toxoplasma gondii —*see* Toxoplasma
  trachea, chronic J42
  trematode NEC —*see* Infestation, fluke
  trench fever A79.0
  Treponema pallidum —*see* Syphilis
  Trichinella (spiralis) B75
  Trichomonas A59.9
    cervix A59.09
    intestine A07.8
    prostate A59.02
    specified site NEC A59.8
    urethra A59.03
    urogenitalis A59.00
    vagina A59.01
    vulva A59.01
  Trichophyton, trichophytic —*see*
      Dermatophytosis
  Trichosporon (beigelii) cutaneum B36.2
  Trichostrongylus B81.2
  Trichuris (trichiura) B79
  Trombicula (irritans) B88.0
  Trypanosoma
    brucei
      gambiense B56.0
      rhodesiense B56.1
    cruzi —*see* Chagas' disease
  tubal —*see* Salpingo-oophoritis
  tuberculous
    latent (LTBI) Z22.7
    NEC —*see* Tuberculosis
  tubo-ovarian —*see* Salpingo-oophoritis
  tunica vaginalis N49.1
  tunnel T80.212
  tympanic membrane NEC —*see* Myringitis
  typhoid (abortive) (ambulant) (bacillus) —*see*
      Typhoid

Infection, infected, infective *(Continued)*
  typhus A75.9
    flea-borne A75.2
    mite-borne A75.3
    recrudescent A75.1
    tick-borne A77.9
      African A77.1
      North Asian A77.2
  umbilicus L08.82
  ureter —*see* Ureteritis
  urethra —*see* Urethritis
  urinary (tract) N39.0
    bladder —*see* Cystitis
    complicating
      pregnancy O23.4- •
        specified type NEC O23.3- •
    kidney —*see* Infection, kidney
    newborn P39.3
    puerperal (postpartum) O86.20
    tuberculous A18.13
    urethra —*see* Urethritis
  uterus, uterine —*see* Endometritis
  vaccination T88.0
  vaccinia not from vaccination B08.011
  vagina (acute) —*see* Vaginitis
  varicella B01.9
  varicose veins —*see* Varix
  vas deferens NEC N49.1
  vesical —*see* Cystitis
  Vibrio
    cholerae A00.0
      El Tor A00.1
    parahaemolyticus (food poisoning)
        A05.3
    vulnificus
      as cause of disease classified elsewhere
          B96.82
      foodborne intoxication A05.5
  Vincent's (gum) (mouth) (tonsil) A69.1
  virus, viral NOS B34.9
    adenovirus
      as cause of disease classified elsewhere
          B97.0
    unspecified nature or site B34.0
    arborvirus, arbovirus arthropod-borne
        A94
    as cause of disease classified elsewhere
        B97.89
      adenovirus B97.0
      coronavirus B97.29
        SARS-associated B97.21
      coxsackievirus B97.11
      echovirus B97.12
      enterovirus B97.10
        coxsackievirus B97.11
        echovirus B97.12
        specified NEC B97.19
      human
        immunodeficiency, type 2 (HIV 2)
            B97.35
        metapneumovirus B97.81
        T-cell lymphotropic,
            type I (HTLV-I) B97.33
            type II (HTLV-II) B97.34
      papillomavirus B97.7
      parvovirus B97.6
      reovirus B97.5
      respiratory syncytial (RSV) —*see* Infection
          virus, respiratory syncytial (RSV)
      retrovirus B97.30
        human
          immunodeficiency, type 2 (HIV 2)
              B97.35
          T-cell lymphotropic,
              type I (HTLV-I) B97.33
              type II (HTLV-II) B97.34
        lentivirus B97.31
        oncovirus B97.32
        specified NEC B97.39
      specified NEC B97.89
    central nervous system A89
      atypical A81.9
        specified NEC A81.89
      enterovirus NEC A88.8
        meningitis A87.0
      slow virus A81.9
        specified NEC A81.89
      specified NEC A88.8
    chest J98.8
    cotia B08.8
    COVID-19 U07.1

Infection, infected, infective (Continued)
  virus, viral (Continued)
    coxsackie —see also Infection, coxsackie B34.1
      as cause of disease classified elsewhere
        B97.11
      ECHO
        as cause of disease classified elsewhere
          B97.12
      unspecified nature or site B34.1
    encephalitis, tick-borne A84.9
    enterovirus, as cause of disease classified
        elsewhere B97.10
      coxsackievirus B97.11
      echovirus B97.12
      specified NEC B97.19
    exanthem NOS B09
    human metapneumovirus as cause of disease
        classified elsewhere B97.81
    human papilloma as cause of disease
        classified elsewhere B97.7
    intestine —see Enteritis, viral
    respiratory syncytial (RSV) —see Infection
        virus, respiratory syncytial (RSV)
      bronchiolitis J21.0
      bronchitis J20.5
      bronchopneumonia J12.1
      otitis media H65.- ● [B97.4]
      pneumonia J12.1
      upper respiratory infection J06.9
          [B97.4]
    rhinovirus
      as cause of disease classified elsewhere
        B97.89
      unspecified nature or site B34.8
    slow A81.9
      specified NEC A81.89
    specified type NEC B33.8
      as cause of disease classified elsewhere
        B97.89
      unspecified nature or site B34.8
    unspecified nature or site B34.9
    West Nile —see Virus, West Nile
    vulva (acute) —see Vulvitis
  West Nile —see Virus, West Nile
  whipworm B79
  worms B83.9
    specified type NEC B83.8
  Wuchereria (bancrofti) B74.0
    malayi B74.1
    yatapoxvirus B08.70
      specified NEC B08.79
  yeast (see also Candidiasis) B37.9
  yellow fever —see Fever, yellow
  Yersinia
    enterocolitica (intestinal) A04.6
    pestis —see Plague
    pseudotuberculosis A28.2
  Zeis' gland —see Hordeolum
  Zika virus A92.5
    congenital P35.4
  zoonotic bacterial NOS A28.9
  Zopfia senegalensis B47.0
Infective, infectious —see condition
Infertility
  female N97.9
    age-related N97.8
    associated with
      anovulation N97.0
      cervical (mucus) disease or anomaly N88.3
      congenital anomaly
        cervix N88.3
        fallopian tube N97.1
        uterus N97.2
        vagina N97.8
      dysmucorrhea N88.3
      fallopian tube disease or anomaly
        N97.1
      pituitary-hypothalamic origin
        E23.0
      specified origin NEC N97.8
      Stein-Leventhal syndrome E28.2
      uterine disease or anomaly N97.2
      vaginal disease or anomaly N97.8
    due to
      cervical anomaly N88.3
      fallopian tube anomaly N97.1
      ovarian failure E28.39
      Stein-Leventhal syndrome
        E28.2
      uterine anomaly N97.2
      vaginal anomaly N97.8

Infertility (Continued)
  femalel (Continued)
    nonimplantation N97.2
    origin
      cervical N88.3
      tubal (block) (occlusion) (stenosis)
        N97.1
      uterine N97.2
      vaginal N97.8
  male N46.9
    azoospermia N46.01
      extratesticular cause N46.029
        drug therapy N46.021
        efferent duct obstruction N46.023
        infection N46.022
        radiation N46.024
        specified cause NEC N46.029
        systemic disease N46.025
      oligospermia N46.11
        extratesticular cause N46.129
          drug therapy N46.121
          efferent duct obstruction N46.123
          infection N46.122
          radiation N46.124
          specified cause NEC N46.129
          systemic disease N46.125
    specified type NEC N46.8
Infestation B88.9
  Acanthocheilonema (perstans) (streptocerca)
      B74.4
  Acariasis B88.0
    demodex folliculorum B88.0
    sarcoptes scabiei B86
    trombiculae B88.0
  Agamofilaria streptocerca B74.4
  Ancylostoma, ankylostoma (braziliense)
      (caninum) (ceylanicum) (duodenale) B76.0
    americanum B76.1
    new world B76.1
  Anisakis larvae, anisakiasis B81.0
  arthropod NEC B88.2
  Ascaris lumbricoides —see Ascariasis
  Balantidium coli A07.0
  beef tapeworm B68.1
  Bothriocephalus (latus) B70.0
    larval B70.1
  broad tapeworm B70.0
    larval B70.1
  Brugia (malayi) B74.1
    timori B74.2
  candiru B88.8
  Capillaria
    hepatica B83.8
    philippinensis B81.1
  cat liver fluke B66.0
  cestodes B71.9
    diphyllobothrium —see Infestation,
        diphyllobothrium
    dipylidiasis B71.1
    hymenolepiasis B71.0
    specified type NEC B71.8
  chigger B88.0
  chigo, chigoe B88.1
  Clonorchis (sinensis) (liver) B66.1
  coccidial A07.3
  crab-lice B85.3
  Cysticercus cellulosae —see Cysticercosis
  Demodex (folliculorum) B88.0
  Dermanyssus gallinae B88.0
  Dermatobia (hominis) —see Myiasis
  Dibothriocephalus (latus) B70.0
    larval B70.1
  Dicrocoelium dendriticum B66.2
  Diphyllobothrium (adult) (latum) (intestinal)
      (pacificum) B70.0
    larval B70.1
  Diplogonoporus (grandis) B71.8
  Dipylidium caninum B67.4
  Distoma hepaticum B66.3
  dog tapeworm B67.4
  Dracunculus medinensis B72
  dragon worm B72
  dwarf tapeworm B71.0
  Echinococcus —see Echinococcus
  Echinostomum ilocanum B66.8
  Entamoeba (histolytica) —see Infection, Ameba
  Enterobius vermicularis B80
  eyelid
    in (due to)
      leishmaniasis B55.1
      loiasis B74.3

Infestation (Continued)
  eyelid (Continued)
    in (due to) (Continued)
      onchocerciasis B73.09
      phthiriasis B85.3
      parasitic NOS B89
  eyeworm B74.3
  Fasciola (gigantica) (hepatica) (indica) B66.3
  Fasciolopsis (buski) (intestine) B66.5
  filarial B74.9
    bancroftian B74.0
    conjunctiva B74.9
    due to
      Acanthocheilonema (perstans)
        (streptocerca) B74.4
      Brugia (malayi) B74.1
        timori B74.2
      Dracunculus medinensis B72
      guinea worm B72
      loa loa B74.3
      Mansonella (ozzardi) (perstans)
        (streptocerca) B74.4
      Onchocerca volvulus B73.00
        eye B73.00
        eyelid B73.09
      Wuchereria (bancrofti) B74.0
    Malayan B74.1
    ozzardi B74.4
    specified type NEC B74.8
  fish tapeworm B70.0
    larval B70.1
  fluke B66.9
    blood NOS —see Schistosomiasis
    cat liver B66.0
    intestinal B66.5
    lancet B66.2
    liver (sheep) B66.3
      cat B66.0
      Chinese B66.1
      due to clonorchiasis B66.1
      oriental B66.1
    lung (oriental) B66.4
    sheep liver B66.3
    specified type NEC B66.8
  fly larvae —see Myiasis
  Gasterophilus (intestinalis) —see Myiasis
  Gastrodiscoides hominis B66.8
  Giardia lamblia A07.1
  Gnathostoma (spinigerum) B83.1
  Gongylonema B83.8
  guinea worm B72
  helminth B83.9
    angiostrongyliasis B83.2
      intestinal B81.3
    gnathostomiasis B83.1
    hirudiniasis, internal B83.4
    intestinal B82.0
      angiostrongyliasis B81.3
      anisakiasis B81.0
      ascariasis —see Ascariasis
      capillariasis B81.1
      cysticercosis —see Cysticercosis
      diphyllobothriasis —see Infestation,
          diphyllobothriasis
      dracunculiasis B72
      echinococcus —see Echinococcosis
      enterobiasis B80
      filariasis —see Infestation, filarial
      fluke —see Infestation, fluke
      hookworm —see Infestation, hookworm
      mixed (types classifiable to more than one of
          the titles B65.0-B81.3 and B81.8) B81.4
      onchocerciasis —see Onchocerciasis
      schistosomiasis —see Infestation,
          schistosoma
      specified
        cestode NEC —see Infestation, cestode
          type NEC B81.8
      strongyloidiasis —see Strongyloidiasis
      taenia —see Infestation, taenia
      trichinellosis B75
      trichostrongyliasis B81.2
      trichuriasis B79
    specified type NEC B83.8
    syngamiasis B83.3
    visceral larva migrans B83.0
  Heterophyes (heterophyes) B66.8
  hookworm B76.9
    ancylostomiasis B76.0
    necatoriasis B76.1
    specified type NEC B76.8

▶ New   ⇨ Revised   ~~deleted~~ Deleted   ● Use Additional Character(s)

Infestation (Continued)
Hymenolepis (diminuta) (nana) B71.0
intestinal NEC B82.9
leeches (aquatic) (land) —see Hirudiniasis
Leishmania —see Leishmaniasis
lice, louse —see Infestation, Pediculus
Linguatula B88.8
Liponyssoides sanguineus B88.0
Loa loa B74.3
    conjunctival B74.3
    eyelid B74.3
louse —see Infestation, Pediculus
maggots —see Myiasis
Mansonella (ozzardi) (perstans) (streptocerca)
    B74.4
Medina (worm) B72
Metagonimus (yokogawai) B66.8
microfilaria streptocerca —see Onchocerciasis
    eye B73.00
    eyelid B73.09
mites B88.9
    scabic B86
Monilia (albicans) —see Candidiasis
mouth B37.0
Necator americanus B76.1
nematode NEC (intestinal) B82.0
    Ancylostoma B76.0
    conjunctiva NEC B83.9
    Enterobius vermicularis B80
    Gnathostoma spinigerum B83.1
    physaloptera B80
    specified NEC B81.8
    trichostrongylus B81.2
    trichuris (trichuria) B79
Oesophagostomum (apiostomum) B81.8
Oestrus ovis —see also Myiasis B87.9
Onchocerca (volvulus) —see Onchocerciasis
Opisthorchis (felineus) (viverrini) B66.0
orbit, parasitic NOS B89
Oxyuris vermicularis B80
Paragonimus (westermani) B66.4
parasite, parasitic B89
    eyelid B89
    intestinal NOS B82.9
    mouth B37.0
    skin B88.9
    tongue B37.0
Parastrongylus
    cantonensis B83.2
    costaricensis B81.3
Pediculus B85.2
    body B85.1
    capitis (humanus) (any site) B85.0
    corporis (humanus) (any site)
        B85.1
    head B85.0
    mixed (classifiable to more than one of the
        titles B85.0-B85.3) B85.4
    pubis (any site) B85.3
Pentastoma B88.8
pest Z59.19
Phthirus (pubis) (any site) B85.3
    with any infestation classifiable to B85.0-B85.2
        B85.4
pinworm B80
pork tapeworm (adult) B68.0
protozoal NEC B64
    intestinal A07.9
        specified NEC A07.8
    specified NEC B60.8
pubic, louse B85.3
rat tapeworm B71.0
red bug B88.0
roundworm (large) NEC B82.0
    Ascariasis —see also Ascariasis B77.9
sandflea B88.1
Sarcoptes scabiei B86
scabies B86
Schistosoma B65.9
    bovis B65.8
    cercariae B65.3
    haematobium B65.0
    intercalatum B65.8
    japonicum B65.2
    mansoni B65.1
    mattheei B65.8
    mekongi B65.8
    specified type NEC B65.8
    spindale B65.8
screw worms —see Myiasis
skin NOS B88.9

Infestation (Continued)
Sparganum (mansoni) (proliferum) (baxteri)
    B70.1
    larval B70.1
specified type NEC B88.8
Spirometra larvae B70.1
Stellantchasmus falcatus B66.8
Strongyloides stercoralis —see Strongyloidiasis
Taenia B68.9
    diminuta B71.0
    echinococcus —see Echinococcus
    mediocanellata B68.1
    nana B71.0
    saginata B68.1
    solium (intestinal form) B68.0
        larval form —see Cysticercosis
Taeniarhynchus saginatus B68.1
tapeworm B71.9
    beef B68.1
    broad B70.0
        larval B70.1
    dog B67.4
    dwarf B71.0
    fish B70.0
        larval B70.1
    pork B68.0
    rat B71.0
Ternidens diminutus B81.8
Tetranychus molestissimus B88.0
threadworm B80
tongue B37.0
Toxocara (canis) (cati) (felis) B83.0
trematode(s) NEC —see Infestation, fluke
Trichinella (spiralis) B75
Trichocephalus B79
Trichomonas —see Trichomoniasis
Trichostrongylus B81.2
Trichuris (trichiura) B79
Trombicula (irritans) B88.0
Tunga penetrans B88.1
Uncinaria americana B76.1
Vandellia cirrhosa B88.8
whipworm B79
worms B83.9
    intestinal B82.0
Wuchereria (bancrofti) B74.0
Infiltrate, infiltration
amyloid (generalized) (localized) —see
    Amyloidosis
calcareous NEC R89.7
    localized —see Degeneration, by site
calcium salt R89.7
cardiac
    fatty —see Degeneration, myocardial
    glycogenic E74.02 [143]
corneal —see Edema, cornea
eyelid —see Inflammation, eyelid
glycogen, glycogenic —see Disease, glycogen
    storage
heart, cardiac
    fatty —see Degeneration, myocardial
    glycogenic E74.02 [143]
inflammatory in vitreous H43.89
kidney N28.89
leukemic —see Leukemia
liver K76.89
    fatty —see Fatty, liver NEC
    glycogen —see also Disease, glycogen storage
        E74.03 [K77]
lung R91.8
    eosinophilic —see Eosinophilia, pulmonary
lymphatic —see also Leukemia, lymphatic
    C91.9-●
    gland I88.9
muscle, fatty M62.89
myocardium, myocardial
    fatty —see Degeneration, myocardial
    glycogenic E74.02 [143]
on chest x-ray R91.8
pulmonary R91.8
    with eosinophilia —see Eosinophilia,
        pulmonary
skin (lymphocytic) L98.6
thymus (gland) (fatty) E32.8
urine R39.0
vesicant agent
    antineoplastic chemotherapy T80.810
    other agent NEC T80.818
vitreous body H43.89
Infirmity R68.89
senile R54

Inflammation, inflamed, inflammatory (with
    exudation)
abducent (nerve) —see Strabismus, paralytic,
    sixth nerve
accessory sinus (chronic) —see Sinusitis
adrenal (gland) E27.8
alveoli, teeth M27.3
    scorbutic E54
anal canal, anus K62.89
antrum (chronic) —see Sinusitis, maxillary
appendix —see Appendicitis
arachnoid —see Meningitis
areola N61.0
    puerperal, postpartum or gestational —see
        Infection, nipple
areolar tissue NOS L08.9
artery —see Arteritis
auditory meatus (external) —see Otitis, externa
Bartholin's gland N75.8
bile duct (common) (hepatic) or passage —see
    Cholangitis
bladder —see Cystitis
bone —see Osteomyelitis
brain —see also Encephalitis
    membrane —see Meningitis
breast N61.0
    puerperal, postpartum, gestational —see
        Mastitis, obstetric
broad ligament —see Disease, pelvis,
    inflammatory
bronchi —see Bronchitis
catarrhal J00
cecum —see Appendicitis
cerebral —see also Encephalitis
    membrane —see Meningitis
cerebrospinal
    meningococcal A39.0
cervix (uteri) —see Cervicitis
chest J98.8
chorioretinal H30.9-●
    cyclitis —see Cyclitis
    disseminated H30.10-●
        generalized H30.13-●
        peripheral H30.12-●
        posterior pole H30.11-●
    epitheliopathy —see Epitheliopathy
    focal H30.00-●
        juxtapapillary H30.01-●
        macular H30.04-●
        paramacular —see Inflammation,
            chorioretinal, focal, macular
        peripheral H30.03-●
        posterior pole H30.02-●
    specified type NEC H30.89-●
choroid —see Inflammation, chorioretinal
chronic, postmastoidectomy cavity —see
    Complications, postmastoidectomy,
    inflammation
colon —see Enteritis
connective tissue (diffuse) NEC —see Disorder,
    soft tissue, specified type NEC
cornea —see Keratitis
corpora cavernosa N48.29
cranial nerve —see Disorder, nerve, cranial
Douglas' cul-de-sac or pouch (chronic)
    N73.0
due to device, implant or graft —see also
    Complications, by site and type, infection
    or inflammation
    arterial graft T82.7
    breast (implant) T85.79
    catheter T85.79
        dialysis (renal) T82.7
            intraperitoneal T85.71
        infusion T82.7
            cranial T85.735
            intrathecal T85.735
            spinal (epidural) (subdural) T85.735
            subarachnoid T85.735
        urinary T83.518
            cystostomy T83.510
            Hopkins T83.518
            ileostomy T83.518
            nephrostomy T83.512
            specified NEC T83.518
            urethral indwelling T83.511
            urostomy T83.518
    electronic (electrode) (pulse generator)
        (stimulator)
        bone T84.7
        cardiac T82.7

Inflammation, inflamed, inflammatory (Continued)
  due to device, implant or graft (Continued)
    electronic (Continued)
      nervous system T85.738
        brain T85.731
        cranial nerve T85.732
        gastric nerve T85.732
        neurostimulator generator T85.734
        peripheral nerve T85.732
        sacral nerve T85.732
        spinal cord T85.733
        vagal nerve T85.732
      urinary T83.590
    fixation, internal (orthopedic) NEC —see
      Complication, fixation device, infection
    gastrointestinal (bile duct) (esophagus)
      T85.79
      neurostimulator electrode (lead) T85.732
    genital NEC T83.69
    heart NEC T82.7
      valve (prosthesis) T82.6
        graft T82.7
    joint prosthesis —see Complication, joint
      prosthesis, infection
    ocular (corneal graft) (orbital implant) NEC
      T85.79
    orthopedic NEC T84.7
    penile (cylinder) (pump) (reservoir)
      T83.61
    specified NEC T85.79
    testicular T83.62
    urinary NEC T83.598
      ileal conduit stent T83.593
      implanted neurostimulation T83.590
      implanted sphincter T83.591
      indwelling ureteral stent T83.592
      nephroureteral stent T83.593
      specified stent NEC T83.593
    vascular NEC T82.7
    ventricular intracranial (communicating)
      shunt T85.730
  duodenum K29.80
    with bleeding K29.81
  dura mater —see Meningitis
  ear (middle) —see also Otitis, media
    external —see Otitis, externa
    inner —see subcategory H83.0
  epididymis —see Epididymitis
  esophagus —see Esophagitis
  ethmoidal (sinus) (chronic) —see Sinusitis,
    ethmoidal
  eustachian tube (catarrhal) —see Salpingitis,
    eustachian
  eyelid H01.9
    abscess —see Abscess, eyelid
    blepharitis —see Blepharitis
    chalazion —see Chalazion
    dermatosis (noninfectious) —see Dermatosis,
      eyelid
    hordeolum —see Hordeolum
    specified NEC H01.8
  fallopian tube —see Salpingo-oophoritis
  fascia —see Myositis
  follicular, pharynx J31.2
  frontal (sinus) (chronic) —see Sinusitis, frontal
  gallbladder —see Cholecystitis
  gastric —see Gastritis
  gastrointestinal —see Enteritis
  genital organ (internal) (diffuse)
    female —see Disease, pelvis, inflammatory
    male N49.9
      multiple sites N49.8
      specified NEC N49.8
  gland (lymph) —see Lymphadenitis
  glottis —see Laryngitis
  granular, pharynx J31.2
  gum K05.10
    nonplaque induced K05.11
    plaque induced K05.10
  heart —see Carditis
  hepatic duct —see Cholangitis
  ileoanal (internal) pouch K91.850
  ileum —see also Enteritis
    regional or terminal —see Enteritis, regional
  intestinal pouch K91.850
  intestine (any part) —see Enteritis
  jaw (acute) (bone) (chronic) (lower)
    (suppurative) (upper) M27.2
  joint NEC —see Arthritis
    sacroiliac M46.1
  kidney —see Nephritis

Inflammation, inflamed, inflammatory (Continued)
  knee (joint) M13.169
    tuberculous A18.02
  labium (majus) (minus) —see Vulvitis
  lacrimal
    gland —see Dacryoadenitis
    passages (duct) (sac) —see also Dacryocystitis
      canaliculitis —see Canaliculitis, lacrimal
  larynx —see Laryngitis
  leg NOS L08.9
  lip K13.0
  liver (capsule) —see also Hepatitis
    chronic K73.9
    suppurative K75.0
  lung (acute) —see also Pneumonia
    chronic J98.4
  lymphatic vessel —see Lymphangitis
  lymph gland or node —see Lymphadenitis
  maxilla, maxillary M27.2
    sinus (chronic) —see Sinusitis, maxillary
  membranes of brain or spinal cord —see
    Meningitis
  meninges —see Meningitis
  mouth K12.1
  muscle —see Myositis
  myocardium —see Myocarditis
  nasal sinus (chronic) —see Sinusitis
  nasopharynx —see Nasopharyngitis
  navel L08.82
  nerve NEC —see Neuritis
  nipple N61.0
    puerperal, postpartum or gestational —see
      Infection, nipple
  nose —see Rhinitis
  oculomotor (nerve) —see Strabismus, paralytic,
    third nerve
  optic nerve —see Neuritis, optic
  orbit (chronic) H05.10
    acute H05.00
      abscess —see Abscess, orbit
      cellulitis —see Cellulitis, orbit
      osteomyelitis —see Osteomyelitis, orbit
      periostitis —see Periostitis, orbital
      tenonitis —see Tenonitis, eye
    granuloma —see Granuloma, orbit
    myositis —see Myositis, orbital
  ovary —see Salpingo-oophoritis
  oviduct —see Salpingo-oophoritis
  pancreas (acute) —see Pancreatitis
  parametrium N73.0
  parotid region L08.9
  pelvis, female —see Disease, pelvis,
    inflammatory
  penis (corpora cavernosa) N48.29
  perianal K62.89
  pericardium —see Pericarditis
  perineum (female) (male) L08.9
  perirectal K62.89
  peritoneum —see Peritonitis
  periuterine —see Disease, pelvis, inflammatory
  perivesical —see Cystitis
  petrous bone (acute) (chronic) —see Petrositis
  pharynx (acute) —see Pharyngitis
  pia mater —see Meningitis
  pleura —see Pleurisy
  polyp, colon —see also Polyp, colon,
    inflammatory K51.40
  prostate —see also Prostatitis
    specified type NEC N41.8
  rectosigmoid —see Rectosigmoiditis
  rectum —see also Proctitis K62.89
  respiratory, upper —see also Infection,
    respiratory, upper J06.9
    acute, due to radiation J70.0
    chronic, due to external agent —see condition,
      respiratory, chronic, due to
    due to
      chemicals, gases, fumes or vapors
        (inhalation) J68.2
      radiation J70.1
  retina —see Chorioretinitis
  retrocecal —see Appendicitis
  retroperitoneal —see Peritonitis
  salivary duct or gland (any) (suppurative) —see
    Sialoadenitis
  scorbutic, alveoli, teeth E54
  scrotum N49.2
  seminal vesicle —see Vesiculitis
  sigmoid —see Enteritis
  sinus —see Sinusitis
  Skene's duct or gland —see Urethritis

Inflammation, inflamed, inflammatory (Continued)
  skin L08.9
  spermatic cord N49.1
  sphenoidal (sinus) —see Sinusitis, sphenoidal
  spinal
    cord —see Encephalitis
    membrane —see Meningitis
    nerve —see Disorder, nerve
  spine —see Spondylopathy, inflammatory
  spleen (capsule) D73.89
  stomach —see Gastritis
  subcutaneous tissue L08.9
  suprarenal (gland) E27.8
  synovial —see Tenosynovitis
  tendon (sheath) NEC —see Tenosynovitis
  testis —see Orchitis
  throat (acute) —see Pharyngitis
  thymus (gland) E32.8
  thyroid (gland) —see Thyroiditis
  tongue K14.0
  tonsil —see Tonsillitis
  trachea —see Tracheitis
  trochlear (nerve) —see Strabismus, paralytic,
    fourth nerve
  tubal —see Salpingo-oophoritis
  tuberculous NEC —see Tuberculosis
  tubo-ovarian —see Salpingo-oophoritis
  tunica vaginalis N49.1
  tympanic membrane —see Tympanitis
  umbilicus, umbilical L08.82
  uterine ligament —see Disease, pelvis,
    inflammatory
  uterus (catarrhal) —see Endometritis
  uveal tract (anterior) NOS —see also Iridocyclitis
    posterior —see Chorioretinitis
  vagina —see Vaginitis
  vas deferens N49.1
  vein —see also Phlebitis
    intracranial or intraspinal (septic) G08
    thrombotic I80.9
      leg —see Phlebitis, leg
      lower extremity —see Phlebitis, leg
  vocal cord J38.3
  vulva —see Vulvitis
  Wharton's duct (suppurative) —see Sialoadenitis
Inflation, lung, imperfect (newborn) —see
  Atelectasis
Influenza (bronchial) (epidemic) (respiratory
  (upper)) (unidentified influenza virus) J11.1
  with
    digestive manifestations J11.2
    encephalopathy J11.81
    enteritis J11.2
    gastroenteritis J11.2
    gastrointestinal manifestations J11.2
    laryngitis J11.1
    myocarditis J11.82
    otitis media J11.83
    pharyngitis J11.1
    pneumonia J11.00
      specified type J11.08
    respiratory manifestations NEC J11.1
    specified manifestation NEC J11.89
  A (non-novel) J10-●
  A/H5N1 —see also Influenza, due to, identified
    novel influenza A virus J09.X2
  avian —see also Influenza, due to, identified
    novel influenza A virus J09.X2
  B J10-●
  bird —see also Influenza, due to, identified novel
    influenza A virus J09.X2
  C J10-●
  novel (2009) H1N1 influenza —see also Influenza,
    due to, identified influenza virus NEC
    J10.1
  novel influenza A/H1N1 —see also Influenza,
    due to, identified influenza virus NEC J10.1
  due to
    avian (see also Influenza, due to, identified
      novel influenza A virus) J09.X2
    identified influenza virus NEC J10.1
      with
        digestive manifestations J10.2
        encephalopathy J10.81
        enteritis J10.2
        gastroenteritis J10.2
        gastrointestinal manifestations J10.2
        laryngitis J10.1
        myocarditis J10.82
        otitis media J10.83
        pharyngitis J10.1

Influenza *(Continued)*
due to *(Continued)*
identified influenza virus *(Continued)*
with *(Continued)*
pneumonia (unspecified type) J10.00
with same identified influenza virus J10.01
specified type NEC J10.08
respiratory manifestations NEC J10.1
specified manifestation NEC J10.89
identified novel influenza A virus J09.X2
with
digestive manifestations J09.X3
encephalopathy J09.X9
enteritis J09.X3
gastroenteritis J09.X3
gastrointestinal manifestations J09.X3
laryngitis J09.X2
myocarditis J09.X9
otitis media J09.X9
pharyngitis J09.X2
pneumonia J09.X1
respiratory manifestations NEC J09.X2
specified manifestation NEC J09.X9
upper respiratory symptoms J09.X2
of other animal origin, not bird or swine *(see also* Influenza, due to, identified novel influenza A virus) J09.X2
swine (viruses that normally cause infections in pigs) —*see also* Influenza, due to, identified novel influenza A virus J09.X2
Influenza-like disease —*see* Influenza
Influenzal —*see* Influenza
Infraction, Freiberg's (metatarsal head) —*see* Osteochondrosis, juvenile, metatarsus
Infraeruption of tooth (teeth) M26.34
Infusion complication, misadventure, or reaction —*see* Complications, infusion
Ingestion
chemical —*see* Table of Drugs and Chemicals, by substance, poisoning
drug or medicament
correct substance properly administered —*see* Table of Drugs and Chemicals, by drug, adverse effect
overdose or wrong substance given or taken —*see* Table of Drugs and Chemicals, by drug, poisoning
foreign body —*see* Foreign body, alimentary tract
multiple drug —*see* Table of Drugs and Chemicals, multiple
tularemia A21.3
Ingrowing
hair (beard) L73.1
nail (finger) (toe) L60.0
Inguinal —*see also* condition
testicle Q53.9
bilateral Q53.212
unilateral Q53.112
Inhalant-induced
anxiety disorder F18.980
depressive disorder F18.94
major neurocognitive disorder F18.97
mild neurocognitive disorder F18.988
psychotic disorder F18.959
Inhalation
anthrax A22.1
flame T27.3
food or foreign body —*see* Foreign body, by site
gases, fumes, or vapors T59.9-•
specified agent NEC —*see* Table of Drugs and Chemicals, by substance T59.89-•
liquid or vomitus —*see* Asphyxia
meconium (newborn) P24.00
with
with respiratory symptoms P24.01
pneumonia (pneumonitis) P24.01
mucus —*see* Asphyxia, mucus
oil or gasoline (causing suffocation) —*see* Foreign body, by site
smoke T59.81-•
with respiratory conditions J70.5
due to chemicals, gases, fumes and vapors J68.9
steam *(see also* Burn, respiratory tract) T59.9-•

Inhalation *(Continued)*
stomach contents or secretions —*see* Foreign body, by site
due to anesthesia (general) (local) or other sedation T88.59
in labor and delivery O74.0
in pregnancy O29.01-•
postpartum, puerperal O89.01
Inhibition, orgasm
female F52.31
male F52.32
Inhibitor, systemic lupus erythematosus (presence of) D68.62
Iniencephalus, iniencephaly Q00.2
Injection, traumatic jet (air) (industrial) (water) (paint or dye) T70.4
Injury —*see also* specified injury type T14.90
abdomen, abdominal S39.91
blood vessel —*see* Injury, blood vessel, abdomen
cavity —*see* Injury, intra-abdominal
contusion S30.1
internal —*see* Injury, intra-abdominal
intra-abdominal organ —*see* Injury, intra-abdominal
nerve —*see* Injury, nerve, abdomen
open —*see* Wound, open, abdomen
specified NEC S39.81
superficial —*see* Injury, superficial, abdomen
Achilles tendon S86.00-•
laceration S86.02-•
specified type NEC S86.09-•
strain S86.01-•
acoustic, resulting in deafness —*see* Injury, nerve, acoustic
adrenal (gland) S37.819
contusion S37.812
laceration S37.813
specified type NEC S37.818
alveolar (process) S09.93
ankle S99.91-•
contusion —*see* Contusion, ankle
dislocation —*see* Dislocation, ankle
fracture —*see* Fracture, ankle
nerve —*see* Injury, nerve, ankle
open —*see* Wound, open, ankle
specified type NEC S99.81-•
sprain —*see* Sprain, ankle
superficial —*see* Injury, superficial, ankle
anterior chamber, eye —*see* Injury, eye, specified site NEC
anus —*see* Injury, abdomen
aorta (thoracic) S25.00
abdominal S35.00
laceration (minor) (superficial) S35.01
major S35.02
specified type NEC S35.09
laceration (minor) (superficial) S25.01
major S25.02
specified type NEC S25.09
arm (upper) S49.9-•
blood vessel —*see* Injury, blood vessel, arm
contusion —*see* Contusion, arm, upper
fracture —*see* Fracture, humerus
lower —*see* Injury, forearm
muscle —*see* Injury, muscle, shoulder
nerve —*see* Injury, nerve, arm
open —*see* Wound, open, arm
specified type NEC S49.8-•
superficial —*see* Injury, superficial, arm
artery (complicating trauma) —*see also* Injury, blood vessel, by site
cerebral or meningeal —*see* Injury, intracranial
auditory canal (external) (meatus) S09.91
auricle, auris, ear S09.91
axilla —*see* Injury, shoulder
back —*see* Injury, back, lower
bile duct S36.13
birth —*see also* Birth, injury P15.9
bladder (sphincter) S37.20
at delivery O71.5
contusion S37.22
laceration S37.23
obstetrical trauma O71.5
specified type NEC S37.29
blast (air) (hydraulic) (immersion) (underwater) NEC T14.8
acoustic nerve trauma —*see* Injury, nerve, acoustic
bladder —*see* Injury, bladder

Injury *(Continued)*
blast *(Continued)*
brain —*see* Concussion
primary, specified NEC S06.8A-•
colon —*see* Injury, intestine, large, blast injury
ear (primary) S09.31-•
secondary S09.39-•
generalized T70.8
lung —*see* Injury, intrathoracic, lung, blast injury
multiple body organs T70.8
peritoneum S36.81
rectum S36.61
retroperitoneum S36.898
small intestine S36.419
duodenum S36.410
specified site NEC S36.418
specified
intra-abdominal organ NEC S36.898
pelvic organ NEC S37.899
blood vessel NEC T14.8
abdomen S35.9-•
aorta —*see* Injury, aorta, abdominal
celiac artery —*see* Injury, blood vessel, celiac artery
iliac vessel —*see* Injury, blood vessel, iliac
laceration S35.91
mesenteric vessel —*see* Injury, mesenteric
portal vein —*see* Injury, blood vessel, portal vein
renal vessel —*see* Injury, blood vessel, renal
specified vessel NEC S35.8X-•
splenic vessel —*see* Injury, blood vessel, splenic
vena cava —*see* Injury, vena cava, inferior
ankle —*see* Injury, blood vessel, foot
aorta (abdominal) (thoracic) —*see* Injury, aorta
arm (upper) NEC S45.90-•
forearm —*see* Injury, blood vessel, forearm
laceration S45.91-•
specified
site NEC S45.80-•
laceration S45.81-•
specified type NEC S45.89-•
type NEC S45.99-•
superficial vein S45.30-•
laceration S45.31-•
specified type NEC S45.39-•
axillary
artery S45.00-•
laceration S45.01-•
specified type NEC S45.09-•
vein S45.20-•
laceration S45.21-•
specified type NEC S45.29-•
azygos vein —*see* Injury, blood vessel, thoracic, specified site NEC
brachial
artery S45.10-•
laceration S45.11-•
specified type NEC S45.19-•
vein S45.20-•
laceration S45.219
specified type NEC S45.29-•
carotid artery (common) (external) (internal, extracranial) S15.00-•
internal, intracranial S06.8-•
laceration (minor) (superficial) S15.01-•
major S15.02-•
specified type NEC S15.09-•
celiac artery S35.219
branch S35.299
laceration (minor) (superficial) S35.291
major S35.292
specified NEC S35.298
laceration (minor) (superficial) S35.211
major S35.212
specified type NEC S35.218
cerebral —*see* Injury, intracranial
deep plantar —*see* Injury, blood vessel, plantar artery
digital (hand) —*see* Injury, blood vessel, finger
dorsal
artery (foot) S95.00-•
laceration S95.01-•
specified type NEC S95.09-•
vein (foot) S95.20-•
laceration S95.21-•
specified type NEC S95.29-•

Injury (Continued)
  blood vessel (Continued)
    due to accidental laceration during
        procedure —see Laceration, accidental
        complicating surgery
    extremity —see Injury, blood vessel, limb
    femoral
      artery (common) (superficial) S75.00-●
        laceration (minor) (superficial) S75.01-●
          major S75.02-●
        specified type NEC S75.09-●
      vein (hip level) (thigh level) S75.10-●
        laceration (minor) (superficial) S75.11-●
          major S75.12-●
        specified type NEC S75.19-●
    finger S65.50-●
      index S65.50-●
        laceration S65.51-●
        specified type NEC S65.59-●
      little S65.50-●
        laceration S65.51-●
        specified type NEC S65.59-●
      middle S65.50-●
        laceration S65.51-●
        specified type NEC S65.59-●
      specified type NEC S65.59-●
      thumb —see Injury, blood vessel, thumb
    foot S95.90-●
      dorsal
        artery —see Injury, blood vessel, dorsal,
            artery
        vein —see Injury, blood vessel, dorsal,
            vein
      laceration S95.91-●
      plantar artery —see Injury, blood vessel,
          plantar artery
      specified
        site NEC S95.80-●
          laceration S95.81-●
          specified type NEC S95.89-●
        specified type NEC S95.99-●
    forearm S55.90-●
      laceration S55.91-●
      radial artery —see Injury, blood vessel,
          radial artery
      specified
        site NEC S55.80-●
          laceration S55.81-●
          specified type NEC S55.89-●
        type NEC S55.99-●
      ulnar artery —see Injury, blood vessel, ulnar
          artery
      vein S55.20-●
        laceration S55.21-●
        specified type NEC S55.29-●
    gastric
      artery —see Injury, mesenteric, artery,
          branch
      vein —see Injury, blood vessel, abdomen
    gastroduodenal artery —see Injury,
        mesenteric, artery, branch
    greater saphenous vein (lower leg level)
        S85.30-●
      hip (and thigh) level S75.20-●
        laceration (minor) (superficial) S75.21-●
          major S75.22-●
        specified type NEC S75.29-●
      laceration S85.31-●
      specified type NEC S85.39-●
    hand (level) S65.90-●
      finger —see Injury, blood vessel, finger
      laceration S65.91-●
      palmar arch —see Injury, blood vessel,
          palmar arch
      radial artery —see Injury, blood vessel,
          radial artery, hand
      specified
        site NEC S65.80-●
          laceration S65.81-●
          specified type NEC S65.89-●
        type NEC S65.99-●
      thumb —see Injury, blood vessel, thumb
      ulnar artery —see Injury, blood vessel, ulnar
          artery, hand
    head S09.0
      intracranial —see Injury, intracranial
      multiple S09.0
    hepatic
      artery —see Injury, mesenteric, artery
      vein —see Injury, vena cava, inferior

Injury (Continued)
  blood vessel (Continued)
    hip S75.90-●
      femoral artery —see Injury, blood vessel,
          femoral, artery
      femoral vein —see Injury, blood vessel,
          femoral, vein
      greater saphenous vein —see Injury, blood
          vessel, greater saphenous, hip level
      laceration S75.91-●
      specified
        site NEC S75.80-●
          laceration S75.81-●
          specified type NEC S75.89-●
        type NEC S75.99-●
    hypogastric (artery) (vein) —see Injury, blood
        vessel, iliac
    iliac S35.5-●
      artery S35.51-●
      specified vessel NEC S35.5-●
      uterine vessel —see Injury, blood vessel,
          uterine
      vein S35.51-●
    innominate —see Injury, blood vessel, thoracic,
        innominate
    intercostal (artery) (vein) —see Injury, blood
        vessel, thoracic, intercostal
    jugular vein (external) S15.20-●
      internal S15.30-●
        laceration (minor) (superficial) S15.31-●
          major S15.32-●
        specified type NEC S15.39-●
      laceration (minor) (superficial) S15.21-●
        major S15.22-●
      specified type NEC S15.29-●
    leg (level) (lower) S85.90-●
      greater saphenous —see Injury, blood
          vessel, greater saphenous
      laceration S85.91-●
      lesser saphenous —see Injury, blood vessel,
          lesser saphenous
      peroneal artery —see Injury, blood vessel,
          peroneal artery
      popliteal
        artery —see Injury, blood vessel,
            popliteal, artery
        vein —see Injury, blood vessel, popliteal,
            vein
      specified
        site NEC S85.80-●
          laceration S85.81-●
          specified type NEC S85.89-●
        type NEC S85.99-●
      thigh —see Injury, blood vessel, hip
      tibial artery —see Injury, blood vessel, tibial
          artery
    lesser saphenous vein (lower leg level)
        S85.40-●
      laceration S85.41-●
      specified type NEC S85.49-●
    limb
      lower —see Injury, blood vessel, leg
      upper —see Injury, blood vessel, arm
    lower back —see Injury, blood vessel,
        abdomen
    specified NEC —see Injury, blood vessel,
        abdomen, specified, site NEC
    mammary (artery) (vein) —see Injury, blood
        vessel, thoracic, specified site NEC
    mesenteric (inferior) (superior)
      artery —see Injury, mesenteric, artery
      vein —see Injury, mesenteric, vein
    neck S15.9
      specified site NEC S15.8
    ovarian (artery) (vein) —see subcategory
        S35.8
    palmar arch (superficial) S65.20-●
      deep S65.30-●
        laceration S65.31-●
        specified type NEC S65.39-●
      laceration S65.21-●
      specified type NEC S65.29-●
    pelvis —see Injury, blood vessel, abdomen
      specified NEC —see Injury, blood vessel,
          abdomen, specified, site NEC
    peroneal artery S85.20-●
      laceration S85.21-●
      specified type NEC S85.29-●
    plantar artery (deep) (foot) S95.10-●
      laceration S95.11-●
      specified type NEC S95.19-●

Injury (Continued)
  blood vessel (Continued)
    popliteal
      artery S85.00-●
        laceration S85.01-●
        specified type NEC S85.09-●
      vein S85.50-●
        laceration S85.51-●
        specified type NEC S85.59-●
    portal vein S35.319
      laceration S35.311
      specified type NEC S35.318
    precerebral —see Injury, blood vessel, neck
    pulmonary (artery) (vein) —see Injury, blood
        vessel, thoracic, pulmonary
    radial artery (forearm level) S55.10-●
      hand and wrist (level) S65.10-●
        laceration S65.11-●
        specified type NEC S65.19-●
      laceration S55.11-●
      specified type NEC S55.19-●
    renal
      artery S35.40-●
        laceration S35.41-●
        specified NEC S35.49-●
      vein S35.40-●
        laceration S35.41-●
        specified NEC S35.49-●
    saphenous vein (greater) (lower leg
        level) —see Injury, blood vessel, greater
        saphenous
      hip and thigh level —see Injury, blood
          vessel, greater saphenous, hip level
      lesser —see Injury, blood vessel, lesser
          saphenous
    shoulder
      specified NEC —see Injury, blood vessel,
          arm, specified site NEC
      superficial vein —see Injury, blood vessel,
          arm, superficial vein
    specified NEC T14.8
    splenic
      artery —see Injury, blood vessel, celiac
          artery, branch
      vein S35.329
        laceration S35.321
        specified NEC S35.328
    subclavian —see Injury, blood vessel, thoracic,
        innominate
    thigh —see Injury, blood vessel, hip
    thoracic S25.90
      aorta S25.00
        laceration (minor) (superficial)
            S25.01
          major S25.02
        specified type NEC S25.09
      azygos vein —see Injury, blood vessel,
          thoracic, specified, site NEC
      innominate
        artery S25.10-●
          laceration (minor) (superficial)
              S25.11-●
            major S25.12-●
          specified type NEC S25.19-●
        vein S25.30-●
          laceration (minor) (superficial)
              S25.31-●
            major S25.32-●
          specified type NEC S25.39-●
      intercostal S25.50-●
        laceration S25.51-●
        specified type NEC S25.59-●
      laceration S25.91
      mammary vessel —see Injury, blood vessel,
          thoracic, specified, site NEC
      pulmonary S25.40-●
        laceration (minor) (superficial) S25.41-●
          major S25.42-●
        specified type NEC S25.49-●
      specified
        site NEC S25.80-●
          laceration S25.81-●
          specified type NEC S25.89-●
        type NEC S25.99
      subclavian —see Injury, blood vessel,
          thoracic, innominate
      vena cava (superior) S25.20
        laceration (minor) (superficial)
            S25.21
          major S25.22
        specified type NEC S25.29

njury *(Continued)*
  blood vessel *(Continued)*
    thumb S65.40-●
      laceration S65.41-●
      specified type NEC S65.49-●
    tibial artery S85.10-●
      anterior S85.13-●
        laceration S85.14-●
        specified injury NEC S85.15-●
      laceration S85.11-●
      posterior S85.16-●
        laceration S85.17-●
        specified injury NEC S85.18-●
      specified injury NEC S85.12-●
    ulnar artery (forearm level) S55.00-●
      hand and wrist (level) S65.00-●
        laceration S65.01-●
        specified type NEC S65.09-●
      laceration S55.01-●
      specified type NEC S55.09-●
    upper arm (level) —*see* Injury, blood vessel,
        arm
      superficial vein —*see* Injury, blood vessel,
          arm, superficial vein
    uterine S35.5-●
      artery S35.53-●
      vein S35.53-●
    vena cava —*see* Injury, vena cava
    vertebral artery S15.10-●
      laceration (minor) (superficial)
          S15.11-●
        major S15.12-●
      specified type NEC S15.19-●
    wrist (level) —*see* Injury, blood vessel,
        hand
  brachial plexus S14.3
    newborn P14.3
  brain (traumatic) S06.9-●
    diffuse (axonal) S06.2X-●
    focal S06.30-●
  brainstem S06.38-●
  breast NOS S29.9
  broad ligament —*see* Injury, pelvic organ,
      specified site NEC
  bronchus, bronchi —*see* Injury, intrathoracic,
      bronchus
  brow S09.90
  buttock S39.92
  canthus, eye S05.90
  cardiac plexus —*see* Injury, nerve, thorax,
      sympathetic
  cauda equina S34.3
  cavernous sinus —*see* Injury, intracranial
  cecum —*see* Injury, colon
  celiac ganglion or plexus —*see* Injury, nerve,
      lumbosacral, sympathetic
  cerebellum —*see* Injury, intracranial
  cerebral —*see* Injury, intracranial
  cervix (uteri) —*see* Injury, uterus
  cheek (wall) S09.93
  chest —*see* Injury, thorax
  childbirth (newborn) —*see also* Birth, injury
    maternal NEC O71.9
  chin S09.93
  choroid (eye) —*see* Injury, eye, specified site
      NEC
  clitoris S39.94
  coccyx —*see also* Injury, back, lower
    complicating delivery O71.6
  colon —*see* Injury, intestine, large
  common bile duct —*see* Injury, liver
  conjunctiva (superficial) —*see* Injury, eye,
      conjunctiva
  conus medullaris —*see* Injury, spinal, sacral
  cord
    spermatic (pelvic region) S37.898
      scrotal region S39.848
    spinal —*see* Injury, spinal cord, by region
  cornea —*see* Injury, eye, specified site NEC
    abrasion —*see* Injury, eye, cornea,
        abrasion
  cortex (cerebral) —*see also* Injury, intracranial
    visual —*see* Injury, nerve, optic
  costal region NEC S29.9
  costochondral NEC S29.9
  cranial
    cavity —*see* Injury, intracranial
    nerve —*see* Injury, nerve, cranial
  crushing —*see* Crush
  cutaneous sensory nerve
  cystic duct —*see* Injury, liver

Injury *(Continued)*
  deep tissue —*see* Contusion, by site
    meaning pressure ulcer —*see* Ulcer, pressure
        L89 with final character .6
  delivery (newborn) P15.9
    maternal NEC O71.9
  Descemet's membrane —*see* Injury, eyeball,
      penetrating
  diaphragm —*see* Injury, intrathoracic, diaphragm
  duodenum —*see* Injury, intestine, small,
      duodenum
  ear (auricle) (external) (canal) S09.91
    abrasion —*see* Abrasion, ear
    bite —*see* Bite, ear
    blister —*see* Blister, ear
    bruise —*see* Contusion, ear
    contusion —*see* Contusion, ear
    external constriction —*see* Constriction,
        external, ear
    hematoma —*see* Hematoma, ear
    inner —*see* Injury, ear, middle
    laceration —*see* Laceration, ear
    middle S09.30-●
      blast —*see* Injury, blast, ear
      specified NEC S09.39-●
    puncture —*see* Puncture, ear
    superficial —*see* Injury, superficial, ear
  eighth cranial nerve (acoustic or auditory) —*see*
      Injury, nerve, acoustic
  elbow S59.90-●
    contusion —*see* Contusion, elbow
    dislocation —*see* Dislocation, elbow
    fracture —*see* Fracture, ulna, upper
        end
    open —*see* Wound, open, elbow
    specified NEC S59.80-●
    sprain —*see* Sprain, elbow
    superficial —*see* Injury, superficial,
        elbow
  eleventh cranial nerve (accessory) —*see* Injury,
      nerve, accessory
  epididymis S39.94
  epigastric region S39.91
  epiglottis NEC S19.89
  esophageal plexus —*see* Injury, nerve, thorax,
      sympathetic
  esophagus (thoracic part) —*see also* Injury,
      intrathoracic, esophagus
    cervical NEC S19.85
  eustachian tube S09.30-●
  eye S05.9-●
    avulsion S05.7-●
    ball —*see* Injury, eyeball
    conjunctiva S05.0-●
    cornea
      abrasion S05.0-●
    laceration S05.3-●
      with prolapse S05.2-●
    lacrimal apparatus S05.8X-●
    orbit penetration S05.4-●
    specified site NEC S05.8X-●
  eyeball S05.8X-●
    contusion S05.1-●
    penetrating S05.6-●
      with
        foreign body S05.5-●
        prolapse or loss of intraocular tissue
            S05.2-●
      without prolapse or loss of intraocular
          tissue S05.3-●
    specified type NEC S05.8-●
  eyebrow S09.93
  eyelid S09.93
    abrasion —*see* Abrasion, eyelid
    contusion —*see* Contusion, eyelid
    open —*see* Wound, open, eyelid
  face S09.93
  fallopian tube S37.509
    bilateral S37.502
      blast injury S37.512
      contusion S37.522
      laceration S37.532
      specified type NEC S37.592
    blast injury (primary) S37.519
      bilateral S37.512
      secondary —*see* Injury, fallopian tube,
          specified type NEC
      unilateral S37.511
    contusion S37.529
      bilateral S37.522
      unilateral S37.521

Injury *(Continued)*
  fallopian tube *(Continued)*
    laceration S37.539
      bilateral S37.532
      unilateral S37.531
    specified type NEC S37.599
      bilateral S37.592
      unilateral S37.591
    unilateral S37.501
      blast injury S37.511
      contusion S37.521
      laceration S37.531
      specified type NEC S37.591
  fascia —*see* Injury, muscle
  fifth cranial nerve (trigeminal) —*see* Injury,
      nerve, trigeminal
  finger (nail) S69.9-●
    blood vessel —*see* Injury, blood vessel, finger
    contusion —*see* Contusion, finger
    dislocation —*see* Dislocation, finger
    fracture —*see* Fracture, finger
    muscle —*see* Injury, muscle, finger
    nerve —*see* Injury, nerve, digital, finger
    open —*see* Wound, open, finger
    specified NEC S69.8-●
    sprain —*see* Sprain, finger
    superficial —*see* Injury, superficial, finger
  first cranial nerve (olfactory) —*see* Injury, nerve,
      olfactory
  flank —*see* Injury, abdomen
  foot S99.92-●
    blood vessel —*see* Injury, blood vessel,
        foot
    contusion —*see* Contusion, foot
    dislocation —*see* Dislocation, foot
    fracture —*see* Fracture, foot
    muscle —*see* Injury, muscle, foot
    open —*see* Wound, open, foot
    specified type NEC S99.82-●
    sprain —*see* Sprain, foot
    superficial —*see* Injury, superficial, foot
  forceps NOS P15.9
  forearm S59.91-●
    blood vessel —*see* Injury, blood vessel,
        forearm
    contusion —*see* Contusion, forearm
    fracture —*see* Fracture, forearm
    muscle —*see* Injury, muscle, forearm
    nerve —*see* Injury, nerve, forearm
    open —*see* Wound, open, forearm
    specified NEC S59.81-●
    superficial —*see* Injury, superficial, forearm
  forehead S09.90
  fourth cranial nerve (trochlear) —*see* Injury,
      nerve, trochlear
  gallbladder S36.129
    contusion S36.122
    laceration S36.123
    specified NEC S36.128
  ganglion
    celiac, coeliac —*see* Injury, nerve, lumbosacral,
        sympathetic
    gasserian —*see* Injury, nerve, trigeminal
    stellate —*see* Injury, nerve, thorax,
        sympathetic
    thoracic sympathetic —*see* Injury, nerve,
        thorax, sympathetic
  gasserian ganglion —*see* Injury, nerve, trigeminal
  gastric artery —*see* Injury, blood vessel, celiac
      artery, branch
  gastroduodenal artery —*see* Injury, blood vessel,
      celiac artery, branch
  gastrointestinal tract —*see* Injury,
      intra-abdominal
    with open wound into abdominal cavity —*see*
        Wound, open, with penetration into
        peritoneal cavity
    colon —*see* Injury, intestine, large
    rectum —*see* Injury, intestine, large, rectum
      with open wound into abdominal cavity
          S36.61
    small intestine —*see* Injury, intestine, small
    specified site NEC —*see* Injury, intra-
        abdominal, specified, site NEC
    stomach —*see* Injury, stomach
  genital organ(s)
    external S39.94
      specified NEC S39.848
    internal S37.90
      fallopian tube —*see* Injury, fallopian tube
      ovary —*see* Injury, ovary

Injury *(Continued)*
   genital organ(s) *(Continued)*
      internal *(Continued)*
         prostate —*see* Injury, prostate
         seminal vesicle —*see* Injury, pelvis, organ,
            specified site NEC
         uterus —*see* Injury, uterus
         vas deferens —*see* Injury, pelvis, organ,
            specified site NEC
      obstetrical trauma O71.9
   gland
      lacrimal laceration —*see* Injury, eye, specified
         site NEC
      salivary S09.93
      thyroid NEC S19.84
   globe (eye) S05.90
      specified NEC S05.8X-●
   groin —*see* Injury, abdomen
   gum S09.90
   hand S69.9-●
      blood vessel —*see* Injury, blood vessel, hand
      contusion —*see* Contusion, hand
      fracture —*see* Fracture, hand
      muscle —*see* Injury, muscle, hand
      nerve —*see* Injury, nerve, hand
      open —*see* Wound, open, hand
      specified NEC S69.8-●
      sprain —*see* Sprain, hand
      superficial —*see* Injury, superficial, hand
   head S09.90
      with loss of consciousness S06.9-●
      specified NEC S09.8-●
   heart (traumatic) S26.90
      with hemopericardium S26.00
         contusion S26.01
         laceration (mild) S26.020
            major S26.022
            moderate S26.021
         specified type NEC S26.09
      without hemopericardium S26.10
         contusion S26.11
         laceration S26.12
         specified type NEC S26.19
      contusion S26.91
      laceration S26.92
      non-traumatic (acute) (chronic) (non-ischemic)
         I5A
      specified type NEC S26.99
   heel —*see* Injury, foot
   hepatic
      artery —*see* Injury, blood vessel, celiac artery,
         branch
      duct —*see* Injury, liver
      vein —*see* Injury, vena cava, inferior
   hip S79.91-●
      blood vessel —*see* Injury, blood vessel, hip
      contusion —*see* Contusion, hip
      dislocation —*see* Dislocation, hip
      fracture —*see* Fracture, femur, neck
      muscle —*see* Injury, muscle, hip
      nerve —*see* Injury, nerve, hip
      open —*see* Wound, open, hip
      specified NEC S79.81-●
      sprain —*see* Sprain, hip
      superficial —*see* Injury, superficial, hip
   hymen S39.94
   hypogastric
      blood vessel —*see* Injury, blood vessel, iliac
      plexus —*see* Injury, nerve, lumbosacral,
         sympathetic
   ileum —*see* Injury, intestine, small
   iliac region S39.91
   instrumental (during surgery) —*see* Laceration,
      accidental complicating surgery
      birth injury —*see* Birth, injury
      nonsurgical —*see* Injury, by site
      obstetrical O71.9
         bladder O71.5
         cervix O71.3
         high vaginal O71.4
         perineal NOS O70.9
         urethra O71.5
         uterus O71.5
            with rupture or perforation O71.1
   internal T14.8
      aorta —*see* Injury, aorta
      bladder (sphincter) —*see* Injury, bladder
         with
            ectopic or molar pregnancy O08.6
         following ectopic or molar pregnancy O08.6
         obstetrical trauma O71.5

Injury *(Continued)*
   internal *(Continued)*
      bronchus, bronchi —*see* Injury, intrathoracic,
         bronchus
      cecum —*see* Injury, intestine, large
      cervix (uteri) —*see also* Injury, uterus
         with ectopic or molar pregnancy O08.6
         following ectopic or molar pregnancy
            O08.6
         obstetrical trauma O71.3
      chest —*see* Injury, intrathoracic
      gastrointestinal tract —*see* Injury,
         intra-abdominal
      heart —*see* Injury, heart
      intestine NEC —*see* Injury, intestine
      intrauterine —*see* Injury, uterus
      mesentery —*see* Injury, intra-abdominal,
         specified, site NEC
      pelvis, pelvic (organ) S37.90
         following ectopic or molar pregnancy
            (subsequent episode) O08.6
         obstetrical trauma NEC O71.5
            rupture or perforation O71.1
         specified NEC S39.83
      rectum —*see* Injury, intestine, large, rectum
      stomach —*see* Injury, stomach
      ureter —*see* Injury, ureter
      urethra (sphincter) following ectopic or molar
         pregnancy O08.6
      uterus —*see* Injury, uterus
   interscapular area —*see* Injury, thorax
   intestine
      large S36.509
         ascending (right) S36.500
            blast injury (primary) S36.510
               secondary S36.590
            contusion S36.520
            laceration S36.530
            specified type NEC S36.590
         blast injury (primary) S36.519
            ascending (right) S36.510
            descending (left) S36.512
            rectum S36.61
            sigmoid S36.513
            specified site NEC S36.518
            transverse S36.511
         contusion S36.529
            ascending (right) S36.520
            descending (left) S36.522
            rectum S36.62
            sigmoid S36.523
            specified site NEC S36.528
            transverse S36.521
         descending (left) S36.502
            blast injury (primary) S36.512
               secondary S36.592
            contusion S36.522
            laceration S36.532
            specified type NEC S36.592
         laceration S36.539
            ascending (right) S36.530
            descending (left) S36.532
            rectum S36.63
            sigmoid S36.533
            specified site NEC S36.538
            transverse S36.531
         rectum S36.60
            blast injury (primary) S36.61
               secondary S36.69
            contusion S36.62
            laceration S36.63
            specified type NEC S36.69
         sigmoid S36.503
            blast injury (primary) S36.513
               secondary S36.593
            contusion S36.523
            laceration S36.533
            specified type NEC S36.593
         specified
            site NEC S36.508
               blast injury (primary)
                  S36.518
                  secondary S36.598
               contusion S36.528
               laceration S36.538
               specified type NEC S36.598
            type NEC S36.599
               ascending (right) S36.590
               descending (left) S36.592
               rectum S36.69
               sigmoid S36.593

Injury *(Continued)*
   intestine *(Continued)*
      large *(Continued)*
         specified *(Continued)*
            type *(Continued)*
               specified site NEC S36.598
               transverse S36.591
         transverse S36.501
            blast injury (primary) S36.511
               secondary S36.591
            contusion S36.521
            laceration S36.531
            specified type NEC S36.591
      small S36.409
         blast injury (primary) S36.419
            duodenum S36.410
            secondary S36.490
               duodenum S36.490
               specified site NEC S36.498
            specified site NEC S36.418
         contusion S36.429
            duodenum S36.420
            specified site NEC S36.428
         duodenum S36.400
            blast injury (primary) S36.410
               secondary S36.490
            contusion S36.420
            laceration S36.430
            specified NEC S36.490
         laceration S36.439
            duodenum S36.430
            specified site NEC S36.438
         specified
            site NEC S36.408
            type NEC S36.499
               duodenum S36.490
               specified site NEC
                  S36.498
   intra-abdominal S36.90
      adrenal gland —*see* Injury, adrenal gland
      bladder —*see* Injury, bladder
      colon —*see* Injury, intestine, large
      contusion S36.92
      fallopian tube —*see* Injury, fallopian tube
      gallbladder —*see* Injury, gallbladder
      intestine —*see* Injury, intestine
      kidney —*see* Injury, kidney
      laceration S36.93
      liver —*see* Injury, liver
      ovary —*see* Injury, ovary
      pancreas —*see* Injury, pancreas
      pelvic NOS S37.90
      peritoneum —*see* Injury, intra-abdominal,
         specified, site NEC
      prostate —*see* Injury, prostate
      rectum —*see* Injury, intestine, large, rectum
      retroperitoneum —*see* Injury, intra-
         abdominal, specified, site NEC
      seminal vesicle —*see* Injury, pelvis, organ,
         specified site NEC
      small intestine —*see* Injury, intestine, small
      specified
         pelvic S37.90
            specified
               site NEC S37.899
                  specified type NEC S37.898
               type NEC S37.99
         site NEC S36.899
            contusion S36.892
            laceration S36.893
            specified type NEC S36.898
         type NEC S36.99
      spleen —*see* Injury, spleen
      stomach —*see* Injury, stomach
      ureter —*see* Injury, ureter
      urethra —*see* Injury, urethra
      uterus —*see* Injury, uterus
      vas deferens —*see* Injury, pelvis, organ,
         specified site NEC
   intracranial (traumatic) *(see also,* if applicable,
      Compression, brain, traumatic) S06.9-●
      cerebellar hemorrhage, traumatic —*see* Injury,
         intracranial, focal
      cerebral edema, traumatic S06.1X-●
         diffuse S06.1X-●
         focal S06.1X-●
      diffuse (axonal) S06.2X-●
      epidural hemorrhage (traumatic) S06.4X-●
      focal brain injury S06.30-●
         contusion —*see* Contusion, cerebral
         laceration —*see* Laceration, cerebral

Injury *(Continued)*
  intracranial *(Continued)*
    intracerebral hemorrhage, traumatic
      S06.36-●
      left side S06.35-●
      right side S06.34-●
      specified NEC S06.89-●
    subarachnoid hemorrhage, traumatic
      S06.6X-●
    subdural hemorrhage, traumatic S06.5X-●
  intraocular —*see* Injury, eyeball, penetrating
  intrathoracic S27.9
    bronchus S27.409
      bilateral S27.402
      blast injury (primary) S27.419
        bilateral S27.412
        secondary —*see* Injury, intrathoracic,
          bronchus, specified type NEC
        unilateral S27.411
      contusion S27.429
        bilateral S27.422
        unilateral S27.421
      laceration S27.439
        bilateral S27.432
        unilateral S27.431
      specified type NEC S27.499
        bilateral S27.492
        unilateral S27.491
      unilateral S27.401
    diaphragm S27.809
      contusion S27.802
      laceration S27.803
      specified type NEC S27.808
    esophagus (thoracic) S27.819
      contusion S27.812
      laceration S27.813
      specified type NEC S27.818
    heart —*see* Injury, heart
    hemopneumothorax S27.2
    hemothorax S27.1
    lung S27.309
      aspiration J69.0
      bilateral S27.302
      blast injury (primary) S27.319
        bilateral S27.312
        secondary —*see* Injury, intrathoracic,
          lung, specified type NEC
        unilateral S27.311
      contusion S27.329
        bilateral S27.322
        unilateral S27.321
      laceration S27.339
        bilateral S27.332
        unilateral S27.331
      specified type NEC S27.399
        bilateral S27.392
        unilateral S27.391
      unilateral S27.301
    pleura S27.60
      laceration S27.63
      specified type NEC S27.69
    pneumothorax S27.0
    specified organ NEC S27.899
      contusion S27.892
      laceration S27.893
      specified type NEC S27.898
    thoracic duct —*see* Injury, intrathoracic,
      specified organ NEC
    thymus gland —*see* Injury, intrathoracic,
      specified organ NEC
    trachea, thoracic S27.50
      blast (primary) S27.51
      contusion S27.52
      laceration S27.53
      specified type NEC S27.59
  iris —*see* Injury, eye, specified site NEC
    penetrating —*see* Injury, eyeball,
      penetrating
  jaw S09.93
  jejunum —*see* Injury, intestine, small
  joint NOS T14.8
    old or residual —*see* Disorder, joint, specified
      type NEC
  kidney S37.00-●
    acute (nontraumatic) N17.9
    contusion —*see* Contusion, kidney
    laceration —*see* Laceration, kidney
    specified NEC S37.09-●
  knee S89.9-●
    contusion —*see* Contusion, knee
    dislocation —*see* Dislocation, knee

Injury *(Continued)*
  knee *(Continued)*
    meniscus (lateral) (medial) —*see* Sprain, knee,
      specified site NEC
      old injury or tear —*see* Derangement, knee,
        meniscus, due to old injury
    open —*see* Wound, open, knee
    specified NEC S89.8-●
    sprain —*see* Sprain, knee
    superficial —*see* Injury, superficial, knee
  labium (majus) (minus) S39.94
  labyrinth, ear S09.30-●
  lacrimal apparatus, duct, gland, or sac —*see*
    Injury, eye, specified site NEC
  larynx NEC S19.81
  leg (lower) S89.9-●
    blood vessel —*see* Injury, blood vessel, leg
    contusion —*see* Contusion, leg
    fracture —*see* Fracture, leg
    muscle —*see* Injury, muscle, leg
    nerve —*see* Injury, nerve, leg
    open —*see* Wound, open, leg
    specified NEC S89.8-●
    superficial —*see* Injury, superficial, leg
  lens, eye —*see* Injury, eye, specified site NEC
    penetrating —*see* Injury, eyeball, penetrating
  limb NEC T14.8
  lip S09.93
  liver S36.119
    contusion S36.112
    laceration S36.113
      major (stellate) S36.116
      minor S36.114
      moderate S36.115
    specified NEC S36.118
  lower back S39.92
    specified NEC S39.82
  lumbar, lumbosacral (region) S39.92
    plexus —*see* Injury, lumbosacral plexus
  lumbosacral plexus S34.4
  lung —*see also* Injury, intrathoracic, lung
    aspiration J69.0
    dabbing (related) U07.0
    electronic cigarette (related) U07.0
    EVALI - [e-cigarette, or vaping, product use
      associated] U07.0
    transfusion-related (TRALI) J95.84
    vaping (associated) (device) (product) (use)
      U07.0
  lymphatic thoracic duct —*see* Injury,
    intrathoracic, specified organ NEC
  malar region S09.93
  mastoid region S09.90
  maxilla S09.93
  mediastinum —*see* Injury, intrathoracic, specified
    organ NEC
  membrane, brain —*see* Injury, intracranial
  meningeal artery —*see* Injury, intracranial,
    subdural hemorrhage
  meninges (cerebral) —*see* Injury, intracranial
  mesenteric
    artery
      branch S35.299
        laceration (minor) (superficial) S35.291
          major S35.292
          specified NEC S35.298
      inferior S35.239
        laceration (minor) (superficial) S35.231
          major S35.232
          specified NEC S35.238
      superior S35.229
        laceration (minor) (superficial) S35.221
          major S35.222
          specified NEC S35.228
      plexus (inferior) (superior) —*see* Injury, nerve,
        lumbosacral, sympathetic
    vein
      inferior S35.349
        laceration S35.341
        specified NEC S35.348
      superior S35.339
        laceration S35.331
        specified NEC S35.338
  mesentery —*see* Injury, intra-abdominal,
    specified site NEC
  mesosalpinx —*see* Injury, pelvic organ, specified
    site NEC
  middle ear S09.30-●
  midthoracic region NOS S29.9
  mouth S09.93
  multiple NOS T07

Injury *(Continued)*
  muscle (and fascia) (and tendon)
    abdomen S39.001
      laceration S39.021
      specified type NEC S39.091
      strain S39.011
    abductor
      thumb, forearm level —*see* Injury, muscle,
        thumb, abductor
    adductor
      thigh S76.20-●
        laceration S76.22-●
        specified type NEC S76.29-●
        strain S76.21-●
    ankle —*see* Injury, muscle, foot
    anterior muscle group, at leg level (lower)
      S86.20-●
      laceration S86.22-●
      specified type NEC S86.29-●
      strain S86.21-●
    arm (upper) —*see* Injury, muscle, shoulder
    biceps (parts NEC) S46.20-●
      laceration S46.22-●
      long head S46.10-●
        laceration S46.12-●
        specified type NEC S46.19-●
        strain S46.11-●
      specified type NEC S46.29-●
      strain S46.21-●
    extensor
      finger(s) (other than thumb) —*see* Injury,
        muscle, finger by site, extensor
      forearm level, specified NEC —*see* Injury,
        muscle, forearm, extensor
      thumb —*see* Injury, muscle, thumb,
        extensor
      toe (large) (ankle level) (foot level) —*see*
        Injury, muscle, toe, extensor
    finger
      extensor (forearm level) S56.40-●
        hand level S66.309
          laceration S66.329
          specified type NEC S66.399
          strain S66.319
        laceration S56.429
        specified type NEC S56.499
        strain S56.419
      flexor (forearm level) S56.10-●
        hand level S66.109
          laceration S66.129
          specified type NEC S66.199
          strain S66.119
        laceration S56.129
        specified type NEC S56.199
        strain S56.119
    index
      extensor (forearm level)
        hand level S66.308
          laceration S66.32-●
          specified type NEC S66.39-●
          strain S66.31-●
        specified type NEC S56.492-●
      flexor (forearm level)
        hand level S66.108
          laceration S66.12-●
          specified type NEC S66.19-●
          strain S66.11-●
        specified type NEC S56.19-●
        strain S56.11-●
      intrinsic S66.50-●
        laceration S66.52-●
        specified type NEC S66.59-●
        strain S66.51-●
    intrinsic S66.509
      laceration S66.529
      specified type NEC S66.599
      strain S66.519
    little
      extensor (forearm level)
        hand level S66.30-●
          laceration S66.32-●
          specified type NEC S66.39-●
          strain S66.31-●
        laceration S56.42-●
        specified type NEC S56.49-●
        strain S56.41-●
      flexor (forearm level)
        hand level S66.10-●
          laceration S66.12-●
          specified type NEC S66.19-●
          strain S66.11-●

Injury *(Continued)*
muscle *(Continued)*
finger *(Continued)*
little *(Continued)*
flexor *(Continued)*
laceration S56.12-●
specified type NEC S56.19-●
strain S56.11-●
intrinsic S66.50-●
laceration S66.52-●
specified type NEC S66.59-●
strain S66.51-●
middle
extensor (forearm level)
hand level S66.30-●
laceration S66.32-●
specified type NEC
S66.39-●
strain S66.31-●
laceration S56.42-●
specified type NEC
S56.49-●
strain S56.41-●
flexor (forearm level)
hand level S66.10-●
laceration S66.12-●
specified type NEC
S66.19-●
strain S66.11-●
laceration S56.12-●
specified type NEC S56.19-●
strain S56.11-●
intrinsic S66.50-●
laceration S66.52-●
specified type NEC S66.59-●
strain S66.51-●
ring
extensor (forearm level)
hand level S66.30-●
laceration S66.32-●
specified type NEC S66.39-●
strain S66.31-●
laceration S56.42-●
specified type NEC S56.49-●
strain S56.41-●
flexor (forearm level)
hand level S66.10-●
laceration S66.12-●
specified type NEC S66.19-●
strain S66.11-●
laceration S56.12-●
specified type NEC S56.19-●
strain S56.11-●
intrinsic S66.50-●
laceration S66.52-●
specified type NEC S66.59-●
strain S66.51-●
flexor
finger(s) (other than thumb) — *see* Injury,
muscle, finger
forearm level, specified NEC —
see Injury, muscle, forearm,
flexor
thumb —*see* Injury, muscle, thumb, flexor
toe (long) (ankle level) (foot level) —*see*
Injury, muscle, toe, flexor
foot S96.90-●
intrinsic S96.20-●
laceration S96.22-●
specified type NEC S96.29-●
strain S96.21-●
laceration S96.92-●
long extensor, toe —*see* Injury, muscle, toe,
extensor
long flexor, toe —*see* Injury, muscle, toe,
flexor
specified
site NEC S96.80-●
laceration S96.82-●
specified type NEC S96.89-●
strain S96.81-●
type NEC S96.99-●
strain S96.91-●
forearm (level) S56.90-●
extensor S56.50-●
laceration S56.52-●
specified type NEC S56.59-●
strain S56.51-●
flexor S56.20-●
laceration S56.22-●
specified type NEC S56.29-●
strain S56.21-●

Injury *(Continued)*
muscle *(Continued)*
forearm *(Continued)*
laceration S56.92-●
specified S56.99-●
site NEC S56.80-●
laceration S56.82-●
strain S56.81-●
type NEC S56.89-●
strain S56.91-●
hand (level) S66.90-●
laceration S66.92-●
specified
site NEC S66.80-●
laceration S66.82-●
specified type NEC S66.89-●
strain S66.81-●
type NEC S66.99-●
strain S66.91-●
head S09.10
laceration S09.12
specified type NEC S09.19
strain S09.11
hip NEC S76.00-●
laceration S76.02-●
specified type NEC S76.09-●
strain S76.01-●
intrinsic
ankle and foot level —*see* Injury, muscle,
foot, intrinsic
finger (other than thumb) —*see* Injury,
muscle, finger by site, intrinsic
foot (level) —*see* Injury, muscle, foot,
intrinsic
thumb —*see* Injury, muscle, thumb, intrinsic
leg (level) (lower) S86.90-●
Achilles tendon —*see* Injury, Achilles
tendon
anterior muscle group —*see* Injury, muscle,
anterior muscle group
laceration S86.92-●
peroneal muscle group —*see* Injury, muscle,
peroneal muscle group
posterior muscle group —*see* Injury, muscle,
posterior muscle group, leg level
specified
site NEC S86.80-●
laceration S86.82-●
specified type NEC S86.89-●
strain S86.81-●
type NEC S86.99-●
strain S86.91-●
long
extensor toe, at ankle and foot level —*see*
Injury, muscle, toe, extensor
flexor, toe, at ankle and foot level —*see*
Injury, muscle, toe, flexor
head, biceps —*see* Injury, muscle, biceps,
long head
lower back S39.002
laceration S39.022
specified type NEC S39.092
strain S39.012
neck (level) S16.9
laceration S16.2
specified type NEC S16.8
strain S16.1
pelvis S39.003
laceration S39.023
specified type NEC S39.093
strain S39.013
peroneal muscle group, at leg level (lower)
S86.30-●
laceration S86.32-●
specified type NEC S86.39-●
strain S86.31-●
posterior muscle (group)
leg level (lower) S86.10-●
laceration S86.12-●
specified type NEC S86.19-●
strain S86.11-●
thigh level S76.30-●
laceration S76.32-●
specified type NEC S76.39-●
strain S76.31-●
quadriceps (thigh) S76.10-●
laceration S76.12-●
specified type NEC S76.19-●
strain S76.11-●
shoulder S46.90-●
laceration S46.92-●
rotator cuff —*see* Injury, rotator cuff

Injury *(Continued)*
muscle *(Continued)*
forearm *(Continued)*
specified site NEC S46.80-●
laceration S46.82-●
specified type NEC S46.89-●
strain S46.81-●
specified type NEC S46.99-●
strain S46.91-●
thigh NEC (level) S76.90-●
adductor —*see* Injury, muscle, adductor,
thigh
laceration S76.92-●
posterior muscle (group) —*see* Injury,
muscle, posterior muscle, thigh
level
quadriceps —*see* Injury, muscle,
quadriceps
specified
site NEC S76.80-●
laceration S76.82-●
specified type NEC S76.89-●
strain S76.81-●
type NEC S76.99-●
strain S76.91-●
thorax (level) S29.009
back wall S29.002
front wall S29.001
laceration S29.029
back wall S29.022
front wall S29.021
specified type NEC S29.099
back wall S29.092
front wall S29.091
strain S29.019
back wall S29.012
front wall S29.011
thumb
abductor (forearm level) S56.30-●
laceration S56.32-●
specified type NEC S56.39-●
strain S56.31-●
extensor (forearm level) S56.30-●
hand level S66.20-●
laceration S66.22-●
specified type NEC S66.29-●
strain S66.21-●
laceration S56.32-●
specified type NEC S56.39-●
strain S56.31-●
flexor (forearm level) S56.00-●
hand level S66.00-●
laceration S66.02-●
specified type NEC S66.09-●
strain S66.01-●
laceration S56.02-●
specified type NEC S56.09-●
strain S56.01-●
wrist level —*see* Injury, muscle, thumb,
flexor, hand level
intrinsic S66.40-●
laceration S66.42-●
specified type NEC S66.49-●
strain S66.41-●
toe —*see also* Injury, muscle, foot
extensor, long S96.10-●
laceration S96.12-●
specified type NEC S96.19-●
strain S96.11-●
flexor, long S96.00-●
laceration S96.02-●
specified type NEC S96.09-●
strain S96.01-●
triceps S46.30-●
laceration S46.32-●
specified type NEC S46.39-●
strain S46.31-●
wrist (and hand) level —*see* Injury, muscle,
hand
musculocutaneous nerve —*see* Injury, nerve,
musculocutaneous
myocardial (acute) (chronic) (non-ischemic)
(non-traumatic) I5A
traumatic —*see* Injury, heart
myocardium —*see also* Injury, heart
non-traumatic —*see* Injury, myocardial
nape —*see* Injury, neck
nasal (septum) (sinus) S09.92
nasopharynx S09.92
neck S19.9
specified NEC S19.80
specified site NEC S19.89

▶ New   ⇒ Revised   ~~deleted~~ Deleted   ● Use Additional Character(s)

▷ New   ⇒ Revised   ~~deleted~~ Deleted   ● Use Additional Character(s)

Injury (Continued)
  nerve (Continued)
    trochlear S04.2-●
      contusion S04.2-●
      laceration S04.2-●
      specified type NEC S04.2-●
    twelfth cranial (hypoglossal) —see Injury,
        nerve, hypoglossal
    ulnar (forearm level) S54.0-●
      arm (upper) (level) S44.0-●
      hand (level) S64.0-●
      wrist (level) —see Injury, nerve, ulnar, hand
    vagus S04.89-●
      specified type NEC S04.89-●
    wrist (level) —see Injury, nerve, hand
  ninth cranial nerve (glossopharyngeal) —see
      Injury, nerve, glossopharyngeal
  nose (septum) S09.92
  obstetrical O71.9
    specified NEC O71.89
  occipital (region) (scalp) S09.90
    lobe —see Injury, intracranial
  optic chiasm S04.02
  optic radiation S04.03-●
  optic tract and pathways S04.03-●
  orbit, orbital (region) —see Injury, eye
    penetrating (with foreign body) —see Injury,
        eye, orbit, penetrating
    specified NEC —see Injury, eye, specified site
        NEC
  ovary, ovarian S37.409
    bilateral S37.402
      contusion S37.422
      laceration S37.432
      specified type NEC S37.492
    blood vessel —see Injury, blood vessel, ovarian
    contusion S37.429
      bilateral S37.422
      unilateral S37.421
    laceration S37.439
      bilateral S37.432
      unilateral S37.431
    specified type NEC S37.499
      bilateral S37.492
      unilateral S37.491
    unilateral S37.401
      contusion S37.421
      laceration S37.431
      specified type NEC S37.491
  palate (hard) (soft) S09.93
  pancreas S36.209
    body S36.201
      contusion S36.221
      laceration S36.231
        major S36.261
        minor S36.241
        moderate S36.251
      specified type NEC S36.291
    contusion S36.229
    head S36.200
      contusion S36.220
      laceration S36.230
        major S36.260
        minor S36.240
        moderate S36.250
      specified type NEC S36.290
    laceration S36.239
      major S36.269
      minor S36.249
      moderate S36.259
    specified type NEC S36.299
    tail S36.202
      contusion S36.222
      laceration S36.232
        major S36.262
        minor S36.242
        moderate S36.252
      specified type NEC S36.292
  parietal (region) (scalp) S09.90
    lobe —see Injury, intracranial
  patellar ligament (tendon) S76.10-●
    laceration S76.12-●
    specified NEC S76.19-●
    strain S76.11-●
  pelvis, pelvic (floor) S39.93
    complicating delivery O70.1
    joint or ligament, complicating delivery O71.6
    organ S37.90
      with ectopic or molar pregnancy
          O08.6
      complication of abortion —see Abortion

Injury (Continued)
  pelvis, pelvic (Continued)
    organ (Continued)
      contusion S37.92
      following ectopic or molar pregnancy O08.6
      laceration S37.93
      obstetrical trauma NEC O71.5
      specified
        site NEC S37.899
          contusion S37.892
          laceration S37.893
          specified type NEC S37.898
        type NEC S37.99
    specified NEC S39.83
  penis S39.94
  perineum S39.94
  peritoneum S36.81
    laceration S36.893
  periurethral tissue —see Injury, urethra
    complicating delivery O71.82
  phalanges
    foot —see Injury, foot
    hand —see Injury, hand
  pharynx NEC S19.85
  pleura —see Injury, intrathoracic, pleura
  plexus
    brachial —see Injury, brachial plexus
    cardiac —see Injury, nerve, thorax,
        sympathetic
    celiac, coeliac —see Injury, nerve, lumbosacral,
        sympathetic
    esophageal —see Injury, nerve, thorax,
        sympathetic
    hypogastric —see Injury, nerve, lumbosacral,
        sympathetic
    lumbar, lumbosacral —see Injury, lumbosacral
        plexus
    mesenteric —see Injury, nerve, lumbosacral,
        sympathetic
    pulmonary —see Injury, nerve, thorax,
        sympathetic
  postcardiac surgery (syndrome) I97.0
  prepuce S39.94
  pressure
    injury —see Ulcer, pressure, by site
  prostate S37.829
    contusion S37.822
    laceration S37.823
    specified type NEC S37.828
  pubic region S39.94
  pudendum S39.94
  pulmonary plexus —see Injury, nerve, thorax,
      sympathetic
  rectovaginal septum NEC S39.83
  rectum —see Injury, intestine, large, rectum
  retina —see Injury, eye, specified site
      NEC
    penetrating —see Injury, eyeball, penetrating
  retroperitoneal —see Injury, intra-abdominal,
      specified site NEC
  rotator cuff (muscle(s)) (tendon(s)) S46.00-●
    laceration S46.02-●
    specified type NEC S46.09-●
    strain S46.01-●
  round ligament —see Injury, pelvic organ,
      specified site NEC
  sacral plexus —see Injury, lumbosacral
      plexus
  salivary duct or gland S09.93
  scalp S09.90
    newborn (birth injury) P12.9
      due to monitoring (electrode) (sampling
          incision) P12.4
      specified NEC P12.89
        caput succedaneum P12.81
  scapular region —see Injury, shoulder
  sclera —see Injury, eye, specified site NEC
    penetrating —see Injury, eyeball, penetrating
  scrotum S39.94
  second cranial nerve (optic) —see Injury, nerve,
      optic
  seminal vesicle —see Injury, pelvic organ,
      specified site NEC
  seventh cranial nerve (facial) —see Injury, nerve,
      facial
  shoulder S49.9-●
    blood vessel —see Injury, blood vessel,
        arm
    contusion —see Contusion, shoulder
    dislocation —see Dislocation, shoulder
    fracture —see Fracture, shoulder

Injury (Continued)
  shoulder (Continued)
    muscle —see Injury, muscle, shoulder
    nerve —see Injury, nerve, shoulder
    open —see Wound, open, shoulder
    specified type NEC S49.8-●
    sprain —see Sprain, shoulder girdle
    superficial —see Injury, superficial,
        shoulder
  sinus
    cavernous —see Injury, intracranial
    nasal S09.92
  sixth cranial nerve (abducent) —see Injury, nerve,
      abducens
  skeleton, birth injury P13.9
    specified part NEC P13.8
  skin NEC T14.8
    surface intact —see Injury, superficial
  skull NEC S09.90
  specified NEC T14.8
  spermatic cord (pelvic region) S37.898
    scrotal region S39.848
  spinal (cord)
    cervical (neck) S14.109
      anterior cord syndrome S14.139
        C1 level S14.131
        C2 level S14.132
        C3 level S14.133
        C4 level S14.134
        C5 level S14.135
        C6 level S14.136
        C7 level S14.137
        C8 level S14.138
      Brown-Séquard syndrome S14.149
        C1 level S14.141
        C2 level S14.142
        C3 level S14.143
        C4 level S14.144
        C5 level S14.145
        C6 level S14.146
        C7 level S14.147
        C8 level S14.148
      C1 level S14.101
      C2 level S14.102
      C3 level S14.103
      C4 level S14.104
      C5 level S14.105
      C6 level S14.106
      C7 level S14.107
      C8 level S14.108
      central cord syndrome
          S14.129
        C1 level S14.121
        C2 level S14.122
        C3 level S14.123
        C4 level S14.124
        C5 level S14.125
        C6 level S14.126
        C7 level S14.127
        C8 level S14.128
      complete lesion S14.119
        C1 level S14.111
        C2 level S14.112
        C3 level S14.113
        C4 level S14.114
        C5 level S14.115
        C6 level S14.116
        C7 level S14.117
        C8 level S14.118
      concussion S14.0
      edema S14.0
      incomplete lesion specified NEC
          S14.159
        C1 level S14.151
        C2 level S14.152
        C3 level S14.153
        C4 level S14.154
        C5 level S14.155
        C6 level S14.156
        C7 level S14.157
        C8 level S14.158
      posterior cord syndrome S14.159
        C1 level S14.151
        C2 level S14.152
        C3 level S14.153
        C4 level S14.154
        C5 level S14.155
        C6 level S14.156
        C7 level S14.157
        C8 level S14.158
    dorsal —see Injury, spinal, thoracic

Injury *(Continued)*
  spinal *(Continued)*
    lumbar S34.109
      complete lesion S34.119
        L1 level S34.111
        L2 level S34.112
        L3 level S34.113
        L4 level S34.114
        L5 level S34.115
      concussion S34.01
      edema S34.01
      incomplete lesion S34.129
        L1 level S34.121
        L2 level S34.122
        L3 level S34.123
        L4 level S34.124
        L5 level S34.125
      L1 level S34.101
      L2 level S34.102
      L3 level S34.103
      L4 level S34.104
      L5 level S34.105
    nerve root NEC
      cervical —*see* Injury, nerve, spinal, root,
        cervical
      dorsal —*see* Injury, nerve, spinal, root, dorsal
      lumbar S34.21
      sacral S34.22
      thoracic —*see* Injury, nerve, spinal, root,
        dorsal
    plexus
      brachial —*see* Injury, brachial
        plexus
      lumbosacral —*see* Injury, lumbosacral
        plexus
    sacral S34.139
      complete lesion S34.131
      incomplete lesion S34.132
    thoracic S24.109
      anterior cord syndrome S24.139
        T1 level S24.131
        T2-T6 level S24.132
        T7-T10 level S24.133
        T11-T12 level S24.134
      Brown-Séquard syndrome
        S24.149
        T1 level S24.141
        T2-T6 level S24.142
        T7-T10 level S24.143
        T11-T12 level S24.144
      complete lesion S24.119
        T1 level S24.111
        T2-T6 level S24.112
        T7-T10 level S24.113
        T11-T12 level S24.114
      concussion S24.0
      edema S24.0
      incomplete lesion specified NEC S24.159
        T1 level S24.151
        T2-T6 level S24.152
        T7-T10 level S24.153
        T11-T12 level S24.154
      posterior cord syndrome S24.159
        T1 level S24.151
        T2-T6 level S24.152
        T7-T10 level S24.153
        T11-T12 level S24.154
      T1 level S24.101
      T2-T6 level S24.102
      T7-T10 level S24.103
      T11-T12 level S24.104
  splanchnic nerve —*see* Injury, nerve,
    lumbosacral, sympathetic
  spleen S36.00
    contusion S36.029
      major S36.021
      minor S36.020
    laceration S36.039
      major (massive) (stellate) S36.032
      moderate S36.031
      superficial (capsular) (minor) S36.030
    specified type NEC S36.09
  splenic artery —*see* Injury, blood vessel, celiac
    artery, branch
  stellate ganglion —*see* Injury, nerve, thorax,
    sympathetic
  sternal region S29.9
  stomach S36.30
    contusion S36.32
    laceration S36.33
    specified type NEC S36.39

Injury *(Continued)*
  subconjunctival —*see* Injury, eye, conjunctiva
  subcutaneous NEC T14.8
  submaxillary region S09.93
  submental region S09.93
  subungual
    fingers —*see* Injury, hand
    toes —*see* Injury, foot
  superficial NEC T14.8
    abdomen, abdominal (wall) S30.92
      abrasion S30.811
      bite S30.871
        insect S30.861
      contusion S30.1
      external constriction S30.841
      foreign body S30.851
    abrasion —*see* Abrasion, by site
    adnexa, eye NEC —*see* Injury, eye, specified
      site NEC
    alveolar process —*see* Injury, superficial, oral
      cavity
    ankle S90.91-●
      abrasion —*see* Abrasion, ankle
      bite —*see* Bite, ankle
      blister —*see* Blister, ankle
      contusion —*see* Contusion, ankle
      external constriction —*see* Constriction,
        external, ankle
      foreign body —*see* Foreign body,
        superficial, ankle
    anus S30.98
    arm (upper) S40.92-●
      abrasion —*see* Abrasion, arm
      bite —*see* Bite, superficial, arm
      blister —*see* Blister, arm (upper)
      contusion —*see* Contusion, arm
      external constriction —*see* Constriction,
        external, arm
      foreign body —*see* Foreign body,
        superficial, arm
    auditory canal (external) (meatus) —*see* Injury,
      superficial, ear
    auricle —*see* Injury, superficial, ear
    axilla —*see* Injury, superficial, arm
    back —*see also* Injury, superficial, thorax, back
      lower S30.91
        abrasion S30.810
        contusion S30.0
        external constriction S30.840
        superficial
          bite NEC S30.870
            insect S30.860
          foreign body S30.850
    bite NEC —*see* Bite, superficial NEC, by site
    blister —*see* Blister, by site
    breast S20.10-●
      abrasion —*see* Abrasion, breast
      bite —*see* Bite, superficial, breast
      contusion —*see* Contusion, breast
      external constriction —*see* Constriction,
        external, breast
      foreign body —*see* Foreign body,
        superficial, breast
    brow —*see* Injury, superficial, head, specified
      NEC
    buttock S30.91
    calf —*see* Injury, superficial, leg
    canthus, eye —*see* Injury, superficial,
      periocular area
    cheek (external) —*see* Injury, superficial, head,
      specified NEC
      internal —*see* Injury, superficial, oral
        cavity
    chest wall —*see* Injury, superficial, thorax
    chin —*see* Injury, superficial, head NEC
    clitoris S30.95
    conjunctiva —*see* Injury, eye, conjunctiva
      with foreign body (in conjunctival sac) —*see*
        Foreign body, conjunctival sac
      contusion —*see* Contusion, by site
    costal region —*see* Injury, superficial, thorax
    digit(s)
      hand —*see* Injury, superficial, finger
    ear (auricle) (canal) (external) S00.40-●
      abrasion —*see* Abrasion, ear
      bite —*see* Bite, superficial, ear
      contusion —*see* Contusion, ear
      external constriction —*see* Constriction,
        external, ear
      foreign body —*see* Foreign body,
        superficial, ear

Injury *(Continued)*
  superficial *(Continued)*
    elbow S50.90-●
      abrasion —*see* Abrasion, elbow
      bite —*see* Bite, superficial, elbow
      blister —*see* Blister, elbow
      contusion —*see* Contusion, elbow
      external constriction —*see* Constriction,
        external, elbow
      foreign body —*see* Foreign body,
        superficial, elbow
    epididymis S30.94
    epigastric region S30.92
    epiglottis —*see* Injury, superficial, throat
    esophagus
      cervical —*see* Injury, superficial,
        throat
    external constriction —*see* Constriction,
      external, by site
    extremity NEC T14.8
    eyeball NEC —*see* Injury, eye, specified site
      NEC
    eyebrow —*see* Injury, superficial, periocular
      area
    eyelid S00.20-●
      abrasion —*see* Abrasion, eyelid
      bite —*see* Bite, superficial, eyelid
      contusion —*see* Contusion, eyelid
      external constriction —*see* Constriction,
        external, eyelid
      foreign body —*see* Foreign body,
        superficial, eyelid
    face NEC —*see* Injury, superficial, head,
      specified NEC
    finger(s) S60.949
      abrasion —*see* Abrasion, finger
      bite —*see* Bite, superficial, finger
      blister —*see* Blister, finger
      contusion —*see* Contusion, finger
      external constriction —*see* Constriction,
        external, finger
      foreign body —*see* Foreign body,
        superficial, finger
      index S60.94-●
      insect bite —*see* Bite, by site, superficial,
        insect
      little S60.94-●
      middle S60.94-●
      ring S60.94-●
    flank S30.92
    foot S90.92-●
      abrasion —*see* Abrasion, foot
      bite —*see* Bite, foot
      blister —*see* Blister, foot
      contusion —*see* Contusion, foot
      external constriction —*see* Constriction,
        external, foot
      foreign body —*see* Foreign body,
        superficial, foot
    forearm S50.91-●
      abrasion —*see* Abrasion, forearm
      bite —*see* Bite, forearm, superficial
      blister —*see* Blister, forearm
      contusion —*see* Contusion, forearm
      elbow only —*see* Injury, superficial, elbow
      external constriction —*see* Constriction,
        external, forearm
      foreign body —*see* Foreign body,
        superficial, forearm
    forehead —*see* Injury, superficial, head NEC
    foreign body —*see* Foreign body, superficial
    genital organs, external
      female S30.97
      male S30.96
    globe (eye) —*see* Injury, eye, specified site
      NEC
    groin S30.92
    gum —*see* Injury, superficial, oral
      cavity
    hand S60.92-●
      abrasion —*see* Abrasion, hand
      bite —*see* Bite, superficial, hand
      contusion —*see* Contusion, hand
      external constriction —*see* Constriction,
        external, hand
      foreign body —*see* Foreign body,
        superficial, hand
    head S00.90
      ear —*see* Injury, superficial, ear
      eyelid —*see* Injury, superficial, eyelid
      nose S00.30

Injury *(Continued)*
  superficial *(Continued)*
    head *(Continued)*
      oral cavity S00.502
      scalp S00.00
      specified site NEC S00.80
    heel —*see* Injury, superficial, foot
    hip S70.91-●
      abrasion —*see* Abrasion, hip
      bite —*see* Bite, superficial, hip
      blister —*see* Blister, hip
      contusion —*see* Contusion, hip
      external constriction —*see* Constriction, external, hip
      foreign body —*see* Foreign body, superficial, hip
    iliac region —*see* Injury, superficial, abdomen
    inguinal region —*see* Injury, superficial, abdomen
    insect bite —*see* Bite, by site, superficial, insect
    interscapular region —*see* Injury, superficial, thorax, back
    jaw —*see* Injury, superficial, head, specified NEC
    knee S80.91-●
      abrasion —*see* Abrasion, knee
      bite —*see* Bite, superficial, knee
      blister —*see* Blister, knee
      contusion —*see* Contusion, knee
      external constriction —*see* Constriction, external, knee
      foreign body —*see* Foreign body, superficial, knee
    labium (majus) (minus) S30.95
    lacrimal (apparatus) (gland) (sac) —*see* Injury, eye, specified site NEC
    larynx —*see* Injury, superficial, throat
    leg (lower) S80.92-●
      abrasion —*see* Abrasion, leg
      bite —*see* Bite, superficial, leg
      contusion —*see* Contusion, leg
      external constriction —*see* Constriction, external, leg
      foreign body —*see* Foreign body, superficial, leg
      knee —*see* Injury, superficial, knee
    limb NEC T14.8
    lip S00.501
    lower back S30.91
    lumbar region S30.91
    malar region —*see* Injury, superficial, head, specified NEC
    mammary —*see* Injury, superficial, breast
    mastoid region —*see* Injury, superficial, head, specified NEC
    mouth —*see* Injury, superficial, oral cavity
    muscle NEC T14.8
    nail NEC T14.8
      finger —*see* Injury, superficial, finger
      toe —*see* Injury, superficial, toe
    nasal (septum) —*see* Injury, superficial, nose
    neck S10.90
      specified site NEC S10.80
    nose (septum) S00.30
    occipital region —*see* Injury, superficial, scalp
    oral cavity S00.502
    orbital region —*see* Injury, superficial, periocular area
    palate —*see* Injury, superficial, oral cavity
    palm —*see* Injury, superficial, hand
    parietal region —*see* Injury, superficial, scalp
    pelvis S30.91
      girdle —*see* Injury, superficial, hip
    penis S30.93
    perineum
      female S30.95
      male S30.91
    periocular area S00.20-●
      abrasion —*see* Abrasion, eyelid
      bite —*see* Bite, superficial, eyelid
      contusion —*see* Contusion, eyelid
      external constriction —*see* Constriction, external, eyelid
      foreign body —*see* Foreign body, superficial, eyelid
    phalanges
      finger —*see* Injury, superficial, finger
      toe —*see* Injury, superficial, toe
    pharynx —*see* Injury, superficial, throat
    pinna —*see* Injury, superficial, ear

Injury *(Continued)*
  superficial *(Continued)*
    popliteal space —*see* Injury, superficial, knee
    prepuce S30.93
    pubic region S30.91
    pudendum
      female S30.97
      male S30.96
    sacral region S30.91
    scalp S00.00
    scapular region —*see* Injury, superficial, shoulder
    sclera —*see* Injury, eye, specified site NEC
    scrotum S30.94
    shin —*see* Injury, superficial, leg
    shoulder S40.91-●
      abrasion —*see* Abrasion, shoulder
      bite —*see* Bite, superficial, shoulder
      blister —*see* Blister, shoulder
      contusion —*see* Contusion, shoulder
      external constriction —*see* Constriction, external, shoulder
      foreign body —*see* Foreign body, superficial, shoulder
    skin NEC T14.8
    sternal region —*see* Injury, superficial, thorax, front
    subconjunctival —*see* Injury, eye, specified site NEC
    subcutaneous NEC T14.8
    submaxillary region —*see* Injury, superficial, head, specified NEC
    submental region —*see* Injury, superficial, head, specified NEC
    subungual
      finger(s) —*see* Injury, superficial, finger
      toe(s) —*see* Injury, superficial, toe
    supraclavicular fossa —*see* Injury, superficial, neck
    supraorbital —*see* Injury, superficial, head, specified NEC
    temple —*see* Injury, superficial, head, specified NEC
    temporal region —*see* Injury, superficial, head, specified NEC
    testis S30.94
    thigh S70.92-●
      abrasion —*see* Abrasion, thigh
      bite —*see* Bite, superficial, thigh
      blister —*see* Blister, thigh
      contusion —*see* Contusion, thigh
      external constriction —*see* Constriction, external, thigh
      foreign body —*see* Foreign body, superficial, thigh
    thorax, thoracic (wall) S20.90
      abrasion —*see* Abrasion, thorax
      back S20.40-●
      bite —*see* Bite, thorax, superficial
      blister —*see* Blister, thorax
      contusion —*see* Contusion, thorax
      external constriction —*see* Constriction, external, thorax
      foreign body —*see* Foreign body, superficial, thorax
      front S20.30-●
    throat S10.10
      abrasion S10.11
      bite S10.17
        insect S10.16
      blister S10.12
      contusion S10.0
      external constriction S10.14
      foreign body S10.15
    thumb S60.93-●
      abrasion —*see* Abrasion, thumb
      bite —*see* Bite, superficial, thumb
      blister —*see* Blister, thumb
      contusion —*see* Contusion, thumb
      external constriction —*see* Constriction, external, thumb
      foreign body —*see* Foreign body, superficial, thumb
      insect bite —*see* Bite, by site, superficial, insect
      specified type NEC S60.39-●
    toe(s) S90.93-●
      abrasion —*see* Abrasion, toe
      bite —*see* Bite, toe
      blister —*see* Blister, toe
      contusion —*see* Contusion, toe

Injury *(Continued)*
  superficial *(Continued)*
    toe(s) *(Continued)*
      external constriction —*see* Constriction, external, toe
      foreign body —*see* Foreign body, superficial, toe
      great S90.93-●
    tongue —*see* Injury, superficial, oral cavity
    tooth, teeth —*see* Injury, superficial, oral cavity
    trachea S10.10
    tunica vaginalis S30.94
    tympanum, tympanic membrane —*see* Injury, superficial, ear
    uvula —*see* Injury, superficial, oral cavity
    vagina S30.95
    vocal cords —*see* Injury, superficial, throat
    vulva S30.95
    wrist S60.91-●
  supraclavicular region —*see* Injury, neck
  supraorbital S09.93
  suprarenal gland (multiple) —*see* Injury, adrenal
  surgical complication (external or internal site) —*see* Laceration, accidental complicating surgery
  temple S09.90
  temporal region S09.90
  tendon —*see also* Injury, muscle, by site
    abdomen —*see* Injury, muscle, abdomen
    Achilles —*see* Injury, Achilles tendon
    lower back —*see* Injury, muscle, lower back
    pelvic organs —*see* Injury, muscle, pelvis
  tenth cranial nerve (pneumogastric or vagus) —*see* Injury, nerve, vagus
  testis S39.94
  thigh S79.92-●
    blood vessel —*see* Injury, blood vessel, hip
    contusion —*see* Contusion, thigh
    fracture —*see* Fracture, femur
    muscle —*see* Injury, muscle, thigh
    nerve —*see* Injury, nerve, thigh
    open —*see* Wound, open, thigh
    specified NEC S79.82-●
    superficial —*see* Injury, superficial, thigh
  third cranial nerve (oculomotor) —*see* Injury, nerve, oculomotor
  thorax, thoracic S29.9
    blood vessel —*see* Injury, blood vessel, thorax
    cavity —*see* Injury, intrathoracic
    dislocation —*see* Dislocation, thorax
    external (wall) S29.9
      contusion —*see* Contusion, thorax
      nerve —*see* Injury, nerve, thorax
      open —*see* Wound, open, thorax
      specified NEC S29.8
      sprain —*see* Sprain, thorax
      superficial —*see* Injury, superficial, thorax
    fracture —*see* Fracture, thorax
    internal —*see* Injury, intrathoracic
    intrathoracic organ —*see* Injury, intrathoracic
    sympathetic ganglion —*see* Injury, nerve, thorax, sympathetic
  throat —*see also* Injury, neck S19.9
  thumb S69.9-●
    blood vessel —*see* Injury, blood vessel, thumb
    contusion —*see* Contusion, thumb
    dislocation —*see* Dislocation, thumb
    fracture —*see* Fracture, thumb
    muscle —*see* Injury, muscle, thumb
    nerve —*see* Injury, nerve, digital, thumb
    open —*see* Wound, open, thumb
    specified NEC S69.8-●
    sprain —*see* Sprain, thumb
    superficial —*see* Injury, superficial, thumb
  thymus (gland) —*see* Injury, intrathoracic, specified organ NEC
  thyroid (gland) NEC S19.84
  toe S99.92-●
    contusion —*see* Contusion, toe
    dislocation —*see* Dislocation, toe
    fracture —*see* Fracture, toe
    muscle —*see* Injury, muscle, toe
    open —*see* Wound, open, toe
    specified type NEC S99.82-●
    sprain —*see* Sprain, toe
    superficial —*see* Injury, superficial, toe
  tongue S09.93
  tonsil S09.93
  tooth S09.93

▶ New   ⇒ Revised   ~~deleted~~ Deleted   ● Use Additional Character(s)

Injury (Continued)
  trachea (cervical) NEC S19.82
    thoracic —see Injury, intrathoracic, trachea,
      thoracic
  transfusion-related acute lung (TRALI)
    J95.84
  tunica vaginalis S39.94
  twelfth cranial nerve (hypoglossal) —see Injury,
    nerve, hypoglossal
  ureter S37.10
    contusion S37.12
    laceration S37.13
    specified type NEC S37.19
  urethra (sphincter) S37.30
    at delivery O71.5
    contusion S37.32
    laceration S37.33
    specified type NEC S37.38
  urinary organ S37.899
    contusion S37.92
    laceration S37.93
    specified
      site NEC S37.899
        contusion S37.892
        laceration S37.893
        specified type NEC S37.898
      type NEC S37.99
  uterus, uterine S37.60
    with ectopic or molar pregnancy O08.6
    blood vessel —see Injury, blood vessel, iliac
    contusion S37.62
    laceration S37.63
      cervix at delivery O71.3
    rupture associated with obstetrics —see
      Rupture, uterus
    specified type NEC S37.69
  uvula S09.93
  vagina S39.93
    abrasion S30.814
    bite S31.45
      insect S30.864
      superficial NEC S30.874
    contusion S30.23
    crush S38.03
    during delivery —see Laceration, vagina,
      during delivery
    external constriction S30.844
    insect bite S30.864
    laceration S31.41
      with foreign body S31.42
    open wound S31.40
    puncture S31.43
      with foreign body S31.44
    superficial S30.95
      foreign body S30.854
  vas deferens —see Injury, pelvic organ, specified
    site NEC
  vascular NEC T14.8
  vein —see Injury, blood vessel
  vena cava (superior) S25.20
    inferior S35.10
      laceration (minor) (superficial) S35.11
        major S35.12
      specified type NEC S35.19
    laceration (minor) (superficial) S25.21
      major S25.22
    specified type NEC S25.29
  vesical (sphincter) —see Injury, bladder
  visual cortex S04.04-●
  vitreous (humor) S05.90
    specified NEC S05.8X-●
  vocal cord NEC S19.83
  vulva S39.94
    abrasion S30.814
    bite S31.45
      insect S30.864
      superficial NEC S30.874
    contusion S30.23
    crush S38.03
    during delivery —see Laceration, perineum,
      female, during delivery
    external constriction S30.844
    insect bite S30.864
    laceration S31.41
      with foreign body S31.42
    open wound S31.40
    puncture S31.43
      with foreign body S31.44
    superficial S30.95
      foreign body S30.854
  whiplash (cervical spine) S13.4

Injury (Continued)
  wrist S69.9-●
    blood vessel —see Injury, blood vessel,
      hand
    contusion —see Contusion, wrist
    dislocation —see Dislocation, wrist
    fracture —see Fracture, wrist
    muscle —see Injury, muscle, hand
    nerve —see Injury, nerve, hand
    open —see Wound, open, wrist
    specified NEC S69.8-●
    sprain —see Sprain, wrist
    superficial —see Injury, superficial, wrist
Inoculation —see also Vaccination
  complication or reaction —see Complications,
    vaccination
Insanity, insane —see also Psychosis
  adolescent —see Schizophrenia
  confusional F28
    acute or subacute F05
  delusional F22
  senile F03
Insect
  bite —see Bite, by site, superficial, insect
  venomous, poisoning NEC (by) —see Venom,
    arthropod
Insecurity
  financial Z59.86
  food Z59.41
  transportation Z59.82
Insensitivity
  adrenocorticotropin hormone (ACTH) E27.49
  androgen E34.50
    complete E34.51
    partial E34.52
Insertion
  cord (umbilical) lateral or velamentous
    O43.12-●
  intrauterine contraceptive device (encounter
    for) —see Intrauterine contraceptive
    device
Insolation (sunstroke) T67.01
Insomnia (organic) G47.00
  without objective findings F51.02
  adjustment F51.02
  adjustment disorder F51.02
  behavioral, of childhood Z73.819
    combined type Z73.812
    limit setting type Z73.811
    sleep-onset association type Z73.810
  childhood Z73.819
  chronic F51.04
    somatized tension F51.04
  conditioned F51.04
  due to
    alcohol
      abuse F10.182
      dependence F10.282
      use F10.982
    amphetamines
      abuse F15.182
      dependence F15.282
      use F15.982
    anxiety disorder F51.05
    caffeine
      abuse F15.182
      dependence F15.282
      use F15.982
    cocaine
      abuse F14.182
      dependence F14.282
      use F14.982
    depression F51.05
    drug NEC
      abuse F19.182
      dependence F19.282
      use F19.982
    medical condition G47.01
    mental disorder NEC F51.05
    opioid
      abuse F11.182
      dependence F11.282
      use F11.982
    psychoactive substance NEC
      abuse F19.182
      dependence F19.282
      use F19.982
    sedative, hypnotic, or anxiolytic
      abuse F13.182
      dependence F13.282
      use F13.982

Insomnia (Continued)
  due to (Continued)
    stimulant NEC
      abuse F15.182
      dependence F15.282
      use F15.982
  fatal familial (FFI) A81.83
  idiopathic F51.01
  learned F51.3
  nonorganic origin F51.01
  not due to a substance or known physiological
    condition F51.01
    specified NEC F51.09
  paradoxical F51.03
  primary F51.01
  psychiatric F51.05
  psychophysiologic F51.04
  related to psychopathology F51.05
  short-term F51.02
  specified NEC G47.09
  stress-related F51.02
  transient F51.02
Inspiration
  food or foreign body —see Foreign body, by site
  mucus —see Asphyxia, mucus
Inspissated bile syndrome (newborn) P59.1
Instability
  emotional (excessive) F60.3
  housing
    housed Z59.819
      with risk of homelessness Z59.811
      homelessness in past 12 months Z59.812
  joint (post-traumatic) M25.30
    ankle M25.37-●
    due to old ligament injury —see Disorder,
      ligament
    elbow M25.32-●
    flail —see Flail, joint
    foot M25.37-●
    hand M25.34-●
    hip M25.35-●
    knee M25.36-●
    lumbosacral —see subcategory M53.2
    prosthesis —see Complications, joint
      prosthesis, mechanical, displacement,
      by site
    sacroiliac —see subcategory M53.2
    secondary to
      old ligament injury —see Disorder,
        ligament
      removal of joint prosthesis M96.89
    shoulder (region) M25.31-●
    specified site NEC M25.39
    spine —see subcategory M53.2
    wrist M25.33-●
  knee (chronic) M23.5-●
  lumbosacral —see subcategory M53.2
  nervous F48.8
  personality (emotional) F60.3
  spine —see Instability, joint, spine
  vasomotor R55
Institutional syndrome (childhood) F94.2
Institutionalization, affecting child Z62.22
  disinhibited attachment F94.2
Insufficiency, insufficient
  accommodation, old age H52.4
  adrenal (gland) E27.40
    primary E27.1
  adrenocortical E27.40
    drug-induced E27.3
    iatrogenic E27.3
    primary E27.1
  anatomic crown height K08.89
  anterior (occlusal) guidance M26.54
  anus K62.89
  aortic (valve) I35.1
    with
      mitral (valve) disease I08.0
        with tricuspid (valve) disease I08.3
      stenosis I35.2
      tricuspid (valve) disease I08.2
        with mitral (valve) disease I08.3
    congenital Q23.1
    rheumatic I06.1
      with
        mitral (valve) disease I08.0
          with tricuspid (valve) disease I08.3
        stenosis I06.2
          with mitral (valve) disease I08.0
            with tricuspid (valve) disease
              I08.3

Insufficiency, insufficient (Continued)
aortic (Continued)
rheumatic (Continued)
with (Continued)
tricuspid (valve) disease I08.2
with mitral (valve) disease I08.3
specified cause NEC I35.1
syphilitic A52.03
arterial I77.1
basilar G45.0
carotid (hemispheric) G45.1
cerebral I67.81
coronary (acute or subacute) I24.89
mesenteric K55.1
peripheral I73.9
precerebral (multiple) (bilateral) G45.2
vertebral G45.0
arteriovenous I99.8
biliary K83.8
cardiac —see also Insufficiency, myocardial
due to presence of (cardiac) prosthesis
I97.11-●
postprocedural I97.11-●
cardiorenal, hypertensive I13.2
cardiovascular —see Disease, cardiovascular
cerebrovascular (acute) I67.81
with transient focal neurological signs and
symptoms G45.8
circulatory NEC I99.8
newborn P29.89
clinical crown length K08.89
convergence H51.11
coronary (acute or subacute) I24.89
chronic or with a stated duration of over 4
weeks I25.89
corticoadrenal E27.40
primary E27.1
dietary E63.9
divergence H51.8
food T73.0
gastroesophageal K22.89
gonadal
ovary E28.39
testis E29.1
▶ health insurance coverage Z59.71
heart —see also Insufficiency, myocardial
newborn P29.0
valve —see Endocarditis
hepatic —see Failure, hepatic
idiopathic autonomic G90.09
interocclusal distance of fully erupted teeth
(ridge) M26.36
kidney N28.9
acute N28.9
chronic N18.9
lacrimal (secretion) H04.12-●
passages —see Stenosis, lacrimal
liver —see Failure, hepatic
lung —see Insufficiency, pulmonary
mental (congenital) —see Disability,
intellectual
mesenteric K55.1
mitral (valve) I34.0
with
aortic valve disease I08.0
with tricuspid (valve) disease
I08.3
obstruction or stenosis I05.2
with aortic valve disease I08.0
tricuspid (valve) disease I08.1
with aortic (valve) disease I08.3
congenital Q23.3
rheumatic I05.1
with
aortic valve disease I08.0
with tricuspid (valve) disease I08.3
obstruction or stenosis I05.2
with aortic valve disease I08.0
with tricuspid (valve) disease I08.3
tricuspid (valve) disease I08.1
with aortic (valve) disease I08.3
active or acute I01.1
with chorea, rheumatic (Sydenham's)
I02.0
specified cause, except rheumatic I34.0
muscle —see also Disease, muscle
heart —see Insufficiency, myocardial
ocular NEC H50.9
myocardial, myocardium (with
arteriosclerosis) —see also Failure,
heart I50.9

Insufficiency, insufficient (Continued)
myocardial, myocardium (Continued)
with
rheumatic fever (conditions in I00) I09.0
active, acute or subacute I01.2
with chorea I02.0
chronic I09.0
inactive or quiescent (with chorea) I09.0
congenital Q24.8
hypertensive —see Hypertension, heart
newborn P29.0
rheumatic I09.0
active, acute, or subacute I01.2
syphilitic A52.06
nourishment (see also Nutrition deficient) T73.0
pancreatic K86.89
exocrine K86.81
parathyroid (gland) E20.9
peripheral vascular (arterial) I73.9
pituitary E23.0
placental (mother) O36.51-●
platelets D69.6
prenatal care affecting management of
pregnancy O09.3-●
progressive pluriglandular E31.0
pulmonary J98.4
acute, following surgery (nonthoracic) J95.2
thoracic J95.1
chronic, following surgery J95.3
following
shock J98.4
trauma J98.4
newborn P28.89
valve I37.1
with stenosis I37.2
congenital Q22.2
rheumatic I09.89
with aortic, mitral or tricuspid (valve)
disease I08.8
pyloric K31.89
renal (acute) N28.9
chronic N18.9
respiratory R06.89
newborn P28.5
rotation —see Malrotation
sleep syndrome F51.12
▶ social insurance Z59.71
suprarenal E27.40
primary E27.1
tarso-orbital fascia, congenital Q10.3
testis E29.1
thyroid (gland) (acquired) E03.9
congenital E03.1
tricuspid (valve) (rheumatic) I07.1
with
aortic (valve) disease I08.2
with mitral (valve) disease I08.3
mitral (valve) disease I08.1
with aortic (valve) disease I08.3
obstruction or stenosis I07.2
with aortic (valve) disease I08.2
with mitral (valve) disease I08.3
congenital Q22.8
nonrheumatic I36.1
with stenosis I36.2
urethral sphincter R32
valve, valvular (heart) I38
aortic —see Insufficiency, aortic (valve)
mitral —see Insufficiency, mitral (valve)
pulmonary —see Insufficiency, pulmonary, valve
tricuspid —see Insufficiency, tricuspid (valve)
congenital Q24.8
vascular I99.8
intestine K55.9
acute —see also Ischemia, intestine, acute
K55.059
mesenteric K55.1
peripheral I73.9
renal —see Hypertension, kidney
velopharyngeal
acquired K13.79
congenital Q38.8
venous (chronic) (peripheral) I87.2
ventricular —see Insufficiency, myocardial
▶ welfare support Z59.72
Insufflation, fallopian Z31.41
Insular —see condition
Insulinoma
pancreas
benign D13.7
malignant C25.4
uncertain behavior D37.8

Insulinoma (Continued)
specified site
benign —see Neoplasm, by site, benign
malignant —see Neoplasm, by site, malignant
uncertain behavior —see Neoplasm, by site,
uncertain behavior
unspecified site
benign D13.7
malignant C25.4
uncertain behavior D37.8
Insuloma —see Insulinoma
Interference
balancing side M26.56
non-working side M26.56
Intermenstrual —see condition
Intermittent —see condition
Internal —see condition
Interrogation
cardiac defibrillator (automatic) (implantable)
Z45.02
cardiac pacemaker Z45.018
cardiac (event) (loop) recorder Z45.09
infusion pump (implanted) (intrathecal) Z45.1
neurostimulator Z46.2
Interruption
aortic arch Q25.21
phase-shift, sleep cycle —see Disorder, sleep,
circadian rhythm
sleep phase-shift, or 24 hour sleep-wake cycle —
see Disorder, sleep, circadian rhythm
Interstitial —see condition
Intertrigo L30.4
labialis K13.0
Intervertebral disc —see condition
Intestine, intestinal —see condition
Intolerance
carbohydrate K90.49
disaccharide, hereditary E73.0
fat NEC K90.49
pancreatic K90.3
food K90.49
dietary counseling and surveillance Z71.3
fructose E74.10
hereditary E74.12
glucose(-galactose) E74.39
gluten K90.01
lactose E73.9
specified NEC E73.8
lysine E72.3
milk NEC K90.49
lactose E73.9
orthostatic, chronic G90.A
protein K90.49
starch NEC K90.49
sucrose (-isomaltose) E74.31
Intoxicated NEC (without dependence) —see
Alcohol, intoxication
Intoxication
acid (see also Acidosis) E87.29
alcoholic (acute) (without dependence) —see
Alcohol, intoxication
alimentary canal K52.1
amphetamine (without dependence) —see also
Abuse, drug, stimulant, with intoxication
stimulant NEC F15.10
with
anxiety disorder F15.180
intoxication F15.129
with
delirium F15.121
perceptual disturbance F15.122
with dependence —see Dependence, drug,
stimulant, with intoxication
anxiolytic (acute) (without dependence) —see
Abuse, drug, sedative, with intoxication
with dependence —see Dependence, drug,
sedative, with intoxication
caffeine F15.929
with dependence —see Dependence, drug,
stimulant, with intoxication
cannabinoids (acute) (without dependence) —see
Use, cannabis, with intoxication
with
abuse —see Abuse, drug, cannabis, with
intoxication
dependence —see Dependence, drug,
cannabis, with intoxication
chemical —see Table of Drugs and
Chemicals
via placenta or breast milk —see Absorption,
chemical, through placenta

▶ New   ⟹ Revised   ~~deleted~~ Deleted   ● Use Additional Character(s)

Irritable, irritability R45.4
  bladder N32.89
  bowel (syndrome) K58.9
    with
      constipation K58.1
      diarrhea K58.0
    mixed K58.2
    psychogenic F45.8
    specified NEC K58.8
  bronchial —see Bronchitis
  cerebral, in newborn P91.3
  colon —see also Irritable, bowel K58.9
    with diarrhea K58.0
    psychogenic F45.8
  duodenum K59.89
  heart (psychogenic) F45.8
  hip —see Derangement, joint, specified type
      NEC, hip
  ileum K59.89
  infant R68.12
  jejunum K59.89
  rectum K59.89
  stomach K31.89
    psychogenic F45.8
  sympathetic G90.89
  urethra N36.8
  without diarrhea K58.9
Irritation
  anus K62.89
  axillary nerve G54.0
  bladder N32.89
  brachial plexus G54.0
  bronchial —see Bronchitis
  cervical plexus G54.2
  cervix —see Cervicitis
  choroid, sympathetic —see Endophthalmitis
  cranial nerve —see Disorder, nerve, cranial
  gastric K31.89
    psychogenic F45.8
  globe, sympathetic —see Uveitis, sympathetic
  labyrinth —see subcategory H83.2
  lumbosacral plexus G54.1
  meninges (traumatic) —see Injury, intracranial
    nontraumatic —see Meningismus
  nerve —see Disorder, nerve
  nervous R45.0
  penis N48.89
  perineum NEC L29.3
  peripheral autonomic nervous system
      G90.89
  peritoneum —see Peritonitis
  pharynx J39.2
  plantar nerve —see Lesion, nerve, plantar
  spinal (cord) (traumatic) —see also Injury, spinal
      cord, by region
    nerve G58.9
      root NEC —see Radiculopathy
    nontraumatic —see Myelopathy
  stomach K31.89
    psychogenic F45.8
  sympathetic nerve NEC G90.89
  ulnar nerve —see Lesion, nerve, ulnar
  vagina N89.8
Ischemia, ischemic I99.8
  bowel (transient)
    acute —see also Ischemia, intestine, acute
        K55.059
    chronic K55.1
    due to mesenteric artery insufficiency K55.1
  brain —see Ischemia, cerebral
  cardiac (see Disease, heart, ischemic)
  cardiomyopathy I25.5
  cerebral (chronic) (generalized) I67.82
    arteriosclerotic I67.2
    intermittent G45.9
    newborn P91.0
    recurrent focal G45.8
    transient G45.9
  colon chronic (due to mesenteric artery
      insufficiency) K55.1
  coronary —see Disease, heart, ischemic
  demand (coronary) —see also Angina I24.89
    with myocardial infarction I21.A1
    resulting in myocardial infarction I21.A1
  heart (chronic or with a stated duration of over 4
      weeks) I25.9
    acute or with a stated duration of 4 weeks or
        less I24.9
    subacute I24.9

Ischemia, ischemic (Continued)
  infarction, muscle —see Infarct, muscle
  intestine (large) (small) (transient) K55.9
    acute K55.059
      diffuse K55.052
      focal K55.051
      large K55.039
        diffuse K55.032
        focal K55.031
      small K55.019
        diffuse K55.012
        focal K55.011
    chronic K55.1
    due to mesenteric artery insufficiency
        K55.1
  IST (inappropriate sinus tachycardia, so stated)
      I47.11
  kidney N28.0
  limb, critical —see Arteriosclerosis, with critical
      limb ischemia
  limb-threatening, chronic —see Arteriosclerosis,
      with critical limb ischemia
  mesenteric, acute —see also Ischemia, intestine,
      acute K55.059
  muscle, traumatic T79.6
  myocardium, myocardial (chronic or with
      a stated duration of over 4 weeks)
      I25.9
    acute, without myocardial infarction
        I51.3
    silent (asymptomatic) I25.6
    transient of newborn P29.4
  renal N28.0
  retina, retinal —see Occlusion, artery,
      retina
  small bowel
    acute K55.019
      diffuse K55.012
      focal K55.011
    chronic K55.1
    due to mesenteric artery insufficiency
        K55.1
  spinal cord G95.11
  subendocardial —see Insufficiency,
      coronary
  supply (coronary) —see also Angina
      I25.9
    due to vasospasm I20.1
Ischial spine —see condition
Ischialgia —see Sciatica
Ischiopagus Q89.4
Ischium, ischial —see condition
Ischuria R34
Iselin's disease or osteochondrosis —see
    Osteochondrosis, juvenile,
    metatarsus
Islands of
  parotid tissue in
    lymph nodes Q38.6
    neck structures Q38.6
  submaxillary glands in
    fascia Q38.6
    lymph nodes Q38.6
    neck muscles Q38.6
Islet cell tumor, pancreas D13.7
Isoimmunization NEC —see also Incompatibility
    affecting management of pregnancy (ABO) (with
        hydrops fetalis) O36.11-●
      anti-A sensitization O36.11-●
      anti-B sensitization O36.19-●
      anti-c sensitization O36.09-●
      anti-C sensitization O36.09-●
      anti-e sensitization O36.09-●
      anti-E sensitization O36.09-●
      Rh NEC O36.09-●
        anti-D antibody O36.01-●
      specified NEC O36.19-●
    newborn P55.9
      with
        hydrops fetalis P56.0
        kernicterus P57.0
      ABO (blood groups) P55.1
      Rhesus (Rh) factor P55.0
      specified type NEC P55.8
Isolation, isolated
  dwelling Z59.89
  family Z63.79
  social Z60.4
Isoleucinosis E71.19

Isomerism atrial appendages (with asplenia or
    polysplenia) Q20.6
Isosporiasis, isosporosis A07.3
Isovaleric acidemia E71.110
Issue of
  medical certificate Z02.79
    for disability determination Z02.71
  repeat prescription (appliance) (glasses)
      (medicinal substance, medicament,
      medicine) Z76.0
    contraception —see Contraception
Itch, itching —see also Pruritus
  baker's L23.6
  barber's B35.0
  bricklayer's L24.5
  cheese B88.0
  clam digger's B65.3
  coolie B76.9
  copra B88.0
  dew B76.9
  dhobi B35.6
  filarial —see Infestation, filarial
  grain B88.0
  grocer's B88.0
  ground B76.9
  harvest B88.0
  jock B35.6
  Malabar B35.5
    beard B35.0
    foot B35.3
    scalp B35.0
  meaning scabies B86
  Norwegian B86
  perianal L29.0
  poultrymen's B88.0
  sarcoptic B86
  scabies B86
  scrub B88.0
  straw B88.0
  swimmer's B65.3
  water B76.9
  winter L29.89
Ivemark's syndrome (asplenia with congenital
    heart disease) Q89.01
Ivory bones Q78.2
Ixodiasis NEC B88.8

J

Jaccoud's syndrome —see Arthropathy,
    postrheumatic, chronic
Jackson's
  membrane Q43.3
  paralysis or syndrome G83.89
  veil Q43.3
Jacquet's dermatitis (diaper dermatitis) L22
Jadassohn-Pellizari's disease or anetoderma
    L90.2
Jadassohn's
  blue nevus —see Nevus
  intraepidermal epithelioma —see Neoplasm,
      skin, benign
Jaffe-Lichtenstein (-Uehlinger) syndrome —see
    Dysplasia, fibrous, bone NEC
Jakob-Creutzfeldt disease or syndrome —see
    Creutzfeldt-Jakob disease or syndrome
Jaksch-Luzet disease D64.89
Jamaican
  neuropathy G92.8
  paraplegic tropical ataxic-spastic syndrome
      G92.8
Janet's disease F48.8
Janiceps Q89.4
Jansky-Bielschowsky amaurotic idiocy
    E75.4
Japanese
  B-type encephalitis A83.0
  river fever A75.3
Jaundice (yellow) R17
  acholuric (familial) (splenomegalic) —see also
      Spherocytosis
    acquired D59.8
  breast-milk (inhibitor) P59.3
  catarrhal (acute) B15.9
    with hepatic coma B15.0
  cholestatic (benign) R17

▶ New   ⇒ Revised   ~~deleted~~ Deleted   ● Use Additional Character(s)

Jaundice *(Continued)*
  due to or associated with
    delayed conjugation P59.8
      associated with (due to) preterm delivery P59.0
      preterm delivery P59.0
    epidemic (catarrhal) B15.9
      with hepatic coma B15.0
      leptospiral A27.0
      spirochetal A27.0
    familial nonhemolytic (congenital) (Gilbert) E80.4
      Crigler-Najjar E80.5
    febrile (acute) B15.9
      with hepatic coma B15.0
      leptospiral A27.0
      spirochetal A27.0
    hematogenous D59.9
    hemolytic (acquired) D59.9
      congenital —*see* Spherocytosis
    hemorrhagic (acute) (leptospiral) (spirochetal) A27.0
    infectious (acute) (subacute) B15.9
      with hepatic coma B15.0
      leptospiral A27.0
      spirochetal A27.0
    leptospiral (hemorrhagic) A27.0
    malignant (without coma) K72.90
      with coma K72.91
    neonatal —*see* Jaundice, newborn
    newborn P59.9
      due to or associated with
        ABO
          antibodies P55.1
          incompatibility, maternal/fetal P55.1
          isoimmunization P55.1
        absence or deficiency of enzyme system for bilirubin conjugation (congenital) P59.8
        bleeding P58.1
        breast milk inhibitors to conjugation P59.3
          associated with preterm delivery P59.0
        bruising P58.0
        Crigler-Najjar syndrome E80.5
        delayed conjugation P59.8
          associated with preterm delivery P59.0
        drugs or toxins
          given to newborn P58.42
          transmitted from mother P58.41
        excessive hemolysis P58.9
          due to
            bleeding P58.1
            bruising P58.0
            drugs or toxins
              given to newborn P58.42
              transmitted from mother P58.41
            infection P58.2
            polycythemia P58.3
            swallowed maternal blood P58.5
          specified type NEC P58.8
        galactosemia E74.21
        Gilbert syndrome E80.4
        hemolytic disease P55.9
          ABO isoimmunization P55.1
          Rh isoimmunization P55.0
          specified NEC P55.8
        hepatocellular damage P59.20
          specified NEC P59.29
        hereditary hemolytic anemia P58.8
        hypothyroidism, congenital E03.1
        incompatibility, maternal/fetal NOS P55.9
        infection P58.2
        inspissated bile syndrome P59.1
        isoimmunization NOS P55.9
        mucoviscidosis E84.9
        polycythemia P58.3
        preterm delivery P59.0
        Rh
          antibodies P55.0
          incompatibility, maternal/fetal P55.0
          isoimmunization P55.0
        specified cause NEC P59.8
        swallowed maternal blood P58.5
        spherocytosis (congenital) D58.0
      nonhemolytic congenital familial (Gilbert) E80.4
    nuclear, newborn —*see also* Kernicterus of newborn P57.9

Jaundice *(Continued)*
  obstructive —*see also* Obstruction, bile duct K83.1
  post-immunization —*see* Hepatitis, viral, type, B
  post-transfusion —*see* Hepatitis, viral, type, B
  regurgitation —*see also* Obstruction, bile duct K83.1
  serum (homologous) (prophylactic) (therapeutic) —*see* Hepatitis, viral, type, B
  spirochetal (hemorrhagic) A27.0
  symptomatic R17
    newborn P59.9
Jaw —*see* condition
Jaw-winking phenomenon or syndrome Q07.8
Jealousy
  alcoholic F10.988
  childhood F93.8
  sibling F93.8
Jejunitis —*see* Enteritis
Jejunostomy status Z93.4
Jejunum, jejunal —*see* condition
Jensen's disease —*see* Inflammation, chorioretinal, focal, juxtapapillary
Jerks, myoclonic G25.3
Jervell-Lange-Nielsen syndrome I45.81
Jeune's disease Q77.2
Jigger disease B88.1
Job's syndrome (chronic granulomatous disease) D71
Joint —*see also* condition
  mice —*see* Loose, body, joint
    knee M23.4-•
Jordan's anomaly or syndrome D72.0
Joseph-Diamond-Blackfan anemia (congenital hypoplastic) D61.01
Jungle yellow fever A95.0
Jüngling's disease —*see* Sarcoidosis
Juvenile —*see* condition

K

Kahler's disease C90.0-•
Kakke E51.11
Kala-azar B55.0
Kallmann's syndrome E23.0
Kanner's syndrome (autism) —*see* Psychosis, childhood
Kaposi's
  dermatosis (xeroderma pigmentosum) Q82.1
  lichen ruber L44.0
    acuminatus L44.0
  sarcoma
    colon C46.4
    connective tissue C46.1
    gastrointestinal organ C46.4
    lung C46.5-•
    lymph node (multiple) C46.3
    palate (hard) (soft) C46.2
    rectum C46.4
    skin (multiple sites) C46.0
    specified site NEC C46.7
    stomach C46.4
    unspecified site C46.9
  varicelliform eruption B00.0
    vaccinia T88.1
Kartagener's syndrome or triad (sinusitis, bronchiectasis, situs inversus) Q89.3
Karyotype
  with abnormality except iso (Xq) Q96.2
  45,X Q96.0
  46,X
    iso (Xq) Q96.1
  46,XX Q98.3
    with streak gonads Q50.32
    hermaphrodite (true) Q99.1
    male Q98.3
  46,XY
    with streak gonads Q56.1
    female Q97.3
    hermaphrodite (true) Q99.1
  47,XXX Q97.0
  47,XXY Q98.0
  47,XYY Q98.5

Kaschin-Beck disease —*see* Disease, Kaschin-Beck
Katayama's disease or fever B65.2
Kawasaki's syndrome M30.3
Kayser-Fleischer ring (cornea) (pseudosclerosis) H18.04-•
Kaznelson's syndrome (congenital hypoplastic anemia) D61.01
Kearns-Sayre syndrome H49.81-•
Kedani fever A75.3
Kelis L91.0
Kelly (-Patterson) syndrome (sideropenic dysphagia) D50.1
Keloid, cheloid L91.0
  acne L73.0
  Addison's L94.0
  cornea —*see* Opacity, cornea
  Hawkin's L91.0
  scar L91.0
Keloma L91.0
Kenya fever A77.1
Keratectasia —*see also* Ectasia, cornea
  congenital Q13.4
Keratinization of alveolar ridge mucosa
  excessive K13.23
  minimal K13.22
Keratinized residual ridge mucosa
  excessive K13.23
  minimal K13.22
Keratitis (nodular) (nonulcerative) (simple) (zonular) H16.9
  with ulceration (central) (marginal) (perforated) (ring) —*see* Ulcer, cornea
  actinic —*see* Photokeratitis
  arborescens (herpes simplex) B00.52
  areolar H16.11-•
  bullosa H16.8
  deep H16.309
    specified type NEC H16.399
  dendritic (a) (herpes simplex) B00.52
  disciform (is) (herpes simplex) B00.52
    varicella B01.81
  filamentary H16.12-•
  gonococcal (congenital or prenatal) A54.33
  herpes, herpetic (simplex) B00.52
    zoster B02.33
  in (due to)
    acanthamebiasis B60.13
    adenovirus B30.0
    exanthema —*see also* Exanthem B09
    herpes (simplex) virus B00.52
    measles B05.81
    syphilis A50.31
    tuberculosis A18.52
    zoster B02.33
  interstitial (nonsyphilitic) H16.30-•
    diffuse H16.32-•
    herpes, herpetic (simplex) B00.52
      zoster B02.33
    sclerosing H16.33-•
    specified type NEC H16.39-•
    syphilitic (congenital) (late) A50.31
    tuberculous A18.52
  macular H16.11-•
  nummular H16.11-•
  oyster shuckers' H16.8
  parenchymatous —*see* Keratitis, interstitial
  petrificans H16.8
  postmeasles B05.81
  punctata
    leprosa A30.9 *[H16.14-•]*
    syphilitic (profunda) A50.31
  punctate H16.14-•
  purulent H16.8
  rosacea L71.8
  sclerosing H16.33-•
  specified type NEC H16.8
  stellate H16.11-•
  striate H16.11-•
  superficial H16.10-•
    with conjunctivitis —*see* Keratoconjunctivitis
    due to light —*see* Photokeratitis
  suppurative H16.8
  syphilitic (congenital) (prenatal) A50.31
  trachomatous A71.1
    sequelae B94.0
  tuberculous A18.52
  vesicular H16.8
  xerotic —*see also* Keratomalacia H16.8
    vitamin A deficiency E50.4

Keratoacanthoma L85.8
Keratocele —see Descemetocele
Keratoconjunctivitis H16.20-●
　Acanthamoeba B60.13
　adenoviral B30.0
　epidemic B30.0
　exposure H16.21-●
　herpes, herpetic (simplex) B00.52
　　zoster B02.33
　in exanthema —see also Exanthem B09
　infectious B30.0
　lagophthalmic —see Keratoconjunctivitis,
　　specified type NEC
　neurotrophic H16.23-●
　phlyctenular H16.25-●
　postmeasles B05.81
　shipyard B30.0
　sicca (Sjogren's) M35.0-●
　　not Sjogren's H16.22-●
　specified type NEC H16.29-●
　tuberculous (phlyctenular) A18.52
　vernal H16.26-●
Keratoconus H18.60-●
　congenital Q13.4
　stable H18.61-●
　unstable H18.62-●
Keratocyst (dental) (odontogenic) —see Cyst,
　calcifying odontogenic
Keratoderma, keratodermia (congenital) (palmaris
　et plantaris) (symmetrical) Q82.8
　acquired L85.1
　　in diseases classified elsewhere L86
　climactericum L85.1
　gonococcal A54.89
　gonorrheal A54.89
　punctata L85.2
　Reiter's —see Reiter's disease
Keratodermatocele —see Descemetocele
Keratoglobus H18.79
　congenital Q15.8
　　with glaucoma Q15.0
Keratohemia —see Pigmentation, cornea, stromal
Keratoiritis —see also Iridocyclitis
　syphilitic A50.39
　tuberculous A18.54
Keratoma L57.0
　palmaris and plantaris hereditarium Q82.8
　senile L57.0
Keratomalacia H18.44-●
　vitamin A deficiency E50.4
Keratomegaly Q13.4
Keratomycosis B49
　nigrans, nigricans (palmaris) B36.1
Keratopathy H18.9
　band H18.42-●
　bullous H18.1-●
　bullous (aphakic), following cataract surgery
　　H59.01-●
Keratoscleritis, tuberculous A18.52
Keratosis L57.0
　actinic L57.0
　arsenical L85.8
　congenital, specified NEC Q80.8
　female genital NEC N94.89
　follicularis Q82.8
　　acquired L11.0
　　congenita Q82.8
　　et parafollicularis in cutem penetrans L87.0
　　spinulosa (decalvans) Q82.8
　　vitamin A deficiency E50.8
　gonococcal A54.89
　lichenoid L82.0
　male genital (external) N50.89
　nigricans L83
　obturans, external ear (canal) —see
　　Cholesteatoma, external ear
　palmaris et plantaris (inherited) (symmetrical)
　　Q82.8
　　acquired L85.1
　penile N48.89
　pharynx J39.2
　pilaris, acquired L85.8
　punctata (palmaris et plantaris) L85.2
　scrotal N50.89
　seborrheic L82.1
　　inflamed L82.0
　senile L57.0
　solar L57.0
　tonsillaris J35.8
　vagina N89.4
　vegetans Q82.8

Keratosis (Continued)
　vitamin A deficiency E50.8
　vocal cord J38.3
Kerato-uveitis —see Iridocyclitis
Kerion (celsi) B35.0
Kernicterus of newborn (not due to
　　isoimmunization) P57.9
　due to isoimmunization (conditions in
　　P55.0-P55.9) P57.0
　specified type NEC P57.8
Kerunoparalysis T75.09
▶Keraunoparalysis T75.09
Keshan disease E59
Ketoacidosis E87.29
　diabetic —see Diabetes, by type, with
　　ketoacidosis
Ketonuria R82.4
Ketosis NEC E88.89
　diabetic —see Diabetes, by type, with
　　ketoacidosis
Kew Garden fever A79.1
Kidney —see condition
Kienböck's disease —see also Osteochondrosis,
　　juvenile, hand, carpal lunate
　adult M93.1
Kimmelstiel (-Wilson) disease —see Diabetes,
　　Kimmelstiel (-Wilson) disease
Kimura disease D21.9
　specified site (see Neoplasm, connective tissue
　　benign)
Kink, kinking
　artery I77.1
　hair (acquired) L67.8
　ileum or intestine —see Obstruction,
　　intestine
　Lane's —see Obstruction, intestine
　organ or site, congenital NEC —see Anomaly,
　　by site
　ureter (pelvic junction) N13.5
　　with
　　　hydronephrosis N13.1
　　　　with infection N13.6
　　　pyelonephritis (chronic) N11.1
　　congenital Q62.39
　vein(s) I87.8
　　caval I87.1
　　peripheral I87.1
Kinnier Wilson's disease (hepatolenticular
　　degeneration) E83.01
Kissing spine M48.20
　cervical region M48.22
　cervicothoracic region M48.23
　lumbar region M48.26
　lumbosacral region M48.27
　occipito-atlanto-axial region M48.21
　thoracic region M48.24
　thoracolumbar region M48.25
Klatskin's tumor C24.0
Klauder's disease A26.8
Klebs' disease —see also Glomerulonephritis
　N05-●
Klebsiella (K.) pneumoniae, as cause of disease
　classified elsewhere B96.1
Kleeblattschaedel skull Q75.051
Klein (e)-Levin syndrome G47.13
Kleptomania F63.2
Klinefelter's syndrome Q98.4
　karyotype 47,XXY Q98.0
　male with more than two X chromosomes Q98.1
Klippel-Feil deficiency, disease, or syndrome
　　(brevicollis) Q76.1
Klippel's disease I67.2
Klippel-Trenaunay (-Weber) syndrome Q87.2
Klumpke (-Déjerine) palsy, paralysis (birth)
　　(newborn) P14.1
Knee —see condition
Knock knee (acquired) M21.06-●
　congenital Q74.1
Knot(s)
　intestinal, syndrome (volvulus) K56.2
　surfer S89.8-●
　umbilical cord (true) O69.2
Knotting (of)
　hair L67.8
　intestine K56.2
Knuckle pad (Garrod's) M72.1
Koch's
　infection —see Tuberculosis
　relapsing fever A68.9
Koch-Weeks' conjunctivitis —see Conjunctivitis,
　　acute, mucopurulent

Köebner's syndrome Q81.8
Köenig's disease (osteochondritis dissecans) —see
　　Osteochondritis, dissecans
Köhler-Pellegrini-Steida disease or syndrome
　　(calcification, knee joint) —see Bursitis, tibial
　　collateral
▶Köhler-Pellegrini-Stieda disease or syndrome
　　(calcification, knee joint) —see Bursitis, tibial
　　collateral
Köhler's disease
　patellar —see Osteochondrosis, juvenile, patella
　tarsal navicular —see Osteochondrosis, juvenile,
　　tarsus
Koilonychia L60.3
　congenital Q84.6
Kojevnikov's, epilepsy —see Kozhevnikof's
　　epilepsy
Koplik's spots B05.9
Kopp's asthma E32.8
Korsakoff's (Wernicke) disease, psychosis or
　　syndrome (alcoholic) F10.96
　with dependence F10.26
　drug-induced
　　due to drug abuse —see Abuse, drug, by type,
　　　with amnestic disorder
　　due to drug dependence —see Dependence,
　　　drug, by type, with amnestic disorder
　nonalcoholic F04
Korsakov's disease, psychosis or syndrome —see
　　Korsakoff's disease
Korsakow's disease, psychosis or syndrome —see
　　Korsakoff's disease
Kostmann's disease or syndrome (infantile genetic
　　agranulocytosis) —see Agranulocytosis
Kozhevnikof's epilepsy G40.109
　intractable G40.119
　　with status epilepticus G40.111
　　without status epilepticus G40.119
　not intractable G40.109
　　with status epilepticus G40.101
　　without status epilepticus G40.109
Krabbe's
　disease E75.23
　syndrome, congenital muscle hypoplasia
　　Q79.8
Kraepelin-Morel disease —see Schizophrenia
Kraft-Weber-Dimitri disease Q85.89
Kraurosis
　ani K62.89
　penis N48.0
　vagina N89.8
　vulva N90.4
Kreotoxism A05.9
Krukenberg's
　spindle —see Pigmentation, cornea, posterior
　tumor C79.6-●
Kufs' disease E75.4
Kugelberg-Welander disease G12.1
Kuhnt-Junius degeneration —see also
　　Degeneration, macula H35.32-●
Kümmell's disease or spondylitis —see
　　Spondylopathy, traumatic
Kupffer cell sarcoma C22.3
Kuru A81.81
Kussmaul's
　disease M30.0
　respiration E87.29
　　in diabetic acidosis —see Diabetes, by type,
　　　with ketoacidosis
Kwashiorkor E40
　marasmic, marasmus type E42
Kyasanur Forest disease A98.2
Kyphoscoliosis, kyphoscoliotic (acquired) —see
　　also Scoliosis M41.9
　congenital Q67.5
　heart (disease) I27.1
　sequelae of rickets E64.3
　tuberculous A18.01
Kyphosis, kyphotic (acquired) M40.209
　cervical region M40.202
　cervicothoracic region M40.203
　congenital Q76.419
　　cervical region Q76.412
　　cervicothoracic region Q76.413
　　occipito-atlanto-axial region Q76.411
　　thoracic region Q76.414
　　thoracolumbar region Q76.415
　Morquio-Brailsford type (spinal) —see also
　　　subcategory M49.8 E76.219
　postlaminectomy M96.3
　postradiation therapy M96.2

Kyphosis, kyphotic (Continued)
  postural (adolescent) M40.00
    cervicothoracic region M40.03
    thoracic region M40.04
    thoracolumbar region M40.05
  secondary NEC M40.10
    cervical region M40.12
    cervicothoracic region M40.13
    thoracic region M40.14
    thoracolumbar region M40.15
  sequelae of rickets E64.3
  specified type NEC M40.299
    cervical region M40.292
    cervicothoracic region M40.293
    thoracic region M40.294
    thoracolumbar region M40.295
  syphilitic, congenital A50.56
    thoracic region M40.204
    thoracolumbar region M40.205
  tuberculous A18.01
Kyrle disease L87.0

L

Labia, labium —see condition
Labile
  blood pressure R09.89
  vasomotor system I73.9
Labioglossal paralysis G12.29
Labium leporinum —see Cleft, lip
Labor —see Delivery
Labored breathing —see Hyperventilation
Labyrinthitis (circumscribed) (destructive)
    (diffuse) (inner ear) (latent) (purulent)
    (suppurative) (see also subcategory)
    H83.0
  syphilitic A52.79
Laceration
  with abortion —see Abortion, by type,
    complicated by laceration of pelvic organs
  abdomen, abdominal
    wall S31.119
      with
        foreign body S31.129
        penetration into peritoneal cavity S31.619
          with foreign body S31.629
      epigastric region S31.112
        with
          foreign body S31.122
          penetration into peritoneal cavity
            S31.612
            with foreign body S31.622
      left
        lower quadrant S31.114
          with
            foreign body S31.124
            penetration into peritoneal cavity
              S31.614
              with foreign body S31.624
        upper quadrant S31.111
          with
            foreign body S31.121
            penetration into peritoneal cavity
              S31.611
              with foreign body S31.621
      periumbilic region S31.115
        with
          foreign body S31.125
          penetration into peritoneal cavity
            S31.615
            with foreign body S31.625
      right
        lower quadrant S31.113
          with
            foreign body S31.123
            penetration into peritoneal cavity
              S31.613
              with foreign body S31.623
        upper quadrant S31.110
          with
            foreign body S31.120
            penetration into peritoneal cavity
              S31.610
              with foreign body S31.620
  accidental, complicating surgery —see
    Complications, surgical, accidental
    puncture or laceration
  Achilles tendon S86.02-●

Laceration (Continued)
  adrenal gland S37.813
  alveolar (process) —see Laceration, oral cavity
  ankle S91.01-●
    with
      foreign body S91.02-●
  antecubital space —see Laceration, elbow
  anus (sphincter) S31.831
    with
      ectopic or molar pregnancy O08.6
      foreign body S31.832
    complicating delivery —see Delivery,
      complicated, by, laceration, anus
      (sphincter)
    following ectopic or molar pregnancy O08.6
    nontraumatic, nonpuerperal —see Fissure,
      anus
  arm (upper) S41.11-●
    with foreign body S41.12-●
    lower —see Laceration, forearm
  auditory canal (external) (meatus) —see
    Laceration, ear
  auricle, ear —see Laceration, ear
  axilla —see Laceration, arm
  back —see also Laceration, thorax, back
    lower S31.010
      with
        foreign body S31.020
          with penetration into retroperitoneal
            space S31.021
        penetration into retroperitoneal space
          S31.011
  bile duct S36.13
  bladder S37.23
    with ectopic or molar pregnancy O08.6
    following ectopic or molar pregnancy O08.6
    obstetrical trauma O71.5
  blood vessel —see Injury, blood vessel
  bowel —see also Laceration, intestine
    with ectopic or molar pregnancy O08.6
    complicating abortion —see Abortion, by type,
      complicated by, specified condition NEC
    following ectopic or molar pregnancy O08.6
    obstetrical trauma O71.5
  brain (any part) (cortex) (diffuse) (membrane) —
      see also Injury, intracranial, diffuse
    during birth P10.8
      with hemorrhage P10.1
    focal —see Injury, intracranial, focal brain
      injury
  brainstem S06.38-●
  breast S21.01-●
    with foreign body S21.02-●
  broad ligament S37.893
    with ectopic or molar pregnancy O08.6
    following ectopic or molar pregnancy O08.6
    laceration syndrome N83.8
    obstetrical trauma O71.6
    syndrome (laceration) N83.8
  buttock S31.801
    with foreign body S31.802
    left S31.821
      with foreign body S31.822
    right S31.811
      with foreign body S31.812
  calf —see Laceration, leg
  canaliculus lacrimalis —see Laceration,
    eyelid
  canthus, eye —see Laceration, eyelid
  capsule, joint —see Sprain
  causing eversion of cervix uteri (old) N86
  central (perineal), complicating delivery O70.9
  cerebellum, traumatic S06.37-●
  cerebral S06.33-●
    during birth P10.8
      with hemorrhage P10.1
    left side S06.32-●
    right side S06.31-●
  cervix (uteri)
    with ectopic or molar pregnancy O08.6
    following ectopic or molar pregnancy O08.6
    nonpuerperal, nontraumatic N88.1
    obstetrical trauma (current) O71.3
    old (postpartal) N88.1
    traumatic S37.63
  cheek (external) S01.41-●
    with foreign body S01.42-●
    internal —see Laceration, oral cavity
  chest wall —see Laceration, thorax
  chin —see Laceration, head, specified site
    NEC

Laceration (Continued)
  chordae tendinae NEC I51.1
    concurrent with acute myocardial
      infarction —see Infarct, myocardium
    following acute myocardial infarction (current
      complication) I23.4
  clitoris —see Laceration, vulva
  colon —see Laceration, intestine, large, colon
  common bile duct S36.13
  cortex (cerebral) —see Injury, intracranial, diffuse
  costal region —see Laceration, thorax
  cystic duct S36.13
  diaphragm S27.803
  digit(s)
    foot —see Laceration, toe
    hand —see Laceration, finger
  duodenum S36.430
  ear (canal) (external) S01.31-●
    with foreign body S01.32-●
    drum S09.2-●
  elbow S51.01-●
    with
      foreign body S51.02-●
  epididymis —see Laceration, testis
  epigastric region —see Laceration, abdomen,
    wall, epigastric region
  esophagus K22.89
    traumatic
      cervical S11.21
        with foreign body S11.22
      thoracic S27.813
  eye (ball) S05.3-●
    with prolapse or loss of intraocular tissue
      S05.2-●
    penetrating S05.6-●
  eyebrow —see Laceration, eyelid
  eyelid S01.11-●
    with foreign body S01.12-●
  face NEC —see Laceration, head, specified site
    NEC
  fallopian tube S37.539
    bilateral S37.532
    unilateral S37.531
  finger(s) S61.219
    with
      damage to nail S61.319
        with
          foreign body S61.329
      foreign body S61.229
    index S61.218
      with
        damage to nail S61.318
          with
            foreign body S61.328
        foreign body S61.228
      left S61.211
        with
          damage to nail S61.311
            with
              foreign body S61.321
          foreign body S61.221
      right S61.210
        with
          damage to nail S61.310
            with
              foreign body S61.320
          foreign body S61.220
    little S61.218
      with
        damage to nail S61.318
          with
            foreign body S61.328
        foreign body S61.228
      left S61.217
        with
          damage to nail S61.317
            with
              foreign body S61.327
          foreign body S61.227
      right S61.216
        with
          damage to nail S61.316
            with
              foreign body S61.326
          foreign body S61.226
    middle S61.218
      with
        damage to nail S61.318
          with
            foreign body S61.328
        foreign body S61.228

Laceration (Continued)
  finger(s) (Continued)
    middle (Continued)
      left S61.213
        with
          damage to nail S61.313
            with
              foreign body S61.323
          foreign body S61.223
      right S61.212
        with
          damage to nail S61.312
            with
              foreign body S61.322
          foreign body S61.222
    ring S61.218
      with
        damage to nail S61.318
          with
            foreign body S61.328
        foreign body S61.228
      left S61.215
        with
          damage to nail S61.315
            with
              foreign body S61.325
          foreign body S61.225
      right S61.214
        with
          damage to nail S61.314
            with
              foreign body S61.324
          foreign body S61.224
  flank S31.119
    with foreign body S31.129
  foot (except toe(s) alone) S91.319
    with foreign body S91.329
    left S91.312
      with foreign body S91.322
    right S91.311
      with foreign body S91.321
    toe —see Laceration, toe
  forearm S51.819
    with
      foreign body S51.829
    elbow only —see Laceration,
      elbow
    left S51.812
      with
        foreign body S51.822
    right S51.811
      with
        foreign body S51.821
  forehead S01.81
    with foreign body S01.82
  fourchette O70.0
    with ectopic or molar pregnancy
      O08.6
    complicating delivery O70.0
    following ectopic or molar pregnancy O08.6
  gallbladder S36.123
  genital organs, external
    female S31.512
      with foreign body S31.522
      vagina —see Laceration, vagina
      vulva —see Laceration, vulva
    male S31.511
      with foreign body S31.521
      penis —see Laceration, penis
      scrotum —see Laceration, scrotum
      testis —see Laceration, testis
  groin —see Laceration, abdomen, wall
  gum —see Laceration, oral cavity
  hand S61.419
    with
      foreign body S61.429
    finger —see Laceration, finger
    left S61.412
      with
        foreign body S61.422
    right S61.411
      with
        foreign body S61.421
    thumb —see Laceration, thumb
  head S01.91
    with foreign body S01.92
    cheek —see Laceration, cheek
    ear —see Laceration, ear
    eyelid —see Laceration, eyelid
    lip —see Laceration, lip
    nose —see Laceration, nose

Laceration (Continued)
  head (Continued)
    oral cavity —see Laceration, oral
      cavity
    scalp S01.01
      with foreign body S01.02
    specified site NEC S01.81
      with foreign body S01.82
    temporomandibular area —see Laceration,
      cheek
  heart —see Injury, heart, laceration
  heel —see Laceration, foot
  hepatic duct S36.13
  hip S71.019
    with foreign body S71.029
    left S71.012
      with foreign body S71.022
    right S71.011
      with foreign body S71.021
  hymen —see Laceration, vagina
  hypochondrium —see Laceration, abdomen,
    wall
  hypogastric region —see Laceration, abdomen,
    wall
  ileum S36.438
  inguinal region —see Laceration, abdomen, wall
  instep —see Laceration, foot
  internal organ —see Injury, by site
  interscapular region —see Laceration, thorax,
    back
  intestine
    large
      colon S36.539
        ascending S36.530
        descending S36.532
        sigmoid S36.533
        specified site NEC S36.538
      rectum S36.63
        transverse S36.531
    small S36.439
      duodenum S36.430
      specified site NEC S36.438
  intra-abdominal organ S36.93
    intestine —see Laceration, intestine
    liver —see Laceration, liver
    pancreas —see Laceration, pancreas
    peritoneum S36.81
    specified site NEC S36.893
    spleen —see Laceration, spleen
    stomach —see Laceration, stomach
  intracranial NEC —see also Injury, intracranial,
    diffuse
    birth injury P10.9
  jaw —see Laceration, head, specified site NEC
  jejunum S36.438
  joint capsule —see Sprain, by site
  kidney S37.03-●
    major (greater than 3 cm) (massive) (stellate)
      S37.06-●
    minor (less than 1 cm) S37.04-●
    moderate (1 to 3 cm) S37.05-●
    multiple S37.06-●
  knee S81.01-●
    with foreign body S81.02-●
  labium (majus) (minus) —see Laceration, vulva
  lacrimal duct —see Laceration, eyelid
  large intestine —see Laceration, intestine, large
  larynx S11.011
    with foreign body S11.012
  leg (lower) S81.819
    with foreign body S81.829
    foot —see Laceration, foot
    knee —see Laceration, knee
    left S81.812
      with foreign body S81.822
    right S81.811
      with foreign body S81.821
    upper —see Laceration, thigh
  ligament —see Sprain
  lip S01.511
    with foreign body S01.521
  liver S36.113
    major (stellate) S36.116
    minor S36.114
    moderate S36.115
  loin —see Laceration, abdomen, wall
  lower back —see Laceration, back, lower
  lumbar region —see Laceration, back, lower
  lung S27.339
    bilateral S27.332
    unilateral S27.331

Laceration (Continued)
  malar region —see Laceration, head, specified
    site NEC
  mammary —see Laceration, breast
  mastoid region —see Laceration, head, specified
    site NEC
  meninges —see Injury, intracranial, diffuse
  meniscus —see Tear, meniscus
  mesentery S36.893
  mesosalpinx S37.893
  mouth —see Laceration, oral cavity
  muscle —see Injury, muscle, by site, laceration
  nail
    finger —see Laceration, finger, with damage
      to nail
    toe —see Laceration, toe, with damage to nail
  nasal (septum) (sinus) —see Laceration, nose
  nasopharynx —see Laceration, head, specified
    site NEC
  neck S11.91
    with foreign body S11.92
    involving
      cervical esophagus S11.21
        with foreign body S11.22
      larynx —see Laceration, larynx
      pharynx —see Laceration, pharynx
      thyroid gland —see Laceration, thyroid
        gland
      trachea —see Laceration, trachea
    specified site NEC S11.81
      with foreign body S11.82
  nerve —see Injury, nerve
  nose (septum) (sinus) S01.21
    with foreign body S01.22
  ocular NOS S05.3-●
    adnexa NOS S01.11-●
  oral cavity S01.512
    with foreign body S01.522
  orbit (eye) —see Wound, open, ocular, orbit
  ovary S37.439
    bilateral S37.432
    unilateral S37.431
  palate —see Laceration, oral cavity
  palm —see Laceration, hand
  pancreas S36.239
    body S36.231
      major S36.261
      minor S36.241
      moderate S36.251
    head S36.230
      major S36.260
      minor S36.240
      moderate S36.250
    major S36.269
    minor S36.249
    moderate S36.259
    tail S36.232
      major S36.262
      minor S36.242
      moderate S36.252
  pelvic S31.010
    with
      foreign body S31.020
        penetration into retroperitoneal cavity
          S31.021
      penetration into retroperitoneal cavity
        S31.011
    floor —see also Laceration, back, lower
      with ectopic or molar pregnancy
        O08.6
      complicating delivery O70.1
      following ectopic or molar pregnancy
        O08.6
      old (postpartal) N81.89
    organ S37.93
      with ectopic or molar pregnancy
        O08.6
      adrenal gland S37.813
      bladder S37.23
      fallopian tube —see Laceration, fallopian
        tube
      following ectopic or molar pregnancy
        O08.6
      kidney —see Laceration, kidney
      obstetrical trauma O71.5
      ovary —see Laceration, ovary
      prostate S37.823
      specified site NEC S37.893
      ureter S37.13
      urethra S37.33
      uterus S37.63

▶ New   ⇒ Revised   ~~deleted~~ Deleted   ● Use Additional Character(s)

Laceration *(Continued)*
penis S31.21
  with foreign body S31.22
perineum
  female S31.41
    with
      ectopic or molar pregnancy O08.6
      foreign body S31.42
    during delivery O70.9
      first degree O70.0
      fourth degree O70.3
      second degree O70.1
      third degree —*see also* Delivery,
        complicated, by, laceration,
        perineum, third degree
        O70.20
    old (postpartal) N81.89
    postpartal N81.89
    secondary (postpartal) O90.1
  male S31.119
    with foreign body S31.129
periocular area (with or without lacrimal
  passages) —*see* Laceration, eyelid
peritoneum S36.893
periumbilic region —*see* Laceration, abdomen,
  wall, periumbilic
periurethral tissue —*see* Laceration, urethra
phalanges
  finger —*see* Laceration, finger
  toe —*see* Laceration, toe
pharynx S11.21
  with foreign body S11.22
pinna —*see* Laceration, ear
popliteal space —*see* Laceration, knee
prepuce —*see* Laceration, penis
prostate S37.823
pubic region S31.119
  with foreign body S31.129
pudendum —*see* Laceration, genital organs,
  external
rectovaginal septum —*see* Laceration, vagina
rectum S36.63
retroperitoneum S36.893
round ligament S37.893
sacral region —*see* Laceration, back, lower
sacroiliac region —*see* Laceration, back,
  lower
salivary gland —*see* Laceration, oral cavity
scalp S01.01
  with foreign body S01.02
scapular region —*see* Laceration, shoulder
scrotum S31.31
  with foreign body S31.32
seminal vesicle S37.893
shin —*see* Laceration, leg
shoulder S41.019
  with foreign body S41.029
  left S41.012
    with foreign body S41.022
  right S41.011
    with foreign body S41.021
small intestine —*see* Laceration, intestine, small
spermatic cord —*see* Laceration, testis
spinal cord (meninges) —*see also* Injury, spinal
  cord, by region
  due to injury at birth P11.5
  newborn (birth injury) P11.5
spleen S36.039
  major (massive) (stellate) S36.032
  moderate S36.031
  superficial (minor) S36.030
sternal region —*see* Laceration, thorax, front
stomach S36.33
submaxillary region —*see* Laceration, head,
  specified site NEC
submental region —*see* Laceration, head,
  specified site NEC
subungual
  finger(s) —*see* Laceration, finger, with damage
    to nail
  toe(s) —*see* Laceration, toe, with damage to
    nail
suprarenal gland —*see* Laceration, adrenal gland
temple, temporal region —*see* Laceration, head,
  specified site NEC
temporomandibular area —*see* Laceration, cheek
tendon —*see* Injury, muscle, by site,
  laceration
  Achilles S86.02-●
tentorium cerebelli —*see* Injury, intracranial,
  diffuse

Laceration *(Continued)*
testis S31.31
  with foreign body S31.32
thigh S71.11-●
  with foreign body S71.12-●
thorax, thoracic (wall) S21.91
  with foreign body S21.92
    back S21.22-●
      with penetration into thoracic cavity
        S21.42-●
    front S21.12-●
      with penetration into thoracic cavity
        S21.32-●
  back S21.21-●
    with
      foreign body S21.22-●
        with penetration into thoracic cavity
          S21.42-●
      penetration into thoracic cavity S21.41-●
  breast —*see* Laceration, breast
  front S21.11-●
    with
      foreign body S21.12-●
        with penetration into thoracic cavity
          S21.32-●
      penetration into thoracic cavity S21.31-●
thumb S61.019
  with
    damage to nail S61.119
      with
        foreign body S61.129
    foreign body S61.029
  left S61.012
    with
      damage to nail S61.112
        with
          foreign body S61.122
      foreign body S61.022
  right S61.011
    with
      damage to nail S61.111
        with
          foreign body S61.121
      foreign body S61.021
thyroid gland S11.11
  with foreign body S11.12
toe(s) S91.119
  with
    damage to nail S91.219
      with
        foreign body S91.229
    foreign body S91.129
  great S91.113
    with
      damage to nail S91.213
        with
          foreign body S91.223
      foreign body S91.123
    left S91.112
      with
        damage to nail S91.212
          with
            foreign body S91.222
        foreign body S91.122
    right S91.111
      with
        damage to nail S91.211
          with
            foreign body S91.221
        foreign body S91.121
  lesser S91.116
    with
      damage to nail S91.216
        with
          foreign body S91.226
      foreign body S91.126
    left S91.115
      with
        damage to nail S91.215
          with
            foreign body S91.225
        foreign body S91.125
    right S91.114
      with
        damage to nail S91.214
          with
            foreign body S91.224
        foreign body S91.124
tongue —*see* Laceration, oral cavity
trachea S11.021
  with foreign body S11.022

Laceration *(Continued)*
tunica vaginalis —*see* Laceration, testis
tympanum, tympanic membrane —*see*
  Laceration, ear, drum
umbilical region S31.115
  with foreign body S31.125
ureter S37.13
urethra S37.33
  with or following ectopic or molar pregnancy
    O08.6
  obstetrical trauma O71.5
urinary organ NEC S37.893
uterus S37.63
  with ectopic or molar pregnancy O08.6
  following ectopic or molar pregnancy O08.6
  nonpuerperal, nontraumatic N85.8
  obstetrical trauma NEC O71.81
  old (postpartal) N85.8
uvula —*see* Laceration, oral cavity
vagina S31.41
  with
    ectopic or molar pregnancy O08.6
    foreign body S31.42
  during delivery O71.4
    with perineal laceration —*see* Laceration,
      perineum, female, during delivery
  following ectopic or molar pregnancy
    O08.6
  nonpuerperal, nontraumatic N89.8
  old (postpartal) N89.8
vas deferens S37.893
vesical —*see* Laceration, bladder
vocal cords S11.031
  with foreign body S11.032
vulva S31.41
  with
    ectopic or molar pregnancy O08.6
    foreign body S31.42
  complicating delivery O70.0
  following ectopic or molar pregnancy O08.6
  nonpuerperal, nontraumatic N90.89
  old (postpartal) N90.89
wrist S61.519
  with
    foreign body S61.529
  left S61.512
    with
      foreign body S61.522
  right S61.511
    with
      foreign body S61.521
Lack of
  achievement in school Z55.3
  adequate
    food Z59.48
    intermaxillary vertical dimension of fully
      erupted teeth M26.36
    sleep Z72.820
  air conditioning Z59.11
  appetite *(see* Anorexia) R63.0
  awareness R41.9
  basic services in physical environment Z58.81
  care
    in home Z74.2
    of infant (at or after birth) T76.02
      confirmed T74.02
  cognitive functions R41.9
  coordination R27.9
    ataxia R27.0
    specified type NEC R27.8
  development (physiological) R62.50
    failure to thrive (child over 28 days old)
      R62.51
      adult R62.7
      newborn P92.6
    short stature R62.52
    specified type NEC R62.59
  electricity services Z59.12
  emotional support Z60.8
  energy R53.83
  financial resources Z59.6
  food Z59.48
  gas services Z59.12
  growth R62.52
  heating Z59.11
  housing (permanent) (temporary) Z59.00
    adequate Z59.10
  learning experiences in childhood Z62.898
  leisure time (affecting life-style) Z73.2
  material resources due to limited financial
    resources, specified NEC Z59.87

Lack of *(Continued)*
  memory —*see also* Amnesia
    mild, following organic brain damage F06.8
  oil services Z59.12
  ovulation N97.0
  parental supervision or control of child Z62.0
  person able to render necessary care Z74.2
  physical exercise Z72.3
  play experience in childhood Z62.898
  posterior occlusal support M26.57
  relaxation (affecting life-style) Z73.2
  safe drinking water Z58.6
  sexual
    desire F52.0
    enjoyment F52.1
  shelter Z59.02
  sleep (adequate) Z72.820
  supervision of child by parent Z62.0
  support, posterior occlusal M26.57
  transportation Z59.82
  water T73.1
    safe drinking Z58.6
    services Z59.12
Lacrimal —*see* condition
Lacrimation, abnormal —*see* Epiphora
Lacrimonasal duct —*see* condition
Lactate, elevated —*see* Acidosis, lactic
Lactation, lactating (breast) (puerperal, postpartum)
  associated
    cracked nipple O92.13
    retracted nipple O92.03
  defective O92.4
  disorder NEC O92.79
  excessive O92.6
  failed (complete) O92.3
    partial O92.4
  mastitis NEC —*see* Mastitis, obstetric
  mother (care and/or examination) Z39.1
  nonpuerperal N64.3
Lacticemia, excessive *(see also* Acidosis) E87.20
Lacunar skull Q75.8
Laennec's cirrhosis K70.30
  with ascites K70.31
  nonalcoholic K74.69
Lafora disease (see also Epilepsy, progressive, Lafora) G40.C09
Lag, lid (nervous) —*see* Retraction, lid
Lagophthalmos (eyelid) (nervous) H02.209
  bilateral, upper and lower eyelids H02.20C
  cicatricial H02.219
    bilateral, upper and lower eyelids H02.21C
    left H02.216
      lower H02.215
      upper H02.214
      upper and lower eyelids H02.21B
    right H02.213
      lower H02.212
      upper H02.211
      upper and lower eyelids H02.21A
  keratoconjunctivitis —*see* Keratoconjunctivitis
  left H02.206
    lower H02.205
    upper H02.204
    upper and lower eyelids H02.20B
  mechanical H02.229
    bilateral, upper and lower eyelids H02.22C
    left H02.226
      lower H02.225
      upper H02.224
      upper and lower eyelids H02.22B
    right H02.223
      lower H02.222
      upper H02.221
      upper and lower eyelids H02.22A
  paralytic H02.239
    bilateral, upper and lower eyelids H02.23C
    left H02.236
      lower H02.235
      upper H02.234
      upper and lower eyelids H02.23B
    right H02.233
      lower H02.232
      upper H02.231
      upper and lower eyelids H02.23A
  right H02.203
    lower H02.202
    upper H02.201
    upper and lower eyelids H02.20A
Laki-Lorand factor deficiency —*see* Defect, coagulation, specified type NEC

Lalling F80.0
Lambert-Eaton syndrome —*see* Syndrome, Lambert-Eaton
Lambliasis, lambliosis A07.1
Landau-Kleffner syndrome —*see* Epilepsy, specified NEC
Landouzy-Déjérine dystrophy or facioscapulohumeral atrophy G71.02
Landouzy's disease (icterohemorrhagic leptospirosis) A27.0
Landry-Guillain-Barré, syndrome or paralysis G61.0
Landry's disease or paralysis G61.0
Lane's
  band Q43.3
  kink —*see* Obstruction, intestine
  syndrome K90.2
Langdon Down's syndrome —*see* Trisomy, 21
Lapsed immunization schedule status Z28.3
Large
  baby (regardless of gestational age) (4000g to 4499g) P08.1
  ear, congenital Q17.1
  physiological cup Q14.2
  stature R68.89
Large-for-dates NEC (infant) (4000g to 4499g) P08.1
  affecting management of pregnancy O36.6-●
  exceptionally (4500g or more) P08.0
Larsen-Johansson disease or osteochondrosis — *see* Osteochondrosis, juvenile, patella
Larsen's syndrome (flattened facies and multiple congenital dislocations) Q74.8
Larva migrans
  cutaneous B76.9
    Ancylostoma B76.0
  visceral B83.0
Laryngeal —*see* condition
Laryngismus (stridulus) J38.5
  congenital P28.89
  diphtheritic A36.2
Laryngitis (acute) (edematous) (fibrinous) (infective) (infiltrative) (malignant) (membranous) (phlegmonous) (pneumococcal) (pseudomembranous) (septic) (subglottic) (suppurative) (ulcerative) J04.0
  with
    influenza, flu, or grippe —*see* Influenza, with, laryngitis
    tracheitis (acute) —*see* Laryngotracheitis
  atrophic J37.0
  catarrhal J37.0
  chronic J37.0
    with tracheitis (chronic) J37.1
  diphtheritic A36.2
  due to external agent —*see* Inflammation, respiratory, upper, due to
  Hemophilus influenzae J04.0
  H. influenzae J04.0
  hypertrophic J37.0
  influenzal —*see* Influenza, with, respiratory manifestations NEC
  obstructive J05.0
  sicca J37.0
  spasmodic J05.0
    acute J04.0
  streptococcal J04.0
  stridulous J05.0
  syphilitic (late) A52.73
    congenital A50.59 *[J99]*
      early A50.03 *[J99]*
  tuberculous A15.5
  Vincent's A69.1
Laryngocele (congenital) (ventricular) Q31.3
Laryngofissure J38.7
  congenital Q31.8
Laryngomalacia (congenital) Q31.5
Laryngopharyngitis (acute) J06.0
  chronic J37.0
  due to external agent —*see* Inflammation, respiratory, upper, due to
Laryngoplegia J38.00
  bilateral J38.02
  unilateral J38.01
Laryngoptosis J38.7
Laryngospasm J38.5
Laryngostenosis J38.6
Laryngotracheitis (acute) (Infectional) (infective) (viral) J04.2
  atrophic J37.1
  catarrhal J37.1
  chronic J37.1

Laryngotracheitis *(Continued)*
  diphtheritic A36.2
  due to external agent —*see* Inflammation, respiratory, upper, due to
  Hemophilus influenzae J04.2
  hypertrophic J37.1
  influenzal —*see* Influenza, with, respiratory manifestations NEC
  pachydermic J38.7
  sicca J37.1
  spasmodic J38.5
    acute J05.0
  streptococcal J04.2
  stridulous J38.5
  syphilitic (late) A52.73
    congenital A50.59 *[J99]*
      early A50.03 *[J99]*
  tuberculous A15.5
  Vincent's A69.1
Laryngotracheobronchitis —*see* Bronchitis
Larynx, laryngeal —*see* condition
Lassa fever A96.2
Lassitude —*see* Weakness
Late
  talker R62.0
  walker R62.0
Late effect(s) —*see* Sequelae
Latent —*see* condition
Laterocession —*see* Lateroversion
Lateroflexion —*see* Lateroversion
Lateroversion
  cervix —*see* Lateroversion, uterus
  uterus, uterine (cervix) (postinfectional) (postpartal, old) N85.4
    congenital Q51.818
    in pregnancy or childbirth O34.59-●
Lathyrism —*see* Poisoning, food, noxious, plant
Launois' syndrome (pituitary gigantism) E22.0
Launois-Bensaude adenolipomatosis E88.89
Laurence-Moon syndrome Q87.84
Lax, laxity —*see also* Relaxation
  ligament (ous) —*see also* Disorder, ligament
    familial M35.7
    knee —*see* Derangement, knee
  skin (acquired) L57.4
    congenital Q82.8
Laxative habit F55.2
Lazy leukocyte syndrome D70.8
Lead miner's lung J63.6
Leak, leakage
  air NEC J93.82
    postprocedural J95.812
  amniotic fluid —*see* Rupture, membranes, premature
  blood (microscopic), fetal, into maternal circulation affecting management of pregnancy —*see* Pregnancy, complicated by
  cerebrospinal fluid G96.00
    cranial
      postoperative G96.08
      specified NEC G96.08
      spontaneous G96.01
      traumatic G96.08
    from spinal (lumbar) puncture G97.0
    spinal
      postoperative G96.09
      post-traumatic G96.09
      specified NEC G96.09
      spontaneous G96.02
    spontaneous
      from
        skull base G96.01
      spine G96.02
  CSF —*see* Leak, cerebrospinal fluid
  device, implant or graft —*see also* Complications, by site and type, mechanical
    arterial graft NEC —*see* Complication, vascular, graft, mechanical, leakage T82.838
    breast (implant) T85.43
    catheter NEC T85.638
      dialysis (renal) T82.43
        intraperitoneal T85.631
      infusion NEC T82.534
        spinal (epidural) (subdural) T85.630
      urinary T83.038
        cystostomy T83.030
        Hopkins T83.038
        ileostomy T83.038
        indwelling T83.031

▶ New   ⇒ Revised   ~~deleted~~ Deleted   ● Use Additional Character(s)

Leak, leakage *(Continued)*
 device, implant or graft *(Continued)*
  catheter *(Continued)*
   urinary *(Continued)*
    nephrostomy T83.032
    specified NEC T83.038
    urostomy T83.038
  gastrointestinal —*see* Complications, prosthetic device, mechanical, gastrointestinal device
  genital NEC T83.498
   penile prosthesis (cylinder) (implanted) (pump) (reservoir) T83.490
   testicular prosthesis T83.491
  heart NEC —*see* Complication, cardiovascular device, mechanical
  joint prosthesis —*see* Complications, joint prosthesis, mechanical, specified NEC, by site
  ocular NEC —*see* Complications, prosthetic device, mechanical, ocular device
  orthopedic NEC —*see* Complication, orthopedic, device, mechanical
  persistent air J93.82
  specified NEC T85.638
  urinary NEC —*see also* Complication, genitourinary, device, urinary, mechanical
   graft T83.23
  vascular NEC —*see* Complication, cardiovascular device, mechanical
  ventricular intracranial shunt T85.03
 urine —*see* Incontinence
Leaky heart —*see* Endocarditis
Learning defect (specific) F81.9
Leather bottle stomach C16.9
Leber's
 congenital amaurosis H35.50
 optic atrophy (hereditary) H47.22
Lederer's anemia D59.19
Leeches (external) —*see* Hirudiniasis
Leg —*see* condition
Legg (-Calvé)-Perthes disease, syndrome or osteochondrosis M91.1-●
Legionellosis A48.1
 nonpneumonic A48.2
Legionnaires'
 disease A48.1
  nonpneumonic A48.2
 pneumonia A48.1
Leigh's disease G31.82
Leiner's disease L21.1
Leiofibromyoma —*see* Leiomyoma
Leiomyoblastoma —*see* Neoplasm, connective tissue, benign
Leiomyofibroma —*see also* Neoplasm, connective tissue, benign
 uterus (cervix) (corpus) D25.9
Leiomyoma —*see also* Neoplasm, connective tissue, benign
 bizarre —*see* Neoplasm, connective tissue, benign
 cellular —*see* Neoplasm, connective tissue, benign
 epithelioid —*see* Neoplasm, connective tissue, benign
 uterus (cervix) (corpus) D25.9
  intramural D25.1
  submucous D25.0
  subserosal D25.2
 vascular —*see* Neoplasm, connective tissue, benign
Leiomyoma, leiomyomatosis (intravascular) — *see* Neoplasm, connective tissue, uncertain behavior
Leiomyosarcoma —*see also* Neoplasm, connective tissue, malignant
 epithelioid —*see* Neoplasm, connective tissue, malignant
 myxoid —*see* Neoplasm, connective tissue, malignant
Leishmaniasis B55.9
 American (mucocutaneous) B55.2
  cutaneous B55.1
 Asian Desert B55.1
 Brazilian B55.2
 cutaneous (any type) B55.1
 dermal —*see also* Leishmaniasis, cutaneous
  post-kala-azar B55.0
 eyelid B55.1
 infantile B55.0

Leishmaniasis *(Continued)*
 Mediterranean B55.0
 mucocutaneous (American) (New World) B55.2
 naso-oral B55.2
 nasopharyngeal B55.2
 old world B55.1
 tegumentaria diffusa B55.1
 visceral B55.0
Leishmanoid, dermal —*see also* Leishmaniasis, cutaneous
 post-kala-azar B55.0
Lenegre's disease I44.2
Lengthening, leg —*see* Deformity, limb, unequal length
Lennert's lymphoma —*see* Lymphoma, Lennert's
Lennox-Gastaut syndrome G40.812
 intractable G40.814
  with status epilepticus G40.813
  without status epilepticus G40.814
 not intractable G40.812
  with status epilepticus G40.811
  without status epilepticus G40.812
Lens —*see* condition
Lenticonus (anterior) (posterior) (congenital) Q12.8
Lenticular degeneration, progressive E83.01
Lentiglobus (posterior) (congenital) Q12.8
Lentigo (congenital) L81.4
 maligna —*see also* Melanoma, in situ
  melanoma —*see* Melanoma
Lentivirus, as cause of disease classified elsewhere B97.31
Leontiasis
 ossium M85.2
 syphilitic (late) A52.78
  congenital A50.59
Lepothrix A48.8
Lepra —*see* Leprosy
Leprechaunism E34.8
Leprosy A30.-●
 with muscle disorder A30.9 *[M63.80]*
  ankle A30.9 *[M63.87-●]*
  foot A30.9 *[M63.87-●]*
  forearm A30.9 *[M63.83-●]*
  hand A30.9 *[M63.84-●]*
  lower leg A30.9 *[M63.86-●]*
  multiple sites A30.9 *[M63.89]*
  pelvic region A30.9 *[M63.85-●]*
  shoulder region A30.9 *[M63.81-●]*
  specified site NEC A30.9 *[M63.88]*
  thigh A30.9 *[M63.85-●]*
  upper arm A30.9 *[M63.82-●]*
 anesthetic A30.9
 BB A30.3
 BL A30.4
 borderline (infiltrated) (neuritic) A30.3
  lepromatous A30.4
  tuberculoid A30.2
 BT A30.2
 dimorphous (infiltrated) (neuritic) A30.3
 I A30.0
 indeterminate (macular) (neuritic) A30.0
 lepromatous (diffuse) (infiltrated) (macular) (neuritic) (nodular) A30.5
 LL A30.5
 macular (early) (neuritic) (simple) A30.9
 maculoanesthetic A30.9
 mixed A30.3
 neural A30.9
 nodular A30.5
 primary neuritic A30.3
 specified type NEC A30.8
 TT A30.1
 tuberculoid (major) (minor) A30.1
Leptocytosis, hereditary D56.9
Leptomeningitis (chronic) (circumscribed) (hemorrhagic) (nonsuppurative) —*see* Meningitis
Leptomeningopathy G96.198
Leptospiral —*see* condition
Leptospirochetal —*see* condition
Leptospirosis A27.9
 canicola A27.89
 due to Leptospira interrogans serovar icterohaemorrhagiae A27.0
 icterohemorrhagica A27.0
 pomona A27.89
 Weil's disease A27.0
Leptus dermatitis B88.0
Leriche's syndrome (aortic bifurcation occlusion) I74.09
Leri's pleonosteosis Q78.8

Leri-Weill syndrome Q77.8
Lermoyez' syndrome —*see* Vertigo, peripheral NEC
Lesch-Nyhan syndrome E79.1
Leser-Trélat disease L82.1
 inflamed L82.0
Lesion(s) (nontraumatic)
 abducens nerve —*see* Strabismus, paralytic, sixth nerve
 alveolar process K08.9
 angiocentric immunoproliferative D47.Z9
 anorectal K62.9
 aortic (valve) I35.9
 auditory nerve —*see* subcategory H93.3
 basal ganglion G25.9
 bile duct —*see* Disease, bile duct
 biomechanical M99.9
  specified type NEC M99.89
   abdomen M99.89
   acromioclavicular M99.87
   cervical region M99.81
   cervicothoracic M99.81
   costochondral M99.88
   costovertebral M99.88
   head region M99.80
   hip M99.85
   lower extremity M99.86
   lumbar region M99.83
   lumbosacral M99.83
   occipitocervical M99.80
   pelvic region M99.85
   pubic M99.85
   rib cage M99.88
   sacral region M99.84
   sacrococcygeal M99.84
   sacroiliac M99.84
   specified NEC M99.89
   sternochondral M99.88
   sternoclavicular M99.87
   thoracic region M99.82
   thoracolumbar M99.82
   upper extremity M99.87
 bladder N32.9
 bone —*see* Disorder, bone
 brachial plexus G54.0
 brain G93.9
  congenital Q04.9
  vascular I67.9
   degenerative I67.9
   hypertensive I67.4
 buccal cavity K13.79
 calcified —*see* Calcification
 cameron —*see* Ulcer, stomach
 canthus —*see* Disorder, eyelid
 carate —*see* Pinta, lesions
 cardia K31.9
 cardiac —*see also* Disease, heart I51.9
  congenital Q24.9
  valvular —*see* Endocarditis
 cauda equina G83.4
 cecum K63.9
 cerebral —*see* Lesion, brain
 cerebrovascular I67.9
  degenerative I67.9
  hypertensive I67.4
 cervical (nerve) root NEC G54.2
 chiasmal —*see* Disorder, optic, chiasm
 chorda tympani G51.8
 coin, lung R91.1
 colon K63.9
 combined periodontic - endodontic K05.5
 congenital —*see* Anomaly, by site
 conjunctiva H11.9
 conus medullaris —*see* Injury, conus medullaris
 coronary artery —*see* Ischemia, heart
 cranial nerve G52.9
  eighth —*see* Disorder, ear
  eleventh G52.9
  fifth G50.9
  first G52.0
  fourth —*see* Strabismus, paralytic, fourth nerve
  seventh G51.9
  sixth —*see* Strabismus, paralytic, sixth nerve
  tenth G52.2
  twelfth G52.3
 cystic —*see* Cyst
 degenerative —*see* Degeneration
 duodenum K31.9

Lesion *(Continued)*
  edentulous (alveolar) ridge, associated with
      trauma, due to traumatic occlusion K06.2
  en coup de sabre L94.1
  eyelid —*see* Disorder, eyelid
  gasserian ganglion G50.8
  gastric K31.9
  gastroduodenal K31.9
  gastrointestinal K63.9
  gingiva, associated with trauma K06.2
  glomerular
    focal and segmental —*see also* N00-N07 with
      fourth character .1 N05.1
    minimal change —*see also* N00-N07 with
      fourth character .0 N05.0
  heart (organic) —*see* Disease, heart
  hyperchromic, due to pinta (carate) A67.1
  hyperkeratotic —*see* Hyperkeratosis
  hypothalamic E23.7
  ileocecal K63.9
  ileum K63.9
  iliohypogastric nerve G57.8-●
  inflammatory —*see* Inflammation
  intestine K63.9
  intracerebral —*see* Lesion, brain
  intrachiasmal (optic) —*see* Disorder, optic,
    chiasm
  intracranial, space-occupying R90.0
  joint —*see* Disorder, joint
    sacroiliac (old) M53.3
  keratotic —*see* Keratosis
  kidney —*see* Disease, renal
  laryngeal nerve (recurrent) G52.2
  lip K13.0
  liver K76.9
  lumbosacral
    plexus G54.1
    root (nerve) NEC G54.4
  lung (coin) R91.1
  maxillary sinus J32.0
  mitral I05.9
  Morel-Lavallée —*see* Hematoma,
    by site
  motor cortex NEC G93.89
  mouth K13.79
  nerve G58.9
    femoral G57.2-●
    median G56.1-●
      carpal tunnel syndrome —*see* Syndrome,
        carpal tunnel
    plantar G57.6-●
    popliteal (lateral) G57.3-●
      medial G57.4-●
    radial G56.3-●
    sciatic G57.0-●
    spinal —*see* Injury, nerve, spinal
    ulnar G56.2-●
  nervous system, congenital Q07.9
  nonallopathic —*see* Lesion, biomechanical
  nose (internal) J34.89
  obstructive —*see* Obstruction
  obturator nerve G57.8-●
  oral mucosa K13.70
  organ or site NEC —*see* Disease, by site
  osteolytic —*see* Osteolysis
  peptic K27.9
  periodontal, due to traumatic occlusion K05.5
  pharynx J39.2
  pigment, pigmented (skin) L81.9
  pinta —*see* Pinta, lesions
  polypoid —*see* Polyp
  prechiasmal (optic) —*see* Disorder, optic, chiasm
  primary —*see also* Syphilis, primary A51.0
    carate A67.0
    pinta A67.0
    yaws A66.0
  pulmonary J98.4
    valve I37.9
  pylorus K31.9
  rectosigmoid K63.9
  retina, retinal H35.9
  sacroiliac (joint) (old) M53.3
  salivary gland K11.9
    benign lymphoepithelial K11.8
  saphenous nerve G57.8-●
  sciatic nerve G57.0-●
  secondary —*see* Syphilis, secondary
  shoulder (region) M75.9-●
    specified NEC M75.8-●
  sigmoid K63.9
  sinus (accessory) (nasal) J34.89

Lesion *(Continued)*
  skin L98.9
    suppurative L08.0
  SLAP S43.43-●
  spinal cord G95.9
    congenital Q06.9
  spleen D73.89
  stomach K31.9
  superior glenoid labrum S43.43-●
  syphilitic —*see* Syphilis
  tertiary —*see* Syphilis, tertiary
  thoracic root (nerve) NEC G54.3
  tonsillar fossa J35.9
  tooth, teeth K08.9
    white spot
      chewing surface K02.51
      pit and fissure surface K02.51
      smooth surface K02.61
  traumatic —*see* specific type of injury by site
  tricuspid (valve) I07.9
    nonrheumatic I36.9
  trigeminal nerve G50.9
  ulcerated or ulcerative —*see* Ulcer, skin
  uterus N85.9
  vagina N89.8
  vulva N90.89
  vagus nerve G52.2
  valvular —*see* Endocarditis
  vascular I99.9
    affecting central nervous system I67.9
    following trauma NEC T14.8
    umbilical cord, complicating delivery O69.5
  warty —*see* Verruca
  white spot (tooth)
    chewing surface K02.51
    pit and fissure surface K02.51
    smooth surface K02.61
Less than a high school diploma Z55.5
Lethargic —*see* condition
Lethargy R53.83
Letterer-Siwe's disease C96.0
Leukemia, leukemic C95.9-●
  acute basophilic C94.8-●
  acute bilineal C95.0-●
  acute erythroid C94.0-●
  acute lymphoblastic C91.0-●
  acute megakaryoblastic C94.2-●
  acute megakaryocytic C94.2-●
  acute mixed lineage C95.0-●
  acute monoblastic (monoblastic/monocytic)
    C93.0-●
  acute monocytic (monoblastic/monocytic)
    C93.0-●
  acute myeloblastic (minimal differentiation)
    (with maturation) C92.0-●
  acute myeloid, NOS C92.0-●
    with
      11q23-abnormality C92.6-●
      dysplasia of remaining hematopoesis and/
        or myelodysplastic disease in its
        history C92.A-●
      multilineage dysplasia C92.A-●
      variation of MLL-gene C92.6-●
    M6 (a)(b) C94.0-●
    M7 C94.2-●
  acute myelomonocytic C92.5-●
  acute promyelocytic C92.4-●
  adult T-cell (HTLV-1-associated) (acute variant)
    (chronic variant) (lymphomatoid variant)
    (smouldering variant) C91.5-●
  aggressive NK-cell C94.8-●
  AML (1/ETO) (M0) (M1) (M2) (without a FAB
    classification) C92.0-●
  AML M3 C92.4-●
  AML M4 (Eo with inv(16) or t(16;16)) C92.5-●
  AML M5 C93.0-●
  AML M5a C93.0-●
  AML M5b C93.0-●
  AML Me with t (15;17) and variants C92.4-●
  atypical chronic myeloid, BCR/ABL-negative
    C92.2-●
  biphenotypic acute C95.0-●
  blast cell C95.0-●
  Burkitt-type, mature B-cell C91.A-●
  chronic eosinophilic (*see also* Syndrome,
    hypereosinophilic, myeloid) C94.8-●
  chronic lymphocytic, of B-cell type C91.1-●
  chronic monocytic C93.1-●
  chronic myelogenous (Philadelphia chromosome
    (Ph1) positive) (t(9;22)) (q34;q11) (with crisis
    of blast cells) C92.1-●

Leukemia, leukemic *(Continued)*
  chronic myeloid, BCR/ABL-positive C92.1-●
    atypical, BCR/ABL-negative C92.2-●
  chronic myelomonocytic C93.1-●
  chronic neutrophilic D47.1
  CMML (-1) (-2) (with eosinophilia) C93.1-●
  granulocytic —*see also* Category C92 C92.9-●
  hairy-cell C91.4-●
  juvenile myelomonocytic C93.3-●
  lymphoid C91.9-●
    specified NEC C91.Z-●
  mast cell C94.3-●
  mature B-cell, Burkitt-type C91.A-●
  monocytic (subacute) C93.9-●
    specified NEC C93.Z-●
  myelogenous —*see also* Category
    C92 C92.9-●
  myeloid C92.9-●
    specified NEC C92.Z-●
  plasma cell C90.1-●
  plasmacytic C90.1-●
  prolymphocytic
    of B-cell type C91.3-●
    of T-cell type C91.6-●
  specified NEC C94.8-●
  stem cell, of unclear lineage C95.0-●
  subacute lymphocytic C91.9-●
  T-cell large granular lymphocytic C91.Z-●
  unspecified cell type C95.9-●
    acute C95.0-●
    chronic C95.1-●
Leukemoid reaction —*see also* Reaction, leukemoid
  D72.823-●
Leukoaraiosis (hypertensive) I67.81
Leukoariosis —*see* Leukoaraiosis
Leukocoria —*see* Disorder, globe, degenerated
  condition, leucocoria
Leukocytopenia D72.819
Leukocytosis D72.829
  eosinophilic D72.19
Leukoderma, leukodermia NEC L81.5
  syphilitic A51.39
    late A52.79
Leukodystrophy G31.80
Leukoedema, oral epithelium K13.29
Leukoencephalitis G04.81
  with vanishing white matter disease G11.6
  acute (subacute) hemorrhagic G36.1
    postimmunization or postvaccinal G04.02
  LMNB1-related autosomal dominant G90.B
  metachromatic E75.25
  pol III-related G11.5
  postinfectious G04.01
  subacute sclerosing A81.1
  van Bogaert's (sclerosing) A81.1
Leukoencephalopathy —*see also* Encephalopathy
  G93.49
  with calcifications and cysts G93.43
  adult-onset, with axonal spheroids (and
    pigmented glia) G93.44
  Binswanger's I67.3
  heroin vapor G92.8
  ~~megaloencephalic, with subcortical cysts G93.42~~
  ▶ megalencephalic , with subcortical cysts
    G93.42
  metachromatic E75.25
  multifocal (progressive) A81.2
  postimmunization and postvaccinal G04.02
  progressive multifocal A81.2
  reversible, posterior G93.6
  van Bogaert's (sclerosing) A81.1
  vascular, progressive I67.3
Leukoerythroblastosis D75.9
Leukokeratosis —*see also* Leukoplakia
  mouth K13.21
  nicotina palati K13.24
  oral mucosa K13.21
  tongue K13.21
  vocal cord J38.3
Leukokraurosis vulva (e) N90.4
Leukoma (cornea) —*see also* Opacity, cornea
  adherent H17.0-●
  interfering with central vision —*see* Opacity,
    cornea, central
Leukomalacia, cerebral, newborn P91.2
  periventricular P91.2
Leukomelanopathy, hereditary D72.0
Leukonychia (punctata) (striata) L60.8
  congenital Q84.4
Leukopathia unguium L60.8
  congenital Q84.4

▶ New   ⇒ Revised   ~~deleted~~ Deleted   ● Use Additional Character(s)

Leukopenia D72.819
  basophilic D72.818
  chemotherapy (cancer) induced D70.1
  congenital D70.0
  cyclic D70.0
  drug induced NEC D70.2
    due to cytoreductive cancer chemotherapy
      D70.1
  eosinophilic D72.818
  familial D70.0
  infantile genetic D70.0
  malignant D70.9
  periodic D70.0
  transitory neonatal P61.5
Leukopenic —see condition
Leukoplakia
  anus K62.89
  bladder (postinfectional) N32.89
  buccal K13.21
  cervix (uteri) N88.0
  esophagus K22.89
  gingiva K13.21
  hairy (oral mucosa) (tongue) K13.3
  kidney (pelvis) N28.89
  larynx J38.7
  lip K13.21
  mouth K13.21
  oral epithelium, including tongue (mucosa)
    K13.21
  palate K13.21
  pelvis (kidney) N28.89
  penis (infectional) N48.0
  rectum K62.89
  syphilitic (late) A52.79
  tongue K13.21
  ureter (postinfectional) N28.89
  urethra (postinfectional) N36.8
  uterus N85.8
  vagina N89.4
  vocal cord J38.3
  vulva N90.4
Leukorrhea N89.8
  due to Trichomonas (vaginalis) A59.00
  trichomonal A59.00
Leukosarcoma C85.9
Levocardia (isolated) Q24.1
  with situs inversus Q89.3
Levotransposition Q20.5
Lev's disease or syndrome (acquired complete
    heart block) I44.2
Levulosuria —see Fructosuria
Levurid L30.2
Lewy body (ies) (disease) G31.83
Leyden-Möbius dystrophy —see Dystrophy,
    Leyden-Möbius
Leydig cell
  carcinoma
    specified site —see Neoplasm, malignant, by
      site
    unspecified site
      female C56.9-●
      male C62.9-●
  tumor
    benign
      specified site —see Neoplasm, benign, by
        site
      unspecified site
        female D27.-●
        male D29.2-●
    malignant
      specified site —see Neoplasm, malignant,
        by site
      unspecified site
        female C56.-●
        male C62.9-●
    specified site —see Neoplasm, uncertain
        behavior, by site
    unspecified site
      female D39.1-●
      male D40.1-●
Leydig-Sertoli cell tumor
  specified site —see Neoplasm, benign, by site
  unspecified site
    female D27.-●
    male D29.2-●
LGMD —see Dystrophy, muscular, limb-girdle
LGSIL (Low grade squamous intraepithelial lesion
    on cytologic smear of)
  anus R85.612
  cervix R87.612
  vagina R87.622

Liar, pathologic F60.2
Libido
  decreased R68.82
Libman-Sacks disease M32.11
Lice (infestation) B85.2
  body (Pediculus corporis) B85.1
  crab B85.3
  head (Pediculus capitis) B85.0
  mixed (classifiable to more than one of the titles
    B85.0-B85.3) B85.4
  pubic (Phthirus pubis) B85.3
Lichen L28.0
  albus L90.0
    penis N48.0
    vulva N90.4
  amyloidosis E85.4 [L99]
  atrophicus L90.0
    penis N48.0
    vulva N90.4
  congenital Q82.8
  myxedematosus L98.5
  nitidus L44.1
  pilaris Q82.8
    acquired L85.8
  planopilaris L66.10
    classic L66.11
    follicular L66.11
    specified NEC L66.19
  planus (chronicus) L43.9
    annularis L43.8
    bullous L43.1
    follicular L66.11
    hypertrophic L43.0
    moniliformis L44.3
    of Wilson L43.9
    specified NEC L43.8
    subacute (active) L43.3
    tropicus L43.3
  ruber
    acuminatus L44.0
    moniliformis L44.3
    planus L43.9
  sclerosus (et atrophicus) L90.0
    penis N48.0
    vulva N90.4
  scrofulosus (primary) (tuberculous) A18.4
  simplex (chronicus) (circumscriptus) L28.0
  striatus L44.2
  urticatus L28.2
Lichenification L28.0
Lichenoid keratosis —see Keratosis, lichenoid
Lichenoides tuberculosis (primary) A18.4
Lichtheim's disease or syndrome D51.0
Lien migrans D73.89
Ligament —see condition
Light
  for gestational age —see Light for dates
  headedness R42
Light-for-dates (infant) P05.00
  with weight of
    499 grams or less P05.01
    500-749 grams P05.02
    750-999 grams P05.03
    1000-1249 grams P05.04
    1250-1499 grams P05.05
    1500-1749 grams P05.06
    1750-1999 grams P05.07
    2000-2499 grams P05.08
    2500 grams and over P05.09
  affecting management of pregnancy O36.59-●
  and small-for-dates —see Small for dates
  specified NEC P05.09
Lightning (effects) (stroke) (struck by) T75.00
  burn —see Burn
  foot E53.8
  shock T75.01
  specified effect NEC T75.09
Lightwood-Albright syndrome N25.89
Lightwood's disease or syndrome (renal tubular
    acidosis) N25.89
Lignac (-de Toni) (-Fanconi) (-Debré) disease or
    syndrome E72.09
  with cystinosis E72.04
Ligneous thyroiditis E06.5
Likoff's syndrome I20.89
Limb —see condition
Limbic epilepsy personality syndrome
    F07.0
Limitation, limited
  activities due to disability Z73.6
  cardiac reserve —see Disease, heart

Limitation, limited (Continued)
  eye muscle duction, traumatic —see Strabismus,
    mechanical
  mandibular range of motion M26.52
Lindau (-von Hippel) disease Q85.83
Line(s)
  Beau's L60.4
  Harris' —see Arrest, epiphyseal
  Hudson's (cornea) —see Pigmentation, cornea,
    anterior
  Stähli's (cornea) —see Pigmentation, cornea,
    anterior
Linea corneae senilis —see Change, cornea, senile
Lingua
  geographica K14.1
  nigra (villosa) K14.3
  plicata K14.5
  tylosis K13.29
Lingual —see condition
Linguatulosis B88.8
Linitis (gastric) plastica C16.9
Lip —see condition
Lipedema —see Edema
Lipemia —see also Hyperlipidemia
  retina, retinalis E78.3
Lipidosis E75.6
  cerebral (infantile) (juvenile) (late) E75.4
  cerebroretinal E75.4
  cerebroside E75.22
  cholesterol (cerebral) E75.5
  glycolipid E75.21
  hepatosplenomegalic E78.3
  sphingomyelin —see Niemann-Pick disease or
    syndrome
  sulfatide E75.29
Lipoadenoma —see Neoplasm, benign, by site
Lipoblastoma —see Lipoma
Lipoblastomatosis —see Lipoma
Lipochondrodystrophy E76.01
Lipochrome histiocytosis (familial) D71
Lipodermatosclerosis —(see also Insufficiency,
    venous) M79.3
  with
    varicose veins - see Varix, leg, with,
      inflammation
    ulcerated - see Varix, leg, with, ulcer, with
      inflammation by site
  ulcerated —see Ulcer, by site
Lipodystrophia progressiva E88.1
Lipodystrophy (progressive) E88.1
  insulin E88.1
  intestinal K90.81
  mesenteric K65.4
Lipofibroma —see Lipoma
Lipofuscinosis, neuronal (with ceroidosis) E75.4
Lipogranuloma, sclerosing L92.8
Lipogranulomatosis E78.89
Lipoid —see also condition
  histiocytosis D76.3
    essential E75.29
  nephrosis N04.9
  proteinosis of Urbach E78.89
Lipoidemia —see Hyperlipidemia
Lipoidosis —see Lipidosis
Lipoma D17.9
  fetal D17.9
    fat cell D17.9
  infiltrating D17.9
  intramuscular D17.9
  pleomorphic D17.9
  site classification
    arms (skin) (subcutaneous) D17.2-●
    connective tissue D17.30
      intra-abdominal D17.5
      intrathoracic D17.4
      peritoneum D17.79
      retroperitoneum D17.79
      specified site NEC D17.39
      spermatic cord D17.6
    face (skin) (subcutaneous) D17.0
    genitourinary organ NEC D17.72
    head (skin) (subcutaneous) D17.0
    intra-abdominal D17.5
    intrathoracic D17.4
    kidney D17.71
    legs (skin) (subcutaneous) D17.2-●
    neck (skin) (subcutaneous) D17.0
    peritoneum D17.79
    retroperitoneum D17.79
    skin D17.30
      specified site NEC D17.39

▶ New   ⇒ Revised   ~~deleted~~ Deleted   ● Use Additional Character(s)

Lyme disease A69.20
Lymph
  gland or node —*see* condition
  scrotum —*see* Infestation, filarial
Lymphadenitis I88.9
  with ectopic or molar pregnancy O08.0
  acute L04.9
    axilla L04.2
    face L04.0
    head L04.0
    hip L04.3
    limb
      lower L04.3
      upper L04.2
    neck L04.0
    shoulder L04.2
    specified site NEC L04.8
    trunk L04.1
  anthracosis (occupational) J60
  any site, except mesenteric I88.9
    chronic I88.1
    subacute I88.1
  breast
    gestational —*see* Mastitis, obstetric
    puerperal, postpartum (nonpurulent) O91.22
  chancroidal (congenital) A57
  chronic I88.1
    mesenteric I88.0
  due to
    Brugia (malayi) B74.1
      timori B74.2
    chlamydial lymphogranuloma A55
    diphtheria (toxin) A36.89
    lymphogranuloma venereum A55
    Wuchereria bancrofti B74.0
  following ectopic or molar pregnancy O08.0
  gonorrheal A54.89
  infective —*see* Lymphadenitis, acute
  mesenteric (acute) (chronic) (nonspecific)
      (subacute) I88.0
    due to Salmonella typhi A01.09
    tuberculous A18.39
  mycobacterial A31.8
  purulent —*see* Lymphadenitis, acute
  pyogenic —*see* Lymphadenitis, acute
  regional, nonbacterial I88.8
  septic —*see* Lymphadenitis, acute
  subacute, unspecified site I88.1
  suppurative —*see* Lymphadenitis, acute
  syphilitic (early) (secondary) A51.49
    late A52.79
  tuberculous —*see* Tuberculosis, lymph gland
  venereal (chlamydial) A55
Lymphadenoid goiter E06.3
Lymphadenopathy (generalized) R59.1
  angioimmunoblastic, with dysproteinemia
      (AILD) C86.5-●
  due to toxoplasmosis (acquired) B58.89
    congenital (acute) (subacute) (chronic) P37.1
  localized R59.0
  syphilitic (early) (secondary) A51.49
Lymphadenosis R59.1
Lymphangiectasis I89.0
  conjunctiva H11.89
  postinfectional I89.0
  scrotum I89.0
Lymphangiectatic elephantiasis, nonfilarial I89.0
Lymphangioendothelioma D18.1
  malignant —*see* Neoplasm, connective tissue,
      malignant
Lymphangioleiomyomatosis J84.81
Lymphangioma D18.1
  capillary D18.1
  cavernous D18.1
  cystic D18.1
  malignant —*see* Neoplasm, connective tissue,
      malignant
Lymphangiomyoma D18.1
Lymphangiomyomatosis J84.81
Lymphangiosarcoma —*see* Neoplasm, connective
    tissue, malignant
Lymphangitis I89.1
  with
    abscess - code by site under Abscess
    cellulitis - code by site under Cellulitis
    ectopic or molar pregnancy O08.0
  acute L03.91
    abdominal wall L03.321
    ankle —*see* Lymphangitis, acute, lower limb
    arm —*see* Lymphangitis, acute, upper limb
    auricle (ear) —*see* Lymphangitis, acute, ear

Lymphangitis (*Continued*)
  acute (*Continued*)
    axilla L03.12-●
    back (any part) L03.322
    buttock L03.327
    cervical (meaning neck) L03.222
    cheek (external) L03.212
    chest wall L03.323
    digit
      finger —*see* Lymphangitis, acute, finger
      toe —*see* Lymphangitis, acute, toe
    ear (external) H60.1-●
    external auditory canal —*see* Lymphangitis,
        acute, ear
    eyelid —*see* Abscess, eyelid
    face NEC L03.212
    finger (intrathecal) (periosteal) (subcutaneous)
        (subcuticular) L03.02-●
    foot —*see* Lymphangitis, acute, lower limb
    gluteal (region) L03.327
    groin L03.324
    hand —*see* Lymphangitis, acute, upper limb
    head NEC L03.891
      face (any part, except ear, eye and nose)
          L03.212
    heel —*see* Lymphangitis, acute, lower limb
    hip —*see* Lymphangitis, acute, lower limb
    jaw (region) L03.212
    knee —*see* Lymphangitis, acute, lower limb
    leg —*see* Lymphangitis, acute, lower limb
    lower limb L03.12-●
      toe —*see* Lymphangitis, acute, toe
    navel L03.326
    neck (region) L03.222
    orbit, orbital —*see* Cellulitis, orbit
    pectoral (region) L03.323
    perineal, perineum L03.325
    scalp (any part) L03.891
    shoulder —*see* Lymphangitis, acute, upper
        limb
    specified site NEC L03.898
    thigh —*see* Lymphangitis, acute, lower limb
    thumb (intrathecal) (periosteal)
        (subcutaneous) (subcuticular) —*see*
        Lymphangitis, acute, finger
    toe (intrathecal) (periosteal) (subcutaneous)
        (subcuticular) L03.04-●
    trunk L03.329
      abdominal wall L03.321
      back (any part) L03.322
      buttock L03.327
      chest wall L03.323
      groin L03.324
      perineal, perineum L03.325
      umbilicus L03.326
    umbilicus L03.326
    upper limb L03.12-●
      axilla —*see* Lymphangitis, acute, axilla
      finger —*see* Lymphangitis, acute, finger
      thumb —*see* Lymphangitis, acute, finger
      wrist —*see* Lymphangitis, acute, upper
          limb
  breast
    gestational —*see* Mastitis, obstetric
  chancroidal A57
  chronic (any site) I89.1
  due to
    Brugia (malayi) B74.1
      timori B74.2
    Wuchereria bancrofti B74.0
  following ectopic or molar pregnancy
      O08.89
  penis
    acute N48.29
    gonococcal (acute) (chronic) A54.09
  puerperal, postpartum, childbirth O86.89
  strumous, tuberculous A18.2
  subacute (any site) I89.1
  tuberculous —*see* Tuberculosis, lymph gland
Lymphatic (vessel) —*see* condition
Lymphatism E32.8
Lymphectasia I89.0
Lymphedema (acquired) —*see also* Elephantiasis
  congenital Q82.0
  hereditary (chronic) (idiopathic) Q82.0
  postmastectomy I97.2
  praecox I89.0
  secondary I89.0
  surgical NEC I97.89
    postmastectomy (syndrome) I97.2
Lymphoblastic —*see* condition

Lymphoblastoma (diffuse) —*see* Lymphoma,
    lymphoblastic (diffuse)
  giant follicular —*see* Lymphoma, lymphoblastic
      (diffuse)
  macrofollicular —*see* Lymphoma, lymphoblastic
      (diffuse)
Lymphocele I89.8
Lymphocytic
  chorioencephalitis (acute) (serous) A87.2
  choriomeningitis (acute) (serous) A87.2
  meningoencephalitis A87.2
Lymphocytoma, benign cutis L98.8
Lymphocytopenia D72.810
Lymphocytosis (symptomatic) D72.820
  infectious (acute) B33.8
Lymphoepithelioma —*see* Neoplasm, malignant,
    by site
Lymphogranuloma (malignant) —*see also*
    Lymphoma, Hodgkin
  chlamydial A55
  inguinale A55
  venereum (any site) (chlamydial) (with stricture
      of rectum) A55
Lymphogranulomatosis (malignant) —*see also*
    Lymphoma, Hodgkin
  benign (Boeck's sarcoid) (Schaumann's) D86.1
Lymphohistiocytosis, hemophagocytic (familial)
    D76.1
Lymphoid —*see* condition
Lymphoma (of) (malignant) C85.90
  adult T-cell (HTLV-1-associated) (acute variant)
      (chronic variant) (lymphomatoid variant)
      (smouldering variant) C91.5-●
  anaplastic large cell
    ALK-negative C84.7-●
    ALK-positive C84.6-●
    breast implant associated (BIA-ALCL) C84.7A
    CD30-positive C84.6-●
    primary cutaneous C86.6-●
  angioimmunoblastic T-cell C86.5-●
  BALT C88.8-●
  B-cell C85.1-●
  B-precursor C83.5-●
  blastic NK-cell C86.4-●
  blastic plasmacytoid dendritic cell neoplasm
      (BPDCN) C86.4-●
  brain, primary —*see* Lymphoma, primary central
      nervous system
  bronchial-associated lymphoid tissue
      [BALT-lymphoma] C88.8-●
  Burkitt (atypical) C83.7-●
  Burkitt-like C83.7-●
  central nervous system, primary —*see*
      Lymphoma, primary central nervous
      system
  centrocytic C83.1-●
  cutaneous follicle center C82.6-●
  cutaneous T-cell C84.A-●
  diffuse follicle center C82.5-●
  diffuse large cell C83.3-●
    anaplastic C83.3-●
    B-cell C83.3-●
    CD30-positive C83.3-●
    centroblastic C83.3-●
  extranodal and solid organ sites NEC
      C83.398
    immunoblastic C83.3-●
    plasmablastic C83.3-●
  primary central nervous system (brain)
      (meninges) (PCNSL) (spinal cord)
      C83.390
    subtype not specified C83.3-●
    T-cell rich C83.3-●
  enteropathy-type (associated) (intestinal) T-cell
      C86.2-●
  extranodal marginal zone B-cell lymphoma of
      mucosa-associated lymphoid tissue
      [MALT-lymphoma] C88.4-●
  extranodal NK/T-cell, nasal type C86.0-●
  follicular C82.9-●
    grade
      I C82.0-●
      II C82.1-●
      III C82.2-●
      IIIa C82.3-●
      IIIb C82.4-●
      specified NEC C82.8-●
  hepatosplenic T-cell (alpha-beta) (gamma-delta)
      C86.1-●
  histiocytic C85.9-●
    true C96.A

Malaria, malarial (Continued)
    subtertian (fever) —see Malaria, falciparum
    tertian (benign) —see also Malaria, vivax
        malignant B50.9
    tropical B50.9
    typhoid B54
    vivax B51.9
        with
            complications NEC B51.8
            ruptured spleen B51.0
Malassez's disease (cystic) N50.89
Malassimilation K90.9
Mal de los pintos —see Pinta
Mal de mer T75.3
Maldescent, testis Q53.9
    bilateral Q53.20
        abdominal Q53.211
        perineal Q53.22
    unilateral Q53.10
        abdominal Q53.111
        perineal Q53.12
Maldevelopment —see also Anomaly
    brain Q07.9
    colon Q43.9
    hip Q74.2
        congenital dislocation Q65.2
            bilateral Q65.1
            unilateral Q65.0-●
    mastoid process Q75.8
    middle ear Q16.4
        except ossicles Q16.4
        ossicles Q16.3
    ossicles Q16.3
    spine Q76.49
    toe Q74.2
Male type pelvis Q74.2
    with disproportion (fetopelvic) O33.3
        causing obstructed labor O65.3
Malformation (congenital) —see also Anomaly
    adrenal gland Q89.1
    affecting multiple systems with skeletal changes
        NEC Q87.5
    alimentary tract Q45.9
        specified type NEC Q45.8
        upper Q40.9
            specified type NEC Q40.8
    aorta Q25.40
        absence Q25.41
        aneurysm, congenital Q25.43
        aplasia Q25.41
        atresia Q25.29
            aortic arch Q25.21
        coarctation (preductal) (postductal) Q25.1
        dilatation, congenital Q25.44
        hypoplasia Q25.42
        patent ductus arteriosus Q25.0
        specified type NEC Q25.49
        stenosis Q25.1
            supravalvular Q25.3
    aortic valve Q23.9
        ▥specified NEC Q23.88
    arteriovenous, aneurysmatic (congenital) Q27.30
        brain Q28.2
            ruptured I60.8
                intracerebral I61.8
                intraparenchymal I61.8
                intraventricular I61.5
                subarachnoid I60.8
        cerebral (see Malformation, arteriovenous,
            brain) Q28.2
        peripheral Q27.30
            congenital Q27.33
            digestive system —see Angiodysplasia
            lower limb Q27.32
            other specified site Q27.39
            renal vessel Q27.34
            upper limb Q27.31
        precerebral vessels (nonruptured) Q28.0
    auricle
        ear (congenital) Q17.3
            acquired H61.119
                left H61.112
                    with right H61.113
                right H61.111
                    with left H61.113
    bile duct Q44.5
    bladder Q64.79
        aplasia Q64.5
        diverticulum Q64.6
        exstrophy —see Exstrophy, bladder
        neck obstruction Q64.31

Malformation (Continued)
    bone Q79.9
        face Q75.9
            specified type NEC Q75.8
        skull Q75.9
            specified type NEC Q75.8
    brain (multiple) Q04.9
        arteriovenous Q28.2
        specified type NEC Q04.8
    branchial cleft Q18.2
    breast Q83.9
        specified type NEC Q83.8
    broad ligament Q50.6
    bronchus Q32.4
    bursa Q79.9
    cardiac
        chambers Q20.9
            specified type NEC Q20.8
        septum Q21.9
            specified type NEC Q21.8
    cerebral Q04.9
        vessels Q28.3
    cervix uteri Q51.9
        specified type NEC Q51.828
    Chiari
        Type I G93.5
        Type II Q07.01
    choroid (congenital) Q14.3
        plexus Q07.8
    circulatory system Q28.9
    cochlea Q16.5
    cornea Q13.4
    coronary vessels Q24.5
    corpus callosum (congenital) Q04.0
    diaphragm Q79.1
    digestive system NEC, specified type NEC
        Q45.8
    dura Q07.9
        brain Q04.9
        spinal Q06.9
    ear Q17.9
        causing impairment of hearing Q16.9
        external Q17.9
            accessory auricle Q17.0
            causing impairment of hearing Q16.9
                absence of
                    auditory canal Q16.1
                    auricle Q16.0
            macrotia Q17.1
            microtia Q17.2
            misplacement Q17.4
            misshapen NEC Q17.3
            prominence Q17.5
            specified type NEC Q17.8
        inner Q16.5
        middle Q16.4
            absence of eustachian tube Q16.2
            ossicles (fusion) Q16.3
        ossicles Q16.3
        specified type NEC Q17.8
    epididymis Q55.4
    esophagus Q39.9
        specified type NEC Q39.8
    eye Q15.9
        lid Q10.3
        specified NEC Q15.8
    fallopian tube Q50.6
    genital organ —see Anomaly, genitalia
    great
        artery Q25.9
            aorta —see Malformation, aorta
            pulmonary artery —see Malformation,
                pulmonary, artery
            specified type NEC Q25.8
        vein Q26.9
            anomalous
                portal venous connection Q26.5
                pulmonary venous connection Q26.4
                    partial Q26.3
                    total Q26.2
            persistent left superior vena cava Q26.1
            portal vein-hepatic artery fistula Q26.6
            specified type NEC Q26.8
            vena cava stenosis, congenital Q26.0
    gum Q38.6
    hair Q84.2
    heart Q24.9
        specified type NEC Q24.8
    integument Q84.9
        specified type NEC Q84.8
    internal ear Q16.5

Malformation (Continued)
    intestine Q43.9
        specified type NEC Q43.8
    iris Q13.2
    joint Q74.9
        ankle Q74.2
        lumbosacral Q76.49
        sacroiliac Q74.2
        specified type NEC Q74.8
    kidney Q63.9
        accessory Q63.0
        giant Q63.3
        horseshoe Q63.1
        hydronephrosis Q62.0
        malposition Q63.2
        specified type NEC Q63.8
    lacrimal apparatus Q10.6
    lingual Q38.3
    lip Q38.0
    liver Q44.70
    lung Q33.9
    meninges or membrane (congenital) Q07.9
        cerebral Q04.8
        spinal (cord) Q06.9
    middle ear Q16.4
        ossicles Q16.3
    mitral valve Q23.9
        ▥specified NEC Q23.88
    Mondini's (congenital) (malformation, cochlea)
        Q16.5
    mouth (congenital) Q38.6
    multiple types NEC Q89.7
    musculoskeletal system Q79.9
    myocardium Q24.8
    nail Q84.6
    nervous system (central) Q07.9
    nose Q30.9
        specified type NEC Q30.8
    optic disc Q14.2
    orbit Q10.7
    ovary Q50.39
    palate Q38.5
    parathyroid gland Q89.2
    pelvic organs or tissues NEC
        in pregnancy or childbirth O34.8-●
            causing obstructed labor O65.5
    penis Q55.69
        aplasia Q55.5
        curvature (lateral) Q55.61
        hypoplasia Q55.62
    pericardium Q24.8
    peripheral vascular system Q27.9
        specified type NEC Q27.8
    pharynx Q38.8
    precerebral vessels Q28.1
    prostate Q55.4
    pulmonary
        arteriovenous Q25.72
        artery Q25.9
            atresia Q25.5
            specified type NEC Q25.79
            stenosis Q25.6
        valve Q22.3
    renal artery Q27.2
    respiratory system Q34.9
    retina Q14.1
    scrotum —see Malformation, testis and scrotum
    seminal vesicles Q55.4
    sense organs NEC Q07.9
    skin Q82.9
    specified NEC Q89.8
    spinal
        cord Q06.9
        nerve root Q07.8
    spine Q76.49
        kyphosis —see Kyphosis, congenital
        lordosis —see Lordosis, congenital
    spleen Q89.09
    stomach Q40.3
        specified type NEC Q40.2
    teeth, tooth K00.9
    tendon Q79.9
    testis and scrotum Q55.20
        aplasia Q55.0
        hypoplasia Q55.1
        polyorchism Q55.21
        retractile testis Q55.22
        scrotal transposition Q55.23
        specified NEC Q55.29
    thorax, bony Q76.9
    throat Q38.8

▶ New   ➡ Revised   ~~deleted~~ Deleted   ● Use Additional Character(s)

Malformation (Continued)
  thyroid gland Q89.2
  tongue (congenital) Q38.3
    hypertrophy Q38.2
    tie Q38.1
  trachea Q32.1
  tricuspid valve Q22.9
    specified type NEC Q22.8
  umbilical cord NEC (complicating delivery)
    O69.89
  umbilicus Q89.9
  ureter Q62.8
    agenesis Q62.4
    duplication Q62.5
    malposition —see Malposition, congenital,
      ureter
    obstructive defect —see Defect, obstructive,
      ureter
    vesico-uretero-renal reflux Q62.7
  urethra Q64.79
    aplasia Q64.5
    duplication Q64.74
    posterior valves Q64.2
    prolapse Q64.71
    stricture Q64.32
  urinary system Q64.9
  uterus Q51.9
    specified type NEC Q51.818
  vagina Q52.4
  vascular system, peripheral Q27.9
  vas deferens Q55.4
    atresia Q55.3
  venous —see Anomaly, vein(s)
  vulva Q52.70
Malfunction —see also Dysfunction
  cardiac electronic device T82.119
    electrode T82.110
    pulse generator T82.111
    specified type NEC T82.118
  catheter device NEC T85.618
    cystostomy T83.010
    dialysis (renal) (vascular) T82.41
      intraperitoneal T85.611
    infusion NEC T82.514
      cranial (see also Complication(s), catheter,
        cranial infusion, mechanical)
        T85.690
      epidural (see also Complication(s), catheter,
        cranial infusion, mechanical)
        T85.690
      intrathecal (see also Complication(s),
        catheter, cranial infusion, mechanical)
        T85.690
      spinal (see also Complication(s), catheter,
        cranial infusion, mechanical) T85.690
      subarachnoid (see also Complication(s),
        catheter, cranial infusion, mechanical)
        T85.690
      subdural (see also Complication(s), catheter,
        cranial infusion, mechanical) T85.690
    urinary —see also Breakdown, device, catheter
      T83.018
  colostomy K94.03
    valve K94.03
  cystostomy (stoma) N99.512
    catheter T83.010
  enteric stoma K94.13
  enterostomy K94.13
  esophagostomy K94.33
  gastroenteric K31.89
  gastrostomy K94.23
  ileostomy K94.13
    valve K94.13
  intrathecal infusion pump T85.615
  jejunostomy K94.13
  nervous system device, implant or graft,
    specified NEC T85.615
  pacemaker —see Malfunction, cardiac electronic
    device
  prosthetic device, internal —see Complications,
    prosthetic device, by site, mechanical
  tracheostomy J95.03
  urinary device NEC —see Complication,
    genitourinary, device, urinary, mechanical
  valve
    colostomy K94.03
    heart T82.09
    ileostomy K94.13
  vascular graft or shunt NEC —see Complication,
    cardiovascular device, mechanical, vascular
  ventricular (communicating shunt) T85.01

Malherbe's tumor —see Neoplasm, skin, benign
Malibu disease L98.8-●
Malignancy —see also Neoplasm, malignant, by site
  unspecified site (primary) C80.1
Malignant —see condition
Malingerer, malingering Z76.5
Mallet finger (acquired) —see Deformity, finger,
  mallet finger
  congenital Q74.0
  sequelae of rickets E64.3
Malleus A24.0
Mallory's bodies R89.7
Mallory-Weiss syndrome K22.6
Malnutrition E46
  degree
    first E44.1
    mild (protein) E44.1
    moderate (protein) E44.0
    second E44.0
    severe (protein-energy) E43
    ▶with
      ▶kwashiorkor E40
      ▶marasmus E41
      intermediate form E42
        with
          kwashiorkor E42
          marasmus E41
    third E43
  following gastrointestinal surgery K91.2
  intrauterine
    light-for-dates —see Light for dates
    small-for-dates —see Small for dates
  lack of care, or neglect (child) (infant) T76.02
    confirmed T74.02
  malignant E40
  protein E46
    calorie E46
      mild E44.1
      moderate E44.0
      severe E43
      ▶with
        ▶kwashiorkor E40
        ▶marasmus E41
        intermediate form E42
          with
            kwashiorkor (and marasmus) E42
            marasmus E41
    energy E46
      mild E44.1
      moderate E44.0
      severe E43
      ▶with
        ▶kwashiorkor E40
        ▶marasmus E41
        intermediate form E42
          with
            kwashiorkor (and marasmus) E42
            marasmus E41
    severe (protein-energy) E43
      with
      ⏩kwashiorkor E40
        ▶with marasmus E42
        marasmus E41
    ▶intermediate form E42
      ▶with
        ▶kwashiorkor (and marasmus) E42
        ▶marasmus E41
Malocclusion (teeth) M26.4
  Angle's M26.219
    class I M26.211
    class II M26.212
    class III M26.213
  due to
    abnormal swallowing M26.59
    mouth breathing M26.59
    tongue, lip or finger habits M26.59
  temporomandibular (joint) M26.69
Malposition
  cervix —see Malposition, uterus
  congenital
    adrenal (gland) Q89.1
    alimentary tract Q45.8
      lower Q43.8
      upper Q40.8
    aorta Q25.49
    appendix Q43.8
    arterial trunk Q20.0
    artery (peripheral) Q27.8
      coronary Q24.5
      digestive system Q27.8
      lower limb Q27.8

Malposition (Continued)
  congenital (Continued)
    artery (Continued)
      pulmonary Q25.79
      specified site NEC Q27.8
      upper limb Q27.8
    auditory canal Q17.8
      causing impairment of hearing Q16.9
    auricle (ear) Q17.4
      causing impairment of hearing Q16.9
      cervical Q18.2
    biliary duct or passage Q44.5
    bladder (mucosa) —see Exstrophy, bladder
    brachial plexus Q07.8
    brain tissue Q04.8
    breast Q83.8
    bronchus Q32.4
    cecum Q43.8
    clavicle Q74.0
    colon Q43.8
    digestive organ or tract NEC Q45.8
      lower Q43.8
      upper Q40.8
    ear (auricle) (external) Q17.4
      ossicles Q16.3
    endocrine (gland) NEC Q89.2
    epiglottis Q31.8
    eustachian tube Q17.8
    eye Q15.8
    facial features Q18.8
    fallopian tube Q50.6
    finger(s) Q68.1
      supernumerary Q69.0
    foot Q66.9-●
    gallbladder Q44.1
    gastrointestinal tract Q45.8
    genitalia, genital organ(s) or tract
      female Q52.8
        external Q52.79
        internal NEC Q52.8
      male Q55.8
    glottis Q31.8
    hand Q68.1
    heart Q24.8
      dextrocardia Q24.0
        with complete transposition of viscera
          Q89.3
    hepatic duct Q44.5
    hip (joint) Q65.89
    intestine (large) (small) Q43.8
      with anomalous adhesions, fixation or
        malrotation Q43.3
    joint NEC Q68.8
    kidney Q63.2
    larynx Q31.8
    limb Q68.8
      lower Q68.8
      upper Q68.8
    liver Q44.79
    lung (lobe) Q33.8
    nail(s) Q84.6
    nerve Q07.8
    nervous system NEC Q07.8
    nose, nasal (septum) Q30.8
    organ or site not listed —see Anomaly, by site
    ovary Q50.39
    pancreas Q45.3
    parathyroid (gland) Q89.2
    patella Q74.1
    peripheral vascular system Q27.8
    pituitary (gland) Q89.2
    respiratory organ or system NEC Q34.8
    rib (cage) Q76.6
      supernumerary in cervical region Q76.5
    scapula Q74.0
    shoulder Q74.0
    spinal cord Q06.8
    spleen Q89.09
    sternum NEC Q76.7
    stomach Q40.2
    symphysis pubis Q74.2
    thymus (gland) Q89.2
    thyroid (gland) (tissue) Q89.2
      cartilage Q31.8
    toe(s) Q66.9-●
      supernumerary Q69.2
    tongue Q38.3
    trachea Q32.1
    ureter Q62.60
      deviation Q62.61
      displacement Q62.62

Malposition *(Continued)*
 congenital *(Continued)*
  ureter *(Continued)*
   ectopia Q62.63
   specified type NEC Q62.69
  uterus Q51.818
  vein(s) (peripheral) Q27.8
   great Q26.8
  vena cava (inferior) (superior) Q26.8
 device, implant or graft —*see also* Complications, by site and type, mechanical T85.628
  arterial graft NEC —*see* Complication, cardiovascular device, mechanical, vascular
  breast (implant) T85.42
  catheter NEC T85.628
   cystostomy T83.020
   dialysis (renal) T82.42
    intraperitoneal T85.621
   infusion NEC T82.524
    spinal (epidural) (subdural) T85.620
   urinary —*see also* Displacement, device, catheter, urinary T83.028
  electronic (electrode) (pulse generator) (stimulator)
   bone T84.320
   cardiac T82.129
    electrode T82.120
    pulse generator T82.121
    specified type NEC T82.128
   nervous system —*see* Complication, prosthetic device, mechanical, electronic nervous system stimulator
   urinary —*see* Complication, genitourinary, device, urinary, mechanical
  fixation, internal (orthopedic) NEC — *see* Complication, fixation device, mechanical
  gastrointestinal —*see* Complications, prosthetic device, mechanical, gastrointestinal device
  genital NEC T83.428
   intrauterine contraceptive device (string) T83.32
   penile prosthesis (cylinder) (implanted) (pump) (reservoir) T83.420
   testicular prosthesis T83.421
  heart NEC —*see* Complication, cardiovascular device, mechanical
  joint prosthesis —*see* Complication, joint prosthesis, mechanical
  ocular NEC —*see* Complications, prosthetic device, mechanical, ocular device
  orthopedic NEC —*see* Complication, orthopedic, device, mechanical
  specified NEC T85.628
  urinary NEC —*see also* Complication, genitourinary, device, urinary, mechanical
   graft T83.22
  vascular NEC —*see* Complication, cardiovascular device, mechanical
  ventricular intracranial shunt T85.02
 fetus —*see* Pregnancy, complicated by (management affected by), presentation, fetal
 gallbladder K82.8
 gastrointestinal tract, congenital Q45.8
 heart, congenital NEC Q24.8
 joint prosthesis —*see* Complications, joint prosthesis, mechanical, displacement, by site
 stomach K31.89
  congenital Q40.2
 tooth, teeth, fully erupted M26.30
 uterus (acute) (acquired) (adherent) (asymptomatic) (postinfectional) (postpartal, old) N85.4
  anteflexion or anteversion N85.4
   congenital Q51.818
  flexion N85.4
   lateral —*see* Lateroversion, uterus
  inversion N85.5
  lateral (flexion) (version) —*see* Lateroversion, uterus
  in pregnancy or childbirth — *see* subcategory O34.5
  retroflexion or retroversion —*see* Retroversion, uterus

Malposture R29.3
Malrotation
 cecum Q43.3
 colon Q43.3
 intestine Q43.3
 kidney Q63.2
Malta fever —*see* Brucellosis
Maltreatment
 adult
  abandonment
   confirmed T74.01
   suspected T76.01
  bullying
   confirmed T74.31
   suspected T76.31
  confirmed T74.91
  financial
   confirmed T74.A1
   suspected T76.A1
  history of Z91.419
  intimidation (through social media)
   confirmed T74.31
   suspected T76.31
  neglect
   confirmed T74.01
   suspected T76.01
  physical abuse
   confirmed T74.11
   suspected T76.11
  psychological abuse
   confirmed T74.31
   history of Z91.411
   suspected T76.31
  sexual abuse
   confirmed T74.21
   suspected T76.21
  suspected T76.91
  threatened abuse (harm) (physical violence) (sexual abuse)
   confirmed T74.31
   suspected T76.31
 child
  abandonment
   confirmed T74.02
   suspected T76.02
  bullying
   confirmed T74.32
   suspected T76.32
  confirmed T74.92
  financial
   confirmed T74.A2
   suspected T76.A2
  history of —*see* History, personal (of), abuse
  intimidation (through social media)
   confirmed T74.32
   suspected T76.32
  neglect
   confirmed T74.02
   history of —*see* History, personal (of), abuse
   suspected T76.02
  physical abuse
   confirmed T74.12
   history of —*see* History, personal (of), abuse
   suspected T76.12
  psychological abuse
   confirmed T74.32
   history of —*see* History, personal (of), abuse
   suspected T76.32
  sexual abuse
   confirmed T74.22
   history of —*see* History, personal (of), abuse
   suspected T76.22
  suspected T76.92
  threatened abuse (harm) (physical violence) (sexual abuse)
   confirmed T74.31
   suspected T76.31
 personal history of Z91.89
Maltworker's lung J67.4
Malunion, fracture —*see* Fracture, by site
Mammillitis N61.0
 puerperal, postpartum O91.02
Mammitis —*see* Mastitis
Mammogram (examination) Z12.39
 routine Z12.31
Mammoplasia N62

Management (of)
 bone conduction hearing device (implanted) Z45.320
 cardiac pacemaker NEC Z45.018
 cerebrospinal fluid drainage device Z45.41
 cochlear device (implanted) Z45.321
 contraceptive Z30.9
  specified NEC Z30.8
 implanted device Z45.9
  specified NEC Z45.89
 infusion pump Z45.1
 procreative Z31.9
  male factor infertility in female Z31.81
  specified NEC Z31.89
 prosthesis (external) —*see also* Fitting Z44.9
  implanted Z45.9
   specified NEC Z45.89
 renal dialysis catheter Z49.01
 vascular access device Z45.2
Mangled —*see* specified injury by site
Mania (monopolar) —*see also* Disorder, mood, manic episode
 with psychotic symptoms F30.2
 without psychotic symptoms F30.10
  mild F30.11
  moderate F30.12
  severe F30.13
 Bell's F30.8
 chronic (recurrent) F31.89
 hysterical F44.89
 puerperal F30.8
 recurrent F31.89
Manic depression F31.9
Manic-depressive insanity, psychosis, or syndrome —*see* Disorder, bipolar
Mannosidosis E77.1
Mansonelliasis, mansonellosis B74.4
Manson's
 disease B65.1
 schistosomiasis B65.1
Manual —*see* condition
Maple-bark-stripper's lung (disease) J67.6
Maple-syrup-urine disease E71.0
Marable's syndrome (celiac artery compression) I77.4
Marasmus E41
 due to malnutrition E41
 intestinal E41
 nutritional E41
 senile R54
 tuberculous NEC —*see* Tuberculosis
Marble
 bones Q78.2
 skin R23.8
Marburg virus disease A98.3
March
 fracture —*see* Fracture, traumatic, stress, by site
 hemoglobinuria D59.6
Marchesani (-Weill) **syndrome** Q87.0
Marchiafava (-Bignami) **syndrome or disease** G37.1
Marchiafava-Micheli syndrome D59.5
Marcus Gunn's syndrome Q07.8
Marfan syndrome —*see* Syndrome, Marfan
Marie-Bamberger disease —*see* Osteoarthropathy, hypertrophic, specified NEC
Marie-Charcot-Tooth neuropathic muscular atrophy G60.0
Marie's
 cerebellar ataxia (late-onset) G11.2
 disease or syndrome (acromegaly) E22.0
Marie-Strümpell arthritis, disease or spondylitis —*see* Spondylitis, ankylosing
Marion's disease (bladder neck obstruction) N32.0
Marital conflict Z63.0
Mark
 port wine Q82.5
 raspberry Q82.5
 strawberry Q82.5
 stretch L90.6
 tattoo L81.8
Marker heterochromatin —*see* Extra, marker chromosomes
Maroteaux-Lamy syndrome (mild) (severe) E76.29
Marrow (bone)
 arrest D61.9
 poor function D75.89
Marseilles fever A77.1
Marsh fever —*see* Malaria

Marshall's (hidrotic) ectodermal dysplasia
Q82.4
Marsh's disease (exophthalmic goiter) E05.00
with storm E05.01
Masculinization (female) with adrenal
hyperplasia E25.9
congenital E25.0
Masculinovoblastoma D27.-●
Masochism (sexual) F65.51
Mason's lung J62.8
Mass
abdominal R19.00
epigastric R19.06
generalized R19.07
left lower quadrant R19.04
left upper quadrant R19.02
periumbilic R19.05
right lower quadrant R19.03
right upper quadrant R19.01
specified site NEC R19.09
breast —*see also* Lump, breast N63.0
chest R22.2
cystic —*see* Cyst
ear H93.8-●
head R22.0
intra-abdominal (diffuse) (generalized) —*see*
Mass, abdominal
kidney N28.89
liver R16.0
localized (skin) R22.9
chest R22.2
head R22.0
limb
lower R22.4-●
upper R22.3-●
neck R22.1
trunk R22.2
lung R91.8
malignant —*see* Neoplasm, malignant, by
site
neck R22.1
pelvic (diffuse) (generalized) —*see* Mass,
abdominal
specified organ NEC —*see* Disease, by site
splenic R16.1
substernal thyroid —*see* Goiter
superficial (localized) R22.9
umbilical (diffuse) (generalized) R19.09
Massive —*see* condition
Mast cell
disease, systemic tissue D47.02
leukemia C94.3-●
neoplasm
malignant C96.20
specified type NEC C96.29
of uncertain behavior NEC D47.09
sarcoma C96.22
tumor D47.09
Mastalgia N64.4
Masters-Allen syndrome N83.8
Mastitis (acute) (diffuse) (nonpuerperal) (subacute)
N61.0
with abscess N61.1
chronic (cystic) —*see* Mastopathy, cystic
cystic (Schimmelbusch's type) —*see* Mastopathy,
cystic
fibrocystic —*see* Mastopathy, cystic
granulomatous N61.2-●
infective N61.0
newborn P39.0
interstitial, gestational or puerperal —*see*
Mastitis, obstetric
neonatal (noninfective) P83.4
infective P39.0
obstetric (interstitial) (nonpurulent)
associated with
lactation O91.23
pregnancy O91.21-●
puerperium O91.22
purulent
associated with
lactation O91.13
pregnancy O91.11-●
puerperium O91.12
periductal —*see* Ectasia, mammary duct
phlegmonous —*see* Mastopathy, cystic
plasma cell —*see* Ectasia, mammary duct
without abscess N61.0
Mastocytoma (extracutaneous) D47.09
malignant C96.29
solitary D47.01

Mastocytosis D47.09
aggressive systemic C96.21
cutaneous (diffuse) (maculopapular) D47.01
congenital Q82.2
of neonatal onset Q82.2
of newborn onset Q82.2
indolent systemic D47.02
isolated bone marrow D47.02
malignant C96.29
systemic (indolent) (smoldering)
with an associated hematological
non-mast cell lineage disease (SM-
AHNMD) D47.02
Mastodynia N64.4
Mastoid —*see* condition
Mastoidalgia —*see* subcategory H92.0
Mastoiditis (coalescent) (hemorrhagic)
(suppurative) H70.9-●
acute, subacute H70.00-●
complicated NEC H70.09-●
subperiosteal H70.01-●
chronic (necrotic) (recurrent) H70.1-●
in (due to)
infectious disease NEC B99 [H75.0-●]
parasitic disease NEC B89 [H75.0-●]
tuberculosis A18.03
petrositis —*see* Petrositis
postauricular fistula —*see* Fistula, postauricular
specified NEC H70.89-●
tuberculous A18.03
Mastopathy, mastopathia N64.9
chronica cystica —*see* Mastopathy, cystic
cystic (chronic) (diffuse) N60.1
with epithelial proliferation N60.3-●
diffuse cystic —*see* Mastopathy, cystic
~~estrogenic, oestrogenica N64.89~~
▶estrogenic, oestrogenica, oestrogenic N64.89
ovarian origin N64.89
Mastoplasia, mastoplastia N62
Masturbation (excessive) F98.8
Maternal care (for) —*see* Pregnancy (complicated
by) (management affected by)
Mathieu's disease (leptospiral jaundice) A27.0
Mauclaire's disease or osteochondrosis —*see*
Osteochondrosis, juvenile, hand, metacarpal
Maxcy's disease A75.2
Maxilla, maxillary —*see* condition
May (-Hegglin) anomaly or syndrome D72.0
McArdle (-Schmid)(-Pearson) disease
(glycogen storage) E74.04
McCune-Albright syndrome Q78.1
McQuarrie's syndrome (idiopathic familial
hypoglycemia) E16.2
ME/CFS (myalgic encephalomyelitis/chronic
fatigue syndrome) G93.32
Meadow's syndrome Q86.1
Measles (black) (hemorrhagic) (suppressed) B05.9
with
complications NEC B05.89
encephalitis B05.0
intestinal complications B05.4
keratitis (keratoconjunctivitis) B05.81
meningitis B05.1
otitis media B05.3
pneumonia B05.2
French —*see* Rubella
German —*see* Rubella
Liberty —*see* Rubella
Meatitis, urethral —*see* Urethritis
Meatus, meatal —*see* condition
Meat-wrappers' asthma J68.9
Meckel-Gruber syndrome Q61.9
Meckel's diverticulitis, diverticulum (displaced)
(hypertrophic) Q43.0
Meconium
ileus, newborn P76.0
in cystic fibrosis E84.11
meaning meconium plug (without cystic
fibrosis) P76.0
obstruction, newborn P76.0
due to fecaliths P76.0
in mucoviscidosis E84.11
peritonitis P78.0
plug syndrome (newborn) NEC P76.0
MED13L (mediator complex subunit 13L)
syndrome Q87.85
Median —*see also* condition
arcuate ligament syndrome I77.4
bar (prostate) (vesical orifice) —*see* Hyperplasia,
prostate
rhomboid glossitis K14.2

Mediastinal shift R93.89
Mediastinitis (acute) (chronic) J98.51
syphilitic A52.73
tuberculous A15.8
Mediastinopericarditis —*see also* Pericarditis
acute I30.9
adhesive I31.0
chronic I31.8
rheumatic I09.2
Mediastinum, mediastinal —*see* condition
Mediator complex subunit 13L (MED13L)
syndrome Q87.85
Medicine poisoning —*see* Table of Drugs and
Chemicals, by drug, poisoning
Mediterranean
fever —*see* Brucellosis
familial M04.1
tick A77.1
kala-azar B55.0
leishmaniasis B55.0
tick fever A77.1
Medulla —*see* condition
Medullary cystic kidney Q61.5
Medullated fibers
optic (nerve) Q14.8
retina Q14.1
Medulloblastoma
desmoplastic C71.6
specified site —*see* Neoplasm, malignant, by site
unspecified site C71.6
Medulloepithelioma —*see also* Neoplasm,
malignant, by site
teratoid —*see* Neoplasm, malignant, by site
Medullomyoblastoma
specified site —*see* Neoplasm, malignant, by site
unspecified site C71.6
Meekeren-Ehlers-Danlos syndrome —*see also*
Syndrome, Ehlers-Danlos Q79.6
Megacolon (acquired) (functional) (not
Hirschsprung's disease) (in) K59.39
Chagas' disease B57.32
congenital, congenitum (aganglionic) Q43.1
Hirschsprung's (disease) Q43.1
toxic NEC K59.31
~~due to Clostridium difficile~~
~~not specified as recurrent A04.72~~
~~recurrent A04.71~~
▶due to
▶Clostridioides difficile
▶not specified as recurrent A04.72
▶recurrent A04.71
▶Clostridium difficile
▶not specified as recurrent A04.72
▶recurrent A04.71
Megaesophagus (functional) K22.0
congenital Q39.5
in (due to) Chagas' disease B57.31
Megalencephaly Q04.5
Megalerythema (epidemic) B08.3
Megaloappendix Q43.8
Megalocephalus, megalocephaly NEC Q75.3
Megalocornea Q15.8
with glaucoma Q15.0
Megalocytic anemia D53.1
Megalodactylia (fingers) (thumbs) (congenital)
Q74.0
toes Q74.2
Megaloduodenum Q43.8
Megaloesophagus (functional) K22.0
congenital Q39.5
Megalogastria (acquired) K31.89
congenital Q40.2
Megalophthalmos Q11.3
Megalopsia H53.15
Megalosplenia —*see* Splenomegaly
Megaloureter N28.82
congenital Q62.2
Megarectum K62.89
Megasigmoid K59.39
congenital Q43.2
Megaureter N28.82
congenital Q62.2
Megavitamin-B6 syndrome E67.2
Megrim —*see* Migraine
Meibomian
cyst, infected —*see* Hordeolum
gland —*see* condition
sty, stye —*see* Hordeolum
Meibomitis —*see* Hordeolum
Meige-Milroy disease (chronic hereditary edema)
Q82.0

Meige's syndrome Q82.0
Melalgia, nutritional E53.8
Melancholia F32.A
  climacteric (single episode) F32.89
    recurrent episode F33.8
  hypochondriac F45.29
  intermittent (single episode) F32.89
    recurrent episode F33.8
  involutional (single episode) F32.89
    recurrent episode F33.8
  menopausal (single episode) F32.89
    recurrent episode F33.8
  puerperal F32.89
  reactive (emotional stress or trauma) F32.3
  recurrent F33.9
  senile F03
  stuporous (single episode) F32.89
    recurrent episode F33.8
Melanemia R79.89
Melanoameloblastoma —see Neoplasm, bone,
    benign
Melanoblastoma —see Melanoma
Melanocarcinoma —see Melanoma
Melanocytoma, eyeball D31.9-●
Melanocytosis, neurocutaneous Q82.8
Melanoderma, melanodermia L81.4
Melanodontia, infantile K03.89
Melanodontoclasia K03.89
Melanoepithelioma —see Melanoma
Melanoma (malignant) C43.9
  acral lentiginous, malignant —see Melanoma,
    skin, by site
  amelanotic —see Melanoma, skin, by site
  balloon cell —see Melanoma, skin, by site
  benign —see Nevus
  desmoplastic, malignant —see Melanoma, skin,
    by site
  epithelioid cell —see Melanoma, skin, by site
    with spindle cell, mixed —see Melanoma,
      skin, by site
  in
    giant pigmented nevus —see Melanoma, skin,
      by site
    Hutchinson's melanotic freckle —see
      Melanoma, skin, by site
    junctional nevus —see Melanoma, skin, by site
    precancerous melanosis —see Melanoma, skin,
      by site
  in situ D03.9
    abdominal wall D03.59
    ala nasi D03.39
    ankle D03.7-●
    anus, anal (margin) (skin) D03.51
    arm D03.6-●
    auditory canal D03.2-●
    auricle (ear) D03.2-●
    auricular canal (external) D03.2-●
    axilla, axillary fold D03.59
    back D03.59
    breast D03.52
    brow D03.39
    buttock D03.59
    canthus (eye) D03.1-●
    cheek (external) D03.39
    chest wall D03.59
    chin D03.39
    choroid D03.8
    conjunctiva D03.8
    ear (external) D03.2-●
    external meatus (ear) D03.2-●
    eye D03.8
    eyebrow D03.39
    eyelid (lower) (upper) D03.1-●
    face D03.30
      specified NEC D03.39
    female genital organ (external) NEC D03.8
    finger D03.6-●
    flank D03.59
    foot D03.7-●
    forearm D03.6-●
    forehead D03.39
    foreskin D03.8
    gluteal region D03.59
    groin D03.59
    hand D03.6-●
    heel D03.7-●
    helix D03.2-●
    hip D03.7-●
    interscapular region D03.59
    iris D03.8
    jaw D03.39

Melanoma (Continued)
  in situ (Continued)
    knee D03.7-●
    labium (majus) (minus) D03.8
    lacrimal gland D03.8
    leg D03.7-●
    lip (lower) (upper) D03.0
    lower limb NEC D03.7-●
    male genital organ (external) NEC D03.8
    nail D03.9
      finger D03.6-●
      toe D03.7-●
    neck D03.4
    nose (external) D03.39
    orbit D03.8
    penis D03.8
    perianal skin D03.51
    perineum D03.51
    pinna D03.2-●
    popliteal fossa or space D03.7-●
    prepuce D03.8
    pudendum D03.8
    retina D03.8
    retrobulbar D03.8
    scalp D03.4
    scrotum D03.8
    shoulder D03.6-●
    specified site NEC D03.8
    submammary fold D03.52
    temple D03.39
    thigh D03.7-●
    toe D03.7-●
    trunk NEC D03.59
    umbilicus D03.59
    upper limb NEC D03.6-●
    vulva D03.8
  juvenile —see Nevus
  malignant, of soft parts except skin —see
    Neoplasm, connective tissue, malignant
  metastatic
    breast C79.81
    genital organ C79.82
    specified site NEC C79.89
  neurotropic, malignant —see Melanoma, skin,
    by site
  nodular —see Melanoma, skin, by site
  regressing, malignant —see Melanoma, skin,
    by site
  skin C43.9
    abdominal wall C43.59
    ala nasi C43.31
    ankle C43.7-●
    anus, anal (skin) C43.51
    arm C43.6-●
    auditory canal (external) C43.2-●
    auricle (ear) C43.2-●
    auricular canal (external) C43.2-●
    axilla, axillary fold C43.59
    back C43.59
    breast (female) (male) C43.52
    brow C43.39
    buttock C43.59
    canthus (eye) C43.1-●
    cheek (external) C43.39
    chest wall C43.59
    chin C43.39
    ear (external) C43.2-●
    elbow C43.6-●
    external meatus (ear) C43.2-●
    eyebrow C43.39
    eyelid (lower) (upper) C43.1-●
    face C43.30
      specified NEC C43.39
    female genital organ (external) NEC
      C51.9
    finger C43.6-●
    flank C43.59
    foot C43.7-●
    forearm C43.6-●
    forehead C43.39
    foreskin C60.0
    glabella C43.39
    gluteal region C43.59
    groin C43.59
    hand C43.6-●
    heel C43.7-●
    helix C43.2-●
    hip C43.7-●
    interscapular region C43.59
    jaw (external) C43.39
    knee C43.7-●

Melanoma (Continued)
  skin (Continued)
    labium C51.9
      majus C51.0
      minus C51.1
    leg C43.7-●
    lip (lower) (upper) C43.0
    lower limb NEC C43.7-●
    male genital organ (external) NEC C63.9
    nail
      finger C43.6-●
      toe C43.7-●
    nasolabial groove C43.39
    nates C43.59
    neck C43.4
    nose (external) C43.31
    overlapping site C43.8
    palpebra C43.1-●
    penis C60.9
    perianal skin C43.51
    perineum C43.51
    pinna C43.2-●
    popliteal fossa or space C43.7-●
    prepuce C60.0
    pudendum C51.9
    scalp C43.4
    scrotum C63.2
    shoulder C43.6-●
    skin NEC C43.9
    submammary fold C43.52
    temple C43.39
    thigh C43.7-●
    toe C43.7-●
    trunk NEC C43.59
    umbilicus C43.59
    upper limb NEC C43.6-●
    vulva C51.9
      overlapping sites C51.8
  spindle cell
    with epithelioid, mixed —see Melanoma, skin,
      by site
    type A C69.4-●
    type B C69.4-●
  superficial spreading —see Melanoma, skin, by
    site
Melanosarcoma —see also Melanoma
  epithelioid cell —see Melanoma
Melanosis L81.4
  addisonian E27.1
    tuberculous A18.7
  adrenal E27.1
  colon K63.89
  conjunctiva —see Pigmentation, conjunctiva
    congenital Q13.89
  cornea (presenile) (senile) —see also
      Pigmentation, cornea
    congenital Q13.4
  eye NEC H57.89
    congenital Q15.8
  lenticularis progressiva Q82.1
  liver K76.89
  precancerous —see also Melanoma, in situ
    malignant melanoma in —see Melanoma
  Riehl's L81.4
  sclera H15.89
    congenital Q13.89
  suprarenal E27.1
  tar L81.4
  toxic L81.4
Melanuria R82.998
MELAS syndrome E88.41
Melasma L81.1
  adrenal (gland) E27.1
  suprarenal (gland) E27.1
Melena K92.1
  with ulcer - code by site under Ulcer, with
      hemorrhage K27.4
  due to swallowed maternal blood P78.2
  newborn, neonatal P54.1
    due to swallowed maternal blood P78.2
Meleney's
  gangrene (cutaneous) —see Ulcer, skin
  ulcer (chronic undermining) —see Ulcer, skin
Melioidosis A24.9
  acute A24.1
  chronic A24.2
  fulminating A24.1
  pneumonia A24.1
  pulmonary (chronic) A24.2
    acute A24.1
    subacute A24.2

▶ New   ⇒ Revised   ~~deleted~~ Deleted   ● Use Additional Character(s)

Melioidosis *(Continued)*
    sepsis A24.1
    specified NEC A24.3
    subacute A24.2
Melitensis, febris A23.0
Melkersson (-Rosenthal) syndrome G51.2
Mellitus, diabetes —*see* Diabetes
Melorheostosis (bone) —*see* Disorder, bone,
        density and structure, specified NEC
Meloschisis Q18.4
Melotia Q17.4
Membrana
    capsularis lentis posterior Q13.89
    epipapillaris Q14.2
Membranacea placenta O43.19-●
Membranaceous uterus N85.8
Membrane(s), membranous —*see also* condition
    cyclitic —*see* Membrane, pupillary
    folds, congenital —*see* Web
    Jackson's Q43.3
    over face of newborn P28.9
    premature rupture —*see* Rupture, membranes,
        premature
    pupillary H21.4-●
        persistent Q13.89
    retained (with hemorrhage) (complicating
        delivery) O72.2
        without hemorrhage O73.1
    secondary cataract —*see* Cataract, secondary
    unruptured (causing asphyxia) —*see* Asphyxia,
        newborn
    vitreous —*see* Opacity, vitreous, membranes and
        strands
Membranitis —*see* Chorioamnionitis
Memory disturbance, lack or loss —*see also*
        Amnesia
    mild, following organic brain damage F06.8
Menadione deficiency E56.1
Menarche
    delayed E30.0
    precocious E30.1
Mendacity, pathologic F60.2
Mendelson's syndrome (due to anesthesia) J95.4
    in labor and delivery O74.0
    in pregnancy O29.01-●
    obstetric O74.0
    postpartum, puerperal O89.01
Ménétrier's disease or syndrome K29.60
    with bleeding K29.61
Ménière's disease, syndrome or vertigo H81.0-●
Meninges, meningeal —*see* condition
Meningioma —*see also* Neoplasm, meninges,
        benign
    angioblastic —*see* Neoplasm, meninges, benign
    angiomatous —*see* Neoplasm, meninges, benign
    atypical —*see* Neoplasm, meninges, uncertain
        behavior
    endotheliomatous —*see* Neoplasm, meninges,
        benign
    fibroblastic —*see* Neoplasm, meninges, benign
    fibrous —*see* Neoplasm, meninges, benign
    hemangioblastic —*see* Neoplasm, meninges,
        benign
    hemangiopericytic —*see* Neoplasm, meninges,
        benign
    malignant —*see* Neoplasm, meninges, malignant
    meningiothelial —*see* Neoplasm, meninges,
        benign
    meningotheliomatous —*see* Neoplasm,
        meninges, benign
    mixed —*see* Neoplasm, meninges, benign
    multiple —*see* Neoplasm, meninges, uncertain
        behavior
    papillary —*see* Neoplasm, meninges, uncertain
        behavior
    psammomatous —*see* Neoplasm, meninges,
        benign
    syncytial —*see* Neoplasm, meninges, benign
    transitional —*see* Neoplasm, meninges, benign
Meningiomatosis (diffuse) —*see* Neoplasm,
        meninges, uncertain behavior
Meningism —*see* Meningismus
Meningismus (infectional) (pneumococcal) R29.1
    due to serum or vaccine R29.1
    influenzal —*see* Influenza, with, manifestations
        NEC
Meningitis (basal) (basic) (brain) (cerebral)
    (cervical) (congestive) (diffuse) (hemorrhagic)
    infantile) (membranous) (metastatic)
    (nonspecific) (pontine) (progressive) (simple)
    (spinal) (subacute) (sympathetic) (toxic) G03.9

Meningitis *(Continued)*
    abacterial G03.0
    actinomycotic A42.81
    adenoviral A87.1
    arbovirus A87.8
    aseptic (acute) G03.0
    bacterial G00.9
        Escherichia coli (E. coli) G00.8
        Friedländer (bacillus) G00.8
        gram-negative G00.9
        H. influenzae G00.0
        Klebsiella G00.8
        pneumococcal G00.1
        specified organism NEC G00.8
        staphylococcal G00.3
        streptococcal (acute) G00.2
    benign recurrent (Mollaret) G03.2
    candidal B37.5
    caseous (tuberculous) A17.0
    cerebrospinal A39.0
    chronic NEC G03.1
    clear cerebrospinal fluid NEC G03.0
    coxsackievirus A87.0
    cryptococcal B45.1
    diplococcal (gram positive) A39.0
    echovirus A87.0
    enteroviral A87.0
    eosinophilic B83.2
    epidemic NEC A39.0
    Escherichia coli (E. coli) G00.8
    fibrinopurulent G00.9
        specified organism NEC G00.8
    Friedländer (bacillus) G00.8
    gonococcal A54.81
    gram-negative cocci G00.9
    gram-positive cocci G00.9
    Haemophilus (influenzae) G00.0
    H. influenzae G00.0
    in (due to)
        adenovirus A87.1
        African trypanosomiasis B56.9 *[G02]*
        anthrax A22.8
        bacterial disease NEC A48.8 *[G01]*
        Chagas' disease (chronic) B57.41
        chickenpox B01.0
        coccidioidomycosis B38.4
        Diplococcus pneumoniae G00.1
        enterovirus A87.0
        herpes (simplex) virus B00.3
            zoster B02.1
        infectious mononucleosis B27.92
        leptospirosis A27.81
        Listeria monocytogenes A32.11
        Lyme disease A69.21
        measles B05.1
        mumps (virus) B26.1
        neurosyphilis (late) A52.13
        parasitic disease NEC B89 *[G02]*
        poliovirus A80.9 *[G02]*
        preventive immunization, inoculation or
            vaccination G03.8
        rubella B06.02
        Salmonella infection A02.21
        specified cause NEC G03.8
        Streptococcal pneumoniae G00.1
        typhoid fever A01.01
        varicella B01.0
        viral disease NEC A87.8
        whooping cough A37.90
        zoster B02.1
    infectious G00.9
    influenzal (H. influenzae) G00.0
    Klebsiella G00.8
    leptospiral (aseptic) A27.81
    lymphocytic (acute) (benign) (serous) A87.2
    meningococcal A39.0
    Mima polymorpha G00.8
    Mollaret (benign recurrent) G03.2
    monilial B37.5
    mycotic NEC B49 *[G02]*
    Neisseria A39.0
    nonbacterial G03.0
    nonpyogenic NEC G03.0
    ossificans G96.198
    pneumococcal streptococcus pneumoniae G00.1
    poliovirus A80.9 *[G02]*
    postmeasles B05.1
    purulent G00.9
        specified organism NEC G00.8
    pyogenic G00.9
        specified organism NEC G00.8

Meningitis *(Continued)*
    Salmonella (arizonae) (Cholerae-Suis)
        (enteritidis) (typhimurium) A02.21
    septic G00.9
        specified organism NEC G00.8
    serosa circumscripta NEC G03.0
    serous NEC G93.2
    specified organism NEC G00.8
    sporotrichosis B42.81
    staphylococcal G00.3
    sterile G03.0
    Streptococcal (acute) G00.2
        pneumoniae G00.1
    suppurative G00.9
        specified organism NEC G00.8
    syphilitic (late) (tertiary) A52.13
        acute A51.41
        congenital A50.41
        secondary A51.41
    Torula histolytica (cryptococcal) B45.1
    traumatic (complication of injury) T79.8
    tuberculous A17.0
    typhoid A01.01
    viral NEC A87.9
    Yersinia pestis A20.3
Meningocele (spinal) —*see also* Spina bifida
    with hydrocephalus —*see* Spina bifida, by site,
        with hydrocephalus
    acquired (traumatic) G96.198
    cerebral —*see* Encephalocele
Meningocerebritis —*see* Meningoencephalitis
Meningococcemia A39.4
    acute A39.2
    chronic A39.3
Meningococcus, meningococcal —*see also*
        condition A39.9
    adrenalitis, hemorrhagic A39.1
    carrier (suspected) of Z22.31
    meningitis (cerebrospinal) A39.0
Meningoencephalitis —*see also* Encephalitis
        G04.90
    acute NEC —*see also* Encephalitis, viral A86
    bacterial NEC G04.2
    California A83.5
    diphasic A84.1
    eosinophilic B83.2
    epidemic A39.81
    herpesviral, herpetic B00.4
        due to herpesvirus 6 B10.01
        due to herpesvirus 7 B10.09
        specified NEC B10.09
    in (due to)
        blastomycosis NEC B40.81
        diseases classified elsewhere G05.3
        free-living amebae B60.2
        Hemophilus influenzae (H. influenzae)
            G00.0
        herpes B00.4
            due to herpesvirus 6 B10.01
            due to herpesvirus 7 B10.09
            specified NEC B10.09
        H. influenzae G00.0
        Lyme disease A69.22
        mercury —*see* subcategory T56.1
        mumps B26.2
        Naegleria (amebae) (organisms) (fowleri)
            B60.2
        Parastrongylus cantonensis B83.2
        toxoplasmosis (acquired) B58.2
            congenital P37.1
    infectious (acute) (viral) A86
    influenzal (H. influenzae) G00.0
    Listeria monocytogenes A32.12
    lymphocytic (serous) A87.2
    mumps B26.2
    parasitic NEC B89 *[G05.3]*
    pneumococcal G04.2
    primary amebic B60.2
    specific (syphilitic) A52.14
    specified organism NEC G04.81
    staphylococcal G04.2
    streptococcal G04.2
    syphilitic A52.14
    toxic NEC G92.8
        due to mercury —*see* subcategory
            T56.1
    tuberculous A17.82
    virus NEC A86
Meningoencephalocele —*see also* Encephalocele
    syphilitic A52.19
        congenital A50.49

Meningoencephalomyelitis —see also
    Meningoencephalitis
  acute NEC (viral) A86
    disseminated G04.00
      postimmunization or postvaccination G04.02
      postinfectious G04.01
  due to
    actinomycosis A42.82
    Torula B45.1
    Toxoplasma or toxoplasmosis (acquired) B58.2
      congenital P37.1
  postimmunization or postvaccination G04.02
Meningoencephalomyelopathy G96.9
Meningoencephalopathy G96.9
Meningomyelitis —see also Meningoencephalitis
  bacterial NEC G04.2
  blastomycotic NEC B40.81
  cryptococcal B45.1
  in diseases classified elsewhere G05.4
  meningococcal A39.81
  syphilitic A52.14
  tuberculous A17.82
Meningomyelocele —see also Spina bifida
  syphilitic A52.19
Meningomyeloneuritis —see Meningoencephalitis
Meningoradiculitis —see Meningitis
Meningovascular —see condition
Menkes' disease or syndrome E83.09
  meaning maple-syrup-urine disease E71.0
Menometrorrhagia N92.1
Menopause, menopausal (asymptomatic) (state)
  Z78.0
  arthritis (any site) NEC —see Arthritis, specified
    form NEC
  bleeding N92.4
  depression (single episode) F32.89
    agitated (single episode) F32.2
      recurrent episode F33.9
    psychotic (single episode) F32.89
      zrecurrent episode F33.8
    recurrent episode F33.9
    melancholia (single episode) F32.89
      recurrent episode F33.8
  paranoid state F22
  postirradiation (postprocedural)
    asymptomatic E89.40
    symptomatic E89.41
  premature E28.319
    asymptomatic E28.319
      postirradiation E89.40
      postsurgical E89.40
    symptomatic E28.310
      postirradiation E89.41
      postsurgical E89.41
  psychosis NEC F28
  symptomatic N95.1
  toxic polyarthritis NEC —see Arthritis, specified
    form NEC
Menorrhagia (primary) N92.0
  climacteric N92.4
    menopausal N92.4
  menopausal N92.4
  perimenopausal N92.4
  postclimacteric N95.0
  postmenopausal N95.0
  preclimacteric or premenopausal N92.4
  pubertal (menses retained) N92.2
Menostaxis N92.0
Menses, retention N94.89
Menstrual —see Menstruation
Menstruation
  absent —see Amenorrhea
  anovulatory N97.0
  cycle, irregular N92.6
  delayed N91.0
  disorder N93.9
    psychogenic F45.8
  during pregnancy O20.8
  excessive (with regular cycle) N92.0
    with irregular cycle N92.1
    at puberty N92.2
  frequent N92.0
  infrequent —see Oligomenorrhea
  irregular N92.6
    specified NEC N92.5
  latent N92.5
  membranous N92.5
  painful —see also Dysmenorrhea N94.6
    primary N94.4
    psychogenic F45.8
    secondary N94.5

Menstruation (Continued)
  passage of clots N92.0
  precocious E30.1
  protracted N92.5
  rare —see Oligomenorrhea
  retained N94.89
  retrograde N92.5
  scanty —see Oligomenorrhea
  suppression N94.89
  vicarious (nasal) N94.89
Mental —see also condition
  deficiency —see Disability, intellectual
  deterioration —see Psychosis
  disorder —see Disorder, mental
  exhaustion F48.8
  insufficiency (congenital) —see Disability,
    intellectual
  observation without need for further medical
    care Z03.89
  retardation —see Disability, intellectual
  subnormality —see Disability, intellectual
  upset —see Disorder, mental
Meralgia paresthetica G57.1-•
Mercurial —see condition
Mercurialism —see subcategory T56.1
MERRF syndrome (myoclonic epilepsy associated
  with ragged-red fiber) E88.42
Merkel cell tumor —see Carcinoma, Merkel cell
Merocele —see Hernia, femoral
Meromelia
  lower limb —see Defect, reduction, lower
    limb
    intercalary
      femur —see Defect, reduction, lower limb,
        specified type NEC
      tibiofibular (complete) (incomplete) —see
        Defect, reduction, lower limb
  upper limb —see Defect, reduction, upper
    limb
    intercalary, humeral, radioulnar —see
      Agenesis, arm, with hand present
Merzbacher-Pelizaeus disease E75.27
Mesaortitis —see Aortitis
Mesarteritis —see Arteritis
Mesencephalitis —see Encephalitis
Mesenchymoma —see also Neoplasm, connective
  tissue, uncertain behavior
  benign —see Neoplasm, connective tissue,
    benign
  malignant —see Neoplasm, connective tissue,
    malignant
Mesenteritis
  retractile K65.4
  sclerosing K65.4
Mesentery, mesenteric —see condition
Mesiodens, mesiodentes K00.1
Mesio-occlusion M26.213
Mesocolon —see condition
Mesonephroma (malignant) —see Neoplasm,
  malignant, by site
  benign —see Neoplasm, benign, by site
Mesophlebitis —see Phlebitis
Mesostromal dysgenesia Q13.89
Mesothelioma (malignant) C45.9
  benign
    mesentery D19.1
    mesocolon D19.1
    omentum D19.1
    peritoneum D19.1
    pleura D19.0
    specified site NEC D19.7
    unspecified site D19.9
  biphasic C45.9
    benign
      mesentery D19.1
      mesocolon D19.1
      omentum D19.1
      peritoneum D19.1
      pleura D19.0
      specified site NEC D19.7
      unspecified site D19.9
  cystic D48.4
  epithelioid C45.9
    benign
      mesentery D19.1
      mesocolon D19.1
      omentum D19.1
      peritoneum D19.1
      pleura D19.0
      specified site NEC D19.7
      unspecified site D19.9

Mesothelioma (Continued)
  fibrous C45.9
    benign
      mesentery D19.1
      mesocolon D19.1
      omentum D19.1
      peritoneum D19.1
      pleura D19.0
      specified site NEC D19.7
      unspecified site D19.9
  site classification
    liver C45.7
    lung C45.7
    mediastinum C45.7
    mesentery C45.1
    mesocolon C45.1
    omentum C45.1
    pericardium C45.2
    peritoneum C45.1
    pleura C45.0
      parietal C45.0
    retroperitoneum C45.7
    specified site NEC C45.7
    unspecified C45.9
Metabolic syndrome E88.810
Metagonimiasis B66.8
Metagonimus infestation (intestine)
  B66.8
Metal
  pigmentation L81.8
  polisher's disease J62.8
Metamorphopsia H53.15
Metaplasia
  apocrine (breast) —see Dysplasia, mammary,
    specified type NEC
  cervix (squamous) —see Dysplasia, cervix
  endometrium (squamous) (uterus) N85.8
  esophagus K22.7-•
  gastric intestinal K31.A0
    with dysplasia K31.A29
      high grade K31.A22
      low grade K31.A21
    indefinite for dysplasia K31.A0
    without dysplasia K31.A19
      involving
        antrum K31.A11
        body (corpus) K31.A12
        cardia K31.A14
        fundus K31.A13
        multiple sites K31.A15
  kidney (pelvis) (squamous) N28.89
  myelogenous D73.1
  myeloid (agnogenic) (megakaryocytic) D73.1
  spleen D73.1
  squamous cell, bladder N32.89
Metastasis, metastatic
  abscess —see Abscess
  calcification E83.59
  cancer
    from specified site —see Neoplasm, malignant,
      by site
    to specified site —see Neoplasm, secondary,
      by site
  deposits (in) —see Neoplasm, secondary, by site
  disease (see also Neoplasm, secondary, by site)
    C79.9
  spread (to) —see Neoplasm, secondary, by site
Metastrongyliasis B83.8
Metatarsalgia M77.4-•
  anterior G57.6-•
  Morton's G57.6-•
Metatarsus, metatarsal —see also condition
  adductus, congenital Q66.22-•
  valgus (abductus), congenital Q66.6
  varus (congenital) Q66.22-•
    primus Q66.21-•
Methadone use —see Use, opioid
Methemoglobinemia D74.9
  acquired (with sulfhemoglobinemia) D74.8
  congenital D74.0
  enzymatic (congenital) D74.0
  Hb M disease D74.0
  hereditary D74.0
  toxic D74.8
Methemoglobinuria —see Hemoglobinuria
Methioninemia E72.19
Methylmalonic acidemia E71.120
Metritis (catarrhal) (hemorrhagic) (septic)
  (suppurative) —see also Endometritis
  cervical —see Cervicitis
Metropathia hemorrhagica N93.8

▶ New   ⇒ Revised   ~~deleted~~ Deleted   • Use Additional Character(s)

Metroperitonitis —*see* Peritonitis, pelvic, female
Metrorrhagia N92.1
    climacteric N92.4
    menopausal N92.4
    perimenopausal N92.4
    postpartum NEC (atonic) (following delivery of placenta) O72.1
        delayed or secondary O72.2
    preclimacteric or premenopausal N92.4
    psychogenic F45.8
Metrorrhexis —*see* Rupture, uterus
Metrosalpingitis N70.91
Metrostaxis N93.8
Metrovaginitis —*see* Endometritis
Meyer-Schwickerath and Weyers syndrome Q87.0
Meynert's amentia (nonalcoholic) F04
    alcoholic F10.96
        with dependence F10.26
Mibelli's disease (porokeratosis) Q82.8
Mice, joint —*see* Loose, body, joint
    knee M23.4
Micrencephalon, micrencephaly Q02
Microalbuminuria R80.9
Microaneurysm, retinal —*see also* Disorder, retina, microaneurysms
    diabetic —*see* E08-E13 with .31
Microangiopathy (peripheral) I73.9
    thrombotic M31.10
        hematopoietic stem cell transplantation-associated [HSCT-TMA] M31.11
Microcalcifications, breast R92.0
Microcephalus, microcephalic, microcephaly Q02
    due to toxoplasmosis (congenital) P37.1
Microcheilia Q18.7
Microcolon (congenital) Q43.8
Microcornea (congenital) Q13.4
Microcytic —*see* condition D57.40
Microdeletions NEC Q93.88
Microdontia K00.2
Microdrepanocytosis D57.40
    with
        acute chest syndrome D57.411
        cerebral vascular involvement D57.413
        crisis (painful) D57.419
            with specified complication NEC D57.418
        pain (vaso-occlusive) D57.419
        splenic sequestration D57.412
Microembolism
    atherothrombotic —*see* Atheroembolism
    retinal —*see* Occlusion, artery, retina
Microencephalon Q02
Microfilaria streptocerca infestation —*see* Onchocerciasis
Microgastria (congenital) Q40.2
Microgenia M26.06
Microgenitalia, congenital
    female Q52.8
    male Q55.8
Microglioma —*see* Lymphoma, non-Hodgkin, specified NEC
Microglossia (congenital) Q38.3
Micrognathia, micrognathism (congenital) (mandibular) (maxillary) M26.09
Microgyria (congenital) Q04.3
Microinfarct of heart —*see* Insufficiency, coronary
Microlentia (congenital) Q12.8
Microlithiasis, alveolar, pulmonary J84.02
Micromastia N64.82
Micromyelia (congenital) Q06.8
Micropenis Q55.62
Microphakia (congenital) Q12.8
Microphthalmos, microphthalmia (congenital) Q11.2
    due to toxoplasmosis P37.1
Micropsia H53.15
Microscopic polyangiitis (polyarteritis) M31.7
Microsporidiosis B60.8
    intestinal A07.8
Microsporon furfur infestation B36.0
Microsporosis —*see also* Dermatophytosis
    nigra B36.1
Microstomia (congenital) Q18.5
Microtia (congenital) (external ear) Q17.2
Microtropia H50.40
Microvillus inclusion disease (MVD) (MVID) Q43.8
Micturition
    disorder NEC —*see also* Difficulty, micturition R39.198
        psychogenic F45.8
    frequency R35.0
        psychogenic F45.8

Micturition (*Continued*)
    hesitancy R39.11
    incomplete emptying R39.14
    nocturnal R35.1
    painful R30.9
        dysuria R30.0
        psychogenic F45.8
        tenesmus R30.1
    poor stream R39.12
    position dependent R39.192
    split stream R39.13
    straining R39.16
    urgency R39.15
Mid plane —*see* condition
Middle
    ear —*see* condition
    lobe (right) syndrome J98.19
Miescher's elastoma L87.2
Mietens' syndrome Q87.2
Migraine (idiopathic) G43.909
    with refractory migraine G43.919
        with status migrainosus G43.911
        without status migrainosus G43.919
    with aura (acute-onset) (prolonged) (typical) (without headache) G43.109
        with refractory migraine G43.119
            with status migrainosus G43.111
            without status migrainosus G43.119
        chronic G43.E09
            with refractory migraine G43.E19
                with status migrainosus G43.E11
                without status migrainosus G43.E19
            intractable
                with status migrainosus G43.E11
                without status migrainosus G43.E19
            not intractable
                with status migrainosus G43.E01
                without status migrainosus G43.E09
            without refractory migraine G43.E09
                with status migrainosus G43.E01
                without status migrainosus G43.E09
        intractable G43.119
            with status migrainosus G43.111
            without status migrainosus G43.119
        not intractable G43.109
            with status migrainosus G43.101
            without status migrainosus G43.109
        persistent G43.509
            with cerebral infarction G43.609
                with refractory migraine G43.619
                    with status migrainosus G43.611
                    without status migrainosus G43.619
                intractable G43.619
                    with status migrainosus G43.611
                    without status migrainosus G43.619
                not intractable G43.609
                    with status migrainosus G43.601
                    without status migrainosus G43.609
                without refractory migraine G43.609
                    with status migrainosus G43.601
                    without status migrainosus G43.609
            without cerebral infarction G43.509
                with refractory migraine G43.519
                    with status migrainosus G43.511
                    without status migrainosus G43.519
                intractable G43.519
                    with status migrainosus G43.511
                    without status migrainosus G43.519
                not intractable G43.509
                    with status migrainosus G43.501
                    without status migrainosus G43.509
                without refractory migraine G43.509
                    with status migrainosus G43.501
                    without status migrainosus G43.509
            without mention of refractory migraine G43.109
                with status migrainosus G43.101
                without status migrainosus G43.109
        abdominal G43.D0
            with refractory migraine G43.D1
            intractable G43.D1
            not intractable G43.D0
            without refractory migraine G43.D0
        basilar —*see* Migraine, with aura
        classical —*see* Migraine, with aura
        common —*see* Migraine, without aura
        complicated G43.109
        equivalents —*see* Migraine, with aura
        familiar —*see* Migraine, hemiplegic

Migraine (*Continued*)
    hemiplegic G43.409
        with refractory migraine G43.419
            with status migrainosus G43.411
            without status migrainosus G43.419
        intractable G43.419
            with status migrainosus G43.411
            without status migrainosus G43.419
        not intractable G43.409
            with status migrainosus G43.401
            without status migrainosus G43.409
        without refractory migraine G43.409
            with status migrainosus G43.401
            without status migrainosus G43.409
    intractable G43.919
        with status migrainosus G43.911
        without status migrainosus G43.919
    menstrual G43.829
        with refractory migraine G43.839
            with status migrainosus G43.831
            without status migrainosus G43.839
        intractable G43.839
            with status migrainosus G43.831
            without status migrainosus G43.839
        not intractable G43.829
            with status migrainosus G43.821
            without status migrainosus G43.829
        without refractory migraine G43.829
            with status migrainosus G43.821
            without status migrainosus G43.829
    menstrually related —*see* Migraine, menstrual
    not intractable G43.909
        with status migrainosus G43.901
        without status migrainosus G43.909
    ophthalmoplegic G43.B0
        with refractory migraine G43.B1
        intractable G43.B1
        not intractable G43.B0
        without refractory migraine G43.B0
    persistent aura (with, without) cerebral infarction —*see* Migraine, with aura, persistent
    preceded or accompanied by transient focal neurological phenomena —*see* Migraine, with aura
    pre-menstrual —*see* Migraine, menstrual
    pure menstrual —*see* Migraine, menstrual
    retinal —*see* Migraine, with aura
    specified NEC G43.809
        intractable G43.819
            with status migrainosus G43.811
            without status migrainosus G43.819
        not intractable G43.809
            with status migrainosus G43.801
            without status migrainosus G43.809
    sporadic —*see* Migraine, hemiplegic
    transformed —*see* Migraine, without aura, chronic
    triggered seizures —*see* Migraine, with aura
    without aura G43.009
        with refractory migraine G43.019
            with status migrainosus G43.011
            without status migrainosus G43.019
        chronic G43.709
            with refractory migraine G43.719
                with status migrainosus G43.711
                without status migrainosus G43.719
            intractable
                with status migrainosus G43.711
                without status migrainosus G43.719
            not intractable
                with status migrainosus G43.701
                without status migrainosus G43.709
            without refractory migraine G43.709
                with status migrainosus G43.701
                without status migrainosus G43.709
        intractable
            with status migrainosus G43.011
            without status migrainosus G43.019
        not intractable
            with status migrainosus G43.001
            without status migrainosus G43.009
        without mention of refractory migraine G43.009
            with status migrainosus G43.001
            without status migrainosus G43.009
        without refractory migraine G43.909
            with status migrainosus G43.901
            without status migrainosus G43.909
Migrant, social Z59.00
Migration, anxiety concerning Z60.3

Migratory, migrating —see also condition
   person Z59.00
   testis Q55.29
Mikity-Wilson disease or syndrome P27.0
Mikulicz' disease or syndrome K11.8
Miliaria L74.3
   alba L74.1
   apocrine L75.2
   crystallina L74.1
   profunda L74.2
   rubra L74.0
   tropicalis L74.2
Miliary —see condition
Milium L72.0
   colloid L57.8
Milk
   crust L21.0
   excessive secretion O92.6
   poisoning —see Poisoning, food, noxious
   retention O92.79
   sickness —see Poisoning, food, noxious
   spots I31.0
Milk-alkali disease or syndrome E83.52
Milk-leg (deep vessels) (nonpuerperal) —see
   Embolism, vein, lower extremity
   complicating pregnancy O22.3-●
   puerperal, postpartum, childbirth O87.1
Milkman's disease or syndrome M83.8
Milky urine —see Chyluria
Millard-Gubler (-Foville) paralysis or syndrome
   G46.3
Millar's asthma J38.5
Miller-Fisher syndrome G61.0
Mills' disease —see Hemiplegia
Millstone maker's pneumoconiosis J62.8
Milroy's disease (chronic hereditary edema) Q82.0
Minamata disease T56.1-●
Miners' asthma or lung J60
Minkowski-Chauffard syndrome —see
   Spherocytosis
Minor —see condition
Minor's disease (hematomyelia) G95.19
Minot's disease (hemorrhagic disease), newborn
   P53
Minot-von Willebrand-Jurgens disease or
   syndrome (angiohemophilia) —see Disease,
   von Willebrand
Minus (and plus) hand (intrinsic) —see Deformity,
   limb, specified type NEC, forearm
Miosis (pupil) H57.03
Mirizzi's syndrome (hepatic duct stenosis) K83.1
Mirror writing F81.0
MIS-A M35.81
MIS-C M35.81
Misadventure (of) (prophylactic) (therapeutic) —see
   also Complications T88.9
   administration of insulin (by accident) —see
     subcategory T38.3
   infusion —see Complications, infusion
   local applications (of fomentations, plasters, etc.)
     T88.9
     burn or scald —see Burn
     specified NEC T88.8
   medical care (early) (late) T88.9
     adverse effect of drugs or chemicals —see
       Table of Drugs and Chemicals
▶   burn or scald —see Burn
▶   specified NEC T88.8
   medical care (early) (late)
     burn or scald —see Burn
     specified NEC T88.8
   specified NEC T88.8
   surgical procedure (early) (late) —see
     Complications, surgical procedure
   transfusion —see Complications, transfusion
   vaccination or other immunological
     procedure —see Complications, vaccination
Miscarriage O03.9
Misdirection, aqueous H40.83-●
Misperception, sleep state F51.02
Misplaced, misplacement
   ear Q17.4
   kidney (acquired) N28.89
     congenital Q63.2
   organ or site, congenital NEC —see Malposition,
     congenital
Missed
   abortion O02.1
   delivery O36.4
Missing —see also Absence
   string of intrauterine contraceptive device T83.32

Misuse of drugs F19.99
Mitchell's disease (erythromelalgia) I73.81
Mite(s) (infestation) B88.9
   diarrhea B88.0
   grain (itch) B88.0
   hair follicle (itch) B88.0
   in sputum B88.0
Mitral —see condition
Mittelschmerz N94.0
Mixed —see condition
MMN (multifocal motor neuropathy) G61.82
MNGIE (Mitochondrial Neurogastrointestinal
   Encephalopathy) syndrome E88.49
Mobile, mobility
   cecum Q43.3
   excessive —see Hypermobility
   gallbladder, congenital Q44.1
   kidney N28.89
   organ or site, congenital NEC —see Malposition,
     congenital
Mobitz heart block (atrioventricular) I44.1
Moebius, Möbius
   disease (ophthalmoplegic migraine) —see
     Migraine, ophthalmoplegic
   syndrome Q87.0
     congenital oculofacial paralysis (with other
       anomalies) Q87.0
     ophthalmoplegic migraine —see Migraine,
       ophthalmoplegic
Moeller's glossitis K14.0
MOGAD (myelin oligodendrocyte glycoprotein
   antibody disease) G37.81
Mohr's syndrome (Types I and II) Q87.0
Mola destruens D39.2
Molar pregnancy O02.0
Molarization of premolars K00.2
Molding, head (during birth) - omit code
Mole (pigmented) —see also Nevus
   blood O02.0
   Breus' O02.0
   cancerous —see Melanoma
   carneous O02.0
   destructive D39.2
   fleshy O02.0
   hydatid, hydatidiform (benign) (complicating
     pregnancy) (delivered) (undelivered) O01.9
     classical O01.0
     complete O01.0
     incomplete O01.1
     invasive D39.2
     malignant D39.2
     partial O01.1
   intrauterine O02.0
   invasive (hydatidiform) D39.2
   malignant
     meaning
       malignant hydatidiform mole D39.2
       melanoma —see Melanoma
   nonhydatidiform O02.0
   nonpigmented —see Nevus
   pregnancy NEC O02.0
   skin —see Nevus
   tubal O00.10-
     with intrauterine pregnancy O00.11-
   vesicular —see Mole, hydatidiform
Molimen, molimina (menstrual) N94.3
Molluscum contagiosum (epitheliale) B08.1
Mönckeberg's arteriosclerosis, disease, or
   sclerosis —see Arteriosclerosis, extremities
Mondini's malformation (cochlea) Q16.5
Mondor's disease I80.8
Monge's disease T70.29
Monilethrix (congenital) Q84.1
Moniliasis —see also Candidiasis B37.9
   neonatal P37.5
Monitoring (encounter for)
   therapeutic drug level Z51.81
Monkey malaria B53.1
Monkeypox B04
Monoarthritis M13.10
   ankle M13.17-●
   elbow M13.12-●
   foot joint M13.17-●
   hand joint M13.14-●
   hip M13.15-●
   knee M13.16-●
   shoulder M13.11-●
   wrist M13.13-●
Monoblastic —see condition
Monochromat (ism), monochromatopsia
   (acquired) (congenital) H53.51

Monocytic —see condition
Monocytopenia D72.818
Monocytosis (symptomatic) D72.821
Monomania —see Psychosis
Mononeuritis G58.9
   cranial nerve —see Disorder, nerve, cranial
   femoral nerve G57.2-●
   lateral
     cutaneous nerve of thigh G57.1-●
     popliteal nerve G57.3-●
   lower limb G57.9-●
     specified nerve NEC G57.8-●
   medial popliteal nerve G57.4-●
   median nerve G56.1-●
   multiplex G58.7
   plantar nerve G57.6-●
   posterior tibial nerve G57.5-●
   radial nerve G56.3-●
   sciatic nerve G57.0-●
   specified NEC G58.8
   tibial nerve G57.4-●
   ulnar nerve G56.2-●
   upper limb G56.9-●
     specified nerve NEC G56.8-●
   vestibular —see subcategory H93.3
Mononeuropathy G58.9
   carpal tunnel syndrome —see Syndrome, carpal
     tunnel
   diabetic NEC —see E08-E13 with .41
   femoral nerve —see Lesion, nerve, femoral
   ilioinguinal nerve G57.8-●
   in diseases classified elsewhere —see category G59
   intercostal G58.0
   lower limb G57.9-●
     causalgia —see Causalgia, lower limb
     femoral nerve —see Lesion, nerve, femoral
     meralgia paresthetica G57.1-●
     plantar nerve —see Lesion, nerve, plantar
     popliteal nerve —see Lesion, nerve, popliteal
     sciatic nerve —see Lesion, nerve, sciatic
     specified NEC G57.8-●
     tarsal tunnel syndrome —see Syndrome, tarsal
       tunnel
   median nerve —see Lesion, nerve, median
   multiplex G58.7
   obturator nerve G57.8-●
   popliteal nerve —see Lesion, nerve, popliteal
   radial nerve —see Lesion, nerve, radial
   saphenous nerve G57.8-●
   specified NEC G58.8
   tarsal tunnel syndrome —see Syndrome, tarsal
     tunnel
   tuberculous A17.83
   ulnar nerve —see Lesion, nerve, ulnar
   upper limb G56.9-●
     carpal tunnel syndrome —see Syndrome,
       carpal tunnel
     causalgia —see Causalgia
     median nerve —see Lesion, nerve, median
     radial nerve —see Lesion, nerve, radial
     specified site NEC G56.8-●
     ulnar nerve —see Lesion, nerve, ulnar
Mononucleosis, infectious B27.90
   with
     complication NEC B27.99
     meningitis B27.92
     polyneuropathy B27.91
   cytomegaloviral B27.10
     with
       complication NEC B27.19
       meningitis B27.12
       polyneuropathy B27.11
   Epstein-Barr (virus) B27.00
     with
       complication NEC B27.09
       meningitis B27.02
       polyneuropathy B27.01
   gammaherpesviral B27.00
     with
       complication NEC B27.09
       meningitis B27.02
       polyneuropathy B27.01
   specified NEC B27.80
     with
       complication NEC B27.89
       meningitis B27.82
       polyneuropathy B27.81
Monoparesis —see Monoplegia
Monoplegia G83.3-●
   congenital (cerebral) G80.8
     spastic G80.1

M

Monoplegia (Continued)
  embolic (current episode) I63.4-•
  following
    cerebrovascular disease
      cerebral infarction
        lower limb I69.34-•
        upper limb I69.33-•
      intracerebral hemorrhage
        lower limb I69.14-•
        upper limb I69.13-•
      lower limb I69.94-•
      nontraumatic intracranial hemorrhage NEC
        lower limb I69.24-•
        upper limb I69.23-•
      specified disease NEC
        lower limb I69.84-•
        upper limb I69.83-•
      stroke NOS
        lower limb I69.34-•
        upper limb I69.33-•
      subarachnoid hemorrhage
        lower limb I69.04-•
        upper limb I69.03-•
    upper limb I69.93-•
  hysterical (transient) F44.4
  lower limb G83.1-•
  psychogenic (conversion reaction) F44.4
  thrombotic (current episode) I63.3-•
  transient R29.818
  upper limb G83.2-•
Monorchism, monorchidism Q55.0
Monosomy —see also Deletion, chromosome
  Q93.9
  specified NEC Q93.89
  whole chromosome
    meiotic nondisjunction Q93.0
    mitotic nondisjunction Q93.1
    mosaicism Q93.1
  X Q96.9
Monster, monstrosity (single) Q89.7
  acephalic Q00.0
  twin Q89.4
Monteggia's fracture (-dislocation) S52.27-•
Mooren's ulcer (cornea) —see Ulcer, cornea,
  Mooren's
Moore's syndrome —see Epilepsy, specified NEC
Mooser-Neill reaction A75.2
Mooser's bodies A75.2
Morbidity not stated or unknown R69
Morbilli —see Measles
Morbus —see also Disease
  angelicus, anglorum E55.0
  Beigel B36.2
  caducus —see Epilepsy
  celiacus K90.0
  comitialis —see Epilepsy
  cordis —see also Disease, heart I51.9
    valvulorum —see Endocarditis
  coxae senilis M16.9
    tuberculous A18.02
  hemorrhagicus neonatorum P53
  maculosus neonatorum P54.5
Morel (-Stewart)(-Morgagni) **syndrome** M85.2
Morel-Kraepelin disease —see Schizophrenia
Morel-Moore syndrome M85.2
Morgagni's
  cyst, organ, hydatid, or appendage
    female Q50.5
    male (epididymal) Q55.4
      testicular Q55.29
  syndrome M85.2
Morgagni-Stewart-Morel syndrome M85.2
Morgagni-Stokes-Adams syndrome I45.9
Morgagni-Turner (-Albright) **syndrome** Q96.9
Moria F07.0
Moron (I.Q. 50-69) F70
Morphea L94.0
Morphinism (without remission) F11.20
  with remission F11.21
Morphinomania (without remission) F11.20
  with remission F11.21
Morquio (-Ullrich)(-Brailsford) **disease or**
  syndrome —see Mucopolysaccharidosis
Mortification (dry) (moist) —see Gangrene
Morton's metatarsalgia (neuralgia)(neuroma)
  (syndrome) G57.6
Morvan's disease or syndrome G60.8
Mosaicism, mosaic (autosomal) (chromosomal)
  45,X/46,XX Q96.3
  45,X/other cell lines NEC with abnormal sex
    chromosome Q96.4

Mosaicism, mosaic (Continued)
  sex chromosome
    female Q97.8
    lines with various numbers of X chromosomes
      Q97.2
    male Q98.7
  XY Q96.3
Moschowitz' disease M31.19
Mother yaw A66.0
Motion sickness (from travel, any vehicle) (from
  roundabouts or swings) T75.3
Mottled, mottling, teeth (enamel) (endemic)
  (nonendemic) K00.3
Mounier-Kuhn syndrome Q32.4
  with bronchiectasis J47.9
    exacerbation (acute) J47.1
    lower respiratory infection J47.0
  acquired J98.09
    with bronchiectasis J47.9
      with
        exacerbation (acute) J47.1
        lower respiratory infection J47.0
Mountain
  sickness T70.29
    with polycythemia , acquired (acute) D75.1
  tick fever A93.2
Mouse, joint —see Loose, body, joint
  knee M23.4-•
Mouth —see condition
Movable
  coccyx —see subcategory M53.2
  kidney N28.89
    congenital Q63.8
  spleen D73.89
Movements, dystonic R25.8
Moyamoya disease I67.5
Mpox B04
MRSA (Methicillin resistant Staphylococcus
  aureus)
  infection A49.02
    as the cause of diseases classified elsewhere
      B95.62
  sepsis A41.02
MSD (multiple sulfatase deficiency) E75.26
MSSA (Methicillin susceptible Staphylococcus
  aureus)
  infection A49.01
    as the cause of diseases classified elsewhere
      B95.61
  sepsis A41.01
Mucha-Habermann disease L41.0
Mucinosis (cutaneous) (focal) (papular) (reticular
  erythematous) (skin) L98.5
  oral K13.79
Mucocele
  appendix K38.8
  buccal cavity K13.79
  gallbladder K82.1
  lacrimal sac, chronic H04.43-•
  nasal sinus J34.1
  nose J34.1
  salivary gland (any) K11.6
  sinus (accessory) (nasal) J34.1
  turbinate (bone) (middle) (nasal) J34.1
  uterus N85.8
Mucolipidosis
  I E77.1
  II, III E77.0
  IV E75.11
Mucopolysaccharidosis E76.3
  beta-gluduronidase deficiency E76.29
  cardiopathy E76.3 [I52]
  Hunter's syndrome E76.1
  Hurler's syndrome E76.01
  Hurler-Scheie syndrome E76.02
  Maroteaux-Lamy syndrome E76.29
  Morquio syndrome E76.219
    A E76.210
    B E76.211
    classic E76.210
  Sanfilippo syndrome E76.22
  Scheie's syndrome E76.03
  specified NEC E76.29
  type
    I
      Hurler's syndrome E76.01
      Hurler-Scheie syndrome E76.02
      Scheie's syndrome E76.03
    II E76.1
    III E76.22
    IV E76.219

Mucopolysaccharidosis (Continued)
  type (Continued)
    IVA E76.210
    IVB E76.211
    VI E76.29
    VII E76.29
Mucormycosis B46.5
  cutaneous B46.3
  disseminated B46.4
  gastrointestinal B46.2
  generalized B46.4
  pulmonary B46.0
  rhinocerebral B46.1
  skin B46.3
  subcutaneous B46.3
Mucositis (ulcerative) K12.30
  due to drugs NEC K12.32
  gastrointestinal K92.81
  mouth (oral) (oropharyngeal) K12.30
    due to antineoplastic therapy
      K12.31
    due to drugs NEC K12.32
    due to radiation K12.33
    specified NEC K12.39
    viral K12.39
  nasal J34.81
  oral cavity —see Mucositis, mouth
  oral soft tissues —see Mucositis, mouth
  vagina and vulva N76.81
Mucositis necroticans agranulocytica —see
  Agranulocytosis
Mucous —see also condition
  patches (syphilitic) A51.39
    congenital A50.07
Mucoviscidosis E84.9
  with meconium obstruction E84.11
Mucus
  asphyxia or suffocation —see Asphyxia, mucus
  in stool R19.5
  plug —see Asphyxia, mucus
Muguet B37.0
Mulberry molars (congenital syphilis) A50.52
Müllerian mixed tumor
  specified site —see Neoplasm, malignant, by site
  unspecified site C54.9
Multicystic kidney (development) Q61.4
Multiparity (grand) Z64.1
  affecting management of pregnancy, labor and
    delivery (supervision only)
      O09.4-•
  requiring contraceptive management —see
    Contraception
Multipartita placenta O43.19-•
Multiple, multiplex —see also condition
  digits (congenital) Q69.9
  endocrine neoplasia —see Neoplasia, endocrine,
    multiple [MEN]
  personality F44.81
Multisystem inflammatory syndrome (in adults)
  (in children) M35.81
Mumps B26.9
  arthritis B26.85
  complication NEC B26.89
  encephalitis B26.2
  hepatitis B26.81
  meningitis (aseptic) B26.1
  meningoencephalitis B26.2
  myocarditis B26.82
  oophoritis B26.89
  orchitis B26.0
  pancreatitis B26.3
  polyneuropathy B26.84
Mumu —see also Infestation, filarial B74.9 [N51]
Münchhausen's syndrome —see Disorder,
  factitious
Münchmeyer's syndrome —see Myositis,
  ossificans, progressiva
Mural —see condition
Murmur (cardiac) (heart) (organic) R01.1
  abdominal R19.15
  aortic (valve) —see Endocarditis, aortic
  benign R01.0
  diastolic —see Endocarditis
  Flint I35.1
  functional R01.0
  Graham Steell I37.1
  innocent R01.0
  mitral (valve) —see Insufficiency, mitral
  nonorganic R01.0
  presystolic, mitral —see Insufficiency, mitral
  pulmonic (valve) I37.8

Murmur (Continued)
- systolic R01.1
- tricuspid (valve) I07.9
- valvular —see Endocarditis
Murri's disease (intermittent hemoglobinuria) D59.6
Muscle, muscular —see also condition
- carnitine (palmityltransferase) deficiency E71.314
Musculoneuralgia —see Neuralgia
Mushroom-workers' (pickers') disease or lung J67.5
Mushrooming hip —see Derangement, joint, specified NEC, hip
Mutation(s)
- factor V Leiden D68.51
- surfactant, of lung J84.83
- prothrombin gene D68.52
Mutism —see also Aphasia
- deaf (acquired) (congenital) NEC H91.3
- elective (adjustment reaction) (childhood) F94.0
- hysterical F44.4
- selective (childhood) F94.0
MVD (microvillus inclusion disease) Q43.8
MVID (microvillus inclusion disease) Q43.8
Myalgia M79.10
- auxiliary muscles, head and neck M79.12
- epidemic (cervical) B33.0
- mastication muscle M79.11
- site specified NEC M79.18
- traumatic NEC T14.8
Myasthenia G70.9
- congenital G70.2
- cordis —see Failure, heart
- developmental G70.2
- gravis G70.00
  - with exacerbation (acute) G70.01
  - in crisis G70.01
  - neonatal, transient P94.0
  - pseudoparalytica G70.00
    - with exacerbation (acute) G70.01
    - in crisis G70.01
- stomach, psychogenic F45.8
- syndrome
  - in
    - diabetes mellitus —see E08-E13 with .44
    - neoplastic disease —see also Neoplasm D49.9 [G73.3]
    - pernicious anemia D51.0 [G73.3]
    - thyrotoxicosis E05.90 [G73.3]
      - with thyroid storm E05.91 [G73.3]
Myasthenic M62.81
Mycelium infection B49
Mycetismus —see Poisoning, food, noxious, mushroom
Mycetoma B47.9
- actinomycotic B47.1
- bone (mycotic) B47.9 [M90.80]
- eumycotic B47.0
- foot B47.9
  - actinomycotic B47.1
  - mycotic B47.0
- madurae NEC B47.9
  - mycotic B47.0
- maduromycotic B47.0
- mycotic B47.0
- nocardial B47.1
Mycobacteriosis —see Mycobacterium
Mycobacterium, mycobacterial (infection) A31.9
- anonymous A31.9
- atypical A31.9
  - cutaneous A31.1
  - pulmonary A31.0
    - tuberculous —see Tuberculosis, pulmonary
  - specified site NEC A31.8
- avium (intracellulare complex) A31.0
- balnei A31.1
- Battey A31.0
- chelonei A31.8
- cutaneous A31.1
- extrapulmonary systemic A31.8
- fortuitum A31.8
- intracellulare (Battey bacillus) A31.0
- kakaferifu A31.8
- kansasii (yellow bacillus) A31.0
- kasongo A31.8
- leprae —see also Leprosy A30.9
- luciflavum A31.1
- marinum (M. balnei) A31.1
- nonspecific —see Mycobacterium, atypical
- pulmonary (atypical) A31.0
  - tuberculous —see Tuberculosis, pulmonary
- scrofulaceum A31.8

Mycobacterium, mycobacterial (Continued)
- simiae A31.8
- systemic, extrapulmonary A31.8
- szulgai A31.8
- terrae A31.8
- triviale A31.8
- tuberculosis (human, bovine) —see Tuberculosis
- ulcerans A31.1
- xenopi A31.8
Mycoplasma (M.) pneumoniae, as cause of disease classified elsewhere B96.0
Mycosis, mycotic B49
- cutaneous NEC B36.9
- ear B36.9
  - in
    - aspergillosis B44.89
    - candidiasis B37.84
    - moniliasis B37.84
- fungoides (extranodal) (solid organ) C84.0-●
- mouth B37.0
- nails B35.1
- opportunistic B48.8
- skin NEC B36.9
- specified NEC B48.8
- stomatitis B37.0
- vagina, vaginitis (candidal) (acute) B37.31
  - chronic (recurrent) B37.32
Mydriasis (pupil) H57.04
Myelatelia Q06.1
Myelinolysis, pontine, central G37.2
Myelitis (acute) (ascending) (childhood) (chronic) (descending) (diffuse) (disseminated) (idiopathic) (pressure) (progressive) (spinal cord) (subacute) —see also Encephalitis G04.91
- flaccid G04.82
- herpes simplex B00.82
- herpes zoster B02.24
- in diseases classified elsewhere G05.4
- necrotizing, subacute G37.4
- optic neuritis in G36.0
- postchickenpox B01.12
- postherpetic B02.24
- postimmunization G04.02
- postinfectious NEC G04.89
- postvaccinal G04.02
- specified NEC G04.89
- syphilitic (transverse) A52.14
- toxic G92.9
- transverse (in demyelinating diseases of central nervous system) G37.3
- tuberculous A17.82
- varicella B01.12
Myeloblastic —see condition
Myeloblastoma
- granular cell —see also Neoplasm, connective tissue
  - malignant —see Neoplasm, connective tissue, malignant
  - tongue D10.1
Myelocele —see Spina bifida
Myelocystocele —see Spina bifida
Myelocytic —see condition
Myelodysplasia D46.9
- specified NEC D46.Z
- spinal cord (congenital) Q06.1
Myelodysplastic syndrome (see also Syndrome, myelodysplastic) D46.9
- with
  - 5q deletion D46.C
  - isolated del (5q) chromosomal abnormality C46.C
  - ▶ pancytopenia, acquired —see Syndrome, myelodysplastic, pancytopenia
  - specified NEC D46.Z
Myeloencephalitis —see Encephalitis
Myelofibrosis D75.81
- with myeloid metaplasia D47.4
- acute C94.4-●
- idiopathic (chronic) D47.4
- primary D47.1
- secondary D75.81
  - in myeloproliferative disease D47.4
Myelogenous —see condition
Myeloid —see condition
Myelokathexis D70.9
Myeloleukodystrophy E75.29
Myelolipoma —see Lipoma
Myeloma (multiple) C90.0-●
- monostotic C90.3
  - plasma cell C90.0-●
- plasma cell C90.0-●
- solitary —see also Plasmacytoma, solitary C90.3-●

Myelomalacia G95.89
Myelomatosis C90.0-●
Myelomeningitis —see Meningoencephalitis
Myelomeningocele (spinal cord) —see Spina bifida
Myelo-osteo-musculodysplasia hereditaria Q79.8
Myelopathic
- anemia D64.89
- muscle atrophy —see Atrophy, muscle, spinal
- pain syndrome G89.0
Myelopathy (spinal cord) G95.9
- drug-induced G95.89
- in (due to)
  - degeneration or displacement, intervertebral disc NEC —see Disorder, disc, with, myelopathy
  - disease classified elsewhere G99.2
  - infection —see Encephalitis
  - intervertebral disc disorder —see also Disorder, disc, with, myelopathy
  - mercury —see subcategory T56.1
  - neoplastic disease —see also Neoplasm D49.9 [G99.2]
  - pernicious anemia D51.0 [G99.2]
  - spondylosis —see Spondylosis, with myelopathy NEC
- necrotic (subacute) (vascular) G95.19
- radiation-induced G95.89
- spondylogenic NEC —see Spondylosis, with myelopathy NEC
- toxic G95.89
- transverse, acute G37.3
- vascular G95.19
- vitamin B12 E53.8 [G32.0]
Myelophthisis D61.82
Myeloradiculitis G04.91
Myeloradiculodysplasia (spinal) Q06.1
Myelosarcoma C92.3-●
Myelosclerosis D75.89
- with myeloid metaplasia D47.4
- disseminated, of nervous system G35
- megakaryocytic D47.4
  - with myeloid metaplasia D47.4
Myelosis
- acute C92.0-●
- aleukemic C92.9-●
- chronic D47.1
- erythremic (acute) C94.0-●
- megakaryocytic C94.2-●
- nonleukemic D72.828
- subacute C92.9-●
Myiasis (cavernous) B87.9
- aural B87.4
- creeping B87.0
- cutaneous B87.0
- dermal B87.0
- ear (external) (middle) B87.4
- eye B87.2
- genitourinary B87.81
- intestinal B87.82
- laryngeal B87.3
- nasopharyngeal B87.3
- ocular B87.2
- orbit B87.2
- skin B87.0
- specified site NEC B87.89
- traumatic B87.1
- wound B87.1
Myoadenoma, prostate —see Hyperplasia, prostate
Myoblastoma
- granular cell —see also Neoplasm, connective tissue, benign
  - malignant —see Neoplasm, connective tissue, malignant
  - tongue D10.1
Myocardial —see condition
Myocardiopathy (congestive) (constrictive) (familial) (hypertrophic nonobstructive) (idiopathic) (infiltrative) (obstructive) (primary) (restrictive) (sporadic) —see also Cardiomyopathy I42.9
- alcoholic I42.6
- cobalt-beer I42.6
- glycogen storage E74.02 [I43]
- hypertrophic obstructive I42.1
- in (due to)
  - beriberi E51.12
  - cardiac glycogenosis E74.02 [I43]
  - Friedreich's ataxia G11.11 [I43]

▶ New   ➡ Revised   ~~deleted~~ Deleted   ● Use Additional Character(s)

Myocardiopathy (Continued)
in (Continued)
myotonia atrophica G71.11 [I43]
progressive muscular dystrophy (see also Dystrophy, muscular, by type) G71.03 [I43]
obscure (African) I42.8
secondary I42.9
thyrotoxic E05.90 [I43]
with storm E05.91 [I43]
toxic NEC I42.7
Myocarditis (with arteriosclerosis) (chronic) (fibroid) (interstitial) (old) (progressive) (senile) I51.4
with
rheumatic fever (conditions in I00) I09.0
active —see Myocarditis, acute, rheumatic
inactive or quiescent (with chorea) I09.0
active I40.9
rheumatic I01.2
with chorea (acute) (rheumatic) (Sydenham's) I02.0
acute or subacute (interstitial) I40.9
due to
streptococcus (beta-hemolytic) I01.2
idiopathic I40.1
rheumatic I01.2
with chorea (acute) (rheumatic) (Sydenham's) I02.0
specified NEC I40.8
aseptic of newborn B33.22
bacterial (acute) I40.0
Coxsackie (virus) B33.22
diphtheritic A36.81
eosinophilic I40.1
epidemic of newborn (Coxsackie) B33.22
Fiedler's (acute) (isolated) I40.1
giant cell (acute) (subacute) I40.1
gonococcal A54.83
granulomatous (idiopathic) (isolated) (nonspecific) I40.1
hypertensive —see Hypertension, heart
idiopathic (granulomatous) I40.1
in (due to)
diphtheria A36.81
epidemic louse-borne typhus A75.0 [I41]
Lyme disease A69.29
sarcoidosis D86.85
scarlet fever A38.1
toxoplasmosis (acquired) B58.81
typhoid A01.02
typhus NEC A75.9 [I41]
infective I40.0
influenzal —see Influenza, with, myocarditis
isolated (acute) I40.1
meningococcal A39.52
mumps B26.82
nonrheumatic, active I40.9
parenchymatous I40.9
pneumococcal I40.0
rheumatic (chronic) (inactive) (with chorea) I09.0
active or acute I01.2
with chorea (acute) (rheumatic) (Sydenham's) I02.0
rheumatoid —see Rheumatoid, carditis
septic I40.0
staphylococcal I40.0
suppurative I40.0
syphilitic (chronic) A52.06
toxic I40.8
rheumatic —see Myocarditis, acute, rheumatic
tuberculous A18.84
typhoid A01.02
valvular —see Endocarditis
virus, viral I40.0
of newborn (Coxsackie) B33.22
Myocardium, myocardial —see condition
Myocardosis —see Cardiomyopathy
Myoclonus, myoclonic, myoclonia (familial) (essential) (multifocal) (simplex) G25.3
drug-induced G25.3
epilepsy —see also Epilepsy, generalized, specified NEC G40.4-●
familial (progressive) see Epilepsy, myoclonus
epileptica (see also Epilepsy, myoclonus) G40.409
with status epilepticus G40.401
facial G51.3-●
familial progressive G25.3
epilepsy —see Epilepsy, myoclonus, progressive
Friedreich's G25.3
jerks G25.3

Myoclonus, myoclonic, myoclonia (Continued)
Lafora - see Epilepsy, myoclonus, progressive, Lafora
massive G25.3
palatal G25.3
pharyngeal G25.3
Myocytolysis I51.5
Myodiastasis —see Diastasis, muscle
Myoendocarditis —see Endocarditis
Myoepithelioma —see Neoplasm, benign, by site
Myofasciitis (acute) —see Myositis
Myofibroma —see also Neoplasm, connective tissue, benign
uterus (cervix) (corpus) —see Leiomyoma
Myofibromatosis D48.19
infantile Q89.8
Myofibrosis M62.89
heart —see Myocarditis
scapulohumeral —see Lesion, shoulder, specified NEC
Myofibrositis M79.7
scapulohumeral —see Lesion, shoulder, specified NEC
Myoglobulinuria, myoglobinuria (primary) R82.1
Myokymia, facial G51.4
Myolipoma —see Lipoma
Myoma —see also Neoplasm, connective tissue, benign
malignant —see Neoplasm, connective tissue, malignant
prostate D29.1
uterus (cervix) (corpus) —see Leiomyoma
Myomalacia M62.89
Myometritis —see Endometritis
Myometrium —see condition
Myonecrosis, clostridial A48.0
Myopathy G72.9
acute
necrotizing G72.81
quadriplegic G72.81
alcoholic G72.1
benign congenital G71.20
central core G71.29
centronuclear G71.228
autosomal (dominant) (recessive) G71.228
other specified NEC G71.228
congenital (benign) G71.20
critical illness G72.81
distal G71.09
drug-induced G72.0
endocrine NEC E34.9 [G73.7]
extraocular muscles H05.82-●
facioscapulohumeral G71.02
hereditary G71.9
specified NEC G71.8
hyaline body G71.29
myosin storage G71.29
immune NEC G72.49
in (due to)
Addison's disease E27.1 [G73.7]
alcohol G72.1
amyloidosis E85.0 [G73.7]
cretinism E00.9 [G73.7]
Cushing's syndrome E24.9 [G73.7]
drugs G72.0
endocrine disease NEC E34.9 [G73.7]
giant cell arteritis M31.6 [G73.7]
glycogen storage disease E74.00 [G73.7]
hyperadrenocorticism E24.9 [G73.7]
hyperparathyroidism NEC E21.3 [G73.7]
hypoparathyroidism E20.9 [G73.7]
hypopituitarism E23.0 [G73.7]
hypothyroidism E03.9 [G73.7]
infectious disease NEC B99 [G73.7]
lipid storage disease E75.6 [G73.7]
metabolic disease NEC E88.9 [G73.7]
myxedema E03.9 [G73.7]
parasitic disease NEC B89 [G73.7]
polyarteritis nodosa M30.0 [G73.7]
rheumatoid arthritis —see Rheumatoid, myopathy
sarcoidosis D86.87
scleroderma M34.82
sicca syndrome M35.03
Sjögren's syndrome M35.03
systemic lupus erythematosus M32.19
thyrotoxicosis (hyperthyroidism) E05.90 [G73.7]
with thyroid storm E05.91 [G73.7]
toxic agent NEC G72.2
inflammatory NEC G72.49
intensive care (ICU) G72.81

Myopathy (Continued)
limb-girdle —see Dystrophy, muscular, limb-girdle
mitochondrial NEC G71.3
Miyoshi, type 3 G71.035
myosin storage G71.29
mytonic, proximal (PROMM) G71.11
myotubular (centronuclear) G71.220
X-linked G71.220
nemaline G71.21
ocular G71.09
oculopharyngeal G71.09
of critical illness G72.81
primary G71.9
specified NEC G71.8
progressive NEC G72.89
proximal myotonic (PROMM) G71.11
rod (body) G71.21
scapulohumeral G71.02
specified NEC G72.89
toxic G72.2
Myopericarditis —see also Pericarditis
chronic rheumatic I09.2
Myopia (axial) (congenital) H52.1-●
degenerative (malignant) H44.20
with
choroidal neovascularization H44.2A-●
foveoschisis H44.2D-●
macular hole H44.2B-●
retinal detachment H44.2C-●
specified maculopathy NEC H44.2E-●
bilateral H44.23
left eye H44.22
right eye H44.21
malignant —see also Myopia, degenerative H44.2-●
pernicious —see also Myopia, degenerative H44.2-●
progressive high (degenerative) —see also Myopia, degenerative H44.2-●
Myosarcoma —see Neoplasm, connective tissue, malignant
Myosis (pupil) H57.03
stromal (endolymphatic) D39.0
Myositis M60.9
clostridial A48.0
due to posture —see Myositis, specified type NEC
epidemic B33.0
fibrosa or fibrous (chronic), Volkmann's T79.6
foreign body granuloma —see Granuloma, foreign body
in (due to)
bilharziasis B65.9 [M63.8-●]
cysticercosis B69.81
leprosy A30.9 [M63.8-●]
mycosis B49 [M63.8-●]
sarcoidosis D86.87
schistosomiasis B65.9 [M63.8-●]
syphilis
late A52.78
secondary A51.49
toxoplasmosis (acquired) B58.82
trichinellosis B75 [M63.8-●]
tuberculosis A18.09
inclusion body [IBM] G72.41
infective M60.009
arm M60.002
left M60.001
right M60.000
leg M60.005
left M60.004
right M60.003
lower limb M60.005
ankle M60.07-●
foot M60.07-●
lower leg M60.06-●
thigh M60.05-●
toe M60.07-●
multiple sites M60.09
specified site NEC M60.08
upper limb M60.002
finger M60.04-●
forearm M60.03-●
hand M60.04-●
shoulder region M60.01-●
upper arm M60.02-●
interstitial M60.10
ankle M60.17-●
foot M60.17-●
forearm M60.13-●
hand M60.14-●

Myositis (Continued)
  interstitial (Continued)
    lower leg M60.16-●
    multiple sites M60.19
    shoulder region M60.11-●
    specified site NEC M60.18
    thigh M60.15-●
    upper arm M60.12-●
  mycotic B49 [M63.8-●]
  ossificans or ossifying (circumscripta) —see also
      Ossification, muscle, specified NEC
    in (due to)
      burns M61.30
        ankle M61.37-●
        foot M61.37-●
        forearm M61.33-●
        hand M61.34-●
        lower leg M61.36-●
        multiple sites M61.39
        pelvic region M61.35-●
        shoulder region M61.31-●
        specified site NEC M61.38
        thigh M61.35-●
        upper arm M61.32-●
      quadriplegia or paraplegia M61.20
        ankle M61.27-●
        foot M61.27-●
        forearm M61.23-●
        hand M61.24-●
        lower leg M61.26-●
        multiple sites M61.29
        pelvic region M61.25-●
        shoulder region M61.21-●
        specified site NEC M61.28
        thigh M61.25-●
        upper arm M61.22-●
  progressiva M61.10
    ankle M61.17-●
    finger M61.14-●
    foot M61.17-●
    forearm M61.13-●
    hand M61.14-●
    lower leg M61.16-●
    multiple sites M61.19
    pelvic region M61.15-●
    shoulder region M61.11-●
    specified site NEC M61.18
    thigh M61.15-●
    toe M61.17-●
    upper arm M61.12-●
  traumatica M61.00
    ankle M61.07-●
    foot M61.07-●
    forearm M61.03-●
    hand M61.04-●
    lower leg M61.06-●
    multiple sites M61.09
    pelvic region M61.05-●
    shoulder region M61.01-●
    specified site NEC M61.08
    thigh M61.05-●
    upper arm M61.02-●
  purulent —see Myositis, infective
  specified type NEC M60.80
    ankle M60.87-●
    foot M60.87-●
    forearm M60.83-●
    hand M60.84-●
    lower leg M60.86-●
    multiple sites M60.89
    pelvic region M60.85-●
    shoulder region M60.81-●
    specified site NEC M60.88
    thigh M60.85-●
    upper arm M60.82-●
  suppurative —see Myositis, infective
  traumatic (old) —see Myositis, specified type
      NEC
Myospasia impulsiva F95.2
Myotonia (acquisita) (intermittens) M62.89
  atrophica G71.11
  chondrodystrophic G71.13
  congenita (acetazolamide responsive)
      (dominant) (recessive) G71.12
  drug-induced G71.14
  dystrophica G71.11
  fluctuans G71.19
  levior G71.12
  permanens G71.19
  symptomatic G71.19
Myotonic pupil —see Anomaly, pupil, function,
    tonic pupil

Myriapodiasis B88.2
Myringitis H73.2-●
  with otitis media —see Otitis, media
  acute H73.00-●
    bullous H73.01-●
    specified NEC H73.09-●
  bullous —see Myringitis, acute, bullous
  chronic H73.1-●
Mysophobia F40.228
Mytilotoxism —see Poisoning, fish
Myxadenitis labialis K13.0
Myxedema (adult) (idiocy) (infantile) (juvenile) —
      see also Hypothyroidism E03.9
  circumscribed E05.90
    with storm E05.91
  coma E03.5
  congenital E00.1
  cutis L98.5
  localized (pretibial) E05.90
    with storm E05.91
  papular L98.5
Myxochondrosarcoma —see Neoplasm, cartilage,
    malignant
Myxofibroma —see Neoplasm, connective tissue,
    benign
  odontogenic —see Cyst, calcifying odontogenic
Myxofibrosarcoma —see Neoplasm, connective
    tissue, malignant
Myxolipoma D17.9
Myxoliposarcoma —see Neoplasm, connective
    tissue, malignant
Myxoma —see also Neoplasm, connective tissue,
    benign
  nerve sheath —see Neoplasm, nerve, benign
  odontogenic —see Cyst, calcifying odontogenic
Myxosarcoma —see Neoplasm, connective tissue,
    malignant

——————— N ———————

Naegeli's
  disease Q82.8
  leukemia, monocytic C93.1-●
Naegleriasis (with meningoencephalitis)
    B60.2
Naffziger's syndrome G54.0
Naga sore —see Ulcer, skin
Nägele's pelvis M95.5
  with disproportion (fetopelvic) O33.0
    causing obstructed labor O65.0
Nail —see also condition
  biting F98.8
  patella syndrome Q87.2
Nanism, nanosomia —see Dwarfism
Nanophyetiasis B66.8
Nanukayami A27.89
Napkin rash L22
Narcolepsy G47.419
  with cataplexy G47.411
  in conditions classified elsewhere G47.429
    with cataplexy G47.421
Narcosis R06.89
Narcotism —see Dependence
NARP (Neuropathy, Ataxia and Retinitis
    pigmentosa) syndrome E88.49
Narrow
  anterior chamber angle H40.03-●
  gingival width (of periodontal soft tissue)
      K05.5
  pelvis —see Contraction, pelvis
Narrowing —see also Stenosis
  artery I77.1
    auditory, internal I65.8
    basilar —see Occlusion, artery, basilar
    carotid —see Occlusion, artery, carotid
  ▶ caudal septum, fixed, lower lateral cartilage,
        alar rim and nasal sill J34.8211
    cerebellar —see Occlusion, artery, cerebellar
    cerebral —see Occlusion artery, cerebral
    choroidal —see Occlusion, artery, precerebral,
        specified NEC
    communicating posterior —see
        Occlusion, artery, precerebral, specified
        NEC
    coronary —see also Disease, heart, ischemic,
        atherosclerotic
      congenital Q24.5
        syphilitic A50.54 [I52]
      due to syphilis NEC A52.06

Narrowing (Continued)
  artery (Continued)
    hypophyseal —see Occlusion, artery,
        precerebral, specified NEC
    pontine —see Occlusion, artery, precerebral,
        specified NEC
    precerebral —see Occlusion, artery, precerebral
    vertebral —see Occlusion, artery, vertebral
  auditory canal (external) —see Stenosis, external
      ear canal
  eustachian tube —see Obstruction, eustachian
      tube
  eyelid —see Disorder, eyelid function
  larynx J38.6
  mesenteric artery —see also Ischemia, intestine,
      acute K55.059
  palate M26.89
  palpebral fissure —see Disorder, eyelid function
  ureter N13.5
    with infection N13.6
  urethra —see Stricture, urethra
Narrowness, abnormal, eyelid Q10.3
Nasal —see condition
Nasolachrymal, nasolacrimal —see condition
Nasopharyngeal —see also condition
  pituitary gland Q89.2
  torticollis M43.6
Nasopharyngitis (acute) (infective) (streptococcal)
    (subacute) J00
  chronic (suppurative) (ulcerative) J31.1
Nasopharynx, nasopharyngeal —see condition
Natal tooth, teeth K00.6
Nausea (without vomiting) R11.0
  with vomiting R11.2
  gravidarum —see Hyperemesis, gravidarum
  marina T75.3
  navalis T75.3
Navel —see condition
Neapolitan fever —see Brucellosis
Near drowning T75.1
Nearsightedness —see Myopia
Near-syncope R55
Nebula, cornea —see Opacity, cornea
Necator americanus infestation B76.1
Necatoriasis B76.1
Neck —see condition
Necrobiosis R68.89
  lipoidica NEC L92.1
    with diabetes —see E08-E13 with .620
Necrolysis, toxic epidermal L51.2
  due to drug
    correct substance properly administered —see
        Table of Drugs and Chemicals, by drug,
        adverse effect
    overdose or wrong substance given or
        taken —see Table of Drugs and
        Chemicals, by drug, poisoning
Necrophilia F65.89
Necrosis, necrotic (ischemic) —see also Gangrene
  adrenal (capsule) (gland) E27.49
  amputation stump (surgical) (late) T87.50
    arm T87.5-●
    leg T87.5-●
  antrum J32.0
  aorta (hyaline) —see also Aneurysm, aorta
    cystic medial —see Dissection, aorta
  artery I77.5
  bladder (aseptic) (sphincter) N32.89
  bone —see also Osteonecrosis M87.9
    aseptic or avascular —see Osteonecrosis
      idiopathic M87.00
    ethmoid J32.2
    jaw M27.2
    tuberculous —see Tuberculosis, bone
  brain I67.89
  breast (aseptic) (fat) (segmental) N64.1
  bronchus J98.09
  central nervous system NEC I67.89
  cerebellar I67.89
  cerebral I67.89
  colon —see also Infarct, intestine K55.049
  cornea H18.89-●
  cortical (acute) (renal) N17.1
  cystic medial (aorta) —see Dissection, aorta
  dental pulp K04.1
  esophagus K22.89
  ethmoid (bone) J32.2
  eyelid —see Disorder, eyelid, degenerative
  fat, fatty (generalized) —see also Disorder, soft
      tissue, specified type NEC
    abdominal wall K65.4
    breast (aseptic) (segmental) N64.1

▶ New   ⇒ Revised   ~~deleted~~ Deleted   ● Use Additional Character(s)

Necrosis, necrotic *(Continued)*
  fat, fatty *(Continued)*
    localized —*see* Degeneration, by site, fatty
    mesentery K65.4
    omentum K65.4
    pancreas K86.89
    peritoneum K65.4
    skin (subcutaneous), newborn P83.0
    subcutaneous, due to birth injury P15.6
  gallbladder —*see* Cholecystitis, acute
  heart —*see* Infarct, myocardium
  hip, aseptic or avascular —*see* Osteonecrosis, by type, femur
  intestine (acute) (hemorrhagic) (massive) —*see also* Infarct, intestine K55.069
  jaw M27.2
  kidney (bilateral) N28.0
    acute N17.9
    cortical (acute) (bilateral) N17.1
      with ectopic or molar pregnancy O08.4
    medullary (bilateral) (in acute renal failure) (papillary) N17.2
    papillary (bilateral) (in acute renal failure) N17.2
    tubular N17.0
      with ectopic or molar pregnancy O08.4
      complicating
        abortion —*see* Abortion, by type, complicated by, tubular necrosis
        ectopic or molar pregnancy O08.4
        pregnancy —*see* Pregnancy, complicated by, diseases of, specified type or system NEC
      following ectopic or molar pregnancy O08.4
      traumatic T79.5
  larynx J38.7
  liver (with hepatic failure) (cell) —*see* Failure, hepatic
    hemorrhagic, central K76.2
  lung J85.0
  lymphatic gland —*see* Lymphadenitis, acute
  mammary gland (fat) (segmental) N64.1
  mastoid (chronic) —*see* Mastoiditis, chronic
  medullary (acute) (renal) N17.2
  mesentery —*see also* Infarct, intestine K55.069
    fat K65.4
  mitral valve —*see* Insufficiency, mitral
  myocardium, myocardial —*see* Infarct, myocardium
▶ nasal septum, head of the inferior turbinate and the upper lateral cartilage J34.8201
  nose J34.0
  omentum (with mesenteric infarction) —*see also* Infarct, intestine K55.069
    fat K65.4
  orbit, orbital —*see* Osteomyelitis, orbit
  ossicles, ear —*see* Abnormal, ear ossicles
  ovary N70.92
  pancreas (aseptic) (duct) (fat) K86.89
    acute (infective) —*see* Pancreatitis, acute
    infective —*see* Pancreatitis, acute
  papillary (acute) (renal) N17.2
  perineum N90.89
  peritoneum (with mesenteric infarction) —*see also* Infarct, intestine K55.069
    fat K65.4
  pharynx J02.9
    in granulocytopenia —*see* Neutropenia
    Vincent's A69.1
  phosphorus —*see* subcategory T54.2
  pituitary (gland) E23.0
    postpartum O99.285
    Sheehan O99.285
  pressure —*see* Ulcer, pressure, by site
  pulmonary J85.0
  pulp (dental) K04.1
  radiation —*see* Necrosis, by site
  radium —*see* Necrosis, by site
  renal —*see* Necrosis, kidney
  sclera H15.89
  scrotum N50.89
  skin or subcutaneous tissue NEC I96
  spine, spinal (column) —*see also* Osteonecrosis, by type, vertebra
    cord G95.19
  spleen D73.5
  stomach K31.89
  stomatitis (ulcerative) A69.0
  subcutaneous fat, newborn P83.88
  subendocardial (acute) I21.4
    chronic I25.89

Necrosis, necrotic *(Continued)*
  suprarenal (capsule) (gland) E27.49
  testis N50.89
  thymus (gland) E32.8
  tonsil J35.8
  trachea J39.8
  tuberculous NEC —*see* Tuberculosis
  tubular (acute) (anoxic) (renal) (toxic) N17.0
    postprocedural N99.0
  vagina N89.8
  vertebra —*see also* Osteonecrosis, by type, vertebra
    tuberculous A18.01
  vulva N90.89
  X-ray —*see* Necrosis, by site
Necrospermia —*see* Infertility, male
Need (for)
  care provider because of (of)
    assistance with personal care Z74.1
    continuous supervision required Z74.3
    impaired mobility Z74.09
    no other household member able to render care Z74.2
    specified reason NEC Z74.8
  immunization —*see* Vaccination
  vaccination —*see* Vaccination
Neglect
  adult
    confirmed T74.01
    history of Z91.412
    suspected T76.01
  child (childhood)
    confirmed T74.02
    history of Z62.812
    suspected T76.02
  emotional, in childhood Z62.898
  hemispatial R41.4
  left-sided R41.4
  sensory R41.4
  visuospatial R41.4
Neisserian infection NEC —*see* Gonococcus
Nelaton's syndrome G60.8
Nelson's syndrome E24.1
Nematodiasis (intestinal) B82.0
  Ancylostoma B76.0
Neonatal —*see also* Newborn
  acne L70.4
  bradycardia P29.12
  screening, abnormal findings on —*see* Abnormal, neonatal screening
  tachycardia P29.11
  tooth, teeth K00.6
Neonatorum —*see* condition
Neoplasia
  endocrine, multiple (MEN) E31.20
    type I E31.21
    type IIA E31.22
    type IIB E31.23
  intraepithelial (histologically confirmed)
    anal (AIN) (histologically confirmed) K62.82
      grade I K62.82
      grade II K62.82
      severe D01.3
    cervical glandular (histologically confirmed) D06.9
    cervix (uteri) (CIN) (histologically confirmed) N87.9
      glandular D06.9
      grade I N87.0
      grade II N87.1
      grade III (severe dysplasia) —*see also* Carcinoma, cervix uteri, in situ D06.9
    prostate (histologically confirmed) (PIN) N42.31
      grade I N42.31
      grade II N42.31
      grade III (severe dysplasia) D07.5
    vagina (histologically confirmed) (VAIN) N89.3
      grade I N89.0
      grade II N89.1
      grade III (severe dysplasia) D07.2
    vulva (histologically confirmed) (VIN) N90.3
      grade I N90.0
      grade II N90.1
      grade III (severe dysplasia) D07.1
Neoplasm, neoplastic —*see also* Table of Neoplasms
  lipomatous, benign —*see* Lipoma
  malignant mast cell C96.20
    specified type NEC C96.29

Neoplasm, neoplastic *(Continued)*
  mast cell, of uncertain behavior NEC D47.09
  myelodysplastic/myeloproliferative, unclassifiable C94.6
Neovascularization
  ciliary body —*see* Disorder, iris, vascular
  cornea H16.40-●
    deep H16.44-●
    ghost vessels —*see* Ghost, vessels
    localized H16.43-●
    pannus —*see* Pannus
  iris —*see* Disorder, iris, vascular
  retina H35.05-●
Nephralgia N23
Nephritis, nephritic (albuminuric) (azotemic) (congenital) (disseminated) (epithelial) (familial) (focal) (granulomatous) (hemorrhagic) (infantile) (nonsuppurative, excretory) (uremic) N05.9
  with
    C3
      glomerulonephritis N05.A
      glomerulopathy N05.A
        with dense deposit disease N05.6
    dense deposit disease N05.6
    diffuse
      crescentic glomerulonephritis N05.7
      endocapillary proliferative glomerulonephritis N05.4
      membranous glomerulonephritis N05.2
      mesangial proliferative glomerulonephritis N05.3
      mesangiocapillary glomerulonephritis N05.5
    edema —*see* Nephrosis
    focal and segmental glomerular lesions N05.1
    foot process disease N04.9
    glomerular lesion
      diffuse sclerosing N05.8
      hypocomplementemic —*see* Nephritis, membranoproliferative
      IgA —*see* Nephropathy, IgA
      lobular, lobulonodular —*see* Nephritis, membranoproliferative
      nodular —*see* Nephritis, membranoproliferative
    lesion of
      glomerulonephritis, proliferative N05.8
      renal necrosis N05.9
    minor glomerular abnormality N05.0
    specified morphological changes NEC N05.8
  acute N00.9
    with
      C3
        glomerulonephritis N00.A
        glomerulopathy N00.A
          with dense deposit disease N00.6
      dense deposit disease N00.6
      diffuse
        crescentic glomerulonephritis N00.7
        endocapillary proliferative glomerulonephritis N00.4
        membranous glomerulonephritis N00.2
        mesangial proliferative glomerulonephritis N00.3
        mesangiocapillary glomerulonephritis N00.5
      focal and segmental glomerular lesions N00.1
      minor glomerular abnormality N00.0
      specified morphological changes NEC N00.8
  amyloid E85.4 *[N08]*
  antiglomerular basement membrane (anti-GBM) antibody NEC
    in Goodpasture's syndrome M31.0
  antitubular basement membrane (tubulo-interstitial) NEC N12
    toxic —*see* Nephropathy, toxic
  arteriolar —*see* Hypertension, kidney
  arteriosclerotic —*see* Hypertension, kidney
  ascending —*see* Nephritis, tubulo-interstitial
  atrophic N03.9
  Balkan (endemic) N15.0
  calculus, calculus —*see* Calculus, kidney
  cardiac —*see* Hypertension, kidney
  cardiovascular —*see* Hypertension, kidney

Nephritis, nephritic *(Continued)*
chronic N03.9
with
C3
glomerulonephritis N03.A
glomerulopathy N03.A
with dense deposit disease N03.6
dense deposit disease N03.6
diffuse
crescentic glomerulonephritis N03.7
endocapillary proliferative
glomerulonephritis N03.4
membranous glomerulonephritis N03.2
mesangial proliferative
glomerulonephritis N03.3
mesangiocapillary glomerulonephritis
N03.5
focal and segmental glomerular lesions
N03.1
minor glomerular abnormality
N03.0
specified morphological changes
NEC N03.8
arteriosclerotic —*see* Hypertension,
kidney
cirrhotic N26.9
complicating pregnancy O26.83-●
croupous N00.9
degenerative —*see* Nephrosis
diffuse sclerosing N05.8
due to
diabetes mellitus —*see* E08-E13 with .21
subacute bacterial endocarditis I33.0
systemic lupus erythematosus (chronic)
M32.14
typhoid fever A01.09
gonococcal (acute) (chronic) A54.21
hypocomplementemic —*see* Nephritis,
membranoproliferative
IgA —*see* Nephropathy, IgA
immune complex (circulating) NEC N05.8
infective —*see* Nephritis, tubulo-interstitial
interstitial —*see* Nephritis, tubulo-interstitial
lead N14.3
membranoproliferative (diffuse) (type 1 or
3) —*see also* N00-N07 with fourth character
.5 N05.5
type 2 —*see also* N00-N07 with fourth
character .6 N05.6
minimal change N05.0
necrotic, necrotizing NEC —*see also* N00-N07
with fourth character .8 N05.8
nephrotic —*see* Nephrosis
nodular —*see* Nephritis, membranoproliferative
polycystic Q61.3
adult type Q61.2
autosomal
dominant Q61.2
recessive NEC Q61.19
childhood type NEC Q61.19
infantile type NEC Q61.19
poststreptococcal N05.9
acute N00.9
chronic N03.9
rapidly progressive N01.9
proliferative NEC —*see also* N00-N07 with fourth
character .8 N05.8
purulent —*see* Nephritis, tubulo-interstitial
rapidly progressive N01.9
with
C3
glomerulonephritis N01.A
glomerulopathy N01.A
with dense deposit disease N01.6
dense deposit disease N01.6
diffuse
crescentic glomerulonephritis N01.7
endocapillary proliferative
glomerulonephritis N01.4
membranous glomerulonephritis N01.2
mesangial proliferative
glomerulonephritis N01.3
mesangiocapillary glomerulonephritis
N01.5
focal and segmental glomerular lesions
N01.1
minor glomerular abnormality N01.0
specified morphological changes NEC
N01.8
salt losing or wasting NEC N28.89
saturnine N14.3

Nephritis, nephritic *(Continued)*
sclerosing, diffuse N05.8
septic —*see* Nephritis, tubulo-interstitial
specified pathology NEC —*see also* N00-N07
with fourth character .8 N05.8
subacute N01.9
suppurative —*see* Nephritis, tubulo-interstitial
syphilitic (late) A52.75
congenital A50.59 *[N08]*
early (secondary) A51.44
toxic —*see* Nephropathy, toxic
tubal, tubular —*see* Nephritis, tubulo-interstitial
tuberculous A18.11
tubulo-interstitial (in) N12
acute (infectious) N10
chronic (infectious) N11.9
nonobstructive N11.8
reflux-associated N11.0
obstructive N11.1
specified NEC N11.8
due to
brucellosis A23.9 *[N16]*
cryoglobulinemia D89.1 *[N16]*
glycogen storage disease E74.00 *[N16]*
Sjögren's syndrome M35.04
vascular —*see* Hypertension, kidney
war N00.9
Nephroblastoma (epithelial) (mesenchymal) C64-●
Nephrocalcinosis E83.59 *[N29]*
Nephrocystitis, pustular —*see* Nephritis,
tubulo-interstitial
Nephrolithiasis (congenital) (pelvis) (recurrent) —
see also Calculus, kidney
Nephroma C64-●
mesoblastic D41.0-●
Nephronephritis —*see* Nephrosis
Nephronophthisis Q61.5
Nephropathia epidemica A98.5
Nephropathy —*see also* Nephritis N28.9
with
edema —*see* Nephrosis
glomerular lesion —*see* Glomerulonephritis
amyloid, hereditary E85.0
analgesic N14.0
with medullary necrosis, acute N17.2
Balkan (endemic) N15.0
chemical —*see* Nephropathy, toxic
contrast-induced N14.11
contrast medium, radiography N14.11
diabetic —*see* E08-E13 with .21
drug-induced N14.2
contrast-induced N14.11
specified NEC N14.19
focal and segmental hyalinosis or sclerosis N02.1
heavy metal-induced N14.3
hereditary NEC N07.9
with
C3
glomerulonephritis N07.A
glomerulopathy N07.A
with dense deposit disease N07.6
dense deposit disease N07.6
diffuse
crescentic glomerulonephritis N07.7
endocapillary proliferative
glomerulonephritis N07.4
membranous glomerulonephritis N07.2
mesangial proliferative
glomerulonephritis N07.3
mesangiocapillary glomerulonephritis
N07.5
focal and segmental glomerular lesions
N07.1
minor glomerular abnormality N07.0
specified morphological changes NEC
N07.8
hypercalcemic N25.89
hypertensive —*see* Hypertension, kidney
hypokalemic (vacuolar) N25.89
IgA IgA N02.B-●
with glomerular lesion N02.B1
focal and segmental hyalinosis or sclerosis
N02.B2
membranoproliferative (diffuse) N02.B3
membranous (diffuse) N02.B4
mesangial proliferative (diffuse) N02.B5
mesangiocapillary (diffuse) N02.B6
proliferative NEC N02.B9
specified pathology NEC N02.B9
lead N14.3
membranoproliferative (diffuse) N02.5

Nephropathy *(Continued)*
membranous (diffuse) N02.20
with
nephrotic syndrome N04.20
primary N04.21
secondary N04.22
idiopathic, with nephrotic syndrome N04.21
primary N06.21
with nephrotic syndrome N04.21
secondary N06.22
with nephrotic syndrome N04.22
mesangial (IgA/IgG) —*see* Nephropathy, IgA
proliferative (diffuse) N02.3
mesangiocapillary (diffuse) N02.5
obstructive N13.8
phenacetin N17.2
phosphate-losing N25.0
potassium depletion N25.89
pregnancy-related O26.83-●
proliferative NEC (see also N00-N07 with fourth
character .8) N05.8
protein-losing N25.89
saturnine N14.3
sickle-cell D57.-● *[N08]*
toxic NEC N14.4
due to
drugs N14.2
analgesic N14.0
specified NEC N14.19
heavy metals N14.3
vasomotor N17.0
water-losing N25.89
Nephroptosis N28.83
Nephropyosis —*see* Abscess, kidney
Nephrorrhagia N28.89
Nephrosclerosis (arteriolar) (arteriosclerotic)
(chronic) (hyaline) —*see also* Hypertension,
kidney
hyperplastic —*see* Hypertension, kidney
senile N26.9
Nephrosis, nephrotic (Epstein's) (syndrome)
(congenital) N04.9
with
foot process disease N04.9
glomerular lesion N04.1
hypocomplementemic N04.5
acute N04.9
anoxic —*see* Nephrosis, tubular
chemical —*see* Nephrosis, tubular
cholemic K76.7
diabetic —*see* E08-E13 with .21
Finnish type (congenital) Q89.8
hemoglobin N10
hemoglobinuric —*see* Nephrosis, tubular
in
amyloidosis E85.4 *[N08]*
diabetes mellitus —*see* E08-E13 with .21
epidemic hemorrhagic fever A98.5
malaria (malariae) B52.0
ischemic —*see* Nephrosis, tubular
lipoid N04.9
lower nephron —*see* Nephrosis, tubular
malarial (malariae) B52.0
minimal change N04.0
myoglobin N10
necrotizing —*see* Nephrosis, tubular
osmotic (sucrose) N25.89
radiation N04.9
syphilitic (late) A52.75
toxic —*see* Nephrosis, tubular
tubular (acute) N17.0
postprocedural N99.0
radiation N04.9
Nephrosonephritis, hemorrhagic (endemic)
A98.5
Nephrostomy
attention to Z43.6
status Z93.6
Nerve —*see also* condition
injury —*see* Injury, nerve, by body site
Nerves R45.0
Nervous —*see also* condition R45.0
heart F45.8
stomach F45.8
tension R45.0
Nervousness R45.0
Nesidioblastoma
pancreas D13.7
specified site NEC —*see* Neoplasm, benign, by
site
unspecified site D13.7

Nettleship's syndrome —*see* Urticaria pigmentosa
Neumann's disease or syndrome L10.1
Neuralgia, neuralgic (acute) M79.2
  accessory (nerve) G52.8
  acoustic (nerve) —*see* subcategory H93.3
  auditory (nerve) —*see* subcategory H93.3
  ciliary G44.009
    intractable G44.001
    not intractable G44.009
  cranial
    nerve —*see also* Disorder, nerve, cranial
      fifth or trigeminal —*see* Neuralgia,
        trigeminal
    postherpetic, postzoster B02.29
  ear —*see* subcategory H92.0
  facialis vera G51.1
  Fothergill's —*see* Neuralgia, trigeminal
  glossopharyngeal (nerve) G52.1
  Horton's G44.099
    intractable G44.091
    not intractable G44.099
  Hunt's B02.21
  hypoglossal (nerve) G52.3
  infraorbital —*see* Neuralgia, trigeminal
  malarial —*see* Malaria
  migrainous G44.009
    intractable G44.001
    not intractable G44.009
  Morton's G57.6-●
  nerve, cranial —*see* Disorder, nerve, cranial
  nose G52.0
  occipital M54.81
  olfactory G52.0
  penis N48.9
  perineum R10.2
  postherpetic NEC B02.29
    trigeminal B02.22
  pubic region R10.2
  scrotum R10.2
  Sluder's G44.89
  specified nerve NEC G58.8
  spermatic cord R10.2
  sphenopalatine (ganglion) G90.09
  trifacial —*see* Neuralgia, trigeminal
  trigeminal G50.0
    postherpetic, postzoster B02.22
  vagus (nerve) G52.2
  writer's F48.8
    organic G25.89
Neurapraxia —*see* Injury, nerve
Neurasthenia F48.8
  cardiac F45.8
  gastric F45.8
  heart F45.8
Neurilemmoma —*see also* Neoplasm, nerve, benign
  acoustic (nerve) D33.3
  malignant —*see also* Neoplasm, nerve, malignant
    acoustic (nerve) C72.4
Neurilemmosarcoma —*see* Neoplasm, nerve,
  malignant
Neurinoma —*see* Neoplasm, nerve, benign
Neurinomatosis —*see* Neoplasm, nerve, uncertain
  behavior
Neuritis (rheumatoid) M79.2
  abducens (nerve) —*see* Strabismus, paralytic,
    sixth nerve
  accessory (nerve) G52.8
  acoustic (nerve) —*see also* subcategory H93.3
    in (due to)
      infectious disease NEC B99 [H94.0-●]
      parasitic disease NEC B89 [H94.0-●]
      syphilitic A52.15
  alcoholic G62.1
    with psychosis —*see* Psychosis, alcoholic
  amyloid, any site E85.4 [G63]
  auditory (nerve) —*see* subcategory H93.3
  brachial —*see* Radiculopathy
    due to displacement, intervertebral disc —*see*
      Disorder, disc, cervical, with neuritis
  cranial nerve
    due to Lyme disease A69.22
    eighth or acoustic or auditory —*see*
      subcategory H93.3
    eleventh or accessory G52.8
    fifth or trigeminal G50.-●
    first or olfactory G52.0
    fourth or trochlear —*see* Strabismus, paralytic,
      fourth nerve
    second or optic —*see* Neuritis, optic
    seventh or facial G51.8
      newborn (birth injury) P11.3

Neuritis (Continued)
  cranial nerve (Continued)
    sixth or abducent —*see* Strabismus, paralytic,
      sixth nerve
    tenth or vagus G52.2
    third or oculomotor —*see* Strabismus,
      paralytic, third nerve
    twelfth or hypoglossal G52.3
  Déjérine-Sottas G60.0
  diabetic (mononeuropathy) —*see* E08-E13 with
    .41
    polyneuropathy —*see* E08-E13 with .42
  due to
    beriberi E51.11
    displacement, prolapse or rupture,
      intervertebral disc —*see* Disorder, disc,
      with, radiculopathy
    herniation, nucleus pulposus M51.9 [G55]
  endemic E51.11
  facial G51.8
    newborn (birth injury) P11.3
  general —*see* Polyneuropathy
  geniculate ganglion G51.1
    due to herpes (zoster) B02.21
  gouty —*see also* Gout, by type M10.9 [G63]
  hypoglossal (nerve) G52.3
  ilioinguinal (nerve) G57.9-●
  infectious (multiple) NEC G61.0
  interstitial hypertrophic progressive G60.0
  lumbar M54.16
  lumbosacral M54.17
  multiple —*see also* Polyneuropathy
    endemic E51.11
    infective, acute G61.0
  multiplex endemica E51.11
  nerve root —*see* Radiculopathy
  oculomotor (nerve) —*see* Strabismus, paralytic,
    third nerve
  olfactory nerve G52.0
  optic (nerve) (hereditary) (sympathetic)
    H46.9
    with demyelination G36.0
      in myelitis G36.0
    nutritional H46.2
    papillitis —*see* Papillitis, optic
    retrobulbar H46.1-●
    specified type NEC H46.8
    toxic H46.3
  peripheral (nerve) G62.9
    multiple —*see* Polyneuropathy
    single —*see* Mononeuritis
  pneumogastric (nerve) G52.2
  postherpetic, postzoster B02.29
  progressive hypertrophic interstitial G60.0
  retrobulbar —*see also* Neuritis, optic, retrobulbar
    in (due to)
      late syphilis A52.15
      meningococcal infection A39.82
    meningococcal A39.82
    syphilitic A52.15
  sciatic (nerve) —*see also* Sciatica
    due to displacement of intervertebral disc —
      see Disorder, disc, with, radiculopathy
  serum —*see also* Reaction, serum T80.69
  shoulder-girdle G54.5
  specified nerve NEC G58.8
  spinal (nerve) root —*see* Radiculopathy
  syphilitic A52.15
  thenar (median) G56.1-●
  thoracic M54.14
  toxic NEC G62.2
  trochlear (nerve) —*see* Strabismus, paralytic,
    fourth nerve
  vagus (nerve) G52.2
Neuroastrocytoma —*see* Neoplasm, uncertain
  behavior, by site
Neuroavitaminosis E56.9 [G99.8]
Neuroblastoma
  olfactory C30.0
  specified site —*see* Neoplasm, malignant, by site
  unspecified site C74.90
Neurochorioretinitis —*see* Chorioretinitis
Neurocirculatory asthenia F45.8
Neurocysticercosis B69.0
Neurocytoma —*see* Neoplasm, benign, by site
Neurodermatitis (circumscribed) (circumscripta)
  (local) L28.0
  atopic L20.81
  diffuse (Brocq) L20.81
  disseminated L20.81
Neuroencephalomyelopathy, optic G36.0

Neuroepithelioma —*see also* Neoplasm, malignant,
  by site
  olfactory C30.0
Neurofibroma —*see also* Neoplasm, nerve, benign
  melanotic —*see* Neoplasm, nerve, benign
  multiple —*see* Neurofibromatosis
  plexiform —*see* Neoplasm, nerve, benign
Neurofibromatosis (multiple) (nonmalignant)
  Q85.00
  acoustic Q85.02
  malignant —*see* Neoplasm, nerve, malignant
  specified NEC Q85.09
  type 1 (von Recklinghausen) Q85.01
  type 2 Q85.02
Neurofibrosarcoma —*see* Neoplasm, nerve,
  malignant
Neurogenic —*see also* condition
  bladder —*see also* Dysfunction, bladder,
    neuromuscular N31.9
    cauda equina syndrome G83.4
  bowel NEC K59.2
  heart F45.8
Neuroglioma —*see* Neoplasm, uncertain behavior,
  by site
Neurolabyrinthitis (of Dix and Hallpike) —*see*
  Neuronitis, vestibular
Neurolathyrism —*see* Poisoning, food, noxious,
  plant
Neuroleprosy A30.9
Neuroma —*see also* Neoplasm, nerve, benign
  acoustic (nerve) D33.3
  amputation (stump) (traumatic) (surgical
    complication) (late) T87.3-●
    arm T87.3-●
    leg T87.3-●
  digital (toe) G57.6-●
  interdigital G58.8
    lower limb toe G57.8-●
    upper limb G56.8-●
  intermetatarsal G57.8-●
  Morton's G57.6-●
  nonneoplastic
    arm G56.9-●
    leg G57.9-●
    lower extremity G57.9-●
    upper extremity G56.9-●
  optic (nerve) D33.3
  plantar G57.6-●
  plexiform —*see* Neoplasm, nerve,
    benign
  surgical (nonneoplastic)
    arm G56.9-●
    leg G57.9-●
    lower extremity G57.9-●
    upper extremity G56.9-●
Neuromyalgia —*see* Neuralgia
Neuromyasthenia (epidemic) (postinfectious)
  G93.39
Neuromyelitis G36.9
  ascending G61.0
  optica G36.0
Neuromyopathy G70.9
  paraneoplastic (*see also*, Neoplasm, by site, if
    known) D49.9 [G13.0]
Neuromyotonia (Isaacs) G71.19
Neuronevus —*see* Nevus
Neuronitis G58.9
  ascending (acute) G57.2-●
  vestibular H81.2-●
Neuroparalytic —*see* condition
Neuropathy, neuropathic G62.9
  acute motor G62.81
  alcoholic G62.1
    with psychosis —*see* Psychosis, alcoholic
  arm G56.9-●
  autonomic, peripheral —*see* Neuropathy,
    peripheral, autonomic
  axillary G56.9-●
  bladder N31.9
    atonic (motor) (sensory) N31.2
    autonomous N31.2
    flaccid N31.2
    nonreflex N31.2
    reflex N31.1
    uninhibited N31.0
  brachial plexus G54.0
  cervical plexus G54.2
  chronic
    progressive segmentally demyelinating
      G62.89
    relapsing demyelinating G62.89

Neuropathy, neuropathic *(Continued)*
  Déjérine-Sottas G60.0
  diabetic —*see* E08-E13 with .40
    mononeuropathy —*see* E08-E13 with .41
    polyneuropathy —*see* E08-E13 with .42
  entrapment G58.9
    iliohypogastric nerve G57.8-●
    ilioinguinal nerve G57.8-●
    lateral cutaneous nerve of thigh
        G57.1-●
    median nerve G56.0-●
    obturator nerve G57.8-●
    peroneal nerve G57.3-●
    posterior tibial nerve G57.5-●
    saphenous nerve G57.8-●
    ulnar nerve G56.2-●
  facial nerve G51.9
  hereditary G60.9
    motor and sensory (types I-IV) G60.0
    sensory G60.8
    specified NEC G60.8
  hypertrophic G60.0
    Charcot-Marie-Tooth G60.0
    Déjérine-Sottas G60.0
    interstitial progressive G60.0
    of infancy G60.0
    Refsum G60.1
  idiopathic G60.9
    progressive G60.3
    specified NEC G60.8
  in association with hereditary ataxia G60.2
  intercostal G58.0
  ischemic —*see* Disorder, nerve
  Jamaica (ginger) G62.2
  leg NEC G57.9-●
  lower extremity G57.9-●
  lumbar plexus G54.1
  median nerve G56.1-●
  motor and sensory —*see also* Polyneuropathy
    hereditary (types I-IV) G60.0
  multifocal motor (MMN) G61.82
  multiple (acute) (chronic) —*see* Polyneuropathy
  optic (nerve) —*see also* Neuritis, optic
    ischemic H47.01-●
  paraneoplastic (sensorial) (Denny Brown) *(see
    also,* Neoplasm, by site, if known) D49.9
    [G13.0]
  peripheral (nerve) —*see also* Polyneuropathy
    G62.9
    autonomic G90.9
      idiopathic G90.09
      in (due to)
        amyloidosis E85.4 *[G99.0]*
        diabetes mellitus —*see* E08-E13 with .43
        endocrine disease NEC E34.9 *[G99.0]*
        gout M10.00 *[G99.0]*
        hyperthyroidism E05.90 *[G99.0]*
          with thyroid storm E05.91 *[G99.0]*
        metabolic disease NEC E88.9
          [G99.0]
    idiopathic G60.9
      progressive G60.3
    in (due to)
      antitetanus serum G62.0
      arsenic G62.2
      drugs NEC G62.0
      lead G62.2
      organophosphate compounds G62.2
      toxic agent NEC G62.2
  plantar nerves G57.6-●
  progressive
    hypertrophic interstitial G60.0
    inflammatory G62.81
  radicular NEC —*see* Radiculopathy
  sacral plexus G54.1
  sciatic G57.0-●
  serum G61.1
  toxic NEC G62.2
  trigeminal sensory G50.8
  ulnar nerve G56.2-●
  uremic N18.9 *[G63]*
  vitamin B12 E53.8 *[G63]*
    with anemia (pernicious) D51.0 *[G63]*
      due to dietary deficiency D51.3 *[G63]*
Neurophthisis —*see also* Disorder, nerve
  peripheral, diabetic —*see* E08-E13 with .42
Neuroretinitis —*see* Chorioretinitis
Neuroretinopathy, hereditary optic H47.22
Neurosarcoma —*see* Neoplasm, nerve,
    malignant
Neurosclerosis —*see* Disorder, nerve

Neurosis, neurotic F48.9
  anankastic F42.8
  anxiety (state) F41.1
    panic type F41.0
  asthenic F48.8
  bladder F45.8
  cardiac (reflex) F45.8
  cardiovascular F45.8
  character F60.9
  colon F45.8
  compensation F68.10
  compulsive, compulsion F42.8
  conversion F44.9
  craft F48.8
  cutaneous F45.8
  depersonalization F48.1
  depressive (reaction) (type) F34.1
  environmental F48.8
  excoriation L98.1
  fatigue F48.8
  functional —*see* Disorder, somatoform
  gastric F45.8
  gastrointestinal F45.8
  heart F45.8
  hypochondriacal F45.21
  hysterical F44.9
  incoordination F45.8
    larynx F45.8
    vocal cord F45.8
  intestine F45.8
  larynx (sensory) F45.8
    hysterical F44.4
  mixed NEC F48.8
  musculoskeletal F45.8
  obsessional F42.8
  obsessive-compulsive F42.8
  occupational F48.8
  ocular NEC F45.8
  organ —*see* Disorder, somatoform
  pharynx F45.8
  phobic F40.9
  posttraumatic (situational) F43.10
    acute F43.11
    chronic F43.12
  psychasthenic (type) F48.8
  railroad F48.8
  rectum F45.8
  respiratory F45.8
  rumination F45.8
  sexual F65.9
  situational F48.8
  social F40.10
    generalized F40.11
  specified type NEC F48.8
  state F48.9
    with depersonalization episode F48.1
  stomach F45.8
  traumatic F43.10
    acute F43.11
    chronic F43.12
  vasomotor F45.8
  visceral F45.8
  war F48.8
Neurospongioblastosis diffusa Q85.1
Neurosyphilis (arrested) (early) (gumma) (late)
    (latent) (recurrent) (relapse) A52.3
  with ataxia (cerebellar) (locomotor) (spastic)
    (spinal) A52.19
  aneurysm (cerebral) A52.05
  arachnoid (adhesive) A52.13
  arteritis (any artery) (cerebral) A52.04
  asymptomatic A52.2
  congenital A50.40
  dura (mater) A52.13
  general paresis A52.17
  hemorrhagic A52.05
  juvenile (asymptomatic) (meningeal)
    A50.40
  leptomeninges (aseptic) A52.13
  meningeal, meninges (adhesive) A52.13
  meningitis A52.13
  meningovascular (diffuse) A52.13
  optic atrophy A52.15
  parenchymatous (degenerative) A52.19
  paresis, paretic A52.17
    juvenile A50.45
  remission in (sustained) A52.3
  serological (without symptoms) A52.2
  specified nature or site NEC A52.19
  tabes, tabetic (dorsalis) A52.11
    juvenile A50.45

Neurosyphilis *(Continued)*
  taboparesis (taboparetic) A52.17
    juvenile A50.45
  thrombosis (cerebral) A52.05
  vascular (cerebral) NEC A52.05
Neurothekeoma —*see* Neoplasm, nerve, benign
Neurotic —*see* Neurosis
Neurotoxemia —*see* Toxemia
Neutroclusion M26.211
Neutropenia, neutropenic (chronic) (genetic)
    (idiopathic) (immune) (infantile) (malignant)
    (pernicious) (splenic) D70.9
▶benign ethnic —*see* Phenotype, Duffy, null
  congenital (primary) D70.0
  cyclic D70.4
  cytoreductive cancer chemotherapy sequela
    D70.1
  drug-induced D70.2
    due to cytoreductive cancer chemotherapy
      D70.1
  due to infection D70.3
  fever D70.9
  neonatal, transitory (isoimmune) (maternal
    transfer) P61.5
  periodic D70.4
  secondary (cyclic) (periodic) (splenic) D70.4
    drug-induced D70.2
      due to cytoreductive cancer chemotherapy
        D70.1
  specified NEC D70.8
  toxic D70.8
Neutrophilia, hereditary giant D72.0
Nevocarcinoma —*see* Melanoma
Nevus D22.9
  achromic —*see* Neoplasm, skin, benign
  amelanotic —*see* Neoplasm, skin, benign
  angiomatous D18.00
    intra-abdominal D18.03
    intracranial D18.02
    skin D18.01
    specified site NEC D18.09
  araneus I78.1
  balloon cell —*see* Neoplasm, skin, benign
  bathing trunk D48.5
  blue —*see* Neoplasm, skin, benign
    cellular —*see* Neoplasm, skin, benign
    giant —*see* Neoplasm, skin, benign
    Jadassohn's —*see* Neoplasm, skin, benign
    malignant —*see* Melanoma
  capillary D18.00
    intra-abdominal D18.03
    intracranial D18.02
    skin D18.01
    specified site NEC D18.09
  cavernous D18.00
    intra-abdominal D18.03
    intracranial D18.02
    skin D18.01
    specified site NEC D18.09
  cellular —*see* Neoplasm, skin, benign
    blue —*see* Neoplasm, skin, benign
  choroid D31.3-●
  comedonicus Q82.5
  conjunctiva D31.0-●
  dermal —*see* Neoplasm, skin, benign
    with epidermal nevus —*see* Neoplasm, skin,
      benign
  dysplastic —*see* Neoplasm, skin, benign
  eye D31.9-●
  flammeus Q82.5
  hemangiomatous D18.00
    intra-abdominal D18.03
    intracranial D18.02
    skin D18.01
    specified site NEC D18.09
  iris D31.4-●
  lacrimal gland D31.5-●
  lymphatic D18.1
  magnocellular
    specified site —*see* Neoplasm, benign, by site
    unspecified site D31.40
  malignant —*see* Melanoma
  meaning hemangioma D18.00
    intra-abdominal D18.03
    intracranial D18.02
    skin D18.01
    specified site NEC D18.09
  mouth (mucosa) D10.30
    specified site NEC D10.39
    white sponge Q38.6
  multiplex Q85.1

Nevus (Continued)
non-neoplastic I78.1
oral mucosa D10.30
    specified site NEC D10.39
    white sponge Q38.6
orbit D31.6-●
pigmented
    giant —see also Neoplasm, skin, uncertain
        behavior D48.5
    malignant melanoma in —see Melanoma
portwine Q82.5
retina D31.2-●
retrobulbar D31.6-●
sanguineous Q82.5
senile I78.1
skin D22.9
    abdominal wall D22.5
    ala nasi D22.39
    ankle D22.7-●
    anus, anal D22.5
    arm D22.6-●
    auditory canal (external) D22.2-●
    auricle (ear) D22.2-●
    auricular canal (external) D22.2-●
    axilla, axillary fold D22.5
    back D22.5
    breast D22.5
    brow D22.39
    buttock D22.5
    canthus (eye) D22.1-●
    cheek (external) D22.39
    chest wall D22.5
    chin D22.39
    ear (external) D22.2-●
    external meatus (ear) D22.2-●
    eyebrow D22.39
    eyelid (lower) (upper) D22.1-●
    face D22.30
        specified NEC D22.39
    female genital organ (external) NEC D28.0
    finger D22.6-●
    flank D22.5
    foot D22.7-●
    forearm D22.6-●
    forehead D22.39
    foreskin D29.0
    genital organ (external) NEC
        female D28.0
        male D29.9
    gluteal region D22.5
    groin D22.5
    hand D22.6-●
    heel D22.7-●
    helix D22.2-●
    hip D22.7-●
    interscapular region D22.5
    jaw D22.39
    knee D22.7-●
    labium (majus) (minus) D28.0
    leg D22.7-●
    lip (lower) (upper) D22.0
    lower limb D22.7-●
    male genital organ (external) D29.9
    nail D22.9
        finger D22.6-●
        toe D22.7-●
    nasolabial groove D22.39
    nates D22.5
    neck D22.4
    nose (external) D22.39
    palpebra D22.1-●
    penis D29.0
    perianal skin D22.5
    perineum D22.5
    pinna D22.2-●
    popliteal fossa or space D22.7-●
    prepuce D29.0
    pudendum D28.0
    scalp D22.4
    scrotum D29.4
    shoulder D22.6-●
    submammary fold D22.5
    temple D22.39
    thigh D22.7-●
    toe D22.7-●
    trunk NEC D22.5
    umbilicus D22.5
    upper limb D22.6-●
    vulva D28.0
specified site NEC —see Neoplasm, benign, by
    site

Nevus (Continued)
spider I78.1
stellar I78.1
strawberry Q82.5
Sutton's benign D22.9
unius lateris Q82.5
Unna's Q82.5
vascular Q82.5
verrucous Q82.5
Newborn (infant) (liveborn) (singleton)
Z38.2
abstinence syndrome P96.1
acne L70.4
affected by
    abnormalities of membranes P02.9
        specified NEC P02.8
    abruptio placenta P02.1
    amino-acid metabolic disorder, transitory
        P74.4
    amniocentesis (while in utero) P00.6
    amnionitis P02.78
    apparent life threatening event (ALTE)
        R68.13
    bleeding (into)
        cerebral cortex P52.22
        germinal matrix P52.0
        ventricles P52.1
    breech delivery P03.0
    cardiac arrest P29.81
    cardiomyopathy I42.8
        congenital I42.4
    cerebral ischemia P91.0
    Cesarean delivery P03.4
    chemotherapy agents P04.11
    chorioamnionitis P02.78
    cocaine (crack) P04.41
    complications of labor and delivery P03.9
        specified NEC P03.89
    compression of umbilical cord NEC P02.5
    contracted pelvis P03.1
    cyanosis P28.2
    delivery P03.9
        Cesarean P03.4
        forceps P03.2
        vacuum extractor P03.3
    drugs of addiction P04.40
        cocaine P04.41
        hallucinogens P04.42
        specified drug NEC P04.49
    entanglement (knot) in umbilical cord P02.5
    environmental chemicals P04.6
    fetal (intrauterine)
        growth retardation P05.9
        inflammatory response syndrome (FIRS)
            P02.70
        malnutrition not light or small for
            gestational age P05.2
    FIRS (fetal inflammatory response syndrome)
        P02.70
    forceps delivery P03.2
    heart rate abnormalities
        bradycardia P29.12
        intrauterine P03.819
            before onset of labor P03.810
            during labor P03.811
        tachycardia P29.11
    hemorrhage (antepartum) P02.1
        cerebellar (nontraumatic) P52.6
        intracerebral (nontraumatic) P52.4
        intracranial (nontraumatic) P52.9
            specified NEC P52.8
        intraventricular (nontraumatic) P52.3
            grade 1 P52.0
            grade 2 P52.1
            grade 3 P52.21
            grade 4 P52.22
        posterior fossa (nontraumatic) P52.6
        subarachnoid (nontraumatic) P52.5
        subependymal P52.0
            with intracerebral extension P52.22
            with intraventricular extension P52.1
                with enlargment of ventricles P52.21
            without intraventricular extension
                P52.0
    hypoxic ischemic encephalopathy [HIE]
        P91.60
        mild P91.61
        moderate P91.62
        severe P91.63
    induction of labor P03.89
    intestinal perforation P78.0

Newborn (Continued)
affected by (Continued)
    intrauterine (fetal) blood loss P50.9
        due to (from)
            cut end of co-twin cord P50.5
            hemorrhage into
                co-twin P50.3
                maternal circulation P50.4
            placenta P50.2
            ruptured cord blood P50.1
            vasa previa P50.0
        specified NEC P50.8
    intrauterine (fetal) hemorrhage P50.9
    intrauterine (in utero) procedure P96.5
    malpresentation (malposition) NEC P03.1
    maternal (complication of) (use of)
        alcohol P04.3
        amphetamines P04.16
        analgesia (maternal) P04.0
        anesthesia (maternal) P04.0
        anticonvulsants P04.13
        antidepressants P04.15
        antineoplastic chemotherapy P04.11
        anxiolytics P04.1A
        blood loss P02.1
        cannabis P04.81
        circulatory disease P00.3
        condition P00.9
            specified NEC P00.89
        cytotoxic drugs P04.12
        delivery P03.9
            Cesarean P03.4
            forceps P03.2
            vacuum extractor P03.3
        diabetes mellitus (pre-existing) P70.1
        disorder P00.9
            specified NEC P00.89
        drugs (addictive) (illegal) NEC P04.49
        ectopic pregnancy P01.4
        gestational diabetes P70.0
        group B streptococcus (GBS) colonization
            (positive) P00.82
        hemorrhage P02.1
        hypertensive disorder P00.0
        incompetent cervix P01.0
        infectious disease P00.2
        injury P00.5
        labor and delivery P03.9
        malpresentation before labor P01.7
        maternal death P01.6
        medical procedure P00.7
        medication P04.19
            specified type NEC P04.18
        multiple pregnancy P01.5
        nutritional disorder P00.4
        oligohydramnios P01.2
        opiates P04.14
            administered for procedures during
                pregnancy or labor and delivery
                P04.0
        parasitic disease P00.2
        periodontal disease P00.81
        placenta previa P02.0
        polyhydramnios P01.3
        precipitate delivery P03.5
        pregnancy P01.9
            specified P01.8
        premature rupture of membranes P01.1
        renal disease P00.1
        respiratory disease P00.3
        sedative-hypnotics P04.17
        surgical procedure P00.6
        tranquilizers administered for procedures
            during pregnancy or labor and
            delivery P04.0
        urinary tract disease P00.1
        uterine contraction (abnormal) P03.6
    meconium peritonitis P78.0
    medication (legal) (maternal use) (prescribed)
        P04.19
    membrane abnormalities P02.9
        specified NEC P02.8
    membranitis P02.78
    methamphetamine(s) P04.49
    mixed metabolic and respiratory acidosis P84
    neonatal abstinence syndrome P96.1
    noxious substances transmitted via placenta
        or breast milk P04.9
        cannabis P04.81
        specified NEC P04.89
    nutritional supplements P04.5

Newborn *(Continued)*
  affected by *(Continued)*
    placenta previa P02.0
    placental
      abnormality (functional) (morphological)
        P02.20
        specified NEC P02.29
      dysfunction P02.29
      infarction P02.29
      insufficiency P02.29
      separation NEC P02.1
      transfusion syndromes P02.3
    placentitis P02.78
    precipitate delivery P03.5
    prolapsed cord P02.4
    respiratory arrest P28.81
    slow intrauterine growth P05.9
    tobacco P04.2
    twin to twin transplacental transfusion P02.3
    umbilical cord (tightly) around neck P02.5
    umbilical cord condition P02.60
      short cord P02.65
      specified NEC P02.69
    uterine contractions (abnormal) P03.6
    vasa previa P02.69
      from intrauterine blood loss P50.0
  apnea *(see also* Apnea, newborn) P28.40
    obstructive P28.42
    primary *(see also* Apnea, newborn, sleep,
      primary) P28.30
    sleep (central) (obstructive) (primary) *(see also*
      Apnea, newborn, sleep, primary)
      P28.30
  born in hospital Z38.00
    by cesarean Z38.01
  born outside hospital Z38.1
  breast buds P96.89
  breast engorgement P83.4
  check-up *—see* Newborn, examination
  convulsion P90
  dehydration P74.1
  examination
    8 to 28 days old Z00.111
    under 8 days old Z00.110
  fever P81.9
    environmentally-induced P81.0
  hyperbilirubinemia P59.9
    of prematurity P59.0
  hypernatremia P74.21
  hyponatremia P74.22
  infection P39.9
    candidal P37.5
    specified NEC P39.8
    urinary tract P39.3
  jaundice P59.9
    due to
      breast milk inhibitor P59.3
      hepatocellular damage P59.20
        specified NEC P59.29
      preterm delivery P59.0
    of prematurity P59.0
    specified NEC P59.8
  late metabolic acidosis P74.0
  mastitis P39.0
    infective P39.0
    noninfective P83.4
  multiple born NEC Z38.8
    born in hospital Z38.68
      by cesarean Z38.69
    born outside hospital Z38.7
  omphalitis P38.9
    with mild hemorrhage P38.1
    without hemorrhage P38.9
  post-term P08.21
  prolonged gestation (over 42 completed weeks)
    P08.22
  quadruplet Z38.8
    born in hospital Z38.63
      by cesarean Z38.64
    born outside hospital Z38.7
  quintuplet Z38.8
    born in hospital Z38.65
      by cesarean Z38.66
    born outside hospital Z38.7
  seizure P90
  sepsis (congenital) P36.9
    due to
      anaerobes NEC P36.5
      Escherichia coli P36.4
      Staphylococcus P36.30
        aureus P36.2
        specified NEC P36.39

Newborn *(Continued)*
  sepsis *(Continued)*
    due to *(Continued)*
      Streptococcus P36.10
        group B P36.0
        specified NEC P36.19
      specified NEC P36.8
  triplet Z38.8
    born in hospital Z38.61
      by cesarean Z38.62
    born outside hospital Z38.7
  twin Z38.5
    born in hospital Z38.30
      by cesarean Z38.31
    born outside hospital Z38.4
  vomiting P92.09
    bilious P92.01
  weight check Z00.111
Newcastle conjunctivitis or disease B30.8
Nezelof's syndrome (pure alymphocytosis) D81.4
Niacin (amide) deficiency E52
Nicolas (-Durand)-Favre disease A55
Nicotine *—see* Tobacco
Nicotinic acid deficiency E52
Niemann-Pick disease or syndrome E75.249
  specified NEC E75.248
  type
    A E75.240
    A/B E75.244
    B E75.241
    C E75.242
    D E75.243
Night
  blindness *—see* Blindness, night
  sweats R61
  terrors (child) F51.4
Nightmares (REM sleep type) F51.5
NIHSS (National Institutes of Health Stroke Scale)
  score R29.7-●
Nipple *—see* condition
Nisbet's chancre A57
Nishimoto (-Takeuchi) disease I67.5
Nitritoid crisis or reaction *—see* Crisis, nitritoid
Nitrosohemoglobinemia D74.8
Njovera A65
~~No general equivalence degree (GED) Z55.5~~
▶ No
  ▶ general equivalence degree (GED) Z55.5
  ▶ health insurance coverage Z59.71
Nocardiosis, nocardiasis A43.9
  cutaneous A43.1
  lung A43.0
  pneumonia A43.0
  pulmonary A43.0
  specified site NEC A43.8
Nocturia R35.1
  psychogenic F45.8
Nocturnal *—see* condition
Nodal rhythm I49.8
Node(s) *—see also* Nodule
  Bouchard's (with arthropathy) M15.2
  Haygarth's M15.8
  Heberden's (with arthropathy) M15.1
  larynx J38.7
  lymph *—see* condition
  milker's B08.03
  Osler's I33.0
  Schmorl's *—see* Schmorl's disease
  singer's J38.2
  teacher's J38.2
  tuberculous *—see* Tuberculosis, lymph gland
  vocal cord J38.2
Nodule(s), nodular
  actinomycotic *—see* Actinomycosis
  breast NEC *—see* Lump, breast N63.0
  colloid (cystic), thyroid E04.1
  cutaneous *—see* Swelling, localized
  endometrial (stromal) D26.1
  Haygarth's M15.8
  inflammatory *—see* Inflammation
  juxta-articular
    syphilitic A52.77
    yaws A66.7
  larynx J38.7
  lung, solitary (subsegmental branch of the
    bronchial tree) R91.1
    multiple R91.8
  milker's B08.03
  prostate N40.2
    with lower urinary tract symptoms (LUTS) N40.3
    without lower urinary tract symptoms (LUTS)
      N40.2

Nodule(s), nodular *(Continued)*
  pulmonary, solitary (subsegmental branch of the
    bronchial tree) R91.1
  retrocardiac R09.89
  rheumatoid M06.30
    ankle M06.37-●
    elbow M06.32-●
    foot joint M06.37-●
    hand joint M06.34-●
    hip M06.35-●
    knee M06.36-●
    multiple site M06.39
    shoulder M06.31-●
    vertebra M06.38
    wrist M06.33-●
  scrotum (inflammatory) N49.2
  singer's J38.2
  solitary, lung (subsegmental branch of the
    bronchial tree) R91.1
    multiple R91.8
  subcutaneous *—see* Swelling, localized
  teacher's J38.2
  thyroid (cold) (gland) (nontoxic) E04.1
    with thyrotoxicosis E05.20
      with thyroid storm E05.21
    toxic or with hyperthyroidism E05.20
      with thyroid storm E05.21
  vocal cord J38.2
Noma (gangrenous) (hospital) (infective)
    A69.0
  auricle I96
  mouth A69.0
  pudendi N76.89
  vulvae N76.89
Nomad, nomadism Z59.00
NOMID (neonatal onset multisystemic
    inflammatory disorder) M04.2
Nonadherence to medical treatment, specified
    NEC Z91.199
  due to
    financial hardship Z91.190
    specified reason NEC Z91.198
Nonautoimmune hemolytic anemia D59.4
  drug-induced D59.2
Nonclosure *—see also* Imperfect, closure
  ductus arteriosus (Botallo's) Q25.0
  foramen
    botalli Q21.12
    ovale Q21.12
Noncompliance Z91.199
  with
    caregiver
      with patient's
        dietary regimen
          due to
            financial hardship Z91.A10
            specified reason NEC Z91.A18
        medical treatment and regimen
          financial hardship Z91.A91
          specified reason NEC Z91.A98
        medication regimen
          due to financial hardship Z91.A41
          specified reason NEC Z91.A48
        renal dialysis
          financial hardship Z91.A51
          specified reason NEC Z91.A58
    dialysis Z91.158
      due to financial hardship Z91.151
    dietary regimen Z91.119
      due to
        financial hardship Z91.110
        specified reason NEC Z91.118
    medical treatment, specified NEC Z91.199
      due to
        financial hardship Z91.190
        specified reason NEC Z91.198
    medication regimen Z91.148
      due to financial hardship Z91.151
      underdosing *—see also* Table of Drugs and
        Chemicals, categories T36-T50, with
        final character 6 Z91.148
      intentional NEC Z91.128
        by caregiver
          due to
            financial hardship Z91.A20
            specified reason NEC Z91.A28
          due to financial hardship of
            patient Z91.120
      unintentional NEC Z91.138
        by caregiver Z91.A3
    renal dialysis Z91.158
      due to financial hardship Z91.151

▶ New   ⟹ Revised   ~~deleted~~ Deleted   ● Use Additional Character(s)

Nondescent (congenital) —*see also* Malposition, congenital
  cecum Q43.3
  colon Q43.3
  testicle Q53.9
    bilateral Q53.20
      abdominal Q53.211
      perineal Q53.22
    unilateral Q53.10
      abdominal Q53.111
      perineal Q53.12
Nondevelopment
  brain Q02
    part of Q04.3
  heart Q24.8
  organ or site, congenital NEC —*see* Hypoplasia
Nonengagement
  head NEC O32.4
    in labor, causing obstructed labor O64.8
Nonexanthematous tick fever A93.2
Nonexpansion, lung (newborn) P28.0
Nonfunctioning
  cystic duct —*see also* Disease, gallbladder K82.8
  gallbladder —*see also* Disease, gallbladder K82.8
  kidney N28.9
  labyrinth —*see* subcategory H83.2
Non-Hodgkin lymphoma NEC —*see* Lymphoma, non-Hodgkin
Nonimplantation, ovum N97.2
Noninsufflation, fallopian tube N97.1
Non-ketotic hyperglycinemia E72.51
Nonne-Milroy syndrome Q82.0
Nonovulation N97.0
Non-palpable testicle(s)
  bilateral R39.84
  unilateral R39.83
Nonpatent fallopian tube N97.1
Nonpneumatization, lung NEC P28.0
Nonrotation —*see* Malrotation
Nonsecretion, urine —*see* Anuria
Nonunion
  fracture —*see* Fracture, by site
  joint, following fusion or arthrodesis M96.0
  organ or site, congenital NEC —*see* Imperfect, closure
  symphysis pubis, congenital Q74.2
Nonvisualization, gallbladder R93.2
Nonvital, nonvitalized tooth K04.99
Non-working side interference M26.56
Noonan's syndrome Q87.19
Normocytic anemia (infectional) due to blood loss (chronic) D50.0
  acute D62
Norrie's disease (congenital) Q15.8
North American blastomycosis B40.9
Norwegian itch B86
Nose, nasal —*see* condition
Nosebleed R04.0
Nose-picking F98.8
Nosomania F45.21
Nosophobia F45.22
Nostalgia F43.20
Notch of iris Q13.2
Notching nose, congenital (tip) Q30.2
Nothnagel's
  syndrome —*see* Strabismus, paralytic, third nerve
  vasomotor acroparesthesia I73.89
Novy's relapsing fever A68.9
  louse-borne A68.0
  tick-borne A68.1
Noxious
  foodstuffs, poisoning by —*see* Poisoning, food, noxious, plant
  substances transmitted through placenta or breast milk P04.9
Nucleus pulposus —*see* condition
Numbness R20.0
Nuns' knee —*see* Bursitis, prepatellar
Nursemaid's elbow S53.03-●
Nutcracker esophagus K22.4
Nutmeg liver K76.1
Nutrient element deficiency E61.9
  specified NEC E61.8
Nutrition deficient or insufficient —*see also* Malnutrition E63.9
  due to
    insufficient food T73.0
    lack of
      care (child) T76.02
        adult T76.01
      food T73.0

Nutrition deficient or insufficient *(Continued)*
  specific element deficiency —*see* Nutrient element deficiency, or by element
  sequelae —*see* Sequelae, nutritional deficiency
  specified NEC E63.8
Nutritional stunting E45
Nyctalopia (night blindness) —*see* Blindness, night
Nycturia R35.1
  psychogenic F45.8
Nymphomania F52.8
Nystagmus H55.00
  benign paroxysmal —*see* Vertigo, benign paroxysmal
  central positional H81.4
  congenital H55.01
  dissociated H55.04
  latent H55.02
  miners' H55.09
  positional
    benign paroxysmal H81.4
    central H81.4
  specified form NEC H55.09
  visual deprivation H55.03

—————— O ——————

Obermeyer's relapsing fever (European) A68.0
Obesity E66.9
  with alveolar hypoventilation E66.2
  adrenal E27.8
▶class
  ▶1 E66.811
  ▶2 E66.812
  ▶3 E66.813
  complicating
    childbirth O99.214
    pregnancy O99.21-●
    puerperium O99.215
⇒constitutional E66.89
  dietary counseling and surveillance Z71.3
  drug-induced E66.1
  due to
    ▶disruption of MC4R pathway E88.82
    drug E66.1
    excess calories E66.09
      morbid E66.01
      severe E66.01
    ▶gene mutation
    ▶leptin (LEP) E88.82
    ▶leptin receptor (LEPR) E88.82
    ▶melanocortin 4 Receptor (MC4R) E88.82
    ▶nuclear receptor coactivator 1 (NCOA1) E88.82
    ▶proopiomelanocortin (POMC) E88.82
    ▶proprotein convertase subtilisin/kexin type 1 (PCSK1) E88.82
    ▶src homology 2B adaptor signaling protein (SH2B1) E88.82
⇒endocrine E66.89
⇒endogenous E66.89
  exogenous E66.09
⇒familial E66.89
⇒glandular E66.89
  hypothyroid —*see* Hypothyroidism
  hypoventilation syndrome (OHS) E66.2
  morbid E66.01
    with
      alveolar hypoventilation E66.2
      obesity hypoventilation syndrome (OHS) E66.2
    due to excess calories E66.01
  nutritional E66.09
  pituitary E23.6
  severe E66.01
⇒specified type NEC E66.89
Oblique —*see* condition
Obliteration
  appendix (lumen) K38.8
  artery I77.1
  bile duct (noncalculous) K83.1
  common duct (noncalculous) K83.1
  cystic duct —*see* Obstruction, gallbladder
  disease, arteriolar I77.1
  endometrium N85.8
  eye, anterior chamber —*see* Disorder, globe, hypotony
  fallopian tube N97.1

Obliteration *(Continued)*
  lymphatic vessel I89.0
    due to mastectomy I97.2
  organ or site, congenital NEC —*see* Atresia, by site
  ureter N13.5
    with infection N13.6
  urethra —*see* Stricture, urethra
  vein I87.8
  vestibule (oral) K08.89
Observation (following) (for) (without need for further medical care) Z04.9
  accident NEC Z04.3
    at work Z04.2
    transport Z04.1
  adverse effect of drug Z03.6
  alleged rape or sexual assault (victim), ruled out
    adult Z04.41
    child Z04.42
  criminal assault Z04.89
  development state
    adolescent Z00.3
    period of rapid growth in childhood Z00.2
    puberty Z00.3
  disease, specified NEC Z03.89
  following work accident Z04.2
  forced sexual exploitation Z04.81
  forced labor exploitation Z04.82
  growth and development state —*see* Observation, development state
  injuries (accidental) NEC —*see also* Observation, accident
  newborn (for)
    suspected condition, related to exposure from the mother or birth process — *see* Newborn, affected by, maternal
    ruled out Z05.9
      cardiac Z05.0
      connective tissue Z05.73
      gastrointestinal Z05.5
      genetic Z05.41
      genitourinary Z05.6
      immunologic Z05.43
      infectious Z05.1
      metabolic Z05.42
      musculoskeletal Z05.72
      neurological Z05.2
      respiratory Z05.3
      skin and subcutaneous tissue Z05.71
      specified condition NEC Z05.89
  postpartum
    immediately after delivery Z39.0
    routine follow-up Z39.2
  pregnancy (normal) (without complication) Z34.9-●
    high risk O09.9-●
  suicide attempt, alleged NEC Z03.89
    self-poisoning Z03.6
  suspected, ruled out —*see also* Suspected condition, ruled out
    abuse, physical
      adult Z04.71
      child Z04.72
    accident at work Z04.2
    adult battering victim Z04.71
    child battering victim Z04.72
    condition NEC Z03.89
      newborn —*see also* Observation, newborn (for), suspected condition, ruled out Z05.9
    drug poisoning or adverse effect Z03.6
    exposure (to)
      anthrax Z03.810
      biological agent NEC Z03.818
    foreign body
      aspirated (inhaled) Z03.822
      ingested Z03.821
      inserted (injected), in (eye) (orifice) (skin) Z03.823
    inflicted injury NEC Z04.89
    suicide attempt, alleged Z03.89
      self-poisoning Z03.6
    toxic effects from ingested substance (drug) (poison) Z03.6
  toxic effects from ingested substance (drug) (poison) Z03.6
Obsession, obsessional state F42.8
  mixed thoughts and acts F42.2
Obsessive-compulsive neurosis or reaction F42.8

Obstetric embolism, septic —*see* Embolism, obstetric, septic

Obstetrical trauma (complicating delivery) O71.9
  with or following ectopic or molar pregnancy O08.6
  specified type NEC O71.89
Obstipation —see Constipation
Obstruction, obstructed, obstructive
  airway J98.8
    with
      allergic alveolitis J67.9
      asthma J45.909
        with
          exacerbation (acute) J45.901
          status asthmaticus J45.902
      bronchiectasis J47.9
        with
          exacerbation (acute) J47.1
          lower respiratory infection J47.0
      bronchitis (chronic) J44.89
      emphysema J43.9
    chronic J44.9
      with
        allergic alveolitis —see Pneumonitis, hypersensitivity
        bronchiectasis J47.9
          with
            exacerbation (acute) J47.1
            lower respiratory infection J47.0
    due to
      foreign body —see Foreign body, by site, causing asphyxia
      inhalation of fumes or vapors J68.9
      laryngospasm J38.5
  ampulla of Vater K83.1
  aortic (heart) (valve) —see Stenosis, aortic
  aortoiliac I74.09
  aqueduct of Sylvius G91.1
    congenital Q03.0
      with spina bifida —see Spina bifida, by site, with hydrocephalus
  Arnold-Chiari —see Arnold-Chiari disease
  artery (see also Atherosclerosis, artery) I70.9
    basilar (complete) (partial) —see Occlusion, artery, basilar
    carotid (complete) (partial) —see Occlusion, artery, carotid
    cerebellar —see Occlusion, artery, cerebellar
    cerebral (anterior) (middle) (posterior) —see Occlusion, artery, cerebral
    precerebral —see Occlusion, artery, precerebral
    renal N28.0
    retinal NEC —see Occlusion, artery, retina
    stent —see Restenosis, stent
    vertebral (complete) (partial) —see Occlusion, artery, vertebral
  band (intestinal) —see also Obstruction, intestine, specified NEC K56.699
  bile duct or passage (common) (hepatic) (noncalculous) K83.1
    with calculus K80.51
    congenital (causing jaundice) Q44.3
  biliary (duct) (tract) K83.1
    gallbladder K82.0
  bladder-neck (acquired) N32.0
    congenital Q64.31
    due to hyperplasia (hypertrophy) of prostate —see Hyperplasia, prostate
  bowel —see Obstruction, intestine
  bronchus J98.09
  canal, ear —see Stenosis, external ear canal
  cardia K22.2
  caval veins (inferior) (superior) I87.1
  cecum —see Obstruction, intestine
  circulatory I99.8
  colon —see Obstruction, intestine
  common duct (noncalculous) K83.1
  coronary (artery) —see Occlusion, coronary
  cystic duct —see also Obstruction, gallbladder
    with calculus K80.21
  device, implant or graft —see also Complications, by site and type, mechanical T85.698
    arterial graft NEC —see Complication, cardiovascular device, mechanical, vascular
    catheter NEC T85.628
      cystostomy T83.090
      dialysis (renal) T82.49
        intraperitoneal T85.691
      Hopkins T83.098
      ileostomy T83.098
      infusion NEC T82.594
        spinal (epidural) (subdural) T85.690

Obstruction, obstructed, obstructive (Continued)
  device, implant or graft (Continued)
    catheter (Continued)
      nephrostomy T83.092
      urethral indwelling T83.091
      urinary T83.098
      urostomy T83.098
    due to infection T85.79
    gastrointestinal —see Complications, prosthetic device, mechanical, gastrointestinal device
    genital NEC T83.498
      intrauterine contraceptive device T83.39
      penile prosthesis (cylinder) (implanted) (pump) (reservoir) T83.490
      testicular prosthesis T83.491
    heart NEC —see Complication, cardiovascular device, mechanical
    joint prosthesis —see Complications, joint prosthesis, mechanical, specified NEC, by site
    orthopedic NEC —see Complication, orthopedic, device, mechanical
    specified NEC T85.628
    urinary NEC —see also Complication, genitourinary, device, urinary, mechanical
      graft T83.29
    vascular NEC —see Complication, cardiovascular device, mechanical
    ventricular intracranial shunt T85.09
  due to foreign body accidentally left in operative wound T81.529
  duodenum K31.5
  ejaculatory duct N50.89
  esophagus K22.2
  eustachian tube (complete) (partial) H68.10-●
    cartilagenous (extrinsic) H68.13-●
      intrinsic H68.12-●
    osseous H68.11-●
  fallopian tube (bilateral) N97.1
  fecal K56.41
    with hernia —see Hernia, by site, with obstruction
  foramen of Monro (congenital) Q03.8
    with spina bifida —see Spina bifida, by site, with hydrocephalus
  foreign body —see Foreign body
  gallbladder K82.0
    with calculus, stones K80.21
    congenital Q44.1
  gastric outlet K31.1
  gastrointestinal —see Obstruction, intestine
  hepatic K76.89
    duct (noncalculous) K83.1
  hepatobiliary K83.1
  ileum —see Obstruction, intestine
  iliofemoral (artery) I74.5
  intestine K56.609
    complete K56.601
    incomplete K56.600
    partial K56.600
    with
      adhesions (intestinal) (peritoneal) K56.50
        complete K56.52
        incomplete K56.51
        partial K56.51
    adynamic K56.0
    by gallstone K56.3
    congenital (small) Q41.9
      large Q42.9
        specified part NEC Q42.8
    neurogenic K56.0
      Hirschsprung's disease or megacolon Q43.1
    newborn P76.9
      due to
        fecaliths P76.8
        inspissated milk P76.2
        meconium (plug) P76.0
          in mucoviscidosis E84.11
      specified NEC P76.8
    postoperative K91.30
      complete K91.32
      incomplete K91.31
      partial K91.31
    reflex K56.0
    specified NEC K56.699
      complete K56.691
      incomplete K56.690
      partial K56.690
    volvulus K56.2
  intracardiac ball valve prosthesis T82.09

Obstruction, obstructed, obstructive (Continued)
  jejunum —see Obstruction, intestine
  joint prosthesis —see Complications, joint prosthesis, mechanical, specified NEC, by site
  kidney (calices) (see also Hydronephrosis) N28.89
  labor —see Delivery
  lacrimal (passages) (duct)
    by
      dacryolith —see Dacryolith
      stenosis —see Stenosis, lacrimal
    congenital Q10.5
    neonatal H04.53-●
  lacrimonasal duct —see Obstruction, lacrimal
  lacteal, with steatorrhea K90.2
  laryngitis —see Laryngitis
  larynx NEC J38.6
    congenital Q31.8
  lung J98.4
    disease, chronic J44.9
  lymphatic I89.0
  meconium (plug)
    newborn P76.0
      due to fecaliths P76.0
      in mucoviscidosis E84.11
  mitral —see Stenosis, mitral
  nasal J34.89
  nasolacrimal duct —see also Obstruction, lacrimal
    congenital Q10.5
  nasopharynx J39.2
  nose J34.89
  organ or site, congenital NEC —see Atresia, by site
  pancreatic duct K86.89
  parotid duct or gland K11.8
  pelviureteral junction N13.5
    with hydronephrosis N13.0
    congenital Q62.39
  pharynx J39.2
  portal (circulation) (vein) I81
  prostate —see also Hyperplasia, prostate
    valve (urinary) N32.0
  pulmonary valve (heart) I37.0
  pyelonephritis (chronic) N11.1
  pylorus
    adult K31.1
    congenital or infantile Q40.0
  rectosigmoid —see Obstruction, intestine
  rectum K62.4
  renal (see also Hydronephrosis) N28.89
    outflow N13.8
    pelvis, congenital Q62.39
  respiratory J98.8
    chronic J44.9
  retinal (vessels) H34.9
  salivary duct (any) K11.8
    with calculus K11.5
  sigmoid —see Obstruction, intestine
  sinus (accessory) (nasal) J34.89
  Stensen's duct K11.8
  stomach NEC K31.89
    acute K31.0
    congenital Q40.2
    due to pylorospasm K31.3
  submandibular duct K11.8
  submaxillary gland K11.8
    with calculus K11.5
  thoracic duct I89.0
  thrombotic —see Thrombosis
  trachea J39.8
  tracheostomy airway J95.03
  tricuspid (valve) —see Stenosis, tricuspid
  upper respiratory, congenital Q34.8
  ureter (functional) (pelvic junction) NEC N13.5
    with
      hydronephrosis N13.1
        with infection N13.6
        congenital Q62.39
      pyelonephritis (chronic) N11.1
    congenital Q62.39
    due to calculus —see Calculus, ureter
  urethra NEC N36.8
    congenital Q64.39
  urinary (moderate) N13.9
    due to hyperplasia (hypertrophy) of prostate —see Hyperplasia, prostate
    organ or tract (lower) N13.9
    prostatic valve N32.0
    specified NEC N13.8
  uropathy N13.9
  uterus N85.8
  vagina N89.5

▶ New   ⇒ Revised   ~~deleted~~ Deleted   ● Use Additional Character(s)

Obstruction, obstructed, obstructive *(Continued)*
  valvular —*see* Endocarditis
  vein, venous I87.1
    caval (inferior) (superior) I87.1
      thrombotic —*see* Thrombosis
    vena cava (inferior) (superior) I87.1
  vesical NEC N32.0
  vesicourethral orifice N32.0
    congenital Q64.31
  vessel NEC I99.8
    stent —*see* Restenosis, stent
Obturator —*see* condition
Occlusal wear, teeth K03.0
Occlusio pupillae —*see* Membrane, pupillary
Occlusion, occluded
  anus K62.4
    congenital Q42.3
      with fistula Q42.2
  aortoiliac (chronic) I74.09
  aqueduct of Sylvius G91.1
    congenital Q03.0
      with spina bifida —*see* Spina bifida, by site,
        with hydrocephalus
  artery —*see also* Atherosclerosis, artery I70.9
    auditory, internal I65.8
    basilar I65.1
      with
        infarction I63.22
          due to
            embolism I63.12
            thrombosis I63.02
    brain or cerebral I66.9
      with infarction (due to) I63.5-●
        embolism I63.4-●
        thrombosis I63.3-●
    carotid I65.2-●
      with
        infarction I63.23-●
          due to
            embolism I63.13-●
            thrombosis I63.03-●
    cerebellar (anterior inferior) (posterior
      inferior) (superior) I66.3
      with infarction I63.54-●
        due to
          embolism I63.44-●
          thrombosis I63.34-●
    cerebral I66.9
      with infarction I63.50
        due to
          embolism I63.40
            specified NEC I63.49
          thrombosis I63.30
            specified NEC I63.39
      anterior I66.1-●
        with infarction I63.52-●
          due to
            embolism I63.42-●
            thrombosis I63.32-●
      middle I66.0-●
        with infarction I63.51-●
          due to
            embolism I63.41-●
            thrombosis I63.31-●
      posterior I66.2-●
        with infarction I63.53-●
          due to
            embolism I63.43-●
            thrombosis I63.33-●
      specified NEC I66.8
        with infarction I63.59
          due to
            embolism I63.4-●
            thrombosis I63.3-●
    choroidal (anterior) —*see* Occlusion,
      artery, cerebral, specified NEC
    communicating posterior —*see* Occlusion,
      artery, precerebral, specified NEC
    complete
      coronary I25.82
      extremities I70.92
    coronary (acute) (thrombotic) (without
      myocardial infarction) I24.0
      with myocardial infarction —*see* Infarction,
        myocardium
      chronic total I25.82
      complete I25.82
      healed or old I25.2
      total (chronic) I25.82
    hypophyseal —*see* Occlusion, artery,
      precerebral, specified NEC
    iliac I74.5

Occlusion, occluded *(Continued)*
  artery *(Continued)*
    lower extremities due to stenosis or stricture
      I77.1
    mesenteric (embolic) (thrombotic) —*see also*
      Infarct, intestine K55.069
    perforating —*see* Occlusion, artery, cerebral,
      specified NEC
    peripheral I77.9
      thrombotic or embolic I74.4
    pontine —*see* Occlusion, artery, precerebral,
      specified NEC
    precerebral I65.9
      with infarction I63.20
        due to
          embolism I63.10
            specified NEC I63.19
          thrombosis I63.00
            specified NEC I63.09
        specified NEC I63.29
      basilar —*see* Occlusion, artery, basilar
      carotid —*see* Occlusion, artery, carotid
      puerperal O88.23
      specified NEC I65.8
        with infarction I63.29
          due to
            embolism I63.19
            thrombosis I63.09
      vertebral —*see* Occlusion, artery, vertebral
    renal N28.0
    retinal
      branch H34.23-●
      central H34.1-●
      partial H34.21-●
      transient H34.0-●
    spinal —*see* Occlusion, artery, precerebral,
      vertebral
    total (chronic)
      coronary I25.82
      extremities I70.92
    vertebral I65.0-●
      with
        infarction I63.21-●
          due to
            embolism I63.11-●
            thrombosis I63.01-●
  basilar artery —*see* Occlusion, artery, basilar
  bile duct (common) (hepatic) (noncalculous)
    K83.1
  bowel —*see* Obstruction, intestine
  carotid (artery) (common) (internal) —*see*
    Occlusion, artery, carotid
  centric (of teeth) M26.59
    maximum intercuspation discrepancy
      M26.55
  cerebellar (artery) —*see* Occlusion, artery,
    cerebellar
  cerebral (artery) —*see* Occlusion, artery, cerebral
  cerebrovascular —*see also* Occlusion, artery,
    cerebral
    with infarction I63.5-●
  cervical canal —*see* Stricture, cervix
  cervix (uteri) —*see* Stricture, cervix
  choanal Q30.0
  choroidal (artery) —*see* Occlusion, artery,
    precerebral, specified NEC
  colon —*see* Obstruction, intestine
  communicating posterior artery —*see* Occlusion,
    artery, precerebral, specified NEC
  coronary (artery) (vein) (thrombotic) —*see also*
    Infarct, myocardium
    chronic total I25.82
    healed or old I25.2
    not resulting in infarction I24.0
    total (chronic) I25.82
  cystic duct —*see* Obstruction, gallbladder
  embolic —*see* Embolism
  fallopian tube N97.1
    congenital Q50.6
  gallbladder —*see also* Obstruction, gallbladder
    congenital (causing jaundice) Q44.1
  gingiva, traumatic K06.2
  hymen N89.6
    congenital Q52.3
  hypophyseal (artery) —*see* Occlusion, artery,
    precerebral, specified NEC
  iliac artery I74.5
  intestine —*see* Obstruction, intestine
  lacrimal passages —*see* Obstruction, lacrimal
  lung J98.4
  lymph or lymphatic channel I89.0
  mammary duct N64.89

Occlusion, occluded *(Continued)*
  mesenteric artery (embolic) (thrombotic) —*see
    also* Infarct, intestine K55.069
  nose J34.89
    congenital Q30.0
  organ or site, congenital NEC —*see* Atresia, by
    site
  oviduct N97.1
    congenital Q50.6
  peripheral arteries
    due to stricture or stenosis I77.1
    upper extremity I74.2
  pontine (artery) —*see* Occlusion, artery,
    precerebral, specified NEC
  posterior lingual, of mandibular teeth M26.29
  precerebral artery —*see* Occlusion, artery,
    precerebral
  punctum lacrimale —*see* Obstruction, lacrimal
  pupil —*see* Membrane, pupillary
  pylorus, adult —*see also* Stricture, pylorus K31.1
  renal artery N28.0
  retina, retinal
    artery —*see* Occlusion, artery, retinal
    vein (central) H34.81-●
      engorgement H34.82-●
      tributary H34.83-●
    vessels H34.9
  spinal artery —*see* Occlusion, artery, precerebral,
    vertebral
  teeth (mandibular) (posterior lingual) M26.29
  thoracic duct I89.0
  thrombotic —*see* Thrombosis, artery
  traumatic
    edentulous (alveolar) ridge K06.2
    gingiva K06.2
    periodontal K05.5
  tubal N97.1
  ureter (complete) (partial) N13.5
    congenital Q62.10
  ureteropelvic junction N13.5
    congenital Q62.11
  ureterovesical orifice N13.5
    congenital Q62.12
  urethra —*see* Stricture, urethra
  uterus N85.8
  vagina N89.5
  vascular NEC I99.8
  vein —*see* Thrombosis
    retinal —*see* Occlusion, retinal, vein
  vena cava (inferior) (superior) —*see* Embolism,
    vena cava
  ventricle (brain) NEC G91.1
  vertebral (artery) —*see* Occlusion, artery,
    vertebral
  vessel (blood) I99.8
  vulva N90.5
Occult
  blood in feces (stools) R19.5
Occupational
  problems NEC Z56.89
Ochlophobia —*see* Agoraphobia
Ochronosis (endogenous) E70.29
Ocular muscle —*see* condition
Oculogyric crisis or disturbance H51.8
  psychogenic F45.8
Oculomotor syndrome H51.9
Oculopathy
  syphilitic NEC A52.71
    congenital
      early A50.01
      late A50.30
    early (secondary) A51.43
    late A52.71
Oddi's sphincter spasm K83.4
Odontalgia K08.89
Odontoameloblastoma —*see* Cyst, calcifying
  odontogenic
Odontoclasia K03.89
Odontodysplasia, regional K00.4
Odontogenesis imperfecta K00.5
Odontoma (ameloblastic) (complex) (compound)
  (fibroameloblastic) —*see* Cyst, calcifying
  odontogenic
Odontomyelitis (closed) (open) K04.01
  irreversible K04.02
  reversible K04.01
Odontorrhagia K08.89
Odontosarcoma, ameloblastic C41.1
  upper jaw (bone) C41.0
Oestriasis —*see* Myiasis
Oguchi's disease H53.63
Ohara's disease —*see* Tularemia

OHS (obesity hypoventilation syndrome) E66.2
Oidiomycosis —see Candidiasis
Oidium albicans infection —see Candidiasis
Old (previous) myocardial infarction
I25.2
Old age (without mention of debility) R54-●
dementia F03
Olfactory —see condition
Oligemia —see Anemia
Oligoastrocytoma
specified site —see Neoplasm, malignant, by site
unspecified site C71.9
Oligocythemia D64.9
Oligodendroblastoma
specified site —see Neoplasm, malignant
unspecified site C71.9
Oligodendroglioma
anaplastic type
specified site —see Neoplasm, malignant, by site
unspecified site C71.9
specified site —see Neoplasm, malignant, by site
unspecified site C71.9
Oligodontia —see Anodontia
Oligoencephalon Q02
Oligohidrosis L74.4
Oligohydramnios O41.0-●
Oligohydrosis L74.4
Oligomenorrhea N91.5
primary N91.3
secondary N91.4
Oligophrenia —see also Disability, intellectual
phenylpyruvic E70.0
Oligospermia N46.11
due to
drug therapy N46.121
efferent duct obstruction N46.123
infection N46.122
radiation N46.124
specified cause NEC N46.129
systemic disease N46.125
Oligotrichia —see Alopecia
Oliguria R34
with, complicating or following ectopic or molar
pregnancy O08.4
postprocedural N99.0
puerperal O90.49
Ollier's disease Q78.4
~~Omenotocele —see Hernia, abdomen, specified
site NEC~~
► Omentocele —see Hernia, abdomen, specified site
NEC
Omentitis —see Peritonitis
Omentum, omental —see condition
Omphalitis (congenital) (newborn) P38.9
with mild hemorrhage P38.1
without hemorrhage P38.9
not of newborn L08.82
tetanus A33
Omphalocele Q79.2
Omphalomesenteric duct, persistent Q43.0
Omphalorrhagia, newborn P51.9
Omsk hemorrhagic fever A98.1
Onanism (excessive) F98.8
Onchocerciasis, onchocercosis B73.1
with
eye disease B73.00
endophthalmitis B73.01
eyelid B73.09
glaucoma B73.02
specified NEC B73.09
eye NEC B73.00
eyelid B73.09
Oncocytoma —see Neoplasm, benign, by site
Oncovirus, as cause of disease classified
elsewhere B97.32
Ondine's curse —see Apnea, sleep
Oneirophrenia F23
Onychauxis L60.2
congenital Q84.5
Onychia —see also Cellulitis, digit
with lymphangitis —see Lymphangitis, acute,
digit
candidal B37.2
dermatophytic B35.1
Onychitis —see also Cellulitis, digit
with lymphangitis —see Lymphangitis, acute,
digit
Onychocryptosis L60.0
Onychodystrophy L60.3
congenital Q84.6

Onychogryphosis, onychogryposis L60.2
Onycholysis L60.1
Onychomadesis L60.8
Onychomalacia L60.3
Onychomycosis (finger) (toe) B35.1
Onycho-osteodysplasia Q87.2
Onychophagia F98.8
Onychophosis L60.8
Onychoptosis L60.8
Onychorrhexis L60.3
congenital Q84.6
Onychoschizia L60.3
Onyxis (finger) (toe) L60.0
Onyxitis —see also Cellulitis, digit
with lymphangitis —see Lymphangitis, acute,
digit
Oophoritis (cystic) (infectional) (interstitial) N70.92
with salpingitis N70.93
acute N70.02
with salpingitis N70.03
chronic N70.12
with salpingitis N70.13
complicating abortion —see Abortion, by type,
complicated by, oophoritis
Oophorocele N83.4-●
Opacity, opacities
cornea H17.-●
central H17.1-●
congenital Q13.3
degenerative —see Degeneration, cornea
hereditary —see Dystrophy, cornea
inflammatory —see Keratitis
minor H17.81-●
peripheral H17.82-●
sequelae of trachoma (healed) B94.0
specified NEC H17.89
enamel (teeth) (fluoride) (nonfluoride) K00.3
lens —see Cataract
snowball —see Deposit, crystalline
vitreous (humor) NEC H43.39-●
congenital Q14.0
membranes and strands H43.31-●
Opalescent dentin (hereditary) K00.5
Open, opening
abnormal, organ or site, congenital —see
Imperfect, closure
angle with
borderline
findings
high risk H40.02-●
low risk H40.01-●
intraocular pressure H40.00-●
cupping of discs H40.01-●
glaucoma (primary) —see Glaucoma, open
angle
bite
anterior M26.220
posterior M26.221
false —see Imperfect, closure
margin on tooth restoration K08.51
restoration margins of tooth K08.51
wound —see Wound, open
Operational fatigue F48.8
Operative —see condition
Operculitis —see Periodontitis
Operculum —see Break, retina
Ophiasis L63.2
Ophthalmia —see also Conjunctivitis H10.9
actinic rays —see Photokeratitis
allergic (acute) —see Conjunctivitis, acute, atopic
blennorrhagic (gonococcal) (neonatorum) A54.31
diphtheritic A36.86
Egyptian A71.1
electrica —see Photokeratitis
gonococcal (neonatorum) A54.31
metastatic —see Endophthalmitis, purulent
migraine —see Migraine, ophthalmoplegic
neonatorum, newborn P39.1
gonococcal A54.31
nodosa H16.24-●
purulent —see Conjunctivitis, acute,
mucopurulent
spring —see Conjunctivitis, acute, atopic
sympathetic —see Uveitis, sympathetic
Ophthalmitis —see Ophthalmia
Ophthalmocele (congenital) Q15.8
Ophthalmoneuromyelitis G36.0
Ophthalmoplegia —see also Strabismus, paralytic
anterior internuclear —see Ophthalmoplegia,
internuclear
ataxia-areflexia G61.0

Ophthalmoplegia (Continued)
diabetic —see E08-E13 with .39
exophthalmic E05.00
with thyroid storm E05.01
external H49.88-●
progressive H49.4-●
with pigmentary retinopathy —see Kearns-
Sayre syndrome
total H49.3-●
internal (complete) (total) H52.51-●
internuclear H51.2-●
migraine —see Migraine, ophthalmoplegic
Parinaud's H49.88-●
progressive external —see Ophthalmoplegia,
external, progressive
supranuclear, progressive G23.1
total (external) —see Ophthalmoplegia, external,
total
Opioid(s)
abuse —see Abuse, drug, opioids
dependence —see Dependence, drug, opioids
induced, without use disorder
anxiety disorder F11.988
delirium F11.921
depressive disorder F11.94
sexual dysfunction F11.981
sleep disorder F11.982
Opisthognathism M26.09
Opisthorchiasis (felineus) (viverrini) B66.0
Opitz' disease D73.2
Opiumism —see Dependence, drug, opioid
Oppenheim's disease G70.2
Oppenheim-Urbach disease (necrobiosis lipoidica
diabeticorum) —see E08-E13 with .620
Optic nerve —see condition
Orbit —see condition
Orchioblastoma C62.9-●
Orchitis (gangrenous) (nonspecific) (septic)
(suppurative) N45.2
blennorrhagic (gonococcal) (acute) (chronic)
A54.23
chlamydial A56.19
filarial —see also Infestation, filarial B74.9 [N51]
gonococcal (acute) (chronic) A54.23
mumps B26.0
syphilitic A52.76
tuberculous A18.15
Orf (virus disease) B08.02
Organic —see also condition
brain syndrome F09
heart —see Disease, heart
mental disorder F09
psychosis F09
Orgasm
anejaculatory N53.13
Oriental
bilharziasis B65.2
schistosomiasis B65.2
Orifice —see condition
Origin of both great vessels from right ventricle
Q20.1
Ormond's disease (with ureteral obstruction) N13.5
with infection N13.6
Ornithine metabolism disorder E72.4
Ornithinemia (Type I) (Type II) E72.4
Ornithosis A70
Orotaciduria, oroticaciduria (congenital)
(hereditary) (pyrimidine deficiency) E79.89
anemia D53.0
Orthodontics
adjustment Z46.4
fitting Z46.4
Orthopnea R06.01
Orthopoxvirus B08.09
Os, uterus —see condition
Osgood-Schlatter disease or osteochondrosis
M92.52-●
Osler (-Weber)-Rendu disease I78.0
Osler's nodes I33.0
Osmidrosis L75.0
Osseous —see condition
Ossification
artery —see Arteriosclerosis
auricle (ear) —see Disorder, pinna, specified type
NEC
bronchial J98.09
cardiac —see Degeneration, myocardial
cartilage (senile) —see Disorder, cartilage,
specified type NEC
coronary (artery) —see Disease, heart, ischemic,
atherosclerotic

Ossification *(Continued)*
  diaphragm J98.6
  ear, middle —*see* Otosclerosis
  falx cerebri G96.198
  fontanel, premature Q75.009
  heart —*see also* Degeneration, myocardial
    valve —*see* Endocarditis
  larynx J38.7
  ligament —*see* Disorder, tendon, specified type
    NEC
    posterior longitudinal —*see* Spondylopathy,
      specified NEC
  meninges (cerebral) (spinal) G96.198
  multiple, eccentric centers —*see* Disorder, bone,
    development or growth
  muscle —*see also* Calcification, muscle
    due to burns —*see* Myositis, ossificans, in,
      burns
    paralytic —*see* Myositis, ossificans, in,
      quadriplegia
    progressive —*see* Myositis, ossificans,
      progressiva
    specified NEC M61.50
      ankle M61.57-●
      foot M61.57-●
      forearm M61.53-●
      hand M61.54-●
      lower leg M61.56-●
      multiple sites M61.59
      pelvic region M61.55-●
      shoulder region M61.51-●
      specified site NEC M61.58
      thigh M61.55-●
      upper arm M61.52-●
    traumatic —*see* Myositis, ossificans,
      traumatica
  myocardium, myocardial —*see* Degeneration,
    myocardial
  penis N48.89
  periarticular —*see* Disorder, joint, specified type
    NEC
  pinna —*see* Disorder, pinna, specified type NEC
  rider's bone —*see* Ossification, muscle, specified
    NEC
  sclera H15.89
  subperiosteal, post-traumatic M89.8X-●
  tendon —*see* Disorder, tendon, specified
    type NEC
  trachea J39.8
  tympanic membrane —*see* Disorder, tympanic
    membrane, specified NEC
  vitreous (humor) —*see* Deposit, crystalline
Osteitis —*see also* Osteomyelitis
  alveolar M27.3
  condensans M85.30
    ankle M85.37-●
    foot M85.37-●
    forearm M85.33-●
    hand M85.34-●
    lower leg M85.36-●
    multiple site M85.39
    neck M85.38
    rib M85.38
    shoulder M85.31-●
    skull M85.38
    specified site NEC M85.38
    thigh M85.35-●
    toe M85.37-●
    upper arm M85.32-●
    vertebra M85.38
  deformans (*see also* Paget's disease, bone) M88.9
    in (due to)
      malignant neoplasm of bone (*see also*,
        Neoplasm, malignant, by site)
        C41.9 *[M90.60]*
      neoplastic disease (*see also* Neoplasm,
        by type and site) D49.9 *[M90.60]*
        carpus D49.2 *[M90.64-●]*
        clavicle D49.2 *[M90.61-●]*
        femur D49.2 *[M90.65-●]*
        fibula D49.2 *[M90.66-●]*
        finger D49.2 *[M90.64-●]*
        humerus D49.2 *[M90.62-●]*
        ilium D49.2 *[M90.65-●]*
        ischium D49.2 *[M90.65-●]*
        metacarpus D49.2 *[M90.64-●]*
        metatarsus D49.2 *[M90.67-●]*
        multiple sites D49.89 *[M90.69]*
        neck D49.2 *[M90.68]*
        pubic ramus D49.2 *[M90.68]*
        radius D49.2 *[M90.63-●]*

Osteitis *(Continued)*
  deformans *(Continued)*
    in (due to) *(Continued)*
      neoplastic disease *(Continued)*
        rib D49.2 *[M90.68]*
        scapula D49.2 *[M90.61-●]*
        skull D49.2 *[M90.68]*
        tarsus D49.2 *[M90.67-●]*
        tibia D49.2 *[M90.66-●]*
        toe D49.2 *[M90.67-●]*
        ulna D49.2 *[M90.63-●]*
        vertebra D49.2 *[M90.68]*
      skull M88.0
    specified NEC —*see* Paget's disease, bone,
      by site
    vertebra M88.1
  due to yaws A66.6
  fibrosa NEC —*see* Cyst, bone, by site
    circumscripta —*see* Dysplasia, fibrous, bone
      NEC
    cystica (generalisata) E21.0
    disseminata Q78.1
    osteoplastica E21.0
  fragilitans Q78.0
  Garr's (sclerosing) —*see* Osteomyelitis, specified
    type NEC
  jaw (acute) (chronic) (lower) (suppurative)
    (upper) M27.2
  parathyroid E21.0
  petrous bone (acute) (chronic) —*see* Petrositis
  sclerotic, nonsuppurative —*see* Osteomyelitis,
    specified type NEC
  tuberculosa A18.09
    cystica D86.89
    multiplex cystoides D86.89
Osteoarthritis M19.90
  ankle M19.07-●
    post-traumatic M19.17-●
    primary M19.07-●
    secondary M19.27-●
  elbow M19.02-●
    post-traumatic M19.12-●
    primary M19.02-●
    secondary M19.22-●
  foot joint M19.07-●
    post-traumatic M19.17-●
    primary M19.07-●
    secondary M19.27-●
  generalized (multiple joints) M15.9
    erosive M15.4
    primary M15.0
    specified NEC M15.8
  hand joint M19.04-●
    first carpometacarpal joint M18.9-●
      post-traumatic —*see* Osteoarthritis,
        post-traumatic NEC, hand joint, first
        carpometacarpal joint
      primary —*see* Osteoarthritis, primary, hand
        joint, first carpometacarpal joint
      secondary —*see* Osteoarthritis, secondary,
        hand joint, first carpometacarpal
        joint
    post-traumatic M19.14-●
    primary M19.04-●
    secondary M19.24-●
  hip M16.9
    bilateral M16.0
      due to hip dysplasia M16.2
      post-traumatic M16.4
      secondary M16.6
    due to hip dysplasia (unilateral)
      M16.3-●
      bilateral M16.2
    post-traumatic —*see* Osteoarthritis, post-
      traumatic, hip
    primary M16.1-●
      bilateral M16.0
    secondary —*see* Osteoarthritis, secondary,
      hip
    unilateral M16.1-●
      due to hip dysplasia M16.3-●
      post-traumatic M16.5-●
      primary M16.1-●
      secondary NEC M16.7
  interphalangeal
    distal (Heberden) M15.1
    proximal (Bouchard) M15.2
  knee M17.9
    bilateral M17.0
      post-traumatic M17.2
      secondary M17.4

Osteoarthritis *(Continued)*
  knee *(Continued)*
      post-traumatic —*see* Osteoarthritis, post-
        traumatic, knee
      primary M17.1-●
        bilateral M17.0
      secondary —*see* Osteoarthritis, secondary,
        knee
      unilateral M17.1-●
        post-traumatic M17.3-●
        primary M17.1-●
        secondary NEC M17.5
  post-traumatic NEC M19.92
    ankle M19.17-●
    elbow M19.12-●
    foot joint M19.17-●
    hand joint M19.14-●
      first carpometacarpal joint M18.3-●
        bilateral M18.2
    hip M16.5-●
      bilateral M16.4
    knee M17.3-●
      bilateral M17.2
    shoulder M19.11-●
    specified site NEC M19.19
    wrist M19.13-●
  primary M19.91
    ankle M19.07-●
    elbow M19.02-●
    foot joint M19.07-●
    hand joint M19.04-●
      first carpometacarpal joint M18.1-●
        bilateral M18.0
    hip M16.1-●
      bilateral M16.0
    knee M17.1-●
      bilateral M17.0
    multiple sites M15.9
    shoulder M19.01-●
    specified site NEC M19.09
    spine —*see* Spondylosis
    wrist M19.03-●
  secondary M19.93
    ankle M19.27-●
    elbow M19.22-●
    foot joint M19.27-●
    hand joint M19.24-●
      first carpometacarpal joint M18.5-●
        bilateral M18.4
    hip M16.7-●
      bilateral M16.6
    knee M17.5-●
      bilateral M17.4
    multiple M15.3
    shoulder M19.21-●
    specified site NEC M19.29
    spine —*see* Spondylosis
    wrist M19.23-●
  shoulder M19.01-●
    post-traumatic M19.11-●
    primary M19.01-●
    secondary M19.21-●
  specified site NEC M19.09
  spine —*see* Spondylosis
  wrist M19.03-●
    first carpometacarpal joint —*see* Osteoarthritis,
      hand joint, first carpometacarpal joint
    post-traumatic M19.13-●
    primary M19.03-●
    secondary M19.23-●
Osteoarthropathy (hypertrophic) M19.90
  ankle —*see* Osteoarthritis, primary, ankle
  elbow —*see* Osteoarthritis, primary, elbow
  foot joint —*see* Osteoarthritis, primary, foot
  hand joint —*see* Osteoarthritis, primary, hand
    joint
  knee joint —*see* Osteoarthritis, primary, knee
  multiple site —*see* Osteoarthritis, primary,
    multiple joint
  pulmonary —*see also* Osteoarthropathy, specified
    type NEC
    hypertrophic —*see* Osteoarthropathy,
      hypertrophic, specified type
      NEC
  secondary —*see* Osteoarthropathy, specified type
    NEC
  secondary hypertrophic —*see* Osteoarthropathy,
    specified type NEC
  shoulder —*see* Osteoarthritis, primary, shoulder
  specified joint NEC —*see* Osteoarthritis, primary,
    specified joint NEC

▶ New　⇒ Revised　~~deleted~~ Deleted　● Use Additional Character(s)

Osteochondrosis *(Continued)*
  Sinding-Larsen —*see* Osteochondrosis, juvenile, patella
    adult M42.10
      cervical region M42.12
      cervicothoracic region M42.13
      lumbar region M42.16
      lumbosacral region M42.17
      multiple sites M42.19
      occipito-atlanto-axial region M42.11
      sacrococcygeal region M42.18
      thoracic region M42.14
      thoracolumbar region M42.15
    juvenile —*see* Osteochondrosis, juvenile, spine
  symphysis pubis (juvenile) M91.0
  syphilitic (congenital) A50.02
  talus (juvenile) —*see* Osteochondrosis, juvenile, tarsus
  tarsus (navicular) (juvenile) —*see* Osteochondrosis, juvenile, tarsus
  tibia (proximal) (tubercle) (juvenile) —*see* Osteochondrosis, juvenile, tibia
  tuberculous —*see* Tuberculosis, bone
  ulna (lower) (juvenile) —*see* Osteochondrosis, juvenile, ulna
  van Neck's M91.0
  vertebral —*see* Osteochondrosis, spine
Osteoclastoma D48.0
  malignant —*see* Neoplasm, bone, malignant
Osteodynia —*see* Disorder, bone, specified type NEC
Osteodystrophy Q78.9
  azotemic N25.0
  congenital Q78.9
  parathyroid, secondary E21.1
  renal N25.0
Osteofibroma —*see* Neoplasm, bone, benign
Osteofibrosarcoma —*see* Neoplasm, bone, malignant
Osteogenesis imperfecta Q78.0
Osteogenic —*see* condition
Osteolysis M89.50
  carpus M89.54-●
  clavicle M89.51-●
  femur M89.55-●
  fibula M89.56-●
  finger M89.54-●
  humerus M89.52-●
  ilium M89.58
  ischium M89.58
  joint prosthesis (periprosthetic) —*see* Complications, joint prosthesis, mechanical, periprosthetic, osteolysis, by site
  metacarpus M89.54-●
  metatarsus M89.57-●
  multiple sites M89.59
  neck M89.58
  periprosthetic —*see* Complications, joint prosthesis, mechanical, periprosthetic, osteolysis, by site
  pubic ramus M89.58
  radius M89.53-●
  rib M89.58
  scapula M89.51-●
  skull M89.58
  tarsus M89.57-●
  tibia M89.56-●
  toe M89.57-●
  ulna M89.53-●
  vertebra M89.58
Osteoma —*see also* Neoplasm, bone, benign
  osteoid —*see also* Neoplasm, bone, benign
    giant —*see* Neoplasm, bone, benign
Osteomalacia M83.9
  adult M83.9
    drug-induced NEC M83.5
    due to
      malabsorption (postsurgical) M83.2
      malnutrition M83.3
    specified NEC M83.8
  aluminium-induced M83.4
  infantile —*see* Rickets
  juvenile —*see* Rickets
  oncogenic E83.89
  pelvis M83.8
  puerperal M83.0
  senile M83.1
  vitamin-D-resistant in adults E83.31 *[M90.8-●]*
    carpus E83.31 *[M90.84-●]*
    clavicle E83.31 *[M90.81-●]*
    femur E83.31 *[M90.85-●]*

Osteomalacia *(Continued)*
  vitamin-D-resistant in adults *(Continued)*
    fibula E83.31 *[M90.86-●]*
    finger E83.31 *[M90.84-●]*
    humerus E83.31 *[M90.82-●]*
    ilium E83.31 *[M90.88]*
    ischium E83.31 *[M90.88]*
    metacarpus E83.31 *[M90.84-●]*
    metatarsus E83.31 *[M90.87-●]*
    multiple sites E83.31 *[M90.89]*
    neck E83.31 *[M90.88]*
    pubic ramus E83.31 *[M90.88]*
    radius E83.31 *[M90.83-●]*
    rib E83.31 *[M90.88]*
    scapula E83.31 *[M90.819]*
    skull E83.31 *[M90.88]*
    tarsus E83.31 *[M90.879]*
    tibia E83.31 *[M90.869]*
    toe E83.31 *[M90.879]*
    ulna E83.31 *[M90.839]*
    vertebra E83.31 *[M90.88]*
Osteomyelitis (general) (infective) (localized) (neonatal) (purulent) (septic) (staphylococcal) (streptococcal) (suppurative) (with periostitis) M86.9
  acute M86.10
    carpus M86.14-●
    clavicle M86.11-●
    femur M86.15-●
    fibula M86.16-●
    finger M86.14-●
    hematogenous M86.00
      carpus M86.04-●
      clavicle M86.01-●
      femur M86.05-●
      fibula M86.06-●
      finger M86.04-●
      humerus M86.02-●
      ilium M86.08
      ischium M86.08
      mandible M27.2
      metacarpus M86.04-●
      metatarsus M86.07-●
      multiple sites M86.09
      neck M86.08
      orbit H05.02-●
      petrous bone —*see* Petrositis
      radius M86.03-●
      rib M86.08
      scapula M86.01-●
      skull M86.08
      tarsus M86.07-●
      tibia M86.06-●
      toe M86.07-●
      ulna M86.03-●
      vertebra —*see* Osteomyelitis, vertebra
    humerus M86.12-●
    ilium M86.18
    ischium M86.18
    mandible M27.2
    metacarpus M86.14-●
    metatarsus M86.17-●
    multiple sites M86.19
    neck M86.18
    orbit H05.02-●
    petrous bone —*see* Petrositis
    radius M86.13-●
    rib M86.18
    scapula M86.11-●
    skull M86.18
    tarsus M86.17-●
    tibia M86.16-●
    toe M86.17-●
    ulna M86.13-●
    vertebra —*see* Osteomyelitis, vertebra
  chronic (or old) M86.60
    with draining sinus M86.40
      carpus M86.44-●
      clavicle M86.41-●
      femur M86.45-●
      fibula M86.46-●
      finger M86.44-●
      humerus M86.42-●
      ilium M86.48
      ischium M86.48
      mandible M27.2
      metacarpus M86.44-●
      metatarsus M86.47-●
      multiple sites M86.49
      neck M86.48
      orbit H05.02-●

Osteomyelitis *(Continued)*
  chronic *(Continued)*
    with draining sinus *(Continued)*
      petrous bone —*see* Petrositis
      pubic ramus M86.48
      radius M86.43-●
      rib M86.48
      scapula M86.41-●
      skull M86.48
      tarsus M86.47-●
      tibia M86.46-●
      toe M86.47-●
      ulna M86.43-●
      vertebra —*see* Osteomyelitis, vertebra
    carpus M86.64-●
    clavicle M86.61-●
    femur M86.65-●
    fibula M86.66-●
    finger M86.64-●
    hematogenous NEC M86.50
      carpus M86.54-●
      clavicle M86.51-●
      femur M86.55-●
      fibula M86.56-●
      finger M86.54-●
      humerus M86.52-●
      ilium M86.58
      ischium M86.58
      mandible M27.2
      metacarpus M86.54-●
      metatarsus M86.57-●
      multifocal M86.30
        carpus M86.34-●
        clavicle M86.31-●
        femur M86.35-●
        fibula M86.36-●
        finger M86.34-●
        humerus M86.32-●
        ilium M86.38
        ischium M86.38
        metacarpus M86.34-●
        metatarsus M86.37-●
        multiple sites M86.39
        neck M86.38
        pubic ramus M86.38
        radius M86.33-●
        rib M86.38
        scapula M86.31-●
        skull M86.38
        tarsus M86.37-●
        tibia M86.36-●
        toe M86.37-●
        ulna M86.33-●
        vertebra —*see* Osteomyelitis, vertebra
      multiple sites M86.59
      neck M86.58
      orbit H05.02-●
      petrous bone —*see* Petrositis
      pubic ramus M86.58
      radius M86.53-●
      rib M86.58
      scapula M86.51-●
      skull M86.58
      tarsus M86.57-●
      tibia M86.56-●
      toe M86.57-●
      ulna M86.53-●
      vertebra —*see* Osteomyelitis, vertebra
    humerus M86.62-●
    ilium M86.659
    ischium M86.659
    mandible M27.2
    metacarpus M86.64-●
    metatarsus M86.67-●
    multifocal —*see* Osteomyelitis, chronic, hematogenous, multifocal
    multiple sites M86.69
    neck M86.68
    orbit H05.02-●
    petrous bone —*see* Petrositis
    radius M86.63-●
    rib M86.68
    scapula M86.61-●
    skull M86.68
    tarsus M86.67-●
    tibia M86.66-●
    toe M86.67-●
    ulna M86.63-●
    vertebra —*see* Osteomyelitis, vertebra
  echinococcal B67.2
  Garr's —*see* Osteomyelitis, specified type NEC

▶ New   ⇒ Revised   ~~deleted~~ Deleted   ● Use Additional Character(s)

Osteophyte M25.70
  ankle M25.77-●
  elbow M25.72-●
  foot joint M25.77-●
  hand joint M25.74-●
  hip M25.75-●
  knee M25.76-●
  shoulder M25.71-●
  spine M25.78
  vertebrae M25.78
  wrist M25.73-●
Osteopoikilosis Q78.8
Osteoporosis (female) (male) M81.0
  with current pathological fracture M80.00
  age-related M81.0
    with current pathologic fracture M80.00
      carpus M80.04-●
      clavicle M80.01-●
      femur M80.05-●
      fibula M80.06-●
      finger M80.04-●
      hip M80.05-●
      humerus M80.02-●
      ilium M80.0A
      ischium M80.0A
      metacarpus M80.04-●
      metatarsus M80.07-●
      pelvis M80.0B
      pubis ramus M80.0A
      radius M80.03-●
      rib(s) M80.0A
      scapula M80.01-●
      site specified NEC M80.0A
      specified site NEC M80.0A
      tarsus M80.07-●
      tibia M80.06-●
      toe M80.07-●
      ulna M80.03-●
      vertebra M80.08
  disuse M81.8
    with current pathological fracture
      M80.80
      carpus M80.84-●
      clavicle M80.81-●
      fibula M80.86-●
      finger M80.84-●
      humerus M80.82-●
      ilium M80.8A
      ischium M80.8A
      metacarpus M80.84-●
      metatarsus M80.87-●
      pelvis M80.8B
      pubis ramus M80.8A
      radius M80.83-●
      scapula M80.81-●
      site specified NEC M80.8A
      tarsus M80.87-●
      tibia M80.86-●
      toe M80.87-●
      ulna M80.83-●
      vertebra M80.88
  drug-induced —see Osteoporosis, specified type
      NEC
  idiopathic —see Osteoporosis, specified type
      NEC
  involutional —see Osteoporosis, age-related
  Lequesne M81.6
  localized M81.6
  postmenopausal M81.0
    with pathological fracture M80.00
      carpus M80.04-●
      clavicle M80.01-●
      femur M80.85-●
      fibula M80.06-●
      finger M80.04-●
      hip M80.85-●
      humerus M80.02-●
      ilium M80.0A
      ischium M80.0A
      metacarpus M80.04-●
      metatarsus M80.07-●
      pelvis M80.0B
      pubis ramus M80.0A
      radius M80.03-●
      scapula M80.01-●
      site specified NEC M80.0A
      tarsus M80.07-●
      tibia M80.06-●
      toe M80.07-●
      ulna M80.03-●
      vertebra M80.08

Osteoporosis (Continued)
  postoophorectomy —see Osteoporosis, specified
      type NEC
  postsurgical malabsorption —see Osteoporosis,
      specified type NEC
  post-traumatic —see Osteoporosis, specified type
      NEC
  senile —see Osteoporosis, age-related
  specified type NEC M81.8
    with pathological fracture M80.80
      carpus M80.84-●
      clavicle M80.81-●
      femur M80.85-●
      fibula M80.86-●
      finger M80.84-●
      hip M80.85-●
      humerus M80.82-●
      ilium M80.8A
      ischium M80.8A
      metacarpus M80.84-●
      metatarsus M80.87-●
      pelvis M80.8B
      radius M80.83-●
      pubis ramus M80.8A
      scapula M80.81-●
      site specified NEC M80.8A
      tarsus M80.87-●
      tibia M80.86-●
      toe M80.87-●
      ulna M80.83-●
      vertebra M80.88
Osteopsathyrosis (idiopathica) Q78.0
Osteoradionecrosis, jaw (acute) (chronic) (lower)
    (suppurative) (upper) M27.2
Osteosarcoma (any form) —see Neoplasm, bone,
    malignant
Osteosclerosis Q78.2
  acquired M85.8-●
  congenita Q77.4
  fragilitas (generalisata) Q78.2
  myelofibrosis D75.81
Osteosclerotic anemia D64.89
Osteosis
  cutis L94.2
  renal fibrocystic N25.0
Österreicher-Turner syndrome Q87.2
Ostium
  atrioventriculare commune Q21.23
  primum (arteriosum) (defect) (persistent) Q21.20
  secundum (arteriosum) (defect) (patent)
      (persistent) Q21.11
Ostrum-Furst syndrome Q75.8
Otalgia —see subcategory H92.0
Otitis (acute) H66.90
  with effusion —see also Otitis, media,
      nonsuppurative
    purulent —see Otitis, media, suppurative
  adhesive —see subcategory H74.1
  chronic —see also Otitis, media, chronic
    with effusion —see also Otitis, media,
        nonsuppurative, chronic
  externa H60.9-●
    abscess —see Abscess, ear, external
    acute (noninfective) H60.50-●
      actinic H60.51-●
      chemical H60.52-●
      contact H60.53-●
      eczematoid H60.54-●
      infective —see Otitis, externa, infective
      reactive H60.55-●
      specified NEC H60.59-●
    cellulitis —see Cellulitis, ear
    chronic H60.6-●
    diffuse —see Otitis, externa, infective, diffuse
    hemorrhagic —see Otitis, externa, infective,
        hemorrhagic
    in (due to)
      aspergillosis B44.89
      candidiasis B37.84
      erysipelas A46 [H62.40]
      herpes (simplex) virus infection B00.1
        zoster B02.8
      impetigo L01.00 [H62.40]
      infectious disease NEC B99 [H62.4-●]
      mycosis NEC B36.9 [H62.40]
      parasitic disease NEC B89 [H62.40]
      viral disease NEC B34.9 [H62.40]
      zoster B02.8
    infective NEC H60.39-●
      abscess —see Abscess, ear, external
      cellulitis —see Cellulitis, ear

Otitis (Continued)
  externa (Continued)
    infective (Continued)
      diffuse H60.31-●
      hemorrhagic H60.32-●
      swimmer's ear —see Swimmer's, ear
    malignant H60.2-●
    mycotic NEC B36.9 [H62.40]
      in
        aspergillosis B44.89
        candidiasis B37.84
        moniliasis B37.84
    necrotizing —see Otitis, externa,
        malignant
    Pseudomonas aeruginosa —see Otitis, externa,
        malignant
    reactive —see Otitis, externa, acute,
        reactive
    specified NEC —see subcategory H60.8
    tropical NEC B36.9 [H62.40]
      in
        aspergillosis B44.89
        candidiasis B37.84
        moniliasis B37.84
  insidiosa —see Otosclerosis
  interna —see subcategory H83.0
  media (hemorrhagic) (staphylococcal)
      (streptococcal) H66.9-●
    with effusion (nonpurulent) —see Otitis,
        media, nonsuppurative
    acute, subacute H66.90
      allergic —see Otitis, media, nonsuppurative,
          acute, allergic
      exudative —see Otitis, media, suppurative,
          acute
      mucoid —see Otitis, media,
          nonsuppurative, acute
      necrotizing —see also Otitis, media,
          suppurative, acute
        in
          measles B05.3
          scarlet fever A38.0
      nonsuppurative NEC —see Otitis, media,
          nonsuppurative, acute
      purulent —see Otitis, media, suppurative,
          acute
      sanguinous —see Otitis, media,
          nonsuppurative, acute
      secretory —see Otitis, media,
          nonsuppurative, acute, serous
      seromucinous —see Otitis, media,
          nonsuppurative, acute
      serous —see Otitis, media, nonsuppurative,
          acute, serous
      suppurative —see Otitis, media,
          suppurative, acute
    allergic —see Otitis, media,
        nonsuppurative
    catarrhal —see Otitis, media,
        nonsuppurative
    chronic H66.90
      with effusion (nonpurulent) —see Otitis,
          media, nonsuppurative, chronic
      allergic —see Otitis, media, nonsuppurative,
          chronic, allergic
      benign suppurative —see Otitis, media,
          suppurative, chronic, tubotympanic
      catarrhal —see Otitis, media,
          nonsuppurative, chronic, serous
      exudative —see Otitis, media, suppurative,
          chronic
      mucinous —see Otitis, media,
          nonsuppurative, chronic, mucoid
      mucoid —see Otitis, media,
          nonsuppurative, chronic, mucoid
      nonsuppurative NEC —see Otitis, media,
          nonsuppurative, chronic
      purulent —see Otitis, media, suppurative,
          chronic
      secretory —see Otitis, media,
          nonsuppurative, chronic, mucoid
      seromucinous —see Otitis, media,
          nonsuppurative, chronic
      serous —see Otitis, media, nonsuppurative,
          chronic, serous
      suppurative —see Otitis, media,
          suppurative, chronic
      transudative —see Otitis, media,
          nonsuppurative, chronic, mucoid
    exudative —see Otitis, media,
        nonsuppurative

Otitis *(Continued)*
  media *(Continued)*
    in (due to) (with)
      influenza —*see* Influenza, with, otitis media
      measles B05.3
      scarlet fever A38.0
      tuberculosis A18.6
      viral disease NEC B34.- ● *[H67.-●]*
    mucoid —*see* Otitis, media, nonsuppurative
    nonsuppurative H65.9-●
      acute or subacute NEC H65.19-●
        allergic H65.11-●
          recurrent H65.11-●
        recurrent H65.19-●
        secretory —*see* Otitis, media,
          nonsuppurative, serous
        serous H65.0-●
          recurrent H65.0-●
      chronic H65.49-●
        allergic H65.41-●
        mucoid H65.3-●
        serous H65.2-●
      postmeasles B05.3
      purulent —*see* Otitis, media, suppurative
      secretory —*see* Otitis, media, nonsuppurative
      seromucinous —*see* Otitis, media,
        nonsuppurative
      serous —*see* Otitis, media, nonsuppurative
      suppurative H66.4-●
        acute H66.00-●
          with rupture of ear drum H66.01-●
          recurrent H66.00-●
            with rupture of ear drum
              H66.01-●
        chronic —*see also* subcategory H66.3
          atticoantral H66.2-●
          benign —*see* Otitis, media, suppurative,
            chronic, tubotympanic
          tubotympanic H66.1-●
      transudative —*see* Otitis, media,
        nonsuppurative
      tuberculous A18.6
Otocephaly Q18.2
Otolith syndrome —*see* subcategory H81.8
Otomycosis (diffuse) NEC B36.9 *[H62.40]*
  in
    aspergillosis B44.89
    candidiasis B37.84
    moniliasis B37.84
Otoporosis —*see* Otosclerosis
Otorrhagia (nontraumatic) H92.2-●
  traumatic - code by Type of injury
Otorrhea H92.1-●
  cerebrospinal (fluid) G96.01
    postoperative G96.08
    specified NEC G96.08
    spontaneous G96.01
    traumatic G96.08
Otosclerosis (general) H80.9-●
  cochlear (endosteal) H80.2-●
  involving
    otic capsule —*see* Otosclerosis, cochlear
    oval window
      nonobliterative H80.0-●
      obliterative H80.1-●
    round window —*see* Otosclerosis, cochlear
  nonobliterative —*see* Otosclerosis, involving,
    oval window, nonobliterative
  obliterative —*see* Otosclerosis, involving, oval
    window, obliterative
  specified NEC H80.8-●
Otospongiosis —*see* Otosclerosis
Otto's disease or pelvis M24.7
Outcome of delivery Z37.9
  multiple births Z37.9
    all liveborn Z37.50
      quadruplets Z37.52
      quintuplets Z37.53
      sextuplets Z37.54
      specified number NEC Z37.59
      triplets Z37.51
    all stillborn Z37.7
    some liveborn Z37.60
      quadruplets Z37.62
      quintuplets Z37.63
      sextuplets Z37.64
      specified number NEC Z37.69
      triplets Z37.61
  single NEC Z37.9
    liveborn Z37.0
    stillborn Z37.1

Outcome of delivery *(Continued)*
  twins NEC Z37.9
    both liveborn Z37.2
    both stillborn Z37.4
    one liveborn, one stillborn Z37.3
Outlet —*see* condition
Ovalocytosis (congenital) (hereditary) —*see*
  Elliptocytosis
Ovarian —*see* Condition
Ovariocele N83.4-●
Ovaritis (cystic) —*see* Oophoritis
Ovary, ovarian —*see also* condition
  resistant syndrome E28.39
  vein syndrome N13.8
Overactive —*see also* Hyperfunction
  adrenal cortex NEC E27.0
  bladder N32.81
  hypothalamus E23.3
  thyroid —*see* Hyperthyroidism
Overactivity R46.3
  child —*see* Disorder, attention-deficit hyperactivity
Overbite (deep) (excessive) (horizontal) (vertical)
  M26.29
Overbreathing —*see* Hyperventilation
Overconscientious personality F60.5
Overdevelopment —*see* Hypertrophy
Overdistension —*see* Distension
Overdose, overdosage (drug) —*see* Table of Drugs
  and Chemicals, by drug, poisoning
Overeating R63.2
  nonorganic origin F50.89
  psychogenic F50.89
Overexertion (effects) (exhaustion) T73.3
Overexposure (effects) T73.9
  exhaustion T73.2
Overfeeding —*see* Overeating
  newborn P92.4
Overfill, endodontic M27.52
Overgrowth
  bacterial
    small intestinal K63.8219
      fungal K63.822
      hydrogen-subtype K63.8211
      hydrogen sulfide-subtype K63.8212
  bone - see Hypertrophy, bone
    intestinal methanogen K63.829
Overhanging of dental restorative material
  (unrepairable) K08.52
Overheated (places) (effects) —*see* Heat
Overjet (excessive horizontal) M26.23
Overlaid, overlying (suffocation) —
  see Asphyxia, traumatic, due to mechanical
  threat
Overlap, excessive horizontal (teeth) M26.23
Overl apping toe (acquired) —*see also* Deformity,
  toe, specified NEC
  congenital (fifth toe) Q66.89
Overload
  circulatory, due to transfusion (blood) (blood
    components) (TACO) E87.71
  fluid E87.70
    due to transfusion (blood) (blood
      components) E87.71
    specified NEC E87.79
  iron, due to repeated red blood cell transfusions
    E83.111
  potassium (K) E87.5
  sodium (Na) E87.0
Overnutrition —*see* Hyperalimentation
Overproduction —*see also* Hypersecretion
  ACTH E27.0
  catecholamine E27.5
  growth hormone E22.0
Overprotection, child by parent Z62.1
Overriding
  aorta Q25.49
  finger (acquired) —*see* Deformity, finger
    congenital Q68.1
  toe (acquired) —*see also* Deformity, toe, specified
    NEC
    congenital Q66.89
Overstrained R53.83
  heart —*see* Hypertrophy, cardiac
Overuse, muscle NEC M70.8-●
Overweight E66.3
Overworked R53.83
Oviduct —*see* condition
Ovotestis Q56.0
Ovulation (cycle)
  failure or lack of N97.0
  pain N94.0

Ovum —*see* condition
Owren's disease or syndrome (parahemophilia)
  D68.2
Ox heart —*see* Hypertrophy, cardiac
Oxalosis E72.53
Oxaluria E72.53
Oxycephaly, oxycephalic Q75.009
  syphilitic, congenital A50.02
Oxyuriasis B80
Oxyuris vermicularis (infestation) B80
Ozena J31.0

P

Pachyderma, pachydermia L85.9
  larynx (verrucosa) J38.7
Pachydermatocele (congenital) Q82.8
Pachydermoperiostosis —*see also*
  Osteoarthropathy, hypertrophic, specified
  type NEC
  clubbed nail M89.40 *[L62]*
Pachygyria Q04.3
Pachymeningitis (adhesive) (basal) (brain)
  (cervical) (chronic) (circumscribed) (external)
  (fibrous) (hemorrhagic) (hypertrophic)
  (internal) (purulent) (spinal) (suppurative) —
  see Meningitis
Pachyonychia (congenital) Q84.5
Pacinian tumor —*see* Neoplasm, skin, benign
Pad, knuckle or Garrod's M72.1
Paget-Schroetter syndrome I82.890
Paget's disease
  with infiltrating duct carcinoma —*see* Neoplasm,
    breast, malignant
  bone M88.9
    carpus M88.84-●
    clavicle M88.81-●
    femur M88.85-●
    fibula M88.86-●
    finger M88.84-●
    humerus M88.82-●
    ilium M88.88
    in neoplastic disease —*see* Osteitis, deformans,
      in neoplastic disease
    ischium M88.88
    metacarpus M88.84-●
    metatarsus M88.87-●
    multiple sites M88.89
    neck M88.88
    pubic ramus M88.88
    radius M88.83-●
    rib M88.88
    scapula M88.81-●
    skull M88.0
    specified NEC M88.88
    tarsus M88.87-●
    tibia M88.86-●
    toe M88.87-●
    ulna M88.83-●
    vertebra M88.1
  breast (female) C50.01-●
    male C50.02-●
  extramammary —*see also* Neoplasm, skin,
    malignant
    anus C21.0
      margin C44.590
      skin C44.590
  intraductal carcinoma —*see* Neoplasm, breast,
    malignant
  malignant —*see* Neoplasm, skin, malignant
    breast (female) C50.01-●
      male C50.02-●
    unspecified site (female) C50.01-●
      male C50.02-●
  mammary —*see* Paget's disease, breast
  nipple —*see* Paget's disease, breast
  osteitis deformans —*see* Paget's disease,
    bone
Pain(s) —*see also* Painful R52
  abdominal R10.9
    colic R10.83
    generalized R10.84
      with acute abdomen R10.0
    lower R10.30
      left quadrant R10.32
      pelvic or perineal R10.2
      periumbilical R10.33
      right quadrant R10.31

Pain *(Continued)*
  abdominal *(Continued)*
    rebound —*see* Tenderness, abdominal,
      rebound
    severe with abdominal rigidity R10.0
    tenderness —*see* Tenderness, abdominal
    upper R10.10
      epigastric R10.13
      left quadrant R10.12
      right quadrant R10.11
  acute R52
    due to trauma G89.11
    neoplasm related G89.3
    postprocedural NEC G89.18
    post-thoracotomy G89.12
    specified by site — code to Pain, by site
  adnexa (uteri) R10.2
  anginoid —*see* Pain, precordial
  anus K62.89
  arm —*see* Pain, limb, upper
  axillary (axilla) M79.62-●
  back (postural) M54.9
  bladder R39.89
    associated with micturition —*see* Micturition,
      painful
    chronic R39.82
  bone —*see* Disorder, bone, specified type NEC
  breast N64.4
  broad ligament R10.2
  cancer associated (acute) (chronic) G89.3
  cecum —*see* Pain, abdominal
  cervicobrachial M53.1
  chest (central) R07.9
    anterior wall R07.89
    atypical R07.89
    ischemic I20.9
    musculoskeletal R07.89
    non-cardiac R07.89
    on breathing R07.1
    pleurodynia R07.81
    precordial R07.2
    wall (anterior) R07.89
  chronic G89.29
    associated with significant psychosocial
      dysfunction G89.4
    due to trauma G89.21
    neoplasm related G89.3
    postoperative NEC G89.28
    postprocedural NEC G89.28
    post-thoracotomy G89.22
    specified NEC G89.29
  coccyx M53.3
  colon —*see* Pain, abdominal
  coronary —*see* Angina
  costochondral R07.1
  diaphragm R07.1
  due to cancer G89.3
  due to device, implant or graft —*see also*
    Complications, by site and type, specified
    NEC T85.848
    arterial graft NEC T82.848
    breast (implant) T85.848
    catheter NEC T85.848
      dialysis (renal) T82.848
        intraperitoneal T85.848
      infusion NEC T82.848
        spinal (epidural) (subdural) T85.840
      urinary (indwelling) T83.84
    electronic (electrode) (pulse generator)
      (stimulator)
      bone T84.84
      cardiac T82.847
      nervous system (brain) (peripheral nerve)
        (spinal) T85.840
      urinary T83.84
    fixation, internal (orthopedic) NEC T84.84
    gastrointestinal (bile duct) (esophagus)
      T85.848
    genital NEC T83.84
    heart NEC T82.847
    infusion NEC T85.848
    joint prosthesis T84.84
    ocular (corneal graft) (orbital implant) NEC
      T85.848
    orthopedic NEC T84.84
    specified NEC T85.848
    urinary NEC T83.84
    vascular NEC T82.848
    ventricular intracranial shunt T85.840
  due to malignancy (primary) (secondary) G89.3
  ear —*see* subcategory H92.0

Pain *(Continued)*
  epigastric, epigastrium R10.13
  eye —*see* Pain, ocular
  face, facial R51.9
    atypical G50.1
  female genital organs NEC N94.89
  finger —*see* Pain, limb, upper
  flank —*see* Pain, abdominal
  foot —*see* Pain, limb, lower
  gallbladder K82.9
  gas (intestinal) R14.1
  gastric —*see* Pain, abdominal
  generalized NOS R52
  genital organ
    female N94.89
    male N50.89
  groin —*see* Pain, abdominal, lower
  hand —*see* Pain, limb, upper
  head —*see* Headache
  heart —*see* Pain, precordial
  infra-orbital —*see* Neuralgia, trigeminal
  intercostal R07.82
  intermenstrual N94.0
  jaw R68.84
  joint M25.50
    ankle M25.57-●
    elbow M25.52-●
    finger M25.54-●
    foot M25.57-●
    hand M25.54-●
    hip M25.55-●
    knee M25.56-●
    shoulder M25.51-●
    specified site NEC M25.59
    toe M25.57-●
    wrist M25.53-●
  kidney N23
  laryngeal R07.0
  leg —*see* Pain, limb, lower
  limb M79.609
    lower M79.60-●
      foot M79.67-●
      lower leg M79.66-●
      thigh M79.65-●
      toe M79.67-●
    upper M79.60-●
      axilla M79.62-●
      finger M79.64-●
      forearm M79.63-●
      hand M79.64-●
      upper arm M79.62-●
  loin M54.50
  low back M54.50
    specified NEC M54.59
    vertebral end plate M54.51
    vertebrogenic M54.51
  lumbar region M54.50
    vertebral end plate M54.51
    vertebrogenic M54.51
  mandibular R68.84
  mastoid —*see* subcategory H92.0
  maxilla R68.84
  menstrual —*see also* Dysmenorrhea N94.6
  metacarpophalangeal (joint) —*see* Pain, joint,
    hand
  metatarsophalangeal (joint) —*see* Pain, joint, foot
  mouth K13.79
  muscle —*see* Myalgia
  musculoskeletal —*see also* Pain, by site M79.18
  myofascial M79.18
  nasal J34.89
  nasopharynx J39.2
  neck NEC M54.2
  nerve NEC —*see* Neuralgia
  neuromuscular —*see* Neuralgia
  nose J34.89
  ocular H57.1-●
  ophthalmic —*see* Pain, ocular
  orbital region —*see* Pain, ocular
  ovary N94.89
  ovulation N94.0
  pelvic (female) R10.2
  penis N48.89
  pericardial —*see* Pain, precordial
  perineal, perineum R10.2
  pharynx J39.2
  pleura, pleural, pleuritic R07.81
  postoperative NOS G89.18
  postprocedural NOS G89.18
  post-thoracotomy G89.12

Pain *(Continued)*
  precordial (region) R07.2
  premenstrual N94.3
  psychogenic (persistent) (any site) F45.41
  radicular (spinal) —*see* Radiculopathy
  rectum K62.89
  respiration R07.1
  retrosternal R07.2
  rheumatoid, muscular —*see* Myalgia
  rib R07.81
  root (spinal) —*see* Radiculopathy
  round ligament (stretch) R10.2
  sacroiliac M53.3
  sciatic —*see* Sciatica
  scrotum N50.82
  seminal vesicle N50.89
  shoulder M25.51-●
  spermatic cord N50.89
  spinal root —*see* Radiculopathy
  spine M54.9
    cervical M54.2
    low back M54.50
      with sciatica M54.4-●
      vertebral end plate —*see* Pain,
        vertebrogenic
    thoracic M54.6
  stomach —*see* Pain, abdominal
  substernal R07.2
  temporomandibular (joint) M26.62-●
  testis N50.81-●
  thoracic spine M54.6
    with radicular and visceral pain M54.14
  throat R07.0
  tibia —*see* Pain, limb, lower
  toe —*see* Pain, limb, lower
  tongue K14.6
  tooth K08.89
  trigeminal —*see* Neuralgia, trigeminal
  tumor associated G89.3
  ureter N23
  urinary (organ) (system) N23
  uterus NEC N94.89
  vagina R10.2
  vertebrogenic M54.89
    low back M54.51
    lumbar M54.51
    syndrome M54.89
  vesical R39.89
    associated with micturition —*see* Micturition,
      painful
  vulva R10.2
Painful —*see also* Pain
  coitus
    female N94.10
    male N53.12
    psychogenic F52.6
  ejaculation (semen) N53.12
    psychogenic F52.6
  erection —*see* Priapism
  feet syndrome E53.8
  joint replacement (hip) (knee) T84.84
  menstruation —*see* Dysmenorrhea
    psychogenic F45.8
  micturition —*see* Micturition, painful
  respiration R07.1
  scar NEC L90.5
  wire sutures T81.89
Painter's colic —*see* subcategory T56.0
Palate —*see* condition
Palatoplegia K13.79
Palatoschisis —*see* Cleft, palate
Palilalia R48.8
Palliative care Z51.5
Pallor R23.1
  optic disc, temporal —*see* Atrophy, optic
Palmar —*see also* condition
  fascia —*see* condition
Palpable
  cecum K63.89
  kidney N28.89
  ovary N83.8
  prostate N42.9
  spleen —*see* Splenomegaly
Palpitations (heart) R00.2
  psychogenic F45.8
Palsy —*see also* Paralysis G83.9
  atrophic diffuse (progressive) G12.22
  Bell's —*see also* Palsy, facial
    newborn P11.3
  brachial plexus NEC G54.0
    newborn (birth injury) P14.3

Palsy (Continued)
  brain —see Palsy, cerebral
  bulbar (progressive) (chronic) G12.22
    of childhood (Fazio-Londe) G12.1
    pseudo NEC G12.29
    supranuclear (progressive) G23.1
  cerebral (congenital) G80.9
    ataxic G80.4
    athetoid G80.3
    choreathetoid G80.3
    diplegic G80.8
      spastic G80.1
    dyskinetic G80.3
      athetoid G80.3
      choreathetoid G80.3
      distonic G80.3
    dystonic G80.3
    hemiplegic G80.8
      spastic G80.2
    mixed G80.8
    monoplegic G80.8
      spastic G80.1
    paraplegic G80.8
      spastic G80.1
    quadriplegic G80.8
      spastic G80.0
    spastic G80.1
      diplegic G80.1
      hemiplegic G80.2
      monoplegic G80.1
      quadriplegic G80.0
      specified NEC G80.1
      tetrapelgic G80.0
    specified NEC G80.8
    syphilitic A52.12
      congenital A50.49
    tetraplegic G80.8
      spastic G80.0
  cranial nerve —see also Disorder, nerve, cranial
    multiple G52.7
      in
        infectious disease B99 [G53]
        neoplastic disease —see also Neoplasm
          D49.9 [G53]
        parasitic disease B89 [G53]
        sarcoidosis D86.82
  creeping G12.22
  diver's T70.3
  Erb's P14.0
  facial G51.0
    newborn (birth injury) P11.3
  glossopharyngeal G52.1
  Klumpke (-Déjérine) P14.1
  lead —see subcategory T56.0
  median nerve (tardy) G56.1-●
  nerve G58.9
    specified NEC G58.8
  peroneal nerve (acute) (tardy) G57.3-●
  progressive supranuclear G23.1
  pseudobulbar NEC G12.29
  radial nerve (acute) G56.3-●
  seventh nerve —see also Palsy, facial
    newborn P11.3
  shaking —see Parkinsonism
  spastic (cerebral) (spinal) G80.1
  ulnar nerve (tardy) G56.2-●
  wasting G12.29
Paludism —see Malaria
Panangiitis M30.0
Panaris, panaritium —see also Cellulitis, digit
  with lymphangitis —see Lymphangitis, acute,
    digit
Panarteritis nodosa M30.0
  brain or cerebral I67.7
Pancake heart R93.1
  with cor pulmonale (chronic) I27.81
Pancarditis (acute) (chronic) I51.89
  rheumatic I09.89
    active or acute I01.8
Pancoast's syndrome or tumor C34.1-●
Pancolitis - see also Colitis
  ulcerative (chronic) K51.00
    with
      complication K51.019
        abscess K51.014
        fistula K51.013
        obstruction K51.012
        rectal bleeding K51.011
        specified complication NEC K51.018
Pancreas, pancreatic —see condition

Pancreatitis (annular) (apoplectic) (calcareous)
    (edematous) (hemorrhagic) (malignant)
    (subacute) (suppurative) K85.90
  with necrosis (uninfected) K85.91
    infected K85.92
  acute (without necrosis or infection)
      K85.90
    with necrosis (uninfected) K85.91
      infected K85.92
    alcohol induced (without necrosis or
        infection) K85.20
      with necrosis (uninfected) K85.21
        infected K85.22
    biliary (without necrosis or infection) K85.10

      with necrosis (uninfected) K85.11
        infected K85.12
    drug induced (without necrosis or infection)
        K85.30
      with necrosis (uninfected) K85.31
        infected K85.32
    gallstone (without necrosis or infection)
        K85.10
      with necrosis (uninfected) K85.11
        infected K85.12
    idiopathic (without necrosis or infection)
        K85.00
      with necrosis (uninfected) K85.01
        infected K85.02
    specified NEC (without necrosis or infection)
        K85.80
      with necrosis (uninfected) K85.81
        infected K85.82
  chronic (infectious) K86.1
    alcohol-induced K86.0
    recurrent K86.1
    relapsing K86.1
  cystic (chronic) K86.1
  cytomegaloviral B25.2
  fibrous (chronic) K86.1
  gallstone (without necrosis or infection) K85.10

      with necrosis (uninfected) K85.11
        infected K85.12
  gangrenous —see Pancreatitis, acute
  interstitial (chronic) K86.1
    acute —see also Pancreatitis, acute K85.80
  mumps B26.3
  recurrent
    acute —see Pancreatitis, acute by type
    chronic
    relapsing, chronic K86.1
  syphilitic A52.74
Pancreatoblastoma —see Neoplasm, pancreas,
  malignant
Pancreolithiasis K86.89
Pancytolysis D75.89
Pancytopenia (acquired) D61.818
  with
    malformations D61.09
    ⇒ myelodysplastic syndrome —see Syndrome,
      myelodysplastic, pancytopenia
      (acquired)
  antineoplastic chemotherapy induced D61.810
  congenital D61.09
  drug-induced NEC D61.811
  ▶ Fanconi D61.03
PANDAS (pediatric autoimmune neuropsychiatric
    disorders associated with streptococcal
    infections syndrome) D89.89
Panencephalitis, subacute, sclerosing A81.1
Panhematopenia D61.9
  congenital D61.09
  constitutional D61.09
  splenic, primary D73.1
Panhemocytopenia D61.9
  congenital D61.09
  constitutional D61.09
Panhypogonadism E29.1
Panhypopituitarism E23.0
  prepubertal E23.0
Panic (attack) (state) F41.0
  reaction to exceptional stress (transient) F43.0
Panmyelopathy, familial, constitutional D61.09
Panmyelophthisis D61.82
  congenital D61.09
Panmyelosis (acute) (with myelofibrosis) C94.4-●
Panner's disease —see Osteochondrosis, juvenile,
  humerus
Panneuritis endemica E51.11

Panniculitis (nodular) (nonsuppurative) M79.3
  back M54.00
    cervical region M54.02
    cervicothoracic region M54.03
    lumbar region M54.06
    lumbosacral region M54.07
    multiple sites M54.09
    occipito-atlanto-axial region M54.01
    sacrococcygeal region M54.08
    thoracic region M54.04
    thoracolumbar region M54.05
  lupus L93.2
  mesenteric K65.4
  neck M54.02
    cervicothoracic region M54.03
    occipito-atlanto-axial region M54.01
  relapsing M35.6
Panniculus adiposus (abdominal) E65
Pannus (allergic) (cornea) (degenerativus) (keratic)
    H16.42-●
  abdominal (symptomatic) E65
  trachomatosus, trachomatous (active) A71.1
Panophthalmitis H44.01-●
Pansinusitis (chronic) (hyperplastic) (nonpurulent)
    (purulent) J32.4
  acute J01.40
    recurrent J01.41
  tuberculous A15.8
Pansynostosis Q75.052
Panuveitis (sympathetic) H44.11-●
Panvalvular disease I08.9
  specified NEC I08.8
PAPA (pyogenic arthritis, pyoderma gangrenosum,
    and acne syndrome) M04.8
Papanicolaou smear, cervix Z12.4
  as part of routine gynecological examination
      Z01.419
    with abnormal findings Z01.411
  for suspected neoplasm Z12.4
  nonspecific abnormal finding R87.619
  routine Z01.419
    with abnormal findings Z01.411
Papilledema (choked disc) H47.10
  associated with
    decreased ocular pressure H47.12
    increased intracranial pressure H47.11
    retinal disorder H47.13
  Foster-Kennedy syndrome H47.14-●
Papillitis H46.00
  anus K62.89
  chronic lingual K14.4
  necrotizing, kidney N17.2
  optic H46.0-●
  rectum K62.89
  renal, necrotizing N17.2
  tongue K14.0
Papilloma —see also Neoplasm, benign, by site
  acuminatum (female) (male) (anogenital)
    A63.0
  basal cell L82.1
    inflamed L82.0
  benign pinta (primary) A67.0
  bladder (urinary) (transitional cell) D41.4
  choroid plexus (lateral ventricle) (third ventricle)
    D33.0
    anaplastic C71.5
    fourth ventricle D33.1
    malignant C71.5
  renal pelvis (transitional cell) D41.1-●
    benign D30.1-●
  Schneiderian
    specified site —see Neoplasm, benign, by site
    unspecified site D14.0
  serous surface
    borderline malignancy
      specified site —see Neoplasm, uncertain
        behavior, by site
      unspecified site D39.10
    specified site —see Neoplasm, benign, by site
    unspecified site D27.9
  transitional (cell)
    bladder (urinary) D41.4
    inverted type —see Neoplasm, uncertain
      behavior, by site
    renal pelvis D41.1-●
    ureter D41.2-●
  ureter (transitional cell) D41.2-●
    benign D30.2-●
  urothelial —see Neoplasm, uncertain behavior,
    by site

▶ New   ⇒ Revised   ~~deleted~~ Deleted   ● Use Additional Character(s)

Papilloma *(Continued)*
villous —*see* Neoplasm, uncertain behavior, by site
adenocarcinoma in —*see* Neoplasm, malignant, by site
in situ —*see* Neoplasm, in situ
yaws, plantar or palmar A66.1
Papillomata, multiple, of yaws A66.1
Papillomatosis —*see also* Neoplasm, benign, by site
confluent and reticulated L83
cystic, breast —*see* Mastopathy, cystic
ductal, breast —*see* Mastopathy, cystic
intraductal (diffuse) —*see* Neoplasm, benign, by site
subareolar duct D24-●
Papillomavirus, as cause of disease classified elsewhere B97.7
Papillon-Léage and Psaume syndrome Q87.0
Papule(s) R23.8
carate (primary) A67.0
fibrous, of nose D22.39
Gottron's L94.4
pinta (primary) A67.0
Papulosis
▒lymphomatoid C86.6-●
malignant I77.89
Papyraceous fetus O31.0-●
Para-albuminemia E88.09
Paracephalus Q89.7
Parachute mitral valve Q23.2
Paracoccidioidomycosis B41.9
disseminated B41.7
generalized B41.7
mucocutaneous-lymphangitic B41.8
pulmonary B41.0
specified NEC B41.8
visceral B41.8
Paradentosis K05.4
Paraffinoma T88.8
Paraganglioma D44.7
adrenal D35.0-●
malignant C74.1-●
aortic body D44.7
malignant C75.5
carotid body D44.6
malignant C75.4
chromaffin —*see also* Neoplasm, benign, by site
malignant —*see* Neoplasm, malignant, by site
extra-adrenal D44.7
malignant C75.5
specified site —*see* Neoplasm, malignant, by site
unspecified site C75.5
specified site —*see* Neoplasm, uncertain behavior, by site
unspecified site D44.7
gangliocytic D13.2
specified site —*see* Neoplasm, benign, by site
unspecified site D13.2
glomus jugulare D44.7
malignant C75.5
jugular D44.7
malignant C75.5
specified site —*see* Neoplasm, malignant, by site
unspecified site C75.5
nonchromaffin D44.7
malignant C75.5
specified site —*see* Neoplasm, malignant, by site
unspecified site C75.5
specified site —*see* Neoplasm, uncertain behavior, by site
unspecified site D44.7
parasympathetic D44.7
specified site —*see* Neoplasm, uncertain behavior, by site
unspecified site D44.7
specified site —*see* Neoplasm, uncertain behavior, by site
sympathetic D44.7
specified site —*see* Neoplasm, uncertain behavior, by site
unspecified site D44.7
unspecified site D44.7
Parageusia R43.2
psychogenic F45.8
Paragonimiasis B66.4

Paragranuloma, Hodgkin —*see* Lymphoma, Hodgkin, specified NEC
Parahemophilia —*see also* Defect, coagulation D68.2
Parakeratosis R23.4
variegata L41.0
Paralysis, paralytic (complete) (incomplete) G83.9
with
syphilis A52.17
abducens, abducent (nerve) —*see* Strabismus, paralytic, sixth nerve
abductor, lower extremity G57.9-●
accessory nerve G52.8
accommodation —*see also* Paresis, of accommodation
hysterical F44.89
acoustic nerve (except Deafness) —*see* subcategory H93.3
agitans —*see also* Parkinsonism G20.C
arteriosclerotic G21.4
alternating (oculomotor) G83.89
amyotrophic G12.21
ankle G57.9-●
anus (sphincter) K62.89
arm —*see* Monoplegia, upper limb
ascending (spinal), acute G61.0
association G12.29
asthenic bulbar G70.00
with exacerbation (acute) G70.01
in crisis G70.01
ataxic (hereditary) G11.9
general (syphilitic) A52.17
atrophic G58.9
infantile, acute —*see* Poliomyelitis, paralytic
progressive G12.22
spinal (acute) —*see* Poliomyelitis, paralytic
axillary G54.0
Babinski-Nageotte's G83.89
Bell's G51.0
newborn P11.3
Benedikt's G46.3
birth injury P14.9
spinal cord P11.5
bladder (neurogenic) (sphincter) N31.2
bowel, colon or intestine K56.0
brachial plexus G54.0
birth injury P14.3
newborn (birth injury) P14.3
brain G83.9
diplegia G83.0
triplegia G83.89
bronchial J98.09
Brown-Séquard G83.81
bulbar (chronic) (progressive) G12.22
infantile —*see* Poliomyelitis, paralytic
poliomyelitic —*see* Poliomyelitis, paralytic
pseudo G12.29
bulbospinal G70.00
with exacerbation (acute) G70.01
in crisis G70.01
cardiac —*see also* Failure, heart I50.9
cerebrocerebellar, diplegic G80.1
cervical
plexus G54.2
sympathetic G90.09
Céstan-Chenais G46.3
Charcot-Marie-Tooth type G60.0
Clark's G80.9
colon K56.0
compressed air T70.3
compression
arm G56.9-●
leg G57.9-●
lower extremity G57.9-●
upper extremity G56.9-●
congenital (cerebral) —*see* Palsy, cerebral
conjugate movement (gaze) (of eye) H51.0
cortical (nuclear) (supranuclear) H51.0
cordis —*see* Failure, heart
cranial or cerebral nerve G52.9
creeping G12.22
crossed leg G83.89
crutch —*see* Injury, brachial plexus
deglutition R13.0
hysterical F44.4
dementia A52.17
descending (spinal) NEC G12.29
diaphragm (flaccid) J98.6
due to accidental dissection of phrenic nerve during procedure —*see* Puncture, accidental complicating surgery

Paralysis, paralytic *(Continued)*
digestive organs NEC K59.89
diplegic —*see* Diplegia
divergence (nuclear) H51.8
diver's T70.3
Duchenne's
birth injury P14.0
due to or associated with
motor neuron disease G12.22
muscular dystrophy G71.01
due to intracranial or spinal birth injury —*see* Palsy, cerebral
embolic (current episode) I63.4-●
Erb (-Duchenne) (birth) (newborn) P14.0
Erb's syphilitic spastic spinal A52.17
esophagus K22.89
eye muscle (extrinsic) H49.9
intrinsic —*see also* Paresis, of accommodation
facial (nerve) G51.0
birth injury P11.3
congenital P11.3
following operation NEC —*see* Puncture, accidental complicating surgery
newborn (birth injury) P11.3
familial (recurrent) (periodic) G72.3
spastic G11.4
fauces J39.2
finger G56.9-●
gait R26.1
gastric nerve (nondiabetic) G52.2
gaze, conjugate H51.0
general (progressive) (syphilitic) A52.17
juvenile A50.45
glottis J38.00
bilateral J38.02
unilateral J38.01
gluteal G54.1
Gubler (-Millard) G46.3
hand —*see* Monoplegia, upper limb
heart —*see* Arrest, cardiac
hemiplegic —*see* Hemiplegia
hyperkalemic periodic (familial) G72.3
hypoglossal (nerve) G52.3
hypokalemic periodic G72.3
hysterical F44.4
ileus K56.0
infantile —*see also* Poliomyelitis, paralytic A80.30
bulbar —*see* Poliomyelitis, paralytic
cerebral —*see* Palsy, cerebral
spastic —*see* Palsy, cerebral, spastic
infective —*see* Poliomyelitis, paralytic
inferior nuclear G83.9
internuclear —*see* Ophthalmoplegia, internuclear
intestine K56.0
iris H57.09
due to diphtheria (toxin) A36.89
ischemic, Volkmann's (complicating trauma) T79.6
Jackson's G83.89
jake —*see* Poisoning, food, noxious, plant
Jamaica ginger (jake) G62.2
juvenile general A50.45
Klumpke (-Déjérine) (birth) (newborn) P14.1
labioglossal (laryngeal) (pharyngeal) G12.29
Landry's G61.0
laryngeal nerve (recurrent) (superior) (unilateral) J38.00
bilateral J38.02
unilateral J38.01
larynx J38.00
bilateral J38.02
due to diphtheria (toxin) A36.2
unilateral J38.01
lateral G12.23
lead —*see* subcategory T56.0
left side —*see* Hemiplegia
leg G83.1-●
both —*see* Paraplegia
crossed G83.89
hysterical F44.4
psychogenic F44.4
transient or transitory R29.818
traumatic NEC —*see* Injury, nerve, leg
levator palpebrae superioris —*see* Blepharoptosis, paralytic
limb —*see* Monoplegia
lip K13.0
Lissauer's A52.17
lower limb —*see* Monoplegia, lower limb
both —*see* Paraplegia

Paralysis, paralytic *(Continued)*
  lung J98.4
  median nerve G56.1-●
  medullary (tegmental) G83.89
  mesencephalic NEC G83.89
    tegmental G83.89
  middle alternating G83.89
  Millard-Gubler-Foville G46.3
  monoplegic —*see* Monoplegia
  motor G83.9
  muscle, muscular NEC G72.89
    due to nerve lesion G58.9
    eye (extrinsic) H49.9
      intrinsic —*see* Paresis, of accommodation
      oblique —*see* Strabismus, paralytic, fourth
        nerve
    iris sphincter H21.9
    ischemic (Volkmann's) (complicating trauma)
      T79.6
    progressive G12.21
    progressive, spinal G12.25
    pseudohypertrophic G71.02
    spinal progressive G12.25
  musculocutaneous nerve G56.9-●
  musculospiral G56.9-●
  nerve —*see also* Disorder, nerve
    abducent —*see* Strabismus, paralytic, sixth
      nerve
    accessory G52.8
    auditory (except Deafness) —*see* subcategory
      H93.3
    birth injury P14.9
    cranial or cerebral G52.9
    facial G51.0
      birth injury P11.3
      congenital P11.3
      newborn (birth injury) P11.3
    fourth or trochlear —*see* Strabismus, paralytic,
      fourth nerve
    newborn (birth injury) P14.9
    oculomotor —*see* Strabismus, paralytic, third
      nerve
    phrenic (birth injury) P14.2
    radial G56.3-●
    seventh or facial G51.0
      newborn (birth injury) P11.3
    sixth or abducent —*see* Strabismus, paralytic,
      sixth nerve
    syphilitic A52.15
    third or oculomotor —*see* Strabismus,
      paralytic, third nerve
    trigeminal G50.9
    trochlear —*see* Strabismus, paralytic, fourth
      nerve
    ulnar G56.2-●
  normokalemic periodic G72.3
  ocular H49.9
    alternating G83.89
  oculofacial, congenital (Moebius) Q87.0
  oculomotor (external bilateral) (nerve) —*see*
    Strabismus, paralytic, third nerve
  palate (soft) K13.79
  paratrigeminal G50.9
  periodic (familial) (hyperkalemic) (hypokalemic)
    (myotonic) (normokalemic) (potassium
    sensitive) (secondary) G72.3
  peripheral autonomic nervous system —*see*
    Neuropathy, peripheral, autonomic
  peroneal (nerve) G57.3-●
  pharynx J39.2
  phrenic nerve G56.8-●
  plantar nerve(s) G57.6-●
  pneumogastric nerve G52.2
  poliomyelitis (current) —*see* Poliomyelitis,
    paralytic
  popliteal nerve G57.3-●
  postepileptic transitory G83.84
  progressive (atrophic) (bulbar) (spinal) G12.22
    general A52.17
    infantile acute —*see* Poliomyelitis, paralytic
    supranuclear G23.1
  pseudobulbar G12.29
  pseudohypertrophic (muscle) (*see also*
    Dystrophy, muscular, by type, if applicable)
    G71.09
  psychogenic F44.4
  quadriceps G57.9-●
  quadriplegic —*see* Tetraplegia
  radial nerve G56.3-●
  rectus muscle (eye) H49.9
  recurrent isolated sleep G47.53

Paralysis, paralytic *(Continued)*
  respiratory (muscle) (system) (tract) R06.81
    center NEC G93.89
    congenital P28.89
    newborn P28.89
  right side —*see* Hemiplegia
  saturnine —*see* subcategory T56.0
  sciatic nerve G57.0-●
  senile G83.9
  shaking —*see* Parkinsonism
  shoulder G56.9-●
  sleep, recurrent isolated G47.53
  spastic G83.9
    cerebral —*see* Palsy, cerebral, spastic
    congenital (cerebral) —*see* Palsy, cerebral, spastic
    familial G11.4
    hereditary G11.4
    quadriplegic G80.0
    syphilitic (spinal) A52.17
  sphincter, bladder —*see* Paralysis, bladder
  spinal (cord) G83.9
    accessory nerve G52.8
    acute —*see* Poliomyelitis, paralytic
    ascending acute G61.0
    atrophic (acute) —*see also* Poliomyelitis,
      paralytic
      spastic, syphilitic A52.17
    congenital NEC —*see* Palsy, cerebral
    hereditary G95.89
    infantile —*see* Poliomyelitis, paralytic
    progressive G12.21
    muscle G12.25
    sequelae NEC G83.89
  sternomastoid G52.8
  stomach K31.84
    diabetic —*see* Diabetes, by type, with
      gastroparesis
    nerve G52.2
      diabetic —*see* Diabetes, by type, with
        gastroparesis
  stroke —*see* Infarct, brain
  ~~subcapsularis G56.8-●~~
  ▶subscapularis G56.8-●
  supranuclear (progressive) G23.1
  ⇒sympathetic G90.89
    cervical G90.09
    nervous system —*see* Neuropathy, peripheral,
      autonomic
  syndrome G83.9
    specified NEC G83.89
  syphilitic spastic spinal (Erb's) A52.17
  thigh G57.9-●
  throat J39.2
    diphtheritic A36.0
    muscle J39.2
  thrombotic (current episode) I63.3-●
  thumb G56.9-●
  tick —*see* Toxicity, venom, arthropod, specified
    NEC
  Todd's (postepileptic transitory paralysis) G83.84
  toe G57.6-●
  tongue K14.8
  transient R29.5
    arm or leg NEC R29.818
    traumatic NEC —*see* Injury, nerve
  trapezius G52.8
  traumatic, transient NEC —*see* Injury, nerve
  trembling —*see* Parkinsonism
  triceps brachii G56.9-●
  trigeminal nerve G50.9
  trochlear (nerve) —*see* Strabismus, paralytic,
    fourth nerve
  ulnar nerve G56.2-●
  upper limb —*see* Monoplegia, upper limb
  uremic N18.9 *[G99.8]*
  uveoparotitic D86.89
  uvula K13.79
    postdiphtheritic A36.0
  vagus nerve G52.2
  ⇒vasomotor NEC G90.89
  velum palati K13.79
  vesical —*see* Paralysis, bladder
  vestibular nerve (except Vertigo) —*see*
    subcategory H93.3
  vocal cords J38.00
    bilateral J38.02
    unilateral J38.01
  Volkmann's (complicating trauma) T79.6
  wasting G12.29
  Weber's G46.3
  wrist G56.9-●

Paramedial urethrovesical orifice
  Q64.79
Paramenia N92.6
Parametritis —*see also* Disease, pelvis,
  inflammatory N73.2
  acute N73.0
  complicating abortion —*see* Abortion, by type,
    complicated by, parametritis
Parametrium, parametric —*see* condition
Paramnesia —*see* Amnesia
Paramolar K00.1
Paramyloidosis E85.89
Paramyoclonus multiplex G25.3
Paramyotonia (congenita) G71.19
Parangi —*see* Yaws
Paranoia (querulans) F22
  senile F03
Paranoid
  dementia (senile) F03
    praecox —*see* Schizophrenia
  personality F60.0
  psychosis (climacteric) (involutional)
    (menopausal) F22
    psychogenic (acute) F23
    senile F03
  reaction (acute) F23
    chronic F22
  schizophrenia F20.0
  state (climacteric) (involutional) (menopausal)
    (simple) F22
    senile F03
  tendencies F60.0
  traits F60.0
  trends F60.0
  type, psychopathic personality F60.0
Paraparesis —*see* Paraplegia
Paraphasia R47.02
Paraphilia F65.9
Paraphimosis (congenital) N47.2
  chancroidal A57
Paraphrenia, paraphrenic (late) F22
  schizophrenia F20.0
Paraplegia (lower) G82.20
  ataxic —*see* Degeneration, combined, spinal
    cord
  complete G82.21
  congenital (cerebral) G80.8
    spastic G80.1
  familial spastic G11.4
  functional (hysterical) F44.4
  hereditary, spastic G11.4
  hysterical F44.4
  incomplete G82.22
  Pott's A18.01
  psychogenic F44.4
  spastic
    Erb's spinal, syphilitic A52.17
    hereditary G11.4
    tropical G04.1
  syphilitic (spastic) A52.17
  traumatic
    current injury - code to injury with seventh
      character A
      sequela of previous injury - code to injury
        with seventh character S
  tropical spastic G04.1
Parapoxvirus B08.60
  specified NEC B08.69
Paraproteinemia D89.2
  benign (familial) D89.2
  monoclonal D47.2
  secondary to malignant disease
    D47.2
Parapsoriasis L41.9
  en plaques L41.4
  guttata L41.1
  large plaque L41.4
  retiform, retiformis L41.5
  small plaque L41.3
  specified NEC L41.8
  varioliformis (acuta) L41.0
Parasitic —*see also* condition
  disease NEC B89
  stomatitis B37.0
  sycosis (beard) (scalp) B35.0
  twin Q89.4
Parasitism B89
  intestinal B82.9
  skin B88.9
  specified —*see* Infestation
Parasitophobia F40.218

▶ New   ⇒ Revised   ~~deleted~~ Deleted   ● Use Additional Character(s)

Parasomnia G47.50
  due to
    alcohol
      abuse F10.182
      dependence F10.282
      use F10.982
    amphetamines
      abuse F15.182
      dependence F15.282
      use F15.982
    caffeine
      abuse F15.182
      dependence F15.282
      use F15.982
    cocaine
      abuse F14.182
      dependence F14.282
      use F14.982
    drug NEC
      abuse F19.182
      dependence F19.282
      use F19.982
    opioid
      abuse F11.182
      dependence F11.282
      use F11.982
    psychoactive substance NEC
      abuse F19.182
      dependence F19.282
      use F19.982
    sedative, hypnotic, or anxiolytic
      abuse F13.182
      dependence F13.282
      use F13.982
    stimulant NEC
      abuse F15.182
      dependence F15.282
      use F15.982
  in conditions classified elsewhere G47.54
  nonorganic origin F51.8
  organic G47.50
  specified NEC G47.59
Paraspadias Q54.9
Paraspasmus facialis G51.8
Parasuicide (attempt)
  history of (personal) Z91.51
    in family Z81.8
Parathyroid gland —see condition
Parathyroid tetany E20.9
Paratrachoma A74.0
Paratyphilitis —see Appendicitis
Paratyphoid (fever) —see Fever, paratyphoid
Paratyphus —see Fever, paratyphoid
Paraurethral duct Q64.79
Paraurethritis —see also Urethritis
  gonococcal (acute) (chronic) (with abscess) A54.1
Paravaccinia NEC B08.04
Paravaginitis —see Vaginitis
Parencephalitis —see also Encephalitis
  sequelae G09
Parent-child conflict —see Conflict, parent-child
  estrangement NEC Z62.890
Paresis —see also Paralysis
  accommodation —see Paresis, of accommodation
  Bernhardt's G57.1-●
  bladder (sphincter) —see also Paralysis, bladder
    tabetic A52.17
  bowel, colon or intestine K56.0
  extrinsic muscle, eye H49.9
  general (progressive) (syphilitic) A52.17
    juvenile A50.45
  heart —see Failure, heart
  insane (syphilitic) A52.17
  juvenile (general) A50.45
  of accommodation H52.52-●
  peripheral progressive (idiopathic) G60.3
  pseudohypertrophic (see also Dystrophy, muscular, by type, if applicable) G71.09
  senile G83.9
  syphilitic (general) A52.17
    congenital A50.45
  vesical NEC N31.2
Paresthesia —see also Disturbance, sensation, skin R20.2
  Bernhardt G57.1-●
Paretic —see condition
Parinaud's
  conjunctivitis H10.89
  oculoglandular syndrome H10.89
  ophthalmoplegia H49.88

Parkinsonism (idiopathic) (primary) G20.C
  with neurogenic orthostatic hypotension (symptomatic) G90.3
  arteriosclerotic G21.4
  dementia (see also Dementia, in, diseases specified elsewhere) G20.C [F02.80]
    with behavioral disturbance (see also Dementia, in, diseases specified elsewhere) G20.C [F02.81-●]
  due to
    drugs NEC G21.19
      neuroleptic G21.11
    medication-induced NEC G21.19
    neuroleptic induced G21.11
  postencephalitic G21.3
  secondary G21.9
    due to
      arteriosclerosis G21.4
      drugs NEC G21.19
        neuroleptic G21.11
      encephalitis G21.3
      external agents NEC G21.2
      syphilis A52.19
    specified NEC G21.8
  syphilitic A52.19
  treatment-induced NEC G21.19
  vascular G21.4
Parkinson's disease, syndrome or tremor —see Parkinsonism
Parodontitis —see Periodontitis
Parodontosis K05.4
Paronychia —see also Cellulitis, digit
  with lymphangitis —see Lymphangitis, acute, digit
  candidal (chronic) B37.2
  tuberculous (primary) A18.4
Parorexia (psychogenic) F50.89
Parosmia R43.1
  psychogenic F45.8
Parotid gland —see condition
Parotitis, parotiditis (allergic) (nonspecific toxic) (purulent) (septic) (suppurative) —see also Sialoadenitis
  epidemic —see Mumps
  infectious —see Mumps
  postoperative K91.89
  surgical K91.89
Parrot fever A70
Parrot's disease (early congenital syphilitic pseudoparalysis) A50.02
Parry-Romberg syndrome G51.8
Parry's disease or syndrome E05.00
  with thyroid storm E05.01
Pars planitis —see Cyclitis
Parsonage (-Aldren)-Turner syndrome G54.5
Parson's disease (exophthalmic goiter) E05.00
  with thyroid storm E05.01
Particolored infant Q82.8
Parturition —see Delivery
Parulis K04.7
  with sinus K04.6
Parvovirus, as cause of disease classified elsewhere B97.6
Pasini and Pierini's atrophoderma L90.3
Passage
  false, urethra N36.5
  meconium (newborn) during delivery P03.82
  of sounds or bougies —see Attention to, artificial, opening
Passive —see condition
  smoking Z77.22
Past due on rent or mortgage Z59.81- ●
Pasteurella septica A28.0
Pasteurellosis —see Infection, Pasteurella
PAT (paroxysmal atrial tachycardia) I47.19
Patau's syndrome —see Trisomy, 13
Patches
  mucous (syphilitic) A51.39
    congenital A50.07
  smokers' (mouth) K13.24
Patellar —see condition
Patent —see also Imperfect, closure
  canal of Nuck Q52.4
  cervix N88.3
  ductus arteriosus or Botallo's Q25.0
  foramen
    botalli Q21.12
    ovale Q21.12
  interauricular septum Q21.19
  interventricular septum Q21.0
  omphalomesenteric duct Q43.0

Patent (Continued)
  os (uteri) —see Patent, cervix
  ostium secundum (type II) Q21.11
  urachus Q64.4
  vitelline duct Q43.0
Paterson (-Brown)(-Kelly) syndrome or web D50.1
Pathologic, pathological —see also condition
  asphyxia R09.01
  fire-setting F63.1
  gambling F63.0
  ovum O02.0
  resorption, tooth K03.3
  stealing F63.2
Pathology (of) —see Disease
  periradicular, associated with previous endodontic treatment NEC M27.59
Pattern, sleep-wake, irregular G47.23
Patulous —see also Imperfect, closure (congenital)
  alimentary tract Q45.8
    lower Q43.8
    upper Q40.8
  eustachian tube H69.0-●
Pause, sinoatrial I49.5
Paxton's disease B36.2
Pearl(s)
  enamel K00.2
  Epstein's K09.8
Pearl-worker's disease —see Osteomyelitis, specified type NEC
Pectenosis K62.4
Pectoral —see condition
Pectus
  carinatum (congenital) Q67.7
    acquired M95.4
    rachitic sequelae (late effect) E64.3
  excavatum (congenital) Q67.6
    acquired M95.4
    rachitic sequelae (late effect) E64.3
  recurvatum (congenital) Q67.6
Pedatrophia E41
Pederosis F65.4
Pediatric inflammatory multisystem syndrome M35.81
Pediculosis (infestation) B85.2
  capitis (head-louse) (any site) B85.0
  corporis (body-louse) (any site) B85.1
  eyelid B85.0
  mixed (classifiable to more than one of the titles B85.0-B85.3) B85.4
  pubis (pubic louse) (any site) B85.3
  vestimenti B85.1
  vulvae B85.3
Pediculus (infestation) —see Pediculosis
Pedophilia F65.4
Peg-shaped teeth K00.2
Pelade —see Alopecia, areata
Pelger-Huët anomaly or syndrome D72.0
Peliosis (rheumatica) D69.0
  hepatis K76.4
    with toxic liver disease K71.8
Pelizaeus-Merzbacher disease E75.27
Pellagra (alcoholic) E52
  with
    polyneuropathy E52 [G63]
Pellagra-cerebellar-ataxia-renal aminoaciduria syndrome E72.02
Pellegrini (-Stieda) disease or syndrome —see Bursitis, tibial collateral
Pellizzi's syndrome E34.8
Pel's crisis A52.11
Pelvic —see also condition
  examination (periodic) (routine) Z01.419
    with abnormal findings Z01.411
  kidney, congenital Q63.2
Pelviolithiasis —see Calculus, kidney
Pelviperitonitis —see also Peritonitis, pelvic
  gonococcal A54.24
  puerperal O85
Pelvis —see condition or type
Pemphigoid L12.9
  benign, mucous membrane L12.1
  bullous L12.0
  cicatricial L12.1
  juvenile L12.2
  ocular L12.1
  specified NEC L12.8
Pemphigus L10.9
  benign familial (chronic) Q82.8
  Brazilian L10.3
  circinatus L13.0
  conjunctiva L12.1

Pemphigus *(Continued)*
  drug-induced L10.5
  erythematosus L10.4
  foliaceous L10.2
  gangrenous —*see* Gangrene
  neonatorum L01.03
  ocular L12.1
  paraneoplastic L10.81
  specified NEC L10.89
  syphilitic (congenital) A50.06
  vegetans L10.1
  vulgaris L10.0
  wildfire L10.3
Pendred's syndrome E07.1
Pendulous
  abdomen, in pregnancy —*see* Pregnancy, complicated by, abnormal, pelvic organs or tissues NEC
  breast N64.89
Penetrating wound —*see also* Puncture
  with internal injury —*see* Injury, by site
  eyeball —*see* Puncture, eyeball
  orbit (with or without foreign body) —*see* Puncture, orbit
  uterus by instrument with or following ectopic or molar pregnancy O08.6
Penicillosis B48.4
Penis —*see* condition
Penitis N48.29
Pentalogy of Fallot Q21.8
Pentasomy X syndrome Q97.1
Pentosuria (essential) E74.89
Percreta placenta O43.23-●
Peregrinating patient —*see* Disorder, factitious
Perforation, perforated (nontraumatic) (of)
  accidental during procedure (blood vessel) (nerve) (organ) —*see* Complication, accidental puncture or laceration
  antrum —*see* Sinusitis, maxillary
  appendix K35.22
    with localized peritonitis K35.32
  atrial septum, multiple Q21.19
  attic, ear —*see* Perforation, tympanum, attic
  bile duct (common) (hepatic) K83.2
    cystic K82.2
  bladder (urinary)
    with or following ectopic or molar pregnancy O08.6
    obstetrical trauma O71.5
    traumatic S37.29
      at delivery O71.5
  bowel K63.1
    with or following ectopic or molar pregnancy O08.6
    newborn P78.0
    obstetrical trauma O71.5
    traumatic —*see* Laceration, intestine
  broad ligament N83.8
    with or following ectopic or molar pregnancy O08.6
    obstetrical trauma O71.6
  by
    device, implant or graft —*see also* Complications, by site and type, mechanical T85.628
      arterial graft NEC —*see* Complication, cardiovascular device, mechanical, vascular
      breast (implant) T85.49
      catheter NEC T85.698
        cystostomy T83.090
        dialysis (renal) T82.49
          intraperitoneal T85.691
        infusion NEC T82.594
          spinal (epidural) (subdural) T85.690
        urinary —*see also* Complications, catheter, urinary T83.098
      electronic (electrode) (pulse generator) (stimulator)
        bone T84.390
        cardiac T82.199
          electrode T82.190
          pulse generator T82.191
          specified type NEC T82.198
        nervous system —*see* Complication, prosthetic device, mechanical, electronic nervous system stimulator
        urinary —*see* Complication, genitourinary, device, urinary, mechanical

Perforation, perforated *(Continued)*
  by *(Continued)*
    device, implant or graft *(Continued)*
      fixation, internal (orthopedic) NEC —*see* Complication, fixation device, mechanical
      gastrointestinal —*see* Complications, prosthetic device, mechanical, gastrointestinal device
      genital NEC T83.498
        intrauterine contraceptive device T83.39
        penile prosthesis T83.490
      heart NEC —*see* Complication, cardiovascular device, mechanical
      joint prosthesis —*see* Complications, joint prosthesis, mechanical, specified NEC, by site
      ocular NEC —*see* Complications, prosthetic device, mechanical, ocular device
      orthopedic NEC —*see* Complication, orthopedic, device, mechanical
      specified NEC T85.628
      urinary NEC —*see also* Complication, genitourinary, device, urinary, mechanical
      graft T83.29
      vascular NEC —*see* Complication, cardiovascular device, mechanical
      ventricular intracranial shunt T85.09
    foreign body left accidentally in operative wound T81.539
    instrument (any) during a procedure, accidental —*see* Puncture, accidental complicating surgery
  cecum K35.22
    with localized peritonitis K35.32
  cervix (uteri) N88.8
    with or following ectopic or molar pregnancy O08.6
    obstetrical trauma O71.3
  colon K63.1
    newborn P78.0
    obstetrical trauma O71.5
    traumatic —*see* Laceration, intestine, large
  common duct (bile) K83.2
  cornea (due to ulceration) —*see* Ulcer, cornea, perforated
  cystic duct K82.2
  diverticulum (intestine) K57.80
    with bleeding K57.81
    large intestine K57.20
      with
        bleeding K57.21
        small intestine K57.40
          with bleeding K57.41
    small intestine K57.00
      with
        bleeding K57.01
        large intestine K57.40
          with bleeding K57.41
  ear drum —*see* Perforation, tympanum
  esophagus K22.3
  ethmoidal sinus —*see* Sinusitis, ethmoidal
  frontal sinus —*see* Sinusitis, frontal
  gallbladder K82.2
  heart valve —*see* Endocarditis
  ileum K63.1
    newborn P78.0
    obstetrical trauma O71.5
    traumatic —*see* Laceration, intestine, small
  instrumental, surgical (accidental) (blood vessel) (nerve) (organ) —*see* Puncture, accidental complicating surgery
  intestine NEC K63.1
    with ectopic or molar pregnancy O08.6
    newborn P78.0
    obstetrical trauma O71.5
    traumatic —*see* Laceration, intestine
    ulcerative NEC K63.1
      newborn P78.0
  jejunum, jejunal K63.1
    obstetrical trauma O71.5
    traumatic —*see* Laceration, intestine, small
    ulcer —*see* Ulcer, gastrojejunal, with perforation
  joint prosthesis —*see* Complications, joint prosthesis, mechanical, specified NEC, by site
  mastoid (antrum) (cell) —*see* Disorder, mastoid, specified NEC
  maxillary sinus —*see* Sinusitis, maxillary

Perforation, perforated *(Continued)*
  membrana tympani —*see* Perforation, tympanum
  nasal
    septum J34.89
      congenital Q30.3
      syphilitic A52.73
    sinus J34.89
      congenital Q30.8
      due to sinusitis —*see* Sinusitis
  palate —*see also* Cleft, palate Q35.9
    syphilitic A52.79
  palatine vault —*see also* Cleft, palate, hard Q35.1
    syphilitic A52.79
      congenital A50.59
  pars flaccida (ear drum) —*see* Perforation, tympanum, attic
  pelvic
    floor S31.030
      with
        ectopic or molar pregnancy O08.6
        penetration into retroperitoneal space S31.031
        retained foreign body S31.040
          with penetration into retroperitoneal space S31.041
      following ectopic or molar pregnancy O08.6
      obstetrical trauma O70.1
    organ S37.99
      adrenal gland S37.818
      bladder —*see* Perforation, bladder
      fallopian tube S37.599
        bilateral S37.592
        unilateral S37.591
      kidney S37.09-●
      obstetrical trauma O71.5
      ovary S37.499
        bilateral S37.492
        unilateral S37.491
      prostate S37.828
      specified organ NEC S37.898
      ureter —*see* Perforation, ureter
      urethra —*see* Perforation, urethra
      uterus —*see* Perforation, uterus
  perineum —*see* Laceration, perineum
  pharynx J39.2
  rectum K63.1
    newborn P78.0
    obstetrical trauma O71.5
    traumatic S36.63
  root canal space due to endodontic treatment M27.51
  sigmoid K63.1
    newborn P78.0
    obstetrical trauma O71.5
    traumatic S36.533
  sinus (accessory) (chronic) (nasal) J34.89
  sphenoidal sinus —*see* Sinusitis, sphenoidal
  surgical (accidental) (by instrument) (blood vessel) (nerve) (organ) —*see* Puncture, accidental complicating surgery
  traumatic
    external —*see* Puncture
    eye —*see* Puncture, eyeball
    internal organ —*see* Injury, by site
  tympanum, tympanic (membrane) (persistent post-traumatic) (postinflammatory) H72.9-●
    attic H72.1-●
      multiple —*see* Perforation, tympanum, multiple
      total —*see* Perforation, tympanum, total
    central H72.0-●
      multiple —*see* Perforation, tympanum, multiple
      total —*see* Perforation, tympanum, total
    marginal NEC —*see* subcategory H72.2
    multiple H72.81-●
    pars flaccida —*see* Perforation, tympanum, attic
    total H72.82-●
    traumatic, current episode S09.2-●
  typhoid, gastrointestinal —*see* Typhoid
  ulcer —*see* Ulcer, by site, with perforation
  ureter N28.89
    traumatic S37.19
  urethra N36.8
    with ectopic or molar pregnancy O08.6
    following ectopic or molar pregnancy O08.6

▶ New   ⇒ Revised   ~~deleted~~ Deleted   ● Use Additional Character(s)

Perforation, perforated *(Continued)*
  urethra *(Continued)*
    obstetrical trauma O71.5
    traumatic S37.39
      at delivery O71.5
  uterus
    with ectopic or molar pregnancy O08.6
    by intrauterine contraceptive device T83.39
    following ectopic or molar pregnancy O08.6
    obstetrical trauma O71.1
    traumatic S37.69
      obstetric O71.1
  uvula K13.79
    syphilitic A52.79
  vagina
    obstetrical trauma O71.4
    other trauma - *see* Puncture, vagina
Periadenitis mucosa necrotica recurrens
  K12.0
Periappendicitis (acute) —*see* Appendicitis
Periarteritis nodosa (disseminated) (infectious)
  (necrotizing) M30.0
Periarthritis (joint) —*see also* Enthesopathy
  Duplay's M75.0-•
  gonococcal A54.42
  humeroscapularis —*see* Capsulitis, adhesive
  scapulohumeral —*see* Capsulitis, adhesive
  shoulder —*see* Capsulitis, adhesive
  wrist M77.2-•
Periarthrosis (angioneural) —*see* Enthesopathy
Pericapsulitis, adhesive (shoulder) —*see*
  Capsulitis, adhesive
Pericarditis (with decompensation) (with effusion)
  I31.9
  with rheumatic fever (conditions in I00)
    active —*see* Pericarditis, rheumatic
    inactive or quiescent I09.2
  acute (hemorrhagic) (nonrheumatic) (Sicca)
    I30.9
    with chorea (acute) (rheumatic) (Sydenham's)
      I02.0
    benign I30.8
    nonspecific I30.0
    rheumatic I01.0
      with chorea (acute) (Sydenham's) I02.0
  adhesive or adherent (chronic) (external)
    (internal) I31.0
    acute —*see* Pericarditis, acute
    rheumatic I09.2
  bacterial (acute) (subacute) (with serous or
    seropurulent effusion) I30.1
  calcareous I31.1
  cholesterol (chronic) I31.8
    acute I30.9
  chronic (nonrheumatic) I31.9
    rheumatic I09.2
  constrictive (chronic) I31.1
  coxsackie B33.23
  fibrinocaseous (tuberculous) A18.84
  fibrinopurulent I30.1
  fibrinous I30.8
  fibrous I31.0
  gonococcal A54.83
  idiopathic I30.0
  in systemic lupus erythematosus M32.12
  infective I30.1
  meningococcal A39.53
  neoplastic (chronic) I31.8
    acute I30.9
  obliterans, obliterating I31.0
  plastic I31.0
  pneumococcal I30.1
  postinfarction I24.1
  purulent I30.1
  rheumatic (active) (acute) (with effusion) (with
    pneumonia) I01.0
    with chorea (acute) (rheumatic) (Sydenham's)
      I02.0
    chronic or inactive (with chorea) I09.2
  rheumatoid —*see* Rheumatoid, carditis
  septic I30.1
  serofibrinous I30.8
  staphylococcal I30.1
  streptococcal I30.1
  suppurative I30.1
  syphilitic A52.06
  tuberculous A18.84
  uremic N18.9 *[I32]*
  viral I30.1
Pericardium, pericardial —*see* condition
Pericellulitis —*see* Cellulitis

Pericementitis (chronic) (suppurative) —*see also*
  Periodontitis
  acute K05.20
    generalized —*see* Periodontitis, aggressive,
      generalized
    localized —*see* Periodontitis, aggressive,
      localized
Perichondritis
  auricle —*see* Perichondritis, ear
  bronchus J98.09
  ear (external) H61.00-•
    acute H61.01-•
    chronic H61.02-•
    external auditory canal —*see* Perichondritis, ear
  larynx J38.7
    syphilitic A52.73
    typhoid A01.09
  nose J34.89
  pinna —*see* Perichondritis, ear
  trachea J39.8
Periclasia K05.4
Pericoronitis —*see* Periodontitis
Pericystitis N30.90
  with hematuria N30.91
Peridiverticulitis (intestine) K57.92
  cecum —*see* Diverticulitis, intestine, large
  colon —*see* Diverticulitis, intestine, large
  duodenum —*see* Diverticulitis, intestine, small
  intestine —*see* Diverticulitis, intestine
  jejunum —*see* Diverticulitis, intestine, small
  rectosigmoid —*see* Diverticulitis, intestine, large
  rectum —*see* Diverticulitis, intestine, large
  sigmoid —*see* Diverticulitis, intestine, large
Periendocarditis —*see* Endocarditis
Periepididymitis N45.1
Perifolliculitis L01.02
  abscedens, caput, scalp L66.3
  capitis, abscedens (et suffodiens) L66.3
  superficial pustular L01.02
Perihepatitis K65.8
Perilabyrinthitis (acute) —*see* subcategory H83.0
Perimeningitis —*see* Meningitis
Perimetritis —*see* Endometritis
Perimetrosalpingitis —*see* Salpingo-oophoritis
Perineocele N81.81
Perinephric, perinephritic —*see* condition
Perinephritis —*see also* Infection, kidney
  purulent —*see* Abscess, kidney
Perineum, perineal —*see* condition
Perineuritis NEC —*see* Neuralgia
Periodic —*see* condition
Periodontitis (chronic) (complex) (compound)
  (local) (simplex) K05.30
  acute K05.20
    generalized K05.229
      moderate K05.222
      severe K05.223
      slight K05.221
    localized K05.219
      moderate K05.212
      severe K05.213
      slight K05.211
  aggressive K05.20
    generalized K05.229
      moderate K05.222
      severe K05.223
      slight K05.221
    localized K05.219
      moderate K05.212
      severe K05.213
      slight K05.211
  apical K04.5
    acute (pulpal origin) K04.4
  generalized K05.329
    moderate K05.322
    severe K05.323
    slight K05.321
  localized K05.319
    moderate K05.312
    severe K05.313
    slight K05.311
Periodontoclasia K05.4
Periodontosis (juvenile) K05.4
Periods —*see also* Menstruation
  heavy N92.0
  irregular N92.6
  shortened intervals (irregular) N92.1
Perionychia —*see also* Cellulitis, digit
  with lymphangitis —*see* Lymphangitis, acute,
    digit
Perioophoritis —*see* Salpingo-oophoritis

Periorchitis N45.2
Periosteum, periosteal —*see* condition
Periostitis (albuminosa) (circumscribed)
  (diffuse) (infective) (monomelic) —*see also*
  Osteomyelitis
  alveolar M27.3
  alveolodental M27.3
  dental M27.3
  gonorrheal A54.43
  jaw (lower) (upper) M27.2
  orbit H05.03-•
  syphilitic A52.77
    congenital (early) A50.02 *[M90.80]*
    secondary A51.46
  tuberculous —*see* Tuberculosis, bone
  yaws (hypertrophic) (early) (late) A66.6
    [M90.80]
Periostosis (hyperplastic) —*see also* Disorder, bone,
  specified type NEC
  with osteomyelitis —*see* Osteomyelitis, specified
    type NEC
Peripartum
  cardiomyopathy O90.3
Periphlebitis —*see* Phlebitis
Periproctitis K62.89
Periprostatitis —*see* Prostatitis
Perirectal —*see* condition
Perirenal —*see* condition
Perisalpingitis —*see* Salpingo-oophoritis
Perisplenitis (infectional) D73.89
Peristalsis, visible or reversed R19.2
Peritendinitis —*see* Enthesopathy
Peritoneum, peritoneal —*see* condition
Peritonitis (adhesive) (bacterial) (fibrinous)
  (hemorrhagic) (idiopathic) (localized)
  (perforative) (primary) (with adhesions) (with
  effusion) K65.9
  with or following
    abscess K65.1
    appendicitis
      with perforation or rupture K35.32
      generalized (*see also* Appendicitis) K35.209
      localized (*see also* Appendicitis) K35.30
    diverticular disease (intestine) K57.80
      with bleeding K57.81
    ectopic or molar pregnancy O08.0
    large intestine K57.20
      with
        bleeding K57.21
        small intestine K57.40
          with bleeding K57.41
    small intestine K57.00
      with
        bleeding K57.01
        large intestine K57.40
          with bleeding K57.41
  acute (generalized) K65.0
  aseptic T81.61
  bile, biliary K65.3
  chemical T81.61
  chlamydial A74.81
  chronic proliferative K65.8
  complicating abortion —*see* Abortion, by type,
    complicated by, pelvic peritonitis
  congenital P78.1
  diaphragmatic K65.0
  diffuse K65.0
  diphtheritic A36.89
  disseminated K65.0
  due to
    bile K65.3
    foreign
      body or object accidentally left during
        a procedure (instrument) (sponge)
        (swab) T81.599
      substance accidentally left during a
        procedure (chemical) (powder) (talc)
        T81.61
    talc T81.61
    urine K65.8
  eosinophilic K65.8
    acute K65.0
  fibrocaseous (tuberculous) A18.31
  fibropurulent K65.0
  following ectopic or molar pregnancy O08.0
  general (ized) K65.0
  gonococcal A54.85
  meconium (newborn) P78.0
  neonatal P78.1
    meconium P78.0
  pancreatic K65.0

Peritonitis *(Continued)*
  paroxysmal, familial E85.0
    benign E85.0
  pelvic
    female N73.5
      acute N73.3
      chronic N73.4
        with adhesions N73.6
    male K65.0
  periodic, familial E85.0
  proliferative, chronic K65.8
  puerperal, postpartum, childbirth O85
  purulent K65.0
  septic K65.0
  specified NEC K65.8
  spontaneous bacterial K65.2
  subdiaphragmatic K65.0
  subphrenic K65.0
  suppurative K65.0
  syphilitic A52.74
    congenital (early) A50.08 *[K67]*
  talc T81.61
  tuberculous A18.31
  urine K65.8
Peritonsillar —*see* condition
Peritonsillitis J36
Perityphlitis *(see also* Cecitis) K37
Periureteritis N28.89
Periurethral —*see* condition
Periurethritis (gangrenous) —*see* Urethritis
Periuterine —*see* condition
Perivaginitis —*see* Vaginitis
Perivasculitis, retinal H35.06-●
Perivasitis (chronic) N49.1
Perivesiculitis (seminal) —*see* Vesiculitis
Perlèche NEC K13.0
  due to
    candidiasis B37.83
    moniliasis B37.83
    riboflavin deficiency E53.0
    vitamin B2 (riboflavin) deficiency E53.0
Pernicious —*see* condition
Pernio, perniosis T69.1
Perpetrator (of abuse) —*see* Index to External
  Causes of Injury, Perpetrator
Persecution
  delusion F22
  social Z60.5
Perseveration (tonic) R48.8
Persistence, persistent (congenital)
  anal membrane Q42.3
    with fistula Q42.2
  arteria stapedia Q16.3
  atrioventricular canal Q21.20
  branchial cleft NOS Q18.2
    cyst Q18.0
    fistula Q18.0
    sinus Q18.0
  bulbus cordis in left ventricle Q21.8
  canal of Cloquet Q14.0
  capsule (opaque) Q12.8
  cilioretinal artery or vein Q14.8
  cloaca Q43.7
  communication —*see* Fistula, congenital
  convolutions
    aortic arch Q25.46
    fallopian tube Q50.6
    oviduct Q50.6
    uterine tube Q50.6
  double aortic arch Q25.45
  ductus arteriosus (Botalli) Q25.0
  fetal
    circulation P29.38
    form of cervix (uteri) Q51.828
    hemoglobin, hereditary (HPFH) D56.4
  foramen
    Botalli Q21.12
    ovale Q21.12
  Gartner's duct Q52.4
  hemoglobin, fetal (hereditary) (HPFH) D56.4
  hyaloid
    artery (generally incomplete) Q14.0
    system Q14.8
  hymen, in pregnancy or childbirth —*see*
    Pregnancy, complicated by, abnormal,
    vulva
  lanugo Q84.2
  left
    posterior cardinal vein Q26.8
    root with right arch of aorta Q25.49
    superior vena cava Q26.1

Persistence, persistent *(Continued)*
  Meckel's diverticulum Q43.0
    malignant —*see* Table of Neoplasms, small
      intestine, malignant
  mucosal disease (middle ear) —*see* Otitis, media,
    suppurative, chronic, tubotympanic
  nail(s), anomalous Q84.6
  omphalomesenteric duct Q43.0
  organ or site not listed —*see* Anomaly, by site
  ostium
    atrioventriculare commune Q21.23
    primum Q21.20
    secundum Q21.11
  ovarian rests in fallopian tube Q50.6
  pancreatic tissue in intestinal tract Q43.8
  primary (deciduous)
    teeth K00.6
    vitreous hyperplasia Q14.0
  pupillary membrane Q13.89
  rhesus (Rh)titer —*see* Complication(s),
    transfusion, incompatibility reaction, Rh
    (factor)
  right aortic arch Q25.47
  sinus
    urogenitalis
      female Q52.8
      male Q55.8
    venosus with imperfect incorporation in right
      auricle Q26.8
  thymus (gland) (hyperplasia) E32.0
  thyroglossal duct Q89.2
  thyrolingual duct Q89.2
  truncus arteriosus or communis Q20.0
  tunica vasculosa lentis Q12.2
  umbilical sinus Q64.4
  urachus Q64.4
  vitelline duct Q43.0
Person (with)
  admitted for clinical research, as a control subject
    (normal comparison) (participant) Z00.6
  awaiting admission to adequate facility
    elsewhere Z75.1
  concern (normal) about sick person in family
    Z63.6
  consulting on behalf of another Z71.0
  feigning illness Z76.5
  living (in)
    without
      adequate housing (heating) (space) Z59.10
      air conditioning Z59.11
      environmental temperature Z59.11
      heating Z59.11
      space Z59.19
      housing (permanent) (temporary) Z59.00
      person able to render necessary care Z74.2
      shelter Z59.02
    alone Z60.2
    boarding school Z59.3
    residential institution Z59.3
  on waiting list Z75.1
  sick or handicapped in family Z63.6
Personality (disorder) F60.9
  accentuation of traits (type A pattern) Z73.1
  affective F34.0
  aggressive F60.3
  amoral F60.2
  anacastic, anankastic F60.5
  antisocial F60.2
  anxious F60.6
  asocial F60.2
  asthenic F60.7
  avoidant F60.6
  borderline F60.3
  change due to organic condition (enduring)
    F07.0
  compulsive F60.5
  cycloid F34.0
  cyclothymic F34.0
  dependent F60.7
  depressive F34.1
  dissocial F60.2
  dual F44.81
  eccentric F60.89
  emotionally unstable F60.3
  expansive paranoid F60.0
  explosive F60.3
  fanatic F60.0
  haltlose type F60.89
  histrionic F60.4
  hyperthymic F34.0
  hypothymic F34.1

Personality *(Continued)*
  hysterical F60.4
  immature F60.89
  inadequate F60.7
  labile (emotional) F60.3
  mixed (nonspecific) F60.89
  morally defective F60.2
  multiple F44.81
  narcissistic F60.81
  obsessional F60.5
  obsessive (-compulsive) F60.5
  organic F07.0
  overconscientious F60.5
  paranoid F60.0
  passive (-dependent) F60.7
  passive-aggressive F60.89
  pathologic F60.9
  pattern defect or disturbance F60.9
  pseudopsychopathic (organic) F07.0
  pseudoretarded (organic) F07.0
  psychoinfantile F60.4
  psychoneurotic NEC F60.89
  psychopathic F60.2
  querulant F60.0
  sadistic F60.89
  schizoid F60.1
  self-defeating F60.89
  sensitive paranoid F60.0
  sociopathic (amoral) (antisocial) (asocial)
    (dissocial) F60.2
  specified NEC F60.89
  type A Z73.1
  unstable (emotional) F60.3
Perthes' disease —*see* Legg-Calvé-Perthes disease
Pertussis *(see also* Whooping cough) A37.90
Perversion, perverted
  appetite F50.89
    psychogenic F50.89
  function
    pituitary gland E23.2
      posterior lobe E22.2
  sense of smell and taste R43.8
    psychogenic F45.8
  sexual —*see* Deviation, sexual
Pervious, congenital —*see also* Imperfect, closure
  ductus arteriosus Q25.0
Pes (congenital) —*see also* Talipes
  acquired —*see also* Deformity, limb, foot,
    specified NEC
    planus —*see* Deformity, limb, flat foot
  adductus Q66.89
  cavus Q66.7-●
  deformity NEC, acquired —*see* Deformity, limb,
    foot, specified NEC
  planus (acquired) (any degree) —*see also*
    Deformity, limb, flat foot
    rachitic sequelae (late effect) E64.3
  valgus Q66.6
Pest, pestis —*see* Plague
Petechia, petechiae R23.3
  newborn P54.5
Petechial typhus A75.9
Peter's anomaly Q13.4
Petit mal seizure —*see* Epilepsy, childhood,
  absence
Petit's hernia —*see* Hernia, abdomen, specified
  site NEC
Petrellidosis B48.2
Petrositis H70.20-●
  acute H70.21-●
  chronic H70.22-●
Peutz-Jeghers disease or syndrome Q85.89
Peyronie's disease N48.6
PFAPA (periodic fever, aphthous stomatitis,
  pharyngitis, and adenopathy syndrome)
  M04.8
Pfeiffer's disease —*see* Mononucleosis, infectious
Phagedena (dry) (moist) (sloughing) —*see also*
  Gangrene
  geometric L88
  penis N48.29
  tropical —*see* Ulcer, skin
  vulva N76.6
Phagedenic —*see* condition
Phakoma H35.89
Phakomatosis —*see also* specific eponymous
  syndromes Q85.9
  Bourneville's Q85.1
  specified NEC Q85.89
Phantom limb syndrome (without pain) G54.7
  with pain G54.6

Pharyngeal pouch syndrome D82.1
Pharyngitis (acute) (catarrhal) (gangrenous)
(infective) (malignant) (membranous)
(phlegmonous) (pseudomembranous)
(simple) (subacute) (suppurative) (ulcerative)
(viral) J02.9
with influenza, flu, or grippe —see Influenza,
with, pharyngitis
aphthous B08.5
atrophic J31.2
chlamydial A56.4
chronic (atrophic) (granular) (hypertrophic)
J31.2
coxsackievirus B08.5
diphtheritic A36.0
enteroviral vesicular B08.5
follicular (chronic) J31.2
fusospirochetal A69.1
gonococcal A54.5
granular (chronic) J31.2
herpesviral B00.2
hypertrophic J31.2
infectional, chronic J31.2
influenzal —see Influenza, with, respiratory
manifestations NEC
lymphonodular, acute (enteroviral) B08.8
pneumococcal J02.8
purulent J02.9
putrid J02.9
septic J02.0
sicca J31.2
specified organism NEC J02.8
staphylococcal J02.8
streptococcal J02.0
syphilitic, congenital (early) A50.03
tuberculous A15.8
vesicular, enteroviral B08.5
viral NEC J02.8
Pharyngoconjunctivitis, viral B30.2
Pharyngolaryngitis (acute) J06.0
chronic J37.0
Pharyngoplegia J39.2
Pharyngotonsillitis, herpesviral B00.2
Pharyngotracheitis, chronic J42
Pharynx, pharyngeal —see condition
Phelan-McDermid syndrome Q93.52
Phencyclidine-induced
anxiety disorder F16.980
bipolar and related disorder F16.94
depressive disorder F16.94
psychotic disorder F16.959
Phenomenon
Arthus' —see Arthus' phenomenon
jaw-winking Q07.8
lupus erythematosus (LE) cell M32.9
Raynaud's (secondary) I73.00
with gangrene I73.01
vasomotor R55
vasospastic I73.9
vasovagal R55
Wenckebach's I44.1
▶Phenotype
  ▶Duffy
    ▶a positive Z67.A2
    ▶a and b positive Z67.A4
    ▶b positive Z67.A3
    ▶Fy (a+b-) Z67.A2
    ▶Fy (a-b-) Z67.A1
    ▶Fy (a-b+) Z67.A3
    ▶Fy (a+b+) Z67.A4
    ▶null Z67.A1
Phenylketonuria E70.1
classical E70.0
maternal E70.1
Pheochromoblastoma
specified site —see Neoplasm, malignant, by
site
unspecified site C74.10
Pheochromocytoma
malignant
specified site —see Neoplasm, malignant, by
site
unspecified site C74.10
specified site —see Neoplasm, benign, by site
unspecified site D35.00
Pheohyphomycosis —see Chromomycosis
Pheomycosis —see Chromomycosis
Phimosis (congenital) (due to infection) N47.1
chancroidal A57
Phlebectasia —see also Varix
congenital Q27.4

Phlebitis (infective) (pyemic) (septic) (suppurative)
I80.9
antepartum —see Thrombophlebitis,
antepartum
blue —see Phlebitis, leg, deep
breast, superficial I80.8
calf muscular vein (NOS) I80.25-●
cavernous (venous) sinus —see Phlebitis,
intracranial (venous) sinus
cerebral (venous) sinus —see Phlebitis,
intracranial (venous) sinus
chest wall, superficial I80.8
cranial (venous) sinus —see Phlebitis,
intracranial (venous) sinus
deep (vessels) —see Phlebitis, leg, deep
due to implanted device —see Complications, by
site and type, specified NEC
during or resulting from a procedure T81.72
femoral vein (superficial) I80.1-●
femoropopliteal vein I80.0-●
gastrocnemial vein I80.25-●
gestational —see Phlebopathy, gestational
hepatic veins I80.8
iliac vein (common) (external) (internal)
I80.21-●
iliofemoral —see Phlebitis, femoral vein
intracranial (venous) sinus (any) G08
nonpyogenic I67.6
intraspinal venous sinuses and veins G08
nonpyogenic G95.19
lateral (venous) sinus —see Phlebitis, intracranial
(venous) sinus
leg I80.3
antepartum —see Thrombophlebitis,
antepartum
deep (vessels) NEC I80.20-●
iliac I80.21-●
popliteal vein I80.22-●
specified vessel NEC I80.29-●
tibial vein (anterior) (posterior) I80.23-●
femoral vein (superficial) I80.1-●
superficial (vessels) I80.0-●
longitudinal sinus —see Phlebitis, intracranial
(venous) sinus
lower limb —see Phlebitis, leg
migrans, migrating (superficial) I82.1
pelvic
with ectopic or molar pregnancy O08.0
following ectopic or molar pregnancy
O08.0
puerperal, postpartum O87.1
peroneal vein I80.24-●
popliteal vein —see Phlebitis, leg, deep, popliteal
portal (vein) K75.1
postoperative T81.72
pregnancy —see Thrombophlebitis, antepartum
puerperal, postpartum, childbirth O87.0
deep O87.1
pelvic O87.1
superficial O87.0
retina —see Vasculitis, retina
saphenous (accessory) (great) (long) (small) —see
Phlebitis, leg, superficial
sinus (meninges) —see Phlebitis, intracranial
(venous) sinus
soleal vein I80.25-●
specified site NEC I80.8
syphilitic A52.09
tibial vein —see Phlebitis, leg, deep, tibial
ulcerative I80.9
leg —see Phlebitis, leg
umbilicus I80.8
uterus (septic) —see Endometritis
varicose (leg) (lower limb) —see Varix, leg, with,
inflammation
Phlebofibrosis I87.8
Phleboliths I87.8
Phlebopathy
gestational O22.9-●
puerperal O87.9
Phlebosclerosis I87.8
Phlebothrombosis —see also Thrombosis
antepartum —see Thrombophlebitis,
antepartum
pregnancy —see Thrombophlebitis, antepartum
puerperal —see Thrombophlebitis, puerperal
Phlebotomus fever A93.1
Phlegmasia
alba dolens O87.1
nonpuerperal —see Phlebitis, femoral vein
cerulea dolens —see Phlebitis, leg, deep

Phlegmon —see Abscess
Phlegmonous —see condition
Phlyctenulosis (allergic) (keratoconjunctivitis)
(nontuberculous) —see also
Keratoconjunctivitis
cornea —see Keratoconjunctivitis
tuberculous A18.52
Phobia, phobic F40.9
animal F40.218
spiders F40.210
examination F40.298
reaction F40.9
simple F40.298
social F40.10
generalized F40.11
specific (isolated) F40.298
animal F40.218
spiders F40.210
blood F40.230
injection F40.231
injury F40.233
men F40.290
natural environment F40.228
thunderstorms F40.220
situational F40.248
bridges F40.242
closed in spaces F40.240
flying F40.243
heights F40.241
specified focus NEC F40.298
transfusion F40.231
women F40.291
specified NEC F40.8
medical care NEC F40.232
state F40.9
Phocas' disease —see Mastopathy, cystic
Phocomelia Q73.1
lower limb —see Agenesis, leg, with foot
present
upper limb —see Agenesis, arm, with hand
present
Phoria H50.50
Phosphate-losing tubular disorder
N25.0
Phosphatemia E83.39
Phosphaturia E83.39
Photodermatitis (sun) L56.8
chronic L57.8
due to drug L56.8
light other than sun L59.8
Photokeratitis H16.13-●
Photophobia H53.14-●
Photophthalmia —see Photokeratitis
Photopsia H53.19
Photoretinitis —see Retinopathy, solar
Photosensitivity, photosensitization (sun) skin
L56.8
light other than sun L59.8
Phrenitis —see Encephalitis
Phrynoderma (vitamin A deficiency)
E50.8
Phthiriasis (pubis) B85.3
with any infestation classifiable to B85.0-B85.2
B85.4
Phthirus infestation —see Phthiriasis
Phthisis —see also Tuberculosis
bulbi (infectional) —see Disorder, globe,
degenerated condition, atrophy
eyeball (due to infection) —see Disorder, globe,
degenerated condition, atrophy
PHTS Q85.81
Phycomycosis —see Zygomycosis
Physalopteriasis B81.8
Physical restraint status Z78.1
Phytobezoar T18.9
intestine T18.3
stomach T18.2
Pian —see Yaws
Pianoma A66.1
Pica F50.89
⬛in adults (in remission) F50.83
⬛infant or child (in remission) F98.3
Picking, nose F98.8
Pick-Niemann disease —see Niemann-Pick disease
or syndrome
Pick's
cerebral atrophy (see also Dementia, in, diseases
specified elsewhere) G31.01 [F02.80]
with behavioral disturbance (see also
Dementia, in, diseases specified
elsewhere) G31.01 [F02.81-●]

Pick's *(Continued)*
    disease or syndrome (brain) *(see also* Dementia, in, diseases specified elsewhere) G31.01 *[F02.80]*
        with behavioral disturbance *(see also* Dementia, in, diseases specified elsewhere) G31.01 *[F02.81-●]*
        brain *(see also* Dementia, in, diseases specified elsewhere) G31.01 *[F02.80]*
            with behavioral disturbance *(see also* Dementia, in, diseases specified elsewhere) G31.01 *[F02.81-●]*
        pericardium (pericardial pseudocirrhosis of liver) I31.1
    syndrome
        brain *(see also* Dementia, in, diseases specified elsewhere) G31.01 *[F02.80]*
            with behavioral disturbance *(see also* Dementia, in, diseases specified elsewhere) G31.01 *[F02.81-●]*
        of heart (pericardial pseudocirrhosis of liver) I31.1
Pickwickian syndrome E66.2
Piebaldism E70.39
Piedra (beard) (scalp) B36.8
    black B36.3
    white B36.2
Pierre Robin deformity or syndrome Q87.0
Pierson's disease or osteochondrosis M91.0
Pig-bel A05.2
Pigeon
    breast or chest (acquired) M95.4
        congenital Q67.7
        rachitic sequelae (late effect) E64.3
    breeder's disease or lung J67.2
    fancier's disease or lung J67.2
    toe —*see* Deformity, toe, specified NEC
Pigmentation (abnormal) (anomaly) L81.9
    conjunctiva H11.13-●
    cornea (anterior) H18.01-●
        posterior H18.05-●
        stromal H18.06-●
    diminished melanin formation NEC L81.6
    iron L81.8
    lids, congenital Q82.8
    limbus corneae —*see* Pigmentation, cornea
    metals L81.8
    optic papilla, congenital Q14.2
    retina, congenital (grouped) (nevoid) Q14.1
    scrotum, congenital Q82.8
    tattoo L81.8
Piles —*see also* Hemorrhoids K64.9
Pili
    annulati or torti (congenital) Q84.1
    incarnati L73.1
Pill roller hand (intrinsic) —*see* Parkinsonism
Pilomatrixoma —*see* Neoplasm, skin, benign
    malignant —*see* Neoplasm, skin, malignant
Pilonidal —*see* condition
Pimple R23.8
PIMS M35.81
PIN —*see* Neoplasia, intraepithelial, prostate
Pinched nerve —*see* Neuropathy, entrapment
Pindborg tumor —*see* Cyst, calcifying odontogenic
Pineal body or gland —*see* condition
Pinealoblastoma C75.3
Pinealoma D44.5
    malignant C75.3
Pineoblastoma C75.3
Pineocytoma D44.5
Pinguecula H11.15-●
Pingueculitis H10.81-●
Pinhole meatus —*see also* Stricture, urethra N35.919
Pink
    disease —*see* subcategory T56.1
    eye —*see* Conjunctivitis, acute, mucopurulent
Pinkus' disease (lichen nitidus) L44.1
Pinpoint
    meatus —*see* Stricture, urethra
    os (uteri) —*see* Stricture, cervix
Pins and needles R20.2
Pinta A67.9
    cardiovascular lesions A67.2
    chancre (primary) A67.0
    erythematous plaques A67.1
    hyperchromic lesions A67.1
    hyperkeratosis A67.1
    lesions A67.9
        cardiovascular A67.2
        hyperchromic A67.1

Pinta *(Continued)*
    lesions *(Continued)*
        intermediate A67.1
        late A67.2
        mixed A67.3
        primary A67.0
        skin (achromic) (cicatricial) (dyschromic) A67.2
            hyperchromic A67.1
            mixed (achromic and hyperchromic) A67.3
    papule (primary) A67.0
    skin lesions (achromic) (cicatricial) (dyschromic) A67.2
        hyperchromic A67.1
        mixed (achromic and hyperchromic) A67.3
    vitiligo A67.2
Pintids A67.1
Pinworm (disease) (infection) (infestation) B80
Piroplasmosis *(see also* Babesiosis) B60.00
    specified NEC B60.09
Pistol wound —*see* Gunshot wound
Pitchers' elbow —*see* Derangement, joint, specified type NEC, elbow
Pithecoid pelvis Q74.2
    with disproportion (fetopelvic) O33.0
        causing obstructed labor O65.0
Pithiatism F48.8
Pitted —*see* Pitting
Pitting —*see also* Edema R60.9
    lip R60.0
    nail L60.8
    teeth K00.4
Pituitary gland —*see* condition
Pituitary-snuff-taker's disease J67.8
Pityriasis (capitis) L21.0
    alba L30.5
    circinata (et maculata) L42
    furfuracea L21.0
    Hebra's L26
    lichenoides L41.0
        chronica L41.1
        et varioliformis (acuta) L41.0
    maculata (et circinata) L30.5
    nigra B36.1
    pilaris, Hebra's L44.0
    rosea L42
    rotunda L44.8
    rubra (Hebra) pilaris L44.0
    simplex L30.5
    specified type NEC L30.5
    streptogenes L30.5
    versicolor (scrotal) B36.0
Placenta, placental —*see* Pregnancy, complicated by (care of) (management affected by), specified condition
Placentitis O41.14-●
Plagiocephaly Q67.3
    non-deformational
        anterior Q75.021
        posterior Q75.04-●
Plague A20.9
    abortive A20.8
    ambulatory A20.8
    asymptomatic A20.8
    bubonic A20.0
    cellulocutaneous A20.1
    cutaneobubonic A20.1
    lymphatic gland A20.0
    meningitis A20.3
    pharyngeal A20.2
    pneumonic (primary) (secondary) A20.2
    pulmonary, pulmonic A20.2
    septicemic A20.7
    tonsillar A20.8
        septicemic A20.7
Planning, family
    contraception Z30.9
    procreation Z31.69
Plaque(s)
    artery, arterial —*see* Arteriosclerosis
    calcareous —*see* Calcification
    coronary, lipid rich I25.83
    epicardial I31.8
    erythematous, of pinta A67.1
    Hollenhorst's —*see* Occlusion, artery, retina
    lipid rich, coronary I25.83
    pleural (without asbestos) J92.9
        with asbestos J92.0
    tongue K13.29

Plasmacytoma C90.3-●
    extramedullary C90.2-●
    medullary C90.0-●
    solitary C90.3-●
Plasmacytopenia D72.818
Plasmacytosis D72.822
Plaster ulcer —*see* Ulcer, pressure, by site
Plateau iris syndrome (post-iridectomy) (postprocedural) (without glaucoma)H21.82
    with glaucoma H40.22-●
Platybasia Q75.8
Platyonychia (congenital) Q84.6
    acquired L60.8
Platypelloid pelvis M95.5
    with disproportion (fetopelvic) O33.0
        causing obstructed labor O65.0
    congenital Q74.2
Platyspondylisis Q76.49
Plaut (-Vincent) disease —*see also* Vincent's A69.1
Plethora R23.2
    newborn P61.1
Pleura, pleural —*see* condition
Pleuralgia R07.81
Pleurisy (acute) (adhesive) (chronic) (costal) (diaphragmatic) (double) (dry) (fibrinous) (fibrous) (interlobar) (latent) (plastic) (primary) (residual) (sicca) (sterile) (subacute) (unresolved) R09.1
    with
        adherent pleura J86.0
        effusion J90
            chylous, chyliform J94.0
            tuberculous (non primary) A15.6
                primary (progressive) A15.7
            tuberculosis —*see* Pleurisy, tuberculous (non primary)
    encysted —*see* Pleurisy, with effusion
    exudative —*see* Pleurisy, with effusion
    fibrinopurulent, fibropurulent —*see* Pyothorax
    hemorrhagic —*see* Hemothorax
    pneumococcal J90
    purulent —*see* Pyothorax
    septic —*see* Pyothorax
    serofibrinous —*see* Pleurisy, with effusion
    seropurulent —*see* Pyothorax
    serous —*see* Pleurisy, with effusion
    staphylococcal J86.9
    streptococcal J90
    suppurative —*see* Pyothorax
    traumatic (post) (current) —*see* Injury, intrathoracic, pleura
    tuberculous (with effusion) (non primary) A15.6
        primary (progressive) A15.7
Pleuritis sicca —*see* Pleurisy
Pleurobronchopneumonia —*see* Pneumonia, broncho
Pleurodynia R07.81
    epidemic B33.0
    viral B33.0
Pleuropericarditis —*see also* Pericarditis
    acute I30.9
Pleuropneumonia (acute) (bilateral) (double) (septic) —*see also* Pneumonia J18.8
    chronic —*see* Fibrosis, lung
Pleuro-pneumonia-like-organism (PPLO), as cause of disease classified elsewhere B96.0
Pleurorrhea —*see* Pleurisy, with effusion
Plexitis, brachial G54.0
Plica
    polonica B85.0
    syndrome, knee M67.5
    tonsil J35.8
Plicated tongue K14.5
Plug
    bronchus NEC J98.09
    meconium (newborn) NEC syndrome P76.0
    mucus —*see* Asphyxia, mucus
Plumbism —*see* subcategory T56.0
Plummer's disease E05.20
    with thyroid storm E05.21
Plummer-Vinson syndrome D50.1
Pluricarential syndrome of infancy E40
Plus (and minus) hand (intrinsic) —*see* Deformity, limb, specified type NEC, forearm
PMEI (polymorphic epilepsy in infancy) G40.83-●
Pneumathemia —*see* Air, embolism
Pneumatic hammer (drill) syndrome T75.21
Pneumatocele (lung) J98.4
    intracranial G93.89
    tension J98.8

Pneumatosis
  cystoides intestinalis K63.89
  intestinalis K63.89
  peritonei K66.8
Pneumaturia R39.89
Pneumoblastoma —see Neoplasm, lung,
    malignant
Pneumocephalus G93.89
Pneumococcemia A40.3
Pneumococcus, pneumococcal —see condition
Pneumoconiosis (due to) (inhalation of) J64
  with tuberculosis (any type in A15) J65
  aluminum J63.0
  asbestos J61
  bagasse, bagassosis J67.1
  bauxite J63.1
  beryllium J63.2
  coal miners' (simple) J60
  coalworkers' (simple) J60
  collier's J60
  cotton dust J66.0
  diatomite (diatomaceous earth) J62.8
  dust
    inorganic NEC J63.6
    lime J62.8
    marble J62.8
    organic NEC J66.8
  fumes or vapors (from silo) J68.9
  graphite J63.3
  grinder's J62.8
  kaolin J62.8
  mica J62.8
  millstone maker's J62.8
  mineral fibers NEC J61
  miner's J60
  moldy hay J67.0
  potter's J62.8
  rheumatoid —see Rheumatoid, lung
  sandblaster's J62.8
  silica, silicate NEC J62.8
    with carbon J60
  stonemason's J62.8
  talc (dust) J62.0
Pneumocystis carinii pneumonia B59
Pneumocystis jiroveci (pneumonia) B59
Pneumocystosis (with pneumonia) B59
Pneumohemopericardium I31.2
Pneumohemothorax J94.2
  traumatic S27.2
Pneumohydropericardium —see Pericarditis
Pneumohydrothorax —see Hydrothorax
Pneumomediastinum J98.2
  congenital or perinatal P25.2
Pneumomycosis B49 [J99]
Pneumonia (acute) (double) (migratory) (purulent)
    (septic) (unresolved) J18.9
  with
    influenza —see Influenza, with,
        pneumonia
    lung abscess J85.1
      due to specified organism —see Pneumonia,
          in (due to)
  2019 (novel) coronavirus J12.82
  adenoviral J12.0
  adynamic J18.2
  alba A50.04
  allergic (see also Pneumonitis, hypersensitivity)
      J82.89
  alveolar —see Pneumonia, lobar
  anaerobes J15.8
  anthrax A22.1
  apex, apical —see Pneumonia, lobar
  Ascaris B77.81
  aspiration J69.0
    due to
      aspiration of microorganisms
        bacterial J15.9
        viral J12.9
      food (regurgitated) J69.0
      gastric secretions J69.0
      milk (regurgitated) J69.0
      oils, essences J69.1
      solids, liquids NEC J69.8
      vomitus J69.0
    newborn P24.81
      amniotic fluid (clear) P24.11
      blood P24.21
      food (regurgitated) P24.31
      liquor (amnii) P24.11
      meconium P24.01
      milk P24.31

Pneumonia (Continued)
  aspiration (Continued)
    newborn (Continued)
      mucus P24.11
      specified NEC P24.81
      stomach contents P24.31
    postprocedural J95.4
  atypical NEC J18.9
  bacillus J15.9
    specified NEC J15.8
  bacterial J15.9
    specified NEC J15.8
  Bacteroides (fragilis) (oralis) (melaninogenicus)
      J15.8
  basal, basic, basilar —see Pneumonia, by type
  bronchiolitis obliterans organized (BOOP)
      J84.89
  broncho-, bronchial (confluent) (croupous)
      (diffuse) (disseminated) (hemorrhagic)
      (involving lobes) (lobar) (terminal) J18.0
    allergic (see also Pneumonitis,
        hypersensitivity) J82.89
    aspiration —see Pneumonia, aspiration
    bacterial J15.9
      specified NEC J15.8
    chronic —see Fibrosis, lung
    diplococcal J13
    Eaton's agent J15.7
    Escherichia coli (E. coli) J15.5
    Friedländer's bacillus J15.0
    Hemophilus influenzae J14
    hypostatic J18.2
    inhalation —see also Pneumonia, aspiration
      due to fumes or vapors (chemical) J68.0
      of oils or essences J69.1
    Klebsiella (pneumoniae) J15.0
    lipid, lipoid J69.1
      endogenous J84.89
    Mycoplasma (pneumoniae) J15.7
    pleuro-pneumonia-like-organisms (PPLO)
        J15.7
    pneumococcal J13
    Proteus J15.69
    Pseudomonas J15.1
    Serratia marcescens J15.69
    specified organism NEC J16.8
    staphylococcal —see Pneumonia,
        staphylococcal
    streptococcal NEC J15.4
      group B J15.3
      pneumoniae J13
    viral, virus —see Pneumonia, viral
  Butyrivibrio (fibriosolvens) J15.8
  Candida B37.1
  caseous —see Tuberculosis, pulmonary
  catarrhal —see Pneumonia, broncho
  chlamydial J16.0
    congenital P23.1
  cholesterol J84.89
  cirrhotic (chronic) —see Fibrosis, lung
  Clostridium (haemolyticum) (novyi) J15.8
  confluent —see Pneumonia, broncho
  congenital (infective) P23.9
    due to
      bacterium NEC P23.6
      Chlamydia P23.1
      Escherichia coli P23.4
      Haemophilus influenzae P23.6
      infective organism NEC P23.8
      Klebsiella pneumoniae P23.6
      Mycoplasma P23.6
      Pseudomonas P23.5
      Staphylococcus P23.2
      Streptococcus (except group B) P23.6
        group B P23.3
      viral agent P23.0
    specified NEC P23.8
  coronavirus (novel) (disease) 2019 J12.82
  COVID-19 J12.82
  croupous —see Pneumonia, lobar
  cryptogenic organizing J84.116
  cytomegalic inclusion B25.0
  cytomegaloviral B25.0
  deglutition —see Pneumonia, aspiration
  desquamative interstitial J84.117
  diffuse —see Pneumonia, broncho
  diplococcal, diplococcus (broncho-) (lobar) J13
  disseminated (focal) —see Pneumonia, broncho
  Eaton's agent J15.7
  embolic, embolism —see Embolism, pulmonary
  Enterobacter J15.69

Pneumonia (Continued)
  eosinophilic J82.81
    acute J82.82
    chronic J82.81
  Escherichia coli (E. coli) J15.5
  Eubacterium J15.8
  fibrinous —see Pneumonia, lobar
  fibroid, fibrous (chronic) —see Fibrosis, lung
  Friedländer's bacillus J15.0
  Fusobacterium (nucleatum) J15.8
  gangrenous J85.0
  giant cell (measles) B05.2
  gonococcal A54.84
  gram-negative bacteria NEC J15.69
    anaerobic J15.8
  Hemophilus influenzae (broncho) (lobar) J14
  human metapneumovirus J12.3
  hypostatic (broncho) (lobar) J18.2
  in (due to)
    Acinetobacter baumannii J15.61
    actinomycosis A42.0
    adenovirus J12.0
    anthrax A22.1
    ascariasis B77.81
    aspergillosis B44.9
    Bacillus anthracis A22.1
    Bacterium anitratum J15.69
    candidiasis B37.1
    chickenpox B01.2
    Chlamydia J16.0
      neonatal P23.1
    coccidioidomycosis B38.2
      acute B38.0
      chronic B38.1
    cytomegalovirus disease B25.0
    Diplococcus (pneumoniae) J13
    Eaton's agent J15.7
    Enterobacter J15.69
    Escherichia coli (E. coli) J15.5
    Friedländer's bacillus J15.0
    fumes and vapors (chemical) (inhalation)
        J68.0
    gonorrhea A54.84
    Hemophilus influenzae (H. influenzae) J14
    Herellea J15.69
    histoplasmosis B39.2
      acute B39.0
      chronic B39.1
    human metapneumovirus J12.3
    Klebsiella (pneumoniae) J15.0
    measles B05.2
    Mycoplasma (pneumoniae) J15.7
    nocardiosis, nocardiasis A43.0
    ornithosis A70
    parainfluenza virus J12.2
    pleuro-pneumonia-like-organism (PPLO)
        J15.7
    pneumococcus J13
    pneumocystosis (Pneumocystis carinii)
        (Pneumocystis jiroveci) B59
    Proteus J15.69
    Pseudomonas NEC J15.1
      pseudomallei A24.1
    psittacosis A70
    Q fever A78
    respiratory syncytial virus (RSV) J12.1
    rheumatic fever I00 [I17]
    rubella B06.81
    Salmonella (infection) A02.22
      typhi A01.03
    schistosomiasis B65.9 [J17]
    Serratia marcescens J15.69
    specified
      bacterium NEC J15.8
      organism NEC J16.8
    spirochetal NEC A69.8
    Staphylococcus J15.20
      aureus (methicillin susceptible) (MSSA)
          J15.211
        methicillin resistant (MRSA)
            J15.212
      specified NEC J15.29
    Streptococcus J15.4
      group B J15.3
      pneumoniae J13
      specified NEC J15.4
    toxoplasmosis B58.3
    tularemia A21.2
    typhoid (fever) A01.03
    varicella B01.2
    virus —see Pneumonia, viral

Pneumonia (*Continued*)
in (due to) (*Continued*)
whooping cough A37.91
due to
Bordetella parapertussis A37.11
Bordetella pertussis A37.01
specified NEC A37.81
Yersinia pestis A20.2
inhalation of food or vomit —*see* Pneumonia,
aspiration
interstitial J84.9
chronic J84.111
desquamative J84.117
due to
collagen vascular disease J84.178
known underlying cause J84.178
idiopathic NOS J84.111
in disease classified elsewhere J84.178
lymphocytic (due to collagen vascular
disease) (in diseases classified elsewhere)
J84.178
lymphoid J84.2
non-specific J84.89
due to
collagen vascular disease J84.178
known underlying cause J84.178
idiopathic J84.113
in diseases classified elsewhere J84.178
plasma cell B59
pseudomonas J15.1
usual J84.112
due to collagen vascular disease J84.178
idiopathic J84.112
in diseases classified elsewhere J84.178
Klebsiella (pneumoniae) J15.0
lipid, lipoid (exogenous) J69.1
endogenous J84.89
lobar (disseminated) (double) (interstitial) J18.1
bacterial J15.9
specified NEC J15.8
chronic —*see* Fibrosis, lung
Escherichia coli (E. coli) J15.5
Friedländer's bacillus J15.0
Hemophilus influenzae J14
hypostatic J18.2
Klebsiella (pneumoniae) J15.0
pneumococcal J13
Proteus J15.69
Pseudomonas J15.1
specified organism NEC J16.8
staphylococcal —*see* Pneumonia,
staphylococcal
streptococcal NEC J15.4
Streptococcus pneumoniae J13
viral, virus —*see* Pneumonia, viral
lobular —*see* Pneumonia, broncho
Löffler's J82.89
lymphoid interstitial J84.2
massive —*see* Pneumonia, lobar
meconium P24.01
MRSA (Methicillin resistant Staphylococcus
aureus) J15.212
MSSA (methicillin susceptible Staphylococcus
aureus) J15.211
multilobar —*see* Pneumonia, by type
Mycoplasma (pneumoniae) J15.7
necrotic J85.0
neonatal P23.9
aspiration —*see* Aspiration, by substance, with
pneumonia
nitrogen dioxide J68.0
organizing J84.89
due to
collagen vascular disease J84.178
known underlying cause J84.178
in diseases classified elsewhere J84.178
orthostatic J18.2
parainfluenza virus J12.2
parenchymatous —*see* Fibrosis, lung
passive J18.2
patchy —*see* Pneumonia, broncho
Peptococcus J15.8
Peptostreptococcus J15.8
plasma cell (of infants) B59
pleurolobar —*see* Pneumonia, lobar
pleuro-pneumonia-like organism (PPLO) J15.7
pneumococcal (broncho) (lobar) J13
Pneumocystis (carinii) (jiroveci) B59
postinfectional NEC B99 *[J17]*
postmeasles B05.2
Proteus J15.69

Pneumonia (*Continued*)
Pseudomonas J15.1
psittacosis A70
radiation J70.0
respiratory syncytial virus (RSV) J12.1
resulting from a procedure J95.89
rheumatic I00 *[J17]*
Salmonella (arizonae) (cholerae-suis) (enteritidis)
(typhimurium) A02.22
typhi A01.03
typhoid fever A01.03
SARS-associated coronavirus J12.81
SARS-CoV-2 J12.82
segmented, segmental —*see* Pneumonia,
broncho- •
Serratia marcescens J15.69
specified NEC J18.8
bacterium NEC J15.8
organism NEC J16.8
virus NEC J12.89
spirochetal NEC A69.8
staphylococcal (broncho) (lobar) J15.20
aureus (methicillin susceptible) (MSSA)
J15.211
methicillin resistant (MRSA) J15.212
specified NEC J15.29
static, stasis J18.2
streptococcal NEC (broncho) (lobar) J15.4
group
A J15.4
B J15.3
specified NEC J15.4
Streptococcus pneumoniae J13
syphilitic, congenital (early) A50.04
traumatic (complication) (early) (secondary)
T79.8
tuberculous (any) —*see* Tuberculosis, pulmonary
tularemic A21.2
varicella B01.2
Veillonella J15.8
ventilator associated J95.851
viral, virus (broncho) (interstitial) (lobar) J12.9
adenoviral J12.0
congenital P23.0
human metapneumovirus J12.3
parainfluenza J12.2
respiratory syncytial (RSV) J12.1
SARS-associated coronavirus J12.81
specified NEC J12.89
white (congenital) A50.04
Pneumonic —*see* condition
Pneumonitis (acute) (primary) (*see also* Pneumonia)
J98.4
air-conditioner J67.7
allergic (due to) J67.9
organic dust NEC J67.8
red cedar dust J67.8
sequoiosis J67.8
wood dust J67.8
aspiration J69.0
due to
anesthesia J95.4
during
labor and delivery O74.0
pregnancy O29.01- •
puerperium O89.01
fumes or gases J68.0
obstetric O74.0
chemical (due to gases, fumes or vapors)
(inhalation) J68.0
due to anesthesia J95.4
cholesterol J84.89
chronic —*see* Fibrosis, lung
congenital rubella P35.0
crack (cocaine) J68.0
due to
beryllium J68.0
cadmium J68.0
crack (cocaine) J68.0
detergent J69.8
fluorocarbon-polymer J68.0
food, vomit (aspiration) J69.0
fumes or vapors J68.0
gases, fumes or vapors (inhalation) J68.0
inhalation
blood J69.8
essences J69.1
food (regurgitated), milk, vomit J69.0
oils, essences J69.1
saliva J69.1
solids, liquids NEC J69.8

Pneumonitis (*Continued*)
due to (*Continued*)
manganese J68.0
nitrogen dioxide J68.0
oils, essences J69.1
solids, liquids NEC J69.8
toxoplasmosis (acquired) B58.3
congenital P37.1
vanadium J68.0
ventilator J95.851
eosinophilic J82.81
acute J82.82
chronic J82.81
hypersensitivity J67.9
air conditioner lung J67.7
bagassosis J67.1
bird fancier's lung J67.2
farmer's lung J67.0
maltworker's lung J67.4
maple bark-stripper's lung J67.6
mushroom worker's lung J67.5
specified organic dust NEC J67.8
suberosis J67.3
interstitial (chronic) J84.89
acute J84.114
lymphoid J84.2
non-specific J84.89
idiopathic J84.113
lymphoid, interstitial J84.2
meconium P24.01
noninfectious J98.4
postanesthetic J95.4
correct substance properly administered —*see*
Table of Drugs and Chemcials, by drug,
adverse effect
in labor and delivery O74.0
in pregnancy O29.01- •
obstetric O74.0
overdose or wrong substance given or taken
(by accident) —*see* Table of Drugs and
Chemicals, by drug, poisoning
postpartum, puerperal O89.01
postoperative J95.4
obstetric O74.0
radiation J70.0
rubella, congenital P35.0
specified NEC J98.4
ventilation (air-conditioning) J67.7
ventilator associated J95.851
wood-dust J67.8
Pneumoconiosis —*see* Pneumoconiosis
Pneumoparotid K11.8
Pneumopathy NEC J98.4
alveolar J84.09
due to organic dust NEC J66.8
parietoalveolar J84.09
Pneumopericarditis —*see also* Pericarditis
acute I30.9
Pneumopericardium —*see also* Pericarditis
congenital P25.3
newborn P25.3
traumatic (post) —*see* Injury, heart
Pneumophagia (psychogenic) F45.8
Pneumopleurisy, pneumopleuritis —*see also*
Pneumonia J18.8
Pneumopyopericardium I30.1
Pneumopyothorax —*see* Pyopneumothorax
with fistula J86.0
Pneumorrhagia —*see also* Hemorrhage, lung
tuberculous —*see* Tuberculosis,
pulmonary
Pneumothorax NOS J93.9
acute J93.83
chronic J93.81
congenital P25.1
perinatal period P25.1
postprocedural J95.811
specified NEC J93.83
spontaneous NOS J93.83
newborn P25.1
primary J93.11
secondary J93.12
tension J93.0
tense valvular, infectional J93.0
tension (spontaneous) J93.0
traumatic S27.0
with hemothorax S27.2
tuberculous —*see* Tuberculosis, pulmonary
Podagra —*see also* Gout M10.9
Podencephalus Q01.9
Poikilocytosis R71.8

▶ New ⟹ Revised ~~deleted~~ Deleted • Use Additional Character(s)

Poikiloderma L81.6
  Civatte's L57.3
  congenital Q82.8
  vasculare atrophicans L94.5
Poikilodermatomyositis M33.10
  with
    myopathy M33.12
    respiratory involvement M33.11
    specified organ involvement NEC M33.19
      amyopathic M33.13
      without myopathy M33.13
Pointed ear (congenital) Q17.3
Poison ivy, oak, sumac or other plant dermatitis
    (allergic) (contact) L23.7
Poisoning (acute) —see also Table of Drugs and
    Chemicals
  algae and toxins T65.82-●
  Bacillus B (aertrycke) (cholerae (suis))
      (paratyphosus) (suipestifer) A02.9
    botulinus A05.1
  bacterial toxins A05.9
  berries, noxious —see Poisoning, food, noxious,
      berries
  botulism A05.1
  ciguatera fish T61.0-●
  Clostridium botulinum A05.1
  death-cap (Amanita phalloides) (Amanita
      verna) —see Poisoning, food, noxious,
      mushrooms
  drug —see Table of Drugs and Chemicals, by
      drug, poisoning
  epidemic, fish (noxious) —see Poisoning, seafood
    bacterial A05.9
  fava bean D55.0
  fish (noxious) T61.9-●
    bacterial —see Intoxication, foodborne, by
        agent
    ciguatera fish —see Poisoning, ciguatera fish
    scombroid fish —see Poisoning, scombroid
        fish
    specified type NEC T61.77-●
  food NEC A05.9
    bacterial —see Intoxication, foodborne, by
        agent
    due to
      Bacillus (aertrycke) (choleraesuis)
          (paratyphosus) (suipestifer) A02.9
        botulinus A05.1
      Clostridium (perfringens) (Welchii)
          A05.2
      salmonella (aertrycke) (choleraesuis)
          (enteritidis) (gallinarum) (paratyphi)
          (suipestifer) A02.9
        with
          gastroenteritis A02.0
          sepsis A02.1
      staphylococcus A05.0
      Vibrio
        parahaemolyticus A05.3
        vulnificus A05.5
    noxious or naturally toxic T62.9-●
      berries —see subcategory T62.1-●
      fish —see Poisoning, seafood
      mushrooms —see subcategory T62.0X-●
      plants NEC —see subcategory T62.2X-●
      seafood —see Poisoning, seafood
      specified NEC —see subcategory
          T62.8X-●
  ichthyotoxism —see Poisoning, seafood
  kreotoxism, food A05.9
  latex T65.81-●
  lead T56.0-●
  mushroom —see Poisoning, food, noxious,
      mushroom
  mussels —see also Poisoning, shellfish
    bacterial —see Intoxication, foodborne, by
        agent
  nicotine (tobacco) T65.2-●
  noxious foodstuffs —see Poisoning, food,
      noxious
  plants, noxious —see Poisoning, food, noxious,
      plants NEC
  ptomaine —see Poisoning, food
  radiation J70.0
  Salmonella (arizonae) (cholerae-suis) (enteritidis)
      (typhimurium) A02.9
  scombroid fish T61.1-●
  seafood (noxious) T61.9-●
    bacterial —see Intoxication, foodborne, by
        agent
    fish —see Poisoning, fish

Poisoning (Continued)
  seafood (Continued)
    shellfish —see Poisoning, shellfish
      specified NEC —see subcategory T61.8X-●
    shellfish (amnesic) (azaspiracid) (diarrheic)
        (neurotoxic) (noxious) (paralytic) T61.78-●
      bacterial —see Intoxication, foodborne, by
          agent
      ciguatera mollusk —see Poisoning, ciguatera
          fish
  specified substance NEC T65.891
  Staphylococcus, food A05.0
  tobacco (nicotine) T65.2-●
  water E87.79
Poker spine —see Spondylitis, ankylosing
Poland syndrome Q79.8
Polioencephalitis (acute) (bulbar) A80.9
  inferior G12.22
  influenzal —see Influenza, with, encephalopathy
  superior hemorrhagic (acute) (Wernicke's) E51.2
  Wernicke's E51.2
Polioencephalomyelitis (acute) (anterior) A80.9
  with beriberi E51.2
Polioencephalopathy, superior hemorrhagic
    E51.2
  with
    beriberi E51.11
    pellagra E52
Poliomeningoencephalitis —see
    Meningoencephalitis
Poliomyelitis (acute) (anterior) (epidemic) A80.9
  with paralysis (bulbar) —see Poliomyelitis,
      paralytic
  abortive A80.4
  ascending (progressive) —see Poliomyelitis,
      paralytic
  bulbar (paralytic) —see Poliomyelitis, paralytic
  congenital P35.8
  nonepidemic A80.9
  nonparalytic A80.4
  paralytic A80.30
    specified NEC A80.39
    vaccine-associated A80.0
    wild virus
      imported A80.1
      indigenous A80.2
  spinal, acute A80.9
Poliosis (eyebrow) (eyelashes) L67.1
  circumscripta, acquired L67.1
Pollakiuria R35.0
  psychogenic F45.8
Pollinosis J30.1
Pollitzer's disease L73.2
Polyadenitis —see also Lymphadenitis
  malignant A20.0
Polyalgia M79.89
Polyangiitis M30.0
  microscopic M31.7
  overlap syndrome M30.8
Polyarteritis
  microscopic M31.7
  nodosa M30.0
    with lung involvement M30.1
    juvenile M30.2
    related condition NEC M30.8
Polyarthralgia —see Pain, joint
Polyarthritis, polyarthropathy —see also Arthritis
    M13.0
  due to or associated with other specified
      conditions —see Arthritis
  epidemic (Australian) (with exanthema)
      B33.1
  infective —see Arthritis, pyogenic or pyemic
  inflammatory M06.4
  juvenile (chronic) (seronegative) M08.3
  migratory M13.8-●
  rheumatic, acute —see Fever, rheumatic
Polyarthrosis M15.9
  post-traumatic M15.3
  primary M15.0
  specified NEC M15.8
Polycarential syndrome of infancy E40
Polychondritis (atrophic) (chronic) —see also
    Disorder, cartilage, specified type NEC
  relapsing M94.1
Polycoria Q13.2
Polycystic (disease)
  degeneration, kidney Q61.3
    autosomal dominant (adult type) Q61.2
    autosomal recessive (infantile type) NEC
        Q61.19

Polycystic (Continued)
  kidney Q61.3
    autosomal
      dominant Q61.2
      recessive NEC Q61.19
    autosomal dominant (adult type) Q61.2
    autosomal recessive (childhood type) NEC
        Q61.19
    infantile type NEC Q61.19
  liver Q44.6
  lung J98.4
    congenital Q33.0
  ovary, ovaries E28.2
  spleen Q89.09
Polycythemia (secondary) D75.1
  acquired D75.1
  benign (familial) D75.0
  due to
    donor twin P61.1
    erythropoietin D75.1
    fall in plasma volume D75.1
    high altitude D75.1
    maternal-fetal transfusion P61.1
    stress D75.1
  emotional D75.1
  erythropoietin D75.1
  familial (benign) D75.0
  Gaisböck's (hypertonica) D75.1
  high altitude D75.1
  hypertonica D75.1
  hypoxemic D75.1
  neonatorum P61.1
  nephrogenous D75.1
  relative D75.1
  secondary D75.1
  spurious D75.1
  stress D75.1
  vera D45
Polycytosis cryptogenica D75.1
Polydactylism, polydactyly Q69.9
  toes Q69.2
Polydipsia R63.1
Polydystrophy, pseudo-Hurler E77.0
Polyembryoma —see Neoplasm, malignant, by site
Polyglandular
  deficiency E31.0
  dyscrasia E31.9
  dysfunction E31.9
  syndrome E31.8
Polyhydramnios O40.-●
Polymastia Q83.1
Polymenorrhea N92.0
Polymyalgia M35.3
  arteritica, giant cell M31.5
  rheumatica M35.3
    with giant cell arteritis M31.5
Polymyositis (acute) (chronic) (hemorrhagic)
    M33.20
  with
    myopathy M33.22
    respiratory involvement M33.21
    skin involvement —see Dermatopolymyositis
    specified organ involvement NEC M33.29
  ossificans (generalisata) (progressiva) —see
      Myositis, ossificans, progressiva
Polyneuritis, polyneuritic —see also
    Polyneuropathy
  acute (post-)infective G61.0
  alcoholic G62.1
  cranialis G52.7
  demyelinating, chronic inflammatory (CIDP)
      G61.81
  diabetic —see Diabetes, polyneuropathy
  diphtheritic A36.83
  due to lack of vitamin NEC E56.9 [G63]
  endemic E51.11
  erythredema —see subcategory T56.1
  febrile, acute G61.0
  hereditary ataxic G60.1
  idiopathic, acute G61.0
  infective (acute) G61.0
  inflammatory, chronic demyelinating (CIDP)
      G61.81
  nutritional E63.9 [G63]
  postinfective (acute) G61.0
  specified NEC G62.89
Polyneuropathy (peripheral) G62.9
  alcoholic G62.1
  amyloid (Portuguese) E85.1 [G63]
    transthyretin-related (ATTR) familial
        E85.1

Polyneuropathy (Continued)
  arsenical E85.1 [G63]
  critical illness G62.81
  demyelinating, chronic inflammatory (CIDP)
    G61.81
  diabetic —see Diabetes, polyneuropathy
  drug-induced G62.0
  hereditary G60.9
    specified NEC G60.8
  idiopathic G60.9
    progressive G60.3
  in (due to)
    alcohol G62.1
      sequelae G65.2
    amyloidosis, familial (Portuguese) E85.1 [G63]
    antitetanus serum G61.1
    arsenic G62.2
      sequelae G65.2
    avitaminosis NEC E56.9 [G63]
    beriberi E51.11
    collagen vascular disease NEC M35.9 [G63]
    deficiency (of)
      B (-complex) vitamins E53.9 [G63]
      vitamin B6 E53.1 [G63]
    diabetes —see Diabetes, polyneuropathy
    diphtheria A36.83
    drug or medicament G62.0
      correct substance properly administered —
        see Table of Drugs and Chemicals, by
        drug, adverse effect
      overdose or wrong substance given or
        taken —see Table of Drugs and
        Chemicals, by drug, poisoning
    endocrine disease NEC E34.9 [G63]
    herpes zoster B02.23
    hypoglycemia E16.2 [G63]
    infectious
      disease NEC B99 [G63]
      mononucleosis B27.91
    lack of vitamin NEC E56.9 [G63]
    lead G62.2
      sequelae G65.2
    leprosy A30.9 [G63]
    Lyme disease A69.22
    metabolic disease NEC E88.9 [G63]
    microscopic polyangiitis M31.7 [G63]
    mumps B26.84
    neoplastic disease —see also Neoplasm D49.9
      [G63]
    nutritional deficiency NEC E63.9 [G63]
    organophosphate compounds G62.2
      sequelae G65.2
    parasitic disease NEC B89 [G63]
    pellagra E52 [G63]
    polyarteritis nodosa M30.0
    porphyria E80.20 [G63]
    radiation G62.82
    rheumatoid arthritis —see Rheumatoid,
      polyneuropathy
    sarcoidosis D86.89
    serum G61.1
    syphilis (late) A52.15
      congenital A50.43
    systemic
      connective tissue disorder M35.9 [G63]
      lupus erythematosus M32.19
    toxic agent NEC G62.2
      sequelae G65.2
    transthyretin-related (ATTR) familial amyloid
      E85.1
      triorthocresyl phosphate G62.2
        sequelae G65.2
      tuberculosis A17.89
      uremia N18.9 [G63]
      vitamin B12 deficiency E53.8 [G63]
        with anemia (pernicious) D51.0 [G63]
          due to dietary deficiency D51.3 [G63]
      zoster B02.23
  inflammatory G61.9
    chronic demyelinating (CIDP) G61.81
    sequelae G65.1
    specified NEC G61.89
  lead G62.2
    sequelae G65.2
  nutritional NEC E63.9 [G63]
  postherpetic (zoster) B02.23
  progressive G60.3
  radiation-induced G62.82
  sensory (hereditary) (idiopathic) G60.8
  specified NEC G62.89
  syphilitic (late) A52.15
    congenital A50.43

Polyopia H53.8
Polyorchism, polyorchidism Q55.21
Polyosteoarthritis —see also Osteoarthritis,
    generalized M15.9- ●
  post-traumatic M15.3
  specified NEC M15.8
Polyostotic fibrous dysplasia Q78.1
Polyotia Q17.0
Polyp, polypus
  accessory sinus J33.8
  adenocarcinoma in —see Neoplasm, malignant,
    by site
  adenocarcinoma in situ in —see Neoplasm, in
    situ, by site
  adenoid tissue J33.0
  adenomatous —see also Neoplasm, benign, by
    site
    adenocarcinoma in —see Neoplasm,
      malignant, by site
    adenocarcinoma in situ in —see Neoplasm, in
      situ, by site
    carcinoma in —see Neoplasm, malignant, by
      site
    carcinoma in situ in —see Neoplasm, in situ,
      by site
    multiple —see Neoplasm, benign
      adenocarcinoma in —see Neoplasm,
        malignant, by site
      adenocarcinoma in situ in —see Neoplasm,
        in situ, by site
  antrum J33.8
  anus, anal (canal) K62.0
  Bartholin's gland N84.3
  bladder D41.4
  carcinoma in —see Neoplasm, malignant, by
    site
  carcinoma in situ in —see Neoplasm, in situ, by
    site
  cecum D12.0
  cervix (uteri) N84.1
    in pregnancy or childbirth —see Pregnancy,
      complicated by, abnormal, cervix
    mucous N84.1
    nonneoplastic N84.1
  choanal J33.0
  cholesterol K82.4
  clitoris N84.3
  colon K63.5
    adenomatous D12.6
      ascending D12.6
      cecum D12.0
      descending D12.4
    ascending K63.5
      sigmoid D12.5
      transverse D12.3
    cecum K63.5
    descending K63.5
    inflammatory K51.40
      with
        abscess K51.414
        complication K51.419
          specified NEC K51.418
        fistula K51.413
        intestinal obstruction K51.412
        rectal bleeding K51.411
    sigmoid D12.5
    transverse D12.3
  corpus uteri N84.0
  dental K04.01
    irreversible K04.02
    reversible K04.01
  duodenum K31.7
  ear (middle) H74.4- ●
  endometrium N84.0
  esophageal K22.81
  esophagogastric junction K22.82
  ethmoidal (sinus) J33.8
  fallopian tube N84.8
  female genital tract N84.9
    specified NEC N84.8
  frontal (sinus) J33.8
  gallbladder K82.4
  gingiva, gum K06.8
  hyperplastic, (any site) K63.5
  labia, labium (majus) (minus) N84.3
  larynx (mucous) J38.1
    adenomatous D14.1
  malignant —see Neoplasm, malignant, by
    site
  maxillary (sinus) J33.8
  middle ear —see Polyp, ear (middle)
  myometrium N84.0

Polyp, polypus (Continued)
  nares
    anterior J33.9
    posterior J33.0
  nasal (mucous) J33.9
    cavity J33.0
    septum J33.0
  nasopharyngeal J33.0
  nose (mucous) J33.9
  oviduct N84.8
  pharynx J39.2
  placenta O90.89
  prostate —see Enlargement, enlarged, prostate
  pudenda, pudendum N84.3
  pulpal (dental) K04.01
    irreversible K04.02
    reversible K04.01
  rectum (nonadenomatous) K62.1
    adenomatous —see Polyp, adenomatous
  septum (nasal) J33.0
  sinus (accessory) (ethmoidal) (frontal)
    (maxillary) (sphenoidal) J33.8
  sphenoidal (sinus) J33.8
  stomach K31.7
    adenomatous D13.1
  tube, fallopian N84.8
  turbinate, mucous membrane J33.8
  umbilical, newborn P83.6
  ureter N28.89
  urethra N36.2
  uterus (body) (corpus) (mucous) N84.0
    cervix N84.1
    in pregnancy or childbirth —see Pregnancy,
      complicated by, tumor, uterus
  vagina N84.2
  vocal cord (mucous) J38.1
  vulva N84.3
Polyphagia R63.2
Polyploidy Q92.7
Polypoid —see condition
Polyposis —see also Polyp
  adenomatous D13.91
  coli (adenomatous) D12.6
    adenocarcinoma in C18.9
    adenocarcinoma in situ in —see Neoplasm, in
      situ, by site
    carcinoma in C18.9
  colon (adenomatous) D12.6
  familial D12.6
    adenocarcinoma in situ in —see Neoplasm, in
      situ, by site
  intestinal D12.6
    adenomatous D13.91
  malignant lymphomatous C83.1
  multiple, adenomatous —see also Neoplasm,
    benign D36.9
Polyradiculitis —see Polyneuropathy
Polyradiculoneuropathy (acute) (postinfective)
    (segmentally demyelinating) G61.0
Polyserositis
  due to pericarditis I31.1
  pericardial I31.1
  periodic, familial E85.0
  tuberculous A19.9
    acute A19.1
    chronic A19.8
Polysplenia syndrome Q89.09
Polysyndactyly —see also Syndactylism, syndactyly
    Q70.4
Polytrichia L68.3
Polyunguia Q84.6
Polyuria R35.89
  nocturnal R35.81
  psychogenic F45.8
  specified NEC R35.89
Pompe's disease (glycogen storage) E74.02
Pompholyx L30.1
Poncet's disease (tuberculous rheumatism) A18.09
Pond fracture —see Fracture, skull
Ponos B55.0
Pons, pontine —see condition
Poor
  aesthetic of existing restoration of tooth K08.56
  contractions, labor O62.2
  gingival margin to tooth restoration K08.51
  personal hygiene R46.0
  prenatal care, affecting management of
    pregnancy —see Pregnancy, complicated by,
      insufficient, prenatal care
  sucking reflex (newborn) R29.2
  urinary stream R39.12
  vision NEC H54.7

▶ New   ⟫ Revised   ~~deleted~~ Deleted   ● Use Additional Character(s)

Pregnancy *(Continued)*
  complicated by *(Continued)*
    abnormal, abnormality *(Continued)*
      pelvic organs O34.9-●
        specified NEC O34.8-●
          causing obstructed labor O65.5
      pelvis (bony) (major) NEC O33.0
      perineum O34.7-●
      position
        placenta O44.0-●
          with hemorrhage O44.1-●
        uterus O34.59-●
      uterus O34.59-●
        causing obstructed labor O65.5
        congenital O34.0-●
      vagina O34.6-●
        causing obstructed labor O65.5
      vulva O34.7-●
        causing obstructed labor O65.5
    abruptio placentae —*see* Abruptio placentae
    abscess or cellulitis
      bladder O23.1-●
      breast O91.11-●
      genital organ or tract O23.9-●
    abuse
      physical O9A.31-●
      psychological O9A.51-●
      sexual O9A.41-●
    adverse effect anesthesia O29.9-●
      aspiration pneumonitis O29.01-●
      cardiac arrest O29.11-●
      cardiac complication NEC O29.19-●
      cardiac failure O29.12-●
      central nervous system complication NEC
        O29.29-●
      cerebral anoxia O29.21-●
      failed or difficult intubation O29.6-●
      inhalation of stomach contents or secretions
        NOS O29.01-●
      local, toxic reaction O29.3X
      Mendelson's syndrome O29.01-●
      pressure collapse of lung O29.02-●
      pulmonary complications NEC O29.09-●
      specified NEC O29.8X
      spinal and epidural type NEC O29.5X
        induced headache O29.4-●
    albuminuria —*see also* Proteinuria, gestational
      O12.1-●
    alcohol use O99.31-●
    amnionitis O41.12-●
    anaphylactoid syndrome of pregnancy
      O88.01-●
    anemia (conditions in D50-D64) (pre-existing)
      O99.01-●
    ▶complicating childbirth O99.02
      complicating the puerperium O99.03
    antepartum hemorrhage O46.9-●
      with coagulation defect —*see* Hemorrhage,
        antepartum, with coagulation defect
      specified NEC O46.8X-●
    appendicitis O99.61-●
    atrophy (yellow) (acute) liver (subacute)
      O26.61-●
    bariatric surgery status O99.84-●
    bicornis or bicornuate uterus O34.0-●
    biliary tract problems O26.61-●
    breech presentation O32.1
    cardiovascular diseases (conditions in I00-I09,
      I20-I52, I70-I99) O99.41-●
    cerebrovascular disorders (conditions in
      I60-I69) O99.41-●
    cervical shortening O26.87-●
    cervicitis O23.51-●
    cesarean scar defect (isthmocele) O34.22
    chloasma (gravidarum) O26.89-●
    cholecystitis O26.64-●
    cholestasis (intrahepatic) O26.61-●
    chorioamnionitis O41.12-●
    circulatory system disorder (conditions in
      I00-I09, I20-I99, O99.41-●)
    compound presentation O32.6
    conjoined twins O30.02-●
    connective system disorders (conditions in
      M00-M99) O99.891
    contracted pelvis (general) O33.1
      inlet O33.2
      outlet O33.3
    convulsions (eclamptic) (uremic) —*see also*
      Eclampsia O15.9-●
    cracked nipple O92.11-●
    cystitis O23.1-●

Pregnancy *(Continued)*
  complicated by *(Continued)*
    cystocele O34.8-●
    death of fetus (near term) O36.4
      early pregnancy O02.1
      of one fetus or more in multiple gestation
        O31.2-●
    deciduitis O41.14-●
    decreased fetal movement O36.81-●
    dental problems O99.61-●
    diabetes (mellitus) O24.91-●
      gestational (pregnancy induced) —*see*
        Diabetes, gestational
      pre-existing O24.31-●
        specified NEC O24.81-●
        type 1 O24.01-●
        type 2 O24.11-●
    digestive system disorders (conditions in
      K00-K93) O99.61-●
    diseases of —*see* Pregnancy, complicated by,
      specified body system disease
      biliary tract O26.61-●
      blood NEC (conditions in D65-D77)
        O99.11-●
      liver O26.61-●
      specified NEC O99.891
    disorders of —*see* Pregnancy, complicated by,
      specified body system disorder
      amniotic fluid and membranes O41.9-●
        specified NEC O41.8X-●
      biliary tract O26.61-●
      ear and mastoid process (conditions in
        H60-H95) O99.891
      eye and adnexa (conditions in H00-H59)
        O99.891
      liver O26.61-●
      skin (conditions in L00-L99) O99.71-●
      specified NEC O99.891
    displacement, uterus NEC O34.59-●
      causing obstructed labor O65.5
    disproportion (due to) O33.9
      fetal (ascites) (hydrops)
        (meningomyelocele) (sacral teratoma)
        (tumor) deformities NEC O33.7
      generally contracted pelvis O33.1
      hydrocephalic fetus O33.6
      inlet contraction of pelvis O33.2
      mixed maternal and fetal origin O33.4
      specified NEC O33.8
    double uterus O34.0-●
      causing obstructed labor O65.5
    drug use (conditions in F11-F19) O99.32-●
    eclampsia, eclamptic (coma) (convulsions)
      (delirium) (nephritis) (uremia) (*see also*
      Eclampsia) O15-●
    ectopic pregnancy —*see* Pregnancy, ectopic
    edema O12.0-●
      with
        gestational hypertension, mild —*see also*
          Pre-eclampsia O14.0-●
        proteinuria O12.2-●
    effusion, amniotic fluid —*see* Pregnancy,
      complicated by, premature rupture of
      membranes
    elderly
      multigravida O09.52-●
      primigravida O09.51-●
    embolism —*see also* Embolism, obstetric,
      pregnancy O88.-●
    endocrine diseases NEC O99.28-●
    endometritis O86.12
    excessive weight gain O26.0-●
    exhaustion O26.81-●
      during labor and delivery O75.81
    face presentation O32.3
    failed induction of labor O61.9
    failed or difficult intubation for anesthesia
      O29.6-●
      instrumental O61.1
      mechanical O61.1
      medical O61.0
      specified NEC O61.8
      surgical O61.1
    false labor (pains) O47.9
      at or after 37 completed weeks of
        pregnancy O47.1
      before 37 completed weeks of pregnancy
        O47.0-●
    fatigue O26.81-●
      during labor and delivery O75.81
    fatty metamorphosis of liver O26.61-●

Pregnancy *(Continued)*
  complicated by *(Continued)*
    female genital mutilation O34.8-● [*N90.81-*●]
    fetal (maternal care for)
      abnormality or damage O35.9
        acid-base balance O68
        specified type NEC O35.8
      acidemia O68
      acidosis O68
      agenesis of corpus callosum O35.01
      alkalosis O68
      anemia and thrombocytopenia O36.82-●
      anencephaly O35.02
      bradycardia O36.83-●
      cardiac anomalies O35.B
      central nervous system malformation or
        damage O35.00
        specified type NEC O35.09
      choroid plexus cysts O35.03
      chromosomal abnormality (conditions in
        Q90-Q99) O35.10
        sex chromosome O35.15
        specified NEC O35.19
        Trisomy 13 O35.11
        Trisomy 18 O35.12
        Trisomy 21 O35.13
        Turner Syndrome O35.14
      conjoined twins O30.02-●
      damage from
        amniocentesis O35.7
        biopsy procedures O35.7
        drug addiction O35.5
        hematological investigation O35.7
        intrauterine contraceptive device O35.7
        maternal
          alcohol addiction O35.4
          cytomegalovirus infection O35.3
          disease NEC O35.8
          drug addiction O35.5
          listeriosis O35.8
          rubella O35.3
          toxoplasmosis O35.8
          viral infection O35.3
        medical procedure NEC O35.7
        radiation O35.6
      death (near term) O36.4
        early pregnancy O02.1
      decreased movement O36.81-●
      depressed heart rate tones O36.83-●
      disproportion due to deformity (fetal)
        O33.7
      encephalocele O35.04
      excessive growth (large for dates) O36.6-●
      facial anomalies O35.A
      gastrointestinal anomalies O35.D
      genitourinary anomalies O35.E
      growth retardation O36.59-●
        light for dates O36.59-●
        small for dates O36.59-●
      heart rate irregularity (abnormal
        variability) (bradycardia)
        (decelerations) (tachycardia) O36.83-●
      hereditary disease O35.2
      holoprosencephaly O35.05
      hydrocephalus O35.06
      hydrocephaly O35.06
      intrauterine death O36.4
      microcephaly O35.07
      musculoskeletal anomalies
        lower extremities O35.H
        trunk O35.F
        upper extremities O35.G
      non-reassuring heart rate or rhythm
        O36.83-●
      poor growth O36.59-●
        light for dates O36.59-●
        small for dates O36.59-●
      problem O36.9-●
        specified NEC O36.89-●
      pulmonary anomalies O35.C
      reduction (elective) O31.3-●
      selective termination O31.3-●
      spina bifida O35.08
      thrombocytopenia O36.82-●
    fibroid (tumor) (uterus) O34.1-●
    fissure of nipple O92.11-●
    gallstones O99.61-●
    gastric banding status O99.84-●
    gastric bypass status O99.84-●
    genital herpes (asymptomatic) (history of)
      (inactive) O98.3-●

▶ New   ⟹ Revised   ~~deleted~~ Deleted   ● Use Additional Character(s)

▷ New   ⇒ Revised   ~~deleted~~ Deleted   • Use Additional Character(s)

Pregnancy (Continued)
  complicated by (Continued)
    preterm labor (Continued)
      without delivery O60.00
        second trimester O60.02
        third trimester O60.03
    previous history of —see Pregnancy,
        supervision of, high-risk
    prolapse, uterus O34.52-●
    proteinuria (gestational) —see also Proteinuria,
        gestational O12.1-●
      with edema O12.2-●
    pruritic urticarial papules and plaques of
        pregnancy (PUPPP) O26.86
    pruritus (neurogenic) O26.89-●
    psychosis or psychoneurosis (puerperal)
        F53.1
    ptyalism O26.89-●
    PUPPP (pruritic urticarial papules and
        plaques of pregnancy) O26.86
    pyelitis O23.0-●
    recurrent pregnancy loss O26.2-●
    renal disease or failure NEC O26.83-●
      with secondary hypertension, pre-
          existing —see Hypertension,
          complicating, pregnancy, pre-existing,
          secondary
        hypertensive, pre-existing —see
          Hypertension, complicating,
          pregnancy, pre-existing, with, renal
          disease
    respiratory condition (conditions in J00-J99)
        O99.51-●
    retained, retention
      dead ovum O02.0
      intrauterine contraceptive device
          O26.3-●
    retroversion, uterus O34.53-●
    Rh immunization, incompatibility or
        sensitization NEC O36.09-●
      anti-D antibody O36.01-●
    rupture
      amnion (premature) —see also Pregnancy,
          complicated by, premature rupture of
          membranes O42-●
      membranes (premature) —see also
          Pregnancy, complicated by, premature
          rupture of membranes O42-●
      uterus (during labor) O71.1
        before onset of labor O71.0-●
    salivation (excessive) O26.89-●
    salpingitis O23.52-●
    salpingo-oophoritis O23.52-●
    sepsis (conditions in A40, A41) O98.81-●
    size date discrepancy (uterine) O26.84-●
    skin condition (conditions in L00-L99)
        O99.71-●
    smoking (tobacco) O99.33-●
    social problem O09.7-●
    specified condition NEC O26.89-●
    spotting O26.85-●
    streptococcus group B (GBS) carrier state
        O99.820
    subluxation of symphysis (pubis) O26.71-●
    syphilis (conditions in A50-A53) O98.11-●
    threatened
      abortion O20.0
      labor O47.9
        at or after 37 completed weeks of
            gestation O47.1
        before 37 completed weeks of gestation
            O47.0-●
    thrombophlebitis (superficial) O22.2-●
    thrombosis O22.9-●
      cerebral venous O22.5-●
      cerebrovenous sinus O22.5-●
      deep O22.3-●
    tobacco use disorder (smoking) O99.33-●
    torsion of uterus O34.59-●
    toxemia O14.9-●
    transverse lie or presentation O32.2
    tuberculosis (conditions in A15-A19) O98.01-●
    tumor (benign)
      cervix O34.4-●
        malignant O9A.11-●
      uterus O34.1-●
    unstable lie O32.0
    upper respiratory infection O99.51-●
    urethritis O23.2-●
    uterine size date discrepancy O26.84-●
    vaginitis or vulvitis O23.59-●

Pregnancy (Continued)
  complicated by (Continued)
    varicose veins (lower extremities) O22.0-●
      genitals O22.1-●
      legs O22.0-●
      perineal O22.1-●
      vaginal or vulval O22.1-●
    venereal disease NEC (conditions in A63.8)
        O98.31-●
    venous disorders O22.9-●
      specified NEC O22.8X-●
    very young mother —see Pregnancy,
        complicated by, young mother
    viral diseases (conditions in A80-B09, B25-B34)
        O98.51-●
    vomiting O21.9
      due to diseases classified elsewhere O21.8
      hyperemesis gravidarum (mild) —see
          also Hyperemesis, gravidarum
          O21.0-●
      late (occurring after 20 weeks of gestation)
          O21.2
    young mother
      multigravida O09.62-●
      primigravida O09.61-●
  concealed O09.3-●
  continuing following
    elective fetal reduction of one or more fetus
        O31.3-●
    intrauterine death of one or more fetus
        O31.2-●
    spontaneous abortion of one or more fetus
        O31.1-●
  cornual O00.80
    with intrauterine pregnancy O00.81
  ectopic (ruptured) O00.90
    with intrauterine pregnancy O00.91
    abdominal O00.00
      with
        intrauterine pregnancy O00.01
        viable fetus O36.7-●
    cervical O00.80
      with intrauterine pregnancy O00.81
    complicated (by) O08.9
      afibrinogenemia O08.1
      cardiac arrest O08.81
      chemical damage of pelvic organ(s) O08.6
      circulatory collapse O08.3
      defibrination syndrome O08.1
      electrolyte imbalance O08.5
      embolism (amniotic fluid) (blood clot)
          (pulmonary) (septic) O08.2
      endometritis O08.0
      genital tract and pelvic infection O08.0
      hemorrhage (delayed) (excessive) O08.1
      infection
        genital tract or pelvic O08.0
        kidney 008.83
        urinary tract O08.83
      intravascular coagulation O08.1
      laceration of pelvic organ(s) O08.6
      metabolic disorder O08.5
      oliguria O08.4
      oophoritis O08.0
      parametritis O08.0
      pelvic peritonitis O08.0
      perforation of pelvic organ(s) O08.6
      renal failure or shutdown O08.4
      salpingitis or salpingo-oophoritis
          O08.0
      sepsis O08.82
      shock O08.3
        septic O08.82
      specified condition NEC O08.89
      tubular necrosis (renal) O08.4
      uremia O08.4
      urinary infection O08.83
      venous complication NEC O08.7
        embolism O08.2
    cornual O00.80
      with intrauterine pregnancy O00.81
    intraligamentous O00.80
      with intrauterine pregnancy O00.81
    mural O00.80
      with intrauterine pregnancy O00.81
    ovarian O00.20-●
      with intrauterine pregnancy O00.21-●
    specified site NEC O00.80
      with intrauterine pregnancy O00.81
    tubal (ruptured) O00.10-●
      with intrauterine pregnancy O00.11-●

Pregnancy (Continued)
  examination (normal) Z34.9-●
    first Z34.0-●
    high-risk —see Pregnancy, supervision of,
        high-risk
    specified Z34.8-●
  extrauterine —see Pregnancy, ectopic
  fallopian O00.10-●
    with intrauterine pregnancy O00.11-●
  false F45.8
  gestational carrier Z33.3
  heptachorionic, hepta-amniotic (septuplets)
      O30.83-●
  hexachorionic, hexa-amniotic (sextuplets)
      O30.83-●
  hidden O09.3-●
  high-risk —see Pregnancy, supervision of,
      high-risk
  incidental finding Z33.1
  interstitial O00.80
    with intrauterine pregnancy O00.81
  intraligamentous O00.80
    with intrauterine pregnancy O00.81
  intramural O00.80
    with intrauterine pregnancy O00.81
  intraperitoneal O00.00
    with intrauterine pregnancy O00.01
  isthmian O00.10-●
    with intrauterine pregnancy O00.11-●
  mesometric (mural) O00.80
    with intrauterine pregnancy O00.81
  molar NEC O02.0
    complicated (by) O08.9
      afibrinogenemia O08.1
      cardiac arrest O08.81
      chemical damage of pelvic organ(s)
          O08.6
      circulatory collapse O08.3
      defibrination syndrome O08.1
      electrolyte imbalance O08.5
      embolism (amniotic fluid) (blood clot)
          (pulmonary) (septic) O08.2
      endometritis O08.0
      genital tract and pelvic infection O08.0
      hemorrhage (delayed) (excessive) O08.1
      infection
        genital tract or pelvic O08.0
        kidney O08.83
        urinary tract O08.83
      intravascular coagulation O08.1
      laceration of pelvic organ(s) O08.6
      metabolic disorder O08.5
      oliguria O08.4
      oophoritis O08.0
      parametritis O08.0
      pelvic peritonitis O08.0
      perforation of pelvic organ(s) O08.6
      renal failure or shutdown O08.4
      salpingitis or salpingo-oophoritis O08.0
      sepsis O08.82
      shock O08.3
        septic O08.82
      specified condition NEC O08.89
      tubular necrosis (renal) O08.4
      uremia O08.4
      urinary infection O08.83
      venous complication NEC O08.7
        embolism O08.2
    hydatidiform —see also Mole, hydatidiform
        O01.9-●
  multiple (gestation) O30.9-●
    greater than quadruplets —see Pregnancy,
        multiple (gestation), specified NEC
    specified NEC O30.80-●
      with
        two or more monoamniotic fetuses
            O30.82-●
        two or more monochorionic fetuses
            O30.81-●
      number of chorions and amnions are both
          equal to the number of fetuses
          O30.83-●
      two or more monoamniotic fetuses
          O30.82-●
      two or more monochorionic fetuses
          O30.81-●
      unable to determine number of placenta
          and number of amniotic sacs O30.89-●
      unspecified number of placenta and
          unspecified number of amniotic sacs
          O30.80-●

▷ New   ⇒ Revised   ~~deleted~~ Deleted   ● Use Additional Character(s)

Presence *(Continued)*
  cardioverter-defibrillator (ICD) Z95.810
  cerebrospinal fluid drainage device Z98.2
  cochlear implant (functional) Z96.21
  contact lens (es) Z97.3
  coronary artery graft or prosthesis Z95.5
  CRT-D (cardiac resynchronization therapy
      defibrillator) Z95.810
  CRT-P (cardiac resynchronization therapy
      pacemaker) Z95.0
  cardioverter-defibrillator (ICD) Z95.810
  CSF shunt Z98.2
  dental prosthesis device Z97.2
  dentures Z97.2
  device (external) NEC Z97.8
    cardiac NEC Z95.818
    heart assist Z95.811
    implanted (functional) Z96.9
      specified NEC Z96.89
    prosthetic Z97.8
  ear implant Z96.20
    cochlear implant Z96.21
    myringotomy tube Z96.22
    specified type NEC Z96.29
  elbow-joint implant (functional) (prosthesis)
      Z96.62-●
  endocrine implant (functional) NEC Z96.49
  eustachian tube stent or device (functional)
      Z96.29
  external hearing-aid or device Z97.4
  finger-joint implant (functional) (prosthetic)
      Z96.69-●
  functional implant Z96.9
    specified NEC Z96.89
  graft
    cardiac NEC Z95.818
    vascular NEC Z95.828
  hearing-aid or device (external) Z97.4
    implant (bone) (cochlear) (functional) Z96.21
  heart assist device Z95.811
  heart valve implant (functional) Z95.2
    prosthetic Z95.2
    specified type NEC Z95.4
    xenogenic Z95.3
  hip-joint implant (functional) (prosthesis)
      Z96.64-●
  ICD (cardioverter-defibrillator) Z95.810
  implanted device (artificial) (functional)
      (prosthetic) Z96.9
    automatic cardiac defibrillator (with
        synchronous cardiac pacemaker)Z95.810
    cardiac pacemaker Z95.0
    cochlear Z96.21
    dental Z96.5
    heart Z95.812
    heart valve Z95.2
      prosthetic Z95.2
      specified NEC Z95.4
      xenogenic Z95.3
    insulin pump Z96.41
    intraocular lens Z96.1
    joint Z96.60
      ankle Z96.66-●
      elbow Z96.62-●
      finger Z96.69-●
      hip Z96.64-●
    Pknee Z96.65-●
      shoulder Z96.61-●
      specified NEC Z96.698
      wrist Z96.63-●
    larynx Z96.3
    myringotomy tube Z96.22
    otological Z96.20
      cochlear Z96.21
      eustachian stent Z96.29
      myringotomy Z96.22
      specified NEC Z96.29
      stapes Z96.29
    skin Z96.81
    skull plate Z96.7
    specified NEC Z96.89
    urogenital Z96.0
  insulin pump (functional) Z96.41
  intestinal bypass or anastomosis Z98.0
  intraocular lens (functional) Z96.1
  intrauterine contraceptive device (IUD) Z97.5
  intravascular implant (functional) (prosthetic)
      NEC Z95.9
    coronary artery Z95.5
    defibrillator (with synchronous cardiac
        pacemaker) Z95.810
    peripheral vessel (with angioplasty) Z95.820

Presence *(Continued)*
  joint implant (prosthetic) (any) Z96.60
    ankle —*see* Presence, ankle joint implant
    elbow —*see* Presence, elbow joint implant
    finger —*see* Presence, finger joint implant
    hip —*see* Presence, hip joint implant
    knee —*see* Presence, knee joint implant
    shoulder —*see* Presence, shoulder joint
        implant
    specified joint NEC Z96.698
    wrist —*see* Presence, wrist joint implant
  knee-joint implant (functional) (prosthesis)
      Z96.65-●
  laryngeal implant (functional) Z96.3
  mandibular implant (dental) Z96.5
  myringotomy tube(s) Z96.22
  neurostimulator (brain) (gastric) (peripheral
      nerve) (sacral nerve) (spinal cord) (vagus
      nerve) Z96.82
  orthopedic-joint implant (prosthetic) (any) —*see*
      Presence, joint implant
  otological implant (functional) Z96.29
  shoulder-joint implant (functional) (prosthesis)
      Z96.61-●
  skull-plate implant Z96.7
  spectacles Z97.3
  stapes implant (functional) Z96.29
  systemic lupus erythematosus [SLE] inhibitor
      D68.62
  tendon implant (functional) (graft) Z96.7
  tooth root(s) implant Z96.5
  ureteral stent Z96.0
  urethral stent Z96.0
  urogenital implant (functional) Z96.0
  vascular implant or device Z95.9
    access port device Z95.828
    specified type NEC Z95.828
  wrist-joint implant (functional) (prosthesis)
      Z96.63-●
Presenile —*see also* condition
  dementia F03
  premature aging E34.8
Presentation, fetal —*see* Delivery, complicated by,
    malposition
Prespondylolisthesis (congenital) Q76.2
Pressure
  area, skin —*see* Ulcer, pressure, by site
  brachial plexus G54.0
  brain G93.5
    injury at birth NEC P11.1
  cerebral —*see* Pressure, brain
  chest R07.89
  cone, tentorial G93.5
  hyposystolic —*see also* Hypotension
    incidental reading, without diagnosis of
        hypotension R03.1
  increased
    intracranial, benign G93.2
      injury at birth P11.0
    intraocular H40.05-●
  injury —*see* Ulcer, pressure, by site
  lumbosacral plexus G54.1
  mediastinum J98.59
  necrosis (chronic) —*see* Ulcer, pressure, by
      site
  parental, inappropriate (excessive) Z62.6
  sore (chronic) —*see* Ulcer, pressure, by site
  spinal cord G95.20
  ulcer (chronic) —*see* Ulcer, pressure, by site
  venous, increased I87.8
Pre-syncope R55
Preterm
  delivery (see also Pregnancy, complicated by,
      preterm labor) O60.10
  labor —*see* Pregnancy, complicated by, preterm
      labor
  newborn (infant) P07.30
    gestational age
      28 completed weeks (28 weeks, 0 days
          through 28 weeks, 6 days) P07.31
      29 completed weeks (29 weeks, 0 days
          through 29 weeks, 6 days) P07.32
      30 completed weeks (30 weeks, 0 days
          through 30 weeks, 6 days) P07.33
      31 completed weeks (31 weeks, 0 days
          through 31 weeks, 6 days) P07.34
      32 completed weeks (32 weeks, 0 days
          through 32 weeks, 6 days) P07.35
      33 completed weeks (33 weeks, 0 days
          through 33 weeks, 6 days) P07.36
      34 completed weeks (34 weeks, 0 days
          through 34 weeks, 6 days) P07.37

Preterm *(Continued)*
  newborn *(Continued)*
    gestational age *(Continued)*
      35 completed weeks (35 weeks, 0 days
          through 35 weeks, 6 days) P07.38
      36 completed weeks (36 weeks, 0 days
          through 36 weeks, 6 days) P07.39
Previa
  placenta (total) (without hemorrhage)
      O44.0-●
    with hemorrhage O44.1-●
    complete O44.0-●
      with hemorrhage O44.1-●
    low —*see also* Delivery, complicated, by,
        placenta, low O44.4-●
      with hemorrhage O44.5-●
    marginal O44.2-●
      with hemorrhage O44.3-●
    partial O44.2-●
      with hemorrhage O44.3-●
  vasa O69.4
Priapism N48.30
  due to
    disease classified elsewhere N48.32
    drug N48.33
    specified cause NEC N48.39
    trauma N48.31
Prickling sensation (skin) R20.2
Prickly heat L74.0
Primary —*see* condition
Primigravida
  elderly, affecting management of pregnancy,
      labor and delivery (supervision only) —
      see Pregnancy, complicated by, elderly,
      primigravida
  older, affecting management of pregnancy,
      labor and delivery (supervision only) —
      see Pregnancy, complicated by, elderly,
      primigravida
  very young, affecting management of pregnancy,
      labor and delivery (supervision only) —*see*
      Pregnancy, complicated by, young mother,
      primigravida
Primipara
  elderly, affecting management of pregnancy,
      labor and delivery (supervision only) —
      see Pregnancy, complicated by, elderly,
      primigravida
  older, affecting management of pregnancy,
      labor and delivery (supervision only) —
      see Pregnancy, complicated by, elderly,
      primigravida
  very young, affecting management of pregnancy,
      labor and delivery (supervision only) —*see*
      Pregnancy, complicated by, young mother,
      primigravida
Primus varus (bilateral) Q66.21-●
PRIND (Prolonged reversible ischemic neurologic
    deficit) I63.9
Pringle's disease (tuberous sclerosis)Q85.1
Prinzmetal angina I20.1
Prizefighter ear —*see* Cauliflower ear
Problem (with) (related to)
  academic Z55.8
  acculturation Z60.3
  adjustment (to)
    change of job Z56.1
    life-cycle transition Z60.0
    pension Z60.0
    retirement Z60.0
  adopted child Z62.821
  alcoholism in family Z63.72
  atypical parenting situation Z62.9
  bankruptcy Z59.89
  behavioral (adult) F69
    drug seeking Z76.5
  birth of sibling affecting child Z62.898
  care (of)
    provider dependency Z74.9
      specified NEC Z74.8
    sick or handicapped person in family or
        household Z63.6
  child
    abuse (affecting the child) —*see* Maltreatment,
        child
    custody or support proceedings Z65.3
    in
      care of non-parental family member Z62.23
      custody of
        grandparent Z62.23
        non-parental relative Z62.23
        non-relative guardian Z62.24

Problem *(Continued)*
  child *(Continued)*
    in *(Continued)*
      foster care Z62.21
      kinship care Z62.23
      welfare
        custody Z62.21
        guardianship Z62.21
    leaving living situation without permission Z62.892
    living in
      group home Z62.22
      orphanage Z62.22
  child-rearing Z62.9
    specified NEC Z62.898
  communication (developmental) F80.9
  completing medical forms Z55.6
  conflict or discord (with)
    boss Z56.4
    classmates Z55.4
    counselor Z64.4
    employer Z56.4
    family Z63.9
      specified NEC Z63.8
    probation officer Z64.4
    social worker Z64.4
    teachers Z55.4
    workmates Z56.4
  conviction in legal proceedings Z65.0
    with imprisonment Z65.1
  counselor Z64.4
  creditors Z59.89
  digestive K92.9
  drug addict in family Z63.72
  ear —*see* Disorder, ear
  economic Z59.9
    affecting care Z59.9
    specified NEC Z59.89
    strain Z59.86
  education Z55.9
    specified NEC Z55.8
  employment Z56.9
    change of job Z56.1
    discord Z56.4
    environment Z56.5
    sexual harassment Z56.81
    specified NEC Z56.89
    stress NEC Z56.6
    stressful schedule Z56.3
    threat of job loss Z56.2
    unemployment Z56.0
  enuresis, child F98.0
  eye H57.9
  failed examinations (school) Z55.2
  falling Z91.81
  family —*see also* Disruption, family Z63.9-●
    specified NEC Z63.8
  feeding (elderly) (infant) NOS R63.39
    newborn P92.9
      breast P92.5
      overfeeding P92.4
      slow P92.2
      specified NEC P92.8
      underfeeding P92.3
    nonorganic F50.89
  finance Z59.9
    specified NEC Z59.89
  foreclosure on loan Z59.89
  foster child Z62.822
  frightening experience(s) in childhood Z62.898
  genital NEC
    female N94.9
    male N50.9
  health care Z75.9
    specified NEC Z75.8
  health literacy Z55.6
  hearing —*see* Deafness
  homelessness Z59.00
  housing Z59.9
    inadequate Z59.10
    isolated Z59.89
    specified NEC Z59.89
  identity (of childhood) F93.8
  illegitimate pregnancy (unwanted) Z64.0
  illiteracy Z55.0
  impaired mobility Z74.09
  imprisonment or incarceration Z65.1
  inadequate teaching affecting education Z55.8
  inappropriate (excessive) parental pressure Z62.6
  influencing health status NEC Z78.9
  in-law Z63.1
  institutionalization, affecting child Z62.22

Problem *(Continued)*
  intrafamilial communication Z63.8
  jealousy, child F93.8
  landlord Z59.2
  language (developmental) F80.9
  learning (developmental) F81.9
  legal Z65.3
    conviction without imprisonment Z65.0
    imprisonment Z65.1
    release from prison Z65.2
  life-management Z73.9
    specified NEC Z73.89
  life-style Z72.9
    gambling Z72.6
    high-risk sexual behavior (heterosexual) Z72.51
      bisexual Z72.53
      homosexual Z72.52
    inappropriate eating habits Z72.4
    self-damaging behavior NEC Z72.89
    specified NEC Z72.89
    tobacco use Z72.0
  literacy Z55.9
    low level Z55.0
    specified NEC Z55.8
  living alone Z60.2
  lodgers Z59.2
  loss of love relationship in childhood Z62.898
  marital Z63.0
    involving
      divorce Z63.5
      estrangement Z63.5
      gender identity F66
  mastication K08.89
  medical
    care, within family Z63.6
    facilities Z75.9
      specified NEC Z75.8
  mental F48.9
  money Z59.86
  multiparity Z64.1
  negative life events in childhood Z62.9
    altered pattern of family relationships Z62.898
    frightening experience Z62.898
    loss of
      love relationship Z62.898
      self-esteem Z62.898
    physical abuse (alleged) —*see* Maltreatment, child
    removal from home Z62.29
    specified event NEC Z62.898
  neighbor Z59.2
  neurological NEC R29.818
  new step-parent affecting child Z62.898
  none (feared complaint unfounded) Z71.1
  occupational NEC Z56.89
  parent-child —*see* Conflict, parent-child
  personal hygiene Z91.89
  personality F69
  phase-of-life transition, adjustment Z60.0
  presence of sick or disabled person
    in family or household Z63.79
    needing care Z63.6
  primary support group (family) Z63.9
    specified NEC Z63.8
  probation officer Z64.4
  psychiatric F99
  psychosexual (development) F66
  psychosocial Z65.9
    religious or spiritual Z65.8
    specified NEC Z65.8
  related to physical environment, specified NEC Z58.89
  relationship Z63.9
    childhood F93.8
  release from prison Z65.2
    religious or spiritual Z65.8
  removal from home affecting child Z62.29
  seeking and accepting known hazardous and harmful
    behavioral or psychological interventions Z65.8
    chemical, nutritional or physical interventions Z65.8
  sexual function (nonorganic) F52.9
  sight H54.7
  sleep disorder, child F51.9
  smell —*see* Disturbance, sensation, smell
  social
    environment Z60.9
      specified NEC Z60.8
    exclusion and rejection Z60.4
    worker Z64.4

Problem *(Continued)*
  speech R47.9
    developmental F80.9
    specified NEC R47.89
  swallowing —*see* Dysphagia
  taste —*see* Disturbance, sensation, taste
  tic, child F95.0
  underachievement in school Z55.3
  unemployment Z56.0
    threatened Z56.2
  unwanted pregnancy Z64.0
  upbringing Z62.9
    specified NEC Z62.898
  urinary N39.9
  voice production R47.89
  work schedule (stressful) Z56.3
Procedure (surgical)
  converted
    arthroscopic to open Z53.33
    laparoscopic to open Z53.31
    specified procedure NEC to open Z53.39
    thoracoscopic to open Z53.32
  for purpose other than remedying health state Z41.9
    specified NEC Z41.8
  not done Z53.9
    because of
      administrative reasons Z53.8
      contraindication Z53.09
        smoking Z53.01
      patient's decision Z53.20
        for reasons of belief or group pressure Z53.1
        left against medical advice (AMA) Z53.29
        left without being seen Z53.21
        specified reason NEC Z53.29
      specified reason NEC Z53.8
Procidentia (uteri) N81.3
Proctalgia K62.89
  fugax K59.4
  spasmodic K59.4
Proctitis K62.89
  amebic (acute) A06.0
  chlamydial A56.3
  gonococcal A54.6
  granulomatous —*see* Enteritis, regional, large intestine
  herpetic A60.1
  radiation K62.7
  tuberculous A18.32
  ulcerative (chronic) K51.20
    with
      complication K51.219
        abscess K51.214
        fistula K51.213
        obstruction K51.212
        rectal bleeding K51.211
        specified NEC K51.218
Proctocele
  female (without uterine prolapse) N81.6
    with uterine prolapse N81.2
      complete N81.3
  male K62.3
Proctocolitis
  allergic K52.29
  food-induced eosinophilic K52.29
  food protein-induced K52.29
  milk protein-induced K52.29
  mucosal —*see* Rectosigmoiditis, ulcerative
Proctoptosis K62.3
Proctorrhagia K62.5
Proctosigmoiditis K63.89
  ulcerative (chronic) —*see* Rectosigmoiditis, ulcerative
Proctospasm K59.4
  psychogenic F45.8
Profichet's disease —*see* Disorder, soft tissue, specified type NEC
Progeria E34.8
Prognathism (mandibular) (maxillary) M26.19
Progonoma (melanotic) —*see* Neoplasm, benign, by site
Progressive —*see* condition
Prolactinoma
  specified site —*see* Neoplasm, benign, by site
  unspecified site D35.2
Prolapse, prolapsed
  anus, anal (canal) (sphincter) K62.2
  arm or hand O32.2
    causing obstructed labor O64.4

Prolapse, prolapsed (Continued)
bladder (mucosa) (sphincter) (acquired)
   congenital Q79.4
   female —see Cystocele
   male N32.89
breast implant (prosthetic) T85.49
cecostomy K94.09
cecum K63.4
cervix, cervical (hypertrophied) N81.2
   anterior lip, obstructing labor O65.5
   congenital Q51.828
   postpartal, old N81.2
   stump N81.85
ciliary body (traumatic) —see Laceration,
   eye(ball), with prolapse or loss of
   interocular tissue
colon (pedunculated) K63.4
colostomy K94.09
disc (intervertebral) —see Displacement,
   intervertebral disc
eye implant (orbital) T85.398
   lens (ocular) —see Complications, intraocular
    lens
fallopian tube N83.4-●
gastric (mucosa) K31.89
genital, female N81.9
   specified NEC N81.89
globe, nontraumatic —see Luxation, globe
ileostomy bud K94.19
intervertebral disc —see Displacement,
   intervertebral disc
intestine (small) K63.4
iris (traumatic) —see Laceration, eye(ball), with
   prolapse or loss of interocular tissue
   nontraumatic H21.89
kidney N28.83
   congenital Q63.2
laryngeal muscles or ventricle J38.7
liver K76.89
meatus urinarius N36.8
mitral (valve) I34.1
ocular lens implant —see Complications,
   intraocular lens
organ or site, congenital NEC —see Malposition,
   congenital
ovary N83.4-●
pelvic floor, female N81.89
perineum, female N81.89
rectum (mucosa) (sphincter) K62.3
   due to trichuris trichuria B79
spleen D73.89
stomach K31.89
umbilical cord
   complicating delivery O69.0
urachus, congenital Q64.4
ureter N28.89
   with obstruction N13.5
    with infection N13.6
ureterovesical orifice N28.89
urethra (acquired) (infected) (mucosa)
   N36.8
   congenital Q64.71
urinary meatus N36.8
   congenital Q64.72
uterovaginal N81.4
   complete N81.3
   incomplete N81.2
uterus (with prolapse of vagina) N81.4
   complete N81.3
   congenital Q51.818
   first degree N81.2
   in pregnancy or childbirth —see Pregnancy,
    complicated by, abnormal, uterus
   incomplete N81.2
   postpartal (old) N81.4
   second degree N81.2
   third degree N81.3
uveal (traumatic) —see Laceration, eye(ball),
   with prolapse or loss of interocular
   tissue
vagina (anterior) (wall) —see Cystocele
   with prolapse of uterus N81.4
    complete N81.3
    incomplete N81.2
   posterior wall N81.6
   posthysterectomy N99.3
vitreous (humor) H43.0-●
   in wound —see Laceration, eye(ball), with
    prolapse or loss of interocular
    tissue
womb —see Prolapse, uterus

Prolapsus, female N81.9
   specified NEC N81.89
Proliferation(s)
primary cutaneous CD30-positive large T-cell
   C86.6-●
   prostate, atypical small acinar N42.32
Proliferative —see condition
Prolonged, prolongation (of)
   bleeding (time) (idiopathic) R79.1
   coagulation (time) R79.1
   gestation (over 42 completed weeks)
    mother O48.1
    newborn P08.22
   interval I44.0
   labor O63.9
    first stage O63.0
    second stage O63.1
   partial thromboplastin time (PTT) R79.1
   pregnancy (more than 42 weeks gestation) O48.1
   prothrombin time R79.1
   QT interval R94.31
   uterine00000 contractions in labor O62.4
Prominence, prominent
   ischial spine or sacral promontory with
    disproportion (fetopelvic) O33.0
    causing obstructed labor O65.0
   auricle (congenital) (ear) Q17.5
   nose (congenital) acquired M95.0
Promiscuity —see High, risk, sexual behavior
Pronation
   ankle —see Deformity, limb, foot, specified
    NEC
   foot —see also Deformity, limb, foot, specified
    NEC
    congenital Q74.2
Prophylactic
   administration of
    antibiotics, long-term Z79.2
     short-term use - omit code
    drug —see also Long-term (current) drug
     therapy (use of) Z79.899-●
   medication Z79.899
   organ removal (for neoplasia management)
    Z40.00
    breast Z40.01
    fallopian tube(s) Z40.03
     with ovary(s) Z40.02
    ovary(s) Z40.02
    specified site NEC Z40.09
   surgery Z40.9
    for risk factors related to malignant
     neoplasm —see Prophylactic, organ
     removal
    specified NEC Z40.8
   vaccination Z23
Propionic acidemia E71.121
Proptosis (ocular) —see also Exophthalmos
   thyroid —see Hyperthyroidism, with goiter
Prosecution, anxiety concerning Z65.3
Prosopagnosia R48.3
Prostadynia N42.81
Prostate, prostatic —see condition
Prostatism —see Hyperplasia, prostate
Prostatitis (congestive) (suppurative) (with cystitis)
   N41.9
   acute N41.0
   cavitary N41.8
   chronic N41.1
   diverticular N41.8
   due to Trichomonas (vaginalis) A59.02
   fibrous N41.1
   gonococcal (acute) (chronic) A54.22
   granulomatous N41.4
   hypertrophic N41.1
   subacute N41.1
   trichomonal A59.02
   tuberculous A18.14
Prostatocystitis N41.3
Prostatorrhea N42.89
Prostatosis N42.82
Prostration R53.83
   heat —see also Heat, exhaustion
    anhydrotic T67.3
    due to
     salt (and water) depletion T67.4
     water depletion T67.3
   nervous F48.8
   senile R54
Protanomaly (anomalous trichromat) H53.54
Protanopia (complete) (incomplete) H53.54
Protection (against) (from) —see Prophylactic

Protein
   deficiency NEC —see Malnutrition
   malnutrition —see Malnutrition
   sickness —see also Reaction, serum T80.69
Proteinemia R77.9
Proteinosis
   alveolar (pulmonary) J84.01
   lipid or lipoid (of Urbach) E78.89
Proteinuria R80.9
   Bence Jones R80.3
   complicating pregnancy —see Proteinuria,
    gestational
   gestational
    complicating
     childbirth O12.14
     pregnancy O12.1-●
      with edema O12.2-●
     puerperium O12.15
   idiopathic R80.0
   isolated R80.0
    with glomerular lesion N06.9
     C3
      glomerulonephritis N06.A
      glomerulopathy N06.A
       with dense deposit disease N06.6
     dense deposit disease N06.6
     diffuse
      crescentic glomerulonephritis
       N06.7
      endocapillary proliferative
       glomerulonephritis N06.4
      mesangiocapillary glomerulonephritis
       N06.5
     focal and segmental hyalinosis or sclerosis
      N06.1
     membranous (diffuse) (see also
      Nephropathy, membranous) N06.2
     mesangial proliferative (diffuse) N06.3
     with diffuse membranous
      glomerulonephritis N06.29
     minimal change N06.0
     specified pathology NEC N06.8
   orthostatic R80.2
    with glomerular lesion —see Proteinuria,
     isolated, with glomerular lesion
   persistent R80.1
    with glomerular lesion —see Proteinuria,
     isolated, with glomerular lesion
   postural R80.2
    with glomerular lesion —see Proteinuria,
     isolated, with glomerular lesion
   pre-eclamptic —see Pre-eclampsia
   puerperal O12.15
   specified type NEC R80.8
Proteolysis, pathologic D65
Proteus (mirabilis) (morganii), as cause of disease
   classified elsewhere B96.4
Prothrombin gene mutation D68.52
Protoporphyria, erythropoietic E80.0
Protozoal —see also condition
   disease B64
   specified NEC B60.8
Protrusion, protrusio
   acetabuli M24.7
   acetabulum (into pelvis) M24.7
   device, implant or graft —see also Complications,
    by site and type, mechanical T85.698
    arterial graft NEC —see Complication,
     cardiovascular device, mechanical,
     vascular
    breast (implant) T85.49
    catheter NEC T85.698
     cystostomy T83.090
     dialysis (renal) T82.49
      intraperitoneal T85.691
     infusion NEC T82.594
      spinal (epidural) (subdural) T85.690
     urinary —see also Complications, catheter,
      urinary T83.098
    electronic (electrode) (pulse generator)
     (stimulator)
     bone T84.390
     nervous system —see Complication,
      prosthetic device, mechanical,
      electronic nervous system stimulator
    fixation, internal (orthopedic) NEC —
     see Complication, fixation device,
     mechanical
    gastrointestinal —see Complications,
     prosthetic device, mechanical,
     gastrointestinal device

▶ New   ⇒ Revised   deleted Deleted   ● Use Additional Character(s)

Protrusion, protrusio (Continued)
  device, implant or graft (Continued)
    genital NEC T83.498
      intrauterine contraceptive device T83.39
      penile prosthesis (cylinder) (implanted)
        (pump) (reservoir) T83.490
      testicular prosthesis T83.491
    heart NEC —see Complication, cardiovascular
      device, mechanical
    joint prosthesis —see Complications, joint
      prosthesis, mechanical, specified NEC,
      by site
    ocular NEC —see Complications, prosthetic
      device, mechanical, ocular device
    orthopedic NEC —see Complication,
      orthopedic, device, mechanical
    specified NEC T85.628
    urinary NEC —see also Complication,
      genitourinary, device, urinary,
      mechanical
      graft T83.29
    vascular NEC —see Complication,
      cardiovascular device, mechanical
    ventricular intracranial shunt T85.09
  intervertebral disc —see Displacement,
    intervertebral disc
  joint prosthesis —see Complications, joint
    prosthesis, mechanical, specified NEC, by
    site
  nucleus pulposus —see Displacement,
    intervertebral disc
Prune belly (syndrome) Q79.4
Prurigo (ferox) (gravis) (Hebrae) (Hebra's) (mitis)
  (simplex) L28.2
  Besnier's L20.0
  estivalis L56.4
  nodularis L28.1
  psychogenic F45.8
Pruritus, pruritic (essential) L29.9
  ani, anus L29.0
    psychogenic F45.8
  anogenital L29.3
    psychogenic F45.8
  cholestatic L29.81
  due to onchocerca volvulus B73.1
  gravidarum —see Pregnancy, complicated by,
    specified pregnancy-related condition
    NEC
  hiemalis L29.89
  neurogenic (any site) F45.8
  perianal L29.0
  psychogenic (any site) F45.8
  scroti, scrotum L29.1
    psychogenic F45.8
  senile, senilis L29.89
  specified NEC L29.89
    psychogenic F45.8
  Trichomonas A59.9
  vulva, vulvae L29.2
    psychogenic F45.8
Pseudarthrosis, pseudoarthrosis (bone) —see
  Nonunion, fracture
  clavicle, congenital Q74.0
  joint, following fusion or arthrodesis M96.0
Pseudoaneurysm —see Aneurysm
Pseudoangina (pectoris) —see Angina
Pseudoangioma I81
Pseudoarteriosus Q28.8
Pseudoarthrosis —see Pseudarthrosis
Pseudobulbar affect (PBA) F48.2
Pseudochromhidrosis L67.8
Pseudocirrhosis, liver, pericardial I31.1
Pseudocowpox B08.03
Pseudocoxalgia M91.3-●
Pseudocroup J38.5
Pseudo-Cushing's syndrome, alcohol-induced
  E24.4
Pseudocyesis F45.8
Pseudocyst
  lung J98.4
  pancreas K86.3
  retina —see Cyst, retina
Pseudoelephantiasis neuroarthritica Q82.0
Pseudoexfoliation, capsule (lens) —see Cataract,
  specified NEC
Pseudofolliculitis barbae L73.1
Pseudoglioma H44.89
Pseudohemophilia (Bernuth's) (hereditary) (type
  B) —see Disease, von Willebrand
  Type A D69.8
  vascular D69.8

Pseudohermaphroditism Q56.3
  adrenal E25.8
  female (see also Disorder, adrenogenital) Q56.2
    with adrenocortical disorder E25.8
    without adrenocortical disorder Q56.2
    adrenal (congenital) E25.0
  male (see also Disorder, adrenogenital) Q56.1
    with
      adrenocortical disorder E25.8
      androgen resistance E34.51
      cleft scrotum Q56.1
      feminizing testis E34.51
      5-alpha-reductase deficiency E29.1
    without gonadal disorder Q56.1
    adrenal E25.8
Pseudo-Hurler's polydystrophy E77.0
Pseudohydrocephalus G93.2
Pseudohypertrophic muscular dystrophy (Erb's)
  G71.02
Pseudohypertrophy, muscle (see also Dystrophy,
  muscular, by type, if applicable) G71.09
Pseudohypoparathyroidism E20.1
Pseudoinsomnia F51.03
Pseudoleukemia, infantile D64.89
Pseudomembranous —see condition
Pseudomeningocele (cerebral) (infective) (post-
  traumatic) G96.198
  postprocedural (spinal) G97.82
Pseudomenses (newborn) P54.6
Pseudomenstruation (newborn) P54.6
Pseudomonas
  aeruginosa, as cause of disease classified
    elsewhere B96.5
  mallei infection A24.0
    as cause of disease classified elsewhere B96.5
  pseudomallei, as cause of disease classified
    elsewhere B96.5
Pseudomyotonia G71.19
Pseudomyxoma peritonei C78.6
Pseudoneuritis, optic (nerve) (disc) (papilla),
  congenital Q14.2
Pseudo-obstruction intestine (acute) (chronic)
  (idiopathic) (intermittent secondary)
  (primary) K59.89
  colonic K59.81
Pseudopapilledema H47.33-●
  congenital Q14.2
Pseudoparalysis
  arm or leg R29.818
  atonic, congenital P94.2
Pseudopelade L66.0
Pseudophakia Z96.1
Pseudopolyarthritis, rhizomelic M35.3
Pseudopolycythemia D75.1
Pseudopseudohypoparathyroidism E20.1
Pseudopterygium H11.81-●
Pseudoptosis (eyelid) —see Blepharochalasis
Pseudopuberty, precocious
  female heterosexual E25.8
  male isosexual E25.8
Pseudorickets (renal) N25.0
Pseudorubella B08.20
Pseudosclerema, newborn P83.88
Pseudosclerosis (brain)
  Jakob's —see Creutzfeldt-Jakob disease or
    syndrome
  of Westphal (Strüümpell) E83.01
  spastic —see Creutzfeldt-Jakob disease or
    syndrome
Pseudotetanus —see Convulsions
Pseudotetany R29.0
  hysterical F44.5
Pseudotruncus arteriosus Q25.49
Pseudotuberculosis A28.2
  enterocolitis A04.8
  pasteurella (infection) A28.0
Pseudotumor G93.2
  cerebri G93.2
  orbital H05.11-●
Pseudoxanthoma elasticum Q82.8
Psilosis (sprue) (tropical) K90.1
  nontropical K90.0
Psittacosis A70
Psoitis M60.88
Psoriasis L40.9
  arthropathic L40.50
    arthritis mutilans L40.52
    distal interphalangeal L40.51
    juvenile L40.54
    other specified L40.59
    spondylitis L40.53

Psoriasis (Continued)
  buccal K13.29
  flexural L40.8
  guttate L40.4
  mouth K13.29
  nummular L40.0
  plaque L40.0
  psychogenic F54
  pustular (generalized) L40.1
    palmaris et plantaris L40.3
  specified NEC L40.8
  vulgaris L40.0
Psychasthenia F48.8
Psychiatric disorder or problem F99
Psychogenic —see also condition
  factors associated with physical conditions F54
Psychological and behavioral factors affecting
  medical condition F59
Psychoneurosis, psychoneurotic —see also Neurosis
  anxiety (state) F41.1
  depersonalization F48.1
  hypochondriacal F45.21
  hysteria F44.9
  neurasthenic F48.8
  personality NEC F60.89
Psychopathy, psychopathic
  affectionless F94.2
  autistic F84.5
  constitution, post-traumatic F07.81
  personality —see Disorder, personality
  sexual —see Deviation, sexual
  state F60.2
Psychosexual identity disorder of childhood F64.2
Psychosis, psychotic F29
  acute (transient) F23
    hysterical F44.9
  affective —see Disorder, mood
  alcoholic F10.959
    with
      abuse F10.159
      anxiety disorder F10.980
        with
          abuse F10.180
          dependence F10.280
      delirium tremens F10.231
      delusions F10.950
        with
          abuse F10.150
          dependence F10.250
      dementia F10.97
        with dependence F10.27
      dependence F10.259
      hallucinosis F10.951
        with
          abuse F10.151
          dependence F10.251
      mood disorder F10.94
        with
          abuse F10.14
          dependence F10.24
      paranoia F10.950
        with
          abuse F10.150
          dependence F10.250
      persisting amnesia F10.96
        with dependence F10.26
    amnestic confabulatory F10.96
      with dependence F10.26
    delirium tremens F10.231
    Korsakoff's, Korsakov's, Korsakow's F10.26
    paranoid type F10.950
      with
        abuse F10.150
        dependence F10.250
  anergastic —see Psychosis, organic
  arteriosclerotic (simple type) (uncomplicated)
    (see also Dementia, vascular) F01.50
    with behavioral disturbance —see Dementia,
      vascular
  childhood F84.0
    atypical F84.8
  climacteric —see Psychosis, involutional
  confusional F29
    acute or subacute F05
    reactive F23
  cycloid F23
  depressive —see Disorder, depressive
  disintegrative (childhood) F84.3
  drug-induced —see F11-F19 with .x59
    paranoid and hallucinatory states —see
      F11-F19 with .x50 or .x51

Psychosis, psychotic *(Continued)*
  due to or associated with
    addiction, drug —*see* F11-F19 with .X59
    dependence
      alcohol F10.259
      drug —*see* F11-F19 with .x59
    epilepsy F06.8
    Huntington's chorea F06.8
    ischemia, cerebrovascular (generalized) F06.8
    multiple sclerosis F06.8
    physical disease F06.8
    presenile dementia F03
    senile dementia F03
    vascular disease (arteriosclerotic) (cerebral)
        (see also Dementia, vascular)* F01.50
      with behavioral disturbance —*see*
          Dementia, vascular
  epileptic F06.8
  episode F23
    due to or associated with physical condition
        F06.8
  exhaustive F43.0
  hallucinatory, chronic F28
  hypomanic F30.8
  hysterical (acute) F44.9
  induced F24
  infantile F84.0
    atypical F84.8
  infective (acute) (subacute) F05
  involutional F28
    depressive —*see* Disorder, depressive
    melancholic —*see* Disorder, depressive
    paranoid (state) F22
  Korsakoff's, Korsakov's, Korsakow's
      (nonalcoholic) F04
    alcoholic F10.96
      in dependence F10.26
    induced by other psychoactive substance —*see*
        categories F11-F19 with .5x
  mania, manic (single episode) F30.2
    recurrent type F31.89
  manic-depressive —*see* Disorder, bipolar
  menopausal —*see* Psychosis, involutional
  mixed schizophrenic and affective F25.8
  multi-infarct (cerebrovascular) *(see also*
      Dementia, vascular)* F01.50
    with behavioral disturbance —*see* Dementia,
        vascular
  nonorganic F29
    specified NEC F28
  organic F09
    due to or associated with
      arteriosclerosis (cerebral) —*see* Psychosis,
          arteriosclerotic
      cerebrovascular disease, arteriosclerotic —
          see Psychosis, arteriosclerotic
      childbirth —*see* Psychosis, puerperal
      Creutzfeldt-Jakob disease or syndrome —
          see Creutzfeldt-Jakob disease or
          syndrome
      dependence, alcohol F10.259
      disease
        alcoholic liver F10.259
        brain, arteriosclerotic —*see* Psychosis,
            arteriosclerotic
        cerebrovascular *(see also* Dementia,
            vascular)* F01.50
          with behavioral disturbance —*see*
              Dementia, vascular
        Creutzfeldt-Jakob —*see* Creutzfeldt-
            Jakob disease or syndrome
        endocrine or metabolic F06.8
          acute or subacute F05
        liver, alcoholic F10.259
      epilepsy transient (acute) F05
      infection
        brain (intracranial) F06.8
          acute or subacute F05
      intoxication
        alcoholic (acute) F10.259
        drug F11-F19 with .x59
      ischemia, cerebrovascular (generalized) —
          see Psychosis, arteriosclerotic
      puerperium —*see* Psychosis,
          puerperal
      trauma, brain (birth) (from electric current)
          (surgical) F06.8
        acute or subacute F05
  infective F06.8
    acute or subacute F05
  post-traumatic F06.8
    acute or subacute F05

Psychosis, psychotic *(Continued)*
  paranoiac F22
  paranoid (climacteric) (involutional)
      (menopausal) F22
    psychogenic (acute) F23
    schizophrenic F20.0
    senile F03
  postpartum F53.1
  presbyophrenic (type) F03
  presenile F03
  psychogenic (paranoid) F23
    depressive F32.3
  puerperal F53.1
    specified type —*see* Psychosis, by type
  reactive (brief) (transient) (emotional stress)
      (psychological trauma) F23
    depressive F32.3
      recurrent F33.3
    excitative type F30.8
  schizoaffective F25.9
    depressive type F25.1
    manic type F25.0
  schizophrenia, schizophrenic —*see*
      Schizophrenia
  schizophrenia-like, in epilepsy F06.2
  schizophreniform F20.81
    affective type F25.9
    brief F23
    confusional type F23
    mixed type F25.0
  senile NEC F03
    depressed or paranoid type F03
    simple deterioration F03
    specified type — code to condition
  shared F24
  situational (reactive) F23
  symbiotic (childhood) F84.3
  symptomatic F09
Psychosomatic —*see* Disorder, psychosomatic
Psychosyndrome, organic F07.9
Psychotic episode due to or associated with
    physical condition F06.8
Pterygium (eye) H11.00-●
  amyloid H11.01-●
  central H11.02-●
  colli Q18.3
  double H11.03-●
  peripheral
    progressive H11.05-●
    stationary H11.04-●
  recurrent H11.06-●
Ptilosis (eyelid) —*see* Madarosis
Ptomaine (poisoning) —*see* Poisoning, food
Ptosis —*see also* Blepharoptosis
  adiposa (false) —*see* Blepharoptosis
  breast N64.81
  brow H57.81-●
  cecum K63.4
  colon K63.4
  congenital (eyelid) Q10.0
    specified site NEC —*see* Anomaly, by site
  eyebrow H57.81-●
  eyelid —*see* Blepharoptosis
    congenital Q10.0
  gastric K31.89
  intestine K63.4
  kidney N28.83
  liver K76.89
  renal N28.83
  splanchnic K63.4
  spleen D73.89
  stomach K31.89
  viscera K63.4
PTP D69.51
Ptyalism (periodic) K11.7
  hysterical F45.8
  pregnancy —*see* Pregnancy, complicated by,
      specified pregnancy-related condition NEC
  psychogenic F45.8
Ptyalolithiasis K11.5
Pubarche, precocious E30.1
Pubertas praecox E30.1
Puberty (development state) Z00.3
  bleeding (excessive) N92.2
  delayed E30.0
  precocious (constitutional) (cryptogenic)
      (idiopathic) E30.1
    central E22.8
    due to
      ovarian hyperfunction E28.1
        estrogen E28.0
      testicular hyperfunction E29.0

Puberty *(Continued)*
  premature E30.1
    due to
      adrenal cortical hyperfunction E25.8
      pineal tumor E34.8
      pituitary (anterior) hyperfunction E22.8
Puckering, macula —*see* Degeneration, macula,
    puckering
Pudenda, pudendum —*see* condition
Puente's disease (simple glandular cheilitis) K13.0
Puerperal, puerperium (complicated by,
    complications)
  abnormal glucose (tolerance test) O99.815
  abscess
    areola O91.02
      associated with lactation O91.03
    Bartholin's gland O86.19
    breast O91.12
      associated with lactation O91.13
    cervix (uteri) O86.11
    genital organ NEC O86.19
    kidney O86.21
    mammary O91.12
      associated with lactation O91.13
    nipple O91.02
      associated with lactation O91.03
    peritoneum O85
    subareolar O91.12
      associated with lactation O91.13
    urinary tract —*see* Puerperal, infection,
        urinary
    uterus O86.12
    vagina (wall) O86.13
    vaginorectal O86.13
    vulvovaginal gland O86.13
  adnexitis O86.19
  afibrinogenemia, or other coagulation defect
      O72.3
  albuminuria (acute) (subacute) —*see* Proteinuria,
      gestational
  alcohol use O99.315
  anemia O90.81
    pre-existing (pre-pregnancy) O99.03
  anesthetic death O89.8
  apoplexy O99.43
  bariatric surgery status O99.845
  blood disorder NEC O99.13
  blood dyscrasia O72.3
  cardiomyopathy O90.3
  cerebrovascular disorder (conditions in I60-I69)
      O99.43
  cervicitis O86.11
  circulatory system disorder O99.43
  coagulopathy (any) O99.13
    with hemorrhage O72.3
  complications O90.9
    specified NEC O90.89
  convulsions —*see* Eclampsia
  cystitis O86.22
  cystopyelitis O86.29
  delirium NEC F05
  diabetes O24.93
    gestational —*see* Puerperal, gestational
        diabetes
    pre-existing O24.33
      specified NEC O24.83
      type 1 O24.03
      type 2 O24.13
  digestive system disorder O99.63
  disease O90.9
    breast NEC O92.29
    cerebrovascular (acute) O99.43
    nonobstetric NEC O99.893
    tubo-ovarian O86.19
    Valsuani's O99.03
  disorder O90.9
    biliary tract O26.63
    lactation O92.70
    liver O26.63
    nonobstetric NEC O99.893
  disruption
    cesarean wound O90.0
    episiotomy wound O90.1
    perineal laceration wound O90.1
  drug use O99.325
  eclampsia (with pre-existing hypertension)
      O15.2
  embolism (pulmonary) (blood clot) —*see*
      Embolism, obstetric, puerperal
  endocrine, nutritional or metabolic disease NEC
      O99.285
  endophlebitis —*see* Puerperal, phlebitis

Puerperal, puerperium (*Continued*)
endotrachelitis O86.11
failure
lactation (complete) O92.3
partial O92.4
renal, acute O90.49
fever (of unknown origin) O86.4
septic O85
fissure, nipple O92.12
associated with lactation O92.13
fistula
breast (due to mastitis) O91.12
associated with lactation O91.13
nipple O91.02
associated with lactation O91.03
galactophoritis O91.22
associated with lactation O91.23
galactorrhea O92.6
gastric banding status O99.845
gastric bypass status O99.83
gastrointestinal disease NEC O99.63
gestational
diabetes O24.439
diet controlled O24.430
insulin (and diet) controlled O24.434
oral drug controlled (antidiabetic)
(hypoglycemic) O24.435
edema O12.05
with proteinuria O12.25
proteinuria O12.15
gonorrhea O98.23
hematoma, subdural O99.43
hemiplegia, cerebral O99.355-●
due to cerebrovascular disorder O99.43
hemorrhage O72.1
brain O99.43
bulbar O99.43
cerebellar O99.43
cerebral O99.43
cortical O99.43
delayed or secondary O72.2
extradural O99.43
internal capsule O99.43
intracranial O99.43
intrapontine O99.43
meningeal O99.43
pontine O99.43
retained placenta O72.0
subarachnoid O99.43
subcortical O99.43
subdural O99.43
third stage O72.0
uterine, delayed O72.2
ventricular O99.43
hemorrhoids O87.2
hepatorenal syndrome O90.41
hypertension —*see* Hypertension, complicating,
puerperium
hypertrophy, breast O92.29
induration breast (fibrous) O92.29
infection O86.4
cervix O86.11
generalized O85
genital tract NEC O86.19
obstetric surgical wound O86.09
kidney (bacillus coli) O86.21
maternal O98.93
carrier state NEC O99.835
gonorrhea O98.23
human immunodeficiency virus (HIV) O98.73
protozoal O98.63
sexually transmitted NEC O98.33
specified NEC O98.83
streptococcus group B (GBS) carrier state
O99.825
syphilis O98.13
tuberculosis O98.03
viral hepatitis O98.43
viral NEC O98.53
nipple O91.02
associated with lactation O91.03
peritoneum O85
renal O86.21
specified NEC O86.89
urinary (asymptomatic) (tract) NEC O86.20
bladder O86.22
kidney O86.21
specified site NEC O86.29
urethra O86.22
vagina O86.13
vein —*see* Puerperal, phlebitis
ischemia, cerebral O99.43

Puerperal, puerperium (*Continued*)
lymphangitis O86.89
breast O91.22
associated with lactation O91.23
malignancy O9A.13
malnutrition O25.3
mammillitis O91.02
associated with lactation O91.03
mammitis O91.22
associated with lactation O91.23
mania F30.8
mastitis O91.22
associated with lactation O91.23
purulent O91.12
associated with lactation O91.13
melancholia —*see* Disorder, depressive
mental disorder NEC O99.345
metroperitonitis O85
metrorrhagia —*see* Hemorrhage, postpartum
metrosalpingitis O86.19
metrovaginitis O86.13
milk leg O87.1
monoplegia, cerebral O99.43
mood disturbance O90.6
necrosis, liver (acute) (subacute)
(conditions in subcategory K72.0) O26.63
with renal failure O90.49
nervous system disorder O99.355
neuritis O90.89
obesity (pre-existing prior to pregnancy) O99.215
obesity surgery status O99.845
occlusion, precerebral artery O99.43
paralysis
bladder (sphincter) O90.89
cerebral O99.43
paralytic stroke O99.43
parametritis O85
paravaginitis O86.13
pelviperitonitis O85
perimetritis O86.12
perimetrosalpingitis O86.19
perinephritis O86.21
periphlebitis —*see* Puerperal phlebitis
peritoneal infection O85
peritonitis (pelvic) O85
perivaginitis O86.13
phlebitis O87.0
deep O87.1
pelvic O87.1
superficial O87.0
phlebothrombosis, deep O87.1
phlegmasia alba dolens O87.1
placental polyp O90.89
pneumonia, embolic —*see* Embolism, obstetric,
puerperal
pre-eclampsia —*see* Pre-eclampsia
psychosis F53.1
pyelitis O86.21
pyelocystitis O86.29
pyelonephritis O86.21
pyelonephrosis O86.21
pyemia O85
pyocystitis O86.29
pyohemia O85
pyometra O86.12
pyonephritis O86.21
pyosalpingitis O86.19
pyrexia (of unknown origin) O86.4
renal
disease NEC O90.89
failure O90.49
respiratory disease NEC O99.53
retention
decidua —*see* Retention, decidua
placenta O72.0
secundines —*see* Retention, secundines
retrated nipple O92.02
salpingo-ovaritis O86.19
salpingoperitonitis O85
secondary perineal tear O90.1
~~sepsis O85~~
sepsis (pelvic) O85
septic thrombophlebitis O86.81
skin disorder NEC O99.73
specified condition NEC O99.893
stroke O99.43
subinvolution (uterus) O90.89
subluxation of symphysis (pubis) O26.73
suppuration —*see* Puerperal, abscess
tetanus A34
thelitis O91.02
associated with lactation O91.03

Puerperal, puerperium (*Continued*)
thrombocytopenia O72.3
thrombophlebitis (superficial) O87.0
deep O87.1
pelvic O87.1
septic O86.81
thrombosis (venous) —*see* Thrombosis,
puerperal
thyroiditis O90.5
toxemia (eclamptic) (pre-eclamptic)
(with convulsions) O15.2
trauma, non-obstetric O9A.23
caused by abuse (physical) (suspected)
O9A.33
confirmed O9A.33
psychological (suspected) O9A.53
confirmed O9A.53
sexual (suspected) O9A.43
confirmed O9A.43
uremia (due to renal failure) O90.49
urethritis O86.22
vaginitis O86.13
varicose veins (legs) O87.4
vulva or perineum O87.8
venous O87.9
vulvitis O86.19
vulvovaginitis O86.13
white leg O87.1
Puerperium —*see* Puerperal
Pulmolithiasis J98.4
Pulmonary —*see* condition
Pulpitis (acute) (anachoretic) (chronic)
(hyperplastic) (putrescent) (suppurative)
(ulcerative) K04.01
irreversible K04.02
reversible K04.01
Pulpless tooth K04.99
Pulse
alternating R00.8
bigeminal R00.8
fast R00.0
feeble, rapid due to shock following injury T79.4
rapid R00.0
weak R09.89
Pulsus alternans or trigeminus R00.8
Punch drunk F07.81
Punctum lacrimale occlusion —*see* Obstruction,
lacrimal
Puncture
abdomen, abdominal
wall S31.139
with
foreign body S31.149
penetration into peritoneal cavity S31.639
with foreign body S31.649
epigastric region S31.132
with
foreign body S31.142
penetration into peritoneal cavity S31.632
with foreign body S31.642
left
lower quadrant S31.134
with
foreign body S31.144
penetration into peritoneal cavity
S31.634
with foreign body S31.644
upper quadrant S31.131
with
foreign body S31.141
penetration into peritoneal cavity
S31.631
with foreign body S31.641
periumbilic region S31.135
with
foreign body S31.145
penetration into peritoneal cavity
S31.635
with foreign body S31.645
right
lower quadrant S31.133
with
foreign body S31.143
penetration into peritoneal cavity
S31.633
with foreign body S31.643
upper quadrant S31.130
with
foreign body S31.140
penetration into peritoneal cavity
S31.630
with foreign body S31.640

Puncture *(Continued)*
  accidental, complicating surgery —*see*
    Complication, accidental puncture or
    laceration
  alveolar (process) —*see* Puncture, oral cavity
  ankle S91.039
    with
      foreign body S91.049
    left S91.032
      with
        foreign body S91.042
    right S91.031
      with
        foreign body S91.041
  anus S31.833
    with foreign body S31.834
  arm (upper) S41.139
    with foreign body S41.149
    left S41.132
      with foreign body S41.142
    lower —*see* Puncture, forearm
    right S41.131
      with foreign body S41.141
  auditory canal (external) (meatus) —*see*
    Puncture, ear
  auricle, ear —*see* Puncture, ear
  axilla —*see* Puncture, arm
  back —*see also* Puncture, thorax, back
    lower S31.030
      with
        foreign body S31.040
          with penetration into retroperitoneal
            space S31.041
          penetration into retroperitoneal space
            S31.031
  bladder (traumatic) S37.29
    nontraumatic N32.89
  breast S21.039
    with foreign body S21.049
    left S21.032
      with foreign body S21.042
    right S21.031
      with foreign body S21.041
  buttock S31.803
    with foreign body S31.804
    left S31.823
      with foreign body S31.824
    right S31.813
      with foreign body S31.814
  by
    device, implant or graft —*see* Complications,
      by site and type, mechanical
    foreign body left accidentally in operative
      wound T81.539
    instrument (any) during a procedure,
      accidental —*see* Puncture, accidental
      complicating surgery
  calf —*see* Puncture, leg
  canaliculus lacrimalis —*see* Puncture,
    eyelid
  canthus, eye —*see* Puncture, eyelid
  cervical esophagus S11.23
    with foreign body S11.24
  cheek (external) S01.439
    with foreign body S01.449
    internal —*see* Puncture, oral cavity
    left S01.432
      with foreign body S01.442
    right S01.431
      with foreign body S01.441
  chest wall —*see* Puncture, thorax
  chin —*see* Puncture, head, specified site
    NEC
  clitoris —*see* Puncture, vulva
  costal region —*see* Puncture, thorax
  digit(s)
    foot —*see* Puncture, toe
    hand —*see* Puncture, finger
  ear (canal) (external) S01.339
    with foreign body S01.349
    drum S09.2-●
    left S01.332
      with foreign body S01.342
    right S01.331
      with foreign body S01.341
  elbow S51.039
    with
      foreign body S51.049
    left S51.032
      with
        foreign body S51.042

Puncture *(Continued)*
  elbow *(Continued)*
    right S51.031
      with
        foreign body S51.041
  epididymis —*see* Puncture, testis
  epigastric region —*see* Puncture, abdomen, wall,
    epigastric
  epiglottis S11.83
    with foreign body S11.84
  esophagus
    cervical S11.23
      with foreign body S11.24
    thoracic S27.818
  eyeball S05.6-●
    with foreign body S05.5-●
  eyebrow —*see* Puncture, eyelid
  eyelid S01.13-●
    with foreign body S01.14-●
    left S01.132
      with foreign body S01.142
    right S01.131
      with foreign body S01.141
  face NEC —*see* Puncture, head, specified site
    NEC
  finger(s) S61.239
    with
      damage to nail S61.339
        with
          foreign body S61.349
      foreign body S61.249
    index S61.238
      with
        damage to nail S61.338
          with
            foreign body S61.348
        foreign body S61.248
    left S61.231
      with
        damage to nail S61.331
          with
            foreign body S61.341
        foreign body S61.241
    right S61.230
      with
        damage to nail S61.330
          with
            foreign body S61.340
        foreign body S61.240
    little S61.238
      with
        damage to nail S61.338
          with
            foreign body S61.348
        foreign body S61.248
    left S61.237
      with
        damage to nail S61.337
          with
            foreign body S61.347
        foreign body S61.247
    right S61.236
      with
        damage to nail S61.336
          with
            foreign body S61.346
        foreign body S61.246
    middle S61.238
      with
        damage to nail S61.338
          with
            foreign body S61.348
        foreign body S61.248
    left S61.233
      with
        damage to nail S61.333
          with
            foreign body S61.343
        foreign body S61.243
    right S61.232
      with
        damage to nail S61.332
          with
            foreign body S61.342
        foreign body S61.242
    ring S61.238
      with
        damage to nail S61.338
          with
            foreign body S61.348
        foreign body S61.248

Puncture *(Continued)*
  finger(s) *(Continued)*
    ring *(Continued)*
      left S61.235
        with
          damage to nail S61.335
            with
              foreign body S61.345
          foreign body S61.245
      right S61.234
        with
          damage to nail S61.334
            with
              foreign body S61.344
          foreign body S61.244
  flank S31.139
    with foreign body S31.149
  foot (except toe(s) alone) S91.339
    with foreign body S91.349
    left S91.332
      with foreign body S91.342
    right S91.331
      with foreign body S91.341
    toe —*see* Puncture, toe
  forearm S51.839
    with
      foreign body S51.849
    elbow only —*see* Puncture, elbow
    left S51.832
      with
        foreign body S51.842
    right S51.831
      with
        foreign body S51.841
  forehead —*see* Puncture, head, specified site
    NEC
  genital organs, external
    female S31.532
      with foreign body S31.542
      vagina —*see* Puncture, vagina
      vulva —*see* Puncture, vulva
    male S31.531
      with foreign body S31.541
      penis —*see* Puncture, penis
      scrotum —*see* Puncture, scrotum
      testis —*see* Puncture, testis
  groin —*see* Puncture, abdomen, wall
  gum —*see* Puncture, oral cavity
  hand S61.439
    with
      foreign body S61.449
    finger —*see* Puncture, finger
    left S61.432
      with
        foreign body S61.442
    right S61.431
      with
        foreign body S61.441
    thumb —*see* Puncture, thumb
  head S01.93
    with foreign body S01.94
    cheek —*see* Puncture, cheek
    ear —*see* Puncture, ear
    eyelid —*see* Puncture, eyelid
    lip —*see* Puncture, oral cavity
    nose —*see* Puncture, nose
    oral cavity —*see* Puncture, oral cavity
    scalp S01.03
      with foreign body S01.04
    specified site NEC S01.83
      with foreign body S01.84
    temporomandibular area —*see* Puncture,
      cheek
  heart S26.99
    with hemopericardium S26.09
    without hemopericardium S26.19
  heel —*see* Puncture, foot
  hip S71.039
    with foreign body S71.049
    left S71.032
      with foreign body S71.042
    right S71.031
      with foreign body S71.041
  hymen —*see* Puncture, vagina
  hypochondrium —*see* Puncture, abdomen, wall
  hypogastric region —*see* Puncture, abdomen,
    wall
  inguinal region —*see* Puncture, abdomen, wall
  instep —*see* Puncture, foot
  internal organs —*see* Injury, by site
  interscapular region —*see* Puncture, thorax, back

▶ New   ⇒ Revised   ~~deleted~~ Deleted   ● Use Additional Character(s)

Puncture *(Continued)*
  intestine
    large
      colon S36.599
        ascending S36.590
        descending S36.592
        sigmoid S36.593
        specified site NEC S36.598
        transverse S36.591
      rectum S36.69
    small S36.499
      duodenum S36.490
      specified site NEC S36.498
  intra-abdominal organ S36.99
    gallbladder S36.128
    intestine —*see* Puncture, intestine
    liver S36.118
    pancreas —*see* Puncture, pancreas
    peritoneum S36.81
    specified site NEC S36.898
    spleen S36.09
    stomach S36.39
  jaw —*see* Puncture, head, specified site NEC
  knee S81.039
    with foreign body S81.049
    left S81.032
      with foreign body S81.042
    right S81.031
      with foreign body S81.041
  labium (majus) (minus) —*see* Puncture, vulva
  lacrimal duct —*see* Puncture, eyelid
  larynx S11.013
    with foreign body S11.014
  leg (lower) S81.839
    with foreign body S81.849
    foot —*see* Puncture, foot
    knee —*see* Puncture, knee
    left S81.832
      with foreign body S81.842
    right S81.831
      with foreign body S81.841
    upper —*see* Puncture, thigh
  lip S01.531
    with foreign body S01.541
  loin —*see* Puncture, abdomen, wall
  lower back —*see* Puncture, back, lower
  lumbar region —*see* Puncture, back, lower
  malar region —*see* Puncture, head, specified site NEC
  mammary —*see* Puncture, breast
  mastoid region —*see* Puncture, head, specified site NEC
  mouth —*see* Puncture, oral cavity
  nail
    finger —*see* Puncture, finger, with damage to nail
    toe —*see* Puncture, toe, with damage to nail
  nasal (septum) (sinus) —*see* Puncture, nose
  nasopharynx —*see* Puncture, head, specified site NEC
  neck S11.93
    with foreign body S11.94
    involving
      cervical esophagus —*see* Puncture, cervical esophagus
      larynx —*see* Puncture, larynx
      pharynx —*see* Puncture, pharynx
      thyroid gland —*see* Puncture, thyroid gland
      trachea —*see* Puncture, trachea
    specified site NEC S11.83
      with foreign body S11.84
  nose (septum) (sinus) S01.23
    with foreign body S01.24
  ocular —*see* Puncture, eyeball - oral cavity S01.532
    with foreign body S01.542
  orbit S05.4-●
  palate —*see* Puncture, oral cavity
  palm —*see* Puncture, hand
  pancreas S36.299
    body S36.291
    head S36.290
    tail S36.292
  pelvis —*see* Puncture, back, lower
  penis S31.23
    with foreign body S31.24
  perineum
    female S31.43
      with foreign body S31.44
    male S31.139
      with foreign body S31.149

Puncture *(Continued)*
  periocular area (with or without lacrimal passages) —*see* Puncture, eyelid
  phalanges
    finger —*see* Puncture, finger
    toe —*see* Puncture, toe
  pharynx S11.23
    with foreign body S11.24
  pinna —*see* Puncture, ear
  popliteal space —*see* Puncture, knee
  prepuce —*see* Puncture, penis
  pubic region S31.139
    with foreign body S31.149
  pudendum —*see* Puncture, genital organs, external
  rectovaginal septum —*see* Puncture, vagina
  sacral region —*see* Puncture, back, lower
  sacroiliac region —*see* Puncture, back, lower
  salivary gland —*see* Puncture, oral cavity
  scalp S01.03
    with foreign body S01.04
  scapular region —*see* Puncture, shoulder
  scrotum S31.33
    with foreign body S31.34
  shin —*see* Puncture, leg
  shoulder S41.039
    with foreign body S41.049
    left S41.032
      with foreign body S41.042
    right S41.031
      with foreign body S41.041
  spermatic cord —*see* Puncture, testis
  sternal region —*see* Puncture, thorax, front
  submaxillary region —*see* Puncture, head, specified site NEC
  submental region —*see* Puncture, head, specified site NEC
  subungual
    finger(s) —*see* Puncture, finger, with damage to nail
    toe —*see* Puncture, toe, with damage to nail
  supraclavicular fossa —*see* Puncture, neck, specified site NEC
  temple, temporal region —*see* Puncture, head, specified site NEC
  temporomandibular area —*see* Puncture, cheek
  testis S31.33
    with foreign body S31.34
  thigh S71.139
    with foreign body S71.149
    left S71.132
      with foreign body S71.142
    right S71.131
      with foreign body S71.141
  thorax, thoracic (wall) S21.93
    with foreign body S21.94
    back S21.23-●
      with
        foreign body S21.24-●
          with penetration S21.44
        penetration S21.43
    breast —*see* Puncture, breast
    front S21.13-●
      with
        foreign body S21.14-●
          with penetration S21.34
        penetration S21.33
  throat —*see* Puncture, neck
  thumb S61.039
    with
      damage to nail S61.139
        with
          foreign body S61.149
      foreign body S61.049
    left S61.032
      with
        damage to nail S61.132
          with
            foreign body S61.142
        foreign body S61.042
    right S61.031
      with
        damage to nail S61.131
          with
            foreign body S61.141
        foreign body S61.041
  thyroid gland S11.13
    with foreign body S11.14

Puncture *(Continued)*
  toe(s) S91.139
    with
      damage to nail S91.239
        with
          foreign body S91.249
      foreign body S91.149
    great S91.133
      with
        damage to nail S91.233
          with
            foreign body S91.243
        foreign body S91.143
      left S91.132
        with
          damage to nail S91.232
            with
              foreign body S91.242
          foreign body S91.142
      right S91.131
        with
          damage to nail S91.231
            with
              foreign body S91.241
          foreign body S91.141
    lesser S91.136
      with
        damage to nail S91.236
          with
            foreign body S91.246
        foreign body S91.146
      left S91.135
        with
          damage to nail S91.235
            with
              foreign body S91.245
          foreign body S91.145
      right S91.134
        with
          damage to nail S91.234
            with
              foreign body S91.244
          foreign body S91.144
  tongue —*see* Puncture, oral cavity
  trachea S11.023
    with foreign body S11.024
  tunica vaginalis —*see* Puncture, testis
  tympanum, tympanic membrane S09.2-●
  umbilical region S31.135
    with foreign body S31.145
  uvula —*see* Puncture, oral cavity
  vagina S31.43
    with foreign body S31.44
  vocal cords S11.033
    with foreign body S11.034
  vulva S31.43
    with foreign body S31.44
  wrist S61.539
    with
      foreign body S61.549
    left S61.532
      with
        foreign body S61.542
    right S61.531
      with
        foreign body S61.541
PUO (pyrexia of unknown origin) R50.9
Pupillary membrane (persistent) Q13.89
Pupillotonia —*see* Anomaly, pupil, function, tonic pupil
Purpura D69.2
  abdominal D69.0
  allergic D69.0
  anaphylactoid D69.0
  annularis telangiectodes L81.7
  arthritic D69.0
  autoerythrocyte sensitization D69.2
  autoimmune D69.0
  bacterial D69.0
  Bateman's (senile) D69.2
  capillary fragility (hereditary) (idiopathic) D69.8
  cryoglobulinemic D89.1
  Devil's pinches D69.2
  fibrinolytic —*see* Fibrinolysis
  fulminans, fulminous D65
  gangrenous D65
  hemorrhagic, hemorrhagica D69.3
    not due to thrombocytopenia D69.0
  Henoch (-Schönlein) (allergic) D69.0
  hypergammaglobulinemic (benign) (Waldenström's) D89.0

Purpura (Continued)
idiopathic (thrombocytopenic) D69.3
nonthrombocytopenic D69.0
immune thrombocytopenic D69.3
infectious D69.0
malignant D69.0
neonatorum P54.5
nervosa D69.0
newborn P54.5
nonthrombocytopenic D69.2
hemorrhagic D69.0
idiopathic D69.0
nonthrombopenic D69.2
peliosis rheumatica D69.0
posttransfusion (post-transfusion) (from (fresh)
whole blood or blood products) D69.51
primary D69.49
red cell membrane sensitivity D69.2
rheumatica D69.0
Schönlein (-Henoch) (allergic) D69.0
scorbutic E54 [D77]
senile D69.2
simplex D69.2
symptomatica D69.0
telangiectasia annularis L81.7
thrombocytopenic D69.49
congenital D69.42
hemorrhagic D69.3
hereditary D69.42
idiopathic D69.3
immune D69.3
neonatal, transitory P61.0
thrombotic M31.19
thrombohemolytic —see Fibrinolysis
thrombolytic —see Fibrinolysis
thrombopenic D69.49
thrombotic, thrombocytopenic
M31.19
toxic D69.0
vascular D69.0
visceral symptoms D69.0
Purpuric spots R23.3
Purulent —see condition
Pus
in
stool R19.5
urine N39.0
tube (rupture) —see Salpingo-oophoritis
Pustular rash L08.0
Pustule (nonmalignant) L08.9
malignant A22.0
Pustulosis palmaris et plantaris
L40.3
Putnam (-Dana) disease or syndrome —see
Degeneration, combined
Putrescent pulp (dental) K04.1
Pyarthritis, pyarthrosis —see Arthritis, pyogenic
or pyemic
tuberculous —see Tuberculosis, joint
Pyelectasis —see Hydronephrosis
Pyelitis (congenital) (uremic) —see also
Pyelonephritis
with
calculus —see category N20
with hydronephrosis N13.6
contracted kidney N11.9
acute N10
chronic N11.9
with calculus —see category N20
with hydronephrosis N13.6
cystica N28.84
puerperal (postpartum) O86.21
tuberculous A18.11
Pyelocystitis —see Pyelonephritis
Pyelonephritis —see also Nephritis,
tubulo-interstitial
with
calculus —see category N20
with hydronephrosis N13.6
contracted kidney N11.9
acute N10
calculus —see category N20
with hydronephrosis N13.6
chronic N11.9
with calculus —see category N20
with hydronephrosis N13.6
associated with ureteral obstruction or
stricture N11.1
nonobstructive N11.8
with reflux (vesicoureteral) N11.0
obstructive N11.1
specified NEC N11.8

Pyelonephritis (Continued)
in (due to)
brucellosis A23.9 [N16]
cryoglobulinemia (mixed) D89.1 [N16]
cystinosis E72.04
diphtheria A36.84
glycogen storage disease E74.09 [N16]
leukemia NEC C95.9-● [N16]
lymphoma NEC C85.90 [N16]
multiple myeloma C90.0-● [N16]
obstruction N11.1
Salmonella infection A02.25
sarcoidosis D86.84
sepsis A41.9 [N16]
Sjögren's disease M35.04
toxoplasmosis B58.83
transplant rejection T86.91 [N16]
Wilson's disease E83.01 [N16]
nonobstructive N12
with reflux (vesicoureteral) N11.0
chronic N11.8
syphilitic A52.75
Pyelonephrosis (obstructive) N11.1
chronic N11.9
Pyelophlebitis I80.8
Pyeloureteritis cystica N28.85
Pyemia, pyemic (fever) (infection) (purulent) —see
also Sepsis
joint —see Arthritis, pyogenic or pyemic
liver K75.1
pneumococcal A40.3
portal K75.1
postvaccinal T88.0
puerperal, postpartum, childbirth O85
specified organism NEC A41.89
tuberculous —see Tuberculosis, miliary
Pygopagus Q89.4
Pyknoepilepsy (idiopathic) —see Pyknolepsy
Pyknolepsy G40.A09
intractable G40.A19
with status epilepticus G40.A11
without status epilepticus G40.A19
not intractable G40.A09
with status epilepticus G40.A01
without status epilepticus G40.A09
Pylephlebitis K75.1
Pyle's syndrome Q78.5
Pylethrombophlebitis K75.1
Pylethrombosis K75.1
Pyloritis K29.90
with bleeding K29.91
Pylorospasm (reflex) NEC K31.3
congenital or infantile Q40.0
neurotic F45.8
newborn Q40.0
psychogenic F45.8
Pylorus, pyloric —see condition
Pyoarthrosis —see Arthritis, pyogenic or pyemic
Pyocele
mastoid —see Mastoiditis, acute
sinus (accessory) —see Sinusitis
turbinate (bone) J32.9
urethra —see also Urethritis N34.0
Pyocolpos —see Vaginitis
Pyocystitis N30.80
with hematuria N30.81
Pyoderma, pyodermia L08.0
gangrenosum L88
newborn P39.4
phagedenic L88
vegetans L08.81
Pyodermatitis L08.0
vegetans L08.81
Pyogenic —see condition
Pyohydronephrosis N13.6
Pyometra, pyometrium, pyometritis —see
Endometritis
Pyomyositis (tropical) —see Myositis,
infective
Pyonephritis N12
Pyonephrosis N13.6
tuberculous A18.11
Pyo-oophoritis —see Salpingo-oophoritis
Pyo-ovarium —see Salpingo-oophoritis
Pyopericarditis, pyopericardium I30.1
Pyophlebitis —see Phlebitis
Pyopneumopericardium I30.1
Pyopneumothorax (infective) J86.9
with fistula J86.0
tuberculous NEC A15.6
Pyosalpinx, pyosalpingitis —see also
Salpingo-oophoritis

Pyothorax J86.9
with fistula J86.0
tuberculous NEC A15.6
Pyoureter N28.89
tuberculous A18.11
Pyramidopallidonigral syndrome G20.C
Pyrexia (of unknown origin) R50.9
atmospheric T67.01
during labor NEC O75.2
heat T67.01
newborn P81.9
environmentally-induced P81.0
persistent R50.9
puerperal O86.4
Pyroglobulinemia NEC E88.09
Pyromania F63.1
Pyrosis R12
Pyuria (bacterial) R82.81

—————— Q ——————

Q fever A78
with pneumonia A78
Quadricuspid aortic valve Q23.88
Quadrilateral fever A78
Quadriparesis —see Quadriplegia
meaning muscle weakness M62.81
Quadriplegia G82.50-●
complete
C1-C4 level G82.51
C5-C7 level G82.53
congenital (cerebral) (spinal) G80.8
spastic G80.0
embolic (current episode) I63.4-●
functional R53.2
incomplete
C1-C4 level G82.52
C5-C7 level G82.54
thrombotic (current episode) I63.3-●
traumatic — code to injury with seventh
character S
current episode —see Injury, spinal (cord),
cervical
Quadruplet, pregnancy —see Pregnancy,
quadruplet
Quarrelsomeness F60.3
Queensland fever A77.3
Quervain's disease M65.4
thyroid E06.1
Queyrat's erythroplasia D07.4
penis D07.4
specified site —see Neoplasm, skin, in situ
unspecified site D07.4
Quincke's disease or edema T78.3
hereditary D84.1
Quinsy (gangrenous) J36
Quintan fever A79.0
Quintuplet, pregnancy —see Pregnancy, quintuplet

—————— R ——————

Rabbit fever —see Tularemia
Rabies A82.9
contact Z20.3
exposure to Z20.3
inoculation reaction —see Complications,
vaccination
sylvatic A82.0
urban A82.1
Rachischisis —see Spina bifida
Rachitic —see also condition
deformities of spine (late effect) (sequelae) E64.3
pelvis (late effect) (sequelae) E64.3
with disproportion (fetopelvic) O33.0
causing obstructed labor O65.0
Rachitis, rachitism (acute) (tarda) —see also Rickets
renalis N25.0
sequelae E64.3
Radial nerve —see condition
Radiation
burn —see Burn
effects NOS T66
sickness NOS T66
therapy, encounter for Z51.0
Radiculitis (pressure) (vertebrogenic) —see
Radiculopathy

Radiculomyelitis —*see also* Encephalitis
  toxic, due to
    Clostridium tetani A35
    Corynebacterium diphtheriae A36.82
Radiculopathy M54.10
  cervical region M54.12
  cervicothoracic region M54.13
  due to
    disc disorder
      C3 M50.11
      C4 M50.11
      C5 M50.121
      C6 M50.122
      C7 M50.123
      C8 M50.13
    displacement of intervertebral disc —*see*
      Disorder, disc, with, radiculopathy
  leg M54.1-●
  lumbar region M54.16
  lumbosacral region M54.17
  occipito-atlanto-axial region M54.11
  postherpetic B02.29
  sacrococcygeal region M54.18
  syphilitic A52.11
  thoracic region (with visceral pain) M54.14
  thoracolumbar region M54.15
Radiodermal burns (acute, chronic, or
    occupational) —*see* Burn
Radiodermatitis L58.9
  acute L58.0
  chronic L58.1
Radiotherapy session Z51.0
RAEB (refractory anemia with excess blasts) D46.2-●
Rage, meaning rabies —*see* Rabies
Ragpicker's disease A22.1
Ragsorter's disease A22.1
Raillietiniasis B71.8
Railroad neurosis F48.8
Railway spine F48.8
Raised —*see also* Elevated
  antibody titer R76.0
Rake teeth, tooth M26.39
Rales R09.89
Ramifying renal pelvis Q63.8
Ramsay-Hunt disease or syndrome —*see also*
    Hunt's disease B02.21
  meaning, dyssynergia cerebellaris myoclonica
    G11.19
Ranula K11.6
  congenital Q38.4
Rape
  adult
    confirmed T74.21
    suspected T76.21
  alleged, observation or examination, ruled out
    adult Z04.41
    child Z04.42
  child
    confirmed T74.22
    suspected T76.22
Rapid
  feeble pulse, due to shock, following injury T79.4
  heart (beat) R00.0
    psychogenic F45.8
  second stage (delivery) O62.3
  time-zone change syndrome G47.25
Rarefaction, bone —*see* Disorder, bone, density
    and structure, specified NEC
Rash (toxic) R21
  canker A38.9
  diaper L22
  drug (internal use) L27.0
    contact —*see also* Dermatitis, due to, drugs,
      external L25.1
  following immunization T88.1
  food —*see* Dermatitis, due to, food
  heat L74.0
  napkin (psoriasiform) L22
  nettle —*see* Urticaria
  pustular L08.0
  rose R21
    epidemic B06.9
  scarlet A38.9
  serum —*see also* Reaction, serum T80.69
  wandering tongue K14.1
Rasmussen aneurysm —*see* Tuberculosis,
    pulmonary
Rasmussen encephalitis G04.81
Rat-bite fever A25.9
  due to Streptobacillus moniliformis A25.1
  spirochetal (morsus muris) A25.0

Rathke's pouch tumor D44.3
Raymond (-Céstan) syndrome I65.8
Raynaud's disease, phenomenon or syndrome
    (secondary) I73.00
  with gangrene (symmetric) I73.01
RDS (newborn) (type I) P22.0
  type II P22.1
Reaction —*see also* Disorder
  adaptation —*see* Disorder, adjustment
  adjustment (anxiety) (conduct disorder)
    (depressiveness) (distress) —*see* Disorder,
      adjustment
    with
      mutism, elective (child) (adolescent)
        F94.0
  adverse
    food (any) (ingested) NEC T78.1
      anaphylactic —*see* Shock, anaphylactic, due
        to food
  anaphylactoid —*see* Shock, anaphylactic
  affective —*see* Disorder, mood
  allergic —*see* Allergy
  anaphylactic —*see* Shock, anaphylactic
  anesthesia —*see* Anesthesia, complication
  antitoxin (prophylactic) (therapeutic) —*see*
    Complications, vaccination
  anxiety F41.1
  Arthus —*see* Arthus' phenomenon
  asthenic F48.8
  combat and operational stress F43.0
  compulsive F42.8
  conversion F44.9
  crisis, acute F43.0
  deoxyribonuclease (DNA) (DNase)
    hypersensitivity D69.2
  depressive (single episode) F32.9
    affective (single episode) F31.4
      recurrent episode F33.9
    neurotic F34.1
    psychoneurotic F34.1
    psychotic F32.3
    recurrent —*see* Disorder, depressive, recurrent
  dissociative F44.9
  drug NEC T88.7
    addictive —*see* Dependence, drug
      transmitted via placenta or breast milk —
        see Absorption, drug, addictive,
          through placenta
    allergic —*see* Allergy, drug
    lichenoid L43.2
    newborn P93.8
      gray baby syndrome P93.0
    overdose or poisoning (by accident) —*see*
      Table of Drugs and Chemicals, by drug,
        poisoning
    photoallergic L56.1
    phototoxic L56.0
    withdrawal —*see* Dependence, by drug, with,
      withdrawal
      infant of dependent mother P96.1
      newborn P96.1
    wrong substance given or taken (by
      accident) —*see* Table of Drugs and
        Chemicals, by drug, poisoning
  fear F40.9
    child (abnormal) F93.8
  febrile nonhemolytic transfusion (FNHTR)
    R50.84
  fluid loss, cerebrospinal G97.1
  foreign
    body NEC —*see* Granuloma, foreign body
    in operative wound (inadvertently left) —
      see Foreign body, accidentally left
        during a procedure
    substance accidentally left during a procedure
      (chemical) (powder) (talc) T81.60
      aseptic peritonitis T81.61
      body or object (instrument) (sponge)
        (swab) —*see* Foreign body,
          accidentally left during a
            procedure
      specified reaction NEC T81.69
  grief —*see* Disorder, adjustment
  Herxheimer's R68.89
  hyperkinetic —*see* Hyperkinesia
  hypochondriacal F45.20
  hypoglycemic, due to insulin E16.0
    with coma (diabetic) —*see* Diabetes, coma
    nondiabetic E15
  therapeutic misadventure —*see* subcategory
    T38.3

Reaction *(Continued)*
  hypomanic F30.8
  hysterical F44.9
  immunization —*see* Complications, vaccination
  incompatibility
    ABO blood group (infusion) (transfusion) —
      see Complication(s), transfusion,
        incompatibility reaction, ABO
      delayed serologic T80.39
    minor blood group (Duffy) (E) (K) (Kell)
      (Kidd) (Lewis) (M) (N) (P) (S)
        T80.89
    Rh (factor) (infusion) (transfusion) —
      see Complication(s), transfusion,
        incompatibility reaction, Rh (factor)
  inflammatory —*see* Infection
  infusion —*see* Complications, infusion
  inoculation (immune serum) —*see*
    Complications, vaccination
  insulin T38.3-●
  involutional psychotic —*see* Disorder, depressive
  leukemoid D72.823
    basophilic D72.823
    lymphocytic D72.823
    monocytic D72.823
    myelocytic D72.823
    neutrophilic D72.823
  LSD (acute)
    due to drug abuse —*see* Abuse, drug,
      hallucinogen
    due to drug dependence —*see* Dependence,
      drug, hallucinogen
  lumbar puncture G97.1
  manic-depressive —*see* Disorder, bipolar
  neurasthenic F48.8
  neurogenic —*see* Neurosis
  neurotic F48.9
  neurotic-depressive F34.1
  nitritoid —*see* Crisis, nitritoid - obsessive-
    compulsive F42
  nonspecific
    to
      cell mediated immunity measurement
        of gamma interferon antigen
        response without active tuberculosis
        R76.12
      QuantiFERON-TB test (QFT) without active
        tuberculosis R76.12
      tuberculin test —*see also* Reaction,
        tuberculin skin test R76.11
  obsessive-compulsive F42.8
  organic, acute or subacute —*see* Delirium
  paranoid (acute) F23
    chronic F22
    senile F03
  passive dependency F60.7
  phobic F40.9
  post-traumatic stress, uncomplicated Z73.3
  psychogenic F99
  psychoneurotic —*see also* Neurosis
    compulsive F42.8
    depersonalization F48.1
    depressive F34.1
    hypochondriacal F45.20
    neurasthenic F48.8
    obsessive F42.8
  psychophysiologic —*see* Disorder,
    somatoform
  psychosomatic —*see* Disorder, somatoform
  psychotic —*see* Psychosis
  scarlet fever toxin —*see* Complications,
    vaccination
  schizophrenic F23
    acute (brief) (undifferentiated) F23
    latent F21
    undifferentiated (acute) (brief) F23
  serological for syphilis —*see* Serology for syphilis
  serum T80.69
    anaphylactic (immediate) —*see also* Shock,
      anaphylactic T80.59
    specified reaction NEC
      due to
        administration of blood and blood
          products T80.61
        immunization T80.62
        serum specified NEC T80.69
        vaccination T80.62
  situational —*see* Disorder, adjustment
  somatization —*see* Disorder, somatoform
  spinal puncture G97.1
    dural G97.1

Reaction *(Continued)*
 stress (severe) F43.9
  acute (agitation) ("daze") (disorientation)
    (disturbance of consciousness) (flight
    reaction) (fugue) F43.0
   specified NEC F43.89
  surgical procedure —*see* Complications, surgical
    procedure
  tetanus antitoxin —*see* Complications,
    vaccination
  toxic, to local anesthesia T81.59
   in labor and delivery O74.4
   in pregnancy O29.3X-●
   postpartum, puerperal O89.3
  toxin-antitoxin —*see* Complications, vaccination
  transfusion (blood) (bone marrow)
    (lymphocytes) (allergic) —*see*
    Complications, transfusion
  tuberculin skin test, abnormal R76.11
  vaccination (any) —*see* Complications,
    vaccination
  withdrawing, child or adolescent F93.8
Reactive airway disease —*see* Asthma
Reactive depression —*see* Reaction, depressive
Rearrangement
 chromosomal
  balanced (in) Q95.9
   abnormal individual (autosomal) Q95.2
    non-sex (autosomal) chromosomes
      Q95.2
    sex/non-sex chromosomes Q95.3
   specified NEC Q95.8
Recalcitrant patient —*see* Noncompliance
Recanalization, thrombus —*see* Thrombosis
Recession, receding
 chamber angle (eye) H21.55-●
 chin M26.09
 gingival (postinfective) (postoperative)
  generalized K06.020
   minimal K06.021
   moderate K06.022
   severe K06.023
  localized K06.010
   minimal K06.011
   moderate K06.012
   severe K06.013
Recklinghausen's disease Q85.01
 bones E21.0
Reclus' disease (cystic) —*see* Mastopathy, cystic
Recrudescence
 deficit
  cerebral infarction - see Sequelae, infarction,
    cerebral
  stroke - see Sequelae, infarction, cerebral
 sequelae
  cerebral infarction - see Sequelae, infarction,
    cerebral
  stroke - see Sequelae, infarction, cerebral
Recrudescent typhus (fever) A75.1
Recruitment, auditory H93.21-●
Rectalgia K62.89
Rectitis K62.89
Rectocele
 female (without uterine prolapse) N81.6
  with uterine prolapse N81.4
   complete N81.3
   incomplete N81.2
  in pregnancy —*see* Pregnancy, complicated by,
    abnormal, pelvic organs or tissues NEC
 male K62.3
Rectosigmoid junction —*see* condition
Rectosigmoiditis K63.89
 ulcerative (chronic) K51.30
  with
   complication K51.319
    abscess K51.314
    fistula K51.313
    obstruction K51.312
    rectal bleeding K51.311
    specified NEC K51.318
Rectourethral —*see* condition
Rectovaginal —*see* condition
Rectovesical —*see* condition
Rectum, rectal —*see* condition
Recurrent —*see* condition
 pregnancy loss —*see* Loss (of), pregnancy,
   recurrent
Red bugs B88.0
Red-cedar lung or pneumonitis J67.8
Red tide —*see also* Table of Drugs and Chemicals
   T65.82-●

Reduced
 mobility Z74.09
 ventilatory or vital capacity R94.2
Redundant, redundancy
 anus (congenital) Q43.8
 clitoris N90.89
 colon (congenital) Q43.8
 foreskin (congenital) N47.8
 intestine (congenital) Q43.8
 labia N90.69
 organ or site, congenital NEC —*see* Accessory
 panniculus (abdominal) E65
 prepuce (congenital) N47.8
 pylorus K31.89
 rectum (congenital) Q43.8
 scrotum N50.89
 sigmoid (congenital) Q43.8
 skin L98.7
  and subcutaneous tissue L98.7
  of face L57.4
   eyelids —*see* Blepharochalasis
 stomach K31.89
Reduplication —*see* Duplication
Reflex R29.2
 hyperactive gag J39.2
 pupillary, abnormal —*see* Anomaly, pupil,
   function
 vasoconstriction I73.9
 vasovagal R55
Reflux K21.9
 acid K21.9
 esophageal K21.9
  with esophagitis (without bleeding) K21.00
   with bleeding K21.01
  newborn P78.83
 gastroesophageal K21.9
  with esophagitis (without bleeding) K21.00
   with bleeding K21.01
 mitral —*see* Insufficiency, mitral
 ureteral —*see* Reflux, vesicoureteral
 vesicoureteral (with scarring) N13.70
  with
   nephropathy N13.729
    with hydroureter N13.739
     bilateral N13.732
     unilateral N13.731
    without hydroureter N13.729
     bilateral N13.722
     unilateral N13.721
   bilateral N13.722
   unilateral N13.721
   pyelonephritis (chronic) N11.0
  without nephropathy N13.71
  congenital Q62.7
Reforming, artificial openings —*see* Attention to,
   artificial, opening
Refractive error —*see* Disorder, refraction
Refsum's disease or syndrome G60.1
Refusal of
 food, psychogenic F50.89
 treatment (because of) Z53.20
  left against medical advice (AMA) Z53.29
  left without being seen Z53.21
  patient's decision NEC Z53.29
  reasons of belief or group pressure Z53.1
Regional —*see* condition
Regurgitation R11.10
 aortic (valve) —*see* Insufficiency, aortic
 food —*see also* Vomiting
  with reswallowing —*see* Rumination
  newborn P92.1
 gastric contents —*see* Vomiting
 heart —*see* Endocarditis
 mitral (valve) —*see* Insufficiency, mitral
  congenital Q23.3
 myocardial —*see* Endocarditis
 pulmonary (valve) (heart) I37.1
  congenital Q22.2
  syphilitic A52.03
 tricuspid —*see* Insufficiency, tricuspid
 valve, valvular —*see* Endocarditis
  congenital Q24.8
 vesicoureteral —*see* Reflux, vesicoureteral
Reichmann's disease or syndrome K31.89
Reifenstein syndrome E34.52
Reinsertion
 implantable subdermal contraceptive Z30.46
 intrauterine contraceptive device Z30.433
Reiter's disease, syndrome, or urethritis M02.30
 ankle M02.37-●
 elbow M02.32-●

Reiter's disease, syndrome, or urethritis *(Continued)*
 foot joint M02.37-●
 hand joint M02.34-●
 hip M02.35-●
 knee M02.36-●
 multiple site M02.39
 shoulder M02.31-●
 vertebra M02.38
 wrist M02.33-●
Rejection
 food, psychogenic F50.89
 transplant T86.91
  bone T86.830
   marrow T86.01
  cornea T86.840-●
  heart T86.21
   with lung(s) T86.31
  intestine T86.850
  kidney T86.11
  liver T86.41
  lung(s) T86.810
   with heart T86.31
  organ (immune or nonimmune cause) T86.91
  pancreas T86.890
  skin (allograft) (autograft) T86.820
  specified NEC T86.890
  stem cell (peripheral blood) (umbilical cord)
    T86.5
Relapsing fever A68.9
 Carter's (Asiatic) A68.1
 Dutton's (West African) A68.1
 Koch's A68.9
 louse-borne (epidemic) A68.0
 Novy's (American) A68.1
 Obermeyers's (European) A68.0
 Spirillum A68.9
 tick-borne (endemic) A68.1
Relationship
 occlusal
  open anterior M26.220
  open posterior M26.221
Relaxation
 anus (sphincter) K62.89
  psychogenic F45.8
 arch (foot) —*see also* Deformity, limb, flat foot
 back ligaments —*see* Instability, joint, spine
 bladder (sphincter) N31.2
 cardioesophageal K21.9
 cervix —*see* Incompetency, cervix
 diaphragm J98.6
 joint (capsule) (ligament) (paralytic) —*see* Flail,
   joint
  congenital NEC Q74.8
 lumbosacral (joint) —*see* subcategory M53.2
 pelvic floor N81.89
 perineum N81.89
 posture R29.3
 rectum (sphincter) K62.89
 sacroiliac (joint) —*see* subcategory M53.2
 scrotum N50.89
 urethra (sphincter) N36.44
 vesical N31.2
Release from prison, anxiety concerning Z65.2
Remains
 canal of Cloquet Q14.0
 capsule (opaque) Q14.8
Remittent fever (malarial) B54
Remnant
 canal of Cloquet Q14.0
 capsule (opaque) Q14.8
 cervix, cervical stump (acquired) (postoperative)
   N88.8
 cystic duct, postcholecystectomy K91.5
 fingernail L60.8
  congenital Q84.6
 meniscus, knee —*see* Derangement, knee,
   meniscus, specified NEC
 thyroglossal duct Q89.2
 tonsil J35.8
  infected (chronic) J35.01
 urachus Q64.4
Removal (from) (of)
 artificial
  arm Z44.00-●
   complete Z44.01-●
   partial Z44.02-●
  eye Z44.2-●
  leg Z44.10-●
   complete Z44.11-●
   partial Z44.12-●
 breast implant Z45.81

▶ New   ⟹ Revised   ~~deleted~~ Deleted   ● Use Additional Character(s)

Removal *(Continued)*
  cardiac pulse generator (battery) (end-of-life)
    Z45.010
  catheter (urinary) (indwelling) Z46.6
    from artificial opening —*see* Attention to,
      artificial, opening
    non-vascular Z46.82
    vascular NEC Z45.2
  device Z46.9
    contraceptive Z30.432
      implantable subdermal Z30.46
    implanted NEC Z45.89
    specified NEC Z46.89
  drains Z48.03
  dressing (nonsurgical) Z48.00
    surgical Z48.01
  external
    fixation device — code to fracture with
      seventh character D
    prosthesis, prosthetic device Z44.9
      breast Z44.3-●
      specified NEC Z44.8
  home in childhood (to foster home or institution)
    Z62.29
  ileostomy Z43.2
  insulin pump Z46.81
  myringotomy device (stent) (tube) Z45.82
  nervous system device NEC Z46.2
    brain neuropacemaker Z46.2
    visual substitution device Z46.2
      implanted Z45.31
  non-vascular catheter Z46.82
  organ, prophylactic (for neoplasia
    management) —*see* Prophylactic, organ
    removal
  orthodontic device Z46.4
  staples Z48.02
  stent
    ureteral Z46.6
  suture Z48.02
  urinary device Z46.6
  vascular access device or catheter Z45.2
Ren
  arcuatus Q63.1
  mobile, mobilis N28.89
    congenital Q63.8
  unguliformis Q63.1
Renal —*see* condition
Rendu-Osler-Weber disease or syndrome I78.0
Reninoma D41.0-●
Renon-Delille syndrome E23.3
Reovirus, as cause of disease classified elsewhere
  B97.5
Repeated falls NEC R29.6
Replaced chromosome by dicentric ring Q93.2
Replacement by artificial or mechanical device or
    prosthesis of
  bladder Z96.0
  blood vessel NEC Z95.828
  bone NEC Z96.7
  cochlea Z96.21
  coronary artery Z95.5
  eustachian tube Z96.29
  eye globe Z97.0
  heart Z95.812
    valve Z95.2
      prosthetic Z95.2
      specified NEC Z95.4
      xenogenic Z95.3
  intestine Z96.89
  joint Z96.60
    hip —*see* Presence, hip joint implant
    knee —*see* Presence, knee joint implant
    specified site NEC Z96.698
  larynx Z96.3
  lens Z96.1
  limb(s) —*see* Presence, artificial, limb
  mandible NEC (for tooth root implant(s)) Z96.5
  organ NEC Z96.89
  peripheral vessel NEC Z95.828
  stapes Z96.29
  teeth Z97.2
  tendon Z96.7
  tissue NEC Z96.89
  tooth root(s) Z96.5
  vessel NEC Z95.828
    coronary (artery) Z95.5
Request for expert evidence Z04.89
Reserve, decreased or low
  cardiac —*see* Disease, heart
  kidney N28.89

Residing
  in place not meant for human habitation
    (abandoned building) (car) (park)
    (sidewalk) Z59.02
  on the street Z59.02
Residual —*see also* condition
  ovary syndrome N99.83
  state, schizophrenic F20.5
  urine R39.198
Resistance, resistant (to)
  activated protein C D68.51
  insulin E88.819
    complicating pregnancy O26.89-●
    specified type NEC E88.818
  organism(s)
    to
      drug Z16.30
        aminoglycosides Z16.29
        amoxicillin Z16.11
        ampicillin Z16.11
        antibiotic(s) Z16.20
          multiple Z16.24
          specified NEC Z16.29
        antifungal Z16.32
        antimicrobial (single) Z16.30
          multiple Z16.35
          specified NEC Z16.39
        antimycobacterial (single) Z16.341
          multiple Z16.342
        antiparasitic Z16.31
        antiviral Z16.33
        beta lactam antibiotics Z16.10
          specified NEC Z16.19
        carbapenem Z16.13
        cephalosporins Z16.19
        extended beta lactamase (ESBL)
          Z16.12
        fluoroquinolones Z16.23
        macrolides Z16.29
        methicillin —*see* MRSA
        multiple drugs (MDRO)
          antibiotics Z16.24
          antimicrobial Z16.35
          antimycobacterials Z16.342
        penicillins Z16.11
        quinine (and related compounds) Z16.31
        quinolones Z16.23
        sulfonamides Z16.29
        tetracyclines Z16.29
        tuberculostatics (single) Z16.341
          multiple Z16.342
        vancomycin Z16.21
          related antibiotics Z16.22
  thyroid hormone E07.89
Resorption
  dental (roots) K03.3
    alveoli M26.79
  teeth (external) (internal) (pathological) (roots)
    K03.3
Respiration
  Cheyne-Stokes R06.3
  decreased due to shock, following injury
    T79.4
  disorder of, psychogenic F45.8
  insufficient, or poor R06.89
    newborn P28.5
  painful R07.1
  sighing, psychogenic F45.8
Respiratory —*see also* condition
  distress syndrome (newborn) (type I) P22.0
    type II P22.1
  syncytial virus, as cause of disease classified
    elsewhere (*see also* Virus, respiratory
    syncytial (RSV)) B97.4
Respite care Z75.5
Response (drug)
  photoallergic L56.1
  phototoxic L56.0
Restenosis
  stent
    vascular
      end stent
        adjacent to stent —*see* Arteriosclerosis
      within the stent
        coronary T82.855
        peripheral T82.856
    in stent
      coronary vessel T82.855
      peripheral vessel T82.856
Restless legs (syndrome) G25.81
Restlessness R45.1

Restoration (of)
  dental
    aesthetically inadequate or displeasing K08.56
    defective K08.50
      specified NEC K08.59
    failure of marginal integrity K08.51
    failure of periodontal anatomical intergrity
      K08.54
  organ continuity from previous sterilization
    (tuboplasty) (vasoplasty) Z31.0
    aftercare Z31.42
  tooth (existing)
    contours biologically incompatible with oral
      health K08.54
    open margins K08.51
    overhanging K08.52
    poor aesthetic K08.56
    poor gingival margins K08.51
    unsatisfactory, of tooth K08.50
      specified NEC K08.59
Restorative material (dental)
  allergy to K08.55
  fractured K08.539
    with loss of material K08.531
    without loss of material K08.530
  unrepairable overhanging of K08.52
Restriction of housing space Z59.19
Rests, ovarian, in fallopian tube Q50.6
Restzustand (schizophrenic) F20.5
Retained —*see also* Retention
  cholelithiasis following cholecystectomy K91.86
  foreign body fragments (type of) Z18.9
    acrylics Z18.2
    animal quill(s) or spines Z18.31
    cement Z18.83
    concrete Z18.83
    crystalline Z18.83
    depleted isotope Z18.09
    depleted uranium Z18.01
    diethylhexyl phthalates Z18.2
    glass Z18.81
    isocyanate Z18.2
    magnetic metal Z18.11
    metal Z18.10
    nonmagnetic metal Z18.12
    nontherapeutic radioactive Z18.09
    organic NEC Z18.39
    plastic Z18.2
    quill(s) (animal) Z18.31
    radioactive (nontherapeutic) NEC Z18.09
    specified NEC Z18.89
    spine(s) (animal) Z18.31
    stone Z18.83
    tooth (teeth) Z18.32
    wood Z18.33
  fragments (type of) Z18.9
    acrylics Z18.2
    animal quill(s) or spines Z18.31
    cement Z18.83
    concrete Z18.83
    crystalline Z18.83
    depleted isotope Z18.09
    depleted uranium Z18.01
    diethylhexyl phthalates Z18.2
    glass Z18.81
    isocyanate Z18.2
    magnetic metal Z18.11
    metal Z18.10
    nonmagnectic metal Z18.12
    nontherapeutic radioactive Z18.09
    organic NEC Z18.39
    plastic Z18.2
    quill(s) (animal) Z18.31
    radioactive (nontherapeutic) NEC Z18.09
    specified NEC Z18.89
    spine(s) (animal) Z18.31
    stone Z18.83
    tooth (teeth) Z18.32
    wood Z18.33
  gallstones, following cholecystectomy K91.86
Retardation
  development, developmental, specific —*see*
    Disorder, developmental
  endochondral bone growth —*see* Disorder, bone,
    development or growth
  growth R62.50
    due to malnutrition E45
  mental —*see* Disability, intellectual
  motor function, specific F82
  physical (child) R62.52
    due to malnutrition E45

▶ New   ⇒ Revised   ~~deleted~~ Deleted   ● Use Additional Character(s)

Rheumatic *(Continued)*
　torticollis M43.6
　typhoid fever A01.09
Rheumatism (articular) (neuralgic) (nonarticular)
　　M79.0
　gout —*see* Arthritis, rheumatoid
　intercostal, meaning Tietze's disease M94.0
　palindromic (any site) M12.30
　　ankle M12.37-●
　　elbow M12.32-●
　　foot joint M12.37-●
　　hand joint M12.34-●
　　hip M12.35-●
　　knee M12.36-●
　　multiple site M12.39
　　shoulder M12.31-●
　　specified joint NEC M12.38
　　vertebrae M12.38
　　wrist M12.33-●
　sciatic M54.4-●
Rheumatoid —*see also* condition
　arthritis —*see also* Arthritis, rheumatoid
　　with involvement of organs NEC M05.60
　　　ankle M05.67-●
　　　elbow M05.62-●
　　　foot joint M05.67-●
　　　hand joint M05.64-●
　　　hip M05.65-●
　　　knee M05.66-●
　　　multiple site M05.69
　　　shoulder M05.61-●
　　　vertebra —*see* Spondylitis, ankylosing
　　　wrist M05.63-●
　　seronegative —*see* Arthritis, rheumatoid,
　　　　seronegative
　　seropositive —*see* Arthritis, rheumatoid,
　　　　seropositive
　carditis M05.30
　　ankle M05.37-●
　　elbow M05.32-●
　　foot joint M05.37-●
　　hand joint M05.34-●
　　hip M05.35-●
　　knee M05.36-●
　　multiple site M05.39
　　shoulder M05.31-●
　　vertebra —*see* Spondylitis, ankylosing
　　wrist M05.33-●
　endocarditis —*see* Rheumatoid, carditis
　lung (disease) M05.10
　　ankle M05.17-●
　　elbow M05.12-●
　　foot joint M05.17-●
　　hand joint M05.14-●
　　hip M05.15-●
　　knee M05.16-●
　　multiple site M05.19
　　shoulder M05.11-●
　　vertebra —*see* Spondylitis, ankylosing
　　wrist M05.13-●
　myocarditis —*see* Rheumatoid, carditis
　myopathy M05.40
　　ankle M05.47-●
　　elbow M05.42-●
　　foot joint M05.47-●
　　hand joint M05.44-●
　　hip M05.45-●
　　knee M05.46-●
　　multiple site M05.49
　　shoulder M05.41-●
　　vertebra —*see* Spondylitis, ankylosing
　　wrist M05.43-●
　pericarditis —*see* Rheumatoid, carditis
　polyarthritis —*see* Arthritis, rheumatoid
　polyneuropathy M05.50
　　ankle M05.57-●
　　elbow M05.52-●
　　foot joint M05.57-●
　　hand joint M05.54-●
　　hip M05.55-●
　　knee M05.56-●
　　multiple site M05.59
　　shoulder M05.51-●
　　vertebra —*see* Spondylitis, ankylosing
　　wrist M05.53-●
　vasculitis M05.20
　　ankle M05.27-●
　　elbow M05.22-●
　　foot joint M05.27-●
　　hand joint M05.24-●
　　hip M05.25-●

Rheumatoid *(Continued)*
　vasculitis *(Continued)*
　　knee M05.26-●
　　multiple site M05.29
　　shoulder M05.21-●
　　vertebra —*see* Spondylitis, ankylosing
　　wrist M05.23-●
Rhinitis (atrophic) (catarrhal) (chronic) (croupous)
　　(fibrinous) (granulomatous) (hyperplastic)
　　(hypertrophic) (membranous) (obstructive)
　　(purulent) (suppurative) (ulcerative) J31.0
　with
　　sore throat —*see* Nasopharyngitis
　acute J00
　allergic J30.9
　　with asthma J45.909
　　　with
　　　　exacerbation (acute) J45.901
　　　　status asthmaticus J45.902
　　　due to
　　　　food J30.5
　　　　pollen J30.1
　　nonseasonal J30.89
　　perennial J30.89
　　seasonal NEC J30.2
　　specified NEC J30.89
　infective J00
　pneumococcal J00
　syphilitic A52.73
　　congenital A50.05 [J99]
　tuberculous A15.8
　vasomotor J30.0
Rhinoantritis (chronic) —*see* Sinusitis, maxillary
Rhinodacryolith —*see* Dacryolith
Rhinolith (nasal sinus) J34.89
Rhinomegaly J34.89
Rhinopharyngitis (acute) (subacute) —*see also*
　　Nasopharyngitis
　chronic J31.1
　destructive ulcerating A66.5
　mutilans A66.5
Rhinophyma L71.1
Rhinorrhea J34.89
　cerebrospinal (fluid) G96.01
　　postoperative G96.08
　　specified NEC G96.08
　　spontaneous G96.01
　　traumatic G96.08
　paroxysmal —*see* Rhinitis, allergic
　spasmodic —*see* Rhinitis, allergic
Rhinosalpingitis —*see* Salpingitis, eustachian
Rhinoscleroma A48.8
Rhinosinusitis —*see* Sinusitis
Rhinosporidiosis B48.1
Rhinovirus infection NEC B34.8
Rhizomelic chondrodysplasia punctata E71.540
Rhythm
　atrioventricular nodal I49.8
　disorder I49.9
　　coronary sinus I49.8
　　ectopic I49.8
　　nodal I49.8
　escape I49.9
　heart, abnormal I49.9
　idioventricular I44.2
　nodal I49.8
　sleep, inversion G47.2-●
　　nonorganic origin —*see* Disorder, sleep,
　　　circadian rhythm, psychogenic
Rhytidosis facialis L98.8
Rib —*see also* condition
　cervical Q76.5
Riboflavin deficiency E53.0
Rice bodies —*see also* Loose, body, joint
　knee M23.4-●
Richter syndrome —*see* Leukemia, chronic
　　lymphocytic, B-cell type
Richter's hernia —*see* Hernia, abdomen, with
　　obstruction
Ricinism —*see* Poisoning, food, noxious, plant
Rickets (active) (acute) (adolescent) (chest wall)
　　(congenital) (current) (infantile) (intestinal) E55.0
　adult —*see* Osteomalacia
　celiac K90.0
　hypophosphatemic with nephrotic-glycosuric
　　dwarfism E72.09
　inactive E64.3
　kidney N25.0
　renal N25.0
　sequelae, any E64.3
　vitamin-D-resistant E83.31 [M90.80]

Rickettsia 364D/R. philipii (Pacific Coast tick
　　fever) A77.8
Rickettsial disease A79.9
　specified type NEC A79.89
Rickettsialpox (Rickettsia akari) A79.1
Rickettsiosis A79.9
　due to
　　Ehrlichia sennetsu A79.81
　　Neorickettsia sennetsu A79.81
　　Rickettsia akari (rickettsialpox) A79.1
　specified type NEC A79.89
　tick-borne A77.9
　vesicular A79.1
Rider's bone —*see* Ossification, muscle, specified
　　NEC
Ridge, alveolus —*see also* condition
　flabby K06.8
Ridged ear, congenital Q17.3
Riedel's
　lobe, liver Q44.79
　struma, thyroiditis or disease E06.5
~~Rieger's anomaly or syndrome Q13.81~~
▶ Rieger anomaly or syndrome Q13.81
Riehl's melanosis L81.4
Rietti-Greppi-Micheli anemia D56.9
Rieux's hernia —*see* Hernia, abdomen, specified
　　site NEC
Riga (-Fede) disease K14.0
Riggs' disease —*see* Periodontitis
Right aortic arch Q25.47
Right middle lobe syndrome J98.11
Rigid, rigidity —*see also* condition
　abdominal R19.30
　　with severe abdominal pain R10.0
　　epigastric R19.36
　　generalized R19.37
　　left lower quadrant R19.34
　　left upper quadrant R19.32
　　periumbilic R19.35
　　right lower quadrant R19.33
　　right upper quadrant R19.31
　articular, multiple, congenital Q68.8
　cervix (uteri) in pregnancy —*see* Pregnancy,
　　complicated by, abnormal, cervix
　hymen (acquired) (congenital) N89.6
　nuchal R29.1
　pelvic floor in pregnancy —*see* Pregnancy,
　　complicated by, abnormal, pelvic organs or
　　tissues NEC
　perineum or vulva in pregnancy —*see*
　　Pregnancy, complicated by, abnormal,
　　vulva
　spine —*see* Dorsopathy, specified NEC
　vagina in pregnancy —*see* Pregnancy,
　　complicated by, abnormal, vagina
Rigors R68.89
　with fever R50.9
Riley-Day syndrome G90.1
RIND (reversible ischemic neurologic deficit)
　　I63.9
Ring(s)
　aorta (vascular) Q25.45
　Bandl's O62.4
　contraction, complicating delivery O62.4
　esophageal, lower (muscular) K22.2
　Fleischer's (cornea) H18.04-●
　hymenal, tight (acquired) (congenital) N89.6
　Kayser-Fleischer (cornea) H18.04-●
　retraction, uterus, pathological O62.4
　Schatzki's (esophagus) (lower) K22.2
　　congenital Q39.3
　Soemmerring's —*see* Cataract, secondary
　vascular (congenital) Q25.8
　　aorta Q25.45
Ringed hair (congenital) Q84.1
Ringworm B35.9
　beard B35.0
　black dot B35.0
　body B35.4
　Burmese B35.5
　corporeal B35.4
　foot B35.3
　groin B35.6
　hand B35.2
　honeycomb B35.0
　nails B35.1
　perianal (area) B35.6
　scalp B35.0
　specified NEC B35.8
　Tokelau B35.5
Rise, venous pressure I87.8

Rising, PSA following treatment for malignant
  neoplasm of prostate R97.21
Risk
  for
    dental caries Z91.849
    high Z91.843
    low Z91.841
    moderate Z91.842
    homelessness, imminent Z59.811
  suffocation (smothering) under another while
    sleeping Z72.823
  suicidal
    meaning personal history of attempted
      suicide Z91.51
    meaning suicidal ideation —see Ideation,
      suicidal
Ritter's disease L00
Rivalry, sibling Z62.891
Rivalta's disease A42.2
River blindness B73.01
Robert's pelvis Q74.2
  with disproportion (fetopelvic) O33.0
    causing obstructed labor O65.0
Robin (-Pierre) syndrome Q87.0
~~Robinow-Silvermann-Smith syndrome Q87.19~~
▶Robinow-Silverman-Smith syndrome
  Q87.19
Robinson's (hidrotic) ectodermal dysplasia or
  syndrome Q82.4
Robles' disease B73.01
Rocky Mountain (spotted) fever A77.0
Roetheln —see Rubella
Roger's disease Q21.0
Rokitansky-Aschoff sinuses (gallbladder)
  K82.8
Rolando's fracture (displaced) S62.22-●
  nondisplaced S62.22-●
Romano-Ward (prolonged QT interval) syndrome
  I45.81
Romberg's disease or syndrome G51.8
Roof, mouth —see condition
Rosacea L71.9
  acne L71.9
  keratitis L71.8
  specified NEC L71.8
Rosary, rachitic E55.0
Rose
  cold J30.1
  fever J30.1
  rash R21
    epidemic B06.9
Rosenbach's erysipeloid A26.0
Rosenthal's disease or syndrome D68.1
Roseola B09
  infantum B08.20
    due to human herpesvirus 6 B08.21
    due to human herpesvirus 7 B08.22
Ross River disease or fever B33.1
Rossbach's disease K31.89
  psychogenic F45.8
Rostan's asthma (cardiac) —see Failure, ventricular,
  left
Rotation
  anomalous, incomplete or insufficient, intestine
    Q43.3
  cecum (congenital) Q43.3
  colon (congenital) Q43.3
  spine, incomplete or insufficient —see
    Dorsopathy, deforming, specified
    NEC
  tooth, teeth, fully erupted M26.35
  vertebra, incomplete or insufficient —see
    Dorsopathy, deforming, specified
    NEC
Rotes Quérol disease or syndrome —see
  Hyperostosis, ankylosing
Roth (-Bernhardt) disease or syndrome —see
  Meralgia paraesthetica
Rothmund (-Thomson) syndrome Q82.8
Rotor's disease or syndrome E80.6
Round
  back (with wedging of vertebrae) —see Kyphosis
    sequelae (late effect) of rickets E64.3
  worms (large) (infestation) NEC B82.0
    Ascariasis —see also Ascariasis B77.9
Roussy-Lévy syndrome G60.0
Rubella (German measles) B06.9
  complication NEC B06.09
    neurological B06.00
  congenital P35.0
  contact Z20.4
  exposure to Z20.4

Rubella (Continued)
  maternal
    care for (suspected) damage to fetus O35.3
    manifest rubella in infant P35.0
    suspected damage to fetus affecting
      management of pregnancy O35.3
  specified complications NEC B06.89
Rubeola (meaning measles) —see Measles
  meaning rubella —see Rubella
Rubeosis, iris —see Disorder, iris, vascular
Rubinstein-Taybi syndrome Q87.2
Rudimentary (congenital) —see also Agenesis
  arm —see Defect, reduction, upper limb
  bone Q79.9
  cervix uteri Q51.828
  eye Q11.2
  lobule of ear Q17.3
  patella Q74.1
  respiratory organs in thoracopagus Q89.4
  tracheal bronchus Q32.4
  uterus Q51.818
    in male Q56.1
  vagina Q52.0
Ruled out condition —see Observation, suspected
Rumination R11.10
  with nausea R11.2
  ~~disorder of infancy F98.21~~
  ▶disorder of infancy or childhood (in remission)
    F98.21
  ▶in adults (in remission) F50.84
  neurotic F42.8
  newborn P92.1
  obsessional F42.8
  psychogenic F42.8
Runaway [from current living environment]
  Z62.892
Runeberg's disease D51.0
Runny nose R09.89
Running out of money Z59.86
Rupia (syphilitic) A51.39
  congenital A50.06
  tertiary A52.79
Rupture, ruptured
  abscess (spontaneous) - code by site under
    Abscess
  aneurysm —see Aneurysm
  anus (sphincter) —see Laceration, anus
  aorta, aortic I71.8
    abdominal I71.30
      infrarenal I71.33
      juxtarenal I71.32
      pararenal I71.31
    arch I71.12
    ascending I71.11
    descending I71.8
      abdominal I71.30
      thoracic I71.13
    syphilitic A52.01
    thoracoabdominal I71.50
      paravisceral I71.52
      supraceliac I71.51
    thorax, thoracic I71.10
    transverse I71.12
    traumatic —see Injury, aorta, laceration, major
    valve or cusp —see also Endocarditis, aortic I35.8
  appendix (with peritonitis) (see also Appendicitis)
    K35.32
    with localized peritonitis (see also
      Appendicitis) K35.32
  arteriovenous fistula, brain —see Fistula,
    arteriovenous, brain, ruptured
  artery I77.2
    brain —see Hemorrhage, intracranial,
      intracerebral
    coronary —see Infarct, myocardium
    heart —see Infarct, myocardium
    pulmonary I28.8
    traumatic (complication) —see Injury, blood
      vessel
  bile duct (common) (hepatic) K83.2
    cystic K82.2
  bladder (sphincter) (nontraumatic)
    (spontaneous) N32.89
    following ectopic or molar pregnancy O08.6
    obstetrical trauma O71.5
    traumatic S37.29
  blood vessel —see also Hemorrhage
    brain —see Hemorrhage, intracranial,
      intracerebral
    heart —see Infarct, myocardium
    traumatic (complication) —see Injury, blood
      vessel, laceration, major, by site

Rupture, ruptured (Continued)
  bone —see Fracture
  bowel (nontraumatic) K63.1
  brain
    aneurysm (congenital) —see also Hemorrhage,
      intracranial, subarachnoid
      syphilitic A52.05
    hemorrhagic —see Hemorrhage, intracranial,
      intracerebral
  capillaries I78.8
  cardiac (auricle) (ventricle) (wall) I23.3
    with hemopericardium I23.0
    infectional I40.9
    traumatic —see Injury, heart
  cartilage (articular) (current) —
    see also Sprain
    knee S83.3-●
    semilunar —see Tear, meniscus
  cecum (with peritonitis) K65.0
    with peritoneal abscess K35.33
    traumatic S36.598
  celiac artery, traumatic —see Injury, blood vessel,
    celiac artery, laceration, major
  cerebral aneurysm (congenital) (see Hemorrhage,
    intracranial, subarachnoid)
  cervix (uteri)
    with ectopic or molar pregnancy O08.6
    following ectopic or molar pregnancy O08.6
    obstetrical trauma O71.3
    traumatic S37.69
  chordae tendineae NEC I51.1
    concurrent with acute myocardial
      infarction —see Infarct, myocardium
    following acute myocardial infarction (current
      complication) I23.4
  choroid (direct) (indirect) (traumatic)
    H31.32-●
  circle of Willis I60.6
  colon (nontraumatic) K63.1
    traumatic —see Injury, intestine, large
  cornea (traumatic) —see Injury, eye, laceration
  coronary (artery) (thrombotic) —see Infarct,
    myocardium
  corpus luteum (infected) (ovary) N83.1-●
  cyst —see Cyst
  cystic duct K82.2
  Descemet's membrane —see Change, corneal
    membrane, Descemet's, rupture
    traumatic —see Injury, eye, laceration
  diaphragm, traumatic —see Injury, intrathoracic,
    diaphragm
  disc —see Rupture, intervertebral disc
  diverticulum (intestine) K57.80
    with bleeding K57.81
    bladder N32.3
    large intestine K57.20
      with
        bleeding K57.21
        small intestine K57.40
          with bleeding K57.41
    small intestine K57.00
      with
        bleeding K57.01
        large intestine K57.40
          with bleeding K57.41
  duodenal stump K31.89
  ear drum (nontraumatic) —see also Perforation,
    tympanum
    traumatic S09.2-●
      due to blast injury —see Injury,
        blast, ear
  esophagus K22.3
  eye (without prolapse or loss of intraocular
    tissue) —see Injury, eye, laceration
  fallopian tube NEC (nonobstetric)
    (nontraumatic) N83.8
    due to pregnancy O00.10-●
      with intrauterine pregnancy O00.11-●
  fontanel P13.1
  gallbladder K82.2
    traumatic S36.128
  gastric —see also Rupture, stomach
    vessel K92.2
  globe (eye) (traumatic) —see Injury, eye,
    laceration
  ▶nontraumatic (see also Disorder, globe) H44.89
  graafian follicle (hematoma) N83.0-●
  heart —see Rupture, cardiac
  hymen (nontraumatic) (nonintentional)
    N89.8
  internal organ, traumatic —see Injury,
    by site

▶ New   ⇒ Revised   ~~deleted~~ Deleted   ● Use Additional Character(s)

Rupture, ruptured *(Continued)*
  intervertebral disc —*see* Displacement,
    intervertebral disc
    traumatic —*see* Rupture, traumatic,
      intervertebral disc
  intestine NEC (nontraumatic) K63.1
    traumatic —*see* Injury, intestine
  iris —*see also* Abnormality, pupillary
    traumatic —*see* Injury, eye, laceration
  joint capsule, traumatic —*see* Sprain
  kidney (traumatic) S37.06-●
    birth injury P15.8
    nontraumatic N28.89
  lacrimal duct (traumatic) —*see* Injury, eye,
    specified site NEC
  lens (cataract) (traumatic) —*see* Cataract,
    traumatic
  ligament, traumatic —*see* Rupture, traumatic,
    ligament, by site
  liver S36.116
    birth injury P15.0
  lymphatic vessel I89.8
  marginal sinus (placental) (with hemorrhage) —
    see Hemorrhage, antepartum, specified
    cause NEC
  membrana tympani (nontraumatic) —*see*
    Perforation, tympanum
  membranes (spontaneous)
    artificial
      delayed delivery following O75.5
    delayed delivery following —*see* Pregnancy,
      complicated by, premature rupture of
      membranes
  meningeal artery I60.8
  meniscus (knee) —*see also* Tear, meniscus
    old —*see* Derangement, meniscus
    site other than knee - code as Sprain
  mesenteric artery, traumatic —*see* Injury,
    mesenteric, artery, laceration, major
  mesentery (nontraumatic) K66.8
    traumatic —*see* Injury, intra-abdominal,
      specified, site NEC
  mitral (valve) I34.89
  muscle (traumatic) —*see also* Strain
    diastasis —*see* Diastasis, muscle
    nontraumatic M62.10
      ankle M62.17-●
      foot M62.17-●
      forearm M62.13-●
      hand M62.14-●
      lower leg M62.16-●
      pelvic region M62.15-●
      shoulder region M62.11-●
      specified site NEC M62.18
      thigh M62.15-●
      upper arm M62.12-●
    traumatic —*see* Strain, by site
  musculotendinous junction NEC,
    nontraumatic —*see* Rupture, tendon,
    spontaneous
  mycotic aneurysm causing cerebral
    hemorrhage —*see* Hemorrhage,
    intracranial, subarachnoid
  myocardium, myocardial —*see* Rupture,
    cardiac
    traumatic —*see* Injury, heart
  nontraumatic, meaning hernia —*see*
    Hernia
  obstructed —*see* Hernia, by site, obstructed
  operation wound —*see* Disruption, wound,
    operation
  ovary, ovarian N83.8
    corpus luteum cyst N83.1-●
    follicle (graafian) N83.0-●
  oviduct (nonobstetric) (nontraumatic) N83.8
    due to pregnancy O00.10-●
      with intrauterine pregnancy O00.11-●
  pancreas (nontraumatic) K86.89
    traumatic S36.299
  papillary muscle NEC I51.2
    following acute myocardial infarction (current
      complication) I23.5
  pelvic
    floor, complicating delivery O70.1
    organ NEC, obstetrical trauma O71.5
  perineum (nonobstetric) (nontraumatic) N90.89
    complicating delivery —*see* Delivery,
      complicated, by, laceration, anus
      (sphincter)
  postoperative wound —*see* Disruption, wound,
    operation
  prostate (traumatic) S37.828

Rupture, ruptured *(Continued)*
  pulmonary
    artery I28.8
    valve (heart) I37.8
    vein I28.8
    vessel I28.8
  pus tube —*see* Salpingitis
  pyosalpinx —*see* Salpingitis
  rectum (nontraumatic) K63.1
    traumatic S36.69
  retina, retinal (traumatic) (without
    detachment) —*see also* Break, retina
    with detachment —*see* Detachment,
      retina, with retinal, break
  rotator cuff (nontraumatic) M75.10-●
    complete M75.12-●
    incomplete M75.11-●
  sclera —*see* Injury, eye, laceration
  sigmoid (nontraumatic) K63.1
    traumatic S36.593
  spinal cord —*see also* Injury, spinal cord, by
    region
    due to injury at birth P11.5
    newborn (birth injury) P11.5
  spleen (traumatic) S36.09
    birth injury P15.1
    congenital (birth injury) P15.1
    due to P. vivax malaria B51.0
    nontraumatic D73.5
    spontaneous D73.5
  splenic vein R58
    traumatic —*see* Injury, blood vessel,
      splenic vein
  stomach (nontraumatic) (spontaneous)
    K31.89
    traumatic S36.39
  supraspinatus (complete) (incomplete)
    (nontraumatic) —*see* Tear, rotator cuff
  symphysis pubis
    obstetric O71.6
    traumatic S33.4
  synovium (cyst) M66.10
    ankle M66.17-●
    elbow M66.12-●
    finger M66.14-●
    foot M66.17-●
    forearm M66.13-●
    hand M66.14-●
    pelvic region M66.15-●
    shoulder region M66.11-●
    specified site NEC M66.18
    thigh M66.15-●
    toe M66.17-●
    upper arm M66.12-●
    wrist M66.13-●
  tendon (traumatic) —*see* Strain
    nontraumatic (spontaneous) M66.9
      ankle M66.87-●
      extensor M66.20
        ankle M66.27-●
        foot M66.27-●
        forearm M66.23-●
        hand M66.24-●
        lower leg M66.26-●
        multiple sites M66.29
        pelvic region M66.25-●
        shoulder region M66.21-●
        specified site NEC M66.28
        thigh M66.25-●
        upper arm M66.22-●
      flexor M66.30
        ankle M66.37-●
        foot M66.37-●
        forearm M66.33-●
        hand M66.34-●
        lower leg M66.36-●
        multiple sites M66.39
        pelvic region M66.35-●
        shoulder region M66.31-●
        specified site NEC M66.38
        thigh M66.35-●
        upper arm M66.32-●
      foot M66.87-●
      forearm M66.83-●
      hand M66.84-●
      lower leg M66.86-●
      multiple sites M66.89
      pelvic region M66.85-●
      shoulder region M66.81-●
      specified
        site NEC M66.88
        tendon M66.80

Rupture, ruptured *(Continued)*
  tendon *(Continued)*
    nontraumatic *(Continued)*
      thigh M66.85-●
      upper arm M66.82-●
  thoracic duct I89.8
  tonsil J35.8
  traumatic
    aorta —*see* Injury, aorta, laceration, major
    diaphragm —*see* Injury, intrathoracic,
      diaphragm
    external site —*see* Wound, open, by site
    eye —*see* Injury, eye, laceration
    internal organ —*see* Injury, by site
    intervertebral disc
      cervical S13.0
      lumbar S33.0
      thoracic S23.0
    kidney S37.06-●
    ligament —*see also* Sprain
      ankle —*see* Sprain, ankle
      carpus —*see* Rupture, traumatic, ligament,
        wrist
      collateral (hand) —*see* Rupture, traumatic,
        ligament, finger, collateral
      finger (metacarpophalangeal)
        (interphalangeal) S63.40-●
        collateral S63.41-●
          index S63.41-●
          little S63.41-●
          middle S63.41-●
          ring S63.41-●
        index S63.40-●
        little S63.40-●
        middle S63.40-●
        palmar S63.42-●
          index S63.42-●
          little S63.42-●
          middle S63.42-●
          ring S63.42-●
        ring S63.40-●
        specified site NEC S63.499
          index S63.49-●
          little S63.49-●
          middle S63.49-●
          ring S63.49-●
        volar plate S63.43-●
          index S63.43-●
          little S63.43-●
          middle S63.43-●
          ring S63.43-●
      foot —*see* Sprain, foot
      radial collateral S53.2-●
      radiocarpal —*see* Rupture, traumatic,
        ligament, wrist, radiocarpal
      ulnar collateral S53.3-●
      ulnocarpal —*see* Rupture, traumatic,
        ligament, wrist, ulnocarpal
      wrist S63.30-●
        collateral S63.31-●
        radiocarpal S63.32-●
        specified site NEC S63.39-●
        ulnocarpal (palmar) S63.33-●
    liver S36.116
    membrana tympani —*see* Rupture, ear drum,
      traumatic
    muscle or tendon —*see* Strain
    myocardium —*see* Injury, heart
    pancreas S36.299
    rectum S36.69
    sigmoid S36.593
    spleen S36.09
    stomach S36.39
    symphysis pubis S33.4
    tympanum, tympanic (membrane) —*see*
      Rupture, ear drum, traumatic
    ureter S37.19
    uterus S37.69
    vagina —*see* Injury, vagina
    vena cava —*see* Injury, vena cava, laceration,
      major
  tricuspid (heart) (valve) I07.8
  tube, tubal (nonobstetric) (nontraumatic) N83.8
    abscess —*see* Salpingitis
    due to pregnancy O00.10-●
      with intrauterine pregnancy O00.11-●
  tympanum, tympanic (membrane)
    (nontraumatic) —*see also* Perforation,
    tympanic membrane H72.9-●
    traumatic —*see* Rupture, ear drum, traumatic
  umbilical cord, complicating delivery
    O69.89

▶ New   ⇒ Revised   ~~deleted~~ Deleted   ● Use Additional Character(s)

Rupture, ruptured (Continued)
ureter (traumatic) S37.19
nontraumatic N28.89
urethra (nontraumatic) N36.8
with ectopic or molar pregnancy O08.6
following ectopic or molar pregnancy O08.6
obstetrical trauma O71.5
traumatic S37.39
uterosacral ligament (nonobstetric)
(nontraumatic) N83.8
uterus (traumatic) S37.69
before labor O71.0-●
during or after labor O71.1
nonpuerperal, nontraumatic N85.8
pregnant (during labor) O71.1
before labor O71.0-●
vagina —see Injury, vagina
valve, valvular (heart) —see Endocarditis
varicose vein —see Varix
varix —see Varix
vena cava R58
traumatic —see Injury, vena cava, laceration,
major
vesical (urinary) N32.89
vessel (blood) R58
pulmonary I28.8
traumatic —see Injury, blood vessel
viscus R19.8
vulva complicating delivery O70.0
Russell-Silver syndrome Q87.19
Russian spring-summer type encephalitis A84.0
Rust's disease (tuberculous cervical spondylitis)
A18.01
Ruvalcaba-Myhre-Smith syndrome E71.440
Rytand-Lipsitch syndrome I44.2

——————— S ———————

Saber, sabre shin or tibia (syphilitic) A50.56
[M90.8-●]
Sac lacrimal —see condition
Saccharomyces infection B37.9
Saccharopinuria E72.3
Saccular —see condition
Sacculation
aorta (nonsyphilitic) —see Aneurysm, aorta
bladder N32.3
intralaryngeal (congenital) (ventricular) Q31.3
larynx (congenital) (ventricular) Q31.3
organ or site, congenital —see Distortion
pregnant uterus —see Pregnancy, complicated by,
abnormal, uterus
ureter N28.89
urethra N36.1
vesical N32.3
Sachs' amaurotic familial idiocy or disease E75.02
Sachs-Tay disease E75.02
Sacks-Libman disease M32.11
Sacralgia M53.3
Sacralization Q76.49
Sacrodynia M53.3
Sacroiliac joint —see condition
Sacroiliitis NEC M46.1
Sacrum —see condition
Saddle
back —see Lordosis
embolus
abdominal aorta I74.01
pulmonary artery I26.92
with acute cor pulmonale I26.02
injury — code to condition
nose M95.0
due to syphilis A50.57
Sadism (sexual) F65.52
Sadness, postpartal O90.6
Sadomasochism F65.50
Saemisch's ulcer (cornea) —see Ulcer, cornea,
central
Sagging
skin and subcutaneous tissue (following bariatric
surgery weight loss) (following dietary
weight loss) L98.7
Sahib disease B55.0
Sailors' skin L57.8
Saint
Anthony's fire —see Erysipelas
triad —see Hernia, diaphragm
Vitus' dance —see Chorea, Sydenham's

Salaam
attack(s) —see Epilepsy, spasms
tic R25.8
Salicylism
abuse F55.8
overdose or wrong substance given —see
Table of Drugs and Chemicals, by drug,
poisoning
Salivary duct or gland —see condition
Salivation, excessive K11.7
Salmonella —see Infection, Salmonella
Salmonellosis A02.0
Salpingitis (catarrhal) (fallopian tube) (nodular)
(pseudofollicular) (purulent) (septic)
N70.91
with oophoritis N70.93
acute N70.01
with oophoritis N70.03
chlamydial A56.11
chronic N70.11
with oophoritis N70.13
complicating abortion —see Abortion, by type,
complicated by, salpingitis
ear —see Salpingitis, eustachian
eustachian (tube) H68.00-●
acute H68.01-●
chronic H68.02-●
follicularis N70.11
with oophoritis N70.13
gonococcal (acute) (chronic) A54.24
interstitial, chronic N70.11
with oophoritis N70.13
isthmica nodosa N70.11
with oophoritis N70.13
specific (gonococcal) (acute) (chronic) A54.24
tuberculous (acute) (chronic) A18.17
venereal (gonococcal) (acute) (chronic)
A54.24
Salpingocele N83.4-●
Salpingo-oophoritis (catarrhal) (purulent)
(ruptured) (septic) (suppurative) N70.93
acute N70.03
with ectopic or molar pregnancy O08.0
following ectopic or molar pregnancy
O08.0
gonococcal A54.24
chronic N70.13
following ectopic or molar pregnancy O08.0
gonococcal (acute) (chronic) A54.24
puerperal O86.19
specific (gonococcal) (acute) (chronic) A54.24
subacute N70.03
tuberculous (acute) (chronic) A18.17
venereal (gonococcal) (acute) (chronic) A54.24
Salpingo-ovaritis —see Salpingo-oophoritis
Salpingoperitonitis —see Salpingo-oophoritis
Salzmann's nodular dystrophy —see Degeneration,
cornea, nodular
Sampson's cyst or tumor N80.10-●
San Joaquin (Valley) fever B38.0
Sandblaster's asthma, lung or pneumoconiosis
J62.8
Sander's disease (paranoia) F22
Sandfly fever A93.1
Sandhoff's disease E75.01
Sanfilippo (Type B) (Type C) (Type D) syndrome
E76.22
Sanger-Brown ataxia G11.2
Sao Paulo fever or typhus A77.0
Saponification, mesenteric K65.8
Sarcocele (benign)
syphilitic A52.76
congenital A50.59
Sarcocystosis A07.8
Sarcoepiplocele —see Hernia
Sarcoepiplomphalocele Q79.2
Sarcoglycanopathy G71.0340
alpha G71.0341
beta G71.0342
delta G71.0349
gamma G71.0349
Sarcoid —see also Sarcoidosis
arthropathy D86.86
Boeck's D86.9
Darier-Roussy D86.3
iridocyclitis D86.83
meningitis D86.81
myocarditis D86.85
myositis D86.87
pyelonephritis D86.84
Spiegler-Fendt L08.89

Sarcoidosis D86.9
with
cranial nerve palsies D86.82
hepatic granuloma D86.89
polyarthritis D86.86
tubulo-interstitial nephropathy D86.84
combined sites NEC D86.89
lung D86.0
and lymph nodes D86.2
lymph nodes D86.1
and lung D86.2
meninges D86.81
skin D86.3
specified type NEC D86.89
Sarcoma (of) —see also Neoplasm, connective
tissue, malignant
alveolar soft part —see Neoplasm, connective
tissue, malignant
ameloblastic C41.1
upper jaw (bone) C41.0
botryoid —see Neoplasm, connective tissue,
malignant
botryoides —see Neoplasm, connective tissue,
malignant
cerebellar C71.6
circumscribed (arachnoidal) C71.6
circumscribed (arachnoidal) cerebellar
C71.6
clear cell —see also Neoplasm, connective tissue,
malignant
kidney C64.-●
dendritic cells (accessory cells) C96.4
embryonal —see Neoplasm, connective tissue,
malignant
endometrial (stromal) C54.1
isthmus C54.0
epithelioid (cell) —see Neoplasm, connective
tissue, malignant
Ewing's —see Neoplasm, bone, malignant
follicular dendritic cell C96.4
germinoblastic (diffuse) —see Lymphoma,
diffuse, large cell
follicular —see Lymphoma, follicular,
specified NEC
giant cell (except of bone) —see also Neoplasm,
connective tissue, malignant
bone —see Neoplasm, bone, malignant
glomoid —see Neoplasm, connective tissue,
malignant
granulocytic C92.3-●
hemangioendothelial —see Neoplasm,
connective tissue, malignant
hemorrhagic, multiple —see Sarcoma, Kaposi's
histiocytic C96.A
Hodgkin —see Lymphoma, Hodgkin
immunoblastic (diffuse) —see Lymphoma,
diffuse large cell
interdigitating dendritic cell C96.4
Kaposi's
colon C46.4
connective tissue C46.1
gastrointestinal organ C46.4
lung C46.5-●
lymph node(s) C46.3
palate (hard) (soft) C46.2
rectum C46.4
skin C46.0
specified site NEC C46.7
stomach C46.4
unspecified site C46.9
Kupffer cell C22.3
Langerhans cell C96.4
leptomeningeal —see Neoplasm, meninges,
malignant
liver NEC C22.4
lymphangioendothelial —see Neoplasm,
connective tissue, malignant
lymphoblastic —see Lymphoma, lymphoblastic
(diffuse)
lymphocytic —see Lymphoma, small cell B-cell
mast cell C96.22
melanotic —see Melanoma
meningeal —see Neoplasm, meninges,
malignant
meningothelial —see Neoplasm, meninges,
malignant
mesenchymal —see also Neoplasm, connective
tissue, malignant
mixed —see Neoplasm, connective tissue,
malignant
mesothelial —see Mesothelioma

▶ New   ⇒ Revised   ~~deleted~~ Deleted   ● Use Additional Character(s)

Sarcoma *(Continued)*
  monstrocellular
    specified site —*see* Neoplasm, malignant, by
        site
    unspecified site C71.9
  myeloid C92.3-●
  neurogenic —*see* Neoplasm, nerve, malignant
  odontogenic C41.1
    upper jaw (bone) C41.0
  osteoblastic —*see* Neoplasm, bone, malignant
  osteogenic —*see also* Neoplasm, bone, malignant
    juxtacortical —*see* Neoplasm, bone, malignant
    periosteal —*see* Neoplasm, bone, malignant
  periosteal —*see also* Neoplasm, bone, malignant
    osteogenic —*see* Neoplasm, bone, malignant
  pleomorphic cell —*see* Neoplasm, connective
        tissue, malignant
  reticulum cell (diffuse) —*see* Lymphoma, diffuse
        large cell
    nodular —*see* Lymphoma, follicular
    pleomorphic cell type —*see* Lymphoma,
        diffuse large cell
  rhabdoid —*see* Neoplasm, malignant, by site
  round cell —*see* Neoplasm, connective tissue,
        malignant
  small cell —*see* Neoplasm, connective tissue,
        malignant
  soft tissue —*see* Neoplasm, connective tissue,
        malignant
  spindle cell —*see* Neoplasm, connective tissue,
        malignant
  stromal (endometrial) C54.1
    isthmus C54.0
  synovial —*see also* Neoplasm, connective tissue,
        malignant
    biphasic —*see* Neoplasm, connective tissue,
        malignant
    epithelioid cell —*see* Neoplasm, connective
        tissue, malignant
    spindle cell —*see* Neoplasm, connective tissue,
        malignant
Sarcomatosis
  meningeal —*see* Neoplasm, meninges, malignant
  specified site NEC —*see* Neoplasm, connective
        tissue, malignant
  unspecified site C80.1
Sarcopenia (age-related) M62.84
Sarcosinemia E72.59
Sarcosporidiosis (intestinal) A07.8
SARS-CoV-2 —*see also* COVID-19
  sequelae (post acute) U09.9
Satiety, early R68.81
Saturnine —*see* condition
Saturnism
  overdose or wrong substance given or taken —
        see Table of Drugs and Chemicals, by drug,
        poisoning
Satyriasis F52.8
Sauriasis —*see* Ichthyosis
SBE (subacute bacterial endocarditis) I33.0
Scabies (any site) B86
Scabs R23.4
Scaglietti-Dagnini syndrome E22.0
Scald —*see* Burn
Scalenus anticus (anterior) syndrome G54.0
Scales R23.4
Scaling, skin R23.4
Scalp —*see* condition
Scapegoating affecting child Z62.3
Scaphocephaly, non-deformational Q75.01
Scapulalgia M89.8X1
Scapulohumeral myopathy G71.02
Scar, scarring —*see also* Cicatrix L90.5
  adherent L90.5
  atrophic L90.5
  cervix
    in pregnancy or childbirth —*see* Pregnancy,
        complicated by, abnormal cervix
  cheloid L91.0
  chorioretinal H31.00-●
    posterior pole macula H31.01-●
    postsurgical H59.81-●
    solar retinopathy H31.02-●
    specified type NEC H31.09-●
  choroid —*see* Scar, chorioretinal
  conjunctiva H11.24-●
  cornea H17.9
    xerophthalmic —*see also* Opacity, cornea
        vitamin A deficiency E50.6
  defect (isthmocele) O34.22
  duodenum, obstructive K31.5

Scar, scarring *(Continued)*
  hypertrophic L91.0
  keloid L91.0
  labia N90.89
  lung (base) J98.4
  macula —*see* Scar, chorioretinal, posterior pole
  muscle M62.89
  myocardium, myocardial I25.2
  painful L90.5
  posterior pole (eye) —*see* Scar, chorioretinal,
        posterior pole
  retina —*see* Scar, chorioretinal
  trachea J39.8
  transmural uterine, in pregnancy O34.29
  uterus N85.8
    in pregnancy O34.29
  vagina N89.8
    postoperative N99.2
  vulva N90.89
Scarabiasis B88.2
Scarlatina (anginosa) (maligna) A38.9
  myocarditis (acute) A38.1
    old —*see* Myocarditis
  otitis media A38.0
  ulcerosa A38.8
Scarlet fever (albuminuria) (angina) A38.9
Schamberg's disease (progressive pigmentary
        dermatosis) L81.7
Schatzki's ring (acquired) (esophagus) (lower)
        K22.2
  congenital Q39.3
Schaufenster krankheit I20.89
Schaumann's
  benign lymphogranulomatosis D86.1
  disease or syndrome —*see* Sarcoidosis
Scheie's syndrome E76.03
Schenck's disease B42.1
Scheuermann's disease or osteochondrosis —*see*
        Osteochondrosis, juvenile, spine
Schilder (-Flatau) disease G37.0
Schilling-type monocytic leukemia C93.0-●
Schimmelbusch's disease, cystic mastitis, or
        hyperplasia —*see* Mastopathy, cystic
Schistosoma infestation —*see* Infestation,
        Schistosoma
Schistosomiasis B65.9
  with muscle disorder B65.9 *[M63.80]*
    ankle B65.9 *[M63.87-●]*
    foot B65.9 *[M63.87-●]*
    forearm B65.9 *[M63.83-●]*
    hand B65.9 *[M63.84-●]*
    lower leg B65.9 *[M63.86-●]*
    multiple sites B65.9 *[M63.89]*
    pelvic region B65.9 *[M63.85-●]*
    shoulder region B65.9 *[M63.81-●]*
    specified site NEC B65.9 *[M63.88]*
    thigh B65.9 *[M63.85-●]*
    upper arm B65.9 *[M63.82-●]*
  Asiatic B65.2
  bladder B65.0
  chestermani B65.8
  colon B65.1
  cutaneous B65.3
  due to
    S. haematobium B65.0
    S. japonicum B65.2
    S. mansoni B65.1
    S. mattheii B65.8
  Eastern B65.2
  genitourinary tract B65.0
  intestinal B65.1
  lung NEC B65.9 *[J99]*
    pneumonia B65.9 *[J17]*
  Manson's (intestinal) B65.1
  oriental B65.2
  pulmonary NEC B65.9 *[J99]*
    pneumonia B65.9
  Schistosoma
    haematobium B65.0
    japonicum B65.2
    mansoni B65.1
  specified type NEC B65.8
  urinary B65.0
  vesical B65.0
Schizencephaly Q04.6
Schizoaffective psychosis F25.9
Schizodontia K00.2
Schizoid personality F60.1
Schizophrenia, schizophrenic F20.9
  acute (brief) (undifferentiated) F23
  atypical (form) F20.3

Schizophrenia, schizophrenic *(Continued)*
  borderline F21
  catalepsy F20.2
  catatonic (type) (excited) (withdrawn) F20.2
  cenesthopathic, cenesthesiopathic F20.89
  childhood type F20.9
  chronic undifferentiated F20.9
  cyclic F25.0
  disorganized (type) F20.1
  flexibilitas cerea F20.2
  hebephrenic (type) F20.1
  incipient F21
  latent F21
  negative type F20.5
  paranoid (type) F20.0
  paraphrenic F20.0
  post-psychotic depression F32.89
  prepsychotic F21
  prodromal F21
  pseudoneurotic F21
  pseudopsychopathic F21
  reaction F23
  residual (state) (type) F20.5
  restzustand F20.5
  schizoaffective (type) —*see* Psychosis,
        schizoaffective
  simple (type) F20.89
  simplex F20.89
  specified type NEC F20.89
  spectrum and other psychotic disorder F29
    specified NEC F28
  stupor F20.2
  syndrome of childhood F84.5
  undifferentiated (type) F20.3
    chronic F20.5
Schizothymia (persistent) F60.1
Schlatter-Osgood disease or osteochondrosis
        M92.52-●
Schlatter's tibia —*see* Osteochondrosis, juvenile,
        tibia
Schmidt's syndrome (polyglandular, autoimmune)
        E31.0
Schmincke's carcinoma or tumor —*see* Neoplasm,
        nasopharynx, malignant
Schmitz (-Stutzer) dysentery A03.0
Schmorl's disease or nodes
  lumbar region M51.46
  lumbosacral region M51.47
  sacrococcygeal region M53.3
  thoracic region M51.44
  thoracolumbar region M51.45
Schneiderian
  papilloma —*see* Neoplasm, nasopharynx benign
    specified site —*see* Neoplasm, benign, by site
    unspecified site D14.0
  specified site —*see* Neoplasm, malignant, by site
    unspecified site C30.0
▶ Scholte's syndrome (malignant carcinoid)
        E34.09
Scholz (-Bielchowsky-Henneberg) disease or
        syndrome E75.25
Schönlein (-Henoch) disease or purpura (primary)
        (rheumatic) D69.0
Schottmuller's disease A01.4
Schroeder's syndrome (endocrine hypertensive)
        E27.0
Schüller-Christian disease or syndrome C96.5
Schultze's type acroparesthesia, simple I73.89
Schultz's disease or syndrome —*see*
        Agranulocytosis
Schwalbe-Ziehen-Oppenheim disease G24.1
Schwannoma —*see also* Neoplasm, nerve, benign
  malignant —*see also* Neoplasm, nerve, malignant
    with rhabdomyoblastic differentiation —*see*
        Neoplasm, nerve, malignant
  melanocytic —*see* Neoplasm, nerve, benign
  pigmented —*see* Neoplasm, nerve, benign
Schwannomatosis Q85.03
Schwartz (-Jampel) syndrome G71.13
Schwartz-Bartter syndrome E22.2
~~Schweninger-Buzzi anetoderma L98.1~~
▶ Schweninger-Buzzi anetoderma L90.1
Sciatic —*see* condition
Sciatica (infective) M54.3-●
  with lumbago M54.4-●
    due to intervertebral disc disorder —*see*
        Disorder, disc, with, radiculopathy
  due to displacement of intervertebral disc
        (with lumbago) —*see* Disorder, disc, with,
        radiculopathy
  wallet M54.3-●

Scimitar syndrome Q26.8
Sclera —see condition
Sclerectasia H15.84-●
Scleredema
  adultorum —see Sclerosis, systemic
  Buschke's —see Sclerosis, systemic
  newborn P83.0
Sclerema (adiposum) (edematosum) (neonatorum)
    (newborn) P83.0
  adultorum —see Sclerosis, systemic
Scleriasis —see Scleroderma
Scleritis H15.00-●
  with corneal involvement H15.04-●
  anterior H15.01-●
  brawny H15.02-●
  in (due to) zoster B02.34
  posterior H15.03-●
  specified type NEC H15.09-●
  syphilitic A52.71
  tuberculous (nodular) A18.51
Sclerochoroiditis H31.8
Scleroconjunctivitis —see Scleritis
Sclerocystic ovary syndrome E28.2
Sclerodactyly, sclerodactylia L94.3
Scleroderma, sclerodermia (acrosclerotic) (diffuse)
    (generalized) (progressive) (pulmonary) —see
    also Sclerosis, systemic M34.9-●
  circumscribed L94.0
  linear L94.1
  localized L94.0
  newborn P83.88
  systemic M34.9
Sclerokeratitis H16.8
  tuberculous A18.52
Scleroma nasi A48.8
Scleromalacia (perforans) H15.05-●
Scleromyxedema L98.5
Sclérose en plaques G35
Sclerosis, sclerotic
  adrenal (gland) E27.8
  Alzheimer's —see Disease, Alzheimer's
  amyotrophic (lateral) G12.21
  aorta, aortic I70.0
    valve —see Endocarditis, aortic
  artery, arterial, arteriolar, arteriovascular —see
      Arteriosclerosis
  ascending multiple G35
  brain (generalized) (lobular) G37.9
    artery, arterial I67.2
    diffuse G37.0
    disseminated G35
    insular G35
    Krabbe's E75.23
    miliary G35
    multiple G35
    presenile (Alzheimer's) —see Disease,
        Alzheimer's, early onset
    senile (arteriosclerotic) I67.2
    stem, multiple G35
    tuberous Q85.1
  bulbar, multiple G35
  bundle of His I44.39
  cardiac —see Disease, heart, ischemic,
      atherosclerotic
  cardiorenal —see Hypertension, cardiorenal
  cardiovascular —see also Disease,
      cardiovascular
    renal —see Hypertension, cardiorenal
  cerebellar —see Sclerosis, brain
  cerebral —see Sclerosis, brain
  cerebrospinal (disseminated) (multiple) G35
  cerebrovascular I67.2
  choroid —see Degeneration, choroid
  combined (spinal cord) —see also Degeneration,
      combined
    multiple G35
  concentric (Balo) G37.5
  cornea —see Opacity, cornea
  coronary (artery) I25.10
    with angina pectoris —see Arteriosclerosis,
        coronary (artery),
  corpus cavernosum
    female N90.89
    male N48.6
  diffuse (brain) (spinal cord) G37.0
  disseminated G35
  dorsal G35
  dorsolateral (spinal cord) —see Degeneration,
      combined
  endometrium N85.5
  extrapyramidal G25.9

Sclerosis, sclerotic (Continued)
  eye, nuclear (senile) —see Cataract, senile,
      nuclear
  focal and segmental (glomerular) —see also
      N00-N07 with fourth character .1 N05.1
  Friedreich's (spinal cord) G11.11
  funicular (spermatic cord) N50.89
  general (vascular) —see Arteriosclerosis
  gland (lymphatic) I89.8
  hepatic K74.1
    alcoholic K70.2
  hereditary
    cerebellar G11.9
    spinal (Friedreich's ataxia) G11.11
  hippocampal G93.81
  insular G35
  kidney —see Sclerosis, renal
  larynx J38.7
  lateral (amyotrophic) (descending) (spinal)
      G12.21
    primary G12.23
  lens, senile nuclear —see Cataract, senile, nuclear
  liver K74.1
    with fibrosis K74.2
      alcoholic K70.2
    alcoholic K70.2
    cardiac K76.1
  lung —see Fibrosis, lung
  mastoid —see Mastoiditis, chronic
  mesial temporal G93.81
  mitral I05.8
  Mönckeberg's (medial) —see Arteriosclerosis,
      extremities
  multiple (brain stem) (cerebral) (generalized)
      (spinal cord) G35
  myocardium, myocardial —see Disease, heart,
      ischemic, atherosclerotic
  nuclear (senile), eye —see Cataract, senile,
      nuclear
  ovary N83.8
  pancreas K86.89
  penis N48.6
  peripheral arteries —see Arteriosclerosis,
      extremities
  plaques G35
  pluriglandular E31.8
  polyglandular E31.8
  posterolateral (spinal cord) —see Degeneration,
      combined
  presenile (Alzheimer's) —see Disease,
      Alzheimer's, early onset
  primary, lateral G12.23
  progressive, systemic M34.0
  pulmonary —see Fibrosis, lung
    artery I27.0
    valve (heart) —see Endocarditis, pulmonary
  renal N26.9
    with
      cystine storage disease E72.09
      hypertensive heart disease (conditions in
          I11) —see Hypertension, cardiorenal
      arteriolar (hyaline) (hyperplastic) —see
          Hypertension, kidney
  retina (senile) (vascular) H35.00
  senile (vascular) —see Arteriosclerosis
  spinal (cord) (progressive) G95.89
    ascending G61.0
    combined —see also Degeneration, combined
      multiple G35
      syphilitic A52.11
    disseminated G35
    dorsolateral —see Degeneration, combined
    hereditary (Friedreich's) (mixed form) G11.11
    lateral (amyotrophic) G12.21
      progressive G12.23
    multiple G35
    posterior (syphilitic) A52.11
  stomach K31.89
  subendocardial, congenital I42.4
  systemic M34.9
    with
      lung involvement M34.81
      myopathy M34.82
      polyneuropathy M34.83
    drug-induced M34.2
    due to chemicals NEC M34.2
    progressive M34.0
    specified NEC M34.89
  temporal (mesial) G93.81
  tricuspid (heart) (valve) I07.8
  tuberous (brain) Q85.1

Sclerosis, sclerotic (Continued)
  tympanic membrane —see Disorder, tympanic
      membrane, specified NEC
  valve, valvular (heart) —see Endocarditis
  vascular —see Arteriosclerosis
  vein I87.8
Scoliosis (acquired) (postural) M41.9
  adolescent (idiopathic) —see Scoliosis,
      idiopathic, adolescent
  congenital Q67.5
    due to bony malformation Q76.3
    failure of segmentation (hemivertebra)
        Q76.3
    hemivertebra fusion Q76.3
    postural Q67.5
  degenerative M41.5-●
  idiopathic M41.20
    adolescent M41.129
      cervical region M41.122
      cervicothoracic region M41.123
      lumbar region M41.126
      lumbosacral region M41.127
      thoracic region M41.124
      thoracolumbar region
          M41.125
    cervical region M41.22
    cervicothoracic region M41.23
    infantile M41.00
      cervical region M41.02
      cervicothoracic region M41.03
      lumbar region M41.06
      lumbosacral region M41.07
      sacrococcygeal region M41.08
      thoracic region M41.04
      thoracolumbar region M41.05
    juvenile M41.119
      cervical region M41.112
      cervicothoracic region M41.113
      lumbar region M41.116
      lumbosacral region M41.117
      thoracic region M41.114
      thoracolumbar region M41.115
    lumbar region M41.26
    lumbosacral region M41.27
    thoracic region M41.24
    thoracolumbar region M41.25
  infantile —see Scoliosis, idiopathic, infantile
  neuromuscular M41.40
    cervical region M41.42
    cervicothoracic region M41.43
    lumbar region M41.46
    lumbosacral region M41.47
    occipito-atlanto-axial region M41.41
    thoracic region M41.44
    thoracolumbar region M41.45
  paralytic —see Scoliosis, neuromuscular
  postprocedural M96.89
  postradiation therapy M96.5
  rachitic (late effect or sequelae) E64.3 [M49.80]
    cervical region E64.3 [M49.82]
    cervicothoracic region E64.3 [M49.83]
    lumbar region E64.3 [M49.86]
    lumbosacral region E64.3 [M49.87]
    multiple sites E64.3 [M49.89]
    occipito-atlanto-axial region E64.3 [M49.81]
    sacrococcygeal region E64.3 [M49.88]
    thoracic region E64.3 [M49.84]
    thoracolumbar region E64.3 [M49.85]
  sciatic M54.4-●
  secondary (to) NEC M41.50
    cerebral palsy, Friedreich's ataxia,
        poliomyelitis, neuromuscular
        disorders —see Scoliosis,
        neuromuscular
    cervical region M41.52
    cervicothoracic region M41.53
    lumbar region M41.56
    lumbosacral region M41.57
    thoracic region M41.54
    thoracolumbar region M41.55
  specified form NEC M41.80
    cervical region M41.82
    cervicothoracic region M41.83
    lumbar region M41.86
    lumbosacral region M41.87
    thoracic region M41.84
    thoracolumbar region M41.85
  thoracogenic M41.30
    thoracic region M41.34
    thoracolumbar region M41.35
  tuberculous A18.01

▶ New   ⇒ Revised   ~~deleted~~ Deleted   ● Use Additional Character(s)

Scoliotic pelvis
- with disproportion (fetopelvic) O33.0
  - causing obstructed labor O65.0

Scorbutus, scorbutic —*see also* Scurvy
- anemia D53.2

Score, NIHSS (National Institutes of Health Stroke Scale) R29.7-●

Scotoma (arcuate) (Bjerrum) (central) (ring) —*see also* Defect, visual field, localized, scotoma
- scintillating H53.12-●

Scratch —*see* Abrasion

Scratchy throat R09.89

Screening (for) Z13.9
- alcoholism Z13.33
- anemia Z13.0
- anomaly, congenital Z13.89
- antenatal, of mother —*see also* Encounter, antenatal Z36.9
- arterial hypertension Z13.6
- arthropod-borne viral disease NEC Z11.59
- autism Z13.41
- bacteriuria, asymptomatic Z13.89
  - specified NEC Z13.39
- behavioral disorder Z13.30
- brain injury, traumatic Z13.850
- bronchitis, chronic Z13.83
- brucellosis Z11.2
- cardiovascular disorder Z13.6
- cataract Z13.5
- chlamydial diseases Z11.8
- cholera Z11.0
- chromosomal abnormalities (nonprocreative) NEC Z13.79
- colonoscopy Z12.11
- congenital
  - dislocation of hip Z13.89
  - eye disorder Z13.5
  - malformation or deformation Z13.89
- contamination NEC Z13.88
- coronavirus (disease) (novel) 2019 Z11.52
- COVID-19 Z11.52
- cystic fibrosis Z13.228
- dengue fever Z11.59
- dental disorder Z13.84
- depression (adult) (adolescent) (child) Z13.31
  - maternal Z13.32
  - perinatal Z13.32
- developmental
  - delays Z13.40
    - global (milestones) Z13.42
    - specified NEC Z13.49
  - handicap Z13.42
    - in early childhood Z13.42
- diabetes mellitus Z13.1
- diphtheria Z11.2
- disability, intellectual Z13.39
- disease or disorder Z13.9
  - bacterial NEC Z11.2
    - intestinal infectious Z11.0
    - respiratory tuberculosis Z11.1
  - behavioral Z13.30
    - specified NEC Z13.39
  - developmental delays Z13.40
    - global (milestones) Z13.42
    - specified NEC Z13.49
  - mental health and behavioral Z13.30
    - specified NEC Z13.39
  - blood or blood-forming organ Z13.0
  - cardiovascular Z13.6
  - Chagas' Z11.6
  - chlamydial Z11.8
  - coronavirus (novel) 2019 Z11.52
  - COVID-19 Z11.52
  - dental Z13.89
  - digestive tract NEC Z13.818
    - lower GI Z13.811
    - upper GI Z13.810
  - ear Z13.5
  - endocrine Z13.29
  - eye Z13.5
  - genitourinary Z13.89
  - heart Z13.6
  - human immunodeficiency virus (HIV) infection Z11.4
  - immunity Z13.0
  - infection
    - intestinal Z11.0
      - specified NEC Z11.6
    - infectious Z11.9
  - metabolic Z13.228
  - neurological Z13.89

Screening *(Continued)*
- disease or disorder *(Continued)*
  - nutritional Z13.21
    - metabolic Z13.228
      - lipoid disorders Z13.220
  - protozoal Z11.6
    - intestinal Z11.0
  - respiratory Z13.83
  - rheumatic Z13.828
  - rickettsial Z11.8
  - sexually-transmitted NEC Z11.3
    - human immunodeficiency virus (HIV) Z11.4
  - sickle-cell (trait) Z13.0
  - skin Z13.89
  - specified NEC Z13.89
  - spirochetal Z11.8
  - thyroid Z13.29
  - vascular Z13.6
  - venereal Z11.3
  - viral NEC Z11.59
    - coronavirus (disease) (novel) 2019 Z11.52
    - COVID-19 Z11.52
    - human immunodeficiency virus (HIV) Z11.4
    - intestinal Z11.0
    - SARS-CoV-2 Z11.52
- elevated titer Z13.89
- emphysema Z13.83
- encephalitis, viral (mosquito- or tick-borne) Z11.59
- exposure to contaminants (toxic) Z13.88
- fever
  - dengue Z11.59
  - hemorrhagic Z11.59
  - yellow Z11.59
- filariasis Z11.6
- galactosemia Z13.228
- gastrointestinal condition Z13.818
- genetic (nonprocreative)- for procreative management —*see* Testing, genetic, for procreative management
  - disease carrier status (nonprocreative) Z13.71
  - specified NEC (nonprocreative) Z13.79
- genitourinary condition Z13.89
- glaucoma Z13.5
- gonorrhea Z11.3
- gout Z13.89
- helminthiasis (intestinal) Z11.6
- hematopoietic malignancy Z12.89
- hemoglobinopathies NEC Z13.0
- hemorrhagic fever Z11.59
- Hodgkin disease Z12.89
- human immunodeficiency virus (HIV) Z11.4
- human papillomavirus Z11.51
- hypertension Z13.6
- infant or child (over 28 days old) Z00.129
  - with abnormal findings Z00.121
- immunity disorders Z13.0
- infection
  - mycotic Z11.8
  - parasitic Z11.8
- ingestion of radioactive substance Z13.88
- intellectual disability Z13.39
- intestinal
  - helminthiasis Z11.6
  - infectious disease Z11.0
- leishmaniasis Z11.6
- leprosy Z11.2
- leptospirosis Z11.8
- leukemia Z12.89
- lymphoma Z12.89
- malaria Z11.6
- malnutrition Z13.29
  - metabolic Z13.228
  - nutritional Z13.21
- measles Z11.59
- mental health disorder Z13.30
  - specified NEC Z13.39
- metabolic errors, inborn Z13.228
- multiphasic Z13.89
- musculoskeletal disorder Z13.828
  - osteoporosis Z13.820
- mycoses Z11.8
- myocardial infarction (acute) Z13.6
- neoplasm (malignant) (of) Z12.9
  - bladder Z12.6
  - blood Z12.89
  - breast Z12.39
    - routine mammogram Z12.31
  - cervix Z12.4

Screening *(Continued)*
- neoplasm *(Continued)*
  - colon Z12.11
  - genitourinary organs NEC Z12.79
    - bladder Z12.6
    - cervix Z12.4
    - ovary Z12.73
    - prostate Z12.5
    - testis Z12.71
    - vagina Z12.72
  - hematopoietic system Z12.89
  - intestinal tract Z12.10
    - colon Z12.11
    - rectum Z12.12
    - small intestine Z12.13
  - lung Z12.2
  - lymph (glands) Z12.89
  - nervous system Z12.82
  - oral cavity Z12.81
  - prostate Z12.5
  - rectum Z12.12
  - respiratory organs Z12.2
  - skin Z12.83
  - small intestine Z12.13
  - specified site NEC Z12.89
  - stomach Z12.0
- nephropathy Z13.89
- nervous system disorders NEC Z13.858
- neurological condition Z13.89
- osteoporosis Z13.820
- parasitic infestation Z11.9
  - specified NEC Z11.8
- phenylketonuria Z13.228
- plague Z11.2
- poisoning (chemical) (heavy metal) Z13.88
- poliomyelitis Z11.59
- postnatal, chromosomal abnormalities Z13.89
- prenatal, of mother —*see also* Encounter, antenatal Z36.9
- protozoal disease Z11.6
  - intestinal Z11.0
- pulmonary tuberculosis Z11.1
- radiation exposure Z13.88
- respiratory condition Z13.83
- respiratory tuberculosis Z11.1
- rheumatoid arthritis Z13.828
- rubella Z11.59
- SARS-CoV-2 Z11.52
- schistosomiasis Z11.6
- sexually-transmitted disease NEC Z11.3
  - human immunodeficiency virus (HIV) Z11.4
- sickle-cell disease or trait Z13.0
- skin condition Z13.89
- sleeping sickness Z11.6
- special Z13.9
  - specified NEC Z13.89
- syphilis Z11.3
- tetanus Z11.2
- trachoma Z11.8
- traumatic brain injury Z13.850
- trypanosomiasis Z11.6
- tuberculosis, respiratory Z11.1
  - active Z11.1
  - latent Z11.7
- venereal disease Z11.3
- viral encephalitis (mosquito- or tick-borne) Z11.59
- whooping cough Z11.2
- worms, intestinal Z11.6
- yaws Z11.8
- yellow fever Z11.59

Scrofula, scrofulosis (tuberculosis of cervical lymph glands) A18.2

Scrofulide (primary) (tuberculous) A18.4

Scrofuloderma, scrofulodermia (any site) (primary) A18.4

Scrofulosus lichen (primary) (tuberculous) A18.4

Scrofulous —*see* condition

Scrotal tongue K14.5

Scrotum —*see* condition

Scurvy, scorbutic E54
- anemia D53.2
- gum E54
- infantile E54
- rickets E55.0 *[M90.80]*

Sealpox B08.62

Seasickness T75.3

Seatworm (infection) (infestation) B80

Sebaceous —*see also* condition
- cyst —*see* Cyst, sebaceous

Seborrhea, seborrheic L21.9
  capillitii R23.8
  capitis L21.0
  dermatitis L21.9
    infantile L21.1
  eczema L21.9
    infantile L21.1
  sicca L21.0
Seckel's syndrome Q87.19
Seclusion, pupil —see Membrane, pupillary
Second hand tobacco smoke exposure (acute)
  (chronic) Z77.22
  in the perinatal period P96.81
Secondary
  dentin (in pulp) K04.3
  neoplasm, secondaries —see Table of Neoplasms,
    secondary
Secretion
  antidiuretic hormone, inappropriate E22.2
  catecholamine, by pheochromocytoma (see also
    Pheochromocytoma, by type) E27.5
  hormone
    antidiuretic, inappropriate (syndrome) E22.2
    by
      carcinoid tumor (see also Tumor, carcinoid)
        E34.09
      pheochromocytoma (see also
        Pheochromocytoma, by type) E27.5
    ectopic NEC E34.2
  urinary
    excessive R35.89
    suppression R34
Section
  nerve, traumatic —see Injury, nerve
Sedative, hypnotic, or anxiolytic-induced
  anxiety disorder F13.980
  bipolar and related disorder F13.94
  delirium F13.921
  depressive disorder F13.94
  major neurocognitive disorder F13.97
  mild neurocognitive disorder F13.988
  psychotic disorder F13.959
  sexual dysfunction F13.981
  sleep disorder F13.982
Segmentation, incomplete (congenital) —see also
  Fusion
  bone NEC Q78.8
  lumbosacral (joint) (vertebra) Q76.49
SEID (systemic exertion intolerance disease)
  G93.32
Seitelberger's syndrome (infantile neuraxonal
  dystrophy) G31.89
Seizure(s) —see also Convulsions R56.9
  absence G40.A-●
  akinetic —see Epilepsy, generalized, specified
    NEC
  atonic —see Epilepsy, generalized, specified NEC
  autonomic (hysterical) F44.5
  convulsive —see Convulsions
  cortical (focal) (motor) —see Epilepsy,
    localization-related, symptomatic, with
    simple partial seizures
  disorder —see also Epilepsy G40.909
  due to stroke —see Sequelae (of), disease,
    cerebrovascular, by type, specified NEC
  epileptic —see Epilepsy
  febrile (simple) R56.00
    with status epilepticus G40.901
    complex (atypical) (complicated) R56.01
      with status epilepticus G40.901
  grand mal G40.409
    intractable G40.419
      with status epilepticus G40.411
      without status epilepticus G40.419
    not intractable G40.409
      with status epilepticus G40.401
      without status epilepticus G40.409
  heart —see Disease, heart
  hysterical F44.5
  intractable G40.919
    with status epilepticus G40.911
  Jacksonian (focal) (motor type) (sensory
    type) —see Epilepsy, localization-related,
    symptomatic, with simple partial seizures
  newborn P90
  nonspecific epileptic
    atonic —see Epilepsy, generalized, specified
      NEC
    clonic —see Epilepsy, generalized, specified
      NEC

Seizure (Continued)
  nonspecific epileptic (Continued)
    myoclonic —see Epilepsy, generalized,
      specified NEC
    tonic —see Epilepsy, generalized, specified
      NEC
    tonic-clonic —see Epilepsy, generalized,
      specified NEC
  partial, developing into secondarily generalized
    seizures
    complex —see Epilepsy, localization-related,
      symptomatic, with complex partial
      seizures
    simple —see Epilepsy, localization-related,
      symptomatic, with simple partial
      seizures
  petit mal G40.A-●
    intractable G40.A1-●
      with status epilepticus G40.A11
      without status epilepticus G40.A19
    not intractable G40.A0 -●
      with status epilepticus G40.A01
      without status epilepticus G40.A01
  post traumatic R56.1
  recurrent G40.909
  specified NEC G40.89
  uncinate —see Epilepsy, localization-related,
    symptomatic, with complex partial
    seizures
Selenium deficiency, dietary E59
Self-damaging behavior (life-style) Z72.89
Self-harm (attempted)
  history (personal)
    in family Z81.8
    nonsuicidal Z91.52
    suicidal Z91.51
  nonsuicidal R45.88
Self-injury, nonsuicidal R45.88
  personal history Z91.52
Self-mutilation (attempted)
  history (personal)
    in family Z81.8
    nonsuicidal Z91.52
    suicidal Z91.51
  nonsuicidal R45.88
Self-poisoning
  history (personal)
    in family Z81.8
  observation following (alleged) attempt Z03.6
Semicoma R40.1
Seminal vesiculitis N49.0
Seminoma C62.9-●
  specified site —see Neoplasm, malignant, by site
Senear-Usher disease or syndrome L10.4
Senectus R54
Senescence (without mention of psychosis) R54
Senile, senility —see also condition R41.81
  with
    acute confusional state F05
    mental changes NOS F03
    psychosis NEC —see Psychosis, senile
  asthenia R54
  cervix (atrophic) N88.8
  debility R54
  endometrium (atrophic) N85.8
  fallopian tube (atrophic) —see Atrophy, fallopian
    tube
  heart (failure) R54
  ovary (atrophic) —see Atrophy, ovary
  premature E34.8
  vagina, vaginitis (atrophic) N95.2
  wart L82.1
Sensation
  burning (skin) R20.8
    tongue K14.6
  foreign body R09.A0
    eye H57.8A-●
    globus R09.A2
    nose R09.A1
    specified site NEC R09.A9
    throat R09.A2
  loss of R20.8
  prickling (skin) R20.2
  tingling (skin) R20.2
Sense loss
  smell —see Disturbance, sensation, smell
  taste —see Disturbance, sensation, taste
  touch R20.8
Sensibility disturbance (cortical) (deep)
  (vibratory) R20.9

Sensitive, sensitivity —see also Allergy
  carotid sinus G90.01
  child (excessive) F93.8
  cold, autoimmune D59.12
  dentin K03.89
  gluten (non-celiac) K90.41
  latex Z91.040
  methemoglobin D74.8
  tuberculin, without clinical or radiological
    symptoms R76.11
  visual
    glare H53.71
    impaired contrast H53.72
Sensitiver Beziehungswahn F22
Sensitization, auto-erythrocytic D69.2
Separation
  anxiety, abnormal (of childhood) F93.0
  apophysis, traumatic - code as Fracture, by site
  choroid —see Detachment, choroid
  epiphysis, epiphyseal
    nontraumatic —see also Osteochondropathy,
      specified type NEC
      upper femoral —see Slipped, epiphysis,
        upper femoral
    traumatic - code as Fracture, by site
  fracture —see Fracture
  infundibulum cardiac from right ventricle by a
    partition Q24.3
  joint (traumatic) (current) - code by site under
    Dislocation
  muscle (nontraumatic) —see Diastasis, muscle
  pubic bone, obstetrical trauma O71.6
  retina, retinal —see Detachment, retina
  symphysis pubis, obstetrical trauma O71.6
  tracheal ring, incomplete, congenital Q32.1
Sepsis (generalized) (unspecified organism) A41.9
  with
    organ dysfunction (acute) (multiple) R65.20
      with septic shock R65.21
  Acinetobacter baumannii A41.54
  actinomycotic A42.7
  adrenal hemorrhage syndrome (meningococcal)
    A39.1
  anaerobic A41.4
  Bacillus anthracis A22.7
  Brucella —see also Brucellosis A23.9
  candidal B37.7
  Cronobacter A41.59
  cryptogenic A41.9
  due to device, implant or graft T85.79
    arterial graft NEC T82.7
    breast (implant) T85.79
    catheter NEC T85.79
      dialysis (renal) T82.7
        intraperitoneal T85.71
      infusion NEC T82.7
        spinal (cranial) (epidural) (intrathecal)
          (spinal) (subarachnoid) (subdural)
          T85.735
      urethral indwelling T83.511
      urinary T83.518
    ectopic or molar pregnancy O08.82
    electronic (electrode) (pulse generator)
      (stimulator)
      bone T84.7
      cardiac T82.7
      nervous system T85.738
        brain T85.731
        neurostimulator generator T85.734
        peripheral nerve T85.732
        spinal cord T85.733
      urinary T83.590
    fixation, internal (orthopedic) —see
      Complication, fixation device, infection
    gastrointestinal (bile duct) (esophagus) T85.79
      neurostimulator electrode (lead) T85.732
    genital T83.69
    heart NEC T82.7
      valve (prosthesis) T82.6
        graft T82.7
    joint prosthesis —see Complication, joint
      prosthesis, infection
    ocular (corneal graft) (orbital implant) T85.79
    orthopedic NEC T84.7
      fixation device, internal —see Complication,
        fixation device, infection
    specified NEC T85.79
    vascular T82.7
    ventricular intracranial (communicating)
      shunt T85.730

Sepsis (Continued)
during labor O75.3
Enterococcus A41.81
Erysipelothrix (rhusiopathiae) (erysipeloid)
 A26.7
Escherichia coli (E. coli) A41.51
extraintestinal yersiniosis A28.2
following
 abortion (subsequent episode) O08.0
  current episode —see Abortion
 ectopic or molar pregnancy O08.82
 immunization T88.0
 infusion, therapeutic injection or transfusion
  NEC T80.29
 obstetrical procedure O86.04
gangrenous A41.9
gonococcal A54.86
Gram-negative (organism) A41.50
 anaerobic A41.4
Haemophilus influenzae A41.3
herpesviral B00.7
intra-abdominal K65.1
intraocular —see Endophthalmitis, purulent
Listeria monocytogenes A32.7
localized — code to specific localized infection
 in operation wound T81.49
 skin —see Abscess
malleus A24.0
melioidosis A24.1
meningeal —see Meningitis
meningococcal A39.4
 acute A39.2
 chronic A39.3
MRSA (Methicillin resistant Staphylococcus
 aureus) A41.02
MSSA (Methicillin susceptible Staphylococcus
 aureus) A41.01
newborn P36.9
 due to
  anaerobes NEC P36.5
  Escherichia coli P36.4
  Staphylococcus P36.30
   aureus P36.2
   specified NEC P36.39
  Streptococcus P36.10
   group B P36.0
   specified NEC P36.19
 specified NEC P36.8
other gram-negative A41.59
Pasteurella multocida A28.0
pelvic, puerperal, postpartum, childbirth O85
pneumococcal A40.3
postprocedural T81.44
Pseudomonas (pseudomonas aeruginosa) A41.52
puerperal, postpartum, childbirth (pelvic) O85
Salmonella (arizonae) (cholerae-suis) (enteritidis)
 (typhimurium) A02.1
Serratia A41.53
severe R65.20
 with septic shock R65.21
Shigella (see also Dysentery, bacillary) A03.9
skin, localized —see Abscess
specified organism NEC A41.89
Staphylococcus, staphylococcal A41.2
 aureus (methicillin susceptible) (MSSA) A41.01
  methicillin resistant (MRSA) A41.02
 coagulase-negative A41.1
 specified NEC A41.1
Streptococcus, streptococcal A40.9
 agalactiae A40.1
 group
  A A40.0
  B A40.1
  D A41.81
 neonatal P36.10
  group B P36.0
  specified NEC P36.19
 pneumoniae A40.3
 pyogenes A40.0
 specified NEC A40.8
tracheostomy stoma J95.02
tularemic A21.7
umbilical, umbilical cord (newborn) —see Sepsis,
 newborn
Yersinia pestis A20.7
Septate —see Septum
Septic —see condition
arm —see Cellulitis, upper limb
 with lymphangitis —see Lymphangitis, acute,
  upper limb

Septic (Continued)
embolus —see Embolism
finger —see Cellulitis, digit
 with lymphangitis —see Lymphangitis, acute,
  digit
foot —see Cellulitis, lower limb
 with lymphangitis —see Lymphangitis, acute,
  lower limb
gallbladder (acute) K81.0
hand —see Cellulitis, upper limb
 with lymphangitis —see Lymphangitis, acute,
  upper limb
joint —see Arthritis, pyogenic or pyemic
leg —see Cellulitis, lower limb
 with lymphangitis —see Lymphangitis, acute,
  lower limb
nail —see also Cellulitis, digit
 with lymphangitis —see Lymphangitis, acute,
  digit
sore —see also Abscess
 throat J02.0
  streptococcal J02.0
spleen (acute) D73.89
teeth, tooth (pulpal origin) K04.4
throat —see Pharyngitis
thrombus —see Thrombosis
toe —see Cellulitis, digit
 with lymphangitis —see Lymphangitis, acute,
  digit
tonsils, chronic J35.01
 with adenoiditis J35.03
uterus —see Endometritis
Septicemia A41.9
meaning sepsis —see Sepsis
Septum, septate (congenital) —see also Anomaly,
 by site
anal Q42.3
 with fistula Q42.2
aqueduct of Sylvius Q03.0
 with spina bifida —see Spina bifida, by site,
  with hydrocephalus
uterus (complete) (partial) Q51.28
 complete Q51.21
 partial Q51.22
 specified NEC Q51.28
vagina Q52.10
 in pregnancy —see Pregnancy, complicated by,
  abnormal vagina
  causing obstructed labor O65.5
 longitudinal Q52.129
  microperforate
   left side Q52.124
   right side Q52.123
  nonobstruction Q52.120
  obstructing Q52.129
   left side Q52.122
   right side Q52.121
 transverse Q52.11
Sequelae (of) —see also condition
abscess, intracranial or intraspinal (conditions in
 G06) G09
amputation — code to injury with seventh
 character S
burn and corrosion — code to injury with
 seventh character S
calcium deficiency E64.8
cerebrovascular disease —see Sequelae, disease,
 cerebrovascular
childbirth O94
contusion — code to injury with seventh
 character S
corrosion —see Sequelae, burn and corrosion
COVID-19 (post acute) U09.9
crushing injury — code to injury with seventh
 character S
disease
 cerebrovascular I69.90
  alteration of sensation I69.998
  aphasia I69.920
  apraxia I69.990
  ataxia I69.993
  cognitive deficits I69.91
  disturbance of vision I69.998
  dysarthria I69.922
  dysphagia I69.991
  dysphasia I69.921
  facial droop I69.992
  facial weakness I69.992
  fluency disorder I69.923
  hemiplegia I69.95-●

Sequelae (Continued)
disease (Continued)
 cerebrovascular (Continued)
  hemorrhage
   intracerebral —see Sequelae, hemorrhage,
    intracerebral
   intracranial, nontraumatic NEC —see
    Sequelae, hemorrhage, intracranial,
    nontraumatic
   subarachnoid —see Sequelae,
    hemorrhage, subarachnoid
  language deficit I69.928
  monoplegia
   lower limb I69.94-●
   upper limb I69.93-●
  paralytic syndrome I69.96-●
  specified effect NEC I69.998
  specified type NEC I69.80
   alteration of sensation I69.898
   aphasia I69.820
   apraxia I69.890
   ataxia I69.893
   cognitive deficits I69.81
   disturbance of vision I69.898
   dysarthria I69.822
   dysphagia I69.891
   dysphasia I69.821
   facial droop I69.892
   facial weakness I69.892
   fluency disorder I69.823
   hemiplegia I69.85-●
   language deficit I69.828
   monoplegia
    lower limb I69.84-●
    upper limb I69.83-●
   paralytic syndrome I69.86-●
   specified effect NEC I69.898
  speech deficit I69.928
  speech deficit I69.828
  stroke NOS —see Sequelae, stroke NOS
dislocation — code to injury with seventh
 character S
encephalitis or encephalomyelitis (conditions in
 G04) G09
 in infectious disease NEC B94.8
 viral B94.1
external cause — code to injury with seventh
 character S
foreign body entering natural orifice — code to
 injury with seventh character S
fracture — code to injury with seventh character
 S
frostbite — code to injury with seventh character
 S
Hansen's disease B92
hemorrhage
 intracerebral I69.10
  alteration of sensation I69.198
  aphasia I69.120
  apraxia I69.190
  ataxia I69.193
  cognitive deficits I69.11
  disturbance of vision I69.198
  dysarthria I69.122
  dysphagia I69.191
  dysphasia I69.121
  facial droop I69.192
  facial weakness I69.192
  fluency disorder I69.123
  hemiplegia I69.15-●
  language deficit NEC I69.128
  monoplegia
   lower limb I69.14-●
   upper limb I69.13-●
  paralytic syndrome I69.16-●
  specified effect NEC I69.198
  speech deficit NEC I69.128
 intracranial, nontraumatic NEC I69.20
  alteration of sensation I69.298
  aphasia I69.220
  apraxia I69.290
  ataxia I69.293
  cognitive deficits I69.21
  disturbance of vision I69.298
  dysarthria I69.222
  dysphagia I69.291
  dysphasia I69.221
  facial droop I69.292
  facial weakness I69.292
  fluency disorder I69.223

Sequelae *(Continued)*
  hemorrhage *(Continued)*
    intracranial, nontraumatic *(Continued)*
      hemiplegia I69.25-●
      language deficit NEC I69.228
      monoplegia
        lower limb I69.24-●
        upper limb I69.23-●
      paralytic syndrome I69.26-●
      specified effect NEC I69.298
      speech deficit NEC I69.228
    subarachnoid I69.00
      alteration of sensation I69.098
      aphasia I69.020
      apraxia I69.090
      ataxia I69.093
      cognitive deficits —*see* subcategory I69.01-●
      disturbance of vision I69.098
      dysarthria I69.022
      dysphagia I69.091
      dysphasia I69.021
      facial droop I69.092
      facial weakness I69.092
      fluency disorder I69.023
      hemiplegia I69.05-●
      language deficit NEC I69.028
      monoplegia
        lower limb I69.04-●
        upper limb I69.03-●
      paralytic syndrome I69.06-●
      specified effect NEC I69.098
      speech deficit NEC I69.028
  hepatitis, viral B94.2
  hyperalimentation E68
  infarction
    cerebral I69.30
      alteration of sensation I69.398
      aphasia I69.320
      apraxia I69.390
      ataxia I69.393
      cognitive deficits I69.31
      disturbance of vision I69.398
      dysarthria I69.322
      dysphagia I69.391
      dysphasia I69.321
      facial droop I69.392
      facial weakness I69.392
      fluency disorder I69.323
      hemiplegia I69.35-●
      language deficit NEC I69.328
      monoplegia
        lower limb I69.34-●
        upper limb I69.33-●
      paralytic syndrome I69.36-●
      specified effect NEC I69.398
      speech deficit NEC I69.328
  infection, pyogenic, intracranial or intraspinal G09
  infectious disease B94.9
    specified NEC B94.8
  injury — code to injury with seventh character S
  leprosy B92
  meningitis
    bacterial (conditions in G00) G09
    other or unspecified cause (conditions in G03) G09
  muscle (and tendon) injury — code to injury with seventh character S
  myelitis —*see* Sequelae, encephalitis
  niacin deficiency E64.8
  nutritional deficiency E64.9
    specified NEC E64.8
  obstetrical condition O94
  parasitic disease B94.9
  phlebitis or thrombophlebitis of intracranial or intraspinal venous sinuses and veins (conditions in G08) G09
  poisoning — code to poisoning with seventh character S
    nonmedicinal substance —*see* Sequelae, toxic effect, nonmedicinal substance
  poliomyelitis (acute) B91
  pregnancy O94
  protein-energy malnutrition E64.0
  puerperium O94
  rickets E64.3
  SARS-CoV-2 (post acute) U09.9
  selenium deficiency E64.8
  sprain and strain — code to injury with seventh character S

Sequelae *(Continued)*
  stroke NOS I69.30
    alteration in sensation I69.398
    aphasia I69.320
    apraxia I69.390
    ataxia I69.393
    cognitive deficits I69.31
    disturbance of vision I69.398
    dysarthria I69.322
    dysphagia I69.391
    dysphasia I69.321
    facial droop I69.392
    facial weakness I69.392
    hemiplegia I69.35-●
    language deficit NEC I69.328
    monoplegia
      lower limb I69.34-●
      upper limb I69.33-●
    paralytic syndrome I69.36-●
    specified effect NEC I69.398
    speech deficit NEC I69.328
  tendon and muscle injury — code to injury with seventh character S
  thiamine deficiency E64.8
  trachoma B94.0
  tuberculosis B90.9
    bones and joints B90.2
    central nervous system B90.0
    genitourinary B90.1
    pulmonary (respiratory) B90.9
    specified organs NEC B90.8
  viral
    encephalitis B94.1
    hepatitis B94.2
  vitamin deficiency NEC E64.8
    A E64.1
    B E64.8
    C E64.2
  wound, open — code to injury with seventh character S
Sequestration —*see also* Sequestrum
  disc —*see* Displacement, intervertebral disc
  lung, congenital Q33.2
Sequestrum
  bone —*see* Osteomyelitis, chronic
  dental M27.2
  jaw bone M27.2
  orbit —*see* Osteomyelitis, orbit
  sinus (accessory) (nasal) —*see* Sinusitis
Sequoiosis lung or pneumonitis J67.8
Serology for syphilis
  doubtful
    with signs or symptoms - code by site and stage under Syphilis
    follow-up of latent syphilis —*see* Syphilis, latent
  negative, with signs or symptoms — code by site and stage under Syphilis
  positive A53.0
    with signs or symptoms - code by site and stage under Syphilis
  reactivated A53.0
Seroma —*see also* Hematoma
  postprocedural —*see* Complication, postprocedural, seroma
  traumatic, secondary and recurrent T79.2
Seropurulent —*see* condition
Serositis, multiple K65.8
  pericardial I31.1
  peritoneal K65.8
Serous —*see* condition
Sertoli cell
  adenoma
    specified site —*see* Neoplasm, benign, by site
    unspecified site
      female D27.9
      male D29.20
  carcinoma
    specified site —*see* Neoplasm, malignant, by site
    unspecified site (male) C62.9-●
      female C56.9
  tumor
    with lipid storage
      specified site —*see* Neoplasm, benign, by site
      unspecified site
        female D27.9
        male D29.20
    specified site —*see* Neoplasm, benign, by site
    unspecified site
      female D27.9
      male D29.20

Sertoli-Leydig cell tumor —*see* Neoplasm, benign, by site
  specified site —*see* Neoplasm, benign, by site
  unspecified site
    female D27.9
    male D29.20
Serum
  allergy, allergic reaction —*see also* Reaction, serum T80.69
    shock —*see also* Shock, anaphylactic T80.59
  arthritis —*see also* Reaction, serum T80.69
  complication or reaction NEC —*see also* Reaction, serum T80.69
  disease NEC —*see also* Reaction, serum T80.69
  hepatitis —*see also* Hepatitis, viral, type B carrier (suspected) of B18.1
  intoxication —*see also* Reaction, serum T80.69
  neuritis —*see also* Reaction, serum T80.69
  neuropathy G61.1
  poisoning NEC —*see also* Reaction, serum T80.69
  rash NEC —*see also* Reaction, serum T80.69
  reaction NEC —*see also* Reaction, serum T80.69
  sickness NEC —*see also* Reaction, serum T80.69
  urticaria —*see also* Reaction, serum T80.69
Sesamoiditis M25.8-●
Sever's disease or osteochondrosis —*see* Osteochondrosis, juvenile, tarsus
Severe sepsis R65.20
  with septic shock R65.21
Sex
  chromosome mosaics Q97.8
    lines with various numbers of X chromosomes Q97.2
  education Z70.8
  reassignment surgery status Z87.890
Sextuplet pregnancy —*see* Pregnancy, sextuplet
Sexual
  function, disorder of (psychogenic) F52.9
  immaturity (female) (male) E30.0
  impotence (psychogenic) organic origin NEC — *see* Dysfunction, sexual, male
  precocity (constitutional) (cryptogenic) (female) (idiopathic) (male) E30.1
Sexuality, pathologic —*see* Deviation, sexual
Sézary disease C84.1-●
Shadow, lung R91.8
Shaking palsy or paralysis —*see* Parkinsonism
Shallowness, acetabulum —*see* Derangement, joint, specified type NEC, hip
Shaver's disease J63.1
Sheath (tendon) —*see* condition
Sheathing, retinal vessels H35.01-●
Shedding
  nail L60.8
  premature, primary (deciduous) teeth K00.6
Sheehan's disease or syndrome E23.0
Shelf, rectal K62.89
Shell teeth K00.5
Shellshock (current) F43.0
  lasting state —*see* Disorder, post-traumatic stress
Shield kidney Q63.1
Shift
  auditory threshold (temporary) H93.24-●
  mediastinal R93.89
Shifting sleep-work schedule (affecting sleep) G47.26
Shiga (-Kruse) dysentery A03.0
Shiga's bacillus A03.0
Shigella (dysentery) —*see* Dysentery, bacillary
Shigellosis A03.9
  Group A A03.0
  Group B A03.1
  Group C A03.2
  Group D A03.3
Shin splints S86.89
Shingles —*see* Herpes, zoster
Shipyard disease or eye B30.0
Shirodkar suture, in pregnancy —*see* Pregnancy, complicated by, incompetent cervix
Shock R57.9
  with ectopic or molar pregnancy O08.3
  adrenal (cortical) (Addisonian) E27.2
  adverse food reaction (anaphylactic) —*see* Shock, anaphylactic, due to food
  allergic —*see* Shock, anaphylactic

▶ New   ➡ Revised   ~~deleted~~ Deleted   ● Use Additional Character(s)

Sickness *(Continued)*
  aviator's T70.29
  balloon T70.29
  car T75.3
  compressed air T70.3
  decompression T70.3
  green D50.8
  milk —*see* Poisoning, food, noxious
  motion T75.3
  mountain T70.29
    acute D75.1
  protein —*see also* Reaction, serum T80.69
  radiation T66
  roundabout (motion) T75.3
  sea T75.3
  serum NEC —*see also* Reaction, serum T80.69
  sleeping (African) B56.9
    by Trypanosoma B56.9
      brucei
        gambiense B56.0
        rhodesiense B56.1
      East African B56.1
      Gambian B56.0
      Rhodesian B56.1
      West African B56.0
  swing (motion) T75.3
  train (railway) (travel) T75.3
  travel (any vehicle) T75.3
Sideropenia —*see* Anemia, iron deficiency
Siderosilicosis J62.8
Siderosis (lung) J63.4
  brain G93.89
  eye (globe) —*see* Disorder, globe, degenerative,
    siderosis
Siemens' syndrome (ectodermal dysplasia)
    Q82.8
Sighing R06.89
  psychogenic F45.8
Sigmoid —*see also* condition
  flexure —*see* condition
  kidney Q63.1
Sigmoiditis —*see also* Enteritis K52.9
  infectious A09
  noninfectious K52.9
Silfversköld's syndrome Q78.9
Silicosiderosis J62.8
Silicosis, silicotic (simple) (complicated) J62.8
  with tuberculosis J65
Silicotuberculosis J65
Silo-fillers' disease J68.8
  bronchitis J68.0
  pneumonitis J68.0
  pulmonary edema J68.1
Silver's syndrome Q87.19
Simian malaria B53.1
Simmonds' cachexia or disease E23.0
Simons' disease or syndrome (progressive
    lipodystrophy) E88.1
Simple, simplex —*see* condition
Simulation, conscious (of illness) Z76.5
Simultanagnosia (asimultagnosia) R48.3
Sin Nombre virus disease (Hantavirus) (cardio)-
    pulmonary syndrome) B33.4
Sinding-Larsen disease or osteochondrosis —*see*
    Osteochondrosis, juvenile, patella
Singapore hemorrhagic fever A91
Singer's node or nodule J38.2
Single
  atrium Q21.20
  coronary artery Q24.5
  umbilical artery Q27.0
  ventricle Q20.4
Singultus R06.6
  epidemicus B33.0
Sinus —*see also* Fistula
  abdominal K63.89
  arrest I45.5
  arrhythmia I49.8
  bradycardia R00.1
  branchial cleft (internal) (external) Q18.0
  coccygeal —*see* Sinus, pilonidal
  dental K04.6
  dermal (congenital) Q06.8
    with abscess Q06.8
    coccygeal, pilonidal —*see* Sinus,
      coccygeal
  infected, skin NEC L08.89
  marginal, ruptured or bleeding —*see*
    Hemorrhage, antepartum, specified cause
    NEC
  medial, face and neck Q18.8

Sinus *(Continued)*
  pause I45.5
  pericranii Q01.9
  pilonidal (infected) (rectum) L05.92
    with abscess L05.02
  preauricular Q18.1
  rectovaginal N82.3
  Rokitansky-Aschoff (gallbladder) K82.8
  sacrococcygeal (dermoid) (infected) —*see* Sinus,
    pilonidal
  tachycardia R00.0
    paroxysmal I47.19
  tarsi syndrome M25.57-•
  testis N50.89
  tract (postinfective) —*see* Fistula
  urachus Q64.4
Sinusitis (accessory) (chronic) (hyperplastic)
    (nasal) (nonpurulent) (purulent) J32.9
  acute J01.90
    ethmoidal J01.20
      recurrent J01.21
    frontal J01.10
      recurrent J01.11
    involving more than one sinus, other than
      pansinusitis J01.80
      recurrent J01.81
    maxillary J01.00
      recurrent J01.01
    pansinusitis J01.40
      recurrent J01.41
    recurrent J01.91
    specified NEC J01.80
      recurrent J01.81
    sphenoidal J01.30
      recurrent J01.31
  allergic —*see* Rhinitis, allergic
  due to high altitude T70.1
  ethmoidal J32.2
    acute J01.20
      recurrent J01.21
  frontal J32.1
    acute J01.10
      recurrent J01.11
  influenzal —*see* Influenza, with, respiratory
    manifestations NEC
  involving more than one sinus but not
      pansinusitis J32.8
    acute J01.80
      recurrent J01.81
  maxillary J32.0
    acute J01.00
      recurrent J01.01
  sphenoidal J32.3
    acute J01.30
      recurrent J01.31
  tuberculous, any sinus A15.8
Sinusitis-bronchiectasis-situs inversus
    (syndrome) (triad) Q89.3
Sipple's syndrome E31.22
Sirenomelia (syndrome) Q87.2
Siriasis T67.01
Sirkari's disease B55.0
Siti A65
Situation, psychiatric F99
Situational
  disturbance (transient) —*see* Disorder,
    adjustment
    acute F43.0
  maladjustment —*see* Disorder, adjustment
  reaction —*see* Disorder, adjustment
    acute F43.0
Situs inversus or transversus (abdominalis)
    (thoracis) Q89.3
Sixth disease B08.20
  due to human herpesvirus 6 B08.21
  due to human herpesvirus 7 B08.22
Sjögren-Larsson syndrome Q87.19
Sjögren's syndrome or disease —*see* Syndrome,
    Sjogren
Skeletal —*see* condition
Skene's gland —*see* condition
Skenitis —*see* Urethritis
Skerljevo A65
Skevas-Zerfus disease —*see* Toxicity, venom,
    marine animal, sea anemone
Skin —*see also* condition
  clammy R23.1
  donor —*see* Donor, skin
  dry L85.3
  hidebound M35.9
Slate-dressers' or slate-miners' lung J62.8

Sleep
  apnea —*see* Apnea, sleep
  deprivation Z72.820
  disorder or disturbance G47.9
    child F51.9
    nonorganic origin F51.9
    specified NEC G47.8
  disturbance G47.9
    nonorganic origin F51.9
  drunkenness F51.9
  rhythm inversion G47.2-•
  terrors F51.4
  walking F51.3
    hysterical F44.89
Sleep hygiene
  abuse Z72.821
  inadequate Z72.821
  poor Z72.821
Sleeping sickness —*see* Sickness, sleeping
Sleeplessness —*see* Insomnia
  menopausal N95.11
Sleep-wake schedule disorder G47.20
Slim disease (in HIV infection) B20
Slipped, slipping
  epiphysis (traumatic) —*see also*
    Osteochondropathy, specified type
    NEC
    capital femoral (traumatic) [SCFE]
      acute (on chronic) S79.01-•
      nontraumatic M93.00-•
    current traumatic - code as Fracture, by site
    upper femoral (nontraumatic) [SUFE]
      M93.00-•
      acute M93.01-•
        on chronic M93.03-•
      chronic M93.02-•
  intervertebral disc —*see* Displacement,
    intervertebral disc
  ligature, umbilical P51.8
  patella —*see* Disorder, patella, derangement NEC
  rib M89.8X8
  sacroiliac joint —*see* subcategory M53.2
  tendon —*see* Disorder, tendon
  ulnar nerve, nontraumatic —*see* Lesion, nerve,
    ulnar
  vertebra NEC —*see* Spondylolisthesis
Slocumb's syndrome E27.0
Sloughing (multiple) (phagedena) (skin) —*see also*
    Gangrene
  abscess —*see* Abscess
  appendix K38.8
  fascia —*see* Disorder, soft tissue, specified type
    NEC
  scrotum N50.89
  tendon —*see* Disorder, tendon
  transplanted organ —*see* Rejection, transplant
  ulcer —*see* Ulcer, skin
Slow
  feeding, newborn P92.2
  flow syndrome, coronary I20.89
  heart(beat) R00.1
Slowing, urinary stream R39.198
Sluder's neuralgia (syndrome) G44.89
Slurred, slurring speech R47.81
Small (ness)
  for gestational age —*see* Small for dates
  introitus, vagina N89.6
  kidney (unknown cause) N27.9
    bilateral N27.1
    unilateral N27.0
  ovary (congenital) Q50.39
  pelvis
    with disproportion (fetopelvic) O33.1
      causing obstructed labor O65.1
  uterus N85.8
  white kidney N03.9
Small-and-light-for-dates —*see* Small for dates
Small-for-dates (infant) P05.10
  with weight of
    499 grams or less P05.11
    500-749 grams P05.12
    750-999 grams P05.13
    1000-1249 grams P05.14
    1250-1499 grams P05.15
    1500-1749 grams P05.16
    1750-1999 grams P05.17
    2000-2499 grams P05.18
    2500 grams and over P05.19
  specified NEC P05.19
Smallpox B03
Smearing, fecal R15.1

► New   ⇒ Revised   ~~deleted~~ Deleted   • Use Additional Character(s)

SMEI (severe myoclonic epilepsy in infancy)
   G40.83-●
Smith-Lemli-Opitz syndrome E78.72
Smith's fracture S52.54-●
Smoker —see Dependence, drug, nicotine
Smoker's
   bronchitis J41.0
   cough J41.0
   palate K13.24
   throat J31.2
   tongue K13.24
Smoking
   passive Z77.22
Smothering spells R06.81
Snaggle teeth, tooth M26.39
Snapping
   finger —see Trigger finger
   hip —see Derangement, joint, specified type
      NEC, hip
      involving the iliotibial band M76.3-●
   knee —see Derangement, knee
      involving the iliotibial band M76.3-●
Sneddon-Wilkinson disease or syndrome
   (sub-corneal pustular dermatosis)
   L13.1
Sneezing (intractable) R06.7
Sniffing
   cocaine
      abuse —see Abuse, drug, cocaine
      dependence —see Dependence, drug, cocaine
   gasoline
      abuse —see Abuse, drug, inhalant
      dependence —see Dependence, drug, inhalant
   glue (airplane)
      abuse —see Abuse, drug, inhalant
      drug dependence —see Dependence, drug,
         inhalant
Sniffles
   newborn P28.89
Snoring R06.83
Snow blindness —see Photokeratitis
Snuffles (non-syphilitic) R06.5
   newborn P28.89
   syphilitic (infant) A50.05 [J99]
Social
   exclusion Z60.4
      due to discrimination or persecution
         (perceived) Z60.5
   migrant Z59.00
      acculturation difficulty Z60.3
   rejection Z60.4
      due to discrimination or persecution Z60.5
   role conflict NEC Z73.5
   skills inadequacy NEC Z73.4
   transplantation Z60.3
Sodoku A25.0
Soemmering's ring —see Cataract, secondary
Soft —see also condition
   nails L60.3
Softening
   bone —see Osteomalacia
   brain (necrotic) (progressive) G93.89
      congenital Q04.8
      embolic I63.4-●
      hemorrhagic —see Hemorrhage, intracranial,
         intracerebral
      occlusive I63.5-●
      thrombotic I63.3-●
   cartilage M94.2-●
      patella M22.4-●
   cerebellar —see Softening, brain
   cerebral —see Softening, brain
   cerebrospinal —see Softening, brain
   myocardial, heart —see Degeneration,
      myocardial
   spinal cord G95.89
   stomach K31.89
Soldier's
   heart F45.8
   patches I31.0
Solitary
   cyst, kidney N28.1
   kidney, congenital Q60.0
Solvent abuse —see Abuse, drug, inhalant
   dependence —see Dependence, drug, inhalant
Somatization reaction, somatic reaction —see
   Disorder, somatoform
Somnambulism F51.3
   hysterical F44.89
Somnolence R40.0
   nonorganic origin F51.11

Sonne dysentery A03.3
Soor B37.0
Sore
   bed —see Ulcer, pressure, by site
   chiclero B55.1
   Delhi B55.1
   desert —see Ulcer, skin
   eye H57.1-●
   Lahore B55.1
   mouth K13.79
      canker K12.0
   muscle M79.10
   Naga —see Ulcer, skin
   of skin —see Ulcer, skin - oriental B55.1
   pressure —see Ulcer, pressure, by site
   skin L98.9
   soft A57
   throat (acute) —see also Pharyngitis
      with influenza, flu, or grippe —see Influenza,
         with, respiratory manifestations NEC
      chronic J31.2
      coxsackie (virus) B08.5
      diphtheritic A36.0
      herpesviral B00.2
      influenzal —see Influenza, with, respiratory
         manifestations NEC
      septic J02.0
      streptococcal (ulcerative) J02.0
      viral NEC J02.8
         coxsackie B08.5
   tropical —see Ulcer, skin
   veldt —see Ulcer, skin
Soto's syndrome (cerebral gigantism) Q87.3
South African cardiomyopathy syndrome I42.8
Southeast Asian hemorrhagic fever A91
Spacing
   abnormal, tooth, teeth, fully erupted M26.30
   excessive, tooth, fully erupted M26.32
Spade-like hand (congenital) Q68.1
Spading nail L60.8
   congenital Q84.6
Spanish collar N47.1
Sparganosis B70.1
Spasm(s), spastic, spasticity —see also condition
   R25.2
   accommodation —see Spasm, of accommodation
   ampulla of Vater K83.4
   anus, ani (sphincter) (reflex) K59.4
      psychogenic F45.8
   artery I73.9
      cerebral G45.9
   Bell's G51.3-●
   bladder (sphincter, external or internal) N32.89
      psychogenic F45.8
   bronchus, bronchiole J98.01
   cardia K22.0
   cardiac I20.1
   carpopedal —see Tetany
   cerebral (arteries) (vascular) G45.9
   cervix, complicating delivery O62.4
   ciliary body (of accommodation) —see Spasm, of
      accommodation
   colon —see also Irritable, bowel K58.9
      with diarrhea K58.0
      psychogenic F45.8
   common duct K83.8
   compulsive —see Tic
   conjugate H51.8
   coronary (artery) I20.1
   diaphragm (reflex) R06.6
      epidemic B33.0
      psychogenic F45.8
   duodenum K59.89
   epidemic diaphragmatic (transient) B33.0
   esophagus (diffuse) K22.4
      psychogenic F45.8
   facial G51.3-●
   fallopian tube N83.8
   gastrointestinal (tract) K31.89
      psychogenic F45.8
   glottis J38.5
      hysterical F44.4
      psychogenic F45.8
         conversion reaction F44.4
      reflex through recurrent laryngeal nerve J38.5
   habit —see Tic
   heart I20.1
   hemifacial (clonic) G51.3-●
   hourglass —see Contraction, hourglass
   hysterical F44.4
   infantile —see Epilepsy, spasms

Spasm (Continued)
   inferior oblique, eye H51.8
   intestinal —see also Syndrome, irritable bowel
      K58.9
      psychogenic F45.8
   larynx, laryngeal J38.5
      hysterical F44.4
      psychogenic F45.8
         conversion reaction F44.4
   levator palpebrae superioris —see Disorder,
      eyelid function
   muscle NEC M62.838
      back M62.830
   nerve, trigeminal G51.0
   nervous F45.8
   nodding F98.4
   occupational F48.8
   oculogyric H51.8
      psychogenic F45.8
   of accommodation H52.53-●
   ophthalmic artery —see Occlusion, artery, retina
   perineal, female N94.89
   peroneo-extensor —see also Deformity, limb, flat
      foot
   pharynx (reflex) J39.2
      hysterical F45.8
      psychogenic F45.8
   psychogenic F45.8
   pylorus NEC K31.3
      adult hypertrophic K31.89
      congenital or infantile Q40.0
      psychogenic F45.8
   rectum (sphincter) K59.4
      psychogenic F45.8
   retinal (artery) —see Occlusion, artery, retina
   sigmoid —see also Syndrome, irritable bowel
      K58.9
      psychogenic F45.8
   sphincter of Oddi K83.4
   stomach K31.89
      neurotic F45.8
   throat J39.2
      hysterical F45.8
      psychogenic F45.8
   tic F95.9
      chronic F95.1
      transient of childhood F95.0
   tongue K14.8
   torsion (progressive) G24.1
   trigeminal nerve —see Neuralgia, trigeminal
   ureter N13.5
   urethra (sphincter) N35.919
   uterus N85.8
      complicating labor O62.4
   vagina N94.2
      psychogenic F52.5
   vascular I73.9
   vasomotor I73.9
   vein NEC I87.8
   viscera —see Pain, abdominal
Spasmodic —see condition
Spasmophilia —see Tetany
Spasmus nutans F98.4
Spastic, spasticity —see also Spasm
   child (cerebral) (congenital) (paralysis) G80.1
Speaker's throat R49.8
Specific, specified —see condition
Speech
   defect, disorder, disturbance, impediment —see
      Disorder, speech R47.9
      psychogenic, in childhood and adolescence
         F98.8
      slurring R47.81
      specified NEC R47.89
Spells, transient oxygen desaturation of newborn
   (see also Apnea, newborn) P28.40
   during sleep (see also Apnea, newborn, sleep,
      primary) P28.30
Spencer's disease A08.19
Spens' syndrome (syncope with heart block) I45.9
Sperm counts (fertility testing) Z31.41
   postvasectomy Z30.8
      reversal Z31.42
Spermatic cord —see condition
Spermatocele N43.40
   congenital Q55.4
   multiple N43.42
   single N43.41
Spermatocystitis N49.0
Spermatocytoma C62.9-●
   specified site —see Neoplasm, malignant, by site

Spermatorrhea N50.89
Sphacelus —see Gangrene
Sphenoidal —see condition
Sphenoiditis (chronic) —see Sinusitis, sphenoidal
Sphenopalatine ganglion neuralgia G90.09
Sphericity, increased, lens (congenital) Q12.4
Spherocytosis (congenital) (familial) (hereditary)
    D58.0
    hemoglobin disease D58.0
    sickle-cell (disease) D57.8-●
Spherophakia Q12.4
Sphincter —see condition
Sphincteritis, sphincter of Oddi —see Cholangitis
Sphingolipidosis E75.3
    specified NEC E75.29
Sphingomyelinosis E75.3
Spicule tooth K00.2
Spider
    bite —see Toxicity, venom, spider
        nonvenomous —see Bite, by site, superficial,
            insect
    fingers —see Syndrome, Marfan
    nevus I78.1
    toes —see Syndrome, Marfan
    vascular I78.1
Spiegler-Fendt
    benign lymphocytoma L98.8
    sarcoid L08.89
Spielmeyer-Vogt disease E75.4
Spina bifida (aperta) Q05.9
    with hydrocephalus NEC Q05.4
    cervical Q05.5
        with hydrocephalus Q05.0
    dorsal Q05.6
        with hydrocephalus Q05.1
    lumbar Q05.7
        with hydrocephalus Q05.2
    lumbosacral Q05.7
        with hydrocephalus Q05.2
    occulta Q76.0
    sacral Q05.8
        with hydrocephalus Q05.3
    thoracic Q05.6
        with hydrocephalus Q05.1
    thoracolumbar Q05.6
        with hydrocephalus Q05.1
Spindle, Krukenberg's —see Pigmentation, cornea,
    posterior
Spine, spinal —see condition
Spiradenoma (eccrine) —see Neoplasm, skin, benign
Spirillosis A25.0
Spirillum
    minus A25.0
    obermeieri infection A68.0
Spirochetal —see condition
Spirochetosis A69.9
    arthritic, arthritica A69.9
    bronchopulmonary A69.8
    icterohemorrhagic A27.0
    lung A69.8
Spirometrosis B70.1
Spitting blood —see Hemoptysis
Splanchnoptosis K63.4
Spleen, splenic —see condition
Splenectasis —see Splenomegaly
Splenitis (interstitial) (malignant) (nonspecific)
    D73.89
    malarial —see also Malaria B54 [D77]
    tuberculous A18.85
Splenocele D73.89
Splenomegaly, splenomegalia (Bengal)
    (cryptogenic) (idiopathic) (tropical) R16.1
    with hepatomegaly R16.2
    cirrhotic D73.2
    congenital Q89.09
    congestive, chronic D73.2
    Egyptian B65.1
    Gaucher's E75.22
    malarial —see also Malaria B54 [D77]
    neutropenic D73.81
    Niemann-Pick —see Niemann-Pick disease or
        syndrome
    siderotic D73.2
    syphilitic A52.79
        congenital (early) A50.08 [D77]
Splenopathy D73.9
Splenoptosis D73.89
Splenosis D73.89
Splinter —see Foreign body, superficial, by site
Split, splitting
    foot Q72.7-●
    hand Q71.6

Split, splitting (Continued)
    heart sounds R01.2
    lip, congenital —see Cleft, lip
    nails L60.3
    urinary stream R39.13
Spondylarthrosis —see Spondylosis
Spondylitis (chronic) —see also Spondylopathy,
    inflammatory
    ankylopoietica —see Spondylitis, ankylosing
    ankylosing (chronic) M45.9
        with lung involvement M45.9 [J99]
        cervical region M45.2
        cervicothoracic region M45.3
        juvenile M08.1
        lumbar region M45.6
        lumbosacral region M45.7
        multiple sites M45.0
        occipito-atlanto-axial region M45.1
        sacrococcygeal region M45.8
        thoracic region M45.4
        thoracolumbar region M45.5
    atrophic (ligamentous) —see Spondylitis,
        ankylosing
    deformans (chronic) —see Spondylosis
    gonococcal A54.41
    gouty —see also Gout, by type, vertebrae M10.08
    in (due to)
        brucellosis A23.9 [M49.80]
            cervical region A23.9 [M49.82]
            cervicothoracic region A23.9 [M49.83]
            lumbar region A23.9 [M49.86]
            lumbosacral region A23.9 [M49.87]
            multiple sites A23.9 [M49.89]
            occipito-atlanto-axial region A23.9 [M49.81]
            sacrococcygeal region A23.9 [M49.88]
            thoracic region A23.9 [M49.84]
            thoracolumbar region A23.9 [M49.85]
        enterobacteria —see also subcategory M49.8
            A04.9
        tuberculosis A18.01
    infectious NEC —see Spondylopathy, infective
    juvenile ankylosing (chronic) M08.1
    Kümmell's —see Spondylopathy, traumatic
    Marie-Strümpell —see Spondylitis, ankylosing
    muscularis —see Spondylopathy, specified
        NEC
    psoriatic L40.53
    rheumatoid —see Spondylitis, ankylosing
    rhizomelica —see Spondylitis, ankylosing
    sacroiliac NEC M46.1
    senescent, senile —see Spondylosis
    traumatic (chronic) or post-traumatic —see
        Spondylopathy, traumatic
    tuberculous A18.01
    typhosa A01.05
Spondyloarthritis
    axial —see also Spondylitis, ankylosing
        non-radiographic M45.A0
            cervical M45.A2
            cervicothoracic M45.A3
            lumbar M45.A6
            lumbosacral M45.A7
            multiple sites M45.AB
            occipito-atlanto-axial region M45.A1
            sacral and sacrococcygeal M45.A8
            thoracic M45.A4
            thoracolumbar M45.A5
Spondylolisthesis (acquired) (degenerative) M43.10
    with disproportion (fetopelvic) O33.0
        causing obstructed labor O65.0
    cervical region M43.12
    cervicothoracic region M43.13
    congenital Q76.2
    lumbar region M43.16
    lumbosacral region M43.17
    multiple sites M43.19
    occipito-atlanto-axial region M43.11
    sacrococcygeal region M43.18
    thoracic region M43.14
    thoracolumbar region M43.15
    traumatic (old) M43.10
        acute
            fifth cervical (displaced) S12.430
                nondisplaced S12.431
                specified type NEC (displaced) S12.450
                    nondisplaced S12.451
                type III S12.44
            fourth cervical (displaced) S12.330
                nondisplaced S12.331
                specified type NEC (displaced) S12.350
                    nondisplaced S12.351
                type III S12.34

Spondylolisthesis (Continued)
    traumatic (Continued)
        acute (Continued)
            second cervical (displaced) S12.130
                nondisplaced S12.131
                specified type NEC (displaced) S12.150
                    nondisplaced S12.151
                type III S12.14
            seventh cervical (displaced) S12.630
                nondisplaced S12.631
                specified type NEC (displaced) S12.650
                    nondisplaced S12.651
                type III S12.64
            sixth cervical (displaced) S12.530
                nondisplaced S12.531
                specified type NEC (displaced) S12.550
                    nondisplaced S12.551
                type III S12.54
            third cervical (displaced) S12.230
                nondisplaced S12.231
                specified type NEC (displaced)
                    S12.250
                    nondisplaced S12.251
                type III S12.24
Spondylolysis (acquired) M43.00
    cervical region M43.02
    cervicothoracic region M43.03
    congenital Q76.2
    lumbar region M43.06
    lumbosacral region M43.07
        with disproportion (fetopelvic) O33.0
            causing obstructed labor O65.8
    multiple sites M43.09
    occipito-atlanto-axial region M43.01
    sacrococcygeal region M43.08
    thoracic region M43.04
    thoracolumbar region M43.05
Spondylopathy M48.9
    infective NEC M46.50
        cervical region M46.52
        cervicothoracic region M46.53
        lumbar region M46.56
        lumbosacral region M46.57
        multiple sites M46.59
        occipito-atlanto-axial region M46.51
        sacrococcygeal region M46.58
        thoracic region M46.54
        thoracolumbar region M46.55
    inflammatory M46.90
        cervical region M46.92
        cervicothoracic region M46.93
        lumbar region M46.96
        lumbosacral region M46.97
        multiple sites M46.99
        occipito-atlanto-axial region M46.91
        sacrococcygeal region M46.98
        specified type NEC M46.80
            cervical region M46.82
            cervicothoracic region M46.83
            lumbar region M46.86
            lumbosacral region M46.87
            multiple sites M46.89
            occipito-atlanto-axial region M46.81
            sacrococcygeal region M46.88
            thoracic region M46.84
            thoracolumbar region M46.85
        thoracic region M46.94
        thoracolumbar region M46.95
    neuropathic, in
        syringomyelia and syringobulbia G95.0
        tabes dorsalis A52.11
    specified NEC —see subcategory M48.8
    traumatic M48.30
        cervical region M48.32
        cervicothoracic region M48.33
        lumbar region M48.36
        lumbosacral region M48.37
        occipito-atlanto-axial region M48.31
        sacrococcygeal region M48.38
        thoracic region M48.34
        thoracolumbar region M48.35
Spondylosis M47.9
    with
        disproportion (fetopelvic) O33.0
            causing obstructed labor O65.0
        myelopathy NEC M47.10
            cervical region M47.12
            cervicothoracic region M47.13
            lumbar region M47.16
            occipito-atlanto-axial region M47.11
            thoracic region M47.14
            thoracolumbar region M47.15

Spondylosis *(Continued)*
  with *(Continued)*
    radiculopathy M47.20
      cervical region M47.22
      cervicothoracic region M47.23
      lumbar region M47.26
      lumbosacral region M47.27
      occipito-atlanto-axial region M47.21
      sacrococcygeal region M47.28
      thoracic region M47.24
      thoracolumbar region M47.25
    without myelopathy or radiculopathy M47.819
      cervical region M47.812
      cervicothoracic region M47.813
      lumbar region M47.816
      lumbosacral region M47.817
      occipito-atlanto-axial region M47.811
      sacrococcygeal region M47.818
      thoracic region M47.814
      thoracolumbar region M47.815
    specified NEC M47.899
      cervical region M47.892
      cervicothoracic region M47.893
      facet joint M47.819
      lumbar region M47.896
      lumbosacral region M47.897
      occipito-atlanto-axial region M47.891
      sacrococcygeal region M47.898
      thoracic region M47.894
      thoracolumbar region M47.895
  traumatic —*see* Spondylopathy, traumatic
Sponge
  inadvertently left in operation wound —*see*
      Foreign body, accidentally left during a
      procedure
  kidney (medullary) Q61.5
Sponge-diver's disease —*see* Toxicity, venom,
    marine animal, sea anemone
Spongioblastoma (any type) —*see* Neoplasm,
    malignant, by site
  specified site —*see* Neoplasm, malignant, by site
  unspecified site C71.9
Spongioneuroblastoma —*see* Neoplasm,
    malignant, by site
Spontaneous —*see also* condition
  fracture (cause unknown) —*see* Fracture,
    pathological
Spoon nail L60.3
  congenital Q84.6
Sporadic —*see* condition
Sporothrix schenckii infection —*see* Sporotrichosis
Sporotrichosis B42.9
  arthritis B42.82
  disseminated B42.7
  generalized B42.7
  lymphocutaneous (fixed) (progressive)
      B42.1
  pulmonary B42.0
  specified NEC B42.89
Spots, spotting (in) (of)
  Bitot's —*see also* Pigmentation, conjunctiva
    in the young child E50.1
      vitamin A deficiency E50.1
  café, au lait L81.3
  Cayenne pepper I78.1
  cotton wool, retina —*see* Occlusion, artery, retina
  de Morgan's (senile angiomas) I78.1
  Fuchs' black (myopic) —*see also* Myopia,
    degenerative H44.2-●
  intermenstrual (regular) N92.0
    irregular N92.1
  Koplik's B05.9
  liver L81.4
  pregnancy O26.85-●
  purpuric R23.3
  ruby I78.1
Spotted fever —*see* Fever, spotted A77.9
Sprain (joint) (ligament)
  acromioclavicular joint or ligament S43.5-●
  ankle S93.40-●
    calcaneofibular ligament S93.41-●
    deltoid ligament S93.42-●
    internal collateral ligament —*see* Sprain,
      ankle, specified ligament NEC
    specified ligament NEC S93.49-●
    talofibular ligament —*see* Sprain, ankle,
      specified ligament NEC
    tibiofibular ligament S93.43-●
  anterior longitudinal, cervical S13.4
  atlas, atlanto-axial, atlanto-occipital S13.4
  breast bone —*see* Sprain, sternum
  calcaneofibular —*see* Sprain, ankle

Sprain *(Continued)*
  carpal —*see* Sprain, wrist
  carpometacarpal —*see* Sprain, hand, specified
      site NEC
  cartilage
    costal S23.41
    semilunar (knee) —*see* Sprain, knee, specified
        site NEC
      with current tear —*see* Tear, meniscus
    thyroid region S13.5
    xiphoid —*see* Sprain, sternum
  cervical, cervicodorsal, cervicothoracic S13.4
  chondrosternal S23.421
  coracoclavicular S43.8-●
  coracohumeral S43.41-●
  coronary, knee —*see* Sprain, knee, specified site
      NEC
  costal cartilage S23.41
  cricoarytenoid articulation or ligament S13.5
  cricothyroid articulation S13.5
  cruciate, knee —*see* Sprain, knee, cruciate
  deltoid, ankle —*see* Sprain, ankle
  dorsal (spine) S23.3
  elbow S53.40-●
    radial collateral ligament S53.43-●
    radiohumeral S53.41-●
    rupture
      radial collateral ligament —*see* Rupture,
          traumatic, ligament, radial collateral
      ulnar collateral ligament —*see* Rupture,
          traumatic, ligament, ulnar collateral
    specified type NEC S53.49-●
    ulnar collateral ligament S53.44-●
    ulnohumeral S53.42-●
  femur, head —*see* Sprain, hip
  fibular collateral, knee —*see* Sprain, knee,
      collateral
  fibulocalcaneal —*see* Sprain, ankle
  finger(s) S63.61-●
    index S63.61-●
    interphalangeal (joint) S63.63-●
      index S63.63-●
      little S63.63-●
      middle S63.63-●
      ring S63.63-●
    little S63.61-●
    metacarpophalangeal (joint) S63.65-●
    middle S63.61-●
    ring S63.61-●
    specified site NEC S63.69-●
      index S63.69-●
      little S63.69-●
      middle S63.69-●
      ring S63.69-●
  foot S93.60-●
    specified ligament NEC S93.69-●
    tarsal ligament S93.61-●
    tarsometatarsal ligament S93.62-●
    toe —*see* Sprain, toe
  hand S63.9-●
    finger —*see* Sprain, finger
    specified site NEC —*see* subcategory
        S63.8
    thumb —*see* Sprain, thumb
  head S03.9
  hip S73.10-●
    iliofemoral ligament S73.11-●
    ischiocapsular (ligament) S73.12-●
    specified NEC S73.19-●
  iliofemoral —*see* Sprain, hip
  innominate
    acetabulum —*see* Sprain, hip
    sacral junction S33.6
  internal
    collateral, ankle —*see* Sprain, ankle
    semilunar cartilage —*see* Sprain, knee,
        specified site NEC
  interphalangeal
    finger —*see* Sprain, finger, interphalangeal
        (joint)
    toe —*see* Sprain, toe, interphalangeal joint
  ischiocapsular —*see* Sprain, hip
  ischiofemoral —*see* Sprain, hip
  jaw (articular disc) (cartilage) (meniscus) S03.4-●
    old M26.69
  knee S83.9-●
    collateral ligament S83.40-●
      lateral (fibular) S83.42-●
      medial (tibial) S83.41-●
    cruciate ligament S83.50-●
      anterior S83.51-●
      posterior S83.52-●

Sprain *(Continued)*
  knee *(Continued)*
    lateral (fibular) collateral ligament S83.42-●
    medial (tibial) collateral ligament S83.41-●
    patellar ligament S76.11-●
    specified site NEC S83.8X-●
    superior tibiofibular joint (ligament) S83.6-●
  lateral collateral, knee —*see* Sprain, knee, collateral
  lumbar (spine) S33.5
  lumbosacral S33.9
  mandible (articular disc) S03.4-●
    old M26.69
  medial collateral, knee —*see* Sprain, knee,
      collateral
  meniscus
    jaw S03.4-●
      old M26.69
    knee —*see* Sprain, knee, specified site NEC
      with current tear —*see* Tear, meniscus
        old —*see* Derangement, knee, meniscus,
            due to old tear
    mandible S03.4-●
      old M26.69
  metacarpal (distal) (proximal) —*see* Sprain,
      hand, specified site NEC
  metacarpophalangeal —*see* Sprain, finger,
      metacarpophalangeal (joint)
  metatarsophalangeal —*see* Sprain, toe,
      metatarsophalangeal joint
  midcarpal —*see* Sprain, hand, specified site NEC
  midtarsal —*see* Sprain, foot, specified site NEC
  neck S13.9
    anterior longitudinal cervical ligament S13.4
    atlanto-axial joint S13.4
    atlanto-occipital joint S13.4
    cervical spine S13.4
    cricoarytenoid ligament S13.5
    cricothyroid ligament S13.5
    specified site NEC S13.8
    thyroid region (cartilage) S13.5
  nose S03.8
  orbicular, hip —*see* Sprain, hip
  patella —*see* Sprain, knee, specified site NEC
  patellar ligament S76.11-●
  pelvis NEC S33.8
  phalanx
    finger —*see* Sprain, finger
    toe —*see* Sprain, toe
  pubofemoral —*see* Sprain, hip
  radiocarpal —*see* Sprain, wrist
  radiohumeral —*see* Sprain, elbow
  radius, collateral —*see* Rupture, traumatic,
      ligament, radial collateral
  rib (cage) S23.41
  rotator cuff (capsule) S43.42-●
  sacroiliac (region)
    chronic or old —*see* subcategory M53.2
    joint S33.6
  scaphoid (hand) —*see* Sprain, hand, specified
      site NEC
  scapula (r) —*see* Sprain, shoulder girdle,
      specified site NEC
  semilunar cartilage (knee) —*see* Sprain, knee,
      specified site NEC
    with current tear —*see* Tear, meniscus
      old —*see* Derangement, knee, meniscus,
          due to old tear
  shoulder joint S43.40-●
    acromioclavicular joint (ligament) —*see*
        Sprain, acromioclavicular joint
    blade —*see* Sprain, shoulder, girdle, specified
        site NEC
    coracoclavicular joint (ligament) —*see* Sprain,
        coracoclavicular joint
    coracohumeral ligament —*see* Sprain,
        coracohumeral joint
    girdle S43.9-●
      specified site NEC S43.8-●
    rotator cuff —*see* Sprain, rotator cuff
    specified site NEC S43.49-●
    sternoclavicular joint (ligament) —*see* Sprain,
        sternoclavicular joint
  spine
    cervical S13.4
    lumbar S33.5
    thoracic S23.3
  sternoclavicular joint S43.6-●
  sternum S23.429
    chondrosternal S23.421
    specified site NEC S23.428
  ▶sternoclavicular (joint) (ligament)
      S43.6-●

Sprain *(Continued)*
  symphysis
    jaw S03.4-●
      old M26.69
    mandibular S03.4-●
      old M26.69
  talofibular —*see* Sprain, ankle
  tarsal —*see* Sprain, foot, specified site
    NEC
  tarsometatarsal —*see* Sprain, foot, specified site
    NEC
  temporomandibular S03.4-●
    old M26.69
  thorax S23.9
    ribs S23.41
    specified site NEC S23.8
    spine S23.3
    sternum —*see* Sprain, sternum
  thumb S63.60-●
    interphalangeal (joint) S63.62-●
    metacarpophalangeal (joint) S63.64-●
    specified site NEC S63.68-●
  thyroid cartilage or region S13.5
  tibia (proximal end) —*see* Sprain, knee, specified
    site NEC
  tibial collateral, knee —*see* Sprain, knee,
    collateral
  tibiofibular
    distal —*see* Sprain, ankle
    superior —*see* Sprain, knee, specified site
      NEC
  toe(s) S93.50-●
    great S93.50-●
    interphalangeal joint S93.51-●
      great S93.51-●
      lesser S93.51-●
    lesser S93.50-●
    metatarsophalangeal joint S93.52-●
      great S93.52-●
      lesser S93.52-●
  ulna, collateral —*see* Rupture, traumatic,
    ligament, ulnar collateral
  ulnohumeral —*see* Sprain, elbow
  wrist S63.50-●
    carpal S63.51-●
    radiocarpal S63.52-●
    specified site NEC S63.59-●
  xiphoid cartilage —*see* Sprain, sternum
Sprengel's deformity (congenital) Q74.0
Sprue (tropical) K90.1
  celiac K90.0
  idiopathic K90.49
  meaning thrush B37.0
  nontropical K90.0
Spur, bone —*see also* Enthesopathy
  calcaneal M77.3-●
  iliac crest M76.2-●
  nose (septum) J34.89
Spurway's syndrome Q78.0
Sputum
  abnormal (amount) (color) (odor) (purulent)
    R09.3
  blood-stained R04.2
  excessive (cause unknown) R09.3
Squamous —*see also* condition
  epithelium in
    cervical canal (congenital) Q51.828
    uterine mucosa (congenital) Q51.818
Squashed nose M95.0
  congenital Q67.4
Squeeze, diver's T70.3
Squint —*see also* Strabismus
  accommodative —*see* Strabismus, convergent
    concomitant
SSADHD (succinic semialdehyde dehydrogenase
  deficiency) E72.81
St. Hubert's disease A82.9
Stab —*see also* Laceration
  internal organs —*see* Injury, by site
Stafne's cyst or cavity M27.0
Staggering gait R26.0
  hysterical F44.4
Staghorn calculus —*see* Calculus, kidney
Stähli's line (cornea) (pigment) —*see* Pigmentation,
  cornea, anterior
Stain, staining
  meconium (newborn) P96.83
  port wine Q82.5
  tooth, teeth (hard tissues) (extrinsic)
    K03.6

Stain, staining *(Continued)*
  tooth, teeth *(Continued)*
    due to
      accretions K03.6
      deposits (betel) (black) (green) (materia
        alba) (orange) (soft) (tobacco)
        K03.6
      metals (copper) (silver) K03.7
      nicotine K03.6
      pulpal bleeding K03.7
      tobacco K03.6
    intrinsic K00.8
Stammering —*see also* Disorder, fluency
  F80.81
Standstill
  auricular I45.5
  cardiac —*see* Arrest, cardiac
  sinoatrial I45.5
  ventricular —*see* Arrest, cardiac
Stannosis J63.5
Stanton's disease —*see* Melioidosis
Staphylitis (acute) (catarrhal) (chronic)
  (gangrenous) (membranous) (suppurative)
  (ulcerative) K12.2
Staphylococcal scalded skin syndrome L00
Staphylococcemia A41.2
Staphylococcus, staphylococcal —*see also*
  condition
  as cause of disease classified elsewhere B95.8
    aureus (methicillin susceptible) (MSSA)
      B95.61
      methicillin resistant (MRSA) B95.62
  specified NEC, as cause of disease classified
    elsewhere B95.7
Staphyloma (sclera)
  cornea H18.72-●
  equatorial H15.81-●
  localized (anterior) H15.82-●
  posticum H15.83-●
  ring H15.85-●
Stargardt's disease —*see* Dystrophy, retina
Starvation (inanition) (due to lack of food) T73.0
  edema —*see* Malnutrition, severe
Stasis
  bile (noncalculous) K83.1
  bronchus J98.09
    with infection —*see* Bronchitis
  cardiac —*see* Failure, heart, congestive
  cecum K59.89
  colon K59.89
  dermatitis I87.2
    with
      varicose ulcer —*see* Varix, leg, with ulcer,
        with inflammation
      varicose veins —*see* Varix, leg, with,
        inflammation
    due to postthrombotic syndrome —*see*
      Syndrome, postthrombotic
  duodenal K31.5
  eczema —*see* Varix, leg, with, inflammation
  edema —*see* Hypertension, venous (chronic),
    idiopathic
  foot T69.0-●
  ileocecal coil K59.89
  ileum K59.89
  intestinal K59.89
  jejunum K59.89
  kidney N19
  liver (cirrhotic) K76.1
  lymphatic I89.8
  pneumonia J18.2
  pulmonary —*see* Edema, lung
  rectal K59.89
  renal N19
    tubular N17.0
  ulcer —*see* Varix, leg, with, ulcer
    without varicose veins (*see also* Ulcer, by site)
      87.2
  urine —*see* Retention, urine
  venous I87.8
State (of)
  affective and paranoid, mixed, organic psychotic
    F06.8
  agitated R45.1
    acute reaction to stress F43.0
  anxiety (neurotic) F41.1
  apprehension F41.1
  burn-out Z73.0
  climacteric, female Z78.0
    symptomatic N95.1

State *(Continued)*
  compulsive F42.8
    mixed with obsessional thoughts F42.2
  confusional (psychogenic) F44.89
    acute —*see also* Delirium
      with
        arteriosclerotic dementia (*see also*
          Dementia, vascular) F01.50
          with behavioral disturbance —*see*
            Dementia, vascular F01.51
        senility or dementia F05
    alcoholic F10.231
    epileptic F05
    reactive (from emotional stress, psychological
      trauma) F44.89
    subacute —*see* Delirium
  convulsive —*see* Convulsions
  crisis F43.0
  depressive F32.A
    neurotic F34.1
  dissociative F44.9
  emotional shock (stress) R45.7
  hypercoagulation —*see* Hypercoagulable
  locked-in G83.5
  menopausal Z78.0
    symptomatic N95.1
  neurotic F48.9
    with depersonalization F48.1
  obsessional F42.8
  oneiroid (schizophrenia-like) F23
  organic
    hallucinatory (nonalcoholic) F06.0
    paranoid (-hallucinatory) F06.2
  panic F41.0
  paranoid F22
    climacteric F22
    involutional F22
    menopausal F22
    organic F06.2
    senile F03
    simple F22
  persistent vegetative R40.3
  phobic F40.9
  postleukotomy F07.0
  pregnant
    gestational carrier Z33.3
    incidental Z33.1
  psychogenic, twilight F44.89
  psychopathic (constitutional) F60.2
  psychotic, organic —*see also* Psychosis, organic
    mixed paranoid and affective F06.8
    senile or presenile F03
    transient NEC F06.8
      with
        depression F06.31
        hallucinations F06.0
  residual schizophrenic F20.5
  restlessness R45.1
  stress (emotional) R45.7
  tension (mental) F48.9
    specified NEC F48.8
  transient organic psychotic NEC F06.8
    depressive type F06.31
    hallucinatory type F06.0
  twilight
    epileptic F05
    psychogenic F44.89
  vegetative, persistent R40.3
  vital exhaustion Z73.0
  withdrawal —*see* Withdrawal, state
Status (post) —*see also* Presence (of)
  absence, epileptic —*see* Epilepsy, by type, with
    status epilepticus
  administration of tPA (rtPA) in a different facility
    within the last 24 hours prior to admission
    to the current facility Z92.82
  adrenalectomy (unilateral) (bilateral) E89.6
  anastomosis Z98.0
  anginosus I20.9
  angioplasty (peripheral) Z98.62
    with implant Z95.820
    coronary artery Z98.61
      with implant Z95.5
  aortocoronary bypass Z95.1
  arthrodesis Z98.1
  artificial opening (of) Z93.9
    gastrointestinal tract Z93.4
    specified NEC Z93.8
    urinary tract Z93.6
    vagina Z93.8

▶ New   ⇒ Revised   ~~deleted~~ Deleted   ● Use Additional Character(s)

Status (Continued)

asthmaticus —see Asthma, by type, with status
asthmaticus
awaiting organ transplant Z76.82
bariatric surgery Z98.84
bed confinement Z74.01
bleb, filtering (vitreous), after glaucoma surgery
Z98.83
breast implant Z98.82
removal Z98.86
cataract extraction Z98.4-●
cholecystectomy Z90.49
clitorectomy N90.811
with excision of labia minora N90.812
colectomy (complete) (partial) Z90.49
colonization —see Carrier (suspected) of
colostomy Z93.3
▸combined receptor
▸negative
hormone receptor negative with human
epidermal growth factor receptor 2
negative Z17.421
hormone receptor negative with human
epidermal growth factor receptor 2
positive Z17.420
▸positive
hormone receptor positive with human
epidermal growth factor receptor 2
negative Z17.411
hormone receptor positive with human
epidermal growth factor receptor 2
positive Z17.410
convulsivus idiopathicus —see Epilepsy, by type,
with status epilepticus
coronary artery angioplasty —see Status,
angioplasty, coronary artery
coronary artery bypass graft Z95.1
cystectomy (urinary bladder) Z90.6
cystostomy Z93.50
appendico-vesicostomy Z93.52
cutaneous Z93.51
specified NEC Z93.59
delinquent immunization Z28.3
dental Z98.818
crown Z98.811
fillings Z98.811
restoration Z98.811
sealant Z98.810
specified NEC Z98.818
deployment (current) (military) Z56.82
dialysis (hemodialysis) (peritoneal) Z99.2
do not resuscitate (DNR) Z66
donor —see Donor
embedded fragments —see Retained, foreign
body fragments (type of)
embedded splinter —see Retained, foreign body
fragments (type of)
enterostomy Z93.4
epileptic, epilepticus —see also Epilepsy, by type,
with status epilepticus G40.901
estrogen receptor
negative Z17.1
positive Z17.0
female genital cutting —see Female genital
mutilation status
female genital mutilation —see Female genital
mutilation status
filtering (vitreous) bleb after glaucoma surgery
Z98.83
gastrectomy (complete) (partial) Z90.3
gastric banding Z98.84
gastric bypass for obesity Z98.84
gastrostomy Z93.1
▸human epidermal growth factor 2 receptor
▸negative Z17.32
▸positive Z17.31
human immunodeficiency virus (HIV) infection,
asymptomatic Z21
⇒hysterectomy (complete) (total) Z90.710
partial (with remaining cervical stump)
Z90.711
⇒ileostomy (ileal pouch) (Kock pouch) Z93.2
implant
breast Z98.82
infibulation N90.813
intestinal bypass Z98.0
jejunostomy Z93.4
lapsed immunization schedule Z28.3
laryngectomy Z90.02
lymphaticus E32.8

Status (Continued)

malignancy
castrate resistant prostate Z19.2
hormone resistant Z19.2
hormone sensitive Z19.1
marmoratus G80.3
mastectomy (unilateral) (bilateral) Z90.1-●
military deployment status (current)
Z56.82
in theater or in support of military war,
peacekeeping and humanitarian
operations Z56.82
nephrectomy (unilateral) (bilateral) Z90.5
nephrostomy Z93.6
obesity surgery Z98.84
oophorectomy
bilateral Z90.722
unilateral Z90.721
organ replacement
by artificial or mechanical device or prosthesis
of
artery Z95.828
bladder Z96.0
blood vessel Z95.828
breast Z97.8
eye globe Z97.0
heart Z95.812
valve Z95.2
intestine Z97.8
joint Z96.60
hip —see Presence, hip joint implant
knee —see Presence, knee joint implant
specified site NEC Z96.698
kidney Z97.8
larynx Z96.3
lens Z96.1
limbs —see Presence, artificial, limb
liver Z97.8
lung Z97.8
pancreas Z97.8
by organ transplant (heterologous)
(homologous) —see Transplant
pacemaker
brain Z96.89
cardiac Z95.0
specified NEC Z96.89
pancreatectomy Z90.410
complete Z90.410
partial Z90.411
total Z90.410
pneumonectomy (complete) (partial) Z90.2
pneumothorax, therapeutic Z98.3
postcommotio cerebri F07.81
postoperative (postprocedural) NEC
Z98.890
breast implant Z98.82
dental Z98.818
crown Z98.811
fillings Z98.811
restoration Z98.811
sealant Z98.810
specified NEC Z98.818
pneumothorax, therapeutic Z98.3
uterine scar Z98.891
postpartum (routine follow-up) Z39.2
care immediately after delivery Z39.0
postsurgical (postprocedural) NEC
Z98.890
pneumothorax, therapeutic Z98.3
pregnancy, incidental Z33.1
▸progesterone receptor
▸negative Z17.22
▸positive Z17.21
prosthesis coronary angioplasty Z95.5
pseudophakia Z96.1
renal dialysis (hemodialysis) (peritoneal) Z99.2
retained foreign body —see Retained, foreign
body fragments (type of)
reversed jejunal transposition (for bypass Z98.0
salpingo-oophorectomy
bilateral Z90.722
unilateral Z90.721
sex reassignment surgery status Z87.890
shunt
arteriovenous (for dialysis) Z99.2
cerebrospinal fluid Z98.2
ventricular (communicating) (for drainage)
Z98.2
splenectomy Z90.81
thymicolymphaticus E32.8

Status (Continued)

thymicus E32.8
thymolymphaticus E32.8
thyroidectomy (hypothyroidism) E89.0
tooth (teeth) extraction —see also Absence, teeth,
acquired K08.409
tPA (rtPA) administration in a different facility
within the last 24 hours prior to admission
to current facility Z92.82
tracheostomy Z93.0
transplant —see Transplant
organ removed Z98.85
tubal ligation Z98.51
underimmunization Z28.3
ureterostomy Z93.6
urethrostomy Z93.6
vagina, artificial Z93.8
vasectomy Z98.52
wheelchair confinement Z99.3
Stealing
child problem F91.8
in company with others Z72.810
pathological (compulsive) F63.2
Steam burn —see Burn
Steatocystoma multiplex L72.2
Steatohepatitis (nonalcoholic) (NASH) K75.81
Steatoma L72.3
eyelid (cystic) —see Dermatosis, eyelid
infected —see Hordeolum
Steatorrhea (chronic) K90.9
with lacteal obstruction K90.2
idiopathic (adult) (infantile) K90.9
pancreatic K90.3
primary K90.0
tropical K90.1
Steatosis E88.89
heart —see Degeneration, myocardial
kidney N28.89
liver NEC K76.0
Steele-Richardson-Olszewski disease or
syndrome G23.1
⇒Steinbrocker's syndrome G90.89
Steinert's disease G71.11
Stein-Leventhal syndrome E28.2
Stein's syndrome E28.2
STEMI —see also Infarct, myocardium, ST elevation
I21.3
Stenocardia I20.89
Stenocephaly Q75.8
Stenosis, stenotic (cicatricial) —see also Stricture
ampulla of Vater K83.1
anus, anal (canal) (sphincter) K62.4
and rectum K62.4
congenital Q42.3
with fistula Q42.2
aorta (ascending) (supraventricular) (congenital)
Q25.1
arteriosclerotic I70.0
calcified I70.0
supravalvular Q25.3
aortic (valve) I35.0
with insufficiency I35.2
congenital Q23.0
rheumatic I06.0
with
incompetency, insufficiency or
regurgitation I06.2
with mitral (valve) disease I08.0
with tricuspid (valve) disease I08.3
mitral (valve) disease I08.0
with tricuspid (valve) disease I08.3
tricuspid (valve) disease I08.3
with mitral (valve) disease I08.3
specified cause NEC I35.0
syphilitic A52.03
aqueduct of Sylvius (congenital) Q03.0
with spina bifida —see Spina bifida,
by site, with hydrocephalus
acquired G91.1
artery NEC —see also Arteriosclerosis I77.1
⇒celiac (compression) I77.4
▸arteriosclerotic I70.8
▸atherosclerosis I70.8
cerebral —see Occlusion, artery, cerebral
extremities —see Arteriosclerosis, extremities
precerebral —see Occlusion, artery,
precerebral
pulmonary (congenital) Q25.6
acquired I28.8
renal I70.1

Stenosis, stenotic *(Continued)*
  artery *(Continued)*
    stent
      coronary T82.855
      peripheral T82.856
  bile duct (common) (hepatic) K83.1
    congenital Q44.3
  bladder-neck (acquired) N32.0
    congenital Q64.31
  brain G93.89
  bronchus J98.09
    congenital Q32.3
    syphilitic A52.72
  cardia (stomach) K22.2
    congenital Q39.3
  cardiovascular —*see* Disease, cardiovascular
  caudal M48.08
  cervix, cervical (canal) N88.2
    congenital Q51.828
    in pregnancy or childbirth —*see* Pregnancy,
      complicated by, abnormal cervix
  colon —*see also* Obstruction, intestine
    congenital Q42.9
      specified NEC Q42.8
  colostomy K94.03
  common (bile) duct K83.1
    congenital Q44.3
  coronary (artery) —*see* Disease, heart, ischemic,
    atherosclerotic
  cystic duct —*see* Obstruction, gallbladder
  due to presence of device, implant or graft —*see*
    also Complications, by site and type,
    specified NEC T85.858
    arterial graft NEC T82.858
    breast (implant) T85.858
    catheter T85.858
      dialysis (renal) T82.858
        intraperitoneal T85.858
      infusion NEC T82.858
        spinal (epidural) (subdural)
          T85.850
      urinary (indwelling) T83.85
    fixation, internal (orthopedic) NEC
      T84.85
    gastrointestinal (bile duct) (esophagus)
      T85.858
    genital NEC T83.85
    heart NEC T82.857
    joint prosthesis T84.85
    ocular (corneal graft) (orbital implant) NEC
      T85.858
    orthopedic NEC T84.85
    specified NEC T85.858
    urinary NEC T83.85
    vascular NEC T82.858
    ventricular intracranial shunt
      T85.850
  duodenum K31.5
    congenital Q41.0
  ejaculatory duct NEC N50.89
  endocervical os —*see* Stenosis, cervix
  enterostomy K94.13
  esophagus K22.2
    congenital Q39.3
    syphilitic A52.79
      congenital A50.59 *[K23]*
  eustachian tube —*see* Obstruction, eustachian
    tube
  external ear canal (acquired) H61.30-●
    congenital Q16.1
    due to
      inflammation H61.32-●
      trauma H61.31-●
    postprocedural H95.81-●
    specified cause NEC H61.39-●
  gallbladder —*see* Obstruction, gallbladder
  glottis J38.6
  heart valve (*see also* Endocarditis) I38
  aortic —*see* Stenosis, aortic
    congenital Q24.8
    mitral —*see* Stenosis, mitral
    pulmonary —*see* Stenosis, pulmonary,
      valve
    tricuspid —*see* Stenosis, tricuspid Q22.4
  hepatic duct K83.1
  hymen N89.6
  hypertrophic subaortic (idiopathic) I42.1
  ileum —*see also* Obstruction, intestine, specified
    NEC K56.699
    congenital Q41.2
  infundibulum cardia Q24.3

Stenosis, stenotic *(Continued)*
  intervertebral foramina —*see also* Lesion,
    biomechanical, specified NEC
    connective tissue M99.79
      abdomen M99.79
      cervical region M99.71
      cervicothoracic M99.71
      head region M99.70
      lumbar region M99.73
      lumbosacral M99.73
      occipitocervical M99.70
      sacral region M99.74
      sacrococcygeal M99.74
      sacroiliac M99.74
      specified NEC M99.79
      thoracic region M99.72
      thoracolumbar M99.72
    disc M99.79
      abdomen M99.79
      cervical region M99.71
      cervicothoracic M99.71
      head region M99.70
      lower extremity M99.76
      lumbar region M99.73
      lumbosacral M99.73
      occipitocervical M99.70
      pelvic M99.75
      rib cage M99.78
      sacral region M99.74
      sacrococcygeal M99.74
      sacroiliac M99.74
      specified NEC M99.79
      thoracic region M99.72
      thoracolumbar M99.72
      upper extremity M99.77
    osseous M99.69
      abdomen M99.69
      cervical region M99.61
      cervicothoracic M99.61
      head region M99.60
      lower extremity M99.66
      lumbar region M99.63
      lumbosacral M99.63
      occipitocervical M99.60
      pelvic M99.65
      rib cage M99.68
      sacral region M99.64
      sacrococcygeal M99.64
      sacroiliac M99.64
      specified NEC M99.69
      thoracic region M99.62
      thoracolumbar M99.62
      upper extremity M99.67
    subluxation —*see* Stenosis, intervertebral
      foramina, osseous
  intestine —*see also* Obstruction, intestine
    congenital (small) Q41.9
      large Q42.9
        specified NEC Q42.8
      specified NEC Q41.8
  jejunum —*see also* Obstruction, intestine,
    specified NEC K56.699
    congenital Q41.1
  lacrimal (passage)
    canaliculi H04.54-●
    congenital Q10.5
    duct H04.55-●
    punctum H04.56-●
    sac H04.57-●
  lacrimonasal duct —*see* Stenosis, lacrimal, duct
    congenital Q10.5
  larynx J38.6
    congenital NEC Q31.8
      subglottic Q31.1
    syphilitic A52.73
      congenital A50.59 *[J99]*
  mitral (chronic) (inactive) (valve) I05.0
    with
      aortic valve disease I08.0
      incompetency, insufficiency or
        regurgitation I05.2
    active or acute I01.1
      with rheumatic or Sydenham's chorea I02.0
    congenital Q23.2
    specified cause, except rheumatic I34.2
    syphilitic A52.03
  myocardium, myocardial —*see also*
    Degeneration, myocardial
    hypertrophic subaortic (idiopathic) I42.1
  nares (anterior) (posterior) J34.89
    congenital Q30.0

Stenosis, stenotic *(Continued)*
  nasal duct —*see also* Stenosis, lacrimal, duct
    congenital Q10.5
  nasolacrimal duct —*see also* Stenosis, lacrimal,
    duct
    congenital Q10.5
  neural canal —*see also* Lesion, biomechanical,
    specified NEC
    connective tissue M99.49
      abdomen M99.49
      cervical region M99.41
      cervicothoracic M99.41
      head region M99.40
      lower extremity M99.46
      lumbar region M99.43
      lumbosacral M99.43
      occipitocervical M99.40
      pelvic M99.45
      rib cage M99.48
      sacral region M99.44
      sacrococcygeal M99.44
      sacroiliac M99.44
      specified NEC M99.49
      thoracic region M99.42
      thoracolumbar M99.42
      upper extremity M99.47
    intervertebral disc M99.59
      abdomen M99.59
      cervical region M99.51
      cervicothoracic M99.51
      head region M99.50
      lower extremity M99.56
      lumbar region M99.53
      lumbosacral M99.53
      occipitocervical M99.50
      pelvic M99.55
      rib cage M99.58
      sacral region M99.54
      sacrococcygeal M99.54
      sacroiliac M99.54
      specified NEC M99.59
      thoracic region M99.52
      thoracolumbar M99.52
      upper extremity M99.57
    osseous M99.39
      abdomen M99.39
      cervical region M99.31
      cervicothoracic M99.31
      head region M99.30
      lower extremity M99.36
      lumbar region M99.33
      lumbosacral M99.33
      occipitocervical M99.30
      pelvic M99.35
      rib cage M99.38
      sacral region M99.34
      sacrococcygeal M99.34
      sacroiliac M99.34
      specified NEC M99.39
      thoracic region M99.32
      thoracolumbar M99.32
      upper extremity M99.37
    subluxation M99.29
      cervical region M99.21
      cervicothoracic M99.21
      head region M99.20
      lower extremity M99.26
      lumbar region M99.23
      lumbosacral M99.23
      occipitocervical M99.20
      pelvic M99.25
      rib cage M99.28
      sacral region M99.24
      sacrococcygeal M99.24
      sacroiliac M99.24
      specified NEC M99.29
      thoracic region M99.22
      thoracolumbar M99.22
      upper extremity M99.27
  organ or site, congenital NEC —*see* Atresia, by
    site
  papilla of Vater K83.1
  pulmonary (artery) (congenital) Q25.6
    with ventricular septal defect, transposition of
      aorta, and hypertrophy of right ventricle
      Q21.3
    acquired I28.8
    in tetralogy of Fallot Q21.3
    infundibular Q24.3
    subvalvular Q24.3
    supravalvular Q25.6

Stenosis, stenotic *(Continued)*
  pulmonary *(Continued)*
    valve I37.0
      with insufficiency I37.2
      congenital Q22.1
      rheumatic I09.89
        with aortic, mitral or tricuspid (valve)
          disease I08.8
    vein, acquired I28.8
    vessel NEC I28.8
  pulmonic (congenital) Q22.1
    infundibular Q24.3
    subvalvular Q24.3
  pylorus (hypertrophic) (acquired) K31.1
    adult K31.1
    congenital Q40.0
    infantile Q40.0
  rectum (sphincter) —*see* Stricture, rectum
  renal artery I70.1
    congenital Q27.1
  salivary duct (any) K11.8
  sphincter of Oddi K83.1
  spinal M48.00
    cervical region M48.02
    cervicothoracic region M48.03
    lumbar region (NOS) (without neurogenic
      claudication) M48.061
      with neurogenic claudication M48.062
    lumbosacral region M48.07
    occipito-atlanto-axial region M48.01
    sacrococcygeal region M48.08
    thoracic region M48.04
    thoracolumbar region M48.05
  stent
    vascular
      end stent
        adjacent to stent —*see* Arteriosclerosis
        within the stent
          coronary T82.855
          peripheral T82.856
      in stent
        coronary vessel T82.855
        peripheral vessel T82.856
  stomach, hourglass K31.2
  subaortic (congenital) Q24.4
    hypertrophic (idiopathic) I42.1
  subglottic J38.6
    congenital Q31.1
    postprocedural J95.5
  trachea J39.8
    congenital Q32.1
    syphilitic A52.73
    tuberculous NEC A15.5
  tracheostomy J95.03
  tricuspid (valve) I07.0
    with
      aortic (valve) disease I08.2
      incompetency, insufficiency or
        regurgitation I07.2
        with aortic (valve) disease I08.2
          with mitral (valve) disease I08.3
      mitral (valve) disease I08.1
        with aortic (valve) disease I08.3
    congenital Q22.4
    nonrheumatic I36.0
      with insufficiency I36.2
  tubal N97.1
  ureter —*see* Atresia, ureter
  ureteropelvic junction, congenital
    Q62.11
  ureterovesical orifice, congenital Q62.12
  urethra (valve) —*see also* Stricture, urethra
    congenital Q64.32
  urinary meatus, congenital Q64.33
  vagina N89.5
    congenital Q52.4
    in pregnancy —*see* Pregnancy, complicated by,
      abnormal vagina
      causing obstructed labor O65.5
  valve (cardiac) (heart) —*see also* Endocarditis
    I38
    congenital Q24.8
      aortic Q23.0
      mitral Q23.2
      pulmonary Q22.1
      tricuspid Q22.4
  vena cava (inferior) (superior) I87.1
    congenital Q26.0
  vesicourethral orifice Q64.31
  vulva N90.5
Stent jail T82.897

Stercolith (impaction) K56.41
  appendix K38.1
Stercoraceous, stercoral ulcer K63.3
  anus or rectum K62.6
Stereotypies NEC F98.4
Sterility —*see* Infertility
Sterilization —*see* Encounter (for), sterilization
Sternalgia —*see* Angina
Sternopagus Q89.4
Sternum bifidum Q76.7
Steroid
  effects (adverse) (adrenocortical) (iatrogenic)
    cushingoid Q24.2
      correct substance properly administered —
        see Table of Drugs and Chemicals, by
        drug, adverse effect
      overdose or wrong substance given or
        taken —*see* Table of Drugs and
        Chemicals, by drug, poisoning
    diabetes —*see* category E09
      correct substance properly administered —
        see Table of Drugs and Chemicals, by
        drug, adverse effect
      overdose or wrong substance given or
        taken —*see* Table of Drugs and
        Chemicals, by drug, poisoning
    fever R50.2
    insufficiency E27.3
      correct substance properly administered —
        see Table of Drugs and Chemicals, by
        drug, adverse effect
      overdose or wrong substance given or
        taken —*see* Table of Drugs and
        Chemicals, by drug, poisoning
  responder H40.04-●
Stevens-Johnson disease or syndrome L51.1
  toxic epidermal necrolysis overlap L51.3
Stewart-Morel syndrome M85.2
Sticker's disease B08.3
Sticky eye —*see* Conjunctivitis, acute,
  mucopurulent
Stieda's disease —*see* Bursitis, tibial collateral
Stiff neck —*see* Torticollis
Stiff-man syndrome G25.82
Stiffness, joint NEC M25.60-●
  ankle M25.67-●
  ankylosis —*see* Ankylosis, joint
  contracture —*see* Contraction, joint
  elbow M25.62-●
  foot M25.67-●
  hand M25.64-●
  hip M25.65-●
  knee M25.66-●
  shoulder M25.61-●
  specified site NEC M25.69
  wrist M25.63-●
Stigmata congenital syphilis A50.59
Stillbirth P95
Still-Felty syndrome —*see* Felty's syndrome
Still's disease or syndrome (juvenile) M08.20
  adult-onset M06.1
  ankle M08.27-●
  elbow M08.22-●
  foot joint M08.27-●
  hand joint M08.24-●
  hip M08.25-●
  knee M08.26-●
  multiple site M08.29
  shoulder M08.21-●
  specified site NEC M08.2A
  vertebra M08.28
  wrist M08.23-●
Stimulation, ovary E28.1
Sting (venomous) (with allergic or anaphylactic
  shock) —*see* Table of Drugs and Chemicals, by
  animal or substance, poisoning
Stippled epiphyses Q78.8
Stitch
  abscess T81.41
  burst (in operation wound) —*see* Disruption,
    wound, operation
Stokes-Adams disease or syndrome I45.9
Stokes' disease E05.00
  with thyroid storm E05.01
Stokvis (-Talma) disease D74.8
Stoma malfunction
  colostomy K94.03
  enterostomy K94.13
  gastrostomy K94.23
  ileostomy K94.13
  tracheostomy J95.03

Stomach —*see* condition
Stomatitis (denture) (ulcerative) K12.1
  angular K13.0
    due to dietary or vitamin deficiency E53.0
  aphthous K12.0
  bovine B08.61
  candidal B37.0
  catarrhal K12.1
  diphtheritic A36.89
  due to
    dietary deficiency E53.0
    thrush B37.0
    vitamin deficiency
      B group NEC E53.9
      B2 (riboflavin) E53.0
  epidemic B08.8
  epizootic B08.8
  follicular K12.1
  gangrenous A69.0
  Geotrichum B48.3
  herpesviral, herpetic B00.2
  herpetiformis K12.0
  malignant K12.1
  membranous acute K12.1
  monilial B37.0
  mycotic B37.0
  necrotizing ulcerative A69.0
  parasitic B37.0
  septic K12.1
  spirochetal A69.1
  suppurative (acute) K12.2
  ulceromembranous A69.1
  vesicular K12.1
    with exanthem (enteroviral) B08.4
    virus disease A93.8
  Vincent's A69.1
Stomatocytosis D58.8
Stomatomycosis B37.0
Stomatorrhagia K13.79
Stone(s) —*see also* Calculus
  bladder (diverticulum) N21.0
  cystine E72.09
  heart syndrome I50.1
  kidney N20.0
  prostate N42.0
  pulpal (dental) K04.2
  renal N20.0
  salivary gland or duct (any) K11.5
  urethra (impacted) N21.1
  urinary (duct) (impacted) (passage) N20.9
    bladder (diverticulum) N21.0
    lower tract N21.9
    specified NEC N21.8
  xanthine E79.82 *[N22]*
Stonecutter's lung J62.8
Stonemason's asthma, disease, lung or
  pneumoconiosis J62.8
Stoppage
  heart —*see* Arrest, cardiac
  urine —*see* Retention, urine
Storm, thyroid —*see* Thyrotoxicosis
Strabismus (congenital) (nonparalytic)
  H50.9
  concomitant H50.40
    convergent —*see* Strabismus, convergent
      concomitant
    divergent —*see* Strabismus, divergent
      concomitant
  convergent concomitant H50.00
    accommodative component H50.43
    alternating H50.05
      with
        A pattern H50.06
        specified nonconcomitances NEC
          H50.08
        V pattern H50.07
    monocular H50.01-●
      with
        A pattern H50.02-●
        specified nonconcomitances NEC
          H50.04-●
        V pattern H50.03-●
    intermittent H50.31-●
      alternating H50.32
  cyclotropia H50.41
  divergent concomitant H50.10
    alternating H50.15
      with
        A pattern H50.16
        specified nonconcomitances NEC H50.18
        V pattern H50.17

Strabismus *(Continued)*
  divergent concomitant *(Continued)*
    monocular H50.11-●
      with
        A pattern H50.12-●
          specified noncomitances NEC H50.14-●
          V pattern H50.13-●
        intermittent H50.33-●
          alternating H50.34
  Duane's syndrome H50.81-●
  due to adhesions, scars H50.69
  heterophoria H50.50
    alternating H50.55
    cyclophoria H50.54
    esophoria H50.51
    exophoria H50.52
    vertical H50.53
  heterotropia H50.40
    intermittent H50.30
  hypertropia H50.2-●
  hypotropia —*see* Hypertropia
  latent H50.50
  mechanical H50.60
    Brown's sheath syndrome H50.61-●
    specified type NEC H50.69
  monofixation syndrome H50.42
  paralytic H49.9
    abducens nerve H49.2-●
    fourth nerve H49.1-●
    Kearns-Sayre syndrome H49.81-●
    ophthalmoplegia (external)
      progressive H49.4-●
        with pigmentary retinopathy H49.81-●
      total H49.3-●
    sixth nerve H49.2-●
    specified type NEC H49.88-●
    third nerve H49.0-●
    trochlear nerve H49.1-●
  specified type NEC H50.89
  vertical H50.2-●
Strain
  back S39.012
  cervical S16.1
  eye NEC —*see* Disturbance, vision, subjective
  heart —*see* Disease, heart
  low back S39.012
  mental NOS Z73.3
    work-related Z56.6
  muscle (tendon) —*see* Injury, muscle, by site,
      strain
  neck S16.1
  physical NOS Z73.3
    work-related Z56.6
  postural —*see also* Disorder, soft tissue, due to
      use
  psychological NEC Z73.3
  tendon —*see* Injury, muscle, by site, strain
Straining, on urination R39.16
Strand, vitreous —*see* Opacity, vitreous,
      membranes and strands
Strangulation, strangulated —*see also* Asphyxia,
      traumatic
  appendix K38.8
  bladder-neck N32.0
  bowel or colon K56.2
  food or foreign body —*see* Foreign body, by site
  hemorrhoids —*see* Hemorrhoids, with
      complication
  hernia —*see also* Hernia, by site, with obstruction
    with gangrene —*see* Hernia, by site, with
        gangrene
  intestine (large) (small) K56.2
    with hernia —*see also* Hernia, by site, with
        obstruction
      with gangrene —*see* Hernia, by site, with
          gangrene
  mesentery K56.2
  mucus —*see* Asphyxia, mucus
  omentum K56.2
  organ or site, congenital NEC —*see* Atresia, by
      site
  ovary —*see* Torsion, ovary
  penis N48.89
    foreign body T19.4
  rupture —*see* Hernia, by site, with obstruction
  stomach due to hernia —*see also* Hernia, by site,
      with obstruction
    with gangrene —*see* Hernia, by site, with
        gangrene
  vesicourethral orifice N32.0
Strangury R30.0
Straw itch B88.0

Strawberry
  gallbladder K82.4
  mark Q82.5
  tongue (red) (white) K14.3
Streak(s)
  macula, angioid H35.33
  ovarian Q50.32
Strephosymbolia F81.0
  secondary to organic lesion R48.8
Streptobacillary fever A25.1
Streptobacillosis A25.1
Streptobacillus moniliformis A25.1
Streptococcus, streptococcal —*see also* condition
  as cause of disease classified elsewhere
      B95.5
  group
    A, as cause of disease classified elsewhere
        B95.0
    B, as cause of disease classified elsewhere
        B95.1
    D, as cause of disease classified elsewhere
        B95.2
  pneumoniae, as cause of disease classified
      elsewhere B95.3
  specified NEC, as cause of disease classified
      elsewhere B95.4
Streptomycosis B47.1
Streptotrichosis A48.8
Stress F43.9
  family —*see* Disruption, family
  fetal P84
    complicating pregnancy O77.9
      due to drug administration O77.1
  mental NEC Z73.3
    work-related Z56.6
  physical NEC Z73.3
    work-related Z56.6
  polycythemia D75.1
  reaction —*see also* Reaction, stress F43.9
  work schedule Z56.3
Stretching, nerve —*see* Injury, nerve
Striae albicantes, atrophicae or distensae (cutis)
      L90.6
Stricture —*see also* Stenosis
  ampulla of Vater K83.1
  anus (sphincter) K62.4
    congenital Q42.3
      with fistula Q42.2
    infantile Q42.3
      with fistula Q42.2
  aorta (ascending) (congenital) Q25.1
    arteriosclerotic I70.0
    calcified I70.0
    supravalvular, congenital Q25.3
  aortic (valve) —*see* Stenosis, aortic
  aqueduct of Sylvius (congenital) Q03.0
    with spina bifida —*see* Spina bifida, by site,
        with hydrocephalus
    acquired G91.1
  artery I77.1
    basilar —*see* Occlusion, artery, basilar
    carotid —*see* Occlusion, artery, carotid
    ⇒celiac (compression) I77.4
      ▸arteriosclerotic I70.8
      ▸atherosclerosis I70.8
    congenital (peripheral) Q27.8
      cerebral Q28.3
      coronary Q24.5
      digestive system Q27.8
      lower limb Q27.8
      retinal Q14.1
      specified site NEC Q27.8
      umbilical Q27.0
      upper limb Q27.8
    coronary —*see* Disease, heart, ischemic,
        atherosclerotic
      congenital Q24.5
    precerebral —*see* Occlusion, artery,
        precerebral
    pulmonary (congenital) Q25.6
      acquired I28.8
    renal I70.1
    vertebral —*see* Occlusion, artery, vertebral
  auditory canal (external) (congenital)
    acquired —*see* Stenosis, external ear canal
  bile duct (common) (hepatic) K83.1
    congenital Q44.3
    postoperative K91.89
  bladder N32.89
    neck N32.0
  bowel —*see* Obstruction, intestine
  brain G93.89

Stricture *(Continued)*
  bronchus J98.09
    congenital Q32.3
    syphilitic A52.72
  cardia (stomach) K22.2
    congenital Q39.3
  cardiac —*see also* Disease, heart
    orifice (stomach) K22.2
  cecum —*see* Obstruction, intestine
  cervix, cervical (canal) N88.2
    congenital Q51.828
    in pregnancy —*see* Pregnancy, complicated by,
        abnormal cervix
      causing obstructed labor O65.5
  colon —*see also* Obstruction, intestine
    congenital Q42.9
    specified NEC Q42.8
  colostomy K94.03
  common (bile) duct K83.1
  coronary (artery) —*see* Disease, heart, ischemic,
      atherosclerotic
  cystic duct —*see* Obstruction,
      gallbladder
  digestive organs NEC, congenital Q45.8
  duodenum K31.5
    congenital Q41.0
  ear canal (external) (congenital) Q16.1
    acquired —*see* Stricture, auditory canal,
        acquired
  ejaculatory duct N50.89
  enterostomy K94.13
  esophagus K22.2
    congenital Q39.3
    syphilitic A52.79
      congenital A50.59 [K23]
  eustachian tube —*see also* Obstruction,
      eustachian tube
    congenital Q17.8
  fallopian tube N97.1
    gonococcal A54.24
    tuberculous A18.17
  gallbladder —*see* Obstruction, gallbladder
  glottis J38.6
  heart —*see also* Disease, heart
    valve (see also Endocarditis) I38
      aortic Q23.0
      mitral Q23.2
      pulmonary Q22.1
      tricuspid Q22.4
  hepatic duct K83.1
  hourglass, of stomach K31.2
  hymen N89.6
  hypopharynx J39.2
  ileum —*see also* Obstruction, intestine, specified
      NEC K56.699
    congenital Q41.2
  intestine —*see also* Obstruction, intestine
    congenital (small) Q41.9
      large Q42.9
        specified NEC Q42.8
      specified NEC Q41.8
    ischemic K55.1
  jejunum —*see also* Obstruction, intestine,
      specified NEC K56.699
    congenital Q41.1
  lacrimal passages —*see also* Stenosis, lacrimal
    congenital Q10.5
  larynx J38.6
    congenital NEC Q31.8
      subglottic Q31.1
    syphilitic A52.73
      congenital A50.59 [J99]
  meatus
    ear (congenital) Q16.1
      acquired —*see* Stricture, auditory canal,
          acquired
    osseous (ear) (congenital) Q16.1
      acquired —*see* Stricture, auditory canal,
          acquired
    urinarius —*see also* Stricture, urethra
      congenital Q64.33
  mitral (valve) —*see* Stenosis, mitral
  myocardium, myocardial I51.5
    hypertrophic subaortic (idiopathic) I42.1
  nares (anterior) (posterior) J34.89
    congenital Q30.0
  nasal duct —*see also* Stenosis, lacrimal,
      duct
    congenital Q10.5
  nasolacrimal duct —*see also* Stenosis, lacrimal,
      duct
    congenital Q10.5

▶ New   ⇒ Revised   ~~deleted~~ Deleted   ● Use Additional Character(s)

Subcortical —see condition
Subcostal syndrome, nerve compression —see
    Mononeuropathy, upper limb, specified site
    NEC
Subcutaneous, subcuticular —see condition
Subdural —see condition
Subendocardium —see condition
Subependymoma
    specified site —see Neoplasm, uncertain
        behavior, by site
    unspecified site D43.2
Suberosis J67.3
Subglossitis —see Glossitis
Subhemophilia D66
Subinvolution
    breast (postlactational) (postpuerperal) N64.89
    puerperal O90.89
    uterus (chronic) (nonpuerperal) N85.3
        puerperal O90.89
Sublingual —see condition
Sublinguitis —see Sialoadenitis
Subluxatable hip Q65.6
Subluxation —see also Dislocation
    acromioclavicular S43.11-●
    ankle S93.0-●
    atlantoaxial, recurrent M43.4
        with myelopathy M43.3
    carpometacarpal (joint) NEC S63.05-●
        thumb S63.04-●
    complex, vertebral —see Complex,
        subluxation
    congenital —see also Malposition, congenital
        hip —see Dislocation, hip, congenital, partial
        joint (excluding hip)
            lower limb Q68.8
            shoulder Q68.8
            upper limb Q68.8
    elbow (traumatic) S53.10-●
        anterior S53.11-●
        lateral S53.14-●
        medial S53.13-●
        posterior S53.12-●
        specified type NEC S53.19-●
    finger S63.20-●
        index S63.20-●
        interphalangeal S63.22-●
            distal S63.24-●
                index S63.24-●
                little S63.24-●
                middle S63.24-●
                ring S63.24-●
            index S63.22-●
            little S63.22-●
            middle S63.22-●
            proximal S63.23-●
                index S63.23-●
                little S63.23-●
                middle S63.23-●
                ring S63.23-●
            ring S63.22-●
        little S63.20-●
        metacarpophalangeal S63.21-●
            index S63.21-●
            little S63.21-●
            middle S63.21-●
            ring S63.21-●
        middle S63.20-●
        ring S63.20-●
    foot S93.30-●
        specified site NEC S93.33-●
        tarsal joint S93.31-●
        tarsometatarsal joint S93.32-●
        toe —see Subluxation, toe
    hip S73.00-●
        anterior S73.03-●
            obturator S73.02-●
        central S73.04-●
        posterior S73.01-●
    interphalangeal (joint)
        finger S63.22-●
            distal joint S63.24-●
                index S63.24-●
                little S63.24-●
                middle S63.24-●
                ring S63.24-●
            index S63.22-●
            little S63.22-●
            middle S63.22-●
            proximal joint S63.23-●
                index S63.23-●
                little S63.23-●

Subluxation (Continued)
    interphalangeal (Continued)
        finger (Continued)
            proximal joint (Continued)
                middle S63.23-●
                ring S63.23-●
            ring S63.22-●
        thumb S63.12-●
        toe S93.13-●
            great S93.13-●
            lesser S93.13-●
    joint prosthesis —see Complications, joint
        prosthesis, mechanical, displacement, by
        site
    knee S83.10-●
        cap —see Subluxation, patella
        patella —see Subluxation, patella
        proximal tibia
            anteriorly S83.11-●
            laterally S83.14-●
            medially S83.13-●
            posteriorly S83.12-●
        specified type NEC S83.19-●
    lens —see Dislocation, lens, partial
    ligament, traumatic —see Sprain, by site
    metacarpal (bone)
        proximal end S63.06-●
    metacarpophalangeal (joint)
        finger S63.21-●
        index S63.21-●
        little S63.21-●
        middle S63.21-●
        ring S63.21-●
        thumb S63.11-●
    metatarsophalangeal joint S93.14-●
        great toe S93.14-●
        lesser toe S93.14-●
    midcarpal (joint) S63.03-●
    patella S83.00-●
        lateral S83.01-●
        recurrent (nontraumatic) —see Dislocation,
            patella, recurrent, incomplete
        specified type NEC S83.09-●
    pathological —see Dislocation, pathological
    radial head S53.00-●
        anterior S53.01-●
        nursemaid's elbow S53.03-●
        posterior S53.02-●
        specified type NEC S53.09-●
    radiocarpal (joint) S63.02-●
    radioulnar (joint)
        distal S63.01-●
        proximal —see Subluxation, elbow
    shoulder
        congenital Q68.8
        girdle S43.30-●
            scapula S43.31-●
            specified site NEC S43.39-●
        traumatic S43.00-●
            anterior S43.01-●
            inferior S43.03-●
            posterior S43.02-●
            specified type NEC S43.08-●
    sternoclavicular (joint) S43.20-●
        anterior S43.21-●
        posterior S43.22-●
    symphysis (pubis) —see also Dislocation,
        symphysis pubis
    thumb S63.103
        interphalangeal joint —see Subluxation,
            interphalangeal (joint), thumb
        metacarpophalangeal joint —see Subluxation,
            metacarpophalangeal (joint), thumb
    toe(s) S93.10-●
        great S93.10-●
            interphalangeal joint S93.13-●
            metatarsophalangeal joint S93.14-●
        interphalangeal joint S93.13-●
        lesser S93.10-●
            interphalangeal joint S93.13-●
            metatarsophalangeal joint S93.14-●
        metatarsophalangeal joint S93.149
    ulnohumeral joint —see Subluxation, elbow
    vertebral
        recurrent NEC —see subcategory
            M43.5
        traumatic
            cervical S13.100
                atlantoaxial joint S13.120
                atlantooccipital joint S13.110
                atloidooccipital joint S13.110

Subluxation (Continued)
    vertebral (Continued)
        traumatic (Continued)
            cervical (Continued)
                joint between
                    C0 and C1 S13.110
                    C1 and C2 S13.120
                    C2 and C3 S13.130
                    C3 and C4 S13.140
                    C4 and C5 S13.150
                    C5 and C6 S13.160
                    C6 and C7 S13.170
                    C7 and T1 S13.180
                occipitoatloid joint S13.110
            lumbar S33.100
                joint between
                    L1 and L2 S33.110
                    L2 and L3 S33.120
                    L3 and L4 S33.130
                    L4 and L5 S33.140
            thoracic S23.100
                joint between
                    T1 and T2 S23.110
                    T2 and T3 S23.120
                    T3 and T4 S23.122
                    T4 and T5 S23.130
                    T5 and T6 S23.132
                    T6 and T7 S23.140
                    T7 and T8 S23.142
                    T8 and T9 S23.150
                    T9 and T10 S23.152
                    T10 and T11 S23.160
                    T11 and T12 S23.162
                    T12 and L1 S23.170
    ulna
        distal end S63.07-●
        proximal end —see Subluxation, elbow
    wrist (carpal bone) S63.00-●
        carpometacarpal joint —see Subluxation,
            carpometacarpal (joint)
        distal radioulnar joint —see Subluxation,
            radioulnar (joint), distal
        metacarpal bone, proximal —see Subluxation,
            metacarpal (bone), proximal end
        midcarpal —see Subluxation, midcarpal
            (joint)
        radiocarpal joint —see Subluxation,
            radiocarpal (joint)
        recurrent —see Dislocation, recurrent, wrist
        specified site NEC S63.09-●
        ulna —see Subluxation, ulna, distal end
Submaxillary —see condition
Submersion (fatal) (nonfatal) T75.1
Submucous —see condition
Subnormal, subnormality
    accommodation (old age) H52.4
    mental —see Disability, intellectual
    temperature (accidental) T68
Subphrenic —see condition
Subscapular nerve —see condition
Subseptus uterus Q51.28
Subsiding appendicitis K36
Substance (other psychoactive) -induced
    anxiety disorder F19.980
    bipolar and related disorder F19.94
    delirium F19.921
    depressive disorder F19.94
    major neurocognitive disorder F19.97
    mild neurocognitive disorder F19.988
    obsessive-compulsive and related disorder
        F19.988
    psychotic disorder F19.959
    sexual dysfunction F19.981
    sleep disorder F19.982
Substernal thyroid E04.9
    congenital Q89.2
Substitution disorder F44.9
Subtentorial —see condition
Subthyroidism (acquired) —see also
    Hypothyroidism
    congenital E03.1
Succenturiate placenta O43.19-●
Sucking thumb, child (excessive) F98.8
Sudamen, sudamina L74.1
Sudanese kala-azar B55.0
Sudden
    hearing loss —see Deafness, sudden
    heart failure —see Failure, heart
Sudeck's atrophy, disease, or syndrome —see
    Algoneurodystrophy
Suffocation —see Asphyxia, traumatic

▶ New   ➡ Revised   ~~deleted~~ Deleted   ● Use Additional Character(s)

Sugar
  blood
    high (transient) R73.9
    low (transient) E16.2
  in urine R81
Suicide, suicidal (attempted) T14.91
  by poisoning —*see* Table of Drugs and Chemicals
  history of (personal) Z91.51
    in family Z81.8
  ideation —*see* Ideation, suicidal
  risk
    meaning personal history of attempted
        suicide Z91.51
    meaning suicidal ideation —*see* Ideation,
        suicidal
  tendencies
    meaning personal history of attempted
        suicide Z91.51
    meaning suicidal ideation —*see* Ideation,
        suicidal
  trauma —*see* nature of injury by site
Suipestifer infection —*see* Infection, salmonella
Sulfhemoglobinemia, sulphemoglobinemia
    (acquired) (with methemoglobinemia) D74.8
Sumatran mite fever A75.3
Summer —*see* condition
Sunburn L55.9
  due to
    tanning bed (acute) L56.8
      chronic L57.8
    ultraviolet radiation (acute) L56.8
      chronic L57.8
  first degree L55.0
  second degree L55.1
  third degree L55.2
SUNCT (short lasting unilateral neuralgiform
    headache with conjunctival injection and
    tearing) G44.059
  intractable G44.051
  not intractable G44.059
Sundowning F05
Sunken acetabulum —*see* Derangement, joint,
    specified type NEC, hip
Sunstroke T67.01
  specified NEC T67.09
Superfecundation —*see* Pregnancy, multiple
Superfetation —*see* Pregnancy, multiple
Superinvolution (uterus) N85.8
Supernumerary (congenital)
  aortic cusps Q23.88
  auditory ossicles Q16.3
  bone Q79.8
  breast Q83.1
  carpal bones Q74.0
  cusps, heart valve NEC Q24.8
    aortic Q23.88
    mitral Q23.2
    pulmonary Q22.3
  digit(s) Q69.9
  ear (lobule) Q17.0
  fallopian tube Q50.6
  finger Q69.0
  hymen Q52.4
  kidney Q63.0
  lacrimonasal duct Q10.6
  lobule (ear) Q17.0
  mitral cusps Q23.2
  muscle Q79.8
  nipple(s) Q83.3
  organ or site not listed —*see* Accessory
  ossicles, auditory Q16.3
  ovary Q50.31
  oviduct Q50.6
  pulmonary, pulmonic cusps Q22.3
  rib Q76.6
    cervical or first (syndrome) Q76.5
  roots (of teeth) K00.2
  spleen Q89.09
  tarsal bones Q74.2
  teeth K00.1
  testis Q55.29
  thumb Q69.1
  toe Q69.2
  uterus Q51.28
  vagina Q52.1
  vertebra Q76.49
Supervision (of)
  contraceptive —*see* Prescription, contraceptives
  dietary (for) Z71.3
    allergy (food) Z71.3
    colitis Z71.3

Supervision (*Continued*)
  dietary (*Continued*)
    diabetes mellitus Z71.3
    food allergy or intolerance Z71.3
    gastritis Z71.3
    hypercholesterolemia Z71.3
    hypoglycemia Z71.3
    intolerance (food) Z71.3
    obesity Z71.3
    specified NEC Z71.3
  healthy infant or child Z76.2
    foundling Z76.1
  high-risk pregnancy —*see* Pregnancy,
      supervision of, high, risk
  lactation Z39.1
  pregnancy —*see* Pregnancy, supervision of
Supplemental teeth K00.1
Suppression
  binocular vision H53.34
  lactation O92.5
  menstruation N94.89
  ovarian secretion E28.39
  renal N28.9
  urine, urinary secretion R34
Suppuration, suppurative —*see also* condition
  accessory sinus (chronic) —*see* Sinusitis
  adrenal gland
  antrum (chronic) —*see* Sinusitis, maxillary
  bladder —*see* Cystitis
  brain G06.0
    sequelae G09
  breast N61.1
    puerperal, postpartum or gestational —*see*
        Mastitis, obstetric, purulent
  dental periosteum M27.3
  ear (middle) —*see also* Otitis, media
    external NEC —*see* Otitis, externa, infective
    internal —*see* subcategory H83.0
  ethmoidal (chronic) (sinus) —*see* Sinusitis,
      ethmoidal
  fallopian tube —*see* Salpingo-oophoritis
  frontal (chronic) (sinus) —*see* Sinusitis, frontal
  gallbladder (acute) K81.0
  gum K05.20
    generalized —*see* Periodontitis, aggressive,
        generalized
    localized —*see* Periodontitis, aggressive,
        localized
  intracranial G06.0
  joint —*see* Arthritis, pyogenic or pyemic
  labyrinthine —*see* subcategory H83.0
  lung —*see* Abscess, lung
  mammary gland N61.1
    puerperal, postpartum O91.12
      associated with lactation O91.13
  maxilla, maxillary M27.2
    sinus (chronic) —*see* Sinusitis, maxillary
  muscle —*see* Myositis, infective
  nasal sinus (chronic) —*see* Sinusitis
  pancreas, acute —*see also* Pancreatitis, acute K85.80
  parotid gland —*see* Sialoadenitis
  pelvis, pelvic
    female —*see* Disease, pelvis, inflammatory
    male K65.0
  pericranial —*see* Osteomyelitis
  salivary duct or gland (any) —*see* Sialoadenitis
  sinus (accessory) (chronic) (nasal) —*see* Sinusitis
  sphenoidal sinus (chronic) —*see* Sinusitis,
      sphenoidal
  thymus (gland) E32.1
  thyroid (gland) E06.0
  tonsil —*see* Tonsillitis
  uterus —*see* Endometritis
Supraeruption of tooth (teeth) M26.34
Supraglottitis J04.30
  with obstruction J04.31
Suprarenal (gland) —*see* condition
Suprascapular nerve —*see* condition
Suprasellar —*see* condition
Surfer's knots or nodules S89.8-●
Surgical
  emphysema T81.82
  procedures, complication or misadventure —*see*
      Complications, surgical procedures
  shock T81.10
Surveillance (of) (for) —*see also* Observation
  alcohol abuse Z71.41
  contraceptive —*see* Prescription, contraceptives
  dietary Z71.3
  drug abuse Z71.51
  neoplasm —*see* Screening, neoplasm

Susceptibility to disease, genetic Z15.89
  malignant neoplasm Z15.09
    breast Z15.01
    endometrium Z15.04
    ovary Z15.02
    prostate Z15.03
    specified NEC Z15.09
  multiple endocrine neoplasia Z15.81
Suspected condition, ruled out —*see also*
    Observation, suspected
  amniotic cavity and membrane Z03.71
  cervical shortening Z03.75
  fetal anomaly Z03.73
  fetal growth Z03.74
  maternal and fetal conditions NEC
      Z03.79
  newborn —*see also* Observation, newborn,
      suspected condition ruled out Z05.9
  oligohydramnios Z03.71
  placental problem Z03.72
  polyhydramnios Z03.71
Suspended uterus
  in pregnancy or childbirth —*see* Pregnancy,
      complicated by, abnormal uterus
Sutton's nevus D22.9
Suture
  burst (in operation wound) T81.31
    external operation wound T81.31
    internal operation wound T81.329
  inadvertently left in operation wound —*see*
      Foreign body, accidentally left during a
      procedure
  removal Z48.02
Swab inadvertently left in operation wound —
    see Foreign body, accidentally left during a
    procedure
Swallowed, swallowing
  difficulty —*see* Dysphagia
  foreign body —*see* Foreign body, alimentary tract
Swan-neck deformity (finger) —*see* Deformity,
    finger, swan-neck
Swearing, compulsive F42.8
  in Gilles de la Tourette's syndrome F95.2
Sweat, sweats
  fetid L75.0
  night R61
Sweating, excessive R61
Sweeley-Klionsky disease E75.21
Sweet's disease or dermatosis L98.2
Swelling (of) R60.9
  abdomen, abdominal (not referable to any
      particular organ) —*see* Mass, abdominal
  ankle —*see* Effusion, joint, ankle
  arm M79.89
    forearm M79.89
  breast —*see also* Lump, breast N63.0
  Calabar B74.3
  cervical gland R59.0
  chest, localized R22.2
  ear H93.8-●
  extremity (lower) (upper) —*see* Disorder, soft
      tissue, specified type NEC
  finger M79.89
  foot M79.89
  glands R59.9
    generalized R59.1
    localized R59.0
  hand M79.89
  head (localized) R22.0
  inflammatory —*see* Inflammation
  intra-abdominal —*see* Mass, abdominal
  joint —*see* Effusion, joint
  leg M79.89
    lower M79.89
  limb —*see* Disorder, soft tissue, specified type
      NEC
  localized (skin) R22.9
    chest R22.2
    head R22.0
    limb
      lower —*see* Mass, localized, limb, lower
      upper —*see* Mass, localized, limb, upper
    neck R22.1
    trunk R22.2
  neck (localized) R22.1
  pelvic —*see* Mass, abdominal
  scrotum N50.89
  splenic —*see* Splenomegaly
  testis N50.89
  toe M79.89
  umbilical R19.09

▶ New   ⇒ Revised   ~~deleted~~ Deleted   • Use Additional Character(s)

Syndrome *(Continued)*
  Boder-Sedgewick G11.3
  Boerhaave's K22.3
  Borjeson Forssman Lehmann Q89.8
  Bouillaud's I01.9
  Bourneville (-Pringle) Q85.1
  Bouveret (-Hoffman) I47.9
  brachial plexus G54.0
  bradycardia-tachycardia I49.5
  brain (nonpsychotic) F09
    with psychosis, psychotic reaction F09
    acute or subacute —*see* Delirium
    congenital —*see* Disability, intellectual
    organic F09
      post-traumatic (nonpsychotic) F07.81
        psychotic F09
      personality change F07.0
      postcontusional F07.81
      post-traumatic, nonpsychotic F07.81
      psycho-organic F09
      psychotic F06.8
  brain stem stroke G46.3
  Brandt's (acrodermatitis enteropathica) E83.2
  broad ligament laceration N83.8
  Brock's J98.11
  bronchiolitis obliterans *(see also* Bronchiolitis, obliterative) J44.81
  bronze baby P83.88
  Brown-Sequard G83.81
  Brugada I49.8
  bubbly lung P27.0
  Buchem's M85.2
  Budd-Chiari I82.0
  bulbar (progressive) G12.22
  Bürger-Grütz E78.3
  Burke's K86.89
  Burnett's (milk-alkali) E83.52
  burning feet E53.9
  Bywaters' T79.5
  Call-Fleming I67.841
  carbohydrate-deficient glycoprotein (CDGS) E77.8
  carcinogenic thrombophlebitis I82.1
  carcinoid E34.00
    heart E34.01
    specified NEC E34.09
  cardiac asthma I50.1
  cardiacos negros I27.0
  cardiofaciocutaneous Q87.89
  cardiopulmonary-obesity E66.2
  cardiorenal —*see* Hypertension, cardiorenal
  cardiorespiratory distress (idiopathic), newborn P22.0
  cardiovascular renal —*see* Hypertension, cardiorenal
  carotid
    artery (hemispheric) (internal) G45.1
    body G90.01
    sinus G90.01
  carpal tunnel G56.0-●
  Cassidy (-Scholte) E34.09
  cat-cry Q93.4
  cat eye Q92.8
  cauda equina G83.4
  causalgia —*see* Causalgia
  celiac K90.0
    artery compression I77.4
    axis I77.4
  central pain G89.0
  cerebellar
    hereditary G11.9
    stroke G46.4
  cerebellomedullary malformation —*see* Spina bifida
  cerebral
    artery
      anterior G46.1
      middle G46.0
      posterior G46.2
    gigantism E22.0
  cervical (root) M53.1
    disc —*see* Disorder, disc, cervical, with neuritis
    fusion Q76.1
    posterior, sympathicus M53.0
    rib Q76.5
    sympathetic paralysis G90.2
  cervicobrachial (diffuse) M53.1
  cervicocranial M53.0
  cervicodorsal outlet G54.2
  cervicothoracic outlet *(see also* Syndrome, thoracic outlet) G54.0
  Céstan (-Raymond) I65.8

Syndrome *(Continued)*
  Charcot's (angina cruris) (intermittent claudication) I73.9
  Charcot-Weiss-Baker G90.09
  CHARGE Q89.8
  Chédiak-Higashi (-Steinbrinck) E70.330
  chest wall R07.1
  Chiari's (hepatic vein thrombosis) I82.0
  Chilaiditi's Q43.3
  child maltreatment —*see* Maltreatment, child
  chondrocostal junction M94.0
  chondroectodermal dysplasia Q77.6
  chromosome 4 short arm deletion Q93.3
  chromosome 5 short arm deletion Q93.4
  chronic
    infantile neurological, cutaneous and articular (CINCA) M04.2
    pain G89.4
      personality F68.8
  Churg-Strauss M30.1
  Clarke-Hadfield K86.89
  Clerambault's automatism G93.89
  Clouston's (hidrotic ectodermal dysplasia) Q82.4
  clumsiness, clumsy child F82
  cluster headache G44.009
    intractable G44.001
    not intractable G44.009
  Coffin-Lowry Q89.8
  cold injury (newborn) P80.0
  combined immunity deficiency D81.9
  compartment (deep) (posterior) (traumatic) T79.A0
    abdomen T79.A3
    lower extremity (hip, buttock, thigh, leg, foot, toes) T79.A2
    nontraumatic
      abdomen M79.A3
      lower extremity (hip, buttock, thigh, leg, foot, toes) M79.A2-●
      specified site NEC M79.A9
      upper extremity (shoulder, arm, forearm, wrist, hand, fingers) M79.A1-●
    postprocedural —*see* Syndrome compartment, nontraumatic
    specified site NEC T79.A9
    upper extremity (shoulder, arm, forearm, wrist, hand, fingers) T79.A1
  complex regional pain —*see* Syndrome, pain, complex regional
  compression T79.5
    anterior spinal —*see* Syndrome, anterior, spinal artery, compression
    cauda equina G83.4
    celiac artery I77.4
    vertebral artery M47.029
      cervical region M47.022
      occipito-atlanto-axial region M47.021
  concussion F07.81
  congenital
    affecting multiple systems NEC Q87.89
    central alveolar hypoventilation G47.35
    facial diplegia Q87.0
    muscular hypertrophy-cerebral Q87.89
    oculo-auriculovertebral Q87.0
    oculofacial diplegia (Moebius) Q87.0
    rubella (manifest) P35.0
  congestion-fibrosis (pelvic), female N94.89
  congestive dysmenorrhea N94.6
  Conn's E26.01
  connective tissue M35.9
    overlap NEC M35.1
  conus medullaris G95.81
  cord
    anterior G83.82
    posterior G83.83
  coronary
    acute NEC I24.9
    insufficiency or intermediate I20.0
    slow flow I20.89
  Costen's (complex) M26.69
  costochondral junction M94.0
  costoclavicular G54.0
  costovertebral E22.0
  Cowden
    PTEN related Q85.81
    specified NEC Q85.82
  craniovertebral M53.0
  Creutzfeldt-Jakob —*see* Creutzfeldt-Jakob disease or syndrome
  cri-du-chat Q93.4
  crib death R99

Syndrome *(Continued)*
  cricopharyngeal —*see* Dysphagia
  croup J05.0
  CRPS I —*see* Syndrome, pain, complex regional I
  crush T79.5
  cubital tunnel —*see* Lesion, nerve, ulnar
  Curschmann (-Batten) (-Steinert) G71.11
  Cushing's E24.9
    alcohol-induced E24.4
    drug-induced E24.2
    due to
      alcohol
        drugs E24.2
      ectopic ACTH E24.3
      overproduction of pituitary ACTH E24.0
      overdose or wrong substance given or taken —*see* Table of Drugs and Chemicals, by drug, poisoning
    pituitary-dependent E24.0
    specified type NEC E24.8
  cryopyrin-associated periodic M04.2
  cryptophthalmos Q87.0
  cystic duct stump K91.5
  cytokine release D89.839
    grade 1 D89.831
    grade 2 D89.832
    grade 3 D89.833
    grade 4 D89.834
    grade 5 D89.835
  Dana-Putnam D51.0
  Danbolt (-Cross) (acrodermatitis enteropathica) E83.2
  Dandy-Walker Q03.1
    with spina bifida Q07.01
  Danlos' *(see also* Syndrome, Ehlers-Danlos) Q79.60
  defibrination —*see also* Fibrinolysis
    with
      antepartum hemorrhage —*see* Hemorrhage, antepartum, with coagulation defect
      intrapartum hemorrhage —*see* Hemorrhage, complicating, delivery
    newborn P60
    postpartum O72.3
  Degos' I77.8
  Déjérine-Roussy G89.0
  delayed sleep phase G47.21
  demyelinating G37.9
  dependence —*see* F10-F19 with fourth character .2
  depersonalization (-derealization) F48.1
  De Quervain E34.51
  de Toni-Fanconi (-Debré) E72.09
    with cystinosis E72.04
  de Vivo syndrome E74.810
  diabetes mellitus-hypertension-nephrosis —*see* Diabetes, nephrosis
  diabetes mellitus in newborn infant P70.2
  diabetes-nephrosis —*see* Diabetes, nephrosis
  diabetic amyotrophy —*see* Diabetes, amyotrophy
  dialysis associated steal T82.898-●
  Diamond-Blackfan D61.01
  Diamond-Gardener D69.2
  DIC (diffuse or disseminated intravascular coagulopathy) D65
  di George's D82.1
  Dighton's Q78.0
  disequilibrium E87.8
  Döhle body-panmyelopathic D72.0
  dorsolateral medullary G46.4
  double athetosis G80.3
  Down *(see also* Down syndrome) Q90.9
  Dravet (intractable) G40.834
    with status epilepticus G40.833
    without status epilepticus G40.834
  Dresbach's (elliptocytosis) D58.1
  DRESS (drug rash with eosinophilia and systemic symptoms) D72.12
  Dressler's (postmyocardial infarction) I24.1
    postcardiotomy I97.0
  drug rash with eosinophilia and systemic symptoms (DRESS) D72.12
  drug withdrawal, infant of dependent mother P96.1
  dry eye H04.12-●
  due to abnormality
    chromosomal Q99.9
      sex
        female phenotype Q97.9
        male phenotype Q98.9
        specified NEC Q99.8

Syndrome *(Continued)*
  dumping (postgastrectomy) K91.1
    nonsurgical K31.89
  Dupré's (meningism) R29.1
  dysmetabolic X E88.810
  dyspraxia, developmental F82
  Eagle-Barrett Q79.4
  Eaton-Lambert —*see* Syndrome, Lambert-Eaton
  Ebstein's Q22.5
  ectopic ACTH E24.3
  eczema-thrombocytopenia D82.0
  Eddowes' Q78.0
  effort (psychogenic) F45.8
  Ehlers-Danlos Q79.60
    classical (cEDS) (classical EDS) Q79.61
    hypermobile (hEDS) (hypermobile EDS) Q79.62
    specified NEC Q79.69
    vascular (vascular EDS) (vEDS) Q79.63
  Eisenmenger's I27.83
  Ekman's Q78.0
  electric feet E53.8
  Ellis-van Creveld Q77.6
  empty nest Z60.0
  endocrine-hypertensive E27.0
  entrapment —*see* Neuropathy, entrapment
  eosinophilia-myalgia M35.89
  epileptic —*see also* Epilepsy, by type
    absence G40.A09
      intractable G40.A19
        with status epilepticus G40.A11
        without status epilepticus G40.A19
      not intractable G40.A09
        with status epilepticus G40.A01
        without status epilepticus G40.A09
  Erdheim-Chester (ECD) E88.89
  Erdheim's E22.0
  erythrocyte fragmentation D59.4
  Evans D69.41
  exhaustion F48.8
  extrapyramidal G25.9
    specified NEC G25.89
  eye retraction —*see* Strabismus
  eyelid-malar-mandible Q87.0
  Faber's D50.9
  facet M47.89-•
  facet joint (*see also* Spondylosis) M47.819
  facial pain, paroxysmal G50.0
  Fallot's Q21.3
  familial cold autoinflammatory M04.2
  familial eczema-thrombocytopenia (Wiskott-Aldrich) D82.0
  Fanconi (-de Toni) (-Debré) E72.09
    with cystinosis E72.04
  ~~Fanconi's (anemia) (congenital pancytopenia) D61.09~~
  fatigue
    chronic G93.32
    postviral G93.31
    psychogenic F48.8
  faulty bowel habit K59.39
  Feil-Klippel (brevicollis) Q76.1
  Felty's —*see* Felty's syndrome
  fertile eunuch E23.0
  fetal
    alcohol (dysmorphic) Q86.0
    hydantoin Q86.1
  Fiedler's I40.1
  first arch Q87.0
  fish odor E72.89
  Fisher's G61.0
  Fitzhugh-Curtis
    due to
      Chlamydia trachomatis A74.81
      ~~Neisseria gonorrhorea (gonococcal peritonitis) A54.85~~
      ▶Neisseria gonorrhea (gonococcal peritonitis) A54.85
  Fitz's —*see also* Pancreatitis, acute K85.80
  Flajani (-Basedow) E05.00
    with thyroid storm E05.01
  flatback —*see* Flatback syndrome
  floppy
    baby P94.2
    iris (intraoperative) (IFIS) H21.81
    mitral valve I34.1
  flush E34.09
  Foix-Alajouanine G95.19
  Fong's Q87.2
  food protein-induced enterocolitis (FPIES) K52.21
  foramen magnum G93.5

Syndrome *(Continued)*
  Foster-Kennedy H47.14-•
  Foville's (peduncular) G46.3
  fragile X Q99.2
  Franceschetti Q75.4
  Frey's
    auriculotemporal G50.8
    hyperhidrosis L74.52
  Friderichsen-Waterhouse A39.1
  Froin's G95.89
  frontal lobe F07.0
  Fukuhara E88.49
  functional
    bowel K59.9
    prepubertal castrate E29.1
  Gaisböck's D75.1
  ganglion (basal ganglia brain) G25.9
    geniculi G51.1
  Gardner-Diamond D69.2
  gastroesophageal
    junction K22.0
    laceration-hemorrhage K22.6
  gastrojejunal loop obstruction K91.89
  Gee-Herter-Heubner K90.0
  Gelineau's G47.419
    with cataplexy G47.411
  genito-anorectal A55
  Gerstmann-Sträussler-Scheinker (GSS) A81.82
  Gianotti-Crosti L44.4
  giant platelet (Bernard-Soulier) D69.1
  Gilles de la Tourette's F95.2
  Glass Q87.89
  Gleich's D72.118
  goiter-deafness E07.1
  Goldberg Q89.8
  Goldberg-Maxwell E34.51
  Good's D83.8
  Gopalan' (burning feet) E53.8
  Gorlin's Q87.89
  Gougerot-Blum L81.7
  Gouley's I31.1
  Gower's R55
  gray or grey (newborn) P93.0
    platelet D69.1
  Gubler-Millard G46.3
  Guillain-Barré (-Strohl) G61.0
  gustatory sweating G50.8
  Hadfield-Clarke K86.89
  hair tourniquet —*see* Constriction, external, by site
  Hamman's J98.19
  hand-foot L27.1
  hand-shoulder G90.89
  hantavirus (cardio)-pulmonary (HPS) (HCPS) B33.4
  happy puppet Q93.51
  Harada's H30.81-•
  Hayem-Faber D50.9
  headache NEC G44.89
    complicated NEC G44.59
  Heberden's I20.89
  Hedinger's E34.01
  Hegglin's D72.0
  HELLP (hemolysis, elevated liver enzymes and low platelet count) O14.2-•
    complicating
      childbirth O14.24
        puerperium O14.25
  hemolytic-uremic D59.30
    atypical D59.39
      genetic D59.32
      hereditary D59.32
      infection-associated D59.31
      secondary D59.39
      specified NEC D59.39
    due to genetic disorder D59.32
    familial D59.32
    hereditary D59.32
    infection-associated D59.31
    secondary D59.39
    Shiga toxin-producing E. coli [STEC] related D59.31
    specified NEC D59.39
    typical D59.31
  hemophagocytic, infection-associated D76.2
  Henoch-Schönlein D69.0
  hepatic flexure K59.89
  hepatopulmonary K76.81
  hepatorenal K76.7
    following delivery O90.41
    postoperative or postprocedural K91.83
    postpartum, puerperal O90.41

Syndrome *(Continued)*
  hepatourologic K76.7
  hereditary alpha tryptasemia D89.44
  Herter (-Gee) (nontropical sprue) K90.0
  Heubner-Herter K90.0
  Heyd's K76.7
  Hilger's G90.09
  histamine-like (fish poisoning) —*see* Poisoning, fish
  histiocytic D76.3
  histiocytosis NEC D76.3
  HIV infection, acute B20
  Hoffmann-Werdnig G12.0
  Hollander-Simons E88.1
  Hoppe-Goldflam G70.00
    with exacerbation (acute) G70.01
    in crisis G70.01
  Horner's G90.2
  hungry bone E83.81
  hunterian glossitis D51.0
  Hunt's (herpetic geniculate ganglionitis) (neuralgia) B02.21
    dyssynergia cerebellaris myoclonica G11.19
  Hutchinson's triad A50.53
  hyperabduction G54.0
  hyperammonemia-hyperornithinemia-homocitrullinemia E72.4
  hypereosinophilic (HES) D72.119
    idiopathic (IHES) D72.110
    lymphocytic variant (LHES) D72.111
    myeloid D72.118
    specified NEC D72.118
  hyperimmunoglobulin D M04.1
  hyperimmunoglobulin E (IgE) D82.4
  hyperkalemic E87.5
  hyperkinetic —*see* Hyperkinesia
  hypermobility M35.7
  hypernatremia E87.0
  hyperosmolarity (*see also*, Diabetes, by type, with hyperosmolarity) E87.0
  hyperperfusion G97.82
  hypersplenic D73.1
  hypertransfusion, newborn P61.1
  hyperventilation F45.8
  hyperviscosity (of serum)
    polycythemic D75.1
    sclerothymic D58.8
  hypoglycemic (familial) (neonatal) E16.2
  hypokalemic E87.6
  hyponatremic E87.1
  hypopituitarism E23.0
  hypoplastic left-heart Q23.4
  hypopotassemia E87.6
  hyposmolality E87.1
  hypotension, maternal O26.5-•
  hypothenar hammer I73.89
  hypoventilation, obesity (OHS) E66.2
  ICF (intravascular coagulation-fibrinolysis) D65
  idiopathic
    cardiorespiratory distress, newborn P22.0
    nephrotic (infantile) N04.9
  iliotibial band M76.3-•
  immobility, immobilization (paraplegic) M62.3
  immune effector cell-associated neurotoxicity (ICANS) G92.00
    grade
      1 G92.01
      2 G92.02
      3 G92.03
      4 G92.04
      5 G92.05
      unspecified G92.00
  immune reconstitution D89.3
  immune reconstitution inflammatory [IRIS] D89.3
  immunity deficiency, combined D81.9
  immunodeficiency
    acquired —*see* Human, immunodeficiency virus (HIV) disease
    combined D81.9
  impending coronary I20.0
  impingement, shoulder M75.4-•
  inappropriate secretion of antidiuretic hormone E22.2
  infant
    gestational diabetes P70.0
    of diabetic mother P70.1
  infantilism (pituitary) E23.0
  inferior vena cava I87.1
  inspissated bile (newborn) P59.1
  institutional (childhood) F94.2
  insufficient sleep F51.12

▶ New   ⟹ Revised   ~~deleted~~ Deleted   • Use Additional Character(s)

Syndrome *(Continued)*
  insulin resistance
    type A E88.811
    type B E88.818
  intermediate coronary (artery) I20.0
  interspinous ligament —*see* Spondylopathy,
    specified NEC
  intestinal
    ➡carcinoid E34.09
    knot K56.2
  intravascular coagulation-fibrinolysis (ICF) D65
  iodine-deficiency, congenital E00.9
    type
      mixed E00.2
      myxedematous E00.1
      neurological E00.0
  IRDS (idiopathic respiratory distress, newborn)
    P22.0
  irritable
    bowel K58.9
      with
        constipation K58.1
        diarrhea K58.0
      mixed K58.2
      psychogenic F45.8
      specified NEC K58.8
    heart (psychogenic) F45.8
    weakness F48.8
  ischemic
    bowel (transient) K55.9
      chronic K55.1
      due to mesenteric artery insufficiency K55.1
    steal T82.898
  IVC (intravascular coagulopathy) D65
  Ivemark's Q89.01
  Jaccoud's —*see* Arthropathy, postrheumatic,
    chronic
  Jackson's G83.89
  Jakob-Creutzfeldt —*see* Creutzfeldt-Jakob
    disease or syndrome
  jaw-winking Q07.8
  Jervell-Lange-Nielsen I45.81
  jet lag G47.25
  Job's D71
  Joseph-Diamond-Blackfan D61.01
  jugular foramen G52.7
  Kabuki Q89.8
  Kanner's (autism) F84.0
  Kartagener's Q89.3
  Kelly's D50.1
  Kimmelstiel-Wilson —*see* Diabetes, specified
    type, with Kimmelstiel-Wilson disease
  ▶Kleefstra Q87.86
  Klein (e)-Levine G47.13
  Klippel-Feil (brevicollis) Q76.1
  ~~Köhler-Pellegrini-Steida —see Bursitis, tibial collateral~~
  ▶Köhler-Pellegrini-Stieda —*see* Bursitis, tibial
    collateral
  König's K59.89
  Korsakoff (-Wernicke) (nonalcoholic) F04
    alcoholic F10.26
  Kostmann's D70.0
  Krabbe's congenital muscle hypoplasia Q79.8
  labyrinthine —*see* subcategory H83.2
  lacunar NEC G46.7
  Lambert-Eaton G70.80
    in
      neoplastic disease G73.1
      specified disease NEC G70.81
  Landau-Kleffner —*see* Epilepsy, specified NEC
  Larsen's Q74.8
  ▶Lassueur Graham-Little Piccardi L66.19
  lateral
    cutaneous nerve of thigh G57.1-●
    medullary G46.4
  Launois' E22.0
  Laurence-Moon Q87.84
  lazy
    leukocyte D70.8
    posture M62.3
  ~~Lemierre I80.8~~
  ▶Lemierre I80.8
  Lennox-Gastaut G40.812
    intractable G40.814
      with status epilepticus G40.813
      without status epilepticus G40.814
    not intractable G40.812
      with status epilepticus G40.811
      without status epilepticus G40.812
  lenticular, progressive E83.01
  Leopold-Levi's E05.90

Syndrome *(Continued)*
  Lev's I44.2
  Li-Fraumeni Z15.01
  Lichtheim's D51.0
  Lightwood's N25.89
  Lignac (de Toni) (-Fanconi) (-Debré) E72.09
    with cystinosis E72.04
  Likoff's I20.89
  limbic epilepsy personality F07.0
  liver-kidney K76.7
  lobotomy F07.0
  Löffler's J82.89
  long arm 18 or 21 deletion Q93.89
  long QT I45.81
  Louis-Barré G11.3
  low
    atmospheric pressure T70.29
    back M54.50
    output (cardiac) I50.9
  lower radicular, newborn (birth injury) P14.8
  Luetscher's (dehydration) E86.0
  Lupus anticoagulant D68.62
  Lutembacher's Q21.19
  macrophage activation D76.1
    due to infection D76.2
  magnesium-deficiency R29.0
  Majeed M04.8
  Mal de Debarquement R42
  malabsorption K90.9
    postsurgical K91.2
  malformation, congenital, due to
    alcohol Q86.0
    exogenous cause NEC Q86.8
    hydantoin Q86.1
    warfarin Q86.2
  malignant
    ➡carcinoid E34.00
    neuroleptic G21.0
  Mallory-Weiss K22.6
  mandibulofacial dysostosis Q75.4
  manic-depressive —*see* Disorder, bipolar
  maple-syrup-urine E71.0
  Marable's I77.4
  Marfan Q87.40
    with
      cardiovascular manifestations Q87.418
        aortic dilation Q87.410
      ocular manifestations Q87.42
      skeletal manifestations Q87.43
  Marie's (acromegaly) E22.0
  mast cell activation —*see* Activation, mast cell
  maternal hypotension —*see* Syndrome,
    hypotension, maternal
  May (-Hegglin) D72.0
  McArdle (-Schmidt) (-Pearson) E74.04
  McQuarrie's E16.2
  meconium plug (newborn) P76.0
  MED13L (mediator complex subunit 13L) Q87.85
  median arcuate ligament I77.4
  mediator complex subunit 13L (MED13L) Q87.85
  Meekeren-Ehlers-Danlos Q79.6
  megavitamin-B6 E67.2
  Meige G24.4
  MELAS E88.41
  Mendelson's O74.0
  MERRF (myoclonic epilepsy associated with
    ragged-red fibers) E88.42
  mesenteric
    artery (superior) K55.1
    vascular insufficiency K55.1
  metabolic E88.810
  ➡metastatic carcinoid E34.00
  micrognathia-glossoptosis Q87.0
  midbrain NEC G93.89
  middle lobe (lung) J98.19
  middle radicular G54.0
  migraine —*see also* Migraine G43.909-●
  Mikulicz' K11.8
  milk-alkali E83.52
  Millard-Gubler G46.3
  Miller-Dieker Q93.88
  Miller-Fisher G61.0
  Minkowski-Chauffard D58.0
  Mirizzi's K83.1
  MNGIE (Mitochondrial Neurogastrointestinal
    Encephalopathy) E88.49
  Möbius, ophthalmoplegic migraine —*see*
    Migraine, ophthalmoplegic
  monofixation H50.42
  Morel-Moore M85.2
  Morel-Morgagni M85.2
  Morgagni (-Morel) (-Stewart) M85.2

Syndrome *(Continued)*
  Morgagni-Adams-Stokes I45.9
  Mounier-Kuhn Q32.4
    with bronchiectasis J47.9
      with
        exacerbation (acute) J47.1
        lower respiratory infection J47.0
    acquired J98.09
      with bronchiectasis J47.9
        with
          exacerbation (acute) J47.1
          lower respiratory infection J47.0
  Muckle-Wells M04.2
  mucocutaneous lymph node (acute febrile)
    (MCLS) M30.3
  multiple endocrine neoplasia (MEN) —*see*
    Neoplasia, endocrine, multiple (MEN}
  multiple operations —*see* Disorder, factitious
  multisystem inflammatory (in adults) (in
    children) M35.81
  myasthenic G70.9
    in
      diabetes mellitus —*see* Diabetes,
        amyotrophy
      endocrine disease NEC E34.9 *[G73.3]*
      neoplastic disease —*see also* Neoplasm
        D49.9 *[G73.3]*
      thyrotoxicosis (hyperthyroidism) E05.90
        [G73.3]
      with thyroid storm E05.91 *[G73.3]*
  myelodysplastic D46.9
    with
      5q deletion D46.C
      isolated del (5q) chromosomal abnormality
        D46.C
      multilineage dysplasia D46.A
        with ringed sideroblasts D46.B
    lesions, low grade D46.20
    specified NEC D46.Z
  myeloid hypereosinophilic D72.118
  myelopathic pain G89.0
  myeloproliferative (chronic) D47.1
  myofascial pain M79.18
  Naffziger's G54.0
  nail patella Q87.2
  NARP (Neuropathy, Ataxia and Retinitis
    pigmentosa) E88.49
  neonatal abstinence P96.1
  nephritic —*see also* Nephritis
    with edema —*see* Nephrosis
    acute N00.9
    chronic N03.9
    rapidly progressive N01.9
  nephrotic (congenital) —*see also* Nephrosis N04.9
    with
      C3
        glomerulonephritis N04.A
        glomerulopathy N04.A
          with dense deposit disease N04.6
      dense deposit disease N04.6
      diffuse
        crescentic glomerulonephritis N04.7
        endocapillary proliferative
          glomerulonephritis N04.4
        membranous glomerulonephritis N04.20
        mesangial proliferative
          glomerulonephritis N04.3
        mesangiocapillary glomerulonephritis
          N04.5
      focal and segmental glomerular lesions
        N04.1
      minor glomerular abnormality N04.0
      specified morphological changes NEC
        N04.8
    diabetic —*see* Diabetes, nephrosis
    specified type NEC with diffuse membranous
      glomerulonephritis N04.29
  neurologic neglect R41.4
  Nezelof's D81.4
  Nonne-Milroy-Meige Q82.0
  Nothnagel's vasomotor acroparesthesia I73.89
  obesity hypoventilation (OHS) E66.2
  obliterans
    bronchiolitis (see also Bronchiolitis,
      obliterative) J44.81
  oculomotor H51.9
  Ogilvie K59.81
  Oliver-McFarlane Q87.89
  ophthalmoplegia-cerebellar ataxia —*see*
    Strabismus, paralytic, third nerve
  oral allergy T78.1
  oral-facial-digital Q87.0

Syndrome *(Continued)*
  organic
    affective F06.30
    amnesic (not alcohol- or drug-induced) F04
    brain F09
    depressive F06.31
    hallucinosis F06.0
    personality F07.0
  Ormond's N13.5
  oro-facial-digital Q87.0
  os trigonum Q68.8
  Osler-Weber-Rendu I78.0
  osteoporosis-osteomalacia M83.8
  Osterreicher-Turner Q87.2
  otolith —*see* subcategory H81.8
  oto-palatal-digital Q87.0
  outlet (thoracic) (*see also* Syndrome, thoracic
      outlet) G54.0
  ovary
    polycystic E28.2
    resistant E28.39
    sclerocystic E28.2
  Owren's D68.2
  Paget-Schroetter I82.890
  pain —*see also* Pain
    complex regional I G90.50
      lower limb G90.52-●
      specified site NEC G90.59
      upper limb G90.51-●
    complex regional II —*see* Causalgia
  painful
    bruising D69.2
    feet E53.8
    prostate N42.81
  paralysis agitans —*see* Parkinsonism
  paralytic G83.9
    specified NEC G83.89
  Parinaud's H51.0
  parkinsonian —*see* Parkinsonism
  Parkinson's —*see* Parkinsonism
  paroxysmal facial pain G50.0
  Parry's E05.00
    with thyroid storm E05.01
  Parsonage (-Aldren)-Turner G54.5
  patella clunk M25.86-●
  Paterson (-Brown) (-Kelly) D50.1
  pectoral girdle I77.89
  pectoralis minor I77.89
  pediatric autoimmune neuropsychiatric
      disorders associated with streptococcal
      infections (PANDAS) D89.89
  pediatric inflammatory multisystem M35.81
  Pelger-Huet D72.0
  pellagra-cerebellar ataxia-renal aminoaciduria
      E72.02
  pellagroid E52
  Pellegrini-Stieda —*see* Bursitis, tibial collateral
  pelvic congestion-fibrosis, female N94.89
  penta X Q97.1
  peptic ulcer —*see* Ulcer, peptic
  perabduction I77.89
  periodic fever M04.1
  periodic fever, aphthous stomatitis, pharyngitis,
      and adenopathy [PFAPA] M04.8
  periodic headache, in adults and children —*see*
      Headache, periodic syndromes in adults
      and children
  periurethral fibrosis N13.5
  Peutz-Jeghers Q85.89
  phantom limb (without pain) G54.7
    with pain G54.6
  pharyngeal pouch D82.1
  Phelan-McDermid Q93.52
  Pick's —*see* Disease, Pick's
  Pickwickian E66.2
  PIE (pulmonary infiltration with eosinophilia)
      J82.89
  pigmentary pallidal degeneration (progressive)
      G23.0
  pineal E34.8
  pituitary E22.0
  placental transfusion —*see* Pregnancy, complicated
      by, placental transfusion syndromes
  plantar fascia M72.2
  plateau iris (post-iridectomy) (postprocedural)
      H21.82
  Plummer-Vinson D50.1
  pluricarential of infancy E40
  plurideficiency E40
  pluriglandular (compensatory) E31.8
    autoimmune E31.0
  pneumatic hammer T75.21

Syndrome *(Continued)*
  polyangiitis overlap M30.8
  polycarential of infancy E40
  polyglandular E31.8
    autoimmune E31.0
  polysplenia Q89.09
  pontine NEC G93.89
  popliteal
    artery entrapment I77.89
    web Q87.89
  postbacterial fatigue G93.39
  postcardiac injury
    postcardiotomy I97.0
    postmyocardial infarction I24.1
  postcardiotomy I97.0
  post chemoembolization — code to associated
      conditions
  postcholecystectomy K91.5
  postcommissurotomy I97.0
  postconcussional F07.81
  postcontusional F07.81
  post-COVID (-19) U09.9
  postencephalitic F07.89
  post endometrial ablation N99.85
  posterior
    cervical sympathetic M53.0
    cord G83.83
    fossa compression G93.5
    reversible encephalopathy (PRES) I67.83
  postgastrectomy (dumping) K91.1
  postgastric surgery K91.1
  postinfarction I24.1
  postinfectious fatigue G93.39
  postlaminectomy NEC M96.1
  postleukotomy F07.0
  postmastectomy lymphedema I97.2
  postmyocardial infarction I24.1
  postoperative NEC T81.9
    blind loop K90.2
  postpartum panhypopituitary (Sheehan)
      E23.0
  postpolio (myelitic) G14
  postthrombotic I87.009
    with
      inflammation I87.02-●
        with ulcer I87.03-●
      specified complication NEC I87.09-●
      ulcer I87.01-●
        with inflammation I87.03-●
    asymptomatic I87.00-●
  postural
    orthostatic tachycardia [POTS] G90.A
    tachycardia G90.A
  postvagotomy K91.1
  postvalvulotomy I97.0
  postviral NEC G93.31
    fatigue G93.31
  Potain's K31.0
  potassium intoxication E87.5
  Prader-Willi Q87.11
  Prader-Willi-like Q87.19
  precerebral artery (multiple) (bilateral)
      G45.2
  preinfarction I20.0
  preleukemic D46.9
  premature senility E34.8
  premenstrual dysphoric F32.81
  premenstrual tension N94.3
  Prinzmetal-Massumi R07.1
  prune belly Q79.4
  pseudocarpal tunnel (sublimis) —*see* Syndrome,
      carpal tunnel
  pseudoparalytica G70.00
    with exacerbation (acute) G70.01
    in crisis G70.01
  pseudo-Turner's Q87.19
  psycho-organic (nonpsychotic severity) F07.9
    acute or subacute F05
    depressive type F06.31
    hallucinatory type F06.0
    nonpsychotic severity F07.0
    specified NEC F07.89
  PTEN (hamartoma) tumor Q85.81
  pulmonary
    arteriosclerosis I27.0
    dysmaturity (Wilson-Mikity) P27.0
    hypoperfusion (idiopathic) P22.0
    renal (hemorrhagic) (Goodpasture's)
        M31.0
  pure
    motor lacunar G46.5
    sensory lacunar G46.6

Syndrome *(Continued)*
  Putnam-Dana D51.0
  pyogenic arthritis, pyoderma gangrenosum, and
      acne [PAPA] M04.8
  pyramidopallidonigral G20.C
  pyriformis —*see* Lesion, nerve, sciatic
  QT interval prolongation I45.81
  radicular NEC —*see* Radiculopathy
    upper limbs, newborn (birth injury) P14.3
  rapid time-zone change G47.25
  Rasmussen G04.81
  Raymond (-Céstan) I65.8
  Raynaud's I73.00
    with gangrene I73.01
  RDS (respiratory distress syndrome, newborn)
      P22.0
  reactive airways dysfunction J68.3
  Refsum's G60.1
  Reifenstein E34.52
  renal glomerulohyalinosis-diabetic —*see*
      Diabetes, nephrosis
  Rendu-Osler-Weber I78.0
  residual ovary N99.83
  resistant ovary E28.39
  respiratory
    distress
      acute J80
        adult J80
        child J80
        idiopathic J84.114
      newborn (idiopathic) (type I) P22.0
        type II P22.1
  restless legs G25.81
  restrictive allograft J4A.0
  retinoblastoma (familial) C69.2
  retroperitoneal fibrosis K68.2
  retroviral seroconversion (acute) Z21
  Reye's G93.7
  Richter —*see* Leukemia, chronic lymphocytic,
      B-cell type
  Ridley's I50.1
  right
    heart, hypoplastic Q22.6
    ventricular obstruction —*see* Failure, heart,
        right
  Romano-Ward (prolonged QT interval)
      I45.81
  rotator cuff, shoulder —*see also* Tear, rotator cuff
      M75.10-●
  Rotes Quérol —*see* Hyperostosis, ankylosing
  Roth —*see* Meralgia paresthetica
  rubella (congenital) P35.0
  Ruvalcaba-Myhre-Smith E71.440
  Rytand-Lipsitch I44.2
  salt
    depletion E87.1
      due to heat NEC T67.8
        causing heat exhaustion or prostration
            T67.4
    low E87.1
  salt-losing N28.89
  SATB2-associated Q87.89
  Scaglietti-Dagnini E22.0
  scalenus anticus (anterior) G54.0
  scapulocostal —*see* Mononeuropathy, upper
      limb, specified site NEC
  scapuloperoneal G71.09
  schizophrenic, of childhood NEC F20.9
  Schnitzler D47.2
  Scholte's E34.09
  Schroeder's E27.0
  Schüller-Christian C96.5
  Schwachman (-Diamond) D61.02
  Schwartz (-Jampel) G71.13
  Schwartz-Bartter E22.2
  scimitar Q26.8
  sclerocystic ovary E28.2
  Seitelberger's G31.89
  septicemic adrenal hemorrhage A39.1
  seroconversion, retroviral (acute) Z21
  serotonin G90.81
  serous meningitis G93.2
  severe acute respiratory (SARS) J12.81
  coronavirus 2 -*see also* COVID-19 U07.1
    pneumonia J12.82
  shaken infant T74.4
  shock (traumatic) T79.4
    kidney N17.0
      following crush injury T79.5
    toxic A48.3
  shock-lung J80
  Shone's — code to specific anomalies

Syndrome *(Continued)*
  short
    bowel K90.829
      with
        colon in continuity K90.821
        ileocolonic anastomosis K90.821
        without colon in continuity K90.822
      gut —*see* Syndrome, short, bowel
    rib Q77.2
  shoulder-hand —*see* Algoneurodystrophy
  Schwachman (-Diamond) D61.02
  sicca —*see* Syndrome, Sjögren
  sick
    cell E87.1
    sinus I49.5
  sick-euthyroid E07.81
  sideropenic D50.1
  Siemens' ectodermal dysplasia Q82.4
  Silfversköld's Q78.9
  Simons' E88.1
  sinus tarsi M25.57-●
  sinusitis-bronchiectasis-situs inversus Q89.3
  Sipple's E31.22
  sirenomelia Q87.2
  Sjögren M35.00
    with
      central nervous system involvement
        M35.07
      dental involvement M35.0C
      gastrointestinal involvement M35.08
      glomerular disease M35.0A
      inflammatory arthritis M35.05
      keratoconjunctivitis M35.01
      lung involvement M35.02
      myopathy M35.03
      peripheral nervous system involvement
        M35.06
      renal tubular acidosis M35.04
      specified organ involvement, NEC M35.09
      tubulo-interstitial nephropathy M35.04
      vasculitis M35.0B
  Slocumb's E27.0
  slow flow, coronary I20.89
  Sluder's G44.89
  Smith-Magenis Q93.88
  Sneddon-Wilkinson L13.1
  Snyder-Robinson Q87.89
  Sotos' Q87.3
  South African cardiomyopathy I42.8
  spasmodic
    upward movement, eyes H51.8
    winking F95.8
  Spen's I45.9
  splenic
    agenesis Q89.01
    flexure K59.89
    neutropenia D73.81
  Spurway's Q78.0
  staphylococcal scalded skin L00
  steal
    arteriovenous T82.898-●
    ischemic T82.898-●
    subclavian G45.8
  Stein-Leventhal E28.2
  Stein's E28.2
  Stevens-Johnson syndrome L51.1
    toxic epidermal necrolysis overlap L51.3
  Stewart-Morel M85.2
  Stickler Q89.8
  stiff baby Q89.8
  stiff man G25.82
  Still-Felty —*see* Felty's syndrome
  Stokes (-Adams) I45.9
  stone heart I50.1
  straight back, congenital Q76.49
  Sturge-Weber (-Dimitri) Q85.89
  subclavian steal G45.8
  subcoracoid-pectoralis minor G54.0
  subcostal nerve compression I77.89
  subphrenic interposition Q43.3
  superior
    cerebellar artery I63.89
    mesenteric artery K55.1
    semi-circular canal dehiscence H83.8X-●
    vena cava I87.1
  supine hypotensive (maternal) —*see* Syndrome,
    hypotension, maternal
  suprarenal cortical E27.0
  supraspinatus —*see also* Tear, rotator cuff
    M75.10-●
  Susac G93.49
  swallowed blood P78.2

Syndrome *(Continued)*
  sweat retention L74.0
  Swyer Q99.1
  Symond's G93.2
  sympathetic
    cervical paralysis G90.2
    pelvic, female N94.89
  systemic inflammatory response (SIRS), of
    non-infectious origin (without organ
    dysfunction) R65.10
    with acute organ dysfunction R65.11
  tachycardia-bradycardia I49.5
  takotsubo I51.81
  TAR (thrombocytopenia with absent radius)
    Q87.2
  tarsal tunnel G57.5-●
  teething K00.7
  tegmental G93.89
  telangiectasic-pigmentation-cataract Q82.8
  temporal pyramidal apex —*see* Otitis, media,
    suppurative, acute
  temporomandibular joint-pain-dysfunction
    M26.62-●
  Terry's —*see also* Myopia, degenerative H44.2-●
  testicular feminization —*see also* Syndrome,
    androgen insensitivity E34.51
  thalamic pain (hyperesthetic) G89.0
  thoracic outlet (compression) G54.0
    ▶ arterial I77.89
    ▶ neurogenic G54.0
    ▶ venous I87.1
  ▥ Thorson-Björck E34.09
  thrombocytopenia with absent radius (TAR)
    Q87.2
  thrombosis with thrombocytopenia D75.84
  thyroid-adrenocortical insufficiency E31.0
  tibial
    anterior M76.81-●
    posterior M76.82-●
  Tietze's M94.0
  time-zone (rapid) G47.25
  Toni-Fanconi E72.09
    with cystinosis E72.04
  Touraine's Q79.8
  tourniquet —*see* Constriction, external, by site
  toxic shock A48.3
  transient left ventricular apical ballooning I51.81
  traumatic vasospastic T75.22
  Treacher Collins Q75.4
  triple X, female Q97.0
  trisomy Q92.9
    13 Q91.7
      meiotic nondisjunction Q91.4
      mitotic nondisjunction Q91.5
      mosaicism Q91.5
      translocation Q91.6
    18 Q91.3
      meiotic nondisjunction Q91.0
      mitotic nondisjunction Q91.1
      mosaicism Q91.1
      translocation Q91.2
  trisomy Q92.9
    20 (q)(p) Q92.8
    21 Q90.9
      meiotic nondisjunction Q90.0
      mitotic nondisjunction Q90.1
      mosaicism Q90.1
      translocation Q90.2
    22 Q92.8
  tropical wet feet T69.0-●
  Trousseau's I82.1
  tumor lysis (following antineoplastic
    chemotherapy) (spontaneous) NEC E88.3
  tumor necrosis factor receptor associated
    periodic (TRAPS) M04.1
  Twiddler's (due to)
    automatic implantable defibrillator T82.198
    cardiac pacemaker T82.198
  Unverricht (-Lundborg) —*see* Epilepsy,
    generalized, idiopathic
  upward gaze H51.8
  uremia, chronic —*see also* Disease, kidney,
    chronic N18.9
  urethral N34.3
  urethro-oculo-articular —*see* Reiter's disease
  urohepatic K76.7
  vago-hypoglossal G52.7
  van Buchem's M85.2
  van der Hoeve's Q78.0
  vascular NEC in cerebrovascular disease G46.8
  vasoconstriction, reversible cerebrovascular
    I67.841

Syndrome *(Continued)*
  vasomotor I73.9
  vasospastic (traumatic) T75.22
  vasovagal R55
  VATER Q87.2
  velo-cardio-facial Q93.81
  vena cava (inferior) (superior) (obstruction) I87.1
  vertebral
    artery G45.0
      compression —*see* Syndrome, anterior,
        spinal artery, compression
      steal G45.0
    vertebro-basilar artery G45.0
  vertebrogenic (pain) (*see also* Pain, vertebrogenic)
    M54.89
  vertiginous —*see* Disorder, vestibular function
  Vinson-Plummer D50.1
  virus B34.9
  visceral larva migrans B83.0
  visual disorientation H53.8
  vitamin B6 deficiency E53.1
  vitreal corneal H59.01-●
  vitreous (touch) H59.01-●
  Vogt-Koyanagi H20.82-●
  Volkmann's T79.6
  von Hippel-Lindau Q85.83
  von Schroetter's I82.890
  von Willebrand (-Jürgen) —*see* Disease, von
    Willebrand
  acquired (*see also* Disease, von Willebrand)
    D68.04
  Waldenström-Kjellberg D50.1
  Wallenberg's G46.3
  wasting (syndrome) due to underlying condition
    E88.A
  water retention E87.79
  Waterhouse (-Friderichsen) A39.1
  Weber-Gubler G46.3
  Weber-Leyden G46.3
  Weber's G46.3
  Wegener's M31.30
    with
      kidney involvement M31.31
      lung involvement M31.30
        with kidney involvement M31.31
  Weingarten's (tropical eosinophilia) J82.89
  Weiss-Baker G90.09
  Werdnig-Hoffman G12.0
  Wermer's E31.21
  Werner's E34.8
  Wernicke-Korsakoff (nonalcoholic) F04
    alcoholic F10.26
  West's —*see* Epilepsy, spasms
  Westphal-Strümpell E83.01
  wet
    feet (maceration) (tropical) T69.0-●
    lung, newborn P22.1
  whiplash S13.4
  whistling face Q87.0
  Wilkie's K55.1
  Wilkinson-Sneddon L13.1
  Willebrand (-Jürgens) —*see* Disease, von
    Willebrand
  Williams Q93.82
  Wilson's (hepatolenticular degeneration) E83.01
  Wiskott-Aldrich D82.0
  withdrawal —*see* Withdrawal, state
    drug
      infant of dependent mother P96.1
      therapeutic use, newborn P96.2
  Woakes' (ethmoiditis) J33.1
  Wright's (hyperabduction) G54.0
  X I20.9
  XXXX Q97.1
  XXXXX Q97.1
  XXXXY Q98.1
  XXY Q98.0
  Yao M04.8
  yellow nail L60.5
  Zahorsky's B08.5
  Zellweger syndrome E71.510
  Zellweger-like syndrome E71.541
Synechia (anterior) (iris) (posterior) (pupil) —*see
    also* Adhesions, iris
  intra-uterine (traumatic) N85.6
Synesthesia R20.8
Syngamiasis, syngamosis B83.3
Synodontia K00.2
Synorchidism, synorchism Q55.1
Synostosis (congenital) Q78.8
  astragalo-scaphoid Q74.2
  radioulnar Q74.0

Synovial sarcoma —*see* Neoplasm, connective
   tissue, malignant
Synovioma (malignant) —*see also* Neoplasm,
   connective tissue, malignant
   benign —*see* Neoplasm, connective tissue, benign
Synoviosarcoma —*see* Neoplasm, connective
   tissue, malignant
Synovitis —*see also* Tenosynovitis M65.90
  ankle and foot M65.97-●
  arm, upper M65.92-●
  crepitant
    hand M70.0-●
    wrist M70.03-●
  forearm M65.93-●
  gonococcal A54.49
  gouty —*see* Gout
  hand M65.94-●
  in (due to)
    crystals M65.8-●
    gonorrhea A54.49
    syphilis (late) A52.78
    use, overuse, pressure —*see* Disorder, soft
      tissue, due to use
  infective NEC —*see* Tenosynovitis, infective NEC
  leg, lower M65.96-●
  multiple sites, unspecified type M65.99
  shoulder M65.91-●
  specified NEC —*see* Tenosynovitis, specified
    type NEC
  specified site, unspecified type M65.98
  syphilitic A52.78
    congenital (early) A50.02
  thigh M65.95-●
  toxic —*see* Synovitis, transient
  transient M67.3-●
    ankle M67.37-●
    elbow M67.32-●
    foot joint M67.37-●
    hand joint M67.34-●
    hip M67.35-●
    knee M67.36-●
    multiple site M67.39
    pelvic region M67.35-●
    shoulder M67.31-●
    specified joint NEC M67.38
    wrist M67.33-●
  traumatic, current —*see* Sprain
  tuberculous —*see* Tuberculosis, synovitis
  villonodular (pigmented) M12.2-●
    ankle M12.27-●
    elbow M12.22-●
    foot joint M12.27-●
    hand joint M12.24-●
    hip M12.25-●
    knee M12.26-●
    multiple site M12.29
    pelvic region M12.25-●
    shoulder M12.21-●
    specified joint NEC M12.28
    vertebrae M12.28
    wrist M12.23-●
Syphilid A51.39
  congenital A50.06
  newborn A50.06
  tubercular (late) A52.79
Syphilis, syphilitic (acquired) A53.9
  abdomen (late) A52.79
  acoustic nerve A52.15
  adenopathy (secondary) A51.49
  adrenal (gland) (with cortical hypofunction) A52.79
  age under 2 years NOS —*see also* Syphilis,
    congenital, early
    acquired A51.9
  alopecia (secondary) A51.32
  anemia (late) A52.79 [D63.8]
  aneurysm (aorta) (ruptured) A52.01
    central nervous system A52.05
    congenital A50.54 [I79.0]
  anus (late) A52.74
    primary A51.1
    secondary A51.39
  aorta (arch) (abdominal) (thoracic) A52.02
    aneurysm A52.01
  aortic (insufficiency) (regurgitation)
    (stenosis) A52.03
    aneurysm A52.01
  arachnoid (adhesive) (cerebral) (spinal) A52.13
  asymptomatic —*see* Syphilis, latent
  ataxia (locomotor) A52.11
  atrophoderma maculatum A51.39
  auricular fibrillation A52.06
  bladder (late) A52.76

Syphilis, syphilitic (Continued)
  bone A52.77
    secondary A51.46
  brain A52.17
  breast (late) A52.79
  bronchus (late) A52.72
  bubo (primary) A51.0
  bulbar palsy A52.19
  bursa (late) A52.78
  cardiac decompensation A52.06
  cardiovascular A52.00
  central nervous system (late) (recurrent)
    (relapse) (tertiary) A52.3
    with
      ataxia A52.11
      general paralysis A52.17
        juvenile A50.45
      paresis (general) A52.17
        juvenile A50.45
      tabes (dorsalis) A52.11
        juvenile A50.45
      taboparesis A52.17
        juvenile A50.45
    aneurysm A52.05
    congenital A50.40
    juvenile A50.40
    remission in (sustained) A52.3
    serology doubtful, negative, or positive A52.3
    specified nature or site NEC A52.19
    vascular A52.05
  cerebral A52.17
    meningovascular A52.13
    nerves (multiple palsies) A52.15
    sclerosis A52.17
    thrombosis A52.05
  cerebrospinal (tabetic type) A52.12
  cerebrovascular A52.05
  cervix (late) A52.76
  chancre (multiple) A51.0
    extragenital A51.2
    Rollet's A51.0
  Charcot's joint A52.16
  chorioretinitis A51.43
    congenital A50.01
    late A52.71
    prenatal A50.01
  choroiditis —*see* Syphilitic chorioretinitis
  choroidoretinitis —*see* Syphilitic chorioretinitis
  ciliary body (secondary) A51.43
    late A52.71
  colon (late) A52.74
  combined spinal sclerosis A52.11
  condyloma (latum) A51.31
  congenital A50.9
    with
      paresis (general) A50.45
      tabes (dorsalis) A50.45
      taboparesis A50.45
    chorioretinitis, choroiditis A50.01 [H32]
    early, or less than 2 years after birth NEC A50.2
      with manifestations —*see* Syphilis,
        congenital, early, symptomatic
      latent (without manifestations) A50.1
        negative spinal fluid test A50.1
        serology positive A50.1
      symptomatic A50.09
        cutaneous A50.06
        mucocutaneous A50.07
        oculopathy A50.01
        osteochondropathy A50.02
        pharyngitis A50.03
        pneumonia A50.04
        rhinitis A50.05
        visceral A50.08
    interstitial keratitis A50.31
    juvenile neurosyphilis A50.45
    late, or 2 years or more after birth NEC A50.7
      chorioretinitis, choroiditis A50.32
      interstitial keratitis A50.31
      juvenile neurosyphilis A50.45
      latent (without manifestations) A50.6
        negative spinal fluid test A50.6
        serology positive A50.6
      symptomatic or with manifestations NEC
        A50.59
        arthropathy A50.55
        cardiovascular A50.54
        Clutton's joints A50.51
        Hutchinson's teeth A50.52
        Hutchinson's triad A50.53
        osteochondropathy A50.56
        saddle nose A50.57

Syphilis, syphilitic (Continued)
  conjugal A53.9
    tabes A52.11
  conjunctiva (late) A52.71
  contact Z20.2
  cord bladder A52.19
  cornea, late A52.71
  coronary (artery) (sclerosis) A52.06
  coryza, congenital A50.05
  cranial nerve A52.15
    multiple palsies A52.15
  cutaneous —*see* Syphilis, skin
  dacryocystitis (late) A52.71
  degeneration, spinal cord A52.12
  dementia paralytica A52.17
    juvenilis A50.45
  destruction of bone A52.77
  dilatation, aorta A52.01
  due to blood transfusion A53.9
  dura mater A52.13
  ear A52.79
    inner A52.79
      nerve (eighth) A52.15
      neurorecurrence A52.15
  early A51.9
    cardiovascular A52.00
    central nervous system A52.3
    latent (without manifestations) (less than 2
      years after infection) A51.5
      negative spinal fluid test A51.5
      serological relapse after treatment A51.5
      serology positive A51.5
    relapse (treated, untreated) A51.9
    skin A51.39
    symptomatic A51.9
      extragenital chancre A51.2
      primary, except extragenital chancre A51.0
      secondary —*see also* Syphilis, secondary
        A51.39
        relapse (treated, untreated) A51.49
      ulcer A51.39
  eighth nerve (neuritis) A52.15
  endemic A65
  endocarditis A52.03
    aortic A52.03
    pulmonary A52.03
  epididymis (late) A52.76
  epiglottis (late) A52.73
  epiphysitis (congenital) (early) A50.02
  episcleritis (late) A52.71
  esophagus A52.79
  eustachian tube A52.73
  exposure to Z20.2
  eye A52.71
  eyelid (late) (with gumma) A52.71
  fallopian tube (late) A52.76
  fracture A52.77
  gallbladder (late) A52.74
  gastric (polyposis) (late) A52.74
  general A53.9
    paralysis A52.17
      juvenile A50.45
  genital (primary) A51.0
  glaucoma A52.71
  gumma NEC A52.79
    cardiovascular system A52.00
    central nervous system A52.3
    congenital A50.59
  heart (block) (decompensation) (disease) (failure)
    A52.06 [I52]
    valve NEC A52.03
  hemianesthesia A52.19
  hemianopsia A52.71
  hemiparesis A52.17
  hemiplegia A52.17
  hepatic artery A52.09
  hepatis A52.74
  hepatomegaly, congenital A50.08
  hereditaria tarda —*see* Syphilis, congenital, late
  hereditary —*see* Syphilis, congenital
  Hutchinson's teeth A50.52
  hyalitis A52.71
  inactive —*see* Syphilis, latent
  infantum —*see* Syphilis, congenital
  inherited —*see* Syphilis, congenital
  internal ear A52.79
  intestine (late) A52.74
  iris, iritis (secondary) A51.43
    late A52.71
  joint (late) A52.77
  keratitis (congenital) (interstitial) (late) A50.31
  kidney (late) A52.75

▶ New   ⇒ Revised   ~~deleted~~ Deleted   ● Use Additional Character(s)

Syphilis, syphilitic *(Continued)*
lacrimal passages (late) A52.71
larynx (late) A52.73
late A52.9
  cardiovascular A52.00
  central nervous system A52.3
  kidney A52.75
  latent or 2 years or more after infection
    (without manifestations) A52.8
    negative spinal fluid test A52.8
    serology positive A52.8
  paresis A52.17
  specified site NEC A52.79
  symptomatic or with manifestations A52.79
  tabes A52.11
latent A53.0
  with signs or symptoms - code by site and
    stage under Syphilis
  central nervous system A52.2
  date of infection unspecified A53.0
  early, or less than 2 years after infection A51.5
  follow-up of latent syphilis A53.0
    date of infection unspecified A53.0
    late, or 2 years or more after infection A52.8
  late, or 2 years or more after infection A52.8
  positive serology (only finding) A53.0
    date of infection unspecified A53.0
    early, or less than 2 years after infection A51.5
    late, or 2 years or more after infection A52.8
lens (late) A52.71
leukoderma A51.39
  late A52.79
lienitis A52.79
lip A51.39
  chancre (primary) A51.2
  late A52.79
Lissauer's paralysis A52.17
liver A52.74
locomotor ataxia A52.11
lung A52.72
lymph gland (early) (secondary) A51.49
  late A52.79
lymphadenitis (secondary) A51.49
macular atrophy of skin A51.39
  striated A52.79
mediastinum (late) A52.73
meninges (adhesive) (brain) (spinal cord) A52.13
meningitis A52.13
  acute (secondary) A51.41
  congenital A50.41
meningoencephalitis A52.14
meningovascular A52.13
  congenital A50.41
mesarteritis A52.09
  brain A52.04
middle ear A52.77
mitral stenosis A52.03
monoplegia A52.17
mouth (secondary) A51.39
  late A52.79
mucocutaneous (secondary) A51.39
  late A52.79
mucous
  membrane (secondary) A51.39
    late A52.79
  patches A51.39
    congenital A50.07
mulberry molars A50.52
muscle A52.78
myocardium A52.06
nasal sinus (late) A52.73
neonatorum —*see* Syphilis, congenital
nephrotic syndrome (secondary) A51.44
nerve palsy (any cranial nerve) A52.15
  multiple A52.15
nervous system, central A52.3
neuritis A52.15
  acoustic A52.15
neurorecidive of retina A52.19
neuroretinitis A52.19
newborn —*see* Syphilis, congenital
nodular superficial (late) A52.79
nonvenereal A65
nose (late) A52.73
  saddle back deformity A50.57
occlusive arterial disease A52.09
oculopathy A52.71
ophthalmic (late) A52.71
optic nerve (atrophy) (neuritis) (papilla) A52.15
orbit (late) A52.71
organic A53.9
osseous (late) A52.77

Syphilis, syphilitic *(Continued)*
osteochondritis (congenital) (early) A50.02
  [M90.80]
osteoporosis A52.77
ovary (late) A52.76
oviduct (late) A52.76
palate (late) A52.79
pancreas (late) A52.74
paralysis A52.17
  general A52.17
    juvenile A50.45
paresis (general) A52.17
  juvenile A50.45
paresthesia A52.19
Parkinson's disease or syndrome A52.19
paroxysmal tachycardia A52.06
pemphigus (congenital) A50.06
penis (chancre) A51.0
  late A52.76
pericardium A52.06
perichondritis, larynx (late) A52.73
periosteum (late) A52.77
  congenital (early) A50.02 [M90.80]
  early (secondary) A51.46
peripheral nerve A52.79
petrous bone (late) A52.77
pharynx (late) A52.73
  secondary A51.39
pituitary (gland) A52.79
pleura (late) A52.73
pneumonia, white A50.04
pontine lesion A52.17
portal vein A52.09
primary A51.0
  anal A51.1
  and secondary —*see* Syphilis, secondary
  central nervous system A52.3
  extragenital chancre NEC A51.2
  fingers A51.2
  genital A51.0
  lip A51.2
  specified site NEC A51.2
  tonsils A51.2
prostate (late) A52.76
ptosis (eyelid) A52.71
pulmonary (late) A52.72
  artery A52.09
pyelonephritis (late) A52.75
recently acquired, symptomatic A51.9
rectum (late) A52.74
respiratory tract (late) A52.73
retina, late A52.71
retrobulbar neuritis A52.15
salpingitis A52.76
sclera (late) A52.71
sclerosis
  cerebral A52.17
  coronary A52.06
  multiple A52.11
scotoma (central) A52.71
scrotum (late) A52.76
secondary (and primary) A51.49
  adenopathy A51.49
  anus A51.39
  bone A51.46
  chorioretinitis, choroiditis A51.43
  hepatitis A51.45
  liver A51.45
  lymphadenitis A51.49
  meningitis (acute) A51.41
  mouth A51.39
  mucous membranes A51.39
  periosteum, periostitis A51.46
  pharynx A51.39
  relapse (treated, untreated) A51.49
  skin A51.39
  specified form NEC A51.49
  tonsil A51.39
  ulcer A51.39
  viscera NEC A51.49
  vulva A51.39
seminal vesicle (late) A52.76
seronegative with signs or symptoms - code by
  site and stage under Syphilis
seropositive
  with signs or symptoms - code by site and
    stage under Syphilis
  follow-up of latent syphilis —*see* Syphilis,
    latent
  only finding —*see* Syphilis, latent
seventh nerve (paralysis) A52.15
sinus, sinusitis (late) A52.73

Syphilis, syphilitic *(Continued)*
skeletal system A52.77
skin (with ulceration) (early) (secondary) A51.39
  late or tertiary A52.79
small intestine A52.74
spastic spinal paralysis A52.17
spermatic cord (late) A52.76
spinal (cord) A52.12
spleen A52.79
splenomegaly A52.79
spondylitis A52.77
staphyloma A52.71
stigmata (congenital) A50.59
stomach A52.74
synovium A52.78
tabes dorsalis (late) A52.11
  juvenile A50.45
tabetic type A52.11
  juvenile A50.45
taboparesis A52.17
  juvenile A50.45
tachycardia A52.06
tendon (late) A52.78
tertiary A52.9
  with symptoms NEC A52.79
  cardiovascular A52.00
  central nervous system A52.3
  multiple NEC A52.79
  specified site NEC A52.79
testis A52.76
thorax A52.73
throat A52.73
thymus (gland) (late) A52.79
thyroid (late) A52.79
tongue (late) A52.79
tonsil (lingual) (late) A52.73
  primary A51.2
  secondary A51.39
trachea (late) A52.73
tunica vaginalis (late) A52.76
ulcer (any site) (early) (secondary) A51.39
  late A52.79
  perforating A52.79
    foot A52.11
urethra (late) A52.76
urogenital (late) A52.76
uterus (late) A52.76
uveal tract (secondary) A51.43
  late A52.71
uveitis (secondary) A51.43
  late A52.71
uvula (late) (perforated) A52.79
vagina A51.0
  late A52.76
valvulitis NEC A52.03
vascular A52.00
  brain (cerebral) A52.05
ventriculi A52.74
vesicae urinariae (late) A52.76
viscera (abdominal) (late) A52.74
  secondary A51.49
vitreous (opacities) (late) A52.71
  hemorrhage A52.71
vulva A51.0
  late A52.76
  secondary A51.39
Syphiloma A52.79
  cardiovascular system A52.00
  central nervous system A52.3
  circulatory system A52.00
  congenital A50.59
Syphilophobia F45.29
Syringadenoma —*see also* Neoplasm, skin, benign
  papillary —*see* Neoplasm, skin, benign
Syringobulbia G95.0
Syringocystadenoma —*see* Neoplasm, skin, benign
  papillary —*see* Neoplasm, skin, benign
Syringoma —*see also* Neoplasm, skin, benign
  chondroid —*see* Neoplasm, skin, benign
Syringomyelia G95.0
Syringomyelitis —*see* Encephalitis
Syringomyelocele —*see* Spina bifida
Syringopontia G95.0
System, systemic —*see also* condition
  disease, combined —*see* Degeneration, combined
  inflammatory response syndrome (SIRS) of
    non-infectious origin (without organ
    dysfunction) R65.10
    with acute organ dysfunction R65.11
  lupus erythematosus M32.9
    inhibitor present D68.62
Systemic exertion intolerance disease [SEID] G93.32

▶ New   ⇛ Revised   ~~deleted~~ Deleted   ● Use Additional Character(s)

T

Tabacism, tabacosis, tabagism —see also Poisoning,
    tobacco
    meaning dependence (without remission)
        F17.200
        with
            disorder F17.299
                in remission F17.211
                specified disorder NEC F17.298
                withdrawal F17.203
Tabardillo A75.9
    flea-borne A75.2
    louse-borne A75.0
Tabes, tabetic A52.10
    with
        central nervous system syphilis A52.10
        Charcot's joint A52.16
        cord bladder A52.19
        crisis, viscera (any) A52.19
        paralysis, general A52.17
        paresis (general) A52.17
        perforating ulcer (foot) A52.19
    arthropathy (Charcot) A52.16
    bladder A52.19
    bone A52.11
    cerebrospinal A52.12
    congenital A50.45
    conjugal A52.10
    dorsalis A52.11
        juvenile A50.49
    juvenile A50.49
    latent A52.19
    mesenterica A18.39
    paralysis, insane, general A52.17
    spasmodic A52.17
    syphilis (cerebrospinal) A52.12
Taboparalysis A52.17
Taboparesis (remission) A52.17
    juvenile A50.45
TAC (trigeminal autonomic cephalgia) NEC
    G44.099
    intractable G44.091
    not intractable G44.099
Tache noir S60.22-●
Tachyalimentation K91.2
Tachyarrhythmia, tachyrhythmia —see
    Tachycardia
Tachycardia R00.0
    atrial (paroxysmal) I47.19
    auricular I47.19
    AV nodal re-entry (re-entrant) I47.19
    junctional (paroxysmal) I47.19
    newborn P29.11
    nodal (paroxysmal) I47.19
    non-paroxysmal AV nodal I45.89
    paroxysmal (sustained) (nonsustained) I47.9
        with sinus bradycardia I49.5
        atrial (PAT) I47.19
        atrioventricular (AV) (re-entrant) I47.19
            psychogenic F54
        junctional I47.19
            ectopic I47.19
        nodal I47.19
        psychogenic (atrial) (supraventricular)
            (ventricular) F54
        supraventricular (sustained) I47.10
            psychogenic F54
        ventricular I47.20
            psychogenic F54
            specified type NEC I47.29
    psychogenic F45.8
    sick sinus I49.5
    sinoauricular NOS R00.0
        Inappropriate, so stated (IST) I47.11
        paroxysmal I47.19
    sinus [sinusal] NOS R00.0
        paroxysmal I47.10
    supraventricular I47.10
    ventricular (paroxysmal) (sustained) I47.20
        psychogenic F54
        specified type NEC I47.29
Tachygastria K31.89
Tachypnea R06.82
    hysterical F45.8
    newborn (idiopathic) (transitory) P22.1
    psychogenic F45.8
    transitory, of newborn P22.1
TACO (transfusion associated circulatory overload)
    E87.71
TAD (transfusion-associated dyspnea) J95.87

Taenia (infection) (infestation) B68.9
    diminuta B71.0
    echinococcal infestation B67.90
    mediocanellata B68.1
    nana B71.0
    saginata B68.1
    solium (intestinal form) B68.0
        larval form —see Cysticercosis
Taeniasis (intestine) —see Taenia
Tag (hypertrophied skin) (infected) L91.8
    adenoid J35.8
    anus K64.4
    hemorrhoidal K64.4
    hymen N89.8
    perineal N90.89
    preauricular Q17.0
    sentinel K64.4
    skin L91.8
        accessory (congenital) Q82.8
        anus K64.4
        congenital Q82.8
        preauricular Q17.0
    tonsil J35.8
    urethra, urethral N36.8
    vulva N90.89
Tahyna fever B33.8
Takahara's disease E80.3
Takayasu's disease or syndrome M31.4
Talaromycosis B48.4
Talcosis (pulmonary) J62.0
Talipes (congenital) Q66.89
    acquired, planus —see Deformity, limb, flat foot
    asymmetric Q66.89
    calcaneovalgus Q66.4-●
    calcaneovarus Q66.1-●
    calcaneus Q66.89
    cavus Q66.7-●
    equinovalgus Q66.6
    equinovarus Q66.0-●
    equinus Q66.89
    percavus Q66.7-●
    planovalgus Q66.6
    planus (acquired) (any degree) —see also
        Deformity, limb, flat foot
        congenital Q66.5-●
        due to rickets (sequelae) E64.3
    valgus Q66.6
    varus Q66.3-●
Tall stature, constitutional E34.4
Talma's disease M62.89
Talon noir S90.3-●
    hand S60.22-●
    heel S90.3-●
    toe S90.1-●
Tamponade, heart I31.4
Tanapox (virus disease) B08.71
Tangier disease E78.6
Tantrum, child problem F91.8
Tapeworm (infection) (infestation) —see Infestation,
    tapeworm
Tapia's syndrome G52.7
TAR (thrombocytopenia with absent radius)
    syndrome Q87.2
Tarral-Besnier disease L44.0
Tarsal tunnel syndrome —see Syndrome, tarsal tunnel
Tarsalgia —see Pain, limb, lower
Tarsitis (eyelid) H01.8
    syphilitic A52.71
    tuberculous A18.4
Tartar (teeth) (dental calculus) K03.6
Tattoo (mark) L81.8
Tauri's disease E74.09
Taurodontism K00.2
Taussig-Bing syndrome Q20.1
Taybi's syndrome Q87.2
Tay-Sachs amaurotic familial idiocy or disease
    E75.02
TBI (traumatic brain injury) S06.9
Teacher's node or nodule J38.2
Tear, torn (traumatic) —see also Laceration
    with abortion —see Abortion
    annular fibrosis M51.35
    anus, anal (sphincter) S31.831
        complicating delivery
            with third degree perineal laceration —
                see also Delivery, complicated, by,
                laceration, perineum, third degree
                O70.20
                with mucosa O70.3
            without third degree perineal laceration O70.4
    nontraumatic (healed) (old) K62.81

Tear, torn (Continued)
    articular cartilage, old —see Derangement, joint,
        articular cartilage, by site
    bladder
        with ectopic or molar pregnancy O08.6
        following ectopic or molar pregnancy O08.6
        obstetrical O71.5
        traumatic —see Injury, bladder
    bowel
        with ectopic or molar pregnancy O08.6
        following ectopic or molar pregnancy O08.6
        obstetrical trauma O71.5
    broad ligament
        with ectopic or molar pregnancy O08.6
        following ectopic or molar pregnancy O08.6
        obstetrical trauma O71.6
    bucket handle (knee) (meniscus) —see Tear,
        meniscus
    capsule, joint —see Sprain
    cartilage —see also Sprain
        articular, old —see Derangement, joint,
            articular cartilage, by site
    cervix
        with ectopic or molar pregnancy O08.6
        following ectopic or molar pregnancy O08.6
        obstetrical trauma (current) O71.3
        old N88.1
        traumatic —see Injury, uterus
    dural G97.41
        nontraumatic G96.11
    internal organ —see Injury, by site
    knee cartilage
        articular (current) S83.3-●
        old —see Derangement, knee, meniscus, due
            to old tear
    ligament —see Sprain
    meniscus (knee) (current injury) S83.209
        bucket-handle S83.20-●
        lateral
            bucket-handle S83.25-●
            complex S83.27-●
            peripheral S83.26-●
            specified type NEC S83.28-●
        medial
            bucket-handle S83.21-●
            complex S83.23-●
            peripheral S83.22-●
            specified type NEC S83.24-●
        old —see Derangement, knee, meniscus, due
            to old tear
        site other than knee - code as Sprain
        specified type NEC S83.20-●
    muscle —see Strain
    pelvic
        floor, complicating delivery O70.1
        organ NEC, obstetrical trauma O71.5
            with ectopic or molar pregnancy O08.6
            following ectopic or molar pregnancy O08.6
    perineal, secondary O90.1
    periurethral tissue, obstetrical trauma O71.82
        with ectopic or molar pregnancy O08.6
        following ectopic or molar pregnancy O08.6
    rectovaginal septum —see Laceration, vagina
    retina, retinal (without detachment)
        (horseshoe) —see also Break, retina,
        horseshoe
        with detachment —see Detachment, retina,
            with retinal, break
    rotator cuff (nontraumatic) M75.10-●
        complete M75.12-●
        incomplete M75.11-●
        traumatic S46.01-●
            capsule S43.42-●
    semilunar cartilage, knee —see Tear, meniscus
    supraspinatus (complete) (incomplete)
        (nontraumatic) —see also Tear, rotator cuff
        M75.10-●
    tendon —see Strain
    tentorial, at birth P10.4
    umbilical cord
        complicating delivery O69.89
    urethra
        with ectopic or molar pregnancy O08.6
        following ectopic or molar pregnancy O08.6
        obstetrical trauma O71.5
    uterus —see Injury, uterus
    vagina —see Laceration, vagina
    vessel, from catheter —see Puncture, accidental
        complicating surgery
    vulva, complicating delivery O70.0
Tear-stone —see Dacryolith

▶ New   ⇒ Revised   deleted Deleted   ● Use Additional Character(s)

Teeth —see also condition
  grinding
    psychogenic F45.8
    sleep related G47.63
Teething (syndrome) K00.7
Telangiectasia, telangiectasis (verrucous) I78.1
  ataxic (cerebellar) (Louis-Bar) G11.3
  familial I78.0
  hemorrhagic, hereditary (congenital) (senile) I78.0
  hereditary, hemorrhagic (congenital) (senile) I78.0
  juxtafoveal H35.07-●
  macular H35.07-●
  macularis eruptiva perstans D47.01
  parafoveal H35.07-●
  retinal (idiopathic) (juxtafoveal) (macular)
    (parafoveal) H35.07-●
  spider I78.1
Telephone scatologia F65.89
Telescoped bowel or intestine K56.1
  congenital Q43.8
Temperature
  body, high (of unknown origin) R50.9
  cold, trauma from T69.9
    newborn P80.0
    specified effect NEC T69.8
Temple —see condition
Temporal —see condition
Temporomandibular joint pain-dysfunction
    syndrome M26.62-●
Temporosphenoidal —see condition
Tendency
  bleeding —see Defect, coagulation
  suicide
    meaning personal history of attempted
      suicide Z91.51
    meaning suicidal ideation —see Ideation,
      suicidal
  to fall R29.6
Tenderness, abdominal R10.819
  epigastric R10.816
  generalized R10.817
  left lower quadrant R10.814
  left upper quadrant R10.812
  periumbilic R10.815
  rebound R10.829
    epigastric R10.826
    generalized R10.827
    left lower quadrant R10.824
    left upper quadrant R10.822
    periumbilic R10.825
    right lower quadrant R10.823
    right upper quadrant R10.821
  right lower quadrant R10.813
  right upper quadrant R10.811
Tendinitis, tendonitis —see also Enthesopathy
  Achilles M76.6-●
  adhesive —see Tenosynovitis, specified type NEC
    shoulder —see Capsulitis, adhesive
  bicipital M75.2-●
  calcific M65.2-●
    ankle M65.27-●
    foot M65.27-●
    forearm M65.23-●
    hand M65.24-●
    lower leg M65.26-●
    multiple sites M65.29
    pelvic region M65.25-●
    shoulder M75.3-●
    specified site NEC M65.28
    thigh M65.25-●
    upper arm M65.22-●
  due to use, overuse, pressure —see also Disorder,
    soft tissue, due to use
    specified NEC —see Disorder, soft tissue, due
      to use, specified NEC
  gluteal M76.0-●
  patellar M76.5-●
  peroneal M76.7-●
  psoas M76.1-●
  tibial (posterior) M76.82-●
    anterior M76.81-●
  trochanteric —see Bursitis, hip, trochanteric
Tendon —see condition
Tendosynovitis —see Tenosynovitis
Tenesmus (rectal) R19.8
  vesical R30.1
Tennis elbow —see Epicondylitis, lateral
Tenonitis —see also Tenosynovitis
  eye (capsule) H05.04-●
Tenontosynovitis —see Tenosynovitis
Tenontothecitis —see Tenosynovitis

Tenophyte —see Disorder, synovium, specified
    type NEC
Tenosynovitis —see also Synovitis M65.90
  adhesive —see Tenosynovitis, specified type NEC
    shoulder —see Capsulitis, adhesive
  bicipital (calcifying) —see Tendinitis,
    bicipital
  gonococcal A54.49
  in (due to)
    crystals M65.8-●
    gonorrhea A54.49
    syphilis (late) A52.78
    use, overuse, pressure —see also Disorder, soft
      tissue, due to use
      specified NEC —see Disorder, soft tissue,
        due to use, specified NEC
  infective NEC M65.1-●
    ankle M65.17-●
    foot M65.17-●
    forearm M65.13-●
    hand M65.14-●
    lower leg M65.16-●
    multiple sites M65.19
    pelvic region M65.15-●
    shoulder region M65.11-●
    specified site NEC M65.18
    thigh M65.15-●
    upper arm M65.12-●
  radial styloid M65.4
  shoulder region M65.81-●
    adhesive —see Capsulitis, adhesive
  specified type NEC M65.88-●
    ankle M65.87-●
    foot M65.87-●
    forearm M65.83-●
    hand M65.84-●
    lower leg M65.86-●
    multiple sites M65.89
    pelvic region M65.85-●
    shoulder region M65.81-●
    specified site NEC M65.88
    thigh M65.85-●
    upper arm M65.82-●
  tuberculous —see Tuberculosis, tenosynovitis
Tenovaginitis —see Tenosynovitis
Tension
  arterial, high —see also Hypertension
    without diagnosis of hypertension R03.0
  headache G44.209
    intractable G44.201
    not intractable G44.209
  nervous R45.0
  pneumothorax J93.0
  premenstrual N94.3
  state (mental) F48.9
Tentorium —see condition
Teratencephalus Q89.8
Teratism Q89.7
Teratoblastoma (malignant) —see Neoplasm,
    malignant, by site
Teratocarcinoma —see also Neoplasm, malignant,
    by site
  liver C22.7
Teratoma (solid) —see also Neoplasm, uncertain
    behavior, by site
  with embryonal carcinoma, mixed —see
    Neoplasm, malignant, by site
  with malignant transformation —see Neoplasm,
    malignant, by site
  adult (cystic) —see Neoplasm, benign, by site
  benign —see Neoplasm, benign, by site
  combined with choriocarcinoma —see
    Neoplasm, malignant, by site
  cystic (adult) —see Neoplasm, benign, by site
  differentiated —see Neoplasm, benign, by site
  embryonal —see also Neoplasm, malignant, by
    site
    liver C22.7
  immature —see Neoplasm, malignant, by site
  liver C22.7
    adult, benign, cystic, differentiated type or
      mature D13.4
  malignant —see also Neoplasm, malignant, by site
    anaplastic —see Neoplasm, malignant, by site
    intermediate —see Neoplasm, malignant, by
      site
    specified site —see Neoplasm, malignant,
      by site
    unspecified site C62.90
  undifferentiated —see Neoplasm, malignant,
    by site

Teratoma (Continued)
  mature —see Neoplasm, uncertain behavior, by
    site
    malignant —see Neoplasm, by site, malignant,
      by site
  ovary D27.-●
    embryonal, immature or malignant C56-●
  solid —see Neoplasm, uncertain behavior, by site
  testis C62.9-●
    adult, benign, cystic, differentiated type or
      mature D29.2-●
    scrotal C62.1-●
    undescended C62.0-●
Termination
  anomalous —see also Malposition, congenital
    right pulmonary vein Q26.3
  pregnancy, elective Z33.2
Ternidens diminutus infestation B81.8
Ternidensiasis B81.8
Terror(s) night (child) F51.4
Terrorism, victim of Z65.4
Terry's syndrome —see also Myopia, degenerative
    H44.2-●
Tertiary —see condition
Test, tests, testing (for)
  adequacy (for dialysis)
    hemodialysis Z49.31
    peritoneal Z49.32
  blood pressure Z01.30
    abnormal reading —see Blood, pressure
  blood typing Z01.83
    Rh typing Z01.83
  blood-alcohol Z02.83
    positive —see Findings, abnormal, in blood
  blood-drug Z02.83
    positive —see Findings, abnormal, in blood
  cardiac pulse generator (battery) Z45.010
  fertility Z31.41
  genetic
    disease carrier status for procreative
      management
      female Z31.430
      male Z31.440
    male partner of patient with recurrent
      pregnancy loss Z31.441
    procreative management NEC
      female Z31.438
      male Z31.448
  hearing Z01.10
    with abnormal findings NEC Z01.118
    infant or child (over 28 days old) Z00.129
      with abnormal findings Z00.121
  HIV (human immunodeficiency virus)
    nonconclusive (in infants) R75
    positive Z21
    seropositive Z21
  immunity status Z01.84
  intelligence NEC Z01.89
  laboratory (as part of a general medical
      examination) Z00.00
    with abnormal finding Z00.01
    for medicolegal reason NEC Z04.89
  male partner of patient with recurrent pregnancy
      loss Z31.441
  Mantoux (for tuberculosis) Z11.1
    abnormal result R76.11
  pregnancy, positive first pregnancy —see
    Pregnancy, normal, first
  procreative Z31.49
    fertility Z31.41
  skin, diagnostic
    allergy Z01.82
      special screening examination —see
        Screening, by name of disease
    Mantoux Z11.1
    tuberculin Z11.1
  specified NEC Z01.89
  tuberculin Z11.1
    abnormal result R76.11
  vision Z01.00
    with abnormal findings Z01.01
    following failed vision screening Z01.020
      with abnormal findings Z01.021
    infant or child (over 28 days old) Z00.129
      with abnormal findings Z00.121
  Wassermann Z11.3
    positive —see Serology for syphilis, positive
Testicle, testicular, testis —see also condition
  feminization syndrome —see also Syndrome,
    androgen insensitivity E34.51
  migrans Q55.29

Tetanus, tetanic (cephalic) (convulsions) A35
    with
        abortion A34
        ectopic or molar pregnancy O08.0
    following ectopic or molar pregnancy O08.0
    inoculation reaction (due to serum) —*see*
        Complications, vaccination
    neonatorum A33
    obstetrical A34
    puerperal, postpartum, childbirth A34
Tetany (due to) R29.0
    alkalosis E87.3
    associated with rickets E55.0
    convulsions R29.0
        hysterical F44.5
    functional (hysterical) F44.5
    hyperkinetic R29.0
        hysterical F44.5
    hyperpnea R06.4
        hysterical F44.5
        psychogenic F45.8
    hyperventilation —*see also* Hyperventilation R06.4
        hysterical F44.5
    neonatal (without calcium or magnesium
        deficiency) P71.3
    parathyroid (gland) E20.9
    parathyroprival E89.2
    post- (para)thyroidectomy E89.2
    postoperative E89.2
    pseudotetany R29.0
    psychogenic (conversion reaction) F44.5
Tetralogy of Fallot Q21.3
Tetraplegia (chronic) —*see also* Quadriplegia G82.50-●
Thailand hemorrhagic fever A91
Thalassanemia —*see* Thalassemia
Thalassemia (anemia) (disease) D56.9
    with other hemoglobinopathy D56.8
    alpha (major) (severe) (triple gene defect) D56.0
        minor D56.3
        silent carrier D56.3
        trait D56.3
    beta (severe) D56.1
        homozygous D56.1
        major D56.1
        minor D56.3
        trait D56.3
    delta-beta (homozygous) D56.2
        minor D56.3
        trait D56.3
    dominant D56.8
    hemoglobin
        C D56.8
        E-beta D56.5
    intermedia D56.1
    major D56.1
    minor D56.3
    mixed D56.8
    sickle-cell —*see* Disease, sickle-cell, thalassemia
    specified type NEC D56.8
    trait D56.3
    variants D56.8
Thanatophoric dwarfism or short stature Q77.1
Thaysen-Gee disease (nontropical sprue) K90.0
Thaysen's disease K90.0
Thecoma D27-●
    luteinized D27-●
    malignant C56-●
Thelarche, premature E30.8
Thelaziasis B83.2
Thelitis N61.0
    puerperal, postpartum or gestational —*see*
        Infection, nipple
Therapeutic —*see* condition
Therapy
    drug, long-term (current) (prophylactic)
        agents affecting estrogen receptors and
            estrogen levels NEC Z79.818
        anastrozole (Arimidex) Z79.811
        antibiotics Z79.2
            short-term use - omit code
        anticoagulants Z79.01
        anti-inflammatory Z79.1
        antiplatelet Z79.02
        antithrombotics Z79.02
        aromatase inhibitors Z79.811
        aspirin Z79.82
        birth control pill or patch Z79.3
        bisphosphonates Z79.83
        contraceptive, oral Z79.3
        drug, specified NEC Z79.899
        estrogen receptor downregulators Z79.818

Therapy *(Continued)*
    drug, long-term *(Continued)*
        Evista Z79.810
        exemestane (Aromasin) Z79.811
        Fareston Z79.810
        fulvestrant (Faslodex) Z79.818
        gonadotropin-releasing hormone (GnRH)
            agonist Z79.818
        goserelin acetate (Zoladex) Z79.818
        hormone replacement Z79.890
        insulin Z79.4
        letrozole (Femara) Z79.811
        leuprolide acetate (leuprorelin) (Lupron)
            Z79.818
        megestrol acetate (Megace) Z79.818
        methadone
            for pain management Z79.891
            maintenance therapy F11.20
        Nolvadex Z79.810
        opiate analgesic Z79.891
        oral antidiabetic Z79.84
        oral contraceptive Z79.3
        oral hypoglycemic Z79.84
        raloxifene (Evista) Z79.810
        selective estrogen receptor modulators
            (SERMs) Z79.810
        short term - omit code
        steroids
            inhaled Z79.51
            systemic Z79.52
        tamoxifen (Nolvadex) Z79.810
        toremifene (Fareston) Z79.810
Thermic —*see* condition
Thermography (abnormal) —*see also* Abnormal,
        diagnostic imaging R93.89
    breast R92.8
Thermoplegia T67.01
Thesaurismosis, glycogen —*see* Disease, glycogen
        storage
Thiamin deficiency E51.9
    specified NEC E51.8
Thiaminic deficiency with beriberi E51.11
Thibierge-Weissenbach syndrome —*see* Sclerosis,
        systemic
Thickening
    bone —*see* Hypertrophy, bone
    breast N64.59
    endometrium R93.89
    epidermal L85.9
        specified NEC L85.8
    hymen N89.6
    larynx J38.7
    nail L60.2
        congenital Q84.5
    periosteal —*see* Hypertrophy, bone
    pleura J92.9
        with asbestos J92.0
    skin R23.4
    subepiglottic J38.7
    tongue K14.8
    valve, heart —*see* Endocarditis
Thigh —*see* condition
Thinning vertebra —*see* Spondylopathy, specified
        NEC
Thirst, excessive R63.1
    due to deprivation of water T73.1
Thomsen disease G71.12
Thoracic —*see also* condition
    kidney Q63.2
▸outlet syndrome (*see also* Syndrome, thoracic
        outlet) G54.0
Thoracogastroschisis (congenital) Q79.8
Thoracopagus Q89.4
Thorax —*see* condition
Thorn's syndrome N28.89
▸Thorson-Björck syndrome E34.09
Threadworm (infection) (infestation) B80
Threatened
    abortion O20.0
        with subsequent abortion O03.9
▸abuse (harm)
        ▸adult —*see* Maltreatment, adult, threatened
            abuse
        ▸child —*see* Maltreatment, child, threatened
            abuse
    job loss, anxiety concerning Z56.2
    labor (without delivery) O47.9
        at or after 37 completed weeks of gestation
            O47.1
        before 37 completed weeks of gestation
            O47.0-●

Threatened *(Continued)*
    loss of job, anxiety concerning Z56.2
    miscarriage O20.0
    unemployment, anxiety concerning Z56.2
Three-day fever A93.1
Threshers' lung J67.0
Thrix annulata (congenital) Q84.1
Throat —*see* condition
Thrombasthenia (Glanzmann) (hemorrhagic)
        (hereditary) D69.1
Thromboangiitis I73.1
    obliterans (general) I73.1
        cerebral I67.89
        vessels
            brain I67.89
            spinal cord I67.89
Thromboarteritis —*see* Arteritis
Thromboasthenia (Glanzmann) (hemorrhagic)
        (hereditary) D69.1
Thrombocytasthenia (Glanzmann) D69.1
Thrombocythemia (hemorrhagic) (see also
        Thrombocytosis) D75.839
    essential D47.3
    idiopathic D47.3
    primary D47.3
Thrombocytopathy (dystrophic) (granulopenic)
        D69.1
Thrombocytopenia, thrombocytopenic D69.6
    with absent radius (TAR) Q87.2
    congenital D69.42
    dilutional D69.59
    due to
        drugs D69.59
        extracorporeal circulation of blood D69.59
        (massive)blood transfusion D69.59
        platelet alloimmunization D69.59
    essential D69.3
    heparin-associated D75.821
    heparin induced (HIT) D75.829
    delayed-onset D75.828
    immune-mediated D75.822
    non-immune D75.821
    persisting D75.828
    syndrome
        autoimmune D75.828
        specified NEC D75.828
        spontaneous (without heparin exposure)
            D75.84
    type 1 D75.821
    type 2 D75.822
    hereditary D69.42
    idiopathic D69.3
    neonatal, transitory P61.0
        due to
            exchange transfusion P61.0
            idiopathic maternal thrombocytopenia P61.0
            isoimmunization P61.0
    primary NEC D69.49
        idiopathic D69.3
    puerperal, postpartum O72.3
    secondary D69.59
    transient neonatal P61.0
    vaccine-induced thrombotic D75.84
Thrombocytosis D75.839
    essential D47.3
    idiopathic D47.3
    primary D47.3
    reactive D75.838
    secondary D75.838
    specified NEC D75.838
Thromboembolism —*see* Embolism
Thrombopathy (Bernard-Soulier) D69.1
    constitutional —*see* Disease, von Willebrand
    Willebrand-Jurgens —*see* Disease, von
        Willebrand
Thrombopenia —*see* Thrombocytopenia
Thrombophilia D68.59
    primary NEC D68.59
    secondary NEC D68.69
    specified NEC D68.69
Thrombophlebitis I80.9
    antepartum O22.2-●
        deep O22.3-●
        superficial O22.2-●
    calf muscular vein (NOS) I80.25-●
    cavernous (venous) sinus G08
        complicating pregnancy O22.5-●
        nonpyogenic I67.6
    cerebral (sinus) (vein) G08
        nonpyogenic I67.6
        sequelae G09

▶ New   ⇒ Revised   ~~deleted~~ Deleted   ● Use Additional Character(s)

Thrombophlebitis (Continued)
  due to implanted device —see Complications, by
      site and type, specified NEC
  during or resulting from a procedure NEC
      T81.72
  femoral vein (superficial) I80.1-●
  femoropopliteal vein I80.0-●
  gastrocnemial vein I80.25-●
  hepatic (vein) I80.8
  idiopathic, recurrent I82.1
  iliac vein (common) (external) (internal) I80.21-●
  iliofemoral I80.1-●
  intracranial venous sinus (any) G08
      nonpyogenic I67.6
      sequelae G09
  intraspinal venous sinuses and veins G08
      nonpyogenic G95.19
  lateral (venous) sinus G08
      nonpyogenic I67.6
  leg I80.3
      superficial I80.0-●
  longitudinal (venous) sinus G08
      nonpyogenic I67.6
  lower extremity I80.299
  migrans, migrating I82.1
  pelvic
      with ectopic or molar pregnancy O08.0
      following ectopic or molar pregnancy O08.0
      puerperal O87.1
  peroneal vein I80.24-●
  popliteal vein —see Phlebitis, leg, deep, popliteal
  portal (vein) K75.1
  postoperative T81.72
  pregnancy —see Thrombophlebitis, antepartum
  puerperal, postpartum, childbirth O87.0
      deep O87.1
      pelvic O87.1
      septic O86.81
      superficial O87.0
  saphenous (greater) (lesser) I80.0-●
  sinus (intracranial) G08
      nonpyogenic I67.6
  soleal vein I80.25-●
  specified site NEC I80.8
  tibial vein (anterior) (posterior) I80.23-●
Thrombosis, thrombotic (bland) (multiple)
      (progressive) (silent) (vessel) I82.90
  anal K64.5
  antepartum —see Thrombophlebitis, antepartum
  aorta, aortic I74.10
      abdominal I74.09
          saddle I74.01
      bifurcation I74.09
      saddle I74.01
      specified site NEC I74.19
      terminal I74.09
      thoracic I74.11
      valve —see Endocarditis, aortic
  apoplexy I63.3-●
  artery, arteries (postinfectional) I74.9
      auditory, internal —see Occlusion, artery,
          precerebral, specified NEC
      basilar —see Occlusion, artery, basilar
      carotid (common) (internal) —see Occlusion,
          artery, carotid
      cerebellar (anterior inferior) (posterior
          inferior) (superior) —see Occlusion,
          artery, cerebellar
      cerebral —see Occlusion, artery, cerebral
      choroidal (anterior) —see Occlusion, artery,
          precerebral, specified NEC
      communicating, posterior —see Occlusion,
          artery, precerebral, specified NEC
      coronary —see also Infarct, myocardium
          not resulting in infarction I24.0
      hepatic I74.8
      hypophyseal —see Occlusion, artery,
          precerebral, specified NEC
      iliac I74.5
      limb I74.4
          lower I74.3
          upper I74.2
      meningeal, anterior or posterior —see
          Occlusion, artery, cerebral, specified NEC
      mesenteric (with gangrene) —see also Infarct,
          intestine K55.069
      ophthalmic —see Occlusion, artery, retina
      pontine —see Occlusion, artery, precerebral,
          specified NEC
      precerebral —see Occlusion, artery,
          precerebral

Thrombosis, thrombotic (Continued)
  artery, arteries (Continued)
      pulmonary (iatrogenic) —see Embolism,
          pulmonary
      renal N28.0
      retinal —see Occlusion, artery, retina
      spinal, anterior or posterior G95.11
      traumatic NEC T14.8
      vertebral —see Occlusion, artery, vertebral
  atrium, auricular —see also Infarct, myocardium
      following acute myocardial infarction (current
          complication) I23.6
      not resulting in infarction I51.3
      old I51.3
  basilar (artery) —see Occlusion, artery, basilar
  brain (artery) (stem) —see also Occlusion, artery,
      cerebral
      due to syphilis A52.05
      puerperal O99.43
      ▶sinus —see Thrombosis, intracranial, venous
          sinus
  capillary I78.8
  cardiac —see also Infarct, myocardium
      not resulting in infarction I51.3
      valve —see Endocarditis
      old I51.3
  carotid (artery) (common) (internal) —see
      Occlusion, artery, carotid
  ▶cavernous (venous) sinus —see Thrombosis,
      intracranial, venous sinus
  cerebellar artery (anterior inferior) (posterior
      inferior) (superior) I66.3
  cerebral (artery) —see Occlusion, artery,
      cerebral
  ▶cerebrovenous sinus —see also Thrombosis,
      intracranial, venous sinus
      puerperium O87.3
  chronic I82.91
  coronary (artery) (vein) —see also Infarct,
      myocardium
      not resulting in infarction I24.0
  corpus cavernosum N48.89
  cortical I66.9
  deep —see Embolism, vein, lower extremity
  due to device, implant or graft —see also
      Complications, by site and type, specified
      NEC T85.868
      arterial graft NEC T82.868
      breast (implant) T85.868
      catheter NEC T85.868
          dialysis (renal) T82.868
              intraperitoneal T85.868
          infusion NEC T82.868
              spinal (epidural) (subdural) T85.860
          urinary (indwelling) T83.86
      electronic (electrode) (pulse generator)
          (stimulator)
          bone T84.86
          cardiac T82.867
          nervous system (brain) (peripheral nerve)
              (spinal) T85.860
          urinary T83.86
      fixation, internal (orthopedic) NEC T84.86
      gastrointestinal (bile duct) (esophagus)
          T85.868
      genital NEC T83.86
      heart T82.867
      joint prosthesis T84.86
      ocular (corneal graft) (orbital implant) NEC
          T85.868
      orthopedic NEC T84.86
      specified NEC T85.868
      urinary NEC T83.86
      vascular NEC T82.868
      ventricular intracranial shunt T85.860
  during the puerperium —see Thrombosis,
      puerperal
  endocardial —see also Infarct, myocardium
      not resulting in infarction I51.3
  eye —see Occlusion, retina
  genital organ
      female NEC N94.89
          pregnancy —see Thrombophlebitis,
              antepartum
      male N50.1
  gestational —see Phlebopathy, gestational
  heart (chamber) —see also Infarct, myocardium
      not resulting in infarction I51.3
      old I51.3
  hepatic (vein) I82.0
      artery I74.8

Thrombosis, thrombotic (Continued)
  history (of) Z86.718
  intestine (with gangrene) —see also Infarct,
      intestine K55.069
  intracardiac NEC (apical) (atrial) (auricular)
      (ventricular) (old) I51.3
  intracranial (arterial) I66.9
      venous sinus (any) G08
          ▶nonpyogenic I67.6
          nonpyogenic origin I67.6
          puerperium O87.3
  intramural —see also Infarct, myocardium
      not resulting in infarction I51.3
      old I51.3
  intraspinal venous sinuses and veins G08
      nonpyogenic G95.19
  kidney (artery) N28.0
  ▶lateral (venous) sinus —see Thrombosis,
      intracranial, venous sinus
  leg —see Thrombosis, vein, lower extremity
      arterial I74.3
  liver (venous) I82.0
      artery I74.8
      portal vein I81
  ▶longitudinal (venous) sinus —see Thrombosis,
      intracranial, venous sinus
  lower limb —see Thrombosis, vein, lower
      extremity
  lung (iatrogenic) (postoperative) —see Embolism,
      pulmonary
  meninges (brain) (arterial) I66.8
  mesenteric (artery) (with gangrene) —see also
      Infarct, intestine K55.069
      vein (inferior) (superior) K55.0-●
  mitral I34.89
  mural —see also Infarct, myocardium
      due to syphilis A52.06
      not resulting in infarction I51.3
      old I51.3
  omentum (with gangrene) —see also Infarct,
      intestine K55.069
  ophthalmic —see Occlusion, retina
  pampiniform plexus (male) N50.1
  parietal —see also Infarct, myocardium
      not resulting in infarction I24.0
  penis, superficial vein N48.81
  perianal venous K64.5
  peripheral arteries I74.4
      upper I74.2
  personal history (of) Z86.718
  portal I81
      due to syphilis A52.09
  puerperal, postpartum O87.0
      brain (artery) O99.43
          venous (sinus) O87.3
      cardiac O99.43
      cerebral (artery) O99.43
          venous (sinus) O87.3
      superficial O87.0
  pulmonary (artery) (iatrogenic) (postoperative)
      (vein) —see Embolism, pulmonary
  renal (artery) N28.0
      vein I82.3
  resulting from presence of device, implant or
      graft —see Complications, by site and type,
      specified NEC
  retina, retinal —see Occlusion, retina
  scrotum N50.1
  seminal vesicle N50.1
  sigmoid (venous) sinus —see Thrombosis,
      intracranial venous sinus
  ▶sinus, intracranial (any) —see Thrombosis,
      intracranial, venous sinus
  specified site NEC I82.890
      chronic I82.891
  spermatic cord N50.1
  spinal cord (arterial) G95.11
      due to syphilis A52.09
      pyogenic origin G06.1
  spleen, splenic D73.5
      artery I74.8
  testis N50.1
  traumatic NEC T14.8
  tricuspid I07.8
  tumor —see Neoplasm, by site
  tunica vaginalis N50.1
  umbilical cord (vessels), complicating delivery
      O69.5
  vas deferens N50.1

Thrombosis, thrombotic *(Continued)*
  vein (acute) I82.90
    antecubital I82.61-•
      chronic I82.71-•
    axillary I82.A1-•
      chronic I82.A2-•
    basilic I82.61-•
      chronic I82.71-•
    brachial I82.62-•
      chronic I82.72-•
    brachiocephalic (innominate) I82.290
      chronic I82.291
    calf muscular I82.46-•
      chronic I82.56-•
    cerebral, nonpyogenic I67.6
    cephalic I82.61-•
      chronic I82.71-•
    chronic I82.91
    deep (DVT) I82.40-•
      calf I82.4Z-•
        chronic I82.5Z-•
      lower leg I82.4Z-•
        chronic I82.5Z-•
      thigh I82.4Y-•
        chronic I82.5Y-•
      upper leg I82.4Y•
        chronic I82.5Y-•
    femoral I82.41-•
      chronic I82.51-•
    iliac (iliofemoral) I82.42-•
      chronic I82.52-•
    innominate I82.290
      chronic I82.291
    internal jugular I82.C1-•
      chronic I82.C2-•
    lower extremity
      deep I82.40-•
        chronic I82.50-•
        specified NEC I82.49-•
          chronic NEC I82.59-•
      distal
        deep I82.4Z-•
      proximal
        deep I82.4Y-•
          chronic I82.5Y-•
      superficial I82.81-•
    perianal K64.5
    peroneal I82.45-•
      chronic I82.55-•
    popliteal I82.43-•
      chronic I82.53-•
    radial I82.62-•
      chronic I82.72-•
    renal I82.3
    saphenous (greater) (lesser) I82.81-•
    specified NEC I82.890
      chronic NEC I82.891
    subclavian I82.B1-•
      chronic I82.B2-•
    thoracic NEC I82.290
      chronic I82.291
    tibial I82.44-•
      chronic I82.54-•
    ulnar I82.62-•
      chronic I82.72-•
    upper extremity I82.60-•
      chronic I82.70-•
      deep I82.62-•
        chronic I82.72-•
      superficial I82.61-•
        chronic I82.71-•
  vena cava
    inferior I82.220
      chronic I82.221
    superior I82.210
      chronic I82.211
  venous, perianal K64.5
  ventricle —*see also* Infarct, myocardium
    following acute myocardial infarction (current
      complication) I23.6
    not resulting in infarction I24.0
    old I51.3
Thrombus —*see* Thrombosis
Thrush —*see also* Candidiasis
  newborn P37.5
  oral B37.0
  vaginal (acute) B37.31
    chronic (recurrent) B37.32
Thumb —*see also* condition
  sucking (child problem) F98.8
Thymitis E32.8

Thymoma —*see also* Neoplasm, thymus, by type
  malignant C37
  metaplastic C37
  microscopic D15.0
  sclerosing C37
  type A C37
  type AB C37
  type B1 C37
  type B2 C37
  type B3 C37
Thymus, thymic (gland) —*see* condition
Thyrocele —*see* Goiter
Thyroglossal —*see also* condition
  cyst Q89.2
  duct, persistent Q89.2
Thyroid (gland) (body) —*see also* condition
  hormone resistance E07.89
  lingual Q89.2
  nodule (cystic) (nontoxic) (single) E04.1
Thyroiditis E06.9
  acute (nonsuppurative) (pyogenic) (suppurative)
    E06.0
  autoimmune E06.3
  chronic (nonspecific) (sclerosing) E06.5
    with thyrotoxicosis, transient E06.2
    fibrous E06.5
    lymphadenoid E06.3
    lymphocytic E06.3
    lymphoid E06.3
  de Quervain's E06.1
  drug-induced E06.4
  fibrous (chronic) E06.5
  giant-cell (follicular) E06.1
  granulomatous (de Quervain) (subacute)
    E06.1
  Hashimoto's (struma lymphomatosa) E06.3
  iatrogenic E06.4
  ligneous E06.5
  lymphocytic (chronic) E06.3
  lymphoid E06.3
  lymphomatous E06.3
  nonsuppurative E06.1
  postpartum, puerperal O90.5
  pseudotuberculous E06.1
  pyogenic E06.0
  radiation E06.4
  Riedel's E06.5
  subacute (granulomatous) E06.1
  suppurative E06.0
  tuberculous A18.81
  viral E06.1
  woody E06.5
Thyrolingual duct, persistent Q89.2
Thyromegaly E01.0
Thyrotoxic
  crisis —*see* Thyrotoxicosis
  heart disease or failure —*see also* Thyrotoxicosis
    E05.90 [143]
    with thyroid storm E05.91 [143]
  storm —*see* Thyrotoxicosis
Thyrotoxicosis (recurrent) E05.90
  with
    goiter (diffuse) E05.00
      with thyroid storm E05.01
      adenomatous uninodular E05.10
        with thyroid storm E05.11
      multinodular E05.20
        with thyroid storm E05.21
      nodular E05.20
        with thyroid storm E05.21
      uninodular E05.10
        with thyroid storm E05.11
    infiltrative
      dermopathy E05.00
        with thyroid storm E05.01
      ophthalmopathy E05.00
        with thyroid storm E05.01
    single thyroid nodule E05.10
      with thyroid storm E05.11
    thyroid storm E05.91
  due to
    ectopic thyroid nodule or tissue E05.30
      with thyroid storm E05.31
    ingestion of (excessive) thyroid material
      E05.40
      with thyroid storm E05.41
    overproduction of thyroid-stimulating
      hormone E05.80
      with thyroid storm E05.81
    specified cause NEC E05.80
      with thyroid storm E05.81

Thyrotoxicosis *(Continued)*
  factitia E05.40
    with thyroid storm E05.41
  heart —*see also* Failure, heart, high-output E05.90
    [143]
    with thyroid storm —*see also* Failure, heart,
      high-output E05.91 [143]
    failure —*see also* Failure, heart, high-output
      E05.90 [143]
  neonatal (transient) P72.1
  transient with chronic thyroiditis E06.2
Tibia vara M92.51-•
Tic (disorder) F95.9
  breathing F95.8
  child problem F95.0
  compulsive F95.1
  de la Tourette F95.2
  degenerative (generalized) (localized) G25.69
    facial G25.69
  disorder
    chronic
      motor F95.1
      vocal F95.1
    combined vocal and multiple motor F95.2
    transient F95.0
  douloureux G50.0
    atypical G50.1
    postherpetic, postzoster B02.22
  drug-induced G25.61
  eyelid F95.8
  habit F95.9
    chronic F95.1
    transient of childhood F95.0
  lid, transient of childhood F95.0
  motor-verbal F95.2
  occupational F48.8
  orbicularis F95.8
    transient of childhood F95.0
  organic origin G25.69
  postchoreic G25.69
  provisional F95.0
  psychogenic, compulsive F95.1
  salaam R25.8
  spasm (motor or vocal) F95.9
    chronic F95.1
    transient of childhood F95.0
  specified NEC F95.8
Tick-borne —*see* condition
Tietze's disease or syndrome M94.0
Tight, tightness
  anus K62.89
  chest R07.89
  fascia (lata) M62.89
  foreskin (congenital) N47.1
  hymen, hymenal ring N89.6
  introitus (acquired) (congenital) N89.6
  rectal sphincter K62.89
  tendon —*see* Short, tendon
  urethral sphincter N35.919
Tilting vertebra —*see* Dorsopathy, deforming,
  specified NEC
Timidity, child F93.8
Tin-miner's lung J63.5
Tinea (intersecta) (tarsi) B35.9
  amiantacea L44.8
  asbestina B35.0
  barbae B35.0
  beard B35.0
  black dot B35.0
  blanca B36.2
  capitis B35.0
  corporis B35.4
  cruris B35.6
  flava B36.0
  foot B35.3
  furfuracea B36.0
  imbricata (Tokelau) B35.5
  kerion B35.0
  manuum B35.2
  microsporic —*see* Dermatophytosis
  nigra B36.1
  nodosa —*see* Piedra
  pedis B35.3
  scalp B35.0
  specified NEC B35.8
  sycosis B35.0
  tonsurans B35.0
  trichophytic —*see* Dermatophytosis
  unguium B35.1
  versicolor B36.0
Tingling sensation (skin) R20.2

Tinnitus NOS H93.1-●
  audible H93.1-●
  aurium H93.1-●
  pulsatile H93.A-●
  subjective H93.1-●
Tipped tooth (teeth) M26.33
Tipping
  pelvis M95.5
    with disproportion (fetopelvic) O33.0
      causing obstructed labor O65.0
  tooth (teeth), fully erupted M26.33
Tiredness R53.83
Tissue —see condition
Tobacco (nicotine)
  abuse —see Tobacco, use
  dependence —see Dependence, drug, nicotine
  harmful use Z72.0
  heart —see Tobacco, toxic effect
  maternal use, affecting newborn P04.2
  toxic effect —see Table of Drugs and Chemicals,
      by substance, poisoning
    chewing tobacco —see Table of Drugs
        and Chemicals, by substance, poisoning
    cigarettes —see Table of Drugs and Chemicals,
        by substance, poisoning
  use Z72.0
    complicating
      childbirth O99.334
      pregnancy O99.33-●
      puerperium O99.335
    counseling and surveillance Z71.6
    history Z87.891
  withdrawal state —see also Dependence, drug,
      nicotine F17.203
Tocopherol deficiency E56.0
Todd's
  cirrhosis K74.3
  paralysis (postepileptic) (transitory) G83.84
Toe —see condition
Toilet, artificial opening —see Attention to,
    artificial, opening
Tokelau (ringworm) B35.5
Tollwut —see Rabies
Tommaselli's disease R31.9
  correct substance properly administered —see
      Table of Drugs and Chemicals, by drug,
      adverse effect
  overdose or wrong substance given or taken —
      see Table of Drugs and Chemicals, by drug,
      poisoning
Tongue —see also condition
  tie Q38.1
Tonic pupil —see Anomaly, pupil, function, tonic
    pupil
Toni-Fanconi syndrome (cystinosis) E72.09
  with cystinosis E72.04
Tonsil —see condition
Tonsillitis (acute) (catarrhal) (croupous) (follicular)
    (gangrenous) (infective) (lacunar) (lingual)
    (malignant) (membranous) (parenchymatous)
    (phlegmonous) (pseudomembranous)
    (purulent) (septic) (subacute) (suppurative)
    (toxic) (ulcerative) (vesicular) (viral) J03.90
  chronic J35.01
    with adenoiditis J35.03
  diphtheritic A36.0
  hypertrophic J35.01
    with adenoiditis J35.03
  recurrent J03.91
  specified organism NEC J03.80
    recurrent J03.81
  staphylococcal J03.80
    recurrent J03.81
  streptococcal J03.00
    recurrent J03.01
  tuberculous A15.8
  Vincent's A69.1
Tooth, teeth —see condition
Toothache K08.89
Topagnosis R20.8
Tophi —see Gout, chronic
TORCH infection —see Infection, congenital
  without active infection P00.2
Torn —see Tear
Tornwaldt's cyst or disease J39.2
Torsades de pointes I47.21
Torsion
  accessory tube —see Torsion, fallopian tube
  adnexa (female) —see Torsion, fallopian tube
  aorta, acquired I77.1
  appendix epididymis N44.04

Torsion (Continued)
  appendix testis N44.03
  bile duct (common) (hepatic) K83.8
    congenital Q44.5
  bowel, colon or intestine K56.2
  cervix —see Malposition, uterus
  cystic duct K82.8
  dystonia —see Dystonia, torsion
  epididymis (appendix) N44.04
  fallopian tube N83.52-●
    with ovary N83.53
  gallbladder K82.8
    congenital Q44.1
  hydatid of Morgagni
    female N83.52-●
    male N44.03
  kidney (pedicle) (leading to infarction)
      N28.0
  Meckel's diverticulum (congenital) Q43.0
    malignant —see Table of Neoplasms, small
        intestine, malignant
  mesentery K56.2
  omentum K56.2
  organ or site, congenital NEC —see Anomaly,
      by site
  ovary (pedicle) N83.51-●
    with fallopian tube N83.53
    congenital Q50.2
  oviduct —see Torsion, fallopian tube
  penis (acquired) N48.82
    congenital Q55.63
  spasm —see Dystonia, torsion
  spermatic cord N44.02
    extravaginal N44.01
    intravaginal N44.02
  spleen D73.5
  testis, testicle N44.00
    appendix N44.03
  tibia —see Deformity, limb, specified type NEC,
      lower leg
  uterus —see Malposition, uterus
Torticollis (intermittent) (spastic) M43.6
  congenital (sternomastoid) Q68.0
  due to birth injury P15.8
  hysterical F44.4
  ocular R29.891
  psychogenic F45.8
    conversion reaction F44.4
  rheumatic M43.6
  rheumatoid M06.88
  spasmodic G24.3
  traumatic, current S13.4
Tortipelvis G24.1
Tortuous
  aortic arch Q25.46
  artery I77.1
  organ or site, congenital NEC —see Distortion
  retinal vessel, congenital Q14.1
  ureter N13.8
  urethra N36.8
  vein —see Varix
Torture, victim of Z65.4
Torula, torular (histolytica) (infection) —see
    Cryptococcosis
Torulosis —see Cryptococcosis
Torus (mandibularis) (palatinus) M27.0
  fracture —see Fracture, by site, torus
Touraine's syndrome Q79.8
Tourette's syndrome F95.2
Tourniquet syndrome —see Constriction, external,
    by site
Tower skull Q75.009
  with exophthalmos Q87.0
Toxemia R68.89
  bacterial —see Sepsis
  burn —see Burn
  eclamptic (with pre-existing hypertension) —see
      Eclampsia
  erysipelatous —see Erysipelas
  fatigue R68.89
  food —see Poisoning, food
  gastrointestinal K52.1
  intestinal K52.1
  kidney —see Uremia
  malarial —see Malaria
  myocardial —see Myocarditis, toxic
  of pregnancy —see Pre-eclampsia
  pre-eclamptic —see Pre-eclampsia
  small intestine K52.1
  staphylococcal, due to food A05.0
  stasis R68.89

Toxemia (Continued)
  uremic —see Uremia
  urinary —see Uremia
Toxemica cerebropathia psychica (nonalcoholic)
    F04
  alcoholic —see Alcohol, amnestic disorder
Toxic (poisoning) —see also condition
    T65.91
  effect —see Table of Drugs and Chemicals, by
      substance, poisoning
  shock syndrome A48.3
  thyroid (gland) —see Thyrotoxicosis
Toxicemia —see Toxemia
Toxicity —see Table of Drugs and Chemicals, by
    substance, poisoning
  fava bean D55.0
  food, noxious —see Poisoning, food
  from drug or nonmedicinal substance —see Table
      of Drugs and Chemicals, by drug
Toxicosis —see also Toxemia
  capillary, hemorrhagic D69.0
Toxinfection, gastrointestinal K52.1
Toxocariasis B83.0
Toxoplasma, toxoplasmosis (acquired) B58.9
  with
    hepatitis B58.1
    meningoencephalitis B58.2
    ocular involvement B58.00
    other organ involvement B58.89
    pneumonia, pneumonitis B58.3
  congenital (acute) (subacute) (chronic)
      P37.1
  maternal, manifest toxoplasmosis in infant
      (acute) (subacute) (chronic) P37.1
tPA (rtPA) administation in a different facility
    within the last 24 hours prior to admission to
    current facility Z92.82
Trabeculation, bladder N32.89
Trachea —see condition
Tracheitis (catarrhal) (infantile) (membranous)
    (plastic) (septal) (suppurative) (viral) J04.10
  with
    bronchitis (15 years of age and above) J40
      acute or subacute —see Bronchitis,
          acute
      chronic J42
      tuberculous NEC A15.5
      under 15 years of age J20.9
    laryngitis (acute) J04.2
      chronic J37.1
      tuberculous NEC A15.5
  acute J04.10
    with obstruction J04.11
  chronic J42
    with
      bronchitis (chronic) J42
      laryngitis (chronic) J37.1
  diphtheritic (membranous) A36.89
  due to external agent —see Inflammation,
      respiratory, upper, due to
  syphilitic A52.73
  tuberculous A15.5
Trachelitis (nonvenereal) —see Cervicitis
Tracheobronchial —see condition
Tracheobronchitis (15 years of age and above) —
    see also Bronchitis
  due to
    Bordetella bronchiseptica A37.80
      with pneumonia A37.81
    Francisella tularensis A21.8
Tracheobronchomegaly Q32.4
  with bronchiectasis J47.9
    with
      exacerbation (acute) J47.1
      lower respiratory infection J47.0
  acquired J98.09
    with bronchiectasis J47.9
      with
        exacerbation (acute) J47.1
        lower respiratory infection J47.0
Tracheobronchopneumonitis —see Pneumonia,
    broncho-●
Tracheocele (external) (internal) J39.8
  congenital Q32.1
Tracheomalacia J39.8
  congenital Q32.0
Tracheopharyngitis (acute) J06.9
  chronic J42
  due to external agent —see Inflammation,
      respiratory, upper, due to
Tracheostenosis J39.8

Tracheostomy
complication —*see* Complication, tracheostomy
status Z93.0
attention to Z43.0
malfunctioning J95.03
Trachoma, trachomatous A71.9
active (stage) A71.1
contraction of conjunctiva A71.1
dubium A71.0
healed or sequelae B94.0
initial (stage) A71.0
pannus A71.1
Türck's J37.0
Traction, vitreomacular H43.82-●
Train sickness T75.3
Trait(s)
Hb-S D57.3
hemoglobin
abnormal NEC D58.2
with thalassemia D56.3
C —*see* Disease, hemoglobin C
S (Hb-S) D57.3
Lepore D56.3
personality, accentuated Z73.1
sickle-cell D57.3
with elliptocytosis or spherocytosis D57.3
type A personality Z73.1
Tramp Z59.00
Trance R41.89
hysterical F44.89
Transaminasemia R74.01
Transection
abdomen (partial) S38.3
aorta (incomplete) —*see also* Injury, aorta
complete —*see* Injury, aorta, laceration, major
carotid artery (incomplete) —*see also* Injury, blood vessel, carotid, laceration
complete —*see* Injury, blood vessel, carotid, laceration, major
celiac artery (incomplete) S35.211
branch (incomplete) S35.291
complete S35.292
complete S35.212
innominate
artery (incomplete) —*see also* Injury, blood vessel, thoracic, innominate, artery, laceration
complete —*see* Injury, blood vessel, thoracic, innominate, artery, laceration, major
vein (incomplete) —*see also* Injury, blood vessel, thoracic, innominate, vein, laceration
complete —*see* Injury, blood vessel, thoracic, innominate, vein, laceration, major
jugular vein (external) (incomplete) —*see also* Injury, blood vessel, jugular vein, laceration
complete —*see* Injury, blood vessel, jugular vein, laceration, major
internal (incomplete) —*see also* Injury, blood vessel, jugular vein, internal, laceration
complete —*see* Injury, blood vessel, jugular vein, internal, laceration, major
mesenteric artery (incomplete) —*see also* Injury, mesenteric, artery, laceration
complete —*see* Injury, mesenteric artery, laceration, major
pulmonary vessel (incomplete) —*see also* Injury, blood vessel, thoracic, pulmonary, laceration
complete —*see* Injury, blood vessel, thoracic, pulmonary, laceration, major
subclavian —*see* Transection, innominate
vena cava (incomplete) —*see also* Injury, vena cava
complete —*see* Injury, vena cava, laceration, major
vertebral artery (incomplete) —*see also* Injury, blood vessel, vertebral, laceration
complete —*see* Injury, blood vessel, vertebral, laceration, major
Transfusion
associated (red blood cell) hemochromatosis E83.111
blood
ABO incompatible —*see* Complication(s), transfusion, incompatibility reaction, ABO
minor blood group (Duffy) (E) (K) (Kell) (Kidd) (Lewis) (M) (N) (P) (S) T80.89
reaction or complication —*see* Complications, transfusion

Transfusion *(Continued)*
fetomaternal (mother) —*see* Pregnancy, complicated by, placenta, transfusion syndrome
maternofetal (mother) —*see* Pregnancy, complicated by, placenta, transfusion syndrome
placental (syndrome) (mother) —*see* Pregnancy, complicated by, placenta, transfusion syndrome
reaction (adverse) —*see* Complications, transfusion
related acute lung injury (TRALI) J95.84
twin-to-twin —*see* Pregnancy, complicated by, placenta, transfusion syndrome, fetus to fetus
Transgender F64.0
Transient (meaning homeless) —*see also* condition Z59.00
Translocation
balanced autosomal Q95.9
in normal individual Q95.0
chromosomes NEC Q99.8
balanced and insertion in normal individual Q95.0
Down's syndrome Q90.2
trisomy
13 Q91.6
18 Q91.2
21 Q90.2
Translucency, iris —*see* Degeneration, iris
Transmission of chemical substances through the placenta —*see* Absorption, chemical, through placenta
Transparency, lung, unilateral J43.0
Transplant (ed) (status) Z94.9
awaiting organ Z76.82
bone Z94.6
marrow Z94.81
candidate Z76.82
complication —*see* Complication, transplant
cornea Z94.7
heart Z94.1
and lung(s) Z94.3
valve Z95.2
prosthetic Z95.2
specified NEC Z95.4
xenogenic Z95.3
intestine Z94.82
kidney Z94.0
liver Z94.4
lung(s) Z94.2
and heart Z94.3
organ (failure) (infection) (rejection)Z94.9
removal status Z98.85
pancreas Z94.83
skin Z94.5
social Z60.3
specified organ or tissue NEC Z94.89
stem cells Z94.84
tissue Z94.9
Transplants, ovarian, endometrial N80.10-●
Transposed —*see* Transposition
Transposition (congenital) —*see also* Malposition, congenital
abdominal viscera Q89.3
aorta (dextra) Q20.3
appendix Q43.8
colon Q43.8
corrected Q20.5
great vessels (complete) (partial) Q20.3
heart Q24.0
with complete transposition of viscera Q89.3
intestine (large) (small) Q43.8
reversed jejunal (for bypass) (status) Z98.0
scrotum Q55.23
stomach Q40.2
with general transposition of viscera Q89.3
tooth, teeth, fully erupted M26.30
vessels, great (complete) (partial) Q20.3
viscera (abdominal) (thoracic) Q89.3
Transsexualism F64.0
Transverse —*see also* condition
arrest (deep), in labor O64.0
lie (mother) O32.2
causing obstructed labor O64.8
Transvestism, transvestitism (dual-role) F64.1
fetishistic F65.1
Trapped placenta (with hemorrhage) O72.0
without hemorrhage O73.0
TRAPS (tumor necrosis factor receptor associated periodic syndrome) M04.1

Trauma, traumatism —*see also* Injury
acoustic —*see* subcategory H83.3
birth —*see* Birth, injury
complicating ectopic or molar pregnancy O08.6
during delivery O71.9
following ectopic or molar pregnancy O08.6
non-accidental —*see* Abuse, physical
obstetric O71.9
specified NEC O71.89
occlusal
primary K08.81
secondary K08.82
Traumatic —*see also* condition
brain injury S06.9
Treacher Collins syndrome Q75.4
Treitz's hernia —*see* Hernia, abdomen, specified site NEC
Trematode infestation —*see* Infestation, fluke
Trematodiasis —*see* Infestation, fluke
Trembling paralysis —*see* Parkinsonism
Tremor(s) R25.1
drug induced G25.1
essential (benign) G25.0
familial G25.0
hereditary G25.0
hysterical F44.4
intention G25.2
medication induced postural G25.1
mercurial —*see* subcategory T56.1
Parkinson's —*see* Parkinsonism
psychogenic (conversion reaction) F44.4
senilis R54
specified type NEC G25.2
Trench
fever A79.0
foot —*see* Immersion, foot
mouth A69.1
Treponema pallidum infection —*see* Syphilis
Treponematosis
due to
T. pallidum —*see* Syphilis
T. pertenue —*see* Yaws
Triad
Hutchinson's (congenital syphilis) A50.53
Kartagener's Q89.3
Saint's —*see* Hernia, diaphragm
Trichiasis (eyelid) H02.059
with entropion —*see* Entropion
left H02.056
lower H02.055
upper H02.054
right H02.053
lower H02.052
upper H02.051
Trichinella spiralis (infection) (infestation) B75
Trichinellosis, trichiniasis, trichinelliasis, trichinosis B75
with muscle disorder B75 [M63.80]
ankle B75 [M63.87-●]
foot B75 [M63.87-●]
forearm B75 [M63.83-●]
hand B75 [M63.84-●]
lower leg B75 [M63.86-●]
multiple sites B75 [M63.89]
pelvic region B75 [M63.85-●]
shoulder region B75 [M63.81-●]
specified site NEC B75 [M63.88]
thigh B75 [M63.85-●]
upper arm B75 [M63.82-●]
Trichobezoar T18.9
intestine T18.3
stomach T18.2
Trichocephaliasis, trichocephalosis B79
Trichocephalus infestation B79
Trichoclasis L67.8
Trichoepithelioma —*see also* Neoplasm, skin, benign
malignant —*see* Neoplasm, skin, malignant
Trichofolliculoma —*see* Neoplasm, skin, benign
Tricholemmoma —*see* Neoplasm, skin, benign
Trichomoniasis A59.9
bladder A59.03
cervix A59.09
intestinal A07.8
prostate A59.02
seminal vesicles A59.09
specified site NEC A59.8
urethra A59.03
urogenitalis A59.00
vagina A59.01
vulva A59.01

▶ New   ⇒ Revised   ~~deleted~~ Deleted   ● Use Additional Character(s)

Trichomycosis
  axillaris A48.8
  nodosa, nodularis B36.8
Trichonodosis L67.8
Trichophytid, trichophyton infection —*see*
  Dermatophytosis
Trichophytobezoar T18.9
  intestine T18.3
  stomach T18.2
Trichophytosis —*see* Dermatophytosis
Trichoptilosis L67.8
Trichorrhexis (nodosa) (invaginata) L67.0
Trichosis axillaris A48.8
Trichosporosis nodosa B36.2
Trichostasis spinulosa (congenital) Q84.1
Trichostrongyliasis, trichostrongylosis (small
  intestine) B81.2
Trichostrongylus infection B81.2
Trichotillomania F63.3
Trichromat, trichromatopsia, anomalous
  (congenital) H53.55
Trichuriasis B79
Trichuris trichiura (infection) (infestation) (any
  site) B79
Tricuspid (valve) —*see* condition
Trifid —*see also* Accessory
  kidney (pelvis) Q63.8
  tongue Q38.3
Trigeminal neuralgia —*see* Neuralgia, trigeminal
Trigeminy R00.8
Trigger finger (acquired) M65.30
  congenital Q74.0
  index finger M65.32-●
  little finger M65.35-●
  middle finger M65.33-●
  ring finger M65.34-●
  thumb M65.31-●
Trigonitis (bladder) (chronic)
  (pseudomembranous) N30.30
  with hematuria N30.31
Trigonocephaly Q75.03
Trilocular heart —*see* Cor triloculare
Trimethylaminuria E72.52
Tripartite placenta O43.19-●
Triphalangeal thumb Q74.0
Triple —*see also* Accessory
  kidneys Q63.0
▶negative breast cancer (TNBC) Z17.421
  uteri Q51.818
  X, female Q97.0
Triple I O41.12-●
Triplegia G83.89
  congenital G80.8
Triplet (newborn) —*see also* Newborn, triplet
  complicating pregnancy —*see* Pregnancy, triplet
Triplication —*see* Accessory
Triploidy Q92.7
Trismus R25.2
  neonatorum A33
  newborn A33
Trisomy (syndrome) Q92.9
  13 (partial) Q91.7
    meiotic nondisjunction Q91.4
    mitotic nondisjunction Q91.5
    mosaicism Q91.5
    translocation Q91.6
  18 (partial) Q91.3
    meiotic nondisjunction Q91.0
    mitotic nondisjunction Q91.1
    mosaicism Q91.1
    translocation Q91.2
  20 Q92.8
  21 (partial) Q90.9
    meiotic nondisjunction Q90.0
    mitotic nondisjunction Q90.1
    mosaicism Q90.1
    translocation Q90.2
  22 Q92.8
  autosomes Q92.9
  chromosome specified NEC Q92.8
    partial Q92.2
      due to unbalanced translocation Q92.5
    specified NEC Q92.8
    whole (nonsex chromosome)
      meiotic nondisjunction Q92.0
      mitotic nondisjunction Q92.1
      mosaicism Q92.1
  due to
    dicentrics —*see* Extra, marker chromosomes
    extra rings —*see* Extra, marker chromosomes
    isochromosomes —*see* Extra, marker
      chromosomes

Trisomy (Continued)
  specified NEC Q92.8
  whole chromosome Q92.9
    meiotic nondisjunction Q92.0
    mitotic nondisjunction Q92.1
    mosaicism Q92.1
    partial Q92.9
    specified NEC Q92.8
Tritanomaly, tritanopia H53.55
Trombiculosis, trombiculiasis, trombidiosis B88.0
Trophedema (congenital) (hereditary) Q82.0
Trophoblastic disease —*see also* Mole,
  hydatidiform O01.9
Tropholymphedema Q82.0
Trophoneurosis NEC G96.89
  disseminated M34.9
Tropical —*see* condition
Trouble —*see also* Disease
  heart —*see* Disease, heart
  kidney —*see* Disease, renal
  nervous R45.0
  sinus —*see* Sinusitis
Trousseau's syndrome (thrombophlebitis migrans)
  I82.1
Truancy, childhood
  from school Z72.810
Truncus
  arteriosus (persistent) Q20.0
  communis Q20.0
Trunk —*see* condition
Trypanosomiasis
  African B56.9
    by Trypanosoma brucei
      gambiense B56.0
      rhodesiense B56.1
  American —*see* Chagas' disease
  Brazilian —*see* Chagas' disease
  by Trypanosoma
    brucei gambiense B56.0
    brucei rhodesiense B56.1
    cruzi —*see* Chagas' disease
  gambiensis, Gambian B56.0
  rhodesiensis, Rhodesian B56.1
  South American —*see* Chagas' disease
  where
    African trypanosomiasis is prevalent B56.9
    Chagas' disease is prevalent B57.2
Tryptasemia, hereditary alpha D89.44
T-shaped incisors K00.2
Tsutsugamushi (disease) (fever) A75.3
Tube, tubal, tubular —*see* condition
Tubercle —*see also* Tuberculosis
  brain, solitary A17.81
  Darwin's Q17.8
  Ghon, primary infection A15.7
Tuberculid, tuberculide (indurating,
  subcutaneous) (lichenoid) (miliary)
  (papulonecrotic) (primary) (skin) A18.4
Tuberculoma —*see also* Tuberculosis
  brain A17.81
  meninges (cerebral) (spinal) A17.1
  spinal cord A17.81
Tuberculosis, tubercular, tuberculous
  (calcification) (calcified) (caseous)
  (chromogenic acid-fast bacilli) (degeneration)
  (fibrocaseous) (fistula) (interstitial)
  (isolated circumscribed lesions) (necrosis)
  (parenchymatous) (ulcerative) A15.9
  with pneumoconiosis (any condition in J60-J64)
    J65
  abdomen (lymph gland) A18.39
  abscess (respiratory) A15.9
    bone A18.03
      hip A18.02
      knee A18.02
      sacrum A18.01
      specified site NEC A18.03
      spinal A18.01
      vertebra A18.01
    brain A17.81
    breast A18.89
    Cowper's gland A18.15
    dura (mater) (cerebral) (spinal) A17.81
    epidural (cerebral) (spinal) A17.81
    female pelvis A18.17
    frontal sinus A15.8
    genital organs NEC A18.10
    genitourinary A18.10
    gland (lymphatic) —*see* Tuberculosis, lymph
      gland
    hip A18.02
    intestine A18.32

Tuberculosis, tubercular, tuberculous (Continued)
  abscess (Continued)
    ischiorectal A18.32
    joint NEC A18.02
      hip A18.02
      knee A18.02
      specified NEC A18.02
      vertebral A18.01
    kidney A18.11
    knee A18.02
    latent Z22.7
    lumbar (spine) A18.01
    lung —*see* Tuberculosis, pulmonary
    meninges (cerebral) (spinal) A17.0
    muscle A18.09
    perianal (fistula) A18.32
    perinephritic A18.11
    perirectal A18.32
    rectum A18.32
    retropharyngeal A15.8
    sacrum A18.01
    scrofulous A18.2
    scrotum A18.15
    skin (primary) A18.4
    spinal cord A17.81
    spine or vertebra (column) A18.01
    subdiaphragmatic A18.31
    testis A18.15
    urinary A18.13
    uterus A18.17
  accessory sinus —*see* Tuberculosis, sinus
  Addison's disease A18.7
  adenitis —*see* Tuberculosis, lymph gland
  adenoids A15.8
  adenopathy —*see* Tuberculosis, lymph gland
  adherent pericardium A18.84
  adnexa (uteri) A18.17
  adrenal (capsule) (gland) A18.7
  alimentary canal A18.32
  anemia A18.89
  ankle (joint) (bone) A18.02
  anus A18.32
  apex, apical —*see* Tuberculosis, pulmonary
  appendicitis, appendix A18.32
  arachnoid A17.0
  artery, arteritis A18.89
    cerebral A18.89
  arthritis (chronic) (synovial) A18.02
    spine or vertebra (column) A18.01
  articular —*see* Tuberculosis, joint
  ascites A18.31
  asthma —*see* Tuberculosis, pulmonary
  axilla, axillary (gland) A18.2
  bladder A18.12
  bone A18.03
    hip A18.02
    knee A18.02
    limb NEC A18.03
    sacrum A18.01
    spine or vertebral column A18.01
  bowel (miliary) A18.32
  brain A17.81
  breast A18.89
  broad ligament A18.17
  bronchi, bronchial, bronchus A15.5
    ectasia, ectasis (bronchiectasis) —*see*
      Tuberculosis, pulmonary
    fistula A15.5
      primary (progressive) A15.7
    gland or node A15.4
      primary (progressive) A15.7
    lymph gland or node A15.4
      primary (progressive) A15.7
  bronchiectasis —*see* Tuberculosis, pulmonary
  bronchitis A15.5
  bronchopleural A15.6
  bronchopneumonia, bronchopneumonic —*see*
    Tuberculosis, pulmonary
  bronchorrhagia A15.5
  bronchotracheal A15.5
  bronze disease A18.7
  buccal cavity A18.83
  bulbourethral gland A18.15
  bursa A18.09
  cachexia A15.9
  cardiomyopathy A18.84
  caries —*see* Tuberculosis, bone
  cartilage A18.02
    intervertebral A18.01
  catarrhal —*see* Tuberculosis, respiratory
  cecum A18.32
  cellulitis (primary) A18.4

Tuberculosis, tubercular, tuberculous (Continued)
cerebellum A17.81
cerebral, cerebrum A17.81
cerebrospinal A17.81
  meninges A17.0
cervical (lymph gland or node) A18.2
cervicitis, cervix (uteri) A18.16
chest —see Tuberculosis, respiratory
chorioretinitis A18.53
choroid, choroiditis A18.53
ciliary body A18.54
colitis A18.32
collier's J65
colliquativa (primary) A18.4
colon A18.32
complex, primary A15.7
congenital P37.0
conjunctiva A18.59
connective tissue (systemic) A18.89
contact Z20.1
cornea (ulcer) A18.52
Cowper's gland A18.15
coxae A18.02
coxalgia A18.02
cul-de-sac of Douglas A18.17
curvature, spine A18.01
cutis (colliquativa) (primary) A18.4
cyst, ovary A18.18
cystitis A18.12
dactylitis A18.03
diarrhea A18.32
diffuse —see Tuberculosis, miliary
digestive tract A18.32
disseminated —see Tuberculosis, miliary
duodenum A18.32
dura (mater) (cerebral) (spinal) A17.0
  abscess (cerebral) (spinal) A17.81
dysentery A18.32
ear (inner) (middle) A18.6
  bone A18.03
  external (primary) A18.4
  skin (primary) A18.4
elbow A18.02
emphysema —see Tuberculosis, pulmonary
empyema A15.6
encephalitis A17.82
endarteritis A18.89
endocarditis A18.84
  aortic A18.84
  mitral A18.84
  pulmonary A18.84
  tricuspid A18.84
endocrine glands NEC A18.82
endometrium A18.17
enteric, enterica, enteritis A18.32
enterocolitis A18.32
epididymis, epididymitis A18.15
epidural abscess (cerebral) (spinal) A17.81
epiglottis A15.5
episcleritis A18.51
erythema (induratum) (nodosum) (primary)
  A18.4
esophagus A18.83
eustachian tube A18.6
exposure (to) Z20.1
exudative —see Tuberculosis, pulmonary
eye A18.50
eyelid (primary) (lupus) A18.4
fallopian tube (acute) (chronic) A18.17
fascia A18.09
fauces A15.8
female pelvic inflammatory disease A18.17
finger A18.03
first infection A15.7
gallbladder A18.83
ganglion A18.09
gastritis A18.83
gastrocolic fistula A18.32
gastroenteritis A18.32
gastrointestinal tract A18.32
general, generalized —see Tuberculosis, miliary
genital organs A18.10
genitourinary A18.10
genu A18.02
glandula suprarenalis A18.7
glandular, general A18.2
glottis A15.5
grinder's J65
gum A18.83
hand A18.03
heart A18.84

Tuberculosis, tubercular, tuberculous (Continued)
hematogenous —see Tuberculosis, miliary
hemoptysis —see Tuberculosis, pulmonary
hemorrhage NEC —see Tuberculosis, pulmonary
hemothorax A15.6
hepatitis A18.83
hilar lymph nodes A15.4
  primary (progressive) A15.7
hip (joint) (disease) (bone) A18.02
hydropneumothorax A15.6
hydrothorax A15.6
hypoadrenalism A18.7
hypopharynx A15.8
ileocecal (hyperplastic) A18.32
ileocolitis A18.32
ileum A18.32
iliac spine (superior) A18.03
immunological findings only A15.7
indurativa (primary) A18.4
infantile A15.7
infection A15.9
  without clinical manifestations A15.7
infraclavicular gland A18.2
inguinal gland A18.2
inguinalis A18.2
intestine (any part) A18.32
iridocyclitis A18.54
iris, iritis A18.54
ischiorectal A18.32
jaw A18.03
jejunum A18.32
joint A18.02
  vertebral A18.01
keratitis (interstitial) A18.52
keratoconjunctivitis A18.52
kidney A18.11
knee (joint) A18.02
kyphosis, kyphoscoliosis A18.01
laryngitis A15.5
larynx A15.5
latent Z22.7
leptomeninges, leptomeningitis (cerebral)
  (spinal) A17.0
lichenoides (primary) A18.4
linguae A18.83
lip A18.83
liver A18.83
lordosis A18.01
lung —see Tuberculosis, pulmonary
lupus vulgaris A18.4
lymph gland or node (peripheral) A18.2
  abdomen A18.39
  bronchial A15.4
    primary (progressive) A15.7
  cervical A18.2
  hilar A15.4
    primary (progressive) A15.7
  intrathoracic A15.4
    primary (progressive) A15.7
  mediastinal A15.4
    primary (progressive) A15.7
  mesenteric A18.39
  retroperitoneal A18.39
  tracheobronchial A15.4
    primary (progressive) A15.7
lymphadenitis —see Tuberculosis, lymph gland
lymphangitis —see Tuberculosis, lymph gland
lymphatic (gland) (vessel) —see Tuberculosis,
  lymph gland
mammary gland A18.89
marasmus A15.9
mastoiditis A18.03
mediastinal lymph gland or node A15.4
  primary (progressive) A15.7
mediastinitis A15.8
  primary (progressive) A15.7
mediastinum A15.8
  primary (progressive) A15.7
medulla A17.81
melanosis, Addisonian A18.7
meninges, meningitis (basilar) (cerebral)
  (cerebrospinal) (spinal) A17.0
meningoencephalitis A17.82
mesentery, mesenteric (gland or node) A18.39
miliary A19.9
  acute A19.2
    multiple sites A19.1
    single specified site A19.0
  chronic A19.8
  specified NEC A19.8
millstone makers' J65

Tuberculosis, tubercular, tuberculous (Continued)
miner's J65
molder's J65
mouth A18.83
multiple A19.9
  acute A19.1
  chronic A19.8
muscle A18.09
myelitis A17.82
myocardium, myocarditis A18.84
nasal (passage) (sinus) A15.8
nasopharynx A15.8
neck gland A18.2
nephritis A18.11
nerve (mononeuropathy) A17.83
nervous system A17.9
nose (septum) A15.8
ocular A18.50
omentum A18.31
oophoritis (acute) (chronic) A18.17
optic (nerve trunk) (papilla) A18.59
orbit A18.59
orchitis A18.15
organ, specified NEC A18.89
osseous —see Tuberculosis, bone
osteitis —see Tuberculosis, bone
osteomyelitis —see Tuberculosis, bone
otitis media A18.6
ovary, ovaritis (acute) (chronic) A18.17
oviduct (acute) (chronic) A18.17
pachymeningitis A17.0
palate (soft) A18.83
pancreas A18.83
papulonecrotic (a) (primary) A18.4
parathyroid glands A18.82
paronychia (primary) A18.4
parotid gland or region A18.83
pelvis (bony) A18.03
penis A18.15
peribronchitis A15.5
pericardium, pericarditis A18.84
perichondritis, larynx A15.5
periostitis —see Tuberculosis, bone
perirectal fistula A18.32
peritoneum NEC A18.31
peritonitis A18.31
pharynx, pharyngitis A15.8
phlyctenulosis (keratoconjunctivitis) A18.52
phthisis NEC —see Tuberculosis, pulmonary
pituitary gland A18.82
pleura, pleural, pleurisy, pleuritis (fibrinous)
  (obliterative) (purulent) (simple plastic)
  (with effusion) A15.6
  primary (progressive) A15.7
pneumonia, pneumonic —see Tuberculosis,
  pulmonary
pneumothorax (spontaneous) (tense valvular) —
  see Tuberculosis, pulmonary
polyneuropathy A17.89
polyserositis A19.9
  acute A19.1
  chronic A19.8
potter's J65
prepuce A18.15
primary (complex) A15.7
proctitis A18.32
prostate, prostatitis A18.14
pulmonalis —see Tuberculosis, pulmonary
pulmonary (cavitated) (fibrotic) (infiltrative)
  (nodular) A15.0
  childhood type or first infection A15.7
  primary (complex) A15.7
pyelitis A18.11
pyelonephritis A18.11
pyemia —see Tuberculosis, miliary
pyonephrosis A18.11
pyopneumothorax A15.6
pyothorax A15.6
rectum (fistula) (with abscess) A18.32
reinfection stage —see Tuberculosis, pulmonary
renal A18.11
renis A18.11
respiratory A15.9
  primary A15.7
  specified site NEC A15.8
retina, retinitis A18.53
retroperitoneal (lymph gland or node) A18.39
rheumatism NEC A18.09
rhinitis A15.8
sacroiliac (joint) A18.01
sacrum A18.01

▶ New   ⇒ Revised   ~~deleted~~ Deleted   ● Use Additional Character(s)

Tuberculosis, tubercular, tuberculous *(Continued)*
  salivary gland A18.83
  salpingitis (acute) (chronic) A18.17
  sandblaster's J65
  sclera A18.51
  scoliosis A18.01
  scrofulous A18.2
  scrotum A18.15
  seminal tract or vesicle A18.15
  senile A15.9
  septic —*see* Tuberculosis, miliary
  shoulder (joint) A18.02
    blade A18.03
  sigmoid A18.32
  sinus (any nasal) A15.8
    bone A18.03
    epididymis A18.15
  skeletal NEC A18.03
  skin (any site) (primary) A18.4
  small intestine A18.32
  soft palate A18.83
  spermatic cord A18.15
  spine, spinal (column) A18.01
    cord A17.81
    medulla A17.81
    membrane A17.0
    meninges A17.0
  spleen, splenitis A18.85
  spondylitis A18.01
  sternoclavicular joint A18.02
  stomach A18.83
  stonemason's J65
  subcutaneous tissue (cellular) (primary) A18.4
  subcutis (primary) A18.4
  subdeltoid bursa A18.83
  submaxillary (region) A18.83
  supraclavicular gland A18.2
  suprarenal (capsule) (gland) A18.7
  swelling, joint —*see also* category M01 *(see also* Tuberculosis, joint) A18.02
  symphysis pubis A18.02
  synovitis A18.09
    articular A18.02
    spine or vertebra A18.01
  systemic —*see* Tuberculosis, miliary
  tarsitis A18.4
  tendon (sheath) —*see* Tuberculosis, tenosynovitis
  tenosynovitis A18.09
    spine or vertebra A18.01
  testis A18.15
  throat A15.8
  thymus gland A18.82
  thyroid gland A18.81
  tongue A18.83
  tonsil, tonsillitis A15.8
  trachea, tracheal A15.5
    lymph gland or node A15.4
      primary (progressive) A15.7
  tracheobronchial A15.5
    lymph gland or node A15.4
      primary (progressive) A15.7
  tubal (acute) (chronic) A18.17
  tunica vaginalis A18.15
  ulcer (skin) (primary) A18.4
    bowel or intestine A18.32
    specified NEC - code under Tuberculosis, by site
  unspecified site A15.9
  ureter A18.11
  urethra, urethral (gland) A18.13
  urinary organ or tract A18.13
  uterus A18.17
  uveal tract A18.54
  uvula A18.83
  vagina A18.18
  vas deferens A18.15
  verruca, verrucosa (cutis) (primary) A18.4
  vertebra (column) A18.01
  vesiculitis A18.15
  vulva A18.18
  wrist (joint) A18.02
Tuberculum
  Carabelli —*see* Note at K00.2
  occlusal —*see* Note at K00.2
  paramolare K00.2
~~Tuberosity, entire maxillary M26.07~~
▶ Tuberosity, entire maxillary M26.07
Tuberous sclerosis (brain) Q85.1
Tubo-ovarian —*see* condition
Tuboplasty, after previous sterilization Z31.0
  aftercare Z31.42

Tubotympanitis, catarrhal (chronic) —*see* Otitis, media, nonsuppurative, chronic, serous
Tularemia A21.9
  with
    conjunctivitis A21.1
    pneumonia A21.2
  abdominal A21.3
  bronchopneumonic A21.2
  conjunctivitis A21.1
  cryptogenic A21.3
  enteric A21.3
  gastrointestinal A21.3
  generalized A21.7
  ingestion A21.3
  intestinal A21.3
  oculoglandular A21.1
  ophthalmic A21.1
  pneumonia (any), pneumonic A21.2
  pulmonary A21.2
  sepsis A21.7
  specified NEC A21.8
  typhoidal A21.7
  ulceroglandular A21.0
Tularensis conjunctivitis A21.1
Tumefaction —*see also* Swelling
  liver —*see* Hypertrophy, liver
Tumor —*see also* Neoplasm, unspecified behavior, by site
  acinar cell —*see* Neoplasm, uncertain behavior, by site
  acinic cell —*see* Neoplasm, uncertain behavior, by site
  adenocarcinoid —*see* Neoplasm, malignant, by site
  adenomatoid —*see also* Neoplasm, benign, by site
    odontogenic —*see* Cyst, calcifying odontogenic
  adnexal (skin) —*see* Neoplasm, skin, benign, by site
  adrenal
    cortical (benign) D35.0-•
      malignant C74.0-•
    rest —*see* Neoplasm, benign, by site
  alpha-cell
    malignant
      pancreas C25.4
      specified site NEC —*see* Neoplasm, malignant, by site
      unspecified site C25.4
    pancreas D13.7
    specified site NEC —*see* Neoplasm, benign, by site
    unspecified site D13.7
  aneurysmal —*see* Aneurysm
  aortic body D44.7
    malignant C75.5
  Askin's —*see* Neoplasm, connective tissue, malignant
  basal cell —*see also* Neoplasm, skin, uncertain behavior D48.5
  Bednar —*see* Neoplasm, skin, malignant
  benign (unclassified) —*see* Neoplasm, benign, by site
  beta-cell
    malignant
      pancreas C25.4
      specified site NEC —*see* Neoplasm, malignant, by site
      unspecified site C25.4
    pancreas D13.7
    specified site NEC —*see* Neoplasm, benign, by site
    unspecified site D13.7
  Brenner D27.9
    borderline malignancy D39.1-•
    malignant C56-•
    proliferating D39.1
  bronchial alveolar, intravascular D38.1
  Brooke's —*see* Neoplasm, skin, benign
  brown fat —*see* Lipoma
  Burkitt —*see* Lymphoma, Burkitt
  calcifying epithelial odontogenic —*see* Cyst, calcifying odontogenic
  carcinoid D3A.00
    benign D3A.00
      appendix D3A.020
      ascending colon D3A.022
      bronchus (lung) D3A.090
      cecum D3A.021
      colon D3A.029

Tumor *(Continued)*
  carcinoid *(Continued)*
    benign *(Continued)*
      descending colon D3A.024
      duodenum D3A.010
      foregut NOS D3A.094
      hindgut NOS D3A.096
      ileum D3A.012
      jejunum D3A.011
      kidney D3A.093
      large intestine D3A.029
      lung (bronchus) D3A.090
      midgut NOS D3A.095
      rectum D3A.026
      sigmoid colon D3A.025
      small intestine D3A.019
      specified NEC D3A.098
      stomach D3A.092
      thymus D3A.091
      transverse colon D3A.023
    malignant C7A.00
      appendix C7A.020
      ascending colon C7A.022
      bronchus (lung) C7A.090
      cecum C7A.021
      colon C7A.029
      descending colon C7A.024
      duodenum C7A.010
      foregut NOS C7A.094
      hindgut NOS C7A.096
      ileum C7A.012
      jejunum C7A.011
      kidney C7A.093
      large intestine C7A.029
      lung (bronchus) C7A.090
      midgut NOS C7A.095
      rectum C7A.026
      sigmoid colon C7A.025
      small intestine C7A.019
      specified NEC C7A.098
      stomach C7A.092
      thymus C7A.091
      transverse colon C7A.023
    ~~mesentery metastasis C7B.04~~
    ▶ mesentery metastasis C7B.04
    secondary C7B.00
      bone C7B.03
      distant lymph nodes C7B.01
      liver C7B.02
      peritoneum C7B.04
      specified NEC C7B.09
  carotid body D44.6
    malignant C75.4
  cells —*see also* Neoplasm, unspecified behavior, by site
    benign —*see* Neoplasm, benign, by site
    malignant —*see* Neoplasm, malignant, by site
    uncertain whether benign or malignant —*see* Neoplasm, uncertain behavior, by site
  cervix, in pregnancy or childbirth —*see* Pregnancy, complicated by, tumor, cervix
  chondromatous giant cell —*see* Neoplasm, bone, benign
  chromaffin —*see also* Neoplasm, benign, by site
    malignant —*see* Neoplasm, malignant, by site
  Cock's peculiar L72.3
  Codman's —*see* Neoplasm, bone, benign
  dentigerous, mixed —*see* Cyst, calcifying odontogenic
  dermoid —*see* Neoplasm, benign, by site
    with malignant transformation C56-•
  desmoid (extra-abdominal) —*see also* Neoplasm, connective tissue, uncertain behavior
    abdominal —*see* Neoplasm, connective tissue, uncertain behavior
  embolus —*see* Neoplasm, secondary, by site
  embryonal (mixed) —*see also* Neoplasm, uncertain behavior, by site
    liver C22.7
  endodermal sinus
    specified site —*see* Neoplasm, malignant, by site
    unspecified site
      female C56.-•
      male C62.90
  epithelial
    benign —*see* Neoplasm, benign, by site
    malignant —*see* Neoplasm, malignant, by site
  Ewing's —*see* Neoplasm, bone, malignant, by site
  fatty —*see* Lipoma
  fibroid —*see* Leiomyoma

Tumor *(Continued)*
  G cell
    malignant
      pancreas C25.4
      specified site NEC —*see* Neoplasm,
        malignant, by site
      unspecified site C25.4
    specified site —*see* Neoplasm, uncertain
      behavior, by site
    unspecified site D37.8
  germ cell —*see also* Neoplasm, malignant, by site
    mixed —*see* Neoplasm, malignant,
      by site
  ghost cell, odontogenic —*see* Cyst, calcifying
    odontogenic
  giant cell —*see also* Neoplasm, uncertain
    behavior, by site
    bone D48.0
      malignant —*see* Neoplasm, bone, malignant
    chondromatous —*see* Neoplasm, bone, benign
    malignant —*see* Neoplasm, malignant,
      by site
    soft parts —*see* Neoplasm, connective tissue,
      uncertain behavior
      malignant —*see* Neoplasm, connective
        tissue, malignant
  glomus D18.00
    intra-abdominal D18.03
    intracranial D18.02
    jugulare D44.7
      malignant C75.5
    skin D18.01
    specified site NEC D18.09
  gonadal stromal —*see* Neoplasm, uncertain
    behavior, by site
  granular cell —*see also* Neoplasm, connective
    tissue, benign
    malignant —*see* Neoplasm, connective tissue,
      malignant
  granulosa cell D39.1-●
    juvenile D39.1-●
    malignant C56-●
  granulosa cell-theca cell D39.1-●
    malignant C56-●
  Grawitz's C64-●
  hemorrhoidal —*see* Hemorrhoids
  hilar cell D27-●
  hilus cell D27-●
  Hurthle cell (benign) D34
    malignant C73
  hydatid —*see* Echinococcus
  hypernephroid —*see also* Neoplasm, uncertain
    behavior, by site
  interstitial cell —*see also* Neoplasm, uncertain
    behavior, by site
    benign —*see* Neoplasm, benign, by site
    malignant —*see* Neoplasm, malignant,
      by site
  intravascular bronchial alveolar D38.1
  islet cell —*see* Neoplasm, benign, by site
    malignant —*see* Neoplasm, malignant, by site
      pancreas C25.4
      specified site NEC —*see* Neoplasm,
        malignant, by site
      unspecified site C25.4
    pancreas D13.7
    specified site NEC —*see* Neoplasm, benign,
      by site
    unspecified site D13.7
  juxtaglomerular D41.0-●
  Klatskin's C24.0
  Krukenberg's C79.6-●
  Leydig cell —*see* Neoplasm, uncertain behavior,
    by site
    benign —*see* Neoplasm, benign, by site
      specified site —*see* Neoplasm, benign, by
        site
      unspecified site
        female D27.9
        male D29.20
    malignant —*see* Neoplasm, malignant, by site
      specified site —*see* Neoplasm, malignant,
        by site
      unspecified site
        female C56.9
        male C62.90
    specified site —*see* Neoplasm, uncertain
      behavior, by site
    unspecified site
      female D39.10
      male D40.10

Tumor *(Continued)*
  lipid cell, ovary D27-●
  lipoid cell, ovary D27-●
  malignant —*see also* Neoplasm, malignant, by
    site C80.1
    fusiform cell (type) C80.1
    giant cell (type) C80.1
    localized, plasma cell —*see* Plasmacytoma,
      solitary
    mixed NEC C80.1
    small cell (type) C80.1
    spindle cell (type) C80.1
    unclassified C80.1
  mast cell D47.09
  melanotic, neuroectodermal —*see* Neoplasm,
    benign, by site
  Merkel cell —*see* Carcinoma, Merkel cell
  mesenchymal
    malignant —*see* Neoplasm, connective tissue,
      malignant
    mixed —*see* Neoplasm, connective tissue,
      uncertain behavior
  mesodermal, mixed —*see also* Neoplasm,
    malignant, by site
    liver C22.4
  mesonephric —*see also* Neoplasm, uncertain
    behavior, by site
    malignant —*see* Neoplasm, malignant, by site
  metastatic
    from specified site —*see* Neoplasm, malignant,
      by site
    of specified site —*see* Neoplasm, malignant,
      by site
    to specified site —*see* Neoplasm, secondary,
      by site
  mixed NEC —*see also* Neoplasm, benign, by site
    malignant —*see* Neoplasm, malignant, by site
  mucinous of low malignant potential
    specified site —*see* Neoplasm, malignant, by
      site
    unspecified site C56.9
  mucocarcinoid
    specified site —*see* Neoplasm, malignant, by
      site
    unspecified site C18.1
  mucoepidermoid —*see* Neoplasm, uncertain
    behavior, by site
  Müllerian, mixed
    specified site —*see* Neoplasm, malignant, by
      site
    unspecified site C54.9
  myoepithelial —*see* Neoplasm, benign,
    by site
  neuroectodermal (peripheral) —*see* Neoplasm,
    malignant, by site
    primitive
      specified site —*see* Neoplasm, malignant,
        by site
      unspecified site C71.9
  neuroendocrine D3A.8
    malignant poorly differentiated C7A.1
    secondary NEC C7B.8
    specified NEC C7A.8
  neurogenic olfactory C30.0
  nonencapsulated sclerosing C73
  odontogenic (adenomatoid) (benign) (calcifying
    epithelial) (keratocystic) (squamous) —*see*
    Cyst, calcifying odontogenic
    malignant C41.1
      upper jaw (bone) C41.0
  ovarian stromal D39.1-●
  ovary, in pregnancy —*see* Pregnancy,
    complicated by
  pacinian —*see* Neoplasm, skin, benign
  Pancoast's —*see* Pancoast's syndrome
  papillary —*see also* Papilloma
    cystic D37.9
    mucinous of low malignant potential C56-●
      specified site —*see* Neoplasm, malignant,
        by site
      unspecified site C56.9
    serous of low malignant potential
      specified site —*see* Neoplasm, malignant,
        by site
      unspecified site C56.9
  pelvic, in pregnancy or childbirth —*see*
    Pregnancy, complicated by
  phantom F45.8
  phyllodes D48.6-●
    benign D24-●
    malignant —*see* Neoplasm, breast, malignant

Tumor *(Continued)*
  Pindborg —*see* Cyst, calcifying odontogenic
  placental site trophoblastic D39.2
  plasma cell (malignant) (localized) —*see*
    Plasmacytoma, solitary
  polyvesicular vitelline
    specified site —*see* Neoplasm, malignant, by
      site
    unspecified site
      female C56.9
      male C62.90
  Pott's puffy —*see* Osteomyelitis, specified NEC
  Rathke's pouch D44.3
  retinal anlage —*see* Neoplasm, benign, by site
  ~~salivary gland type, mixed —see Neoplasm,~~
    ~~salivary gland, benign~~
    ~~malignant —see Neoplasm, salivary gland,~~
    ~~malignant~~
  ▶salivary gland or duct type, mixed —*see*
    Neoplasm, salivary gland or duct, benign
    ▶malignant —*see* Neoplasm, salivary gland or
      duct, malignant
  Sampson's N80.10-●
  Schmincke's —*see* Neoplasm, nasopharynx,
    malignant
  sclerosing stromal D27-●
  sebaceous —*see* Cyst, sebaceous
  secondary —*see* Neoplasm, secondary, by
    site
    carcinoid C7B.00
      bone C7B.03
      distant lymph nodes C7B.01
      liver C7B.02
      peritoneum C7B.04
      specified NEC C7B.09
    neuroendocrine NEC C7B.8
  serous of low malignant potential
    specified site —*see* Neoplasm, malignant, by
      site
    unspecified site C56.9
  Sertoli cell —*see* Neoplasm, benign, by site
    with lipid storage
      specified site —*see* Neoplasm, benign, by
        site
      unspecified site
        female D27.9
        male D29.20
    specified site —*see* Neoplasm, benign, by site
    unspecified site
      female D27.9
      male D29.20
  Sertoli-Leydig cell —*see* Neoplasm, benign, by
    site
    specified site —*see* Neoplasm, benign, by site
    unspecified site
      female D27.9
      male D29.20
  sex cord(-stromal) —*see* Neoplasm, uncertain
    behavior, by site
    with annular tubules D39.1-●
  skin appendage —*see* Neoplasm, skin,
    benign
  smooth muscle —*see* Neoplasm, connective
    tissue, uncertain behavior
  soft tissue
    benign —*see* Neoplasm, connective tissue,
      benign
    malignant —*see* Neoplasm, connective tissue,
      malignant
  sternomastoid (congenital) Q68.0
  stromal
    endometrial D39.0
    gastric D48.19
      benign D21.4
      ➡malignant C49.A2
      uncertain behavior D48.19
    gastrointestinal C49.A-●
      benign D21.4
      esophagus C49.A1
      large intestine C49.A4
      malignant C49.A0
        colon C49.A4
        duodenum C49.A3
        esophagus C49.A1
        ileum C49.A3
        jejunum C49.A3
        Meckel diverticulum C49.A3
        large intestine C49.A4
        omentum C49.A9
        peritoneum C49.A9
        rectum C49.A5

Tumor *(Continued)*
  stromal *(Continued)*
    gastrointestinal *(Continued)*
      malignant *(Continued)*
        small intestine C49.A3
        specified site NEC C49.A9
        stomach C49.A2
      rectum C49.A5
      small intestine C49.A3
      specified site NEC C49.A9
      stomach C49.A2
      uncertain behavior D48.19
    intestine
      benign D21.4
      malignant
        large C49.A4
        small C49.A3
      uncertain behavior D48.19
    ovarian D39.1-●
    stomach C49.A2
      benign D21.4
      malignant C49.A2
      uncertain behavior D48.19
  sweat gland —*see also* Neoplasm, skin, uncertain behavior
    benign —*see* Neoplasm, skin, benign
    malignant —*see* Neoplasm, skin, malignant
  syphilitic, brain A52.17
  testicular D40.10
  testicular stromal D40.1-●
  theca cell D27.-●
  theca cell-granulosa cell D39.1-●
  Triton, malignant —*see* Neoplasm, nerve, malignant
  trophoblastic, placental site D39.2
  turban D23.4
  uterus (body), in pregnancy or childbirth —*see* Pregnancy, complicated by, tumor, uterus
  vagina, in pregnancy or childbirth —*see* Pregnancy, complicated by
  varicose —*see* Varix
  von Recklinghausen's —*see* Neurofibromatosis
  vulva or perineum, in pregnancy or childbirth —*see* Pregnancy, complicated by
    causing obstructed labor O65.5
  Warthin's —*see* Neoplasm, salivary gland or duct, benign
  Wilms' C64-●
  yolk sac —*see* Neoplasm, malignant, by site
    specified site —*see* Neoplasm, malignant, by site
    unspecified site
      female C56.9
      male C62.90
Tumor lysis syndrome (following antineoplastic chemotherapy) (spontaneous) NEC E88.3
Tumorlet —*see* Neoplasm, uncertain behavior, by site
Tungiasis B88.1
Tunica vasculosa lentis Q12.2
Turban tumor D23.4
Türck's trachoma J37.0
Turner-Kieser syndrome Q87.2
Turner-like syndrome Q87.19
Turner's
  hypoplasia (tooth) K00.4
  syndrome Q96.9
    specified NEC Q96.8
  tooth K00.4
Turner-Ullrich syndrome Q96.9
Tussis convulsiva —*see* Whooping cough
Twiddler's syndrome (due to)
  automatic implantable defibrillator T82.198
  cardiac pacemaker T82.198
Twilight state
  epileptic F05
  psychogenic F44.89
Twin (newborn) —*see also* Newborn, twin
  conjoined Q89.4
  pregnancy —*see* Pregnancy, twin
Twinning, teeth K00.2
Twist, twisted
  bowel, colon or intestine K56.2
  hair (congenital) Q84.1
  mesentery K56.2
  omentum K56.2
  organ or site, congenital NEC —*see* Anomaly, by site
  ovarian pedicle —*see* Torsion, ovary

Twitching R25.3
Tylosis (acquired) L84
  buccalis K13.29
  linguae K13.29
  palmaris et plantaris (congenital) (inherited) Q82.8
    acquired L85.1
Tympanism R14.0
Tympanites (abdominal) (intestinal) R14.0
Tympanitis —*see* Myringitis
Tympanosclerosis —*see* subcategory H74.0
Tympanum —*see* condition
Tympany
  abdomen R14.0
  chest R09.89
Type A behavior pattern Z73.1
Typhlitis —*see* Cecitis
Typhoenteritis —*see* Typhoid
Typhoid (abortive) (ambulant) (any site) (clinical) (fever) (hemorrhagic) (infection) (intermittent) (malignant) (rheumatic) (Widal negative) A01.00
  with pneumonia A01.03
  abdominal A01.09
  arthritis A01.04
  carrier (suspected) of Z22.0
  cholecystitis (current) A01.09
  endocarditis A01.02
  heart involvement A01.02
  inoculation reaction —*see* Complications, vaccination
  meningitis A01.01
  mesenteric lymph nodes A01.09
  myocarditis A01.02
  Orientia Tsutsugamushi (scrub typhus) A75.3
  osteomyelitis A01.05
  perichondritis, larynx A01.09
  pneumonia A01.03
  specified NEC A01.09
  spine A01.05
  ulcer (perforating) A01.09
Typhomalaria (fever) —*see* Malaria
Typhomania A01.00
Typhoperitonitis A01.09
Typhus (fever) A75.9
  abdominal, abdominalis —*see* Typhoid
  African tick A77.1
  amarillic A95.9
  brain A75.9 *[G94]*
  cerebral A75.9 *[G94]*
  classical A75.0
  due to Rickettsia
    prowazekii A75.0
      recrudescent A75.1
    tsutsugamushi A75.3
    typhi A75.2
  endemic (flea-borne) A75.2
  epidemic (louse-borne) A75.0
  exanthematic NEC A75.0
  exanthematicus SAI A75.0
    brillii SAI A75.1
    mexicanus SAI A75.2
    typhus murinus A75.2
  flea-borne A75.2
  India tick A77.1
  Kenya (tick) A77.1
  louse-borne A75.0
  Mexican A75.2
  mite-borne A75.3
  murine A75.2
  North Asian tick-borne A77.2
  petechial A75.9
  Queensland tick A77.3
  rat A75.2
  recrudescent A75.1
  recurrens —*see* Fever, relapsing
  Sao Paulo A77.0
  scrub (China) (India) (Malaysia) (New Guinea) A75.3
  shop (of Malaysia) A75.2
  Siberian tick A77.2
  tick-borne A77.9
  tropical (mite-borne) A75.3
Tyrosinemia E70.21
  newborn, transitory P74.5
Tyrosinosis E70.21
Tyrosinuria E70.29

——————— U ———————

Uhl's anomaly or disease Q24.8
Ulcer, ulcerated, ulcerating, ulceration, ulcerative
  alveolar process M27.3
  amebic (intestine) A06.1
    skin A06.7
  anastomotic —*see* Ulcer, gastrojejunal
  anorectal K62.6
  antral —*see* Ulcer, stomach
  anus (sphincter) (solitary) K62.6
  aorta —*see* Aneurysm
  aphthous (oral) (recurrent) K12.0
    genital organ(s)
      female N76.6
      male N50.89
  artery I77.2
  atrophic —*see* Ulcer, skin
    decubitus —*see* Ulcer, pressure, by site
  back L98.429
    with
      bone involvement without evidence of necrosis L98.426
      bone necrosis L98.424
      exposed fat layer L98.422
      muscle involvement without evidence of necrosis L98.425
      muscle necrosis L98.423
      skin breakdown only L98.421
      specified severity NEC L98.428
  Barrett's (esophagus) K22.10
    with bleeding K22.11
  bile duct (common) (hepatic) K83.8
  bladder (solitary) (sphincter) NEC N32.89
    bilharzial B65.9 *[N33]*
    in schistosomiasis (bilharzial) B65.9 *[N33]*
    submucosal —*see* Cystitis, interstitial
    tuberculous A18.12
  bleeding K27.4
  bone —*see* Osteomyelitis, specified type NEC
  bowel —*see* Ulcer, intestine
  breast N61.1
  bronchus J98.09
  buccal (cavity) (traumatic) K12.1
  Buruli A31.1
  buttock L98.419
    with
      bone involvement without evidence of necrosis L98.416
      bone necrosis L98.414
      exposed fat layer L98.412
      muscle involvement without evidence of necrosis L98.415
      muscle necrosis L98.413
      skin breakdown only L98.411
      specified severity NEC L98.418
  cameron - see Ulcer, stomach
  cancerous —*see* Neoplasm, malignant, by site
  cardia K22.10
    with bleeding K22.11
  cardioesophageal (peptic) K22.10
    with bleeding K22.11
  cecum —*see* Ulcer, intestine
  cervix (uteri) (decubitus) (trophic) N86
    with cervicitis N72
  chancroidal A57
  chiclero B55.1
  chronic (cause unknown) —*see* Ulcer, skin
  Cochin-China B55.1
  colon —*see* Ulcer, intestine
  conjunctiva H10.89
  cornea H16.00-●
    with hypopyon H16.03-●
    central H16.01-●
    dendritic (herpes simplex) B00.52
    marginal H16.04-●
    Mooren's H16.05-●
    mycotic H16.06-●
    perforated H16.07-●
    ring H16.02-●
    tuberculous (phlyctenular) A18.52
  corpus cavernosum (chronic) N48.5
  crural —*see* Ulcer, lower limb
  Curling's —*see* Ulcer, peptic, acute
  Cushing's —*see* Ulcer, peptic, acute
  cystic duct K82.8
  cystitis (interstitial) —*see* Cystitis, interstitial
  decubitus —*see* Ulcer, pressure, by site
  dendritic, cornea (herpes simplex) B00.52
  diabetes, diabetic —*see* Diabetes, ulcer

Ulcer, ulcerated, ulcerating, ulceration,
   ulcerative — *(Continued)*
  Dieulafoy's K25.0
  due to
    infection NEC —*see* Ulcer, skin
    radiation NEC L59.8
    trophic disturbance (any region) —*see* Ulcer,
      skin
    X-ray L58.1
  duodenum, duodenal (eroded) (peptic)
    K26.9
    with
      hemorrhage K26.4
        and perforation K26.6
      perforation K26.5
    acute K26.3
      with
        hemorrhage K26.0
          and perforation K26.2
        perforation K26.1
    chronic (erosive) K26.7
      with
        hemorrhage K26.4
          and perforation K26.6
        perforation K26.5
  dysenteric A09
  elusive —*see* Cystitis, interstitial
  endocarditis (acute) (chronic) (subacute) I28.8
  epiglottis J38.7
  esophagus (peptic) K22.10
    with bleeding K22.11
    due to
      aspirin K22.10
        with bleeding K22.11
      gastrointestinal reflux disease (without
        bleeding) K21.00
        with bleeding K21.01
      ingestion of chemical or medicament
        K22.10
        with bleeding K22.11
    fungal K22.10
      with bleeding K22.11
    infective K22.10
      with bleeding K22.11
    varicose —*see* Varix, esophagus
  eyelid (region) H01.8
  fauces J39.2
  Fenwick (-Hunner) (solitary) —*see* Cystitis,
    interstitial
  fistulous —*see* Ulcer, skin
  foot (indolent) (trophic) —*see* Ulcer, lower limb
  frambesial, initial A66.0
  frenum (tongue) K14.0
  gallbladder or duct K82.8
  gangrenous —*see* Gangrene
  gastric —*see* Ulcer, stomach
  gastrocolic —*see* Ulcer, gastrojejunal
  gastroduodenal —*see* Ulcer, peptic
  gastroesophageal —*see* Ulcer, stomach
  gastrointestinal —*see* Ulcer, gastrojejunal
  gastrojejunal (peptic) K28.9
    with
      hemorrhage K28.4
        and perforation K28.6
      perforation K28.5
    acute K28.3
      with
        hemorrhage K28.0
          and perforation K28.2
        perforation K28.1
    chronic K28.7
      with
        hemorrhage K28.4
          and perforation K28.6
        perforation K28.5
  gastrojejunocolic —*see* Ulcer, gastrojejunal
  gingiva K06.8
  gingivitis K05.10
    nonplaque induced K05.11
    plaque induced K05.10
  glottis J38.7
  granuloma of pudenda A58
  gum K06.8
  gumma, due to yaws A66.4
  heel —*see* Ulcer, lower limb
  hemorrhoid —*see also* Hemorrhoids, by degree
    K64.8
  Hunner's —*see* Cystitis, interstitial
  hypopharynx J39.2
  hypopyon (chronic) (subacute) —*see* Ulcer,
    cornea, with hypopyon
  hypostaticum —*see* Ulcer, varicose

Ulcer, ulcerated, ulcerating, ulceration,
   ulcerative — *(Continued)*
  ileum —*see* Ulcer, intestine
  intestine, intestinal K63.3
    with perforation K63.1
    amebic A06.1
    duodenal —*see* Ulcer, duodenum
    granulocytopenic (with hemorrhage) —*see*
      Neutropenia
    marginal —*see* Ulcer, gastrojejunal
    perforating K63.1
      newborn P78.0
    primary, small intestine K63.3
    rectum K62.6
    stercoraceous, stercoral K63.3
    tuberculous A18.32
    typhoid (fever) —*see* Typhoid
    varicose I86.8
  jejunum, jejunal —*see* Ulcer, gastrojejunal
  keratitis —*see* Ulcer, cornea
  knee —*see* Ulcer, lower limb
  labium (majus) (minus) N76.6
  laryngitis —*see* Laryngitis
  larynx (aphthous) (contact) J38.7
    diphtheritic A36.2
  leg —*see* Ulcer, lower limb
  lip K13.0
  Lipschütz's N76.6
  lower limb (atrophic) (chronic) (neurogenic)
    (perforating) (pyogenic) (trophic) (tropical)
    L97.909
    with
      bone involvement without evidence of
        necrosis L97.906
      bone necrosis L97.904
      exposed fat layer L97.902
      muscle involvement without evidence of
        necrosis L97.905
      muscle necrosis L97.903
      skin breakdown only L97.901
      specified severity NEC L97.908
    ankle L97.309
      with
        bone involvement without evidence of
          necrosis L97.306
        bone necrosis L97.304
        exposed fat layer L97.302
        muscle involvement without evidence of
          necrosis L97.305
        muscle necrosis L97.303
        skin breakdown only L97.301
        specified severity NEC L97.308
      left L97.329
        with
          bone involvement without evidence of
            necrosis L97.326
          bone necrosis L97.324
          exposed fat layer L97.322
          muscle involvement without evidence
            of necrosis L97.325
          muscle necrosis L97.323
          skin breakdown only L97.321
          specified severity NEC L97.328
      right L97.319
        with
          bone involvement without evidence of
            necrosis L97.316
          bone necrosis L97.314
          exposed fat layer L97.312
          muscle involvement without evidence
            of necrosis
            L97.315
          muscle necrosis L97.313
          skin breakdown only L97.311
          specified severity NEC L97.318
    calf L97.209
      with
        bone involvement without evidence of
          necrosis L97.206
        bone necrosis L97.204
        exposed fat layer L97.202
        muscle involvement without evidence of
          necrosis L97.205
        muscle necrosis L97.203
        skin breakdown only L97.201
        specified severity NEC
          L97.208
      left L97.229
        with
          bone involvement without evidence of
            necrosis L97.226
          bone necrosis L97.224

Ulcer, ulcerated, ulcerating, ulceration,
   ulcerative — *(Continued)*
  lower limb *(Continued)*
    calf *(Continued)*
      left *(Continued)*
        with *(Continued)*
          exposed fat layer L97.222
          muscle involvement without evidence
            of necrosis L97.225
          muscle necrosis L97.223
          skin breakdown only L97.221
          specified severity NEC
            L97.228
      right L97.219
        with
          bone involvement without evidence of
            necrosis L97.216
          bone necrosis L97.214
          exposed fat layer L97.212
          muscle involvement without evidence
            of necrosis L97.215
          muscle necrosis L97.213
          skin breakdown only L97.211
          specified severity NEC L97.218
    decubitus —*see* Ulcer, pressure, by site
    foot specified NEC L97.509
      with
        bone involvement without evidence of
          necrosis L97.506
        bone necrosis L97.504
        exposed fat layer L97.502
        muscle involvement without evidence of
          necrosis L97.505
        muscle necrosis L97.503
        skin breakdown only L97.501
        specified severity NEC L97.508
      left L97.529
        with
          bone involvement without evidence of
            necrosis L97.526
          bone necrosis L97.524
          exposed fat layer L97.522
          muscle involvement without evidence
            of necrosis L97.525
          muscle necrosis L97.523
          skin breakdown only L97.521
          specified severity NEC L97.528
      right L97.519
        with
          bone involvement without evidence of
            necrosis L97.516
          bone necrosis L97.514
          exposed fat layer L97.512
          muscle involvement without evidence
            of necrosis L97.515
          muscle necrosis L97.513
          skin breakdown only L97.511
          specified severity NEC L97.518
    heel L97.409
      with
        bone involvement without evidence of
          necrosis L97.406
        bone necrosis L97.404
        exposed fat layer L97.402
        muscle involvement without evidence of
          necrosis L97.405
        muscle necrosis L97.403
        skin breakdown only L97.401
        specified severity NEC L97.408
      left L97.429
        with
          bone involvement without evidence of
            necrosis L97.426
          bone necrosis L97.424
          exposed fat layer L97.422
          muscle involvement without evidence
            of necrosis L97.425
          muscle necrosis L97.423
          skin breakdown only L97.421
          specified severity NEC L97.428
      right L97.419
        with
          bone involvement without evidence of
            necrosis L97.416
          bone necrosis L97.414
          exposed fat layer L97.412
          muscle involvement without evidence
            of necrosis L97.415
          muscle necrosis L97.413
          skin breakdown only L97.411
          specified severity NEC
            L97.418

▶ New   ➡ Revised   ~~deleted~~ Deleted   ● Use Additional Character(s)

Ulcer, ulcerated, ulcerating, ulceration, ulcerative — (Continued)
lower limb (Continued)
  left L97.929
    with
      bone involvement without evidence of necrosis L97.926
      bone necrosis L97.924
      exposed fat layer L97.922
      muscle involvement without evidence of necrosis L97.925
      muscle necrosis L97.923
      skin breakdown only L97.921
      specified severity NEC L97.928
  lower leg NOS L97.909
    with
      bone involvement without evidence of necrosis L97.906
      bone necrosis L97.904
      exposed fat layer L97.902
      muscle involvement without evidence of necrosis L97.905
      muscle necrosis L97.903
      skin breakdown only L97.901
      specified severity NEC L97.908
  left L97.929
    with
      bone involvement without evidence of necrosis L97.926
      bone necrosis L97.924
      exposed fat layer L97.922
      muscle involvement without evidence of necrosis L97.925
      muscle necrosis L97.923
      skin breakdown only L97.921
      specified severity NEC L97.928
  right L97.919
    with
      bone involvement without evidence of necrosis L97.916
      bone necrosis L97.914
      exposed fat layer L97.912
      muscle involvement without evidence of necrosis L97.915
      muscle necrosis L97.913
      skin breakdown only L97.911
      specified severity NEC L97.918
  specified site NEC L97.809
    with
      bone involvement without evidence of necrosis L97.806
      bone necrosis L97.804
      exposed fat layer L97.802
      muscle involvement without evidence of necrosis L97.805
      muscle necrosis L97.803
      skin breakdown only L97.801
      specified severity NEC L97.808
  left L97.829
    with
      bone involvement without evidence of necrosis L97.826
      bone necrosis L97.824
      exposed fat layer L97.822
      muscle involvement without evidence of necrosis L97.825
      muscle necrosis L97.823
      skin breakdown only L97.821
      specified severity NEC L97.828
  right L97.819
    with
      bone involvement without evidence of necrosis L97.816
      bone necrosis L97.814
      exposed fat layer L97.812
      muscle involvement without evidence of necrosis L97.815
      muscle necrosis L97.813
      skin breakdown only L97.811
      specified severity NEC L97.818
  midfoot L97.409
    with
      bone involvement without evidence of necrosis L97.406
      bone necrosis L97.404
      exposed fat layer L97.402
      muscle involvement without evidence of necrosis L97.405
      muscle necrosis L97.403
      skin breakdown only L97.401
      specified severity NEC L97.408

Ulcer, ulcerated, ulcerating, ulceration, ulcerative — (Continued)
lower limb (Continued)
  midfoot (Continued)
    left L97.429
      with
        bone involvement without evidence of necrosis L97.426
        bone necrosis L97.424
        exposed fat layer L97.422
        muscle involvement without evidence of necrosis L97.425
        muscle necrosis L97.423
        skin breakdown only L97.421
        specified severity NEC L97.428
    right L97.419
      with
        bone involvement without evidence of necrosis L97.416
        bone necrosis L97.414
        exposed fat layer L97.412
        muscle involvement without evidence of necrosis L97.415
        muscle necrosis L97.413
        skin breakdown only L97.411
        specified severity NEC L97.418
  right L97.919
    with
      bone involvement without evidence of necrosis L97.916
      bone necrosis L97.914
      exposed fat layer L97.912
      muscle involvement without evidence of necrosis L97.915
      muscle necrosis L97.913
      skin breakdown only L97.911
      specified severity NEC L97.918
  thigh L97.109
    with
      bone involvement without evidence of necrosis L97.106
      bone necrosis L97.104
      exposed fat layer L97.102
      muscle involvement without evidence of necrosis L97.105
      muscle necrosis L97.103
      skin breakdown only L97.101
      specified severity NEC L97.108
  left L97.129
    with
      bone involvement without evidence of necrosis L97.126
      bone necrosis L97.124
      exposed fat layer L97.122
      muscle involvement without evidence of necrosis L97.125
      muscle necrosis L97.123
      skin breakdown only L97.121
      specified severity NEC L97.128
  right L97.119
    with
      bone involvement without evidence of necrosis L97.116
      bone necrosis L97.114
      exposed fat layer L97.112
      muscle involvement without evidence of necrosis L97.115
      muscle necrosis L97.113
      skin breakdown only L97.111
      specified severity NEC L97.118
  toe L97.509
    with
      bone involvement without evidence of necrosis L97.506
      bone necrosis L97.504
      exposed fat layer L97.502
      muscle involvement without evidence of necrosis L97.505
      muscle necrosis L97.503
      skin breakdown only L97.501
      specified severity NEC L97.508
  left L97.529
    with
      bone involvement without evidence of necrosis L97.526
      bone necrosis L97.524
      exposed fat layer L97.522
      muscle involvement without evidence of necrosis L97.525
      muscle necrosis L97.523
      skin breakdown only L97.521
      specified severity NEC L97.528

Ulcer, ulcerated, ulcerating, ulceration, ulcerative — (Continued)
lower limb (Continued)
  toe (Continued)
    right L97.519
      with
        bone involvement without evidence of necrosis L97.516
        bone necrosis L97.514
        exposed fat layer L97.512
        muscle involvement without evidence of necrosis L97.515
        muscle necrosis L97.513
        skin breakdown only L97.511
        specified severity NEC L97.518
  leprous A30.1
  syphilitic A52.19
  varicose —see Varix, leg, with, ulcer
luetic —see Ulcer, syphilitic
lung J98.4
  tuberculous —see Tuberculosis, pulmonary
malignant —see Neoplasm, malignant, by site
marginal NEC —see Ulcer, gastrojejunal
meatus (urinarius) N34.2
Meckel's diverticulum Q43.0
  malignant —see Table of Neoplasms, small intestine, malignant
Meleney's (chronic undermining) —see Ulcer, skin
Mooren's (cornea) —see Ulcer, cornea, Mooren's
mycobacterial (skin) A31.1
nasopharynx J39.2
neck, uterus N86
neurogenic NEC —see Ulcer, skin
nose, nasal (passage) (infective) (septum) J34.0
  skin —see Ulcer, skin
  spirochetal A69.8
  varicose (bleeding) I86.8
oral mucosa (traumatic) K12.1
palate (soft) K12.1
penis (chronic) N48.5
peptic (site unspecified) K27.9
  with
    hemorrhage K27.4
      and perforation K27.6
    perforation K27.5
  acute K27.3
    with
      hemorrhage K27.0
        and perforation K27.2
      perforation K27.1
  chronic K27.7
    with
      hemorrhage K27.4
        and perforation K27.6
      perforation K27.5
  esophagus K22.10
    with bleeding K22.11
  newborn P78.82
perforating K27.5
  skin —see Ulcer, skin
peritonsillar J35.8
phagedenic (tropical) —see Ulcer, skin
pharynx J39.2
phlebitis —see Phlebitis
plaster —see Ulcer, pressure, by site
popliteal space —see Ulcer, lower limb
postpyloric —see Ulcer, duodenum
prepuce N47.7
prepyloric —see Ulcer, stomach
pressure (pressure area) L89.9-●
  ankle L89.5-●
  back L89.1-●
  buttock L89.3-●
  coccyx L89.15-●
  contiguous site of back, buttock, hip L89.4-●
  elbow L89.0-●
  face L89.81-●
  head L89.81-●
  heel L89.6-●
  hip L89.2-●
  sacral region (tailbone) L89.15-●
  specified site NEC L89.89-●
  stage 1 (healing) (pre-ulcer skin changes limited to persistent focal edema)
    ankle L89.5-●
    back L89.1-●
    buttock L89.3-●
    coccyx L89.15-●
    contiguous site of back, buttock, hip L89.4-●
    elbow L89.0-●

Ulcer, ulcerated, ulcerating, ulceration,
   ulcerative — (Continued)
  pressure (Continued)
   stage 1 (Continued)
    face L89.81-●
    head L89.81-●
    heel L89.6-●
    hip L89.2-●
    sacral region (tailbone) L89.15-●
    specified site NEC L89.89-●
   stage 2 (healing) (abrasion, blister, partial
    thickness skin loss involving epidermis
    and/or dermis)
    ankle L89.5-●
    back L89.1-●
    buttock L89.3-●
    coccyx L89.15-●
    contiguous site of back, buttock, hip L89.4-●
    elbow L89.0-●
    face L89.81-●
    head L89.81-●
    heel L89.6-●
    hip L89.2-●
    sacral region (tailbone) L89.15-●
    specified site NEC L89.89-●
   stage 3 (healing) (full thickness skin loss
    involving damage or necrosis of
    subcutaneous tissue)
    ankle L89.5-●
    back L89.1-●
    buttock L89.3-●
    coccyx L89.15-●
    contiguous site of back, buttock, hip
     L89.4-●
    elbow L89.0-●
    face L89.81-●
    head L89.81-●
    heel L89.6-●
    hip L89.2-●
    sacral region (tailbone) L89.15-●
    specified site NEC L89.89-●
   stage 4 (healing) (necrosis of soft tissues
    through to underlying muscle, tendon,
    or bone)
    ankle L89.5-●
    back L89.1-●
    buttock L89.3-●
    coccyx L89.15-●
    contiguous site of back, buttock, hip
     L89.4-●
    elbow L89.0-●
    face L89.81-●
    head L89.81-●
    heel L89.6-●
    hip L89.2-●
    sacral region (tailbone) L89.15-●
    specified site NEC L89.89-●
   unspecified stage
    ankle L89.5-●
    back L89.1-●
    buttock L89.3-●
    coccyx L89.15-●
    contiguous site of back, buttock, hip
     L89.4-●
    elbow L89.0-●
    face L89.81-●
    head L89.81-●
    heel L89.6-●
    hip L89.2-●
    sacral region (tailbone) L89.15-●
    specified site NEC L89.89-●
   unstageable
    ankle L89.5-●
    back L89.1-●
    buttock L89.3-●
    coccyx L89.15-●
    contiguous site of back, buttock, hip
     L89.4-●
    elbow L89.0-●
    face L89.81-●
    head L89.81-●
    heel L89.6-●
    hip L89.2-●
    sacral region (tailbone) L89.15-●
    specified site NEC L89.89-●
  primary of intestine K63.3
   with perforation K63.1
  prostate N41.9
  pyloric —see Ulcer, stomach
  rectosigmoid K63.3
   with perforation K63.1

Ulcer, ulcerated, ulcerating, ulceration,
   ulcerative — (Continued)
  rectum (sphincter) (solitary) K62.6
   stercoraceous, stercoral K62.6
  retina —see Inflammation, chorioretinal
  rodent —see also Neoplasm, skin, malignant
  sclera —see Scleritis
  scrofulous (tuberculous) A18.2
  scrotum N50.89
   tuberculous A18.15
   varicose I86.1
  seminal vesicle N50.89
  sigmoid —see Ulcer, intestine
  skin (atrophic) (chronic) (neurogenic) (non-
   healing) (perforating) (pyogenic) (trophic)
   (tropical) L98.499
   with gangrene —see Gangrene
   amebic A06.7
   back —see Ulcer, back
   buttock —see Ulcer, buttock
   decubitus —see Ulcer, pressure
   lower limb —see Ulcer, lower limb
   mycobacterial A31.1
   specified site NEC L98.499
    with
     bone involvement without evidence of
      necrosis L98.496
     bone necrosis L98.494
     exposed fat layer L98.492
     muscle involvement without evidence of
      necrosis L98.495
     muscle necrosis L98.493
     skin breakdown only L98.491
     specified severity NEC L98.498
   tuberculous (primary) A18.4
   varicose —see Ulcer, varicose
  sloughing —see Ulcer, skin
  solitary, anus or rectum (sphincter) K62.6
  sore throat J02.9
   streptococcal J02.0
  spermatic cord N50.89
  spine (tuberculous) A18.01
  stasis (venous) —see Varix, leg, with, ulcer
   without varicose veins (see also Ulcer, by site)
    I87.2
  stercoraceous, stercoral K63.3
   with perforation K63.1
   anus or rectum K62.6
  stoma, stomal —see Ulcer, gastrojejunal
  stomach (eroded) (peptic) (round) K25.9
   with
    hemorrhage K25.4
     and perforation K25.6
    perforation K25.5
   acute K25.3
    with
     hemorrhage K25.0
      and perforation K25.2
     perforation K25.1
   chronic K25.7
    with
     hemorrhage K25.4
      and perforation K25.6
     perforation K25.5
  stomal —see Ulcer, gastrojejunal
  stomatitis K12.1
  stress —see Ulcer, peptic
  strumous (tuberculous) A18.2
  submucosal, bladder —see Cystitis,
   interstitial
  syphilitic (any site) (early) (secondary)
   A51.39
   late A52.79
   perforating A52.79
    foot A52.11
  testis N50.89
  thigh —see Ulcer, lower limb
  throat J39.2
   diphtheritic A36.0
  toe —see Ulcer, lower limb
  tongue (traumatic) K14.0
  tonsil J35.8
   diphtheritic A36.0
  trachea J39.8
  trophic —see Ulcer, skin
  tropical —see Ulcer, skin
  tuberculous —see Tuberculosis, ulcer
  tunica vaginalis N50.89
  turbinate J34.89
  typhoid (perforating) —see Typhoid
  unspecified site —see Ulcer, skin

Ulcer, ulcerated, ulcerating, ulceration,
   ulcerative — (Continued)
  urethra (meatus) —see Urethritis
  uterus N85.8
   cervix N86
    with cervicitis N72
   neck N86
    with cervicitis N72
  vagina N76.5
   in Behçet's disease M35.2 [N77.0]
   pessary N89.8
  valve, heart I33.0
  varicose (lower limb, any part) —see also Varix,
   leg, with, ulcer
   broad ligament I86.2
   esophagus —see Varix, esophagus
   inflamed or infected —see Varix, leg, with
    ulcer, with inflammation
   nasal septum I86.8
   perineum I86.3
   scrotum I86.1
   specified site NEC I86.8
   sublingual I86.0
   vulva I86.3
  vas deferens N50.89
  vulva (acute) (infectional) N76.6
   in (due to)
    Behçet's disease M35.2 [N77.0]
    herpesviral (herpes simplex) infection A60.04
    tuberculosis A18.18
  vulvobuccal, recurring N76.6
  X-ray L58.1
  yaws A66.4
Ulcerosa scarlatina A38.8
Ulcus —see also Ulcer
  cutis tuberculosum A18.4
  duodeni —see Ulcer, duodenum
  durum (syphilitic) A51.0
   extragenital A51.2
  gastrojejunale —see Ulcer, gastrojejunal
  hypostaticum —see Ulcer, varicose
  molle (cutis) (skin) A57
  serpens corneae —see Ulcer, cornea, central
  ventriculi —see Ulcer, stomach
Ulegyria Q04.8
Ulerythema
  ophryogenes, congenital Q84.2
  sycosiforme L73.8
Ullrich(-Bonnevie)(-Turner) syndrome —see also
  Turner's syndrome Q87.19
Ullrich-Feichtiger syndrome Q87.0
Ulnar —see condition
Ulorrhagia, ulorrhea K06.8
Umbilicus, umbilical —see condition
Unable to
  make ends meet Z59.86
  obtain
   adequate
    childcare due to limited financial resources,
     specified NEC Z59.87
    clothing due to limited financial resources,
     specified NEC Z59.87
    utilities due to limited financial resources,
     specified NEC Z59.87
   basic
    needs due to limited financial resources,
     specified NEC Z59.87
   services in physical environment Z58.81
   internet service, due to unavailability in
    geographic area Z58.81
   telephone service, due to unavailability in
    geographic area Z58.81
   utilities, due to inadequate physical
    environment Z58.81
Unacceptable
  contours of tooth K08.54
  morphology of tooth K08.54
Unaffordable transportation Z59.82
Unavailability (of)
  bed at medical facility Z75.1
  health service-related agencies Z75.4
  medical facilities (at) Z75.3
   due to
    investigation by social service agency Z75.2
    lack of services at home Z75.0
    remoteness from facility Z75.3
    waiting list Z75.1
   home Z75.0
   outpatient clinic Z75.3
  schooling Z55.1
  social service agencies Z75.4

▶ New   ⇒ Revised   ~~deleted~~ Deleted   ● Use Additional Character(s)

Uncinaria americana infestation B76.1
Uncinariasis B76.9
Uncongenial work Z56.5
Unconscious (ness) —*see* Coma
Underachievement in school Z55.3
Underdevelopment —*see also* Undeveloped
  nose Q30.1
  sexual E30.0
Underdosing —*see also* Table of Drugs and
    Chemicals, categories T36-T50, with final
    character 6 Z91.14
  intentional NEC Z91.128
    due to financial hardship of patient Z91.120
  unintentional NEC Z91.138
    due to patient's age related debility Z91.130
Underfeeding, newborn P92.3
Underfill, endodontic M27.53
Underimmunization status Z28.3
Undernourishment —*see* Malnutrition
Undernutrition —*see* Malnutrition
Under observation —*see* Observation
Underweight R63.6
  for gestational age —*see* Light for dates
Underwood's disease P83.0
Undescended —*see also* Malposition, congenital
  cecum Q43.3
  colon Q43.3
  testicle —*see* Cryptorchid
Undeveloped, undevelopment —*see also*
    Hypoplasia
  brain (congenital) Q02
  cerebral (congenital) Q02
  heart Q24.8
  lung Q33.6
  testis E29.1
  uterus E30.0
Undiagnosed (disease) R69
Undulant fever —*see* Brucellosis
Unemployment, anxiety concerning Z56.0
  threatened Z56.2
Unequal length (acquired) (limb) —*see also*
    Deformity, limb, unequal length
  leg —*see also* Deformity, limb, unequal length
    congenital Q72.9- ●
Unextracted dental root K08.3
Unguis incarnatus L60.0
Unhappiness R45.2
Unicornate uterus Q51.4
  in pregnancy or childbirth O34.00
▶ Unicuspid aortic valve (at birth) (congenital)
    Q23.81
Unilateral —*see also* condition
  development, breast N64.89
  organ or site, congenital NEC —*see* Agenesis,
    by site
Unilocular heart Q20.8
Union, abnormal —*see also* Fusion
  larynx and trachea Q34.8
Universal mesentery Q43.3
Unreliable transportation Z59.82
Unrepairable overhanging of dental restorative
    materials K08.52
Unroofed coronary sinus Q21.13
Unsafe transportation Z59.82
Unsatisfactory
  restoration of tooth K08.50
    specified NEC K08.59
  sample of cytologic smear
    anus R85.615
    cervix R87.615
    vagina R87.625
  surroundings Z59.19
    work Z56.5
Unsoundness of mind —*see* Psychosis
Unstable
  back NEC —*see* Instability, joint, spine
  hip (congenital) Q65.6
    acquired —*see* Derangement, joint, specified
      type NEC, hip
  joint —*see* Instability, joint
    secondary to removal of joint prosthesis
      M96.89
  lie (mother) O32.0
  lumbosacral joint (congenital) —*see* subcategory
    M53.2
  sacroiliac —*see* subcategory M53.2
  spine NEC —*see* Instability, joint, spine
Unsteadiness on feet R26.81
Untruthfulness, child problem F91.8
Unverricht(-Lundborg) disease or epilepsy —*see*
    Epilepsy, generalized, idiopathic

Unwanted
  multiple moves in the last 12 months Z59.81- ●
  pregnancy Z64.0
Upbringing, institutional Z62.22
  away from parents NEC Z62.29
  in care of non-parental family member
    Z62.21
  in foster care Z62.21
  in orphanage or group home Z62.22
  in welfare custody Z62.21
Upper respiratory —*see* condition
Upset
  gastric K30
  gastrointestinal K30
    psychogenic F45.8
  intestinal (large) (small) K59.9
    psychogenic F45.8
  menstruation N93.9
  mental F48.9
  stomach K30
    psychogenic F45.8
Urachus —*see also* condition
  patent or persistent Q64.4
Urbach-Oppenheim disease (necrobiosis lipoidica
    diabeticorum) —*see* E08-E13 with .620
Urbach's lipoid proteinosis E78.89
Urbach-Wiethe disease E78.89
Urban yellow fever A95.1
Urea
  blood, high —*see* Uremia
  cycle metabolism disorder —*see* Disorder, urea
    cycle metabolism
Uremia, uremic N19
  with
    ectopic or molar pregnancy O08.4
    polyneuropathy N18.9 *[G63]*
  chronic NOS —*see also* Disease, kidney, chronic
    N18.9
    due to hypertension —*see* Hypertensive,
      kidney
  complicating
    ectopic or molar pregnancy O08.4
  congenital P96.0
  extrarenal R39.2
  following ectopic or molar pregnancy O08.4
  newborn P96.0
  prerenal R39.2
Ureter, ureteral —*see* condition
Ureteralgia N23
Ureterectasis —*see* Hydroureter
Ureteritis N28.89
  cystica N28.86
  due to calculus N20.1
    with calculus, kidney N20.2
      with hydronephrosis N13.2
  gonococcal (acute) (chronic) A54.21
  nonspecific N28.89
Ureterocele N28.89
  congenital (orthotopic) Q62.31
    ectopic Q62.32
Ureterolith, ureterolithiasis —*see* Calculus, ureter
Ureterostomy
  attention to Z43.6
  status Z93.6
Urethra, urethral —*see* condition
Urethralgia R39.89
Urethritis (anterior) (posterior) N34.2
  calculous N21.1
  candidal B37.41
  chlamydial A56.01
  diplococcal (gonococcal) A54.01
    with abscess (accessory gland) (periurethral)
      A54.1
  gonococcal A54.01
    with abscess (accessory gland) (periurethral)
      A54.1
  nongonococcal N34.1
    Reiter's —*see* Reiter's disease
  nonspecific N34.1
  nonvenereal N34.1
  postmenopausal N34.2
  puerperal O86.22
  Reiter's —*see* Reiter's disease
  specified NEC N34.2
  trichomonal or due to Trichomonas (vaginalis)
    A59.03
Urethrocele N81.0
  with
    cystocele —*see* Cystocele
    prolapse of uterus —*see* Prolapse, uterus
Urethrolithiasis (with colic or infection) N21.1

Urethrorectal —*see* condition
Urethrorrhagia N36.8
Urethrorrhea R36.9
Urethrostomy
  attention to Z43.6
  status Z93.6
Urethrotrigonitis —*see* Trigonitis
Urethrovaginal —*see* condition
Urgency
  fecal R15.2
  hypertensive —*see* Hypertension
  urinary R39.15
Urhidrosis, uridrosis L74.8
Uric acid in blood (increased) E79.0
Uricacidemia (asymptomatic) E79.0
Uricemia (asymptomatic) E79.0
Uricosuria R82.998
Urinary —*see* condition
Urination
  frequent R35.0
  painful R30.9
Urine
  blood in —*see* Hematuria
  discharge, excessive R35.89
  enuresis, nonorganic origin F98.0
  extravasation R39.0
  frequency R35.0
  incontinence R32
    nonorganic origin F98.0
  intermittent stream R39.198
  pus in N39.0
  retention or stasis R33.9
    organic R33.8
      drug-induced R33.0
    psychogenic F45.8
  secretion
    deficient R34
    excessive R35.89
    frequency R35.0
  stream
    intermittent R39.198
    slowing R39.198
    splitting R39.13
    weak R39.12
Urinemia —*see* Uremia
Urinoma, urethra N36.8
Uroarthritis, infectious (Reiter's) —*see* Reiter's
    disease
Urodialysis R34
Urolithiasis —*see* Calculus, urinary
Uronephrosis —*see* Hydronephrosis
Uropathy N39.9
  obstructive N13.9
    specified NEC N13.8
  reflux N13.9
    specified NEC N13.8
  vesicoureteral reflux-associated —*see* Reflux,
    vesicoureteral
Urosepsis — code to condition
Urticaria L50.9
  with angioneurotic edema T78.3
    hereditary D84.1
  allergic L50.0
  cholinergic L50.5
  chronic L50.8
  cold, familial L50.2
  contact L50.6
  dermatographic L50.3
  due to
    cold or heat L50.2
    drugs L50.0
    food L50.0
    inhalants L50.0
    plants L50.6
    serum —*see also* Reaction, serum T80.69
  factitial L50.3
  familial cold M04.2
  giant T78.3
    hereditary D84.1
  gigantea T78.3
  idiopathic L50.1
  larynx T78.3
    hereditary D84.1
  neonatorum P83.88
  nonallergic L50.1
  papulosa (Hebra) L28.2
  pigmentosa D47.01
    congenital Q82.2
    of neonatal onset Q82.2
    of newborn onset Q82.2
  recurrent periodic L50.8

Urticaria *(Continued)*
  serum —*see also* Reaction, serum T80.69
  solar L56.3
  specified type NEC L50.8
  thermal (cold) (heat) L50.2
  vibratory L50.4
  xanthelasmoidea —*see* Urticaria pigmentosa
Use (of)
▶alcohol *(see also* Alcohol, alcoholic, by disorder)
    F10.90
  with
   ▶anxiety disorder F10.980
    intoxication F10.929
    sleep disorder F10.982
    withdrawal F10.939
     with
      perceptual disturbance
       F10.932
     delirium F10.931
     uncomplicated F10.930
   harmful —*see* Abuse, alcohol
   in remission F10.91
  amphetamines —*see* Use, stimulant NEC
  caffeine —*see* Use, stimulant NEC
  cannabis F12.90
   with
    anxiety disorder F12.980
    intoxication F12.929
     with
      delirium F12.921
      perceptual disturbance F12.922
     uncomplicated F12.920
    other specified disorder F12.988
    psychosis F12.959
     delusions F12.950
     hallucinations F12.951
    unspecified disorder F12.99
    withdrawal F12.93
   in remission F12.91
  cocaine F14.90
   with
    anxiety disorder F14.980
    intoxication F14.929
     with
      delirium F14.921
      perceptual disturbance F14.922
     uncomplicated F14.920
    other specified disorder F14.988
    psychosis F14.959
     delusions F14.950
     hallucinations F14.951
    sexual dysfunction F14.981
    sleep disorder F14.982
    unspecified disorder F14.99
    withdrawal F14.93
   harmful —*see* Abuse, drug, cocaine
   in remission F14.91
  drug(s) NEC F19.90
   with sleep disorder F19.982
   harmful —*see* Abuse, drug, by type
  hallucinogen NEC F16.90
   with
    anxiety disorder F16.980
    intoxication F16.929
     with
      delirium F16.921
     uncomplicated F16.920
    mood disorder F16.94
    other specified disorder F16.988
    perception disorder (flashbacks) F16.983
    psychosis F16.959
     delusions F16.950
     hallucinations F16.951
    unspecified disorder F16.99
   harmful —*see* Abuse, drug, hallucinogen NEC
   in remission F16.91
  inhalants F18.90
   with
    anxiety disorder F18.980
    intoxication F18.929
     with delirium F18.921
     uncomplicated F18.920
    mood disorder F18.94
    other specified disorder F18.988
    persisting dementia F18.97
    psychosis F18.959
     delusions F18.950
     hallucinations F18.951
    unspecified disorder F18.99
   harmful —*see* Abuse, drug, inhalant
   in remission F18.91

Use *(Continued)*
  methadone —*see* Use, opioid
  nonprescribed drugs F19.90
   harmful —*see* Abuse, non-psychoactive
    substance
  opioid F11.90
   with
    disorder F11.99
     mood F11.94
     sleep F11.982
     specified type NEC F11.988
    intoxication F11.929
     with
      delirium F11.921
      perceptual disturbance F11.922
     uncomplicated F11.920
    opioid-associated amnestic syndrome
     F11.988
    withdrawal F11.93
   harmful —*see* Abuse, drug, opioid
   in remission F11.91
  patent medicines F19.90
   harmful —*see* Abuse, non-psychoactive
    substance
  psychoactive drug NEC F19.90
   with
    anxiety disorder F19.980
    intoxication F19.929
     with
      delirium F19.921
      perceptual disturbance F19.922
     uncomplicated F19.920
    mood disorder F19.94
    other specified disorder F19.988
    persisting
     amnestic disorder F19.96
     dementia F19.97
    psychosis F19.959
     delusions F19.950
     hallucinations F19.951
    sexual dysfunction F19.981
    sleep disorder F19.982
    unspecified disorder F19.99
    withdrawal F19.939
     with
      delirium F19.931
      perceptual disturbance F19.932
     uncomplicated F19.930
   harmful —*see* Abuse, drug NEC, psychoactive
    NEC
   in remission F19.91
  sedative, hypnotic, or anxiolytic F13.90
   with
    anxiety disorder F13.980
    intoxication F13.929
     with
      delirium F13.921
     uncomplicated F13.920
    other specified disorder F13.988
    persisting
     amnestic disorder F13.96
     dementia F13.97
    psychosis F13.959
     delusions F13.950
     hallucinations F13.951
    sexual dysfunction F13.981
    sleep disorder F13.982
    unspecified disorder F13.99
   harmful —*see* Abuse, drug, sedative, hypnotic,
    or anxiolytic
   in remission F13.91
  stimulant NEC F15.90
   with
    anxiety disorder F15.980
    intoxication F15.929
     with
      delirium F15.921
      perceptual disturbance F15.922
     uncomplicated F15.920
    mood disorder F15.94
    other specified disorder F15.988
    psychosis F15.959
     delusions F15.950
     hallucinations F15.951
    sexual dysfunction F15.981
    sleep disorder F15.982
    unspecified disorder F15.99
    withdrawal F15.93
   harmful —*see* Abuse, drug, stimulant
    NEC
   in remission F15.91

Use *(Continued)*
  tobacco Z72.0
   with dependence —*see* Dependence,
    drug, nicotine
   volatile solvents —*see also* Use, inhalant F18.90
    harmful —*see* Abuse, drug, inhalant
Usher-Senear disease or syndrome L10.4
Uta B55.1
Uteromegaly N85.2
Uterovaginal —*see* condition
Uterovesical —*see* condition
Uveal —*see* condition
Uveitis (anterior) —*see also* Iridocyclitis
  acute —*see* Iridocyclitis, acute
  chronic —*see* Iridocyclitis, chronic
  due to toxoplasmosis (acquired) B58.09
   congenital P37.1
  granulomatous —*see* Iridocyclitis, chronic
  heterochromic —*see* Cyclitis, Fuchs'
   heterochromic
  lens-induced —*see* Iridocyclitis,
   lens-induced
  posterior —*see* Chorioretinitis
  sympathetic H44.13-●
  syphilitic (secondary) A51.43
   congenital (early) A50.01
   late A52.71
  tuberculous A18.54
Uveoencephalitis —*see* Inflammation, chorioretinal
Uveokeratitis —*see* Iridocyclitis
Uveoparotitis D86.89
Uvula —*see* condition
Uvulitis (acute) (catarrhal) (chronic) (membranous)
  (suppurative) (ulcerative) K12.2

——————— V ———————

Vaccination (prophylactic)
  complication or reaction —*see* Complications,
   vaccination
  delayed Z28.9
  encounter for Z23
  not done —*see* Immunization, not done, because
   (of)
Vaccinia (generalized) (localized) T88.1
  without vaccination B08.011
  congenital P35.8
Vacuum, in sinus (accessory) (nasal) J34.89
Vagabond, vagabondage Z59.00
Vagabond's disease B85.1
Vagina, vaginal —*see* condition
Vaginalitis (tunica) (testis) N49.1
Vaginismus (reflex) N94.2
  functional F52.5
  nonorganic F52.5
  psychogenic F52.5
  secondary N94.2
Vaginitis (acute) (circumscribed) (diffuse)
  (emphysematous) (nonvenereal) (ulcerative)
  N76.0
  with ectopic or molar pregnancy O08.0
  amebic A06.82
  atrophic, postmenopausal N95.2
  bacterial N76.0
  blennorrhagic (gonococcal) A54.02
  candidal (acute) B37.31
  chronic (recurrent) B37.32
  chlamydial A56.02
  chronic N76.1
  due to Trichomonas (vaginalis) A59.01
  following ectopic or molar pregnancy O08.0
  gonococcal A54.02
   with abscess (accessory gland) (periurethral)
    A54.1
  granuloma A58
  in (due to)
   candidiasis (acute) B37.31
   chronic (recurrent) B37.32
   herpesviral (herpes simplex) infection A60.04
   pinworm infection B80 *[N77.1]*
   monilial (acute) B37.31
   chronic (recurrent) B37.32
  mycotic (candidal) (acute) B37.31
   chronic (recurrent) B37.32
  postmenopausal atrophic N95.2
  puerperal (postpartum) O86.13
  senile (atrophic) N95.2
  subacute or chronic N76.1

Vasospasm (vasoconstriction) (*see also* Angiospasm)
 I73.9
  cerebral (cerebrovascular) (artery) I67.848
   reversible I67.841
  coronary I20.1
  nerve
   arm —*see* Mononeuropathy, upper limb
   brachial plexus G54.0
   cervical plexus G54.2
   leg —*see* Mononeuropathy, lower limb
  peripheral NOS I73.9
  retina (artery) —*see* Occlusion, artery, retina
Vasospastic —*see* condition
Vasovagal attack (paroxysmal) R55
  psychogenic F45.8
VATER syndrome Q87.2
Vater's ampulla —*see* condition
Vegetation, vegetative
  adenoid (nasal fossa) J35.8
  endocarditis (acute) (any valve) (subacute) I33.0
  heart (mycotic) (valve) I33.0
Veil
  Jackson's Q43.3
Vein, venous —*see* condition
Veldt sore —*see* Ulcer, skin
Velpeau's hernia —*see* Hernia, femoral
Venereal
  bubo A55
  disease A64
  granuloma inguinale A58
  lymphogranuloma (Durand-Nicolas-Favre) A55
Venofibrosis I87.8
Venom, venomous —*see* Table of Drugs and
  Chemicals, by animal or substance, poisoning
Venous —*see* condition
Ventilator lung, newborn P27.8
Ventral —*see* condition
Ventricle, ventricular —*see also* condition
  escape I49.3
  inversion Q20.5
Ventriculitis (cerebral) —*see also* Encephalitis
  G04.90
Ventriculostomy status Z98.2
Vernet's syndrome G52.7
Verneuil's disease (syphilitic bursitis) A52.78
Verruca (due to HPV) (filiformis) (simplex) (viral)
  (vulgaris) B07.9
  acuminata A63.0
  necrogenica (primary) (tuberculosa) A18.4
  plana B07.8
  plantaris B07.0
  seborrheica L82.1
   inflamed L82.0
  senile (seborrheic) L82.1
   inflamed L82.0
  tuberculosa (primary) A18.4
  venereal A63.0
Verrucosities —*see* Verruca
Verruga peruana, peruviana A44.1
Version
  cervix —*see* Malposition, uterus
  uterus (postinfectional) (postpartal, old) —*see*
   Malposition, uterus
Vertebra, vertebral —*see* condition
Vertical talus (congenital) Q66.80
  left foot Q66.82
  right foot Q66.81
Vertigo R42
  auditory —*see* Vertigo, aural
  aural H81.31-●
  benign paroxysmal (positional) H81.1-●
  central (origin) H81.4
  cerebral H81.4
  Dix and Hallpike (epidemic) —*see* Neuronitis,
   vestibular
  due to infrasound T75.23
  epidemic A88.1
   Dix and Hallpike —*see* Neuronitis, vestibular
   Pedersen's —*see* Neuronitis, vestibular
   vestibular neuronitis —*see* Neuronitis,
    vestibular
  hysterical F44.89
  infrasound T75.23
  labyrinthine —*see* subcategory H81.0
  laryngeal R05.4
  malignant positional H81.4
  Ménière's —*see* subcategory H81.40
  menopausal N95.11
  otogenic —*see* Vertigo, aural
  paroxysmal positional, benign —*see* Vertigo,
   benign paroxysmal

Vertigo (*Continued*)
  Pedersen's (epidemic) —*see* Neuronitis,
   vestibular
  peripheral NEC H81.39-●
  positional
   benign paroxysmal —*see* Vertigo, benign
    paroxysmal
   malignant H81.4
Very-low-density-lipoprotein-type (VLDL)
  hyperlipoproteinemia E78.1
Vesania —*see* Psychosis
Vesical —*see* condition
Vesicle
  cutaneous R23.8
  seminal —*see* condition
  skin R23.8
Vesicocolic —*see* condition
Vesicoperineal —*see* condition
Vesicorectal —*see* condition
Vesicourethrorectal —*see* condition
Vesicovaginal —*see* condition
Vesicular —*see* condition
Vesiculitis (seminal) N49.0
  amebic A06.82
  gonorrheal (acute) (chronic) A54.23
  trichomonal A59.09
  tuberculous A18.15
Vestibulitis (ear) —*see also* subcategory
  H83.0
  nose (external) J34.89
  vulvar N94.810
Vestibulopathy, acute peripheral (recurrent) —*see*
  Neuronitis, vestibular
Vestige, vestigial —*see also* Persistence
  branchial Q18.0
  structures in vitreous Q14.0
Vibration
  adverse effects T75.20
   pneumatic hammer syndrome T75.21
   specified effect NEC T75.29
   vasospastic syndrome T75.22
   vertigo from infrasound T75.23
  exposure (occupational) Z57.7
  vertigo T75.23
Vibriosis A28.9
Victim (of)
  crime Z65.4
  disaster Z65.5
  terrorism Z65.4
  torture Z65.4
  war Z65.5
Vidal's disease L28.0
Villaret's syndrome G52.7
Villous —*see* condition
VIN —*see* Neoplasia, intraepithelial, vulva
Vincent's infection (angina) (gingivitis)
  A69.1
  stomatitis NEC A69.1
Vinson-Plummer disease or syndrome D50.1
Violence, physical R45.6
Viosterol deficiency —*see* Deficiency, calciferol
Vipoma —*see* Neoplasm, malignant, by site
Viremia B34.9
Virilism (adrenal) E25.9
  congenital E25.0
Virilization (female) (suprarenal) E25.9
  congenital E25.0
  isosexual E28.2
Virulent bubo A57
Virus, viral —*see also* condition
  as cause of disease classified elsewhere
   B97.89
   respiratory syncytial virus (RSV) —*see* Virus,
    infection, respiratory syncytial (RSV)
  cytomegalovirus B25.9
  human immunodeficiency (HIV) —*see* Human,
   immunodeficiency virus (HIV) disease
  infection —*see* Infection, virus
  respiratory syncytial (RSV)
   as cause of disease classified elsewhere B97.4
   bronchiolitis J21.0
   bronchitis J20.5
   bronchopneumonia J12.1
   otitis media H65-● [B97.4]
   pneumonia J12.1
   upper respiratory infection J06.9 [B97.4]
  specified NEC B34.8
  swine influenza (viruses that normally cause
   infections in pigs) —*see also* Influenza, due
   to, identified novel influenza A virus
   J09.X2

Virus, viral (*Continued*)
  West Nile (fever) A92.30
   with
    complications NEC A92.39
    cranial nerve disorders A92.32
    encephalitis A92.31
    encephalomyelitis A92.31
    neurologic manifestation NEC A92.32
    optic neuritis A92.32
    polyradiculitis A92.32
Viscera, visceral —*see* condition
Visceroptosis K63.4
Visible peristalsis R19.2
Vision, visual
  binocular, suppression H53.34
  blurred, blurring H53.8
   hysterical F44.6
  defect, defective NEC H54.7
  disorientation (syndrome) H53.8
  disturbance H53.9
   hysterical F44.6
  double H53.2
  examination Z01.00
   with abnormal findings Z01.01
   following failed vision screening Z01.020
    with abnormal findings Z01.021
  field, limitation (defect) —*see* Defect, visual field
  hallucinations R44.1
  halos H53.19
  loss —*see* Loss, vision
   sudden —*see* Disturbance, vision, subjective,
    loss, sudden
  low (both eyes) —*see* Low, vision
  perception, simultaneous without fusion H53.33
Vitality, lack or want of R53.83
  newborn P96.89
Vitamin deficiency —*see* Deficiency, vitamin
Vitelline duct, persistent Q43.0
Vitiligo L80
  eyelid H02.739
   left H02.736
    lower H02.735
    upper H02.734
   right H02.733
    lower H02.732
    upper H02.731
  pinta A67.2
  vulva N90.89
Vitreal corneal syndrome H59.01-●
Vitreoretinopathy, proliferative —*see also*
  Retinopathy, proliferative
  with retinal detachment —*see* Detachment,
   retina, traction
Vitreous —*see also* condition
  touch syndrome —*see* Complication,
   postprocedural, following cataract surgery
Vocal cord —*see* condition
Vogt-Koyanagi syndrome H20.82-●
Vogt's disease or syndrome G80.3
Vogt-Spielmeyer amaurotic idiocy or disease
  E75.4
Voice
  change R49.9
   specified NEC R49.8
  loss —*see* Aphonia
Volhynian fever A79.0
Volkmann's ischemic contracture or paralysis
  (complicating trauma) T79.6
Volvulus (bowel) (colon) (intestine) K56.2
  with perforation K56.2
  congenital Q43.8
  duodenum K31.5
  fallopian tube —*see* Torsion, fallopian tube
  oviduct —*see* Torsion, fallopian tube
  stomach (due to absence of gastrocolic ligament)
   K31.89
Vomiting R11.10
  with nausea R11.2
  without nausea R11.11
  asphyxia —*see* Foreign body, by site, causing
   asphyxia, gastric contents
  bilious (cause unknown) R11.14
   following gastro-intestinal surgery K91.0
   in newborn P92.01
  blood —*see* Hematemesis
  causing asphyxia, choking, or suffocation —*see*
   Foreign body, by site
  cyclical, in migraine G43.A0
   with refractory migraine G43.A1
   intractable G43.A1
   not intractable G43.A0

Vomiting (Continued)
  cyclical, in migraine (Continued)
    psychogenic F50.89
    without refractory migraine G43.A0
  cyclical syndrome NOS (unrelated to migraine) R53.1
    persistent R11.15
  ~~fecal mater R11.13~~
  ▶fecal matter R11.13
  following gastrointestinal surgery K91.0
    psychogenic F50.89
  functional K31.89
  hysterical F50.89
  nervous F50.89
  neurotic F50.89
  newborn NEC P92.09
    bilious P92.01
  periodic R11.10
    psychogenic F50.89
  projectile R11.12
  psychogenic F50.89
  uremic —see Uremia
Vomito negro —see Fever, yellow
Von Bezold's abscess —see Mastoiditis, acute
Von Economo-Cruchet disease A85.8
Von Eulenburg's disease G71.19
Von Gierke's disease E74.01
Von Hippel (-Lindau) disease or syndrome Q85.83
Von Jaksch's anemia or disease D64.89
Von Recklinghausen
  disease (neurofibromatosis) Q85.01
    bones E21.0
Von Schroetter's syndrome I82.890
Von Willebrand (-Jurgens)(-Minot) disease or syndrome —see Disease, von Willebrand
Von Zumbusch's disease L40.1
Voyeurism F65.3
Vrolik's disease Q78.0
Vulva —see condition
Vulvismus N94.2
Vulvitis (acute) (allergic) (atrophic) (hypertrophic) (intertriginous) (senile) N76.2
  with ectopic or molar pregnancy O08.0
  adhesive, congenital Q52.79
  blennorrhagic (gonococcal) A54.02
  candidal (acute) B37.31
    chronic (recurrent) B37.32
  chlamydial A56.02
  due to Haemophilus ducreyi A57
  following ectopic or molar pregnancy O08.0
  gonococcal A54.02
    with abscess (accessory gland) (periurethral) A54.1
  herpesviral A60.04
  leukoplakic N90.4
  monilial (acute) B37.31
    chronic (recurrent) B37.32
  puerperal (postpartum) O86.19
  subacute or chronic N76.3
  syphilitic (early) A51.0
    late A52.76
  trichomonal A59.01
  tuberculous A18.18
Vulvodynia N94.819
  specified NEC N94.818
Vulvorectal —see condition
Vulvovaginitis (acute) —see Vaginitis

W

Waiting list, person on Z75.1
  for organ transplant Z76.82
  undergoing social agency investigation Z75.2
Waldenström
  hypergammaglobulinemia D89.0
  ⟹syndrome or macroglobulinemia C88.0-●
Waldenström-Kjellberg syndrome D50.1
Walking
  difficulty R26.2
    psychogenic F44.4
  sleep F51.3
    hysterical F44.89
Wall, abdominal —see condition
Wallenberg's disease or syndrome G46.3
Wallgren's disease I87.8
Wandering
  gallbladder, congenital Q44.1
  in diseases classified elsewhere Z91.83

Wandering (Continued)
  kidney, congenital Q63.8
  organ or site, congenital NEC —see Malposition, congenital, by site
  pacemaker (heart) I49.8
  spleen D73.89
War neurosis F48.8
Wart (due to HPV) (filiform) (infectious) (viral) B07.9
  anogenital region (venereal) A63.0
  common B07.8
  external genital organs (venereal) A63.0
  flat B07.8
  Hassal-Henle's (of cornea) H18.49
  Peruvian A44.1
  plantar B07.0
  prosector (tuberculous) A18.4
  seborrheic L82.1
    inflamed L82.0
  senile (seborrheic) L82.1
    inflamed L82.0
  tuberculous A18.4
  venereal A63.0
⟹**Warthin's tumor** —see Neoplasm, salivary gland or duct, benign
Wassilieff's disease A27.0
Wasting
  disease (syndrome) E88.A
  due to
    malnutrition E43
      with marasmus E41
    underlying condition E88.A
  extreme (due to malnutrition) E43
    with marasmus E41
  muscle NEC —see Atrophy, muscle
Water
  clefts (senile cataract) —see Cataract, senile, incipient
  deprivation of T73.1
  intoxication E87.79
  itch B76.9
  lack of T73.1
    safe drinking Z58.6
  loading E87.70
  on
    brain —see Hydrocephalus
    chest J94.8
  poisoning E87.79
Waterbrash R12
Waterhouse(-Friderichsen) syndrome or disease (meningococcal) A39.1
Water-losing nephritis N25.89
Watermelon stomach K31.819
  with hemorrhage K31.811
  without hemorrhage K31.819
Watsoniasis B66.8
Wax in ear —see Impaction, cerumen
Weak, weakening, weakness (generalized) R53.1
  arches (acquired) —see also Deformity, limb, flat foot
  bladder (sphincter) R32
  facial R29.810
    following
      cerebrovascular disease I69.992
        cerebral infarction I69.392
        intracerebral hemorrhage I69.192
        nontraumatic intracranial hemorrhage NEC I69.292
        specified disease NEC I69.892
        stroke I69.392
        subarachnoid hemorrhage I69.092
  foot (double) —see also Weak, arches
  heart, cardiac —see Failure, heart
  mind F70
  muscle M62.81
  myocardium —see Failure, heart
  newborn P96.89
  pelvic fundus N81.89
  pubocervical tissue N81.82
  rectovaginal tissue N81.83
  senile R54
  urinary stream R39.12
  valvular —see Endocarditis
Wear, worn (with normal or routine use)
  articular bearing surface of internal joint prosthesis —see Complications, joint prosthesis, mechanical, wear of articular bearing surfaces, by site
  device, implant or graft —see Complications, by site, mechanical complication
  tooth, teeth (approximal) (hard tissues) (interproximal) (occlusal) K03.0

Weather, weathered
  effects of
    cold T69.9
      specified effect NEC T69.8
    hot —see Heat
    skin L57.8
Weaver's syndrome Q87.3
Web, webbed (congenital)
  duodenal Q43.8
  esophagus Q39.4
  fingers Q70.1
  larynx (glottic) (subglottic) Q31.0
  neck (pterygium colli) Q18.3
  Paterson-Kelly D50.1
  popliteal syndrome Q87.89
  toes Q70.3
Weber-Christian disease M35.6
Weber-Cockayne syndrome (epidermolysis bullosa) Q81.8
Weber-Gubler syndrome G46.3
Weber-Leyden syndrome G46.3
Weber-Osler syndrome I78.0
Weber's paralysis or syndrome G46.3
Wedge-shaped or wedging vertebra —see Collapse, vertebra NEC
Wegener's granulomatosis or syndrome M31.30
  with
    kidney involvement M31.31
    lung involvement M31.30
      with kidney involvement M31.31
Wegner's disease A50.02
Weight
  1000-2499 grams at birth (low) —see Low, birthweight
  999 grams or less at birth (extremely low) —see Low, birthweight, extreme
  and length below 10th percentile for gestational age P05.1-●
  below but length above 10th percentile for gestational age P05.0-●
  gain (abnormal) (excessive) R63.5
    in pregnancy —see Pregnancy, complicated by, excessive weight gain
    low —see Pregnancy, complicated by, insufficient, weight gain
  loss (abnormal) (cause unknown) R63.4
Weightlessness (effect of) T75.82
Weil (l)-Marchesani syndrome Q87.19
Weil's disease A27.0
Weingarten's syndrome J82.89
Weir Mitchell's disease I73.81
Weiss-Baker syndrome G90.09
Wells' disease L98.3
Wen —see Cyst, sebaceous
Wenckebach's block or phenomenon I44.1
Werdnig-Hoffmann syndrome (muscular atrophy) G12.0
Werlhof's disease D69.3
Werner-His disease A79.0
Werner's disease or syndrome E31.21
Werner's disease or syndrome E34.8
Wernicke-Korsakoff's syndrome or psychosis (alcoholic) F10.96
  with dependence F10.26
  drug-induced
    due to drug abuse —see Abuse, drug, by type, with amnestic disorder
    due to drug dependence —see Dependence, drug, by type, with amnestic disorder
  nonalcoholic F04
Wernicke-Posadas disease B38.9
Wernicke's
  developmental aphasia F80.2
  disease or syndrome E51.2
  encephalopathy E51.2
  polioencephalitis, superior E51.2
West African fever B50.8
Westphal-Strümpell syndrome E83.01
West's syndrome —see Epilepsy, spasms
Wet
  feet, tropical (maceration) (syndrome) —see Immersion, foot
  lung (syndrome), newborn P22.1
Wharton's duct —see condition
Wheal —see Urticaria
Wheezing R06.2
Whiplash injury S13.4
Whipple's disease —see also subcategory M14.8-● K90.81
Whipworm (disease) (infection) (infestation) B79
Whistling face Q87.0

▶ New   ⇒ Revised   ~~deleted~~ Deleted   ● Use Additional Character(s)

W

Wound, open *(Continued)*
  phalanges
    finger —*see* Wound, open, finger
    toe —*see* Wound, open, toe
  pharynx S11.20
  pinna —*see* Wound, open, ear
  popliteal space —*see* Wound, open, knee
  prepuce —*see* Wound, open, penis
  pubic region —*see* Wound, open, back, lower
  pudendum —*see* Wound, open, genital organs,
    external
  puncture wound —*see* Puncture
  rectovaginal septum —*see* Wound, open, vagina
  right
    lower quadrant S31.103
      with penetration into peritoneal cavity
        S31.603
      bite —*see* Bite, abdomen, wall, right, lower
        quadrant
      laceration —*see* Laceration, abdomen, wall,
        right, lower quadrant
      puncture —*see* Puncture, abdomen, wall,
        right, lower quadrant
    upper quadrant S31.100
      with penetration into peritoneal cavity
        S31.600
      bite —*see* Bite, abdomen, wall, right, upper
        quadrant
      laceration —*see* Laceration, abdomen, wall,
        right, upper quadrant
      puncture —*see* Puncture, abdomen, wall,
        right, upper quadrant
  sacral region —*see* Wound, open, back, lower
  sacroiliac region —*see* Wound, open, back,
    lower
  salivary gland —*see* Wound, open, oral cavity
  scalp S01.00
    bite S01.05
    laceration —*see* Laceration, scalp
    puncture —*see* Puncture, scalp
  scalpel, newborn (birth injury) P15.8
  scapular region —*see* Wound, open, shoulder
  sclera —*see* Wound, open, ocular
  scrotum S31.30
    with amputation —*see* Amputation, traumatic,
      scrotum
    bite S31.35
    laceration —*see* Laceration, scrotum
    puncture —*see* Puncture, scrotum
  shin —*see* Wound, open, leg
  shoulder S41.00-●
    with amputation —*see* Amputation, traumatic,
      arm
    bite —*see* Bite, shoulder
    laceration —*see* Laceration, shoulder
    puncture —*see* Puncture, shoulder
  skin NOS T14.8
  spermatic cord —*see* Wound, open, testis
  sternal region —*see* Wound, open, thorax, front
    wall
  submaxillary region —*see* Wound, open, head,
    specified site NEC
  submental region —*see* Wound, open, head,
    specified site NEC
  subungual
    finger(s) —*see* Wound, open, finger
    toe(s) —*see* Wound, open, toe
  supraclavicular region —*see* Wound, open, neck,
    specified site NEC
  temple, temporal region —*see* Wound, open,
    head, specified site NEC
  temporomandibular area —*see* Wound, open,
    cheek
  testis S31.30
    with amputation —*see* Amputation, traumatic,
      testes
    bite S31.35
    laceration —*see* Laceration, testis
    puncture —*see* Puncture, testis
  thigh S71.10-●
    with amputation —*see* Amputation, traumatic,
      hip
    bite —*see* Bite, thigh
    laceration —*see* Laceration, thigh
    puncture —*see* Puncture, thigh
  thorax, thoracic (wall) S21.90
    back S21.20-●
      with penetration S21.40
    bite —*see* Bite, thorax
    breast —*see* Wound, open, breast

Wound, open *(Continued)*
  thorax, thoracic *(Continued)*
    front S21.10-●
      with penetration S21.30
    laceration —*see* Laceration, thorax
    puncture —*see* Puncture, thorax
  throat —*see* Wound, open, neck
  thumb S61.009
    with
      amputation —*see* Amputation, traumatic,
        thumb
      damage to nail S61.109
    bite —*see* Bite, thumb
    laceration —*see* Laceration, thumb
    left S61.002
      with
        damage to nail S61.102
      puncture —*see* Puncture, thumb
    right S61.001
      with
        damage to nail S61.101
  thyroid (gland) —*see* Wound, open, neck, thyroid
  toe(s) S91.109
    with
      amputation —*see* Amputation, traumatic,
        toe
      damage to nail S91.209
    bite —*see* Bite, toe
    great S91.103
      with
        damage to nail S91.203
      left S91.102
        with
          damage to nail S91.202
      right S91.101
        with
          damage to nail S91.201
      laceration —*see* Laceration, toe
    lesser S91.106
      with
        damage to nail S91.206
      left S91.105
        with
          damage to nail S91.205
      right S91.104
        with
          damage to nail S91.204
    puncture —*see* Puncture, toe
  tongue —*see* Wound, open, oral cavity
  trachea (cervical region) —*see* Wound, open,
    neck, trachea
  tunica vaginalis —*see* Wound, open, testis
  tympanum, tympanic membrane S09.2-●
    laceration —*see* Laceration, ear, drum
    puncture —*see* Puncture, tympanum
  umbilical region —*see* Wound, open, abdomen,
    wall, periumbilic region
  uvula —*see* Wound, open, oral cavity
  vagina S31.40
    bite S31.45
    laceration —*see* Laceration, vagina
    puncture —*see* Puncture, vagina
  vitreous (humor) —*see* Wound, open, ocular
  vocal cord S11.039
    bite —*see* Bite, vocal cord
    laceration S11.031
      with foreign body S11.032
    puncture S11.033
      with foreign body S11.034
  vulva S31.40
    with amputation —*see* Amputation, traumatic,
      vulva
    bite S31.45
    laceration —*see* Laceration, vulva
    puncture —*see* Puncture, vulva
  wrist S61.50-●
    bite —*see* Bite, wrist
    laceration —*see* Laceration, wrist
    puncture —*see* Puncture, wrist
Wound, superficial —*see* Injury *(see also* specified
  injury type)
Wright's syndrome G54.0
Wrist —*see* condition
Wrong drug (by accident) (given in error) —
  see Table of Drugs and Chemicals, by
  drug, poisoning
Wry neck —*see* Torticollis
Wuchereria (bancrofti) **infestation** B74.0
Wuchereriasis B74.0
Wuchernde Struma Langhans C73

X

Xanthelasma (eyelid) (palpebrarum) H02.60
  left H02.66
    lower H02.65
    upper H02.64
  right H02.63
    lower H02.62
    upper H02.61
Xanthelasmatosis (essential) E78.2
Xanthinuria, hereditary E79.82
Xanthoastrocytoma
  specified site —*see* Neoplasm, malignant, by site
  unspecified site C71.9
Xanthofibroma —*see* Neoplasm, connective tissue,
  benign
Xanthogranuloma D76.3
Xanthoma(s), xanthomatosis (primary) (familial)
  (hereditary) E75.5
  with
    hyperlipoproteinemia
      Type I E78.3
      Type III E78.2
      Type IV E78.1
      Type V E78.3
  bone (generalisata) C96.5
  cerebrotendinous E75.5
  cutaneotendinous E75.5
  disseminatum (skin) E78.2
  eruptive E78.2
  hypercholesterinemic E78.00
  hypercholesterolemic E78.00
  hyperlipidemic E78.5
  joint E75.5
  multiple (skin) E78.2
  tendon (sheath) E75.5
  tuberosum E78.2
  tuberous E78.2
  tubo-eruptive E78.2
  verrucous, oral mucosa K13.4
Xanthosis R23.8
Xenophobia F40.10
Xeroderma —*see also* Ichthyosis
  acquired L85.0
  eyelid H01.149
    left H01.146
      lower H01.145
      upper H01.144
    right H01.143
      lower H01.142
      upper H01.141
  pigmentosum Q82.1
  vitamin A deficiency E50.8
Xerophthalmia (vitamin A deficiency) E50.7
  unrelated to vitamin A deficiency —*see*
    Keratoconjunctivitis
Xerosis
  conjunctiva H11.14-●
    with Bitot's spots —*see also* Pigmentation,
      conjunctiva
      vitamin A deficiency E50.1
    vitamin A deficiency E50.0
  cornea H18.89-●
    with ulceration —*see* Ulcer, cornea
      vitamin A deficiency E50.3
    vitamin A deficiency E50.2
  cutis (dry skin) L85.3
  skin L85.3
Xerostomia K11.7
Xiphopagus Q89.4
XO syndrome Q96.9
X-ray (of)
  abnormal findings —*see* Abnormal, diagnostic
    imaging
  breast (mammogram) (routine) Z12.31
  chest
    routine (as part of a general medical
      examination) Z00.00
      with abnormal findings Z00.01
  routine (as part of a general medical
    examination) Z00.00
    with abnormal findings Z00.01
XXXXY syndrome Q98.1
XXY syndrome Q98.0

ICD-10-CM
Table of Neoplasms

ICD-10-CM

Table of Neoplasms

TON

The list below gives the code numbers for neoplasms by anatomical site. For each site there are six possible code numbers according to whether the neoplasm in question is malignant, benign, in situ, of uncertain behavior, or of unspecified nature. The description of the neoplasm will often indicate which of the six columns is appropriate; e.g., malignant melanoma of skin, benign fibroadenoma of breast, carcinoma in situ of cervix uteri.

Where such descriptors are not present, the remainder of the Index should be consulted where guidance is given to the appropriate column for each morphological (histological) variety listed; e.g., Mesonephroma—*see Neoplasm, malignant;* Embryoma—*see also Neoplasm, uncertain behavior;* Disease, Bowen's—*see Neoplasm, skin, in situ.* However, the guidance in the Index can be overridden if one of the descriptors mentioned above is present; e.g., malignant adenoma of colon is coded to C18.9 and not to D12.6 as the adjective "Malignant" overrides the Index entry 'Adenoma—*see also Neoplasm, benign.*'

Codes listed with a dash -, following the code have a required additional character for laterality. The Tablular must be reviewed for the complete code.

	Malignant Primary	Malignant Secondary	Ca in situ	Benign	Uncertain Behavior	Unspecified Behavior
Neoplasm, neoplastic	C80.1	C79.9	D09.9	D36.9	D48.9	D49.9
abdomen, abdominal	C76.2	C79.8-●	D09.8	D36.7	D48.7	D49.89
cavity	C76.2	C79.8-●	D09.8	D36.7	D48.7	D49.89
organ	C76.2	C79.8-●	D09.8	D36.7	D48.7	D49.89
viscera	C76.2	C79.8-●	D09.8	D36.7	D48.7	D49.89
wall—*see also Neoplasm, abdomen, wall, skin*	C44.509	C79.2-●	D04.5	D23.5	D48.5	D49.2
connective tissue	C49.4	C79.8-●	—	D21.4	D48.1	D49.2
skin	C44.509					
basal cell carcinoma	C44.519	—	—	—	—	—
specified type NEC	C44.599	—	—	—	—	—
squamous cell carcinoma	C44.529	—	—	—	—	—
abdominopelvic	C76.8	C79.8-●	—	D36.7	D48.7	D49.89
accessory sinus—*see Neoplasm, sinus*						
acoustic nerve	C72.4-●	C79.49	—	D33.3	D43.3	D49.7
adenoid (pharynx) (tissue)	C11.1	C79.89	D00.08	D10.6	D37.05	D49.0
adipose tissue—*see also Neoplasm, connective tissue*	C49.4	C79.89	—	D21.9	D48.1	D49.2
adnexa (uterine)	C57.4	C79.89	D07.39	D28.7	D39.8	D49.59
adrenal	C74.9-●	C79.7-●	D09.3	D35.0-●	D44.1-●	D49.7
capsule	C74.9-●	C79.7-●	D09.3	D35.0-●	D44.1-●	D49.7
cortex	C74.0-●	C79.7-●	D09.3	D35.0-●	D44.1-●	D49.7
gland	C74.9-●	C79.7-●	D09.3	D35.0-●	D44.1-●	D49.7
medulla	C74.1-●	C79.7-●	D09.3	D35.0-●	D44.1-●	D49.7
ala nasi (external)—*see also Neoplasm, skin, nose*	C44.301	C79.2	D04.39	D23.39	D48.5	D49.2
alimentary canal or tract NEC	C26.9	C78.80	D01.9	D13.99	D37.9	D49.0
alveolar	C03.9	C79.89	D00.03	D10.39	D37.09	D49.0
mucosa	C03.9	C79.89	D00.03	D10.39	D37.09	D49.0
lower	C03.1	C79.89	D00.03	D10.39	D37.09	D49.0
upper	C03.0	C79.89	D00.03	D10.39	D37.09	D49.0
ridge or process	C41.1	C79.51	—	D16.5-●	D48.0	D49.2
carcinoma	C03.9	C79.8-●	—	—	—	—
lower	C03.1	C79.8-●	—	—	—	—
upper	C03.0	C79.8-●	—	—	—	—
lower	C41.1	C79.51	—	D16.5-●	D48.0	D49.2
mucosa	C03.9	C79.89	D00.03	D10.39	D37.09	D49.0
lower	C03.1	C79.89	D00.03	D10.39	D37.09	D49.0
upper	C03.0	C79.89	D00.03	D10.39	D37.09	D49.0
upper	C41.0	C79.51	—	D16.4-●	D48.0	D49.2
sulcus	C06.1	C79.89	D00.02	D10.39	D37.09	D49.0
alveolus	C03.9	C79.89	D00.03	D10.39	D37.09	D49.0
lower	C03.1	C79.89	D00.03	D10.39	D37.09	D49.0
upper	C03.0	C79.89	D00.03	D10.39	D37.09	D49.0
ampulla of Vater	C24.1	C78.89	D01.5	D13.5	D37.6	D49.0
ankle NEC	C76.5-●	C79.89	D04.7-●	D36.7	D48.7	D49.89
anorectum, anorectal (junction)	C21.8	C78.5	D01.3	D12.9	D37.8	D49.0
antecubital fossa or space	C76.4-●	C79.89	D04.6-●	D36.7	D48.7	D49.89
antrum (Highmore) (maxillary)	C31.0	C78.39	D02.3	D14.0	D38.5	D49.1
pyloric	C16.3	C78.89	D00.2	D13.1	D37.1	D49.0
tympanicum	C30.1	C78.39	D02.3	D14.0	D38.5	D49.1
anus, anal	C21.0	C78.5	D01.3	D12.9	D37.8	D49.0
canal	C21.1	C78.5	D01.3	D12.9	D37.8	D49.0
cloacogenic zone	C21.2	C78.5	D01.3	D12.9	D37.8	D49.0
margin—*see also Neoplasm, anus, skin*	C44.500	C79.2	D04.5	D23.5	D48.5	D49.2
overlapping lesion with rectosigmoid junction or rectum	C21.8	—	—	—	—	—
skin	C44.500	C79.2	D04.5	D23.5	D48.5	D49.2
basal cell carcinoma	C44.510	—	—	—	—	—
specified type NEC	C44.590	—	—	—	—	—
squamous cell carcinoma	C44.520	—	—	—	—	—
sphincter	C21.1	C78.5	D01.3	D12.9	D37.8	D49.0
aorta (thoracic)	C49.3	C79.89	—	D21.3	D48.1	D49.2
abdominal	C49.4	C79.89	—	D21.4	D48.1	D49.2
aortic body	C75.5	C79.89	—	D35.6	D44.7	D49.7
aponeurosis	C49.9	C79.89	—	D21.9	D48.1	D49.2
palmar	C49.1-●	C79.89	—	D21.1-●	D48.1	D49.2
plantar	C49.2-●	C79.89	—	D21.2-●	D48.1	D49.2

TABLE OF NEOPLASMS

	Malignant Primary	Malignant Secondary	Ca in situ	Benign	Uncertain Behavior	Unspecified Behavior
appendix	C18.1	C78.5	D01.0	D12.1	D37.3	D49.0
arachnoid	C70.9	C79.49	—	D32.9	D42.9	D49.7
cerebral	C70.0	C79.32	—	D32.0	D42.0	D49.7
spinal	C70.1	C79.49	—	D32.1	D42.1	D49.7
areola	C50.0-•	C79.81	D05.-•	D24.-•	D48.6-•	D49.3
arm NEC	C76.4-•	C79.89	D04.6-•	D36.7	D48.7	D49.89
artery — see Neoplasm, connective tissue						
aryepiglottic fold	C13.1	C79.89	D00.08	D10.7	D37.05	D49.0
hypopharyngeal aspect	C13.1	C79.89	D00.08	D10.7	D37.05	D49.0
laryngeal aspect	C32.1	C78.39	D02.0	D14.1	D38.0	D49.1
marginal zone	C13.1	C79.89	D00.08	D10.7	D37.05	D49.0
arytenoid (cartilage)	C32.3	C78.39	D02.0	D14.1	D38.0	D49.1
fold — see Neoplasm, aryepiglottic						
associated with transplanted organ	C80.2	—	—	—	—	—
atlas	C41.2	C79.51	—	D16.6	D48.0	D49.2
atrium, cardiac	C38.0	C79.89	—	D15.1	D48.7	D49.89
auditory						
canal (external) (skin)	C44.20-•	C79.2	D04.2-•	D23.2-•	D48.5	D49.2
internal	C30.1	C78.39	D02.3	D14.0	D38.5	D49.1
nerve	C72.4-•	C79.49	—	D33.3	D43.3	D49.7
tube	C30.1	C78.39	D02.3	D14.0	D38.5	D49.1
opening	C11.2	C79.89	D00.08	D10.6	D37.05	D49.0
auricle, ear — see also Neoplasm, skin, ear	C44.20-•	C79.2	D04.2-•	D23.2-•	D48.5	D49.2
auricular canal (external) — see also Neoplasm, skin, ear	C44.20-•	C79.2	D04.2-•	D23.2-•	D48.5	D49.2
internal	C30.1	C78.39	D02.3	D14.0	D38.5	D49.2
autonomic nerve or nervous system NEC (see Neoplasm, nerve, peripheral)						
axilla, axillary	C76.1	C79.89	D09.8	D36.7	D48.7	D49.89
fold — see also Neoplasm, skin, trunk	C44.509	C79.2	D04.5	D23.5	D48.5	D49.2
back NEC	C76.8	C79.89	D04.5	D36.7	D48.7	D49.89
Bartholin's gland	C51.0	C79.82	D07.1	D28.0	D39.8	D49.59
basal ganglia	C71.0	C79.31	—	D33.0	D43.0	D49.6
basis pedunculi	C71.7	C79.31	—	D33.1	D43.1	D49.6
bile or biliary (tract)	C24.9	C78.89	D01.5	D13.5	D37.6	D49.0
canaliculi (biliferi) (intrahepatic)	C22.1	C78.7	D01.5	D13.4	D37.6	D49.0
canals, interlobular	C22.1	C78.89	D01.5	D13.4	D37.6	D49.0

	Malignant Primary	Malignant Secondary	Ca in situ	Benign	Uncertain Behavior	Unspecified Behavior
bile or biliary (Continued)						
duct or passage (common) (cystic) (extrahepatic)	C24.0	C78.89	D01.5	D13.5	D37.6	D49.0
interlobular	C22.1	C78.89	D01.5	D13.4	D37.6	D49.0
intrahepatic	C22.1	C78.7	D01.5	D13.4	D37.6	D49.0
and extrahepatic	C24.8	C78.89	D01.5	D13.5	D37.6	D49.0
bladder (urinary)	C67.9	C79.11	D09.0	D30.3	D41.4	D49.4
dome	C67.1	C79.11	D09.0	D30.3	D41.4	D49.4
neck	C67.5	C79.11	D09.0	D30.3	D41.4	D49.4
orifice	C67.9	C79.11	D09.0	D30.3	D41.4	D49.4
ureteric	C67.6	C79.11	D09.0	D30.3	D41.4	D49.4
urethral	C67.5	C79.11	D09.0	D30.3	D41.4	D49.4
overlapping lesion	C67.8	—	—	—	—	—
sphincter	C67.8	C79.11	D09.0	D30.3	D41.4	D49.4
trigone	C67.0	C79.11	D09.0	D30.3	D41.4	D49.4
urachus	C67.7	C79.11	D09.0	D30.3	D41.4	D49.4
wall	C67.9	C79.11	D09.0	D30.3	D41.4	D49.4
anterior	C67.3	C79.11	D09.0	D30.3	D41.4	D49.4
lateral	C67.2	C79.11	D09.0	D30.3	D41.4	D49.4
posterior	C67.4	C79.11	D09.0	D30.3	D41.4	D49.4
blood vessel — see Neoplasm, connective tissue						
bone (periosteum)	C41.9	C79.51	—	D16.9-•	D48.0	D49.2
acetabulum	C41.4	C79.51	—	D16.8-•	D48.0	D49.2
ankle	C40.3-•	C79.51	—	D16.3-•	—	—
arm NEC	C40.0-•	C79.51	—	D16.0-•	—	—
astragalus	C40.3-•	C79.51	—	D16.3-•	—	—
atlas	C41.2	C79.51	—	D16.6-•	D48.0	D49.2
axis	C41.2	C79.51	—	D16.6-•	D48.0	D49.2
back NEC	C41.2	C79.51	—	D16.6-•	D48.0	D49.2
calcaneus	C40.3-•	C79.51	—	D16.3-•	—	—
calvarium	C41.0	C79.51	—	D16.4-•	D48.0	D49.2
carpus (any)	C40.1-•	C79.51	—	D16.1-•	—	—
cartilage NEC	C41.9	C79.51	—	D16.9-•	D48.0	D49.2
clavicle	C41.3	C79.51	—	D16.7-•	D48.0	D49.2
clivus	C41.0	C79.51	—	D16.4-•	D48.0	D49.2
coccygeal vertebra	C41.4	C79.51	—	D16.8-•	D48.0	D49.2
coccyx	C41.4	C79.51	—	D16.8-•	D48.0	D49.2
costal cartilage	C41.3	C79.51	—	D16.7-•	D48.0	D49.2
costovertebral joint	C41.3	C79.51	—	D16.7-•	D48.0	D49.2
cranial	C41.0	C79.51	—	D16.4-•	D48.0	D49.2
cuboid	C40.3-•	C79.51	—	D16.3-•	—	—
cuneiform	C41.9	C79.51	—	D16.9-•	D48.0	D49.2
elbow	C40.0-•	C79.51	—	D16.0-•	—	—

◀ New ◀ Revised ~~deleted~~ Deleted • Use Additional Character(s)

	Malignant Primary	Malignant Secondary	Ca in situ	Benign	Uncertain Behavior	Unspecified Behavior
bone *(Continued)*						
ethmoid (labyrinth)	C41.0	C79.51	—	D16.4-●	D48.0	D49.2
face	C41.0	C79.51	—	D16.4-●	D48.0	D49.2
femur (any part)	C40.2-●	C79.51	—	D16.2-●	—	—
fibula (any part)	C40.2-●	C79.51	—	D16.2-●	—	—
finger (any)	C40.1-●	C79.51	—	D16.1-●	—	—
foot	C40.3-●	C79.51	—	D16.3-●	—	—
forearm	C40.0-●	C79.51	—	D16.0-●	—	—
frontal	C41.0	C79.51	—	D16.4-●	D48.0	D49.2
hand	C40.1-●	C79.51	—	D16.1-●	—	—
heel	C40.3-●	C79.51	—	D16.3-●	—	—
hip	C41.4	C79.51	—	D16.8-●	D48.0	D49.2
humerus (any part)	C40.0-●	C79.51	—	D16.0-●	—	—
hyoid	C41.0	C79.51	—	D16.4-●	D48.0	D49.2
ilium	C41.4	C79.51	—	D16.8-●	D48.0	D49.2
innominate	C41.4	C79.51	—	D16.8-●	D48.0	D49.2
intervertebral cartilage or disc	C41.2	C79.51	—	D16.6-●	D48.0	D49.2
ischium	C41.4	C79.51	—	D16.8-●	D48.0	D49.2
jaw (lower)	C41.1	C79.51	—	D16.5-●	D48.0	D49.2
knee	C40.2-●	C79.51	—	D16.2-●	—	—
leg NEC	C40.2-●	C79.51	—	D16.2-●	—	—
limb NEC	C40.9-●	C79.51	—	D16.9-●	—	—
lower (long bones)	C40.2-●	C79.51	—	D16.2-●	—	—
short bones	C40.3-●	C79.51	—	D16.3-●	—	—
upper (long bones)	C40.0-●	C79.51	—	D16.0-●	—	—
short bones	C40.1-●	C79.51	—	D16.1-●	—	—
malar	C41.0	C79.51	—	D16.4-●	D48.0	D49.2
mandible	C41.1	C79.51	—	D16.5-●	D48.0	D49.2
marrow NEC (any bone)	C96.9	C79.52	—	—	D47.9	D49.89
mastoid	C41.0	C79.51	—	D16.4-●	D48.0	D49.2
maxilla, maxillary (superior)	C41.0	C79.51	—	D16.4-●	D48.0	D49.2
inferior	C41.1	C79.51	—	D16.5-●	D48.0	D49.2
metacarpus (any)	C40.1-●	C79.51	—	D16.1-●	—	—
metatarsus (any)	C40.3-●	C79.51	—	D16.3-●	—	—
overlapping sites	C40.8-●	—	—	—	—	—
navicular						
ankle	C40.3-●	C79.51	—	—	—	—
hand	C40.1-●	C79.51	—	—	—	—
nose, nasal	C41.0	C79.51	—	D16.4-●	D48.0	D49.2
occipital	C41.0	C79.51	—	D16.4-●	D48.0	D49.2
orbit	C41.0	C79.51	—	D16.4-●	D48.0	D49.2
parietal	C41.0	C79.51	—	D16.4-●	D48.0	D49.2
patella	C40.2-●	C79.51	—	—	—	—
pelvic	C41.4	C79.51	—	D16.8	D48.0	D49.2

	Malignant Primary	Malignant Secondary	Ca in situ	Benign	Uncertain Behavior	Unspecified Behavior
bone *(Continued)*						
phalanges						
foot	C40.3-●	C79.51	—	—	—	—
hand	C40.1-●	C79.51	—	—	—	—
pubic	C41.4	C79.51	—	D16.8	D48.0	D49.2
radius (any part)	C40.0-●	C79.51	—	D16.0-●	—	—
rib	C41.3	C79.51	—	D16.7	D48.0	D49.2
sacral vertebra	C41.4	C79.51	—	D16.8	D48.0	D49.2
sacrum	C41.4	C79.51	—	D16.8	D48.0	D49.2
scaphoid	—	—	—	—	—	—
of ankle	C40.3-●	C79.51	—	—	—	—
of hand	C40.1-●	C79.51	—	—	—	—
scapula (any part)	C40.0-●	C79.51	—	D16.0-●	—	—
sella turcica	C41.0	C79.51	—	D16.4-●	D48.0	D49.2
shoulder	C40.0-●	C79.51	—	D16.0-●	—	—
skull	C41.0	C79.51	—	D16.4-●	D48.0	D49.2
sphenoid	C41.0	C79.51	—	D16.4-●	D48.0	D49.2
spine, spinal (column)	C41.2	C79.51	—	D16.6	D48.0	D49.2
coccyx	C41.4	C79.51	—	D16.8	D48.0	D49.2
sacrum	C41.4	C79.51	—	D16.8	D48.0	D49.2
sternum	C41.3	C79.51	—	D16.7	D48.0	D49.2
tarsus (any)	C40.3-●	C79.51	—	—	—	—
temporal	C41.0	C79.51	—	D16.4-●	D48.0	D49.2
thumb	C40.1-●	C79.51	—	—	—	—
tibia (any part)	C40.2-●	C79.51	—	—	—	—
toe (any)	C40.3-●	C79.51	—	—	—	—
trapezium	C40.1-●	C79.51	—	—	—	—
trapezoid	C40.1-●	C79.51	—	—	—	—
turbinate	C41.0	C79.51	—	D16.4-●	D48.0	D49.2
ulna (any part)	C40.0-●	C79.51	—	D16.0-●	—	—
unciform	C40.1-●	C79.51	—	—	—	—
vertebra (column)	C41.2	C79.51	—	D16.6	D48.0	D49.2
coccyx	C41.4	C79.51	—	D16.8	D48.0	D49.2
sacrum	C41.4	C79.51	—	D16.8	D48.0	D49.2
vomer	C41.0	C79.51	—	D16.4-●	D48.0	D49.2
wrist	C40.1-●	C79.51	—	—	—	—
xiphoid process	C41.3	C79.51	—	D16.7	D48.0	D49.2
zygomatic	C41.0	C79.51	—	D16.4-●	D48.0	D49.2
book-leaf (mouth)	C06.89	C79.89	D00.00	D10.39	D37.09	D49.0
bowel — *see Neoplasm, intestine*						
brachial plexus	C47.1-●	C79.89	—	D36.12	D48.2	D49.2
brain NEC	C71.9	C79.31	—	D33.2	D43.2	D49.6
basal ganglia	C71.0	C79.31	—	D33.0	D43.0	D49.6
cerebellopontine angle	C71.6	C79.31	—	D33.1	D43.1	D49.6

	Malignant Primary	Malignant Secondary	Ca in situ	Benign	Uncertain Behavior	Unspecified Behavior
brain NEC *(Continued)*						
cerebellum NOS	C71.6	C79.31	—	D33.1	D43.1	D49.6
cerebrum	C71.0	C79.31	—	D33.0	D43.0	D49.6
choroid plexus	C71.7	C79.31	—	D33.1	D43.1	D49.6
corpus callosum	C71.8	C79.31	—	D33.2	D43.2	D49.6
corpus striatum	C71.0	C79.31	—	D33.0	D43.0	D49.6
cortex (cerebral)	C71.0	C79.31	—	D33.0	D43.0	D49.6
frontal lobe	C71.1	C79.31	—	D33.0	D43.0	D49.6
globus pallidus	C71.0	C79.31	—	D33.0	D43.0	D49.6
hippocampus	C71.2	C79.31	—	D33.0	D43.0	D49.6
hypothalamus	C71.0	C79.31	—	D33.0	D43.0	D49.6
internal capsule	C71.0	C79.31	—	D33.0	D43.0	D49.6
medulla oblongata	C71.7	C79.31	—	D33.1	D43.1	D49.6
meninges	C70.0	C79.32	—	D32.0	D42.0	D49.7
midbrain	C71.7	C79.31	—	D33.1	D43.1	D49.6
occipital lobe	C71.4	C79.31	—	D33.0	D43.0	D49.6
overlapping lesion	C71.8	C79.31	—	—	—	—
parietal lobe	C71.3	C79.31	—	D33.0	D43.0	D49.6
peduncle	C71.7	C79.31	—	D33.1	D43.1	D49.6
pons	C71.7	C79.31	—	D33.1	D43.1	D49.6
stem	C71.7	C79.31	—	D33.1	D43.1	D49.6
tapetum	C71.8	C79.31	—	D33.2	D43.2	D49.6
temporal lobe	C71.2	C79.31	—	D33.0	D43.0	D49.6
thalamus	C71.0	C79.31	—	D33.0	D43.0	D49.6
uncus	C71.2	C79.31	—	D33.0	D43.0	D49.6
ventricle (floor)	C71.5	C79.31	—	D33.0	D43.0	D49.6
fourth	C71.7	C79.31	—	D33.1	D43.1	D49.6
branchial (cleft) (cyst) (vestiges)	C10.4	C79.89	D00.08	D10.5	D37.05	D49.0
breast (connective tissue) (glandular tissue) (soft parts)	C50.9-●	C79.81	D05.-●	D24.-●	D48.6-●	D49.3
areola	C50.0-●	C79.81	D05.-●	D24.-●	D48.6-●	D49.3
axillary tail	C50.6-●	C79.81	D05.-●	D24.-●	D48.6-●	D49.3
central portion	C50.1-●	C79.81	D05.-●	D24.-●	D48.6-●	D49.3
inner	C50.8-●	C79.81	D05.-●	D24.-●	D48.6-●	D49.3
lower	C50.8-●	C79.81	D05.-●	D24.-●	D48.6-●	D49.3
lower-inner quadrant	C50.3-●	C79.81	D05.-●	D24.-●	D48.6-●	D49.3
lower-outer quadrant	C50.5-●	C79.81	D05.-●	D24.-●	D48.6-●	D49.3
mastectomy site (skin) — *see also Neoplasm, breast, skin*	C44.501	C79.2	—	—	—	—
specified as breast tissue	C50.8-●	C79.81	—	—	—	—
midline	C50.8-●	C79.81	D05.-●	D24.-●	D48.6-●	D49.3
nipple	C50.0-●	C79.81	D05.-●	D24.-●	D48.6-●	D49.3
outer	C50.8-●	C79.81	D05.-●	D24.-●	D48.6-●	D49.3
overlapping lesion	C50.8-●	—	—	—	—	—

	Malignant Primary	Malignant Secondary	Ca in situ	Benign	Uncertain Behavior	Unspecified Behavior
breast *(Continued)*						
skin	C44.501	C79.2	D04.5	D23.5	D48.5	D49.2
basal cell carcinoma	C44.511	—	—	—	—	—
specified type NEC	C44.591	—	—	—	—	—
squamous cell carcinoma	C44.521	—	—	—	—	—
tail (axillary)	C50.6-●	C79.81	D05.-●	D24.-●	D48.6-●	D49.3
upper	C50.8-●	C79.81	D05.-●	D24.-●	D48.6-●	D49.3
upper-inner quadrant	C50.2-●	C79.81	D05.-●	D24.-●	D48.6-●	D49.3
upper-outer quadrant	C50.4-●	C79.81	D05.-●	D24.-●	D48.6-●	D49.3
broad ligament	C57.1	C79.82	D07.39	D28.2	D39.8	D49.59
bronchiogenic, bronchogenic (lung)	C34.9-●	C78.0-●	D02.2-●	D14.3-●	D38.1	D49.1
bronchiole	C34.9-●	C78.0-●	D02.2-●	D14.3-●	D38.1	D49.1
bronchus	C34.9-●	C78.0-●	D02.2-●	D14.3-●	D38.1	D49.1
carina	C34.0-●	C78.0-●	D02.2-●	D14.3-●	D38.1	D49.1
lower lobe of lung	C34.3-●	C78.0-●	D02.2-●	D14.3-●	D38.1	D49.1
main	C34.0-●	C78.0-●	D02.2-●	D14.3-●	D38.1	D49.1
middle lobe of lung	C34.2	C78.0-●	D02.21	D14.31	D38.1	D49.1
overlapping lesion	C34.8-●	—	—	—	—	—
upper lobe of lung	C34.1-●	C78.0-●	D02.2-●	D14.3-●	D38.1	D49.1
brow	C44.309	C79.2	D04.39	D23.39	D48.5	D49.2
basal cell carcinoma	C44.319	—	—	—	—	—
specified type NEC	C44.399	—	—	—	—	—
squamous cell carcinoma	C44.329	—	—	—	—	—
buccal (cavity)	C06.9	C79.89	D00.00	D10.39	D37.09	D49.0
commissure	C06.0	C79.89	D00.02	D10.39	D37.09	D49.0
groove (lower) (upper)	C06.1	C79.89	D00.02	D10.39	D37.09	D49.0
mucosa	C06.0	C79.89	D00.02	D10.39	D37.09	D49.0
sulcus (lower) (upper)	C06.1	C79.89	D00.02	D10.39	D37.09	D49.0
bulbourethral gland	C68.0	C79.19	D09.19	D30.4	D41.3	D49.59
bursa — *see Neoplasm, connective tissue*						
buttock NEC	C76.3	C79.89	D04.5	D36.7	D48.7	D49.89
calf	C76.5-●	C79.89	D04.7-●	D36.7	D48.7	D49.89
calvarium	C41.0	C79.51	—	D16.4-●	D48.0	D49.2
calyx, renal	C65.-●	C79.0-●	D09.19	D30.1-●	D41.1-●	D49.51-●
canal						
anal	C21.1	C78.5	D01.3	D12.9	D37.8	D49.0
auditory (external) — *see also Neoplasm, skin, ear*	C44.20-●	C79.2	D04.2-●	D23.2-●	D48.5	D49.2
auricular (external) — *see also Neoplasm, skin, ear*	C44.20-●	C79.2	D04.2-●	D23.2-●	D48.5	D49.2
canaliculi, biliary (biliferi) (intrahepatic)	C22.1	C78.7	D01.5	D13.4	D37.6	D49.0

◀ New ◀ Revised ~~deleted~~ Deleted ● Use Additional Character(s)

	Malignant Primary	Malignant Secondary	Ca in situ	Benign	Uncertain Behavior	Unspecified Behavior
canthus (eye) (inner) (outer)	C44.10-●	C79.2	D04.1-●	D23.1-●	D48.5	D49.2
basal cell carcinoma	C44.11-●	—	—	—	—	—
sebaceous cell	C44.13-●	—	—	—	—	—
specified type NEC	C44.19-●	—	—	—	—	—
squamous cell carcinoma	C44.12-●	—	—	—	—	—
capillary — see Neoplasm, connective tissue						
caput coli	C18.0	C78.5	D01.0	D12.0	D37.4	D49.0
carcinoid — see Tumor, carcinoid						
cardia (gastric)	C16.0	C78.89	D00.2	D13.1	D37.1	D49.0
cardiac orifice (stomach)	C16.0	C78.89	D00.2	D13.1	D37.1	D49.0
cardio-esophageal junction	C16.0	C78.89	D00.2	D13.1	D37.1	D49.0
cardio-esophagus	C16.0	C78.89	D00.2	D13.1	D37.1	D49.0
carina (bronchus)	C34.0-●	C78.0-●	D02.2-●	D14.3-●	D38.1	D49.1
carotid (artery)	C49.0	C79.89	—	D21.0	D48.1	D49.2
body	C75.4	C79.89	—	D35.5	D44.6	D49.7
carpus (any bone)	C40.1-●	C79.51	—	D16.1-●	—	—
cartilage (articular) (joint) NEC — see also Neoplasm, bone	C41.9	C79.51	—	D16.9-●	D48.0	D49.2
arytenoid	C32.3	C78.39	D02.0	D14.1	D38.0	D49.1
auricular	C49.0	C79.89	—	D21.0	D48.1	D49.2
bronchi	C34.0-●	C78.39	—	D14.3-●	D38.1	D49.1
costal	C41.3	C79.51	—	D16.7	D48.0	D49.2
cricoid	C32.3	C78.39	D02.0	D14.1	D38.0	D49.1
cuneiform	C32.3	C78.39	D02.0	D14.1	D38.0	D49.1
ear (external)	C49.0	C79.89	—	D21.0	D48.1	D49.2
ensiform	C41.3	C79.51	—	D16.7	D48.0	D49.2
epiglottis	C32.1	C78.39	D02.0	D14.1	D38.0	D49.1
anterior surface	C10.1	C79.89	D00.08	D10.5	D37.05	D49.0
eyelid	C49.0	C79.89	—	D21.0	D48.1	D49.2
intervertebral	C41.2	C79.51	—	D16.6	D48.0	D49.2
larynx, laryngeal	C32.3	C78.39	D02.0	D14.1	D38.0	D49.1
nose, nasal	C30.0	C78.39	D02.3	D14.0	D38.5	D49.1
pinna	C49.0	C79.89	—	D21.0	D48.1	D49.2
rib	C41.3	C79.51	—	D16.7	D48.0	D49.2
semilunar (knee)	C40.2-●	C79.51	—	D16.2-●	D48.0	D49.2
thyroid	C32.3	C78.39	D02.0	D14.1	D38.0	D49.1
trachea	C33	C78.39	D02.1	D14.2	D38.1	D49.1
cauda equina	C72.1	C79.49	—	D33.4	D43.4	D49.7
cavity						
buccal	C06.9	C79.89	D00.00	D10.30	D37.09	D49.0
nasal	C30.0	C78.39	D02.3	D14.0	D38.5	D49.1
oral	C06.9	C79.89	D00.00	D10.30	D37.09	D49.0

	Malignant Primary	Malignant Secondary	Ca in situ	Benign	Uncertain Behavior	Unspecified Behavior
cavity (Continued)						
peritoneal	C48.2	C78.6	—	D20.1	D48.4	D49.0
tympanic	C30.1	C78.39	D02.3	D14.0	D38.5	D49.1
cecum	C18.0	C78.5	D01.0	D12.0	D37.4	D49.0
central nervous system	C72.9	C79.40	—	—	—	—
cerebellopontine (angle)	C71.6	C79.31	—	D33.1	D43.1	D49.6
cerebellum, cerebellar	C71.6	C79.31	—	D33.1	D43.1	D49.6
cerebrum, cerebra (cortex) (hemisphere) (white matter)	C71.0	C79.31	—	D33.0	D43.0	D49.6
meninges	C70.0	C79.32	—	D32.0	D42.0	D49.7
peduncle	C71.7	C79.31	—	D33.1	D43.1	D49.6
ventricle	C71.5	C79.31	—	D33.0	D43.0	D49.6
fourth	C71.7	C79.31	—	D33.1	D43.1	D49.6
cervical region	C76.0	C79.89	D09.8	D36.7	D48.7	D49.89
cervix (cervical) (uteri) (uterus)	C53.9	C79.82	D06.9	D26.0	D39.0	D49.59
canal	C53.0	C79.82	D06.0	D26.0	D39.0	D49.59
endocervix (canal) (gland)	C53.0	C79.82	D06.0	D26.0	D39.0	D49.59
exocervix	C53.1	C79.82	D06.1	D26.0	D39.0	D49.59
external os	C53.1	C79.82	D06.1	D26.0	D39.0	D49.59
internal os	C53.0	C79.82	D06.0	D26.0	D39.0	D49.59
nabothian gland	C53.0	C79.82	D06.0	D26.0	D39.0	D49.59
overlapping lesion	C53.8	—	—	—	—	—
squamocolumnar junction	C53.8	C79.82	D06.7	D26.0	D39.0	D49.59
stump	C53.8	C79.82	D06.7	D26.0	D39.0	D49.59
cheek	C76.0	C79.89	D09.8	D36.7	D48.7	D49.89
external	C44.309	C79.2	D04.39	D23.39	D48.5	D49.2
basal cell carcinoma	C44.319	—	—	—	—	—
specified type NEC	C44.399	—	—	—	—	—
squamous cell carcinoma	C44.329	—	—	—	—	—
inner aspect	C06.0	C79.89	D00.02	D10.39	D37.09	D49.0
internal	C06.0	C79.89	D00.02	D10.39	D37.09	D49.0
mucosa	C06.0	C79.89	D00.02	D10.39	D37.09	D49.0
chest (wall) NEC	C76.1	C79.89	D09.8	D36.7	D48.7	D49.89
chiasma opticum	C72.3-●	C79.49	—	D33.3	D43.3	D49.7
chin	C44.309	C79.2	D04.39	D23.39	D48.5	D49.2
basal cell carcinoma	C44.319	—	—	—	—	—
specified type NEC	C44.399	—	—	—	—	—
squamous cell carcinoma	C44.329	—	—	—	—	—
choana	C11.3	C79.89	D00.08	D10.6	D37.05	D49.0
cholangiole	C22.1	C78.89	D01.5	D13.4	D37.6	D49.0
choledochal duct	C24.0	C78.89	D01.5	D13.5	D37.6	D49.0
choroid	C69.3-●	C79.49	D09.2-●	D31.3-●	D48.7	D49.81
plexus	C71.5	C79.31	—	D33.0	D43.0	D49.6
ciliary body	C69.4-●	C79.49	D09.2-●	D31.4-●	D48.7	D49.89

TABLE OF NEOPLASMS

	Malignant Primary	Malignant Secondary	Ca in situ	Benign	Uncertain Behavior	Unspecified Behavior
clavicle	C41.3	C79.51	—	D16.7	D48.0	D49.2
clitoris	C51.2	C79.82	D07.1	D28.0	D39.8	D49.59
clivus	C41.0	C79.51	—	D16.4-•	D48.0	D49.2
cloacogenic zone	C21.2	C78.5	D01.3	D12.9	D37.8	D49.0
coccygeal						
body or glomus	C49.5	C79.89	—	D21.5	D48.1	D49.2
vertebra	C41.4	C79.51	—	D16.8	D48.0	D49.2
coccyx	C41.4	C79.51	—	D16.8	D48.0	D49.2
colon — see also Neoplasm, intestine, large	C18.9	C78.5	—	—	—	—
with rectum	C19	C78.5	D01.1	D12.7	D37.5	D49.0
column, spinal — see Neoplasm, spine						
columnella — see also Neoplasm, skin, face	C44.390	C79.2	D04.39	D23.39	D48.5	D49.2
commissure						
labial, lip	C00.6	C79.89	D00.01	D10.39	D37.01	D49.0
laryngeal	C32.0	C78.39	D02.0	D14.1	D38.0	D49.1
common (bile) duct	C24.0	C78.89	D01.5	D13.5	D37.6	D49.0
concha — see also Neoplasm, skin, ear	C44.20-•	C79.2	D04.2-•	D23.2-•	D48.5	D49.2
nose	C30.0	C78.39	D02.3	D14.0	D38.5	D49.1
conjunctiva	C69.0-•	C79.49	D09.2-•	D31.0-•	D48.7	D49.89
connective tissue NEC	C49.9	C79.89	—	D21.9	D48.1	D49.2

Note: For neoplasms of connective tissue (blood vessel, bursa, fascia, ligament, muscle, peripheral nerves, sympathetic and parasympathetic nerves and ganglia, synovia, tendon, etc.) or of morphological types that indicate connective tissue, code according to the list under "Neoplasm, connective tissue." For sites that do not appear in this list, code to neoplasm of that site; e.g., fibrosarcoma, pancreas (C25.9).

Note: Morphological types that indicate connective tissue appear in their proper place in the alphabetic index with the instruction "*see Neoplasm, connective tissue ....*"

	Malignant Primary	Malignant Secondary	Ca in situ	Benign	Uncertain Behavior	Unspecified Behavior
abdomen	C49.4	C79.89	—	D21.4	D48.1	D49.2
abdominal wall	C49.4	C79.89	—	D21.4	D48.1	D49.2
ankle	C49.2-•	C79.89	—	D21.2-•	D48.1	D49.2
antecubital fossa or space	C49.1-•	C79.89	—	D21.1-•	D48.1	D49.2
arm	C49.1-•	C79.89	—	D21.1-•	D48.1	D49.2
auricle (ear)	C49.0	C79.89	—	D21.0	D48.1	D49.2
axilla	C49.3	C79.89	—	D21.3	D48.1	D49.2
back	C49.6	C79.89	—	D21.6	D48.1	D49.2
breast — see Neoplasm, breast						
buttock	C49.5	C79.89	—	D21.5	D48.1	D49.2
calf	C49.2-•	C79.89	—	D21.2-•	D48.1	D49.2
cervical region	C49.0	C79.89	—	D21.0	D48.1	D49.2

connective tissue NEC (Continued)

	Malignant Primary	Malignant Secondary	Ca in situ	Benign	Uncertain Behavior	Unspecified Behavior
cheek	C49.0	C79.89	—	D21.0	D48.1	D49.2
chest (wall)	C49.3	C79.89	—	D21.3	D48.1	D49.2
chin	C49.0	C79.89	—	D21.0	D48.1	D49.2
diaphragm	C49.3	C79.89	—	D21.3	D48.1	D49.2
ear (external)	C49.0	C79.89	—	D21.0	D48.1	D49.2
elbow	C49.1-•	C79.89	—	D21.1-•	D48.1	D49.2
extrarectal	C49.5	C79.89	—	D21.5	D48.1	D49.2
extremity	C49.9	C79.89	—	D21.9	D48.1	D49.2
lower	C49.2-•	C79.89	—	D21.2-•	D48.1	D49.2
upper	C49.1-•	C79.89	—	D21.1-•	D48.1	D49.2
eyelid	C49.0	C79.89	—	D21.0	D48.1	D49.2
face	C49.0	C79.89	—	D21.0	D48.1	D49.2
finger	C49.1-•	C79.89	—	D21.1-•	D48.1	D49.2
flank	C49.6	C79.89	—	D21.6	D48.1	D49.2
foot	C49.2-•	C79.89	—	D21.2-•	D48.1	D49.2
forearm	C49.1-•	C79.89	—	D21.1-•	D48.1	D49.2
forehead	C49.0	C79.89	—	D21.0	D48.1	D49.2
gastric	C49.4	C79.89	—	D21.4	D48.1	D49.2
gastrointestinal	C49.4	C79.89	—	D21.4	D48.1	D49.2
gluteal region	C49.5	C79.89	—	D21.5	D48.1	D49.2
great vessels NEC	C49.3	C79.89	—	D21.3	D48.1	D49.2
groin	C49.5	C79.89	—	D21.5	D48.1	D49.2
hand	C49.1-•	C79.89	—	D21.1-•	D48.1	D49.2
head	C49.0	C79.89	—	D21.0	D48.1	D49.2
heel	C49.2-•	C79.89	—	D21.2-•	D48.1	D49.2
hip	C49.2-•	C79.89	—	D21.2-•	D48.1	D49.2
hypochondrium	C49.4	C79.89	—	D21.4	D48.1	D49.2
iliopsoas muscle	C49.5	C79.89	—	D21.5	D48.1	D49.2
infraclavicular region	C49.3	C79.89	—	D21.3	D48.1	D49.2
inguinal (canal) (region)	C49.5	C79.89	—	D21.5	D48.1	D49.2
intestinal	C49.4	C79.89	—	D21.4	D48.1	D49.2
intrathoracic	C49.3	C79.89	—	D21.3	D48.1	D49.2
ischiorectal fossa	C49.5	C79.89	—	D21.5	D48.1	D49.2
jaw	C03.9	C79.89	D00.03	D10.39	D48.1	D49.0
knee	C49.2-•	C79.89	—	D21.2-•	D48.1	D49.2
leg	C49.2-•	C79.89	—	D21.2-•	D48.1	D49.2
limb NEC	C49.9	C79.89	—	D21.9	D48.1	D49.2
lower	C49.2-•	C79.89	—	D21.2-•	D48.1	D49.2
upper	C49.1-•	C79.89	—	D21.1-•	D48.1	D49.2
nates	C49.5	C79.89	—	D21.5	D48.1	D49.2
neck	C49.0	C79.89	—	D21.0	D48.1	D49.2
orbit	C69.6-•	C79.49	D09.2-•	D31.6-•	D48.1	D49.89
overlapping lesion	C49.8	—	—	—	—	—

◀ New   ◀ Revised   deleted Deleted   • Use Additional Character(s)

connective tissue NEC *(Continued)*	Malignant Primary	Malignant Secondary	Ca in situ	Benign	Uncertain Behavior	Unspecified Behavior
pararectal	C49.5	C79.89	—	D21.5	D48.1	D49.2
para-urethral	C49.5	C79.89	—	D21.5	D48.1	D49.2
paravaginal	C49.5	C79.89	—	D21.5	D48.1	D49.2
pelvis (floor)	C49.5	C79.89	—	D21.5	D48.1	D49.2
pelvo-abdominal	C49.8	C79.89	—	D21.6	D48.1	D49.2
perineum	C49.5	C79.89	—	D21.5	D48.1	D49.2
perirectal (tissue)	C49.5	C79.89	—	D21.5	D48.1	D49.2
periurethral (tissue)	C49.5	C79.89	—	D21.5	D48.1	D49.2
popliteal fossa or space	C49.2-●	C79.89	—	D21.2-●	D48.1	D49.2
presacral	C49.5	C79.89	—	D21.5	D48.1	D49.2
psoas muscle	C49.4	C79.89	—	D21.4	D48.1	D49.2
pterygoid fossa	C49.0	C79.89	—	D21.0	D48.1	D49.2
rectovaginal septum or wall	C49.5	C79.89	—	D21.5	D48.1	D49.2
rectovesical	C49.5	C79.89	—	D21.5	D48.1	D49.2
retroperitoneum	C48.0	C78.6	—	D20.0	D48.3	D49.0
sacrococcygeal region	C49.5	C79.89	—	D21.5	D48.1	D49.2
scalp	C49.0	C79.89	—	D21.0	D48.1	D49.2
scapular region	C49.3	C79.89	—	D21.3	D48.1	D49.2
shoulder	C49.1-●	C79.89	—	D21.1-●	D48.1	D49.2
skin (dermis) NEC — *see also Neoplasm, skin, by site*	C44.90	C79.2	D04.9	D23.9	D48.5	D49.2
stomach	C49.4	C79.89	—	D21.4	D48.1	D49.2
submental	C49.0	C79.89	—	D21.0	D48.1	D49.2
supraclavicular region	C49.0	C79.89	—	D21.0	D48.1	D49.2
temple	C49.0	C79.89	—	D21.0	D48.1	D49.2
temporal region	C49.0	C79.89	—	D21.0	D48.1	D49.2
thigh	C49.2-●	C79.89	—	D21.2-●	D48.1	D49.2
thoracic (duct) (wall)	C49.3	C79.89	—	D21.3	D48.1	D49.2
thorax	C49.3	C79.89	—	D21.3	D48.1	D49.2
thumb	C49.1-●	C79.89	—	D21.1-●	D48.1	D49.2
toe	C49.2-●	C79.89	—	D21.2-●	D48.1	D49.2
trunk	C49.6	C79.89	—	D21.6	D48.1	D49.2
umbilicus	C49.4	C79.89	—	D21.4	D48.1	D49.2
vesicorectal	C49.5	C79.89	—	D21.5	D48.1	D49.2
wrist	C49.1-●	C79.89	—	D21.1-●	D48.1	D49.2
conus medullaris	C72.0	C79.49	—	D33.4	D43.4	D49.7
cord (true) (vocal)	C32.0	C78.39	D02.0	D14.1	D38.0	D49.1
false	C32.1	C78.39	D02.0	D14.1	D38.0	D49.1
spermatic	C63.1-●	C79.82	D07.69	D29.8	D40.8	D49.59
spinal (cervical) (lumbar) (thoracic)	C72.0	C79.49	—	D33.4	D43.4	D49.7
cornea (limbus)	C69.1-●	C79.49	D09.2-●	D31.1-●	D48.7	D49.89
corpus						

corpus *(Continued)*	Malignant Primary	Malignant Secondary	Ca in situ	Benign	Uncertain Behavior	Unspecified Behavior
albicans	C56.-●	C79.6-●	D07.39	D27.-●	D39.1-●	D49.59
callosum, brain	C71.0	C79.31	—	D33.2	D43.2	D49.6
cavernosum	C60.2	C79.82	D07.4	D29.0	D40.8	D49.59
gastric	C16.2	C78.89	D00.2	D13.1	D37.1	D49.0
overlapping sites	C54.8	—	—	—	—	—
penis	C60.2	C79.82	D07.4	D29.0	D40.8	D49.59
striatum, cerebrum	C71.0	C79.31	—	D33.0	D43.0	D49.6
uteri	C54.9	C79.82	D07.0	D26.1	D39.0	D49.59
isthmus	C54.0	C79.82	D07.0	D26.1	D39.0	D49.59
cortex						
adrenal	C74.0-●	C79.7-●	D09.3	D35.0-●	D44.1-●	D49.7
cerebral	C71.0	C79.31	—	D33.0	D43.0	D49.6
costal cartilage	C41.3	C79.51	—	D16.7	D48.0	D49.2
costovertebral joint	C41.3	C79.51	—	D16.7	D48.0	D49.2
Cowper's gland	C68.0	C79.19	D09.19	D30.4	D41.3	D49.59
cranial (fossa, any)	C71.9	C79.31	—	D33.2	D43.2	D49.6
meninges	C70.0	C79.32	—	D32.0	D42.0	D49.7
nerve	C72.50	C79.49	—	D33.3	D43.3	D49.7
specified NEC	C72.59	C79.49	—	D33.3	D43.3	D49.7
craniobuccal pouch	C75.2	C79.89	D09.3	D35.2	D44.3	D49.7
craniopharyngeal (duct) (pouch)	C75.2	C79.89	D09.3	D35.3	D44.4	D49.7
cricoid	C13.0	C79.89	D00.08	D10.7	D37.05	D49.0
cartilage	C32.3	C78.39	D02.0	D14.1	D38.0	D49.1
cricopharynx	C13.0	C79.89	D00.08	D10.7	D37.05	D49.0
crypt of Morgagni	C21.8	C78.5	D01.3	D12.9	D37.8	D49.0
crystalline lens	C69.4-●	C79.49	D09.2-●	D31.4-●	D48.7	D49.89
cul-de-sac (Douglas')	C48.1	C78.6	—	D20.1	D48.4	D49.0
cuneiform cartilage	C32.3	C78.39	D02.0	D14.1	D38.0	D49.1
cutaneous — *see Neoplasm, skin*						
cutis — *see Neoplasm, skin*						
cystic (bile) duct (common)	C24.0	C78.89	D01.5	D13.5	D37.6	D49.0
dermis — *see Neoplasm, skin*						
diaphragm	C49.3	C79.89	—	D21.3	D48.1	D49.2
digestive organs, system, tube, or tract NEC	C26.9	C78.89	D01.9	D13.99	D37.9	D49.0
disc, intervertebral	C41.2	C79.51	—	D16.6	D48.0	D49.2
disease, generalized	C80.0	—	—	—	—	—
disseminated	C80.0	—	—	—	—	—
Douglas' cul-de-sac or pouch	C48.1	C78.6	—	D20.1	D48.4	D49.0
duodenojejunal junction	C17.8	C78.4	D01.49	D13.39	D37.2	D49.0
duodenum	C17.0	C78.4	D01.49	D13.2	D37.2	D49.0

TABLE OF NEOPLASMS

	Malignant Primary	Malignant Secondary	Ca in situ	Benign	Uncertain Behavior	Unspecified Behavior
dura (cranial) (mater)	C70.9	C79.49	—	D32.9	D42.9	D49.7
cerebral	C70.0	C79.32	—	D32.0	D42.0	D49.7
spinal	C70.1	C79.49	—	D32.1	D42.1	D49.7
ear (external) — see also Neoplasm, skin, ear	C44.20-●	C79.2	D04.2-●	D23.2-●	D48.5	D49.2
auricle or auris — see also Neoplasm, skin, ear	C44.20-●	C79.2	D04.2-●	D23.2-●	D48.5	D49.2
canal, external — see also Neoplasm, skin, ear	C44.20-●	C79.2	D04.2-●	D23.2-●	D48.5	D49.2
cartilage	C49.0	C79.89	—	D21.0	D48.1	D49.2
external meatus — see also Neoplasm, skin, ear	C44.20-●	C79.2	D04.2-●	D23.2-●	D48.5	D49.2
inner	C30.1	C78.39	D02.3	D14.0	D38.5	D49.1
lobule — see also Neoplasm, skin, ear	C44.20-●	C79.2	D04.2-●	D23.2-●	D48.5	D49.2
middle	C30.1	C78.39	D02.3	D14.0	D38.5	D49.1
overlapping lesion with accessory sinuses	C31.8	—	—	—	—	—
skin	C44.20-●	C79.2	D04.2-●	D23.2-●	D48.5	D49.2
basal cell carcinoma	C44.21-●	—	—	—	—	—
specified type NEC	C44.29-●	—	—	—	—	—
squamous cell carcinoma	C44.22-●	—	—	—	—	—
earlobe	C44.20-●	C79.2	D04.2-●	D23.2-●	D48.5	D49.2
basal cell carcinoma	C44.21-●	—	—	—	—	—
specified type NEC	C44.29-●	—	—	—	—	—
squamous cell carcinoma	C44.22-●	—	—	—	—	—
ejaculatory duct	C63.7	C79.82	D07.69	D29.8	D40.8	D49.59
elbow NEC	C76.4-●	C79.89	D04.6-●	D36.7	D48.7	D49.89
endocardium	C38.0	C79.89		D15.1	D48.7	D49.89
endocervix (canal) (gland)	C53.0	C79.82	D06.0	D26.0	D39.0	D49.59
endocrine gland NEC	C75.9	C79.89	D09.3	D35.9	D44.9	D49.7
pluriglandular	C75.8	C79.89	D09.3	D35.7	D44.9	D49.7
endometrium (gland) (stroma)	C54.1	C79.82	D07.0	D26.1	D39.0	D49.59
ensiform cartilage	C41.3	C79.51		D16.7	D48.0	D49.2
enteric — see Neoplasm, intestine						
ependyma (brain)	C71.5	C79.31	—	D33.0	D43.0	D49.6
fourth ventricle	C71.7	C79.31	—	D33.1	D43.1	D49.6
epicardium	C38.0	C79.89		D15.1	D48.7	D49.89
epididymis	C63.0-●	C79.82	D07.69	D29.3-●	D40.8	D49.59
epidural	C72.9	C79.49	—	D33.9	D43.9	D49.7
epiglottis	C32.1	C78.39	D02.0	D14.1	D38.0	D49.1
anterior aspect or surface	C10.1	C79.89	D00.08	D10.5	D37.05	D49.0
cartilage	C32.3	C78.39	D02.0	D14.1	D38.0	D49.1
free border (margin)	C10.1	C79.89	D00.08	D10.5	D37.05	D49.0

	Malignant Primary	Malignant Secondary	Ca in situ	Benign	Uncertain Behavior	Unspecified Behavior
junctional region	C10.8	C79.89	D00.08	D10.5	D37.05	D49.0
posterior (laryngeal) surface	C32.1	C78.39	D02.0	D14.1	D38.0	D49.1
suprahyoid portion	C32.1	C78.39	D02.0	D14.1	D38.0	D49.1
esophagogastric junction	C16.0	C78.89	D00.2	D13.1	D37.1	D49.0
esophagus	C15.9	C78.89	D00.1	D13.0	D37.8	D49.0
abdominal	C15.5	C78.89	D00.1	D13.0	D37.8	D49.0
cervical	C15.3	C78.89	D00.1	D13.0	D37.8	D49.0
distal (third)	C15.5	C78.89	D00.1	D13.0	D37.8	D49.0
lower (third)	C15.5	C78.89	D00.1	D13.0	D37.8	D49.0
middle (third)	C15.4	C78.89	D00.1	D13.0	D37.8	D49.0
overlapping lesion	C15.8	—	—	—	—	—
proximal (third)	C15.3	C78.89	D00.1	D13.0	D37.8	D49.0
thoracic	C15.4	C78.89	D00.1	D13.0	D37.8	D49.0
upper (third)	C15.3	C78.89	D00.1	D13.0	D37.8	D49.0
ethmoid (sinus)	C31.1	C78.39	D02.3	D14.0	D38.5	D49.1
bone or labyrinth	C41.0	C79.51	—	D16.4-●	D48.0	D49.2
eustachian tube	C30.1	C78.39	D02.3	D14.0	D38.5	D49.1
exocervix	C53.1	C79.82	D06.1	D26.0	D39.0	D49.59
external						
meatus (ear) — see also Neoplasm, skin, ear	C44.20-●	C79.2	D04.2-●	D23.2-●	D48.5	D49.2
os, cervix uteri	C53.1	C79.82	D06.1	D26.0	D39.0	D49.59
extradural	C72.9	C79.49	—	D33.9	D43.9	D49.7
extrahepatic (bile) duct	C24.0	C78.89	D01.5	D13.5	D37.6	D49.0
overlapping lesion with gallbladder	C24.8	—	—	—	—	—
extraocular muscle	C69.6-●	C79.49	D09.2-●	D31.6-●	D48.7	D49.89
extrarectal	C76.3	C79.89	D09.8	D36.7	D48.7	D49.89
extremity	C76.8	C79.89	D04.8	D36.7	D48.7	D49.89
lower	C76.5-●	C79.89	D04.7-●	D36.7	D48.7	D49.89
upper	C76.4-●	C79.89	D04.6-●	D36.7	D48.7	D49.89
eye NEC	C69.9-●	C79.49	D09.2	D31.9	D48.7	D49.89
overlapping sites	C69.8	—	—	—	—	—
eyeball	C69.9-●	C79.49	D09.2-●	D31.9-●	D48.7	D49.89
eyebrow	C44.309	C79.2	D04.39	D23.39	D48.5	D49.2
basal cell carcinoma	C44.319	—	—	—	—	—
specified type NEC	C44.399	—	—	—	—	—
squamous cell carcinoma	C44.329	—	—	—	—	—
eyelid (lower) (skin) (upper)	C44.10-●	—	—	—	—	—
basal cell carcinoma	C44.11-●	—	—	—	—	—
cartilage	C49.0	C79.89	—	D21.0	D48.1	D49.2
sebaceous cell	C44.13-●	—	—	—	—	—
specified type NEC	C44.19-●	—	—	—	—	—
squamous cell carcinoma	C44.12-●	—	—	—	—	—

◀ New   ◀ Revised   ~~deleted~~ Deleted   ● Use Additional Character(s)

	Malignant Primary	Malignant Secondary	Ca in situ	Benign	Uncertain Behavior	Unspecified Behavior
face NEC	C76.0	C79.89	D04.39	D36.7	D48.7	D49.89
fallopian tube (accessory)	C57.0-●	C79.82	D07.39	D28.2	D39.8	D49.59
falx (cerebella) (cerebri)	C70.0	C79.32	—	D32.0	D42.0	D49.7
fascia — see also Neoplasm, connective tissue						
palmar	C49.1-●	C79.89	—	D21.1-●	D48.1	D49.2
plantar	C49.2-●	C79.89	—	D21.2-●	D48.1	D49.2
fatty tissue — see Neoplasm, connective tissue						
fauces, faucial NEC	C10.9	C79.89	D00.08	D10.5	D37.05	D49.0
pillars	C09.1	C79.89	D00.08	D10.5	D37.05	D49.0
tonsil	C09.9	C79.89	D00.08	D10.4	D37.05	D49.0
femur (any part)	C40.2-●	—	—	D16.2-●	—	—
fetal membrane	C58	C79.82	D07.0	D26.7	D39.2	D49.59
fibrous tissue — see Neoplasm, connective tissue						
fibula (any part)	C40.2-●	C79.51	—	D16.2-●	—	—
filum terminale	C72.0	C79.49	—	D33.4	D43.4	D49.7
finger NEC	C76.4-●	C79.89	D04.6-●	D36.7	D48.7	D49.89
flank NEC	C76.8	C79.89	D04.5	D36.7	D48.7	D49.89
follicle, nabothian	C53.0	C79.82	D06.0	D26.0	D39.0	D49.59
foot NEC	C76.5-●	C79.89	D04.7-●	D36.7	D48.7	D49.89
forearm NEC	C76.4-●	C79.89	D04.6-●	D36.7	D48.7	D49.89
forehead (skin)	C44.309	C79.2	D04.39	D23.39	D48.5	D49.2
basal cell carcinoma	C44.319	—	—	—	—	—
specified type NEC	C44.399	—	—	—	—	—
squamous cell carcinoma	C44.329	—	—	—	—	—
foreskin	C60.0	C79.82	D07.4	D29.0	D40.8	D49.59
fornix						
pharyngeal	C11.3	C79.89	D00.08	D10.6	D37.05	D49.0
vagina	C52	C79.82	D07.2	D28.1	D39.8	D49.59
fossa (of)						
anterior (cranial)	C71.9	C79.31	—	D33.2	D43.2	D49.6
cranial	C71.9	C79.31	—	D33.2	D43.2	D49.6
ischiorectal	C76.3	C79.89	D09.8	D36.7	D48.7	D49.89
middle (cranial)	C71.9	C79.31	—	D33.2	D43.2	D49.6
piriform	C12	C79.89	D00.08	D10.7	D37.05	D49.0
pituitary	C75.1	C79.89	D09.3	D35.2	D44.3	D49.7
posterior (cranial)	C71.9	C79.31	—	D33.2	D43.2	D49.6
pterygoid	C49.0	C79.89	—	D21.0	D48.1	D49.2
pyriform	C12	C79.89	D00.08	D10.7	D37.05	D49.0
Rosenmuller	C11.2	C79.89	D00.08	D10.6	D37.05	D49.0
tonsillar	C09.0	C79.89	D00.08	D10.5	D37.05	D49.0
fourchette	C51.9	C79.82	D07.1	D28.0	D39.8	D49.59
frenulum						
labii — see Neoplasm, lip, internal						
linguae	C02.2	C79.89	D00.07	D10.1	D37.02	D49.0
frontal						
bone	C41.0	C79.51	—	D16.4-●	D48.0	D49.2
lobe, brain	C71.1	C79.31	—	D33.0	D43.0	D49.6
pole	C71.1	C79.31	—	D33.0	D43.0	D49.6
sinus	C31.2	C78.39	D02.3	D14.0	D38.5	D49.1
fundus						
stomach	C16.1	C78.89	D00.2	D13.1	D37.1	D49.0
uterus	C54.3	C79.82	D07.0	D26.1	D39.0	D49.59
gall duct (extrahepatic)	C24.0	C78.89	D01.5	D13.5	D37.6	D49.0
intrahepatic	C22.1	C78.7	D01.5	D13.4	D37.6	D49.0
gallbladder	C23	C78.89	D01.5	D13.5	D37.6	D49.0
overlapping lesion with extrahepatic bile ducts	C24.8	—	—	—	—	—
ganglia — see also Neoplasm, nerve, peripheral	C47.9	C79.89	—	D36.10	D48.2	D49.2
basal	C71.0	C79.31	—	D33.0	D43.0	D49.6
cranial nerve	C72.50	C79.49	—	D33.3	D43.3	D49.7
Gartner's duct	C52	C79.82	D07.2	D28.1	D39.8	D49.59
gastric — see Neoplasm, stomach						
gastrocolic	C26.9	C78.89	D01.9	D13.99	D37.9	D49.0
gastroesophageal junction	C16.0	C78.89	D00.2	D13.1	D37.1	D49.0
gastrointestinal (tract) NEC	C26.9	C78.89	D01.9	D13.99	D37.9	D49.0
generalized	C80.0	—	—	—	—	—
genital organ or tract						
female NEC	C57.9	C79.82	D07.30	D28.9	D39.9	D49.59
overlapping lesion	C57.8	—	—	—	—	—
specified site NEC	C57.7	C79.82	D07.39	D28.7	D39.8	D49.59
male NEC	C63.9	C79.82	D07.60	D29.9	D40.9	D49.59
overlapping lesion	C63.8	—	—	—	—	—
specified site NEC	C63.7	C79.82	D07.69	D29.8	D40.8	D49.59
genitourinary tract						
female	C57.9	C79.82	D07.30	D28.9	D39.9	D49.59
male	C63.9	C79.82	D07.60	D29.9	D40.9	D49.59
gingiva (alveolar) (marginal)	C03.9	C79.89	D00.03	D10.39	D37.09	D49.0
lower	C03.1	C79.89	D00.03	D10.39	D37.09	D49.0
mandibular	C03.1	C79.89	D00.03	D10.39	D37.09	D49.0
maxillary	C03.0	C79.89	D00.03	D10.39	D37.09	D49.0
upper	C03.0	C79.89	D00.03	D10.39	D37.09	D49.0

◀ New ◀ Revised ~~deleted~~ Deleted ● Use Additional Character(s)

TABLE OF NEOPLASMS

	Malignant Primary	Malignant Secondary	Ca in situ	Benign	Uncertain Behavior	Unspecified Behavior
gland, glandular (lymphatic) (system) — *see also Neoplasm, lymph gland*						
endocrine NEC	C75.9	C79.89	D09.3	D35.9	D44.9	D49.7
salivary — *see Neoplasm, salivary gland*						
glans penis	C60.1	C79.82	D07.4	D29.0	D40.8	D49.59
globus pallidus	C71.0	C79.31	—	D33.0	D43.0	D49.6
glomus						
coccygeal	C49.5	C79.89	—	D21.5	D48.1	D49.2
jugularis	C75.5	C79.89	—	D35.6	D44.7	D49.7
glosso-epiglottic fold(s)	C10.1	C79.89	D00.08	D10.5	D37.05	D49.0
glossopalatine fold	C09.1	C79.89	D00.08	D10.5	D37.05	D49.0
glossopharyngeal sulcus	C09.0	C79.89	D00.08	D10.5	D37.05	D49.0
glottis	C32.0	C78.39	D02.0	D14.1	D38.0	D49.1
gluteal region	C76.3	C79.89	D04.5	D36.7	D48.7	D49.89
great vessels NEC	C49.3	C79.89	—	D21.3	D48.1	D49.2
groin NEC	C76.3	C79.89	D04.5	D36.7	D48.7	D49.89
gum	C03.9	C79.89	D00.03	D10.39	D37.09	D49.0
lower	C03.1	C79.89	D00.03	D10.39	D37.09	D49.0
upper	C03.0	C79.89	D00.03	D10.39	D37.09	D49.0
hand NEC	C76.4-●	C79.89	D04.6-●	D36.7	D48.7	D49.89
head NEC	C76.0	C79.89	D04.4	D36.7	D48.7	D49.89
heart	C38.0	C79.89	—	D15.1	D48.7	D49.89
heel NEC	C76.5-●	C79.89	D04.7-●	D36.7	D48.7	D49.89
helix — *see also Neoplasm, skin, ear*	C44.20-●	C79.2	D04.2-●	D23.2-●	D48.5	D49.2
hematopoietic, hemopoietic tissue NEC	C96.9	—	—	—	—	—
specified NEC	C96.Z	—	—	—	—	—
hemisphere, cerebral	C71.0	C79.31	—	D33.0	D43.0	D49.6
hemorrhoidal zone	C21.1	C78.5	D01.3	D12.9	D37.8	D49.0
hepatic — *see also Index to disease, by histology*	C22.9	C78.7	D01.5	D13.4	D37.6	D49.0
duct (bile)	C24.0	C78.89	D01.5	D13.5	D37.6	D49.0
flexure (colon)	C18.3	C78.5	D01.0	D12.3	D37.4	D49.0
primary	C22.8	C78.7	D01.5	D13.4	D37.6	D49.0
hepatobiliary	C24.9	C79.89	D01.5	D13.5	D37.6	D49.0
hepatoblastoma	C22.2	C78.7	D01.5	D13.4	D37.6	D49.0
hepatoma	C22.0	C78.7	D01.5	D13.4	D37.6	D49.0
hilus of lung	C34.0-●	C78.0-●	D02.2-●	D14.3-●	D38.1	D49.1
hip NEC	C76.5-●	C79.89	D04.7-●	D36.7	D48.7	D49.89
hippocampus, brain	C71.2	C79.31	—	D33.0	D43.0	D49.6
humerus (any part)	C40.0-●	C79.51	—	D16.0-●	—	—
hymen	C52	C79.82	D07.2	D28.1	D39.8	D49.59

	Malignant Primary	Malignant Secondary	Ca in situ	Benign	Uncertain Behavior	Unspecified Behavior
hypopharynx, hypopharyngeal NEC	C13.9	C79.89	D00.08	D10.7	D37.05	D49.0
overlapping lesion	C13.8	—	—	—	—	—
postcricoid region	C13.0	C79.89	D00.08	D10.7	D37.05	D49.0
posterior wall	C13.2	C79.89	D00.08	D10.7	D37.05	D49.0
pyriform fossa (sinus)	C12	C79.89	D00.08	D10.7	D37.05	D49.0
hypophysis	C75.1	C79.89	D09.3	D35.2	D44.3	D49.7
hypothalamus	C71.0	C79.31	—	D33.0	D43.0	D49.6
ileocecum, ileocecal (coil) (junction) (valve)	C18.0	C78.5	D01.0	D12.0	D37.4	D49.0
ileum	C17.2	C78.4	D01.49	D13.39	D37.2	D49.0
ilium	C41.4	C79.51	—	D16.8	D48.0	D49.2
immunoproliferative NEC	C88.9	—	—	—	—	—
infraclavicular (region)	C76.1	C79.89	D04.5	D36.7	D48.7	D49.89
inguinal (region)	C76.3	C79.89	D04.5	D36.7	D48.7	D49.89
insula	C71.0	C79.31	—	D33.0	D43.0	D49.6
insular tissue (pancreas)	C25.4	C78.89	D01.7	D13.7	D37.8	D49.0
brain	C71.0	C79.31	—	D33.0	D43.0	D49.6
interarytenoid fold	C13.1	C79.89	D00.08	D10.7	D37.05	D49.0
hypopharyngeal aspect	C13.1	C79.89	D00.08	D10.7	D37.05	D49.0
laryngeal aspect	C32.1	C78.39	D02.0	D14.1	D38.0	D49.1
marginal zone	C13.1	C79.89	D00.08	D10.7	D37.05	D49.0
interdental papillae	C03.9	C79.89	D00.03	D10.39	D37.09	D49.0
lower	C03.1	C79.89	D00.03	D10.39	D37.09	D49.0
upper	C03.0	C79.89	D00.03	D10.39	D37.09	D49.0
internal						
capsule	C71.0	C79.31	—	D33.0	D43.0	D49.6
os (cervix)	C53.0	C79.82	D06.0	D26.0	D39.0	D49.59
intervertebral cartilage or disc	C41.2	C79.51	—	D16.6	D48.0	D49.2
intestine, intestinal	C26.0	C78.80	D01.40	D13.99	D37.8	D49.0
large	C18.9	C78.5	D01.0	D12.6	D37.4	D49.0
appendix	C18.1	C78.5	D01.0	D12.1	D37.3	D49.0
caput coli	C18.0	C78.5	D01.0	D12.0	D37.4	D49.0
cecum	C18.0	C78.5	D01.0	D12.0	D37.4	D49.0
colon	C18.9	C78.5	D01.0	D12.6	D37.4	D49.0
and rectum	C19	C78.5	D01.1	D12.7	D37.5	D49.0
ascending	C18.2	C78.5	D01.0	D12.2	D37.4	D49.0
caput	C18.0	C78.5	D01.0	D12.0	D37.4	D49.0
descending	C18.6	C78.5	D01.0	D12.4	D37.4	D49.0
distal	C18.6	C78.5	D01.0	D12.4	D37.4	D49.0
left	C18.6	C78.5	D01.0	D12.4	D37.4	D49.0
overlapping lesion	C18.8	—	—	—	—	—
pelvic	C18.7	C78.5	D01.0	D12.5	D37.4	D49.0
right	C18.2	C78.5	D01.0	D12.2	D37.4	D49.0

◀ New   ◀ Revised   ~~deleted~~ Deleted   ● Use Additional Character(s)

TABLE OF NEOPLASMS

	Malignant Primary	Malignant Secondary	Ca in situ	Benign	Uncertain Behavior	Unspecified Behavior
intestine, intestinal *(Continued)*						
large *(Continued)*						
colon *(Continued)*						
sigmoid (flexure)	C18.7	C78.5	D01.0	D12.5	D37.4	D49.0
transverse	C18.4	C78.5	D01.0	D12.3	D37.4	D49.0
hepatic flexure	C18.3	C78.5	D01.0	D12.3	D37.4	D49.0
ileocecum, ileocecal (coil) (valve)	C18.0	C78.5	D01.0	D12.0	D37.4	D49.0
overlapping lesion	C18.8	—	—	—	—	—
sigmoid flexure (lower) (upper)	C18.7	C78.5	D01.0	D12.5	D37.4	D49.0
splenic flexure	C18.5	C78.5	D01.0	D12.3	D37.4	D49.0
small	C17.9	C78.4	D01.40	D13.30	D37.2	D49.0
duodenum	C17.0	C78.4	D01.49	D13.2	D37.2	D49.0
ileum	C17.2	C78.4	D01.49	D13.39	D37.2	D49.0
jejunum	C17.1	C78.4	D01.49	D13.39	D37.2	D49.0
overlapping lesion	C17.8	—	—	—	—	—
tract NEC	C26.0	C78.89	D01.40	D13.99	D37.8	D49.0
intra-abdominal	C76.2	C79.89	D09.8	D36.7	D48.7	D49.89
intracranial NEC	C71.9	C79.31	—	D33.2	D43.2	D49.6
intrahepatic (bile) duct	C22.1	C78.7	D01.5	D13.4	D37.6	D49.0
intraocular	C69.9-●	C79.49	D09.2-●	D31.9-●	D48.7	D49.89
intraorbital	C69.6-●	C79.49	D09.2-●	D31.6-●	D48.7	D49.89
intrasellar	C75.1	C79.89	D09.3	D35.2	D44.3	D49.7
intrathoracic (cavity) (organs)	C76.1	C79.89	D09.8	D15.9	D48.7	D49.89
specified NEC	C76.1	C79.89	D09.8	D15.7	—	—
iris	C69.4-●	C79.49	D09.2-●	D31.4-●	D48.7	D49.89
ischiorectal (fossa)	C76.3	C79.89	D09.8	D36.7	D48.7	D49.89
ischium	C41.4	C79.51	—	D16.8	D48.0	D49.2
island of Reil	C71.0	C79.31	—	D33.0	D43.0	D49.6
islands or islets of Langerhans	C25.4	C78.89	D01.7	D13.7	D37.8	D49.0
isthmus uteri	C54.0	C79.82	D07.0	D26.1	D39.0	D49.59
jaw	C76.0	C79.89	D09.8	D36.7	D48.7	D49.89
bone	C41.1	C79.51	—	D16.5-●	D48.0	D49.2
lower	C41.1	C79.51	—	D16.5-●	—	—
upper	C41.0	C79.51	—	D16.4-●	—	—
carcinoma (any type) (lower) (upper)	C76.0	C79.89	—	—	—	—
skin — *see also* Neoplasm, skin, face	C44.309	C79.2	D04.39	D23.39	D48.5	D49.2
soft tissues	C03.9	C79.89	D00.03	D10.39	D37.09	D49.0
lower	C03.1	C79.89	D00.03	D10.39	D37.09	D49.0
upper	C03.0	C79.89	D00.03	D10.39	D37.09	D49.0
jejunum	C17.1	C78.4	D01.49	D13.39	D37.2	D49.0
joint NEC — *see also* Neoplasm, bone	C41.9	C79.51	—	D16.9-●	D48.0	D49.2
acromioclavicular	C40.0-●	C79.51	—	D16.0-●	—	—
bursa or synovial membrane — *see* Neoplasm, connective tissue						
costovertebral	C41.3	C79.51	—	D16.7	D48.0	D49.2
sternocostal	C41.3	C79.51	—	D16.7	D48.0	D49.2
temporomandibular	C41.1	C79.51	—	D16.5-●	D48.0	D49.2
junction						
anorectal	C21.8	C78.5	D01.3	D12.9	D37.8	D49.0
cardioesophageal	C16.0	C78.89	D00.2	D13.1	D37.1	D49.0
esophagogastric	C16.0	C78.89	D00.2	D13.1	D37.1	D49.0
gastroesophageal	C16.0	C78.89	D00.2	D13.1	D37.1	D49.0
hard and soft palate	C05.9	C79.89	D00.00	D10.39	D37.09	D49.0
ileocecal	C18.0	C78.5	D01.0	D12.0	D37.4	D49.0
pelvirectal	C19	C78.5	D01.1	D12.7	D37.5	D49.0
pelviureteric	C65.-●	C79.0-●	D09.19	D30.1-●	D41.1-●	D49.59
rectosigmoid	C19	C78.5	D01.1	D12.7	D37.5	D49.0
squamocolumnar, of cervix	C53.8	C79.82	D06.7	D26.0	D39.0	D49.59
Kaposi's sarcoma — *see* Kaposi's, sarcoma						
kidney (parenchymal)	C64.-●	C79.0-●	D09.19	D30.0-●	D41.0-●	D49.51-●
calyx	C65.-●	C79.0-●	D09.19	D30.1-●	D41.1-●	D49.51-●
hilus	C65.-●	C79.0-●	D09.19	D30.1-●	D41.1-●	D49.51-●
pelvis	C65.-●	C79.0-●	D09.19	D30.1-●	D41.1-●	D49.51-●
knee NEC	C76.5-●	C79.89	D04.7-●	D36.7	D48.7	D49.89
labia (skin)	C51.9	C79.82	D07.1	D28.0	D39.8	D49.59
majora	C51.0	C79.82	D07.1	D28.0	D39.8	D49.59
minora	C51.1	C79.82	D07.1	D28.0	D39.8	D49.59
labial — *see also* Neoplasm, lip	C00.9	C79.89	D00.01	D10.0	D37.01	D49.0
sulcus (lower) (upper)	C06.1	C79.89	D00.02	D10.39	D37.09	D49.0
labium (skin)	C51.9	C79.82	D07.1	D28.0	D39.8	D49.59
majus	C51.0	C79.82	D07.1	D28.0	D39.8	D49.59
minus	C51.1	C79.82	D07.1	D28.0	D39.8	D49.59
lacrimal						
canaliculi	C69.5-●	C79.49	D09.2-●	D31.5-●	D48.7	D49.89
duct (nasal)	C69.5-●	C79.49	D09.2-●	D31.5-●	D48.7	D49.89
gland	C69.5-●	C79.49	D09.2-●	D31.5-●	D48.7	D49.89
punctum	C69.5-●	C79.49	D09.2-●	D31.5-●	D48.7	D49.89
sac	C69.5-●	C79.49	D09.2-●	D31.5-●	D48.7	D49.89
Langerhans, islands or islets	C25.4	C78.89	D01.7	D13.7	D37.8	D49.0
laryngopharynx	C13.9	C79.89	D00.08	D10.7	D37.05	D49.0

	Malignant Primary	Malignant Secondary	Ca in situ	Benign	Uncertain Behavior	Unspecified Behavior
larynx, laryngeal NEC	C32.9	C78.39	D02.0	D14.1	D38.0	D49.1
aryepiglottic fold	C32.1	C78.39	D02.0	D14.1	D38.0	D49.1
cartilage (arytenoid) (cricoid) (cuneiform) (thyroid)	C32.3	C78.39	D02.0	D14.1	D38.0	D49.1
commissure (anterior) (posterior)	C32.0	C78.39	D02.0	D14.1	D38.0	D49.1
extrinsic NEC	C32.1	C78.39	D02.0	D14.1	D38.0	D49.1
meaning hypopharynx	C13.9	C79.89	D00.08	D10.7	D37.05	D49.0
interarytenoid fold	C32.1	C78.39	D02.0	D14.1	D38.0	D49.1
intrinsic	C32.0	C78.39	D02.0	D14.1	D38.0	D49.1
overlapping lesion	C32.8	—	—	—	—	—
ventricular band	C32.1	C78.39	D02.0	D14.1	D38.0	D49.1
leg NEC	C76.5-●	C79.89	D04.7-●	D36.7	D48.7	D49.89
lens, crystalline	C69.4-●	C79.49	D09.2-●	D31.4-●	D48.7	D49.89
lid (lower) (upper)	C44.10-●	C79.2	D04.1-●	D23.1-●	D48.5	D49.2
basal cell carcinoma	C44.11-●	—	—	—	—	—
sebaceous cell	C44.13-●	—	—	—	—	—
specified type NEC	C44.19-●	—	—	—	—	—
squamous cell carcinoma	C44.12-●	—	—	—	—	—
ligament — see also Neoplasm, connective tissue						
broad	C57.1	C79.82	D07.39	D28.2	D39.8	D49.59
Mackenrodt's	C57.7	C79.82	D07.39	D28.7	D39.8	D49.59
non-uterine — see Neoplasm, connective tissue						
round	C57.2	C79.82	—	D28.2	D39.8	D49.59
sacro-uterine	C57.3	C79.82	—	D28.2	D39.8	D49.59
uterine	C57.3	C79.82	—	D28.2	D39.8	D49.59
utero-ovarian	C57.7	C79.82	D07.39	D28.2	D39.8	D49.59
uterosacral	C57.3	C79.82	—	D28.2	D39.8	D49.59
limb	C76.8	C79.89	D04.8	D36.7	D48.7	D49.89
lower	C76.5-●	C79.89	D04.7-●	D36.7	D48.7	D49.89
upper	C76.4-●	C79.89	D04.6-●	D36.7	D48.7	D49.89
limbus of cornea	C69.1-●	C79.49	D09.2-●	D31.1-●	D48.7	D49.89
lingual NEC — see also Neoplasm, tongue	C02.9	C79.89	D00.07	D10.1	D37.02	D49.0
lingula, lung	C34.1-●	C78.0-●	D02.2-●	D14.3-●	D38.1	D49.1
lip	C00.9	C79.89	D00.01	D10.0	D37.01	D49.0
buccal aspect — see Neoplasm, lip, internal						
commissure	C00.6	C79.89	D00.01	D10.0	D37.01	D49.0
external	C00.2	C79.89	D00.01	D10.0	D37.01	D49.0
lower	C00.1	C79.89	D00.01	D10.0	D37.01	D49.0
upper	C00.0	C79.89	D00.01	D10.0	D37.01	D49.0
frenulum — see Neoplasm, lip, internal						

	Malignant Primary	Malignant Secondary	Ca in situ	Benign	Uncertain Behavior	Unspecified Behavior
lip (Continued)						
inner aspect — see Neoplasm, lip, internal						
internal	C00.5	C79.89	D00.01	D10.0	D37.01	D49.0
lower	C00.4	C79.89	D00.01	D10.0	D37.01	D49.0
upper	C00.3	C79.89	D00.01	D10.0	D37.01	D49.0
lipstick area	C00.2	C79.89	D00.01	D10.0	D37.01	D49.0
lower	C00.1	C79.89	D00.01	D10.0	D37.01	D49.0
upper	C00.0	C79.89	D00.01	D10.0	D37.01	D49.0
lower	C00.1	C79.89	D00.01	D10.0	D37.01	D49.0
internal	C00.4	C79.89	D00.01	D10.0	D37.01	D49.0
mucosa — see Neoplasm, lip, internal						
oral aspect — see Neoplasm, lip, internal						
overlapping lesion	C00.8	—	—	—	—	—
with oral cavity or pharynx	C14.8	—	—	—	—	—
skin (commissure) (lower) (upper)	C44.00	C79.2	D04.0	D23.0	D48.5	D49.2
basal cell carcinoma	C44.01	—	—	—	—	—
specified type NEC	C44.09	—	—	—	—	—
squamous cell carcinoma	C44.02	—	—	—	—	—
upper	C00.0	C79.89	D00.01	D10.0	D37.01	D49.0
internal	C00.3	C79.89	D00.01	D10.0	D37.01	D49.0
vermilion border	C00.2	C79.89	D00.01	D10.0	D37.01	D49.0
lower	C00.1	C79.89	D00.01	D10.0	D37.01	D49.0
upper	C00.0	C79.89	D00.01	D10.0	D37.01	D49.0
lipomatous — see Lipoma, by site						
liver — see also Index to disease, by histology	C22.9	C78.7	D01.5	D13.4	D37.6	D49.0
primary	C22.8	C78.7	D01.5	D13.4	D37.6	D49.0
lumbosacral plexus	C47.5	C79.89	—	D36.16	D48.2	D49.2
lung	C34.9-●	C78.0-●	D02.2-●	D14.3-●	D38.1	D49.1
azygos lobe	C34.1-●	C78.0-●	D02.2-●	D14.3-●	D38.1	D49.1
carina	C34.0-●	C78.0-●	D02.2-●	D14.3-●	D38.1	D49.1
hilus	C34.0-●	C78.0-●	D02.2-●	D14.3-●	D38.1	D49.1
linqula	C34.1-●	C78.0-●	D02.2-●	D14.3-●	D38.1	D49.1
lobe NEC	C34.9-●	C78.0-●	D02.2-●	D14.3-●	D38.1	D49.1
lower lobe	C34.3-●	C78.0-●	D02.2-●	D14.3-●	D38.1	D49.1
main bronchus	C34.0-●	C78.0-●	D02.2-●	D14.3-●	D38.1	D49.1
mesothelioma — see Mesothelioma						
middle lobe	C34.2	C78.0-●	D02.21	D14.31	D38.1	D49.1
overlapping lesion	C34.8-●	—	—	—	—	—
upper lobe	C34.1-●	C78.0-●	D02.2-●	D14.3-●	D38.1	D49.1

◀ New   ◀ Revised   ~~deleted~~ Deleted   ● Use Additional Character(s)

	Malignant Primary	Malignant Secondary	Ca in situ	Benign	Uncertain Behavior	Unspecified Behavior
lymph, lymphatic channel NEC	C49.9	C79.89	—	D21.9	D48.1	D49.2
gland (secondary)	—	C77.9	—	D36.0	D48.7	D49.89
abdominal	—	C77.2	—	D36.0	D48.7	D49.89
aortic	—	C77.2	—	D36.0	D48.7	D49.89
arm	—	C77.3	—	D36.0	D48.7	D49.89
auricular (anterior) (posterior)	—	C77.0	—	D36.0	D48.7	D49.89
axilla, axillary	—	C77.3	—	D36.0	D48.7	D49.89
brachial	—	C77.3	—	D36.0	D48.7	D49.89
bronchial	—	C77.1	—	D36.0	D48.7	D49.89
bronchopulmonary	—	C77.1	—	D36.0	D48.7	D49.89
celiac	—	C77.2	—	D36.0	D48.7	D49.89
cervical	—	C77.0	—	D36.0	D48.7	D49.89
cervicofacial	—	C77.0	—	D36.0	D48.7	D49.89
Cloquet	—	C77.4	—	D36.0	D48.7	D49.89
colic	—	C77.2	—	D36.0	D48.7	D49.89
common duct	—	C77.2	—	D36.0	D48.7	D49.89
cubital	—	C77.3	—	D36.0	D48.7	D49.89
diaphragmatic	—	C77.1	—	D36.0	D48.7	D49.89
epigastric, inferior	—	C77.1	—	D36.0	D48.7	D49.89
epitrochlear	—	C77.3	—	D36.0	D48.7	D49.89
esophageal	—	C77.1	—	D36.0	D48.7	D49.89
face	—	C77.0	—	D36.0	D48.7	D49.89
femoral	—	C77.4	—	D36.0	D48.7	D49.89
gastric	—	C77.2	—	D36.0	D48.7	D49.89
groin	—	C77.4	—	D36.0	D48.7	D49.89
head	—	C77.0	—	D36.0	D48.7	D49.89
hepatic	—	C77.2	—	D36.0	D48.7	D49.89
hilar (pulmonary)	—	C77.1	—	D36.0	D48.7	D49.89
splenic	—	C77.2	—	D36.0	D48.7	D49.89
hypogastric	—	C77.5	—	D36.0	D48.7	D49.89
ileocolic	—	C77.2	—	D36.0	D48.7	D49.89
iliac	—	C77.5	—	D36.0	D48.7	D49.89
infraclavicular	—	C77.3	—	D36.0	D48.7	D49.89
inguina, inguinal	—	C77.4	—	D36.0	D48.7	D49.89
innominate	—	C77.1	—	D36.0	D48.7	D49.89
intercostal	—	C77.1	—	D36.0	D48.7	D49.89
intestinal	—	C77.2	—	D36.0	D48.7	D49.89
intrabdominal	—	C77.2	—	D36.0	D48.7	D49.89
intrapelvic	—	C77.5	—	D36.0	D48.7	D49.89
intrathoracic	—	C77.1	—	D36.0	D48.7	D49.89
jugular	—	C77.0	—	D36.0	D48.7	D49.89
leg	—	C77.4	—	D36.0	D48.7	D49.89
limb						
lower	—	C77.4	—	D36.0	D48.7	D49.89
upper	—	C77.3	—	D36.0	D48.7	D49.89
lymph, lymphatic channel NEC (Continued)						
gland (Continued)						
lower limb	—	C77.4	—	D36.0	D48.7	D49.89
lumbar	—	C77.2	—	D36.0	D48.7	D49.89
mandibular	—	C77.0	—	D36.0	D48.7	D49.89
mediastinal	—	C77.1	—	D36.0	D48.7	D49.89
mesenteric (inferior) (superior)	—	C77.2	—	D36.0	D48.7	D49.89
midcolic	—	C77.2	—	D36.0	D48.7	D49.89
multiple sites in categories C77.0 - C77.5	—	C77.8	—	D36.0	D48.7	D49.89
neck	—	C77.0	—	D36.0	D48.7	D49.89
obturator	—	C77.5	—	D36.0	D48.7	D49.89
occipital	—	C77.0	—	D36.0	D48.7	D49.89
pancreatic	—	C77.2	—	D36.0	D48.7	D49.89
para-aortic	—	C77.2	—	D36.0	D48.7	D49.89
paracervical	—	C77.5	—	D36.0	D48.7	D49.89
parametrial	—	C77.5	—	D36.0	D48.7	D49.89
parasternal	—	C77.1	—	D36.0	D48.7	D49.89
parotid	—	C77.0	—	D36.0	D48.7	D49.89
pectoral	—	C77.3	—	D36.0	D48.7	D49.89
pelvic	—	C77.5	—	D36.0	D48.7	D49.89
peri-aortic	—	C77.2	—	D36.0	D48.7	D49.89
peripancreatic	—	C77.2	—	D36.0	D48.7	D49.89
popliteal	—	C77.4	—	D36.0	D48.7	D49.89
porta hepatis	—	C77.2	—	D36.0	D48.7	D49.89
portal	—	C77.2	—	D36.0	D48.7	D49.89
preauricular	—	C77.0	—	D36.0	D48.7	D49.89
prelaryngeal	—	C77.0	—	D36.0	D48.7	D49.89
presymphysial	—	C77.5	—	D36.0	D48.7	D49.89
pretracheal	—	C77.0	—	D36.0	D48.7	D49.89
primary (any site) NEC	C96.9	—	—	—	—	—
pulmonary (hiler)	—	C77.1	—	D36.0	D48.7	D49.89
pyloric	—	C77.2	—	D36.0	D48.7	D49.89
retroperitoneal	—	C77.2	—	D36.0	D48.7	D49.89
retropharyngeal	—	C77.0	—	D36.0	D48.7	D49.89
Rosenmuller's	—	C77.4	—	D36.0	D48.7	D49.89
sacral	—	C77.5	—	D36.0	D48.7	D49.89
scalene	—	C77.0	—	D36.0	D48.7	D49.89
site NEC	—	C77.9	—	D36.0	D48.7	D49.89
splenic (hilar)	—	C77.2	—	D36.0	D48.7	D49.89
subclavicular	—	C77.3	—	D36.0	D48.7	D49.89
subinguinal	—	C77.4	—	D36.0	D48.7	D49.89

TABLE OF NEOPLASMS

	Malignant Primary	Malignant Secondary	Ca in situ	Benign	Uncertain Behavior	Unspecified Behavior
lymph, lymphatic channel NEC *(Continued)*						
gland *(Continued)*						
sublingual	—	C77.0	—	D36.0	D48.7	D49.89
submandibular	—	C77.0	—	D36.0	D48.7	D49.89
submaxillary	—	C77.0	—	D36.0	D48.7	D49.89
submental	—	C77.0	—	D36.0	D48.7	D49.89
subscapular	—	C77.3	—	D36.0	D48.7	D49.89
supraclavicular	—	C77.0	—	D36.0	D48.7	D49.89
thoracic	—	C77.1	—	D36.0	D48.7	D49.89
tibial	—	C77.4	—	D36.0	D48.7	D49.89
tracheal	—	C77.1	—	D36.0	D48.7	D49.89
tracheobronchial	—	C77.1	—	D36.0	D48.7	D49.89
upper limb	—	C77.3	—	D36.0	D48.7	D49.89
Virchow's	—	C77.0	—	D36.0	D48.7	D49.89
node — *see also Neoplasm, lymph gland*						
primary NEC	C96.9	—	—	—	—	—
vessel — *see also Neoplasm, connective tissue*	C49.9	C79.89	—	D21.9	D48.1	D49.2
Mackenrodt's ligament	C57.7	C79.82	D07.39	D28.7	D39.8	D49.59
malar	C41.0	C79.51	—	D16.4-•	D48.0	D49.2
region — *see Neoplasm, cheek*						
mammary gland — *see Neoplasm, breast*						
mandible	C41.1	C79.51	—	D16.5-•	D48.0	D49.2
alveolar						
mucosa (carcinoma)	C03.1	C79.89	D00.03	D10.39	D37.09	D49.0
ridge or process	C41.1	C79.51	—	D16.5-•	D48.0	D49.2
marrow (bone) NEC	C96.9	C79.52	—	—	D47.9	D49.89
mastectomy site (skin) — *see also Neoplasm, breast, skin*	C44.501	C79.2	—	—	—	—
specified as breast tissue	C50.8-•	C79.81	—	—	—	—
mastoid (air cells) (antrum) (cavity)	C30.1	C78.39	D02.3	D14.0	D38.5	D49.1
bone or process	C41.0	C79.51	—	D16.4-•	D48.0	D49.2
maxilla, maxillary (superior)	C41.0	C79.51	—	D16.4-•	D48.0	D49.2
alveolar						
mucosa	C03.0	C79.89	D00.03	D10.39	D37.09	D49.0
ridge or process (carcinoma)	C41.0	C79.51	—	D16.4-•	D48.0	D49.2
antrum	C31.0	C78.39	D02.3	D14.0	D38.5	D49.1
carcinoma	C03.0	C79.51				
inferior — *see Neoplasm, mandible*						
sinus	C31.0	C78.39	D02.3	D14.0	D38.5	D49.1

	Malignant Primary	Malignant Secondary	Ca in situ	Benign	Uncertain Behavior	Unspecified Behavior
meatus external (ear) — *see also Neoplasm, skin, ear*	C44.20-•	C79.2	D04.2-•	D23.2-•	D48.5	D49.2
Meckel diverticulum, malignant	C17.3	C78.4	D01.49	D13.39	D37.2	D49.0
mediastinum, mediastinal	C38.3	C78.1	—	D15.2	D38.3	D49.89
anterior	C38.1	C78.1	—	D15.2	D38.3	D49.89
posterior	C38.2	C78.1	—	D15.2	D38.3	D49.89
medulla						
adrenal	C74.1-•	C79.7-•	D09.3	D35.0-•	D44.1-•	D49.7
oblongata	C71.7	C79.31	—	D33.1	D43.1	D49.6
meibomian gland	C44.10-•	C79.2	D04.1-•	D23.1-•	D48.5	D49.2
basal cell carcinoma	C44.11-•	—	—	—	—	—
sebaceous cell	C44.13-•	—	—	—	—	—
specified type NEC	C44.19-•	—	—	—	—	—
squamous cell carcinoma	C44.12-•	—	—	—	—	—
melanoma — *see Melanoma*						
meninges	C70.9	C79.49	—	D32.9	D42.9	D49.7
brain	C70.0	C79.32	—	D32.0	D42.0	D49.7
cerebral	C70.0	C79.32	—	D32.0	D42.0	D49.7
crainial	C70.0	C79.32	—	D32.0	D42.0	D49.7
intracranial	C70.0	C79.32	—	D32.0	D42.0	D49.7
spinal (cord)	C70.1	C79.49	—	D32.1	D42.1	D49.7
meniscus, knee joint (lateral) (medial)	C40.2-•	C79.51	—	D16.2-•	D48.0	D49.2
Merkel cell — *see Carcinoma, Merkel cell*						
mesentery, mesenteric	C48.1	C78.6	—	D20.1	D48.4	D49.0
mesoappendix	C48.1	C78.6	—	D20.1	D48.4	D49.0
mesocolon	C48.1	C78.6	—	D20.1	D48.4	D49.0
mesopharynx — *see Neoplasm, oropharynx*						
mesosalpinx	C57.1	C79.82	D07.39	D28.2	D39.8	D49.59
mesothelial tissue — *see Mesothelioma*						
mesothelioma — *see Mesothelioma*						
mesovarium	C57.1	C79.82	D07.39	D28.2	D39.8	D49.59
metacarpus (any bone)	C40.1-•	C79.51	—	D16.1-•	—	—
metastatic NEC — *see also Neoplasm, by site, secondary*	—	C79.9	—	—	—	—
metatarsus (any bone)	C40.3-•	C79.51	—	D16.3-•	—	—
midbrain	C71.7	C79.31	—	D33.1	D43.1	D49.6
milk duct — *see Neoplasm, breast*						
mons						
pubis	C51.9	C79.82	D07.1	D28.0	D39.8	D49.59
veneris	C51.9	C79.82	D07.1	D28.0	D39.8	D49.59

◀ New ◀ Revised ~~deleted~~ Deleted • Use Additional Character(s)

	Malignant Primary	Malignant Secondary	Ca in situ	Benign	Uncertain Behavior	Unspecified Behavior
motor tract	C72.9	C79.49	—	D33.9	D43.9	D49.7
brain	C71.9	C79.31	—	D33.2	D43.2	D49.6
cauda equina	C72.1	C79.49	—	D33.4	D43.4	D49.7
spinal	C72.0	C79.49	—	D33.4	D43.4	D49.7
mouth	C06.9	C79.89	D00.00	D10.30	D37.09	D49.0
book-leaf	C06.89	C79.89				
floor	C04.9	C79.89	D00.06	D10.2	D37.09	D49.0
anterior portion	C04.0	C79.89	D00.06	D10.2	D37.09	D49.0
lateral portion	C04.1	C79.89	D00.06	D10.2	D37.09	D49.0
overlapping lesion	C04.8	—	—	—	—	—
overlapping NEC	C06.80	—	—	—	—	—
roof	C05.9	C79.89	D00.00	D10.39	D37.09	D49.0
specified part NEC	C06.89	C79.89	D00.00	D10.39	D37.09	D49.0
vestibule	C06.1	C79.89	D00.00	D10.39	D37.09	D49.0
mucosa						
alveolar (ridge or process)	C03.9	C79.89	D00.03	D10.39	D37.09	D49.0
lower	C03.1	C79.89	D00.03	D10.39	D37.09	D49.0
upper	C03.0	C79.89	D00.03	D10.39	D37.09	D49.0
buccal	C06.0	C79.89	D00.02	D10.39	D37.09	D49.0
cheek	C06.0	C79.89	D00.02	D10.39	D37.09	D49.0
lip — see Neoplasm, lip, internal						
nasal	C30.0	C78.39	D02.3	D14.0	D38.5	D49.1
oral	C06.0	C79.89	D00.02	D10.39	D37.09	D49.0
Mullerian duct						
female	C57.7	C79.82	D07.39	D28.7	D39.8	D49.59
male	C63.7	C79.82	D07.69	D29.8	D40.8	D49.59
muscle — see also Neoplasm, connective tissue						
extraocular	C69.6-●	C79.49	D09.2-●	D31.6-●	D48.7	D49.89
myocardium	C38.0	C79.89	—	D15.1	D48.7	D49.89
myometrium	C54.2	C79.82	D07.0	D26.1	D39.0	D49.59
myopericardium	C38.0	C79.89	—	D15.1	D48.7	D49.89
nabothian gland (follicle)	C53.0	C79.82	D06.0	D26.0	D39.0	D49.59
nail — see also Neoplasm, skin, limb	C44.90	C79.2	D04.9	D23.9	D48.5	D49.2
finger — see also Neoplasm, skin, limb, upper	C44.60-●	C79.2	D04.6-●	D23.6-●	D48.5	D49.2
toe — see also Neoplasm, skin, limb, lower	C44.70-●	C79.2	D04.7-●	D23.7-●	D48.5	D49.2
nares, naris (anterior) (posterior)	C30.0	C78.39	D02.3	D14.0	D38.5	D49.1
nasal — see Neoplasm, nose						
nasolabial groove — see also Neoplasm, skin, face	C44.309	C79.2	D04.39	D23.39	D48.5	D49.2
nasolacrimal duct	C69.5-●	C79.49	D09.2-●	D31.5-●	D48.7	D49.89
nasopharynx, nasopharyngeal	C11.9	C79.89	D00.08	D10.6	D37.05	D49.0
floor	C11.3	C79.89	D00.08	D10.6	D37.05	D49.0
overlapping lesion	C11.8	—	—	—	—	—
roof	C11.0	C79.89	D00.08	D10.6	D37.05	D49.0
wall	C11.9	C79.89	D00.08	D10.6	D37.05	D49.0
anterior	C11.3	C79.89	D00.08	D10.6	D37.05	D49.0
lateral	C11.2	C79.89	D00.08	D10.6	D37.05	D49.0
posterior	C11.1	C79.89	D00.08	D10.6	D37.05	D49.0
superior	C11.0	C79.89	D00.08	D10.6	D37.05	D49.0
nates — see also Neoplasm, skin, trunk	C44.509	C79.2	D04.5	D23.5	D48.5	D49.2
neck NEC	C76.0	C79.89	D09.8	D36.7	D48.7	D49.89
skin	C44.40	—	—	—	—	—
basal cell carcinoma	C44.41	—	—	—	—	—
specified type NEC	C44.49	—	—	—	—	—
squamous cell carcinoma	C44.42	—	—	—	—	—
nerve (ganglion)	C47.9	C79.89	—	D36.10	D48.2	D49.2
abducens	C72.59	C79.49	—	D33.3	D43.3	D49.7
accessory (spinal)	C72.59	C79.49	—	D33.3	D43.3	D49.7
acoustic	C72.4-●	C79.49	—	D33.3	D43.3	D49.7
auditory	C72.4-●	C79.49	—	D33.3	D43.3	D49.7
autonomic NEC — see also Neoplasm, nerve, peripheral	C47.9	C79.89	—	D36.10	D48.2	D49.2
brachial	C47.1-●	C79.89	—	D36.12	D48.2	D49.2
cranial	C72.50	C79.49	—	D33.3	D43.3	D49.7
specified NEC	C72.59	C79.49	—	D33.3	D43.3	D49.7
facial	C72.59	C79.49	—	D33.3	D43.3	D49.7
femoral	C47.2-●	C79.89	—	D36.13	D48.2	D49.2
ganglion NEC — see also Neoplasm, nerve, peripheral	C47.9	C79.89	—	D36.10	D48.2	D49.2
glossopharyngeal	C72.59	C79.49	—	D33.3	D43.3	D49.7
hypoglossal	C72.59	C79.49	—	D33.3	D43.3	D49.7
intercostal	C47.3	C79.89	—	D36.14	D48.2	D49.2
lumbar	C47.6	C79.89	—	D36.17	D48.2	D49.2
median	C47.1-●	C79.89	—	D36.12	D48.2	D49.2
obturator	C47.2-●	C79.89	—	D36.13	D48.2	D49.2
oculomotor	C72.59	C79.49	—	D33.3	D43.3	D49.7
olfactory	C72.2-●	C79.49	—	D33.3	D43.3	D49.7
optic	C72.3-●	C79.49	—	D33.3	D43.3	D49.7
parasympathetic NEC	C47.9	C79.89	—	D36.10	D48.2	D49.2
peripheral NEC	C47.9	C79.89	—	D36.10	D48.2	D49.2
abdomen	C47.4	C79.89	—	D36.15	D48.2	D49.2
abdominal wall	C47.4	C79.89	—	D36.15	D48.2	D49.2

◀ New ◀ Revised ~~deleted~~ Deleted ● Use Additional Character(s)

TABLE OF NEOPLASMS

nerve (Continued)	Malignant Primary	Malignant Secondary	Ca in situ	Benign	Uncertain Behavior	Unspecified Behavior
peripheral NEC (Continued)						
ankle	C47.2-●	C79.89	—	D36.13	D48.2	D49.2
antecubital fossa or space	C47.1-●	C79.89	—	D36.12	D48.2	D49.2
arm	C47.1-●	C79.89	—	D36.12	D48.2	D49.2
auricle (ear)	C47.0	C79.89	—	D36.11	D48.2	D49.2
axilla	C47.3	C79.89	—	D36.12	D48.2	D49.2
back	C47.6	C79.89	—	D36.17	D48.2	D49.2
buttock	C47.5	C79.89	—	D36.16	D48.2	D49.2
calf	C47.2-●	C79.89	—	D36.13	D48.2	D49.2
cervical region	C47.0	C79.89	—	D36.11	D48.2	D49.2
cheek	C47.0	C79.89	—	D36.11	D48.2	D49.2
chest (wall)	C47.3	C79.89	—	D36.14	D48.2	D49.2
chin	C47.0	C79.89	—	D36.11	D48.2	D49.2
ear (external)	C47.0	C79.89	—	D36.11	D48.2	D49.2
elbow	C47.1-●	C79.89	—	D36.12	D48.2	D49.2
extrarectal	C47.5	C79.89	—	D36.16	D48.2	D49.2
extremity	C47.9	C79.89	—	D36.10	D48.2	D49.2
lower	C47.2-●	C79.89	—	D36.13	D48.2	D49.2
upper	C47.1-●	C79.89	—	D36.12	D48.2	D49.2
eyelid	C47.0	C79.89	—	D36.11	D48.2	D49.2
face	C47.0	C79.89	—	D36.11	D48.2	D49.2
finger	C47.1-●	C79.89	—	D36.12	D48.2	D49.2
flank	C47.6	C79.89	—	D36.17	D48.2	D49.2
foot	C47.2-●	C79.89	—	D36.13	D48.2	D49.2
forearm	C47.1-●	C79.89	—	D36.12	D48.2	D49.2
forehead	C47.0	C79.89	—	D36.11	D48.2	D49.2
gluteal region	C47.5	C79.89	—	D36.16	D48.2	D49.2
groin	C47.5	C79.89	—	D36.16	D48.2	D49.2
hand	C47.1-●	C79.89	—	D36.12	D48.2	D49.2
head	C47.0	C79.89	—	D36.11	D48.2	D49.2
heel	C47.2-●	C79.89	—	D36.13	D48.2	D49.2
hip	C47.2-●	C79.89	—	D36.13	D48.2	D49.2
infraclavicular region	C47.3	C79.89	—	D36.14	D48.2	D49.2
inguinal (canal) (region)	C47.5	C79.89	—	D36.16	D48.2	D49.2
intrathoracic	C47.3	C79.89	—	D36.14	D48.2	D49.2
ischiorectal fossa	C47.5	C79.89	—	D36.16	D48.2	D49.2
knee	C47.2-●	C79.89	—	D36.13	D48.2	D49.2
leg	C47.2-●	C79.89	—	D36.13	D48.2	D49.2
limb NEC	C47.9	C79.89	—	D36.10	D48.2	D49.2
lower	C47.2-●	C79.89	—	D36.13	D48.2	D49.2
upper	C47.1-●	C79.89	—	D36.12	D48.2	D49.2
nates	C47.5	C79.89	—	D36.16	D48.2	D49.2
neck	C47.0	C79.89	—	D36.11	D48.2	D49.2

nerve (Continued)	Malignant Primary	Malignant Secondary	Ca in situ	Benign	Uncertain Behavior	Unspecified Behavior
peripheral NEC (Continued)						
orbit	C69.6-●	C79.49	—	D31.6-●	D48.7	D49.2
pararectal	C47.5	C79.89	—	D36.16	D48.2	D49.2
paraurethral	C47.5	C79.89	—	D36.16	D48.2	D49.2
paravaginal	C47.5	C79.89	—	D36.16	D48.2	D49.2
pelvis (floor)	C47.5	C79.89	—	D36.16	D48.2	D49.2
pelvoabdominal	C47.8	C79.89	—	D36.17	D48.2	D49.2
perineum	C47.5	C79.89	—	D36.16	D48.2	D49.2
perirectal (tissue)	C47.5	C79.89	—	D36.16	D48.2	D49.2
periurethral (tissue)	C47.5	C79.89	—	D36.16	D48.2	D49.2
popliteal fossa or space	C47.2-●	C79.89	—	D36.13	D48.2	D49.2
presacral	C47.5	C79.89	—	D36.16	D48.2	D49.2
pterygoid fossa	C47.0	C79.89	—	D36.11	D48.2	D49.2
rectovaginal septum or wall	C47.5	C79.89	—	D36.16	D48.2	D49.2
rectovesical	C47.5	C79.89	—	D36.16	D48.2	D49.2
sacrococcygeal region	C47.5	C79.89	—	D36.16	D48.2	D49.2
scalp	C47.0	C79.89	—	D36.11	D48.2	D49.2
scapular region	C47.3	C79.89	—	D36.14	D48.2	D49.2
shoulder	C47.1-●	C79.89	—	D36.12	D48.2	D49.2
submental	C47.0	C79.89	—	D36.11	D48.2	D49.2
supraclavicular region	C47.0	C79.89	—	D36.11	D48.2	D49.2
temple	C47.0	C79.89	—	D36.11	D48.2	D49.2
temporal region	C47.0	C79.89	—	D36.11	D48.2	D49.2
thigh	C47.2-●	C79.89	—	D36.13	D48.2	D49.2
thoracic (duct) (wall)	C47.3	C79.89	—	D36.14	D48.2	D49.2
thorax	C47.3	C79.89	—	D36.14	D48.2	D49.2
thumb	C47.1-●	C79.89	—	D36.12	D48.2	D49.2
toe	C47.2-●	C79.89	—	D36.13	D48.2	D49.2
trunk	C47.6	C79.89	—	D36.17	D48.2	D49.2
umbilicus	C47.4	C79.89	—	D36.15	D48.2	D49.2
vesicorectal	C47.5	C79.89	—	D36.16	D48.2	D49.2
wrist	C47.1-●	C79.89	—	D36.12	D48.2	D49.2
radial	C47.1-●	C79.89	—	D36.12	D48.2	D49.2
sacral	C47.5	C79.89	—	D36.16	D48.2	D49.2
sciatic	C47.2-●	C79.89	—	D36.13	D48.2	D49.2
spinal NEC	C47.9	C79.89	—	D36.10	D48.2	D49.2
accessory	C72.59	C79.49	—	D33.3	D43.3	D49.7
sympathetic NEC — see also Neoplasm, nerve, peripheral	C47.9	C79.89	—	D36.10	D48.2	D49.2
trigeminal	C72.59	C79.49	—	D33.3	D43.3	D49.7
trochlear	C72.59	C79.49	—	D33.3	D43.3	D49.7
ulnar	C47.1-●	C79.89	—	D36.12	D48.2	D49.2
vagus	C72.59	C79.49	—	D33.3	D43.3	D49.7

◀ New ◀ Revised ~~deleted~~ Deleted ● Use Additional Character(s)

	Malignant Primary	Malignant Secondary	Ca in situ	Benign	Uncertain Behavior	Unspecified Behavior
nervous system (central)	C72.9	C79.40	—	D33.9	D43.9	D49.7
autonomic — see Neoplasm, nerve, peripheral						
parasympathetic — see Neoplasm, nerve, peripheral						
specified site NEC	—	C79.49	—	D33.7	D43.8	—
sympathetic — see Neoplasm, nerve, peripheral						
nevus — see Nevus						
nipple	C50.0-•	C79.81	D05.-•	D24.-•	—	—
nose, nasal	C76.0	C79.89	D09.8	D36.7	D48.7	D49.89
ala (external) (nasi) — see also Neoplasm, nose, skin	C44.301	C79.2	D04.39	D23.39	D48.5	D49.2
bone	C41.0	C79.51	—	D16.4-•	D48.0	D49.2
cartilage	C30.0	C78.39	D02.3	D14.0	D38.5	D49.1
cavity	C30.0	C78.39	D02.3	D14.0	D38.5	D49.1
choana	C11.3	C79.89	D00.08	D10.6	D37.05	D49.0
external (skin) — see also Neoplasm, nose, skin	C44.301	C79.2	D04.39	D23.39	D48.5	D49.2
fossa	C30.0	C78.39	D02.3	D14.0	D38.5	D49.1
internal	C30.0	C78.39	D02.3	D14.0	D38.5	D49.1
mucosa	C30.0	C78.39	D02.3	D14.0	D38.5	D49.1
septum	C30.0	C78.39	D02.3	D14.0	D38.5	D49.1
posterior margin	C11.3	C79.89	D00.08	D10.6	D37.05	D49.0
sinus — see Neoplasm, sinus						
skin	C44.301	C79.2	D04.39	D23.39	D48.5	D49.2
basal cell carcinoma	C44.311	—	—	—	—	—
specified type NEC	C44.391	—	—	—	—	—
squamous cell carcinoma	C44.321	—	—	—	—	—
turbinate (mucosa)	C30.0	C78.39	D02.3	D14.0	D38.5	D49.1
bone	C41.0	C79.51	—	D16.4-•	D48.0	D49.2
vestibule	C30.0	C78.39	D02.3	D14.0	D38.5	D49.1
nostril	C30.0	C78.39	D02.3	D14.0	D38.5	D49.1
nucleus pulposus	C41.2	C79.51	—	D16.6	D48.0	D49.2
occipital						
bone	C41.0	C79.51	—	D16.4-•	D48.0	D49.2
lobe or pole, brain	C71.4	C79.31	—	D33.0	D43.0	D49.6
odontogenic — see Neoplasm, jaw, bone						
olfactory nerve or bulb	C72.2-•	C79.49	—	D33.3	D43.3	D49.7
olive (brain)	C71.7	C79.31	—	D33.1	D43.1	D49.6
omentum	C48.1	C78.6	—	D20.1	D48.4	D49.0
operculum (brain)	C71.0	C79.31	—	D33.0	D43.0	D49.6
optic nerve, chiasm, or tract	C72.3-•	C79.49	—	D33.3	D43.3	D49.7

	Malignant Primary	Malignant Secondary	Ca in situ	Benign	Uncertain Behavior	Unspecified Behavior
oral (cavity)	C06.9	C79.89	D00.00	D10.30	D37.09	D49.0
ill-defined	C14.8	C79.89	D00.00	D10.30	D37.09	D49.0
mucosa	C06.0	C79.89	D00.02	D10.39	D37.09	D49.0
orbit	C69.6-•	C79.49	D09.2-•	D31.6-•	D48.7	D49.89
autonomic nerve	C69.6-•	C79.49	—	D31.6-•	D48.7	D49.2
bone	C41.0	C79.51	—	D16.4-•	D48.0	D49.2
eye	C69.6-•	C79.49	D09.2-•	D31.6-•	D48.7	D49.89
peripheral nerves	C69.6-•	C79.49	—	D31.6-•	D48.7	D49.2
soft parts	C69.6-•	C79.49	D09.2-•	D31.6-•	D48.7	D49.89
organ of Zuckerkandl	C75.5	C79.89	—	D35.6	D44.7	D49.7
oropharynx	C10.9	C79.89	D00.08	D10.5	D37.05	D49.0
branchial cleft (vestige)	C10.4	C79.89	D00.08	D10.5	D37.05	D49.0
junctional region	C10.8	C79.89	D00.08	D10.5	D37.05	D49.0
lateral wall	C10.2	C79.89	D00.08	D10.5	D37.05	D49.0
overlapping lesion	C10.8	—	—	—	—	—
pillars or fauces	C09.1	C79.89	D00.08	D10.5	D37.05	D49.0
posterior wall	C10.3	C79.89	D00.08	D10.5	D37.05	D49.0
vallecula	C10.0	C79.89	D00.08	D10.5	D37.05	D49.0
os						
external	C53.1	C79.82	D06.1	D26.0	D39.0	D49.59
internal	C53.0	C79.82	D06.0	D26.0	D39.0	D49.59
ovary	C56.-•	C79.6-•	D07.39	D27.-•	D39.1-•	D49.59
oviduct	C57.0-•	C79.82	D07.39	D28.2	D39.8	D49.59
palate	C05.9	C79.89	D00.00	D10.39	D37.09	D49.0
hard	C05.0	C79.89	D00.05	D10.39	D37.09	D49.0
junction of hard and soft palate	C05.9	C79.89	D00.00	D10.39	D37.09	D49.0
overlapping lesions	C05.8	—	—	—	—	—
soft	C05.1	C79.89	D00.04	D10.39	D37.09	D49.0
nasopharyngeal surface	C11.3	C79.89	D00.08	D10.6	D37.05	D49.0
posterior surface	C11.3	C79.89	D00.08	D10.6	D37.05	D49.0
superior surface	C11.3	C79.89	D00.08	D10.6	D37.05	D49.0
palatoglossal arch	C09.1	C79.89	D00.00	D10.5	D37.09	D49.0
palatopharyngeal arch	C09.1	C79.89	D00.00	D10.5	D37.09	D49.0
pallium	C71.0	C79.31	—	D33.0	D43.0	D49.6
palpebra	C44.10-•	C79.2	D04.1-•	D23.1-•	D48.5	D49.2
basal cell carcinoma	C44.11-•	—	—	—	—	—
sebaceous cell	C44.13-•	—	—	—	—	—
specified type NEC	C44.19-•	—	—	—	—	—
squamous cell carcinoma	C44.12-•	—	—	—	—	—
pancreas	C25.9	C78.89	D01.7	D13.6	D37.8	D49.0
body	C25.1	C78.89	D01.7	D13.6	D37.8	D49.0
duct (of Santorini) (of Wirsung)	C25.3	C78.89	D01.7	D13.6	D37.8	D49.0
ectopic tissue	C25.7	C78.89	—	D13.6	D37.8	D49.0
head	C25.0	C78.89	D01.7	D13.6	D37.8	D49.0

◀ New   ◀ Revised   deleted Deleted   • Use Additional Character(s)

	Malignant Primary	Malignant Secondary	Ca in situ	Benign	Uncertain Behavior	Unspecified Behavior
pancreas *(Continued)*						
islet cells	C25.4	C78.89	D01.7	D13.7	D37.8	D49.0
neck	C25.7	C78.89	D01.7	D13.6	D37.8	D49.0
overlapping lesion	C25.8	—	—	—	—	—
tail	C25.2	C78.89	D01.7	D13.6	D37.8	D49.0
para-aortic body	C75.5	C79.89	—	D35.6	D44.7	D49.7
paraganglion NEC	C75.5	C79.89	—	D35.6	D44.7	D49.7
parametrium	C57.3	C79.82	—	D28.2	D39.8	D49.59
paranephric	C48.0	C78.6	—	D20.0	D48.3	D49.0
pararectal	C76.3	C79.89	—	D36.7	D48.7	D49.89
parasagittal (region)	C76.0	C79.89	D09.8	D36.7	D48.7	D49.89
parasellar	C72.9	C79.49	—	D33.9	D43.8	D49.7
parathyroid (gland)	C75.0	C79.89	D09.3	D35.1	D44.2	D49.7
paraurethral	C76.3	C79.89	—	D36.7	D48.7	D49.89
gland	C68.1	C79.19	D09.19	D30.8	D41.8	D49.59
paravaginal	C76.3	C79.89	—	D36.7	D48.7	D49.89
parenchyma, kidney	C64.-●	C79.0-●	D09.19	D30.0-●	D41.0-●	D49.51-●
parietal						
bone	C41.0	C79.51	—	D16.4-●	D48.0	D49.2
lobe, brain	C71.3	C79.31	—	D33.0	D43.0	D49.6
paroophoron	C57.1	C79.82	D07.39	D28.2	D39.8	D49.59
parotid (duct) (gland)	C07	C79.89	D00.00	D11.0	D37.030	D49.0
parovarium	C57.1	C79.82	D07.39	D28.2	D39.8	D49.59
patella	C40.20	C79.51	—	—	—	—
peduncle, cerebral	C71.7	C79.31	—	D33.1	D43.1	D49.6
pelvirectal junction	C19	C78.5	D01.1	D12.7	D37.5	D49.0
pelvis, pelvic	C76.3	C79.89	D09.8	D36.7	D48.7	D49.89
bone	C41.4	C79.51	—	D16.8	D48.0	D49.2
floor	C76.3	C79.89	D09.8	D36.7	D48.7	D49.89
renal	C65.-●	C79.0-●	D09.19	D30.1-●	D41.1-●	D49.51-●
viscera	C76.3	C79.89	D09.8	D36.7	D48.7	D49.89
wall	C76.3	C79.89	D09.8	D36.7	D48.7	D49.89
pelvo-abdominal	C76.8	C79.89	D09.8	D36.7	D48.7	D49.89
penis	C60.9	C79.82	D07.4	D29.0	D40.8	D49.59
body	C60.2	C79.82	D07.4	D29.0	D40.8	D49.59
corpus (cavernosum)	C60.2	C79.82	D07.4	D29.0	D40.8	D49.59
glans	C60.1	C79.82	D07.4	D29.0	D40.8	D49.59
overlapping sites	C60.8	—	—	—	—	—
skin NEC	C60.9	C79.82	D07.4	D29.0	D40.8	D49.59
periadrenal (tissue)	C48.0	C78.6	—	D20.0	D48.3	D49.0
perianal (skin) — *see also* Neoplasm, anus, skin	C44.500	C79.2	D04.5	D23.5	D48.5	D49.2
pericardium	C38.0	C79.89	—	D15.1	D48.7	D49.89
perinephric	C48.0	C78.6	—	D20.0	D48.3	D49.0
perineum	C76.3	C79.89	D09.8	D36.7	D48.7	D49.89
periodontal tissue NEC	C03.9	C79.89	D00.03	D10.39	D37.09	D49.0
periosteum — *see Neoplasm, bone*						
peripancreatic	C48.0	C78.6	—	D20.0	D48.3	D49.0
peripheral nerve NEC	C47.9	C79.89	—	D36.10	D48.2	D49.2
perirectal (tissue)	C76.3	C79.89	—	D36.7	D48.7	D49.89
perirenal (tissue)	C48.0	C78.6	—	D20.0	D48.3	D49.0
peritoneum, peritoneal (cavity)	C48.2	C78.6	—	D20.1	D48.4	D49.0
benign mesothelial tissue — *see* Mesothelioma, benign						
overlapping lesion	C48.8	—	—	—	—	—
with digestive organs	C26.9					
parietal	C48.1	C78.6	—	D20.1	D48.4	D49.0
pelvic	C48.1	C78.6	—	D20.1	D48.4	D49.0
specified part NEC	C48.1	C78.6	—	D20.1	D48.4	D49.0
peritonsillar (tissue)	C76.0	C79.89	D09.8	D36.7	D48.7	D49.89
periurethral tissue	C76.3	C79.89	—	D36.7	D48.7	D49.89
phalanges						
foot	C40.3-●	C79.51	—	D16.3-●	—	—
hand	C40.1-●	C79.51	—	D16.1-●	—	—
pharynx, pharyngeal	C14.0	C79.89	D00.08	D10.9	D37.05	D49.0
bursa	C11.1	C79.89	D00.08	D10.6	D37.05	D49.0
fornix	C11.3	C79.89	D00.08	D10.6	D37.05	D49.0
recess	C11.2	C79.89	D00.08	D10.6	D37.05	D49.0
region	C14.0	C79.89	D00.08	D10.9	D37.05	D49.0
tonsil	C11.1	C79.89	D00.08	D10.6	D37.05	D49.0
wall (lateral) (posterior)	C14.0	C79.89	D00.08	D10.9	D37.05	D49.0
pia mater	C70.9	C79.40	—	D32.9	D42.9	D49.7
cerebral	C70.0	C79.32	—	D32.0	D42.0	D49.7
cranial	C70.0	C79.32	—	D32.0	D42.0	D49.7
spinal	C70.1	C79.49	—	D32.1	D42.1	D49.7
pillars of fauces	C09.1	C79.89	D00.08	D10.5	D37.05	D49.0
pineal (body) (gland)	C75.3	C79.89	D09.3	D35.4	D44.5	D49.7
pinna (ear) NEC — *see also* Neoplasm, skin, ear	C44.20-●	C79.2	D04.2-●	D23.2-●	D48.5	D49.2
piriform fossa or sinus	C12	C79.89	D00.08	D10.7	D37.05	D49.0
pituitary (body) (fossa) (gland) (lobe)	C75.1	C79.89	D09.3	D35.2	D44.3	D49.7
placenta	C58	C79.82	D07.0	D26.7	D39.2	D49.59
pleura, pleural (cavity)	C38.4	C78.2	—	D19.0	D38.2	D49.1
overlapping lesion with heart or mediastinum	C38.8	—	—	—	—	—
parietal	C38.4	C78.2	—	D19.0	D38.2	D49.1
visceral	C38.4	C78.2	—	D19.0	D38.2	D49.1

◀ New   ◀ Revised   ~~deleted~~ Deleted   ● Use Additional Character(s)

	Malignant Primary	Malignant Secondary	Ca in situ	Benign	Uncertain Behavior	Unspecified Behavior
plexus						
brachial	C47.1-●	C79.89	—	D36.12	D48.2	D49.2
cervical	C47.0	C79.89	—	D36.11	D48.2	D49.2
choroid	C71.5	C79.31	—	D33.0	D43.0	D49.6
lumbosacral	C47.5	C79.89	—	D36.16	D48.2	D49.2
sacral	C47.5	C79.89	—	D36.16	D48.2	D49.2
pluriendocrine	C75.8	C79.89	D09.3	D35.7	D44.9	D49.7
pole						
frontal	C71.1	C79.31	—	D33.0	D43.0	D49.6
occipital	C71.4	C79.31	—	D33.0	D43.0	D49.6
pons (varolii)	C71.7	C79.31	—	D33.1	D43.1	D49.6
popliteal fossa or space	C76.5-●	C79.89	D04.7-●	D36.7	D48.7	D49.89
postcricoid (region)	C13.0	C79.89	D00.08	D10.7	D37.05	D49.0
posterior fossa (cranial)	C71.9	C79.31	—	D33.2	D43.2	D49.6
postnasal space	C11.9	C79.89	D00.08	D10.6	D37.05	D49.0
prepuce	C60.0	C79.82	D07.4	D29.0	D40.8	D49.59
prepylorus	C16.4	C78.89	D00.2	D13.1	D37.1	D49.0
presacral (region)	C76.3	C79.89	—	D36.7	D48.7	D49.89
prostate (gland)	C61	C79.82	D07.5	D29.1	D40.0	D49.59
utricle	C68.0	C79.19	D09.19	D30.4	D41.3	D49.59
pterygoid fossa	C49.0	C79.89	—	D21.0	D48.1	D49.2
pubic bone	C41.4	C79.51	—	D16.8	D48.0	D49.2
pudenda, pudendum (female)	C51.9	C79.82	D07.1	D28.0	D39.8	D49.59
pulmonary — see also Neoplasm, lung	C34.9-●	C78.0-●	D02.2-●	D14.3-●	D38.1	D49.1
putamen	C71.0	C79.31	—	D33.0	D43.0	D49.6
pyloric						
antrum	C16.3	C78.89	D00.2	D13.1	D37.1	D49.0
canal	C16.4	C78.89	D00.2	D13.1	D37.1	D49.0
pylorus	C16.4	C78.89	D00.2	D13.1	D37.1	D49.0
pyramid (brain)	C71.7	C79.31	—	D33.1	D43.1	D49.6
pyriform fossa or sinus	C12	C79.89	D00.08	D10.7	D37.05	D49.0
radius (any part)	C40.0-●	C79.51	—	D16.0-●	—	—
Rathke's pouch	C75.1	C79.89	D09.3	D35.2	D44.3	D49.7
rectosigmoid (junction)	C19	C78.5	D01.1	D12.7	D37.5	D49.0
overlapping lesion with anus or rectum	C21.8	—	—	—	—	—
rectouterine pouch	C48.1	C78.6	—	D20.1	D48.4	D49.0
rectovaginal septum or wall	C76.3	C79.89	D09.8	D36.7	D48.7	D49.89
rectovesical septum	C76.3	C79.89	D09.8	D36.7	D48.7	D49.89
rectum (ampulla)	C20	C78.5	D01.2	D12.8	D37.5	D49.0
and colon	C19	C78.5	D01.1	D12.7	D37.5	D49.0
overlapping lesion with anus or rectosigmoid junction	C21.8	—	—	—	—	—
renal	C64.-●	C79.0-●	D09.19	D30.0-●	D41.0-●	D49.51-●
calyx	C65.-●	C79.0-●	D09.19	D30.1-●	D41.1-●	D49.51-●
hilus	C65.-●	C79.0-●	D09.19	D30.1-●	D41.1-●	D49.51-●
parenchyma	C64.-●	C79.0-●	D09.19	D30.0-●	D41.0-●	D49.51-●
pelvis	C65.-●	C79.0-●	D09.19	D30.1-●	D41.1-●	D49.51-●
respiratory						
organs or system NEC	C39.9	C78.30	D02.4	D14.4	D38.6	D49.1
tract NEC	C39.9	C78.30	D02.4	D14.4	D38.5	D49.1
upper	C39.0	C78.30	D02.4	D14.4	D38.5	D49.1
retina	C69.2-●	C79.49	D09.2-●	D31.2-●	D48.7	D49.81
retrobulbar	C69.6-●	C79.49	—	D31.6-●	D48.7	D49.89
retrocecal	C48.0	C78.6	—	D20.0	D48.3	D49.0
retromolar (area) (triangle) (trigone)	C06.2	C79.89	D00.00	D10.39	D37.09	D49.0
retro-orbital	C76.0	C79.89	D09.8	D36.7	D48.7	D49.89
retroperitoneal (space) (tissue)	C48.0	C78.6	—	D20.0	D48.3	D49.0
retroperitoneum	C48.0	C78.6	—	D20.0	D48.3	D49.0
retropharyngeal	C14.0	C79.89	D00.08	D10.9	D37.05	D49.0
retrovesical (septum)	C76.3	C79.89	D09.8	D36.7	D48.7	D49.89
rhinencephalon	C71.0	C79.31	—	D33.0	D43.0	D49.6
rib	C41.3	C79.51	—	D16.7	D48.0	D49.2
Rosenmuller's fossa	C11.2	C79.89	D00.08	D10.6	D37.05	D49.0
round ligament	C57.2	C79.82	—	D28.2	D39.8	D49.59
sacrococcyx, sacrococcygeal	C41.4	C79.51	—	D16.8	D48.0	D49.2
region	C76.3	C79.89	D09.8	D36.7	D48.7	D49.89
sacrouterine ligament	C57.3	C79.82	—	D28.2	D39.8	D49.59
sacrum, sacral (vertebra)	C41.4	C79.51	—	D16.8	D48.0	D49.2
salivary gland or duct (major)	C08.9	C79.89	D00.00	D11.9	D37.039	D49.0
minor NEC	C06.9	C79.89	D00.00	D10.39	D37.04	D49.0
overlapping lesion	C08.9	—	—	—	—	—
parotid	C07	C79.89	D00.00	D11.0	D37.030	D49.0
pluriglandular	C08.9	C79.89	D00.00	D11.9	D37.039	D49.0
sublingual	C08.1	C79.89	D00.00	D11.7	D37.031	D49.0
submandibular	C08.0	C79.89	D00.00	D11.7	D37.032	D49.0
submaxillary	C08.0	C79.89	D00.00	D11.7	D37.032	D49.0
salpinx (uterine)	C57.0-●	C79.82	D07.39	D28.2	D39.8	D49.59
Santorini's duct	C25.3	C78.89	D01.7	D13.6	D37.8	D49.0
scalp	C44.40	C79.2	D04.4	D23.4	D48.5	D49.2
basal cell carcinoma	C44.41	—	—	—	—	—
specified type NEC	C44.49	—	—	—	—	—
squamous cell carcinoma	C44.42	—	—	—	—	—
scapula (any part)	C40.0-●	C79.51	—	D16.0-●	—	—
scapular region	C76.1	C79.89	D09.8	D36.7	D48.7	D49.89

	Malignant Primary	Malignant Secondary	Ca in situ	Benign	Uncertain Behavior	Unspecified Behavior
scar NEC — *see also Neoplasm, skin, by site*	C44.90	C79.2	D04.9	D23.9	D48.5	D49.2
sciatic nerve	C47.2-●	C79.89	—	D36.13	D48.2	D49.2
sclera	C69.4-●	C79.49	D09.2-●	D31.4-●	D48.7	D49.89
scrotum (skin)	C63.2	C79.82	D07.61	D29.4	D40.8	D49.59
sebaceous gland — *see Neoplasm, skin*						
sella turcica	C75.1	C79.89	D09.3	D35.2	D44.3	D49.7
bone	C41.0	C79.51	—	D16.4-●	D48.0	D49.2
semilunar cartilage (knee)	C40.2-●	C79.51	—	D16.2-●	D48.0	D49.2
seminal vesicle	C63.7	C79.82	D07.69	D29.8	D40.8	D49.59
septum						
nasal	C30.0	C78.39	D02.3	D14.0	D38.5	D49.1
posterior margin	C11.3	C79.89	D00.08	D10.6	D37.05	D49.0
rectovaginal	C76.3	C79.89	D09.8	D36.7	D48.7	D49.89
rectovesical	C76.3	C79.89	D09.8	D36.7	D48.7	D49.89
urethrovaginal	C57.9	C79.82	D07.30	D28.9	D39.9	D49.59
vesicovaginal	C57.9	C79.82	D07.30	D28.9	D39.9	D49.59
shoulder NEC	C76.4-●	C79.89	D04.6-●	D36.7	D48.7	D49.89
sigmoid flexure (lower) (upper)	C18.7	C78.5	D01.0	D12.5	D37.4	D49.0
sinus (accessory)	C31.9	C78.39	D02.3	D14.0	D38.5	D49.1
bone (any)	C41.0	C79.51	—	D16.4-●	D48.0	D49.2
ethmoidal	C31.1	C78.39	D02.3	D14.0	D38.5	D49.1
frontal	C31.2	C78.39	D02.3	D14.0	D38.5	D49.1
maxillary	C31.0	C78.39	D02.3	D14.0	D38.5	D49.1
nasal, paranasal NEC	C31.9	C78.39	D02.3	D14.0	D38.5	D49.1
overlapping lesion	C31.8	—				
pyriform	C12	C79.89	D00.08	D10.7	D37.05	D49.0
sphenoid	C31.3	C78.39	D02.3	D14.0	D38.5	D49.1
skeleton, skeletal NEC	C41.9	C79.51	—	D16.9-●	D48.0	D49.2
Skene's gland	C68.1	C79.19	D09.19	D30.8	D41.8	D49.59
skin NOS	C44.90	C79.2	D04.9	D23.9	D48.5	D49.2
abdominal wall	C44.509	C79.2	D04.5	D23.5	D48.5	D49.2
basal cell carcinoma	C44.519	—	—	—	—	—
specified type NEC	C44.599	—	—	—	—	—
squamous cell carcinoma	C44.529	—	—	—	—	—
ala nasi — *see also Neoplasm, nose, skin*	C44.301	C79.2	D04.39	D23.39	D48.5	D49.2
ankle — *see also skin, limb, lower*	C44.70-●	C79.2	D04.7-●	D23.7-●	D48.5	D49.2
antecubital space — *see also Neoplasm, skin, limb, upper*	C44.60-●	C79.2	D04.6-●	D23.6-●	D48.5	D49.2

	Malignant Primary	Malignant Secondary	Ca in situ	Benign	Uncertain Behavior	Unspecified Behavior
skin NOS *(Continued)*						
anus	C44.500	C79.2	D04.5	D23.5	D48.5	D49.2
basal cell carcinoma	C44.510	—	—	—	—	—
specified type NEC	C44.590	—	—	—	—	—
squamous cell carcinoma	C44.520	—	—	—	—	—
arm — *see also Neoplasm, skin, limb, upper*	C44.60-●	C79.2	D04.6-●	D23.6-●	D48.5	D49.2
auditory canal (external) — *see also Neoplasm, skin, ear*	C44.20-●	C79.2	D04.2-●	D23.2-●	D48.5	D49.2
auricle (ear) — *see also Neoplasm, skin, ear*	C44.20-●	C79.2	D04.2-●	D23.2-●	D48.5	D49.2
auricular canal (external) — *see also Neoplasm, skin, ear*	C44.20-●	C79.2	D04.2-●	D23.2-●	D48.5	D49.2
axilla, axillary fold — *see also Neoplasm, skin, trunk*	C44.509	C79.2	D04.5	D23.5	D48.5	D49.2
back — *see also Neoplasm, skin, trunk*	C44.509	C79.2	D04.5	D23.5	D48.5	D49.2
basal cell carcinoma	C44.91					
breast	C44.501	C79.2	D04.5	D23.5	D48.5	D49.2
basal cell carcinoma	C44.511	—	—	—	—	—
specified type NEC	C44.591	—	—	—	—	—
squamous cell carcinoma	C44.521	—	—	—	—	—
brow — *see also Neoplasm, skin, face*	C44.309	C79.2	D04.39	D23.39	D48.5	D49.2
buttock — *see also Neoplasm, skin, trunk*	C44.509	C79.2	D04.5	D23.5	D48.5	D49.2
calf — *see also Neoplasm, skin, limb, lower*	C44.70-●	C79.2	D04.7-●	D23.7-●	D48.5	D49.2
canthus (eye) (inner) (outer)	C44.10-●	C79.2	D04.1-●	D23.1-●	D48.5	D49.2
basal cell carcinoma	C44.11-●	—	—	—	—	—
sebaceous cell	C44.13-●	—	—	—	—	—
specified type NEC	C44.19-●	—	—	—	—	—
squamous cell carcinoma	C44.12-●	—	—	—	—	—
cervical region — *see also Neoplasm, skin, neck*	C44.40	C79.2	D04.4	D23.4	D48.5	D49.2
cheek (external) — *see also Neoplasm, skin, face*	C44.309	C79.2	D04.39	D23.39	D48.5	D49.2
chest (wall) — *see also Neoplasm, skin, trunk*	C44.509	C79.2	D04.5	D23.5	D48.5	D49.2
chin — *see also Neoplasm, skin, face*	C44.309	C79.2	D04.39	D23.39	D48.5	D49.2
clavicular area — *see also Neoplasm, skin, trunk*	C44.509	C79.2	D04.5	D23.5	D48.5	D49.2
clitoris	C51.2	C79.82	D07.1	D28.0	D39.8	D49.59

◀ New ◀ Revised ~~deleted~~ Deleted ● Use Additional Character(s)

skin NOS (Continued)

	Malignant Primary	Malignant Secondary	Ca in situ	Benign	Uncertain Behavior	Unspecified Behavior
columnella — see also Neoplasm, skin, face	C44.309	C79.2	D04.39	D23.39	D48.5	D49.2
concha — see also Neoplasm, skin, ear	C44.20-●	C79.2	D04.2-●	D23.2-●	D48.5	D49.2
ear (external)	C44.20-●	C79.2	D04.2-●	D23.2-●	D48.5	D49.2
basal cell carcinoma	C44.21-●	—	—	—	—	—
specified type NEC	C44.29-●	—	—	—	—	—
squamous cell carcinoma	C44.22-●	—	—	—	—	—
elbow — see also Neoplasm, skin, limb, upper	C44.60-●	C79.2	D04.6-●	D23.6-●	D48.5	D49.2
eyebrow — see also Neoplasm, skin, face	C44.309	C79.2	D04.39	D23.39	D48.5	D49.2
eyelid	C44.10-●	C79.2	D04.1-●	D23.1-●	D48.5	D49.2
basal cell carcinoma	C44.11-●	—	—	—	—	—
sebaceous cell	C44.13-●	—	—	—	—	—
specified type NEC	C44.19-●	—	—	—	—	—
squamous cell carcinoma	C44.12-●	—	—	—	—	—
face NOS	C44.300	C79.2	D04.30	D23.30	D48.5	D49.2
basal cell carcinoma	C44.310	—	—	—	—	—
specified type NEC	C44.390	—	—	—	—	—
squamous cell carcinoma	C44.320	—	—	—	—	—
female genital organs (external)	C51.9	C79.82	D07.1	D28.0	D39.8	D49.59
clitoris	C51.2	C79.82	D07.1	D28.0	D39.8	D49.59
labium NEC	C51.9	C79.82	D07.1	D28.0	D39.8	D49.59
majus	C51.0	C79.82	D07.1	D28.0	D39.8	D49.59
minus	C51.1	C79.82	D07.1	D28.0	D39.8	D49.59
pudendum	C51.9	C79.82	D07.1	D28.0	D39.8	D49.59
vulva	C51.9	C79.82	D07.1	D28.0	D39.8	D49.59
finger — see also Neoplasm, skin, limb, upper	C44.60-●	C79.2	D04.6-●	D23.6-●	D48.5	D49.2
flank — see also Neoplasm, skin, trunk	C44.509	C79.2	D04.5	D23.5	D48.5	D49.2
foot — see also Neoplasm, skin, limb, lower	C44.70-●	C79.2	D04.7-●	D23.7-●	D48.5	D49.2
forearm — see also Neoplasm, skin, limb, upper	C44.60-●	C79.2	D04.6-●	D23.6-●	D48.5	D49.2
forehead — see also Neoplasm, skin, face	C44.309	C79.2	D04.39	D23.39	D48.5	D49.2
glabella — see also Neoplasm, skin, face	C44.309	C79.2	D04.39	D23.39	D48.5	D49.2
gluteal region — see also Neoplasm, skin, trunk	C44.509	C79.2	D04.5	D23.5	D48.5	D49.2
groin — see also Neoplasm, skin, trunk	C44.509	C79.2	D04.5	D23.5	D48.5	D49.2

skin NOS (Continued)

	Malignant Primary	Malignant Secondary	Ca in situ	Benign	Uncertain Behavior	Unspecified Behavior
hand — see also Neoplasm, skin, limb, upper	C44.60-●	C79.2	D04.6-●	D23.6-●	D48.5	D49.2
head NEC — see also Neoplasm, skin, scalp	C44.40	C79.2	D04.4	D23.4	D48.5	D49.2
heel — see also Neoplasm, skin, limb, lower	C44.70-●	C79.2	D04.7-●	D23.7-●	D48.5	D49.2
helix — see also Neoplasm, skin, ear	C44.20-●	C79.2	D04.2-●	D23.2-●	D48.5	D49.2
hip — see also Neoplasm, skin, limb, lower	C44.70-●	C79.2	D04.7-●	D23.7-●	D48.5	D49.2
infraclavicular region — see also Neoplasm, skin, trunk	C44.509	C79.2	D04.5	D23.5	D48.5	D49.2
inguinal region — see also Neoplasm, skin, trunk	C44.509	C79.2	D04.5	D23.5	D48.5	D49.2
jaw — see also Neoplasm, skin, face	C44.309	C79.2	D04.39	D23.39	D48.5	D49.2
Kaposi's sarcoma — see Kaposi's, sarcoma, skin						
knee — see also Neoplasm, skin, limb, lower	C44.70-●	C79.2	D04.7-●	D23.7-●	D48.5	D49.2
labia						
majora	C51.0	C79.82	D07.1	D28.0	D39.8	D49.59
minora	C51.1	C79.82	D07.1	D28.0	D39.8	D49.59
leg — see also Neoplasm, skin, limb, lower	C44.70-●	C79.2	D04.7-●	D23.7-●	D48.5	D49.2
lid (lower) (upper)	C44.10-●	C79.2	D04.1-●	D23.1-●	D48.5	D49.2
basal cell carcinoma	C44.11-●	—	—	—	—	—
sebaceous cell	C44.13-●	—	—	—	—	—
specified type NEC	C44.19-●	—	—	—	—	—
squamous cell carcinoma	C44.12-●	—	—	—	—	—
limb NEC	C44.90	C79.2	D04.9	D23.9	D48.5	D49.2
basal cell carcinoma	C44.91					
lower	C44.70-●	C79.2	D04.7-●	D23.7-●	D48.5	D49.2
basal cell carcinoma	C44.71-●	—	—	—	—	—
specified type NEC	C44.79-●	—	—	—	—	—
squamous cell carcinoma	C44.72-●	—	—	—	—	—
upper	C44.60-●	C79.2	D04.6-●	D23.6-●	D48.5	D49.2
basal cell carcinoma	C44.61-●	—	—	—	—	—
specified type NEC	C44.69-●	—	—	—	—	—
squamous cell carcinoma	C44.62-●	—	—	—	—	—
lip (lower) (upper)	C44.00	C79.2	D04.0	D23.0	D48.5	D49.2
basal cell carcinoma	C44.01	—	—	—	—	—
specified type NEC	C44.09	—	—	—	—	—
squamous cell carcinoma	C44.02	—	—	—	—	—

◀ New ◀ Revised ~~deleted~~ Deleted ● Use Additional Character(s)

skin NOS (Continued)	Malignant Primary	Malignant Secondary	Ca in situ	Benign	Uncertain Behavior	Unspecified Behavior
male genital organs	C63.9	C79.82	D07.60	D29.9	D40.8	D49.59
penis	C60.9	C79.82	D07.4	D29.0	D40.8	D49.59
prepuce	C60.0	C79.82	D07.4	D29.0	D40.8	D49.59
scrotum	C63.2	C79.82	D07.61	D29.4	D40.8	D49.59
mastectomy site (skin) — see also Neoplasm, skin, breast	C44.501	C79.2	—	—	—	—
specified as breast tissue	C50.8-●	C79.81	—	—	—	—
meatus, acoustic (external) — see also Neoplasm, skin, ear	C44.20-●	C79.2	D04.2-●	D23.2-●	D48.5	D49.2
melanotic — see Melanoma						
Merkel cell — see Carcinoma, Merkel cell						
nates — see also Neoplasm, skin, trunk	C44.509	C79.2	D04.5	D23.5	D48.5	D49.2
neck	C44.40	C79.2	D04.4	D23.4	D48.5	D49.2
basal cell carcinoma	C44.41	—	—	—	—	—
specified type NEC	C44.49	—	—	—	—	—
squamous cell carcinoma	C44.42	—	—	—	—	—
nevus — see Nevus, skin						
nose (external) — see also Neoplasm, nose, skin	C44.301	C79.2	D04.39	D23.39	D48.5	D49.2
overlapping lesion	C44.80					
basal cell carcinoma	C44.81	—	—	—	—	—
specified type NEC	C44.89	—	—	—	—	—
squamous cell carcinoma	C44.82	—	—	—	—	—
palm — see also Neoplasm, skin, limb, upper	C44.60-●	C79.2	D04.6-●	D23.6-●	D48.5	D49.2
palpebra	C44.10-●	C79.2	D04.1-●	D23.1-●	D48.5	D49.2
basal cell carcinoma	C44.11-●	—	—	—	—	—
sebaceous cell	C44.13-●	—	—	—	—	—
specified type NEC	C44.19-●	—	—	—	—	—
squamous cell carcinoma	C44.12-●	—	—	—	—	—
penis NEC	C60.9	C79.82	D07.4	D29.0	D40.8	D49.59
perianal — see also Neoplasm, skin, anus	C44.500	C79.2	D04.5	D23.5	D48.5	D49.2
perineum — see also Neoplasm, skin, anus	C44.500	C79.2	D04.5	D23.5	D48.5	D49.2
pinna — see also Neoplasm, skin, ear	C44.20-●	C79.2	D04.2-●	D23.2-●	D48.5	D49.2
plantar — see also Neoplasm, skin, limb, lower	C44.70-●	C79.2	D04.7-●	D23.7-●	D48.5	D49.2
popliteal fossa or space — see also Neoplasm, skin, limb, lower	C44.70-●	C79.2	D04.7-●	D23.7-●	D48.5	D49.2

skin NOS (Continued)	Malignant Primary	Malignant Secondary	Ca in situ	Benign	Uncertain Behavior	Unspecified Behavior
prepuce	C60.0	C79.82	D07.4	D29.0	D40.8	D49.59
pubes — see also Neoplasm, skin, trunk	C44.509	C79.2	D04.5	D23.5	D48.5	D49.2
sacrococcygeal region — see also Neoplasm, skin, trunk	C44.509	C79.2	D04.5	D23.5	D48.5	D49.2
scalp	C44.40	C79.2	D04.4	D23.4	D48.5	D49.2
basal cell carcinoma	C44.41	—	—	—	—	—
specified type NEC	C44.49	—	—	—	—	—
squamous cell carcinoma	C44.42	—	—	—	—	—
scapular region — see also Neoplasm, skin, trunk	C44.509	C79.2	D04.5	D23.5	D48.5	D49.2
scrotum	C63.2	C79.82	D07.61	D29.4	D40.8	D49.59
shoulder — see also Neoplasm, skin, limb, upper	C44.60-●	C79.2	D04.6-●	D23.6-●	D48.5	D49.2
sole (foot) — see also Neoplasm, skin, limb, lower	C44.70-●	C79.2	D04.7-●	D23.7-●	D48.5	D49.2
specified sites NEC	C44.80	C79.2	D04.8	D23.9	D48.5	D49.2
basal cell carcinoma	C44.81	—	—	—	—	—
specified type NEC	C44.89	—	—	—	—	—
squamous cell carcinoma	C44.82	—	—	—	—	—
specified type NEC	C44.99	—	—	—	—	—
squamous cell carcinoma	C44.92	—	—	—	—	—
submammary fold — see also Neoplasm, skin, trunk	C44.509	C79.2	D04.5	D23.5	D48.5	D49.2
supraclavicular region — see also Neoplasm, skin, neck	C44.40	C79.2	D04.4	D23.4	D48.5	D49.2
temple — see also Neoplasm, skin, face	C44.309	C79.2	D04.39	D23.39	D48.5	D49.2
thigh — see also Neoplasm, skin, limb, lower	C44.70-●	C79.2	D04.7-●	D23.7-●	D48.5	D49.2
thoracic wall — see also Neoplasm, skin, trunk	C44.509	C79.2	D04.5	D23.5	D48.5	D49.2
thumb — see also Neoplasm, skin, limb, upper	C44.60-●	C79.2	D04.6-●	D23.6-●	D48.5	D49.2
toe — see also Neoplasm, skin, limb, lower	C44.70-●	C79.2	D04.7-●	D23.7-●	D48.5	D49.2
tragus — see also Neoplasm, skin, ear	C44.20-●	C79.2	D04.2-●	D23.2-●	D48.5	D49.2
trunk	C44.509	C79.2	D04.5	D23.5	D48.5	D49.2
basal cell carcinoma	C44.519	—	—	—	—	—
specified type NEC	C44.599	—	—	—	—	—
squamous cell carcinoma	C44.529	—	—	—	—	—
umbilicus — see also Neoplasm, skin, trunk	C44.509	C79.2	D04.5	D23.5	D48.5	D49.2

◀ New ◀ Revised ~~deleted~~ Deleted ● Use Additional Character(s)

	Malignant Primary	Malignant Secondary	Ca in situ	Benign	Uncertain Behavior	Unspecified Behavior
skin NOS *(Continued)*						
vulva	C51.9	C79.82	D07.1	D28.0	D39.8	D49.59
overlapping lesion	C51.8	—	—	—	—	—
wrist — *see also Neoplasm, skin, limb, upper*	C44.60-●	C79.2	D04.6-●	D23.6-●	D48.5	D49.2
skull	C41.0	C79.51	—	D16.4-●	D48.0	D49.2
soft parts or tissues — *see Neoplasm, connective tissue*						
specified site NEC	C76.8	C79.89	D09.8	D36.7	D48.7	D49.89
spermatic cord	C63.1-●	C79.82	D07.69	D29.8	D40.8	D49.59
sphenoid	C31.3	C78.39	D02.3	D14.0	D38.5	D49.1
bone	C41.0	C79.51	—	D16.4-●	D48.0	D49.2
sinus	C31.3	C78.39	D02.3	D14.0	D38.5	D49.1
sphincter						
anal	C21.1	C78.5	D01.3	D12.9	D37.8	D49.0
of Oddi	C24.0	C78.89	D01.5	D13.5	D37.6	D49.0
spine, spinal (column)	C41.2	C79.51	—	D16.6	D48.0	D49.2
bulb	C71.7	C79.31	—	D33.1	D43.1	D49.6
coccyx	C41.4	C79.51	—	D16.8	D48.0	D49.2
cord (cervical) (lumbar) (sacral) (thoracic)	C72.0	C79.49	—	D33.4	D43.4	D49.7
dura mater	C70.1	C79.49	—	D32.1	D42.1	D49.7
lumbosacral	C41.2	C79.51	—	D16.6	D48.0	D49.2
marrow NEC	C96.9	C79.52	—	—	D47.9	D49.89
membrane	C70.1	C79.49	—	D32.1	D42.1	D49.7
meninges	C70.1	C79.49	—	D32.1	D42.1	D49.7
nerve (root)	C47.9	C79.89	—	D36.10	D48.2	D49.2
pia mater	C70.1	C79.49	—	D32.1	D42.1	D49.7
root	C47.9	C79.89	—	D36.10	D48.2	D49.2
sacrum	C41.4	C79.51	—	D16.8	D48.0	D49.2
spleen, splenic NEC	C26.1	C78.89	D01.7	D13.99	D37.8	D49.0
flexure (colon)	C18.5	C78.5	D01.0	D12.3	D37.4	D49.0
stem, brain	C71.7	C79.31	—	D33.1	D43.1	D49.6
Stensen's duct	C07	C79.89	D00.00	D11.0	D37.030	D49.0
sternum	C41.3	C79.51	—	D16.7	D48.0	D49.2
stomach	C16.9	C78.89	D00.2	D13.1	D37.1	D49.0
antrum (pyloric)	C16.3	C78.89	D00.2	D13.1	D37.1	D49.0
body	C16.2	C78.89	D00.2	D13.1	D37.1	D49.0
cardia	C16.0	C78.89	D00.2	D13.1	D37.1	D49.0
cardiac orifice	C16.0	C78.89	D00.2	D13.1	D37.1	D49.0
corpus	C16.2	C78.89	D00.2	D13.1	D37.1	D49.0
fundus	C16.1	C78.89	D00.2	D13.1	D37.1	D49.0
greater curvature NEC	C16.6	C78.89	D00.2	D13.1	D37.1	D49.0
lesser curvature NEC	C16.5	C78.89	D00.2	D13.1	D37.1	D49.0

	Malignant Primary	Malignant Secondary	Ca in situ	Benign	Uncertain Behavior	Unspecified Behavior
stomach *(Continued)*						
overlapping lesion	C16.8	—	—	—	—	—
prepylorus	C16.4	C78.89	D00.2	D13.1	D37.1	D49.0
pylorus	C16.4	C78.89	D00.2	D13.1	D37.1	D49.0
wall NEC	C16.9	C78.89	D00.2	D13.1	D37.1	D49.0
anterior NEC	C16.8	C78.89	D00.2	D13.1	D37.1	D49.0
posterior NEC	C16.8	C78.89	D00.2	D13.1	D37.1	D49.0
stroma, endometrial	C54.1	C79.82	D07.0	D26.1	D39.0	D49.59
stump, cervical	C53.8	C79.82	D06.7	D26.0	D39.0	D49.59
subcutaneous (nodule) (tissue) NEC — *see Neoplasm, connective tissue*						
subdural	C70.9	C79.32	—	D32.9	D42.9	D49.7
subglottis, subglottic	C32.2	C78.39	D02.0	D14.1	D38.0	D49.1
sublingual	C04.9	C79.89	D00.06	D10.2	D37.09	D49.0
gland or duct	C08.1	C79.89	D00.00	D11.7	D37.031	D49.0
submandibular gland	C08.0	C79.89	D00.00	D11.7	D37.032	D49.0
submaxillary gland or duct	C08.0	C79.89	D00.00	D11.7	D37.032	D49.0
submental	C76.0	C79.89	D09.8	D36.7	D48.7	D49.89
subpleural	C34.9-●	C78.0-●	D02.2-●	D14.3-●	D38.1	D49.1
substernal	C38.1	C78.1	—	D15.2	D38.3	D49.89
sudoriferous, sudoriparous gland, site unspecified	C44.90	C79.2	D04.9	D23.9	D48.5	D49.2
specified site — *see Neoplasm, skin*						
supraclavicular region	C76.0	C79.89	D09.8	D36.7	D48.7	D49.89
supraglottis	C32.1	C78.39	D02.0	D14.1	D38.0	D49.1
suprarenal	C74.9-●	C79.7-●	D09.3	D35.0-●	D44.1-●	D49.7
capsule	C74.9-●	C79.7-●	D09.3	D35.0-●	D44.1-●	D49.7
cortex	C74.0-●	C79.7-●	D09.3	D35.0-●	D44.1-●	D49.7
gland	C74.9-●	C79.7-●	D09.3	D35.0-●	D44.1-●	D49.7
medulla	C74.1-●	C79.7-●	D09.3	D35.0-●	D44.1-●	D49.7
suprasellar (region)	C71.9	C79.31	—	D33.2	D43.2	D49.6
supratentorial (brain) NEC	C71.0	C79.31	—	D33.0	D43.0	D49.6
sweat gland (apocrine) (eccrine), site unspecified	C44.90	C79.2	D04.9	D23.9	D48.5	D49.2
specified site — *see Neoplasm, skin*						
sympathetic nerve or nervous system NEC	C47.9	C79.89	—	D36.10	D48.2	D49.2
symphysis pubis	C41.4	C79.51	—	D16.8	D48.0	D49.2
synovial membrane — *see Neoplasm, connective tissue*						
tapetum, brain	C71.8	C79.31	—	D33.2	D43.2	D49.6

◄ New ◄ Revised ~~deleted~~ Deleted ● Use Additional Character(s)

TABLE OF NEOPLASMS

TABLE OF NEOPLASMS

	Malignant Primary	Malignant Secondary	Ca in situ	Benign	Uncertain Behavior	Unspecified Behavior
tarsus (any bone)	C40.3-●	C79.51	—	D16.3-●	—	—
temple (skin) — see also Neoplasm, skin, face	C44.309	C79.2	D04.39	D23.39	D48.5	D49.2
temporal						
bone	C41.0	C79.51	—	D16.4-●	D48.0	D49.2
lobe or pole	C71.2	C79.31	—	D33.0	D43.0	D49.6
region	C76.0	C79.89	D09.8	D36.7	D48.7	D49.89
skin — see also Neoplasm, skin, face	C44.309	C79.2	D04.39	D23.39	D48.5	D49.2
tendon (sheath) — see Neoplasm, connective tissue						
tentorium (cerebelli)	C70.0	C79.32	—	D32.0	D42.0	D49.7
testis, testes	C62.9-●	C79.82	D07.69	D29.2-●	D40.1-●	D49.59
descended	C62.1-●	C79.82	D07.69	D29.2-●	D40.1-●	D49.59
ectopic	C62.0-●	C79.82	D07.69	D29.2-●	D40.1-●	D49.59
retained	C62.0-●	C79.82	D07.69	D29.2-●	D40.1-●	D49.59
scrotal	C62.1-●	C79.82	D07.69	D29.2-●	D40.1-●	D49.59
undescended	C62.0-●	C79.82	D07.69	D29.2-●	D40.1-●	D49.59
unspecified whether descended or undescended	C62.9-●	C79.82	D07.69	D29.2-●	D40.1-●	D49.59
thalamus	C71.0	C79.31	—	D33.0	D43.0	D49.6
thigh NEC	C76.5-●	C79.89	D04.7-●	D36.7	D48.7	D49.89
thorax, thoracic (cavity) (organs NEC)	C76.1	C79.89	D09.8	D36.7	D48.7	D49.89
duct	C49.3	C79.89	—	D21.3	D48.1	D49.2
wall NEC	C76.1	C79.89	D09.8	D36.7	D48.7	D49.89
throat	C14.0	C79.89	D00.08	D10.9	D37.05	D49.0
thumb NEC	C76.4-●	C79.89	D04.6-●	D36.7	D48.7	D49.89
thymus (gland)	C37	C79.89	D09.3	D15.0	D38.4	D49.89
thyroglossal duct	C73	C79.89	D09.3	D34	D44.0	D49.7
thyroid (gland)	C73	C79.89	D09.3	D34	D44.0	D49.7
cartilage	C32.3	C78.39	D02.0	D14.1	D38.0	D49.1
tibia (any part)	C40.2-●	C79.51	—	D16.2-●	—	—
toe NEC	C76.5-●	C79.89	D04.7-●	D36.7	D48.7	D49.89
tongue	C02.9	C79.89	D00.07	D10.1	D37.02	D49.0
anterior (two-thirds) NEC	C02.3	C79.89	D00.07	D10.1	D37.02	D49.0
dorsal surface	C02.0	C79.89	D00.07	D10.1	D37.02	D49.0
ventral surface	C02.2	C79.89	D00.07	D10.1	D37.02	D49.0
base (dorsal surface)	C01	C79.89	D00.07	D10.1	D37.02	D49.0
border (lateral)	C02.1	C79.89	D00.07	D10.1	D37.02	D49.0
dorsal surface NEC	C02.0	C79.89	D00.07	D10.1	D37.02	D49.0
fixed part NEC	C01	C79.89	D00.07	D10.1	D37.02	D49.0
foreamen cecum	C02.0	C79.89	D00.07	D10.1	D37.02	D49.0
frenulum linguae	C02.2	C79.89	D00.07	D10.1	D37.02	D49.0

	Malignant Primary	Malignant Secondary	Ca in situ	Benign	Uncertain Behavior	Unspecified Behavior
tongue (Continued)						
junctional zone	C02.8	C79.89	D00.07	D10.1	D37.02	D49.0
margin (lateral)	C02.1	C79.89	D00.07	D10.1	D37.02	D49.0
midline NEC	C02.0	C79.89	D00.07	D10.1	D37.02	D49.0
mobile part NEC	C02.3	C79.89	D00.07	D10.1	D37.02	D49.0
overlapping lesion	C02.8	—	—	—	—	—
posterior (third)	C01	C79.89	D00.07	D10.1	D37.02	D49.0
root	C01	C79.89	D00.07	D10.1	D37.02	D49.0
surface (dorsal)	C02.0	C79.89	D00.07	D10.1	D37.02	D49.0
base	C01	C79.89	D00.07	D10.1	D37.02	D49.0
ventral	C02.2	C79.89	D00.07	D10.1	D37.02	D49.0
tip	C02.1	C79.89	D00.07	D10.1	D37.02	D49.0
tonsil	C02.4	C79.89	D00.07	D10.1	D37.02	D49.0
tonsil	C09.9	C79.89	D00.08	D10.4	D37.05	D49.0
fauces, faucial	C09.9	C79.89	D00.08	D10.4	D37.05	D49.0
lingual	C02.4	C79.89	D00.07	D10.1	D37.02	D49.0
overlapping sites	C09.8	—	—	—	—	—
palatine	C09.9	C79.89	D00.08	D10.4	D37.05	D49.0
pharyngeal	C11.1	C79.89	D00.08	D10.6	D37.05	D49.0
pillar (anterior) (posterior)	C09.1	C79.89	D00.08	D10.5	D37.05	D49.0
tonsillar fossa	C09.0	C79.89	D00.08	D10.5	D37.05	D49.0
tooth socket NEC	C03.9	C79.89	D00.03	D10.39	D37.09	D49.0
trachea (cartilage) (mucosa)	C33	C78.39	D02.1	D14.2	D38.1	D49.1
overlapping lesion with bronchus or lung	C34.8-●	—	—	—	—	—
tracheobronchial	C34.8-●	C78.39	D02.1	D14.2	D38.1	D49.1
overlapping lesion with lung	C34.8-●	—	—	—	—	—
tragus — see also Neoplasm, skin, ear	C44.20-●	C79.2	D04.2-●	D23.2-●	D48.5	D49.2
trunk NEC	C76.8	C79.89	D04.5	D36.7	D48.7	D49.89
tubo-ovarian	C57.8	C79.82	D07.39	D28.7	D39.8	D49.59
tunica vaginalis	C63.7	C79.82	D07.69	D29.8	D40.8	D49.59
turbinate (bone)	C41.0	C79.51	—	D16.4-●	D48.0	D49.2
nasal	C30.0	C78.39	D02.3	D14.0	D38.5	D49.1
tympanic cavity	C30.1	C78.39	D02.3	D14.0	D38.5	D49.1
ulna (any part)	C40.0-●	C79.51	—	D16.0-●	—	—
umbilicus, umbilical — see also Neoplasm, skin, trunk	C44.509	C79.2	D04.5	D23.5	D48.5	D49.2
uncus, brain	C71.2	C79.31	—	D33.0	D43.0	D49.6
unknown site or unspecified	C80.1	C79.9	D09.9	D36.9	D48.9	D49.9
urachus	C67.7	C79.11	D09.0	D30.3	D41.4	D49.4
ureter, ureteral	C66.-●	C79.19	D09.19	D30.2-●	D41.2-●	D49.59
orifice (bladder)	C67.6	C79.11	D09.0	D30.3	D41.4	D49.4
ureter-bladder (junction)	C67.6	C79.11	D09.0	D30.3	D41.4	D49.4

◀ New   ◀ Revised   ~~deleted~~ Deleted   ● Use Additional Character(s)

TABLE OF NEOPLASMS

	Malignant Primary	Malignant Secondary	Ca in situ	Benign	Uncertain Behavior	Unspecified Behavior
urethra, urethral (gland)	C68.0	C79.19	D09.19	D30.4	D41.3	D49.59
orifice, internal	C67.5	C79.11	D09.0	D30.3	D41.4	D49.4
urethrovaginal (septum)	C57.9	C79.82	D07.30	D28.9	D39.8	D49.59
urinary organ or system	C68.9	C79.10	D09.10	D30.9	D41.9	D49.59
bladder — see Neoplasm, bladder						
overlapping lesion	C68.8	—	—	—	—	—
specified sites NEC	C68.8	C79.19	D09.19	D30.8	D41.8	D49.59
utero-ovarian	C57.8	C79.82	D07.39	D28.7	D39.8	D49.59
ligament	C57.1	C79.82	D07.39	D28.2	D39.8	D49.59
uterosacral ligament	C57.3	C79.82	—	D28.2	D39.8	D49.59
uterus, uteri, uterine	C55	C79.82	D07.0	D26.9	D39.0	D49.59
adnexa NEC	C57.4	C79.82	D07.39	D28.7	D39.8	D49.59
body	C54.9	C79.82	D07.0	D26.1	D39.0	D49.59
cervix	C53.9	C79.82	D06.9	D26.0	D39.0	D49.59
cornu	C54.9	C79.82	D07.0	D26.1	D39.0	D49.59
corpus	C54.9	C79.82	D07.0	D26.1	D39.0	D49.59
endocervix (canal) (gland)	C53.0	C79.82	D06.0	D26.0	D39.0	D49.59
endometrium	C54.1	C79.82	D07.0	D26.1	D39.0	D49.59
exocervix	C53.1	C79.82	D06.1	D26.0	D39.0	D49.59
external os	C53.1	C79.82	D06.1	D26.0	D39.0	D49.59
fundus	C54.3	C79.82	D07.0	D26.1	D39.0	D49.59
internal os	C53.0	C79.82	D06.0	D26.0	D39.0	D49.59
isthmus	C54.0	C79.82	D07.0	D26.1	D39.0	D49.59
ligament	C57.3	C79.82	—	D28.2	D39.8	D49.59
broad	C57.1	C79.82	D07.39	D28.2	D39.8	D49.59
round	C57.2	C79.82	—	D28.2	D39.8	D49.59
lower segment	C54.0	C79.82	D07.0	D26.1	D39.0	D49.59
myometrium	C54.2	C79.82	D07.0	D26.1	D39.0	D49.59
overlapping sites	C54.8	—	—	—	—	—
squamocolumnar junction	C53.8	C79.82	D06.7	D26.0	D39.0	D49.59
tube	C57.0-●	C79.82	D07.39	D28.2	D39.8	D49.59
utricle, prostatic	C68.0	C79.19	D09.19	D30.4	D41.3	D49.59
uveal tract	C69.4-●	C79.49	D09.2-●	D31.4-●	D48.7	D49.89
uvula	C05.2	C79.89	D00.04	D10.39	D37.09	D49.0
vagina, vaginal (fornix) (vault) (wall)	C52	C79.82	D07.2	D28.1	D39.8	D49.59
vaginovesical	C57.9	C79.82	D07.30	D28.9	D39.9	D49.59
septum	C57.9	C79.82	D07.30	D28.9	D39.9	D49.59
vallecula (epigiottis)	C10.0	C79.89	D00.08	D10.5	D37.05	D49.0
vas deferens	C63.1-●	C79.82	D07.69	D29.8	D40.8	D49.59
vascular — see Neoplasm, connective tissue						

	Malignant Primary	Malignant Secondary	Ca in situ	Benign	Uncertain Behavior	Unspecified Behavior
Vater's ampulla	C24.1	C78.89	D01.5	D13.5	D37.6	D49.0
vein, venous — see Neoplasm, connective tissue						
vena cava (abdominal) (inferior)	C49.4	C79.89	—	D21.4	D48.1	D49.2
superior	C49.3	C79.89	—	D21.3	D48.1	D49.2
ventricle (cerebral) (floor) (lateral) (third)	C71.5	C79.31	—	D33.0	D43.0	D49.6
cardiac (left) (right)	C38.0	C79.89	—	D15.1	D48.7	D49.89
fourth	C71.7	C79.31	—	D33.1	D43.1	D49.6
ventricular band of larynx	C32.1	C78.39	D02.0	D14.1	D38.0	D49.1
ventriculus — see Neoplasm, stomach						
vermillion border — see Neoplasm, lip						
vermis, cerebellum	C71.6	C79.31	—	D33.1	D43.1	D49.6
vertebra (column)	C41.2	C79.51	—	D16.6	D48.0	D49.2
coccyx	C41.4	C79.51	—	D16.8-●	D48.0	D49.2
marrow NEC	C96.9	C79.52	—	—	D47.9	D49.89
sacrum	C41.4	C79.51	—	D16.8-●	D48.0	D49.2
vesical — see Neoplasm, bladder						
vesicle, seminal	C63.7	C79.82	D07.69	D29.8	D40.8	D49.59
vesicocervical tissue	C57.9	C79.82	D07.30	D28.9	D39.9	D49.59
vesicorectal	C76.3	C79.82	D09.8	D36.7	D48.7	D49.89
vesicovaginal	C57.9	C79.82	D07.30	D28.9	D39.9	D49.59
septum	C57.9	C79.82	D07.30	D28.9	D39.8	D49.59
vessel (blood) — see Neoplasm, connective tissue						
vestibular gland, greater	C51.0	C79.82	D07.1	D28.0	D39.8	D49.59
vestibule						
mouth	C06.1	C79.89	D00.00	D10.39	D37.09	D49.0
nose	C30.0	C78.39	D02.3	D14.0	D38.5	D49.1
Virchow's gland	C77.0	C77.0	—	D36.0	D48.7	D49.89
viscera NEC	C76.8	C79.89	D09.8	D36.7	D48.7	D49.89
vocal cords (true)	C32.0	C78.39	D02.0	D14.1	D38.0	D49.1
false	C32.1	C78.39	D02.0	D14.1	D38.0	D49.1
vomer	C41.0	C79.51	—	D16.4-●	D48.0	D49.2
vulva	C51.9	C79.82	D07.1	D28.0	D39.8	D49.59
vulvovaginal gland	C51.0	C79.82	D07.1	D28.0	D39.8	D49.59
Waldeyer's ring	C14.2	C79.89	D00.08	D10.9	D37.05	D49.0
Wharton's duct	C08.0	C79.89	D00.00	D11.7	D37.032	D49.0
white matter (central) (cerebral)	C71.0	C79.31	—	D33.0	D43.0	D49.6
windpipe	C33	C78.39	D02.1	D14.2	D38.1	D49.1

TABLE OF NEOPLASMS

	Malignant Primary	Malignant Secondary	Ca in situ	Benign	Uncertain Behavior	Unspecified Behavior
Wirsung's duct	C25.3	C78.89	D01.7	D13.6	D37.8	D49.0
wolffian (body) (duct)						
female	C57.7	C79.82	D07.39	D28.7	D39.8	D49.59
male	C63.7	C79.82	D07.69	D29.8	D40.8	D49.59

	Malignant Primary	Malignant Secondary	Ca in situ	Benign	Uncertain Behavior	Unspecified Behavior
womb — *see Neoplasm, uterus*						
wrist NEC	C76.4-●	C79.89	D04.6-●	D36.7	D48.7	D49.89
xiphoid process	C41.3	C79.51	—	D16.7	D48.0	D49.2
Zuckerkandl organ	C75.5	C79.89	—	D35.6	D44.7	D49.7

◀ New   ◀ Revised   ~~deleted~~ Deleted   ● Use Additional Character(s)

TABLE OF NEOPLASMS

ICD-10-CM
Table of Drugs and Chemicals

	External Cause (T-Code)					
Substance	Poisoning, Accidental (Unintentional)	Poisoning, Intentional Self-Harm	Poisoning, Assault	Poisoning, Undetermined	Adverse Effect	Underdosing
#						
1-propanol	T51.3X1	T51.3X2	T51.3X3	T51.3X4	—	—
2-propanol	T51.2X1	T51.2X2	T51.2X3	T51.2X4	—	—
2,4-D (dichlorophen-oxyacetic acid)	T60.3X1	T60.3X2	T60.3X3	T60.3X4	—	—
2,4-toluene diisocyanate	T65.0X1	T65.0X2	T65.0X3	T65.0X4	—	—
2,4,5-T (trichloro-phenoxyacetic acid)	T60.1X1	T60.1X2	T60.1X3	T60.1X4	—	—
3,4-methylenedioxy-methamphetamine	T43.641	T43.642	T43.643	T43.644	—	—
14-hydroxydihydro-morphinone	T40.2X1	T40.2X2	T40.2X3	T40.2X4	T40.2X5	T40.2X6
A						
ABOB	T37.5X1	T37.5X2	T37.5X3	T37.5X4	T37.5X5	T37.5X6
Abrine	T62.2X1	T62.2X2	T62.2X3	T62.2X4	—	—
Abrus (seed)	T62.2X1	T62.2X2	T62.2X3	T62.2X4	—	—
Absinthe	T51.0X1	T51.0X2	T51.0X3	T51.0X4	—	—
beverage	T51.0X1	T51.0X2	T51.0X3	T51.0X4	—	—
Acaricide	T60.8X1	T60.8X2	T60.8X3	T60.8X4	—	—
Acebutolol	T44.7X1	T44.7X2	T44.7X3	T44.7X4	T44.7X5	T44.7X6
Acecarbromal	T42.6X1	T42.6X2	T42.6X3	T42.6X4	T42.6X5	T42.6X6
Aceclidine	T44.1X1	T44.1X2	T44.1X3	T44.1X4	T44.1X5	T44.1X6
Acedapsone	T37.0X1	T37.0X2	T37.0X3	T37.0X4	T37.0X5	T37.0X6
Acefylline piperazine	T48.6X1	T48.6X2	T48.6X3	T48.6X4	T48.6X5	T48.6X6
Acemorphan	T40.2X1	T40.2X2	T40.2X3	T40.2X4	T40.2X5	T40.2X6
Acenocoumarin	T45.511	T45.512	T45.513	T45.514	T45.515	T45.516
Acenocoumarol	T45.511	T45.512	T45.513	T45.514	T45.515	T45.516
Acepifylline	T48.6X1	T48.6X2	T48.6X3	T48.6X4	T48.6X5	T48.6X6
Acepromazine	T43.3X1	T43.3X2	T43.3X3	T43.3X4	T43.3X5	T43.3X6
Acesulfamethoxypyridazine	T37.0X1	T37.0X2	T37.0X3	T37.0X4	T37.0X5	T37.0X6
Acetal	T52.8X1	T52.8X2	T52.8X3	T52.8X4	—	—
Acetaldehyde (vapor)	T52.8X1	T52.8X2	T52.8X3	T52.8X4	—	—
liquid	T65.891	T65.892	T65.893	T65.894	—	—
P-Acetamidophenol	T39.1X1	T39.1X2	T39.1X3	T39.1X4	T39.1X5	T39.1X6
Acetaminophen	T39.1X1	T39.1X2	T39.1X3	T39.1X4	T39.1X5	T39.1X6
Acetaminosalol	T39.1X1	T39.1X2	T39.1X3	T39.1X4	T39.1X5	T39.1X6
Acetanilide	T39.1X1	T39.1X2	T39.1X3	T39.1X4	T39.1X5	T39.1X6
Acetarsol	T37.3X1	T37.3X2	T37.3X3	T37.3X4	T37.3X5	T37.3X6
Acetazolamide	T50.2X1	T50.2X2	T50.2X3	T50.2X4	T50.2X5	T50.2X6
Acetiamine	T45.2X1	T45.2X2	T45.2X3	T45.2X4	T45.2X5	T45.2X6
Acetic						
acid	T54.2X1	T54.2X2	T54.2X3	T54.2X4	—	—
with sodium acetate (ointment)	T49.3X1	T49.3X2	T49.3X3	T49.3X4	T49.3X5	T49.3X6

	External Cause (T-Code)					
Substance	Poisoning, Accidental (Unintentional)	Poisoning, Intentional Self-Harm	Poisoning, Assault	Poisoning, Undetermined	Adverse Effect	Underdosing
Acetic (Continued)						
acid (Continued)						
ester (solvent) (vapor)	T52.8X1	T52.8X2	T52.8X3	T52.8X4	—	—
irrigating solution	T50.3X1	T50.3X2	T50.3X3	T50.3X4	T50.3X5	T50.3X6
medicinal (lotion)	T49.2X1	T49.2X2	T49.2X3	T49.2X4	T49.2X5	T49.2X6
anhydride	T65.891	T65.892	T65.893	T65.894	—	—
ether (vapor)	T52.8X1	T52.8X2	T52.8X3	T52.8X4	—	—
Acetohexamide	T38.3X1	T38.3X2	T38.3X3	T38.3X4	T38.3X5	T38.3X6
Acetohydroxamic acid	T50.991	T50.992	T50.993	T50.994	T50.995	T50.996
Acetomenaphthone	T45.7X1	T45.7X2	T45.7X3	T45.7X4	T45.7X5	T45.7X6
Acetomorphine	T40.1X1	T40.1X2	T40.1X3	T40.1X4	—	—
Acetone (oils)	T52.4X1	T52.4X2	T52.4X3	T52.4X4	—	—
chlorinated	T52.4X1	T52.4X2	T52.4X3	T52.4X4	—	—
vapor	T52.4X1	T52.4X2	T52.4X3	T52.4X4	—	—
Acetonitrile	T52.8X1	T52.8X2	T52.8X3	T52.8X4	—	—
Acetophenazine	T43.3X1	T43.3X2	T43.3X3	T43.3X4	T43.3X5	T43.3X6
Acetophenetedin	T39.1X1	T39.1X2	T39.1X3	T39.1X4	T39.1X5	T39.1X6
Acetophenone	T52.4X1	T52.4X2	T52.4X3	T52.4X4	—	—
Acetorphine	T40.2X1	T40.2X2	T40.2X3	T40.2X4	—	—
Acetosulfone (sodium)	T37.1X1	T37.1X2	T37.1X3	T37.1X4	T37.1X5	T37.1X6
Acetrizoate (sodium)	T50.8X1	T50.8X2	T50.8X3	T50.8X4	T50.8X5	T50.8X6
Acetylcarbromal	T42.6X1	T42.6X2	T42.6X3	T42.6X4	T42.6X5	T42.6X6
Acetrizoic acid	T50.8X1	T50.8X2	T50.8X3	T50.8X4	T50.8X5	T50.8X6
Acetyl						
bromide	T53.6X1	T53.6X2	T53.6X3	T53.6X4	—	—
chloride	T53.6X1	T53.6X2	T53.6X3	T53.6X4	—	—
Acetylcholine						
chloride	T44.1X1	T44.1X2	T44.1X3	T44.1X4	T44.1X5	T44.1X6
derivative	T44.1X1	T44.1X2	T44.1X3	T44.1X4	T44.1X5	T44.1X6
Acetylcysteine	T48.4X1	T48.4X2	T48.4X3	T48.4X4	T48.4X5	T48.4X6
Acetyldigitoxin	T46.0X1	T46.0X2	T46.0X3	T46.0X4	T46.0X5	T46.0X6
Acetyldigoxin	T46.0X1	T46.0X2	T46.0X3	T46.0X4	T46.0X5	T46.0X6
Acetyldihydrocodeine	T40.2X1	T40.2X2	T40.2X3	T40.2X4	—	—
Acetyldihydrocodeinone	T40.2X1	T40.2X2	T40.2X3	T40.2X4	—	—
Acetylene (gas)	T59.891	T59.892	T59.893	T59.894		
dichloride	T53.6X1	T53.6X2	T53.6X3	T53.6X4	—	—
incomplete combustion of	T58.11	T58.12	T58.13	T58.14		
industrial	T59.891	T59.892	T59.893	T59.894		
tetrachloride	T53.6X1	T53.6X2	T53.6X3	T53.6X4	—	—
vapor	T53.6X1	T53.6X2	T53.6X3	T53.6X4	—	—
Acetylphenylhydrazine	T39.8X1	T39.8X2	T39.8X3	T39.8X4	T39.8X5	T39.8X6
Acetylpheneturide	T42.6X1	T42.6X2	T42.6X3	T42.6X4	T42.6X5	T42.6X6

◀ New   ◀ Revised   ~~deleted~~ Deleted

Substance	Poisoning, Accidental (Unintentional)	Poisoning, Intentional Self-Harm	Poisoning, Assault	Poisoning, Undetermined	Adverse Effect	Underdosing
Acetylsalicylic acid (salts)	T39.011	T39.012	T39.013	T39.014	T39.015	T39.016
enteric coated	T39.011	T39.012	T39.013	T39.014	T39.015	T39.016
Acetylsulfamethoxypyridazine	T37.0X1	T37.0X2	T37.0X3	T37.0X4	T37.0X5	T37.0X6
Achromycin	T36.4X1	T36.4X2	T36.4X3	T36.4X4	T36.4X5	T36.4X6
ophthalmic preparation	T49.5X1	T49.5X2	T49.5X3	T49.5X4	T49.5X5	T49.5X6
topical NEC	T49.0X1	T49.0X2	T49.0X3	T49.0X4	T49.0X5	T49.0X6
Aciclovir	T37.5X1	T37.5X2	T37.5X3	T37.5X4	T37.5X5	T37.5X6
Acid (corrosive) NEC	T54.2X1	T54.2X2	T54.2X3	T54.2X4	—	—
Acidifying agent NEC	T50.901	T50.902	T50.903	T50.904	T50.905	T50.906
Acipimox	T46.6X1	T46.6X2	T46.6X3	T46.6X4	T46.6X5	T46.6X6
Acitretin	T50.991	T50.992	T50.993	T50.994	T50.995	T50.996
Aclarubicin	T45.1X1	T45.1X2	T45.1X3	T45.1X4	T45.1X5	T45.1X6
Aclatonium napadisilate	T48.1X1	T48.1X2	T48.1X3	T48.1X4	T48.1X5	T48.1X6
Aconite (wild)	T46.991	T46.992	T46.993	T46.994	T46.995	T46.996
Aconitine	T46.991	T46.992	T46.993	T46.994	T46.995	T46.996
Aconitum ferox	T46.991	T46.992	T46.993	T46.994	T46.995	T46.996
Acridine	T65.6X1	T65.6X2	T65.6X3	T65.6X4	—	—
vapor	T59.891	T59.892	T59.893	T59.894	—	—
Acriflavine	T37.91	T37.92	T37.93	T37.94	T37.95	T37.96
Acriflavinium chloride	T49.0X1	T49.0X2	T49.0X3	T49.0X4	T49.0X5	T49.0X6
Acrinol	T49.0X1	T49.0X2	T49.0X3	T49.0X4	T49.0X5	T49.0X6
Acrisorcin	T49.0X1	T49.0X2	T49.0X3	T49.0X4	T49.0X5	T49.0X6
Acrivastine	T45.0X1	T45.0X2	T45.0X3	T45.0X4	T45.0X5	T45.0X6
Acrolein (gas)	T59.891	T59.892	T59.893	T59.894	—	—
liquid	T54.1X1	T54.1X2	T54.1X3	T54.1X4	—	—
Acrylamide	T65.891	T65.892	T65.893	T65.894	—	—
Acrylic resin	T49.3X1	T49.3X2	T49.3X3	T49.3X4	T49.3X5	T49.3X6
Acrylonitrile	T65.891	T65.892	T65.893	T65.894	—	—
Actaea spicata	T62.2X1	T62.2X2	T62.2X3	T62.2X4	—	—
berry	T62.1X1	T62.1X2	T62.1X3	T62.1X4	—	—
Acterol	T37.3X1	T37.3X2	T37.3X3	T37.3X4	T37.3X5	T37.3X6
ACTH	T38.811	T38.812	T38.813	T38.814	T38.815	T38.816
Actinomycin C	T45.1X1	T45.1X2	T45.1X3	T45.1X4	T45.1X5	T45.1X6
Actinomycin D	T45.1X1	T45.1X2	T45.1X3	T45.1X4	T45.1X5	T45.1X6
Activated charcoal — see also Charcoal, medicinal	T47.6X1	T47.6X2	T47.6X3	T47.6X4	T47.6X5	T47.6X6
Acyclovir	T37.5X1	T37.5X2	T37.5X3	T37.5X4	T37.5X5	T37.5X6
Adenine	T45.2X1	T45.2X2	T45.2X3	T45.2X4	T45.2X5	T45.2X6
arabinoside	T37.5X1	T37.5X2	T37.5X3	T37.5X4	T37.5X5	T37.5X6
Adenosine (phosphate)	T46.2X1	T46.2X2	T46.2X3	T46.2X4	T46.2X5	T46.2X6
ADH	T38.891	T38.892	T38.893	T38.894	T38.895	T38.896
Adhesive NEC	T65.891	T65.892	T65.893	T65.894	—	—

Substance	Poisoning, Accidental (Unintentional)	Poisoning, Intentional Self-Harm	Poisoning, Assault	Poisoning, Undetermined	Adverse Effect	Underdosing
Adicillin	T36.0X1	T36.0X2	T36.0X3	T36.0X4	T36.0X5	T36.0X6
Adiphenine	T44.3X1	T44.3X2	T44.3X3	I44.3X4	T44.3X5	T44.3X6
Adipiodone	T50.8X1	T50.8X2	T50.8X3	T50.8X4	T50.8X5	T50.8X6
Adjunct, pharmaceutical	T50.901	T50.902	T50.903	T50.904	T50.905	T50.906
Adrenal (extract, cortex or medulla) (glucocorticoids) (hormones) (mineralo corticoids)	T38.0X1	T38.0X2	T38.0X3	T38.0X4	T38.0X5	T38.0X6
ENT agent	T49.6X1	T49.6X2	T49.6X3	T49.6X4	T49.6X5	T49.6X6
ophthalmic preparation	T49.5X1	T49.5X2	T49.5X3	T49.5X4	T49.5X5	T49.5X6
topical NEC	T49.0X1	T49.0X2	T49.0X3	T49.0X4	T49.0X5	T49.0X6
Adrenaline	T44.5X1	T44.5X2	T44.5X3	T44.5X4	T44.5X5	T44.5X6
Adrenalin — see Adrenaline						
Adrenergic NEC	T44.901	T44.902	T44.903	T44.904	T44.905	T44.906
blocking agent NEC	T44.8X1	T44.8X2	T44.8X3	T44.8X4	T44.8X5	T44.8X6
beta, heart	T44.7X1	T44.7X2	T44.7X3	T44.7X4	T44.7X5	T44.7X6
specified NEC	T44.991	T44.992	T44.993	T44.994	T44.995	T44.996
Adrenochrome						
(mono) semicarbazone	T46.991	T46.992	T46.993	T46.994	T46.995	T46.996
derivative	T46.991	T46.992	T46.993	T46.994	T46.995	T46.996
Adrenocorticotrophic hormone	T38.811	T38.812	T38.813	T38.814	T38.815	T38.816
Adrenocorticotrophin	T38.811	T38.812	T38.813	T38.814	T38.815	T38.816
Adriamycin	T45.1X1	T45.1X2	T45.1X3	T45.1X4	T45.1X5	T45.1X6
Aerosol spray NEC	T65.91	T65.92	T65.93	T65.94	—	—
Aerosporin	T36.8X1	T36.8X2	T36.8X3	T36.8X4	T36.8X5	T36.8X6
ENT agent	T49.6X1	T49.6X2	T49.6X3	T49.6X4	T49.6X5	T49.6X6
ophthalmic preparation	T49.5X1	T49.5X2	T49.5X3	T49.5X4	T49.5X5	T49.5X6
topical NEC	T49.0X1	T49.0X2	T49.0X3	T49.0X4	T49.0X5	T49.0X6
Aethusa cynapium	T62.2X1	T62.2X2	T62.2X3	T62.2X4		
Afghanistan black	T40.711	T40.712	T40.713	T40.714	T40.715	T40.716
Aflatoxin	T64.01	T64.02	T64.03	T64.04	—	—
Afloqualone	T42.8X1	T42.8X2	T42.8X3	T42.8X4	T42.8X5	T42.8X6
African boxwood	T62.2X1	T62.2X2	T62.2X3	T62.2X4	—	—
Agar	T47.4X1	T47.4X2	T47.4X3	T47.4X4	T47.4X5	T47.4X6
Agonist						
predominantly						
alpha-adrenoreceptor	T44.4X1	T44.4X2	T44.4X3	T44.4X4	T44.4X5	T44.4X6
beta-adrenoreceptor	T44.5X1	T44.5X2	T44.5X3	T44.5X4	T44.5X5	T44.5X6
Agricultural agent NEC	T65.91	T65.92	T65.93	T65.94	—	—
Agrypnal	T42.3X1	T42.3X2	T42.3X3	T42.3X4	T42.3X5	T42.3X6
AHLG	T50.Z11	T50.Z12	T50.Z13	T50.Z14	T50.Z15	T50.Z16
Air contaminant(s), source/type NOS	T65.91	T65.92	T65.93	T65.94	—	—

◀ New ◀ Revised ~~deleted~~ Deleted

Substance	External Cause (T-Code)					
	Poisoning, Accidental (Unintentional)	Poisoning, Intentional Self-Harm	Poisoning, Assault	Poisoning, Undetermined	Adverse Effect	Underdosing
Ajmaline	T46.2X1	T46.2X2	T46.2X3	T46.2X4	T46.2X5	T46.2X6
Akritoin	T37.8X1	T37.8X2	T37.8X3	T37.8X4	T37.8X5	T37.8X6
Akee	T62.1X1	T62.1X2	T62.1X3	T62.1X4	—	—
Akrinol	T49.0X1	T49.0X2	T49.0X3	T49.0X4	T49.0X5	T49.0X6
Alacepril	T46.4X1	T46.4X2	T46.4X3	T46.4X4	T46.4X5	T46.4X6
Alantolactone	T37.4X1	T37.4X2	T37.4X3	T37.4X4	T37.4X5	T37.4X6
Albamycin	T36.8X1	T36.8X2	T36.8X3	T36.8X4	T36.8X5	T36.8X6
Albendazole	T37.4X1	T37.4X2	T37.4X3	T37.4X4	T37.4X5	T37.4X6
Albumin						
bovine	T45.8X1	T45.8X2	T45.8X3	T45.8X4	T45.8X5	T45.8X6
human serum	T45.8X1	T45.8X2	T45.8X3	T45.8X4	T45.8X5	T45.8X6
salt-poor	T45.8X1	T45.8X2	T45.8X3	T45.8X4	T45.8X5	T45.8X6
normal human serum	T45.8X1	T45.8X2	T45.8X3	T45.8X4	T45.8X5	T45.8X6
Albuterol	T48.6X1	T48.6X2	T48.6X3	T48.6X4	T48.6X5	T48.6X6
Albutoin	T42.0X1	T42.0X2	T42.0X3	T42.0X4	T42.0X5	T42.0X6
Alclometasone	T49.0X1	T49.0X2	T49.0X3	T49.0X4	T49.0X5	T49.0X6
Alcohol	T51.91	T51.92	T51.93	T51.94	—	—
absolute	T51.0X1	T51.0X2	T51.0X3	T51.0X4	—	—
beverage	T51.0X1	T51.0X2	T51.0X3	T51.0X4	—	—
allyl	T51.8X1	T51.8X2	T51.8X3	T51.8X4	—	—
amyl	T51.3X1	T51.3X2	T51.3X3	T51.3X4	—	—
antifreeze	T51.1X1	T51.1X2	T51.1X3	T51.1X4	—	—
beverage	T51.0X1	T51.0X2	T51.0X3	T51.0X4	—	—
butyl	T51.3X1	T51.3X2	T51.3X3	T51.3X4	—	—
dehydrated	T51.0X1	T51.0X2	T51.0X3	T51.0X4	—	—
beverage	T51.0X1	T51.0X2	T51.0X3	T51.0X4	—	—
denatured	T51.0X1	T51.0X2	T51.0X3	T51.0X4	—	—
deterrent NEC	T50.6X1	T50.6X2	T50.6X3	T50.6X4	T50.6X5	T50.6X6
diagnostic (gastric function)	T50.8X1	T50.8X2	T50.8X3	T50.8X4	T50.8X5	T50.8X6
ethyl	T51.0X1	T51.0X2	T51.0X3	T51.0X4	—	—
beverage	T51.0X1	T51.0X2	T51.0X3	T51.0X4	—	—
grain	T51.0X1	T51.0X2	T51.0X3	T51.0X4	—	—
beverage	T51.0X1	T51.0X2	T51.0X3	T51.0X4	—	—
industrial	T51.0X1	T51.0X2	T51.0X3	T51.0X4	—	—
isopropyl	T51.2X1	T51.2X2	T51.2X3	T51.2X4	—	—
methyl	T51.1X1	T51.1X2	T51.1X3	T51.1X4	—	—
preparation for consumption	T51.0X1	T51.0X2	T51.0X3	T51.0X4	—	—
propyl	T51.3X1	T51.3X2	T51.3X3	T51.3X4	—	—
secondary	T51.2X1	T51.2X2	T51.2X3	T51.2X4	—	—
radiator	T51.1X1	T51.1X2	T51.1X3	T51.1X4	—	—
rubbing	T51.2X1	T51.2X2	T51.2X3	T51.2X4	—	—
specified type NEC	T51.8X1	T51.8X2	T51.8X3	T51.8X4	—	—

Substance	External Cause (T-Code)					
	Poisoning, Accidental (Unintentional)	Poisoning, Intentional Self-Harm	Poisoning, Assault	Poisoning, Undetermined	Adverse Effect	Underdosing
Alcohol (Continued)						
surgical	T51.0X1	T51.0X2	T51.0X3	T51.0X4	—	—
vapor (from any type of Alcohol)	T59.891	T59.892	T59.893	T59.894	—	—
wood	T51.1X1	T51.1X2	T51.1X3	T51.1X4	—	—
Alcuronium (chloride)	T48.1X1	T48.1X2	T48.1X3	T48.1X4	T48.1X5	T48.1X6
Aldactone	T50.0X1	T50.0X2	T50.0X3	T50.0X4	T50.0X5	T50.0X6
Aldesulfone sodium	T37.1X1	T37.1X2	T37.1X3	T37.1X4	T37.1X5	T37.1X6
Aldicarb	T60.0X1	T60.0X2	T60.0X3	T60.0X4	—	—
Aldomet	T46.5X1	T46.5X2	T46.5X3	T46.5X4	T46.5X5	T46.5X6
Aldosterone	T50.0X1	T50.0X2	T50.0X3	T50.0X4	T50.0X5	T50.0X6
Aldrin (dust)	T60.1X1	T60.1X2	T60.1X3	T60.1X4	—	—
Aleve — see Naproxen						
Alexitol sodium	T47.1X1	T47.1X2	T47.1X3	T47.1X4	T47.1X5	T47.1X6
Alfacalcidol	T45.2X1	T45.2X2	T45.2X3	T45.2X4	T45.2X5	T45.2X6
Alfadolone	T41.1X1	T41.1X2	T41.1X3	T41.1X4	T41.1X5	T41.1X6
Alfaxalone	T41.1X1	T41.1X2	T41.1X3	T41.1X4	T41.1X5	T41.1X6
Alfentanil	T40.411	T40.412	T40.413	T40.414	T40.415	T40.416
Alfuzosin (hydrochloride)	T44.8X1	T44.8X2	T44.8X3	T44.8X4	T44.8X5	T44.8X6
Algae (harmful) (toxin)	T65.821	T65.822	T65.823	T65.824	—	—
Algeldrate	T47.1X1	T47.1X2	T47.1X3	T47.1X4	T47.1X5	T47.1X6
Algin	T47.8X1	T47.8X2	T47.8X3	T47.8X4	T47.8X5	T47.8X6
Alglucerase	T45.3X1	T45.3X2	T45.3X3	T45.3X4	T45.3X5	T45.3X6
Alidase	T45.3X1	T45.3X2	T45.3X3	T45.3X4	T45.3X5	T45.3X6
Alimemazine	T43.3X1	T43.3X2	T43.3X3	T43.3X4	T43.3X5	T43.3X6
Aliphatic thiocyanates	T65.0X1	T65.0X2	T65.0X3	T65.0X4	—	—
Alizapride	T45.0X1	T45.0X2	T45.0X3	T45.0X4	T45.0X5	T45.0X6
Alkali (caustic)	T54.3X1	T54.3X2	T54.3X3	T54.3X4	—	—
Alkalizing agent NEC	T50.901	T50.902	T50.903	T50.904	T50.905	T50.906
Alkaline antiseptic solution (aromatic)	T49.6X1	T49.6X2	T49.6X3	T49.6X4	T49.6X5	T49.6X6
Alkalinizing agents (medicinal)	T50.901	T50.902	T50.903	T50.904	T50.905	T50.906
Alka-seltzer	T39.011	T39.012	T39.013	T39.014	T39.015	T39.016
Alkavervir	T46.5X1	T46.5X2	T46.5X3	T46.5X4	T46.5X5	T46.5X6
Alkonium (bromide)	T49.0X1	T49.0X2	T49.0X3	T49.0X4	T49.0X5	T49.0X6
Alkylating drug NEC	T45.1X1	T45.1X2	T45.1X3	T45.1X4	T45.1X5	T45.1X6
antimyeloproliferative	T45.1X1	T45.1X2	T45.1X3	T45.1X4	T45.1X5	T45.1X6
lymphatic	T45.1X1	T45.1X2	T45.1X3	T45.1X4	T45.1X5	T45.1X6
Alkylisocyanate	T65.0X1	T65.0X2	T65.0X3	T65.0X4	—	—
Allantoin	T49.411	T49.412	T49.413	T49.414	T49.415	T49.416
Allegron	T43.0X1	T43.0X2	T43.0X3	T43.0X4	T43.0X5	T43.0X6
Allethrin	T49.0X1	T49.0X2	T49.0X3	T49.0X4	T49.0X5	T49.0X6
Allobarbital	T42.3X1	T42.3X2	T42.3X3	T42.3X4	T42.3X5	T42.3X6

TABLE OF DRUGS AND CHEMICALS

Substance	Poisoning, Accidental (Unintentional)	Poisoning, Intentional Self-Harm	Poisoning, Assault	Poisoning, Undetermined	Adverse Effect	Underdosing
			External Cause (T-Code)			
Allopurinol	T50.4X1	T50.4X2	T50.4X3	T50.4X4	T50.4X5	T50.4X6
Allyl						
alcohol	T51.8X1	T51.8X2	T51.8X3	T51.8X4	—	—
disulfide	T46.6X1	T46.6X2	T46.6X3	T46.6X4	T46.6X5	T46.6X6
Allylestrenol	T38.5X1	T38.5X2	T38.5X3	T38.5X4	T38.5X5	T38.5X6
Allylisopropylacetylurea	T42.6X1	T42.6X2	T42.6X3	T42.6X4	T42.6X5	T42.6X6
Allylisopropylmalonylurea	T42.3X1	T42.3X2	T42.3X3	T42.3X4	T42.3X5	T42.3X6
Allylthiourea	T49.3X1	T49.3X2	T49.3X3	T49.3X4	T49.3X5	T49.3X6
Allyltribromide	T42.6X1	T42.6X2	T42.6X3	T42.6X4	T42.6X5	T42.6X6
Allypropymal	T42.3X1	T42.3X2	T42.3X3	T42.3X4	T42.3X5	T42.3X6
Almagate	T47.1X1	T47.1X2	T47.1X3	T47.1X4	T47.1X5	T47.1X6
Almasilate	T47.1X1	T47.1X2	T47.1X3	T47.1X4	T47.1X5	T47.1X6
Almitrine	T50.7X1	T50.7X2	T50.7X3	T50.7X4	T50.7X5	T50.7X6
Aloes	T47.2X1	T47.2X2	T47.2X3	T47.2X4	T47.2X5	T47.2X6
Aloglutamol	T47.1X1	T47.1X2	T47.1X3	T47.1X4	T47.1X5	T47.1X6
Aloin	T47.2X1	T47.2X2	T47.2X3	T47.2X4	T47.2X5	T47.2X6
Aloxidone	T42.2X1	T42.2X2	T42.2X3	T42.2X4	T42.2X5	T42.2X6
Alpha						
acetyldigoxin	T46.0X1	T46.0X2	T46.0X3	T46.0X4	T46.0X5	T46.0X6
adrenergic blocking drug	T44.6X1	T44.6X2	T44.6X3	T44.6X4	T44.6X5	T44.6X6
amylase	T45.3X1	T45.3X2	T45.3X3	T45.3X4	T45.3X5	T45.3X6
tocoferol (acetate)	T45.2X1	T45.2X2	T45.2X3	T45.2X4	T45.2X5	T45.2X6
tocopherol	T45.2X1	T45.2X2	T45.2X3	T45.2X4	T45.2X5	T45.2X6
Alphadolone	T41.1X1	T41.1X2	T41.1X3	T41.1X4	T41.1X5	T41.1X6
Alphaprodine	T40.491	T40.492	T40.493	T40.494	T40.495	T40.496
Alphaxalone	T41.1X1	T41.1X2	T41.1X3	T41.1X4	T41.1X5	T41.1X6
Alprazolam	T42.4X1	T42.4X2	T42.4X3	T42.4X4	T42.4X5	T42.4X6
Alprenolol	T44.7X1	T44.7X2	T44.7X3	T44.7X4	T44.7X5	T44.7X6
Alprostadil	T46.7X1	T46.7X2	T46.7X3	T46.7X4	T46.7X5	T46.7X6
Alsactide	T38.811	T38.812	T38.813	T38.814	T38.815	T38.816
Alseroxylon	T46.5X1	T46.5X2	T46.5X3	T46.5X4	T46.5X5	T46.5X6
Alteplase	T45.611	T45.612	T45.613	T45.614	T45.615	T45.616
Altizide	T50.2X1	T50.2X2	T50.2X3	T50.2X4	T50.2X5	T50.2X6
Altretamine	T45.1X1	T45.1X2	T45.1X3	T45.1X4	T45.1X5	T45.1X6
Alum (medicinal)	T49.4X1	T49.4X2	T49.4X3	T49.4X4	T49.4X5	T49.4X6
nonmedicinal (ammonium) (potassium)	T56.891	T56.892	T56.893	T56.894	—	—
Aluminium, aluminum						
acetate	T49.2X1	T49.2X2	T49.2X3	T49.2X4	T49.2X5	T49.2X6
solution	T49.0X1	T49.0X2	T49.0X3	T49.0X4	T49.0X5	T49.0X6
aspirin	T39.011	T39.012	T39.013	T39.014	T39.015	T39.016
bis (acetylsalicylate)	T39.011	T39.012	T39.013	T39.014	T39.015	T39.016

Substance	Poisoning, Accidental (Unintentional)	Poisoning, Intentional Self-Harm	Poisoning, Assault	Poisoning, Undetermined	Adverse Effect	Underdosing
			External Cause (T-Code)			
Aluminium, aluminum (Continued)						
carbonate (gel, basic)	T47.1X1	T47.1X2	T47.1X3	T47.1X4	T47.1X5	T47.1X6
chlorhydroxide-complex	T47.1X1	T47.1X2	T47.1X3	T47.1X4	T47.1X5	T47.1X6
chloride	T49.2X1	T49.2X2	T49.2X3	T49.2X4	T49.2X5	T49.2X6
clofibrate	T46.6X1	T46.6X2	T46.6X3	T46.6X4	T46.6X5	T46.6X6
diacetate	T49.2X1	T49.2X2	T49.2X3	T49.2X4	T49.2X5	T49.2X6
glycinate	T47.1X1	T47.1X2	T47.1X3	T47.1X4	T47.1X5	T47.1X6
hydroxide (gel)	T47.1X1	T47.1X2	T47.1X3	T47.1X4	T47.1X5	T47.1X6
hydroxide-magnesium carb. gel	T47.1X1	T47.1X2	T47.1X3	T47.1X4	T47.1X5	T47.1X6
magnesium silicate	T47.1X1	T47.1X2	T47.1X3	T47.1X4	T47.1X5	T47.1X6
nicotinate	T46.7X1	T46.7X2	T46.7X3	T46.7X4	T46.7X5	T46.7X6
ointment (surgical) (topical)	T49.3X1	T49.3X2	T49.3X3	T49.3X4	T49.3X5	T49.3X6
phosphate	T47.1X1	T47.1X2	T47.1X3	T47.1X4	T47.1X5	T47.1X6
salicylate	T39.091	T39.092	T39.093	T39.094	T39.095	T39.096
silicate	T47.1X1	T47.1X2	T47.1X3	T47.1X4	T47.1X5	T47.1X6
sodium silicate	T47.1X1	T47.1X2	T47.1X3	T47.1X4	T47.1X5	T47.1X6
subacetate	T49.2X1	T49.2X2	T49.2X3	T49.2X4	T49.2X5	T49.2X6
sulfate	T49.0X1	T49.0X2	T49.0X3	T49.0X4	T49.0X5	T49.0X6
tannate	T47.6X1	T47.6X2	T47.6X3	T47.6X4	T47.6X5	T47.6X6
topical NEC	T49.3X1	T49.3X2	T49.3X3	T49.3X4	T49.3X5	T49.3X6
Alurate	T42.3X1	T42.3X2	T42.3X3	T42.3X4	T42.3X5	T42.3X6
Alverine	T44.3X1	T44.3X2	T44.3X3	T44.3X4	T44.3X5	T44.3X6
Alvodine	T40.2X1	T40.2X2	T40.2X3	T40.2X4	T40.2X5	T40.2X6
Amanita phalloides	T62.0X1	T62.0X2	T62.0X3	T62.0X4	—	—
Amanitine	T62.0X1	T62.0X2	T62.0X3	T62.0X4	—	—
Amantadine	T42.8X1	T42.8X2	T42.8X3	T42.8X4	T42.8X5	T42.8X6
Ambazone	T49.6X1	T49.6X2	T49.6X3	T49.6X4	T49.6X5	T49.6X6
Ambenonium (chloride)	T44.0X1	T44.0X2	T44.0X3	T44.0X4	T44.0X5	T44.0X6
Ambroxol	T48.4X1	T48.4X2	T48.4X3	T48.4X4	T48.4X5	T48.4X6
Ambuphylline	T48.6X1	T48.6X2	T48.6X3	T48.6X4	T48.6X5	T48.6X6
Ambutonium bromide	T44.3X1	T44.3X2	T44.3X3	T44.3X4	T44.3X5	T44.3X6
Amcinonide	T49.0X1	T49.0X2	T49.0X3	T49.0X4	T49.0X5	T49.0X6
Amdinocilline	T36.0X1	T36.0X2	T36.0X3	T36.0X4	T36.0X5	T36.0X6
Ametazole	T50.8X1	T50.8X2	T50.8X3	T50.8X4	T50.8X5	T50.8X6
Amethocaine	T41.3X1	T41.3X2	T41.3X3	T41.3X4	T41.3X5	T41.3X6
regional	T41.3X1	T41.3X2	T41.3X3	T41.3X4	T41.3X5	T41.3X6
spinal	T41.3X1	T41.3X2	T41.3X3	T41.3X4	T41.3X5	T41.3X6
Amethopterin	T45.1X1	T45.1X2	T45.1X3	T45.1X4	T45.1X5	T45.1X6
Amezinium metilsulfate	T44.991	T44.992	T44.993	T44.994	T44.995	T44.996
Amfebutamone	T43.291	T43.292	T43.293	T43.294	T43.295	T43.296
Amfepramone	T50.5X1	T50.5X2	T50.5X3	T50.5X4	T50.5X5	T50.5X6

◀ New ◀ Revised ~~deleted~~ Deleted

Substance	Poisoning, Accidental (Unintentional)	Poisoning, Intentional Self-Harm	Poisoning, Assault	Poisoning, Undetermined	Adverse Effect	Underdosing
Amfetamine	T43.621	T43.622	T43.623	T43.624	T43.625	T43.626
Amfetaminil	T43.621	T43.622	T43.623	T43.624	T43.625	T43.626
Amfomycin	T36.8X1	T36.8X2	T36.8X3	T36.8X4	T36.8X5	T36.8X6
Amidefrine mesilate	T48.5X1	T48.5X2	T48.5X3	T48.5X4	T48.5X5	T48.5X6
Amidone	T40.3X1	T40.3X2	T40.3X3	T40.3X4	T40.3X5	T40.3X6
Amidopyrine	T39.2X1	T39.2X2	T39.2X3	T39.2X4	T39.2X5	T39.2X6
Amidotrizoate	T50.8X1	T50.8X2	T50.8X3	T50.8X4	T50.8X5	T50.8X6
Amiflamine	T43.1X1	T43.1X2	T43.1X3	T43.1X4	T43.1X5	T43.1X6
Amikacin	T36.5X1	T36.5X2	T36.5X3	T36.5X4	T36.5X5	T36.5X6
Amikhelline	T46.3X1	T46.3X2	T46.3X3	T46.3X4	T46.3X5	T46.3X6
Amiloride	T50.2X1	T50.2X2	T50.2X3	T50.2X4	T50.2X5	T50.2X6
Aminacrine	T49.0X1	T49.0X2	T49.0X3	T49.0X4	T49.0X5	T49.0X6
Amineptine	T43.011	T43.012	T43.013	T43.014	T43.015	T43.016
Aminitrozole	T37.3X1	T37.3X2	T37.3X3	T37.3X4	T37.3X5	T37.3X6
Aminoacetic acid (derivatives)	T50.3X1	T50.3X2	T50.3X3	T50.3X4	T50.3X5	T50.3X6
Amino acids	T50.3X1	T50.3X2	T50.3X3	T50.3X4	T50.3X5	T50.3X6
Aminoacridine	T49.0X1	T49.0X2	T49.0X3	T49.0X4	T49.0X5	T49.0X6
Aminobenzoic acid (-p)	T49.3X1	T49.3X2	T49.3X3	T49.3X4	T49.3X5	T49.3X6
4-Aminobutyric acid	T43.8X1	T43.8X2	T43.8X3	T43.8X4	T43.8X5	T43.8X6
Aminocaproic acid	T45.621	T45.622	T45.623	T45.624	T45.625	T45.626
Aminofenazone	T39.2X1	T39.2X2	T39.2X3	T39.2X4	T39.2X5	T39.2X6
Aminoethylisothiourium	T45.8X1	T45.8X2	T45.8X3	T45.8X4	T45.8X5	T45.8X6
Aminoglutethimide	T45.1X1	T45.1X2	T45.1X3	T45.1X4	T45.1X5	T45.1X6
Aminohippuric acid	T50.8X1	T50.8X2	T50.8X3	T50.8X4	T50.8X5	T50.8X6
Aminomethylbenzoic acid	T45.691	T45.692	T45.693	T45.694	T45.695	T45.696
Aminometradine	T50.2X1	T50.2X2	T50.2X3	T50.2X4	T50.2X5	T50.2X6
Aminopentamide	T44.3X1	T44.3X2	T44.3X3	T44.3X4	T44.3X5	T44.3X6
Aminophenazone	T39.2X1	T39.2X2	T39.2X3	T39.2X4	T39.2X5	T39.2X6
Aminophenol	T54.0X1	T54.0X2	T54.0X3	T54.0X4	—	—
4-Aminophenol derivatives	T39.1X1	T39.1X2	T39.1X3	T39.1X4	T39.1X5	T39.1X6
Aminophenylpyridone	T43.591	T43.592	T43.593	T43.594	T43.595	T43.596
Aminophylline	T48.6X1	T48.6X2	T48.6X3	T48.6X4	T48.6X5	T48.6X6
Aminopterin sodium	T45.1X1	T45.1X2	T45.1X3	T45.1X4	T45.1X5	T45.1X6
Aminopyrine	T39.2X1	T39.2X2	T39.2X3	T39.2X4	T39.2X5	T39.2X6
8-Aminoquinoline drugs	T37.2X1	T37.2X2	T37.2X3	T37.2X4	T37.2X5	T37.2X6
Aminorex	T50.5X1	T50.5X2	T50.5X3	T50.5X4	T50.5X5	T50.5X6
Aminosalicylic acid	T37.1X1	T37.1X2	T37.1X3	T37.1X4	T37.1X5	T37.1X6
Aminosalylum	T37.1X1	T37.1X2	T37.1X3	T37.1X4	T37.1X5	T37.1X6
Amiodarone	T46.2X1	T46.2X2	T46.2X3	T46.2X4	T46.2X5	T46.2X6
Amiphenazole	T50.7X1	T50.7X2	T50.7X3	T50.7X4	T50.7X5	T50.7X6
Amiquinsin	T46.5X1	T46.5X2	T46.5X3	T46.5X4	T46.5X5	T46.5X6
Amisometradine	T50.2X1	T50.2X2	T50.2X3	T50.2X4	T50.2X5	T50.2X6
Amisulpride	T43.591	T43.592	T43.593	T43.594	T43.595	T43.596
Amitriptyline	T43.021	T43.022	T43.023	T43.024	T43.025	T43.026
Amitriptylinoxide	T43.021	T43.022	T43.023	T43.024	T43.025	T43.026
Amlexanox	T48.6X1	T48.6X2	T48.6X3	T48.6X4	T48.6X5	T48.6X6
Ammonia (fumes) (gas) (vapor)	T59.891	T59.892	T59.893	T59.894	—	—
aromatic spirit	T48.991	T48.992	T48.993	T48.994	T48.995	T48.996
liquid (household)	T54.3X1	T54.3X2	T54.3X3	T54.3X4	—	—
Ammoniated mercury	T49.0X1	T49.0X2	T49.0X3	T49.0X4	T49.0X5	T49.0X6
Ammonium						
acid tartrate	T49.5X1	T49.5X2	T49.5X3	T49.5X4	T49.5X5	T49.5X6
bromide	T42.6X1	T42.6X2	T42.6X3	T42.6X4	T42.6X5	T42.6X6
carbonate	T54.3X1	T54.3X2	T54.3X3	T54.3X4	—	—
chloride	T50.991	T50.992	T50.993	T50.994	T50.995	T50.996
expectorant	T48.4X1	T48.4X2	T48.4X3	T48.4X4	T48.4X5	T48.4X6
compounds (household) NEC	T54.3X1	T54.3X2	T54.3X3	T54.3X4	—	—
fumes (any usage)	T59.891	T59.892	T59.893	T59.894	—	—
industrial	T54.3X1	T54.3X2	T54.3X3	T54.3X4	—	—
ichthyosulronate	T49.4X1	T49.4X2	T49.4X3	T49.4X4	T49.4X5	T49.4X6
mandelate	T37.91	T37.92	T37.93	T37.94	T37.95	T37.96
sulfamate	T60.3X1	T60.3X2	T60.3X3	T60.3X4	—	—
sulfonate resin	T47.8X1	T47.8X2	T47.8X3	T47.8X4	T47.8X5	T47.8X6
Amobarbital (sodium)	T42.3X1	T42.3X2	T42.3X3	T42.3X4	T42.3X5	T42.3X6
Amodiaquine	T37.2X1	T37.2X2	T37.2X3	T37.2X4	T37.2X5	T37.2X6
Amopyroquin(e)	T37.2X1	T37.2X2	T37.2X3	T37.2X4	T37.2X5	T37.2X6
Amoxapine	T43.011	T43.012	T43.013	T43.014	T43.015	T43.016
Amoxicillin	T36.0X1	T36.0X2	T36.0X3	T36.0X4	T36.0X5	T36.0X6
Amperozide	T43.591	T43.592	T43.593	T43.594	T43.595	T43.596
Amphenidone	T43.591	T43.592	T43.593	T43.594	T43.595	T43.596
Amphetamine NEC	T43.621	T43.622	T43.623	T43.624	T43.625	T43.626
Amphomycin	T36.8X1	T36.8X2	T36.8X3	T36.8X4	T36.8X5	T36.8X6
Amphotalide	T37.4X1	T37.4X2	T37.4X3	T37.4X4	T37.4X5	T37.4X6
Amphotericin B	T36.7X1	T36.7X2	T36.7X3	T36.7X4	T36.7X5	T36.7X6
topical	T49.0X1	T49.0X2	T49.0X3	T49.0X4	T49.0X5	T49.0X6
Ampicillin	T36.0X1	T36.0X2	T36.0X3	T36.0X4	T36.0X5	T36.0X6
Amprotropine	T44.3X1	T44.3X2	T44.3X3	T44.3X4	T44.3X5	T44.3X6
Amsacrine	T45.1X1	T45.1X2	T45.1X3	T45.1X4	T45.1X5	T45.1X6
Amygdaline	T62.2X1	T62.2X2	T62.2X3	T62.2X4	—	—
Amyl						
acetate	T52.8X1	T52.8X2	T52.8X3	T52.8X4	—	—
vapor	T59.891	T59.892	T59.893	T59.894	—	—
alcohol	T51.3X1	T51.3X2	T51.3X3	T51.3X4	—	—
chloride	T53.6X1	T53.6X2	T53.6X3	T53.6X4	—	—

TABLE OF DRUGS AND CHEMICALS

Substance	Poisoning, Accidental (Unintentional)	Poisoning, Intentional Self-Harm	Poisoning, Assault	Poisoning, Undetermined	Adverse Effect	Underdosing
Amyl (Continued)						
formate	T52.8X1	T52.8X2	T52.8X3	T52.8X4	—	—
nitrite	T46.3X1	T46.3X2	T46.3X3	T46.3X4	T46.3X5	T46.3X6
propionate	T65.891	T65.892	T65.893	T65.894	—	—
Amylase	T47.5X1	T47.5X2	T47.5X3	T47.5X4	T47.5X5	T47.5X6
Amyleine, regional	T41.3X1	T41.3X2	T41.3X3	T41.3X4	T41.3X5	T41.3X6
Amylene						
dichloride	T53.6X1	T53.6X2	T53.6X3	T53.6X4	—	—
hydrate	T51.3X1	T51.3X2	T51.3X3	T51.3X4	—	—
Amylmetacresol	T49.6X1	T49.6X2	T49.6X3	T49.6X4	T49.6X5	T49.6X6
Amylobarbitone	T42.3X1	T42.3X2	T42.3X3	T42.3X4	T42.3X5	T42.3X6
Amylocaine, regional	T41.3X1	T41.3X2	T41.3X3	T41.3X4	T41.3X5	T41.3X6
infiltration (subcutaneous)	T41.3X1	T41.3X2	T41.3X3	T41.3X4	T41.3X5	T41.3X6
nerve block (peripheral) (plexus)	T41.3X1	T41.3X2	T41.3X3	T41.3X4	T41.3X5	T41.3X6
spinal	T41.3X1	T41.3X2	T41.3X3	T41.3X4	T41.3X5	T41.3X6
topical (surface)	T41.3X1	T41.3X2	T41.3X3	T41.3X4	T41.3X5	T41.3X6
Amylopectin	T47.6X1	T47.6X2	T47.6X3	T47.6X4	T47.6X5	T47.6X6
Amytal (sodium)	T42.3X1	T42.3X2	T42.3X3	T42.3X4	T42.3X5	T42.3X6
Anabolic steroid	T38.7X1	T38.7X2	T38.7X3	T38.7X4	T38.7X5	T38.7X6
Analeptic NEC	T50.7X1	T50.7X2	T50.7X3	T50.7X4	T50.7X5	T50.7X6
Analgesic	T39.91	T39.92	T39.93	T39.94	T39.95	T39.96
anti-inflammatory NEC	T39.91	T39.92	T39.93	T39.94	T39.95	T39.96
propionic acid derivative	T39.311	T39.312	T39.313	T39.314	T39.315	T39.316
antirheumatic NEC	T39.4X1	T39.4X2	T39.4X3	T39.4X4	T39.4X5	T39.4X6
aromatic NEC	T39.1X1	T39.1X2	T39.1X3	T39.1X4	T39.1X5	T39.1X6
narcotic NEC	T40.601	T40.602	T40.603	T40.604	T40.605	T40.606
combination	T40.601	T40.602	T40.603	T40.604	T40.605	T40.606
obstetric	T40.601	T40.602	T40.603	T40.604	T40.605	T40.606
non-narcotic NEC	T39.91	T39.92	T39.93	T39.94	T39.95	T39.96
combination	T39.91	T39.92	T39.93	T39.94	T39.95	T39.96
pyrazole	T39.2X1	T39.2X2	T39.2X3	T39.2X4	T39.2X5	T39.2X6
specified NEC	T39.8X1	T39.8X2	T39.8X3	T39.8X4	T39.8X5	T39.8X6
Analgin	T39.2X1	T39.2X2	T39.2X3	T39.2X4	T39.2X5	T39.2X6
Anamirta cocculus	T62.1X1	T62.1X2	T62.1X3	T62.1X4	—	—
Ancillin	T36.0X1	T36.0X2	T36.0X3	T36.0X4	T36.0X5	T36.0X6
Ancrod	T45.691	T45.692	T45.693	T45.694	T45.695	T45.696
Androgen	T38.7X1	T38.7X2	T38.7X3	T38.7X4	T38.7X5	T38.7X6
Androgen-estrogen mixture	T38.7X1	T38.7X2	T38.7X3	T38.7X4	T38.7X5	T38.7X6
Androstalone	T38.7X1	T38.7X2	T38.7X3	T38.7X4	T38.7X5	T38.7X6
Androstanolone	T38.7X1	T38.7X2	T38.7X3	T38.7X4	T38.7X5	T38.7X6
Androsterone	T38.7X1	T38.7X2	T38.7X3	T38.7X4	T38.7X5	T38.7X6

Substance	Poisoning, Accidental (Unintentional)	Poisoning, Intentional Self-Harm	Poisoning, Assault	Poisoning, Undetermined	Adverse Effect	Underdosing
Anemone pulsatilla	T62.2X1	T62.2X2	T62.2X3	T62.2X4	—	—
Anesthesia						
caudal	T41.3X1	T41.3X2	T41.3X3	T41.3X4	T41.3X5	T41.3X6
endotracheal	T41.0X1	T41.0X2	T41.0X3	T41.0X4	T41.0X5	T41.0X6
epidural	T41.3X1	T41.3X2	T41.3X3	T41.3X4	T41.3X5	T41.3X6
inhalation	T41.0X1	T41.0X2	T41.0X3	T41.0X4	T41.0X5	T41.0X6
local	T41.3X1	T41.3X2	T41.3X3	T41.3X4	T41.3X5	T41.3X6
mucosal	T41.3X1	T41.3X2	T41.3X3	T41.3X4	T41.3X5	T41.3X6
muscle relaxation	T48.1X1	T48.1X2	T48.1X3	T48.1X4	T48.1X5	T48.1X6
nerve blocking	T41.3X1	T41.3X2	T41.3X3	T41.3X4	T41.3X5	T41.3X6
plexus blocking	T41.3X1	T41.3X2	T41.3X3	T41.3X4	T41.3X5	T41.3X6
potentiated	T41.201	T41.202	T41.203	T41.204	T41.205	T41.206
rectal	T41.201	T41.202	T41.203	T41.204	T41.205	T41.206
general	T41.201	T41.202	T41.203	T41.204	T41.205	T41.206
local	T41.3X1	T41.3X2	T41.3X3	T41.3X4	T41.3X5	T41.3X6
regional	T41.3X1	T41.3X2	T41.3X3	T41.3X4	T41.3X5	T41.3X6
surface	T41.3X1	T41.3X2	T41.3X3	T41.3X4	T41.3X5	T41.3X6
Anesthetic NEC — see also Anesthesia	T41.41	T41.42	T41.43	T41.44	T41.45	T41.46
with muscle relaxant	T41.201	T41.202	T41.203	T41.204	T41.205	T41.206
general	T41.201	T41.202	T41.203	T41.204	T41.205	T41.206
local	T41.3X1	T41.3X2	T41.3X3	T41.3X4	T41.3X5	T41.3X6
gaseous NEC	T41.0X1	T41.0X2	T41.0X3	T41.0X4	T41.0X5	T41.0X6
general NEC	T41.201	T41.202	T41.203	T41.204	T41.205	T41.206
halogenated hydrocarbon derivatives NEC	T41.0X1	T41.0X2	T41.0X3	T41.0X4	T41.0X5	T41.0X6
infiltration NEC	T41.3X1	T41.3X2	T41.3X3	T41.3X4	T41.3X5	T41.3X6
intravenous NEC	T41.1X1	T41.1X2	T41.1X3	T41.1X4	T41.1X5	T41.1X6
local NEC	T41.3X1	T41.3X2	T41.3X3	T41.3X4	T41.3X5	T41.3X6
rectal	T41.201	T41.202	T41.203	T41.204	T41.205	T41.206
general	T41.201	T41.202	T41.203	T41.204	T41.205	T41.206
local	T41.3X1	T41.3X2	T41.3X3	T41.3X4	T41.3X5	T41.3X6
regional NEC	T41.3X1	T41.3X2	T41.3X3	T41.3X4	T41.3X5	T41.3X6
spinal NEC	T41.3X1	T41.3X2	T41.3X3	T41.3X4	T41.3X5	T41.3X6
thiobarbiturate	T41.1X1	T41.1X2	T41.1X3	T41.1X4	T41.1X5	T41.1X6
topical	T41.3X1	T41.3X2	T41.3X3	T41.3X4	T41.3X5	T41.3X6
Aneurine	T45.2X1	T45.2X2	T45.2X3	T45.2X4	T45.2X5	T45.2X6
Angio-Conray	T50.8X1	T50.8X2	T50.8X3	T50.8X4	T50.8X5	T50.8X6
Angiotensin	T44.5X1	T44.5X2	T44.5X3	T44.5X4	T44.5X5	T44.5X6
Angiotensinamide	T44.991	T44.992	T44.993	T44.994	T44.995	T44.996
Anhydrohydroxy-progesterone	T38.5X1	T38.5X2	T38.5X3	T38.5X4	T38.5X5	T38.5X6
Anhydron	T50.2X1	T50.2X2	T50.2X3	T50.2X4	T50.2X5	T50.2X6
Anileridine	T40.491	T40.492	T40.493	T40.494	T40.495	T40.496

◄ New ◄ Revised ~~deleted~~ Deleted

	External Cause (T-Code)					
Substance	Poisoning, Accidental (Unintentional)	Poisoning, Intentional Self-Harm	Poisoning, Assault	Poisoning, Undetermined	Adverse Effect	Underdosing
Aniline (dye) (liquid)	T65.3X1	T65.3X2	T65.3X3	T65.3X4	—	—
analgesic	T39.1X1	T39.1X2	T39.1X3	T39.1X4	T39.1X5	T39.1X6
derivatives, therapeutic NEC	T39.1X1	T39.1X2	T39.1X3	T39.1X4	T39.1X5	T39.1X6
vapor	T65.3X1	T65.3X2	T65.3X3	T65.3X4	—	—
Anise oil	T47.5X1	T47.5X2	T47.5X3	T47.5X4	T47.5X5	T47.5X6
Aniscoropine	T44.3X1	T44.3X2	T44.3X3	T44.3X4	T44.3X5	T44.3X6
Anisidine	T65.3X1	T65.3X2	T65.3X3	T65.3X4	—	—
Anisindione	T45.511	T45.512	T45.513	T45.514	T45.515	T45.516
Anisotropine methyl-bromide	T44.3X1	T44.3X2	T44.3X3	T44.3X4	T44.3X5	T44.3X6
Anistreplase	T45.611	T45.612	T45.613	T45.614	T45.615	T45.616
Anorexiant (central)	T50.5X1	T50.5X2	T50.5X3	T50.5X4	T50.5X5	T50.5X6
Anorexic agents	T50.5X1	T50.5X2	T50.5X3	T50.5X4	T50.5X5	T50.5X6
Ansamycin	T36.6X1	T36.6X2	T36.6X3	T36.6X4	T36.6X5	T36.6X6
Ant (bite) (sting)	T63.421	T63.422	T63.423	T63.424	—	—
Antabuse	T50.6X1	T50.6X2	T50.6X3	T50.6X4	T50.6X5	T50.6X6
Ant poison — see Insecticide						
Antacid NEC	T47.1X1	T47.1X2	T47.1X3	T47.1X4	T47.1X5	T47.1X6
Antagonist						
Aldosterone	T50.0X1	T50.0X2	T50.0X3	T50.0X4	T50.0X5	T50.0X6
alpha-adrenoreceptor	T44.6X1	T44.6X2	T44.6X3	T44.6X4	T44.6X5	T44.6X6
anticoagulant	T45.7X1	T45.7X2	T45.7X3	T45.7X4	T45.7X5	T45.7X6
beta-adrenoreceptor	T44.7X1	T44.7X2	T44.7X3	T44.7X4	T44.7X5	T44.7X6
extrapyramidal NEC	T44.3X1	T44.3X2	T44.3X3	T44.3X4	T44.3X5	T44.3X6
folic acid	T45.1X1	T45.1X2	T45.1X3	T45.1X4	T45.1X5	T45.1X6
H2 receptor	T47.0X1	T47.0X2	T47.0X3	T47.0X4	T47.0X5	T47.0X6
heavy metal	T45.8X1	T45.8X2	T45.8X3	T45.8X4	T45.8X5	T45.8X6
narcotic analgesic	T50.7X1	T50.7X2	T50.7X3	T50.7X4	T50.7X5	T50.7X6
opiate	T50.7X1	T50.7X2	T50.7X3	T50.7X4	T50.7X5	T50.7X6
pyrimidine	T45.1X1	T45.1X2	T45.1X3	T45.1X4	T45.1X5	T45.1X6
serotonin	T46.5X1	T46.5X2	T46.5X3	T46.5X4	T46.5X5	T46.5X6
Antazolin(e)	T45.0X1	T45.0X2	T45.0X3	T45.0X4	T45.0X5	T45.0X6
Anterior pituitary hormone NEC	T38.811	T38.812	T38.813	T38.814	T38.815	T38.816
Anthelmintic NEC	T37.4X1	T37.4X2	T37.4X3	T37.4X4	T37.4X5	T37.4X6
Anthiolimine	T37.4X1	T37.4X2	T37.4X3	T37.4X4	T37.4X5	T37.4X6
Anthralin	T49.4X1	T49.4X2	T49.4X3	T49.4X4	T49.4X5	T49.4X6
Anthramycin	T45.1X1	T45.1X2	T45.1X3	T45.1X4	T45.1X5	T45.1X6
Antiadrenergic NEC	T44.8X1	T44.8X2	T44.8X3	T44.8X4	T44.8X5	T44.8X6
Antiallergic NEC	T45.0X1	T45.0X2	T45.0X3	T45.0X4	T45.0X5	T45.0X6
Anti-anemic (drug) (preparation)	T45.8X1	T45.8X2	T45.8X3	T45.8X4	T45.8X5	T45.8X6
Antiandrogen NEC	T38.6X1	T38.6X2	T38.6X3	T38.6X4	T38.6X5	T38.6X6
Antianxiety drug NEC	T43.501	T43.502	T43.503	T43.504	T43.505	T43.506
Antiaris toxicaria	T65.891	T65.892	T65.893	T65.894	—	—

	External Cause (T-Code)					
Substance	Poisoning, Accidental (Unintentional)	Poisoning, Intentional Self-Harm	Poisoning, Assault	Poisoning, Undetermined	Adverse Effect	Underdosing
Antiarteriosclerotic drug	T46.6X1	T46.6X2	T46.6X3	T46.6X4	T46.6X5	T46.6X6
Antiasthmatic drug NEC	T48.6X1	T48.6X2	T48.6X3	T48.6X4	T48.6X5	T48.6X6
Antibiotic NEC	T36.91	T36.92	T36.93	T36.94	T36.95	T36.96
aminoglycoside	T36.5X1	T36.5X2	T36.5X3	T36.5X4	T36.5X5	T36.5X6
anticancer	T45.1X1	T45.1X2	T45.1X3	T45.1X4	T45.1X5	T45.1X6
antifungal	T36.7X1	T36.7X2	T36.7X3	T36.7X4	T36.7X5	T36.7X6
antimycobacterial	T36.5X1	T36.5X2	T36.5X3	T36.5X4	T36.5X5	T36.5X6
antineoplastic	T45.1X1	T45.1X2	T45.1X3	T45.1X4	T45.1X5	T45.1X6
cephalosporin (group)	T36.1X1	T36.1X2	T36.1X3	T36.1X4	T36.1X5	T36.1X6
chloramphenicol (group)	T36.2X1	T36.2X2	T36.2X3	T36.2X4	T36.2X5	T36.2X6
ENT	T49.6X1	T49.6X2	T49.6X3	T49.6X4	T49.6X5	T49.6X6
eye	T49.5X1	T49.5X2	T49.5X3	T49.5X4	T49.5X5	T49.5X6
fungicidal (local)	T49.0X1	T49.0X2	T49.0X3	T49.0X4	T49.0X5	T49.0X6
intestinal	T36.8X1	T36.8X2	T36.8X3	T36.8X4	T36.8X5	T36.8X6
b-lactam NEC	T36.1X1	T36.1X2	T36.1X3	T36.1X4	T36.1X5	T36.1X6
local	T49.0X1	T49.0X2	T49.0X3	T49.0X4	T49.0X5	T49.0X6
macrolides	T36.3X1	T36.3X2	T36.3X3	T36.3X4	T36.3X5	T36.3X6
polypeptide	T36.8X1	T36.8X2	T36.8X3	T36.8X4	T36.8X5	T36.8X6
specified NEC	T36.8X1	T36.8X2	T36.8X3	T36.8X4	T36.8X5	T36.8X6
tetracycline (group)	T36.4X1	T36.4X2	T36.4X3	T36.4X4	T36.4X5	T36.4X6
throat	T49.6X1	T49.6X2	T49.6X3	T49.6X4	T49.6X5	T49.6X6
Anticancer agents NEC	T45.1X1	T45.1X2	T45.1X3	T45.1X4	T45.1X5	T45.1X6
Anticholesterolemic drug NEC	T46.6X1	T46.6X2	T46.6X3	T46.6X4	T46.6X5	T46.6X6
Anticholinergic NEC	T44.3X1	T44.3X2	T44.3X3	T44.3X4	T44.3X5	T44.3X6
Anticholinesterase	T44.0X1	T44.0X2	T44.0X3	T44.0X4	T44.0X5	T44.0X6
organophosphorus	T44.0X1	T44.0X2	T44.0X3	T44.0X4	T44.0X5	T44.0X6
insecticide	T60.0X1	T60.0X2	T60.0X3	T60.0X4	—	—
nerve gas	T59.891	T59.892	T59.893	T59.894	—	—
reversible	T44.0X1	T44.0X2	T44.0X3	T44.0X4	T44.0X5	T44.0X6
ophthalmological	T49.5X1	T49.5X2	T49.5X3	T49.5X4	T49.5X5	T49.5X6
Anticoagulant NEC	T45.511	T45.512	T45.513	T45.514	T45.515	T45.516
Antagonist	T45.7X1	T45.7X2	T45.7X3	T45.7X4	T45.7X5	T45.7X6
Anti-common-cold drug NEC	T48.5X1	T48.5X2	T48.5X3	T48.5X4	T48.5X5	T48.5X6
Anticonvulsant	T42.71	T42.72	T42.73	T42.74	T42.75	T42.76
barbiturate	T42.3X1	T42.3X2	T42.3X3	T42.3X4	T42.3X5	T42.3X6
combination (with barbiturate)	T42.3X1	T42.3X2	T42.3X3	T42.3X4	T42.3X5	T42.3X6
hydantoin	T42.0X1	T42.0X2	T42.0X3	T42.0X4	T42.0X5	T42.0X6
hypnotic NEC	T42.6X1	T42.6X2	T42.6X3	T42.6X4	T42.6X5	T42.6X6
oxazolidinedione	T42.2X1	T42.2X2	T42.2X3	T42.2X4	T42.2X5	T42.2X6
pyrimidinedione	T42.6X1	T42.6X2	T42.6X3	T42.6X4	T42.6X5	T42.6X6
specified NEC	T42.6X1	T42.6X2	T42.6X3	T42.6X4	T42.6X5	T42.6X6
succinimide	T42.2X1	T42.2X2	T42.2X3	T42.2X4	T42.2X5	T42.2X6

TABLE OF DRUGS AND CHEMICALS

Substance	External Cause (T-Code)					
	Poisoning, Accidental (Unintentional)	Poisoning, Intentional Self-Harm	Poisoning, Assault	Poisoning, Undetermined	Adverse Effect	Underdosing
Anti-D immunoglobulin (human)	T50.Z11	T50.Z12	T50.Z13	T50.Z14	T50.Z15	T50.Z16
Antidepressant NEC	T43.201	T43.202	T43.203	T43.204	T43.205	T43.206
monoamine oxidase inhibitor	T43.1X1	T43.1X2	T43.1X3	T43.1X4	T43.1X5	T43.1X6
selective serotonin norepinephrine reuptake inhibitor	T43.211	T43.212	T43.213	T43.214	T43.215	T43.216
selective serotonin reuptake inhibitor	T43.221	T43.222	T43.223	T43.224	T43.225	T43.226
specified NEC	T43.291	T43.292	T43.293	T43.294	T43.295	T43.296
tetracyclic	T43.021	T43.022	T43.023	T43.024	T43.025	T43.026
triazolopyridine	T43.221	T43.222	T43.223	T43.224	T43.225	T43.226
tricyclic	T43.011	T43.012	T43.013	T43.014	T43.015	T43.016
Antidiabetic NEC	T38.3X1	T38.3X2	T38.3X3	T38.3X4	T38.3X5	T38.3X6
biguanide	T38.3X1	T38.3X2	T38.3X3	T38.3X4	T38.3X5	T38.3X6
and sulfonyl combined	T38.3X1	T38.3X2	T38.3X3	T38.3X4	T38.3X5	T38.3X6
combined	T38.3X1	T38.3X2	T38.3X3	T38.3X4	T38.3X5	T38.3X6
sulfonylurea	T38.3X1	T38.3X2	T38.3X3	T38.3X4	T38.3X5	T38.3X6
Antidiarrheal drug NEC	T47.6X1	T47.6X2	T47.6X3	T47.6X4	T47.6X5	T47.6X6
absorbent	T47.6X1	T47.6X2	T47.6X3	T47.6X4	T47.6X5	T47.6X6
Antidiphtheria serum	T50.Z11	T50.Z12	T50.Z13	T50.Z14	T50.Z15	T50.Z16
Antidiuretic hormone	T38.891	T38.892	T38.893	T38.894	T38.895	T38.896
Antidote NEC	T50.6X1	T50.6X2	T50.6X3	T50.6X4	T50.6X5	T50.6X6
heavy metal	T45.8X1	T45.8X2	T45.8X3	T45.8X4	T45.8X5	T45.8X6
Antidysrhythmic NEC	T46.2X1	T46.2X2	T46.2X3	T46.2X4	T46.2X5	T46.2X6
Antiemetic drug	T45.0X1	T45.0X2	T45.0X3	T45.0X4	T45.0X5	T45.0X6
Antiepilepsy agent	T42.71	T42.72	T42.73	T42.74	T42.75	T42.76
combination	T42.5X1	T42.5X2	T42.5X3	T42.5X4	T42.5X5	T42.5X6
mixed	T42.5X1	T42.5X2	T42.5X3	T42.5X4	T42.5X5	T42.5X6
specified, NEC	T42.6X1	T42.6X2	T42.6X3	T42.6X4	T42.6X5	T42.6X6
Antiestrogen NEC	T38.6X1	T38.6X2	T38.6X3	T38.6X4	T38.6X5	T38.6X6
Antifertility pill	T38.4X1	T38.4X2	T38.4X3	T38.4X4	T38.4X5	T38.4X6
Antifibrinolytic drug	T45.621	T45.622	T45.623	T45.624	T45.625	T45.626
Antifilarial drug	T37.4X1	T37.4X2	T37.4X3	T37.4X4	T37.4X5	T37.4X6
Antiflatulent	T47.5X1	T47.5X2	T47.5X3	T47.5X4	T47.5X5	T47.5X6
Antifreeze	T65.91	T65.92	T65.93	T65.94	—	—
alcohol	T51.1X1	T51.1X2	T51.1X3	T51.1X4	—	—
ethylene glycol	T51.8X1	T51.8X2	T51.8X3	T51.8X4	—	—
Antifungal						
antibiotic (systemic)	T36.7X1	T36.7X2	T36.7X3	T36.7X4	T36.7X5	T36.7X6
anti-infective NEC	T37.91	T37.92	T37.93	T37.94	T37.95	T37.96
disinfectant, local	T49.0X1	T49.0X2	T49.0X3	T49.0X4	T49.0X5	T49.0X6
nonmedicinal (spray)	T60.3X1	T60.3X2	T60.3X3	T60.3X4	—	—
topical	T49.0X1	T49.0X2	T49.0X3	T49.0X4	T49.0X5	T49.0X6

Substance	External Cause (T-Code)					
	Poisoning, Accidental (Unintentional)	Poisoning, Intentional Self-Harm	Poisoning, Assault	Poisoning, Undetermined	Adverse Effect	Underdosing
Anti-gastric-secretion drug NEC	T47.1X1	T47.1X2	T47.1X3	T47.1X4	T47.1X5	T47.1X6
Antigonadotrophin NEC	T38.6X1	T38.6X2	T38.6X3	T38.6X4	T38.6X5	T38.6X6
Antihallucinogen	T43.501	T43.502	T43.503	T43.504	T43.505	T43.506
Antihelmintics	T37.4X1	T37.4X2	T37.4X3	T37.4X4	T37.4X5	T37.4X6
Antihemophilic						
factor	T45.8X1	T45.8X2	T45.8X3	T45.8X4	T45.8X5	T45.8X6
fraction	T45.8X1	T45.8X2	T45.8X3	T45.8X4	T45.8X5	T45.8X6
globulin concentrate	T45.7X1	T45.7X2	T45.7X3	T45.7X4	T45.7X5	T45.7X6
human plasma	T45.8X1	T45.8X2	T45.8X3	T45.8X4	T45.8X5	T45.8X6
plasma, dried	T45.7X1	T45.7X2	T45.7X3	T45.7X4	T45.7X5	T45.7X6
Antihemorrhoidal preparation	T49.2X1	T49.2X2	T49.2X3	T49.2X4	T49.2X5	T49.2X6
Antiheparin drug	T45.7X1	T45.7X2	T45.7X3	T45.7X4	T45.7X5	T45.7X6
Antihistamine	T45.0X1	T45.0X2	T45.0X3	T45.0X4	T45.0X5	T45.0X6
Antihookworm drug	T37.4X1	T37.4X2	T37.4X3	T37.4X4	T37.4X5	T37.4X6
Anti-human lymphocytic globulin	T50.Z11	T50.Z12	T50.Z13	T50.Z14	T50.Z15	T50.Z16
Antihyperlipidemic drug	T46.6X1	T46.6X2	T46.6X3	T46.6X4	T46.6X5	T46.6X6
Antihypertensive drug NEC	T46.5X1	T46.5X2	T46.5X3	T46.5X4	T46.5X5	T46.5X6
Anti-infective NEC	T37.91	T37.92	T37.93	T37.94	T37.95	T37.96
anthelmintic	T37.4X1	T37.4X2	T37.4X3	T37.4X4	T37.4X5	T37.4X6
antibiotics	T36.91	T36.92	T36.93	T36.94	T36.95	T36.96
specified NEC	T36.8X1	T36.8X2	T36.8X3	T36.8X4	T36.8X5	T36.8X6
antimalarial	T37.2X1	T37.2X2	T37.2X3	T37.2X4	T37.2X5	T37.2X6
antimycobacterial NEC	T37.1X1	T37.1X2	T37.1X3	T37.1X4	T37.1X5	T37.1X6
antibiotics	T36.5X1	T36.5X2	T36.5X3	T36.5X4	T36.5X5	T36.5X6
antiprotozoal NEC	T37.3X1	T37.3X2	T37.3X3	T37.3X4	T37.3X5	T37.3X6
blood	T37.2X1	T37.2X2	T37.2X3	T37.2X4	T37.2X5	T37.2X6
antiviral	T37.5X1	T37.5X2	T37.5X3	T37.5X4	T37.5X5	T37.5X6
arsenical	T37.8X1	T37.8X2	T37.8X3	T37.8X4	T37.8X5	T37.8X6
bismuth, local	T49.0X1	T49.0X2	T49.0X3	T49.0X4	T49.0X5	T49.0X6
ENT	T49.6X1	T49.6X2	T49.6X3	T49.6X4	T49.6X5	T49.6X6
eye NEC	T49.5X1	T49.5X2	T49.5X3	T49.5X4	T49.5X5	T49.5X6
heavy metals NEC	T37.8X1	T37.8X2	T37.8X3	T37.8X4	T37.8X5	T37.8X6
local NEC	T49.0X1	T49.0X2	T49.0X3	T49.0X4	T49.0X5	T49.0X6
specified NEC	T49.0X1	T49.0X2	T49.0X3	T49.0X4	T49.0X5	T49.0X6
mixed	T37.91	T37.92	T37.93	T37.94	T37.95	T37.96
ophthalmic preparation	T49.5X1	T49.5X2	T49.5X3	T49.5X4	T49.5X5	T49.5X6
topical NEC	T49.0X1	T49.0X2	T49.0X3	T49.0X4	T49.0X5	T49.0X6
Anti-inflammatory drug NEC	T49.0X1	T49.0X2	T49.0X3	T49.0X4	T49.0X5	T49.0X6
local	T49.0X1	T49.0X2	T49.0X3	T49.0X4	T49.0X5	T49.0X6
nonsteroidal NEC	T39.391	T39.392	T39.393	T39.394	T39.395	T39.396
propionic acid derivative	T39.311	T39.312	T39.313	T39.314	T39.315	T39.316
specified NEC	T39.391	T39.392	T39.393	T39.394	T39.395	T39.396

◀ New ◀ Revised ~~deleted~~ Deleted

Substance	External Cause (T-Code)					
	Poisoning, Accidental (Unintentional)	Poisoning, Intentional Self-Harm	Poisoning, Assault	Poisoning, Undetermined	Adverse Effect	Underdosing
Antikaluretic	T50.3X1	T50.3X2	T50.3X3	T50.3X4	T50.3X5	T50.3X6
Antiknock (tetraethyl lead)	T56.0X1	T56.0X2	T56.0X3	T56.0X4	—	—
Antilipemic drug NEC	T46.6X1	T46.6X2	T46.6X3	T46.6X4	T46.6X5	T46.6X6
Antimalarial	T37.2X1	T37.2X2	T37.2X3	T37.2X4	T37.2X5	T37.2X6
prophylactic NEC	T37.2X1	T37.2X2	T37.2X3	T37.2X4	T37.2X5	T37.2X6
pyrimidine derivative	T37.2X1	T37.2X2	T37.2X3	T37.2X4	T37.2X5	T37.2X6
Antimetabolite	T45.1X1	T45.1X2	T45.1X3	T45.1X4	T45.1X5	T45.1X6
Antimitotic agent	T45.1X1	T45.1X2	T45.1X3	T45.1X4	T45.1X5	T45.1X6
Antimony (compounds) (vapor) NEC	T56.891	T56.892	T56.893	T56.894	—	—
anti-infectives	T37.8X1	T37.8X2	T37.8X3	T37.8X4	T37.8X5	T37.8X6
dimercaptosuccinate	T37.3X1	T37.3X2	T37.3X3	T37.3X4	T37.3X5	T37.3X6
hydride	T56.891	T56.892	T56.893	T56.894	—	—
pesticide (vapor)	T60.8X1	T60.8X2	T60.8X3	T60.8X4	—	—
potassium (sodium) tartrate	T37.8X1	T37.8X2	T37.8X3	T37.8X4	T37.8X5	T37.8X6
sodium dimercaptosuccinate	T37.3X1	T37.3X2	T37.3X3	T37.3X4	T37.3X5	T37.3X6
tartrated	T37.8X1	T37.8X2	T37.8X3	T37.8X4	T37.8X5	T37.8X6
Antimuscarinic NEC	T44.3X1	T44.3X2	T44.3X3	T44.3X4	T44.3X5	T44.3X6
Antimycobacterial drug NEC	T37.1X1	T37.1X2	T37.1X3	T37.1X4	T37.1X5	T37.1X6
antibiotics	T36.5X1	T36.5X2	T36.5X3	T36.5X4	T36.5X5	T36.5X6
combination	T37.1X1	T37.1X2	T37.1X3	T37.1X4	T37.1X5	T37.1X6
Antinausea drug	T45.0X1	T45.0X2	T45.0X3	T45.0X4	T45.0X5	T45.0X6
Antinematode drug	T37.4X1	T37.4X2	T37.4X3	T37.4X4	T37.4X5	T37.4X6
Antineoplastic NEC	T45.1X1	T45.1X2	T45.1X3	T45.1X4	T45.1X5	T45.1X6
alkaloidal	T45.1X1	T45.1X2	T45.1X3	T45.1X4	T45.1X5	T45.1X6
antibiotics	T45.1X1	T45.1X2	T45.1X3	T45.1X4	T45.1X5	T45.1X6
combination	T45.1X1	T45.1X2	T45.1X3	T45.1X4	T45.1X5	T45.1X6
estrogen	T38.5X1	T38.5X2	T38.5X3	T38.5X4	T38.5X5	T38.5X6
steroid	T38.7X1	T38.7X2	T38.7X3	T38.7X4	T38.7X5	T38.7X6
Antiparasitic drug (systemic)	T37.91	T37.92	T37.93	T37.94	T37.95	T37.96
local	T49.0X1	T49.0X2	T49.0X3	T49.0X4	T49.0X5	T49.0X6
specified NEC	T37.8X1	T37.8X2	T37.8X3	T37.8X4	T37.8X5	T37.8X6
Antiparkinsonism drug NEC	T42.8X1	T42.8X2	T42.8X3	T42.8X4	T42.8X5	T42.8X6
Antiperspirant NEC	T49.2X1	T49.2X2	T49.2X3	T49.2X4	T49.2X5	T49.2X6
Antiphlogistic NEC	T39.4X1	T39.4X2	T39.4X3	T39.4X4	T39.4X5	T39.4X6
Antiplatyhelmintic drug	T37.4X1	T37.4X2	T37.4X3	T37.4X4	T37.4X5	T37.4X6
Antiprotozoal drug NEC	T37.3X1	T37.3X2	T37.3X3	T37.3X4	T37.3X5	T37.3X6
blood	T37.2X1	T37.2X2	T37.2X3	T37.2X4	T37.2X5	T37.2X6
local	T49.0X1	T49.0X2	T49.0X3	T49.0X4	T49.0X5	T49.0X6
Antipruritic drug NEC	T49.1X1	T49.1X2	T49.1X3	T49.1X4	T49.1X5	T49.1X6
Antipsychotic drug	T43.501	T43.502	T43.503	T43.504	T43.505	T43.506
specified NEC	T43.591	T43.592	T43.593	T43.594	T43.595	T43.596

Substance	External Cause (T-Code)					
	Poisoning, Accidental (Unintentional)	Poisoning, Intentional Self-Harm	Poisoning, Assault	Poisoning, Undetermined	Adverse Effect	Underdosing
Antipyretic	T39.91	T39.92	T39.93	T39.94	T39.95	T39.96
specified NEC	T39.8X1	T39.8X2	T39.8X3	T39.8X4	T39.8X5	T39.8X6
Antipyrine	T39.2X1	T39.2X2	T39.2X3	T39.2X4	T39.2X5	T39.2X6
Antirabies hyperimmune serum	T50.Z11	T50.Z12	T50.Z13	T50.Z14	T50.Z15	T50.Z16
Antirheumatic NEC	T39.4X1	T39.4X2	T39.4X3	T39.4X4	T39.4X5	T39.4X6
Antirigidity drug NEC	T42.8X1	T42.8X2	T42.8X3	T42.8X4	T42.8X5	T42.8X6
Antischistosomal drug	T37.4X1	T37.4X2	T37.4X3	T37.4X4	T37.4X5	T37.4X6
Antiscorpion sera	T50.Z11	T50.Z12	T50.Z13	T50.Z14	T50.Z15	T50.Z16
Antiseborrheics	T49.4X1	T49.4X2	T49.4X3	T49.4X4	T49.4X5	T49.4X6
Antiseptics (external) (medicinal)	T49.0X1	T49.0X2	T49.0X3	T49.0X4	T49.0X5	T49.0X6
Antistine	T45.0X1	T45.0X2	T45.0X3	T45.0X4	T45.0X5	T45.0X6
Antitapeworm drug	T37.4X1	T37.4X2	T37.4X3	T37.4X4	T37.4X5	T37.4X6
Antitetanus immunoglobulin	T50.Z11	T50.Z12	T50.Z13	T50.Z14	T50.Z15	T50.Z16
Antithrombotic	T45.521	T45.522	T45.523	T45.524	T45.525	T45.526
Antithyroid drug NEC	T38.2X1	T38.2X2	T38.2X3	T38.2X4	T38.2X5	T38.2X6
Antitoxin	T50.Z11	T50.Z12	T50.Z13	T50.Z14	T50.Z15	T50.Z16
diphtheria	T50.Z11	T50.Z12	T50.Z13	T50.Z14	T50.Z15	T50.Z16
gas gangrene	T50.Z11	T50.Z12	T50.Z13	T50.Z14	T50.Z15	T50.Z16
tetanus	T50.Z11	T50.Z12	T50.Z13	T50.Z14	T50.Z15	T50.Z16
Antitoxin, any	T50.901	T50.902	T50.903	T50.904	T50.905	T50.906
Antitrichomonal drug	T37.3X1	T37.3X2	T37.3X3	T37.3X4	T37.3X5	T37.3X6
Antituberculars	T37.1X1	T37.1X2	T37.1X3	T37.1X4	T37.1X5	T37.1X6
antibiotics	T36.5X1	T36.5X2	T36.5X3	T36.5X4	T36.5X5	T36.5X6
Antitussive NEC	T48.3X1	T48.3X2	T48.3X3	T48.3X4	T48.3X5	T48.3X6
codeine mixture	T40.2X1	T40.2X2	T40.2X3	T40.2X4	T40.2X5	T40.2X6
opiate	T40.2X1	T40.2X2	T40.2X3	T40.2X4	T40.2X5	T40.2X6
Antivaricose drug	T46.8X1	T46.8X2	T46.8X3	T46.8X4	T46.8X5	T46.8X6
Antivenin, antivenom (sera)	T50.Z11	T50.Z12	T50.Z13	T50.Z14	T50.Z15	T50.Z16
crotaline	T50.Z11	T50.Z12	T50.Z13	T50.Z14	T50.Z15	T50.Z16
spider bite	T50.Z11	T50.Z12	T50.Z13	T50.Z14	T50.Z15	T50.Z16
Antivertigo drug	T45.0X1	T45.0X2	T45.0X3	T45.0X4	T45.0X5	T45.0X6
Antiviral drug NEC	T37.5X1	T37.5X2	T37.5X3	T37.5X4	T37.5X5	T37.5X6
eye	T49.5X1	T49.5X2	T49.5X3	T49.5X4	T49.5X5	T49.5X6
Antiwhipworm drug	T37.4X1	T37.4X2	T37.4X3	T37.4X4	T37.4X5	T37.4X6
Ant poisons—see Pesticides						
Antrol—see also by specific chemical substance	T60.91	T60.92	T60.93	T60.94	—	—
fungicide	T60.91	T60.92	T60.93	T60.94	—	—
ANTU (alpha naphthylthiourea)	T60.4X1	T60.4X2	T60.4X3	T60.4X4	—	—
Apalcillin	T36.0X1	T36.0X2	T36.0X3	T36.0X4	T36.0X5	T36.0X6
APC	T48.5X1	T48.5X2	T48.5X3	T48.5X4	T48.5X5	T48.5X6
Aplonidine	T44.4X1	T44.4X2	T44.4X3	T44.4X4	T44.4X5	T44.4X6
Apomorphine	T47.7X1	T47.7X2	T47.7X3	T47.7X4	T47.7X5	T47.7X6

TABLE OF DRUGS AND CHEMICALS

Substance	Poisoning, Accidental (Unintentional)	Poisoning, Intentional Self-Harm	Poisoning, Assault	Poisoning, Undetermined	Adverse Effect	Underdosing
Appetite depressants, central	T50.5X1	T50.5X2	T50.5X3	T50.5X4	T50.5X5	T50.5X6
Apraclonidine (hydrochloride)	T44.4X1	T44.4X2	T44.4X3	T44.4X4	T44.4X5	T44.4X6
Apresoline	T46.5X1	T46.5X2	T46.5X3	T46.5X4	T46.5X5	T46.5X6
Aprindine	T46.2X1	T46.2X2	T46.2X3	T46.2X4	T46.2X5	T46.2X6
Aprobarbital	T42.3X1	T42.3X2	T42.3X3	T42.3X4	T42.3X5	T42.3X6
Apronalide	T42.6X1	T42.6X2	T42.6X3	T42.6X4	T42.6X5	T42.6X6
Aprotinin	T45.621	T45.622	T45.623	T45.624	T45.625	T45.626
Aptocaine	T41.3X1	T41.3X2	T41.3X3	T41.3X4	T41.3X5	T41.3X6
Aqua fortis	T54.2X1	T54.2X2	T54.2X3	T54.2X4	—	—
Ara-A	T37.5X1	T37.5X2	T37.5X3	T37.5X4	T37.5X5	T37.5X6
Ara-C	T45.1X1	T45.1X2	T45.1X3	T45.1X4	T45.1X5	T45.1X6
Arachis oil	T49.3X1	T49.3X2	T49.3X3	T49.3X4	T49.3X5	T49.3X6
cathartic	T47.4X1	T47.4X2	T47.4X3	T47.4X4	T47.4X5	T47.4X6
Aralen	T37.2X1	T37.2X2	T37.2X3	T37.2X4	T37.2X5	T37.2X6
Arecoline	T44.1X1	T44.1X2	T44.1X3	T44.1X4	T44.1X5	T44.1X6
Arginine	T50.991	T50.992	T50.993	T50.994	T50.995	T50.996
glutamate	T50.991	T50.992	T50.993	T50.994	T50.995	T50.996
Argyrol	T49.0X1	T49.0X2	T49.0X3	T49.0X4	T49.0X5	T49.0X6
ENT agent	T49.6X1	T49.6X2	T49.6X3	T49.6X4	T49.6X5	T49.6X6
ophthalmic preparation	T49.5X1	T49.5X2	T49.5X3	T49.5X4	T49.5X5	T49.5X6
Aristocort	T38.0X1	T38.0X2	T38.0X3	T38.0X4	T38.0X5	T38.0X6
ENT agent	T49.6X1	T49.6X2	T49.6X3	T49.6X4	T49.6X5	T49.6X6
ophthalmic preparation	T49.5X1	T49.5X2	T49.5X3	T49.5X4	T49.5X5	T49.5X6
topical NEC	T49.0X1	T49.0X2	T49.0X3	T49.0X4	T49.0X5	T49.0X6
Aromatics, corrosive	T54.1X1	T54.1X2	T54.1X3	T54.1X4	—	—
disinfectants	T54.1X1	T54.1X2	T54.1X3	T54.1X4	—	—
Arsenate of lead	T57.0X1	T57.0X2	T57.0X3	T57.0X4	—	—
herbicide	T57.0X1	T57.0X2	T57.0X3	T57.0X4	—	—
Arsenic, arsenicals (compounds) (dust) (vapor) NEC	T57.0X1	T57.0X2	T57.0X3	T57.0X4	—	—
anti-infectives	T37.8X1	T37.8X2	T37.8X3	T37.8X4	T37.8X5	T37.8X6
pesticide (dust) (fumes)	T57.0X1	T57.0X2	T57.0X3	T57.0X4	—	—
Arsine (gas)	T57.0X1	T57.0X2	T57.0X3	T57.0X4	—	—
Arsphenamine (silver)	T37.8X1	T37.8X2	T37.8X3	T37.8X4	T37.8X5	T37.8X6
Arsthinol	T37.3X1	T37.3X2	T37.3X3	T37.3X4	T37.3X5	T37.3X6
Artane	T44.3X1	T44.3X2	T44.3X3	T44.3X4	T44.3X5	T44.3X6
Arthropod (venomous) NEC	T63.481	T63.482	T63.483	T63.484	—	—
Articaine	T41.3X1	T41.3X2	T41.3X3	T41.3X4	T41.3X5	T41.3X6
Asbestos	T57.8X1	T57.8X2	T57.8X3	T57.8X4	—	—
Ascaridole	T37.4X1	T37.4X2	T37.4X3	T37.4X4	T37.4X5	T37.4X6
Ascorbic acid	T45.2X1	T45.2X2	T45.2X3	T45.2X4	T45.2X5	T45.2X6
Asiaticoside	T49.0X1	T49.0X2	T49.0X3	T49.0X4	T49.0X5	T49.0X6
Asparaginase	T45.1X1	T45.1X2	T45.1X3	T45.1X4	T45.1X5	T45.1X6
Aspidium (oleoresin)	T37.4X1	T37.4X2	T37.4X3	T37.4X4	T37.4X5	T37.4X6
Aspirin (aluminum) (soluble)	T39.011	T39.012	T39.013	T39.014	T39.015	T39.016
Aspoxicillin	T36.0X1	T36.0X2	T36.0X3	T36.0X4	T36.0X5	T36.0X6
Astemizole	T45.0X1	T45.0X2	T45.0X3	T45.0X4	T45.0X5	T45.0X6
Astringent (local)	T49.2X1	T49.2X2	T49.2X3	T49.2X4	T49.2X5	T49.2X6
specified NEC	T49.2X1	T49.2X2	T49.2X3	T49.2X4	T49.2X5	T49.2X6
Astromicin	T36.5X1	T36.5X2	T36.5X3	T36.5X4	T36.5X5	T36.5X6
Ataractic drug NEC	T43.501	T43.502	T43.503	T43.504	T43.505	T43.506
Atenolol	T44.7X1	T44.7X2	T44.7X3	T44.7X4	T44.7X5	T44.7X6
Atonia drug, intestinal	T47.4X1	T47.4X2	T47.4X3	T47.4X4	T47.4X5	T47.4X6
Atophan	T50.4X1	T50.4X2	T50.4X3	T50.4X4	T50.4X5	T50.4X6
Atracurium besilate	T48.1X1	T48.1X2	T48.1X3	T48.1X4	T48.1X5	T48.1X6
Atropine	T44.3X1	T44.3X2	T44.3X3	T44.3X4	T44.3X5	T44.3X6
derivative	T44.3X1	T44.3X2	T44.3X3	T44.3X4	T44.3X5	T44.3X6
methonitrate	T44.3X1	T44.3X2	T44.3X3	T44.3X4	T44.3X5	T44.3X6
Attapulgite	T47.6X1	T47.6X2	T47.6X3	T47.6X4	T47.6X5	T47.6X6
Attenuvax	T50.991	T50.992	T50.993	T50.994	T50.995	T50.996
Auramine	T65.891	T65.892	T65.893	T65.894	—	—
dye	T65.6X1	T65.6X2	T65.6X3	T65.6X4	—	—
fungicide	T60.3X1	T60.3X2	T60.3X3	T60.3X4	—	—
Auranofin	T39.4X1	T39.4X2	T39.4X3	T39.4X4	T39.4X5	T39.4X6
Aurantiin	T46.991	T46.992	T46.993	T46.994	T46.995	T46.996
Aureomycin	T36.4X1	T36.4X2	T36.4X3	T36.4X4	T36.4X5	T36.4X6
ophthalmic preparation	T49.5X1	T49.5X2	T49.5X3	T49.5X4	T49.5X5	T49.5X6
topical NEC	T49.0X1	T49.0X2	T49.0X3	T49.0X4	T49.0X5	T49.0X6
Aurothioglucose	T39.4X1	T39.4X2	T39.4X3	T39.4X4	T39.4X5	T39.4X6
Aurothioglycanide	T39.4X1	T39.4X2	T39.4X3	T39.4X4	T39.4X5	T39.4X6
Aurothiomalate sodium	T39.4X1	T39.4X2	T39.4X3	T39.4X4	T39.4X5	T39.4X6
Aurotioprol	T39.4X1	T39.4X2	T39.4X3	T39.4X4	T39.4X5	T39.4X6
Automobile fuel	T52.0X1	T52.0X2	T52.0X3	T52.0X4	—	—
Autonomic nervous system agent NEC	T44.901	T44.902	T44.903	T44.904	T44.905	T44.906
Avlosulfon	T37.1X1	T37.1X2	T37.1X3	T37.1X4	T37.1X5	T37.1X6
Avomine	T42.6X1	T42.6X2	T42.6X3	T42.6X4	T42.6X5	T42.6X6
Axerophthol	T45.2X1	T45.2X2	T45.2X3	T45.2X4	T45.2X5	T45.2X6
Azacitidine	T45.1X1	T45.1X2	T45.1X3	T45.1X4	T45.1X5	T45.1X6
Azacyclonol	T43.591	T43.592	T43.593	T43.594	T43.595	T43.596
Azadirachta	T60.2X1	T60.2X2	T60.2X3	T60.2X4	—	—
Azanidazole	T37.3X1	T37.3X2	T37.3X3	T37.3X4	T37.3X5	T37.3X6
Azapetine	T46.7X1	T46.7X2	T46.7X3	T46.7X4	T46.7X5	T46.7X6
Azapropazone	T39.2X1	T39.2X2	T39.2X3	T39.2X4	T39.2X5	T39.2X6

◀ New ◀ Revised ~~deleted~~ Deleted

Substance	Poisoning, Accidental (Unintentional)	Poisoning, Intentional Self-Harm	Poisoning, Assault	Poisoning, Undetermined	Adverse Effect	Underdosing
Azaribine	T45.1X1	T45.1X2	T45.1X3	T45.1X4	T45.1X5	T45.1X6
Azaserine	T45.1X1	T45.1X2	T45.1X3	T45.1X4	T45.1X5	T45.1X6
Azatadine	T45.0X1	T45.0X2	T45.0X3	T45.0X4	T45.0X5	T45.0X6
Azatepa	T45.1X1	T45.1X2	T45.1X3	T45.1X4	T45.1X5	T45.1X6
Azathioprine	T45.1X1	T45.1X2	T45.1X3	T45.1X4	T45.1X5	T45.1X6
Azelaic acid	T49.0X1	T49.0X2	T49.0X3	T49.0X4	T49.0X5	T49.0X6
Azelastine	T45.0X1	T45.0X2	T45.0X3	T45.0X4	T45.0X5	T45.0X6
Azidocillin	T36.0X1	T36.0X2	T36.0X3	T36.0X4	T36.0X5	T36.0X6
Azidothymidine	T37.5X1	T37.5X2	T37.5X3	T37.5X4	T37.5X5	T37.5X6
Azinphos (ethyl) (methyl)	T60.0X1	T60.0X2	T60.0X3	T60.0X4	—	—
Aziridine (chelating)	T54.1X1	T54.1X2	T54.1X3	T54.1X4	—	—
Azithromycin	T36.3X1	T36.3X2	T36.3X3	T36.3X4	T36.3X5	T36.3X6
Azlocillin	T36.01	T36.02	T36.03	T36.04	T36.05	T36.06
Azobenzene smoke	T65.3X1	T65.3X2	T65.3X3	T65.3X4	—	—
acaricide	T60.8X1	T60.8X2	T60.8X3	T60.8X4	—	—
Azosulfamide	T37.0X1	T37.0X2	T37.0X3	T37.0X4	T37.0X5	T37.0X6
AZT	T37.5X1	T37.5X2	T37.5X3	T37.5X4	T37.5X5	T37.5X6
Aztreonam	T36.1X1	T36.1X2	T36.1X3	T36.1X4	T36.1X5	T36.1X6
Azulfidine	T37.0X1	T37.0X2	T37.0X3	T37.0X4	T37.0X5	T37.0X6
Azuresin	T50.8X1	T50.8X2	T50.8X3	T50.8X4	T50.8X5	T50.8X6
B						
Bacampicillin	T36.0X1	T36.0X2	T36.0X3	T36.0X4	T36.0X5	T36.0X6
Bacillus						
lactobacillus	T47.8X1	T47.8X2	T47.8X3	T47.8X4	T47.8X5	T47.8X6
subtilis	T47.6X1	T47.6X2	T47.6X3	T47.6X4	T47.6X5	T47.6X6
Bacimycin	T49.0X1	T49.0X2	T49.0X3	T49.0X4	T49.0X5	T49.0X6
ophthalmic preparation	T49.5X1	T49.5X2	T49.5X3	T49.5X4	T49.5X5	T49.5X6
Bacitracin zinc	T49.0X1	T49.0X2	T49.0X3	T49.0X4	T49.0X5	T49.0X6
with neomycin	T49.0X1	T49.0X2	T49.0X3	T49.0X4	T49.0X5	T49.0X6
ENT agent	T49.6X1	T49.6X2	T49.6X3	T49.6X4	T49.6X5	T49.6X6
ophthalmic preparation	T49.5X1	T49.5X2	T49.5X3	T49.5X4	T49.5X5	T49.5X6
topical NEC	T49.0X1	T49.0X2	T49.0X3	T49.0X4	T49.0X5	T49.0X6
Baclofen	T42.8X1	T42.8X2	T42.8X3	T42.8X4	T42.8X5	T42.8X6
Baking soda	T50.991	T50.992	T50.993	T50.994	T50.995	T50.996
BAL	T45.8X1	T45.8X2	T45.8X3	T45.8X4	T45.8X5	T45.8X6
Bambuterol	T48.6X1	T48.6X2	T48.6X3	T48.6X4	T48.6X5	T48.6X6
Bamethan (sulfate)	T46.7X1	T46.7X2	T46.7X3	T46.7X4	T46.7X5	T46.7X6
Bamifylline	T48.6X1	T48.6X2	T48.6X3	T48.6X4	T48.6X5	T48.6X6
Bamipine	T45.0X1	T45.0X2	T45.0X3	T45.0X4	T45.0X5	T45.0X6
Baneberry — see Actaea spicata						
Banewort — see Belladonna						

Substance	Poisoning, Accidental (Unintentional)	Poisoning, Intentional Self-Harm	Poisoning, Assault	Poisoning, Undetermined	Adverse Effect	Underdosing
Barbenyl	T42.3X1	T42.3X2	T42.3X3	T42.3X4	T42.3X5	T42.3X6
Barbexaclone	T42.6X1	T42.6X2	T42.6X3	T42.6X4	T42.6X5	T42.6X6
Barbital	T42.3X1	T42.3X2	T42.3X3	T42.3X4	T42.3X5	T42.3X6
sodium	T42.3X1	T42.3X2	T42.3X3	T42.3X4	T42.3X5	T42.3X6
Barbitone	T42.3X1	T42.3X2	T42.3X3	T42.3X4	T42.3X5	T42.3X6
Barbiturate NEC	T42.3X1	T42.3X2	T42.3X3	T42.3X4	T42.3X5	T42.3X6
with tranquilizer	T42.3X1	T42.3X2	T42.3X3	T42.3X4	T42.3X5	T42.3X6
anesthetic (intravenous)	T41.1X1	T41.1X2	T41.1X3	T41.1X4	T41.1X5	T41.1X6
Barium (carbonate) (chloride) (sulfite)	T57.8X1	T57.8X2	T57.8X3	T57.8X4		
diagnostic agent	T50.8X1	T50.8X2	T50.8X3	T50.8X4	T50.8X5	T50.8X6
pesticide	T60.4X1	T60.4X2	T60.4X3	T60.4X4	—	—
rodenticide	T60.4X1	T60.4X2	T60.4X3	T60.4X4	—	—
sulfate (medicinal)	T50.8X1	T50.8X2	T50.8X3	T50.8X4	T50.8X5	T50.8X6
Barrier cream	T49.3X1	T49.3X2	T49.3X3	T49.3X4	T49.3X5	T49.3X6
Basic fuchsin	T49.0X1	T49.0X2	T49.0X3	T49.0X4	T49.0X5	T49.0X6
Battery acid or fluid	T54.2X1	T54.2X2	T54.2X3	T54.2X4		
Bay rum	T51.8X1	T51.8X2	T51.8X3	T51.8X4	—	—
BCG (vaccine)	T50.A91	T50.A92	T50.A93	T50.A94	T50.A95	T50.A96
BCNU	T45.1X1	T45.1X2	T45.1X3	T45.1X4	T45.1X5	T45.1X6
Bearsfoot	T62.2X1	T62.2X2	T62.2X3	T62.2X4	—	—
Beclamide	T42.6X1	T42.6X2	T42.6X3	T42.6X4	T42.6X5	T42.6X6
Beclomethasone	T44.5X1	T44.5X2	T44.5X3	T44.5X4	T44.5X5	T44.5X6
Bee (sting) (venom)	T63.441	T63.442	T63.443	T63.444	—	—
Befunolol	T49.5X1	T49.5X2	T49.5X3	T49.5X4	T49.5X5	T49.5X6
Bekanamycin	T36.5X1	T36.5X2	T36.5X3	T36.5X4	T36.5X5	T36.5X6
Belladonna — see also Nightshade						
alkaloids	T44.3X1	T44.3X2	T44.3X3	T44.3X4	T44.3X5	T44.3X6
extract	T44.3X1	T44.3X2	T44.3X3	T44.3X4	T44.3X5	T44.3X6
herb	T44.3X1	T44.3X2	T44.3X3	T44.3X4	T44.3X5	T44.3X6
Bemegride	T50.7X1	T50.7X2	T50.7X3	T50.7X4	T50.7X5	T50.7X6
Benactyzine	T44.3X1	T44.3X2	T44.3X3	T44.3X4	T44.3X5	T44.3X6
Benadryl	T45.0X1	T45.0X2	T45.0X3	T45.0X4	T45.0X5	T45.0X6
Benaprizine	T44.3X1	T44.3X2	T44.3X3	T44.3X4	T44.3X5	T44.3X6
Benazepril	T46.4X1	T46.4X2	T46.4X3	T46.4X4	T46.4X5	T46.4X6
Bencyclane	T46.7X1	T46.7X2	T46.7X3	T46.7X4	T46.7X5	T46.7X6
Bendazol	T46.3X1	T46.3X2	T46.3X3	T46.3X4	T46.3X5	T46.3X6
Bendrofluazide	T50.2X1	T50.2X2	T50.2X3	T50.2X4	T50.2X5	T50.2X6
Bendroflumethiazide	T50.2X1	T50.2X2	T50.2X3	T50.2X4	T50.2X5	T50.2X6
Benemid	T50.4X1	T50.4X2	T50.4X3	T50.4X4	T50.4X5	T50.4X6
Benethamine penicillin	T36.0X1	T36.0X2	T36.0X3	T36.0X4	T36.0X5	T36.0X6
Benisone	T49.0X1	T49.0X2	T49.0X3	T49.0X4	T49.0X5	T49.0X6

◄ New ◖ Revised ~~deleted~~ Deleted

Substance	Poisoning, Accidental (Unintentional)	Poisoning, Intentional Self-Harm	Poisoning, Assault	Poisoning, Undetermined	Adverse Effect	Underdosing
Benexate	T47.1X1	T47.1X2	T47.1X3	T47.1X4	T47.1X5	T47.1X6
Benfluorex	T46.6X1	T46.6X2	T46.6X3	T46.6X4	T46.6X5	T46.6X6
Benfotiamine	T45.2X1	T45.2X2	T45.2X3	T45.2X4	T45.2X5	T45.2X6
Benomyl	T60.0X1	T60.0X2	T60.0X3	T60.0X4	—	—
Benoquin	T49.8X1	T49.8X2	T49.8X3	T49.8X4	T49.8X5	T49.8X6
Benoxinate	T41.3X1	T41.3X2	T41.3X3	T41.3X4	T41.3X5	T41.3X6
Benperidol	T43.4X1	T43.4X2	T43.4X3	T43.4X4	T43.4X5	T43.4X6
Benproperine	T48.3X1	T48.3X2	T48.3X3	T48.3X4	T48.3X5	T48.3X6
Benserazide	T42.8X1	T42.8X2	T42.8X3	T42.8X4	T42.8X5	T42.8X6
Bentazepam	T42.4X1	T42.4X2	T42.4X3	T42.4X4	T42.4X5	T42.4X6
Bentiromide	T50.8X1	T50.8X2	T50.8X3	T50.8X4	T50.8X5	T50.8X6
Bentonite	T49.3X1	T49.3X2	T49.3X3	T49.3X4	T49.3X5	T49.3X6
Benzalbutyramide	T46.6X1	T46.6X2	T46.6X3	T46.6X4	T46.6X5	T46.6X6
Benzalkonium (chloride)	T49.0X1	T49.0X2	T49.0X3	T49.0X4	T49.0X5	T49.0X6
ophthalmic preparation	T49.5X1	T49.5X2	T49.5X3	T49.5X4	T49.5X5	T49.5X6
Benzamine	T41.3X1	T41.3X2	T41.3X3	T41.3X4	T41.3X5	T41.3X6
lactate	T49.1X1	T49.1X2	T49.1X3	T49.1X4	T49.1X5	T49.1X6
Benzamidosalicylate (calcium)	T37.1X1	T37.1X2	T37.1X3	T37.1X4	T37.1X5	T37.1X6
Benzamphetamine	T50.5X1	T50.5X2	T50.5X3	T50.5X4	T50.5X5	T50.5X6
Benzapril hydrochloride	T46.5X1	T46.5X2	T46.5X3	T46.5X4	T46.5X5	T46.5X6
Benzathine benzylpenicillin	T36.0X1	T36.0X2	T36.0X3	T36.0X4	T36.0X5	T36.0X6
Benzathine penicillin	T36.0X1	T36.0X2	T36.0X3	T36.0X4	T36.0X5	T36.0X6
Benzatropine	T42.8X1	T42.8X2	T42.8X3	T42.8X4	T42.8X5	T42.8X6
Benzbromarone	T50.4X1	T50.4X2	T50.4X3	T50.4X4	T50.4X5	T50.4X6
Benzcarbimine	T45.1X1	T45.1X2	T45.1X3	T45.1X4	T45.1X5	T45.1X6
Benzedrex	T44.991	T44.992	T44.993	T44.994	T44.995	T44.996
Benzedrine (amphetamine)	T43.621	T43.622	T43.623	T43.624	T43.625	T43.626
Benzenamine	T65.3X1	T65.3X2	T65.3X3	T65.3X4	—	—
Benzene	T52.1X1	T52.1X2	T52.1X3	T52.1X4	—	—
homologues (acetyl) (dimethyl) (methyl) (solvent)	T52.2X1	T52.2X2	T52.2X3	T52.2X4	—	—
Benzethonium (chloride)	T49.0X1	T49.0X2	T49.0X3	T49.0X4	T49.0X5	T49.0X6
Benzfetamine	T50.5X1	T50.5X2	T50.5X3	T50.5X4	T50.5X5	T50.5X6
Benzhexol	T44.3X1	T44.3X2	T44.3X3	T44.3X4	T44.3X5	T44.3X6
Benzhydramine (chloride)	T45.0X1	T45.0X2	T45.0X3	T45.0X4	T45.0X5	T45.0X6
Benzidine	T65.891	T65.892	T65.893	T65.894	—	—
Benzilonium bromide	T44.3X1	T44.3X2	T44.3X3	T44.3X4	T44.3X5	T44.3X6
Benzimidazole	T60.3X1	T60.3X2	T60.3X3	T60.3X4	—	—
Benzin(e) — see Ligroin						
Benziodarone	T46.3X1	T46.3X2	T46.3X3	T46.3X4	T46.3X5	T46.3X6
Benznidazole	T37.3X1	T37.3X2	T37.3X3	T37.3X4	T37.3X5	T37.3X6
Benzocaine	T41.3X1	T41.3X2	T41.3X3	T41.3X4	T41.3X5	T41.3X6

Substance	Poisoning, Accidental (Unintentional)	Poisoning, Intentional Self-Harm	Poisoning, Assault	Poisoning, Undetermined	Adverse Effect	Underdosing
Benzoctamine	T43.0X1	T43.0X2	T43.0X3	T43.0X4	T43.0X5	T43.0X6
Benzodiapin	T42.4X1	T42.4X2	T42.4X3	T42.4X4	T42.4X5	T42.4X6
Benzodiazepine NEC	T42.4X1	T42.4X2	T42.4X3	T42.4X4	T42.4X5	T42.4X6
Benzoic acid	T49.0X1	T49.0X2	T49.0X3	T49.0X4	T49.0X5	T49.0X6
with salicylic acid	T49.0X1	T49.0X2	T49.0X3	T49.0X4	T49.0X5	T49.0X6
Benzoin (tincture)	T48.5X1	T48.5X2	T48.5X3	T48.5X4	T48.5X5	T48.5X6
Benzol (benzene)	T52.1X1	T52.1X2	T52.1X3	T52.1X4	—	—
vapor	T52.0X1	T52.0X2	T52.0X3	T52.0X4	—	—
Benzomorphan	T40.2X1	T40.2X2	T40.2X3	T40.2X4	T40.2X5	T40.2X6
Benzonatate	T48.3X1	T48.3X2	T48.3X3	T48.3X4	T48.3X5	T48.3X6
Benzophenones	T49.3X1	T49.3X2	T49.3X3	T49.3X4	T49.3X5	T49.3X6
Benzopyrone	T46.991	T46.992	T46.993	T46.994	T46.995	T46.996
Benzothiadiazides	T50.2X1	T50.2X2	T50.2X3	T50.2X4	T50.2X5	T50.2X6
Benzoxonium chloride	T49.0X1	T49.0X2	T49.0X3	T49.0X4	T49.0X5	T49.0X6
Benzoyl peroxide	T49.0X1	T49.0X2	T49.0X3	T49.0X4	T49.0X5	T49.0X6
Benzoylpas calcium	T37.1X1	T37.1X2	T37.1X3	T37.1X4	T37.1X5	T37.1X6
Benzperidin	T43.591	T43.592	T43.593	T43.594	T43.595	T43.596
Benzperidol	T43.591	T43.592	T43.593	T43.594	T43.595	T43.596
Benzphetamine	T50.5X1	T50.5X2	T50.5X3	T50.5X4	T50.5X5	T50.5X6
Benzpyrinium bromide	T44.1X1	T44.1X2	T44.1X3	T44.1X4	T44.1X5	T44.1X6
Benzquinamide	T45.0X1	T45.0X2	T45.0X3	T45.0X4	T45.0X5	T45.0X6
Benzthiazide	T50.2X1	T50.2X2	T50.2X3	T50.2X4	T50.2X5	T50.2X6
Benztropine						
anticholinergic	T44.3X1	T44.3X2	T44.3X3	T44.3X4	T44.3X5	T44.3X6
antiparkinson	T42.8X1	T42.8X2	T42.8X3	T42.8X4	T42.8X5	T42.8X6
Benzydamine	T49.0X1	T49.0X2	T49.0X3	T49.0X4	T49.0X5	T49.0X6
Benzyl						
acetate	T52.8X1	T52.8X2	T52.8X3	T52.8X4	—	—
alcohol	T49.0X1	T49.0X2	T49.0X3	T49.0X4	T49.0X5	T49.0X6
benzoate	T49.0X1	T49.0X2	T49.0X3	T49.0X4	T49.0X5	T49.0X6
Benzoic acid	T49.0X1	T49.0X2	T49.0X3	T49.0X4	T49.0X5	T49.0X6
morphine	T40.2X1	T40.2X2	T40.2X3	T40.2X4	—	—
nicotinate	T46.6X1	T46.6X2	T46.6X3	T46.6X4	T46.6X5	T46.6X6
penicillin	T36.0X1	T36.0X2	T36.0X3	T36.0X4	T36.0X5	T36.0X6
Benzylhydrochlorthia-zide	T50.2X1	T50.2X2	T50.2X3	T50.2X4	T50.2X5	T50.2X6
Benzylpenicillin	T36.0X1	T36.0X2	T36.0X3	T36.0X4	T36.0X5	T36.0X6
Benzylthiouracil	T38.2X1	T38.2X2	T38.2X3	T38.2X4	T38.2X5	T38.2X6
Bephenium hydroxy-naphthoate	T37.4X1	T37.4X2	T37.4X3	T37.4X4	T37.4X5	T37.4X6
Bepridil	T46.1X1	T46.1X2	T46.1X3	T46.1X4	T46.1X5	T46.1X6
Bergamot oil	T65.891	T65.892	T65.893	T65.894	—	—
Bergapten	T50.991	T50.992	T50.993	T50.994	T50.995	T50.996
Berries, poisonous	T62.1X1	T62.1X2	T62.1X3	T62.1X4		

◀ New　◀ Revised　~~deleted~~ Deleted

Substance	Poisoning, Accidental (Unintentional)	Poisoning, Intentional Self-Harm	Poisoning, Assault	Poisoning, Undetermined	Adverse Effect	Underdosing
Beryllium (compounds)	T56.7X1	T56.7X2	T56.7X3	T56.7X4	—	—
b-acetyldigoxin	T46.0X1	T46.0X2	T46.0X3	T46.0X4	T46.0X5	T46.0X6
beta adrenergic blocking agent, heart	T44.7X1	T44.7X2	T44.7X3	T44.7X4	T44.7X5	T44.7X6
b-benzalbutyramide	T46.6X1	T46.6X2	T46.6X3	T46.6X4	T46.6X5	T46.6X6
Betacarotene	T45.2X1	T45.2X2	T45.2X3	T45.2X4	T45.2X5	T45.2X6
b-eucaine	T49.1X1	T49.1X2	T49.1X3	T49.1X4	T49.1X5	T49.1X6
Beta-Chlor	T42.6X1	T42.6X2	T42.6X3	T42.6X4	T42.6X5	T42.6X6
b-galactosidase	T47.5X1	T47.5X2	T47.5X3	T47.5X4	T47.5X5	T47.5X6
Betahistine	T46.7X1	T46.7X2	T46.7X3	T46.7X4	T46.7X5	T46.7X6
Betaine	T47.5X1	T47.5X2	T47.5X3	T47.5X4	T47.5X5	T47.5X6
Betamethasone	T49.0X1	T49.0X2	T49.0X3	T49.0X4	T49.0X5	T49.0X6
topical	T49.0X1	T49.0X2	T49.0X3	T49.0X4	T49.0X5	T49.0X6
Betamicin	T36.8X1	T36.8X2	T36.8X3	T36.8X4	T36.8X5	T36.8X6
Betanidine	T46.5X1	T46.5X2	T46.5X3	T46.5X4	T46.5X5	T46.5X6
b-sitosterol(s)	T46.6X1	T46.6X2	T46.6X3	T46.6X4	T46.6X5	T46.6X6
Betaxolol	T44.7X1	T44.7X2	T44.7X3	T44.7X4	T44.7X5	T44.7X6
Betazole	T50.8X1	T50.8X2	T50.8X3	T50.8X4	T50.8X5	T50.8X6
Bethanechol	T44.1X1	T44.1X2	T44.1X3	T44.1X4	T44.1X5	T44.1X6
chloride	T44.1X1	T44.1X2	T44.1X3	T44.1X4	T44.1X5	T44.1X6
Bethanidine	T46.5X1	T46.5X2	T46.5X3	T46.5X4	T46.5X5	T46.5X6
Betoxycaine	T41.3X1	T41.3X2	T41.3X3	T41.3X4	T41.3X5	T41.3X6
Betula oil	T49.3X1	T49.3X2	T49.3X3	T49.3X4	T49.3X5	T49.3X6
Bevantolol	T44.7X1	T44.7X2	T44.7X3	T44.7X4	T44.7X5	T44.7X6
Bevonium metilsulfate	T44.3X1	T44.3X2	T44.3X3	T44.3X4	T44.3X5	T44.3X6
Bezafibrate	T46.6X1	T46.6X2	T46.6X3	T46.6X4	T46.6X5	T46.6X6
Bezitramide	T40.491	T40.492	T40.493	T40.494	T40.495	T40.496
BHA	T50.991	T50.992	T50.993	T50.994	T50.995	T50.996
Bhang	T40.711	T40.712	T40.713	T40.714	T40.715	T40.716
BHC (medicinal)	T49.0X1	T49.0X2	T49.0X3	T49.0X4	T49.0X5	T49.0X6
nonmedicinal (vapor)	T53.6X1	T53.6X2	T53.6X3	T53.6X4	—	—
Bialamicol	T37.3X1	T37.3X2	T37.3X3	T37.3X4	T37.3X5	T37.3X6
Bibenzonium bromide	T48.3X1	T48.3X2	T48.3X3	T48.3X4	T48.3X5	T48.3X6
Bibrocathol	T49.5X1	T49.5X2	T49.5X3	T49.5X4	T49.5X5	T49.5X6
Bichloride of mercury — see Mercury, chloride						
Bichromates (calcium) (potassium) (sodium) (crystals)	T57.8X1	T57.8X2	T57.8X3	T57.8X4	—	—
fumes	T56.2X1	T56.2X2	T56.2X3	T56.2X4	—	—
Biclotymol	T49.6X1	T49.6X2	T49.6X3	T49.6X4	T49.6X5	T49.6X6
Bicuculline	T50.7X1	T50.7X2	T50.7X3	T50.7X4	T50.7X5	T50.7X6
Bifemelane	T43.291	T43.292	T43.293	T43.294	T43.295	T43.296
Biguanide derivatives, oral	T38.3X1	T38.3X2	T38.3X3	T38.3X4	T38.3X5	T38.3X6

Substance	Poisoning, Accidental (Unintentional)	Poisoning, Intentional Self-Harm	Poisoning, Assault	Poisoning, Undetermined	Adverse Effect	Underdosing
Biligrafin	T50.8X1	T50.8X2	T50.8X3	T50.8X4	T50.8X5	T50.8X6
Bile salts	T47.5X1	T47.5X2	T47.5X3	T47.5X4	T47.5X5	T47.5X6
Bilopaque	T50.8X1	T50.8X2	T50.8X3	T50.8X4	T50.8X5	T50.8X6
Binifibrate	T46.6X1	T46.6X2	T46.6X3	T46.6X4	T46.6X5	T46.6X6
Binitrobenzol	T65.3X1	T65.3X2	T65.3X3	T65.3X4	—	—
Bioflavonoid(s)	T46.991	T46.992	T46.993	T46.994	T46.995	T46.996
Biological substance NEC	T50.901	T50.902	T50.903	T50.904	T50.905	T50.906
Biotin	T45.2X1	T45.2X2	T45.2X3	T45.2X4	T45.2X5	T45.2X6
Biperiden	T44.3X1	T44.3X2	T44.3X3	T44.3X4	T44.3X5	T44.3X6
Bisacodyl	T47.2X1	T47.2X2	T47.2X3	T47.2X4	T47.2X5	T47.2X6
Bisbentiamine	T45.2X1	T45.2X2	T45.2X3	T45.2X4	T45.2X5	T45.2X6
Bisbutiamine	T45.2X1	T45.2X2	T45.2X3	T45.2X4	T45.2X5	T45.2X6
Bisdequalinium (salts) (diacetate)	T49.6X1	T49.6X2	T49.6X3	T49.6X4	T49.6X5	T49.6X6
Bishydroxycoumarin	T45.511	T45.512	T45.513	T45.514	T45.515	T45.516
Bismarsen	T37.8X1	T37.8X2	T37.8X3	T37.8X4	T37.8X5	T37.8X6
Bismuth salts	T47.6X1	T47.6X2	T47.6X3	T47.6X4	T47.6X5	T47.6X6
aluminate	T47.1X1	T47.1X2	T47.1X3	T47.1X4	T47.1X5	T47.1X6
anti-infectives	T37.8X1	T37.8X2	T37.8X3	T37.8X4	T37.8X5	T37.8X6
formic iodide	T49.0X1	T49.0X2	T49.0X3	T49.0X4	T49.0X5	T49.0X6
glycolylarsenate	T49.0X1	T49.0X2	T49.0X3	T49.0X4	T49.0X5	T49.0X6
nonmedicinal (compounds) NEC	T65.91	T65.92	T65.93	T65.94	—	—
subcarbonate	T47.6X1	T47.6X2	T47.6X3	T47.6X4	T47.6X5	T47.6X6
subsalicylate	T37.8X1	T37.8X2	T37.8X3	T37.8X4	T37.8X5	T37.8X6
sulfarsphenamine	T37.8X1	T37.8X2	T37.8X3	T37.8X4	T37.8X5	T37.8X6
Bisoprolol	T44.7X1	T44.7X2	T44.7X3	T44.7X4	T44.7X5	T44.7X6
Bisoxatin	T47.2X1	T47.2X2	T47.2X3	T47.2X4	T47.2X5	T47.2X6
Bisulepin (hydrochloride)	T45.0X1	T45.0X2	T45.0X3	T45.0X4	T45.0X5	T45.0X6
Bithionol	T37.8X1	T37.8X2	T37.8X3	T37.8X4	T37.8X5	T37.8X6
anthelminthic	T37.4X1	T37.4X2	T37.4X3	T37.4X4	T37.4X5	T37.4X6
Bitolterol	T48.6X1	T48.6X2	T48.6X3	T48.6X4	T48.6X5	T48.6X6
Bitoscanate	T37.4X1	T37.4X2	T37.4X3	T37.4X4	T37.4X5	T37.4X6
Bitter almond oil	T62.8X1	T62.8X2	T62.8X3	T62.8X4	—	—
Bittersweet	T62.2X1	T62.2X2	T62.2X3	T62.2X4	—	—
Black						
flag	T60.91	T60.92	T60.93	T60.94	—	—
henbane	T62.2X1	T62.2X2	T62.2X3	T62.2X4	—	—
leaf (40)	T60.91	T60.92	T60.93	T60.94	—	—
widow spider (bite)	T63.311	T63.312	T63.313	T63.314	—	—
antivenin	T50.Z11	T50.Z12	T50.Z13	T50.Z14	T50.Z15	T50.Z16
Blast furnace gas (carbon monoxide from)	T58.8X1	T58.8X2	T58.8X3	T58.8X4		
Bleach	T54.91	T54.92	T54.93	T54.94	—	—

◀ New   ◀ Revised   ~~deleted~~ Deleted

Substance	External Cause (T-Code)					
	Poisoning, Accidental (Unintentional)	Poisoning, Intentional Self-Harm	Poisoning, Assault	Poisoning, Undetermined	Adverse Effect	Underdosing
Bleaching agent (medicinal)	T49.4X1	T49.4X2	T49.4X3	T49.4X4	T49.4X5	T49.4X6
Bleomycin	T45.1X1	T45.1X2	T45.1X3	T45.1X4	T45.1X5	T45.1X6
Blockain	T41.3X1	T41.3X2	T41.3X3	T41.3X4	T41.3X5	T41.3X6
infiltration (subcutaneous)	T41.3X1	T41.3X2	T41.3X3	T41.3X4	T41.3X5	T41.3X6
nerve block (peripheral) (plexus)	T41.3X1	T41.3X2	T41.3X3	T41.3X4	T41.3X5	T41.3X6
topical (surface)	T41.3X1	T41.3X2	T41.3X3	T41.3X4	T41.3X5	T41.3X6
Blockers, calcium channel	T46.1X1	T46.1X2	T46.1X3	T46.1X4	T46.1X5	T46.1X6
Blood (derivatives) (natural) (plasma) (whole)	T45.8X1	T45.8X2	T45.8X3	T45.8X4	T45.8X5	T45.8X6
dried	T45.8X1	T45.8X2	T45.8X3	T45.8X4	T45.8X5	T45.8X6
drug affecting NEC	T45.91	T45.92	T45.93	T45.94	T45.95	T45.96
expander NEC	T45.8X1	T45.8X2	T45.8X3	T45.8X4	T45.8X5	T45.8X6
fraction NEC	T45.8X1	T45.8X2	T45.8X3	T45.8X4	T45.8X5	T45.8X6
substitute (macromolecular)	T45.8X1	T45.8X2	T45.8X3	T45.8X4	T45.8X5	T45.8X6
Blue velvet	T40.2X1	T40.2X2	T40.2X3	T40.2X4	—	—
Bone meal	T62.8X1	T62.8X2	T62.8X3	T62.8X4	—	—
Bonine	T45.0X1	T45.0X2	T45.0X3	T45.0X4	T45.0X5	T45.0X6
Bopindolol	T44.7X1	T44.7X2	T44.7X3	T44.7X4	T44.7X5	T44.7X6
Boracic acid	T49.0X1	T49.0X2	T49.0X3	T49.0X4	T49.0X5	T49.0X6
ENT agent	T49.6X1	T49.6X2	T49.6X3	T49.6X4	T49.6X5	T49.6X6
ophthalmic preparation	T49.5X1	T49.5X2	T49.5X3	T49.5X4	T49.5X5	T49.5X6
Borane complex	T57.8X1	T57.8X2	T57.8X3	T57.8X4	—	—
Borate(s)	T57.8X1	T57.8X2	T57.8X3	T57.8X4	—	—
buffer	T50.991	T50.992	T50.993	T50.994	T50.995	T50.996
cleanser	T54.91	T54.92	T54.93	T54.94	—	—
sodium	T57.8X1	T57.8X2	T57.8X3	T57.8X4	—	—
Borax (cleanser)	T54.91	T54.92	T54.93	T54.94	—	—
Bordeaux mixture	T60.3X1	T60.3X2	T60.3X3	T60.3X4	—	—
Boric acid	T49.0X1	T49.0X2	T49.0X3	T49.0X4	T49.0X5	T49.0X6
ENT agent	T49.6X1	T49.6X2	T49.6X3	T49.6X4	T49.6X5	T49.6X6
ophthalmic preparation	T49.5X1	T49.5X2	T49.5X3	T49.5X4	T49.5X5	T49.5X6
Bornaprine	T44.3X1	T44.3X2	T44.3X3	T44.3X4	T44.3X5	T44.3X6
Boron	T57.8X1	T57.8X2	T57.8X3	T57.8X4	—	—
hydride NEC	T57.8X1	T57.8X2	T57.8X3	T57.8X4	—	—
fumes or gas	T57.8X1	T57.8X2	T57.8X3	T57.8X4	—	—
trifluoride	T59.891	T59.892	T59.893	T59.894	—	—
Botox	T48.291	T48.292	T48.293	T48.294	T48.295	T48.296
Botulinus anti-toxin (type A, B)	T50.Z11	T50.Z12	T50.Z13	T50.Z14	T50.Z15	T50.Z16
Brake fluid vapor	T59.891	T59.892	T59.893	T59.894	—	—
Brallobarbital	T42.3X1	T42.3X2	T42.3X3	T42.3X4	T42.3X5	T42.3X6
Bran (wheat)	T47.4X1	T47.4X2	T47.4X3	T47.4X4	T47.4X5	T47.4X6
Brass (fumes)	T56.891	T56.892	T56.893	T56.894	—	—

Substance	External Cause (T-Code)					
	Poisoning, Accidental (Unintentional)	Poisoning, Intentional Self-Harm	Poisoning, Assault	Poisoning, Undetermined	Adverse Effect	Underdosing
Brasso	T52.0X1	T52.0X2	T52.0X3	T52.0X4	—	—
Bretylium tosilate	T46.2X1	T46.2X2	T46.2X3	T46.2X4	T46.2X5	T46.2X6
Brevital (sodium)	T41.1X1	T41.1X2	T41.1X3	T41.1X4	T41.1X5	T41.1X6
Brinase	T45.3X1	T45.3X2	T45.3X3	T45.3X4	T45.3X5	T45.3X6
British antilewisite	T45.8X1	T45.8X2	T45.8X3	T45.8X4	T45.8X5	T45.8X6
Brodifacoum	T60.4X1	T60.4X2	T60.4X3	T60.4X4	—	—
Bromal (hydrate)	T42.6X1	T42.6X2	T42.6X3	T42.6X4	T42.6X5	T42.6X6
Bromazepam	T42.4X1	T42.4X2	T42.4X3	T42.4X4	T42.4X5	T42.4X6
Bromazine	T45.0X1	T45.0X2	T45.0X3	T45.0X4	T45.0X5	T45.0X6
Brombenzylcyanide	T59.3X1	T59.3X2	T59.3X3	T59.3X4	—	—
Bromelains	T45.3X1	T45.3X2	T45.3X3	T45.3X4	T45.3X5	T45.3X6
Bromethalin	T60.4X1	T60.4X2	T60.4X3	T60.4X4	—	—
Bromhexine	T48.4X1	T48.4X2	T48.4X3	T48.4X4	T48.4X5	T48.4X6
Bromide salts	T42.6X1	T42.6X2	T42.6X3	T42.6X4	T42.6X5	T42.6X6
Bromindione	T45.511	T45.512	T45.513	T45.514	T45.515	T45.516
Bromine						
compounds (medicinal)	T42.6X1	T42.6X2	T42.6X3	T42.6X4	T42.6X5	T42.6X6
sedative	T42.6X1	T42.6X2	T42.6X3	T42.6X4	T42.6X5	T42.6X6
vapor	T59.891	T59.892	T59.893	T59.894	—	—
Bromisovalum	T42.6X1	T42.6X2	T42.6X3	T42.6X4	T42.6X5	T42.6X6
Bromisoval	T42.6X1	T42.6X2	T42.6X3	T42.6X4	T42.6X5	T42.6X6
Bromobenzylcyanide	T59.3X1	T59.3X2	T59.3X3	T59.3X4	—	—
Bromochlorosalicylani-lide	T49.0X1	T49.0X2	T49.0X3	T49.0X4	T49.0X5	T49.0X6
Bromocriptine	T42.8X1	T42.8X2	T42.8X3	T42.8X4	T42.8X5	T42.8X6
Bromodiphenhydramine	T45.0X1	T45.0X2	T45.0X3	T45.0X4	T45.0X5	T45.0X6
Bromoform	T42.6X1	T42.6X2	T42.6X3	T42.6X4	T42.6X5	T42.6X6
Bromophenol blue reagent	T50.991	T50.992	T50.993	T50.994	T50.995	T50.996
Bromopride	T47.8X1	T47.8X2	T47.8X3	T47.8X4	T47.8X5	T47.8X6
Bromosalicylchloranitide	T49.0X1	T49.0X2	T49.0X3	T49.0X4	T49.0X5	T49.0X6
Bromosalicylhydroxamic acid	T37.1X1	T37.1X2	T37.1X3	T37.1X4	T37.1X5	T37.1X6
Bromo-seltzer	T39.1X1	T39.1X2	T39.1X3	T39.1X4	T39.1X5	T39.1X6
Bromoxynil	T60.3X1	T60.3X2	T60.3X3	T60.3X4	—	—
Bromperidol	T43.4X1	T43.4X2	T43.4X3	T43.4X4	T43.4X5	T43.4X6
Brompheniramine	T45.0X1	T45.0X2	T45.0X3	T45.0X4	T45.0X5	T45.0X6
Bromsulfophthalein	T50.8X1	T50.8X2	T50.8X3	T50.8X4	T50.8X5	T50.8X6
Bromural	T42.6X1	T42.6X2	T42.6X3	T42.6X4	T42.6X5	T42.6X6
Bromvaletone	T42.6X1	T42.6X2	T42.6X3	T42.6X4	T42.6X5	T42.6X6
Bronchodilator NEC	T48.6X1	T48.6X2	T48.6X3	T48.6X4	T48.6X5	T48.6X6
Brotizolam	T42.4X1	T42.4X2	T42.4X3	T42.4X4	T42.4X5	T42.4X6
Brovincamine	T46.7X1	T46.7X2	T46.7X3	T46.7X4	T46.7X5	T46.7X6
Brown spider (bite) (venom)	T63.391	T63.392	T63.393	T63.394	—	—

◀ New   ◀ Revised   ~~deleted~~ Deleted

Substance	Poisoning, Accidental (Unintentional)	Poisoning, Intentional Self-Harm	Poisoning, Assault	Poisoning, Undetermined	Adverse Effect	Underdosing
Brown recluse spider (bite) (venom)	T63.331	T63.332	T63.333	T63.334	—	—
Broxaterol	T48.6X1	T48.6X2	T48.6X3	T48.6X4	T48.6X5	T48.6X6
Broxuridine	T45.1X1	T45.1X2	T45.1X3	T45.1X4	T45.1X5	T45.1X6
Broxyquinoline	T37.8X1	T37.8X2	T37.8X3	T37.8X4	T37.8X5	T37.8X6
Bruceine	T48.291	T48.292	T48.293	T48.294	T48.295	T48.296
Brucia	T62.2X1	T62.2X2	T62.2X3	T62.2X4	—	—
Brucine	T65.1X1	T65.1X2	T65.1X3	T65.1X4	—	—
Brunswick green — see Copper						
Bruten — see Ibuprofen						
Bryonia	T47.2X1	T47.2X2	T47.2X3	T47.2X4	T47.2X5	T47.2X6
Buclizine	T45.0X1	T45.0X2	T45.0X3	T45.0X4	T45.0X5	T45.0X6
Buclosamide	T49.0X1	T49.0X2	T49.0X3	T49.0X4	T49.0X5	T49.0X6
Budesonide	T44.5X1	T44.5X2	T44.5X3	T44.5X4	T44.5X5	T44.5X6
Budralazine	T46.5X1	T46.5X2	T46.5X3	T46.5X4	T46.5X5	T46.5X6
Bufferin	T39.011	T39.012	T39.013	T39.014	T39.015	T39.016
Buflomedil	T46.7X1	T46.7X2	T46.7X3	T46.7X4	T46.7X5	T46.7X6
Buformin	T38.3X1	T38.3X2	T38.3X3	T38.3X4	T38.3X5	T38.3X6
Bufotenine	T40.991	T40.992	T40.993	T40.994	—	—
Bufrolin	T48.6X1	T48.6X2	T48.6X3	T48.6X4	T48.6X5	T48.6X6
Bufylline	T48.6X1	T48.6X2	T48.6X3	T48.6X4	T48.6X5	T48.6X6
Bulk filler	T50.5X1	T50.5X2	T50.5X3	T50.5X4	T50.5X5	T50.5X6
cathartic	T47.4X1	T47.4X2	T47.4X3	T47.4X4	T47.4X5	T47.4X6
Bumetanide	T50.1X1	T50.1X2	T50.1X3	T50.1X4	T50.1X5	T50.1X6
Bunaftine	T46.2X1	T46.2X2	T46.2X3	T46.2X4	T46.2X5	T46.2X6
Bunamiodyl	T50.8X1	T50.8X2	T50.8X3	T50.8X4	T50.8X5	T50.8X6
Bunazosin	T44.6X1	T44.6X2	T44.6X3	T44.6X4	T44.6X5	T44.6X6
Bunitrolol	T44.7X1	T44.7X2	T44.7X3	T44.7X4	T44.7X5	T44.7X6
Buphenine	T46.7X1	T46.7X2	T46.7X3	T46.7X4	T46.7X5	T46.7X6
Bupivacaine	T41.3X1	T41.3X2	T41.3X3	T41.3X4	T41.3X5	T41.3X6
infiltration (subcutaneous)	T41.3X1	T41.3X2	T41.3X3	T41.3X4	T41.3X5	T41.3X6
nerve block (peripheral) (plexus)	T41.3X1	T41.3X2	T41.3X3	T41.3X4	T41.3X5	T41.3X6
spinal	T41.3X1	T41.3X2	T41.3X3	T41.3X4	T41.3X5	T41.3X6
Bupranolol	T44.7X1	T44.7X2	T44.7X3	T44.7X4	T44.7X5	T44.7X6
Buprenorphine	T40.491	T40.492	T40.493	T40.494	T40.495	T40.496
Bupropion	T43.291	T43.292	T43.293	T43.294	T43.295	T43.296
Burimamide	T47.1X1	T47.1X2	T47.1X3	T47.1X4	T47.1X5	T47.1X6
Buserelin	T38.891	T38.892	T38.893	T38.894	T38.895	T38.896
Buspirone	T43.591	T43.592	T43.593	T43.594	T43.595	T43.596
Busulfan, busulphan	T45.1X1	T45.1X2	T45.1X3	T45.1X4	T45.1X5	T45.1X6
Butabarbital (sodium)	T42.3X1	T42.3X2	T42.3X3	T42.3X4	T42.3X5	T42.3X6
Butabarbitone	T42.3X1	T42.3X2	T42.3X3	T42.3X4	T42.3X5	T42.3X6

Substance	Poisoning, Accidental (Unintentional)	Poisoning, Intentional Self-Harm	Poisoning, Assault	Poisoning, Undetermined	Adverse Effect	Underdosing
Butabarpal	T42.3X1	T42.3X2	T42.3X3	T42.3X4	T42.3X5	T42.3X6
Butacaine	T41.3X1	T41.3X2	T41.3X3	T41.3X4	T41.3X5	T41.3X6
Butalamine	T46.7X1	T46.7X2	T46.7X3	T46.7X4	T46.7X5	T46.7X6
Butalbital	T42.3X1	T42.3X2	T42.3X3	T42.3X4	T42.3X5	T42.3X6
Butallylonal	T42.3X1	T42.3X2	T42.3X3	T42.3X4	T42.3X5	T42.3X6
Butamben	T41.3X1	T41.3X2	T41.3X3	T41.3X4	T41.3X5	T41.3X6
Butamirate	T48.3X1	T48.3X2	T48.3X3	T48.3X4	T48.3X5	T48.3X6
Butane (distributed in mobile container)	T59.891	T59.892	T59.893	T59.894	—	—
distributed through pipes	T59.891	T59.892	T59.893	T59.894	—	—
incomplete combustion	T58.11	T58.12	T58.13	T58.14	—	—
Butanilicaine	T41.3X1	T41.3X2	T41.3X3	T41.3X4	T41.3X5	T41.3X6
Butanol	T51.3X1	T51.3X2	T51.3X3	T51.3X4		
Butanone, 2-butanone	T52.4X1	T52.4X2	T52.4X3	T52.4X4	—	—
Butantrone	T49.4X1	T49.4X2	T49.4X3	T49.4X4	T49.4X5	T49.4X6
Butaperazine	T43.3X1	T43.3X2	T43.3X3	T43.3X4	T43.3X5	T43.3X6
Butazolidin	T39.2X1	T39.2X2	T39.2X3	T39.2X4	T39.2X5	T39.2X6
Butetamate	T48.6X1	T48.6X2	T48.6X3	T48.6X4	T48.6X5	T48.6X6
Butethal	T42.3X1	T42.3X2	T42.3X3	T42.3X4	T42.3X5	T42.3X6
Butethamate	T44.3X1	T44.3X2	T44.3X3	T44.3X4	T44.3X5	T44.3X6
Buthalitone (sodium)	T41.1X1	T41.1X2	T41.1X3	T41.1X4	T41.1X5	T41.1X6
Butisol (sodium)	T42.3X1	T42.3X2	T42.3X3	T42.3X4	T42.3X5	T42.3X6
Butizide	T50.2X1	T50.2X2	T50.2X3	T50.2X4	T50.2X5	T50.2X6
Butobarbital	T42.3X1	T42.3X2	T42.3X3	T42.3X4	T42.3X5	T42.3X6
sodium	T42.3X1	T42.3X2	T42.3X3	T42.3X4	T42.3X5	T42.3X6
Butobarbitone	T42.3X1	T42.3X2	T42.3X3	T42.3X4	T42.3X5	T42.3X6
Butoconazole (nitrate)	T49.0X1	T49.0X2	T49.0X3	T49.0X4	T49.0X5	T49.0X6
Butorphanol	T40.491	T40.492	T40.493	T40.494	T40.495	T40.496
Butriptyline	T43.011	T43.012	T43.013	T43.014	T43.015	T43.016
Butropium bromide	T44.3X1	T44.3X2	T44.3X3	T44.3X4	T44.3X5	T44.3X6
Buttercups	T62.2X1	T62.2X2	T62.2X3	T62.2X4	—	—
Butter of antimony — see Antimony						
Butyl						
acetate (secondary)	T52.8X1	T52.8X2	T52.8X3	T52.8X4	—	—
alcohol	T51.3X1	T51.3X2	T51.3X3	T51.3X4	—	—
aminobenzoate	T41.3X1	T41.3X2	T41.3X3	T41.3X4	T41.3X5	T41.3X6
butyrate	T52.8X1	T52.8X2	T52.8X3	T52.8X4	—	—
carbinol	T51.3X1	T51.3X2	T51.3X3	T51.3X4	—	—
carbitol	T52.3X1	T52.3X2	T52.3X3	T52.3X4	—	—
cellosolve	T52.3X1	T52.3X2	T52.3X3	T52.3X4	—	—
chloral (hydrate)	T42.6X1	T42.6X2	T42.6X3	T42.6X4	T42.6X5	T42.6X6
formate	T52.8X1	T52.8X2	T52.8X3	T52.8X4	—	—

TABLE OF DRUGS AND CHEMICALS

TABLE OF DRUGS AND CHEMICALS

Substance	Poisoning, Accidental (Unintentional)	Poisoning, Intentional Self-Harm	Poisoning, Assault	Poisoning, Undetermined	Adverse Effect	Underdosing
Butyl *(Continued)*						
lactate	T52.8X1	T52.8X2	T52.8X3	T52.8X4	—	—
propionate	T52.8X1	T52.8X2	T52.8X3	T52.8X4	—	—
scopolamine bromide	T44.3X1	T44.3X2	T44.3X3	T44.3X4	T44.3X5	T44.3X6
thiobarbital sodium	T41.1X1	T41.1X2	T41.1X3	T41.1X4	T41.1X5	T41.1X6
Butylated hydroxy-anisole	T50.991	T50.992	T50.993	T50.994	T50.995	T50.996
Butylchloral hydrate	T42.6X1	T42.6X2	T42.6X3	T42.6X4	T42.6X5	T42.6X6
Butyltoluene	T52.2X1	T52.2X2	T52.2X3	T52.2X4	—	—
Butyn	T41.3X1	T41.3X2	T41.3X3	T41.3X4	T41.3X5	T41.3X6
Butyrophenone (-based tranquilizers)	T43.4X1	T43.4X2	T43.4X3	T43.4X4	T43.4X5	T43.4X6
C						
Cabergoline	T42.8X1	T42.8X2	T42.8X3	T42.8X4	T42.8X5	T42.8X6
Cacodyl, cacodylic acid	T57.0X1	T57.0X2	T57.0X3	T57.0X4	—	—
Cactinomycin	T45.1X1	T45.1X2	T45.1X3	T45.1X4	T45.1X5	T45.1X6
Cade oil	T49.4X1	T49.4X2	T49.4X3	T49.4X4	T49.4X5	T49.4X6
Cadexomer iodine	T49.0X1	T49.0X2	T49.0X3	T49.0X4	T49.0X5	T49.0X6
Cadmium (chloride) (fumes) (oxide)	T56.3X1	T56.3X2	T56.3X3	T56.3X4	—	—
sulfide (medicinal) NEC	T49.4X1	T49.4X2	T49.4X3	T49.4X4	T49.4X5	T49.4X6
Cadralazine	T46.5X1	T46.5X2	T46.5X3	T46.5X4	T46.5X5	T46.5X6
Caffeine	T43.611	T43.612	T43.613	T43.614	T43.615	T43.616
Calabar bean	T62.2X1	T62.2X2	T62.2X3	T62.2X4	—	—
Caladium seguinum	T62.2X1	T62.2X2	T62.2X3	T62.2X4	—	—
Calamine (lotion)	T49.3X1	T49.3X2	T49.3X3	T49.3X4	T49.3X5	T49.3X6
Calcifediol	T45.2X1	T45.2X2	T45.2X3	T45.2X4	T45.2X5	T45.2X6
Calciferol	T45.2X1	T45.2X2	T45.2X3	T45.2X4	T45.2X5	T45.2X6
Calcitonin	T50.991	T50.992	T50.993	T50.994	T50.995	T50.996
Calcitriol	T45.2X1	T45.2X2	T45.2X3	T45.2X4	T45.2X5	T45.2X6
Calcium	T50.3X1	T50.3X2	T50.3X3	T50.3X4	T50.3X5	T50.3X6
actylsalicylate	T39.011	T39.012	T39.013	T39.014	T39.015	T39.016
benzamidosalicylate	T37.1X1	T37.1X2	T37.1X3	T37.1X4	T37.1X5	T37.1X6
bromide	T42.6X1	T42.6X2	T42.6X3	T42.6X4	T42.6X5	T42.6X6
bromolactobionate	T42.6X1	T42.6X2	T42.6X3	T42.6X4	T42.6X5	T42.6X6
carbaspirin	T39.011	T39.012	T39.013	T39.014	T39.015	T39.016
carbimide	T50.6X1	T50.6X2	T50.6X3	T50.6X4	T50.6X5	T50.6X6
carbonate	T47.1X1	T47.1X2	T47.1X3	T47.1X4	T47.1X5	T47.1X6
chloride	T50.991	T50.992	T50.993	T50.994	T50.995	T50.996
anhydrous	T50.991	T50.992	T50.993	T50.994	T50.995	T50.996
cyanide	T57.8X1	T57.8X2	T57.8X3	T57.8X4	—	—
dioctyl sulfosuccinate	T47.4X1	T47.4X2	T47.4X3	T47.4X4	T47.4X5	T47.4X6
disodium edathamil	T45.8X1	T45.8X2	T45.8X3	T45.8X4	T45.8X5	T45.8X6

Substance	Poisoning, Accidental (Unintentional)	Poisoning, Intentional Self-Harm	Poisoning, Assault	Poisoning, Undetermined	Adverse Effect	Underdosing
Calcium *(Continued)*						
disodium edetate	T45.8X1	T45.8X2	T45.8X3	T45.8X4	T45.8X5	T45.8X6
dobesilate	T46.991	T46.992	T46.993	T46.994	T46.995	T46.996
EDTA	T45.8X1	T45.8X2	T45.8X3	T45.8X4	T45.8X5	T45.8X6
ferrous citrate	T45.4X1	T45.4X2	T45.4X3	T45.4X4	T45.4X5	T45.4X6
folinate	T45.8X1	T45.8X2	T45.8X3	T45.8X4	T45.8X5	T45.8X6
glubionate	T50.3X1	T50.3X2	T50.3X3	T50.3X4	T50.3X5	T50.3X6
gluconate	T50.3X1	T50.3X2	T50.3X3	T50.3X4	T50.3X5	T50.3X6
gluconogalactogluconate	T50.3X1	T50.3X2	T50.3X3	T50.3X4	T50.3X5	T50.3X6
hydrate, hydroxide	T54.3X1	T54.3X2	T54.3X3	T54.3X4	—	—
hypochlorite	T54.3X1	T54.3X2	T54.3X3	T54.3X4	—	—
iodide	T48.4X1	T48.4X2	T48.4X3	T48.4X4	T48.4X5	T48.4X6
ipodate	T50.8X1	T50.8X2	T50.8X3	T50.8X4	T50.8X5	T50.8X6
lactate	T50.3X1	T50.3X2	T50.3X3	T50.3X4	T50.3X5	T50.3X6
leucovorin	T45.8X1	T45.8X2	T45.8X3	T45.8X4	T45.8X5	T45.8X6
mandelate	T37.91	T37.92	T37.93	T37.94	T37.95	T37.96
oxide	T54.3X1	T54.3X2	T54.3X3	T54.3X4	—	—
pantothenate	T45.2X1	T45.2X2	T45.2X3	T45.2X4	T45.2X5	T45.2X6
phosphate	T50.3X1	T50.3X2	T50.3X3	T50.3X4	T50.3X5	T50.3X6
salicylate	T39.091	T39.092	T39.093	T39.094	T39.095	T39.096
salts	T50.3X1	T50.3X2	T50.3X3	T50.3X4	T50.3X5	T50.3X6
Calculus-dissolving drug	T50.991	T50.992	T50.993	T50.994	T50.995	T50.996
Calomel	T49.0X1	T49.0X2	T49.0X3	T49.0X4	T49.0X5	T49.0X6
Caloric agent	T50.3X1	T50.3X2	T50.3X3	T50.3X4	T50.3X5	T50.3X6
Calusterone	T38.7X1	T38.7X2	T38.7X3	T38.7X4	T38.7X5	T38.7X6
Camazepam	T42.4X1	T42.4X2	T42.4X3	T42.4X4	T42.4X5	T42.4X6
Camomile	T49.0X1	T49.0X2	T49.0X3	T49.0X4	T49.0X5	T49.0X6
Camoquin	T37.2X1	T37.2X2	T37.2X3	T37.2X4	T37.2X5	T37.2X6
Camphor						
insecticide	T60.2X1	T60.2X2	T60.2X3	T60.2X4	—	—
medicinal	T49.8X1	T49.8X2	T49.8X3	T49.8X4	T49.8X5	T49.8X6
Camylofin	T44.3X1	T44.3X2	T44.3X3	T44.3X4	T44.3X5	T44.3X6
Cancer chemotherapy drug regimen	T45.1X1	T45.1X2	T45.1X3	T45.1X4	T45.1X5	T45.1X6
Candeptin	T49.0X1	T49.0X2	T49.0X3	T49.0X4	T49.0X5	T49.0X6
Candicidin	T49.0X1	T49.0X2	T49.0X3	T49.0X4	T49.0X5	T49.0X6
Cannabinoids, synthetic	T40.721	T40.722	T40.723	T40.724	T40.725	T40.726
Cannabinol	T40.711	T40.712	T40.713	T40.714	T40.715	T40.716
Cannabis (derivatives)	T40.711	T40.712	T40.713	T40.714	T40.715	T40.716
Canned heat	T51.1X1	T51.1X2	T51.1X3	T51.1X4	—	—
Canrenoic acid	T50.0X1	T50.0X2	T50.0X3	T50.0X4	T50.0X5	T50.0X6
Canrenone	T50.0X1	T50.0X2	T50.0X3	T50.0X4	T50.0X5	T50.0X6

◀ New   ◀ Revised   ~~deleted~~ Deleted

Substance	Poisoning, Accidental (Unintentional)	Poisoning, Intentional Self-Harm	Poisoning, Assault	Poisoning, Undetermined	Adverse Effect	Underdosing
External Cause (T-Code)						
Cantharides, cantharidin, cantharis	T49.8X1	T49.8X2	T49.8X3	T49.8X4	T49.8X5	T49.8X6
Canthaxanthin	T50.991	T50.992	T50.993	T50.994	T50.995	T50.996
Capillary-active drug NEC	T46.901	T46.902	T46.903	T46.904	T46.905	T46.906
Capreomycin	T36.8X1	T36.8X2	T36.8X3	T36.8X4	T36.8X5	T36.8X6
Capsicum	T49.4X1	T49.4X2	T49.4X3	T49.4X4	T49.4X5	T49.4X6
Captafol	T60.3X1	T60.3X2	T60.3X3	T60.3X4	—	—
Captan	T60.3X1	T60.3X2	T60.3X3	T60.3X4	—	—
Captodiame, captodiamine	T43.591	T43.592	T43.593	T43.594	T43.595	T43.596
Captopril	T46.4X1	T46.4X2	T46.4X3	T46.4X4	T46.4X5	T46.4X6
Caramiphen	T44.3X1	T44.3X2	T44.3X3	T44.3X4	T44.3X5	T44.3X6
Carazolol	T44.7X1	T44.7X2	T44.7X3	T44.7X4	T44.7X5	T44.7X6
Carbachol	T44.1X1	T44.1X2	T44.1X3	T44.1X4	T44.1X5	T44.1X6
Carbacrylamine (resin)	T50.3X1	T50.3X2	T50.3X3	T50.3X4	T50.3X5	T50.3X6
Carbamate (insecticide)	T60.0X1	T60.0X2	T60.0X3	T60.0X4	—	—
Carbamate (sedative)	T42.6X1	T42.6X2	T42.6X3	T42.6X4	T42.6X5	T42.6X6
herbicide	T60.0X1	T60.0X2	T60.0X3	T60.0X4	—	—
insecticide	T60.0X1	T60.0X2	T60.0X3	T60.0X4	—	—
Carbamazepine	T42.1X1	T42.1X2	T42.1X3	T42.1X4	T42.1X5	T42.1X6
Carbamide	T47.3X1	T47.3X2	T47.3X3	T47.3X4	T47.3X5	T47.3X6
peroxide	T49.0X1	T49.0X2	T49.0X3	T49.0X4	T49.0X5	T49.0X6
topical	T49.8X1	T49.8X2	T49.8X3	T49.8X4	T49.8X5	T49.8X6
Carbamylcholine chloride	T44.1X1	T44.1X2	T44.1X3	T44.1X4	T44.1X5	T44.1X6
Carbaril	T60.0X1	T60.0X2	T60.0X3	T60.0X4	—	—
Carbarsone	T37.3X1	T37.3X2	T37.3X3	T37.3X4	T37.3X5	T37.3X6
Carbaryl	T60.0X1	T60.0X2	T60.0X3	T60.0X4	—	—
Carbaspirin	T39.011	T39.012	T39.013	T39.014	T39.015	T39.016
Carbazochrome (salicylate) (sodium sulfonate)	T49.4X1	T49.4X2	T49.4X3	T49.4X4	T49.4X5	T49.4X6
Carbenicillin	T36.0X1	T36.0X2	T36.0X3	T36.0X4	T36.0X5	T36.0X6
Carbenoxolone	T47.1X1	T47.1X2	T47.1X3	T47.1X4	T47.1X5	T47.1X6
Carbetapentane	T48.3X1	T48.3X2	T48.3X3	T48.3X4	T48.3X5	T48.3X6
Carbethyl salicylate	T39.091	T39.092	T39.093	T39.094	T39.095	T39.096
Carbidopa (with levodopa)	T42.8X1	T42.8X2	T42.8X3	T42.8X4	T42.8X5	T42.8X6
Carbimazole	T38.2X1	T38.2X2	T38.2X3	T38.2X4	T38.2X5	T38.2X6
Carbinol	T51.1X1	T51.1X2	T51.1X3	T51.1X4	—	—
Carbinoxamine	T45.0X1	T45.0X2	T45.0X3	T45.0X4	T45.0X5	T45.0X6
Carbiphene	T39.8X1	T39.8X2	T39.8X3	T39.8X4	T39.8X5	T39.8X6
Carbitol	T52.3X1	T52.3X2	T52.3X3	T52.3X4	—	—
Carbocaine	T41.3X1	T41.3X2	T41.3X3	T41.3X4	T41.3X5	T41.3X6
infiltration (subcutaneous)	T41.3X1	T41.3X2	T41.3X3	T41.3X4	T41.3X5	T41.3X6
nerve block (peripheral) (plexus)	T41.3X1	T41.3X2	T41.3X3	T41.3X4	T41.3X5	T41.3X6
topical (surface)	T41.3X1	T41.3X2	T41.3X3	T41.3X4	T41.3X5	T41.3X6

Substance	Poisoning, Accidental (Unintentional)	Poisoning, Intentional Self-Harm	Poisoning, Assault	Poisoning, Undetermined	Adverse Effect	Underdosing
External Cause (T-Code)						
Carbo medicinalis	T47.6X1	T47.6X2	T47.6X3	T47.6X4	T47.6X5	T47.6X6
Carbomycin	T36.8X1	T36.8X2	T36.8X3	T36.8X4	T36.8X5	T36.8X6
Carbocisteine	T48.4X1	T48.4X2	T48.4X3	T48.4X4	T48.4X5	T48.4X6
Carbocromen	T46.3X1	T46.3X2	T46.3X3	T46.3X4	T46.3X5	T46.3X6
Carbol fuchsin	T49.0X1	T49.0X2	T49.0X3	T49.0X4	T49.0X5	T49.0X6
Carbolic acid — see also Phenol	T54.0X1	T54.0X2	T54.0X3	T54.0X4	—	—
Carbolonium (bromide)	T48.1X1	T48.1X2	T48.1X3	T48.1X4	T48.1X5	T48.1X6
Carbon						
bisulfide (liquid)	T65.4X1	T65.4X2	T65.4X3	T65.4X4	—	—
vapor	T65.4X1	T65.4X2	T65.4X3	T65.4X4	—	—
dioxide (gas)	T59.7X1	T59.7X2	T59.7X3	T59.7X4	—	—
medicinal	T41.5X1	T41.5X2	T41.5X3	T41.5X4	T41.5X5	T41.5X6
nonmedicinal	T59.7X1	T59.7X2	T59.7X3	T59.7X4	—	—
snow	T49.4X1	T49.4X2	T49.4X3	T49.4X4	T49.4X5	T49.4X6
disulfide (liquid)	T65.4X1	T65.4X2	T65.4X3	T65.4X4	—	—
vapor	T65.4X1	T65.4X2	T65.4X3	T65.4X4	—	—
monoxide (from incomplete combustion)	T58.91	T58.92	T58.93	T58.94	—	—
blast furnace gas	T58.8X1	T58.8X2	T58.8X3	T58.8X4		
butane (distributed in mobile container)	T58.11	T58.12	T58.13	T58.14		
distributed through pipes	T58.11	T58.12	T58.13	T58.14		
charcoal fumes	T58.2X1	T58.2X2	T58.2X3	T58.2X4		
coal	T58.2X1	T58.2X2	T58.2X3	T58.2X4		
coke (in domestic stoves, fireplaces)	T58.2X1	T58.2X2	T58.2X3	T58.2X4	—	—
gas (piped)	T58.11	T58.12	T58.13	T58.14	—	—
solid (in domestic stoves, fireplaces)	T58.2X1	T58.2X2	T58.2X3	T58.2X4	—	—
exhaust gas (motor) not in transit	T58.01	T58.02	T58.03	T58.04	—	—
combustion engine, any not in watercraft	T58.01	T58.02	T58.03	T58.04		
farm tractor, not in transit	T58.01	T58.02	T58.03	T58.04		
gas engine	T58.01	T58.02	T58.03	T58.04		
motor pump	T58.01	T58.02	T58.03	T58.04		
motor vehicle, not in transit	T58.01	T58.02	T58.03	T58.04		
fuel (in domestic use)	T58.2X1	T58.2X2	T58.2X3	T58.2X4		
gas (piped)	T58.11	T58.12	T58.13	T58.14	—	—
in mobile container	T58.11	T58.12	T58.13	T58.14	—	—
utility	T58.11	T58.12	T58.13	T58.14	—	—
in mobile container	T58.11	T58.12	T58.13	T58.14	—	—
piped (natural)	T58.11	T58.12	T58.13	T58.14		

Substance	Poisoning, Accidental (Unintentional)	Poisoning, Intentional Self-Harm	Poisoning, Assault	Poisoning, Undetermined	Adverse Effect	Underdosing
Carbon *(Continued)*						
monoxide *(Continued)*						
illuminating gas	T58.11	T58.12	T58.13	T58.14	—	—
industrial fuels or gases, any	T58.8X1	T58.8X2	T58.8X3	T58.8X4	—	—
kerosene (in domestic stoves, fireplaces)	T58.2X1	T58.2X2	T58.2X3	T58.2X4	—	—
kiln gas or vapor	T58.8X1	T58.8X2	T58.8X3	T58.8X4	—	—
motor exhaust gas, not in transit	T58.01	T58.02	T58.03	T58.04	—	—
piped gas (manufactured) (natural)	T58.11	T58.12	T58.13	T58.14	—	—
producer gas	T58.8X1	T58.8X2	T58.8X3	T58.8X4	—	—
propane (distributed in mobile container)	T58.11	T58.12	T58.13	T58.14	—	—
distributed through pipes	T58.11	T58.12	T58.13	T58.14	—	—
specified source NEC	T58.8X1	T58.8X2	T58.8X3	T58.8X4	—	—
stove gas	T58.11	T58.12	T58.13	T58.14	—	—
piped	T58.11	T58.12	T58.13	T58.14	—	—
utility gas	T58.11	T58.12	T58.13	T58.14	—	—
piped	T58.11	T58.12	T58.13	T58.14	—	—
water gas	T58.11	T58.12	T58.13	T58.14	—	—
wood (in domestic stoves, fireplaces)	T58.2X1	T58.2X2	T58.2X3	T58.2X4	—	—
tetrachloride (vapor) NEC	T53.0X1	T53.0X2	T53.0X3	T53.0X4	—	—
liquid (cleansing agent) NEC	T53.0X1	T53.0X2	T53.0X3	T53.0X4	—	—
solvent	T53.0X1	T53.0X2	T53.0X3	T53.0X4	—	—
Carbonic acid gas	T59.7X1	T59.7X2	T59.7X3	T59.7X4	—	—
anhydrase inhibitor NEC	T50.2X1	T50.2X2	T50.2X3	T50.2X4	T50.2X5	T50.2X6
Carbophenothion	T60.0X1	T60.0X2	T60.0X3	T60.0X4	—	—
Carboplatin	T45.1X1	T45.1X2	T45.1X3	T45.1X4	T45.1X5	T45.1X6
Carboprost	T48.0X1	T48.0X2	T48.0X3	T48.0X4	T48.0X5	T48.0X6
Carboquone	T45.1X1	T45.1X2	T45.1X3	T45.1X4	T45.1X5	T45.1X6
Carbowax	T49.3X1	T49.3X2	T49.3X3	T49.3X4	T49.3X5	T49.3X6
Carboxymethyl-cellulose	T47.4X1	T47.4X2	T47.4X3	T47.4X4	T47.4X5	T47.4X6
S-Carboxymethyl-cysteine	T48.4X1	T48.4X2	T48.4X3	T48.4X4	T48.4X5	T48.4X6
Carbrital	T42.3X1	T42.3X2	T42.3X3	T42.3X4	T42.3X5	T42.3X6
Carbromal	T42.6X1	T42.6X2	T42.6X3	T42.6X4	T42.6X5	T42.6X6
Carbutamide	T38.3X1	T38.3X2	T38.3X3	T38.3X4	T38.3X5	T38.3X6
Carbuterol	T48.6X1	T48.6X2	T48.6X3	T48.6X4	T48.6X5	T48.6X6
Cardiac						
depressants	T46.2X1	T46.2X2	T46.2X3	T46.2X4	T46.2X5	T46.2X6
rhythm regulator	T46.2X1	T46.2X2	T46.2X3	T46.2X4	T46.2X5	T46.2X6
specified NEC	T46.2X1	T46.2X2	T46.2X3	T46.2X4	T46.2X5	T46.2X6

Substance	Poisoning, Accidental (Unintentional)	Poisoning, Intentional Self-Harm	Poisoning, Assault	Poisoning, Undetermined	Adverse Effect	Underdosing
Cardiografin	T50.8X1	T50.8X2	T50.8X3	T50.8X4	T50.8X5	T50.8X6
Cardio-green	T50.8X1	T50.8X2	T50.8X3	T50.8X4	T50.8X5	T50.8X6
Cardiotonic (glycoside) NEC	T46.0X1	T46.0X2	T46.0X3	T46.0X4	T46.0X5	T46.0X6
Cardiovascular drug NEC	T46.901	T46.902	T46.903	T46.904	T46.905	T46.906
Cardrase	T50.2X1	T50.2X2	T50.2X3	T50.2X4	T50.2X5	T50.2X6
Carfusin	T49.0X1	T49.0X2	T49.0X3	T49.0X4	T49.0X5	T49.0X6
Carfecillin	T36.0X1	T36.0X2	T36.0X3	T36.0X4	T36.0X5	T36.0X6
Carfenazine	T43.3X1	T43.3X2	T43.3X3	T43.3X4	T43.3X5	T43.3X6
Carindacillin	T36.0X1	T36.0X2	T36.0X3	T36.0X4	T36.0X5	T36.0X6
Carisoprodol	T42.8X1	T42.8X2	T42.8X3	T42.8X4	T42.8X5	T42.8X6
Carmellose	T47.4X1	T47.4X2	T47.4X3	T47.4X4	T47.4X5	T47.4X6
Carminative	T47.5X1	T47.5X2	T47.5X3	T47.5X4	T47.5X5	T47.5X6
Carmofur	T45.1X1	T45.1X2	T45.1X3	T45.1X4	T45.1X5	T45.1X6
Carmustine	T45.1X1	T45.1X2	T45.1X3	T45.1X4	T45.1X5	T45.1X6
Carotene	T45.2X1	T45.2X2	T45.2X3	T45.2X4	T45.2X5	T45.2X6
Carphenazine	T43.3X1	T43.3X2	T43.3X3	T43.3X4	T43.3X5	T43.3X6
Carpipramine	T42.4X1	T42.4X2	T42.4X3	T42.4X4	T42.4X5	T42.4X6
Carprofen	T39.311	T39.312	T39.313	T39.314	T39.315	T39.316
Carpronium chloride	T44.3X1	T44.3X2	T44.3X3	T44.3X4	T44.3X5	T44.3X6
Carrageenan	T47.8X1	T47.8X2	T47.8X3	T47.8X4	T47.8X5	T47.8X6
Carteolol	T44.7X1	T44.7X2	T44.7X3	T44.7X4	T44.7X5	T44.7X6
Carter's Little Pills	T47.2X1	T47.2X2	T47.2X3	T47.2X4	T47.2X5	T47.2X6
Cascara (sagrada)	T47.2X1	T47.2X2	T47.2X3	T47.2X4	T47.2X5	T47.2X6
Cassava	T62.2X1	T62.2X2	T62.2X3	T62.2X4	—	—
Castellani's paint	T49.0X1	T49.0X2	T49.0X3	T49.0X4	T49.0X5	T49.0X6
Castor						
bean	T62.2X1	T62.2X2	T62.2X3	T62.2X4	—	—
oil	T47.2X1	T47.2X2	T47.2X3	T47.2X4	T47.2X5	T47.2X6
Catalase	T45.3X1	T45.3X2	T45.3X3	T45.3X4	T45.3X5	T45.3X6
Caterpillar (sting)	T63.431	T63.432	T63.433	T63.434	—	—
Catha (edulis) (tea)	T43.691	T43.692	T43.693	T43.694	—	—
Cathartic NEC	T47.4X1	T47.4X2	T47.4X3	T47.4X4	T47.4X5	T47.4X6
anthacene derivative	T47.2X1	T47.2X2	T47.2X3	T47.2X4	T47.2X5	T47.2X6
bulk	T47.4X1	T47.4X2	T47.4X3	T47.4X4	T47.4X5	T47.4X6
contact	T47.2X1	T47.2X2	T47.2X3	T47.2X4	T47.2X5	T47.2X6
emollient NEC	T47.4X1	T47.4X2	T47.4X3	T47.4X4	T47.4X5	T47.4X6
irritant NEC	T47.2X1	T47.2X2	T47.2X3	T47.2X4	T47.2X5	T47.2X6
mucilage	T47.4X1	T47.4X2	T47.4X3	T47.4X4	T47.4X5	T47.4X6
saline	T47.3X1	T47.3X2	T47.3X3	T47.3X4	T47.3X5	T47.3X6
vegetable	T47.2X1	T47.2X2	T47.2X3	T47.2X4	T47.2X5	T47.2X6
Cathine	T50.5X1	T50.5X2	T50.5X3	T50.5X4	T50.5X5	T50.5X6
Cathomycin	T36.8X1	T36.8X2	T36.8X3	T36.8X4	T36.8X5	T36.8X6

◄ New ◀ Revised ~~deleted~~ Deleted

Substance	Poisoning, Accidental (Unintentional)	Poisoning, Intentional Self-Harm	Poisoning, Assault	Poisoning, Undetermined	Adverse Effect	Underdosing
Cation exchange resin	T50.3X1	T50.3X2	T50.3X3	T50.3X4	T50.3X5	T50.3X6
Caustic(s) NEC	T54.91	T54.92	T54.93	T54.94	—	—
alkali	T54.3X1	T54.3X2	T54.3X3	T54.3X4	—	—
hydroxide	T54.3X1	T54.3X2	T54.3X3	T54.3X4	—	—
potash	T54.3X1	T54.3X2	T54.3X3	T54.3X4	—	—
soda	T54.3X1	T54.3X2	T54.3X3	T54.3X4	—	—
specified NEC	T54.91	T54.92	T54.93	T54.94	—	—
Ceepryn	T49.0X1	T49.0X2	T49.0X3	T49.0X4	T49.0X5	T49.0X6
ENT agent	T49.6X1	T49.6X2	T49.6X3	T49.6X4	T49.6X5	T49.6X6
lozenges	T49.6X1	T49.6X2	T49.6X3	T49.6X4	T49.6X5	T49.6X6
Cefacetrile	T36.1X1	T36.1X2	T36.1X3	T36.1X4	T36.1X5	T36.1X6
Cefaclor	T36.1X1	T36.1X2	T36.1X3	T36.1X4	T36.1X5	T36.1X6
Cefadroxil	T36.1X1	T36.1X2	T36.1X3	T36.1X4	T36.1X5	T36.1X6
Cefalexin	T36.1X1	T36.1X2	T36.1X3	T36.1X4	T36.1X5	T36.1X6
Cefaloglycin	T36.1X1	T36.1X2	T36.1X3	T36.1X4	T36.1X5	T36.1X6
Cefaloridine	T36.1X1	T36.1X2	T36.1X3	T36.1X4	T36.1X5	T36.1X6
Cefalosporins	T36.1X1	T36.1X2	T36.1X3	T36.1X4	T36.1X5	T36.1X6
Cefalotin	T36.1X1	T36.1X2	T36.1X3	T36.1X4	T36.1X5	T36.1X6
Cefamandole	T36.1X1	T36.1X2	T36.1X3	T36.1X4	T36.1X5	T36.1X6
Cefamycin antibiotic	T36.1X1	T36.1X2	T36.1X3	T36.1X4	T36.1X5	T36.1X6
Cefapirin	T36.1X1	T36.1X2	T36.1X3	T36.1X4	T36.1X5	T36.1X6
Cefatrizine	T36.1X1	T36.1X2	T36.1X3	T36.1X4	T36.1X5	T36.1X6
Cefazedone	T36.1X1	T36.1X2	T36.1X3	T36.1X4	T36.1X5	T36.1X6
Cefazolin	T36.1X1	T36.1X2	T36.1X3	T36.1X4	T36.1X5	T36.1X6
Cefbuperazone	T36.1X1	T36.1X2	T36.1X3	T36.1X4	T36.1X5	T36.1X6
Cefetamet	T36.1X1	T36.1X2	T36.1X3	T36.1X4	T36.1X5	T36.1X6
Cefixime	T36.1X1	T36.1X2	T36.1X3	T36.1X4	T36.1X5	T36.1X6
Cefmenoxime	T36.1X1	T36.1X2	T36.1X3	T36.1X4	T36.1X5	T36.1X6
Cefmetazole	T36.1X1	T36.1X2	T36.1X3	T36.1X4	T36.1X5	T36.1X6
Cefminox	T36.1X1	T36.1X2	T36.1X3	T36.1X4	T36.1X5	T36.1X6
Cefonicid	T36.1X1	T36.1X2	T36.1X3	T36.1X4	T36.1X5	T36.1X6
Cefoperazone	T36.1X1	T36.1X2	T36.1X3	T36.1X4	T36.1X5	T36.1X6
Ceforanide	T36.1X1	T36.1X2	T36.1X3	T36.1X4	T36.1X5	T36.1X6
Cefotaxime	T36.1X1	T36.1X2	T36.1X3	T36.1X4	T36.1X5	T36.1X6
Cefotetan	T36.1X1	T36.1X2	T36.1X3	T36.1X4	T36.1X5	T36.1X6
Cefotiam	T36.1X1	T36.1X2	T36.1X3	T36.1X4	T36.1X5	T36.1X6
Cefoxitin	T36.1X1	T36.1X2	T36.1X3	T36.1X4	T36.1X5	T36.1X6
Cefpimizole	T36.1X1	T36.1X2	T36.1X3	T36.1X4	T36.1X5	T36.1X6
Cefpiramide	T36.1X1	T36.1X2	T36.1X3	T36.1X4	T36.1X5	T36.1X6
Cefradine	T36.1X1	T36.1X2	T36.1X3	T36.1X4	T36.1X5	T36.1X6
Cefroxadine	T36.1X1	T36.1X2	T36.1X3	T36.1X4	T36.1X5	T36.1X6
Cefsulodin	T36.1X1	T36.1X2	T36.1X3	T36.1X4	T36.1X5	T36.1X6

Substance	Poisoning, Accidental (Unintentional)	Poisoning, Intentional Self-Harm	Poisoning, Assault	Poisoning, Undetermined	Adverse Effect	Underdosing
Ceftazidime	T36.1X1	T36.1X2	T36.1X3	T36.1X4	T36.1X5	T36.1X6
Cefteram	T36.1X1	T36.1X2	T36.1X3	T36.1X4	T36.1X5	T36.1X6
Ceftezole	T36.1X1	T36.1X2	T36.1X3	T36.1X4	T36.1X5	T36.1X6
Ceftizoxime	T36.1X1	T36.1X2	T36.1X3	T36.1X4	T36.1X5	T36.1X6
Ceftriaxone	T36.1X1	T36.1X2	T36.1X3	T36.1X4	T36.1X5	T36.1X6
Cefuroxime	T36.1X1	T36.1X2	T36.1X3	T36.1X4	T36.1X5	T36.1X6
Cefuzonam	T36.1X1	T36.1X2	T36.1X3	T36.1X4	T36.1X5	T36.1X6
Celestone	T38.0X1	T38.0X2	T38.0X3	T38.0X4	T38.0X5	T38.0X6
topical	T49.0X1	T49.0X2	T49.0X3	T49.0X4	T49.0X5	T49.0X6
Celiprolol	T44.7X1	T44.7X2	T44.7X3	T44.7X4	T44.7X5	T44.7X6
Cellosolve	T52.91	T52.92	T52.93	T52.94	—	—
Cell stimulants and proliferants	T49.8X1	T49.8X2	T49.8X3	T49.8X4	T49.8X5	T49.8X6
Cellulose						
cathartic	T47.4X1	T47.4X2	T47.4X3	T47.4X4	T47.4X5	T47.4X6
hydroxyethyl	T47.4X1	T47.4X2	T47.4X3	T47.4X4	T47.4X5	T47.4X6
nitrates (topical)	T49.3X1	T49.3X2	T49.3X3	T49.3X4	T49.3X5	T49.3X6
oxidized	T49.4X1	T49.4X2	T49.4X3	T49.4X4	T49.4X5	T49.4X6
Centipede (bite)	T63.411	T63.412	T63.413	T63.414	—	—
Central nervous system						
depressants	T42.71	T42.72	T42.73	T42.74	T42.75	T42.76
anesthetic (general) NEC	T41.201	T41.202	T41.203	T41.204	T41.205	T41.206
gases NEC	T41.0X1	T41.0X2	T41.0X3	T41.0X4	T41.0X5	T41.0X6
intravenous	T41.1X1	T41.1X2	T41.1X3	T41.1X4	T41.1X5	T41.1X6
barbiturates	T42.3X1	T42.3X2	T42.3X3	T42.3X4	T42.3X5	T42.3X6
benzodiazepines	T42.4X1	T42.4X2	T42.4X3	T42.4X4	T42.4X5	T42.4X6
bromides	T42.6X1	T42.6X2	T42.6X3	T42.6X4	T42.6X5	T42.6X6
cannabis sativa	T40.711	T40.712	T40.713	T40.714	T40.715	T40.716
chloral hydrate	T42.6X1	T42.6X2	T42.6X3	T42.6X4	T42.6X5	T42.6X6
ethanol	T51.0X1	T51.0X2	T51.0X3	T51.0X4	—	—
hallucinogenics	T40.901	T40.902	T40.903	T40.904	T40.905	T40.906
hypnotics	T42.71	T42.72	T42.73	T42.74	T42.75	T42.76
specified NEC	T42.6X1	T42.6X2	T42.6X3	T42.6X4	T42.6X5	T42.6X6
muscle relaxants	T42.8X1	T42.8X2	T42.8X3	T42.8X4	T42.8X5	T42.8X6
paraldehyde	T42.6X1	T42.6X2	T42.6X3	T42.6X4	T42.6X5	T42.6X6
sedatives; sedative-hypnotics	T42.71	T42.72	T42.73	T42.74	T42.75	T42.76
mixed NEC	T42.6X1	T42.6X2	T42.6X3	T42.6X4	T42.6X5	T42.6X6
specified NEC	T42.6X1	T42.6X2	T42.6X3	T42.6X4	T42.6X5	T42.6X6
muscle-tone depressants	T42.8X1	T42.8X2	T42.8X3	T42.8X4	T42.8X5	T42.8X6
stimulants	T43.601	T43.602	T43.603	T43.604	T43.605	T43.606
amphetamines	T43.621	T43.622	T43.623	T43.624	T43.625	T43.626
analeptics	T50.7X1	T50.7X2	T50.7X3	T50.7X4	T50.7X5	T50.7X6

TABLE OF DRUGS AND CHEMICALS

Substance	Poisoning, Accidental (Unintentional)	Poisoning, Intentional Self-Harm	Poisoning, Assault	Poisoning, Undetermined	Adverse Effect	Underdosing
Central nervous system (Continued)						
stimulants (Continued)						
antidepressants	T43.201	T43.202	T43.203	T43.204	T43.205	T43.206
opiate antagonists	T50.7X1	T50.7X2	T50.7X3	T50.7X4	T50.7X5	T50.7X6
specified NEC	T43.691	T43.692	T43.693	T43.694	T43.695	T43.696
Cephalexin	T36.1X1	T36.1X2	T36.1X3	T36.1X4	T36.1X5	T36.1X6
Cephaloglycin	T36.1X1	T36.1X2	T36.1X3	T36.1X4	T36.1X5	T36.1X6
Cephaloridine	T36.1X1	T36.1X2	T36.1X3	T36.1X4	T36.1X5	T36.1X6
Cephalosporins	T36.1X1	T36.1X2	T36.1X3	T36.1X4	T36.1X5	T36.1X6
N (adicillin)	T36.0X1	T36.0X2	T36.0X3	T36.0X4	T36.0X5	T36.0X6
Cephalothin	T36.1X1	T36.1X2	T36.1X3	T36.1X4	T36.1X5	T36.1X6
Cephalotin	T36.1X1	T36.1X2	T36.1X3	T36.1X4	T36.1X5	T36.1X6
Cephradine	T36.1X1	T36.1X2	T36.1X3	T36.1X4	T36.1X5	T36.1X6
Cerbera (odallam)	T62.2X1	T62.2X2	T62.2X3	T62.2X4	—	—
Cerberin	T46.0X1	T46.0X2	T46.0X3	T46.0X4	T46.0X5	T46.0X6
Cerebral stimulants	T43.601	T43.602	T43.603	T43.604	T43.605	T43.606
psychotherapeutic	T43.601	T43.602	T43.603	T43.604	T43.605	T43.606
specified NEC	T43.691	T43.692	T43.693	T43.694	T43.695	T43.696
Cerium oxalate	T45.0X1	T45.0X2	T45.0X3	T45.0X4	T45.0X5	T45.0X6
Cerous oxalate	T45.0X1	T45.0X2	T45.0X3	T45.0X4	T45.0X5	T45.0X6
Ceruletide	T50.8X1	T50.8X2	T50.8X3	T50.8X4	T50.8X5	T50.8X6
Cetalkonium (chloride)	T49.0X1	T49.0X2	T49.0X3	T49.0X4	T49.0X5	T49.0X6
Cethexonium chloride	T49.0X1	T49.0X2	T49.0X3	T49.0X4	T49.0X5	T49.0X6
Cetiedil	T46.7X1	T46.7X2	T46.7X3	T46.7X4	T46.7X5	T46.7X6
Cetirizine	T45.0X1	T45.0X2	T45.0X3	T45.0X4	T45.0X5	T45.0X6
Cetomacrogol	T50.991	T50.992	T50.993	T50.994	T50.995	T50.996
Cetotiamine	T45.2X1	T45.2X2	T45.2X3	T45.2X4	T45.2X5	T45.2X6
Cetoxime	T45.0X1	T45.0X2	T45.0X3	T45.0X4	T45.0X5	T45.0X6
Cetraxate	T47.1X1	T47.1X2	T47.1X3	T47.1X4	T47.1X5	T47.1X6
Cetrimide	T49.0X1	T49.0X2	T49.0X3	T49.0X4	T49.0X5	T49.0X6
Cetrimonium (bromide)	T49.0X1	T49.0X2	T49.0X3	T49.0X4	T49.0X5	T49.0X6
Cetylpyridinium chloride	T49.0X1	T49.0X2	T49.0X3	T49.0X4	T49.0X5	T49.0X6
ENT agent	T49.6X1	T49.6X2	T49.6X3	T49.6X4	T49.6X5	T49.6X6
lozenges	T49.6X1	T49.6X2	T49.6X3	T49.6X4	T49.6X5	T49.6X6
Cevadillasee Sabadilla						
Cevitamic acid	T45.2X1	T45.2X2	T45.2X3	T45.2X4	T45.2X5	T45.2X6
Chalk, precipitated	T47.1X1	T47.1X2	T47.1X3	T47.1X4	T47.1X5	T47.1X6
Chamomile	T49.0X1	T49.0X2	T49.0X3	T49.0X4	T49.0X5	T49.0X6
Ch'an su	T46.0X1	T46.0X2	T46.0X3	T46.0X4	T46.0X5	T46.0X6
Charcoal	T47.6X1	T47.6X2	T47.6X3	T47.6X4	T47.6X5	T47.6X6
activated — see also Charcoal, medicinal	T47.6X1	T47.6X2	T47.6X3	T47.6X4	T47.6X5	T47.6X6

Substance	Poisoning, Accidental (Unintentional)	Poisoning, Intentional Self-Harm	Poisoning, Assault	Poisoning, Undetermined	Adverse Effect	Underdosing
Charcoal (Continued)						
fumes (Carbon monoxide)	T58.2X1	T58.2X2	T58.2X3	T58.2X4	—	—
industrial	T58.8X1	T58.8X2	T58.8X3	T58.8X4	—	—
medicinal (activated)	T47.6X1	T47.6X2	T47.6X3	T47.6X4	T47.6X5	T47.6X6
antidiarrheal	T47.6X1	T47.6X2	T47.6X3	T47.6X4	T47.6X5	T47.6X6
poison control	T47.8X1	T47.8X2	T47.8X3	T47.8X4	T47.8X5	T47.8X6
specified use other than for diarrhea	T47.8X1	T47.8X2	T47.8X3	T47.8X4	T47.8X5	T47.8X6
topical	T49.8X1	T49.8X2	T49.8X3	T49.8X4	T49.8X5	T49.8X6
Chaulmosulfone	T37.1X1	T37.1X2	T37.1X3	T37.1X4	T37.1X5	T37.1X6
Chelating agent NEC	T50.6X1	T50.6X2	T50.6X3	T50.6X4	T50.6X5	T50.6X6
Chelidonium majus	T62.2X1	T62.2X2	T62.2X3	T62.2X4	—	—
Chemical substance NEC	T65.91	T65.92	T65.93	T65.94	—	—
Chenodeoxycholic acid	T47.5X1	T47.5X2	T47.5X3	T47.5X4	T47.5X5	T47.5X6
Chenodiol	T47.5X1	T47.5X2	T47.5X3	T47.5X4	T47.5X5	T47.5X6
Chenopodium	T37.4X1	T37.4X2	T37.4X3	T37.4X4	T37.4X5	T37.4X6
Cherry laurel	T62.2X1	T62.2X2	T62.2X3	T62.2X4	—	—
Chinidin(e)	T46.2X1	T46.2X2	T46.2X3	T46.2X4	T46.2X5	T46.2X6
Chiniofon	T37.8X1	T37.8X2	T37.8X3	T37.8X4	T37.8X5	T37.8X6
Chlophedianol	T48.3X1	T48.3X2	T48.3X3	T48.3X4	T48.3X5	T48.3X6
Chloral	T42.6X1	T42.6X2	T42.6X3	T42.6X4	T42.6X5	T42.6X6
derivative	T42.6X1	T42.6X2	T42.6X3	T42.6X4	T42.6X5	T42.6X6
hydrate	T42.6X1	T42.6X2	T42.6X3	T42.6X4	T42.6X5	T42.6X6
Chloralamide	T42.6X1	T42.6X2	T42.6X3	T42.6X4	T42.6X5	T42.6X6
Chloralodol	T42.6X1	T42.6X2	T42.6X3	T42.6X4	T42.6X5	T42.6X6
Chloralose	T60.4X1	T60.4X2	T60.4X3	T60.4X4	—	—
Chlorambucil	T45.1X1	T45.1X2	T45.1X3	T45.1X4	T45.1X5	T45.1X6
Chloramine	T57.8X1	T57.8X2	T57.8X3	T57.8X4	—	—
T	T49.0X1	T49.0X2	T49.0X3	T49.0X4	T49.0X5	T49.0X6
topical	T49.0X1	T49.0X2	T49.0X3	T49.0X4	T49.0X5	T49.0X6
Chloramphenicol	T36.2X1	T36.2X2	T36.2X3	T36.2X4	T36.2X5	T36.2X6
ENT agent	T49.6X1	T49.6X2	T49.6X3	T49.6X4	T49.6X5	T49.6X6
ophthalmic preparation	T49.5X1	T49.5X2	T49.5X3	T49.5X4	T49.5X5	T49.5X6
topical NEC	T49.0X1	T49.0X2	T49.0X3	T49.0X4	T49.0X5	T49.0X6
Chlorate (potassium) (sodium) NEC	T60.3X1	T60.3X2	T60.3X3	T60.3X4	—	—
herbicide	T60.3X1	T60.3X2	T60.3X3	T60.3X4	—	—
Chlorazanil	T50.2X1	T50.2X2	T50.2X3	T50.2X4	T50.2X5	T50.2X6
Chlorbenzene, chlorbenzol	T53.7X1	T53.7X2	T53.7X3	T53.7X4	—	—
Chlorbenzoxamine	T44.3X1	T44.3X2	T44.3X3	T44.3X4	T44.3X5	T44.3X6
Chlorbutol	T42.6X1	T42.6X2	T42.6X3	T42.6X4	T42.6X5	T42.6X6
Chlorcyclizine	T45.0X1	T45.0X2	T45.0X3	T45.0X4	T45.0X5	T45.0X6

◀ New ◀ Revised ~~deleted~~ Deleted

Substance	Poisoning, Accidental (Unintentional)	Poisoning, Intentional Self-Harm	Poisoning, Assault	Poisoning, Undetermined	Adverse Effect	Underdosing
Chlordan(e) (dust)	T60.1X1	T60.1X2	T60.1X3	T60.1X4	—	—
Chlordantoin	T49.0X1	T49.0X2	T49.0X3	T49.0X4	T49.0X5	T49.0X6
Chlordiazepoxide	T42.4X1	T42.4X2	T42.4X3	T42.4X4	T42.4X5	T42.4X6
Chlordiethyl benzamide	T49.3X1	T49.3X2	T49.3X3	T49.3X4	T49.3X5	T49.3X6
Chloresium	T49.8X1	T49.8X2	T49.8X3	T49.8X4	T49.8X5	T49.8X6
Chlorethiazol	T42.6X1	T42.6X2	T42.6X3	T42.6X4	T42.6X5	T42.6X6
Chlorethyl — see Ethyl, chloride						
Chloretone	T42.6X1	T42.6X2	T42.6X3	T42.6X4	T42.6X5	T42.6X6
Chlorex	T53.6X1	T53.6X2	T53.6X3	T53.6X4	—	—
insecticide	T60.1X1	T60.1X2	T60.1X3	T60.1X4	—	—
Chlorfenvinphos	T60.0X1	T60.0X2	T60.0X3	T60.0X4	—	—
Chlorhexadol	T42.6X1	T42.6X2	T42.6X3	T42.6X4	T42.6X5	T42.6X6
Chlorhexamide	T45.1X1	T45.1X2	T45.1X3	T45.1X4	T45.1X5	T45.1X6
Chlorhexidine	T49.0X1	T49.0X2	T49.0X3	T49.0X4	T49.0X5	T49.0X6
Chlorhydroxyquinolin	T49.0X1	T49.0X2	T49.0X3	T49.0X4	T49.0X5	T49.0X6
Chloride of lime (bleach)	T54.3X1	T54.3X2	T54.3X3	T54.3X4	—	—
Chlorimipramine	T43.011	T43.012	T43.013	T43.014	T43.015	T43.016
Chlorinated						
camphene	T53.6X1	T53.6X2	T53.6X3	T53.6X4	—	—
diphenyl	T53.7X1	T53.7X2	T53.7X3	T53.7X4	—	—
hydrocarbons NEC	T53.91	T53.92	T53.93	T53.94	—	—
solvents	T53.91	T53.92	T53.93	T53.94	—	—
lime (bleach)	T54.3X1	T54.3X2	T54.3X3	T54.3X4	—	—
and boric acid solution	T49.0X1	T49.0X2	T49.0X3	T49.0X4	T49.0X5	T49.0X6
naphthalene (insecticide)	T60.1X1	T60.1X2	T60.1X3	T60.1X4	—	—
industrial (non-pesticide)	T53.7X1	T53.7X2	T53.7X3	T53.7X4	—	—
pesticide NEC	T60.8X1	T60.8X2	T60.8X3	T60.8X4	—	—
soda — see also Sodium hypochlorite						
solution	T49.0X1	T49.0X2	T49.0X3	T49.0X4	T49.0X5	T49.0X6
Chlorine (fumes) (gas)	T59.4X1	T59.4X2	T59.4X3	T59.4X4	—	—
bleach	T54.3X1	T54.3X2	T54.3X3	T54.3X4	—	—
compound gas NEC	T59.4X1	T59.4X2	T59.4X3	T59.4X4	—	—
disinfectant	T59.4X1	T59.4X2	T59.4X3	T59.4X4	—	—
releasing agents NEC	T59.4X1	T59.4X2	T59.4X3	T59.4X4	—	—
Chlorisondamine chloride	T46.991	T46.992	T46.993	T46.994	T46.995	T46.996
Chlormadinone	T38.5X1	T38.5X2	T38.5X3	T38.5X4	T38.5X5	T38.5X6
Chlormephos	T60.0X1	T60.0X2	T60.0X3	T60.0X4	—	—
Chlormerodrin	T50.2X1	T50.2X2	T50.2X3	T50.2X4	T50.2X5	T50.2X6
Chlormethiazole	T42.6X1	T42.6X2	T42.6X3	T42.6X4	T42.6X5	T42.6X6
Chlormethine	T45.1X1	T45.1X2	T45.1X3	T45.1X4	T45.1X5	T45.1X6
Chlormethylenecycline	T36.4X1	T36.4X2	T36.4X3	T36.4X4	T36.4X5	T36.4X6

Substance	Poisoning, Accidental (Unintentional)	Poisoning, Intentional Self-Harm	Poisoning, Assault	Poisoning, Undetermined	Adverse Effect	Underdosing
Chlormezanone	T42.6X1	T42.6X2	T42.6X3	T42.6X4	T42.6X5	T42.6X6
Chloroacetic acid	T60.3X1	T60.3X2	T60.3X3	T60.3X4	—	—
Chloroacetone	T59.3X1	T59.3X2	T59.3X3	T59.3X4	—	—
Chloroacetophenone	T59.3X1	T59.3X2	T59.3X3	T59.3X4	—	—
Chloroaniline	T53.7X1	T53.7X2	T53.7X3	T53.7X4	—	—
Chlorobenzene, chlorobenzol	T53.7X1	T53.7X2	T53.7X3	T53.7X4	—	—
Chlorobromomethane (fire extinguisher)	T53.6X1	T53.6X2	T53.6X3	T53.6X4	—	—
Chlorobutanol	T49.0X1	T49.0X2	T49.0X3	T49.0X4	T49.0X5	T49.0X6
Chlorocresol	T49.0X1	T49.0X2	T49.0X3	T49.0X4	T49.0X5	T49.0X6
Chlorodehydro-methyltestosterone	T38.7X1	T38.7X2	T38.7X3	T38.7X4	T38.7X5	T38.7X6
Chlorodinitrobenzene	T53.7X1	T53.7X2	T53.7X3	T53.7X4	—	—
dust or vapor	T53.7X1	T53.7X2	T53.7X3	T53.7X4	—	—
Chlorodiphenyl	T53.7X1	T53.7X2	T53.7X3	T53.7X4	—	—
Chloroethane — see Ethyl, chloride						
Chloroethylene	T53.6X1	T53.6X2	T53.6X3	T53.6X4	—	—
Chlorofluorocarbons	T53.5X1	T53.5X2	T53.5X3	T53.5X4	—	—
Chloroform (fumes) (vapor)	T53.1X1	T53.1X2	T53.1X3	T53.1X4	—	—
anesthetic	T41.0X1	T41.0X2	T41.0X3	T41.0X4	T41.0X5	T41.0X6
solvent	T53.1X1	T53.1X2	T53.1X3	T53.1X4	—	—
water, concentrated	T41.0X1	T41.0X2	T41.0X3	T41.0X4	T41.0X5	T41.0X6
Chloroguanide	T37.2X1	T37.2X2	T37.2X3	T37.2X4	T37.2X5	T37.2X6
Chloromycetin	T36.2X1	T36.2X2	T36.2X3	T36.2X4	T36.2X5	T36.2X6
ENT agent	T49.6X1	T49.6X2	T49.6X3	T49.6X4	T49.6X5	T49.6X6
ophthalmic preparation	T49.5X1	T49.5X2	T49.5X3	T49.5X4	T49.5X5	T49.5X6
otic solution	T49.6X1	T49.6X2	T49.6X3	T49.6X4	T49.6X5	T49.6X6
topical NEC	T49.0X1	T49.0X2	T49.0X3	T49.0X4	T49.0X5	T49.0X6
Chloronitrobenzene	T53.7X1	T53.7X2	T53.7X3	T53.7X4	—	—
dust or vapor	T53.7X1	T53.7X2	T53.7X3	T53.7X4	—	—
Chlorophacinone	T60.4X1	T60.4X2	T60.4X3	T60.4X4	—	—
Chlorophenol	T53.7X1	T53.7X2	T53.7X3	T53.7X4	—	—
Chlorophenothane	T60.1X1	T60.1X2	T60.1X3	T60.1X4	—	—
Chlorophyll	T50.991	T50.992	T50.993	T50.994	T50.995	T50.996
Chloropicrin (fumes)	T53.6X1	T53.6X2	T53.6X3	T53.6X4	—	—
fumigant	T60.8X1	T60.8X2	T60.8X3	T60.8X4	—	—
fungicide	T60.3X1	T60.3X2	T60.3X3	T60.3X4	—	—
pesticide	T60.8X1	T60.8X2	T60.8X3	T60.8X4	—	—
Chloroprocaine	T41.3X1	T41.3X2	T41.3X3	T41.3X4	T41.3X5	T41.3X6
infiltration (subcutaneous)	T41.3X1	T41.3X2	T41.3X3	T41.3X4	T41.3X5	T41.3X6
nerve block (peripheral) (plexus)	T41.3X1	T41.3X2	T41.3X3	T41.3X4	T41.3X5	T41.3X6
spinal	T41.3X1	T41.3X2	T41.3X3	T41.3X4	T41.3X5	T41.3X6

◀ New ◀ Revised ~~deleted~~ Deleted

	External Cause (T-Code)					
Substance	Poisoning, Accidental (Unintentional)	Poisoning, Intentional Self-Harm	Poisoning, Assault	Poisoning, Undetermined	Adverse Effect	Underdosing
Chloroptic	T49.5X1	T49.5X2	T49.5X3	T49.5X4	T49.5X5	T49.5X6
Chloropurine	T45.1X1	T45.1X2	T45.1X3	T45.1X4	T45.1X5	T45.1X6
Chloropyramine	T45.0X1	T45.0X2	T45.0X3	T45.0X4	T45.0X5	T45.0X6
Chloropyrifos	T60.0X1	T60.0X2	T60.0X3	T60.0X4	—	—
Chloropyrilene	T45.0X1	T45.0X2	T45.0X3	T45.0X4	T45.0X5	T45.0X6
Chloroquine	T37.2X1	T37.2X2	T37.2X3	T37.2X4	T37.2X5	T37.2X6
Chlorothalonil	T60.3X1	T60.3X2	T60.3X3	T60.3X4	—	—
Chlorothen	T45.0X1	T45.0X2	T45.0X3	T45.0X4	T45.0X5	T45.0X6
Chlorothiazide	T50.2X1	T50.2X2	T50.2X3	T50.2X4	T50.2X5	T50.2X6
Chlorothymol	T49.4X1	T49.4X2	T49.4X3	T49.4X4	T49.4X5	T49.4X6
Chlorotrianisene	T38.5X1	T38.5X2	T38.5X3	T38.5X4	T38.5X5	T38.5X6
Chlorovinyldichloro-arsine, not in war	T57.0X1	T57.0X2	T57.0X3	T57.0X4	—	—
Chloroxine	T49.4X1	T49.4X2	T49.4X3	T49.4X4	T49.4X5	T49.4X6
Chloroxylenol	T49.0X1	T49.0X2	T49.0X3	T49.0X4	T49.0X5	T49.0X6
Chlorphenamine	T45.0X1	T45.0X2	T45.0X3	T45.0X4	T45.0X5	T45.0X6
Chlorphenesin	T42.8X1	T42.8X2	T42.8X3	T42.8X4	T42.8X5	T42.8X6
topical (antifungal)	T49.0X1	T49.0X2	T49.0X3	T49.0X4	T49.0X5	T49.0X6
Chlorpheniramine	T45.0X1	T45.0X2	T45.0X3	T45.0X4	T45.0X5	T45.0X6
Chlorphenoxamine	T45.0X1	T45.0X2	T45.0X3	T45.0X4	T45.0X5	T45.0X6
Chlorphentermine	T50.5X1	T50.5X2	T50.5X3	T50.5X4	T50.5X5	T50.5X6
Chlorprocaine — see Chloroprocaine						
Chlorproguanil	T37.2X1	T37.2X2	T37.2X3	T37.2X4	T37.2X5	T37.2X6
Chlorpromazine	T43.3X1	T43.3X2	T43.3X3	T43.3X4	T43.3X5	T43.3X6
Chlorpropamide	T38.3X1	T38.3X2	T38.3X3	T38.3X4	T38.3X5	T38.3X6
Chlorprothixene	T43.4X1	T43.4X2	T43.4X3	T43.4X4	T43.4X5	T43.4X6
Chlorquinaldol	T49.0X1	T49.0X2	T49.0X3	T49.0X4	T49.0X5	T49.0X6
Chlorquinol	T49.0X1	T49.0X2	T49.0X3	T49.0X4	T49.0X5	T49.0X6
Chlortalidone	T50.2X1	T50.2X2	T50.2X3	T50.2X4	T50.2X5	T50.2X6
Chlortetracycline	T36.4X1	T36.4X2	T36.4X3	T36.4X4	T36.4X5	T36.4X6
Chlorthalidone	T50.2X1	T50.2X2	T50.2X3	T50.2X4	T50.2X5	T50.2X6
Chlorthiophos	T60.0X1	T60.0X2	T60.0X3	T60.0X4	—	—
Chlorotrianisene	T38.5X1	T38.5X2	T38.5X3	T38.5X4	T38.5X5	T38.5X6
Chlor-Trimeton	T45.0X1	T45.0X2	T45.0X3	T45.0X4	T45.0X5	T45.0X6
Chlorthion	T60.0X1	T60.0X2	T60.0X3	T60.0X4	—	—
Chlorzoxazone	T42.8X1	T42.8X2	T42.8X3	T42.8X4	T42.8X5	T42.8X6
Choke damp	T59.7X1	T59.7X2	T59.7X3	T59.7X4	—	—
Cholagogues	T47.5X1	T47.5X2	T47.5X3	T47.5X4	T47.5X5	T47.5X6
Cholebrine	T50.8X1	T50.8X2	T50.8X3	T50.8X4	T50.8X5	T50.8X6
Cholecalciferol	T45.2X1	T45.2X2	T45.2X3	T45.2X4	T45.2X5	T45.2X6
Cholecystokinin	T50.8X1	T50.8X2	T50.8X3	T50.8X4	T50.8X5	T50.8X6
Cholera vaccine	T50.A91	T50.A92	T50.A93	T50.A94	T50.A95	T50.A96

	External Cause (T-Code)					
Substance	Poisoning, Accidental (Unintentional)	Poisoning, Intentional Self-Harm	Poisoning, Assault	Poisoning, Undetermined	Adverse Effect	Underdosing
Choleretic	T47.5X1	T47.5X2	T47.5X3	T47.5X4	T47.5X5	T47.5X6
Cholesterol-lowering agents	T46.6X1	T46.6X2	T46.6X3	T46.6X4	T46.6X5	T46.6X6
Cholestyramine (resin)	T46.6X1	T46.6X2	T46.6X3	T46.6X4	T46.6X5	T46.6X6
Cholic acid	T47.5X1	T47.5X2	T47.5X3	T47.5X4	T47.5X5	T47.5X6
Choline	T48.6X1	T48.6X2	T48.6X3	T48.6X4	T48.6X5	T48.6X6
chloride	T50.991	T50.992	T50.993	T50.994	T50.995	T50.996
dihydrogen citrate	T50.991	T50.992	T50.993	T50.994	T50.995	T50.996
salicylate	T39.091	T39.092	T39.093	T39.094	T39.095	T39.096
theophyllinate	T48.6X1	T48.6X2	T48.6X3	T48.6X4	T48.6X5	T48.6X6
Cholinergic (drug) NEC	T44.1X1	T44.1X2	T44.1X3	T44.1X4	T44.1X5	T44.1X6
muscle tone enhancer	T44.1X1	T44.1X2	T44.1X3	T44.1X4	T44.1X5	T44.1X6
organophosphorus	T44.0X1	T44.0X2	T44.0X3	T44.0X4	T44.0X5	T44.0X6
insecticide	T60.0X1	T60.0X2	T60.0X3	T60.0X4	—	—
nerve gas	T59.891	T59.892	T59.893	T59.894	—	—
trimethyl ammonium propanediol	T44.1X1	T44.1X2	T44.1X3	T44.1X4	T44.1X5	T44.1X6
Cholinesterase reactivator	T50.6X1	T50.6X2	T50.6X3	T50.6X4	T50.6X5	T50.6X6
Cholografin	T50.8X1	T50.8X2	T50.8X3	T50.8X4	T50.8X5	T50.8X6
Chorionic gonadotropin	T38.891	T38.892	T38.893	T38.894	T38.895	T38.896
Chromate	T56.2X1	T56.2X2	T56.2X3	T56.2X4	—	—
dust or mist	T56.2X1	T56.2X2	T56.2X3	T56.2X4	—	—
lead — see also Lead	T56.0X1	T56.0X2	T56.0X3	T56.0X4	—	—
paint	T56.0X1	T56.0X2	T56.0X3	T56.0X4	—	—
Chromic						
acid	T56.2X1	T56.2X2	T56.2X3	T56.2X4	—	—
dust or mist	T56.2X1	T56.2X2	T56.2X3	T56.2X4	—	—
phosphate 32P	T45.1X1	T45.1X2	T45.1X3	T45.1X4	T45.1X5	T45.1X6
Chromium	T56.2X1	T56.2X2	T56.2X3	T56.2X4	—	—
compounds — see Chromate						
sesquioxide	T50.8X1	T50.8X2	T50.8X3	T50.8X4	T50.8X5	T50.8X6
Chromomycin A3	T45.1X1	T45.1X2	T45.1X3	T45.1X4	T45.1X5	T45.1X6
Chromonar	T46.3X1	T46.3X2	T46.3X3	T46.3X4	T46.3X5	T46.3X6
Chromyl chloride	T56.2X1	T56.2X2	T56.2X3	T56.2X4	—	—
Chrysarobin	T49.4X1	T49.4X2	T49.4X3	T49.4X4	T49.4X5	T49.4X6
Chrysazin	T47.2X1	T47.2X2	T47.2X3	T47.2X4	T47.2X5	T47.2X6
Chymar	T45.3X1	T45.3X2	T45.3X3	T45.3X4	T45.3X5	T45.3X6
ophthalmic preparation	T49.5X1	T49.5X2	T49.5X3	T49.5X4	T49.5X5	T49.5X6
Chymopapain	T45.3X1	T45.3X2	T45.3X3	T45.3X4	T45.3X5	T45.3X6
Chymotrypsin	T45.3X1	T45.3X2	T45.3X3	T45.3X4	T45.3X5	T45.3X6
ophthalmic preparation	T49.5X1	T49.5X2	T49.5X3	T49.5X4	T49.5X5	T49.5X6
Cianidanol	T50.991	T50.992	T50.993	T50.994	T50.995	T50.996
Cianopramine	T43.011	T43.012	T43.013	T43.014	T43.015	T43.016
Cibenzoline	T46.2X1	T46.2X2	T46.2X3	T46.2X4	T46.2X5	T46.2X6

◀ New ◀ Revised ~~deleted~~ Deleted

	External Cause (T-Code)					
Substance	Poisoning, Accidental (Unintentional)	Poisoning, Intentional Self-Harm	Poisoning, Assault	Poisoning, Undetermined	Adverse Effect	Underdosing
Ciclacillin	T36.0X1	T36.0X2	T36.0X3	T36.0X4	T36.0X5	T36.0X6
Ciclobarbital — see Hexobarbital						
Ciclonicate	T46.7X1	T46.7X2	T46.7X3	T46.7X4	T46.7X5	T46.7X6
Ciclopirox (olamine)	T49.0X1	T49.0X2	T49.0X3	T49.0X4	T49.0X5	T49.0X6
Ciclosporin	T45.1X1	T45.1X2	T45.1X3	T45.1X4	T45.1X5	T45.1X6
Cicuta maculata or virosa	T62.2X1	T62.2X2	T62.2X3	T62.2X4	—	—
Cicutoxin	T62.2X1	T62.2X2	T62.2X3	T62.2X4	—	—
Cigarette lighter fluid	T52.0X1	T52.0X2	T52.0X3	T52.0X4	—	—
Cigarettes (tobacco)	T65.221	T65.222	T65.223	T65.224	—	—
Ciguatoxin	T61.01	T61.02	T61.03	T61.04	—	—
Cilazapril	T46.4X1	T46.4X2	T46.4X3	T46.4X4	T46.4X5	T46.4X6
Cimetidine	T47.0X1	T47.0X2	T47.0X3	T47.0X4	T47.0X5	T47.0X6
Cimetropium bromide	T44.3X1	T44.3X2	T44.3X3	T44.3X4	T44.3X5	T44.3X6
Cinchocaine	T41.3X1	T41.3X2	T41.3X3	T41.3X4	T41.3X5	T41.3X6
topical (surface)	T41.3X1	T41.3X2	T41.3X3	T41.3X4	T41.3X5	T41.3X6
Cinchona	T37.2X1	T37.2X2	T37.2X3	T37.2X4	T37.2X5	T37.2X6
Cinchonine alkaloids	T37.2X1	T37.2X2	T37.2X3	T37.2X4	T37.2X5	T37.2X6
Cinchophen	T50.4X1	T50.4X2	T50.4X3	T50.4X4	T50.4X5	T50.4X6
Cinepazide	T46.7X1	T46.7X2	T46.7X3	T46.7X4	T46.7X5	T46.7X6
Cinnamedrine	T48.5X1	T48.5X2	T48.5X3	T48.5X4	T48.5X5	T48.5X6
Cinnarizine	T45.0X1	T45.0X2	T45.0X3	T45.0X4	T45.0X5	T45.0X6
Cinoxacin	T37.8X1	T37.8X2	T37.8X3	T37.8X4	T37.8X5	T37.8X6
Ciprofibrate	T46.6X1	T46.6X2	T46.6X3	T46.6X4	T46.6X5	T46.6X6
Ciprofloxacin	T36.8X1	T36.8X2	T36.8X3	T36.8X4	T36.8X5	T36.8X6
Cisapride	T47.8X1	T47.8X2	T47.8X3	T47.8X4	T47.8X5	T47.8X6
Cisplatin	T45.1X1	T45.1X2	T45.1X3	T45.1X4	T45.1X5	T45.1X6
Citalopram	T43.221	T43.222	T43.223	T43.224	T43.225	T43.226
Citanest	T41.3X1	T41.3X2	T41.3X3	T41.3X4	T41.3X5	T41.3X6
infiltration (subcutaneous)	T41.3X1	T41.3X2	T41.3X3	T41.3X4	T41.3X5	T41.3X6
nerve block (peripheral) (plexus)	T41.3X1	T41.3X2	T41.3X3	T41.3X4	T41.3X5	T41.3X6
Citric acid	T47.5X1	T47.5X2	T47.5X3	T47.5X4	T47.5X5	T47.5X6
Citrovorum (factor)	T45.8X1	T45.8X2	T45.8X3	T45.8X4	T45.8X5	T45.8X6
Claviceps purpurea	T62.2X1	T62.2X2	T62.2X3	T62.2X4	—	—
Clavulanic acid	T36.1X1	T36.1X2	T36.1X3	T36.1X4	T36.1X5	T36.1X6
Cleaner, cleansing agent, type not specified	T65.891	T65.892	T65.893	T65.894	—	—
of paint or varnish	T52.91	T52.92	T52.93	T52.94	—	—
specified type NEC	T65.891	T65.892	T65.893	T65.894	—	—
Clebopride	T47.8X1	T47.8X2	T47.8X3	T47.8X4	T47.8X5	T47.8X6
Clefamide	T37.3X1	T37.3X2	T37.3X3	T37.3X4	T37.3X5	T37.3X6
Clemastine	T45.0X1	T45.0X2	T45.0X3	T45.0X4	T45.0X5	T45.0X6
Clematis vitalba	T62.2X1	T62.2X2	T62.2X3	T62.2X4	—	—

	External Cause (T-Code)					
Substance	Poisoning, Accidental (Unintentional)	Poisoning, Intentional Self-Harm	Poisoning, Assault	Poisoning, Undetermined	Adverse Effect	Underdosing
Clemizole	T45.0X1	T45.0X2	T45.0X3	T45.0X4	T45.0X5	T45.0X6
penicillin	T36.0X1	T36.0X2	T36.0X3	T36.0X4	T36.0X5	T36.0X6
Clenbuterol	T48.6X1	T48.6X2	T48.6X3	T48.6X4	T48.6X5	T48.6X6
Clidinium bromide	T44.3X1	T44.3X2	T44.3X3	T44.3X4	T44.3X5	T44.3X6
Clindamycin	T36.8X1	T36.8X2	T36.8X3	T36.8X4	T36.8X5	T36.8X6
Clinofibrate	T46.6X1	T46.6X2	T46.6X3	T46.6X4	T46.6X5	T46.6X6
Clioquinol	T37.8X1	T37.8X2	T37.8X3	T37.8X4	T37.8X5	T37.8X6
Cliradon	T40.2X1	T40.2X2	T40.2X3	T40.2X4	—	—
Clobazam	T42.4X1	T42.4X2	T42.4X3	T42.4X4	T42.4X5	T42.4X6
Clobenzorex	T50.5X1	T50.5X2	T50.5X3	T50.5X4	T50.5X5	T50.5X6
Clobetasol	T49.0X1	T49.0X2	T49.0X3	T49.0X4	T49.0X5	T49.0X6
Clobetasone	T49.0X1	T49.0X2	T49.0X3	T49.0X4	T49.0X5	T49.0X6
Clobutinol	T48.3X1	T48.3X2	T48.3X3	T48.3X4	T48.3X5	T48.3X6
Clocapramine	T43.0X1	T43.0X2	T43.0X3	T43.0X4	T43.0X5	T43.0X6
Clocortolone	T38.0X1	T38.0X2	T38.0X3	T38.0X4	T38.0X5	T38.0X6
Clodantoin	T49.0X1	T49.0X2	T49.0X3	T49.0X4	T49.0X5	T49.0X6
Clodronic acid	T50.991	T50.992	T50.993	T50.994	T50.995	T50.996
Clofazimine	T37.1X1	T37.1X2	T37.1X3	T37.1X4	T37.1X5	T37.1X6
Clofedanol	T48.3X1	T48.3X2	T48.3X3	T48.3X4	T48.3X5	T48.3X6
Clofenamide	T50.2X1	T50.2X2	T50.2X3	T50.2X4	T50.2X5	T50.2X6
Clofenotane	T49.0X1	T49.0X2	T49.0X3	T49.0X4	T49.0X5	T49.0X6
Clofezone	T39.2X1	T39.2X2	T39.2X3	T39.2X4	T39.2X5	T39.2X6
Clofibrate	T46.6X1	T46.6X2	T46.6X3	T46.6X4	T46.6X5	T46.6X6
Clofibride	T46.6X1	T46.6X2	T46.6X3	T46.6X4	T46.6X5	T46.6X6
Cloforex	T50.5X1	T50.5X2	T50.5X3	T50.5X4	T50.5X5	T50.5X6
Clomacran	T43.0X1	T43.0X2	T43.0X3	T43.0X4	T43.0X5	T43.0X6
Clomethiazole	T42.6X1	T42.6X2	T42.6X3	T42.6X4	T42.6X5	T42.6X6
Clometocillin	T36.0X1	T36.0X2	T36.0X3	T36.0X4	T36.0X5	T36.0X6
Clomifene	T38.5X1	T38.5X2	T38.5X3	T38.5X4	T38.5X5	T38.5X6
Clomiphene	T38.5X1	T38.5X2	T38.5X3	T38.5X4	T38.5X5	T38.5X6
Clomipramine	T43.011	T43.012	T43.013	T43.014	T43.015	T43.016
Clomocycline	T36.4X1	T36.4X2	T36.4X3	T36.4X4	T36.4X5	T36.4X6
Clonazepam	T42.4X1	T42.4X2	T42.4X3	T42.4X4	T42.4X5	T42.4X6
Clonidine	T46.5X1	T46.5X2	T46.5X3	T46.5X4	T46.5X5	T46.5X6
Clonixin	T39.8X1	T39.8X2	T39.8X3	T39.8X4	T39.8X5	T39.8X6
Clopamide	T50.2X1	T50.2X2	T50.2X3	T50.2X4	T50.2X5	T50.2X6
Clopenthixol	T43.4X1	T43.4X2	T43.4X3	T43.4X4	T43.4X5	T43.4X6
Cloperastine	T48.3X1	T48.3X2	T48.3X3	T48.3X4	T48.3X5	T48.3X6
Clophedianol	T48.3X1	T48.3X2	T48.3X3	T48.3X4	T48.3X5	T48.3X6
Cloponone	T36.2X1	T36.2X2	T36.2X3	T36.2X4	T36.2X5	T36.2X6
Cloprednol	T38.0X1	T38.0X2	T38.0X3	T38.0X4	T38.0X5	T38.0X6
Cloral betaine	T42.6X1	T42.6X2	T42.6X3	T42.6X4	T42.6X5	T42.6X6

◄ New ◄ Revised ~~deleted~~ Deleted

Substance	Poisoning, Accidental (Unintentional)	Poisoning, Intentional Self-Harm	Poisoning, Assault	Poisoning, Undetermined	Adverse Effect	Underdosing
Cloramfenicol	T36.2X1	T36.2X2	T36.2X3	T36.2X4	T36.2X5	T36.2X6
Clorazepate (dipotassium)	T42.4X1	T42.4X2	T42.4X3	T42.4X4	T42.4X5	T42.4X6
Clorexolone	T50.2X1	T50.2X2	T50.2X3	T50.2X4	T50.2X5	T50.2X6
Clorox (bleach)	T54.91	T54.92	T54.93	T54.94	—	—
Clorfenamine	T45.0X1	T45.0X2	T45.0X3	T45.0X4	T45.0X5	T45.0X6
Clorgiline	T43.1X1	T43.1X2	T43.1X3	T43.1X4	T43.1X5	T43.1X6
Clorotepine	T44.3X1	T44.3X2	T44.3X3	T44.3X4	T44.3X5	T44.3X6
Clorprenaline	T48.6X1	T48.6X2	T48.6X3	T48.6X4	T48.6X5	T48.6X6
Clortermine	T50.5X1	T50.5X2	T50.5X3	T50.5X4	T50.5X5	T50.5X6
Clotiapine	T43.591	T43.592	T43.593	T43.594	T43.595	T43.596
Clotiazepam	T42.4X1	T42.4X2	T42.4X3	T42.4X4	T42.4X5	T42.4X6
Clotibric acid	T46.6X1	T46.6X2	T46.6X3	T46.6X4	T46.6X5	T46.6X6
Clotrimazole	T49.0X1	T49.0X2	T49.0X3	T49.0X4	T49.0X5	T49.0X6
Cloxacillin	T36.0X1	T36.0X2	T36.0X3	T36.0X4	T36.0X5	T36.0X6
Cloxazolam	T42.4X1	T42.4X2	T42.4X3	T42.4X4	T42.4X5	T42.4X6
Cloxiquine	T49.0X1	T49.0X2	T49.0X3	T49.0X4	T49.0X5	T49.0X6
Clozapine	T42.4X1	T42.4X2	T42.4X3	T42.4X4	T42.4X5	T42.4X6
Coagulant NEC	T45.7X1	T45.7X2	T45.7X3	T45.7X4	T45.7X5	T45.7X6
Coal (carbon monoxide from) — see also Carbon, monoxide, coal	T58.2X1	T58.2X2	T58.2X3	T58.2X4	—	—
oil — see Kerosene						
tar	T49.1X1	T49.1X2	T49.1X3	T49.1X4	T49.1X5	T49.1X6
fumes	T59.891	T59.892	T59.893	T59.894	—	—
medicinal (ointment)	T49.4X1	T49.4X2	T49.4X3	T49.4X4	T49.4X5	T49.4X6
analgesics NEC	T39.2X1	T39.2X2	T39.2X3	T39.2X4	T39.2X5	T39.2X6
naphtha (solvent)	T52.0X1	T52.0X2	T52.0X3	T52.0X4		
Cobalamine	T45.2X1	T45.2X2	T45.2X3	T45.2X4	T45.2X5	T45.2X6
Cobalt (nonmedicinal) (fumes) (industrial)	T56.891	T56.892	T56.893	T56.894		
medicinal (trace) (chloride)	T45.8X1	T45.8X2	T45.8X3	T45.8X4	T45.8X5	T45.8X6
Cobra (venom)	T63.041	T63.042	T63.043	T63.044		
Coca (leaf)	T40.5X1	T40.5X2	T40.5X3	T40.5X4	T40.5X5	T40.5X6
Cocaine	T40.5X1	T40.5X2	T40.5X3	T40.5X4	T40.5X5	T40.5X6
topical anesthetic	T41.3X1	T41.3X2	T41.3X3	T41.3X4	T41.3X5	T41.3X6
Cocarboxylase	T45.3X1	T45.3X2	T45.3X3	T45.3X4	T45.3X5	T45.3X6
Coccidioidin	T50.8X1	T50.8X2	T50.8X3	T50.8X4	T50.8X5	T50.8X6
Cocculus indicus	T62.1X1	T62.1X2	T62.1X3	T62.1X4		
Cochineal	T65.6X1	T65.6X2	T65.6X3	T65.6X4		
medicinal products	T50.991	T50.992	T50.993	T50.994	T50.995	T50.996
Codeine	T40.2X1	T40.2X2	T40.2X3	T40.2X4	T40.2X5	T40.2X6
Cod-liver oil	T45.2X1	T45.2X2	T45.2X3	T45.2X4	T45.2X5	T45.2X6

Substance	Poisoning, Accidental (Unintentional)	Poisoning, Intentional Self-Harm	Poisoning, Assault	Poisoning, Undetermined	Adverse Effect	Underdosing
Coenzyme A	T50.991	T50.992	T50.993	T50.994	T50.995	T50.996
Coffee	T62.8X1	T62.8X2	T62.8X3	T62.8X4	—	—
Cogalactoisomerase	T50.991	T50.992	T50.993	T50.994	T50.995	T50.996
Cogentin	T44.3X1	T44.3X2	T44.3X3	T44.3X4	T44.3X5	T44.3X6
Coke fumes or gas (carbon monoxide)	T58.2X1	T58.2X2	T58.2X3	T58.2X4		
industrial use	T58.8X1	T58.8X2	T58.8X3	T58.8X4	—	—
Colace	T47.4X1	T47.4X2	T47.4X3	T47.4X4	T47.4X5	T47.4X6
Colaspase	T45.1X1	T45.1X2	T45.1X3	T45.1X4	T45.1X5	T45.1X6
Colchicine	T50.4X1	T50.4X2	T50.4X3	T50.4X4	T50.4X5	T50.4X6
Colchicum	T62.2X1	T62.2X2	T62.2X3	T62.2X4	—	—
Cold cream	T49.3X1	T49.3X2	T49.3X3	T49.3X4	T49.3X5	T49.3X6
Colecalciferol	T45.2X1	T45.2X2	T45.2X3	T45.2X4	T45.2X5	T45.2X6
Colestipol	T46.6X1	T46.6X2	T46.6X3	T46.6X4	T46.6X5	T46.6X6
Colestyramine	T46.6X1	T46.6X2	T46.6X3	T46.6X4	T46.6X5	T46.6X6
Colimycin	T36.8X1	T36.8X2	T36.8X3	T36.8X4	T36.8X5	T36.8X6
Colistimethate	T36.8X1	T36.8X2	T36.8X3	T36.8X4	T36.8X5	T36.8X6
Colistin	T36.8X1	T36.8X2	T36.8X3	T36.8X4	T36.8X5	T36.8X6
sulfate (eye preparation)	T49.5X1	T49.5X2	T49.5X3	T49.5X4	T49.5X5	T49.5X6
Collagen	T50.991	T50.992	T50.993	T50.994	T50.995	T50.996
Collagenase	T49.4X1	T49.4X2	T49.4X3	T49.4X4	T49.4X5	T49.4X6
Collodion	T49.3X1	T49.3X2	T49.3X3	T49.3X4	T49.3X5	T49.3X6
Colocynth	T47.2X1	T47.2X2	T47.2X3	T47.2X4	T47.2X5	T47.2X6
Colophony adhesive	T49.3X1	T49.3X2	T49.3X3	T49.3X4	T49.3X5	T49.3X6
Colorant — see also Dye	T50.991	T50.992	T50.993	T50.994	T50.995	T50.996
Coloring matter — see Dye(s)						
Combustion gas (after combustion) — see Carbon, monoxide						
prior to combustion	T59.891	T59.892	T59.893	T59.894	—	—
Compazine	T43.3X1	T43.3X2	T43.3X3	T43.3X4	T43.3X5	T43.3X6
Compound						
42 (warfarin)	T60.4X1	T60.4X2	T60.4X3	T60.4X4	—	—
269 (endrin)	T60.1X1	T60.1X2	T60.1X3	T60.1X4	—	—
497 (dieldrin)	T60.1X1	T60.1X2	T60.1X3	T60.1X4	—	—
1080 (sodium fluoroacetate)	T60.4X1	T60.4X2	T60.4X3	T60.4X4	—	—
3422 (parathion)	T60.0X1	T60.0X2	T60.0X3	T60.0X4	—	—
3911 (phorate)	T60.0X1	T60.0X2	T60.0X3	T60.0X4	—	—
3956 (toxaphene)	T60.1X1	T60.1X2	T60.1X3	T60.1X4	—	—
4049 (malathion)	T60.0X1	T60.0X2	T60.0X3	T60.0X4	—	—
4069 (malathion)	T60.0X1	T60.0X2	T60.0X3	T60.0X4	—	—
4124 (dicapthon)	T60.0X1	T60.0X2	T60.0X3	T60.0X4	—	—

◀ New ◀ Revised ~~deleted~~ Deleted

	External Cause (T-Code)					
Substance	Poisoning, Accidental (Unintentional)	Poisoning, Intentional Self-Harm	Poisoning, Assault	Poisoning, Undetermined	Adverse Effect	Underdosing
Compound *(Continued)*						
E (cortisone)	T38.0X1	T38.0X2	T38.0X3	T38.0X4	T38.0X5	T38.0X6
F (hydrocortisone)	T38.0X1	T38.0X2	T38.0X3	T38.0X4	T38.0X5	T38.0X6
Congener, anabolic	T38.7X1	T38.7X2	T38.7X3	T38.7X4	T38.7X5	T38.7X6
Congo red	T50.8X1	T50.8X2	T50.8X3	T50.8X4	T50.8X5	T50.8X6
Coniine, conine	T62.2X1	T62.2X2	T62.2X3	T62.2X4	—	—
Conium (maculatum)	T62.2X1	T62.2X2	T62.2X3	T62.2X4	—	—
Conjugated estrogenic substances	T38.5X1	T38.5X2	T38.5X3	T38.5X4	T38.5X5	T38.5X6
Contac	T48.5X1	T48.5X2	T48.5X3	T48.5X4	T48.5X5	T48.5X6
Contact lens solution	T49.5X1	T49.5X2	T49.5X3	T49.5X4	T49.5X5	T49.5X6
Contraceptive (oral)	T38.4X1	T38.4X2	T38.4X3	T38.4X4	T38.4X5	T38.4X6
vaginal	T49.8X1	T49.8X2	T49.8X3	T49.8X4	T49.8X5	T49.8X6
Contrast medium, radiography	T50.8X1	T50.8X2	T50.8X3	T50.8X4	T50.8X5	T50.8X6
Convallaria glycosides	T46.0X1	T46.0X2	T46.0X3	T46.0X4	T46.0X5	T46.0X6
Convallaria majalis	T62.2X1	T62.2X2	T62.2X3	T62.2X4	—	—
berry	T62.1X1	T62.1X2	T62.1X3	T62.1X4	—	—
Copper (dust) (fumes) (nonmedicinal) NEC	T56.4X1	T56.4X2	T56.4X3	T56.4X4		
arsenate, arsenite	T57.0X1	T57.0X2	T57.0X3	T57.0X4	—	—
insecticide	T60.2X1	T60.2X2	T60.2X3	T60.2X4	—	—
emetic	T47.7X1	T47.7X2	T47.7X3	T47.7X4	T47.7X5	T47.7X6
fungicide	T60.3X1	T60.3X2	T60.3X3	T60.3X4	—	—
gluconate	T49.0X1	T49.0X2	T49.0X3	T49.0X4	T49.0X5	T49.0X6
insecticide	T60.2X1	T60.2X2	T60.2X3	T60.2X4	—	—
medicinal (trace)	T45.8X1	T45.8X2	T45.8X3	T45.8X4	T45.8X5	T45.8X6
oleate	T49.0X1	T49.0X2	T49.0X3	T49.0X4	T49.0X5	T49.0X6
sulfate	T56.4X1	T56.4X2	T56.4X3	T56.4X4	—	—
cupric	T56.4X1	T56.4X2	T56.4X3	T56.4X4	—	—
fungicide	T60.3X1	T60.3X2	T60.3X3	T60.3X4	—	—
medicinal						
ear	T49.6X1	T49.6X2	T49.6X3	T49.6X4	T49.6X5	T49.6X6
emetic	T47.7X1	T47.7X2	T47.7X3	T47.7X4	T47.7X5	T47.7X6
eye	T49.5X1	T49.5X2	T49.5X3	T49.5X4	T49.5X5	T49.5X6
cuprous	T56.4X1	T56.4X2	T56.4X3	T56.4X4	—	—
fungicide	T60.3X1	T60.3X2	T60.3X3	T60.3X4	—	—
medicinal						
ear	T49.6X1	T49.6X2	T49.6X3	T49.6X4	T49.6X5	T49.6X6
emetic	T47.7X1	T47.7X2	T47.7X3	T47.7X4	T47.7X5	T47.7X6
eye	T49.5X1	T49.5X2	T49.5X3	T49.5X4	T49.5X5	T49.5X6
Copperhead snake (bite) (venom)	T63.061	T63.062	T63.063	T63.064	—	—
Coral (sting)	T63.691	T63.692	T63.693	T63.694	—	—
snake (bite) (venom)	T63.021	T63.022	T63.023	T63.024	—	—

	External Cause (T-Code)					
Substance	Poisoning, Accidental (Unintentional)	Poisoning, Intentional Self-Harm	Poisoning, Assault	Poisoning, Undetermined	Adverse Effect	Underdosing
Corbadrine	T49.6X1	T49.6X2	T49.6X3	T49.6X4	T49.6X5	T49.6X6
Cordran	T49.0X1	T49.0X2	T49.0X3	T49.0X4	T49.0X5	T49.0X6
Cordite	T65.891	T65.892	T65.893	T65.894	—	—
vapor	T59.891	T59.892	T59.893	T59.894	—	—
Corn cures	T49.4X1	T49.4X2	T49.4X3	T49.4X4	T49.4X5	T49.4X6
Cornhusker's lotion	T49.3X1	T49.3X2	T49.3X3	T49.3X4	T49.3X5	T49.3X6
Corn starch	T49.3X1	T49.3X2	T49.3X3	T49.3X4	T49.3X5	T49.3X6
Coronary vasodilator NEC	T46.3X1	T46.3X2	T46.3X3	T46.3X4	T46.3X5	T46.3X6
Corrosive NEC	T54.91	T54.92	T54.93	T54.94	—	—
acid NEC	T54.2X1	T54.2X2	T54.2X3	T54.2X4	—	—
aromatics	T54.1X1	T54.1X2	T54.1X3	T54.1X4	—	—
disinfectant	T54.1X1	T54.1X2	T54.1X3	T54.1X4	—	—
fumes NEC	T54.91	T54.92	T54.93	T54.94	—	—
specified NEC	T54.91	T54.92	T54.93	T54.94	—	—
sublimate	T56.1X1	T56.1X2	T56.1X3	T56.1X4	—	—
Cortate	T38.0X1	T38.0X2	T38.0X3	T38.0X4	T38.0X5	T38.0X6
Cort-Dome	T38.0X1	T38.0X2	T38.0X3	T38.0X4	T38.0X5	T38.0X6
ENT agent	T49.6X1	T49.6X2	T49.6X3	T49.6X4	T49.6X5	T49.6X6
ophthalmic preparation	T49.5X1	T49.5X2	T49.5X3	T49.5X4	T49.5X5	T49.5X6
topical NEC	T49.0X1	T49.0X2	T49.0X3	T49.0X4	T49.0X5	T49.0X6
Cortef	T38.0X1	T38.0X2	T38.0X3	T38.0X4	T38.0X5	T38.0X6
ENT agent	T49.6X1	T49.6X2	T49.6X3	T49.6X4	T49.6X5	T49.6X6
ophthalmic preparation	T49.5X1	T49.5X2	T49.5X3	T49.5X4	T49.5X5	T49.5X6
topical NEC	T49.0X1	T49.0X2	T49.0X3	T49.0X4	T49.0X5	T49.0X6
Corticosteroid	T38.0X1	T38.0X2	T38.0X3	T38.0X4	T38.0X5	T38.0X6
ENT agent	T49.6X1	T49.6X2	T49.6X3	T49.6X4	T49.6X5	T49.6X6
mineral	T50.0X1	T50.0X2	T50.0X3	T50.0X4	T50.0X5	T50.0X6
ophthalmic	T49.5X1	T49.5X2	T49.5X3	T49.5X4	T49.5X5	T49.5X6
topical NEC	T49.0X1	T49.0X2	T49.0X3	T49.0X4	T49.0X5	T49.0X6
Corticotropin	T38.811	T38.812	T38.813	T38.814	T38.815	T38.816
Cortisol	T49.0X1	T49.0X2	T49.0X3	T49.0X4	T49.0X5	T49.0X6
ENT agent	T49.6X1	T49.6X2	T49.6X3	T49.6X4	T49.6X5	T49.6X6
ophthalmic preparation	T49.5X1	T49.5X2	T49.5X3	T49.5X4	T49.5X5	T49.5X6
topical NEC	T49.0X1	T49.0X2	T49.0X3	T49.0X4	T49.0X5	T49.0X6
Cortisone (acetate)	T38.0X1	T38.0X2	T38.0X3	T38.0X4	T38.0X5	T38.0X6
ENT agent	T49.6X1	T49.6X2	T49.6X3	T49.6X4	T49.6X5	T49.6X6
ophthalmic preparation	T49.5X1	T49.5X2	T49.5X3	T49.5X4	T49.5X5	T49.5X6
topical NEC	T49.0X1	T49.0X2	T49.0X3	T49.0X4	T49.0X5	T49.0X6
Cortivazol	T38.0X1	T38.0X2	T38.0X3	T38.0X4	T38.0X5	T38.0X6
Cortogen	T38.0X1	T38.0X2	T38.0X3	T38.0X4	T38.0X5	T38.0X6
ENT agent	T49.6X1	T49.6X2	T49.6X3	T49.6X4	T49.6X5	T49.6X6
ophthalmic preparation	T49.5X1	T49.5X2	T49.5X3	T49.5X4	T49.5X5	T49.5X6

TABLE OF DRUGS AND CHEMICALS

Substance	Poisoning, Accidental (Unintentional)	Poisoning, Intentional Self-Harm	Poisoning, Assault	Poisoning, Undetermined	Adverse Effect	Underdosing
Cortone	T38.0X1	T38.0X2	T38.0X3	T38.0X4	T38.0X5	T38.0X6
ENT agent	T49.6X1	T49.6X2	T49.6X3	T49.6X4	T49.6X5	T49.6X6
ophthalmic preparation	T49.5X1	T49.5X2	T49.5X3	T49.5X4	T49.5X5	T49.5X6
Cortril	T38.0X1	T38.0X2	T38.0X3	T38.0X4	T38.0X5	T38.0X6
ENT agent	T49.6X1	T49.6X2	T49.6X3	T49.6X4	T49.6X5	T49.6X6
ophthalmic preparation	T49.5X1	T49.5X2	T49.5X3	T49.5X4	T49.5X5	T49.5X6
topical NEC	T49.0X1	T49.0X2	T49.0X3	T49.0X4	T49.0X5	T49.0X6
Corynebacterium parvum	T45.1X1	T45.1X2	T45.1X3	T45.1X4	T45.1X5	T45.1X6
Cosmetic preparation	T49.8X1	T49.8X2	T49.8X3	T49.8X4	T49.8X5	T49.8X6
Cosmetics	T49.8X1	T49.8X2	T49.8X3	T49.8X4	T49.8X5	T49.8X6
Cosyntropin	T38.811	T38.812	T38.813	T38.814	T38.815	T38.816
Cotarnine	T45.7X1	T45.7X2	T45.7X3	T45.7X4	T45.7X5	T45.7X6
Co-trimoxazole	T36.8X1	T36.8X2	T36.8X3	T36.8X4	T36.8X5	T36.8X6
Cottonseed oil	T49.3X1	T49.3X2	T49.3X3	T49.3X4	T49.3X5	T49.3X6
Cough mixture (syrup)	T48.4X1	T48.4X2	T48.4X3	T48.4X4	T48.4X5	T48.4X6
containing opiates	T40.2X1	T40.2X2	T40.2X3	T40.2X4	T40.2X5	T40.2X6
expectorants	T48.4X1	T48.4X2	T48.4X3	T48.4X4	T48.4X5	T48.4X6
Coumadin	T45.511	T45.512	T45.513	T45.514	T45.515	T45.516
rodenticide	T60.4X1	T60.4X2	T60.4X3	T60.4X4	—	—
Coumaphos	T60.0X1	T60.0X2	T60.0X3	T60.0X4	—	—
Coumarin	T45.511	T45.512	T45.513	T45.514	T45.515	T45.516
Coumetarol	T45.511	T45.512	T45.513	T45.514	T45.515	T45.516
Cowbane	T62.2X1	T62.2X2	T62.2X3	T62.2X4	—	—
Cozyme	T45.2X1	T45.2X2	T45.2X3	T45.2X4	T45.2X5	T45.2X6
Crack	T40.5X1	T40.5X2	T40.5X3	T40.5X4	—	—
Crataegus extract	T46.0X1	T46.0X2	T46.0X3	T46.0X4	T46.0X5	T46.0X6
Creolin	T54.1X1	T54.1X2	T54.1X3	T54.1X4	—	—
disinfectant	T54.1X1	T54.1X2	T54.1X3	T54.1X4	—	—
Creosol (compound)	T49.0X1	T49.0X2	T49.0X3	T49.0X4	T49.0X5	T49.0X6
Creosote (coal tar) (beechwood)	T49.0X1	T49.0X2	T49.0X3	T49.0X4	T49.0X5	T49.0X6
medicinal (expectorant)	T48.4X1	T48.4X2	T48.4X3	T48.4X4	T48.4X5	T48.4X6
syrup	T48.4X1	T48.4X2	T48.4X3	T48.4X4	T48.4X5	T48.4X6
Cresol(s)	T49.0X1	T49.0X2	T49.0X3	T49.0X4	T49.0X5	T49.0X6
and soap solution	T49.0X1	T49.0X2	T49.0X3	T49.0X4	T49.0X5	T49.0X6
Cresyl acetate	T49.0X1	T49.0X2	T49.0X3	T49.0X4	T49.0X5	T49.0X6
Cresylic acid	T49.0X1	T49.0X2	T49.0X3	T49.0X4	T49.0X5	T49.0X6
Crimidine	T60.4X1	T60.4X2	T60.4X3	T60.4X4	—	—
Croconazole	T37.8X1	T37.8X2	T37.8X3	T37.8X4	T37.8X5	T37.8X6
Cromoglicic acid	T48.6X1	T48.6X2	T48.6X3	T48.6X4	T48.6X5	T48.6X6
Cromolyn	T48.6X1	T48.6X2	T48.6X3	T48.6X4	T48.6X5	T48.6X6
Cromonar	T46.3X1	T46.3X2	T46.3X3	T46.3X4	T46.3X5	T46.3X6

Substance	Poisoning, Accidental (Unintentional)	Poisoning, Intentional Self-Harm	Poisoning, Assault	Poisoning, Undetermined	Adverse Effect	Underdosing
Cropropamide	T39.8X1	T39.8X2	T39.8X3	T39.8X4	T39.8X5	T39.8X6
with crotethamide	T50.7X1	T50.7X2	T50.7X3	T50.7X4	T50.7X5	T50.7X6
Crotamiton	T49.0X1	T49.0X2	T49.0X3	T49.0X4	T49.0X5	T49.0X6
Crotethamide	T39.8X1	T39.8X2	T39.8X3	T39.8X4	T39.8X5	T39.8X6
with cropropamide	T50.7X1	T50.7X2	T50.7X3	T50.7X4	T50.7X5	T50.7X6
Croton (oil)	T47.2X1	T47.2X2	T47.2X3	T47.2X4	T47.2X5	T47.2X6
chloral	T42.6X1	T42.6X2	T42.6X3	T42.6X4	T42.6X5	T42.6X6
Crude oil	T52.0X1	T52.0X2	T52.0X3	T52.0X4	—	—
Cryogenine	T39.8X1	T39.8X2	T39.8X3	T39.8X4	T39.8X5	T39.8X6
Cryolite (vapor)	T60.1X1	T60.1X2	T60.1X3	T60.1X4	—	—
insecticide	T60.1X1	T60.1X2	T60.1X3	T60.1X4	—	—
Cryptenamine (tannates)	T46.5X1	T46.5X2	T46.5X3	T46.5X4	T46.5X5	T46.5X6
Crystal violet	T49.0X1	T49.0X2	T49.0X3	T49.0X4	T49.0X5	T49.0X6
Cuckoopint	T62.2X1	T62.2X2	T62.2X3	T62.2X4	—	—
Cumetharol	T45.511	T45.512	T45.513	T45.514	T45.515	T45.516
Cupric						
acetate	T60.3X1	T60.3X2	T60.3X3	T60.3X4	—	—
acetoarsenite	T57.0X1	T57.0X2	T57.0X3	T57.0X4	—	—
arsenate	T57.0X1	T57.0X2	T57.0X3	T57.0X4	—	—
gluconate	T49.0X1	T49.0X2	T49.0X3	T49.0X4	T49.0X5	T49.0X6
oleate	T49.0X1	T49.0X2	T49.0X3	T49.0X4	T49.0X5	T49.0X6
sulfate	T56.4X1	T56.4X2	T56.4X3	T56.4X4		
Cuprous sulfate — see also Copper, sulfate	T56.4X1	T56.4X2	T56.4X3	T56.4X4	—	—
Curare, curarine	T48.1X1	T48.1X2	T48.1X3	T48.1X4	T48.1X5	T48.1X6
Cyamemazine	T43.3X1	T43.3X2	T43.3X3	T43.3X4	T43.3X5	T43.3X6
Cyamopsis tetragono-loba	T46.6X1	T46.6X2	T46.6X3	T46.6X4	T46.6X5	T46.6X6
Cyanacetyl hydrazide	T37.1X1	T37.1X2	T37.1X3	T37.1X4	T37.1X5	T37.1X6
Cyanic acid (gas)	T59.891	T59.892	T59.893	T59.894		
Cyanide(s) (compounds) (potassium) (sodium) NEC	T65.0X1	T65.0X2	T65.0X3	T65.0X4	—	—
dust or gas (inhalation) NEC	T57.3X1	T57.3X2	T57.3X3	T57.3X4	—	—
fumigant	T65.0X1	T65.0X2	T65.0X3	T65.0X4	—	—
hydrogen	T57.3X1	T57.3X2	T57.3X3	T57.3X4	—	—
mercuric — see Mercury						
pesticide (dust) (fumes)	T65.0X1	T65.0X2	T65.0X3	T65.0X4	—	—
Cyanoacrylate adhesive	T49.3X1	T49.3X2	T49.3X3	T49.3X4	T49.3X5	T49.3X6
Cyanocobalamin	T45.8X1	T45.8X2	T45.8X3	T45.8X4	T45.8X5	T45.8X6
Cyanogen (chloride) (gas) NEC	T59.891	T59.892	T59.893	T59.894	—	—
Cyclacillin	T36.0X1	T36.0X2	T36.0X3	T36.0X4	T36.0X5	T36.0X6
Cyclaine	T41.3X1	T41.3X2	T41.3X3	T41.3X4	T41.3X5	T41.3X6
Cyclamate	T50.991	T50.992	T50.993	T50.994	T50.995	T50.996

◄ New ◄ Revised ~~deleted~~ Deleted

Substance	Poisoning, Accidental (Unintentional)	Poisoning, Intentional Self-Harm	Poisoning, Assault	Poisoning, Undetermined	Adverse Effect	Underdosing
Cyclamen europaeum	T62.2X1	T62.2X2	T62.2X3	T62.2X4	—	—
Cyclandelate	T46.7X1	T46.7X2	T46.7X3	T46.7X4	T46.7X5	T46.7X6
Cyclazocine	T50.7X1	T50.7X2	T50.7X3	T50.7X4	T50.7X5	T50.7X6
Cyclizine	T45.0X1	T45.0X2	T45.0X3	T45.0X4	T45.0X5	T45.0X6
Cyclobarbital	T42.3X1	T42.3X2	T42.3X3	T42.3X4	T42.3X5	T42.3X6
Cyclobarbitone	T42.3X1	T42.3X2	T42.3X3	T42.3X4	T42.3X5	T42.3X6
Cyclobenzaprine	T48.1X1	T48.1X2	T48.1X3	T48.1X4	T48.1X5	T48.1X6
Cyclodrine	T44.3X1	T44.3X2	T44.3X3	T44.3X4	T44.3X5	T44.3X6
Cycloguanil embonate	T37.2X1	T37.2X2	T37.2X3	T37.2X4	T37.2X5	T37.2X6
Cycloheptadiene	T43.291	T43.292	T43.293	T43.294	T43.295	T43.296
Cyclohexane	T52.8X1	T52.8X2	T52.8X3	T52.8X4	—	—
Cyclohexanol	T51.8X1	T51.8X2	T51.8X3	T51.8X4	—	—
Cyclohexanone	T52.4X1	T52.4X2	T52.4X3	T52.4X4	—	—
Cycloheximide	T60.3X1	T60.3X2	T60.3X3	T60.3X4	—	—
Cyclohexyl acetate	T52.8X1	T52.8X2	T52.8X3	T52.8X4	—	—
Cycloleucin	T45.1X1	T45.1X2	T45.1X3	T45.1X4	T45.1X5	T45.1X6
Cyclomethycaine	T41.3X1	T41.3X2	T41.3X3	T41.3X4	T41.3X5	T41.3X6
Cyclopentamine	T44.4X1	T44.4X2	T44.4X3	T44.4X4	T44.4X5	T44.4X6
Cyclopenthiazide	T50.2X1	T50.2X2	T50.2X3	T50.2X4	T50.2X5	T50.2X6
Cyclopentolate	T44.3X1	T44.3X2	T44.3X3	T44.3X4	T44.3X5	T44.3X6
Cyclophosphamide	T45.1X1	T45.1X2	T45.1X3	T45.1X4	T45.1X5	T45.1X6
Cycloplegic drug	T49.5X1	T49.5X2	T49.5X3	T49.5X4	T49.5X5	T49.5X6
Cyclopropane	T41.291	T41.292	T41.293	T41.294	T41.295	T41.296
Cyclopyrabital	T39.8X1	T39.8X2	T39.8X3	T39.8X4	T39.8X5	T39.8X6
Cycloserine	T37.1X1	T37.1X2	T37.1X3	T37.1X4	T37.1X5	T37.1X6
Cyclosporin	T45.1X1	T45.1X2	T45.1X3	T45.1X4	T45.1X5	T45.1X6
Cyclothiazide	T50.2X1	T50.2X2	T50.2X3	T50.2X4	T50.2X5	T50.2X6
Cycrimine	T44.3X1	T44.3X2	T44.3X3	T44.3X4	T44.3X5	T44.3X6
Cyhalothrin	T60.1X1	T60.1X2	T60.1X3	T60.1X4	—	—
Cymarin	T46.0X1	T46.0X2	T46.0X3	T46.0X4	T46.0X5	T46.0X6
Cypermethrin	T60.1X1	T60.1X2	T60.1X3	T60.1X4	—	—
Cyphenothrin	T60.2X1	T60.2X2	T60.2X3	T60.2X4	—	—
Cyproheptadine	T45.0X1	T45.0X2	T45.0X3	T45.0X4	T45.0X5	T45.0X6
Cyprolidol	T43.291	T43.292	T43.293	T43.294	T43.295	T43.296
Cyproterone	T38.6X1	T38.6X2	T38.6X3	T38.6X4	T38.6X5	T38.6X6
Cysteamine	T50.6X1	T50.6X2	T50.6X3	T50.6X4	T50.6X5	T50.6X6
Cytarabine	T45.1X1	T45.1X2	T45.1X3	T45.1X4	T45.1X5	T45.1X6
Cytisus						
laburnum	T62.2X1	T62.2X2	T62.2X3	T62.2X4	—	—
scoparius	T62.2X1	T62.2X2	T62.2X3	T62.2X4	—	—
Cytochrome C	T47.5X1	T47.5X2	T47.5X3	T47.5X4	T47.5X5	T47.5X6
Cytomel	T38.1X1	T38.1X2	T38.1X3	T38.1X4	T38.1X5	T38.1X6

Substance	Poisoning, Accidental (Unintentional)	Poisoning, Intentional Self-Harm	Poisoning, Assault	Poisoning, Undetermined	Adverse Effect	Underdosing
Cytosine arabinoside	T45.1X1	T45.1X2	T45.1X3	T45.1X4	T45.1X5	T45.1X6
Cytoxan	T45.1X1	T45.1X2	T45.1X3	T45.1X4	T45.1X5	T45.1X6
Cytozyme	T45.7X1	T45.7X2	T45.7X3	T45.7X4	T45.7X5	T45.7X6
2,4-D	T60.3X1	T60.3X2	T60.3X3	T60.3X4	—	—
D						
Dacarbazine	T45.1X1	T45.1X2	T45.1X3	T45.1X4	T45.1X5	T45.1X6
Dactinomycin	T45.1X1	T45.1X2	T45.1X3	T45.1X4	T45.1X5	T45.1X6
DADPS	T37.1X1	T37.1X2	T37.1X3	T37.1X4	T37.1X5	T37.1X6
Dakin's solution	T49.0X1	T49.0X2	T49.0X3	T49.0X4	T49.0X5	T49.0X6
Dalapon (sodium)	T60.3X1	T60.3X2	T60.3X3	T60.3X4	—	—
Dalmane	T42.4X1	T42.4X2	T42.4X3	T42.4X4	T42.4X5	T42.4X6
Danazol	T38.6X1	T38.6X2	T38.6X3	T38.6X4	T38.6X5	T38.6X6
Danilone	T45.511	T45.512	T45.513	T45.514	T45.515	T45.516
Danthron	T47.2X1	T47.2X2	T47.2X3	T47.2X4	T47.2X5	T47.2X6
Dantrolene	T42.8X1	T42.8X2	T42.8X3	T42.8X4	T42.8X5	T42.8X6
Dantron	T47.2X1	T47.2X2	T47.2X3	T47.2X4	T47.2X5	T47.2X6
Daphne (gnidium) (mezereum)	T62.2X1	T62.2X2	T62.2X3	T62.2X4	—	—
berry	T62.1X1	T62.1X2	T62.1X3	T62.1X4	—	—
Dapsone	T37.1X1	T37.1X2	T37.1X3	T37.1X4	T37.1X5	T37.1X6
Daraprim	T37.2X1	T37.2X2	T37.2X3	T37.2X4	T37.2X5	T37.2X6
Darnel	T62.2X1	T62.2X2	T62.2X3	T62.2X4	—	—
Darvon	T39.8X1	T39.8X2	T39.8X3	T39.8X4	T39.8X5	T39.8X6
Daunomycin	T45.1X1	T45.1X2	T45.1X3	T45.1X4	T45.1X5	T45.1X6
Daunorubicin	T45.1X1	T45.1X2	T45.1X3	T45.1X4	T45.1X5	T45.1X6
DBI	T38.3X1	T38.3X2	T38.3X3	T38.3X4	T38.3X5	T38.3X6
D-Con	T60.91	T60.92	T60.93	T60.94	—	—
insecticide	T60.2X1	T60.2X2	T60.2X3	T60.2X4	—	—
rodenticide	T60.4X1	T60.4X2	T60.4X3	T60.4X4	—	—
DDAVP	T38.891	T38.892	T38.893	T38.894	T38.895	T38.896
DDE (bis(chlorophenyl)-dichloroethylene)	T60.2X1	T60.2X2	T60.2X3	T60.2X4	—	—
DDS	T37.1X1	T37.1X2	T37.1X3	T37.1X4	T37.1X5	T37.1X6
DDT (dust)	T60.1X1	T60.1X2	T60.1X3	T60.1X4	—	—
Deadly nightshade — see also Belladonna	T62.2X1	T62.2X2	T62.2X3	T62.2X4	—	—
berry	T62.1X1	T62.1X2	T62.1X3	T62.1X4	—	—
Deamino-D-arginine vasopressin	T38.891	T38.892	T38.893	T38.894	T38.895	T38.896
Deanol (aceglumate)	T50.991	T50.992	T50.993	T50.994	T50.995	T50.996
Debrisoquine	T46.5X1	T46.5X2	T46.5X3	T46.5X4	T46.5X5	T46.5X6
Decaborane	T57.8X1	T57.8X2	T57.8X3	T57.8X4	—	—
fumes	T59.891	T59.892	T59.893	T59.894	—	—

TABLE OF DRUGS AND CHEMICALS

Substance	Poisoning, Accidental (Unintentional)	Poisoning, Intentional Self-Harm	Poisoning, Assault	Poisoning, Undetermined	Adverse Effect	Underdosing
Decadron	T38.0X1	T38.0X2	T38.0X3	T38.0X4	T38.0X5	T38.0X6
ENT agent	T49.6X1	T49.6X2	T49.6X3	T49.6X4	T49.6X5	T49.6X6
ophthalmic preparation	T49.5X1	T49.5X2	T49.5X3	T49.5X4	T49.5X5	T49.5X6
topical NEC	T49.0X1	T49.0X2	T49.0X3	T49.0X4	T49.0X5	T49.0X6
Decahydronaphthalene	T52.8X1	T52.8X2	T52.8X3	T52.8X4	—	—
Decalin	T52.8X1	T52.8X2	T52.8X3	T52.8X4	—	—
Decamethonium (bromide)	T48.1X1	T48.1X2	T48.1X3	T48.1X4	T48.1X5	T48.1X6
Decholin	T47.5X1	T47.5X2	T47.5X3	T47.5X4	T47.5X5	T47.5X6
Declomycin	T36.4X1	T36.4X2	T36.4X3	T36.4X4	T36.4X5	T36.4X6
Decongestant, nasal (mucosa)	T48.5X1	T48.5X2	T48.5X3	T48.5X4	T48.5X5	T48.5X6
combination	T48.5X1	T48.5X2	T48.5X3	T48.5X4	T48.5X5	T48.5X6
Deet	T60.8X1	T60.8X2	T60.8X3	T60.8X4	—	—
Deferoxamine	T45.8X1	T45.8X2	T45.8X3	T45.8X4	T45.8X5	T45.8X6
Deflazacort	T38.0X1	T38.0X2	T38.0X3	T38.0X4	T38.0X5	T38.0X6
Deglycyrrhizinized extract of licorice	T48.4X1	T48.4X2	T48.4X3	T48.4X4	T48.4X5	T48.4X6
Dehydrocholic acid	T47.5X1	T47.5X2	T47.5X3	T47.5X4	T47.5X5	T47.5X6
Dehydroemetine	T37.3X1	T37.3X2	T37.3X3	T37.3X4	T37.3X5	T37.3X6
Dekalin	T52.8X1	T52.8X2	T52.8X3	T52.8X4	—	—
Delalutin	T38.5X1	T38.5X2	T38.5X3	T38.5X4	T38.5X5	T38.5X6
Delphinium	T62.2X1	T62.2X2	T62.2X3	T62.2X4	—	—
Deltasone	T38.0X1	T38.0X2	T38.0X3	T38.0X4	T38.0X5	T38.0X6
Deltra	T38.0X1	T38.0X2	T38.0X3	T38.0X4	T38.0X5	T38.0X6
Delvinal	T42.3X1	T42.3X2	T42.3X3	T42.3X4	T42.3X5	T42.3X6
Delorazepam	T42.4X1	T42.4X2	T42.4X3	T42.4X4	T42.4X5	T42.4X6
Deltamethrin	T60.1X1	T60.1X2	T60.1X3	T60.1X4	—	—
Demecarium (bromide)	T49.5X1	T49.5X2	T49.5X3	T49.5X4	T49.5X5	T49.5X6
Demeclocycline	T36.4X1	T36.4X2	T36.4X3	T36.4X4	T36.4X5	T36.4X6
Demecolcine	T45.1X1	T45.1X2	T45.1X3	T45.1X4	T45.1X5	T45.1X6
Demegestone	T38.5X1	T38.5X2	T38.5X3	T38.5X4	T38.5X5	T38.5X6
Demelanizing agents	T49.8X1	T49.8X2	T49.8X3	T49.8X4	T49.8X5	T49.8X6
Demephion -O and -S	T60.0X1	T60.0X2	T60.0X3	T60.0X4	—	—
Demerol	T40.2X1	T40.2X2	T40.2X3	T40.2X4	T40.2X5	T40.2X6
Demethylchlortetracycline	T36.4X1	T36.4X2	T36.4X3	T36.4X4	T36.4X5	T36.4X6
Demethyltetracycline	T36.4X1	T36.4X2	T36.4X3	T36.4X4	T36.4X5	T36.4X6
Demeton -O and -S	T60.0X1	T60.0X2	T60.0X3	T60.0X4	—	—
Demulcent (external)	T49.3X1	T49.3X2	T49.3X3	T49.3X4	T49.3X5	T49.3X6
specified NEC	T49.3X1	T49.3X2	T49.3X3	T49.3X4	T49.3X5	T49.3X6
Demulen	T38.4X1	T38.4X2	T38.4X3	T38.4X4	T38.4X5	T38.4X6
Denatured alcohol	T51.0X1	T51.0X2	T51.0X3	T51.0X4	—	—
Dendrid	T49.5X1	T49.5X2	T49.5X3	T49.5X4	—	T49.5X6
Dental drug, topical application NEC	T49.7X1	T49.7X2	T49.7X3	T49.7X4	T49.7X5	T49.7X6

Substance	Poisoning, Accidental (Unintentional)	Poisoning, Intentional Self-Harm	Poisoning, Assault	Poisoning, Undetermined	Adverse Effect	Underdosing
Dentifrice	T49.7X1	T49.7X2	T49.7X3	T49.7X4	T49.7X5	T49.7X6
Deodorant spray (feminine hygiene)	T49.8X1	T49.8X2	T49.8X3	T49.8X4	T49.8X5	T49.8X6
Deoxycortone	T50.0X1	T50.0X2	T50.0X3	T50.0X4	T50.0X5	T50.0X6
2-Deoxy-5-fluorouridine	T45.1X1	T45.1X2	T45.1X3	T45.1X4	T45.1X5	T45.1X6
5-Deoxy-5-fluorouridine	T45.1X1	T45.1X2	T45.1X3	T45.1X4	T45.1X5	T45.1X6
Deoxyribonuclease (pancreatic)	T45.3X1	T45.3X2	T45.3X3	T45.3X4	T45.3X5	T45.3X6
Depilatory	T49.4X1	T49.4X2	T49.4X3	T49.4X4	T49.4X5	T49.4X6
Deprenalin	T42.8X1	T42.8X2	T42.8X3	T42.8X4	T42.8X5	T42.8X6
Deprenyl	T42.8X1	T42.8X2	T42.8X3	T42.8X4	T42.8X5	T42.8X6
Depressant, appetite	T50.5X1	T50.5X2	T50.5X3	T50.5X4	T50.5X5	T50.5X6
Depressant						
appetite, central	T50.5X1	T50.5X2	T50.5X3	T50.5X4	T50.5X5	T50.5X6
cardiac	T46.2X1	T46.2X2	T46.2X3	T46.2X4	T46.2X5	T46.2X6
central nervous system (anesthetic) — see also Central nervous system, depressants	T42.71	T42.72	T42.73	T42.74	T42.75	T42.76
general anesthetic	T41.201	T41.202	T41.203	T41.204	T41.205	T41.206
muscle tone	T42.8X1	T42.8X2	T42.8X3	T42.8X4	T42.8X5	T42.8X6
muscle tone, central	T42.8X1	T42.8X2	T42.8X3	T42.8X4	T42.8X5	T42.8X6
psychotherapeutic	T43.501	T43.502	T43.503	T43.504	T43.505	T43.506
Deptropine	T45.0X1	T45.0X2	T45.0X3	T45.0X4	T45.0X5	T45.0X6
Dequalinium (chloride)	T49.0X1	T49.0X2	T49.0X3	T49.0X4	T49.0X5	T49.0X6
Derris root	T60.2X1	T60.2X2	T60.2X3	T60.2X4	—	—
Deserpidine	T43.011	T43.012	T43.013	T43.014	T43.015	T43.016
Desferrioxamine	T45.8X1	T45.8X2	T45.8X3	T45.8X4	T45.8X5	T45.8X6
Desipramine	T43.0X1	T43.0X2	T43.0X3	T43.0X4	T43.0X5	T43.0X6
Deslanoside	T46.0X1	T46.0X2	T46.0X3	T46.0X4	T46.0X5	T46.0X6
Desloughing agent	T49.4X1	T49.4X2	T49.4X3	T49.4X4	T49.4X5	T49.4X6
Desmethylimipramine	T43.011	T43.012	T43.013	T43.014	T43.015	T43.016
Desmopressin	T38.891	T38.892	T38.893	T38.894	T38.895	T38.896
Desocodeine	T40.2X1	T40.2X2	T40.2X3	T40.2X4	T40.2X5	T40.2X6
Desogestrel	T38.5X1	T38.5X2	T38.5X3	T38.5X4	T38.5X5	T38.5X6
Desomorphine	T40.2X1	T40.2X2	T40.2X3	T40.2X4	—	—
Desonide	T49.0X1	T49.0X2	T49.0X3	T49.0X4	T49.0X5	T49.0X6
Desoximetasone	T49.0X1	T49.0X2	T49.0X3	T49.0X4	T49.0X5	T49.0X6
Desoxycorticosteroid	T50.0X1	T50.0X2	T50.0X3	T50.0X4	T50.0X5	T50.0X6
Desoxycortone	T50.0X1	T50.0X2	T50.0X3	T50.0X4	T50.0X5	T50.0X6
Desoxyephedrine	T43.651	T43.652	T43.653	T43.654	T43.655	T43.656
Detaxtran	T46.6X1	T46.6X2	T46.6X3	T46.6X4	T46.6X5	T46.6X6
Detergent	T49.2X1	T49.2X2	T49.2X3	T49.2X4	T49.2X5	T49.2X6
external medication	T49.2X1	T49.2X2	T49.2X3	T49.2X4	T49.2X5	T49.2X6
local	T49.2X1	T49.2X2	T49.2X3	T49.2X4	T49.2X5	T49.2X6

◀ New ◀ Revised ~~deleted~~ Deleted

	External Cause (T-Code)					
Substance	Poisoning, Accidental (Unintentional)	Poisoning, Intentional Self-Harm	Poisoning, Assault	Poisoning, Undetermined	Adverse Effect	Underdosing
Detergent *(Continued)*						
medicinal	T49.2X1	T49.2X2	T49.2X3	T49.2X4	T49.2X5	T49.2X6
nonmedicinal	T55.1X1	T55.1X2	T55.1X3	T55.1X4	—	—
specified NEC	T55.1X1	T55.1X2	T55.1X3	T55.1X4	T55.1X5	T55.1X6
Deterrent, alcohol	T50.6X1	T50.6X2	T50.6X3	T50.6X4	T50.6X5	T50.6X6
Detoxifying agent	T50.6X1	T50.6X2	T50.6X3	T50.6X4	T50.6X5	T50.6X6
Detrothyronine	T38.1X1	T38.1X2	T38.1X3	T38.1X4	T38.1X5	T38.1X6
Dettol (external medication)	T49.0X1	T49.0X2	T49.0X3	T49.0X4	T49.0X5	T49.0X6
Dexamethasone	T38.0X1	T38.0X2	T38.0X3	T38.0X4	T38.0X5	T38.0X6
ENT agent	T49.6X1	T49.6X2	T49.6X3	T49.6X4	T49.6X5	T49.6X6
ophthalmic preparation	T49.5X1	T49.5X2	T49.5X3	T49.5X4	T49.5X5	T49.5X6
topical NEC	T49.0X1	T49.0X2	T49.0X3	T49.0X4	T49.0X5	T49.0X6
Dexamfetamine	T43.621	T43.622	T43.623	T43.624	T43.625	T43.626
Dexamphetamine	T43.621	T43.622	T43.623	T43.624	T43.625	T43.626
Dexbrompheniramine	T45.0X1	T45.0X2	T45.0X3	T45.0X4	T45.0X5	T45.0X6
Dexchlorpheniramine	T45.0X1	T45.0X2	T45.0X3	T45.0X4	T45.0X5	T45.0X6
Dexedrine	T43.621	T43.622	T43.623	T43.624	T43.625	T43.626
Dexetimide	T44.3X1	T44.3X2	T44.3X3	T44.3X4	T44.3X5	T44.3X6
Dexfenfluramine	T50.5X1	T50.5X2	T50.5X3	T50.5X4	T50.5X5	T50.5X6
Dexpanthenol	T45.2X1	T45.2X2	T45.2X3	T45.2X4	T45.2X5	T45.2X6
Dextran (40) (70) (150)	T45.8X1	T45.8X2	T45.8X3	T45.8X4	T45.8X5	T45.8X6
Dextriferron	T45.4X1	T45.4X2	T45.4X3	T45.4X4	T45.4X5	T45.4X6
Dextroamphetamine	T43.621	T43.622	T43.623	T43.624	T43.625	T43.626
Dextro calcium pantothenate	T45.2X1	T45.2X2	T45.2X3	T45.2X4	T45.2X5	T45.2X6
Dextromethorphan	T48.3X1	T48.3X2	T48.3X3	T48.3X4	T48.3X5	T48.3X6
Dextromoramide	T40.491	T40.492	T40.493	T40.494	—	—
topical	T49.8X1	T49.8X2	T49.8X3	T49.8X4	T49.8X5	T49.8X6
Dextro pantothenyl alcohol	T45.2X1	T45.2X2	T45.2X3	T45.2X4	T45.2X5	T45.2X6
Dextropropoxyphene	T40.491	T40.492	T40.493	T40.494	T40.495	T40.496
Dextrorphan	T40.2X1	T40.2X2	T40.2X3	T40.2X4	T40.2X5	T40.2X6
Dextrose	T50.3X1	T50.3X2	T50.3X3	T50.3X4	T50.3X5	T50.3X6
concentrated solution, intravenous	T46.8X1	T46.8X2	T46.8X3	T46.8X4	T46.8X5	T46.8X6
Dextrothyroxin	T38.1X1	T38.1X2	T38.1X3	T38.1X4	T38.1X5	T38.1X6
Dextrothyroxine sodium	T38.1X1	T38.1X2	T38.1X3	T38.1X4	T38.1X5	T38.1X6
DFP	T44.0X1	T44.0X2	T44.0X3	T44.0X4	T44.0X5	T44.0X6
DHE	T37.3X1	T37.3X2	T37.3X3	T37.3X4	T37.3X5	T37.3X6
45	T46.5X1	T46.5X2	T46.5X3	T46.5X4	T46.5X5	T46.5X6
Diabinese	T38.3X1	T38.3X2	T38.3X3	T38.3X4	T38.3X5	T38.3X6
Diacetone alcohol	T52.4X1	T52.4X2	T52.4X3	T52.4X4	—	—
Diacetyl monoxime	T50.991	T50.992	T50.993	T50.994	—	—
Diacetylmorphine	T40.1X1	T40.1X2	T40.1X3	T40.1X4	—	—

	External Cause (T-Code)					
Substance	Poisoning, Accidental (Unintentional)	Poisoning, Intentional Self-Harm	Poisoning, Assault	Poisoning, Undetermined	Adverse Effect	Underdosing
Diachylon plaster	T49.4X1	T49.4X2	T49.4X3	T49.4X4	T49.4X5	T49.4X6
Diaethylstilboestrolum	T38.5X1	T38.5X2	T38.5X3	T38.5X4	T38.5X5	T38.5X6
Diagnostic agent NEC	T50.8X1	T50.8X2	T50.8X3	T50.8X4	T50.8X5	T50.8X6
Dial (soap)	T49.2X1	T49.2X2	T49.2X3	T49.2X4	T49.2X5	T49.2X6
sedative	T42.3X1	T42.3X2	T42.3X3	T42.3X4	T42.3X5	T42.3X6
Dialkyl carbonate	T52.91	T52.92	T52.93	T52.94	—	—
Diallylbarbituric acid	T42.3X1	T42.3X2	T42.3X3	T42.3X4	T42.3X5	T42.3X6
Diallymal	T42.3X1	T42.3X2	T42.3X3	T42.3X4	T42.3X5	T42.3X6
Dialysis solution (intraperitoneal)	T50.3X1	T50.3X2	T50.3X3	T50.3X4	T50.3X5	T50.3X6
Diaminodiphenylsulfone	T37.1X1	T37.1X2	T37.1X3	T37.1X4	T37.1X5	T37.1X6
Diamorphine	T40.1X1	T40.1X2	T40.1X3	T40.1X4	—	—
Diamox	T50.2X1	T50.2X2	T50.2X3	T50.2X4	T50.2X5	T50.2X6
Diamthazole	T49.0X1	T49.0X2	T49.0X3	T49.0X4	T49.0X5	T49.0X6
Dianthone	T47.2X1	T47.2X2	T47.2X3	T47.2X4	T47.2X5	T47.2X6
Diaphenylsulfone	T37.0X1	T37.0X2	T37.0X3	T37.0X4	T37.0X5	T37.0X6
Diasone (sodium)	T37.1X1	T37.1X2	T37.1X3	T37.1X4	T37.1X5	T37.1X6
Diastase	T47.5X1	T47.5X2	T47.5X3	T47.5X4	T47.5X5	T47.5X6
Diatrizoate	T50.8X1	T50.8X2	T50.8X3	T50.8X4	T50.8X5	T50.8X6
Diazepam	T42.4X1	T42.4X2	T42.4X3	T42.4X4	T42.4X5	T42.4X6
Diazinon	T60.0X1	T60.0X2	T60.0X3	T60.0X4	—	—
Diazomethane (gas)	T59.891	T59.892	T59.893	T59.894	—	—
Diazoxide	T46.5X1	T46.5X2	T46.5X3	T46.5X4	T46.5X5	T46.5X6
Dibekacin	T36.5X1	T36.5X2	T36.5X3	T36.5X4	T36.5X5	T36.5X6
Dibenamine	T44.6X1	T44.6X2	T44.6X3	T44.6X4	T44.6X5	T44.6X6
Dibenzepin	T43.011	T43.012	T43.013	T43.014	T43.015	T43.016
Dibenzheptropine	T45.0X1	T45.0X2	T45.0X3	T45.0X4	T45.0X5	T45.0X6
Dibenzyline	T44.6X1	T44.6X2	T44.6X3	T44.6X4	T44.6X5	T44.6X6
Diborane (gas)	T59.891	T59.892	T59.893	T59.894	—	—
Dibromochloropropane	T60.8X1	T60.8X2	T60.8X3	T60.8X4	—	—
Dibromodulcitol	T45.1X1	T45.1X2	T45.1X3	T45.1X4	T45.1X5	T45.1X6
Dibromoethane	T53.6X1	T53.6X2	T53.6X3	T53.6X4	—	—
Dibromomannitol	T45.1X1	T45.1X2	T45.1X3	T45.1X4	T45.1X5	T45.1X6
Dibromopropamidine isethionate	T49.0X1	T49.0X2	T49.0X3	T49.0X4	T49.0X5	T49.0X6
Dibrompropamidine	T49.0X1	T49.0X2	T49.0X3	T49.0X4	T49.0X5	T49.0X6
Dibucaine	T41.3X1	T41.3X2	T41.3X3	T41.3X4	T41.3X5	T41.3X6
topical (surface)	T41.3X1	T41.3X2	T41.3X3	T41.3X4	T41.3X5	T41.3X6
Dibunate sodium	T48.3X1	T48.3X2	T48.3X3	T48.3X4	T48.3X5	T48.3X6
Dibutoline sulfate	T44.3X1	T44.3X2	T44.3X3	T44.3X4	T44.3X5	T44.3X6
Dicamba	T60.3X1	T60.3X2	T60.3X3	T60.3X4	—	—
Dicapthon	T60.0X1	T60.0X2	T60.0X3	T60.0X4	—	—
Dichlobenil	T60.3X1	T60.3X2	T60.3X3	T60.3X4	—	—
Dichlone	T60.3X1	T60.3X2	T60.3X3	T60.3X4	—	—

TABLE OF DRUGS AND CHEMICALS

	External Cause (T-Code)					
Substance	Poisoning, Accidental (Unintentional)	Poisoning, Intentional Self-Harm	Poisoning, Assault	Poisoning, Undetermined	Adverse Effect	Underdosing
Dichloralphenozone	T42.6X1	T42.6X2	T42.6X3	T42.6X4	T42.6X5	T42.6X6
Dichlorbenzidine	T65.3X1	T65.3X2	T65.3X3	T65.3X4	—	—
Dichlorhydrin	T52.8X1	T52.8X2	T52.8X3	T52.8X4	—	—
Dichlorhydroxyquinoline	T37.8X1	T37.8X2	T37.8X3	T37.8X4	T37.8X5	T37.8X6
Dichlorobenzene	T53.7X1	T53.7X2	T53.7X3	T53.7X4	—	—
Dichlorobenzyl alcohol	T49.6X1	T49.6X2	T49.6X3	T49.6X4	T49.6X5	T49.6X6
Dichlorodifluoromethane	T53.5X1	T53.5X2	T53.5X3	T53.5X4	—	—
Dichloroethane	T52.8X1	T52.8X2	T52.8X3	T52.8X4	—	—
Sym-Dichloroethyl ether	T53.6X1	T53.6X2	T53.6X3	T53.6X4	—	—
Dichloroethyl sulfide, not in war	T59.891	T59.892	T59.893	T59.894	—	—
Dichloroethylene	T53.6X1	T53.6X2	T53.6X3	T53.6X4	—	—
Dichloroformoxine, not in war	T59.891	T59.892	T59.893	T59.894	—	—
Dichlorohydrin, alpha-dichlorohydrin	T52.8X1	T52.8X2	T52.8X3	T52.8X4	—	—
Dichloromethane (solvent)	T53.4X1	T53.4X2	T53.4X3	T53.4X4	—	—
vapor	T53.4X1	T53.4X2	T53.4X3	T53.4X4	—	—
Dichloronaphthoquinone	T60.3X1	T60.3X2	T60.3X3	T60.3X4	—	—
Dichlorophen	T37.4X1	T37.4X2	T37.4X3	T37.4X4	T37.4X5	T37.4X6
2,4-Dichlorophenoxy-acetic acid	T60.3X1	T60.3X2	T60.3X3	T60.3X4	—	—
Dichloropropene	T60.3X1	T60.3X2	T60.3X3	T60.3X4	—	—
Dichloropropionic acid	T60.3X1	T60.3X2	T60.3X3	T60.3X4	—	—
Dichlorphenamide	T50.2X1	T50.2X2	T50.2X3	T50.2X4	T50.2X5	T50.2X6
Dichlorvos	T60.0X1	T60.0X2	T60.0X3	T60.0X4	—	—
Diclofenac	T39.391	T39.392	T39.393	T39.394	T39.395	T39.396
Diclofenamide	T50.2X1	T50.2X2	T50.2X3	T50.2X4	T50.2X5	T50.2X6
Diclofensine	T43.291	T43.292	T43.293	T43.294	T43.295	T43.296
Diclonixine	T39.8X1	T39.8X2	T39.8X3	T39.8X4	T39.8X5	T39.8X6
Dicloxacillin	T36.0X1	T36.0X2	T36.0X3	T36.0X4	T36.0X5	T36.0X6
Dicophane	T49.0X1	T49.0X2	T49.0X3	T49.0X4	T49.0X5	T49.0X6
Dicoumarol, dicoumarin, dicumarol	T45.511	T45.512	T45.513	T45.514	T45.515	T45.516
Dicrotophos	T60.0X1	T60.0X2	T60.0X3	T60.0X4	—	—
Dicyanogen (gas)	T65.0X1	T65.0X2	T65.0X3	T65.0X4	—	—
Dicyclomine	T44.3X1	T44.3X2	T44.3X3	T44.3X4	T44.3X5	T44.3X6
Dicycloverine	T44.3X1	T44.3X2	T44.3X3	T44.3X4	T44.3X5	T44.3X6
Dideoxycytidine	T37.5X1	T37.5X2	T37.5X3	T37.5X4	T37.5X5	T37.5X6
Dideoxyinosine	T37.5X1	T37.5X2	T37.5X3	T37.5X4	T37.5X5	T37.5X6
Dieldrin (vapor)	T60.1X1	T60.1X2	T60.1X3	T60.1X4	—	—
Diemal	T42.3X1	T42.3X2	T42.3X3	T42.3X4	T42.3X5	T42.3X6
Dienestrol	T38.5X1	T38.5X2	T38.5X3	T38.5X4	T38.5X5	T38.5X6
Dienoestrol	T38.5X1	T38.5X2	T38.5X3	T38.5X4	T38.5X5	T38.5X6
Dietetic drug NEC	T50.901	T50.902	T50.903	T50.904	T50.905	T50.906
Diethazine	T42.8X1	T42.8X2	T42.8X3	T42.8X4	T42.8X5	T42.8X6

	External Cause (T-Code)					
Substance	Poisoning, Accidental (Unintentional)	Poisoning, Intentional Self-Harm	Poisoning, Assault	Poisoning, Undetermined	Adverse Effect	Underdosing
Diethyl						
barbituric acid	T42.3X1	T42.3X2	T42.3X3	T42.3X4	T42.3X5	T42.3X6
carbamazine	T37.4X1	T37.4X2	T37.4X3	T37.4X4	T37.4X5	T37.4X6
carbinol	T51.3X1	T51.3X2	T51.3X3	T51.3X4	—	—
carbonate	T52.8X1	T52.8X2	T52.8X3	T52.8X4	—	—
ether (vapor) — see also Ether	T41.0X1	T41.0X2	T41.0X3	T41.0X4	T41.0X5	T41.0X6
oxide	T52.8X1	T52.8X2	T52.8X3	T52.8X4	—	—
propion	T50.5X1	T50.5X2	T50.5X3	T50.5X4	T50.5X5	T50.5X6
stilbestrol	T38.5X1	T38.5X2	T38.5X3	T38.5X4	T38.5X5	T38.5X6
toluamide (nonmedicinal)	T60.8X1	T60.8X2	T60.8X3	T60.8X4	—	—
medicinal	T49.3X1	T49.3X2	T49.3X3	T49.3X4	T49.3X5	T49.3X6
Diethylcarbamazine	T37.4X1	T37.4X2	T37.4X3	T37.4X4	T37.4X5	T37.4X6
Diethylene						
dioxide	T52.8X1	T52.8X2	T52.8X3	T52.8X4	—	—
glycol (monoacetate) (monobutyl ether) (monoethyl ether)	T52.3X1	T52.3X2	T52.3X3	T52.3X4	—	—
Diethylhexylphthalate	T65.891	T65.892	T65.893	T65.894	—	—
Diethylpropion	T50.5X1	T50.5X2	T50.5X3	T50.5X4	T50.5X5	T50.5X6
Diethylstilbestrol	T38.5X1	T38.5X2	T38.5X3	T38.5X4	T38.5X5	T38.5X6
Diethylstilboestrol	T38.5X1	T38.5X2	T38.5X3	T38.5X4	T38.5X5	T38.5X6
Diethylsulfone-diethylmethane	T42.6X1	T42.6X2	T42.6X3	T42.6X4	T42.6X5	T42.6X6
Diethyltoluamide	T49.0X1	T49.0X2	T49.0X3	T49.0X4	T49.0X5	T49.0X6
Diethyltryptamine (DET)	T40.991	T40.992	T40.993	T40.994	—	—
Difebarbamate	T42.3X1	T42.3X2	T42.3X3	T42.3X4	T42.3X5	T42.3X6
Difencloxazine	T40.2X1	T40.2X2	T40.2X3	T40.2X4	T40.2X5	T40.2X6
Difenidol	T45.0X1	T45.0X2	T45.0X3	T45.0X4	T45.0X5	T45.0X6
Difenoxin	T47.6X1	T47.6X2	T47.6X3	T47.6X4	T47.6X5	T47.6X6
Difetarsone	T37.3X1	T37.3X2	T37.3X3	T37.3X4	T37.3X5	T37.3X6
Diffusin	T45.3X1	T45.3X2	T45.3X3	T45.3X4	T45.3X5	T45.3X6
Diflorasone	T49.0X1	T49.0X2	T49.0X3	T49.0X4	T49.0X5	T49.0X6
Diflubenzuron	T60.1X1	T60.1X2	T60.1X3	T60.1X4	—	—
Diflos	T44.0X1	T44.0X2	T44.0X3	T44.0X4	T44.0X5	T44.0X6
Diflucortolone	T49.0X1	T49.0X2	T49.0X3	T49.0X4	T49.0X5	T49.0X6
Diflunisal	T39.091	T39.092	T39.093	T39.094	T39.095	T39.096
Difluoromethyldopa	T42.8X1	T42.8X2	T42.8X3	T42.8X4	T42.8X5	T42.8X6
Difluorophate	T44.0X1	T44.0X2	T44.0X3	T44.0X4	T44.0X5	T44.0X6
Digestant NEC	T47.5X1	T47.5X2	T47.5X3	T47.5X4	T47.5X5	T47.5X6
Digitalin(e)	T46.0X1	T46.0X2	T46.0X3	T46.0X4	T46.0X5	T46.0X6
Digitalis (leaf) (glycoside)	T46.0X1	T46.0X2	T46.0X3	T46.0X4	T46.0X5	T46.0X6
lanata	T46.0X1	T46.0X2	T46.0X3	T46.0X4	T46.0X5	T46.0X6
purpurea	T46.0X1	T46.0X2	T46.0X3	T46.0X4	T46.0X5	T46.0X6
Digitoxin	T46.0X1	T46.0X2	T46.0X3	T46.0X4	T46.0X5	T46.0X6

◀ New　◀ Revised　~~deleted~~ Deleted

Substance	External Cause (T-Code) Poisoning, Accidental (Unintentional)	Poisoning, Intentional Self-Harm	Poisoning, Assault	Poisoning, Undetermined	Adverse Effect	Underdosing
Digitoxose	T46.0X1	T46.0X2	T46.0X3	T46.0X4	T46.0X5	T46.0X6
Digoxin	T46.0X1	T46.0X2	T46.0X3	T46.0X4	T46.0X5	T46.0X6
Digoxine	T46.0X1	T46.0X2	T46.0X3	T46.0X4	T46.0X5	T46.0X6
Dihydralazine	T46.5X1	T46.5X2	T46.5X3	T46.5X4	T46.5X5	T46.5X6
Dihydrazine	T46.5X1	T46.5X2	T46.5X3	T46.5X4	T46.5X5	T46.5X6
Dihydrocodeinone	T40.2X1	T40.2X2	T40.2X3	T40.2X4	T40.2X5	T40.2X6
Dihydroergocornine	T46.7X1	T46.7X2	T46.7X3	T46.7X4	T46.7X5	T46.7X6
Dihydroergocristine (mesilate)	T46.7X1	T46.7X2	T46.7X3	T46.7X4	T46.7X5	T46.7X6
Dihydroergokryptine	T46.7X1	T46.7X2	T46.7X3	T46.7X4	T46.7X5	T46.7X6
Dihydroergotamine	T46.5X1	T46.5X2	T46.5X3	T46.5X4	T46.5X5	T46.5X6
Dihydroergotoxine	T46.7X1	T46.7X2	T46.7X3	T46.7X4	T46.7X5	T46.7X6
mesilate	T46.7X1	T46.7X2	T46.7X3	T46.7X4	T46.7X5	T46.7X6
Dihydrohydroxycodein-one	T40.2X1	T40.2X2	T40.2X3	T40.2X4	T40.2X5	T40.2X6
Dihydrohydroxymorphinone	T40.2X1	T40.2X2	T40.2X3	T40.2X4	T40.2X5	T40.2X6
Dihydroisocodeine	T40.2X1	T40.2X2	T40.2X3	T40.2X4	T40.2X5	T40.2X6
Dihydromorphine	T40.2X1	T40.2X2	T40.2X3	T40.2X4	—	—
Dihydromorphinone	T40.2X1	T40.2X2	T40.2X3	T40.2X4	T40.2X5	T40.2X6
Dihydrostreptomycin	T36.5X1	T36.5X2	T36.5X3	T36.5X4	T36.5X5	T36.5X6
Dihydrotachysterol	T45.2X1	T45.2X2	T45.2X3	T45.2X4	T45.2X5	T45.2X6
Dihydroxyaluminum aminoacetate	T47.1X1	T47.1X2	T47.1X3	T47.1X4	T47.1X5	T47.1X6
Dihydroxyaluminum sodium carbonate	T47.1X1	T47.1X2	T47.1X3	T47.1X4	T47.1X5	T47.1X6
Dihydroxyanthraquinone	T47.2X1	T47.2X2	T47.2X3	T47.2X4	T47.2X5	T47.2X6
Dihydroxycodeinone	T40.2X1	T40.2X2	T40.2X3	T40.2X4	T40.2X5	T40.2X6
Dihydroxypropyl theophylline	T50.2X1	T50.2X2	T50.2X3	T50.2X4	T50.2X5	T50.2X6
Diiodohydroxyquin	T37.8X1	T37.8X2	T37.8X3	T37.8X4	T37.8X5	T37.8X6
topical	T49.0X1	T49.0X2	T49.0X3	T49.0X4	T49.0X5	T49.0X6
Diiodohydroxyquinoline	T37.8X1	T37.8X2	T37.8X3	T37.8X4	T37.8X5	T37.8X6
Diiodotyrosine	T38.2X1	T38.2X2	T38.2X3	T38.2X4	T38.2X5	T38.2X6
Diisopromine	T44.3X1	T44.3X2	T44.3X3	T44.3X4	T44.3X5	T44.3X6
Diisopropylamine	T46.3X1	T46.3X2	T46.3X3	T46.3X4	T46.3X5	T46.3X6
Diisopropylfluorophosphonate	T44.0X1	T44.0X2	T44.0X3	T44.0X4	T44.0X5	T44.0X6
Dilantin	T42.0X1	T42.0X2	T42.0X3	T42.0X4	T42.0X5	T42.0X6
Dilaudid	T40.2X1	T40.2X2	T40.2X3	T40.2X4	T40.2X5	T40.2X6
Dilazep	T46.3X1	T46.3X2	T46.3X3	T46.3X4	T46.3X5	T46.3X6
Dill	T47.5X1	T47.5X2	T47.5X3	T47.5X4	T47.5X5	T47.5X6
Diloxanide	T37.3X1	T37.3X2	T37.3X3	T37.3X4	T37.3X5	T37.3X6
Diltiazem	T46.1X1	T46.1X2	T46.1X3	T46.1X4	T46.1X5	T46.1X6
Dimazole	T49.0X1	T49.0X2	T49.0X3	T49.0X4	T49.0X5	T49.0X6
Dimefline	T50.7X1	T50.7X2	T50.7X3	T50.7X4	T50.7X5	T50.7X6
Dimefox	T60.0X1	T60.0X2	T60.0X3	T60.0X4	—	—
Dimemorfan	T48.3X1	T48.3X2	T48.3X3	T48.3X4	T48.3X5	T48.3X6
Dimenhydrinate	T45.0X1	T45.0X2	T45.0X3	T45.0X4	T45.0X5	T45.0X6
Dimercaprol (British anti-lewisite)	T45.8X1	T45.8X2	T45.8X3	T45.8X4	T45.8X5	T45.8X6
Dimercaptopropanol	T45.8X1	T45.8X2	T45.8X3	T45.8X4	T45.8X5	T45.8X6
Dimestrol	T38.5X1	T38.5X2	T38.5X3	T38.5X4	T38.5X5	T38.5X6
Dimetane	T45.0X1	T45.0X2	T45.0X3	T45.0X4	T45.0X5	T45.0X6
Dimethicone	T47.1X1	T47.1X2	T47.1X3	T47.1X4	T47.1X5	T47.1X6
Dimethindene	T45.0X1	T45.0X2	T45.0X3	T45.0X4	T45.0X5	T45.0X6
Dimethisoquin	T49.1X1	T49.1X2	T49.1X3	T49.1X4	T49.1X5	T49.1X6
Dimethisterone	T38.5X1	T38.5X2	T38.5X3	T38.5X4	T38.5X5	T38.5X6
Dimethoate	T60.0X1	T60.0X2	T60.0X3	T60.0X4	—	—
Dimethocaine	T41.3X1	T41.3X2	T41.3X3	T41.3X4	T41.3X5	T41.3X6
Dimethoxanate	T48.3X1	T48.3X2	T48.3X3	T48.3X4	T48.3X5	T48.3X6
Dimethyl						
arsine, arsinic acid	T57.0X1	T57.0X2	T57.0X3	T57.0X4	—	—
carbinol	T51.2X1	T51.2X2	T51.2X3	T51.2X4	—	—
carbonate	T52.8X1	T52.8X2	T52.8X3	T52.8X4	—	—
diguanide	T38.3X1	T38.3X2	T38.3X3	T38.3X4	T38.3X5	T38.3X6
ketone	T52.4X1	T52.4X2	T52.4X3	T52.4X4	—	—
vapor	T52.4X1	T52.4X2	T52.4X3	T52.4X4	—	—
meperidine	T40.2X1	T40.2X2	T40.2X3	T40.2X4	T40.2X5	T40.2X6
parathion	T60.0X1	T60.0X2	T60.0X3	T60.0X4	—	—
phthlate	T49.3X1	T49.3X2	T49.3X3	T49.3X4	T49.3X5	T49.3X6
polysiloxane	T47.8X1	T47.8X2	T47.8X3	T47.8X4	T47.8X5	T47.8X6
sulfate (fumes)	T59.891	T59.892	T59.893	T59.894	—	—
liquid	T65.891	T65.892	T65.893	T65.894	—	—
sulfoxide (nonmedicinal)	T52.8X1	T52.8X2	T52.8X3	T52.8X4	—	—
medicinal	T49.4X1	T49.4X2	T49.4X3	T49.4X4	T49.4X5	T49.4X6
tryptamine	T40.991	T40.992	T40.993	T40.994	—	—
tubocurarine	T48.1X1	T48.1X2	T48.1X3	T48.1X4	T48.1X5	T48.1X6
Dimethylamine sulfate	T49.4X1	T49.4X2	T49.4X3	T49.4X4	T49.4X5	T49.4X6
Dimethylformamide	T52.8X1	T52.8X2	T52.8X3	T52.8X4	—	—
Dimethyltubocurarinium chloride	T48.1X1	T48.1X2	T48.1X3	T48.1X4	T48.1X5	T48.1X6
Dimeticone	T47.1X1	T47.1X2	T47.1X3	T47.1X4	T47.1X5	T47.1X6
Dimetilan	T60.0X1	T60.0X2	T60.0X3	T60.0X4	—	—
Dimetindene	T45.0X1	T45.0X2	T45.0X3	T45.0X4	T45.0X5	T45.0X6
Dimetotiazine	T43.3X1	T43.3X2	T43.3X3	T43.3X4	T43.3X5	T43.3X6
Dimorpholamine	T50.7X1	T50.7X2	T50.7X3	T50.7X4	T50.7X5	T50.7X6
Dimoxyline	T46.3X1	T46.3X2	T46.3X3	T46.3X4	T46.3X5	T46.3X6
Dinitrobenzene	T65.3X1	T65.3X2	T65.3X3	T65.3X4	—	—
vapor	T59.891	T59.892	T59.893	T59.894	—	—

TABLE OF DRUGS AND CHEMICALS

TABLE OF DRUGS AND CHEMICALS

	External Cause (T-Code)					
Substance	Poisoning, Accidental (Unintentional)	Poisoning, Intentional Self-Harm	Poisoning, Assault	Poisoning, Undetermined	Adverse Effect	Underdosing
Dinitrobenzol	T65.3X1	T65.3X2	T65.3X3	T65.3X4	—	—
vapor	T59.891	T59.892	T59.893	T59.894	—	—
Dinitrobutylphenol	T65.3X1	T65.3X2	T65.3X3	T65.3X4	—	—
Dinitro (-ortho-)cresol (pesticide) (spray)	T65.3X1	T65.3X2	T65.3X3	T65.3X4	—	—
Dinitrocyclohexylphenol	T65.3X1	T65.3X2	T65.3X3	T65.3X4	—	—
Dinitrophenol	T65.3X1	T65.3X2	T65.3X3	T65.3X4	—	—
Dinoprost	T48.0X1	T48.0X2	T48.0X3	T48.0X4	T48.0X5	T48.0X6
Dinoprostone	T48.0X1	T48.0X2	T48.0X3	T48.0X4	T48.0X5	T48.0X6
Dinoseb	T60.3X1	T60.3X2	T60.3X3	T60.3X4	—	—
Dioctyl sulfosuccinate (calcium) (sodium)	T47.4X1	T47.4X2	T47.4X3	T47.4X4	T47.4X5	T47.4X6
Diodone	T50.8X1	T50.8X2	T50.8X3	T50.8X4	T50.8X5	T50.8X6
Diodoquin	T37.8X1	T37.8X2	T37.8X3	T37.8X4	T37.8X5	T37.8X6
Dionin	T40.2X1	T40.2X2	T40.2X3	T40.2X4	T40.2X5	T40.2X6
Diosmin	T46.991	T46.992	T46.993	T46.994	T46.995	T46.996
Dioxane	T52.8X1	T52.8X2	T52.8X3	T52.8X4	—	—
Dioxathion	T60.0X1	T60.0X2	T60.0X3	T60.0X4	—	—
Dioxin	T53.7X1	T53.7X2	T53.7X3	T53.7X4	—	—
Dioxopromethazine	T43.3X1	T43.3X2	T43.3X3	T43.3X4	T43.3X5	T43.3X6
Dioxyline	T46.3X1	T46.3X2	T46.3X3	T46.3X4	T46.3X5	T46.3X6
Dipentene	T52.8X1	T52.8X2	T52.8X3	T52.8X4	—	—
Diperodon	T41.3X1	T41.3X2	T41.3X3	T41.3X4	T41.3X5	T41.3X6
Diphacinone	T60.4X1	T60.4X2	T60.4X3	T60.4X4	—	—
Diphemanil	T44.3X1	T44.3X2	T44.3X3	T44.3X4	T44.3X5	T44.3X6
metilsulfate	T44.3X1	T44.3X2	T44.3X3	T44.3X4	T44.3X5	T44.3X6
Diphenadione	T45.511	T45.512	T45.513	T45.514	T45.515	T45.516
rodenticide	T60.4X1	T60.4X2	T60.4X3	T60.4X4	—	—
Diphenhydramine	T45.0X1	T45.0X2	T45.0X3	T45.0X4	T45.0X5	T45.0X6
Diphenidol	T45.0X1	T45.0X2	T45.0X3	T45.0X4	T45.0X5	T45.0X6
Diphenoxylate	T47.6X1	T47.6X2	T47.6X3	T47.6X4	T47.6X5	T47.6X6
Diphenylamine	T65.3X1	T65.3X2	T65.3X3	T65.3X4	—	—
Diphenylbutazone	T39.2X1	T39.2X2	T39.2X3	T39.2X4	T39.2X5	T39.2X6
Diphenylchloroarsine, not in war	T57.0X1	T57.0X2	T57.0X3	T57.0X4	—	—
Diphenylhydantoin	T42.0X1	T42.0X2	T42.0X3	T42.0X4	T42.0X5	T42.0X6
Diphenylmethane dye	T52.1X1	T52.1X2	T52.1X3	T52.1X4	—	—
Diphenylpyraline	T45.0X1	T45.0X2	T45.0X3	T45.0X4	T45.0X5	T45.0X6
Diphtheria						
antitoxin	T50.Z11	T50.Z12	T50.Z13	T50.Z14	T50.Z15	T50.Z16
toxoid	T50.A91	T50.A92	T50.A93	T50.A94	T50.A95	T50.A96
with tetanus toxoid	T50.A21	T50.A22	T50.A23	T50.A24	T50.A25	T50.A26
with pertussis component	T50.A11	T50.A12	T50.A13	T50.A14	T50.A15	T50.A16

	External Cause (T-Code)					
Substance	Poisoning, Accidental (Unintentional)	Poisoning, Intentional Self-Harm	Poisoning, Assault	Poisoning, Undetermined	Adverse Effect	Underdosing
Diphtheria *(Continued)*						
vaccine (combination)	T50.A91	T50.A92	T50.A93	T50.A94	T50.A95	T50.A96
combination						
including pertussis	T50.A11	T50.A12	T50.A13	T50.A14	T50.A15	T50.A16
without pertussis	T50.A21	T50.A22	T50.A23	T50.A24	T50.A25	T50.A26
Diphylline	T50.2X1	T50.2X2	T50.2X3	T50.2X4	T50.2X5	T50.2X6
Dipipanone	T40.491	T40.492	T40.493	T40.494	—	—
Dipivefrine	T49.5X1	T49.5X2	T49.5X3	T49.5X4	T49.5X5	T49.5X6
Diplovax	T50.B91	T50.B92	T50.B93	T50.B94	T50.B95	T50.B96
Diprophylline	T50.2X1	T50.2X2	T50.2X3	T50.2X4	T50.2X5	T50.2X6
Dipropyline	T48.291	T48.292	T48.293	T48.294	T48.295	T48.296
Dipyridamole	T46.3X1	T46.3X2	T46.3X3	T46.3X4	T46.3X5	T46.3X6
Dipyrone	T39.2X1	T39.2X2	T39.2X3	T39.2X4	T39.2X5	T39.2X6
Diquat (dibromide)	T60.3X1	T60.3X2	T60.3X3	T60.3X4	—	—
Disinfectant	T65.891	T65.892	T65.893	T65.894	—	—
alkaline	T54.3X1	T54.3X2	T54.3X3	T54.3X4	—	—
aromatic	T54.1X1	T54.1X2	T54.1X3	T54.1X4	—	—
intestinal	T37.8X1	T37.8X2	T37.8X3	T37.8X4	T37.8X5	T37.8X6
Disipal	T42.8X1	T42.8X2	T42.8X3	T42.8X4	T42.8X5	T42.8X6
Disodium edetate	T50.6X1	T50.6X2	T50.6X3	T50.6X4	T50.6X5	T50.6X6
Disoprofol	T41.291	T41.292	T41.293	T41.294	T41.295	T41.296
Disopyramide	T46.2X1	T46.2X2	T46.2X3	T46.2X4	T46.2X5	T46.2X6
Distigmine (bromide)	T44.0X1	T44.0X2	T44.0X3	T44.0X4	T44.0X5	T44.0X6
Disulfamide	T50.2X1	T50.2X2	T50.2X3	T50.2X4	T50.2X5	T50.2X6
Disulfanilamide	T37.0X1	T37.0X2	T37.0X3	T37.0X4	T37.0X5	T37.0X6
Disulfiram	T50.6X1	T50.6X2	T50.6X3	T50.6X4	T50.6X5	T50.6X6
Disulfoton	T60.0X1	T60.0X2	T60.0X3	T60.0X4	—	—
Dithiazanine iodide	T37.4X1	T37.4X2	T37.4X3	T37.4X4	T37.4X5	T37.4X6
Dithiocarbamate	T60.0X1	T60.0X2	T60.0X3	T60.0X4	—	—
Dithranol	T49.4X1	T49.4X2	T49.4X3	T49.4X4	T49.4X5	T49.4X6
Diucardin	T50.2X1	T50.2X2	T50.2X3	T50.2X4	T50.2X5	T50.2X6
Diupres	T50.2X1	T50.2X2	T50.2X3	T50.2X4	T50.2X5	T50.2X6
Diuretic NEC	T50.2X1	T50.2X2	T50.2X3	T50.2X4	T50.2X5	T50.2X6
benzothiadiazine	T50.2X1	T50.2X2	T50.2X3	T50.2X4	T50.2X5	T50.2X6
carbonic acid anhydrase inhibitors	T50.2X1	T50.2X2	T50.2X3	T50.2X4	T50.2X5	T50.2X6
furfuryl NEC	T50.2X1	T50.2X2	T50.2X3	T50.2X4	T50.2X5	T50.2X6
loop (high-ceiling)	T50.1X1	T50.1X2	T50.1X3	T50.1X4	T50.1X5	T50.1X6
mercurial NEC	T50.2X1	T50.2X2	T50.2X3	T50.2X4	T50.2X5	T50.2X6
osmotic	T50.2X1	T50.2X2	T50.2X3	T50.2X4	T50.2X5	T50.2X6
purine NEC	T50.2X1	T50.2X2	T50.2X3	T50.2X4	T50.2X5	T50.2X6
saluretic NEC	T50.2X1	T50.2X2	T50.2X3	T50.2X4	T50.2X5	T50.2X6

◀ New ◀ Revised ~~deleted~~ Deleted

Substance	Poisoning, Accidental (Unintentional)	Poisoning, Intentional Self-Harm	Poisoning, Assault	Poisoning, Undetermined	Adverse Effect	Underdosing
Diuretic NEC *(Continued)*						
sulfonamide	T50.2X1	T50.2X2	T50.2X3	T50.2X4	T50.2X5	T50.2X6
thiazide NEC	T50.2X1	T50.2X2	T50.2X3	T50.2X4	T50.2X5	T50.2X6
xanthine	T50.2X1	T50.2X2	T50.2X3	T50.2X4	T50.2X5	T50.2X6
Diurgin	T50.2X1	T50.2X2	T50.2X3	T50.2X4	T50.2X5	T50.2X6
Diuril	T50.2X1	T50.2X2	T50.2X3	T50.2X4	T50.2X5	T50.2X6
Diuron	T60.3X1	T60.3X2	T60.3X3	T60.3X4	—	—
Divalproex	T42.6X1	T42.6X2	T42.6X3	T42.6X4	T42.6X5	T42.6X6
Divinyl ether	T41.0X1	T41.0X2	T41.0X3	T41.0X4	T41.0X5	T41.0X6
Dixanthogen	T49.0X1	T49.0X2	T49.0X3	T49.0X4	T49.0X5	T49.0X6
Dixyrazine	T43.3X1	T43.3X2	T43.3X3	T43.3X4	T43.3X5	T43.3X6
D-lysergic acid diethylamide	T40.8X1	T40.8X2	T40.8X3	T40.8X4	—	—
DMCT	T36.4X1	T36.4X2	T36.4X3	T36.4X4	T36.4X5	T36.4X6
DMSO — *see Dimethyl, sulfoxide*						
DNBP	T60.3X1	T60.3X2	T60.3X3	T60.3X4	—	—
DNOC	T65.3X1	T65.3X2	T65.3X3	T65.3X4	—	—
DOCA	T38.0X1	T38.0X2	T38.0X3	T38.0X4	T38.0X5	T38.0X6
Dobutamine	T44.5X1	T44.5X2	T44.5X3	T44.5X4	T44.5X5	T44.5X6
Docusate sodium	T47.4X1	T47.4X2	T47.4X3	T47.4X4	T47.4X5	T47.4X6
Dodicin	T49.0X1	T49.0X2	T49.0X3	T49.0X4	T49.0X5	T49.0X6
Dofamium chloride	T49.0X1	T49.0X2	T49.0X3	T49.0X4	T49.0X5	T49.0X6
Dolophine	T40.3X1	T40.3X2	T40.3X3	T40.3X4	T40.3X5	T40.3X6
Doloxene	T39.8X1	T39.8X2	T39.8X3	T39.8X4	T39.8X5	T39.8X6
Domestic gas (after combustion) — *see Gas, utility*						
prior to combustion	T59.891	T59.892	T59.893	T59.894	—	—
Domiodol	T48.4X1	T48.4X2	T48.4X3	T48.4X4	T48.4X5	T48.4X6
Domiphen (bromide)	T49.0X1	T49.0X2	T49.0X3	T49.0X4	T49.0X5	T49.0X6
Domperidone	T45.0X1	T45.0X2	T45.0X3	T45.0X4	T45.0X5	T45.0X6
Dopa	T42.8X1	T42.8X2	T42.8X3	T42.8X4	T42.8X5	T42.8X6
Dopamine	T44.991	T44.992	T44.993	T44.994	T44.995	T44.996
Doriden	T42.6X1	T42.6X2	T42.6X3	T42.6X4	T42.6X5	T42.6X6
Dormiral	T42.3X1	T42.3X2	T42.3X3	T42.3X4	T42.3X5	T42.3X6
Dormison	T42.6X1	T42.6X2	T42.6X3	T42.6X4	T42.6X5	T42.6X6
Dornase	T48.4X1	T48.4X2	T48.4X3	T48.4X4	T48.4X5	T48.4X6
Dorsacaine	T41.3X1	T41.3X2	T41.3X3	T41.3X4	T41.3X5	T41.3X6
Dosulepin	T43.011	T43.012	T43.013	T43.014	T43.015	T43.016
Dothiepin	T43.011	T43.012	T43.013	T43.014	T43.015	T43.016
Doxantrazole	T48.6X1	T48.6X2	T48.6X3	T48.6X4	T48.6X5	T48.6X6
Doxapram	T50.7X1	T50.7X2	T50.7X3	T50.7X4	T50.7X5	T50.7X6
Doxazosin	T44.6X1	T44.6X2	T44.6X3	T44.6X4	T44.6X5	T44.6X6
Doxepin	T43.011	T43.012	T43.013	T43.014	T43.015	T43.016
Doxifluridine	T45.1X1	T45.1X2	T45.1X3	T45.1X4	T45.1X5	T45.1X6
Doxorubicin	T45.1X1	T45.1X2	T45.1X3	T45.1X4	T45.1X5	T45.1X6
Doxycycline	T36.4X1	T36.4X2	T36.4X3	T36.4X4	T36.4X5	T36.4X6
Doxylamine	T45.0X1	T45.0X2	T45.0X3	T45.0X4	T45.0X5	T45.0X6
Dramamine	T45.0X1	T45.0X2	T45.0X3	T45.0X4	T45.0X5	T45.0X6
Drano (drain cleaner)	T54.3X1	T54.3X2	T54.3X3	T54.3X4	—	—
Dressing, live pulp	T49.7X1	T49.7X2	T49.7X3	T49.7X4	T49.7X5	T49.7X6
Drocode	T40.2X1	T40.2X2	T40.2X3	T40.2X4	T40.2X5	T40.2X6
Dromoran	T40.2X1	T40.2X2	T40.2X3	T40.2X4	T40.2X5	T40.2X6
Dromostanolone	T38.7X1	T38.7X2	T38.7X3	T38.7X4	T38.7X5	T38.7X6
Dronabinol	T40.711	T40.712	T40.713	T40.714	T40.715	T40.716
Droperidol	T43.591	T43.592	T43.593	T43.594	T43.595	T43.596
Dropropizine	T48.3X1	T48.3X2	T48.3X3	T48.3X4	T48.3X5	T48.3X6
Drostanolone	T38.7X1	T38.7X2	T38.7X3	T38.7X4	T38.7X5	T38.7X6
Drotaverine	T44.3X1	T44.3X2	T44.3X3	T44.3X4	T44.3X5	T44.3X6
Drotrecogin alfa	T45.511	T45.512	T45.513	T45.514	T45.515	T45.516
Drug NEC	T50.901	T50.902	T50.903	T50.904	T50.905	T50.906
specified NEC	T50.991	T50.992	T50.993	T50.994	T50.995	T50.996
DTIC	T45.1X1	T45.1X2	T45.1X3	T45.1X4	T45.1X5	T45.1X6
Duboisine	T44.3X1	T44.3X2	T44.3X3	T44.3X4	T44.3X5	T44.3X6
Dulcolax	T47.2X1	T47.2X2	T47.2X3	T47.2X4	T47.2X5	T47.2X6
Duponol (C) (EP)	T49.2X1	T49.2X2	T49.2X3	T49.2X4	T49.2X5	T49.2X6
Durabolin	T38.7X1	T38.7X2	T38.7X3	T38.7X4	T38.7X5	T38.7X6
Dyclone	T41.3X1	T41.3X2	T41.3X3	T41.3X4	T41.3X5	T41.3X6
Dyclonine	T41.3X1	T41.3X2	T41.3X3	T41.3X4	T41.3X5	T41.3X6
Dydrogesterone	T38.5X1	T38.5X2	T38.5X3	T38.5X4	T38.5X5	T38.5X6
Dye NEC	T65.6X1	T65.6X2	T65.6X3	T65.6X4	—	—
antiseptic	T49.0X1	T49.0X2	T49.0X3	T49.0X4	T49.0X5	T49.0X6
diagnostic agents	T50.8X1	T50.8X2	T50.8X3	T50.8X4	T50.8X5	T50.8X6
pharmaceutical NEC	T50.901	T50.902	T50.903	T50.904	T50.905	T50.906
Dyflos	T44.0X1	T44.0X2	T44.0X3	T44.0X4	T44.0X5	T44.0X6
Dymelor	T38.3X1	T38.3X2	T38.3X3	T38.3X4	T38.3X5	T38.3X6
Dynamite	T65.3X1	T65.3X2	T65.3X3	T65.3X4	—	—
fumes	T59.891	T59.892	T59.893	T59.894	—	—
Dyphylline	T44.3X1	T44.3X2	T44.3X3	T44.3X4	T44.3X5	T44.3X6
E						
Ear drug NEC	T49.6X1	T49.6X2	T49.6X3	T49.6X4	T49.6X5	T49.6X6
Ear preparations	T49.6X1	T49.6X2	T49.6X3	T49.6X4	T49.6X5	T49.6X6
Econazole	T49.0X1	T49.0X2	T49.0X3	T49.0X4	T49.0X5	T49.0X6
Ecothiopate iodide	T49.5X1	T49.5X2	T49.5X3	T49.5X4	T49.5X5	T49.5X6
Echothiophate, echothiopate, ecothiopate	T49.5X1	T49.5X2	T49.5X3	T49.5X4	T49.5X5	T49.5X6

	External Cause (T-Code)					
Substance	Poisoning, Accidental (Unintentional)	Poisoning, Intentional Self-Harm	Poisoning, Assault	Poisoning, Undetermined	Adverse Effect	Underdosing
Ecstasy	T43.641	T43.642	T43.643	T43.644	—	—
Ectylurea	T42.6X1	T42.6X2	T42.6X3	T42.6X4	T42.6X5	T42.6X6
Edathamil disodium	T45.8X1	T45.8X2	T45.8X3	T45.8X4	T45.8X5	T45.8X6
Edecrin	T50.1X1	T50.1X2	T50.1X3	T50.1X4	T50.1X5	T50.1X6
Edetate, disodium (calcium)	T45.8X1	T45.8X2	T45.8X3	T45.8X4	T45.8X5	T45.8X6
Edoxudine	T49.5X1	T49.5X2	T49.5X3	T49.5X4	T49.5X5	T49.5X6
Edrophonium	T44.0X1	T44.0X2	T44.0X3	T44.0X4	T44.0X5	T44.0X6
chloride	T44.0X1	T44.0X2	T44.0X3	T44.0X4	T44.0X5	T44.0X6
EDTA	T50.6X1	T50.6X2	T50.6X3	T50.6X4	T50.6X5	T50.6X6
Eflornithine	T37.2X1	T37.2X2	T37.2X3	T37.2X4	T37.2X5	T37.2X6
Efloxate	T46.3X1	T46.3X2	T46.3X3	T46.3X4	T46.3X5	T46.3X6
Elase	T49.8X1	T49.8X2	T49.8X3	T49.8X4	T49.8X5	T49.8X6
Elastase	T47.5X1	T47.5X2	T47.5X3	T47.5X4	T47.5X5	T47.5X6
Elaterium	T47.2X1	T47.2X2	T47.2X3	T47.2X4	T47.2X5	T47.2X6
Elcatonin	T50.991	T50.992	T50.993	T50.994	T50.995	T50.996
Elder	T62.2X1	T62.2X2	T62.2X3	T62.2X4	—	—
berry (unripe)	T62.1X1	T62.1X2	T62.1X3	T62.1X4	—	—
Electrolyte balance drug	T50.3X1	T50.3X2	T50.3X3	T50.3X4	T50.3X5	T50.3X6
Electrolytes NEC	T50.3X1	T50.3X2	T50.3X3	T50.3X4	T50.3X5	T50.3X6
Electrolytic agent NEC	T50.3X1	T50.3X2	T50.3X3	T50.3X4	T50.3X5	T50.3X6
Elemental diet	T50.901	T50.902	T50.903	T50.904	T50.905	T50.906
Elliptinium acetate	T45.1X1	T45.1X2	T45.1X3	T45.1X4	T45.1X5	T45.1X6
Embramine	T45.0X1	T45.0X2	T45.0X3	T45.0X4	T45.0X5	T45.0X6
Emepronium (salts)	T44.3X1	T44.3X2	T44.3X3	T44.3X4	T44.3X5	T44.3X6
bromide	T44.3X1	T44.3X2	T44.3X3	T44.3X4	T44.3X5	T44.3X6
Emetic NEC	T47.7X1	T47.7X2	T47.7X3	T47.7X4	T47.7X5	T47.7X6
Emetine	T37.3X1	T37.3X2	T37.3X3	T37.3X4	T37.3X5	T37.3X6
Emollient NEC	T49.3X1	T49.3X2	T49.3X3	T49.3X4	T49.3X5	T49.3X6
Emorfazone	T39.8X1	T39.8X2	T39.8X3	T39.8X4	T39.8X5	T39.8X6
Emylcamate	T43.591	T43.592	T43.593	T43.594	T43.595	T43.596
Enalapril	T46.4X1	T46.4X2	T46.4X3	T46.4X4	T46.4X5	T46.4X6
Enalaprilat	T46.4X1	T46.4X2	T46.4X3	T46.4X4	T46.4X5	T46.4X6
Encainide	T46.2X1	T46.2X2	T46.2X3	T46.2X4	T46.2X5	T46.2X6
Endocaine	T41.3X1	T41.3X2	T41.3X3	T41.3X4	T41.3X5	T41.3X6
Endosulfan	T60.2X1	T60.2X2	T60.2X3	T60.2X4	—	—
Endothall	T60.3X1	T60.3X2	T60.3X3	T60.3X4	—	—
Endralazine	T46.5X1	T46.5X2	T46.5X3	T46.5X4	T46.5X5	T46.5X6
Endrin	T60.1X1	T60.1X2	T60.1X3	T60.1X4	—	—
Enflurane	T41.0X1	T41.0X2	T41.0X3	T41.0X4	T41.0X5	T41.0X6
Enhexymal	T42.3X1	T42.3X2	T42.3X3	T42.3X4	T42.3X5	T42.3X6
Enocitabine	T45.1X1	T45.1X2	T45.1X3	T45.1X4	T45.1X5	T45.1X6
Enovid	T38.4X1	T38.4X2	T38.4X3	T38.4X4	T38.4X5	T38.4X6

	External Cause (T-Code)					
Substance	Poisoning, Accidental (Unintentional)	Poisoning, Intentional Self-Harm	Poisoning, Assault	Poisoning, Undetermined	Adverse Effect	Underdosing
Enoxacin	T36.8X1	T36.8X2	T36.8X3	T36.8X4	T36.8X5	T36.8X6
Enoxaparin (sodium)	T45.511	T45.512	T45.513	T45.514	T45.515	T45.516
Enpiprazole	T43.591	T43.592	T43.593	T43.594	T43.595	T43.596
Enprofylline	T48.6X1	T48.6X2	T48.6X3	T48.6X4	T48.6X5	T48.6X6
Enprostil	T47.1X1	T47.1X2	T47.1X3	T47.1X4	T47.1X5	T47.1X6
ENT preparations (anti-infectives)	T49.6X1	T49.6X2	T49.6X3	T49.6X4	T49.6X5	T49.6X6
Enviomycin	T36.8X1	T36.8X2	T36.8X3	T36.8X4	T36.8X5	T36.8X6
Enzodase	T45.3X1	T45.3X2	T45.3X3	T45.3X4	T45.3X5	T45.3X6
Enzyme NEC	T45.3X1	T45.3X2	T45.3X3	T45.3X4	T45.3X5	T45.3X6
depolymerizing	T49.8X1	T49.8X2	T49.8X3	T49.8X4	T49.8X5	T49.8X6
fibrolytic	T45.3X1	T45.3X2	T45.3X3	T45.3X4	T45.3X5	T45.3X6
gastric	T47.5X1	T47.5X2	T47.5X3	T47.5X4	T47.5X5	T47.5X6
intestinal	T47.5X1	T47.5X2	T47.5X3	T47.5X4	T47.5X5	T47.5X6
local action	T49.4X1	T49.4X2	T49.4X3	T49.4X4	T49.4X5	T49.4X6
proteolytic	T49.4X1	T49.4X2	T49.4X3	T49.4X4	T49.4X5	T49.4X6
thrombolytic	T45.3X1	T45.3X2	T45.3X3	T45.3X4	T45.3X5	T45.3X6
EPAB	T41.3X1	T41.3X2	T41.3X3	T41.3X4	T41.3X5	T41.3X6
Epanutin	T42.0X1	T42.0X2	T42.0X3	T42.0X4	T42.0X5	T42.0X6
Ephedra	T44.991	T44.992	T44.993	T44.994	T44.995	T44.996
Ephedrine	T44.991	T44.992	T44.993	T44.994	T44.995	T44.996
Epichlorhydrin, epichlorohydrin	T52.8X1	T52.8X2	T52.8X3	T52.8X4	—	—
Epicillin	T36.0X1	T36.0X2	T36.0X3	T36.0X4	T36.0X5	T36.0X6
Epiestriol	T38.5X1	T38.5X2	T38.5X3	T38.5X4	T38.5X5	T38.5X6
Epilim — see Sodium, valproate						
Epimestrol	T38.5X1	T38.5X2	T38.5X3	T38.5X4	T38.5X5	T38.5X6
Epinephrine	T44.5X1	T44.5X2	T44.5X3	T44.5X4	T44.5X5	T44.5X6
Epirubicin	T45.1X1	T45.1X2	T45.1X3	T45.1X4	T45.1X5	T45.1X6
Epitiostanol	T38.7X1	T38.7X2	T38.7X3	T38.7X4	T38.7X5	T38.7X6
Epitizide	T50.2X1	T50.2X2	T50.2X3	T50.2X4	T50.2X5	T50.2X6
EPN	T60.0X1	T60.0X2	T60.0X3	T60.0X4	—	—
EPO	T45.8X1	T45.8X2	T45.8X3	T45.8X4	T45.8X5	T45.8X6
Epoetin alpha	T45.8X1	T45.8X2	T45.8X3	T45.8X4	T45.8X5	T45.8X6
Epomediol	T50.991	T50.992	T50.993	T50.994	T50.995	T50.996
Epoprostenol	T45.521	T45.522	T45.523	T45.524	T45.525	T45.526
Epoxy resin	T65.891	T65.892	T65.893	T65.894	—	—
Eprazinone	T48.4X1	T48.4X2	T48.4X3	T48.4X4	T48.4X5	T48.4X6
Epsilon amino-caproic acid	T45.621	T45.622	T45.623	T45.624	T45.625	T45.626
Epsom salt	T47.3X1	T47.3X2	T47.3X3	T47.3X4	T47.3X5	T47.3X6
Eptazocine	T40.491	T40.492	T40.493	T40.494	T40.495	T40.496
Equanil	T43.591	T43.592	T43.593	T43.594	T43.595	T43.596
Equisetum	T62.2X1	T62.2X2	T62.2X3	T62.2X4	—	—
diuretic	T50.2X1	T50.2X2	T50.2X3	T50.2X4	T50.2X5	T50.2X6

◀ New   ◀ Revised   ~~deleted~~ Deleted

Substance	Poisoning, Accidental (Unintentional)	Poisoning, Intentional Self-Harm	Poisoning, Assault	Poisoning, Undetermined	Adverse Effect	Underdosing
Ergobasine	T48.0X1	T48.0X2	T48.0X3	T48.0X4	T48.0X5	T48.0X6
Ergocalciferol	T45.2X1	T45.2X2	T45.2X3	T45.2X4	T45.2X5	T45.2X6
Ergoloid mesylates	T46.7X1	T46.7X2	T46.7X3	T46.7X4	T46.7X5	T46.7X6
Ergometrine	T48.0X1	T48.0X2	T48.0X3	T48.0X4	T48.0X5	T48.0X6
Ergonovine	T48.0X1	T48.0X2	T48.0X3	T48.0X4	T48.0X5	T48.0X6
Ergot NEC	T64.81	T64.82	T64.83	T64.84	—	—
derivative	T48.0X1	T48.0X2	T48.0X3	T48.0X4	T48.0X5	T48.0X6
medicinal (alkaloids)	T48.0X1	T48.0X2	T48.0X3	T48.0X4	T48.0X5	T48.0X6
prepared	T48.0X1	T48.0X2	T48.0X3	T48.0X4	T48.0X5	T48.0X6
Ergotamine	T46.5X1	T46.5X2	T46.5X3	T46.5X4	T46.5X5	T46.5X6
Ergotocine	T48.0X1	T48.0X2	T48.0X3	T48.0X4	T48.0X5	T48.0X6
Ergotrate	T48.0X1	T48.0X2	T48.0X3	T48.0X4	T48.0X5	T48.0X6
Eritrityl tetranitrate	T46.3X1	T46.3X2	T46.3X3	T46.3X4	T46.3X5	T46.3X6
Erythrityl tetranitrate	T46.3X1	T46.3X2	T46.3X3	T46.3X4	T46.3X5	T46.3X6
Erythrol tetranitrate	T46.3X1	T46.3X2	T46.3X3	T46.3X4	T46.3X5	T46.3X6
Erythromycin (salts)	T36.3X1	T36.3X2	T36.3X3	T36.3X4	T36.3X5	T36.3X6
ophthalmic preparation	T49.5X1	T49.5X2	T49.5X3	T49.5X4	T49.5X5	T49.5X6
topical NEC	T49.0X1	T49.0X2	T49.0X3	T49.0X4	T49.0X5	T49.0X6
Erythropoietin	T45.8X1	T45.8X2	T45.8X3	T45.8X4	T45.8X5	T45.8X6
human	T45.8X1	T45.8X2	T45.8X3	T45.8X4	T45.8X5	T45.8X6
Escin	T46.991	T46.992	T46.993	T46.994	T46.995	T46.996
Esculin	T45.2X1	T45.2X2	T45.2X3	T45.2X4	T45.2X5	T45.2X6
Esculoside	T45.2X1	T45.2X2	T45.2X3	T45.2X4	T45.2X5	T45.2X6
ESDT (ether-soluble tar distillate)	T49.1X1	T49.1X2	T49.1X3	T49.1X4	T49.1X5	T49.1X6
Eserine	T49.5X1	T49.5X2	T49.5X3	T49.5X4	T49.5X5	T49.5X6
Esflurbiprofen	T39.311	T39.312	T39.313	T39.314	T39.315	T39.316
Eskabarb	T42.3X1	T42.3X2	T42.3X3	T42.3X4	T42.3X5	T42.3X6
Eskalith	T43.8X1	T43.8X2	T43.8X3	T43.8X4	T43.8X5	T43.8X6
Esmolol	T44.7X1	T44.7X2	T44.7X3	T44.7X4	T44.7X5	T44.7X6
Estanozolol	T38.7X1	T38.7X2	T38.7X3	T38.7X4	T38.7X5	T38.7X6
Estazolam	T42.4X1	T42.4X2	T42.4X3	T42.4X4	T42.4X5	T42.4X6
Estradiol	T38.5X1	T38.5X2	T38.5X3	T38.5X4	T38.5X5	T38.5X6
with testosterone	T38.7X1	T38.7X2	T38.7X3	T38.7X4	T38.7X5	T38.7X6
benzoate	T38.5X1	T38.5X2	T38.5X3	T38.5X4	T38.5X5	T38.5X6
Estramustine	T45.1X1	T45.1X2	T45.1X3	T45.1X4	T45.1X5	T45.1X6
Estriol	T38.5X1	T38.5X2	T38.5X3	T38.5X4	T38.5X5	T38.5X6
Estrogen	T38.5X1	T38.5X2	T38.5X3	T38.5X4	T38.5X5	T38.5X6
with progesterone	T38.5X1	T38.5X2	T38.5X3	T38.5X4	T38.5X5	T38.5X6
conjugated	T38.5X1	T38.5X2	T38.5X3	T38.5X4	T38.5X5	T38.5X6
Estrone	T38.5X1	T38.5X2	T38.5X3	T38.5X4	T38.5X5	T38.5X6
Estropipate	T38.5X1	T38.5X2	T38.5X3	T38.5X4	T38.5X5	T38.5X6

Substance	Poisoning, Accidental (Unintentional)	Poisoning, Intentional Self-Harm	Poisoning, Assault	Poisoning, Undetermined	Adverse Effect	Underdosing
Etacrynate sodium	T50.1X1	T50.1X2	T50.1X3	T50.1X4	T50.1X5	T50.1X6
Etacrynic acid	T50.1X1	T50.1X2	T50.1X3	T50.1X4	T50.1X5	T50.1X6
Etafedrine	T48.6X1	T48.6X2	T48.6X3	T48.6X4	T48.6X5	T48.6X6
Etafenone	T46.3X1	T46.3X2	T46.3X3	T46.3X4	T46.3X5	T46.3X6
Etambutol	T37.1X1	T37.1X2	T37.1X3	T37.1X4	T37.1X5	T37.1X6
Etamiphyllin	T48.6X1	T48.6X2	T48.6X3	T48.6X4	T48.6X5	T48.6X6
Etamivan	T50.7X1	T50.7X2	T50.7X3	T50.7X4	T50.7X5	T50.7X6
Etamsylate	T45.7X1	T45.7X2	T45.7X3	T45.7X4	T45.7X5	T45.7X6
Etebenecid	T50.4X1	T50.4X2	T50.4X3	T50.4X4	T50.4X5	T50.4X6
Ethacridine	T49.0X1	T49.0X2	T49.0X3	T49.0X4	T49.0X5	T49.0X6
Ethacrynic acid	T50.1X1	T50.1X2	T50.1X3	T50.1X4	T50.1X5	T50.1X6
Ethadione	T42.2X1	T42.2X2	T42.2X3	T42.2X4	T42.2X5	T42.2X6
Ethambutol	T37.1X1	T37.1X2	T37.1X3	T37.1X4	T37.1X5	T37.1X6
Ethamide	T50.2X1	T50.2X2	T50.2X3	T50.2X4	T50.2X5	T50.2X6
Ethamivan	T50.7X1	T50.7X2	T50.7X3	T50.7X4	T50.7X5	T50.7X6
Ethamsylate	T45.7X1	T45.7X2	T45.7X3	T45.7X4	T45.7X5	T45.7X6
Ethanol	T51.0X1	T51.0X2	T51.0X3	T51.0X4	—	—
beverage	T51.0X1	T51.0X2	T51.0X3	T51.0X4	—	—
Ethanolamine oleate	T46.8X1	T46.8X2	T46.8X3	T46.8X4	T46.8X5	T46.8X6
Ethaverine	T44.3X1	T44.3X2	T44.3X3	T44.3X4	T44.3X5	T44.3X6
Ethchlorvynol	T42.6X1	T42.6X2	T42.6X3	T42.6X4	T42.6X5	T42.6X6
Ethebenecid	T50.4X1	T50.4X2	T50.4X3	T50.4X4	T50.4X5	T50.4X6
Ether (vapor)	T41.0X1	T41.0X2	T41.0X3	T41.0X4	T41.0X5	T41.0X6
anesthetic	T41.0X1	T41.0X2	T41.0X3	T41.0X4	T41.0X5	T41.0X6
divinyl	T41.0X1	T41.0X2	T41.0X3	T41.0X4	T41.0X5	T41.0X6
ethyl (medicinal)	T41.0X1	T41.0X2	T41.0X3	T41.0X4	T41.0X5	T41.0X6
nonmedicinal	T52.8X1	T52.8X2	T52.8X3	T52.8X4	—	—
petroleum—see Ligroin						
solvent	T52.8X1	T52.8X2	T52.8X3	T52.8X4	—	—
Ethiazide	T50.2X1	T50.2X2	T50.2X3	T50.2X4	T50.2X5	T50.2X6
Ethidium chloride (vapor)	T59.891	T59.892	T59.893	T59.894	—	—
Ethinamate	T42.6X1	T42.6X2	T42.6X3	T42.6X4	T42.6X5	T42.6X6
Ethinylestradiol, ethinyloestradiol	T38.5X1	T38.5X2	T38.5X3	T38.5X4	T38.5X5	T38.5X6
with						
levonorgestrel	T38.4X1	T38.4X2	T38.4X3	T38.4X4	T38.4X5	T38.4X6
norethisterone	T38.4X1	T38.4X2	T38.4X3	T38.4X4	T38.4X5	T38.4X6
Ethiodized oil (131 I)	T50.8X1	T50.8X2	T50.8X3	T50.8X4	T50.8X5	T50.8X6
Ethion	T60.0X1	T60.0X2	T60.0X3	T60.0X4	—	—
Ethionamide	T37.1X1	T37.1X2	T37.1X3	T37.1X4	T37.1X5	T37.1X6
Ethioniamide	T37.1X1	T37.1X2	T37.1X3	T37.1X4	T37.1X5	T37.1X6
Ethisterone	T38.5X1	T38.5X2	T38.5X3	T38.5X4	T38.5X5	T38.5X6
Ethobral	T42.3X1	T42.3X2	T42.3X3	T42.3X4	T42.3X5	T42.3X6

TABLE OF DRUGS AND CHEMICALS

Substance	External Cause (T-Code) Poisoning, Accidental (Unintentional)	Poisoning, Intentional Self-Harm	Poisoning, Assault	Poisoning, Undetermined	Adverse Effect	Underdosing
Ethocaine (infiltration) (topical)	T41.3X1	T41.3X2	T41.3X3	T41.3X4	T41.3X5	T41.3X6
nerve block (peripheral) (plexus)	T41.3X1	T41.3X2	T41.3X3	T41.3X4	T41.3X5	T41.3X6
spinal	T41.3X1	T41.3X2	T41.3X3	T41.3X4	T41.3X5	T41.3X6
Ethoheptazine	T40.491	T40.492	T40.493	T40.494	T40.495	T40.496
Ethopropazine	T44.3X1	T44.3X2	T44.3X3	T44.3X4	T44.3X5	T44.3X6
Ethosuximide	T42.2X1	T42.2X2	T42.2X3	T42.2X4	T42.2X5	T42.2X6
Ethotoin	T42.0X1	T42.0X2	T42.0X3	T42.0X4	T42.0X5	T42.0X6
Ethoxazene	T37.91	T37.92	T37.93	T37.94	T37.95	T37.96
Ethoxazorutoside	T46.991	T46.992	T46.993	T46.994	T46.995	T46.996
2-Ethoxyethanol	T52.3X1	T52.3X2	T52.3X3	T52.3X4	—	—
Ethoxzolamide	T50.2X1	T50.2X2	T50.2X3	T50.2X4	T50.2X5	T50.2X6
Ethyl						
acetate	T52.8X1	T52.8X2	T52.8X3	T52.8X4	—	—
alcohol	T51.0X1	T51.0X2	T51.0X3	T51.0X4	—	—
beverage	T51.0X1	T51.0X2	T51.0X3	T51.0X4	—	—
aldehyde (vapor)	T59.891	T59.892	T59.893	T59.894	—	—
liquid	T52.8X1	T52.8X2	T52.8X3	T52.8X4		
aminobenzoate	T41.3X1	T41.3X2	T41.3X3	T41.3X4	T41.3X5	T41.3X6
aminophenothiazine	T43.3X1	T43.3X2	T43.3X3	T43.3X4	T43.3X5	T43.3X6
benzoate	T52.8X1	T52.8X2	T52.8X3	T52.8X4	—	—
biscoumacetate	T45.511	T45.512	T45.513	T45.514	T45.515	T45.516
bromide (anesthetic)	T41.0X1	T41.0X2	T41.0X3	T41.0X4	T41.0X5	T41.0X6
carbamate	T45.1X1	T45.1X2	T45.1X3	T45.1X4	T45.1X5	T45.1X6
carbinol	T51.3X1	T51.3X2	T51.3X3	T51.3X4	—	—
carbonate	T52.8X1	T52.8X2	T52.8X3	T52.8X4	—	—
chaulmoograte	T37.1X1	T37.1X2	T37.1X3	T37.1X4	T37.1X5	T37.1X6
chloride (anesthetic)	T41.0X1	T41.0X2	T41.0X3	T41.0X4	T41.0X5	T41.0X6
anesthetic (local)	T41.3X1	T41.3X2	T41.3X3	T41.3X4	T41.3X5	T41.3X6
inhaled	T41.0X1	T41.0X2	T41.0X3	T41.0X4	T41.0X5	T41.0X6
local	T49.4X1	T49.4X2	T49.4X3	T49.4X4	T49.4X5	T49.4X6
solvent	T53.6X1	T53.6X2	T53.6X3	T53.6X4	—	—
dibunate	T48.3X1	T48.3X2	T48.3X3	T48.3X4	T48.3X5	T48.3X6
dichloroarsine (vapor)	T57.0X1	T57.0X2	T57.0X3	T57.0X4	—	—
estranol	T38.7X1	T38.7X2	T38.7X3	T38.7X4	T38.7X5	T38.7X6
ether — see also Ether	T52.8X1	T52.8X2	T52.8X3	T52.8X4	—	—
formate NEC (solvent)	T52.0X1	T52.0X2	T52.0X3	T52.0X4	—	—
fumarate	T49.4X1	T49.4X2	T49.4X3	T49.4X4	T49.4X5	T49.4X6
hydroxyisobutyrate NEC (solvent)	T52.8X1	T52.8X2	T52.8X3	T52.8X4	—	—
iodoacetate	T59.3X1	T59.3X2	T59.3X3	T59.3X4	—	—
lactate NEC (solvent)	T52.8X1	T52.8X2	T52.8X3	T52.8X4	—	—
loflazepate	T42.4X1	T42.4X2	T42.4X3	T42.4X4	T42.4X5	T42.4X6

Substance	External Cause (T-Code) Poisoning, Accidental (Unintentional)	Poisoning, Intentional Self-Harm	Poisoning, Assault	Poisoning, Undetermined	Adverse Effect	Underdosing
Ethyl (Continued)						
mercuric chloride	T56.1X1	T56.1X2	T56.1X3	T56.1X4	—	—
methylcarbinol	T51.8X1	T51.8X2	T51.8X3	T51.8X4	—	—
morphine	T40.2X1	T40.2X2	T40.2X3	T40.2X4	T40.2X5	T40.2X6
noradrenaline	T48.6X1	T48.6X2	T48.6X3	T48.6X4	T48.6X5	T48.6X6
oxybutyrate NEC (solvent)	T52.8X1	T52.8X2	T52.8X3	T52.8X4	—	—
Ethylene (gas)	T59.891	T59.892	T59.893	T59.894		
anesthetic (general)	T41.0X1	T41.0X2	T41.0X3	T41.0X4	T41.0X5	T41.0X6
chlorohydrin	T52.8X1	T52.8X2	T52.8X3	T52.8X4	—	—
vapor	T53.6X1	T53.6X2	T53.6X3	T53.6X4	—	—
dichloride	T52.8X1	T52.8X2	T52.8X3	T52.8X4	—	—
vapor	T53.6X1	T53.6X2	T53.6X3	T53.6X4	—	—
dinitrate	T52.3X1	T52.3X2	T52.3X3	T52.3X4		
glycol(s)	T52.8X1	T52.8X2	T52.8X3	T52.8X4		
dinitrate	T52.3X1	T52.3X2	T52.3X3	T52.3X4		
monobutyl ether	T52.3X1	T52.3X2	T52.3X3	T52.3X4		
imine	T54.1X1	T54.1X2	T54.1X3	T54.1X4		
oxide (fumigant) (nonmedicinal)	T59.891	T59.892	T59.893	T59.894	—	—
medicinal	T49.0X1	T49.0X2	T49.0X3	T49.0X4	T49.0X5	T49.0X6
Ethylenediamine theophylline	T48.6X1	T48.6X2	T48.6X3	T48.6X4	T48.6X5	T48.6X6
Ethylenediaminetetra-acetic acid	T50.6X1	T50.6X2	T50.6X3	T50.6X4	T50.6X5	T50.6X6
Ethylenedinitrilotetra-acetate	T50.6X1	T50.6X2	T50.6X3	T50.6X4	T50.6X5	T50.6X6
Ethylestrenol	T38.7X1	T38.7X2	T38.7X3	T38.7X4	T38.7X5	T38.7X6
Ethylhydroxycellulose	T47.4X1	T47.4X2	T47.4X3	T47.4X4	T47.4X5	T47.4X6
Ethylidene						
chloride NEC	T53.6X1	T53.6X2	T53.6X3	T53.6X4	—	—
diacetate	T60.3X1	T60.3X2	T60.3X3	T60.3X4	—	—
dicoumarin	T45.511	T45.512	T45.513	T45.514	T45.515	T45.516
dicoumarol	T45.511	T45.512	T45.513	T45.514	T45.515	T45.516
diethyl ether	T52.0X1	T52.0X2	T52.0X3	T52.0X4	—	—
Ethylmorphine	T40.2X1	T40.2X2	T40.2X3	T40.2X4	T40.2X5	T40.2X6
Ethylnorepinephrine	T48.6X1	T48.6X2	T48.6X3	T48.6X4	T48.6X5	T48.6X6
Ethylparachlorophen-oxyisobutyrate	T46.6X1	T46.6X2	T46.6X3	T46.6X4	T46.6X5	T46.6X6
Ethynodiol	T38.4X1	T38.4X2	T38.4X3	T38.4X4	T38.4X5	T38.4X6
with mestranol diacetate	T38.4X1	T38.4X2	T38.4X3	T38.4X4	T38.4X5	T38.4X6
Etidocaine	T41.3X1	T41.3X2	T41.3X3	T41.3X4	T41.3X5	T41.3X6
infiltration (subcutaneous)	T41.3X1	T41.3X2	T41.3X3	T41.3X4	T41.3X5	T41.3X6
nerve (peripheral) (plexus)	T41.3X1	T41.3X2	T41.3X3	T41.3X4	T41.3X5	T41.3X6
Etidronate	T50.991	T50.992	T50.993	T50.994	T50.995	T50.996
Etidronic acid (disodium salt)	T50.991	T50.992	T50.993	T50.994	T50.995	T50.996
Etifoxine	T42.6X1	T42.6X2	T42.6X3	T42.6X4	T42.6X5	T42.6X6

◀ New ◀ Revised ~~deleted~~ Deleted

Substance	Poisoning, Accidental (Unintentional)	Poisoning, Intentional Self-Harm	Poisoning, Assault	Poisoning, Undetermined	Adverse Effect	Underdosing
Etilefrine	T44.4X1	T44.4X2	T44.4X3	T44.4X4	T44.4X5	T44.4X6
Etilfen	T42.3X1	T42.3X2	T42.3X3	T42.3X4	T42.3X5	T42.3X6
Etinodiol	T38.4X1	T38.4X2	T38.4X3	T38.4X4	T38.4X5	T38.4X6
Etiroxate	T46.6X1	T46.6X2	T46.6X3	T46.6X4	T46.6X5	T46.6X6
Etizolam	T42.4X1	T42.4X2	T42.4X3	T42.4X4	T42.4X5	T42.4X6
Etodolac	T39.391	T39.392	T39.393	T39.394	T39.395	T39.396
Etofamide	T37.3X1	T37.3X2	T37.3X3	T37.3X4	T37.3X5	T37.3X6
Etofibrate	T46.6X1	T46.6X2	T46.6X3	T46.6X4	T46.6X5	T46.6X6
Etofylline	T46.7X1	T46.7X2	T46.7X3	T46.7X4	T46.7X5	T46.7X6
clofibrate	T46.6X1	T46.6X2	T46.6X3	T46.6X4	T46.6X5	T46.6X6
Etoglucid	T45.1X1	T45.1X2	T45.1X3	T45.1X4	T45.1X5	T45.1X6
Etomidate	T41.1X1	T41.1X2	T41.1X3	T41.1X4	T41.1X5	T41.1X6
Etomide	T39.8X1	T39.8X2	T39.8X3	T39.8X4	T39.8X5	T39.8X6
Etomidoline	T44.3X1	T44.3X2	T44.3X3	T44.3X4	T44.3X5	T44.3X6
Etoposide	T45.1X1	T45.1X2	T45.1X3	T45.1X4	T45.1X5	T45.1X6
Etorphine	T40.2X1	T40.2X2	T40.2X3	T40.2X4	T40.2X5	T40.2X6
Etoval	T42.3X1	T42.3X2	T42.3X3	T42.3X4	T42.3X5	T42.3X6
Etozolin	T50.1X1	T50.1X2	T50.1X3	T50.1X4	T50.1X5	T50.1X6
Etretinate	T50.991	T50.992	T50.993	T50.994	T50.995	T50.996
Etryptamine	T43.691	T43.692	T43.693	T43.694	T43.695	T43.696
Etybenzatropine	T44.3X1	T44.3X2	T44.3X3	T44.3X4	T44.3X5	T44.3X6
Etynodiol	T38.4X1	T38.4X2	T38.4X3	T38.4X4	T38.4X5	T38.4X6
Eucaine	T41.3X1	T41.3X2	T41.3X3	T41.3X4	T41.3X5	T41.3X6
Eucalyptus oil	T49.7X1	T49.7X2	T49.7X3	T49.7X4	T49.7X5	T49.7X6
Eucatropine	T49.5X1	T49.5X2	T49.5X3	T49.5X4	T49.5X5	T49.5X6
Eucodal	T40.2X1	T40.2X2	T40.2X3	T40.2X4	T40.2X5	T40.2X6
Euneryl	T42.3X1	T42.3X2	T42.3X3	T42.3X4	T42.3X5	T42.3X6
Euphthalmine	T44.3X1	T44.3X2	T44.3X3	T44.3X4	T44.3X5	T44.3X6
Eurax	T49.0X1	T49.0X2	T49.0X3	T49.0X4	T49.0X5	T49.0X6
Euresol	T49.4X1	T49.4X2	T49.4X3	T49.4X4	T49.4X5	T49.4X6
Euthroid	T38.1X1	T38.1X2	T38.1X3	T38.1X4	T38.1X5	T38.1X6
Evans blue	T50.8X1	T50.8X2	T50.8X3	T50.8X4	T50.8X5	T50.8X6
Evipal	T42.3X1	T42.3X2	T42.3X3	T42.3X4	T42.3X5	T42.3X6
sodium	T41.1X1	T41.1X2	T41.1X3	T41.1X4	T41.1X5	T41.1X6
Evipan	T42.3X1	T42.3X2	T42.3X3	T42.3X4	T42.3X5	T42.3X6
sodium	T41.1X1	T41.1X2	T41.1X3	T41.1X4	T41.1X5	T41.1X6
Exalamide	T49.0X1	T49.0X2	T49.0X3	T49.0X4	T49.0X5	T49.0X6
Exalgin	T39.1X1	T39.1X2	T39.1X3	T39.1X4	T39.1X5	T39.1X6
Excipients, pharmaceutical	T50.901	T50.902	T50.903	T50.904	T50.905	T50.906
Exhaust gas (engine) (motor vehicle)	T58.01	T58.02	T58.03	T58.04	—	—
Ex-Lax (phenolphthalein)	T47.2X1	T47.2X2	T47.2X3	T47.2X4	T47.2X5	T47.2X6
Expectorant NEC	T48.4X1	T48.4X2	T48.4X3	T48.4X4	T48.4X5	T48.4X6

Substance	Poisoning, Accidental (Unintentional)	Poisoning, Intentional Self-Harm	Poisoning, Assault	Poisoning, Undetermined	Adverse Effect	Underdosing
Extended insulin zinc suspension	T38.3X1	T38.3X2	T38.3X3	T38.3X4	T38.3X5	T38.3X6
External medications (skin) (mucous membrane)	T49.91	T49.92	T49.93	T49.94	T49.95	T49.96
dental agent	T49.7X1	T49.7X2	T49.7X3	T49.7X4	T49.7X5	T49.7X6
ENT agent	T49.6X1	T49.6X2	T49.6X3	T49.6X4	T49.6X5	T49.6X6
ophthalmic preparation	T49.5X1	T49.5X2	T49.5X3	T49.5X4	T49.5X5	T49.5X6
specified NEC	T49.8X1	T49.8X2	T49.8X3	T49.8X4	T49.8X5	T49.8X6
Extrapyramidal antagonist NEC	T44.3X1	T44.3X2	T44.3X3	T44.3X4	T44.3X5	T44.3X6
Eye agents (anti-infective)	T49.5X1	T49.5X2	T49.5X3	T49.5X4	T49.5X5	T49.5X6
Eye drug NEC	T49.5X1	T49.5X2	T49.5X3	T49.5X4	T49.5X5	T49.5X6
F						
FAC (fluorouracil + doxorubicin + cyclophosphamide)	T45.1X1	T45.1X2	T45.1X3	T45.1X4	T45.1X5	T45.1X6
Factor						
I (fibrinogen)	T45.8X1	T45.8X2	T45.8X3	T45.8X4	T45.8X5	T45.8X6
III (thromboplastin)	T45.8X1	T45.8X2	T45.8X3	T45.8X4	T45.8X5	T45.8X6
VIII (antihemophilic Factor) (Concentrate)	T45.8X1	T45.8X2	T45.8X3	T45.8X4	T45.8X5	T45.8X6
IX complex	T45.7X1	T45.7X2	T45.7X3	T45.7X4	T45.7X5	T45.7X6
human	T45.8X1	T45.8X2	T45.8X3	T45.8X4	T45.8X5	T45.8X6
Famotidine	T47.0X1	T47.0X2	T47.0X3	T47.0X4	T47.0X5	T47.0X6
Fat suspension, intravenous	T50.991	T50.992	T50.993	T50.994	T50.995	T50.996
Fazadinium bromide	T48.1X1	T48.1X2	T48.1X3	T48.1X4	T48.1X5	T48.1X6
Febarbamate	T42.3X1	T42.3X2	T42.3X3	T42.3X4	T42.3X5	T42.3X6
Fecal softener	T47.4X1	T47.4X2	T47.4X3	T47.4X4	T47.4X5	T47.4X6
Fedrilate	T48.3X1	T48.3X2	T48.3X3	T48.3X4	T48.3X5	T48.3X6
Felodipine	T46.1X1	T46.1X2	T46.1X3	T46.1X4	T46.1X5	T46.1X6
Felypressin	T38.891	T38.892	T38.893	T38.894	T38.895	T38.896
Femoxetine	T43.221	T43.222	T43.223	T43.224	T43.225	T43.226
Fenalcomine	T46.3X1	T46.3X2	T46.3X3	T46.3X4	T46.3X5	T46.3X6
Fenamisal	T37.1X1	T37.1X2	T37.1X3	T37.1X4	T37.1X5	T37.1X6
Fenazone	T39.2X1	T39.2X2	T39.2X3	T39.2X4	T39.2X5	T39.2X6
Fenbendazole	T37.4X1	T37.4X2	T37.4X3	T37.4X4	T37.4X5	T37.4X6
Fenbutrazate	T50.5X1	T50.5X2	T50.5X3	T50.5X4	T50.5X5	T50.5X6
Fencamfamine	T43.691	T43.692	T43.693	T43.694	T43.695	T43.696
Fendiline	T46.1X1	T46.1X2	T46.1X3	T46.1X4	T46.1X5	T46.1X6
Fenetylline	T43.691	T43.692	T43.693	T43.694	T43.695	T43.696
Fenflumizole	T39.391	T39.392	T39.393	T39.394	T39.395	T39.396
Fenfluramine	T50.5X1	T50.5X2	T50.5X3	T50.5X4	T50.5X5	T50.5X6
Fenobarbital	T42.3X1	T42.3X2	T42.3X3	T42.3X4	T42.3X5	T42.3X6
Fenofibrate	T46.6X1	T46.6X2	T46.6X3	T46.6X4	T46.6X5	T46.6X6
Fenoprofen	T39.311	T39.312	T39.313	T39.314	T39.315	T39.316
Fenoterol	T48.6X1	T48.6X2	T48.6X3	T48.6X4	T48.6X5	T48.6X6

TABLE OF DRUGS AND CHEMICALS

Substance	Poisoning, Accidental (Unintentional)	Poisoning, Intentional Self-Harm	Poisoning, Assault	Poisoning, Undetermined	Adverse Effect	Underdosing
				External Cause (T-Code)		
Fenoverine	T44.3X1	T44.3X2	T44.3X3	T44.3X4	T44.3X5	T44.3X6
Fenoxazoline	T48.5X1	T48.5X2	T48.5X3	T48.5X4	T48.5X5	T48.5X6
Fenproporex	T50.5X1	T50.5X2	T50.5X3	T50.5X4	T50.5X5	T50.5X6
Fenquizone	T50.2X1	T50.2X2	T50.2X3	T50.2X4	T50.2X5	T50.2X6
Fentanyl (analogs)	T40.411	T40.412	T40.413	T40.414	T40.415	T40.416
Fentazin	T43.3X1	T43.3X2	T43.3X3	T43.3X4	T43.3X5	T43.3X6
Fenthion	T60.0X1	T60.0X2	T60.0X3	T60.0X4	—	—
Fenticlor	T49.0X1	T49.0X2	T49.0X3	T49.0X4	T49.0X5	T49.0X6
Fenylbutazone	T39.2X1	T39.2X2	T39.2X3	T39.2X4	T39.2X5	T39.2X6
Feprazone	T39.2X1	T39.2X2	T39.2X3	T39.2X4	T39.2X5	T39.2X6
Fer de lance (bite) (venom)	T63.061	T63.062	T63.063	T63.064	—	—
Ferric — see also Iron						
chloride	T45.4X1	T45.4X2	T45.4X3	T45.4X4	T45.4X5	T45.4X6
citrate	T45.4X1	T45.4X2	T45.4X3	T45.4X4	T45.4X5	T45.4X6
hydroxide						
colloidal	T45.4X1	T45.4X2	T45.4X3	T45.4X4	T45.4X5	T45.4X6
polymaltose	T45.4X1	T45.4X2	T45.4X3	T45.4X4	T45.4X5	T45.4X6
pyrophosphate	T45.4X1	T45.4X2	T45.4X3	T45.4X4	T45.4X5	T45.4X6
Ferritin	T45.4X1	T45.4X2	T45.4X3	T45.4X4	T45.4X5	T45.4X6
Ferrocholinate	T45.4X1	T45.4X2	T45.4X3	T45.4X4	T45.4X5	T45.4X6
Ferrodextrane	T45.4X1	T45.4X2	T45.4X3	T45.4X4	T45.4X5	T45.4X6
Ferropolimaler	T45.4X1	T45.4X2	T45.4X3	T45.4X4	T45.4X5	T45.4X6
Ferrous — see also Iron						
phosphate	T45.4X1	T45.4X2	T45.4X3	T45.4X4	T45.4X5	T45.4X6
salt	T45.4X1	T45.4X2	T45.4X3	T45.4X4	T45.4X5	T45.4X6
with folic acid	T45.4X1	T45.4X2	T45.4X3	T45.4X4	T45.4X5	T45.4X6
Ferrous fumarate, gluconate, lactate, salt NEC, sulfate (medicinal)	T45.4X1	T45.4X2	T45.4X3	T45.4X4	T45.4X5	T45.4X6
Ferrovanadium (fumes)	T59.891	T59.892	T59.893	T59.894	—	—
Ferrum — see Iron						
Fertilizers NEC	T65.891	T65.892	T65.893	T65.894	—	—
with herbicide mixture	T60.3X1	T60.3X2	T60.3X3	T60.3X4	—	—
Fetoxilate	T47.6X1	T47.6X2	T47.6X3	T47.6X4	T47.6X5	T47.6X6
Fiber, dietary	T47.4X1	T47.4X2	T47.4X3	T47.4X4	T47.4X5	T47.4X6
Fibrinogen (human)	T45.8X1	T45.8X2	T45.8X3	T45.8X4	T45.8X5	T45.8X6
Fibrinolysin (human)	T45.691	T45.692	T45.693	T45.694	T45.695	T45.696
Fibrinolysis						
affecting drug	T45.601	T45.602	T45.603	T45.604	T45.605	T45.606
inhibitor NEC	T45.621	T45.622	T45.623	T45.624	T45.625	T45.626
Fibrinolytic drug	T45.611	T45.612	T45.613	T45.614	T45.615	T45.616
Filix mas	T37.4X1	T37.4X2	T37.4X3	T37.4X4	T37.4X5	T37.4X6
Filtering cream	T49.3X1	T49.3X2	T49.3X3	T49.3X4	T49.3X5	T49.3X6

Substance	Poisoning, Accidental (Unintentional)	Poisoning, Intentional Self-Harm	Poisoning, Assault	Poisoning, Undetermined	Adverse Effect	Underdosing
				External Cause (T-Code)		
Fiorinal	T39.011	T39.012	T39.013	T39.014	T39.015	T39.016
Firedamp	T59.891	T59.892	T59.893	T59.894	—	—
Fish, noxious, nonbacterial	T61.91	T61.92	T61.93	T61.94	—	—
ciguatera	T61.01	T61.02	T61.03	T61.04	—	—
scombroid	T61.11	T61.12	T61.13	T61.14	—	—
shell	T61.781	T61.782	T61.783	T61.784	—	—
specified NEC	T61.771	T61.772	T61.773	T61.774	—	—
Flagyl	T37.3X1	T37.3X2	T37.3X3	T37.3X4	T37.3X5	T37.3X6
Flavine adenine dinucleotide	T45.2X1	T45.2X2	T45.2X3	T45.2X4	T45.2X5	T45.2X6
Flavodic acid	T46.991	T46.992	T46.993	T46.994	T46.995	T46.996
Flavoxate	T44.3X1	T44.3X2	T44.3X3	T44.3X4	T44.3X5	T44.3X6
Flaxedil	T48.1X1	T48.1X2	T48.1X3	T48.1X4	T48.1X5	T48.1X6
Flaxseed (medicinal)	T49.3X1	T49.3X2	T49.3X3	T49.3X4	T49.3X5	T49.3X6
Flecainide	T46.2X1	T46.2X2	T46.2X3	T46.2X4	T46.2X5	T46.2X6
Fleroxacin	T36.8X1	T36.8X2	T36.8X3	T36.8X4	T36.8X5	T36.8X6
Floctafenine	T39.8X1	T39.8X2	T39.8X3	T39.8X4	T39.8X5	T39.8X6
Flomax	T44.6X1	T44.6X2	T44.6X3	T44.6X4	T44.6X5	T44.6X6
Flomoxef	T36.1X1	T36.1X2	T36.1X3	T36.1X4	T36.1X5	T36.1X6
Flopropione	T44.3X1	T44.3X2	T44.3X3	T44.3X4	T44.3X5	T44.3X6
Florantyrone	T47.5X1	T47.5X2	T47.5X3	T47.5X4	T47.5X5	T47.5X6
Floraquin	T37.8X1	T37.8X2	T37.8X3	T37.8X4	T37.8X5	T37.8X6
Florinef	T38.0X1	T38.0X2	T38.0X3	T38.0X4	T38.0X5	T38.0X6
ENT agent	T49.6X1	T49.6X2	T49.6X3	T49.6X4	T49.6X5	T49.6X6
ophthalmic preparation	T49.5X1	T49.5X2	T49.5X3	T49.5X4	T49.5X5	T49.5X6
topical NEC	T49.0X1	T49.0X2	T49.0X3	T49.0X4	T49.0X5	T49.0X6
Flowers of sulfur	T49.4X1	T49.4X2	T49.4X3	T49.4X4	T49.4X5	T49.4X6
Floxuridine	T45.1X1	T45.1X2	T45.1X3	T45.1X4	T45.1X5	T45.1X6
Fluanisone	T43.4X1	T43.4X2	T43.4X3	T43.4X4	T43.4X5	T43.4X6
Flubendazole	T37.4X1	T37.4X2	T37.4X3	T37.4X4	T37.4X5	T37.4X6
Fluclorolone acetonide	T49.0X1	T49.0X2	T49.0X3	T49.0X4	T49.0X5	T49.0X6
Flucloxacillin	T36.0X1	T36.0X2	T36.0X3	T36.0X4	T36.0X5	T36.0X6
Fluconazole	T37.8X1	T37.8X2	T37.8X3	T37.8X4	T37.8X5	T37.8X6
Flucytosine	T37.8X1	T37.8X2	T37.8X3	T37.8X4	T37.8X5	T37.8X6
Fludeoxyglucose (18F)	T50.8X1	T50.8X2	T50.8X3	T50.8X4	T50.8X5	T50.8X6
Fludiazepam	T42.4X1	T42.4X2	T42.4X3	T42.4X4	T42.4X5	T42.4X6
Fludrocortisone	T50.0X1	T50.0X2	T50.0X3	T50.0X4	T50.0X5	T50.0X6
ENT agent	T49.6X1	T49.6X2	T49.6X3	T49.6X4	T49.6X5	T49.6X6
ophthalmic preparation	T49.5X1	T49.5X2	T49.5X3	T49.5X4	T49.5X5	T49.5X6
topical NEC	T49.0X1	T49.0X2	T49.0X3	T49.0X4	T49.0X5	T49.0X6
Fludroxycortide	T49.0X1	T49.0X2	T49.0X3	T49.0X4	T49.0X5	T49.0X6
Flufenamic acid	T39.391	T39.392	T39.393	T39.394	T39.395	T39.396
Fluindione	T45.511	T45.512	T45.513	T45.514	T45.515	T45.516

◀ New   ◀ Revised   ~~deleted~~ Deleted

Substance	Poisoning, Accidental (Unintentional)	Poisoning, Intentional Self-Harm	Poisoning, Assault	Poisoning, Undetermined	Adverse Effect	Underdosing
Flumequine	T37.8X1	T37.8X2	T37.8X3	T37.8X4	T37.8X5	T37.8X6
Flumethasone	T49.0X1	T49.0X2	T49.0X3	T49.0X4	T49.0X5	T49.0X6
Flumethiazide	T50.2X1	T50.2X2	T50.2X3	T50.2X4	T50.2X5	T50.2X6
Flumidin	T37.5X1	T37.5X2	T37.5X3	T37.5X4	T37.5X5	T37.5X6
Flunarizine	T46.7X1	T46.7X2	T46.7X3	T46.7X4	T46.7X5	T46.7X6
Flunidazole	T37.8X1	T37.8X2	T37.8X3	T37.8X4	T37.8X5	T37.8X6
Flunisolide	T48.6X1	T48.6X2	T48.6X3	T48.6X4	T48.6X5	T48.6X6
Flunitrazepam	T42.4X1	T42.4X2	T42.4X3	T42.4X4	T42.4X5	T42.4X6
Fluocinolone (acetonide)	T49.0X1	T49.0X2	T49.0X3	T49.0X4	T49.0X5	T49.0X6
Fluocinonide	T49.0X1	T49.0X2	T49.0X3	T49.0X4	T49.0X5	T49.0X6
Fluocortin (butyl)	T49.0X1	T49.0X2	T49.0X3	T49.0X4	T49.0X5	T49.0X6
Fluocortolone	T49.0X1	T49.0X2	T49.0X3	T49.0X4	T49.0X5	T49.0X6
Fluohydrocortisone	T38.0X1	T38.0X2	T38.0X3	T38.0X4	T38.0X5	T38.0X6
ENT agent	T49.6X1	T49.6X2	T49.6X3	T49.6X4	T49.6X5	T49.6X6
ophthalmic preparation	T49.5X1	T49.5X2	T49.5X3	T49.5X4	T49.5X5	T49.5X6
topical NEC	T49.0X1	T49.0X2	T49.0X3	T49.0X4	T49.0X5	T49.0X6
Fluonid	T49.0X1	T49.0X2	T49.0X3	T49.0X4	T49.0X5	T49.0X6
Fluopromazine	T43.3X1	T43.3X2	T43.3X3	T43.3X4	T43.3X5	T43.3X6
Fluoroacetate	T60.8X1	T60.8X2	T60.8X3	T60.8X4	—	—
Fluorescein	T50.8X1	T50.8X2	T50.8X3	T50.8X4	T50.8X5	T50.8X6
Fluorhydrocortisone	T50.0X1	T50.0X2	T50.0X3	T50.0X4	T50.0X5	T50.0X6
Fluoride (nonmedicinal) (pesticide) (sodium) NEC	T60.8X1	T60.8X2	T60.8X3	T60.8X4		
hydrogen — see Hydrofluoric acid						
medicinal NEC	T50.991	T50.992	T50.993	T50.994	T50.995	T50.996
dental use	T49.7X1	T49.7X2	T49.7X3	T49.7X4	T49.7X5	T49.7X6
not pesticide NEC	T54.91	T54.92	T54.93	T54.94	—	—
stannous	T49.7X1	T49.7X2	T49.7X3	T49.7X4	T49.7X5	T49.7X6
Fluorinated corticosteroids	T38.0X1	T38.0X2	T38.0X3	T38.0X4	T38.0X5	T38.0X6
Fluorine (gas)	T59.5X1	T59.5X2	T59.5X3	T59.5X4		
salt — see Fluoride(s)						
Fluoristan	T49.7X1	T49.7X2	T49.7X3	T49.7X4	T49.7X5	T49.7X6
Fluormetholone	T49.0X1	T49.0X2	T49.0X3	T49.0X4	T49.0X5	T49.0X6
Fluoroacetate	T60.8X1	T60.8X2	T60.8X3	T60.8X4	—	—
Fluorocarbon monomer	T53.6X1	T53.6X2	T53.6X3	T53.6X4	—	—
Fluorocytosine	T37.8X1	T37.8X2	T37.8X3	T37.8X4	T37.8X5	T37.8X6
Fluorodeoxyuridine	T45.1X1	T45.1X2	T45.1X3	T45.1X4	T45.1X5	T45.1X6
Fluorometholone	T49.0X1	T49.0X2	T49.0X3	T49.0X4	T49.0X5	T49.0X6
ophthalmic preparation	T49.5X1	T49.5X2	T49.5X3	T49.5X4	T49.5X5	T49.5X6
Fluorophosphate insecticide	T60.0X1	T60.0X2	T60.0X3	T60.0X4	—	—
Fluorosol	T46.3X1	T46.3X2	T46.3X3	T46.3X4	T46.3X5	T46.3X6
Fluorouracil	T45.1X1	T45.1X2	T45.1X3	T45.1X4	T45.1X5	T45.1X6
Fluorphenylalanine	T49.5X1	T49.5X2	T49.5X3	T49.5X4	T49.5X5	T49.5X6
Fluothane	T41.0X1	T41.0X2	T41.0X3	T41.0X4	T41.0X5	T41.0X6
Fluoxetine	T43.221	T43.222	T43.223	T43.224	T43.225	T43.226
Fluoxymesterone	T38.7X1	T38.7X2	T38.7X3	T38.7X4	T38.7X5	T38.7X6
Flupenthixol	T43.4X1	T43.4X2	T43.4X3	T43.4X4	T43.4X5	T43.4X6
Flupentixol	T43.4X1	T43.4X2	T43.4X3	T43.4X4	T43.4X5	T43.4X6
Fluphenazine	T43.3X1	T43.3X2	T43.3X3	T43.3X4	T43.3X5	T43.3X6
Fluprednidene	T49.0X1	T49.0X2	T49.0X3	T49.0X4	T49.0X5	T49.0X6
Fluprednisolone	T38.0X1	T38.0X2	T38.0X3	T38.0X4	T38.0X5	T38.0X6
Fluradoline	T39.8X1	T39.8X2	T39.8X3	T39.8X4	T39.8X5	T39.8X6
Flurandrenolide	T49.0X1	T49.0X2	T49.0X3	T49.0X4	T49.0X5	T49.0X6
Flurandrenolone	T49.0X1	T49.0X2	T49.0X3	T49.0X4	T49.0X5	T49.0X6
Flurazepam	T42.4X1	T42.4X2	T42.4X3	T42.4X4	T42.4X5	T42.4X6
Flurbiprofen	T39.311	T39.312	T39.313	T39.314	T39.315	T39.316
Flurobate	T49.0X1	T49.0X2	T49.0X3	T49.0X4	T49.0X5	T49.0X6
Flurotyl	T43.291	T43.292	T43.293	T43.294	T43.295	T43.296
Fluroxene	T41.0X1	T41.0X2	T41.0X3	T41.0X4	T41.0X5	T41.0X6
Fluspirilene	T43.591	T43.592	T43.593	T43.594	T43.595	T43.596
Flutamide	T38.6X1	T38.6X2	T38.6X3	T38.6X4	T38.6X5	T38.6X6
Flutazolam	T42.4X1	T42.4X2	T42.4X3	T42.4X4	T42.4X5	T42.4X6
Fluticasone propionate	T38.0X1	T38.0X2	T38.0X3	T38.0X4	T38.0X5	T38.0X6
Flutoprazepam	T42.4X1	T42.4X2	T42.4X3	T42.4X4	T42.4X5	T42.4X6
Flutropium bromide	T48.6X1	T48.6X2	T48.6X3	T48.6X4	T48.6X5	T48.6X6
Fluvoxamine	T43.221	T43.222	T43.223	T43.224	T43.225	T43.226
Folacin	T45.8X1	T45.8X2	T45.8X3	T45.8X4	T45.8X5	T45.8X6
Folic acid	T45.8X1	T45.8X2	T45.8X3	T45.8X4	T45.8X5	T45.8X6
with ferrous salt	T45.2X1	T45.2X2	T45.2X3	T45.2X4	T45.2X5	T45.2X6
antagonist	T45.1X1	T45.1X2	T45.1X3	T45.1X4	T45.1X5	T45.1X6
Folinic acid	T45.8X1	T45.8X2	T45.8X3	T45.8X4	T45.8X5	T45.8X6
Folium stramoniae	T48.6X1	T48.6X2	T48.6X3	T48.6X4	T48.6X5	T48.6X6
Follicle-stimulating hormone, human	T38.811	T38.812	T38.813	T38.814	T38.815	T38.816
Folpet	T60.3X1	T60.3X2	T60.3X3	T60.3X4	—	—
Fominoben	T48.3X1	T48.3X2	T48.3X3	T48.3X4	T48.3X5	T48.3X6
Food, foodstuffs, noxious, nonbacterial, NEC	T62.91	T62.92	T62.93	T62.94	—	—
berries	T62.1X1	T62.1X2	T62.1X3	T62.1X4	—	—
fish — see also Fish	T61.91	T61.92	T61.93	T61.94	—	—
mushrooms	T62.0X1	T62.0X2	T62.0X3	T62.0X4	—	—
plants	T62.2X1	T62.2X2	T62.2X3	T62.2X4	—	—
seafood	T61.91	T61.92	T61.93	T61.94	—	—
specified NEC	T61.8X1	T61.8X2	T61.8X3	T61.8X4	—	—
seeds	T62.2X1	T62.2X2	T62.2X3	T62.2X4	—	—

TABLE OF DRUGS AND CHEMICALS

◀ New   ◀ Revised   ~~deleted~~ Deleted

TABLE OF DRUGS AND CHEMICALS

Substance	Poisoning, Accidental (Unintentional)	Poisoning, Intentional Self-Harm	Poisoning, Assault	Poisoning, Undetermined	Adverse Effect	Underdosing
Food, foodstuffs, noxious, nonbacterial, NEC *(Continued)*						
shellfish	T61.781	T61.782	T61.783	T61.784	—	—
specified NEC	T62.8X1	T62.8X2	T62.8X3	T62.8X4	—	—
Fool's parsley	T62.2X1	T62.2X2	T62.2X3	T62.2X4	—	—
Formaldehyde (solution), gas or vapor	T59.2X1	T59.2X2	T59.2X3	T59.2X4	—	—
fungicide	T60.3X1	T60.3X2	T60.3X3	T60.3X4	—	—
Formalin	T59.2X1	T59.2X2	T59.2X3	T59.2X4	—	—
fungicide	T60.3X1	T60.3X2	T60.3X3	T60.3X4	—	—
vapor	T59.2X1	T59.2X2	T59.2X3	T59.2X4	—	—
Formic acid	T54.2X1	T54.2X2	T54.2X3	T54.2X4	—	—
vapor	T59.891	T59.892	T59.893	T59.894	—	—
Foscarnet sodium	T37.5X1	T37.5X2	T37.5X3	T37.5X4	T37.5X5	T37.5X6
Fosfestrol	T38.5X1	T38.5X2	T38.5X3	T38.5X4	T38.5X5	T38.5X6
Fosfomycin	T36.8X1	T36.8X2	T36.8X3	T36.8X4	T36.8X5	T36.8X6
Fosfonet sodium	T37.5X1	T37.5X2	T37.5X3	T37.5X4	T37.5X5	T37.5X6
Fosinopril	T46.4X1	T46.4X2	T46.4X3	T46.4X4	T46.4X5	T46.4X6
sodium	T46.4X1	T46.4X2	T46.4X3	T46.4X4	T46.4X5	T46.4X6
Fowler's solution	T57.0X1	T57.0X2	T57.0X3	T57.0X4	—	—
Foxglove	T62.2X1	T62.2X2	T62.2X3	T62.2X4	—	—
Framycetin	T36.5X1	T36.5X2	T36.5X3	T36.5X4	T36.5X5	T36.5X6
Frangula	T47.2X1	T47.2X2	T47.2X3	T47.2X4	T47.2X5	T47.2X6
extract	T47.2X1	T47.2X2	T47.2X3	T47.2X4	T47.2X5	T47.2X6
Frei antigen	T50.8X1	T50.8X2	T50.8X3	T50.8X4	T50.8X5	T50.8X6
Freon	T53.5X1	T53.5X2	T53.5X3	T53.5X4	—	—
Fructose	T50.3X1	T50.3X2	T50.3X3	T50.3X4	T50.3X5	T50.3X6
Frusemide	T50.1X1	T50.1X2	T50.1X3	T50.1X4	T50.1X5	T50.1X6
FSH	T38.811	T38.812	T38.813	T38.814	T38.815	T38.816
Ftorafur	T45.1X1	T45.1X2	T45.1X3	T45.1X4	T45.1X5	T45.1X6
Fuel						
automobile	T52.0X1	T52.0X2	T52.0X3	T52.0X4	—	—
exhaust gas, not in transit	T58.01	T58.02	T58.03	T58.04	—	—
vapor NEC	T52.0X1	T52.0X2	T52.0X3	T52.0X4	—	—
gas (domestic use) — *see also Carbon, monoxide, fuel, utility*	T59.891	T59.892	T59.893	T59.894	—	—
utility	T59.891	T59.892	T59.893	T59.894	—	—
in mobile container	T59.891	T59.892	T59.893	T59.894	—	—
incomplete combustion of — *see Carbon, monoxide, fuel, utility*						
piped (natural)	T59.891	T59.892	T59.893	T59.894	—	—
industrial, incomplete combustion	T58.8X1	T58.8X2	T58.8X3	T58.8X4	—	—

Substance	Poisoning, Accidental (Unintentional)	Poisoning, Intentional Self-Harm	Poisoning, Assault	Poisoning, Undetermined	Adverse Effect	Underdosing
Fugillin	T36.8X1	T36.8X2	T36.8X3	T36.8X4	T36.8X5	T36.8X6
Fulminate of mercury	T56.1X1	T56.1X2	T56.1X3	T56.1X4	—	—
Fulvicin	T36.7X1	T36.7X2	T36.7X3	T36.7X4	T36.7X5	T36.7X6
Fumadil	T36.8X1	T36.8X2	T36.8X3	T36.8X4	T36.8X5	T36.8X6
Fumagillin	T36.8X1	T36.8X2	T36.8X3	T36.8X4	T36.8X5	T36.8X6
Fumaric acid	T49.4X1	T49.4X2	T49.4X3	T49.4X4	T49.4X5	T49.4X6
Fumes (from)	T59.91	T59.92	T59.93	T59.94	—	—
carbon monoxide — *see Carbon, monoxide*						
charcoal (domestic use) — *see Charcoal, fumes*						
chloroform — *see Chloroform*						
coke (in domestic stoves, fireplaces) — *see Coke, fumes*						
corrosive NEC	T54.91	T54.92	T54.93	T54.94	—	—
ether — *see Ether*						
freons	T53.5X1	T53.5X2	T53.5X3	T53.5X4	—	—
hydrocarbons	T59.891	T59.892	T59.893	T59.894	—	—
petroleum (liquefied)	T59.891	T59.892	T59.893	T59.894	—	—
distributed through pipes (pure or mixed with air)	T59.891	T59.892	T59.893	T59.894	—	—
lead — *see Lead*						
metal — *see Metals, or the specified metal*						
nitrogen dioxide	T59.0X1	T59.0X2	T59.0X3	T59.0X4	—	—
pesticides — *see Pesticide*						
petroleum (liquefied)	T59.891	T59.892	T59.893	T59.894	—	—
distributed through pipes (pure or mixed with air)	T59.891	T59.892	T59.893	T59.894	—	—
polyester	T59.891	T59.892	T59.893	T59.894	—	—
specified source NEC — *see also substance specified*	T59.891	T59.892	T59.893	T59.894	—	—
sulfur dioxide	T59.1X1	T59.1X2	T59.1X3	T59.1X4	—	—
Fumigant NEC	T60.91	T60.92	T60.93	T60.94	—	—
Fungi, noxious, used as food	T62.0X1	T62.0X2	T62.0X3	T62.0X4	—	—
Fungicide NEC (nonmedicinal)	T60.3X1	T60.3X2	T60.3X3	T60.3X4	—	—
Fungizone	T36.7X1	T36.7X2	T36.7X3	T36.7X4	T36.7X5	T36.7X6
topical	T49.0X1	T49.0X2	T49.0X3	T49.0X4	T49.0X5	T49.0X6
Furacin	T49.0X1	T49.0X2	T49.0X3	T49.0X4	T49.0X5	T49.0X6
Furadantin	T37.91	T37.92	T37.93	T37.94	T37.95	T37.96
Furazolidone	T37.8X1	T37.8X2	T37.8X3	T37.8X4	T37.8X5	T37.8X6
Furazolium chloride	T49.0X1	T49.0X2	T49.0X3	T49.0X4	T49.0X5	T49.0X6
Furfural	T52.8X1	T52.8X2	T52.8X3	T52.8X4	—	—

◀ New ◀ Revised ~~deleted~~ Deleted

Substance	Poisoning, Accidental (Unintentional)	Poisoning, Intentional Self-Harm	Poisoning, Assault	Poisoning, Undetermined	Adverse Effect	Underdosing
Furnace (coal burning) (domestic), gas from industrial	T58.2X1	T58.2X2	T58.2X3	T58.2X4	—	—
industrial	T58.8X1	T58.8X2	T58.8X3	T58.8X4	—	—
Furniture polish	T65.891	T65.892	T65.893	T65.894	—	—
Furosemide	T50.1X1	T50.1X2	T50.1X3	T50.1X4	T50.1X5	T50.1X6
Furoxone	T37.91	T37.92	T37.93	T37.94	T37.95	T37.96
Fursultiamine	T45.2X1	T45.2X2	T45.2X3	T45.2X4	T45.2X5	T45.2X6
Fusafungine	T36.8X1	T36.8X2	T36.8X3	T36.8X4	T36.8X5	T36.8X6
Fusel oil (any) (amyl) (butyl) (propyl), vapor	T51.3X1	T51.3X2	T51.3X3	T51.3X4		
Fusidate (ethanolamine) (sodium)	T36.8X1	T36.8X2	T36.8X3	T36.8X4	T36.8X5	T36.8X6
Fusidic acid	T36.8X1	T36.8X2	T36.8X3	T36.8X4	T36.8X5	T36.8X6
Fytic acid, nonasodium	T50.6X1	T50.6X2	T50.6X3	T50.6X4	T50.6X5	T50.6X6
G						
GABA	T43.8X1	T43.8X2	T43.8X3	T43.8X4	T43.8X5	T43.8X6
Gadolinium	T56.821	T56.822	T56.823	T56.824	T56.825	—
Gadopentetic acid	T50.8X1	T50.8X2	T50.8X3	T50.8X4	T50.8X5	T50.8X6
Galactose	T50.3X1	T50.3X2	T50.3X3	T50.3X4	T50.3X5	T50.3X6
b-Galactosidase	T47.5X1	T47.5X2	T47.5X3	T47.5X4	T47.5X5	T47.5X6
Galantamine	T44.0X1	T44.0X2	T44.0X3	T44.0X4	T44.0X5	T44.0X6
Gallamine (triethiodide)	T48.1X1	T48.1X2	T48.1X3	T48.1X4	T48.1X5	T48.1X6
Gallium citrate	T50.991	T50.992	T50.993	T50.994	T50.995	T50.996
Gallopamil	T46.1X1	T46.1X2	T46.1X3	T46.1X4	T46.1X5	T46.1X6
Gamboge	T47.2X1	T47.2X2	T47.2X3	T47.2X4	T47.2X5	T47.2X6
Gamimune	T50.Z11	T50.Z12	T50.Z13	T50.Z14	T50.Z15	T50.Z16
Gamma-aminobutyric acid	T43.8X1	T43.8X2	T43.8X3	T43.8X4	T43.8X5	T43.8X6
Gamma-benzene hexachloride (medicinal)	T49.0X1	T49.0X2	T49.0X3	T49.0X4	T49.0X5	T49.0X6
nonmedicinal, vapor	T53.6X1	T53.6X2	T53.6X3	T53.6X4	—	—
Gamma-BHC (medicinal) — see also Gamma-benzene hexachloride	T49.0X1	T49.0X2	T49.0X3	T49.0X4	T49.0X5	T49.0X6
Gamma globulin	T50.Z11	T50.Z12	T50.Z13	T50.Z14	T50.Z15	T50.Z16
Gamulin	T50.Z11	T50.Z12	T50.Z13	T50.Z14	T50.Z15	T50.Z16
Ganciclovir (sodium)	T37.5X1	T37.5X2	T37.5X3	T37.5X4	T37.5X5	T37.5X6
Ganglionic blocking drug NEC	T44.2X1	T44.2X2	T44.2X3	T44.2X4	T44.2X5	T44.2X6
specified NEC	T44.2X1	T44.2X2	T44.2X3	T44.2X4	T44.2X5	T44.2X6
Ganja	T40.711	T40.712	T40.713	T40.714	T40.715	T40.716
Garamycin	T36.5X1	T36.5X2	T36.5X3	T36.5X4	T36.5X5	T36.5X6
ophthalmic preparation	T49.5X1	T49.5X2	T49.5X3	T49.5X4	T49.5X5	T49.5X6
topical NEC	T49.0X1	T49.0X2	T49.0X3	T49.0X4	T49.0X5	T49.0X6
Gardenal	T42.3X1	T42.3X2	T42.3X3	T42.3X4	T42.3X5	T42.3X6

Substance	Poisoning, Accidental (Unintentional)	Poisoning, Intentional Self-Harm	Poisoning, Assault	Poisoning, Undetermined	Adverse Effect	Underdosing
Gardepanyl	T42.3X1	T42.3X2	T42.3X3	T42.3X4	T42.3X5	T42.3X6
Gas NEC	T59.91	T59.92	T59.93	T59.94	—	—
acetylene	T59.891	T59.892	T59.893	T59.894	—	—
incomplete combustion of	T58.11	T58.12	T58.13	T58.14		
air contaminants, source or type not specified	T59.91	T59.92	T59.93	T59.94	—	—
anesthetic	T41.0X1	T41.0X2	T41.0X3	T41.0X4	T41.0X5	T41.0X6
blast furnace	T58.8X1	T58.8X2	T58.8X3	T58.8X4	—	—
butane — see Butane						
carbon monoxide — see Carbon, monoxide						
chlorine	T59.4X1	T59.4X2	T59.4X3	T59.4X4	—	—
coal	T58.2X1	T58.2X2	T58.2X3	T58.2X4	—	—
cyanide	T57.3X1	T57.3X2	T57.3X3	T57.3X4	—	—
dicyanogen	T65.0X1	T65.0X2	T65.0X3	T65.0X4	—	—
domestic — see Domestic gas	T57.91	T57.92	T57.93	T57.94		
exhaust	T57.91	T57.92	T57.93	T57.94		
from utility (for cooking, heating, or lighting) (after combustion) — see Carbon, monoxide, fuel, utility						
prior to combustion	T59.891	T59.892	T59.893	T59.894	—	—
from wood or coal-burning stove or fireplace	T57.91	T57.92	T57.93	T57.94	—	—
fuel (domestic use) (after combustion) — see also Carbon, monoxide, fuel	T57.91	T57.92	T57.93	T57.94	—	—
industrial use	T58.8X1	T58.8X2	T58.8X3	T58.8X4	—	—
prior to combustion	T59.891	T59.892	T59.893	T59.894	—	—
utility	T59.891	T59.892	T59.893	T59.894	—	—
in mobile container	T59.891	T59.892	T59.893	T59.894	—	—
incomplete combustion of — see Carbon, monoxide, fuel, utility						
piped (natural)	T59.891	T59.892	T59.893	T59.894	—	—
garage	T58.01	T58.02	T58.03	T58.04		
hydrocarbon NEC	T59.891	T59.892	T59.893	T59.894	—	—
incomplete combustion of — see Carbon, monoxide, fuel, utility						
liquefied — see Butane						
piped	T59.891	T59.892	T59.893	T59.894	—	—
hydrocyanic acid	T65.0X1	T65.0X2	T65.0X3	T65.0X4	—	—

TABLE OF DRUGS AND CHEMICALS

Substance	Poisoning, Accidental (Unintentional)	Poisoning, Intentional Self-Harm	Poisoning, Assault	Poisoning, Undetermined	Adverse Effect	Underdosing
Gas NEC *(Continued)*						
illuminating (after combustion)	T58.11	T58.12	T58.13	T58.14	—	—
prior to combustion	T59.891	T59.892	T59.893	T59.894	—	—
incomplete combustion, any — see Carbon, monoxide						
kiln	T58.8X1	T58.8X2	T58.8X3	T58.8X4	—	—
lacrimogenic	T59.3X1	T59.3X2	T59.3X3	T59.3X4	—	—
liquefied petroleum — see Butane						
marsh	T59.891	T59.892	T59.893	T59.894	—	—
motor exhaust, not in transit	T58.01	T58.02	T58.03	T58.04	—	—
mustard, not in war	T59.891	T59.892	T59.893	T59.894	—	—
natural	T59.891	T59.892	T59.893	T59.894	—	—
nerve, not in war	T59.91	T59.92	T59.93	T59.94	—	—
oil	T52.0X1	T52.0X2	T52.0X3	T52.0X4	—	—
petroleum (liquefied) (distributed in mobile containers)	T59.891	T59.892	T59.893	T59.894	—	—
piped (pure or mixed with air)	T59.891	T59.892	T59.893	T59.894	—	—
piped (manufactured) (natural) NEC	T59.891	T59.892	T59.893	T59.894	—	—
producer	T58.8X1	T58.8X2	T58.8X3	T58.8X4	—	—
propane — see Propane						
refrigerant (chlorofluoro-carbon)	T53.5X1	T53.5X2	T53.5X3	T53.5X4	—	—
not chlorofluoro-carbon	T59.891	T59.892	T59.893	T59.894	—	—
sewer	T59.91	T59.92	T59.93	T59.94	—	—
specified source NEC	T59.91	T59.92	T59.93	T59.94	—	—
stove (after combustion)	T58.11	T58.12	T58.13	T58.14	—	—
tear	T59.3X1	T59.3X2	T59.3X3	T59.3X4	—	—
therapeutic	T41.5X1	T41.5X2	T41.5X3	T41.5X4	T41.5X5	T41.5X6
utility (for cooking, heating, or lighting) (piped) NEC	T59.891	T59.892	T59.893	T59.894	—	—
in mobile container	T59.891	T59.892	T59.893	T59.894	—	—
incomplete combustion of — see Carbon, monoxide, fuel, utility						
piped (natural)	T59.891	T59.892	T59.893	T59.894	—	—
water	T58.11	T58.12	T58.13	T58.14	—	—
incomplete combustion of — see Carbon, monoxide, fuel, utility						

Substance	Poisoning, Accidental (Unintentional)	Poisoning, Intentional Self-Harm	Poisoning, Assault	Poisoning, Undetermined	Adverse Effect	Underdosing
Gaseous substance — *see Gas*						
Gasoline	T52.0X1	T52.0X2	T52.0X3	T52.0X4	—	—
vapor	T52.0X1	T52.0X2	T52.0X3	T52.0X4	—	—
Gastric enzymes	T47.5X1	T47.5X2	T47.5X3	T47.5X4	T47.5X5	T47.5X6
Gastrografin	T50.8X1	T50.8X2	T50.8X3	T50.8X4	T50.8X5	T50.8X6
Gastrointestinal drug	T47.91	T47.92	T47.93	T47.94	T47.95	T47.96
biological	T47.8X1	T47.8X2	T47.8X3	T47.8X4	T47.8X5	T47.8X6
specified NEC	T47.8X1	T47.8X2	T47.8X3	T47.8X4	T47.8X5	T47.8X6
Gaultheria procumbens	T62.2X1	T62.2X2	T62.2X3	T62.2X4	—	—
Gelatin (intravenous)	T45.8X1	T45.8X2	T45.8X3	T45.8X4	T45.8X5	T45.8X6
absorbable (sponge)	T45.7X1	T45.7X2	T45.7X3	T45.7X4	T45.7X5	T45.7X6
Gefarnate	T44.3X1	T44.3X2	T44.3X3	T44.3X4	T44.3X5	T44.3X6
Gelfilm	T49.8X1	T49.8X2	T49.8X3	T49.8X4	T49.8X5	T49.8X6
Gelfoam	T45.7X1	T45.7X2	T45.7X3	T45.7X4	T45.7X5	T45.7X6
Gelsemine	T50.991	T50.992	T50.993	T50.994	T50.995	T50.996
Gelsemium (sempervirens)	T62.2X1	T62.2X2	T62.2X3	T62.2X4	—	—
Gemeprost	T48.0X1	T48.0X2	T48.0X3	T48.0X4	T48.0X5	T48.0X6
Gemfibrozil	T46.6X1	T46.6X2	T46.6X3	T46.6X4	T46.6X5	T46.6X6
Gemonil	T42.3X1	T42.3X2	T42.3X3	T42.3X4	T42.3X5	T42.3X6
Gentamicin	T36.5X1	T36.5X2	T36.5X3	T36.5X4	T36.5X5	T36.5X6
ophthalmic preparation	T49.5X1	T49.5X2	T49.5X3	T49.5X4	T49.5X5	T49.5X6
topical NEC	T49.0X1	T49.0X2	T49.0X3	T49.0X4	T49.0X5	T49.0X6
Gentian	T47.5X1	T47.5X2	T47.5X3	T47.5X4	T47.5X5	T47.5X6
violet	T49.0X1	T49.0X2	T49.0X3	T49.0X4	T49.0X5	T49.0X6
Gepefrine	T44.4X1	T44.4X2	T44.4X3	T44.4X4	T44.4X5	T44.4X6
Gestonorone caproate	T38.5X1	T38.5X2	T38.5X3	T38.5X4	T38.5X5	T38.5X6
Gexane	T49.0X1	T49.0X2	T49.0X3	T49.0X4	T49.0X5	T49.0X6
Gila monster (venom)	T63.111	T63.112	T63.113	T63.114	—	—
Ginger	T47.5X1	T47.5X2	T47.5X3	T47.5X4	T47.5X5	T47.5X6
Jamaica — *see Jamaica, ginger*						
Gitalin	T46.0X1	T46.0X2	T46.0X3	T46.0X4	T46.0X5	T46.0X6
amorphous	T46.0X1	T46.0X2	T46.0X3	T46.0X4	T46.0X5	T46.0X6
Gitaloxin	T46.0X1	T46.0X2	T46.0X3	T46.0X4	T46.0X5	T46.0X6
Gitoxin	T46.0X1	T46.0X2	T46.0X3	T46.0X4	T46.0X5	T46.0X6
Glafenine	T39.8X1	T39.8X2	T39.8X3	T39.8X4	T39.8X5	T39.8X6
Glandular extract (medicinal) NEC	T50.Z91	T50.Z92	T50.Z93	T50.Z94	T50.Z95	T50.Z96
Glaucarubin	T37.3X1	T37.3X2	T37.3X3	T37.3X4	T37.3X5	T37.3X6
Glibenclamide	T38.3X1	T38.3X2	T38.3X3	T38.3X4	T38.3X5	T38.3X6
Glibornuride	T38.3X1	T38.3X2	T38.3X3	T38.3X4	T38.3X5	T38.3X6
Gliclazide	T38.3X1	T38.3X2	T38.3X3	T38.3X4	T38.3X5	T38.3X6
Glimidine	T38.3X1	T38.3X2	T38.3X3	T38.3X4	T38.3X5	T38.3X6

◀ New ◀ Revised ~~deleted~~ Deleted

Substance	Poisoning, Accidental (Unintentional)	Poisoning, Intentional Self-Harm	Poisoning, Assault	Poisoning, Undetermined	Adverse Effect	Underdosing
Glipizide	T38.3X1	T38.3X2	T38.3X3	T38.3X4	T38.3X5	T38.3X6
Gliquidone	T38.3X1	T38.3X2	T38.3X3	T38.3X4	T38.3X5	T38.3X6
Glisolamide	T38.3X1	T38.3X2	T38.3X3	T38.3X4	T38.3X5	T38.3X6
Glisoxepide	T38.3X1	T38.3X2	T38.3X3	T38.3X4	T38.3X5	T38.3X6
Globin zinc insulin	T38.3X1	T38.3X2	T38.3X3	T38.3X4	T38.3X5	T38.3X6
Globulin						
antilymphocytic	T50.Z11	T50.Z12	T50.Z13	T50.Z14	T50.Z15	T50.Z16
antirhesus	T50.Z11	T50.Z12	T50.Z13	T50.Z14	T50.Z15	T50.Z16
antivenin	T50.Z11	T50.Z12	T50.Z13	T50.Z14	T50.Z15	T50.Z16
antiviral	T50.Z11	T50.Z12	T50.Z13	T50.Z14	T50.Z15	T50.Z16
Glucagon	T38.3X1	T38.3X2	T38.3X3	T38.3X4	T38.3X5	T38.3X6
Glucocorticoids	T38.0X1	T38.0X2	T38.0X3	T38.0X4	T38.0X5	T38.0X6
Glucocorticosteroid	T38.0X1	T38.0X2	T38.0X3	T38.0X4	T38.0X5	T38.0X6
Gluconic acid	T50.991	T50.992	T50.993	T50.994	T50.995	T50.996
Glucosamine sulfate	T39.4X1	T39.4X2	T39.4X3	T39.4X4	T39.4X5	T39.4X6
Glucose	T50.3X1	T50.3X2	T50.3X3	T50.3X4	T50.3X5	T50.3X6
with sodium chloride	T50.3X1	T50.3X2	T50.3X3	T50.3X4	T50.3X5	T50.3X6
Glucosulfone sodium	T37.1X1	T37.1X2	T37.1X3	T37.1X4	T37.1X5	T37.1X6
Glucurolactone	T47.8X1	T47.8X2	T47.8X3	T47.8X4	T47.8X5	T47.8X6
Glue NEC	T52.8X1	T52.8X2	T52.8X3	T52.8X4	—	—
Glutamic acid	T47.5X1	T47.5X2	T47.5X3	T47.5X4	T47.5X5	T47.5X6
Glutaral (medicinal)	T49.0X1	T49.0X2	T49.0X3	T49.0X4	T49.0X5	T49.0X6
nonmedicinal	T65.891	T65.892	T65.893	T65.894	—	—
Glutaraldehyde (nonmedicinal)	T65.891	T65.892	T65.893	T65.894	—	—
medicinal	T49.0X1	T49.0X2	T49.0X3	T49.0X4	T49.0X5	T49.0X6
Glutathione	T50.6X1	T50.6X2	T50.6X3	T50.6X4	T50.6X5	T50.6X6
Glutethimide	T42.6X1	T42.6X2	T42.6X3	T42.6X4	T42.6X5	T42.6X6
Glyburide	T38.3X1	T38.3X2	T38.3X3	T38.3X4	T38.3X5	T38.3X6
Glycerin	T47.4X1	T47.4X2	T47.4X3	T47.4X4	T47.4X5	T47.4X6
Glycerol	T47.4X1	T47.4X2	T47.4X3	T47.4X4	T47.4X5	T47.4X6
borax	T49.6X1	T49.6X2	T49.6X3	T49.6X4	T49.6X5	T49.6X6
intravenous	T50.3X1	T50.3X2	T50.3X3	T50.3X4	T50.3X5	T50.3X6
iodinated	T48.4X1	T48.4X2	T48.4X3	T48.4X4	T48.4X5	T48.4X6
Glycerophosphate	T50.991	T50.992	T50.993	T50.994	T50.995	T50.996
Glyceryl						
gualacolate	T48.4X1	T48.4X2	T48.4X3	T48.4X4	T48.4X5	T48.4X6
nitrate	T46.3X1	T46.3X2	T46.3X3	T46.3X4	T46.3X5	T46.3X6
triacetate (topical)	T49.0X1	T49.0X2	T49.0X3	T49.0X4	T49.0X5	T49.0X6
trinitrate	T46.3X1	T46.3X2	T46.3X3	T46.3X4	T46.3X5	T46.3X6
Glycine	T50.3X1	T50.3X2	T50.3X3	T50.3X4	T50.3X5	T50.3X6
Glyclopyramide	T38.3X1	T38.3X2	T38.3X3	T38.3X4	T38.3X5	T38.3X6
Glycobiarsol	T37.3X1	T37.3X2	T37.3X3	T37.3X4	T37.3X5	T37.3X6

Substance	Poisoning, Accidental (Unintentional)	Poisoning, Intentional Self-Harm	Poisoning, Assault	Poisoning, Undetermined	Adverse Effect	Underdosing
Glycols (ether)	T52.3X1	T52.3X2	T52.3X3	T52.3X4	—	—
Glyconiazide	T37.1X1	T37.1X2	T37.1X3	T37.1X4	T37.1X5	T37.1X6
Glycopyrrolate	T44.3X1	T44.3X2	T44.3X3	T44.3X4	T44.3X5	T44.3X6
Glycopyrronium	T44.3X1	T44.3X2	T44.3X3	T44.3X4	T44.3X5	T44.3X6
bromide	T44.3X1	T44.3X2	T44.3X3	T44.3X4	T44.3X5	T44.3X6
Glycoside, cardiac (stimulant)	T46.0X1	T46.0X2	T46.0X3	T46.0X4	T46.0X5	T46.0X6
Glycyclamide	T38.3X1	T38.3X2	T38.3X3	T38.3X4	T38.3X5	T38.3X6
Glycyrrhiza extract	T48.4X1	T48.4X2	T48.4X3	T48.4X4	T48.4X5	T48.4X6
Glycyrrhizic acid	T48.4X1	T48.4X2	T48.4X3	T48.4X4	T48.4X5	T48.4X6
Glycyrrhizinate potassium	T48.4X1	T48.4X2	T48.4X3	T48.4X4	T48.4X5	T48.4X6
Glymidine sodium	T38.3X1	T38.3X2	T38.3X3	T38.3X4	T38.3X5	T38.3X6
Glyphosate	T60.3X1	T60.3X2	T60.3X3	T60.3X4	—	—
Glyphylline	T48.6X1	T48.6X2	T48.6X3	T48.6X4	T48.6X5	T48.6X6
Gold						
colloidal (I98Au)	T45.1X1	T45.1X2	T45.1X3	T45.1X4	T45.1X5	T45.1X6
salts	T39.4X1	T39.4X2	T39.4X3	T39.4X4	T39.4X5	T39.4X6
Golden sulfide of antimony	T56.891	T56.892	T56.893	T56.894	—	—
Goldylocks	T62.2X1	T62.2X2	T62.2X3	T62.2X4	—	—
Gonadal tissue extract	T38.901	T38.902	T38.903	T38.904	T38.905	T38.906
female	T38.5X1	T38.5X2	T38.5X3	T38.5X4	T38.5X5	T38.5X6
male	T38.7X1	T38.7X2	T38.7X3	T38.7X4	T38.7X5	T38.7X6
Gonadorelin	T38.891	T38.892	T38.893	T38.894	T38.895	T38.896
Gonadotropin	T38.891	T38.892	T38.893	T38.894	T38.895	T38.896
chorionic	T38.891	T38.892	T38.893	T38.894	T38.895	T38.896
pituitary	T38.811	T38.812	T38.813	T38.814	T38.815	T38.816
Goserelin	T45.1X1	T45.1X2	T45.1X3	T45.1X4	T45.1X5	T45.1X6
Grain alcohol	T51.0X1	T51.0X2	T51.0X3	T51.0X4	—	—
Gramicidin	T49.0X1	T49.0X2	T49.0X3	T49.0X4	T49.0X5	T49.0X6
Granisetron	T45.0X1	T45.0X2	T45.0X3	T45.0X4	T45.0X5	T45.0X6
Gratiola officinalis	T62.2X1	T62.2X2	T62.2X3	T62.2X4	—	—
Grease	T65.891	T65.892	T65.893	T65.894		
Green hellebore	T62.2X1	T62.2X2	T62.2X3	T62.2X4	—	
Green soap	T49.2X1	T49.2X2	T49.2X3	T49.2X4	T49.2X5	T49.2X6
Grifulvin	T36.7X1	T36.7X2	T36.7X3	T36.7X4	T36.7X5	T36.7X6
Griseofulvin	T36.7X1	T36.7X2	T36.7X3	T36.7X4	T36.7X5	T36.7X6
Growth hormone	T38.811	T38.812	T38.813	T38.814	T38.815	T38.816
Guaiacol derivatives	T48.4X1	T48.4X2	T48.4X3	T48.4X4	T48.4X5	T48.4X6
Guaiac reagent	T50.991	T50.992	T50.993	T50.994	T50.995	T50.996
Guaifenesin	T48.4X1	T48.4X2	T48.4X3	T48.4X4	T48.4X5	T48.4X6
Guaimesal	T48.4X1	T48.4X2	T48.4X3	T48.4X4	T48.4X5	T48.4X6
Guaiphenesin	T48.4X1	T48.4X2	T48.4X3	T48.4X4	T48.4X5	T48.4X6
Guamecycline	T36.4X1	T36.4X2	T36.4X3	T36.4X4	T36.4X5	T36.4X6

TABLE OF DRUGS AND CHEMICALS

Substance	External Cause (T-Code)					
	Poisoning, Accidental (Unintentional)	Poisoning, Intentional Self-Harm	Poisoning, Assault	Poisoning, Undetermined	Adverse Effect	Underdosing
Guanabenz	T46.5X1	T46.5X2	T46.5X3	T46.5X4	T46.5X5	T46.5X6
Guanacline	T46.5X1	T46.5X2	T46.5X3	T46.5X4	T46.5X5	T46.5X6
Guanadrel	T46.5X1	T46.5X2	T46.5X3	T46.5X4	T46.5X5	T46.5X6
Guanatol	T37.2X1	T37.2X2	T37.2X3	T37.2X4	T37.2X5	T37.2X6
Guanethidine	T46.5X1	T46.5X2	T46.5X3	T46.5X4	T46.5X5	T46.5X6
Guanfacine	T46.5X1	T46.5X2	T46.5X3	T46.5X4	T46.5X5	T46.5X6
Guano	T65.891	T65.892	T65.893	T65.894	—	—
Guanochlor	T46.5X1	T46.5X2	T46.5X3	T46.5X4	T46.5X5	T46.5X6
Guanoclor	T46.5X1	T46.5X2	T46.5X3	T46.5X4	T46.5X5	T46.5X6
Guanoctine	T46.5X1	T46.5X2	T46.5X3	T46.5X4	T46.5X5	T46.5X6
Guanoxabenz	T46.5X1	T46.5X2	T46.5X3	T46.5X4	T46.5X5	T46.5X6
Guanoxan	T46.5X1	T46.5X2	T46.5X3	T46.5X4	T46.5X5	T46.5X6
Guar gum (medicinal)	T46.6X1	T46.6X2	T46.6X3	T46.6X4	T46.6X5	T46.6X6
H						
Hachimycin	T36.7X1	T36.7X2	T36.7X3	T36.7X4	T36.7X5	T36.7X6
Hair						
dye	T49.4X1	T49.4X2	T49.4X3	T49.4X4	T49.4X5	T49.4X6
preparation NEC	T49.4X1	T49.4X2	T49.4X3	T49.4X4	T49.4X5	T49.4X6
Halazepam	T42.4X1	T42.4X2	T42.4X3	T42.4X4	T42.4X5	T42.4X6
Halcinolone	T49.0X1	T49.0X2	T49.0X3	T49.0X4	T49.0X5	T49.0X6
Halcinonide	T49.0X1	T49.0X2	T49.0X3	T49.0X4	T49.0X5	T49.0X6
Halethazole	T49.0X1	T49.0X2	T49.0X3	T49.0X4	T49.0X5	T49.0X6
Hallucinogen NOS	T40.901	T40.902	T40.903	T40.904	T40.905	T40.906
specified NEC	T40.991	T40.992	T40.993	T40.994	T40.995	T40.996
Halofantrine	T37.2X1	T37.2X2	T37.2X3	T37.2X4	T37.2X5	T37.2X6
Halofenate	T46.6X1	T46.6X2	T46.6X3	T46.6X4	T46.6X5	T46.6X6
Halometasone	T49.0X1	T49.0X2	T49.0X3	T49.0X4	T49.0X5	T49.0X6
Haloperidol	T43.4X1	T43.4X2	T43.4X3	T43.4X4	T43.4X5	T43.4X6
Haloprogin	T49.0X1	T49.0X2	T49.0X3	T49.0X4	T49.0X5	T49.0X6
Halotex	T49.0X1	T49.0X2	T49.0X3	T49.0X4	T49.0X5	T49.0X6
Halothane	T41.0X1	T41.0X2	T41.0X3	T41.0X4	T41.0X5	T41.0X6
Haloxazolam	T42.4X1	T42.4X2	T42.4X3	T42.4X4	T42.4X5	T42.4X6
Halquinols	T49.0X1	T49.0X2	T49.0X3	T49.0X4	T49.0X5	T49.0X6
Hamamelis	T49.2X1	T49.2X2	T49.2X3	T49.2X4	T49.2X5	T49.2X6
Haptendextran	T45.8X1	T45.8X2	T45.8X3	T45.8X4	T45.8X5	T45.8X6
Harmonyl	T46.5X1	T46.5X2	T46.5X3	T46.5X4	T46.5X5	T46.5X6
Hartmann's solution	T50.3X1	T50.3X2	T50.3X3	T50.3X4	T50.3X5	T50.3X6
Hashish	T40.711	T40.712	T40.713	T40.714	T40.715	T40.716
Hawaiian Woodrose seeds	T40.991	T40.992	T40.993	T40.994	—	—
HCB	T60.3X1	T60.3X2	T60.3X3	T60.3X4	—	—
HCH	T53.6X1	T53.6X2	T53.6X3	T53.6X4	—	—
medicinal	T49.0X1	T49.0X2	T49.0X3	T49.0X4	T49.0X5	T49.0X6

Substance	External Cause (T-Code)					
	Poisoning, Accidental (Unintentional)	Poisoning, Intentional Self-Harm	Poisoning, Assault	Poisoning, Undetermined	Adverse Effect	Underdosing
HCN	T57.3X1	T57.3X2	T57.3X3	T57.3X4	—	—
Headache cures, drugs, powders NEC	T50.901	T50.902	T50.903	T50.904	T50.905	T50.906
Heavenly Blue (morning glory)	T40.991	T40.992	T40.993	T40.994	—	—
Heavy metal antidote	T45.8X1	T45.8X2	T45.8X3	T45.8X4	T45.8X5	T45.8X6
Hedaquinium	T49.0X1	T49.0X2	T49.0X3	T49.0X4	T49.0X5	T49.0X6
Hedge hyssop	T62.2X1	T62.2X2	T62.2X3	T62.2X4	—	—
Heet	T49.8X1	T49.8X2	T49.8X3	T49.8X4	T49.8X5	T49.8X6
Helium	T48.991	T48.992	T48.993	T48.994	T48.995	T48.996
Helenin	T37.4X1	T37.4X2	T37.4X3	T37.4X4	T37.4X5	T37.4X6
Hellebore (black) (green) (white)	T62.2X1	T62.2X2	T62.2X3	T62.2X4	—	—
Helium (nonmedicinal) NEC	T59.891	T59.892	T59.893	T59.894	—	—
medicinal	T48.991	T48.992	T48.993	T48.994	T48.995	T48.996
Hematin	T45.8X1	T45.8X2	T45.8X3	T45.8X4	T45.8X5	T45.8X6
Hematinic preparation	T45.8X1	T45.8X2	T45.8X3	T45.8X4	T45.8X5	T45.8X6
Hemlock	T62.2X1	T62.2X2	T62.2X3	T62.2X4	—	—
Hemostatic	T45.621	T45.622	T45.623	T45.624	T45.625	T45.626
drug, systemic	T45.621	T45.622	T45.623	T45.624	T45.625	T45.626
Hemostyptic	T49.4X1	T49.4X2	T49.4X3	T49.4X4	T49.4X5	T49.4X6
Henbane	T62.2X1	T62.2X2	T62.2X3	T62.2X4	—	—
Heparin (sodium)	T45.511	T45.512	T45.513	T45.514	T45.515	T45.516
action reverser	T45.7X1	T45.7X2	T45.7X3	T45.7X4	T45.7X5	T45.7X6
Heparin-fraction	T45.511	T45.512	T45.513	T45.514	T45.515	T45.516
Heparinoid (systemic)	T45.511	T45.512	T45.513	T45.514	T45.515	T45.516
Hepatic secretion stimulant	T47.8X1	T47.8X2	T47.8X3	T47.8X4	T47.8X5	T47.8X6
Hepatitis B						
immune globulin	T50.Z11	T50.Z12	T50.Z13	T50.Z14	T50.Z15	T50.Z16
vaccine	T50.B91	T50.B92	T50.B93	T50.B94	T50.B95	T50.B96
Hepronicate	T46.7X1	T46.7X2	T46.7X3	T46.7X4	T46.7X5	T46.7X6
Heptabarb	T42.3X1	T42.3X2	T42.3X3	T42.3X4	T42.3X5	T42.3X6
Heptabarbitone	T42.3X1	T42.3X2	T42.3X3	T42.3X4	T42.3X5	T42.3X6
Heptabarbital	T42.3X1	T42.3X2	T42.3X3	T42.3X4	T42.3X5	T42.3X6
Heptachlor	T60.1X1	T60.1X2	T60.1X3	T60.1X4	—	—
Heptalgin	T40.2X1	T40.2X2	T40.2X3	T40.2X4	T40.2X5	T40.2X6
Heptaminol	T46.3X1	T46.3X2	T46.3X3	T46.3X4	T46.3X5	T46.3X6
Herbicide NEC	T60.3X1	T60.3X2	T60.3X3	T60.3X4	—	—
Heroin	T40.1X1	T40.1X2	T40.1X3	T40.1X4	—	—
Herplex	T49.5X1	T49.5X2	T49.5X3	T49.5X4	T49.5X5	T49.5X6
HES	T45.8X1	T45.8X2	T45.8X3	T45.8X4	T45.8X5	T45.8X6
Hesperidin	T46.991	T46.992	T46.993	T46.994	T46.995	T46.996
Hetacillin	T36.0X1	T36.0X2	T36.0X3	T36.0X4	T36.0X5	T36.0X6

◀ New   ◀ Revised   ~~deleted~~ Deleted

Substance	External Cause (T-Code) Poisoning, Accidental (Unintentional)	Poisoning, Intentional Self-Harm	Poisoning, Assault	Poisoning, Undetermined	Adverse Effect	Underdosing
Hetastarch	T45.8X1	T45.8X2	T45.8X3	T45.8X4	T45.8X5	T45.8X6
HETP	T60.0X1	T60.0X2	T60.0X3	T60.0X4	—	—
Hexachlorobenzene (vapor)	T60.3X1	T60.3X2	T60.3X3	T60.3X4	—	—
Hexachlorocyclohexane	T53.6X1	T53.6X2	T53.6X3	T53.6X4	—	—
Hexachlorophene	T49.0X1	T49.0X2	T49.0X3	T49.0X4	T49.0X5	T49.0X6
Hexadiline	T46.3X1	T46.3X2	T46.3X3	T46.3X4	T46.3X5	T46.3X6
Hexadimethrine (bromide)	T45.7X1	T45.7X2	T45.7X3	T45.7X4	T45.7X5	T45.7X6
Hexadylamine	T46.3X1	T46.3X2	T46.3X3	T46.3X4	T46.3X5	T46.3X6
Hexaethyl tetraphosphate	T60.0X1	T60.0X2	T60.0X3	T60.0X4	—	—
Hexafluorenium bromide	T48.1X1	T48.1X2	T48.1X3	T48.1X4	T48.1X5	T48.1X6
Hexafluorodiethyl ether	T43.291	T43.292	T43.293	T43.294	T43.295	T43.296
Hexafluronium (bromide)	T48.1X1	T48.1X2	T48.1X3	T48.1X4	T48.1X5	T48.1X6
Hexahydrobenzol	T52.8X1	T52.8X2	T52.8X3	T52.8X4	—	—
Hexahydrocresol(s)	T51.8X1	T51.8X2	T51.8X3	T51.8X4	—	—
arsenide	T57.0X1	T57.0X2	T57.0X3	T57.0X4	—	—
arseniurated	T57.0X1	T57.0X2	T57.0X3	T57.0X4	—	—
cyanide	T57.3X1	T57.3X2	T57.3X3	T57.3X4	—	—
gas	T59.891	T59.892	T59.893	T59.894	—	—
Fluoride (liquid)	T57.8X1	T57.8X2	T57.8X3	T57.8X4	—	—
vapor	T59.891	T59.892	T59.893	T59.894	—	—
phophorated	T60.0X1	T60.0X2	T60.0X3	T60.0X4	—	—
sulfate	T57.8X1	T57.8X2	T57.8X3	T57.8X4	—	—
sulfide (gas)	T59.6X1	T59.6X2	T59.6X3	T59.6X4	—	—
arseniurated	T57.0X1	T57.0X2	T57.0X3	T57.0X4	—	—
sulfurated	T57.8X1	T57.8X2	T57.8X3	T57.8X4	—	—
Hexahydrophenol	T51.8X1	T51.8X2	T51.8X3	T51.8X4	—	—
Hexa-germ	T49.2X1	T49.2X2	T49.2X3	T49.2X4	T49.2X5	T49.2X6
Hexalen	T51.8X1	T51.8X2	T51.8X3	T51.8X4	—	—
Hexamethonium bromide	T44.2X1	T44.2X2	T44.2X3	T44.2X4	T44.2X5	T44.2X6
Hexamethylene	T52.8X1	T52.8X2	T52.8X3	T52.8X4	—	—
Hexamethylmelamine	T45.1X1	T45.1X2	T45.1X3	T45.1X4	T45.1X5	T45.1X6
Hexamidine	T49.0X1	T49.0X2	T49.0X3	T49.0X4	T49.0X5	T49.0X6
Hexamine (mandelate)	T37.8X1	T37.8X2	T37.8X3	T37.8X4	T37.8X5	T37.8X6
Hexanone, 2-hexanone	T52.4X1	T52.4X2	T52.4X3	T52.4X4	—	—
Hexanuorenium	T48.1X1	T48.1X2	T48.1X3	T48.1X4	T48.1X5	T48.1X6
Hexapropymate	T42.6X1	T42.6X2	T42.6X3	T42.6X4	T42.6X5	T42.6X6
Hexasonium iodide	T44.3X1	T44.3X2	T44.3X3	T44.3X4	T44.3X5	T44.3X6
Hexcarbacholine bromide	T48.1X1	T48.1X2	T48.1X3	T48.1X4	T48.1X5	T48.1X6
Hexemal	T42.3X1	T42.3X2	T42.3X3	T42.3X4	T42.3X5	T42.3X6
Hexestrol	T38.5X1	T38.5X2	T38.5X3	T38.5X4	T38.5X5	T38.5X6
Hexethal (sodium)	T42.3X1	T42.3X2	T42.3X3	T42.3X4	T42.3X5	T42.3X6
Hexetidine	T37.8X1	T37.8X2	T37.8X3	T37.8X4	T37.8X5	T37.8X6

Substance	External Cause (T-Code) Poisoning, Accidental (Unintentional)	Poisoning, Intentional Self-Harm	Poisoning, Assault	Poisoning, Undetermined	Adverse Effect	Underdosing
Hexobarbital	T42.3X1	T42.3X2	T42.3X3	T42.3X4	T42.3X5	T42.3X6
rectal	T41.291	T41.292	T41.293	T41.294	T41.295	T41.296
sodium	T41.1X1	T41.1X2	T41.1X3	T41.1X4	T41.1X5	T41.1X6
Hexobendine	T46.3X1	T46.3X2	T46.3X3	T46.3X4	T46.3X5	T46.3X6
Hexocyclium	T44.3X1	T44.3X2	T44.3X3	T44.3X4	T44.3X5	T44.3X6
metilsulfate	T44.3X1	T44.3X2	T44.3X3	T44.3X4	T44.3X5	T44.3X6
Hexoestrol	T38.5X1	T38.5X2	T38.5X3	T38.5X4	T38.5X5	T38.5X6
Hexone	T52.4X1	T52.4X2	T52.4X3	T52.4X4	—	—
Hexoprenaline	T48.6X1	T48.6X2	T48.6X3	T48.6X4	T48.6X5	T48.6X6
Hexylcaine	T41.3X1	T41.3X2	T41.3X3	T41.3X4	T41.3X5	T41.3X6
Hexylresorcinol	T52.2X1	T52.2X2	T52.2X3	T52.2X4	—	—
HGH (human growth hormone)	T38.811	T38.812	T38.813	T38.814	T38.815	T38.816
Hinkle's pills	T47.2X1	T47.2X2	T47.2X3	T47.2X4	T47.2X5	T47.2X6
Histalog	T50.8X1	T50.8X2	T50.8X3	T50.8X4	T50.8X5	T50.8X6
Histamine (phosphate)	T50.8X1	T50.8X2	T50.8X3	T50.8X4	T50.8X5	T50.8X6
Histoplasmin	T50.8X1	T50.8X2	T50.8X3	T50.8X4	T50.8X5	T50.8X6
Holly berries	T62.2X1	T62.2X2	T62.2X3	T62.2X4	—	—
Homatropine	T44.3X1	T44.3X2	T44.3X3	T44.3X4	T44.3X5	T44.3X6
methylbromide	T44.3X1	T44.3X2	T44.3X3	T44.3X4	T44.3X5	T44.3X6
Homochlorcyclizine	T45.0X1	T45.0X2	T45.0X3	T45.0X4	T45.0X5	T45.0X6
Homosalate	T49.3X1	T49.3X2	T49.3X3	T49.3X4	T49.3X5	T49.3X6
Homo-tet	T50.Z11	T50.Z12	T50.Z13	T50.Z14	T50.Z15	T50.Z16
Hormone	T38.801	T38.802	T38.803	T38.804	T38.805	T38.806
adrenal cortical steroids	T38.0X1	T38.0X2	T38.0X3	T38.0X4	T38.0X5	T38.0X6
androgenic	T38.7X1	T38.7X2	T38.7X3	T38.7X4	T38.7X5	T38.7X6
anterior pituitary NEC	T38.811	T38.812	T38.813	T38.814	T38.815	T38.816
antidiabetic agents	T38.3X1	T38.3X2	T38.3X3	T38.3X4	T38.3X5	T38.3X6
antidiuretic	T38.891	T38.892	T38.893	T38.894	T38.895	T38.896
cancer therapy	T45.1X1	T45.1X2	T45.1X3	T45.1X4	T45.1X5	T45.1X6
follicle stimulating	T38.811	T38.812	T38.813	T38.814	T38.815	T38.816
gonadotropic	T38.891	T38.892	T38.893	T38.894	T38.895	T38.896
pituitary	T38.811	T38.812	T38.813	T38.814	T38.815	T38.816
growth	T38.811	T38.812	T38.813	T38.814	T38.815	T38.816
luteinizing	T38.811	T38.812	T38.813	T38.814	T38.815	T38.816
ovarian	T38.5X1	T38.5X2	T38.5X3	T38.5X4	T38.5X5	T38.5X6
oxytocic	T48.0X1	T48.0X2	T48.0X3	T48.0X4	T48.0X5	T48.0X6
parathyroid (derivatives)	T50.991	T50.992	T50.993	T50.994	T50.995	T50.996
pituitary (posterior) NEC	T38.891	T38.892	T38.893	T38.894	T38.895	T38.896
anterior	T38.811	T38.812	T38.813	T38.814	T38.815	T38.816
specified, NEC	T38.891	T38.892	T38.893	T38.894	T38.895	T38.896
thyroid	T38.1X1	T38.1X2	T38.1X3	T38.1X4	T38.1X5	T38.1X6
Hornet (sting)	T63.451	T63.452	T63.453	T63.454	—	—

◀ New   ◀ Revised   ~~deleted~~ Deleted

TABLE OF DRUGS AND CHEMICALS

Substance	External Cause (T-Code)					
	Poisoning, Accidental (Unintentional)	Poisoning, Intentional Self-Harm	Poisoning, Assault	Poisoning, Undetermined	Adverse Effect	Underdosing
Horse anti-human lymphocytic serum	T50.Z11	T50.Z12	T50.Z13	T50.Z14	T50.Z15	T50.Z16
Horticulture agent NEC	T65.91	T65.92	T65.93	T65.94	—	—
with pesticide	T60.91	T60.92	T60.93	T60.94	—	—
Human						
albumin	T45.8X1	T45.8X2	T45.8X3	T45.8X4	T45.8X5	T45.8X6
growth hormone (HGH)	T38.811	T38.812	T38.813	T38.814	T38.815	T38.816
immune serum	T50.Z11	T50.Z12	T50.Z13	T50.Z14	T50.Z15	T50.Z16
Hyaluronidase	T45.3X1	T45.3X2	T45.3X3	T45.3X4	T45.3X5	T45.3X6
Hyazyme	T45.3X1	T45.3X2	T45.3X3	T45.3X4	T45.3X5	T45.3X6
Hycodan	T40.2X1	T40.2X2	T40.2X3	T40.2X4	T40.2X5	T40.2X6
Hydantoin derivative NEC	T42.0X1	T42.0X2	T42.0X3	T42.0X4	T42.0X5	T42.0X6
Hydeltra	T38.0X1	T38.0X2	T38.0X3	T38.0X4	T38.0X5	T38.0X6
Hydergine	T44.6X1	T44.6X2	T44.6X3	T44.6X4	T44.6X5	T44.6X6
Hydrabamine penicillin	T36.0X1	T36.0X2	T36.0X3	T36.0X4	T36.0X5	T36.0X6
Hydralazine	T46.5X1	T46.5X2	T46.5X3	T46.5X4	T46.5X5	T46.5X6
Hydrargaphen	T49.0X1	T49.0X2	T49.0X3	T49.0X4	T49.0X5	T49.0X6
Hydrargyri amino-chloridum	T49.0X1	T49.0X2	T49.0X3	T49.0X4	T49.0X5	T49.0X6
Hydrastine	T48.291	T48.292	T48.293	T48.294	T48.295	T48.296
Hydrazine	T54.1X1	T54.1X2	T54.1X3	T54.1X4	—	—
monoamine oxidase inhibitors	T43.1X1	T43.1X2	T43.1X3	T43.1X4	T43.1X5	T43.1X6
Hydrazoic acid, azides	T54.2X1	T54.2X2	T54.2X3	T54.2X4	—	—
Hydriodic acid	T48.4X1	T48.4X2	T48.4X3	T48.4X4	T48.4X5	T48.4X6
Hydrocarbon gas	T59.891	T59.892	T59.893	T59.894	—	—
incomplete combustion of — see Carbon, monoxide, fuel, utility						
liquefied (mobile container)	T59.891	T59.892	T59.893	T59.894	—	—
piped (natural)	T59.891	T59.892	T59.893	T59.894	—	—
Hydrochloric acid (liquid)	T54.2X1	T54.2X2	T54.2X3	T54.2X4	—	—
medicinal (digestant)	T47.5X1	T47.5X2	T47.5X3	T47.5X4	T47.5X5	T47.5X6
vapor	T59.891	T59.892	T59.893	T59.894	—	—
Hydrochlorothiazide	T50.2X1	T50.2X2	T50.2X3	T50.2X4	T50.2X5	T50.2X6
Hydrocodone	T40.2X1	T40.2X2	T40.2X3	T40.2X4	T40.2X5	T40.2X6
Hydrocortisone (derivatives)	T38.0X1	T38.0X2	T38.0X3	T38.0X4	T38.0X5	T38.0X6
aceponate	T49.0X1	T49.0X2	T49.0X3	T49.0X4	T49.0X5	T49.0X6
ENT agent	T49.6X1	T49.6X2	T49.6X3	T49.6X4	T49.6X5	T49.6X6
ophthalmic preparation	T49.5X1	T49.5X2	T49.5X3	T49.5X4	T49.5X5	T49.5X6
topical NEC	T49.0X1	T49.0X2	T49.0X3	T49.0X4	T49.0X5	T49.0X6
Hydrocortone	T38.0X1	T38.0X2	T38.0X3	T38.0X4	T38.0X5	T38.0X6
ENT agent	T49.6X1	T49.6X2	T49.6X3	T49.6X4	T49.6X5	T49.6X6
ophthalmic preparation	T49.5X1	T49.5X2	T49.5X3	T49.5X4	T49.5X5	T49.5X6
topical NEC	T49.0X1	T49.0X2	T49.0X3	T49.0X4	T49.0X5	T49.0X6

Substance	External Cause (T-Code)					
	Poisoning, Accidental (Unintentional)	Poisoning, Intentional Self-Harm	Poisoning, Assault	Poisoning, Undetermined	Adverse Effect	Underdosing
Hydrocyanic acid (liquid)	T57.3X1	T57.3X2	T57.3X3	T57.3X4	—	—
gas	T65.0X1	T65.0X2	T65.0X3	T65.0X4	—	—
Hydroflumethiazide	T50.2X1	T50.2X2	T50.2X3	T50.2X4	T50.2X5	T50.2X6
Hydrofluoric acid (liquid)	T54.2X1	T54.2X2	T54.2X3	T54.2X4	—	—
vapor	T59.891	T59.892	T59.893	T59.894	—	—
Hydrogen	T59.891	T59.892	T59.893	T59.894	—	—
arsenide	T57.0X1	T57.0X2	T57.0X3	T57.0X4	—	—
arseniureted	T57.0X1	T57.0X2	T57.0X3	T57.0X4	—	—
chloride	T57.8X1	T57.8X2	T57.8X3	T57.8X4	—	—
cyanide (salts)	T57.3X1	T57.3X2	T57.3X3	T57.3X4	—	—
gas	T57.3X1	T57.3X2	T57.3X3	T57.3X4	—	—
Fluoride	T59.5X1	T59.5X2	T59.5X3	T59.5X4	—	—
vapor	T59.5X1	T59.5X2	T59.5X3	T59.5X4	—	—
peroxide	T49.0X1	T49.0X2	T49.0X3	T49.0X4	T49.0X5	T49.0X6
phosphureted	T57.1X1	T57.1X2	T57.1X3	T57.1X4	—	—
sulfide	T59.6X1	T59.6X2	T59.6X3	T59.6X4	—	—
arseniureted	T57.0X1	T57.0X2	T57.0X3	T57.0X4	—	—
sulfureted	T59.6X1	T59.6X2	T59.6X3	T59.6X4	—	—
Hydromethylpyridine	T46.7X1	T46.7X2	T46.7X3	T46.7X4	T46.7X5	T46.7X6
Hydromorphinol	T40.2X1	T40.2X2	T40.2X3	T40.2X4	—	—
Hydromorphinone	T40.2X1	T40.2X2	T40.2X3	T40.2X4	T40.2X5	T40.2X6
Hydromorphone	T40.2X1	T40.2X2	T40.2X3	T40.2X4	T40.2X5	T40.2X6
Hydromox	T50.2X1	T50.2X2	T50.2X3	T50.2X4	T50.2X5	T50.2X6
Hydrophilic lotion	T49.3X1	T49.3X2	T49.3X3	T49.3X4	T49.3X5	T49.3X6
Hydroquinidine	T46.2X1	T46.2X2	T46.2X3	T46.2X4	T46.2X5	T46.2X6
Hydroquinone	T52.2X1	T52.2X2	T52.2X3	T52.2X4	—	—
vapor	T59.891	T59.892	T59.893	T59.894	—	—
Hydrosulfuric acid (gas)	T59.6X1	T59.6X2	T59.6X3	T59.6X4	—	—
Hydrotalcite	T47.1X1	T47.1X2	T47.1X3	T47.1X4	T47.1X5	T47.1X6
Hydrous wool fat	T49.3X1	T49.3X2	T49.3X3	T49.3X4	T49.3X5	T49.3X6
Hydroxide, caustic	T54.3X1	T54.3X2	T54.3X3	T54.3X4	—	—
Hydroxocobalamin	T45.8X1	T45.8X2	T45.8X3	T45.8X4	T45.8X5	T45.8X6
Hydroxyamphetamine	T49.5X1	T49.5X2	T49.5X3	T49.5X4	T49.5X5	T49.5X6
Hydroxycarbamide	T45.1X1	T45.1X2	T45.1X3	T45.1X4	T45.1X5	T45.1X6
Hydroxychloroquine	T37.8X1	T37.8X2	T37.8X3	T37.8X4	T37.8X5	T37.8X6
Hydroxydihydrocodeinone	T40.2X1	T40.2X2	T40.2X3	T40.2X4	T40.2X5	T40.2X6
Hydroxyestrone	T38.5X1	T38.5X2	T38.5X3	T38.5X4	T38.5X5	T38.5X6
Hydroxyethyl starch	T45.8X1	T45.8X2	T45.8X3	T45.8X4	T45.8X5	T45.8X6
Hydroxymethylpentanone	T52.4X1	T52.4X2	T52.4X3	T52.4X4	—	—
Hydroxyphenamate	T43.591	T43.592	T43.593	T43.594	T43.595	T43.596
Hydroxyphenylbutazone	T39.2X1	T39.2X2	T39.2X3	T39.2X4	T39.2X5	T39.2X6

◄ New ◄ Revised ~~deleted~~ Deleted

	External Cause (T-Code)					
Substance	Poisoning, Accidental (Unintentional)	Poisoning, Intentional Self-Harm	Poisoning, Assault	Poisoning, Undetermined	Adverse Effect	Underdosing
Hydroxyprogesterone	T38.5X1	T38.5X2	T38.5X3	T38.5X4	T38.5X5	T38.5X6
caproate	T38.5X1	T38.5X2	T38.5X3	T38.5X4	T38.5X5	T38.5X6
Hydroxyquinoline (derivatives) NEC	T37.8X1	T37.8X2	T37.8X3	T37.8X4	T37.8X5	T37.8X6
Hydroxystilbamidine	T37.3X1	T37.3X2	T37.3X3	T37.3X4	T37.3X5	T37.3X6
Hydroxytoluene (nonmedicinal)	T54.0X1	T54.0X2	T54.0X3	T54.0X4	—	—
medicinal	T49.0X1	T49.0X2	T49.0X3	T49.0X4	T49.0X5	T49.0X6
Hydroxyurea	T45.1X1	T45.1X2	T45.1X3	T45.1X4	T45.1X5	T45.1X6
Hydroxyzine	T43.591	T43.592	T43.593	T43.594	T43.595	T43.596
antiallergic	T45.0X1	T45.0X2	T45.0X3	T45.0X4	T45.0X5	T45.0X6
Hyoscine	T44.3X1	T44.3X2	T44.3X3	T44.3X4	T44.3X5	T44.3X6
Hyoscyamine	T44.3X1	T44.3X2	T44.3X3	T44.3X4	T44.3X5	T44.3X6
Hyoscyamus	T44.3X1	T44.3X2	T44.3X3	T44.3X4	T44.3X5	T44.3X6
dry extract	T44.3X1	T44.3X2	T44.3X3	T44.3X4	T44.3X5	T44.3X6
Hypaque	T50.8X1	T50.8X2	T50.8X3	T50.8X4	T50.8X5	T50.8X6
Hypertussis	T50.Z11	T50.Z12	T50.Z13	T50.Z14	T50.Z15	T50.Z16
Hypnotic	T42.71	T42.72	T42.73	T42.74	T42.75	T42.76
anticonvulsant	T42.71	T42.72	T42.73	T42.74	T42.75	T42.76
specified NEC	T42.6X1	T42.6X2	T42.6X3	T42.6X4	T42.6X5	T42.6X6
Hypochlorite	T49.0X1	T49.0X2	T49.0X3	T49.0X4	T49.0X5	T49.0X6
Hypophysis, posterior	T38.891	T38.892	T38.893	T38.894	T38.895	T38.896
Hypotensive NEC	T46.5X1	T46.5X2	T46.5X3	T46.5X4	T46.5X5	T46.5X6
Hypromellose	T49.5X1	T49.5X2	T49.5X3	T49.5X4	T49.5X5	T49.5X6
Ibacitabine	T37.5X1	T37.5X2	T37.5X3	T37.5X4	T37.5X5	T37.5X6
Ibopamine	T44.991	T44.992	T44.993	T44.994	T44.995	T44.996
Ibufenac	T39.311	T39.312	T39.313	T39.314	T39.315	T39.316
Ibuprofen	T39.311	T39.312	T39.313	T39.314	T39.315	T39.316
Ibuproxam	T39.311	T39.312	T39.313	T39.314	T39.315	T39.316
Ibuterol	T48.6X1	T48.6X2	T48.6X3	T48.6X4	T48.6X5	T48.6X6
Ichthammol	T49.0X1	T49.0X2	T49.0X3	T49.0X4	T49.0X5	T49.0X6
Ichthyol	T49.4X1	T49.4X2	T49.4X3	T49.4X4	T49.4X5	T49.4X6
Idarubicin	T45.1X1	T45.1X2	T45.1X3	T45.1X4	T45.1X5	T45.1X6
Idrocilamide	T42.8X1	T42.8X2	T42.8X3	T42.8X4	T42.8X5	T42.8X6
Ifenprodil	T46.7X1	T46.7X2	T46.7X3	T46.7X4	T46.7X5	T46.7X6
Ifosfamide	T45.1X1	T45.1X2	T45.1X3	T45.1X4	T45.1X5	T45.1X6
Iletin	T38.3X1	T38.3X2	T38.3X3	T38.3X4	T38.3X5	T38.3X6
Ilex	T62.2X1	T62.2X2	T62.2X3	T62.2X4	—	—
Illuminating gas (after combustion)	T58.11	T58.12	T58.13	T58.14	—	—
prior to combustion	T59.891	T59.892	T59.893	T59.894	—	—
Ilopan	T45.2X1	T45.2X2	T45.2X3	T45.2X4	T45.2X5	T45.2X6

	External Cause (T-Code)					
Substance	Poisoning, Accidental (Unintentional)	Poisoning, Intentional Self-Harm	Poisoning, Assault	Poisoning, Undetermined	Adverse Effect	Underdosing
Iloprost	T46.7X1	T46.7X2	T46.7X3	T46.7X4	T46.7X5	T46.7X6
Ilotycin	T36.3X1	T36.3X2	T36.3X3	T36.3X4	T36.3X5	T36.3X6
ophthalmic preparation	T49.5X1	T49.5X2	T49.5X3	T49.5X4	T49.5X5	T49.5X6
topical NEC	T49.0X1	T49.0X2	T49.0X3	T49.0X4	T49.0X5	T49.0X6
Imidazole-4-carboxamide	T45.1X1	T45.1X2	T45.1X3	T45.1X4	T45.1X5	T45.1X6
Imipenem	T36.0X1	T36.0X2	T36.0X3	T36.0X4	T36.0X5	T36.0X6
Imipramine	T43.011	T43.012	T43.013	T43.014	T43.015	T43.016
Iminostilbene	T42.1X1	T42.1X2	T42.1X3	T42.1X4	T42.1X5	T42.1X6
Immu-G	T50.Z11	T50.Z12	T50.Z13	T50.Z14	T50.Z15	T50.Z16
Immuglobin	T50.Z11	T50.Z12	T50.Z13	T50.Z14	T50.Z15	T50.Z16
Immune						
checkpoint inhibitors	T45.AX1	T45.AX2	T45.AX3	T45.AX4	T45.AX5	T45.AX6
globulin	T50.Z11	T50.Z12	T50.Z13	T50.Z14	T50.Z15	T50.Z16
serum globulin	T50.Z11	T50.Z12	T50.Z13	T50.Z14	T50.Z15	T50.Z16
Immunoglobin human (intravenous) (normal)	T50.Z11	T50.Z12	T50.Z13	T50.Z14	T50.Z15	T50.Z16
unmodified	T50.Z11	T50.Z12	T50.Z13	T50.Z14	T50.Z15	T50.Z16
Immunostimulant drug	T45.AX1	T45.AX2	T45.AX3	T45.AX4	T45.AX5	T45.AX6
Immunosuppressive drug	T45.1X1	T45.1X2	T45.1X3	T45.1X4	T45.1X5	T45.1X6
Immu-tetanus	T50.Z11	T50.Z12	T50.Z13	T50.Z14	T50.Z15	T50.Z16
Indalpine	T43.221	T43.222	T43.223	T43.224	T43.225	T43.226
Indanazoline	T48.5X1	T48.5X2	T48.5X3	T48.5X4	T48.5X5	T48.5X6
Indandione (derivatives)	T45.511	T45.512	T45.513	T45.514	T45.515	T45.516
Indapamide	T46.5X1	T46.5X2	T46.5X3	T46.5X4	T46.5X5	T46.5X6
Indendione (derivatives)	T45.511	T45.512	T45.513	T45.514	T45.515	T45.516
Indenolol	T44.7X1	T44.7X2	T44.7X3	T44.7X4	T44.7X5	T44.7X6
Inderal	T44.7X1	T44.7X2	T44.7X3	T44.7X4	T44.7X5	T44.7X6
Indian						
hemp	T40.711	T40.712	T40.713	T40.714	T40.715	T40.716
tobacco	T62.2X1	T62.2X2	T62.2X3	T62.2X4	—	—
Indigo carmine	T50.8X1	T50.8X2	T50.8X3	T50.8X4	T50.8X5	T50.8X6
Indobufen	T45.521	T45.522	T45.523	T45.524	T45.525	T45.526
Indocin	T39.2X1	T39.2X2	T39.2X3	T39.2X4	T39.2X5	T39.2X6
Indocyanine green	T50.8X1	T50.8X2	T50.8X3	T50.8X4	T50.8X5	T50.8X6
Indometacin	T39.391	T39.392	T39.393	T39.394	T39.395	T39.396
Indomethacin	T39.391	T39.392	T39.393	T39.394	T39.395	T39.396
farnesil	T39.4X1	T39.4X2	T39.4X3	T39.4X4	T39.4X5	T39.4X6
Indoramin	T44.6X1	T44.6X2	T44.6X3	T44.6X4	T44.6X5	T44.6X6
Industrial						
alcohol	T51.0X1	T51.0X2	T51.0X3	T51.0X4	—	—
fumes	T59.891	T59.892	T59.893	T59.894	—	—
solvents (fumes) (vapors)	T52.91	T52.92	T52.93	T52.94	—	—
Influenza vaccine	T50.B91	T50.B92	T50.B93	T50.B94	T50.B95	T50.B96

TABLE OF DRUGS AND CHEMICALS

Substance	External Cause (T-Code)					
	Poisoning, Accidental (Unintentional)	Poisoning, Intentional Self-Harm	Poisoning, Assault	Poisoning, Undetermined	Adverse Effect	Underdosing
Ingested substance NEC	T65.91	T65.92	T65.93	T65.94	—	—
INH	T37.1X1	T37.1X2	T37.1X3	T37.1X4	T37.1X5	T37.1X6
Inhalation, gas (noxious) — see Gas						
Inhibitor						
angiotensin-converting enzyme	T46.4X1	T46.4X2	T46.4X3	T46.4X4	T46.4X5	T46.4X6
carbonic anhydrase	T50.2X1	T50.2X2	T50.2X3	T50.2X4	T50.2X5	T50.2X6
fibrinolysis	T45.621	T45.622	T45.623	T45.624	T45.625	T45.626
monoamine oxidase NEC	T43.1X1	T43.1X2	T43.1X3	T43.1X4	T43.1X5	T43.1X6
hydrazine	T43.1X1	T43.1X2	T43.1X3	T43.1X4	T43.1X5	T43.1X6
postsynaptic	T43.8X1	T43.8X2	T43.8X3	T43.8X4	T43.8X5	T43.8X6
prothrombin synthesis	T45.511	T45.512	T45.513	T45.514	T45.515	T45.516
Ink	T65.891	T65.892	T65.893	T65.894	—	—
Inorganic substance NEC	T57.91	T57.92	T57.93	T57.94	—	—
Inosine pranobex	T37.5X1	T37.5X2	T37.5X3	T37.5X4	T37.5X5	T37.5X6
Inositol	T50.991	T50.992	T50.993	T50.994	T50.995	T50.996
nicotinate	T46.7X1	T46.7X2	T46.7X3	T46.7X4	T46.7X5	T46.7X6
Inproquone	T45.1X1	T45.1X2	T45.1X3	T45.1X4	T45.1X5	T45.1X6
Insect (sting), venomous	T63.481	T63.482	T63.483	T63.484	—	—
ant	T63.421	T63.422	T63.423	T63.424	—	—
bee	T63.441	T63.442	T63.443	T63.444	—	—
caterpillar	T63.431	T63.432	T63.433	T63.434	—	—
hornet	T63.451	T63.452	T63.453	T63.454	—	—
wasp	T63.461	T63.462	T63.463	T63.464	—	—
Insecticide NEC	T60.91	T60.92	T60.93	T60.94	—	—
carbamate	T60.0X1	T60.0X2	T60.0X3	T60.0X4	—	—
chlorinated	T60.1X1	T60.1X2	T60.1X3	T60.1X4	—	—
mixed	T60.91	T60.92	T60.93	T60.94	—	—
organochlorine	T60.1X1	T60.1X2	T60.1X3	T60.1X4	—	—
organophosphorus	T60.0X1	T60.0X2	T60.0X3	T60.0X4	—	—
Insular tissue extract	T38.3X1	T38.3X2	T38.3X3	T38.3X4	T38.3X5	T38.3X6
Insulin (amorphous) (globin) (isophane) (Lente) (NPH) (Semilente) (Ultralente)	T38.3X1	T38.3X2	T38.3X3	T38.3X4	T38.3X5	T38.3X6
defalan	T38.3X1	T38.3X2	T38.3X3	T38.3X4	T38.3X5	T38.3X6
human	T38.3X1	T38.3X2	T38.3X3	T38.3X4	T38.3X5	T38.3X6
injection, soluble	T38.3X1	T38.3X2	T38.3X3	T38.3X4	T38.3X5	T38.3X6
biphasic	T38.3X1	T38.3X2	T38.3X3	T38.3X4	T38.3X5	T38.3X6
intermediate acting	T38.3X1	T38.3X2	T38.3X3	T38.3X4	T38.3X5	T38.3X6
protamine zinc	T38.3X1	T38.3X2	T38.3X3	T38.3X4	T38.3X5	T38.3X6
slow acting	T38.3X1	T38.3X2	T38.3X3	T38.3X4	T38.3X5	T38.3X6

Substance	External Cause (T-Code)					
	Poisoning, Accidental (Unintentional)	Poisoning, Intentional Self-Harm	Poisoning, Assault	Poisoning, Undetermined	Adverse Effect	Underdosing
zinc						
protamine injection	T38.3X1	T38.3X2	T38.3X3	T38.3X4	T38.3X5	T38.3X6
suspension (amorphous) (crystalline)	T38.3X1	T38.3X2	T38.3X3	T38.3X4	T38.3X5	T38.3X6
Interferon (alpha) (beta) (gamma)	T37.5X1	T37.5X2	T37.5X3	T37.5X4	T37.5X5	T37.5X6
Intestinal motility control drug	T47.6X1	T47.6X2	T47.6X3	T47.6X4	T47.6X5	T47.6X6
biological	T47.8X1	T47.8X2	T47.8X3	T47.8X4	T47.8X5	T47.8X6
Intranarcon	T41.1X1	T41.1X2	T41.1X3	T41.1X4	T41.1X5	T41.1X6
Intravenous						
amino acids	T50.991	T50.992	T50.993	T50.994	T50.995	T50.996
fat suspension	T50.991	T50.992	T50.993	T50.994	T50.995	T50.996
Inulin	T50.8X1	T50.8X2	T50.8X3	T50.8X4	T50.8X5	T50.8X6
Invert sugar	T50.3X1	T50.3X2	T50.3X3	T50.3X4	T50.3X5	T50.3X6
Inza — see Naproxen						
Iobenzamic acid	T50.8X1	T50.8X2	T50.8X3	T50.8X4	T50.8X5	T50.8X6
Iocarmic acid	T50.8X1	T50.8X2	T50.8X3	T50.8X4	T50.8X5	T50.8X6
Iocetamic acid	T50.8X1	T50.8X2	T50.8X3	T50.8X4	T50.8X5	T50.8X6
Iodamide	T50.8X1	T50.8X2	T50.8X3	T50.8X4	T50.8X5	T50.8X6
Iodide NEC — see also Iodine	T49.0X1	T49.0X2	T49.0X3	T49.0X4	T49.0X5	T49.0X6
mercury (ointment)	T49.0X1	T49.0X2	T49.0X3	T49.0X4	T49.0X5	T49.0X6
methylate	T49.0X1	T49.0X2	T49.0X3	T49.0X4	T49.0X5	T49.0X6
potassium (expectorant) NEC	T48.4X1	T48.4X2	T48.4X3	T48.4X4	T48.4X5	T48.4X6
Iodinated						
contrast medium	T50.8X1	T50.8X2	T50.8X3	T50.8X4	T50.8X5	T50.8X6
glycerol	T48.4X1	T48.4X2	T48.4X3	T48.4X4	T48.4X5	T48.4X6
human serum albumin (131I)	T50.8X1	T50.8X2	T50.8X3	T50.8X4	T50.8X5	T50.8X6
Iodine (antiseptic, external) (tincture) NEC	T49.0X1	T49.0X2	T49.0X3	T49.0X4	T49.0X5	T49.0X6
125 — see also Radiation sickness, and Exposure to radioactive isotopes						
therapeutic	T50.991	T50.992	T50.993	T50.994	T50.995	T50.996
131 — see also Radiation sickness, and Exposure to radioactive isotopes						
therapeutic	T38.2X1	T38.2X2	T38.2X3	T38.2X4	T38.2X5	T38.2X6
diagnostic	T50.8X1	T50.8X2	T50.8X3	T50.8X4	T50.8X5	T50.8X6
for thyroid conditions (antithyroid)	T38.2X1	T38.2X2	T38.2X3	T38.2X4	T38.2X5	T38.2X6
solution	T49.0X1	T49.0X2	T49.0X3	T49.0X4	T49.0X5	T49.0X6
vapor	T59.891	T59.892	T59.893	T59.894	—	—
Iodipamide	T50.8X1	T50.8X2	T50.8X3	T50.8X4	T50.8X5	T50.8X6
Iodized (poppy seed) oil	T50.8X1	T50.8X2	T50.8X3	T50.8X4	T50.8X5	T50.8X6
Iodobismitol	T37.8X1	T37.8X2	T37.8X3	T37.8X4	T37.8X5	T37.8X6

◀ New   ◀ Revised   ~~deleted~~ Deleted

	External Cause (T-Code)					
Substance	Poisoning, Accidental (Unintentional)	Poisoning, Intentional Self-Harm	Poisoning, Assault	Poisoning, Undetermined	Adverse Effect	Underdosing
Iodochlorhydroxyquin	T37.8X1	T37.8X2	T37.8X3	T37.8X4	T37.8X5	T37.8X6
topical	T49.0X1	T49.0X2	T49.0X3	T49.0X4	T49.0X5	T49.0X6
Iodochlorhydroxyquino-line	T37.8X1	T37.8X2	T37.8X3	T37.8X4	T37.8X5	T37.8X6
Iodocholesterol (131I)	T50.8X1	T50.8X2	T50.8X3	T50.8X4	T50.8X5	T50.8X6
Iodoform	T49.0X1	T49.0X2	T49.0X3	T49.0X4	T49.0X5	T49.0X6
Iodohippuric acid	T50.8X1	T50.8X2	T50.8X3	T50.8X4	T50.8X5	T50.8X6
Iodopanoic acid	T50.8X1	T50.8X2	T50.8X3	T50.8X4	T50.8X5	T50.8X6
Iodophthalein (sodium)	T50.8X1	T50.8X2	T50.8X3	T50.8X4	T50.8X5	T50.8X6
Iodopyracet	T50.8X1	T50.8X2	T50.8X3	T50.8X4	T50.8X5	T50.8X6
Iodoquinol	T37.8X1	T37.8X2	T37.8X3	T37.8X4	T37.8X5	T37.8X6
Iodoxamic acid	T50.8X1	T50.8X2	T50.8X3	T50.8X4	T50.8X5	T50.8X6
Iofendylate	T50.8X1	T50.8X2	T50.8X3	T50.8X4	T50.8X5	T50.8X6
Ioglycamic acid	T50.8X1	T50.8X2	T50.8X3	T50.8X4	T50.8X5	T50.8X6
Iohexol	T50.8X1	T50.8X2	T50.8X3	T50.8X4	T50.8X5	T50.8X6
Ion exchange resin						
anion	T47.8X1	T47.8X2	T47.8X3	T47.8X4	T47.8X5	T47.8X6
cation	T50.3X1	T50.3X2	T50.3X3	T50.3X4	T50.3X5	T50.3X6
cholestyramine	T46.6X1	T46.6X2	T46.6X3	T46.6X4	T46.6X5	T46.6X6
intestinal	T47.8X1	T47.8X2	T47.8X3	T47.8X4	T47.8X5	T47.8X6
Iopamidol	T50.8X1	T50.8X2	T50.8X3	T50.8X4	T50.8X5	T50.8X6
Iopanoic acid	T50.8X1	T50.8X2	T50.8X3	T50.8X4	T50.8X5	T50.8X6
Iophenoic acid	T50.8X1	T50.8X2	T50.8X3	T50.8X4	T50.8X5	T50.8X6
Iopodate, sodium	T50.8X1	T50.8X2	T50.8X3	T50.8X4	T50.8X5	T50.8X6
Iopodic acid	T50.8X1	T50.8X2	T50.8X3	T50.8X4	T50.8X5	T50.8X6
Iopromide	T50.8X1	T50.8X2	T50.8X3	T50.8X4	T50.8X5	T50.8X6
Iopydol	T50.8X1	T50.8X2	T50.8X3	T50.8X4	T50.8X5	T50.8X6
Iotalamic acid	T50.8X1	T50.8X2	T50.8X3	T50.8X4	T50.8X5	T50.8X6
Iothalamate	T50.8X1	T50.8X2	T50.8X3	T50.8X4	T50.8X5	T50.8X6
Iothiouracil	T38.2X1	T38.2X2	T38.2X3	T38.2X4	T38.2X5	T38.2X6
Iotrol	T50.8X1	T50.8X2	T50.8X3	T50.8X4	T50.8X5	T50.8X6
Iotrolan	T50.8X1	T50.8X2	T50.8X3	T50.8X4	T50.8X5	T50.8X6
Iotroxate	T50.8X1	T50.8X2	T50.8X3	T50.8X4	T50.8X5	T50.8X6
Iotroxic acid	T50.8X1	T50.8X2	T50.8X3	T50.8X4	T50.8X5	T50.8X6
Ioversol	T50.8X1	T50.8X2	T50.8X3	T50.8X4	T50.8X5	T50.8X6
Ioxaglate	T50.8X1	T50.8X2	T50.8X3	T50.8X4	T50.8X5	T50.8X6
Ioxaglic acid	T50.8X1	T50.8X2	T50.8X3	T50.8X4	T50.8X5	T50.8X6
Ioxitalamic acid	T50.8X1	T50.8X2	T50.8X3	T50.8X4	T50.8X5	T50.8X6
Ipecac	T47.7X1	T47.7X2	T47.7X3	T47.7X4	T47.7X5	T47.7X6
Ipecacuanha	T48.4X1	T48.4X2	T48.4X3	T48.4X4	T48.4X5	T48.4X6
Ipodate, calcium	T50.8X1	T50.8X2	T50.8X3	T50.8X4	T50.8X5	T50.8X6
Ipral	T42.3X1	T42.3X2	T42.3X3	T42.3X4	T42.3X5	T42.3X6
Ipratropium (bromide)	T48.6X1	T48.6X2	T48.6X3	T48.6X4	T48.6X5	T48.6X6

	External Cause (T-Code)					
Substance	Poisoning, Accidental (Unintentional)	Poisoning, Intentional Self-Harm	Poisoning, Assault	Poisoning, Undetermined	Adverse Effect	Underdosing
Ipriflavone	T46.3X1	T46.3X2	T46.3X3	T46.3X4	T46.3X5	T46.3X6
Iprindole	T43.011	T43.012	T43.013	T43.014	T43.015	T43.016
Iproclozide	T43.1X1	T43.1X2	T43.1X3	T43.1X4	T43.1X5	T43.1X6
Iprofenin	T50.8X1	T50.8X2	T50.8X3	T50.8X4	T50.8X5	T50.8X6
Iproheptine	T49.2X1	T49.2X2	T49.2X3	T49.2X4	T49.2X5	T49.2X6
Iproniazid	T43.1X1	T43.1X2	T43.1X3	T43.1X4	T43.1X5	T43.1X6
Iproplatin	T45.1X1	T45.1X2	T45.1X3	T45.1X4	T45.1X5	T45.1X6
Iproveratril	T46.1X1	T46.1X2	T46.1X3	T46.1X4	T46.1X5	T46.1X6
Iron (compounds) (medicinal) NEC	T45.4X1	T45.4X2	T45.4X3	T45.4X4	T45.4X5	T45.4X6
ammonium	T45.4X1	T45.4X2	T45.4X3	T45.4X4	T45.4X5	T45.4X6
dextran injection	T45.4X1	T45.4X2	T45.4X3	T45.4X4	T45.4X5	T45.4X6
nonmedicinal	T56.891	T56.892	T56.893	T56.894	—	—
salts	T45.4X1	T45.4X2	T45.4X3	T45.4X4	T45.4X5	T45.4X6
sorbitex	T45.4X1	T45.4X2	T45.4X3	T45.4X4	T45.4X5	T45.4X6
sorbitol citric acid complex	T45.4X1	T45.4X2	T45.4X3	T45.4X4	T45.4X5	T45.4X6
Irrigating fluid (vaginal)	T49.8X1	T49.8X2	T49.8X3	T49.8X4	T49.8X5	T49.8X6
eye	T49.5X1	T49.5X2	T49.5X3	T49.5X4	T49.5X5	T49.5X6
Isepamicin	T36.5X1	T36.5X2	T36.5X3	T36.5X4	T36.5X5	T36.5X6
Isoaminile (citrate)	T48.3X1	T48.3X2	T48.3X3	T48.3X4	T48.3X5	T48.3X6
Isoamyl nitrite	T46.3X1	T46.3X2	T46.3X3	T46.3X4	T46.3X5	T46.3X6
Isobenzan	T60.1X1	T60.1X2	T60.1X3	T60.1X4	—	—
Isobutyl acetate	T52.8X1	T52.8X2	T52.8X3	T52.8X4	—	—
Isocarboxazid	T43.1X1	T43.1X2	T43.1X3	T43.1X4	T43.1X5	T43.1X6
Isoconazole	T49.0X1	T49.0X2	T49.0X3	T49.0X4	T49.0X5	T49.0X6
Isocyanate	T65.0X1	T65.0X2	T65.0X3	T65.0X4	—	—
Isoephedrine	T44.991	T44.992	T44.993	T44.994	T44.995	T44.996
Isoetarine	T48.6X1	T48.6X2	T48.6X3	T48.6X4	T48.6X5	T48.6X6
Isoethadione	T42.2X1	T42.2X2	T42.2X3	T42.2X4	T42.2X5	T42.2X6
Isoetharine	T44.5X1	T44.5X2	T44.5X3	T44.5X4	T44.5X5	T44.5X6
Isoflurane	T41.0X1	T41.0X2	T41.0X3	T41.0X4	T41.0X5	T41.0X6
Isoflurophate	T44.0X1	T44.0X2	T44.0X3	T44.0X4	T44.0X5	T44.0X6
Isomaltose, ferric complex	T45.4X1	T45.4X2	T45.4X3	T45.4X4	T45.4X5	T45.4X6
Isometheptene	T44.3X1	T44.3X2	T44.3X3	T44.3X4	T44.3X5	T44.3X6
Isoniazid	T37.1X1	T37.1X2	T37.1X3	T37.1X4	T37.1X5	T37.1X6
with						
rifampicin	T36.6X1	T36.6X2	T36.6X3	T36.6X4	T36.6X5	T36.6X6
thioacetazone	T37.1X1	T37.1X2	T37.1X3	T37.1X4	T37.1X5	T37.1X6
Isonicotinic acid hydrazide	T37.1X1	T37.1X2	T37.1X3	T37.1X4	T37.1X5	T37.1X6
Isonipecaine	T40.491	T40.492	T40.493	T40.494	T40.495	T40.496
Isopentaquine	T37.2X1	T37.2X2	T37.2X3	T37.2X4	T37.2X5	T37.2X6
Isophane insulin	T38.3X1	T38.3X2	T38.3X3	T38.3X4	T38.3X5	T38.3X6
Isophorone	T65.891	T65.892	T65.893	T65.894	—	—

TABLE OF DRUGS AND CHEMICALS

◀ New   ◀ Revised   ~~deleted~~ Deleted

TABLE OF DRUGS AND CHEMICALS

Substance	Poisoning, Accidental (Unintentional)	Poisoning, Intentional Self-Harm	Poisoning, Assault	Poisoning, Undetermined	Adverse Effect	Underdosing
Isophosphamide	T45.1X1	T45.1X2	T45.1X3	T45.1X4	T45.1X5	T45.1X6
Isopregnenone	T38.5X1	T38.5X2	T38.5X3	T38.5X4	T38.5X5	T38.5X6
Isoprenaline	T48.6X1	T48.6X2	T48.6X3	T48.6X4	T48.6X5	T48.6X6
Isopromethazine	T43.3X1	T43.3X2	T43.3X3	T43.3X4	T43.3X5	T43.3X6
Isopropamide	T44.3X1	T44.3X2	T44.3X3	T44.3X4	T44.3X5	T44.3X6
iodide	T44.3X1	T44.3X2	T44.3X3	T44.3X4	T44.3X5	T44.3X6
Isopropanol	T51.2X1	T51.2X2	T51.2X3	T51.2X4	—	—
Isopropyl						
acetate	T52.8X1	T52.8X2	T52.8X3	T52.8X4	—	—
alcohol	T51.2X1	T51.2X2	T51.2X3	T51.2X4	—	—
medicinal	T49.4X1	T49.4X2	T49.4X3	T49.4X4	T49.4X5	T49.4X6
ether	T52.8X1	T52.8X2	T52.8X3	T52.8X4	—	—
Isopropylaminophena-zone	T39.2X1	T39.2X2	T39.2X3	T39.2X4	T39.2X5	T39.2X6
Isoproterenol	T48.6X1	T48.6X2	T48.6X3	T48.6X4	T48.6X5	T48.6X6
Isosorbide dinitrate	T46.3X1	T46.3X2	T46.3X3	T46.3X4	T46.3X5	T46.3X6
Isothipendyl	T45.0X1	T45.0X2	T45.0X3	T45.0X4	T45.0X5	T45.0X6
Isotretinoin	T50.991	T50.992	T50.993	T50.994	T50.995	T50.996
Isoxazolyl penicillin	T36.0X1	T36.0X2	T36.0X3	T36.0X4	T36.0X5	T36.0X6
Isoxicam	T39.391	T39.392	T39.393	T39.394	T39.395	T39.396
Isoxsuprine	T46.7X1	T46.7X2	T46.7X3	T46.7X4	T46.7X5	T46.7X6
Ispagula	T47.4X1	T47.4X2	T47.4X3	T47.4X4	T47.4X5	T47.4X6
husk	T47.4X1	T47.4X2	T47.4X3	T47.4X4	T47.4X5	T47.4X6
Isradipine	T46.1X1	T46.1X2	T46.1X3	T46.1X4	T46.1X5	T46.1X6
I-thyroxine sodium	T38.1X1	T38.1X2	T38.1X3	T38.1X4	T38.1X5	T38.1X6
Itraconazole	T37.8X1	T37.8X2	T37.8X3	T37.8X4	T37.8X5	T37.8X6
Itramin tosilate	T46.3X1	T46.3X2	T46.3X3	T46.3X4	T46.3X5	T46.3X6
Ivermectin	T37.4X1	T37.4X2	T37.4X3	T37.4X4	T37.4X5	T37.4X6
Izoniazid	T37.1X1	T37.1X2	T37.1X3	T37.1X4	T37.1X5	T37.1X6
with thioacetazone	T37.1X1	T37.1X2	T37.1X3	T37.1X4	T37.1X5	T37.1X6

J

Substance	Poisoning, Accidental (Unintentional)	Poisoning, Intentional Self-Harm	Poisoning, Assault	Poisoning, Undetermined	Adverse Effect	Underdosing
Jalap	T47.2X1	T47.2X2	T47.2X3	T47.2X4	T47.2X5	T47.2X6
Jamaica						
dogwood (bark)	T39.8X1	T39.8X2	T39.8X3	T39.8X4	T39.8X5	T39.8X6
ginger	T65.891	T65.892	T65.893	T65.894	—	—
root	T62.2X1	T62.2X2	T62.2X3	T62.2X4	—	—
Jatropha	T62.2X1	T62.2X2	T62.2X3	T62.2X4	—	—
curcas	T62.2X1	T62.2X2	T62.2X3	T62.2X4	—	—
Jectofer	T45.4X1	T45.4X2	T45.4X3	T45.4X4	T45.4X5	T45.4X6
Jellyfish (sting)	T63.621	T63.622	T63.623	T63.624	—	—
Jequirity (bean)	T62.2X1	T62.2X2	T62.2X3	T62.2X4	—	—
Jimson weed (stramonium)	T62.2X1	T62.2X2	T62.2X3	T62.2X4	—	—
seeds	T62.2X1	T62.2X2	T62.2X3	T62.2X4	—	—

Substance	Poisoning, Accidental (Unintentional)	Poisoning, Intentional Self-Harm	Poisoning, Assault	Poisoning, Undetermined	Adverse Effect	Underdosing
Josamycin	T36.3X1	T36.3X2	T36.3X3	T36.3X4	T36.3X5	T36.3X6
Juniper tar	T49.1X1	T49.1X2	T49.1X3	T49.1X4	T49.1X5	T49.1X6

K

Substance	Poisoning, Accidental (Unintentional)	Poisoning, Intentional Self-Harm	Poisoning, Assault	Poisoning, Undetermined	Adverse Effect	Underdosing
Kallidinogenase	T46.7X1	T46.7X2	T46.7X3	T46.7X4	T46.7X5	T46.7X6
Kallikrein	T46.7X1	T46.7X2	T46.7X3	T46.7X4	T46.7X5	T46.7X6
Kanamycin	T36.5X1	T36.5X2	T36.5X3	T36.5X4	T36.5X5	T36.5X6
Kantrex	T36.5X1	T36.5X2	T36.5X3	T36.5X4	T36.5X5	T36.5X6
Kaolin	T47.6X1	T47.6X2	T47.6X3	T47.6X4	T47.6X5	T47.6X6
light	T47.6X1	T47.6X2	T47.6X3	T47.6X4	T47.6X5	T47.6X6
Karaya (gum)	T47.4X1	T47.4X2	T47.4X3	T47.4X4	T47.4X5	T47.4X6
Kebuzone	T39.2X1	T39.2X2	T39.2X3	T39.2X4	T39.2X5	T39.2X6
Kelevan	T60.1X1	T60.1X2	T60.1X3	T60.1X4	—	—
Kemithal	T41.1X1	T41.1X2	T41.1X3	T41.1X4	T41.1X5	T41.1X6
Kenacort	T38.0X1	T38.0X2	T38.0X3	T38.0X4	T38.0X5	T38.0X6
Keratolytic drug NEC	T49.4X1	T49.4X2	T49.4X3	T49.4X4	T49.4X5	T49.4X6
anthracene	T49.4X1	T49.4X2	T49.4X3	T49.4X4	T49.4X5	T49.4X6
Keratoplastic NEC	T49.4X1	T49.4X2	T49.4X3	T49.4X4	T49.4X5	T49.4X6
Kerosene, kerosine (fuel) (solvent) NEC	T52.0X1	T52.0X2	T52.0X3	T52.0X4	—	—
insecticide	T52.0X1	T52.0X2	T52.0X3	T52.0X4	—	—
vapor	T52.0X1	T52.0X2	T52.0X3	T52.0X4	—	—
Ketamine	T41.291	T41.292	T41.293	T41.294	T41.295	T41.296
Ketazolam	T42.4X1	T42.4X2	T42.4X3	T42.4X4	T42.4X5	T42.4X6
Ketazon	T39.2X1	T39.2X2	T39.2X3	T39.2X4	T39.2X5	T39.2X6
Ketobemidone	T40.491	T40.492	T40.493	T40.494	—	—
Ketoconazole	T49.0X1	T49.0X2	T49.0X3	T49.0X4	T49.0X5	T49.0X6
Ketols	T52.4X1	T52.4X2	T52.4X3	T52.4X4	—	—
Ketone oils	T52.4X1	T52.4X2	T52.4X3	T52.4X4	—	—
Ketoprofen	T39.311	T39.312	T39.313	T39.314	T39.315	T39.316
Ketorolac	T39.8X1	T39.8X2	T39.8X3	T39.8X4	T39.8X5	T39.8X6
Ketotifen	T45.0X1	T45.0X2	T45.0X3	T45.0X4	T45.0X5	T45.0X6
Khat	T43.691	T43.692	T43.693	T43.694	—	—
Khellin	T46.3X1	T46.3X2	T46.3X3	T46.3X4	T46.3X5	T46.3X6
Khelloside	T46.3X1	T46.3X2	T46.3X3	T46.3X4	T46.3X5	T46.3X6
Kiln gas or vapor (carbon monoxide)	T58.8X1	T58.8X2	T58.8X3	T58.8X4	—	—
Kitasamycin	T36.3X1	T36.3X2	T36.3X3	T36.3X4	T36.3X5	T36.3X6
Konsyl	T47.4X1	T47.4X2	T47.4X3	T47.4X4	T47.4X5	T47.4X6
Kosam seed	T62.2X1	T62.2X2	T62.2X3	T62.2X4	—	—
Krait (venom)	T63.091	T63.092	T63.093	T63.094	—	—
Kwell (insecticide)	T60.1X1	T60.1X2	T60.1X3	T60.1X4	—	—
anti-infective (topical)	T49.0X1	T49.0X2	T49.0X3	T49.0X4	T49.0X5	T49.0X6

◀ New ◀ Revised ~~deleted~~ Deleted

Substance	Poisoning, Accidental (Unintentional)	Poisoning, Intentional Self-Harm	Poisoning, Assault	Poisoning, Undetermined	Adverse Effect	Underdosing
L						
Labetalol	T44.8X1	T44.8X2	T44.8X3	T44.8X4	T44.8X5	T44.8X6
Laburnum (seeds)	T62.2X1	T62.2X2	T62.2X3	T62.2X4	—	—
leaves	T62.2X1	T62.2X2	T62.2X3	T62.2X4	—	—
Lachesine	T49.5X1	T49.5X2	T49.5X3	T49.5X4	T49.5X5	T49.5X6
Lacidipine	T46.5X1	T46.5X2	T46.5X3	T46.5X4	T46.5X5	T46.5X6
Lacquer	T65.6X1	T65.6X2	T65.6X3	T65.6X4	—	—
Lacrimogenic gas	T59.3X1	T59.3X2	T59.3X3	T59.3X4		
Lactated potassic saline	T50.3X1	T50.3X2	T50.3X3	T50.3X4	T50.3X5	T50.3X6
Lactic acid	T49.8X1	T49.8X2	T49.8X3	T49.8X4	T49.8X5	T49.8X6
Lactobacillus						
acidophilus	T47.6X1	T47.6X2	T47.6X3	T47.6X4	T47.6X5	T47.6X6
compound	T47.6X1	T47.6X2	T47.6X3	T47.6X4	T47.6X5	T47.6X6
bifidus, lyophilized	T47.6X1	T47.6X2	T47.6X3	T47.6X4	T47.6X5	T47.6X6
bulgaricus	T47.6X1	T47.6X2	T47.6X3	T47.6X4	T47.6X5	T47.6X6
sporogenes	T47.6X1	T47.6X2	T47.6X3	T47.6X4	T47.6X5	T47.6X6
Lactoflavin	T45.2X1	T45.2X2	T45.2X3	T45.2X4	T45.2X5	T45.2X6
Lactose (as excipient)	T50.901	T50.902	T50.903	T50.904	T50.905	T50.906
Lactuca (virosa) (extract)	T42.6X1	T42.6X2	T42.6X3	T42.6X4	T42.6X5	T42.6X6
Lactucarium	T42.6X1	T42.6X2	T42.6X3	T42.6X4	T42.6X5	T42.6X6
Lactulose	T47.3X1	T47.3X2	T47.3X3	T47.3X4	T47.3X5	T47.3X6
Laevo — see Levo-						
Lanatosides	T46.0X1	T46.0X2	T46.0X3	T46.0X4	T46.0X5	T46.0X6
Lanolin	T49.3X1	T49.3X2	T49.3X3	T49.3X4	T49.3X5	T49.3X6
Largactil	T43.3X1	T43.3X2	T43.3X3	T43.3X4	T43.3X5	T43.3X6
Larkspur	T62.2X1	T62.2X2	T62.2X3	T62.2X4	—	—
Laroxyl	T43.011	T43.012	T43.013	T43.014	T43.015	T43.016
Lassar's paste	T49.4X1	T49.4X2	T49.4X3	T49.4X4	T49.4X5	T49.4X6
Lasix	T50.1X1	T50.1X2	T50.1X3	T50.1X4	T50.1X5	T50.1X6
Latamoxef	T36.1X1	T36.1X2	T36.1X3	T36.1X4	T36.1X5	T36.1X6
Latex	T65.811	T65.812	T65.813	T65.814	—	—
Lathyrus (seed)	T62.2X1	T62.2X2	T62.2X3	T62.2X4	—	—
Laudanum	T40.0X1	T40.0X2	T40.0X3	T40.0X4	T40.0X5	T40.0X6
Laudexium	T48.1X1	T48.1X2	T48.1X3	T48.1X4	T48.1X5	T48.1X6
Laughing gas	T41.0X1	T41.0X2	T41.0X3	T41.0X4	T41.0X5	T41.0X6
Laurel, black or cherry	T62.2X1	T62.2X2	T62.2X3	T62.2X4	—	—
Laurolinium	T49.0X1	T49.0X2	T49.0X3	T49.0X4	T49.0X5	T49.0X6
Lauryl sulfoacetate	T49.2X1	T49.2X2	T49.2X3	T49.2X4	T49.2X5	T49.2X6

Substance	Poisoning, Accidental (Unintentional)	Poisoning, Intentional Self-Harm	Poisoning, Assault	Poisoning, Undetermined	Adverse Effect	Underdosing
Laxative NEC	T47.4X1	T47.4X2	T47.4X3	T47.4X4	T47.4X5	T47.4X6
osmotic	T47.3X1	T47.3X2	T47.3X3	T47.3X4	T47.3X5	T47.3X6
saline	T47.3X1	T47.3X2	T47.3X3	T47.3X4	T47.3X5	T47.3X6
stimulant	T47.2X1	T47.2X2	T47.2X3	T47.2X4	T47.2X5	T47.2X6
L-dopa	T42.8X1	T42.8X2	T42.8X3	T42.8X4	T42.8X5	T42.8X6
Lead (dust) (fumes) (vapor) NEC	T56.0X1	T56.0X2	T56.0X3	T56.0X4	—	—
acetate	T49.2X1	T49.2X2	T49.2X3	T49.2X4	T49.2X5	T49.2X6
alkyl (fuel additive)	T56.0X1	T56.0X2	T56.0X3	T56.0X4	—	—
anti-infectives	T37.8X1	T37.8X2	T37.8X3	T37.8X4	T37.8X5	T37.8X6
antiknock compound (tetraethyl)	T56.0X1	T56.0X2	T56.0X3	T56.0X4	—	—
arsenate, arsenite (dust) (herbicide) (insecticide) (vapor)	T57.0X1	T57.0X2	T57.0X3	T57.0X4	—	—
carbonate	T56.0X1	T56.0X2	T56.0X3	T56.0X4	—	—
paint	T56.0X1	T56.0X2	T56.0X3	T56.0X4	—	—
chromate	T56.0X1	T56.0X2	T56.0X3	T56.0X4	—	—
paint	T56.0X1	T56.0X2	T56.0X3	T56.0X4	—	—
dioxide	T56.0X1	T56.0X2	T56.0X3	T56.0X4	—	—
inorganic	T56.0X1	T56.0X2	T56.0X3	T56.0X4	—	—
iodide	T56.0X1	T56.0X2	T56.0X3	T56.0X4	—	—
pigment (paint)	T56.0X1	T56.0X2	T56.0X3	T56.0X4	—	—
monoxide (dust)	T56.0X1	T56.0X2	T56.0X3	T56.0X4	—	—
paint	T56.0X1	T56.0X2	T56.0X3	T56.0X4	—	—
organic	T56.0X1	T56.0X2	T56.0X3	T56.0X4	—	—
oxide	T56.0X1	T56.0X2	T56.0X3	T56.0X4	—	—
paint	T56.0X1	T56.0X2	T56.0X3	T56.0X4	—	—
paint	T56.0X1	T56.0X2	T56.0X3	T56.0X4	—	—
salts	T56.0X1	T56.0X2	T56.0X3	T56.0X4	—	—
specified compound NEC	T56.0X1	T56.0X2	T56.0X3	T56.0X4	—	—
tetra-ethyl	T56.0X1	T56.0X2	T56.0X3	T56.0X4	—	—
Lebanese red	T40.711	T40.712	T40.713	T40.714	T40.715	T40.716
Lefetamine	T39.8X1	T39.8X2	T39.8X3	T39.8X4	T39.8X5	T39.8X6
Lenperone	T43.4X1	T43.4X2	T43.4X3	T43.4X4	T43.4X5	T43.4X6
Lente lietin (insulin)	T38.3X1	T38.3X2	T38.3X3	T38.3X4	T38.3X5	T38.3X6
Leptazol	T50.7X1	T50.7X2	T50.7X3	T50.7X4	T50.7X5	T50.7X6
Leptophos	T60.0X1	T60.0X2	T60.0X3	T60.0X4	—	—
Leritine	T40.2X1	T40.2X2	T40.2X3	T40.2X4	T40.2X5	T40.2X6
Letosteine	T48.4X1	T48.4X2	T48.4X3	T48.4X4	T48.4X5	T48.4X6
Letter	T38.1X1	T38.1X2	T38.1X3	T38.1X4	T38.1X5	T38.1X6
Lettuce opium	T42.6X1	T42.6X2	T42.6X3	T42.6X4	T42.6X5	T42.6X6
Leucinocaine	T41.3X1	T41.3X2	T41.3X3	T41.3X4	T41.3X5	T41.3X6

◀ New   ◀ Revised   ~~deleted~~ Deleted

TABLE OF DRUGS AND CHEMICALS

Substance	Poisoning, Accidental (Unintentional)	Poisoning, Intentional Self-Harm	Poisoning, Assault	Poisoning, Undetermined	Adverse Effect	Underdosing
Leucocianidol	T46.991	T46.992	T46.993	T46.994	T46.995	T46.996
Leucovorin (factor)	T45.8X1	T45.8X2	T45.8X3	T45.8X4	T45.8X5	T45.8X6
Leukeran	T45.1X1	T45.1X2	T45.1X3	T45.1X4	T45.1X5	T45.1X6
Leuprolide	T38.891	T38.892	T38.893	T38.894	T38.895	T38.896
Levalbuterol	T48.6X1	T48.6X2	T48.6X3	T48.6X4	T48.6X5	T48.6X6
Levallorphan	T50.7X1	T50.7X2	T50.7X3	T50.7X4	T50.7X5	T50.7X6
Levamisole	T37.4X1	T37.4X2	T37.4X3	T37.4X4	T37.4X5	T37.4X6
Levanil	T42.6X1	T42.6X2	T42.6X3	T42.6X4	T42.6X5	T42.6X6
Levarterenol	T44.4X1	T44.4X2	T44.4X3	T44.4X4	T44.4X5	T44.4X6
Levdropropizine	T48.3X1	T48.3X2	T48.3X3	T48.3X4	T48.3X5	T48.3X6
Levobunolol	T49.5X1	T49.5X2	T49.5X3	T49.5X4	T49.5X5	T49.5X6
Levocabastine (hydrochloride)	T45.0X1	T45.0X2	T45.0X3	T45.0X4	T45.0X5	T45.0X6
Levocarnitine	T50.991	T50.992	T50.993	T50.994	T50.995	T50.996
Levodopa	T42.8X1	T42.8X2	T42.8X3	T42.8X4	T42.8X5	T42.8X6
with carbidopa	T42.8X1	T42.8X2	T42.8X3	T42.8X4	T42.8X5	T42.8X6
Levo-dromoran	T40.2X1	T40.2X2	T40.2X3	T40.2X4	T40.2X5	T40.2X6
Levoglutamide	T50.991	T50.992	T50.993	T50.994	T50.995	T50.996
Levoid	T38.1X1	T38.1X2	T38.1X3	T38.1X4	T38.1X5	T38.1X6
Levo-iso-methadone	T40.3X1	T40.3X2	T40.3X3	T40.3X4	T40.3X5	T40.3X6
Levomepromazine	T43.3X1	T43.3X2	T43.3X3	T43.3X4	T43.3X5	T43.3X6
Levonordefrin	T49.6X1	T49.6X2	T49.6X3	T49.6X4	T49.6X5	T49.6X6
Levonorgestrel	T38.4X1	T38.4X2	T38.4X3	T38.4X4	T38.4X5	T38.4X6
with ethinylestradiol	T38.5X1	T38.5X2	T38.5X3	T38.5X4	T38.5X5	T38.5X6
Levopromazine	T43.3X1	T43.3X2	T43.3X3	T43.3X4	T43.3X5	T43.3X6
Levoprome	T42.6X1	T42.6X2	T42.6X3	T42.6X4	T42.6X5	T42.6X6
Levopropoxyphene	T40.491	T40.492	T40.493	T40.494	T40.495	T40.496
Levopropylhexedrine	T50.5X1	T50.5X2	T50.5X3	T50.5X4	T50.5X5	T50.5X6
Levoproxyphylline	T48.6X1	T48.6X2	T48.6X3	T48.6X4	T48.6X5	T48.6X6
Levorphanol	T40.491	T40.492	T40.493	T40.494	T40.495	T40.496
Levothyroxine	T38.1X1	T38.1X2	T38.1X3	T38.1X4	T38.1X5	T38.1X6
sodium	T38.1X1	T38.1X2	T38.1X3	T38.1X4	T38.1X5	T38.1X6
Levsin	T44.3X1	T44.3X2	T44.3X3	T44.3X4	T44.3X5	T44.3X6
Levulose	T50.3X1	T50.3X2	T50.3X3	T50.3X4	T50.3X5	T50.3X6
Lewisite (gas), not in war	T57.0X1	T57.0X2	T57.0X3	T57.0X4	—	—
Librium	T42.4X1	T42.4X2	T42.4X3	T42.4X4	T42.4X5	T42.4X6
Lidex	T49.0X1	T49.0X2	T49.0X3	T49.0X4	T49.0X5	T49.0X6
Lidocaine	T41.3X1	T41.3X2	T41.3X3	T41.3X4	T41.3X5	T41.3X6
regional	T41.3X1	T41.3X2	T41.3X3	T41.3X4	T41.3X5	T41.3X6
spinal	T41.3X1	T41.3X2	T41.3X3	T41.3X4	T41.3X5	T41.3X6
Lidofenin	T50.8X1	T50.8X2	T50.8X3	T50.8X4	T50.8X5	T50.8X6
Lidoflazine	T46.1X1	T46.1X2	T46.1X3	T46.1X4	T46.1X5	T46.1X6
Lighter fluid	T52.0X1	T52.0X2	T52.0X3	T52.0X4	—	—

Substance	Poisoning, Accidental (Unintentional)	Poisoning, Intentional Self-Harm	Poisoning, Assault	Poisoning, Undetermined	Adverse Effect	Underdosing
Lignin hemicellulose	T47.6X1	T47.6X2	T47.6X3	T47.6X4	T47.6X5	T47.6X6
Lignocaine	T41.3X1	T41.3X2	T41.3X3	T41.3X4	T41.3X5	T41.3X6
regional	T41.3X1	T41.3X2	T41.3X3	T41.3X4	T41.3X5	T41.3X6
spinal	T41.3X1	T41.3X2	T41.3X3	T41.3X4	T41.3X5	T41.3X6
Ligroin(e) (solvent)	T52.0X1	T52.0X2	T52.0X3	T52.0X4	—	—
vapor	T59.891	T59.892	T59.893	T59.894	—	—
Ligustrum vulgare	T62.2X1	T62.2X2	T62.2X3	T62.2X4		
Lily of the valley	T62.2X1	T62.2X2	T62.2X3	T62.2X4		
Lime (chloride)	T54.3X1	T54.3X2	T54.3X3	T54.3X4		
Limonene	T52.8X1	T52.8X2	T52.8X3	T52.8X4		
Lincomycin	T36.8X1	T36.8X2	T36.8X3	T36.8X4	T36.8X5	T36.8X6
Lindane (insecticide) (nonmedicinal) (vapor)	T53.6X1	T53.6X2	T53.6X3	T53.6X4	—	—
medicinal	T49.0X1	T49.0X2	T49.0X3	T49.0X4	T49.0X5	T49.0X6
Liniments NEC	T49.91	T49.92	T49.93	T49.94	T49.95	T49.96
Linoleic acid	T46.6X1	T46.6X2	T46.6X3	T46.6X4	T46.6X5	T46.6X6
Linolenic acid	T46.6X1	T46.6X2	T46.6X3	T46.6X4	T46.6X5	T46.6X6
Linseed	T47.4X1	T47.4X2	T47.4X3	T47.4X4	T47.4X5	T47.4X6
Liothyronine	T38.1X1	T38.1X2	T38.1X3	T38.1X4	T38.1X5	T38.1X6
Liotrix	T38.1X1	T38.1X2	T38.1X3	T38.1X4	T38.1X5	T38.1X6
Lipancreatin	T47.5X1	T47.5X2	T47.5X3	T47.5X4	T47.5X5	T47.5X6
Lipo-alprostadil	T46.7X1	T46.7X2	T46.7X3	T46.7X4	T46.7X5	T46.7X6
Lipo-Lutin	T38.5X1	T38.5X2	T38.5X3	T38.5X4	T38.5X5	T38.5X6
Lipotropic drug NEC	T50.901	T50.902	T50.903	T50.904	T50.905	T50.906
Liquefied petroleum gases	T59.891	T59.892	T59.893	T59.894	—	—
piped (pure or mixed with air)	T59.891	T59.892	T59.893	T59.894	—	—
Liquid						
paraffin	T47.4X1	T47.4X2	T47.4X3	T47.4X4	T47.4X5	T47.4X6
petrolatum	T47.4X1	T47.4X2	T47.4X3	T47.4X4	T47.4X5	T47.4X6
topical	T49.3X1	T49.3X2	T49.3X3	T49.3X4	T49.3X5	T49.3X6
specified NEC	T65.891	T65.892	T65.893	T65.894	—	—
substance	T65.91	T65.92	T65.93	T65.94		
Liquor creosolis compositus	T65.891	T65.892	T65.893	T65.894		
Liquorice	T48.4X1	T48.4X2	T48.4X3	T48.4X4	T48.4X5	T48.4X6
extract	T47.8X1	T47.8X2	T47.8X3	T47.8X4	T47.8X5	T47.8X6
Lirugen	T50.991	T50.992	T50.993	T50.994	T50.995	T50.996
Lisinopril	T46.4X1	T46.4X2	T46.4X3	T46.4X4	T46.4X5	T46.4X6
Lisuride	T42.8X1	T42.8X2	T42.8X3	T42.8X4	T42.8X5	T42.8X6
Lithane	T43.8X1	T43.8X2	T43.8X3	T43.8X4	T43.8X5	T43.8X6
Lithium	T56.891	T56.892	T56.893	T56.894	—	—
gluconate	T43.591	T43.592	T43.593	T43.594	T43.595	T43.596
salts (carbonate)	T43.591	T43.592	T43.593	T43.594	T43.595	T43.596

◀ New ◀ Revised deleted Deleted

Substance	External Cause (T-Code)					
	Poisoning, Accidental (Unintentional)	Poisoning, Intentional Self-Harm	Poisoning, Assault	Poisoning, Undetermined	Adverse Effect	Underdosing
Lithonate	T43.8X1	T43.8X2	T43.8X3	T43.8X4	T43.8X5	T43.8X6
Liver						
extract	T45.8X1	T45.8X2	T45.8X3	T45.8X4	T45.8X5	T45.8X6
for parenteral use	T45.8X1	T45.8X2	T45.8X3	T45.8X4	T45.8X5	T45.8X6
fraction 1	T45.8X1	T45.8X2	T45.8X3	T45.8X4	T45.8X5	T45.8X6
hydrolysate	T45.8X1	T45.8X2	T45.8X3	T45.8X4	T45.8X5	T45.8X6
Lizard (bite) (venom)	T63.121	T63.122	T63.123	T63.124	—	—
LMD	T45.8X1	T45.8X2	T45.8X3	T45.8X4	T45.8X5	T45.8X6
Lobelia	T62.2X1	T62.2X2	T62.2X3	T62.2X4	—	—
Lobeline	T50.7X1	T50.7X2	T50.7X3	T50.7X4	T50.7X5	T50.7X6
Local action drug NEC	T49.8X1	T49.8X2	T49.8X3	T49.8X4	T49.8X5	T49.8X6
Locorten	T49.0X1	T49.0X2	T49.0X3	T49.0X4	T49.0X5	T49.0X6
Lofepramine	T43.011	T43.012	T43.013	T43.014	T43.015	T43.016
Lolium temulentum	T62.2X1	T62.2X2	T62.2X3	T62.2X4	—	—
Lomotil	T47.6X1	T47.6X2	T47.6X3	T47.6X4	T47.6X5	T47.6X6
Lomustine	T45.1X1	T45.1X2	T45.1X3	T45.1X4	T45.1X5	T45.1X6
Lonidamine	T45.1X1	T45.1X2	T45.1X3	T45.1X4	T45.1X5	T45.1X6
Loperamide	T47.6X1	T47.6X2	T47.6X3	T47.6X4	T47.6X5	T47.6X6
Loprazolam	T42.4X1	T42.4X2	T42.4X3	T42.4X4	T42.4X5	T42.4X6
Lorajmine	T46.2X1	T46.2X2	T46.2X3	T46.2X4	T46.2X5	T46.2X6
Loratidine	T45.0X1	T45.0X2	T45.0X3	T45.0X4	T45.0X5	T45.0X6
Lorazepam	T42.4X1	T42.4X2	T42.4X3	T42.4X4	T42.4X5	T42.4X6
Lorcainide	T46.2X1	T46.2X2	T46.2X3	T46.2X4	T46.2X5	T46.2X6
Lormetazepam	T42.4X1	T42.4X2	T42.4X3	T42.4X4	T42.4X5	T42.4X6
Lotions NEC	T49.91	T49.92	T49.93	T49.94	T49.95	T49.96
Lotusate	T42.3X1	T42.3X2	T42.3X3	T42.3X4	T42.3X5	T42.3X6
Lovastatin	T46.6X1	T46.6X2	T46.6X3	T46.6X4	T46.6X5	T46.6X6
Loxapine	T43.591	T43.592	T43.593	T43.594	T43.595	T43.596
Lowila	T49.2X1	T49.2X2	T49.2X3	T49.2X4	T49.2X5	T49.2X6
Lozenges (throat)	T49.6X1	T49.6X2	T49.6X3	T49.6X4	T49.6X5	T49.6X6
LSD	T40.8X1	T40.8X2	T40.8X3	T40.8X4	—	—
L-Tryptophan — see Amino acid						
Lubricant, eye	T49.5X1	T49.5X2	T49.5X3	T49.5X4	T49.5X5	T49.5X6
Lubricating oil NEC	T52.0X1	T52.0X2	T52.0X3	T52.0X4	—	—
Lucanthone	T37.4X1	T37.4X2	T37.4X3	T37.4X4	T37.4X5	T37.4X6
Luminal	T42.3X1	T42.3X2	T42.3X3	T42.3X4	T42.3X5	T42.3X6
Lung irritant (gas) NEC	T59.91	T59.92	T59.93	T59.94	—	—
Luteinizing hormone	T38.811	T38.812	T38.813	T38.814	T38.815	T38.816
Lutocylol	T38.5X1	T38.5X2	T38.5X3	T38.5X4	T38.5X5	T38.5X6
Lutromone	T38.5X1	T38.5X2	T38.5X3	T38.5X4	T38.5X5	T38.5X6
Lututrin	T48.291	T48.292	T48.293	T48.294	T48.295	T48.296
Lye (Concentrated)	T54.3X1	T54.3X2	T54.3X3	T54.3X4	—	—

Substance	External Cause (T-Code)					
	Poisoning, Accidental (Unintentional)	Poisoning, Intentional Self-Harm	Poisoning, Assault	Poisoning, Undetermined	Adverse Effect	Underdosing
Lygranum (skin test)	T50.8X1	T50.8X2	T50.8X3	T50.8X4	T50.8X5	T50.8X6
Lymecycline	T36.4X1	T36.4X2	T36.4X3	T36.4X4	T36.4X5	T36.4X6
Lymphogranuloma venereum antigen	T50.8X1	T50.8X2	T50.8X3	T50.8X4	T50.8X5	T50.8X6
Lynestrenol	T38.4X1	T38.4X2	T38.4X3	T38.4X4	T38.4X5	T38.4X6
Lypressin	T38.891	T38.892	T38.893	T38.894	T38.895	T38.896
Lyovac Sodium Edecrin	T50.1X1	T50.1X2	T50.1X3	T50.1X4	T50.1X5	T50.1X6
Lysergic acid diethylamide	T40.8X1	T40.8X2	T40.8X3	T40.8X4	—	—
Lysergide	T40.8X1	T40.8X2	T40.8X3	T40.8X4	—	—
Lysine vasopressin	T38.891	T38.892	T38.893	T38.894	T38.895	T38.896
Lysol	T54.1X1	T54.1X2	T54.1X3	T54.1X4	—	—
Lysozyme	T49.0X1	T49.0X2	T49.0X3	T49.0X4	T49.0X5	T49.0X6
Lytta (vitatta)	T49.8X1	T49.8X2	T49.8X3	T49.8X4	T49.8X5	T49.8X6
M						
Mace	T59.3X1	T59.3X2	T59.3X3	T59.3X4	—	—
Macrogol	T50.991	T50.992	T50.993	T50.994	T50.995	T50.996
Macrolide						
anabolic drug	T38.7X1	T38.7X2	T38.7X3	T38.7X4	T38.7X5	T38.7X6
antibiotic	T36.3X1	T36.3X2	T36.3X3	T36.3X4	T36.3X5	T36.3X6
Mafenide	T49.0X1	T49.0X2	T49.0X3	T49.0X4	T49.0X5	T49.0X6
Magaldrate	T47.1X1	T47.1X2	T47.1X3	T47.1X4	T47.1X5	T47.1X6
Magic mushroom	T40.991	T40.992	T40.993	T40.994	—	—
Magnamycin	T36.8X1	T36.8X2	T36.8X3	T36.8X4	T36.8X5	T36.8X6
Magnesia magma	T47.1X1	T47.1X2	T47.1X3	T47.1X4	T47.1X5	T47.1X6
Magnesium NEC	T56.891	T56.892	T56.893	T56.894	—	—
carbonate	T47.1X1	T47.1X2	T47.1X3	T47.1X4	T47.1X5	T47.1X6
citrate	T47.4X1	T47.4X2	T47.4X3	T47.4X4	T47.4X5	T47.4X6
hydroxide	T47.1X1	T47.1X2	T47.1X3	T47.1X4	T47.1X5	T47.1X6
oxide	T47.1X1	T47.1X2	T47.1X3	T47.1X4	T47.1X5	T47.1X6
peroxide	T49.0X1	T49.0X2	T49.0X3	T49.0X4	T49.0X5	T49.0X6
salicylate	T39.091	T39.092	T39.093	T39.094	T39.095	T39.096
silicofluoride	T50.3X1	T50.3X2	T50.3X3	T50.3X4	T50.3X5	T50.3X6
sulfate	T47.4X1	T47.4X2	T47.4X3	T47.4X4	T47.4X5	T47.4X6
thiosulfate	T45.0X1	T45.0X2	T45.0X3	T45.0X4	T45.0X5	T45.0X6
trisilicate	T47.1X1	T47.1X2	T47.1X3	T47.1X4	T47.1X5	T47.1X6
Malathion (medicinal)	T49.0X1	T49.0X2	T49.0X3	T49.0X4	T49.0X5	T49.0X6
insecticide	T60.0X1	T60.0X2	T60.0X3	T60.0X4	—	—
Male fern extract	T37.4X1	T37.4X2	T37.4X3	T37.4X4	T37.4X5	T37.4X6
M-AMSA	T45.1X1	T45.1X2	T45.1X3	T45.1X4	T45.1X5	T45.1X6
Mandelic acid	T37.8X1	T37.8X2	T37.8X3	T37.8X4	T37.8X5	T37.8X6
Manganese (dioxide) (salts)	T57.2X1	T57.2X2	T57.2X3	T57.2X4	—	—
medicinal	T50.991	T50.992	T50.993	T50.994	T50.995	T50.996

◀ New ◀ Revised ~~deleted~~ Deleted

Substance	External Cause (T-Code)					
	Poisoning, Accidental (Unintentional)	Poisoning, Intentional Self-Harm	Poisoning, Assault	Poisoning, Undetermined	Adverse Effect	Underdosing
Mannitol	T47.3X1	T47.3X2	T47.3X3	T47.3X4	T47.3X5	T47.3X6
hexanitrate	T46.3X1	T46.3X2	T46.3X3	T46.3X4	T46.3X5	T46.3X6
Mannomustine	T45.1X1	T45.1X2	T45.1X3	T45.1X4	T45.1X5	T45.1X6
MAO inhibitors	T43.1X1	T43.1X2	T43.1X3	T43.1X4	T43.1X5	T43.1X6
Mapharsen	T37.8X1	T37.8X2	T37.8X3	T37.8X4	T37.8X5	T37.8X6
Maphenide	T49.0X1	T49.0X2	T49.0X3	T49.0X4	T49.0X5	T49.0X6
Maprotiline	T43.021	T43.022	T43.023	T43.024	T43.025	T43.026
Marcaine	T41.3X1	T41.3X2	T41.3X3	T41.3X4	T41.3X5	T41.3X6
infiltration (subcutaneous)	T41.3X1	T41.3X2	T41.3X3	T41.3X4	T41.3X5	T41.3X6
nerve block (peripheral) (plexus)	T41.3X1	T41.3X2	T41.3X3	T41.3X4	T41.3X5	T41.3X6
Marezine	T45.0X1	T45.0X2	T45.0X3	T45.0X4	T45.0X5	T45.0X6
Marihuana	T40.711	T40.712	T40.713	T40.714	T40.715	T40.716
Marijuana	T40.711	T40.712	T40.713	T40.714	T40.715	T40.716
Marine (sting)	T63.691	T63.692	T63.693	T63.694	—	—
animals (sting)	T63.691	T63.692	T63.693	T63.694	—	—
plants (sting)	T63.711	T63.712	T63.713	T63.714	—	—
Marplan	T43.1X1	T43.1X2	T43.1X3	T43.1X4	T43.1X5	T43.1X6
Marsh gas	T59.891	T59.892	T59.893	T59.894	—	—
Marsilid	T43.1X1	T43.1X2	T43.1X3	T43.1X4	T43.1X5	T43.1X6
Matulane	T45.1X1	T45.1X2	T45.1X3	T45.1X4	T45.1X5	T45.1X6
Mazindol	T50.5X1	T50.5X2	T50.5X3	T50.5X4	T50.5X5	T50.5X6
MCPA	T60.3X1	T60.3X2	T60.3X3	T60.3X4	—	—
MDMA	T43.641	T43.642	T43.643	T43.644	—	—
Meadow saffron	T62.2X1	T62.2X2	T62.2X3	T62.2X4	—	—
Measles virus vaccine (attenuated)	T50.B91	T50.B92	T50.B93	T50.B94	T50.B95	T50.B96
Meat, noxious	T62.8X1	T62.8X2	T62.8X3	T62.8X4	—	—
Meballymal	T42.3X1	T42.3X2	T42.3X3	T42.3X4	T42.3X5	T42.3X6
Mebanazine	T43.1X1	T43.1X2	T43.1X3	T43.1X4	T43.1X5	T43.1X6
Mebaral	T42.3X1	T42.3X2	T42.3X3	T42.3X4	T42.3X5	T42.3X6
Mebendazole	T37.4X1	T37.4X2	T37.4X3	T37.4X4	T37.4X5	T37.4X6
Mebeverine	T44.3X1	T44.3X2	T44.3X3	T44.3X4	T44.3X5	T44.3X6
Mebhydrolin	T45.0X1	T45.0X2	T45.0X3	T45.0X4	T45.0X5	T45.0X6
Mebumal	T42.3X1	T42.3X2	T42.3X3	T42.3X4	T42.3X5	T42.3X6
Mebutamate	T43.591	T43.592	T43.593	T43.594	T43.595	T43.596
Mecamylamine	T44.2X1	T44.2X2	T44.2X3	T44.2X4	T44.2X5	T44.2X6
Mechlorethamine	T45.1X1	T45.1X2	T45.1X3	T45.1X4	T45.1X5	T45.1X6
Mecillinam	T36.0X1	T36.0X2	T36.0X3	T36.0X4	T36.0X5	T36.0X6
Meclizine (hydrochloride)	T45.0X1	T45.0X2	T45.0X3	T45.0X4	T45.0X5	T45.0X6
Meclocycline	T36.4X1	T36.4X2	T36.4X3	T36.4X4	T36.4X5	T36.4X6
Meclofenamate	T39.391	T39.392	T39.393	T39.394	T39.395	T39.396
Meclofenamic acid	T39.391	T39.392	T39.393	T39.394	T39.395	T39.396

Substance	External Cause (T-Code)					
	Poisoning, Accidental (Unintentional)	Poisoning, Intentional Self-Harm	Poisoning, Assault	Poisoning, Undetermined	Adverse Effect	Underdosing
Meclofenoxate	T43.691	T43.692	T43.693	T43.694	T43.695	T43.696
Meclozine	T45.0X1	T45.0X2	T45.0X3	T45.0X4	T45.0X5	T45.0X6
Mecobalamin	T45.8X1	T45.8X2	T45.8X3	T45.8X4	T45.8X5	T45.8X6
Mecoprop	T60.3X1	T60.3X2	T60.3X3	T60.3X4	—	—
Mecrilate	T49.3X1	T49.3X2	T49.3X3	T49.3X4	T49.3X5	T49.3X6
Mecysteine	T48.4X1	T48.4X2	T48.4X3	T48.4X4	T48.4X5	T48.4X6
Medazepam	T42.4X1	T42.4X2	T42.4X3	T42.4X4	T42.4X5	T42.4X6
Medicament NEC	T50.901	T50.902	T50.903	T50.904	T50.905	T50.906
Medinal	T42.3X1	T42.3X2	T42.3X3	T42.3X4	T42.3X5	T42.3X6
Medomin	T42.3X1	T42.3X2	T42.3X3	T42.3X4	T42.3X5	T42.3X6
Medrogestone	T38.5X1	T38.5X2	T38.5X3	T38.5X4	T38.5X5	T38.5X6
Medroxalol	T44.8X1	T44.8X2	T44.8X3	T44.8X4	T44.8X5	T44.8X6
Medroxyprogesterone acetate (depot)	T38.5X1	T38.5X2	T38.5X3	T38.5X4	T38.5X5	T38.5X6
Medrysone	T49.0X1	T49.0X2	T49.0X3	T49.0X4	T49.0X5	T49.0X6
Mefenamic acid	T39.391	T39.392	T39.393	T39.394	T39.395	T39.396
Mefenorex	T50.5X1	T50.5X2	T50.5X3	T50.5X4	T50.5X5	T50.5X6
Mefloquine	T37.2X1	T37.2X2	T37.2X3	T37.2X4	T37.2X5	T37.2X6
Mefruside	T50.2X1	T50.2X2	T50.2X3	T50.2X4	T50.2X5	T50.2X6
Megahallucinogen	T40.901	T40.902	T40.903	T40.904	T40.905	T40.906
Megestrol	T38.5X1	T38.5X2	T38.5X3	T38.5X4	T38.5X5	T38.5X6
Meglumine						
antimoniate	T37.8X1	T37.8X2	T37.8X3	T37.8X4	T37.8X5	T37.8X6
diatrizoate	T50.8X1	T50.8X2	T50.8X3	T50.8X4	T50.8X5	T50.8X6
iodipamide	T50.8X1	T50.8X2	T50.8X3	T50.8X4	T50.8X5	T50.8X6
iotroxate	T50.8X1	T50.8X2	T50.8X3	T50.8X4	T50.8X5	T50.8X6
MEK (methyl ethyl ketone)	T52.4X1	T52.4X2	T52.4X3	T52.4X4	—	—
Meladrazine	T44.3X1	T44.3X2	T44.3X3	T44.3X4	T44.3X5	T44.3X6
Meladinin	T49.3X1	T49.3X2	T49.3X3	T49.3X4	T49.3X5	T49.3X6
Melaleuca alternifolia oil	T49.0X1	T49.0X2	T49.0X3	T49.0X4	T49.0X5	T49.0X6
Melanizing agents	T49.3X1	T49.3X2	T49.3X3	T49.3X4	T49.3X5	T49.3X6
Melanocyte-stimulating hormone	T38.891	T38.892	T38.893	T38.894	T38.895	T38.896
Melarsonyl potassium	T37.3X1	T37.3X2	T37.3X3	T37.3X4	T37.3X5	T37.3X6
Melarsoprol	T37.3X1	T37.3X2	T37.3X3	T37.3X4	T37.3X5	T37.3X6
Melia azedarach	T62.2X1	T62.2X2	T62.2X3	T62.2X4	—	—
Melitracen	T43.011	T43.012	T43.013	T43.014	T43.015	T43.016
Mellaril	T43.3X1	T43.3X2	T43.3X3	T43.3X4	T43.3X5	T43.3X6
Meloxine	T49.3X1	T49.3X2	T49.3X3	T49.3X4	T49.3X5	T49.3X6
Melperone	T43.4X1	T43.4X2	T43.4X3	T43.4X4	T43.4X5	T43.4X6
Melphalan	T45.1X1	T45.1X2	T45.1X3	T45.1X4	T45.1X5	T45.1X6
Memantine	T43.8X1	T43.8X2	T43.8X3	T43.8X4	T43.8X5	T43.8X6

◀ New ◀ Revised ~~deleted~~ Deleted

Substance	Poisoning, Accidental (Unintentional)	Poisoning, Intentional Self-Harm	Poisoning, Assault	Poisoning, Undetermined	Adverse Effect	Underdosing
External Cause (T-Code)						
Menadiol	T45.7X1	T45.7X2	T45.7X3	T45.7X4	T45.7X5	T45.7X6
sodium sulfate	T45.7X1	T45.7X2	T45.7X3	T45.7X4	T45.7X5	T45.7X6
Menadione	T45.7X1	T45.7X2	T45.7X3	T45.7X4	T45.7X5	T45.7X6
sodium bisulfite	T45.7X1	T45.7X2	T45.7X3	T45.7X4	T45.7X5	T45.7X6
Menaphthone	T45.7X1	T45.7X2	T45.7X3	T45.7X4	T45.7X5	T45.7X6
Menaquinone	T45.7X1	T45.7X2	T45.7X3	T45.7X4	T45.7X5	T45.7X6
Menatetrenone	T45.7X1	T45.7X2	T45.7X3	T45.7X4	T45.7X5	T45.7X6
Meningococcal vaccine	T50.A91	T50.A92	T50.A93	T50.A94	T50.A95	T50.A96
Menningovax (-AC) (-C)	T50.A91	T50.A92	T50.A93	T50.A94	T50.A95	T50.A96
Menotropins	T38.811	T38.812	T38.813	T38.814	T38.815	T38.816
Menthol	T48.5X1	T48.5X2	T48.5X3	T48.5X4	T48.5X5	T48.5X6
Mepacrine	T37.2X1	T37.2X2	T37.2X3	T37.2X4	T37.2X5	T37.2X6
Meparfynol	T42.6X1	T42.6X2	T42.6X3	T42.6X4	T42.6X5	T42.6X6
Mepartricin	T36.7X1	T36.7X2	T36.7X3	T36.7X4	T36.7X5	T36.7X6
Mepazine	T43.3X1	T43.3X2	T43.3X3	T43.3X4	T43.3X5	T43.3X6
Mepenzolate	T44.3X1	T44.3X2	T44.3X3	T44.3X4	T44.3X5	T44.3X6
bromide	T44.3X1	T44.3X2	T44.3X3	T44.3X4	T44.3X5	T44.3X6
Meperidine	T40.491	T40.492	T40.493	T40.494	T40.495	T40.496
Mephebarbital	T42.3X1	T42.3X2	T42.3X3	T42.3X4	T42.3X5	T42.3X6
Mephenamin(e)	T42.8X1	T42.8X2	T42.8X3	T42.8X4	T42.8X5	T42.8X6
Mephenesin	T42.8X1	T42.8X2	T42.8X3	T42.8X4	T42.8X5	T42.8X6
Mephenhydramine	T45.0X1	T45.0X2	T45.0X3	T45.0X4	T45.0X5	T45.0X6
Mephenoxalone	T42.8X1	T42.8X2	T42.8X3	T42.8X4	T42.8X5	T42.8X6
Mephentermine	T44.991	T44.992	T44.993	T44.994	T44.995	T44.996
Mephenytoin	T42.0X1	T42.0X2	T42.0X3	T42.0X4	T42.0X5	T42.0X6
with phenobarbital	T42.3X1	T42.3X2	T42.3X3	T42.3X4	T42.3X5	T42.3X6
Mephobarbital	T42.3X1	T42.3X2	T42.3X3	T42.3X4	T42.3X5	T42.3X6
Mephosfolan	T60.0X1	T60.0X2	T60.0X3	T60.0X4	—	—
Mepindolol	T44.7X1	T44.7X2	T44.7X3	T44.7X4	T44.7X5	T44.7X6
Mepiperphenidol	T44.3X1	T44.3X2	T44.3X3	T44.3X4	T44.3X5	T44.3X6
Mepitiostane	T38.7X1	T38.7X2	T38.7X3	T38.7X4	T38.7X5	T38.7X6
Mepivacaine	T41.3X1	T41.3X2	T41.3X3	T41.3X4	T41.3X5	T41.3X6
epidural	T41.3X1	T41.3X2	T41.3X3	T41.3X4	T41.3X5	T41.3X6
Meprednisone	T38.0X1	T38.0X2	T38.0X3	T38.0X4	T38.0X5	T38.0X6
Meprobam	T43.591	T43.592	T43.593	T43.594	T43.595	T43.596
Meprobamate	T43.591	T43.592	T43.593	T43.594	T43.595	T43.596
Meproscillarin	T46.0X1	T46.0X2	T46.0X3	T46.0X4	T46.0X5	T46.0X6
Meprylcaine	T41.3X1	T41.3X2	T41.3X3	T41.3X4	T41.3X5	T41.3X6
Meptazinol	T39.8X1	T39.8X2	T39.8X3	T39.8X4	T39.8X5	T39.8X6
Mepyramine	T45.0X1	T45.0X2	T45.0X3	T45.0X4	T45.0X5	T45.0X6
Mequitazine	T43.3X1	T43.3X2	T43.3X3	T43.3X4	T43.3X5	T43.3X6
Meralluride	T50.2X1	T50.2X2	T50.2X3	T50.2X4	T50.2X5	T50.2X6

Substance	Poisoning, Accidental (Unintentional)	Poisoning, Intentional Self-Harm	Poisoning, Assault	Poisoning, Undetermined	Adverse Effect	Underdosing
External Cause (T-Code)						
Merbaphen	T50.2X1	T50.2X2	T50.2X3	T50.2X4	T50.2X5	T50.2X6
Merbromin	T49.0X1	T49.0X2	T49.0X3	T49.0X4	T49.0X5	T49.0X6
Mercaptobenzothiazole salts	T49.0X1	T49.0X2	T49.0X3	T49.0X4	T49.0X5	T49.0X6
Mercaptomerin	T50.2X1	T50.2X2	T50.2X3	T50.2X4	T50.2X5	T50.2X6
Mercaptopurine	T45.1X1	T45.1X2	T45.1X3	T45.1X4	T45.1X5	T45.1X6
Mercumatilin	T50.2X1	T50.2X2	T50.2X3	T50.2X4	T50.2X5	T50.2X6
Mercuramide	T50.2X1	T50.2X2	T50.2X3	T50.2X4	T50.2X5	T50.2X6
Mercurochrome	T49.0X1	T49.0X2	T49.0X3	T49.0X4	T49.0X5	T49.0X6
Mercurophylline	T50.2X1	T50.2X2	T50.2X3	T50.2X4	T50.2X5	T50.2X6
Mercury, mercurial, mercuric, mercurous (compounds) (cyanide) (fumes) (nonmedicinal) (vapor) NEC	T56.1X1	T56.1X2	T56.1X3	T56.1X4	—	—
ammoniated	T49.0X1	T49.0X2	T49.0X3	T49.0X4	T49.0X5	T49.0X6
anti-infective						
local	T49.0X1	T49.0X2	T49.0X3	T49.0X4	T49.0X5	T49.0X6
systemic	T37.8X1	T37.8X2	T37.8X3	T37.8X4	T37.8X5	T37.8X6
topical	T49.0X1	T49.0X2	T49.0X3	T49.0X4	T49.0X5	T49.0X6
chloride (ammoniated)	T49.0X1	T49.0X2	T49.0X3	T49.0X4	T49.0X5	T49.0X6
fungicide	T56.1X1	T56.1X2	T56.1X3	T56.1X4	—	—
diuretic NEC	T50.2X1	T50.2X2	T50.2X3	T50.2X4	T50.2X5	T50.2X6
fungicide	T56.1X1	T56.1X2	T56.1X3	T56.1X4	—	—
organic (fungicide)	T56.1X1	T56.1X2	T56.1X3	T56.1X4	—	—
oxide, yellow	T49.0X1	T49.0X2	T49.0X3	T49.0X4	T49.0X5	T49.0X6
Mersalyl	T50.2X1	T50.2X2	T50.2X3	T50.2X4	T50.2X5	T50.2X6
Merthiolate	T49.0X1	T49.0X2	T49.0X3	T49.0X4	T49.0X5	T49.0X6
ophthalmic preparation	T49.5X1	T49.5X2	T49.5X3	T49.5X4	T49.5X5	T49.5X6
Meruvax	T50.B91	T50.B92	T50.B93	T50.B94	T50.B95	T50.B96
Mesalazine	T47.8X1	T47.8X2	T47.8X3	T47.8X4	T47.8X5	T47.8X6
Mescal buttons	T40.991	T40.992	T40.993	T40.994	—	—
Mescaline	T40.991	T40.992	T40.993	T40.994	—	—
Mesna	T48.4X1	T48.4X2	T48.4X3	T48.4X4	T48.4X5	T48.4X6
Mesoglycan	T46.6X1	T46.6X2	T46.6X3	T46.6X4	T46.6X5	T46.6X6
Mesoridazine	T43.3X1	T43.3X2	T43.3X3	T43.3X4	T43.3X5	T43.3X6
Mestanolone	T38.7X1	T38.7X2	T38.7X3	T38.7X4	T38.7X5	T38.7X6
Mesterolone	T38.7X1	T38.7X2	T38.7X3	T38.7X4	T38.7X5	T38.7X6
Mestranol	T38.5X1	T38.5X2	T38.5X3	T38.5X4	T38.5X5	T38.5X6
Mesulergine	T42.8X1	T42.8X2	T42.8X3	T42.8X4	T42.8X5	T42.8X6
Mesulfen	T49.0X1	T49.0X2	T49.0X3	T49.0X4	T49.0X5	T49.0X6
Mesuximide	T42.2X1	T42.2X2	T42.2X3	T42.2X4	T42.2X5	T42.2X6
Metabutethamine	T41.3X1	T41.3X2	T41.3X3	T41.3X4	T41.3X5	T41.3X6
Metacresylacetate	T49.0X1	T49.0X2	T49.0X3	T49.0X4	T49.0X5	T49.0X6
Metacycline	T36.4X1	T36.4X2	T36.4X3	T36.4X4	T36.4X5	T36.4X6

◀ New ◀ Revised ~~deleted~~ Deleted

TABLE OF DRUGS AND CHEMICALS

Substance	External Cause (T-Code)					
	Poisoning, Accidental (Unintentional)	Poisoning, Intentional Self-Harm	Poisoning, Assault	Poisoning, Undetermined	Adverse Effect	Underdosing
Metaldehyde (snail killer) NEC	T60.8X1	T60.8X2	T60.8X3	T60.8X4	—	—
Metals (heavy) (nonmedicinal)	T56.91	T56.92	T56.93	T56.94	—	—
dust, fumes, or vapor NEC	T56.91	T56.92	T56.93	T56.94	—	—
gadolinium	T56.821	T56.822	T56.823	T56.824	T56.825	—
light NEC	T56.91	T56.92	T56.93	T56.94	—	—
dust, fumes, or vapor NEC	T56.91	T56.92	T56.93	T56.94	—	—
specified NEC	T56.891	T56.892	T56.893	T56.894	—	—
thallium	T56.811	T56.812	T56.813	T56.814	—	—
Metamfetamine	T43.651	T43.652	T43.652	T43.654	T43.655	T43.656
Metamizole sodium	T39.2X1	T39.2X2	T39.2X3	T39.2X4	T39.2X5	T39.2X6
Metampicillin	T36.0X1	T36.0X2	T36.0X3	T36.0X4	T36.0X5	T36.0X6
Metamucil	T47.4X1	T47.4X2	T47.4X3	T47.4X4	T47.4X5	T47.4X6
Metaphen	T49.0X1	T49.0X2	T49.0X3	T49.0X4	T49.0X5	T49.0X6
Metandienone	T38.7X1	T38.7X2	T38.7X3	T38.7X4	T38.7X5	T38.7X6
Metandrostenolone	T38.7X1	T38.7X2	T38.7X3	T38.7X4	T38.7X5	T38.7X6
Metaphos	T60.0X1	T60.0X2	T60.0X3	T60.0X4	—	—
Metapramine	T43.011	T43.012	T43.013	T43.014	T43.015	T43.016
Metaproterenol	T48.291	T48.292	T48.293	T48.294	T48.295	T48.296
Metaraminol	T44.4X1	T44.4X2	T44.4X3	T44.4X4	T44.4X5	T44.4X6
Metaxalone	T42.8X1	T42.8X2	T42.8X3	T42.8X4	T42.8X5	T42.8X6
Metenolone	T38.7X1	T38.7X2	T38.7X3	T38.7X4	T38.7X5	T38.7X6
Metergoline	T42.8X1	T42.8X2	T42.8X3	T42.8X4	T42.8X5	T42.8X6
Metescufylline	T46.991	T46.992	T46.993	T46.994	T46.995	T46.996
Meteteoin	T42.0X1	T42.0X2	T42.0X3	T42.0X4	T42.0X5	T42.0X6
Metformin	T38.3X1	T38.3X2	T38.3X3	T38.3X4	T38.3X5	T38.3X6
Methacholine	T44.1X1	T44.1X2	T44.1X3	T44.1X4	T44.1X5	T44.1X6
Methacycline	T36.4X1	T36.4X2	T36.4X3	T36.4X4	T36.4X5	T36.4X6
Methadone	T40.3X1	T40.3X2	T40.3X3	T40.3X4	T40.3X5	T40.3X6
Methallenestril	T38.5X1	T38.5X2	T38.5X3	T38.5X4	T38.5X5	T38.5X6
Methallenoestril	T38.5X1	T38.5X2	T38.5X3	T38.5X4	T38.5X5	T38.5X6
Methamphetamine	T43.651	T43.652	T43.652	T43.654	T43.655	T43.656
Methampyrone	T39.2X1	T39.2X2	T39.2X3	T39.2X4	T39.2X5	T39.2X6
Methandienone	T38.7X1	T38.7X2	T38.7X3	T38.7X4	T38.7X5	T38.7X6
Methandriol	T38.7X1	T38.7X2	T38.7X3	T38.7X4	T38.7X5	T38.7X6
Methandrostenolone	T38.7X1	T38.7X2	T38.7X3	T38.7X4	T38.7X5	T38.7X6
Methane	T59.891	T59.892	T59.893	T59.894	—	—
Methanethiol	T59.891	T59.892	T59.893	T59.894	—	—
Methaniazide	T37.1X1	T37.1X2	T37.1X3	T37.1X4	T37.1X5	T37.1X6
Methanol (vapor)	T51.1X1	T51.1X2	T51.1X3	T51.1X4	—	—
Methantheline	T44.3X1	T44.3X2	T44.3X3	T44.3X4	T44.3X5	T44.3X6
Methanthelinium bromide	T44.3X1	T44.3X2	T44.3X3	T44.3X4	T44.3X5	T44.3X6
Methaphenilene	T45.0X1	T45.0X2	T45.0X3	T45.0X4	T45.0X5	T45.0X6

Substance	External Cause (T-Code)					
	Poisoning, Accidental (Unintentional)	Poisoning, Intentional Self-Harm	Poisoning, Assault	Poisoning, Undetermined	Adverse Effect	Underdosing
Methapyrilene	T45.0X1	T45.0X2	T45.0X3	T45.0X4	T45.0X5	T45.0X6
Methaqualone (compound)	T42.6X1	T42.6X2	T42.6X3	T42.6X4	T42.6X5	T42.6X6
Metharbital	T42.3X1	T42.3X2	T42.3X3	T42.3X4	T42.3X5	T42.3X6
Methazolamide	T50.2X1	T50.2X2	T50.2X3	T50.2X4	T50.2X5	T50.2X6
Methdilazine	T43.3X1	T43.3X2	T43.3X3	T43.3X4	T43.3X5	T43.3X6
Methedrine	T43.651	T43.652	T43.652	T43.654	T43.655	T43.656
Methenamine (mandelate)	T37.8X1	T37.8X2	T37.8X3	T37.8X4	T37.8X5	T37.8X6
Methenolone	T38.7X1	T38.7X2	T38.7X3	T38.7X4	T38.7X5	T38.7X6
Methergine	T48.0X1	T48.0X2	T48.0X3	T48.0X4	T48.0X5	T48.0X6
Methetoin	T42.0X1	T42.0X2	T42.0X3	T42.0X4	T42.0X5	T42.0X6
Methiacil	T38.2X1	T38.2X2	T38.2X3	T38.2X4	T38.2X5	T38.2X6
Methicillin	T36.0X1	T36.0X2	T36.0X3	T36.0X4	T36.0X5	T36.0X6
Methimazole	T38.2X1	T38.2X2	T38.2X3	T38.2X4	T38.2X5	T38.2X6
Methiodal sodium	T50.8X1	T50.8X2	T50.8X3	T50.8X4	T50.8X5	T50.8X6
Methionine	T50.991	T50.992	T50.993	T50.994	T50.995	T50.996
Methisazone	T37.5X1	T37.5X2	T37.5X3	T37.5X4	T37.5X5	T37.5X6
Methisoprinol	T37.5X1	T37.5X2	T37.5X3	T37.5X4	T37.5X5	T37.5X6
Methitural	T42.3X1	T42.3X2	T42.3X3	T42.3X4	T42.3X5	T42.3X6
Methixene	T44.3X1	T44.3X2	T44.3X3	T44.3X4	T44.3X5	T44.3X6
Methobarbital, methobarbitone	T42.3X1	T42.3X2	T42.3X3	T42.3X4	T42.3X5	T42.3X6
Methocarbamol	T42.8X1	T42.8X2	T42.8X3	T42.8X4	T42.8X5	T42.8X6
skeletal muscle relaxant	T48.1X1	T48.1X2	T48.1X3	T48.1X4	T48.1X5	T48.1X6
Methohexital	T41.1X1	T41.1X2	T41.1X3	T41.1X4	T41.1X5	T41.1X6
Methohexitone	T41.1X1	T41.1X2	T41.1X3	T41.1X4	T41.1X5	T41.1X6
Methoin	T42.0X1	T42.0X2	T42.0X3	T42.0X4	T42.0X5	T42.0X6
Methopholine	T39.8X1	T39.8X2	T39.8X3	T39.8X4	T39.8X5	T39.8X6
Methopromazine	T43.3X1	T43.3X2	T43.3X3	T43.3X4	T43.3X5	T43.3X6
Methorate	T48.3X1	T48.3X2	T48.3X3	T48.3X4	T48.3X5	T48.3X6
Methoserpidine	T46.5X1	T46.5X2	T46.5X3	T46.5X4	T46.5X5	T46.5X6
Methotrexate	T45.1X1	T45.1X2	T45.1X3	T45.1X4	T45.1X5	T45.1X6
Methotrimeprazine	T43.3X1	T43.3X2	T43.3X3	T43.3X4	T43.3X5	T43.3X6
Methoxa-Dome	T49.3X1	T49.3X2	T49.3X3	T49.3X4	T49.3X5	T49.3X6
Methoxamine	T44.4X1	T44.4X2	T44.4X3	T44.4X4	T44.4X5	T44.4X6
Methoxsalen	T50.991	T50.992	T50.993	T50.994	T50.995	T50.996
Methoxyaniline	T65.3X1	T65.3X2	T65.3X3	T65.3X4	—	—
Methoxybenzyl penicillin	T36.0X1	T36.0X2	T36.0X3	T36.0X4	T36.0X5	T36.0X6
Methoxychlor	T53.7X1	T53.7X2	T53.7X3	T53.7X4	—	—
Methoxy-DDT	T53.7X1	T53.7X2	T53.7X3	T53.7X4	—	—
2-Methoxyethanol	T52.3X1	T52.3X2	T52.3X3	T52.3X4	—	—
Methoxyflurane	T41.0X1	T41.0X2	T41.0X3	T41.0X4	T41.0X5	T41.0X6
Methoxyphenamine	T48.6X1	T48.6X2	T48.6X3	T48.6X4	T48.6X5	T48.6X6
Methoxypromazine	T43.3X1	T43.3X2	T43.3X3	T43.3X4	T43.3X5	T43.3X6

◀ New ◀ Revised ~~deleted~~ Deleted

	External Cause (T-Code)					
Substance	Poisoning, Accidental (Unintentional)	Poisoning, Intentional Self-Harm	Poisoning, Assault	Poisoning, Undetermined	Adverse Effect	Underdosing
5-Methoxypsoralen (5-MOP)	T50.991	T50.992	T50.993	T50.994	T50.995	T50.996
8-Methoxypsoralen (8-MOP)	T50.991	T50.992	T50.993	T50.994	T50.995	T50.996
Methscopolamine bromide	T44.3X1	T44.3X2	T44.3X3	T44.3X4	T44.3X5	T44.3X6
Methsuximide	T42.2X1	T42.2X2	T42.2X3	T42.2X4	T42.2X5	T42.2X6
Methyclothiazide	T50.2X1	T50.2X2	T50.2X3	T50.2X4	T50.2X5	T50.2X6
Methyl						
acetate	T52.4X1	T52.4X2	T52.4X3	T52.4X4	—	—
acetone	T52.4X1	T52.4X2	T52.4X3	T52.4X4	—	—
acrylate	T65.891	T65.892	T65.893	T65.894	—	—
alcohol	T51.1X1	T51.1X2	T51.1X3	T51.1X4	—	—
aminophenol	T65.3X1	T65.3X2	T65.3X3	T65.3X4	—	—
amphetamine	T43.651	T43.652	T43.652	T43.654	T43.655	T43.656
androstanolone	T38.7X1	T38.7X2	T38.7X3	T38.7X4	T38.7X5	T38.7X6
atropine	T44.3X1	T44.3X2	T44.3X3	T44.3X4	T44.3X5	T44.3X6
benzene	T52.2X1	T52.2X2	T52.2X3	T52.2X4	—	—
benzoate	T52.8X1	T52.8X2	T52.8X3	T52.8X4	—	—
benzol	T52.2X1	T52.2X2	T52.2X3	T52.2X4	—	—
bromide (gas)	T59.891	T59.892	T59.893	T59.894	—	—
fumigant	T60.8X1	T60.8X2	T60.8X3	T60.8X4	—	—
butanol	T51.3X1	T51.3X2	T51.3X3	T51.3X4	—	—
carbinol	T51.1X1	T51.1X2	T51.1X3	T51.1X4	—	—
carbonate	T52.8X1	T52.8X2	T52.8X3	T52.8X4	—	—
CCNU	T45.1X1	T45.1X2	T45.1X3	T45.1X4	T45.1X5	T45.1X6
cellosolve	T52.91	T52.92	T52.93	T52.94	—	—
cellulose	T47.4X1	T47.4X2	T47.4X3	T47.4X4	T47.4X5	T47.4X6
chloride (gas)	T59.891	T59.892	T59.893	T59.894	—	—
chloroformate	T59.3X1	T59.3X2	T59.3X3	T59.3X4	—	—
cyclohexane	T52.8X1	T52.8X2	T52.8X3	T52.8X4	—	—
cyclohexanol	T51.8X1	T51.8X2	T51.8X3	T51.8X4	—	—
cyclohexanone	T52.8X1	T52.8X2	T52.8X3	T52.8X4	—	—
cyclohexyl acetate	T52.8X1	T52.8X2	T52.8X3	T52.8X4	—	—
demeton	T60.0X1	T60.0X2	T60.0X3	T60.0X4	—	—
dihydromorphinone	T40.2X1	T40.2X2	T40.2X3	T40.2X4	T40.2X5	T40.2X6
ergometrine	T48.0X1	T48.0X2	T48.0X3	T48.0X4	T48.0X5	T48.0X6
ergonovine	T48.0X1	T48.0X2	T48.0X3	T48.0X4	T48.0X5	T48.0X6
ethyl ketone	T52.4X1	T52.4X2	T52.4X3	T52.4X4	—	—
glucamine antimonate	T37.8X1	T37.8X2	T37.8X3	T37.8X4	T37.8X5	T37.8X6
hydrazine	T65.891	T65.892	T65.893	T65.894	—	—
iodide	T65.891	T65.892	T65.893	T65.894	—	—
isobutyl ketone	T52.4X1	T52.4X2	T52.4X3	T52.4X4	—	—
isothiocyanate	T60.3X1	T60.3X2	T60.3X3	T60.3X4	—	—
mercaptan	T59.891	T59.892	T59.893	T59.894	—	—

	External Cause (T-Code)					
Substance	Poisoning, Accidental (Unintentional)	Poisoning, Intentional Self-Harm	Poisoning, Assault	Poisoning, Undetermined	Adverse Effect	Underdosing
Methyl (Continued)						
morphine NEC	T40.2X1	T40.2X2	T40.2X3	T40.2X4	T40.2X5	T40.2X6
nicotinate	T49.4X1	T49.4X2	T49.4X3	T49.4X4	T49.4X5	T49.4X6
paraben	T49.0X1	T49.0X2	T49.0X3	T49.0X4	T49.0X5	T49.0X6
parafynol	T42.6X1	T42.6X2	T42.6X3	T42.6X4	T42.6X5	T42.6X6
parathion	T60.0X1	T60.0X2	T60.0X3	T60.0X4	—	—
peridol	T43.4X1	T43.4X2	T43.4X3	T43.4X4	T43.4X5	T43.4X6
phenidate	T43.631	T43.632	T43.633	T43.634	T43.635	T43.636
prednisolone	T38.0X1	T38.0X2	T38.0X3	T38.0X4	T38.0X5	T38.0X6
ENT agent	T49.6X1	T49.6X2	T49.6X3	T49.6X4	T49.6X5	T49.6X6
ophthalmic preparation	T49.5X1	T49.5X2	T49.5X3	T49.5X4	T49.5X5	T49.5X6
topical NEC	T49.0X1	T49.0X2	T49.0X3	T49.0X4	T49.0X5	T49.0X6
propylcarbinol	T51.3X1	T51.3X2	T51.3X3	T51.3X4	—	—
rosaniline NEC	T49.0X1	T49.0X2	T49.0X3	T49.0X4	T49.0X5	T49.0X6
salicylate	T49.2X1	T49.2X2	T49.2X3	T49.2X4	T49.2X5	T49.2X6
sulfate (fumes)	T59.891	T59.892	T59.893	T59.894	—	—
liquid	T52.8X1	T52.8X2	T52.8X3	T52.8X4	—	—
sulfonal	T42.6X1	T42.6X2	T42.6X3	T42.6X4	T42.6X5	T42.6X6
testosterone	T38.7X1	T38.7X2	T38.7X3	T38.7X4	T38.7X5	T38.7X6
thiouracil	T38.2X1	T38.2X2	T38.2X3	T38.2X4	T38.2X5	T38.2X6
Methylamphetamine	T43.651	T43.652	T43.652	T43.654	T43.655	T43.656
Methylated spirit	T51.1X1	T51.1X2	T51.1X3	T51.1X4	—	—
Methylatropine nitrate	T44.3X1	T44.3X2	T44.3X3	T44.3X4	T44.3X5	T44.3X6
Methylbenactyzium bromide	T44.3X1	T44.3X2	T44.3X3	T44.3X4	T44.3X5	T44.3X6
Methylbenzethonium chloride	T49.0X1	T49.0X2	T49.0X3	T49.0X4	T49.0X5	T49.0X6
Methylcellulose	T47.4X1	T47.4X2	T47.4X3	T47.4X4	T47.4X5	T47.4X6
laxative	T47.4X1	T47.4X2	T47.4X3	T47.4X4	T47.4X5	T47.4X6
Methylchlorophenoxy-acetic acid	T60.3X1	T60.3X2	T60.3X3	T60.3X4	—	—
Methyldopa	T46.5X1	T46.5X2	T46.5X3	T46.5X4	T46.5X5	T46.5X6
Methyldopate	T46.5X1	T46.5X2	T46.5X3	T46.5X4	T46.5X5	T46.5X6
Methylene						
blue	T50.6X1	T50.6X2	T50.6X3	T50.6X4	T50.6X5	T50.6X6
chloride or dichloride (solvent) NEC	T53.4X1	T53.4X2	T53.4X3	T53.4X4	—	—
Methylenedioxyamphet-amine	T43.621	T43.622	T43.623	T43.624	T43.625	T43.626
Methylenedioxymethamphetamine	T43.641	T43.642	T43.643	T43.644	—	—
Methylergometrine	T48.0X1	T48.0X2	T48.0X3	T48.0X4	T48.0X5	T48.0X6
Methylergonovine	T48.0X1	T48.0X2	T48.0X3	T48.0X4	T48.0X5	T48.0X6
Methylestrenolone	T38.5X1	T38.5X2	T38.5X3	T38.5X4	T38.5X5	T38.5X6
Methylethyl cellulose	T50.991	T50.992	T50.993	T50.994	T50.995	T50.996
Methylhexabital	T42.3X1	T42.3X2	T42.3X3	T42.3X4	T42.3X5	T42.3X6
Methylmorphine	T40.2X1	T40.2X2	T40.2X3	T40.2X4	T40.2X5	T40.2X6

◀ New ◀ Revised ~~deleted~~ Deleted

Substance	Poisoning, Accidental (Unintentional)	Poisoning, Intentional Self-Harm	Poisoning, Assault	Poisoning, Undetermined	Adverse Effect	Underdosing
Methylparaben (ophthalmic)	T49.5X1	T49.5X2	T49.5X3	T49.5X4	T49.5X5	T49.5X6
Methylparafynol	T42.6X1	T42.6X2	I42.6X3	T42.6X4	T42.6X5	T42.6X6
Methylpentynol, methylpenthynol	T42.6X1	T42.6X2	T42.6X3	T42.6X4	T42.6X5	T42.6X6
Methylphenidate	T43.631	T43.632	T43.633	T43.634	T43.635	T43.636
Methylphenobarbital	T42.3X1	T42.3X2	T42.3X3	T42.3X4	T42.3X5	T42.3X6
Methylpolysiloxane	T47.1X1	T47.1X2	T47.1X3	T47.1X4	T47.1X5	T47.1X6
Methylprednisolone — see Methyl, prednisolone						
Methylrosaniline	T49.0X1	T49.0X2	T49.0X3	T49.0X4	T49.0X5	T49.0X6
Methylrosanilinium chloride	T49.0X1	T49.0X2	T49.0X3	T49.0X4	T49.0X5	T49.0X6
Methyltestosterone	T38.7X1	T38.7X2	T38.7X3	T38.7X4	T38.7X5	T38.7X6
Methylthionine chloride	T50.6X1	T50.6X2	T50.6X3	T50.6X4	T50.6X5	T50.6X6
Methylthioninium chloride	T50.6X1	T50.6X2	T50.6X3	T50.6X4	T50.6X5	T50.6X6
Methylthiouracil	T38.2X1	T38.2X2	T38.2X3	T38.2X4	T38.2X5	T38.2X6
Methyprylon	T42.6X1	T42.6X2	T42.6X3	T42.6X4	T42.6X5	T42.6X6
Methysergide	T46.5X1	T46.5X2	T46.5X3	T46.5X4	T46.5X5	T46.5X6
Metiamide	T47.1X1	T47.1X2	T47.1X3	T47.1X4	T47.1X5	T47.1X6
Meticillin	T36.0X1	T36.0X2	T36.0X3	T36.0X4	T36.0X5	T36.0X6
Meticrane	T50.2X1	T50.2X2	T50.2X3	T50.2X4	T50.2X5	T50.2X6
Metildigoxin	T46.0X1	T46.0X2	T46.0X3	T46.0X4	T46.0X5	T46.0X6
Metipranolol	T49.5X1	T49.5X2	T49.5X3	T49.5X4	T49.5X5	T49.5X6
Metirosine	T46.5X1	T46.5X2	T46.5X3	T46.5X4	T46.5X5	T46.5X6
Metisazone	T37.5X1	T37.5X2	T37.5X3	T37.5X4	T37.5X5	T37.5X6
Metixene	T44.3X1	T44.3X2	T44.3X3	T44.3X4	T44.3X5	T44.3X6
Metizoline	T48.5X1	T48.5X2	T48.5X3	T48.5X4	T48.5X5	T48.5X6
Metoclopramide	T45.0X1	T45.0X2	T45.0X3	T45.0X4	T45.0X5	T45.0X6
Metofenazate	T43.3X1	T43.3X2	T43.3X3	T43.3X4	T43.3X5	T43.3X6
Metofoline	T39.8X1	T39.8X2	T39.8X3	T39.8X4	T39.8X5	T39.8X6
Metolazone	T50.2X1	T50.2X2	T50.2X3	T50.2X4	T50.2X5	T50.2X6
Metopon	T40.2X1	T40.2X2	T40.2X3	T40.2X4	T40.2X5	T40.2X6
Metoprine	T45.1X1	T45.1X2	T45.1X3	T45.1X4	T45.1X5	T45.1X6
Metoprolol	T44.7X1	T44.7X2	T44.7X3	T44.7X4	T44.7X5	T44.7X6
Metrifonate	T60.0X1	T60.0X2	T60.0X3	T60.0X4	—	—
Metrizamide	T50.8X1	T50.8X2	T50.8X3	T50.8X4	T50.8X5	T50.8X6
Metrizoic acid	T50.8X1	T50.8X2	T50.8X3	T50.8X4	T50.8X5	T50.8X6
Metronidazole	T37.8X1	T37.8X2	T37.8X3	T37.8X4	T37.8X5	T37.8X6
Metycaine	T41.3X1	T41.3X2	T41.3X3	T41.3X4	T41.3X5	T41.3X6
infiltration (subcutaneous)	T41.3X1	T41.3X2	T41.3X3	T41.3X4	T41.3X5	T41.3X6
nerve block (peripheral) (plexus)	T41.3X1	T41.3X2	T41.3X3	T41.3X4	T41.3X5	T41.3X6
topical (surface)	T41.3X1	T41.3X2	T41.3X3	T41.3X4	T41.3X5	T41.3X6
Metyrapone	T50.8X1	T50.8X2	T50.8X3	T50.8X4	T50.8X5	T50.8X6
Mevinphos	T60.0X1	T60.0X2	T60.0X3	T60.0X4	—	—

Substance	Poisoning, Accidental (Unintentional)	Poisoning, Intentional Self-Harm	Poisoning, Assault	Poisoning, Undetermined	Adverse Effect	Underdosing
Mexazolam	T42.4X1	T42.4X2	T42.4X3	T42.4X4	T42.4X5	T42.4X6
Mexenone	T49.3X1	T49.3X2	T49.3X3	T49.3X4	T49.3X5	T49.3X6
Mexiletine	T46.2X1	T46.2X2	T46.2X3	T46.2X4	T46.2X5	T46.2X6
Mezereon	T62.2X1	T62.2X2	T62.2X3	T62.2X4	—	—
berries	T62.1X1	T62.1X2	T62.1X3	T62.1X4	—	—
Mezlocillin	T36.0X1	T36.0X2	T36.0X3	T36.0X4	T36.0X5	T36.0X6
Mianserin	T43.021	T43.022	T43.023	T43.024	T43.025	T43.026
Micatin	T49.0X1	T49.0X2	T49.0X3	T49.0X4	T49.0X5	T49.0X6
Miconazole	T49.0X1	T49.0X2	T49.0X3	T49.0X4	T49.0X5	T49.0X6
Micronomicin	T36.5X1	T36.5X2	T36.5X3	T36.5X4	T36.5X5	T36.5X6
Midazolam	T42.4X1	T42.4X2	T42.4X3	T42.4X4	T42.4X5	T42.4X6
Midecamycin	T36.3X1	T36.3X2	T36.3X3	T36.3X4	T36.3X5	T36.3X6
Mifepristone	T38.6X1	T38.6X2	T38.6X3	T38.6X4	T38.6X5	T38.6X6
Milk of magnesia	T47.1X1	T47.1X2	T47.1X3	T47.1X4	T47.1X5	T47.1X6
Millipede (tropical) (venomous)	T63.411	T63.412	T63.413	T63.414	—	—
Miltown	T43.591	T43.592	T43.593	T43.594	T43.595	T43.596
Milverine	T44.3X1	T44.3X2	T44.3X3	T44.3X4	T44.3X5	T44.3X6
Minaprine	T43.291	T43.292	T43.293	T43.294	T43.295	T43.296
Minaxolone	T41.291	T41.292	T41.293	T41.294	T41.295	T41.296
Mineral						
acids	T54.2X1	T54.2X2	T54.2X3	T54.2X4	—	—
oil (laxative) (medicinal)	T47.4X1	T47.4X2	T47.4X3	T47.4X4	T47.4X5	T47.4X6
emulsion	T47.2X1	T47.2X2	T47.2X3	T47.2X4	T47.2X5	T47.2X6
nonmedicinal	T52.0X1	T52.0X2	T52.0X3	T52.0X4	—	—
topical	T49.3X1	T49.3X2	T49.3X3	T49.3X4	T49.3X5	T49.3X6
salt NEC	T50.3X1	T50.3X2	T50.3X3	T50.3X4	T50.3X5	T50.3X6
spirits	T52.0X1	T52.0X2	T52.0X3	T52.0X4	—	—
Mineralocorticosteroid	T50.0X1	T50.0X2	T50.0X3	T50.0X4	T50.0X5	T50.0X6
Minocycline	T36.4X1	T36.4X2	T36.4X3	T36.4X4	T36.4X5	T36.4X6
Minoxidil	T46.7X1	T46.7X2	T46.7X3	T46.7X4	T46.7X5	T46.7X6
Miokamycin	T36.3X1	T36.3X2	T36.3X3	T36.3X4	T36.3X5	T36.3X6
Miotic drug	T49.5X1	T49.5X2	T49.5X3	T49.5X4	T49.5X5	T49.5X6
Mipafox	T60.0X1	T60.0X2	T60.0X3	T60.0X4	—	—
Mirex	T60.1X1	T60.1X2	T60.1X3	T60.1X4	—	—
Mirtazapine	T43.021	T43.022	T43.023	T43.024	T43.025	T43.026
Misonidazole	T37.3X1	T37.3X2	T37.3X3	T37.3X4	T37.3X5	T37.3X6
Misoprostol	T47.1X1	T47.1X2	T47.1X3	T47.1X4	T47.1X5	T47.1X6
Mithramycin	T45.1X1	T45.1X2	T45.1X3	T45.1X4	T45.1X5	T45.1X6
Mitobronitol	T45.1X1	T45.1X2	T45.1X3	T45.1X4	T45.1X5	T45.1X6
Mitoguazone	T45.1X1	T45.1X2	T45.1X3	T45.1X4	T45.1X5	T45.1X6
Mitolactol	T45.1X1	T45.1X2	T45.1X3	T45.1X4	T45.1X5	T45.1X6
Mitomycin	T45.1X1	T45.1X2	T45.1X3	T45.1X4	T45.1X5	T45.1X6

◄ New   ◄ Revised   deleted Deleted

Substance	Poisoning, Accidental (Unintentional)	Poisoning, Intentional Self-Harm	Poisoning, Assault	Poisoning, Undetermined	Adverse Effect	Underdosing
Mitopodozide	T45.1X1	T45.1X2	T45.1X3	T45.1X4	T45.1X5	T45.1X6
Mitotane	T45.1X1	T45.1X2	T45.1X3	T45.1X4	T45.1X5	T45.1X6
Mitoxantrone	T45.1X1	T45.1X2	T45.1X3	T45.1X4	T45.1X5	T45.1X6
Mivacurium chloride	T48.1X1	T48.1X2	T48.1X3	T48.1X4	T48.1X5	T48.1X6
Miyari bacteria	T47.6X1	T47.6X2	T47.6X3	T47.6X4	T47.6X5	T47.6X6
Moclobemide	T43.1X1	T43.1X2	T43.1X3	T43.1X4	T43.1X5	T43.1X6
Moderil	T46.5X1	T46.5X2	T46.5X3	T46.5X4	T46.5X5	T46.5X6
Mofebutazone	T39.2X1	T39.2X2	T39.2X3	T39.2X4	T39.2X5	T39.2X6
Mogadon — see Nitrazepam						
Molindone	T43.591	T43.592	T43.593	T43.594	T43.595	T43.596
Molsidomine	T46.3X1	T46.3X2	T46.3X3	T46.3X4	T46.3X5	T46.3X6
Mometasone	T49.0X1	T49.0X2	T49.0X3	T49.0X4	T49.0X5	T49.0X6
Monistat	T49.0X1	T49.0X2	T49.0X3	T49.0X4	T49.0X5	T49.0X6
Monkshood	T62.2X1	T62.2X2	T62.2X3	T62.2X4	—	—
Monoamine oxidase inhibitor NEC	T43.1X1	T43.1X2	T43.1X3	T43.1X4	T43.1X5	T43.1X6
hydrazine	T43.1X1	T43.1X2	T43.1X3	T43.1X4	T43.1X5	T43.1X6
Monobenzone	T49.4X1	T49.4X2	T49.4X3	T49.4X4	T49.4X5	T49.4X6
Monochloroacetic acid	T60.3X1	T60.3X2	T60.3X3	T60.3X4	—	—
Monochlorobenzene	T53.7X1	T53.7X2	T53.7X3	T53.7X4	—	—
Monoethanolamine	T46.8X1	T46.8X2	T46.8X3	T46.8X4	T46.8X5	T46.8X6
oleate	T46.8X1	T46.8X2	T46.8X3	T46.8X4	T46.8X5	T46.8X6
Monooctanoin	T50.991	T50.992	T50.993	T50.994	T50.995	T50.996
Monophenylbutazone	T39.2X1	T39.2X2	T39.2X3	T39.2X4	T39.2X5	T39.2X6
Monosodium glutamate	T65.891	T65.892	T65.893	T65.894	—	—
Monosulfiram	T49.0X1	T49.0X2	T49.0X3	T49.0X4	T49.0X5	T49.0X6
Monoxide, carbon — see Carbon, monoxide	T57.91	T57.92	T57.93	T57.94	—	—
Monoxidine hydrochloride	T46.1X1	T46.1X2	T46.1X3	T46.1X4	T46.1X5	T46.1X6
Monuron	T60.3X1	T60.3X2	T60.3X3	T60.3X4	—	—
Moperone	T43.4X1	T43.4X2	T43.4X3	T43.4X4	T43.4X5	T43.4X6
Mopidamol	T45.1X1	T45.1X2	T45.1X3	T45.1X4	T45.1X5	T45.1X6
MOPP (mechlorethamine + vincristine + prednisone + procarbazine)	T45.1X1	T45.1X2	T45.1X3	T45.1X4	T45.1X5	T45.1X6
Morfin	T40.2X1	T40.2X2	T40.2X3	T40.2X4	T40.2X5	T40.2X6
Morinamide	T37.1X1	T37.1X2	T37.1X3	T37.1X4	T37.1X5	T37.1X6
Morning glory seeds	T40.991	T40.992	T40.993	T40.994	—	—
Moroxydine	T37.5X1	T37.5X2	T37.5X3	T37.5X4	T37.5X5	T37.5X6
Morphazinamide	T37.1X1	T37.1X2	T37.1X3	T37.1X4	T37.1X5	T37.1X6
Morphine	T40.2X1	T40.2X2	T40.2X3	T40.2X4	T40.2X5	T40.2X6
antagonist	T50.7X1	T50.7X2	T50.7X3	T50.7X4	T50.7X5	T50.7X6
Morpholinylethylmorphine	T40.2X1	T40.2X2	T40.2X3	T40.2X4	—	—
Morsuximide	T42.2X1	T42.2X2	T42.2X3	T42.2X4	T42.2X5	T42.2X6

Substance	Poisoning, Accidental (Unintentional)	Poisoning, Intentional Self-Harm	Poisoning, Assault	Poisoning, Undetermined	Adverse Effect	Underdosing
Mosapramine	T43.591	T43.592	T43.593	T43.594	T43.595	T43.596
Moth balls — see also Pesticide	T60.2X1	T60.2X2	T60.2X3	T60.2X4	—	—
naphthalene	T60.2X1	T60.2X2	T60.2X3	T60.2X4	—	—
paradichlorobenzene	T60.1X1	T60.1X2	T60.1X3	T60.1X4	—	—
Motor exhaust gas	T58.01	T58.02	T58.03	T58.04	—	—
Mouthwash (antiseptic) (zinc chloride)	T49.6X1	T49.6X2	T49.6X3	T49.6X4	T49.6X5	T49.6X6
Moxastine	T45.0X1	T45.0X2	T45.0X3	T45.0X4	T45.0X5	T45.0X6
Moxaverine	T44.3X1	T44.3X2	T44.3X3	T44.3X4	T44.3X5	T44.3X6
Moxifensine	T43.291	T43.292	T43.293	T43.294	T43.295	T43.296
Moxisylyte	T46.7X1	T46.7X2	T46.7X3	T46.7X4	T46.7X5	T46.7X6
Mucilage, plant	T47.4X1	T47.4X2	T47.4X3	T47.4X4	T47.4X5	T47.4X6
Mucolytic drug	T48.4X1	T48.4X2	T48.4X3	T48.4X4	T48.4X5	T48.4X6
Mucomyst	T48.4X1	T48.4X2	T48.4X3	T48.4X4	T48.4X5	T48.4X6
Mucous membrane agents (external)	T49.91	T49.92	T49.93	T49.94	T49.95	T49.96
specified NEC	T49.8X1	T49.8X2	T49.8X3	T49.8X4	T49.8X5	T49.8X6
Multiple unspecified drugs, medicaments and biological substances	T50.911	T50.912	T50.913	T50.914	T50.915	T50.916
Mumps						
immune globulin (human)	T50.Z11	T50.Z12	T50.Z13	T50.Z14	T50.Z15	T50.Z16
skin test antigen	T50.8X1	T50.8X2	T50.8X3	T50.8X4	T50.8X5	T50.8X6
vaccine	T50.B91	T50.B92	T50.B93	T50.B94	T50.B95	T50.B96
Mumpsvax	T50.B91	T50.B92	T50.B93	T50.B94	T50.B95	T50.B96
Mupirocin	T49.0X1	T49.0X2	T49.0X3	T49.0X4	T49.0X5	T49.0X6
Muriatic acid — see Hydrochloric acid						
Muromonab-CD3	T45.1X1	T45.1X2	T45.1X3	T45.1X4	T45.1X5	T45.1X6
Muscle relaxant — see Relaxant, muscle						
Muscle-action drug NEC	T48.201	T48.202	T48.203	T48.204	T48.205	T48.206
Muscle affecting agents NEC	T48.201	T48.202	T48.203	T48.204	T48.205	T48.206
oxytocic	T48.0X1	T48.0X2	T48.0X3	T48.0X4	T48.0X5	T48.0X6
relaxants	T48.201	T48.202	T48.203	T48.204	T48.205	T48.206
central nervous system	T42.8X1	T42.8X2	T42.8X3	T42.8X4	T42.8X5	T42.8X6
skeletal	T48.1X1	T48.1X2	T48.1X3	T48.1X4	T48.1X5	T48.1X6
smooth	T44.3X1	T44.3X2	T44.3X3	T44.3X4	T44.3X5	T44.3X6
Muscle-tone depressant, central NEC	T42.8X1	T42.8X2	T42.8X3	T42.8X4	T42.8X5	T42.8X6
specified NEC	T42.8X1	T42.8X2	T42.8X3	T42.8X4	T42.8X5	T42.8X6
Mushroom, noxious	T62.0X1	T62.0X2	T62.0X3	T62.0X4	—	—
Mussel, noxious	T61.781	T61.782	T61.783	T61.784	—	—

TABLE OF DRUGS AND CHEMICALS

Substance	External Cause (T-Code)					
	Poisoning, Accidental (Unintentional)	Poisoning, Intentional Self-Harm	Poisoning, Assault	Poisoning, Undetermined	Adverse Effect	Underdosing
Mustard (emetic)	T47.7X1	T47.7X2	T47.7X3	T47.7X4	T47.7X5	T47.7X6
black	T47.7X1	T47.7X2	T47.7X3	T47.7X4	T47.7X5	T47.7X6
gas, not in war	T59.91	T59.92	T59.93	T59.94	—	—
nitrogen	T45.1X1	T45.1X2	T45.1X3	T45.1X4	T45.1X5	T45.1X6
Mustine	T45.1X1	T45.1X2	T45.1X3	T45.1X4	T45.1X5	T45.1X6
M-vac	T45.1X1	T45.1X2	T45.1X3	T45.1X4	T45.1X5	T45.1X6
Mycifradin	T36.5X1	T36.5X2	T36.5X3	T36.5X4	T36.5X5	T36.5X6
topical	T49.0X1	T49.0X2	T49.0X3	T49.0X4	T49.0X5	T49.0X6
Mycitracin	T36.8X1	T36.8X2	T36.8X3	T36.8X4	T36.8X5	T36.8X6
ophthalmic preparation	T49.5X1	T49.5X2	T49.5X3	T49.5X4	T49.5X5	T49.5X6
Mycostatin	T36.7X1	T36.7X2	T36.7X3	T36.7X4	T36.7X5	T36.7X6
topical	T49.0X1	T49.0X2	T49.0X3	T49.0X4	T49.0X5	T49.0X6
Mycotoxins	T64.81	T64.82	T64.83	T64.84	—	—
aflatoxin	T64.01	T64.02	T64.03	T64.04	—	—
specified NEC	T64.81	T64.82	T64.83	T64.84	—	—
Mydriacyl	T44.3X1	T44.3X2	T44.3X3	T44.3X4	T44.3X5	T44.3X6
Mydriatic drug	T49.5X1	T49.5X2	T49.5X3	T49.5X4	T49.5X5	T49.5X6
Myelobromal	T45.1X1	T45.1X2	T45.1X3	T45.1X4	T45.1X5	T45.1X6
Myleran	T45.1X1	T45.1X2	T45.1X3	T45.1X4	T45.1X5	T45.1X6
Myochrysin(e)	T39.2X1	T39.2X2	T39.2X3	T39.2X4	T39.2X5	T39.2X6
Myoneural blocking agents	T48.1X1	T48.1X2	T48.1X3	T48.1X4	T48.1X5	T48.1X6
Myralact	T49.0X1	T49.0X2	T49.0X3	T49.0X4	T49.0X5	T49.0X6
Myristica fragrans	T62.2X1	T62.2X2	T62.2X3	T62.2X4	—	—
Myristicin	T65.891	T65.892	T65.893	T65.894	—	—
Mysoline	T42.3X1	T42.3X2	T42.3X3	T42.3X4	T42.3X5	T42.3X6

N

Substance						
Nabilone	T40.711	T40.712	T40.713	T40.714	T40.715	T40.716
Nabumetone	T39.391	T39.392	T39.393	T39.394	T39.395	T39.396
Nadolol	T44.7X1	T44.7X2	T44.7X3	T44.7X4	T44.7X5	T44.7X6
Nafcillin	T36.0X1	T36.0X2	T36.0X3	T36.0X4	T36.0X5	T36.0X6
Nafoxidine	T38.6X1	T38.6X2	T38.6X3	T38.6X4	T38.6X5	T38.6X6
Naftazone	T46.991	T46.992	T46.993	T46.994	T46.995	T46.996
Naftidrofuryl (oxalate)	T46.7X1	T46.7X2	T46.7X3	T46.7X4	T46.7X5	T46.7X6
Naftifine	T49.0X1	T49.0X2	T49.0X3	T49.0X4	T49.0X5	T49.0X6
Nail polish remover	T52.91	T52.92	T52.93	T52.94	—	—
Nalbuphine	T40.491	T40.492	T40.493	T40.494	T40.495	T40.496
Naled	T60.0X1	T60.0X2	T60.0X3	T60.0X4	—	—
Nalidixic acid	T37.8X1	T37.8X2	T37.8X3	T37.8X4	T37.8X5	T37.8X6
Nalorphine	T50.7X1	T50.7X2	T50.7X3	T50.7X4	T50.7X5	T50.7X6
Naloxone	T50.7X1	T50.7X2	T50.7X3	T50.7X4	T50.7X5	T50.7X6
Naltrexone	T50.7X1	T50.7X2	T50.7X3	T50.7X4	T50.7X5	T50.7X6
Namenda	T43.8X1	T43.8X2	T43.8X3	T43.8X4	T43.8X5	T43.8X6

Substance	External Cause (T-Code)					
	Poisoning, Accidental (Unintentional)	Poisoning, Intentional Self-Harm	Poisoning, Assault	Poisoning, Undetermined	Adverse Effect	Underdosing
Nandrolone	T38.7X1	T38.7X2	T38.7X3	T38.7X4	T38.7X5	T38.7X6
Naphazoline	T48.5X1	T48.5X2	T48.5X3	T48.5X4	T48.5X5	T48.5X6
Naphtha (painters') (petroleum)	T52.0X1	T52.0X2	T52.0X3	T52.0X4	—	—
solvent	T52.0X1	T52.0X2	T52.0X3	T52.0X4	—	—
vapor	T52.0X1	T52.0X2	T52.0X3	T52.0X4	—	—
Naphthalene (non-chlorinated)	T60.2X1	T60.2X2	T60.2X3	T60.2X4	—	—
chlorinated	T60.1X1	T60.1X2	T60.1X3	T60.1X4	—	—
vapor	T60.1X1	T60.1X2	T60.1X3	T60.1X4	—	—
insecticide or moth repellent	T60.2X1	T60.2X2	T60.2X3	T60.2X4	—	—
chlorinated	T60.1X1	T60.1X2	T60.1X3	T60.1X4	—	—
vapor	T60.2X1	T60.2X2	T60.2X3	T60.2X4	—	—
chlorinated	T60.1X1	T60.1X2	T60.1X3	T60.1X4	—	—
Naphthol	T65.891	T65.892	T65.893	T65.894	—	—
Naphthylamine	T65.891	T65.892	T65.893	T65.894	—	—
Naphthylthiourea (ANTU)	T60.4X1	T60.4X2	T60.4X3	T60.4X4	—	—
Naprosyn — see Naproxen						
Naproxen	T39.311	T39.312	T39.313	T39.314	T39.315	T39.316
Narcotic (drug)	T40.601	T40.602	T40.603	T40.604	T40.605	T40.606
analgesic NEC	T40.601	T40.602	T40.603	T40.604	T40.605	T40.606
antagonist	T50.7X1	T50.7X2	T50.7X3	T50.7X4	T50.7X5	T50.7X6
specified NEC	T40.691	T40.692	T40.693	T40.694	T40.695	T40.696
synthetic	T40.491	T40.492	T40.493	T40.494	T40.495	T40.496
Narcotine	T48.3X1	T48.3X2	T48.3X3	T48.3X4	T48.3X5	T48.3X6
Nardil	T43.1X1	T43.1X2	T43.1X3	T43.1X4	T43.1X5	T43.1X6
Nasal drug NEC	T49.6X1	T49.6X2	T49.6X3	T49.6X4	T49.6X5	T49.6X6
Natamycin	T49.0X1	T49.0X2	T49.0X3	T49.0X4	T49.0X5	T49.0X6
Natrium cyanide — see Cyanide(s)						
Natural gas	T59.891	T59.892	T59.893	T59.894	—	—
incomplete combustion	T57.91	T57.92	T57.93	T57.94	—	—
Natural						
blood (product)	T45.8X1	T45.8X2	T45.8X3	T45.8X4	T45.8X5	T45.8X6
gas (piped)	T59.891	T59.892	T59.893	T59.894	—	—
incomplete combustion	T58.11	T58.12	T58.13	T58.14	—	—
Nealbarbital	T42.3X1	T42.3X2	T42.3X3	T42.3X4	T42.3X5	T42.3X6
Nectadon	T48.3X1	T48.3X2	T48.3X3	T48.3X4	T48.3X5	T48.3X6
Nedocromil	T48.6X1	T48.6X2	T48.6X3	T48.6X4	T48.6X5	T48.6X6
Nefopam	T39.8X1	T39.8X2	T39.8X3	T39.8X4	T39.8X5	T39.8X6
Nematocyst (sting)	T63.691	T63.692	T63.693	T63.694	—	—
Nembutal	T42.3X1	T42.3X2	T42.3X3	T42.3X4	T42.3X5	T42.3X6
Nemonapride	T43.591	T43.592	T43.593	T43.594	T43.595	T43.596
Neoarsphenamine	T37.8X1	T37.8X2	T37.8X3	T37.8X4	T37.8X5	T37.8X6

◀ New　◀ Revised　~~deleted~~ Deleted

Substance	External Cause (T-Code)					
	Poisoning, Accidental (Unintentional)	Poisoning, Intentional Self-Harm	Poisoning, Assault	Poisoning, Undetermined	Adverse Effect	Underdosing
Neocinchophen	T50.4X1	T50.4X2	T50.4X3	T50.4X4	T50.4X5	T50.4X6
Neomycin (derivatives)	T36.5X1	T36.5X2	T36.5X3	T36.5X4	T36.5X5	T36.5X6
with						
bacitracin	T49.0X1	T49.0X2	T49.0X3	T49.0X4	T49.0X5	T49.0X6
neostigmine	T44.0X1	T44.0X2	T44.0X3	T44.0X4	T44.0X5	T44.0X6
ENT agent	T49.6X1	T49.6X2	T49.6X3	T49.6X4	T49.6X5	T49.6X6
ophthalmic preparation	T49.5X1	T49.5X2	T49.5X3	T49.5X4	T49.5X5	T49.5X6
topical NEC	T49.0X1	T49.0X2	T49.0X3	T49.0X4	T49.0X5	T49.0X6
Neonal	T42.3X1	T42.3X2	T42.3X3	T42.3X4	T42.3X5	T42.3X6
Neoprontosil	T37.0X1	T37.0X2	T37.0X3	T37.0X4	T37.0X5	T37.0X6
Neosalvarsan	T37.8X1	T37.8X2	T37.8X3	T37.8X4	T37.8X5	T37.8X6
Neosilversalvarsan	T37.8X1	T37.8X2	T37.8X3	T37.8X4	T37.8X5	T37.8X6
Neosporin	T36.8X1	T36.8X2	T36.8X3	T36.8X4	T36.8X5	T36.8X6
ENT agent	T49.6X1	T49.6X2	T49.6X3	T49.6X4	T49.6X5	T49.6X6
opthalmic preparation	T49.5X1	T49.5X2	T49.5X3	T49.5X4	T49.5X5	T49.5X6
topical NEC	T49.0X1	T49.0X2	T49.0X3	T49.0X4	T49.0X5	T49.0X6
Neostigmine bromide	T44.0X1	T44.0X2	T44.0X3	T44.0X4	T44.0X5	T44.0X6
Neraval	T42.3X1	T42.3X2	T42.3X3	T42.3X4	T42.3X5	T42.3X6
Neravan	T42.3X1	T42.3X2	T42.3X3	T42.3X4	T42.3X5	T42.3X6
Nerium oleander	T62.2X1	T62.2X2	T62.2X3	T62.2X4	—	—
Nerve gas, not in war	T59.91	T59.92	T59.93	T59.94	—	—
Nesacaine	T41.3X1	T41.3X2	T41.3X3	T41.3X4	T41.3X5	T41.3X6
infiltration (subcutaneous)	T41.3X1	T41.3X2	T41.3X3	T41.3X4	T41.3X5	T41.3X6
nerve block (peripheral) (plexus)	T41.3X1	T41.3X2	T41.3X3	T41.3X4	T41.3X5	T41.3X6
Netilmicin	T36.5X1	T36.5X2	T36.5X3	T36.5X4	T36.5X5	T36.5X6
Neurobarb	T42.3X1	T42.3X2	T42.3X3	T42.3X4	T42.3X5	T42.3X6
Neuroleptic drug NEC	T43.501	T43.502	T43.503	T43.504	T43.505	T43.506
Neuromuscular blocking drug	T48.1X1	T48.1X2	T48.1X3	T48.1X4	T48.1X5	T48.1X6
Neutral insulin injection	T38.3X1	T38.3X2	T38.3X3	T38.3X4	T38.3X5	T38.3X6
Neutral spirits	T51.0X1	T51.0X2	T51.0X3	T51.0X4	—	—
beverage	T51.0X1	T51.0X2	T51.0X3	T51.0X4	—	—
Niacin	T46.7X1	T46.7X2	T46.7X3	T46.7X4	T46.7X5	T46.7X6
Niacinamide	T45.2X1	T45.2X2	T45.2X3	T45.2X4	T45.2X5	T45.2X6
Nialamide	T43.1X1	T43.1X2	T43.1X3	T43.1X4	T43.1X5	T43.1X6
Niaprazine	T42.6X1	T42.6X2	T42.6X3	T42.6X4	T42.6X5	T42.6X6
Nicametate	T46.7X1	T46.7X2	T46.7X3	T46.7X4	T46.7X5	T46.7X6
Nicardipine	T46.1X1	T46.1X2	T46.1X3	T46.1X4	T46.1X5	T46.1X6
Nicergoline	T46.7X1	T46.7X2	T46.7X3	T46.7X4	T46.7X5	T46.7X6
Nickel (carbonyl) (tetra-carbonyl) (fumes) (vapor)	T56.891	T56.892	T56.893	T56.894	—	—

Substance	External Cause (T-Code)					
	Poisoning, Accidental (Unintentional)	Poisoning, Intentional Self-Harm	Poisoning, Assault	Poisoning, Undetermined	Adverse Effect	Underdosing
Nickelocene	T56.891	T56.892	T56.893	T56.894	—	—
Niclosamide	T37.4X1	T37.4X2	T37.4X3	T37.4X4	T37.4X5	T37.4X6
Nicofuranose	T46.7X1	T46.7X2	T46.7X3	T46.7X4	T46.7X5	T46.7X6
Nicomorphine	T40.2X1	T40.2X2	T40.2X3	T40.2X4	—	—
Nicorandil	T46.3X1	T46.3X2	T46.3X3	T46.3X4	T46.3X5	T46.3X6
Nicotiana (plant)	T62.2X1	T62.2X2	T62.2X3	T62.2X4	—	—
Nicotinamide	T45.2X1	T45.2X2	T45.2X3	T45.2X4	T45.2X5	T45.2X6
Nicotine (insecticide) (spray) (sulfate) NEC	T60.2X1	T60.2X2	T60.2X3	T60.2X4	—	—
from tobacco	T65.291	T65.292	T65.293	T65.294	—	—
cigarettes	T65.221	T65.222	T65.223	T65.224	—	—
not insecticide	T65.291	T65.292	T65.293	T65.294	—	—
Nicotinic acid	T46.7X1	T46.7X2	T46.7X3	T46.7X4	T46.7X5	T46.7X6
Nicotinyl alcohol	T46.7X1	T46.7X2	T46.7X3	T46.7X4	T46.7X5	T46.7X6
Nicoumalone	T45.511	T45.512	T45.513	T45.514	T45.515	T45.516
Nifedipine	T46.1X1	T46.1X2	T46.1X3	T46.1X4	T46.1X5	T46.1X6
Nifenazone	T39.2X1	T39.2X2	T39.2X3	T39.2X4	T39.2X5	T39.2X6
Nifuraldezone	T37.91	T37.92	T37.93	T37.94	T37.95	T37.96
Nifuratel	T37.8X1	T37.8X2	T37.8X3	T37.8X4	T37.8X5	T37.8X6
Nifurtimox	T37.3X1	T37.3X2	T37.3X3	T37.3X4	T37.3X5	T37.3X6
Nifurtoinol	T37.8X1	T37.8X2	T37.8X3	T37.8X4	T37.8X5	T37.8X6
Nightshade, deadly (solanum)— see also Belladonna	T62.2X1	T62.2X2	T62.2X3	T62.2X4	—	—
berry	T62.1X1	T62.1X2	T62.1X3	T62.1X4	—	—
Nikethamide	T50.7X1	T50.7X2	T50.7X3	T50.7X4	T50.7X5	T50.7X6
Nilstat	T36.7X1	T36.7X2	T36.7X3	T36.7X4	T36.7X5	T36.7X6
topical	T49.0X1	T49.0X2	T49.0X3	T49.0X4	T49.0X5	T49.0X6
Nilutamide	T38.6X1	T38.6X2	T38.6X3	T38.6X4	T38.6X5	T38.6X6
Nimesulide	T39.391	T39.392	T39.393	T39.394	T39.395	T39.396
Nimetazepam	T42.4X1	T42.4X2	T42.4X3	T42.4X4	T42.4X5	T42.4X6
Nimodipine	T46.1X1	T46.1X2	T46.1X3	T46.1X4	T46.1X5	T46.1X6
Nimorazole	T37.3X1	T37.3X2	T37.3X3	T37.3X4	T37.3X5	T37.3X6
Nimustine	T45.1X1	T45.1X2	T45.1X3	T45.1X4	T45.1X5	T45.1X6
Niridazole	T37.4X1	T37.4X2	T37.4X3	T37.4X4	T37.4X5	T37.4X6
Nisentil	T40.2X1	T40.2X2	T40.2X3	T40.2X4	T40.2X5	T40.2X6
Nisoldipine	T46.1X1	T46.1X2	T46.1X3	T46.1X4	T46.1X5	T46.1X6
Nitramine	T65.3X1	T65.3X2	T65.3X3	T65.3X4	—	—
Nitrate, organic	T46.3X1	T46.3X2	T46.3X3	T46.3X4	T46.3X5	T46.3X6
Nitrazepam	T42.4X1	T42.4X2	T42.4X3	T42.4X4	T42.4X5	T42.4X6
Nitrefazole	T50.6X1	T50.6X2	T50.6X3	T50.6X4	T50.6X5	T50.6X6
Nitrendipine	T46.1X1	T46.1X2	T46.1X3	T46.1X4	T46.1X5	T46.1X6

◀ New ◀ Revised ~~deleted~~ Deleted

Substance	Poisoning, Accidental (Unintentional)	Poisoning, Intentional Self-Harm	Poisoning, Assault	Poisoning, Undetermined	Adverse Effect	Underdosing
External Cause (T-Code)						
Nitric						
acid (liquid)	T54.2X1	T54.2X2	T54.2X3	T54.2X4	—	—
vapor	T59.891	T59.892	T59.893	T59.894	—	—
oxide (gas)	T59.0X1	T59.0X2	T59.0X3	T59.0X4	—	—
Nitrimidazine	T37.3X1	T37.3X2	T37.3X3	T37.3X4	T37.3X5	T37.3X6
Nitrite, amyl (medicinal) (vapor)	T46.3X1	T46.3X2	T46.3X3	T46.3X4	T46.3X5	T46.3X6
Nitroaniline	T65.3X1	T65.3X2	T65.3X3	T65.3X4	—	—
vapor	T59.891	T59.892	T59.893	T59.894	—	—
Nitrobenzene, nitrobenzol	T65.3X1	T65.3X2	T65.3X3	T65.3X4	—	—
vapor	T65.3X1	T65.3X2	T65.3X3	T65.3X4	—	—
Nitrocellulose	T65.891	T65.892	T65.893	T65.894	—	—
lacquer	T65.891	T65.892	T65.893	T65.894	—	—
Nitrodiphenyl	T65.3X1	T65.3X2	T65.3X3	T65.3X4	—	—
Nitrofural	T49.0X1	T49.0X2	T49.0X3	T49.0X4	T49.0X5	T49.0X6
Nitrofurantoin	T37.8X1	T37.8X2	T37.8X3	T37.8X4	T37.8X5	T37.8X6
Nitrofurazone	T49.0X1	T49.0X2	T49.0X3	T49.0X4	T49.0X5	T49.0X6
Nitrogen	T59.0X1	T59.0X2	T59.0X3	T59.0X4	—	—
mustard	T45.1X1	T45.1X2	T45.1X3	T45.1X4	T45.1X5	T45.1X6
Nitroglycerin, nitro-glycerol (medicinal)	T46.3X1	T46.3X2	T46.3X3	T46.3X4	T46.3X5	T46.3X6
nonmedicinal	T65.5X1	T65.5X2	T65.5X3	T65.5X4	—	—
fumes	T65.5X1	T65.5X2	T65.5X3	T65.5X4	—	—
Nitroglycol	T52.3X1	T52.3X2	T52.3X3	T52.3X4	—	—
Nitrohydrochloric acid	T54.2X1	T54.2X2	T54.2X3	T54.2X4	—	—
Nitromersol	T49.0X1	T49.0X2	T49.0X3	T49.0X4	T49.0X5	T49.0X6
Nitronaphthalene	T65.891	T65.892	T65.893	T65.894	—	—
Nitrophenol	T54.0X1	T54.0X2	T54.0X3	T54.0X4	—	—
Nitropropane	T52.8X1	T52.8X2	T52.8X3	T52.8X4	—	—
Nitroprusside	T46.5X1	T46.5X2	T46.5X3	T46.5X4	T46.5X5	T46.5X6
Nitrosodimethylamine	T65.3X1	T65.3X2	T65.3X3	T65.3X4	—	—
Nitrothiazol	T37.4X1	T37.4X2	T37.4X3	T37.4X4	T37.4X5	T37.4X6
Nitrotoluene, nitrotoluol	T65.3X1	T65.3X2	T65.3X3	T65.3X4	—	—
vapor	T65.3X1	T65.3X2	T65.3X3	T65.3X4	—	—
Nitrous						
acid (liquid)	T54.2X1	T54.2X2	T54.2X3	T54.2X4	—	—
fumes	T59.891	T59.892	T59.893	T59.894	—	—
ether spirit	T46.3X1	T46.3X2	T46.3X3	T46.3X4	T46.3X5	T46.3X6
oxide	T41.0X1	T41.0X2	T41.0X3	T41.0X4	T41.0X5	T41.0X6
Nitroxoline	T37.8X1	T37.8X2	T37.8X3	T37.8X4	T37.8X5	T37.8X6
Nitrozone	T49.0X1	T49.0X2	T49.0X3	T49.0X4	T49.0X5	T49.0X6
Nizatidine	T47.0X1	T47.0X2	T47.0X3	T47.0X4	T47.0X5	T47.0X6

Substance	Poisoning, Accidental (Unintentional)	Poisoning, Intentional Self-Harm	Poisoning, Assault	Poisoning, Undetermined	Adverse Effect	Underdosing
External Cause (T-Code)						
Nizofenone	T43.8X1	T43.8X2	T43.8X3	T43.8X4	T43.8X5	T43.8X6
Noctec	T42.6X1	T42.6X2	T42.6X3	T42.6X4	T42.6X5	T42.6X6
Noludar	T42.6X1	T42.6X2	T42.6X3	T42.6X4	T42.6X5	T42.6X6
Noptil	T42.3X1	T42.3X2	T42.3X3	T42.3X4	T42.3X5	T42.3X6
Nomegestrol	T38.5X1	T38.5X2	T38.5X3	T38.5X4	T38.5X5	T38.5X6
Nomifensine	T43.291	T43.292	T43.293	T43.294	T43.295	T43.296
Nonoxinol	T49.8X1	T49.8X2	T49.8X3	T49.8X4	T49.8X5	T49.8X6
Nonylphenoxy (polyethoxy-ethanol)	T49.8X1	T49.8X2	T49.8X3	T49.8X4	T49.8X5	T49.8X6
Noptil	T42.3X1	T42.3X2	T42.3X3	T42.3X4	T42.3X5	T42.3X6
Noradrenaline	T44.4X1	T44.4X2	T44.4X3	T44.4X4	T44.4X5	T44.4X6
Noramidopyrine	T39.2X1	T39.2X2	T39.2X3	T39.2X4	T39.2X5	T39.2X6
methanesulfonate sodium	T39.2X1	T39.2X2	T39.2X3	T39.2X4	T39.2X5	T39.2X6
Norbormide	T60.4X1	T60.4X2	T60.4X3	T60.4X4	—	—
Nordazepam	T42.4X1	T42.4X2	T42.4X3	T42.4X4	T42.4X5	T42.4X6
Norepinephrine	T44.4X1	T44.4X2	T44.4X3	T44.4X4	T44.4X5	T44.4X6
Norethandrolone	T38.7X1	T38.7X2	T38.7X3	T38.7X4	T38.7X5	T38.7X6
Norethindrone	T38.4X1	T38.4X2	T38.4X3	T38.4X4	T38.4X5	T38.4X6
Norethisterone (acetate) (enantate)	T38.4X1	T38.4X2	T38.4X3	T38.4X4	T38.4X5	T38.4X6
with ethinylestradiol	T38.5X1	T38.5X2	T38.5X3	T38.5X4	T38.5X5	T38.5X6
Noretynodrel	T38.5X1	T38.5X2	T38.5X3	T38.5X4	T38.5X5	T38.5X6
Norfenefrine	T44.4X1	T44.4X2	T44.4X3	T44.4X4	T44.4X5	T44.4X6
Norfloxacin	T36.8X1	T36.8X2	T36.8X3	T36.8X4	T36.8X5	T36.8X6
Norgestrel	T38.4X1	T38.4X2	T38.4X3	T38.4X4	T38.4X5	T38.4X6
Norgestrienone	T38.4X1	T38.4X2	T38.4X3	T38.4X4	T38.4X5	T38.4X6
Norlestrin	T38.4X1	T38.4X2	T38.4X3	T38.4X4	T38.4X5	T38.4X6
Norlutin	T38.4X1	T38.4X2	T38.4X3	T38.4X4	T38.4X5	T38.4X6
Normal serum albumin (human), salt-poor	T45.8X1	T45.8X2	T45.8X3	T45.8X4	T45.8X5	T45.8X6
Normethandrone	T38.5X1	T38.5X2	T38.5X3	T38.5X4	T38.5X5	T38.5X6
Normison—*see* Benzodiazepines						
Normorphine	T40.2X1	T40.2X2	T40.2X3	T40.2X4	—	—
Norpseudoephedrine	T50.5X1	T50.5X2	T50.5X3	T50.5X4	T50.5X5	T50.5X6
Nortestosterone (furanpropionate)	T38.7X1	T38.7X2	T38.7X3	T38.7X4	T38.7X5	T38.7X6
Nortriptyline	T43.011	T43.012	T43.013	T43.014	T43.015	T43.016
Noscapine	T48.3X1	T48.3X2	T48.3X3	T48.3X4	T48.3X5	T48.3X6
Nose preparations	T49.6X1	T49.6X2	T49.6X3	T49.6X4	T49.6X5	T49.6X6
Novobiocin	T36.5X1	T36.5X2	T36.5X3	T36.5X4	T36.5X5	T36.5X6
Novocain (infiltration) (topical)	T41.3X1	T41.3X2	T41.3X3	T41.3X4	T41.3X5	T41.3X6
nerve block (peripheral) (plexus)	T41.3X1	T41.3X2	T41.3X3	T41.3X4	T41.3X5	T41.3X6
spinal	T41.3X1	T41.3X2	T41.3X3	T41.3X4	T41.3X5	T41.3X6

◀ New ◀ Revised ~~deleted~~ Deleted

Substance	External Cause (T-Code) Poisoning, Accidental (Unintentional)	Poisoning, Intentional Self-Harm	Poisoning, Assault	Poisoning, Undetermined	Adverse Effect	Underdosing
Noxious foodstuff	T62.91	T62.92	T62.93	T62.94	—	—
specified NEC	T62.8X1	T62.8X2	T62.8X3	T62.8X4	—	—
Noxiptiline	T43.011	T43.012	T43.013	T43.014	T43.015	T43.016
Noxytiolin	T49.0X1	T49.0X2	T49.0X3	T49.0X4	T49.0X5	T49.0X6
NPH Iletin (insulin)	T38.3X1	T38.3X2	T38.3X3	T38.3X4	T38.3X5	T38.3X6
Numorphan	T40.2X1	T40.2X2	T40.2X3	T40.2X4	T40.2X5	T40.2X6
Nunol	T42.3X1	T42.3X2	T42.3X3	T42.3X4	T42.3X5	T42.3X6
Nupercaine (spinal anesthetic)	T41.3X1	T41.3X2	T41.3X3	T41.3X4	T41.3X5	T41.3X6
topical (surface)	T41.3X1	T41.3X2	T41.3X3	T41.3X4	T41.3X5	T41.3X6
Nutmeg oil (liniment)	T49.3X1	T49.3X2	T49.3X3	T49.3X4	T49.3X5	T49.3X6
Nutritional supplement	T50.901	T50.902	T50.903	T50.904	T50.905	T50.906
Nux vomica	T65.1X1	T65.1X2	T65.1X3	T65.1X4	—	—
Nydrazid	T37.1X1	T37.1X2	T37.1X3	T37.1X4	T37.1X5	T37.1X6
Nylidrin	T46.7X1	T46.7X2	T46.7X3	T46.7X4	T46.7X5	T46.7X6
Nystatin	T36.7X1	T36.7X2	T36.7X3	T36.7X4	T36.7X5	T36.7X6
topical	T49.0X1	T49.0X2	T49.0X3	T49.0X4	T49.0X5	T49.0X6
Nytol	T45.0X1	T45.0X2	T45.0X3	T45.0X4	T45.0X5	T45.0X6
O						
Obidoxime chloride	T50.6X1	T50.6X2	T50.6X3	T50.6X4	T50.6X5	T50.6X6
Octafonium (chloride)	T49.3X1	T49.3X2	T49.3X3	T49.3X4	T49.3X5	T49.3X6
Octamethyl pyrophos-phoramide	T60.0X1	T60.0X2	T60.0X3	T60.0X4	—	—
Octanoin	T50.991	T50.992	T50.993	T50.994	T50.995	T50.996
Octatropine methyl-bromide	T44.3X1	T44.3X2	T44.3X3	T44.3X4	T44.3X5	T44.3X6
Octotiamine	T45.2X1	T45.2X2	T45.2X3	T45.2X4	T45.2X5	T45.2X6
Octoxinol (9)	T49.8X1	T49.8X2	T49.8X3	T49.8X4	T49.8X5	T49.8X6
Octreotide	T38.991	T38.992	T38.993	T38.994	T38.995	T38.996
Octyl nitrite	T46.3X1	T46.3X2	T46.3X3	T46.3X4	T46.3X5	T46.3X6
Oestradiol	T38.5X1	T38.5X2	T38.5X3	T38.5X4	T38.5X5	T38.5X6
Oestriol	T38.5X1	T38.5X2	T38.5X3	T38.5X4	T38.5X5	T38.5X6
Oestrogen	T38.5X1	T38.5X2	T38.5X3	T38.5X4	T38.5X5	T38.5X6
Oestrone	T38.5X1	T38.5X2	T38.5X3	T38.5X4	T38.5X5	T38.5X6
Ofloxacin	T36.8X1	T36.8X2	T36.8X3	T36.8X4	T36.8X5	T36.8X6
Oil (of)	T65.891	T65.892	T65.893	T65.894	—	—
bitter almond	T62.8X1	T62.8X2	T62.8X3	T62.8X4	—	—
cloves	T49.7X1	T49.7X2	T49.7X3	T49.7X4	T49.7X5	T49.7X6
colors	T65.6X1	T65.6X2	T65.6X3	T65.6X4	—	—
fumes	T59.891	T59.892	T59.893	T59.894	—	—
lubricating	T52.0X1	T52.0X2	T52.0X3	T52.0X4	—	—
Niobe	T52.8X1	T52.8X2	T52.8X3	T52.8X4	—	—

Substance	External Cause (T-Code) Poisoning, Accidental (Unintentional)	Poisoning, Intentional Self-Harm	Poisoning, Assault	Poisoning, Undetermined	Adverse Effect	Underdosing
Oil (of) *(Continued)*						
vitriol (liquid)	T54.2X1	T54.2X2	T54.2X3	T54.2X4	—	—
fumes	T54.2X1	T54.2X2	T54.2X3	T54.2X4	—	—
wintergreen (bitter) NEC	T49.3X1	T49.3X2	T49.3X3	T49.3X4	T49.3X5	T49.3X6
Oily preparation (for skin)	T49.3X1	T49.3X2	T49.3X3	T49.3X4	T49.3X5	T49.3X6
Ointment NEC	T49.3X1	T49.3X2	T49.3X3	T49.3X4	T49.3X5	T49.3X6
Olanzapine	T43.591	T43.592	T43.593	T43.594	T43.595	T43.596
Oleander	T62.2X1	T62.2X2	T62.2X3	T62.2X4	—	—
Oleandomycin	T36.3X1	T36.3X2	T36.3X3	T36.3X4	T36.3X5	T36.3X6
Oleandrin	T46.0X1	T46.0X2	T46.0X3	T46.0X4	T46.0X5	T46.0X6
Oleic acid	T46.6X1	T46.6X2	T46.6X3	T46.6X4	T46.6X5	T46.6X6
Oleovitamin A	T45.2X1	T45.2X2	T45.2X3	T45.2X4	T45.2X5	T45.2X6
Oleum ricini	T47.2X1	T47.2X2	T47.2X3	T47.2X4	T47.2X5	T47.2X6
Olive oil (medicinal) NEC	T47.4X1	T47.4X2	T47.4X3	T47.4X4	T47.4X5	T47.4X6
Olivomycin	T45.1X1	T45.1X2	T45.1X3	T45.1X4	T45.1X5	T45.1X6
Olsalazine	T47.8X1	T47.8X2	T47.8X3	T47.8X4	T47.8X5	T47.8X6
Omeprazole	T47.1X1	T47.1X2	T47.1X3	T47.1X4	T47.1X5	T47.1X6
OMPA	T60.0X1	T60.0X2	T60.0X3	T60.0X4	—	—
Ondansetron	T45.0X1	T45.0X2	T45.0X3	T45.0X4	T45.0X5	T45.0X6
Oncovin	T45.1X1	T45.1X2	T45.1X3	T45.1X4	T45.1X5	T45.1X6
Ophthaine	T41.3X1	T41.3X2	T41.3X3	T41.3X4	T41.3X5	T41.3X6
Ophthetic	T41.3X1	T41.3X2	T41.3X3	T41.3X4	T41.3X5	T41.3X6
Opiate NEC	T40.601	T40.602	T40.603	T40.604	T40.605	T40.606
antagonists	T50.7X1	T50.7X2	T50.7X3	T50.7X4	T50.7X5	T50.7X6
Opioid NEC	T40.2X1	T40.2X2	T40.2X3	T40.2X4	T40.2X5	T40.2X6
Opipramol	T43.011	T43.012	T43.013	T43.014	T43.015	T43.016
Opium alkaloids (total)	T40.0X1	T40.0X2	T40.0X3	T40.0X4	T40.0X5	T40.0X6
standardized powdered	T40.0X1	T40.0X2	T40.0X3	T40.0X4	T40.0X5	T40.0X6
tincture (camphorated)	T40.0X1	T40.0X2	T40.0X3	T40.0X4	T40.0X5	T40.0X6
Oracon	T38.4X1	T38.4X2	T38.4X3	T38.4X4	T38.4X5	T38.4X6
Oragrafin	T50.8X1	T50.8X2	T50.8X3	T50.8X4	T50.8X5	T50.8X6
Oral contraceptives	T38.4X1	T38.4X2	T38.4X3	T38.4X4	T38.4X5	T38.4X6
Oral rehydration salts	T50.3X1	T50.3X2	T50.3X3	T50.3X4	T50.3X5	T50.3X6
Orazamide	T50.991	T50.992	T50.993	T50.994	T50.995	T50.996
Orciprenaline	T48.291	T48.292	T48.293	T48.294	T48.295	T48.296
Organidin	T48.4X1	T48.4X2	T48.4X3	T48.4X4	T48.4X5	T48.4X6
Organonitrate NEC	T46.3X1	T46.3X2	T46.3X3	T46.3X4	T46.3X5	T46.3X6
Organophosphates	T60.0X1	T60.0X2	T60.0X3	T60.0X4	—	—
Orimune	T50.B91	T50.B92	T50.B93	T50.B94	T50.B95	T50.B96
Orinase	T38.3X1	T38.3X2	T38.3X3	T38.3X4	T38.3X5	T38.3X6
Ormeloxifene	T38.6X1	T38.6X2	T38.6X3	T38.6X4	T38.6X5	T38.6X6

◄ New ◄ Revised ~~deleted~~ Deleted

TABLE OF DRUGS AND CHEMICALS

Substance	Poisoning, Accidental (Unintentional)	Poisoning, Intentional Self-Harm	Poisoning, Assault	Poisoning, Undetermined	Adverse Effect	Underdosing
Ornidazole	T37.3X1	T37.3X2	T37.3X3	T37.3X4	T37.3X5	T37.3X6
Ornithine aspartate	T50.991	T50.992	T50.993	T50.994	T50.995	T50.996
Ornoprostil	T47.1X1	T47.1X2	T47.1X3	T47.1X4	T47.1X5	T47.1X6
Orphenadrine (hydrochloride)	T42.8X1	T42.8X2	T42.8X3	T42.8X4	T42.8X5	T42.8X6
Ortal (sodium)	T42.3X1	T42.3X2	T42.3X3	T42.3X4	T42.3X5	T42.3X6
Orthoboric acid	T49.0X1	T49.0X2	T49.0X3	T49.0X4	T49.0X5	T49.0X6
ENT agent	T49.6X1	T49.6X2	T49.6X3	T49.6X4	T49.6X5	T49.6X6
ophthalmic preparation	T49.5X1	T49.5X2	T49.5X3	T49.5X4	T49.5X5	T49.5X6
Orthocaine	T41.3X1	T41.3X2	T41.3X3	T41.3X4	T41.3X5	T41.3X6
Orthodichlorobenzene	T53.7X1	T53.7X2	T53.7X3	T53.7X4	—	—
Ortho-Novum	T38.4X1	T38.4X2	T38.4X3	T38.4X4	T38.4X5	T38.4X6
Orthotolidine (reagent)	T54.2X1	T54.2X2	T54.2X3	T54.2X4	—	—
Osmic acid (liquid)	T54.2X1	T54.2X2	T54.2X3	T54.2X4	—	—
fumes	T54.2X1	T54.2X2	T54.2X3	T54.2X4	—	—
Osmotic diuretics	T50.2X1	T50.2X2	T50.2X3	T50.2X4	T50.2X5	T50.2X6
Otilonium bromide	T44.3X1	T44.3X2	T44.3X3	T44.3X4	T44.3X5	T44.3X6
Otorhinolaryngological drug NEC	T49.6X1	T49.6X2	T49.6X3	T49.6X4	T49.6X5	T49.6X6
Ouabain(e)	T46.0X1	T46.0X2	T46.0X3	T46.0X4	T46.0X5	T46.0X6
Ovarian						
hormone	T38.5X1	T38.5X2	T38.5X3	T38.5X4	T38.5X5	T38.5X6
stimulant	T38.5X1	T38.5X2	T38.5X3	T38.5X4	T38.5X5	T38.5X6
Ovral	T38.4X1	T38.4X2	T38.4X3	T38.4X4	T38.4X5	T38.4X6
Ovulen	T38.4X1	T38.4X2	T38.4X3	T38.4X4	T38.4X5	T38.4X6
Oxacillin	T36.0X1	T36.0X2	T36.0X3	T36.0X4	T36.0X5	T36.0X6
Oxalic acid	T54.2X1	T54.2X2	T54.2X3	T54.2X4	—	—
ammonium salt	T50.991	T50.992	T50.993	T50.994	T50.995	T50.996
Oxamniquine	T37.4X1	T37.4X2	T37.4X3	T37.4X4	T37.4X5	T37.4X6
Oxanamide	T43.591	T43.592	T43.593	T43.594	T43.595	T43.596
Oxandrolone	T38.7X1	T38.7X2	T38.7X3	T38.7X4	T38.7X5	T38.7X6
Oxantel	T37.4X1	T37.4X2	T37.4X3	T37.4X4	T37.4X5	T37.4X6
Oxapium iodide	T44.3X1	T44.3X2	T44.3X3	T44.3X4	T44.3X5	T44.3X6
Oxaprotiline	T43.021	T43.022	T43.023	T43.024	T43.025	T43.026
Oxaprozin	T39.311	T39.312	T39.313	T39.314	T39.315	T39.316
Oxatomide	T45.0X1	T45.0X2	T45.0X3	T45.0X4	T45.0X5	T45.0X6
Oxazepam	T42.4X1	T42.4X2	T42.4X3	T42.4X4	T42.4X5	T42.4X6
Oxazimedrine	T50.5X1	T50.5X2	T50.5X3	T50.5X4	T50.5X5	T50.5X6
Oxazolam	T42.4X1	T42.4X2	T42.4X3	T42.4X4	T42.4X5	T42.4X6
Oxazolidine derivatives	T42.2X1	T42.2X2	T42.2X3	T42.2X4	T42.2X5	T42.2X6
Oxazolidinedione (derivative)	T42.2X1	T42.2X2	T42.2X3	T42.2X4	T42.2X5	T42.2X6
Ox bile extract	T47.5X1	T47.5X2	T47.5X3	T47.5X4	T47.5X5	T47.5X6
Oxcarbazepine	T42.1X1	T42.1X2	T42.1X3	T42.1X4	T42.1X5	T42.1X6
Oxedrine	T44.4X1	T44.4X2	T44.4X3	T44.4X4	T44.4X5	T44.4X6
Oxeladin (citrate)	T48.3X1	T48.3X2	T48.3X3	T48.3X4	T48.3X5	T48.3X6
Oxendolone	T38.5X1	T38.5X2	T38.5X3	T38.5X4	T38.5X5	T38.5X6
Oxetacaine	T41.3X1	T41.3X2	T41.3X3	T41.3X4	T41.3X5	T41.3X6
Oxethazine	T41.3X1	T41.3X2	T41.3X3	T41.3X4	T41.3X5	T41.3X6
Oxetorone	T39.8X1	T39.8X2	T39.8X3	T39.8X4	T39.8X5	T39.8X6
Oxiconazole	T49.0X1	T49.0X2	T49.0X3	T49.0X4	T49.0X5	T49.0X6
Oxidizing agent NEC	T54.91	T54.92	T54.93	T54.94	—	—
Oxipurinol	T50.4X1	T50.4X2	T50.4X3	T50.4X4	T50.4X5	T50.4X6
Oxitriptan	T43.291	T43.292	T43.293	T43.294	T43.295	T43.296
Oxitropium bromide	T48.6X1	T48.6X2	T48.6X3	T48.6X4	T48.6X5	T48.6X6
Oxodipine	T46.1X1	T46.1X2	T46.1X3	T46.1X4	T46.1X5	T46.1X6
Oxolamine	T48.3X1	T48.3X2	T48.3X3	T48.3X4	T48.3X5	T48.3X6
Oxolinic acid	T37.8X1	T37.8X2	T37.8X3	T37.8X4	T37.8X5	T37.8X6
Oxomemazine	T43.3X1	T43.3X2	T43.3X3	T43.3X4	T43.3X5	T43.3X6
Oxophenarsine	T37.3X1	T37.3X2	T37.3X3	T37.3X4	T37.3X5	T37.3X6
Oxprenolol	T44.7X1	T44.7X2	T44.7X3	T44.7X4	T44.7X5	T44.7X6
Oxsoralen	T49.3X1	T49.3X2	T49.3X3	T49.3X4	T49.3X5	T49.3X6
Oxtriphylline	T48.6X1	T48.6X2	T48.6X3	T48.6X4	T48.6X5	T48.6X6
Oxybate sodium	T41.291	T41.292	T41.293	T41.294	T41.295	T41.296
Oxybuprocaine	T41.3X1	T41.3X2	T41.3X3	T41.3X4	T41.3X5	T41.3X6
Oxybutynin	T44.3X1	T44.3X2	T44.3X3	T44.3X4	T44.3X5	T44.3X6
Oxychlorosene	T49.0X1	T49.0X2	T49.0X3	T49.0X4	T49.0X5	T49.0X6
Oxycodone	T40.2X1	T40.2X2	T40.2X3	T40.2X4	T40.2X5	T40.2X6
Oxyfedrine	T46.3X1	T46.3X2	T46.3X3	T46.3X4	T46.3X5	T46.3X6
Oxygen	T41.5X1	T41.5X2	T41.5X3	T41.5X4	T41.5X5	T41.5X6
Oxylone	T49.0X1	T49.0X2	T49.0X3	T49.0X4	T49.0X5	T49.0X6
ophthalmic preparation	T49.5X1	T49.5X2	T49.5X3	T49.5X4	T49.5X5	T49.5X6
Oxymesterone	T38.7X1	T38.7X2	T38.7X3	T38.7X4	T38.7X5	T38.7X6
Oxymetazoline	T48.5X1	T48.5X2	T48.5X3	T48.5X4	T48.5X5	T48.5X6
Oxymetholone	T38.7X1	T38.7X2	T38.7X3	T38.7X4	T38.7X5	T38.7X6
Oxymorphone	T40.2X1	T40.2X2	T40.2X3	T40.2X4	T40.2X5	T40.2X6
Oxypertine	T43.591	T43.592	T43.593	T43.594	T43.595	T43.596
Oxyphenbutazone	T39.2X1	T39.2X2	T39.2X3	T39.2X4	T39.2X5	T39.2X6
Oxyphencyclimine	T44.3X1	T44.3X2	T44.3X3	T44.3X4	T44.3X5	T44.3X6
Oxyphenisatine	T47.2X1	T47.2X2	T47.2X3	T47.2X4	T47.2X5	T47.2X6
Oxyphenonium bromide	T44.3X1	T44.3X2	T44.3X3	T44.3X4	T44.3X5	T44.3X6
Oxypolygelatin	T45.8X1	T45.8X2	T45.8X3	T45.8X4	T45.8X5	T45.8X6
Oxyquinoline (derivatives)	T37.8X1	T37.8X2	T37.8X3	T37.8X4	T37.8X5	T37.8X6
Oxytetracycline	T36.4X1	T36.4X2	T36.4X3	T36.4X4	T36.4X5	T36.4X6
Oxytocic drug NEC	T48.0X1	T48.0X2	T48.0X3	T48.0X4	T48.0X5	T48.0X6
Oxytocin (synthetic)	T48.0X1	T48.0X2	T48.0X3	T48.0X4	T48.0X5	T48.0X6
Ozone	T59.891	T59.892	T59.893	T59.894	—	—

◀ New ▷ Revised deleted Deleted

Substance	Poisoning, Accidental (Unintentional)	Poisoning, Intentional Self-Harm	Poisoning, Assault	Poisoning, Undetermined	Adverse Effect	Underdosing
P						
PABA	T49.3X1	T49.3X2	T49.3X3	T49.3X4	T49.3X5	T49.3X6
Packed red cells	T45.8X1	T45.8X2	T45.8X3	T45.8X4	T45.8X5	T45.8X6
Padimate	T49.3X1	T49.3X2	T49.3X3	T49.3X4	T49.3X5	T49.3X6
Paint NEC	T65.6X1	T65.6X2	T65.6X3	T65.6X4	—	—
cleaner	T52.91	T52.92	T52.93	T52.94	—	—
fumes NEC	T59.891	T59.892	T59.893	T59.894	—	—
lead (fumes)	T56.0X1	T56.0X2	T56.0X3	T56.0X4		—
solvent NEC	T52.8X1	T52.8X2	T52.8X3	T52.8X4	—	—
stripper	T52.8X1	T52.8X2	T52.8X3	T52.8X4	—	—
Palfium	T40.2X1	T40.2X2	T40.2X3	T40.2X4	—	—
Palm kernel oil	T50.991	T50.992	T50.993	T50.994	T50.995	T50.996
Paludrine	T37.2X1	T37.2X2	T37.2X3	T37.2X4	T37.2X5	T37.2X6
PAM (pralidoxime)	T50.6X1	T50.6X2	T50.6X3	T50.6X4	T50.6X5	T50.6X6
Pamaquine (naphthoute)	T37.2X1	T37.2X2	T37.2X3	T37.2X4	T37.2X5	T37.2X6
Panadol	T39.1X1	T39.1X2	T39.1X3	T39.1X4	T39.1X5	T39.1X6
Pancreatic						
digestive secretion stimulant	T47.8X1	T47.8X2	T47.8X3	T47.8X4	T47.8X5	T47.8X6
dornase	T45.3X1	T45.3X2	T45.3X3	T45.3X4	T45.3X5	T45.3X6
Pancreatin	T47.5X1	T47.5X2	T47.5X3	T47.5X4	T47.5X5	T47.5X6
Pancrelipase	T47.5X1	T47.5X2	T47.5X3	T47.5X4	T47.5X5	T47.5X6
Pancuronium (bromide)	T48.1X1	T48.1X2	T48.1X3	T48.1X4	T48.1X5	T48.1X6
Pangamic acid	T45.2X1	T45.2X2	T45.2X3	T45.2X4	T45.2X5	T45.2X6
Panthenol	T45.2X1	T45.2X2	T45.2X3	T45.2X4	T45.2X5	T45.2X6
topical	T49.8X1	T49.8X2	T49.8X3	T49.8X4	T49.8X5	T49.8X6
Pantopon	T40.0X1	T40.0X2	T40.0X3	T40.0X4	T40.0X5	T40.0X6
Pantothenic acid	T45.2X1	T45.2X2	T45.2X3	T45.2X4	T45.2X5	T45.2X6
Panwarfin	T45.511	T45.512	T45.513	T45.514	T45.515	T45.516
Papain	T47.5X1	T47.5X2	T47.5X3	T47.5X4	T47.5X5	T47.5X6
digestant	T47.5X1	T47.5X2	T47.5X3	T47.5X4	T47.5X5	T47.5X6
Papaveretum	T40.0X1	T40.0X2	T40.0X3	T40.0X4	T40.0X5	T40.0X6
Papaverine	T44.3X1	T44.3X2	T44.3X3	T44.3X4	T44.3X5	T44.3X6
Para-acetamidophenol	T39.1X1	T39.1X2	T39.1X3	T39.1X4	T39.1X5	T39.1X6
Para-aminobenzoic acid	T49.3X1	T49.3X2	T49.3X3	T49.3X4	T49.3X5	T49.3X6
Para-aminophenol derivatives	T39.1X1	T39.1X2	T39.1X3	T39.1X4	T39.1X5	T39.1X6
Para-aminosalicylic acid	T37.1X1	T37.1X2	T37.1X3	T37.1X4	T37.1X5	T37.1X6
Paracetaldehyde	T42.6X1	T42.6X2	T42.6X3	T42.6X4	T42.6X5	T42.6X6
Paracetamol	T39.1X1	T39.1X2	T39.1X3	T39.1X4	T39.1X5	T39.1X6
Parachlorophenol (camphorated)	T49.0X1	T49.0X2	T49.0X3	T49.0X4	T49.0X5	T49.0X6
Paracodin	T40.2X1	T40.2X2	T40.2X3	T40.2X4	T40.2X5	T40.2X6
Paradione	T42.2X1	T42.2X2	T42.2X3	T42.2X4	T42.2X5	T42.2X6

Substance	Poisoning, Accidental (Unintentional)	Poisoning, Intentional Self-Harm	Poisoning, Assault	Poisoning, Undetermined	Adverse Effect	Underdosing
Paraffin(s) (wax)	T52.0X1	T52.0X2	T52.0X3	T52.0X4	—	—
liquid (medicinal)	T47.4X1	T47.4X2	T47.4X3	T47.4X4	T47.4X5	T47.4X6
nonmedicinal	T52.0X1	T52.0X2	T52.0X3	T52.0X4	—	—
Paraformaldehyde	T60.3X1	T60.3X2	T60.3X3	T60.3X4	—	—
Paraldehyde	T42.6X1	T42.6X2	T42.6X3	T42.6X4	T42.6X5	T42.6X6
Paramethadione	T42.2X1	T42.2X2	T42.2X3	T42.2X4	T42.2X5	T42.2X6
Paramethasone	T38.0X1	T38.0X2	T38.0X3	T38.0X4	T38.0X5	T38.0X6
acetate	T49.0X1	T49.0X2	T49.0X3	T49.0X4	T49.0X5	T49.0X6
Paraoxon	T60.0X1	T60.0X2	T60.0X3	T60.0X4	—	—
Paraquat	T60.3X1	T60.3X2	T60.3X3	T60.3X4	—	—
Parasympatholytic NEC	T44.3X1	T44.3X2	T44.3X3	T44.3X4	T44.3X5	T44.3X6
Parasympathomimetic drug NEC	T44.1X1	T44.1X2	T44.1X3	T44.1X4	T44.1X5	T44.1X6
Parathion	T60.0X1	T60.0X2	T60.0X3	T60.0X4	—	—
Parathormone	T50.991	T50.992	T50.993	T50.994	T50.995	T50.996
Parathyroid extract	T50.991	T50.992	T50.993	T50.994	T50.995	T50.996
Paratyphoid vaccine	T50.A91	T50.A92	T50.A93	T50.A94	T50.A95	T50.A96
Paredrine	T44.4X1	T44.4X2	T44.4X3	T44.4X4	T44.4X5	T44.4X6
Paregoric	T40.0X1	T40.0X2	T40.0X3	T40.0X4	T40.0X5	T40.0X6
Pargyline	T46.5X1	T46.5X2	T46.5X3	T46.5X4	T46.5X5	T46.5X6
Paris green	T57.0X1	T57.0X2	T57.0X3	T57.0X4	—	—
insecticide	T57.0X1	T57.0X2	T57.0X3	T57.0X4	—	—
Parnate	T43.1X1	T43.1X2	T43.1X3	T43.1X4	T43.1X5	T43.1X6
Paromomycin	T36.5X1	T36.5X2	T36.5X3	T36.5X4	T36.5X5	T36.5X6
Paroxypropione	T45.1X1	T45.1X2	T45.1X3	T45.1X4	T45.1X5	T45.1X6
Parzone	T40.2X1	T40.2X2	T40.2X3	T40.2X4	T40.2X5	T40.2X6
PAS	T37.1X1	T37.1X2	T37.1X3	T37.1X4	T37.1X5	T37.1X6
Pasiniazid	T37.1X1	T37.1X2	T37.1X3	T37.1X4	T37.1X5	T37.1X6
PBB (polybrominated biphenyls)	T65.891	T65.892	T65.893	T65.894	—	—
PCB	T65.891	T65.892	T65.893	T65.894	—	—
PCP						
meaning pentachlorophenol	T60.1X1	T60.1X2	T60.1X3	T60.1X4	—	—
fungicide	T60.3X1	T60.3X2	T60.3X3	T60.3X4	—	—
herbicide	T60.3X1	T60.3X2	T60.3X3	T60.3X4	—	—
insecticide	T60.1X1	T60.1X2	T60.1X3	T60.1X4	—	—
meaning phencyclidine	T40.991	T40.992	T40.993	T40.994		
Peach kernel oil (emulsion)	T47.4X1	T47.4X2	T47.4X3	T47.4X4	T47.4X5	T47.4X6
Peanut oil (emulsion) NEC	T47.4X1	T47.4X2	T47.4X3	T47.4X4	T47.4X5	T47.4X6
topical	T49.3X1	T49.3X2	T49.3X3	T49.3X4	T49.3X5	T49.3X6
Pearly Gates (morning glory seeds)	T40.991	T40.992	T40.993	T40.994		
Pecazine	T43.3X1	T43.3X2	T43.3X3	T43.3X4	T43.3X5	T43.3X6
Pectin	T47.6X1	T47.6X2	T47.6X3	T47.6X4	T47.6X5	T47.6X6

TABLE OF DRUGS AND CHEMICALS

TABLE OF DRUGS AND CHEMICALS

Substance	Poisoning, Accidental (Unintentional)	Poisoning, Intentional Self-Harm	Poisoning, Assault	Poisoning, Undetermined	Adverse Effect	Underdosing
Pefloxacin	T37.8X1	T37.8X2	T37.8X3	T37.8X4	T37.8X5	T37.8X6
Pegademase, bovine	T50.Z91	T50.Z92	T50.Z93	I50.Z94	T50.Z95	T50.Z96
Pelletierine tannate	T37.4X1	T37.4X2	T37.4X3	T37.4X4	T37.4X5	T37.4X6
Pemirolast (potassium)	T48.6X1	T48.6X2	T48.6X3	T48.6X4	T48.6X5	T48.6X6
Pemoline	T50.7X1	T50.7X2	T50.7X3	T50.7X4	T50.7X5	T50.7X6
Pempidine	T44.2X1	T44.2X2	T44.2X3	T44.2X4	T44.2X5	T44.2X6
Penamecillin	T36.0X1	T36.0X2	T36.0X3	T36.0X4	T36.0X5	T36.0X6
Penbutolol	T44.7X1	T44.7X2	T44.7X3	T44.7X4	T44.7X5	T44.7X6
Penethamate	T36.0X1	T36.0X2	T36.0X3	T36.0X4	T36.0X5	T36.0X6
Penfluridol	T43.591	T43.592	T43.593	T43.594	T43.595	T43.596
Penflutizide	T50.2X1	T50.2X2	T50.2X3	T50.2X4	T50.2X5	T50.2X6
Pengitoxin	T46.0X1	T46.0X2	T46.0X3	T46.0X4	T46.0X5	T46.0X6
Penicillamine	T50.6X1	T50.6X2	T50.6X3	T50.6X4	T50.6X5	T50.6X6
Penicillin (any)	T36.0X1	T36.0X2	T36.0X3	T36.0X4	T36.0X5	T36.0X6
Penicillinase	T45.3X1	T45.3X2	T45.3X3	T45.3X4	T45.3X5	T45.3X6
Penicilloyl polylysine	T50.8X1	T50.8X2	T50.8X3	T50.8X4	T50.8X5	T50.8X6
Penimepicycline	T36.4X1	T36.4X2	T36.4X3	T36.4X4	T36.4X5	T36.4X6
Pentachloroethane	T53.6X1	T53.6X2	T53.6X3	T53.6X4	—	—
Pentachloronaphthalene	T53.7X1	T53.7X2	T53.7X3	T53.7X4	—	—
Pentachlorophenol (pesticide)	T60.1X1	T60.1X2	T60.1X3	T60.1X4	—	—
fungicide	T60.3X1	T60.3X2	T60.3X3	T60.3X4	—	—
herbicide	T60.3X1	T60.3X2	T60.3X3	T60.3X4	—	—
insecticide	T60.1X1	T60.1X2	T60.1X3	T60.1X4	—	—
Pentaerythritol tetranitrate	T46.3X1	T46.3X2	T46.3X3	T46.3X4	T46.3X5	T46.3X6
Pentaerythritol	T46.3X1	T46.3X2	T46.3X3	T46.3X4	T46.3X5	T46.3X6
chloral	T42.6X1	T42.6X2	T42.6X3	T42.6X4	T42.6X5	T42.6X6
tetranitrate NEC	T46.3X1	T46.3X2	T46.3X3	T46.3X4	T46.3X5	T46.3X6
Pentagastrin	T50.8X1	T50.8X2	T50.8X3	T50.8X4	T50.8X5	T50.8X6
Pentalin	T53.6X1	T53.6X2	T53.6X3	T53.6X4	—	—
Pentamethonium bromide	T44.2X1	T44.2X2	T44.2X3	T44.2X4	T44.2X5	T44.2X6
Pentamidine	T37.3X1	T37.3X2	T37.3X3	T37.3X4	T37.3X5	T37.3X6
Pentanol	T51.3X1	T51.3X2	T51.3X3	T51.3X4	—	—
Pentapyrrolinium (bitartrate)	T44.2X1	T44.2X2	T44.2X3	T44.2X4	T44.2X5	T44.2X6
Pentaquine	T37.2X1	T37.2X2	T37.2X3	T37.2X4	T37.2X5	T37.2X6
Pentazocine	T40.491	T40.492	T40.493	T40.494	T40.495	T40.496
Pentetrazole	T50.7X1	T50.7X2	T50.7X3	T50.7X4	T50.7X5	T50.7X6
Penthienate bromide	T44.3X1	T44.3X2	T44.3X3	T44.3X4	T44.3X5	T44.3X6
Pentifylline	T46.7X1	T46.7X2	T46.7X3	T46.7X4	T46.7X5	T46.7X6
Pentobarbital	T42.3X1	T42.3X2	T42.3X3	T42.3X4	T42.3X5	T42.3X6
sodium	T42.3X1	T42.3X2	T42.3X3	T42.3X4	T42.3X5	T42.3X6
Pentobarbitone	T42.3X1	T42.3X2	T42.3X3	T42.3X4	T42.3X5	T42.3X6
Pentolonium tartrate	T44.2X1	T44.2X2	T44.2X3	T44.2X4	T44.2X5	T44.2X6

Substance	Poisoning, Accidental (Unintentional)	Poisoning, Intentional Self-Harm	Poisoning, Assault	Poisoning, Undetermined	Adverse Effect	Underdosing
Pentosan polysulfate (sodium)	T39.8X1	T39.8X2	T39.8X3	T39.8X4	T39.8X5	T39.8X6
Pentostatin	T45.1X1	T45.1X2	T45.1X3	T45.1X4	T45.1X5	T45.1X6
Pentothal	T41.1X1	T41.1X2	T41.1X3	T41.1X4	T41.1X5	T41.1X6
Pentoxifylline	T46.7X1	T46.7X2	T46.7X3	T46.7X4	T46.7X5	T46.7X6
Pentoxyverine	T48.3X1	T48.3X2	T48.3X3	T48.3X4	T48.3X5	T48.3X6
Pentrinat	T46.3X1	T46.3X2	T46.3X3	T46.3X4	T46.3X5	T46.3X6
Pentylenetetrazole	T50.7X1	T50.7X2	T50.7X3	T50.7X4	T50.7X5	T50.7X6
Pentylsalicylamide	T37.1X1	T37.1X2	T37.1X3	T37.1X4	T37.1X5	T37.1X6
Pentymal	T42.3X1	T42.3X2	T42.3X3	T42.3X4	T42.3X5	T42.3X6
Peplomycin	T45.1X1	T45.1X2	T45.1X3	T45.1X4	T45.1X5	T45.1X6
Peppermint (oil)	T47.5X1	T47.5X2	T47.5X3	T47.5X4	T47.5X5	T47.5X6
Pepsin	T47.5X1	T47.5X2	T47.5X3	T47.5X4	T47.5X5	T47.5X6
digestant	T47.5X1	T47.5X2	T47.5X3	T47.5X4	T47.5X5	T47.5X6
Pepstatin	T47.1X1	T47.1X2	T47.1X3	T47.1X4	T47.1X5	T47.1X6
Peptavlon	T50.8X1	T50.8X2	T50.8X3	T50.8X4	T50.8X5	T50.8X6
Perazine	T43.3X1	T43.3X2	T43.3X3	T43.3X4	T43.3X5	T43.3X6
Percaine (spinal)	T41.3X1	T41.3X2	T41.3X3	T41.3X4	T41.3X5	T41.3X6
topical (surface)	T41.3X1	T41.3X2	T41.3X3	T41.3X4	T41.3X5	T41.3X6
Perchloroethylene	T53.3X1	T53.3X2	T53.3X3	T53.3X4	—	—
medicinal	T37.4X1	T37.4X2	T37.4X3	T37.4X4	T37.4X5	T37.4X6
vapor	T53.3X1	T53.3X2	T53.3X3	T53.3X4	—	—
Percodan	T40.2X1	T40.2X2	T40.2X3	T40.2X4	T40.2X5	T40.2X6
Percogesic — see also Acetaminophen	T45.0X1	T45.0X2	T45.0X3	T45.0X4	T45.0X5	T45.0X6
Percorten	T38.0X1	T38.0X2	T38.0X3	T38.0X4	T38.0X5	T38.0X6
Pergolide	T42.8X1	T42.8X2	T42.8X3	T42.8X4	T42.8X5	T42.8X6
Pergonal	T38.811	T38.812	T38.813	T38.814	T38.815	T38.816
Perhexilene	T46.3X1	T46.3X2	T46.3X3	T46.3X4	T46.3X5	T46.3X6
Perhexiline (maleate)	T46.3X1	T46.3X2	T46.3X3	T46.3X4	T46.3X5	T46.3X6
Periactin	T45.0X1	T45.0X2	T45.0X3	T45.0X4	T45.0X5	T45.0X6
Periciazine	T43.3X1	T43.3X2	T43.3X3	T43.3X4	T43.3X5	T43.3X6
Periclor	T42.6X1	T42.6X2	T42.6X3	T42.6X4	T42.6X5	T42.6X6
Perindopril	T46.4X1	T46.4X2	T46.4X3	T46.4X4	T46.4X5	T46.4X6
Perisoxal	T39.8X1	T39.8X2	T39.8X3	T39.8X4	T39.8X5	T39.8X6
Peritrate	T46.3X1	T46.3X2	T46.3X3	T46.3X4	T46.3X5	T46.3X6
Peritoneal dialysis solution	T50.3X1	T50.3X2	T50.3X3	T50.3X4	T50.3X5	T50.3X6
Perlapine	T42.4X1	T42.4X2	T42.4X3	T42.4X4	T42.4X5	T42.4X6
Permanganate	T65.891	T65.892	T65.893	T65.894	—	—
Permethrin	T60.1X1	T60.1X2	T60.1X3	T60.1X4	—	—
Pernocton	T42.3X1	T42.3X2	T42.3X3	T42.3X4	T42.3X5	T42.3X6
Pernoston	T42.3X1	T42.3X2	T42.3X3	T42.3X4	T42.3X5	T42.3X6
Peronine	T40.2X1	T40.2X2	T40.2X3	T40.2X4	—	—
Perphenazine	T43.3X1	T43.3X2	T43.3X3	T43.3X4	T43.3X5	T43.3X6

◀ New   ◀ Revised   ~~deleted~~ Deleted

Substance	Poisoning, Accidental (Unintentional)	Poisoning, Intentional Self-Harm	Poisoning, Assault	Poisoning, Undetermined	Adverse Effect	Underdosing
Pertofrane	T43.011	T43.012	T43.013	T43.014	T43.015	T43.016
Pertussis						
immune serum (human)	T50.Z11	T50.Z12	T50.Z13	T50.Z14	T50.Z15	T50.Z16
vaccine (with diphtheria toxoid) (with tetanus toxoid)	T50.A11	T50.A12	T50.A13	T50.A14	T50.A15	T50.A16
Peruvian balsam	T49.0X1	T49.0X2	T49.0X3	T49.0X4	T49.0X5	T49.0X6
Peruvoside	T46.0X1	T46.0X2	T46.0X3	T46.0X4	T46.0X5	T46.0X6
Pesticide (dust) (fumes) (vapor) NEC	T60.91	T60.92	T60.93	T60.94	—	—
arsenic	T57.0X1	T57.0X2	T57.0X3	T57.0X4	—	—
chlorinated	T60.1X1	T60.1X2	T60.1X3	T60.1X4	—	—
cyanide	T65.0X1	T65.0X2	T65.0X3	T65.0X4	—	—
kerosene	T52.0X1	T52.0X2	T52.0X3	T52.0X4	—	—
mixture (of compounds)	T60.91	T60.92	T60.93	T60.94	—	—
naphthalene	T60.2X1	T60.2X2	T60.2X3	T60.2X4	—	—
organochlorine (compounds)	T60.1X1	T60.1X2	T60.1X3	T60.1X4	—	—
petroleum (distillate) (products) NEC	T60.8X1	T60.8X2	T60.8X3	T60.8X4	—	—
specified ingredient NEC	T60.8X1	T60.8X2	T60.8X3	T60.8X4	—	—
strychnine	T65.1X1	T65.1X2	T65.1X3	T65.1X4	—	—
thallium	T60.4X1	T60.4X2	T60.4X3	T60.4X4	—	—
Pethidine	T40.491	T40.492	T40.493	T40.494	T40.495	T40.496
Petrichloral	T42.6X1	T42.6X2	T42.6X3	T42.6X4	T42.6X5	T42.6X6
Petrol	T52.0X1	T52.0X2	T52.0X3	T52.0X4	—	—
vapor	T52.0X1	T52.0X2	T52.0X3	T52.0X4	—	—
Petrolatum	T49.3X1	T49.3X2	T49.3X3	T49.3X4	T49.3X5	T49.3X6
hydrophilic	T49.3X1	T49.3X2	T49.3X3	T49.3X4	T49.3X5	T49.3X6
liquid	T47.4X1	T47.4X2	T47.4X3	T47.4X4	T47.4X5	T47.4X6
topical	T49.3X1	T49.3X2	T49.3X3	T49.3X4	T49.3X5	T49.3X6
nonmedicinal	T52.0X1	T52.0X2	T52.0X3	T52.0X4	—	—
red veterinary	T49.3X1	T49.3X2	T49.3X3	T49.3X4	T49.3X5	T49.3X6
white	T49.3X1	T49.3X2	T49.3X3	T49.3X4	T49.3X5	T49.3X6
Petroleum (products) NEC	T52.0X1	T52.0X2	T52.0X3	T52.0X4	—	—
benzine(s) — see Ligroin						
ether — see Ligroin						
jelly — see Petrolatum						
naphtha — see Ligroin						
pesticide	T60.8X1	T60.8X2	T60.8X3	T60.8X4	—	—
solids	T52.0X1	T52.0X2	T52.0X3	T52.0X4	—	—
solvents	T52.0X1	T52.0X2	T52.0X3	T52.0X4	—	—
vapor	T52.0X1	T52.0X2	T52.0X3	T52.0X4	—	—
Peyote	T40.991	T40.992	T40.993	T40.994	—	—
Phanodorm, phanodorn	T42.3X1	T42.3X2	T42.3X3	T42.3X4	T42.3X5	T42.3X6

Substance	Poisoning, Accidental (Unintentional)	Poisoning, Intentional Self-Harm	Poisoning, Assault	Poisoning, Undetermined	Adverse Effect	Underdosing
Phanquinone	T37.3X1	T37.3X2	T37.3X3	T37.3X4	T37.3X5	T37.3X6
Phanquone	T37.3X1	T37.3X2	T37.3X3	T37.3X4	T37.3X5	T37.3X6
Pharmaceutical						
adjunct NEC	T50.901	T50.902	T50.903	T50.904	T50.905	T50.906
excipient NEC	T50.901	T50.902	T50.903	T50.904	T50.905	T50.906
sweetener	T50.901	T50.902	T50.903	T50.904	T50.905	T50.906
viscous agent	T50.901	T50.902	T50.903	T50.904	T50.905	T50.906
Phemitone	T42.3X1	T42.3X2	T42.3X3	T42.3X4	T42.3X5	T42.3X6
Phenacaine	T41.3X1	T41.3X2	T41.3X3	T41.3X4	T41.3X5	T41.3X6
Phenacemide	T42.6X1	T42.6X2	T42.6X3	T42.6X4	T42.6X5	T42.6X6
Phenacetin	T39.1X1	T39.1X2	T39.1X3	T39.1X4	T39.1X5	T39.1X6
Phenadoxone	T40.2X1	T40.2X2	T40.2X3	T40.2X4	—	—
Phenaglycodol	T43.591	T43.592	T43.593	T43.594	T43.595	T43.596
Phenantoin	T42.0X1	T42.0X2	T42.0X3	T42.0X4	T42.0X5	T42.0X6
Phenaphthazine reagent	T50.991	T50.992	T50.993	T50.994	T50.995	T50.996
Phenazocine	T40.491	T40.492	T40.493	T40.494	T40.495	T40.496
Phenazone	T39.2X1	T39.2X2	T39.2X3	T39.2X4	T39.2X5	T39.2X6
Phenazopyridine	T39.8X1	T39.8X2	T39.8X3	T39.8X4	T39.8X5	T39.8X6
Phenbenicillin	T36.0X1	T36.0X2	T36.0X3	T36.0X4	T36.0X5	T36.0X6
Phenbutrazate	T50.5X1	T50.5X2	T50.5X3	T50.5X4	T50.5X5	T50.5X6
Phencyclidine	T40.991	T40.992	T40.993	T40.994	T40.995	T40.996
Phendimetrazine	T50.5X1	T50.5X2	T50.5X3	T50.5X4	T50.5X5	T50.5X6
Phenelzine	T43.1X1	T43.1X2	T43.1X3	T43.1X4	T43.1X5	T43.1X6
Phenemal	T42.3X1	T42.3X2	T42.3X3	T42.3X4	T42.3X5	T42.3X6
Phenergan	T42.6X1	T42.6X2	T42.6X3	T42.6X4	T42.6X5	T42.6X6
Pheneticillin	T36.0X1	T36.0X2	T36.0X3	T36.0X4	T36.0X5	T36.0X6
Pheneturide	T42.6X1	T42.6X2	T42.6X3	T42.6X4	T42.6X5	T42.6X6
Phenformin	T38.3X1	T38.3X2	T38.3X3	T38.3X4	T38.3X5	T38.3X6
Phenglutarimide	T44.3X1	T44.3X2	T44.3X3	T44.3X4	T44.3X5	T44.3X6
Phenicarbazide	T39.8X1	T39.8X2	T39.8X3	T39.8X4	T39.8X5	T39.8X6
Phenindamine	T45.0X1	T45.0X2	T45.0X3	T45.0X4	T45.0X5	T45.0X6
Phenindione	T45.511	T45.512	T45.513	T45.514	T45.515	T45.516
Pheniprazine	T43.1X1	T43.1X2	T43.1X3	T43.1X4	T43.1X5	T43.1X6
Pheniramine	T45.0X1	T45.0X2	T45.0X3	T45.0X4	T45.0X5	T45.0X6
Phenisatin	T47.2X1	T47.2X2	T47.2X3	T47.2X4	T47.2X5	T47.2X6
Phenmetrazine	T50.5X1	T50.5X2	T50.5X3	T50.5X4	T50.5X5	T50.5X6
Phenobal	T42.3X1	T42.3X2	T42.3X3	T42.3X4	T42.3X5	T42.3X6
Phenobarbital	T42.3X1	T42.3X2	T42.3X3	T42.3X4	T42.3X5	T42.3X6
with						
mephenytoin	T42.3X1	T42.3X2	T42.3X3	T42.3X4	T42.3X5	T42.3X6
phenytoin	T42.3X1	T42.3X2	T42.3X3	T42.3X4	T42.3X5	T42.3X6
sodium	T42.3X1	T42.3X2	T42.3X3	T42.3X4	T42.3X5	T42.3X6

◀ New ◀ Revised ~~deleted~~ Deleted

Substance	External Cause (T-Code) Poisoning, Accidental (Unintentional)	Poisoning, Intentional Self-Harm	Poisoning, Assault	Poisoning, Undetermined	Adverse Effect	Underdosing
Phenobarbitone	T42.3X1	T42.3X2	T42.3X3	T42.3X4	T42.3X5	T42.3X6
Phenobutiodil	T50.8X1	T50.8X2	T50.8X3	T50.8X4	T50.8X5	T50.8X6
Phenoctide	T49.0X1	T49.0X2	T49.0X3	T49.0X4	T49.0X5	T49.0X6
Phenol	T49.0X1	T49.0X2	T49.0X3	T49.0X4	T49.0X5	T49.0X6
disinfectant	T54.0X1	T54.0X2	T54.0X3	T54.0X4	—	—
in oil injection	T46.8X1	T46.8X2	T46.8X3	T46.8X4	T46.8X5	T46.8X6
medicinal	T49.1X1	T49.1X2	T49.1X3	T49.1X4	T49.1X5	T49.1X6
nonmedicinal NEC	T54.0X1	T54.0X2	T54.0X3	T54.0X4	—	—
pesticide	T60.8X1	T60.8X2	T60.8X3	T60.8X4	—	—
red	T50.8X1	T50.8X2	T50.8X3	T50.8X4	T50.8X5	T50.8X6
Phenolic preparation	T49.1X1	T49.1X2	T49.1X3	T49.1X4	T49.1X5	T49.1X6
Phenolphthalein	T47.2X1	T47.2X2	T47.2X3	T47.2X4	T47.2X5	T47.2X6
Phenolsulfonphthalein	T50.8X1	T50.8X2	T50.8X3	T50.8X4	T50.8X5	T50.8X6
Phenomorphan	T40.2X1	T40.2X2	T40.2X3	T40.2X4	—	—
Phenonyl	T42.3X1	T42.3X2	T42.3X3	T42.3X4	T42.3X5	T42.3X6
Phenoperidine	T40.491	T40.492	T40.493	T40.494	—	—
Phenopyrazone	T46.991	T46.992	T46.993	T46.994	T46.995	T46.996
Phenoquin	T50.4X1	T50.4X2	T50.4X3	T50.4X4	T50.4X5	T50.4X6
Phenothiazine (psychotropic) NEC	T43.3X1	T43.3X2	T43.3X3	T43.3X4	T43.3X5	T43.3X6
insecticide	T60.2X1	T60.2X2	T60.2X3	T60.2X4	—	—
Phenothrin	T49.0X1	T49.0X2	T49.0X3	T49.0X4	T49.0X5	T49.0X6
Phenoxybenzamine	T46.7X1	T46.7X2	T46.7X3	T46.7X4	T46.7X5	T46.7X6
Phenoxyethanol	T49.0X1	T49.0X2	T49.0X3	T49.0X4	T49.0X5	T49.0X6
Phenoxymethyl penicillin	T36.0X1	T36.0X2	T36.0X3	T36.0X4	T36.0X5	T36.0X6
Phenprobamate	T42.8X1	T42.8X2	T42.8X3	T42.8X4	T42.8X5	T42.8X6
Phenprocoumon	T45.511	T45.512	T45.513	T45.514	T45.515	T45.516
Phensuximide	T42.2X1	T42.2X2	T42.2X3	T42.2X4	T42.2X5	T42.2X6
Phentermine	T50.5X1	T50.5X2	T50.5X3	T50.5X4	T50.5X5	T50.5X6
Phenthicillin	T36.0X1	T36.0X2	T36.0X3	T36.0X4	T36.0X5	T36.0X6
Phentolamine	T46.7X1	T46.7X2	T46.7X3	T46.7X4	T46.7X5	T46.7X6
Phenyl						
butazone	T39.2X1	T39.2X2	T39.2X3	T39.2X4	T39.2X5	T39.2X6
enediamine	T65.3X1	T65.3X2	T65.3X3	T65.3X4	—	—
hydrazine	T65.3X1	T65.3X2	T65.3X3	T65.3X4	—	—
antineoplastic	T45.1X1	T45.1X2	T45.1X3	T45.1X4	T45.1X5	T45.1X6
mercuric compounds — see Mercury						
salicylate	T49.3X1	T49.3X2	T49.3X3	T49.3X4	T49.3X5	T49.3X6
Phenylalanine mustard	T45.1X1	T45.1X2	T45.1X3	T45.1X4	T45.1X5	T45.1X6
Phenylbutazone	T39.2X1	T39.2X2	T39.2X3	T39.2X4	T39.2X5	T39.2X6
Phenylenediamine	T65.3X1	T65.3X2	T65.3X3	T65.3X4	—	—
Phenylephrine	T44.4X1	T44.4X2	T44.4X3	T44.4X4	T44.4X5	T44.4X6

Substance	External Cause (T-Code) Poisoning, Accidental (Unintentional)	Poisoning, Intentional Self-Harm	Poisoning, Assault	Poisoning, Undetermined	Adverse Effect	Underdosing
Phenylethylbiguanide	T38.3X1	T38.3X2	T38.3X3	T38.3X4	T38.3X5	T38.3X6
Phenylmercuric						
acetate	T49.0X1	T49.0X2	T49.0X3	T49.0X4	T49.0X5	T49.0X6
borate	T49.0X1	T49.0X2	T49.0X3	T49.0X4	T49.0X5	T49.0X6
nitrate	T49.0X1	T49.0X2	T49.0X3	T49.0X4	T49.0X5	T49.0X6
Phenylmethylbarbitone	T42.3X1	T42.3X2	T42.3X3	T42.3X4	T42.3X5	T42.3X6
Phenylpropanol	T47.5X1	T47.5X2	T47.5X3	T47.5X4	T47.5X5	T47.5X6
Phenylpropanolamine	T44.991	T44.992	T44.993	T44.994	T44.995	T44.996
Phenylsulfthion	T60.0X1	T60.0X2	T60.0X3	T60.0X4	—	—
Phenyltoloxamine	T45.0X1	T45.0X2	T45.0X3	T45.0X4	T45.0X5	T45.0X6
Phenyramidol, phenyramidon	T39.8X1	T39.8X2	T39.8X3	T39.8X4	T39.8X5	T39.8X6
Phenytoin	T42.0X1	T42.0X2	T42.0X3	T42.0X4	T42.0X5	T42.0X6
with Phenobarbital	T42.3X1	T42.3X2	T42.3X3	T42.3X4	T42.3X5	T42.3X6
pHisoHex	T49.2X1	T49.2X2	T49.2X3	T49.2X4	T49.2X5	T49.2X6
Pholcodine	T48.3X1	T48.3X2	T48.3X3	T48.3X4	T48.3X5	T48.3X6
Pholedrine	T46.991	T46.992	T46.993	T46.994	T46.995	T46.996
Phorate	T60.0X1	T60.0X2	T60.0X3	T60.0X4	—	—
Phosdrin	T60.0X1	T60.0X2	T60.0X3	T60.0X4	—	—
Phosfolan	T60.0X1	T60.0X2	T60.0X3	T60.0X4	—	—
Phosgene (gas)	T59.891	T59.892	T59.893	T59.894		
Phosphamidon	T60.0X1	T60.0X2	T60.0X3	T60.0X4	—	—
Phosphate	T65.891	T65.892	T65.893	T65.894		
laxative	T47.4X1	T47.4X2	T47.4X3	T47.4X4	T47.4X5	T47.4X6
organic	T60.0X1	T60.0X2	T60.0X3	T60.0X4	—	—
solvent	T52.91	T52.92	T52.93	T52.94		
tricresyl	T65.891	T65.892	T65.893	T65.894	—	—
Phosphine	T57.1X1	T57.1X2	T57.1X3	T57.1X4		
fumigant	T57.1X1	T57.1X2	T57.1X3	T57.1X4	—	—
Phospholine	T49.5X1	T49.5X2	T49.5X3	T49.5X4	T49.5X5	T49.5X6
Phosphoric acid	T54.2X1	T54.2X2	T54.2X3	T54.2X4	—	—
Phosphorus (compound) NEC	T57.1X1	T57.1X2	T57.1X3	T57.1X4		
pesticide	T60.0X1	T60.0X2	T60.0X3	T60.0X4	—	—
Phthalates	T65.891	T65.892	T65.893	T65.894		
Phthalic anhydride	T65.891	T65.892	T65.893	T65.894		
Phthalimidoglutarimide	T42.6X1	T42.6X2	T42.6X3	T42.6X4	T42.6X5	T42.6X6
Phthalylsulfathiazole	T37.0X1	T37.0X2	T37.0X3	T37.0X4	T37.0X5	T37.0X6
Phylloquinone	T45.7X1	T45.7X2	T45.7X3	T45.7X4	T45.7X5	T45.7X6
Physeptone	T40.3X1	T40.3X2	T40.3X3	T40.3X4	T40.3X5	T40.3X6
Physostigma venenosum	T62.2X1	T62.2X2	T62.2X3	T62.2X4	—	—
Physostigmine	T49.5X1	T49.5X2	T49.5X3	T49.5X4	T49.5X5	T49.5X6
Phytolacca decandra	T62.2X1	T62.2X2	T62.2X3	T62.2X4	—	—
berries	T62.1X1	T62.1X2	T62.1X3	T62.1X4	—	—

◄ New ◄ Revised ~~deleted~~ Deleted

Substance	External Cause (T-Code)					
	Poisoning, Accidental (Unintentional)	Poisoning, Intentional Self-Harm	Poisoning, Assault	Poisoning, Undetermined	Adverse Effect	Underdosing
Phytomenadione	T45.7X1	T45.7X2	T45.7X3	T45.7X4	T45.7X5	T45.7X6
Phytonadione	T45.7X1	T45.7X2	T45.7X3	T45.7X4	T45.7X5	T45.7X6
Picoperine	T48.3X1	T48.3X2	T48.3X3	T48.3X4	T48.3X5	T48.3X6
Picosulfate (sodium)	T47.2X1	T47.2X2	T47.2X3	T47.2X4	T47.2X5	T47.2X6
Picric (acid)	T54.2X1	T54.2X2	T54.2X3	T54.2X4	—	—
Picrotoxin	T50.7X1	T50.7X2	T50.7X3	T50.7X4	T50.7X5	T50.7X6
Piketoprofen	T49.0X1	T49.0X2	T49.0X3	T49.0X4	T49.0X5	T49.0X6
Pilocarpine	T44.1X1	T44.1X2	T44.1X3	T44.1X4	T44.1X5	T44.1X6
Pilocarpus (jaborandi) extract	T44.1X1	T44.1X2	T44.1X3	T44.1X4	T44.1X5	T44.1X6
Pilsicainide (hydrochloride)	T46.2X1	T46.2X2	T46.2X3	T46.2X4	T46.2X5	T46.2X6
Pimaricin	T36.7X1	T36.7X2	T36.7X3	T36.7X4	T36.7X5	T36.7X6
Pimeclone	T50.7X1	T50.7X2	T50.7X3	T50.7X4	T50.7X5	T50.7X6
Pimelic ketone	T52.8X1	T52.8X2	T52.8X3	T52.8X4	—	—
Pimethixene	T45.0X1	T45.0X2	T45.0X3	T45.0X4	T45.0X5	T45.0X6
Piminodine	T40.2X1	T40.2X2	T40.2X3	T40.2X4	T40.2X5	T40.2X6
Pimozide	T43.591	T43.592	T43.593	T43.594	T43.595	T43.596
Pinacidil	T46.5X1	T46.5X2	T46.5X3	T46.5X4	T46.5X5	T46.5X6
Pinaverium bromide	T44.3X1	T44.3X2	T44.3X3	T44.3X4	T44.3X5	T44.3X6
Pinazepam	T42.4X1	T42.4X2	T42.4X3	T42.4X4	T42.4X5	T42.4X6
Pindolol	T44.7X1	T44.7X2	T44.7X3	T44.7X4	T44.7X5	T44.7X6
Pindone	T60.4X1	T60.4X2	T60.4X3	T60.4X4	—	—
Pine oil (disinfectant)	T65.891	T65.892	T65.893	T65.894	—	—
Pinkroot	T37.4X1	T37.4X2	T37.4X3	T37.4X4	T37.4X5	T37.4X6
Pipadone	T40.2X1	T40.2X2	T40.2X3	T40.2X4	—	—
Pipamazine	T45.0X1	T45.0X2	T45.0X3	T45.0X4	T45.0X5	T45.0X6
Pipamperone	T43.4X1	T43.4X2	T43.4X3	T43.4X4	T43.4X5	T43.4X6
Pipazetate	T48.3X1	T48.3X2	T48.3X3	T48.3X4	T48.3X5	T48.3X6
Pipemidic acid	T37.8X1	T37.8X2	T37.8X3	T37.8X4	T37.8X5	T37.8X6
Pipenzolate bromide	T44.3X1	T44.3X2	T44.3X3	T44.3X4	T44.3X5	T44.3X6
Piperacetazine	T43.3X1	T43.3X2	T43.3X3	T43.3X4	T43.3X5	T43.3X6
Piperacillin	T36.0X1	T36.0X2	T36.0X3	T36.0X4	T36.0X5	T36.0X6
Piperazine	T37.4X1	T37.4X2	T37.4X3	T37.4X4	T37.4X5	T37.4X6
estrone sulfate	T38.5X1	T38.5X2	T38.5X3	T38.5X4	T38.5X5	T38.5X6
Piper cubeba	T62.2X1	T62.2X2	T62.2X3	T62.2X4	—	—
Piperidione	T48.3X1	T48.3X2	T48.3X3	T48.3X4	—	—
Piperidolate	T44.3X1	T44.3X2	T44.3X3	T44.3X4	T44.3X5	T44.3X6
Piperocaine	T41.3X1	T41.3X2	T41.3X3	T41.3X4	T41.3X5	T41.3X6
infiltration (subcutaneous)	T41.3X1	T41.3X2	T41.3X3	T41.3X4	T41.3X5	T41.3X6
nerve block (peripheral) (plexus)	T41.3X1	T41.3X2	T41.3X3	T41.3X4	T41.3X5	T41.3X6
topical (surface)	T41.3X1	T41.3X2	T41.3X3	T41.3X4	T41.3X5	T41.3X6
Piperonyl butoxide	T60.8X1	T60.8X2	T60.8X3	T60.8X4	—	—
Pipethanate	T44.3X1	T44.3X2	T44.3X3	T44.3X4	T44.3X5	T44.3X6

Substance	External Cause (T-Code)					
	Poisoning, Accidental (Unintentional)	Poisoning, Intentional Self-Harm	Poisoning, Assault	Poisoning, Undetermined	Adverse Effect	Underdosing
Pipobroman	T45.1X1	T45.1X2	T45.1X3	T45.1X4	T45.1X5	T45.1X6
Pipofezine	T43.0X1	T43.0X2	T43.0X3	T43.0X4	T43.0X5	T43.0X6
Pipotiazine	T43.3X1	T43.3X2	T43.3X3	T43.3X4	T43.3X5	T43.3X6
Pipoxizine	T45.0X1	T45.0X2	T45.0X3	T45.0X4	T45.0X5	T45.0X6
Pipradrol	T43.691	T43.692	T43.693	T43.694	T43.695	T43.696
Piprinhydrinate	T45.0X1	T45.0X2	T45.0X3	T45.0X4	T45.0X5	T45.0X6
Pirarubicin	T45.1X1	T45.1X2	T45.1X3	T45.1X4	T45.1X5	T45.1X6
Pirazinamide	T37.1X1	T37.1X2	T37.1X3	T37.1X4	T37.1X5	T37.1X6
Pirbuterol	T48.6X1	T48.6X2	T48.6X3	T48.6X4	T48.6X5	T48.6X6
Pirenzepine	T47.1X1	T47.1X2	T47.1X3	T47.1X4	T47.1X5	T47.1X6
Piretanide	T50.1X1	T50.1X2	T50.1X3	T50.1X4	T50.1X5	T50.1X6
Piribedil	T42.8X1	T42.8X2	T42.8X3	T42.8X4	T42.8X5	T42.8X6
Piridoxilate	T46.3X1	T46.3X2	T46.3X3	T46.3X4	T46.3X5	T46.3X6
Piritramide	T40.491	T40.492	T40.493	T40.494	—	—
Pirlindole	T43.0X1	T43.0X2	T43.0X3	T43.0X4	T43.0X5	T43.0X6
Piromidic acid	T37.8X1	T37.8X2	T37.8X3	T37.8X4	T37.8X5	T37.8X6
Piroxicam	T39.391	T39.392	T39.393	T39.394	T39.395	T39.396
beta-cyclodextrin complex	T39.8X1	T39.8X2	T39.8X3	T39.8X4	T39.8X5	T39.8X6
Pirozadil	T46.6X1	T46.6X2	T46.6X3	T46.6X4	T46.6X5	T46.6X6
Piscidia (bark) (erythrina)	T39.8X1	T39.8X2	T39.8X3	T39.8X4	T39.8X5	T39.8X6
Pitch	T65.891	T65.892	T65.893	T65.894	—	—
Pitkin's solution	T41.3X1	T41.3X2	T41.3X3	T41.3X4	T41.3X5	T41.3X6
Pitocin	T48.0X1	T48.0X2	T48.0X3	T48.0X4	T48.0X5	T48.0X6
Pitressin (tannate)	T38.891	T38.892	T38.893	T38.894	T38.895	T38.896
Pituitary extracts (posterior)	T38.891	T38.892	T38.893	T38.894	T38.895	T38.896
anterior	T38.811	T38.812	T38.813	T38.814	T38.815	T38.816
Pituitrin	T38.891	T38.892	T38.893	T38.894	T38.895	T38.896
Pivampicillin	T36.0X1	T36.0X2	T36.0X3	T36.0X4	T36.0X5	T36.0X6
Pivmecillinam	T36.0X1	T36.0X2	T36.0X3	T36.0X4	T36.0X5	T36.0X6
Placental hormone	T38.891	T38.892	T38.893	T38.894	T38.895	T38.896
Placidyl	T42.6X1	T42.6X2	T42.6X3	T42.6X4	T42.6X5	T42.6X6
Plague vaccine	T50.A91	T50.A92	T50.A93	T50.A94	T50.A95	T50.A96
Plant						
food or fertilizer NEC	T65.891	T65.892	T65.893	T65.894	—	—
containing herbicide	T60.3X1	T60.3X2	T60.3X3	T60.3X4	—	—
noxious, used as food	T62.2X1	T62.2X2	T62.2X3	T62.2X4	—	—
berries	T62.1X1	T62.1X2	T62.1X3	T62.1X4	—	—
seeds	T62.2X1	T62.2X2	T62.2X3	T62.2X4	—	—
specified type NEC	T62.2X1	T62.2X2	T62.2X3	T62.2X4	—	—
Plasma	T45.8X1	T45.8X2	T45.8X3	T45.8X4	T45.8X5	T45.8X6
expander NEC	T45.8X1	T45.8X2	T45.8X3	T45.8X4	T45.8X5	T45.8X6
protein fraction (human)	T45.8X1	T45.8X2	T45.8X3	T45.8X4	T45.8X5	T45.8X6

◄ New   ◄ Revised   ~~deleted~~ Deleted

TABLE OF DRUGS AND CHEMICALS

Substance	External Cause (T-Code)					
	Poisoning, Accidental (Unintentional)	Poisoning, Intentional Self-Harm	Poisoning, Assault	Poisoning, Undetermined	Adverse Effect	Underdosing
Plasmanate	T45.8X1	T45.8X2	T45.8X3	T45.8X4	T45.8X5	T45.8X6
Plasminogen (tissue) activator	T45.611	T45.612	T45.613	T45.614	T45.615	T45.616
Plaster dressing	T49.3X1	T49.3X2	T49.3X3	T49.3X4	T49.3X5	T49.3X6
Plastic dressing	T49.3X1	T49.3X2	T49.3X3	T49.3X4	T49.3X5	T49.3X6
Plegicil	T43.3X1	T43.3X2	T43.3X3	T43.3X4	T43.3X5	T43.3X6
Plicamycin	T45.1X1	T45.1X2	T45.1X3	T45.1X4	T45.1X5	T45.1X6
Podophyllotoxin	T49.8X1	T49.8X2	T49.8X3	T49.8X4	T49.8X5	T49.8X6
Podophyllum (resin)	T49.4X1	T49.4X2	T49.4X3	T49.4X4	T49.4X5	T49.4X6
Poison NEC	T65.91	T65.92	T65.93	T65.94	—	—
Poisonous berries	T62.1X1	T62.1X2	T62.1X3	T62.1X4	—	—
Pokeweed (any part)	T62.2X1	T62.2X2	T62.2X3	T62.2X4	—	—
Poldine metilsulfate	T44.3X1	T44.3X2	T44.3X3	T44.3X4	T44.3X5	T44.3X6
Polidexide (sulfate)	T46.6X1	T46.6X2	T46.6X3	T46.6X4	T46.6X5	T46.6X6
Polidocanol	T46.8X1	T46.8X2	T46.8X3	T46.8X4	T46.8X5	T46.8X6
Poliomyelitis vaccine	T50.B91	T50.B92	T50.B93	T50.B94	T50.B95	T50.B96
Polish (car) (floor) (furniture) (metal) (porcelain) (silver)	T65.891	T65.892	T65.893	T65.894	—	—
abrasive	T65.891	T65.892	T65.893	T65.894	—	—
porcelain	T65.891	T65.892	T65.893	T65.894	—	—
Poloxalkol	T47.4X1	T47.4X2	T47.4X3	T47.4X4	T47.4X5	T47.4X6
Poloxamer	T47.4X1	T47.4X2	T47.4X3	T47.4X4	T47.4X5	T47.4X6
Polyaminostyrene resins	T50.3X1	T50.3X2	T50.3X3	T50.3X4	T50.3X5	T50.3X6
Polycarbophil	T47.4X1	T47.4X2	T47.4X3	T47.4X4	T47.4X5	T47.4X6
Polychlorinated biphenyl	T65.891	T65.892	T65.893	T65.894	—	—
Polycycline	T36.4X1	T36.4X2	T36.4X3	T36.4X4	T36.4X5	T36.4X6
Polyester fumes	T59.891	T59.892	T59.893	T59.894	—	—
Polyester resin hardener	T52.91	T52.92	T52.93	T52.94	—	—
fumes	T59.891	T59.892	T59.893	T59.894	—	—
Polyestradiol phosphate	T38.5X1	T38.5X2	T38.5X3	T38.5X4	T38.5X5	T38.5X6
Polyethanolamine alkyl sulfate	T49.2X1	T49.2X2	T49.2X3	T49.2X4	T49.2X5	T49.2X6
Polyethylene adhesive	T49.3X1	T49.3X2	T49.3X3	T49.3X4	T49.3X5	T49.3X6
Polyferose	T45.4X1	T45.4X2	T45.4X3	T45.4X4	T45.4X5	T45.4X6
Polygeline	T45.8X1	T45.8X2	T45.8X3	T45.8X4	T45.8X5	T45.8X6
Polymyxin	T36.8X1	T36.8X2	T36.8X3	T36.8X4	T36.8X5	T36.8X6
B	T36.8X1	T36.8X2	T36.8X3	T36.8X4	T36.8X5	T36.8X6
ENT agent	T49.6X1	T49.6X2	T49.6X3	T49.6X4	T49.6X5	T49.6X6
ophthalmic preparation	T49.5X1	T49.5X2	T49.5X3	T49.5X4	T49.5X5	T49.5X6
topical NEC	T49.0X1	T49.0X2	T49.0X3	T49.0X4	T49.0X5	T49.0X6
E sulfate (eye preparation)	T49.5X1	T49.5X2	T49.5X3	T49.5X4	T49.5X5	T49.5X6
Polynoxylin	T49.0X1	T49.0X2	T49.0X3	T49.0X4	T49.0X5	T49.0X6
Polyoestradiol phosphate	T38.5X1	T38.5X2	T38.5X3	T38.5X4	T38.5X5	T38.5X6
Polyoxymethyleneurea	T49.0X1	T49.0X2	T49.0X3	T49.0X4	T49.0X5	T49.0X6

Substance	External Cause (T-Code)					
	Poisoning, Accidental (Unintentional)	Poisoning, Intentional Self-Harm	Poisoning, Assault	Poisoning, Undetermined	Adverse Effect	Underdosing
Polysilane	T47.8X1	T47.8X2	T47.8X3	T47.8X4	T47.8X5	T47.8X6
Polytetrafluoroethylene (inhaled)	T59.891	T59.892	T59.893	T59.894	—	—
Polythiazide	T50.2X1	T50.2X2	T50.2X3	T50.2X4	T50.2X5	T50.2X6
Polyvidone	T45.8X1	T45.8X2	T45.8X3	T45.8X4	T45.8X5	T45.8X6
Polyvinylpyrrolidone	T45.8X1	T45.8X2	T45.8X3	T45.8X4	T45.8X5	T45.8X6
Pontocaine (hydrochloride) (infiltration) (topical)	T41.3X1	T41.3X2	T41.3X3	T41.3X4	T41.3X5	T41.3X6
nerve block (peripheral) (plexus)	T41.3X1	T41.3X2	T41.3X3	T41.3X4	T41.3X5	T41.3X6
spinal	T41.3X1	T41.3X2	T41.3X3	T41.3X4	T41.3X5	T41.3X6
Porfiromycin	T45.1X1	T45.1X2	T45.1X3	T45.1X4	T45.1X5	T45.1X6
Posterior pituitary hormone NEC	T38.891	T38.892	T38.893	T38.894	T38.895	T38.896
Pot	T40.711	T40.712	T40.713	T40.714	T40.715	T40.716
Potash (caustic)	T54.3X1	T54.3X2	T54.3X3	T54.3X4	—	—
Potassic saline injection (lactated)	T50.3X1	T50.3X2	T50.3X3	T50.3X4	T50.3X5	T50.3X6
Potassium (salts) NEC	T50.3X1	T50.3X2	T50.3X3	T50.3X4	T50.3X5	T50.3X6
aminobenzoate	T45.8X1	T45.8X2	T45.8X3	T45.8X4	T45.8X5	T45.8X6
aminosalicylate	T37.1X1	T37.1X2	T37.1X3	T37.1X4	T37.1X5	T37.1X6
antimony 'tartrate'	T37.8X1	T37.8X2	T37.8X3	T37.8X4	T37.8X5	T37.8X6
arsenite (solution)	T57.0X1	T57.0X2	T57.0X3	T57.0X4	—	—
bichromate	T56.2X1	T56.2X2	T56.2X3	T56.2X4	—	—
bisulfate	T47.3X1	T47.3X2	T47.3X3	T47.3X4	T47.3X5	T47.3X6
bromide	T42.6X1	T42.6X2	T42.6X3	T42.6X4	T42.6X5	T42.6X6
canrenoate	T50.0X1	T50.0X2	T50.0X3	T50.0X4	T50.0X5	T50.0X6
carbonate	T54.3X1	T54.3X2	T54.3X3	T54.3X4	—	—
chlorate NEC	T65.891	T65.892	T65.893	T65.894	—	—
chloride	T50.3X1	T50.3X2	T50.3X3	T50.3X4	T50.3X5	T50.3X6
citrate	T50.991	T50.992	T50.993	T50.994	T50.995	T50.996
cyanide	T65.0X1	T65.0X2	T65.0X3	T65.0X4	—	—
ferric hexacyanoferrate (medicinal)	T50.6X1	T50.6X2	T50.6X3	T50.6X4	T50.6X5	T50.6X6
nonmedicinal	T65.891	T65.892	T65.893	T65.894	—	—
Fluoride	T57.8X1	T57.8X2	T57.8X3	T57.8X4	—	—
glucaldrate	T47.1X1	T47.1X2	T47.1X3	T47.1X4	T47.1X5	T47.1X6
hydroxide	T54.3X1	T54.3X2	T54.3X3	T54.3X4	—	—
iodate	T49.0X1	T49.0X2	T49.0X3	T49.0X4	T49.0X5	T49.0X6
iodide	T48.4X1	T48.4X2	T48.4X3	T48.4X4	T48.4X5	T48.4X6
nitrate	T57.8X1	T57.8X2	T57.8X3	T57.8X4	—	—
oxalate	T65.891	T65.892	T65.893	T65.894	—	—
perchlorate (nonmedicinal) NEC	T65.891	T65.892	T65.893	T65.894	—	—
antithyroid	T38.2X1	T38.2X2	T38.2X3	T38.2X4	T38.2X5	T38.2X6
medicinal	T38.2X1	T38.2X2	T38.2X3	T38.2X4	T38.2X5	T38.2X6

◀ New ◀ Revised ~~deleted~~ Deleted

	External Cause (T-Code)					
Substance	Poisoning, Accidental (Unintentional)	Poisoning, Intentional Self-Harm	Poisoning, Assault	Poisoning, Undetermined	Adverse Effect	Underdosing
Permanganate (nonmedicinal)	T65.891	T65.892	T65.893	T65.894	—	—
medicinal	T49.0X1	T49.0X2	T49.0X3	T49.0X4	T49.0X5	T49.0X6
sulfate	T47.2X1	T47.2X2	T47.2X3	T47.2X4	T47.2X5	T47.2X6
Potassium-removing resin	T50.3X1	T50.3X2	T50.3X3	T50.3X4	T50.3X5	T50.3X6
Potassium-retaining drug	T50.3X1	T50.3X2	T50.3X3	T50.3X4	T50.3X5	T50.3X6
Povidone	T45.8X1	T45.8X2	T45.8X3	T45.8X4	T45.8X5	T45.8X6
iodine	T49.0X1	T49.0X2	T49.0X3	T49.0X4	T49.0X5	T49.0X6
Practolol	T44.7X1	T44.7X2	T44.7X3	T44.7X4	T44.7X5	T44.7X6
Prajmalium bitartrate	T46.2X1	T46.2X2	T46.2X3	T46.2X4	T46.2X5	T46.2X6
Pralidoxime (iodide)	T50.6X1	T50.6X2	T50.6X3	T50.6X4	T50.6X5	T50.6X6
chloride	T50.6X1	T50.6X2	T50.6X3	T50.6X4	T50.6X5	T50.6X6
Pramiverine	T44.3X1	T44.3X2	T44.3X3	T44.3X4	T44.3X5	T44.3X6
Pramocaine	T49.1X1	T49.1X2	T49.1X3	T49.1X4	T49.1X5	T49.1X6
Pramoxine	T49.1X1	T49.1X2	T49.1X3	T49.1X4	T49.1X5	T49.1X6
Prasterone	T38.7X1	T38.7X2	T38.7X3	T38.7X4	T38.7X5	T38.7X6
Pravastatin	T46.6X1	T46.6X2	T46.6X3	T46.6X4	T46.6X5	T46.6X6
Prazepam	T42.4X1	T42.4X2	T42.4X3	T42.4X4	T42.4X5	T42.4X6
Praziquantel	T37.4X1	T37.4X2	T37.4X3	T37.4X4	T37.4X5	T37.4X6
Prazitone	T43.291	T43.292	T43.293	T43.294	T43.295	T43.296
Prazosin	T44.6X1	T44.6X2	T44.6X3	T44.6X4	T44.6X5	T44.6X6
Prednicarbate	T49.0X1	T49.0X2	T49.0X3	T49.0X4	T49.0X5	T49.0X6
Prednimustine	T45.1X1	T45.1X2	T45.1X3	T45.1X4	T45.1X5	T45.1X6
Prednisolone	T38.0X1	T38.0X2	T38.0X3	T38.0X4	T38.0X5	T38.0X6
ENT agent	T49.6X1	T49.6X2	T49.6X3	T49.6X4	T49.6X5	T49.6X6
ophthalmic preparation	T49.5X1	T49.5X2	T49.5X3	T49.5X4	T49.5X5	T49.5X6
steaglate	T49.0X1	T49.0X2	T49.0X3	T49.0X4	T49.0X5	T49.0X6
topical NEC	T49.0X1	T49.0X2	T49.0X3	T49.0X4	T49.0X5	T49.0X6
Prednisone	T38.0X1	T38.0X2	T38.0X3	T38.0X4	T38.0X5	T38.0X6
Prednylidene	T38.0X1	T38.0X2	T38.0X3	T38.0X4	T38.0X5	T38.0X6
Pregnandiol	T38.5X1	T38.5X2	T38.5X3	T38.5X4	T38.5X5	T38.5X6
Pregneninolone	T38.5X1	T38.5X2	T38.5X3	T38.5X4	T38.5X5	T38.5X6
Preludin	T43.691	T43.692	T43.693	T43.694	T43.695	T43.696
Premarin	T38.5X1	T38.5X2	T38.5X3	T38.5X4	T38.5X5	T38.5X6
Premedication anesthetic	T41.201	T41.202	T41.203	T41.204	T41.205	T41.206
Prenalterol	T44.5X1	T44.5X2	T44.5X3	T44.5X4	T44.5X5	T44.5X6
Prenoxdiazine	T48.3X1	T48.3X2	T48.3X3	T48.3X4	T48.3X5	T48.3X6
Prenylamine	T46.3X1	T46.3X2	T46.3X3	T46.3X4	T46.3X5	T46.3X6
Preparation, local	T49.4X1	T49.4X2	T49.4X3	T49.4X4	T49.4X5	T49.4X6
Preparation H	T49.8X1	T49.8X2	T49.8X3	T49.8X4	T49.8X5	T49.8X6
Preservative (nonmedicinal)	T65.891	T65.892	T65.893	T65.894	—	—
medicinal	T50.901	T50.902	T50.903	T50.904	T50.905	T50.906
wood	T60.91	T60.92	T60.93	T60.94	—	—

	External Cause (T-Code)					
Substance	Poisoning, Accidental (Unintentional)	Poisoning, Intentional Self-Harm	Poisoning, Assault	Poisoning, Undetermined	Adverse Effect	Underdosing
Prethcamide	T50.7X1	T50.7X2	T50.7X3	T50.7X4	T50.7X5	T50.7X6
Pride of China	T62.2X1	T62.2X2	T62.2X3	T62.2X4	—	—
Pridinol	T44.3X1	T44.3X2	T44.3X3	T44.3X4	T44.3X5	T44.3X6
Prifinium bromide	T44.3X1	T44.3X2	T44.3X3	T44.3X4	T44.3X5	T44.3X6
Prilocaine	T41.3X1	T41.3X2	T41.3X3	T41.3X4	T41.3X5	T41.3X6
infiltration (subcutaneous)	T41.3X1	T41.3X2	T41.3X3	T41.3X4	T41.3X5	T41.3X6
nerve block (peripheral) (plexus)	T41.3X1	T41.3X2	T41.3X3	T41.3X4	T41.3X5	T41.3X6
regional	T41.3X1	T41.3X2	T41.3X3	T41.3X4	T41.3X5	T41.3X6
Primaquine	T37.2X1	T37.2X2	T37.2X3	T37.2X4	T37.2X5	T37.2X6
Primidone	T42.6X1	T42.6X2	T42.6X3	T42.6X4	T42.6X5	T42.6X6
Primula (veris)	T62.2X1	T62.2X2	T62.2X3	T62.2X4	—	—
Prinadol	T40.2X1	T40.2X2	T40.2X3	T40.2X4	T40.2X5	T40.2X6
Priscol, Priscoline	T44.6X1	T44.6X2	T44.6X3	T44.6X4	T44.6X5	T44.6X6
Pristinamycin	T36.3X1	T36.3X2	T36.3X3	T36.3X4	T36.3X5	T36.3X6
Privet	T62.2X1	T62.2X2	T62.2X3	T62.2X4	—	—
berries	T62.1X1	T62.1X2	T62.1X3	T62.1X4	—	—
Privine	T44.4X1	T44.4X2	T44.4X3	T44.4X4	T44.4X5	T44.4X6
Pro-Banthine	T44.3X1	T44.3X2	T44.3X3	T44.3X4	T44.3X5	T44.3X6
Probarbital	T42.3X1	T42.3X2	T42.3X3	T42.3X4	T42.3X5	T42.3X6
Probenecid	T50.4X1	T50.4X2	T50.4X3	T50.4X4	T50.4X5	T50.4X6
Probucol	T46.6X1	T46.6X2	T46.6X3	T46.6X4	T46.6X5	T46.6X6
Procainamide	T46.2X1	T46.2X2	T46.2X3	T46.2X4	T46.2X5	T46.2X6
Procaine	T41.3X1	T41.3X2	T41.3X3	T41.3X4	T41.3X5	T41.3X6
benzylpenicillin	T36.0X1	T36.0X2	T36.0X3	T36.0X4	T36.0X5	T36.0X6
nerve block (peripheral) (plexus)	T41.3X1	T41.3X2	T41.3X3	T41.3X4	T41.3X5	T41.3X6
penicillin G	T36.0X1	T36.0X2	T36.0X3	T36.0X4	T36.0X5	T36.0X6
regional	T41.3X1	T41.3X2	T41.3X3	T41.3X4	T41.3X5	T41.3X6
spinal	T41.3X1	T41.3X2	T41.3X3	T41.3X4	T41.3X5	T41.3X6
Procalmidol	T43.591	T43.592	T43.593	T43.594	T43.595	T43.596
Procarbazine	T45.1X1	T45.1X2	T45.1X3	T45.1X4	T45.1X5	T45.1X6
Procaterol	T44.5X1	T44.5X2	T44.5X3	T44.5X4	T44.5X5	T44.5X6
Prochlorperazine	T43.3X1	T43.3X2	T43.3X3	T43.3X4	T43.3X5	T43.3X6
Procyclidine	T44.3X1	T44.3X2	T44.3X3	T44.3X4	T44.3X5	T44.3X6
Producer gas	T58.8X1	T58.8X2	T58.8X3	T58.8X4	—	—
Profadol	T40.491	T40.492	T40.493	T40.494	T40.495	T40.496
Profenamine	T44.3X1	T44.3X2	T44.3X3	T44.3X4	T44.3X5	T44.3X6
Profenil	T44.3X1	T44.3X2	T44.3X3	T44.3X4	T44.3X5	T44.3X6
Proflavine	T49.0X1	T49.0X2	T49.0X3	T49.0X4	T49.0X5	T49.0X6
Progabide	T42.6X1	T42.6X2	T42.6X3	T42.6X4	T42.6X5	T42.6X6
Progestin	T38.5X1	T38.5X2	T38.5X3	T38.5X4	T38.5X5	T38.5X6
oral contraceptive	T38.4X1	T38.4X2	T38.4X3	T38.4X4	T38.4X5	T38.4X6

TABLE OF DRUGS AND CHEMICALS

Substance	Poisoning, Accidental (Unintentional)	Poisoning, Intentional Self-Harm	Poisoning, Assault	Poisoning, Undetermined	Adverse Effect	Underdosing
Progesterone	T38.5X1	T38.5X2	T38.5X3	T38.5X4	T38.5X5	T38.5X6
Progestogen NEC	T38.5X1	T38.5X2	T38.5X3	T38.5X4	T38.5X5	T38.5X6
Progestone	T38.5X1	T38.5X2	T38.5X3	T38.5X4	T38.5X5	T38.5X6
Proglumide	T47.1X1	T47.1X2	T47.1X3	T47.1X4	T47.1X5	T47.1X6
Proguanil	T37.2X1	T37.2X2	T37.2X3	T37.2X4	T37.2X5	T37.2X6
Prolactin	T38.811	T38.812	T38.813	T38.814	T38.815	T38.816
Prolintane	T43.691	T43.692	T43.693	T43.694	T43.695	T43.696
Proloid	T38.1X1	T38.1X2	T38.1X3	T38.1X4	T38.1X5	T38.1X6
Proluton	T38.5X1	T38.5X2	T38.5X3	T38.5X4	T38.5X5	T38.5X6
Promacetin	T37.1X1	T37.1X2	T37.1X3	T37.1X4	T37.1X5	T37.1X6
Promazine	T43.3X1	T43.3X2	T43.3X3	T43.3X4	T43.3X5	T43.3X6
Promedol	T40.2X1	T40.2X2	T40.2X3	T40.2X4	—	—
Promegestone	T38.5X1	T38.5X2	T38.5X3	T38.5X4	T38.5X5	T38.5X6
Promethazine (teoclate)	T43.3X1	T43.3X2	T43.3X3	T43.3X4	T43.3X5	T43.3X6
Promin	T37.1X1	T37.1X2	T37.1X3	T37.1X4	T37.1X5	T37.1X6
Pronase	T45.3X1	T45.3X2	T45.3X3	T45.3X4	T45.3X5	T45.3X6
Pronestyl (hydrochloride)	T46.2X1	T46.2X2	T46.2X3	T46.2X4	T46.2X5	T46.2X6
Pronetalol	T44.7X1	T44.7X2	T44.7X3	T44.7X4	T44.7X5	T44.7X6
Prontosil	T37.0X1	T37.0X2	T37.0X3	T37.0X4	T37.0X5	T37.0X6
Propachlor	T60.3X1	T60.3X2	T60.3X3	T60.3X4	—	—
Propafenone	T46.2X1	T46.2X2	T46.2X3	T46.2X4	T46.2X5	T46.2X6
Propallylonal	T42.3X1	T42.3X2	T42.3X3	T42.3X4	T42.3X5	T42.3X6
Propamidine	T49.0X1	T49.0X2	T49.0X3	T49.0X4	T49.0X5	T49.0X6
Propane (distributed in mobile container)	T59.891	T59.892	T59.893	T59.894	—	—
distributed through pipes	T59.891	T59.892	T59.893	T59.894	—	—
incomplete combustion	T57.11	T57.12	T57.13	T57.14	—	—
Propanidid	T41.291	T41.292	T41.293	T41.294	T41.295	T41.296
Propanil	T60.3X1	T60.3X2	T60.3X3	T60.3X4	—	—
1-Propanol	T51.3X1	T51.3X2	T51.3X3	T51.3X4	—	—
2-Propanol	T51.2X1	T51.2X2	T51.2X3	T51.2X4	—	—
Propantheline	T44.3X1	T44.3X2	T44.3X3	T44.3X4	T44.3X5	T44.3X6
bromide	T44.3X1	T44.3X2	T44.3X3	T44.3X4	T44.3X5	T44.3X6
Proparacaine	T41.3X1	T41.3X2	T41.3X3	T41.3X4	T41.3X5	T41.3X6
Propatylnitrate	T46.3X1	T46.3X2	T46.3X3	T46.3X4	T46.3X5	T46.3X6
Propicillin	T36.0X1	T36.0X2	T36.0X3	T36.0X4	T36.0X5	T36.0X6
Propiolactone	T49.0X1	T49.0X2	T49.0X3	T49.0X4	T49.0X5	T49.0X6
Propiomazine	T45.0X1	T45.0X2	T45.0X3	T45.0X4	T45.0X5	T45.0X6
Propionaldehyde (medicinal)	T42.6X1	T42.6X2	T42.6X3	T42.6X4	T42.6X5	T42.6X6
Propionate (calcium) (sodium)	T49.0X1	T49.0X2	T49.0X3	T49.0X4	T49.0X5	T49.0X6
Propion gel	T49.0X1	T49.0X2	T49.0X3	T49.0X4	T49.0X5	T49.0X6

Substance	Poisoning, Accidental (Unintentional)	Poisoning, Intentional Self-Harm	Poisoning, Assault	Poisoning, Undetermined	Adverse Effect	Underdosing
Propitocaine	T41.3X1	T41.3X2	T41.3X3	T41.3X4	T41.3X5	T41.3X6
infiltration (subcutaneous)	T41.3X1	T41.3X2	T41.3X3	T41.3X4	T41.3X5	T41.3X6
nerve block (peripheral) (plexus)	T41.3X1	T41.3X2	T41.3X3	T41.3X4	T41.3X5	T41.3X6
Propofol	T41.291	T41.292	T41.293	T41.294	T41.295	T41.296
Propoxur	T60.0X1	T60.0X2	T60.0X3	T60.0X4	—	—
Propoxycaine	T41.3X1	T41.3X2	T41.3X3	T41.3X4	T41.3X5	T41.3X6
infiltration (subcutaneous)	T41.3X1	T41.3X2	T41.3X3	T41.3X4	T41.3X5	T41.3X6
nerve block (peripheral) (plexus)	T41.3X1	T41.3X2	T41.3X3	T41.3X4	T41.3X5	T41.3X6
topical (surface)	T41.3X1	T41.3X2	T41.3X3	T41.3X4	T41.3X5	T41.3X6
Propoxyphene	T40.491	T40.492	T40.493	T40.494	T40.495	T40.496
Propranolol	T44.7X1	T44.7X2	T44.7X3	T44.7X4	T44.7X5	T44.7X6
Propyl						
alcohol	T51.3X1	T51.3X2	T51.3X3	T51.3X4	—	—
carbinol	T51.3X1	T51.3X2	T51.3X3	T51.3X4	—	—
hexadrine	T44.4X1	T44.4X2	T44.4X3	T44.4X4	T44.4X5	T44.4X6
iodone	T50.8X1	T50.8X2	T50.8X3	T50.8X4	T50.8X5	T50.8X6
thiouracil	T38.2X1	T38.2X2	T38.2X3	T38.2X4	T38.2X5	T38.2X6
Propylaminophenothiazine	T43.3X1	T43.3X2	T43.3X3	T43.3X4	T43.3X5	T43.3X6
Propylene	T59.891	T59.892	T59.893	T59.894	—	—
Propylhexedrine	T48.5X1	T48.5X2	T48.5X3	T48.5X4	T48.5X5	T48.5X6
Propyliodone	T50.8X1	T50.8X2	T50.8X3	T50.8X4	T50.8X5	T50.8X6
Propylthiouracil	T38.2X1	T38.2X2	T38.2X3	T38.2X4	T38.2X5	T38.2X6
Propylparaben (ophthalmic)	T49.5X1	T49.5X2	T49.5X3	T49.5X4	T49.5X5	T49.5X6
Propyphenazone	T39.2X1	T39.2X2	T39.2X3	T39.2X4	T39.2X5	T39.2X6
Proquazone	T39.391	T39.392	T39.393	T39.394	T39.395	T39.396
Proscillaridin	T46.0X1	T46.0X2	T46.0X3	T46.0X4	T46.0X5	T46.0X6
Prostacyclin	T45.521	T45.522	T45.523	T45.524	T45.525	T45.526
Prostaglandin (I2)	T45.521	T45.522	T45.523	T45.524	T45.525	T45.526
E1	T46.7X1	T46.7X2	T46.7X3	T46.7X4	T46.7X5	T46.7X6
E2	T48.0X1	T48.0X2	T48.0X3	T48.0X4	T48.0X5	T48.0X6
F2 alpha	T48.0X1	T48.0X2	T48.0X3	T48.0X4	T48.0X5	T48.0X6
Prostigmin	T44.0X1	T44.0X2	T44.0X3	T44.0X4	T44.0X5	T44.0X6
Prosultiamine	T45.2X1	T45.2X2	T45.2X3	T45.2X4	T45.2X5	T45.2X6
Protamine sulfate	T45.7X1	T45.7X2	T45.7X3	T45.7X4	T45.7X5	T45.7X6
zinc insulin	T38.3X1	T38.3X2	T38.3X3	T38.3X4	T38.3X5	T38.3X6
Protease	T47.5X1	T47.5X2	T47.5X3	T47.5X4	T47.5X5	T47.5X6
Protectant, skin NEC	T49.3X1	T49.3X2	T49.3X3	T49.3X4	T49.3X5	T49.3X6
Protein hydrolysate	T50.991	T50.992	T50.993	T50.994	T50.995	T50.996
Prothiaden — see Dothiepin hydrochloride						
Prothionamide	T37.1X1	T37.1X2	T37.1X3	T37.1X4	T37.1X5	T37.1X6

◀ New   ◀ Revised   ~~deleted~~ Deleted

Substance	Poisoning, Accidental (Unintentional)	Poisoning, Intentional Self-Harm	Poisoning, Assault	Poisoning, Undetermined	Adverse Effect	Underdosing
Prothipendyl	T43.591	T43.592	T43.593	T43.594	T43.595	T43.596
Prothoate	T60.0X1	T60.0X2	T60.0X3	T60.0X4	—	—
Prothrombin						
activator	T45.7X1	T45.7X2	T45.7X3	T45.7X4	T45.7X5	T45.7X6
synthesis inhibitor	T45.511	T45.512	T45.513	T45.514	T45.515	T45.516
Protionamide	T37.1X1	T37.1X2	T37.1X3	T37.1X4	T37.1X5	T37.1X6
Protirelin	T38.891	T38.892	T38.893	T38.894	T38.895	T38.896
Protokylol	T48.6X1	T48.6X2	T48.6X3	T48.6X4	T48.6X5	T48.6X6
Protopam	T50.6X1	T50.6X2	T50.6X3	T50.6X4	T50.6X5	T50.6X6
Protoveratrine(s) (A) (B)	T46.5X1	T46.5X2	T46.5X3	T46.5X4	T46.5X5	T46.5X6
Protriptyline	T43.011	T43.012	T43.013	T43.014	T43.015	T43.016
Provera	T38.5X1	T38.5X2	T38.5X3	T38.5X4	T38.5X5	T38.5X6
Provitamin A	T45.2X1	T45.2X2	T45.2X3	T45.2X4	T45.2X5	T45.2X6
Proxibarbal	T42.3X1	T42.3X2	T42.3X3	T42.3X4	T42.3X5	T42.3X6
Proxymetacaine	T41.3X1	T41.3X2	T41.3X3	T41.3X4	T41.3X5	T41.3X6
Proxyphylline	T48.6X1	T48.6X2	T48.6X3	T48.6X4	T48.6X5	T48.6X6
Prozac — see Fluoxetine hydrochloride						
Prunus						
laurocerasus	T62.2X1	T62.2X2	T62.2X3	T62.2X4	—	—
virginiana	T62.2X1	T62.2X2	T62.2X3	T62.2X4	—	—
Prussian blue						
commercial	T65.891	T65.892	T65.893	T65.894	—	—
therapeutic	T50.6X1	T50.6X2	T50.6X3	T50.6X4	T50.6X5	T50.6X6
Prussic acid	T65.0X1	T65.0X2	T65.0X3	T65.0X4	—	—
vapor	T57.3X1	T57.3X2	T57.3X3	T57.3X4	—	—
Pseudoephedrine	T44.991	T44.992	T44.993	T44.994	T44.995	T44.996
Psilocin	T40.991	T40.992	T40.993	T40.994	—	—
Psilocybin	T40.991	T40.992	T40.993	T40.994	—	—
Psilocybine	T40.991	T40.992	T40.993	T40.994	—	—
Psoralene (nonmedicinal)	T65.891	T65.892	T65.893	T65.894	—	—
Psoralens (medicinal)	T50.991	T50.992	T50.993	T50.994	T50.995	T50.996
PSP (phenolsulfonphthalein)	T50.8X1	T50.8X2	T50.8X3	T50.8X4	T50.8X5	T50.8X6
Psychodysleptic drug NOS	T40.901	T40.902	T40.903	T40.904	T40.905	T40.906
specified NEC	T40.991	T40.992	T40.993	T40.994	T40.995	T40.996
Psychostimulant	T43.601	T43.602	T43.603	T43.604	T43.605	T43.606
amphetamine	T43.621	T43.622	T43.623	T43.624	T43.625	T43.626
caffeine	T43.611	T43.612	T43.613	T43.614	T43.615	T43.616
methylphenidate	T43.631	T43.632	T43.633	T43.634	T43.635	T43.636
specified NEC	T43.691	T43.692	T43.693	T43.694	T43.695	T43.696
Psychotherapeutic drug NEC	T43.91	T43.92	T43.93	T43.94	T43.95	T43.96
antidepressants — see also Antidepressant	T43.201	T43.202	T43.203	T43.204	T43.205	T43.206

Substance	Poisoning, Accidental (Unintentional)	Poisoning, Intentional Self-Harm	Poisoning, Assault	Poisoning, Undetermined	Adverse Effect	Underdosing
Psychotherapeutic drug NEC (Continued)						
specified NEC	T43.8X1	T43.8X2	T43.8X3	T43.8X4	T43.8X5	T43.8X6
tranquilizers NEC	T43.501	T43.502	T43.503	T43.504	T43.505	T43.506
Psychotomimetic agents	T40.901	T40.902	T40.903	T40.904	T40.905	T40.906
Psychotropic drug NEC	T43.91	T43.92	T43.93	T43.94	T43.95	T43.96
specified NEC	T43.8X1	T43.8X2	T43.8X3	T43.8X4	T43.8X5	T43.8X6
Psyllium hydrophilic mucilloid	T47.4X1	T47.4X2	T47.4X3	T47.4X4	T47.4X5	T47.4X6
Pteroylglutamic acid	T45.8X1	T45.8X2	T45.8X3	T45.8X4	T45.8X5	T45.8X6
Pteroyltriglutamate	T45.1X1	T45.1X2	T45.1X3	T45.1X4	T45.1X5	T45.1X6
PTFE — see Polytetrafluoroethylene						
Pulp						
devitalizing paste	T49.7X1	T49.7X2	T49.7X3	T49.7X4	T49.7X5	T49.7X6
dressing	T49.7X1	T49.7X2	T49.7X3	T49.7X4	T49.7X5	T49.7X6
Pulsatilla	T62.2X1	T62.2X2	T62.2X3	T62.2X4	—	—
Pumpkin seed extract	T37.4X1	T37.4X2	T37.4X3	T37.4X4	T37.4X5	T37.4X6
Purex (bleach)	T54.91	T54.92	T54.93	T54.94	—	—
Purgative NEC — see also Cathartic	T47.4X1	T47.4X2	T47.4X3	T47.4X4	T47.4X5	T47.4X6
Purine analogue (antineoplastic)	T45.1X1	T45.1X2	T45.1X3	T45.1X4	T45.1X5	T45.1X6
Purine diuretics	T50.2X1	T50.2X2	T50.2X3	T50.2X4	T50.2X5	T50.2X6
Purinethol	T45.1X1	T45.1X2	T45.1X3	T45.1X4	T45.1X5	T45.1X6
PVP	T45.8X1	T45.8X2	T45.8X3	T45.8X4	T45.8X5	T45.8X6
Pyrabital	T39.8X1	T39.8X2	T39.8X3	T39.8X4	T39.8X5	T39.8X6
Pyramidon	T39.2X1	T39.2X2	T39.2X3	T39.2X4	T39.2X5	T39.2X6
Pyrantel	T37.4X1	T37.4X2	T37.4X3	T37.4X4	T37.4X5	T37.4X6
Pyrathiazine	T45.0X1	T45.0X2	T45.0X3	T45.0X4	T45.0X5	T45.0X6
Pyrazinamide	T37.1X1	T37.1X2	T37.1X3	T37.1X4	T37.1X5	T37.1X6
Pyrazinoic acid (amide)	T37.1X1	T37.1X2	T37.1X3	T37.1X4	T37.1X5	T37.1X6
Pyrazole (derivatives)	T39.2X1	T39.2X2	T39.2X3	T39.2X4	T39.2X5	T39.2X6
Pyrazolone analgesic NEC	T39.2X1	T39.2X2	T39.2X3	T39.2X4	T39.2X5	T39.2X6
Pyrethrin, pyrethrum (nonmedicinal)	T60.2X1	T60.2X2	T60.2X3	T60.2X4	—	—
Pyrethrum extract	T49.0X1	T49.0X2	T49.0X3	T49.0X4	T49.0X5	T49.0X6
Pyribenzamine	T45.0X1	T45.0X2	T45.0X3	T45.0X4	T45.0X5	T45.0X6
Pyridine	T52.8X1	T52.8X2	T52.8X3	T52.8X4	—	—
aldoxime methiodide	T50.6X1	T50.6X2	T50.6X3	T50.6X4	T50.6X5	T50.6X6
aldoxime methyl chloride	T50.6X1	T50.6X2	T50.6X3	T50.6X4	T50.6X5	T50.6X6
vapor	T59.891	T59.892	T59.893	T59.894	—	—
Pyridium	T39.8X1	T39.8X2	T39.8X3	T39.8X4	T39.8X5	T39.8X6
Pyridostigmine bromide	T44.0X1	T44.0X2	T44.0X3	T44.0X4	T44.0X5	T44.0X6
Pyridoxal phosphate	T45.2X1	T45.2X2	T45.2X3	T45.2X4	T45.2X5	T45.2X6

TABLE OF DRUGS AND CHEMICALS

Substance	Poisoning, Accidental (Unintentional)	Poisoning, Intentional Self-Harm	Poisoning, Assault	Poisoning, Undetermined	Adverse Effect	Underdosing
Pyridoxine	T45.2X1	T45.2X2	T45.2X3	T45.2X4	T45.2X5	T45.2X6
Pyrilamine	T45.0X1	T45.0X2	T45.0X3	T45.0X4	T45.0X5	T45.0X6
Pyrimethamine	T37.2X1	T37.2X2	T37.2X3	T37.2X4	T37.2X5	T37.2X6
with sulfadoxine	T37.2X1	T37.2X2	T37.2X3	T37.2X4	T37.2X5	T37.2X6
Pyrimidine antagonist	T45.1X1	T45.1X2	T45.1X3	T45.1X4	T45.1X5	T45.1X6
Pyriminil	T60.4X1	T60.4X2	T60.4X3	T60.4X4	—	—
Pyrithione zinc	T49.4X1	T49.4X2	T49.4X3	T49.4X4	T49.4X5	T49.4X6
Pyrithyldione	T42.6X1	T42.6X2	T42.6X3	T42.6X4	T42.6X5	T42.6X6
Pyrogallic acid	T49.0X1	T49.0X2	T49.0X3	T49.0X4	T49.0X5	T49.0X6
Pyrogallol	T49.0X1	T49.0X2	T49.0X3	T49.0X4	T49.0X5	T49.0X6
Pyroxylin	T49.3X1	T49.3X2	T49.3X3	T49.3X4	T49.3X5	T49.3X6
Pyrrobutamine	T45.0X1	T45.0X2	T45.0X3	T45.0X4	T45.0X5	T45.0X6
Pyrrolizidine alkaloids	T62.8X1	T62.8X2	T62.8X3	T62.8X4	—	—
Pyrvinium chloride	T37.4X1	T37.4X2	T37.4X3	T37.4X4	T37.4X5	T37.4X6
PZI	T38.3X1	T38.3X2	T38.3X3	T38.3X4	T38.3X5	T38.3X6
Q						
Quaalude	T42.6X1	T42.6X2	T42.6X3	T42.6X4	T42.6X5	T42.6X6
Quarternary ammonium						
anti-infective	T49.0X1	T49.0X2	T49.0X3	T49.0X4	T49.0X5	T49.0X6
ganglion blocking	T44.2X1	T44.2X2	T44.2X3	T44.2X4	T44.2X5	T44.2X6
parasympatholytic	T44.3X1	T44.3X2	T44.3X3	T44.3X4	T44.3X5	T44.3X6
Quazepam	T42.4X1	T42.4X2	T42.4X3	T42.4X4	T42.4X5	T42.4X6
Quicklime	T54.3X1	T54.3X2	T54.3X3	T54.3X4	—	—
Quillaja extract	T48.4X1	T48.4X2	T48.4X3	T48.4X4	T48.4X5	T48.4X6
Quinacrine	T37.2X1	T37.2X2	T37.2X3	T37.2X4	T37.2X5	T37.2X6
Quinaglute	T46.2X1	T46.2X2	T46.2X3	T46.2X4	T46.2X5	T46.2X6
Quinalbarbital	T42.3X1	T42.3X2	T42.3X3	T42.3X4	T42.3X5	T42.3X6
Quinalbarbitone sodium	T42.3X1	T42.3X2	T42.3X3	T42.3X4	T42.3X5	T42.3X6
Quinalphos	T60.0X1	T60.0X2	T60.0X3	T60.0X4	—	—
Quinapril	T46.4X1	T46.4X2	T46.4X3	T46.4X4	T46.4X5	T46.4X6
Quinestradiol	T38.5X1	T38.5X2	T38.5X3	T38.5X4	T38.5X5	T38.5X6
Quinestradol	T38.5X1	T38.5X2	T38.5X3	T38.5X4	T38.5X5	T38.5X6
Quinestrol	T38.5X1	T38.5X2	T38.5X3	T38.5X4	T38.5X5	T38.5X6
Quinethazone	T50.2X1	T50.2X2	T50.2X3	T50.2X4	T50.2X5	T50.2X6
Quingestanol	T38.4X1	T38.4X2	T38.4X3	T38.4X4	T38.4X5	T38.4X6
Quinidine	T46.2X1	T46.2X2	T46.2X3	T46.2X4	T46.2X5	T46.2X6
Quinine	T37.2X1	T37.2X2	T37.2X3	T37.2X4	T37.2X5	T37.2X6
Quiniobine	T37.8X1	T37.8X2	T37.8X3	T37.8X4	T37.8X5	T37.8X6
Quinisocaine	T49.1X1	T49.1X2	T49.1X3	T49.1X4	T49.1X5	T49.1X6
Quinocide	T37.2X1	T37.2X2	T37.2X3	T37.2X4	T37.2X5	T37.2X6
Quinoline (derivatives) NEC	T37.8X1	T37.8X2	T37.8X3	T37.8X4	T37.8X5	T37.8X6

Substance	Poisoning, Accidental (Unintentional)	Poisoning, Intentional Self-Harm	Poisoning, Assault	Poisoning, Undetermined	Adverse Effect	Underdosing
Quinupramine	T43.011	T43.012	T43.013	T43.014	T43.015	T43.016
Quotane	T41.3X1	T41.3X2	T41.3X3	T41.3X4	T41.3X5	T41.3X6
R						
Rabies						
immune globulin (human)	T50.Z11	T50.Z12	T50.Z13	T50.Z14	T50.Z15	T50.Z16
vaccine	T50.B91	T50.B92	T50.B93	T50.B94	T50.B95	T50.B96
Racemoramide	T40.2X1	T40.2X2	T40.2X3	T40.2X4	—	—
Racemorphan	T40.2X1	T40.2X2	T40.2X3	T40.2X4	T40.2X5	T40.2X6
Racepinefrin	T44.5X1	T44.5X2	T44.5X3	T44.5X4	T44.5X5	T44.5X6
Raclopride	T43.591	T43.592	T43.593	T43.594	T43.595	T43.596
Radiator alcohol	T51.1X1	T51.1X2	T51.1X3	T51.1X4	—	—
Radioactive drug NEC	T50.8X1	T50.8X2	T50.8X3	T50.8X4	T50.8X5	T50.8X6
Radio-opaque (drugs) (materials)	T50.8X1	T50.8X2	T50.8X3	T50.8X4	T50.8X5	T50.8X6
Ramifenazone	T39.2X1	T39.2X2	T39.2X3	T39.2X4	T39.2X5	T39.2X6
Ramipril	T46.4X1	T46.4X2	T46.4X3	T46.4X4	T46.4X5	T46.4X6
Ranitidine	T47.0X1	T47.0X2	T47.0X3	T47.0X4	T47.0X5	T47.0X6
Ranunculus	T62.2X1	T62.2X2	T62.2X3	T62.2X4	—	—
Rat poison NEC	T60.4X1	T60.4X2	T60.4X3	T60.4X4	—	—
Rattlesnake (venom)	T63.011	T63.012	T63.013	T63.014		
Raubasine	T46.7X1	T46.7X2	T46.7X3	T46.7X4	T46.7X5	T46.7X6
Raudixin	T46.5X1	T46.5X2	T46.5X3	T46.5X4	T46.5X5	T46.5X6
Rautensin	T46.5X1	T46.5X2	T46.5X3	T46.5X4	T46.5X5	T46.5X6
Rautina	T46.5X1	T46.5X2	T46.5X3	T46.5X4	T46.5X5	T46.5X6
Rautotal	T46.5X1	T46.5X2	T46.5X3	T46.5X4	T46.5X5	T46.5X6
Rauwiloid	T46.5X1	T46.5X2	T46.5X3	T46.5X4	T46.5X5	T46.5X6
Rauwoldin	T46.5X1	T46.5X2	T46.5X3	T46.5X4	T46.5X5	T46.5X6
Rauwolfia (alkaloids)	T46.5X1	T46.5X2	T46.5X3	T46.5X4	T46.5X5	T46.5X6
Razoxane	T45.1X1	T45.1X2	T45.1X3	T45.1X4	T45.1X5	T45.1X6
Realgar	T57.0X1	T57.0X2	T57.0X3	T57.0X4	—	—
Recombinant (R) — see specific protein						
Red blood cells, packed	T45.8X1	T45.8X2	T45.8X3	T45.8X4	T45.8X5	T45.8X6
Red squill (scilliroside)	T60.4X1	T60.4X2	T60.4X3	T60.4X4	—	—
Reducing agent, industrial NEC	T65.891	T65.892	T65.893	T65.894	—	—
Refrigerant gas (chlorofluoro-carbon)	T53.5X1	T53.5X2	T53.5X3	T53.5X4	—	—
not chlorofluoro-carbon	T59.891	T59.892	T59.893	T59.894	—	—
Regroton	T50.2X1	T50.2X2	T50.2X3	T50.2X4	T50.2X5	T50.2X6
Rehydration salts (oral)	T50.3X1	T50.3X2	T50.3X3	T50.3X4	T50.3X5	T50.3X6
Rela	T42.8X1	T42.8X2	T42.8X3	T42.8X4	T42.8X5	T42.8X6

◄ New ◄ Revised ~~deleted~~ Deleted

Substance	Poisoning, Accidental (Unintentional)	Poisoning, Intentional Self-Harm	Poisoning, Assault	Poisoning, Undetermined	Adverse Effect	Underdosing
Relaxant, muscle						
anesthetic	T48.1X1	T48.1X2	T48.1X3	T48.1X4	T48.1X5	T48.1X6
central nervous system	T42.8X1	T42.8X2	T42.8X3	T42.8X4	T42.8X5	T42.8X6
skeletal NEC	T48.1X1	T48.1X2	T48.1X3	T48.1X4	T48.1X5	T48.1X6
smooth NEC	T44.3X1	T44.3X2	T44.3X3	T44.3X4	T44.3X5	T44.3X6
Remoxipride	T43.591	T43.592	T43.593	T43.594	T43.595	T43.596
Renese	T50.2X1	T50.2X2	T50.2X3	T50.2X4	T50.2X5	T50.2X6
Renografin	T50.8X1	T50.8X2	T50.8X3	T50.8X4	T50.8X5	T50.8X6
Replacement solution	T50.3X1	T50.3X2	T50.3X3	T50.3X4	T50.3X5	T50.3X6
Reproterol	T48.6X1	T48.6X2	T48.6X3	T48.6X4	T48.6X5	T48.6X6
Rescinnamine	T46.5X1	T46.5X2	T46.5X3	T46.5X4	T46.5X5	T46.5X6
Reserpin(e)	T46.5X1	T46.5X2	T46.5X3	T46.5X4	T46.5X5	T46.5X6
Resorcin, resorcinol (nonmedicinal)	T65.891	T65.892	T65.893	T65.894	—	—
medicinal	T49.4X1	T49.4X2	T49.4X3	T49.4X4	T49.4X5	T49.4X6
Respaire	T48.4X1	T48.4X2	T48.4X3	T48.4X4	T48.4X5	T48.4X6
Respiratory drug NEC	T48.901	T48.902	T48.903	T48.904	T48.905	T48.906
antiasthmatic NEC	T48.6X1	T48.6X2	T48.6X3	T48.6X4	T48.6X5	T48.6X6
anti-common-cold NEC	T48.5X1	T48.5X2	T48.5X3	T48.5X4	T48.5X5	T48.5X6
expectorant NEC	T48.4X1	T48.4X2	T48.4X3	T48.4X4	T48.4X5	T48.4X6
stimulant	T48.901	T48.902	T48.903	T48.904	T48.905	T48.906
Retinoic acid	T49.0X1	T49.0X2	T49.0X3	T49.0X4	T49.0X5	T49.0X6
Retinol	T45.2X1	T45.2X2	T45.2X3	T45.2X4	T45.2X5	T45.2X6
Rh (D) immune globulin (human)	T50.Z11	T50.Z12	T50.Z13	T50.Z14	T50.Z15	T50.Z16
Rhodine	T39.011	T39.012	T39.013	T39.014	T39.015	T39.016
RhoGAM	T50.Z11	T50.Z12	T50.Z13	T50.Z14	T50.Z15	T50.Z16
Rhubarb						
dry extract	T47.2X1	T47.2X2	T47.2X3	T47.2X4	T47.2X5	T47.2X6
tincture, compound	T47.2X1	T47.2X2	T47.2X3	T47.2X4	T47.2X5	T47.2X6
Ribavirin	T37.5X1	T37.5X2	T37.5X3	T37.5X4	T37.5X5	T37.5X6
Riboflavin	T45.2X1	T45.2X2	T45.2X3	T45.2X4	T45.2X5	T45.2X6
Ribostamycin	T36.5X1	T36.5X2	T36.5X3	T36.5X4	T36.5X5	T36.5X6
Ricin	T62.2X1	T62.2X2	T62.2X3	T62.2X4	—	—
Ricinus communis	T62.2X1	T62.2X2	T62.2X3	T62.2X4	—	—
Rickettsial vaccine NEC	T50.A91	T50.A92	T50.A93	T50.A94	T50.A95	T50.A96
Rifabutin	T36.6X1	T36.6X2	T36.6X3	T36.6X4	T36.6X5	T36.6X6
Rifamide	T36.6X1	T36.6X2	T36.6X3	T36.6X4	T36.6X5	T36.6X6
Rifampicin	T36.6X1	T36.6X2	T36.6X3	T36.6X4	T36.6X5	T36.6X6
with isoniazid	T37.1X1	T37.1X2	T37.1X3	T37.1X4	T37.1X5	T37.1X6
Rifampin	T36.6X1	T36.6X2	T36.6X3	T36.6X4	T36.6X5	T36.6X6
Rifamycin	T36.6X1	T36.6X2	T36.6X3	T36.6X4	T36.6X5	T36.6X6
Rifaximin	T36.6X1	T36.6X2	T36.6X3	T36.6X4	T36.6X5	T36.6X6
Rimantadine	T37.5X1	T37.5X2	T37.5X3	T37.5X4	T37.5X5	T37.5X6
Rimazolium metilsulfate	T39.8X1	T39.8X2	T39.8X3	T39.8X4	T39.8X5	T39.8X6
Rimifon	T37.1X1	T37.1X2	T37.1X3	T37.1X4	T37.1X5	T37.1X6
Rimiterol	T48.6X1	T48.6X2	T48.6X3	T48.6X4	T48.6X5	T48.6X6
Ringer (lactate) solution	T50.3X1	T50.3X2	T50.3X3	T50.3X4	T50.3X5	T50.3X6
Ristocetin	T36.8X1	T36.8X2	T36.8X3	T36.8X4	T36.8X5	T36.8X6
Ritalin	T43.631	T43.632	T43.633	T43.634	T43.635	T43.636
Ritodrine	T44.5X1	T44.5X2	T44.5X3	T44.5X4	T44.5X5	T44.5X6
Roach killer — see Insecticide						
Rociverine	T44.3X1	T44.3X2	T44.3X3	T44.3X4	T44.3X5	T44.3X6
Rocky Mountain spotted fever vaccine	T50.A91	T50.A92	T50.A93	T50.A94	T50.A95	T50.A96
Rodenticide NEC	T60.4X1	T60.4X2	T60.4X3	T60.4X4	—	—
Rohypnol	T42.4X1	T42.4X2	T42.4X3	T42.4X4	T42.4X5	T42.4X6
Rokitamycin	T36.3X1	T36.3X2	T36.3X3	T36.3X4	T36.3X5	T36.3X6
Rolaids	T47.1X1	T47.1X2	T47.1X3	T47.1X4	T47.1X5	T47.1X6
Rolitetracycline	T36.4X1	T36.4X2	T36.4X3	T36.4X4	T36.4X5	T36.4X6
Romilar	T48.3X1	T48.3X2	T48.3X3	T48.3X4	T48.3X5	T48.3X6
Ronifibrate	T46.6X1	T46.6X2	T46.6X3	T46.6X4	T46.6X5	T46.6X6
Rosaprostol	T47.1X1	T47.1X2	T47.1X3	T47.1X4	T47.1X5	T47.1X6
Rose bengal sodium (131I)	T50.8X1	T50.8X2	T50.8X3	T50.8X4	T50.8X5	T50.8X6
Rose water ointment	T49.3X1	T49.3X2	T49.3X3	T49.3X4	T49.3X5	T49.3X6
Rosoxacin	T37.8X1	T37.8X2	T37.8X3	T37.8X4	T37.8X5	T37.8X6
Rotenone	T60.2X1	T60.2X2	T60.2X3	T60.2X4	—	—
Rotoxamine	T45.0X1	T45.0X2	T45.0X3	T45.0X4	T45.0X5	T45.0X6
Rough-on-rats	T60.4X1	T60.4X2	T60.4X3	T60.4X4	—	—
Roxatidine	T47.0X1	T47.0X2	T47.0X3	T47.0X4	T47.0X5	T47.0X6
Roxithromycin	T36.3X1	T36.3X2	T36.3X3	T36.3X4	T36.3X5	T36.3X6
Rt-PA	T45.611	T45.612	T45.613	T45.614	T45.615	T45.616
Rubbing alcohol	T51.2X1	T51.2X2	T51.2X3	T51.2X4	—	—
Rubefacient	T49.4X1	T49.4X2	T49.4X3	T49.4X4	T49.4X5	T49.4X6
Rubella vaccine	T50.B91	T50.B92	T50.B93	T50.B94	T50.B95	T50.B96
Rubelogen	T50.B91	T50.B92	T50.B93	T50.B94	T50.B95	T50.B96
Rubeovax	T50.991	T50.992	T50.993	T50.994	T50.995	T50.996
Rubidium chloride Rb82	T50.8X1	T50.8X2	T50.8X3	T50.8X4	T50.8X5	T50.8X6
Rubidomycin	T45.1X1	T45.1X2	T45.1X3	T45.1X4	T45.1X5	T45.1X6
Rue	T62.2X1	T62.2X2	T62.2X3	T62.2X4	—	—
Rufocromomycin	T45.1X1	T45.1X2	T45.1X3	T45.1X4	T45.1X5	T45.1X6
Russel's viper venin	T45.7X1	T45.7X2	T45.7X3	T45.7X4	T45.7X5	T45.7X6
Ruta (graveolens)	T62.2X1	T62.2X2	T62.2X3	T62.2X4	—	—
Rutinum	T46.991	T46.992	T46.993	T46.994	T46.995	T46.996
Rutoside	T46.991	T46.992	T46.993	T46.994	T46.995	T46.996

◀ New   ◀ Revised   ~~deleted~~ Deleted

TABLE OF DRUGS AND CHEMICALS

Substance	External Cause (T-Code)					
	Poisoning, Accidental (Unintentional)	Poisoning, Intentional Self-Harm	Poisoning, Assault	Poisoning, Undetermined	Adverse Effect	Underdosing
S						
Sabadilla (plant)	T62.2X1	T62.2X2	T62.2X3	T62.2X4	—	—
pesticide	T60.2X1	T60.2X2	T60.2X3	T60.2X4	—	—
Saccharated iron oxide	T45.8X1	T45.8X2	T45.8X3	T45.8X4	T45.8X5	T45.8X6
Saccharin	T50.901	T50.902	T50.903	T50.904	T50.905	T50.906
Saccharomyces boulardii	T47.6X1	T47.6X2	T47.6X3	T47.6X4	T47.6X5	T47.6X6
Safflower oil	T46.6X1	T46.6X2	T46.6X3	T46.6X4	T46.6X5	T46.6X6
Safrazine	T43.1X1	T43.1X2	T43.1X3	T43.1X4	T43.1X5	T43.1X6
Salazosulfapyridine	T37.0X1	T37.0X2	T37.0X3	T37.0X4	T37.0X5	T37.0X6
Salbutamol	T48.6X1	T48.6X2	T48.6X3	T48.6X4	T48.6X5	T48.6X6
Salicylamide	T39.091	T39.092	T39.093	T39.094	T39.095	T39.096
Salicylate NEC	T39.091	T39.092	T39.093	T39.094	T39.095	T39.096
methyl	T49.3X1	T49.3X2	T49.3X3	T49.3X4	T49.3X5	T49.3X6
theobromine calcium	T50.2X1	T50.2X2	T50.2X3	T50.2X4	T50.2X5	T50.2X6
Salicylazosulfapyridine	T37.0X1	T37.0X2	T37.0X3	T37.0X4	T37.0X5	T37.0X6
Salicylhydroxamic acid	T49.0X1	T49.0X2	T49.0X3	T49.0X4	T49.0X5	T49.0X6
Salicylic acid	T49.4X1	T49.4X2	T49.4X3	T49.4X4	T49.4X5	T49.4X6
with benzoic acid	T49.4X1	T49.4X2	T49.4X3	T49.4X4	T49.4X5	T49.4X6
congeners	T39.091	T39.092	T39.093	T39.094	T39.095	T39.096
derivative	T39.091	T39.092	T39.093	T39.094	T39.095	T39.096
salts	T39.091	T39.092	T39.093	T39.094	T39.095	T39.096
Salinazid	T37.1X1	T37.1X2	T37.1X3	T37.1X4	T37.1X5	T37.1X6
Salmeterol	T48.6X1	T48.6X2	T48.6X3	T48.6X4	T48.6X5	T48.6X6
Salol	T49.3X1	T49.3X2	T49.3X3	T49.3X4	T49.3X5	T49.3X6
Salsalate	T39.091	T39.092	T39.093	T39.094	T39.095	T39.096
Salt substitute	T50.901	T50.902	T50.903	T50.904	T50.905	T50.906
Salt-replacing drug	T50.901	T50.902	T50.903	T50.904	T50.905	T50.906
Salt-retaining mineralocorticoid	T50.0X1	T50.0X2	T50.0X3	T50.0X4	T50.0X5	T50.0X6
Saluretic NEC	T50.2X1	T50.2X2	T50.2X3	T50.2X4	T50.2X5	T50.2X6
Saluron	T50.2X1	T50.2X2	T50.2X3	T50.2X4	T50.2X5	T50.2X6
Salvarsan 606 (neosilver) (silver)	T37.8X1	T37.8X2	T37.8X3	T37.8X4	T37.8X5	T37.8X6
Sambucus canadensis	T62.2X1	T62.2X2	T62.2X3	T62.2X4	—	—
berry	T62.1X1	T62.1X2	T62.1X3	T62.1X4	—	—
Sandril	T46.5X1	T46.5X2	T46.5X3	T46.5X4	T46.5X5	T46.5X6
Sanguinaria canadensis	T62.2X1	T62.2X2	T62.2X3	T62.2X4	—	—
Saniflush (cleaner)	T54.2X1	T54.2X2	T54.2X3	T54.2X4	—	—
Santonin	T37.4X1	T37.4X2	T37.4X3	T37.4X4	T37.4X5	T37.4X6
Santyl	T49.8X1	T49.8X2	T49.8X3	T49.8X4	T49.8X5	T49.8X6
Saralasin	T46.5X1	T46.5X2	T46.5X3	T46.5X4	T46.5X5	T46.5X6
Sarcolysin	T45.1X1	T45.1X2	T45.1X3	T45.1X4	T45.1X5	T45.1X6
Sarkomycin	T45.1X1	T45.1X2	T45.1X3	T45.1X4	T45.1X5	T45.1X6
Saroten	T43.011	T43.012	T43.013	T43.014	T43.015	T43.016

Substance	External Cause (T-Code)					
	Poisoning, Accidental (Unintentional)	Poisoning, Intentional Self-Harm	Poisoning, Assault	Poisoning, Undetermined	Adverse Effect	Underdosing
Saturnine — *see* Lead						
Savin (oil)	T49.4X1	T49.4X2	T49.4X3	T49.4X4	T49.4X5	T49.4X6
Scammony	T47.2X1	T47.2X2	T47.2X3	T47.2X4	T47.2X5	T47.2X6
Scarlet red	T49.8X1	T49.8X2	T49.8X3	T49.8X4	T49.8X5	T49.8X6
Scheele's green	T57.0X1	T57.0X2	T57.0X3	T57.0X4	—	—
insecticide	T57.0X1	T57.0X2	T57.0X3	T57.0X4	—	—
Schizontozide (blood) (tissue)	T37.2X1	T37.2X2	T37.2X3	T37.2X4	T37.2X5	T37.2X6
Schradan	T60.0X1	T60.0X2	T60.0X3	T60.0X4	—	—
Schweinfurth green	T57.0X1	T57.0X2	T57.0X3	T57.0X4	—	—
insecticide	T57.0X1	T57.0X2	T57.0X3	T57.0X4	—	—
Scilla, rat poison	T60.4X1	T60.4X2	T60.4X3	T60.4X4	—	—
Scillaren	T60.4X1	T60.4X2	T60.4X3	T60.4X4	—	—
Sclerosing agent	T46.8X1	T46.8X2	T46.8X3	T46.8X4	T46.8X5	T46.8X6
Scombrotoxin	T61.11	T61.12	T61.13	T61.14	—	—
Scopolamine	T44.3X1	T44.3X2	T44.3X3	T44.3X4	T44.3X5	T44.3X6
Scopolia extract	T44.3X1	T44.3X2	T44.3X3	T44.3X4	T44.3X5	T44.3X6
Scouring powder	T65.891	T65.892	T65.893	T65.894	—	—
Sea						
anemone (sting)	T63.631	T63.632	T63.633	T63.634	—	—
cucumber (sting)	T63.691	T63.692	T63.693	T63.694	—	—
snake (bite) (venom)	T63.091	T63.092	T63.093	T63.094	—	—
urchin spine (puncture)	T63.691	T63.692	T63.693	T63.694	—	—
Seafood	T61.91	T61.92	T61.93	T61.94	—	—
specified NEC	T61.8X1	T61.8X2	T61.8X3	T61.8X4	—	—
Secbutabarbital	T42.3X1	T42.3X2	T42.3X3	T42.3X4	T42.3X5	T42.3X6
Secbutabarbitone	T42.3X1	T42.3X2	T42.3X3	T42.3X4	T42.3X5	T42.3X6
Secnidazole	T37.3X1	T37.3X2	T37.3X3	T37.3X4	T37.3X5	T37.3X6
Secobarbital	T42.3X1	T42.3X2	T42.3X3	T42.3X4	T42.3X5	T42.3X6
Seconal	T42.3X1	T42.3X2	T42.3X3	T42.3X4	T42.3X5	T42.3X6
Secretin	T50.8X1	T50.8X2	T50.8X3	T50.8X4	T50.8X5	T50.8X6
Sedative NEC	T42.71	T42.72	T42.73	T42.74	T42.75	T42.76
mixed NEC	T42.6X1	T42.6X2	T42.6X3	T42.6X4	T42.6X5	T42.6X6
Sedormid	T42.6X1	T42.6X2	T42.6X3	T42.6X4	T42.6X5	T42.6X6
Seed disinfectant or dressing	T60.8X1	T60.8X2	T60.8X3	T60.8X4	—	—
Seeds (poisonous)	T62.2X1	T62.2X2	T62.2X3	T62.2X4	—	—
Selegiline	T42.8X1	T42.8X2	T42.8X3	T42.8X4	T42.8X5	T42.8X6
Selenium NEC	T56.891	T56.892	T56.893	T56.894	—	—
disulfide or sulfide	T49.4X1	T49.4X2	T49.4X3	T49.4X4	T49.4X5	T49.4X6
fumes	T59.891	T59.892	T59.893	T59.894	—	—
sulfide	T49.4X1	T49.4X2	T49.4X3	T49.4X4	T49.4X5	T49.4X6
Selenomethionine (75Se)	T50.8X1	T50.8X2	T50.8X3	T50.8X4	T50.8X5	T50.8X6
Selsun	T49.4X1	T49.4X2	T49.4X3	T49.4X4	T49.4X5	T49.4X6

◀ New   ◀ Revised   ~~deleted~~ Deleted

Substance	Poisoning, Accidental (Unintentional)	Poisoning, Intentional Self-Harm	Poisoning, Assault	Poisoning, Undetermined	Adverse Effect	Underdosing
	External Cause (T-Code)					
Semustine	T45.1X1	T45.1X2	T45.1X3	T45.1X4	T45.1X5	T45.1X6
Senega syrup	T48.4X1	T48.4X2	T48.4X3	T48.4X4	T48.4X5	T48.4X6
Senna	T47.2X1	T47.2X2	T47.2X3	T47.2X4	T47.2X5	T47.2X6
Sennoside A+B	T47.2X1	T47.2X2	T47.2X3	T47.2X4	T47.2X5	T47.2X6
Septisol	T49.2X1	T49.2X2	T49.2X3	T49.2X4	T49.2X5	T49.2X6
Seractide	T38.811	T38.812	T38.813	T38.814	T38.815	T38.816
Serax	T42.4X1	T42.4X2	T42.4X3	T42.4X4	T42.4X5	T42.4X6
Serenesil	T42.6X1	T42.6X2	T42.6X3	T42.6X4	T42.6X5	T42.6X6
Serenium (hydrochloride)	T37.91	T37.92	T37.93	T37.94	T37.95	T37.96
Serepax — see Oxazepam						
Sermorelin	T38.891	T38.892	T38.893	T38.894	T38.895	T38.896
Sernyl	T41.1X1	T41.1X2	T41.1X3	T41.1X4	T41.1X5	T41.1X6
Serotonin	T50.991	T50.992	T50.993	T50.994	T50.995	T50.996
Serpasil	T46.5X1	T46.5X2	T46.5X3	T46.5X4	T46.5X5	T46.5X6
Serrapeptase	T45.3X1	T45.3X2	T45.3X3	T45.3X4	T45.3X5	T45.3X6
Serum						
antibotulinus	T50.Z11	T50.Z12	T50.Z13	T50.Z14	T50.Z15	T50.Z16
anticytotoxic	T50.Z11	T50.Z12	T50.Z13	T50.Z14	T50.Z15	T50.Z16
antidiphtheria	T50.Z11	T50.Z12	T50.Z13	T50.Z14	T50.Z15	T50.Z16
antimeningococcus	T50.Z11	T50.Z12	T50.Z13	T50.Z14	T50.Z15	T50.Z16
anti-Rh	T50.Z11	T50.Z12	T50.Z13	T50.Z14	T50.Z15	T50.Z16
anti-snake-bite	T50.Z11	T50.Z12	T50.Z13	T50.Z14	T50.Z15	T50.Z16
antitetanic	T50.Z11	T50.Z12	T50.Z13	T50.Z14	T50.Z15	T50.Z16
antitoxic	T50.Z11	T50.Z12	T50.Z13	T50.Z14	T50.Z15	T50.Z16
complement (inhibitor)	T45.8X1	T45.8X2	T45.8X3	T45.8X4	T45.8X5	T45.8X6
convalescent	T50.Z11	T50.Z12	T50.Z13	T50.Z14	T50.Z15	T50.Z16
hemolytic complement	T45.8X1	T45.8X2	T45.8X3	T45.8X4	T45.8X5	T45.8X6
immune (human)	T50.Z11	T50.Z12	T50.Z13	T50.Z14	T50.Z15	T50.Z16
protective NEC	T50.Z11	T50.Z12	T50.Z13	T50.Z14	T50.Z15	T50.Z16
Setastine	T45.0X1	T45.0X2	T45.0X3	T45.0X4	T45.0X5	T45.0X6
Setoperone	T43.591	T43.592	T43.593	T43.594	T43.595	T43.596
Sewer gas	T59.91	T59.92	T59.93	T59.94	—	—
Shampoo	T55.0X1	T55.0X2	T55.0X3	T55.0X4	—	—
Shellfish, noxious, nonbacterial	T61.781	T61.782	T61.783	T61.784	—	—
Sildenafil	T46.7X1	T46.7X2	T46.7X3	T46.7X4	T46.7X5	T46.7X6
Silibinin	T50.991	T50.992	T50.993	T50.994	T50.995	T50.996
Silicone NEC	T65.891	T65.892	T65.893	T65.894	—	—
medicinal	T49.3X1	T49.3X2	T49.3X3	T49.3X4	T49.3X5	T49.3X6
Silvadene	T49.0X1	T49.0X2	T49.0X3	T49.0X4	T49.0X5	T49.0X6
Silver	T49.0X1	T49.0X2	T49.0X3	T49.0X4	T49.0X5	T49.0X6
anti-infectives	T49.0X1	T49.0X2	T49.0X3	T49.0X4	T49.0X5	T49.0X6
arsphenamine	T37.8X1	T37.8X2	T37.8X3	T37.8X4	T37.8X5	T37.8X6

Substance	Poisoning, Accidental (Unintentional)	Poisoning, Intentional Self-Harm	Poisoning, Assault	Poisoning, Undetermined	Adverse Effect	Underdosing
	External Cause (T-Code)					
Silver (Continued)						
colloidal	T49.0X1	T49.0X2	T49.0X3	T49.0X4	T49.0X5	T49.0X6
nitrate	T49.0X1	T49.0X2	T49.0X3	T49.0X4	T49.0X5	T49.0X6
ophthalmic preparation	T49.5X1	T49.5X2	T49.5X3	T49.5X4	T49.5X5	T49.5X6
toughened (keratolytic)	T49.4X1	T49.4X2	T49.4X3	T49.4X4	T49.4X5	T49.4X6
nonmedicinal (dust)	T56.891	T56.892	T56.893	T56.894	—	—
protein	T49.5X1	T49.5X2	T49.5X3	T49.5X4	T49.5X5	T49.5X6
salvarsan	T37.8X1	T37.8X2	T37.8X3	T37.8X4	T37.8X5	T37.8X6
sulfadiazine	T49.4X1	T49.4X2	T49.4X3	T49.4X4	T49.4X5	T49.4X6
Silymarin	T50.991	T50.992	T50.993	T50.994	T50.995	T50.996
Simaldrate	T47.1X1	T47.1X2	T47.1X3	T47.1X4	T47.1X5	T47.1X6
Simazine	T60.3X1	T60.3X2	T60.3X3	T60.3X4	—	—
Simethicone	T47.1X1	T47.1X2	T47.1X3	T47.1X4	T47.1X5	T47.1X6
Simfibrate	T46.6X1	T46.6X2	T46.6X3	T46.6X4	T46.6X5	T46.6X6
Simvastatin	T46.6X1	T46.6X2	T46.6X3	T46.6X4	T46.6X5	T46.6X6
Sincalide	T50.8X1	T50.8X2	T50.8X3	T50.8X4	T50.8X5	T50.8X6
Sinequan	T43.011	T43.012	T43.013	T43.014	T43.015	T43.016
Singoserp	T46.5X1	T46.5X2	T46.5X3	T46.5X4	T46.5X5	T46.5X6
Sintrom	T45.511	T45.512	T45.513	T45.514	T45.515	T45.516
Sisomicin	T36.5X1	T36.5X2	T36.5X3	T36.5X4	T36.5X5	T36.5X6
Sitosterols	T46.6X1	T46.6X2	T46.6X3	T46.6X4	T46.6X5	T46.6X6
Skeletal muscle relaxants	T48.1X1	T48.1X2	T48.1X3	T48.1X4	T48.1X5	T48.1X6
Skin						
agents (external)	T49.91	T49.92	T49.93	T49.94	T49.95	T49.96
specified NEC	T49.8X1	T49.8X2	T49.8X3	T49.8X4	T49.8X5	T49.8X6
test antigen	T50.8X1	T50.8X2	T50.8X3	T50.8X4	T50.8X5	T50.8X6
Sleep-eze	T45.0X1	T45.0X2	T45.0X3	T45.0X4	T45.0X5	T45.0X6
Sleeping draught, pill	T42.71	T42.72	T42.73	T42.74	T42.75	T42.76
Smallpox vaccine	T50.B11	T50.B12	T50.B13	T50.B14	T50.B15	T50.B16
Smelter fumes NEC	T56.91	T56.92	T56.93	T56.94	—	—
Smog	T59.1X1	T59.1X2	T59.1X3	T59.1X4	—	—
Smoke NEC	T59.811	T59.812	T59.813	T59.814	—	—
Smooth muscle relaxant	T44.3X1	T44.3X2	T44.3X3	T44.3X4	T44.3X5	T44.3X6
Snail killer NEC	T60.8X1	T60.8X2	T60.8X3	T60.8X4	—	—
Snake venom or bite	T63.001	T63.002	T63.003	T63.004	—	—
hemocoagulase	T45.7X1	T45.7X2	T45.7X3	T45.7X4	T45.7X5	T45.7X6
Snuff	T65.211	T65.212	T65.213	T65.214	—	—
Soap (powder) (product)	T55.0X1	T55.0X2	T55.0X3	T55.0X4	—	—
enema	T47.4X1	T47.4X2	T47.4X3	T47.4X4	T47.4X5	T47.4X6
medicinal, soft	T49.2X1	T49.2X2	T49.2X3	T49.2X4	T49.2X5	T49.2X6
superfatted	T49.2X1	T49.2X2	T49.2X3	T49.2X4	T49.2X5	T49.2X6
Sobrerol	T48.4X1	T48.4X2	T48.4X3	T48.4X4	T48.4X5	T48.4X6

TABLE OF DRUGS AND CHEMICALS

Substance	Poisoning, Accidental (Unintentional)	Poisoning, Intentional Self-Harm	Poisoning, Assault	Poisoning, Undetermined	Adverse Effect	Underdosing
Soda (caustic)	T54.3X1	T54.3X2	T54.3X3	T54.3X4	—	—
bicarb	T47.1X1	T47.1X2	T47.1X3	T47.1X4	T47.1X5	T47.1X6
chlorinated — see Sodium, hypochlorite						
Sodium						
acetosulfone	T37.1X1	T37.1X2	T37.1X3	T37.1X4	T37.1X5	T37.1X6
acetrizoate	T50.8X1	T50.8X2	T50.8X3	T50.8X4	T50.8X5	T50.8X6
acid phosphate	T50.3X1	T50.3X2	T50.3X3	T50.3X4	T50.3X5	T50.3X6
alginate	T47.8X1	T47.8X2	T47.8X3	T47.8X4	T47.8X5	T47.8X6
amidotrizoate	T50.8X1	T50.8X2	T50.8X3	T50.8X4	T50.8X5	T50.8X6
aminopterin	T45.1X1	T45.1X2	T45.1X3	T45.1X4	T45.1X5	T45.1X6
amylosulfate	T47.8X1	T47.8X2	T47.8X3	T47.8X4	T47.8X5	T47.8X6
amytal	T42.3X1	T42.3X2	T42.3X3	T42.3X4	T42.3X5	T42.3X6
antimony gluconate	T37.3X1	T37.3X2	T37.3X3	T37.3X4	T37.3X5	T37.3X6
arsenate	T57.0X1	T57.0X2	T57.0X3	T57.0X4	—	—
aurothiomalate	T39.4X1	T39.4X2	T39.4X3	T39.4X4	T39.4X5	T39.4X6
aurothiosulfate	T39.4X1	T39.4X2	T39.4X3	T39.4X4	T39.4X5	T39.4X6
barbiturate	T42.3X1	T42.3X2	T42.3X3	T42.3X4	T42.3X5	T42.3X6
basic phosphate	T47.4X1	T47.4X2	T47.4X3	T47.4X4	T47.4X5	T47.4X6
bicarbonate	T47.1X1	T47.1X2	T47.1X3	T47.1X4	T47.1X5	T47.1X6
bichromate	T57.8X1	T57.8X2	T57.8X3	T57.8X4	—	—
biphosphate	T50.3X1	T50.3X2	T50.3X3	T50.3X4	T50.3X5	T50.3X6
bisulfate	T65.891	T65.892	T65.893	T65.894	—	—
borate						
cleanser	T57.8X1	T57.8X2	T57.8X3	T57.8X4	—	—
eye	T49.5X1	T49.5X2	T49.5X3	T49.5X4	T49.5X5	T49.5X6
therapeutic	T49.8X1	T49.8X2	T49.8X3	T49.8X4	T49.8X5	T49.8X6
bromide	T42.6X1	T42.6X2	T42.6X3	T42.6X4	T42.6X5	T42.6X6
cacodylate (nonmedicinal) NEC	T50.8X1	T50.8X2	T50.8X3	T50.8X4	T50.8X5	T50.8X6
anti-infective	T37.8X1	T37.8X2	T37.8X3	T37.8X4	T37.8X5	T37.8X6
herbicide	T60.3X1	T60.3X2	T60.3X3	T60.3X4	—	—
calcium edetate	T45.8X1	T45.8X2	T45.8X3	T45.8X4	T45.8X5	T45.8X6
carbonate NEC	T54.3X1	T54.3X2	T54.3X3	T54.3X4	—	—
chlorate NEC	T65.891	T65.892	T65.893	T65.894	—	—
herbicide	T54.91	T54.92	T54.93	T54.94	—	—
chloride	T50.3X1	T50.3X2	T50.3X3	T50.3X4	T50.3X5	T50.3X6
with glucose	T50.3X1	T50.3X2	T50.3X3	T50.3X4	T50.3X5	T50.3X6
chromate	T65.891	T65.892	T65.893	T65.894	—	—
citrate	T50.991	T50.992	T50.993	T50.994	T50.995	T50.996
cromoglicate	T48.6X1	T48.6X2	T48.6X3	T48.6X4	T48.6X5	T48.6X6
cyanide	T65.0X1	T65.0X2	T65.0X3	T65.0X4	—	—
cyclamate	T50.3X1	T50.3X2	T50.3X3	T50.3X4	T50.3X5	T50.3X6

Substance	Poisoning, Accidental (Unintentional)	Poisoning, Intentional Self-Harm	Poisoning, Assault	Poisoning, Undetermined	Adverse Effect	Underdosing
Sodium (Continued)						
dehydrocholate	T45.8X1	T45.8X2	T45.8X3	T45.8X4	T45.8X5	T45.8X6
diatrizoate	T50.8X1	T50.8X2	T50.8X3	T50.8X4	T50.8X5	T50.8X6
dibunate	T48.4X1	T48.4X2	T48.4X3	T48.4X4	T48.4X5	T48.4X6
dioctyl sulfosuccinate	T47.4X1	T47.4X2	T47.4X3	T47.4X4	T47.4X5	T47.4X6
dipantoyl ferrate	T45.8X1	T45.8X2	T45.8X3	T45.8X4	T45.8X5	T45.8X6
edetate	T45.8X1	T45.8X2	T45.8X3	T45.8X4	T45.8X5	T45.8X6
ethacrynate	T50.1X1	T50.1X2	T50.1X3	T50.1X4	T50.1X5	T50.1X6
feredetate	T45.8X1	T45.8X2	T45.8X3	T45.8X4	T45.8X5	T45.8X6
Fluoride — see Fluoride						
fluoroacetate (dust) (pesticide)	T60.4X1	T60.4X2	T60.4X3	T60.4X4	—	—
free salt	T50.3X1	T50.3X2	T50.3X3	T50.3X4	T50.3X5	T50.3X6
fusidate	T36.8X1	T36.8X2	T36.8X3	T36.8X4	T36.8X5	T36.8X6
glucaldrate	T47.1X1	T47.1X2	T47.1X3	T47.1X4	T47.1X5	T47.1X6
glucosulfone	T37.1X1	T37.1X2	T37.1X3	T37.1X4	T37.1X5	T37.1X6
glutamate	T45.8X1	T45.8X2	T45.8X3	T45.8X4	T45.8X5	T45.8X6
hydrogen carbonate	T50.3X1	T50.3X2	T50.3X3	T50.3X4	T50.3X5	T50.3X6
hydroxide	T54.3X1	T54.3X2	T54.3X3	T54.3X4	—	—
hypochlorite (bleach) NEC	T54.3X1	T54.3X2	T54.3X3	T54.3X4	—	—
disinfectant	T54.3X1	T54.3X2	T54.3X3	T54.3X4	—	—
medicinal (anti-infective) (external)	T49.0X1	T49.0X2	T49.0X3	T49.0X4	T49.0X5	T49.0X6
vapor	T54.3X1	T54.3X2	T54.3X3	T54.3X4	—	—
hyposulfite	T49.0X1	T49.0X2	T49.0X3	T49.0X4	T49.0X5	T49.0X6
indigotin disulfonate	T50.8X1	T50.8X2	T50.8X3	T50.8X4	T50.8X5	T50.8X6
iodide	T50.991	T50.992	T50.993	T50.994	T50.995	T50.996
I-131	T50.8X1	T50.8X2	T50.8X3	T50.8X4	T50.8X5	T50.8X6
therapeutic	T38.2X1	T38.2X2	T38.2X3	T38.2X4	T38.2X5	T38.2X6
iodohippurate (131I)	T50.8X1	T50.8X2	T50.8X3	T50.8X4	T50.8X5	T50.8X6
iopodate	T50.8X1	T50.8X2	T50.8X3	T50.8X4	T50.8X5	T50.8X6
iothalamate	T50.8X1	T50.8X2	T50.8X3	T50.8X4	T50.8X5	T50.8X6
iron edetate	T45.4X1	T45.4X2	T45.4X3	T45.4X4	T45.4X5	T45.4X6
lactate (compound solution)	T45.8X1	T45.8X2	T45.8X3	T45.8X4	T45.8X5	T45.8X6
lauryl (sulfate)	T49.2X1	T49.2X2	T49.2X3	T49.2X4	T49.2X5	T49.2X6
(L)-triiodothyronine	T38.1X1	T38.1X2	T38.1X3	T38.1X4	T38.1X5	T38.1X6
magnesium citrate	T50.991	T50.992	T50.993	T50.994	T50.995	T50.996
mersalate	T50.2X1	T50.2X2	T50.2X3	T50.2X4	T50.2X5	T50.2X6
metasilicate	T65.891	T65.892	T65.893	T65.894	—	—
metrizoate	T50.8X1	T50.8X2	T50.8X3	T50.8X4	T50.8X5	T50.8X6
monofluoroacetate (pesticide)	T60.1X1	T60.1X2	T60.1X3	T60.1X4	—	—
morrhuate	T46.8X1	T46.8X2	T46.8X3	T46.8X4	T46.8X5	T46.8X6
nafcillin	T36.0X1	T36.0X2	T36.0X3	T36.0X4	T36.0X5	T36.0X6

◀ New ◀ Revised ~~deleted~~ Deleted

Substance	Poisoning, Accidental (Unintentional)	Poisoning, Intentional Self-Harm	Poisoning, Assault	Poisoning, Undetermined	Adverse Effect	Underdosing
Sodium *(Continued)*						
nitrate (oxidizing agent)	T65.891	T65.892	T65.893	T65.894	—	—
nitrite	T50.6X1	T50.6X2	T50.6X3	T50.6X4	T50.6X5	T50.6X6
nitroferricyanide	T46.5X1	T46.5X2	T46.5X3	T46.5X4	T46.5X5	T46.5X6
nitroprusside	T46.5X1	T46.5X2	T46.5X3	T46.5X4	T46.5X5	T46.5X6
oxalate	T65.891	T65.892	T65.893	T65.894	—	—
oxide/peroxide	T65.891	T65.892	T65.893	T65.894	—	—
oxybate	T41.291	T41.292	T41.293	T41.294	T41.295	T41.296
para-aminohippurate	T50.8X1	T50.8X2	T50.8X3	T50.8X4	T50.8X5	T50.8X6
perborate (nonmedicinal) NEC	T65.891	T65.892	T65.893	T65.894	—	—
medicinal	T49.0X1	T49.0X2	T49.0X3	T49.0X4	T49.0X5	T49.0X6
soap	T55.0X1	T55.0X2	T55.0X3	T55.0X4		
percarbonate — see Sodium, perborate						
pertechnetate Tc99m	T50.8X1	T50.8X2	T50.8X3	T50.8X4	T50.8X5	T50.8X6
phosphate						
cellulose	T45.8X1	T45.8X2	T45.8X3	T45.8X4	T45.8X5	T45.8X6
dibasic	T47.2X1	T47.2X2	T47.2X3	T47.2X4	T47.2X5	T47.2X6
monobasic	T47.2X1	T47.2X2	T47.2X3	T47.2X4	T47.2X5	T47.2X6
phytate	T50.6X1	T50.6X2	T50.6X3	T50.6X4	T50.6X5	T50.6X6
picosulfate	T47.2X1	T47.2X2	T47.2X3	T47.2X4	T47.2X5	T47.2X6
polyhydroxyaluminium monocarbonate	T47.1X1	T47.1X2	T47.1X3	T47.1X4	T47.1X5	T47.1X6
polystyrene sulfonate	T50.3X1	T50.3X2	T50.3X3	T50.3X4	T50.3X5	T50.3X6
propionate	T49.0X1	T49.0X2	T49.0X3	T49.0X4	T49.0X5	T49.0X6
propyl hydroxybenzoate	T50.991	T50.992	T50.993	T50.994	T50.995	T50.996
psylliate	T46.8X1	T46.8X2	T46.8X3	T46.8X4	T46.8X5	T46.8X6
removing resins	T50.3X1	T50.3X2	T50.3X3	T50.3X4	T50.3X5	T50.3X6
salicylate	T39.091	T39.092	T39.093	T39.094	T39.095	T39.096
salt NEC	T50.3X1	T50.3X2	T50.3X3	T50.3X4	T50.3X5	T50.3X6
selenate	T60.2X1	T60.2X2	T60.2X3	T60.2X4	—	—
stibogluconate	T37.3X1	T37.3X2	T37.3X3	T37.3X4	T37.3X5	T37.3X6
sulfate	T47.4X1	T47.4X2	T47.4X3	T47.4X4	T47.4X5	T47.4X6
sulfoxone	T37.1X1	T37.1X2	T37.1X3	T37.1X4	T37.1X5	T37.1X6
tetradecyl sulfate	T46.8X1	T46.8X2	T46.8X3	T46.8X4	T46.8X5	T46.8X6
thiopental	T41.1X1	T41.1X2	T41.1X3	T41.1X4	T41.1X5	T41.1X6
thiosalicylate	T39.091	T39.092	T39.093	T39.094	T39.095	T39.096
thiosulfate	T50.6X1	T50.6X2	T50.6X3	T50.6X4	T50.6X5	T50.6X6
tolbutamide	T38.3X1	T38.3X2	T38.3X3	T38.3X4	T38.3X5	T38.3X6
l-triiodothyronine	T38.1X1	T38.1X2	T38.1X3	T38.1X4	T38.1X5	T38.1X6
tyropanoate	T50.8X1	T50.8X2	T50.8X3	T50.8X4	T50.8X5	T50.8X6
valproate	T42.6X1	T42.6X2	T42.6X3	T42.6X4	T42.6X5	T42.6X6
versenate	T50.6X1	T50.6X2	T50.6X3	T50.6X4	T50.6X5	T50.6X6

Substance	Poisoning, Accidental (Unintentional)	Poisoning, Intentional Self-Harm	Poisoning, Assault	Poisoning, Undetermined	Adverse Effect	Underdosing
Sodium-free salt	T50.901	T50.902	T50.903	T50.904	T50.905	T50.906
Sodium-removing resin	T50.3X1	T50.3X2	T50.3X3	T50.3X4	T50.3X5	T50.3X6
Soft soap	T55.0X1	T55.0X2	T55.0X3	T55.0X4	—	—
Solanine	T62.2X1	T62.2X2	T62.2X3	T62.2X4	—	—
berries	T62.1X1	T62.1X2	T62.1X3	T62.1X4	—	—
Solanum dulcamara	T62.2X1	T62.2X2	T62.2X3	T62.2X4	—	—
berries	T62.1X1	T62.1X2	T62.1X3	T62.1X4	—	—
Solapsone	T37.1X1	T37.1X2	T37.1X3	T37.1X4	T37.1X5	T37.1X6
Solar lotion	T49.3X1	T49.3X2	T49.3X3	T49.3X4	T49.3X5	T49.3X6
Solasulfone	T37.1X1	T37.1X2	T37.1X3	T37.1X4	T37.1X5	T37.1X6
Soldering fluid	T65.891	T65.892	T65.893	T65.894	—	—
Solid substance	T65.91	T65.92	T65.93	T65.94	—	—
specified NEC	T65.891	T65.892	T65.893	T65.894	—	—
Solvent, industrial NEC	T52.91	T52.92	T52.93	T52.94	—	—
naphtha	T52.0X1	T52.0X2	T52.0X3	T52.0X4	—	—
petroleum	T52.0X1	T52.0X2	T52.0X3	T52.0X4	—	—
specified NEC	T52.8X1	T52.8X2	T52.8X3	T52.8X4	—	—
Soma	T42.8X1	T42.8X2	T42.8X3	T42.8X4	T42.8X5	T42.8X6
Somatorelin	T38.891	T38.892	T38.893	T38.894	T38.895	T38.896
Somatostatin	T38.991	T38.992	T38.993	T38.994	T38.995	T38.996
Somatotropin	T38.811	T38.812	T38.813	T38.814	T38.815	T38.816
Somatrem	T38.811	T38.812	T38.813	T38.814	T38.815	T38.816
Somatropin	T38.811	T38.812	T38.813	T38.814	T38.815	T38.816
Sominex	T45.0X1	T45.0X2	T45.0X3	T45.0X4	T45.0X5	T45.0X6
Somnos	T42.6X1	T42.6X2	T42.6X3	T42.6X4	T42.6X5	T42.6X6
Somonal	T42.3X1	T42.3X2	T42.3X3	T42.3X4	T42.3X5	T42.3X6
Soneryl	T42.3X1	T42.3X2	T42.3X3	T42.3X4	T42.3X5	T42.3X6
Soothing syrup	T50.901	T50.902	T50.903	T50.904	T50.905	T50.906
Sopor	T42.6X1	T42.6X2	T42.6X3	T42.6X4	T42.6X5	T42.6X6
Soporific	T42.71	T42.72	T42.73	T42.74	T42.75	T42.76
Soporific drug	T42.71	T42.72	T42.73	T42.74	T42.75	T42.76
specified type NEC	T42.6X1	T42.6X2	T42.6X3	T42.6X4	T42.6X5	T42.6X6
Sorbide nitrate	T46.3X1	T46.3X2	T46.3X3	T46.3X4	T46.3X5	T46.3X6
Sorbitol	T47.4X1	T47.4X2	T47.4X3	T47.4X4	T47.4X5	T47.4X6
Sotalol	T44.7X1	T44.7X2	T44.7X3	T44.7X4	T44.7X5	T44.7X6
Sotradecol	T46.8X1	T46.8X2	T46.8X3	T46.8X4	T46.8X5	T46.8X6
Soysterol	T46.6X1	T46.6X2	T46.6X3	T46.6X4	T46.6X5	T46.6X6
Spacoline	T44.3X1	T44.3X2	T44.3X3	T44.3X4	T44.3X5	T44.3X6
Spanish fly	T49.8X1	T49.8X2	T49.8X3	T49.8X4	T49.8X5	T49.8X6
Sparine	T43.3X1	T43.3X2	T43.3X3	T43.3X4	T43.3X5	T43.3X6
Sparteine	T48.0X1	T48.0X2	T48.0X3	T48.0X4	T48.0X5	T48.0X6

◀ New ◀ Revised ~~deleted~~ Deleted

Substance	External Cause (T-Code)					
	Poisoning, Accidental (Unintentional)	Poisoning, Intentional Self-Harm	Poisoning, Assault	Poisoning, Undetermined	Adverse Effect	Underdosing
Spasmolytic						
anticholinergics	T44.3X1	T44.3X2	T44.3X3	T44.3X4	T44.3X5	T44.3X6
autonomic	T44.3X1	T44.3X2	T44.3X3	T44.3X4	T44.3X5	T44.3X6
bronchial NEC	T48.6X1	T48.6X2	T48.6X3	T48.6X4	T48.6X5	T48.6X6
quaternary ammonium	T44.3X1	T44.3X2	T44.3X3	T44.3X4	T44.3X5	T44.3X6
skeletal muscle NEC	T48.1X1	T48.1X2	T48.1X3	T48.1X4	T48.1X5	T48.1X6
Spectinomycin	T36.5X1	T36.5X2	T36.5X3	T36.5X4	T36.5X5	T36.5X6
Speed	T43.651	T43.652	T43.652	T43.654	T43.655	T43.656
Spermicide	T49.8X1	T49.8X2	T49.8X3	T49.8X4	T49.8X5	T49.8X6
Spider (bite) (venom)	T63.391	T63.392	T63.393	T63.394	—	—
antivenin	T50.Z11	T50.Z12	T50.Z13	T50.Z14	T50.Z15	T50.Z16
Spigelia (root)	T37.4X1	T37.4X2	T37.4X3	T37.4X4	T37.4X5	T37.4X6
Spindle inactivator	T50.4X1	T50.4X2	T50.4X3	T50.4X4	T50.4X5	T50.4X6
Spiperone	T43.4X1	T43.4X2	T43.4X3	T43.4X4	T43.4X5	T43.4X6
Spiramycin	T36.3X1	T36.3X2	T36.3X3	T36.3X4	T36.3X5	T36.3X6
Spirapril	T46.4X1	T46.4X2	T46.4X3	T46.4X4	T46.4X5	T46.4X6
Spirilene	T43.591	T43.592	T43.593	T43.594	T43.595	T43.596
Spirit(s) (neutral) NEC	T51.0X1	T51.0X2	T51.0X3	T51.0X4	—	—
beverage	T51.0X1	T51.0X2	T51.0X3	T51.0X4	—	—
industrial	T51.0X1	T51.0X2	T51.0X3	T51.0X4	—	—
mineral	T52.0X1	T52.0X2	T52.0X3	T52.0X4	—	—
of salt — see Hydrochloric acid						
surgical	T51.0X1	T51.0X2	T51.0X3	T51.0X4	—	—
Spironolactone	T50.0X1	T50.0X2	T50.0X3	T50.0X4	T50.0X5	T50.0X6
Spiroperidol	T43.4X1	T43.4X2	T43.4X3	T43.4X4	T43.4X5	T43.4X6
Sponge, absorbable (gelatin)	T45.7X1	T45.7X2	T45.7X3	T45.7X4	T45.7X5	T45.7X6
Sporostacin	T49.0X1	T49.0X2	T49.0X3	T49.0X4	T49.0X5	T49.0X6
Spray (aerosol)	T65.91	T65.92	T65.93	T65.94	—	—
cosmetic	T65.891	T65.892	T65.893	T65.894	—	—
medicinal NEC	T50.901	T50.902	T50.903	T50.904	T50.905	T50.906
pesticides — see Pesticide						
specified content — see specific substance						
Spurge flax	T62.2X1	T62.2X2	T62.2X3	T62.2X4	—	—
Spurges	T62.2X1	T62.2X2	T62.2X3	T62.2X4	—	—
Sputum viscosity-lowering drug	T48.4X1	T48.4X2	T48.4X3	T48.4X4	T48.4X5	T48.4X6
Squill	T46.0X1	T46.0X2	T46.0X3	T46.0X4	T46.0X5	T46.0X6
rat poison	T60.4X1	T60.4X2	T60.4X3	T60.4X4	—	—
Squirting cucumber (cathartic)	T47.2X1	T47.2X2	T47.2X3	T47.2X4	T47.2X5	T47.2X6
Stains	T65.6X1	T65.6X2	T65.6X3	T65.6X4	—	—
Stannous fluoride	T49.7X1	T49.7X2	T49.7X3	T49.7X4	T49.7X5	T49.7X6
Stanolone	T38.7X1	T38.7X2	T38.7X3	T38.7X4	T38.7X5	T38.7X6

Substance	External Cause (T-Code)					
	Poisoning, Accidental (Unintentional)	Poisoning, Intentional Self-Harm	Poisoning, Assault	Poisoning, Undetermined	Adverse Effect	Underdosing
Stanozolol	T38.7X1	T38.7X2	T38.7X3	T38.7X4	T38.7X5	T38.7X6
Staphisagria or stavesacre (pediculicide)	T49.0X1	T49.0X2	T49.0X3	T49.0X4	T49.0X5	T49.0X6
Starch	T50.901	T50.902	T50.903	T50.904	T50.905	T50.906
Stelazine	T43.3X1	T43.3X2	T43.3X3	T43.3X4	T43.3X5	T43.3X6
Stemetil	T43.3X1	T43.3X2	T43.3X3	T43.3X4	T43.3X5	T43.3X6
Stepronin	T48.4X1	T48.4X2	T48.4X3	T48.4X4	T48.4X5	T48.4X6
Sterculia	T47.4X1	T47.4X2	T47.4X3	T47.4X4	T47.4X5	T47.4X6
Sternutator gas	T59.891	T59.892	T59.893	T59.894	—	—
Steroid	T38.0X1	T38.0X2	T38.0X3	T38.0X4	T38.0X5	T38.0X6
anabolic	T38.7X1	T38.7X2	T38.7X3	T38.7X4	T38.7X5	T38.7X6
androgenic	T38.7X1	T38.7X2	T38.7X3	T38.7X4	T38.7X5	T38.7X6
antineoplastic, hormone	T38.7X1	T38.7X2	T38.7X3	T38.7X4	T38.7X5	T38.7X6
estrogen	T38.5X1	T38.5X2	T38.5X3	T38.5X4	T38.5X5	T38.5X6
ENT agent	T49.6X1	T49.6X2	T49.6X3	T49.6X4	T49.6X5	T49.6X6
ophthalmic preparation	T49.5X1	T49.5X2	T49.5X3	T49.5X4	T49.5X5	T49.5X6
topical NEC	T49.0X1	T49.0X2	T49.0X3	T49.0X4	T49.0X5	T49.0X6
Stibine	T56.891	T56.892	T56.893	T56.894	—	—
Stibogluconate	T37.3X1	T37.3X2	T37.3X3	T37.3X4	T37.3X5	T37.3X6
Stibophen	T37.4X1	T37.4X2	T37.4X3	T37.4X4	T37.4X5	T37.4X6
Stilbamidine (isetionate)	T37.3X1	T37.3X2	T37.3X3	T37.3X4	T37.3X5	T37.3X6
Stilbestrol	T38.5X1	T38.5X2	T38.5X3	T38.5X4	T38.5X5	T38.5X6
Stilboestrol	T38.5X1	T38.5X2	T38.5X3	T38.5X4	T38.5X5	T38.5X6
Stimulant						
central nervous system — see also Psychostimulant	T43.601	T43.602	T43.603	T43.604	T43.605	T43.606
analeptics	T50.7X1	T50.7X2	T50.7X3	T50.7X4	T50.7X5	T50.7X6
opiate antagonist	T50.7X1	T50.7X2	T50.7X3	T50.7X4	T50.7X5	T50.7X6
psychotherapeutic NEC — see also Psychotherapeutic drug	T43.601	T43.602	T43.603	T43.604	T43.605	T43.606
specified NEC	T43.691	T43.692	T43.693	T43.694	T43.695	T43.696
respiratory	T48.901	T48.902	T48.903	T48.904	T48.905	T48.906
Stone-dissolving drug	T50.901	T50.902	T50.903	T50.904	T50.905	T50.906
Storage battery (cells) (acid)	T54.2X1	T54.2X2	T54.2X3	T54.2X4	—	—
Stovaine	T41.3X1	T41.3X2	T41.3X3	T41.3X4	T41.3X5	T41.3X6
infiltration (subcutaneous)	T41.3X1	T41.3X2	T41.3X3	T41.3X4	T41.3X5	T41.3X6
nerve block (peripheral) (plexus)	T41.3X1	T41.3X2	T41.3X3	T41.3X4	T41.3X5	T41.3X6
spinal	T41.3X1	T41.3X2	T41.3X3	T41.3X4	T41.3X5	T41.3X6
topical (surface)	T41.3X1	T41.3X2	T41.3X3	T41.3X4	T41.3X5	T41.3X6
Stovarsal	T37.8X1	T37.8X2	T37.8X3	T37.8X4	T37.8X5	T37.8X6
Stove gas — see Gas, stove	T57.91	T57.92	T57.93	T57.94	—	—

◀ New ◀ Revised ~~deleted~~ Deleted

Substance	External Cause (T-Code)					
	Poisoning, Accidental (Unintentional)	Poisoning, Intentional Self-Harm	Poisoning, Assault	Poisoning, Undetermined	Adverse Effect	Underdosing
Stoxil	T49.5X1	T49.5X2	T49.5X3	T49.5X4	T49.5X5	T49.5X6
Stramonium	T48.6X1	T48.6X2	T48.6X3	T48.6X4	T48.6X5	T48.6X6
natural state	T62.2X1	T62.2X2	T62.2X3	T62.2X4	—	—
Streptodornase	T45.3X1	T45.3X2	T45.3X3	T45.3X4	T45.3X5	T45.3X6
Streptoduocin	T36.5X1	T36.5X2	T36.5X3	T36.5X4	T36.5X5	T36.5X6
Streptokinase	T45.611	T45.612	T45.613	T45.614	T45.615	T45.616
Streptomycin (derivative)	T36.5X1	T36.5X2	T36.5X3	T36.5X4	T36.5X5	T36.5X6
Streptonivicin	T36.5X1	T36.5X2	T36.5X3	T36.5X4	T36.5X5	T36.5X6
Streptovarycin	T36.5X1	T36.5X2	T36.5X3	T36.5X4	T36.5X5	T36.5X6
Streptozocin	T45.1X1	T45.1X2	T45.1X3	T45.1X4	T45.1X5	T45.1X6
Streptozotocin	T45.1X1	T45.1X2	T45.1X3	T45.1X4	T45.1X5	T45.1X6
Stripper (paint) (solvent)	T52.8X1	T52.8X2	T52.8X3	T52.8X4	—	—
Strobane	T60.1X1	T60.1X2	T60.1X3	T60.1X4	—	—
Strofantina	T46.0X1	T46.0X2	T46.0X3	T46.0X4	T46.0X5	T46.0X6
Strophanthin (g) (k)	T46.0X1	T46.0X2	T46.0X3	T46.0X4	T46.0X5	T46.0X6
Strophanthus	T46.0X1	T46.0X2	T46.0X3	T46.0X4	T46.0X5	T46.0X6
Strophantin	T46.0X1	T46.0X2	T46.0X3	T46.0X4	T46.0X5	T46.0X6
Strophantin-g	T46.0X1	T46.0X2	T46.0X3	T46.0X4	T46.0X5	T46.0X6
Strychnine (nonmedicinal) (pesticide) (salts)	T65.1X1	T65.1X2	T65.1X3	T65.1X4	—	—
medicinal	T48.291	T48.292	T48.293	T48.294	T48.295	T48.296
Strychnos (ignatii) — *see* Strychnine						
Styramate	T42.8X1	T42.8X2	T42.8X3	T42.8X4	T42.8X5	T42.8X6
Styrene	T65.891	T65.892	T65.893	T65.894	—	—
Succinimide, antiepileptic or anticonvulsant	T42.2X1	T42.2X2	T42.2X3	T42.2X4	T42.2X5	T42.2X6
mercuric — *see* Mercury						
Succinylcholine	T48.1X1	T48.1X2	T48.1X3	T48.1X4	T48.1X5	T48.1X6
Succinylsulfathiazole	T37.0X1	T37.0X2	T37.0X3	T37.0X4	T37.0X5	T37.0X6
Sucralfate	T47.1X1	T47.1X2	T47.1X3	T47.1X4	T47.1X5	T47.1X6
Sucrose	T50.3X1	T50.3X2	T50.3X3	T50.3X4	T50.3X5	T50.3X6
Sufentanil	T40.411	T40.412	T40.413	T40.414	T40.415	T40.416
Sulbactam	T36.0X1	T36.0X2	T36.0X3	T36.0X4	T36.0X5	T36.0X6
Sulbenicillin	T36.0X1	T36.0X2	T36.0X3	T36.0X4	T36.0X5	T36.0X6
Sulbentine	T49.0X1	T49.0X2	T49.0X3	T49.0X4	T49.0X5	T49.0X6
Sulfacetamide	T49.0X1	T49.0X2	T49.0X3	T49.0X4	T49.0X5	T49.0X6
ophthalmic preparation	T49.5X1	T49.5X2	T49.5X3	T49.5X4	T49.5X5	T49.5X6
Sulfachlorpyridazine	T37.0X1	T37.0X2	T37.0X3	T37.0X4	T37.0X5	T37.0X6
Sulfacitine	T37.0X1	T37.0X2	T37.0X3	T37.0X4	T37.0X5	T37.0X6
Sulfadiasulfone sodium	T37.0X1	T37.0X2	T37.0X3	T37.0X4	T37.0X5	T37.0X6
Sulfadiazine	T37.0X1	T37.0X2	T37.0X3	T37.0X4	T37.0X5	T37.0X6
silver (topical)	T49.0X1	T49.0X2	T49.0X3	T49.0X4	T49.0X5	T49.0X6

Substance	External Cause (T-Code)					
	Poisoning, Accidental (Unintentional)	Poisoning, Intentional Self-Harm	Poisoning, Assault	Poisoning, Undetermined	Adverse Effect	Underdosing
Sulfadimethoxine	T37.0X1	T37.0X2	T37.0X3	T37.0X4	T37.0X5	T37.0X6
Sulfadimidine	T37.0X1	T37.0X2	T37.0X3	T37.0X4	T37.0X5	T37.0X6
Sulfadoxine	T37.0X1	T37.0X2	T37.0X3	T37.0X4	T37.0X5	T37.0X6
with pyrimethamine	T37.2X1	T37.2X2	T37.2X3	T37.2X4	T37.2X5	T37.2X6
Sulfaethidole	T37.0X1	T37.0X2	T37.0X3	T37.0X4	T37.0X5	T37.0X6
Sulfafurazole	T37.0X1	T37.0X2	T37.0X3	T37.0X4	T37.0X5	T37.0X6
Sulfaguanidine	T37.0X1	T37.0X2	T37.0X3	T37.0X4	T37.0X5	T37.0X6
Sulfalene	T37.0X1	T37.0X2	T37.0X3	T37.0X4	T37.0X5	T37.0X6
Sulfaloxate	T37.0X1	T37.0X2	T37.0X3	T37.0X4	T37.0X5	T37.0X6
Sulfaloxic acid	T37.0X1	T37.0X2	T37.0X3	T37.0X4	T37.0X5	T37.0X6
Sulfamazone	T39.2X1	T39.2X2	T39.2X3	T39.2X4	T39.2X5	T39.2X6
Sulfamerazine	T37.0X1	T37.0X2	T37.0X3	T37.0X4	T37.0X5	T37.0X6
Sulfameter	T37.0X1	T37.0X2	T37.0X3	T37.0X4	T37.0X5	T37.0X6
Sulfamethazine	T37.0X1	T37.0X2	T37.0X3	T37.0X4	T37.0X5	T37.0X6
Sulfamethizole	T37.0X1	T37.0X2	T37.0X3	T37.0X4	T37.0X5	T37.0X6
Sulfamethoxazole	T37.0X1	T37.0X2	T37.0X3	T37.0X4	T37.0X5	T37.0X6
with trimethoprim	T36.8X1	T36.8X2	T36.8X3	T36.8X4	T36.8X5	T36.8X6
Sulfamethoxydiazine	T37.0X1	T37.0X2	T37.0X3	T37.0X4	T37.0X5	T37.0X6
Sulfamethoxypyridazine	T37.0X1	T37.0X2	T37.0X3	T37.0X4	T37.0X5	T37.0X6
Sulfamethylthiazole	T37.0X1	T37.0X2	T37.0X3	T37.0X4	T37.0X5	T37.0X6
Sulfametoxydiazine	T37.0X1	T37.0X2	T37.0X3	T37.0X4	T37.0X5	T37.0X6
Sulfamidopyrine	T39.2X1	T39.2X2	T39.2X3	T39.2X4	T39.2X5	T39.2X6
Sulfamonomethoxine	T37.0X1	T37.0X2	T37.0X3	T37.0X4	T37.0X5	T37.0X6
Sulfamoxole	T37.0X1	T37.0X2	T37.0X3	T37.0X4	T37.0X5	T37.0X6
Sulfamylon	T49.0X1	T49.0X2	T49.0X3	T49.0X4	T49.0X5	T49.0X6
Sulfan blue (diagnostic dye)	T50.8X1	T50.8X2	T50.8X3	T50.8X4	T50.8X5	T50.8X6
Sulfanilamide	T37.0X1	T37.0X2	T37.0X3	T37.0X4	T37.0X5	T37.0X6
Sulfanilylguanidine	T37.0X1	T37.0X2	T37.0X3	T37.0X4	T37.0X5	T37.0X6
Sulfaperin	T37.0X1	T37.0X2	T37.0X3	T37.0X4	T37.0X5	T37.0X6
Sulfaphenazole	T37.0X1	T37.0X2	T37.0X3	T37.0X4	T37.0X5	T37.0X6
Sulfaphenylthiazole	T37.0X1	T37.0X2	T37.0X3	T37.0X4	T37.0X5	T37.0X6
Sulfaproxyline	T37.0X1	T37.0X2	T37.0X3	T37.0X4	T37.0X5	T37.0X6
Sulfapyridine	T37.0X1	T37.0X2	T37.0X3	T37.0X4	T37.0X5	T37.0X6
Sulfapyrimidine	T37.0X1	T37.0X2	T37.0X3	T37.0X4	T37.0X5	T37.0X6
Sulfarsphenamine	T37.8X1	T37.8X2	T37.8X3	T37.8X4	T37.8X5	T37.8X6
Sulfasalazine	T37.0X1	T37.0X2	T37.0X3	T37.0X4	T37.0X5	T37.0X6
Sulfasuxidine	T37.0X1	T37.0X2	T37.0X3	T37.0X4	T37.0X5	T37.0X6
Sulfasymazine	T37.0X1	T37.0X2	T37.0X3	T37.0X4	T37.0X5	T37.0X6
Sulfated amylopectin	T47.8X1	T47.8X2	T47.8X3	T47.8X4	T47.8X5	T47.8X6
Sulfathiazole	T37.0X1	T37.0X2	T37.0X3	T37.0X4	T37.0X5	T37.0X6
Sulfatostearate	T49.2X1	T49.2X2	T49.2X3	T49.2X4	T49.2X5	T49.2X6
Sulfinpyrazone	T50.4X1	T50.4X2	T50.4X3	T50.4X4	T50.4X5	T50.4X6

◄ New   ◄ Revised   ~~deleted~~ Deleted

	External Cause (T-Code)					
Substance	Poisoning, Accidental (Unintentional)	Poisoning, Intentional Self-Harm	Poisoning, Assault	Poisoning, Undetermined	Adverse Effect	Underdosing
Sulfiram	T49.0X1	T49.0X2	T49.0X3	T49.0X4	T49.0X5	T49.0X6
Sulfisomidine	T37.0X1	T37.0X2	T37.0X3	T37.0X4	T37.0X5	T37.0X6
Sulfisoxazole	T37.0X1	T37.0X2	T37.0X3	T37.0X4	T37.0X5	T37.0X6
ophthalmic preparation	T49.5X1	T49.5X2	T49.5X3	T49.5X4	T49.5X5	T49.5X6
Sulfobromophthalein (sodium)	T50.8X1	T50.8X2	T50.8X3	T50.8X4	T50.8X5	T50.8X6
Sulfobromphthalein	T50.8X1	T50.8X2	T50.8X3	T50.8X4	T50.8X5	T50.8X6
Sulfogaiacol	T48.4X1	T48.4X2	T48.4X3	T48.4X4	T48.4X5	T48.4X6
Sulfomyxin	T36.8X1	T36.8X2	T36.8X3	T36.8X4	T36.8X5	T36.8X6
Sulfonal	T42.6X1	T42.6X2	T42.6X3	T42.6X4	T42.6X5	T42.6X6
Sulfonamide NEC	T37.0X1	T37.0X2	T37.0X3	T37.0X4	T37.0X5	T37.0X6
eye	T49.5X1	T49.5X2	T49.5X3	T49.5X4	T49.5X5	T49.5X6
Sulfonazide	T37.1X1	T37.1X2	T37.1X3	T37.1X4	T37.1X5	T37.1X6
Sulfones	T37.1X1	T37.1X2	T37.1X3	T37.1X4	T37.1X5	T37.1X6
Sulfonethylmethane	T42.6X1	T42.6X2	T42.6X3	T42.6X4	T42.6X5	T42.6X6
Sulfonmethane	T42.6X1	T42.6X2	T42.6X3	T42.6X4	T42.6X5	T42.6X6
Sulfonphthal, sulfonphthol	T50.8X1	T50.8X2	T50.8X3	T50.8X4	T50.8X5	T50.8X6
Sulfonylurea derivatives, oral	T38.3X1	T38.3X2	T38.3X3	T38.3X4	T38.3X5	T38.3X6
Sulforidazine	T43.3X1	T43.3X2	T43.3X3	T43.3X4	T43.3X5	T43.3X6
Sulfoxone	T37.1X1	T37.1X2	T37.1X3	T37.1X4	T37.1X5	T37.1X6
Sulfur, sulfurated, sulfuric, sulfurous, sulfuryl (compounds NEC) (medicinal)	T49.4X1	T49.4X2	T49.4X3	T49.4X4	T49.4X5	T49.4X6
acid	T54.2X1	T54.2X2	T54.2X3	T54.2X4	—	—
dioxide (gas)	T59.1X1	T59.1X2	T59.1X3	T59.1X4	—	—
ether — see Ether(s)						
hydrogen	T59.6X1	T59.6X2	T59.6X3	T59.6X4	—	—
medicinal (keratolytic) (ointment) NEC	T49.4X1	T49.4X2	T49.4X3	T49.4X4	T49.4X5	T49.4X6
ointment	T49.0X1	T49.0X2	T49.0X3	T49.0X4	T49.0X5	T49.0X6
pesticide (vapor)	T60.91	T60.92	T60.93	T60.94	—	—
vapor NEC	T59.891	T59.892	T59.893	T59.894	—	—
Sulfuric acid	T54.2X1	T54.2X2	T54.2X3	T54.2X4	—	—
Sulglicotide	T47.1X1	T47.1X2	T47.1X3	T47.1X4	T47.1X5	T47.1X6
Sulindac	T39.391	T39.392	T39.393	T39.394	T39.395	T39.396
Sulisatin	T47.2X1	T47.2X2	T47.2X3	T47.2X4	T47.2X5	T47.2X6
Sulisobenzone	T49.3X1	T49.3X2	T49.3X3	T49.3X4	T49.3X5	T49.3X6
Sulkowitch's reagent	T50.8X1	T50.8X2	T50.8X3	T50.8X4	T50.8X5	T50.8X6
Sulmetozine	T44.3X1	T44.3X2	T44.3X3	T44.3X4	T44.3X5	T44.3X6
Suloctidil	T46.7X1	T46.7X2	T46.7X3	T46.7X4	T46.7X5	T46.7X6
Sulph — see also Sulf-						
Sulphadiazine	T37.0X1	T37.0X2	T37.0X3	T37.0X4	T37.0X5	T37.0X6
Sulphadimethoxine	T37.0X1	T37.0X2	T37.0X3	T37.0X4	T37.0X5	T37.0X6

	External Cause (T-Code)					
Substance	Poisoning, Accidental (Unintentional)	Poisoning, Intentional Self-Harm	Poisoning, Assault	Poisoning, Undetermined	Adverse Effect	Underdosing
Sulphadimidine	T37.0X1	T37.0X2	T37.0X3	T37.0X4	T37.0X5	T37.0X6
Sulphadione	T37.1X1	T37.1X2	T37.1X3	T37.1X4	T37.1X5	T37.1X6
Sulphafurazole	T37.0X1	T37.0X2	T37.0X3	T37.0X4	T37.0X5	T37.0X6
Sulphamethizole	T37.0X1	T37.0X2	T37.0X3	T37.0X4	T37.0X5	T37.0X6
Sulphamethoxazole	T37.0X1	T37.0X2	T37.0X3	T37.0X4	T37.0X5	T37.0X6
Sulphan blue	T50.8X1	T50.8X2	T50.8X3	T50.8X4	T50.8X5	T50.8X6
Sulphaphenazole	T37.0X1	T37.0X2	T37.0X3	T37.0X4	T37.0X5	T37.0X6
Sulphapyridine	T37.0X1	T37.0X2	T37.0X3	T37.0X4	T37.0X5	T37.0X6
Sulphasalazine	T37.0X1	T37.0X2	T37.0X3	T37.0X4	T37.0X5	T37.0X6
Sulphinpyrazone	T50.4X1	T50.4X2	T50.4X3	T50.4X4	T50.4X5	T50.4X6
Sulpiride	T43.591	T43.592	T43.593	T43.594	T43.595	T43.596
Sulprostone	T48.0X1	T48.0X2	T48.0X3	T48.0X4	T48.0X5	T48.0X6
Sulpyrine	T39.2X1	T39.2X2	T39.2X3	T39.2X4	T39.2X5	T39.2X6
Sultamicillin	T36.0X1	T36.0X2	T36.0X3	T36.0X4	T36.0X5	T36.0X6
Sulthiame	T42.6X1	T42.6X2	T42.6X3	T42.6X4	T42.6X5	T42.6X6
Sultiame	T42.6X1	T42.6X2	T42.6X3	T42.6X4	T42.6X5	T42.6X6
Sultopride	T43.591	T43.592	T43.593	T43.594	T43.595	T43.596
Sumatriptan	T39.8X1	T39.8X2	T39.8X3	T39.8X4	T39.8X5	T39.8X6
Sunflower seed oil	T46.6X1	T46.6X2	T46.6X3	T46.6X4	T46.6X5	T46.6X6
Superinone	T48.4X1	T48.4X2	T48.4X3	T48.4X4	T48.4X5	T48.4X6
Suprofen	T39.311	T39.312	T39.313	T39.314	T39.315	T39.316
Suramin (sodium)	T37.4X1	T37.4X2	T37.4X3	T37.4X4	T37.4X5	T37.4X6
Surfacaine	T41.3X1	T41.3X2	T41.3X3	T41.3X4	T41.3X5	T41.3X6
Surital	T41.1X1	T41.1X2	T41.1X3	T41.1X4	T41.1X5	T41.1X6
Sutilains	T45.3X1	T45.3X2	T45.3X3	T45.3X4	T45.3X5	T45.3X6
Suxamethonium (chloride)	T48.1X1	T48.1X2	T48.1X3	T48.1X4	T48.1X5	T48.1X6
Suxethonium (chloride)	T48.1X1	T48.1X2	T48.1X3	T48.1X4	T48.1X5	T48.1X6
Suxibuzone	T39.2X1	T39.2X2	T39.2X3	T39.2X4	T39.2X5	T39.2X6
Sweet oil (birch)	T49.3X1	T49.3X2	T49.3X3	T49.3X4	T49.3X5	T49.3X6
Sweet niter spirit	T46.3X1	T46.3X2	T46.3X3	T46.3X4	T46.3X5	T46.3X6
Sweetener	T50.901	T50.902	T50.903	T50.904	T50.905	T50.906
Sym-dichloroethyl ether	T53.6X1	T53.6X2	T53.6X3	T53.6X4	—	—
Sympatholytic NEC	T44.8X1	T44.8X2	T44.8X3	T44.8X4	T44.8X5	T44.8X6
haloalkylamine	T44.8X1	T44.8X2	T44.8X3	T44.8X4	T44.8X5	T44.8X6
Sympathomimetic NEC	T44.901	T44.902	T44.903	T44.904	T44.905	T44.906
anti-common-cold	T48.5X1	T48.5X2	T48.5X3	T48.5X4	T48.5X5	T48.5X6
bronchodilator	T48.6X1	T48.6X2	T48.6X3	T48.6X4	T48.6X5	T48.6X6
specified NEC	T44.991	T44.992	T44.993	T44.994	T44.995	T44.996
Synagis	T50.B91	T50.B92	T50.B93	T50.B94	T50.B95	T50.B96
Synalar	T49.0X1	T49.0X2	T49.0X3	T49.0X4	T49.0X5	T49.0X6
Synthetic cannabinoids	T40.721	T40.722	T40.723	T40.724	T40.725	T40.726
Synthroid	T38.1X1	T38.1X2	T38.1X3	T38.1X4	T38.1X5	T38.1X6

◄ New ◄◄ Revised ~~deleted~~ Deleted

TABLE OF DRUGS AND CHEMICALS

Substance	Poisoning, Accidental (Unintentional)	Poisoning, Intentional Self-Harm	Poisoning, Assault	Poisoning, Undetermined	Adverse Effect	Underdosing
Syntocinon	T48.0X1	T48.0X2	T48.0X3	T48.0X4	T48.0X5	T48.0X6
Syrosingopine	T46.5X1	T46.5X2	T46.5X3	T46.5X4	T46.5X5	T46.5X6
Systemic drug	T45.91	T45.92	T45.93	T45.94	T45.95	T45.96
specified NEC	T45.8X1	T45.8X2	T45.8X3	T45.8X4	T45.8X5	T45.8X6
2,4,5-T	T60.3X1	T60.3X2	T60.3X3	T60.3X4	—	—

T

Substance	Poisoning, Accidental (Unintentional)	Poisoning, Intentional Self-Harm	Poisoning, Assault	Poisoning, Undetermined	Adverse Effect	Underdosing
Tablets — see also specified substance	T50.901	T50.902	T50.903	T50.904	T50.905	T50.906
Tace	T38.5X1	T38.5X2	T38.5X3	T38.5X4	T38.5X5	T38.5X6
Tacrine	T44.0X1	T44.0X2	T44.0X3	T44.0X4	T44.0X5	T44.0X6
Tadalafil	T46.7X1	T46.7X2	T46.7X3	T46.7X4	T46.7X5	T46.7X6
Talampicillin	T36.0X1	T36.0X2	T36.0X3	T36.0X4	T36.0X5	T36.0X6
Talbutal	T42.3X1	T42.3X2	T42.3X3	T42.3X4	T42.3X5	T42.3X6
Talc powder	T49.3X1	T49.3X2	T49.3X3	T49.3X4	T49.3X5	T49.3X6
Talcum	T49.3X1	T49.3X2	T49.3X3	T49.3X4	T49.3X5	T49.3X6
Taleranol	T38.6X1	T38.6X2	T38.6X3	T38.6X4	T38.6X5	T38.6X6
Tamoxifen	T38.6X1	T38.6X2	T38.6X3	T38.6X4	T38.6X5	T38.6X6
Tamsulosin	T44.6X1	T44.6X2	T44.6X3	T44.6X4	T44.6X5	T44.6X6
Tandearil, tanderil	T39.2X1	T39.2X2	T39.2X3	T39.2X4	T39.2X5	T39.2X6
Tannic acid	T49.2X1	T49.2X2	T49.2X3	T49.2X4	T49.2X5	T49.2X6
medicinal (astringent)	T49.2X1	T49.2X2	T49.2X3	T49.2X4	T49.2X5	T49.2X6
Tannin — see Tannic acid						
Tansy	T62.2X1	T62.2X2	T62.2X3	T62.2X4	—	—
TAO	T36.3X1	T36.3X2	T36.3X3	T36.3X4	T36.3X5	T36.3X6
Tapazole	T38.2X1	T38.2X2	T38.2X3	T38.2X4	T38.2X5	T38.2X6
Tar NEC	T52.0X1	T52.0X2	T52.0X3	T52.0X4	—	—
camphor	T60.1X1	T60.1X2	T60.1X3	T60.1X4	—	—
distillate	T49.1X1	T49.1X2	T49.1X3	T49.1X4	T49.1X5	T49.1X6
fumes	T59.891	T59.892	T59.893	T59.894	—	—
medicinal	T49.1X1	T49.1X2	T49.1X3	T49.1X4	T49.1X5	T49.1X6
ointment	T49.1X1	T49.1X2	T49.1X3	T49.1X4	T49.1X5	T49.1X6
Taractan	T43.591	T43.592	T43.593	T43.594	T43.595	T43.596
Tarantula (venomous)	T63.321	T63.322	T63.323	T63.324	—	—
Tartar emetic	T37.8X1	T37.8X2	T37.8X3	T37.8X4	T37.8X5	T37.8X6
Tartaric acid	T65.891	T65.892	T65.893	T65.894	—	—
Tartrated antimony (anti-infective)	T37.8X1	T37.8X2	T37.8X3	T37.8X4	T37.8X5	T37.8X6
Tartrate, laxative	T47.4X1	T47.4X2	T47.4X3	T47.4X4	T47.4X5	T47.4X6
Tauromustine	T45.1X1	T45.1X2	T45.1X3	T45.1X4	T45.1X5	T45.1X6
TCA — see Trichloroacetic acid						
TCDD	T53.7X1	T53.7X2	T53.7X3	T53.7X4	—	—
TDI (vapor)	T65.0X1	T65.0X2	T65.0X3	T65.0X4	—	—
Tear						
gas	T59.3X1	T59.3X2	T59.3X3	T59.3X4	—	—
solution	T49.5X1	T49.5X2	T49.5X3	T49.5X4	T49.5X5	T49.5X6
Teclothiazide	T50.2X1	T50.2X2	T50.2X3	T50.2X4	T50.2X5	T50.2X6
Teclozan	T37.3X1	T37.3X2	T37.3X3	T37.3X4	T37.3X5	T37.3X6
Tegafur	T45.1X1	T45.1X2	T45.1X3	T45.1X4	T45.1X5	T45.1X6
Tegretol	T42.1X1	T42.1X2	T42.1X3	T42.1X4	T42.1X5	T42.1X6
Teicoplanin	T36.8X1	T36.8X2	T36.8X3	T36.8X4	T36.8X5	T36.8X6
Telepaque	T50.8X1	T50.8X2	T50.8X3	T50.8X4	T50.8X5	T50.8X6
Tellurium	T56.891	T56.892	T56.893	T56.894	—	—
fumes	T56.891	T56.892	T56.893	T56.894	—	—
TEM	T45.1X1	T45.1X2	T45.1X3	T45.1X4	T45.1X5	T45.1X6
Temazepam	T42.4X1	T42.4X2	T42.4X3	T42.4X4	T42.4X5	T42.4X6
Temocillin	T36.0X1	T36.0X2	T36.0X3	T36.0X4	T36.0X5	T36.0X6
Tenamfetamine	T43.621	T43.622	T43.623	T43.624	T43.625	T43.626
Teniposide	T45.1X1	T45.1X2	T45.1X3	T45.1X4	T45.1X5	T45.1X6
Tenitramine	T46.3X1	T46.3X2	T46.3X3	T46.3X4	T46.3X5	T46.3X6
Tenoglicin	T48.4X1	T48.4X2	T48.4X3	T48.4X4	T48.4X5	T48.4X6
Tenonitrozole	T37.3X1	T37.3X2	T37.3X3	T37.3X4	T37.3X5	T37.3X6
Tenoxicam	T39.391	T39.392	T39.393	T39.394	T39.395	T39.396
TEPA	T45.1X1	T45.1X2	T45.1X3	T45.1X4	T45.1X5	T45.1X6
TEPP	T60.0X1	T60.0X2	T60.0X3	T60.0X4	—	—
Teprotide	T46.5X1	T46.5X2	T46.5X3	T46.5X4	T46.5X5	T46.5X6
Terazosin	T44.6X1	T44.6X2	T44.6X3	T44.6X4	T44.6X5	T44.6X6
Terbufos	T60.0X1	T60.0X2	T60.0X3	T60.0X4	—	—
Terbutaline	T48.6X1	T48.6X2	T48.6X3	T48.6X4	T48.6X5	T48.6X6
Terconazole	T49.0X1	T49.0X2	T49.0X3	T49.0X4	T49.0X5	T49.0X6
Terfenadine	T45.0X1	T45.0X2	T45.0X3	T45.0X4	T45.0X5	T45.0X6
Teriparatide (acetate)	T50.991	T50.992	T50.993	T50.994	T50.995	T50.996
Terizidone	T37.1X1	T37.1X2	T37.1X3	T37.1X4	T37.1X5	T37.1X6
Terlipressin	T38.891	T38.892	T38.893	T38.894	T38.895	T38.896
Terodiline	T46.3X1	T46.3X2	T46.3X3	T46.3X4	T46.3X5	T46.3X6
Teroxalene	T37.4X1	T37.4X2	T37.4X3	T37.4X4	T37.4X5	T37.4X6
Terpin(cis) hydrate	T48.4X1	T48.4X2	T48.4X3	T48.4X4	T48.4X5	T48.4X6
Terramycin	T36.4X1	T36.4X2	T36.4X3	T36.4X4	T36.4X5	T36.4X6
Tertatolol	T44.7X1	T44.7X2	T44.7X3	T44.7X4	T44.7X5	T44.7X6
Tessalon	T48.3X1	T48.3X2	T48.3X3	T48.3X4	T48.3X5	T48.3X6
Testolactone	T38.7X1	T38.7X2	T38.7X3	T38.7X4	T38.7X5	T38.7X6
Testosterone	T38.7X1	T38.7X2	T38.7X3	T38.7X4	T38.7X5	T38.7X6
Tetanus toxoid or vaccine	T50.A91	T50.A92	T50.A93	T50.A94	T50.A95	T50.A96
antitoxin	T50.Z11	T50.Z12	T50.Z13	T50.Z14	T50.Z15	T50.Z16
immune globulin (human)	T50.Z11	T50.Z12	T50.Z13	T50.Z14	T50.Z15	T50.Z16

TABLE OF DRUGS AND CHEMICALS

Substance	External Cause (T-Code)					
	Poisoning, Accidental (Unintentional)	Poisoning, Intentional Self-Harm	Poisoning, Assault	Poisoning, Undetermined	Adverse Effect	Underdosing
Tetanus toxoid or vaccine *(Continued)*						
toxoid	T50.A91	T50.A92	T50.A93	T50.A94	T50.A95	T50.A96
with diphtheria toxoid	T50.A21	T50.A22	T50.A23	T50.A24	T50.A25	T50.A26
with pertussis	T50.A11	T50.A12	T50.A13	T50.A14	T50.A15	T50.A16
Tetrabenazine	T43.591	T43.592	T43.593	T43.594	T43.595	T43.596
Tetracaine	T41.3X1	T41.3X2	T41.3X3	T41.3X4	T41.3X5	T41.3X6
nerve block (peripheral) (plexus)	T41.3X1	T41.3X2	T41.3X3	T41.3X4	T41.3X5	T41.3X6
regional	T41.3X1	T41.3X2	T41.3X3	T41.3X4	T41.3X5	T41.3X6
spinal	T41.3X1	T41.3X2	T41.3X3	T41.3X4	T41.3X5	T41.3X6
Tetrachlorethylene — *see Tetrachloroethylene*						
Tetrachlormethiazide	T50.2X1	T50.2X2	T50.2X3	T50.2X4	T50.2X5	T50.2X6
2,3,7,8-Tetrachlorodibenzo-p-dioxin	T53.7X1	T53.7X2	T53.7X3	T53.7X4	—	—
Tetrachloroethane	T53.6X1	T53.6X2	T53.6X3	T53.6X4	—	—
vapor	T53.6X1	T53.6X2	T53.6X3	T53.6X4	—	—
paint or varnish	T53.6X1	T53.6X2	T53.6X3	T53.6X4	—	—
Tetrachloroethylene (liquid)	T53.3X1	T53.3X2	T53.3X3	T53.3X4	—	—
medicinal	T37.4X1	T37.4X2	T37.4X3	T37.4X4	T37.4X5	T37.4X6
vapor	T53.3X1	T53.3X2	T53.3X3	T53.3X4	—	—
Tetrachloromethane — *see Carbon tetrachloride*						
Tetracosactide	T38.811	T38.812	T38.813	T38.814	T38.815	T38.816
Tetracosactrin	T38.811	T38.812	T38.813	T38.814	T38.815	T38.816
Tetracycline	T36.4X1	T36.4X2	T36.4X3	T36.4X4	T36.4X5	T36.4X6
ophthalmic preparation	T49.5X1	T49.5X2	T49.5X3	T49.5X4	T49.5X5	T49.5X6
topical NEC	T49.0X1	T49.0X2	T49.0X3	T49.0X4	T49.0X5	T49.0X6
Tetradifon	T60.8X1	T60.8X2	T60.8X3	T60.8X4	—	—
Tetradotoxin	T61.771	T61.772	T61.773	T61.774	—	—
Tetraethyl						
lead	T56.0X1	T56.0X2	T56.0X3	T56.0X4	—	—
pyrophosphate	T60.0X1	T60.0X2	T60.0X3	T60.0X4	—	—
Tetraethylammonium chloride	T44.2X1	T44.2X2	T44.2X3	T44.2X4	T44.2X5	T44.2X6
Tetraethylthiuram disulfide	T50.6X1	T50.6X2	T50.6X3	T50.6X4	T50.6X5	T50.6X6
Tetrahydroaminoacridine	T44.0X1	T44.0X2	T44.0X3	T44.0X4	T44.0X5	T44.0X6
Tetrahydrocannabinol	T40.711	T40.712	T40.713	T40.714	T40.715	T40.716
Tetrahydrofuran	T52.8X1	T52.8X2	T52.8X3	T52.8X4	—	—
Tetrahydronaphthalene	T52.8X1	T52.8X2	T52.8X3	T52.8X4	—	—
Tetrahydrozoline	T49.5X1	T49.5X2	T49.5X3	T49.5X4	T49.5X5	T49.5X6
Tetralin	T52.8X1	T52.8X2	T52.8X3	T52.8X4	—	—
Tetramethrin	T60.2X1	T60.2X2	T60.2X3	T60.2X4	—	—

Substance	External Cause (T-Code)					
	Poisoning, Accidental (Unintentional)	Poisoning, Intentional Self-Harm	Poisoning, Assault	Poisoning, Undetermined	Adverse Effect	Underdosing
Tetramethylthiuram (disulfide) NEC	T60.3X1	T60.3X2	T60.3X3	T60.3X4	—	—
medicinal	T49.0X1	T49.0X2	T49.0X3	T49.0X4	T49.0X5	T49.0X6
Tetramisole	T37.4X1	T37.4X2	T37.4X3	T37.4X4	T37.4X5	T37.4X6
Tetranicotinoyl fructose	T46.7X1	T46.7X2	T46.7X3	T46.7X4	T46.7X5	T46.7X6
Tetronal	T42.6X1	T42.6X2	T42.6X3	T42.6X4	T42.6X5	T42.6X6
Tetrazepam	T42.4X1	T42.4X2	T42.4X3	T42.4X4	T42.4X5	T42.4X6
Tetryl	T65.3X1	T65.3X2	T65.3X3	T65.3X4	—	—
Tetrylammonium chloride	T44.2X1	T44.2X2	T44.2X3	T44.2X4	T44.2X5	T44.2X6
Tetryzoline	T49.5X1	T49.5X2	T49.5X3	T49.5X4	T49.5X5	T49.5X6
Thalidomide	T45.1X1	T45.1X2	T45.1X3	T45.1X4	T45.1X5	T45.1X6
Thallium (compounds) (dust) NEC	T56.811	T56.812	T56.813	T56.814	—	—
pesticide	T60.4X1	T60.4X2	T60.4X3	T60.4X4	—	—
THC	T40.711	T40.712	T40.713	T40.714	T40.715	T40.716
Thebacon	T48.3X1	T48.3X2	T48.3X3	T48.3X4	T48.3X5	T48.3X6
Thebaine	T40.2X1	T40.2X2	T40.2X3	T40.2X4	T40.2X5	T40.2X6
Thenoic acid	T49.6X1	T49.6X2	T49.6X3	T49.6X4	T49.6X5	T49.6X6
Thenyldiamine	T45.0X1	T45.0X2	T45.0X3	T45.0X4	T45.0X5	T45.0X6
Theobromine (calcium salicylate)	T48.6X1	T48.6X2	T48.6X3	T48.6X4	T48.6X5	T48.6X6
sodium salicylate	T48.6X1	T48.6X2	T48.6X3	T48.6X4	T48.6X5	T48.6X6
Theophyllamine	T48.6X1	T48.6X2	T48.6X3	T48.6X4	T48.6X5	T48.6X6
Theophylline	T48.6X1	T48.6X2	T48.6X3	T48.6X4	T48.6X5	T48.6X6
aminobenzoic acid	T48.6X1	T48.6X2	T48.6X3	T48.6X4	T48.6X5	T48.6X6
ethylenediamine	T48.6X1	T48.6X2	T48.6X3	T48.6X4	T48.6X5	T48.6X6
piperazine p-amino-benzoate	T48.6X1	T48.6X2	T48.6X3	T48.6X4	T48.6X5	T48.6X6
Thiabendazole	T37.4X1	T37.4X2	T37.4X3	T37.4X4	T37.4X5	T37.4X6
Thialbarbital	T41.1X1	T41.1X2	T41.1X3	T41.1X4	T41.1X5	T41.1X6
Thiamazole	T38.2X1	T38.2X2	T38.2X3	T38.2X4	T38.2X5	T38.2X6
Thiambutosine	T37.1X1	T37.1X2	T37.1X3	T37.1X4	T37.1X5	T37.1X6
Thiamine	T45.2X1	T45.2X2	T45.2X3	T45.2X4	T45.2X5	T45.2X6
Thiamphenicol	T36.2X1	T36.2X2	T36.2X3	T36.2X4	T36.2X5	T36.2X6
Thiamylal	T41.1X1	T41.1X2	T41.1X3	T41.1X4	T41.1X5	T41.1X6
sodium	T41.1X1	T41.1X2	T41.1X3	T41.1X4	T41.1X5	T41.1X6
Thiazesim	T43.291	T43.292	T43.293	T43.294	T43.295	T43.296
Thiazides (diuretics)	T50.2X1	T50.2X2	T50.2X3	T50.2X4	T50.2X5	T50.2X6
Thiazinamium metilsulfate	T43.3X1	T43.3X2	T43.3X3	T43.3X4	T43.3X5	T43.3X6
Thiethylperazine	T43.3X1	T43.3X2	T43.3X3	T43.3X4	T43.3X5	T43.3X6
Thimerosal	T49.0X1	T49.0X2	T49.0X3	T49.0X4	T49.0X5	T49.0X6
ophthalmic preparation	T49.5X1	T49.5X2	T49.5X3	T49.5X4	T49.5X5	T49.5X6
Thioacetazone	T37.1X1	T37.1X2	T37.1X3	T37.1X4	T37.1X5	T37.1X6
with isoniazid	T37.1X1	T37.1X2	T37.1X3	T37.1X4	T37.1X5	T37.1X6
Thiobarbital sodium	T41.1X1	T41.1X2	T41.1X3	T41.1X4	T41.1X5	T41.1X6

◀ New ◀ Revised ~~deleted~~ Deleted

Substance	Poisoning, Accidental (Unintentional)	Poisoning, Intentional Self-Harm	Poisoning, Assault	Poisoning, Undetermined	Adverse Effect	Underdosing
Thiobarbiturate anesthetic	T41.1X1	T41.1X2	T41.1X3	T41.1X4	T41.1X5	T41.1X6
Thiobismol	T37.8X1	T37.8X2	T37.8X3	T37.8X4	T37.8X5	T37.8X6
Thiobutabarbital sodium	T41.1X1	T41.1X2	T41.1X3	T41.1X4	T41.1X5	T41.1X6
Thiocarbamate (insecticide)	T60.0X1	T60.0X2	T60.0X3	T60.0X4	—	—
Thiocarbamide	T38.2X1	T38.2X2	T38.2X3	T38.2X4	T38.2X5	T38.2X6
Thiocarbarsone	T37.8X1	T37.8X2	T37.8X3	T37.8X4	T37.8X5	T37.8X6
Thiocarlide	T37.1X1	T37.1X2	T37.1X3	T37.1X4	T37.1X5	T37.1X6
Thioctamide	T50.991	T50.992	T50.993	T50.994	T50.995	T50.996
Thioctic acid	T50.991	T50.992	T50.993	T50.994	T50.995	T50.996
Thiofos	T60.0X1	T60.0X2	T60.0X3	T60.0X4	—	—
Thioglycolate	T49.4X1	T49.4X2	T49.4X3	T49.4X4	T49.4X5	T49.4X6
Thioglycolic acid	T65.891	T65.892	T65.893	T65.894	—	—
Thioguanine	T45.1X1	T45.1X2	T45.1X3	T45.1X4	T45.1X5	T45.1X6
Thiomercaptomerin	T50.2X1	T50.2X2	T50.2X3	T50.2X4	T50.2X5	T50.2X6
Thiomerin	T50.2X1	T50.2X2	T50.2X3	T50.2X4	T50.2X5	T50.2X6
Thiomersal	T49.0X1	T49.0X2	T49.0X3	T49.0X4	T49.0X5	T49.0X6
Thionazin	T60.0X1	T60.0X2	T60.0X3	T60.0X4	—	—
Thiopental (sodium)	T41.1X1	T41.1X2	T41.1X3	T41.1X4	T41.1X5	T41.1X6
Thiopentone (sodium)	T41.1X1	T41.1X2	T41.1X3	T41.1X4	T41.1X5	T41.1X6
Thiopropazate	T43.3X1	T43.3X2	T43.3X3	T43.3X4	T43.3X5	T43.3X6
Thioproperazine	T43.3X1	T43.3X2	T43.3X3	T43.3X4	T43.3X5	T43.3X6
Thioridazine	T43.3X1	T43.3X2	T43.3X3	T43.3X4	T43.3X5	T43.3X6
Thiosinamine	T49.3X1	T49.3X2	T49.3X3	T49.3X4	T49.3X5	T49.3X6
Thiotepa	T45.1X1	T45.1X2	T45.1X3	T45.1X4	T45.1X5	T45.1X6
Thiothixene	T43.4X1	T43.4X2	T43.4X3	T43.4X4	T43.4X5	T43.4X6
Thiouracil (benzyl) (methyl) (propyl)	T38.2X1	T38.2X2	T38.2X3	T38.2X4	T38.2X5	T38.2X6
Thiourea	T38.2X1	T38.2X2	T38.2X3	T38.2X4	T38.2X5	T38.2X6
Thiphenamil	T44.3X1	T44.3X2	T44.3X3	T44.3X4	T44.3X5	T44.3X6
Thiram	T60.3X1	T60.3X2	T60.3X3	T60.3X4	—	—
medicinal	T49.2X1	T49.2X2	T49.2X3	T49.2X4	T49.2X5	T49.2X6
Thonzylamine (systemic)	T45.0X1	T45.0X2	T45.0X3	T45.0X4	T45.0X5	T45.0X6
mucosal decongestant	T48.5X1	T48.5X2	T48.5X3	T48.5X4	T48.5X5	T48.5X6
Thorazine	T43.3X1	T43.3X2	T43.3X3	T43.3X4	T43.3X5	T43.3X6
Thorium dioxide suspension	T50.8X1	T50.8X2	T50.8X3	T50.8X4	T50.8X5	T50.8X6
Thornapple	T62.2X1	T62.2X2	T62.2X3	T62.2X4	—	—
Throat drug NEC	T49.6X1	T49.6X2	T49.6X3	T49.6X4	T49.6X5	T49.6X6
Thrombin	T45.7X1	T45.7X2	T45.7X3	T45.7X4	T45.7X5	T45.7X6
Thrombolysin	T45.611	T45.612	T45.613	T45.614	T45.615	T45.616
Thromboplastin	T45.7X1	T45.7X2	T45.7X3	T45.7X4	T45.7X5	T45.7X6
Thurfyl nicotinate	T46.7X1	T46.7X2	T46.7X3	T46.7X4	T46.7X5	T46.7X6
Thymol	T49.0X1	T49.0X2	T49.0X3	T49.0X4	T49.0X5	T49.0X6
Thymopentin	T37.5X1	T37.5X2	T37.5X3	T37.5X4	T37.5X5	T37.5X6
Thymoxamine	T46.7X1	T46.7X2	T46.7X3	T46.7X4	T46.7X5	T46.7X6
Thymus extract	T38.891	T38.892	T38.893	T38.894	T38.895	T38.896
Thyreotrophic hormone	T38.811	T38.812	T38.813	T38.814	T38.815	T38.816
Thyroglobulin	T38.1X1	T38.1X2	T38.1X3	T38.1X4	T38.1X5	T38.1X6
Thyroid (hormone)	T38.1X1	T38.1X2	T38.1X3	T38.1X4	T38.1X5	T38.1X6
Thyrolar	T38.1X1	T38.1X2	T38.1X3	T38.1X4	T38.1X5	T38.1X6
Thyrotrophin	T38.811	T38.812	T38.813	T38.814	T38.815	T38.816
Thyrotropic hormone	T38.811	T38.812	T38.813	T38.814	T38.815	T38.816
Thyroxine	T38.1X1	T38.1X2	T38.1X3	T38.1X4	T38.1X5	T38.1X6
Tiabendazole	T37.4X1	T37.4X2	T37.4X3	T37.4X4	T37.4X5	T37.4X6
Tiamizide	T50.2X1	T50.2X2	T50.2X3	T50.2X4	T50.2X5	T50.2X6
Tianeptine	T43.291	T43.292	T43.293	T43.294	T43.295	T43.296
Tiapamil	T46.1X1	T46.1X2	T46.1X3	T46.1X4	T46.1X5	T46.1X6
Tiapride	T43.591	T43.592	T43.593	T43.594	T43.595	T43.596
Tiaprofenic acid	T39.311	T39.312	T39.313	T39.314	T39.315	T39.316
Tiaramide	T39.8X1	T39.8X2	T39.8X3	T39.8X4	T39.8X5	T39.8X6
Ticarcillin	T36.0X1	T36.0X2	T36.0X3	T36.0X4	T36.0X5	T36.0X6
Ticlatone	T49.0X1	T49.0X2	T49.0X3	T49.0X4	T49.0X5	T49.0X6
Ticlopidine	T45.521	T45.522	T45.523	T45.524	T45.525	T45.526
Ticrynafen	T50.1X1	T50.1X2	T50.1X3	T50.1X4	T50.1X5	T50.1X6
Tidiacic	T50.991	T50.992	T50.993	T50.994	T50.995	T50.996
Tiemonium	T44.3X1	T44.3X2	T44.3X3	T44.3X4	T44.3X5	T44.3X6
iodide	T44.3X1	T44.3X2	T44.3X3	T44.3X4	T44.3X5	T44.3X6
Tienilic acid	T50.1X1	T50.1X2	T50.1X3	T50.1X4	T50.1X5	T50.1X6
Tifenamil	T44.3X1	T44.3X2	T44.3X3	T44.3X4	T44.3X5	T44.3X6
Tigan	T45.0X1	T45.0X2	T45.0X3	T45.0X4	T45.0X5	T45.0X6
Tigloidine	T44.3X1	T44.3X2	T44.3X3	T44.3X4	T44.3X5	T44.3X6
Tilactase	T47.5X1	T47.5X2	T47.5X3	T47.5X4	T47.5X5	T47.5X6
Tiletamine	T41.291	T41.292	T41.293	T41.294	T41.295	T41.296
Tilidine	T40.441	T40.442	T40.443	T40.444	—	—
Timepidium bromide	T44.3X1	T44.3X2	T44.3X3	T44.3X4	T44.3X5	T44.3X6
Timiperone	T43.4X1	T43.4X2	T43.4X3	T43.4X4	T43.4X5	T43.4X6
Timolol	T44.7X1	T44.7X2	T44.7X3	T44.7X4	T44.7X5	T44.7X6
Tin (chloride) (dust) (oxide) NEC	T56.6X1	T56.6X2	T56.6X3	T56.6X4	—	—
anti-infectives	T37.8X1	T37.8X2	T37.8X3	T37.8X4	T37.8X5	T37.8X6
Tincture, iodine — see Iodine						
Tindal	T43.3X1	T43.3X2	T43.3X3	T43.3X4	T43.3X5	T43.3X6
Tinidazole	T37.3X1	T37.3X2	T37.3X3	T37.3X4	T37.3X5	T37.3X6
Tinoridine	T39.8X1	T39.8X2	T39.8X3	T39.8X4	T39.8X5	T39.8X6
Tiocarlide	T37.1X1	T37.1X2	T37.1X3	T37.1X4	T37.1X5	T37.1X6
Tioclomarol	T45.511	T45.512	T45.513	T45.514	T45.515	T45.516

Substance	Poisoning, Accidental (Unintentional)	Poisoning, Intentional Self-Harm	Poisoning, Assault	Poisoning, Undetermined	Adverse Effect	Underdosing
Tioconazole	T49.0X1	T49.0X2	T49.0X3	T49.0X4	T49.0X5	T49.0X6
Tioguanine	T45.1X1	T45.1X2	T45.1X3	T45.1X4	T45.1X5	T45.1X6
Tiopronin	T50.991	T50.992	T50.993	T50.994	T50.995	T50.996
Tiotixene	T43.4X1	T43.4X2	T43.4X3	T43.4X4	T43.4X5	T43.4X6
Tioxolone	T49.4X1	T49.4X2	T49.4X3	T49.4X4	T49.4X5	T49.4X6
Tipepidine	T48.3X1	T48.3X2	T48.3X3	T48.3X4	T48.3X5	T48.3X6
Tiquizium bromide	T44.3X1	T44.3X2	T44.3X3	T44.3X4	T44.3X5	T44.3X6
Tiratricol	T38.1X1	T38.1X2	T38.1X3	T38.1X4	T38.1X5	T38.1X6
Tisopurine	T50.4X1	T50.4X2	T50.4X3	T50.4X4	T50.4X5	T50.4X6
Titanium (compounds) (vapor)	T56.891	T56.892	T56.893	T56.894	—	—
dioxide	T49.3X1	T49.3X2	T49.3X3	T49.3X4	T49.3X5	T49.3X6
ointment	T49.3X1	T49.3X2	T49.3X3	T49.3X4	T49.3X5	T49.3X6
oxide	T49.3X1	T49.3X2	T49.3X3	T49.3X4	T49.3X5	T49.3X6
tetrachloride	T56.891	T56.892	T56.893	T56.894	—	—
Titanocene	T56.891	T56.892	T56.893	T56.894	—	—
Titroid	T38.1X1	T38.1X2	T38.1X3	T38.1X4	T38.1X5	T38.1X6
Tizanidine	T42.8X1	T42.8X2	T42.8X3	T42.8X4	T42.8X5	T42.8X6
TMTD	T60.3X1	T60.3X2	T60.3X3	T60.3X4		
TNT (fumes)	T65.3X1	T65.3X2	T65.3X3	T65.3X4		
Toadstool	T62.0X1	T62.0X2	T62.0X3	T62.0X4	—	—
Tobacco NEC	T65.291	T65.292	T65.293	T65.294		
cigarettes	T65.221	T65.222	T65.223	T65.224		
Indian	T62.2X1	T62.2X2	T62.2X3	T62.2X4	—	—
smoke, second-hand	T65.221	T65.222	T65.223	T65.224		—
Tobramycin	T36.5X1	T36.5X2	T36.5X3	T36.5X4	T36.5X5	T36.5X6
Tocainide	T46.2X1	T46.2X2	T46.2X3	T46.2X4	T46.2X5	T46.2X6
Tocoferol	T45.2X1	T45.2X2	T45.2X3	T45.2X4	T45.2X5	T45.2X6
Tocopherol	T45.2X1	T45.2X2	T45.2X3	T45.2X4	T45.2X5	T45.2X6
acetate	T45.2X1	T45.2X2	T45.2X3	T45.2X4	T45.2X5	T45.2X6
Tocosamine	T48.0X1	T48.0X2	T48.0X3	T48.0X4	T48.0X5	T48.0X6
Todralazine	T46.5X1	T46.5X2	T46.5X3	T46.5X4	T46.5X5	T46.5X6
Tofisopam	T42.4X1	T42.4X2	T42.4X3	T42.4X4	T42.4X5	T42.4X6
Tofranil	T43.011	T43.012	T43.013	T43.014	T43.015	T43.016
Toilet deodorizer	T65.891	T65.892	T65.893	T65.894	—	—
Tolamolol	T44.7X1	T44.7X2	T44.7X3	T44.7X4	T44.7X5	T44.7X6
Tolazamide	T38.3X1	T38.3X2	T38.3X3	T38.3X4	T38.3X5	T38.3X6
Tolazoline	T46.7X1	T46.7X2	T46.7X3	T46.7X4	T46.7X5	T46.7X6
Tolbutamide (sodium)	T38.3X1	T38.3X2	T38.3X3	T38.3X4	T38.3X5	T38.3X6
Tolciclate	T49.0X1	T49.0X2	T49.0X3	T49.0X4	T49.0X5	T49.0X6
Tolmetin	T39.391	T39.392	T39.393	T39.394	T39.395	T39.396
Tolnaftate	T49.0X1	T49.0X2	T49.0X3	T49.0X4	T49.0X5	T49.0X6
Tolonidine	T46.5X1	T46.5X2	T46.5X3	T46.5X4	T46.5X5	T46.5X6

Substance	Poisoning, Accidental (Unintentional)	Poisoning, Intentional Self-Harm	Poisoning, Assault	Poisoning, Undetermined	Adverse Effect	Underdosing
Toloxatone	T42.6X1	T42.6X2	T42.6X3	T42.6X4	T42.6X5	T42.6X6
Tolperisone	T44.3X1	T44.3X2	T44.3X3	T44.3X4	T44.3X5	T44.3X6
Tolserol	T42.8X1	T42.8X2	T42.8X3	T42.8X4	T42.8X5	T42.8X6
Toluene (liquid)	T52.2X1	T52.2X2	T52.2X3	T52.2X4	—	—
diisocyanate	T65.0X1	T65.0X2	T65.0X3	T65.0X4	—	—
Toluidine	T65.891	T65.892	T65.893	T65.894	—	—
vapor	T59.891	T59.892	T59.893	T59.894	—	—
Toluol (liquid)	T52.2X1	T52.2X2	T52.2X3	T52.2X4	—	—
vapor	T52.2X1	T52.2X2	T52.2X3	T52.2X4	—	—
Toluylenediamine	T65.3X1	T65.3X2	T65.3X3	T65.3X4	—	—
Tolylene-2,4-diisocyanate	T65.0X1	T65.0X2	T65.0X3	T65.0X4	—	—
Tonic NEC	T50.901	T50.902	T50.903	T50.904	T50.905	T50.906
Topical action drug NEC	T49.91	T49.92	T49.93	T49.94	T49.95	T49.96
ear, nose or throat	T49.6X1	T49.6X2	T49.6X3	T49.6X4	T49.6X5	T49.6X6
eye	T49.5X1	T49.5X2	T49.5X3	T49.5X4	T49.5X5	T49.5X6
skin	T49.91	T49.92	T49.93	T49.94	T49.95	T49.96
specified NEC	T49.8X1	T49.8X2	T49.8X3	T49.8X4	T49.8X5	T49.8X6
Toquizine	T44.3X1	T44.3X2	T44.3X3	T44.3X4	T44.3X5	T44.3X6
Toremifene	T38.6X1	T38.6X2	T38.6X3	T38.6X4	T38.6X5	T38.6X6
Tosylchloramide sodium	T49.8X1	T49.8X2	T49.8X3	T49.8X4	T49.8X5	T49.8X6
Toxaphene (dust) (spray)	T60.1X1	T60.1X2	T60.1X3	T60.1X4	—	—
Toxin, diphtheria (Schick Test)	T50.8X1	T50.8X2	T50.8X3	T50.8X4	T50.8X5	T50.8X6
Toxoid						
combined	T50.A21	T50.A22	T50.A23	T50.A24	T50.A25	T50.A26
diphtheria	T50.A91	T50.A92	T50.A93	T50.A94	T50.A95	T50.A96
tetanus	T50.A91	T50.A92	T50.A93	T50.A94	T50.A95	T50.A96
Trace element NEC	T45.8X1	T45.8X2	T45.8X3	T45.8X4	T45.8X5	T45.8X6
Tractor fuel NEC	T52.0X1	T52.0X2	T52.0X3	T52.0X4	—	—
Tragacanth	T50.991	T50.992	T50.993	T50.994	T50.995	T50.996
Tramadol	T40.421	T40.422	T40.423	T40.424	T40.425	T40.426
Tramazoline	T48.5X1	T48.5X2	T48.5X3	T48.5X4	T48.5X5	T48.5X6
Tranexamic acid	T45.621	T45.622	T45.623	T45.624	T45.625	T45.626
Tranilast	T45.0X1	T45.0X2	T45.0X3	T45.0X4	T45.0X5	T45.0X6
Tranquilizer NEC	T43.501	T43.502	T43.503	T43.504	T43.505	T43.506
with hypnotic or sedative	T42.6X1	T42.6X2	T42.6X3	T42.6X4	T42.6X5	T42.6X6
benzodiazepine NEC	T42.4X1	T42.4X2	T42.4X3	T42.4X4	T42.4X5	T42.4X6
butyrophenone NEC	T43.4X1	T43.4X2	T43.4X3	T43.4X4	T43.4X5	T43.4X6
carbamate	T43.591	T43.592	T43.593	T43.594	T43.595	T43.596
dimethylamine	T43.3X1	T43.3X2	T43.3X3	T43.3X4	T43.3X5	T43.3X6
ethylamine	T43.3X1	T43.3X2	T43.3X3	T43.3X4	T43.3X5	T43.3X6
hydroxyzine	T43.591	T43.592	T43.593	T43.594	T43.595	T43.596
major NEC	T43.501	T43.502	T43.503	T43.504	T43.505	T43.506

◀ New ◀ Revised ~~deleted~~ Deleted

Substance	Poisoning, Accidental (Unintentional)	Poisoning, Intentional Self-Harm	Poisoning, Assault	Poisoning, Undetermined	Adverse Effect	Underdosing
Tranquilizer NEC *(Continued)*						
penothiazine NEC	T43.3X1	T43.3X2	T43.3X3	T43.3X4	T43.3X5	T43.3X6
phenothiazine-based	T43.3X1	T43.3X2	T43.3X3	T43.3X4	T43.3X5	T43.3X6
piperazine NEC	T43.3X1	T43.3X2	T43.3X3	T43.3X4	T43.3X5	T43.3X6
piperidine	T43.3X1	T43.3X2	T43.3X3	T43.3X4	T43.3X5	T43.3X6
propylamine	T43.3X1	T43.3X2	T43.3X3	T43.3X4	T43.3X5	T43.3X6
specified NEC	T43.591	T43.592	T43.593	T43.594	T43.595	T43.596
thioxanthene NEC	T43.591	T43.592	T43.593	T43.594	T43.595	T43.596
Tranxene	T42.4X1	T42.4X2	T42.4X3	T42.4X4	T42.4X5	T42.4X6
Tranylcypromine	T43.1X1	T43.1X2	T43.1X3	T43.1X4	T43.1X5	T43.1X6
Trapidil	T46.3X1	T46.3X2	T46.3X3	T46.3X4	T46.3X5	T46.3X6
Trasentine	T44.3X1	T44.3X2	T44.3X3	T44.3X4	T44.3X5	T44.3X6
Travert	T50.3X1	T50.3X2	T50.3X3	T50.3X4	T50.3X5	T50.3X6
Trazodone	T43.211	T43.212	T43.213	T43.214	T43.215	T43.216
Trecator	T37.1X1	T37.1X2	T37.1X3	T37.1X4	T37.1X5	T37.1X6
Treosulfan	T45.1X1	T45.1X2	T45.1X3	T45.1X4	T45.1X5	T45.1X6
Tretamine	T45.1X1	T45.1X2	T45.1X3	T45.1X4	T45.1X5	T45.1X6
Tretinoin	T49.0X1	T49.0X2	T49.0X3	T49.0X4	T49.0X5	T49.0X6
Tretoquinol	T48.6X1	T48.6X2	T48.6X3	T48.6X4	T48.6X5	T48.6X6
Triacetin	T49.0X1	T49.0X2	T49.0X3	T49.0X4	T49.0X5	T49.0X6
Triacetoxyanthracene	T49.4X1	T49.4X2	T49.4X3	T49.4X4	T49.4X5	T49.4X6
Triacetyloleandomycin	T36.3X1	T36.3X2	T36.3X3	T36.3X3	T36.3X5	T36.3X6
Triamcinolone	T38.0X1	T38.0X2	T38.0X3	T38.0X4	T38.0X5	T38.0X6
ENT agent	T49.6X1	T49.6X2	T49.6X3	T49.6X4	T49.6X5	T49.6X6
hexacetonide	T49.0X1	T49.0X2	T49.0X3	T49.0X4	T49.0X5	T49.0X6
ophthalmic preparation	T49.5X1	T49.5X2	T49.5X3	T49.5X4	T49.5X5	T49.5X6
topical NEC	T49.0X1	T49.0X2	T49.0X3	T49.0X4	T49.0X5	T49.0X6
Triampyzine	T44.3X1	T44.3X2	T44.3X3	T44.3X4	T44.3X5	T44.3X6
Triamterene	T50.2X1	T50.2X2	T50.2X3	T50.2X4	T50.2X5	T50.2X6
Triazine (herbicide)	T60.3X1	T60.3X2	T60.3X3	T60.3X4	—	—
Triaziquone	T45.1X1	T45.1X2	T45.1X3	T45.1X4	T45.1X5	T45.1X6
Triazolam	T42.4X1	T42.4X2	T42.4X3	T42.4X4	T42.4X5	T42.4X6
Triazole (herbicide)	T60.3X1	T60.3X2	T60.3X3	T60.3X4	—	—
Tribenoside	T46.991	T46.992	T46.993	T46.994	T46.995	T46.996
Tribromacetaldehyde	T42.6X1	T42.6X2	T42.6X3	T42.6X4	T42.6X5	T42.6X6
Tribromoethanol, rectal	T41.291	T41.292	T41.293	T41.294	T41.295	T41.296
Tribromomethane	T42.6X1	T42.6X2	T42.6X3	T42.6X4	T42.6X5	T42.6X6
Trichlorethane	T53.2X1	T53.2X2	T53.2X3	T53.2X4	—	—
Trichlorethylene	T53.2X1	T53.2X2	T53.2X3	T53.2X4	—	—
Trichlorfon	T60.0X1	T60.0X2	T60.0X3	T60.0X4	—	—
Trichlormethiazide	T50.2X1	T50.2X2	T50.2X3	T50.2X4	T50.2X5	T50.2X6
Trichlormethine	T45.1X1	T45.1X2	T45.1X3	T45.1X4	T45.1X5	T45.1X6

Substance	Poisoning, Accidental (Unintentional)	Poisoning, Intentional Self-Harm	Poisoning, Assault	Poisoning, Undetermined	Adverse Effect	Underdosing
Trichloroacetic acid, Trichloracetic acid	T54.2X1	T54.2X2	T54.2X3	T54.2X4	—	—
medicinal	T49.4X1	T49.4X2	T49.4X3	T49.4X4	T49.4X5	T49.4X6
Trichloroethane	T53.2X1	T53.2X2	T53.2X3	T53.2X4	—	—
Trichloroethanol	T42.6X1	T42.6X2	T42.6X3	T42.6X4	T42.6X5	T42.6X6
Trichloroethylene (liquid) (vapor)	T53.2X1	T53.2X2	T53.2X3	T53.2X4	—	—
anesthetic (gas)	T41.0X1	T41.0X2	T41.0X3	T41.0X4	T41.0X5	T41.0X6
vapor NEC	T53.2X1	T53.2X2	T53.2X3	T53.2X4	—	—
Trichloroethyl phosphate	T42.6X1	T42.6X2	T42.6X3	T42.6X4	T42.6X5	T42.6X6
Trichlorofluoromethane NEC	T53.5X1	T53.5X2	T53.5X3	T53.5X4	—	—
Trichloronate	T60.0X1	T60.0X2	T60.0X3	T60.0X4	—	—
2,4,5-Trichlorophen-oxyacetic acid	T60.3X1	T60.3X2	T60.3X3	T60.3X4	—	—
Trichloropropane	T53.6X1	T53.6X2	T53.6X3	T53.6X4	—	—
Trichlorotriethylamine	T45.1X1	T45.1X2	T45.1X3	T45.1X4	T45.1X5	T45.1X6
Trichomonacides NEC	T37.3X1	T37.3X2	T37.3X3	T37.3X4	T37.3X5	T37.3X6
Trichomycin	T36.7X1	T36.7X2	T36.7X3	T36.7X4	T36.7X5	T36.7X6
Triclobisonium chloride	T49.0X1	T49.0X2	T49.0X3	T49.0X4	T49.0X5	T49.0X6
Triclocarban	T49.0X1	T49.0X2	T49.0X3	T49.0X4	T49.0X5	T49.0X6
Triclofos	T42.6X1	T42.6X2	T42.6X3	T42.6X4	T42.6X5	T42.6X6
Triclosan	T49.0X1	T49.0X2	T49.0X3	T49.0X4	T49.0X5	T49.0X6
Tricresyl phosphate	T65.891	T65.892	T65.893	T65.894	—	—
solvent	T52.91	T52.92	T52.93	T52.94	—	—
Tricyclamol chloride	T44.3X1	T44.3X2	T44.3X3	T44.3X4	T44.3X5	T44.3X6
Tridesilon	T49.0X1	T49.0X2	T49.0X3	T49.0X4	T49.0X5	T49.0X6
Tridihexethyl iodide	T44.3X1	T44.3X2	T44.3X3	T44.3X4	T44.3X5	T44.3X6
Tridione	T42.2X1	T42.2X2	T42.2X3	T42.2X4	T42.2X5	T42.2X6
Trientine	T45.8X1	T45.8X2	T45.8X3	T45.8X4	T45.8X5	T45.8X6
Triethanolamine NEC	T54.3X1	T54.3X2	T54.3X3	T54.3X4	—	—
detergent	T54.3X1	T54.3X2	T54.3X3	T54.3X4	—	—
trinitrate (biphosphate)	T46.3X1	T46.3X2	T46.3X3	T46.3X4	T46.3X5	T46.3X6
Triethanomelamine	T45.1X1	T45.1X2	T45.1X3	T45.1X4	T45.1X5	T45.1X6
Triethylenemelamine	T45.1X1	T45.1X2	T45.1X3	T45.1X4	T45.1X5	T45.1X6
Triethylenephosphoramide	T45.1X1	T45.1X2	T45.1X3	T45.1X4	T45.1X5	T45.1X6
Triethylenethiophosphoramide	T45.1X1	T45.1X2	T45.1X3	T45.1X4	T45.1X5	T45.1X6
Trifluoperazine	T43.3X1	T43.3X2	T43.3X3	T43.3X4	T43.3X5	T43.3X6
Trifluoroethyl vinyl ether	T41.0X1	T41.0X2	T41.0X3	T41.0X4	T41.0X5	T41.0X6
Trifluperidol	T43.4X1	T43.4X2	T43.4X3	T43.4X4	T43.4X5	T43.4X6
Triflupromazine	T43.3X1	T43.3X2	T43.3X3	T43.3X4	T43.3X5	T43.3X6
Trifluridine	T37.5X1	T37.5X2	T37.5X3	T37.5X4	T37.5X5	T37.5X6
Triflusal	T45.521	T45.522	T45.523	T45.524	T45.525	T45.526
Trihexyphenidyl	T44.3X1	T44.3X2	T44.3X3	T44.3X4	T44.3X5	T44.3X6
Triiodothyronine	T38.1X1	T38.1X2	T38.1X3	T38.1X4	T38.1X5	T38.1X6

◀ New ◀ Revised ~~deleted~~ Deleted

Substance	External Cause (T-Code) Poisoning, Accidental (Unintentional)	Poisoning, Intentional Self-Harm	Poisoning, Assault	Poisoning, Undetermined	Adverse Effect	Underdosing
Trilene	T41.0X1	T41.0X2	T41.0X3	T41.0X4	T41.0X5	T41.0X6
Trilostane	T38.991	T38.992	T38.993	T38.994	T38.995	T38.996
Trimebutine	T44.3X1	T44.3X2	T44.3X3	T44.3X4	T44.3X5	T44.3X6
Trimecaine	T41.3X1	T41.3X2	T41.3X3	T41.3X4	T41.3X5	T41.3X6
Trimeprazine (tartrate)	T44.3X1	T44.3X2	T44.3X3	T44.3X4	T44.3X5	T44.3X6
Trimetaphan camsilate	T44.2X1	T44.2X2	T44.2X3	T44.2X4	T44.2X5	T44.2X6
Trimetazidine	T46.7X1	T46.7X2	T46.7X3	T46.7X4	T46.7X5	T46.7X6
Trimethadione	T42.2X1	T42.2X2	T42.2X3	T42.2X4	T42.2X5	T42.2X6
Trimethaphan	T44.2X1	T44.2X2	T44.2X3	T44.2X4	T44.2X5	T44.2X6
Trimethidinium	T44.2X1	T44.2X2	T44.2X3	T44.2X4	T44.2X5	T44.2X6
Trimethobenzamide	T45.0X1	T45.0X2	T45.0X3	T45.0X4	T45.0X5	T45.0X6
Trimethoprim	T37.8X1	T37.8X2	T37.8X3	T37.8X4	T37.8X5	T37.8X6
with sulfamethoxazole	T36.8X1	T36.8X2	T36.8X3	T36.8X4	T36.8X5	T36.8X6
Trimethylcarbinol	T51.3X1	T51.3X2	T51.3X3	T51.3X4	—	—
Trimethylpsoralen	T49.3X1	T49.3X2	T49.3X3	T49.3X4	T49.3X5	T49.3X6
Trimeton	T45.0X1	T45.0X2	T45.0X3	T45.0X4	T45.0X5	T45.0X6
Trimetrexate	T45.1X1	T45.1X2	T45.1X3	T45.1X4	T45.1X5	T45.1X6
Trimipramine	T43.011	T43.012	T43.013	T43.014	T43.015	T43.016
Trimustine	T45.1X1	T45.1X2	T45.1X3	T45.1X4	T45.1X5	T45.1X6
Trinitrine	T46.3X1	T46.3X2	T46.3X3	T46.3X4	T46.3X5	T46.3X6
Trinitrobenzol	T65.3X1	T65.3X2	T65.3X3	T65.3X4	—	—
Trinitrophenol	T65.3X1	T65.3X2	T65.3X3	T65.3X4	—	—
Trinitrotoluene (fumes)	T65.3X1	T65.3X2	T65.3X3	T65.3X4	—	—
Trional	T42.6X1	T42.6X2	T42.6X3	T42.6X4	T42.6X5	T42.6X6
Triorthocresyl phosphate	T65.891	T65.892	T65.893	T65.894	—	—
Trioxide of arsenic	T57.0X1	T57.0X2	T57.0X3	T57.0X4	—	—
Trioxysalen	T49.4X1	T49.4X2	T49.4X3	T49.4X4	T49.4X5	T49.4X6
Tripamide	T50.2X1	T50.2X2	T50.2X3	T50.2X4	T50.2X5	T50.2X6
Triparanol	T46.6X1	T46.6X2	T46.6X3	T46.6X4	T46.6X5	T46.6X6
Tripelennamine	T45.0X1	T45.0X2	T45.0X3	T45.0X4	T45.0X5	T45.0X6
Triperiden	T44.3X1	T44.3X2	T44.3X3	T44.3X4	T44.3X5	T44.3X6
Triperidol	T43.4X1	T43.4X2	T43.4X3	T43.4X4	T43.4X5	T43.4X6
Triphenylphosphate	T65.891	T65.892	T65.893	T65.894	—	—
Triple						
bromides	T42.6X1	T42.6X2	T42.6X3	T42.6X4	T42.6X5	T42.6X6
carbonate	T47.1X1	T47.1X2	T47.1X3	T47.1X4	T47.1X5	T47.1X6
vaccine						
DPT	T50.A11	T50.A12	T50.A13	T50.A14	T50.A15	T50.A16
including pertussis	T50.A11	T50.A12	T50.A13	T50.A14	T50.A15	T50.A16
MMR	T50.B91	T50.B92	—	—	—	—
Triprolidine	T45.0X1	T45.0X2	T45.0X3	T45.0X4	T45.0X5	T45.0X6
Trisodium hydrogen edetate	T50.6X1	T50.6X2	T50.6X3	T50.6X4	T50.6X5	T50.6X6

Substance	External Cause (T-Code) Poisoning, Accidental (Unintentional)	Poisoning, Intentional Self-Harm	Poisoning, Assault	Poisoning, Undetermined	Adverse Effect	Underdosing
Trisoralen	T49.3X1	T49.3X2	T49.3X3	T49.3X4	T49.3X5	T49.3X6
Trisulfapyrimidines	T37.0X1	T37.0X2	T37.0X3	T37.0X4	T37.0X5	T37.0X6
Trithiozine	T44.3X1	T44.3X2	T44.3X3	T44.3X4	T44.3X5	T44.3X6
Tritiozine	T44.3X1	T44.3X2	T44.3X3	T44.3X4	T44.3X5	T44.3X6
Tritoqualine	T45.0X1	T45.0X2	T45.0X3	T45.0X4	T45.0X5	T45.0X6
Trofosfamide	T45.1X1	T45.1X2	T45.1X3	T45.1X4	T45.1X5	T45.1X6
Troleandomycin	T36.3X1	T36.3X2	T36.3X3	T36.3X4	T36.3X5	T36.3X6
Trolnitrate (phosphate)	T46.3X1	T46.3X2	T46.3X3	T46.3X4	T46.3X5	T46.3X6
Tromantadine	T37.5X1	T37.5X2	T37.5X3	T37.5X4	T37.5X5	T37.5X6
Trometamol	T50.2X1	T50.2X2	T50.2X3	T50.2X4	T50.2X5	T50.2X6
Tromethamine	T50.2X1	T50.2X2	T50.2X3	T50.2X4	T50.2X5	T50.2X6
Tronothane	T41.3X1	T41.3X2	T41.3X3	T41.3X4	T41.3X5	T41.3X6
Tropacine	T44.3X1	T44.3X2	T44.3X3	T44.3X4	T44.3X5	T44.3X6
Tropatepine	T44.3X1	T44.3X2	T44.3X3	T44.3X4	T44.3X5	T44.3X6
Tropicamide	T44.3X1	T44.3X2	T44.3X3	T44.3X4	T44.3X5	T44.3X6
Trospium chloride	T44.3X1	T44.3X2	T44.3X3	T44.3X4	T44.3X5	T44.3X6
Troxerutin	T46.991	T46.992	T46.993	T46.994	T46.995	T46.996
Troxidone	T42.2X1	T42.2X2	T42.2X3	T42.2X4	T42.2X5	T42.2X6
Tryparsamide	T37.3X1	T37.3X2	T37.3X3	T37.3X4	T37.3X5	T37.3X6
Trypsin	T45.3X1	T45.3X2	T45.3X3	T45.3X4	T45.3X5	T45.3X6
Tryptizol	T43.011	T43.012	T43.013	T43.014	T43.015	T43.016
TSH	T38.811	T38.812	T38.813	T38.814	T38.815	T38.816
Tuaminoheptane	T48.5X1	T48.5X2	T48.5X3	T48.5X4	T48.5X5	T48.5X6
Tuberculin, purified protein derivative (PPD)	T50.8X1	T50.8X2	T50.8X3	T50.8X4	T50.8X5	T50.8X6
Tubocurare	T48.1X1	T48.1X2	T48.1X3	T48.1X4	T48.1X5	T48.1X6
Tubocurarine (chloride)	T48.1X1	T48.1X2	T48.1X3	T48.1X4	T48.1X5	T48.1X6
Tulobuterol	T48.6X1	T48.6X2	T48.6X3	T48.6X4	T48.6X5	T48.6X6
Turpentine (spirits of)	T52.8X1	T52.8X2	T52.8X3	T52.8X4	—	—
vapor	T52.8X1	T52.8X2	T52.8X3	T52.8X4	—	—
Tybamate	T43.591	T43.592	T43.593	T43.594	T43.595	T43.596
Tyloxapol	T48.4X1	T48.4X2	T48.4X3	T48.4X4	T48.4X5	T48.4X6
Tymazoline	T48.5X1	T48.5X2	T48.5X3	T48.5X4	T48.5X5	T48.5X6
Typhoid-paratyphoid vaccine	T50.A91	T50.A92	T50.A93	T50.A94	T50.A95	T50.A96
Typhus vaccine	T50.A91	T50.A92	T50.A93	T50.A94	T50.A95	T50.A96
Tyropanoate	T50.8X1	T50.8X2	T50.8X3	T50.8X4	T50.8X5	T50.8X6
Tyrothricin	T49.6X1	T49.6X2	T49.6X3	T49.6X4	T49.6X5	T49.6X6
ENT agent	T49.6X1	T49.6X2	T49.6X3	T49.6X4	T49.6X5	T49.6X6
ophthalmic preparation	T49.5X1	T49.5X2	T49.5X3	T49.5X4	T49.5X5	T49.5X6

U

Substance	External Cause (T-Code) Poisoning, Accidental (Unintentional)	Poisoning, Intentional Self-Harm	Poisoning, Assault	Poisoning, Undetermined	Adverse Effect	Underdosing
Ufenamate	T39.391	T39.392	T39.393	T39.394	T39.395	T39.396
Ultraviolet light protectant	T49.3X1	T49.3X2	T49.3X3	T49.3X4	T49.3X5	T49.3X6

◀ New ◀ Revised ~~deleted~~ Deleted

	External Cause (T-Code)					
Substance	Poisoning, Accidental (Unintentional)	Poisoning, Intentional Self-Harm	Poisoning, Assault	Poisoning, Undetermined	Adverse Effect	Underdosing
Undecenoic acid	T49.0X1	T49.0X2	T49.0X3	T49.0X4	T49.0X5	T49.0X6
Undecoylium	T49.0X1	T49.0X2	T49.0X3	T49.0X4	T49.0X5	T49.0X6
Undecylenic acid (derivatives)	T49.0X1	T49.0X2	T49.0X3	T49.0X4	T49.0X5	T49.0X6
Unna's boot	T49.3X1	T49.3X2	T49.3X3	T49.3X4	T49.3X5	T49.3X6
Unsaturated fatty acid	T46.6X1	T46.6X2	T46.6X3	T46.6X4	T46.6X5	T46.6X6
Uracil mustard	T45.1X1	T45.1X2	T45.1X3	T45.1X4	T45.1X5	T45.1X6
Uramustine	T45.1X1	T45.1X2	T45.1X3	T45.1X4	T45.1X5	T45.1X6
Urapidil	T46.5X1	T46.5X2	T46.5X3	T46.5X4	T46.5X5	T46.5X6
Urari	T48.1X1	T48.1X2	T48.1X3	T48.1X4	T48.1X5	T48.1X6
Urate oxidase	T50.4X1	T50.4X2	T50.4X3	T50.4X4	T50.4X5	T50.4X6
Urea	T47.3X1	T47.3X2	T47.3X3	T47.3X4	T47.3X5	T47.3X6
peroxide	T49.0X1	T49.0X2	T49.0X3	T49.0X4	T49.0X5	T49.0X6
stibamine	T37.4X1	T37.4X2	T37.4X3	T37.4X4	T37.4X5	T37.4X6
topical	T49.8X1	T49.8X2	T49.8X3	T49.8X4	T49.8X5	T49.8X6
Urethane	T45.1X1	T45.1X2	T45.1X3	T45.1X4	T45.1X5	T45.1X6
Urginea (maritima) (scilla) —see Squill						
Uric acid metabolism drug NEC	T50.4X1	T50.4X2	T50.4X3	T50.4X4	T50.4X5	T50.4X6
Uricosuric agent	T50.4X1	T50.4X2	T50.4X3	T50.4X4	T50.4X5	T50.4X6
Urinary anti-infective	T37.8X1	T37.8X2	T37.8X3	T37.8X4	T37.8X5	T37.8X6
Urofollitropin	T38.811	T38.812	T38.813	T38.814	T38.815	T38.816
Urokinase	T45.611	T45.612	T45.613	T45.614	T45.615	T45.616
Urokon	T50.8X1	T50.8X2	T50.8X3	T50.8X4	T50.8X5	T50.8X6
Ursodeoxycholic acid	T50.991	T50.992	T50.993	T50.994	T50.995	T50.996
Ursodiol	T50.991	T50.992	T50.993	T50.994	T50.995	T50.996
Urtica	T62.2X1	T62.2X2	T62.2X3	T62.2X4	—	—
Utility gas—see Gas, utility						
V						
Vaccine NEC	T50.Z91	T50.Z92	T50.Z93	T50.Z94	T50.Z95	T50.Z96
antineoplastic	T50.Z91	T50.Z92	T50.Z93	T50.Z94	T50.Z95	T50.Z96
bacterial NEC	T50.A91	T50.A92	T50.A93	T50.A94	T50.A95	T50.A96
with						
other bacterial component	T50.A91	T50.A92	T50.A93	T50.A94	T50.A95	T50.A96
pertussis component	T50.A91	T50.A92	T50.A93	T50.A94	T50.A95	T50.A96
viral-rickettsial component	T50.A91	T50.A92	T50.A93	T50.A94	T50.A95	T50.A96
mixed NEC	T50.A91	T50.A92	T50.A93	T50.A94	T50.A95	T50.A96
BCG	T50.A91	T50.A92	T50.A93	T50.A94	T50.A95	T50.A96
cholera	T50.A91	T50.A92	T50.A93	T50.A94	T50.A95	T50.A96
diphtheria	T50.A91	T50.A92	T50.A93	T50.A94	T50.A95	T50.A96
with tetanus	T50.A21	T50.A22	T50.A23	T50.A24	T50.A25	T50.A26
and pertussis	T50.A11	T50.A12	T50.A13	T50.A14	T50.A15	T50.A16

	External Cause (T-Code)					
Substance	Poisoning, Accidental (Unintentional)	Poisoning, Intentional Self-Harm	Poisoning, Assault	Poisoning, Undetermined	Adverse Effect	Underdosing
Vaccine NEC *(Continued)*						
influenza	T50.B91	T50.B92	T50.B93	T50.B94	T50.B95	T50.B96
measles	T50.B91	T50.B92	T50.B93	T50.B94	T50.B95	T50.B96
with mumps and rubella	T50.B91	T50.B92	T50.B93	T50.B94	T50.B95	T50.B96
meningococcal	T50.A91	T50.A92	T50.A93	T50.A94	T50.A95	T50.A96
mumps	T50.B91	T50.B92	T50.B93	T50.B94	T50.B95	T50.B96
paratyphoid	T50.A91	T50.A92	T50.A93	T50.A94	T50.A95	T50.A96
pertussis	T50.A11	T50.A12	T50.A13	T50.A14	T50.A15	T50.A16
with diphtheria	T50.A11	T50.A12	T50.A13	T50.A14	T50.A15	T50.A16
and tetanus	T50.A11	T50.A12	T50.A13	T50.A14	T50.A15	T50.A16
plague	T50.A91	T50.A92	T50.A93	T50.A94	T50.A95	T50.A96
poliomyelitis	T50.B91	T50.B92	T50.B93	T50.B94	T50.B95	T50.B96
poliovirus	T50.B91	T50.B92	T50.B93	T50.B94	T50.B95	T50.B96
rabies	T50.B91	T50.B92	T50.B93	T50.B94	T50.B95	T50.B96
respiratory syncytial virus	T50.B91	T50.B92	T50.B93	T50.B94	T50.B95	T50.B96
rickettsial NEC	T50.A91	T50.A92	T50.A93	T50.A94	T50.A95	T50.A96
with						
bacterial component	T50.A21	T50.A22	T50.A23	T50.A24	T50.A25	T50.A26
Rocky Mountain spotted fever	T50.A91	T50.A92	T50.A93	T50.A94	T50.A95	T50.A96
rubella	T50.B91	T50.B92	T50.B93	T50.B94	T50.B95	T50.B96
sabin oral	T50.B91	T50.B92	T50.B93	T50.B94	T50.B95	T50.B96
smallpox	T50.B11	T50.B12	T50.B13	T50.B14	T50.B15	T50.B16
TAB	T50.A91	T50.A92	T50.A93	T50.A94	T50.A95	T50.A96
tetanus	T50.A91	T50.A92	T50.A93	T50.A94	T50.A95	T50.A96
typhoid	T50.A91	T50.A92	T50.A93	T50.A94	T50.A95	T50.A96
typhus	T50.A91	T50.A92	T50.A93	T50.A94	T50.A95	T50.A96
viral NEC	T50.B91	T50.B92	T50.B93	T50.B94	T50.B95	T50.B96
yellow fever	T50.B91	T50.B92	T50.B93	T50.B94	T50.B95	T50.B96
Vaccinia immune globulin	T50.Z11	T50.Z12	T50.Z13	T50.Z14	T50.Z15	T50.Z16
Vaginal contraceptives	T49.8X1	T49.8X2	T49.8X3	T49.8X4	T49.8X5	T49.8X6
Valerian						
root	T42.6X1	T42.6X2	T42.6X3	T42.6X4	T42.6X5	T42.6X6
tincture	T42.6X1	T42.6X2	T42.6X3	T42.6X4	T42.6X5	T42.6X6
Valethamate bromide	T44.3X1	T44.3X2	T44.3X3	T44.3X4	T44.3X5	T44.3X6
Valisone	T49.0X1	T49.0X2	T49.0X3	T49.0X4	T49.0X5	T49.0X6
Valium	T42.4X1	T42.4X2	T42.4X3	T42.4X4	T42.4X5	T42.4X6
Valmid	T42.6X1	T42.6X2	T42.6X3	T42.6X4	T42.6X5	T42.6X6
Valnoctamide	T42.6X1	T42.6X2	T42.6X3	T42.6X4	T42.6X5	T42.6X6
Valproate (sodium)	T42.6X1	T42.6X2	T42.6X3	T42.6X4	T42.6X5	T42.6X6
Valproic acid	T42.6X1	T42.6X2	T42.6X3	T42.6X4	T42.6X5	T42.6X6
Valpromide	T42.6X1	T42.6X2	T42.6X3	T42.6X4	T42.6X5	T42.6X6
Vanadium	T56.891	T56.892	T56.893	T56.894	—	—

TABLE OF DRUGS AND CHEMICALS

Substance	Poisoning, Accidental (Unintentional)	Poisoning, Intentional Self-Harm	Poisoning, Assault	Poisoning, Undetermined	Adverse Effect	Underdosing
Vancomycin	T36.8X1	T36.8X2	T36.8X3	T36.8X4	T36.8X5	T36.8X6
Vapor—see also Gas	T59.91	T59.92	T59.93	T59.94	—	—
kiln (carbon monoxide)	T58.8X1	T58.8X2	T58.8X3	T58.8X4	—	—
lead—see Lead						
specified source NEC	T59.891	T59.892	T59.893	T59.894	—	—
Vardenafil	T46.7X1	T46.7X2	T46.7X3	T46.7X4	T46.7X5	T46.7X6
Varicose reduction drug	T46.8X1	T46.8X2	T46.8X3	T46.8X4	T46.8X5	T46.8X6
Varnish	T65.4X1	T65.4X2	T65.4X3	T65.4X4	—	—
cleaner	T52.91	T52.92	T52.93	T52.94	—	—
Vaseline	T49.3X1	T49.3X2	T49.3X3	T49.3X4	T49.3X5	T49.3X6
Vasodilan	T46.7X1	T46.7X2	T46.7X3	T46.7X4	T46.7X5	T46.7X6
Vasodilator						
coronary NEC	T46.3X1	T46.3X2	T46.3X3	T46.3X4	T46.3X5	T46.3X6
peripheral NEC	T46.7X1	T46.7X2	T46.7X3	T46.7X4	T46.7X5	T46.7X6
Vasopressin	T38.891	T38.892	T38.893	T38.894	T38.895	T38.896
Vasopressor drugs	T38.891	T38.892	T38.893	T38.894	T38.895	T38.896
Vecuronium bromide	T48.1X1	T48.1X2	T48.1X3	T48.1X4	T48.1X5	T48.1X6
Vegetable extract, astringent	T49.2X1	T49.2X2	T49.2X3	T49.2X4	T49.2X5	T49.2X6
Venlafaxine	T43.211	T43.212	T43.213	T43.214	T43.215	T43.216
Venom, venomous (bite) (sting)	T63.91	T63.92	T63.93	T63.94	—	—
amphibian NEC	T63.831	T63.832	T63.833	T63.834	—	—
animal NEC	T63.891	T63.892	T63.893	T63.894	—	—
ant	T63.421	T63.422	T63.423	T63.424	—	—
arthropod NEC	T63.481	T63.482	T63.483	T63.484	—	—
bee	T63.441	T63.442	T63.443	T63.444	—	—
centipede	T63.411	T63.412	T63.413	T63.414	—	—
fish	T63.591	T63.592	T63.593	T63.594	—	—
frog	T63.811	T63.812	T63.813	T63.814	—	—
hornet	T63.451	T63.452	T63.453	T63.454	—	—
insect NEC	T63.481	T63.482	T63.483	T63.484	—	—
lizard	T63.121	T63.122	T63.123	T63.124	—	—
marine						
animals	T63.691	T63.692	T63.693	T63.694	—	—
bluebottle	T63.611	T63.612	T63.613	T63.614	—	—
jellyfish NEC	T63.621	T63.622	T63.623	T63.624	—	—
Portuguese Man-o-war	T63.611	T63.612	T63.613	T63.614	—	—
sea anemone	T63.631	T63.632	T63.633	T63.634	—	—
specified NEC	T63.691	T63.692	T63.693	T63.694	—	—
fish	T63.591	T63.592	T63.593	T63.594	—	—
plants	T63.711	T63.712	T63.713	T63.714	—	—
sting ray	T63.511	T63.512	T63.513	T63.514	—	—

Substance	Poisoning, Accidental (Unintentional)	Poisoning, Intentional Self-Harm	Poisoning, Assault	Poisoning, Undetermined	Adverse Effect	Underdosing
Venom, venomous (Continued)						
millipede (tropical)	T63.411	T63.412	T63.413	T63.414	—	—
plant NEC	T63.791	T63.792	T63.793	T63.794	—	—
marine	T63.711	T63.712	T63.713	T63.714	—	—
reptile	T63.191	T63.192	T63.193	T63.194	—	—
gila monster	T63.111	T63.112	T63.113	T63.114	—	—
lizard NEC	T63.121	T63.122	T63.123	T63.124	—	—
scorpion	T63.2X1	T63.2X2	T63.2X3	T63.2X4	—	—
snake	T63.001	T63.002	T63.003	T63.004	—	—
African NEC	T63.081	T63.082	T63.083	T63.084	—	—
American (North) (South) NEC	T63.061	T63.062	T63.063	T63.064	—	—
Asian	T63.081	T63.082	T63.083	T63.084	—	—
Australian	T63.071	T63.072	T63.073	T63.074	—	—
cobra	T63.041	T63.042	T63.043	T63.044	—	—
coral snake	T63.021	T63.022	T63.023	T63.024	—	—
rattlesnake	T63.011	T63.012	T63.013	T63.014	—	—
specified NEC	T63.091	T63.092	T63.093	T63.094	—	—
taipan	T63.031	T63.032	T63.033	T63.034	—	—
specified NEC	T63.891	T63.892	T63.893	T63.894	—	—
spider	T63.301	T63.302	T63.303	T63.304	—	—
black widow	T63.311	T63.312	T63.313	T63.314	—	—
brown recluse	T63.331	T63.332	T63.333	T63.334	—	—
specified NEC	T63.391	T63.392	T63.393	T63.394	—	—
tarantula	T63.321	T63.322	T63.323	T63.324	—	—
sting ray	T63.511	T63.512	T63.513	T63.514	—	—
toad	T63.821	T63.822	T63.823	T63.824	—	—
wasp	T63.461	T63.462	T63.463	T63.464	—	—
Venous sclerosing drug NEC	T46.8X1	T46.8X2	T46.8X3	T46.8X4	T46.8X5	T46.8X6
Ventolin—see Albuterol						
Verapamil	T46.1X1	T46.1X2	T46.1X3	T46.1X4	T46.1X5	T46.1X6
Veramon	T42.3X1	T42.3X2	T42.3X3	T42.3X4	T42.3X5	T42.3X6
Veratrine	T46.5X1	T46.5X2	T46.5X3	T46.5X4	T46.5X5	T46.5X6
Veratrum						
album	T62.2X1	T62.2X2	T62.2X3	T62.2X4	—	—
alkaloids	T46.5X1	T46.5X2	T46.5X3	T46.5X4	T46.5X5	T46.5X6
viride	T62.2X1	T62.2X2	T62.2X3	T62.2X4	—	—
Verdigris	T60.3X1	T60.3X2	T60.3X3	T60.3X4	—	—
Veronal	T42.3X1	T42.3X2	T42.3X3	T42.3X4	T42.3X5	T42.3X6
Veroxil	T37.4X1	T37.4X2	T37.4X3	T37.4X4	T37.4X5	T37.4X6
Versenate	T50.6X1	T50.6X2	T50.6X3	T50.6X4	T50.6X5	T50.6X6

◀ New ◀ Revised ~~deleted~~ Deleted

Substance	Poisoning, Accidental (Unintentional)	Poisoning, Intentional Self-Harm	Poisoning, Assault	Poisoning, Undetermined	Adverse Effect	Underdosing
Versidyne	T39.8X1	T39.8X2	T39.8X3	T39.8X4	T39.8X5	T39.8X6
Vetrabutine	T48.0X1	T48.0X2	T48.0X3	T48.0X4	T48.0X5	T48.0X6
Vidarabine	T37.5X1	T37.5X2	T37.5X3	T37.5X4	T37.5X5	T37.5X6
Vienna						
green	T57.0X1	T57.0X2	T57.0X3	T57.0X4	—	—
insecticide	T60.2X1	T60.2X2	T60.2X3	T60.2X4	—	—
red	T57.0X1	T57.0X2	T57.0X3	T57.0X4	—	—
pharmaceutical dye	T50.991	T50.992	T50.993	T50.994	T50.995	T50.996
Vigabatrin	T42.6X1	T42.6X2	T42.6X3	T42.6X4	T42.6X5	T42.6X6
Viloxazine	T43.291	T43.292	T43.293	T43.294	T43.295	T43.296
Viminol	T39.8X1	T39.8X2	T39.8X3	T39.8X4	T39.8X5	T39.8X6
Vinbarbital, vinbarbitone	T42.3X1	T42.3X2	T42.3X3	T42.3X4	T42.3X5	T42.3X6
Vinblastine	T45.1X1	T45.1X2	T45.1X3	T45.1X4	T45.1X5	T45.1X6
Vinburnine	T46.7X1	T46.7X2	T46.7X3	T46.7X4	T46.7X5	T46.7X6
Vincamine	T45.1X1	T45.1X2	T45.1X3	T45.1X4	T45.1X5	T45.1X6
Vincristine	T45.1X1	T45.1X2	T45.1X3	T45.1X4	T45.1X5	T45.1X6
Vindesine	T45.1X1	T45.1X2	T45.1X3	T45.1X4	T45.1X5	T45.1X6
Vinesthene, vinethene	T41.0X1	T41.0X2	T41.0X3	T41.0X4	T41.0X5	T41.0X6
Vinorelbine tartrate	T45.1X1	T45.1X2	T45.1X3	T45.1X4	T45.1X5	T45.1X6
Vinpocetine	T46.7X1	T46.7X2	T46.7X3	T46.7X4	T46.7X5	T46.7X6
Vinyl						
acetate	T65.891	T65.892	T65.893	T65.894	—	—
bital	T42.3X1	T42.3X2	T42.3X3	T42.3X4	T42.3X5	T42.3X6
bromide	T65.891	T65.892	T65.893	T65.894	—	—
chloride	T59.891	T59.892	T59.893	T59.894	—	—
ether	T41.0X1	T41.0X2	T41.0X3	T41.0X4	T41.0X5	T41.0X6
Vinylbital	T42.3X1	T42.3X2	T42.3X3	T42.3X4	T42.3X5	T42.3X6
Vinylidene chloride	T65.891	T65.892	T65.893	T65.894	—	—
Vioform	T37.8X1	T37.8X2	T37.8X3	T37.8X4	T37.8X5	T37.8X6
topical	T49.0X1	T49.0X2	T49.0X3	T49.0X4	T49.0X5	T49.0X6
Viomycin	T36.8X1	T36.8X2	T36.8X3	T36.8X4	T36.8X5	T36.8X6
Viosterol	T45.2X1	T45.2X2	T45.2X3	T45.2X4	T45.2X5	T45.2X6
Viper (venom)	T63.091	T63.092	T63.093	T63.094	—	—
Viprynium	T37.4X1	T37.4X2	T37.4X3	T37.4X4	T37.4X5	T37.4X6
Viquidil	T46.7X1	T46.7X2	T46.7X3	T46.7X4	T46.7X5	T46.7X6
Viral vaccine NEC	T50.B91	T50.B92	T50.B93	T50.B94	T50.B95	T50.B96
Virginiamycin	T36.8X1	T36.8X2	T36.8X3	T36.8X4	T36.8X5	T36.8X6
Virugon	T37.5X1	T37.5X2	T37.5X3	T37.5X4	T37.5X5	T37.5X6
Viscous agent	T50.901	T50.902	T50.903	T50.904	T50.905	T50.906
Visine	T49.5X1	T49.5X2	T49.5X3	T49.5X4	T49.5X5	T49.5X6
Visnadine	T46.3X1	T46.3X2	T46.3X3	T46.3X4	T46.3X5	T46.3X6

Substance	Poisoning, Accidental (Unintentional)	Poisoning, Intentional Self-Harm	Poisoning, Assault	Poisoning, Undetermined	Adverse Effect	Underdosing
Vitamin NEC	T45.2X1	T45.2X2	T45.2X3	T45.2X4	T45.2X5	T45.2X6
A	T45.2X1	T45.2X2	T45.2X3	T45.2X4	T45.2X5	T45.2X6
B NEC	T45.2X1	T45.2X2	T45.2X3	T45.2X4	T45.2X5	T45.2X6
nicotinic acid	T46.7X1	T46.7X2	T46.7X3	T46.7X4	T46.7X5	T46.7X6
B1	T45.2X1	T45.2X2	T45.2X3	T45.2X4	T45.2X5	T45.2X6
B2	T45.2X1	T45.2X2	T45.2X3	T45.2X4	T45.2X5	T45.2X6
B6	T45.2X1	T45.2X2	T45.2X3	T45.2X4	T45.2X5	T45.2X6
B12	T45.2X1	T45.2X2	T45.2X3	T45.2X4	T45.2X5	T45.2X6
B15	T45.2X1	T45.2X2	T45.2X3	T45.2X4	T45.2X5	T45.2X6
C	T45.2X1	T45.2X2	T45.2X3	T45.2X4	T45.2X5	T45.2X6
D	T45.2X1	T45.2X2	T45.2X3	T45.2X4	T45.2X5	T45.2X6
D2	T45.2X1	T45.2X2	T45.2X3	T45.2X4	T45.2X5	T45.2X6
D3	T45.2X1	T45.2X2	T45.2X3	T45.2X4	T45.2X5	T45.2X6
E	T45.2X1	T45.2X2	T45.2X3	T45.2X4	T45.2X5	T45.2X6
E acetate	T45.2X1	T45.2X2	T45.2X3	T45.2X4	T45.2X5	T45.2X6
hematopoietic	T45.8X1	T45.8X2	T45.8X3	T45.8X4	T45.8X5	T45.8X6
K NEC	T45.7X1	T45.7X2	T45.7X3	T45.7X4	T45.7X5	T45.7X6
K1	T45.7X1	T45.7X2	T45.7X3	T45.7X4	T45.7X5	T45.7X6
K2	T45.7X1	T45.7X2	T45.7X3	T45.7X4	T45.7X5	T45.7X6
PP	T45.2X1	T45.2X2	T45.2X3	T45.2X4	T45.2X5	T45.2X6
ulceroprotectant	T47.1X1	T47.1X2	T47.1X3	T47.1X4	T47.1X5	T47.1X6
Vleminckx's solution	T49.4X1	T49.4X2	T49.4X3	T49.4X4	T49.4X5	T49.4X6
Voltaren — see Diclofenac sodium						
W						
Warfarin	T45.511	T45.512	T45.513	T45.514	T45.515	T45.516
rodenticide	T60.4X1	T60.4X2	T60.4X3	T60.4X4	—	—
sodium	T45.511	T45.512	T45.513	T45.514	T45.515	T45.516
Wasp (sting)	T63.461	T63.462	T63.463	T63.464	—	—
Water						
balance drug	T50.3X1	T50.3X2	T50.3X3	T50.3X4	T50.3X5	T50.3X6
distilled	T50.3X1	T50.3X2	T50.3X3	T50.3X4	T50.3X5	T50.3X6
gas — see Gas, water						
incomplete combustion of — see Carbon, monoxide, fuel, utility						
hemlock	T62.2X1	T62.2X2	T62.2X3	T62.2X4	—	—
moccasin (venom)	T63.061	T63.062	T63.063	T63.064	—	—
purified	T50.3X1	T50.3X2	T50.3X3	T50.3X4	T50.3X5	T50.3X6
Wax (paraffin) (petroleum)	T52.0X1	T52.0X2	T52.0X3	T52.0X4	—	—
automobile	T65.891	T65.892	T65.893	T65.894	—	—
floor	T52.0X1	T52.0X2	T52.0X3	T52.0X4	—	—

◄ New   ◄ Revised   ~~deleted~~ Deleted

TABLE OF DRUGS AND CHEMICALS

Substance	Poisoning, Accidental (Unintentional)	Poisoning, Intentional Self-Harm	Poisoning, Assault	Poisoning, Undetermined	Adverse Effect	Underdosing
	External Cause (T-Code)					
Weed killers NEC	T60.3X1	T60.3X2	T60.3X3	T60.3X4	—	—
Welldorm	T42.6X1	T42.6X2	T42.6X3	T42.6X4	T42.6X5	T42.6X6
White						
arsenic	T57.0X1	T57.0X2	T57.0X3	T57.0X4	—	—
hellebore	T62.2X1	T62.2X2	T62.2X3	T62.2X4	—	—
lotion (keratolytic)	T49.4X1	T49.4X2	T49.4X3	T49.4X4	T49.4X5	T49.4X6
spirit	T52.0X1	T52.0X2	T52.0X3	T52.0X4	—	—
Whitewash	T65.891	T65.892	T65.893	T65.894	—	—
Whole blood (human)	T45.8X1	T45.8X2	T45.8X3	T45.8X4	T45.8X5	T45.8X6
Wild						
black cherry	T62.2X1	T62.2X2	T62.2X3	T62.2X4	—	—
poisonous plants NEC	T62.2X1	T62.2X2	T62.2X3	T62.2X4	—	—
Window cleaning fluid	T65.891	T65.892	T65.893	T65.894		
Wintergreen (oil)	T49.3X1	T49.3X2	T49.3X3	T49.3X4	T49.3X5	T49.3X6
Wisterine	T62.2X1	T62.2X2	T62.2X3	T62.2X4		
Witch hazel	T49.2X1	T49.2X2	T49.2X3	T49.2X4	T49.2X5	T49.2X6
Wood alcohol or spirit	T51.1X1	T51.1X2	T51.1X3	T51.1X4	—	—
Wool fat (hydrous)	T49.3X1	T49.3X2	T49.3X3	T49.3X4	T49.3X5	T49.3X6
Woorali	T48.1X1	T48.1X2	T48.1X3	T48.1X4	T48.1X5	T48.1X6
Wormseed, American	T37.4X1	T37.4X2	T37.4X3	T37.4X4	T37.4X5	T37.4X6
X						
Xamoterol	T44.5X1	T44.5X2	T44.5X3	T44.5X4	T44.5X5	T44.5X6
Xanthine diuretics	T50.2X1	T50.2X2	T50.2X3	T50.2X4	T50.2X5	T50.2X6
Xanthinol nicotinate	T46.7X1	T46.7X2	T46.7X3	T46.7X4	T46.7X5	T46.7X6
Xanthotoxin	T49.3X1	T49.3X2	T49.3X3	T49.3X4	T49.3X5	T49.3X6
Xantinol nicotinate	T46.7X1	T46.7X2	T46.7X3	T46.7X4	T46.7X5	T46.7X6
Xantocillin	T36.0X1	T36.0X2	T36.0X3	T36.0X4	T36.0X5	T36.0X6
Xenon (127Xe) (133Xe)	T50.8X1	T50.8X2	T50.8X3	T50.8X4	T50.8X5	T50.8X6
Xenysalate	T49.4X1	T49.4X2	T49.4X3	T49.4X4	T49.4X5	T49.4X6
Xibornol	T37.8X1	T37.8X2	T37.8X3	T37.8X4	T37.8X5	T37.8X6
Xigris	T45.511	T45.512	T45.513	T45.514	T45.515	T45.516
Xipamide	T50.2X1	T50.2X2	T50.2X3	T50.2X4	T50.2X5	T50.2X6
Xylene (vapor)	T52.2X1	T52.2X2	T52.2X3	T52.2X4	—	—
Xylocaine (infiltration) (topical)	T41.3X1	T41.3X2	T41.3X3	T41.3X4	T41.3X5	T41.3X6
nerve block (peripheral) (plexus)	T41.3X1	T41.3X2	T41.3X3	T41.3X4	T41.3X5	T41.3X6
spinal	T41.3X1	T41.3X2	T41.3X3	T41.3X4	T41.3X5	T41.3X6
Xylol (vapor)	T52.2X1	T52.2X2	T52.2X3	T52.2X4	—	—
Xylometazoline	T48.5X1	T48.5X2	T48.5X3	T48.5X4	T48.5X5	T48.5X6

Substance	Poisoning, Accidental (Unintentional)	Poisoning, Intentional Self-Harm	Poisoning, Assault	Poisoning, Undetermined	Adverse Effect	Underdosing
	External Cause (T-Code)					
Y						
Yeast	T45.2X1	T45.2X2	T45.2X3	T45.2X4	T45.2X5	T45.2X6
dried	T45.2X1	T45.2X2	T45.2X3	T45.2X4	T45.2X5	T45.2X6
Yellow						
fever vaccine	T50.B91	T50.B92	T50.B93	T50.B94	T50.B95	T50.B96
jasmine	T62.2X1	T62.2X2	T62.2X3	T62.2X4	—	—
phenolphthalein	T47.2X1	T47.2X2	T47.2X3	T47.2X4	T47.2X5	T47.2X6
Yew	T62.2X1	T62.2X2	T62.2X3	T62.2X4	—	—
Yohimbic acid	T40.991	T40.992	T40.993	T40.994	T40.995	T40.996
Z						
Zactane	T39.8X1	T39.8X2	T39.8X3	T39.8X4	T39.8X5	T39.8X6
Zalcitabine	T37.5X1	T37.5X2	T37.5X3	T37.5X4	T37.5X5	T37.5X6
Zaroxolyn	T50.2X1	T50.2X2	T50.2X3	T50.2X4	T50.2X5	T50.2X6
Zephiran (topical)	T49.0X1	T49.0X2	T49.0X3	T49.0X4	T49.0X5	T49.0X6
ophthalmic preparation	T49.5X1	T49.5X2	T49.5X3	T49.5X4	T49.5X5	T49.5X6
Zeranol	T38.7X1	T38.7X2	T38.7X3	T38.7X4	T38.7X5	T38.7X6
Zerone	T51.1X1	T51.1X2	T51.1X3	T51.1X4	—	—
Zidovudine	T37.5X1	T37.5X2	T37.5X3	T37.5X4	T37.5X5	T37.5X6
Zimeldine	T43.221	T43.222	T43.223	T43.224	T43.225	T43.226
Zinc (compounds) (fumes) (vapor) NEC	T56.5X1	T56.5X2	T56.5X3	T56.5X4	—	—
anti-infectives	T49.0X1	T49.0X2	T49.0X3	T49.0X4	T49.0X5	T49.0X6
antivaricose	T46.8X1	T46.8X2	T46.8X3	T46.8X4	T46.8X5	T46.8X6
bacitracin	T49.0X1	T49.0X2	T49.0X3	T49.0X4	T49.0X5	T49.0X6
chloride (mouthwash)	T49.6X1	T49.6X2	T49.6X3	T49.6X4	T49.6X5	T49.6X6
chromate	T56.5X1	T56.5X2	T56.5X3	T56.5X4	—	—
gelatin	T49.3X1	T49.3X2	T49.3X3	T49.3X4	T49.3X5	T49.3X6
oxide	T49.3X1	T49.3X2	T49.3X3	T49.3X4	T49.3X5	T49.3X6
plaster	T49.3X1	T49.3X2	T49.3X3	T49.3X4	T49.3X5	T49.3X6
peroxide	T49.0X1	T49.0X2	T49.0X3	T49.0X4	T49.0X5	T49.0X6
pesticides	T56.5X1	T56.5X2	T56.5X3	T56.5X4	—	—
phosphide	T60.4X1	T60.4X2	T60.4X3	T60.4X4	—	—
pyrithionate	T49.4X1	T49.4X2	T49.4X3	T49.4X4	T49.4X5	T49.4X6
stearate	T49.3X1	T49.3X2	T49.3X3	T49.3X4	T49.3X5	T49.3X6
sulfate	T49.5X1	T49.5X2	T49.5X3	T49.5X4	T49.5X5	T49.5X6
ENT agent	T49.6X1	T49.6X2	T49.6X3	T49.6X4	T49.6X5	T49.6X6
ophthalmic solution	T49.5X1	T49.5X2	T49.5X3	T49.5X4	T49.5X5	T49.5X6
topical NEC	T49.0X1	T49.0X2	T49.0X3	T49.0X4	T49.0X5	T49.0X6
undecylenate	T49.0X1	T49.0X2	T49.0X3	T49.0X4	T49.0X5	T49.0X6

◄ New   ◄ Revised   ~~deleted~~ Deleted

Substance	Poisoning, Accidental (Unintentional)	Poisoning, Intentional Self-Harm	Poisoning, Assault	Poisoning, Undetermined	Adverse Effect	Underdosing
Zineb	T60.0X1	T60.0X2	T60.0X3	T60.0X4	—	—
Zinostatin	T45.1X1	T45.1X2	T45.1X3	T45.1X4	T45.1X5	T45.1X6
Zipeprol	T48.3X1	T48.3X2	T48.3X3	T48.3X4	T48.3X5	T48.3X6
Zofenopril	T46.4X1	T46.4X2	T46.4X3	T46.4X4	T46.4X5	T46.4X6
Zolpidem	T42.6X1	T42.6X2	T42.6X3	T42.6X4	T42.6X5	T42.6X6
Zomepirac	T39.391	T39.392	T39.393	T39.394	T39.395	T39.396
Zopiclone	T42.6X1	T42.6X2	T42.6X3	T42.6X4	T42.6X5	T42.6X6

Substance	Poisoning, Accidental (Unintentional)	Poisoning, Intentional Self-Harm	Poisoning, Assault	Poisoning, Undetermined	Adverse Effect	Underdosing
Zorubicin	T45.1X1	T45.1X2	T45.1X3	T45.1X4	T45.1X5	T45.1X6
Zotepine	T43.591	T43.592	T43.593	T43.594	T43.595	T43.596
Zovant	T45.511	T45.512	T45.513	T45.514	T45.515	T45.516
Zoxazolamine	T42.8X1	T42.8X2	T42.8X3	T42.8X4	T42.8X5	T42.8X6
Zuclopenthixol	T43.4X1	T43.4X2	T43.4X3	T43.4X4	T43.4X5	T43.4X6
Zygadenus (venenosus)	T62.2X1	T62.2X2	T62.2X3	T62.2X4	—	—
Zyprexa	T43.591	T43.592	T43.593	T43.594	T43.595	T43.596

TABLE OF DRUGS AND CHEMICALS

ECI

External Cause
of Injuries Index

A

Abandonment (causing exposure to weather conditions) (with intent to injure or kill) NEC X58

Abuse (adult) (child) (mental) (physical) (sexual) X58

Accident (to) X58
aircraft (in transit) (powered) —*see also* Accident, transport, aircraft
due to, caused by cataclysm —*see* Forces of nature, by type
animal-drawn vehicle —*see* Accident, transport, animal-drawn vehicle occupant
animal-rider —*see* Accident, transport, animal-rider
automobile —*see* Accident, transport, car occupant
bare foot water skiier V94.4
boat, boating —*see also* Accident, watercraft
striking swimmer
powered V94.11
unpowered V94.12
bus —*see* Accident, transport, bus occupant
cable car, not on rails V98.0
on rails —*see* Accident, transport, streetcar occupant
car —*see* Accident, transport, car occupant
caused by, due to
animal NEC W64
chain hoist W24.0
cold (excessive) —*see* Exposure, cold
corrosive liquid, substance —*see* Table of Drugs and Chemicals
cutting or piercing instrument —*see* Contact, with, by type of instrument
drive belt W24.0
electric
current —*see* Exposure, electric current
motor —*see also* Contact, with, by type of machine W31.3
current (of) W86.8
environmental factor NEC X58
explosive material —*see* Explosion
fire, flames —*see* Exposure, fire
firearm missile —*see* Discharge, firearm by type
heat (excessive) —*see* Heat
hot —*see* Contact, with, hot
ignition —*see* Ignition
lifting device W24.0
lightning —*see* subcategory T75.0
causing fire —*see* Exposure, fire
machine, machinery —*see* Contact, with, by type of machine
natural factor NEC X58
pulley (block) W24.0
radiation —*see* Radiation
steam X13.1
inhalation X13.0
pipe X16
thunderbolt —*see* subcategory T75.0
causing fire —*see* Exposure, fire
transmission device W24.1
coach —*see* Accident, transport, bus occupant
coal car —*see* Accident, transport, industrial vehicle occupant
diving —*see also* Fall, into, water
with
drowning or submersion —*see* Drowning
forklift —*see* Accident, transport, industrial vehicle occupant
heavy transport vehicle NOS —*see* Accident, transport, truck occupant
ice yacht V98.2
in
medical, surgical procedure
as, or due to misadventure —*see* Misadventure
causing an abnormal reaction or later complication without mention of misadventure —*see also* Complication of or following, by type of procedure Y84.9
land yacht V98.1
late effect of —*see* W00-X58 with 7th character S
logging car —*see* Accident, transport, industrial vehicle occupant

Accident *(Continued)*
machine, machinery —*see also* Contact, with, by type of machine
on board watercraft V93.69
explosion —*see* Explosion, in, watercraft
fire —*see* Burn, on board watercraft
powered craft V93.63
ferry boat V93.61
fishing boat V93.62
jet ski V93.63
liner V93.61
merchant ship V93.60
passenger ship V93.61
sailboat V93.64
mine tram —*see* Accident, transport, industrial vehicle occupant
mobility scooter (motorized) —*see* Accident, transport, pedestrian, conveyance, specified type NEC
motor scooter —*see* Accident, transport, motorcycle
motor vehicle NOS (traffic) —*see also* Accident, transport V89.2
nontraffic V89.0
three-wheeled NOS —*see* Accident, transport, three-wheeled motor vehicle occupant
motorcycle NOS —*see* Accident, transport, motorcycle
nonmotor vehicle NOS (nontraffic) —*see also* Accident, transport V89.1
traffic NOS V89.3
nontraffic (victim's mode of transport NOS) V88.9
collision (between) V88.7
bus and truck V88.5
car and:
bus V88.3
pickup V88.2
three-wheeled motor vehicle V88.0
train V88.6
truck V88.4
two-wheeled motor vehicle V88.0
van V88.2
specified vehicle NEC and:
three-wheeled motor vehicle V88.1
two-wheeled motor vehicle V88.1
known mode of transport —*see* Accident, transport, by type of vehicle
noncollision V88.8
on board watercraft V93.89
powered craft V93.83
ferry boat V93.81
fishing boat V93.82
jet ski V93.83
liner V93.81
merchant ship V93.80
passenger ship V93.81
unpowered craft V93.88
canoe V93.85
inflatable V93.86
in tow
recreational V94.31
specified NEC V94.32
kayak V93.85
sailboat V93.84
surf-board V93.88
water skis V93.87
windsurfer V93.88
parachutist V97.29
entangled in object V97.21
injured on landing V97.22
pedal cycle —*see* Accident, transport, pedal cyclist
pedestrian (on foot)
with
another pedestrian W51
with fall W03
due to ice or snow W00.0
on pedestrian conveyance NEC V00.09
rider of
hoverboard V00.038
Segway V00.038
standing
electric scooter V00.031
micro-mobility pedestrian conveyance NEC V00.038
roller skater (in-line) V00.01
skate boarder V00.02
transport vehicle —*see* Accident, transport
on pedestrian conveyance —*see* Accident, transport, pedestrian, conveyance

Accident *(Continued)*
pick-up truck or van —*see* Accident, transport, pickup truck occupant
quarry truck —*see* Accident, transport, industrial vehicle occupant
railway vehicle (any) (in motion) —*see* Accident, transport, railway vehicle occupant
due to cataclysm —*see* Forces of nature, by type
scooter (non-motorized) —*see* Accident, transport, pedestrian, conveyance, scooter
sequelae of —*see* W00-X58 with 7th character S
skateboard —*see* Accident, transport, pedestrian, conveyance, skateboard
ski (ing) —*see* Accident, transport, pedestrian, conveyance
lift V98.3
specified cause NEC X58
streetcar —*see* Accident, transport, streetcar occupant
traffic (victim's mode of transport NOS) V87.9
collision (between) V87.7
bus and truck V87.5
car and:
bus V87.3
pickup V87.2
three-wheeled motor vehicle V87.0
train V87.6
truck V87.4
two-wheeled motor vehicle V87.0
van V87.2
specified vehicle NEC V86.39
and
three-wheeled motor vehicle V87.1
two-wheeled motor vehicle V87.1
driver V86.09
person on outside V86.29
passenger V86.19
while boarding or alighting V86.49
known mode of transport —*see* Accident, transport, by type of vehicle
noncollision V87.8
transport (involving injury to) V99
18 wheeler —*see* Accident, transport, truck occupant
agricultural vehicle occupant (nontraffic) V84.9
driver V84.5
hanger-on V84.7
passenger V84.6
traffic V84.3
driver V84.0
hanger-on V84.2
passenger V84.1
while boarding or alighting V84.4
aircraft NEC V97.89
military NEC V97.818
with civilian aircraft V97.810
civilian injured by V97.811
occupant injured (in)
nonpowered craft accident V96.9
balloon V96.00
collision V96.03
crash V96.01
explosion V96.05
fire V96.04
forced landing V96.02
specified type NEC V96.09
glider V96.20
collision V96.23
crash V96.21
explosion V96.25
fire V96.24
forced landing V96.22
specified type NEC V96.29
hang glider V96.10
collision V96.13
crash V96.11
explosion V96.15
fire V96.14
forced landing V96.12
specified type NEC V96.19
specified craft NEC V96.8
powered craft accident V95.9
fixed wing NEC
commercial V95.30
collision V95.33
crash V95.31

▶ New   ⇒ Revised   ~~deleted~~ Deleted   ● Use Additional Character(s)

Accident (Continued)
  transport (Continued)
    aircraft (Continued)
      occupant injured (Continued)
        powered craft accident Continued)
          fixed wing (Continued)
            commercial I70.521 (Continued)
              explosion V95.35
              fire V95.34
              forced landing V95.32
              specified type NEC V95.39
            private V95.20
              collision V95.23
              crash V95.21
              explosion V95.25
              fire V95.24
              forced landing V95.22
              specified type NEC V95.29
          glider V95.10
            collision V95.13
            crash V95.11
            explosion V95.15
            fire V95.14
            forced landing V95.12
            specified type NEC V95.19
          helicopter V95.00
            collision V95.03
            crash V95.01
            explosion V95.05
            fire V95.04
            forced landing V95.02
            specified type NEC V95.09
          spacecraft V95.40
            collision V95.43
            crash V95.41
            explosion V95.45
            fire V95.44
            forced landing V95.42
            specified type NEC V95.49
          specified craft NEC V95.8
          ultralight V95.10
            collision V95.13
            crash V95.11
            explosion V95.15
            fire V95.14
            forced landing V95.12
            specified type NEC V95.19
        specified accident NEC V97.0
        while boarding or alighting
          V97.1
      person (injured by)
        falling from, in or on aircraft V97.0
        machinery on aircraft V97.89
        on ground with aircraft involvement
          V97.39
        rotating propeller V97.32
        struck by object falling from aircraft
          V97.31
        sucked into aircraft jet V97.33
        while boarding or alighting aircraft
          V97.1
      airport (battery-powered) passenger
        vehicle —see Accident, transport,
        industrial vehicle occupant
    all-terrain vehicle occupant (nontraffic)
      V86.95
      driver V86.55
      dune buggy —see Accident, transport, dune
        buggy occupant
      hanger-on V86.75
      passenger V86.65
      snowmobile —see Accident, transport,
        snowmobile occupant
      specified type NEC V86.99
        driver V86.59
        passenger V86.69
        person on outside V86.79
      traffic V86.35
        driver V86.05
        hanger-on V86.25
        passenger V86.15
      while boarding or alighting V86.45
    ambulance occupant (traffic) V86.31
      driver V86.01
      hanger-on V86.21
      nontraffic V86.91
        driver V86.51
        hanger-on V86.71
        passenger V86.61
      passenger V86.11
      while boarding or alighting V86.41

Accident (Continued)
  transport (Continued)
    animal-drawn vehicle occupant (in) V80.929
      collision (with)
        animal V80.12
          being ridden V80.711
        animal-drawn vehicle V80.721
        bus V80.42
        car V80.42
        fixed or stationary object V80.82
        military vehicle V80.920
        nonmotor vehicle V80.791
        pedal cycle V80.22
        pedestrian V80.12
        pickup V80.42
        railway train or vehicle V80.62
        specified motor vehicle NEC V80.52
        streetcar V80.731
        truck V80.42
        two-or three-wheeled motor vehicle
          V80.32
        van V80.42
      noncollision V80.02
      specified circumstance NEC V80. 928
    animal-rider V80.919
      collision (with)
        animal V80.11
          being ridden V80.710
        animal-drawn vehicle V80.720
        bus V80.41
        car V80.41
        fixed or stationary object V80.81
        military vehicle V80.910
        nonmotor vehicle V80.790
        pedal cycle V80.21
        pedestrian V80.11
        pickup V80.41
        railway train or vehicle V80.61
        specified motor vehicle NEC V80.51
        streetcar V80.730
        truck V80.41
        two- or three-wheeled motor vehicle
          V80.31
        van V80.41
      noncollision V80.018
        specified as horse rider V80.010
      specified circumstance NEC V80.918
    armored car —see Accident, transport, truck
      occupant
    battery-powered truck (baggage) (mail) —see
      Accident, transport, industrial vehicle
      occupant
    bus occupant V79.9
      collision (with)
        animal (traffic) V70.9
          being ridden (traffic) V76.9
            nontraffic V76.3
            while boarding or alighting V76.4
          nontraffic V70.3
          while boarding or alighting V70.4
        animal-drawn vehicle (traffic) V76.9
          nontraffic V76.3
          while boarding or alighting V76.4
        bus (traffic) V74.9
          nontraffic V74.3
          while boarding or alighting V74.4
        car (traffic) V73.9
          nontraffic V73.3
          while boarding or alighting V73.4
        motor vehicle NOS (traffic) V79.60
          nontraffic V79.20
          specified type NEC (traffic) V79.69
            nontraffic V79.29
        pedal cycle (traffic) V71.9
          nontraffic V71.3
          while boarding or alighting V71.4
        pickup truck (traffic) V73.9
          nontraffic V73.3
          while boarding or alighting V73.4
        railway vehicle (traffic) V75.9
          nontraffic V75.3
          while boarding or alighting V75.4
        specified vehicle NEC (traffic) V76.9
          nontraffic V76.3
          while boarding or alighting V76.4
        stationary object (traffic) V77.9
          nontraffic V77.3
          while boarding or alighting V77.4
        streetcar (traffic) V76.9
          nontraffic V76.3
          while boarding or alighting V76.4

Accident (Continued)
  transport (Continued)
    bus occupant (Continued)
      collision (Continued)
        three wheeled motor vehicle (traffic)
          V72.9
          nontraffic V72.3
          while boarding or alighting V72.4
        truck (traffic) V74.9
          nontraffic V74.3
          while boarding or alighting V74.4
        two wheeled motor vehicle (traffic) V72.9
          nontraffic V72.3
          while boarding or alighting V72.4
        van (traffic) V73.9
          nontraffic V73.3
          while boarding or alighting V73.4
      driver
        collision (with)
          animal (traffic) V70.5
            being ridden (traffic) V76.5
              nontraffic V76.0
            nontraffic V70.0
          animal-drawn vehicle (traffic)
            V76.5
            nontraffic V76.0
          bus (traffic) V74.5
            nontraffic V74.0
          car (traffic) V73.5
            nontraffic V73.0
          motor vehicle NOS (traffic) V79.40
            nontraffic V79.00
            specified type NEC (traffic) V79.49
              nontraffic V79.09

          pedal cycle (traffic) V71.5
            nontraffic V71.0
          pickup truck (traffic) V73.5
            nontraffic V73.0
          railway vehicle (traffic) V75.5
            nontraffic V75.0
          specified vehicle NEC (traffic)
            V76.5
            nontraffic V76.0
          stationary object (traffic) V77.5
            nontraffic V77.0
          streetcar (traffic) V76.5
            nontraffic V76.0
          three wheeled motor vehicle (traffic)
            V72.5
            nontraffic V72.0
          truck (traffic) V74.5
            nontraffic V74.0
          two wheeled motor vehicle (traffic)
            V72.5
            nontraffic V72.0
          van (traffic) V73.5
            nontraffic V73.0
        noncollision accident (traffic) V78.5
          nontraffic V78.0
      hanger-on
        collision (with)
          animal (traffic) V70.7
            being ridden (traffic) V76.7
              nontraffic V76.2
            nontraffic V70.2
          animal-drawn vehicle (traffic)
            V76.7
            nontraffic V76.2
          bus (traffic) V74.7
            nontraffic V74.2
          car (traffic) V73.7
            nontraffic V73.2
          pedal cycle (traffic) V71.7
            nontraffic V71.2
          pickup truck (traffic) V73.7
            nontraffic V73.2
          railway vehicle (traffic) V75.7
            nontraffic V75.2
          specified vehicle NEC (traffic)
            V76.7
            nontraffic V76.2
          stationary object (traffic) V77.7
            nontraffic V77.2
          streetcar (traffic) V76.7
            nontraffic V76.2
          three wheeled motor vehicle (traffic)
            V72.7
            nontraffic V72.2
          truck (traffic) V74.7
            nontraffic V74.2

Accident *(Continued)*
  transport *(Continued)*
    bus occupant *(Continued)*
      hanger-on *(Continued)*
        collision *(Continued)*
          two wheeled motor vehicle (traffic) V72.7
            nontraffic V72.2
          van (traffic) V73.7
            nontraffic V73.2
        noncollision accident (traffic) V78.7
          nontraffic V78.2
      noncollision accident (traffic) V78.9
        nontraffic V78.3
        while boarding or alighting V78.4
      nontraffic V79.3
      passenger
        collision (with)
          animal (traffic) V70.6
            being ridden (traffic) V76.6
              nontraffic V76.1
            nontraffic V70.1
          animal-drawn vehicle (traffic) V76.6
            nontraffic V76.1
          bus (traffic) V74.6
            nontraffic V74.1
          car (traffic) V73.6
            nontraffic V73.1
          motor vehicle NOS (traffic) V79.50
            nontraffic V79.10
            specified type NEC (traffic) V79.59
              nontraffic V79.19
          pedal cycle (traffic) V71.6
            nontraffic V71.1
          pickup truck (traffic) V73.6
            nontraffic V73.1
          railway vehicle (traffic) V75.6
            nontraffic V75.1
          specified vehicle NEC (traffic) V76.6
            nontraffic V76.1
          stationary object (traffic) V77.6
            nontraffic V77.1
          streetcar (traffic) V76.6
            nontraffic V76.1
          three wheeled motor vehicle (traffic) V72.6
            nontraffic V72.1
          truck (traffic) V74.6
            nontraffic V74.1
          two wheeled motor vehicle (traffic) V72.6
            nontraffic V72.1
          van (traffic) V73.6
            nontraffic V73.1
        noncollision accident (traffic) V78.6
          nontraffic V78.1
      specified type NEC V79.88
        military vehicle V79.81
    cable car, not on rails V98.0
      on rails —*see* Accident, transport, streetcar occupant
    car occupant V49.9
      ambulance occupant —*see* Accident, transport, ambulance occupant
      collision (with)
        animal (traffic) V40.9
          being ridden (traffic) V46.9
            nontraffic V46.3
            while boarding or alighting V46.4
          nontraffic V40.3
          while boarding or alighting V40.4
        animal-drawn vehicle (traffic) V46.9
          nontraffic V46.3
          while boarding or alighting V46.4
        bus (traffic) V44.9
          nontraffic V44.3
          while boarding or alighting V44.4
        car (traffic) V43.92
          nontraffic V43.32
          while boarding or alighting V43.42
        motor vehicle NOS (traffic) V49.60
          nontraffic V49.20
          specified type NEC (traffic) V49.69
            nontraffic V49.29
        pedal cycle (traffic) V41.9
          nontraffic V41.3
          while boarding or alighting V41.4
        pickup truck (traffic) V43.93
          nontraffic V43.33
          while boarding or alighting V43.43

Accident *(Continued)*
  transport *(Continued)*
    car occupant *(Continued)*
      collision *(Continued)*
        railway vehicle (traffic) V45.9
          nontraffic V45.3
          while boarding or alighting V45.4
        specified vehicle NEC (traffic) V46.9
          nontraffic V46.3
          while boarding or alighting V46.4
        sport utility vehicle (traffic) V43.91
          nontraffic V43.31
          while boarding or alighting V43.41
        stationary object (traffic) V47.9
          nontraffic V47.3
          while boarding or alighting V47.4
        streetcar (traffic) V46.9
          nontraffic V46.3
          while boarding or alighting V46.4
        three wheeled motor vehicle (traffic) V42.9
          nontraffic V42.3
          while boarding or alighting V42.4
        truck (traffic) V44.9
          nontraffic V44.3
          while boarding or alighting V44.4
        two wheeled motor vehicle (traffic) V42.9
          nontraffic V42.3
          while boarding or alighting V42.4
        van (traffic) V43.94
          nontraffic V43.34
          while boarding or alighting V43.44
      driver
        collision (with)
          animal (traffic) V40.5
            being ridden (traffic) V46.5
              nontraffic V46.0
            nontraffic V40.0
          animal-drawn vehicle (traffic) V46.5
            nontraffic V46.0
          bus (traffic) V44.5
            nontraffic V44.0
          car (traffic) V43.52
            nontraffic V43.02
          motor vehicle NOS (traffic) V49.40
            nontraffic V49.00
            specified type NEC (traffic) V49.49
              nontraffic V49.09
          pedal cycle (traffic) V41.5
            nontraffic V41.0
          pickup truck (traffic) V43.53
            nontraffic V43.03
          railway vehicle (traffic) V45.5
            nontraffic V45.0
          specified vehicle NEC (traffic) V46.5
            nontraffic V46.0
          sport utility vehicle (traffic) V43.51
            nontraffic V43.01
          stationary object (traffic) V47.5
            nontraffic V47.0
          streetcar (traffic) V46.5
            nontraffic V46.0
          three wheeled motor vehicle (traffic) V42.5
            nontraffic V42.0
          truck (traffic) V44.5
            nontraffic V44.0
          two wheeled motor vehicle (traffic) V42.5
            nontraffic V42.0
          van (traffic) V43.54
            nontraffic V43.04
        noncollision accident (traffic) V48.5
          nontraffic V48.0
      hanger-on
        collision (with)
          animal (traffic) V40.7
            being ridden (traffic) V46.7
              nontraffic V46.2
            nontraffic V40.2
          animal-drawn vehicle (traffic) V46.7
            nontraffic V46.2
          bus (traffic) V44.7
            nontraffic V44.2
          car (traffic) V43.72
            nontraffic V43.22
          pedal cycle (traffic) V41.7
            nontraffic V41.2
          pickup truck (traffic) V43.73
            nontraffic V43.23

Accident *(Continued)*
  transport *(Continued)*
    car occupant *(Continued)*
      hanger-on *(Continued)*
        collision *(Continued)*
          railway vehicle (traffic) V45.7
            nontraffic V45.2
          specified vehicle NEC (traffic) V46.7
            nontraffic V46.2
          sport utility vehicle (traffic) V43.71
            nontraffic V43.21
          stationary object (traffic) V47.7
            nontraffic V47.2
          streetcar (traffic) V46.7
            nontraffic V46.2
          three wheeled motor vehicle (traffic) V42.7
            nontraffic V42.2
          truck (traffic) V44.7
            nontraffic V44.2
          two wheeled motor vehicle (traffic) V42.7
            nontraffic V42.2
          van (traffic) V43.74
            nontraffic V43.24
        noncollision accident (traffic) V48.7
          nontraffic V48.2
      noncollision accident (traffic) V48.9
        nontraffic V48.3
        while boarding or alighting V48.4
      nontraffic V49.3
      passenger
        collision (with)
          animal (traffic) V40.6
            being ridden (traffic) V46.6
              nontraffic V46.1
            nontraffic V40.1
          animal-drawn vehicle (traffic) V46.6
            nontraffic V46.1
          bus (traffic) V44.6
            nontraffic V44.1
          car (traffic) V43.62
            nontraffic V43.12
          motor vehicle NOS (traffic) V49.50
            nontraffic V49.10
            specified type NEC (traffic) V49.59
              nontraffic V49.19
          pedal cycle (traffic) V41.6
            nontraffic V41.1
          pickup truck (traffic) V43.63
            nontraffic V43.13
          railway vehicle (traffic) V45.6
            nontraffic V45.1
          specified vehicle NEC (traffic) V46.6
            nontraffic V46.1
          sport utility vehicle (traffic) V43.61
            nontraffic V43.11
          stationary object (traffic) V47.6
            nontraffic V47.1
          streetcar (traffic) V46.6
            nontraffic V46.1
          three wheeled motor vehicle (traffic) V42.6
            nontraffic V42.1
          truck (traffic) V44.6
            nontraffic V44.1
          two wheeled motor vehicle (traffic) V42.6
            nontraffic V42.1
          van (traffic) V43.64
            nontraffic V43.14
        noncollision accident (traffic) V48.6
          nontraffic V48.1
      specified type NEC V49.88
        military vehicle V49.81
    coal car —*see* Accident, transport, industrial vehicle occupant
    construction vehicle occupant (nontraffic) V85.9
      driver V85.5
      hanger-on V85.7
      passenger V85.6
      traffic V85.3
        driver V85.0
        hanger-on V85.2
        passenger V85.1
      while boarding or alighting V85.4
    dirt bike rider (nontraffic) V86.96
      driver V86.56
      hanger-on V86.76
      passenger V86.66

▶ New ➡ Revised ~~deleted~~ Deleted ● Use Additional Character(s)

Accident *(Continued)*
  transport *(Continued)*
    dirt bike rider *(Continued)*
      traffic V86.36
        driver V86.06
        hanger-on V86.26
        passenger V86.16
      while boarding or alighting V86.46
    due to cataclysm —*see* Forces of nature, by
      type
    dune buggy occupant (nontraffic) V86.93
      driver V86.53
      hanger-on V86.73
      passenger V86.63
      traffic V86.33
        driver V86.03
        hanger-on V86.23
        passenger V86.13
      while boarding or alighting V86.43
    e-bicycle —*see* Accident, transport, electric
      (assisted) bicyclist
    e-bike —*see* Accident, transport, electric
      (assisted) bicyclist
    electric (assisted) bicyclist V29.91
      collision (with)
        animal (traffic) V20.91
          being ridden (traffic) V26.91
            nontraffic V26.21
              while boarding or alighting
                V26.31
          nontraffic V20.21
          while boarding or alighting V20.31
        animal-drawn vehicle (traffic) V26.91
          nontraffic V26.21
          while boarding or alighting V26.31
        bus (traffic) V24.91
          nontraffic V24.21
          while boarding or alighting V24.31
        car (traffic) V23.91
          nontraffic V23.21
          while boarding or alighting V23.31
        motor vehicle NOS (traffic) V29.601
          nontraffic V29.201
          specified type NEC (traffic) V29.691
            nontraffic V29.291
        pedal cycle (traffic) V21.91
          nontraffic V21.21
          while boarding or alighting V21.31
        pedestrian V20.91
          nontraffic V20.01
          while boarding or alighting V20.31
        pickup truck (traffic) V23.91
          nontraffic V23.21
          while boarding or alighting V23.31
        railway vehicle (traffic) V25.91
          nontraffic V25.21
          while boarding or alighting V25.31
        specified vehicle NEC (traffic) V26.91
          nontraffic V26.21
          while boarding or alighting V26.31
        stationary object (traffic) V27.91
          nontraffic V27.21
          while boarding or alighting V27.31
        streetcar (traffic) V26.91
          nontraffic V26.21
          while boarding or alighting V26.31
        three wheeled motor vehicle (traffic)
          V22.91
          nontraffic V22.21
          while boarding or alighting V22.31
        truck (traffic) V24.91
          nontraffic V24.21
          while boarding or alighting V24.31
        two wheeled motor vehicle (traffic)
          V22.91
          nontraffic V22.21
          while boarding or alighting V22.31
        van (traffic) V23.91
          nontraffic V23.21
          while boarding or alighting V23.31
      driver
        collision (with)
          animal (traffic) V20.41
            being ridden (traffic) V26.41
              nontraffic V26.01
            nontraffic V20.01
          animal-drawn vehicle (traffic)
            V26.41
            nontraffic V26.01
          bus (traffic) V24.41
            nontraffic V24.01

Accident *(Continued)*
  transport *(Continued)*
    bus occupant *(Continued)*
      driver *(Continued)*
        collision *(Continued)*
          car (traffic) V23.41
            nontraffic V23.01
          motor vehicle NOS (traffic) V29.401
            nontraffic V29.001
            specified type NEC (traffic) V29.491
              nontraffic V29.091
          pedal cycle (traffic) V21.41
            nontraffic V21.01
          pedestrian
            nontraffic V20.01
            traffic V20.41
          pickup truck (traffic) V23.41
            nontraffic V23.01
          railway vehicle (traffic) V25.41
            nontraffic V25.01
          specified vehicle NEC (traffic) V26.41
            nontraffic V26.01
          stationary object (traffic) V27.41
            nontraffic V27.01
          streetcar (traffic) V26.41
            nontraffic V26.01
          three wheeled motor vehicle (traffic)
            V22.41
            nontraffic V22.01
          truck (traffic) V24.41
            nontraffic V24.01
          two wheeled motor vehicle (traffic)
            V22.41
            nontraffic V22.01
          van (traffic) V23.41
            nontraffic V23.01
        noncollision accident (traffic) V28.41
          nontraffic V28.01
      noncollision accident (traffic) V28.91
        nontraffic V28.21
        while boarding or alighting V28.31
      nontraffic V29.31
      passenger
        collision (with)
          animal (traffic) V20.51
            being ridden (traffic) V26.51
              nontraffic V26.11
            nontraffic V20.11
          animal-drawn vehicle (traffic) V26.51
            nontraffic V26.11
          bus (traffic) V24.51
            nontraffic V24.11
          car (traffic) V23.51
            nontraffic V23.11
          motor vehicle NOS (traffic) V29.501
            nontraffic V29.101
            specified type NEC (traffic) V29.591
              nontraffic V29.191
          pedal cycle (traffic) V21.51
            nontraffic V21.11
          pedestrian
            nontraffic V20.11
            traffic V20.51
          pickup truck (traffic) V23.51
            nontraffic V23.11
          railway vehicle (traffic) V25.51
            nontraffic 25.11
          specified vehicle NEC (traffic) V26.51
            nontraffic V26.11
          stationary object (traffic) V27.51
            nontraffic V27.11
          streetcar (traffic) V26.51
            nontraffic V26.11
          three wheeled motor vehicle (traffic)
            V22.51
            nontraffic V22.11
          truck (traffic) V24.51
            nontraffic V24.11
          two wheeled motor vehicle (traffic)
            V22.51
            nontraffic V22.11
          van (traffic) V23.51
            nontraffic V23.11
        noncollision accident (traffic) V28.51
          nontraffic V28.11
      specified type NEC V29.881
        military V29.811
    forklift —*see* Accident, transport,
      industrial vehicle occupant
    go cart —*see* Accident, transport, all-terrain
      vehicle occupant

Accident *(Continued)*
  transport *(Continued)*
    golf cart —*see* Accident, transport,
      all-terrain vehicle occupant
    heavy transport vehicle occupant —
      see Accident, transport, truck occupant
    hoverboard V00.848
    ice yacht V98.2
    industrial vehicle occupant (nontraffic) V83.9
      driver V83.5
      hanger-on V83.7
      passenger V83.6
      traffic V83.3
        driver V83.0
        hanger-on V83.2
        passenger V83.1
      while boarding or alighting V83.4
    interurban electric car —*see* Accident,
      transport, streetcar
    land yacht V98.1
    logging car —*see* Accident, transport,
      industrial vehicle occupant
    military vehicle occupant (traffic) V86.34
      driver V86.04
      hanger-on V86.24
      nontraffic V86.94
        driver V86.54
        hanger-on V86.74
        passenger V86.64
      passenger V86.14
      while boarding or alighting V86.44
    mine tram —*see* Accident, transport, industrial
      vehicle occupant
    motor vehicle NEC occupant (traffic) V89.2
    motorcoach —*see* Accident, transport,
      bus occupant
    motor/cross bike rider —*see also* Accident,
      transport, dirt bike rider V86.96
    motorcycle V29.99
      collision (with)
        animal (traffic) V20.99
          being ridden (traffic) V26.99
            nontraffic V26.29
              while boarding or alighting V26.39
          nontraffic V20.29
          while boarding or alighting V20.39
        animal-drawn vehicle (traffic) V26.99
          nontraffic V26.29
          while boarding or alighting V26.39
        bus (traffic) V24.99
          nontraffic V24.29
          while boarding or alighting V24.39
        car (traffic) V23.99
          nontraffic V23.29
          while boarding or alighting V23.39
        motor vehicle NOS (traffic) V29.608
          nontraffic V29.208
          specified type NEC (traffic) V29.698
            nontraffic V29.298
        pedal cycle (traffic) V21.99
          nontraffic V21.29
          while boarding or alighting V21.39
        pickup truck (traffic) V23.99
          nontraffic V23.29
          while boarding or alighting V23.39
        railway vehicle (traffic) V25.99
          nontraffic V25.29
          while boarding or alighting V25.39
        specified vehicle NEC (traffic) V26.99
          nontraffic V26.29
          while boarding or alighting V26.39
        stationary object (traffic) V27.99
          nontraffic V27.29
          while boarding or alighting V27.39
        streetcar (traffic) V26.99
          nontraffic V26.29
          while boarding or alighting V26.39
        three wheeled motor vehicle (traffic)
          V22.99
          nontraffic V22.29
          while boarding or alighting V22.39
        truck (traffic) V24.99
          nontraffic V24.29
          while boarding or alighting V24.39
        two wheeled motor vehicle (traffic)
          V22.99
          nontraffic V22.29
          while boarding or alighting V22.39
        van (traffic) V23.99
          nontraffic V23.29
          while boarding or alighting V23.39

Accident (Continued)
  transport (Continued)
    motorcycle (Continued)
      driver (Continued)
        collision (with)
          animal (traffic) V20.49
            being ridden (traffic) V26.49
              nontraffic V26.09
            nontraffic V20.09
          animal-drawn vehicle (traffic) V26.49
            nontraffic V26.09
          bus (traffic) V24.49
            nontraffic V24.09
          car (traffic) V23.49
            nontraffic V23.09
          motor vehicle NOS (traffic) V29.408
            nontraffic V29.008
            specified type NEC (traffic) V29.498
              nontraffic V29.098
          pedal cycle (traffic) V21.49
            nontraffic V21.09
          pedestrian
            nontraffic V20.09
            traffic V20.49
          pickup truck (traffic) V23.49
            nontraffic V23.09
          railway vehicle (traffic) V25.49
            nontraffic V25.09
          specified vehicle NEC (traffic) V26.49
            nontraffic V26.09
          stationary object (traffic) V27.49
            nontraffic V27.09
          streetcar (traffic) V26.49
            nontraffic V26.09
          three wheeled motor vehicle (traffic) V22.49
            nontraffic V22.09
          truck (traffic) V24.49
            nontraffic V24.09
          two wheeled motor vehicle (traffic) V22.49
            nontraffic V22.09
          van (traffic) V23.49
            nontraffic V23.09
        noncollision accident (traffic) V28.49
          nontraffic V28.09
      noncollision accident (traffic) V28.99
        nontraffic V28.29
        while boarding or alighting V28.39
      nontraffic V29.39
      passenger
        collision (with)
          animal (traffic) V20.59
            being ridden (traffic) V26.59
              nontraffic V26.19
            nontraffic V20.19
          animal-drawn vehicle (traffic) V26.59
            nontraffic V26.19
          bus (traffic) V24.59
            nontraffic V24.19
          car (traffic) V23.59
            nontraffic V23.19
          motor vehicle NOS (traffic) V29.508
            nontraffic V29.108
            specified type NEC (traffic) V29.598
              nontraffic V29.198
          pedal cycle (traffic) V21.59
            nontraffic V21.19
          pedestrian
            nontraffic V20.19
            traffic V20.59
          pickup truck (traffic) V23.59
            nontraffic V23.19
          railway vehicle (traffic) V25.59
            nontraffic V25.19
          specified vehicle NEC (traffic) V26.59
            nontraffic V26.19
          stationary object (traffic) V27.59
            nontraffic V27.19
          streetcar (traffic) V26.59
            nontraffic V26.19
          three wheeled motor vehicle (traffic) V22.59
            nontraffic V22.19
          truck (traffic) V24.59
            nontraffic V24.19
          two wheeled motor vehicle (traffic) V22.59
            nontraffic V22.19

Accident (Continued)
  transport (Continued)
    motorcycle (Continued)
      passenger (Continued)
        collision (Continued)
          van (traffic) V23.59
            nontraffic V23.19
        noncollision accident (traffic) V28.59
          nontraffic V28.19
      specified type NEC V29.888
        military vehicle V29.818
    occupant (of)
      aircraft (powered) V95.9
        fixed wing
          commercial —see Accident, transport, aircraft, occupant, powered, fixed wing, commercial
          private —see Accident, transport, aircraft, occupant, powered, fixed wing, private
        nonpowered V96.9
        specified NEC V95.8
      airport battery-powered vehicle —see Accident, transport, industrial vehicle occupant
      all-terrain vehicle (ATV) —see Accident, transport, all-terrain vehicle occupant
      animal-drawn vehicle —see Accident, transport, animal-drawn vehicle occupant
      automobile —see Accident, transport, car occupant
      balloon V96.00
      battery-powered vehicle —see Accident, transport, industrial vehicle occupant
      bicycle —see Accident, transport, pedal cyclist
        motorized —see Accident, transport, motorcycle rider
      boat NEC —see Accident, watercraft
      bulldozer —see Accident, transport, construction vehicle occupant
      bus —see Accident, transport, bus occupant
      cable car (on rails) —see also Accident, transport, streetcar occupant
        not on rails V98.0
      car —see also Accident, transport, car occupant
        cable (on rails) —see also Accident, transport, streetcar occupant
          not on rails V98.0
      coach —see Accident, transport, bus occupant
      coal-car —see Accident, transport, industrial vehicle occupant
      digger —see Accident, transport, construction vehicle occupant
      dump truck —see Accident, transport, construction vehicle occupant
      earth-leveler —see Accident, transport, construction vehicle occupant
      farm machinery (self-propelled) —see Accident, transport, agricultural vehicle occupant
      forklift —see Accident, transport, industrial vehicle occupant
      glider (unpowered) V96.20
        hang V96.10
        powered (microlight) (ultralight) —see Accident, transport, aircraft, occupant, powered, glider
      glider (unpowered) NEC V96.20
      hang-glider V96.10
      harvester —see Accident, transport, agricultural vehicle occupant
      heavy (transport) vehicle —see Accident, transport, truck occupant
      helicopter —see Accident, transport, aircraft, occupant, helicopter
      ice-yacht V98.2
      kite (carrying person) V96.8
      land-yacht V98.1
      logging car —see Accident, transport, industrial vehicle occupant
      mechanical shovel —see Accident, transport, construction vehicle occupant
      microlight —see Accident, transport, aircraft, occupant, powered, glider
      minibus —see Accident, transport, pickup truck occupant

Accident (Continued)
  transport (Continued)
    occupant (Continued)
      minivan —see Accident, transport, pickup truck occupant
      moped —see Accident, transport, motorcycle
      motor scooter —see Accident, transport, motorcycle
      motorcycle (with sidecar) —see Accident, transport, motorcycle
      off-road motor-vehicle —see also Accident, transport, all-terrain vehicle occupant V86.99
      pedal cycle —see also Accident, transport, pedal cyclist
      pick-up (truck) —see Accident, transport, pickup truck occupant
      railway (train) (vehicle) (subterranean) (elevated) —see Accident, transport, railway vehicle occupant
      rickshaw —see Accident, transport, pedal cycle
        pedal driven —see Accident, transport, pedal cyclist
      road-roller —see Accident, transport, construction vehicle occupant
      ship NOS V94.9
      ski-lift (chair) (gondola) V98.3
      snowmobile —see Accident, transport, snowmobile occupant
      spacecraft, spaceship —see Accident, transport, aircraft, occupant, spacecraft
      sport utility vehicle —see Accident, transport, pickup truck occupant
      streetcar (interurban) (operating on public street or highway) —see Accident, transport, streetcar occupant
      SUV —see Accident, transport, pickup truck occupant
      téléférique V98.0
      three-wheeled vehicle (motorized) —see also Accident, transport, three-wheeled motor vehicle occupant
        nonmotorized —see Accident, transport, pedal cycle
      tractor (farm) (and trailer) —see Accident, transport, agricultural vehicle occupant
      train —see Accident, transport, railway vehicle occupant
      tram —see Accident, transport, streetcar occupant
        in mine or quarry —see Accident, transport, industrial vehicle occupant
      tricycle —see Accident, transport, pedal cycle
        motorized —see Accident, transport, three-wheeled motor vehicle
      trolley —see Accident, transport, streetcar occupant
        in mine or quarry —see Accident, transport, industrial vehicle occupant
      tub, in mine or quarry —see Accident, transport, industrial vehicle occupant
      ultralight —see Accident, transport, aircraft, occupant, powered, glider
      van —see Accident, transport, van occupant
      vehicle NEC V89.9
        heavy transport —see Accident, transport, truck occupant
        motor (traffic) NEC V89.2
          nontraffic NEC V89.0
      watercraft NOS V94.9
        causing drowning —see Drowning, resulting from accident to boat
      off-road motor-vehicle —see also Accident, transport, all-terrain vehicle occupant V86.99
    parachutist V97.29
      after accident to aircraft —see Accident, transport, aircraft
      entangled in object V97.21
      injured on landing V97.22

▶ New   ⟹ Revised   ~~deleted~~ Deleted   • Use Additional Character(s)

Accident *(Continued)*
  transport *(Continued)*
    pedal cyclist V19.9
      collision (with)
        animal (traffic) V10.9
          being ridden (traffic) V16.9
            nontraffic V16.2
            while boarding or alighting
              V16.3
          nontraffic V10.2
          while boarding or alighting V10.3
        animal-drawn vehicle (traffic) V16.9
          nontraffic V16.2
          while boarding or alighting V16.3
        bus (traffic) V14.9
          nontraffic V14.2
          while boarding or alighting V14.3
        car (traffic) V13.9
          nontraffic V13.2
          while boarding or alighting V13.3
        motor vehicle NOS (traffic) V19.60
          nontraffic V19.20
          specified type NEC (traffic) V19.69
            nontraffic V19.29
        pedal cycle (traffic) V11.9
          nontraffic V11.2
          while boarding or alighting V11.3
        pickup truck (traffic) V13.9
          nontraffic V13.2
          while boarding or alighting V13.3
        railway vehicle (traffic) V15.9
          nontraffic V15.2
          while boarding or alighting V15.3
        specified vehicle NEC (traffic) V16.9
          nontraffic V16.2
          while boarding or alighting V16.3
        stationary object (traffic) V17.9
          nontraffic V17.2
          while boarding or alighting V17.3
        streetcar (traffic) V16.9
          nontraffic V16.2
          while boarding or alighting V16.3
        three wheeled motor vehicle (traffic)
          V12.9
          nontraffic V12.2
          while boarding or alighting V12.3
        truck (traffic) V14.9
          nontraffic V14.2
          while boarding or alighting V14.3
        two wheeled motor vehicle (traffic)
          V12.9
          nontraffic V12.2
          while boarding or alighting V12.3
        van (traffic) V13.9
          nontraffic V13.2
          while boarding or alighting V13.3
      driver
        collision (with)
          animal (traffic) V10.4
            being ridden (traffic) V16.4
              nontraffic V16.0
            nontraffic V10.828
          animal-drawn vehicle (traffic) V16.4
            nontraffic V16.0
          bus (traffic) V14.4
            nontraffic V14.0
          car (traffic) V13.4
            nontraffic V13.0
          motor vehicle NOS (traffic) V19.40
            nontraffic V19.00
            specified type NEC (traffic)
              V19.49
              nontraffic V19.09
          pedal cycle (traffic) V11.4
            nontraffic V11.0
          pickup truck (traffic) V13.4
            nontraffic V13.0
          railway vehicle (traffic) V15.4
            nontraffic V15.0
          specified vehicle NEC (traffic)
            V16.4
            nontraffic V16.0
          stationary object (traffic) V17.4
            nontraffic V17.0
          streetcar (traffic) V16.4
            nontraffic V16.0
          three wheeled motor vehicle (traffic)
            V12.4
            nontraffic V12.0
          truck (traffic) V14.4
            nontraffic V14.0

Accident *(Continued)*
  transport *(Continued)*
    parachutist *(Continued)*
      driver *(Continued)*
        collision *(Continued)*
          two wheeled motor vehicle (traffic)
            V12.4
            nontraffic V12.0
          van (traffic) V13.4
            nontraffic V13.0
        noncollision accident (traffic) V18.4
          nontraffic V18.0
      noncollision accident (traffic) V18.9
        nontraffic V18.2
        while boarding or alighting V18.3
      nontraffic V19.3
      passenger
        collision (with)
          animal (traffic) V10.5
            being ridden (traffic) V16.5
              nontraffic V16.1
            nontraffic V10.1
          animal-drawn vehicle (traffic) V16.5
            nontraffic V16.1

          bus (traffic) V14.5
            nontraffic V14.1
          car (traffic) V13.5
            nontraffic V13.1
          motor vehicle NOS (traffic) V19.50
            nontraffic V19.10
            specified type NEC (traffic) V19.59
              nontraffic V19.19
          pedal cycle (traffic) V11.5
            nontraffic V11.1
          pickup truck (traffic) V13.5
            nontraffic V13.1
          railway vehicle (traffic) V15.5
            nontraffic V15.1
          specified vehicle NEC (traffic) V16.5
            nontraffic V16.1
          stationary object (traffic) V17.5
            nontraffic V17.1
          streetcar (traffic) V16.5
            nontraffic V16.1
          three wheeled motor vehicle (traffic)
            V12.5
            nontraffic V12.1
          truck (traffic) V14.5
            nontraffic V14.1
          two wheeled motor vehicle (traffic)
            V12.5
            nontraffic V12.1
          van (traffic) V13.5
            nontraffic V13.1
        noncollision accident (traffic) V18.5
          nontraffic V18.1
      specified type NEC V19.88
      military vehicle V19.81
    pedestrian
      conveyance (occupant) V09.9
        baby stroller V00.828
          collision (with) V09.9
            animal being ridden or animal
              drawn vehicle V06.99
              nontraffic V06.09
              traffic V06.19
            bus or heavy transport V04.99
              nontraffic V04.09
              traffic V04.19
            car V03.99
              nontraffic V03.09
              traffic V03.19
            pedal cycle V01.99
              nontraffic V01.09
              traffic V01.19
            pick-up truck or van V03.99
              nontraffic V03.09
              traffic V03.19
            railway (train) (vehicle)
              V05.99
              nontraffic V05.09
              traffic V05.19
            stationary object V00.822
            streetcar V06.99
              nontraffic V06.09
              traffic V06.19
            two- or three-wheeled motor
              vehicle V02.99
              nontraffic V02.09
              traffic V02.19

Accident *(Continued)*
  transport *(Continued)*
    pedestrian *(Continued)*
      conveyance *(Continued)*
        baby stroller *(Continued)*
          collision *(Continued)*
            vehicle V09.9
              animal-drawn V06.99
                nontraffic V06.09
                traffic V06.19
              motor
                nontraffic V09.00
                traffic V09.20
          fall V00.821
          nontraffic V09.1
            involving motor vehicle NEC
              V09.00
          traffic V09.3
            involving motor vehicle NEC
              V09.20
        flat-bottomed NEC V00.388
          collision (with) V09.9
            animal being ridden or animal
              drawn vehicle V06.99
              nontraffic V06.09
              traffic V06.19
            bus or heavy transport V04.99
              nontraffic V04.09
              traffic V04.19
            car V03.99
              nontraffic V03.09
              traffic V03.19
            pedal cycle V01.99
              nontraffic V01.09
              traffic V01.19
            pick-up truck or van V03.99
              nontraffic V03.09
              traffic V03.19
            railway (train) (vehicle) V05.99
              nontraffic V05.09
              traffic V05.19
            stationary object V00.382
            streetcar V06.99
              nontraffic V06.09
              traffic V06.19
            two-or three-wheeled motor vehicle
              V02.99
              nontraffic V02.09
              traffic V02.19
            vehicle V09.9
              animal-drawn V06.99
                nontraffic V06.09
                traffic V06.19
              motor
                nontraffic V09.00
                traffic V09.20
          fall V00.381
          nontraffic V09.1
            involving motor vehicle NEC V09.00
          snow
            board —*see* Accident, transport,
              pedestrian, conveyance, snow
              board
            ski —*see* Accident, transport,
              pedestrian, conveyance, skis
              (snow)
          traffic V09.3
            involving motor vehicle NEC
              V09.20
        gliding type NEC V00.288
          collision (with) V09.9
            animal being ridden or animal
              drawn vehicle V06.99
              nontraffic V06.09
              traffic V06.19
            bus or heavy transport
              V04.99
              nontraffic V04.09
              traffic V04.19
            car V03.99
              nontraffic V03.09
              traffic V03.19
            pedal cycle V01.99
              nontraffic V01.09
              traffic V01.19
            pick-up truck or van V03.99
              nontraffic V03.09
              traffic V03.19
            railway (train) (vehicle) V05.99
              nontraffic V05.09
              traffic V05.19

Accident (Continued)
  transport (Continued)
    pedestrian (Continued)
      conveyance (Continued)
        gliding type (Continued)
          collision (Continued)
            stationary object V00.282
            streetcar V06.99
              nontraffic V06.09
              traffic V06.19
            two- or three-wheeled motor
                vehicle V02.99
              nontraffic V02.09
              traffic V02.19
            vehicle V09.9
              animal-drawn V06.99
                nontraffic V06.09
                traffic V06.19
              motor
                nontraffic V09.00
                traffic V09.20
          fall V00.281
          heelies —see Accident, transport,
              pedestrian, conveyance,
              heelies
          hoverboard
            collision with
              animal being ridden or animal
                  drawn vehicle V06.938
                nontraffic V06.038
                traffic V06.138
              bus or heavy transport
                  V04.938
                nontraffic V04.038
                traffic V04.138
              car V03.938
                nontraffic V03.038
                traffic V03.138
              pedal cycle V01.938
                nontraffic V01.038
                traffic V01.138
              pick-up or van V03.938
                nontraffic V03.038
                traffic V03.138
              railway (train) (vehicle) V05.938
                nontraffic V05.038
                traffic V05.138
              streetcar V06.938
                nontraffic V06.038
                traffic V06.138
              three-wheeled motor vehicle
                  V02.938
                nontraffic V02.038
                traffic V02.138
              two-wheeled motor vehicle
                  V02.938
                nontraffic V02.038
                traffic V02.138
              vehicle, nonmotor, specified NEC
                  V06.938
                nontraffic V06.038
                traffic V06.138
            fall V00.848
          ice skate —see Accident, transport,
              pedestrian, conveyance, ice skate
          nontraffic V09.1
            involving motor vehicle NEC
                V09.00
          Segway
            collision with
              animal being ridden or animal
                  drawn vehicle V06.938
                nontraffic V06.038
                traffic V06.138
              bus or heavy transport V04.938
                nontraffic V04.038
                traffic V04.138
              car V03.938
                nontraffic V03.038
                traffic V03.138
              pedal cycle V01.938
                nontraffic V01.038
                traffic V01.138
              pick-up or van V03.038
                nontraffic V01.038
                traffic V03.138
              railway (train) (vehicle) V05.938
                nontraffic V05.038
                traffic V05.138
              streetcar V06.938
                nontraffic V06.038
                traffic V06.138

Accident (Continued)
  transport (Continued)
    pedestrian (Continued)
      conveyance (Continued)
        gliding type (Continued)
          Segway (Continued)
            collision with (Continued)
              three-wheeled motor vehicle
                  V02.938
                nontraffic V02.038
                traffic V02.138
              two-wheeled motor vehicle
                  V02.938
                nontraffic V02.038
                traffic V02.138
              vehicle, nonmotor, specified NEC
                  V06.938
                nontraffic V06.038
                traffic V06.138
            fall V00.848
          sled —see Accident, transport,
              pedestrian, conveyance, sled
          standing
            electric scooter
              collision with
                animal being ridden or animal
                    drawn vehicle
                    V06.931
                  nontraffic V06.031
                  traffic V06.131
                bus or heavy transport
                    V04.931
                  nontraffic V04.031
                  traffic V04.131
                car V03.931
                  nontraffic V03.031
                  traffic V03.131
                pedal cycle V01.931
                  nontraffic V01.031
                  traffic V01.131
                pick-up or van V03.931
                  nontraffic V03.031
                  traffic V03.131
                railway (train) (vehicle)
                    V05.931
                  nontraffic V05.031
                  traffic V05.131
                streetcar V06.931
                  nontraffic V06.031
                  traffic V06.131
                three-wheeled motor vehicle
                    V02.931
                  nontraffic V02.031
                  traffic V02.131
                two-wheeled motor vehicle
                    V02.931
                  nontraffic V02.031
                  traffic V02.131
                vehicle, nonmotor, specified
                    NEC V06.931
                  nontraffic V06.031
                  traffic V06.131
              fall V00.841
            micro-mobility pedestrian
                conveyance
              collision with
                animal being ridden or animal
                    drawn vehicle
                    V06.938
                  nontraffic V06.038
                  traffic V06.138
                bus or heavy transport
                    V04.938
                  nontraffic V04.038
                  traffic V04.138
                car V03.938
                  nontraffic V03.038
                  traffic V03.138
                pedal cycle V01.938
                  nontraffic V01.038
                  traffic V01.138
                pick-up or van V03.938
                  nontraffic V03.038
                  traffic V03.138
                railway (train) (vehicle)
                    V05.938
                  nontraffic V05.038
                  traffic V05.138
                stationary object V00.842
                streetcar V06.938
                  nontraffic V06.038
                  traffic V06.138

Accident (Continued)
  transport (Continued)
    pedestrian (Continued)
      conveyance (Continued)
        gliding type (Continued)
          standing (Continued)
            micro-mobility pedestrian
                conveyance —(Continued)
              collision with (Continued)
                three-wheeled motor vehicle
                    V02.938
                  nontraffic V02.038
                  traffic V02.138
                two-wheeled motor vehicle
                    V02.938
                  nontraffic V02.038
                  traffic V02.138
                vehicle, nonmotor, specified
                    NEC V06.938
                  nontraffic V06.038
                  traffic V06.138
              fall V00.848
              traffic V09.3
                involving motor vehicle NEC
                    V09.20
              wheelies —see Accident, transport,
                  pedestrian, conveyance,
                  heelies
          heelies V00.158
            colliding with stationary object
                V00.152
            fall V00.151
          ice skates V00.218
            collision (with) V09.9
              animal being ridden or animal
                  drawn vehicle V06.99
                nontraffic V06.09
                traffic V06.19
              bus or heavy transport V04.99
                nontraffic V04.09
                traffic V04.19
              car V03.99
                nontraffic V03.09
                traffic V03.19
              pedal cycle V01.99
                nontraffic V01.09
                traffic V01.19
              pick-up truck or van V03.99
                nontraffic V03.09
                traffic V03.19
              railway (train) (vehicle) V05.99
                nontraffic V05.09
                traffic V05.19
              stationary object V00.212
              streetcar V06.99
                nontraffic V06.09
                traffic V06.19
              two- or three-wheeled motor
                  vehicle V02.99
                nontraffic V02.09
                traffic V02.19
              vehicle V09.9
                animal-drawn V06.99
                  nontraffic V06.09
                  traffic V06.19
                motor
                  nontraffic V09.00
                  traffic V09.20
            fall V00.211
            nontraffic V09.1
              involving motor vehicle NEC
                  V09.00
            traffic V09.3
              involving motor vehicle NEC
                  V09.20
          motorized mobility scooter V00.838
            collision with stationary object
                V00.832
            fall from V00.831
            nontraffic V09.1
              involving motor vehicle V09.00
                military V09.01
                specified type NEC V09.09
          roller skates (non in-line) V00.128
            collision (with) V09.9
              animal being ridden or animal
                  drawn vehicle V06.91
                nontraffic V06.01
                traffic V06.11
              bus or heavy transport V04.91
                nontraffic V04.01
                traffic V04.11

▶ New   ⇛ Revised   ~~deleted~~ Deleted   ● Use Additional Character(s)

Accident *(Continued)*
  transport *(Continued)*
    pedestrian *(Continued)*
      conveyance *(Continued)*
        roller skates *(Continued)*
          collision *(Continued)*
            car V03.91
              nontraffic V03.01
              traffic V03.11
            pedal cycle V01.91
              nontraffic V01.01
              traffic V01.11
            pick-up truck or van V03.91
              nontraffic V03.01
              traffic V03.11
            railway (train) (vehicle)
                V05.91
              nontraffic V05.01
              traffic V05.11
            stationary object V00.122
            streetcar V06.91
              nontraffic V06.01
              traffic V06.11
            two- or three-wheeled motor
                vehicle V02.91
              nontraffic V02.01
              traffic V02.11
            vehicle V09.9
              animal-drawn V06.91
                nontraffic V06.01
                traffic V06.11
              motor
                nontraffic V09.00
                traffic V09.20
          fall V00.121
          in-line V00.118
            collision —*see also* Accident,
                transport, pedestrian,
                conveyance occupant, roller
                skates, collision
              with stationary object
                V00.112
            fall V00.111
          nontraffic V09.1
            involving motor vehicle NEC
                V09.00
          traffic V09.3
            involving motor vehicle NEC
                V09.20
        rolling shoes V00.158
          colliding with stationary object
              V00.152
          fall V00.151
        rolling type NEC V00.188
          collision (with) V09.9
            animal being ridden or animal
                drawn vehicle V06.99
              nontraffic V06.09
              traffic V06.19
            bus or heavy transport
                V04.99
              nontraffic V04.09
              traffic V04.19
            car V03.99
              nontraffic V03.09
              traffic V03.19
            pedal cycle V01.99
              nontraffic V01.09
              traffic V01.19
            pick-up truck or van
                V03.99
              nontraffic V03.09
              traffic V03.19
            railway (train) (vehicle)
                V05.99
              nontraffic V05.09
              traffic V05.19
            stationary object V00.182
            streetcar V06.99
              nontraffic V06.09
              traffic V06.19
            two- or three-wheeled motor
                vehicle V02.99
              nontraffic V02.09
              traffic V02.19
            vehicle V09.9
              animal-drawn V06.99
                nontraffic V06.09
                traffic V06.19
              motor
                nontraffic V09.00
                traffic V09.20

Accident *(Continued)*
  transport *(Continued)*
    pedestrian *(Continued)*
      conveyance *(Continued)*
        rolling type *(Continued)*
          fall V00.181
          in-line roller skate —*see* Accident,
              transport, pedestrian,
              conveyance, roller skate, in-line
          nontraffic V09.1
            involving motor vehicle NEC
                V09.00
          roller skate —*see* Accident, transport,
              pedestrian, conveyance, roller
              skate
          scooter (non-motorized) —*see*
              Accident, transport, pedestrian,
              conveyance, scooter
          skateboard —*see* Accident, transport,
              pedestrian, conveyance,
              skateboard
          traffic V09.3
            involving motor vehicle NEC
                V09.20
        scooter (non-motorized) V00.148
          collision (with) V09.9
            animal being ridden or
                animal drawn vehicle
                V06.99
              nontraffic V06.09
              traffic V06.19
            bus or heavy transport
                V04.99
              nontraffic V04.09
              traffic V04.19
            car V03.99
              nontraffic V03.09
              traffic V03.19
            pedal cycle V01.99
              nontraffic V01.09
              traffic V01.19
            pick-up truck or van
                V03.99
              nontraffic V03.09
              traffic V03.19
            railway (train) (vehicle)
                V05.99
              nontraffic V05.09
              traffic V05.19
            stationary object V00.142
            streetcar V06.99
              nontraffic V06.09
              traffic V06.19
            two- or three-wheeled motor
                vehicle V02.99
              nontraffic V02.09
              traffic V02.19
            vehicle V09.9
              animal-drawn V06.99
                nontraffic V06.09
                traffic V06.19
              motor
                nontraffic V09.00
                traffic V09.20
          fall V00.141
          nontraffic V09.1
            involving motor vehicle NEC
                V09.00
          traffic V09.3
            involving motor vehicle NEC
                V09.20
        skateboard V00.138
          collision (with) V09.9
            animal being ridden or animal
                drawn vehicle V06.92
              nontraffic V06.02
              traffic V06.12
            bus or heavy transport V04.92
              nontraffic V04.02
              traffic V04.12
            car V03.92
              nontraffic V03.02
              traffic V03.12
            pedal cycle V01.92
              nontraffic V01.02
              traffic V01.12
            pick-up truck or van V03.92
              nontraffic V03.02
              traffic V03.12
            railway (train) (vehicle) V05.92
              nontraffic V05.02
              traffic V05.12

Accident *(Continued)*
  transport *(Continued)*
    pedestrian *(Continued)*
      conveyance *(Continued)*
        skateboard *(Continued)*
          collision *(Continued)*
            stationary object V00.132
            streetcar V06.92
              nontraffic V06.02
              traffic V06.12
            two- or three-wheeled motor
                vehicle V02.92
              nontraffic V02.02
              traffic V02.12
            vehicle V09.9
              animal-drawn V06.92
                nontraffic V06.02
                traffic V06.12
              motor
                nontraffic V09.00
                traffic V09.20
          fall V00.131
          nontraffic V09.1
            involving motor vehicle NEC
                V09.00
          traffic V09.3
            involving motor vehicle NEC
                V09.20
        skis (snow) V00.328
          collision (with) V09.9
            animal being ridden or animal
                drawn vehicle V06.99
              nontraffic V06.09
              traffic V06.19
            bus or heavy transport V04.99
              nontraffic V04.09
              traffic V04.19
            car V03.99
              nontraffic V03.09
              traffic V03.19
            pedal cycle V01.99
              nontraffic V01.09
              traffic V01.19
            pick-up truck or van V03.99
              nontraffic V03.09
              traffic V03.19
            railway (train) (vehicle) V05.99
              nontraffic V05.09
              traffic V05.19
            stationary object V00.322
            streetcar V06.99
              nontraffic V06.09
              traffic V06.19
            two- or three-wheeled motor
                vehicle V02.99
              nontraffic V02.09
              traffic V02.19
            vehicle V09.9
              animal-drawn V06.99
                nontraffic V06.09
                traffic V06.19
              motor
                nontraffic V09.00
                traffic V09.20
          fall V00.321
          nontraffic V09.1
            involving motor vehicle NEC
                V09.00
          traffic V09.3
            involving motor vehicle NEC
                V09.20
        sled V00.228
          collision (with) V09.9
            animal being ridden or animal
                drawn vehicle V06.99
              nontraffic V06.09
              traffic V06.19
            bus or heavy transport V04.99
              nontraffic V04.09
              traffic V04.19
            car V03.99
              nontraffic V03.09
              traffic V03.19
            pedal cycle V01.99
              nontraffic V01.09
              traffic V01.19
            pick-up truck or van V03.99
              nontraffic V03.09
              traffic V03.19
            railway (train) (vehicle) V05.99
              nontraffic V05.09
              traffic V05.19

A

Accident (Continued)
  transport (Continued)
    pedestrian (Continued)
      conveyance (Continued)
        sled (Continued)
          collision (Continued)
            stationary object V00.222
            streetcar V06.99
              nontraffic V06.09
              traffic V06.19
            two- or three-wheeled motor
              vehicle V02.99
              nontraffic V02.09
              traffic V02.19
            vehicle V09.9
              animal-drawn V06.99
                nontraffic V06.09
                traffic V06.19
              motor
                nontraffic V09.00
                traffic V09.20
          fall V00.221
          nontraffic V09.1
            involving motor vehicle NEC
              V09.00
          traffic V09.3
            involving motor vehicle NEC
              V09.20
        snow board V00.318
          collision (with) V09.9
            animal being ridden or animal
              drawn vehicle V06.99
              nontraffic V06.09
              traffic V06.19
            bus or heavy transport V04.99
              nontraffic V04.09
              traffic V04.19
            car V03.99
              nontraffic V03.09
              traffic V03.19
            pedal cycle V01.99
              nontraffic V01.09
              traffic V01.19
            pick-up truck or van V03.99
              nontraffic V03.09
              traffic V03.19
            railway (train) (vehicle) V05.99
              nontraffic V05.09
              traffic V05.19
            stationary object V00.312
            streetcar V06.99
              nontraffic V06.09
              traffic V06.19
            two- or three-wheeled motor
              vehicle V02.99
              nontraffic V02.09
              traffic V02.19
            vehicle V09.9
              animal-drawn V06.99
                nontraffic V06.09
                traffic V06.19
              motor
                nontraffic V09.00
                traffic V09.20
          fall V00.311
          nontraffic V09.1
            involving motor vehicle NEC V09.00
          traffic V09.3
            involving motor vehicle NEC V09.20
        specified type NEC V00.898
          collision (with) V09.9
            animal being ridden or animal
              drawn vehicle V06.99
              nontraffic V06.09
              traffic V06.19
            bus or heavy transport V04.99
              nontraffic V04.09
              traffic V04.19
            car V03.99
              nontraffic V03.09
              traffic V03.19
            pedal cycle V01.99
              nontraffic V01.09
              traffic V01.19
            pick-up truck or van V03.99
              nontraffic V03.09
              traffic V03.19
            railway (train) (vehicle) V05.99
              nontraffic V05.09
              traffic V05.19
            stationary object V00.892

Accident (Continued)
  transport (Continued)
    pedestrian (Continued)
      conveyance (Continued)
        specified type (Continued)
          collision (Continued)
            streetcar V06.99
              nontraffic V06.09
              traffic V06.19
            two- or three-wheeled motor
              vehicle V02.99
              nontraffic V02.09
              traffic V02.19
            vehicle V09.9
              animal-drawn V06.99
                nontraffic V06.09
                traffic V06.19
              motor
                nontraffic V09.00
                traffic V09.20
          fall V00.891
          nontraffic V09.1
            involving motor vehicle NEC
              V09.00
          traffic V09.3
            involving motor vehicle NEC
              V09.20
        traffic V09.3
          involving motor vehicle V09.20
            military V09.21
            specified type NEC V09.29
        wheelchair (powered) V00.818
          collision (with) V09.9
            animal being ridden or animal
              drawn vehicle V06.99
              nontraffic V06.09
              traffic V06.19
            bus or heavy transport V04.99
              nontraffic V04.09
              traffic V04.19
            car V03.99
              nontraffic V03.09
              traffic V03.19
            pedal cycle V01.99
              nontraffic V01.09
              traffic V01.19
            pick-up truck or van V03.99
              nontraffic V03.09
              traffic V03.19
            railway (train) (vehicle) V05.99
              nontraffic V05.09
              traffic V05.19
            stationary object V00.812
            streetcar V06.99
              nontraffic V06.09
              traffic V06.19
            two- or three-wheeled motor
              vehicle V02.99
              nontraffic V02.09
              traffic V02.19
            vehicle V09.9
              animal-drawn V06.99
                nontraffic V06.09
                traffic V06.19
              motor
                nontraffic V09.00
                traffic V09.20
          fall V00.811
          nontraffic V09.1
            involving motor vehicle NEC V09.00
          traffic V09.3
            involving motor vehicle NEC V09.20
        wheeled shoe V00.158
          colliding with stationary object
            V00.152
          fall V00.151
      on foot —see also Accident, pedestrian
        collision (with)
          animal being ridden or animal drawn
            vehicle V06.90
            nontraffic V06.00
            traffic V06.10
          bus or heavy transport V04.90
            nontraffic V04.00
            traffic V04.10
          car V03.90
            nontraffic V03.00
            traffic V03.10
          pedal cycle V01.90
            nontraffic V01.00
            traffic V01.10

Accident (Continued)
  transport (Continued)
    pedestrian (Continued)
      on foot (Continued)
        collision (Continued)
          pick-up truck or van V03.90
            nontraffic V03.00
            traffic V03.10
          railway (train) (vehicle) V05.90
            nontraffic V05.00
            traffic V05.10
          streetcar V06.90
            nontraffic V06.00
            traffic V06.10
          two- or three-wheeled motor vehicle
            V02.90
            nontraffic V02.00
            traffic V02.10
          vehicle V09.9
            animal-drawn V06.90
              nontraffic V06.00
              traffic V06.10
            motor
              nontraffic V09.00
              traffic V09.20
         nontraffic V09.1
          involving motor vehicle V09.00
            military V09.01
            specified type NEC V09.09
        traffic V09.3
          involving motor vehicle V09.20
            military V09.21
            specified type NEC V09.29
      person NEC (unknown way or transportation)
        V99
        collision (between)
          bus (with)
            heavy transport vehicle (traffic) V87.5
              nontraffic V88.5
          car (with)
            nontraffic V88.5
            bus (traffic) V87.3
              nontraffic V88.3
            heavy transport vehicle (traffic) V87.4
              nontraffic V88.4
            pick-up truck or van (traffic) V87.2
              nontraffic V88.2
            train or railway vehicle (traffic) V87.6
              nontraffic V88.6
            two- or three-wheeled motor vehicle
              (traffic) V87.0
              nontraffic V88.0
           motor vehicle (traffic) NEC V87.7
            nontraffic V88.7
           two- or three-wheeled vehicle (with)
            (traffic)
            motor vehicle NEC V87.1
              nontraffic V88.1
          nonmotor vehicle (collision) (noncollision)
            (traffic) V87.9
            nontraffic V88.9
      pickup truck occupant V59.9
        collision (with)
          animal (traffic) V50.9
            being ridden (traffic) V56.9
              nontraffic V56.3
              while boarding or alighting V56.4
            nontraffic V50.3
            while boarding or alighting V50.4
          animal-drawn vehicle (traffic) V56.9
            nontraffic V56.3
            while boarding or alighting V56.4
          bus (traffic) V54.9
            nontraffic V54.3
            while boarding or alighting V54.4
          car (traffic) V53.9
            nontraffic V53.3
            while boarding or alighting V53.4
          motor vehicle NOS (traffic) V59.60
            nontraffic V59.20
            specified type NEC (traffic) V59.69
              nontraffic V59.29
          pedal cycle (traffic) V51.9
            nontraffic V51.3
            while boarding or alighting V51.4
          pickup truck (traffic) V53.9
            nontraffic V53.3
            while boarding or alighting V53.4
          railway vehicle (traffic) V55.9
            nontraffic V55.3
            while boarding or alighting V55.4

▶ New   ⇒ Revised   deleted Deleted   ● Use Additional Character(s)

Accident *(Continued)*
  transport *(Continued)*
    pedestrian *(Continued)*
      pickup truck occupant *(Continued)*
        specified vehicle NEC (traffic) V56.9
          nontraffic V56.3
          while boarding or alighting V56.4
        stationary object (traffic) V57.9
          nontraffic V57.3
          while boarding or alighting V57.4
        streetcar (traffic) V56.9
          nontraffic V56.3
          while boarding or alighting V56.4
        three wheeled motor vehicle (traffic)
          V52.9
          nontraffic V52.3
          while boarding or alighting V52.4
        truck (traffic) V54.9
          nontraffic V54.3
          while boarding or alighting V54.4
        two wheeled motor vehicle (traffic) V52.9
          nontraffic V52.3
          while boarding or alighting V52.4
        van (traffic) V53.9
          nontraffic V53.3
          while boarding or alighting V53.4
      driver
        collision (with)
          animal (traffic) V50.5
            being ridden (traffic) V56.5
              nontraffic V56.0
            nontraffic V50.0
          animal-drawn vehicle (traffic)
            V56.5
            nontraffic V56.0
          bus (traffic) V54.5
            nontraffic V54.0
          car (traffic) V53.5
            nontraffic V53.0
          motor vehicle NOS (traffic) V59.40
            nontraffic V59.00
            specified type NEC (traffic) V59.49
              nontraffic V59.09
          pedal cycle (traffic) V51.5
            nontraffic V51.0
          pickup truck (traffic) V53.5
            nontraffic V53.0
          railway vehicle (traffic) V55.5
            nontraffic V55.0
          specified vehicle NEC (traffic) V56.5
            nontraffic V56.0
          stationary object (traffic) V57.5
            nontraffic V57.0
          streetcar (traffic) V56.5
            nontraffic V56.0
          three wheeled motor vehicle (traffic)
            V52.5
            nontraffic V52.0
          truck (traffic) V54.5
            nontraffic V54.0
          two wheeled motor vehicle (traffic)
            V52.5
            nontraffic V52.0
          van (traffic) V53.5
            nontraffic V53.0
        noncollision accident (traffic) V58.5
          nontraffic V58.0
      hanger-on
        collision (with)
          animal (traffic) V50.7
            being ridden (traffic) V56.7
              nontraffic V56.2
            nontraffic V50.2
          animal-drawn vehicle (traffic) V56.7
            nontraffic V56.2
          bus (traffic) V54.7
            nontraffic V54.2
          car (traffic) V53.7
            nontraffic V53.2
          pedal cycle (traffic) V51.7
            nontraffic V51.2
          pickup truck (traffic) V53.7
            nontraffic V53.2
          railway vehicle (traffic) V55.7
            nontraffic V55.2
          specified vehicle NEC (traffic) V56.7
            nontraffic V56.2
          stationary object (traffic) V57.7
            nontraffic V57.2
          streetcar (traffic) V56.7
            nontraffic V56.2

Accident *(Continued)*
  transport *(Continued)*
    pedestrian *(Continued)*
      hanger-on *(Continued)*
        collision *(Continued)*
          three wheeled motor vehicle (traffic)
            V52.7
            nontraffic V52.2
          truck (traffic) V54.7
            nontraffic V54.2
          two wheeled motor vehicle (traffic)
            V52.7
            nontraffic V52.2
          van (traffic) V53.7
            nontraffic V53.2
        noncollision accident (traffic) V58.7
          nontraffic V58.2
      noncollision accident (traffic) V58.9
        nontraffic V58.3
        while boarding or alighting V58.4
      nontraffic V59.3
      passenger
        collision (with)
          animal (traffic) V50.6
            being ridden (traffic) V56.6
              nontraffic V56.1
            nontraffic V50.1
          animal-drawn vehicle (traffic) V56.6
            nontraffic V56.1
          bus (traffic) V54.6
            nontraffic V54.1
          car (traffic) V53.6
            nontraffic V53.1
          motor vehicle NOS (traffic) V59.50
            nontraffic V59.10
            specified type NEC (traffic) V59.59
              nontraffic V59.19
          pedal cycle (traffic) V51.6
            nontraffic V51.1
          pickup truck (traffic) V53.6
            nontraffic V53.1
          railway vehicle (traffic) V55.6
            nontraffic V55.1
          specified vehicle NEC (traffic) V56.6
            nontraffic V56.1
          stationary object (traffic) V57.6
            nontraffic V57.1
          streetcar (traffic) V56.6
            nontraffic V56.1
          three wheeled motor vehicle (traffic)
            V52.6
            nontraffic V52.1
          truck (traffic) V54.6
            nontraffic V54.1
          two wheeled motor vehicle (traffic)
            V52.6
            nontraffic V52.1
          van (traffic) V53.6
            nontraffic V53.1
        noncollision accident (traffic) V58.6
          nontraffic V58.1
      specified type NEC V59.88
        military vehicle V59.81
      quarry truck —*see* Accident, transport,
        industrial vehicle occupant
      race car —*see* Accident, transport, motor
        vehicle NEC occupant
      railway vehicle occupant V81.9
        collision (with) V81.3
          motor vehicle (non-military) (traffic)
            V81.1
            military V81.83
            nontraffic V81.0
          rolling stock V81.2
          specified object NEC V81.3
        during derailment V81.7
          with antecedent collision —*see* Accident,
            transport, railway vehicle occupant,
            collision
        explosion V81.81
        fall (in railway vehicle) V81.5
          during derailment V81.7
            with antecedent collision —*see*
              Accident, transport, railway
              vehicle occupant, collision
          from railway vehicle V81.6
            during derailment V81.7
              with antecedent collision —*see*
                Accident, transport, railway
                vehicle occupant, collision
        while boarding or alighting V81.4

Accident *(Continued)*
  transport *(Continued)*
    railway vehicle occupan *(Continued)*
      fire V81.81
      object falling onto train V81.82
      specified type NEC V81.89
      while boarding or alighting V81.4
    Segway V00.848
    ski lift V98.3
    snowmobile occupant (nontraffic) V86.92
      driver V86.52
      hanger-on V86.72
      passenger V86.62
      traffic V86.32
        driver V86.02
        hanger-on V86.22
        passenger V86.12
      while boarding or alighting V86.42
    specified NEC V98.8
    sport utility vehicle occupant —*see also*
      Accident, transport, pickup truck
      occupant
    streetcar occupant V82.9
      collision (with) V82.3
        motor vehicle (traffic) V82.1
          nontraffic V82.0
        rolling stock V82.2
      during derailment V82.7
        with antecedent collision —*see* Accident,
          transport, streetcar occupant,
          collision
      fall (in streetcar) V82.5
        during derailment V82.7
          with antecedent collision —*see*
            Accident, transport, streetcar
            occupant, collision
        from streetcar V82.6
          during derailment V82.7
            with antecedent collision —*see*
              Accident, transport, streetcar
              occupant, collision
          while boarding or alighting
            V82.4
      while boarding or alighting V82.4
      specified type NEC V82.8
      while boarding or alighting V82.4
    three-wheeled motor vehicle occupant V39.9
      collision (with)
        animal (traffic) V30.9
          being ridden (traffic) V36.9
            nontraffic V36.3
            while boarding or alighting V36.4
          nontraffic V30.3
          while boarding or alighting V30.4
        animal-drawn vehicle (traffic) V36.9
          nontraffic V36.3
          while boarding or alighting V36.4
        bus (traffic) V34.9
          nontraffic V34.3
          while boarding or alighting V34.4
        car (traffic) V33.9
          nontraffic V33.3
          while boarding or alighting V33.4
        motor vehicle NOS (traffic) V39.60
          nontraffic V39.20
          specified type NEC (traffic) V39.69
            nontraffic V39.29
        pedal cycle (traffic) V31.9
          nontraffic V31.3
          while boarding or alighting
            V31.4
        pickup truck (traffic) V33.9
          nontraffic V33.3
          while boarding or alighting
            V33.4
        railway vehicle (traffic) V35.9
          nontraffic V35.3
          while boarding or alighting V35.4
        specified vehicle NEC (traffic) V36.9
          nontraffic V36.3
          while boarding or alighting V36.4
        stationary object (traffic) V37.9
          nontraffic V37.3
          while boarding or alighting V37.4
        streetcar (traffic) V36.9
          nontraffic V36.3
          while boarding or alighting V36.4
        three wheeled motor vehicle (traffic)
          V32.9
          nontraffic V32.3
          while boarding or alighting V32.4

Accident *(Continued)*
  transport *(Continued)*
    three-wheeled motor vehicle
        occupant—*(Continued)*
      collision *(Continued)*
        truck (traffic) V34.9
          nontraffic V34.3
          while boarding or alighting V34.4
        two wheeled motor vehicle (traffic) V32.9
          nontraffic V32.3
          while boarding or alighting V32.4
        van (traffic) V33.9
          nontraffic V33.3
          while boarding or alighting V33.4
      driver
        collision (with)
          animal (traffic) V30.5
            being ridden (traffic) V36.5
              nontraffic V36.0
            nontraffic V30.0
          animal-drawn vehicle (traffic) V36.5
            nontraffic V36.0
          bus (traffic) V34.5
            nontraffic V34.0
          car (traffic) V33.5
            nontraffic V33.0
          motor vehicle NOS (traffic) V39.40
            nontraffic V39.00
            specified type NEC (traffic) V39.49
              nontraffic V39.09
          pedal cycle (traffic) V31.5
            nontraffic V31.0
          pickup truck (traffic) V33.5
            nontraffic V33.0
          railway vehicle (traffic) V35.5
            nontraffic V35.0
          specified vehicle NEC (traffic)
              V36.5
            nontraffic V36.0
          stationary object (traffic) V37.5
            nontraffic V37.0
          streetcar (traffic) V36.5
            nontraffic V36.0
          three wheeled motor vehicle (traffic)
              V32.5
            nontraffic V32.0
          truck (traffic) V34.5
            nontraffic V34.0
          two wheeled motor vehicle (traffic)
              V32.5
            nontraffic V32.0
          van (traffic) V33.5
            nontraffic V33.0
        noncollision accident (traffic) V38.5
          nontraffic V38.0
      hanger-on
        collision (with)
          animal (traffic) V30.7
            being ridden (traffic) V36.7
              nontraffic V36.2
            nontraffic V30.2
          animal-drawn vehicle (traffic) V36.7
            nontraffic V36.2
          bus (traffic) V34.7
            nontraffic V34.2
          car (traffic) V33.7
            nontraffic V33.2
          pedal cycle (traffic) V31.7
            nontraffic V31.2
          pickup truck (traffic) V33.7
            nontraffic V33.2
          railway vehicle (traffic) V35.7
            nontraffic V35.2
          specified vehicle NEC (traffic) V36.7
            nontraffic V36.2
          stationary object (traffic) V37.7
            nontraffic V37.2
          streetcar (traffic) V36.7
            nontraffic V36.2
          three wheeled motor vehicle (traffic)
              V32.7
            nontraffic V32.2
          truck (traffic) V34.7
            nontraffic V34.2
          two wheeled motor vehicle (traffic)
              V32.7
            nontraffic V32.2
          van (traffic) V33.7
            nontraffic V33.2
        noncollision accident (traffic) V38.7
          nontraffic V38.2

Accident *(Continued)*
  transport *(Continued)*
    three-wheeled motor vehicle
        occupant—*(Continued)*
      noncollision accident (traffic) V38.9
        nontraffic V38.3
        while boarding or alighting V38.4
      nontraffic V39.3
      passenger
        collision (with)
          animal (traffic) V30.6
            being ridden (traffic) V36.6
              nontraffic V36.1
            nontraffic V30.1
          animal-drawn vehicle (traffic) V36.6
            nontraffic V36.1
          bus (traffic) V34.6
            nontraffic V34.1
          car (traffic) V33.6
            nontraffic V33.1
          motor vehicle NOS (traffic) V39.50
            nontraffic V39.10
            specified type NEC (traffic) V39.59
              nontraffic V39.19
          pedal cycle (traffic) V31.6
            nontraffic V31.1
          pickup truck (traffic) V33.6
            nontraffic V33.1
          railway vehicle (traffic) V35.6
            nontraffic V35.1
          specified vehicle NEC (traffic) V36.6
            nontraffic V36.1
          stationary object (traffic) V37.6
            nontraffic V37.1
          streetcar (traffic) V36.6
            nontraffic V36.1
          three wheeled motor vehicle (traffic)
              V32.6
            nontraffic V32.1
          truck (traffic) V34.6
            nontraffic V34.1
          two wheeled motor vehicle (traffic)
              V32.6
            nontraffic V32.1
          van (traffic) V33.6
            nontraffic V33.1
        noncollision accident (traffic) V38.6
          nontraffic V38.1
      specified type NEC V39.89
        military vehicle V39.81
    tractor (farm) (and trailer) —*see* Accident,
        transport, agricultural vehicle occupant
    tram —*see* Accident, transport, streetcar
      in mine or quarry —*see* Accident, transport,
          industrial vehicle occupant
    trolley —*see* Accident, transport, streetcar
      in mine or quarry —*see* Accident, transport,
          industrial vehicle occupant
    truck (heavy) occupant V69.9
      collision (with)
        animal (traffic) V60.9
          being ridden (traffic) V66.9
            nontraffic V66.3
            while boarding or alighting V66.4
          nontraffic V60.3
          while boarding or alighting V60.4
        animal-drawn vehicle (traffic) V66.9
          nontraffic V66.3
          while boarding or alighting V66.4
        bus (traffic) V64.9
          nontraffic V64.3
          while boarding or alighting V64.4
        car (traffic) V63.9
          nontraffic V63.3
          while boarding or alighting V63.4
        motor vehicle NOS (traffic) V69.60
          nontraffic V69.20
          specified type NEC (traffic) V69.69
            nontraffic V69.29
        pedal cycle (traffic) V61.9
          nontraffic V61.3
          while boarding or alighting V61.4
        pickup truck (traffic) V63.9
          nontraffic V63.3
          while boarding or alighting V63.4
        railway vehicle (traffic) V65.9
          nontraffic V65.3
          while boarding or alighting V65.4
        specified vehicle NEC (traffic) V66.9
          nontraffic V66.3
          while boarding or alighting V66.4

Accident *(Continued)*
  transport *(Continued)*
    truck (heavy) occupant *(Continued)*
      collision *(Continued)*
        stationary object (traffic) V67.9
          nontraffic V67.3
          while boarding or alighting V67.4
        streetcar (traffic) V66.9
          nontraffic V66.3
          while boarding or alighting V66.4
        three wheeled motor vehicle (traffic)
            V62.9
          nontraffic V62.3
          while boarding or alighting V62.4
        truck (traffic) V64.9
          nontraffic V64.3
          while boarding or alighting V64.4
        two wheeled motor vehicle (traffic) V62.9
          nontraffic V62.3
          while boarding or alighting V62.4
        van (traffic) V63.9
          nontraffic V63.3
          while boarding or alighting V63.4
      driver
        collision (with)
          animal (traffic) V60.5
            being ridden (traffic) V66.5
              nontraffic V66.0
            nontraffic V60.0
          animal-drawn vehicle (traffic) V66.5
            nontraffic V66.0
          bus (traffic) V64.5
            nontraffic V64.0
          car (traffic) V63.5
            nontraffic V63.0
          motor vehicle NOS (traffic) V69.40
            nontraffic V69.00
            specified type NEC (traffic)
                V69.49
              nontraffic V69.09
          pedal cycle (traffic) V61.5
            nontraffic V61.0
          pickup truck (traffic) V63.5
            nontraffic V63.0
          railway vehicle (traffic) V65.5
            nontraffic V65.0
          specified vehicle NEC (traffic) V66.5
            nontraffic V66.0
          stationary object (traffic) V67.5
            nontraffic V67.0
          streetcar (traffic) V66.5
            nontraffic V66.0
          three wheeled motor vehicle (traffic)
              V62.5
            nontraffic V62.0
          truck (traffic) V64.5
            nontraffic V64.0
          two wheeled motor vehicle (traffic)
              V62.5
            nontraffic V62.0
          van (traffic) V63.5
            nontraffic V63.0
        noncollision accident (traffic) V68.5
          nontraffic V68.0
    dump —*see* Accident, transport,
        construction vehicle occupant
    hanger-on
      collision (with)
        animal (traffic) V60.7
          being ridden (traffic) V66.7
            nontraffic V66.2
          nontraffic V60.2
        animal-drawn vehicle (traffic)
            V66.7
          nontraffic V66.2
        bus (traffic) V64.7
          nontraffic V64.2
        car (traffic) V63.7
          nontraffic V63.2
        pedal cycle (traffic) V61.7
          nontraffic V61.2
        pickup truck (traffic) V63.7
          nontraffic V63.2
        railway vehicle (traffic) V65.7
          nontraffic V65.2
        specified vehicle NEC (traffic) V66.7
          nontraffic V66.2
        stationary object (traffic) V67.7
          nontraffic V67.2
        streetcar (traffic) V66.7
          nontraffic V66.2

▶ New   ⇒ Revised   ~~deleted~~ Deleted   ● Use Additional Character(s)

Accident (Continued)
  transport (Continued)
    truck (heavy) occupant (Continued)
      hanger-on (Continued)
        collision (Continued)
          three wheeled motor vehicle (traffic) V62.7
            nontraffic V62.2
          truck (traffic) V64.7
            nontraffic V64.2
          two wheeled motor vehicle (traffic) V62.7
            nontraffic V62.2
          van (traffic) V63.7
            nontraffic V63.2
        noncollision accident (traffic) V68.7
          nontraffic V68.2
      noncollision accident (traffic) V68.9
        nontraffic V68.3
        while boarding or alighting V68.4
      nontraffic V69.3
      passenger
        collision (with)
          animal (traffic) V60.6
            being ridden (traffic) V66.6
              nontraffic V66.1
            nontraffic V60.1
          animal-drawn vehicle (traffic) V66.6
            nontraffic V66.1
          bus (traffic) V64.6
            nontraffic V64.1
          car (traffic) V63.6
            nontraffic V63.1
          motor vehicle NOS (traffic) V69.50
            nontraffic V69.10
            specified type NEC (traffic) V69.59
              nontraffic V69.19
          pedal cycle (traffic) V61.6
            nontraffic V61.1
          pickup truck (traffic) V63.6
            nontraffic V63.1
          railway vehicle (traffic) V65.6
            nontraffic V65.1
          specified vehicle NEC (traffic) V66.6
            nontraffic V66.1
          stationary object (traffic) V67.6
            nontraffic V67.1
          streetcar (traffic) V66.6
            nontraffic V66.1
          three wheeled motor vehicle (traffic) V62.6
            nontraffic V62.1
          truck (traffic) V64.6
            nontraffic V64.1
          two wheeled motor vehicle (traffic) V62.6
            nontraffic V62.1
          van (traffic) V63.6
            nontraffic V63.1
      noncollision accident (traffic) V68.6
        nontraffic V68.1
    pickup —see Accident, transport, pickup truck occupant
    specified type NEC V69.88
      military vehicle V69.81
    van occupant V59.9
      collision (with)
        animal (traffic) V50.9
          being ridden (traffic) V56.9
            nontraffic V56.3
            while boarding or alighting V56.4
          nontraffic V50.3
          while boarding or alighting V50.4
        animal-drawn vehicle (traffic) V56.9
          nontraffic V56.3
          while boarding or alighting V56.4
        bus (traffic) V54.9
          nontraffic V54.3
          while boarding or alighting V54.4
        car (traffic) V53.9
          nontraffic V53.3
          while boarding or alighting V53.4
        motor vehicle NOS (traffic) V59.60
          nontraffic V59.20
          specified type NEC (traffic) V59.69
           nontraffic V59.29
        pedal cycle (traffic) V51.9
          nontraffic V51.3
          while boarding or alighting V51.4

Accident (Continued)
  transport (Continued)
    van occupant (Continued)
      collision (Continued)
        pickup truck (traffic) V53.9
          nontraffic V53.3
          while boarding or alighting V53.4
        railway vehicle (traffic) V55.9
          nontraffic V55.3
          while boarding or alighting V55.4
        specified vehicle NEC (traffic) V56.9
          nontraffic V56.3
          while boarding or alighting V56.4
        stationary object (traffic) V57.9
          nontraffic V57.3
          while boarding or alighting V57.4
        streetcar (traffic) V56.9
          nontraffic V56.3
          while boarding or alighting V56.4
        three wheeled motor vehicle (traffic) V52.9
          nontraffic V52.3
          while boarding or alighting V52.4
        truck (traffic) V54.9
          nontraffic V54.3
          while boarding or alighting V54.4
        two wheeled motor vehicle (traffic) V52.9
          nontraffic V52.3
          while boarding or alighting V52.4
        van (traffic) V53.9
          nontraffic V53.3
          while boarding or alighting V53.4
      driver
        collision (with)
          animal (traffic) V50.5
           being ridden (traffic) V56.5
            nontraffic V56.0
           nontraffic V50.0
          animal-drawn vehicle (traffic) V56.5
           nontraffic V56.0
          bus (traffic) V54.5
           nontraffic V54.0
          car (traffic) V53.5
           nontraffic V53.0
          motor vehicle NOS (traffic) V59.40
           nontraffic V59.00
           specified type NEC (traffic) V59.49
            nontraffic V59.09
          pedal cycle (traffic) V51.5
           nontraffic V51.0
          pickup truck (traffic) V53.5
           nontraffic V53.0
          railway vehicle (traffic) V55.5
           nontraffic V55.0
          specified vehicle NEC (traffic) V56.5
           nontraffic V56.0
          stationary object (traffic) V57.5
           nontraffic V57.0
          streetcar (traffic) V56.5
           nontraffic V56.0
          three wheeled motor vehicle (traffic) V52.5
           nontraffic V52.0
          truck (traffic) V54.5
           nontraffic V54.0
          two wheeled motor vehicle (traffic) V52.5
           nontraffic V52.0
          van (traffic) V53.5
           nontraffic V53.0
        noncollision accident (traffic) V58.5
          nontraffic V58.0
      hanger-on
        collision (with)
          animal (traffic) V50.7
           being ridden (traffic) V56.7
            nontraffic V56.2
           nontraffic V50.2
          animal-drawn vehicle (traffic) V56.7
           nontraffic V56.2
          bus (traffic) V54.7
           nontraffic V54.2
          car (traffic) V53.7
           nontraffic V53.2
          pedal cycle (traffic) V51.7
           nontraffic V51.2
          pickup truck (traffic) V53.7
           nontraffic V53.2
          railway vehicle (traffic) V55.7
           nontraffic V55.2

Accident (Continued)
  transport (Continued)
    van occupant (Continued)
      hanger-on (Continued)
        collision (Continued)
          specified vehicle NEC (traffic) V56.7
           nontraffic V56.2
          stationary object (traffic) V57.7
           nontraffic V57.2
          streetcar (traffic) V56.7
           nontraffic V56.2
          three wheeled motor vehicle (traffic) V52.7
           nontraffic V52.2
          truck (traffic) V54.7
           nontraffic V54.2
          two wheeled motor vehicle (traffic) V52.7
           nontraffic V52.2
          van (traffic) V53.7
           nontraffic V53.2
        noncollision accident (traffic) V58.7
          nontraffic V58.2
      noncollision accident (traffic) V58.9
        nontraffic V58.3
        while boarding or alighting V58.4
      nontraffic V59.3
      passenger
        collision (with)
          animal (traffic) V50.6
           being ridden (traffic) V56.6
            nontraffic V56.1
           nontraffic V50.1
          animal-drawn vehicle (traffic) V56.6
           nontraffic V56.1
          bus (traffic) V54.6
           nontraffic V54.1
          car (traffic) V53.6
           nontraffic V53.1
          motor vehicle NOS (traffic) V59.50
           nontraffic V59.10
           specified type NEC (traffic) V59.59
            nontraffic V59.19
          pedal cycle (traffic) V51.6
           nontraffic V51.1
          pickup truck (traffic) V53.6
           nontraffic V53.1
          railway vehicle (traffic) V55.6
           nontraffic V55.1
          specified vehicle NEC (traffic) V56.6
           nontraffic V56.1
          stationary object (traffic) V57.6
           nontraffic V57.1
          streetcar (traffic) V56.6
           nontraffic V56.1
          three wheeled motor vehicle (traffic) V52.6
           nontraffic V52.1
          truck (traffic) V54.6
           nontraffic V54.1
          two wheeled motor vehicle (traffic) V52.6
           nontraffic V52.1
          van (traffic) V53.6
           nontraffic V53.1
        noncollision accident (traffic) V58.6
          nontraffic V58.1
      specified type NEC V59.88
        military vehicle V59.81
    watercraft occupant —see Accident, watercraft
    vehicle NEC V89.9
    animal-drawn NEC —see Accident, transport, animal-drawn vehicle occupant
    special
      agricultural —see Accident, transport, agricultural vehicle occupant
      construction —see Accident, transport, construction vehicle occupant
      industrial —see Accident, transport, industrial vehicle occupant
      three-wheeled NEC (motorized) —see Accident, transport, three-wheeled motor vehicle occupant
  watercraft V94.9
    causing
      drowning —see Drowning, due to, accident to, watercraft
      injury NEC V91.89
        crushed between craft and object V91.19
          powered craft V91.13
           ferry boat V91.11
           fishing boat V91.12

Accident *(Continued)*
  watercraft *(Continued)*
    causing *(Continued)*
      injury *(Continued)*
        crushed between craft and
          object— *(Continued)*
          powered craft *(Continued)*
            jet ski V91.13
            liner V91.11
            merchant ship V91.10
            passenger ship V91.11
          unpowered craft V91.18
            canoe V91.15
            inflatable V91.16
            kayak V91.15
            sailboat V91.14
            surf-board V91.18
            windsurfer V91.18
        fall on board V91.29
          powered craft V91.23
            ferry boat V91.21
            fishing boat V91.22
            jet ski V91.23
            liner V91.21
            merchant ship V91.20
            passenger ship V91.21
          unpowered craft
            canoe V91.25
            inflatable V91.26
            kayak V91.25
            sailboat V91.24
        fire on board causing burn V91.09
          powered craft V91.03
            ferry boat V91.01
            fishing boat V91.02
            jet ski V91.03
            liner V91.01
            merchant ship V91.00
            passenger ship V91.01
          unpowered craft V91.08
            canoe V91.05
            inflatable V91.06
            kayak V91.05
            sailboat V91.04
            surf-board V91.08
            water skis V91.07
            windsurfer V91.08
        hit by falling object V91.39
          powered craft V91.33
            ferry boat V91.31
            fishing boat V91.32
            jet skis V91.33
            liner V91.31
            merchant ship V91.30
            passenger ship V91.31
          unpowered craft V91.38
            canoe V91.35
            inflatable V91.36
            kayak V91.35
            sailboat V91.34
            surf-board V91.38
            water skis V91.37
            windsurfer V91.38
        specified type NEC V91.89
          powered craft V91.83
            ferry boat V91.81
            fishing boat V91.82
            jet ski V91.83
            liner V91.81
            merchant ship V91.80
            passenger ship V91.81
          unpowered craft V91.88
            canoe V91.85
            inflatable V91.86
            kayak V91.85
            sailboat V91.84
            surf-board V91.88
            water skis V91.87
            windsurfer V91.88
    due to, caused by cataclysm —*see* Forces of
      nature, by type
    military NEC V94.818
      with civilian watercraft V94.810
      civilian in water injured by V94.811
    nonpowered, struck by
      nonpowered vessel V94.22
      powered vessel V94.21
    specified type NEC V94.89
    striking swimmer
      powered V94.11
      unpowered V94.12

Acid throwing (assault) Y08.89
Activity (involving) (of victim at time of event)
  Y93.9
  aerobic and step exercise (class) Y93.A3
  alpine skiing Y93.23
  animal care NEC Y93.K9
  arts and handcrafts NEC Y93.D9
  athletics NEC Y93.79
  athletics played as a team or group NEC Y93.69
  athletics played individually NEC Y93.59
  baking Y93.G3
  ballet Y93.41
  barbells Y93.B3
  BASE (Building, Antenna, Span, Earth) jumping
    Y93.33
  baseball Y93.64
  basketball Y93.67
  bathing (personal) Y93.E1
  beach volleyball Y93.68
  bike riding Y93.55
  blackout game Y93.85
  boogie boarding Y93.18
  bowling Y93.54
  boxing Y93.71
  brass instrument playing Y93.J4
  building construction Y93.H3
  bungee jumping Y93.34
  calisthenics Y93.A2
  canoeing (in calm and turbulent water) Y93.16
  capture the flag Y93.6A
  cardiorespiratory exercise NEC Y93.A9
  caregiving (providing) NEC Y93.F9
    bathing Y93.F1
    lifting Y93.F2
  cellular
    communication device Y93.C2
    telephone Y93.C2
  challenge course Y93.A5
  cheerleading Y93.45
  choking game Y93.85
  circuit training Y93.A4
  cleaning
    floor Y93.E5
  climbing NEC Y93.39
    mountain Y93.31
    rock Y93.31
    wall Y93.31
  clothing care and maintenance NEC Y93.E9
  combatives Y93.75
  computer
    keyboarding Y93.C1
    technology NEC Y93.C9
  confidence course Y93.A5
  construction (building) Y93.H3
  cooking and baking Y93.G3
  cool down exercises Y93.A2
  cricket Y93.69
  crocheting Y93.D1
  cross country skiing Y93.24
  dancing (all types) Y93.41
  digging
    dirt Y93.H1
  dirt digging Y93.H1
  dishwashing Y93.G1
  diving (platform) (springboard) Y93.12
    underwater Y93.15
  dodge ball Y93.6A
  downhill skiing Y93.23
  drum playing Y93.J2
  dumbbells Y93.B3
  electronic
    devices NEC Y93.C9
      hand held interactive Y93.C2
    game playing (using) (with)
      interactive device Y93.C2
      keyboard or other stationary device Y93.C1
  elliptical machine Y93.A1
  exercise(s)
    machines ((primarily) for)
      cardiorespiratory conditioning Y93.A1
      muscle strengthening Y93.B1
    muscle strengthening (non-machine) NEC
      Y93.B9
  external motion NEC Y93.I9
    rollercoaster Y93.I1
  fainting game Y93.85
  field hockey Y93.65
  figure skating (pairs) (singles) Y93.21
  flag football Y93.62
  floor mopping and cleaning Y93.E5
  food preparation and clean up Y93.G1

Activity *(Continued)*
  football (American) NOS Y93.61
    flag Y93.62
    tackle Y93.61
    touch Y93.62
  four square Y93.6A
  free weights Y93.B3
  frisbee (ultimate) Y93.74
  furniture
    building Y93.D3
    finishing Y93.D3
    repair Y93.D3
  game playing (electronic)
    using interactive device Y93.C2
    using keyboard or other stationary device
      Y93.C1
  gardening Y93.H2
  golf Y93.53
  grass drills Y93.A6
  grilling and smoking food Y93.G2
  grooming and shearing an animal Y93.K3
  guerilla drills Y93.A6
  gymnastics (rhythmic) Y93.43
  hand held interactive electronic device Y93.C2
  handball Y93.73
  handcrafts NEC Y93.D9
  hang gliding Y93.35
  hiking (on level or elevated terrain) Y93.01
  hockey (ice) Y93.22
    field Y93.65
  horseback riding Y93.52
  household (interior) maintenance NEC Y93.E9
  ice NEC Y93.29
    dancing Y93.21
    hockey Y93.22
    skating Y93.21
  inline roller skating Y93.51
  ironing Y93.E4
  judo Y93.75
  jumping (off) NEC Y93.39
    BASE (Building, Antenna, Span, Earth) Y93.33
    bungee Y93.34
    jacks Y93.A2
    rope Y93.56
  jumping jacks Y93.A2
  jumping rope Y93.56
  karate Y93.75
  kayaking (in calm and turbulent water) Y93.16
  keyboarding (computer) Y93.C1
  kickball Y93.6A
  knitting Y93.D1
  lacrosse Y93.65
  land maintenance NEC Y93.H9
  landscaping Y93.H2
  laundry Y93.E2
  machines (exercise)
    primarily for cardiorespiratory conditioning
      Y93.A1
    primarily for muscle strengthening Y93.B1
  maintenance
    exterior building NEC Y93.H9
    household (interior) NEC Y93.E9
    land Y93.H9
    property Y93.H9
  marching (on level or elevated terrain) Y93.01
  martial arts Y93.75
  microwave oven Y93.G3
  milking an animal Y93.K2
  mopping (floor) Y93.E5
  mountain climbing Y93.31
  muscle strengthening
    exercises (non-machine) NEC Y93.B9
    machines Y93.B1
  musical keyboard (electronic) playing Y93.J1
  nordic skiing Y93.24
  obstacle course Y93.A5
  oven (microwave) Y93.G3
  packing up and unpacking in moving to a new
    residence Y93.E6
  parasailing Y93.19
  pass out game Y93.85
  percussion instrument playing NEC Y93.J2
  personal
    bathing and showering Y93.E1
    hygiene NEC Y93.E8
    showering Y93.E1
  physical games generally associated with school
    recess, summer camp and children Y93.6A
  physical training NEC Y93.A9
  piano playing Y93.J1
  pilates Y93.B4

A

Assault *(Continued)*
  steam X98.0
  striking against
    other person Y04.2
    sports equipment Y08.09
      baseball bat Y08.02
      hockey stick Y08.01
  struck by
    sports equipment Y08.09
      baseball bat Y08.02
      hockey stick Y08.01
  submersion —*see* Assault, drowning
  violence Y09
  weapon Y09
    blunt Y00
    cutting or piercing —*see* Assault, cutting or
      piercing instrument
    firearm —*see* Assault, firearm
  wound Y09
    cutting —*see* Assault, cutting or piercing
      instrument
    gunshot —*see* Assault, firearm
    knife X99.1
    piercing —*see* Assault, cutting or piercing
      instrument
    puncture —*see* Assault, cutting or piercing
      instrument
    stab —*see* Assault, cutting or piercing
      instrument
Attack by mammals NEC W55.89
Avalanche —*see* Landslide
Aviator's disease —*see* Air, pressure

B

Barotitis, barodontalgia, barosinusitis,
  barotrauma (otitic) (sinus) —*see* Air, pressure
Battered (baby) (child) (person) (syndrome)
  X58
Bayonet wound W26.1
  in
    legal intervention —*see* Legal, intervention,
      sharp object, bayonet
    war operations —*see* War operations,
      combat
  stated as undetermined whether accidental or
    intentional Y28.8
  suicide (attempt) X78.2
Bean in nose —*see* categories T17 and T18
Bed set on fire NEC —*see* Exposure, fire,
  uncontrolled, building, bed
Beheading (by guillotine)
  homicide X99.9
  legal execution —*see* Legal, intervention
Bending, injury in (prolonged) (static)
  X50.1
Bends —*see* Air, pressure, change
Bite, bitten by
  alligator W58.01
  arthropod (nonvenomous) NEC W57
  bull W55.21
  cat W55.01
  cow W55.21
  crocodile W58.11
  dog W54.0
  goat W55.31
  hoof stock NEC W55.31
  horse W55.11
  human being (accidentally) W50.3
    with intent to injure or kill Y04.1
    as, or caused by, a crowd or human stampede
      (with fall) W52
    assault Y04.1
    homicide (attempt) Y04.1
    in
      fight Y04.1
  insect (nonvenomous) W57
  lizard (nonvenomous) W59.01
  mammal NEC W55.81
    marine W56.31
  marine animal (nonvenomous) W56.81
  millipede W57
  moray eel W56.51
  mouse W53.01
  person(s) (accidentally) W50.3
    with intent to injure or kill Y04.1
    as, or caused by, a crowd or human stampede
      (with fall) W52
    assault Y04.1

Bite, bitten by *(Continued)*
  person(s) *(Continued)*
    homicide (attempt) Y04.1
    in
      fight Y04.1
  pig W55.41
  raccoon W55.51
  rat W53.11
  reptile W59.81
    lizard W59.01
    snake W59.11
    turtle W59.21
      terrestrial W59.81
  rodent W53.81
    mouse W53.01
    rat W53.11
    specified NEC W53.81
    squirrel W53.21
  shark W56.41
  sheep W55.31
  snake (nonvenomous) W59.11
  spider (nonvenomous) W57
  squirrel W53.21
Blast (air) **in war operations** —*see* War operations,
  blast
Blizzard X37.2
Blood alcohol level Y90.9
  20-39mg/100ml Y90.1
  40-59mg/100ml Y90.2
  60-79mg/100ml Y90.3
  80-99mg/100ml Y90.4
  100-119mg/100ml Y90.5
  120-199mg/100ml Y90.6
  200-239mg/100ml Y90.7
  less than 20mg/100ml Y90.0
  presence in blood, level not specified
    Y90.9
Blow X58
  by law-enforcing agent, police (on duty) —*see*
    Legal, intervention, manhandling
    blunt object —*see* Legal, intervention, blunt
      object
Blowing up —*see* Explosion
Brawl (hand) (fists) (foot) Y04.0
Breakage (accidental) (part of)
  ladder (causing fall) W11
  scaffolding (causing fall) W12
Broken
  glass, contact with —*see* Contact, with,
    glass
  power line (causing electric shock) W85
Bumping against, into (accidentally)
  object NEC W22.8
    with fall —*see* Fall, due to, bumping against,
      object
    caused by crowd or human stampede (with
      fall) W52
    sports equipment W21.9
  person(s) W51
    with fall W03
      due to ice or snow W00.0
    assault Y04.2
    caused by, a crowd or human stampede (with
      fall) W52
    homicide (attempt) Y04.2
  sports equipment W21.9
Burn, burned, burning (accidental) (by) (from)
  (on)
  acid NEC —*see* Table of Drugs and
    Chemicals
  bed linen —*see* Exposure, fire, uncontrolled, in
    building, bed
  blowtorch X08.8
    with ignition of clothing NEC X06.2
      nightwear X05
  bonfire, campfire (controlled) —*see also*
    Exposure, fire, controlled, not in
    building
    uncontrolled —*see* Exposure, fire,
      uncontrolled, not in building
  candle X08.8
    with ignition of clothing NEC X06.2
      nightwear X05
  caustic liquid, substance (external) (internal)
    NEC —*see* Table of Drugs and
    Chemicals
  chemical (external) (internal) —*see also* Table of
    Drugs and Chemicals
    in war operations —*see* War operations, fire
  cigar(s) or cigarette(s) X08.8
    with ignition of clothing NEC X06.2
      nightwear X05

Burn, burned, burning *(Continued)*
  clothes, clothing NEC (from controlled fire)
    X06.2
    with conflagration —*see* Exposure, fire,
      uncontrolled, building
    not in building or structure —*see* Exposure,
      fire, uncontrolled, not in building
  cooker (hot) X15.8
    stated as undetermined whether accidental or
      intentional Y27.3
    suicide (attempt) X77.3
  electric blanket X16
  engine (hot) X17
  fire, flames —*see* Exposure, fire
  flare, Very pistol —*see* Discharge, firearm NEC
  heat
    from appliance (electrical) (household) X15.8
      cooker X15.8
      hotplate X15.2
      kettle X15.8
      light bulb X15.8
      saucepan X15.3
      skillet X15.3
      stated as undetermined whether accidental
        or intentional Y27.3
      stove X15.0
      suicide (attempt) X77.3
      toaster X15.1
    in local application or packing during medical
      or surgical procedure
      Y63.5
  heating
    appliance, radiator or pipe X16
  homicide (attempt) —*see* Assault, burning
  hot
    air X14.1
    cooker X15.8
    drink X10.0
    engine X17
    fat X10.2
    fluid NEC X12
    food X10.1
    gases X14.1
    heating appliance X16
    household appliance NEC X15.8
    kettle X15.8
    liquid NEC X12
    machinery X17
    metal (molten) (liquid) NEC X18
    object (not producing fire or flames) NEC X19
    oil (cooking) X10.2
    pipe(s) X16
    radiator X16
    saucepan (glass) (metal) X15.3
    stove (kitchen) X15.0
    substance NEC X19
      caustic or corrosive NEC —*see* Table of
        Drugs and Chemicals
    toaster X15.1
    tool X17
    vapor X13.1
    water (tap) —*see* Contact, with, hot, tap water
  hotplate X15.2
    suicide (attempt) X77.3
  ignition —*see* Ignition
  in war operations —*see* War operations, fire
  inflicted by other person X97
    by hot objects, hot vapor, and steam —*see*
      Assault, burning, hot object
  internal, from swallowed caustic, corrosive
    liquid, substance —*see* Table of Drugs and
    Chemicals
  iron (hot) X15.8
    stated as undetermined whether accidental or
      intentional Y27.3
    suicide (attempt) X77.3
  kettle (hot) X15.8
    stated as undetermined whether accidental or
      intentional Y27.3
    suicide (attempt) X77.3
  lamp (flame) X08.8
    with ignition of clothing NEC X06.2
      nightwear X05
  lighter (cigar) (cigarette) X08.8
    with ignition of clothing NEC X06.2
      nightwear X05
  lightning —*see* subcategory T75.0
    causing fire —*see* Exposure, fire
  liquid (boiling) (hot) NEC X12
    stated as undetermined whether accidental or
      intentional Y27.2
    suicide (attempt) X77.2

▶ New   ⟹ Revised   ~~deleted~~ Deleted   ● Use Additional Character(s)

A & B

Burn, burned, burning (Continued)
local application of externally applied substance
   in medical or surgical care Y63.5
machinery (hot) X17
matches X08.8
  with ignition of clothing NEC X06.2
    nightwear X05
mattress —see Exposure, fire, uncontrolled,
  building, bed
medicament, externally applied Y63.5
metal (hot) (liquid) (molten) NEC X18
nightwear (nightclothes, nightdress, gown,
  pajamas, robe) X05
object (hot) NEC X19
on board watercraft
  due to
    accident to watercraft V91.09
      powered craft V91.03
        ferry boat V91.01
        fishing boat V91.02
        jet ski V91.03
        liner V91.01
        merchant ship V91.00
        passenger ship V91.01
      unpowered craft V91.08
        canoe V91.05
        inflatable V91.06
        kayak V91.05
        sailboat V91.04
        surf-board V91.08
        water skis V91.07
        windsurfer V91.08
    fire on board V93.09
      ferry boat V93.01
      fishing boat V93.02
      jet ski V93.03
      liner V93.01
      merchant ship V93.00
      passenger ship V93.01
      powered craft NEC V93.03
      sailboat V93.04
    specified heat source NEC on board V93.19
      ferry boat V93.11
      fishing boat V93.12
      jet ski V93.13
      liner V93.11
      merchant ship V93.10
      passenger ship V93.11
      powered craft NEC V93.13
      sailboat V93.14
pipe (hot) X16
  smoking X08.8
    with ignition of clothing NEC X06.2
      nightwear X05
powder —see Powder burn
radiator (hot) X16
saucepan (hot) (glass) (metal) X15.3
  stated as undetermined whether accidental or
    intentional Y27.3
  suicide (attempt) X77.3
self-inflicted X76
  stated as undetermined whether accidental or
    intentional Y26
stated as undetermined whether
  accidental or intentional Y27.0
steam X13.1
  pipe X16
    stated as undetermined whether accidental
      or intentional Y27.8
  stated as undetermined whether
    accidental or intentional Y27.0
  suicide (attempt) X77.0
stove (hot) (kitchen) X15.0
  stated as undetermined whether
    accidental or intentional Y27.3
  suicide (attempt) X77.3
substance (hot) NEC X19
  boiling X12
    stated as undetermined whether accidental
      or intentional Y27.2
    suicide (attempt) X77.2
  molten (metal) X18
suicide (attempt) NEC X76
  hot
    household appliance X77.3
    object X77.9
stated as undetermined whether accidental or
  intentional Y27.0
therapeutic misadventure
  heat in local application or packing during
    medical or surgical procedure Y63.5
  overdose of radiation Y63.2

Burn, burned, burning (Continued)
toaster (hot) X15.1
  stated as undetermined whether accidental or
    intentional Y27.3
  suicide (attempt) X77.3
tool (hot) X17
torch, welding X08.8
  with ignition of clothing NEC X06.2
    nightwear X05
trash fire (controlled) —see Exposure, fire,
  controlled, not in building
  uncontrolled —see Exposure, fire,
    uncontrolled, not in building
vapor (hot) X13.1
  stated as undetermined whether accidental or
    intentional Y27.0
  suicide (attempt) X77.0
Very pistol —see Discharge, firearm NEC
Butted by animal W55.82
bull W55.22
cow W55.22
goat W55.32
horse W55.12
pig W55.42
sheep W55.32

C

Caisson disease —see Air, pressure, change
Campfire (exposure to) (controlled) —see also
  Exposure, fire, controlled, not in building
  uncontrolled —see Exposure, fire, uncontrolled,
    not in building
Capital punishment (any means) —see Legal,
  intervention
Car sickness T75.3
Casualty (not due to war) NEC X58
war —see War operations
Cat
bite W55.01
scratch W55.03
Cataclysm, cataclysmic (any injury) NEC —see
  Forces of nature
Catching fire —see Exposure, fire
Caught
between
  folding object W23.0
  objects (moving) W23.0
    and
      machinery —see Contact, with, by
        type of machine
      stationary W23.2
    stationary W23.1
      and moving W23.2
  sliding door and door frame W23.0
by, in
  machinery (moving parts of) —see Contact,
    with, by type of machine
  washing-machine wringer W23.0
under packing crate (due to losing grip) W23.1
Cave-in caused by cataclysmic earth surface
  movement or eruption —see Landslide
Change(s) in air pressure —see Air, pressure,
  change
Choked, choking (on) (any object except food or
  vomitus)
food (bone) (seed) —see categories T17 and T18
vomitus T17.81-•
Civil insurrection —see War operations
Cloudburst (any injury) X37.8
Cold, exposure to (accidental) (excessive) (extreme)
  (natural) (place) NEC —see Exposure, cold
Collapse
building W20.1
  burning (uncontrolled fire) X00.2
dam or man-made structure (causing earth
  movement) X36.0
machinery —see Contact, with, by type of
  machine
structure W20.1
  burning (uncontrolled fire) X00.2
Collision (accidental) NEC —see also Accident,
  transport V89.9
pedestrian W51
  with fall W03
    due to ice or snow W00.0
    involving pedestrian conveyance —see
      Accident, transport, pedestrian,
      conveyance

Collision (Continued)
with fall (Continued)
  and
    crowd or human stampede (with fall) W52
    object W22.8
      with fall —see Fall, due to, bumping
        against, object
  person(s) —see Collision, pedestrian
  transport vehicle NEC V89.9
    and
      avalanche, fallen or not moving —see
        Accident, transport
      falling or moving —see Landslide
      landslide, fallen or not moving —see
        Accident, transport
      falling or moving —see Landslide
    due to cataclysm —see Forces of nature, by
      type
  intentional, purposeful suicide (attempt) —see
    Suicide, collision
Combustion, spontaneous —see Ignition
Complication (delayed) of or following (medical
  or surgical procedure) Y84.9
with misadventure —see Misadventure
amputation of limb(s) Y83.5
anastomosis (arteriovenous) (blood vessel)
  (gastrojejunal) (tendon) (natural or artificial
  material) Y83.2
aspiration (of fluid) Y84.4
  tissue Y84.8
biopsy Y84.8
blood
  sampling Y84.7
  transfusion
    procedure Y84.8
bypass Y83.2
catheterization (urinary) Y84.6
  cardiac Y84.0
colostomy Y83.3
cystostomy Y83.3
dialysis (kidney) Y84.1
drug —see Table of Drugs and Chemicals
due to misadventure —see Misadventure
duodenostomy Y83.3
electroshock therapy Y84.3
external stoma, creation of Y83.3
formation of external stoma Y83.3
gastrostomy Y83.3
graft Y83.2
hypothermia (medically-induced) Y84.8
implant, implantation (of)
  artificial
    internal device (cardiac pacemaker)
      (electrodes in brain) (heart valve
      prosthesis) (orthopedic) Y83.1
    material or tissue (for anastomosis or
      bypass) Y83.2
      with creation of external stoma
        Y83.3
    natural tissues (for anastomosis or bypass)
      Y83.2
      with creation of external stoma Y83.3
infusion
  procedure Y84.8
injection —see Table of Drugs and
  Chemicals
  procedure Y84.8
insertion of gastric or duodenal sound Y84.5
insulin-shock therapy Y84.3
paracentesis (abdominal) (thoracic) (aspirative)
  Y84.4
procedures other than surgical operation —see
  Complication of or following, by type of
  procedure
radiological procedure or therapy Y84.2
removal of organ (partial) (total) NEC Y83.6
sampling
  blood Y84.7
  fluid NEC Y84.4
  tissue Y84.8
shock therapy Y84.3
surgical operation NEC —see also Complication
  of or following, by type of operation Y83.9
  reconstructive NEC Y83.4
  with
    anastomosis, bypass or graft
      Y83.2
    formation of external stoma Y83.3
  specified NEC Y83.8
transfusion —see also Table of Drugs and
  Chemicals
  procedure Y84.8

B & C

Complication *(Continued)*
transplant, transplantation (heart) (kidney)
(liver) (whole organ, any) Y83.Ø
partial organ Y83.4
ureterostomy Y83.3
vaccination —*see also* Table of Drugs and
Chemicals
procedure Y84.8
Compression
divers' squeeze —*see* Air, pressure, change
trachea by
food (lodged in esophagus) —*see* categories
T17 and T18
vomitus (lodged in esophagus) T17.81-●
Conflagration —*see* Exposure, fire, uncontrolled
Constriction (external)
hair W49.Ø1
jewelry W49.Ø4
ring W49.Ø4
rubber band W49.Ø3
specified item NEC W49.Ø9
string W49.Ø2
thread W49.Ø2
Contact (accidental)
with
abrasive wheel (metalworking) W31.1
alligator W58.Ø9
bite W58.Ø1
crushing W58.Ø3
strike W58.Ø2
amphibian W62.9
frog W62.Ø
toad W62.1
animal (nonvenomous) NEC W64
marine W56.89
bite W56.81
dolphin —*see* Contact, with, dolphin
fish NEC —*see* Contact, with, fish
mammal —*see* Contact, with, mammal,
marine
orca —*see* Contact, with, orca
sea lion —*see* Contact, with, sea lion
shark —*see* Contact, with, shark
strike W56.82
animate mechanical force NEC W64
arrow W21.89
not thrown, projected or falling W45.8
arthropods (nonvenomous) W57
axe W27.Ø
band-saw (industrial) W31.2
bayonet —*see* Bayonet wound
bee(s) X58
bench-saw (industrial) W31.2
bird W61.99
bite W61.91
chicken —*see* Contact, with, chicken
duck —*see* Contact, with, duck
goose —*see* Contact, with, goose
macaw —*see* Contact, with, macaw
parrot —*see* Contact, with, parrot
psittacine —*see* Contact, with, psittacine
strike W61.92
turkey —*see* Contact, with, turkey
blender W29.Ø
boiling water X12
stated as undetermined whether accidental
or intentional Y27.2
suicide (attempt) X77.2
bore, earth-drilling or mining (land) (seabed)
W31.Ø
buffalo —*see* Contact, with, hoof stock
NEC
bull W55.29
bite W55.21
gored W55.22
strike W55.22
bumper cars W31.81
camel —*see* Contact, with, hoof stock NEC
can
lid W26.8
opener W27.4
powered W29.Ø
cat W55.Ø9
bite W55.Ø1
scratch W55.Ø3
caterpillar (venomous) X58
centipede (venomous) X58
chain
hoist W24.Ø
agricultural operations W3Ø.89
saw W29.3

Contact *(Continued)*
with *(Continued)*
chicken W61.39
peck W61.33
strike W61.32
chisel W27.Ø
circular saw W31.2
cobra X58
combine (harvester) W3Ø.Ø
conveyer belt W24.1
cooker (hot) X15.8
stated as undetermined whether accidental
or intentional Y27.3
suicide (attempt) X77.3
coral X58
cotton gin W31.82
cow W55.29
bite W55.21
strike W55.22
crane W24.Ø
agricultural operations W3Ø.89
crocodile W58.19
bite W58.11
crushing W58.13
strike W58.12
dagger W26.1
stated as undetermined whether accidental
or intentional Y28.2
suicide (attempt) X78.2
dairy equipment W31.82
dart W21.89
not thrown, projected or falling W45.8
deer —*see* Contact, with, hoof stock
NEC
derrick W24.Ø
agricultural operations W3Ø.89
hay W3Ø.2
dog W54.8
bite W54.Ø
strike W54.1
dolphin W56.Ø9
bite W56.Ø1
strike W56.Ø2
donkey —*see* Contact, with, hoof stock NEC
drill (powered) W29.8
earth (land) (seabed) W31.Ø
nonpowered W27.8
drive belt W24.Ø
agricultural operations W3Ø.89
dry ice —*see* Exposure, cold, man-made
dryer (clothes) (powered) (spin) W29.2
duck W61.69
bite W61.61
strike W61.62
earth(-)
drilling machine (industrial) W31.Ø
scraping machine in stationary use W31.83
edge of stiff paper W26.2
electric
beater W29.Ø
blanket X16
fan W29.2
commercial W31.82
knife W29.1
mixer W29.Ø
elevator (building) W24.Ø
agricultural operations W3Ø.89
grain W3Ø.3
engine(s), hot NEC X17
excavating machine W31.Ø
farm machine W3Ø.9
feces —*see* Contact, with, by type of
animal
fer de lance X58
fish W56.59
bite W56.51
shark —*see* Contact, with, shark
strike W56.52
flying horses W31.81
forging (metalworking) machine W31.1
fork W27.4
forklift (truck) W24.Ø
agricultural operations W3Ø.89
frog W62.Ø
garden
cultivator (powered) W29.3
riding W3Ø.89
fork W27.1
gas turbine W31.3
Gila monster X58
giraffe —*see* Contact, with, hoof stock NEC

Contact *(Continued)*
with *(Continued)*
glass (sharp) (broken) W25
with subsequent fall W18.Ø2
assault X99.Ø
due to fall —*see* Fall, by type
stated as undetermined whether accidental
or intentional Y28. Ø
suicide (attempt) X78.Ø
goat W55.39
bite W55.31
strike W55.32
goose W61.59
bite W61.51
strike W61.52
hand
saw W27.Ø
tool (not powered) NEC W27.8
powered W29.8
harvester W3Ø.Ø
hay-derrick W3Ø.2
heat NEC X19
from appliance (electrical) (household) —
see Contact, with, hot, household
appliance
heating appliance X16
heating
appliance (hot) X16
pad (electric) X16
hedge-trimmer (powered) W29.3
hoe W27.1
hoist (chain) (shaft) NEC W24.Ø
agricultural W3Ø.89
hoof stock NEC W55.39
bite W55.31
strike W55.32
hornet(s) X58
horse W55.19
bite W55.11
strike W55.12
hot
air X14.1
inhalation X14.Ø
cooker X15.8
cooking
pan X15.3
pot X15.3
drinks X1Ø.Ø
engine X17
fats X1Ø.2
fluids NEC X12
assault X98.2
suicide (attempt) X77.2
undetermined whether accidental or
intentional Y27.2
food X1Ø.1
gases X14.1
inhalation X14.Ø
heating appliance X16
household appliance X15.8
assault X98.3
cooker X15.8
hotplate X15.2
kettle X15.8
light bulb X15.8
object NEC X19
assault X98.8
stated as undetermined whether
accidental or intentional Y27.9
suicide (attempt) X77.8
saucepan X15.3
skillet X15.3
stated as undetermined whether
accidental or intentional Y27.3
stove X15.Ø
suicide (attempt) X77.3
toaster X15.1
kettle X15.8
light bulb X15.8
liquid NEC —*see also* Burn X12
drinks X1Ø.Ø
stated as undetermined whether
accidental or intentional Y27.2
suicide (attempt) X77.2
tap water X11.8
stated as undetermined whether
accidental or intentional Y27.1
suicide (attempt) X77.1
machinery X17
metal (molten) (liquid) NEC X18
object (not producing fire or flames) NEC X19

▶ New   ⇒ Revised   ~~deleted~~ Deleted   ● Use Additional Character(s)

Contact (Continued)
  with (Continued)
    hot (Continued)
      oil (cooking) X10.2
      pipe X16
      plate X15.2
      radiator X16
      saucepan (glass) (metal) X15.3
      skillet X15.3
      stove (kitchen) X15.0
      substance NEC X19
      tap-water X11.8
        assault X98.1
        heated on stove X12
          stated as undetermined whether
            accidental or intentional Y27.2
          suicide (attempt) X77.2
        in bathtub X11.0
        running X11.1
        stated as undetermined whether
          accidental or intentional Y27.1
        suicide (attempt) X77.1
      toaster X15.1
      tool X17
      vapors X13.1
        inhalation X13.0
      water (tap) X11.8
        boiling X12
          stated as undetermined whether
            accidental or intentional Y27.2
          suicide (attempt) X77.2
        heated on stove X12
          stated as undetermined whether
            accidental or intentional Y27.2
          suicide (attempt) X77.2
        in bathtub X11.0
        running X11.1
        stated as undetermined whether
          accidental or intentional Y27.1
        suicide (attempt) X77.1
    hotplate X15.2
    ice-pick W27.4
    insect (nonvenomous) NEC W57
    kettle (hot) X15.8
    knife W26.0
      assault X99.1
      electric W29.1
      stated as undetermined whether accidental
        or intentional Y28.1
      suicide (attempt) X78.1
    lathe (metalworking) W31.1
      turnings W45.8
      woodworking W31.2
    lawnmower (powered) (ridden) W28
      causing electrocution W86.8
        suicide (attempt) X83.1
      unpowered W27.1
    lift, lifting (devices) W24.0
      agricultural operations W30.89
      shaft W24.0
    liquefied gas —see Exposure, cold, man-made
    liquid air, hydrogen, nitrogen —see Exposure,
      cold, man-made
    lizard (nonvenomous) W59.09
      bite W59.01
      strike W59.02
    llama —see Contact, with, hoof stock NEC
    macaw W61.19
      bite W61.11
      strike W61.12
    machine, machinery W31.9
      abrasive wheel W31.1
      agricultural including animal-powered W30.9
        combine harvester W30.0
        grain storage elevator W30.3
        hay derrick W30.2
        power take-off device W30.1
        reaper W30.0
        specified NEC W30.89
        thresher W30.0
        transport vehicle, stationary W30.81
      band saw W31.2
      bench saw W31.2
      circular saw W31.2
      commercial NEC W31.82
      drilling, metal (industrial) W31.1
      earth-drilling W31.0
      earthmoving or scraping W31.89
      excavating W31.89
      forging machine W31.1
      gas turbine W31.3

Contact (Continued)
  with (Continued)
    machine, machinery (Continued)
      hot X17
      internal combustion engine W31.3
      land drill W31.0
      lathe W31.1
      lifting (devices) W24.0
      metal drill W31.1
      metalworking (industrial) W31.1
      milling, metal W31.1
      mining W31.0
      molding W31.2
      overhead plane W31.2
      power press, metal W31.1
      prime mover W31.3
      printing W31.89
      radial saw W31.2
      recreational W31.81
      roller-coaster W31.81
      rolling mill, metal W31.1
      sander W31.2
      seabed drill W31.0
      shaft
        hoist W31.0
        lift W31.0
      specified NEC W31.89
      spinning W31.89
      steam engine W31.3
      transmission W24.1
      undercutter W31.0
      water driven turbine W31.3
      weaving W31.89
      woodworking or forming (industrial)
        W31.2
    mammal (feces) (urine) W55.89
      bull —see Contact, with, bull
      cat —see Contact, with, cat
      cow —see Contact, with, cow
      goat —see Contact, with, goat
      hoof stock —see Contact, with, hoof stock
      horse —see Contact, with, horse
      marine W56.39
        dolphin —see Contact, with, dolphin
        orca —see Contact, with, orca
        sea lion —see Contact, with, sea lion
        specified NEC W56.39
          bite W56.31
          strike W56.32
      pig —see Contact, with, pig
      raccoon —see Contact, with, raccoon
      rodent —see Contact, with, rodent
      sheep —see Contact, with, sheep
      specified NEC W55.89
        bite W55.81
        strike W55.82
    marine
      animal W56.89
        bite W56.81
        dolphin —see Contact, with, dolphin
        fish NEC —see Contact, with, fish
        mammal —see Contact, with, mammal,
          marine
        orca —see Contact, with, orca
        sea lion —see Contact, with, sea lion
        shark —see Contact, with, shark
        strike W56.82
    meat
      grinder (domestic) W29.0
        industrial W31.82
        nonpowered W27.4
      slicer (domestic) W29.0
        industrial W31.82
    merry go round W31.81
    metal, (hot) (liquid) (molten) NEC X18
    millipede W57
    nail W45.0
      gun W29.4
    needle (sewing) W27.3
      hypodermic W46.0
        contaminated W46.1
    object (blunt) NEC
      hot NEC X19
      legal intervention —see Legal, intervention,
        blunt object
      sharp NEC W45.8
        inflicted by other person NEC W45.8
          stated as
            intentional homicide (attempt) —see
              Assault, cutting or piercing
              instrument

Contact (Continued)
  with (Continued)
    object (Continued)
      sharp (Continued)
        legal intervention —see Legal,
          intervention, sharp object
        self-inflicted X78.9
    orca W56.29
      bite W56.21
      strike W56.22
    overhead plane W31.2
    paper (as sharp object) W26.2
    paper-cutter W27.5
    parrot W61.09
      bite W61.01
      strike W61.02
    pig W55.49
      bite W55.41
      strike W55.42
    pipe, hot X16
    pitchfork W27.1
    plane (metal) (wood) W27.0
      overhead W31.2
    plant thorns, spines, sharp leaves or other
      mechanisms W60
    powered
      garden cultivator W29.3
      household appliance, implement, or
        machine W29.8
      saw (industrial) W31.2
        hand W29.8
    printing machine W31.89
    psittacine bird W61.29
      bite W61.21
      macaw —see Contact, with, macaw
      parrot —see Contact, with, parrot
      strike W61.22
    pulley (block) (transmission) W24.0
      agricultural operations W30.89
    raccoon W55.59
      bite W55.51
      strike W55.52
    radial-saw (industrial) W31.2
    radiator (hot) X16
    rake W27.1
    rattlesnake X58
    reaper W30.0
    reptile W59.89
      lizard —see Contact, with, lizard
      snake —see Contact, with, snake
      specified NEC W59.89
        bite W59.81
        crushing W59.83
        strike W59.82
      turtle —see Contact, with, turtle
    rivet gun (powered) W29.4
    road scraper —see Accident, transport,
      construction vehicle
    rodent (feces) (urine) W53.89
      bite W53.81
      mouse W53.09
        bite W53.01
      rat W53.19
        bite W53.11
      specified NEC W53.89
        bite W53.81
      squirrel W53.29
        bite W53.21
    roller coaster W31.81
    rope NEC W24.0
      agricultural operations W30.89
    saliva —see Contact, with, by type of animal
    sander W29.8
      industrial W31.2
    saucepan (hot) (glass) (metal) X15.3
    saw W27.0
      band (industrial) W31.2
      bench (industrial) W31.2
      chain W29.3
      hand W27.0
    sawing machine, metal W31.1
    scissors W27.2
    scorpion X58
    screwdriver W27.0
      powered W29.8
    sea
      anemone, cucumber or urchin (spine) X58
      lion W56.19
        bite W56.11
        strike W56.12
    serpent —see Contact, with, snake, by type

Contact *(Continued)*
  with *(Continued)*
    sewing-machine (electric) (powered) W29.2
      not powered W27.8
    shaft (hoist) (lift) (transmission) NEC W24.0
      agricultural W30.89
    shark W56.49
      bite W56.41
      strike W56.42
    sharp object(s) W26.9
      specified NEC W26.8
    shears (hand) W27.2
      powered (industrial) W31.1
        domestic W29.2
    sheep W55.39
      bite W55.31
      strike W55.32
    shovel W27.8
      steam —*see* Accident, transport, construction vehicle
    snake (nonvenomous) W59.19
      bite W59.11
      crushing W59.13
      strike W59.12
    spade W27.1
    spider (venomous) X58
    spin-drier W29.2
    spinning machine W31.89
    splinter W45.8
    sports equipment W21.9
    staple gun (powered) W29.8
    steam X13.1
      engine W31.3
      inhalation X13.0
      pipe X16
      shovel W31.89
    stove (hot) (kitchen) X15.0
    substance, hot NEC X19
      molten (metal) X18
    sword W26.1
      assault X99.2
      stated as undetermined whether accidental or intentional Y28.2
      suicide (attempt) X78.2
    tarantula X58
    thresher W30.0
    tin can lid W26.8
    toad W62.1
    toaster (hot) X15.1
    tool W27.8
      hand (not powered) W27.8
        auger W27.0
        axe W27.0
        can opener W27.4
        chisel W27.0
        fork W27.4
        garden W27.1
        handsaw W27.0
        hoe W27.1
        ice-pick W27.4
        kitchen utensil W27.4
        manual
          lawn mower W27.1
          sewing machine W27.8
        meat grinder W27.4
        needle (sewing) W27.3
          hypodermic W46.0
            contaminated W46.1
        paper cutter W27.5
        pitchfork W27.1
        rake W27.1
        scissors W27.2
        screwdriver W27.0
        specified NEC W27.8
        workbench W27.0
      hot X17
      powered W29.8
        blender W29.0
          commercial W31.82
        can opener W29.0
          commercial W31.82
        chainsaw W29.3
        clothes dryer W29.2
          commercial W31.82
        dishwasher W29.2
          commercial W31.82
        edger W29.3
        electric fan W29.2
          commercial W31.82
        electric knife W29.1

Contact *(Continued)*
  with *(Continued)*
    tool *(Continued)*
      powered *(Continued)*
        food processor W29.0
          commercial W31.82
        garbage disposal W29.0
          commercial W31.82
        garden tool W29.3
        hedge trimmer W29.3
        ice maker W29.0
          commercial W31.82
        kitchen appliance W29.0
          commercial W31.82
        lawn mower W28
        meat grinder W29.0
          commercial W31.82
        mixer W29.0
          commercial W31.82
        rototiller W29.3
        sewing machine W29.2
          commercial W31.82
        washing machine W29.2
          commercial W31.82
    transmission device (belt, cable, chain, gear, pinion, shaft) W24.1
      agricultural operations W30.89
    turbine (gas) (water-driven) W31.3
    turkey W61.49
      peck W61.43
      strike W61.42
    turtle (nonvenomous) W59.29
      bite W59.21
      strike W59.22
      terrestrial W59.89
        bite W59.81
        crushing W59.83
        strike W59.82
    under-cutter W31.0
    urine —*see* Contact, with, by type of animal
    vehicle
      agricultural use (transport) —*see* Accident, transport, agricultural vehicle
        not on public highway W30.81
      industrial use (transport) —*see* Accident, transport, industrial vehicle
        not on public highway W31.83
      off-road use (transport) —*see* Accident, transport, all-terrain or off-road vehicle
        not on public highway W31.83
      special construction use (transport) —*see* Accident, transport, construction vehicle
        not on public highway W31.83
    venomous
      animal X58
      arthropods X58
      lizard X58
      marine animal NEC X58
      marine plant NEC X58
      millipedes (tropical) X58
      plant(s) X58
      snake X58
      spider X58
      viper X58
    washing-machine (powered) W29.2
    wasp X58
    weaving-machine W31.89
    winch W24.0
      agricultural operations W30.89
    wire NEC W24.0
      agricultural operations W30.89
    wood slivers W45.8
    yellow jacket X58
    zebra —*see* Contact, with, hoof stock NEC
  pressure X50.9
  stress X50.9
Coup de soleil X32
Crash
  aircraft (in transit) (powered) V95.9
    balloon V96.01
    fixed wing NEC (private) V95.21
      commercial V95.31
    glider V96.21
      hang V96.11
      powered V95.11
    helicopter V95.01
    in war operations —*see* War operations, destruction of aircraft
    microlight V95.11

Crash *(Continued)*
  aircraft *(Continued)*
    nonpowered V96.9
      specified NEC V96.8
    powered NEC V95.8
    stated as
      homicide (attempt) Y08.81
      suicide (attempt) X83.0
    ultralight V95.11
    spacecraft V95.41
  transport vehicle NEC —*see also* Accident, transport V89.9
    homicide (attempt) Y03.8
    motor NEC (traffic) V89.2
      homicide (attempt) Y03.8
      suicide (attempt) —*see* Suicide, collision
Cruelty (mental) (physical) (sexual) X58
Crushed (accidentally) X58
  between objects (moving) (stationary and moving) W23.0
    stationary W23.1
  by
    alligator W58.03
    avalanche NEC —*see* Landslide
    cave-in W20.0
      caused by cataclysmic earth surface movement —*see* Landslide
    crocodile W58.13
    crowd or human stampede W52
    falling
      aircraft V97.39
        in war operations —*see* War operations, destruction of aircraft
      earth, material W20.0
        caused by cataclysmic earth surface movement —*see* Landslide
      object NEC W20.8
    landslide NEC —*see* Landslide
    lizard (nonvenomous) W59.09
    machinery —*see* Contact, with, by type of machine
    reptile NEC W59.89
    snake (nonvenomous) W59.13
  in
    machinery —*see* Contact, with, by type of machine
Cut, cutting (any part of body) (accidental) —*see also* Contact, with, by object or machine
  during medical or surgical treatment as misadventure —*see* Index to Diseases and Injuries, Complications
  homicide (attempt) —*see* Assault, cutting or piercing instrument
  inflicted by other person —*see* Assault, cutting or piercing instrument
  legal
    execution —*see* Legal, intervention
    intervention —*see* Legal, intervention, sharp object
  machine NEC —*see also* Contact, with, by type of machine W31.9
  self-inflicted —*see* Suicide, cutting or piercing instrument
  suicide (attempt) —*see* Suicide, cutting or piercing instrument
Cyclone (any injury) X37.1

D

Decapitation (accidental circumstances) NEC X58
  homicide X99.9
  legal execution —*see* Legal, intervention
Dehydration from lack of water X58
Deprivation X58
Derailment (accidental)
  railway (rolling stock) (train) (vehicle) (without antecedent collision) V81.7
    with antecedent collision —*see* Accident, transport, railway vehicle occupant
  streetcar (without antecedent collision) V82.7
    with antecedent collision —*see* Accident, transport, streetcar occupant
Descent
  parachute (voluntary) (without accident to aircraft) V97.29
    due to accident to aircraft —*see* Accident, transport, aircraft
Desertion X58

C & D

Destitution X58
Disability, late effect or sequela of injury —*see* Sequelae
Discharge (accidental)
  airgun W34.010
    assault X95.01
    homicide (attempt) X95.01
    stated as undetermined whether accidental or intentional Y24.0
    suicide (attempt) X74.01
  BB gun —*see* Discharge, airgun
  firearm (accidental) W34.00
    assault X95.9
    handgun (pistol) (revolver) W32.0
      assault X93
      homicide (attempt) X93
      legal intervention —*see* Legal, intervention, firearm, handgun
      stated as undetermined whether accidental or intentional Y22
      suicide (attempt) X72
    homicide (attempt) X95.9
    hunting rifle W33.02
      assault X94.1
      homicide (attempt) X94.1
      legal intervention
        injuring
          bystander Y35.032
          law enforcement personnel Y35.031
          suspect Y35.033
          unspecified person Y35.039
      stated as undetermined whether accidental or intentional Y23.1
      suicide (attempt) X73.1
    larger W33.00
      assault X94.9
      homicide (attempt) X94.9
      hunting rifle —*see* Discharge, firearm, hunting rifle
      legal intervention —*see* Legal, intervention, firearm by type of firearm
      machine gun —*see* Discharge, firearm, machine gun
      shotgun —*see* Discharge, firearm, shotgun
      specified NEC W33.09
        assault X94.8
        homicide (attempt) X94.8
        legal intervention
          injuring
            bystander Y35.092
            law enforcement personnel Y35.091
            suspect Y35.093
            unspecified person Y35.099
        stated as undetermined whether accidental or intentional Y23.8
        suicide (attempt) X73.8
      stated as undetermined whether accidental or intentional Y23.9
      suicide (attempt) X73.9
    legal intervention
      injuring
        bystander Y35.002
        law enforcement personnel Y35.001
        suspect Y35.03
        unspecified person Y35.009
      using rubber bullet
        injuring
          bystander Y35.042
          law enforcement personnel Y35.041
          suspect Y35.043
          unspecified person Y35.049
    machine gun W33.03
      assault X94.2
      homicide (attempt) X94.2
      legal intervention —*see* Legal, intervention, firearm, machine gun
      stated as undetermined whether accidental or intentional Y23.3
      suicide (attempt) X73.2
    pellet gun —*see* Discharge, airgun
    shotgun W33.01
      assault X94.0
      homicide (attempt) X94.0
      legal intervention —*see* Legal, intervention, firearm, specified NEC
      stated as undetermined whether accidental or intentional Y23.0
      suicide (attempt) X73.0
    specified NEC W34.09
      assault X95.8
      homicide (attempt) X95.8

Discharge (Continued)
  firearm (Continued)
    specified (Continued)
      legal intervention —*see* Legal, intervention, firearm, specified NEC
      stated as undetermined whether accidental or intentional Y24.8
      suicide (attempt) X74.8
    stated as undetermined whether accidental or intentional Y24.9
    suicide (attempt) X74.9
    Very pistol W34.09
      assault X95.8
      homicide (attempt) X95.8
      stated as undetermined whether accidental or intentional Y24.8
      suicide (attempt) X74.8
  firework(s) W39
    stated as undetermined whether accidental or intentional Y25
  gas-operated gun NEC W34.018
    airgun —*see* Discharge, airgun
    assault X95.09
    homicide (attempt) X95.09
    paintball gun —*see* Discharge, paintball gun
    stated as undetermined whether accidental or intentional Y24.8
    suicide (attempt) X74.09
  gun NEC —*see also* Discharge, firearm NEC
    air —*see* Discharge, airgun
    BB —*see* Discharge, airgun
    for single hand use —*see* Discharge, firearm, handgun
    hand —*see* Discharge, firearm, handgun
    machine —*see* Discharge, firearm, machine gun
    other specified —*see* Discharge, firearm NEC
    paintball —*see* Discharge, paintball gun
    pellet —*see* Discharge, airgun
  handgun —*see* Discharge, firearm, handgun
  machine gun —*see* Discharge, firearm, machine gun
  paintball gun W34.011
    assault X95.02
    homicide (attempt) X95.02
    stated as undetermined whether accidental or intentional Y24.8
    suicide (attempt) X74.02
  pistol —*see* Discharge, firearm, handgun
    flare —*see* Discharge, firearm, Very pistol
    pellet —*see* Discharge, airgun
    Very —*see* Discharge, firearm, Very pistol
  revolver —*see* Discharge, firearm, handgun
  rifle (hunting) —*see* Discharge, firearm, hunting rifle
  shotgun —*see* Discharge, firearm, shotgun
  spring-operated gun NEC W34.018
    assault X95.09
    homicide (attempt) X95.09
    stated as undetermined whether accidental or intentional Y24.8
    suicide (attempt) X74.09
Disease
  Andes W94.11
  aviator's —*see* Air, pressure
  range W94.11
Diver's disease, palsy, paralysis, squeeze —*see* Air, pressure
Diving (into water) —*see* Accident, diving
Dog bite W54.0
Dragged by transport vehicle NEC —*see also* Accident, transport V09.9
Drinking poison (accidental) —*see* Table of Drugs and Chemicals
Dropped (accidentally) **while being carried or supported by other person** W04
Drowning (accidental) W74
  assault X92.9
  due to
    accident (to)
      machinery —*see* Contact, with, by type of machine
      watercraft V90.89
        burning V90.29
          powered V90.23
            fishing boat V90.22
            jet ski V90.23
            merchant ship V90.20
            passenger ship V90.21
          unpowered V90.28
            canoe V90.25
            inflatable V90.26

Drowning (Continued)
  due to (Continued)
    accident (Continued)
      watercraft (Continued)
        burning (Continued)
          unpowered (Continued)
            kayak V90.25
            sailboat V90.24
            water skis V90.27
        crushed V90.39
          powered V90.33
            fishing boat V90.32
            jet ski V90.33
            merchant ship V90.30
            passenger ship V90.31
          unpowered V90.38
            canoe V90.35
            inflatable V90.36
            kayak V90.35
            sailboat V90.34
            water skis V90.37
        overturning V90.09
          powered V90.03
            fishing boat V90.02
            jet ski V90.03
            merchant ship V90.00
            passenger ship V90.01
          unpowered V90.08
            canoe V90.05
            inflatable V90.06
            kayak V90.05
            sailboat V90.04
        sinking V90.19
          powered V90.13
            fishing boat V90.12
            jet ski V90.13
            merchant ship V90.10
            passenger ship V90.11
          unpowered V90.18
            canoe V90.15
            inflatable V90.16
            kayak V90.15
            sailboat V90.14
        specified type NEC V90.89
          powered V90.83
            fishing boat V90.82
            jet ski V90.83
            merchant ship V90.80
            passenger ship V90.81
          unpowered V90.88
            canoe V90.85
            inflatable V90.86
            kayak V90.85
            sailboat V90.84
            water skis V90.87
    avalanche —*see* Landslide
    cataclysmic
      earth surface movement NEC —*see* Forces of nature, earth movement
      storm —*see* Forces of nature, cataclysmic storm
    cloudburst X37.8
    cyclone X37.1
    fall overboard (from) V92.09
      powered craft V92.03
        ferry boat V92.01
        fishing boat V92.02
        jet ski V92.03
        liner V92.01
        merchant ship V92.00
        passenger ship V92.01
      resulting from
        accident to watercraft —*see* Drowning, due to, accident to, watercraft
        being washed overboard (from) V92.29
          powered craft V92.23
            ferry boat V92.21
            fishing boat V92.22
            jet ski V92.23
            liner V92.21
            merchant ship V92.20
            passenger ship V92.21
          unpowered craft V92.28
            canoe V92.25
            inflatable V92.26
            kayak V92.25
            sailboat V92.24
            surf-board V92.28
            water skis V92.27
            windsurfer V92.28

Drowning *(Continued)*
- due to *(Continued)*
  - fall overboard *(Continued)*
    - resulting from *(Continued)*
      - motion of watercraft V92.19
        - powered craft V92.13
          - ferry boat V92.11
          - fishing boat V92.12
          - jet ski V92.13
          - liner V92.11
          - merchant ship V92.10
          - passenger ship V92.11
        - unpowered craft
          - canoe V92.15
          - inflatable V92.16
          - kayak V92.15
          - sailboat V92.14
      - unpowered craft V92.08
        - canoe V92.05
        - inflatable V92.06
        - kayak V92.05
        - sailboat V92.04
        - surf-board V92.08
        - water skis V92.07
        - windsurfer V92.08
  - hurricane X37.0
  - jumping into water from watercraft (involved in accident) —*see also* Drowning, due to, accident to, watercraft
    - without accident to or on watercraft W16.711
  - tidal wave NEC —*see* Forces of nature, tidal wave
  - torrential rain X37.8
- following
  - fall
    - into
      - bathtub W16.211
      - bucket W16.221
      - fountain —*see* Drowning, following, fall, into, water, specified NEC
      - quarry —*see* Drowning, following, fall, into, water, specified NEC
      - reservoir —*see* Drowning, following, fall, into, water, specified NEC
      - swimming-pool W16.011
        - stated as undetermined whether accidental or intentional Y21.3
        - striking
          - bottom W16.021
          - wall W16.031
        - suicide (attempt) X71.2
      - water NOS W16.41
        - natural (lake) (open sea) (river) (stream) (pond) W16.111
          - striking
            - bottom W16.121
            - side W16.131
        - specified NEC W16.311
          - striking
            - bottom W16.321
            - wall W16.331
  - overboard NEC —*see* Drowning, due to, fall overboard
- jump or dive
  - from boat W16.711
    - striking bottom W16.721
  - into
    - fountain —*see* Drowning, following, jump or dive, into, water, specified NEC
    - quarry —*see* Drowning, following, jump or dive, into, water, specified NEC
    - reservoir —*see* Drowning, following, jump or dive, into, water, specified NEC
    - swimming-pool W16.511
      - striking
        - bottom W16.521
        - wall W16.531
      - suicide (attempt) X71.2
    - water NOS W16.91
      - natural (lake) (open sea) (river) (stream) (pond) W16.611
      - specified NEC W16.811
        - striking
          - bottom W16.821
          - wall W16.831
      - striking bottom W16.621
- homicide (attempt) X92.9

Drowning *(Continued)*
- in
  - bathtub (accidental) W65
    - assault X92.0
    - following fall W16.211
      - stated as undetermined whether accidental or intentional Y21.1
    - stated as undetermined whether accidental or intentional Y21.0
    - suicide (attempt) X71.0
  - lake —*see* Drowning, in, natural water
  - natural water (lake) (open sea) (river) (stream) (pond) W69
    - assault X92.3
    - following
      - dive or jump W16.611
        - striking bottom W16.621
      - fall W16.111
        - striking
          - bottom W16.121
          - side W16.131
    - stated as undetermined whether accidental or intentional Y21.4
    - suicide (attempt) X71.3
  - quarry —*see* Drowning, in, specified place NEC
  - quenching tank —*see* Drowning, in, specified place NEC
  - reservoir —*see* Drowning, in, specified place NEC
  - river —*see* Drowning, in, natural water
  - sea —*see* Drowning, in, natural water
  - specified place NEC W73
    - assault X92.8
    - following
      - dive or jump W16.811
        - striking
          - bottom W16.821
          - wall W16.831
      - fall W16.311
        - striking
          - bottom W16.321
          - wall W16.331
    - stated as undetermined whether accidental or intentional Y21.8
    - suicide (attempt) X71.8
  - stream —*see* Drowning, in, natural water
  - swimming-pool W67
    - assault X92.1
      - following fall X92.2
    - following
      - dive or jump W16.511
        - striking
          - bottom W16.521
          - wall W16.531
      - fall W16.011
        - striking
          - bottom W16.021
          - wall W16.031
    - stated as undetermined whether accidental or intentional Y21.2
      - following fall Y21.3
    - suicide (attempt) X71.1
      - following fall X71.2
  - war operations —*see* War operations, restriction of airway
- resulting from accident to watercraft —*see* Drowning, due to, accident, watercraft
- self-inflicted X71.9
- stated as undetermined whether accidental or intentional Y21.9
- suicide (attempt) X71.9

E

Earth (surface) movement NEC —*see* Forces of nature, earth movement
Earth falling (on) W20.0
- caused by cataclysmic earth surface movement or eruption —*see* Landslide
Earthquake (any injury) X34
Effect(s) (adverse) of
- air pressure (any) —*see* Air, pressure
- cold, excessive (exposure to) —*see* Exposure, cold
- heat (excessive) —*see* Heat
- hot place (weather) —*see* Heat

Effect *(Continued)*
- insolation X30
- late —*see* Sequelae
- motion —*see* Motion
- nuclear explosion or weapon in war operations —*see* War operations, nuclear weapon
- radiation —*see* Radiation
- travel —*see* Travel
Electric shock (accidental) (by) (in) —*see* Exposure, electric current
Electrocution (accidental) —*see* Exposure, electric current
Endotracheal tube wrongly placed during anesthetic procedure Y65.3
Entanglement
- in
  - bed linen, causing suffocation —*see* category T71
  - wheel of pedal cycle V19.88
Entry of foreign body or material —*see* Foreign body
Environmental pollution related condition —*see* Z57
Execution, legal (any method) —*see* Legal, intervention
Exhaustion
- cold —*see* Exposure, cold
- due to excessive exertion —*see also* Overexertion X50.9
- heat —*see* Heat
Explosion (accidental) (of) (with secondary fire) W40.9
- acetylene W40.1
- aerosol can W36.1
- air tank (compressed) (in machinery) W36.2
- aircraft (in transit) (powered) NEC V95.9
  - balloon V96.05
  - fixed wing NEC (private) V95.25
    - commercial V95.35
  - glider V96.25
    - hang V96.15
    - powered V95.15
  - helicopter V95.05
  - in war operations —*see* War operations, destruction of aircraft
  - microlight V95.15
  - nonpowered V96.9
    - specified NEC V96.8
  - powered NEC V95.8
  - stated as
    - ▶ homicide (attempt) Y08.81
    - suicide (attempt) X83.0
  - ultralight V95.15
- anesthetic gas in operating room W40.1
- antipersonnel bomb W40.8
  - assault X96.0
  - homicide (attempt) X96.0
  - suicide (attempt) X75
- assault X96.9
- bicycle tire W37.0
- blasting (cap) (materials) W40.0
- boiler (machinery), not on transport vehicle W35
  - on watercraft —*see* Explosion, in, watercraft
- butane W40.1
- caused by other person X96.9
- coal gas W40.1
- detonator W40.0
- dump (munitions) W40.8
- dynamite W40.0
  - in
    - assault X96.8
    - homicide (attempt) X96.8
    - legal intervention
      - injuring
        - bystander Y35.112
        - law enforcement personnel Y35.111
        - suspect Y35.113
        - unspecified person Y35.119
    - suicide (attempt) X75
- explosive (material) W40.9
  - gas W40.1
  - in blasting operation W40.0
  - specified NEC W40.8
    - in
      - assault X96.8
      - homicide (attempt) X96.8
      - legal intervention
        - injuring
          - bystander Y35.192
          - law enforcement personnel Y35.191

▶ New ⬆ Revised ~~deleted~~ Deleted ● Use Additional Character(s)

Explosion (Continued)
  explosive (Continued)
    specified (Continued)
      in (Continued)
        legal intervention (Continued)
          injuring (Continued)
            suspect Y35.193
            unspecified person Y35.199
        suicide (attempt) X75
  factory (munitions) W40.8
  fertilizer bomb W40.8
    assault X96.3
    homicide (attempt) X96.3
    suicide (attempt) X75
  fire-damp W40.1
  firearm (parts) NEC W34.19
    airgun W34.110
    BB gun W34.110
    gas, air or spring-operated gun NEC W34.118
    handgun W32.1
    hunting rifle W33.12
    larger firearm W33.10
      specified NEC W33.19
    machine gun W33.13
    paintball gun W34.111
    pellet gun W34.110
    shotgun W33.11
    Very pistol [flare] W34.19
  fireworks W39
  gas (coal) (explosive) W40.1
    cylinder W36.9
      aerosol can W36.1
      air tank W36.2
      pressurized W36.3
      specified NEC W36.8
  gasoline (fumes) (tank) not in moving motor vehicle W40.1
    bomb W40.8
      assault X96.1
      homicide (attempt) X96.1
      suicide (attempt) X75
    in motor vehicle —see Accident, transport, by type of vehicle
  grain store W40.8
  grenade W40.8
    in
      assault X96.8
      homicide (attempt) X96.8
      legal intervention
        injuring
          bystander Y35.192
          law enforcement personnel Y35.191
          suspect Y35.193
          unspecified person Y35.199
      suicide (attempt) X75
  handgun (parts) —see Explosion, firearm, handgun (parts)
  homicide (attempt) X96.9
    antipersonnel bomb —see Explosion, antipersonnel bomb
    fertilizer bomb —see Explosion, fertilizer bomb
    gasoline bomb —see Explosion, gasoline bomb
    letter bomb —see Explosion, letter bomb
    pipe bomb —see Explosion, pipe bomb
    specified NEC X96.8
  hose, pressurized W37.8
  hot water heater, tank (in machinery) W35
    on watercraft —see Explosion, in, watercraft
  in, on
    dump W40.8
    factory W40.8
    mine (of explosive gases) NEC W40.1
    watercraft V93.59
      powered craft V93.53
        ferry boat V93.51
        fishing boat V93.52
        jet ski V93.53
        liner V93.51
        merchant ship V93.50
        passenger ship V93.51
        sailboat V93.54
  letter bomb W40.8
    assault X96.2
    homicide (attempt) X96.2
    suicide (attempt) X75
  machinery —see also Contact, with, by type of machine
    on board watercraft —see Explosion, in, watercraft
    pressure vessel —see Explosion, by type of vessel

Explosion (Continued)
  methane W40.1
  mine W40.1
  missile NEC W40.8
  mortar bomb W40.8
    in
      assault X96.8
      homicide (attempt) X96.8
      legal intervention
        injuring
          bystander Y35.192
          law enforcement personnel Y35.191
          suspect Y35.193
          unspecified person Y35.199
      suicide (attempt) X75
  munitions (dump) (factory) W40.8
  pipe, pressurized W37.8
    bomb W40.8
      assault X96.4
      homicide (attempt) X96.4
      suicide (attempt) X75
  pressure, pressurized
    cooker W38
    gas tank (in machinery) W36.3
    hose W37.8
    pipe W37.8
    specified device NEC W38
    tire W37.8
      bicycle W37.0
    vessel (in machinery) W38
  propane W40.1
  self-inflicted X75
  shell (artillery) NEC W40.8
    during war operations —see War operations, explosion
    in
      legal intervention
        injuring
          bystander Y35.122
          law enforcement personnel Y35.121
          suspect Y35.123
          unspecified person Y35.129
    war —see War operations, explosion
  spacecraft V95.45
  stated as undetermined whether accidental or intentional Y25
  steam or water lines (in machinery) W37.8
  stove W40.9
  suicide (attempt) X75
  tire, pressurized W37.8
    bicycle W37.0
  undetermined whether accidental or intentional Y25
  vehicle tire NEC W37.8
    bicycle W37.0
  war operations —see War operations, explosion

Exposure (to) X58
  air pressure change —see Air, pressure
  cold (accidental) (excessive) (extreme) (natural) (place) X31
    assault Y08.89
    due to
      man-made conditions W93.8
        dry ice (contact) W93.01
          inhalation W93.02
        liquid air (contact) (hydrogen) (nitrogen) W93.11
          inhalation W93.12
        refrigeration unit (deep freeze) W93.2
      suicide (attempt) X83.2
      weather (conditions) X31
    homicide (attempt) Y08.89
    self-inflicted X83.2
  due to abandonment or neglect X58
  electric current W86.8
    appliance (faulty) W86.8
      domestic W86.0
    caused by other person Y08.89
    conductor (faulty) W86.1
    control apparatus (faulty) W86.1
    electric power generating plant, distribution station W86.1
    electroshock gun —see Exposure, electric current, taser
    high-voltage cable W85
    homicide (attempt) Y08.89
    legal execution —see Legal, intervention, specified means NEC
    lightning —see subcategory T75.0
    live rail W86.8

Exposure (Continued)
  electric current (Continued)
    misadventure in medical or surgical procedure in electroshock therapy Y63.4
    motor (electric) (faulty) W86.8
      domestic W86.0
    self-inflicted X83.1
    specified NEC W86.8
      domestic W86.0
    stun gun —see Exposure, electric current, taser
    suicide (attempt) X83.1
    taser W86.8
      assault Y08.89
      legal intervention —see category Y35
      self-harm (intentional) X83.8
      undetermined intent Y33
    third rail W86.8
    transformer (faulty) W86.1
    transmission lines W85
  environmental tobacco smoke X58
  excessive
    cold —see Exposure, cold
    heat (natural) NEC X30
    man-made W92
  factor(s) NOS X58
    environmental NEC X58
    man-made NEC W99
    natural NEC —see Forces of nature
    specified NEC X58
  fire, flames (accidental) X08.8
    assault X97
    campfire —see Exposure, fire, controlled, not in building
    controlled (in)
      with ignition (of) clothing —see also Ignition, clothes X06.2
        nightwear X05
      bonfire —see Exposure, fire, controlled, not in building
      brazier (in building or structure) —see also Exposure, fire, controlled, building
        not in building or structure —see Exposure, fire, controlled, not in building
      building or structure X02.0
        with
          fall from building X02.3
          from building X02.5
          injury due to building collapse X02.2
          smoke inhalation X02.1
        hit by object from building X02.4
        specified mode of injury NEC X02.8
      fireplace, furnace or stove —see Exposure, fire, controlled, building
      not in building or structure X03.0
        with
          fall X03.3
          smoke inhalation X03.1
        hit by object X03.4
        specified mode of injury NEC X03.8
      trash —see Exposure, fire, controlled, not in building
    fireplace —see Exposure, fire, controlled, building
    fittings or furniture (in building or structure) (uncontrolled) —see Exposure, fire, uncontrolled, building
    forest (uncontrolled) —see Exposure, fire, uncontrolled, not in building
    grass (uncontrolled) —see Exposure, fire, uncontrolled, not in building
    hay (uncontrolled) —see Exposure, fire, uncontrolled, not in building
    homicide (attempt) X97
    ignition of highly flammable material X04
    in, of, on, starting in
      machinery —see Contact, with, by type of machine
      motor vehicle (in motion) —see also Accident, transport, occupant by type of vehicle V87.8
        with collision —see Collision
      railway rolling stock, train, vehicle V81.81
        with collision —see Accident, transport, railway vehicle occupant
      street car (in motion) V82.8
        with collision —see Accident, transport, streetcar occupant
      transport vehicle NEC —see also Accident, transport
        with collision —see Collision

E & F

Exposure (Continued)

  fire, flames (Continued)

    in, of, on, starting in (Continued)

      war operations —see also War operations, fire

        from nuclear explosion —see War operations, nuclear weapons

      watercraft (in transit) (not in transit) V91.09

        localized —see Burn, on board watercraft, due to, fire on board

        powered craft V91.03

          ferry boat V91.01

          fishing boat V91.02

          jet skis V91.03

          liner V91.01

          merchant ship V91.00

          passenger ship V91.01

        unpowered craft V91.08

          canoe V91.05

          inflatable V91.06

          kayak V91.05

          sailboat V91.04

          surf-board V91.08

          waterskis V91.07

          windsurfer V91.08

    lumber (uncontrolled) —see Exposure, fire, uncontrolled, not in building

    mine (uncontrolled) —see Exposure, fire, uncontrolled, not in building

    prairie (uncontrolled) —see Exposure, fire, uncontrolled, not in building

    resulting from

      explosion —see Explosion

      lightning X08.8

    self-inflicted X76

    specified NEC X08.8

    started by other person X97

    stated as undetermined whether accidental or intentional Y26

    stove —see Exposure, fire, controlled, building

    suicide (attempt) X76

    tunnel (uncontrolled) —see Exposure, fire, uncontrolled, not in building

    uncontrolled

      in building or structure X00.0

        with

          fall from building X00.3

          injury due to building collapse X00.2

          jump from building X00.5

          smoke inhalation X00.1

        bed X08.00

          due to

            cigarette X08.01

            specified material NEC X08.09

        furniture NEC X08.20

          due to

            cigarette X08.21

            specified material NEC X08.29

        hit by object from building X00.4

        sofa X08.10

          due to

            cigarette X08.11

            specified material NEC X08.19

        specified mode of injury NEC X00.8

      not in building or structure (any) X01.0

        with

          fall X01.3

          smoke inhalation X01.1

        hit by object X01.4

        specified mode of injury NEC X01.8

    undetermined whether accidental or intentional Y26

  forces of nature NEC —see Forces of nature

  G-forces (abnormal) W49.9

  gravitational forces (abnormal) W49.9

  heat (natural) NEC —see Heat

  high-pressure jet (hydraulic) (pneumatic) W49.9

  hydraulic jet W49.9

  inanimate mechanical force W49.9

  jet, high-pressure (hydraulic) (pneumatic) W49.9

  lightning —see subcategory T75.0

    causing fire —see Exposure, fire

  mechanical forces NEC W49.9

    animate NEC W64

    inanimate NEC W49.9

  noise W42.9

    supersonic W42.0

  noxious substance —see Table of Drugs and Chemicals

  pneumatic jet W49.9

Exposure (Continued)

  prolonged in deep-freeze unit or refrigerator W93.2

  radiation —see Radiation

  smoke —see also Exposure, fire

    tobacco, second hand Z77.22

  specified factors NEC X58

  sunlight X32

    man-made (sun lamp) W89.8

      tanning bed W89.1

  supersonic waves W42.0

  transmission line(s), electric W85

  vibration W49.9

  waves

    infrasound W49.9

    sound W42.9

    supersonic W42.0

  weather NEC —see Forces of nature

External cause status Y99.9

  child assisting in compensated work for family Y99.8

  civilian activity done for financial or other compensation Y99.0

  civilian activity done for income or pay Y99.0

  family member assisting in compensated work for other family member Y99.8

  hobby not done for income Y99.8

  leisure activity Y99.8

  military activity Y99.1

  off-duty activity of military personnel Y99.8

  recreation or sport not for income or while a student Y99.8

  specified NEC Y99.8

  student activity Y99.8

  volunteer activity Y99.2

— F —

Factors, supplemental

  alcohol

    blood level

      less than 20mg/100ml Y90.0

      presence in blood, level not specified Y90.9

      20-39mg/100ml Y90.1

      40-59mg/100ml Y90.2

      60-79mg/100ml Y90.3

      80-99mg/100ml Y90.4

      100-119mg/100ml Y90.5

      120-199mg/100ml Y90.6

      200-239mg/100ml Y90.7

      240mg/100ml or more Y90.8

      presence in blood, but level not specified Y90.9

  environmental-pollution-related condition —see Z57

  nosocomial condition Y95

  work-related condition Y99.0

Failure

  in suture or ligature during surgical procedure Y65.2

  mechanical, of instrument or apparatus (any) (during any medical or surgical procedure) Y65.8

  sterile precautions (during medical and surgical care) —see Misadventure, failure, sterile precautions, by type of procedure

  to

    introduce tube or instrument Y65.4

      endotracheal tube during anesthesia Y65.3

    make curve (transport vehicle) NEC —see Accident, transport

    remove tube or instrument Y65.4

Fall, falling (accidental) W19

  building W20.1

    burning (uncontrolled fire) X00.3

  down

    embankment W17.81

    escalator W10.0

    hill W17.81

    ladder W11

    ramp W10.2

    stairs, steps W10.9

  due to

    bumping against

      object W18.00

        sharp glass W18.02

        specified NEC W18.09

        sports equipment W18.01

Fall, falling (Continued)

  due to (Continued)

    bumping against (Continued)

      person W03

        due to ice or snow W00.0

        on pedestrian conveyance —see Accident, transport, pedestrian, conveyance

    collision with another person W03

      due to ice or snow W00.0

      involving pedestrian conveyance —see Accident, transport, pedestrian, conveyance

    grocery cart tipping over W17.82

    ice or snow W00.9

      from one level to another W00.2

        on stairs or steps W00.1

      involving pedestrian conveyance —see Accident, transport, pedestrian, conveyance

      on same level W00.0

    slipping (on moving sidewalk) W01.0

      with subsequent striking against object W01.10

        furniture W01.190

        sharp object W01.119

          glass W01.110

          power tool or machine W01.111

          specified NEC W01.118

        specified NEC W01.198

    striking against

      object W18.00

        sharp glass W18.02

        specified NEC W18.09

        sports equipment W18.01

      person W03

        due to ice or snow W00.0

        on pedestrian conveyance —see Accident, transport, pedestrian, conveyance

  earth (with asphyxia or suffocation (by pressure)) —see Earth, falling

  from, off, out of

    aircraft NEC (with accident to aircraft NEC) V97.0

      while boarding or alighting V97.1

    balcony W13.0

    bed W06

    boat, ship, watercraft NEC (with drowning or submersion) —see Drowning, due to, fall overboard

      with hitting bottom or object V94.0

    bridge W13.1

    building W13.9

      burning (uncontrolled fire) X00.3

    cavity W17.2

    chair W07

    cherry picker W17.89

    cliff W15

    dock W17.4

    embankment W17.81

    escalator W10.0

    flagpole W13.8

    furniture NEC W08

    grocery cart W17.82

    haystack W17.89

    high place NEC W17.89

      stated as undetermined whether accidental or intentional Y30

    hole W17.2

    incline W10.2

    ladder W11

    lifting device W17.89

    machine, machinery —see also Contact, with, by type of machine

      not in operation W17.89

    manhole W17.1

    mobile elevated work platform [MEWP] W17.89

    motorized mobility scooter W05.2

    one level to another NEC W17.89

      intentional, purposeful, suicide (attempt) X80

      stated as undetermined whether accidental or intentional Y30

    pit W17.2

    playground equipment W09.8

      jungle gym W09.2

      slide W09.0

      swing W09.1

    quarry W17.89

    railing W13.9

    ramp W10.2

    roof W13.2

    scaffolding W12

▶ New   ⇒ Revised   ~~deleted~~ Deleted   ● Use Additional Character(s)

Fall, falling *(Continued)*
 from, off, out of *(Continued)*
  scooter (nonmotorized) W05.1
   motorized mobility W05.2
  sky lift W17.89
  stairs, steps W10.9
   curb W10.1
   due to ice or snow W00.1
   escalator W10.0
   incline W10.2
   ramp W10.2
   sidewalk curb W10.1
   specified NEC W10.8
  Standing
   electric scooter V00.841
   micro-mobility pedestrian conveyance
    V00.848
  stepladder W11
  stool W08
  storm drain W17.1
  streetcar NEC V82.6
   with antecedent collision —*see*
    Accident, transport, streetcar occupant
   while boarding or alighting V82.4
  structure NEC W13.8
   burning (uncontrolled fire) X00.3
  table W08
  toilet W18.11
   with subsequent striking against object
    W18.12
  train NEC V81.6
   during derailment (without antecedent
    collision) V81.7
    with antecedent collision —*see* Accident,
     transport, railway vehicle occupant
   while boarding or alighting V81.4
  transport vehicle after collision —*see* Accident,
   transport, by type of vehicle, collision
  tree W14
  vehicle (in motion) NEC —*see also* Accident,
   transport V89.9
   motor NEC —*see also* Accident, transport,
    occupant, by type of vehicle V87.8
   stationary W17.89
    while boarding or alighting —*see*
     Accident, transport, by type of
     vehicle, while boarding or
     alighting
  viaduct W13.8
  wall W13.8
  watercraft —*see also* Drowning, due to, fall
   overboard
   with hitting bottom or object V94.0
  well W17.0
  wheelchair, non-moving W05.0
   powered —*see* Accident, transport,
    pedestrian, conveyance occupant,
    specified type NEC
  window W13.4
 in, on
  aircraft NEC V97.0
   with accident to aircraft V97.0
   while boarding or alighting V97.1
  bathtub (empty) W18.2
   filled W16.212
    causing drowning W16.211
  escalator W10.0
  incline W10.2
  ladder W11
  machine, machinery —*see* Contact, with, by
   type of machine
  object, edged, pointed or sharp (with cut) —
   see Fall, by type
  playground equipment W09.8
   jungle gym W09.2
   slide W09.0
   swing W09.1
  ramp W10.2
  scaffolding W12
  shower W18.2
   causing drowning W16.211
  staircase, stairs, steps W10.9
   curb W10.1
   due to ice or snow W00.1
   escalator W10.0
   incline W10.2
   specified NEC W10.8
  streetcar (without antecedent collision)
   V82.5
   with antecedent collision —*see* Accident,
    transport, streetcar occupant
   while boarding or alighting V82.4

Fall, falling *(Continued)*
 in, on *(Continued)*
  train (without antecedent collision)
   V81.5
   with antecedent collision —*see* Accident,
    transport, railway vehicle
    occupant
   during derailment (without antecedent
    collision) V81.7
    with antecedent collision —*see* Accident,
     transport, railway vehicle
     occupant
   while boarding or alighting V81.4
  transport vehicle after collision —*see* Accident,
   transport, by type of vehicle,
   collision
  watercraft V93.39
   due to
    accident to craft V91.29
     powered craft V91.23
      ferry boat V91.21
      fishing boat V91.22
      jet ski V91.23
      liner V91.21
      merchant ship V91.20
      passenger ship V91.21
     unpowered craft
      canoe V91.25
      inflatable V91.26
      kayak V91.25
      sailboat V91.24
    powered craft V93.33
     ferry boat V93.31
     fishing boat V93.32
     jet ski V93.33
     liner V93.31
     merchant ship V93.30
     passenger ship V93.31
    unpowered craft V93.38
     canoe V93.35
     inflatable V93.36
     kayak V93.35
     sailboat V93.34
     surf-board V93.38
     windsurfer V93.38
 into
  cavity W17.2
  dock W17.4
  fire —*see* Exposure, fire, by type
  haystack W17.89
  hole W17.2
  manhole W17.1
  moving part of machinery —*see* Contact, with,
   by type of machine
  ocean —*see* Fall, into, water
  opening in surface NEC W17.89
  pit W17.2
  pond —*see* Fall, into, water
  quarry W17.89
  river —*see* Fall, into, water
  shaft W17.89
  storm drain W17.1
  stream —*see* Fall, into, water
  swimming pool —*see also* Fall, into, water, in,
   swimming pool
   empty W17.3
  tank W17.89
  water W16.42
   causing drowning W16.41
   from watercraft —*see* Drowning, due to, fall
    overboard
   hitting diving board W21.4
   in
    bathtub W16.212
     causing drowning W16.211
    bucket W16.222
     causing drowning W16.221
    natural body of water W16.112
     causing drowning W16.111
     striking
      bottom W16.122
       causing drowning W16.121
      side W16.132
       causing drowning W16.131
    specified water NEC W16.312
     causing drowning W16.311
     striking
      bottom W16.322
       causing drowning W16.321
      wall W16.332
       causing drowning
        W16.331

Fall, falling *(Continued)*
 into *(Continued)*
  water *(Continued)*
   in *(Continued)*
    swimming pool W16.012
     causing drowning W16.011
     striking
      bottom W16.022
       causing drowning W16.021
      wall W16.032
       causing drowning W16.031
    utility bucket W16.222
     causing drowning W16.221
   well W17.0
  involving
   bed W06
   chair W07
   furniture NEC W08
   glass —*see* Fall, by type
   playground equipment W09.8
    jungle gym W09.2
    slide W09.0
    swing W09.1
   roller blades —*see* Accident, transport,
    pedestrian, conveyance
   skateboard(s) —*see* Accident, transport,
    pedestrian, conveyance
   skates (ice) (in line) (roller) —*see*
    Accident, transport, pedestrian,
    conveyance
   skis —*see* Accident, transport, pedestrian,
    conveyance
   table W08
   wheelchair, non-moving W05.0
    powered —*see* Accident, transport,
     pedestrian, conveyance, specified
     type NEC
  object —*see* Struck by, object, falling
  off
   toilet W18.11
    with subsequent striking against object
     W18.12
  on same level W18.30
   due to
    specified NEC W18.39
    stepping on an object W18.31
  out of
   bed W06
   building NEC W13.8
   chair W07
   furniture NEC W08
   wheelchair, non-moving W05.0
    powered —*see* Accident, transport,
     pedestrian, conveyance, specified
     type NEC
   window W13.4
  over
   animal W01.0
   cliff W15
   embankment W17.81
   small object W01.0
  rock W20.8
  same level W18.30
   from
    being crushed, pushed, or stepped on
     by a crowd or human stampede W52
    collision, pushing, shoving, by or with
     other person W03
    slipping, stumbling, tripping W01.0
   involving ice or snow W00.0
    involving skates (ice) (roller), skateboard,
     skis —*see* Accident, transport,
     pedestrian, conveyance
  snowslide (avalanche) —*see* Landslide
  stone W20.8
  structure W20.1
   burning (uncontrolled fire) X00.3
  through
   bridge W13.1
   floor W13.3
   roof W13.2
   wall W13.8
   window W13.4
  timber W20.8
  tree (caused by lightning) W20.8
  while being carried or supported by other
   person(s) W04
Fallen on by
 animal (not being ridden) NEC W55.89
Felo-de-se —*see* Suicide
Fight (hand) (fists) (foot) —*see* Assault, fight
Fire (accidental) —*see* Exposure, fire

Firearm discharge —see Discharge, firearm
Fireball effects from nuclear explosion in war operations —see War operations, nuclear weapons
Fireworks (explosion) W39
Flash burns from explosion —see Explosion
Flood (any injury) (caused by) X38
  collapse of man-made structure causing earth movement X36.0
  tidal wave —see Forces of nature, tidal wave
Food (any type) in
  air passages (with asphyxia, obstruction, or suffocation) —see categories T17 and T18
  alimentary tract causing asphyxia (due to compression of trachea) —see categories T17 and T18
Forces of nature X39.8
  avalanche X36.1
    causing transport accident —see Accident, transport, by type of vehicle
  blizzard X37.2
  cataclysmic storm X37.9
    with flood X38
    blizzard X37.2
    cloudburst X37.8
    cyclone X37.1
    dust storm X37.3
    hurricane X37.0
    specified storm NEC X37.8
    storm surge X37.0
    tornado X37.1
    twister X37.1
    typhoon X37.0
  cloudburst X37.8
  cold (natural) X31
  cyclone X37.1
  dam collapse causing earth movement X36.0
  dust storm X37.3
  earth movement X36.1
    caused by dam or structure collapse X36.0
    earthquake X34
  earthquake X34
  flood (caused by) X38
    dam collapse X36.0
    tidal wave —see Forces of nature, tidal wave
  heat (natural) X30
  hurricane X37.0
  landslide X36.1
    causing transport accident —see Accident, transport, by type of vehicle
  lightning —see subcategory T75.0
    causing fire —see Exposure, fire
  mudslide X36.1
    causing transport accident —see Accident, transport, by type of vehicle
  radiation (natural) X39.08
    radon X39.01
  radon X39.01
  specified force NEC X39.8
  storm surge X37.0
  structure collapse causing earth movement X36.0
  sunlight X32
  tidal wave X37.41
    due to
      earthquake X37.41
      landslide X37.43
      storm X37.42
      volcanic eruption X37.41
  tornado X37.1
  tsunami X37.41
  twister X37.1
  typhoon X37.0
  volcanic eruption X35
Foreign body
  aspiration —see Index to Diseases and Injuries, Foreign body, respitory tract
  embedded in skin W45
  entering through
    natural orifice W44.9
      audio device W44.G1
      battery W44.A0
        button W44.A1
        cylindrical W44.A9
        other specified NEC W44.A9
      bezoar W44.F1
        bottle cap W44.E9
        can lid W44.E9
        combination metal and plastic
          jewelry W44.G3
          toy and toy part W44.G2
        dagger W44.H2
        dart W44.H1

Foreign body (Continued)
  entering through (Continued)
    bezoar (Continued)
      ear buds W44.G1
      food W44.F3
      glass W44.C0
        intact W44.C2
          bottle W44.C2
        shard W44.C1
        sharp W44.C1
      hearing aids W44.G1
      insect W44.F4
      knife W44.H2
      magnetic metal W44.D0
        bead W44.D1
        coin W44.D2
        jewelry W44.D4
        object specified NEC W44.D9
        toy W44.D3
      needle (hypodermic) (sewing) W44.H1
      non-magnetic metal W44.E0
        bead W44.E1
        coin W44.E2
        jewelry W44.E4
        object specified NEC W44.E9
        toy W44.E3
      objects of natural or organic material W44.F0
        specified NEC W44.F9
      other
        non-organic objects W44.G0
          specified NEC W44.G9
        sharp object unspecified W44.H0
      plastic
        bead W44.B1
        bottle W44.B5
        coin W44.B2
        jewelry W44.B4
        object W44.B0
          specified NEC W44.B9
        toy and toy part W44.B3
      pull tab W44.E9
      rubber band W44.F2
      safety pin W44.H1
      specified NEC W44.8
      sword W44.H2
    skin W45.8
      can lid W26.8
      nail W45.0
      paper W26.2
      specified NEC W45.8
      splinter W45.8
Forest fire (exposure to) —see Exposure, fire, uncontrolled, not in building
Found injured X58
  from exposure (to) —see Exposure
  on
    highway, road(way), street V89.9
    railway right of way V81.9
Fracture (circumstances unknown or unspecified) X58
  due to specified cause NEC X58
Freezing —see Exposure, cold
Frostbite X31
  due to man-made conditions —see Exposure, cold, man-made
Frozen —see Exposure, cold

G

Gored by bull W55.22
Gunshot wound W34.00

H

Hailstones, injured by X39.8
Hanged herself or himself —see Hanging, self-inflicted
Hanging (accidental) —see also category T71
  legal execution —see Legal, intervention, specified means NEC
Heat (effects of) (excessive) X30
  due to
    man-made conditions W92
      on board watercraft V93.29
        fishing boat V93.22
        merchant ship V93.20

Heat (Continued)
  due to (Continued)
    man-made conditions (Continued)
      on board watercraft (Continued)
        passenger ship V93.21
        sailboat V93.24
        specified powered craft NEC V93.23
    weather (conditions) X30
  from
    electric heating apparatus causing burning X16
    nuclear explosion in war operations — see War operations, nuclear weapons
  inappropriate in local application or packing in medical or surgical procedure Y63.5
Hemorrhage
  delayed following medical or surgical treatment without mention of misadventure —see Index to Diseases and Injuries, Complication(s)
  during medical or surgical treatment as misadventure —see Index to Diseases and Injuries, Complication(s)
High
  altitude (effects) —see Air, pressure, low
  level of radioactivity, effects —see Radiation
  pressure (effects) —see Air, pressure, high
  temperature, effects —see Heat
Hit, hitting (accidental) by —see Struck by
Hitting against —see Striking against
Homicide (attempt) (justifiable) —see Assault
Hot
  place, effects —see also Heat
  weather, effects X30
House fire (uncontrolled) —see Exposure, fire, uncontrolled, building
Humidity, causing problem X39.8
Hunger X58
Hurricane (any injury) X37.0
Hypobarism, hypobaropathy —see Air, pressure, low

I

Ictus
  caloris —see also Heat
  solaris X30
Ignition (accidental) —see also Exposure, fire X08.8
  anesthetic gas in operating room W40.1
  apparel X06.2
    from highly flammable material X04
    nightwear X05
  bed linen (sheets) (spreads) (pillows) (mattress) —see Exposure, fire, uncontrolled, building, bed
  benzine X04
  clothes, clothing NEC (from controlled fire) X06.2
    from
      highly flammable material X04
  ether X04
    in operating room W40.1
  explosive material —see Explosion
  gasoline X04
  jewelry (plastic) (any) X06.0
  kerosene X04
  material
    explosive —see Explosion
    highly flammable with secondary explosion X04
  nightwear X05
  paraffin X04
  petrol X04
Immersion (accidental) —see also Drowning
  hand or foot due to cold (excessive) X31
Implantation of quills of porcupine W55.89
Inanition (from) (hunger) X58
  thirst X58.8
Inappropriate operation performed
  correct operation on wrong side or body part (wrong side) (wrong site) Y65.53
  operation intended for another patient done on wrong patient Y65.52
  wrong operation performed on correct patient Y65.51
Inattention after, at birth (homicidal intent) (infanticidal intent) X58

▶ New   ⇒ Revised   ~~deleted~~ Deleted   ● Use Additional Character(s)

Incident, adverse
device
anesthesiology Y70.8
accessory Y70.2
diagnostic Y70.0
miscellaneous Y70.8
monitoring Y70.0
prosthetic Y70.2
rehabilitative Y70.1
surgical Y70.3
therapeutic Y70.1
cardiovascular Y71.8
accessory Y71.2
diagnostic Y71.0
miscellaneous Y71.8
monitoring Y71.0
prosthetic Y71.2
rehabilitative Y71.1
surgical Y71.3
therapeutic Y71.1
gastroenterology Y73.8
accessory Y73.2
diagnostic Y73.0
miscellaneous Y73.8
monitoring Y73.0
prosthetic Y73.2
rehabilitative Y73.1
surgical Y73.3
therapeutic Y73.1
general
hospital Y74.8
accessory Y74.2
diagnostic Y74.0
miscellaneous Y74.8
monitoring Y74.0
prosthetic Y74.2
rehabilitative Y74.1
surgical Y74.3
therapeutic Y74.1
surgical Y81.8
accessory Y81.2
diagnostic Y81.0
miscellaneous Y81.8
monitoring Y81.0
prosthetic Y81.2
rehabilitative Y81.1
surgical Y81.3
therapeutic Y81.1
gynecological Y76.8
accessory Y76.2
diagnostic Y76.0
miscellaneous Y76.8
monitoring Y76.0
prosthetic Y76.2
rehabilitative Y76.1
surgical Y76.3
therapeutic Y76.1
medical Y82.9
specified type NEC Y82.8
neurological Y75.8
accessory Y75.2
diagnostic Y75.0
miscellaneous Y75.8
monitoring Y75.0
prosthetic Y75.2
rehabilitative Y75.1
surgical Y75.3
therapeutic Y75.1
obstetrical Y76.8
accessory Y76.2
diagnostic Y76.0
miscellaneous Y76.8
monitoring Y76.0
prosthetic Y76.2
rehabilitative Y76.1
surgical Y76.3
therapeutic Y76.1
ophthalmic Y77.8
accessory Y77.2
contact lens (rigid gas permeable)
(soft) (hydrophilic)) Y77.11
diagnostic Y77.0
miscellaneous Y77.8
monitoring Y77.0
prosthetic Y77.2
rehabilitative Y77.19
surgical Y77.3
therapeutic Y77.19
orthopedic Y79.8
accessory Y79.2
diagnostic Y79.0
miscellaneous Y79.8

Incident, adverse *(Continued)*
device *(Continued)*
orthopedic *(Continued)*
monitoring Y79.0
prosthetic Y79.2
rehabilitative Y79.1
surgical Y79.3
therapeutic Y79.1
otorhinolaryngological Y72.8
accessory Y72.2
diagnostic Y72.0
miscellaneous Y72.8
monitoring Y72.0
prosthetic Y72.2
rehabilitative Y72.1
surgical Y72.3
therapeutic Y72.1
personal use Y74.8
accessory Y74.2
diagnostic Y74.0
miscellaneous Y74.8
monitoring Y74.0
prosthetic Y74.2
rehabilitative Y74.1
surgical Y74.3
therapeutic Y74.1
physical medicine Y80.8
accessory Y80.2
diagnostic Y80.0
miscellaneous Y80.8
monitoring Y80.0
prosthetic Y80.2
rehabilitative Y80.1
surgical Y80.3
therapeutic Y80.1
plastic surgical Y81.8
accessory Y81.2
diagnostic Y81.0
miscellaneous Y81.8
monitoring Y81.0
prosthetic Y81.2
rehabilitative Y81.1
surgical Y81.3
therapeutic Y81.1
radiological Y78.8
accessory Y78.2
diagnostic Y78.0
miscellaneous Y78.8
monitoring Y78.0
prosthetic Y78.2
rehabilitative Y78.1
surgical Y78.3
therapeutic Y78.1
urology Y73.8
accessory Y73.2
diagnostic Y73.0
miscellaneous Y73.8
monitoring Y73.0
prosthetic Y73.2
rehabilitative Y73.1
surgical Y73.3
therapeutic Y73.1
Incineration (accidental) —*see* Exposure, fire
Infanticide —*see* Assault
Infrasound waves (causing injury) W49.9
Ingestion
foreign body (causing injury) (with
obstruction) —*see* Foreign body, alimentary
canal
poisonous
plant(s) X58
substance NEC —*see* Table of Drugs and
Chemicals
Inhalation
excessively cold substance, man-made —*see*
Exposure, cold, man-made
food (any type) (into respiratory tract) (with
asphyxia, obstruction respiratory tract,
suffocation) —*see* categories T17
and T18
foreign body —*see* Foreign body, aspiration
gastric contents (with asphyxia, obstruction
respiratory passage, suffocation)
T17.81-●
hot air or gases X14.0
liquid air, hydrogen, nitrogen W93.12
suicide (attempt) X83.2
steam X13.0
assault X98.0
stated as undetermined whether accidental or
intentional Y27.0
suicide (attempt) X77.0

Inhalation *(Continued)*
toxic gas —*see* Table of Drugs and
Chemicals
vomitus (with asphyxia, obstruction respiratory
passage, suffocation) T17.81-●
Injury, injured (accidental(ly)) NOS X58
by, caused by, from
assault —*see* Assault
law-enforcing agent, police, in course of legal
intervention —*see* Legal intervention
suicide (attempt) X83.8
due to, in
civil insurrection —*see* War operations
fight —*see also* Assault, fight Y04.0
war operations —*see* War operations
homicide —*see also* Assault Y09
inflicted (by)
in course of arrest (attempted), suppression
of disturbance, maintenance of order,
by law-enforcing agents —*see* Legal
intervention
other person
stated as
accidental X58
intentional, homicide (attempt) —*see*
Assault
undetermined whether accidental or
intentional Y33
purposely (inflicted) by other person(s) —*see*
Assault
self-inflicted X83.8
stated as accidental X58
specified cause NEC X58
undetermined whether accidental or intentional
Y33
Insolation, effects X30
Insufficient nourishment X58
Interruption of respiration (by)
food (lodged in esophagus) —*see* categories T17
and T18
vomitus (lodged in esophagus) T17.81-●
Intervention, legal —*see* Legal intervention
Intoxication
drug —*see* Table of Drugs and Chemicals
poison —*see* Table of Drugs and
Chemicals

——— **J** ———

Jammed (accidentally)
between objects (moving) (stationary and
moving) W23.0
stationary W23.1
Jumped, jumping
before moving object NEC X81.8
motor vehicle X81.0
subway train X81.1
train X81.1
undetermined whether accidental or
intentional Y31
from
boat (into water) voluntarily,
without accident (to or on boat)
W16.712
with
accident to or on boat —*see* Accident,
watercraft
drowning or submersion W16.711
suicide (attempt) X71.3
striking bottom W16.722
causing drowning W16.721
building —*see also* Jumped, from,
high place W13.9
burning (uncontrolled fire) X00.5
high place NEC W17.89
suicide (attempt) X80
undetermined whether accidental or
intentional Y30
structure —*see also* Jumped, from, high place
W13.9
burning (uncontrolled fire) X00.5
into water W16.92
causing drowning W16.91
from, off watercraft —*see* Jumped, from, boat
in
natural body W16.612
causing drowning W16.611
striking bottom W16.622
causing drowning W16.621

Jumped, jumping (Continued)
  into water (Continued)
    in (Continued)
      specified place NEC W16.812
        causing drowning W16.811
        striking
          bottom W16.822
            causing drowning W16.821
          wall W16.832
            causing drowning W16.831
      swimming pool W16.512
        causing drowning W16.511
        striking
          bottom W16.522
            causing drowning W16.521
          wall W16.532
            causing drowning W16.531
  suicide (attempt) X71.3

K

Kicked by
  animal NEC W55.82
  person(s) (accidentally) W50.1
    with intent to injure or kill Y04.0
    as, or caused by, a crowd or human stampede (with fall) W52
    assault Y04.0
    homicide (attempt) Y04.0
    in
      fight Y04.0
      legal intervention
        injuring
          bystander Y35.812
          law enforcement personnel Y35.811
          suspect Y35.813
          unspecified person Y35.819
Kicking
  against
    object W22.8
      sports equipment W21.9
      stationary W22.09
        sports equipment W21.89
    person —*see* Striking against, person
    sports equipment W21.9
  carpet stretcher with knee X50.3
Killed, killing (accidentally) **NOS** —*see also* Injury X58
  in
    action —*see* War operations
    brawl, fight (hand) (fists) (foot) Y04.0
      by weapon —*see also* Assault
        cutting, piercing —*see* Assault, cutting or piercing instrument
        firearm —*see* Discharge, firearm, by type, homicide
  self
    stated as
      accident NOS X58
      suicide —*see* Suicide
      undetermined whether accidental or intentional Y33
Kneeling (prolonged) (static) X50.1
Knocked down (accidentally) (by) **NOS** X58
  animal (not being ridden) NEC —*see also* Struck by, by type of animal
  crowd or human stampede W52
  person W51
    in brawl, fight Y04.0
  transport vehicle NEC —*see also* Accident, transport V09.9

L

Laceration NEC —*see* Injury
Lack of
  care (helpless person) (infant) (newborn) X58
  food except as result of abandonment or neglect X58
    due to abandonment or neglect X58
  water except as result of transport accident X58
    due to transport accident —*see* Accident, transport, by type
  helpless person, infant, newborn X58

Landslide (falling on transport vehicle) X36.1
  caused by collapse of man-made structure X36.0
Late effect —*see* Sequelae
Legal
  execution (any method) —*see* Legal, intervention
  intervention (by)
    baton —*see* Legal, intervention, blunt object, baton
    bayonet —*see* Legal, intervention, sharp object, bayonet
    blow —*see* Legal, intervention, manhandling
    blunt object
      baton
        injuring
          bystander Y35.312
          law enforcement personnel Y35.311
          suspect Y35.313
          unspecified person Y35.319
      injuring
        bystander Y35.302
        law enforcement personnel Y35.301
        suspect Y35.303
        unspecified person Y35.309
      specified NEC
        injuring
          bystander Y35.392
          law enforcement personnel Y35.391
          suspect Y35.393
          unspecified person Y35.399
      stave
        injuring
          bystander Y35.392
          law enforcement personnel Y35.391
          suspect Y35.393
          unspecified person Y35.399
    bomb —*see* Legal, intervention, explosive
    conducted energy device
      injuring
        bystander Y35.832
        law enforcement personnel Y35.831
        suspect Y35.833
        unspecified person Y35.839
    cutting or piercing instrument —*see* Legal, intervention, sharp object
    dynamite —*see* Legal, intervention, explosive, dynamite
    electroshock device (taser)
      injuring
        bystander Y35.832
        law enforcement personnel Y35.831
        suspect Y35.833
        unspecified person Y35.839
    explosive(s)
      dynamite
        injuring
          bystander Y35.112
          law enforcement personnel Y35.111
          suspect Y35.113
          unspecified person Y35.119
      grenade
        injuring
          bystander Y35.192
          law enforcement personnel Y35.191
          suspect Y35.193
          unspecified person Y35.199
      injuring
        bystander Y35.102
        law enforcement personnel Y35.101
        suspect Y35.103
        unspecified person Y35.109
      mortar bomb
        injuring
          bystander Y35.192
          law enforcement personnel Y35.191
          suspect Y35.193
          unspecified person Y35.199
      shell
        injuring
          bystander Y35.122
          law enforcement personnel Y35.121
          suspect Y35.123
          unspecified person Y35.129
      specified NEC
        injuring
          bystander Y35.192
          law enforcement personnel Y35.191
          suspect Y35.193
          unspecified person Y35.199

Legal (Continued)
  intervention (by) (Continued)
    firearm(s) (discharge)
      handgun
        injuring
          bystander Y35.022
          law enforcement personnel Y35.021
          suspect Y35.023
          unspecified person Y35.029
      injuring
        bystander Y35.002
        law enforcement personnel Y35.001
        suspect Y35.003
        unspecified person Y35.009
      machine gun
        injuring
          bystander Y35.012
          law enforcement personnel Y35.011
          suspect Y35.013
          unspecified person Y35.019
      rifle pellet
        injuring
          bystander Y35.032
          law enforcement personnel Y35.031
          suspect Y35.033
          unspecified person Y35.039
      rubber bullet
        injuring
          bystander Y35.042
          law enforcement personnel Y35.041
          suspect Y35.043
          unspecified person Y35.049
      shotgun —*see* Legal, intervention, firearm, specified NEC
      specified NEC
        injuring
          bystander Y35.092
          law enforcement personnel Y35.091
          suspect Y35.093
          unspecified person Y35.099
    gas (asphyxiation) (poisoning)
      injuring
        bystander Y35.202
        law enforcement personnel Y35.201
        suspect Y35.203
        unspecified person Y35.209
      specified NEC
        injuring
          bystander Y35.292
          law enforcement personnel Y35.291
          suspect Y35.293
          unspecified person Y35.299
      tear gas
        injuring
          bystander Y35.212
          law enforcement personnel Y35.211
          suspect Y35.213
          unspecified person Y35.219
    grenade —*see* Legal, intervention, explosive, grenade
    injuring
      bystander Y35.92
      law enforcement personnel Y35.91
      suspect Y35.93
      unspecified person Y35.99
    late effect (of) —*see* with 7th character S Y35
    manhandling
      injuring
        bystander Y35.812
        law enforcement personnel Y35.811
        suspect Y35.813
        unspecified person Y35.819
    sequelae (of) —*see* with 7th character S Y35
    sharp objects
      bayonet
        injuring
          bystander Y35.412
          law enforcement personnel Y35.411
          suspect Y35.413
          unspecified person Y35.419
      injuring
        bystander Y35.402
        law enforcement personnel Y35.401
        suspect Y35.403
        unspecified person Y35.409
      specified NEC
        injuring
          bystander Y35.492
          law enforcement personnel Y35.491

▶ New   ⇒ Revised   ~~deleted~~ Deleted   ● Use Additional Character(s)

Legal *(Continued)*
  intervention *(Continued)*
    sharp objects *(Continued)*
      specified *(Continued)*
        injuring *(Continued)*
          suspect Y35.493
          unspecified person Y35.499
      specified means NEC
        injuring
          bystander Y35.892
          law enforcement personnel Y35.891
          suspect Y35.893
          unspecified person Y35.899
      stabbing —*see* Legal, intervention, sharp object
      stave —*see* Legal, intervention, blunt object, stave
      stun gun
        injuring
          bystander Y35.832
          law enforcement personnel Y35.831
          suspect Y35.833
          unspecified person Y35.839
      taser
        injuring
          bystander Y35.832
          law enforcement personnel Y35.831
          suspect Y35.833
          unspecified person Y35.839
      tear gas —*see* Legal, intervention, gas, tear gas
      truncheon —*see* Legal, intervention, blunt object, stave
Lifting —*see also* Overexertion
  heavy objects X50.0
  weights X50.0
Lightning (shock) (stroke) (struck by) —*see* subcategory T75.0
  causing fire —*see* Exposure, fire
Loss of control (transport vehicle) NEC —*see* Accident, transport
Lost at sea NOS —*see* Drowning, due to, fall overboard
Low
  pressure (effects) —*see* Air, pressure, low
  temperature (effects) —*see* Exposure, cold
Lying before train, vehicle or other moving object X81.8
  subway train X81.1
  train X81.1
  undetermined whether accidental or intentional Y31
Lynching —*see* Assault

M

Malfunction (mechanism or component) (of)
  firearm
    airgun W34.10
    BB gun W34.110
    gas, air or spring-operated gun NEC W34.118
    handgun W32.1
    hunting rifle W33.12
    larger firearm W33.10
      specified NEC W33.19
    machine gun W33.13
    paintball gun W34.111
    pellet gun W34.110
    shotgun W33.11
    specified NEC W34.19
    Very pistol [flare] W34.19
  handgun —*see* Malfunction, firearm, handgun
Maltreatment —*see* Perpetrator
Mangled (accidentally) NOS X58
Manhandling (in brawl, fight) Y04.0
  legal intervention —*see* Legal, intervention, manhandling
Manslaughter (nonaccidental) —*see* Assault
Mauled by animal NEC W55.89
Medical procedure, complication of (delayed or as an abnormal reaction without mention of misadventure) —*see* Complication of or following, by specified type of procedure
  due to or as a result of misadventure —*see* Misadventure
Melting (due to fire) —*see also* Exposure, fire
  apparel NEC X06.3
  clothes, clothing NEC X06.3
    nightwear X05

Melting *(Continued)*
  fittings or furniture (burning building) (uncontrolled fire) X00.8
  nightwear X05
  plastic jewelry X06.1
Mental cruelty X58
Military operations (injuries to military and civilians occuring during peacetime on military property and during routine military exercises and operations) (by) (from) (involving) Y37.90-●
  air blast Y37.20-●
  aircraft
    destruction —*see* Military operations, destruction of aircraft
    airway restriction —*see* Military operations, restriction of airways
  asphyxiation —*see* Military operations, restriction of airways
  biological weapons Y37.6X-●
  blast Y37.20-●
  blast fragments Y37.20-●
  blast wave Y37.20-●
  blast wind Y37.20-●
  bomb Y37.20-●
    dirty Y37.50-●
    gasoline Y37.31-●
    incendiary Y37.31-●
    petrol Y37.31-●
  bullet Y37.43-●
    incendiary Y37.32-●
    rubber Y37.41-●
  chemical weapons Y37.7X-●
  combat
    hand to hand (unarmed) combat Y37.44-●
    using blunt or piercing object Y37.45-●
  conflagration —*see* Military operations, fire
  conventional warfare NEC Y37.49-●
  depth-charge Y37.01-●
  destruction of aircraft Y37.10-●
    due to
      air to air missile Y37.11-●
      collision with other aircraft Y37.12-●
      detonation (accidental) of onboard munitions and explosives Y37.14-●
      enemy fire or explosives Y37.11-●
      explosive placed on aircraft Y37.11-●
      onboard fire Y37.13-●
      rocket propelled grenade [RPG] Y37.11-●
      small arms fire Y37.11-●
      surface to air missile Y37.11-●
    specified NEC Y37.19-●
  detonation (accidental) of
    onboard marine weapons Y37.05-●
    own munitions or munitions launch device Y37.24-●
  dirty bomb Y37.50-●
  explosion (of) Y37.20-●
    aerial bomb Y37.21-●
    bomb NOS —*see also* Military operations, bomb(s) Y37.20-●
    fragments Y37.20-●
    grenade Y37.29-●
    guided missile Y37.22-●
    improvised explosive device [IED] (person-borne) (roadside) (vehicle-borne) Y37.23-●
    land mine Y37.29-●
    marine mine (at sea) (in harbor) Y37.02-●
    marine weapon Y37.00-●
      specified NEC Y37.09-●
    own munitions or munitions launch device (accidental) Y37.24-●
    sea-based artillery shell Y37.03-●
    specified NEC Y37.29-●
    torpedo Y37.04-●
  fire Y37.30-●
    specified NEC Y37.39-●
  firearms
    discharge Y37.43-●
    pellets Y37.42-●
  flamethrower Y37.33-●
  fragments (from) (of)
    improvised explosive device [IED] (person-borne) (roadside) (vehicle-borne) Y37.26-●
    munitions Y37.25-●
    specified NEC Y37.29-●
    weapons Y37.27-●
  friendly fire Y37.92-●

Melting *(Continued)*
  hand to hand (unarmed) combat Y37.44-●
  hot substances —*see* Military operations, fire
  incendiary bullet Y37.32-●
  nuclear weapon (effects of) Y37.50-●
    acute radiation exposure Y37.54-●
    blast pressure Y37.51-●
    direct blast Y37.51-●
    direct heat Y37.53-●
    fallout exposure Y37.54-●
    fireball Y37.53-●
    indirect blast (struck or crushed by blast debris) (being thrown by blast) Y37.52-●
    ionizing radiation (immediate exposure) Y37.54-●
    nuclear radiation Y37.54-●
    radiation
      ionizing (immediate exposure) Y37.54-●
      nuclear Y37.54-●
      thermal Y37.53-●
    secondary effects Y37.54-●
    specified NEC Y37.59-●
    thermal radiation Y37.53-●
  restriction of air (airway)
    intentional Y37.46-●
    unintentional Y37.47-●
  rubber bullets Y37.41-●
  shrapnel NOS Y37.29-●
  suffocation —*see* Military operations, restriction of airways
  unconventional warfare NEC Y37.7X-●
  underwater blast NOS Y37.00-●
  warfare
    conventional NEC Y37.49-●
    unconventional NEC Y37.7X-●
  weapon of mass destruction [WMD] Y37.91-●
  weapons
    biological weapons Y37.6X-●
    chemical Y37.7X-●
    nuclear (effects of) Y37.50-●
      acute radiation exposure Y37.54-●
      blast pressure Y37.51-●
      direct blast Y37.51-●
      direct heat Y37.53-●
      fallout exposure Y37.54-●
      fireball Y37.53-●
      radiation
        ionizing (immediate exposure) Y37.54-●
        nuclear Y37.54-●
        thermal Y37.53-●
      secondary effects Y37.54-●
      specified NEC Y37.59-●
    of mass destruction [WMD] Y37.91-●
Misadventure(s) to patient(s) during surgical or medical care Y69
  contaminated medical or biological substance (blood, drug, fluid) Y64.9
    administered (by) NEC Y64.9
      immunization Y64.1
      infusion Y64.0
      injection Y64.1
      specified means NEC Y64.8
      transfusion Y64.0
      vaccination Y64.1
  excessive amount of blood or other fluid during transfusion or infusion Y63.0
  failure
    in dosage Y63.9
      electroshock therapy Y63.4
      inappropriate temperature (too hot or too cold) in local application and packing Y63.5
      infusion
        excessive amount of fluid Y63.0
        incorrect dilution of fluid Y63.1
      insulin-shock therapy Y63.4
      nonadministration of necessary drug or biological substance Y63.6
      overdose —*see* Table of Drugs and Chemicals
        radiation, in therapy Y63.2
      radiation
        overdose Y63.2
      specified procedure NEC Y63.8
      transfusion
        excessive amount of blood Y63.0
    mechanical, of instrument or apparatus (any) (during any procedure) Y65.8

L & M

Misadventure(s) to patient(s) during surgical or
  medical care — *(Continued)*
  failure *(Continued)*
    sterile precautions (during procedure) Y62.9
      aspiration of fluid or tissue (by puncture or
        catheterization, except heart) Y62.6
      biopsy (except needle aspiration)
        Y62.8
        needle (aspirating) Y62.6
      blood sampling Y62.6
      catheterization Y62.6
        heart Y62.5
      dialysis (kidney) Y62.2
      endoscopic examination Y62.4
      enema Y62.8
      immunization Y62.3
      infusion Y62.1
      injection Y62.3
      needle biopsy Y62.6
      paracentesis (abdominal) (thoracic)
        Y62.6
      perfusion Y62.2
      puncture (lumbar) Y62.6
      removal of catheter or packing
        Y62.8
      specified procedure NEC Y62.8
      surgical operation Y62.0
      transfusion Y62.1
      vaccination Y62.3
    suture or ligature during surgical procedure
      Y65.2
    to introduce or to remove tube or
      instrument —*see* Failure, to
  hemorrhage —*see* Index to Diseases and Injuries,
    Complication(s)
  inadvertent exposure of patient to radiation
    Y63.3
  inappropriate
    operation performed —*see*
      Inappropriate operation performed
    temperature (too hot or too cold) in
      local application or packing
      Y63.5
  infusion —*see also* Misadventure, by type,
    infusion Y69
    excessive amount of fluid Y63.0
    incorrect dilution of fluid Y63.1
    wrong fluid Y65.1
  mismatched blood in transfusion Y65.0
  nonadministration of necessary drug or
    biological substance Y63.6
  overdose —*see* Table of Drugs and
    Chemicals
    radiation (in therapy) Y63.2
  perforation —*see* Index to Diseases and Injuries,
    Complication(s)
  performance of inappropriate operation —*see*
    Inappropriate operation performed
  puncture —*see* Index to Diseases and Injuries,
    Complication(s)
  specified type NEC Y65.8
    failure
      suture or ligature during surgical operation
        Y65.2
      to introduce or to remove tube or
        instrument —*see* Failure, to
    infusion of wrong fluid Y65.1
    performance of inappropriate operation —*see*
      Inappropriate operation performed
    transfusion of mismatched blood
      Y65.0
    wrong
      fluid in infusion Y65.1
      placement of endotracheal tube
        during anesthetic procedure
        Y65.3
  transfusion —*see* Misadventure, by type,
    transfusion
    excessive amount of blood Y63.0
    mismatched blood Y65.0
  wrong
    drug given in error —*see* Table of Drugs and
      Chemicals
    fluid in infusion Y65.1
    placement of endotracheal tube during
      anesthetic procedure Y65.3
Mismatched blood in transfusion Y65.0
Motion sickness T75.3
Mountain sickness W94.11
Mudslide (of cataclysmic nature) —*see* Landslide
Murder (attempt) —*see* Assault

— **N** —

Nail
  contact with W45.0
    gun W29.4
  embedded in skin W45.0
Neglect (criminal) (homicidal intent) X58
Noise (causing injury) (pollution) W42.9
  supersonic W42.0
Nonadministration (of)
  drug or biological substance (necessary) Y63.6
  surgical and medical care Y66
Nosocomial condition Y95

— **O** —

Object
  falling
    from, in, on, hitting
      machinery —*see* Contact, with, by type of
        machine
    set in motion by
      accidental explosion or rupture of pressure
        vessel W38
      firearm —*see* Discharge, firearm, by type
      machine (ry) —*see* Contact, with, by type of
        machine
Overdose (drug) —*see* Table of Drugs and
  Chemicals
  radiation Y63.2
Overexertion X50.9
  from
    prolonged static or awkward postures X50.1
    repetitive movements X50.3
    specified strenuous movements or postures
      NEC X50.9
    strenuous movement or load X50.0
Overexposure (accidental) (to)
  cold —*see also* Exposure, cold X31
    due to man-made conditions —*see* Exposure,
      cold, man-made
  heat —*see also* Heat X30
  radiation —*see* Radiation
  radioactivity W88.0
  sun (sunburn) X32
  weather NEC —*see* Forces of nature
  wind NEC —*see* Forces of nature
Overheated —*see* Heat
Overturning (accidental)
  machinery —*see* Contact, with, by type of
    machine
  transport vehicle NEC —*see also* Accident,
    transport V89.9
  watercraft (causing drowning, submersion) —
    see also Drowning, due to, accident to,
    watercraft, overturning
    causing injury except drowning or
      submersion —*see* Accident, watercraft,
      causing, injury NEC

— **P** —

Parachute descent (voluntary) (without accident to
  aircraft) V97.29
  due to accident to aircraft —*see* Accident,
    transport, aircraft
Pecked by bird W61.99
Perforation during medical or surgical treatment
  as misadventure —*see* Index to Diseases and
    Injuries, Complication(s)
Perpetrator, perpetration, of assault, maltreatment
  and neglect (by) Y07.9
  acquaintance Y07.54
  aunt Y07.47
  boyfriend
    current Y07.030
    former Y07.031
  brother Y07.410
    stepbrother Y07.435
  child (adopted) (biological) (foster) (in-law)
    (step) Y07.44
  coach Y07.53
  cousin
    female Y07.491
    male Y07.490

Perpetrator, perpetration, of assault, maltreatment
  and neglect *(Continued)*
  daughter (adopted) (biological) (foster) (in-law)
    (step) Y07.44
  daycare provider Y07.519
    at-home
      adult care Y07.512
      childcare Y07.510
    care center
      adult care Y07.513
      childcare Y07.511
  family member NEC Y07.499
  father Y07.11
    adoptive Y07.13
    foster Y07.420
    stepfather Y07.430
  foster father Y07.420
  foster mother Y07.421
  friend Y07.54
  girl friend
    current Y07.040
    former Y07.041
  grandchild (adopted) (biological) (foster)
    (in-law) (step) Y07.45
  granddaughter (adopted) (biological) (foster)
    (in-law) (step) Y07.45
  grandfather Y07.46
  grandmother Y07.46
  grandparent Y07.46
  grandson (adopted) (biological) (foster) (in-law)
    (step) Y07.45
  healthcare provider Y07.529
    mental health Y07.521
    specified NEC Y07.528
  husband
    current Y07.010
    former Y07.011
  instructor Y07.53
  mother Y07.12
    adoptive Y07.14
    foster Y07.421
    stepmother Y07.433
  non-binary
    child (adopted) (biological) (foster) (in-law)
      (step) Y07.44
    grandchild (adopted) (biological) (foster)
      (in-law) (step) Y07.45
    grandparent Y07.46
    parental sibling Y07.47
  nonfamily member Y07.50
    specified NEC Y07.59
  nurse Y07.528
  occupational therapist Y07.528
  parental sibling Y07.47
  partner
    female (dating) (intimate)
      current Y07.040
      former Y07.041
    gender non-conforming
      current Y07.050
      former Y07.051
    male (dating) (intimate)
      current Y07.030
      former Y07.031
    non-binary
      current Y07.050
      former Y07.051
    of parent
      female Y07.434
      male Y07.432
  physical therapist Y07.528
  sister Y07.411
  son (adopted) (biological) (foster) (in-law) (step)
    Y07.44
  speech therapist Y07.528
  stepbrother Y07.435
  stepfather Y07.430
  stepmother Y07.433
  stepsister Y07.436
  teacher Y07.53
  uncle Y07.47
  wife
    current Y07.020
    former Y07.021
Piercing —*see* Contact, with, by type of object or
  machine
Pinched
  between objects (moving) (stationary and
    moving) W23.0
    stationary W23.1

New   Revised   ~~deleted~~ Deleted   ● Use Additional Character(s)

Place of occurrence (Continued)
  residence (Continued)
    institutional (Continued)
      orphanage (Continued)
        specified NEC Y92.118
        swimming pool Y92.115
        yard Y92.116
      prison Y92.149
        bathroom Y92.142
        cell Y92.143
        courtyard Y92.147
        dining room Y92.141
        kitchen Y92.140
        specified NEC Y92.148
        swimming pool Y92.146
      reform school Y92.159
        bathroom Y92.152
        bedroom Y92.153
        dining room Y92.151
        driveway Y92.154
        garage Y92.155
        garden Y92.157
        kitchen Y92.150
        specified NEC Y92.158
        swimming pool Y92.156
        yard Y92.157
      school dormitory Y92.169
        bathroom Y92.162
        bedroom Y92.163
        dining room Y92.161
        kitchen Y92.160
        specified NEC Y92.168
      specified NEC Y92.199
        bathroom Y92.192
        bedroom Y92.193
        dining room Y92.191
        driveway Y92.194
        garage Y92.195
        garden Y92.197
        kitchen Y92.190
        specified NEC Y92.198
        swimming pool Y92.196
        yard Y92.197
    kitchen Y92.000
    mobile home Y92.029
      bathroom Y92.022
      bedroom Y92.023
      dining room Y92.021
      driveway Y92.024
      garage Y92.025
      garden Y92.027
      kitchen Y92.020
      specified NEC Y92.028
      swimming pool Y92.026
      yard Y92.027
    specified place in residence NEC Y92.008
    specified residence type NEC Y92.099
      bathroom Y92.091
      bedroom Y92.092
      driveway Y92.093
      garage Y92.094
      garden Y92.096
      kitchen Y92.090
      specified NEC Y92.098
      swimming pool Y92.095
      yard Y92.096
  restaurant Y92.511
  riding school Y92.39
  river Y92.828
  road Y92.410
  rodeo ring Y92.39
  rugby field Y92.328
  same day surgery center Y92.530
  sand pit Y92.64
  school (private) (public) (state) Y92.219
    college Y92.214
    daycare center Y92.210
    elementary school Y92.211
    high school Y92.213
    kindergarten Y92.211
    middle school Y92.212
    specified NEC Y92.218
    trace school Y92.215
    university Y92.214
    vocational school Y92.215
  sea (shore) Y92.832
  senior citizen center Y92.29
  service area
    airport Y92.520
    bus station Y92.521
    gas station Y92.524

Place of occurrence (Continued)
  service area (Continued)
    highway rest stop Y92.523
    railway station Y92.522
  shipyard Y92.62
  shop(commercial) Y92.513
  sidewalk Y92.480
  silo Y92.79
  skating rink (roller) Y92.331
    ice Y92.330
  slaughter house Y92.86
  soccer field Y92.322
  specified place NEC Y92.89
  sports area Y92.39
    athletic
      court Y92.318
        basketball Y92.310
        specified NEC Y92.318
        squash Y92.311
        tennis Y92.312
      field Y92.328
        baseball Y92.320
        cricket ground Y92.328
        football Y92.321
        hockey Y92.328
        soccer Y92.322
        specified NEC Y92.328
    golf course Y92.39
    gymnasium Y92.39
    riding school Y92.39
    skating rink (roller) Y92.331
      ice Y92.330
    stadium Y92.39
    swimming pool Y92.34
  squash court Y92.311
  stadium Y92.39
  steeplechasing course Y92.39
  store Y92.512
  stream Y92.828
  street and highway Y92.410
    bike path Y92.482
    freeway Y92.411
    highway ramp Y92.415
    interstate highway Y92.411
    local residential or business street Y92.414
    motorway Y92.411
    parking lot Y92.481
    parkway Y92.412
    sidewalk Y92.480
    specified NEC Y92.488
    state road Y92.413
  subway car Y92.816
  supermarket Y92.512
  swamp Y92.828
  swimming pool (public) Y92.34
    private (at) Y92.095
      boarding house Y92.045
      military base Y92.136
      mobile home Y92.026
      nursing home Y92.125
      orphanage Y92.115
      prison Y92.146
      reform school Y92.156
      single family residence Y92.016
  synagogue Y92.22
  tavern
  television station Y92.59
  tennis court Y92.312
  theater Y92.254
  trade area Y92.59
    bank Y92.510
    cafe Y92.511
    casino Y92.59
    garage Y92.59
    hotel Y92.59
    market Y92.512
    office building Y92.59
    radio station Y92.59
    restaurant Y92.511
    shop Y92.513
    shopping mall Y92.59
    store Y92.513
    supermarket Y92.512
    television station Y92.59
    warehouse Y92.59
  trailer park, residential —see Place of occurrence, residence, mobile home
  trailer site NOS Y92.89
  train Y92.815
    station Y92.522
  truck Y92.812

Place of occurrence (Continued)
  tunnel under construction Y92. 69
  university Y92.214
  urgent (health) care center Y92.532
  vehicle (transport) Y92.818
    airplane Y92.813
    boat Y92.814
    bus Y92.811
    car Y92.810
    specified NEC Y92.818
    subway car Y92.816
    train Y92.815
    truck Y92.812
  warehouse Y92.59
  water reservoir Y92.89
  wilderness area Y92.828
    desert Y92.820
    forest Y92.821
    marsh Y92.828
    mountain Y92.828
    prairie Y92.828
    specified NEC Y92.828
    swamp Y92.828
  workshop Y92.69
  yard, private Y92.096
    boarding house Y92.046
    mobile home Y92.027
    single family house Y92.017
  youth center Y92.29
  zoo (zoological garden) Y92.834
Plumbism —see Table of Drugs and Chemicals, lead
Poisoning (accidental) (by) —see also Table of Drugs and Chemicals
  by plant, thorns, spines, sharp leaves or other mechanisms NEC X58
  carbon monoxide
    generated by
      motor vehicle —see Accident, transport
      watercraft (in transit) (not in transit) V93.89
        ferry boat V93.81
        fishing boat V93.82
        jet skis V93.83
        liner V93.81
        merchant ship V93.80
        passenger ship V93.81
        powered craft NEC V93.83
  caused by injection of poisons into skin by plant thorns, spines, sharp leaves X58
    marine or sea plants (venomous) X58
  exhaust gas
    generated by
      motor vehicle —see Accident, transport
      watercraft (in transit) (not in transit) V93.89
        ferry boat V93.81
        fishing boat V93.82
        jet skis V93.83
        liner V93.81
        merchant ship V93.80
        passenger ship V93.81
        powered craft NEC V93.83
  fumes or smoke due to
    explosion —see also Explosion W40.9
    fire —see Exposure, fire
    ignition —see Ignition
  gas
    in legal intervention —see Legal, intervention, gas
    legal execution —see Legal, intervention, gas
  in war operations —see War operations
  legal
    execution —see Legal, Intervention, gas
    intervention
      by gas —see Legal, intervention, gas
      other specified means —see Legal, intervention, specified means NEC
Powder burn (by) (from)
  airgun W34.110
  BB gun W34.110
  firearm NEC W34.19
  gas, air or spring-operated gun NEC W34.118
  handgun W32.1
  hunting rifle W33.12
  larger firearm W33.10
    specified NEC W33.19
  machine gun W33.13
  paintball gun W34.111
  pellet gun W34.110
  shotgun W33.11
  Very pistol [flare] W34.19

▶ New   ➡ Revised   ~~deleted~~ Deleted   ● Use Additional Character(s)

Premature cessation (of) surgical and medical care Y66
Privation (food) (water) X58
Procedure (operation)
  correct, on wrong side or body part (wrong side) (wrong site) Y65.53
  intended for another patient done on wrong patient Y65.52
  performed on patient not scheduled for surgery Y65.52
  performed on wrong patient Y65.52
  wrong, performed on correct patient Y65.51
Prolonged
  sitting in transport vehicle —see Sitting
  stay in
    high altitude as cause of anoxia, barodontalgia, barotitis or hypoxia W94.11
    weightless environment X52
Pulling, excessive —see also Overexertion X50.9
Puncture, puncturing —see also Contact, with, by type of object or machine
  by
    plant thorns, spines, sharp leaves or other mechanisms NEC W60
  during medical or surgical treatment as misadventure —see Index to Diseases and Injuries, Complication(s)
Pushed, pushing (accidental) (injury in)
  by other person(s) (accidental) W51
    with fall W03
      due to ice or snow W00.0
    as, or caused by, a crowd or human stampede (with fall) W52
    before moving object NEC Y02.8
      motor vehicle Y02.0
      subway train Y02.1
      train Y02.1
    from
      high place NEC
        in accidental circumstances W17.89
        stated as
          intentional, homicide (attempt) Y01
          undetermined whether accidental or intentional Y30
      transport vehicle NEC —see also Accident, transport V89.9
        stated as
          intentional, homicide (attempt) Y08.89
    overexertion X50.9

R

Radiation (exposure to)
  arc lamps W89.0
  atomic power plant (malfunction) NEC W88.1
  complication of or abnormal reaction to medical radiotherapy Y84.2
  electromagnetic, ionizing W88.0
  gamma rays W88.1
  in
    war operations (from or following nuclear explosion) —see also War operations
  inadvertent exposure of patient (receiving test or therapy) Y63.3
  infrared (heaters and lamps) W90.1
    excessive heat from W92
  ionized, ionizing (particles, artificially accelerated)
    radioisotopes W88.1
    specified NEC W88.8
    x-rays W88.0
  isotopes, radioactive —see Radiation, radioactive isotopes
  laser(s) W90.2
    in war operations —see War operations
    misadventure in medical care Y63.2
  light sources (man-made visible and ultraviolet) W89.9
    natural X32
    specified NEC W89.8
    tanning bed W89.1
    welding light W89.0
  man-made visible light W89.9
    specified NEC W89.8
    tanning bed W89.1
    welding light W89.0

Radiation (Continued)
  microwave W90.8
  misadventure in medical or surgical procedure Y63.2
  natural NEC X39.08
    radon X39.01
  overdose (in medical or surgical procedure) Y63.2
  radar W90.0
  radioactive isotopes (any) W88.1
    atomic power plant malfunction W88.1
    misadventure in medical or surgical treatment Y63.2
  radiofrequency W90.0
  radium NEC W88.1
  sun X32
  ultraviolet (light) (man-made) W89.9
    natural X32
    specified NEC W89.8
    tanning bed W89.1
    welding light W89.0
  welding arc, torch, or light W89.0
    excessive heat from W92
  x-rays (hard) (soft) W88.0
Range disease W94.11
▶ Rape (attempted) (confirmed) T74.2-●
▶ suspected T76.2-●
Rat bite W53.11
Reaching (prolonged) (static) X50.1
Reaction, abnormal to medical procedure —see also Complication of or following, by type of procedure Y84.9
  with misadventure —see Misadventure
  biologicals —see Table of Drugs and Chemicals
  drugs —see Table of Drugs and Chemicals
  vaccine —see Table of Drugs and Chemicals
Recoil
  airgun W34.110
  BB gun W34.110
  firearm NEC W34.19
  gas, air or spring-operated gun NEC W34.118
  handgun W32.1
  hunting rifle W33.12
  larger firearm W33.10
    specified NEC W33.19
  machine gun W33.13
  paintball gun W34.111
  pellet W34.110
  shotgun W33.11
  Very pistol [flare] W34.19
Reduction in
  atmospheric pressure —see Air, pressure, change
Rock falling on or hitting (accidentally) (person) W20.8
  in cave-in W20.0
Run over (accidentally) (by)
  animal (not being ridden) NEC W55.89
  machinery —see Contact, with, by specified type of machine
  transport vehicle NEC —see also Accident, transport V09.9
    intentional homicide (attempt) Y03.0
    motor NEC V09.20
      intentional homicide (attempt) Y03.0
Running
  before moving object X81.8
    motor vehicle X81.0
Running off, away
  animal (being ridden) —see also Accident, transport V80.918
    not being ridden W55.89
  animal-drawn vehicle NEC —see also Accident, transport V80.928
  highway, road(way), street
    transport vehicle NEC —see also Accident, transport V89.9
Rupture pressurized devices —see Explosion, by type of device

S

Saturnism —see Table of Drugs and Chemicals, lead
Scald, scalding (accidental) (by) (from) (in) X19
  air (hot) X14.1
  gases (hot) X14.1
  homicide (attempt) —see Assault, burning, hot object

Scald, scalding (Continued)
  inflicted by other person
    stated as intentional, homicide (attempt) —see Assault, burning, hot object
  liquid (boiling) (hot) NEC X12
    stated as undetermined whether accidental or intentional Y27.2
    suicide (attempt) X77.2
  local application of externally applied substance in medical or surgical care Y63.5
  metal (molten) (liquid) (hot) NEC X18
    self-inflicted X77.9
    stated as undetermined whether accidental or intentional Y27.8
  steam X13.1
    assault X98.0
    stated as undetermined whether accidental or intentional Y27.0
    suicide (attempt) X77.0
  suicide (attempt) X77.9
  vapor (hot) X13.1
    assault X98.0
    stated as undetermined whether accidental or intentional Y27.0
    suicide (attempt) X77.0
Scratched by
  cat W55.03
  person(s) (accidentally) W50.4
    with intent to injure or kill Y04.0
    as, or caused by, a crowd or human stampede (with fall) W52
    assault Y04.0
    homicide (attempt) Y04.0
    in
      fight Y04.0
      legal intervention
        injuring
          bystander Y35.892
          law enforcement personnel Y35.891
          suspect Y35.893
          unspecified person Y35.899
Seasickness T75.3
Self-harm NEC —see also External cause by type, undetermined whether accidental or intentional
  intentional —see Suicide
  poisoning NEC —see Table of drugs and biologicals, accident
Self-inflicted (injury) NEC —see also External cause by type, undetermined whether accidental or intentional
  intentional —see Suicide
  poisoning NEC —see Table of drugs and biologicals, accident
Sequelae (of)
  accident NEC —see W00-X58 with 7th character S
  assault (homicidal) (any means) —see X92-Y08 with 7th character S
  homicide, attempt (any means) —see X92-Y08 with 7th character S
  injury undetermined whether accidentally or purposely inflicted —see Y21-Y33 with 7th character S
  intentional self-harm (classifiable to X71-X83) —see X71-X83 with 7th character S
  legal intervention (see with 7th character S Y35)
  motor vehicle accident —see V00-V99 with 7th character S
  suicide, attempt (any means) —see X71-X83 with 7th character S
  transport accident —see V00-V99 with 7th character S
  war operations —see War operations
Shock
  electric —see Exposure, electric current
  from electric appliance (any) (faulty) W86.8
    domestic W86.0
    suicide (attempt) X83.1
Shooting, shot (accidental (ly)) —see also Discharge, firearm, by type
  herself or himself —see Discharge, firearm by type, self-inflicted
  homicide (attempt) —see Discharge, firearm by type, homicide
  in war operations —see War operations
  inflicted by other person —see Discharge, firearm by type, homicide
    accidental —see Discharge, firearm, by type of firearm

P, R, & S

Shooting, shot (Continued)
  legal
    execution —*see* Legal, intervention, firearm
    intervention —*see* Legal, intervention, firearm
  self-inflicted —*see* Discharge, firearm by type,
    suicide
    accidental —*see* Discharge, firearm, by type
      of firearm
  suicide (attempt) —*see* Discharge, firearm by
    type, suicide
Shoving (accidentally) **by other person** —*see*
  Pushed, by other person
Sickness
  alpine W94.11
  motion —*see* Motion
  mountain W94.11
Sinking (accidental)
  watercraft (causing drowning, submersion) —
    see also Drowning, due to, accident to,
    watercraft, sinking
  causing injury except drowning or
    submersion —*see* Accident, watercraft,
    causing, injury NEC
Siriasis X32
Sitting (prolonged) (static) X50.1
Slashed wrists —*see* Cut, self-inflicted
Slipping (accidental) (on same level) (with fall)
  W01.0
  without fall W18.40
    due to
      specified NEC W18.49
      stepping from one level to another W18.43
      stepping into hole or opening W18.42
      stepping on object W18.41
  on
    ice W00.0
      with skates —*see* Accident, transport,
        pedestrian, conveyance
    mud W01.0
    oil W01.0
    snow W00.0
      with skis —*see* Accident, transport,
        pedestrian, conveyance
    surface (slippery) (wet) NEC W01.0
Sliver, wood, contact with W45.8
Smoldering (due to fire) —*see* Exposure, fire
Sodomy (attempted) by force T74.2-●
Sound waves (causing injury) W42.9
  supersonic W42.0
Splinter, contact with W45.8
Stab, stabbing —*see* Cut
Standing (prolonged) (static) X50.1
Starvation X58
Status of external cause Y99.9
  child assisting in compensated work for family
    Y99.8
  civilian activity done for financial or other
    compensation Y99.0
  civilian activity done for income or pay Y99.0
  family member assisting in compensated work
    for other family member Y99.8
  hobby not done for income Y99.8
  leisure activity Y99.8
  military activity Y99.1
  off-duty activity of military personnel Y99.8
  recreation or sport not for income or while a
    student Y99.8
  specified NEC Y99.8
  student activity Y99.8
  volunteer activity Y99.2
Stepped on
  by
    animal (not being ridden) NEC W55.89
    crowd or human stampede W52
    person W50.0
Stepping on
  object W22.8
    with fall W18.31
    sports equipment W21.9
    stationary W22.09
      sports equipment W21.89
  person W51
    by crowd or human stampede W52
  sports equipment W21.9
Sting
  arthropod, nonvenomous W57
  insect, nonvenomous W57
Storm (cataclysmic) —*see* Forces of nature,
  cataclysmic storm

Straining, excessive —*see also* Overexertion X50.9
Strangling —*see* Strangulation
Strangulation (accidental) —*see* category T71
Strenuous movements —*see also* Overexertion X50.9
Striking against
  airbag (automobile) W22.10
    driver side W22.11
    front passenger side W22.12
    specified NEC W22.19
  bottom when
    diving or jumping into water (in)
      W16.822
      causing drowning W16.821
      from boat W16.722
        causing drowning W16.721
      natural body W16.622
        causing drowning W16.821
      swimming pool W16.522
        causing drowning W16.521
    falling into water (in) W16.322
      causing drowning W16.321
      fountain —*see* Striking against, bottom
        when, falling into water, specified
        NEC
      natural body W16.122
        causing drowning W16.121
      reservoir —*see* Striking against, bottom
        when, falling into water, specified
        NEC
      specified NEC W16.322
        causing drowning W16.321
      swimming pool W16.022
        causing drowning W16.021
  diving board (swimming-pool) W21.4
  object W22.8
    with
      drowning or submersion —*see* Drowning
      fall —*see* Fall, due to, bumping against,
        object
      caused by crowd or human stampede (with
        fall) W52
      furniture W22.03
      lamppost W22.02
      sports equipment W21.9
      stationary W22.09
        sports equipment W21.89
      wall W22.01
    person(s) W51
      with fall W03
        due to ice or snow W00.0
      as, or caused by, a crowd or human stampede
        (with fall) W52
      assault Y04.2
      homicide (attempt) Y04.2
  sports equipment W21.9
  wall (when) W22.01
    diving or jumping into water (in) W16.832
      causing drowning W16.831
    swimming pool W16.532
      causing drowning W16.531
    falling into water (in) W16.332
      causing drowning W16.331
    fountain —*see* Striking against, wall when,
      falling into water, specified NEC
    natural body W16.132
      causing drowning W16.131
    reservoir —*see* Striking against, wall when,
      falling into water, specified NEC
    specified NEC W16.332
      causing drowning W16.331
    swimming pool W16.032
      causing drowning W16.031
    swimming pool (when) W22.042
      causing drowning W22.041
    diving or jumping into water W16.532
      causing drowning W16.531
    falling into water W16.032
      causing drowning W16.031
Struck (accidentally) **by**
  airbag (automobile) W22.10
    driver side W22.11
    front passenger side W22.12
    specified NEC W22.19
  alligator W58.02
  animal (not being ridden) NEC W55.89
  avalanche —*see* Landslide
  ball (hit) (thrown) W21.00
    assault Y08.09
    baseball W21.03

Struck (Continued)
  ball (Continued)
    basketball W21.05
    football W21.01
    golf ball W21.04
    football W21.01
    soccer W21.02
    softball W21.07
    specified NEC W21.09
    volleyball W21.06
  bat or racquet
    baseball bat W21.11
      assault Y08.02
    golf club W21.13
      assault Y08.09
    specified NEC W21.19
      assault Y08.09
    tennis racquet W21.12
      assault Y08.09
  bullet —*see also* Discharge, firearm by type
    in war operations —*see* War operations
  crocodile W58.12
  dog W54.1
  flare, Very pistol —*see* Discharge, firearm NEC
  hailstones X39.8
  hockey (ice)
    field
      puck W21.221
      stick W21.211
    puck W21.220
    stick W21.210
      assault Y08.01
  landslide —*see* Landslide
  law-enforcement agent (on duty) —*see* Legal,
    intervention, manhandling
    with blunt object —*see* Legal, intervention,
      blunt object
  lightning —*see* subcategory T75.0
    causing fire —*see* Exposure, fire
  machine —*see* Contact, with, by type of machine
  mammal NEC W55.89
    marine W56.32
  marine animal W56.82
  missile
    firearm —*see* Discharge, firearm by type
    in war operations —*see* War operations,
      missile
  object W22.8
    blunt W22.8
      assault Y00
      suicide (attempt) X79
      undetermined whether accidental or
        intentional Y29
    falling W20.8
      from, in, on
        building W20.1
          burning (uncontrolled fire)
            X00.4
        cataclysmic
          earth surface movement NEC —*see*
            Landslide
          storm —*see* Forces of nature,
            cataclysmic storm
        cave-in W20.0
        earthquake X34
        machine (in operation) —*see* Contact,
          with, by type of machine
        structure W20.1
          burning X00.4
        transport vehicle (in motion) —*see*
          Accident, transport, by type of
          vehicle
        watercraft V93.49
          due to
            accident to craft V91.39
              powered craft V91.33
                ferry boat V91.31
                fishing boat V91.32
                jet ski V91.33
                liner V91.31
                merchant ship V91.30
                passenger ship V91.31
              unpowered craft V91.38
                canoe V91.35
                inflatable V91.36
                kayak V91.35
                sailboat V91.34
                surf-board V91.38
                windsurfer V91.38

▶ New   ⇒ Revised   ~~deleted~~ Deleted   ● Use Additional Character(s)

Struck (Continued)
  object (Continued)
    falling (Continued)
      from, in (Continued)
        watercraft (Continued)
          powered craft V93.43
            ferry boat V93.41
            fishing boat V93.42
            jet ski V93.43
            liner V93.41
            merchant ship V93.40
            passenger ship V93.41
          unpowered craft V93.48
            sailboat V93.44
            surf-board V93.48
            windsurfer V93.48
      moving NEC W20.8
      projected W20.8
        assault Y00
        in sports W21.9
          assault Y08.09
          ball W21.00
            baseball W21.03
            basketball W21.05
            football W21.01
            golf ball W21.04
            soccer W21.02
            softball W21.07
            specified NEC W21.09
            volleyball W21.06
          bat or racquet
            baseball bat W21.11
              assault Y08.02
            golf club W21.13
              assault Y08.09-●
            specified NEC W21.19
              assault Y08.09
            tennis racquet W21.12
              assault Y08.09
          hockey (ice)
            field
              puck W21.221
              stick W21.211
            puck W21.220
            stick W21.210
              assault Y08.01
          specified NEC W21.89
      set in motion by explosion —see Explosion
      thrown W20.8
        assault Y00
        in sports W21.9
          assault Y08.09
          ball W21.00
            baseball W21.03
            basketball W21.05
            football W21.01
            golf ball W21.04
            soccer W21.02
            soft ball W21.07
            specified NEC W21.09
            volleyball W21.06
          bat or racquet
            baseball bat W21.11
              assault Y08.02
            golf club W21.13
              assault Y08.09
            specified NEC W21.19
              assault Y08.09
            tennis racquet W21.12
              assault Y08.09
          hockey (ice)
            field
              puck W21.221
              stick W21.211
            puck W21.220
            stick W21.210
              assault Y08.01
          specified NEC W21.89
  other person(s) W50.0
    with
      blunt object W22.8
        intentional, homicide (attempt) Y00
        sports equipment W21.9
        undetermined whether accidental or
          intentional Y29
      fall W03
        due to ice or snow W00.0
    as, or caused by, a crowd or human stampede
      (with fall) W52

Struck (Continued)
  other person(s) (Continued)
    assault Y04.2
    homicide (attempt) Y04.2
    in legal intervention
      injuring
        bystander Y35.812
        law enforcement personnel
          Y35.811
        suspect Y35.813
        unspecified person Y35.819
    sports equipment W21.9
  police (on duty) —see Legal, intervention,
    manhandling
    with blunt object —see Legal, intervention,
      blunt object
  sports equipment W21.9
    assault Y08.09
    ball W21.00
      baseball W21.03
      basketball W21.05
      football W21.01
      golf ball W21.04
      soccer W21.02
      soft ball W21.07
      specified NEC W21.09
      volleyball W21.06
    bat or racquet
      baseball bat W21.11
        assault Y08.02
      golf club W21.13
        assault Y08.09
      specified NEC W21.19
      tennis racquet W21.12
        assault Y08.09
    cleats (shoe) W21.31
    foot wear NEC W21.39
    football helmet W21.81
    hockey
      field
        puck W21.221
        stick W21.211
      puck W21.220
      stick W21.210
        assault Y08.01
    skate blades W21.32
    specified NEC W21.89
      assault Y08.09
  thunderbolt —see subcategory
    T75.0
    causing fire —see Exposure, fire
  transport vehicle NEC —see also Accident,
    transport V09.9
    intentional, homicide (attempt) Y03.0
    motor NEC —see also Accident, transport
      V09.20
    homicide Y03.0
  vehicle (transport) NEC —see Accident,
    transport, by type of vehicle
    stationary (falling from jack,
      hydraulic lift, ramp)
      W20.8
Stumbling
  without fall W18.40
    due to
      specified NEC W18.49
      stepping from one level to another W18.43
      stepping into hole or opening W18.42
      stepping on object W18.41
    over
      animal NEC W01.0
        with fall W18.09
      carpet, rug or (small) object W22.8
        with fall W18.09
      person W51
        with fall W03
          due to ice or snow W00.0
Submersion (accidental) —see Drowning
Suffocation (accidental) (by external means)
  (by pressure) (mechanical) —see also category
  T71
  due to, by
    avalanche —see Landslide
    explosion —see Explosion
    fire —see Exposure, fire
    food, any type (aspiration) (ingestion)
      (inhalation) —see categories T17 and T18
    ignition —see Ignition
    landslide —see Landslide

Suffocation (Continued)
  due to, by (Continued)
    machine (ry) —see Contact, with, by type of
      machine
    vomitus (aspiration) (inhalation)
      T17.81-●
  in
    burning building X00.8
Suicide, suicidal (attempted) (by) X83.8
  blunt object X79
  burning, burns X76
    hot object X77.9
      fluid NEC X77.2
      household appliance X77.3
      specified NEC X77.8
      steam X77.0
      tap water X77.1
      vapors X77.0
  caustic substance —see Table of Drugs and
    Chemicals
  cold, extreme X83.2
  collision of motor vehicle with
    motor vehicle X82.0
    specified NEC X82.8
    train X82.1
    tree X82.2
  crashing of aircraft X83.0
  cut (any part of body) X78.9
  cutting or piercing instrument X78.9
    dagger X78.2
    glass X78.0
    knife X78.1
    specified NEC X78.8
    sword X78.2
  drowning (in) X71.9
    bathtub X71.0
    natural water X71.3
    specified NEC X71.8
    swimming pool X71.1
      following fall X71.2
  electrocution X83.1
  explosive(s) (material) X75
  fire, flames X76
  firearm X74.9
    airgun X74.01
    handgun X72
    hunting rifle X73.1
    larger X73.9
      specified NEC X73.8
    machine gun X73.2
    shotgun X73.0
    specified NEC X74.8
  hanging X83.8
  hot object —see Suicide, burning, hot object
  jumping
    before moving object X81.8
      motor vehicle X81.0
      subway train X81.1
      train X81.1
    from high place X80
  late effect of attempt —see X71-X83 with 7th
    character S
  lying before moving object, train, vehicle
    X81.8
  poisoning —see Table of Drugs and Chemicals
  puncture (any part of body) —see Suicide,
    cutting or piercing instrument
  scald —see Suicide, burning, hot object
  sequelae of attempt —see X71-X83 with 7th
    character S
  sharp object (any) —see Suicide, cutting or
    piercing instrument
  shooting —see Suicide, firearm
  specified means NEC X83.8
  stab (any part of body) —see Suicide, cutting or
    piercing instrument
  steam, hot vapors X77.0
  strangulation X83.8
  submersion —see Suicide, drowning
  suffocation X83.8
  wound NEC X83.8
Sunstroke X32
Supersonic waves (causing injury) W42.0
Surgical procedure, complication of (delayed or
  as an abnormal reaction without mention of
  misadventure) —see also Complication of or
  following, by type of procedure
  due to or as a result of misadventure —see
    Misadventure

S

Swallowed, swallowing
  foreign body —see Foreign body, alimentary
      canal
  poison —see Table of Drugs and Chemicals
  substance
    caustic or corrosive —see Table of Drugs and
        Chemicals
    poisonous —see Table of Drugs and
        Chemicals

— T —

Tackle in sport W03
Terrorism (involving) Y38.80
  biological weapons Y38.6X-●
  chemical weapons Y38.7X-●
  conflagration Y38.3X-●
  drowning and submersion Y38.89-●
  explosion Y38.2X-●
    destruction of aircraft Y38.1X-●
    marine weapons Y38.0X-●
  fire Y38.3X-●
  firearms Y38.4X-●
  hot substances Y38.3X-●
  lasers Y38.89-●
  nuclear weapons Y38.5X-●
  piercing or stabbing instruments
      Y38.89-●
  secondary effects Y38.9X-●
  specified method NEC Y38.89-●
  suicide bomber Y38.81-●
Thirst X58
Threat to breathing
  aspiration —see Aspiration
  due to cave-in, falling earth or substance NEC —
      see category T71
Thrown (accidentally)
  against part (any) of or object in transport
      vehicle (in motion) NEC —see also Accident,
      transport
  from
    high place, homicide (attempt) Y01
    machinery —see Contact, with, by type of
        machine
    transport vehicle NEC —see also Accident,
        transport V89.9
  off —see Thrown, from
Thunderbolt —see subcategory T75.0
  causing fire —see Exposure, fire
Tidal wave (any injury) NEC —see Forces of
    nature, tidal wave
Took
  overdose (drug) —see Table of Drugs and
      Chemicals
  poison —see Table of Drugs and Chemicals
Tornado (any injury) X37.1
Torrential rain (any injury) X37.8
Torture X58
Trampled by animal NEC W55.89
Trapped (accidentally)
  between objects (moving) (stationary and
      moving) —see Caught
  by part (any) of
    electric (assisted) bicycle V29.881
    motorcycle V29.888
    pedal cycle V19.88
    transport vehicle NEC —see also Accident,
        transport V89.9
Travel (effects) (sickness) T75.3
Tree falling on or hitting (accidentally) (person)
    W20.8
Tripping
  without fall W18.40
    due to
      specified NEC W18.49
      stepping from one level to another W18.43
      stepping into hole or opening
          W18.42
      stepping on object W18.41
  over
    animal W01.0
      with fall W01.0
    carpet, rug or (small) object W22.8
      with fall W18.09
    person W51
      with fall W03
        due to ice or snow W00.0

Twisted by person(s) (accidentally) W50.2
  with intent to injure or kill Y04.0
  as, or caused by, a crowd or human stampede
      (with fall) W52
  assault Y04.0
  homicide (attempt) Y04.0
  in
    fight Y04.0
    legal intervention —see Legal, intervention,
        manhandling
Twisting (prolonged) (static) X50.1

— U —

Underdosing of necessary drugs, medicaments or
    biological substances Y63.6
Undetermined intent (contact)
    (exposure)
  automobile collision Y32
  blunt object Y29
  drowning (submersion) (in) Y21.9
    bathtub Y21.0
      after fall Y21.1
    natural water (lake) (ocean) (pond) (river)
        (stream) Y21.4
    specified place NEC Y21.8
    swimming pool Y21.2
      after fall Y21.3
  explosive material Y25
  fall, jump or push from high place
      Y30
  falling, lying or running before moving object
      Y31
  fire Y26
  firearm discharge Y24.9
    airgun (BB) (pellet) Y24.0
    handgun (pistol) (revolver)
        Y22
    hunting rifle Y23.1
    larger Y23.9
      hunting rifle Y23.1
      machine gun Y23.3
      military Y23.2
      shotgun Y23.0
      specified type NEC Y23.8
    machine gun Y23.3
    military Y23.2
    shotgun Y23.0
    specified type NEC Y24.8
    Very pistol Y24.8
  hot object Y27.9
    fluid NEC Y27.2
    household appliance Y27.3
    specified object NEC Y27.8
    steam Y27.0
    tap water Y27.1
    vapor Y27.0
  jump, fall or push from high place Y30
  lying, falling or running before moving object
      Y31
  motor vehicle crash Y32
  push, fall or jump from high place Y30
  running, falling or lying before moving object
      Y31
  sharp object Y28.9
    dagger Y28.2
    glass Y28.0
    knife Y28.1
    specified object NEC Y28.8
    sword Y28.2
  smoke Y26
  specified event NEC Y33
Use of hand as hammer X50.3

— V —

Vibration (causing injury) W49.9
Victim (of)
  avalanche —see Landslide
  earth movements NEC —see Forces of nature,
      earth movement
  earthquake X34
  flood —see Flood
  landslide —see Landslide

Victim (Continued)
  lightning —see subcategory T75.0
    causing fire —see Exposure, fire
  storm (cataclysmic) NEC —see Forces of nature,
      cataclysmic storm
  volcanic eruption X35
Volcanic eruption (any injury) X35
Vomitus, gastric contents in air passages (with
    asphyxia, obstruction or suffocation)
    T17.81-●

— W —

Walked into stationary object (any) W22.09
  furniture W22.03
  lamppost W22.02
  wall W22.01
War operations (injuries to military personnel and
    civilians during war, civil insurrection and
    peacekeeping missions) (by) (from)
    (involving) Y36.90-●
  after cessation of hostilities Y36.89-●
    explosion (of)
      bomb placed during war operations
          Y36.82-●
      mine placed during war operations
          Y36.81-●
      specified NEC Y36.88-●
  air blast Y36.20-●
  aircraft
    destruction —see War operations, destruction
        of aircraft
    airway restriction —see War operations,
        restriction of airways
    asphyxiation —see War operations, restriction of
        airways
  biological weapons Y36.6X-●
  blast Y36.20-●
  blast fragments Y36.20-●
  blast wave Y36.20-●
  blast wind Y36.20-●
  bomb Y36.20-●
    dirty Y36.50-●
    gasoline Y36.31-●
    incendiary Y36.31-●
    petrol Y36.31-●
  bullet Y36.43-●
    incendiary Y36.32-●
    rubber Y36.41-●
  chemical weapons Y36.7X-●
  combat
    hand to hand (unarmed) combat
        Y36.44-●
    using blunt or piercing object Y36.45-●
  conflagration —see War operations, fire
  conventional warfare NEC Y36.49-●
  depth-charge Y36.01-●
  destruction of aircraft Y36.10-●
    due to
      air to air missile Y36.11-●
      collision with other aircraft Y36.12-●
      detonation (accidental) of onboard
          munitions and explosives Y36.14-●
      enemy fire or explosives Y36.11-●
      explosive placed on aircraft Y36.11-●
      onboard fire Y36.13-●
      rocket propelled grenade [RPG]
          Y36.11-●
      small arms fire Y36.11-●
      surface to air missile Y36.11-●
      specified NEC Y36.19-●
  detonation (accidental) of
    onboard marine weapons Y36.05-●
    own munitions or munitions launch device
        Y36.24-●
  dirty bomb Y36.50-●
  explosion (of) Y36.20-●
    aerial bomb Y36.21-●
    after cessation of hostilities
      bomb placed during war operations
          Y36.82-●
      mine placed during war operations
          Y36.81-●
    bomb NOS —see also War operations, bomb(s)
        Y36.20-●
    fragments Y36.20-●
    grenade Y36.29-●

War operations *(Continued)*
  explosion *(Continued)*
    guided missile Y36.22-●
    improvised explosive device [IED]
        (person-borne) (roadside)
        (vehicle-borne) Y36.23-●
    land mine Y36.29-●
    marine mine (at sea) (in harbor) Y36.02-●
    marine weapon Y36.00-●
        specified NEC Y36.09-●
    own munitions or munitions launch
        device (accidental) Y36.24-●
    sea-based artillery shell Y36.03-●
    specified NEC Y36.29-●
    torpedo Y36.04-●
  fire Y36.30-●
    specified NEC Y36.39-●
  firearms
    discharge Y36.43-●
    pellets Y36.42-●
  flamethrower Y36.33-●
  fragments (from) (of)
    improvised explosive device [IED]
        (person-borne) (roadside)
        (vehicle-borne) Y36.26-●
    munitions Y36.25-●
    specified NEC Y36.29-●
    weapons Y36.27-●
  friendly fire Y36.92
  hand to hand (unarmed) combat Y36.44-●
  hot substances —*see* War operations, fire
  incendiary bullet Y36.32-●
  nuclear weapon (effects of) Y36.50-●
    acute radiation exposure Y36.54-●
    blast pressure Y36.51-●

War operations *(Continued)*
  nuclear weapon *(Continued)*
    direct blast Y36.51-●
    direct heat Y36.53-●
    fallout exposure Y36.54-●
    fireball Y36.53-●
    indirect blast (struck or crushed by blast
        debris) (being thrown by blast) Y36.52-●
    ionizing radiation (immediate exposure)
        Y36.54-●
    nuclear radiation Y36.54-●
    radiation
        ionizing (immediate exposure)
            Y36.54-●
        nuclear Y36.54-●
        thermal Y36.53-●
    secondary effects Y36.54-●
    specified NEC Y36.59-●
    thermal radiation Y36.53-●
  restriction of air (airway)
    intentional Y36.46-●
    unintentional Y36.47-●
  rubber bullets Y36.41-●
  shrapnel NOS Y36.29-●
  suffocation —*see* War operations, restriction of
      airways
  unconventional warfare NEC Y36.7X-●
  underwater blast NOS Y36.00-●
  warfare
    conventional NEC Y36.49-●
    unconventional NEC Y36.7X-●
  weapon of mass destruction [WMD] Y36.91
  weapons
    biological weapons Y36.6X-●
    chemical Y36.7X-●

War operations *(Continued)*
  weapons *(Continued)*
    nuclear (effects of) Y36.50-●
        acute radiation exposure Y36.54-●
        blast pressure Y36.51-●
        direct blast Y36.51-●
        direct heat Y36.53-●
        fallout exposure Y36.54-●
        fireball Y36.53-●
        radiation
            ionizing (immediate exposure) Y36.54-●
            nuclear Y36.54-●
            thermal Y36.53-●
        secondary effects Y36.54-●
        specified NEC Y36.59-●
    of mass destruction [WMD] Y36.91-●
Washed
  away by flood —*see* Flood
  off road by storm (transport vehicle) —*see* Forces
      of nature, cataclysmic storm
Weather exposure NEC —*see* Forces of nature
Weightlessness (causing injury) (effects of) (in
      spacecraft, real or simulated) X52
Work related condition Y99.0
Wound (accidental) NEC —*see also* Injury X58
  battle —*see also* War operations Y36.90
  gunshot —*see* Discharge, firearm by type
Wreck transport vehicle NEC —*see also* Accident,
      transport V89.9
Wrong
  device implanted into correct surgical site Y65.51
  fluid in infusion Y65.1
  patient, procedure performed on Y65.52
  procedure (operation) on correct patient Y65.51

W

PART III

ICD-10-CM Tabular List of Diseases and Injuries

CHAPTER 1

CERTAIN INFECTIOUS AND PARASITIC DISEASES (A00-B99)

OGCR Chapter-Specific Coding Guidelines

1. **Chapter 1: Certain Infectious and Parasitic Diseases (A00-B99)**

   a. **Human Immunodeficiency Virus (HIV) Infections**

      1) **Code only confirmed cases**

      Code only confirmed cases of HIV infection/illness. This is an exception to the hospital inpatient guideline Section II, H.

      In this context, "confirmation" does not require documentation of positive serology or culture for HIV; the provider's diagnostic statement that the patient is HIV positive, or has an HIV-related illness is sufficient.

      2) **Selection and sequencing of HIV codes**

         (a) **Patient admitted for HIV-related condition**

         If a patient is admitted for an HIV-related condition, the principal diagnosis should be B20, Human immunodeficiency virus [HIV] disease followed by additional diagnosis codes for all reported HIV-related conditions.

         (b) **Patient with HIV disease admitted for unrelated condition**

         If a patient with HIV disease is admitted for an unrelated condition (such as a traumatic injury), the code for the unrelated condition (e.g., the nature of injury code) should be the principal diagnosis. Other diagnoses would be B20 followed by additional diagnosis codes for all reported HIV-related conditions.

         (c) **Whether the patient is newly diagnosed**

         Whether the patient is newly diagnosed or has had previous admissions/encounters for HIV conditions is irrelevant to the sequencing decision.

         (d) **Asymptomatic human immunodeficiency virus**

         Z21, Asymptomatic human immunodeficiency virus [HIV] infection status, is to be applied when the patient without any documentation of symptoms is listed as being "HIV positive," "known HIV," "HIV test positive," or similar terminology. Do not use this code if the term "AIDS" is used or if the patient is treated for any HIV-related illness or is described as having any condition(s) resulting from his/her HIV positive status; use B20 in these cases.

         (e) **Patients with inconclusive HIV serology**

         Patients with inconclusive HIV serology, but no definitive diagnosis or manifestations of the illness, may be assigned code R75, Inconclusive laboratory evidence of human immunodeficiency virus [HIV].

         (f) **Previously diagnosed HIV-related illness**

         Patients with any known prior diagnosis of an HIV-related illness should be coded to B20. Once a patient has developed an HIV-related illness, the patient should always be assigned code B20 on every subsequent admission/encounter. Patients previously diagnosed with any HIV illness (B20) should never be assigned to R75 or Z21, Asymptomatic human immunodeficiency virus [HIV] infection status.

         (g) **HIV Infection in Pregnancy, Childbirth and the Puerperium**

         During pregnancy, childbirth or the puerperium, a patient admitted (or presenting for a health care encounter) because of an HIV-related illness should receive a principal diagnosis code of O98.7-, Human immunodeficiency [HIV] disease complicating pregnancy, childbirth and the puerperium, followed by B20 and the code(s) for the HIV-related illness(es). Codes from Chapter 15 always take sequencing priority.

         Patients with asymptomatic HIV infection status admitted (or presenting for a health care encounter) during pregnancy, childbirth, or the puerperium should receive codes of O98.7- and Z21.

         (h) **Encounters for testing for HIV**

         If a patient is being seen to determine his/her HIV status, use code Z11.4, Encounter for screening for human immunodeficiency virus [HIV]. Use additional codes for any associated high-risk behavior.

         If a patient with signs or symptoms is being seen for HIV testing, code the signs and symptoms. An additional counseling code Z71.7, Human immunodeficiency virus [HIV] counseling, may be used if counseling is provided during the encounter for the test.

         When a patient returns to be informed of his/her HIV test results and the test result is negative, use code Z71.7, Human immunodeficiency virus [HIV] counseling.

         If the results are positive, see previous guidelines and assign codes as appropriate.

      b. **Infectious agents as the cause of diseases classified to other chapters**

      Certain infections are classified in chapters other than Chapter 1 and no organism is identified as part of the infection code. In these instances, it is necessary to use an additional code from Chapter 1 to identify the organism. A code from category B95, Streptococcus, Staphylococcus, and Enterococcus as the cause of diseases classified to other chapters, B96, Other bacterial agents as the cause of diseases classified to other chapters, or B97, Viral agents as the cause of diseases classified to other chapters, is to be used as an additional code to identify the organism. An instructional note will be found at the infection code advising that an additional organism code is required.

      c. **Infections resistant to antibiotics**

      Many bacterial infections are resistant to current antibiotics. It is necessary to identify all infections documented as antibiotic resistant. Assign a code from category Z16, Resistance to antimicrobial drugs, following the infection code only if the infection code does not identify drug resistance.

      d. **Sepsis, Severe Sepsis, and Septic Shock**

      1) **Coding of Sepsis and Severe Sepsis**

         (a) **Sepsis**

         For a diagnosis of sepsis, assign the appropriate code for the underlying systemic infection. If the type of infection or causal organism is not further specified, assign code A41.9, Sepsis, unspecified organism.

         A code from subcategory R65.2, Severe sepsis, should not be assigned unless severe sepsis or an associated acute organ dysfunction is documented.

         (i) Negative or inconclusive blood cultures and sepsis

         Negative or inconclusive blood cultures do not preclude a diagnosis of sepsis in patients with clinical evidence of the condition, however, the provider should be queried.

         (ii) Urosepsis

         The term urosepsis is a nonspecific term. It is not to be considered synonymous with sepsis. It has no default code in the Alphabetic Index. Should a provider use this term, he/she must be queried for clarification.

         (iii) Sepsis with organ dysfunction

         If a patient has sepsis and associated acute organ dysfunction or multiple organ dysfunction (MOD), follow the instructions for coding severe sepsis.

         (iv) Acute organ dysfunction that is not clearly associated with the sepsis

         If a patient has sepsis and an acute organ dysfunction, but the medical record documentation indicates that the acute organ dysfunction is related to a medical condition other than the sepsis, do not assign a code from subcategory R65.2, Severe sepsis. An acute organ dysfunction must be associated with the sepsis in order to assign the severe sepsis code. If the documentation is not clear as to whether an acute organ dysfunction is related to the sepsis or another medical condition, query the provider.

         (b) **Severe sepsis**

         The coding of severe sepsis requires a minimum of 2 codes: first a code for the underlying systemic infection, followed by a code from subcategory R65.2, Severe sepsis. If the causal organism is not documented, assign code A41.9, Sepsis, unspecified organism, for the infection. Additional code(s) for the associated acute organ dysfunction are also required.

         Due to the complex nature of severe sepsis, some cases may require querying the provider prior to assignment of the codes.

      2) **Septic shock**

         (a) Septic shock generally refers to circulatory failure associated with severe sepsis, and therefore, it represents a type of acute organ dysfunction.

         For all cases of septic shock, the code for the systemic infection should be sequenced first, followed by code R65.21, Severe sepsis with septic shock or code T81.12, Postprocedural septic shock.

Any additional codes for the other acute organ dysfunctions should also be assigned. As noted in the sequencing instructions in the Tabular List, the code for septic shock cannot be assigned as a principal diagnosis.

3) Sequencing of severe sepsis

If severe sepsis is present on admission, and meets the definition of principal diagnosis, the underlying systemic infection should be assigned as principal diagnosis followed by the appropriate code from subcategory R65.2 as required by the sequencing rules in the Tabular List. A code from subcategory R65.2 can never be assigned as a principal diagnosis.

When severe sepsis develops during an encounter (it was not present on admission) the underlying systemic infection and the appropriate code from subcategory R65.2 should be assigned as secondary diagnoses.

Severe sepsis may be present on admission but the diagnosis may not be confirmed until sometime after admission. If the documentation is not clear whether severe sepsis was present on admission, the provider should be queried.

4) Sepsis and severe sepsis with a localized infection

If the reason for admission is both sepsis or severe sepsis and a localized infection, such as pneumonia or cellulitis, a code(s) for the underlying systemic infection should be assigned first and the code for the localized infection should be assigned as a secondary diagnosis. If the patient has severe sepsis, a code from subcategory R65.2 should also be assigned as a secondary diagnosis. If the patient is admitted with a localized infection, such as pneumonia, and sepsis/severe sepsis doesn't develop until after admission, the localized infection should be assigned first, followed by the appropriate sepsis/severe sepsis codes.

5) Sepsis due to a postprocedural infection

(a) Documentation of causal relationship

As with all postprocedural complications, code assignment is based on the provider's documentation of the relationship between the infection and the procedure.

(b) Sepsis due to a postprocedural infection

For infections following a procedure, a code from T81.40, to T81.43. Infection following a procedure, or O86.00 to O86.03, Infection of obstetric surgical wound, that identifies the site of the infection should be coded first, if known. Assign an additional code for sepsis following a procedure (T81.44) or sepsis following an obstetrical procedure (O86.04). Use an additional code to identify the infectious agent. If the patient has severe sepsis the appropriate code from subcategory R65.2 should also be assigned with the additional code(s) for any acute organ dysfunction.

For infections following infusion, transfusion, therapeutic injection, or immunization, a code from subcategory T80.2, Infections following infusion, transfusion, and therapeutic injection, or code T88.0-, Infection following immunization, should be coded first, followed by the code for the specific infection. If the patient has severe sepsis, the appropriate code from subcategory R65.2 should also be assigned, with the additional codes(s) for any acute organ dysfunction.

(c) Postprocedural infection and postprocedural septic shock

If a postprocedural infection has resulted in postprocedural septic shock, assign the codes indicated above for sepsis due to a postprocedural infection, followed by code T81.12-, Postprocedural septic shock. Do not assign code R65.21, Severe sepsis with septic shock. Additional code(s) should be assigned for any acute organ dysfunction.

6) Sepsis and severe sepsis associated with a noninfectious process (condition)

In some cases a noninfectious process (condition), such as trauma, may lead to an infection which can result in sepsis or severe sepsis. If sepsis or severe sepsis is documented as associated with a noninfectious condition, such as a burn or serious injury, and this condition meets the definition for principal diagnosis, the code for the noninfectious condition should be sequenced first, followed by the code for the resulting infection. If severe sepsis is present, a code from subcategory R65.2 should also be assigned with any associated organ dysfunction(s) codes. It is not necessary to assign a code from subcategory R65.1, Systemic inflammatory response syndrome (SIRS) of noninfectious origin, for these cases.

If the infection meets the definition of principal diagnosis it should be sequenced before the noninfectious condition. When both the associated noninfectious condition and the infection meet the definition of principal diagnosis either may be assigned as principal diagnosis.

Only one code from category R65, Symptoms and signs specifically associated with systemic inflammation and infection, should be assigned. Therefore, when a noninfectious condition leads to an infection resulting in severe sepsis, assign the appropriate code from subcategory R65.2, Severe sepsis. Do not additionally assign a code from subcategory R65.1, Systemic inflammatory response syndrome (SIRS) of noninfectious origin.

See Section I.C.18. SIRS due to non-infectious process

7) Sepsis and septic shock complicating abortion, pregnancy, childbirth, and the puerperium

See Section I.C.15. Sepsis and septic shock complicating abortion, pregnancy, childbirth and the puerperium

8) Newborn sepsis

See Section I.C.16. f. Bacterial sepsis of Newborn

e. Methicillin Resistant Staphylococcus aureus (MRSA) Conditions

1) Selection and sequencing of MRSA codes

(a) Combination codes for MRSA infection

When a patient is diagnosed with an infection that is due to methicillin resistant *Staphylococcus aureus* (MRSA), and that infection has a combination code that includes the causal organism (e.g., sepsis, pneumonia) assign the appropriate combination code for the condition (e.g., code A41.02, Sepsis due to Methicillin resistant Staphylococcus aureus or code J15.212, Pneumonia due to Methicillin resistant Staphylococcus aureus). Do not assign code B95.62, Methicillin resistant Staphylococcus aureus infection as the cause of diseases classified elsewhere, as an additional code because the combination code includes the type of infection and the MRSA organism. Do not assign a code from subcategory Z16.11, Resistance to penicillins, as an additional diagnosis.

See Section C.1. for instructions on coding and sequencing of sepsis and severe sepsis.

(b) Other codes for MRSA infection

When there is documentation of a current infection (e.g., wound infection, stitch abscess, urinary tract infection) due to MRSA, and that infection does not have a combination code that includes the causal organism, assign the appropriate code to identify the condition along with code B95.62, Methicillin resistant Staphylococcus aureus infection as the cause of diseases classified elsewhere for the MRSA infection. Do not assign a code from subcategory Z16.11, Resistance to penicillins.

(c) Methicillin susceptible Staphylococcus aureus (MSSA) and MRSA colonization

The condition or state of being colonized or carrying MSSA or MRSA is called colonization or carriage, while an individual person is described as being colonized or being a carrier. Colonization means that MSSA or MSRA is present on or in the body without necessarily causing illness. A positive MRSA colonization test might be documented by the provider as "MRSA screen positive" or "MRSA nasal swab positive".

Assign code Z22.322, Carrier or suspected carrier of Methicillin resistant Staphylococcus aureus, for patients documented as having MRSA colonization. Assign code Z22.321, Carrier or suspected carrier of Methicillin susceptible Staphylococcus aureus, for patient documented as having MSSA colonization. Colonization is not necessarily indicative of a disease process or as the cause of a specific condition the patient may have unless documented as such by the provider.

(d) MRSA colonization and infection

If a patient is documented as having both MRSA colonization and infection during a hospital admission, code Z22.322, Carrier or suspected carrier of Methicillin resistant Staphylococcus aureus, and a code for the MRSA infection may both be assigned.

f. Zika virus infections

1) Code only confirmed cases

Code only a confirmed diagnosis of Zika virus (A92.5, Zika virus disease) as documented by the provider. This is an exception to the hospital inpatient guideline Section II, H.

In this context, "confirmation" does not require documentation of the type of test performed; the physician's diagnostic statement that the condition is confirmed is sufficient. This code should be assigned regardless of the stated mode of transmission.

If the provider documents "suspected", "possible" or "probable" Zika, do not assign code A92.5. Assign a code(s) explaining the reason for encounter (such as fever, rash, or joint pain) or Z20.821, Contact with and (suspected) exposure to Zika virus.

CHAPTER 1

CERTAIN INFECTIOUS AND PARASITIC DISEASES (A00-B99)

Includes   diseases generally recognized as communicable or transmissible

Use additional code to identify resistance to antimicrobial drugs (Z16.-)

Excludes1   certain localized infections - see body system-related chapters

Excludes2   carrier or suspected carrier of infectious disease (Z22.-)

infectious and parasitic diseases complicating pregnancy, childbirth and the puerperium (O98.-)

infectious and parasitic diseases specific to the perinatal period (P35-P39)

influenza and other acute respiratory infections (J00-J22)

This chapter contains the following blocks:

A00-A09	Intestinal infectious diseases
A15-A19	Tuberculosis
A20-A28	Certain zoonotic bacterial diseases
A30-A49	Other bacterial diseases
A50-A64	Infections with a predominantly sexual mode of transmission
A65-A69	Other spirochetal diseases
A70-A74	Other diseases caused by chlamydiae
A75-A79	Rickettsioses
A80-A89	Viral and prion infections of the central nervous system
A90-A99	Arthropod-borne viral fevers and viral hemorrhagic fevers
B00-B09	Viral infections characterized by skin and mucous membrane lesions
B10	Other human herpesviruses
B15-B19	Viral hepatitis
B20	Human immunodeficiency virus [HIV] disease
B25-B34	Other viral diseases
B35-B49	Mycoses
B50-B64	Protozoal diseases
B65-B83	Helminthiases
B85-B89	Pediculosis, acariasis and other infestations
B90-B94	Sequelae of infectious and parasitic diseases
B95-B97	Bacterial and viral infectious agents
B99	Other infectious diseases

INTESTINAL INFECTIOUS DISEASES (A00-A09)

● **A00**   **Cholera**
A serious, often deadly, infectious disease of the small intestine

   A00.0   **Cholera due to Vibrio cholerae 01, biovar cholerae**
     Classical cholera

   A00.1   **Cholera due to Vibrio cholerae 01, biovar eltor**
     Cholera eltor

   A00.9   **Cholera, unspecified**

● **A01**   **Typhoid and paratyphoid fevers**
Caused by Salmonella typhi and Salmonella paratyphi A, B, and C bacteria

   ● **A01.0**   **Typhoid fever**
     Infection due to Salmonella typhi

     A01.00   **Typhoid fever, unspecified**

     A01.01   **Typhoid meningitis**

     A01.02   **Typhoid fever with heart involvement**
       Typhoid endocarditis
       Typhoid myocarditis

     A01.03   **Typhoid pneumonia** 🏷️

     A01.04   **Typhoid arthritis** 🏷️

     A01.05   **Typhoid osteomyelitis**

     A01.09   **Typhoid fever with other complications**

Item 1-1   **Salmonella** is a bacterium that lives in the intestines of fowl and mammals and can spread to humans through improper food preparation and cooking. Salmonellosis is an infection with the bacterium. Symptoms include diarrhea, fever, and abdominal cramps 12 to 72 hours after infection. The illness usually lasts 4 to 7 days, and most persons recover without treatment. The diarrhea may be so severe that the patient needs to be hospitalized. Patients with immunocompromised systems in chronic, ill health are more likely to have the infection invade their bloodstream with life-threatening results. For example, patients with sickle cell disease are more prone to salmonella osteomyelitis than others.

   A01.1   **Paratyphoid fever A**

   A01.2   **Paratyphoid fever B**

   A01.3   **Paratyphoid fever C**

   A01.4   **Paratyphoid fever, unspecified**
     Infection due to Salmonella paratyphi NOS

● **A02**   **Other salmonella infections**

   Includes   infection or foodborne intoxication due to any Salmonella species other than S. typhi and S. paratyphi

   A02.0   **Salmonella enteritis**
     Salmonellosis

   A02.1   **Salmonella sepsis** 🏷️

   ● **A02.2**   **Localized salmonella infections**

     A02.20   **Localized salmonella infection, unspecified**
       Specified in the documentation as localized, but unspecified as to type

     A02.21   **Salmonella meningitis**
       Specified as localized in the meninges

     A02.22   **Salmonella pneumonia** 🏷️
       Specified as localized in the lungs

     A02.23   **Salmonella arthritis** 🏷️
       Specified as localized in the joints

     A02.24   **Salmonella osteomyelitis** 🏷️
       Specified as localized in bone

     A02.25   **Salmonella pyelonephritis**
       Salmonella tubulo-interstitial nephropathy

     A02.29   **Salmonella with other localized infection**
       Specified as localized (because it is still under localized heading) but does not assign into any of the above codes

   A02.8   **Other specified salmonella infections**
     Any specified salmonella infection which does NOT assign into any of the above codes (not specified as localized)

   A02.9   **Salmonella infection, unspecified**
     Unspecified in the documentation as to specific type of salmonella

● **A03**   **Shigellosis**
An infectious disease caused by bacteria (Shigella)

   A03.0   **Shigellosis due to Shigella dysenteriae**
     Group A shigellosis [Shiga-Kruse dysentery]

   A03.1   **Shigellosis due to Shigella flexneri**
     Group B shigellosis

   A03.2   **Shigellosis due to Shigella boydii**
     Group C shigellosis

   A03.3   **Shigellosis due to Shigella sonnei**
     Group D shigellosis

   A03.8   **Other shigellosis**

   A03.9   **Shigellosis, unspecified**
     Bacillary dysentery NOS

● **A04**   **Other bacterial intestinal infections**

   Excludes1   bacterial foodborne intoxications, NEC (A05.-)
     tuberculous enteritis (A18.32)

   A04.0   **Enteropathogenic Escherichia coli infection**
     Pertaining to or producing intestinal disease

   A04.1   **Enterotoxigenic Escherichia coli infection**
     Producing or containing intestinal toxin

Figure 1-1 Electron micrograph of escherichia coli (E. coli) expressing P fimbriae. (Getty Image)

Item 1–2 *Escherichia coli [E. coli]* is a Gram-negative bacterium found in the intestinal tracts of humans and animals and is usually nonpathogenic. Pathogenic strains can cause diarrhea or pyogenic (pus-producing) infections. Can be a threat to food safety.

A04.2   Enteroinvasive Escherichia coli infection
Capable of penetrating and spreading through intestinal mucosal epithelium

A04.3   Enterohemorrhagic Escherichia coli infection
Causing bloody diarrhea, resulting from microorganisms

A04.4   Other intestinal Escherichia coli infections
Escherichia coli enteritis NOS

A04.5   Campylobacter enteritis
Spiral shaped bacterium

A04.6   Enteritis due to Yersinia enterocolitica
> **Excludes1**   extraintestinal yersiniosis (A28.2)

Transmitted by infected food/water and person-to-person contact, affecting intestinal tract

● **A04.7   Enterocolitis due to Clostridium difficile**
▶Clostridioides difficile colitis
Foodborne intoxication by Clostridium difficile
Pseudomembraneous colitis
Marked by fibrinous deposit (false membrane) with enmeshed necrotic cells

     A04.71   Enterocolitis due to Clostridium difficile, recurrent
         Coding Clinic: 2020, Q1, P18

     A04.72   Enterocolitis due to Clostridium difficile, not specified as recurrent

A04.8   Other specified bacterial intestinal infections

A04.9   Bacterial intestinal infection, unspecified
Bacterial enteritis NOS

● **A05   Other bacterial foodborne intoxications, not elsewhere classified**
> **Excludes1**   Clostridium difficile foodborne intoxication and infection (A04.7-)
> Escherichia coli infection (A04.0-A04.4)
> listeriosis (A32.-)
> salmonella foodborne intoxication and infection (A02.-)
> toxic effect of noxious foodstuffs (T61-T62)

A05.0   Foodborne staphylococcal intoxication

A05.1   Botulism food poisoning
Botulism NOS
Classical foodborne intoxication due to Clostridium botulinum
> **Excludes1**   infant botulism (A48.51)
> wound botulism (A48.52)

A05.2   Foodborne Clostridium perfringens [Clostridium welchii] intoxication
Type A causes gas gangrene and necrotizing colitis; major cause of food poisoning in humans
Enteritis necroticans
Pig-bel

A05.3   Foodborne Vibrio parahaemolyticus intoxication
Organism that survives only in high salt environment (halophilic), major cause of gastroenteritis due to consumption of raw or improperly cooked fish/seafood

A05.4   Foodborne Bacillus cereus intoxication
Spore-forming species commonly found in soil, causes food poisoning from formation of intestinal toxins in contaminated foods

A05.5   Foodborne Vibrio vulnificus intoxication
Species that survives in high salt environment (halophilic) with infection by eating raw seafood causes septicemia and cellulitis

A05.8   Other specified bacterial foodborne intoxications

A05.9   Bacterial foodborne intoxication, unspecified

● **A06   Amebiasis**
An intestinal illness caused by the microscopic parasite Entamoeba histolytica
> **Includes**   infection due to Entamoeba histolytica
> **Excludes1**   other protozoal intestinal diseases (A07.-)
> **Excludes2**   acanthamebiasis (B60.1-)
> Naegleriasis (B60.2)

A06.0   Acute amebic dysentery
Acute amebiasis
Intestinal amebiasis NOS

A06.1   Chronic intestinal amebiasis

A06.2   Amebic nondysenteric colitis
Pertaining to single cell microorganism

A06.3   Ameboma of intestine
Tumorlike mass produced by localized inflammation often in intestine
Ameboma NOS

A06.4   Amebic liver abscess
Hepatic amebiasis

A06.5   Amebic lung abscess 🔗
Amebic abscess of lung (and liver)

A06.6   Amebic brain abscess
Amebic abscess of brain (and liver) (and lung)

A06.7   Cutaneous amebiasis

● **A06.8   Amebic infection of other sites**

     A06.81   Amebic cystitis

     A06.82   Other amebic genitourinary infections
         Amebic balanitis
         Amebic vesiculitis
         Amebic vulvovaginitis

         A06.89   Other amebic infections
             Amebic appendicitis
             Amebic splenic abscess

A06.9   Amebiasis, unspecified

● **A07   Other protozoal intestinal diseases**
A07.0   Balantidiasis
Balantidial dysentery
Infection by protozoa that may cause diarrhea and dysentery, with ulceration of colonic mucous membranes

A07.1   Giardiasis [lambliasis]
Common infection in small intestine spread by contaminated food, water, or direct person-to-person contact

A07.2   Cryptosporidiosis 🔗
Human infection with protozoa usually seen as self-limited diarrhea in those who work with cattle

A07.3   Isosporiasis
Human intestinal disease caused by protozoa
Infection due to Isospora belli and Isospora hominis
Intestinal coccidiosis
Isosporosis

A07.4   Cyclosporiasis
Infection by protozoa with most common species infecting humans being C cayetanensis

A07.8 Other specified protozoal intestinal diseases
Intestinal microsporidiosis
Intestinal trichomoniasis
Sarcocystosis
Sarcosporidiosis

A07.9 Protozoal intestinal disease, unspecified
Flagellate diarrhea
Protozoal colitis
Protozoal diarrhea
Protozoal dysentery

● **A08 Viral and other specified intestinal infections**
> **Excludes1** influenza with involvement of gastrointestinal tract (J09.X3, J10.2, J11.2)

A08.0 Rotaviral enteritis

● **A08.1 Acute gastroenteropathy due to Norwalk agent and other small round viruses**

    A08.11 Acute gastroenteropathy due to Norwalk agent
Acute gastroenteropathy due to Norovirus
Acute gastroenteropathy due to Norwalk-like agent

    A08.19 Acute gastroenteropathy due to other small round viruses
Acute gastroenteropathy due to small round virus [SRV] NOS

A08.2 Adenoviral enteritis

● **A08.3 Other viral enteritis**

    A08.31 Calicivirus enteritis

    A08.32 Astrovirus enteritis

    A08.39 Other viral enteritis
Coxsackie virus enteritis
Echovirus enteritis
Enterovirus enteritis NEC
Torovirus enteritis

A08.4 Viral intestinal infection, unspecified
Viral enteritis NOS
Viral gastroenteritis NOS
Viral gastroenteropathy NOS
Coding Clinic: 2016, Q3, P12

A08.8 Other specified intestinal infections

A09 Infectious gastroenteritis and colitis, unspecified
Infectious colitis NOS
Infectious enteritis NOS
Infectious gastroenteritis NOS
> **Excludes1** colitis NOS (K52.9)
> diarrhea NOS (R19.7)
> enteritis NOS (K52.9)
> gastroenteritis NOS (K52.9)
> noninfective gastroenteritis and colitis, unspecified (K52.9)

TUBERCULOSIS (A15–A19)

> **Includes** infections due to Mycobacterium tuberculosis and Mycobacterium bovis
> **Excludes1** congenital tuberculosis (P37.0)
> nonspecific reaction to test for tuberculosis without active tuberculosis (R76.1-)
> pneumoconiosis associated with tuberculosis, any type in A15 (J65)
> positive PPD (R76.11)
> positive tuberculin skin test without active tuberculosis (R76.11)
> sequelae of tuberculosis (B90.-)
> silicotuberculosis (J65)

● **A15 Respiratory tuberculosis**

A15.0 Tuberculosis of lung
Tuberculous bronchiectasis
Chronic dilatation of bronchi
Tuberculous fibrosis of lung
Tuberculous pneumonia
Tuberculous pneumothorax

Figure 1-2 Far advanced bilateral pulmonary tuberculosis before and after 8 months of treatment with streptomycin, PAS, and isoniazid. (Getty Image)

Item 1–3 Tuberculosis is a common and deadly infectious disease caused by the *Mycobacterium tuberculosis* organism. The first tuberculosis infection is called the **primary infection** and most commonly attacks the lungs but can affect the central nervous system, lymphatic system, circulatory system, genitourinary system, bones, joints, and even the skin. A **Ghon** lesion is the **initial lesion.** A **secondary lesion** occurs when the tubercle bacilli are carried to other areas.

Item 1–4 Although it primarily affects the lungs, the bacteria *Mycobacterium tuberculosis* can travel from the pulmonary circulation to virtually any organ in the body, much as a cancer metastasizes to a secondary site. If the immune system becomes compromised by age or disease, what would otherwise be a self-limiting primary tuberculosis in the lungs will develop in other organs. These are known as extrapulmonary sites.

A15.4 Tuberculosis of intrathoracic lymph nodes
Tuberculosis of hilar lymph nodes
Tuberculosis of mediastinal lymph nodes
Tuberculosis of tracheobronchial lymph nodes
> **Excludes1** tuberculosis specified as primary (A15.7)

A15.5 Tuberculosis of larynx, trachea and bronchus
Tuberculosis of bronchus
Tuberculosis of glottis
Tuberculosis of larynx
Tuberculosis of trachea

A15.6 Tuberculous pleurisy
Tuberculosis of pleura
Tuberculous empyema
> **Excludes1** primary respiratory tuberculosis (A15.7)

A15.7 Primary respiratory tuberculosis

A15.8 Other respiratory tuberculosis
Mediastinal tuberculosis
Nasopharyngeal tuberculosis
Tuberculosis of nose
Tuberculosis of sinus [any nasal]

A15.9 Respiratory tuberculosis unspecified

● **A17 Tuberculosis of nervous system**

A17.0 Tuberculous meningitis
Tuberculosis of meninges (cerebral) (spinal)
Tuberculous leptomeningitis
> **Excludes1** tuberculous meningoencephalitis (A17.82)

A17.1 Meningeal tuberculoma
Tuberculoma of meninges (cerebral) (spinal)
> **Excludes2** tuberculoma of brain and spinal cord (A17.81)

● **A17.8 Other tuberculosis of nervous system**

    A17.81 Tuberculoma of brain and spinal cord
Tuberculous abscess of brain and spinal cord

    A17.82 Tuberculous meningoencephalitis
Inflammation of brain and meninges; AKA cerebromeningitis and encephalomeningitis
Tuberculous myelitis

    A17.83 Tuberculous neuritis
Tuberculous mononeuropathy

    A17.89 Other tuberculosis of nervous system
Tuberculous polyneuropathy

A17.9 Tuberculosis of nervous system, unspecified

▶ New   ⇒ Revised   ~~deleted~~ Deleted   Excludes 1   Excludes 2   Includes   Use additional   Code first   Code also   Key words
OGCR Official Guidelines   X Assign placeholder X   ● Use Additional Character(s)   ▶ Manifestation Code   Hierarchical Condition Category   **Coding Clinic**

● **A18   Tuberculosis of other organs**
  ● **A18.0   Tuberculosis of bones and joints**
    A18.01   Tuberculosis of spine
      Pott's disease or curvature of spine
      Tuberculous arthritis
      Tuberculous osteomyelitis of spine
      Tuberculous spondylitis
    A18.02   Tuberculous arthritis of other joints
      Tuberculosis of hip (joint)
      Tuberculosis of knee (joint)
    A18.03   Tuberculosis of other bones
      Tuberculous mastoiditis
      Tuberculous osteomyelitis
    A18.09   Other musculoskeletal tuberculosis
      Tuberculous myositis
      Tuberculous synovitis
      Tuberculous tenosynovitis

  ● **A18.1   Tuberculosis of genitourinary system**
    A18.10   Tuberculosis of genitourinary system, unspecified
    A18.11   Tuberculosis of kidney and ureter
    A18.12   Tuberculosis of bladder
    A18.13   Tuberculosis of other urinary organs
      Tuberculous urethritis
    A18.14   Tuberculosis of prostate   A
    A18.15   Tuberculosis of other male genital organs
    A18.16   Tuberculosis of cervix
    A18.17   Tuberculous female pelvic inflammatory disease
      Tuberculous endometritis
      Tuberculous oophoritis and salpingitis
      Oophoritis = inflammation of ovary
      Salpingitis = inflammation of fallopian tube
    A18.18   Tuberculosis of other female genital organs
      Tuberculous ulceration of vulva

  A18.2   Tuberculous peripheral lymphadenopathy
    Tuberculous adenitis
    Excludes2   tuberculosis of bronchial and mediastinal lymph nodes (A15.4)
      tuberculosis of mesenteric and retroperitoneal lymph nodes (A18.39)
      tuberculous tracheobronchial adenopathy (A15.4)

  ● **A18.3   Tuberculosis of intestines, peritoneum and mesenteric glands**
    A18.31   Tuberculous peritonitis
      Tuberculous ascites
    A18.32   Tuberculous enteritis
      Tuberculosis of anus and rectum
      Tuberculosis of intestine (large) (small)
    A18.39   Retroperitoneal tuberculosis
      Tuberculosis of mesenteric glands
      Tuberculosis of retroperitoneal (lymph glands)

  A18.4   Tuberculosis of skin and subcutaneous tissue
    Erythema induratum, tuberculous
    ⇒Lupus exedens
    Lupus vulgaris NOS
    Lupus vulgaris of eyelid
    Cutaneous tuberculosis characterized by reddish brown plaque on skin surrounded by papules and nodules
    Scrofuloderma
    Type of cutaneous tuberculosis, with direct extension of tuberculosis into skin from underlying structures; AKA tuberculosis colliquativa
    Tuberculosis of external ear
    Excludes2   lupus erythematosus (L93.-)
      systemic lupus erythematosus (M32.-)

  ● **A18.5   Tuberculosis of eye**
    Excludes2   lupus vulgaris of eyelid (A18.4)
    A18.50   Tuberculosis of eye, unspecified
    A18.51   Tuberculous episcleritis
      Inflammation of episclera and adjacent tissues

Item 1-5   Miliary tuberculosis can be a life-threatening condition. If a tuberculous lesion enters a blood vessel, immense dissemination of tuberculous organisms can occur if the immune system is weak. High-risk populations—children under 4 years of age, the elderly, or the immunocompromised—are particularly prone to this type of infection. The lesions will have a millet seedlike appearance on chest x-ray. Bronchial washings and biopsy may aid in diagnosis.

    A18.52   Tuberculous keratitis
      Tuberculous interstitial keratitis
      Tuberculous keratoconjunctivitis (interstitial) (phlyctenular)
      Inflammation of cornea and conjunctiva
    A18.53   Tuberculous chorioretinitis
      Inflammation of choroid and retina; retinochoroiditis
    A18.54   Tuberculous iridocyclitis
      Inflammation of iris and ciliary body
    A18.59   Other tuberculosis of eye
      Tuberculous conjunctivitis

  A18.6   Tuberculosis of (inner) (middle) ear
    Tuberculous otitis media
    Excludes2   tuberculosis of external ear (A18.4)
      tuberculous mastoiditis (A18.03)

  A18.7   Tuberculosis of adrenal glands
    Tuberculous Addison's disease

  ● **A18.8   Tuberculosis of other specified organs**
    A18.81   Tuberculosis of thyroid gland
    A18.82   Tuberculosis of other endocrine glands
      Tuberculosis of pituitary gland
      Tuberculosis of thymus gland
    A18.83   Tuberculosis of digestive tract organs, not elsewhere classified
      Excludes1   tuberculosis of intestine (A18.32)
    A18.84   Tuberculosis of heart
      Tuberculous cardiomyopathy
      Tuberculous endocarditis
      Tuberculous myocarditis
      Tuberculous pericarditis
    A18.85   Tuberculosis of spleen
    A18.89   Tuberculosis of other sites
      Tuberculosis of muscle
      Tuberculous cerebral arteritis

● **A19   Miliary tuberculosis**
    Includes   disseminated tuberculosis
      generalized tuberculosis
      tuberculous polyserositis
  A19.0   Acute miliary tuberculosis of a single specified site
  A19.1   Acute miliary tuberculosis of multiple sites
  A19.2   Acute miliary tuberculosis, unspecified
  A19.8   Other miliary tuberculosis
  A19.9   Miliary tuberculosis, unspecified

CERTAIN ZOONOTIC BACTERIAL DISEASES (A20-A28)

● **A20   Plague**
  Infectious disease caused by a Yersinia pestis bacterium, transmitted by a rodent flea bite or handling of infected animal
    Includes   infection due to Yersinia pestis
  A20.0   Bubonic plague
  A20.1   Cellulocutaneous plague
    Skin and subcutaneous tissue plague
  A20.2   Pneumonic plague 🦠
  A20.3   Plague meningitis
  A20.7   Septicemic plague 🦠
  A20.8   Other forms of plague
    Abortive plague
    Asymptomatic plague
    Pestis minor
    Systemic bacterial disease
  A20.9   Plague, unspecified

CHAPTER 1 (A00-B99)

CHAPTER 1 (A00-B99)

● **A21   Tularemia**
Caused by Francisella tularensis bacterium found in rodents, rabbits, and hares and transmitted to humans by contact with infected animal tissues or by ticks, biting flies, or mosquitoes

> **Includes**   deer-fly fever
> infection due to Francisella tularensis
> rabbit fever

Coding Clinic: 2016, Q4, P25

A21.0   Ulceroglandular tularemia
Most common form of tularemia in humans is painful, swollen, erythematous papule at point of inoculation that ruptures to form shallow ulcer

A21.1   Oculoglandular tularemia
Primary site of entry is conjunctival sac, results in granulomatous corneal lesions
Ophthalmic tularemia

A21.2   Pulmonary tularemia 🐾

A21.3   Gastrointestinal tularemia
Abdominal tularemia

A21.7   Generalized tularemia

A21.8   Other forms of tularemia

A21.9   Tularemia, unspecified

● **A22   Anthrax**
An acute infectious disease caused by the spore-forming Bacillus anthracis; occurs in humans exposed to infected animals or tissue from infected animals

> **Includes**   infection due to Bacillus anthracis

A22.0   Cutaneous anthrax
Malignant carbuncle
Malignant pustule

A22.1   Pulmonary anthrax 🐾
Inhalation anthrax
Ragpicker's disease
Woolsorter's disease

A22.2   Gastrointestinal anthrax

A22.7   Anthrax sepsis 🐾
Infectious bacterial disease

A22.8   Other forms of anthrax
Anthrax meningitis

A22.9   Anthrax, unspecified

● **A23   Brucellosis**

> **Includes**   Malta fever
> Mediterranean fever
> undulant fever

A23.0   Brucellosis due to Brucella melitensis
Resulting in flu-like symptoms that may lead to chronic symptoms that include recurrent fevers, joint pain, and fatigue

A23.1   Brucellosis due to Brucella abortus
Most common cause of brucellosis in humans; AKA Bang bacillus

A23.2   Brucellosis due to Brucella suis
Species found primarily in pigs, rabbits, and reindeer

A23.3   Brucellosis due to Brucella canis
Species that causes respiratory tract infection in humans

A23.8   Other brucellosis

A23.9   Brucellosis, unspecified

Item 1-6   Brucellosis: An infectious disease caused by the bacterium Brucella. Humans are infected by contact with contaminated animals or animal products. In humans brucellosis symptoms that are similar to the flu include fever, sweats, headaches, back pains, and physical weakness. Severe infections of the central nervous system or lining of the heart may occur. Brucellosis can also cause chronic symptoms that include recurrent fevers, joint pain, and fatigue.

● **A24   Glanders and melioidosis**
Infection, usually of rodents, which spreads to other animals and humans, caused by Burkholderia pseudomallei through break in skin contaminated with infested soil or water

A24.0   Glanders
Infection due to Pseudomonas mallei
Malleus

A24.1   Acute and fulminating melioidosis
Melioidosis pneumonia
Melioidosis sepsis

A24.2   Subacute and chronic melioidosis

A24.3   Other melioidosis

A24.9   Melioidosis, unspecified
Infection due to Pseudomonas pseudomallei NOS
Whitmore's disease

● **A25   Rat-bite fevers**
RBF, infectious disease caused by Streptobacillus moniliformis or Spirillum minus.

A25.0   Spirillosis
Any disease condition caused by spirilla
Sodoku

A25.1   Streptobacillosis
Acute, febrile human illness caused by bacteria transmitted by rats in most cases, passed from rodent to human via rodent's urine or mucous secretions; AKA rat fever
Epidemic arthritic erythema
Haverhill fever
Streptobacillary rat-bite fever

A25.9   Rat-bite fever, unspecified

● **A26   Erysipeloid**
Infection with Erysipelothrix rhusiopathiae, occurring often as occupational disease resulting from handling infected fish, shellfish, meat, or poultry

A26.0   Cutaneous erysipeloid
Erythema migrans

A26.7   Erysipelothrix sepsis 🐾

A26.8   Other forms of erysipeloid

A26.9   Erysipeloid, unspecified

● **A27   Leptospirosis**
Occurs most commonly in the tropics

A27.0   Leptospirosis icterohemorrhagica
Leptospiral or spirochetal jaundice (hemorrhagic)
Weil's disease

● **A27.8   Other forms of leptospirosis**

A27.81   Aseptic meningitis in leptospirosis

A27.89   Other forms of leptospirosis

A27.9   Leptospirosis, unspecified

● **A28   Other zoonotic bacterial diseases, not elsewhere classified**

A28.0   Pasteurellosis
Infection of humans or other animals by species of Pasteurella

A28.1   Cat-scratch disease
Cat-scratch fever

A28.2   Extraintestinal yersiniosis
Infection from Yersinia enterocolitica; AKA enteric yersiniosis, intestinal yersiniosis, Yersinia enteritis

> **Excludes1**   enteritis due to Yersinia enterocolitica (A04.6)
> plague (A20.-)

A28.8   Other specified zoonotic bacterial diseases, not elsewhere classified

A28.9   Zoonotic bacterial disease, unspecified

OTHER BACTERIAL DISEASES (A30-A49)

● **A30   Leprosy [Hansen's disease]**
Chronic infectious disease attacking the skin, peripheral nerves, and mucous membranes

> **Includes**   infection due to Mycobacterium leprae
> **Excludes1**   sequelae of leprosy (B92)

A30.0   Indeterminate leprosy
I leprosy

A30.1   Tuberculoid leprosy
TT leprosy

▶ New   ⇒ Revised   ~~deleted~~ Deleted   Excludes 1   Excludes 2   Includes   Use additional   Code first   Code also   Key words
OGCR Official Guidelines   X Assign placeholder X   ● Use Additional Character(s)   ▶ Manifestation Code   🐾 Hierarchical Condition Category   Coding Clinic

A30.2   **Borderline tuberculoid leprosy**
    BT leprosy

A30.3   **Borderline leprosy**
    BB leprosy

A30.4   **Borderline lepromatous leprosy**
    BL leprosy

A30.5   **Lepromatous leprosy**
    LL leprosy

A30.8   **Other forms of leprosy**

A30.9   **Leprosy, unspecified**

● A31   **Infection due to other mycobacteria**
    Excludes2 leprosy (A30.-)
                 tuberculosis (A15-A19)

A31.0   **Pulmonary mycobacterial infection** 🔖
    Infection due to Mycobacterium avium
    Infection due to Mycobacterium intracellulare [Battey bacillus]
    Infection due to Mycobacterium kansasii

A31.1   **Cutaneous mycobacterial infection**
    Buruli ulcer
    Infection due to Mycobacterium marinum
    Infection due to Mycobacterium ulcerans

A31.2   **Disseminated mycobacterium avium-intracellulare complex (DMAC)** 🔖
    MAC sepsis

A31.8   **Other mycobacterial infections**

A31.9   **Mycobacterial infection, unspecified**
    Atypical mycobacterial infection NOS
    Mycobacteriosis NOS

● A32   **Listeriosis**
    Infection caused by Listeria monocytogenes
    Includes listerial foodborne infection
    Excludes1 neonatal (disseminated) listeriosis (P37.2)

A32.0   **Cutaneous listeriosis**

● A32.1   **Listerial meningitis and meningoencephalitis**
    A32.11   **Listerial meningitis**
    A32.12   **Listerial meningoencephalitis**

A32.7   **Listerial sepsis** 🔖

● A32.8   **Other forms of listeriosis**
    A32.81   **Oculoglandular listeriosis**
        Primary infection site is conjunctival sac, which if untreated may result in perforation of cornea and optic atrophy

    A32.82   **Listerial endocarditis**
        Exudative and proliferative inflammatory condition of endocardium caused by listeria bacteria

    A32.89   **Other forms of listeriosis**
        Listerial cerebral arteritis

A32.9   **Listeriosis, unspecified**

A33   **Tetanus neonatorum**   **N**
    Neonate = newborn

A34   **Obstetrical tetanus**   **M**

A35   **Other tetanus**
    Tetanus NOS
    Excludes1 tetanus neonatorum (A33)
                 obstetrical tetanus (A34)

● A36   **Diphtheria**
A36.0   **Pharyngeal diphtheria**
    Diphtheritic membranous angina
    Tonsillar diphtheria

A36.1   **Nasopharyngeal diphtheria**

A36.2   **Laryngeal diphtheria**
    Diphtheritic laryngotracheitis

A36.3   **Cutaneous diphtheria**
    Excludes2 erythrasma (L08.1)

Item 1-7 Diphtheria: *A highly contagious bacterial disease that results in the formation of an adherent membrane in the throat that may lead to suffocation. In its most poisonous form, it attacks the heart and lungs. It is spread by direct physical contact or breathing the aerosolized secretions of infected individuals. The exact location is specified in the codes.*

● A36.8   **Other diphtheria**
    A36.81   **Diphtheritic cardiomyopathy** 🔖
        Diphtheritic myocarditis
    A36.82   **Diphtheritic radiculomyelitis**
    A36.83   **Diphtheritic polyneuritis**
    A36.84   **Diphtheritic tubulo-interstitial nephropathy**
    A36.85   **Diphtheritic cystitis**
    A36.86   **Diphtheritic conjunctivitis**
    A36.89   **Other diphtheritic complications**
        Diphtheritic peritonitis

A36.9   **Diphtheria, unspecified**

● A37   **Whooping cough**
    Pertussis is a highly contagious disease caused by the bacterium Bordetella pertussis and results in a whooping sounding cough.

● A37.0   **Whooping cough due to Bordetella pertussis**
    A37.00   **Whooping cough due to Bordetella pertussis without pneumonia**
        Paroxysmal cough due to Bordetella pertussis without pneumonia
    A37.01   **Whooping cough due to Bordetella pertussis with pneumonia**
        Paroxysmal cough due to Bordetella pertussis without pneumonia

● A37.1   **Whooping cough due to Bordetella parapertussis**
    A37.10   **Whooping cough due to Bordetella parapertussis without pneumonia**
    A37.11   **Whooping cough due to Bordetella parapertussis with pneumonia**

● A37.8   **Whooping cough due to other Bordetella species**
    A37.80   **Whooping cough due to other Bordetella species without pneumonia**
    A37.81   **Whooping cough due to other Bordetella species with pneumonia**

● A37.9   **Whooping cough, unspecified species**
    A37.90   **Whooping cough, unspecified species without pneumonia**
    A37.91   **Whooping cough, unspecified species with pneumonia**

● A38   **Scarlet fever**
    Most commonly caused by the bacteria Streptococcus pneumoniae and Neisseria meningitides
    Includes scarlatina
    Excludes2 streptococcal sore throat (J02.0)

A38.0   **Scarlet fever with otitis media**
A38.1   **Scarlet fever with myocarditis**
A38.8   **Scarlet fever with other complications**
A38.9   **Scarlet fever, uncomplicated**
    Scarlet fever, NOS

● A39   **Meningococcal infection**
    Most commonly caused by the bacteria Streptococcus pneumoniae and Neisseria meningitides

A39.0   **Meningococcal meningitis**
A39.1   **Waterhouse-Friderichsen syndrome** 🔖
    Fulminating complication of meningococcemia
    Meningococcal hemorrhagic adrenalitis
    Meningococcic adrenal syndrome

A39.2   **Acute meningococcemia** 🔖
A39.3   **Chronic meningococcemia** 🔖
A39.4   **Meningococcemia, unspecified** 🔖
● A39.5   **Meningococcal heart disease**
    A39.50   **Meningococcal carditis, unspecified**
    A39.51   **Meningococcal endocarditis**
    A39.52   **Meningococcal myocarditis**
    A39.53   **Meningococcal pericarditis**

CHAPTER 1 (A00-B99)

● **A39.8   Other meningococcal infections**

     A39.81   Meningococcal encephalitis

     A39.82   Meningococcal retrobulbar neuritis

         Optic neuritis in portion of optic nerve posterior to eyeball; AKA postocular optic neuritis

     A39.83   Meningococcal arthritis 🜚

     A39.84   Postmeningococcal arthritis 🜚

     A39.89   Other meningococcal infections

         Meningococcal conjunctivitis

A39.9   Meningococcal infection, unspecified

     Meningococcal disease NOS

● **A40   Streptococcal sepsis**

     Code first

         , if applicable, postprocedural sepsis (T81.44-)

         sepsis due to central venous catheter (T80.211-)

         streptococcal sepsis during labor (O75.3)

         streptococcal sepsis following abortion or ectopic or molar pregnancy (O03.37, O03.87, O04.87, O07.37, O08.82)

         streptococcal sepsis following immunization (T88.0-)

         streptococcal sepsis following infusion, transfusion or therapeutic injection (T80.22-, T80.29-)

     Excludes1   neonatal (P36.0-P36.1)

         puerperal sepsis (O85)

         sepsis due to Streptococcus, group D (A41.81)

A40.0   Sepsis due to streptococcus, group A 🜚

A40.1   Sepsis due to streptococcus, group B 🜚

     Coding Clinic: 2019, Q1, P14

A40.3   Sepsis due to Streptococcus pneumoniae 🜚

     Pneumococcal sepsis

A40.8   Other streptococcal sepsis 🜚

A40.9   Streptococcal sepsis, unspecified 🜚

● **A41   Other sepsis**

     Code first

         , if applicable, postprocedural sepsis (T81.44-)

         sepsis due to central venous catheter (T80.211-)

         sepsis during labor (O75.3)

         sepsis following abortion, ectopic or molar pregnancy (O03.37, O03.87, O04.87, O07.37, O08.82)

         sepsis following immunization (T88.0-)

         sepsis following infusion, transfusion or therapeutic injection (T80.22-, T80.29-)

     Excludes1   bacteremia NOS (R78.81)

         neonatal (P36.-)

         puerperal sepsis (O85)

         streptococcal sepsis (A40.-)

     Excludes2   sepsis (due to) (in) actinomycotic (A42.7)

         sepsis (due to) (in) anthrax (A22.7)

         sepsis (due to) (in) candidal (B37.7)

         sepsis (due to) (in) Erysipelothrix (A26.7)

         sepsis (due to) (in) extraintestinal yersiniosis (A28.2)

         sepsis (due to) (in) gonococcal (A54.86)

         sepsis (due to) (in) herpesviral (B00.7)

         sepsis (due to) (in) listerial (A32.7)

         sepsis (due to) (in) melioidosis (A24.1)

         sepsis (due to) (in) meningococcal (A39.2-A39.4)

         sepsis (due to) (in) plague (A20.7)

         sepsis (due to) (in) tularemia (A21.7)

         toxic shock syndrome (A48.3)

     Coding Clinic: 2022, Q1, P35; 2016, Q1, P39

● **A41.0   Sepsis due to Staphylococcus aureus**

     A41.01   Sepsis due to Methicillin susceptible Staphylococcus aureus 🜚

         MSSA sepsis

         Staphylococcus aureus sepsis NOS

     A41.02   Sepsis due to Methicillin resistant Staphylococcus aureus 🜚

     A41.1   Sepsis due to other specified staphylococcus 🜚

         Coagulase negative staphylococcus sepsis

         Coding Clinic: 2024, Q1, P19

     A41.2   Sepsis due to unspecified staphylococcus 🜚

     A41.3   Sepsis due to Hemophilus influenzae 🜚

     A41.4   Sepsis due to anaerobes 🜚

         Excludes1   gas gangrene (A48.0)

● **A41.5   Sepsis due to other Gram-negative organisms**

     A41.50   Gram-negative sepsis, unspecified 🜚

         Gram-negative sepsis NOS

     A41.51   Sepsis due to Escherichia coli [E. coli] 🜚

         Coding Clinic: 2018, Q1, P16

     A41.52   Sepsis due to Pseudomonas 🜚

         Pseudomonas aeruginosa

     A41.53   Sepsis due to Serratia 🜚

     A41.54   Sepsis due to Acinetobacter baumannii

     A41.59   Other Gram-negative sepsis 🜚

         Coding Clinic: 2019, Q1, P13

● **A41.8   Other specified sepsis**

     A41.81   Sepsis due to Enterococcus 🜚

     A41.89   Other specified sepsis 🜚

         Coding Clinic: 2021, Q1, P33; 2016, Q3, P8-14

     A41.9   Sepsis, unspecified organism 🜚

         Septicemia NOS

         Coding Clinic: 2022, Q2, P5; Q1, P30; 2018, Q4, P18

● **A42   Actinomycosis**

     Excludes1   actinomycetoma (B47.1)

     A42.0   Pulmonary actinomycosis 🜚

     A42.1   Abdominal actinomycosis

     A42.2   Cervicofacial actinomycosis

     A42.7   Actinomycotic sepsis 🜚

● **A42.8   Other forms of actinomycosis**

     A42.81   Actinomycotic meningitis

     A42.82   Actinomycotic encephalitis

     A42.89   Other forms of actinomycosis

     A42.9   Actinomycosis, unspecified

● **A43   Nocardiosis**

     A43.0   Pulmonary nocardiosis 🜚

     A43.1   Cutaneous nocardiosis

     A43.8   Other forms of nocardiosis

     A43.9   Nocardiosis, unspecified

● **A44   Bartonellosis**

     A44.0   Systemic bartonellosis

         Oroya fever

     A44.1   Cutaneous and mucocutaneous bartonellosis

         Verruga peruana

     A44.8   Other forms of bartonellosis

     A44.9   Bartonellosis, unspecified

    A46   Erysipelas

     Excludes1   postpartum or puerperal erysipelas (O86.89)

● **A48   Other bacterial diseases, not elsewhere classified**

     Excludes1   actinomycetoma (B47.1)

     A48.0   Gas gangrene 🜚

         Clostridial cellulitis

         Clostridial myonecrosis

         Coding Clinic: 2017, Q4, P102

     A48.1   Legionnaires' disease 🜚

     A48.2   Nonpneumonic Legionnaires' disease [Pontiac fever]

     A48.3   Toxic shock syndrome 🜚

         Use additional code to identify the organism (B95, B96)

         Excludes1   endotoxic shock NOS (R57.8)

                 sepsis NOS (A41.9)

         Coding Clinic: 2022, Q1, P35

▶ New   ⇒ Revised   ~~deleted~~ Deleted   Excludes 1   Excludes 2   Includes   Use additional   Code first   Code also   Key words

OGCR Official Guidelines   X Assign placeholder X   ● Use Additional Character(s)   ▶ Manifestation Code   🜚 Hierarchical Condition Category   Coding Clinic

A48.4   **Brazilian purpuric fever**
Systemic Hemophilus aegyptius infection

● **A48.5**   **Other specified botulism**
Non-foodborne intoxication due to toxins of
Clostridium botulinum [C. botulinum]

     Excludes1   food poisoning due to toxins of
Clostridium botulinum (A05.1)

     A48.51   **Infant botulism**   P

     A48.52   **Wound botulism**
Non-foodborne botulism NOS
Use additional code for associated wound

A48.8   **Other specified bacterial diseases**

● **A49**   **Bacterial infection of unspecified site**

     Excludes1   bacterial agents as the cause of diseases classified
elsewhere (B95-B96)
chlamydial infection NOS (A74.9)
meningococcal infection NOS (A39.9)
rickettsial infection NOS (A79.9)
spirochetal infection NOS (A69.9)

● **A49.0**   **Staphylococcal infection, unspecified site**

     A49.01   **Methicillin susceptible Staphylococcus aureus
infection, unspecified site**
Methicillin susceptible Staphylococcus aureus
(MSSA) infection
Staphylococcus aureus infection NOS

     A49.02   **Methicillin resistant Staphylococcus aureus
infection, unspecified site**
Methicillin resistant Staphylococcus aureus
(MRSA) infection

A49.1   **Streptococcal infection, unspecified site**

A49.2   **Hemophilus influenzae infection, unspecified site**
Any of seven bacterium of genus Haemophilus

A49.3   **Mycoplasma infection, unspecified site**
*Bacterium of class Mollicutes, unusual group of bacteria
distinguished by absence of cell wall*

A49.8   **Other bacterial infections of unspecified site**

A49.9   **Bacterial infection, unspecified**

     Excludes1   bacteremia NOS (R78.81)

Item 1-8   **Gas gangrene** is a necrotizing subcutaneous infection that will cause tissue death. Patients with poor circulation (e.g., diabetes, peripheral nephropathy) will have low oxygen content in their tissues (hypoxia), which allows the Clostridium bacteria to flourish. Gas gangrene often occurs at the site of a surgical wound or trauma. Onset is sudden and dramatic. Treatment can include debridement, amputation, and/or hyperbaric oxygen treatments.

Figure 1-3   Chancre of primary syphilis. (From James WD, Berger TG, Elston DM: Andrews' Diseases of the Skin: Clinical Dermatology, Philadelphia, Saunders Elsevier, 2006)

Item 1-9   **Syphilis,** also known as lues, is the most serious of the venereal diseases caused by *Treponema pallidum.* The **primary** stage is characterized by an ulceration known as **chancre,** which usually appears on the genitals but can also develop on the anus, lips, tonsils, breasts, or fingers. Syphilis is easy to cure in its early stages. A single intramuscular injection of penicillin will usually cure a person who has had syphilis for less than a year.

The **secondary** stage is characterized by a rash that can affect any area of the body. **Latent** syphilis is divided into **early,** which is diagnosed within two years of infection, and **late,** which is diagnosed two years or more after infection. Additional doses of penicillin or another antibiotic are needed to treat someone who has had syphilis for longer than a year. For those allergic to penicillin, there are other antibiotic treatments. **Congenital** syphilis is also labeled **early** or **late** based on the time of diagnosis.

INFECTIONS WITH A PREDOMINANTLY SEXUAL MODE OF TRANSMISSION (A50-A64)

     Excludes1
nonspecific and nongonococcal urethritis (N34.1)
Reiter's disease (M02.3-)

     Excludes2   human immunodeficiency virus [HIV] disease
(B20)

● **A50**   **Congenital syphilis**

● **A50.0**   **Early congenital syphilis, symptomatic**
Any congenital syphilitic condition specified as early or
manifest less than two years after birth

     A50.01   **Early congenital syphilitic oculopathy**

     A50.02   **Early congenital syphilitic osteochondropathy**

     A50.03   **Early congenital syphilitic pharyngitis**
Early congenital syphilitic laryngitis

     A50.04   **Early congenital syphilitic pneumonia**

     A50.05   **Early congenital syphilitic rhinitis**

     A50.06   **Early cutaneous congenital syphilis**

     A50.07   **Early mucocutaneous congenital syphilis**

     A50.08   **Early visceral congenital syphilis**

     A50.09   **Other early congenital syphilis, symptomatic**

A50.1   **Early congenital syphilis, latent**
Congenital syphilis without clinical manifestations,
with positive serological reaction and negative
spinal fluid test, less than two years after birth

A50.2   **Early congenital syphilis, unspecified**
Congenital syphilis NOS less than two years after birth

● **A50.3**   **Late congenital syphilitic oculopathy**

     Excludes1   Hutchinson's triad (A50.53)

     A50.30   **Late congenital syphilitic oculopathy,
unspecified**

     A50.31   **Late congenital syphilitic interstitial keratitis**

     A50.32   **Late congenital syphilitic chorioretinitis**

     A50.39   **Other late congenital syphilitic oculopathy**

● **A50.4**   **Late congenital neurosyphilis [juvenile neurosyphilis]**
Use additional code to identify any associated mental
disorder

     Excludes1   Hutchinson's triad (A50.53)

     A50.40   **Late congenital neurosyphilis, unspecified**
Juvenile neurosyphilis NOS

     A50.41   **Late congenital syphilitic meningitis**

     A50.42   **Late congenital syphilitic encephalitis**

     A50.43   **Late congenital syphilitic polyneuropathy**

     A50.44   **Late congenital syphilitic optic nerve atrophy**

     A50.45   **Juvenile general paresis**
Dementia paralytica juvenilis
Juvenile taboparetic neurosyphilis

     A50.49   **Other late congenital neurosyphilis**
Juvenile tabes dorsalis

● **A50.5**   **Other late congenital syphilis, symptomatic**
Any congenital syphilitic condition specified as late or
manifest two years or more after birth

     A50.51   **Clutton's joints**

     A50.52   **Hutchinson's teeth**

     A50.53   **Hutchinson's triad**

     A50.54   **Late congenital cardiovascular syphilis**

     A50.55   **Late congenital syphilitic arthropathy**

     A50.56   **Late congenital syphilitic osteochondropathy**

     A50.57   **Syphilitic saddle nose**

     A50.59   **Other late congenital syphilis, symptomatic**

A50.6   **Late congenital syphilis, latent**
Congenital syphilis without clinical manifestations,
with positive serological reaction and negative
spinal fluid test, two years or more after birth.

A50.7   **Late congenital syphilis, unspecified**
Congenital syphilis NOS two years or more after birth.

A50.9   **Congenital syphilis, unspecified**

CHAPTER 1 (A00-B99)

● **A51   Early syphilis**

　　A51.0   Primary genital syphilis
　　　　Syphilitic chancre NOS

　　A51.1   Primary anal syphilis

　　A51.2   Primary syphilis of other sites

　● **A51.3   Secondary syphilis of skin and mucous membranes**

　　　A51.31   Condyloma latum

　　　A51.32   Syphilitic alopecia

　　　A51.39   Other secondary syphilis of skin
　　　　　Syphilitic leukoderma
　　　　　Syphilitic mucous patch

　　　　　Excludes1   late syphilitic leukoderma
　　　　　　　(A52.79)

　● **A51.4   Other secondary syphilis**

　　　A51.41   Secondary syphilitic meningitis

　　　A51.42   Secondary syphilitic female pelvic disease

　　　A51.43   Secondary syphilitic oculopathy
　　　　　Secondary syphilitic chorioretinitis
　　　　　Secondary syphilitic iridocyclitis, iritis
　　　　　Secondary syphilitic uveitis

　　　A51.44   Secondary syphilitic nephritis

　　　A51.45   Secondary syphilitic hepatitis

　　　A51.46   Secondary syphilitic osteopathy

　　　A51.49   Other secondary syphilitic conditions
　　　　　Secondary syphilitic lymphadenopathy
　　　　　Secondary syphilitic myositis

　　A51.5   Early syphilis, latent
　　　　Syphilis (acquired) without clinical manifestations, with
　　　　　positive serological reaction and negative spinal
　　　　　fluid test, less than two years after infection.

　　A51.9   Early syphilis, unspecified

● **A52   Late syphilis**

　● **A52.0   Cardiovascular and cerebrovascular syphilis**

　　　A52.00   Cardiovascular syphilis, unspecified

　　　A52.01   Syphilitic aneurysm of aorta

　　　A52.02   Syphilitic aortitis

　　　A52.03   Syphilitic endocarditis
　　　　　Syphilitic aortic valve incompetence or stenosis
　　　　　Syphilitic mitral valve stenosis
　　　　　Syphilitic pulmonary valve regurgitation

　　　A52.04   Syphilitic cerebral arteritis

　　　A52.05   Other cerebrovascular syphilis
　　　　　Syphilitic cerebral aneurysm (ruptured) (non-
　　　　　　ruptured)
　　　　　Syphilitic cerebral thrombosis

　　　A52.06   Other syphilitic heart involvement
　　　　　Syphilitic coronary artery disease
　　　　　Syphilitic myocarditis
　　　　　Syphilitic pericarditis

　　　A52.09   Other cardiovascular syphilis

　● **A52.1   Symptomatic neurosyphilis**

　　　A52.10   Symptomatic neurosyphilis, unspecified

　　　A52.11   Tabes dorsalis
　　　　　*Cognitive decline with progressive degeneration of
　　　　　posterior columns, roots, and ganglia of spinal
　　　　　cord, occur 15-20 years after initial infection
　　　　　of syphilis; AKA Duchenne disease*
　　　　　Locomotor ataxia (progressive)
　　　　　Tabetic neurosyphilis

　　　A52.12   Other cerebrospinal syphilis

　　　A52.13   Late syphilitic meningitis

　　　A52.14   Late syphilitic encephalitis

　　　A52.15   Late syphilitic neuropathy
　　　　　Late syphilitic acoustic neuritis
　　　　　Late syphilitic optic (nerve) atrophy
　　　　　Late syphilitic polyneuropathy
　　　　　Late syphilitic retrobulbar neuritis

　　　A52.16   Charcôt's arthropathy (tabetic)
　　　　　*Progressive musculoskeletal condition characterized
　　　　　by joint dislocation, fractures, and deformities,
　　　　　results in progressive destruction of bone and
　　　　　soft tissue of weight-bearing joints*

　　　A52.17   General paresis
　　　　　*Chronic meningoencephalitis results in loss of
　　　　　cortical function, or progressive dementia
　　　　　and generalized paralysis, occurring 10-20
　　　　　years after initial infection of syphilis; AKA
　　　　　Bayle disease, dementia paralytica, paralytic
　　　　　dementiaparetic neurosyphilis, syphilitic
　　　　　meningoencephalitis*
　　　　　Dementia paralytica

　　　A52.19   Other symptomatic neurosyphilis
　　　　　Syphilitic parkinsonism

　　A52.2   Asymptomatic neurosyphilis

　　A52.3   Neurosyphilis, unspecified
　　　　Gumma (syphilitic)
　　　　Destructive lesions of syphilis
　　　　Syphilis (late)
　　　　Syphiloma
　　　　Coding Clinic: 2021, Q2, P6

　● **A52.7   Other symptomatic late syphilis**

　　　A52.71   Late syphilitic oculopathy
　　　　　Late syphilitic chorioretinitis
　　　　　Late syphilitic episcleritis

　　　A52.72   Syphilis of lung and bronchus

　　　**A52.73   Symptomatic late syphilis of other respiratory
　　　　　organs**

　　　A52.74   Syphilis of liver and other viscera
　　　　　Late syphilitic peritonitis

　　　A52.75   Syphilis of kidney and ureter
　　　　　Syphilitic glomerular disease

　　　A52.76   Other genitourinary symptomatic late syphilis
　　　　　Late syphilitic female pelvic inflammatory
　　　　　　disease

　　　A52.77   Syphilis of bone and joint

　　　A52.78   Syphilis of other musculoskeletal tissue
　　　　　Late syphilitic bursitis
　　　　　Syphilis [stage unspecified] of bursa
　　　　　Syphilis [stage unspecified] of muscle
　　　　　Syphilis [stage unspecified] of synovium
　　　　　Syphilis [stage unspecified] of tendon

　　　A52.79   Other symptomatic late syphilis
　　　　　Late syphilitic leukoderma
　　　　　Syphilis of adrenal gland
　　　　　Syphilis of pituitary gland
　　　　　Syphilis of thyroid gland
　　　　　Syphilitic splenomegaly

　　　　　Excludes1   syphilitic leukoderma
　　　　　　　(secondary) (A51.39)

　　A52.8   Late syphilis, latent
　　　　Syphilis (acquired) without clinical manifestations, with
　　　　　positive serological reaction and negative spinal
　　　　　fluid test, two years or more after infection

　　A52.9   Late syphilis, unspecified

● **A53   Other and unspecified syphilis**

　　A53.0   Latent syphilis, unspecified as early or late
　　　　Latent syphilis NOS
　　　　Positive serological reaction for syphilis

　　A53.9   Syphilis, unspecified
　　　　Infection due to Treponema pallidum NOS
　　　　Syphilis (acquired) NOS

　　　　Excludes1   syphilis NOS under two years of age
　　　　　　(A50.2)

▶ New   ⇒ Revised   ~~deleted~~ Deleted   Excludes 1   Excludes 2   Includes   Use additional   Code first   Code also   Key words

OGCR Official Guidelines   X Assign placeholder X   ● Use Additional Character(s)   ▶ Manifestation Code   🐾 Hierarchical Condition Category   Coding Clinic

Item 1-10 An STD (sexually transmitted disease) caused by **Neisseria gonorrhoeae** that flourishes in the warm, moist areas of the reproductive tract. Untreated gonorrhea spreads to other parts of the body, causing inflammation of the testes or prostate or pelvic inflammatory disease (PID).

● **A54   Gonococcal infection**
  ● **A54.0   Gonococcal infection of lower genitourinary tract without periurethral or accessory gland abscess**
    Excludes1   gonococcal infection with genitourinary gland abscess (A54.1)
        gonococcal infection with periurethral abscess (A54.1)
    A54.00   Gonococcal infection of lower genitourinary tract, unspecified
    A54.01   Gonococcal cystitis and urethritis, unspecified
    A54.02   Gonococcal vulvovaginitis, unspecified
    A54.03   Gonococcal cervicitis, unspecified
    A54.09   Other gonococcal infection of lower genitourinary tract
  A54.1   Gonococcal infection of lower genitourinary tract with periurethral and accessory gland abscess
    Gonococcal Bartholin's gland abscess
  ● **A54.2   Gonococcal pelviperitonitis and other gonococcal genitourinary infection**
    A54.21   Gonococcal infection of kidney and ureter
    A54.22   Gonococcal prostatitis
    A54.23   Gonococcal infection of other male genital organs
        Gonococcal epididymitis
        Gonococcal orchitis
    A54.24   Gonococcal female pelvic inflammatory disease
        Gonococcal pelviperitonitis
        Excludes1   gonococcal peritonitis (A54.85)
    A54.29   Other gonococcal genitourinary infections
  ● **A54.3   Gonococcal infection of eye**
    A54.30   Gonococcal infection of eye, unspecified
    A54.31   Gonococcal conjunctivitis
        Form of bacterial conjunctivitis contracted by newborns during delivery; AKA neonatal conjunctivitis
        Ophthalmia neonatorum due to gonococcus
    A54.32   Gonococcal iridocyclitis
        Inflammation of iris and of ciliary body due to gonococcal infection
    A54.33   Gonococcal keratitis
        Inflammation of cornea due to gonococcal infection; AKA keratoconjunctivitis, keratopathy
    A54.39   Other gonococcal eye infection
        Gonococcal endophthalmia
  ● **A54.4   Gonococcal infection of musculoskeletal system**
    A54.40   Gonococcal infection of musculoskeletal system, unspecified 🔍
    A54.41   Gonococcal spondylopathy 🔍
        Disorder of vertebrae due to gonococcal infection; AKA rachiopathy
    A54.42   Gonococcal arthritis 🔍
        Excludes2   gonococcal infection of spine (A54.41)
    A54.43   Gonococcal osteomyelitis 🔍
        Excludes2   gonococcal infection of spine (A54.41)
    A54.49   Gonococcal infection of other musculoskeletal tissue 🔍
        Gonococcal bursitis
        Gonococcal myositis
        Gonococcal synovitis
        Gonococcal tenosynovitis
  A54.5   Gonococcal pharyngitis
  A54.6   Gonococcal infection of anus and rectum

  ● **A54.8   Other gonococcal infections**
    A54.81   Gonococcal meningitis
    A54.82   Gonococcal brain abscess
    A54.83   Gonococcal heart infection
        Gonococcal endocarditis
        Gonococcal myocarditis
        Gonococcal pericarditis
    A54.84   Gonococcal pneumonia 🔍
    A54.85   Gonococcal peritonitis 🔍
        Excludes1   gonococcal pelviperitonitis (A54.24)
    A54.86   Gonococcal sepsis 🔍
    A54.89   Other gonococcal infections
        Gonococcal keratoderma
        Gonococcal lymphadenitis
  A54.9   Gonococcal infection, unspecified

A55   Chlamydial lymphogranuloma (venereum)
  Climatic or tropical bubo
  Durand-Nicolas-Favre disease
  Esthiomene
  Lymphogranuloma inguinale

● **A56   Other sexually transmitted chlamydial diseases**
  Includes   sexually transmitted diseases due to Chlamydia trachomatis
  Excludes1   neonatal chlamydial conjunctivitis (P39.1)
    neonatal chlamydial pneumonia (P23.1)
  Excludes2   chlamydial lymphogranuloma (A55)
    conditions classified to A74.-
  ● **A56.0   Chlamydial infection of lower genitourinary tract**
    A56.00   Chlamydial infection of lower genitourinary tract, unspecified
    A56.01   Chlamydial cystitis and urethritis
    A56.02   Chlamydial vulvovaginitis
    A56.09   Other chlamydial infection of lower genitourinary tract
        Chlamydial cervicitis
  ● **A56.1   Chlamydial infection of pelviperitoneum and other genitourinary organs**
    A56.11   Chlamydial female pelvic inflammatory disease
    A56.19   Other chlamydial genitourinary infection
        Chlamydial epididymitis
        Chlamydial orchitis
  A56.2   Chlamydial infection of genitourinary tract, unspecified
  A56.3   Chlamydial infection of anus and rectum
  A56.4   Chlamydial infection of pharynx
  A56.8   Sexually transmitted chlamydial infection of other sites

A57   Chancroid
  Ulcus molle
  Sexually transmitted infection caused by bacteria, Haemophilus ducreyi

A58   Granuloma inguinale
  Chronic, progressive, ulcerative granulomatous disease
  Donovanosis

● **A59   Trichomoniasis**
  Excludes2   intestinal trichomoniasis (A07.8)
  A common STD caused by a parasite, Trichomonas vaginalis
  ● **A59.0   Urogenital trichomoniasis**
    A59.00   Urogenital trichomoniasis, unspecified
        Fluor (vaginalis) due to Trichomonas
        Leukorrhea (vaginalis) due to Trichomonas
    A59.01   Trichomonal vulvovaginitis
    A59.02   Trichomonal prostatitis
    A59.03   Trichomonal cystitis and urethritis
    A59.09   Other urogenital trichomoniasis
        Common sexually transmitted disease (STD) caused by single-celled protozoan parasite; AKA trich
        Trichomonas cervicitis

A59.8 Trichomoniasis of other sites

A59.9 Trichomoniasis, unspecified

● A60 Anogenital herpesviral [herpes simplex] infections

  ● A60.0 Herpesviral infection of genitalia and urogenital tract

  A60.00 Herpesviral infection of urogenital system, unspecified

  A60.01 Herpesviral infection of penis

  A60.02 Herpesviral infection of other male genital organs

  A60.03 Herpesviral cervicitis

  A60.04 Herpesviral vulvovaginitis
  Herpesviral [herpes simplex] ulceration
  Herpesviral [herpes simplex] vaginitis
  Herpesviral [herpes simplex] vulvitis

  A60.09 Herpesviral infection of other urogenital tract
  Coding Clinic: 2020, Q1, P20

  A60.1 Herpesviral infection of perianal skin and rectum

  A60.9 Anogenital herpesviral infection, unspecified

● A63 Other predominantly sexually transmitted diseases, not elsewhere classified

  Excludes2 molluscum contagiosum (B08.1)
             papilloma of cervix (D26.0)

  A63.0 Anogenital (venereal) warts
  Anogenital warts due to (human) papillomavirus [HPV]
  Condyloma acuminatum

  A63.8 Other specified predominantly sexually transmitted diseases

A64 Unspecified sexually transmitted disease

OTHER SPIROCHETAL DISEASES (A65-A69)

  Excludes2 leptospirosis (A27.-)
             syphilis (A50-A53)

A65 Nonvenereal syphilis
  Bejel
  Endemic syphilis
  Njovera

● A66 Yaws
  Endemic, infectious, tropical disease caused by spirochete, spread by direct contact; AKA frambesia, framboesia, frambesia tropica

  Includes bouba
            frambesia (tropica)
            pian

  A66.0 Initial lesions of yaws
  Chancre of yaws
  Frambesia, initial or primary
  Initial frambesial ulcer
  Mother yaw

  A66.1 Multiple papillomata and wet crab yaws
  Frambesioma
  Pianoma
  Plantar or palmar papilloma of yaws

  A66.2 Other early skin lesions of yaws
  Cutaneous yaws, less than five years after infection
  Early yaws (cutaneous)(macular)(maculopapular)(micropapular)(papular)
  Frambeside of early yaws

  A66.3 Hyperkeratosis of yaws
  Hypertrophy of stratum corneum of skin in which there are small, hard, verrucous scales
  Ghoul hand
  Hyperkeratosis, palmar or plantar (early) (late) due to yaws
  Worm-eaten soles

  A66.4 Gummata and ulcers of yaws
  Small, rubbery granuloma with necrotic center and inflamed characteristic of advanced stage of syphilis; AKA syphiloma
  Gummatous frambeside
  Nodular late yaws (ulcerated)

  A66.5 Gangosa
  Manifestation of yaws that develops in the soft palate and spreads eroding bone, cartilage, and soft tissue
  Rhinopharyngitis mutilans

  A66.6 Bone and joint lesions of yaws 🐄
  Yaws ganglion
  Yaws goundou
  Yaws gumma, bone
  Yaws gummatous osteitis or periostitis
  Yaws hydrarthrosis
  Yaws osteitis
  Yaws periostitis (hypertrophic)

  A66.7 Other manifestations of yaws
  Juxta-articular nodules of yaws
  Mucosal yaws

  A66.8 Latent yaws
  Yaws without clinical manifestations, with positive serology

  A66.9 Yaws, unspecified

● A67 Pinta [carate]
  Group of nonvenereal diseases caused by Treponema species

  A67.0 Primary lesions of pinta
  Chancre (primary) of pinta
  Papule (primary) of pinta

  A67.1 Intermediate lesions of pinta
  Erythematous plaques of pinta
  Hyperchromic lesions of pinta
  Hyperkeratosis of pinta
  Pintids

  A67.2 Late lesions of pinta
  Achromic skin lesions of pinta
  Cicatricial skin lesions of pinta
  Dyschromic skin lesions of pinta

  A67.3 Mixed lesions of pinta
  Achromic with hyperchromic skin lesions of pinta [carate]

  A67.9 Pinta, unspecified

● A68 Relapsing fevers
  Includes recurrent fever
  Excludes2 Lyme disease (A69.2-)

  A68.0 Louse-borne relapsing fever
  Relapsing fever due to Borrelia recurrentis

  A68.1 Tick-borne relapsing fever
  Relapsing fever due to any Borrelia species other than Borrelia recurrentis

  A68.9 Relapsing fever, unspecified

● A69 Other spirochetal infections

  A69.0 Necrotizing ulcerative stomatitis
  Cancrum oris
  Fusospirochetal gangrene
  Noma
  Stomatitis gangrenosa

  A69.1 Other Vincent's infections
  Fusospirochetal pharyngitis
  Necrotizing ulcerative (acute) gingivitis
  Necrotizing ulcerative (acute) gingivostomatitis
  Spirochetal stomatitis
  Trench mouth
  Vincent's angina
  Vincent's gingivitis

  ● A69.2 Lyme disease
  Erythema chronicum migrans due to Borrelia burgdorferi

  A69.20 Lyme disease, unspecified
  Coding Clinic: 2021, Q4, P5

  A69.21 Meningitis due to Lyme disease

Item 1-11 Cancrum oris, also known as **noma** or **gangrenous stomatitis,** begins as an ulcer of the gingiva and results in a progressive gangrenous process.

▶ New   ⇛ Revised   ~~deleted~~ Deleted   Excludes 1   Excludes 2   Includes   Use additional   Code first   Code also   Key words

OGCR Official Guidelines   X Assign placeholder X   ● Use Additional Character(s)   ▶ Manifestation Code   🐄 Hierarchical Condition Category   Coding Clinic

A69.22 **Other neurologic disorders in Lyme disease**
        Cranial neuritis
        Meningoencephalitis
        Polyneuropathy

A69.23 **Arthritis due to Lyme disease** 🔗

A69.29 **Other conditions associated with Lyme disease**
        Myopericarditis due to Lyme disease
        Coding Clinic: 2016, Q3, P12

A69.8   **Other specified spirochetal infections**

A69.9   **Spirochetal infection, unspecified**

OTHER DISEASES CAUSED BY CHLAMYDIAE (A70-A74)

Excludes1 sexually transmitted chlamydial diseases
              (A55-A56)

A70 **Chlamydia psittaci infections**
     Ornithosis
     Parrot fever
     Psittacosis

● A71 **Trachoma**
       Excludes1 sequelae of trachoma (B94.0)

A71.0 **Initial stage of trachoma**
        Trachoma dubium

A71.1 **Active stage of trachoma**
        Granular conjunctivitis (trachomatous)
        Trachomatous follicular conjunctivitis
        Trachomatous pannus

A71.9 **Trachoma, unspecified**

● A74 **Other diseases caused by chlamydiae**
       Excludes1 neonatal chlamydial conjunctivitis (P39.1)
                      neonatal chlamydial pneumonia (P23.1)
                      Reiter's disease (M02.3-)
                      sexually transmitted chlamydial diseases
                      (A55-A56)
       Excludes2 chlamydial pneumonia (J16.0)

A74.0 **Chlamydial conjunctivitis**
        Paratrachoma

● A74.8 **Other chlamydial diseases**
         A74.81 **Chlamydial peritonitis**
         A74.89 **Other chlamydial diseases**

A74.9 **Chlamydial infection, unspecified**
        Chlamydiosis NOS

RICKETTSIOSES (A75-A79)

● A75 **Typhus fever**
       Excludes1 rickettsiosis due to Ehrlichia sennetsu (A79.81)

A75.0 **Epidemic louse-borne typhus fever due to Rickettsia
        prowazekii**
        Organisms transmitted between humans via louse
        Classical typhus (fever)
        Epidemic (louse-borne) typhus

A75.1 **Recrudescent typhus [Brill's disease]**
        Brill-Zinsser disease

A75.2 **Typhus fever due to Rickettsia typhi**
        Murine (flea-borne) typhus

A75.3 **Typhus fever due to Rickettsia tsutsugamushi**
        Scrub (mite-borne) typhus
        Tsutsugamushi fever
        Typhus fever due to Orientia Tsutsugamushi (scrub
        typhus)

A75.9 **Typhus fever, unspecified**
        Typhus (fever) NOS

● A77 **Spotted fever [tick-borne rickettsioses]**
A77.0 **Spotted fever due to Rickettsia rickettsii**
        Rocky Mountain spotted fever
        Sao Paulo fever

A77.1 **Spotted fever due to Rickettsia conorii**
        African tick typhus
        Boutonneuse fever
        India tick typhus
        Kenya tick typhus
        Marseilles fever
        Mediterranean tick fever

Item 1-12 Rickettsioses are diseases spread from ticks, lice, fleas, or mites to humans.
  Typhus is spread to humans chiefly by the fleas of rats.
  Endemic identifies a disease as being present in low numbers of humans at all times, whereas **epidemic** identifies a disease as being present in high numbers of humans at a specific time. Morbidity (death) is higher in epidemic diseases.
  Brill's disease, also known as **Brill-Zinsser disease,** is spread from human to human by body lice and also from the lice of flying squirrels. **Scrub typhus** is spread in the same ways as Brill's disease.
  Malaria is spread to humans by mosquitoes.

A77.2 **Spotted fever due to Rickettsia siberica**
        North Asian tick fever
        Siberian tick typhus

A77.3 **Spotted fever due to Rickettsia australis**
        Queensland tick typhus

● A77.4 **Ehrlichiosis**
         Type of tick-borne fever caused by bacteria infection
         Excludes1 anaplasmosis [A. phagocytophilum]
                        (A79.82)
                        rickettsiosis due to Ehrlichia sennetsu (A79.81)
                        Coding Clinic: 2021, Q4, P5

         A77.40 **Ehrlichiosis, unspecified**
                 Coding Clinic: 2021, Q4, P5
     ➥ A77.41 **Ehrlichiosis chaffeensis [E. chaffeensis]**
         A77.49 **Other ehrlichiosis**
                 Ehrlichiosis due to E. ewingii
                 Ehrlichiosis due to E. muris euclairensis

A77.8 **Other spotted fevers**
        Rickettsia 364D/R. philipii (Pacific Coast tick fever)
        Spotted fever due to Rickettsia africae (African tick bite
        fever)
        Spotted fever due to Rickettsia parkeri]

A77.9 **Spotted fever, unspecified**
        Tick-borne typhus NOS

A78 **Q fever**
     Infection due to Coxiella burnetii
     Nine Mile fever
     Quadrilateral fever

● A79 **Other rickettsioses**
A79.0 **Trench fever**
        Quintan fever
        Wolhynian fever

A79.1 **Rickettsialpox due to Rickettsia akari**
        Kew Garden fever
        Vesicular rickettsiosis

● A79.8 **Other specified rickettsioses**
         A79.81 **Rickettsiosis due to Ehrlichia sennetsu**
                 Rickettsiosis due to Neorickettsia sennetsu
         A79.82 **Anaplasmosis [A. phagocytophilum]**
                 Transfusion transmitted A. phagocytophilum
                 Coding Clinic: 2021, Q4, P5
         A79.89 **Other specified rickettsioses**

A79.9 **Rickettsiosis, unspecified**
        Rickettsial infection NOS

VIRAL AND PRION INFECTIONS OF THE CENTRAL NERVOUS SYSTEM (A80-A89)

Excludes1 postpolio syndrome (G14)
              sequelae of poliomyelitis (B91)
              sequelae of viral encephalitis (B94.1)

● A80 **Acute poliomyelitis**
       Excludes1 acute flaccid myelitis (G04.82)
A80.0 **Acute paralytic poliomyelitis, vaccine-associated**
A80.1 **Acute paralytic poliomyelitis, wild virus, imported**
A80.2 **Acute paralytic poliomyelitis, wild virus, indigenous**
● A80.3 **Acute paralytic poliomyelitis, other and unspecified**
         A80.30 **Acute paralytic poliomyelitis, unspecified**
         A80.39 **Other acute paralytic poliomyelitis**
A80.4 **Acute nonparalytic poliomyelitis**
A80.9 **Acute poliomyelitis, unspecified**

CHAPTER 1 (A00-B99)

CHAPTER 1 (A00-B99)

● **A81   Atypical virus infections of central nervous system**

    Includes   diseases of the central nervous system caused by prions

    Use additional , if applicable, code to identify:

      dementia with anxiety (F02.84, F02.A4, F02.B4, F02.C4)

      dementia with behavioral disturbance (F02.81-, F02.A1-, F02.B1-, F02.C1-)

      dementia with mood disturbance (F02.83, F02.A3, F02.B3, F02.C3)

      dementia with psychotic disturbance (F02.82, F02.A2, F02.B2, F02.C2)

      dementia without behavioral disturbance (F02.80, F02.A0, F02.B0, F02.C0)

      mild neurocognitive disorder due to known physiological condition (F06.7-)

● **A81.0   Creutzfeldt-Jakob disease**

    A81.00   Creutzfeldt-Jakob disease, unspecified

        Jakob-Creutzfeldt disease, unspecified

    A81.01   Variant Creutzfeldt-Jakob disease

        vCJD

    A81.09   Other Creutzfeldt-Jakob disease

        CJD

        Familial Creutzfeldt-Jakob disease

        Iatrogenic Creutzfeldt-Jakob disease

        Sporadic Creutzfeldt-Jakob disease

        Subacute spongiform encephalopathy (with dementia)

A81.1   Subacute sclerosing panencephalitis

    Type of viral encephalitis that causes parenchymatous lesions in gray and white matter of brain

    Dawson's inclusion body encephalitis

    Van Bogaert's sclerosing leukoencephalopathy

A81.2   Progressive multifocal leukoencephalopathy

    Group of diseases affecting white matter of brain

    Multifocal leukoencephalopathy NOS

● **A81.8   Other atypical virus infections of central nervous system**

    A81.81   Kuru

    A81.82   Gerstmann-Sträussler-Scheinker syndrome

        GSS syndrome

    A81.83   Fatal familial insomnia

        FFI

    A81.89   Other atypical virus infections of central nervous system

A81.9   Atypical virus infection of central nervous system, unspecified

    Prion diseases of the central nervous system NOS

● **A82   Rabies**

    Viral disease affecting the central nervous system and transmitted from infected mammals to man

    A82.0   Sylvatic rabies

    A82.1   Urban rabies

    A82.9   Rabies, unspecified

● **A83   Mosquito-borne viral encephalitis**

    Inflammation of the brain caused most commonly by Herpes Simplex virus

    Includes   mosquito-borne viral meningoencephalitis

    Excludes2   Venezuelan equine encephalitis (A92.2)

                  West Nile fever (A92.3-)

                  West Nile virus (A92.3-)

    A83.0   Japanese encephalitis

    A83.1   Western equine encephalitis

    A83.2   Eastern equine encephalitis

    A83.3   St. Louis encephalitis

    A83.4   Australian encephalitis

        Kunjin virus disease

Item 1-13   Acute Poliomyelitis: Also called infantile paralysis and is caused by the poliovirus, which enters the body orally and infects the intestinal wall and then enters the blood stream and central nervous system, causing muscle weakness and paralysis. This disease has been nearly eradicated with the polio vaccine.

Item 1-14   Encephalitis is an inflammation of the brain most often caused by a virus but may also be caused by a bacteria and most commonly transmitted by a mosquito. **Myelitis** is an inflammation of the spinal cord that may disrupt CNS function. Untreated myelitis may rapidly lead to permanent damage to the spinal cord. **Encephalomyelitis** is a general term for an inflammation of the brain and spinal cord.

    A83.5   California encephalitis

        California meningoencephalitis

        La Crosse encephalitis

    A83.6   Rocio virus disease

        Mosquito-borne virus

    A83.8   Other mosquito-borne viral encephalitis

    A83.9   Mosquito-borne viral encephalitis, unspecified

● **A84   Tick-borne viral encephalitis**

    Includes   tick-borne viral meningoencephalitis

    A84.0   Far Eastern tick-borne encephalitis [Russian spring-summer encephalitis]

    A84.1   Central European tick-borne encephalitis

    A84.8   Other tick-borne viral encephalitis

      A84.81   Powassan virus disease

      A84.89   Other tick-borne viral encephalitis

         Louping ill

         Code first, if applicable, transfusion related infection (T80.22-)

    A84.9   Tick-borne viral encephalitis, unspecified

● **A85   Other viral encephalitis, not elsewhere classified**

    Includes   specified viral encephalomyelitis NEC

                specified viral meningoencephalitis NEC

    Excludes1   encephalitis due to cytomegalovirus (B25.8)

             encephalitis due to herpesvirus NEC (B10.0-)

             encephalitis due to herpesvirus [herpes simplex] (B00.4)

             encephalitis due to measles virus (B05.0)

             encephalitis due to mumps virus (B26.2)

             encephalitis due to poliomyelitis virus (A80.-)

             encephalitis due to zoster (B02.0)

             lymphocytic choriomeningitis (A87.2)

             myalgic encephalomyelitis (G93.32)

    A85.0   Enteroviral encephalitis

        Enteroviral encephalomyelitis

    A85.1   Adenoviral encephalitis

        Adenoviral meningoencephalitis

    A85.2   Arthropod-borne viral encephalitis, unspecified

      Excludes1   West nile virus with encephalitis (A92.31)

    A85.8   Other specified viral encephalitis

        Encephalitis lethargica

        Von Economo-Cruchet disease

A86   Unspecified viral encephalitis

    Viral encephalomyelitis NOS

    Viral meningoencephalitis NOS

● **A87   Viral meningitis**

    Excludes1   meningitis due to herpesvirus [herpes simplex] (B00.3)

             meningitis due to measles virus (B05.1)

             meningitis due to mumps virus (B26.1)

             meningitis due to poliomyelitis virus (A80.-)

             meningitis due to zoster (B02.1)

    A87.0   Enteroviral meningitis

        Group of common viruses responsible for the majority of viral meningitis

        Coxsackievirus meningitis

        Echovirus meningitis

    A87.1   Adenoviral meningitis

    A87.2   Lymphocytic choriomeningitis

        Lymphocytic meningoencephalitis

    A87.8   Other viral meningitis

    A87.9   Viral meningitis, unspecified

▶ New   ⇒ Revised   ~~deleted~~ Deleted   Excludes 1   Excludes 2   Includes   Use additional   Code first   Code also   Key words

OGCR Official Guidelines   X Assign placeholder X   ● Use Additional Character(s)   ▷ Manifestation Code   🏷 Hierarchical Condition Category   **Coding Clinic**

● **A88 Other viral infections of central nervous system, not elsewhere classified**

>   **Excludes1**   viral encephalitis NOS (A86)
>   viral meningitis NOS (A87.9)

    A88.0 Enteroviral exanthematous fever [Boston exanthem]
        Infectious skin eruption

    A88.1 Epidemic vertigo

    A88.8 Other specified viral infections of central nervous system

A89 Unspecified viral infection of central nervous system

OGCR Section I. C.1.f.

Certain Infectious and Parasitic Diseases (A00-B99)

Zika virus infections

Code only confirmed cases

Code only a confirmed diagnosis of Zika virus (A92.5, Zika virus disease) as documented by the provider. This is an exception to the hospital inpatient guideline Section II, H.

In this context, "confirmation" does not require documentation of the type of test performed; the physician's diagnostic statement that the condition is confirmed is sufficient. This code should be assigned regardless of the stated mode of transmission.

If the provider documents "suspected", "possible" or "probable" Zika, do not assign code A92.5. Assign a code(s) explaining the reason for encounter (such as fever, rash, or joint pain) or Z20.828, Contact with and (suspected) exposure to other viral communicable diseases.

ARTHROPOD-BORNE VIRAL FEVERS AND VIRAL HEMORRHAGIC FEVERS (A90-A99)

A90 Dengue fever [classical dengue]
    Acute, self-limited disease, characterized by fever, prostration, severe muscle pains, headache, rash, lymphadenopathy, and leukopenia, caused by dengue virus; AKA breakbone, dandy

>   **Excludes1**   dengue hemorrhagic fever (A91)

    Coding Clinic: 2016, Q3, P13

A91 Dengue hemorrhagic fever
    Serious follow-up to regular dengue, with symptoms of hemorrhage

● **A92 Other mosquito-borne viral fevers**

>   **Excludes1**   Ross River disease (B33.1)

    A92.0 Chikungunya virus disease
        Transmitted by mosquitoes
        Chikungunya (hemorrhagic) fever

    A92.1 O'nyong-nyong fever
        Acute, nonfatal febrile disease transmitted by mosquitoes, which clinically resembles dengue and chikungunya

    A92.2 Venezuelan equine fever
        Venezuelan equine encephalitis
        Venezuelan equine encephalomyelitis virus disease

    ● **A92.3 West Nile virus infection**
        West Nile fever

        A92.30 West Nile virus infection, unspecified
            West Nile fever NOS
            West Nile fever without complications
            West Nile virus NOS

        A92.31 West Nile virus infection with encephalitis
            West Nile encephalitis
            West Nile encephalomyelitis
            Coding Clinic: 2016, Q3, P13

        A92.32 West Nile virus infection with other neurologic manifestation
            Use additional code to specify the neurologic manifestation

        A92.39 West Nile virus infection with other complications
            Use additional code to specify the other conditions

    A92.4 Rift Valley fever

    A92.5 Zika virus disease
        Zika virus fever
        Zika virus infection
        Zika NOS

>   **Excludes1**   congenital Zika virus disease (P35.4)

        Coding Clinic: 2016, Q4, P4-7, 121

    A92.8 Other specified mosquito-borne viral fevers

    A92.9 Mosquito-borne viral fever, unspecified

● **A93 Other arthropod-borne viral fevers, not elsewhere classified**

    A93.0 Oropouche virus disease
        Tropical viral infection
        Oropouche fever

    A93.1 Sandfly fever
        Pappataci fever
        Phlebotomus fever

    A93.2 Colorado tick fever

    A93.8 Other specified arthropod-borne viral fevers
        Piry virus disease
        Vesicular stomatitis virus disease [Indiana fever]

A94 Unspecified arthropod-borne viral fever
    Arboviral fever NOS
    Arbovirus infection NOS

● **A95 Yellow fever**
    Acute infectious disease transmitted by mosquitoes

    A95.0 Sylvatic yellow fever
        Jungle yellow fever

    A95.1 Urban yellow fever

    A95.9 Yellow fever, unspecified

● **A96 Arenaviral hemorrhagic fever**
    Virus that causes various hemorrhagic fevers

    A96.0 Junin hemorrhagic fever
        Argentinian hemorrhagic fever

    A96.1 Machupo hemorrhagic fever
        Transmitted by contact with infected rodents
        Bolivian hemorrhagic fever

    A96.2 Lassa fever
        Acute type of hemorrhagic fever caused by contact with disease carrying mouse or person

    A96.8 Other arenaviral hemorrhagic fevers

    A96.9 Arenaviral hemorrhagic fever, unspecified

● **A98 Other viral hemorrhagic fevers, not elsewhere classified**

>   **Excludes1**   chikungunya hemorrhagic fever (A92.0)
>   dengue hemorrhagic fever (A91)

    A98.0 Crimean-Congo hemorrhagic fever
        Virus transmitted by ticks and contact with blood, secretions, or fluids from infected humans or animals
        Central Asian hemorrhagic fever

    A98.1 Omsk hemorrhagic fever
        Transmitted to humans by bites of infected ticks or contact with infected muskrats

    A98.2 Kyasanur Forest disease
        Transmitted via infected monkeys, voles, ticks

    A98.3 Marburg virus disease
        Rare, acute, often fatal type of hemorrhagic fever

    A98.4 Ebola virus disease

    A98.5 Hemorrhagic fever with renal syndrome
        Epidemic hemorrhagic fever
        Korean hemorrhagic fever
        Russian hemorrhagic fever
        Hantaan virus disease
        Hantavirus disease with renal manifestations
        Nephropathia epidemica
        Songo fever

>   **Excludes1**   hantavirus (cardio)-pulmonary syndrome (B33.4)

    A98.8 Other specified viral hemorrhagic fevers

A99 Unspecified viral hemorrhagic fever

Figure 1-4 Primary herpes simplex in and around the mouth. The infection is usually acquired from siblings or parents and is readily transmitted to other direct contacts. (Getty Image)

Item 1–15 Herpes is a viral disease for which there is no cure. There are two types of the herpes simplex virus: **Type I** causes **cold sores** or **fever blisters,** and **Type II** causes **genital herpes.** The virus can be spread from a sore on the lips to the genitals or from the genitals to the lips.

VIRAL INFECTIONS CHARACTERIZED BY SKIN AND MUCOUS MEMBRANE LESIONS (B00-B09)

● **B00   Herpesviral [herpes simplex] infections**
> **Excludes1**   congenital herpesviral infections (P35.2)
> **Excludes2**   anogenital herpesviral infection (A60.-)
> gammaherpesviral mononucleosis (B27.0-)
> herpangina (B08.5)

B00.0   Eczema herpeticum
> *Cutaneous eruption caused by herpes simplex virus (HSV) type 1, HSV-2, coxsackievirus A16, or vaccinia virus*
> Kaposi's varicelliform eruption

B00.1   Herpesviral vesicular dermatitis
> *Vesicle formation; characteristics include formation of blisters and scabs on feet and legs*
> Herpes simplex facialis
> Herpes simplex labialis
> Herpes simplex otitis externa
> Vesicular dermatitis of ear
> Vesicular dermatitis of lip

B00.2   Herpesviral gingivostomatitis and pharyngotonsillitis
> *Inflammation involving both gingivae and oral mucosa*
> Herpesviral pharyngitis
> *Inflammation of pharynx and tonsils; AKA tonsillopharyngitis*

B00.3   Herpesviral meningitis

B00.4   Herpesviral encephalitis
> Herpesviral meningoencephalitis
> Simian B disease
> > **Excludes1**   herpesviral encephalitis due to herpesvirus 6 and 7 (B10.01, B10.09)
> > non-simplex herpesviral encephalitis (B10.0-)

● **B00.5   Herpesviral ocular disease**
B00.50   Herpesviral ocular disease, unspecified
B00.51   Herpesviral iridocyclitis
> Herpesviral iritis
> Herpesviral uveitis, anterior
B00.52   Herpesviral keratitis
> Herpesviral keratoconjunctivitis
B00.53   Herpesviral conjunctivitis
B00.59   Other herpesviral disease of eye
> Herpesviral dermatitis of eyelid

B00.7   Disseminated herpesviral disease 🅗
> Herpesviral sepsis

● **B00.8   Other forms of herpesviral infections**
B00.81   Herpesviral hepatitis
B00.82   Herpes simplex myelitis 🅗
B00.89   Other herpesviral infection
> Herpesviral whitlow

B00.9   Herpesviral infection, unspecified
> Herpes simplex infection NOS

● **B01   Varicella [chickenpox]**
> *Very contagious disease caused by the varicella zoster virus that results in an itchy outbreak of skin blisters (varicella). The same virus causes shingles (zoster).*

B01.0   Varicella meningitis

Item 1-16 Zoster: Also known as **shingles** and is caused by the same virus as chickenpox. After exposure, the virus lies dormant in nerve tissue and is activated by factors including aging, stress, suppression of the immune system, and certain medication. It begins as a unilateral rash that leads to blisters and sores on the skin. It may involve the nerve pathways of the eye, forehead, nose, and eyelids and may be very painful with long-term systemic effects.

● **B01.1   Varicella encephalitis, myelitis and encephalomyelitis**
> Postchickenpox encephalitis, myelitis and encephalomyelitis
B01.11   Varicella encephalitis and encephalomyelitis
> Postchickenpox encephalitis and encephalomyelitis
B01.12   Varicella myelitis 🅗
> Postchickenpox myelitis
B01.2   Varicella pneumonia
● **B01.8   Varicella with other complications**
B01.81   Varicella keratitis
B01.89   Other varicella complications
B01.9   Varicella without complication
> Varicella NOS

● **B02   Zoster [herpes zoster]**
> **Includes**   shingles
> zona

B02.0   Zoster encephalitis
> Zoster meningoencephalitis
B02.1   Zoster meningitis
● **B02.2   Zoster with other nervous system involvement**
> Coding Clinic: 2019, Q1, P18
B02.21   Postherpetic geniculate ganglionitis
B02.22   Postherpetic trigeminal neuralgia
B02.23   Postherpetic polyneuropathy
B02.24   Postherpetic myelitis 🅗
> Herpes zoster myelitis
B02.29   Other postherpetic nervous system involvement
> Postherpetic radiculopathy

● **B02.3   Zoster ocular disease**
B02.30   Zoster ocular disease, unspecified
B02.31   Zoster conjunctivitis
B02.32   Zoster iridocyclitis
B02.33   Zoster keratitis
> Herpes zoster keratoconjunctivitis
B02.34   Zoster scleritis
B02.39   Other herpes zoster eye disease
> Zoster blepharitis
B02.7   Disseminated zoster
B02.8   Zoster with other complications
> Herpes zoster otitis externa
B02.9   Zoster without complications
> Zoster NOS

B03   Smallpox
> **Note:** In 1980 the 33rd World Health Assembly declared that smallpox had been eradicated. The classification is maintained for surveillance purposes.

B04   Monkeypox
▶ **Mpox**
> *Disease occurring in captive monkeys and other mammals that may be transmitted to humans, clinically similar to smallpox*
> Coding Clinic: 2022, Q3, P3

Figure 1-5 Photograph of eyelids with marginal blepharitis. (From Hoyt CS, Taylor D: Pediatric Ophthalmology and Strabismus, London, Elsevier Saunders, 2005)

Item 1–17 Blepharitis is a common condition in which the eyelid is swollen and yellow scaling and conjunctivitis develop. Usually the hair on the scalp and brow is involved.

▶ New   ⇒ Revised   ~~deleted~~ Deleted   Excludes 1   Excludes 2   Includes   Use additional   Code first   Code also   Key words
OGCR Official Guidelines   X Assign placeholder X   ● Use Additional Character(s)   ▶ Manifestation Code   🅗 Hierarchical Condition Category   Coding Clinic

● **B05**   **Measles**
> **Includes**   morbilli
> **Excludes1**   subacute sclerosing panencephalitis (A81.1)

B05.0   Measles complicated by encephalitis
> Postmeasles encephalitis

B05.1   Measles complicated by meningitis
> Postmeasles meningitis

B05.2   Measles complicated by pneumonia
> Postmeasles pneumonia

B05.3   Measles complicated by otitis media
> Postmeasles otitis media

B05.4   Measles with intestinal complications

● **B05.8**   Measles with other complications
> **B05.81**   Measles keratitis and keratoconjunctivitis
> **B05.89**   Other measles complications

B05.9   Measles without complication
> Measles NOS

● **B06**   **Rubella [German measles]**
> **Excludes1**   congenital rubella (P35.0)

● **B06.0**   Rubella with neurological complications
> **B06.00**   Rubella with neurological complication, unspecified
> **B06.01**   Rubella encephalitis
> > Rubella meningoencephalitis
> **B06.02**   Rubella meningitis
> **B06.09**   Other neurological complications of rubella

● **B06.8**   Rubella with other complications
> **B06.81**   Rubella pneumonia
> **B06.82**   Rubella arthritis 🦠
> **B06.89**   Other rubella complications

B06.9   Rubella without complication
> Rubella NOS

● **B07**   **Viral warts**
> **Includes**   verruca simplex
> > verruca vulgaris
> > viral warts due to human papillomavirus
> **Excludes2**   anogenital (venereal) warts (A63.0)
> > papilloma of bladder (D41.4)
> > papilloma of cervix (D26.0)
> > papilloma larynx (D14.1)

B07.0   Plantar wart
> Verruca plantaris

B07.8   Other viral warts
> Common wart
> Flat wart
> Verruca plana

B07.9   Viral wart, unspecified

● **B08**   **Other viral infections characterized by skin and mucous membrane lesions, not elsewhere classified**
> **Excludes1**   vesicular stomatitis virus disease (A93.8)

● **B08.0**   Other orthopoxvirus infections
> **Excludes2**   monkeypox (B04)
> ● **B08.01**   Cowpox and vaccinia not from vaccine
> > **B08.010**   Cowpox
> > **B08.011**   Vaccinia not from vaccine
> > > **Excludes1**   vaccinia (from vaccination) (generalized) (T88.1)
> **B08.02**   Orf virus disease
> > Contagious pustular dermatitis
> > Ecthyma contagiosum
> **B08.03**   Pseudocowpox [milker's node]
> **B08.04**   Paravaccinia, unspecified
> **B08.09**   Other orthopoxvirus infections
> > Orthopoxvirus infection NOS

B08.1   Molluscum contagiosum
> *Various skin diseases characterized by soft, rounded, cutaneous lesions*

● **B08.2**   Exanthema subitum [sixth disease] Roseola infantum
> *Acute, short-lived high fever in infants and young children followed by a rash mainly on the trunk, caused by human herpesvirus 6*
> **B08.20**   Exanthema subitum [sixth disease], unspecified Roseola infantum, unspecified   P
> **B08.21**   Exanthema subitum [sixth disease] due to human herpesvirus 6 Roseola infantum due to human herpesvirus 6   P
> > *Virus results in sudden rash; infection results in lifelong persistence*
> **B08.22**   Exanthema subitum [sixth disease] due to human herpesvirus 7 Roseola infantum due to human herpesvirus 7   P

B08.3   Erythema infectiosum [fifth disease]
> *Moderately contagious, epidemic disease in children caused by B19 virus; onset of rash that begins as redness of cheeks, later there is rash on trunk and limbs; when this fades, there may be central clearing that leaves lacelike pattern*

B08.4   Enteroviral vesicular stomatitis with exanthem
> Hand, foot and mouth disease
> *Check your documentation—this code is HAND, foot, and mouth disease. Code B08.8 is foot and mouth disease.*

B08.5   Enteroviral vesicular pharyngitis
> Herpangina

● **B08.6**   Parapoxvirus infections
> **B08.60**   Parapoxvirus infection, unspecified
> **B08.61**   Bovine stomatitis
> **B08.62**   Sealpox
> **B08.69**   Other parapoxvirus infections

● **B08.7**   Yatapoxvirus infections
> **B08.70**   Yatapoxvirus infection, unspecified
> **B08.71**   Tanapox virus disease
> **B08.72**   Yaba pox virus disease
> > Yaba monkey tumor disease
> **B08.79**   Other yatapoxvirus infections

B08.8   Other specified viral infections characterized by skin and mucous membrane lesions
> Enteroviral lymphonodular pharyngitis
> Foot-and-mouth disease
> > *Check your documentation. Code B08.4 is for HAND, foot, and mouth disease.*
> Poxvirus NEC

B09   Unspecified viral infection characterized by skin and mucous membrane lesions
> Viral enanthema NOS
> Viral exanthema NOS

OTHER HUMAN HERPESVIRUSES (B10)

● **B10**   Other human herpesviruses
> **Excludes2**   cytomegalovirus (B25.9)
> > Epstein-Barr virus (B27.0-)
> > herpes NOS (B00.9)
> > herpes simplex (B00.-)
> > herpes zoster (B02.-)
> > human herpesvirus NOS (B00.-)
> > human herpesvirus 1 and 2 (B00.-)
> > human herpesvirus 3 (B01.-, B02.-)
> > human herpesvirus 4 (B27.0-)
> > human herpesvirus 5 (B25.-)
> > varicella (B01.-)
> > zoster (B02.-)
> **Coding Clinic: 2024, Q2, P21**

CHAPTER 1 (A00-B99)

● **B10.0   Other human herpesvirus encephalitis**

     Excludes2   herpes encephalitis NOS (B00.4)
                   herpes simplex encephalitis (B00.4)
                   human herpesvirus encephalitis (B00.4)
                   simian B herpes virus encephalitis (B00.4)

     B10.01   Human herpesvirus 6 encephalitis
              Sudden rash or roseola

     B10.09   Other human herpesvirus encephalitis
              Human herpesvirus 7 encephalitis
              Virus closely related to human herpesvirus 6, but
                 not known to cause any disease
              Coding Clinic: 2024, Q2, P21

● **B10.8   Other human herpesvirus infection**

     B10.81   Human herpesvirus 6 infection
              Causative agent of exanthema subitum that results
                 in sudden rash

     B10.82   Human herpesvirus 7 infection
              Closely related to human herpesvirus 6, but not
                 known cause any disease

     B10.89   Other human herpesvirus infection
              Human herpesvirus 8 infection
              May be the cause of Kaposi sarcoma, a malignant
                 tumor
              Kaposi's sarcoma-associated herpesvirus
                 infection

VIRAL HEPATITIS (B15-B19)

     Excludes1   sequelae of viral hepatitis (B94.2)
     Excludes2   cytomegaloviral hepatitis (B25.1)
                   herpesviral [herpes simplex] hepatitis (B00.81)

● **B15   Acute hepatitis A**

     B15.0   Hepatitis A with hepatic coma

     B15.9   Hepatitis A without hepatic coma
              Hepatitis A (acute) (viral) NOS

● **B16   Acute hepatitis B**

     B16.0   Acute hepatitis B with delta-agent with hepatic coma

     B16.1   Acute hepatitis B with delta-agent without hepatic coma

     B16.2   Acute hepatitis B without delta-agent with hepatic coma

     **B16.9   Acute hepatitis B without delta-agent and without
              hepatic coma**
              Hepatitis B (acute) (viral) NOS
              Coding Clinic: 2016, Q3, P13

● **B17   Other acute viral hepatitis**

     B17.0   Acute delta-(super) infection of hepatitis B carrier

 ● **B17.1   Acute hepatitis C**

     B17.10   Acute hepatitis C without hepatic coma
              Acute hepatitis C NOS

     B17.11   Acute hepatitis C with hepatic coma

     B17.2   Acute hepatitis E

     B17.8   Other specified acute viral hepatitis
              Hepatitis non-A non-B (acute) (viral) NEC

     B17.9   Acute viral hepatitis, unspecified
              Acute hepatitis NOS
              Acute infectious hepatitis NOS

Figure 1-6   Hepatitis B viral infection. **A.** Liver parenchyma showing hepatocytes with diffuse granular cytoplasm, so-called ground glass hepatocytes (H&E). **B.** Immunoperoxidase stains from the same case, showing cytoplasmic inclusions of viral particles. (From Kumar: Robbins and Cotran: Pathologic Basis of Disease, ed 8, Saunders, An Imprint of Elsevier, 2009)

Item 1-18   Hepatitis A (HAV) was formerly called epidemic, infectious, short-incubation, or acute catarrhal jaundice hepatitis. The primary transmission mode is the oral-fecal route. **Hepatitis B (HBV)** was formerly called long-incubation period, serum, or homologous serum hepatitis. Transmission modes are through blood from infected persons and from body fluids of infected mother to neonate. **Hepatitis C (HCV),** caused by the hepatitis C virus, is primarily transfusion associated. **Hepatitis D (HDV),** also called delta hepatitis, is caused by the hepatitis D virus in patients formerly or currently infected with hepatitis B. **Hepatitis E (HEV)** is also called enterically transmitted non-A, non-B hepatitis. The primary transmission mode is the oral-fecal route, usually through contaminated water.

● **B18   Chronic viral hepatitis**

     Includes   Carrier of viral hepatitis

     B18.0   Chronic viral hepatitis B with delta-agent 🏷

     B18.1   Chronic viral hepatitis B without delta-agent 🏷
              Carrier of viral hepatitis B
              Chronic (viral) hepatitis B

     B18.2   Chronic viral hepatitis C 🏷
              Carrier of viral hepatitis C
              Coding Clinic: 2018, Q1, P4; 2017, Q1, P41

     B18.8   Other chronic viral hepatitis 🏷
              Carrier of other viral hepatitis

     B18.9   Chronic viral hepatitis, unspecified 🏷
              Carrier of unspecified viral hepatitis

● **B19   Unspecified viral hepatitis**

     B19.0   Unspecified viral hepatitis with hepatic coma

 ● **B19.1   Unspecified viral hepatitis B**

     **B19.10   Unspecified viral hepatitis B without hepatic
                   coma**
                 Unspecified viral hepatitis B NOS

     B19.11   Unspecified viral hepatitis B with hepatic coma

 ● **B19.2   Unspecified viral hepatitis C**

     **B19.20   Unspecified viral hepatitis C without hepatic
                   coma**
                 Viral hepatitis C NOS

     B19.21   Unspecified viral hepatitis C with hepatic coma

     B19.9   Unspecified viral hepatitis without hepatic coma
              Viral hepatitis NOS

OGCR   Section I. C.1.a.

Certain Infectious and Parasitic Diseases (A00-B99)

a. Human Immunodeficiency Virus (HIV) Infections

   1) Code only confirmed cases

     Code only confirmed cases of HIV infection illness. This is an exception to the hospital inpatient guideline Section II, H.

     In this context, "confirmation" does not require documentation of positive serology or culture for HIV; the provider's diagnostic statement that the patient is HIV positive or has an HIV-related illness is sufficient.

HUMAN IMMUNODEFICIENCY VIRUS [HIV] DISEASE (B20)

B20   Human immunodeficiency virus [HIV] disease 🏷

     Includes   acquired immune deficiency syndrome [AIDS]
                   AIDS-related complex [ARC]
                   HIV infection, symptomatic

     Code first Human immunodeficiency virus [HIV] disease
              complicating pregnancy, childbirth and the puerperium, if
              applicable (O98.7-)

     Use additional code(s) to identify all manifestations of HIV
              infection

     Excludes1   asymptomatic human immunodeficiency virus
                   [HIV] infection status (Z21)
                   exposure to HIV virus (Z20.6)
                   inconclusive serologic evidence of HIV (R75)
          Coding Clinic: 2022, Q1, P36; 2021, Q2, P6; 2019, Q1, P9-11

▶ New   ⇒ Revised   ~~deleted~~ Deleted   Excludes 1   Excludes 2   Includes   Use additional   Code first   Code also   Key words

OGCR Official Guidelines   X Assign placeholder X   ● Use Additional Character(s)   ▌ Manifestation Code   🏷 Hierarchical Condition Category   Coding Clinic

Figure 1-7 Kaposi's sarcoma. There are large confluent hyperpigmented patch-stage lesions with lymphedema. (From Kanski, JJ: Clinical Diagnosis in Ophthalmology, London, Elsevier Mosby, 2006)

Item 1-19 AIDS (acquired immune deficiency syndrome) is caused by **HIV** (human immunodeficiency virus). HIV affects certain white blood cells (T-4 lymphocytes) and destroys the ability of the cells to fight infections, making patients susceptible to a host of infectious diseases (e.g., **Pneumocystis carinii pneumonia [PCP], Kaposi's sarcoma,** and **lymphoma**). **AIDS-related complex (ARC)** is an early stage of AIDS in which tests for HIV are positive but the symptoms are mild.

OTHER VIRAL DISEASES (B25-B34)

● **B25　Cytomegaloviral disease**
　　AKA: HCMV or Human Herpesvirus 5 (HHV-5)
　　Excludes1　congenital cytomegalovirus infection (P35.1)
　　　　　　　　cytomegaloviral mononucleosis (B27.1-)

　B25.0　Cytomegaloviral pneumonitis 🔗

　B25.1　Cytomegaloviral hepatitis 🔗

　B25.2　Cytomegaloviral pancreatitis 🔗

　B25.8　Other cytomegaloviral diseases 🔗
　　　　Cytomegaloviral encephalitis

　B25.9　Cytomegaloviral disease, unspecified 🔗

● **B26　Mumps**
　　Includes　epidemic parotitis
　　　　　　　infectious parotitis
　　Acute, contagious, viral disease

　B26.0　Mumps orchitis

　B26.1　Mumps meningitis

　B26.2　Mumps encephalitis

　B26.3　Mumps pancreatitis

● **B26.8　Mumps with other complications**

　　B26.81　Mumps hepatitis

　　B26.82　Mumps myocarditis

　　B26.83　Mumps nephritis

　　B26.84　Mumps polyneuropathy

　　B26.85　Mumps arthritis 🔗

　　B26.89　Other mumps complications

　B26.9　Mumps without complication
　　　　Mumps NOS
　　　　Mumps parotitis NOS

● **B27　Infectious mononucleosis**
　　Includes　glandular fever
　　　　　　　monocytic angina
　　　　　　　Pfeiffer's disease

● **B27.0　Gammaherpesviral mononucleosis**
　　AKA: Pfeiffer's disease, infective mononucleosis
　　Mononucleosis due to Epstein-Barr virus

　　B27.00　Gammaherpesviral mononucleosis without complication
　　　　　　Infective mononucleosis

　　B27.01　Gammaherpesviral mononucleosis with polyneuropathy

　　B27.02　Gammaherpesviral mononucleosis with meningitis

　　B27.09　Gammaherpesviral mononucleosis with other complications
　　　　　　Hepatomegaly in gammaherpesviral mononucleosis
　　　　　　Coding Clinic: 2024, Q2, P21,22

● **B27.1　Cytomegaloviral mononucleosis**
　　Infectious disease resembling infectious mononucleosis

　　B27.10　Cytomegaloviral mononucleosis without complications

　　B27.11　Cytomegaloviral mononucleosis with polyneuropathy

　　B27.12　Cytomegaloviral mononucleosis with meningitis

　　B27.19　Cytomegaloviral mononucleosis with other complication
　　　　　　Hepatomegaly in cytomegaloviral mononucleosis

● **B27.8　Other infectious mononucleosis**

　　B27.80　Other infectious mononucleosis without complication

　　B27.81　Other infectious mononucleosis with polyneuropathy

　　B27.82　Other infectious mononucleosis with meningitis

　　B27.89　Other infectious mononucleosis with other complication
　　　　　　Hepatomegaly in other infectious mononucleosis

● **B27.9　Infectious mononucleosis, unspecified**

　　B27.90　Infectious mononucleosis, unspecified without complication

　　B27.91　Infectious mononucleosis, unspecified with polyneuropathy

　　B27.92　Infectious mononucleosis, unspecified with meningitis

　　B27.99　Infectious mononucleosis, unspecified with other complication
　　　　　　Hepatomegaly in unspecified infectious mononucleosis

● **B30　Viral conjunctivitis**
　　Excludes1　herpesviral [herpes simplex] ocular disease
　　　　　　　　(B00.5)
　　　　　　　　ocular zoster (B02.3)

　B30.0　Keratoconjunctivitis due to adenovirus
　　　　Epidemic keratoconjunctivitis
　　　　Shipyard eye

　B30.1　Conjunctivitis due to adenovirus
　　　　Acute adenoviral follicular conjunctivitis
　　　　Swimming-pool conjunctivitis

　B30.2　Viral pharyngoconjunctivitis

　B30.3　Acute epidemic hemorrhagic conjunctivitis (enteroviral)
　　　　Conjunctivitis due to coxsackievirus 24
　　　　Conjunctivitis due to enterovirus 70
　　　　Hemorrhagic conjunctivitis (acute)(epidemic)

　B30.8　Other viral conjunctivitis
　　　　Newcastle conjunctivitis

　B30.9　Viral conjunctivitis, unspecified

● **B33　Other viral diseases, not elsewhere classified**

　B33.0　Epidemic myalgia
　　　　Acute infectious disease, caused by group A coxsackie viruses or other enteroviruses with symptoms that include sudden pain in chest or upper abdomen with fever
　　　　Bornholm disease

　B33.1　Ross River disease
　　　　Epidemic polyarthritis and exanthema
　　　　Ross River fever

● **B33.2 Viral carditis**
Coxsackie (virus) carditis
   B33.20 Viral carditis, unspecified
   B33.21 Viral endocarditis
   B33.22 Viral myocarditis
   B33.23 Viral pericarditis
   B33.24 Viral cardiomyopathy
B33.3 Retrovirus infections, not elsewhere classified
Retrovirus infection NOS
B33.4 Hantavirus (cardio)-pulmonary syndrome [HPS] [HCPS]
Hantavirus disease with pulmonary manifestations
Sin nombre virus disease
Use additional code to identify any associated acute kidney failure (N17.9)
   Excludes1 hantavirus disease with renal manifestations (A98.5)
     hemorrhagic fever with renal manifestations (A98.5)
B33.8 Other specified viral diseases
   Excludes1 anogenital human papillomavirus infection (A63.0)
     viral warts due to human papillomavirus infection (B07)

● **B34 Viral infection of unspecified site**
   Excludes1 anogenital human papillomavirus infection (A63.0)
     cytomegaloviral disease NOS (B25.9)
     herpesvirus [herpes simplex] infection NOS (B00.9)
     retrovirus infection NOS (B33.3)
     viral agents as the cause of diseases classified elsewhere (B97.-)
     viral warts due to human papillomavirus infection (B07)
B34.0 Adenovirus infection, unspecified
B34.1 Enterovirus infection, unspecified
Intestinal tract infection
Coxsackievirus infection NOS
Echovirus infection NOS
B34.2 Coronavirus infection, unspecified
   Excludes1 COVID-19 (U07.1)
     pneumonia due to SARS-associated coronavirus (J12.81)
B34.3 Parvovirus infection, unspecified
B34.4 Papovavirus infection, unspecified
B34.8 Other viral infections of unspecified site
B34.9 Viral infection, unspecified
Viremia NOS
Coding Clinic: 2016, Q3, P10

MYCOSES (B35-B49)

   Excludes2 hypersensitivity pneumonitis due to organic dust (J67.-)
     mycosis fungoides (C84.0-)

● **B35 Dermatophytosis**
AKA tinea or ringworm
   Includes favus
     infections due to species of Epidermophyton, Micro-sporum and Trichophyton
     tinea, any type except those in B36.-
B35.0 Tinea barbae and tinea capitis
Beard ringworm
Kerion
Scalp ringworm
Sycosis, mycotic
B35.1 Tinea unguium
White patches or pits on surface or edges of nails, followed by infection under nail plate
Dermatophytic onychia
Dermatophytosis of nail
Onychomycosis
Ringworm of nails

B35.2 Tinea manuum
Tinea of hands
Dermatophytosis of hand
Hand ringworm
B35.3 Tinea pedis
Tinea affecting feet
Athlete's foot
Dermatophytosis of foot
Foot ringworm
B35.4 Tinea corporis
Infecting skin areas other than hands
Ringworm of the body
B35.5 Tinea imbricata
Chronic tropical tinea corporis; AKA Oriental ringworm, tinea inguinalis, tinea cruris
Tokelau
B35.6 Tinea cruris
In groin or perineal area, spreading to adjacent regions; AKA jock itch, eczema marginatum, ringworm of groin, or tinea inguinalis
Dhobi itch
Groin ringworm
Jock itch
B35.8 Other dermatophytoses
Disseminated dermatophytosis
Granulomatous dermatophytosis
B35.9 Dermatophytosis, unspecified
Ringworm NOS

● **B36 Other superficial mycoses**
B36.0 Pityriasis versicolor
Common, chronic, symptomless disorder that includes macular patches of various sizes and shapes; AKA liver spots
Tinea flava
Tinea versicolor
B36.1 Tinea nigra
Minor fungal infection, with dark lesions, usually on skin of hands
Keratomycosis nigricans palmaris
Microsporosis nigra
Pityriasis nigra
B36.2 White piedra
White to light brown nodules on hair of beard, axilla, or groin; AKA trichosporosis
Tinea blanca
B36.3 Black piedra
Characterized by small black or brown nodules on shafts of scalp hair
B36.8 Other specified superficial mycoses
B36.9 Superficial mycosis, unspecified

● **B37 Candidiasis**
   Includes candidosis
     moniliasis
   Excludes1 neonatal candidiasis (P37.5)
B37.0 Candidal stomatitis
Oral thrush
B37.1 Pulmonary candidiasis
Candidal bronchitis
Candidal pneumonia

Figure 1-8 Oral candidiasis (thrush). (From James WD, Berger T, Elston D: Andrews' Diseases of the Skin: Clinical Dermatology, 11e, Saunders, 2011)

Item 1-20 Candidiasis, also called oidiomycosis or moniliasis, is a fungal infection. It most often appears on moist cutaneous areas of the body but can also be responsible for a variety of systemic infections such as endocarditis, meningitis, arthritis, and myositis. Antifungal medications cure most yeast infections.

▶ New ⟹ Revised ~~deleted~~ Deleted | Excludes 1 | Excludes 2 | Includes | Use additional | Code first | Code also | Key words
OGCR Official Guidelines X Assign placeholder X ● Use Additional Character(s) ▶ Manifestation Code ✿ Hierarchical Condition Category **Coding Clinic**

Item 1–21 Bird and bat droppings that fall into the soil give rise to a fungus that can spread airborne spores. When inhaled into the lungs, these spores divide and multiply into lesions. Histoplasmosis capsulatum takes three forms: primary (lodged in the lungs only), chronic (resembles TB), and disseminated (infection has moved to other organs). This is an opportunistic infection in immunosuppressed patients.

B37.2   **Candidiasis of skin and nail**
     Candidal onychia
     Candidal paronychia
     Excludes2   diaper dermatitis (L22)

B37.3   **Candidiasis of vulva and vagina**
     Candidal vulvovaginitis
     Monilial vulvovaginitis
     Vaginal thrush

     B37.31   **Acute candidiasis of vulva and vagina**
         Candidiasis of vulva and vagina NOS

     B37.32   **Chronic candidiasis of vulva and vagina**
         Recurrent candidiasis of vulva and vagina

● B37.4   **Candidiasis of other urogenital sites**

     B37.41   **Candidal cystitis and urethritis**

     B37.42   **Candidal balanitis**
         Male condition only

     B37.49   **Other urogenital candidiasis**
         Candidal pyelonephritis

B37.5   **Candidal meningitis**

B37.6   **Candidal endocarditis**

B37.7   **Candidal sepsis** 🦠
     Disseminated candidiasis systemic candidiasis

● B37.8   **Candidiasis of other sites**

     B37.81   **Candidal esophagitis** 🦠

     B37.82   **Candidal enteritis**
         Candidal proctitis

     B37.83   **Candidal cheilitis**
         Inflammation affecting lip

     B37.84   **Candidal otitis externa**
         Inflammation of external auditory canal

     B37.89   **Other sites of candidiasis**
         Infection manifested by invasive candidiasis
         Candidal osteomyelitis

B37.9   **Candidiasis, unspecified**
     Thrush NOS

● B38   **Coccidioidomycosis**
     Fungal disease; AKA coccidioidosis, coccidioidal granuloma, Posadas, or Posadas-Wernicke disease

     B38.0   **Acute pulmonary coccidioidomycosis** 🦠

     B38.1   **Chronic pulmonary coccidioidomycosis** 🦠

     B38.2   **Pulmonary coccidioidomycosis, unspecified** 🦠

     B38.3   **Cutaneous coccidioidomycosis**

     B38.4   **Coccidioidomycosis meningitis**

     B38.7   **Disseminated coccidioidomycosis**
         Generalized coccidioidomycosis

   ● B38.8   **Other forms of coccidioidomycosis**

     B38.81   **Prostatic coccidioidomycosis**

     B38.89   **Other forms of coccidioidomycosis**

     B38.9   **Coccidioidomycosis, unspecified**

● B39   **Histoplasmosis**
     Infection resulting from inhalation or ingestion of spores; AKA Darling disease

     Code first associated AIDS (B20)

     Use additional code for any associated manifestations, such as:
       endocarditis (I39)
       meningitis (G02)
       pericarditis (I32)
       retinitis (H32)

     B39.0   **Acute pulmonary histoplasmosis capsulati** 🦠

     B39.1   **Chronic pulmonary histoplasmosis capsulati** 🦠

     B39.2   **Pulmonary histoplasmosis capsulati, unspecified** 🦠

B39.3   **Disseminated histoplasmosis capsulati**
     Generalized histoplasmosis capsulati

B39.4   **Histoplasmosis capsulati, unspecified**
     American histoplasmosis

B39.5   **Histoplasmosis duboisii**
     African histoplasmosis

B39.9   **Histoplasmosis, unspecified**

● B40   **Blastomycosis**
     Rare and potentially fatal infection caused by inhaling fungus found in moist soil in temperate climates.

     Excludes1   Brazilian blastomycosis (B41.-)
            keloidal blastomycosis (B48.0)

     B40.0   **Acute pulmonary blastomycosis** 🦠

     B40.1   **Chronic pulmonary blastomycosis** 🦠

     B40.2   **Pulmonary blastomycosis, unspecified** 🦠

     B40.3   **Cutaneous blastomycosis**

     B40.7   **Disseminated blastomycosis**
         Generalized blastomycosis

   ● B40.8   **Other forms of blastomycosis**

     B40.81   **Blastomycotic meningoencephalitis**
         Meningomyelitis due to blastomycosis

     B40.89   **Other forms of blastomycosis**

     B40.9   **Blastomycosis, unspecified**

● B41   **Paracoccidioidomycosis**
     Fungal infection usually chronic that begins in lungs, spreads to mucocutaneous areas which may extend to skin, tonsils, gastrointestinal lymphatics, liver, and spleen; AKA Almeida or Lutz-Splendore-Almeida disease, Brazilian or South American blastomycosis, or paracoccidioidal granuloma

     Includes   Brazilian blastomycosis
            Lutz' disease

     B41.0   **Pulmonary paracoccidioidomycosis** 🦠

     B41.7   **Disseminated paracoccidioidomycosis**
         Generalized paracoccidioidomycosis

     B41.8   **Other forms of paracoccidioidomycosis**

     B41.9   **Paracoccidioidomycosis, unspecified**

● B42   **Sporotrichosis**
     Chronic fungal infection with nodular lesions

     B42.0   **Pulmonary sporotrichosis**

     B42.1   **Lymphocutaneous sporotrichosis**

     B42.7   **Disseminated sporotrichosis**
         Generalized sporotrichosis

   ● B42.8   **Other forms of sporotrichosis**

     B42.81   **Cerebral sporotrichosis**
         Meningitis due to sporotrichosis

     B42.82   **Sporotrichosis arthritis** 🦠

     B42.89   **Other forms of sporotrichosis**

     B42.9   **Sporotrichosis, unspecified**

● B43   **Chromomycosis and pheomycotic abscess**
     Chronic fungal infection of skin, initiated at site of puncture affecting lower limb or foot (mossy foot)

     B43.0   **Cutaneous chromomycosis**
         Dermatitis verrucosa

     B43.1   **Pheomycotic brain abscess**
         Cerebral chromomycosis

     B43.2   **Subcutaneous pheomycotic abscess and cyst**

     B43.8   **Other forms of chromomycosis**

     B43.9   **Chromomycosis, unspecified**

● B44   **Aspergillosis**
     Infection marked by inflammatory lesions in skin, ear, orbit, nasal sinuses, lungs, and occasionally bones and meninges

     Includes   aspergilloma

     B44.0   **Invasive pulmonary aspergillosis** 🦠

     B44.1   **Other pulmonary aspergillosis** 🦠

CHAPTER 1 (A00-B99)

B44.2   **Tonsillar aspergillosis** 🐾

B44.7   **Disseminated aspergillosis** 🐾
       Generalized aspergillosis

● B44.8   **Other forms of aspergillosis**

      B44.81   **Allergic bronchopulmonary aspergillosis** 🐾

      B44.89   **Other forms of aspergillosis** 🐾

B44.9   **Aspergillosis, unspecified** 🐾

● B45   **Cryptococcosis**
     Infection in the immunocompromised and fatal if left untreated; AKA
     torulosis, Buschke, or Busse-Buschke disease

     B45.0   **Pulmonary cryptococcosis** 🐾

     B45.1   **Cerebral cryptococcosis** 🐾
          Cryptococcal meningitis
          Cryptococcosis meningocerebralis

     B45.2   **Cutaneous cryptococcosis** 🐾

     B45.3   **Osseous cryptococcosis** 🐾

     B45.7   **Disseminated cryptococcosis** 🐾
          Generalized cryptococcosis

     B45.8   **Other forms of cryptococcosis** 🐾

     B45.9   **Cryptococcosis, unspecified** 🐾

● B46   **Zygomycosis**
     Fungal infections including subcutaneous lesions and infection of
     sinuses, brain, or lungs

     B46.0   **Pulmonary mucormycosis** 🐾
          Fungal infection affecting lung

     B46.1   **Rhinocerebral mucormycosis** 🐾

     B46.2   **Gastrointestinal mucormycosis** 🐾

     B46.3   **Cutaneous mucormycosis** 🐾
          Subcutaneous mucormycosis

     B46.4   **Disseminated mucormycosis** 🐾
          Generalized mucormycosis

     B46.5   **Mucormycosis, unspecified** 🐾

     B46.8   **Other zygomycoses** 🐾
          Entomophthoromycosis

     B46.9   **Zygomycosis, unspecified** 🐾
          Phycomycosis NOS

● B47   **Mycetoma**
     Slow progressive, destructive fungal infection of cutaneous and
     subcutaneous tissues, fascia, and bone, primarily seen in foot
     (Madura foot) or leg

     B47.0   **Eumycetoma**
          Madura foot, mycotic Maduromycosis

     B47.1   **Actinomycetoma**

     B47.9   **Mycetoma, unspecified**
          Madura foot NOS

● B48   **Other mycoses, not elsewhere classified**

     B48.0   **Lobomycosis**
          Infection with symptoms of red, smooth, hard cutaneous
          nodules resembling keloids
          Keloidal blastomycosis
          Lobo's disease

     B48.1   **Rhinosporidiosis**
          Chronic, localized granulomatous fungal infection, affecting
          mucocutaneous tissues, usually of nose characterized by
          polyps, papillomas, and wartlike lesions

     B48.2   **Allescheriasis**
          Fungal infection
          Infection due to Pseudallescheria boydii
          Excludes1   eumycetoma (B47.0)

     B48.3   **Geotrichosis**
          Fungal infection usually of bronchi, lungs, mouth, or
          intestinal tract
          Geotrichum stomatitis

     B48.4   **Penicillosis** 🐾
          Fungal infection
          Talaromycosis

     B48.8   **Other specified mycoses** 🐾
          Adiaspiromycosis
          Infection of tissue and organs by Alternaria
          Infection of tissue and organs by Drechslera
          Infection of tissue and organs by Fusarium
          Infection of tissue and organs by saprophytic fungi
          NEC

B49   **Unspecified mycosis**
     Fungemia NOS

PROTOZOAL DISEASES (B50-B64)

   Excludes1   amebiasis (A06.-)
               other protozoal intestinal diseases (A07.-)

● B50   **Plasmodium falciparum malaria**
     Severe form of malaria that can be fatal
     Includes   mixed infections of Plasmodium falciparum with
               any other Plasmodium species

     B50.0   **Plasmodium falciparum malaria with cerebral complications**
          Cerebral malaria NOS

     B50.8   **Other severe and complicated Plasmodium falciparum malaria**
          Severe or complicated Plasmodium falciparum malaria
          NOS

     B50.9   **Plasmodium falciparum malaria, unspecified**

● B51   **Plasmodium vivax malaria**
     Includes   mixed infections of Plasmodium vivax with other
               Plasmodium species, except Plasmodium
               falciparum

     Excludes1   plasmodium vivax with Plasmodium falciparum
                (B50.-)

     B51.0   **Plasmodium vivax malaria with rupture of spleen**

     B51.8   **Plasmodium vivax malaria with other complications**

     B51.9   **Plasmodium vivax malaria without complication**
          Plasmodium vivax malaria NOS

● B52   **Plasmodium malariae malaria**
     Causes fever that recurs at approximately three-day intervals (quartan
     fever), longer than two-day (tertian) intervals of other malarial
     parasites
     Includes   mixed infections of Plasmodium malariae
               with other Plasmodium species, except
               Plasmodium falciparum and Plasmodium
               vivax

     Excludes1   plasmodium falciparum (B50.-)
                plasmodium vivax (B51.-)

     B52.0   **Plasmodium malariae malaria with nephropathy**

     B52.8   **Plasmodium malariae malaria with other complications**

     B52.9   **Plasmodium malariae malaria without complication**
          Plasmodium malariae malaria NOS

● B53   **Other specified malaria**

     B53.0   **Plasmodium ovale malaria**
          Least diagnosed type of malaria spread by female mosquitoes
          of rare species
          Excludes1   plasmodium ovale with Plasmodium
                falciparum (B50.-)
                plasmodium ovale with Plasmodium
                malariae (B52.-)
                plasmodium ovale with Plasmodium
                vivax (B51.-)

     B53.1   **Malaria due to simian plasmodia**
          Malaria-like disease (parasite infection)
          Excludes1   malaria due to simian plasmodia with
                Plasmodium falciparum (B50.-)
                malaria due to simian plasmodia with
                Plasmodium malariae (B52.-)
                malaria due to simian plasmodia with
                Plasmodium ovale (B53.0)
                malaria due to simian plasmodia with
                Plasmodium vivax (B51.-)

     B53.8   **Other malaria, not elsewhere classified**

▶ New   ⇒ Revised   ~~deleted~~ Deleted   Excludes 1   Excludes 2   Includes   Use additional   Code first   Code also   Key words

616   OGCR Official Guidelines   X Assign placeholder X   ● Use Additional Character(s)   ▌ Manifestation Code   🐾 Hierarchical Condition Category   Coding Clinic

B54 Unspecified malaria

● B55 Leishmaniasis
Protozoal infection

B55.0 Visceral leishmaniasis
Kala-azar
Post-kala-azar dermal leishmaniasis

B55.1 Cutaneous leishmaniasis

B55.2 Mucocutaneous leishmaniasis

B55.9 Leishmaniasis, unspecified

● B56 African trypanosomiasis
Human African trypanosomiasis (HAT) is transmitted by fly bites

B56.0 Gambiense trypanosomiasis
Infection due to Trypanosoma brucei gambiense
West African sleeping sickness

B56.1 Rhodesiense trypanosomiasis
East African sleeping sickness
Infection due to Trypanosoma brucei rhodesiense

B56.9 African trypanosomiasis, unspecified
Sleeping sickness NOS

● B57 Chagas' disease
Tropical parasitic disease

Includes American trypanosomiasis
infection due to Trypanosoma cruzi

B57.0 Acute Chagas' disease with heart involvement
Acute Chagas' disease with myocarditis

B57.1 Acute Chagas' disease without heart involvement
Acute Chagas' disease NOS

B57.2 Chagas' disease (chronic) with heart involvement
American trypanosomiasis NOS
Chagas' disease (chronic) NOS
Chagas' disease (chronic) with myocarditis
Trypanosomiasis NOS

● B57.3 Chagas' disease (chronic) with digestive system involvement

B57.30 Chagas' disease with digestive system involvement, unspecified

B57.31 Megaesophagus in Chagas' disease

B57.32 Megacolon in Chagas' disease

B57.39 Other digestive system involvement in Chagas' disease

● B57.4 Chagas' disease (chronic) with nervous system involvement

B57.40 Chagas' disease with nervous system involvement, unspecified

B57.41 Meningitis in Chagas' disease

B57.42 Meningoencephalitis in Chagas' disease

B57.49 Other nervous system involvement in Chagas' disease

B57.5 Chagas' disease (chronic) with other organ involvement

● B58 Toxoplasmosis
Infection by protozoon transmitted in cysts in feces of cats

Includes infection due to Toxoplasma gondii

Excludes1 congenital toxoplasmosis (P37.1)

● B58.0 Toxoplasma oculopathy

B58.00 Toxoplasma oculopathy, unspecified

B58.01 Toxoplasma chorioretinitis

B58.09 Other toxoplasma oculopathy
Toxoplasma uveitis

B58.1 Toxoplasma hepatitis

B58.2 Toxoplasma meningoencephalitis 🦠

B58.3 Pulmonary toxoplasmosis 🦠

● B58.8 Toxoplasmosis with other organ involvement

B58.81 Toxoplasma myocarditis

B58.82 Toxoplasma myositis

B58.83 Toxoplasma tubulo-interstitial nephropathy
Toxoplasma pyelonephritis

B58.89 Toxoplasmosis with other organ involvement

B58.9 Toxoplasmosis, unspecified

B59 Pneumocystosis 🦠
Caused by fungus
Pneumonia due to Pneumocystis carinii
Pneumonia due to Pneumocystis jiroveci

● B60 Other protozoal diseases, not elsewhere classified

Excludes1 cryptosporidiosis (A07.2)
intestinal microsporidiosis (A07.8)
isosporiasis (A07.3)

● B60.0 Babesiosis
Tickborne disease caused by microscopic organisms

B60.00 Babesiosis, unspecified
Babesiosis due to unspecified Babesia species
Piroplasmosis, unspecified

B60.01 Babesiosis due to Babesia microti
Infection due to B. microti

B60.02 Babesiosis due to Babesia duncani
Infection due to B. duncani and B. duncani-type species

B60.03 Babesiosis due to Babesia divergens
Babesiosis due to Babesia MO-1
Infection due to B. divergens and B. divergens-like strains

B60.09 Other babesiosis
Babesiosis due to Babesia KO-1
Babesiosis due to Babesia venatorum
Infection due to other Babesia species
Infection due to other protozoa of the order Piroplasmida
Other piroplasmosis

● B60.1 Acanthamebiasis

B60.10 Acanthamebiasis, unspecified

B60.11 Meningoencephalitis due to Acanthamoeba (culbertsoni)

B60.12 Conjunctivitis due to Acanthamoeba

B60.13 Keratoconjunctivitis due to Acanthamoeba

B60.19 Other acanthamebic disease

B60.2 Naegleriasis
Infection with microscopic organisms
Primary amebic meningoencephalitis

B60.8 Other specified protozoal diseases
Microsporidiosis

B64 Unspecified protozoal disease

HELMINTHIASES (B65-B83)

Diseases or infestations caused by parasitic worms

● B65 Schistosomiasis [bilharziasis]
Infection with flukes (flat parasitic worms)

Includes snail fever

B65.0 Schistosomiasis due to Schistosoma haematobium [urinary schistosomiasis]

B65.1 Schistosomiasis due to Schistosoma mansoni [intestinal schistosomiasis]

B65.2 Schistosomiasis due to Schistosoma japonicum
Asiatic schistosomiasis

B65.3 Cercarial dermatitis
Swimmer's itch

Item 1–22 Toxoplasmosis is caused by the protozoa **Toxoplasma gondii,** of which the house cat can be a host. Human infection occurs when contact is made with materials containing the pathogen, such as feces, contaminated soil, or ingestion of infected lamb, goat, or pork. Of the infected, very few have symptoms because a healthy person's immune system keeps the parasite from causing illness. When the immune system is compromised, symptoms may occur. Clinical symptoms include flu-like symptoms, but the disease progresses to include the eyes and the brain in babies.

CHAPTER 1 (A00-B99)

CHAPTER 1 (A00-B99)

B65.8   Other schistosomiasis
Infection due to Schistosoma intercalatum
Infection due to Schistosoma mattheei
Infection due to Schistosoma mekongi

B65.9   Schistosomiasis, unspecified

● **B66   Other fluke infections**
Trematode (parasitic worms)

B66.0   Opisthorchiasis
Infection due to cat liver fluke
Infection due to Opisthorchis (felineus)(viverrini)

B66.1   Clonorchiasis
Chinese liver fluke disease
Infection due to Clonorchis sinensis
Oriental liver fluke disease

B66.2   Dicroceliasis
Liver fluke
Infection due to Dicrocoelium dendriticum
Lancet fluke infection

B66.3   Fascioliasis
Infection due to Fasciola gigantica
Infection due to Fasciola hepatica
Infection due to Fasciola indica
Sheep liver fluke disease

B66.4   Paragonimiasis 🦠
Infection due to Paragonimus species
Lung fluke disease
Pulmonary distomiasis

B66.5   Fasciolopsiasis
Largest intestinal fluke in humans
Infection due to Fasciolopsis buski
Intestinal distomiasis

B66.8   Other specified fluke infections
Echinostomiasis
Heterophyiasis
Metagonimiasis
Nanophyetiasis
Watsoniasis

B66.9   Fluke infection, unspecified

● **B67   Echinococcosis**
Larval forms of tapeworms usually of liver or lungs
Includes   hydatidosis

B67.0   Echinococcus granulosus infection of liver
B67.1   Echinococcus granulosus infection of lung 🦠
B67.2   Echinococcus granulosus infection of bone
● **B67.3   Echinococcus granulosus infection, other and multiple sites**

    B67.31   Echinococcus granulosus infection, thyroid gland
    B67.32   Echinococcus granulosus infection, multiple sites
    B67.39   Echinococcus granulosus infection, other sites

B67.4   Echinococcus granulosus infection, unspecified
Dog tapeworm (infection)

B67.5   Echinococcus multilocularis infection of liver
● **B67.6   Echinococcus multilocularis infection, other and multiple sites**

    B67.61   Echinococcus multilocularis infection, multiple sites
    B67.69   Echinococcus multilocularis infection, other sites

B67.7   Echinococcus multilocularis infection, unspecified
B67.8   Echinococcosis, unspecified, of liver
● **B67.9   Echinococcosis, other and unspecified**

    B67.90   Echinococcosis, unspecified
Echinococcosis NOS
    B67.99   Other echinococcosis

Item 1-23 Echinococcosis: Also known as hydatid disease; is caused by Echinococcus granulosus, E. multilocularis, and E. vogeli tapeworms; and is contracted from infected food. Found in southern South America, the Mediterranean, the Middle East, central Asia, and Africa and uncommon in the United States but has been reported in California, New Mexico, Arizona and Utah. The disease is treated with medication over a long course, as it is resistive.

● **B68   Taeniasis**
Intestinal tapeworm (cestode) infection from raw or undercooked meat of infected animal
Excludes1   cysticercosis (B69.-)

B68.0   Taenia solium taeniasis
Pork tapeworm (infection)

B68.1   Taenia saginata taeniasis
Beef tapeworm (infection)
Infection due to adult tapeworm Taenia saginata

B68.9   Taeniasis, unspecified

● **B69   Cysticercosis**
Systemic illness caused by the larvae of pork tapeworm
Includes   cysticerciasis infection due to larval form of Taenia solium

B69.0   Cysticercosis of central nervous system
B69.1   Cysticercosis of eye
● **B69.8   Cysticercosis of other sites**

    B69.81   Myositis in cysticercosis
    B69.89   Cysticercosis of other sites

B69.9   Cysticercosis, unspecified

● **B70   Diphyllobothriasis and sparganosis**
Infection with tapeworms seen most often from inadequately cooked fish

B70.0   Diphyllobothriasis
Diphyllobothrium (adult) (latum) (pacificum) infection
Fish tapeworm (infection)
Excludes2   larval diphyllobothriasis (B70.1)

B70.1   Sparganosis
Infection with migrating tapeworm larvae, which invade subcutaneous tissues, causing inflammation and fibrosis that resembles cellulitis
Infection due to Sparganum (mansoni) (proliferum)
Infection due to Spirometra larva
Larval diphyllobothriasis
Spirometrosis

● **B71   Other cestode infections**

B71.0   Hymenolepiasis
Intestinal infestation with tapeworms
Dwarf tapeworm infection
Rat tapeworm (infection)

B71.1   Dipylidiasis
Infection with tapeworm common to dogs and cats and seen in children having close contact with infected pets

B71.8   Other specified cestode infections
Infection by the larval stage of a tapeworm, usually through fruit or vegetables
Coenurosis

B71.9   Cestode infection, unspecified
Tapeworm (infection) NOS

B72   Dracunculiasis
Infection with roundworms
Includes   guinea worm infection
infection due to Dracunculus medinensis

● **B73   Onchocerciasis**
Infection with parasitic worm
Includes   onchocerca volvulus infection
onchocercosis
river blindness

● **B73.0   Onchocerciasis with eye disease**

    B73.00   Onchocerciasis with eye involvement, unspecified
    B73.01   Onchocerciasis with endophthalmitis
    B73.02   Onchocerciasis with glaucoma
    B73.09   Onchocerciasis with other eye involvement
Infestation of eyelid due to onchocerciasis

B73.1   Onchocerciasis without eye disease

▶ New   ⇒ Revised   d̶e̶l̶e̶t̶e̶d̶ Deleted   Excludes 1   Excludes 2   Includes   Use additional   Code first   Code also   Key words

OGCR Official Guidelines   X Assign placeholder X   ● Use Additional Character(s)   ▶ Manifestation Code   🦠 Hierarchical Condition Category   Coding Clinic

● **B74   Filariasis**
Infestation with slender threadlike worms
Excludes2   onchocerciasis (B73)
tropical (pulmonary) eosinophilia NOS (J82.89)

B74.0   Filariasis due to Wuchereria bancrofti
Bancroftian elephantiasis
Bancroftian filariasis

B74.1   Filariasis due to Brugia malayi

B74.2   Filariasis due to Brugia timori

B74.3   Loiasis
Infection with round worms growing in subcutaneous connective tissue
Calabar swelling
Eyeworm disease of Africa
Loa loa infection

B74.4   Mansonelliasis
Infection with filarial parasite
Infection due to Mansonella ozzardi
Infection due to Mansonella perstans
Infection due to Mansonella streptocerca

B74.8   Other filariases
Dirofilariasis

B74.9   Filariasis, unspecified

● **B75   Trichinellosis**
Infestation with parasitic roundworms ingested in undercooked contaminated meat
Includes   infection due to Trichinella species trichiniasis

● **B76   Hookworm diseases**
Occurs in hot, humid parts of world where larvae are soil borne, enter digestive tract through skin of feet/legs or in contaminated food/water; AKA ground itch
Includes   uncinariasis

B76.0   Ancylostomiasis
Infection due to Ancylostoma species

B76.1   Necatoriasis
Infection due to Necator americanus

B76.8   Other hookworm diseases

B76.9   Hookworm disease, unspecified
Cutaneous larva migrans NOS

● **B77   Ascariasis**
Infection by roundworm in small intestine
Includes   ascaridiasis
roundworm infection

B77.0   Ascariasis with intestinal complications

● **B77.8   Ascariasis with other complications**
B77.81   Ascariasis pneumonia
B77.89   Ascariasis with other complications

B77.9   Ascariasis, unspecified

● **B78   Strongyloidiasis**
Infection with adult female roundworms
Excludes1   trichostrongyliasis (B81.2)

B78.0   Intestinal strongyloidiasis
B78.1   Cutaneous strongyloidiasis
B78.7   Disseminated strongyloidiasis
B78.9   Strongyloidiasis, unspecified

● **B79   Trichuriasis**
Intestinal infection with roundworms
Includes   trichocephaliasis
whipworm (disease)(infection)

● **B80   Enterobiasis**
Intestinal infection with pinworms
Includes   oxyuriasis
pinworm infection
threadworm infection

● **B81   Other intestinal helminthiases, not elsewhere classified**
Diseases or infestations caused by parasitic worms
Excludes1   angiostrongyliasis due to:
Angiostrongylus cantonensis (B83.2)
Parastrongylus cantonensis (B83.2)

B81.0   Anisakiasis
Roundworm infection via contaminated undercooked infected fish or marine mammals
Infection due to Anisakis larva

B81.1   Intestinal capillariasis
Infestation with of parasites (nematodes)
Capillariasis NOS
Infection due to Capillaria philippinensis
Excludes2   hepatic capillariasis (B83.8)

B81.2   Trichostrongyliasis

B81.3   Intestinal angiostrongyliasis
Angiostrongyliasis due to:
Angiostrongylus costaricensis (B83.2)
Parastrongylus costaricensis (B83.2)

B81.4   Mixed intestinal helminthiases
Infection due to intestinal helminths classified to more than one of the categories B65.0-B81.3 and B81.8
Mixed helminthiasis NOS

B81.8   Other specified intestinal helminthiases
Infection due to Oesophagostomum species [esophagostomiasis]
Infection due to Ternidens diminutus [ternidensiasis]

● **B82   Unspecified intestinal parasitism**
B82.0   Intestinal helminthiasis, unspecified
Infected with worms
B82.9   Intestinal parasitism, unspecified

● **B83   Other helminthiases**
Caused by parasitic worms
Excludes1   capillariasis NOS (B81.1)
Excludes2   intestinal capillariasis (B81.1)

B83.0   Visceral larva migrans
Prolonged migration of nematode larvae
Toxocariasis

B83.1   Gnathostomiasis
Infection with nematode occurring from ingested undercooked fish contaminated with larvae; larvae migrate to subcutaneous tissue or deeper tissues, results are abscesses
Wandering swelling

B83.2   Angiostrongyliasis due to Parastrongylus cantonensis
Nematode infection caused by eating contaminated raw snails, slugs, or paratenic hosts such as prawns or crabs; larval worms migrate to central nervous system resulting in eosinophilic meningitis
Eosinophilic meningoencephalitis due to Parastrongylus cantonensis
Excludes2   intestinal angiostrongyliasis (B81.3)

B83.3   Syngamiasis
Infestation with gapeworm from turkey, pheasant, guinea fowl, goose, and wild birds
Syngamosis

B83.4   Internal hirudiniasis
Infestation by leeches
Excludes2   external hirudiniasis (B88.3)

B83.8   Other specified helminthiases
Parasitic worm infestation
Acanthocephaliasis
Gongylonemiasis
Hepatic capillariasis
Metastrongyliasis
Thelaziasis

B83.9   Helminthiasis, unspecified
Worms NOS
Excludes1   intestinal helminthiasis NOS (B82.0)

CHAPTER 1 (A00-B99)

PEDICULOSIS, ACARIASIS AND OTHER INFESTATIONS (B85-B89)

● **B85   Pediculosis and phthiriasis**
    Infestation of lice

    B85.0   Pediculosis due to Pediculus humanus capitis
            Head-louse infestation

    B85.1   Pediculosis due to Pediculus humanus corporis
            Body-louse infestation

    B85.2   Pediculosis, unspecified

    B85.3   Phthiriasis
            Crab or pubic lice
            Infestation by crab-louse
            Infestation by Phthirus pubis

    B85.4   Mixed pediculosis and phthiriasis
            Infestation classifiable to more than one of the
                categories B85.0-B85.3

B86   Scabies
    Contagious dermatitis caused by mites
    Sarcoptic itch

● **B87   Myiasis**
    Infestation by fly maggots
        Includes   infestation by larva of flies

    B87.0   Cutaneous myiasis
            Creeping myiasis

    B87.1   Wound myiasis
            Traumatic myiasis

    B87.2   Ocular myiasis

    B87.3   Nasopharyngeal myiasis
            Laryngeal myiasis

    B87.4   Aural myiasis

    ● **B87.8   Myiasis of other sites**
            B87.81   Genitourinary myiasis
            B87.82   Intestinal myiasis
            B87.89   Myiasis of other sites

    B87.9   Myiasis, unspecified

● **B88   Other infestations**

    B88.0   Other acariasis
            Acarine dermatitis
            Dermatitis due to Demodex species
            Dermatitis due to Dermanyssus gallinae
            Dermatitis due to Liponyssoides sanguineus
            Trombiculosis
                Excludes2   scabies (B86)

    B88.1   Tungiasis [sandflea infestation]
            Inflammatory skin disease caused by infestation of fleas

    B88.2   Other arthropod infestations
            Scarabiasis

    B88.3   External hirudiniasis
            Leech infestation NOS
                Excludes2   internal hirudiniasis (B83.4)

    B88.8   Other specified infestations
            Infection of topical fresh water fish parasite
            Ichthyoparasitism due to Vandellia cirrhosa
            Linguatulosis
            Porocephaliasis

    B88.9   Infestation, unspecified
            Infestation (skin) NOS
            Infestation by mites NOS
            Skin parasites NOS

B89   Unspecified parasitic disease

SEQUELAE OF INFECTIOUS AND PARASITIC DISEASES (B90-B94)

Note: Categories B90-B94 are to be used to indicate conditions
        in categories A00-B89 as the cause of sequelae, which are
        themselves classified elsewhere. The 'sequelae' include
        conditions specified as such; they also include residuals
        of diseases classifiable to the above categories if there
        is evidence that the disease itself is no longer present.
        Codes from these categories are not to be used for chronic
        infections. Code chronic current infections to active infectious
        disease as appropriate.

*Code first condition resulting from (sequela) the infectious or parasitic
    disease*

● **B90   Sequelae of tuberculosis**
    Condition resulting from tuberculosis

    B90.0   Sequelae of central nervous system tuberculosis
    B90.1   Sequelae of genitourinary tuberculosis
    B90.2   Sequelae of tuberculosis of bones and joints
    B90.8   Sequelae of tuberculosis of other organs
            Excludes2   sequelae of respiratory tuberculosis
                        (B90.9)

    B90.9   Sequelae of respiratory and unspecified tuberculosis
            Sequelae of tuberculosis NOS

B91   Sequelae of poliomyelitis
        Excludes1   postpolio syndrome (G14)

B92   Sequelae of leprosy

● **B94   Sequelae of other and unspecified infectious and parasitic
        diseases**

    B94.0   Sequelae of trachoma
    B94.1   Sequelae of viral encephalitis
    B94.2   Sequelae of viral hepatitis
    **B94.8   Sequelae of other specified infectious and parasitic
            diseases**
            Coding Clinic: 2021, Q4, P102-106; 2021, Q1, P34,37,41,44,46,48

    B94.9   Sequelae of unspecified infectious and parasitic disease
            Excludes2   post COVID-19 condition (U09.9)
            Coding Clinic: 2017, Q4, P109

OGCR Section I.C.1.b.

Certain infectious and parasitic diseases
Infectious agents as the cause of diseases classified to other
chapters
Certain infections are classified in chapters other than Chapter 1
and no organism is identified as part of the infection code. In
these instances, it is necessary to use an additional code from
Chapter 1 to identify the organism. A code from category B95,
Streptococcus, Staphylococcus, and Enterococcus as the cause of
diseases classified to other chapters, B96, Other bacterial agents
as the cause of diseases classified to other chapters, or B97, Viral
agents as the cause of diseases classified to other chapters, is
to be used as an additional code to identify the organism. An
instructional note will be found at the infection code advising
that an additional organism code is required.

BACTERIAL AND VIRAL INFECTIOUS AGENTS (B95-B97)

Note: These categories are provided for use as supplementary or
        additional codes to identify the infectious agent(s) in diseases
        classified elsewhere.
        *Code the disease first, then the bacterium. Do not report codes from
        B95-B97 for sepsis.*

● **B95   Streptococcus, Staphylococcus, and Enterococcus as the cause of
        diseases classified elsewhere**

    **B95.0   Streptococcus, group A, as the cause of diseases
            classified elsewhere**

    **B95.1   Streptococcus, group B, as the cause of diseases
            classified elsewhere**
            Coding Clinic: 2020, Q1, P10; 2019, Q2, P9-10; 2018, Q4, P23

    **B95.2   Enterococcus as the cause of diseases classified
            elsewhere**

▶ New   ⇒ Revised   ~~deleted~~ Deleted   Excludes 1   Excludes 2   Includes   Use additional   Code first   Code also   Key words
OGCR Official Guidelines   X Assign placeholder X   ● Use Additional Character(s)   ▶ Manifestation Code   🕭 Hierarchical Condition Category   Coding Clinic

B95.3   Streptococcus pneumoniae as the cause of diseases classified elsewhere

B95.4   Other streptococcus as the cause of diseases classified elsewhere

B95.5   Unspecified streptococcus as the cause of diseases classified elsewhere

● **B95.6**   Staphylococcus aureus as the cause of diseases classified elsewhere

     B95.61   Methicillin susceptible Staphylococcus aureus infection as the cause of diseases classified elsewhere

         Methicillin susceptible Staphylococcus aureus (MSSA) infection as the cause of diseases classified elsewhere

         Staphylococcus aureus infection NOS as the cause of diseases classified elsewhere

     B95.62   Methicillin resistant Staphylococcus aureus infection as the cause of diseases classified elsewhere

         Methicillin resistant staphylococcus aureus (MRSA) infection as the cause of diseases classified elsewhere

         Coding Clinic: 2016, Q1, P13

B95.7   Other staphylococcus as the cause of diseases classified elsewhere

B95.8   Unspecified staphylococcus as the cause of diseases classified elsewhere

● **B96**   Other bacterial agents as the cause of diseases classified elsewhere

     B96.0   Mycoplasma pneumoniae [M. pneumoniae] as the cause of diseases classified elsewhere

         Pleuro-pneumonia-like-organism [PPLO]

     B96.1   Klebsiella pneumoniae [K. pneumoniae] as the cause of diseases classified elsewhere

● **B96.2**   Escherichia coli [E. coli] as the cause of diseases classified elsewhere

     B96.20   Unspecified Escherichia coli [E. coli] as the cause of diseases classified elsewhere

         Escherichia coli [E. coli] NOS

         Coding Clinic: 2022, Q1, P31; 2018, Q4, P34; 2018, Q1, P16

     B96.21   Shiga toxin-producing Escherichia coli [E. coli] [STEC] O157 as the cause of diseases classified elsewhere

         E. coli O157:H- (nonmotile) with confirmation of Shiga toxin

         E. coli O157 with confirmation of Shiga toxin when H antigen is unknown, or is not H7

         O157:H7 Escherichia coli [E.coli] with or without confirmation of Shiga toxin-production

         Shiga toxin-producing Escherichia coli [E.coli] O157:H7 with or without confirmation of Shiga toxin-production

         STEC O157:H7 with or without confirmation of Shiga toxin-production

     B96.22   Other specified Shiga toxin-producing Escherichia coli [E. coli] [STEC] as the cause of diseases classified elsewhere

         Non-O157 Shiga toxin-producing Escherichia coli [E.coli]

         Non-O157 Shiga toxin-producing Escherichia coli [E.coli] with known O group

     B96.23   Unspecified Shiga toxin-producing Escherichia coli [E. coli] [STEC] as the cause of diseases classified elsewhere

         Shiga toxin-producing Escherichia coli [E. coli] with unspecified O group

         STEC NOS

     B96.29   Other Escherichia coli [E. coli] as the cause of diseases classified elsewhere

         Non-Shiga toxin-producing E. coli

B96.3   Hemophilus influenzae [H. influenzae] as the cause of diseases classified elsewhere

B96.4   Proteus (mirabilis) (morganii) as the cause of diseases classified elsewhere

B96.5   Pseudomonas (aeruginosa) (mallei) (pseudomallei) as the cause of diseases classified elsewhere

     Coding Clinic: 2015, Q1, P18

B96.6   Bacteroides fragilis [B. fragilis] as the cause of diseases classified elsewhere

B96.7   Clostridium perfringens [C. perfringens] as the cause of diseases classified elsewhere

● **B96.8**   Other specified bacterial agents as the cause of diseases classified elsewhere

     B96.81   Helicobacter pylori [H. pylori] as the cause of diseases classified elsewhere

     B96.82   Vibrio vulnificus as the cause of diseases classified elsewhere

     B96.83   Acinetobacter baumannii as the cause of diseases classified elsewhere

     B96.89   Other specified bacterial agents as the cause of diseases classified elsewhere

● **B97**   Viral agents as the cause of diseases classified elsewhere

     B97.0   Adenovirus as the cause of diseases classified elsewhere

● **B97.1**   Enterovirus as the cause of diseases classified elsewhere

     B97.10   Unspecified enterovirus as the cause of diseases classified elsewhere

     B97.11   Coxsackievirus as the cause of diseases classified elsewhere

     B97.12   Echovirus as the cause of diseases classified elsewhere

     B97.19   Other enterovirus as the cause of diseases classified elsewhere

● **B97.2**   Coronavirus as the cause of diseases classified elsewhere

     B97.21   SARS-associated coronavirus as the cause of diseases classified elsewhere

         Excludes1   pneumonia due to SARS-associated coronavirus (J12.81)

     B97.29   Other coronavirus as the cause of diseases classified elsewhere

● **B97.3**   Retrovirus as the cause of diseases classified elsewhere

     Excludes1   human immunodeficiency virus [HIV] disease (B20)

     B97.30   Unspecified retrovirus as the cause of diseases classified elsewhere

     B97.31   Lentivirus as the cause of diseases classified elsewhere

     B97.32   Oncovirus as the cause of diseases classified elsewhere

     B97.33   Human T-cell lymphotrophic virus, type I [HTLV-I] as the cause of diseases classified elsewhere

     B97.34   Human T-cell lymphotrophic virus, type II [HTLV-II] as the cause of diseases classified elsewhere

     B97.35   Human immunodeficiency virus, type 2 [HIV 2] as the cause of diseases classified elsewhere

     B97.39   Other retrovirus as the cause of diseases classified elsewhere

CHAPTER 1 (A00–B99)

N   Newborn Age: 0   **P**   Pediatric Age: 0–17   **M**   Maternity DX: 9–64   **A**   Adult Age: 15–124

Item 1–24 Retrovirus develops by copying its RNA, genetic materials, into the DNA, which then produces new virus particles. It is from the Retroviridae virus family. **Human T-cell lymphotropic virus, Type I (HTLV-I),** is also called human T-cell leukemia virus, Type I, and is a retrovirus thought to cause T-cell leukemia/lymphoma. **Human T-cell lymphotropic virus, Type II (HTLV-II),** is also called human T-cell leukemia virus, Type II, and is a retrovirus associated with hematologic disorders.

HIV-2 is one of the serotypes of HIV and is usually confined to West Africa, whereas **HIV-1** is found worldwide.

B97.4 **Respiratory syncytial** virus as the cause of diseases classified elsewhere

RSV as the cause of diseases classified elsewhere

Code first related disorders, such as:
  otitis media (H65.-)
  upper respiratory infection (J06.9)

Excludes1   acute bronchiolitis due to respiratory syncytial virus (RSV) (J21.0)
acute bronchitis due to respiratory syncytial virus (RSV) (J20.5)
respiratory syncytial virus (RSV) pneumonia (J12.1)

B97.5 **Reovirus** as the cause of diseases classified elsewhere

B97.6 **Parvovirus** as the cause of diseases classified elsewhere

B97.7 **Papillomavirus** as the cause of diseases classified elsewhere

● B97.8 **Other viral agents** as the cause of diseases classified elsewhere

B97.81 **Human metapneumovirus** as the cause of diseases classified elsewhere

B97.89 **Other viral agents** as the cause of diseases classified elsewhere
Coding Clinic: 2016, Q3, P8-10, 14

OTHER INFECTIOUS DISEASES (B99)

● B99 **Other and unspecified infectious diseases**

B99.8 **Other infectious disease**

B99.9 **Unspecified infectious disease**

▶ New   ⇒ Revised   ~~deleted~~ Deleted   Excludes 1   Excludes 2   Includes   Use additional   Code first   Code also   Key words
OGCR Official Guidelines   X Assign placeholder X   ● Use Additional Character(s)   ◗ Manifestation Code   🦫 Hierarchical Condition Category   Coding Clinic

CHAPTER 2

NEOPLASMS (C00-D49)

2. **Chapter 2: Neoplasms (C00-D49)**
General guidelines
Chapter 2 of the ICD-10-CM contains the codes for most benign and all malignant neoplasms. Certain benign neoplasms, such as prostatic adenomas, may be found in the specific body system chapters. To properly code a neoplasm it is necessary to determine from the record if the neoplasm is benign, in-situ, malignant, or of uncertain histologic behavior. If malignant, any secondary (metastatic) sites should also be determined.

Primary malignant neoplasms overlapping site boundaries
A primary malignant neoplasm that overlaps two or more contiguous (next to each other) sites should be classified to the subcategory/code .8 ('overlapping lesion'), unless the combination is specifically indexed elsewhere. For multiple neoplasms of the same site that are not contiguous such as tumors in different quadrants of the same breast, codes for each site should be assigned.

Malignant neoplasm of ectopic tissue
Malignant neoplasms of ectopic tissue are to be coded to the site of origin mentioned, e.g., ectopic pancreatic malignant neoplasms involving the stomach are coded to malignant neoplasm of pancreas, unspecified (C25.9).

The neoplasm table in the Alphabetic Index should be referenced first. However, if the histological term is documented, that term should be referenced first, rather than going immediately to the Neoplasm Table, in order to determine which column in the Neoplasm Table is appropriate. For example, if the documentation indicates "adenoma," refer to the term in the Alphabetic Index to review the entries under this term and the instructional note to "see also neoplasm, by site, benign." The table provides the proper code based on the type of neoplasm and the site. It is important to select the proper column in the table that corresponds to the type of neoplasm. The Tabular List should then be referenced to verify that the correct code has been selected from the table and that a more specific site code does not exist.

See Section I.C.21. Factors influencing health status and contact with health services, Status, for information regarding Z15.0, codes for genetic susceptibility to cancer.

a. Treatment directed at the malignancy
If the treatment is directed at the malignancy, designate the malignancy as the principal diagnosis.

The only exception to this guideline is if a patient admission/encounter is solely for the administration of chemotherapy, immunotherapy or external beam radiation therapy, assign the appropriate Z51.— code as the first-listed or principal diagnosis, and the diagnosis or problem for which the service is being performed as a secondary diagnosis.

b. Treatment of secondary site
When a patient is admitted because of a primary neoplasm with metastasis and treatment is directed toward the secondary site only, the secondary neoplasm is designated as the principal diagnosis even though the primary malignancy is still present.

c. Coding and sequencing of complications
Coding and sequencing of complications associated with the malignancies or with the therapy thereof are subject to the following guidelines:

1) Anemia associated with malignancy
When admission/encounter is for management of an anemia associated with the malignancy, and the treatment is only for anemia, the appropriate code for the malignancy is sequenced as the principal or first-listed diagnosis followed by the appropriate code for the anemia (such as code D63.0, Anemia in neoplastic disease).

2) Anemia associated with chemotherapy, immunotherapy and radiation therapy
When the admission/encounter is for management of an anemia associated with an adverse effect of the administration of chemotherapy or immunotherapy and the only treatment is for the anemia, the anemia code is sequenced first followed by .

the appropriate codes for the neoplasm and the adverse effect (T45.1X5, Adverse effect of antineoplastic and immunosuppressive drugs).

When the admission/encounter is for management of an anemia associated with an adverse effect of radiotherapy, the anemia code should be sequenced first, followed by the appropriate neoplasm code and code Y84.2, Radiological procedure and radiotherapy as the cause of abnormal reaction of the patient, or of later complication, without mention of misadventure at the time of the procedure.

3) Management of dehydration due to the malignancy
When the admission/encounter is for management of dehydration due to the malignancy and only the dehydration is being treated (intravenous rehydration), the dehydration is sequenced first, followed by the code(s) for the malignancy.

4) Treatment of a complication resulting from a surgical procedure
When the admission/encounter is for treatment of a complication resulting from a surgical procedure, designate the complication as the principal or first-listed diagnosis if treatment is directed at resolving the complication.

d. Primary malignancy previously excised
When a primary malignancy has been previously excised or eradicated from its site and there is no further treatment directed to that site and there is no evidence of any existing primary malignancy at that site, a code from category Z85, Personal history of malignant neoplasm, should be used to indicate the former site of the malignancy. Any mention of extension, invasion, or metastasis to another site is coded as a secondary malignant neoplasm to that site. The secondary site may be the principal or first-listed with the Z85 code used as a secondary code.

e. Admissions/Encounters involving chemotherapy, immunotherapy and radiation therapy
1) Episode of care involves surgical removal of neoplasm
When an episode of care involves the surgical removal of a neoplasm, primary or secondary site, followed by adjunct chemotherapy or radiation treatment during the same episode of care, the code for the neoplasm should be assigned as principal or first-listed diagnosis.

2) Patient admission/encounter solely for administration of chemotherapy, immunotherapy and radiation therapy
If a patient admission/encounter is solely for the administration of chemotherapy, immunotherapy or external beam radiation therapy assign code Z51.0, Encounter for antineoplastic radiation therapy, or Z51.11, Encounter for antineoplastic chemotherapy, or Z51.12, Encounter for antineoplastic immunotherapy as the first-listed or principal diagnosis. If a patient receives more than one of these therapies during the same admission more than one of these codes may be assigned, in any sequence.

The malignancy for which the therapy is being administered should be assigned as a secondary diagnosis.

If a patient admission/encounter is for the insertion or implantation of radioactive elements (e.g., brachytherapy) the appropriate code for the malignancy is sequenced as the principal or first-listed diagnosis. Code Z51.0 should not be assigned.

3) Patient admitted for radiation therapy, chemotherapy or immunotherapy and develops complications
When a patient is admitted for the purpose of external beam radiotherapy, immunotherapy or chemotherapy and develops complications such as uncontrolled nausea and vomiting or dehydration, the principal or first-listed diagnosis is Z51.0, Encounter for antineoplastic radiation therapy, or Z51.11, Encounter for antineoplastic chemotherapy, or Z51.12, Encounter for antineoplastic immunotherapy followed by any codes for the complications.

When a patient is admitted for the purpose of insertion or implantation of radioactive elements (e.g., brachytherapy) and develops complications such as uncontrolled nausea and vomiting or dehydration, the principal or first-listed diagnosis is the appropriate code for the malignancy followed by any codes for the complications.

f. Admission/encounter to determine extent of malignancy
When the reason for admission/encounter is to determine the extent of the malignancy, or for a procedure such as paracentesis

or thoracentesis, the primary malignancy or appropriate metastatic site is designated as the principal or first-listed diagnosis, even though chemotherapy or radiotherapy is administered.

g. Symptoms, signs, and abnormal findings listed in Chapter 18 associated with neoplasms

Symptoms, signs, and ill-defined conditions listed in Chapter 18 characteristic of, or associated with, an existing primary or secondary site malignancy cannot be used to replace the malignancy as principal or first-listed diagnosis, regardless of the number of admissions or encounters for treatment and care of the neoplasm.

See Section I.C.21. Factors influencing health status and contact with health services, Encounter for prophylactic organ removal.

h. Admission/encounter for pain control/management

See Section I.C.6. for information on coding admission/encounter for pain control/management.

i. Malignancy in two or more noncontiguous sites

A patient may have more than one malignant tumor in the same organ. These tumors may represent different primaries or metastatic disease, depending on the site. Should the documentation be unclear, the provider should be queried as to the status of each tumor so that the correct codes can be assigned.

j. Disseminated malignant neoplasm, unspecified

Code C80.0, Disseminated malignant neoplasm, unspecified, is for use only in those cases where the patient has advanced metastatic disease and no known primary or secondary sites are specified. It should not be used in place of assigning codes for the primary site and all known secondary sites.

k. Malignant neoplasm without specification of site

Code C80.1, Malignant (primary) neoplasm, unspecified, equates to Cancer, unspecified. This code should only be used when no determination can be made as to the primary site of a malignancy. This code should rarely be used in the inpatient setting.

l. Sequencing of neoplasm codes

1) Encounter for treatment of primary malignancy

If the reason for the encounter is for treatment of a primary malignancy, assign the malignancy as the principal/first-listed diagnosis. The primary site is to be sequenced first, followed by any metastatic sites.

2) Encounter for treatment of secondary malignancy

When an encounter is for a primary malignancy with metastasis and treatment is directed toward the metastatic (secondary) site(s) only, the metastatic site(s) is designated as the principal/first-listed diagnosis. The primary malignancy is coded as an additional code.

3) Malignant neoplasm in a pregnant patient

When a pregnant woman has a malignant neoplasm, a code from subcategory O9A.1-, Malignant neoplasm complicating pregnancy, childbirth, and the puerperium, should be sequenced first, followed by the appropriate code from Chapter 2 to indicate the type of neoplasm.

4) Encounter for complication associated with a neoplasm

When an encounter is for management of a complication associated with a neoplasm, such as dehydration, and the treatment is only for the complication, the complication is coded first, followed by the appropriate code(s) for the neoplasm.

The exception to this guideline is anemia. When the admission/encounter is for management of an anemia associated with the malignancy, and the treatment is only for anemia, the appropriate code for the malignancy is sequenced as the principal or first-listed diagnosis followed by code D63.0, Anemia in neoplastic disease.

5) Complication from surgical procedure for treatment of a neoplasm

When an encounter is for treatment of a complication resulting from a surgical procedure performed for the treatment of the neoplasm, designate the complication as the principal/first-listed diagnosis. See guideline regarding the coding of a current malignancy versus personal history to determine if the code for the neoplasm should also be assigned.

6) Pathologic fracture due to a neoplasm

When an encounter is for a pathological fracture due to a neoplasm, and the focus of treatment is the fracture, a code from subcategory M84.5, Pathological fracture in neoplastic disease, should be sequenced first, followed by the code for the neoplasm.

If the focus of treatment is the neoplasm with an associated pathological fracture, the neoplasm code should be sequenced first, followed by a code from M84.5 for the pathological fracture.

m. Current malignancy versus personal history of malignancy

When a primary malignancy has been excised but further treatment, such as an additional surgery for the malignancy, radiation therapy or chemotherapy is directed to that site, the primary malignancy code should be used until treatment is completed.

When a primary malignancy has been previously excised or eradicated from its site, there is no further treatment (of the malignancy) directed to that site, and there is no evidence of any existing primary malignancy at that site, a code from category Z85, Personal history of malignant neoplasm, should be used to indicate the former site of the malignancy.

Subcategories Z85.0–Z85.7 should only be assigned for the former site of a primary malignancy, not the site of a secondary malignancy. Codes from subcategory Z85.8-, may be assigned for the former site(s) of either a primary or secondary malignancy included in this subcategory.

See Section I.C.21. Factors influencing health status and contact with health services, History (of)

n. Leukemia, Multiple Myeloma, and Malignant Plasma Cell Neoplasms in remission versus personal history

The categories for leukemia, and category C90, Multiple myeloma and malignant plasma cell neoplasms, have codes indicating whether or not the leukemia has achieved remission. There are also codes Z85.6, Personal history of leukemia, and Z85.79, Personal history of other malignant neoplasms of lymphoid, hematopoietic and related tissues. If the documentation is unclear, as to whether the leukemia has achieved remission, the provider should be queried.

See Section I.C.21. Factors influencing health status and contact with health services, History (of)

o. Aftercare following surgery for neoplasm

See Section I.C.21. Factors influencing health status and contact with health services, Aftercare

p. Follow-up care for completed treatment of a malignancy

See Section I.C.21. Factors influencing health status and contact with health services, Follow-up

q. Prophylactic organ removal for prevention of malignancy

See Section I.C. 21, Factors influencing health status and contact with health services, Prophylactic organ removal

r. Malignant neoplasm associated with transplanted organ

A malignant neoplasm of a transplanted organ should be coded as a transplant complication. Assign first the appropriate code from category T86.-, Complications of transplanted organs and tissue, followed by code C80.2, Malignant neoplasm associated with transplanted organ. Use an additional code for the specific malignancy.

Item 2–1 Neoplasm: Neo = new, plasm = growth, development, formation. This new growth (mass, tumor) can be malignant or benign, which is confirmed by the pathology report. Do not assign a code to a neoplasm until you review the pathology report. Certain CPT codes will specify benign or malignant lesion, so be certain the diagnosis code supports the procedure code.

CHAPTER 2

NEOPLASMS (C00-D49)

This chapter contains the following blocks:

C00-C14	Malignant neoplasms of lip, oral cavity and pharynx
C15-C26	Malignant neoplasms of digestive organs
C30-C39	Malignant neoplasms of respiratory and intrathoracic organs
C40-C41	Malignant neoplasms of bone and articular cartilage
C43-C44	Melanoma and other malignant neoplasms of skin
C45-C49	Malignant neoplasms of mesothelial and soft tissue
C50	Malignant neoplasms of breast
C51-C58	Malignant neoplasms of female genital organs
C60-C63	Malignant neoplasms of male genital organs
C64-C68	Malignant neoplasms of urinary tract
C69-C72	Malignant neoplasms of eye, brain and other parts of central nervous system
C73-C75	Malignant neoplasms of thyroid and other endocrine glands
C7A	Malignant neuroendocrine tumors
C7B	Secondary neuroendocrine tumors
C76-C80	Malignant neoplasms of ill-defined, other secondary and unspecified sites
C81-C96	Malignant neoplasms of lymphoid, hematopoietic and related tissue
D00-D09	In situ neoplasms
D10-D36	Benign neoplasms, except benign neuroendocrine tumors
D3A	Benign neuroendocrine tumors
D37-D48	Neoplasms of uncertain behavior, polycythemia vera and myelodysplastic syndromes
D49	Neoplasms of unspecified behavior

Notes: Functional activity

All neoplasms are classified in this chapter, whether they are functionally active or not. An additional code from Chapter 4 may be used, to identify functional activity associated with any neoplasm.

Morphology [Histology]

Chapter 2 classifies neoplasms primarily by site (topography), with broad groupings for behavior, malignant, in situ, benign, etc. The Table of Neoplasms should be used to identify the correct topography code. In a few cases, such as for malignant melanoma and certain neuroendocrine tumors, the morphology (histologic type) is included in the category and codes.

Primary malignant neoplasms overlapping site boundaries

A primary malignant neoplasm that overlaps two or more contiguous (next to each other) sites should be classified to the subcategory/code .8 ("overlapping lesion"), unless the combination is specifically indexed elsewhere. For multiple neoplasms of the same site that are not contiguous, such as tumors in different quadrants of the same breast, codes for each site should be assigned.

Malignant neoplasm of ectopic tissue

Malignant neoplasms of ectopic tissue are to be coded to the site mentioned, e.g., ectopic pancreatic malignant neoplasms are coded to pancreas, unspecified (C25.9).

MALIGNANT NEOPLASMS (C00-C96)

MALIGNANT NEOPLASMS, STATED OR PRESUMED TO BE PRIMARY (OF SPECIFIED SITES), AND CERTAIN SPECIFIED HISTOLOGIES, EXCEPT NEUROENDOCRINE, AND OF LYMPHOID, HEMATOPOIETIC AND RELATED TISSUE (C00-C75)

MALIGNANT NEOPLASMS OF LIP, ORAL CAVITY AND PHARYNX (C00-C14)

● C00   **Malignant neoplasm of lip**
   Use additional code to identify:
      alcohol abuse and dependence (F10.-)
      history of tobacco dependence (Z87.891)
      tobacco dependence (F17.-)
      tobacco use (Z72.0)
   Excludes1   malignant melanoma of lip (C43.0)
         Merkel cell carcinoma of lip (C4A.0)
         other and unspecified malignant neoplasm of skin of lip (C44.0-)

   C00.0   **Malignant neoplasm of external upper lip**
         Malignant neoplasm of lipstick area of upper lip
         Malignant neoplasm of upper lip NOS
         Malignant neoplasm of vermilion border of upper lip

   C00.1   **Malignant neoplasm of external lower lip**
         Malignant neoplasm of lower lip NOS
         Malignant neoplasm of lipstick area of lower lip
         Malignant neoplasm of vermilion border of lower lip

   C00.2   **Malignant neoplasm of external lip, unspecified**
         Malignant neoplasm of vermilion border of lip NOS

   C00.3   **Malignant neoplasm of upper lip, inner aspect**
         Malignant neoplasm of buccal aspect of upper lip
         Malignant neoplasm of frenulum of upper lip
         Malignant neoplasm of mucosa of upper lip
         Malignant neoplasm of oral aspect of upper lip

   C00.4   **Malignant neoplasm of lower lip, inner aspect**
         Malignant neoplasm of buccal aspect of lower lip
         Malignant neoplasm of frenulum of lower lip
         Malignant neoplasm of mucosa of lower lip
         Malignant neoplasm of oral aspect of lower lip

   C00.5   **Malignant neoplasm of lip, unspecified, inner aspect**
         Malignant neoplasm of buccal aspect of lip, unspecified
         Malignant neoplasm of frenulum of lip, unspecified
         Malignant neoplasm of mucosa of lip, unspecified
         Malignant neoplasm of oral aspect of lip, unspecified

   C00.6   **Malignant neoplasm of commissure of lip, unspecified**
         Commissure: Site of union of corresponding parts

   C00.8   **Malignant neoplasm of overlapping sites of lip**

   C00.9   **Malignant neoplasm of lip, unspecified**

Figure 2-1 Anatomical structures of the mouth and lips. **A.** Transitional or vermilion borders. Lips are connected to the gums by frenulum. **B.** Dorsal surface. **C.** Ventral surface.

CHAPTER 2 (C00-D49)

C01   Malignant neoplasm of base of tongue 🦠
Malignant neoplasm of dorsal surface of base of tongue
Malignant neoplasm of fixed part of tongue NOS
Malignant neoplasm of posterior third of tongue
Use additional code to identify:
alcohol abuse and dependence (F10.-)
history of tobacco dependence (Z87.891)
tobacco dependence (F17.-)
tobacco use (Z72.0)

● **C02   Malignant neoplasm of other and unspecified parts of tongue**
Use additional code to identify:
alcohol abuse and dependence (F10.-)
history of tobacco dependence (Z87.891)
tobacco dependence (F17.-)
tobacco use (Z72.0)

C02.0   Malignant neoplasm of dorsal surface of tongue 🦠
Malignant neoplasm of anterior two-thirds of tongue, dorsal surface
Excludes2   malignant neoplasm of dorsal surface of base of tongue (C01)

C02.1   Malignant neoplasm of border of tongue 🦠
Malignant neoplasm of tip of tongue

C02.2   Malignant neoplasm of ventral surface of tongue 🦠
Malignant neoplasm of anterior two-thirds of tongue, ventral surface
Malignant neoplasm of frenulum linguae

C02.3   Malignant neoplasm of anterior two-thirds of tongue, part unspecified 🦠
Malignant neoplasm of middle third of tongue NOS
Malignant neoplasm of mobile part of tongue NOS

C02.4   Malignant neoplasm of lingual tonsil 🦠
Lingual tonsil: Aggregation of lymph follicles at root of tongue
Excludes2   malignant neoplasm of tonsil NOS (C09.9)

C02.8   Malignant neoplasm of overlapping sites of tongue 🦠
Malignant neoplasm of two or more contiguous sites of tongue

C02.9   Malignant neoplasm of tongue, unspecified 🦠

● **C03   Malignant neoplasm of gum**
Includes   malignant neoplasm of alveolar (ridge) mucosa
malignant neoplasm of gingiva
Use additional code to identify:
alcohol abuse and dependence (F10.-)
history of tobacco dependence (Z87.891)
tobacco dependence (F17.-)
tobacco use (Z72.0)
Excludes2   malignant odontogenic neoplasms (C41.0-C41.1)

C03.0   Malignant neoplasm of upper gum 🦠
C03.1   Malignant neoplasm of lower gum 🦠
C03.9   Malignant neoplasm of gum, unspecified 🦠

● **C04   Malignant neoplasm of floor of mouth**
Use additional code to identify:
alcohol abuse and dependence (F10.-)
history of tobacco dependence (Z87.891)
tobacco dependence (F17.-)
tobacco use (Z72.0)

C04.0   Malignant neoplasm of anterior floor of mouth 🦠
Malignant neoplasm of anterior to the premolar-canine junction

C04.1   Malignant neoplasm of lateral floor of mouth 🦠
C04.8   Malignant neoplasm of overlapping sites of floor of mouth 🦠
C04.9   Malignant neoplasm of floor of mouth, unspecified 🦠

● **C05   Malignant neoplasm of palate**
Use additional code to identify:
alcohol abuse and dependence (F10.-)
history of tobacco dependence (Z87.891)
tobacco dependence (F17.-)
tobacco use (Z72.0)
Excludes1   Kaposi's sarcoma of palate (C46.2)

C05.0   Malignant neoplasm of hard palate 🦠
C05.1   Malignant neoplasm of soft palate 🦠
Excludes2   malignant neoplasm of nasopharyngeal surface of soft palate (C11.3)

C05.2   Malignant neoplasm of uvula 🦠
C05.8   Malignant neoplasm of overlapping sites of palate 🦠
C05.9   Malignant neoplasm of palate, unspecified 🦠
Malignant neoplasm of roof of mouth

● **C06   Malignant neoplasm of other and unspecified parts of mouth**
Use additional code to identify:
alcohol abuse and dependence (F10.-)
history of tobacco dependence (Z87.891)
tobacco dependence (F17.-)
tobacco use (Z72.0)

C06.0   Malignant neoplasm of cheek mucosa 🦠
Malignant neoplasm of buccal mucosa NOS
Malignant neoplasm of internal cheek

C06.1   Malignant neoplasm of vestibule of mouth 🦠
Malignant neoplasm of buccal sulcus (upper) (lower)
Malignant neoplasm of labial sulcus (upper) (lower)

C06.2   Malignant neoplasm of retromolar area 🦠
● **C06.8   Malignant neoplasm of overlapping sites of other and unspecified parts of mouth**
C06.80   Malignant neoplasm of overlapping sites of unspecified parts of mouth 🦠
C06.89   Malignant neoplasm of overlapping sites of other parts of mouth 🦠
'book leaf' neoplasm [ventral surface of tongue and floor of mouth]

C06.9   Malignant neoplasm of mouth, unspecified 🦠
Malignant neoplasm of minor salivary gland, unspecified site
Malignant neoplasm of oral cavity NOS

C07   Malignant neoplasm of parotid gland 🦠
Use additional code to identify:
alcohol abuse and dependence (F10.-)
exposure to environmental tobacco smoke (Z77.22)
exposure to tobacco smoke in the perinatal period (P96.81)
history of tobacco dependence (Z87.891)
occupational exposure to environmental tobacco smoke (Z57.31)
tobacco dependence (F17.-)
tobacco use (Z72.0)

Parotid gland
Sublingual gland
Submandibular gland

Figure 2-2 Major salivary glands.

▶ New   ⇒ Revised   ~~deleted~~ Deleted   Excludes 1   Excludes 2   Includes   Use additional   Code first   Code also   Key words
OGCR Official Guidelines   X Assign placeholder X   ● Use Additional Character(s)   ▶ Manifestation Code   🦠 Hierarchical Condition Category   Coding Clinic

● **C08**   **Malignant neoplasm of other and unspecified major salivary glands**

     Includes   malignant neoplasm of salivary ducts

     Use additional code to identify:
       alcohol abuse and dependence (F10.-)
       exposure to environmental tobacco smoke (Z77.22)
       exposure to tobacco smoke in the perinatal period (P96.81)
       history of tobacco dependence (Z87.891)
       occupational exposure to environmental tobacco smoke
         (Z57.31)
       tobacco dependence (F17.-)
       tobacco use (Z72.0)

     Excludes1   malignant neoplasms of specified minor salivary glands which are classified according to their anatomical location

     Excludes2   malignant neoplasms of minor salivary glands NOS (C06.9)
         malignant neoplasm of parotid gland (C07)

   C08.0   **Malignant neoplasm of submandibular gland** 🦠
       Malignant neoplasm of submaxillary gland

   C08.1   **Malignant neoplasm of sublingual gland** 🦠

   C08.9   **Malignant neoplasm of major salivary gland, unspecified** 🦠
       Malignant neoplasm of salivary gland (major) NOS

    ★ **(See Plate 28 of the Anatomy Illustrations.)**

● **C09**   **Malignant neoplasm of tonsil**

     Use additional code to identify:
       alcohol abuse and dependence (F10.-)
       exposure to environmental tobacco smoke (Z77.22)
       exposure to tobacco smoke in the perinatal period (P96.81)
       history of tobacco dependence (Z87.891)
       occupational exposure to environmental tobacco smoke
         (Z57.31)
       tobacco dependence (F17.-)
       tobacco use (Z72.0)

     Excludes2   malignant neoplasm of lingual tonsil (C02.4)
         malignant neoplasm of pharyngeal tonsil (C11.1)

   C09.0   **Malignant neoplasm of tonsillar fossa** 🦠
       Surface of palatine (two masses of lymphatic tissue on sides of throat) tonsils

   C09.1   **Malignant neoplasm of tonsillar pillar (anterior) (posterior)** 🦠
       Extension from palatine (two masses of lymphatic tissue on sides of throat) tonsils

   C09.8   **Malignant neoplasm of overlapping sites of tonsil** 🦠

   C09.9   **Malignant neoplasm of tonsil, unspecified** 🦠
       Malignant neoplasm of tonsil NOS
       Malignant neoplasm of faucial tonsils
       Malignant neoplasm of palatine tonsils

● **C10**   **Malignant neoplasm of oropharynx**
     Area of throat at back of mouth

     Use additional code to identify:
       alcohol abuse and dependence (F10.-)
       exposure to environmental tobacco smoke (Z77.22)
       exposure to tobacco smoke in the perinatal period (P96.81)
       history of tobacco dependence (Z87.891)
       occupational exposure to environmental tobacco smoke
         (Z57.31)
       tobacco dependence (F17.-)
       tobacco use (Z72.0)

     Excludes2   malignant neoplasm of tonsil (C09.-)

   C10.0   **Malignant neoplasm of vallecula** 🦠
       Vallecula, depression or furrow

   C10.1   **Malignant neoplasm of anterior surface of epiglottis** 🦠
       Malignant neoplasm of epiglottis, free border [margin]
       Malignant neoplasm of glossoepiglottic fold(s)

      Excludes2   malignant neoplasm of epiglottis (suprahyoid portion) NOS (C32.1)

   C10.2   **Malignant neoplasm of lateral wall of oropharynx** 🦠

   C10.3   **Malignant neoplasm of posterior wall of oropharynx** 🦠

   C10.4   **Malignant neoplasm of branchial cleft** 🦠
       Congenital slitlike openings formed between branchial arches pharyngeal groove
       Malignant neoplasm of branchial cyst [site of neoplasm]

   C10.8   **Malignant neoplasm of overlapping sites of oropharynx** 🦠
       Malignant neoplasm of junctional region of oropharynx

   C10.9   **Malignant neoplasm of oropharynx, unspecified** 🦠

● **C11**   **Malignant neoplasm of nasopharynx**

     Use additional code to identify:
       exposure to environmental tobacco smoke (Z77.22)
       exposure to tobacco smoke in the perinatal period (P96.81)
       history of tobacco dependence (Z87.891)
       occupational exposure to environmental tobacco smoke
         (Z57.31)
       tobacco dependence (F17.-)
       tobacco use (Z72.0)

   C11.0   **Malignant neoplasm of superior wall of nasopharynx** 🦠
       Part of pharynx that lies above soft palate
       Malignant neoplasm of roof of nasopharynx

   C11.1   **Malignant neoplasm of posterior wall of nasopharynx** 🦠
       Malignant neoplasm of adenoid
       Malignant neoplasm of pharyngeal tonsil

   C11.2   **Malignant neoplasm of lateral wall of nasopharynx** 🦠
       Malignant neoplasm of fossa of Rosenmüller
       Malignant neoplasm of opening of auditory tube
       Malignant neoplasm of pharyngeal recess

   C11.3   **Malignant neoplasm of anterior wall of nasopharynx** 🦠
       Malignant neoplasm of floor of nasopharynx
       Malignant neoplasm of nasopharyngeal (anterior) (posterior) surface of soft palate
       Malignant neoplasm of posterior margin of nasal choana
       Malignant neoplasm of posterior margin of nasal septum

   C11.8   **Malignant neoplasm of overlapping sites of nasopharynx** 🦠

   C11.9   **Malignant neoplasm of nasopharynx, unspecified** 🦠
       Malignant neoplasm of nasopharyngeal wall NOS

● **C12**   **Malignant neoplasm of pyriform sinus** 🦠
     Malignant neoplasm of pyriform fossa

     Use additional code to identify:
       exposure to environmental tobacco smoke (Z77.22)
       exposure to tobacco smoke in the perinatal period (P96.81)
       history of tobacco dependence (Z87.891)
       occupational exposure to environmental tobacco smoke
         (Z57.31)
       tobacco dependence (F17.-)
       tobacco use (Z72.0)

● **C13**   **Malignant neoplasm of hypopharynx**

     Use additional code to identify:
       exposure to environmental tobacco smoke (Z77.22)
       exposure to tobacco smoke in the perinatal period (P96.81)
       history of tobacco dependence (Z87.891)
       occupational exposure to environmental tobacco smoke
         (Z57.31)
       tobacco dependence (F17.-)
       tobacco use (Z72.0)

     Excludes2   malignant neoplasm of pyriform sinus (C12)

   C13.0   **Malignant neoplasm of postcricoid region** 🦠
       Behind the cricoid cartilage of neck

   C13.1   **Malignant neoplasm of aryepiglottic fold, hypopharyngeal aspect** 🦠
       Arytenoepiglottic fold, triangular opening between side of epiglottis and apex of arytenoid cartilage
       Malignant neoplasm of aryepiglottic fold, marginal zone
       Malignant neoplasm of aryepiglottic fold NOS
       Malignant neoplasm of interarytenoid fold, marginal zone
       Malignant neoplasm of interarytenoid fold NOS

      Excludes2   malignant neoplasm of aryepiglottic fold or interarytenoid fold, laryngeal aspect (C32.1)

CHAPTER 2 (C00-D49)

C13.2   Malignant neoplasm of posterior wall of hypopharynx
C13.8   Malignant neoplasm of overlapping sites of hypopharynx
C13.9   Malignant neoplasm of hypopharynx, unspecified
        Malignant neoplasm of hypopharyngeal wall NOS

● C14   Malignant neoplasm of other and ill-defined sites in the lip, oral cavity and pharynx
        Use additional code to identify:
            alcohol abuse and dependence (F10.-)
            exposure to environmental tobacco smoke (Z77.22)
            exposure to tobacco smoke in the perinatal period (P96.81)
            history of tobacco dependence (Z87.891)
            occupational exposure to environmental tobacco smoke (Z57.31)
            tobacco dependence (F17.-)
            tobacco use (Z72.0)
        Excludes1   malignant neoplasm of oral cavity NOS (C06.9)
C14.0   Malignant neoplasm of pharynx, unspecified
C14.2   Malignant neoplasm of Waldeyer's ring
C14.8   Malignant neoplasm of overlapping sites of lip, oral cavity and pharynx
        Primary malignant neoplasm of two or more contiguous sites of lip, oral cavity and pharynx
        Excludes1   'book leaf' neoplasm [ventral surface of tongue and floor of mouth] (C06.89)

MALIGNANT NEOPLASM OF DIGESTIVE ORGANS (C15-C26)

Excludes1   Kaposi's sarcoma of gastrointestinal sites (C46.4)

Excludes2   gastrointestinal stromal tumors (C49.A-)

● C15   Malignant neoplasms of esophagus
        Use additional code to identify:
            alcohol abuse and dependence (F10.-)
C15.3   Malignant neoplasm of upper third of esophagus
C15.4   Malignant neoplasm of middle third of esophagus
C15.5   Malignant neoplasm of lower third of esophagus
        Excludes1   malignant neoplasm of cardio-esophageal junction (C16.0)
        Coding Clinic: 2022, Q3, P10
C15.8   Malignant neoplasm of overlapping sites of esophagus
C15.9   Malignant neoplasm of esophagus, unspecified

● C16   Malignant neoplasm of stomach
        Use additional code to identify:
            alcohol abuse and dependence (F10.-)
        Excludes2   malignant carcinoid tumor of the stomach (C7A.092)
C16.0   Malignant neoplasm of cardia
        Malignant neoplasm of cardiac orifice
        Malignant neoplasm of cardio-esophageal junction
        Malignant neoplasm of esophagus and stomach
        Malignant neoplasm of gastro-esophageal junction
C16.1   Malignant neoplasm of fundus of stomach
C16.2   Malignant neoplasm of body of stomach
C16.3   Malignant neoplasm of pyloric antrum
        Malignant neoplasm of gastric antrum
C16.4   Malignant neoplasm of pylorus
        Malignant neoplasm of prepylorus
        Malignant neoplasm of pyloric canal
C16.5   Malignant neoplasm of lesser curvature of stomach, unspecified
        Malignant neoplasm of lesser curvature of stomach, not classifiable to C16.1-C16.4
C16.6   Malignant neoplasm of greater curvature of stomach, unspecified
        Malignant neoplasm of greater curvature of stomach, not classifiable to C16.0-C16.4
C16.8   Malignant neoplasm of overlapping sites of stomach
C16.9   Malignant neoplasm of stomach, unspecified
        Gastric cancer NOS
C17.0   Malignant neoplasm of duodenum
        First or proximal portion of small intestine, extending from pylorus to jejunum
C17.1   Malignant neoplasm of jejunum
        Second section of small intestine, extending from duodenum to ileum
C17.2   Malignant neoplasm of ileum
        Distal and longest portion of small intestine, extending from jejunum to cecum
        Excludes1   malignant neoplasm of ileocecal valve (C18.0)
C17.3   Meckel's diverticulum, malignant
        Appendage of ileum
        Excludes1   Meckel's diverticulum, congenital (Q43.0)

Figure 2-3   The esophagus is the muscular tube that connects the pharynx and the stomach. The 10 inch (25 cm) long esophagus is divided into three parts: **cervical, thoracic,** and **abdominal.**

Figure 2-4   Parts of the stomach.

Item 2-2   The esophagus opens into the stomach through the **cardiac orifice,** also called the **cardioesophageal junction.** The **cardia** is adjacent to the cardiac orifice. The stomach widens into the **greater** and **lesser curvatures.** The **pyloric antrum** precedes the **pylorus,** which opens to the duodenum.

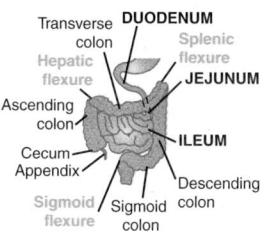

Figure 2-5   Small intestine and colon.

● **C17   Malignant neoplasm of small intestine**

Excludes1   malignant carcinoid tumor of the small intestine (C7A.01)

C17.8   Malignant neoplasm of overlapping sites of small intestine

C17.9   Malignant neoplasm of small intestine, unspecified

● **C18   Malignant neoplasm of colon**

Excludes1   malignant carcinoid tumors of the colon (C7A.02)

C18.0   Malignant neoplasm of cecum
First section of large intestine
Malignant neoplasm of ileocecal valve

C18.1   Malignant neoplasm of appendix
Blind ended tube connected to the cecum; AKA vermiform appendix

C18.2   Malignant neoplasm of ascending colon
Ascending colon is between cecum and right colic flexure

C18.3   Malignant neoplasm of hepatic flexure
A flexure is a bending in a structure or organ. Note the three flexures illustrated in Figure 2–5.

C18.4   Malignant neoplasm of transverse colon
Portion of colon that runs transversely across upper part of abdomen, between right and left colic flexures

C18.5   Malignant neoplasm of splenic flexure
Bend at junction of transverse and descending colon

C18.6   Malignant neoplasm of descending colon
Portion between left colic flexure and sigmoid colon at pelvic brim; AKA iliac colon

C18.7   Malignant neoplasm of sigmoid colon
S-shaped part of colon extending from pelvic brim to third segment of sacrum
Malignant neoplasm of sigmoid (flexure)

Excludes1   malignant neoplasm of rectosigmoid junction (C19)

C18.8   Malignant neoplasm of overlapping sites of colon

C18.9   Malignant neoplasm of colon, unspecified
Malignant neoplasm of large intestine NOS

C19   Malignant neoplasm of rectosigmoid junction
Malignant neoplasm of colon with rectum
Malignant neoplasm of rectosigmoid (colon)

Excludes1   malignant carcinoid tumors of the colon (C7A.02-)

C20   Malignant neoplasm of rectum
Malignant neoplasm of rectal ampulla

Excludes1   malignant carcinoid tumor of the rectum (C7A.026)

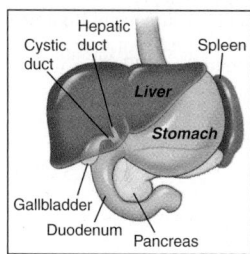

Figure 2-6   Diagram of liver, gallbladder, hepatic duct, pancreas, and spleen. (From Thibodeau and Patton: Anatomy and Physiology, ed 7, Mosby, 2010)

● **C21   Malignant neoplasm of anus and anal canal**

Excludes2   malignant carcinoid tumors of the colon (C7A.02-)
malignant melanoma of anal margin (C43.51)
malignant melanoma of anal skin (C43.51)
malignant melanoma of perianal skin (C43.51)
other and unspecified malignant neoplasm of anal margin (C44.500, C44.510, C44.520, C44.590)
other and unspecified malignant neoplasm of anal skin (C44.500, C44.510, C44.520, C44.590)
other and unspecified malignant neoplasm of perianal skin (C44.500, C44.510, C44.520, C44.590)

C21.0   Malignant neoplasm of anus, unspecified

C21.1   Malignant neoplasm of anal canal
Terminal part of large intestine
Malignant neoplasm of anal sphincter

C21.2   Malignant neoplasm of cloacogenic zone

C21.8   Malignant neoplasm of overlapping sites of rectum, anus and anal canal
Malignant neoplasm of anorectal junction
Malignant neoplasm of anorectum
Primary malignant neoplasm of two or more contiguous sites of rectum, anus and anal canal

● **C22   Malignant neoplasm of liver and intrahepatic bile ducts**
Intrahepatic: Within liver
Use additional code to identify:
alcohol abuse and dependence (F10.-)
hepatitis B (B16.-, B18.0-B18.1) hepatitis C (B17.1-, B18.2)

Excludes1   malignant neoplasm of biliary tract NOS (C24.9)
secondary malignant neoplasm of liver and intrahepatic bile duct (C78.7)

C22.0   Liver cell carcinoma
Hepatocellular carcinoma
Hepatoma

C22.1   Intrahepatic bile duct carcinoma
Cholangiocarcinoma
Adenocarcinoma (cancer that originates in glandular tissue) arising from epithelium of intrahepatic bile ducts

Excludes1   malignant neoplasm of hepatic duct (C24.0)

Coding Clinic: 2023, Q1, P24

C22.2   Hepatoblastoma
Malignant intrahepatic tumor

C22.3   Angiosarcoma of liver
Kupffer cell sarcoma

C22.4   Other sarcomas of liver

C22.7   Other specified carcinomas of liver

Item 2–3   Islets of Langerhans (endocrine producing cells comprising 1% to 2% of the pancreatic mass) make and secrete hormones that regulate the body's production of insulin, glucagon, and stomach acid. Breakdown of the insulin-producing cells can cause diabetes mellitus. Islet cell tumors can be benign or malignant and include glucagonomas, insulinomas, gastrinomas, and neuroendocrine tumor. The neoplasm table must be consulted for the correct neoplasm code.

Figure 2-7   Paranasal sinuses. (From Buck CJ: Step-by-Step Medical Coding, ed 2016, St. Louis, Elsevier, 2016)

CHAPTER 2 (C00-D49)

C22.8   **Malignant neoplasm of liver, primary, unspecified as to type** 🏷️

C22.9   **Malignant neoplasm of liver, not specified as primary or secondary** 🏷️

C23   **Malignant neoplasm of gallbladder** 🏷️

● **C24**   **Malignant neoplasm of other and unspecified parts of biliary tract**

    Excludes1   malignant neoplasm of intrahepatic bile duct (C22.1)

C24.0   **Malignant neoplasm of extrahepatic bile duct** 🏷️
Extrahepatic = outside the liver
Malignant neoplasm of biliary duct or passage NOS
Malignant neoplasm of common bile duct
Malignant neoplasm of cystic duct
Malignant neoplasm of hepatic duct

C24.1   **Malignant neoplasm of ampulla of Vater** 🏷️
Union of pancreatic duct and common bile duct

C24.8   **Malignant neoplasm of overlapping sites of biliary tract** 🏷️
Malignant neoplasm involving both intrahepatic and extrahepatic bile ducts
Primary malignant neoplasm of two or more contiguous sites of biliary tract

C24.9   **Malignant neoplasm of biliary tract, unspecified** 🏷️

● **C25**   **Malignant neoplasm of pancreas**
Check documentation for specific site.
Code also if applicable exocrine pancreatic insufficiency (K86.81)
Use additional code to identify:
  alcohol abuse and dependence (F10.-)

C25.0   **Malignant neoplasm of head of pancreas** 🏷️

C25.1   **Malignant neoplasm of body of pancreas** 🏷️
Coding Clinic: 2018, Q4, P40

C25.2   **Malignant neoplasm of tail of pancreas** 🏷️

C25.3   **Malignant neoplasm of pancreatic duct** 🏷️

C25.4   **Malignant neoplasm of endocrine pancreas** 🏷️
Malignant neoplasm of islets of Langerhans
That part of the pancreas that acts as endocrine gland and consists of islets of Langerhans
    Use additional code to identify any functional activity.

C25.7   **Malignant neoplasm of other parts of pancreas** 🏷️
Malignant neoplasm of neck of pancreas

C25.8   **Malignant neoplasm of overlapping sites of pancreas** 🏷️

C25.9   **Malignant neoplasm of pancreas, unspecified** 🏷️

● **C26**   **Malignant neoplasm of other and ill-defined digestive organs**
    Excludes1   malignant neoplasm of peritoneum and retroperitoneum (C48.-)

C26.0   **Malignant neoplasm of intestinal tract, part unspecified** 🏷️
Malignant neoplasm of intestine NOS

C26.1   **Malignant neoplasm of spleen** 🏷️
    Excludes1   Hodgkin lymphoma (C81.-)
               non-Hodgkin lymphoma (C82-C85)

C26.9   **Malignant neoplasm of ill-defined sites within the digestive system** 🏷️
Malignant neoplasm of alimentary canal or tract NOS
Malignant neoplasm of gastrointestinal tract NOS
    Excludes1   malignant neoplasm of abdominal NOS (C76.2)
               malignant neoplasm of intra-abdominal NOS (C76.2)

MALIGNANT NEOPLASMS OF RESPIRATORY AND INTRATHORACIC ORGANS (C30-C39)

    Includes   malignant neoplasm of middle ear
    Excludes1   mesothelioma (C45.-)

● **C30**   **Malignant neoplasm of nasal cavity and middle ear**

C30.0   **Malignant neoplasm of nasal cavity**
Malignant neoplasm of cartilage of nose
Malignant neoplasm of nasal concha
Malignant neoplasm of internal nose
Malignant neoplasm of septum of nose
Malignant neoplasm of vestibule of nose
Anterior part of nasal cavity
    Excludes1   malignant neoplasm of nasal bone (C41.0)
               malignant neoplasm of nose NOS (C76.0)
               malignant neoplasm of olfactory bulb (C72.2-)
               malignant neoplasm of posterior margin of nasal septum and choana (C11.3)
               malignant melanoma of skin of nose (C43.31)
               malignant neoplasm of turbinates (C41.0)
               other and unspecified malignant neoplasm of skin of nose (C44.301, C44.311, C44.321, C44.391)

C30.1   **Malignant neoplasm of middle ear** 🏷️
Malignant neoplasm of antrum tympanicum
Boney cavity or chamber
Malignant neoplasm of auditory tube
Malignant neoplasm of eustachian tube
Malignant neoplasm of inner ear
Malignant neoplasm of mastoid air cells
Malignant neoplasm of tympanic cavity
    Excludes1   malignant neoplasm of auricular canal (external) (C43.2-, C44.2-)
               malignant neoplasm of bone of ear (meatus) (C41.0)
               malignant neoplasm of cartilage of ear (C49.0)
               malignant melanoma of skin of (external) ear (C43.2-)
               other and unspecified malignant neoplasm of skin of (external) ear (C44.2-)

● **C31**   **Malignant neoplasm of accessory sinuses**
Paired sinuses in bones of face

C31.0   **Malignant neoplasm of maxillary sinus** 🏷️
Malignant neoplasm of antrum (Highmore) (maxillary)

C31.1   **Malignant neoplasm of ethmoidal sinus** 🏷️

C31.2   **Malignant neoplasm of frontal sinus** 🏷️

C31.3   **Malignant neoplasm of sphenoid sinus** 🏷️

C31.8   **Malignant neoplasm of overlapping sites of accessory sinuses** 🏷️

C31.9   **Malignant neoplasm of accessory sinus, unspecified** 🏷️

● **C32**   **Malignant neoplasm of larynx**
Use additional code to identify:
  alcohol abuse and dependence (F10.-)
  exposure to environmental tobacco smoke (Z77.22)
  exposure to tobacco smoke in the perinatal period (P96.81)
  history of tobacco dependence (Z87.891)
  occupational exposure to environmental tobacco smoke (Z57.31)
  tobacco dependence (F17.-)
  tobacco use (Z72.0)

CHAPTER 2 (C00-D49)

▶ New   ➡ Revised   ~~deleted~~ Deleted   Excludes 1   Excludes 2   Includes   Use additional   Code first   Code also   Key words
OGCR Official Guidelines   **X** Assign placeholder X   ● Use Additional Character(s)   ▷ Manifestation Code   🏷️ Hierarchical Condition Category   **Coding Clinic**

C32.0   **Malignant neoplasm of glottis** 🦟
  Vocal apparatus of larynx, consisting of true vocal cords (plicae vocales) and opening between them (rima glottidis)
  Malignant neoplasm of intrinsic larynx
  Malignant neoplasm of laryngeal commissure (anterior) (posterior)
  Malignant neoplasm of vocal cord (true) NOS
  *True vocal cords ("lower vocal folds") produce vocalization when air from the lungs passes between them. Check your documentation. Code C32.1 is for malignant neoplasm of the **false** vocal cords.*

C32.1   **Malignant neoplasm of supraglottis** 🦟
  Area of pharynx above glottis
  Malignant neoplasm of aryepiglottic fold or interarytenoid fold, laryngeal aspect
  Malignant neoplasm of epiglottis (suprahyoid portion) NOS
  Malignant neoplasm of extrinsic larynx
  Malignant neoplasm of false vocal cord
  False vocal cords ("upper vocal folds") are not involved in vocalization. Check your documentation. Code C32.0 is for true vocal cords.
  Malignant neoplasm of posterior (laryngeal) surface of epiglottis
  Malignant neoplasm of ventricular bands
  > **Excludes2**   malignant neoplasm of anterior surface of epiglottis (C10.1)
  > malignant neoplasm of aryepiglottic fold or interarytenoid fold, hypopharyngeal aspect (C13.1)
  > malignant neoplasm of aryepiglottic fold or interarytenoid fold, marginal zone (C13.1)
  > malignant neoplasm of aryepiglottic fold or interarytenoid fold NOS (C13.1)

C32.2   **Malignant neoplasm of subglottis** 🦟
  Lowest part of larynx from just below vocal cords down to top of trachea

C32.3   **Malignant neoplasm of laryngeal cartilage** 🦟
  Cartilages of larynx, including cricoid, thyroid, and epiglottic, and two each of arytenoid, corniculate, and cuneiform

C32.8   **Malignant neoplasm of overlapping sites of larynx** 🦟

C32.9   **Malignant neoplasm of larynx, unspecified** 🦟

C33   **Malignant neoplasm of trachea** 🦟
  Use additional code to identify:
  exposure to environmental tobacco smoke (Z77.22)
  exposure to tobacco smoke in the perinatal period (P96.81)
  history of tobacco dependence (Z87.891)
  occupational exposure to environmental tobacco smoke (Z57.31)
  tobacco dependence (F17.-)
  tobacco use (Z72.0)

● **C34**   **Malignant neoplasm of bronchus and lung**
  Use additional code to identify:
  exposure to environmental tobacco smoke (Z77.22)
  exposure to tobacco smoke in the perinatal period (P96.81)
  history of tobacco dependence (Z87.891)
  occupational exposure to environmental tobacco smoke (Z57.31)
  tobacco dependence (F17.-)
  tobacco use (Z72.0)
  > **Excludes1**   Kaposi's sarcoma of lung (C46.5-)
  > malignant carcinoid tumor of the bronchus and lung (C7A.090)
  Coding Clinic: 2023, Q1, P20

● **C34.0**   Malignant neoplasm of main bronchus
  Malignant neoplasm of carina
  Ridgelike structure
  Malignant neoplasm of hilus (of lung)
  Anatomic depression or pit
  C34.00   Malignant neoplasm of unspecified main bronchus 🦟
  C34.01   Malignant neoplasm of right main bronchus 🦟
  C34.02   Malignant neoplasm of left main bronchus 🦟

● **C34.1**   Malignant neoplasm of upper lobe, bronchus or lung
  C34.10   Malignant neoplasm of unspecified bronchus or lung 🦟
  C34.11   Malignant neoplasm of upper lobe, right bronchus or lung 🦟
  C34.12   Malignant neoplasm of upper lobe, left bronchus or lung 🦟

C34.2   Malignant neoplasm of middle lobe, bronchus or lung 🦟

● **C34.3**   Malignant neoplasm of lower lobe, bronchus or lung
  C34.30   Malignant neoplasm of lower lobe, unspecified bronchus or lung 🦟
  C34.31   Malignant neoplasm of lower lobe, right bronchus or lung 🦟
  C34.32   Malignant neoplasm of lower lobe, left bronchus or lung 🦟

● **C34.8**   Malignant neoplasm of overlapping sites of bronchus and lung
  C34.80   Malignant neoplasm of overlapping sites of unspecified bronchus and lung 🦟
  C34.81   Malignant neoplasm of overlapping sites of right bronchus and lung 🦟
  C34.82   Malignant neoplasm of overlapping sites of left bronchus and lung 🦟

● **C34.9**   Malignant neoplasm of unspecified part of bronchus or lung
  C34.90   Malignant neoplasm of unspecified part of unspecified bronchus or lung 🦟
  Lung cancer NOS
  Coding Clinic: 2022, Q4, P23
  C34.91   Malignant neoplasm of unspecified part of right bronchus or lung 🦟
  C34.92   Malignant neoplasm of unspecified part of left bronchus or lung 🦟

C37   **Malignant neoplasm of thymus** 🦟
  > **Excludes1**   malignant carcinoid tumor of the thymus (C7A.091)

● **C38**   **Malignant neoplasm of heart, mediastinum and pleura**
  > **Excludes1**   mesothelioma (C45.-)

C38.0   **Malignant neoplasm of heart** 🦟
  Malignant neoplasm of pericardium
  > **Excludes1**   malignant neoplasm of great vessels (C49.3)

C38.1   **Malignant neoplasm of anterior mediastinum** 🦟

C38.2   **Malignant neoplasm of posterior mediastinum** 🦟

C38.3   **Malignant neoplasm of mediastinum, part unspecified** 🦟

C38.4   **Malignant neoplasm of pleura** 🦟

C38.8   **Malignant neoplasm of overlapping sites of heart, mediastinum and pleura** 🦟
  Pleura are comprised of serous membrane that lines the thoracic cavity (parietal) and covers the lungs (visceral).

CHAPTER 2 (C00–D49)

● **C39** **Malignant neoplasm of other and ill-defined sites in the respiratory system and intrathoracic organs**
Intrathoracic: within thorax/chest

Use additional code to identify:
  exposure to environmental tobacco smoke (Z77.22)
  exposure to tobacco smoke in the perinatal period (P96.81)
  history of tobacco dependence (Z87.891)
  occupational exposure to environmental tobacco smoke (Z57.31)
  tobacco dependence (F17.-)
  tobacco use (Z72.0)

Excludes1   intrathoracic malignant neoplasm NOS (C76.1)
         thoracic malignant neoplasm NOS (C76.1)

C39.0   **Malignant neoplasm of upper respiratory tract, part unspecified** 🐾

C39.9   **Malignant neoplasm of lower respiratory tract, part unspecified** 🐾
      Malignant neoplasm of respiratory tract NOS

MALIGNANT NEOPLASMS OF BONE AND ARTICULAR CARTILAGE (C40-C41)

Includes   malignant neoplasm of cartilage (articular) (joint)
      malignant neoplasm of periosteum

Excludes1   malignant neoplasm of bone marrow NOS (C96.9)
      malignant neoplasm of synovia (C49.-)

● **C40** **Malignant neoplasm of bone and articular cartilage of limbs**
Use additional code to identify major osseous defect, if applicable (M89.7-)

● C40.0   **Malignant neoplasm of scapula and long bones of upper limb**

C40.00   **Malignant neoplasm of scapula and long bones of unspecified upper limb** 🐾

C40.01   **Malignant neoplasm of scapula and long bones of right upper limb** 🐾

C40.02   **Malignant neoplasm of scapula and long bones of left upper limb** 🐾

● C40.1   **Malignant neoplasm of short bones of upper limb**

C40.10   **Malignant neoplasm of short bones of unspecified upper limb** 🐾

C40.11   **Malignant neoplasm of short bones of right upper limb** 🐾

C40.12   **Malignant neoplasm of short bones of left upper limb** 🐾

● C40.2   **Malignant neoplasm of long bones of lower limb**

C40.20   **Malignant neoplasm of long bones of unspecified lower limb** 🐾

C40.21   **Malignant neoplasm of long bones of right lower limb** 🐾

C40.22   **Malignant neoplasm of long bones of left lower limb** 🐾

● C40.3   **Malignant neoplasm of short bones of lower limb**

C40.30   **Malignant neoplasm of short bones of unspecified lower limb** 🐾

C40.31   **Malignant neoplasm of short bones of right lower limb** 🐾

C40.32   **Malignant neoplasm of short bones of left lower limb** 🐾

● C40.8   **Malignant neoplasm of overlapping sites of bone and articular cartilage of limb**

C40.80   **Malignant neoplasm of overlapping sites of bone and articular cartilage of unspecified limb** 🐾

C40.81   **Malignant neoplasm of overlapping sites of bone and articular cartilage of right limb** 🐾

C40.82   **Malignant neoplasm of overlapping sites of bone and articular cartilage of left limb** 🐾

● C40.9   **Malignant neoplasm of unspecified bones and articular cartilage of limb**

C40.90   **Malignant neoplasm of unspecified bones and articular cartilage of unspecified limb** 🐾

C40.91   **Malignant neoplasm of unspecified bones and articular cartilage of right limb** 🐾

C40.92   **Malignant neoplasm of unspecified bones and articular cartilage of left limb** 🐾

● **C41** **Malignant neoplasm of bone and articular cartilage of other and unspecified sites**

Excludes1   malignant neoplasm of bones of limbs (C40.-)
      malignant neoplasm of cartilage of ear (C49.0)
      malignant neoplasm of cartilage of eyelid (C49.0)
      malignant neoplasm of cartilage of larynx (C32.3)
      malignant neoplasm of cartilage of limbs (C40.-)
      malignant neoplasm of cartilage of nose (C30.0)

C41.0   **Malignant neoplasm of bones of skull and face** 🐾
      Malignant neoplasm of maxilla (superior)
      Malignant neoplasm of orbital bone

Excludes2   carcinoma, any type except intraosseous or odontogenic of:
      maxillary sinus (C31.0)
      upper jaw (C03.0)
      malignant neoplasm of jaw bone (lower) (C41.1)

C41.1   **Malignant neoplasm of mandible** 🐾
      Malignant neoplasm of inferior maxilla
      Malignant neoplasm of lower jaw bone

Excludes2   carcinoma, any type except intraosseous or odontogenic of:
      jaw NOS (C03.9)
      lower (C03.1)
      malignant neoplasm of upper jaw bone (C41.0)

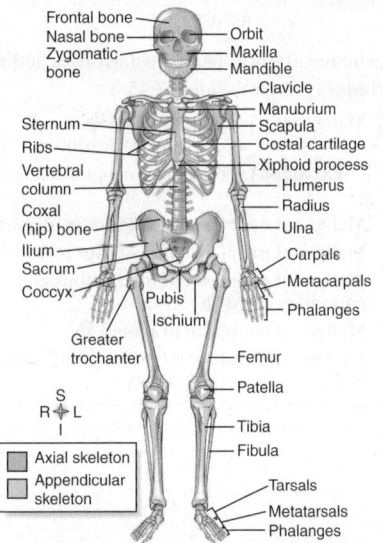

Figure 2-8   Diagram of skeleton of trunk and limbs with bones labeled. (From Thibodeau and Patton: Anatomy and Physiology, ed 7, Mosby, 2010)

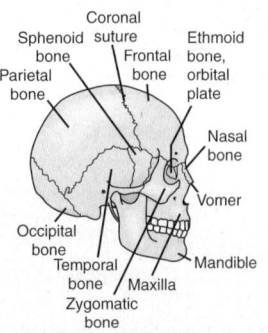

Figure 2-9   Bones of the skull.

▶ New   ⇒ Revised   ~~deleted~~ Deleted   Excludes 1   Excludes 2   Includes   Use additional   Code first   Code also   Key words

632   OGCR Official Guidelines   X Assign placeholder X   ● Use Additional Character(s)   ▶ Manifestation Code   🐾 Hierarchical Condition Category   **Coding Clinic**

C41.2 Malignant neoplasm of vertebral column
     Excludes1 malignant neoplasm of sacrum and coccyx (C41.4)

C41.3 Malignant neoplasm of ribs, sternum and clavicle 🔖

C41.4 Malignant neoplasm of pelvic bones, sacrum and coccyx 🔖

C41.9 Malignant neoplasm of bone and articular cartilage, unspecified 🔖

MELANOMA AND OTHER MALIGNANT NEOPLASMS OF SKIN (C43-C44)

● C43 Malignant melanoma of skin
     Excludes1 melanoma in situ (D03.-)
     Excludes2 malignant melanoma of skin of genital organs (C51-C52, C60.-, C63.-)
           Merkel cell carcinoma (C4A.-)
           sites other than skin-code to malignant neoplasm of the site

C43.0 Malignant melanoma of lip 🔖
     Excludes1 malignant neoplasm of vermilion border of lip (C00.0-C00.2)

● C43.1 Malignant melanoma of eyelid, including canthus
     Canthus: Either corner of eye where upper and lower eyelids meet
     C43.10 Malignant melanoma of unspecified eyelid, including canthus 🔖
     ● C43.11 Malignant melanoma of right eyelid, including canthus 🔖
         C43.111 Malignant melanoma of right upper eyelid, including canthus 🔖
         C43.112 Malignant melanoma of right lower eyelid, including canthus 🔖
     ● C43.12 Malignant melanoma of left eyelid, including canthus 🔖
         C43.121 Malignant melanoma of left upper eyelid, including canthus 🔖
         C43.122 Malignant melanoma of left lower eyelid, including canthus 🔖

● C43.2 Malignant melanoma of ear and external auricular canal
     C43.20 Malignant melanoma of unspecified ear and external auricular canal 🔖
     C43.21 Malignant melanoma of right ear and external auricular canal 🔖
     C43.22 Malignant melanoma of left ear and external auricular canal 🔖

● C43.3 Malignant melanoma of other and unspecified parts of face
     C43.30 Malignant melanoma of unspecified part of face 🔖
     C43.31 Malignant melanoma of nose 🔖
     C43.39 Malignant melanoma of other parts of face 🔖

C43.4 Malignant melanoma of scalp and neck 🔖

Figure 2-10 Malignant melanoma of skin. (Getty Image)

Item 2–4 Malignant melanoma is a serious form of skin cancer that affects the melanocytes (pigment-forming cells) and is caused by ultraviolet (UV) rays from the sun that damage skin. It is most commonly seen in the 40- to 60-year-olds with fair skin, blue or green eyes, and red or blond hair who sunburn easily.

Melanoma can spread very rapidly and is the most deadly form of skin cancer. It is less common than other types of skin cancer. The rate of melanoma is increasing and currently is the leading cause of death from skin disease.

● C43.5 Malignant melanoma of trunk
     Excludes2 malignant neoplasm of anus NOS (C21.0)
           malignant neoplasm of scrotum (C63.2)
     C43.51 Malignant melanoma of anal skin 🔖
         Malignant melanoma of anal margin
         Malignant melanoma of perianal skin
     C43.52 Malignant melanoma of skin of breast 🔖
     C43.59 Malignant melanoma of other part of trunk 🔖

● C43.6 Malignant melanoma of upper limb, including shoulder
     C43.60 Malignant melanoma of upper limb, including shoulder, unspecified side 🔖
     C43.61 Malignant melanoma of right upper limb, including shoulder 🔖
     C43.62 Malignant melanoma of left upper limb, including shoulder 🔖

● C43.7 Malignant melanoma of lower limb, including hip
     C43.70 Malignant melanoma of unspecified lower limb, including hip 🔖
     C43.71 Malignant melanoma of right lower limb, including hip 🔖
     C43.72 Malignant melanoma of left lower limb, including hip 🔖

C43.8 Malignant melanoma of overlapping sites of skin 🔖

C43.9 Malignant melanoma of skin, unspecified 🔖
     Malignant melanoma of unspecified site of skin
     Melanoma (malignant) NOS

● C44 Other and unspecified malignant neoplasm of skin
     Includes malignant neoplasm of sebaceous glands
           malignant neoplasm of sweat glands
     Excludes1 Kaposi's sarcoma of skin (C46.0)
           malignant melanoma of skin (C43.-)
           malignant neoplasm of skin of genital organs (C51-C52, C60.-, C63.2)
           Merkel cell carcinoma (C4A.-)

● C44.0 Other and unspecified malignant neoplasm of skin of lip
     Excludes1 malignant neoplasm of lip (C00.-)
     C44.00 Unspecified malignant neoplasm of skin of lip
     C44.01 Basal cell carcinoma of skin of lip
     C44.02 Squamous cell carcinoma of skin of lip
     C44.09 Other specified malignant neoplasm of skin of lip

● C44.1 Other and unspecified malignant neoplasm of skin of eyelid, including canthus
     Excludes1 connective tissue of eyelid (C49.0)
     ● C44.10 Unspecified malignant neoplasm of skin of eyelid, including canthus
         C44.101 Unspecified malignant neoplasm of skin of unspecified eyelid, including canthus
         ● C44.102 Unspecified malignant neoplasm of skin of right eyelid, including canthus
             C44.1021 Unspecified malignant neoplasm of skin of right upper eyelid, including canthus
             C44.1022 Unspecified malignant neoplasm of skin of right lower eyelid, including canthus
         ● C44.109 Unspecified malignant neoplasm of skin of left eyelid, including canthus
             C44.1091 Unspecified malignant neoplasm of skin of left upper eyelid, including canthus
             C44.1092 Unspecified malignant neoplasm of skin of left lower eyelid, including canthus

● C44.11 Basal cell carcinoma of skin of eyelid, including canthus

  C44.111 Basal cell carcinoma of skin of unspecified eyelid, including canthus

● C44.112 Basal cell carcinoma of skin of right eyelid, including canthus

  C44.1121 Basal cell carcinoma of skin of right upper eyelid, including canthus

  C44.1122 Basal cell carcinoma of skin of right lower eyelid, including canthus

● C44.119 Basal cell carcinoma of skin of left eyelid, including canthus

  C44.1191 Basal cell carcinoma of skin of left upper eyelid, including canthus

  C44.1192 Basal cell carcinoma of skin of left lower eyelid, including canthus

● C44.12 Squamous cell carcinoma of skin of eyelid, including canthus

  C44.121 Squamous cell carcinoma of skin of unspecified eyelid, including canthus

● C44.122 Squamous cell carcinoma of skin of right eyelid, including canthus

  C44.1221 Squamous cell carcinoma of skin of right upper eyelid, including canthus

  C44.1222 Squamous cell carcinoma of skin of right lower eyelid, including canthus

● C44.129 Squamous cell carcinoma of skin of left eyelid, including canthus

  C44.1291 Squamous cell carcinoma of skin of left upper eyelid, including canthus

  C44.1292 Squamous cell carcinoma of skin of left lower eyelid, including canthus

● C44.13 Sebaceous cell carcinoma of skin of eyelid, including canthus

  C44.131 Sebaceous cell carcinoma of skin of unspecified eyelid, including canthus

● C44.132 Sebaceous cell carcinoma of skin of right eyelid, including canthus

  C44.1321 Sebaceous cell carcinoma of skin of right upper eyelid, including canthus

  C44.1322 Sebaceous cell carcinoma of skin of right lower eyelid, including canthus

● C44.139 Sebaceous cell carcinoma of skin of left eyelid, including canthus

  C44.1391 Sebaceous cell carcinoma of skin of left upper eyelid, including canthus

  C44.1392 Sebaceous cell carcinoma of skin of left lower eyelid, including canthus

● C44.19 Other specified malignant neoplasm of skin of eyelid, including canthus

  C44.191 Other specified malignant neoplasm of skin of unspecified eyelid, including canthus

● C44.192 Other specified malignant neoplasm of skin of right eyelid, including canthus

  C44.1921 Other specified malignant neoplasm of skin of right upper eyelid, including canthus

  C44.1922 Other specified malignant neoplasm of skin of right lower eyelid, including canthus

● C44.199 Other specified malignant neoplasm of skin of left eyelid, including canthus

  C44.1991 Other specified malignant neoplasm of skin of left upper eyelid, including canthus

  C44.1992 Other specified malignant neoplasm of skin of left lower eyelid, including canthus

● C44.2 Other and unspecified malignant neoplasm of skin of ear and external auricular canal

  Excludes1   connective tissue of ear (C49.0)

● C44.20 Unspecified malignant neoplasm of skin of ear and external auricular canal

  C44.201 Unspecified malignant neoplasm of skin of unspecified ear and external auricular canal

  C44.202 Unspecified malignant neoplasm of skin of right ear and external auricular canal

  C44.209 Unspecified malignant neoplasm of skin of left ear and external auricular canal

● C44.21 Basal cell carcinoma of skin of ear and external auricular canal

  C44.211 Basal cell carcinoma of skin of unspecified ear and external auricular canal

  C44.212 Basal cell carcinoma of skin of right ear and external auricular canal

  C44.219 Basal cell carcinoma of skin of left ear and external auricular canal

● C44.22 Squamous cell carcinoma of skin of ear and external auricular canal

  C44.221 Squamous cell carcinoma of skin of unspecified ear and external auricular canal

  C44.222 Squamous cell carcinoma of skin of right ear and external auricular canal

  C44.229 Squamous cell carcinoma of skin of left ear and external auricular canal

● C44.29 Other specified malignant neoplasm of skin of ear and external auricular canal

  C44.291 Other specified malignant neoplasm of skin of unspecified ear and external auricular canal

  C44.292 Other specified malignant neoplasm of skin of right ear and external auricular canal

  C44.299 Other specified malignant neoplasm of skin of left ear and external auricular canal

● C44.3 Other and unspecified malignant neoplasm of skin of other and unspecified parts of face

● C44.30 Unspecified malignant neoplasm of skin of other and unspecified parts of face

  C44.300 Unspecified malignant neoplasm of skin of unspecified part of face

  C44.301 Unspecified malignant neoplasm of skin of nose

  C44.309 Unspecified malignant neoplasm of skin of other parts of face

▶ New   ⟹ Revised   ~~deleted~~ Deleted | Excludes 1 | | Excludes 2 | | Includes | | Use additional | | Code first | | Code also | | Key words |

OGCR Official Guidelines   X Assign placeholder X   ● Use Additional Character(s)   ▶ Manifestation Code   🔖 Hierarchical Condition Category   **Coding Clinic**

● C44.31 Basal cell carcinoma of skin of other and unspecified parts of face

    C44.310 Basal cell carcinoma of skin of unspecified parts of face

    C44.311 Basal cell carcinoma of skin of nose

    C44.319 Basal cell carcinoma of skin of other parts of face
        Coding Clinic: 2017, Q1, P4

● C44.32 Squamous cell carcinoma of skin of other and unspecified parts of face

    C44.320 Squamous cell carcinoma of skin of unspecified parts of face

    C44.321 Squamous cell carcinoma of skin of nose

    C44.329 Squamous cell carcinoma of skin of other parts of face

● C44.39 Other specified malignant neoplasm of skin of other and unspecified parts of face

    C44.390 Other specified malignant neoplasm of skin of unspecified parts of face

    C44.391 Other specified malignant neoplasm of skin of nose

    C44.399 Other specified malignant neoplasm of skin of other parts of face

● C44.4 Other and unspecified malignant neoplasm of skin of scalp and neck

    C44.40 Unspecified malignant neoplasm of skin of scalp and neck

    C44.41 Basal cell carcinoma of skin of scalp and neck

    C44.42 Squamous cell carcinoma of skin of scalp and neck

    C44.49 Other specified malignant neoplasm of skin of scalp and neck

● C44.5 Other and unspecified malignant neoplasm of skin of trunk

    Excludes1 anus NOS (C21.0)
            scrotum (C63.2)

● C44.50 Unspecified malignant neoplasm of skin of trunk

    C44.500 Unspecified malignant neoplasm of anal skin
        Unspecified malignant neoplasm of anal margin
        Unspecified malignant neoplasm of perianal skin

    C44.501 Unspecified malignant neoplasm of skin of breast

    C44.509 Unspecified malignant neoplasm of skin of other part of trunk

● C44.51 Basal cell carcinoma of skin of trunk

    C44.510 Basal cell carcinoma of anal skin
        Basal cell carcinoma of anal margin
        Basal cell carcinoma of perianal skin

    C44.511 Basal cell carcinoma of skin of breast

    C44.519 Basal cell carcinoma of skin of other part of trunk

● C44.52 Squamous cell carcinoma of skin of trunk

    C44.520 Squamous cell carcinoma of anal skin
        Squamous cell carcinoma of anal margin
        Squamous cell carcinoma of perianal skin

    C44.521 Squamous cell carcinoma of skin of breast

    C44.529 Squamous cell carcinoma of skin of other part of trunk

● C44.59 Other specified malignant neoplasm of skin of trunk

    C44.590 Other specified malignant neoplasm of anal skin
        Other specified malignant neoplasm of anal margin
        Other specified malignant neoplasm of perianal skin

    C44.591 Other specified malignant neoplasm of skin of breast

    C44.599 Other specified malignant neoplasm of skin of other part of trunk

● C44.6 Other and unspecified malignant neoplasm of skin of upper limb, including shoulder

● C44.60 Unspecified malignant neoplasm of skin of upper limb, including shoulder

    C44.601 Unspecified malignant neoplasm of skin of unspecified upper limb, including shoulder

    C44.602 Unspecified malignant neoplasm of skin of right upper limb, including shoulder

    C44.609 Unspecified malignant neoplasm of skin of left upper limb, including shoulder

● C44.61 Basal cell carcinoma of skin of upper limb, including shoulder

    C44.611 Basal cell carcinoma of skin of unspecified upper limb, including shoulder

    C44.612 Basal cell carcinoma of skin of right upper limb, including shoulder

    C44.619 Basal cell carcinoma of skin of left upper limb, including shoulder

● C44.62 Squamous cell carcinoma of skin of upper limb, including shoulder

    C44.621 Squamous cell carcinoma of skin of unspecified upper limb, including shoulder

    C44.622 Squamous cell carcinoma of skin of right upper limb, including shoulder

    C44.629 Squamous cell carcinoma of skin of left upper limb, including shoulder

● C44.69 Other specified malignant neoplasm of skin of upper limb, including shoulder

    C44.691 Other specified malignant neoplasm of skin of unspecified upper limb, including shoulder

    C44.692 Other specified malignant neoplasm of skin of right upper limb, including shoulder

    C44.699 Other specified malignant neoplasm of skin of left upper limb, including shoulder

● C44.7 Other and unspecified malignant neoplasm of skin of lower limb, including hip

● C44.70 Unspecified malignant neoplasm of skin of lower limb, including hip

    C44.701 Unspecified malignant neoplasm of skin of unspecified lower limb, including hip

    C44.702 Unspecified malignant neoplasm of skin of right lower limb, including hip

    C44.709 Unspecified malignant neoplasm of skin of left lower limb, including hip

● C44.71 Basal cell carcinoma of skin of lower limb, including hip

    C44.711 Basal cell carcinoma of skin of unspecified lower limb, including hip

    C44.712 Basal cell carcinoma of skin of right lower limb, including hip

    C44.719 Basal cell carcinoma of skin of left lower limb, including hip

CHAPTER 2 (C00-D49)

- **C44.72** Squamous cell carcinoma of skin of lower limb, including hip
  - **C44.721** Squamous cell carcinoma of skin of unspecified lower limb, including hip
  - **C44.722** Squamous cell carcinoma of skin of right lower limb, including hip
  - **C44.729** Squamous cell carcinoma of skin of left lower limb, including hip
- **C44.79** Other specified malignant neoplasm of skin of lower limb, including hip
  - **C44.791** Other specified malignant neoplasm of skin of unspecified lower limb, including hip
  - **C44.792** Other specified malignant neoplasm of skin of right lower limb, including hip
  - **C44.799** Other specified malignant neoplasm of skin of left lower limb, including hip
- **C44.8** Other and unspecified malignant neoplasm of overlapping sites of skin
  - **C44.80** Unspecified malignant neoplasm of overlapping sites of skin
  - **C44.81** Basal cell carcinoma of overlapping sites of skin
  - **C44.82** Squamous cell carcinoma of overlapping sites of skin
  - **C44.89** Other specified malignant neoplasm of overlapping sites of skin
- **C44.9** Other and unspecified malignant neoplasm of skin, unspecified
  - **C44.90** Unspecified malignant neoplasm of skin, unspecified
    - Malignant neoplasm of unspecified site of skin
  - **C44.91** Basal cell carcinoma of skin, unspecified
  - **C44.92** Squamous cell carcinoma of skin, unspecified
  - **C44.99** Other specified malignant neoplasm of skin, unspecified

---

MALIGNANT NEOPLASMS OF MESOTHELIAL AND SOFT TISSUE (C45-C49)

- **C45** **Mesothelioma**
  - *Malignant cells develop in protective lining that covers internal organs (mesothelium) caused by exposure to asbestos*
  - **C45.0** Mesothelioma of pleura 🝔
    - **Excludes1** other malignant neoplasm of pleura (C38.4)
    - Coding Clinic: 2017, Q2, P11
  - **C45.1** Mesothelioma of peritoneum 🝔
    - Mesothelioma of cul-de-sac
    - Mesothelioma of mesentery
    - Mesothelioma of mesocolon
    - Mesothelioma of omentum
    - Mesothelioma of peritoneum (parietal) (pelvic)
    - **Excludes1** other malignant neoplasm of soft tissue of peritoneum (C48.-)

Figure 2-11 Kaposi's sarcoma. There are large confluent hyperpigmented patch-stage lesions with lymphedema. (From Goldman L, Ausiello D, Arend W, Armitage J, Clemmons D, Drazen J, Griggs R, et al: Cecil Medicine: Expert Consult, 23e, Saunders, 2007)

- **C45.2** Mesothelioma of pericardium 🝔
  - **Excludes1** other malignant neoplasm of pericardium (C38.0)
- **C45.7** Mesothelioma of other sites 🝔
- **C45.9** Mesothelioma, unspecified 🝔

- **C46** **Kaposi's sarcoma**
  - *Code first any human immunodeficiency virus [HIV] disease (B20)*
  - **C46.0** Kaposi's sarcoma of skin 🝔
  - **C46.1** Kaposi's sarcoma of soft tissue 🝔
    - Kaposi's sarcoma of blood vessel
    - Kaposi's sarcoma of connective tissue
    - Kaposi's sarcoma of fascia
    - Kaposi's sarcoma of ligament
    - Kaposi's sarcoma of lymphatic(s) NEC
    - Kaposi's sarcoma of muscle
    - **Excludes2** Kaposi's sarcoma of lymph glands and nodes (C46.3)
  - **C46.2** Kaposi's sarcoma of palate 🝔
  - **C46.3** Kaposi's sarcoma of lymph nodes 🝔
  - **C46.4** Kaposi's sarcoma of gastrointestinal sites 🝔
  - **C46.5** Kaposi's sarcoma of lung
    - **C46.50** Kaposi's sarcoma of unspecified lung 🝔
    - **C46.51** Kaposi's sarcoma of right lung 🝔
    - **C46.52** Kaposi's sarcoma of left lung 🝔
  - **C46.7** Kaposi's sarcoma of other sites 🝔
  - **C46.9** Kaposi's sarcoma, unspecified 🝔
    - Kaposi's sarcoma of unspecified site

- **C47** **Malignant neoplasm of peripheral nerves and autonomic nervous system**
  - **Includes** malignant neoplasm of sympathetic and parasympathetic nerves and ganglia
  - **Excludes1** Kaposi's sarcoma of soft tissue (C46.1)
  - **C47.0** Malignant neoplasm of peripheral nerves of head, face and neck 🝔
    - **Excludes1** malignant neoplasm of peripheral nerves of orbit (C69.6-)
  - **C47.1** Malignant neoplasm of peripheral nerves of upper limb, including shoulder
    - **C47.10** Malignant neoplasm of peripheral nerves of unspecified upper limb, including shoulder 🝔
    - **C47.11** Malignant neoplasm of peripheral nerves of right upper limb, including shoulder 🝔
    - **C47.12** Malignant neoplasm of peripheral nerves of left upper limb, including shoulder 🝔
  - **C47.2** Malignant neoplasm of peripheral nerves of lower limb, including hip
    - **C47.20** Malignant neoplasm of peripheral nerves of unspecified lower limb, including hip 🝔
    - **C47.21** Malignant neoplasm of peripheral nerves of right lower limb, including hip 🝔
    - **C47.22** Malignant neoplasm of peripheral nerves of left lower limb, including hip 🝔
  - **C47.3** Malignant neoplasm of peripheral nerves of thorax 🝔
  - **C47.4** Malignant neoplasm of peripheral nerves of abdomen 🝔
  - **C47.5** Malignant neoplasm of peripheral nerves of pelvis 🝔
  - **C47.6** Malignant neoplasm of peripheral nerves of trunk, unspecified 🝔
    - Malignant neoplasm of peripheral nerves of unspecified part of trunk
  - **C47.8** Malignant neoplasm of overlapping sites of peripheral nerves and autonomic nervous system 🝔
  - **C47.9** Malignant neoplasm of peripheral nerves and autonomic nervous system, unspecified 🝔
    - Malignant neoplasm of unspecified site of peripheral nerves of autonomic nervous system

Item 2–5 Kaposi's sarcoma is a cancer that causes patches of abnormal tissue to grow under the skin; in the lining of the mouth, nose, and throat; or in other organs, often beginning and spreading to other organs. Patients who have had organ transplants or patients with AIDS are at high risk for this malignancy.

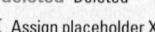

▶ New   ➡ Revised   ~~deleted~~ Deleted   Excludes 1   Excludes 2   Includes   Use additional   Code first   Code also   Key words

636

OGCR Official Guidelines   X Assign placeholder X   ● Use Additional Character(s)   ▌ Manifestation Code   🝔 Hierarchical Condition Category   Coding Clinic

● **C48**   Malignant neoplasm of retroperitoneum and peritoneum
>   **Excludes1**   Kaposi's sarcoma of connective tissue (C46.1)
>   mesothelioma (C45.-)

     C48.0   Malignant neoplasm of retroperitoneum 🔲
>   *Behind/outside of peritoneum*

     C48.1   Malignant neoplasm of specified parts of peritoneum 🔲
>   *Serous membrane lining abdominopelvic walls and covering*
>   *viscera*
>   Malignant neoplasm of cul-de-sac
>   Malignant neoplasm of mesentery
>   Malignant neoplasm of mesocolon
>   Malignant neoplasm of omentum
>   Malignant neoplasm of parietal peritoneum
>   Malignant neoplasm of pelvic peritoneum

     C48.2   Malignant neoplasm of peritoneum, unspecified 🔲

     C48.8   Malignant neoplasm of overlapping sites of
retroperitoneum and peritoneum 🔲

● **C49**   Malignant neoplasm of other connective and soft tissue
>   **Includes**   malignant neoplasm of blood vessel
>   malignant neoplasm of bursa
>   malignant neoplasm of cartilage
>   malignant neoplasm of fascia
>   malignant neoplasm of fat
>   malignant neoplasm of ligament, except uterine
>   malignant neoplasm of lymphatic vessel
>   malignant neoplasm of muscle
>   malignant neoplasm of synovia
>   malignant neoplasm of tendon (sheath)

>   **Excludes1**   malignant neoplasm of cartilage (of):
>   articular (C40-C41)
>   larynx (C32.3)
>   nose (C30.0)
>   malignant neoplasm of connective tissue of breast
>   (C50.-)

>   **Excludes2**   Kaposi's sarcoma of soft tissue (C46.1)
>   malignant neoplasm of heart (C38.0)
>   malignant neoplasm of peripheral nerves and
>   autonomic nervous system (C47.-)
>   malignant neoplasm of peritoneum (C48.2)
>   malignant neoplasm of retroperitoneum (C48.0)
>   malignant neoplasm of uterine ligament (C57.3)
>   mesothelioma (C45.-)

     C49.0   Malignant neoplasm of connective and soft tissue of
head, face and neck 🔲
>   Malignant neoplasm of connective tissue of ear
>   Malignant neoplasm of connective tissue of eyelid
>   **Excludes1**   connective tissue of orbit (C69.6-)

●   **C49.1**   Malignant neoplasm of connective and soft tissue of
upper limb, including shoulder

         C49.10   Malignant neoplasm of connective and soft
tissue of unspecified upper limb, including
shoulder 🔲

         C49.11   Malignant neoplasm of connective and soft
tissue of right upper limb, including
shoulder 🔲

         C49.12   Malignant neoplasm of connective and soft
tissue of left upper limb, including shoulder 🔲

●   **C49.2**   Malignant neoplasm of connective and soft tissue of
lower limb, including hip

         C49.20   Malignant neoplasm of connective and soft
tissue of unspecified lower limb, including
hip 🔲

         C49.21   Malignant neoplasm of connective and soft
tissue of right lower limb, including hip 🔲

         C49.22   Malignant neoplasm of connective and soft
tissue of left lower limb, including hip 🔲

     C49.3   Malignant neoplasm of connective and soft tissue of
thorax 🔲
>   Malignant neoplasm of axilla
>   Malignant neoplasm of diaphragm
>   Malignant neoplasm of great vessels
>   **Excludes1**   malignant neoplasm of breast (C50.-)
>   malignant neoplasm of heart (C38.0)
>   malignant neoplasm of mediastinum
>   (C38.1-C38.3)
>   malignant neoplasm of thymus (C37)

Coding Clinic: 2015, Q3, P19

     C49.4   Malignant neoplasm of connective and soft tissue of
abdomen 🔲
>   Malignant neoplasm of abdominal wall
>   Malignant neoplasm of hypochondrium

Coding Clinic: 2019, Q4, P44

     C49.5   Malignant neoplasm of connective and soft tissue of
pelvis 🔲
>   Malignant neoplasm of buttock
>   Malignant neoplasm of groin
>   Malignant neoplasm of perineum

     C49.6   Malignant neoplasm of connective and soft tissue of
trunk, unspecified 🔲
>   Malignant neoplasm of back NOS

     C49.8   Malignant neoplasm of overlapping sites of connective
and soft tissue 🔲
>   Primary malignant neoplasm of two or more
>   contiguous sites of connective and soft tissue

     C49.9   Malignant neoplasm of connective and soft
tissue, unspecified 🔲

●   **C49.A**   Gastrointestinal stromal tumor
Coding Clinic: 2016, Q4, P8

         C49.A0   Gastrointestinal stromal tumor, unspecified
site 🔲

         C49.A1   Gastrointestinal stromal tumor of esophagus 🔲

         C49.A2   Gastrointestinal stromal tumor of stomach 🔲

         C49.A3   Gastrointestinal stromal tumor of small
intestine 🔲

         C49.A4   Gastrointestinal stromal tumor of large
intestine 🔲

         C49.A5   Gastrointestinal stromal tumor of rectum 🔲

         C49.A9   Gastrointestinal stromal tumor of other sites 🔲

● **C4A**   Merkel cell carcinoma

     C4A.0   Merkel cell carcinoma of lip 🔲
>   **Excludes1**   malignant neoplasm of vermilion border
>   of lip (C00.0-C00.2)

●   **C4A.1**   Merkel cell carcinoma of eyelid, including canthus

         C4A.10   Merkel cell carcinoma of unspecified eyelid,
including canthus 🔲

     ●   **C4A.11**   Merkel cell carcinoma of right eyelid, including
canthus 🔲

             C4A.111   Merkel cell carcinoma of right upper
eyelid, including canthus 🔲

             C4A.112   Merkel cell carcinoma of right lower
eyelid, including canthus 🔲

     ●   **C4A.12**   Merkel cell carcinoma of left eyelid, including
canthus 🔲

             C4A.121   Merkel cell carcinoma of left upper
eyelid, including canthus 🔲

             C4A.122   Merkel cell carcinoma of left lower
eyelid, including canthus 🔲

●   **C4A.2**   Merkel cell carcinoma of ear and external auricular canal

         C4A.20   Merkel cell carcinoma of unspecified ear and
external auricular canal 🔲

         C4A.21   Merkel cell carcinoma of right ear and external
auricular canal 🔲

         C4A.22   Merkel cell carcinoma of left ear and external
auricular canal 🔲

CHAPTER 2 (C00-D49)

● C4A.3 Merkel cell carcinoma of other and unspecified parts of face

    C4A.30 Merkel cell carcinoma of unspecified part of face 🔲

    C4A.31 Merkel cell carcinoma of nose 🔲

    C4A.39 Merkel cell carcinoma of other parts of face 🔲

● C4A.4 Merkel cell carcinoma of scalp and neck 🔲

● C4A.5 Merkel cell carcinoma of trunk

    Excludes2 malignant neoplasm of anus NOS (C21.0)
              malignant neoplasm of scrotum (C63.2)

    C4A.51 Merkel cell carcinoma of anal skin 🔲
        Merkel cell carcinoma of anal margin
        Merkel cell carcinoma of perianal skin

    C4A.52 Merkel cell carcinoma of skin of breast 🔲

    C4A.59 Merkel cell carcinoma of other part of trunk 🔲

● C4A.6 Merkel cell carcinoma of upper limb, including shoulder

    C4A.60 Merkel cell carcinoma of unspecified upper limb, including shoulder 🔲

    C4A.61 Merkel cell carcinoma of right upper limb, including shoulder 🔲

    C4A.62 Merkel cell carcinoma of left upper limb, including shoulder 🔲

● C4A.7 Merkel cell carcinoma of lower limb, including hip

    C4A.70 Merkel cell carcinoma of unspecified lower limb, including hip 🔲

    C4A.71 Merkel cell carcinoma of right lower limb, including hip 🔲

    C4A.72 Merkel cell carcinoma of left lower limb, including hip 🔲

  C4A.8 Merkel cell carcinoma of overlapping sites 🔲

  C4A.9 Merkel cell carcinoma, unspecified 🔲
        Merkel cell carcinoma of unspecified site
        Merkel cell carcinoma NOS

MALIGNANT NEOPLASMS OF BREAST (C50)

● C50 Malignant neoplasm of breast

    Includes connective tissue of breast
              Paget's disease of breast
              Paget's disease of nipple
              Intraductal carcinoma of breast characterized by eczema-like inflammatory skin changes

⇒ Use additional code to identify estrogen, and other hormones and factors receptor status (Z17.0, Z17.1)

    Excludes1 skin of breast (C44.501, C44.511, C44.521, C44.591)

● C50.0 Malignant neoplasm of nipple and areola

  ● C50.01 Malignant neoplasm of nipple and areola, female

    C50.011 Malignant neoplasm of nipple and areola, right female breast 🔲

    C50.012 Malignant neoplasm of nipple and areola, left female breast 🔲

    C50.019 Malignant neoplasm of nipple and areola, unspecified female breast 🔲

  ● C50.02 Malignant neoplasm of nipple and areola, male

    C50.021 Malignant neoplasm of nipple and areola, right male breast 🔲

    C50.022 Malignant neoplasm of nipple and areola, left male breast 🔲

    C50.029 Malignant neoplasm of nipple and areola, unspecified male breast 🔲

● C50.1 Malignant neoplasm of central portion of breast

  ● C50.11 Malignant neoplasm of central portion of breast, female

    C50.111 Malignant neoplasm of central portion of right female breast 🔲

    C50.112 Malignant neoplasm of central portion of left female breast 🔲

    C50.119 Malignant neoplasm of central portion of unspecified female breast 🔲

Figure 2-12 Female breast quadrants and axillary tail.

  ● C50.12 Malignant neoplasm of central portion of breast, male

    C50.121 Malignant neoplasm of central portion of right male breast 🔲

    C50.122 Malignant neoplasm of central portion of left male breast 🔲

    C50.129 Malignant neoplasm of central portion of unspecified male breast 🔲

● C50.2 Malignant neoplasm of upper-inner quadrant of breast

  ● C50.21 Malignant neoplasm of upper-inner quadrant of breast, female

    C50.211 Malignant neoplasm of upper-inner quadrant of right female breast 🔲

    C50.212 Malignant neoplasm of upper-inner quadrant of left female breast 🔲

    C50.219 Malignant neoplasm of upper-inner quadrant of unspecified female breast 🔲

  ● C50.22 Malignant neoplasm of upper-inner quadrant of breast, male

    C50.221 Malignant neoplasm of upper-inner quadrant of right male breast 🔲

    C50.222 Malignant neoplasm of upper-inner quadrant of left male breast 🔲

    C50.229 Malignant neoplasm of upper-inner quadrant of unspecified male breast 🔲

● C50.3 Malignant neoplasm of lower-inner quadrant of breast

  ● C50.31 Malignant neoplasm of lower-inner quadrant of breast, female

    C50.311 Malignant neoplasm of lower-inner quadrant of right female breast 🔲

    C50.312 Malignant neoplasm of lower-inner quadrant of left female breast 🔲

    C50.319 Malignant neoplasm of lower-inner quadrant of unspecified female breast 🔲

  ● C50.32 Malignant neoplasm of lower-inner quadrant of breast, male

    C50.321 Malignant neoplasm of lower-inner quadrant of right male breast 🔲

    C50.322 Malignant neoplasm of lower-inner quadrant of left male breast 🔲

    C50.329 Malignant neoplasm of lower-inner quadrant of unspecified male breast 🔲

● C50.4 Malignant neoplasm of upper-outer quadrant of breast

  ● C50.41 Malignant neoplasm of upper-outer quadrant of breast, female

    C50.411 Malignant neoplasm of upper-outer quadrant of right female breast 🔲

    C50.412 Malignant neoplasm of upper-outer quadrant of left female breast 🔲

    C50.419 Malignant neoplasm of upper-outer quadrant of unspecified female breast 🔲

▶ New   ⇒ Revised   ~~deleted~~ Deleted   Excludes 1   Excludes 2   Includes   Use additional   Code first   Code also   Key words

OGCR Official Guidelines   X Assign placeholder X   ● Use Additional Character(s)   ▷ Manifestation Code   🔲 Hierarchical Condition Category   **Coding Clinic**

● **C50.42** Malignant neoplasm of upper-outer quadrant of breast, male

    C50.421 Malignant neoplasm of upper-outer quadrant of right male breast 🦠

    C50.422 Malignant neoplasm of upper-outer quadrant of left male breast 🦠

    C50.429 Malignant neoplasm of upper-outer quadrant of unspecified male breast 🦠

● **C50.5** Malignant neoplasm of lower-outer quadrant of breast

    ● **C50.51** Malignant neoplasm of lower-outer quadrant of breast, female

       C50.511 Malignant neoplasm of lower-outer quadrant of right female breast 🦠

       C50.512 Malignant neoplasm of lower-outer quadrant of left female breast 🦠

       C50.519 Malignant neoplasm of lower-outer quadrant of unspecified female breast 🦠

    ● **C50.52** Malignant neoplasm of lower-outer quadrant of breast, male

       C50.521 Malignant neoplasm of lower-outer quadrant of right male breast 🦠

       C50.522 Malignant neoplasm of lower-outer quadrant of left male breast 🦠

       C50.529 Malignant neoplasm of lower-outer quadrant of unspecified male breast 🦠

● **C50.6** Malignant neoplasm of axillary tail of breast

    ● **C50.61** Malignant neoplasm of axillary tail of breast, female

       C50.611 Malignant neoplasm of axillary tail of right female breast 🦠

       C50.612 Malignant neoplasm of axillary tail of left female breast 🦠

       C50.619 Malignant neoplasm of axillary tail of unspecified female breast 🦠

    ● **C50.62** Malignant neoplasm of axillary tail of breast, male

       C50.621 Malignant neoplasm of axillary tail of right male breast 🦠

       C50.622 Malignant neoplasm of axillary tail of left male breast 🦠

       C50.629 Malignant neoplasm of axillary tail of unspecified male breast 🦠

● **C50.8** Malignant neoplasm of overlapping sites of breast

    ● **C50.81** Malignant neoplasm of overlapping sites of breast, female

       C50.811 Malignant neoplasm of overlapping sites of right female breast 🦠

       C50.812 Malignant neoplasm of overlapping sites of left female breast 🦠

       C50.819 Malignant neoplasm of overlapping sites of unspecified female breast 🦠

    ● **C50.82** Malignant neoplasm of overlapping sites of breast, male

       C50.821 Malignant neoplasm of overlapping sites of right male breast 🦠

       C50.822 Malignant neoplasm of overlapping sites of left male breast 🦠

       C50.829 Malignant neoplasm of overlapping sites of unspecified male breast 🦠

● **C50.9** Malignant neoplasm of breast of unspecified site

    ● **C50.91** Malignant neoplasm of breast of unspecified site, female

       C50.911 Malignant neoplasm of unspecified site of right female breast 🦠

       C50.912 Malignant neoplasm of unspecified site of left female breast 🦠
         Coding Clinic: 2022, Q3, P11,15

       C50.919 Malignant neoplasm of unspecified site of unspecified female breast 🦠

● **C50.92** Malignant neoplasm of breast of unspecified site, male

    C50.921 Malignant neoplasm of unspecified site of right male breast 🦠

    C50.922 Malignant neoplasm of unspecified site of left male breast 🦠

    C50.929 Malignant neoplasm of unspecified site of unspecified male breast 🦠

MALIGNANT NEOPLASMS OF FEMALE GENITAL ORGANS (C51-C58)

> **Includes**   malignant neoplasm of skin of female genital organs

● C51   Malignant neoplasm of vulva

    Excludes1   carcinoma in situ of vulva (D07.1)

    C51.0   Malignant neoplasm of labium majus 🦠
       Outer folds of skin external female genitalia
       Malignant neoplasm of Bartholin's [greater vestibular] gland

    C51.1   Malignant neoplasm of labium minus 🦠
       Two inner folds surrounding vulva in female genitalia

    C51.2   Malignant neoplasm of clitoris 🦠

    C51.8   Malignant neoplasm of overlapping sites of vulva 🦠

    C51.9   Malignant neoplasm of vulva, unspecified 🦠
       Malignant neoplasm of external female genitalia NOS
       Malignant neoplasm of pudendum

  C52   Malignant neoplasm of vagina 🦠

    Excludes1   carcinoma in situ of vagina (D07.2)

● C53   Malignant neoplasm of cervix uteri

    Excludes1   carcinoma in situ of cervix uteri (D06.-)

    C53.0   Malignant neoplasm of endocervix 🦠
       Inside the cervix

    C53.1   Malignant neoplasm of exocervix 🦠
       Outside the cervix

    C53.8   Malignant neoplasm of overlapping sites of cervix uteri 🦠

    C53.9   Malignant neoplasm of cervix uteri, unspecified 🦠
       Coding Clinic: 2017, Q4, P103

● C54   Malignant neoplasm of corpus uteri

    C54.0   Malignant neoplasm of isthmus uteri 🦠
       Constricted part of uterus between cervix and body
       Malignant neoplasm of lower uterine segment

    C54.1   Malignant neoplasm of endometrium 🦠
       Lining of uterus

    C54.2   Malignant neoplasm of myometrium 🦠
       Middle layer of uterine wall consisting of smooth muscle supporting stromal and vascular tissue

    C54.3   Malignant neoplasm of fundus uteri 🦠
       Top rounded portion of uterus

    C54.8   Malignant neoplasm of overlapping sites of corpus uteri ♀ 🦠
       Main body of uterus
       Coding Clinic: 2023, Q3, P15

    C54.9   Malignant neoplasm of corpus uteri, unspecified 🦠

  C55   Malignant neoplasm of uterus, part unspecified 🦠

Figure 2-13   Cervix uteri.

● **C56   Malignant neoplasm of ovary**
    Use additional code to identify any functional activity

    C56.1   Malignant neoplasm of right ovary 🐾

    C56.2   Malignant neoplasm of left ovary 🐾

    C56.3   Malignant neoplasm of bilateral ovaries

    C56.9   Malignant neoplasm of unspecified ovary 🐾

● **C57   Malignant neoplasm of other and unspecified female genital organs**

  ● **C57.0   Malignant neoplasm of fallopian tube**
      Malignant neoplasm of oviduct
      Malignant neoplasm of uterine tube

      C57.00   Malignant neoplasm of unspecified fallopian tube 🐾

      C57.01   Malignant neoplasm of right fallopian tube 🐾

      C57.02   Malignant neoplasm of left fallopian tube 🐾

  ● **C57.1   Malignant neoplasm of broad ligament**

      C57.10   Malignant neoplasm of unspecified broad ligament 🐾

      C57.11   Malignant neoplasm of right broad ligament 🐾

      C57.12   Malignant neoplasm of left broad ligament 🐾

  ● **C57.2   Malignant neoplasm of round ligament**

      C57.20   Malignant neoplasm of unspecified round ligament 🐾

      C57.21   Malignant neoplasm of right round ligament 🐾

      C57.22   Malignant neoplasm of left round ligament 🐾

    C57.3   Malignant neoplasm of parametrium
      Malignant neoplasm of uterine ligament NOS

    C57.4   Malignant neoplasm of uterine adnexa, unspecified ♀

    C57.7   Malignant neoplasm of other specified female genital organs 🐾
      Malignant neoplasm of wolffian body or duct

    C57.8   Malignant neoplasm of overlapping sites of female genital organs 🐾
      Primary malignant neoplasm of two or more contiguous sites of the female genital organs whose point of origin cannot be determined
      Primary tubo-ovarian malignant neoplasm whose point of origin cannot be determined
      Primary utero-ovarian malignant neoplasm whose point of origin cannot be determined

    C57.9   Malignant neoplasm of female genital organ, unspecified 🐾
      Malignant neoplasm of female genitourinary tract NOS

C58   Malignant neoplasm of placenta 🐾   **M**

    Includes   choriocarcinoma NOS
              chorionepithelioma NOS

    Excludes1   chorioadenoma (destruens) (D39.2)
              hydatidiform mole NOS (O01.9)
              invasive hydatidiform mole (D39.2)
              male choriocarcinoma NOS (C62.9-)
              malignant hydatidiform mole (D39.2)

MALIGNANT NEOPLASMS OF MALE GENITAL ORGANS (C60-C63)

    Includes   malignant neoplasm of skin of male genital organs

● **C60   Malignant neoplasm of penis**

    C60.0   Malignant neoplasm of prepuce 🐾
      Malignant neoplasm of foreskin

    C60.1   Malignant neoplasm of glans penis 🐾

    C60.2   Malignant neoplasm of body of penis 🐾
      Malignant neoplasm of corpus cavernosum

    C60.8   Malignant neoplasm of overlapping sites of penis 🐾

    C60.9   Malignant neoplasm of penis, unspecified 🐾
      Malignant neoplasm of skin of penis NOS

C61   Malignant neoplasm of prostate 🐾
    Use additional , if applicable, code to identify:
      hormone sensitivity status (Z19.1-Z19.2)
      rising PSA following treatment for malignant neoplasm of prostate (R97.21)

    Excludes1   malignant neoplasm of seminal vesicle (C63.7)

● **C62   Malignant neoplasm of testis**
    Use additional code to identify any functional activity.

  ● **C62.0   Malignant neoplasm of undescended testis**
      Malignant neoplasm of ectopic testis
      Malignant neoplasm of retained testis

      C62.00   Malignant neoplasm of unspecified undescended testis 🐾

      C62.01   Malignant neoplasm of undescended right testis 🐾

      C62.02   Malignant neoplasm of undescended left testis 🐾

  ● **C62.1   Malignant neoplasm of descended testis**
      Malignant neoplasm of scrotal testis

      C62.10   Malignant neoplasm of unspecified descended testis, unspecified side 🐾

      C62.11   Malignant neoplasm of descended right testis 🐾

      C62.12   Malignant neoplasm of descended left testis 🐾

  ● **C62.9   Malignant neoplasm of testis, unspecified whether descended or undescended**

      C62.90   Malignant neoplasm of unspecified testis, unspecified whether descended or undescended 🐾
        Malignant neoplasm of testis NOS

      C62.91   Malignant neoplasm of right testis, unspecified whether descended or undescended 🐾

      C62.92   Malignant neoplasm of left testis, unspecified whether descended or undescended 🐾

● **C63   Malignant neoplasm of other and unspecified male genital organs**

  ● **C63.0   Malignant neoplasm of epididymis**

      C63.00   Malignant neoplasm of unspecified epididymis 🐾

      C63.01   Malignant neoplasm of right epididymis 🐾

      C63.02   Malignant neoplasm of left epididymis 🐾

  ● **C63.1   Malignant neoplasm of spermatic cord**

      C63.10   Malignant neoplasm of unspecified spermatic cord 🐾

      C63.11   Malignant neoplasm of right spermatic cord 🐾

      C63.12   Malignant neoplasm of left spermatic cord 🐾

    C63.2   Malignant neoplasm of scrotum 🐾
      Malignant neoplasm of skin of scrotum

    C63.7   Malignant neoplasm of other specified male genital organs 🐾
      Malignant neoplasm of seminal vesicle
      Malignant neoplasm of tunica vaginalis

    C63.8   Malignant neoplasm of overlapping sites of male genital organs 🐾
      Primary malignant neoplasm of two or more contiguous sites of male genital organs whose point of origin cannot be determined

    C63.9   Malignant neoplasm of male genital organ, unspecified 🐾
      Malignant neoplasm of male genitourinary tract NOS

Figure 2-14 Penis and other male genital organs.

▶ New   ⟹ Revised   ~~deleted~~ Deleted   Excludes 1   Excludes 2   Includes   Use additional   Code first   Code also   Key words

OGCR Official Guidelines   X Assign placeholder X   ● Use Additional Character(s)   ) Manifestation Code   🐾 Hierarchical Condition Category   Coding Clinic

MALIGNANT NEOPLASMS OF URINARY TRACT (C64-C68)

● **C64   Malignant neoplasm of kidney, except renal pelvis**

    Excludes1   malignant carcinoid tumor of the kidney (C7A.093)
          malignant neoplasm of renal calyces (C65.-)
          malignant neoplasm of renal pelvis (C65.-)

    C64.1   Malignant neoplasm of right kidney, except renal pelvis 🔧

    C64.2   Malignant neoplasm of left kidney, except renal pelvis 🔧

    C64.9   Malignant neoplasm of unspecified kidney, except renal pelvis 🔧

● **C65   Malignant neoplasm of renal pelvis**

    Includes   malignant neoplasm of pelviureteric junction
          malignant neoplasm of renal calyces

    C65.1   Malignant neoplasm of right renal pelvis 🔧

    C65.2   Malignant neoplasm of left renal pelvis 🔧

    C65.9   Malignant neoplasm of unspecified renal pelvis 🔧

● **C66   Malignant neoplasm of ureter**

    Excludes1   malignant neoplasm of ureteric orifice of bladder (C67.6)

    C66.1   Malignant neoplasm of right ureter 🔧

    C66.2   Malignant neoplasm of left ureter 🔧

    C66.9   Malignant neoplasm of unspecified ureter 🔧

● **C67   Malignant neoplasm of bladder**

    C67.0   Malignant neoplasm of trigone of bladder 🔧
        Triangular area formed by three openings in the floor of urinary bladder

    C67.1   Malignant neoplasm of dome of bladder 🔧
        Vaulted roof
        Coding Clinic: 2023, Q3, P16

    C67.2   Malignant neoplasm of lateral wall of bladder 🔧
        Side walls
        Coding Clinic: 2023, Q3, P16

    C67.3   Malignant neoplasm of anterior wall of bladder 🔧
        Front wall
        Coding Clinic: 2023, Q3, P16

    C67.4   Malignant neoplasm of posterior wall of bladder 🔧
        Back wall

    C67.5   Malignant neoplasm of bladder neck 🔧
        Joining of bladder and urethra
        Malignant neoplasm of internal urethral orifice
        Coding Clinic: 2023, Q3, P16

    C67.6   Malignant neoplasm of ureteric orifice 🔧
        Opening from bladder to ureters

    C67.7   Malignant neoplasm of urachus 🔧
        Embryonic canal that connects the urinary bladder with the structure that forms the umbilical cord (allantois)

    C67.8   Malignant neoplasm of overlapping sites of bladder 🔧

    C67.9   Malignant neoplasm of bladder, unspecified 🔧
        Coding Clinic: 2017, Q1, P6; 2016, Q1, P19

● **C68   Malignant neoplasm of other and unspecified urinary organs**

    Excludes1   malignant neoplasm of female genitourinary tract NOS (C57.9)
          malignant neoplasm of male genitourinary tract NOS (C63.9)

    C68.0   Malignant neoplasm of urethra 🔧
        Excludes1   malignant neoplasm of urethral orifice of bladder (C67.5)

    C68.1   Malignant neoplasm of paraurethral glands 🔧
        Group of glands of female urethra drained by paraurethral ducts; AKA Skene glands, female prostate

    C68.8   Malignant neoplasm of overlapping sites of urinary organs
        Primary malignant neoplasm of two or more contiguous sites of urinary organs whose point of origin cannot be determined

    C68.9   Malignant neoplasm of urinary organ, unspecified 🔧
        Malignant neoplasm of urinary system NOS

MALIGNANT NEOPLASMS OF EYE, BRAIN AND OTHER PARTS OF CENTRAL NERVOUS SYSTEM (C69-C72)

● **C69   Malignant neoplasm of eye and adnexa**

    Excludes1   malignant neoplasm of connective tissue of eyelid (C49.0)
          malignant neoplasm of eyelid (skin) (C43.1-, C44.1-)
          malignant neoplasm of optic nerve (C72.3-)

●   C69.0   Malignant neoplasm of conjunctiva

    C69.00   Malignant neoplasm of unspecified conjunctiva 🔧

    C69.01   Malignant neoplasm of right conjunctiva 🔧

    C69.02   Malignant neoplasm of left conjunctiva 🔧

●   C69.1   Malignant neoplasm of cornea

    C69.10   Malignant neoplasm of unspecified cornea 🔧

    C69.11   Malignant neoplasm of right cornea 🔧

    C69.12   Malignant neoplasm of left cornea 🔧

●   C69.2   Malignant neoplasm of retina

    Excludes1   dark area on retina (D49.81)
          neoplasm of unspecified behavior of retina and choroid (D49.81)
          retinal freckle (D49.81)

    C69.20   Malignant neoplasm of unspecified retina 🔧

    C69.21   Malignant neoplasm of right retina 🔧

    C69.22   Malignant neoplasm of left retina 🔧

●   C69.3   Malignant neoplasm of choroid

    C69.30   Malignant neoplasm of unspecified choroid 🔧

    C69.31   Malignant neoplasm of right choroid 🔧

    C69.32   Malignant neoplasm of left choroid 🔧

●   C69.4   Malignant neoplasm of ciliary body

    C69.40   Malignant neoplasm of unspecified ciliary body 🔧

    C69.41   Malignant neoplasm of right ciliary body 🔧

    C69.42   Malignant neoplasm of left ciliary body 🔧

●   C69.5   Malignant neoplasm of lacrimal gland and duct
        Malignant neoplasm of lacrimal sac
        Malignant neoplasm of nasolacrimal duct

    C69.50   Malignant neoplasm of unspecified lacrimal gland and duct 🔧

    C69.51   Malignant neoplasm of right lacrimal gland and duct 🔧

    C69.52   Malignant neoplasm of left lacrimal gland and duct 🔧

●   C69.6   Malignant neoplasm of orbit
        Malignant neoplasm of connective tissue of orbit
        Malignant neoplasm of extraocular muscle
        Malignant neoplasm of peripheral nerves of orbit
        Malignant neoplasm of retrobulbar tissue
        Malignant neoplasm of retro-ocular tissue

    Excludes1   malignant neoplasm of orbital bone (C41.0)

    C69.60   Malignant neoplasm of unspecified orbit 🔧

    C69.61   Malignant neoplasm of right orbit 🔧

    C69.62   Malignant neoplasm of left orbit 🔧

●   C69.8   Malignant neoplasm of overlapping sites of eye and adnexa

    C69.80   Malignant neoplasm of overlapping sites of unspecified eye and adnexa 🔧

    C69.81   Malignant neoplasm of overlapping sites of right eye and adnexa 🔧

    C69.82   Malignant neoplasm of overlapping sites of left eye and adnexa 🔧

●   C69.9   Malignant neoplasm of unspecified site of eye
        Malignant neoplasm of eyeball

    C69.90   Malignant neoplasm of unspecified site of unspecified eye 🔧

    C69.91   Malignant neoplasm of unspecified site of right eye 🔧

    C69.92   Malignant neoplasm of unspecified site of left eye 🔧

CHAPTER 2 (C00-D49)

● **C70   Malignant neoplasm of meninges**
    C70.0   Malignant neoplasm of cerebral meninges
    C70.1   Malignant neoplasm of spinal meninges
    C70.9   Malignant neoplasm of meninges, unspecified

● **C71   Malignant neoplasm of brain**
    Excludes1   malignant neoplasm of cranial nerves (C72.2-C72.5)
        retrobulbar malignant neoplasm (C69.6-)
    C71.0   Malignant neoplasm of cerebrum, except lobes and ventricles
        Malignant neoplasm of supratentorial NOS
    C71.1   Malignant neoplasm of frontal lobe
    C71.2   Malignant neoplasm of temporal lobe
    C71.3   Malignant neoplasm of parietal lobe
    C71.4   Malignant neoplasm of occipital lobe
    C71.5   Malignant neoplasm of cerebral ventricle
        Excludes1   malignant neoplasm of fourth cerebral ventricle (C71.7)
    C71.6   Malignant neoplasm of cerebellum
    C71.7   Malignant neoplasm of brain stem
        Malignant neoplasm of fourth cerebral ventricle
        Infratentorial malignant neoplasm NOS
    C71.8   Malignant neoplasm of overlapping sites of brain
    C71.9   Malignant neoplasm of brain, unspecified

● **C72   Malignant neoplasm of spinal cord, cranial nerves and other parts of central nervous system**
    Excludes1   malignant neoplasm of meninges (C70.-)
        malignant neoplasm of peripheral nerves and autonomic nervous system (C47.-)
    C72.0   Malignant neoplasm of spinal cord
    C72.1   Malignant neoplasm of cauda equina
        Lower end of spinal column
  ● **C72.2**   Malignant neoplasm of olfactory nerve
        Malignant neoplasm of olfactory bulb
        C72.20   Malignant neoplasm of unspecified olfactory nerve
        C72.21   Malignant neoplasm of right olfactory nerve
        C72.22   Malignant neoplasm of left olfactory nerve
  ● **C72.3**   Malignant neoplasm of optic nerve
        C72.30   Malignant neoplasm of unspecified optic nerve
        C72.31   Malignant neoplasm of right optic nerve
        C72.32   Malignant neoplasm of left optic nerve
  ● **C72.4**   Malignant neoplasm of acoustic nerve
        C72.40   Malignant neoplasm of unspecified acoustic nerve
        C72.41   Malignant neoplasm of right acoustic nerve
        C72.42   Malignant neoplasm of left acoustic nerve
  ● **C72.5**   Malignant neoplasm of other and unspecified cranial nerves
        C72.50   Malignant neoplasm of unspecified cranial nerve
            Malignant neoplasm of cranial nerve NOS
        C72.59   Malignant neoplasm of other cranial nerves
    C72.9   Malignant neoplasm of central nervous system, unspecified
        Malignant neoplasm of unspecified site of central nervous system
        Malignant neoplasm of nervous system NOS

MALIGNANT NEOPLASMS OF THYROID AND OTHER ENDOCRINE GLANDS (C73-C75)

  C73   Malignant neoplasm of thyroid gland
    Use additional code to identify any functional activity

● **C74   Malignant neoplasm of adrenal gland**
  ● **C74.0**   Malignant neoplasm of cortex of adrenal gland
        C74.00   Malignant neoplasm of cortex of unspecified adrenal gland
        C74.01   Malignant neoplasm of cortex of right adrenal gland
        C74.02   Malignant neoplasm of cortex of left adrenal gland
  ● **C74.1**   Malignant neoplasm of medulla of adrenal gland
        Pair of glands situated on top of or above each kidney ("suprarenal")
        C74.10   Malignant neoplasm of medulla of unspecified adrenal gland
        C74.11   Malignant neoplasm of medulla of right adrenal gland
        C74.12   Malignant neoplasm of medulla of left adrenal gland
  ● **C74.9**   Malignant neoplasm of unspecified part of adrenal gland
        C74.90   Malignant neoplasm of unspecified part of unspecified adrenal gland
        C74.91   Malignant neoplasm of unspecified part of right adrenal gland
        C74.92   Malignant neoplasm of unspecified part of left adrenal gland

● **C75   Malignant neoplasm of other endocrine glands and related structures**
    Excludes1   malignant carcinoid tumors (C7A.0-)
        malignant neoplasm of adrenal gland (C74.-)
        malignant neoplasm of endocrine pancreas (C25.4)
        malignant neoplasm of islets of Langerhans (C25.4)
        malignant neoplasm of ovary (C56.-)
        malignant neoplasm of testis (C62.-)
        malignant neoplasm of thymus (C37)
        malignant neoplasm of thyroid gland (C73)
        malignant neuroendocrine tumors (C7A.-)
    C75.0   Malignant neoplasm of parathyroid gland
    C75.1   Malignant neoplasm of pituitary gland
    C75.2   Malignant neoplasm of craniopharyngeal duct
    C75.3   Malignant neoplasm of pineal gland
    C75.4   Malignant neoplasm of carotid body
    C75.5   Malignant neoplasm of aortic body and other paraganglia
    C75.8   Malignant neoplasm with pluriglandular involvement, unspecified
    C75.9   Malignant neoplasm of endocrine gland, unspecified

Figure 2-15   The brain.

▶ New   ⟹ Revised   ~~deleted~~ Deleted   Excludes 1   Excludes 2   Includes   Use additional   Code first   Code also   Key words
OGCR Official Guidelines   X Assign placeholder X   ● Use Additional Character(s)   ▷ Manifestation Code   🐮 Hierarchical Condition Category   Coding Clinic

CHAPTER 2 (C00-D49)

MALIGNANT NEOPLASMS OF ILL-DEFINED, OTHER SECONDARY AND UNSPECIFIED SITES (C76-C80)

● **C76** **Malignant neoplasm of other and ill-defined sites**

Excludes1   malignant neoplasm of female genitourinary tract NOS (C57.9)

malignant neoplasm of male genitourinary tract NOS (C63.9)

malignant neoplasm of lymphoid, hematopoietic and related tissue (C81-C96)

malignant neoplasm of skin (C44.-)

malignant neoplasm of unspecified site NOS (C80.1)

C76.0   Malignant neoplasm of head, face and neck 🔖

Malignant neoplasm of cheek NOS

Malignant neoplasm of nose NOS

C76.1   Malignant neoplasm of thorax 🔖

Intrathoracic malignant neoplasm NOS

Malignant neoplasm of axilla NOS

Thoracic malignant neoplasm NOS

C76.2   Malignant neoplasm of abdomen 🔖

C76.3   Malignant neoplasm of pelvis 🔖

Malignant neoplasm of groin NOS

Malignant neoplasm of sites overlapping systems within the pelvis

Rectovaginal (septum) malignant neoplasm

Between rectum and vagina

Rectovesical (septum) malignant neoplasm

Between rectum and urinary bladder; AKA vesicorectal

● **C76.4**   Malignant neoplasm of upper limb

C76.40   Malignant neoplasm of unspecified upper limb 🔖

C76.41   Malignant neoplasm of right upper limb 🔖

C76.42   Malignant neoplasm of left upper limb 🔖

● **C76.5**   Malignant neoplasm of lower limb

C76.50   Malignant neoplasm of unspecified lower limb 🔖

C76.51   Malignant neoplasm of right lower limb 🔖

C76.52   Malignant neoplasm of left lower limb 🔖

C76.8   Malignant neoplasm of other specified ill-defined sites 🔖

Malignant neoplasm of overlapping ill-defined sites

● **C77** **Secondary and unspecified malignant neoplasm of lymph nodes**

Excludes1   malignant neoplasm of lymph nodes, specified as primary (C81-C86, C88, C96.-)

mesentary metastasis of carcinoid tumor (C7B.04)

secondary carcinoid tumors of distant lymph nodes (C7B.01)

C77.0   Secondary and unspecified malignant neoplasm of lymph nodes of head, face and neck 🔖

Secondary and unspecified malignant neoplasm of supraclavicular lymph nodes

Coding Clinic: 2022, Q3, P15

C77.1   Secondary and unspecified malignant neoplasm of intrathoracic lymph nodes 🔖

C77.2   Secondary and unspecified malignant neoplasm of intra-abdominal lymph nodes 🔖

C77.3   Secondary and unspecified malignant neoplasm of axilla and upper limb lymph nodes 🔖

Secondary and unspecified malignant neoplasm of pectoral lymph nodes

C77.4   Secondary and unspecified malignant neoplasm of inguinal and lower limb lymph nodes 🔖

C77.5   Secondary and unspecified malignant neoplasm of intrapelvic lymph nodes 🔖

C77.8   Secondary and unspecified malignant neoplasm of lymph nodes of multiple regions 🔖

C77.9   Secondary and unspecified malignant neoplasm of lymph node, unspecified 🔖

Item 2–6 The adrenal glands are a pair of glands situated on top of or above each kidney ("suprarenal") and chiefly responsible for regulating the stress response through the synthesis of corticosteroids and catecholamines, including cortisol and adrenaline.

● **C78** **Secondary malignant neoplasm of respiratory and digestive organs**

Excludes1   secondary carcinoid tumors of liver (C7B.02)

secondary carcinoid tumors of peritoneum (C7B.04)

Excludes2   lymph node metastases (C77.0)

Coding Clinic: 2023, Q1, P22

● **C78.0**   Secondary malignant neoplasm of lung

C78.00   Secondary malignant neoplasm of unspecified lung 🔖

Coding Clinic: 2022, Q3, P9

C78.01   Secondary malignant neoplasm of right lung 🔖

Coding Clinic: 2024, Q2, P11; 2023, Q3, P15

C78.02   Secondary malignant neoplasm of left lung 🔖

Coding Clinic: 2023, Q3, P15

C78.1   Secondary malignant neoplasm of mediastinum 🔖

Thoracic cavity between pleural cavities

C78.2   Secondary malignant neoplasm of pleura 🔖

Serous membrane covering lungs and lining thoracic cavity

● **C78.3**   Secondary malignant neoplasm of other and unspecified respiratory organs

C78.30   Secondary malignant neoplasm of unspecified respiratory organ 🔖

C78.39   Secondary malignant neoplasm of other respiratory organs 🔖

C78.4   Secondary malignant neoplasm of small intestine 🔖

C78.5   Secondary malignant neoplasm of large intestine and rectum 🔖

C78.6   Secondary malignant neoplasm of retroperitoneum and peritoneum 🔖

Coding Clinic: 2017, Q2, P12

C78.7   Secondary malignant neoplasm of liver and intrahepatic bile duct 🔖

Coding Clinic: 2024, Q1, P25; 2022, Q3, P15

● **C78.8**   Secondary malignant neoplasm of other and unspecified digestive organs

C78.80   Secondary malignant neoplasm of unspecified digestive organ 🔖

C78.89   Secondary malignant neoplasm of other digestive organs 🔖

Code also exocrine pancreatic insufficiency (K86.81)

● **C79** **Secondary malignant neoplasm of other and unspecified sites**

Excludes1   secondary carcinoid tumors (C7B.-)

secondary neuroendocrine tumors (C7B.-)

Coding Clinic: 2023, Q1, P22

● **C79.0**   Secondary malignant neoplasm of kidney and renal pelvis

C79.00   Secondary malignant neoplasm of unspecified kidney and renal pelvis 🔖

C79.01   Secondary malignant neoplasm of right kidney and renal pelvis 🔖

C79.02   Secondary malignant neoplasm of left kidney and renal pelvis 🔖

● **C79.1**   Secondary malignant neoplasm of bladder and other and unspecified urinary organs

C79.10   Secondary malignant neoplasm of unspecified urinary organs 🔖

C79.11   Secondary malignant neoplasm of bladder 🔖

Excludes2   lymph node metastases (C77.0)

C79.19   Secondary malignant neoplasm of other urinary organs 🔖

C79.2   Secondary malignant neoplasm of skin 🔖

Excludes1   secondary Merkel cell carcinoma (C7B.1)

● **C79.3**   Secondary malignant neoplasm of brain and cerebral meninges

C79.31   Secondary malignant neoplasm of brain 🔖

Coding Clinic: 2022, Q3, P9,11

C79.32   Secondary malignant neoplasm of cerebral meninges 🔖

Coding Clinic: 2020, Q1, P13

CHAPTER 2 (C00-D49)

- **C79.4** Secondary malignant neoplasm of other and unspecified parts of nervous system
  - **C79.40** Secondary malignant neoplasm of unspecified part of nervous system
  - **C79.49** Secondary malignant neoplasm of other parts of nervous system
- **C79.5** Secondary malignant neoplasm of bone and bone marrow
  - **Excludes1** secondary carcinoid tumors of bone (C7B.03)
  - **C79.51** Secondary malignant neoplasm of bone
    - Coding Clinic: 2022, Q3, P15
  - **C79.52** Secondary malignant neoplasm of bone marrow
- **C79.6** Secondary malignant neoplasm of ovary
  - **C79.60** Secondary malignant neoplasm of unspecified ovary
  - **C79.61** Secondary malignant neoplasm of right ovary
  - **C79.62** Secondary malignant neoplasm of left ovary
  - **C79.63** Secondary malignant neoplasm of bilateral ovaries
- **C79.7** Secondary malignant neoplasm of adrenal gland
  - **C79.70** Secondary malignant neoplasm of unspecified adrenal gland
  - **C79.71** Secondary malignant neoplasm of right adrenal gland
  - **C79.72** Secondary malignant neoplasm of left adrenal gland
- **C79.8** Secondary malignant neoplasm of other specified sites
  - **C79.81** Secondary malignant neoplasm of breast
  - **C79.82** Secondary malignant neoplasm of genital organs
    - Coding Clinic: 2023, Q3, P15
  - **C79.89** Secondary malignant neoplasm of other specified sites
    - Coding Clinic: 2017, Q2, P11
- **C79.9** Secondary malignant neoplasm of unspecified site
  - Metastatic cancer NOS
  - Metastatic disease NOS
  - **Excludes1** carcinomatosis NOS (C80.0)
    - generalized cancer NOS (C80.0)
    - malignant (primary) neoplasm of unspecified site (C80.1)
  - Coding Clinic: 2023, Q2, P5

MALIGNANT NEUROENDOCRINE TUMORS (C7A)

- **C7A** Malignant neuroendocrine tumors
  - Code also any associated multiple endocrine neoplasia [MEN] syndromes (E31.2-)
  - Use additional code to identify any associated endocrine syndrome, such as:
    - carcinoid syndrome (E34.00)
  - **Excludes2** malignant pancreatic islet cell tumors (C25.4)
    - Merkel cell carcinoma (C4A.-)
- **C7A.0** Malignant carcinoid tumors
  - **C7A.00** Malignant carcinoid tumor of unspecified site
  - **C7A.01** Malignant carcinoid tumors of the small intestine
    - **C7A.010** Malignant carcinoid tumor of the duodenum
    - **C7A.011** Malignant carcinoid tumor of the jejunum
    - **C7A.012** Malignant carcinoid tumor of the ileum
    - **C7A.019** Malignant carcinoid tumor of the small intestine, unspecified portion

- **C7A.02** Malignant carcinoid tumors of the appendix, large intestine, and rectum
  - **C7A.020** Malignant carcinoid tumor of the appendix
  - **C7A.021** Malignant carcinoid tumor of the cecum
  - **C7A.022** Malignant carcinoid tumor of the ascending colon
  - **C7A.023** Malignant carcinoid tumor of the transverse colon
  - **C7A.024** Malignant carcinoid tumor of the descending colon
  - **C7A.025** Malignant carcinoid tumor of the sigmoid colon
  - **C7A.026** Malignant carcinoid tumor of the rectum
  - **C7A.029** Malignant carcinoid tumor of the large intestine, unspecified portion
    - Malignant carcinoid tumor of the colon NOS
- **C7A.09** Malignant carcinoid tumors of other sites
  - **C7A.090** Malignant carcinoid tumor of the bronchus and lung
  - **C7A.091** Malignant carcinoid tumor of the thymus
  - **C7A.092** Malignant carcinoid tumor of the stomach
  - **C7A.093** Malignant carcinoid tumor of the kidney
  - **C7A.094** Malignant carcinoid tumor of the foregut, unspecified
  - **C7A.095** Malignant carcinoid tumor of the midgut, unspecified
  - **C7A.096** Malignant carcinoid tumor of the hindgut, unspecified
  - **C7A.098** Malignant carcinoid tumors of other sites
- **C7A.1** Malignant poorly differentiated neuroendocrine tumors
  - Malignant poorly differentiated neuroendocrine tumor NOS
  - Malignant poorly differentiated neuroendocrine carcinoma, any site
  - High grade neuroendocrine carcinoma, any site
  - Coding Clinic: 2023, Q1, P21-22
- **C7A.8** Other malignant neuroendocrine tumors
  - Secondary neuroendocrine tumors (C7B)
  - Coding Clinic: 2019, Q3, P7

SECONDARY NEUROENDOCRINE TUMORS (C7B)

- **C7B** Secondary neuroendocrine tumors
  - Use additional code to identify any functional activity
  - **C7B.0** Secondary carcinoid tumors
    - **C7B.00** Secondary carcinoid tumors, unspecified site
    - **C7B.01** Secondary carcinoid tumors of distant lymph nodes
    - **C7B.02** Secondary carcinoid tumors of liver
    - **C7B.03** Secondary carcinoid tumors of bone
    - **C7B.04** Secondary carcinoid tumors of peritoneum
      - Mesentary metastasis of carcinoid tumor
    - **C7B.09** Secondary carcinoid tumors of other sites
  - **C7B.1** Secondary Merkel cell carcinoma
    - Merkel cell carcinoma nodal presentation
    - Merkel cell carcinoma visceral metastatic presentation
  - **C7B.8** Other secondary neuroendocrine tumors
    - Coding Clinic: 2024, Q2, P10; 2023, Q1, P21; 2019, Q3, P7

● **C80** Malignant neoplasm without specification of site

    Excludes1   malignant carcinoid tumor of unspecified site (C7A.00)

                    malignant neoplasm of specified multiple sites-code to each site

    C80.0 Disseminated malignant neoplasm, unspecified 🖱
        Carcinomatosis NOS
        Generalized cancer, unspecified site (primary) (secondary)
        Generalized malignancy, unspecified site (primary) (secondary)

    C80.1 Malignant (primary) neoplasm, unspecified 🖱
        Cancer NOS
        Cancer unspecified site (primary)
        Carcinoma unspecified site (primary)
        Malignancy unspecified site (primary)
        Excludes1   secondary malignant neoplasm of unspecified site (C79.9)

    C80.2 Malignant neoplasm associated with transplanted organ 🖱
        Code first complication of transplanted organ (T86.-)
        Use additional code to identify the specific malignancy

★ **(See Plate 1 of the Anatomy Illustrations.)**

MALIGNANT NEOPLASMS OF LYMPHOID, HEMATOPOIETIC AND RELATED TISSUE (C81-C96)

    Excludes2   Kaposi's sarcoma of lymph nodes (C46.3)
                    secondary and unspecified neoplasm of lymph nodes (C77.-)
                    secondary neoplasm of bone marrow (C79.52)
                    secondary neoplasm of spleen (C78.89)

● **C81** Hodgkin lymphoma
    Form of malignant lymphoma with four types, nodular sclerosis, mixed cellularity, lymphocyte depleted, and lymphocyte predominant
    Excludes1   personal history of Hodgkin lymphoma (Z85.71)

  ● **C81.0** Nodular lymphocyte predominant Hodgkin lymphoma
    Least aggressive, least common, typically no symptoms
    Lymphocytic-histiocytic predominance Hodgkin's disease

    C81.00 Nodular lymphocyte predominant Hodgkin lymphoma, unspecified site 🖱

    C81.01 Nodular lymphocyte predominant Hodgkin lymphoma, lymph nodes of head, face, and neck 🖱

    C81.02 Nodular lymphocyte predominant Hodgkin lymphoma, intrathoracic lymph nodes 🖱

    C81.03 Nodular lymphocyte predominant Hodgkin lymphoma, intra-abdominal lymph nodes 🖱

    C81.04 Nodular lymphocyte predominant Hodgkin lymphoma, lymph nodes of axilla and upper limb 🖱

    C81.05 Nodular lymphocyte predominant Hodgkin lymphoma, lymph nodes of inguinal region and lower limb 🖱

    C81.06 Nodular lymphocyte predominant Hodgkin lymphoma, intrapelvic lymph nodes 🖱

    C81.07 Nodular lymphocyte predominant Hodgkin lymphoma, spleen 🖱

    C81.08 Nodular lymphocyte predominant Hodgkin lymphoma, lymph nodes of multiple sites 🖱

    C81.09 Nodular lymphocyte predominant Hodgkin lymphoma, extranodal and solid organ sites 🖱

  ▶**C81.0A** Nodular lymphocyte predominant Hodgkin lymphoma, in remission

  ● **C81.1** Nodular sclerosis Hodgkin lymphoma
    Nodular sclerosis classical Hodgkin lymphoma
    Moderately aggressive; most common in young adults

    C81.10 Nodular sclerosis Hodgkin lymphoma, unspecified site 🖱

    C81.11 Nodular sclerosis Hodgkin lymphoma, lymph nodes of head, face, and neck 🖱

    C81.12 Nodular sclerosis Hodgkin lymphoma, intrathoracic lymph nodes 🖱

    C81.13 Nodular sclerosis Hodgkin lymphoma, intra-abdominal lymph nodes 🖱

    C81.14 Nodular sclerosis Hodgkin lymphoma, lymph nodes of axilla and upper limb 🖱

    C81.15 Nodular sclerosis Hodgkin lymphoma, lymph nodes of inguinal region and lower limb 🖱

    C81.16 Nodular sclerosis Hodgkin lymphoma, intrapelvic lymph nodes 🖱

    C81.17 Nodular sclerosis Hodgkin lymphoma, spleen 🖱

    C81.18 Nodular sclerosis Hodgkin lymphoma, lymph nodes of multiple sites 🖱

    C81.19 Nodular sclerosis Hodgkin lymphoma, extranodal and solid organ sites 🖱

  ▶**C81.1A** Nodular sclerosis Hodgkin lymphoma, in remission

  ● **C81.2** Mixed cellularity Hodgkin lymphoma
    Mixed cellularity classical Hodgkin lymphoma
    A type of Hodgkin's that is moderately aggressive with mixed cell types

    C81.20 Mixed cellularity Hodgkin lymphoma, unspecified site 🖱

    C81.21 Mixed cellularity Hodgkin lymphoma, lymph nodes of head, face, and neck 🖱

    C81.22 Mixed cellularity Hodgkin lymphoma, intrathoracic lymph nodes 🖱

    C81.23 Mixed cellularity Hodgkin lymphoma, intra-abdominal lymph nodes 🖱

    C81.24 Mixed cellularity Hodgkin lymphoma, lymph nodes of axilla and upper limb 🖱

    C81.25 Mixed cellularity Hodgkin lymphoma, lymph nodes of inguinal region and lower limb 🖱

    C81.26 Mixed cellularity Hodgkin lymphoma, intrapelvic lymph nodes 🖱

    C81.27 Mixed cellularity Hodgkin lymphoma, spleen 🖱

    C81.28 Mixed cellularity Hodgkin lymphoma, lymph nodes of multiple sites 🖱

    C81.29 Mixed cellularity Hodgkin lymphoma, extranodal and solid organ sites 🖱

  ▶**C81.2A** Mixed cellularity Hodgkin lymphoma, in remission

  ● **C81.3** Lymphocyte depleted Hodgkin lymphoma
    Lymphocyte depleted classical Hodgkin lymphoma
    Most aggressive type with poor prognosis

    C81.30 Lymphocyte depleted Hodgkin lymphoma, unspecified site 🖱

    C81.31 Lymphocyte depleted Hodgkin lymphoma, lymph nodes of head, face, and neck 🖱

    C81.32 Lymphocyte depleted Hodgkin lymphoma, intrathoracic lymph nodes 🖱

    C81.33 Lymphocyte depleted Hodgkin lymphoma, intra-abdominal lymph nodes 🖱

    C81.34 Lymphocyte depleted Hodgkin lymphoma, lymph nodes of axilla and upper limb 🖱

C81.35 Lymphocyte depleted Hodgkin lymphoma, lymph nodes of inguinal region and lower limb 🐾

C81.36 Lymphocyte depleted Hodgkin lymphoma, intrapelvic lymph nodes 🐾

C81.37 Lymphocyte depleted Hodgkin lymphoma, spleen 🐾

C81.38 Lymphocyte depleted Hodgkin lymphoma, lymph nodes of multiple sites 🐾

C81.39 Lymphocyte depleted Hodgkin lymphoma, extranodal and solid organ sites 🐾

▶**C81.3A** Lymphocyte depleted Hodgkin lymphoma, in remission

● **C81.4** Lymphocyte-rich Hodgkin lymphoma
Lymphocyte-rich classical Hodgkin lymphoma

> **Excludes1** nodular lymphocyte predominant Hodgkin lymphoma (C81.0-)

C81.40 Lymphocyte-rich Hodgkin lymphoma, unspecified site 🐾

C81.41 Lymphocyte-rich Hodgkin lymphoma, lymph nodes of head, face, and neck 🐾

C81.42 Lymphocyte-rich Hodgkin lymphoma, intrathoracic lymph nodes 🐾

C81.43 Lymphocyte-rich Hodgkin lymphoma, intra-abdominal lymph nodes 🐾

C81.44 Lymphocyte-rich Hodgkin lymphoma, lymph nodes of axilla and upper limb 🐾

C81.45 Lymphocyte-rich Hodgkin lymphoma, lymph nodes of inguinal region and lower limb 🐾

C81.46 Lymphocyte-rich Hodgkin lymphoma, intrapelvic lymph nodes 🐾

C81.47 Lymphocyte-rich Hodgkin lymphoma, spleen 🐾

C81.48 Lymphocyte-rich Hodgkin lymphoma, lymph nodes of multiple sites 🐾

C81.49 Lymphocyte-rich Hodgkin lymphoma, extranodal and solid organ sites 🐾

▶**C81.4A** Lymphocyte-rich Hodgkin lymphoma, in remission

● **C81.7** Other Hodgkin lymphoma
Classical Hodgkin lymphoma NOS
Other classical Hodgkin lymphoma

C81.70 Other Hodgkin lymphoma, unspecified site 🐾

C81.71 Other Hodgkin lymphoma, lymph nodes of head, face, and neck 🐾

C81.72 Other Hodgkin lymphoma, intrathoracic lymph nodes 🐾

C81.73 Other Hodgkin lymphoma, intra-abdominal lymph nodes 🐾

C81.74 Other Hodgkin lymphoma, lymph nodes of axilla and upper limb 🐾

C81.75 Other Hodgkin lymphoma, lymph nodes of inguinal region and lower limb 🐾

C81.76 Other Hodgkin lymphoma, intrapelvic lymph nodes 🐾

C81.77 Other Hodgkin lymphoma, spleen 🐾

C81.78 Other Hodgkin lymphoma, lymph nodes of multiple sites 🐾

C81.79 Other Hodgkin lymphoma, extranodal and solid organ sites 🐾

▶**C81.7A** Other Hodgkin lymphoma, in remission

● **C81.9** Hodgkin lymphoma, unspecified

C81.90 Hodgkin lymphoma, unspecified, unspecified site 🐾

C81.91 Hodgkin lymphoma, unspecified, lymph nodes of head, face, and neck 🐾

C81.92 Hodgkin lymphoma, unspecified, intrathoracic lymph nodes 🐾

C81.93 Hodgkin lymphoma, unspecified, intra-abdominal lymph nodes 🐾

C81.94 Hodgkin lymphoma, unspecified, lymph nodes of axilla and upper limb 🐾

C81.95 Hodgkin lymphoma, unspecified, lymph nodes of inguinal region and lower limb 🐾

C81.96 Hodgkin lymphoma, unspecified, intrapelvic lymph nodes 🐾

C81.97 Hodgkin lymphoma, unspecified, spleen 🐾

C81.98 Hodgkin lymphoma, unspecified, lymph nodes of multiple sites 🐾

C81.99 Hodgkin lymphoma, unspecified, extranodal and solid organ sites 🐾

▶**C81.9A** Hodgkin lymphoma, unspecified, in remission

● **C82** Follicular lymphoma
Group of malignant lymphomas

> **Includes** follicular lymphoma with or without diffuse areas

> **Excludes1** mature T/NK-cell lymphomas (C84.-)
> personal history of non-Hodgkin lymphoma (Z85.72)

● **C82.0** Follicular lymphoma grade I

C82.00 Follicular lymphoma grade I, unspecified site 🐾

C82.01 Follicular lymphoma grade I, lymph nodes of head, face, and neck 🐾

C82.02 Follicular lymphoma grade I, intrathoracic lymph nodes 🐾

C82.03 Follicular lymphoma grade I, intra-abdominal lymph nodes 🐾

C82.04 Follicular lymphoma grade I, lymph nodes of axilla and upper limb 🐾

C82.05 Follicular lymphoma grade I, lymph nodes of inguinal region and lower limb 🐾

C82.06 Follicular lymphoma grade I, intrapelvic lymph nodes 🐾

C82.07 Follicular lymphoma grade I, spleen 🐾

C82.08 Follicular lymphoma grade I, lymph nodes of multiple sites 🐾

C82.09 Follicular lymphoma grade I, extranodal and solid organ sites 🐾

▶**C82.0A** Follicular lymphoma grade I, in remission

● **C82.1** Follicular lymphoma grade II

C82.10 Follicular lymphoma grade II, unspecified site 🐾

C82.11 Follicular lymphoma grade II, lymph nodes of head, face, and neck 🐾

C82.12 Follicular lymphoma grade II, intrathoracic lymph nodes 🐾

C82.13 Follicular lymphoma grade II, intra-abdominal lymph nodes 🐾

C82.14 Follicular lymphoma grade II, lymph nodes of axilla and upper limb 🐾

C82.15 Follicular lymphoma grade II, lymph nodes of inguinal region and lower limb 🐾

C82.16 Follicular lymphoma grade II, intrapelvic lymph nodes 🐾

C82.17 Follicular lymphoma grade II, spleen 🐾

C82.18 Follicular lymphoma grade II, lymph nodes of multiple sites 🐾

C82.19 Follicular lymphoma grade II, extranodal and solid organ sites 🐾

▶**C82.1A** Follicular lymphoma grade II, in remission

● **C82.2** Follicular lymphoma grade III, unspecified

C82.20 Follicular lymphoma grade III, unspecified, unspecified site 🐾

C82.21 Follicular lymphoma grade III, unspecified, lymph nodes of head, face, and neck 🐾

C82.22 Follicular lymphoma grade III, unspecified, intrathoracic lymph nodes 🐾

C82.23 Follicular lymphoma grade III, unspecified, intra-abdominal lymph nodes 🐾

CHAPTER 2 (C00-D49)

C82.24   Follicular lymphoma grade III, unspecified, lymph nodes of axilla and upper limb 🔍

C82.25   Follicular lymphoma grade III, unspecified, lymph nodes of inguinal region and lower limb 🔍

C82.26   Follicular lymphoma grade III, unspecified, intrapelvic lymph nodes 🔍

C82.27   Follicular lymphoma grade III, unspecified, spleen 🔍

C82.28   Follicular lymphoma grade III, unspecified, lymph nodes of multiple sites 🔍

C82.29   Follicular lymphoma grade III, unspecified, extranodal and solid organ sites 🔍

▶ C82.2A   Follicular lymphoma grade III, unspecified, in remission

● C82.3   Follicular lymphoma grade IIIa

C82.30   Follicular lymphoma grade IIIa, unspecified site 🔍

C82.31   Follicular lymphoma grade IIIa, lymph nodes of head, face, and neck 🔍

C82.32   Follicular lymphoma grade IIIa, intrathoracic lymph nodes 🔍

C82.33   Follicular lymphoma grade IIIa, intra-abdominal lymph nodes 🔍

C82.34   Follicular lymphoma grade IIIa, lymph nodes of axilla and upper limb 🔍

C82.35   Follicular lymphoma grade IIIa, lymph nodes of inguinal region and lower limb 🔍

C82.36   Follicular lymphoma grade IIIa, intrapelvic lymph nodes 🔍

C82.37   Follicular lymphoma grade IIIa, spleen 🔍

C82.38   Follicular lymphoma grade IIIa, lymph nodes of multiple sites 🔍

C82.39   Follicular lymphoma grade IIIa, extranodal and solid organ sites 🔍

▶ C82.3A   Follicular lymphoma grade IIIa, in remission

● C82.4   Follicular lymphoma grade IIIb

C82.40   Follicular lymphoma grade IIIb, unspecified site 🔍

C82.41   Follicular lymphoma grade IIIb, lymph nodes of head, face, and neck 🔍

C82.42   Follicular lymphoma grade IIIb, intrathoracic lymph nodes 🔍

C82.43   Follicular lymphoma grade IIIb, intra-abdominal lymph nodes 🔍

C82.44   Follicular lymphoma grade IIIb, lymph nodes of axilla and upper limb 🔍

C82.45   Follicular lymphoma grade IIIb, lymph nodes of inguinal region and lower limb 🔍

C82.46   Follicular lymphoma grade IIIb, intrapelvic lymph nodes 🔍

C82.47   Follicular lymphoma grade IIIb, spleen 🔍

C82.48   Follicular lymphoma grade IIIb, lymph nodes of multiple sites 🔍

C82.49   Follicular lymphoma grade IIIb, extranodal and solid organ sites 🔍

▶ C82.4A   Follicular lymphoma grade IIIb, in remission

● C82.5   Diffuse follicle center lymphoma

C82.50   Diffuse follicle center lymphoma, unspecified site 🔍

C82.51   Diffuse follicle center lymphoma, lymph nodes of head, face, and neck 🔍

C82.52   Diffuse follicle center lymphoma, intrathoracic lymph nodes 🔍

C82.53   Diffuse follicle center lymphoma, intra-abdominal lymph nodes 🔍

C82.54   Diffuse follicle center lymphoma, lymph nodes of axilla and upper limb 🔍

C82.55   Diffuse follicle center lymphoma, lymph nodes of inguinal region and lower limb 🔍

C82.56   Diffuse follicle center lymphoma, intrapelvic lymph nodes 🔍

C82.57   Diffuse follicle center lymphoma, spleen 🔍

C82.58   Diffuse follicle center lymphoma, lymph nodes of multiple sites 🔍

C82.59   Diffuse follicle center lymphoma, extranodal and solid organ sites 🔍

▶ C82.5A   Diffuse follicle center lymphoma, in remission

● C82.6   Cutaneous follicle center lymphoma

C82.60   Cutaneous follicle center lymphoma, unspecified site 🔍

C82.61   Cutaneous follicle center lymphoma, lymph nodes of head, face, and neck 🔍

C82.62   Cutaneous follicle center lymphoma, intrathoracic lymph nodes 🔍

C82.63   Cutaneous follicle center lymphoma, intra-abdominal lymph nodes 🔍

C82.64   Cutaneous follicle center lymphoma, lymph nodes of axilla and upper limb 🔍

C82.65   Cutaneous follicle center lymphoma, lymph nodes of inguinal region and lower limb 🔍

C82.66   Cutaneous follicle center lymphoma, intrapelvic lymph nodes 🔍

C82.67   Cutaneous follicle center lymphoma, spleen 🔍

C82.68   Cutaneous follicle center lymphoma, lymph nodes of multiple sites 🔍

C82.69   Cutaneous follicle center lymphoma, extranodal and solid organ sites 🔍

▶ C82.6A   Cutaneous follicle center lymphoma, in remission

● C82.8   Other types of follicular lymphoma

C82.80   Other types of follicular lymphoma, unspecified site 🔍

C82.81   Other types of follicular lymphoma, lymph nodes of head, face, and neck 🔍

C82.82   Other types of follicular lymphoma, intrathoracic lymph nodes 🔍

C82.83   Other types of follicular lymphoma, intra-abdominal lymph nodes 🔍

C82.84   Other types of follicular lymphoma, lymph nodes of axilla and upper limb 🔍

C82.85   Other types of follicular lymphoma, lymph nodes of inguinal region and lower limb 🔍

C82.86   Other types of follicular lymphoma, intra pelvic lymph nodes 🔍

C82.87   Other types of follicular lymphoma, spleen 🔍

C82.88   Other types of follicular lymphoma, lymph nodes of multiple sites 🔍

C82.89   Other types of follicular lymphoma, extranodal and solid organ sites 🔍

▶ C82.8A   Other types of follicular lymphoma, in remission

● C82.9   Follicular lymphoma, unspecified

C82.90   Follicular lymphoma, unspecified, unspecified site 🔍

C82.91   Follicular lymphoma, unspecified, lymph nodes of head, face, and neck 🔍

C82.92   Follicular lymphoma, unspecified, intrathoracic lymph nodes 🔍

C82.93   Follicular lymphoma, unspecified, intra-abdominal lymph nodes 🔍

C82.94   Follicular lymphoma, unspecified, lymph nodes of axilla and upper limb 🔍

C82.95   Follicular lymphoma, unspecified, lymph nodes of inguinal region and lower limb 🔍

C82.96   Follicular lymphoma, unspecified, intra pelvic lymph nodes 🔍

C82.97   Follicular lymphoma, unspecified, spleen 🔍

C82.98   Follicular lymphoma, unspecified, lymph nodes of multiple sites 🔍

CHAPTER 2 (C00-D49)

C82.99 **Follicular lymphoma, unspecified, extranodal and solid organ sites** 🐾
▶ C82.9A **Follicular lymphoma, unspecified, in remission**

● C83 **Non-follicular lymphoma**
  Excludes1 personal history of non-Hodgkin lymphoma (Z85.72)

● C83.0 **Small cell B-cell lymphoma**
  Lymphoplasmacytic lymphoma
  Nodal marginal zone lymphoma
  Non-leukemic variant of B-CLL
  Splenic marginal zone lymphoma
  Excludes1 chronic lymphocytic leukemia (C91.1)
    mature T/NK-cell lymphomas (C84.-)
    ➡ Waldenström macroglobulinemia (C88.00)
  Coding Clinic: 2023, Q1, P18-19
C83.00 Small cell B-cell lymphoma, unspecified site 🐾
C83.01 Small cell B-cell lymphoma, lymph nodes of head, face, and neck 🐾
C83.02 Small cell B-cell lymphoma, intrathoracic lymph nodes 🐾
C83.03 Small cell B-cell lymphoma, intra-abdominal lymph nodes 🐾
C83.04 Small cell B-cell lymphoma, lymph nodes of axilla and upper limb 🐾
C83.05 Small cell B-cell lymphoma, lymph nodes of inguinal region and lower limb 🐾
C83.06 Small cell B-cell lymphoma, intrapelvic lymph nodes 🐾
C83.07 Small cell B-cell lymphoma, spleen 🐾
C83.08 Small cell B-cell lymphoma, lymph nodes of multiple sites 🐾
C83.09 Small cell B-cell lymphoma, extranodal and solid organ sites 🐾
▶ C83.0A Small cell B-cell lymphoma, in remission

● C83.1 **Mantle cell lymphoma**
  Centrocytic lymphoma
  Malignant lymphomatous polyposis
C83.10 Mantle cell lymphoma, unspecified site 🐾
  Coding Clinic: 2024, Q1, P24
C83.11 Mantle cell lymphoma, lymph nodes of head, face, and neck 🐾
C83.12 Mantle cell lymphoma, intrathoracic lymph nodes 🐾
C83.13 Mantle cell lymphoma, intra-abdominal lymph nodes 🐾
C83.14 Mantle cell lymphoma, lymph nodes of axilla and upper limb 🐾
C83.15 Mantle cell lymphoma, lymph nodes of inguinal region and lower limb 🐾
C83.16 Mantle cell lymphoma, intrapelvic lymph nodes 🐾
C83.17 Mantle cell lymphoma, spleen 🐾
C83.18 Mantle cell lymphoma, lymph nodes of multiple sites 🐾
C83.19 Mantle cell lymphoma, extranodal and solid organ sites 🐾
▶ C83.1A Mantle cell lymphoma, in remission
▶ Centrocytic lymphoma, in remission

● C83.3 **Diffuse large B-cell lymphoma**
  Anaplastic diffuse large B-cell lymphoma
  CD30-positive diffuse large B-cell lymphoma
  Centroblastic diffuse large B-cell lymphoma
  ~~Diffuse large B-cell lymphoma, subtype not specified~~
  Immunoblastic diffuse large B-cell lymphoma
  Plasmablastic diffuse large B-cell lymphoma
  Diffuse large B-cell lymphoma, subtype not specified
  T-cell rich diffuse large B-cell lymphoma
  Excludes1 mediastinal (thymic) large B-cell lymphoma (C85.2-)
    mature T/NK-cell lymphomas (C84.-)
C83.30 Diffuse large B-cell lymphoma, unspecified site 🐾
C83.31 Diffuse large B-cell lymphoma, lymph nodes of head, face, and neck 🐾
C83.32 Diffuse large B-cell lymphoma, intrathoracic lymph nodes 🐾
C83.33 Diffuse large B-cell lymphoma, intra-abdominal lymph nodes 🐾
C83.34 Diffuse large B-cell lymphoma, lymph nodes of axilla and upper limb 🐾
C83.35 Diffuse large B-cell lymphoma, lymph nodes of inguinal region and lower limb 🐾
C83.36 Diffuse large B-cell lymphoma, intrapelvic lymph nodes 🐾
C83.37 Diffuse large B-cell lymphoma, spleen 🐾
C83.38 Diffuse large B-cell lymphoma, lymph nodes of multiple sites 🐾
  Coding Clinic: 2023, Q1, P22
C83.39 Diffuse large B-cell lymphoma, extranodal and solid organ sites 🐾
  Coding Clinic: 2023, Q1, P22
▶ C83.390 Primary central nervous system lymphoma
▶ PCNSL of brain
▶ PCNSL of meninges
▶ PCNSL of spinal cord
▶ PCNSL NOS
  Excludes1 Primary central nervous system lymphoma, Burkitt (C83.79)
▶ Primary central nervous system lymphoma, lymphoblastic (C83.59)
▶ Primary central nervous system lymphoma, other (C83.89)
▶ Primary central nervous system lymphoma, peripheral T-cell (C84.49)
▶ C83.398 Diffuse large B-cell lymphoma of other extranodal and solid organ sites
▶ C83.3A Diffuse large B-cell lymphoma, in remission

● C83.5 **Lymphoblastic (diffuse) lymphoma**
  Highly malignant type of non-Hodgkin lymphoma with diffuse infiltration
  B-precursor lymphoma
  Lymphoblastic B-cell lymphoma
  Lymphoblastic lymphoma NOS
  Lymphoblastic T-cell lymphoma
  T-precursor lymphoma
C83.50 Lymphoblastic (diffuse) lymphoma, unspecified site 🐾
C83.51 Lymphoblastic (diffuse) lymphoma, lymph nodes of head, face, and neck 🐾
C83.52 Lymphoblastic (diffuse) lymphoma, intrathoracic lymph nodes 🐾
C83.53 Lymphoblastic (diffuse) lymphoma, intra-abdominal lymph nodes 🐾
C83.54 Lymphoblastic (diffuse) lymphoma, lymph nodes of axilla and upper limb 🐾
C83.55 Lymphoblastic (diffuse) lymphoma, lymph nodes of inguinal region and lower limb 🐾

C83.56   Lymphoblastic (diffuse) lymphoma, intrapelvic lymph nodes

C83.57   Lymphoblastic (diffuse) lymphoma, spleen

C83.58   Lymphoblastic (diffuse) lymphoma, lymph nodes of multiple sites

C83.59   Lymphoblastic (diffuse) lymphoma, extranodal and solid organ sites

▶ C83.5A   Lymphoblastic (diffuse) lymphoma, in remission

● C83.7   **Burkitt lymphoma**
Form of small cell lymphoma
Atypical Burkitt lymphoma
Burkitt-like lymphoma

    Excludes1   mature B-cell leukemia Burkitt type (C91.A-)

C83.70   Burkitt lymphoma, unspecified site

C83.71   Burkitt lymphoma, lymph nodes of head, face, and neck

C83.72   Burkitt lymphoma, intrathoracic lymph nodes

C83.73   Burkitt lymphoma, intra-abdominal lymph nodes

C83.74   Burkitt lymphoma, lymph nodes of axilla and upper limb

C83.75   Burkitt lymphoma, lymph nodes of inguinal region and lower limb

C83.76   Burkitt lymphoma, intrapelvic lymph nodes

C83.77   Burkitt lymphoma, spleen

C83.78   Burkitt lymphoma, lymph nodes of multiple sites

C83.79   Burkitt lymphoma, extranodal and solid organ sites

▶ C83.7A   Burkitt lymphoma, in remission

● C83.8   **Other non-follicular lymphoma**
Intravascular large B-cell lymphoma
Lymphoid granulomatosis
Primary effusion B-cell lymphoma

    Excludes1   mediastinal (thymic) large B-cell lymphoma (C85.2-)
       T-cell rich B-cell lymphoma (C83.3-)

C83.80   Other non-follicular lymphoma, unspecified site

C83.81   Other non-follicular lymphoma, lymph nodes of head, face, and neck

C83.82   Other non-follicular lymphoma, intrathoracic lymph nodes

C83.83   Other non-follicular lymphoma, intra-abdominal lymph nodes

C83.84   Other non-follicular lymphoma, lymph nodes of axilla and upper limb

C83.85   Other non-follicular lymphoma, lymph nodes of inguinal region and lower limb

C83.86   Other non-follicular lymphoma, intrapelvic lymph nodes

C83.87   Other non-follicular lymphoma, spleen

C83.88   Other non-follicular lymphoma, lymph nodes of multiple sites

C83.89   Other non-follicular lymphoma, extranodal and solid organ sites

▶ C83.8A   Other non-follicular lymphoma, in remission

● C83.9   **Non-follicular (diffuse) lymphoma, unspecified**

C83.90   Non-follicular (diffuse) lymphoma, unspecified, unspecified site

C83.91   Non-follicular (diffuse) lymphoma, unspecified, lymph nodes of head, face, and neck

C83.92   Non-follicular (diffuse) lymphoma, unspecified, intrathoracic lymph nodes

C83.93   Non-follicular (diffuse) lymphoma, unspecified, intra-abdominal lymph nodes

C83.94   Non-follicular (diffuse) lymphoma, unspecified, lymph nodes of axilla and upper limb

C83.95   Non-follicular (diffuse) lymphoma, unspecified, lymph nodes of inguinal region and lower limb

C83.96   Non-follicular (diffuse) lymphoma, unspecified, intrapelvic lymph nodes

C83.97   Non-follicular (diffuse) lymphoma, unspecified, spleen

C83.98   Non-follicular (diffuse) lymphoma, unspecified, lymph nodes of multiple sites

C83.99   Non-follicular (diffuse) lymphoma, unspecified, extranodal and solid organ sites

▶ C83.9A   Non-follicular (diffuse) lymphoma, unspecified, in remission

● C84   **Mature T/NK-cell lymphomas**

    Excludes1   personal history of non-Hodgkin lymphoma (Z85.72)

● C84.0   **Mycosis fungoides**
Chronic or rapidly progressive form of cutaneous T-cell lymphoma; AKA granuloma fungoides

    Excludes1   peripheral T-cell lymphoma, not elsewhere classified (C84.4-)

C84.00   Mycosis fungoides, unspecified site

C84.01   Mycosis fungoides, lymph nodes of head, face, and neck

C84.02   Mycosis fungoides, intrathoracic lymph nodes

C84.03   Mycosis fungoides, intra-abdominal lymph nodes

C84.04   Mycosis fungoides, lymph nodes of axilla and upper limb

C84.05   Mycosis fungoides, lymph nodes of inguinal region and lower limb

C84.06   Mycosis fungoides, intrapelvic lymph nodes

C84.07   Mycosis fungoides, spleen

C84.08   Mycosis fungoides, lymph nodes of multiple sites

C84.09   Mycosis fungoides, extranodal and solid organ sites

▶ C84.0A   Mycosis fungoides, in remission

● C84.1   **Sézary disease**
Type of cutaneous lymphoma affecting T-cells

C84.10   Sézary disease, unspecified site

C84.11   Sézary disease, lymph nodes of head, face, and neck

C84.12   Sézary disease, intrathoracic lymph nodes

C84.13   Sézary disease, intra-abdominal lymph nodes

C84.14   Sézary disease, lymph nodes of axilla and upper limb

C84.15   Sézary disease, lymph nodes of inguinal region and lower limb

C84.16   Sézary disease, intrapelvic lymph nodes

C84.17   Sézary disease, spleen

C84.18   Sézary disease, lymph nodes of multiple sites

C84.19   Sézary disease, extranodal and solid organ sites

▶ C84.1A   Sézary disease, in remission

● C84.4   **Peripheral T-cell lymphoma, not elsewhere classified**
Diverse group of blood carcinomas originating from T-cells, requiring aggressive chemotherapy
Lennert's lymphoma
Lymphoepithelioid lymphoma
Mature T-cell lymphoma, not elsewhere classified

C84.40   Peripheral T-cell lymphoma, not elsewhere classified, unspecified site

C84.41   Peripheral T-cell lymphoma, not elsewhere classified, lymph nodes of head, face, and neck

CHAPTER 2 (C00-D49)

CHAPTER 2 (C00–D49)

C84.42   Peripheral T-cell lymphoma, not elsewhere classified, intrathoracic lymph nodes 🦠

C84.43   Peripheral T-cell lymphoma, not elsewhere classified, intra-abdominal lymph nodes 🦠

C84.44   Peripheral T-cell lymphoma, not elsewhere classified, lymph nodes of axilla and upper limb 🦠

C84.45   Peripheral T-cell lymphoma, not elsewhere classified, lymph nodes of inguinal region and lower limb 🦠

C84.46   Peripheral T-cell lymphoma, not elsewhere classified, intrapelvic lymph nodes 🦠

C84.47   Peripheral T-cell lymphoma, not elsewhere classified, spleen 🦠

C84.48   Peripheral T-cell lymphoma, not elsewhere classified, lymph nodes of multiple sites 🦠

C84.49   Peripheral T-cell lymphoma, not elsewhere classified, extranodal and solid organ sites 🦠

▶C84.4A   Peripheral T-cell lymphoma, not elsewhere classified, in remission

●C84.6   **Anaplastic large cell lymphoma, ALK-positive**
Anaplastic large cell lymphoma, CD30-positive

C84.60   Anaplastic large cell lymphoma, ALK-positive, unspecified site 🦠

C84.61   Anaplastic large cell lymphoma, ALK-positive, lymph nodes of head, face, and neck 🦠

C84.62   Anaplastic large cell lymphoma, ALK-positive, intrathoracic lymph nodes 🦠

C84.63   Anaplastic large cell lymphoma, ALK-positive, intra-abdominal lymph nodes 🦠

C84.64   Anaplastic large cell lymphoma, ALK-positive, lymph nodes of axilla and upper limb 🦠

C84.65   Anaplastic large cell lymphoma, ALK-positive, lymph nodes of inguinal region and lower limb 🦠

C84.66   Anaplastic large cell lymphoma, ALK-positive, intrapelvic lymph nodes 🦠

C84.67   Anaplastic large cell lymphoma, ALK-positive, spleen 🦠

C84.68   Anaplastic large cell lymphoma, ALK-positive, lymph nodes of multiple sites 🦠

C84.69   Anaplastic large cell lymphoma, ALK-positive, extranodal and solid organ sites 🦠

▶C84.6A   Anaplastic large cell lymphoma, ALK-positive, in remission

●C84.7   **Anaplastic large cell lymphoma, ALK-negative**
Excludes1   primary cutaneous CD30-positive T-cell proliferations (C86.6-)

C84.70   Anaplastic large cell lymphoma, ALK-negative, unspecified site 🦠

C84.71   Anaplastic large cell lymphoma, ALK-negative, lymph nodes of head, face, and neck 🦠

C84.72   Anaplastic large cell lymphoma, ALK-negative, intrathoracic lymph nodes 🦠

C84.73   Anaplastic large cell lymphoma, ALK-negative, intra-abdominal lymph nodes 🦠

C84.74   Anaplastic large cell lymphoma, ALK-negative, lymph nodes of axilla and upper limb 🦠

C84.75   Anaplastic large cell lymphoma, ALK-negative, lymph nodes of inguinal region and lower limb 🦠

C84.76   Anaplastic large cell lymphoma, ALK-negative, intrapelvic lymph nodes 🦠

C84.77   Anaplastic large cell lymphoma, ALK-negative, spleen 🦠

C84.78   Anaplastic large cell lymphoma, ALK-negative, lymph nodes of multiple sites 🦠

C84.79   Anaplastic large cell lymphoma, ALK-negative, extranodal and solid organ sites 🦠

C84.7A   Anaplastic large cell lymphoma, ALK-negative, breast
Breast implant associated anaplastic large cell lymphoma (BIA-ALCL)
Use additional code to identify:
breast implant status (Z98.82)
personal history of breast implant removal (Z98.86)

▶C84.7B   Anaplastic large cell lymphoma, ALK-negative, in remission

●C84.9   **Mature T/NK-cell lymphomas, unspecified**
NK/T cell lymphoma NOS
Excludes1   mature T-cell lymphoma, not elsewhere classified (C84.4-)

C84.90   Mature T/NK-cell lymphomas, unspecified, unspecified site 🦠

C84.91   Mature T/NK-cell lymphomas, unspecified, lymph nodes of head, face, and neck 🦠

C84.92   Mature T/NK-cell lymphomas, unspecified, intrathoracic lymph nodes 🦠

C84.93   Mature T/NK-cell lymphomas, unspecified, intra-abdominal lymph nodes 🦠

C84.94   Mature T/NK-cell lymphomas, unspecified, lymph nodes of axilla and upper limb 🦠

C84.95   Mature T/NK-cell lymphomas, unspecified, lymph nodes of inguinal region and lower limb 🦠

C84.96   Mature T/NK-cell lymphomas, unspecified, intrapelvic lymph nodes 🦠

C84.97   Mature T/NK-cell lymphomas, unspecified, spleen 🦠

C84.98   Mature T/NK-cell lymphomas, unspecified, lymph nodes of multiple sites 🦠

C84.99   Mature T/NK-cell lymphomas, unspecified, extranodal and solid organ sites 🦠

▶C84.9A   Mature T/NK-cell lymphomas, unspecified, in remission

●C84.A   **Cutaneous T-cell lymphoma, unspecified**

C84.A0   Cutaneous T-cell lymphoma, unspecified, unspecified site 🦠

C84.A1   Cutaneous T-cell lymphoma, unspecified lymph nodes of head, face, and neck 🦠

C84.A2   Cutaneous T-cell lymphoma, unspecified, intrathoracic lymph nodes 🦠

C84.A3   Cutaneous T-cell lymphoma, unspecified, intra-abdominal lymph nodes 🦠

C84.A4   Cutaneous T-cell lymphoma, unspecified, lymph nodes of axilla and upper limb 🦠

C84.A5   Cutaneous T-cell lymphoma, unspecified, lymph nodes of inguinal region and lower limb 🦠

C84.A6   Cutaneous T-cell lymphoma, unspecified, intrapelvic lymph nodes 🦠

C84.A7   Cutaneous T-cell lymphoma, unspecified, spleen 🦠
Coding Clinic: 2021, Q2, P7

C84.A8   Cutaneous T-cell lymphoma, unspecified, lymph nodes of multiple sites 🦠
Coding Clinic: 2021, Q2, P7

C84.A9   Cutaneous T-cell lymphoma, unspecified, extranodal and solid organ sites 🦠

▶C84.AA   Cutaneous T-cell lymphoma, unspecified, in remission

Item 2–7 Lymphosarcoma, also known as malignant lymphoma, is a cancer of the lymph system exhibiting abnormal cells encompassing an entire lymph node creating a diffuse pattern without any definite organization. Diffuse pattern lymphoma has a more unfavorable survival outlook than those with a follicular or nodular pattern. Reticulosarcoma is the most common aggressive form of non-Hodgkin lymphoma.

● C84.Z   Other mature T/NK-cell lymphomas

   Note: If T-cell lineage or involvement is mentioned in conjunction with a specific lymphoma, code to the more specific description.

   ⇒ **Excludes1**   angioimmunoblastic T-cell lymphoma (C86.5Ø)
   ⇒ blastic NK-cell lymphoma (C86.4Ø)
   ⇒ enteropathy-type T-cell lymphoma (C86.2Ø)
   ⇒ extranodal NK-cell lymphoma, nasal type (C86.ØØ)
   ⇒ hepatosplenic T-cell lymphoma (C86.1Ø)
   ⇒ primary cutaneous CD3Ø-positive T-cell proliferations (C86.6Ø)
   ⇒ subcutaneous panniculitis-like T-cell lymphoma (C86.3Ø)
   T-cell leukemia (C91.1-)

   C84.ZØ   Other mature T/NK-cell lymphomas, unspecified site 🔍

   C84.Z1   Other mature T/NK-cell lymphomas, lymph nodes of head, face, and neck 🔍

   C84.Z2   Other mature T/NK-cell lymphomas, intrathoracic lymph nodes 🔍

   C84.Z3   Other mature T/NK-cell lymphomas, intra-abdominal lymph nodes 🔍

   C84.Z4   Other mature T/NK-cell lymphomas, lymph nodes of axilla and upper limb 🔍

   C84.Z5   Other mature T/NK-cell lymphomas, lymph nodes of inguinal region and lower limb 🔍

   C84.Z6   Other mature T/NK-cell lymphomas, intrapelvic lymph nodes 🔍

   C84.Z7   Other mature T/NK-cell lymphomas, spleen 🔍

   C84.Z8   Other mature T/NK-cell lymphomas, lymph nodes of multiple sites 🔍

   C84.Z9   Other mature T/NK-cell lymphomas, extranodal and solid organ sites 🔍

   ▷ C84.ZA   Other mature T/NK-cell lymphomas, in remission

● C85   Other specified and unspecified types of non-Hodgkin lymphoma

   Excludes1   other specified types of T/NK-cell lymphoma (C86.-)
   personal history of non-Hodgkin lymphoma (Z85.72)

● C85.1   Unspecified B-cell lymphoma

   Note: If B-cell lineage or involvement is mentioned in conjunction with a specific lymphoma, code to the more specific description.

   C85.1Ø   Unspecified B-cell lymphoma, unspecified site 🔍

   C85.11   Unspecified B-cell lymphoma, lymph nodes of head, face, and neck 🔍

   C85.12   Unspecified B-cell lymphoma, intrathoracic lymph nodes 🔍

   C85.13   Unspecified B-cell lymphoma, intra-abdominal lymph nodes 🔍

   C85.14   Unspecified B-cell lymphoma, lymph nodes of axilla and upper limb 🔍

   C85.15   Unspecified B-cell lymphoma, lymph nodes of inguinal region and lower limb 🔍

   C85.16   Unspecified B-cell lymphoma, intrapelvic lymph nodes 🔍

   C85.17   Unspecified B-cell lymphoma, spleen 🔍

   C85.18   Unspecified B-cell lymphoma, lymph nodes of multiple sites 🔍

   C85.19   Unspecified B-cell lymphoma, extranodal and solid organ sites 🔍

   ▷ C85.1A   Unspecified B-cell lymphoma, in remission

● C85.2   Mediastinal (thymic) large B-cell lymphoma

   C85.2Ø   Mediastinal (thymic) large B-cell lymphoma, unspecified site 🔍

   C85.21   Mediastinal (thymic) large B-cell lymphoma, lymph nodes of head, face, and neck 🔍

   C85.22   Mediastinal (thymic) large B-cell lymphoma, intrathoracic lymph nodes 🔍

   C85.23   Mediastinal (thymic) large B-cell lymphoma, intra-abdominal lymph nodes 🔍

   C85.24   Mediastinal (thymic) large B-cell lymphoma, lymph nodes of axilla and upper limb 🔍

   C85.25   Mediastinal (thymic) large B-cell lymphoma, lymph nodes of inguinal region and lower limb 🔍

   C85.26   Mediastinal (thymic) large B-cell lymphoma, intrapelvic lymph nodes 🔍

   C85.27   Mediastinal (thymic) large B-cell lymphoma, spleen 🔍

   C85.28   Mediastinal (thymic) large B-cell lymphoma, lymph nodes of multiple sites 🔍

   C85.29   Mediastinal (thymic) large B-cell lymphoma, extranodal and solid organ sites 🔍

   ▷ C85.2A   Mediastinal (thymic) large B-cell lymphoma, in remission

● C85.8   Other specified types of non-Hodgkin lymphoma

   C85.8Ø   Other specified types of non-Hodgkin lymphoma, unspecified site 🔍

   C85.81   Other specified types of non-Hodgkin lymphoma, lymph nodes of head, face, and neck 🔍

   C85.82   Other specified types of non-Hodgkin lymphoma, intrathoracic lymph nodes 🔍

   C85.83   Other specified types of non-Hodgkin lymphoma, intra-abdominal lymph nodes 🔍

   C85.84   Other specified types of non-Hodgkin lymphoma, lymph nodes of axilla and upper limb 🔍

   C85.85   Other specified types of non-Hodgkin lymphoma, lymph nodes of inguinal region and lower limb 🔍

   C85.86   Other specified types of non-Hodgkin lymphoma, intrapelvic lymph nodes 🔍

   C85.87   Other specified types of non-Hodgkin lymphoma, spleen 🔍

   C85.88   Other specified types of non-Hodgkin lymphoma, lymph nodes of multiple sites 🔍

   C85.89   Other specified types of non-Hodgkin lymphoma, extranodal and solid organ sites 🔍

   ▷ C85.8A   Other specified types of non-Hodgkin lymphoma, in remission

● C85.9   Non-Hodgkin lymphoma, unspecified

   Lymphoma NOS
   Malignant lymphoma NOS
   Non-Hodgkin lymphoma NOS

   C85.9Ø   Non-Hodgkin lymphoma, unspecified, unspecified site 🔍

   C85.91   Non-Hodgkin lymphoma, unspecified, lymph nodes of head, face, and neck 🔍

   C85.92   Non-Hodgkin lymphoma, unspecified, intrathoracic lymph nodes 🔍

   C85.93   Non-Hodgkin lymphoma, unspecified, intra-abdominal lymph nodes 🔍

   C85.94   Non-Hodgkin lymphoma, unspecified, lymph nodes of axilla and upper limb 🔍

   C85.95   Non-Hodgkin lymphoma, unspecified, lymph nodes of inguinal region and lower limb 🔍

   C85.96   Non-Hodgkin lymphoma, unspecified, intrapelvic lymph nodes 🔍

   C85.97   Non-Hodgkin lymphoma, unspecified, spleen 🔍

   C85.98   Non-Hodgkin lymphoma, unspecified, lymph nodes of multiple sites 🔍

CHAPTER 2 (CØØ-D49)

C85.99   **Non-Hodgkin lymphoma, unspecified, extranodal and solid organ sites** 🩺

▶C85.9A   **Non-Hodgkin lymphoma, unspecified, in remission**

● **C86**   **Other specified types of T/NK-cell lymphoma**

   Excludes1   anaplastic large cell lymphoma, ALK negative (C84.7-)
             anaplastic large cell lymphoma, ALK positive (C84.6-)
             mature T/NK-cell lymphomas (C84.-)
             other specified types of non-Hodgkin lymphoma (C85.8-)

C86.0   **Extranodal NK/T-cell lymphoma, nasal type** 🩺

   ▶C86.00   **Extranodal NK/T-cell lymphoma, nasal type not having achieved remission**
     ▶Extranodal NK/T-cell lymphoma, nasal type NOS
     ▶Extranodal NK/T-cell lymphoma, nasal type with failed remission

   ▶C86.01   **Extranodal NK/T-cell lymphoma, nasal type, in remission**

C86.1   **Hepatosplenic T-cell lymphoma** 🩺
   Alpha-beta and gamma delta types

   ▶C86.10   **Hepatosplenic T-cell lymphoma not having achieved remission**
     ▶Hepatosplenic T-cell lymphoma NOS
     ▶Hepatosplenic T-cell lymphoma with failed remission

   ▶C86.11   **Hepatosplenic T-cell lymphoma, in remission**

C86.2   **Enteropathy-type (intestinal) T-cell lymphoma** 🩺
   Enteropathy associated T-cell lymphoma

   ▶C86.20   **Enteropathy-type (intestinal) T-cell lymphoma not having achieved remission**
     ▶Enteropathy associated T-cell lymphoma NOS
     ▶Enteropathy associated T-cell lymphoma not having achieved remission
     ▶Enteropathy associated T-cell lymphoma with failed remission
     ▶Enteropathy-type (intestinal) T-cell lymphoma NOS
     ▶Enteropathy-type (intestinal) T-cell lymphoma with failed remission

   ▶C86.21   **Enteropathy-type (intestinal) T-cell lymphoma, in remission**
     ▶Enteropathy associated T-cell lymphoma, in remission

C86.3   **Subcutaneous panniculitis-like T-cell lymphoma** 🩺

   ▶C86.30   **Subcutaneous panniculitis-like T-cell lymphoma not having achieved remission**
     ▶Subcutaneous panniculitis-like T-cell lymphoma NOS
     ▶Subcutaneous panniculitis-like T-cell lymphoma with failed remission

   ▶C86.3   **Subcutaneous panniculitis-like T-cell lymphoma, in remission**

C86.4   **Blastic NK-cell lymphoma** 🩺
   Blastic plasmacytoid dendritic cell neoplasm (BPDCN)

   ▶C86.40   **Blastic NK-cell lymphoma not having achieved remission**
     ▶Blastic NK-cell lymphoma NOS
     ▶Blastic NK-cell lymphoma with failed remission
     ▶Blastic plasmacytoid dendritic cell neoplasm (BPDCN) NOS
     ▶Blastic plasmacytoid dendritic cell neoplasm (BPDCN) not having achieved remission
     ▶Blastic plasmacytoid dendritic cell neoplasm (BPDCN) with failed remission

   ▶C86.41   **Blastic NK-cell lymphoma, in remission**
     Blastic plasmacytoid dendritic cell neoplasm (BPDCN), in remission

C86.5   **Angioimmunoblastic T-cell lymphoma** 🩺
   Angioimmunoblastic lymphadenopathy with dysproteinemia (AILD)

▶C86.50   **Angioimmunoblastic T-cell lymphoma not having achieved remission**
   ▶Angioimmunoblastic lymphadenopathy with dysproteinemia (AILD) NOS
   ▶Angioimmunoblastic lymphadenopathy with dysproteinemia (AILD) not having achieved remission
   ▶Angioimmunoblastic lymphadenopathy with dysproteinemia (AILD) with failed remission
   ▶Angioimmunoblastic T-cell lymphoma NOS
   ▶Angioimmunoblastic T-cell lymphoma with failed remission

▶C86.51   **Angioimmunoblastic T-cell lymphoma, in remission**
   ▶Angioimmunoblastic lymphadenopathy with dysproteinemia (AILD), in remission

C86.6   **Primary cutaneous CD30-positive T-cell proliferations** 🩺
   Lymphomatoid papulosis
   Primary cutaneous anaplastic large cell lymphoma
   Primary cutaneous CD30-positive large T-cell lymphoma

   ▶C86.60   **Primary cutaneous CD30-positive T-cell proliferations not having achievedremission**
     ▶Lymphomatoid papulosis NOS
     ▶Lymphomatoid papulosis not having achieved remission
     ▶Lymphomatoid papulosis with failed remission
     ▶Primary cutaneous anaplastic large cell lymphoma NOS
     ▶Primary cutaneous anaplastic large cell lymphoma not having achieved remission
     ▶Primary cutaneous anaplastic large cell lymphoma with failed remission
     ▶Primary cutaneous CD30-positive large T-cell lymphoma NOS
     ▶Primary cutaneous CD30-positive large T-cell lymphoma not having achieved remission
     ▶Primary cutaneous CD30-positive large T-cell lymphoma with failed remission
     ▶Primary cutaneous CD30-positive T-cell proliferations NOS
     ▶Primary cutaneous CD30-positive T-cell proliferations with failed remission

   ▶C86.61   **Primary cutaneous CD30-positive T-cell proliferations, in remission**

● **C88**   **Malignant immunoproliferative diseases and certain other B-cell lymphomas**
   Diseases involving immune system

   Excludes1   B-cell lymphoma, unspecified (C85.1-)
             personal history of other malignant neoplasms of lymphoid, hematopoietic and related tissues (Z85.79)

C88.0   **Waldenström's macroglobulinemia** 🩺
   Lymphoplasmacytic lymphoma with IgM-production
   Macroglobulinemia (idiopathic) (primary)

   Excludes1   small cell B-cell lymphoma (C83.0)

   ▶C88.00   **Waldenström macroglobulinemia not having achieved remission**
     ▶Lymphoplasmacytic lymphoma with IgM-production, NOS
     ▶Lymphoplasmacytic lymphoma with IgM-production not having achieved remission
     ▶Lymphoplasmacytic lymphoma with IgM-production with failed remission
     ▶Macroglobulinemia (idiopathic) (primary) NOS
     ▶Macroglobulinemia (idiopathic) (primary) not having achieved remission
     ▶Macroglobulinemia (idiopathic) (primary) with failed remission
     ▶Waldenström macroglobulinemia NOS
     ▶Waldenström macroglobulinemia with failed remission

   ▶C88.01   **Waldenström macroglobulinemia, in remission**

▶ New   ⇒ Revised   ~~deleted~~ Deleted   Excludes 1   Excludes 2   Includes   Use additional   Code first   Code also   Key words

OGCR Official Guidelines   X Assign placeholder X   ● Use Additional Character(s)   ▶ Manifestation Code   🩺 Hierarchical Condition Category   Coding Clinic

C88.2   Heavy chain disease 🔍
     Franklin disease
     Gamma heavy chain disease
     Mu heavy chain disease

▷ **C88.20   Heavy chain disease not having achieved remission**
     ▷ Franklin disease NOS
     Franklin disease not having achieved remission
     ▷ Franklin disease with failed remission
     ▷ Gamma heavy chain disease NOS
     ▷ Gamma heavy chain disease not having achieved remission
     ▷ Gamma heavy chain disease with failed remission
     ▷ Heavy chain disease NOS
     ▷ Heavy chain disease with failed remissionMu heavy chain disease not having achieved remission
     ▷ Mu heavy chain disease NOS
     ▷ Mu heavy chain disease not having achieved remission
     ▷ Mu heavy chain disease with failed remission

▷ **C88.21   Heavy chain disease, in remission**

C88.3   Immunoproliferative small intestinal disease 🔍
     Alpha heavy chain disease
     Mediterranean lymphoma

▷ **C88.30   Immunoproliferative small intestinal disease not having achieved remission**
     ▷ Alpha heavy chain disease NOS
     ▷ Alpha heavy chain disease not having achieved remission
     ▷ Alpha heavy chain disease with failed remission
     ▷ Immunoproliferative small intestinal disease NOS
     ▷ Immunoproliferative small intestinal disease with failed remission
     ▷ Mediterranean lymphoma NOS
     ▷ Mediterranean lymphoma not having achieved remission
     ▷ Mediterranean lymphoma with failed remission

▷ **C88.31   Immunoproliferative small intestinal disease, in remission**

C88.4   Extranodal marginal zone B-cell lymphoma of mucosa-associated lymphoid tissue [MALT-lymphoma] 🔍
     Lymphoma of skin-associated lymphoid tissue [SALT-lymphoma]
     Lymphoma of bronchial-associated lymphoid tissue [BALT-lymphoma]

     Excludes1   high malignant (diffuse large B-cell) lymphoma (C83.3-)

▷ **C88.40   Extranodal marginal zone B-cell lymphoma of mucosa-associated lymphoid tissue[MALT-lymphoma] not having achieved remission**
     ▷ Extranodal marginal zone B-cell lymphoma of mucosa-associated lymphoid tissue [MALT-lymphoma] NOS
     ▷ Extranodal marginal zone B-cell lymphoma of mucosa-associated lymphoid tissue [MALT-lymphoma] with failed remission
     ▷ Lymphoma of bronchial-associated lymphoid tissue [BALT-lymphoma] NOS
     ▷ Lymphoma of bronchial-associated lymphoid tissue [BALT-lymphoma] not having achieved remission
     ▷ Lymphoma of bronchial-associated lymphoid tissue [BALT-lymphoma] with failed remission
     ▷ Lymphoma of skin-associated lymphoid tissue [SALT-lymphoma] NOS
     ▷ Lymphoma of skin-associated lymphoid tissue [SALT-lymphoma] not having achieved remission
     ▷ Lymphoma of skin-associated lymphoid tissue [SALT-lymphoma] with failed remission

▷ **C88.41   Extranodal marginal zone B-cell**

Item 2–8   Multiple myeloma is a cancer of a plasma cell (a type of white blood cell) and is an incurable but treatable disease. Immunoproliferative neoplasm is a term for diseases (mostly cancers) in which the immune system cells proliferate.

C88.8   Other malignant immunoproliferative diseases 🔍

▷ **C88.80   Other malignant immunoproliferative diseases not having achieved remission**
     ▷ Other malignant immunoproliferative diseases NOS
     ▷ Other malignant immunoproliferative diseases with failed remission

▷ **C88.81   Other malignant immunoproliferative diseases, in remission**

C88.9   Malignant immunoproliferative disease, unspecified 🔍
     Immunoproliferative disease NOS

▷ **C88.90   Malignant immunoproliferative disease, unspecified not having achieved remission**
     ▷ Immunoproliferative disease NOS
     ▷ Immunoproliferative disease NOS not having achieved remission
     ▷ Immunoproliferative disease NOS with failed remission
     ▷ Malignant immunoproliferative disease, unspecified NOS
     ▷ Malignant immunoproliferative disease, unspecified with failed remission

▷ **C88.91   Malignant immunoproliferative disease, unspecified, in remission**

● **C90   Multiple myeloma and malignant plasma cell neoplasms**
     Excludes1   personal history of other malignant neoplasms of lymphoid, hematopoietic and related tissues (Z85.79)

● **C90.0   Multiple myeloma**
     Kahler's disease
     Medullary plasmacytoma
     Myelomatosis
     Plasma cell myeloma

     Excludes1   solitary myeloma (C90.3-)
                 solitary plasmacytoma (C90.3-)

     C90.00   Multiple myeloma not having achieved remission 🔍
         Multiple myeloma with failed remission
         Multiple myeloma NOS

     C90.01   Multiple myeloma in remission 🔍

     C90.02   Multiple myeloma in relapse 🔍

● **C90.1   Plasma cell leukemia**
     Rare type of acute leukemia
     Plasmacytic leukemia
     Coding Clinic: 2019, Q2, P30

     C90.10   Plasma cell leukemia not having achieved remission 🔍
         Plasma cell leukemia with failed remission
         Plasma cell leukemia NOS
         Coding Clinic: 2019, Q2, P30

     C90.11   Plasma cell leukemia in remission 🔍

     C90.12   Plasma cell leukemia in relapse 🔍

● **C90.2   Extramedullary plasmacytoma**
     Malignant monoclonal plasma cell tumor growing in soft tissue; AKA plasma cell dyscrasias

     C90.20   Extramedullary plasmacytoma not having achieved remission 🔍
         Extramedullary plasmacytoma with failed remission
         Extramedullary plasmacytoma NOS

     C90.21   Extramedullary plasmacytoma in remission 🔍

     C90.22   Extramedullary plasmacytoma in relapse 🔍

CHAPTER 2 (C00-D49)

- **C90.3 Solitary plasmacytoma**
  Localized malignant plasma cell tumor NOS
  Plasmacytoma NOS
  Solitary myeloma
  - **C90.30 Solitary plasmacytoma not having achieved remission** 🦠
    Solitary plasmacytoma with failed remission
    Solitary plasmacytoma NOS
  - **C90.31 Solitary plasmacytoma in remission** 🦠
  - **C90.32 Solitary plasmacytoma in relapse** 🦠

- **C91 Lymphoid leukemia**
  Type of leukemia affecting circulating cells of lymphoid origin
  Excludes1 personal history of leukemia (Z85.6)
  - **C91.0 Acute lymphoblastic leukemia [ALL]**
    Note: Codes in subcategory C91.0 should only be used for T-cell and B-cell precursor leukemia
    - **C91.00 Acute lymphoblastic leukemia not having achieved remission** 🦠
      Acute lymphoblastic leukemia with failed remission
      Acute lymphoblastic leukemia NOS
      Coding Clinic: 2022, Q1, P16
    - **C91.01 Acute lymphoblastic leukemia, in remission** 🦠
    - **C91.02 Acute lymphoblastic leukemia, in relapse** 🦠
  - **C91.1 Chronic lymphocytic leukemia of B-cell type**
    Lymphoplasmacytic leukemia
    Richter syndrome
    Excludes1 lymphoplasmacytic lymphoma (C83.0-)
    Coding Clinic: 2023, Q1, P18
    - **C91.10 Chronic lymphocytic leukemia of B-cell type not having achieved remission** 🦠
      Chronic lymphocytic leukemia of B-cell type with failed remission
      Chronic lymphocytic leukemia of B-cell type NOS
    - **C91.11 Chronic lymphocytic leukemia of B-cell type in remission** 🦠
    - **C91.12 Chronic lymphocytic leukemia of B-cell type in relapse** 🦠
      Coding Clinic: 2023, Q1, P18
  - **C91.3 Prolymphocytic leukemia of B-cell type**
    Chronic leukemia with symptoms of large number of circulating lymphocytes
    - **C91.30 Prolymphocytic leukemia of B-cell type not having achieved remission** 🦠
      Prolymphocytic leukemia of B-cell type with failed remission
      Prolymphocytic leukemia of B-cell type NOS
    - **C91.31 Prolymphocytic leukemia of B-cell type, in remission** 🦠
    - **C91.32 Prolymphocytic leukemia of B-cell type, in relapse** 🦠
  - **C91.4 Hairy cell leukemia**
    Chronic leukemia with splenomegaly and excessive number of abnormal large mononuclear cells covered by hairlike villi
    Leukemic reticuloendotheliosis
    - **C91.40 Hairy cell leukemia not having achieved remission** 🦠
      Hairy cell leukemia with failed remission
      Hairy cell leukemia NOS
    - **C91.41 Hairy cell leukemia, in remission** 🦠
    - **C91.42 Hairy cell leukemia, in relapse** 🦠

- **C91.5 Adult T-cell lymphoma/leukemia (HTLV-1-associated)**
  Acute variant of adult T-cell lymphoma/leukemia (HTLV-1-associated)
  Chronic variant of adult T-cell lymphoma/leukemia (HTLV-1-associated)
  Lymphomatoid variant of adult T-cell lymphoma/leukemia (HTLV-1-associated)
  Smouldering variant of adult T-cell lymphoma/leukemia (HTLV-1-associated)
  - **C91.50 Adult T-cell lymphoma/leukemia (HTLV-1-associated) not having achieved remission** 🦠 A
    Adult T-cell lymphoma/leukemia (HTLV-1-associated) with failed remission
    Adult T-cell lymphoma/leukemia (HTLV-1-associated) NOS
  - **C91.51 Adult T-cell lymphoma/leukemia (HTLV-1-associated), in remission** 🦠 A
  - **C91.52 Adult T-cell lymphoma/leukemia (HTLV-1-associated), in relapse** 🦠 A
- **C91.6 Prolymphocytic leukemia of T-cell type**
  - **C91.60 Prolymphocytic leukemia of T-cell type not having achieved remission** 🦠
    Prolymphocytic leukemia of T-cell type with failed remission
    Prolymphocytic leukemia of T-cell type NOS
  - **C91.61 Prolymphocytic leukemia of T-cell type, in remission** 🦠
  - **C91.62 Prolymphocytic leukemia of T-cell type, in relapse** 🦠
- **C91.9 Lymphoid leukemia, unspecified**
  - **C91.90 Lymphoid leukemia, unspecified not having achieved remission** 🦠
    Lymphoid leukemia with failed remission
    Lymphoid leukemia NOS
  - **C91.91 Lymphoid leukemia, unspecified, in remission** 🦠
  - **C91.92 Lymphoid leukemia, unspecified, in relapse** 🦠
- **C91.A Mature B-cell leukemia Burkitt-type**
  Excludes1 Burkitt lymphoma (C83.7-)
  - **C91.A0 Mature B-cell leukemia Burkitt-type not having achieved remission** 🦠
    Mature B-cell leukemia Burkitt-type with failed remission
    Mature B-cell leukemia Burkitt-type NOS
  - **C91.A1 Mature B-cell leukemia Burkitt-type, in remission** 🦠
  - **C91.A2 Mature B-cell leukemia Burkitt-type, in relapse** 🦠
- **C91.Z Other lymphoid leukemia**
  T-cell large granular lymphocytic leukemia (associated with rheumatoid arthritis)
  - **C91.Z0 Other lymphoid leukemia not having achieved remission** 🦠
    Other lymphoid leukemia with failed remission
    Other lymphoid leukemia NOS
    Coding Clinic: 2019, Q2, P25
  - **C91.Z1 Other lymphoid leukemia, in remission** 🦠
  - **C91.Z2 Other lymphoid leukemia, in relapse** 🦠
- **C92 Myeloid leukemia**
  Code also, if applicable, pancytopenia (acquired) (D61.818)
  Includes granulocytic leukemia
  myelogenous leukemia
  Excludes1 personal history of leukemia (Z85.6)
  Coding Clinic: 2019, Q1, P16

Item 2-9 Leukemia is a cancer (acute or chronic) of the blood-forming tissues of the bone marrow. Blood cells all start out as stem cells. They mature and become red cells, white cells, or platelets. There are three main types of leukocytes (white cells that fight infection): monocytes, lymphocytes, and granulocytes. **Acute monocytic leukemia** (AML) affects monocytes. **Acute lymphoid leukemia** (ALL) affects lymphocytes, and **acute myeloid leukemia** (AML) affects cells that typically develop into white blood cells (not lymphocytes), though it may develop in other blood cells.

▶ New   ⇒ Revised   ~~deleted~~ Deleted   Excludes 1   Excludes 2   Includes   Use additional   Code first   Code also   Key words
OGCR Official Guidelines   X Assign placeholder X   ● Use Additional Character(s)   ▸ Manifestation Code   🦠 Hierarchical Condition Category   Coding Clinic

● **C92.0**   **Acute myeloblastic leukemia**
Acute myeloblastic leukemia, minimal differentiation
Acute myeloblastic leukemia (with maturation)
Acute myeloblastic leukemia 1/ETO
Acute myeloblastic leukemia M0
Acute myeloblastic leukemia M1
Acute myeloblastic leukemia M2
Acute myeloblastic leukemia with t(8;21)
Acute myeloblastic leukemia (without a FAB classification) NOS
Refractory anemia with excess blasts in transformation [RAEB T]

> **Excludes1**   acute exacerbation of chronic myeloid leukemia (C92.10)
> refractory anemia with excess of blasts not in transformation (D46.2-)

Coding Clinic: 2018, Q4, P87

    C92.00   **Acute myeloblastic leukemia, not having achieved remission** 🔍
Acute myeloblastic leukemia with failed remission
Acute myeloblastic leukemia NOS

    C92.01   **Acute myeloblastic leukemia, in remission** 🔍
Coding Clinic: 2021, Q3, P4

    C92.02   **Acute myeloblastic leukemia, in relapse** 🔍
Coding Clinic: 2023, Q1, P23

● **C92.1**   **Chronic myeloid leukemia, BCR/ABL-positive**
Chronic myelogenous leukemia, Philadelphia chromosome (Ph1) positive
Chronic myelogenous leukemia, t(9;22) (q34;q11)
Chronic myelogenous leukemia with crisis of blast cells

> **Excludes1**   atypical chronic myeloid leukemia BCR/ABL-negative (C92.2-)
> chronic myelomonocytic leukemia (C93.1-)
> chronic myeloproliferative disease (D47.1)

    C92.10   **Chronic myeloid leukemia, BCR/ABL-positive, not having achieved remission** 🔍
Chronic myeloid leukemia, BCR/ABL-positive with failed remission
Chronic myeloid leukemia, BCR/ABL-positive NOS
Coding Clinic: 2017, Q1, P7

    C92.11   **Chronic myeloid leukemia, BCR/ABL-positive, in remission** 🔍

    C92.12   **Chronic myeloid leukemia, BCR/ABL-positive, in relapse** 🔍

● **C92.2**   **Atypical chronic myeloid leukemia, BCR/ABL-negative**

    C92.20   **Atypical chronic myeloid leukemia, BCR/ABL-negative, not having achieved remission** 🔍
Atypical chronic myeloid leukemia, BCR/ABL-negative with failed remission
Atypical chronic myeloid leukemia, BCR/ABL-negative NOS

    C92.21   **Atypical chronic myeloid leukemia, BCR/ABL-negative, in remission** 🔍

    C92.22   **Atypical chronic myeloid leukemia, BCR/ABL-negative, in relapse** 🔍

● **C92.3**   **Myeloid sarcoma**
A malignant tumor of immature myeloid cells
Chloroma
Granulocytic sarcoma

    C92.30   **Myeloid sarcoma, not having achieved remission** 🔍
Myeloid sarcoma with failed remission
Myeloid sarcoma NOS

    C92.31   **Myeloid sarcoma, in remission** 🔍

    C92.32   **Myeloid sarcoma, in relapse** 🔍

● **C92.4**   **Acute promyelocytic leukemia**
AML M3
AML Me with t(15;17) and variants

    C92.40   **Acute promyelocytic leukemia, not having achieved remission** 🔍
Acute promyelocytic leukemia with failed remission
Acute promyelocytic leukemia NOS

    C92.41   **Acute promyelocytic leukemia, in remission** 🔍

    C92.42   **Acute promyelocytic leukemia, in relapse** 🔍

● **C92.5**   **Acute myelomonocytic leukemia**
AML M4
AML M4 Eo with inv(16) or t(16;16)

    C92.50   **Acute myelomonocytic leukemia, not having achieved remission** 🔍
Acute myelomonocytic leukemia with failed remission
Acute myelomonocytic leukemia NOS

    C92.51   **Acute myelomonocytic leukemia, in remission** 🔍

    C92.52   **Acute myelomonocytic leukemia, in relapse** 🔍

● **C92.6**   **Acute myeloid leukemia with 11q23-abnormality**
Acute myeloid leukemia with variation of MLL-gene

    C92.60   **Acute myeloid leukemia with 11q23-abnormality not having achieved remission** 🔍
Acute myeloid leukemia with 11q23-abnormality with failed remission
Acute myeloid leukemia with 11q23-abnormality NOS

    C92.61   **Acute myeloid leukemia with 11q23-abnormality in remission** 🔍

    C92.62   **Acute myeloid leukemia with 11q23-abnormality in relapse** 🔍

● **C92.9**   **Myeloid leukemia, unspecified**

    C92.90   **Myeloid leukemia, unspecified, not having achieved remission** 🔍
Myeloid leukemia, unspecified with failed remission
Myeloid leukemia, unspecified NOS

    C92.91   **Myeloid leukemia, unspecified in remission** 🔍

    C92.92   **Myeloid leukemia, unspecified in relapse** 🔍

● **C92.A**   **Acute myeloid leukemia with multilineage dysplasia**
Acute myeloid leukemia with dysplasia of remaining hematopoesis and/or myelodysplastic disease in its history

    C92.A0   **Acute myeloid leukemia with multilineage dysplasia, not having achieved remission** 🔍
Acute myeloid leukemia with multilineage dysplasia with failed remission
Acute myeloid leukemia with multilineage dysplasia NOS

    C92.A1   **Acute myeloid leukemia with multilineage dysplasia, in remission** 🔍

    C92.A2   **Acute myeloid leukemia with multilineage dysplasia, in relapse** 🔍

● **C92.Z**   **Other myeloid leukemia**

    C92.Z0   **Other myeloid leukemia not having achieved remission** 🔍
Myeloid leukemia NEC with failed remission
Myeloid leukemia NEC

    C92.Z1   **Other myeloid leukemia, in remission** 🔍

    C92.Z2   **Other myeloid leukemia, in relapse** 🔍

● **C93**   **Monocytic leukemia**

> **Includes**   monocytoid leukemia
> **Excludes1**   personal history of leukemia (Z85.6)

● **C93.0**   **Acute monoblastic/monocytic leukemia**
AML M5
AML M5a
AML M5b

CHAPTER 2 (C00-D49)

C93.00 Acute monoblastic/monocytic leukemia, not having achieved remission 🏷
  Acute monoblastic/monocytic leukemia with failed remission
  Acute monoblastic/monocytic leukemia NOS

C93.01 Acute monoblastic/monocytic leukemia, in remission 🏷

C93.02 Acute monoblastic/monocytic leukemia, in relapse 🏷

● **C93.1** Chronic myelomonocytic leukemia
  Chronic monocytic leukemia
  CMML-1
  CMML-2
  CMML with eosinophilia
  Code also, if applicable, eosinophilia (D72.18)

C93.10 Chronic myelomonocytic leukemia not having achieved remission 🏷
  Chronic myelomonocytic leukemia with failed remission
  Chronic myelomonocytic leukemia NOS

C93.11 Chronic myelomonocytic leukemia, in remission 🏷

C93.12 Chronic myelomonocytic leukemia, in relapse 🏷

● **C93.3** Juvenile myelomonocytic leukemia

C93.30 Juvenile myelomonocytic leukemia, not having achieved remission 🏷 P
  Juvenile myelomonocytic leukemia with failed remission
  Juvenile myelomonocytic leukemia NOS

C93.31 Juvenile myelomonocytic leukemia, in remission 🏷 P

C93.32 Juvenile myelomonocytic leukemia, in relapse 🏷 P

● **C93.9** Monocytic leukemia, unspecified

C93.90 Monocytic leukemia, unspecified, not having achieved remission 🏷
  Monocytic leukemia, unspecified with failed remission
  Monocytic leukemia, unspecified NOS

C93.91 Monocytic leukemia, unspecified in remission 🏷

C93.92 Monocytic leukemia, unspecified in relapse 🏷

● **C93.Z** Other monocytic leukemia

C93.Z0 Other monocytic leukemia, not having achieved remission 🏷
  Other monocytic leukemia NOS

C93.Z1 Other monocytic leukemia, in remission 🏷

C93.Z2 Other monocytic leukemia, in relapse 🏷

● **C94** Other leukemias of specified cell type
  Excludes1 leukemic reticuloendotheliosis (C91.4-)
    myelodysplastic syndromes (D46.-)
    personal history of leukemia (Z85.6)
    plasma cell leukemia (C90.1-)

● **C94.0** Acute erythroid leukemia
  Acute myeloid leukemia M6(a)(b)
  Erythroleukemia

C94.00 Acute erythroid leukemia, not having achieved remission 🏷
  Acute erythroid leukemia with failed remission
  Acute erythroid leukemia NOS

C94.01 Acute erythroid leukemia, in remission 🏷

C94.02 Acute erythroid leukemia, in relapse 🏷

● **C94.2** Acute megakaryoblastic leukemia
  Acute myeloid leukemia M7
  Acute megakaryocytic leukemia

C94.20 Acute megakaryoblastic leukemia not having achieved remission 🏷
  Acute megakaryoblastic leukemia with failed remission
  Acute megakaryoblastic leukemia NOS

C94.21 Acute megakaryoblastic leukemia, in remission 🏷

C94.22 Acute megakaryoblastic leukemia, in relapse 🏷

● **C94.3** Mast cell leukemia

C94.30 Mast cell leukemia not having achieved remission 🏷
  Mast cell leukemia with failed remission
  Mast cell leukemia NOS

C94.31 Mast cell leukemia, in remission 🏷

C94.32 Mast cell leukemia, in relapse 🏷

● **C94.4** Acute panmyelosis with myelofibrosis
  Acute myelofibrosis
  Excludes1 myelofibrosis NOS (D75.81)
    secondary myelofibrosis NOS (D75.81)

C94.40 Acute panmyelosis with myelofibrosis not having achieved remission 🏷
  Acute myelofibrosis NOS
  Acute panmyelosis with myelofibrosis with failed remission
  Acute panmyelosis NOS

C94.41 Acute panmyelosis with myelofibrosis, in remission 🏷

C94.42 Acute panmyelosis with myelofibrosis, in relapse 🏷

C94.6 Myelodysplastic disease, not elsewhere classified 🏷
  Myelodysplastic/myeloproliferative neoplasm, unclassifiable
  Myeloproliferative disease, not elsewhere classified

● **C94.8** Other specified leukemias
  Aggressive NK-cell leukemia
  Acute basophilic leukemia
  Code also, if applicable, eosinophilia (D72.18)

C94.80 Other specified leukemias not having achieved remission 🏷
  Other specified leukemia with failed remission
  Other specified leukemias NOS

C94.81 Other specified leukemias, in remission 🏷

C94.82 Other specified leukemias, in relapse 🏷

● **C95** Leukemia of unspecified cell type
  Excludes1 personal history of leukemia (Z85.6)

● **C95.0** Acute leukemia of unspecified cell type
  Acute bilineal leukemia
  Acute mixed lineage leukemia
  Biphenotypic acute leukemia
  Stem cell leukemia of unclear lineage
  Excludes1 acute exacerbation of unspecified chronic leukemia (C95.10)

C95.00 Acute leukemia of unspecified cell type not having achieved remission 🏷
  Acute leukemia of unspecified cell type with failed remission
  Acute leukemia NOS

C95.01 Acute leukemia of unspecified cell type, in remission 🏷

C95.02 Acute leukemia of unspecified cell type, in relapse 🏷

● **C95.1** Chronic leukemia of unspecified cell type

C95.10 Chronic leukemia of unspecified cell type not having achieved remission 🏷
  Chronic leukemia of unspecified cell type with failed remission
  Chronic leukemia NOS

C95.11   Chronic leukemia of unspecified cell type, in remission 🔊

C95.12   Chronic leukemia of unspecified cell type, in relapse 🔊

● **C95.9**   Leukemia, unspecified

    C95.90   Leukemia, unspecified not having achieved remission 🔊
       Leukemia, unspecified with failed remission
       Leukemia NOS

    C95.91   Leukemia, unspecified, in remission 🔊

    C95.92   Leukemia, unspecified, in relapse 🔊

● **C96**   Other and unspecified malignant neoplasms of lymphoid, hematopoietic and related tissue

    Excludes1   personal history of other malignant neoplasms of lymphoid, hematopoietic and related tissues (Z85.79)

    C96.0   Multifocal and multisystemic (disseminated) Langerhans-cell histiocytosis 🔊
       Histiocytosis X, multisystemic
       Letterer-Siwe disease

       Excludes1   adult pulmonary Langerhans cell histiocytosis (J84.82)
              multifocal and unisystemic Langerhans-cell histiocytosis (C96.5)
              unifocal Langerhans-cell histiocytosis (C96.6)

    ● **C96.2**   Malignant mast cell neoplasm

       Excludes1   indolent mastocytosis (D47.02)
              mast cell leukemia (C94.30)
              mastocytosis (congenital) (cutaneous) (Q82.2)

    C96.20   Malignant mast cell neoplasm, unspecified 🔊
    C96.21   Aggressive systemic mastocytosis 🔊
    C96.22   Mast cell sarcoma 🔊
    C96.29   Other malignant mast cell neoplasm 🔊

    C96.4   Sarcoma of dendritic cells (accessory cells) 🔊
       Follicular dendritic cell sarcoma
       Interdigitating dendritic cell sarcoma
       Langerhans cell sarcoma

    C96.5   Multifocal and unisystemic Langerhans-cell histiocytosis 🔊
       Hand-Schüller-Christian disease
       Histiocytosis X, multifocal

       Excludes1   multifocal and multisystemic (disseminated) Langerhans-cell histiocytosis (C96.0)
              unifocal Langerhans-cell histiocytosis (C96.6)

    C96.6   Unifocal Langerhans-cell histiocytosis 🔊
       Eosinophilic granuloma
       Histiocytosis X, unifocal
       Histiocytosis X NOS
       Langerhans-cell histiocytosis NOS

       Excludes1   multifocal and multisysemic (disseminated) Langerhans-cell histiocytosis (C96.0)
              multifocal and unisystemic Langerhans-cell histiocytosis (C96.5)

    C96.9   Malignant neoplasm of lymphoid, hematopoietic and related tissue, unspecified 🔊

    C96.A   Histiocytic sarcoma 🔊
       Malignant histiocytosis

    C96.Z   Other specified malignant neoplasms of lymphoid, hematopoietic and related tissue 🔊

IN SITU NEOPLASMS (D00-D09)

In situ is carcinoma involving cells in localized tissues that has not spread to nearby tissues

    Includes   Bowen's disease
       erythroplasia
       grade III intraepithelial neoplasia
       Queyrat's erythroplasia

● **D00**   Carcinoma in situ of oral cavity, esophagus and stomach

    Excludes1   melanoma in situ (D03.-)

    ● **D00.0**   Carcinoma in situ of lip, oral cavity and pharynx
       Use additional code to identify:
       exposure to environmental tobacco smoke (Z77.22)
       exposure to tobacco smoke in the perinatal period (P96.81)
       history of tobacco dependence (Z87.891)
       occupational exposure to environmental tobacco smoke (Z57.31)
       tobacco dependence (F17.-)
       tobacco use (Z72.0)

       Excludes1   carcinoma in situ of aryepiglottic fold or interarytenoid fold, laryngeal aspect (D02.0)
              carcinoma in situ of epiglottis NOS (D02.0)
              carcinoma in situ of epiglottis suprahyoid portion (D02.0)
              carcinoma in situ of skin of lip (D03.0, D04.0)

    D00.00   Carcinoma in situ of oral cavity, unspecified site
    D00.01   Carcinoma in situ of labial mucosa and vermilion border
    D00.02   Carcinoma in situ of buccal mucosa
    D00.03   Carcinoma in situ of gingiva and edentulous alveolar ridge
    D00.04   Carcinoma in situ of soft palate
    D00.05   Carcinoma in situ of hard palate
    D00.06   Carcinoma in situ of floor of mouth
    D00.07   Carcinoma in situ of tongue
    D00.08   Carcinoma in situ of pharynx
       Carcinoma in situ of aryepiglottic fold NOS
       Carcinoma in situ of hypopharyngeal aspect of aryepiglottic fold
       Carcinoma in situ of marginal zone of aryepiglottic fold

    D00.1   Carcinoma in situ of esophagus
    D00.2   Carcinoma in situ of stomach

● **D01**   Carcinoma in situ of other and unspecified digestive organs

    Excludes1   melanoma in situ (D03.-)

    D01.0   Carcinoma in situ of colon

       Excludes1   carcinoma in situ of rectosigmoid junction (D01.1)

    D01.1   Carcinoma in situ of rectosigmoid junction
    D01.2   Carcinoma in situ of rectum
    D01.3   Carcinoma in situ of anus and anal canal
       Anal intraepithelial neoplasia III [AIN III]
       Severe dysplasia of anus

       Excludes1   anal intraepithelial neoplasia I and II [AIN I and AIN II] (K62.82)
              carcinoma in situ of anal margin (D04.5)
              carcinoma in situ of anal skin (D04.5)
              carcinoma in situ of perianal skin (D04.5)

    ● **D01.4**   Carcinoma in situ of other and unspecified parts of intestine

       Excludes1   carcinoma in situ of ampulla of Vater (D01.5)

    D01.40   Carcinoma in situ of unspecified part of intestine
    D01.49   Carcinoma in situ of other parts of intestine

D01.5   **Carcinoma in situ of liver, gallbladder and bile ducts**
Carcinoma in situ of ampulla of Vater

D01.7   **Carcinoma in situ of other specified digestive organs**
Carcinoma in situ of pancreas

D01.9   **Carcinoma in situ of digestive organ, unspecified**

● **D02**   **Carcinoma in situ of middle ear and respiratory system**
Use additional code to identify:
exposure to environmental tobacco smoke (Z77.22)
exposure to tobacco smoke in the perinatal period (P96.81)
history of tobacco dependence (Z87.891)
occupational exposure to environmental tobacco smoke (Z57.31)
tobacco dependence (F17.-)
tobacco use (Z72.0)

> **Excludes1**   melanoma in situ (D03.-)

D02.0   **Carcinoma in situ of larynx**
Carcinoma in situ of aryepiglottic fold or interarytenoid fold, laryngeal aspect
Carcinoma in situ of epiglottis (suprahyoid portion)

> **Excludes1**   carcinoma in situ of aryepiglottic fold or interarytenoid fold NOS (D00.08)
> carcinoma in situ of hypopharyngeal aspect (D00.08)
> carcinoma in situ of marginal zone (D00.08)

D02.1   **Carcinoma in situ of trachea**

● **D02.2**   **Carcinoma in situ of bronchus and lung**

    D02.20   **Carcinoma in situ of unspecified bronchus and lung**

    D02.21   **Carcinoma in situ of right bronchus and lung**

    D02.22   **Carcinoma in situ of left bronchus and lung**

D02.3   **Carcinoma in situ of other parts of respiratory system**
Carcinoma in situ of accessory sinuses
Carcinoma in situ of middle ear
Carcinoma in situ of nasal cavities

> **Excludes1**   carcinoma in situ of ear (external) (skin) (D04.2-)
> carcinoma in situ of nose NOS (D09.8)
> carcinoma in situ of skin of nose (D04.3)

D02.4   **Carcinoma in situ of respiratory system, unspecified**

● **D03**   **Melanoma in situ**

D03.0   **Melanoma in situ of lip** 🐾

● **D03.1**   **Melanoma in situ of eyelid, including canthus**

    D03.10   **Melanoma in situ of unspecified eyelid, including canthus** 🐾

   ● **D03.11**   **Melanoma in situ of right eyelid, including canthus** 🐾

      D03.111   Melanoma in situ of right upper eyelid, including canthus 🐾

      D03.112   Melanoma in situ of right lower eyelid, including canthus 🐾

   ● **D03.12**   **Melanoma in situ of left eyelid, including canthus** 🐾

      D03.121   Melanoma in situ of left upper eyelid, including canthus 🐾

      D03.122   Melanoma in situ of left lower eyelid, including canthus 🐾

● **D03.2**   **Melanoma in situ of ear and external auricular canal**

    D03.20   **Melanoma in situ of unspecified ear and external auricular canal** 🐾

    D03.21   **Melanoma in situ of right ear and external auricular canal** 🐾

    D03.22   **Melanoma in situ of left ear and external auricular canal** 🐾

● **D03.3**   **Melanoma in situ of other and unspecified parts of face**

    D03.30   **Melanoma in situ of unspecified part of face** 🐾

    D03.39   **Melanoma in situ of other parts of face** 🐾

D03.4   **Melanoma in situ of scalp and neck** 🐾

● **D03.5**   **Melanoma in situ of trunk**

    D03.51   **Melanoma in situ of anal skin** 🐾
Melanoma in situ of anal margin
Melanoma in situ of perianal skin

    D03.52   **Melanoma in situ of breast (skin) (soft tissue)** 🐾

    D03.59   **Melanoma in situ of other part of trunk** 🐾

● **D03.6**   **Melanoma in situ of upper limb, including shoulder**

    D03.60   **Melanoma in situ of unspecified upper limb, including shoulder** 🐾

    D03.61   **Melanoma in situ of right upper limb, including shoulder** 🐾

    D03.62   **Melanoma in situ of left upper limb, including shoulder** 🐾

● **D03.7**   **Melanoma in situ of lower limb, including hip**

    D03.70   **Melanoma in situ of unspecified lower limb, including hip** 🐾

    D03.71   **Melanoma in situ of right lower limb, including hip** 🐾

    D03.72   **Melanoma in situ of left lower limb, including hip** 🐾

D03.8   **Melanoma in situ of other sites** 🐾
Melanoma in situ of scrotum

> **Excludes1**   carcinoma in situ of scrotum (D07.61)

D03.9   **Melanoma in situ, unspecified** 🐾

● **D04**   **Carcinoma in situ of skin**

> **Excludes1**   erythroplasia of Queyrat (penis) NOS (D07.4)
> melanoma in situ (D03.-)

D04.0   **Carcinoma in situ of skin of lip**

> **Excludes2**   carcinoma in situ of vermilion border of lip (D00.01)

● **D04.1**   **Carcinoma in situ of skin of eyelid, including canthus**

    D04.10   **Carcinoma in situ of skin of unspecified eyelid, including canthus**

   ● **D04.11**   **Carcinoma in situ of skin of right eyelid, including canthus**

      D04.111   Carcinoma in situ of skin of right upper eyelid, including canthus

      D04.112   Carcinoma in situ of skin of right lower eyelid, including canthus

   ● **D04.12**   **Carcinoma in situ of skin of left eyelid, including canthus**

      D04.121   Carcinoma in situ of skin of left upper eyelid, including canthus

      D04.122   Carcinoma in situ of skin of left lower eyelid, including canthus

● **D04.2**   **Carcinoma in situ of skin of ear and external auricular canal**

    D04.20   **Carcinoma in situ of skin of unspecified ear and external auricular canal**

    D04.21   **Carcinoma in situ of skin of right ear and external auricular canal**

    D04.22   **Carcinoma in situ of skin of left ear and external auricular canal**

● **D04.3**   **Carcinoma in situ of skin of other and unspecified parts of face**

    D04.30   **Carcinoma in situ of skin of unspecified part of face**

    D04.39   **Carcinoma in situ of skin of other parts of face**

D04.4   **Carcinoma in situ of skin of scalp and neck**

D04.5   **Carcinoma in situ of skin of trunk**
Carcinoma in situ of anal margin
Carcinoma in situ of anal skin
Carcinoma in situ of perianal skin
Carcinoma in situ of skin of breast

> **Excludes1**   carcinoma in situ of anus NOS (D01.3)
> carcinoma in situ of scrotum (D07.61)
> carcinoma in situ of skin of genital organs (D07.-)

▶ New   ⇒ Revised   ~~deleted~~ Deleted   Excludes 1   Excludes 2   Includes   Use additional   Code first   Code also   Key words

OGCR Official Guidelines   X Assign placeholder X   ● Use Additional Character(s)   ▶ Manifestation Code   🐾 Hierarchical Condition Category   Coding Clinic

● D04.6 Carcinoma in situ of skin of upper limb, including shoulder

  D04.60 Carcinoma in situ of skin of unspecified upper limb, including shoulder

  D04.61 Carcinoma in situ of skin of right upper limb, including shoulder

  D04.62 Carcinoma in situ of skin of left upper limb, including shoulder

● D04.7 Carcinoma in situ of skin of lower limb, including hip

  D04.70 Carcinoma in situ of skin of unspecified lower limb, including hip

  D04.71 Carcinoma in situ of skin of right lower limb, including hip

  D04.72 Carcinoma in situ of skin of left lower limb, including hip

  D04.8 Carcinoma in situ of skin of other sites

  D04.9 Carcinoma in situ of skin, unspecified

● D05 Carcinoma in situ of breast

  Excludes1   carcinoma in situ of skin of breast (D04.5)
                  melanoma in situ of breast (skin) (D03.5)
                  Paget's disease of breast or nipple (C50.-)

  ▶ **Excludes2** malignant neoplasm of breast (C50.-)

● D05.0 Lobular carcinoma in situ of breast

  D05.00 Lobular carcinoma in situ of unspecified breast

  D05.01 Lobular carcinoma in situ of right breast

  D05.02 Lobular carcinoma in situ of left breast

● D05.1 Intraductal carcinoma in situ of breast

  D05.10 Intraductal carcinoma in situ of unspecified breast

  D05.11 Intraductal carcinoma in situ of right breast

  D05.12 Intraductal carcinoma in situ of left breast

● D05.8 Other specified type of carcinoma in situ of breast

  D05.80 Other specified type of carcinoma in situ of unspecified breast

  D05.81 Other specified type of carcinoma in situ of right breast

  D05.82 Other specified type of carcinoma in situ of left breast

● D05.9 Unspecified type of carcinoma in situ of breast

  D05.90 Unspecified type of carcinoma in situ of unspecified breast

  D05.91 Unspecified type of carcinoma in situ of right breast

  D05.92 Unspecified type of carcinoma in situ of left breast

● D06 Carcinoma in situ of cervix uteri

  Includes   cervical adenocarcinoma in situ
                 cervical intraepithelial glandular neoplasia
                 cervical intraepithelial neoplasia III [CIN III]
                 severe dysplasia of cervix uteri

  Excludes1 cervical intraepithelial neoplasia II [CIN II] (N87.1)
                 cytologic evidence of malignancy of cervix without histologic confirmation (R87.614)
                 high grade squamous intraepithelial lesion (HGSIL) of cervix (R87.613)
                 melanoma in situ of cervix (D03.5)
                 moderate cervical dysplasia (N87.1)

  D06.0 Carcinoma in situ of endocervix

  D06.1 Carcinoma in situ of exocervix

  D06.7 Carcinoma in situ of other parts of cervix

  D06.9 Carcinoma in situ of cervix, unspecified

● D07 Carcinoma in situ of other and unspecified genital organs

  Excludes1   melanoma in situ of trunk (D03.5)

  D07.0 Carcinoma in situ of endometrium

  D07.1 Carcinoma in situ of vulva
        Severe dysplasia of vulva
        Vulvar intraepithelial neoplasia III [VIN III]

    Excludes1   moderate dysplasia of vulva (N90.1)
                    vulvar intraepithelial neoplasia II [VIN II] (N90.1)

  D07.2 Carcinoma in situ of vagina
        Severe dysplasia of vagina
        Vaginal intraepithelial neoplasia III [VIN III]

    Excludes1   moderate dysplasia of vagina (N89.1)
                    vaginal intraepithelial neoplasia II [VIN II] (N89.1)

● D07.3 Carcinoma in situ of other and unspecified female genital organs

  D07.30 Carcinoma in situ of unspecified female genital organs

  D07.39 Carcinoma in situ of other female genital organs

  D07.4 Carcinoma in situ of penis
        Erythroplasia of Queyrat NOS

  D07.5 Carcinoma in situ of prostate
        Prostatic intraepithelial neoplasia III (PIN III)
        Severe dysplasia of prostate

    Excludes1   dysplasia (mild) (moderate) of prostate (N42.3-)
                    prostatic intraepithelial neoplasia II [PIN II] (N42.3-)

● D07.6 Carcinoma in situ of other and unspecified male genital organs

  D07.60 Carcinoma in situ of unspecified male genital organs

  D07.61 Carcinoma in situ of scrotum

  D07.69 Carcinoma in situ of other male genital organs

● D09 Carcinoma in situ of other and unspecified sites

  Excludes1   melanoma in situ (D03.-)

  D09.0 Carcinoma in situ of bladder

● D09.1 Carcinoma in situ of other and unspecified urinary organs

  D09.10 Carcinoma in situ of unspecified urinary organ

  D09.19 Carcinoma in situ of other urinary organs

● D09.2 Carcinoma in situ of eye

  Excludes1   carcinoma in situ of skin of eyelid (D04.1-)

  D09.20 Carcinoma in situ of unspecified eye

  D09.21 Carcinoma in situ of right eye

  D09.22 Carcinoma in situ of left eye

  D09.3 Carcinoma in situ of thyroid and other endocrine glands

    Excludes1   carcinoma in situ of endocrine pancreas (D01.7)
                    carcinoma in situ of ovary (D07.39)
                    carcinoma in situ of testis (D07.69)

  D09.8 Carcinoma in situ of other specified sites

  D09.9 Carcinoma in situ, unspecified

BENIGN NEOPLASMS, EXCEPT BENIGN NEUROENDOCRINE TUMORS (D10-D36)

● D10 Benign neoplasm of mouth and pharynx

  D10.0 Benign neoplasm of lip
        Benign neoplasm of lip (frenulum) (inner aspect) (mucosa) (vermilion border)

    Excludes1   benign neoplasm of skin of lip (D22.0, D23.0)

  D10.1 Benign neoplasm of tongue
        Benign neoplasm of lingual tonsil

  D10.2 Benign neoplasm of floor of mouth

● D10.3 Benign neoplasm of other and unspecified parts of mouth

  D10.30 Benign neoplasm of unspecified part of mouth

CHAPTER 2 (C00–D49)

D10.39   **Benign neoplasm of other parts of mouth**
Benign neoplasm of minor salivary gland NOS
> **Excludes1**   benign odontogenic neoplasms
> (D16.4-D16.5)
> benign neoplasm of mucosa of
> lip (D10.0)
> benign neoplasm of
> nasopharyngeal surface of
> soft palate (D10.6)

D10.4   **Benign neoplasm of tonsil**
Benign neoplasm of tonsil (faucial) (palatine)
> **Excludes1**   benign neoplasm of lingual tonsil
> (D10.1)
> benign neoplasm of pharyngeal tonsil
> (D10.6)
> benign neoplasm of tonsillar fossa (D10.5)
> benign neoplasm of tonsillar pillars
> (D10.5)

D10.5   **Benign neoplasm of other parts of oropharynx**
Division of pharynx lying between soft palate and upper edge of epiglottis
Benign neoplasm of epiglottis, anterior aspect
Benign neoplasm of tonsillar fossa
Benign neoplasm of tonsillar pillars
Benign neoplasm of vallecula
> **Excludes1**   benign neoplasm of epiglottis NOS
> (D14.1)
> benign neoplasm of epiglottis,
> suprahyoid portion (D14.1)

D10.6   **Benign neoplasm of nasopharynx**
Segment of pharynx that lies above soft palate
Benign neoplasm of pharyngeal tonsil
Benign neoplasm of posterior margin of septum and
choanae

D10.7   **Benign neoplasm of hypopharynx**
Segment of pharynx that lies below upper edge of epiglottis and opens into larynx and esophagus

D10.9   **Benign neoplasm of pharynx, unspecified**

● **D11**   **Benign neoplasm of major salivary glands**
> **Excludes1**   benign neoplasms of specified minor salivary
> glands which are classified according to their
> anatomical location
> benign neoplasms of minor salivary glands NOS
> (D10.39)

D11.0   **Benign neoplasm of parotid gland**

D11.7   **Benign neoplasm of other major salivary glands**
Benign neoplasm of sublingual salivary gland
Benign neoplasm of submandibular salivary gland

D11.9   **Benign neoplasm of major salivary gland, unspecified**

● **D12**   **Benign neoplasm of colon, rectum, anus and anal canal**
> **Excludes2**   benign carcinoid tumors of the large intestine and
> rectum (D3A.02-)
> polyp of colon NOS (K63.5)

Coding Clinic: 2017, Q1, P15; 2015, Q2, P14

D12.0   **Benign neoplasm of cecum**
Benign neoplasm of ileocecal valve

D12.1   **Benign neoplasm of appendix**
> **Excludes1**   benign carcinoid tumor of the appendix
> (D3A.020)

D12.2   **Benign neoplasm of ascending colon**
Coding Clinic: 2018, Q2, P14; 2017, Q1, P15

D12.3   **Benign neoplasm of transverse colon**
Benign neoplasm of hepatic flexure
Benign neoplasm of splenic flexure
> *Flexure is a bending in a structure or organ. Note the three flexures illustrated in Figure 2–17. Hepatic = liver, sigmoid = colon, splenic = spleen.*
Coding Clinic: 2017, Q1, P16

D12.4   **Benign neoplasm of descending colon**
Coding Clinic: 2015, Q2, P14

D12.5   **Benign neoplasm of sigmoid colon**

D12.6   **Benign neoplasm of colon, unspecified**
Adenomatosis of colon
Benign neoplasm of large intestine NOS
Polyposis (hereditary) of colon
> **Excludes1**   inflammatory polyp of colon (K51.4-)
Coding Clinic: 2017, Q1, P8-9

D12.7   **Benign neoplasm of rectosigmoid junction**
Angle where sigmoid colon becomes rectum

D12.8   **Benign neoplasm of rectum**
> **Excludes1**   benign carcinoid tumor of the rectum
> (D3A.026)
Coding Clinic: 2018, Q1, P7

D12.9   **Benign neoplasm of anus and anal canal**
Benign neoplasm of anus NOS
> **Excludes1**   benign neoplasm of anal margin (D22.5,
> D23.5)
> benign neoplasm of anal skin (D22.5,
> D23.5)
> benign neoplasm of perianal skin (D22.5,
> D23.5)

● **D13**   **Benign neoplasm of other and ill-defined parts of digestive system**
> **Excludes1**   benign stromal tumors of digestive system
> (D21.4)

D13.0   **Benign neoplasm of esophagus**

D13.1   **Benign neoplasm of stomach**
> **Excludes1**   benign carcinoid tumor of the stomach
> (D3A.092)

D13.2   **Benign neoplasm of duodenum**
> **Excludes1**   benign carcinoid tumor of the duodenum
> (D3A.010)

Figure 2-16 The esophagus is the muscular tube that connects the pharynx and the stomach. The 10 inch (25 cm) long esophagus is divided into three parts: **cervical, thoracic,** and **abdominal.**

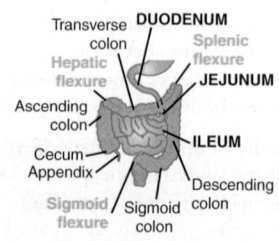

Figure 2-17 Small intestine and colon.

▶ New   ⟹ Revised   ~~deleted~~ Deleted   Excludes 1   Excludes 2   Includes   Use additional   Code first   Code also   Key words

OGCR Official Guidelines   X Assign placeholder X   ● Use Additional Character(s)   ▌ Manifestation Code   ⬙ Hierarchical Condition Category   Coding Clinic

● **D13.3** **Benign neoplasm of other and unspecified parts of small intestine**

     Excludes1   benign carcinoid tumors of the small intestine (D3A.01-)
                 benign neoplasm of ileocecal valve (D12.0)

     D13.30   Benign neoplasm of unspecified part of small intestine

     D13.39   Benign neoplasm of other parts of small intestine

D13.4   **Benign neoplasm of liver**
     Benign neoplasm of intrahepatic bile ducts

D13.5   **Benign neoplasm of extrahepatic bile ducts**
     Extensions of common hepatic bile duct (tube that collects bile from liver)

D13.6   **Benign neoplasm of pancreas**

     Excludes1   benign neoplasm of endocrine pancreas (D13.7)

D13.7   **Benign neoplasm of endocrine pancreas**
     Pancreatic islets: Cells scattered throughout pancreas
     Islet cell tumor
     Benign neoplasm of islets of Langerhans
     Use additional code to identify any functional activity.

D13.9   **Benign neoplasm of ill-defined sites within the digestive system**

     D13.91 Familial adenomatous polyposis
         Code also associated conditions, such as:
            benign neoplasm of colon (D12.6)
            malignant neoplasm of colon (C18.-)

     D13.99 Benign neoplasm of ill-defined sites within the digestive system
         Benign neoplasm of digestive system NOS
         Benign neoplasm of intestine NOS
         Benign neoplasm of spleen

● **D11**   Benign neoplasm of middle ear and respiratory system

     D14.0   **Benign neoplasm of middle ear, nasal cavity and accessory sinuses**
         Benign neoplasm of cartilage of nose

         Excludes1   benign neoplasm of auricular canal (external) (D22.2-, D23.2-)
                 benign neoplasm of bone of ear (D16.4)
                 benign neoplasm of bone of nose (D16.4)
                 benign neoplasm of cartilage of ear (D21.0)
                 benign neoplasm of ear (external) (skin) (D22.2-, D23.2-)
                 benign neoplasm of nose NOS (D36.7)
                 benign neoplasm of skin of nose (D22.39, D23.39)
                 benign neoplasm of olfactory bulb (D33.3)
                 benign neoplasm of posterior margin of septum and choanae (D10.6)
                 polyp of accessory sinus (J33.8)
                 polyp of ear (middle) (H74.4)
                 polyp of nasal (cavity) (J33.-)

     D14.1   **Benign neoplasm of larynx**
         Adenomatous polyp of larynx
         Benign neoplasm of epiglottis (suprahyoid portion)
         Horseshoe-shaped bone in anterior midline of neck between chin and thyroid cartilage

         Excludes1   benign neoplasm of epiglottis, anterior aspect (D10.5)
                 polyp (nonadenomatous) of vocal cord or larynx (J38.1)

     D14.2   **Benign neoplasm of trachea**

     ● **D14.3**   **Benign neoplasm of bronchus and lung**

         Excludes1   benign carcinoid tumor of the bronchus and lung (D3A.090)

         D14.30   Benign neoplasm of unspecified bronchus and lung

         D14.31   Benign neoplasm of right bronchus and lung

         D14.32   Benign neoplasm of left bronchus and lung

     D14.4   **Benign neoplasm of respiratory system, unspecified**

● **D15**   Benign neoplasm of other and unspecified intrathoracic organs

     Excludes1   benign neoplasm of mesothelial tissue (D19.-)

     D15.0   **Benign neoplasm of thymus**

         Excludes1   benign carcinoid tumor of the thymus (D3A.091)

     D15.1   **Benign neoplasm of heart**

         Excludes1   benign neoplasm of great vessels (D21.3)

     D15.2   **Benign neoplasm of mediastinum**

     D15.7   **Benign neoplasm of other specified intrathoracic organs**

     D15.9   **Benign neoplasm of intrathoracic organ, unspecified**

● **D16**   Benign neoplasm of bone and articular cartilage

     Excludes1   benign neoplasm of connective tissue of ear (D21.0)
                 benign neoplasm of connective tissue of eyelid (D21.0)
                 benign neoplasm of connective tissue of larynx (D14.1)
                 benign neoplasm of connective tissue of nose (D14.0)
                 benign neoplasm of synovia (D21.-)

     ● **D16.0**   **Benign neoplasm of scapula and long bones of upper limb**

         D16.00   Benign neoplasm of scapula and long bones of unspecified upper limb

         D16.01   Benign neoplasm of scapula and long bones of right upper limb

         D16.02   Benign neoplasm of scapula and long bones of left upper limb

     ● **D16.1**   **Benign neoplasm of short bones of upper limb**

         D16.10   Benign neoplasm of short bones of unspecified upper limb

         D16.11   Benign neoplasm of short bones of right upper limb

         D16.12   Benign neoplasm of short bones of left upper limb

     ● **D16.2**   **Benign neoplasm of long bones of lower limb**

         D16.20   Benign neoplasm of long bones of unspecified lower limb

         D16.21   Benign neoplasm of long bones of right lower limb

         D16.22   Benign neoplasm of long bones of left lower limb

     ● **D16.3**   **Benign neoplasm of short bones of lower limb**

         D16.30   Benign neoplasm of short bones of unspecified lower limb

         D16.31   Benign neoplasm of short bones of right lower limb

         D16.32   Benign neoplasm of short bones of left lower limb

     D16.4   **Benign neoplasm of bones of skull and face**
         Benign neoplasm of maxilla (superior)
         Benign neoplasm of orbital bone
         Cavity or socket of skull in which eye and its appendages are located
         Keratocyst of maxilla
         Keratocystic odontogenic tumor of maxilla

         Excludes2   benign neoplasm of lower jaw bone (D16.5)

     D16.5   **Benign neoplasm of lower jaw bone**
         Keratocyst of mandible
         Keratocystic odontogenic tumor of mandible

     D16.6   **Benign neoplasm of vertebral column**

         Excludes1   benign neoplasm of sacrum and coccyx (D16.8)

     D16.7   **Benign neoplasm of ribs, sternum and clavicle**

     D16.8   **Benign neoplasm of pelvic bones, sacrum and coccyx**

     D16.9   **Benign neoplasm of bone and articular cartilage, unspecified**

CHAPTER 2 (C00-D49)

● **D17　Benign lipomatous neoplasm**
Slow-growing benign tumors (rubbery masses) of mature fat cells enclosed in a thin fibrous capsule

D17.0　Benign lipomatous neoplasm of skin and subcutaneous tissue of head, face and neck

D17.1　Benign lipomatous neoplasm of skin and subcutaneous tissue of trunk

● **D17.2　Benign lipomatous neoplasm of skin and subcutaneous tissue of limb**

　　D17.20　Benign lipomatous neoplasm of skin and subcutaneous tissue of unspecified limb

　　D17.21　Benign lipomatous neoplasm of skin and subcutaneous tissue of right arm

　　D17.22　Benign lipomatous neoplasm of skin and subcutaneous tissue of left arm

　　D17.23　Benign lipomatous neoplasm of skin and subcutaneous tissue of right leg

　　D17.24　Benign lipomatous neoplasm of skin and subcutaneous tissue of left leg

● **D17.3　Benign lipomatous neoplasm of skin and subcutaneous tissue of other and unspecified sites**

　　D17.30　Benign lipomatous neoplasm of skin and subcutaneous tissue of unspecified sites

　　D17.39　Benign lipomatous neoplasm of skin and subcutaneous tissue of other sites

D17.4　Benign lipomatous neoplasm of intrathoracic organs

D17.5　Benign lipomatous neoplasm of intra-abdominal organs

　　Excludes1　benign lipomatous neoplasm of peritoneum and retroperitoneum (D17.79)

D17.6　Benign lipomatous neoplasm of spermatic cord

● **D17.7　Benign lipomatous neoplasm of other sites**

　　D17.71　Benign lipomatous neoplasm of kidney

　　D17.72　Benign lipomatous neoplasm of other genitourinary organ

　　D17.79　Benign lipomatous neoplasm of other sites
　　　　Benign lipomatous neoplasm of peritoneum
　　　　Benign lipomatous neoplasm of retroperitoneum

D17.9　Benign lipomatous neoplasm, unspecified
　　　Lipoma NOS

● **D18　Hemangioma and lymphangioma, any site**

　　Excludes1　benign neoplasm of glomus jugulare (D35.6)
　　　　　　blue or pigmented nevus (D22.-)
　　　　　　nevus NOS (D22.-)
　　　　　　vascular nevus (Q82.5)

Figure 2-18 Hemangioma of skin and subcutaneous tissue. (Getty Image)

Item 2-10　Hemangiomas are abnormally dense collections of dilated capillaries that occur on the skin or in internal organs. Hemangiomas are both deep and superficial and undergo a rapid growth phase when the size increases rapidly, followed by a rest phase, in which the tumor changes very little, followed by an involutional phase in which the tumor begins to and can disappear altogether. **Lymphangiomas** or cystic hygroma are benign collections of overgrown lymph vessels and, although rare, may occur anywhere but most commonly on the head and neck of children and infants. Visceral organs, lungs, and gastrointestinal tract may also be involved.

● **D18.0　Hemangioma**
Common type of vascular malformation
Angioma NOS
Cavernous nevus

　　D18.00　Hemangioma unspecified site

　　D18.01　Hemangioma of skin and subcutaneous tissue

　　D18.02　Hemangioma of intracranial structures 🐾

　　D18.03　Hemangioma of intra-abdominal structures

　　D18.09　Hemangioma of other sites

D18.1　Lymphangioma, any site
　　Coding Clinic: 2018, Q2, P13

● **D19　Benign neoplasm of mesothelial tissue**
Mesothelial tissue is the membrane lining several body cavities

D19.0　Benign neoplasm of mesothelial tissue of pleura

D19.1　Benign neoplasm of mesothelial tissue of peritoneum

D19.7　Benign neoplasm of mesothelial tissue of other sites

D19.9　Benign neoplasm of mesothelial tissue, unspecified
　　Benign mesothelioma NOS

● **D20　Benign neoplasm of soft tissue of retroperitoneum and peritoneum**

　　Excludes1　benign lipomatous neoplasm of peritoneum and retroperitoneum (D17.79)
　　　　　　benign neoplasm of mesothelial tissue (D19.-)

D20.0　Benign neoplasm of soft tissue of retroperitoneum

D20.1　Benign neoplasm of soft tissue of peritoneum

● **D21　Other benign neoplasms of connective and other soft tissue**

　　Includes　benign neoplasm of blood vessel
　　　　　benign neoplasm of bursa
　　　　　benign neoplasm of cartilage
　　　　　benign neoplasm of fascia
　　　　　benign neoplasm of fat
　　　　　benign neoplasm of ligament, except uterine
　　　　　benign neoplasm of lymphatic channel
　　　　　benign neoplasm of muscle
　　　　　benign neoplasm of synovia
　　　　　benign neoplasm of tendon (sheath)
　　　　　benign stromal tumors

　　Excludes1　benign neoplasm of articular cartilage (D16.-)
　　　　　benign neoplasm of cartilage of larynx (D14.1)
　　　　　benign neoplasm of cartilage of nose (D14.0)
　　　　　benign neoplasm of connective tissue of breast (D24.-)
　　　　　benign neoplasm of peripheral nerves and autonomic nervous system (D36.1-)
　　　　　benign neoplasm of peritoneum (D20.1)
　　　　　benign neoplasm of retroperitoneum (D20.0)
　　　　　benign neoplasm of uterine ligament, any (D28.2)
　　　　　benign neoplasm of vascular tissue (D18.-)
　　　　　hemangioma (D18.0-)
　　　　　lipomatous neoplasm (D17.-)
　　　　　lymphangioma (D18.1)
　　　　　uterine leiomyoma (D25.-)

D21.0　Benign neoplasm of connective and other soft tissue of head, face and neck
　　Benign neoplasm of connective tissue of ear
　　Benign neoplasm of connective tissue of eyelid

　　Excludes1　benign neoplasm of connective tissue of orbit (D31.6-)

● **D21.1　Benign neoplasm of connective and other soft tissue of upper limb, including shoulder**

　　D21.10　Benign neoplasm of connective and other soft tissue of unspecified upper limb, including shoulder

　　D21.11　Benign neoplasm of connective and other soft tissue of right upper limb, including shoulder

　　D21.12　Benign neoplasm of connective and other soft tissue of left upper limb, including shoulder

▶ New　⇒ Revised　~~deleted~~ Deleted　Excludes 1　Excludes 2　Includes　Use additional　Code first　Code also　Key words
OGCR Official Guidelines　X Assign placeholder X　● Use Additional Character(s)　▶ Manifestation Code　🐾 Hierarchical Condition Category　Coding Clinic

- **D21.2** Benign neoplasm of connective and other soft tissue of lower limb, including hip
  - **D21.20** Benign neoplasm of connective and other soft tissue of unspecified lower limb, including hip
  - **D21.21** Benign neoplasm of connective and other soft tissue of right lower limb, including hip
  - **D21.22** Benign neoplasm of connective and other soft tissue of left lower limb, including hip
- **D21.3** Benign neoplasm of connective and other soft tissue of thorax

  Benign neoplasm of axilla
  Benign neoplasm of diaphragm
  Benign neoplasm of great vessels
  - **Excludes1**   benign neoplasm of heart (D15.1)
    benign neoplasm of mediastinum (D15.2)
    benign neoplasm of thymus (D15.0)
- **D21.4** Benign neoplasm of connective and other soft tissue of abdomen

  Benign stromal tumors of abdomen
- **D21.5** Benign neoplasm of connective and other soft tissue of pelvis
  - **Excludes1**   benign neoplasm of any uterine ligament (D28.2)
    uterine leiomyoma (D25.-)
- **D21.6** Benign neoplasm of connective and other soft tissue of trunk, unspecified

  Benign neoplasm of connective and other soft tissue of back NOS
- **D21.9** Benign neoplasm of connective and other soft tissue, unspecified

- **D22** Melanocytic nevi
  - **Includes**   atypical nevus
    blue hairy pigmented nevus
    nevus NOS
  - **D22.0** Melanocytic nevi of lip

    Skin lesions composed of nests of nevus cells with macules/papules
  - **D22.1** Melanocytic nevi of eyelid, including canthus
    - **D22.10** Melanocytic nevi of unspecified eyelid, including canthus
    - **D22.11** Melanocytic nevi of right eyelid, including canthus
      - **D22.111** Melanocytic nevi of right upper eyelid, including canthus
      - **D22.112** Melanocytic nevi of right lower eyelid, including canthus
    - **D22.12** Melanocytic nevi of left eyelid, including canthus
      - **D22.121** Melanocytic nevi of left upper eyelid, including canthus
      - **D22.122** Melanocytic nevi of left lower eyelid, including canthus
  - **D22.2** Melanocytic nevi of ear and external auricular canal
    - **D22.20** Melanocytic nevi of unspecified ear and external auricular canal
    - **D22.21** Melanocytic nevi of right ear and external auricular canal
    - **D22.22** Melanocytic nevi of left ear and external auricular canal
  - **D22.3** Melanocytic nevi of other and unspecified parts of face
    - **D22.30** Melanocytic nevi of unspecified part of face
    - **D22.39** Melanocytic nevi of other parts of face
  - **D22.4** Melanocytic nevi of scalp and neck
  - **D22.5** Melanocytic nevi of trunk

    Melanocytic nevi of anal margin
    Melanocytic nevi of anal skin
    Melanocytic nevi of perianal skin
    Melanocytic nevi of skin of breast

- **D22.6** Melanocytic nevi of upper limb, including shoulder
  - **D22.60** Melanocytic nevi of unspecified upper limb, including shoulder
  - **D22.61** Melanocytic nevi of right upper limb, including shoulder
  - **D22.62** Melanocytic nevi of left upper limb, including shoulder
- **D22.7** Melanocytic nevi of lower limb, including hip
  - **D22.70** Melanocytic nevi of unspecified lower limb, including hip
  - **D22.71** Melanocytic nevi of right lower limb, including hip
  - **D22.72** Melanocytic nevi of left lower limb, including hip
- **D22.9** Melanocytic nevi, unspecified

- **D23** Other benign neoplasms of skin
  - **Includes**   benign neoplasm of hair follicles
    benign neoplasm of sebaceous glands
    benign neoplasm of sweat glands
  - **Excludes1**   benign lipomatous neoplasms of skin (D17.0-D17.3)
  - **Excludes2**   melanocytic nevi (D22.-)
  - **D23.0** Other benign neoplasm of skin of lip
    - **Excludes1**   benign neoplasm of vermilion border of lip (D10.0)
  - **D23.1** Other benign neoplasm of skin of eyelid, including canthus
    - **D23.10** Other benign neoplasm of skin unspecified of eyelid, including canthus
    - **D23.11** Other benign neoplasm of skin of right eyelid, including canthus
      - **D23.111** Other benign neoplasm of skin of right upper eyelid, including canthus
      - **D23.112** Other benign neoplasm of skin of right lower eyelid, including canthus
    - **D23.12** Other benign neoplasm of skin of left eyelid, including canthus
      - **D23.121** Other benign neoplasm of skin of left upper eyelid, including canthus
      - **D23.122** Other benign neoplasm of skin of left lower eyelid, including canthus
  - **D23.2** Other benign neoplasm of skin of ear and external auricular canal
    - **D23.20** Other benign neoplasm of skin of unspecified ear and external auricular canal
    - **D23.21** Other benign neoplasm of skin of right ear and external auricular canal
    - **D23.22** Other benign neoplasm of skin of left ear and external auricular canal
  - **D23.3** Other benign neoplasm of skin of other and unspecified parts of face
    - **D23.30** Other benign neoplasm of skin of unspecified part of face
    - **D23.39** Other benign neoplasm of skin of other parts of face
  - **D23.4** Other benign neoplasm of skin of scalp and neck
  - **D23.5** Other benign neoplasm of skin of trunk

    Other benign neoplasm of anal margin
    Other benign neoplasm of anal skin
    Other benign neoplasm of perianal skin
    Other benign neoplasm of skin of breast
    - **Excludes1**   benign neoplasm of anus NOS (D12.9)
  - **D23.6** Other benign neoplasm of skin of upper limb, including shoulder
    - **D23.60** Other benign neoplasm of skin of unspecified upper limb, including shoulder
    - **D23.61** Other benign neoplasm of skin of right upper limb, including shoulder
    - **D23.62** Other benign neoplasm of skin of left upper limb, including shoulder

CHAPTER 2 (C00-D49)

Item 2–11 Teratoma: terat = monster, oma = mass, tumor. Alternate terms: dermoid cyst of the ovary, ovarian teratoma. Teratomas are neoplasms and arise from germ cells (ovaries in female and testes in male) and can be benign or malignant. Teratomas have been known to contain hair, nails, and teeth, giving them a bizarre ("monster") appearance.

● **D23.7** **Other benign neoplasm of skin of lower limb, including hip**

     D23.70 Other benign neoplasm of skin of unspecified lower limb, including hip

     D23.71 Other benign neoplasm of skin of right lower limb, including hip

     D23.72 Other benign neoplasm of skin of left lower limb, including hip

     D23.9 Other benign neoplasm of skin, unspecified

● **D24** **Benign neoplasm of breast**

     Includes benign neoplasm of connective tissue of breast
             benign neoplasm of soft parts of breast
             fibroadenoma of breast

     Excludes2 adenofibrosis of breast (N60.2)
             benign cyst of breast (N60.-)
             benign mammary dysplasia (N60.-)
             benign neoplasm of skin of breast (D22.5, D23.5)
             fibrocystic disease of breast (N60.-)

     D24.1 Benign neoplasm of right breast
         Coding Clinic: 2017, Q1, P5

     D24.2 Benign neoplasm of left breast

     D24.9 Benign neoplasm of unspecified breast

● **D25** **Leiomyoma of uterus**
     Benign tumors or nodules of the uterine wall

     Includes uterine fibroid
             uterine fibromyoma
             uterine myoma

     D25.0 Submucous leiomyoma of uterus

     D25.1 Intramural leiomyoma of uterus
         Interstitial leiomyoma of uterus

     D25.2 Subserosal leiomyoma of uterus
         Subperitoneal leiomyoma of uterus

     D25.9 Leiomyoma of uterus, unspecified

● **D26** **Other benign neoplasms of uterus**

     D26.0 Other benign neoplasm of cervix uteri

     D26.1 Other benign neoplasm of corpus uteri

     D26.7 Other benign neoplasm of other parts of uterus

     D26.9 Other benign neoplasm of uterus, unspecified

● **D27** **Benign neoplasm of ovary**
     Use additional code to identify any functional activity.

     Excludes2 corpus albicans cyst (N83.2-)
             corpus luteum cyst (N83.1-)
             endometrial cyst (N80.1-)
             follicular (atretic) cyst (N83.0-)
             graafian follicle cyst (N83.0-)
             ovarian cyst NEC (N83.2-)
             ovarian retention cyst (N83.2-)

     D27.0 Benign neoplasm of right ovary

     D27.1 Benign neoplasm of left ovary

     D27.9 Benign neoplasm of unspecified ovary
         Ovarian teratoma

● **D28** **Benign neoplasm of other and unspecified female genital organs**

     Includes adenomatous polyp
             benign neoplasm of skin of female genital organs
             benign teratoma

     Excludes1 epoophoron cyst (Q50.5)
             fimbrial cyst (Q50.4)
             Gartner's duct cyst (Q52.4)
             parovarian cyst (Q50.5)

     D28.0 Benign neoplasm of vulva

     D28.1 Benign neoplasm of vagina

     D28.2 Benign neoplasm of uterine tubes and ligaments
         Benign neoplasm of fallopian tube
         Benign neoplasm of uterine ligament (broad) (round)

     D28.7 Benign neoplasm of other specified female genital organs

     D28.9 Benign neoplasm of female genital organ, unspecified

● **D29** **Benign neoplasm of male genital organs**
     Includes benign neoplasm of skin of male genital organs

     D29.0 Benign neoplasm of penis

     D29.1 Benign neoplasm of prostate
         Excludes1 enlarged prostate (N40.-)

●   **D29.2** Benign neoplasm of testis
         Use additional code to identify any functional activity.

         D29.20 Benign neoplasm of unspecified testis
         D29.21 Benign neoplasm of right testis
         D29.22 Benign neoplasm of left testis

●   **D29.3** Benign neoplasm of epididymis
         D29.30 Benign neoplasm of unspecified epididymis
         D29.31 Benign neoplasm of right epididymis
         D29.32 Benign neoplasm of left epididymis

     D29.4 Benign neoplasm of scrotum
         Benign neoplasm of skin of scrotum

     D29.8 Benign neoplasm of other specified male genital organs
         Benign neoplasm of seminal vesicle
         Benign neoplasm of spermatic cord
         Benign neoplasm of tunica vaginalis

     D29.9 Benign neoplasm of male genital organ, unspecified

● **D30** **Benign neoplasm of urinary organs**

●   **D30.0** Benign neoplasm of kidney
         Excludes1 benign carcinoid tumor of the kidney (D3A.093)
                 benign neoplasm of renal calyces (D30.1-)
                 benign neoplasm of renal pelvis (D30.1-)

         D30.00 Benign neoplasm of unspecified kidney
         D30.01 Benign neoplasm of right kidney
         D30.02 Benign neoplasm of left kidney

●   **D30.1** Benign neoplasm of renal pelvis
         D30.10 Benign neoplasm of unspecified renal pelvis
         D30.11 Benign neoplasm of right renal pelvis
         D30.12 Benign neoplasm of left renal pelvis

●   **D30.2** Benign neoplasm of ureter
         Excludes1 benign neoplasm of ureteric orifice of bladder (D30.3)

         D30.20 Benign neoplasm of unspecified ureter
         D30.21 Benign neoplasm of right ureter
         D30.22 Benign neoplasm of left ureter

     D30.3 Benign neoplasm of bladder
         Benign neoplasm of ureteric orifice of bladder
         Benign neoplasm of urethral orifice of bladder

     D30.4 Benign neoplasm of urethra
         Excludes1 benign neoplasm of urethral orifice of bladder (D30.3)

     D30.8 Benign neoplasm of other specified urinary organs
         Benign neoplasm of paraurethral glands

     D30.9 Benign neoplasm of urinary organ, unspecified
         Benign neoplasm of urinary system NOS

● **D31** **Benign neoplasm of eye and adnexa**
     Excludes1 benign neoplasm of connective tissue of eyelid (D21.0)
             benign neoplasm of optic nerve (D33.3)
             benign neoplasm of skin of eyelid (D22.1-, D23.1-)

●   **D31.0** Benign neoplasm of conjunctiva
         D31.00 Benign neoplasm of unspecified conjunctiva
         D31.01 Benign neoplasm of right conjunctiva
         D31.02 Benign neoplasm of left conjunctiva

▶ New   ⇒ Revised   ~~deleted~~ Deleted   Excludes 1   Excludes 2   Includes   Use additional   Code first   Code also   Key words

664   OGCR Official Guidelines   X Assign placeholder X   ● Use Additional Character(s)   ▶ Manifestation Code   🏷 Hierarchical Condition Category   **Coding Clinic**

● **D31.1**   **Benign neoplasm of cornea**

     D31.10   Benign neoplasm of unspecified cornea

     D31.11   Benign neoplasm of right cornea

     D31.12   Benign neoplasm of left cornea

● **D31.2**   **Benign neoplasm of retina**

     Excludes1   dark area on retina (D49.81)
                 hemangioma of retina (D49.81)
                 neoplasm of unspecified behavior of
                      retina and choroid (D49.81)
                 retinal freckle (D49.81)

     D31.20   Benign neoplasm of unspecified retina

     D31.21   Benign neoplasm of right retina

     D31.22   Benign neoplasm of left retina

● **D31.3**   **Benign neoplasm of choroid**

     D31.30   Benign neoplasm of unspecified choroid

     D31.31   Benign neoplasm of right choroid

     D31.32   Benign neoplasm of left choroid

● **D31.4**   **Benign neoplasm of ciliary body**

     D31.40   Benign neoplasm of unspecified ciliary body

     D31.41   Benign neoplasm of right ciliary body

     D31.42   Benign neoplasm of left ciliary body

● **D31.5**   **Benign neoplasm of lacrimal gland and duct**
       Benign neoplasm of lacrimal sac
       Benign neoplasm of nasolacrimal duct

     D31.50   Benign neoplasm of unspecified lacrimal gland
               and duct

     D31.51   Benign neoplasm of right lacrimal gland and
               duct

     D31.52   Benign neoplasm of left lacrimal gland and
               duct

● **D31.6**   **Benign neoplasm of unspecified site of orbit**
       Benign neoplasm of connective tissue of orbit
       Benign neoplasm of extraocular muscle
       Benign neoplasm of peripheral nerves of orbit
       Benign neoplasm of retrobulbar tissue
       Benign neoplasm of retro-ocular tissue

     Excludes1   benign neoplasm of orbital bone (D16.4)

     D31.60   Benign neoplasm of unspecified site of
               unspecified orbit

     D31.61   Benign neoplasm of unspecified site of right
               orbit

     D31.62   Benign neoplasm of unspecified site of left
               orbit

● **D31.9**   **Benign neoplasm of unspecified part of eye**
       Benign neoplasm of eyeball

     D31.90   Benign neoplasm of unspecified part of
               unspecified eye

     D31.91   Benign neoplasm of unspecified part of right
               eye

     D31.92   Benign neoplasm of unspecified part of left eye

● **D32**   **Benign neoplasm of meninges**

     D32.0   Benign neoplasm of cerebral meninges 🐾

     D32.1   Benign neoplasm of spinal meninges 🐾

     D32.9   Benign neoplasm of meninges, unspecified 🐾
              Meningioma NOS

● **D33**   **Benign neoplasm of brain and other parts of central nervous system**

     Excludes1   angioma (D18.0-)
                 benign neoplasm of meninges (D32.-)
                 benign neoplasm of peripheral nerves and
                    autonomic nervous system (D36.1-)
                 hemangioma (D18.0-)
                 neurofibromatosis (Q85.0-)
                 retro-ocular benign neoplasm (D31.6-)

     D33.0   Benign neoplasm of brain, supratentorial 🐾
              Benign neoplasm of cerebral ventricle
              Benign neoplasm of cerebrum
              Benign neoplasm of frontal lobe
              Benign neoplasm of occipital lobe
              Benign neoplasm of parietal lobe
              Benign neoplasm of temporal lobe

         Excludes1   benign neoplasm of fourth ventricle
                       (D33.1)

     D33.1   Benign neoplasm of brain, infratentorial 🐾
              Benign neoplasm of brain stem
              Benign neoplasm of cerebellum
              Benign neoplasm of fourth ventricle

     D33.2   Benign neoplasm of brain, unspecified 🐾

     D33.3   Benign neoplasm of cranial nerves 🐾
              Benign neoplasm of olfactory bulb

     D33.4   Benign neoplasm of spinal cord 🐾

     D33.7   Benign neoplasm of other specified parts of central
         nervous system 🐾

     D33.9   Benign neoplasm of central nervous
         system, unspecified 🐾
              Benign neoplasm of nervous system (central) NOS

D34   **Benign neoplasm of thyroid gland**
       Use additional code to identify any functional activity.

● **D35**   **Benign neoplasm of other and unspecified endocrine glands**
       Use additional code to identify any functional activity.

     Excludes1   benign neoplasm of endocrine pancreas (D13.7)
                 benign neoplasm of ovary (D27.-)
                 benign neoplasm of testis (D29.2.-)
                 benign neoplasm of thymus (D15.0)

     ● **D35.0**   Benign neoplasm of adrenal gland

         D35.00   Benign neoplasm of unspecified adrenal gland

         D35.01   Benign neoplasm of right adrenal gland

         D35.02   Benign neoplasm of left adrenal gland

     D35.1   Benign neoplasm of parathyroid gland

     D35.2   Benign neoplasm of pituitary gland 🐾

     D35.3   Benign neoplasm of craniopharyngeal duct 🐾

     D35.4   Benign neoplasm of pineal gland 🐾

     D35.5   Benign neoplasm of carotid body

     D35.6   Benign neoplasm of aortic body and other paraganglia
              Benign tumor of glomus jugulare

     D35.7   Benign neoplasm of other specified endocrine glands

     D35.9   Benign neoplasm of endocrine gland, unspecified
              Benign neoplasm of unspecified endocrine gland

● **D36**   **Benign neoplasm of other and unspecified sites**

     D36.0   Benign neoplasm of lymph nodes

         Excludes1   lymphangioma (D18.1)

     ● **D36.1**   Benign neoplasm of peripheral nerves and autonomic nervous system

         Excludes1   benign neoplasm of peripheral nerves of
                     orbit (D31.6-)
                     neurofibromatosis (Q85.0-)

         D36.10   Benign neoplasm of peripheral nerves and
                 autonomic nervous system, unspecified

         D36.11   Benign neoplasm of peripheral nerves and
                 autonomic nervous system of face, head, and
                 neck

         D36.12   Benign neoplasm of peripheral nerves and
                 autonomic nervous system, upper limb,
                 including shoulder

         D36.13   Benign neoplasm of peripheral nerves and
                 autonomic nervous system of lower limb,
                 including hip

         D36.14   Benign neoplasm of peripheral nerves and
                 autonomic nervous system of thorax

         D36.15   Benign neoplasm of peripheral nerves and
                 autonomic nervous system of abdomen

CHAPTER 2 (C00-D49)

D36.16　Benign neoplasm of peripheral nerves and autonomic nervous system of pelvis

D36.17　Benign neoplasm of peripheral nerves and autonomic nervous system of trunk, unspecified

D36.7　Benign neoplasm of other specified sites
Benign neoplasm of nose NOS
Benign neoplasm of back NOS

D36.9　Benign neoplasm, unspecified site

NEOPLASMS OF UNCERTAIN BEHAVIOR, POLYCYTHEMIA VERA AND MYELODYSPLASTIC SYNDROMES (D37-D48)

Note: Categories D37-D44, and D48 classify by site neoplasms of uncertain behavior, i.e., histologic confirmation whether the neoplasm is malignant or benign cannot be made.
Excludes1 neoplasms of unspecified behavior (D49.-)

D37　Neoplasm of uncertain behavior of oral cavity and digestive organs
Excludes1 stromal tumors of uncertain behavior of digestive system (D48.1-)

D37.0　Neoplasm of uncertain behavior of lip, oral cavity and pharynx
Excludes1 neoplasm of uncertain behavior of aryepiglottic fold or interarytenoid fold, laryngeal aspect (D38.0)
neoplasm of uncertain behavior of epiglottis NOS (D38.0)
neoplasm of uncertain behavior of skin of lip (D48.5)
neoplasm of uncertain behavior of suprahyoid portion of epiglottis (D38.0)

D37.01　Neoplasm of uncertain behavior of lip
Neoplasm of uncertain behavior of vermilion border of lip

D37.02　Neoplasm of uncertain behavior of tongue

D37.03　Neoplasm of uncertain behavior of the major salivary glands
D37.030　Neoplasm of uncertain behavior of the parotid salivary glands
D37.031　Neoplasm of uncertain behavior of the sublingual salivary glands
D37.032　Neoplasm of uncertain behavior of the submandibular salivary glands
D37.039　Neoplasm of uncertain behavior of the major salivary glands, unspecified

D37.04　Neoplasm of uncertain behavior of the minor salivary glands
Neoplasm of uncertain behavior of submucosal salivary glands of lip
Neoplasm of uncertain behavior of submucosal salivary glands of cheek
Neoplasm of uncertain behavior of submucosal salivary glands of hard palate
Neoplasm of uncertain behavior of submucosal salivary glands of soft palate

D37.05　Neoplasm of uncertain behavior of pharynx
Neoplasm of uncertain behavior of aryepiglottic fold of pharynx NOS
Neoplasm of uncertain behavior of hypopharyngeal aspect of aryepiglottic fold of pharynx
Neoplasm of uncertain behavior of marginal zone of aryepiglottic fold of pharynx

D37.09　Neoplasm of uncertain behavior of other specified sites of the oral cavity

D37.1　Neoplasm of uncertain behavior of stomach

D37.2　Neoplasm of uncertain behavior of small intestine

D37.3　Neoplasm of uncertain behavior of appendix

D37.4　Neoplasm of uncertain behavior of colon

D37.5　Neoplasm of uncertain behavior of rectum
Neoplasm of uncertain behavior of rectosigmoid junction
Rectosigmoid junction: Angle where sigmoid colon becomes rectum

D37.6　Neoplasm of uncertain behavior of liver, gallbladder and bile ducts
Neoplasm of uncertain behavior of ampulla of Vater
Ampulla of Vater: Enlarged segment of ducts from liver and pancreas at entry point to small intestine

D37.8　Neoplasm of uncertain behavior of other specified digestive organs
Neoplasm of uncertain behavior of anal canal
Neoplasm of uncertain behavior of anal sphincter
Neoplasm of uncertain behavior of anus NOS
Neoplasm of uncertain behavior of esophagus
Neoplasm of uncertain behavior of intestine NOS
Neoplasm of uncertain behavior of pancreas
Excludes1 neoplasm of uncertain behavior of anal margin (D48.5)
neoplasm of uncertain behavior of anal skin (D48.5)
neoplasm of uncertain behavior of perianal skin (D48.5)

D37.9　Neoplasm of uncertain behavior of digestive organ, unspecified

D38　Neoplasm of uncertain behavior of middle ear and respiratory and intrathoracic organs
Excludes1 neoplasm of uncertain behavior of heart (D48.7)

D38.0　Neoplasm of uncertain behavior of larynx
Neoplasm of uncertain behavior of aryepiglottic fold or interarytenoid fold, laryngeal aspect
Neoplasm of uncertain behavior of epiglottis (suprahyoid portion)
Excludes1 neoplasm of uncertain behavior of aryepiglottic fold or interarytenoid fold NOS (D37.05)
neoplasm of uncertain behavior of hypopharyngeal aspect of aryepiglottic fold (D37.05)
neoplasm of uncertain behavior of marginal zone of aryepiglottic fold (D37.05)

D38.1　Neoplasm of uncertain behavior of trachea, bronchus and lung

D38.2　Neoplasm of uncertain behavior of pleura

D38.3　Neoplasm of uncertain behavior of mediastinum

D38.4　Neoplasm of uncertain behavior of thymus

D38.5　Neoplasm of uncertain behavior of other respiratory organs
Neoplasm of uncertain behavior of accessory sinuses
Neoplasm of uncertain behavior of cartilage of nose
Neoplasm of uncertain behavior of middle ear
Neoplasm of uncertain behavior of nasal cavities
Excludes1 neoplasm of uncertain behavior of ear (external) (skin) (D48.5)
neoplasm of uncertain behavior of nose NOS (D48.7)
neoplasm of uncertain behavior of skin of nose (D48.5)

D38.6　Neoplasm of uncertain behavior of respiratory organ, unspecified

D39　Neoplasm of uncertain behavior of female genital organs

D39.0　Neoplasm of uncertain behavior of uterus

D39.1　Neoplasm of uncertain behavior of ovary
Use additional code to identify any functional activity.
D39.10　Neoplasm of uncertain behavior of unspecified ovary
D39.11　Neoplasm of uncertain behavior of right ovary
D39.12　Neoplasm of uncertain behavior of left ovary

D39.2 Neoplasm of uncertain behavior of placentaM
        Chorioadenoma destruens
        Invasive hydatidiform mole
        Malignant hydatidiform mole
        Excludes1   hydatidiform mole NOS (O01.9)
        Coding Clinic: 2023, Q3, P15

D39.8 Neoplasm of uncertain behavior of other specified female genital organs
        Neoplasm of uncertain behavior of skin of female genital organs

D39.9 Neoplasm of uncertain behavior of female genital organ, unspecified

BENIGN NEUROENDOCRINE TUMORS (D3A)

⬤**D3A** Benign neuroendocrine tumors
        Code also any associated multiple endocrine neoplasia [MEN] syndromes (E31.2-)
        Use additional code to identify any associated endocrine syndrome, such as:
           carcinoid syndrome (E34.00)
        Excludes2   benign pancreatic islet cell tumors (D13.7)
   ⬤**D3A.0** Benign carcinoid tumors
        D3A.00 Benign carcinoid tumor of unspecified site
           Carcinoid tumor NOS
     ⬤**D3A.01** Benign carcinoid tumors of the small intestine
           D3A.010 Benign carcinoid tumor of the duodenum
           D3A.011 Benign carcinoid tumor of the jejunum
           D3A.012 Benign carcinoid tumor of the ileum
           D3A.019 Benign carcinoid tumor of the small intestine, unspecified portion
     ⬤**D3A.02** Benign carcinoid tumors of the appendix, large intestine, and rectum
           D3A.020 Benign carcinoid tumor of the appendix
           D3A.021 Benign carcinoid tumor of the cecum
           D3A.022 Benign carcinoid tumor of the ascending colon
           D3A.023 Benign carcinoid tumor of the transverse colon
           D3A.024 Benign carcinoid tumor of the descending colon
           D3A.025 Benign carcinoid tumor of the sigmoid colon
           D3A.026 Benign carcinoid tumor of the rectum
           D3A.029 Benign carcinoid tumor of the large intestine, unspecified portion
              Benign carcinoid tumor of the colon NOS
     ⬤**D3A.09** Benign carcinoid tumors of other sites
           D3A.090 Benign carcinoid tumor of the bronchus and lung
           D3A.091 Benign carcinoid tumor of the thymus
           D3A.092 Benign carcinoid tumor of the stomach
           D3A.093 Benign carcinoid tumor of the kidney
           D3A.094 Benign carcinoid tumor of the foregut, unspecified
           D3A.095 Benign carcinoid tumor of the midgut, unspecified
           D3A.096 Benign carcinoid tumor of the hindgut, unspecified
           D3A.098 Benign carcinoid tumors of other sites
   D3A.8 Other benign neuroendocrine tumors
        Neuroendocrine tumor NOS

Figure 2-19   Major salivary glands.

Parotid gland

Sublingual gland

Submandibular gland

⬤**D40** Neoplasm of uncertain behavior of male genital organs
        D40.0 Neoplasm of uncertain behavior of prostate
   ⬤**D40.1** Neoplasm of uncertain behavior of testis
           D40.10 Neoplasm of uncertain behavior of unspecified testis
           D40.11 Neoplasm of uncertain behavior of right testis
           D40.12 Neoplasm of uncertain behavior of left testis
        D40.8 Neoplasm of uncertain behavior of other specified male genital organs
           Neoplasm of uncertain behavior of skin of male genital organs
        D40.9 Neoplasm of uncertain behavior of male genital organ, unspecified

⬤**D41** Neoplasm of uncertain behavior of urinary organs
   ⬤**D41.0** Neoplasm of uncertain behavior of kidney
        Excludes1   neoplasm of uncertain behavior of renal pelvis (D41.1-)
           D41.00 Neoplasm of uncertain behavior of unspecified kidney
           D41.01 Neoplasm of uncertain behavior of right kidney
           D41.02 Neoplasm of uncertain behavior of left kidney
   ⬤**D41.1** Neoplasm of uncertain behavior of renal pelvis
           D41.10 Neoplasm of uncertain behavior of unspecified renal pelvis
           D41.11 Neoplasm of uncertain behavior of right renal pelvis
           D41.12 Neoplasm of uncertain behavior of left renal pelvis
   ⬤**D41.2** Neoplasm of uncertain behavior of ureter
           D41.20 Neoplasm of uncertain behavior of unspecified ureter
           D41.21 Neoplasm of uncertain behavior of right ureter
           D41.22 Neoplasm of uncertain behavior of left ureter
        D41.3 Neoplasm of uncertain behavior of urethra
        D41.4 Neoplasm of uncertain behavior of bladder
        D41.8 Neoplasm of uncertain behavior of other specified urinary organs
        D41.9 Neoplasm of uncertain behavior of unspecified urinary organ

⬤**D42** Neoplasm of uncertain behavior of meninges
        D42.0 Neoplasm of uncertain behavior of cerebral meninges
        D42.1 Neoplasm of uncertain behavior of spinal meninges
        D42.9 Neoplasm of uncertain behavior of meninges, unspecified

CHAPTER 2 (C00-D49)

- **D43 Neoplasm of uncertain behavior of brain and central nervous system**
  - **Excludes1** neoplasm of uncertain behavior of peripheral nerves and autonomic nervous system (D48.2)
  - **D43.0 Neoplasm of uncertain behavior of brain, supratentorial** 🦠
    - *Superior to tentorium of cerebellum*
    - Neoplasm of uncertain behavior of cerebral ventricle
    - Neoplasm of uncertain behavior of cerebrum
    - Neoplasm of uncertain behavior of frontal lobe
    - Neoplasm of uncertain behavior of occipital lobe
    - Neoplasm of uncertain behavior of parietal lobe
    - Neoplasm of uncertain behavior of temporal lobe
      - **Excludes1** neoplasm of uncertain behavior of fourth ventricle (D43.1)
  - **D43.1 Neoplasm of uncertain behavior of brain, infratentorial** 🦠
    - *Beneath the tentorium of cerebellum*
    - Neoplasm of uncertain behavior of brain stem
    - Neoplasm of uncertain behavior of cerebellum
    - Neoplasm of uncertain behavior of fourth ventricle
    - Coding Clinic: 2023, Q2, P16
  - **D43.2 Neoplasm of uncertain behavior of brain, unspecified** 🦠
  - **D43.3 Neoplasm of uncertain behavior of cranial nerves** 🦠
  - **D43.4 Neoplasm of uncertain behavior of spinal cord** 🦠
  - **D43.8 Neoplasm of uncertain behavior of other specified parts of central nervous system** 🦠
  - **D43.9 Neoplasm of uncertain behavior of central nervous system, unspecified** 🦠
    - Neoplasm of uncertain behavior of nervous system (central) NOS
- **D44 Neoplasm of uncertain behavior of endocrine glands**
  - **Excludes1** multiple endocrine adenomatosis (E31.2-)
    - multiple endocrine neoplasia (E31.2-)
    - neoplasm of uncertain behavior of endocrine pancreas (D37.8)
    - neoplasm of uncertain behavior of ovary (D39.1-)
    - neoplasm of uncertain behavior of testis (D40.1-)
    - neoplasm of uncertain behavior of thymus (D38.4)
  - **D44.0 Neoplasm of uncertain behavior of thyroid gland**
  - **D44.1 Neoplasm of uncertain behavior of adrenal gland**
    - Use additional code to identify any functional activity.
    - **D44.10 Neoplasm of uncertain behavior of unspecified adrenal gland**
    - **D44.11 Neoplasm of uncertain behavior of right adrenal gland**
    - **D44.12 Neoplasm of uncertain behavior of left adrenal gland**
  - **D44.2 Neoplasm of uncertain behavior of parathyroid gland**
  - **D44.3 Neoplasm of uncertain behavior of pituitary gland** 🦠
    - Use additional code to identify any functional activity.
  - **D44.4 Neoplasm of uncertain behavior of craniopharyngeal duct** 🦠
  - **D44.5 Neoplasm of uncertain behavior of pineal gland** 🦠
  - **D44.6 Neoplasm of uncertain behavior of carotid body** 🦠
  - **D44.7 Neoplasm of uncertain behavior of aortic body and other paraganglia** 🦠
    - Coding Clinic: 2016, Q4, P26
  - **D44.9 Neoplasm of uncertain behavior of unspecified endocrine gland**

- **D45 Polycythemia vera** 🦠
  - **Excludes1** familial polycythemia (D75.0)
    - secondary polycythemia (D75.1)
  - *Primary polycythemia. Secondary polycythemia is D75.1. Check your documentation. Polycythemia is caused by too many red blood cells, which increase the thickness of blood (viscosity). This can cause engorgement of the spleen (splenomegaly) with extra RBCs and potential clot formation.*
- **D46 Myelodysplastic syndromes**
  - Use additional code for adverse effect, if applicable, to identify drug (T36-T50 with fifth or sixth character 5)
  - **Excludes2** drug-induced aplastic anemia (D61.1)
  - **D46.0 Refractory anemia without ring sideroblasts, so stated** 🦠
    - Refractory anemia without sideroblasts, without excess of blasts
  - **D46.1 Refractory anemia with ring sideroblasts RARS** 🦠
  - **D46.2 Refractory anemia with excess of blasts [RAEB]**
    - *Form of myelodysplasia with increased immature white blood cells (blasts) in bone marrow*
    - **D46.20 Refractory anemia with excess of blasts, unspecified RAEB NOS** 🦠
    - **D46.21 Refractory anemia with excess of blasts 1 RAEB 1** 🦠
      - *Bone marrow disease which results in insufficient RBCs (anemia) in which level of blasts is less than 10%*
    - **D46.22 Refractory anemia with excess of blasts 2 RAEB 2** 🦠
      - *Bone marrow disease manifested by insufficient numbers of RBCs (anemia) with level of blasts 10-20%*
  - **D46.A Refractory cytopenia with multilineage dysplasia** 🦠
  - **D46.B Refractory cytopenia with multilineage dysplasia and ring sideroblasts** 🦠
    - RCMD RS
  - **D46.C Myelodysplastic syndrome with isolated del(5q) chromosomal abnormality** 🦠
    - Myelodysplastic syndrome with 5q deletion
    - 5q minus syndrome NOS
  - **D46.4 Refractory anemia, unspecified** 🦠
  - **D46.Z Other myelodysplastic syndromes** 🦠
    - **Excludes1** chronic myelomonocytic leukemia (C93.1-)
  - **D46.9 Myelodysplastic syndrome, unspecified** 🦠
    - Myelodysplasia NOS
- **D47 Other neoplasms of uncertain behavior of lymphoid, hematopoietic and related tissue**
  - **D47.0 Mast cell neoplasms of uncertain behavior**
    - **Excludes1** congenital cutaneous mastocytosis (Q82.2)
      - histiocytic neoplasms of uncertain behavior (D47.Z9)
      - malignant mast cell neoplasm (C96.2-)
    - **D47.01 Cutaneous mastocytosis**
      - Diffuse cutaneous mastocytosis
      - Maculopapular cutaneous mastocytosis
      - Solitary mastocytoma
      - Telangiectasia macularis eruptiva perstans
      - Urticaria pigmentosa
      - **Excludes1** congenit[a]l (diffuse) (maculopapular) cutaneous mastocytosis (Q82.2)
        - congenital urticaria pigmentosa (Q82.2)
        - extracutaneous mastocytoma (D47.09)

▶ New ⇒ Revised ~~deleted~~ Deleted Excludes 1 Excludes 2 Includes Use additional Code first Code also Key words
OGCR Official Guidelines X Assign placeholder X ● Use Additional Character(s) ▷ Manifestation Code 🦠 Hierarchical Condition Category Coding Clinic

D47.02 Systemic mastocytosis
Indolent systemic mastocytosis
Isolated bone marrow mastocytosis
Smoldering systemic mastocytosis
Systemic mastocytosis, with an associated hematological non-mast cell lineage disease (SM-AHNMD)

Code also if applicable, any associated hematological non-mast cell lineage disease, such as:
acute myeloid leukemia (C92.6-, C92.A-)
chronic myelomonocytic leukemia (C93.1-)
essential thrombocytosis (D47.3)
hypereosinophilic syndrome (D72.1)
myelodysplastic syndrome (D46.9)
myeloproliferative syndrome (D47.1)
non-Hodgkin lymphoma (C82-C85)
plasma cell myeloma (C90.0-)
polycythemia vera (D45)

Excludes1   aggressive systemic mastocytosis (C96.21)
mast cell leukemia (C94.3-)

D47.09 Other mast cell neoplasms of uncertain behavior
Extracutaneous mastocytoma
Mast cell tumor NOS
Mastocytoma NOS
Mastocytosis NOS

D47.1 Chronic myeloproliferative disease 🔖
Chronic neutrophilic leukemia
Myeloproliferative disease, unspecified

Excludes1   atypical chronic myeloid leukemia BCR/ABL-negative (C92.2-)
chronic myeloid leukemia BCR/ABL-positive (C92.1-)
myelofibrosis NOS (D75.81)
myelophthisic anemia (D61.82)
myelophthisis (D61.82)
secondary myelofibrosis NOS (D75.81)

D47.2 Monoclonal gammopathy
Monoclonal gammopathy of undetermined significance [MGUS]
Coding Clinic: 2021, Q3, P5

D47.3 Essential (hemorrhagic) thrombocythemia 🔖
Essential thrombocytosis
Idiopathic hemorrhagic thrombocythemia
Primary thrombocytosis

Excludes2   reactive thrombocytosis (D75.838)
secondary thrombocytosis (D75.838)
thrombocythemia NOS (D75.839)
thrombocytosis NOS (D75.839)

D47.4 Osteomyelofibrosis 🔖
Chronic idiopathic myelofibrosis
Myelofibrosis (idiopathic) (with myeloid metaplasia)
Myelosclerosis (megakaryocytic) with myeloid metaplasia
Secondary myelofibrosis in myeloproliferative disease

Excludes1   acute myelofibrosis (C94.4-)

D47.9 Neoplasm of uncertain behavior of lymphoid, hematopoietic and related tissue, unspecified 🔖
Lymphoproliferative disease NOS

⬤**D47.Z Other specified neoplasms of uncertain behavior of lymphoid, hematopoietic and related tissue**

D47.Z1 Post-transplant lymphoproliferative disorder (PTLD) 🔖
Code first complications of transplanted organs and tissue (T86.-)

D47.Z2 Castleman disease 🔖
Code also if applicable, human herpesvirus 8 infection (B10.89)

Excludes2   Kaposi's sarcoma (C46.-)
Coding Clinic: 2016, Q4, P8

D47.Z9 Other specified neoplasms of uncertain behavior of lymphoid, hematopoietic and related tissue 🔖
Histiocytic tumors of uncertain behavior

⬤**D48 Neoplasm of uncertain behavior of other and unspecified sites**

Excludes1   neurofibromatosis (nonmalignant) (Q85.0-)

D48.0 Neoplasm of uncertain behavior of bone and articular cartilage

Excludes1   neoplasm of uncertain behavior of cartilage of ear (D48.1-)
neoplasm of uncertain behavior of cartilage of larynx (D38.0)
neoplasm of uncertain behavior of cartilage of nose (D38.5)
neoplasm of uncertain behavior of connective tissue of eyelid (D48.1-)
neoplasm of uncertain behavior of synovia (D48.1-)

⬤**D48.1 Neoplasm of uncertain behavior of connective and other soft tissue**
Neoplasm of uncertain behavior of connective tissue of ear
Neoplasm of uncertain behavior of connective tissue of eyelid
Stromal tumors of uncertain behavior of digestive system

Excludes1   neoplasm of uncertain behavior of articular cartilage (D48.0)
neoplasm of uncertain behavior of cartilage of larynx (D38.0)
neoplasm of uncertain behavior of cartilage of nose (D38.5)
neoplasm of uncertain behavior of connective tissue of breast (D48.6-)

⬤**D48.11 Desmoid tumor**

D48.110 Desmoid tumor of head and neck

D48.111 Desmoid tumor of chest wall

D48.112 Desmoid tumor, intrathoracic

D48.113 Desmoid tumor of abdominal wall

D48.114 Desmoid tumor, intraabdomin
Desmoid tumor of pelvic cavity
Desmoid tumor, peritoneal, retroperitoneal

D48.115 Desmoid tumor of upper extremity and shoulder girdle

D48.116 Desmoid tumor of lower extremity and pelvic girdle
Desmoid tumor of buttock

D48.117 Desmoid tumor of back

D48.118 Desmoid tumor of other site

D48.119 Desmoid tumor of unspecified site

D48.19 Other specified neoplasm of uncertain behavior of connective and other soft tissue

D48.2 Neoplasm of uncertain behavior of peripheral nerves and autonomic nervous system

Excludes1   neoplasm of uncertain behavior of peripheral nerves of orbit (D48.7)

D48.3 Neoplasm of uncertain behavior of retroperitoneum

D48.4 Neoplasm of uncertain behavior of peritoneum

CHAPTER 2 (C00–D49)

D48.5   Neoplasm of uncertain behavior of skin
     Neoplasm of uncertain behavior of anal margin
     Neoplasm of uncertain behavior of anal skin
     Neoplasm of uncertain behavior of perianal skin
     Neoplasm of uncertain behavior of skin of breast
     Excludes1   neoplasm of uncertain behavior of anus
              NOS (D37.8)
              neoplasm of uncertain behavior of skin of
                genital organs (D39.8, D40.8)
              neoplasm of uncertain behavior of
                vermilion border of lip (D37.0)

● **D48.6   Neoplasm of uncertain behavior of breast**
     Neoplasm of uncertain behavior of connective tissue of
        breast
     Cystosarcoma phyllodes
     Excludes1   neoplasm of uncertain behavior of skin of
              breast (D48.5)

     **D48.60   Neoplasm of uncertain behavior of unspecified
               breast**
     D48.61   Neoplasm of uncertain behavior of right breast
     D48.62   Neoplasm of uncertain behavior of left breast

D48.7   Neoplasm of uncertain behavior of other specified sites
     Neoplasm of uncertain behavior of eye
     Neoplasm of uncertain behavior of heart
     Neoplasm of uncertain behavior of peripheral nerves
        of orbit
     Excludes1   neoplasm of uncertain behavior of
              connective tissue (D48.1-)
              neoplasm of uncertain behavior of skin of
                eyelid (D48.5)

D48.9   Neoplasm of uncertain behavior, unspecified

● **D49   Neoplasms of unspecified behavior**
     Note: Category D49 classifies by site neoplasms of unspecified
        morphology and behavior. The term "mass," unless
        otherwise stated, is not to be regarded as a neoplastic growth.
     Includes   'growth' NOS
                 neoplasm NOS
                 new growth NOS
                 tumor NOS
     Excludes1   neoplasms of uncertain behavior (D37-D44, D48)

D49.0   Neoplasm of unspecified behavior of digestive system
     Excludes1   neoplasm of unspecified behavior of
              margin of anus (D49.2)
              neoplasm of unspecified behavior of
                perianal skin (D49.2)
              neoplasm of unspecified behavior of skin
                of anus (D49.2)

D49.1   Neoplasm of unspecified behavior of respiratory system

**D49.2   Neoplasm of unspecified behavior of bone, soft tissue,
         and skin**
     Excludes1   neoplasm of unspecified behavior of anal
              canal (D49.0)
              neoplasm of unspecified behavior of anus
                NOS (D49.0)
              neoplasm of unspecified behavior of bone
                marrow (D49.89)
              neoplasm of unspecified behavior of
                cartilage of larynx (D49.1)
              neoplasm of unspecified behavior of
                cartilage of nose (D49.1)
              neoplasm of unspecified behavior of
                connective tissue of breast (D49.3)
              neoplasm of unspecified behavior of skin
                of genital organs (D49.59)
              neoplasm of unspecified behavior of
                vermilion border of lip (D49.0)

D49.3   Neoplasm of unspecified behavior of breast
     Excludes1   neoplasm of unspecified behavior of skin
              of breast (D49.2)

D49.4   Neoplasm of unspecified behavior of bladder

● **D49.5   Neoplasm of unspecified behavior of other
         genitourinary organs**
     ● **D49.51   Neoplasm of unspecified behavior of kidney**
         **D49.511   Neoplasm of unspecified behavior of
                   right kidney**
                   Coding Clinic: 2016, Q4, P9
         **D49.512   Neoplasm of unspecified behavior of
                   left kidney**
                   Coding Clinic: 2016, Q4, P9
         **D49.519   Neoplasm of unspecified behavior of
                   unspecified kidney**
                   Coding Clinic: 2016, Q4, P9
     **D49.59   Neoplasm of unspecified behavior of other
               genitourinary organ**
              Coding Clinic: 2016, Q4, P9

D49.6   Neoplasm of unspecified behavior of brain 🐾
     Excludes1   neoplasm of unspecified behavior of
              cerebral meninges (D49.7)
              neoplasm of unspecified behavior of
                cranial nerves (D49.7)

**D49.7   Neoplasm of unspecified behavior of endocrine glands
         and other parts of nervous system**
     Excludes1   neoplasm of unspecified behavior
              of peripheral, sympathetic, and
              parasympathetic nerves and ganglia
              (D49.2)

● **D49.8   Neoplasm of unspecified behavior of other specified
         sites**
     Excludes1   neoplasm of unspecified behavior of
              eyelid (skin) (D49.2)
              neoplasm of unspecified behavior of
                eyelid cartilage (D49.2)
              neoplasm of unspecified behavior of great
                vessels (D49.2)
              neoplasm of unspecified behavior of optic
                nerve (D49.7)

     **D49.81   Neoplasm of unspecified behavior of retina and
               choroid**
             Dark area on retina
             Retinal freckle
     **D49.89   Neoplasm of unspecified behavior of other
               specified sites**

D49.9   Neoplasm of unspecified behavior of unspecified site

OGCR Chapter-Specific Coding Guidelines
3. Chapter 3: Disease of the blood and blood-forming organs and certain disorders involving the immune mechanism (D50-D89) Reserved for future guideline expansion

CHAPTER 3

DISEASES OF THE BLOOD AND BLOOD-FORMING ORGANS AND CERTAIN DISORDERS INVOLVING THE IMMUNE MECHANISM (D50-D89)

Excludes2   autoimmune disease (systemic) NOS (M35.9)
certain conditions originating in the perinatal period (P00-P96)
complications of pregnancy, childbirth and the puerperium (O00-O9A)
congenital malformations, deformations and chromosomal abnormalities (Q00-Q99)
endocrine, nutritional and metabolic diseases (E00-E88)
human immunodeficiency virus [HIV] disease (B20)
injury, poisoning and certain other consequences of external causes (S00-T88)
neoplasms (C00-D49)
symptoms, signs and abnormal clinical and laboratory findings, not elsewhere classified (R00-R94)

This chapter contains the following blocks:

D50-D53	Nutritional anemias
D55-D59	Hemolytic anemias
D60-D64	Aplastic and other anemias and other bone marrow failure syndromes
D65-D69	Coagulation defects, purpura and other hemorrhagic conditions
D70-D77	Other disorders of blood and blood-forming organs
D78	Intraoperative and postprocedural complications of the spleen
D80-D89	Certain disorders involving the immune mechanism

NUTRITIONAL ANEMIAS (D50-D53)

● **D50   Iron deficiency anemia**
A disease characterized by a decrease in the number of red cells (hemoglobin) in the blood.

   Includes   asiderotic anemia
hypochromic anemia

   D50.0   Iron deficiency anemia secondary to blood loss (chronic)
Posthemorrhagic anemia (chronic)

     Excludes1   acute posthemorrhagic anemia (D62)
congenital anemia from fetal blood loss (P61.3)

     Coding Clinic: 2019, Q3, P17

   D50.1   Sideropenic dysphagia
Weblike growth of membranes in throat that makes swallowing difficult
Kelly-Paterson syndrome
Plummer-Vinson syndrome

   D50.8   Other iron deficiency anemias
Iron deficiency anemia due to inadequate dietary iron intake

   D50.9   Iron deficiency anemia, unspecified

● **D51   Vitamin B12 deficiency anemia**

   Excludes1   vitamin B12 deficiency (E53.8)

   D51.0   Vitamin B12 deficiency anemia due to intrinsic factor deficiency
Addison anemia
Biermer anemia
Pernicious (congenital) anemia
Congenital intrinsic factor deficiency

   D51.1   Vitamin B12 deficiency anemia due to selective vitamin B12 malabsorption with proteinuria
Imerslund (Gräsbeck) syndrome
Megaloblastic hereditary anemia

   D51.2   Transcobalamin II deficiency

   D51.3   Other dietary vitamin B12 deficiency anemia
Vegan anemia

   D51.8   Other vitamin B12 deficiency anemias

   D51.9   Vitamin B12 deficiency anemia, unspecified

● **D52   Folate deficiency anemia**

   Excludes1   folate deficiency without anemia (E53.8)

   D52.0   Dietary folate deficiency anemia
Nutritional megaloblastic anemia

   D52.1   Drug-induced folate deficiency anemia
Use additional code for adverse effect, if applicable, to identify drug (T36-T50 with fifth or sixth character 5)

   D52.8   Other folate deficiency anemias

   D52.9   Folate deficiency anemia, unspecified
Folic acid deficiency anemia NOS

● **D53   Other nutritional anemias**

   Includes   megaloblastic anemia unresponsive to vitamin B12 or folate therapy

   D53.0   Protein deficiency anemia
Amino-acid deficiency anemia
Orotaciduric anemia

     Excludes1   Lesch-Nyhan syndrome (E79.1)

   D53.1   Other megaloblastic anemias, not elsewhere classified
Megaloblastic anemia NOS

     Excludes1   Di Guglielmo's disease (C94.0)

   D53.2   Scorbutic anemia
Anemia resulting from deficiency of ascorbic acid (vitamin C)

     Excludes1   scurvy (E54)

   D53.8   Other specified nutritional anemias
Anemia associated with deficiency of copper
Anemia associated with deficiency of molybdenum
Anemia associated with deficiency of zinc

     Excludes1   nutritional deficiencies without anemia, such as:
copper deficiency NOS (E61.0)
molybdenum deficiency NOS (E61.5)
zinc deficiency NOS (E60)

   D53.9   Nutritional anemia, unspecified
Simple chronic anemia

     Excludes1   anemia NOS (D64.9)

     Coding Clinic: 2018, Q4, P88

HEMOLYTIC ANEMIAS (D55-D59)

● **D55   Anemia due to enzyme disorders**

   Excludes1   drug-induced enzyme deficiency anemia (D59.2)

   D55.0   Anemia due to glucose-6-phosphate dehydrogenase [G6PD] deficiency 🔗
Favism
G6PD deficiency anemia

     Excludes1   glucose-6-phosphate dehydrogenase (G6PD) deficiency without anemia (D75.A)

   D55.1   Anemia due to other disorders of glutathione metabolism 🔗
Anemia (due to) enzyme deficiencies, except G6PD, related to the hexose monophosphate [HMP] shunt pathway
Anemia (due to) hemolytic nonspherocytic (hereditary), type I

CHAPTER 3 (D50-D89)

- **D55.2 Anemia due to disorders of glycolytic enzymes** 🦠
  - **D55.21 Anemia due to pyruvate kinase deficiency**
    - PK deficiency anemia
    - Pyruvate kinase deficiency anemia
  - **D55.29 Anemia due to other disorders of glycolytic enzymes**
    - Hexokinase deficiency anemia
    - Triose-phosphate isomerase deficiency anemia
    - **Excludes1**   disorders of glycolysis not associated with anemia (E74.81-)
- **D55.3 Anemia due to disorders of nucleotide metabolism** 🦠
- **D55.8 Other anemias due to enzyme disorders** 🦠
- **D55.9 Anemia due to enzyme disorder, unspecified** 🦠

- **D56 Thalassemia**
  - *Hereditary disorders characterized by low production of hemoglobin or excessive destruction of red blood cells*
  - **Excludes1**   sickle-cell thalassemia (D57.4-)
  - **D56.0 Alpha thalassemia** 🦠
    - Alpha thalassemia major
    - Hemoglobin H Constant Spring
    - Hemoglobin H disease
    - Hydrops fetalis due to alpha thalassemia
    - Severe alpha thalassemia
    - Triple gene defect alpha thalassemia
    - Use additional code, if applicable, for hydrops fetalis due to alpha thalassemia (P56.99)
    - **Excludes1**   alpha thalassemia trait or minor (D56.3)
      - asymptomatic alpha thalassemia (D56.3)
      - hydrops fetalis due to isoimmunization (P56.0)
      - hydrops fetalis not due to immune hemolysis (P83.2)
  - **D56.1 Beta thalassemia** 🦠
    - Beta thalassemia major
    - Cooley's anemia
    - Homozygous beta thalassemia
    - Severe beta thalassemia
    - Thalassemia intermedia
    - Thalassemia major
    - **Excludes1**   beta thalassemia minor (D56.3)
      - beta thalassemia trait (D56.3)
      - delta-beta thalassemia (D56.2)
      - hemoglobin E-beta thalassemia (D56.5)
      - sickle-cell beta thalassemia (D57.4-)
  - **D56.2 Delta-beta thalassemia** 🦠
    - Homozygous delta-beta thalassemia
    - **Excludes1**   delta-beta thalassemia minor (D56.3)
      - delta-beta thalassemia trait (D56.3)
  - **D56.3 Thalassemia minor**
    - *Genetic disorders that have in common defective production of hemoglobin*
    - Alpha thalassemia minor
    - Alpha thalassemia silent carrier
    - Alpha thalassemia trait
    - Beta thalassemia minor
    - Beta thalassemia trait
    - Delta-beta thalassemia minor
    - Delta-beta thalassemia trait
    - Thalassemia trait NOS
    - **Excludes1**   alpha thalassemia (D56.0)
      - beta thalassemia (D56.1)
      - delta-beta thalassemia (D56.2)
      - hemoglobin E-beta thalassemia (D56.5)
      - sickle-cell trait (D57.3)
  - **D56.4 Hereditary persistence of fetal hemoglobin [HPFH]** 🦠
    - *Persistent production of hemoglobin*
  - **D56.5 Hemoglobin E-beta thalassemia** 🦠
    - **Excludes1**   beta thalassemia (D56.1)
      - beta thalassemia minor (D56.3)
      - beta thalassemia trait (D56.3)
      - delta-beta thalassemia (D56.2)
      - delta-beta thalassemia trait (D56.3)
      - hemoglobin E disease (D58.2)
      - other hemoglobinopathies (D58.2)
      - sickle-cell beta thalassemia (D57.4-)
  - **D56.8 Other thalassemias** 🦠
    - Dominant thalassemia
    - Hemoglobin C thalassemia
    - Mixed thalassemia
    - Thalassemia with other hemoglobinopathy
    - **Excludes1**   hemoglobin C disease (D58.2)
      - hemoglobin E disease (D58.2)
      - other hemoglobinopathies (D58.2)
      - sickle cell anemia (D57.-)
      - sickle-cell thalassemia (D57.4-)
  - **D56.9 Thalassemia, unspecified**
    - Mediterranean anemia (with other hemoglobinopathy)

- **D57 Sickle-cell disorders**
  - *Inherited disease in which red blood cells, normally disc-shaped, become crescent shaped*
  - Use additional code for any associated fever (R50.81)
  - **Excludes1**   other hemoglobinopathies (D58.-)
  - Coding Clinic: 2022, Q2, P29
  - **D57.0 Hb-SS disease with crisis**
    - Sickle-cell disease with crisis
    - Hb-SS disease with (vaso-occlusive) pain
    - **D57.00 Hb-SS disease with crisis, unspecified** 🦠
      - Hb-SS disease with (painful) crisis NOS
      - Hb-SS disease with (vaso-occlusive) pain NOS
    - **D57.01 Hb-SS disease with acute chest syndrome** 🦠
    - **D57.02 Hb-SS disease with splenic sequestration** 🦠
    - **D57.03 Hb-SS disease with cerebral vascular involvement**
      - Code also, if applicable, cerebral infarction (I63.-)
    - **D57.04 Hb-SS disease with dactylitis**
      - Coding Clinic: 2023, Q4, P7
    - **D57.09 Hb-SS disease with crisis with other specified complication**
      - Use additional code to identify complications, such as:
        - cholelithiasis (K80.-)
        - priapism (N48.32)
  - **D57.1 Sickle-cell disease without crisis Hb-SS disease without crisis** 🦠
    - Sickle-cell anemia NOS
    - Sickle-cell disease NOS
    - Sickle-cell disorder NOS
  - **D57.2 Sickle-cell/Hb-C disease**
    - Hb-SC disease
    - Hb-S/Hb-C disease
    - **D57.20 Sickle-cell/Hb-C disease without crisis** 🦠
    - **D57.21 Sickle-cell/Hb-C disease with crisis**
      - **D57.211 Sickle-cell/Hb-C disease with acute chest syndrome** 🦠
      - **D57.212 Sickle-cell/Hb-C disease with splenic sequestration** 🦠
      - **D57.213 Sickle-cell/Hb-C disease with cerebral vascular involvement**
        - Code also, if applicable, cerebral infarction (I63.-)
      - **D57.214 Sickle-cell/Hb-C disease with dactylitis**
      - **D57.218 Sickle-cell/Hb-C disease with crisis with other specified complication**
        - Use additional code to identify complications, such as:
          - cholelithiasis (K80.-)
          - priapism (N48.32)
      - **D57.219 Sickle-cell/Hb-C disease with crisis, unspecified** 🦠
        - Sickle-cell/Hb-C disease with crisis NOS
        - Sickle-cell/Hb-C disease with (vaso-occlusive) pain NOS

D57.3 Sickle-cell trait 🔖
  Hb-S trait
  Heterozygous hemoglobin S

● **D57.4 Sickle-cell thalassemia**
  Sickle-cell beta thalassemia
  Thalassemia Hb-S disease

  D57.40 Sickle-cell thalassemia without crisis 🔖
    Microdrepanocytosis
    Sickle-cell thalassemia NOS

  ● **D57.41 Sickle-cell thalassemia, unspecified, with crisis**
    Sickle-cell "crisis" is precipitated when abnormally crescent-shaped red blood cells form clots and interrupt blood flow to major organs, causing severe pain and organ damage.
    Sickle-cell thalassemia with (painful) crisis NOS
    Sickle-cell thalassemia with (vaso-occlusive) pain NOS

    D57.411 Sickle-cell thalassemia, unspecified, with acute chest syndrome 🔖

    D57.412 Sickle-cell thalassemia with, unspecified, splenic sequestration 🔖

    D57.413 Sickle-cell thalassemia, unspecified, with cerebral vascular involvement
       Code also, if applicable cerebral infarction (I63.-)

    D57.414 Sickle-cell thalassemia, unspecified, with dactylitis

    D57.418 Sickle-cell thalassemia, unspecified, with crisis with other specified complication
       Use additional code to identify complications, such as:
        cholelithiasis (K80.-)
        priapism (N48.32)

    D57.419 Sickle-cell thalassemia with, unspecified, crisis 🔖
       Sickle-cell thalassemia with (painful) crisis NOS
       Sickle-cell thalassemia with (vaso-occlusive) pain NOS

  D57.42 Sickle-cell thalassemia beta zero without crisis
    HbS-beta zero without crisis
    Sickle-cell beta zero without crisis

  ● **D57.43 Sickle-cell thalassemia beta zero with crisis**
    HbS-beta zero with crisis
    Sickle-cell beta zero with crisis

    D57.431 Sickle-cell thalassemia beta zero with acute chest syndrome
       HbS-beta zero with acute chest syndrome
       Sickle-cell beta zero with acute chest syndrome

    D57.432 Sickle-cell thalassemia beta zero with splenic sequestration
       HbS-beta zero with splenic sequestration
       Sickle-cell beta zero with splenic sequestration

    D57.433 Sickle-cell thalassemia beta zero with cerebral vascular involvement
       HbS-beta zero with cerebral vascular involvement
       Sickle-cell beta zero with cerebral vascular involvement
       Code also, if applicable cerebral infarction (I63.-)

    D57.434 Sickle-cell thalassemia beta zero with dactylitis

    D57.438 Sickle-cell thalassemia beta zero with crisis with other specified complication
       HbS-beta zero with other specified complication
       Sickle-cell beta zero with other specified complication
       Use additional code to identify complications, such as:
        cholelithiasis (K80.-)
        priapism (N48.32)

    D57.439 Sickle-cell thalassemia beta zero with crisis, unspecified
       HbS-beta zero with other specified complication
       Sickle-cell beta zero with crisis unspecified
       Sickle-cell thalassemia beta zero with (painful) crisis NOS
       Sickle-cell thalassemia beta zero with (vaso-occlusive) pain NOS

  D57.44 Sickle-cell thalassemia beta plus without crisis
    HbS-beta plus without crisis
    Sickle-cell beta plus without crisis

  ● **D57.45 Sickle-cell thalassemia beta plus with crisis**
    HbS-beta plus with crisis
    Sickle-cell beta plus with crisis

    D57.451 Sickle-cell thalassemia beta plus with acute chest syndrome
       HbS-beta plus with acute chest syndrome
       Sickle-cell beta plus with acute chest syndrome

    D57.452 Sickle-cell thalassemia beta plus with splenic sequestration
       HbS-beta plus with splenic sequestration
       Sickle-cell beta plus with splenic sequestration

    D57.453 Sickle-cell thalassemia beta plus with cerebral vascular involvement
       HbS-beta plus with cerebral vascular involvement
       Sickle-cell beta plus with cerebral vascular involvement
       Code also, if applicable cerebral infarction (I63.-)

    D57.454 Sickle-cell thalassemia beta plus with dactylitis

    D57.458 Sickle-cell thalassemia beta plus with crisis with other specified complication
       HbS-beta plus with crisis with other specified complication
       Sickle-cell beta plus with crisis with other specified complication
       Use additional code to identify complications, such as:
        cholelithiasis (K80.-)
        priapism (N48.32)

    D57.459 Sickle-cell thalassemia beta plus with crisis, unspecified
       HbS-beta plus with crisis with unspecified complication
       Sickle-cell beta plus with crisis with unspecified complication
       Sickle-cell thalassemia beta plus with (painful) crisis NOS
       Sickle-cell thalassemia beta plus with (vaso-occlusive) pain NOS

CHAPTER 3 (D50-D89)

● **D57.8 Other sickle-cell disorders**
Hb-SD disease
Hb-SE disease

   D57.80 Other sickle-cell disorders without crisis 🅗
●   **D57.81 Other sickle-cell disorders with crisis**

     D57.811 Other sickle-cell disorders with acute chest syndrome 🅗

     D57.812 Other sickle-cell disorders with splenic sequestration 🅗

     D57.813 Other sickle-cell disorders with cerebral vascular involvement

       Code also, if applicable: cerebral infarction (I63.-)

     D57.814 Other sickle-cell disorders with dactylitis

     D57.818 Other sickle-cell disorders with crisis with other specified complication

       Use additional code to identify complications, such as:
       cholelithiasis (K80.-)
       priapism (N48.32)

     D57.819 Other sickle-cell disorders with crisis, unspecified 🅗
       Other sickle-cell disorders with crisis NOS
       Other sickle-cell disorders with (vaso-occlusive) pain NOS

● **D58 Other hereditary hemolytic anemias**
Genetic condition in which bone marrow is unable to compensate for premature destruction of red blood cells

   Excludes1 hemolytic anemia of the newborn (P55.-)

D58.0 Hereditary spherocytosis 🅗
Presence of spherocytes (spherically shaped red blood cells)
Acholuric (familial) jaundice
Congenital (spherocytic) hemolytic icterus
Minkowski-Chauffard syndrome

D58.1 Hereditary elliptocytosis 🅗
Presence of large numbers of elliptocytes in blood
Elliptocytosis (congenital)
Ovalocytosis (congenital) (hereditary)

D58.2 Other hemoglobinopathies 🅗
Abnormal hemoglobin NOS
Congenital Heinz body anemia
Hb-C disease
Hb-D disease
Hb-E disease
Hemoglobinopathy NOS
Unstable hemoglobin hemolytic disease

   Excludes1 familial polycythemia (D75.0)
     Hb-M disease (D74.0)
     hemoglobin E-beta thalassemia (D56.5)
     hereditary persistence of fetal hemoglobin [HPFH] (D56.4)
     high-altitude polycythemia (D75.1)
     methemoglobinemia (D74.-)
     other hemoglobinopathies with thalassemia (D56.8)

D58.8 Other specified hereditary hemolytic anemias 🅗
Stomatocytosis

D58.9 Hereditary hemolytic anemia, unspecified 🅗

● **D59 Acquired hemolytic anemia**

D59.0 Drug-induced autoimmune hemolytic anemia 🅗
Use additional code for adverse effect, if applicable, to identify drug (T36-T50 with fifth or sixth character 5)

D59.1 Other autoimmune hemolytic anemias 🅗
   Excludes2 Evans syndrome (D69.41)
     hemolytic disease of newborn (P55.-)
     paroxysmal cold hemoglobinuria (D59.6)

D59.10 Autoimmune hemolytic anemia, unspecified

D59.11 Warm autoimmune hemolytic anemia
Warm type (primary) (secondary) (symptomatic) autoimmune hemolytic anemia
Warm type autoimmune hemolytic disease

D59.12 Cold autoimmune hemolytic anemia
Chronic cold hemagglutinin disease
Cold agglutinin disease
Cold agglutinin hemoglobinuria
Cold type (primary) (secondary) (symptomatic) autoimmune hemolytic anemia
Cold type autoimmune hemolytic disease

D59.13 Mixed type autoimmune hemolytic anemia
Mixed type autoimmune hemolytic disease
Mixed type, cold and warm, (primary) (secondary) (symptomatic) autoimmune hemolyticanemia

D59.19 Other autoimmune hemolytic anemia

D59.2 Drug-induced nonautoimmune hemolytic anemia 🅗
Drug-induced enzyme deficiency anemia
Use additional code for adverse effect, if applicable, to identify drug (T36-T50 with fifth or sixth character 5)

D59.3 Hemolytic-uremic syndrome 🅗
Code also, if applicable, any associated:
acute kidney failure (N17.-)
chronic kidney disease (N18.-)

D59.30 Hemolytic-uremic syndrome, unspecified
Hemolytic-uremic syndrome NOS

D59.31 Infection-associated hemolytic-uremic syndrome
Shiga toxin-producing E. coli [STEC] related hemolytic uremic syndrome
Typical hemolytic uremic syndrome
Use Additional code to identify associated infection, such as:
E. coli infection (B96.2-)
Human immunodeficiency virus [HIV] disease (B20)
Pneumococcal meningitis (G00.1)
Pneumococcal pneumonia (J13)
Sepsis due to Streptococcus pneumoniae (A40.3)
Shigella dysenteriae (A03.9)
Streptococcus pneumoniae as the cause of diseases classified elsewhere (B95.3)

D59.32 Hereditary hemolytic-uremic syndrome
Atypical hemolytic uremic syndrome with an identified genetic cause
Code also, if applicable:
defects in the complement system (D84.1)
methylmalonic acidemia (E71.120)

D59.39 Other hemolytic-uremic syndrome
Atypical (nongenetic) hemolytic uremic syndrome
Secondary hemolytic-uremic syndrome
Code first, if applicable, any associated:
COVID-19 (U07.1)
complications of kidney transplant (T86.1-)
complications of heart transplant (T86.2-)
complications of liver transplant (T86.4-)
Code also, if applicable, any associated condition, such as:
hypertensive emergency (I16.1)
malignant neoplasm (C00-C96)
systemic lupus erythematosus (M32.-)
Use Additional code, if applicable, for adverse effect to identify drug (T36-T50 with fifth or sixth character 5)
Coding Clinic: 2022, Q4, P6

▶ New   ⇒ Revised   ~~deleted~~ Deleted   Excludes 1   Excludes 2   Includes   Use additional   Code first   Code also   Key words

  OGCR Official Guidelines   X Assign placeholder X   ● Use Additional Character(s)   ▶ Manifestation Code   🅗 Hierarchical Condition Category   Coding Clinic

D59.4   **Other nonautoimmune hemolytic anemias** 🔍
Mechanical hemolytic anemia
Microangiopathic hemolytic anemia
Toxic hemolytic anemia

D59.5   **Paroxysmal nocturnal hemoglobinuria [Marchiafava-Micheli]** 🔍
    Excludes1   hemoglobinuria NOS (R82.3)

D59.6   **Hemoglobinuria due to hemolysis from other external causes** 🔍
Hemoglobinuria from exertion
March hemoglobinuria
Paroxysmal cold hemoglobinuria
Use additional code (Chapter 20) to identify external cause
    Excludes1   hemoglobinuria NOS (R82.3)

D59.8   **Other acquired hemolytic anemias** 🔍

D59.9   **Acquired hemolytic anemia, unspecified** 🔍
Idiopathic hemolytic anemia, chronic

APLASTIC AND OTHER ANEMIAS AND OTHER BONE MARROW FAILURE SYNDROMES (D60-D64)

● **D60**   **Acquired pure red cell aplasia [erythroblastopenia]**
Deficiency of erythroblasts
    Includes   red cell aplasia (acquired) (adult) (with thymoma)
    Excludes1   congenital red cell aplasia (D61.01)

D60.0   **Chronic acquired pure red cell aplasia** 🔍
Lack of development of blood cell

D60.1   **Transient acquired pure red cell aplasia** 🔍

D60.8   **Other acquired pure red cell aplasias** 🔍

D60.9   **Acquired pure red cell aplasia, unspecified** 🔍

● **D61**   **Other aplastic anemias and other bone marrow failure syndromes**
    Excludes2   neutropenia (D70.-)

● **D61.0**   **Constitutional aplastic anemia**
Condition where bone marrow is unable to produce blood cells

   D61.01   **Constitutional (pure) red blood cell aplasia** 🔍
Blackfan-Diamond syndrome
Congenital (pure) red cell aplasia
Familial hypoplastic anemia
Primary (pure) red cell aplasia
Red cell (pure) aplasia of infants
    Excludes1   acquired red cell aplasia (D60.9)

   D61.02   **Shwachman-Diamond syndrome**
Code also, if applicable, associated conditions such as:
acute myeloblastic leukemia (C92.0-)
exocrine pancreatic insufficiency (K86.81)
myelodysplastic syndrome (D46.-)
Use additional code, if applicable, for genetic susceptibility to other malignant neoplasm(Z15.09)

   ▶ **D61.03**   **Fanconi anemia**
▶ Fanconi pancytopenia
▶ Fanconi's anemia
    ▶ **Excludes1**   Fanconi syndrome (E72.0-)

   D61.09   **Other constitutional aplastic anemia** 🔍
~~Fanconi's anemia~~
Pancytopenia with malformations

D61.1   **Drug-induced aplastic anemia** 🔍
Use additional code for adverse effect, if applicable, to identify drug (T36-T50 with fifth or sixth character 5)

D61.2   **Aplastic anemia due to other external agents** 🔍
Code first, if applicable, toxic effects of substances chiefly nonmedicinal as to source (T51-T65)

D61.3   **Idiopathic aplastic anemia** 🔍

● **D61.8**   **Other specified aplastic anemias and other bone marrow failure syndromes**
● **D61.81**   **Pancytopenia**
Marked deficiency of all the blood elements: Red blood cells (erythrocytes), white blood cells (leukocytes), and platelets (thrombocytes). Check laboratory results.
    Excludes1   pancytopenia (due to) (with) aplastic anemia (D61.9)
pancytopenia (due to) (with) bone marrow infiltration (D61.82)
pancytopenia (due to) (with) congenital (pure) red cell aplasia (D61.01)
pancytopenia (due to) (with) hairy cell leukemia (C91.4-)
pancytopenia (due to) (with) human immunodeficiency virus disease (B20.-)
pancytopenia (due to) (with) leukoerythroblastic anemia (D61.82)
pancytopenia (due to) (with) myeloproliferative disease (D47.1)
    Excludes2   pancytopenia (due to) (with) myelodysplastic syndromes (D46.-)

   D61.810   **Antineoplastic chemotherapy induced pancytopenia** 🔍
    Excludes2   aplastic anemia due to antineoplastic chemotherapy (D61.1)

   D61.811   **Other drug-induced pancytopenia** 🔍
    Excludes2   aplastic anemia due to drugs (D61.1)

   D61.818   **Other pancytopenia** 🔍
    Coding Clinic: 2023, Q1, P23; 2019, Q1, P16

   D61.82   **Myelophthisis** 🔍
Leukoerythroblastic anemia
Myelophthisic anemia
Panmyelophthisis
Code also the underlying disorder, such as:
malignant neoplasm of breast (C50.-)
tuberculosis (A15.-)
    Excludes1   idiopathic myelofibrosis (D47.1)
myelofibrosis NOS (D75.81)
myelofibrosis with myeloid metaplasia (D47.4)
primary myelofibrosis (D47.1)
secondary myelofibrosis (D75.81)

   D61.89   **Other specified aplastic anemias and other bone marrow failure syndromes** 🔍

D61.9   **Aplastic anemia, unspecified** 🔍
Hypoplastic anemia NOS
Medullary hypoplasia

D62   **Acute posthemorrhagic anemia**
    Excludes1   anemia due to chronic blood loss (D50.0)
blood loss anemia NOS (D50.0)
congenital anemia from fetal blood loss (P61.3)
Coding Clinic: 2019, Q3, P13,17

CHAPTER 3 (D50-D89)

● **D63**   **Anemia in chronic diseases classified elsewhere**

▷ *D63.0*   *Anemia in neoplastic disease*

    Code first neoplasm (C00-D49)

Excludes1   aplastic anemia due to antineoplastic chemotherapy (D61.1)

Excludes2   anemia due to antineoplastic chemotherapy (D64.81)

OGCR   Section I.C.2.e.2.

> 2) Anemia associated with chemotherapy, immunotherapy and radiation therapy
>
> When the admission/encounter is for management of an anemia associated with an adverse effect of the administration of chemotherapy or immunotherapy and the only treatment is for the anemia, the anemia code is sequenced first followed by the appropriate codes for the neoplasm and the adverse effect (T45.1X5, Adverse effect of antineoplastic and immunosuppressive drugs).

▷ *D63.1*   *Anemia in chronic kidney disease*

    Erythropoietin resistant anemia (EPO resistant anemia)

    Code first underlying chronic kidney disease (CKD) (N18.-)

▷ *D63.8*   *Anemia in other chronic diseases classified elsewhere*

    Code first underlying disease, such as:

       diphyllobothriasis (B70.0)

       hookworm disease (B76.0-B76.9)

       hypothyroidism (E00.0-E03.9)

       malaria (B50.0-B54)

       symptomatic late syphilis (A52.79)

       tuberculosis (A18.89)

● **D64**   **Other anemias**

Excludes1   refractory anemia (D46.-)

    refractory anemia with excess blasts in transformation [RAEB T] (C92.0-)

D64.0   **Hereditary sideroblastic anemia** 🅗

    Abnormal production RBCs (erythrocytes)

    Sex-linked hypochromic sideroblastic anemia

▷ *D64.1*   *Secondary sideroblastic anemia due to disease* 🅗

    Code first underlying disease

D64.2   **Secondary sideroblastic anemia due to drugs and toxins** 🅗

    Code first poisoning due to drug or toxin, if applicable (T36-T65 with fifth or sixth character 1-4)

    Use additional code for adverse effect, if applicable, to identify drug (T36-T50 with fifth or sixth character 5)

D64.3   **Other sideroblastic anemias** 🅗

    Sideroblastic anemia NOS

    Pyridoxine-responsive sideroblastic anemia NEC

D64.4   **Congenital dyserythropoietic anemia**

    Any of several rare hereditary anemias, mostly types of macrocytic anemia

    Dyshematopoietic anemia (congenital)

Excludes1   Blackfan-Diamond syndrome (D61.01)

    Di Guglielmo's disease (C94.0)

● **D64.8**   **Other specified anemias**

D64.81   **Anemia due to antineoplastic chemotherapy**

    Antineoplastic chemotherapy induced anemia

    aplastic anemia due to antineoplastic chemotherapy (D61.1)

Excludes2   anemia in neoplastic disease (D63.0)

    Coding Clinic: 2023, Q3, P4; 2023, Q2, P18; 2021, Q3, P4

D64.89   **Other specified anemias**

    Infantile pseudoleukemia

D64.9   **Anemia, unspecified**

    Coding Clinic: 2018, Q4, P88; 2017, Q1, P7

COAGULATION DEFECTS, PURPURA AND OTHER HEMORRHAGIC CONDITIONS (D65-D69)

D65   **Disseminated intravascular coagulation [defibrination syndrome]** 🅗

    Blood clots form and consume all coagulation proteins and platelets and disrupt normal coagulation, resulting in abnormal bleeding

    Afibrinogenemia, acquired

    Consumption coagulopathy

    COVID-19 associated diffuse or disseminated intravascular coagulopathy

    Diffuse or disseminated intravascular coagulation [DIC]

    Fibrinolytic hemorrhage, acquired

    Fibrinolytic purpura

    Purpura fulminans

    Code also, if applicable, associated condition

Excludes1   disseminated intravascular coagulation (complicating):

    abortion or ectopic or molar pregnancy (O00-O07, O08.1)

    in newborn (P60)

    pregnancy, childbirth and the puerperium (O45.0, O46.0, O67.0, O72.3)

    Coding Clinic: 2022, Q4, P9; 2021, Q1, P39; 2019, Q2, P25

D66   **Hereditary factor VIII deficiency** 🅗

    Inherited coagulation disorder carried by females but most often affecting males

    Classical hemophilia

    Deficiency factor VIII (with functional defect)

    Hemophilia NOS

    Hemophilia A

Excludes1   factor VIII deficiency with vascular defect (D68.0-)

D67   **Hereditary factor IX deficiency** 🅗

    Christmas disease

    Factor IX deficiency (with functional defect)

    Hemophilia B

    Plasma thromboplastin component [PTC] deficiency

● **D68**   **Other coagulation defects**

Excludes1   abnormal coagulation profile NOS (R79.1)

Excludes2   coagulation defects complicating abortion or ectopic or molar pregnancy (O00-O07, O08.1)

    coagulation defects complicating pregnancy, childbirth and the puerperium (O45.0, O46.0, O67.0, O72.3)

    Coding Clinic: 2016, Q1, P14

D68.0   **Von Willebrand disease** 🅗

    Congenital bleeding disorder

Excludes1   capillary fragility (hereditary) (D69.8)

    factor VIII deficiency NOS (D66)

    factor VIII deficiency with functional defect (D66)

D68.00   **Von Willebrand disease, unspecified**

D68.01   **Von Willebrand disease, type 1**

    Partial quantitative deficiency of von Willebrand factor

    Type 1C von Willebrand disease

    Coding Clinic: 2022, Q4, P9

● **D68.02**   **Von Willebrand disease, type 2**

    Qualitative defects of von Willebrand factor

D68.020   **Von Willebrand disease, type 2A**

    Qualitative defects of von Willebrand factor with decreased platelet adhesion and selective deficiency of high-molecular-weight multimers

▶ New   ⇒ Revised   ~~deleted~~ Deleted   Excludes 1   Excludes 2   Includes   Use additional   Code first   Code also   Key words

OGCR Official Guidelines   X Assign placeholder X   ● Use Additional Character(s)   ▷ Manifestation Code   🅗 Hierarchical Condition Category   Coding Clinic

D68.021   **Von Willebrand disease, type 2B**
Qualitative defects of von Willebrand factor with high-molecular-weight von Willebrand factor loss
Qualitative defects of von Willebrand factor with hyper-adhesive forms
Qualitative defects of von Willebrand factor with increased affinity for platelet glycoprotein lb

D68.022   **Von Willebrand disease, type 2M**
Qualitative defects of von Willebrand factor with defective platelet adhesion with anormal size distribution of von Willebrand factor multimers

D68.023   **Von Willebrand disease, type 2N**
Qualitative defects of von Willebrand factor with defective von Willebrand factor to factor VIII binding
Qualitative defects of von Willebrand factor with markedly decreased affinity for factor VIII

D68.029   **Von Willebrand disease, type 2, unspecified**
Qualitative defect in von Willebrand factor function, with no further subtyping

D68.03   **Von Willebrand disease, type 3**
(Near) complete absence of von Willebrand factor
Total quantitative deficiency of von Willebrand factor

D68.04   **Acquired von Willebrand disease**
Acquired von Willebrand syndrome

D68.09   **Other von Willebrand disease**
Platelet-type von Willebrand disease
Pseudo-von Willebrand disease

Code also, if applicable, qualitative platelet defects (D69.1)

D68.1   **Hereditary factor XI deficiency** 🔒
Deficiency of blood coagulation resulting in systemic blood-clotting defect
Hemophilia C
Plasma thromboplastin antecedent [PTA] deficiency
Rosenthal's disease

D68.2   **Hereditary deficiency of other clotting factors** 🔒
Blood clotting disorders caused by hereditary deficiencies of one or more clotting factors
AC globulin deficiency
Congenital afibrinogenemia
Deficiency of factor I [fibrinogen]
Deficiency of factor II [prothrombin]
Deficiency of factor V [labile]
Deficiency of factor VII [stable]
Deficiency of factor X [Stuart-Prower]
Deficiency of factor XII [Hageman]
Deficiency of factor XIII [fibrin stabilizing]
Dysfibrinogenemia (congenital)
Hypoproconvertinemia
Owren's disease
Proaccelerin deficiency

● D68.3   **Hemorrhagic disorder due to circulating anticoagulants**
Blood clotting disorders caused by anticoagulants (warfarin and heparin)

● D68.31   **Hemorrhagic disorder due to intrinsic circulating anticoagulants, antibodies, or inhibitors**

D68.311   **Acquired hemophilia** 🔒
Autoimmune hemophilia
Autoimmune inhibitors to clotting factors
Secondary hemophilia

D68.312   **Antiphospholipid antibody with hemorrhagic disorder** 🔒
Lupus anticoagulant (LAC) with hemorrhagic disorder
Systemic lupus erythematosus [SLE] inhibitor with hemorrhagic disorder

Excludes 1   antiphospholipid antibody, finding without diagnosis (R76.0)
antiphospholipid antibody syndrome (D68.61)
antiphospholipid antibody with hypercoagulable state (D68.61)
lupus anticoagulant (LAC) finding without diagnosis (R76.0)
lupus anticoagulant (LAC) with hypercoagulable state (D68.62)
systemic lupus erythematosus [SLE] inhibitor finding without diagnosis (R76.0)
systemic lupus erythematosus [SLE] inhibitor with hypercoagulable state (D68.62)

D68.318   **Other hemorrhagic disorder due to intrinsic circulating anticoagulants, antibodies, or inhibitors** 🔒
Antithromboplastinemia
Antithromboplastinogenemia
Hemorrhagic disorder due to intrinsic increase in antithrombin
Hemorrhagic disorder due to intrinsic increase in anti-VIIIa
Hemorrhagic disorder due to intrinsic increase in anti-IXa
Hemorrhagic disorder due to intrinsic increase in anti-XIa

D68.32   **Hemorrhagic disorder due to extrinsic circulating anticoagulants** 🔒
Drug-induced hemorrhagic disorder
Hemorrhagic disorder due to increase in anti-IIa
Hemorrhagic disorder due to increase in anti-Xa
Hyperheparinemia

Use additional code for adverse effect, if applicable, to identify drug (T45.515, T45.525)
Coding Clinic: 2021, Q1, P5; 2016, Q1, P14-15

CHAPTER 3 (D50-D89)

D68.4 **Acquired coagulation factor deficiency** 🐾
Deficiency of coagulation factor due to liver disease
Deficiency of coagulation factor due to vitamin K deficiency
> **Excludes1** vitamin K deficiency of newborn (P53)

● D68.5 **Primary thrombophilia**
AKA idiopathic thrombocytopenia, may be acquired or congenital and is a common cause of coagulation disorders.
Primary hypercoagulable states
> **Excludes1** antiphospholipid syndrome (D68.61)
> lupus anticoagulant (D68.62)
> secondary activated protein C resistance (D68.69)
> secondary antiphospholipid antibody syndrome (D68.69)
> secondary lupus anticoagulant with hypercoagulable state (D68.69)
> secondary systemic lupus erythematosus [SLE] inhibitor with hypercoagulable state (D68.69)
> systemic lupus erythematosus [SLE] inhibitor finding without diagnosis (R76.0)
> systemic lupus erythematosus [SLE] inhibitor with hemorrhagic disorder (D68.312)
> thrombotic thrombocytopenic purpura (M31.19)

D68.51 **Activated protein C resistance** 🐾
Factor V Leiden mutation

D68.52 **Prothrombin gene mutation** 🐾

D68.59 **Other primary thrombophilia** 🐾
Antithrombin III deficiency
Hypercoagulable state NOS
Primary hypercoagulable state NEC
Primary thrombophilia NEC
Protein C deficiency
Protein S deficiency
Thrombophilia NOS
Coding Clinic: 2021, Q2, P8-9

● D68.6 **Other thrombophilia**
Other hypercoagulable states
> **Excludes1** diffuse or disseminated intravascular coagulation [DIC] (D65)
> heparin induced thrombocytopenia (HIT) (D75.82-)
> hyperhomocysteinemia (E72.11)

D68.61 **Antiphospholipid syndrome** 🐾
Anticardiolipin syndrome
Antiphospholipid antibody syndrome
> **Excludes1** anti-phospholipid antibody, finding without diagnosis (R76.0)
> anti-phospholipid antibody with hemorrhagic disorder (D68.312)
> lupus anticoagulant syndrome (D68.62)

D68.62 **Lupus anticoagulant syndrome** 🐾
Lupus anticoagulant
Presence of systemic lupus erythematosus [SLE] inhibitor
> **Excludes1** anticardiolipin syndrome (D68.61)
> antiphospholipid syndrome (D68.61)
> lupus anticoagulant (LAC) finding without diagnosis (R76.0)
> lupus anticoagulant (LAC) with hemorrhagic disorder (D68.312)

D68.69 **Other thrombophilia** 🐾
COVID-19 associated hypercoagulability
Hypercoagulable states NEC
Secondary hypercoagulable state NOS
Code also, if applicable, associated condition
Coding Clinic: 2021, Q2, P8

D68.8 **Other specified coagulation defects** 🐾
COVID-19 associated coagulopathy
Code also, if applicable, associated condition
> **Excludes1** hemorrhagic disease of newborn (P53)
Coding Clinic: 2021, Q1, P39-40

D68.9 **Coagulation defect, unspecified** 🐾

● D69 **Purpura and other hemorrhagic conditions**
Group of conditions characterized by small hemorrhages in skin, mucous membranes, or serosal surfaces
> **Excludes1** benign hypergammaglobulinemic purpura (D89.0)
> cryoglobulinemic purpura (D89.1)
> essential (hemorrhagic) thrombocythemia (D47.3)
> hemorrhagic thrombocythemia (D47.3)
> purpura fulminans (D65)
> thrombotic thrombocytopenic purpura (M31.19)
> Waldenström hypergammaglobulinemic purpura (D89.0)

D69.0 **Allergic purpura** 🐾
Allergic vasculitis
Nonthrombocytopenic hemorrhagic purpura
Nonthrombocytopenic idiopathic purpura
Purpura anaphylactoid
Purpura Henoch(-Schönlein)
Purpura rheumatica
Vascular purpura
> **Excludes1** thrombocytopenic hemorrhagic purpura (D69.3)

D69.1 **Qualitative platelet defects** 🐾
Bernard-Soulier [giant platelet] syndrome
Glanzmann's disease
Grey platelet syndrome
Thromboasthenia (hemorrhagic) (hereditary)
Thrombocytopathy
> **Excludes1** hemolytic-uremic syndrome (D59.3-)
> **Excludes2** von Willebrand disease (D68.0-)

D69.2 **Other nonthrombocytopenic purpura** 🐾
Purpura NOS
Purpura simplex
Senile purpura

D69.3 **Immune thrombocytopenic purpura** 🐾
Hemorrhagic (thrombocytopenic) purpura
Idiopathic thrombocytopenic purpura
Tidal platelet dysgenesis

● D69.4 **Other primary thrombocytopenia**
> **Excludes1** transient neonatal thrombocytopenia (P61.0)
> Wiskott-Aldrich syndrome (D82.0)

D69.41 **Evans syndrome** 🐾
Acquired hemolytic anemia and thrombocytopenia

D69.42 **Congenital and hereditary thrombocytopenia purpura** 🐾
Congenital thrombocytopenia
Hereditary thrombocytopenia
Code first congenital or hereditary disorder, such as:
thrombocytopenia with absent radius (TAR syndrome) (Q87.2)

D69.49 **Other primary thrombocytopenia** 🐾
Megakaryocytic hypoplasia
Primary thrombocytopenia NOS

▶ New ⇒ Revised ~~deleted~~ Deleted Excludes 1 Excludes 2 Includes Use additional Code first Code also Key words
OGCR Official Guidelines X Assign placeholder X ● Use Additional Character(s) ▶ Manifestation Code 🐾 Hierarchical Condition Category **Coding Clinic**

● **D69.5**   **Secondary thrombocytopenia**
  Acquired reduction of number of platelets required for blood
  clotting
> **Excludes1**   heparin induced thrombocytopenia (HIT)
> (D75.82-)
> transient thrombocytopenia of newborn
> (P61.0)

   D69.51   **Posttransfusion purpura**
     Posttransfusion purpura from whole blood
     (fresh) or blood products PTP
   D69.59   **Other secondary thrombocytopenia**

D69.6   **Thrombocytopenia, unspecified** 🔏

D69.8   **Other specified hemorrhagic conditions** 🔏
   Capillary fragility (hereditary)
   Vascular pseudohemophilia

D69.9   **Hemorrhagic condition, unspecified** 🔏

OTHER DISORDERS OF BLOOD AND BLOOD-FORMING ORGANS (D70-D77)

● **D70**   **Neutropenia**
   Code also, if applicable, mucositis (J34.81, K12.3-, K92.81,
     N76.81)
   Decrease in number of neutrophils (type of white blood cell)
> **Includes**   agranulocytosis
> decreased absolute neurophile count (ANC)
> **Excludes1**   neutropenic splenomegaly (D73.81)
> transient neonatal neutropenia (P61.5)

D70.0   **Congenital agranulocytosis** 🔏
   Reduced numbers of neutrophils (type of white blood cell)
   Congenital neutropenia
   Infantile genetic agranulocytosis
   Kostmann's disease

D70.1   **Agranulocytosis secondary to cancer chemotherapy** 🔏
   Decreased numbers of granulocytes (type of white blood cell)
   Code also *underlying neoplasm*
   Use additional code for adverse effect, if applicable, to
     identify drug (T45.1X5)

D70.2   **Other drug-induced agranulocytosis** 🔏
   Use additional code for adverse effect, if applicable,
     to identify drug (T36-T50 with fifth or sixth
     character 5)

D70.3   **Neutropenia due to infection** 🔏

D70.4   **Cyclic neutropenia** 🔏
   Chronic neutropenia (low number of type of white blood cell)
   Cyclic hematopoiesis
   Periodic neutropenia

D70.8   **Other neutropenia** 🔏

D70.9   **Neutropenia, unspecified** 🔏
   Coding Clinic: 2019, Q2, P25

D71   **Functional disorders of polymorphonuclear neutrophils** 🔏
   Polymorphonuclear: varying shapes of nucleus; AKA PMNs
   Cell membrane receptor complex [CR3] defect
   Chronic (childhood) granulomatous disease
   Congenital dysphagocytosis
   Progressive septic granulomatosis

● **D72**   **Other disorders of white blood cells**
> **Excludes1**   basophilia (D72.824)
> immunity disorders (D80-D89)
> neutropenia (D70)
> preleukemia (syndrome) (D46.9)

D72.0   **Genetic anomalies of leukocytes** 🔏
   Alder (granulation) (granulocyte) anomaly
   Alder syndrome
   Hereditary leukocytic hypersegmentation
   Hereditary leukocytic hyposegmentation
   Hereditary leukomelanopathy
   May-Hegglin (granulation) (granulocyte) anomaly
   May-Hegglin syndrome
   Pelger-Huët (granulation) (granulocyte) anomaly
   Pelger-Huët syndrome
> **Excludes1**   Chédiak (-Steinbrinck)-Higashi syndrome
> (E70.330)

● **D72.1**   **Eosinophilia**
   Formation and accumulation of high number of white cells in
     blood/tissue
> **Excludes2**   Löffler's syndrome (J82.89)
> pulmonary eosinophilia (J82.-)

D72.10   **Eosinophilia, unspecified**

● **D72.11**   **Hypereosinophilic syndrome [HES]**
   D72.110   **Idiopathic hypereosinophilic**
     syndrome [IHES]
   D72.111   **Lymphocytic Variant**
     Hypereosinophilic Syndrome [LHES]
     Lymphocyte variant
      hypereosinophilia
     Code also, if applicable, any
      associated lymphocytic
      neoplastic disorder
   D72.118   **Other hypereosinophilic syndrome**
     Episodic angioedema with
      eosinophilia
     Gleich's syndrome
   D72.119   **Hypereosinophilic syndrome [HES],**
     unspecified

D72.12   **Drug rash with eosinophilia and systemic**
   symptoms syndrome
   DRESS syndrome
   Use additional code for adverse effect, if
     applicable, to identify drug (T36-T50 with
     fifth or sixth character 5)

▷ **D72.18**   *Eosinophilia in diseases classified elsewhere*
   Code first underlying disease, such as:
     chronic myelomonocytic leukemia (C93.1-)

D72.19   **Other eosinophilia**
   Familial eosinophilia
   Hereditary eosinophilia

● **D72.8**   **Other specified disorders of white blood cells**
> **Excludes1**   leukemia (C91-C95)

● **D72.81**   **Decreased white blood cell count**
> **Excludes1**   neutropenia (D70.-)

   D72.810   **Lymphocytopenia**
     Decreased lymphocytes
     Reduction in number of lympho cytes
      in blood
   D72.818   **Other decreased white blood cell**
     count
     Basophilic leukopenia
     Eosinophilic leukopenia
     Monocytopenia
     Other decreased leukocytes
     Plasmacytopenia
   D72.819   **Decreased white blood cell**
     count, unspecified
     Decreased leukocytes, unspecified
     Leukocytopenia, unspecified
     Leukopenia
> **Excludes1**   malignant leukopenia
> (D70.9)

● **D72.82**   **Elevated white blood cell count**
> **Excludes1**   eosinophilia (D72.1)

   D72.820   **Lymphocytosis (symptomatic)**
     Elevated lymphocytes
     Excess of normal lymphocytes
   D72.821   **Monocytosis (symptomatic)**
> **Excludes1**   infectious
> mononucleosis
> (B27.-)

   D72.822   **Plasmacytosis**
     Presence of excess plasma cells

CHAPTER 3 (D50-D89)

D72.823 **Leukemoid reaction**
Basophilic leukemoid reaction
Leukemoid reaction NOS
Lymphocytic leukemoid reaction
Monocytic leukemoid reaction
Myelocytic leukemoid reaction
Neutrophilic leukemoid reaction

D72.824 **Basophilia**
Increase of basophils in blood

D72.825 **Bandemia**
Bandemia without diagnosis of
specific infection
*Excess number of band cells (immature
white blood cells) released by bone
marrow*

> **Excludes1** confirmed infection
> -code to infection
> leukemia (C91.-,
> C92.-, C93.-,
> C94.-, C95.-)

D72.828 **Other elevated white blood cell count**

D72.829 **Elevated white blood cell count, unspecified**
Elevated leukocytes, unspecified
Leukocytosis, unspecified

D72.89 **Other specified disorders of white blood cells**
Abnormality of white blood cells NEC

D72.9 **Disorder of white blood cells, unspecified**
Abnormal leukocyte differential NOS

● **D73** **Diseases of spleen**

D73.0 **Hyposplenism**
Diminished functioning of spleen
Atrophy of spleen

> **Excludes1** asplenia (congenital) (Q89.01)
> postsurgical absence of spleen (Z90.81)

D73.1 **Hypersplenism**
Accelerated function of spleen

> **Excludes1** neutropenic splenomegaly (D73.81)
> primary splenic neutropenia (D73.81)
> splenitis, splenomegaly in late syphilis
> (A52.79)
> splenitis, splenomegaly in tuberculosis
> (A18.85)
> splenomegaly NOS (R16.1)
> splenomegaly congenital (Q89.0)

D73.2 **Chronic congestive splenomegaly**
Enlargement of spleen

D73.3 **Abscess of spleen**

D73.4 **Cyst of spleen**

D73.5 **Infarction of spleen**
Splenic rupture, nontraumatic
Torsion of spleen

> **Excludes1** rupture of spleen due to Plasmodium
> vivax malaria (B51.0)
> traumatic rupture of spleen (S36.03-)

● D73.8 **Other diseases of spleen**

D73.81 **Neutropenic splenomegaly**
Werner-Schultz disease
*Enlarged spleen responding to inadequate number
of neutrophils*

D73.89 **Other diseases of spleen**
Fibrosis of spleen NOS
Perisplenitis
Splenitis NOS

D73.9 **Disease of spleen, unspecified**

● D74 **Methemoglobinemia**
Excessive methemoglobin (form of hemoglobin)

D74.0 **Congenital methemoglobinemia**
Congenital NADH-methemoglobin reductase
deficiency
Hemoglobin-M [Hb-M] disease
Methemoglobinemia, hereditary

D74.8 **Other methemoglobinemias**
Acquired methemoglobinemia (with
sulfhemoglobinemia)
Toxic methemoglobinemia

D74.9 **Methemoglobinemia, unspecified**

● **D75** **Other and unspecified diseases of blood and blood-forming organs**

> **Excludes2** acute lymphadenitis (L04.-)
> chronic lymphadenitis (I88.1)
> enlarged lymph nodes (R59.-)
> hypergammaglobulinemia NOS (D89.2)
> lymphadenitis NOS (I88.9)
> mesenteric lymphadenitis (acute) (chronic) (I88.0)

D75.0 **Familial erythrocytosis**
*Genetic mutation of gene that results in increased circulating
RBCs*
Benign polycythemia
Familial polycythemia

> **Excludes1** hereditary ovalocytosis (D58.1)

D75.1 **Secondary polycythemia**
Increase in total red cell mass
Acquired polycythemia
Emotional polycythemia
Erythrocytosis NOS
Hypoxemic polycythemia
Nephrogenous polycythemia
Polycythemia due to erythropoietin
Polycythemia due to fall in plasma volume
Polycythemia due to high altitude
Polycythemia due to stress
Polycythemia NOS
Relative polycythemia

> **Excludes1** polycythemia neonatorum (P61.1)
> polycythemia vera (D45)

● D75.8 **Other specified diseases of blood and blood-forming
organs**

▷ D75.81 *Myelofibrosis* 🅗
Replacing bone marrow by fibrous tissue
Myelofibrosis NOS
Secondary myelofibrosis NOS

Code first the underlying disorder, such as:
malignant neoplasm of breast (C50.-)
Use additional code, if applicable,
for associated therapy-related
myelodysplastic syndrome (D46.-)
Use additional code for adverse effect, if
applicable, to identify drug (T45.1X5)

> **Excludes1** acute myelofibrosis (C94.4-)
> idiopathic myelofibrosis (D47.1)
> leukoerythroblastic anemia
> (D61.82)
> myelofibrosis with myeloid
> metaplasia (D47.4)
> myelophthisic anemia (D61.82)
> myelophthisis (D61.82)
> primary myelofibrosis (D47.1)

D75.82 **Heparin induced thrombocytopenia (HIT)** 🅗
Use Additional code, if applicable, for adverse
effect of heparin (T45.515-)

D75.821 **Non-immune heparin-induced
thrombocytopenia**
Non-immune HIT
Type 1 heparin-induced
thrombocytopenia

D75.822 **Immune-mediated heparin-induced
thrombocytopenia**
Immune-mediated HIT
Type 2 heparin-induced
thrombocytopenia

D75.828 **Other heparin-induced thrombocytopenia syndrome**
Autoimmune heparin-induced thrombocytopenia syndrome
Delayed-onset heparin-induced thrombocytopenia
Persisting heparin-induced thrombocytopenia

D75.829 **Heparin-induced thrombocytopenia, unspecified**

● D75.83 **Thrombocytosis**

    Excludes2   essential thrombocythemia (D47.3)

D75.838 **Other thrombocytosis**
Reactive thrombocytosis
Secondary thrombocytosis
Code also, underlying condition, if known and applicable

D75.839 **Thrombocytosis, unspecified**
Thrombocythemia NOS
Thrombocytosis NOS

D75.84 **Other platelet-activating anti-PF4 disorders**
Spontaneous heparin-induced thrombocytopenia syndrome (without heparin exposure)
Thrombosis with thrombocytopenia syndrome
Vaccine-induced thrombotic thrombocytopenia
Use Additional code, if applicable, for adverse effect of other viral vaccine (T50.B95-)

D75.89 **Other specified diseases of blood and blood-forming organs**

D75.9 **Disease of blood and blood-forming organs, unspecified**

D75.A **Glucose-6-phosphate dehydrogenase (G6PD) deficiency without anemia**

    Excludes1   glucose-6-phosphate dehydrogenase (G6PD) deficiency with anemia (D55.0)

● **D76 Other specified diseases with participation of lymphoreticular and reticulohistiocytic tissue**

    Excludes1   (Abt-) Letterer-Siwe disease (C96.0)
eosinophilic granuloma (C96.6)
Hand-Schüller-Christian disease (C96.5)
histiocytic medullary reticulosis (C96.9)
histiocytic sarcoma (C96.A)
histiocytosis X, multifocal (C96.5)
histiocytosis X, unifocal (C96.6)
Langerhans-cell histiocytosis, multifocal (C96.5)
Langerhans-cell histiocytosis NOS (C96.6)
Langerhans-cell histiocytosis, unifocal (C96.6)
leukemic reticuloendotheliosis (C91.4-)
lipomelanotic reticulosis (I89.8)
malignant histiocytosis (C96.A)
malignant reticulosis (C86.0)
nonlipid reticuloendotheliosis (C96.0)

D76.1 **Hemophagocytic lymphohistiocytosis** 🔗
Familial hemophagocytic reticulosis
Histiocytoses of mononuclear phagocytes

D76.2 **Hemophagocytic syndrome, infection-associated** 🔗
Use additional code to identify infectious agent or disease.

D76.3 **Other histiocytosis syndromes** 🔗
Reticulohistiocytoma (giant-cell)
Sinus histiocytosis with massive lymphadenopathy
Xanthogranuloma

▶ **D77 Other disorders of blood and blood-forming organs in diseases classified elsewhere**
Code first underlying disease, such as:
amyloidosis (E85.-)
congenital early syphilis (A50.0-)
echinococcosis (B67.0-B67.9)
malaria (B50.0-B54)
schistosomiasis [bilharziasis] (B65.0-B65.9)
vitamin C deficiency (E54)

    Excludes1   rupture of spleen due to Plasmodium vivax malaria (B51.0)
splenitis, splenomegaly in late syphilis (A52.79)
splenitis, splenomegaly in tuberculosis (A18.85)

INTRAOPERATIVE AND POSTPROCEDURAL COMPLICATIONS OF THE SPLEEN (D78)

● **D78 Intraoperative and postprocedural complications of the spleen**
Coding Clinic: 2016, Q4, P9

● D78.0 **Intraoperative hemorrhage and hematoma of the spleen complicating a procedure**

    Excludes1   intraoperative hemorrhage and hematoma of the spleen due to accidental puncture or laceration during a procedure (D78.1-)

D78.01 **Intraoperative hemorrhage and hematoma of the spleen complicating a procedure on the spleen**

D78.02 **Intraoperative hemorrhage and hematoma of the spleen complicating other procedure**

● D78.1 **Accidental puncture and laceration of the spleen during a procedure**

D78.11 **Accidental puncture and laceration of the spleen during a procedure on the spleen**

D78.12 **Accidental puncture and laceration of the spleen during other procedure**
Coding Clinic: 2022, Q1, P22-23

● D78.2 **Postprocedural hemorrhage of the spleen following a procedure**

D78.21 **Postprocedural hemorrhage of the spleen following a procedure on the spleen**

D78.22 **Postprocedural hemorrhage of the spleen following other procedure**

● D78.3 **Postprocedural hematoma and seroma of the spleen following a procedure**

D78.31 **Postprocedural hematoma of the spleen following a procedure on the spleen**

D78.32 **Postprocedural hematoma of the spleen following other procedure**

D78.33 **Postprocedural seroma of the spleen following a procedure on the spleen**

D78.34 **Postprocedural seroma of the spleen following other procedure**

● D78.8 **Other intraoperative and postprocedural complications of the spleen**
Use additional code, if applicable, to further specify disorder

D78.81 **Other intraoperative complications of the spleen**

D78.89 **Other postprocedural complications of the spleen**

CERTAIN DISORDERS INVOLVING THE IMMUNE MECHANISM (D80-D89)

    Includes   defects in the complement system
immunodeficiency disorders, except human immunodeficiency virus [HIV] disease
sarcoidosis

    Excludes1   autoimmune disease (systemic) NOS (M35.9)
functional disorders of polymorphonuclear neutrophils (D71)
human immunodeficiency virus [HIV] disease (B20)

CHAPTER 3 (D50-D89)

● **D80　Immunodeficiency with predominantly antibody defects**

　D80.0　**Hereditary hypogammaglobulinemia** 🦠
　　　　Autosomal recessive agammaglobulinemia (Swiss type)
　　　　X-linked agammaglobulinemia [Bruton] (with growth hormone deficiency)

　D80.1　**Nonfamilial hypogammaglobulinemia** 🦠
　　　　Abnormally low levels of all classes of immunoglobulins
　　　　Agammaglobulinemia with immunoglobulin-bearing B-lymphocytes
　　　　Common variable agammaglobulinemia [CVAgamma]
　　　　Hypogammaglobulinemia NOS

　D80.2　**Selective deficiency of immunoglobulin A [IgA]** 🦠

　D80.3　**Selective deficiency of immunoglobulin G [IgG] subclasses** 🦠

　D80.4　**Selective deficiency of immunoglobulin M [IgM]** 🦠

　D80.5　**Immunodeficiency with increased immunoglobulin M [IgM]** 🦠

　D80.6　**Antibody deficiency with near-normal immunoglobulins or with hyperimmunoglobulinemia** 🦠
　　　　Abnormally high levels of immunoglobulins in serum

　D80.7　**Transient hypogammaglobulinemia of infancy** 🦠

　D80.8　**Other immunodeficiencies with predominantly antibody defects** 🦠
　　　　Kappa light chain deficiency

　D80.9　**Immunodeficiency with predominantly antibody defects, unspecified** 🦠

● **D81　Combined immunodeficiencies**

　Excludes1　autosomal recessive agammaglobulinemia (Swiss type) (D80.0)

　D81.0　**Severe combined immunodeficiency [SCID] with reticular dysgenesis** 🦠

　D81.1　**Severe combined immunodeficiency [SCID] with low T- and B-cell numbers** 🦠

　D81.2　**Severe combined immunodeficiency [SCID] with low or normal B-cell numbers** 🦠

● D81.3　**Adenosine deaminase [ADA] deficiency** 🦠

　　D81.30　**Adenosine deaminase deficiency, unspecified**
　　　　　ADA deficiency NOS

　　D81.31　**Severe combined immunodeficiency due to adenosine deaminase deficiency**
　　　　　ADA deficiency with SCID
　　　　　Adenosine deaminase [ADA] deficiency with severe combined immunodeficiency

　　D81.32　**Adenosine deaminase 2 deficiency**
　　　　　ADA2 deficiency
　　　　　Adenosine deaminase deficiency type 2
　　　　　Code also, if applicable, any associated manifestations, such as:
　　　　　　polyarteritis nodosa (M30.0)
　　　　　　stroke (I63.-)

　　D81.39　**Other adenosine deaminase deficiency**
　　　　　Adenosine deaminase [ADA] deficiency type 1, NOS
　　　　　Adenosine deaminase [ADA] deficiency type 1, without SCID
　　　　　Adenosine deaminase [ADA] deficiency type 1, without severe combined immunodeficiency
　　　　　Partial ADA deficiency (type 1)
　　　　　Partial adenosine deaminase deficiency (type 1)

　D81.4　**Nezelof's syndrome** 🦠

　D81.5　**Purine nucleoside phosphorylase [PNP] deficiency** 🦠

　D81.6　**Major histocompatibility complex class I deficiency** 🦠
　　　　Bare lymphocyte syndrome

　D81.7　**Major histocompatibility complex class II deficiency** 🦠

● D81.8　**Other combined immunodeficiencies**

　● D81.81　**Biotin-dependent carboxylase deficiency**
　　　　　Multiple carboxylase deficiency

　　　　Excludes1　biotin-dependent carboxylase deficiency due to dietary deficiency of biotin (E53.8)

　　　D81.810　**Biotinidase deficiency**

　　　D81.818　**Other biotin-dependent carboxylase deficiency**
　　　　　　Holocarboxylase synthetase deficiency
　　　　　　Other multiple carboxylase deficiency

　　　D81.819　**Biotin-dependent carboxylase deficiency, unspecified**
　　　　　　Multiple carboxylase deficiency, unspecified

　　D81.82　**Activated Phosphoinositide 3-kinase Delta Syndrome [APDS]**
　　　　　p110d-activating mutation causing senescent T cells, lymphadenopathy, and immunodeficiency [PASLI] disease
　　　　　Code also, if applicable, any associated manifestations, such as:
　　　　　　bronchiectasis (J47.-)
　　　　　　herpes virus infections (B00.-)
　　　　　　other acute respiratory tract infections (J00-J06; J20-J22)
　　　　　　other infections (A00-B99)
　　　　　　pneumonia (J12-J18)

　　D81.89　**Other combined immunodeficiencies** 🦠

　D81.9　**Combined immunodeficiency, unspecified** 🦠
　　　　Severe combined immunodeficiency disorder [SCID] NOS

● **D82　Immunodeficiency associated with other major defects**

　Excludes1　ataxia telangiectasia [Louis-Bar] (G11.3)

　D82.0　**Wiskott-Aldrich syndrome** 🦠
　　　　X-linked immunodeficiency
　　　　Immunodeficiency with thrombocytopenia and eczema

　D82.1　**Di George's syndrome** 🦠
　　　　Congenital disorder with defective development of third and fourth pharyngeal pouches
　　　　Pharyngeal pouch syndrome
　　　　Thymic alymphoplasia
　　　　Thymic aplasia or hypoplasia with immunodeficiency
　　　　Coding Clinic: 2019, Q3, P14

　D82.2　**Immunodeficiency with short-limbed stature** 🦠

　D82.3　**Immunodeficiency following hereditary defective response to Epstein-Barr virus** 🦠
　　　　X-linked lymphoproliferative disease

　D82.4　**Hyperimmunoglobulin E [IgE] syndrome** 🦠
　　　　Suspected genetic defect that produces high levels of antibody immunoglobulin (IgE) that causes skin and lung infections and eczema

　D82.8　**Immunodeficiency associated with other specified major defects** 🦠

　D82.9　**Immunodeficiency associated with major defect, unspecified** 🦠

● **D83　Common variable immunodeficiency**

　D83.0　**Common variable immunodeficiency with predominant abnormalities of B-cell numbers and function** 🦠

　D83.1　**Common variable immunodeficiency with predominant immunoregulatory T-cell disorders** 🦠

　D83.2　**Common variable immunodeficiency with autoantibodies to B- or T-cells** 🦠

　D83.8　**Other common variable immunodeficiencies** 🦠

　D83.9　**Common variable immunodeficiency, unspecified** 🦠

● **D84　Other immunodeficiencies**

　D84.0　**Lymphocyte function antigen-1 [LFA-1] defect** 🦠

● **D84.1 Defects in the complement system** 🔖
C1 esterase inhibitor [C1-INH] deficiency

D84.8 Other specified immunodeficiencies 🔖

▷ *D84.81 Immunodeficiency due to conditions classified elsewhere*

Code first underlying condition, such as:
chromosomal abnormalities (Q90-Q99)
diabetes mellitus (E08-E13)
malignant neoplasms (C00-C96)

Excludes1 *certain disorders involving the immune mechanism (D80-D83, D84.0, D84.1, D84.9)*
human immunodeficiency virus [HIV] disease (B20)

● **D84.82 Immunodeficiency due to drugs and external causes**

D84.821 Immunodeficiency due to drugs
Immunodeficiency due to (current or past) medication

Use additional code for adverse effect if applicable, to identify adverse effect of drug (T36-T50 with fifth or six character 5)

Use additional code, if applicable, for associated long term (current) drug therapy drug or medication such as:
long term (current) drug therapy systemic steroids (Z79.52)
other long term (current) drug therapy (Z79.899)

D84.822 Immunodeficiency due to external causes

Code also, if applicable, radiological procedure and radiotherapy (Y84.2)

Use additional code for external cause such as:
exposure to ionizing radiation (W88)

D84.89 Other immunodeficiencies

D84.9 Immunodeficiency, unspecified 🔖
Immunocompromised NOS
Immunodeficient NOS
Immunosuppressed NOS

● **D86 Sarcoidosis**

D86.0 Sarcoidosis of lung 🔖

D86.1 Sarcoidosis of lymph nodes

D86.2 Sarcoidosis of lung with sarcoidosis of lymph nodes 🔖

D86.3 Sarcoidosis of skin

● **D86.8 Sarcoidosis of other sites**

D86.81 Sarcoid meningitis

D86.82 Multiple cranial nerve palsies in sarcoidosis 🔖

D86.83 Sarcoid iridocyclitis
Rare large tumor with irregular surface of iris

D86.84 Sarcoid pyelonephritis
Systemic disease of unknown etiology characterized by chronic granulomatous inflammation with tissue destruction of pelvis kidney
Tubulo-interstitial nephropathy in sarcoidosis

D86.85 Sarcoid myocarditis

D86.86 Sarcoid arthropathy
Polyarthritis in sarcoidosis

D86.87 Sarcoid myositis
Granumloma of muscle

D86.89 Sarcoidosis of other sites
Hepatic granuloma
Uveoparotid fever [Heerfordt]

D86.9 Sarcoidosis, unspecified

Item 3-1 Sarcoidosis: A symptom of an inflammation producing tiny lumps of cells (granulomas) in various organs, most commonly the lungs and lymph nodes, that affect organ function. Cause is unknown occurring primarily in 20- to 40-year-olds, African-American, especially women, and those of Asian, German, Irish, Scandinavian, and Puerto Rican heritage.

● **D89 Other disorders involving the immune mechanism, not elsewhere classified**

Excludes1 hyperglobulinemia NOS (R77.1)
monoclonal gammopathy (of undetermined significance) (D47.2)

Excludes2 transplant failure and rejection (T86.-)

D89.0 Polyclonal hypergammaglobulinemia
Benign hypergammaglobulinemic purpura
Polyclonal gammopathy NOS

D89.1 Cryoglobulinemia 🔖
Cryoglobulin (proteins) in blood that precipitate temperatures below 98.6° F; usually symptomatic of underlying disease
Cryoglobulinemic purpura
Cryoglobulinemic vasculitis
Essential cryoglobulinemia
Idiopathic cryoglobulinemia
Mixed cryoglobulinemia
Primary cryoglobulinemia
Secondary cryoglobulinemia

D89.2 Hypergammaglobulinemia, unspecified

D89.3 Immune reconstitution syndrome 🔖
Immune reconstitution inflammatory syndrome [IRIS]

Use additional code for adverse effect, if applicable, to identify drug (T36-T50 with fifth or sixth character 5)

● **D89.4 Mast cell activation syndrome and related disorders**

Excludes1 aggressive systemic mastocytosis (C96.21)
congenital cutaneous mastocytosis (Q82.2)
(non-congenital) cutaneous mastocytosis (D47.01)
(indolent) systemic mastocytosis (D47.02)
malignant mast cell neoplasm (C96.2-)
malignant mastocytoma (C96.29)
mast cell leukemia (C94.3-)
mast cell sarcoma (C96.22)
mastocytoma NOS (D47.09)
other mast cell neoplasms of uncertain behavior (D47.09)
systemic mastocytosis associated with a clonal hematologic non-mast cell lineage disease (SM-AHNMD) (D47.02)

Coding Clinic: 2016, Q4, P11

D89.40 Mast cell activation, unspecified 🔖
Mast cell activation disorder, unspecified
Mast cell activation syndrome, NOS

D89.41 Monoclonal mast cell activation syndrome 🔖
Coding Clinic: 2016, Q4, P11

D89.42 Idiopathic mast cell activation syndrome 🔖
Coding Clinic: 2016, Q4, P11

D89.44 Hereditary alpha tryptasemia
Use additional code, if applicable, for:
allergy status, other than to drugs and biological substances (Z91.0-)
personal history of anaphylaxis (Z87.892)

D89.43 Secondary mast cell activation 🔖
Secondary mast cell activation syndrome
Code also underlying etiology, if known
Coding Clinic: 2016, Q4, P11

D89.49 Other mast cell activation disorder 🔖
Other mast cell activation syndrome
Coding Clinic: 2016, Q4, P11

CHAPTER 3 (D50-D89)

● **D89.8   Other specified disorders involving the immune mechanism, not elsewhere classified**

  ● **D89.81   Graft-versus-host disease**

     Code first underlying cause, such as:
       complications of transplanted organs and tissue (T86.-)
       complications of blood transfusion (T80.89)

     Use additional code to identify associated manifestations, such as:
     desquamative dermatitis (L30.8)
     diarrhea (R19.7)
     elevated bilirubin (R17)
     hair loss (L65.9)

     D89.810   Acute graft-versus-host disease 🦠

     D89.811   Chronic graft-versus-host disease 🦠
               Coding Clinic: 2023, Q3, P20

     D89.812   Acute on chronic graft-versus-host disease 🦠

     D89.813   Graft-versus-host disease, unspecified 🦠

   D89.82   Autoimmune lymphoproliferative syndrome [ALPS] 🦠

   D89.84   IgG4-related disease
     Immunoglobulin G4-related disease

● **D89.83   Cytokine release syndrome**   No Exclusions

     Code first underlying cause, such as:
     complications following infusion, transfusion and therapeutic injection (T80.89-)
     complications of transplanted organs and tissue (T86.-)

     Use additional code to identify associated manifestations
     ▶code for adverse effect, if applicable, to identify immune checkpointinhibitors and immunostimulant drugs (T45.AX5)

     D89.831   Cytokine release syndrome, grade 1

     D89.832   Cytokine release syndrome, grade 2

     D89.833   Cytokine release syndrome, grade 3

     D89.834   Cytokine release syndrome, grade 4

     D89.835   Cytokine release syndrome, grade 5

     D89.839   Cytokine release syndrome, grade unspecified

   D89.89   Other specified disorders involving the immune mechanism, not elsewhere classified 🦠

     Excludes1   human immunodeficiency virus disease (B20)

     Coding Clinic: 2017, Q4, P109

D89.9   Disorder involving the immune mechanism, unspecified 🦠
   Immune disease NOS
   Coding Clinic: 2015, Q3, P22

▶ New   ⇒ Revised   ~~deleted~~ Deleted   Excludes 1   Excludes 2   Includes   Use additional   Code first   Code also   Key words

OGCR Official Guidelines   X Assign placeholder X   ● Use Additional Character(s)   ▷ Manifestation Code   🦠 Hierarchical Condition Category   Coding Clinic

CHAPTER 4

ENDOCRINE, NUTRITIONAL AND METABOLIC DISEASES (E00-E89)

OGCR Chapter-Specific Coding Guidelines

4. Chapter 4: Endocrine, Nutritional, and Metabolic Diseases (E00-E89)

  a. Diabetes mellitus

The diabetes mellitus codes are combination codes that include the type of diabetes mellitus, the body system affected, and the complications affecting that body system. As many codes within a particular category as are necessary to describe all of the complications of the disease may be used. They should be sequenced based on the reason for a particular encounter. Assign as many codes from categories E08 – E13 as needed to identify all of the associated conditions that the patient has.

    1) Type of diabetes

The age of a patient is not the sole determining factor, though most type 1 diabetics develop the condition before reaching puberty. For this reason type 1 diabetes mellitus is also referred to as juvenile diabetes.

    2) Type of diabetes mellitus not documented

If the type of diabetes mellitus is not documented in the medical record the default is E11.-, Type 2 diabetes mellitus.

    3) Diabetes mellitus and the use of insulin oral hypoglycemics

If the documentation in a medical record does not indicate the type of diabetes but does indicate that the patient uses insulin, code E11, Type 2 diabetes mellitus, should be assigned. An additional code should be assigned from category Z79 to identify the long-term (current) use of insulin or oral hypoglycemic drugs. If the patient is treated with both oral medications and insulin, only the code for long-term (current) use of insulin should be assigned. Code Z79.4 should not be assigned if insulin is given temporarily to bring a type 2 patient's blood sugar under control during an encounter.

    4) Diabetes mellitus in pregnancy and gestational diabetes

See Section I.C.15. Diabetes mellitus in pregnancy.
See Section I.C.15. Gestational (pregnancy induced) diabetes

    5) Complications due to insulin pump malfunction

      (a) Underdose of insulin due to insulin pump failure

An underdose of insulin due to an insulin pump failure should be assigned to a code from subcategory T85.6, Mechanical complication of other specified internal and external prosthetic devices, implants and grafts, that specifies the type of pump malfunction, as the principal or first-listed code, followed by code T38.3X6-, Underdosing of insulin and oral hypoglycemic [antidiabetic] drugs. Additional codes for the type of diabetes mellitus and any associated complications due to the underdosing should also be assigned.

      (b) Overdose of insulin due to insulin pump failure

The principal or first-listed code for an encounter due to an insulin pump malfunction resulting in an overdose of insulin, should also be T85.6-, Mechanical complication of other specified internal and external prosthetic devices, implants and grafts, followed by code T38.3X1-, Poisoning by insulin and oral hypoglycemic [antidiabetic] drugs, accidental (unintentional).

    6) Secondary diabetes mellitus

Codes under categories E08, Diabetes mellitus due to underlying condition, E09, Drug or chemical induced diabetes mellitus and E13, Other specified diabetes mellitus, identify complications/manifestations associated with secondary diabetes mellitus. Secondary diabetes is always caused by another condition or event (e.g., cystic fibrosis, malignant neoplasm of pancreas, pancreatectomy, adverse effect of drug, or poisoning).

      (a) Secondary diabetes mellitus and the use of insulin or hypoglycemic drugs

For patients with secondary diabetes mellitus who routinely use insulin or oral hypoglycemic drugs, an additional code from category Z79 should be assigned to identify the long-term (current) use of insulin or oral hypoglycemic drugs. If the patient is treated with both oral medications and insulin, only the code for long-term (current) use of insulin should be assigned. Code Z79.4 should not be assigned if insulin is given temporarily to bring a type 2 patient's blood sugar under control during an encounter.

      (b) Assigning and sequencing secondary diabetes codes and its causes

The sequencing of the secondary diabetes codes in relationship to codes for the cause of the diabetes is based on the Tabular List instructions for categories E08, E09 and E13.

        (i) Secondary diabetes mellitus due to pancreatectomy For postpancreatectomy diabetes mellitus (lack of insulin due to the surgical removal of all or part of the pancreas), assign code E89.1, Postprocedural hypoinsulinemia. Assign a code from category E13 and a code from subcategory Z90.41-, Acquired absence of pancreas, as additional codes.

        (ii) Secondary diabetes due to drugs Secondary diabetes may be caused by an adverse effect of correctly administered medications, poisoning or sequela of poisoning.

See Section I.C.19.e for coding of adverse effects and poisoning, and Section I.C.20 for external cause code reporting.

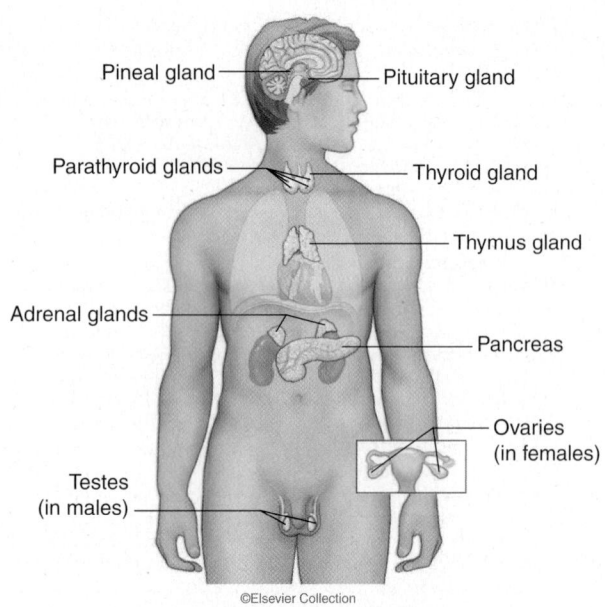

Figure 4-1   The endocrine system. ©Elsevier Collection.

Figure 4-2   Goiter is an enlargement of the thyroid gland.

Item 4–1   Simple goiter indicates no nodules are present. The most common type of goiter is a **diffuse colloidal,** also called a **nontoxic** or **endemic** goiter.

E00.2   **Congenital iodine-deficiency syndrome, mixed type**
Endemic cretinism, mixed type

E00.9   **Congenital iodine-deficiency syndrome, unspecified**
Congenital iodine-deficiency hypothyroidism NOS
Endemic cretinism NOS

● E01   **Iodine-deficiency related thyroid disorders and allied conditions**
Excludes1   congenital iodine-deficiency syndrome (E00.-)
subclinical iodine-deficiency hypothyroidism (E02)

E01.0   **Iodine-deficiency related diffuse (endemic) goiter**
Thyroid gland is enlarged

E01.1   **Iodine-deficiency related multinodular (endemic) goiter**
Iodine-deficiency related nodular goiter

E01.2   **Iodine-deficiency related (endemic) goiter, unspecified**
Endemic goiter NOS

E01.8   **Other iodine-deficiency related thyroid disorders and allied conditions**
Acquired iodine-deficiency hypothyroidism NOS

E02   **Subclinical iodine-deficiency hypothyroidism**
Coding Clinic: 2021, Q1, P8-9

● E03   **Other hypothyroidism**
Excludes1   iodine-deficiency related hypothyroidism (E00-E02)
postprocedural hypothyroidism (E89.0)

E03.0   **Congenital hypothyroidism with diffuse goiter**
Congenital parenchymatous goiter (nontoxic)
Congenital goiter (nontoxic) NOS
Excludes1   transitory congenital goiter with normal function (P72.0)

E03.1   **Congenital hypothyroidism without goiter**
Aplasia of thyroid (with myxedema)
Congenital atrophy of thyroid
Congenital hypothyroidism NOS

E03.2   **Hypothyroidism due to medicaments and other exogenous substances**
Code first poisoning due to drug or toxin, if applicable (T36-T65 with fifth or sixth character 1-4)
Use additional code for adverse effect, if applicable, to identify drug (T36-T50 with fifth or sixth character 5)

E03.3   **Postinfectious hypothyroidism**

E03.4   **Atrophy of thyroid (acquired)**
Excludes1   congenital atrophy of thyroid (E03.1)

E03.5   **Myxedema coma** 🏷
Often fatal complication of long-term hypothyroidism

E03.8   **Other specified hypothyroidism**

E03.9   **Hypothyroidism, unspecified**
Myxedema NOS
Coding Clinic: 2021, Q1, P9

CHAPTER 4

ENDOCRINE, NUTRITIONAL AND METABOLIC DISEASES (E00-E89)

All neoplasms, whether functionally active or not, are classified in Chapter 2. Appropriate codes in this chapter (i.e., E05.8, E07.0, E16-E31, E34.-) may be used as additional codes to indicate either functional activity by neoplasms and ectopic endocrine tissue or hyperfunction and hypofunction of endocrine glands associated with neoplasms and other conditions classified elsewhere.

Excludes1   transitory endocrine and metabolic disorders specific to newborn (P70-P74)

This chapter contains the following blocks:

E00-E07	Disorders of thyroid gland
E08-E13	Diabetes mellitus
E15-E16	Other disorders of glucose regulation and pancreatic internal secretion
E20-E35	Disorders of other endocrine glands
E36	Intraoperative complications of endocrine system
E40-E46	Malnutrition
E50-E64	Other nutritional deficiencies
E65-E68	Overweight, obesity and other hyperalimentation
E70-E88	Metabolic disorders
E89	Postprocedural endocrine and metabolic complications and disorders, not elsewhere classified

DISORDERS OF THYROID GLAND (E00-E07)

● E00   **Congenital iodine-deficiency syndrome**
Use additional code (F70-F79) to identify associated intellectual disabilities.
Excludes1   subclinical iodine-deficiency hypothyroidism (E02)

E00.0   **Congenital iodine-deficiency syndrome, neurological type**
Endemic cretinism, neurological type

E00.1   **Congenital iodine-deficiency syndrome, myxedematous type**
Dry, waxy type of swelling (nonpitting edema) with abnormal deposits of mucin in skin (mucinosis) and other tissues
Endemic hypothyroid cretinism
Endemic cretinism, myxedematous type

Item 4–2   Hypothyroidism is a condition in which there are insufficient levels of thyroxine. **Cretinism** is congenital hypothyroidism, which can result in mental and physical retardation.

▶ New   ⟹ Revised   ~~deleted~~ Deleted   Excludes 1   Excludes 2   Includes   Use additional   Code first   Code also   Key words
OGCR Official Guidelines   X Assign placeholder X   ● Use Additional Character(s)   ▶ Manifestation Code   🏷 Hierarchical Condition Category   Coding Clinic

● **E04   Other nontoxic goiter**

     Excludes1   congenital goiter (NOS) (diffuse)
                   (parenchymatous) (E03.0)
                 iodine-deficiency related goiter (E00-E02)

     E04.0   Nontoxic diffuse goiter
           Thyroid gland is enlarged
           Diffuse (colloid) nontoxic goiter
           Simple nontoxic goiter

     E04.1   Nontoxic single thyroid nodule
           Colloid nodule (cystic) (thyroid)
           Nontoxic uninodular goiter
           Thyroid (cystic) nodule NOS

     E04.2   Nontoxic multinodular goiter
           Enlarged thyroid gland with multiple nodules
           Cystic goiter NOS
           Multinodular (cystic) goiter NOS

     E04.8   Other specified nontoxic goiter

     E04.9   Nontoxic goiter, unspecified
           Goiter NOS
           Nodular goiter (nontoxic) NOS

● **E05   Thyrotoxicosis [hyperthyroidism]**
     Enlarged thyroid gland with multiple nodules

     Excludes1   chronic thyroiditis with transient thyrotoxicosis
                 (E06.2)
                 neonatal thyrotoxicosis (P72.1)

● **E05.0   Thyrotoxicosis with diffuse goiter**
           Exophthalmic or toxic goiter NOS
           Graves' disease
           Toxic diffuse goiter

     E05.00   Thyrotoxicosis with diffuse goiter without thyrotoxic crisis or storm

     E05.01   Thyrotoxicosis with diffuse goiter with thyrotoxic crisis or storm

● **E05.1   Thyrotoxicosis with toxic single thyroid nodule**
           Thyrotoxicosis with toxic uninodular goiter

     E05.10   Thyrotoxicosis with toxic single thyroid nodule without thyrotoxic crisis or storm

     E05.11   Thyrotoxicosis with toxic single thyroid nodule with thyrotoxic crisis or storm

● **E05.2   Thyrotoxicosis with toxic multinodular goiter**
           Toxic nodular goiter NOS

     E05.20   Thyrotoxicosis with toxic multinodular goiter without thyrotoxic crisis or storm

     E05.21   Thyrotoxicosis with toxic multinodular goiter with thyrotoxic crisis or storm

● **E05.3   Thyrotoxicosis from ectopic thyroid tissue**

     E05.30   Thyrotoxicosis from ectopic thyroid tissue without thyrotoxic crisis or storm

     E05.31   Thyrotoxicosis from ectopic thyroid tissue with thyrotoxic crisis or storm

● **E05.4   Thyrotoxicosis factitia**

     E05.40   Thyrotoxicosis factitia without thyrotoxic crisis or storm

     E05.41   Thyrotoxicosis factitia with thyrotoxic crisis or storm

● **E05.8   Other thyrotoxicosis**
           Overproduction of thyroid-stimulating hormone

     E05.80   Other thyrotoxicosis without thyrotoxic crisis or storm

     E05.81   Other thyrotoxicosis with thyrotoxic crisis or storm

● **E05.9   Thyrotoxicosis, unspecified**
           Hyperthyroidism NOS

     E05.90   Thyrotoxicosis, unspecified without thyrotoxic crisis or storm

     E05.91   Thyrotoxicosis, unspecified with thyrotoxic crisis or storm

● **E06   Thyroiditis**
     An inflammation of the thyroid gland which results in an inability to convert iodine into thyroid hormone

     Excludes1   postpartum thyroiditis (O90.5)

     E06.0   Acute thyroiditis
           Abscess of thyroid
           Pyogenic thyroiditis
           Suppurative thyroiditis
           Use additional code (B95-B97) to identify infectious agent.

     E06.1   Subacute thyroiditis
           Inflammation of thyroid gland following viral upper respiratory infection
           de Quervain thyroiditis
           Giant-cell thyroiditis
           Granulomatous thyroiditis
           Nonsuppurative thyroiditis
           Viral thyroiditis

         Excludes1   autoimmune thyroiditis (E06.3)

     E06.2   Chronic thyroiditis with transient thyrotoxicosis
           Chronic inflammation of thyroid gland with intermittent overproduction of thyroid hormone

         Excludes1   autoimmune thyroiditis (E06.3)

     E06.3   Autoimmune thyroiditis
           Hashimoto's thyroiditis
           Hashitoxicosis (transient)
           Lymphadenoid goiter
           Lymphocytic thyroiditis
           Struma lymphomatosa
           Coding Clinic: 2024, Q1, P14

     E06.4   Drug-induced thyroiditis
           Use additional code for adverse effect, if applicable, to identify drug (T36-T50 with fifth or sixth character 5)

     E06.5   Other chronic thyroiditis
           Chronic fibrous thyroiditis
           Chronic thyroiditis NOS
           Ligneous thyroiditis
           Riedel thyroiditis

     E06.9   Thyroiditis, unspecified

Figure 4-3   Graves' disease. In Graves' disease, exophthalmos often looks more pronounced than it actually is because of the extreme lid retraction that may occur. This patient, for instance, had minimal proptosis of the left eye but marked lid retraction. (From Lissauer T, Clayden G, and Craft A: Illustrated Textbook of Paediatrics, Edinburgh, Mosby, 2015)

Item 4–3   Thyrotoxicosis is a condition caused by excessive amounts of the thyroid hormone thyroxine production or hyperthyroidism. **Graves' disease is associated with hyperthyroidism** (known as **Basedow's disease** in Europe).

CHAPTER 4 (E00-E89)

E07 Other disorders of thyroid

E07.0 Hypersecretion of calcitonin
C-cell hyperplasia of thyroid
Hypersecretion of thyrocalcitonin

E07.1 Dyshormogenetic goiter
Group of several types of goiter resulting from enzyme defects in hormone synthesis
▶Dyshormonogenetic goiter
Familial dyshormogenetic goiter
Pendred's syndrome
Excludes1 transitory congenital goiter with normal function (P72.0)

E07.8 Other specified disorders of thyroid
E07.81 Sick-euthyroid syndrome
Euthyroid sick-syndrome
E07.89 Other specified disorders of thyroid
Abnormality of thyroid-binding globulin
Hemorrhage of thyroid
Infarction of thyroid

E07.9 Disorder of thyroid, unspecified
OGCR Section I.C.4.a.

Diabetes mellitus

The diabetes mellitus codes are combination codes that include the type of diabetes mellitus, body system affected, and the complications affecting that body system. As many codes within a particular category as are necessary to describe all of the complications of the disease may be used. They should be sequenced based on the reason for a particular visit. Assign as many codes from categories E08–E13 as needed to identify all of the associated conditions that the patient has.

DIABETES MELLITUS (E08-E13)

A metabolic disease that results in persistent hyperglycemia
Coding Clinic: 2016, Q4, P142

E08 Diabetes mellitus due to underlying condition

Code first the underlying condition, such as:
congenital rubella (P35.0)
Cushing's syndrome (E24.-)
cystic fibrosis (E84.-)
malignant neoplasm (C00-C96)
malnutrition (E40-E46)
pancreatitis and other diseases of the pancreas (K85-K86.-)
Use additional code to identify control using:
▶injectable non-insulin antidiabetic drugs (Z79.85)
insulin (Z79.4)
oral antidiabetic drugs (Z79.84)
oral hypoglycemic drugs (Z79.84)
Excludes1 drug or chemical induced diabetes mellitus (E09.-)
gestational diabetes (O24.4-)
neonatal diabetes mellitus (P70.2)
postpancreatectomy diabetes mellitus (E13.-)
postprocedural diabetes mellitus (E13.-)
secondary diabetes mellitus NEC (E13.-)
type 1 diabetes mellitus (E10.-)
type 2 diabetes mellitus (E11.-)

E08.0 Diabetes mellitus due to underlying condition with hyperosmolarity
E08.00 Diabetes mellitus due to underlying condition with hyperosmolarity without nonketotic hyperglycemic-hyperosmolar coma (NKHHC)
E08.01 Diabetes mellitus due to underlying condition with hyperosmolarity with coma

E08.1 Diabetes mellitus due to underlying condition with ketoacidosis
E08.10 Diabetes mellitus due to underlying condition with ketoacidosis without coma
E08.11 Diabetes mellitus due to underlying condition with ketoacidosis with coma

E08.2 Diabetes mellitus due to underlying condition with kidney complications
E08.21 Diabetes mellitus due to underlying condition with diabetic nephropathy
Diabetes mellitus due to underlying condition with intercapillary glomerulosclerosis
Diabetes mellitus due to underlying condition with intracapillary glomerulonephrosis
Diabetes mellitus due to underlying condition with Kimmelstiel-Wilson disease
E08.22 Diabetes mellitus due to underlying condition with diabetic chronic kidney disease
Use additional code to identify stage of chronic kidney disease (N18.1-N18.6)
E08.29 Diabetes mellitus due to underlying condition with other diabetic kidney complication
Renal tubular degeneration in diabetes mellitus due to underlying condition

E08.3 Diabetes mellitus due to underlying condition with ophthalmic complications
Changes in blood vessels of retina in which blood vessels swell and leak fluid into retinal surface.
Coding Clinic: 2016, Q4, P11
E08.31 Diabetes mellitus due to underlying condition with unspecified diabetic retinopathy
E08.311 Diabetes mellitus due to underlying condition with unspecified diabetic retinopathy with macular edema
E08.319 Diabetes mellitus due to underlying condition with unspecified diabetic retinopathy without macular edema
E08.32 Diabetes mellitus due to underlying condition with mild nonproliferative diabetic retinopathy
Diabetes mellitus due to underlying condition with nonproliferative diabetic retinopathy NOS
One of the following 7th characters is to be assigned to codes in subcategory E08.32 to designate laterality of the disease:

1	right eye
2	left eye
3	bilateral
9	unspecified eye

E08.321 Diabetes mellitus due to underlying condition with mild nonproliferative diabetic retinopathy with macular edema
E08.329 Diabetes mellitus due to underlying condition with mild nonproliferative diabetic retinopathy without macular edema
E08.33 Diabetes mellitus due to underlying condition with moderate nonproliferative diabetic retinopathy
One of the following 7th characters is to be assigned to codes in subcategory E08.33 to designate laterality of the disease:

1	right eye
2	left eye
3	bilateral
9	unspecified eye

E08.331 Diabetes mellitus due to underlying condition with moderate nonproliferative diabetic retinopathy with macular edema
E08.339 Diabetes mellitus due to underlying condition with moderate nonproliferative diabetic retinopathy without macular edema

● **E08.34** **Diabetes mellitus due to underlying condition with severe nonproliferative diabetic retinopathy**

One of the following 7th characters is to be assigned to codes in subcategory E08.34 to designate laterality of the disease:

1	right eye
2	left eye
3	bilateral
9	unspecified eye

●》 *E08.341*   *Diabetes mellitus due to underlying condition with severe nonproliferative diabetic retinopathy with macular edema* 🔍

●》 *E08.349*   *Diabetes mellitus due to underlying condition with severe nonproliferative diabetic retinopathy without macular edema* 🔍

● **E08.35** **Diabetes mellitus due to underlying condition with proliferative diabetic retinopathy**

One of the following 7th characters is to be assigned to codes in subcategory E08.35 to designate laterality of the disease:

1	right eye
2	left eye
3	bilateral
9	unspecified eye

●》 *E08.351*   *Diabetes mellitus due to underlying condition with proliferative diabetic retinopathy with macular edema* 🔍

●》 *E08.352*   *Diabetes mellitus due to underlying condition with proliferative diabetic retinopathy with traction retinal detachment involving the macula* 🔍

●》 *E08.353*   *Diabetes mellitus due to underlying condition with proliferative diabetic retinopathy with traction retinal detachment not involving the macula* 🔍

●》 *E08.354*   *Diabetes mellitus due to underlying condition with proliferative diabetic retinopathy with combined traction retinal detachment and rhegmatogenous retinal detachment* 🔍

●》 *E08.355*   *Diabetes mellitus due to underlying condition with stable proliferative diabetic retinopathy* 🔍

●》 *E08.359*   *Diabetes mellitus due to underlying condition with proliferative diabetic retinopathy without macular edema* 🔍

》 *E08.36*   *Diabetes mellitus due to underlying condition with diabetic cataract* 🔍

X ●》 *E08.37*   *Diabetes mellitus due to underlying condition with diabetic macular edema, resolved following treatment* 🔍

One of the following 7th characters is to be assigned to code E08.37 to designate laterality of the disease:

1	right eye
2	left eye
3	bilateral
9	unspecified eye

》 *E08.39*   *Diabetes mellitus due to underlying condition with other diabetic ophthalmic complication* 🔍

Use additional code to identify manifestation, such as:
diabetic glaucoma (H40-H42)

● **E08.4** **Diabetes mellitus due to underlying condition with neurological complications**

》 *E08.40*   *Diabetes mellitus due to underlying condition with diabetic neuropathy, unspecified* 🔍

》 *E08.41*   *Diabetes mellitus due to underlying condition with diabetic mononeuropathy* 🔍

》 *E08.42*   *Diabetes mellitus due to underlying condition with diabetic polyneuropathy* 🔍
     Diabetes mellitus due to underlying condition with diabetic neuralgia

》 *E08.43*   *Diabetes mellitus due to underlying condition with diabetic autonomic (poly)neuropathy* 🔍
     Diabetes mellitus due to underlying condition with diabetic gastroparesis

》 *E08.44*   *Diabetes mellitus due to underlying condition with diabetic amyotrophy* 🔍

》 *E08.49*   *Diabetes mellitus due to underlying condition with other diabetic neurological complication* 🔍

● **E08.5** **Diabetes mellitus due to underlying condition with circulatory complications**

》 *E08.51*   *Diabetes mellitus due to underlying condition with diabetic peripheral angiopathy without gangrene* 🔍

》 *E08.52*   *Diabetes mellitus due to underlying condition with diabetic peripheral angiopathy with gangrene* 🔍
     Diabetes mellitus due to underlying condition with diabetic gangrene

》 *E08.59*   *Diabetes mellitus due to underlying condition with other circulatory complications* 🔍

● **E08.6** **Diabetes mellitus due to underlying condition with other specified complications**

● **E08.61** **Diabetes mellitus due to underlying condition with diabetic arthropathy**

》 *E08.610*   *Diabetes mellitus due to underlying condition with diabetic neuropathic arthropathy* 🔍
     Diabetes mellitus due to underlying condition with Charcôt's joints

》 *E08.618*   *Diabetes mellitus due to underlying condition with other diabetic arthropathy* 🔍

● **E08.62** **Diabetes mellitus due to underlying condition with skin complications**

》 *E08.620*   *Diabetes mellitus due to underlying condition with diabetic dermatitis* 🔍
     Diabetes mellitus due to underlying condition with diabetic necrobiosis lipoidica

》 *E08.621*   *Diabetes mellitus due to underlying condition with foot ulcer* 🔍
     Use additional code to identify site of ulcer (L97.4-, L97.5-)

》 *E08.622*   *Diabetes mellitus due to underlying condition with other skin ulcer* 🔍
     Use additional code to identify site of ulcer (L97.1-L97.9, L98.41-L98.49)

》 *E08.628*   *Diabetes mellitus due to underlying condition with other skin complications* 🔍

● **E08.63** **Diabetes mellitus due to underlying condition with oral complications**

》 *E08.630*   *Diabetes mellitus due to underlying condition with periodontal disease* 🔍

》 *E08.638*   *Diabetes mellitus due to underlying condition with other oral complications* 🔍

CHAPTER 4 (E00-E89)

● **E08.64** **Diabetes mellitus due to underlying condition with hypoglycemia**
▶ Use additional code for hypoglycemia level, if applicable (E16.A-)

  ▹ *E08.641*   *Diabetes mellitus due to underlying condition with hypoglycemia with coma* 🐾

  ▹ *E08.649*   *Diabetes mellitus due to underlying condition with hypoglycemia without coma* 🐾

  ▹ *E08.65*   *Diabetes mellitus due to underlying condition with hyperglycemia* 🐾

  ▹ *E08.69*   *Diabetes mellitus due to underlying condition with other specified complication* 🐾
            Use additional code to identify complication

▹ *E08.8*   *Diabetes mellitus due to underlying condition with unspecified complications* 🐾

▹ *E08.9*   *Diabetes mellitus due to underlying condition without complications* 🐾

● **E09**   **Drug or chemical induced diabetes mellitus**
    Code first poisoning due to drug or toxin, if applicable (T36-T65 with fifth or sixth character 1-4)
    Use additional code for adverse effect, if applicable, to identify drug (T36-T50 with fifth or sixth character 5)
    Use additional code to identify control using:
    ▶ injectable non-insulin antidiabetic drugs (Z79.85)
      insulin (Z79.4)
      oral antidiabetic drugs (Z79.84)
      oral hypoglycemic drugs (Z79.84)
    Excludes1   diabetes mellitus due to underlying condition (E08.-)
                gestational diabetes (O24.4-)
                neonatal diabetes mellitus (P70.2)
                postpancreatectomy diabetes mellitus (E13.-)
                postprocedural diabetes mellitus (E13.-)
                secondary diabetes mellitus NEC (E13.-)
                type 1 diabetes mellitus (E10.-)
                type 2 diabetes mellitus (E11.-)

● **E09.0**   **Drug or chemical induced diabetes mellitus with hyperosmolarity**
  E09.00   **Drug or chemical induced diabetes mellitus with hyperosmolarity without nonketotic hyperglycemic-hyperosmolar coma (NKHHC)** 🐾
  E09.01   **Drug or chemical induced diabetes mellitus with hyperosmolarity with coma** 🐾

● **E09.1**   **Drug or chemical induced diabetes mellitus with ketoacidosis**
  E09.10   **Drug or chemical induced diabetes mellitus with ketoacidosis without coma** 🐾
  E09.11   **Drug or chemical induced diabetes mellitus with ketoacidosis with coma** 🐾

● **E09.2**   **Drug or chemical induced diabetes mellitus with kidney complications**
  E09.21   **Drug or chemical induced diabetes mellitus with diabetic nephropathy** 🐾
      Drug or chemical induced diabetes mellitus with intercapillary glomerulosclerosis
      Drug or chemical induced diabetes mellitus with intracapillary glomerulonephrosis
      Drug or chemical induced diabetes mellitus with Kimmelstiel-Wilson disease
  E09.22   **Drug or chemical induced diabetes mellitus with diabetic chronic kidney disease** 🐾
      Use additional code to identify stage of chronic kidney disease (N18.1-N18.6)
  E09.29   **Drug or chemical induced diabetes mellitus with other diabetic kidney complication** 🐾
      Drug or chemical induced diabetes mellitus with renal tubular degeneration

● **E09.3**   **Drug or chemical induced diabetes mellitus with ophthalmic complications**
    Coding Clinic: 2016, Q4, P11
  ● **E09.31**   **Drug or chemical induced diabetes mellitus with unspecified diabetic retinopathy**
    E09.311   **Drug or chemical induced diabetes mellitus with unspecified diabetic retinopathy with macular edema** 🐾
    E09.319   **Drug or chemical induced diabetes mellitus with unspecified diabetic retinopathy without macular edema** 🐾

● **E09.32**   **Drug or chemical induced diabetes mellitus with mild nonproliferative diabetic retinopathy**
    Drug or chemical induced diabetes mellitus with nonproliferative diabetic retinopathy NOS
    One of the following 7th characters is to be assigned to codes in subcategory E09.32 to designate laterality of the disease:

1	right eye
2	left eye
3	bilateral
9	unspecified eye

  ● **E09.321**   **Drug or chemical induced diabetes mellitus with mild nonproliferative diabetic retinopathy with macular edema** 🐾
  ● **E09.329**   **Drug or chemical induced diabetes mellitus with mild nonproliferative diabetic retinopathy without macular edema** 🐾

● **E09.33**   **Drug or chemical induced diabetes mellitus with moderate nonproliferative diabetic retinopathy**
    One of the following 7th characters is to be assigned to codes in subcategory E09.33 to designate laterality of the disease:

1	right eye
2	left eye
3	bilateral
9	unspecified eye

  ● **E09.331**   **Drug or chemical induced diabetes mellitus with moderate nonproliferative diabetic retinopathy with macular edema** 🐾
  ● **E09.339**   **Drug or chemical induced diabetes mellitus with moderate nonproliferative diabetic retinopathy without macular edema** 🐾

● **E09.34**   **Drug or chemical induced diabetes mellitus with severe nonproliferative diabetic retinopathy**
    One of the following 7th characters is to be assigned to codes in subcategory E09.34 to designate laterality of the disease:

1	right eye
2	left eye
3	bilateral
9	unspecified eye

  ● **E09.341**   **Drug or chemical induced diabetes mellitus with severe nonproliferative diabetic retinopathy with macular edema** 🐾
  ● **E09.349**   **Drug or chemical induced diabetes mellitus with severe nonproliferative diabetic retinopathy without macular edema** 🐾

● E09.35   **Drug or chemical induced diabetes mellitus with proliferative diabetic retinopathy**

One of the following 7th characters is to be assigned to codes in subcategory E09.35 to designate laterality of the disease:

1	right eye
2	left eye
3	bilateral
9	unspecified eye

● E09.351   **Drug or chemical induced diabetes mellitus with proliferative diabetic retinopathy with macular edema** 🔍

● E09.352   **Drug or chemical induced diabetes mellitus with proliferative diabetic retinopathy with traction retinal** 🔍 **detachment involving the macula**

● E09.353   **Drug or chemical induced diabetes mellitus with proliferative diabetic retinopathy with traction retinal detachment not involving the macula** 🔍

● E09.354   **Drug or chemical induced diabetes mellitus with proliferative diabetic retinopathy with combined traction retinal detachment and rhegmatogenous retinal detachment** 🔍

● E09.355   **Drug or chemical induced diabetes mellitus with stable proliferative diabetic retinopathy** 🔍

● E09.359   **Drug or chemical induced diabetes mellitus with proliferative diabetic retinopathy without macular edema** 🔍

E09.36   **Drug or chemical induced diabetes mellitus with diabetic cataract** 🔍

X ● E09.37   **Drug or chemical induced diabetes mellitus with diabetic macular edema, resolved following treatment** 🔍

One of the following 7th characters is to be assigned to code E09.37 to designate laterality of the disease:

1	right eye
2	left eye
3	bilateral
9	unspecified eye

E09.39   **Drug or chemical induced diabetes mellitus with other diabetic ophthalmic complication** 🔍

Use additional code to identify manifestation, such as:
diabetic glaucoma (H40-H42)

● E09.4   **Drug or chemical induced diabetes mellitus with neurological complications**

E09.40   **Drug or chemical induced diabetes mellitus with neurological complications with diabetic neuropathy, unspecified** 🔍

E09.41   **Drug or chemical induced diabetes mellitus with neurological complications with diabetic mononeuropathy** 🔍

E09.42   **Drug or chemical induced diabetes mellitus with neurological complications with diabetic polyneuropathy** 🔍
Drug or chemical induced diabetes mellitus with diabetic neuralgia

E09.43   **Drug or chemical induced diabetes mellitus with neurological complications with diabetic autonomic (poly)neuropathy** 🔍
Drug or chemical induced diabetes mellitus with diabetic gastroparesis

E09.44   **Drug or chemical induced diabetes mellitus with neurological complications with diabetic amyotrophy** 🔍

E09.49   **Drug or chemical induced diabetes mellitus with neurological complications with other diabetic neurological complication** 🔍

● E09.5   **Drug or chemical induced diabetes mellitus with circulatory complications**

E09.51   **Drug or chemical induced diabetes mellitus with diabetic peripheral angiopathy without gangrene** 🔍

E09.52   **Drug or chemical induced diabetes mellitus with diabetic peripheral angiopathy with gangrene** 🔍
Drug or chemical induced diabetes mellitus with diabetic gangrene

E09.59   **Drug or chemical induced diabetes mellitus with other circulatory complications** 🔍

● E09.6   **Drug or chemical induced diabetes mellitus with other specified complications**

● E09.61   **Drug or chemical induced diabetes mellitus with diabetic arthropathy**

E09.610   **Drug or chemical induced diabetes mellitus with diabetic neuropathic arthropathy** 🔍
Drug or chemical induced diabetes mellitus with Charcôt's joints
Progressive degeneration of weight-bearing joint

E09.618   **Drug or chemical induced diabetes mellitus with other diabetic arthropathy** 🔍

● E09.62   **Drug or chemical induced diabetes mellitus with skin complications**

E09.620   **Drug or chemical induced diabetes mellitus with diabetic dermatitis** 🔍
Drug or chemical induced diabetes mellitus with diabetic necrobiosis lipoidica
Necrotizing skin condition

E09.621   **Drug or chemical induced diabetes mellitus with foot ulcer** 🔍
Use additional code to identify site of ulcer (L97.4-, L97.5-)

E09.622   **Drug or chemical induced diabetes mellitus with other skin ulcer** 🔍
Use additional code to identify site of ulcer (L97.1-L97.9, L98.41-L98.49)

E09.628   **Drug or chemical induced diabetes mellitus with other skin complications** 🔍

● E09.63   **Drug or chemical induced diabetes mellitus with oral complications**

E09.630   **Drug or chemical induced diabetes mellitus with periodontal disease** 🔍

E09.638   **Drug or chemical induced diabetes mellitus with other oral complications** 🔍

● E09.64   **Drug or chemical induced diabetes mellitus with hypoglycemia**

▶ Use additional code for hypoglycemia level, if applicable (E16.A-)

E09.641   **Drug or chemical induced diabetes mellitus with hypoglycemia with coma** 🔍

E09.649   **Drug or chemical induced diabetes mellitus with hypoglycemia without coma** 🔍

E09.65   **Drug or chemical induced diabetes mellitus with hyperglycemia** 🔍

E09.69   **Drug or chemical induced diabetes mellitus with other specified complication** 🔍
Use additional code to identify complication

E09.8   **Drug or chemical induced diabetes mellitus with unspecified complications** 🔍

E09.9   **Drug or chemical induced diabetes mellitus without complications** 🔍

● **E10**   **Type 1 diabetes mellitus**

Includes   brittle diabetes (mellitus)
diabetes (mellitus) due to autoimmune process
diabetes (mellitus) due to immune mediated
pancreatic islet beta-cell destruction
idiopathic diabetes (mellitus)
juvenile onset diabetes (mellitus)
ketosis-prone diabetes (mellitus)

Excludes1   diabetes mellitus due to underlying condition
(E08.-)
drug or chemical induced diabetes mellitus
(E09.-)
gestational diabetes (O24.4-)
hyperglycemia NOS (R73.9)
neonatal diabetes mellitus (P70.2)
postpancreatectomy diabetes mellitus (E13.-)
postprocedural diabetes mellitus (E13.-)
secondary diabetes mellitus NEC (E13.-)
type 2 diabetes mellitus (E11.-)

● **E10.1**   **Type 1 diabetes mellitus with ketoacidosis**
*Acidosis accompanied by accumulation of ketone bodies
(ketosis) in body tissues and fluids*

E10.10   **Type 1 diabetes mellitus with ketoacidosis
without coma** 🦠
Coding Clinic: 2013, Q3, P20

E10.11   **Type 1 diabetes mellitus with ketoacidosis with
coma** 🦠

● **E10.2**   **Type 1 diabetes mellitus with kidney complications**

E10.21   **Type 1 diabetes mellitus with diabetic
nephropathy** 🦠
Type 1 diabetes mellitus with intercapillary
glomerulosclerosis
Type 1 diabetes mellitus with intracapillary
glomerulonephrosis
Type 1 diabetes mellitus with Kimmelstiel-
Wilson disease

E10.22   **Type 1 diabetes mellitus with diabetic chronic
kidney disease** 🦠
Use additional code to identify stage of chronic
kidney disease (N18.1-N18.6)

E10.29   **Type 1 diabetes mellitus with other diabetic
kidney complication** 🦠
Type 1 diabetes mellitus with renal tubular
degeneration
Coding Clinic: 2016, Q1, P13

● **E10.3**   **Type 1 diabetes mellitus with ophthalmic complications**
Coding Clinic: 2016, Q4, P11

● **E10.31**   **Type 1 diabetes mellitus with unspecified
diabetic retinopathy**

E10.311   **Type 1 diabetes mellitus
with unspecified diabetic retinopathy
with macular edema** 🦠

E10.319   **Type 1 diabetes mellitus
with unspecified diabetic retinopathy
without macular edema** 🦠

● **E10.32**   **Type 1 diabetes mellitus with mild
nonproliferative diabetic retinopathy**
Type 1 diabetes mellitus with nonproliferative
diabetic retinopathy NOS

One of the following 7th characters is to be
assigned to codes in subcategory E10.32 to
designate laterality of the disease:

1	right eye
2	left eye
3	bilateral
9	unspecified eye

● **E10.321**   **Type 1 diabetes mellitus with mild
nonproliferative diabetic retinopathy
with macular edema** 🦠

● **E10.329**   **Type 1 diabetes mellitus with mild
nonproliferative diabetic retinopathy
without macular edema** 🦠

● **E10.33**   **Type 1 diabetes mellitus with moderate
nonproliferative diabetic retinopathy**
One of the following 7th characters is to be
assigned to codes in subcategory E10.33 to
designate laterality of the disease:

1	right eye
2	left eye
3	bilateral
9	unspecified eye

● **E10.331**   **Type 1 diabetes mellitus with
moderate nonproliferative diabetic
retinopathy with macular edema** 🦠

● **E10.339**   **Type 1 diabetes mellitus with
moderate nonproliferative diabetic
retinopathy without macular
edema** 🦠

● **E10.34**   **Type 1 diabetes mellitus with severe
nonproliferative diabetic retinopathy**
One of the following 7th characters is to be
assigned to codes in subcategory E10.34 to
designate laterality of the disease:

1	right eye
2	left eye
3	bilateral
9	unspecified eye

● **E10.341**   **Type 1 diabetes mellitus with severe
nonproliferative diabetic retinopathy
with macular edema** 🦠

● **E10.349**   **Type 1 diabetes mellitus with severe
nonproliferative diabetic retinopathy
without macular edema** 🦠

● **E10.35**   **Type 1 diabetes mellitus with proliferative
diabetic retinopathy**
One of the following 7th characters is to be
assigned to codes in subcategory E10.35 to
designate laterality of the disease:

1	right eye
2	left eye
3	bilateral
9	unspecified eye

● **E10.351**   **Type 1 diabetes mellitus with
proliferative diabetic retinopathy
with macular edema** 🦠

● **E10.352**   **Type 1 diabetes mellitus with
proliferative diabetic retinopathy
with traction retinal detachment
involving the macula** 🦠

● **E10.353**   **Type 1 diabetes mellitus with
proliferative diabetic retinopathy
with traction retinal detachment not
involving the macula** 🦠

● **E10.354**   **Type 1 diabetes mellitus with
proliferative diabetic retinopathy
with combined traction retinal
detachment and rhegmatogenous
retinal detachment** 🦠

● **E10.355**   **Type 1 diabetes mellitus with stable
proliferative diabetic retinopathy** 🦠

● **E10.359**   **Type 1 diabetes mellitus with
proliferative diabetic retinopathy
without macular edema** 🦠

E10.36   **Type 1 diabetes mellitus with diabetic
cataract** 🦠

X● **E10.37**   **Type 1 diabetes mellitus with diabetic macular edema, resolved following treatment** 🔖

One of the following 7th characters is to be assigned to code E10.37 to designate laterality of the disease:

1	right eye
2	left eye
3	bilateral
9	unspecified eye

E10.39   **Type 1 diabetes mellitus with other diabetic ophthalmic complication** 🔖

Use additional code to identify manifestation, such as:
diabetic glaucoma (H40-H42)

● **E10.4**   **Type 1 diabetes mellitus with neurological complications**

E10.40   **Type 1 diabetes mellitus with diabetic neuropathy, unspecified** 🔖

E10.41   **Type 1 diabetes mellitus with diabetic mononeuropathy** 🔖

E10.42   **Type 1 diabetes mellitus with diabetic polyneuropathy** 🔖
Type 1 diabetes mellitus with diabetic neuralgia

E10.43   **Type 1 diabetes mellitus with diabetic autonomic (poly)neuropathy** 🔖
Type 1 diabetes mellitus with diabetic gastroparesis

E10.44   **Type 1 diabetes mellitus with diabetic amyotrophy** 🔖

E10.49   **Type 1 diabetes mellitus with other diabetic neurological complication** 🔖

● **E10.5**   **Type 1 diabetes mellitus with circulatory complications**

E10.51   **Type 1 diabetes mellitus with diabetic peripheral angiopathy without gangrene** 🔖

E10.52   **Type 1 diabetes mellitus with diabetic peripheral angiopathy with gangrene** 🔖
Type 1 diabetes mellitus with diabetic gangrene

E10.59   **Type 1 diabetes mellitus with other circulatory complications** 🔖

● **E10.6**   **Type 1 diabetes mellitus with other specified complications**

● **E10.61**   **Type 1 diabetes mellitus with diabetic arthropathy**

E10.610   **Type 1 diabetes mellitus with diabetic neuropathic arthropathy** 🔖
Type 1 diabetes mellitus with Charcôt's joints

E10.618   **Type 1 diabetes mellitus with other diabetic arthropathy** 🔖

● **E10.62**   **Type 1 diabetes mellitus with skin complications**

E10.620   **Type 1 diabetes mellitus with diabetic dermatitis** 🔖
Type 1 diabetes mellitus with diabetic necrobiosis lipoidica

E10.621   **Type 1 diabetes mellitus with foot ulcer** 🔖
Use additional code to identify site of ulcer (L97.4-, L97.5-)

E10.622   **Type 1 diabetes mellitus with other skin ulcer** 🔖
Use additional code to identify site of ulcer (L97.1-L97.9, L98.41-L98.49)

E10.628   **Type 1 diabetes mellitus with other skin complications** 🔖

● **E10.63**   **Type 1 diabetes mellitus with oral complications**

E10.630   **Type 1 diabetes mellitus with periodontal disease** 🔖

E10.638   **Type 1 diabetes mellitus with other oral complications** 🔖

● **E10.64**   **Type 1 diabetes mellitus with hypoglycemia**
▶ Use additional code for hypoglycemia level, if applicable (E16.A-)

E10.641   **Type 1 diabetes mellitus with hypoglycemia with coma** 🔖

E10.649   **Type 1 diabetes mellitus with hypoglycemia without coma** 🔖
Coding Clinic: 2016, Q1, P13

E10.65   **Type 1 diabetes mellitus with hyperglycemia** 🔖
Coding Clinic: 2022, Q1, P29; 2013, Q3, P20

E10.69   **Type 1 diabetes mellitus with other specified complication** 🔖
Use additional code to identify complication
Coding Clinic: 2022, Q1, P29

E10.8   **Type 1 diabetes mellitus with unspecified complications** 🔖

E10.9   **Type 1 diabetes mellitus without complications** 🔖

▶ **E10.A**   **Type 1 diabetes mellitus, presymptomatic**
▶ Early-stage type 1 diabetes mellitus

▶ **E10.A0**   **Type 1 diabetes mellitus, presymptomatic, unspecified**

▶ **E10.A1**   **Type 1 diabetes mellitus, presymptomatic, Stage 1**
▶ Multiple confirmed islet autoantibodies with normoglycemia

▶ **E10.A2**   **Type 1 diabetes mellitus, presymptomatic, Stage 2**
▶ Confirmed islet autoimmunity with dysglycemia

● **E11**   **Type 2 diabetes mellitus**

Includes   diabetes (mellitus) due to insulin secretory defect
diabetes NOS
insulin resistant diabetes (mellitus)

Use additional code to identify control using:
▶ injectable non-insulin antidiabetic drugs (Z79.85)
insulin (Z79.4)
oral antidiabetic drugs (Z79.84)
oral hypoglycemic drugs (Z79.84)

Excludes1   diabetes mellitus due to underlying condition (E08.-)
drug or chemical induced diabetes mellitus (E09.-)
gestational diabetes (O24.4-)
neonatal diabetes mellitus (P70.2)
postpancreatectomy diabetes mellitus (E13.-)
postprocedural diabetes mellitus (E13.-)
secondary diabetes mellitus NEC (E13.-)
type 1 diabetes mellitus (E10.-)
Coding Clinic: 2023, Q2, P10; 2020, Q1, P12; 2016, Q4, P121, Q2, P10

● **E11.0**   **Type 2 diabetes mellitus with hyperosmolarity**

E11.00   **Type 2 diabetes mellitus with hyperosmolarity without nonketotic hyperglycemic-hyperosmolar coma (NKHHC)** 🔖
Coding Clinic: 2022, Q1, P28

E11.01   **Type 2 diabetes mellitus with hyperosmolarity with coma** 🔖

● **E11.1**   **Type 2 diabetes mellitus with ketoacidosis**

E11.10   **Type 2 diabetes mellitus with ketoacidosis without coma** 🔖
Coding Clinic: 2017, Q4, P6

E11.11   **Type 2 diabetes mellitus with ketoacidosis with coma** 🔖

CHAPTER 4 (E00-E89)

● **E11.2** **Type 2 diabetes mellitus with kidney complications**

    E11.21 **Type 2 diabetes mellitus with diabetic nephropathy** 🐾

        Type 2 diabetes mellitus with intercapillary glomerulosclerosis

        Type 2 diabetes mellitus with intracapillary glomerulonephrosis

        Type 2 diabetes mellitus with Kimmelstiel-Wilson disease

        Coding Clinic: 2019, Q3, P3

    E11.22 **Type 2 diabetes mellitus with diabetic chronic kidney disease** 🐾

        Use additional code to identify stage of chronic kidney disease (N18.1-N18.6)

        Coding Clinic: 2022, Q3, P16; 2019, Q3, P3; 2018, Q4, P88; 2016, Q2, P36, Q1, P13

    E11.29 **Type 2 diabetes mellitus with other diabetic kidney complication** 🐾

        Type 2 diabetes mellitus with renal tubular degeneration

● **E11.3** **Type 2 diabetes mellitus with ophthalmic complications**

    Coding Clinic: 2016, Q4, P11

  ● **E11.31** **Type 2 diabetes mellitus with unspecified diabetic retinopathy**

      E11.311 **Type 2 diabetes mellitus with unspecified diabetic retinopathy with macular edema** 🐾

      E11.319 **Type 2 diabetes mellitus with unspecified diabetic retinopathy without macular edema** 🐾

        Coding Clinic: 2013, Q3, P20

  ● **E11.32** **Type 2 diabetes mellitus with mild nonproliferative diabetic retinopathy**

      Type 2 diabetes mellitus with nonproliferative diabetic retinopathy NOS

      One of the following 7th characters is to be assigned to codes in subcategory E11.32 to designate laterality of the disease:

1	right eye
2	left eye
3	bilateral
9	unspecified eye

    ● **E11.321** **Type 2 diabetes mellitus with mild nonproliferative diabetic retinopathy with macular edema** 🐾

    ● **E11.329** **Type 2 diabetes mellitus with mild nonproliferative diabetic retinopathy without macular edema** 🐾

  ● **E11.33** **Type 2 diabetes mellitus with moderate nonproliferative diabetic retinopathy**

      One of the following 7th characters is to be assigned to codes in subcategory E11.33 to designate laterality of the disease:

1	right eye
2	left eye
3	bilateral
9	unspecified eye

    ● **E11.331** **Type 2 diabetes mellitus with moderate nonproliferative diabetic retinopathy with macular edema** 🐾

    ● **E11.339** **Type 2 diabetes mellitus with moderate nonproliferative diabetic retinopathy without macular edema** 🐾

● **E11.34** **Type 2 diabetes mellitus with severe nonproliferative diabetic retinopathy**

    One of the following 7th characters is to be assigned to codes in subcategory E11.34 to designate laterality of the disease:

1	right eye
2	left eye
3	bilateral
9	unspecified eye

  ● **E11.341** **Type 2 diabetes mellitus with severe nonproliferative diabetic retinopathy with macular edema** 🐾

  ● **E11.349** **Type 2 diabetes mellitus with severe nonproliferative diabetic retinopathy without macular edema** 🐾

● **E11.35** **Type 2 diabetes mellitus with proliferative diabetic retinopathy**

    One of the following 7th characters is to be assigned to codes in subcategory E11.35 to designate laterality of the disease:

1	right eye
2	left eye
3	bilateral
9	unspecified eye

  ● **E11.351** **Type 2 diabetes mellitus with proliferative diabetic retinopathy with macular edema** 🐾

  ● **E11.352** **Type 2 diabetes mellitus with proliferative diabetic retinopathy with traction retinal detachment involving the macula** 🐾

  ● **E11.353** **Type 2 diabetes mellitus with proliferative diabetic retinopathy with traction retinal detachment not involving the macula** 🐾

  ● **E11.354** **Type 2 diabetes mellitus with proliferative diabetic retinopathy with combined traction retinal detachment and rhegmatogenous retinal detachment** 🐾

  ● **E11.355** **Type 2 diabetes mellitus with stable proliferative diabetic retinopathy** 🐾

  ● **E11.359** **Type 2 diabetes mellitus with proliferative diabetic retinopathy without macular edema** 🐾

  E11.36 **Type 2 diabetes mellitus with diabetic cataract** 🐾

    Coding Clinic: 2019, Q2, P30-31; 2016, Q2, P36

X ● **E11.37** **Type 2 diabetes mellitus with diabetic macular edema, resolved following treatment** 🐾

    One of the following 7th characters is to be assigned to code E11.37 to designate laterality of the disease:

1	right eye
2	left eye
3	bilateral
9	unspecified eye

  E11.39 **Type 2 diabetes mellitus with other diabetic ophthalmic complication** 🐾

    Use additional code to identify manifestation, such as:

      diabetic glaucoma (H40-H42)

    Coding Clinic: 2023, Q3, P19

● **E11.4** **Type 2 diabetes mellitus with neurological complications**

    Coding Clinic: 2022, Q3, P16

  E11.40 **Type 2 diabetes mellitus with diabetic neuropathy, unspecified** 🐾

▶ New	➡ Revised	~~deleted~~ Deleted	Excludes 1	Excludes 2	Includes	Use additional	Code first	Code also	Key words

OGCR Official Guidelines   X Assign placeholder X   ● Use Additional Character(s)   ▶ Manifestation Code   🐾 Hierarchical Condition Category   Coding Clinic

E11.41   **Type 2 diabetes mellitus with diabetic mononeuropathy** 🔖

E11.42   **Type 2 diabetes mellitus with diabetic polyneuropathy** 🔖
     Type 2 diabetes mellitus with diabetic neuralgia
     Coding Clinic: 2020, Q1, P12; 2016, Q1, P13

E11.43   **Type 2 diabetes mellitus with diabetic autonomic (poly)neuropathy** 🔖
     Type 2 diabetes mellitus with diabetic gastroparesis
     Coding Clinic: 2023, Q2, P9; 2016, Q2, P36

E11.44   **Type 2 diabetes mellitus with diabetic amyotrophy** 🔖
     Coding Clinic: 2022, Q3, P15; 2016, Q2, P36

E11.49   **Type 2 diabetes mellitus with other diabetic neurological complication** 🔖

● **E11.5   Type 2 diabetes mellitus with circulatory complications**

E11.51   **Type 2 diabetes mellitus with diabetic peripheral angiopathy without gangrene** 🔖

E11.52   **Type 2 diabetes mellitus with diabetic peripheral angiopathy with gangrene** 🔖
     Type 2 diabetes mellitus with diabetic gangrene
     Coding Clinic: 2017, Q4, P102

E11.59   **Type 2 diabetes mellitus with other circulatory complications** 🔖

● **E11.6   Type 2 diabetes mellitus with other specified complications**

  ● E11.61   **Type 2 diabetes mellitus with diabetic arthropathy**

     E11.610   **Type 2 diabetes mellitus with diabetic neuropathic arthropathy** 🔖
       Type 2 diabetes mellitus with Charcôt's joints
       Coding Clinic: 2016, Q2, P36

     E11.618   **Type 2 diabetes mellitus with other diabetic arthropathy** 🔖
       Coding Clinic: 2018, Q2, P7; 2016, Q2, P36

  ● E11.62   **Type 2 diabetes mellitus with skin complications**

     E11.620   **Type 2 diabetes mellitus with diabetic dermatitis** 🔖
       Type 2 diabetes mellitus with diabetic necrobiosis lipoidica

     E11.621   **Type 2 diabetes mellitus with foot ulcer** 🔖
       Use additional code to identify site of ulcer (L97.4-, L97.5-)
       Coding Clinic: 2020, Q1, P12; 2016, Q1, P12

     E11.622   **Type 2 diabetes mellitus with other skin ulcer** 🔖
       Use additional code to identify site of ulcer (L97.1-L97.9, L98.41-L98.49)
       Coding Clinic: 2021, Q1, P8; 2017, Q4, P17

     E11.628   **Type 2 diabetes mellitus with other skin complications** 🔖

  ● E11.63   **Type 2 diabetes mellitus with oral complications**

     E11.630   **Type 2 diabetes mellitus with periodontal disease** 🔖

     E11.638   **Type 2 diabetes mellitus with other oral complications** 🔖

  ● E11.64   **Type 2 diabetes mellitus with hypoglycemia**
     ▶ Use additional code for hypoglycemia level, if applicable (E16.A-)

     E11.641   **Type 2 diabetes mellitus with hypoglycemia with coma** 🔖

     E11.649   **Type 2 diabetes mellitus with hypoglycemia without coma** 🔖
       Coding Clinic: 2016, Q3, P42; 2015, Q3, P21

E11.65   **Type 2 diabetes mellitus with hyperglycemia** 🔖
     Coding Clinic: 2023, Q2, P10; 2022, Q1, P28; 2013, Q3, P20

E11.69   **Type 2 diabetes mellitus with other specified complication** 🔖
     Use additional code to identify complication
     Coding Clinic: 2020, Q1, P12; 2016, Q4, P142

● **E11.8   Type 2 diabetes mellitus with unspecified complications** 🔖

● **E11.9   Type 2 diabetes mellitus without complications** 🔖
     Coding Clinic: 2023, Q3, P19; 2016, Q4, P142, Q2, P36

● **E13   Other specified diabetes mellitus**

   Includes   diabetes mellitus due to genetic defects of beta-cell function
     diabetes mellitus due to genetic defects in insulin action
     postpancreatectomy diabetes mellitus
     postprocedural diabetes mellitus
     secondary diabetes mellitus NEC

   Use additional code to identify control using:
   ▶ injectable non-insulin antidiabetic drugs (Z79.85)
     insulin (Z79.4)
     oral antidiabetic drugs (Z79.84)
     oral hypoglycemic drugs (Z79.84)

   Excludes1   diabetes (mellitus) due to autoimmune process (E10.-)
     diabetes (mellitus) due to immune mediated pancreatic islet beta-cell destruction (E10.-)
     diabetes mellitus due to underlying condition (E08.-)
     drug or chemical induced diabetes mellitus (E09.-)
     gestational diabetes (O24.4-)
     neonatal diabetes mellitus (P70.2)
     type 1 diabetes mellitus (E10.-)

● **E13.0   Other specified diabetes mellitus with hyperosmolarity**

     E13.00   **Other specified diabetes mellitus with hyperosmolarity without nonketotic hyperglycemic-hyperosmolar coma (NKHHC)** 🔖

     E13.01   **Other specified diabetes mellitus with hyperosmolarity with coma** 🔖

● **E13.1   Other specified diabetes mellitus with ketoacidosis**

     E13.10   **Other specified diabetes mellitus with ketoacidosis without coma** 🔖
       Coding Clinic: 2016, Q2, P10; 2013, Q1, P26

     E13.11   **Other specified diabetes mellitus with ketoacidosis with coma** 🔖

● **E13.2   Other specified diabetes mellitus with kidney complications**

     E13.21   **Other specified diabetes mellitus with diabetic nephropathy** 🔖
       Other specified diabetes mellitus with intercapillary glomerulosclerosis
       Other specified diabetes mellitus with intracapillary glomerulonephrosis
       Other specified diabetes mellitus with Kimmelstiel-Wilson disease

     E13.22   **Other specified diabetes mellitus with diabetic chronic kidney disease** 🔖
       Use additional code to identify stage of chronic kidney disease (N18.1-N18.6)

     E13.29   **Other specified diabetes mellitus with other diabetic kidney complication** 🔖
       Other specified diabetes mellitus with renal tubular degeneration

- **E13.3** **Other specified diabetes mellitus with ophthalmic complications**
  Coding Clinic: 2016, Q4, P11
  - **E13.31** **Other specified diabetes mellitus with unspecified diabetic retinopathy**
    - **E13.311** Other specified diabetes mellitus with unspecified diabetic retinopathy with macular edema 🔖
    - **E13.319** Other specified diabetes mellitus with unspecified diabetic retinopathy without macular edema 🔖
  - **E13.32** **Other specified diabetes mellitus with mild nonproliferative diabetic retinopathy**
    Other specified diabetes mellitus with nonproliferative diabetic retinopathy NOS
    One of the following 7th characters is to be assigned to codes in subcategory E13.32 to designate laterality of the disease:

1	right eye
2	left eye
3	bilateral
9	unspecified eye

    - **E13.321** Other specified diabetes mellitus with mild nonproliferative diabetic retinopathy with macular edema 🔖
    - **E13.329** Other specified diabetes mellitus with mild nonproliferative diabetic retinopathy without macular edema 🔖
  - **E13.33** **Other specified diabetes mellitus with moderate nonproliferative diabetic retinopathy**
    One of the following 7th characters is to be assigned to codes in subcategory E13.33 to designate laterality of the disease:

1	right eye
2	left eye
3	bilateral
9	unspecified eye

    - **E13.331** Other specified diabetes mellitus with moderate nonproliferative diabetic retinopathy with macular edema 🔖
    - **E13.339** Other specified diabetes mellitus with moderate nonproliferative diabetic retinopathy without macular edema 🔖
  - **E13.34** **Other specified diabetes mellitus with severe nonproliferative diabetic retinopathy**
    One of the following 7th characters is to be assigned to codes in subcategory E13.34 to designate laterality of the disease:

1	right eye
2	left eye
3	bilateral
9	unspecified eye

    - **E13.341** Other specified diabetes mellitus with severe nonproliferative diabetic retinopathy with macular edema 🔖
    - **E13.349** Other specified diabetes mellitus with severe nonproliferative diabetic retinopathy without macular edema 🔖
  - **E13.35** **Other specified diabetes mellitus with proliferative diabetic retinopathy**
    One of the following 7th characters is to be assigned to codes in subcategory E13.35 to designate laterality of the disease:

1	right eye
2	left eye
3	bilateral
9	unspecified eye

    - **E13.351** Other specified diabetes mellitus with proliferative diabetic retinopathy with macular edema 🔖
    - **E13.352** Other specified diabetes mellitus with proliferative diabetic retinopathy with traction retinal detachment involving the macula 🔖
    - **E13.353** Other specified diabetes mellitus with proliferative diabetic retinopathy with traction retinal detachment not involving the macula 🔖
    - **E13.354** Other specified diabetes mellitus with proliferative diabetic retinopathy with combined traction retinal detachment and rhegmatogenous retinal detachment 🔖
    - **E13.355** Other specified diabetes mellitus with stable proliferative diabetic retinopathy 🔖
    - **E13.359** Other specified diabetes mellitus with proliferative diabetic retinopathy without macular edema 🔖
  - **E13.36** Other specified diabetes mellitus with diabetic cataract 🔖
  - X ● **E13.37** Other specified diabetes mellitus with diabetic macular edema, resolved following treatment 🔖
    One of the following 7th characters is to be assigned to code E13.37 to designate laterality of the disease:

1	right eye
2	left eye
3	bilateral
9	unspecified eye

  - **E13.39** Other specified diabetes mellitus with other diabetic ophthalmic complication 🔖
    Use additional code to identify manifestation, such as:
    diabetic glaucoma (H40-H42)
- **E13.4** **Other specified diabetes mellitus with neurological complications**
  - **E13.40** Other specified diabetes mellitus with diabetic neuropathy, unspecified 🔖
  - **E13.41** Other specified diabetes mellitus with diabetic mononeuropathy 🔖
  - **E13.42** Other specified diabetes mellitus with diabetic polyneuropathy 🔖
    Other specified diabetes mellitus with diabetic neuralgia
  - **E13.43** Other specified diabetes mellitus with diabetic autonomic (poly)neuropathy 🔖
    Other specified diabetes mellitus with diabetic gastroparesis
  - **E13.44** Other specified diabetes mellitus with diabetic amyotrophy 🔖
  - **E13.49** Other specified diabetes mellitus with other diabetic neurological complication 🔖
- **E13.5** **Other specified diabetes mellitus with circulatory complications**
  - **E13.51** Other specified diabetes mellitus with diabetic peripheral angiopathy without gangrene 🔖
  - **E13.52** Other specified diabetes mellitus with diabetic peripheral angiopathy with gangrene 🔖
    Other specified diabetes mellitus with diabetic gangrene
  - **E13.59** Other specified diabetes mellitus with other circulatory complications 🔖

▶ New   ⇒ Revised   ~~deleted~~ Deleted   Excludes 1   Excludes 2   Includes   Use additional   Code first   Code also   Key words

OGCR Official Guidelines   X Assign placeholder X   ● Use Additional Character(s)   ▷ Manifestation Code   🔖 Hierarchical Condition Category   Coding Clinic

● **E13.6** **Other specified diabetes mellitus with other specified complications**

  ● **E13.61** **Other specified diabetes mellitus with diabetic arthropathy**

    E13.610 **Other specified diabetes mellitus with diabetic neuropathic arthropathy** 🦠
      Other specified diabetes mellitus with Charcôt's joints

    E13.618 **Other specified diabetes mellitus with other diabetic arthropathy** 🦠

  ● **E13.62** **Other specified diabetes mellitus with skin complications**

    E13.620 **Other specified diabetes mellitus with diabetic dermatitis** 🦠
      Other specified diabetes mellitus with diabetic necrobiosis lipoidica

    E13.621 **Other specified diabetes mellitus with foot ulcer** 🦠
      Use additional code to identify site of ulcer (L97.4-, L97.5-)

    E13.622 **Other specified diabetes mellitus with other skin ulcer** 🦠
      Use additional code to identify site of ulcer (L97.1-L97.9, L98.41-L98.49)

    E13.628 **Other specified diabetes mellitus with other skin complications** 🦠

  ● **E13.63** **Other specified diabetes mellitus with oral complications**

    E13.630 **Other specified diabetes mellitus with periodontal disease** 🦠

    E13.638 **Other specified diabetes mellitus with other oral complications** 🦠

  ● **E13.64** **Other specified diabetes mellitus with hypoglycemia**
    ▶ Use additional code for hypoglycemia level, if applicable (E16.A-)

    E13.641 **Other specified diabetes mellitus with hypoglycemia with coma** 🦠

    E13.649 **Other specified diabetes mellitus with hypoglycemia without coma** 🦠

  E13.65 **Other specified diabetes mellitus with hyperglycemia** 🦠

  E13.69 **Other specified diabetes mellitus with other specified complication** 🦠
    Use additional code to identify complication

E13.8 **Other specified diabetes mellitus with unspecified complications** 🦠

E13.9 **Other specified diabetes mellitus without complications** 🦠

OTHER DISORDERS OF GLUCOSE REGULATION AND PANCREATIC INTERNAL SECRETION (E15-E16)

E15 **Nondiabetic hypoglycemic coma** 🦠
  Includes drug-induced insulin coma in nondiabetic hyperinsulinism with hypoglycemic coma hypoglycemic coma NOS

● **E16** **Other disorders of pancreatic internal secretion**

  E16.0 **Drug-induced hypoglycemia without coma**
    Excludes1 diabetes with hypoglycemia without coma (E09.649)
    ▶ Use additional ~~code for adverse effect, if applicable, to identify drug (T36-T50 with fifth or sixth character 5)~~ code for hypoglycemia level, if applicable (E16.A-)

E16.1 **Other hypoglycemia**
  Functional hyperinsulinism
  Functional nonhyperinsulinemic hypoglycemia
  Hyperinsulinism NOS
  Hyperplasia of pancreatic islet beta cells NOS
    Excludes1 diabetes with hypoglycemia (E08.649, E10.649, E11.649, E13.649)
      hypoglycemia in infant of diabetic mother (P70.1)
      neonatal hypoglycemia (P70.4)
  ▶ Use additional code for hypoglycemia level, if applicable (E16.A-)
  Coding Clinic: 2024, Q2, P10

E16.2 **Hypoglycemia, unspecified**
    Excludes1 diabetes with hypoglycemia (E08.649, E10.649, E11.649, E13.649)
  ▶ Use additional code for hypoglycemia level, if applicable (E16.A-)
  Coding Clinic: 2016, Q3, P42

E16.3 **Increased secretion of glucagon**
  Hyperplasia of pancreatic endocrine cells with glucagon excess

E16.4 **Increased secretion of gastrin**
  Hypergastrinemia
  Hyperplasia of pancreatic endocrine cells with gastrin excess
  Zollinger-Ellison syndrome

E16.8 **Other specified disorders of pancreatic internal secretion**
  Increased secretion from endocrine pancreas of growth hormone-releasing hormone
  Increased secretion from endocrine pancreas of pancreatic polypeptide
  Increased secretion from endocrine pancreas of somatostatin
  Increased secretion from endocrine pancreas of vasoactive-intestinal polypeptide

E16.9 **Disorder of pancreatic internal secretion, unspecified**
  Islet-cell hyperplasia NOS
  Pancreatic endocrine cell hyperplasia NOS

▶ **E16.A** **Hypoglycemia level**

  ▶ **E16.A1** **Hypoglycemia level 1**
    ▶ Decreased blood glucose level 1

  ▶ **E16.A2** **Hypoglycemia level 2**
    ▶ Decreased blood glucose level 2

  ▶ **E16.A3** **Hypoglycemia level 3**
    ▶ Decreased blood glucose level 3

DISORDERS OF OTHER ENDOCRINE GLANDS (E20-E35)

Excludes1 galactorrhea (N64.3)
    gynecomastia (N62)

● **E20** **Hypoparathyroidism**
  Greatly reduced function of parathyroid glands; AKA parathyroid insufficiency
    Excludes1 Di George's syndrome (D82.1)
      postprocedural hypoparathyroidism (E89.2)
      tetany NOS (R29.0)
      transitory neonatal hypoparathyroidism (P71.4)

E20.0 **Idiopathic hypoparathyroidism** 🦠
  Rare condition, unknown cause; short dwarf-like with round face

E20.1 **Pseudohypoparathyroidism**
  Hereditary condition resembling hypoparathyroidism, but caused by inability to respond to parathyroid hormone

CHAPTER 4 (E00–E89)

● **E20.8   Other hypoparathyroidism** 🅒
   ● **E20.81   Hypoparathyroidism due to impaired parathyroid hormone secretion**
     E20.810   Autosomal dominant hypocalcemia
         Autosomal dominant hypocalcemia type 1 (ADH1)
         Autosomal dominant hypocalcemia type 2 (ADH2)
         Code also, if applicable, any associated conditions, such as:
         calculus of kidney (N20.0)
         chronic kidney disease (N18.-)
         respiratory distress (J80, R06.-)
         seizure disorder (G40.-, R56.9)
     E20.811   Secondary hypoparathyroidism in diseases classified elsewhere
         Code first underlying condition, if known
     E20.812   Autoimmune hypoparathyroidism
         Code first, if applicable, underlying condition such as:
         autoimmune polyglandular failure (E31.0)
         Schmidt's syndrome (E31.0)
     E20.818   Other specified hypoparathyroidism due to impaired parathyroid hormonesecretion
         Familial isolated hypoparathyroidism
     E20.819   Hypoparathyroidism due to impaired parathyroid hormone secretion,unspecified
   E20.89   Other specified hypoparathyroidism
     Familial hypoparathyroidism
   E20.9   Hypoparathyroidism, unspecified 🅒
     Parathyroid tetany

● **E21   Hyperparathyroidism and other disorders of parathyroid gland**
   Excludes1   adult osteomalacia (M83.-)
         ectopic hyperparathyroidism (E34.2)
         hungry bone syndrome (E83.81)
         infantile and juvenile osteomalacia (E55.0)
   Excludes2   familial hypocalciuric hypercalcemia (E83.52)
   E21.0   Primary hyperparathyroidism 🅒
     Hyperplasia of parathyroid
     Osteitis fibrosa cystica generalisata [von Recklinghausen's disease of bone]
   E21.1   Secondary hyperparathyroidism, not elsewhere classified 🅒
     Excludes1   secondary hyperparathyroidism of renal origin (N25.81)
   E21.2   Other hyperparathyroidism 🅒
     Tertiary hyperparathyroidism
     Excludes1   familial hypocalciuric hypercalcemia (E83.52)
   E21.3   Hyperparathyroidism, unspecified 🅒
   E21.4   Other specified disorders of parathyroid gland 🅒
   E21.5   Disorder of parathyroid gland, unspecified 🅒

● **E22   Hyperfunction of pituitary gland**
   Excludes1   Cushing's syndrome (E24.-)
         Nelson's syndrome (E24.1)
         overproduction of ACTH not associated with Cushing's disease (E27.0)
         overproduction of pituitary ACTH (E24.0)
         overproduction of thyroid-stimulating hormone (E05.8-)
   E22.0   Acromegaly and pituitary gigantism 🅒
     Chronic disease caused by hypersecretion of growth hormone
     Overproduction of growth hormone
     Excludes1   constitutional gigantism (E34.4)
         constitutional tall stature (E34.4)
         increased secretion from endocrine pancreas of growth hormone-releasing hormone (E16.8)
   E22.1   Hyperprolactinemia 🅒
     Increased levels of prolactin
     Use additional code for adverse effect, if applicable, to identify drug (T36-T50 with fifth or sixth character 5)
   E22.2   Syndrome of inappropriate secretion of antidiuretic hormone 🅒
   E22.8   Other hyperfunction of pituitary gland 🅒
     Central precocious puberty
   E22.9   Hyperfunction of pituitary gland, unspecified 🅒

● **E23   Hypofunction and other disorders of the pituitary gland**
   Includes   the listed conditions whether the disorder is in the pituitary or the hypothalamus
   Excludes1   postprocedural hypopituitarism (E89.3)
   E23.0   Hypopituitarism 🅒
     Fertile eunuch syndrome
     Hypogonadotropic hypogonadism
     Idiopathic growth hormone deficiency
     Isolated deficiency of gonadotropin
     Isolated deficiency of growth hormone
     Isolated deficiency of pituitary hormone
     Kallmann's syndrome
     Lorain-Levi short stature
     Necrosis of pituitary gland (postpartum)
     Panhypopituitarism
     Pituitary cachexia
     Pituitary insufficiency NOS
     Pituitary short stature
     Sheehan's syndrome
     Simmonds' disease
     Coding Clinic: 2024, Q1, P15
   E23.1   Drug-induced hypopituitarism 🅒
     Use additional code for adverse effect, if applicable, to identify drug (T36-T50 with fifth or sixth character 5)
   E23.2   Diabetes insipidus 🅒
     Excludes1   nephrogenic diabetes insipidus (N25.1)

Item 4–5   Hyperadrenalism is overactivity of the adrenal cortex, which secretes corticosteroid hormones. Excessive glucocorticoid hormone results in hyperglycemia **(Cushing's syndrome),** and excessive aldosterone results in **Conn's syndrome. Adrenogenital syndrome** is the result of excessive secretion of androgens, male hormones, which stimulates premature sexual development. **Hypoadrenalism, Addison's disease,** is a condition in which the adrenal glands atrophy.

Figure 4-5 Centripetal and generalized obesity and dorsal kyphosis in a woman with Cushing's disease. (From Salvo SG: Mosby's Pathology for Massage Therapists, St. Louis, MO: Mosby/Elsevier, 2009)

Item 4–4   Hyperparathyroidism is an overactive parathyroid gland that secretes excessive parathormone, causing increased levels of circulating calcium. This results in a loss of calcium in the bone (osteoporosis).
   Hypoparathyroidism is an underactive parathyroid gland that results in decreased levels of circulating calcium. The primary manifestation is **tetany,** a continuous muscle spasm.

Figure 4-4   Tetany caused by hypoparathyroidism.

▶ New   ⇒ Revised   ~~deleted~~ Deleted   Excludes 1   Excludes 2   Includes   Use additional   Code first   Code also   Key words
OGCR Official Guidelines   X Assign placeholder X   ● Use Additional Character(s)   ▶ Manifestation Code   🅒 Hierarchical Condition Category   Coding Clinic

E23.3   **Hypothalamic dysfunction, not elsewhere classified** 🔍
    Excludes1   Prader-Willi syndrome (Q87.11)
                   Russell-Silver syndrome (Q87.19)
    Coding Clinic: 2024, Q1, P15

E23.6   **Other disorders of pituitary gland** 🔍
    Abscess of pituitary
    Adiposogenital dystrophy

E23.7   **Disorder of pituitary gland, unspecified** 🔍

● **E24**   **Cushing's syndrome**
    Excludes1   congenital adrenal hyperplasia (E25.0)

E24.0   **Pituitary-dependent Cushing's disease** 🔍
    Overproduction of pituitary ACTH
    Pituitary-dependent hypercorticalism

E24.1   **Nelson's syndrome** 🔍

E24.2   **Drug-induced Cushing's syndrome** 🔍
    Use additional code for adverse effect, if applicable,
      to identify drug (T36-T50 with fifth or sixth
      character 5)

E24.3   **Ectopic ACTH syndrome** 🔍

E24.4   **Alcohol-induced pseudo-Cushing's syndrome** 🔍

E24.8   **Other Cushing's syndrome** 🔍

E24.9   **Cushing's syndrome, unspecified** 🔍

● **E25**   **Adrenogenital disorders**
    Disorder of production of steroid hormone in adrenal gland
    Includes   adrenogenital syndromes, virilizing or
               feminizing, whether acquired or due to
               adrenal hyperplasia consequent on inborn
               enzyme defects in hormone synthesis
               female adrenal pseudohermaphroditism
               female heterosexual precocious pseudopuberty
               male isosexual precocious pseudopuberty
               male macrogenitosomia praecox
               male sexual precocity with adrenal hyperplasia
               male virilization (female)
    Excludes1   indeterminate sex and pseudohermaphroditism
                   (Q56)
                   chromosomal abnormalities (Q90-Q99)

E25.0   **Congenital adrenogenital disorders associated with enzyme deficiency** 🔍
    Congenital adrenal hyperplasia
    21-Hydroxylase deficiency
    Salt-losing congenital adrenal hyperplasia

E25.8   **Other adrenogenital disorders** 🔍
    Idiopathic adrenogenital disorder
    Use additional code for adverse effect, if applicable,
      to identify drug (T36-T50 with fifth or sixth
      character 5)

E25.9   **Adrenogenital disorder, unspecified** 🔍
    Adrenogenital syndrome NOS

● **E26**   **Hyperaldosteronism**
    Abnormality of electrolyte metabolism caused by excessive secretion
    of aldosterone

● E26.0   **Primary hyperaldosteronism**
    E26.01   **Conn's syndrome** 🔍
         Code also adrenal adenoma (D35.0-)
    E26.02   **Glucocorticoid-remediable aldosteronism** 🔍
         Familial aldosteronism type I
    E26.09   **Other primary hyperaldosteronism** 🔍
         Primary aldosteronism due to adrenal
           hyperplasia (bilateral)

E26.1   **Secondary hyperaldosteronism** 🔍

● E26.8   **Other hyperaldosteronism**
    E26.81   **Bartter's syndrome** 🔍
    E26.89   **Other hyperaldosteronism** 🔍

E26.9   **Hyperaldosteronism, unspecified** 🔍
    Aldosteronism NOS
    Hyperaldosteronism NOS

● **E27**   **Other disorders of adrenal gland**

E27.0   **Other adrenocortical overactivity** 🔍
    Overproduction of ACTH, not associated with
      Cushing's disease
    Premature adrenarche
    Excludes1   Cushing's syndrome (E24.-)

E27.1   **Primary adrenocortical insufficiency** 🔍
    Addison's disease
    Autoimmune adrenalitis
    Excludes1   Addison only phenotype
                  adrenoleukodystrophy (E71.528)
                  amyloidosis (E85.-)
                  tuberculous Addison's disease (A18.7)
                  Waterhouse-Friderichsen syndrome
                    (A39.1)

E27.2   **Addisonian crisis** 🔍
    Acute onset of adrenocortical insufficiency
    Adrenal crisis
    Adrenocortical crisis

E27.3   **Drug-induced adrenocortical insufficiency** 🔍
    Use additional code for adverse effect, if applicable,
      to identify drug (T36-T50 with fifth or sixth
      character 5)

● E27.4   **Other and unspecified adrenocortical insufficiency**
    Excludes1   adrenoleukodystrophy [Addison-
                  Schilder] (E71.528)
                  Waterhouse-Friderichsen syndrome
                    (A39.1)
    E27.40   **Unspecified adrenocortical insufficiency** 🔍
         Adrenocortical insufficiency NOS
         Hypoaldosteronism
         Coding Clinic: 2024, Q1, P15
    E27.49   **Other adrenocortical insufficiency** 🔍
         Adrenal hemorrhage
         Adrenal infarction
         Coding Clinic: 2024, Q1, P15

E27.5   **Adrenomedullary hyperfunction** 🔍
    Adrenomedullary hyperplasia
    Catecholamine hypersecretion

E27.8   **Other specified disorders of adrenal gland** 🔍
    Abnormality of cortisol-binding globulin

E27.9   **Disorder of adrenal gland, unspecified** 🔍

● **E28**   **Ovarian dysfunction**
    Excludes1   isolated gonadotropin deficiency (E23.0)
                  postprocedural ovarian failure (E89.4-)

E28.0   **Estrogen excess**
    Use additional code for adverse effect, if applicable,
      to identify drug (T36-T50 with fifth or sixth
      character 5)

E28.1   **Androgen excess**
    Hypersecretion of ovarian androgens
    Use additional code for adverse effect, if applicable,
      to identify drug (T36-T50 with fifth or sixth
      character 5)

E28.2   **Polycystic ovarian syndrome**
    Sclerocystic ovary syndrome
    Stein-Leventhal syndrome
    Coding Clinic: 2022, Q2, P16

● E28.3   **Primary ovarian failure**
    Excludes1   pure gonadal dysgenesis (Q99.1)
                  Turner's syndrome (Q96.-)
    ● E28.31   **Premature menopause**
         E28.310   **Symptomatic premature menopause** A
            Symptoms such as flushing,
               sleeplessness, headache, lack of
               concentration, associated with
               premature menopause
         E28.319   **Asymptomatic premature menopause**   A
            Premature menopause NOS

CHAPTER 4 (E00–E89)

E28.39   **Other primary ovarian failure**
     Decreased estrogen
     Resistant ovary syndrome

E28.8   **Other ovarian dysfunction**
     Ovarian hyperfunction NOS
     Excludes1   postprocedural ovarian failure (E89.4-)

E28.9   **Ovarian dysfunction, unspecified**

● E29   **Testicular dysfunction**
     Excludes1   androgen insensitivity syndrome (E34.5-)
                azoospermia or oligospermia NOS (N46.0-N46.1)
                isolated gonadotropin deficiency (E23.0)
                Klinefelter's syndrome (Q98.0-Q98.1, Q98.4)

E29.0   **Testicular hyperfunction**
     Hypersecretion of testicular hormones

E29.1   **Testicular hypofunction**
     Defective biosynthesis of testicular androgen NOS
     5-delta-Reductase deficiency (with male pseudohermaphroditism)
     Testicular hypogonadism NOS
     Use additional code for adverse effect, if applicable, to identify drug (T36-T50 with fifth or sixth character 5)
     Excludes1   postprocedural testicular hypofunction (E89.5)

E29.8   **Other testicular dysfunction**

E29.9   **Testicular dysfunction, unspecified**

● E30   **Disorders of puberty, not elsewhere classified**

E30.0   **Delayed puberty**
     Constitutional delay of puberty
     Delayed sexual development

E30.1   **Precocious puberty**   P
     Sexual maturation at earlier age than normal, or before age 8 in girls and 9 in boys, usually hormonal; AKA sexual precocity or pubertas praecox
     Precocious menstruation
     Excludes1   Albright (-McCune) (-Sternberg) syndrome (Q78.1)
                central precocious puberty (E22.8)
                congenital adrenal hyperplasia (E25.0)
                female heterosexual precocious pseudopuberty (E25.-)
                male isosexual precocious pseudopuberty (E25.-)

E30.8   **Other disorders of puberty**   P
     Premature thelarche

E30.9   **Disorder of puberty, unspecified**

● E31   **Polyglandular dysfunction**
     Excludes1   ataxia telangiectasia [Louis-Bar] (G11.3)
                dystrophia myotonica [Steinert] (G71.11)
                pseudohypoparathyroidism (E20.1)

E31.0   **Autoimmune polyglandular failure** 🔖
     Schmidt's syndrome

E31.1   **Polyglandular hyperfunction** 🔖
     Excludes1   multiple endocrine adenomatosis (E31.2-)
                multiple endocrine neoplasia (E31.2-)

● E31.2   **Multiple endocrine neoplasia [MEN] syndromes**
     Adenomatous hyperplasia and malignant tumors in endocrine glands
     Multiple endocrine adenomatosis
     Code also any associated malignancies and other conditions associated with the syndromes

E31.20   **Multiple endocrine neoplasia [MEN] syndrome, unspecified** 🔖
     Multiple endocrine adenomatosis NOS
     Multiple endocrine neoplasia [MEN] syndrome NOS

E31.21   **Multiple endocrine neoplasia [MEN] type I** 🔖
     Wermer's syndrome

E31.22   **Multiple endocrine neoplasia [MEN] type IIA** 🔖
     Sipple's syndrome

E31.23   **Multiple endocrine neoplasia [MEN] type IIB** 🔖

E31.8   **Other polyglandular dysfunction** 🔖

E31.9   **Polyglandular dysfunction, unspecified** 🔖

● E32   **Diseases of thymus**
     Excludes1   aplasia or hypoplasia of thymus with immunodeficiency (D82.1)
                myasthenia gravis (G70.0)

E32.0   **Persistent hyperplasia of thymus** 🔖
     Hypertrophy of thymus

E32.1   **Abscess of thymus** 🔖

E32.8   **Other diseases of thymus** 🔖
     Excludes1   aplasia or hypoplasia with immunodeficiency (D82.1)
                thymoma (D15.0)

E32.9   **Disease of thymus, unspecified** 🔖

● E34   **Other endocrine disorders**
     Excludes1   pseudohypoparathyroidism (E20.1)

E34.0   **Carcinoid syndrome** 🔖
     ~~Note: May be used as an additional code to identify functional activity associated with a carcinoid tumor.~~
     ▶ Code also the underlying disorder, such as:
       ▶ primary neuroendocrine tumors (C7A.-)
       ▶ secondary neuroendocrine tumors (C7B.-)

▶ E34.00   **Carcinoid syndrome, unspecified**
     ▶ Carcinoid disease, unspecified

▶ E34.01   **Carcinoid heart syndrome**
     ▶ Carcinoid heart disease
     ▶ Hedinger syndrome

▶ E34.09   **Other carcinoid syndrome**
     ▶ Carcinoid disease NEC
     ▶ Carcinoid syndrome NEC
     ▶ Other carcinoid disease

E34.1   **Other hypersecretion of intestinal hormones**

E34.2   **Ectopic hormone secretion, not elsewhere classified**
     Excludes1   ectopic ACTH syndrome (E24.3)

E34.3   **Short stature due to endocrine disorder**
     Excludes1   achondroplastic short stature (Q77.4)
                hypochondroplastic short stature (Q77.4)
                nutritional short stature (E45)
                pituitary short stature (E23.0)
                progeria (E34.8)
                renal short stature (N25.0)
                Russell-Silver syndrome (Q87.19)
                short-limbed stature with immunodeficiency (D82.2)
                short stature due to endocrine disorder (E34.3-)
                short stature in specific dysmorphic syndromes - code to syndrome - see Alphabetical Index
                short stature NOS (R62.52)

E34.30   **Short stature due to endocrine disorder, unspecified**

E34.31   **Constitutional short stature**
     Constitutional delay of growth, puberty, or maturation

- **E34.32**   **Genetic causes of short stature**
  - E34.321   **Primary insulin-like growth factor-1 (IGF-1) deficiency**
    - Acid-labile subunit gene (IGFALS) defect
    - Growth hormone gene 1 (GH1) defect with growth hormone neutralizing antibodies
    - Growth hormone insensitivity syndrome (GHIS)
    - Insulin-like growth factor 1 gene (IGF1) defect
    - Laron type short stature
    - Severe primary insulin-like growth factor-1 deficiency (SPIGFD)
    - Signal transducer and activator of transcription 5B gene (STAT5b) defect
  - E34.322   **Insulin-like growth factor-1 (IGF-1) resistance**
    - Genetic syndrome with resistance to insulin-like growth factor-1
    - Insulin-like growth factor-1 receptor (IGF-1R) defect
    - Post-insulin-like growth factor-1 receptor signaling defect
  - E34.328   **Other genetic causes of short stature**
    - Short stature due to ACAN gene variant
    - Short stature due to aggrecan deficiency
    - Short stature due to NPR-2 gene variant
  - E34.329   **Unspecified genetic causes of short stature**
- **E34.39**   **Other short stature due to endocrine disorder**
- E34.4   **Constitutional tall stature**
  - Constitutional gigantism
- **E34.5**   **Androgen insensitivity syndrome**
  - E34.50   **Androgen insensitivity syndrome, unspecified**
    - Androgen insensitivity NOS
  - E34.51   **Complete androgen insensitivity syndrome**
    - Complete androgen insensitivity
    - de Quervain syndrome
    - Goldberg-Maxwell syndrome
  - E34.52   **Partial androgen insensitivity syndrome**
    - Partial androgen insensitivity
    - Reifenstein syndrome
- E34.8   **Other specified endocrine disorders**
  - Pineal gland dysfunction
  - Progeria
  - **Excludes2**   pseudohypoparathyroidism (E20.1)
- E34.9   **Endocrine disorder, unspecified**
  - Endocrine disturbance NOS
  - Hormone disturbance NOS

- **E35**   *Disorders of endocrine glands in diseases classified elsewhere*
  - *Code first underlying disease, such as:*
  - late congenital syphilis of thymus gland [Dubois disease] (A50.9)
  - Use additional code, if applicable, to identify:
  - sequelae of tuberculosis of other organs (B90.8)
  - **Excludes1**   Echinococcus granulosus infection of thyroid gland (B67.3)
    - meningococcal hemorrhagic adrenalitis (A39.1)
    - syphilis of endocrine gland (A52.79)
    - tuberculosis of adrenal gland, except calcification (A18.7)
    - tuberculosis of endocrine gland NEC (A18.82)
    - tuberculosis of thyroid gland (A18.81)
    - Waterhouse-Friderichsen syndrome (A39.1)

INTRAOPERATIVE COMPLICATIONS OF ENDOCRINE SYSTEM (E36)

- **E36**   **Intraoperative complications of endocrine system**
  - **Excludes2**   postprocedural endocrine and metabolic complications and disorders, not elsewhere classified (E89.-)
  - **E36.0**   **Intraoperative hemorrhage and hematoma of an endocrine system organ or structure complicating a procedure**
    - **Excludes1**   intraoperative hemorrhage and hematoma of an endocrine system organ or structure due to accidental puncture or laceration during a procedure (E36.1-)
    - E36.01   **Intraoperative hemorrhage and hematoma of an endocrine system organ or structure complicating an endocrine system procedure**
      - Coding Clinic: 2020, Q1, P19
    - E36.02   **Intraoperative hemorrhage and hematoma of an endocrine system organ or structure complicating other procedure**
  - **E36.1**   **Accidental puncture and laceration of an endocrine system organ or structure during a procedure**
    - E36.11   **Accidental puncture and laceration of an endocrine system organ or structure during an endocrine system procedure**
    - E36.12   **Accidental puncture and laceration of an endocrine system organ or structure during other procedure**
  - E36.8   **Other intraoperative complications of endocrine system**
    - Use additional code, if applicable, to further specify disorder

MALNUTRITION (E40-E46)

- **Excludes1**   intestinal malabsorption (K90.-)
  - sequelae of protein-calorie malnutrition (E64.0)
- **Excludes2**   nutritional anemias (D50-D53)
  - starvation (T73.0)

- E40   **Kwashiorkor**
  - *Malnutrition produced by severe protein deficiency*
  - Severe malnutrition with nutritional edema with dyspigmentation of skin and hair
  - **Excludes1**   marasmic kwashiorkor (E42)
  - Coding Clinic: 22017, Q3, P25
- E41   **Nutritional marasmus**
  - Severe malnutrition with marasmus
  - **Excludes1**   marasmic kwashiorkor (E42)
  - Coding Clinic: 2017, Q3, P24-25
- E42   **Marasmic kwashiorkor**
  - *Severe protein malnutrition*
  - Intermediate form severe protein-calorie malnutrition
  - Severe protein-calorie malnutrition with signs of both kwashiorkor and marasmus
  - Coding Clinic: 2017, Q3, P25
- E43   **Unspecified severe protein-calorie malnutrition**
  - Starvation edema
  - Coding Clinic: 2023, Q4, P15; 2022, Q1, P13; 2020, Q1, P5-6; 2017, Q4, P108-109; 2017, Q3, P25
- **E44**   **Protein-calorie malnutrition of moderate and mild degree**
  - E44.0   **Moderate protein-calorie malnutrition**
  - E44.1   **Mild protein-calorie malnutrition**
- E45   **Retarded development following protein-calorie malnutrition**
  - Nutritional short stature
  - Nutritional stunting
  - Physical retardation due to malnutrition

CHAPTER 4 (E00-E89)

CHAPTER 4 (E00-E89)

E46   Unspecified protein-calorie malnutrition 🕸
      Malnutrition NOS
      Protein-calorie imbalance NOS

    Excludes1   nutritional deficiency NOS (E63.9)

    Coding Clinic: 2017, Q3, P25

OTHER NUTRITIONAL DEFICIENCIES (E50-E64)

    Excludes2   nutritional anemias (D50-D53)

● E50   Vitamin A deficiency
    Excludes1   sequelae of vitamin A deficiency (E64.1)

    E50.0   Vitamin A deficiency with conjunctival xerosis

    E50.1   Vitamin A deficiency with Bitot's spot and conjunctival xerosis
        Bitot's spot in the young child

    E50.2   Vitamin A deficiency with corneal xerosis

    E50.3   Vitamin A deficiency with corneal ulceration and xerosis

    E50.4   Vitamin A deficiency with keratomalacia
        Eye disorder that results in dry cornea caused by vitamin A deficiency

    E50.5   Vitamin A deficiency with night blindness

    E50.6   Vitamin A deficiency with xerophthalmic scars of cornea
        Abnormal dryness and thickening of conjunctiva and cornea due to vitamin A deficiency

    E50.7   Other ocular manifestations of vitamin A deficiency
        Xerophthalmia NOS

    E50.8   Other manifestations of vitamin A deficiency
        Follicular keratosis
        Xeroderma

    E50.9   Vitamin A deficiency, unspecified
        Hypovitaminosis A NOS

● E51   Thiamine deficiency
    Excludes1   sequelae of thiamine deficiency (E64.8)

    ● E51.1   Beriberi

        E51.11   Dry beriberi
            Thiamine deficiency with nervous system manifestation most often caused by excessive alcohol consumption
            Beriberi NOS
            Beriberi with polyneuropathy

        E51.12   Wet beriberi
            Thiamine deficiency with cardiovascular manifestation most often caused by excessive alcohol consumption
            Beriberi with cardiovascular manifestations
            Cardiovascular beriberi
            Shoshin disease

    E51.2   Wernicke's encephalopathy
        Acute disease of brain due to thiamine deficiency most often associated with excessive alcohol consumption

    E51.8   Other manifestations of thiamine deficiency

    E51.9   Thiamine deficiency, unspecified

E52   Niacin deficiency [pellagra]
    Niacin (-tryptophan) deficiency
    Nicotinamide deficiency
    Pellagra (alcoholic)
    Excludes1   sequelae of niacin deficiency (E64.8)

● E53   Deficiency of other B group vitamins
    Excludes1   sequelae of vitamin B deficiency (E64.8)

    E53.0   Riboflavin deficiency
        Ariboflavinosis
        Vitamin B2 deficiency

    E53.1   Pyridoxine deficiency
        Vitamin B6 deficiency
        Excludes1   pyridoxine-responsive sideroblastic anemia (D64.3)

    E53.8   Deficiency of other specified B group vitamins
        Biotin deficiency
        Cyanocobalamin deficiency
        Folate deficiency
        Folic acid deficiency
        Pantothenic acid deficiency
        Vitamin B12 deficiency
        Excludes1   folate deficiency anemia (D52.-)
                   vitamin B12 deficiency anemia (D51.-)

    E53.9   Vitamin B deficiency, unspecified

E54   Ascorbic acid deficiency
    Deficiency of vitamin C
    Scurvy
    Excludes1   scorbutic anemia (D53.2)
              sequelae of vitamin C deficiency (E64.2)

● E55   Vitamin D deficiency
    Excludes1   adult osteomalacia (M83.-)
              osteoporosis (M80.-)
              sequelae of rickets (E64.3)

    E55.0   Rickets, active
        Infantile osteomalacia
        Juvenile osteomalacia
        Softening of bone
        Excludes1   celiac rickets (K90.0)
                 Crohn's rickets (K50.-)
                 hereditary vitamin D-dependent rickets (E83.32)
                 inactive rickets (E64.3)
                 renal rickets (N25.0)
                 sequelae of rickets (E64.3)
                 vitamin D-resistant rickets (E83.31)

    E55.9   Vitamin D deficiency, unspecified
        Avitaminosis D

● E56   Other vitamin deficiencies
    Excludes1   sequelae of other vitamin deficiencies (E64.8)

    E56.0   Deficiency of vitamin E

    E56.1   Deficiency of vitamin K
        Excludes1   deficiency of coagulation factor due to vitamin K deficiency (D68.4)
                 vitamin K deficiency of newborn (P53)

    E56.8   Deficiency of other vitamins

    E56.9   Vitamin deficiency, unspecified

E58   Dietary calcium deficiency
    Excludes1   disorders of calcium metabolism (E83.5-)
              sequelae of calcium deficiency (E64.8)

Item 4–6   Bitot's spots are the result of a buildup of keratin debris found on the superficial surface the conjunctiva; oval, triangular, or irregular in shape; and a sign of vitamin A deficiency and associated with night blindness. The disease may progress to **keratomalacia,** which can result in eventual prolapse of the iris and loss of the lens.

Figure 4-6   Bitot's spot on the conjunctiva.

Figure 4-7   The sharply demarcated, characteristic scaling dermatitis of pellagra. (From James WD, Berger TG, Elston DM: Andrews' Diseases of the Skin: Clinical Dermatology, Philadelphia, Saunders Elsevier, 2006)

Item 4–7   Pellagra is associated with a deficiency of niacin and its precursor, **tryptophan.** Characteristics of the condition include diarrhea, dermatitis on exposed skin surfaces, dementia, and death. It is prevalent in developing countries where nutrition is inadequate. **Beriberi** is associated with thiamine deficiency.

▶ New   ⇒ Revised   ~~deleted~~ Deleted   Excludes 1   Excludes 2   Includes   Use additional   Code first   Code also   Key words

OGCR Official Guidelines   X Assign placeholder X   ● Use Additional Character(s)   ▶ Manifestation Code   🕸 Hierarchical Condition Category   **Coding Clinic**

E59   Dietary selenium deficiency
Keshan disease
> **Excludes1**   sequelae of selenium deficiency (E64.8)

E60   Dietary zinc deficiency

●**E61   Deficiency of other nutrient elements**
Use additional code for adverse effect, if applicable, to identify drug (T36-T50 with fifth or sixth character 5)
> **Excludes1**   disorders of mineral metabolism (E83.-)
> iodine deficiency related thyroid disorders (E00-E02)
> sequelae of malnutrition and other nutritional deficiencies (E64.-)

E61.0   Copper deficiency

E61.1   Iron deficiency
> **Excludes1**   iron deficiency anemia (D50.-)

E61.2   Magnesium deficiency

E61.3   Manganese deficiency

E61.4   Chromium deficiency

E61.5   Molybdenum deficiency

E61.6   Vanadium deficiency

E61.7   Deficiency of multiple nutrient elements

E61.8   Deficiency of other specified nutrient elements

E61.9   Deficiency of nutrient element, unspecified

●**E63   Other nutritional deficiencies**
> **Excludes2**   dehydration (E86.0)
> failure to thrive, adult (R62.7)
> failure to thrive, child (R62.51)
> feeding problems in newborn (P92.-)
> sequelae of malnutrition and other nutritional deficiencies (E64.-)

E63.0   Essential fatty acid [EFA] deficiency

E63.1   Imbalance of constituents of food intake

E63.8   Other specified nutritional deficiencies

E63.9   Nutritional deficiency, unspecified

●**E64   Sequelae of malnutrition and other nutritional deficiencies**
Pathological condition resulting from disease, injury, or other trauma
Note: This category is to be used to indicate conditions in categories E43, E44, E46, E50-E63 as the cause of sequelae, which are themselves classified elsewhere. The "sequelae" include conditions specified as such; they also include the late effects of diseases classifiable to the above categories if the disease itself is no longer present
Code first condition resulting from (sequela) of malnutrition and other nutritional deficiencies

E64.0   Sequelae of protein-calorie malnutrition 🔎
> **Excludes2**   retarded development following protein-calorie malnutrition (E45)

E64.1   Sequelae of vitamin A deficiency

E64.2   Sequelae of vitamin C deficiency

E64.3   Sequelae of rickets

E64.8   Sequelae of other nutritional deficiencies

E64.9   Sequelae of unspecified nutritional deficiency

OVERWEIGHT, OBESITY AND OTHER HYPERALIMENTATION (E65-E68)

E65   Localized adiposity
Fat pad

●**E66   Overweight and obesity**
Code first obesity complicating pregnancy, childbirth and the puerperium, if applicable (O99.21-)
⇒ Use additional code to identify body mass index (BMI), if known, for adults (Z68.1-Z68.45) or pediatrics (Z68.5-)
> **Excludes2**   adiposogenital dystrophy E23.6)
> lipomatosis NOS (E88.2)
> lipomatosis dolorosa [Dercum] (E88.2)
> Prader-Willi syndrome (Q87.11)
Coding Clinic: 2022, Q3, P7; 2018, Q4, P80

●**E66.0   Obesity due to excess calories**

E66.01   Morbid (severe) obesity due to excess calories 🔎
> **Excludes1**   morbid (severe) obesity with alveolar hypoventilation (E66.2)
Coding Clinic: 2022, Q3, P6; 2022, Q2, P9; 2018, Q4, P79

E66.09   Other obesity due to excess calories

E66.1   Drug-induced obesity
Use additional code for adverse effect, if applicable, to identify drug (T36-T50 with fifth or sixth character 5)
Coding Clinic: 2022, Q3, P6

E66.2   Morbid (severe) obesity with alveolar hypoventilation 🔎
Uncommon condition of unknown cause leading to inadequate ventilation in lungs, even though lungs and airways are normal
Obesity hypoventilation syndrome (OHS)
Pickwickian syndrome

E66.3   Overweight

E66.8   Other obesity
▶**E66.81   Obesity class**
▶**E66.811   Obesity, class 1**
▶**E66.812   Obesity, class 2**
▶**E66.813   Obesity, class 3**
▶**E66.89   Other obesity not elsewhere classified**

E66.9   Obesity, unspecified
Obesity NOS
Coding Clinic: 2021, Q2, P10-11

●**E67   Other hyperalimentation**
Ingestion of more than optimal amount of nutrients
> **Excludes1**   hyperalimentation NOS (R63.2)
> sequelae of hyperalimentation (E68)

E67.0   Hypervitaminosis A

E67.1   Hypercarotenemia

E67.2   Megavitamin-B6 syndrome

E67.3   Hypervitaminosis D

E67.8   Other specified hyperalimentation

E68   Sequelae of hyperalimentation
Code first condition resulting from (sequela) of hyperalimentation

METABOLIC DISORDERS (E70-E88)

> **Excludes1**   androgen insensitivity syndrome (E34.5-)
> congenital adrenal hyperplasia (E25.0)
> hemolytic anemias attributable to enzyme disorders (D55.-)
> Marfan syndrome (Q87.4-)
> 5-alpha-reductase deficiency (E29.1)
> **Excludes2**   Ehlers-Danlos syndromes (Q79.6-)

●**E70   Disorders of aromatic amino-acid metabolism**
E70.0   Classical phenylketonuria 🔎
Inherited disorder that increases to harmful levels amino acid phenylalanine

E70.1   Other hyperphenylalaninemias 🔎

●**E70.2   Disorders of tyrosine metabolism**
> **Excludes1**   transitory tyrosinemia of newborn (P74.5)

E70.20   Disorder of tyrosine metabolism, unspecified 🔎
Tyrosine: Nonessential amino acid occurring in most proteins

E70.21   Tyrosinemia 🔎
Congenital amino acid metabolism
Hypertyrosinemia

E70.29   Other disorders of tyrosine metabolism 🔎
Alkaptonuria
Ochronosis

CHAPTER 4 (E00-E89)

● **E70.3   Albinism**
Congenital condition of reduced or absent pigment in eyes, skin, and hair

     E70.30   Albinism, unspecified 🅒

●   E70.31   Ocular albinism

       E70.310   X-linked ocular albinism 🅒

       E70.311   Autosomal recessive ocular albinism 🅒

       E70.318   Other ocular albinism 🅒

       E70.319   Ocular albinism, unspecified 🅒

●   E70.32   Oculocutaneous albinism
Partial or total lack of melanin pigment in eyes

Excludes1   Chediak-Higashi syndrome (E70.330)
Hermansky-Pudlak syndrome (E70.331)

       E70.320   Tyrosinase negative oculocutaneous albinism 🅒
Albinism I
Oculocutaneous albinism ty-neg

       E70.321   Tyrosinase positive oculocutaneous albinism 🅒
Albinism II
Oculocutaneous albinism ty-pos

       E70.328   Other oculocutaneous albinism 🅒
Cross syndrome

       E70.329   Oculocutaneous albinism, unspecified 🅒

●   E70.33   Albinism with hematologic abnormality

       E70.330   Chediak-Higashi syndrome 🅒

       E70.331   Hermansky-Pudlak syndrome 🅒

       E70.338   Other albinism with hematologic abnormality 🅒

       E70.339   Albinism with hematologic abnormality, unspecified 🅒

     E70.39   Other specified albinism 🅒
Piebaldism

● **E70.4   Disorders of histidine metabolism**

     E70.40   Disorders of histidine metabolism, unspecified 🅒

     E70.41   Histidinemia 🅒

     E70.49   Other disorders of histidine metabolism 🅒

   E70.5   Disorders of tryptophan metabolism 🅒

● **E70.8   Other disorders of aromatic amino-acid metabolism** 🅒

     E70.81   Aromatic L-amino acid decarboxylase deficiency
AADC deficiency

     E70.89   Other disorders of aromatic amino-acid metabolism

   E70.9   Disorder of aromatic amino-acid metabolism, unspecified 🅒

● **E71   Disorders of branched-chain amino-acid metabolism and fatty-acid metabolism**

   E71.0   Maple-syrup-urine disease 🅒
Due to defect in amino acid catabolism, causing severe ketoacidosis with smell of maple syrup in urine and on body

● **E71.1   Other disorders of branched-chain amino-acid metabolism**

●   E71.11   Branched-chain organic acidurias

       E71.110   Isovaleric acidemia 🅒

       E71.111   3-methylglutaconic aciduria 🅒

       E71.118   Other branched-chain organic acidurias 🅒

●   E71.12   Disorders of propionate metabolism

       E71.120   Methylmalonic acidemia 🅒

       E71.121   Propionic acidemia 🅒

       E71.128   Other disorders of propionate metabolism 🅒

     E71.19   Other disorders of branched-chain amino-acid metabolism 🅒
Hyperleucine-isoleucinemia
Hypervalinemia

   E71.2   Disorder of branched-chain amino-acid metabolism, unspecified 🅒

● **E71.3   Disorders of fatty-acid metabolism**

Excludes1   peroxisomal disorders (E71.5)
Refsum's disease (G60.1)
Schilder's disease (G37.0)

Excludes2   carnitine deficiency due to inborn error of metabolism (E71.42)

     E71.30   Disorder of fatty-acid metabolism, unspecified

●   E71.31   Disorders of fatty-acid oxidation

       E71.310   Long chain/very long chain acyl CoA dehydrogenase deficiency 🅒
LCAD deficiency
VLCAD deficiency

       E71.311   Medium chain acyl CoA dehydrogenase deficiency 🅒
MCAD deficiency

       E71.312   Short chain acyl CoA dehydrogenase deficiency 🅒
SCAD deficiency

       E71.313   Glutaric aciduria type II 🅒
Glutaric aciduria type II A
Glutaric aciduria type II B
Glutaric aciduria type II C

Excludes1   glutaric aciduria (type 1) NOS (E72.3)

       E71.314   Muscle carnitine palmitoyltransferase deficiency 🅒

       E71.318   Other disorders of fatty-acid oxidation 🅒

     E71.32   Disorders of ketone metabolism 🅒

     E71.39   Other disorders of fatty-acid metabolism 🅒

● **E71.4   Disorders of carnitine metabolism**

Excludes1   muscle carnitine palmitoyltransferase deficiency (E71.314)

     E71.40   Disorder of carnitine metabolism, unspecified 🅒

     E71.41   Primary carnitine deficiency 🅒

     E71.42   Carnitine deficiency due to inborn errors of metabolism 🅒
Code also associated inborn error or metabolism

     E71.43   Iatrogenic carnitine deficiency 🅒
Iatrogenic: Outcomes from activity of physicians
Carnitine deficiency due to hemodialysis
Carnitine deficiency due to Valproic acid therapy

●   E71.44   Other secondary carnitine deficiency

       E71.440   Ruvalcaba-Myhre-Smith syndrome 🅒

       E71.448   Other secondary carnitine deficiency

● **E71.5   Peroxisomal disorders**
Class of conditions which lead to disorders of lipid metabolism

Excludes1   Schilder's disease (G37.0)

     E71.50   Peroxisomal disorder, unspecified 🅒

●   E71.51   Disorders of peroxisome biogenesis
Group 1 peroxisomal disorders

Excludes1   Refsum's disease (G60.1)

       E71.510   Zellweger syndrome 🅒

       E71.511   Neonatal adrenoleukodystrophy 🅒

Excludes1   X-linked adrenoleuko-dystrophy (E71.42-)

       E71.518   Other disorders of peroxisome biogenesis 🅒

▶ New   ⇒ Revised   ~~deleted~~ Deleted   Excludes 1   Excludes 2   Includes   Use additional   Code first   Code also   Key words

704

OGCR Official Guidelines   X Assign placeholder X   ● Use Additional Character(s)   ▶ Manifestation Code   🅒 Hierarchical Condition Category   Coding Clinic

Item 4–8 Leukodystrophy is characterized by degeneration and/or failure of the myelin formation of the central nervous system and sometimes of the peripheral nervous system. The disease is inherited and progressive.

● **E71.52** **X-linked adrenoleukodystrophy**

    E71.520 **Childhood cerebral X-linked adrenoleukodystrophy** 🦠

    E71.521 **Adolescent X-linked adrenoleukodystrophy** 🦠

    E71.522 **Adrenomyeloneuropathy** 🦠

    E71.528 **Other X-linked adrenoleukodystrophy** 🦠

        Addison only phenotype adrenoleukodystrophy

        Addison-Schilder adrenoleukodystrophy

    E71.529 **X-linked adrenoleukodystrophy, unspecified type** 🦠

    E71.53 **Other group 2 peroxisomal disorders** 🦠

● E71.54 **Other peroxisomal disorders**

    E71.540 **Rhizomelic chondrodysplasia punctata** 🦠

        Rare, severe, inherited disorder with limb shortening, bone and cartilage abnormalities, abnormal facial appearance, severe mental retardation, psychomotor retardation, and cataracts

        Excludes1 chondrodysplasia punctata NOS (Q77.3)

    E71.541 **Zellweger-like syndrome** 🦠

    E71.542 **Other group 3 peroxisomal disorders** 🦠

    E71.548 **Other peroxisomal disorders** 🦠

● **E72** **Other disorders of amino-acid metabolism**

    Excludes1 disorders of:

        aromatic amino-acid metabolism (E70.-)

        branched-chain amino-acid metabolism (E71.0-E71.2)

        fatty-acid metabolism (E71.3)

        purine and pyrimidine metabolism (E79.-)

        gout (M1A.-, M10.-)

● **E72.0** **Disorders of amino-acid transport**

    Excludes1 disorders of tryptophan metabolism (E70.5)

    E72.00 **Disorders of amino-acid transport, unspecified** 🦠

    E72.01 **Cystinuria** 🦠

        Hereditary aminoaciduria due to impairment of renal transport with predominant symptom of urinary cystine calculi

    E72.02 **Hartnup's disease** 🦠

        Inborn error of metabolism

    E72.03 **Lowe's syndrome** 🦠

        X-linked disorder with rickets, hydrophthalmia, congenital glaucoma, cataracts, mental retardation, and renal tubule dysfunction

        Use additional code for associated glaucoma (H42)

    E72.04 **Cystinosis** 🦠

        Genetic disease with excessive depostits of amino acid cystine in cells

        Fanconi (-de Toni) (-Debré) syndrome with cystinosis

        Excludes1 Fanconi (-de Toni) (-Debré) syndrome without cystinosis (E72.09)

    E72.09 **Other disorders of amino-acid transport** 🦠

        Fanconi (-de Toni) (-Debré) syndrome, unspecified

● **E72.1** **Disorders of sulfur-bearing amino-acid metabolism**

    Excludes1 cystinosis (E72.04)

        cystinuria (E72.01)

        transcobalamin II deficiency (D51.2)

    E72.10 **Disorders of sulfur-bearing amino-acid metabolism, unspecified** 🦠

    E72.11 **Homocystinuria** 🦠

        Cystathionine synthase deficiency

    E72.12 **Methylenetetrahydrofolate reductase deficiency** 🦠

    E72.19 **Other disorders of sulfur-bearing amino-acid metabolism** 🦠

        Cystathioninuria

        Methioninemia

        Sulfite oxidase deficiency

● **E72.2** **Disorders of urea cycle metabolism**

    Excludes1 disorders of ornithine metabolism (E72.4)

    E72.20 **Disorder of urea cycle metabolism, unspecified** 🦠

        Hyperammonemia

        Elevated levels of ammonia

        Excludes1 hyperammonemia-hyperornithinemia-homocitrullinemia syndrome E72.4

        transient hyperammonemia of newborn (P74.6)

    E72.21 **Argininemia** 🦠

        Disorder in which deficiency of enzyme arginase causes build-up of arginine and ammonia in blood

    E72.22 **Arginosuccinic aciduria** 🦠

        Gene disorder of urea cycle resulting accumulation of ammonia

    E72.23 **Citrullinemia** 🦠

        Urea cycle disorder that causes ammonia and other toxic substances to accumulate in blood

    E72.29 **Other disorders of urea cycle metabolism** 🦠

    E72.3 **Disorders of lysine and hydroxylysine metabolism** 🦠

        Glutaric aciduria NOS

        Glutaric aciduria (type I)

        Hydroxylysinemia

        Hyperlysinemia

        Excludes1 glutaric aciduria type II (E71.313)

        Refsum's disease (G60.1)

        Zellweger syndrome (E71.510)

    E72.4 **Disorders of ornithine metabolism** 🦠

        Hyperammonemia-Hyperornithinemia-Homocitrullinemia syndrome

        Ornithinemia (types I, II)

        Ornithine transcarbamylase deficiency

        Excludes1 hereditary choroidal dystrophy (H31.2-)

● **E72.5** **Disorders of glycine metabolism**

    E72.50 **Disorder of glycine metabolism, unspecified** 🦠

    E72.51 **Non-ketotic hyperglycinemia** 🦠

    E72.52 **Trimethylaminuria** 🦠

    E72.53 **Primary hyperoxaluria** 🦠

        Oxalosis

        Oxaluria

    E72.59 **Other disorders of glycine metabolism** 🦠

        D-glycericacidemia

        Hyperhydroxyprolinemia

        Hyperprolinemia (types I, II)

        Sarcosinemia

- **E72.8** Other specified disorders of amino-acid metabolism 🝐
  - **E72.81** Disorders of gamma aminobutyric acid metabolism 🝐
    - 4-hydroxybutyric aciduria
    - Disorders of GABA metabolism
    - GABA metabolic defect
    - GABA transaminase deficiency
    - GABA-T deficiency
    - Gamma-hydroxybutyric aciduria
    - SSADHD
    - Succinic semialdehyde dehydrogenase deficiency
  - **E72.89** Other specified disorders of amino-acid metabolism 🝐
    - Disorders of beta-amino-acid metabolism
    - Disorders of gamma-glutamyl cycle
  - **E72.9** Disorder of amino-acid metabolism, unspecified 🝐

- **E73** Lactose intolerance
  Intolerance for lactose, due to inherited deficiency of lactase activity in intestinal mucosa
  - **E73.0** Congenital lactase deficiency
  - **E73.1** Secondary lactase deficiency
  - **E73.8** Other lactose intolerance
  - **E73.9** Lactose intolerance, unspecified

- **E74** Other disorders of carbohydrate metabolism
  - **Excludes1** diabetes mellitus (E08-E13)
    - hypoglycemia NOS (E16.2)
    - increased secretion of glucagon (E16.3)
    - mucopolysaccharidosis (E76.0-E76.3)
  - **E74.0** Glycogen storage disease
    - **E74.00** Glycogen storage disease, unspecified 🝐
    - **E74.01** von Gierke's disease 🝐
      - Type I glycogen storage disease
    - **E74.02** Pompe disease 🝐
      - Cardiac glycogenosis
      - Type II glycogen storage disease
    - **E74.03** Cori disease 🝐
      - Forbes' disease
      - Type III glycogen storage disease
    - **E74.04** McArdle disease 🝐
      - Type V glycogen storage disease
    - **E74.05** Lysosome-associated membrane protein 2 [LAMP2] deficiency
      - Danon disease
      - Code also, if applicable, associated manifestations such as:
        - dilated cardiomyopathy (I42.0)
        - obstructive hypertrophic cardiomyopathy (I42.1)
    - **E74.09** Other glycogen storage disease 🝐
      - Andersen disease
      - Glycogen storage disease, types 0, IV, VI-XI
      - Hers disease
      - Liver phosphorylase deficiency
      - Muscle phosphofructokinase deficiency
      - Tauri disease
  - **E74.1** Disorders of fructose metabolism
    - **Excludes1** muscle phosphofructokinase deficiency (E74.09)
    - **E74.10** Disorder of fructose metabolism, unspecified
    - **E74.11** Essential fructosuria
      - Fructokinase deficiency
    - **E74.12** Hereditary fructose intolerance
      - Fructosemia
    - **E74.19** Other disorders of fructose metabolism
      - Fructose-1, 6-diphosphatase deficiency

- **E74.2** Disorders of galactose metabolism
  - **E74.20** Disorders of galactose metabolism, unspecified 🝐
  - **E74.21** Galactosemia 🝐
    Genetic disorders resulting from defective simple sugar (galactose) metabolism
  - **E74.29** Other disorders of galactose metabolism 🝐
    - Galactokinase deficiency
- **E74.3** Other disorders of intestinal carbohydrate absorption
  - **Excludes2** lactose intolerance (E73.-)
  - **E74.31** Sucrase-isomaltase deficiency
    Deficiency in metabolism in intestinal mucosa results in malabsorption of sucrose and starch
  - **E74.39** Other disorders of intestinal carbohydrate absorption
    - Disorder of intestinal carbohydrate absorption NOS
    - Glucose-galactose malabsorption
    - Sucrase deficiency
  - **E74.4** Disorders of pyruvate metabolism and gluconeogenesis 🝐
    - Deficiency of phosphoenolpyruvate carboxykinase
    - Deficiency of pyruvate carboxylase
    - Deficiency of pyruvate dehydrogenase
    - **Excludes1** disorders of pyruvate metabolism and gluconeogenesis with anemia (D55.-)
      - Leigh's syndrome (G31.82)
- **E74.8** Other specified disorders of carbohydrate metabolism 🝐
  - **E74.81** Disorders of glucose transport, not elsewhere classified
    - **E74.810** Glucose transporter protein type 1 deficiency
      - De Vivo syndrome
      - Glucose transport defect, blood-brain barrier
      - GLUT1 deficiency
      - GLUT1 deficiency syndrome 1, infantile onset
      - GLUT1 deficiency syndrome 2, childhood onset
    - **E74.818** Other disorders of glucose transport
      - (Familial) renal glycosuria
    - **E74.819** Disorders of glucose transport, unspecified
  - ▶ **E74.82** Disorders of citrate metabolism
    - ▶ **E74.820** SLC13A5 Citrate Transporter Disorder
    - ▶ **E74.829** Other disorders of citrate metabolism
  - **E74.89** Other specified disorders of carbohydrate metabolism
    - Essential pentosuria
    - Coding Clinic: 2023, Q3, P3
  - **E74.9** Disorder of carbohydrate metabolism, unspecified 🝐
- **E75** Disorders of sphingolipid metabolism and other lipid storage disorders
  - **Excludes1** mucolipidosis, types I-III (E77.0-E77.1)
    - Refsum's disease (G60.1)
- **E75.0** GM2 gangliosidosis
  Rare metabolic disorder that causes destruction of nerve cells of brain and spinal cord
  - **E75.00** GM2 gangliosidosis, unspecified
  - **E75.01** Sandhoff disease
  - **E75.02** Tay-Sachs disease
  - **E75.09** Other GM2 gangliosidosis
    - Adult GM2 gangliosidosis
    - Juvenile GM2 gangliosidosis

▶ New   ⇒ Revised   ~~deleted~~ Deleted   Excludes 1   Excludes 2   Includes   Use additional   Code first   Code also   Key words
OGCR Official Guidelines   X Assign placeholder X   ● Use Additional Character(s)   ▶ Manifestation Code   🝐 Hierarchical Condition Category   Coding Clinic

● **E75.1** **Other and unspecified gangliosidosis**

    E75.10 **Unspecified gangliosidosis**
        Gangliosidosis NOS

    E75.11 **Mucolipidosis IV**
        Disorder with symptoms of psychomotor
        retardation and severe visual impairment

    E75.19 **Other gangliosidosis**
        GM1 gangliosidosis
        GM3 gangliosidosis

● **E75.2** **Other sphingolipidosis**
    Lysosomal (a particle in a cytoplasm cell that contains
    digestive enzymes) storage diseases with symptoms of
    abnormal storage of amino acids

    Excludes1 adrenoleukodystrophy [Addison-
        Schilder] (E71.528)

    E75.21 **Fabry (-Anderson) disease** 🐾

    E75.22 **Gaucher disease** 🐾

    E75.23 **Krabbe disease**

●   **E75.24** **Niemann-Pick disease**
        Acid sphingomyelinase deficiency (ASMD)

        E75.240 **Niemann-Pick disease type A** 🐾
            Acid sphingomyelinase deficiency
              type A (ASMD type A)
            Infantile neurovisceral acid
              sphingomyelinase deficiency

        E75.241 **Niemann-Pick disease type B** 🐾
            Acid sphingomyelinase deficiency
              type B (ASMD type B)
            Chronic visceral acid
              sphingomyelinase deficiency

        E75.242 **Niemann-Pick disease type C** 🐾

        E75.243 **Niemann-Pick disease type D** 🐾

        E75.244 **Niemann-Pick disease type A/B**
            Acid sphingomyelinase deficiency
              type A/B (ASMD type A/B)
            Chronic neurovisceral acid
              sphingomyelinase deficiency

        E75.248 **Other Niemann-Pick disease** 🐾

        E75.249 **Niemann-Pick disease, unspecified** 🐾
            Acid sphingomyelinase deficiency
              (ASMD) NOS

    E75.25 **Metachromatic leukodystrophy**

    E75.26 **Sulfatase deficiency**
        Multiple sulfatase deficiency (MSD)

    E75.27 **Pelizaeus-Merzbacher disease**

    E75.28 **Canavan disease**

    E75.29 **Other sphingolipidosis**
        Farber's syndrome
        Sulfatide lipidosis

  E75.3 **Sphingolipidosis, unspecified** 🐾

  E75.4 **Neuronal ceroid lipofuscinosis**
    Batten disease
    Bielschowsky-Jansky disease
    Kufs disease
    Spielmeyer-Vogt disease

  E75.5 **Other lipid storage disorders**
    Cerebrotendinous cholesterosis [van Bogaert-Scherer-
        Epstein]
    Wolman's disease

  E75.6 **Lipid storage disorder, unspecified**

● **E76** **Disorders of glycosaminoglycan metabolism**

●   **E76.0** **Mucopolysaccharidosis, type I**
    Inborn metabolic disorder of enzymes that break down
    carbohydrates

    E76.01 **Hurler's syndrome** 🐾

    E76.02 **Hurler-Scheie syndrome** 🐾

    E76.03 **Scheie's syndrome** 🐾

  E76.1 **Mucopolysaccharidosis, type II** 🐾
    Inborn metabolic disorder of enzymes that break down
    carbohydrates occurs in 2-4 year old males
    Hunter's syndrome

● **E76.2** **Other mucopolysaccharidoses**

●   **E76.21** **Morquio mucopolysaccharidoses**

    E76.210 **Morquio A mucopolysaccharidoses** 🐾
        Classic Morquio syndrome
        Morquio syndrome A
        Mucopolysaccharidosis, type IVA

    E76.211 **Morquio B mucopolysaccharidoses** 🐾
        Morquio-like
            mucopolysaccharidoses
        Morquio-like syndrome
        Morquio syndrome B
        Mucopolysaccharidosis, type IVB

    E76.219 **Morquio mucopolysaccharidoses,
        unspecified** 🐾
        Morquio syndrome
        Mucopolysaccharidosis, type IV

    E76.22 **Sanfilippo mucopolysaccharidoses** 🐾
        Mucopolysaccharidosis, type III (A) (B) (C) (D)
        Sanfilippo A syndrome
        Sanfilippo B syndrome
        Sanfilippo C syndrome
        Sanfilippo D syndrome

    E76.29 **Other mucopolysaccharidoses** 🐾
        beta-Glucuronidase deficiency
        Maroteaux-Lamy (mild) (severe) syndrome
        Mucopolysaccharidosis, types VI, VII

  E76.3 **Mucopolysaccharidosis, unspecified** 🐾

  E76.8 **Other disorders of glucosaminoglycan metabolism** 🐾

  E76.9 **Glucosaminoglycan metabolism disorder, unspecified** 🐾

● **E77** **Disorders of glycoprotein metabolism**

  E77.0 **Defects in post-translational modification of lysosomal
  enzymes** 🐾
    Mucolipidosis II [I-cell disease]
    Mucolipidosis III [pseudo-Hurler polydystrophy]

  E77.1 **Defects in glycoprotein degradation** 🐾
    Aspartylglucosaminuria
    Fucosidosis
    Mannosidosis
    Sialidosis [mucolipidosis I]

  E77.8 **Other disorders of glycoprotein metabolism** 🐾

  E77.9 **Disorder of glycoprotein metabolism, unspecified** 🐾

● **E78** **Disorders of lipoprotein metabolism and other lipidemias**

    Excludes1 sphingolipidosis (E75.0-E75.3)

●   **E78.0** **Pure hypercholesterolemia**
    Coding Clinic: 2016, Q4, P13

    E78.00 **Pure hypercholesterolemia, unspecified**
        Fredrickson's hyperlipoproteinemia, type IIa
        Hyperbetalipoproteinemia
        Low-density-lipoprotein-type [LDL]
            hyperlipoproteinemia
        (Pure) hypercholesterolemia NOS
        Coding Clinic: 2023, Q2, P9; 2022, Q2, P6; 2016, Q4, P13

    E78.01 **Familial hypercholesterolemia**
        Coding Clinic: 2016, Q4, P13

  E78.1 **Pure hyperglyceridemia**
    Elevated fasting triglycerides
    Endogenous hyperglyceridemia
    Fredrickson's hyperlipoproteinemia, type IV
    Hyperlipidemia, group B
    Hyperprebetalipoproteinemia
    Very-low-density-lipoprotein-type [VLDL]
        hyperlipoproteinemia

CHAPTER 4 (E00-E89)

E78.2   **Mixed hyperlipidemia**
> Broad- or floating-betalipoproteinemia
> Combined hyperlipidemia NOS
> Elevated cholesterol with elevated triglycerides NEC
> Fredrickson's hyperlipoproteinemia, type IIb or III
> Hyperbetalipoproteinemia with prebetalipoproteinemia
> Hypercholesteremia with endogenous hyperglyceridemia
> Hyperlipidemia, group C
> Tubo-eruptive xanthoma
> Xanthoma tuberosum

> **Excludes1**   cerebrotendinous cholesterosis [van Bogaert-Scherer-Epstein] (E75.5)
> familial combined hyperlipidemia (E78.49)
> Coding Clinic: 2023, Q2, P9-10; 2022, Q2, P6-7

E78.3   **Hyperchylomicronemia**
> Chylomicron retention disease
> Fredrickson's hyperlipoproteinemia, type I or V
> Hyperlipidemia, group D
> Mixed hyperglyceridemia

E78.4   **Other hyperlipidemia**

> **E78.41**   **Elevated Lipoprotein(a)**
> > Elevated Lp(a)

> **E78.49**   **Other hyperlipidemia**
> > Familial combined hyperlipidemia

E78.5   **Hyperlipidemia, unspecified**
> Coding Clinic: 2022, Q2, P6

E78.6   **Lipoprotein deficiency**
> Abetalipoproteinemia
> Depressed HDL cholesterol
> High-density lipoprotein deficiency
> Hypoalphalipoproteinemia
> Hypobetalipoproteinemia (familial)
> Lecithin cholesterol acyltransferase deficiency
> Tangier disease

E78.7   **Disorders of bile acid and cholesterol metabolism**

> **Excludes1**   Niemann-Pick disease type C (E75.242)

> **E78.70**   **Disorder of bile acid and cholesterol metabolism, unspecified**

> **E78.71**   **Barth syndrome**

> **E78.72**   **Smith-Lemli-Opitz syndrome**

> **E78.79**   **Other disorders of bile acid and cholesterol metabolism**
> > Coding Clinic: 2023, Q1, P27

E78.8   **Other disorders of lipoprotein metabolism**

> **E78.81**   **Lipoid dermatoarthritis**

> **E78.89**   **Other lipoprotein metabolism disorders**

E78.9   **Disorder of lipoprotein metabolism, unspecified**

E79   **Disorders of purine and pyrimidine metabolism**
Purines, along with pyrimidines, signal RNA and DNA production

> **Excludes1**   Ataxia-telangiectasia (Q87.19)
> Bloom's syndrome (Q82.8)
> Cockayne's syndrome (Q87.19)
> calculus of kidney (N20.0)
> combined immunodeficiency disorders (D81.-)
> Fanconi's anemia (D61.09)
> gout (M1A.-, M10.-)
> orotaciduric anemia (D53.0)
> progeria (E34.8)
> Werner's syndrome (E34.8)
> xeroderma pigmentosum (Q82.1)

E79.0   **Hyperuricemia without signs of inflammatory arthritis and tophaceous disease**
> Asymptomatic hyperuricemia

E79.1   **Lesch-Nyhan syndrome** 🗝
> HGPRT deficiency

E79.2   **Myoadenylate deaminase deficiency** 🗝

E79.8   **Other disorders of purine and pyrimidine metabolism** 🗝

> **E79.81**   **Aicardi-Goutières syndrome**

> **E79.82**   **Hereditary xanthinuria**

> **E79.89**   **Other specified disorders of purine and pyrimidine metabolism**

E79.9   **Disorder of purine and pyrimidine metabolism, unspecified** 🗝

E80   **Disorders of porphyrin and bilirubin metabolism**
Group of chemical compounds in RBCs that combine with iron to form heme

> **Includes**   defects of catalase and peroxidase

E80.0   **Hereditary erythropoietic porphyria** 🗝
> Congenital erythropoietic porphyria
> Erythropoietic protoporphyria

E80.1   **Porphyria cutanea tarda** 🗝

E80.2   **Other and unspecified porphyria**

> **E80.20**   **Unspecified porphyria** 🗝
> > Porphyria NOS

> **E80.21**   **Acute intermittent (hepatic) porphyria** 🗝

> **E80.29**   **Other porphyria** 🗝
> > Hereditary coproporphyria

E80.3   **Defects of catalase and peroxidase** 🗝
> Acatalasia [Takahara]

E80.4   **Gilbert syndrome**

E80.5   **Crigler-Najjar syndrome**

E80.6   **Other disorders of bilirubin metabolism**
> Dubin-Johnson syndrome
> Rotor's syndrome
> Coding Clinic: 2022, Q3, P7

E80.7   **Disorder of bilirubin metabolism, unspecified**

E83   **Disorders of mineral metabolism**

> **Excludes1**   dietary mineral deficiency (E58-E61)
> parathyroid disorders (E20-E21)
> vitamin D deficiency (E55.-)

E83.0   **Disorders of copper metabolism**

> **E83.00**   **Disorder of copper metabolism, unspecified**

> **E83.01**   **Wilson's disease**
> > Code also associated Kayser Fleischer ring (H18.04-)

> **E83.09**   **Other disorders of copper metabolism**
> > Menkes' (kinky hair) (steely hair) disease

E83.1   **Disorders of iron metabolism**

> **Excludes1**   iron deficiency anemia (D50.-)
> sideroblastic anemia (D64.0-D64.3)

> **E83.10**   **Disorder of iron metabolism, unspecified**

> **E83.11**   **Hemochromatosis**

> > **Excludes1**   GALD (P78.84)
> > Gestational alloimmune liver disease (P78.84)
> > Neonatal hemochromatosis (P78.84)

> > **E83.110**   **Hereditary hemochromatosis** 🗝
> > > Bronzed diabetes
> > > Pigmentary cirrhosis (of liver)
> > > Primary (hereditary) hemochromatosis

> > **E83.111**   **Hemochromatosis due to repeated red blood cell transfusions**
> > > Iron overload due to repeated red blood cell transfusions
> > > Transfusion (red blood cell) associated hemochromatosis

> > **E83.118**   **Other hemochromatosis**

> > **E83.119**   **Hemochromatosis, unspecified**

> **E83.19**   **Other disorders of iron metabolism**
> > Use additional code, if applicable, for idiopathic pulmonary hemosiderosis (J84.03)

E83.2   **Disorders of zinc metabolism**
> Acrodermatitis enteropathica

E83.3   **Disorders of phosphorus metabolism and phosphatases**

> **Excludes1**   adult osteomalacia (M83.-)
> osteoporosis (M80.-)

> **E83.30**   **Disorder of phosphorus metabolism, unspecified**

▶ New   ⇒ Revised   ~~deleted~~ Deleted   Excludes 1   Excludes 2   Includes   Use additional   Code first   Code also   Key words

OGCR Official Guidelines   X Assign placeholder X   ● Use Additional Character(s)   ▶ Manifestation Code   🗝 Hierarchical Condition Category   Coding Clinic

E83.31   **Familial hypophosphatemia**
     Vitamin D-resistant osteomalacia
     Vitamin D-resistant rickets
     Excludes1   vitamin D-deficiency rickets (E55.0)

E83.32   **Hereditary vitamin D-dependent rickets (type 1) (type 2)**
     25-hydroxyvitamin D 1-alpha-hydroxylase deficiency
     Pseudovitamin D deficiency
     Vitamin D receptor defect

E83.39   **Other disorders of phosphorus metabolism**
     Acid phosphatase deficiency
     Hypophosphatasia

● E83.4   **Disorders of magnesium metabolism**

E83.40   **Disorders of magnesium metabolism, unspecified**

E83.41   **Hypermagnesemia**
     Coding Clinic: 2016, Q4, P55

E83.42   **Hypomagnesemia**

E83.49   **Other disorders of magnesium metabolism**

● E83.5   **Disorders of calcium metabolism**
     autoimmune hypoparathyroidism (E20.812)
     autosomal dominant hypocalcemia (E20.810)
     Excludes1   chondrocalcinosis (M11.1-M11.2)
         hungry bone syndrome (E83.81)
         hyperparathyroidism (E21.0-E21.3)
         secondary hypoparathyroidism in diseases classified elsewhere (E20.811)

E83.50   **Unspecified disorder of calcium metabolism**

E83.51   **Hypocalcemia**

E83.52   **Hypercalcemia**
     Familial hypocalciuric hypercalcemia

E83.59   **Other disorders of calcium metabolism**
     Idiopathic hypercalciuria

● E83.8   **Other disorders of mineral metabolism**

E83.81   **Hungry bone syndrome**

E83.89   **Other disorders of mineral metabolism**

E83.9   **Disorder of mineral metabolism, unspecified**

● E84   **Cystic fibrosis**
     Includes   mucoviscidosis
     Code also exocrine pancreatic insufficiency (K86.81)

E84.0   **Cystic fibrosis with pulmonary manifestations**
     Use additional code to identify any infectious organism present, such as:
     Pseudomonas (B96.5)
     Coding Clinic: 2021, Q1, P24

● E84.1   **Cystic fibrosis with intestinal manifestations**

E84.11   **Meconium ileus in cystic fibrosis**   **N**
     Excludes1   meconium ileus not due to cystic fibrosis (P76.0)

E84.19   **Cystic fibrosis with other intestinal manifestations**
     Distal intestinal obstruction syndrome

E84.8   **Cystic fibrosis with other manifestations**

E84.9   **Cystic fibrosis, unspecified**

● E85   **Amyloidosis**
     A disorder resulting from the abnormal deposition of a particular protein (amyloid) into tissues of the body
     Excludes2   Alzheimer's disease (G30.0-)

E85.0   **Non-neuropathic heredofamilial amyloidosis**
     Hereditary amyloid nephropathy
     Code also associated disorders, such as: autoinflammatory syndromes (M04.-)
     Excludes2   Transthyretin-related (ATTR) familial amyloid cardiomyopathy (E85.4)

E85.1   **Neuropathic heredofamilial amyloidosis**
     Amyloid polyneuropathy (Portuguese)
     Transthyretin-related (ATTR) familial amyloid polyneuropathy
     Coding Clinic: 2012, Q4, P100

E85.2   **Heredofamilial amyloidosis, unspecified**

E85.3   **Secondary systemic amyloidosis**
     Hemodialysis-associated amyloidosis

E85.4   **Organ-limited amyloidosis**
     Localized amyloidosis
     Transthyretin-related (ATTR) familial amyloid cardiomyopathy

● E85.8   **Other amyloidosis**

E85.81   **Light chain (AL) amyloidosis**
     Coding Clinic: 2024, Q2, P9

E85.82   **Wild-type transthyretin-related (ATTR) amyloidosis**
     Senile systemic amyloidosis (SSA)

E85.89   **Other amyloidosis**

E85.9   **Amyloidosis, unspecified**

● E86   **Volume depletion**
     Excludes1   dehydration of newborn (P74.1)
         postprocedural hypovolemic shock (T81.19)
         traumatic hypovolemic shock (T79.4)
     Excludes2   hypovolemic shock NOS (R57.1)
     Use additional code(s) for any associated disorders of electrolyte and acid-base balance (E87.-)
     Coding Clinic: 2019, Q2, P7

E86.0   **Dehydration**
     Excessive loss of body water
     Coding Clinic: 2019, Q2, P7-8

E86.1   **Hypovolemia**
     Diminished volume of circulating blood
     Depletion of volume of plasma

E86.9   **Volume depletion, unspecified**
     Coding Clinic: 2019, Q2, P7-8

● E87   **Other disorders of fluid, electrolyte and acid-base balance**
     Excludes1   diabetes insipidus (E23.2)
         electrolyte imbalance associated with hyperemesis gravidarum (O21.1)
         electrolyte imbalance following ectopic or molar pregnancy (O08.5)
         familial periodic paralysis (G72.3)
         metabolic acidemia in newborn, unspecified (P19.9)

E87.0   **Hyperosmolality and hypernatremia**
     Sodium [Na] excess
     Sodium [Na] overload
     ~~Excludes1 diabetes with hyperosmolarity (E08, E09, E11, E13 with final characters .00 or .011)~~
     ▶ **Excludes2**   diabetes with hyperosmolarity (E08, ▶E09, E11, E13 with final ▶characters .00 or .01)
     Coding Clinic: 2022, Q1, P29; 2018, Q2, P6

E87.1   **Hypo-osmolality and hyponatremia**
     Sodium [Na] deficiency
     Excludes1   syndrome of inappropriate secretion of antidiuretic hormone (E22.2)
     Coding Clinic: 2018, Q2, P6

Item 4–9   Circulating fluid volume is regulated by the amount of water and sodium ingested, excreted by the kidneys into the urine, and lost through the gastrointestinal tract, lungs, and skin. To maintain blood volume within a normal range, the kidneys regulate the amount of water and sodium lost into the urine. Too much **(fluid overload)** or too little fluid volume **(volume depletion)** will affect blood pressure. Severe cases of vomiting, diarrhea, bleeding, and burns (fluid loss through exposed burn surface area) can contribute to fluid loss. Internal body environment must maintain a precise balance (homeostasis) between too much fluid and too little fluid. This complex balancing mechanism is critical to good health.

CHAPTER 4 (E00-E89)

- **E87.2   Acidosis**
  > **Excludes1**   diabetic acidosis - see categories E08-E10, E11, E13 with ketoacidosis
  - **E87.20   Acidosis, unspecified**
    Lactic acidosis NOS
    Metabolic acidosis NOS
    > Code also, if applicable, respiratory failure with hypercapnia (J96. with 5th character 2)
  - **E87.21   Acute metabolic acidosis**
    Acute lactic acidosis
  - **E87.22   Chronic metabolic acidosis**
    Chronic lactic acidosis
    Code first underlying etiology, if applicable
    Coding Clinic: 2022, Q4, P14
  - **E87.29   Other acidosis**
    Respiratory acidosis NOS
    > **Excludes2**   acute respiratory acidosis (J96.02)
    chronic respiratory acidosis (J96.12)

- **E87.3   Alkalosis**
  Alkalosis NOS
  Metabolic alkalosis
  Respiratory alkalosis

- **E87.4   Mixed disorder of acid-base balance**

- **E87.5   Hyperkalemia**
  Potassium [K] excess
  Potassium [K] overload

- **E87.6   Hypokalemia**
  Potassium [K] deficiency

- **E87.7   Fluid overload**
  > **Excludes1**   edema NOS (R60.9)
  fluid retention (R60.9)
  - **E87.70   Fluid overload, unspecified**
    Coding Clinic: 2023, Q1, P19
  - **E87.71   Transfusion associated circulatory overload**
    Fluid overload due to transfusion (blood) (blood components) TACO
  - **E87.79   Other fluid overload**

- **E87.8   Other disorders of electrolyte and fluid balance, not elsewhere classified**
  Electrolyte imbalance NOS
  Hyperchloremia
  Hypochloremia

- **E88   Other and unspecified metabolic disorders**
  Use additional codes for associated conditions
  > **Excludes1**   histiocytosis X (chronic) (C96.6)
- **E88.0   Disorders of plasma-protein metabolism, not elsewhere classified**
  > **Excludes1**   monoclonal gammopathy (of undetermined significance) (D47.2)
  polyclonal hypergammaglobulinemia (D89.0)
  ⇒ Waldenström macroglobulinemia (C88.00)
  > **Excludes2**   disorder of lipoprotein metabolism (E78.-)
  - **E88.01   Alpha-1-antitrypsin deficiency AAT deficiency** 🦴
  - **E88.02   Plasminogen deficiency**
    Dysplasminogenemia
    Hypoplasminogenemia
    Type 1 plasminogen deficiency
    Type 2 plasminogen deficiency
    > Code also, if applicable, ligneous conjunctivitis (H10.51)
    Use additional code for associated findings, such as:
    hydrocephalus (G91.4)
    otitis media (H67.-)
    respiratory disorder related to plasminogen deficiency (J99)
  - **E88.09   Other disorders of plasma-protein metabolism, not elsewhere classified**
    Bisalbuminemia

- **E88.1   Lipodystrophy, not elsewhere classified**
  Defective fat metabolism resulting in absence of subcutaneous fat
  Lipodystrophy NOS
  > **Excludes1**   Whipple's disease (K90.81)

- **E88.2   Lipomatosis, not elsewhere classified**
  Abnormal tumorlike accumulations of fat in tissue
  Lipomatosis NOS
  Lipomatosis (Check) dolorosa [Dercum]

- **E88.3   Tumor lysis syndrome**
  Tumor lysis syndrome (spontaneous)
  Tumor lysis syndrome following antineoplastic drug chemotherapy
  > Use additional code for adverse effect, if applicable, to identify drug (T45.1X5)
  Coding Clinic: 2019, Q2, P25

- **E88.4   Mitochondrial metabolism disorders**
  Congenital disorder of metabolism
  > **Excludes1**   disorders of pyruvate metabolism (E74.4)
  Kearns-Sayre syndrome (H49.81)
  Leber's disease (H47.22)
  Leigh's encephalopathy (G31.82)
  Mitochondrial myopathy, NEC (G71.3)
  Reye's syndrome (G93.7)
  - **E88.40   Mitochondrial metabolism disorder, unspecified** 🦴
  - **E88.41   MELAS syndrome** 🦴
    Mitochondrial myopathy, encephalopathy, lactic acidosis and stroke-like episodes
  - **E88.42   MERRF syndrome** 🦴
    Myoclonic epilepsy associated with ragged-red fibers
    > Code also progressive myoclonic epilepsy (G40.3-)
  - **E88.43   Disorders of mitochondrial tRNA synthetases**
  - **E88.49   Other mitochondrial metabolism disorders** 🦴

- **E88.8   Other specified metabolic disorders**
  - **E88.81   Metabolic syndrome and other insulin resistance**
    Use additional codes for associated manifestations, such as:
    obesity (E66.-)
    Coding Clinic: 2022, Q3, P6-7
    - **E88.810   Metabolic syndrome**
      Dysmetabolic syndrome
    - **E88.811   Insulin resistance syndrome, Type A**
      Coding Clinic: 2023, Q4, P14
    - **E88.818   Other insulin resistance**
      Insulin resistance syndrome, Type B
    - **E88.819   Insulin resistance, unspecified**
  - ▶ **E88.82   Obesity due to disruption of MC4R pathway**
    ▶ Use additional code, if applicable, to identify associated manifestations, such as polyphagia (R63.2)
    ▶ Use additional code to identify body mass index (BMI), if known (Z68.-)
  - **E88.89   Other specified metabolic disorders** 🦴
    Launois-Bensaude adenolipomatosis
    > **Excludes1**   adult pulmonary Langerhans cell histiocytosis (J84.82)

- **E88.9   Metabolic disorder, unspecified**
- **E88.A   Wasting disease (syndrome) due to underlying condition**
  Cachexia due to underlying condition
  Code first underlying condition
  > **Excludes1**   cachexia NOS (R64)
  nutritional marasmus (E41)
  > **Excludes2**   failure to thrive (R62.51, R62.7)
  Coding Clinic: 2023, Q4, P15

▶ New   ⇒ Revised   ~~deleted~~ Deleted   Excludes 1   Excludes 2   Includes   Use additional   Code first   Code also   Key words

710   OGCR Official Guidelines   X Assign placeholder X   ● Use Additional Character(s)   ▶ Manifestation Code   🦴 Hierarchical Condition Category   Coding Clinic

POSTPROCEDURAL ENDOCRINE AND METABOLIC COMPLICATIONS AND DISORDERS, NOT ELSEWHERE CLASSIFIED (E89)

● **E89   Postprocedural endocrine and metabolic complications and disorders, not elsewhere classified**

Excludes2   intraoperative complications of endocrine system organ or structure (E36.0-, E36.1-, E36.8)

E89.0   Postprocedural hypothyroidism
Postirradiation hypothyroidism
Postsurgical hypothyroidism

E89.1   Postprocedural hypoinsulinemia
Postpancreatectomy hyperglycemia
Postsurgical hypoinsulinemia

▶ *Code first*, *if applicable, diabetes mellitus (postpancreatectomy) (postprocedural) (E13.-)*

Use additional code, if applicable, to identify:
~~diabetes mellitus (postpancreatectomy)~~
~~(postprocedural) (E13.)~~
acquired absence of pancreas (Z90.41-)
insulin use (Z79.4)

Excludes1   transient postprocedural hyperglycemia (R73.9)
transient postprocedural hypoglycemia (E16.2)

E89.2   Postprocedural hypoparathyroidism 🔗
Parathyroprival tetany
Coding Clinic: 2023, Q3, P13

E89.3   Postprocedural hypopituitarism 🔗
Postirradiation hypopituitarism

● **E89.4   Postprocedural ovarian failure**

E89.40   Asymptomatic postprocedural ovarian failure
Postprocedural ovarian failure NOS

E89.41   Symptomatic postprocedural ovarian failure
Symptoms such as flushing, sleeplessness, headache, lack of concentration, associated with postprocedural menopause

E89.5   Postprocedural testicular hypofunction

E89.6   Postprocedural adrenocortical (-medullary) hypofunction 🔗

● **E89.8   Other postprocedural endocrine and metabolic complications and disorders**
Coding Clinic: 2016, Q4, P9

● **E89.81   Postprocedural hemorrhage of an endocrine system organ or structure following a procedure**

E89.810   Postprocedural hemorrhage of an endocrine system organ or structure following an endocrine system procedure

E89.811   Postprocedural hemorrhage of an endocrine system organ or structure following other procedure

● **E89.82   Postprocedural hematoma and seroma of an endocrine system organ or structure**

E89.820   Postprocedural hematoma of an endocrine system organ or structure following an endocrine system procedure

E89.821   Postprocedural hematoma of an endocrine system organ or structure following other procedure

E89.822   Postprocedural seroma of an endocrine system organ or structure following an endocrine system procedure

E89.823   Postprocedural seroma of an endocrine system organ or structure following other procedure 🔗

E89.89   Other postprocedural endocrine and metabolic complications and disorders 🔗

Use additional code, if applicable, to further specify disorder

CHAPTER 4 (E00-E89)

CHAPTER 5

MENTAL, BEHAVIORAL AND NEURODEVELOPMENTAL DISORDERS (F01-F99)

OGCR   Chapter-Specific Coding Guidelines

5. **Chapter 5: Mental, Behavioral and Neurodevelopmental disorders (F01 – F99)**

a. Pain disorders related to psychological factors

Assign code F45.41, for pain that is exclusively related to psychological disorders. As indicated by the Excludes 1 note under category G89, a code from category G89 should not be assigned with code F45.41

Code F45.42, Pain disorders with related psychological factors, should be used with a code from category G89, Pain, not elsewhere classified, if there is documentation of a psychological component for a patient with acute or chronic pain.

See Section I.C.6. Pain

b. Mental and behavioral disorders due to psychoactive substance use

1) In Remission

Selection of codes for "in remission" for categories F10-F19, Mental and behavioral disorders due to psychoactive substance use (categories F10-F19 with -11, -.21) requires the provider's clinical judgment. The appropriate codes for "in remission" are assigned only on the basis of provider documentation (as defined in the Official Guidelines for Coding and Reporting), unless otherwise instructed by the classification.

Mild substance use disorders in early or sustained remission are classified to the appropriate codes for substance abuse in remission, and moderate or severe substance use disorders in early or sustained remission are classified to the appropriate codes for substance dependence in remission.

2) Psychoactive Substance Use, Abuse and Dependence

When the provider documentation refers to use, abuse and dependence of the same substance (e.g., alcohol, opioid, cannabis, etc.), only one code should be assigned to identify the pattern of use based on the following hierarchy:
- If both use and abuse are documented, assign only the code for abuse
- If both abuse and dependence are documented, assign only the code for dependence
- If use, abuse and dependence are all documented, assign only the code for dependence
- If both use and dependence are documented, assign only the code for dependence

3) Psychoactive Substance Use, Unspecified

As with all other unspecified diagnoses, the codes for unspecified psychoactive substance use disorders (F10.9-, F11.9-, F12.9-, F13.9-, F14.9-, F15.9-, F16.9-, F19.9-, F19.9-) should only be assigned based on provider documentation and when they meet the definition of a reportable diagnosis (see Section III, Reporting Additional Diagnoses). These codes are to be used only when the psychoactive substance use is associated with a physical, mental or behavioral disorder, and such a relationship is documented by the provider.

c. Factitious Disorder

Factitious disorder imposed on self or Munchausen's syndrome is a disorder in which a person falsely reports or causes his or her own physical or psychological signs or symptoms. For patients with documented factitious disorder on self or Munchausen's syndrome, assign the appropriate code from subcategory F68.1-, Factitious disorder imposed on self.

Munchausen's syndrome by proxy (MSBP) is a disorder in which a caregiver (perpetrator) falsely reports or causes an illness or injury in another person (victim) under his or her care, such as a child, an elderly adult, or a person who has a disability. The condition is also referred to as "factitious disorder imposed on another" or "factitious disorder by proxy." The perpetrator, not the victim, receives this diagnosis. Assign code F68.A, Factitious disorder imposed on another, to the perpetrator's record. For the victim of a patient suffering from MSBP, assign the appropriate code from categories T74, Adult and child abuse, neglect and other maltreatment, confirmed, or T76, Adult and child abuse, neglect and other maltreatment, suspected.

See Section I.C.19.f. Adult and child abuse, neglect and other maltreatment

CHAPTER 5

MENTAL, BEHAVIORAL AND NEURODEVELOPMENTAL DISORDERS (F01-F99)

Includes   disorders of psychological development

Excludes2   symptoms, signs and abnormal clinical laboratory findings, not elsewhere classified (R00-R99)

This chapter contains the following blocks:

F01-F09	Mental disorders due to known physiological conditions
F10-F19	Mental and behavioral disorders due to psychoactive substance use
F20-F29	Schizophrenia, schizotypal, delusional, and other non-mood psychotic disorders
F30-F39	Mood [affective] disorders
F40-F48	Anxiety, dissociative, stress-related, somatoform and other nonpsychotic mental disorders
F50-F59	Behavioral syndromes associated with physiological disturbances and physical factors
F60-F69	Disorders of adult personality and behavior
F70-F79	Intellectual disabilities
F80-F89	Pervasive and specific developmental disorders
F90-F98	Behavioral and emotional disorders with onset usually occurring in childhood and adolescence
F99	Unspecified mental disorder

MENTAL DISORDERS DUE TO KNOWN PHYSIOLOGICAL CONDITIONS (F01-F09)

This block comprises a range of mental disorders grouped together on the basis of their having in common a demonstrable etiology in cerebral disease, brain injury, or other insult leading to cerebral dysfunction. The dysfunction may be primary, as in diseases, injuries, and insults that affect the brain directly and selectively; or secondary, as in systemic diseases and disorders that attack the brain only as one of the multiple organs or systems of the body that are involved.

● **F01   Vascular dementia**

Vascular dementia as a result of infarction of the brain due to vascular disease, including hypertensive cerebrovascular disease.

Includes   arteriosclerotic dementia

major neurocognitive disorder due to vascular disease
multi-infarct dementia

▶ *Code first, the underlying physiological condition or sequelae of cerebrovascular disease if applicable, any causal condition*

● **F01.5   Vascular dementia, unspecified severity**

  F01.50   Vascular dementia, unspecified severity, without behavioral disturbance, psychotic disturbance, mood disturbance, and anxiety   A

    Major neurocognitive disorder due to vascular disease NOS
    Vascular dementia NOS
    Coding Clinic: 2021, Q2, P4

  ● **F01.51   Vascular dementia, unspecified severity, with behavioral disturbance**   A

▶ New   ⇛ Revised   ~~deleted~~ Deleted   Excludes 1   Excludes 2   Includes   Use additional   Code first   Code also   Key words
OGCR Official Guidelines   X Assign placeholder X   ● Use Additional Character(s)   ▶ Manifestation Code   ℞ Hierarchical Condition Category   Coding Clinic

F01.511   **Vascular dementia, unspecified severity, with agitation**   A

    Major neurocognitive disorder due to vascular disease, unspecified severity, with aberrant motor behavior such as restlessness, rocking, pacing, or exit-seeking

    Major neurocognitive disorder due to vascular disease, unspecified severity, with verbal or physical behaviors such as profanity, shouting, threatening, anger, aggression, combativeness, or violence

    Vascular dementia, unspecified severity, with aberrant motor behavior such as restlessness, rocking, pacing, or exit-seeking

    Vascular dementia, unspecified severity, with verbal or physical behaviors such as profanity, shouting, threatening, anger, aggression, combativeness, or violence

F01.518   **Vascular dementia, unspecified severity, with other behavioral disturbance**   A

    Major neurocognitive disorder due to vascular disease, unspecified severity, with behavioral disturbances such as sleep disturbance, social disinhibition, or sexual disinhibition

    Vascular dementia, unspecified severity, with behavioral disturbances such as sleep disturbance, social disinhibition, or sexual disinhibition

    Use Additional code, if applicable, to identify wandering in vascular dementia (Z91.83)

F01.52   **Vascular dementia, unspecified severity, with psychotic disturbance**   A

    Major neurocognitive disorder due to vascular disease, unspecified severity, with psychotic disturbance such as hallucinations, paranoia, suspiciousness, or delusional state

    Vascular dementia, unspecified severity, with psychotic disturbance such as hallucinations, paranoia, suspiciousness, or delusional state

F01.53   **Vascular dementia, unspecified severity, with mood disturbance**   A

    Major neurocognitive disorder due to vascular disease, unspecified severity, with mood disturbance such as depression, apathy, or anhedonia

    Vascular dementia, unspecified severity, with mood disturbance such as depression, apathy, or anhedonia

F01.54   **Vascular dementia, unspecified severity, with anxiety**   A

    Major neurocognitive disorder due to vascular disease, unspecified severity, with anxiety

● **F01.A**   **Vascular dementia, mild**

    Excludes1   mild neurocognitive disorder due to known physiological condition with or without behavioral disturbance (F06.7-)

F01.A0   **Vascular dementia, mild, without behavioral disturbance, psychotic disturbance, mood disturbance, and anxiety**   A

    Major neurocognitive disorder due to vascular disease, mild, NOS

    Vascular dementia, mild, NOS

● **F01.A1**   **Vascular dementia, mild, with behavioral disturbance**

F01.A11   **Vascular dementia, mild, with agitation**   A

    Major neurocognitive disorder due to vascular disease, mild, with aberrant motor behavior such as restlessness, rocking, pacing, or exit-seeking

    Major neurocognitive disorder due to vascular disease, mild, with verbal or physical behaviors such as profanity, shouting, threatening, anger, aggression, combativeness, or violence

    Vascular dementia, mild, with aberrant motor behavior such as restlessness, rocking, pacing, or exit-seeking

    Vascular dementia, mild, with verbal or physical behaviors such as profanity, shouting, threatening, anger, aggression, combativeness, or violence

F01.A18   **Vascular dementia, mild, with other behavioral disturbance**   A

    Major neurocognitive disorder due to vascular disease, mild, with behavioral disturbances such as sleep disturbance, social disinhibition, or sexual disinhibition

    Vascular dementia, mild, with behavioral disturbances such as sleep disturbance, social disinhibition, or sexual disinhibition

    Use Additional code, if applicable, to identify wandering in vascular dementia (Z91.83)

F01.A2   **Vascular dementia, mild, with psychotic disturbance**   A

    Major neurocognitive disorder due to vascular disease, mild, with psychotic disturbance such as hallucinations, paranoia, suspiciousness, or delusional state

    Vascular dementia, mild, with psychotic disturbance such as hallucinations, paranoia, suspiciousness, or delusional state

F01.A3   **Vascular dementia, mild, with mood disturbance**   A

    Major neurocognitive disorder due to vascular disease, mild, with mood disturbance such as depression, apathy, or anhedonia

    Vascular dementia, mild, with mood disturbance such as depression, apathy, or anhedonia

F01.A4   **Vascular dementia, mild, with anxiety**   A

    Major neurocognitive disorder due to vascular disease, mild, with anxiety

CHAPTER 5 (F01-F99)

● **F01.B   Vascular dementia, moderate**

     F01.B0   Vascular dementia, moderate, without behavioral disturbance, psychotic disturbance, mood disturbance, and anxiety   **A**

         Major neurocognitive disorder due to vascular disease, moderate, NOS

         Vascular dementia, moderate, NOS

   ● **F01.B1   Vascular dementia, moderate, with behavioral disturbance**

         F01.B11   Vascular dementia, moderate, with agitation   **A**

             Major neurocognitive disorder due to vascular disease, moderate, with aberrant motor behavior such as restlessness, rocking, pacing, or exit-seeking

             Major neurocognitive disorder due to vascular disease, moderate, with verbal or physical behaviors such as profanity, shouting, threatening, anger, aggression, combativeness, or violence

             Vascular dementia, moderate, with aberrant motor behavior such as restlessness, rocking, pacing, or exit-seeking

             Vascular dementia, moderate, with verbal or physical behaviors such as profanity, shouting, threatening, anger, aggression, combativeness, or violence

         F01.B18   Vascular dementia, moderate, with other behavioral disturbance   **A**

             Major neurocognitive disorder due to vascular disease, moderate, with behavioral disturbances such as sleep disturbance, social disinhibition, or sexual disinhibition

             Vascular dementia, moderate, with behavioral disturbances such as sleep disturbance, social disinhibition, or sexual disinhibition

         Use Additional code, if applicable, to identify wandering in vascular dementia (Z91.83)

     F01.B2   Vascular dementia, moderate, with psychotic disturbance   **A**

         Major neurocognitive disorder due to vascular disease, moderate, with psychotic disturbance such as hallucinations, paranoia, suspiciousness, or delusional state

         Vascular dementia, moderate, with psychotic disturbance such as hallucinations, paranoia, suspiciousness, or delusional state

     F01.B3   Vascular dementia, moderate, with mood disturbance   **A**

         Major neurocognitive disorder due to vascular disease, moderate, with mood disturbance such as depression, apathy, or anhedonia

         Vascular dementia, moderate, with mood disturbance such as depression, apathy, or anhedonia

     F01.B4   Vascular dementia, moderate, with anxiety   **A**

         Major neurocognitive disorder due to vascular disease, moderate, with anxiety

● **F01.C   Vascular dementia, severe**

     F01.C0   Vascular dementia, severe, without behavioral disturbance, psychotic disturbance, mood disturbance, and anxiety   **A**

         Major neurocognitive disorder due to vascular disease, severe, NOS

         Vascular dementia, severe, NOS

   ● **F01.C1   Vascular dementia, severe, with behavioral disturbance**

         F01.C11   Vascular dementia, severe, with agitation   **A**

             Major neurocognitive disorder due to vascular disease, severe, with aberrant motor behavior such as restlessness, rocking, pacing, or exit-seeking

             Major neurocognitive disorder due to vascular disease, severe, with verbal or physical behaviors such as profanity, shouting, threatening, anger, aggression, combativeness, or violence

             Vascular dementia, severe, with aberrant motor behavior such as restlessness, rocking, pacing, or exit-seeking

             Vascular dementia, severe, with verbal or physical behaviors such as profanity, shouting, threatening, anger, aggression, combativeness, or violence

         F01.C18   Vascular dementia, severe, with other behavioral disturbance   **A**

             Major neurocognitive disorder due to vascular disease, severe, with behavioral disturbances such as sleep disturbance, social disinhibition, or sexual disinhibition

             Vascular dementia, severe, with behavioral disturbances such as sleep disturbance, social disinhibition, or sexual disinhibition

         Use Additional code, if applicable, to identify wandering in vascular dementia (Z91.83)

     F01.C2   Vascular dementia, severe, with psychotic disturbance   **A**

         Major neurocognitive disorder due to vascular disease, severe, with psychotic disturbance such as hallucinations, paranoia, suspiciousness, or delusional state

         Vascular dementia, severe, with psychotic disturbance such as hallucinations, paranoia, suspiciousness, or delusional state

     F01.C3   Vascular dementia, severe, with mood disturbance   **A**

         Major neurocognitive disorder due to vascular disease, severe, with mood disturbance such as depression, apathy, or anhedonia

         Vascular dementia, severe, with mood disturbance such as depression, apathy, or anhedonia

     F01.C4   Vascular dementia, severe, with anxiety   **A**

         Major neurocognitive disorder due to vascular disease, severe, with anxiety

▶ New   ⇒ Revised   ~~deleted~~ Deleted   Excludes 1   Excludes 2   Includes   Use additional   Code first   Code also   Key words

OGCR Official Guidelines   X Assign placeholder X   ● Use Additional Character(s)   ▶ Manifestation Code   Ⓗ Hierarchical Condition Category   Coding Clinic

● **F02**   **Dementia in other diseases classified elsewhere**

     Code first the underlying physiological condition, such as:
       Alzheimer's (G30.-)
       cerebral lipidosis (E75.4)
       Creutzfeldt-Jakob disease (A81.0-)
       dementia with Lewy bodies (G31.83)
       dementia with Parkinsonism (G31.83)
       epilepsy and recurrent seizures (G40.-)
       frontotemporal dementia (G31.09)
       hepatolenticular degeneration (E83.01)
       human immunodeficiency virus [HIV] disease (B20)
       Huntington's disease (G10)
       hypercalcemia (E83.52)
       hypothyroidism, acquired (E00-E03.-)
       intoxications (T36-T65)
       Jakob-Creutzfeldt disease (A81.0-)
       multiple sclerosis (G35)
    ▶ neurocognitive disorder with Lewy bodies (G31.83)
       neurosyphilis (A52.17)
       niacin deficiency [pellagra] (E52)
    ▶ other frontotemporal neurocognitive disorder (G31.90)
       Parkinson's disease (G20.-)
       Pick's disease (G31.01)
       polyarteritis nodosa (M30.0)
       prion disease (A81.9)
       systemic lupus erythematosus (M32.-)
       traumatic brain injury (S06.-)
       trypanosomiasis (B56.-, B57.-)
       vitamin B deficiency (E53.8)

    Includes   Major neurocognitive disorder in other diseases classified elsewhere

    Excludes1   mild neurocognitive disorder due to known physiological condition with or without behavioral disturbance (F06.7-)

    Excludes2   dementia in alcohol and psychoactive substance disorders (F10-F19, with .17, .27, .97)
                vascular dementia (F01.5-, F01.A-, F01.B-, F01.C-)
      Coding Clinic: 2016, Q4, P141

● **F02.8**   **Dementia in other diseases classified elsewhere, unspecified severity**

   ▷ *F02.80*   *Dementia in other diseases classified elsewhere, unspecified severity, without behavioral disturbance, psychotic disturbance, mood disturbance, and anxiety*
         Dementia in other diseases classified elsewhere NOS
         Major neurocognitive disorder in other diseases classified elsewhere NOS
         Coding Clinic: 2024, Q2, P9; 2017, Q1, P43; 2016, Q2, P6

● *F02.81*   *Dementia in other diseases classified elsewhere, unspecified severity, with behavioral disturbance*
      Coding Clinic: 2017, Q2, P8, Q1, P43

   ▷ **F02.811**   **Dementia in other diseases classified elsewhere, unspecified severity, with agitation**
         Dementia in other diseases classified elsewhere, unspecified severity, with aberrant motor behavior such as restlessness, rocking, pacing, or exit-seeking
         Dementia in other diseases classified elsewhere, unspecified severity, with verbal or physical behaviors such as profanity, shouting, threatening, anger, aggression, combativeness, or violence
         Major neurocognitive disorder in other diseases classified elsewhere, unspecified severity, with aberrant motor behavior such as restlessness, rocking, pacing, or exit-seeking
         Major neurocognitive disorder in other diseases classified elsewhere, unspecified severity, with verbal or physical behaviors such as profanity, shouting, threatening, anger, aggression, combativeness, or violence

   ▷ **F02.818**   **Dementia in other diseases classified elsewhere, unspecified severity, with other behavioral disturbance**
         Dementia in other diseases classified elsewhere with sleep disturbance, social disinhibition, or sexual disinhibition
         Major neurocognitive disorder in other diseases classified elsewhere with sleep disturbance, social disinhibition, or sexual disinhibition

      Use Additional code, if applicable, to identify wandering in dementia in conditions classified elsewhere (Z91.83)

   ▷ **F02.82**   **Dementia in other diseases classified elsewhere, unspecified severity, with psychotic disturbance**
         Dementia in other diseases classified elsewhere, unspecified severity, with psychotic disturbance such as hallucinations, paranoia, suspiciousness, or delusional state
         Major neurocognitive disorder in other diseases classified elsewhere, unspecified, with psychotic disturbance such as hallucinations, paranoia, suspiciousness, or delusional state

   ▷ **F02.83**   **Dementia in other diseases classified elsewhere, unspecified severity, with mood disturbance**
         Dementia in other diseases classified elsewhere, unspecified severity, with mood disturbance such as depression, apathy, or anhedonia
         Major neurocognitive disorder in other diseases classified elsewhere unspecified severity, with mood disturbance such as with depression, apathy, or anhedonia

CHAPTER 5 (F01-F99)

▶ **F02.84** **Dementia in other diseases classified elsewhere, unspecified severity, with anxiety**
Major neurocognitive disorder in other diseases classified elsewhere unspecified severity, with anxiety

● **F02.A** **Dementia in other diseases classified elsewhere, mild**

> **Excludes1**   mild neurocognitive disorder due to known physiological condition with or without behavioral disturbance (F06.7-)

▶ **F02.A0** **Dementia in other diseases classified elsewhere, mild, without behavioral disturbance, psychotic disturbance, mood disturbance, and anxiety**
Dementia in other diseases classified elsewhere, mild, NOS
Major neurocognitive disorder in other diseases classified elsewhere, mild, NOS

● **F02.A1** **Dementia in other diseases classified elsewhere, mild, with behavioral disturbance**

> ▶ **F02.A11** **Dementia in other diseases classified elsewhere, mild, with agitation**
Dementia in other diseases classified elsewhere, mild, with aberrant motor behavior such as restlessness, rocking, pacing, or exit-seeking
Dementia in other diseases classified elsewhere, mild, with verbal or physical behaviors such as profanity, shouting, threatening, anger, aggression, combativeness, or violence
Major neurocognitive disorder in other diseases classified elsewhere, mild, with aberrant motor behavior such as restlessness, rocking, pacing, or exit-seeking
Major neurocognitive disorder in other diseases classified elsewhere, mild, with verbal or physical behaviors such as profanity, shouting, threatening, anger, aggression, combativeness, or violence

> ▶ **F02.A18** **Dementia in other diseases classified elsewhere, mild, with other behavioral disturbance**
Dementia in other diseases classified elsewhere, mild, with behavioral disturbances such as sleep disturbance, social disinhibition, or sexual disinhibition
Major neurocognitive disorder in other diseases classified elsewhere, mild, with behavioral disturbances such as sleep disturbance, social disinhibition, or sexual disinhibition

> Use Additional code, if applicable, to identify wandering in dementia in conditions classified elsewhere (Z91.83)

▶ **F02.A2** **Dementia in other diseases classified elsewhere, mild, with psychotic disturbance**
Dementia in other diseases classified elsewhere, mild, with psychotic disturbance such as hallucinations, paranoia, suspiciousness, or delusional state
Major neurocognitive disorder in other diseases classified elsewhere, mild, with psychotic disturbance such as hallucinations, paranoia, suspiciousness, or delusional state

▶ **F02.A3** **Dementia in other diseases classified elsewhere, mild, with mood disturbance**
Dementia in other diseases classified elsewhere, mild, with mood disturbance such as depression, apathy, or anhedonia
Major neurocognitive disorder in other diseases classified elsewhere, mild, with mood disturbance such as depression, apathy, or anhedonia

▶ **F02.A4** **Dementia in other diseases classified elsewhere, mild, with anxiety**
Major neurocognitive disorder in other diseases classified elsewhere, mild, with anxiety

● **F02.B** **Dementia in other diseases classified elsewhere, moderate**

▶ **F02.B0** **Dementia in other diseases classified elsewhere, moderate, without behavioral disturbance, psychotic disturbance, mood disturbance, and anxiety**
Dementia in other diseases classified elsewhere, moderate, NOS
Major neurocognitive disorder in other diseases classified elsewhere, moderate, NOS

● **F02.B1** **Dementia in other diseases classified elsewhere, moderate, with behavioral disturbance**

> ▶ **F02.B11** **Dementia in other diseases classified elsewhere, moderate, with agitation**
Dementia in other diseases classified elsewhere, moderate, with aberrant motor behavior such as restlessness, rocking, pacing, or exit-seeking
Dementia in other diseases classified elsewhere, moderate, with verbal or physical behaviors such as profanity, shouting, threatening, anger, aggression, combativeness, or violence
Major neurocognitive disorder in other diseases classified elsewhere, moderate, with aberrant motor behavior such as restlessness, rocking, pacing, or exit- seeking
Major neurocognitive disorder in other diseases classified elsewhere, moderate, with verbal or physical behaviors such as profanity, shouting, threatening, anger, aggression, combativeness, or violence

> ▶ **F02.B18** **Dementia in other diseases classified elsewhere, moderate, with other behavioral disturbance**
Dementia in other diseases classified elsewhere, moderate, with behavioral disturbances such as sleep disturbance, social disinhibition, or sexual disinhibition
Major neurocognitive disorder in other diseases classified elsewhere, moderate, with behavioral disturbance such as sleep disturbance, social disinhibition, or sexual disinhibition

> Use Additional code, if applicable, to identify wandering in dementia in conditions classified elsewhere (Z91.83)

CHAPTER 5 (F01-F99)

F02.B2　**Dementia in other diseases classified elsewhere, moderate, with psychotic disturbance**
　　　　Dementia in other diseases classified elsewhere, moderate, with psychotic disturbance such as hallucinations, paranoia, suspiciousness, or delusional state
　　　　Major neurocognitive disorder in other diseases classified elsewhere, moderate, with psychotic disturbance such as hallucinations, paranoia, suspiciousness, or delusional state

F02.B3　**Dementia in other diseases classified elsewhere, moderate, with mood disturbance**
　　　　Dementia in other diseases classified elsewhere, moderate, with mood disturbance such as depression, apathy, or anhedonia
　　　　Major neurocognitive disorder in other diseases classified elsewhere, moderate, with mood disturbance such as depression, apathy, or anhedonia

F02.B4　**Dementia in other diseases classified elsewhere, moderate, with anxiety**
　　　　Major neurocognitive disorder in other diseases classified elsewhere, moderate, with anxiety

● **F02.C　Dementia in other diseases classified elsewhere, severe**

F02.C0　**Dementia in other diseases classified elsewhere, severe, without behavioral disturbance, psychotic disturbance, mood disturbance, and anxiety**
　　　　Dementia in other diseases classified elsewhere, severe, NOS
　　　　Major neurocognitive disorder in other diseases classified elsewhere, severe, NOS

● F02.C1　**Dementia in other diseases classified elsewhere, severe, with behavioral disturbance**

F02.C11　**Dementia in other diseases classified elsewhere, severe, with agitation**
　　　　Dementia in other diseases classified elsewhere, severe, with aberrant motor behavior such as restlessness, rocking, pacing, or exit-seeking
　　　　Dementia in other diseases classified elsewhere, severe, with verbal or physical behaviors such as profanity, shouting, threatening, anger, aggression, combativeness, or violence
　　　　Major neurocognitive disorder in other diseases classified elsewhere, severe, with aberrant motor behavior such as restlessness, rocking, pacing, or exit-seeking
　　　　Major neurocognitive disorder in other diseases classified elsewhere, severe, with verbal or physical behaviors such as profanity, shouting, threatening, anger, aggression, combativeness, or violence
　　　　Coding Clinic: 2022, Q4, P15

F02.C18　**Dementia in other diseases classified elsewhere, severe, with other behavioral disturbance**
　　　　Dementia in other diseases classified elsewhere, severe, with behavioral disturbances such as sleep disturbance, social disinhibition, or sexual disinhibition
　　　　Major neurocognitive disorder in other diseases classified elsewhere, severe, with behavioral disturbances such as sleep disturbance, social disinhibition, or sexual disinhibition
　　　　Use Additional code, if applicable, to identify wandering in dementia in conditions classified elsewhere (Z91.83)

F02.C2　**Dementia in other diseases classified elsewhere, severe, with psychotic disturbance**
　　　　Dementia in other diseases classified elsewhere, severe, with psychotic disturbance such as hallucinations, paranoia, suspiciousness, or delusional state
　　　　Major neurocognitive disorder in other diseases classified elsewhere, severe, with psychotic disturbance such as hallucinations, paranoia, suspiciousness, or delusional state

F02.C3　**Dementia in other diseases classified elsewhere, severe, with mood disturbance**
　　　　Dementia in other diseases classified elsewhere, severe, with mood disturbance such as depression, apathy, or anhedonia
　　　　Major neurocognitive disorder in other diseases classified elsewhere, severe, with mood disturbance such as depression, apathy, or anhedonia

F02.C4　**Dementia in other diseases classified elsewhere, severe, with anxiety**
　　　　Major neurocognitive disorder in other diseases classified elsewhere, severe, with anxiety

● **F03　Unspecified dementia**
　　　Major neurocognitive disorder NOS
　　　Presenile dementia NOS
　　　Presenile psychosis NOS
　　　Primary degenerative dementia NOS
　　　Senile dementia NOS
　　　Senile dementia depressed or paranoid type
　　　Senile psychosis NOS
　　　~~Excludes1　senility NOS (R41.81)~~
　　▶ **Excludes2**　dementia with delirium or acute confusional state (F05)
　　　　　　　　mild memory disturbance due to known physiological condition (F06.8)
　　　　　　　　~~senile dementia with delirium or acute confusional state (F05)~~

● **F03.9　Unspecified dementia, unspecified severity**

F03.90　**Unspecified dementia, unspecified severity, without behavioral disturbance, psychotic disturbance, mood disturbance, and anxiety**　A
　　　　Dementia NOS
　　　　Coding Clinic: 2024, Q2, P9; 2021, Q2, P4; 2012, Q4, P92

● F03.91   Unspecified dementia with, unspecified
           severity, behavioral disturbance
           F03.911   Unspecified dementia,
                     unspecified severity, with agitation   A
                     Unspecified dementia, unspecified
                        severity, with aberrant motor
                        behavior such as restlessness,
                        rocking, pacing, or exit-seeking
                     Unspecified dementia, unspecified
                        severity, with verbal or physical
                        behaviors such as profanity,
                        shouting, threatening, anger,
                        aggression, combativeness, or
                        violence
           F03.918   Unspecified dementia, unspecified
                     severity, with other behavioral
                     disturbance   A
                     Unspecified dementia, unspecified
                        severity, with behavioral
                        disturbances such as sleep
                        disturbance, social disinhibition,
                        or sexual disinhibition

                     Use Additional code, if applicable, to identify
                        wandering in unspecified dementia
                        (Z91.83)
   F03.92   Unspecified dementia, unspecified severity,
            with psychotic disturbance   A
            Unspecified dementia, unspecified severity,
               with psychotic disturbance such as
               hallucinations, paranoia, suspiciousness,
               or delusional state
   F03.93   Unspecified dementia, unspecified severity,
            with mood disturbance   A
            Unspecified dementia, unspecified severity,
               with mood disturbance such as
               depression, apathy, or anhedonia
   F03.94   Unspecified dementia, unspecified severity,
            with anxiety   A

● F03.A   Unspecified dementia, mild
          Excludes1   mild neurocognitive disorder due to
                      known physiological condition with
                      or without behavioral disturbance
                      (F06.7-)
   F03.A0   Unspecified dementia, mild, without behavioral
            disturbance, psychotic disturbance, mood
            disturbance, and anxiety   A
            Dementia, mild, NOS
  ● F03.A1   Unspecified dementia, mild, with behavioral
            disturbance
            F03.A11   Unspecified dementia, mild, with
                      agitation   A
                      Unspecified dementia, mild, with
                         aberrant motor behavior such
                         as restlessness, rocking, pacing,
                         or exit-seeking
                      Unspecified dementia, mild, with
                         verbal or physical behaviors
                         such as profanity, shouting,
                         threatening, anger, aggression,
                         combativeness, or violence
            F03.A18   Unspecified dementia, mild,
                      with other behavioral disturbance   A
                      Unspecified dementia, mild, with
                         behavioral disturbances
                         such as sleep disturbance,
                         social disinhibition, or sexual
                         disinhibition

                      Use Additional code, if applicable, to identify
                         wandering in unspecified dementia
                         (Z91.83)

   F03.A2   Unspecified dementia, mild, with psychotic
            disturbance   A
            Unspecified dementia, mild, with psychotic
               disturbance such as hallucinations,
               paranoia, suspiciousness, or delusional
               state
   F03.A3   Unspecified dementia, mild, with mood
            disturbance   A
            Unspecified dementia, mild, with mood
               disturbance such as depression, apathy, or
               anhedonia
   F03.A4   Unspecified dementia, mild, with
            anxiety   A
● F03.B   Unspecified dementia, moderate
   F03.B0   Unspecified dementia, moderate, without
            behavioral disturbance, psychotic disturbance,
            mood disturbance, and anxiety   A
            Dementia, moderate, NOS
  ● F03.B1   Unspecified dementia, moderate, with
            behavioral disturbance
            F03.B11   Unspecified dementia, moderate, with
                      agitation   A
                      Unspecified dementia, moderate,
                         with aberrant motor behavior
                         such as restlessness, rocking,
                         pacing, or exit-seeking
                      Unspecified dementia, moderate,
                         with verbal or physical
                         behaviors such as profanity,
                         shouting, threatening, anger,
                         aggression, combativeness, or
                         violence
            F03.B18   Unspecified dementia, moderate,
                      with other behavioral disturbance   A
                      Unspecified dementia, moderate,
                         with behavioral disturbances
                         such as sleep disturbance,
                         social disinhibition, or sexual
                         disinhibition

                      Use Additional code, if applicable, to identify
                         wandering in unspecified dementia (Z91.83)

   F03.B2   Unspecified dementia, moderate, with psychotic
            disturbance   A
            Unspecified dementia, moderate, with psychotic
               disturbance such as hallucinations,
               paranoia, suspiciousness, or delusional state
   F03.B3   Unspecified dementia, moderate, with mood
            disturbance   A
            Unspecified dementia, moderate, with mood
               disturbance such as depression, apathy, or
               anhedonia
   F03.B4   Unspecified dementia, moderate, with anxiety   A
● F03.C   Unspecified dementia, severe
   F03.C0   Unspecified dementia, severe, without
            behavioral disturbance, psychotic disturbance,
            mood disturbance, and anxiety   A
            Dementia, severe, NOS
  ● F03.C1   Unspecified dementia, severe, with behavioral
            disturbance
            F03.C11   Unspecified dementia, severe, with
                      agitation   A
                      Unspecified dementia, severe, with
                         aberrant motor behavior such
                         as restlessness, rocking, pacing,
                         or exit-seeking
                      Unspecified dementia, severe, with
                         verbal or physical behaviors
                         such as profanity, shouting,
                         threatening, anger, aggression,
                         combativeness, or violence

Item 5-1 Psychosis was a term formerly applied to any mental disorder
but is now restricted to disturbances of a great magnitude in which there is a
personality disintegration and loss of contact with reality.

▶ New   ⇒ Revised   ~~deleted~~ Deleted   Excludes 1   Excludes 2   Includes   Use additional   Code first   Code also   Key words

OGCR Official Guidelines   X Assign placeholder X   ● Use Additional Character(s)   ▶ Manifestation Code   🦢 Hierarchical Condition Category   Coding Clinic

F03.C18   **Unspecified dementia, severe, with other behavioral disturbance**   A

Unspecified dementia, severe, with behavioral disturbances such as sleep disturbance, social disinhibition, or sexual disinhibition

Use Additional code, if applicable, to identify wandering in unspecified dementia (Z91.83)

F03.C2   **Unspecified dementia, severe, with psychotic disturbance**   A

Unspecified dementia, severe, with psychotic disturbance such as hallucinations, paranoia, suspiciousness, or delusional state

F03.C3   **Unspecified dementia, severe, with mood disturbance**   A

Unspecified dementia, severe, with mood disturbance such as depression, apathy, or anhedonia

Coding Clinic: 2023, Q4, P15

F03.C4   **Unspecified dementia, severe, with anxiety**   A

F04   **Amnestic disorder due to known physiological condition**

Korsakov's psychosis or syndrome, nonalcoholic

Code first the underlying physiological condition

Excludes1   amnesia NOS (R41.3)
anterograde amnesia (R41.1)
dissociative amnesia (F44.0)
retrograde amnesia (R41.2)

Excludes2   alcohol-induced or unspecified Korsakov's syndrome (F10.26, F10.96)
Korsakov's syndrome induced by other psychoactive substances (F13.26, F13.96, F19.16, F19.26, F19.96)

F05   **Delirium due to known physiological condition**

Acute or subacute brain syndrome
Acute or subacute confusional state (nonalcoholic)
Acute or subacute infective psychosis
Acute or subacute organic reaction
Acute or subacute psycho-organic syndrome
Delirium of mixed etiology
Delirium superimposed on dementia
Sundowning

Code first the underlying physiological condition, such as:
dementia (F03.9-)

Excludes1   delirium NOS (R41.0)

Excludes2   delirium tremens alcohol-induced or unspecified (F10.231, F10.921)

Coding Clinic: 2019, Q2, P34

● **F06**   **Other mental disorders due to known physiological condition**

Includes   mental disorders due to endocrine disorder
mental disorders due to exogenous hormone
mental disorders due to exogenous toxic substance
mental disorders due to primary cerebral disease
mental disorders due to somatic illness
mental disorders due to systemic disease affecting the brain

Code first the underlying physiological condition

Excludes1   unspecified dementia (F03.0-)

Excludes2   delirium due to known physiological condition (F05)
dementia as classified in F01-F02
other mental disorders associated with alcohol and other psychoactive substances (F10-F19)

F06.0   **Psychotic disorder with hallucinations due to known physiological condition**

Organic hallucinatory state (nonalcoholic)

Excludes2   hallucinations and perceptual disturbance induced by alcohol and other psychoactive substances (F10-F19 with .151, .251, .951)
schizophrenia (F20.-)

F06.1   **Catatonic disorder due to known physiological condition**

Catatonia associated with another mental disorder
Catatonia NOS

Excludes1   catatonic stupor (R40.1)
stupor NOS (R40.1)

Excludes2   catatonic schizophrenia (F20.2)
dissociative stupor (F44.2)

F06.2   **Psychotic disorder with delusions due to known physiological condition**

Paranoid and paranoid-hallucinatory organic states
Schizophrenia-like psychosis in epilepsy

Excludes2   alcohol and drug-induced psychotic disorder (F10-F19 with .150, .250, .950)
brief psychotic disorder (F23)
delusional disorder (F22)
schizophrenia (F20.-)

● **F06.3**   **Mood disorder due to known physiological condition**

Excludes2   mood disorders due to alcohol and other psychoactive substances (F10-F19 with .14, .24, .94)
mood disorders, not due to known physiological condition or unspecified (F30-F39)

F06.30   **Mood disorder due to known physiological condition, unspecified**

F06.31   **Mood disorder due to known physiological condition with depressive features**

Depressive disorder due to known physiological condition, with depressive features

F06.32   **Mood disorder due to known physiological condition with major depressive-like episode**

Depressive disorder due to known physiological condition, with major depressive-like episode

F06.33   **Mood disorder due to known physiological condition with manic features**

Bipolar and related disorder due to a known physiological condition, with manic features
Bipolar and related disorder due to known physiological condition, with manic- or hypomanic-like episodes

F06.34   **Mood disorder due to known physiological condition with mixed features**

Bipolar and related disorder due to known physiological condition, with mixed features
Depressive disorder due to known physiological condition, with mixed features

F06.4   **Anxiety disorder due to known physiological condition**

Excludes2   anxiety disorders due to alcohol and other psychoactive substances (F10-F19 with .180, .280, .980)
anxiety disorders, not due to known physiological condition or unspecified (F40.-, F41.-)

● **F06.7**   **Mild neurocognitive disorder due to known physiological condition**
     Mild neurocognitive impairment due to a known physiological condition

     Code first the underlying physiological condition, such as:
       Alzheimer's disease (G30.-)
       ~~frontotemporal neurocognitive disorder (G31.09)~~
       human immunodeficiency virus [HIV] disease (B20)
       Huntington's disease (G10)
       Neurocognitive disorder with Lewy bodies (G31.83)
       ▶other frontotemporal neurocognitive disorder (G31.09)
       Parkinson's disease (G20.-)
       systemic lupus erythematosus (M32.-)
       traumatic brain injury (S06.-)
       vitamin B deficiency (E53-)

     Excludes1   age related cognitive decline (R41.81)
                  altered mental status (R41.82)
                  cerebral degeneration (G31.9)
                  change in mental status (R41.82)
                  cognitive deficits following (sequelae of) cerebral hemorrhage or infarction (I69.01- I69.11-, I69.21-I69.31-, I69.81-I69.91-)
                  ⇉dementia (F01.-, F02.-, F03.0-)
                  mild cognitive impairment due to unknown or unspecified etiology (G31.84)
                  neurologic neglect syndrome (R41.4)
                  personality change, nonpsychotic (F68.8)

     F06.70   **Mild neurocognitive disorder due to known physiological condition without behavioral disturbance**
         Mild neurocognitive disorder due to known physiological condition, NOS

     F06.71   **Mild neurocognitive disorder due to known physiological condition with behavioral disturbance**

   F06.8   **Other specified mental disorders due to known physiological condition**
     Epileptic psychosis NOS
     Obsessive-compulsive and related disorder due to a known physiological condition
     Organic dissociative disorder
     Organic emotionally labile [asthenic] disorder

● **F07**   **Personality and behavioral disorders due to known physiological condition**

     Code first the underlying physiological condition

   F07.0   **Personality change due to known physiological condition**
     Frontal lobe syndrome
     Limbic epilepsy personality syndrome
     Lobotomy syndrome
     Organic personality disorder
     Organic pseudopsychopathic personality
     Organic pseudoretarded personality
     Postleucotomy syndrome

     Excludes1   mild cognitive impairment (G31.84)
                  postconcussional syndrome (F07.81)
                  postencephalitic syndrome (F07.89)
                  signs and symptoms involving emotional state (R45.-)

     Excludes2   specific personality disorder (F60.-)

● **F07.8**   **Other personality and behavioral disorders due to known physiological condition**

     F07.81   **Postconcussional syndrome**
         Postcontusional syndrome (encephalopathy)
         Post-traumatic brain syndrome, nonpsychotic

         Use additional code to identify associated post-traumatic headache, if applicable (G44.3-)

         Excludes1   current concussion (brain) (S06.0-)
                      postencephalitic syndrome (F07.89)

     F07.89   **Other personality and behavioral disorders due to known physiological condition**
         Postencephalitic syndrome
         Damage to temporal brain lobes with memory loss and abnormal behavior
         Right hemispheric organic affective disorder

   F07.9   **Unspecified personality and behavioral disorder due to known physiological condition**
     Organic psychosyndrome
     Due to exposure to organic solvents

● **F09**   **Unspecified mental disorder due to known physiological condition**
     Mental disorder NOS due to known physiological condition
     Organic brain syndrome NOS
     Organic mental disorder NOS
     Organic psychosis NOS
     Symptomatic psychosis NOS

     Code first the underlying physiological condition

     Excludes1   mild neurocognitive disorder due to known physiological condition (F06.7-)
                  psychosis NOS (F29)

MENTAL AND BEHAVIORAL DISORDERS DUE TO PSYCHOACTIVE SUBSTANCE USE (F10-F19)

● **F10**   **Alcohol related disorders**
     Use additional code for blood alcohol level, if applicable (Y90.-)
     Coding Clinic: 2019, Q3, P8

● **F10.1**   **Alcohol abuse**

     Excludes1   alcohol dependence (F10.2-)
                  alcohol use, unspecified (F10.9-)

     F10.10   **Alcohol abuse, uncomplicated**
         Alcohol use disorder, mild

     F10.11   **Alcohol abuse, in remission**
         Alcohol use disorder, mild, in early remission
         Alcohol use disorder, mild, in sustained remission
         Coding Clinic: 2022, Q1, P25

●   **F10.12**   **Alcohol abuse with intoxication**

     F10.120   **Alcohol abuse with intoxication, uncomplicated** 🕮

     F10.121   **Alcohol abuse with intoxication, delirium** 🕮

     F10.129   **Alcohol abuse with intoxication, unspecified** 🕮

●   **F10.13**   **Alcohol abuse, with withdrawal**

     F10.130   **Alcohol abuse with withdrawal, uncomplicated**

     F10.131   **Alcohol abuse with withdrawal delirium**

     F10.132   **Alcohol abuse with withdrawal with perceptual disturbance**

     F10.139   **Alcohol abuse with withdrawal, unspecified**

     F10.14   **Alcohol abuse with alcohol-induced mood disorder** 🕮
         Alcohol use disorder, mild, with alcohol-induced bipolar or related disorder
         Alcohol use disorder, mild, with alcohol-induced depressive disorder

●   **F10.15**   **Alcohol abuse with alcohol-induced psychotic disorder**

     F10.150   **Alcohol abuse with alcohol-induced psychotic disorder with delusions** 🕮

     F10.151   **Alcohol abuse with alcohol-induced psychotic disorder with hallucinations** 🕮

     F10.159   **Alcohol abuse with alcohol-induced psychotic disorder, unspecified** 🕮

▶ New   ⇉ Revised   ~~deleted~~ Deleted   Excludes 1   Excludes 2   Includes   Use additional   Code first   Code also   Key words

OGCR Official Guidelines   X Assign placeholder X   ● Use Additional Character(s)   ⫶ Manifestation Code   🕮 Hierarchical Condition Category   Coding Clinic

● **F10.18** **Alcohol abuse with other alcohol-induced disorders**
Coding Clinic: 2022, Q1, P33

     F10.180 **Alcohol abuse with alcohol-induced anxiety disorder** 🔗
Coding Clinic: 2022, Q1, P33

     F10.181 **Alcohol abuse with alcohol-induced sexual dysfunction** 🔗

     F10.182 **Alcohol abuse with alcohol-induced sleep disorder** 🔗

     F10.188 **Alcohol abuse with other alcohol-induced disorder** 🔗
Coding Clinic: 2022, Q1, P25

F10.19 **Alcohol abuse with unspecified alcohol-induced disorder** 🔗

● **F10.2** **Alcohol dependence**

     Excludes1 alcohol abuse (F10.1-)
                 alcohol use, unspecified (F10.9-)

     Excludes2 toxic effect of alcohol (T51.0-)

Coding Clinic: 2019, Q3, P8

F10.20 **Alcohol dependence, uncomplicated** 🔗
Alcohol use disorder, moderate
Alcohol use disorder, severe
Coding Clinic: 2020, Q1, P9

F10.21 **Alcohol dependence, in remission** 🔗
Alcohol use disorder, moderate, in early remission
Alcohol use disorder, moderate, in sustained remission
Alcohol use disorder, severe, in early remission
Alcohol use disorder, severe, in sustained remission

● **F10.22** **Alcohol dependence with intoxication**
Acute drunkenness (in alcoholism)

     Excludes2 alcohol dependence with withdrawal (F10.23-)

     F10.220 **Alcohol dependence with intoxication, uncomplicated** 🔗

     F10.221 **Alcohol dependence with intoxication delirium** 🔗

     F10.229 **Alcohol dependence with intoxication, unspecified** 🔗

● **F10.23** **Alcohol dependence with withdrawal**

     Excludes2 alcohol dependence with intoxication (F10.22-)

     F10.230 **Alcohol dependence with withdrawal, uncomplicated** 🔗

     F10.231 **Alcohol dependence with withdrawal delirium** 🔗

     F10.232 **Alcohol dependence with withdrawal with perceptual disturbance** 🔗

     F10.239 **Alcohol dependence with withdrawal, unspecified** 🔗
Coding Clinic: 2015, Q2, P15

F10.24 **Alcohol dependence with alcohol-induced mood disorder** 🔗
Alcohol use disorder, moderate, with alcohol-induced bipolar or related disorder
Alcohol use disorder, moderate, with alcohol-induced depressive disorder
Alcohol use disorder, severe, with alcohol-induced bipolar or related disorder
Alcohol use disorder, severe, with alcohol-induced depressive disorder

● **F10.25** **Alcohol dependence with alcohol-induced psychotic disorder**

     F10.250 **Alcohol dependence with alcohol-induced psychotic disorder with delusions** 🔗

     F10.251 **Alcohol dependence with alcohol-induced psychotic disorder with hallucinations** 🔗

     F10.259 **Alcohol dependence with alcohol-induced psychotic disorder, unspecified** 🔗

F10.26 **Alcohol dependence with alcohol-induced persisting amnestic disorder** 🔗
Alcohol use disorder, moderate, with alcohol-induced major neurocognitive disorder, amnestic-confabulatory type
Alcohol use disorder, severe, with alcohol-induced major neurocognitive disorder, amnestic-confabulatory type

F10.27 **Alcohol dependence with alcohol-induced persisting dementia** 🔗
Alcohol use disorder, moderate, with alcohol-induced major neurocognitive disorder, nonamnestic-confabulatory type
Alcohol use disorder, severe, with alcohol-induced major neurocognitive disorder, nonamnestic-confabulatory type

● **F10.28** **Alcohol dependence with other alcohol-induced disorders**

     F10.280 **Alcohol dependence with alcohol-induced anxiety disorder** 🔗

     F10.281 **Alcohol dependence with alcohol-induced sexual dysfunction** 🔗

     F10.282 **Alcohol dependence with alcohol-induced sleep disorder** 🔗

     F10.288 **Alcohol dependence with other alcohol-induced disorder** 🔗
Alcohol use disorder, moderate, with alcohol-induced mild neurocognitive disorder
Alcohol use disorder, severe, with alcohol-induced mild neurocognitive disorder
Coding Clinic: 2020, Q1, P9

F10.29 **Alcohol dependence with unspecified alcohol-induced disorder** 🔗

● **F10.9** **Alcohol use, unspecified**

     Excludes1 alcohol abuse (F10.1-)
                 alcohol dependence (F10.2-)

F10.90 **Alcohol use, unspecified, uncomplicated**

F10.91 **Alcohol use, unspecified, in remission**

● **F10.92** **Alcohol use, unspecified with intoxication**

     F10.920 **Alcohol use, unspecified with intoxication, uncomplicated** 🔗

     F10.921 **Alcohol use, unspecified with intoxication delirium** 🔗

     F10.929 **Alcohol use, unspecified with intoxication, unspecified** 🔗

● **F10.93** **Alcohol use, unspecified with withdrawal**

     F10.930 **Alcohol use, unspecified with withdrawal, uncomplicated**

     F10.931 **Alcohol use, unspecified with withdrawal delirium**

     F10.932 **Alcohol use, unspecified with withdrawal with perceptual disturbance**

     F10.939 **Alcohol use, unspecified with withdrawal, unspecified**

F10.94 **Alcohol use, unspecified with alcohol-induced mood disorder**
Alcohol-induced bipolar or related disorder, without use disorder
Alcohol-induced depressive disorder, without use disorder

CHAPTER 5 (F01-F99)

● F10.95 Alcohol use, unspecified with alcohol-induced psychotic disorder

    F10.950 Alcohol use, unspecified with alcohol-induced psychotic disorder with delusions 🔖

    F10.951 Alcohol use, unspecified with alcohol-induced psychotic disorder with hallucinations 🔖

    F10.959 Alcohol use, unspecified with alcohol-induced psychotic disorder, unspecified 🔖

      Alcohol-induced psychotic disorder without use disorder

F10.96 Alcohol use, unspecified with alcohol-induced persisting amnestic disorder 🔖

    Alcohol-induced major neurocognitive disorder, amnestic-confabulatory type, without use disorder

F10.97 Alcohol use, unspecified with alcohol-induced persisting dementia 🔖

    Alcohol-induced major neurocognitive disorder, nonamnestic-confabulatory type, without use disorder

● F10.98 Alcohol use, unspecified with other alcohol-induced disorders

    F10.980 Alcohol use, unspecified with alcohol-induced anxiety disorder 🔖

      Alcohol-induced anxiety disorder, without use disorder

    F10.981 Alcohol use, unspecified with alcohol-induced sexual dysfunction 🔖

      Alcohol-induced sexual dysfunction, without use disorder

    F10.982 Alcohol use, unspecified with alcohol-induced sleep disorder 🔖

      Alcohol-induced sleep disorder, without use disorder

    F10.988 Alcohol use, unspecified with other alcohol-induced disorder 🔖

      Alcohol-induced mild neurocognitive disorder, without use disorder

      Coding Clinic: 2019, Q3, P8

F10.99 Alcohol use, unspecified with unspecified alcohol-induced disorder 🔖

● F11 Opioid related disorders

 ● F11.1 Opioid abuse

    Excludes1 opioid dependence (F11.2-)
      opioid use, unspecified (F11.9-)

  F11.10 Opioid abuse, uncomplicated
    Opioid use disorder, mild

  F11.11 Opioid abuse, in remission
    Opioid use disorder, mild, in early remission
    Opioid use disorder, mild, in sustained remission

  ● F11.12 Opioid abuse with intoxication

    F11.120 Opioid abuse with intoxication, uncomplicated 🔖

    F11.121 Opioid abuse with intoxication delirium 🔖

    F11.122 Opioid abuse with intoxication with perceptual disturbance 🔖

    F11.129 Opioid abuse with intoxication, unspecified 🔖

  F11.13 Opioid abuse with withdrawal

  F11.14 Opioid abuse with opioid-induced mood disorder 🔖
    Opioid use disorder, mild, with opioid-induced depressive disorder

● F11.15 Opioid abuse with opioid-induced psychotic disorder

    F11.150 Opioid abuse with opioid-induced psychotic disorder with delusions 🔖

    F11.151 Opioid abuse with opioid-induced psychotic disorder with hallucinations 🔖

    F11.159 Opioid abuse with opioid-induced psychotic disorder, unspecified 🔖

● F11.18 Opioid abuse with other opioid-induced disorder

    F11.181 Opioid abuse with opioid-induced sexual dysfunction 🔖

    F11.182 Opioid abuse with opioid-induced sleep disorder 🔖

    F11.188 Opioid abuse with other opioid-induced disorder 🔖

      Opioid-associated amnestic syndrome with opioid abuse

F11.19 Opioid abuse with unspecified opioid-induced disorder 🔖

● F11.2 Opioid dependence

    Excludes1 opioid abuse (F11.1-)
      opioid use, unspecified (F11.9-)

    Excludes2 opioid poisoning (T40.0—T40.2-)

  F11.20 Opioid dependence, uncomplicated 🔖
    Opioid use disorder, moderate
    Opioid use disorder, severe

  F11.21 Opioid dependence, in remission 🔖
    Opioid use disorder, moderate, in early remission
    Opioid use disorder, moderate, in sustained remission
    Opioid use disorder, severe, in early remission
    Opioid use disorder, severe, in sustained remission

  ● F11.22 Opioid dependence with intoxication

    Excludes1 opioid dependence with withdrawal (F11.23)

    F11.220 Opioid dependence with intoxication, uncomplicated 🔖

    F11.221 Opioid dependence with intoxication delirium 🔖

    F11.222 Opioid dependence with intoxication with perceptual disturbance 🔖

    F11.229 Opioid dependence with intoxication, unspecified 🔖

  F11.23 Opioid dependence with withdrawal 🔖

    Excludes1 opioid dependence with intoxication (F11.22-)

  F11.24 Opioid dependence with opioid-induced mood disorder 🔖
    Opioid use disorder, moderate, with opioid-induced depressive disorder

● F11.25 Opioid dependence with opioid-induced psychotic disorder

    F11.250 Opioid dependence with opioid-induced psychotic disorder with delusions 🔖

    F11.251 Opioid dependence with opioid-induced psychotic disorder with hallucinations 🔖

    F11.259 Opioid dependence with opioid-induced psychotic disorder, unspecified 🔖

● F11.28 Opioid dependence with other opioid-induced disorder

    F11.281 Opioid dependence with opioid-induced sexual dysfunction 🔖

    F11.282 Opioid dependence with opioid-induced sleep disorder 🔖

722

▶ New ⇒ Revised ~~deleted~~ Deleted Excludes 1 Excludes 2 Includes Use additional Code first Code also Key words

OGCR Official Guidelines X Assign placeholder X ● Use Additional Character(s) ▷ Manifestation Code 🔖 Hierarchical Condition Category Coding Clinic

F11.288　Opioid dependence with other opioid-induced disorder 🔊

F11.29　Opioid dependence with unspecified opioid-induced disorder 🔊

● F11.9　Opioid use, unspecified

　　Excludes1　opioid abuse (F11.1-)
　　　　　　　opioid dependence (F11.2-)

F11.90　Opioid use, unspecified, uncomplicated

F11.91　Opioid use, unspecified, in remission

● F11.92　Opioid use, unspecified with intoxication

　　Excludes1　opioid use, unspecified with withdrawal (F11.93)

　F11.920　Opioid use, unspecified with intoxication, uncomplicated 🔊

　F11.921　Opioid use, unspecified with intoxication delirium 🔊
　　　　　　Opioid-induced delirium

　F11.922　Opioid use, unspecified with intoxication with perceptual disturbance 🔊

　F11.929　Opioid use, unspecified with intoxication, unspecified 🔊

F11.93　Opioid use, unspecified with withdrawal 🔊

　　Excludes1　opioid use, unspecified with intoxication (F11.92-)

F11.94　Opioid use, unspecified with opioid-induced mood disorder 🔊
　　　　Opioid-induced depressive disorder, without use disorder

● F11.95　Opioid use, unspecified with opioid-induced psychotic disorder

　F11.950　Opioid use, unspecified with opioid-induced psychotic disorder with delusions 🔊

　F11.951　Opioid use, unspecified with opioid-induced psychotic disorder with hallucinations 🔊

　F11.959　Opioid use, unspecified with opioid-induced psychotic disorder, unspecified 🔊

● F11.98　Opioid use, unspecified with other specified opioid-induced disorder

　F11.981　Opioid use, unspecified with opioid-induced sexual dysfunction 🔊
　　　　　Opioid-induced sexual dysfunction, without use disorder

　F11.982　Opioid use, unspecified with opioid-induced sleep disorder 🔊
　　　　　Opioid-induced sleep disorder, without use disorder

　F11.988　Opioid use, unspecified with other opioid-induced disorder 🔊
　　　　　Opioid-associated amnestic syndrome with opioid abuse
　　　　　Opioid-induced anxiety disorder, without use disorder

F11.99　Opioid use, unspecified with unspecified opioid-induced disorder 🔊

● F12　Cannabis related disorders

　　Includes　marijuana

　　Coding Clinic: 2020, Q1, P8

● F12.1　Cannabis abuse

　　Excludes1　cannabis dependence (F12.2-)
　　　　　　　cannabis use, unspecified (F12.9-)

F12.10　Cannabis abuse, uncomplicated
　　　　Cannabis use disorder, mild

F12.11　Cannabis abuse, in remission
　　　　Cannabis use disorder, mild, in early remission
　　　　Cannabis use disorder, mild, in sustained remission

● F12.12　Cannabis abuse with intoxication

　F12.120　Cannabis abuse with intoxication, uncomplicated 🔊

　F12.121　Cannabis abuse with intoxication delirium 🔊

　F12.122　Cannabis abuse with intoxication with perceptual disturbance 🔊

　F12.129　Cannabis abuse with intoxication, unspecified 🔊

F12.13　Cannabis abuse with withdrawal

● F12.15　Cannabis abuse with psychotic disorder

　F12.150　Cannabis abuse with psychotic disorder with delusions 🔊

　F12.151　Cannabis abuse with psychotic disorder with hallucinations 🔊

　F12.159　Cannabis abuse with psychotic disorder, unspecified 🔊

● F12.18　Cannabis abuse with other cannabis-induced disorder

　F12.180　Cannabis abuse with cannabis-induced anxiety disorder 🔊

　F12.188　Cannabis abuse with other cannabis-induced disorder 🔊
　　　　　Cannabis use disorder, mild, with cannabis-induced sleep disorder
　　　　　Opioid-associated amnestic syndrome with opioid abuse

F12.19　Cannabis abuse with unspecified cannabis-induced disorder 🔊

● F12.2　Cannabis dependence

　　Excludes1　cannabis abuse (F12.1-)
　　　　　　　cannabis use, unspecified (F12.9-)

　　Excludes2　cannabis poisoning (T40.7-)

F12.20　Cannabis dependence, uncomplicated 🔊
　　　　Cannabis use disorder, moderate
　　　　Cannabis use disorder, severe

F12.21　Cannabis dependence, in remission 🔊
　　　　Cannabis use disorder, moderate, in early remission
　　　　Cannabis use disorder, moderate, in sustained remission
　　　　Cannabis use disorder, severe, in early remission
　　　　Cannabis use disorder, severe, in sustained remission

● F12.22　Cannabis dependence with intoxication

　F12.220　Cannabis dependence with intoxication, uncomplicated 🔊

　F12.221　Cannabis dependence with intoxication delirium 🔊

　F12.222　Cannabis dependence with intoxication with perceptual disturbance 🔊

　F12.229　Cannabis dependence with intoxication, unspecified 🔊

F12.23　Cannabis dependence with withdrawal 🔊

● F12.25　Cannabis dependence with psychotic disorder

　F12.250　Cannabis dependence with psychotic disorder with delusions 🔊

　F12.251　Cannabis dependence with psychotic disorder with hallucinations 🔊

　F12.259　Cannabis dependence with psychotic disorder, unspecified 🔊

● F12.28   Cannabis dependence with other cannabis-induced disorder

    F12.280   Cannabis dependence with cannabis-induced anxiety disorder 🐾

    F12.288   Cannabis dependence with other cannabis-induced disorder 🐾
        Cannabis use disorder, moderate, with cannabis-induced sleep disorder
        Cannabis use disorder, severe, with cannabis-induced sleep disorder

    F12.29   Cannabis dependence with unspecified cannabis-induced disorder 🐾

● F12.9   Cannabis use, unspecified
    Excludes1   cannabis abuse (F12.1-)
              cannabis dependence (F12.2-)

    F12.90   Cannabis use, unspecified, uncomplicated
        Coding Clinic: 2023, Q3, P18

    F12.91   Cannabis use, unspecified, in remission

● F12.92   Cannabis use, unspecified with intoxication

    F12.920   Cannabis use, unspecified with intoxication, uncomplicated 🐾

    F12.921   Cannabis use, unspecified with intoxication delirium 🐾

    F12.922   Cannabis use, unspecified with intoxication with perceptual disturbance 🐾

    F12.929   Cannabis use, unspecified with intoxication, unspecified 🐾

    F12.93   Cannabis use, unspecified with withdrawal 🐾

● F12.95   Cannabis use, unspecified with psychotic disorder

    F12.950   Cannabis use, unspecified with psychotic disorder with delusions

    F12.951   Cannabis use, unspecified with psychotic disorder with hallucinations 🐾

    F12.959   Cannabis use, unspecified with psychotic disorder, unspecified 🐾
        Cannabis-induced psychotic disorder, without use disorder

● F12.98   Cannabis use, unspecified with other cannabis-induced disorder

    F12.980   Cannabis use, unspecified with anxiety disorder 🐾
        Cannabis-induced anxiety disorder, without use disorder

    F12.988   Cannabis use, unspecified with other cannabis-induced disorder 🐾
        Cannabis-induced sleep disorder, without use disorder

    F12.99   Cannabis use, unspecified with unspecified cannabis-induced disorder 🐾

● F13   Sedative, hypnotic, or anxiolytic related disorders

● F13.1   Sedative, hypnotic or anxiolytic-related abuse
    Excludes1   sedative, hypnotic or anxiolytic-related dependence (F13.2-)
              sedative, hypnotic, or anxiolytic use, unspecified (F13.9-)

    F13.10   Sedative, hypnotic or anxiolytic abuse, uncomplicated
        Sedative, hypnotic, or anxiolytic use disorder, mild

    F13.11   Sedative, hypnotic or anxiolytic abuse, in remission
        Sedative, hypnotic or anxiolytic use disorder, mild, in early remission
        Sedative, hypnotic or anxiolytic use disorder, mild, in sustained remission

● F13.12   Sedative, hypnotic or anxiolytic abuse with intoxication

    F13.120   Sedative, hypnotic or anxiolytic abuse with intoxication, uncomplicated 🐾

    F13.121   Sedative, hypnotic or anxiolytic abuse with intoxication delirium 🐾

    F13.129   Sedative, hypnotic or anxiolytic abuse with intoxication, unspecified 🐾

● F13.13   Sedative, hypnotic or anxiolytic abuse with withdrawal

    F13.130   Sedative, hypnotic or anxiolytic abuse with withdrawal, uncomplicated

    F13.131   Sedative, hypnotic or anxiolytic abuse with withdrawal delirium

    F13.132   Sedative, hypnotic or anxiolytic abuse with withdrawal with perceptual disturbance

    F13.139   Sedative, hypnotic or anxiolytic abuse with withdrawal, unspecified

    F13.14   Sedative, hypnotic or anxiolytic abuse with sedative, hypnotic or anxiolytic-induced mood disorder 🐾
        Sedative, hypnotic, or anxiolytic use disorder, mild, with sedative, hypnotic, or anxiolytic-induced bipolar or related disorder
        Sedative, hypnotic, or anxiolytic use disorder, mild, with sedative, hypnotic, or anxiolytic-induced depressive disorder

● F13.15   Sedative, hypnotic or anxiolytic abuse with sedative, hypnotic or anxiolytic-induced psychotic disorder

    F13.150   Sedative, hypnotic or anxiolytic abuse with sedative, hypnotic or anxiolytic-induced psychotic disorder with delusions 🐾

    F13.151   Sedative, hypnotic or anxiolytic abuse with sedative, hypnotic or anxiolytic-induced psychotic disorder with hallucinations 🐾

    F13.159   Sedative, hypnotic or anxiolytic abuse with sedative, hypnotic or anxiolytic-induced psychotic disorder, unspecified 🐾

● F13.18   Sedative, hypnotic or anxiolytic abuse with other sedative, hypnotic or anxiolytic-induced disorders

    F13.180   Sedative, hypnotic or anxiolytic abuse with sedative, hypnotic or anxiolytic-induced anxiety disorder 🐾

    F13.181   Sedative, hypnotic or anxiolytic abuse with sedative, hypnotic or anxiolytic-induced sexual dysfunction 🐾

    F13.182   Sedative, hypnotic or anxiolytic abuse with sedative, hypnotic or anxiolytic-induced sleep disorder 🐾

    F13.188   Sedative, hypnotic or anxiolytic abuse with other sedative, hypnotic or anxiolytic-induced disorder 🐾

    F13.19   Sedative, hypnotic or anxiolytic abuse with unspecified sedative, hypnotic or anxiolytic-induced disorder 🐾

● F13.2   Sedative, hypnotic or anxiolytic-related dependence
    Excludes1   sedative, hypnotic or anxiolytic-related abuse (F13.1-)
              sedative, hypnotic, or anxiolytic use, unspecified (F13.9-)
    Excludes2   sedative, hypnotic, or anxiolytic poisoning (T42.-)

    F13.20   Sedative, hypnotic or anxiolytic dependence, uncomplicated 🐾

▶ New   ⇒ Revised   ~~deleted~~ Deleted   Excludes 1   Excludes 2   Includes   Use additional   Code first   Code also   Key words
OGCR Official Guidelines   X Assign placeholder X   ● Use Additional Character(s)   ▶ Manifestation Code   🐾 Hierarchical Condition Category   Coding Clinic

F13.21   **Sedative, hypnotic or anxiolytic dependence, in remission** 🔖
　　Sedative, hypnotic or anxiolytic use disorder, moderate, in early remission
　　Sedative, hypnotic or anxiolytic use disorder, moderate, in sustained remission
　　Sedative, hypnotic or anxiolytic use disorder, severe, in early remission
　　Sedative, hypnotic or anxiolytic use disorder, severe, in sustained remission

●F13.22   **Sedative, hypnotic or anxiolytic dependence with intoxication**
　　Excludes1　sedative, hypnotic or anxiolytic dependence with withdrawal (F13.23-)

F13.220   **Sedative, hypnotic or anxiolytic dependence with intoxication, uncomplicated** 🔖

F13.221   **Sedative, hypnotic or anxiolytic dependence with intoxication delirium** 🔖

F13.229   **Sedative, hypnotic or anxiolytic dependence with intoxication, unspecified** 🔖

●F13.23   **Sedative, hypnotic or anxiolytic dependence with withdrawal**
　　Sedative, hypnotic, or anxiolytic use disorder, moderate
　　Sedative, hypnotic, or anxiolytic use disorder, severe
　　Excludes1　sedative, hypnotic or anxiolytic dependence with intoxication (F13.22-)

F13.230   **Sedative, hypnotic or anxiolytic dependence with withdrawal, uncomplicated** 🔖

F13.231   **Sedative, hypnotic or anxiolytic dependence with withdrawal delirium** 🔖

F13.232   **Sedative, hypnotic or anxiolytic dependence with withdrawal with perceptual disturbance** 🔖
　　Sedative, hypnotic, or anxiolytic withdrawal with perceptual disturbances

F13.239   **Sedative, hypnotic or anxiolytic dependence with withdrawal, unspecified** 🔖
　　Sedative, hypnotic, or anxiolytic withdrawal without perceptual disturbances

F13.24   **Sedative, hypnotic or anxiolytic dependence with sedative, hypnotic or anxiolytic-induced mood disorder** 🔖
　　Sedative, hypnotic, or anxiolytic use disorder, moderate, with sedative, hypnotic, or anxiolytic-induced bipolar or related disorder
　　Sedative, hypnotic, or anxiolytic use disorder, moderate, with sedative, hypnotic, or anxiolytic-induced depressive disorder
　　Sedative, hypnotic, or anxiolytic use disorder, severe, with sedative, hypnotic, or anxiolytic-induced bipolar or related disorder
　　Sedative, hypnotic, or anxiolytic use disorder, severe, with sedative, hypnotic, or anxiolytic-induced depressive disorder

●F13.25   **Sedative, hypnotic or anxiolytic dependence with sedative, hypnotic or anxiolytic-induced psychotic disorder**

F13.250   **Sedative, hypnotic or anxiolytic dependence with sedative, hypnotic or anxiolytic-induced psychotic disorder with delusions** 🔖

F13.251   **Sedative, hypnotic or anxiolytic dependence with sedative, hypnotic or anxiolytic-induced psychotic disorder with hallucinations** 🔖

F13.259   **Sedative, hypnotic or anxiolytic dependence with sedative, hypnotic or anxiolytic-induced psychotic disorder, unspecified** 🔖

F13.26   **Sedative, hypnotic or anxiolytic dependence with sedative, hypnotic or anxiolytic-induced persisting amnestic disorder** 🔖

F13.27   **Sedative, hypnotic or anxiolytic dependence with sedative, hypnotic or anxiolytic-induced persisting dementia** 🔖
　　Sedative, hypnotic, or anxiolytic use disorder, moderate, with sedative, hypnotic, or anxiolytic-induced major neurocognitive disorder
　　Sedative, hypnotic, or anxiolytic use disorder, severe, with sedative, hypnotic, or anxiolytic-induced major neurocognitive disorder

●F13.28   **Sedative, hypnotic or anxiolytic dependence with other sedative, hypnotic or anxiolytic-induced disorders**

F13.280   **Sedative, hypnotic or anxiolytic dependence with sedative, hypnotic or anxiolytic-induced anxiety disorder** 🔖

F13.281   **Sedative, hypnotic or anxiolytic dependence with sedative, hypnotic or anxiolytic-induced sexual dysfunction** 🔖

F13.282   **Sedative, hypnotic or anxiolytic dependence with sedative, hypnotic or anxiolytic-induced sleep disorder** 🔖

F13.288   **Sedative, hypnotic or anxiolytic dependence with other sedative, hypnotic or anxiolytic-induced disorder** 🔖
　　Sedative, hypnotic, or anxiolytic use disorder, moderate, with sedative, hypnotic, or anxiolytic-induced mild neurocognitive disorder
　　Sedative, hypnotic, or anxiolytic use disorder, severe, with sedative, hypnotic, or anxiolytic-induced mild neurocognitive disorder

F13.29   **Sedative, hypnotic or anxiolytic dependence with unspecified sedative, hypnotic or anxiolytic-induced disorder** 🔖

●F13.9   **Sedative, hypnotic or anxiolytic-related use, unspecified**
　　Excludes1　sedative, hypnotic or anxiolytic-related abuse (F13.1-)
　　　　sedative, hypnotic or anxiolytic-related dependence (F13.2-)

F13.90   **Sedative, hypnotic, or anxiolytic use, unspecified, uncomplicated**

F13.91   **Sedative, hypnotic or anxiolytic use, unspecified, in remission**

●F13.92   **Sedative, hypnotic or anxiolytic use, unspecified with intoxication**
　　Excludes1　sedative, hypnotic or anxiolytic use, unspecified with withdrawal (F13.93-)

F13.920   Sedative, hypnotic or anxiolytic
           use, unspecified with intoxication,
           uncomplicated 🐾

F13.921   Sedative, hypnotic or anxiolytic
           use, unspecified with intoxication
           delirium 🐾
                Sedative, hypnotic, or anxiolytic-
                induced delirium

F13.929   Sedative, hypnotic or anxiolytic
           use, unspecified with intoxication,
           unspecified 🐾

● F13.93   Sedative, hypnotic or anxiolytic use,
           unspecified with withdrawal
           Excludes1   sedative, hypnotic or anxiolytic
                       use, unspecified with
                       intoxication (F13.92-)

F13.930   Sedative, hypnotic or anxiolytic
           use, unspecified with withdrawal,
           uncomplicated 🐾

F13.931   Sedative, hypnotic or anxiolytic
           use, unspecified with withdrawal
           delirium 🐾

F13.932   Sedative, hypnotic or anxiolytic
           use, unspecified with withdrawal
           with perceptual
           disturbances 🐾

F13.939   Sedative, hypnotic or anxiolytic
           use, unspecified with withdrawal,
           unspecified 🐾

F13.94   Sedative, hypnotic or anxiolytic
           use, unspecified with sedative, hypnotic or
           anxiolytic-induced mood disorder 🐾
                Sedative, hypnotic, or anxiolytic-induced
                bipolar or related disorder, without use
                disorder
                Sedative, hypnotic, or anxiolytic-induced
                depressive disorder, without use disorder

● F13.95   Sedative, hypnotic or anxiolytic use,
           unspecified with sedative, hypnotic or
           anxiolytic-induced psychotic disorder

F13.950   Sedative, hypnotic or anxiolytic
           use, unspecified with sedative,
           hypnotic or anxiolytic-induced
           psychotic disorder with delusions 🐾

F13.951   Sedative, hypnotic or anxiolytic
           use, unspecified with sedative,
           hypnotic or anxiolytic-induced
           psychotic disorder with
           hallucinations 🐾

F13.959   Sedative, hypnotic or anxiolytic
           use, unspecified with sedative,
           hypnotic or anxiolytic-induced
           psychotic disorder, unspecified 🐾
                Sedative, hypnotic, or anxiolytic-
                induced psychotic disorder,
                without use disorder

F13.96   Sedative, hypnotic or anxiolytic
           use, unspecified with sedative, hypnotic or
           anxiolytic-induced persisting amnestic
           disorder 🐾

F13.97   Sedative, hypnotic or anxiolytic
           use, unspecified with sedative, hypnotic
           or anxiolytic-induced persisting
           dementia 🐾
                Sedative, hypnotic, or anxiolytic-induced
                major neurocognitive disorder, without
                use disorder

● F13.98   Sedative, hypnotic or anxiolytic use,
           unspecified with other sedative, hypnotic or
           anxiolytic-induced disorders

F13.980   Sedative, hypnotic or anxiolytic
           use, unspecified with sedative,
           hypnotic or anxiolytic-induced
           anxiety disorder 🐾
                Sedative, hypnotic, or anxiolytic-
                induced anxiety disorder,
                without use disorder

F13.981   Sedative, hypnotic or anxiolytic
           use, unspecified with sedative,
           hypnotic or anxiolytic-induced sexual
           dysfunction 🐾
                Sedative, hypnotic, or anxiolytic-
                induced sexual dysfunction
                disorder, without use disorder

F13.982   Sedative, hypnotic or anxiolytic
           use, unspecified with sedative,
           hypnotic or anxiolytic-induced sleep
           disorder 🐾
                Sedative, hypnotic, or anxiolytic-
                induced sleep disorder, without
                use disorder

F13.988   Sedative, hypnotic or anxiolytic
           use, unspecified with other sedative,
           hypnotic or anxiolytic-induced
           disorder 🐾
                Sedative, hypnotic, or anxiolytic-
                induced mild neurocognitive
                disorder

F13.99   Sedative, hypnotic or anxiolytic
           use, unspecified with unspecified sedative,
           hypnotic or anxiolytic-induced disorder 🐾

● F14   Cocaine related disorders
        Excludes2   other stimulant-related disorders (F15.-)

● F14.1 Cocaine abuse
         Excludes1   cocaine dependence (F14.2-)
                     cocaine use, unspecified (F14.9-)

F14.10   Cocaine abuse, uncomplicated
                Cocaine use disorder, mild

F14.11   Cocaine abuse, in remission
                Cocaine use disorder, mild, in early remission
                Cocaine use disorder, mild, in sustained
                remission

● F14.12   Cocaine abuse with intoxication

F14.120   Cocaine abuse with intoxication,
           uncomplicated 🐾

F14.121   Cocaine abuse with intoxication with
           delirium 🐾

F14.122   Cocaine abuse with intoxication with
           perceptual disturbance 🐾

F14.129   Cocaine abuse with
           intoxication, unspecified 🐾

F14.13   Cocaine abuse, unspecified with
           withdrawal

F14.14   Cocaine abuse with cocaine-induced mood
           disorder 🐾
                Cocaine use disorder, mild, with cocaine-
                induced bipolar or related disorder
                Cocaine use disorder, mild, with cocaine-
                induced depressive disorder

● F14.15   Cocaine abuse with cocaine-induced psychotic
           disorder

F14.150   Cocaine abuse with cocaine-induced
           psychotic disorder with delusions 🐾

F14.151   Cocaine abuse with cocaine-induced
           psychotic disorder with
           hallucinations 🐾

F14.159   Cocaine abuse with cocaine-induced
           psychotic disorder, unspecified 🐾

▶ New   ⇒ Revised   deleted Deleted   Excludes 1   Excludes 2   Includes   Use additional   Code first   Code also   Key words
OGCR Official Guidelines   X Assign placeholder X   ● Use Additional Character(s)   ▶ Manifestation Code   🐾 Hierarchical Condition Category   Coding Clinic

● **F14.18**   Cocaine abuse with other cocaine-induced disorder

     F14.180   Cocaine abuse with cocaine-induced anxiety disorder 🔎

     F14.181   Cocaine abuse with cocaine-induced sexual dysfunction 🔎

     F14.182   Cocaine abuse with cocaine-induced sleep disorder 🔎

     F14.188   Cocaine abuse with other cocaine-induced disorder 🔎
         Cocaine use disorder, mild, with cocaine-induced obsessive-compulsive or related disorder

   F14.19   Cocaine abuse with unspecified cocaine-induced disorder 🔎

● **F14.2**   Cocaine dependence

     Excludes1   cocaine abuse (F14.1-)
               cocaine use, unspecified (F14.9-)

     Excludes2   cocaine poisoning (T40.5-)

   F14.20   Cocaine dependence, uncomplicated 🔎
         Cocaine use disorder, moderate
         Cocaine use disorder, severe

   F14.21   Cocaine dependence, in remission 🔎
         Cocaine use disorder, moderate, in early remission
         Cocaine use disorder, moderate, in sustained remission
         Cocaine use disorder, severe, in early remission
         Cocaine use disorder, severe, in sustained remission
         Coding Clinic: 2017, Q2, P27

● **F14.22**   Cocaine dependence with intoxication

     Excludes1   cocaine dependence with withdrawal (F14.23)

     F14.220   Cocaine dependence with intoxication, uncomplicated 🔎

     F14.221   Cocaine dependence with intoxication delirium 🔎

     F14.222   Cocaine dependence with intoxication with perceptual disturbance 🔎

     F14.229   Cocaine dependence with intoxication, unspecified 🔎

   F14.23   Cocaine dependence with withdrawal 🔎

     Excludes1   cocaine dependence with intoxication (F14.22-)

   F14.24   Cocaine dependence with cocaine-induced mood disorder 🔎
         Cocaine use disorder, moderate, with cocaine-induced bipolar or related disorder
         Cocaine use disorder, moderate, with cocaine-induced depressive disorder
         Cocaine use disorder, severe, with cocaine-induced bipolar or related disorder
         Cocaine use disorder, severe, with cocaine-induced depressive disorder

● **F14.25**   Cocaine dependence with cocaine-induced psychotic disorder

     F14.250   Cocaine dependence with cocaine-induced psychotic disorder with delusions 🔎

     F14.251   Cocaine dependence with cocaine-induced psychotic disorder with hallucinations 🔎

     F14.259   Cocaine dependence with cocaine-induced psychotic disorder, unspecified 🔎

● **F14.28**   Cocaine dependence with other cocaine-induced disorder

     F14.280   Cocaine dependence with cocaine-induced anxiety disorder 🔎

     F14.281   Cocaine dependence with cocaine-induced sexual dysfunction 🔎

     F14.282   Cocaine dependence with cocaine-induced sleep disorder 🔎

     F14.288   Cocaine dependence with other cocaine-induced disorder 🔎
         Cocaine use disorder, moderate, with cocaine-induced obsessive-compulsive or related disorder
         Cocaine use disorder, severe, with cocaine-induced obsessive-compulsive or related disorder

   F14.29   Cocaine dependence with unspecified cocaine-induced disorder 🔎

● **F14.9**   Cocaine use, unspecified

     Excludes1   cocaine abuse (F14.1-)
               cocaine dependence (F14.2-)

   F14.90   Cocaine use, unspecified, uncomplicated
         Coding Clinic: 2018, Q2, P11

   F14.91   Cocaine use, unspecified, in remission

● **F14.92**   Cocaine use, unspecified with intoxication

     F14.920   Cocaine use, unspecified with intoxication, uncomplicated 🔎

     F14.921   Cocaine use, unspecified with intoxication delirium 🔎

     F14.922   Cocaine use, unspecified with intoxication with perceptual disturbance 🔎

     F14.929   Cocaine use, unspecified with intoxication, unspecified 🔎

   F14.93   Cocaine use, unspecified with withdrawal

   F14.94   Cocaine use, unspecified with cocaine-induced mood disorder 🔎
         Cocaine-induced bipolar or related disorder, without use disorder
         Cocaine-induced depressive disorder, without use disorder

● **F14.95**   Cocaine use, unspecified with cocaine-induced psychotic disorder

     F14.950   Cocaine use, unspecified with cocaine-induced psychotic disorder with delusions 🔎

     F14.951   Cocaine use, unspecified with cocaine-induced psychotic disorder with hallucinations 🔎

     F14.959   Cocaine use, unspecified with cocaine-induced psychotic disorder, unspecified 🔎
         Cocaine-induced psychotic disorder, without use disorder

● **F14.98**   Cocaine use, unspecified with other specified cocaine-induced disorder

     F14.980   Cocaine use, unspecified with cocaine-induced anxiety disorder 🔎
         Cocaine-induced anxiety disorder, without use disorder

     F14.981   Cocaine use, unspecified with cocaine-induced sexual dysfunction 🔎
         Cocaine-induced sexual dysfunction, without use disorder

F14.982   **Cocaine use, unspecified with cocaine-induced sleep disorder** 🐾
      Cocaine-induced sleep disorder, without use disorder

F14.988   **Cocaine use, unspecified with other cocaine-induced disorder** 🐾
      Cocaine-induced obsessive-compulsive or related disorder

F14.99   **Cocaine use, unspecified with unspecified cocaine-induced disorder** 🐾

● **F15**   **Other stimulant related disorders**

   Includes   amphetamine-related disorders
               caffeine

   Excludes2   cocaine-related disorders (F14.-)

● **F15.1**   **Other stimulant abuse**

   Excludes1   other stimulant dependence (F15.2-)
               other stimulant use, unspecified (F15.9-)

F15.10   **Other stimulant abuse, uncomplicated**
      Amphetamine type substance use disorder, mild
      Other or unspecified stimulant use disorder, mild

F15.11   **Other stimulant abuse, in remission**
      Amphetamine type substance use disorder, mild, in early remission
      Amphetamine type substance use disorder, mild, in sustained remission
      Other or unspecified stimulant use disorder, mild, in early remission
      Other or unspecified stimulant use disorder, mild, in sustained remission
      Coding Clinic: 2021, Q3, P8

● F15.12   **Other stimulant abuse with intoxication**

F15.120   **Other stimulant abuse with intoxication, uncomplicated** 🐾

F15.121   **Other stimulant abuse with intoxication delirium** 🐾

F15.122   **Other stimulant abuse with intoxication with perceptual disturbance** 🐾
      Amphetamine or other stimulant use disorder, mild, with amphetamine or other stimulant intoxication, with perceptual disturbances

F15.129   **Other stimulant abuse with intoxication, unspecified** 🐾
      Amphetamine or other stimulant use disorder, mild, with amphetamine or other stimulant intoxication, without perceptual disturbances

F15.13   **Other stimulant abuse with withdrawal**

F15.14   **Other stimulant abuse with stimulant-induced mood disorder** 🐾
      Amphetamine or other stimulant use disorder, mild, with amphetamine or other stimulant-induced bipolar or related disorder
      Amphetamine or other stimulant use disorder, mild, with amphetamine or other stimulant-induced depressive disorder

● F15.15   **Other stimulant abuse with stimulant-induced psychotic disorder**

F15.150   **Other stimulant abuse with stimulant-induced psychotic disorder with delusions** 🐾

F15.151   **Other stimulant abuse with stimulant-induced psychotic disorder with hallucinations** 🐾

F15.159   **Other stimulant abuse with stimulant-induced psychotic disorder, unspecified** 🐾

● F15.18   **Other stimulant abuse with other stimulant-induced disorder**

F15.180   **Other stimulant abuse with stimulant-induced anxiety disorder** 🐾

F15.181   **Other stimulant abuse with stimulant-induced sexual dysfunction** 🐾

F15.182   **Other stimulant abuse with stimulant-induced sleep disorder** 🐾

F15.188   **Other stimulant abuse with other stimulant-induced disorder** 🐾
      Amphetamine or other stimulant use disorder, mild, with amphetamine or other stimulant-induced obsessive-compulsive or related disorder

F15.19   **Other stimulant abuse with unspecified stimulant-induced disorder** 🐾

● **F15.2**   **Other stimulant dependence**

   Excludes1   other stimulant abuse (F15.1-)
               other stimulant use, unspecified (F15.9-)

F15.20   **Other stimulant dependence, uncomplicated** 🐾
      Amphetamine type substance use disorder, moderate
      Amphetamine type substance use disorder, severe
      Other or unspecified stimulant use disorder, moderate
      Other or unspecified stimulant use disorder, severe

F15.21   **Other stimulant dependence, in remission** 🐾
      Amphetamine type substance use disorder, moderate, in early remission
      Amphetamine type substance use disorder, moderate, in sustained remission
      Amphetamine type substance use disorder, severe, in early remission
      Amphetamine type substance use disorder, severe, in sustained remission
      Other or unspecified stimulant use disorder, moderate, in early remission
      Other or unspecified stimulant use disorder, moderate, in sustained remission
      Other or unspecified stimulant use disorder, severe, in early remission
      Other or unspecified stimulant use disorder, severe, in sustained remission

● F15.22   **Other stimulant dependence with intoxication**

   Excludes1   other stimulant dependence with withdrawal (F15.23)

F15.220   **Other stimulant dependence with intoxication, uncomplicated** 🐾

F15.221   **Other stimulant dependence with intoxication delirium** 🐾

F15.222   **Other stimulant dependence with intoxication with perceptual disturbance** 🐾
      Amphetamine or other stimulant use disorder, moderate, with amphetamine or other stimulant intoxication, with perceptual disturbances
      Amphetamine or other stimulant use disorder, severe, with amphetamine or other stimulant intoxication, with perceptual disturbances

F15.229 **Other stimulant dependence with intoxication, unspecified** 🔖
   Amphetamine or other stimulant use disorder, moderate, with amphetamine or other stimulant intoxication, without perceptual disturbances
   Amphetamine or other stimulant use disorder, severe, with amphetamine or other stimulant intoxication, without perceptual disturbances

F15.23 **Other stimulant dependence with withdrawal** 🔖
   Amphetamine or other stimulant withdrawal
   Excludes1 other stimulant dependence with intoxication (F15.22-)

F15.24 **Other stimulant dependence with stimulant-induced mood disorder** 🔖
   Amphetamine or other stimulant use disorder, moderate, with amphetamine or other stimulant-induced bipolar or related disorder
   Amphetamine or other stimulant use disorder, moderate, with amphetamine or other stimulant-induced depressive disorder
   Amphetamine or other stimulant use disorder, severe, with amphetamine or other stimulant-induced bipolar or related disorder
   Amphetamine or other stimulant use disorder, severe, with amphetamine or other stimulant-induced depressive disorder

F15.25 **Other stimulant dependence with stimulant-induced psychotic disorder**
  F15.250 **Other stimulant dependence with stimulant-induced psychotic disorder with delusions** 🔖
  F15.251 **Other stimulant dependence with stimulant-induced psychotic disorder with hallucinations** 🔖
  F15.259 **Other stimulant dependence with stimulant-induced psychotic disorder, unspecified** 🔖

F15.28 **Other stimulant dependence with other stimulant-induced disorder**
  F15.280 **Other stimulant dependence with stimulant-induced anxiety disorder** 🔖
  F15.281 **Other stimulant dependence with stimulant-induced sexual dysfunction** 🔖
  F15.282 **Other stimulant dependence with stimulant-induced sleep disorder** 🔖
  F15.288 **Other stimulant dependence with other stimulant-induced disorder** 🔖
     Amphetamine or other stimulant use disorder, moderate, with amphetamine or other stimulant-induced obsessive-compulsive or related disorder
     Amphetamine or other stimulant use disorder, severe, with amphetamine or other stimulant-induced obsessive-compulsive or related disorder

F15.29 **Other stimulant dependence with unspecified stimulant-induced disorder** 🔖

F15.9 **Other stimulant use, unspecified**
   Excludes1 other stimulant abuse (F15.1-)
        other stimulant dependence (F15.2-)

F15.90 **Other stimulant use, unspecified, uncomplicated**
   Coding Clinic: 2022, Q4, P46

F15.91 **Other stimulant use, unspecified, in remission**

F15.92 **Other stimulant use, unspecified with intoxication**
   Excludes1 other stimulant use, unspecified with withdrawal (F15.93)
  F15.920 **Other stimulant use, unspecified with intoxication, uncomplicated** 🔖
  F15.921 **Other stimulant use, unspecified with intoxication delirium** 🔖
     Amphetamine or other stimulant-induced delirium
  F15.922 **Other stimulant use, unspecified with intoxication with perceptual disturbance** 🔖
  F15.929 **Other stimulant use, unspecified with intoxication, unspecified** 🔖
     Caffeine intoxication

F15.93 **Other stimulant use, unspecified with withdrawal** 🔖
   Caffeine withdrawal
   Excludes1 other stimulant use, unspecified with intoxication (F15.92-)

F15.94 **Other stimulant use, unspecified with stimulant-induced mood disorder** 🔖
   Amphetamine or other stimulant-induced bipolar or related disorder, without use disorder
   Amphetamine or other stimulant-induced depressive disorder, without use disorder

F15.95 **Other stimulant use, unspecified with stimulant-induced psychotic disorder**
  F15.950 **Other stimulant use, unspecified with stimulant-induced psychotic disorder with delusions** 🔖
  F15.951 **Other stimulant use, unspecified with stimulant-induced psychotic disorder with hallucinations** 🔖
  F15.959 **Other stimulant use, unspecified with stimulant-induced psychotic disorder, unspecified** 🔖
     Amphetamine or other stimulant-induced psychotic disorder, without use disorder

F15.98 **Other stimulant use, unspecified with other stimulant-induced disorder**
  F15.980 **Other stimulant use, unspecified with stimulant-induced anxiety disorder** 🔖
     Amphetamine or other stimulant-induced anxiety disorder, without use disorder
     Caffeine-induced anxiety disorder, without use disorder
  F15.981 **Other stimulant use, unspecified with stimulant-induced sexual dysfunction** 🔖
     Amphetamine or other stimulant-induced sexual dysfunction, without use disorder
  F15.982 **Other stimulant use, unspecified with stimulant-induced sleep disorder** 🔖
     Amphetamine or other stimulant-induced sleep disorder, without use disorder
     Caffeine-induced sleep disorder, without use disorder
  F15.988 **Other stimulant use, unspecified with other stimulant-induced disorder** 🔖
     Amphetamine or other stimulant-induced obsessive-compulsive or related disorder, without use disorder

F15.99 **Other stimulant use, unspecified with unspecified stimulant-induced disorder** 🔖

CHAPTER 5 (F01-F99)

● **F16**   **Hallucinogen related disorders**
     Includes   ecstasy
                 PCP
                 phencyclidine

● **F16.1**   **Hallucinogen abuse**
     Excludes1   hallucinogen dependence (F16.2-)
                     hallucinogen use, unspecified (F16.9-)

     F16.10   **Hallucinogen abuse, uncomplicated**
            Other hallucinogen use disorder, mild
            Phencyclidine use disorder, mild
            Coding Clinic: 2018, Q4, P31

     F16.11   **Hallucinogen abuse, in remission**
            Other hallucinogen use disorder, mild, in early remission
            Other hallucinogen use disorder, mild, in sustained remission
            Phencyclidine use disorder, mild, in early remission
            Phencyclidine use disorder, mild, in sustained remission

●   **F16.12**   **Hallucinogen abuse with intoxication**
     F16.120   **Hallucinogen abuse with intoxication, uncomplicated** 🅗
     F16.121   **Hallucinogen abuse with intoxication with delirium** 🅗
     F16.122   **Hallucinogen abuse with intoxication with perceptual disturbance** 🅗
     F16.129   **Hallucinogen abuse with intoxication, unspecified** 🅗

     F16.14   **Hallucinogen abuse with hallucinogen-induced mood disorder** 🅗
            Other hallucinogen use disorder, mild, with other hallucinogen-induced bipolar or related disorder
            Other hallucinogen use disorder, mild, with other hallucinogen-induced depressive disorder
            Phencyclidine use disorder, mild, with phencyclidine-induced bipolar or related disorder
            Phencyclidine use disorder, mild, with phencyclidine-induced depressive disorder

●   **F16.15**   **Hallucinogen abuse with hallucinogen-induced psychotic disorder**
     F16.150   **Hallucinogen abuse with hallucinogen-induced psychotic disorder with delusions** 🅗
     F16.151   **Hallucinogen abuse with hallucinogen-induced psychotic disorder with hallucinations** 🅗
     F16.159   **Hallucinogen abuse with hallucinogen-induced psychotic disorder, unspecified** 🅗

●   **F16.18**   **Hallucinogen abuse with other hallucinogen-induced disorder**
     F16.180   **Hallucinogen abuse with hallucinogen-induced anxiety disorder** 🅗
     F16.183   **Hallucinogen abuse with hallucinogen persisting perception disorder (flashbacks)** 🅗
     F16.188   **Hallucinogen abuse with other hallucinogen-induced disorder** 🅗

     F16.19   **Hallucinogen abuse with unspecified hallucinogen-induced disorder** 🅗

● **F16.2**   **Hallucinogen dependence**
     Excludes1   hallucinogen abuse (F16.1-)
                     hallucinogen use, unspecified (F16.9-)

     F16.20   **Hallucinogen dependence, uncomplicated** 🅗
            Other hallucinogen use disorder, moderate
            Other hallucinogen use disorder, severe
            Phencyclidine use disorder, moderate
            Phencyclidine use disorder, severe

     F16.21   **Hallucinogen dependence, in remission** 🅗
            Other hallucinogen use disorder, moderate, in early remission
            Other hallucinogen use disorder, moderate, in sustained remission
            Other hallucinogen use disorder, severe, in early remission
            Other hallucinogen use disorder, severe, in sustained remission
            Phencyclidine use disorder, moderate, in early remission
            Phencyclidine use disorder, moderate, in sustained remission
            Phencyclidine use disorder, severe, in early remission
            Phencyclidine use disorder, severe, in sustained remission

●   **F16.22**   **Hallucinogen dependence with intoxication**
     F16.220   **Hallucinogen dependence with intoxication, uncomplicated** 🅗
     F16.221   **Hallucinogen dependence with intoxication with delirium** 🅗
     F16.229   **Hallucinogen dependence with intoxication, unspecified** 🅗

     F16.24   **Hallucinogen dependence with hallucinogen-induced mood disorder** 🅗
            Other hallucinogen use disorder, moderate, with other hallucinogen-induced bipolar or related disorder
            Other hallucinogen use disorder, moderate, with other hallucinogen-induced depressive disorder
            Other hallucinogen use disorder, severe, with other hallucinogen-induced bipolar or related disorder
            Other hallucinogen use disorder, severe, with other hallucinogen-induced depressive disorder
            Phencyclidine use disorder, moderate, with phencyclidine-induced bipolar or related disorder
            Phencyclidine use disorder, moderate, with phencyclidine-induced depressive disorder
            Phencyclidine use disorder, severe, with phencyclidine-induced bipolar or related disorder
            Phencyclidine use disorder, severe, with phencyclidine-induced depressive disorder

●   **F16.25**   **Hallucinogen dependence with hallucinogen-induced psychotic disorder**
     F16.250   **Hallucinogen dependence with hallucinogen-induced psychotic disorder with delusions** 🅗
     F16.251   **Hallucinogen dependence with hallucinogen-induced psychotic disorder with hallucinations** 🅗
     F16.259   **Hallucinogen dependence with hallucinogen-induced psychotic disorder, unspecified** 🅗

● **F16.28**   **Hallucinogen dependence with other hallucinogen-induced disorder**
     F16.280   **Hallucinogen dependence with hallucinogen-induced anxiety disorder** 🔍
     F16.283   **Hallucinogen dependence with hallucinogen persisting perception disorder (flashbacks)** 🔍
     F16.288   **Hallucinogen dependence with other hallucinogen-induced disorder** 🔍
   F16.29   **Hallucinogen dependence with unspecified hallucinogen-induced disorder** 🔍

● **F16.9**   **Hallucinogen use, unspecified**
     Excludes1   hallucinogen abuse (F16.1-)
                hallucinogen dependence (F16.2-)
   F16.90   **Hallucinogen use, unspecified, uncomplicated**
   F16.91   **Hallucinogen use, unspecified, in remission**
● **F16.92**   **Hallucinogen use, unspecified with intoxication**
     F16.920   **Hallucinogen use, unspecified with intoxication, uncomplicated** 🔍
     F16.921   **Hallucinogen use, unspecified with intoxication with delirium** 🔍
          Other hallucinogen intoxication delirium
     F16.929   **Hallucinogen use, unspecified with intoxication, unspecified** 🔍
   F16.94   **Hallucinogen use, unspecified with hallucinogen-induced mood disorder** 🔍
          Other hallucinogen-induced bipolar or related disorder, without use disorder
          Other hallucinogen-induced depressive disorder, without use disorder
          Phencyclidine-induced bipolar or related disorder, without use disorder
          Phencyclidine-induced depressive disorder, without use disorder
● **F16.95**   **Hallucinogen use, unspecified with hallucinogen-induced psychotic disorder**
     F16.950   **Hallucinogen use, unspecified with hallucinogen-induced psychotic disorder with delusions** 🔍
     F16.951   **Hallucinogen use, unspecified with hallucinogen-induced psychotic disorder with hallucinations** 🔍
     F16.959   **Hallucinogen use, unspecified with hallucinogen-induced psychotic disorder, unspecified** 🔍
          Other hallucinogen-induced psychotic disorder, without use disorder
          Phencyclidine-induced psychotic disorder, without use disorder
● **F16.98**   **Hallucinogen use, unspecified with other specified hallucinogen-induced disorder**
     F16.980   **Hallucinogen use, unspecified with hallucinogen-induced anxiety disorder** 🔍
          Other hallucinogen-induced anxiety disorder, without use disorder
          Phencyclidine-induced anxiety disorder, without use disorder
     F16.983   **Hallucinogen use, unspecified with hallucinogen persisting perception disorder (flashbacks)** 🔍
     F16.988   **Hallucinogen use, unspecified with other hallucinogen-induced disorder** 🔍
   F16.99   **Hallucinogen use, unspecified with unspecified hallucinogen-induced disorder** 🔍

● **F17**   **Nicotine dependence**
     Excludes1   history of tobacco dependence (Z87.891)
                tobacco use NOS (Z72.0)
     Excludes2   tobacco use (smoking) during pregnancy, childbirth and the puerperium (O99.33-)
                toxic effect of nicotine (T65.2-)
● **F17.2**   **Nicotine dependence**
   ● **F17.20**   **Nicotine dependence, unspecified**
     F17.200   **Nicotine dependence, unspecified, uncomplicated**
          Tobacco use disorder, mild
          Tobacco use disorder, moderate
          Tobacco use disorder, severe
          Coding Clinic: 2016, Q1, P37
     F17.201   **Nicotine dependence, unspecified, in remission**
          Tobacco use disorder, mild, in early remission
          Tobacco use disorder, mild, in sustained remission
          Tobacco use disorder, moderate, in early remission
          Tobacco use disorder, moderate, in sustained remission
          Tobacco use disorder, severe, in early remission
          Tobacco use disorder, severe, in sustained remission
     F17.203   **Nicotine dependence unspecified, with withdrawal**
          Tobacco withdrawal
     F17.208   **Nicotine dependence, unspecified, with other nicotine-induced disorders**
     F17.209   **Nicotine dependence, unspecified, with unspecified nicotine-induced disorders**
   ● **F17.21**   **Nicotine dependence, cigarettes**
     F17.210   **Nicotine dependence, cigarettes, uncomplicated**
          Coding Clinic: 2017, Q2, P28-29
     F17.211   **Nicotine dependence, cigarettes, in remission**
          Tobacco use disorder, cigarettes, mild, in early remission
          Tobacco use disorder, cigarettes, mild, in sustained remission
          Tobacco use disorder, cigarettes, moderate, in early remission
          Tobacco use disorder, cigarettes, moderate, in sustained remission
          Tobacco use disorder, cigarettes, severe, in early remission
          Tobacco use disorder, cigarettes, severe, in sustained remission
     F17.213   **Nicotine dependence, cigarettes, with withdrawal**
     F17.218   **Nicotine dependence, cigarettes, with other nicotine-induced disorders**
     F17.219   **Nicotine dependence, cigarettes, with unspecified nicotine-induced disorders**

CHAPTER 5 (F01-F99)

● **F17.22** Nicotine dependence, chewing tobacco
  F17.220 Nicotine dependence, chewing tobacco, uncomplicated
  F17.221 Nicotine dependence, chewing tobacco, in remission
    Tobacco use disorder, chewing tobacco, mild, in early remission
    Tobacco use disorder, chewing tobacco, mild, in sustained remission
    Tobacco use disorder, chewing tobacco, moderate, in early remission
    Tobacco use disorder, chewing tobacco, moderate, in sustained remission
    Tobacco use disorder, chewing tobacco, severe, in early remission
    Tobacco use disorder, chewing tobacco, severe, in sustained remission
  F17.223 Nicotine dependence, chewing tobacco, with withdrawal
  F17.228 Nicotine dependence, chewing tobacco, with other nicotine-induced disorders
  F17.229 Nicotine dependence, chewing tobacco, with unspecified nicotine-induced disorders
● **F17.29** Nicotine dependence, other tobacco product
  F17.290 Nicotine dependence, other tobacco product, uncomplicated
    Coding Clinic: 2017, Q2, P28-29
  F17.291 Nicotine dependence, other tobacco product, in remission
    Tobacco use disorder, other tobacco product, mild, in early remission
    Tobacco use disorder, other tobacco product, mild, in sustained remission
    Tobacco use disorder, other tobacco product, moderate, in early remission
    Tobacco use disorder, other tobacco product, moderate, in sustained remission
    Tobacco use disorder, other tobacco product, severe, in early remission
    Tobacco use disorder, other tobacco product, severe, in sustained remission
  F17.293 Nicotine dependence, other tobacco product, with withdrawal
  F17.298 Nicotine dependence, other tobacco product, with other nicotine-induced disorders
  F17.299 Nicotine dependence, other tobacco product, with unspecified nicotine-induced disorders

● **F18** Inhalant related disorders
  Includes volatile solvents
● **F18.1** Inhalant abuse
  Excludes1 inhalant dependence (F18.2-)
    inhalant use, unspecified (F18.9-)
  F18.10 Inhalant abuse, uncomplicated
    Inhalant use disorder, mild
  F18.11 Inhalant abuse, in remission
    Inhalant use disorder, mild, in early remission
    Inhalant use disorder, mild, in sustained remission

● **F18.12** Inhalant abuse with intoxication
  F18.120 Inhalant abuse with intoxication, uncomplicated
  F18.121 Inhalant abuse with intoxication delirium
  F18.129 Inhalant abuse with intoxication, unspecified
  F18.14 Inhalant abuse with inhalant-induced mood disorder
    Inhalant use disorder, mild, with inhalant-induced depressive disorder
● **F18.15** Inhalant abuse with inhalant-induced psychotic disorder
  F18.150 Inhalant abuse with inhalant-induced psychotic disorder with delusions
  F18.151 Inhalant abuse with inhalant-induced psychotic disorder with hallucinations
  F18.159 Inhalant abuse with inhalant-induced psychotic disorder, unspecified
  F18.17 Inhalant abuse with inhalant-induced dementia
    Inhalant use disorder, mild, with inhalant-induced major neurocognitive disorder
● **F18.18** Inhalant abuse with other inhalant-induced disorders
  F18.180 Inhalant abuse with inhalant-induced anxiety disorder
  F18.188 Inhalant abuse with other inhalant-induced disorder
    Inhalant use disorder, mild, with inhalant-induced mild neurocognitive disorder
  F18.19 Inhalant abuse with unspecified inhalant-induced disorder
● **F18.2** Inhalant dependence
  Excludes1 inhalant abuse (F18.1-)
    inhalant use, unspecified (F18.9-)
  F18.20 Inhalant dependence, uncomplicated
    Inhalant use disorder, moderate
    Inhalant use disorder, severe
  F18.21 Inhalant dependence, in remission
    Inhalant use disorder, moderate, in early remission
    Inhalant use disorder, moderate, in sustained remission
    Inhalant use disorder, severe, in early remission
    Inhalant use disorder, severe, in sustained remission
● **F18.22** Inhalant dependence with intoxication
  F18.220 Inhalant dependence with intoxication, uncomplicated
  F18.221 Inhalant dependence with intoxication delirium
  F18.229 Inhalant dependence with intoxication, unspecified
  F18.24 Inhalant dependence with inhalant-induced mood disorder
    Inhalant use disorder, moderate, with inhalant-induced depressive disorder
    Inhalant use disorder, severe, with inhalant-induced depressive disorder

● F18.25   **Inhalant dependence with inhalant-induced psychotic disorder**

     F18.250   Inhalant dependence with inhalant-induced psychotic disorder with delusions 🐾

     F18.251   Inhalant dependence with inhalant-induced psychotic disorder with hallucinations 🐾

     F18.259   Inhalant dependence with inhalant-induced psychotic disorder, unspecified 🐾

   F18.27   Inhalant dependence with inhalant-induced dementia 🐾
     Inhalant use disorder, moderate, with inhalant-induced major neurocognitive disorder
     Inhalant use disorder, severe, with inhalant-induced major neurocognitive disorder

● F18.28   **Inhalant dependence with other inhalant-induced disorders**

     F18.280   Inhalant dependence with inhalant-induced anxiety disorder 🐾

     F18.288   Inhalant dependence with other inhalant-induced disorder 🐾
       Inhalant use disorder, moderate, with inhalant-induced mild neurocognitive disorder
       Inhalant use disorder, severe, with inhalant-induced mild neurocognitive disorder

   F18.29   Inhalant dependence with unspecified inhalant-induced disorder 🐾

● F18.9   **Inhalant use, unspecified**

     Excludes1   inhalant abuse (F18.1-)
              inhalant dependence (F18.2-)

   F18.90   Inhalant use, unspecified, uncomplicated

   F18.91   Inhalant use, unspecified, in remission

● F18.92   Inhalant use, unspecified with intoxication

     F18.920   Inhalant use, unspecified with intoxication, uncomplicated 🐾

     F18.921   Inhalant use, unspecified with intoxication with delirium 🐾

     F18.929   Inhalant use, unspecified with intoxication, unspecified 🐾

   F18.94   Inhalant use, unspecified with inhalant-induced mood disorder 🐾
     Inhalant-induced depressive disorder

● F18.95   Inhalant use, unspecified with inhalant-induced psychotic disorder

     F18.950   Inhalant use, unspecified with inhalant-induced psychotic disorder with delusions 🐾

     F18.951   Inhalant use, unspecified with inhalant-induced psychotic disorder with hallucinations 🐾

     F18.959   Inhalant use, unspecified with inhalant-induced psychotic disorder, unspecified 🐾

   F18.97   Inhalant use, unspecified with inhalant-induced persisting dementia 🐾
     Inhalant-induced major neurocognitive disorder

● F18.98   Inhalant use, unspecified with other inhalant-induced disorders

     F18.980   Inhalant use, unspecified with inhalant-induced anxiety disorder 🐾

     F18.988   Inhalant use, unspecified with other inhalant-induced disorder 🐾
       Inhalant-induced mild neurocognitive disorder

   F18.99   Inhalant use, unspecified with unspecified inhalant-induced disorder 🐾

● F19   **Other psychoactive substance related disorders**

     Includes   polysubstance drug use (indiscriminate drug use)

● F19.1   **Other psychoactive substance abuse**

     Excludes1   other psychoactive substance dependence (F19.2-)
              other psychoactive substance use, unspecified (F19.9-)

   F19.10   Other psychoactive substance abuse, uncomplicated
     Other (or unknown) substance use disorder, mild

   F19.11   Other psychoactive substance abuse, in remission
     Other (or unknown) substance use disorder, mild, in early remission
     Other (or unknown) substance use disorder, mild, in sustained remission

● F19.12   Other psychoactive substance abuse with intoxication

     F19.120   Other psychoactive substance abuse with intoxication, uncomplicated 🐾

     F19.121   Other psychoactive substance abuse with intoxication delirium 🐾

     F19.122   Other psychoactive substance abuse with intoxication with perceptual disturbances 🐾

     F19.129   Other psychoactive substance abuse with intoxication, unspecified 🐾

● F19.13   Other psychoactive substance abuse with withdrawal

     F19.130   Other psychoactive substance abuse with withdrawal, uncomplicated

     F19.131   Other psychoactive substance abuse with withdrawal delirium

     F19.132   Other psychoactive substance abuse with withdrawal with perceptual disturbance

     F19.139   Other psychoactive substance abuse with withdrawal, unspecified
       Coding Clinic: 2023, Q3, P16

   F19.14   Other psychoactive substance abuse with psychoactive substance-induced mood disorder 🐾
     Other (or unknown) substance use disorder, mild, with other (or unknown) substance-induced bipolar or related disorder
     Other (or unknown) substance use disorder, mild, with other (or unknown) substance-induced depressive disorder

● F19.15   Other psychoactive substance abuse with psychoactive substance-induced psychotic disorder

     F19.150   Other psychoactive substance abuse with psychoactive substance-induced psychotic disorder with delusions 🐾

     F19.151   Other psychoactive substance abuse with psychoactive substance-induced psychotic disorder with hallucinations 🐾

     F19.159   Other psychoactive substance abuse with psychoactive substance-induced psychotic disorder, unspecified 🐾

   F19.16   Other psychoactive substance abuse with psychoactive substance-induced persisting amnestic disorder 🐾

CHAPTER 5 (F01-F99)

F19.17   Other psychoactive substance abuse with psychoactive substance-induced persisting dementia 🅒
> Other (or unknown) substance use disorder, mild, with other (or unknown) substance-induced major neurocognitive disorder

● F19.18   Other psychoactive substance abuse with other psychoactive substance-induced disorders

    F19.180   Other psychoactive substance abuse with psychoactive substance-induced anxiety disorder 🅒

    F19.181   Other psychoactive substance abuse with psychoactive substance-induced sexual dysfunction 🅒

    F19.182   Other psychoactive substance abuse with psychoactive substance-induced sleep disorder 🅒

    F19.188   Other psychoactive substance abuse with other psychoactive substance-induced disorder 🅒
> Other (or unknown) substance use disorder, mild, with other (or unknown) substance-induced mild neurocognitive disorder
> Other (or unknown) substance use disorder, mild, with other (or unknown) substance-induced obsessive-compulsive or related disorder

F19.19   Other psychoactive substance abuse with unspecified psychoactive substance-induced disorder 🅒

● F19.2   Other psychoactive substance dependence
> **Excludes1**   other psychoactive substance abuse (F19.1-)
> other psychoactive substance use, unspecified (F19.9-)

F19.20   Other psychoactive substance dependence, uncomplicated 🅒
> Other (or unknown) substance use disorder, moderate
> Other (or unknown) substance use disorder, severe

F19.21   Other psychoactive substance dependence, in remission 🅒
> Other (or unknown) substance use disorder, moderate, in early remission
> Other (or unknown) substance use disorder, moderate, in sustained remission
> Other (or unknown) substance use disorder, severe, in early remission
> Other (or unknown) substance use disorder, severe, in sustained remission

● F19.22   Other psychoactive substance dependence with intoxication
> **Excludes1**   other psychoactive substance dependence with withdrawal (F19.23-)

    F19.220   Other psychoactive substance dependence with intoxication, uncomplicated 🅒

    F19.221   Other psychoactive substance dependence with intoxication delirium 🅒

    F19.222   Other psychoactive substance dependence with intoxication with perceptual disturbance 🅒

    F19.229   Other psychoactive substance dependence with intoxication, unspecified 🅒

● F19.23   Other psychoactive substance dependence with withdrawal
> **Excludes1**   other psychoactive substance dependence with intoxication (F19.22-)

    F19.230   Other psychoactive substance dependence with withdrawal, uncomplicated 🅒

    F19.231   Other psychoactive substance dependence with withdrawal delirium 🅒

    F19.232   Other psychoactive substance dependence with withdrawal with perceptual disturbance 🅒

    F19.239   Other psychoactive substance dependence with withdrawal, unspecified 🅒

F19.24   Other psychoactive substance dependence with psychoactive substance-induced mood disorder 🅒
> Other (or unknown) substance use disorder, moderate, with other (or unknown) substance-induced bipolar or related disorder
> Other (or unknown) substance use disorder, moderate, with other (or unknown) substance-induced depressive disorder
> Other (or unknown) substance use disorder, severe, with other (or unknown) substance-induced bipolar or related disorder
> Other (or unknown) substance use disorder, severe, with other (or unknown) substance-induced depressive disorder

● F19.25   Other psychoactive substance dependence with psychoactive substance-induced psychotic disorder

    F19.250   Other psychoactive substance dependence with psychoactive substance-induced psychotic disorder with delusions 🅒

    F19.251   Other psychoactive substance dependence with psychoactive substance-induced psychotic disorder with hallucinations 🅒

    F19.259   Other psychoactive substance dependence with psychoactive substance-induced psychotic disorder, unspecified 🅒

F19.26   Other psychoactive substance dependence with psychoactive substance-induced persisting amnestic disorder 🅒

F19.27   Other psychoactive substance dependence with psychoactive substance-induced persisting dementia 🅒
> Other (or unknown) substance use disorder, moderate, with other (or unknown) substance-induced major neurocognitive disorder
> Other (or unknown) substance use disorder, severe, with other (or unknown) substance-induced major neurocognitive disorder

● F19.28   Other psychoactive substance dependence with other psychoactive substance-induced disorders

    F19.280   Other psychoactive substance dependence with psychoactive substance-induced anxiety disorder 🅒

    F19.281   Other psychoactive substance dependence with psychoactive substance-induced sexual dysfunction 🅒

    F19.282   Other psychoactive substance dependence with psychoactive substance-induced sleep disorder 🅒

▶ New   ⇒ Revised   ~~deleted~~ Deleted   Excludes 1   Excludes 2   Includes   Use additional   Code first   Code also   Key words
OGCR Official Guidelines   X Assign placeholder X   ● Use Additional Character(s)   ▶ Manifestation Code   🅒 Hierarchical Condition Category   **Coding Clinic**

F19.288   Other psychoactive substance dependence with other psychoactive substance-induced disorder 🔍

Other (or unknown) substance use disorder, moderate, with other (or unknown) substance-induced mild neurocognitive disorder

Other (or unknown) substance use disorder, severe, with other (or unknown) substance-induced mild neurocognitive disorder

Other (or unknown) substance use disorder, moderate, with other (or unknown) substance-induced obsessive-compulsive or related disorder

Other (or unknown) substance use disorder, severe, with other (or unknown) substance-induced obsessive-compulsive or related disorder

F19.29   Other psychoactive substance dependence with unspecified psychoactive substance-induced disorder 🔍

● F19.9   Other psychoactive substance use, unspecified

    Excludes1   other psychoactive substance abuse (F19.1-)

                 other psychoactive substance dependence (F19.2-)

F19.90   Other psychoactive substance use, unspecified, uncomplicated

F19.91   Other psychoactive substance use, unspecified, in remission

● F19.92   Other psychoactive substance use, unspecified with intoxication

    Excludes1   other psychoactive substance use, unspecified with withdrawal (F19.93)

    F19.920   Other psychoactive substance use, unspecified with intoxication, uncomplicated 🔍

    F19.921   Other psychoactive substance use, unspecified with intoxication with delirium 🔍

       Other (or unknown) substance-induced delirium

    F19.922   Other psychoactive substance use, unspecified with intoxication with perceptual disturbance 🔍

    F19.929   Other psychoactive substance use, unspecified with intoxication, unspecified 🔍

● F19.93   Other psychoactive substance use, unspecified with withdrawal

    Excludes1   other psychoactive substance use, unspecified with intoxication (F19.92-)

    F19.930   Other psychoactive substance use, unspecified with withdrawal, uncomplicated 🔍

    F19.931   Other psychoactive substance use, unspecified with withdrawal delirium 🔍

    F19.932   Other psychoactive substance use, unspecified with withdrawal with perceptual disturbance 🔍

    F19.939   Other psychoactive substance use, unspecified with withdrawal, unspecified 🔍

F19.94   Other psychoactive substance use, unspecified with psychoactive substance-induced mood disorder 🔍

    Other (or unknown) substance-induced bipolar or related disorder, without use disorder

    Other (or unknown) substance-induced depressive disorder, without use disorder

● F19.95   Other psychoactive substance use, unspecified with psychoactive substance-induced psychotic disorder

    F19.950   Other psychoactive substance use, unspecified with psychoactive substance-induced psychotic disorder with delusions 🔍

    F19.951   Other psychoactive substance use, unspecified with psychoactive substance-induced psychotic disorder with hallucinations 🔍

    F19.959   Other psychoactive substance use, unspecified with psychoactive substance-induced psychotic disorder, unspecified 🔍

       Other or unknown substance-induced psychotic disorder, without use disorder

F19.96   Other psychoactive substance use, unspecified with psychoactive substance-induced persisting amnestic disorder 🔍

F19.97   Other psychoactive substance use, unspecified with psychoactive substance-induced persisting dementia 🔍

    Other (or unknown) substance-induced major neurocognitive disorder, without use disorder

● F19.98   Other psychoactive substance use, unspecified with other psychoactive substance-induced disorders

    F19.980   Other psychoactive substance use, unspecified with psychoactive substance-induced anxiety disorder 🔍

       Other (or unknown) substance-induced anxiety disorder, without use disorder

    F19.981   Other psychoactive substance use, unspecified with psychoactive substance-induced sexual dysfunction 🔍

       Other (or unknown) substance-induced sexual dysfunction, without use disorder

    F19.982   Other psychoactive substance use, unspecified with psychoactive substance-induced sleep disorder 🔍

       Other (or unknown) substance-induced sleep disorder, without use disorder

    F19.988   Other psychoactive substance use, unspecified with other psychoactive substance-induced disorder 🔍

       Other (or unknown) substance-induced mild neurocognitive disorder, without use disorder

       Other (or unknown) substance-induced obsessive-compulsive or related disorder, without use disorder

F19.99   Other psychoactive substance use, unspecified with unspecified psychoactive substance-induced disorder 🔍

SCHIZOPHRENIA, SCHIZOTYPAL, DELUSIONAL, AND OTHER NON-MOOD PSYCHOTIC DISORDERS (F20-F29)

● **F20　Schizophrenia**
Personality disorders characterized by multiple mental and behavioral irregularities (may exhibit disorganized thinking, delusions, and auditory hallucinations)

Excludes1　brief psychotic disorder (F23)
cyclic schizophrenia (F25.0)
mood [affective] disorders with psychotic symptoms (F30.2, F31.2, F31.5, F31.64, F32.3, F33.3)
schizoaffective disorder (F25.-)
schizophrenic reaction NOS (F23)

Excludes2　schizophrenic reaction in:
alcoholism (F10.15-, F10.25-, F10.95-)
brain disease (F06.2)
epilepsy (F06.2)
psychoactive drug use (F11-F19 with .15, .25, .95)
schizotypal disorder (F21)

▶Use additional code, if applicable, to identify:
▶other specified cognitive deficit (R41.84-)
Coding Clinic: 2019, Q2, P32

F20.0　Paranoid schizophrenia 🦠
Paraphrenic schizophrenia
Excludes1　involutional paranoid state (F22)
paranoia (F22)

F20.1　Disorganized schizophrenia 🦠
Hebephrenic schizophrenia
Hebephrenia

F20.2　Catatonic schizophrenia 🦠
Schizophrenic catalepsy
Schizophrenic catatonia
Schizophrenic flexibilitas cerea
Excludes1　catatonic stupor (R40.1)

F20.3　Undifferentiated schizophrenia 🦠
Atypical schizophrenia
Excludes1　acute schizophrenia-like psychotic disorder (F23)
Excludes2　post-schizophrenic depression (F32.89)

F20.5　Residual schizophrenia 🦠
Restzustand (schizophrenic)
Schizophrenic residual state

● **F20.8　Other schizophrenia**
F20.81　Schizophreniform disorder 🦠
Schizophreniform psychosis NOS
F20.89　Other schizophrenia 🦠
Cenesthopathic schizophrenia
Simple schizophrenia

F20.9　Schizophrenia, unspecified 🦠
Coding Clinic: 2019, Q2, P32

F21　Schizotypal disorder
Personality disorder characterized by need for social isolation, odd behavior and thinking, and often unconventional beliefs
Borderline schizophrenia
Latent schizophrenia
Latent schizophrenic reaction
Prepsychotic schizophrenia
Prodromal schizophrenia
Pseudoneurotic schizophrenia
Pseudopsychopathic schizophrenia
Schizotypal personality disorder
Excludes2　Asperger's syndrome (F84.5)
schizoid personality disorder (F60.1)

F22　Delusional disorders 🦠
Delusional dysmorphophobia
Involutional paranoid state
Paranoia
Paranoia querulans
Paranoid psychosis
Paranoid state
Paraphrenia (late)
Sensitiver Beziehungswahn
Excludes1　mood [affective] disorders with psychotic symptoms (F30.2, F31.2, F31.5, F31.64, F32.3, F33.3)
paranoid schizophrenia (F20.0)
Excludes2　paranoid personality disorder (F60.0)
paranoid psychosis, psychogenic (F23)
paranoid reaction (F23)

F23　Brief psychotic disorder
Paranoid reaction
Psychogenic paranoid psychosis
Excludes2　mood [affective] disorders with psychotic symptoms (F30.2, F31.2, F31.5, F31.64, F32.3, F33.3)
Coding Clinic: 2019, Q2, P32

F24　Shared psychotic disorder 🦠
Folie à deux
Induced paranoid disorder
Induced psychotic disorder

● **F25　Schizoaffective disorders**
Mental disorder exhibiting major depressive episode, manic episode, or mixed episode occurs with symptoms of schizophrenia, and mood disorder
Excludes1　mood [affective] disorders with psychotic symptoms (F30.2, F31.2, F31.5, F31.64, F32.3, F33.3)
schizophrenia (F20.-)

F25.0　Schizoaffective disorder, bipolar type 🦠
Cyclic schizophrenia
Schizoaffective disorder, manic type
Schizoaffective disorder, mixed type
Schizoaffective psychosis, bipolar type

F25.1　Schizoaffective disorder, depressive type 🦠
Schizoaffective psychosis, depressive type

F25.8　Other schizoaffective disorders 🦠

F25.9　Schizoaffective disorder, unspecified 🦠
Schizoaffective psychosis NOS

F28　Other psychotic disorder not due to a substance or known physiological condition
Chronic hallucinatory psychosis
Other specified schizophrenia spectrum and other psychotic disorder

F29　Unspecified psychosis not due to a substance or known physiological condition
Psychosis NOS
Unspecified schizophrenia spectrum and other psychotic disorder
Excludes1　mental disorder NOS (F99)
unspecified mental disorder due to known physiological condition (F09)

MOOD [AFFECTIVE] DISORDERS (F30-F39)

● **F30　Manic episode**
Elevated, expansive, or irritable mood
Includes　bipolar disorder, single manic episode
mixed affective episode
Excludes1　bipolar disorder (F31.-)
major depressive disorder, single episode (F32.-)
major depressive disorder, recurrent (F33.-)

▶ New　⟹ Revised　~~deleted~~ Deleted　Excludes 1　Excludes 2　Includes　Use additional　Code first　Code also　Key words
OGCR Official Guidelines　X Assign placeholder X　● Use Additional Character(s)　▶ Manifestation Code　🦠 Hierarchical Condition Category　Coding Clinic

● **F30.1**   Manic episode without psychotic symptoms
     F30.10   Manic episode without psychotic symptoms, unspecified 🔍
     F30.11   Manic episode without psychotic symptoms, mild 🔍
     F30.12   Manic episode without psychotic symptoms, moderate 🔍
     F30.13   Manic episode, severe, without psychotic symptoms 🔍
   F30.2   Manic episode, severe with psychotic symptoms 🔍
      Manic stupor
      Mania with mood-congruent psychotic symptoms
      Mania with mood-incongruent psychotic symptoms
   F30.3   Manic episode in partial remission 🔍
   F30.4   Manic episode in full remission 🔍
   F30.8   Other manic episodes 🔍
      Abnormality of mood resembling mania but less intense
      Hypomania
   F30.9   Manic episode, unspecified 🔍
      Mania NOS

● **F31**   **Bipolar disorder**
    Mood disorders with history of manic, mixed, or hypomanic episodes

    Includes   bipolar I disorder
                  bipolar type I disorder
                  manic-depressive illness
                  manic-depressive psychosis
                  manic-depressive reaction
                  seasonal bipolar disorder

    Excludes1   bipolar disorder, single manic episode (F30.-)
                 major depressive disorder, single episode (F32.-)
                 major depressive disorder, recurrent (F33.-)

    Excludes2   cyclothymia (F34.0)

    Coding Clinic: 2020, Q1, P23

   F31.0   Bipolar disorder, current episode hypomanic 🔍
● **F31.1**   Bipolar disorder, current episode manic without psychotic features
     F31.10   Bipolar disorder, current episode manic without psychotic features, unspecified 🔍
     F31.11   Bipolar disorder, current episode manic without psychotic features, mild 🔍
     F31.12   Bipolar disorder, current episode manic without psychotic features, moderate 🔍
     F31.13   Bipolar disorder, current episode manic without psychotic features, severe 🔍
   F31.2   Bipolar disorder, current episode manic severe with psychotic features 🔍
      Bipolar disorder, current episode manic with mood-congruent psychotic symptoms
      Bipolar disorder, current episode manic with mood-incongruent psychotic symptoms
      Bipolar I disorder, current or most recent episode manic with psychotic features
● **F31.3**   Bipolar disorder, current episode depressed, mild or moderate severity
     F31.30   Bipolar disorder, current episode depressed, mild or moderate severity, unspecified 🔍
     F31.31   Bipolar disorder, current episode depressed, mild 🔍
     F31.32   Bipolar disorder, current episode depressed, moderate 🔍
   F31.4   Bipolar disorder, current episode depressed, severe, without psychotic features 🔍
   F31.5   Bipolar disorder, current episode depressed, severe, with psychotic features 🔍
      Bipolar disorder, current episode depressed with mood-incongruent psychotic symptoms
      Bipolar disorder, current episode depressed with mood-congruent psychotic symptoms
      Bipolar I disorder, current or most recent episode depressed, with psychotic features

● **F31.6**   Bipolar disorder, current episode mixed
     F31.60   Bipolar disorder, current episode mixed, unspecified 🔍
     F31.61   Bipolar disorder, current episode mixed, mild 🔍
     F31.62   Bipolar disorder, current episode mixed, moderate 🔍
     F31.63   Bipolar disorder, current episode mixed, severe, without psychotic features 🔍
     F31.64   Bipolar disorder, current episode mixed, severe, with psychotic features 🔍
      Bipolar disorder, current episode mixed with mood-congruent psychotic symptoms
      Bipolar disorder, current episode mixed with mood-incongruent psychotic symptoms
● **F31.7**   Bipolar disorder, currently in remission
     F31.70   Bipolar disorder, currently in remission, most recent episode unspecified 🔍
     F31.71   Bipolar disorder, in partial remission, most recent episode hypomanic 🔍
     F31.72   Bipolar disorder, in full remission, most recent episode hypomanic 🔍
     F31.73   Bipolar disorder, in partial remission, most recent episode manic 🔍
     F31.74   Bipolar disorder, in full remission, most recent episode manic 🔍
     F31.75   Bipolar disorder, in partial remission, most recent episode depressed 🔍
     F31.76   Bipolar disorder, in full remission, most recent episode depressed 🔍
     F31.77   Bipolar disorder, in partial remission, most recent episode mixed 🔍
     F31.78   Bipolar disorder, in full remission, most recent episode mixed 🔍
● **F31.8**   Other bipolar disorders
     F31.81   Bipolar II disorder 🔍
       Bipolar disorder, type 2
     F31.89   Other bipolar disorder 🔍
       Recurrent manic episodes NOS
   F31.9   Bipolar disorder, unspecified 🔍
      Manic depression
      Coding Clinic: 2020, Q1, P23

● **F32**   **Depressive episode**
    Includes   single episode of agitated depression
                  single episode of depressive reaction
                  single episode of major depression
                  single episode of psychogenic depression
                  single episode of reactive depression
                  single episode of vital depression

    Excludes1   bipolar disorder (F31.-)
                 manic episode (F30.-)
                 recurrent depressive disorder (F33.-)

    Excludes2   adjustment disorder (F43.2)

   F32.0   Major depressive disorder, single episode, mild 🔍
   F32.1   Major depressive disorder, single episode, moderate 🔍
   F32.2   Major depressive disorder, single episode, severe without psychotic features 🔍
   F32.3   Major depressive disorder, single episode, severe with psychotic features 🔍
      Single episode of major depression with mood-congruent psychotic symptoms
      Single episode of major depression with mood-incongruent psychotic symptoms
      Single episode of major depression with psychotic symptoms
      Single episode of psychogenic depressive psychosis
      Single episode of psychotic depression
      Single episode of reactive depressive psychosis
   F32.4   Major depressive disorder, single episode, in partial remission 🔍

CHAPTER 5 (F01-F99)

Figure 5-1   PET scan of depressed individual's brain before and after recovery. (From Fortinash KM: Psychiatric Mental Health Nursing, ed 4, St. Louis, Mosby, 2008)

F32.5   **Major depressive disorder, single episode, in full remission** 🐾

● F32.8   **Other depressive episodes**

     F32.81   **Premenstrual dysphoric disorder**

         Excludes1   premenstrual tension syndrome (N94.3)
         Coding Clinic: 2016, Q4, P14

     F32.89   **Other specified depressive episodes**
         Atypical depression
         Post-schizophrenic depression
         Single episode of 'masked' depression NOS
         Coding Clinic: 2016, Q4, P14

F32.9   **Major depressive disorder, single episode, unspecified**
     Major depression NOS
     Coding Clinic: 2021, Q1, P10

F32.A   **Depression, unspecified**
     Depression NOS
     Depressive disorder NOS
     Coding Clinic: 2023, Q4, P15; 2021, Q4, P10

● F33   **Major depressive disorder, recurrent**

     Includes   recurrent episodes of depressive reaction
         recurrent episodes of endogenous depression
         recurrent episodes of major depression
         recurrent episodes of psychogenic depression
         recurrent episodes of reactive depression
         recurrent episodes of seasonal affective disorder
         recurrent episodes of seasonal depressive disorder
         recurrent episodes of vital depression

     Excludes1   bipolar disorder (F31.-)
         manic episode (F30.-)
     Coding Clinic: 2020, Q1, P23

F33.0   **Major depressive disorder, recurrent, mild** 🐾

F33.1   **Major depressive disorder, recurrent, moderate** 🐾

F33.2   **Major depressive disorder, recurrent, severe without psychotic features** 🐾

F33.3   **Major depressive disorder, recurrent, severe with psychotic symptoms** 🐾
     Endogenous depression with psychotic symptoms
     Major depressive disorder, recurrent, with psychotic features
     Recurrent severe episodes of major depression with mood-congruent psychotic symptoms
     Recurrent severe episodes of major depression with mood-incongruent psychotic symptoms
     Recurrent severe episodes of major depression with psychotic symptoms
     Recurrent severe episodes of psychogenic depressive psychosis
     Recurrent severe episodes of psychotic depression
     Recurrent severe episodes of reactive depressive psychosis

● F33.4   **Major depressive disorder, recurrent, in remission**

     F33.40   **Major depressive disorder, recurrent, in remission, unspecified** 🐾

     F33.41   **Major depressive disorder, recurrent, in partial remission** 🐾

     F33.42   **Major depressive disorder, recurrent, in full remission** 🐾

F33.8   **Other recurrent depressive disorders** 🐾
     Recurrent brief depressive episodes

F33.9   **Major depressive disorder, recurrent, unspecified** 🐾
     Monopolar depression NOS

● F34   **Persistent mood [affective] disorders**

     F34.0   **Cyclothymic disorder**
         Affective personality disorder
         Cycloid personality
         Cyclothymia
         Cyclothymic personality

     F34.1   **Dysthymic disorder**
         Depressive neurosis
         Depressive personality disorder
         Dysthymia
         Neurotic depression
         Persistent anxiety depression
         Persistent depressive disorder

         Excludes2   anxiety depression (mild or not persistent) (F41.8)

● F34.8   **Other persistent mood [affective] disorders**

     F34.81   **Disruptive mood dysregulation disorder** 🐾
         Coding Clinic: 2016, Q4, P14

     F34.89   **Other specified persistent mood disorders** 🐾
         Coding Clinic: 2016, Q4, P14

F34.9   **Persistent mood [affective] disorder, unspecified** 🐾

F39   **Unspecified mood [affective] disorder** 🐾
     Affective psychosis NOS

ANXIETY, DISSOCIATIVE, STRESS-RELATED, SOMATOFORM AND OTHER NONPSYCHOTIC MENTAL DISORDERS (F40-F48)

● F40   **Phobic anxiety disorders**
     Irrational fear with avoidance of the feared subject, activity, or situation even though the individual knows that the reaction is excessive

● F40.0   **Agoraphobia**
     Intense, irrational fear of open spaces

     F40.00   **Agoraphobia, unspecified**

     F40.01   **Agoraphobia with panic disorder**
         Panic disorder with agoraphobia

         Excludes1   panic disorder without agoraphobia (F41.0)

     F40.02   **Agoraphobia without panic disorder**

● F40.1   **Social phobias**
     Anthropophobia
     Social anxiety disorder
     Social anxiety disorder of childhood
     Social neurosis

     F40.10   **Social phobia, unspecified**

     F40.11   **Social phobia, generalized**

● F40.2   **Specific (isolated) phobias**

     Excludes2   dysmorphophobia (nondelusional) (F45.22)
         nosophobia (F45.22)

     ● F40.21   **Animal type phobia**

         F40.210   **Arachnophobia**
             Fear of spiders

         F40.218   **Other animal type phobia**

     ● F40.22   **Natural environment type phobia**

         F40.220   **Fear of thunderstorms**

         F40.228   **Other natural environment type phobia**

● **F40.23**   **Blood, injection, injury type phobia**
     F40.230   **Fear of blood**
     F40.231   **Fear of injections and transfusions**
     F40.232   **Fear of other medical care**
     F40.233   **Fear of injury**

● **F40.24**   **Situational type phobia**
     F40.240   **Claustrophobia**
       Fear of closed spaces
     F40.241   **Acrophobia**
       Fear of heights
     F40.242   **Fear of bridges**
     F40.243   **Fear of flying**
     F40.248   **Other situational type phobia**

● **F40.29**   **Other specified phobia**
     F40.290   **Androphobia**
       Fear of men
     F40.291   **Gynephobia**
       Fear of women
     F40.298   **Other specified phobia**

F40.8   **Other phobic anxiety disorders**
     Phobic anxiety disorder of childhood

F40.9   **Phobic anxiety disorder, unspecified**
     Phobia NOS
     Phobic state NOS

● **F41**   **Other anxiety disorders**
     Excludes2   anxiety in:
         acute stress reaction (F43.0)
         transient adjustment reaction (F43.2)
         neurasthenia (F48.8)
         psychophysiologic disorders (F45.-)
         separation anxiety (F93.0)

F41.0   **Panic disorder [episodic paroxysmal anxiety]**
     Panic attack
     Panic state
     Excludes1   panic disorder with agoraphobia (F40.01)

F41.1   **Generalized anxiety disorder**
     Anxiety neurosis
     Anxiety reaction
     Anxiety state
     Overanxious disorder
     Excludes2   neurasthenia (F48.8)

F41.3   **Other mixed anxiety disorders**

F41.8   **Other specified anxiety disorders**
     Anxiety depression (mild or not persistent)
     Anxiety hysteria
     Mixed anxiety and depressive disorder
     Coding Clinic: 2021, Q1, P11

F41.9   **Anxiety disorder, unspecified**
     Anxiety NOS
     Coding Clinic: 2021, Q1, P11

● **F42**   **Obsessive-compulsive disorder**
     Anxiety disorder with recurrent obsessions or compulsions
     Excludes2   obsessive-compulsive personality (disorder)
         (F60.5)
         obsessive-compulsive symptoms occurring in
           depression (F32-F33)
         obsessive-compulsive symptoms occurring in
           schizophrenia (F20.-)

F42.2   **Mixed obsessional thoughts and acts**
     Coding Clinic: 2016, Q4, P15

F42.3   **Hoarding disorder**
     Coding Clinic: 2016, Q4, P14-15

F42.4   **Excoriation (skin-picking) disorder**
     Excludes1   factitial dermatitis (L98.1)
         other specified behavioral and emotional
           disorders with onset usually
           occurring in early childhood and
           adolescence (F98.8)
     Coding Clinic: 2016, Q4, P14-15

F42.8   **Other obsessive-compulsive disorder**
     Anancastic neurosis
     Obsessive-compulsive neurosis
     Coding Clinic: 2016, Q4, P15

F42.9   **Obsessive-compulsive disorder, unspecified**
     Coding Clinic: 2016, Q4, P15

● **F43**   **Reaction to severe stress and adjustment disorders**
F43.0   **Acute stress reaction**
     Acute crisis reaction
     Acute reaction to stress
     Combat and operational stress reaction
     Combat fatigue
     Crisis state
     Psychic shock

● **F43.1**   **Post-traumatic stress disorder (PTSD)**
     Traumatic neurosis
     F43.10   **Post-traumatic stress disorder, unspecified**
     F43.11   **Post-traumatic stress disorder, acute**
     F43.12   **Post-traumatic stress disorder, chronic**

● **F43.2**   **Adjustment disorders**
     Culture shock
     Grief reaction
     Hospitalism in children
     Excludes2   separation anxiety disorder of childhood
         (F93.0)
     F43.20   **Adjustment disorder, unspecified**
     F43.21   **Adjustment disorder with depressed mood**
     F43.22   **Adjustment disorder with anxiety**
     F43.23   **Adjustment disorder with mixed anxiety and depressed mood**
     F43.24   **Adjustment disorder with disturbance of conduct**
     F43.25   **Adjustment disorder with mixed disturbance of emotions and conduct**
     F43.29   **Adjustment disorder with other symptoms**

● **F43.8**   **Other reactions to severe stress**
     Other specified trauma and stressor-related disorder
     F43.81   **Prolonged grief disorder**
       Complicated grief
       Complicated grief disorder
       Persistent complex bereavement disorder
     F43.89   **Other reactions to severe stress**

F43.9   **Reaction to severe stress, unspecified**
     Trauma and stressor-related disorder, NOS

● **F44**   **Dissociative and conversion disorders**
     Includes   conversion hysteria
         conversion reaction
         hysteria
         hysterical psychosis
     Excludes2   malingering [conscious simulation] (Z76.5)

F44.0   **Dissociative amnesia**
     Sudden loss of memory for personal information
     Excludes1   amnesia NOS (R41.3)
         anterograde amnesia (R41.1)
         dissociative amnesia with dissociative
           fugue (F44.1)
         retrograde amnesia (R41.2)
     Excludes2   alcohol or other psychoactive substance-
         induced amnestic disorder (F10, F13,
         F19 with .26, .96)
         amnestic disorder due to known
           physiological condition (F04)
         postictal amnesia in epilepsy (G40.-)

F44.1   **Dissociative fugue**
     Characterized by episode of sudden, unexpected travel with amnesia for past and partial to total confusion about identity or assumption of new identity
     Dissociative amnesia with dissociative fugue
     Excludes2   postictal fugue in epilepsy (G40.-)

CHAPTER 5 (F01-F99)

CHAPTER 5 (F01-F99)

F44.2   Dissociative stupor
Profound diminution or absence of voluntary movement and responsiveness to external stimuli

    Excludes1   catatonic stupor (R40.1)
                        stupor NOS (R40.1)

    Excludes2   catatonic disorder due to known
                        physiological condition (F06.1)
                        depressive stupor (F32, F33)
                        manic stupor (F30, F31)

F44.4   Conversion disorder with motor symptom or deficit
Conversion disorder with abnormal movement
Conversion disorder with speech symptoms
Conversion disorder with swallowing symptoms
Conversion disorder with weakness/paralysis
Dissociative motor disorders
Psychogenic aphonia
Psychogenic dysphonia

F44.5   Conversion disorder with seizures or convulsions
Conversion disorder with attacks or seizures
Dissociative convulsions
Coding Clinic: 2019, Q1, P19

F44.6   Conversion disorder with sensory symptom or deficit
Conversion disorder with anesthesia or sensory loss
Conversion disorder with special sensory symptoms
Dissociative anesthesia and sensory loss
Psychogenic deafness

F44.7   Conversion disorder with mixed symptom presentation

● **F44.8   Other dissociative and conversion disorders**

    F44.81   Dissociative identity disorder
               Multiple personality disorder

    F44.89   Other dissociative and conversion disorders
               Ganser's syndrome
               Psychogenic confusion
               Psychogenic twilight state
               Trance and possession disorders

F44.9   Dissociative and conversion disorder, unspecified
Dissociative disorder NOS

OGCR Section I.C.5.a.

Pain disorders related to psychological factors
Assign code F45.41, for pain that is exclusively related to psychological disorders. As indicated by the Excludes 1 note under category G89, a code from category G89 should not be assigned with code F45.41 Code F45.42, Pain disorders with related psychological factors, should be used with a code from category G89, Pain, not elsewhere classified, if there is documentation of a psychological component for a patient with acute or chronic pain.
See Section I.C.6. Pain

● **F45   Somatoform disorders**
Mental disorders characterized by symptoms suggesting general medical condition

    Excludes2   dissociative and conversion disorders (F44.-)
                  factitious disorders (F68.1-, F68.A)
                  hair-plucking (F63.3)
                  lalling (F80.0)
                  lisping (F80.0)
                  malingering [conscious simulation] (Z76.5)
                  nail-biting (F98.8)
                  psychological or behavioral factors associated
                     with disorders or diseases classified
                     elsewhere (F54)
                  sexual dysfunction, not due to a substance or
                     known physiological condition (F52.-)
                  thumb-sucking (F98.8)
                  tic disorders (in childhood and adolescence) (F95.-)
                  Tourette's syndrome (F95.2)
                  trichotillomania (F63.3)

F45.0   Somatization disorder
Briquet's disorder
Multiple psychosomatic disorder

F45.1   Undifferentiated somatoform disorder
Somatic symptom disorder
Undifferentiated psychosomatic disorder

● **F45.2   Hypochondriacal disorders**
Persistent, unrealistic preoccupation with possibility of having serious disease

    Excludes2   delusional dysmorphophobia (F22)
                  fixed delusions about bodily functions or
                     shape (F22)

F45.20   Hypochondriacal disorder, unspecified

F45.21   Hypochondriasis
    Hypochondriacal neurosis
    Illness anxiety disorder

F45.22   Body dysmorphic disorder
    ▶Bigorexia
    Dysmorphophobia (nondelusional)
    ▶Muscle dysmorphia
    Nosophobia

F45.29   Other hypochondriacal disorders

● **F45.4   Pain disorders related to psychological factors**

    Excludes1   pain NOS (R52)

F45.41   Pain disorder exclusively related to psychological factors
    Somatoform pain disorder (persistent)

F45.42   Pain disorder with related psychological factors
    Code also associated acute or chronic pain
       (G89.-)

F45.8   Other somatoform disorders
Psychogenic dysmenorrhea
Psychogenic dysphagia, including 'globus hystericus'
Psychogenic pruritus
Psychogenic torticollis
Somatoform autonomic dysfunction
Teeth grinding

    Excludes1   sleep related teeth grinding (G47.63)
Coding Clinic: 2016, Q4, P118

F45.9   Somatoform disorder, unspecified
Psychosomatic disorder NOS

● **F48   Other nonpsychotic mental disorders**

F48.1   Depersonalization-derealization syndrome

F48.2   Pseudobulbar affect
Involuntary emotional expression disorder
Code first underlying cause, if known, such as:
  amyotrophic lateral sclerosis (G12.21)
  multiple sclerosis (G35)
  sequelae of cerebrovascular disease (I69.-)
  sequelae of traumatic intracranial injury (S06.-)

F48.8   Other specified nonpsychotic mental disorders
Dhat syndrome
Neurasthenia
Occupational neurosis, including writer's cramp
Psychasthenia
Psychasthenic neurosis
Psychogenic syncope

F48.9   Nonpsychotic mental disorder, unspecified
Neurosis NOS

BEHAVIORAL SYNDROMES ASSOCIATED WITH PHYSIOLOGICAL DISTURBANCES AND PHYSICAL FACTORS (F50-F59)

● **F50   Eating disorders**

    Excludes1   anorexia NOS (R63.0)
                  feeding problems of newborn (P92.-)
                  polyphagia (R63.2)

    Excludes2   feeding difficulties (R63.3-)
                  feeding disorder in infancy or childhood (F98.2-)

▶ New   ⟱ Revised   ~~deleted~~ Deleted   Excludes 1   Excludes 2   Includes   Use additional   Code first   Code also   Key words

740   OGCR Official Guidelines   X Assign placeholder X   ● Use Additional Character(s)   ◢ Manifestation Code   🅗 Hierarchical Condition Category   Coding Clinic

● **F50.0**   **Anorexia nervosa**
      Excludes1   loss of appetite (R63.0)
               psychogenic loss of appetite (F50.89)
  F50.00   **Anorexia nervosa, unspecified**
  F50.01   **Anorexia nervosa, restricting type**
      ▷**F50.010**   **Anorexia nervosa, restricting type, mild**
          ▷Anorexia nervosa, restricting type, with a body mass index greater than or equal to 17 kg/m2
      ▷**F50.011**   **Anorexia nervosa, restricting type, moderate**
          ▷Anorexia nervosa, restricting type, with a body mass index of 16.0-16.99 kg/m2
      ▷**F50.012**   **Anorexia nervosa, restricting type, severe**
          ▷Anorexia nervosa, restricting type, with a body mass index of 15.0-15.99 kg/m2
      ▷**F50.013**   **Anorexia nervosa, restricting type, extreme**
          ▷Anorexia nervosa, restricting type, with a body mass index of less than 15.0 kg/m2
      ▷**F50.014**   **Anorexia nervosa, restricting type, in remission**
          ▷Anorexia nervosa, restricting type, in full remission
          ▷Anorexia nervosa, restricting type, in partial remission
      ▷**F50.019**   **Anorexia nervosa, restricting type, unspecified**
  F50.02   **Anorexia nervosa, binge eating/purging type**
      Excludes1   bulimia nervosa (F50.02-)
      Coding Clinic: 2022, Q1, P13
      ▷**F50.020**   **Anorexia nervosa, binge eating/purging type, mild**
          ▷Anorexia nervosa, binge eating/purging type, with a body mass index greater thanor equal to 17 kg/m2
      ▷**F50.021**   **Anorexia nervosa, binge eating/purging type, moderate**
          ▷Anorexia nervosa, binge eating/purging type, with a body mass index of 16.0-16.99kg/m2
      ▷**F50.022**   **Anorexia nervosa, binge eating/purging type, severe**
          ▷Anorexia nervosa, binge eating/purging type, with a body mass index of 15.0-15.99kg/m2
      ▷**F50.023**   **Anorexia nervosa, binge eating/purging type, extreme**
          ▷Anorexia nervosa, binge eating/purging type, with a body mass index of less than 15.0 kg/m2
      ▷**F50.024**   **Anorexia nervosa, binge eating/purging type, in remission**
          ▷Anorexia nervosa, binge eating/purging type, in full remission
          ▷Anorexia nervosa, binge eating/purging type, in partial remission
      ▷**F50.029**   **Anorexia nervosa, binge eating/purging type, unspecified**

F50.2   **Bulimia nervosa**
      Bulimia NOS
      Hyperorexia nervosa
    ▷**Excludes1**   anorexia nervosa, binge eating/purging type (F50.02-)
  ▷**F50.20**   **Bulimia nervosa, unspecified**
  ▷**F50.21**   **Bulimia nervosa, mild**
      ▷Bulimia nervosa with 1-3 episodes of inappropriate compensatory behavior per week
  ▷**F50.22**   **Bulimia nervosa, moderate**
      ▷Bulimia nervosa with 4-7 episodes of inappropriate compensatory behavior per week
  ▷**F50.23**   **Bulimia nervosa, severe**
      ▷Bulimia nervosa with 8-13 episodes of inappropriate compensatory behavior per week
  ▷**F50.24**   **Bulimia nervosa, extreme**
      ▷Bulimia nervosa with 14 or more episodes of inappropriate compensatory behavior perweek
  ▷**F50.25**   **Bulimia nervosa, in remission**
      ▷Bulimia nervosa, in full remission
      ▷Bulimia nervosa, in partial remission

● **F50.8**   **Other eating disorders**
      ~~Excludes1~~ ~~pica of infancy and childhood (F98.3)~~
  F50.81   **Binge eating disorder**
      Coding Clinic: 2016, Q4, P15
    ▷**F50.810**   **Binge eating disorder, mild**
      ▷Binge eating disorder with 1-3 binge eating episodes per week
    ▷**F50.811**   **Binge eating disorder, moderate**
      ▷Binge eating disorder with 4-7 binge eating episodes per week
    ▷**F50.812**   **Binge eating disorder, severe**
      ▷Binge eating disorder with 8-13 binge eating episodes per week
    ▷**F50.813**   **Binge eating disorder, extreme**
      ▷Binge eating disorder with 14 or more eating episodes per week
    ▷**F50.814**   **Binge eating disorder, in remission**
      ▷Binge eating disorder, in full remission
      ▷Binge eating disorder, in partial remission
    ▷**F50.819**   **Binge eating disorder, unspecified**
  F50.82   **Avoidant/restrictive food intake disorder**
      ▷Avoidant/restrictive food intake disorder, in remission
  ▷**F50.83**   **Pica in adults**   A
      ▷Pica in adults, in remission
     ▷**Excludes1**   pica in infancy and childhood (F98.3)
  ▷**F50.84**   **Rumination disorder in adults**   A
      ▷Rumination disorder in adults, in remission
     ▷**Excludes1**   rumination disorder in infancy and childhood (F98.21)
  F50.89   **Other specified eating disorder**
      ~~Pica in adults~~
      Psychogenic loss of appetite
      Coding Clinic: 2016, Q4, P16
F50.9   **Eating disorder, unspecified**
      Atypical anorexia nervosa
      Atypical bulimia nervosa
      Feeding or eating disorder, unspecified
      Other specified feeding disorder

CHAPTER 5 (F01-F99)

CHAPTER 5 (F01-F99)

● **F51**   **Sleep disorders not due to a substance or known physiological condition**
     Excludes2   organic sleep disorders (G47.-)

● **F51.0**   **Insomnia not due to a substance or known physiological condition**
     Excludes2   alcohol related insomnia (F10.182, F10.282, F10.982)
         drug-related insomnia (F11.182, F11.282, F11.982, F13.182, F13.282, F13.982, F14.182, F14.282, F14.982, F15.182, F15.282, F15.982, F19.182, F19.282, F19.982)
         insomnia NOS (G47.0-)
         insomnia due to known physiological condition (G47.0-)
         organic insomnia (G47.0-)
         sleep deprivation (Z72.820)

     F51.01   **Primary insomnia**
         Idiopathic insomnia
     F51.02   **Adjustment insomnia**
     F51.03   **Paradoxical insomnia**
     F51.04   **Psychophysiologic insomnia**
     F51.05   **Insomnia due to other mental disorder**
         Code also associated mental disorder
     F51.09   **Other insomnia not due to a substance or known physiological condition**

● **F51.1**   **Hypersomnia not due to a substance or known physiological condition**
     Hypersomnia: Excessive sleeping/sleepiness
     Excludes2   alcohol related hypersomnia (F10.182, F10.282, F10.982)
         drug-related hypersomnia (F11.182, F11.282, F11.982, F13.182, F13.282, F13.982, F14.182, F14.282, F14.982, F15.182, F15.282, F15.982, F19.182, F19.282, F19.982)
         hypersomnia NOS (G47.10)
         hypersomnia due to known physiological condition (G47.10)
         idiopathic hypersomnia (G47.11, G47.12)
         narcolepsy (G47.4-)

     F51.11   **Primary hypersomnia**
     F51.12   **Insufficient sleep syndrome**
         Excludes1   sleep deprivation (Z72.820)
     F51.13   **Hypersomnia due to other mental disorder**
         Code also associated mental disorder
     F51.19   **Other hypersomnia not due to a substance or known physiological condition**

     F51.3   **Sleepwalking [somnambulism]**
         Non-rapid eye movement sleep arousal disorders, sleepwalking type
     F51.4   **Sleep terrors [night terrors]**
         Non-rapid eye movement sleep arousal disorders, sleep terror type
     F51.5   **Nightmare disorder**
         Dream anxiety disorder
     F51.8   **Other sleep disorders not due to a substance or known physiological condition**
     F51.9   **Sleep disorder not due to a substance or known physiological condition, unspecified**
         Emotional sleep disorder NOS

● **F52**   **Sexual dysfunction not due to a substance or known physiological condition**
     Excludes2   Dhat syndrome (F48.8)

     F52.0   **Hypoactive sexual desire disorder**
         Total loss of feeling of sexual pleasure
         Lack or loss of sexual desire
         Male hypoactive sexual desire disorder
         Sexual anhedonia
         Excludes1   decreased libido (R68.82)
     F52.1   **Sexual aversion disorder**
         Sexual aversion and lack of sexual enjoyment

● **F52.2**   **Sexual arousal disorders**
     Failure of genital response
     F52.21   **Male erectile disorder**
         Erectile disorder
         Psychogenic impotence
         Excludes1   impotence of organic origin (N52.-)
           impotence NOS (N52.-)
     F52.22   **Female sexual arousal disorder**
         Female sexual interest/arousal disorder

● **F52.3**   **Orgasmic disorder**
     Inhibited orgasm
     Psychogenic anorgasmy
     F52.31   **Female orgasmic disorder**
     F52.32   **Male orgasmic disorder**
         Delayed ejaculation

     F52.4   **Premature ejaculation**
     F52.5   **Vaginismus not due to a substance or known physiological condition**
         Psychogenic vaginismus
         Excludes2   vaginismus (due to a known physiological condition) (N94.2)
     F52.6   **Dyspareunia not due to a substance or known physiological condition**
         Dyspareunia: Difficult or painful sexual intercourse
         Genito-pelvic pain penetration disorder
         Psychogenic dyspareunia
         Excludes2   dyspareunia (due to a known physiological condition) (N94.1-)
     F52.8   **Other sexual dysfunction not due to a substance or known physiological condition**
         Excessive sexual drive
         Nymphomania
         Satyriasis
     F52.9   **Unspecified sexual dysfunction not due to a substance or known physiological condition**
         Sexual dysfunction NOS

● **F53**   **Mental and behavioral disorders associated with the puerperium, not elsewhere classified**
     Acute mental illness with sudden onset following childbirth with symptoms of affective psychosis, disorientation, and confusion are prevalent
     Excludes1   mood disorders with psychotic features (F30.2, F31.2, F31.5, F31.64, F32.3, F33.3)
         postpartum dysphoria (O90.6)
         psychosis in schizophrenia, schizotypal, delusional, and other psychotic disorders (F20-F29)

     F53.0   **Postpartum depression**   M
         Postnatal depression, NOS
         Postpartum depression, NOS
         Coding Clinic: 2018, Q4, P8

     F53.1   **Puerperal psychosis**   M
         Postpartum psychosis
         Puerperal psychosis, NOS
         Coding Clinic: 2018, Q4, P9

▷ **F54**   *Psychological and behavioral factors associated with disorders or diseases classified elsewhere*
     Psychological factors affecting physical conditions
     Code first the associated physical disorder, such as:
     asthma (J45.-)
     dermatitis (L23-L25)
     gastric ulcer (K25.-)
     mucous colitis (K58.-)
     ulcerative colitis (K51.-)
     urticaria (L50.-)
     Excludes2   tension-type headache (G44.2)

● **F55**   **Abuse of non-psychoactive substances**
     Excludes2   abuse of psychoactive substances (F10-F19)
     F55.0   **Abuse of antacids**
     F55.1   **Abuse of herbal or folk remedies**
         Coding Clinic: 2023, Q3, P16

▶ New   ⇒ Revised   ~~deleted~~ Deleted   Excludes 1   Excludes 2   Includes   Use additional   Code first   Code also   Key words

F55.2   Abuse of laxatives
F55.3   Abuse of steroids or hormones
F55.4   Abuse of vitamins
F55.8   Abuse of other non-psychoactive substances

F59   **Unspecified behavioral syndromes associated with physiological disturbances and physical factors**
Psychogenic physiological dysfunction NOS

DISORDERS OF ADULT PERSONALITY AND BEHAVIOR (F60-F69)

● F60   **Specific personality disorders**
Long-term patterns of thoughts and behaviors causing serious problems with relationships and work

F60.0   **Paranoid personality disorder**
Hostile, devious, and combative response to disappointments
Expansive paranoid personality (disorder)
Fanatic personality (disorder)
Querulant personality (disorder)
Paranoid personality (disorder)
Sensitive paranoid personality (disorder)
Excludes2   paranoia (F22)
paranoia querulans (F22)
paranoid psychosis (F22)
paranoid schizophrenia (F20.0)
paranoid state (F22)

F60.1   **Schizoid personality disorder**
Detachment from social relationships with minimal emotional experiences and expressions
Excludes2   Asperger's syndrome (F84.5)
delusional disorder (F22)
schizoid disorder of childhood (F84.5)
schizophrenia (F20.-)
schizotypal disorder (F21)

F60.2   **Antisocial personality disorder**
Continuous and chronic antisocial behavior
Amoral personality (disorder)
Asocial personality (disorder)
Dissocial personality disorder
Psychopathic personality (disorder)
Sociopathic personality (disorder)
Excludes1   conduct disorders (F91.-)
Excludes2   borderline personality disorder (F60.3)

F60.3   **Borderline personality disorder**
Instability of mood, self-image or sense of self, and interpersonal relationships
Aggressive personality (disorder)
Emotionally unstable personality disorder
Explosive personality (disorder)
Excludes2   antisocial personality disorder (F60.2)

F60.4   **Histrionic personality disorder**
Personality disorder with excessive emotional and attention-seeking behavior
Hysterical personality (disorder)
Psychoinfantile personality (disorder)

F60.5   **Obsessive-compulsive personality disorder**
Anankastic personality (disorder)
Compulsive personality (disorder)
Obsessional personality (disorder)
Excludes2   obsessive-compulsive disorder (F42.-)

F60.6   **Avoidant personality disorder**
Anxious personality disorder

F60.7   **Dependent personality disorder**
Asthenic personality (disorder)
Inadequate personality (disorder)
Passive personality (disorder)

● F60.8   **Other specific personality disorders**
F60.81   **Narcissistic personality disorder**
Vanity, conceit, egotism or indifference to plight of others
F60.89   **Other specific personality disorders**
Eccentric personality disorder
'Haltlose' type personality disorder
Immature personality disorder
Passive-aggressive personality disorder
Psychoneurotic personality disorder
Self-defeating personality disorder

F60.9   **Personality disorder, unspecified**
Character disorder NOS
Character neurosis NOS
Pathological personality NOS

● F63   **Impulse disorders**
Excludes2   habitual excessive use of alcohol or psychoactive substances (F10-F19)
impulse disorders involving sexual behavior (F65.-)

F63.0   **Pathological gambling**
Compulsive gambling
Gambling disorder
Excludes1   gambling and betting NOS (Z72.6)
Excludes2   excessive gambling by manic patients (F30, F31)
gambling in antisocial personality disorder (F60.2)

F63.1   **Pyromania**
Pathological fire-setting
Excludes2   fire-setting (by) (in):
adult with antisocial personality disorder (F60.2)
alcohol or psychoactive substance intoxication (F10-F19)
conduct disorders (F91.-)
mental disorders due to known physiological condition (F01-F09)
schizophrenia (F20.-)

F63.2   **Kleptomania**
Pathological stealing
Excludes1   shoplifting as the reason for observation for suspected mental disorder (Z03.8)
Excludes2   depressive disorder with stealing (F31-F33)
stealing due to underlying mental condition-code to mental condition
stealing in mental disorders due to known physiological condition (F01-F09)

F63.3   **Trichotillomania**
Hair plucking
Excludes2   other stereotyped movement disorder (F98.4)

● F63.8   **Other impulse disorders**
F63.81   **Intermittent explosive disorder**
F63.89   **Other impulse disorders**

F63.9   **Impulse disorder, unspecified**
Impulse control disorder NOS

● F64   **Gender identity disorders**
F64.0   **Transsexualism**
Gender identity disorder in adolescence and adulthood
Gender incongruence in adolescents and adults
Gender identity in adolescents and adults
Transgender
Excludes1   gender identity disorder of childhood (F64.2)
Coding Clinic: 2016, Q4, P16

CHAPTER 5 (F01-F99)

F64.1   **Dual role transvestism**
Use additional code to identify sex reassignment status (Z87.890)
> **Excludes1**   gender identity disorder in childhood (F64.2)

> **Excludes2**   fetishistic transvestism (F65.1)

Coding Clinic: 2016, Q4, P16

F64.2   **Gender identity disorder of childhood**   P
Gender dysphoria in children
Gender incongruence of childhood
> **Excludes1**   gender identity disorder in adolescence and adulthood (F64.0)

> **Excludes2**   sexual maturation disorder (F66)

F64.8   **Other gender identity disorders**
Other specified gender dysphoria

F64.9   **Gender identity disorder, unspecified**
Gender dysphoria, unspecified
Gender incongruence, unspecified
Gender-role disorder NOS

● **F65**   **Paraphilias**

F65.0   **Fetishism**
Intense sexual urges and arousing fantasies using inanimate objects
Fetishistic disorder

F65.1   **Transvestic fetishism**
Intense sexual urges, arousal, or orgasm associated with fantasized/actual cross-dressing
Fetishistic transvestism
Transvestic disorder

F65.2   **Exhibitionism**
Exhibitionistic disorder

F65.3   **Voyeurism**
Sexual urges or arousal involving real or fantasized observation of unsuspecting people who are naked, disrobing, or engaging in sexual activity
Voyeuristic disorder

F65.4   **Pedophilia**
Pedophilic disorder

● **F65.5**   **Sadomasochism**

F65.50   **Sadomasochism, unspecified**

F65.51   **Sexual masochism**
Sexual masochism disorder

F65.52   **Sexual sadism**
Sexual sadism disorder

● **F65.8**   **Other paraphilias**

F65.81   **Frotteurism**
Sexual arousal or orgasm is achieved by rubbing up against another person (or fantasies of), in crowded place with unsuspecting victim
Frotteuristic disorder

F65.89   **Other paraphilias**
Necrophilia
Other specified paraphilic disorder

F65.9   **Paraphilia, unspecified**
Paraphilic disorder, unspecified
Sexual deviation NOS

F66   **Other sexual disorders**
Sexual maturation disorder
Sexual relationship disorder

● **F68**   **Other disorders of adult personality and behavior**

● **F68.1**   **Factitious disorder imposed on self**
Compensation neurosis
Elaboration of physical symptoms for psychological reasons
Hospital hopper syndrome
Münchhausen's syndrome
Peregrinating patient
> **Excludes2**   factitial dermatitis (L98.1)
> person feigning illness (with obvious motivation) (Z76.5)

F68.10   **Factitious disorder imposed on self, unspecified**

F68.11   **Factitious disorder imposed on self with predominantly psychological signs and symptoms**

F68.12   **Factitious disorder imposed on self with predominantly physical signs and symptoms**

F68.13   **Factitious disorder imposed on self with combined psychological and physical signs and symptoms**

F68.8   **Other specified disorders of adult personality and behavior**

F68.A   **Factitious disorder imposed on another**
Factitious disorder by proxy
Münchausen's by proxy

F69   **Unspecified disorder of adult personality and behavior**   A

INTELLECTUAL DISABILITIES (F70-F79)

Code first any associated physical or developmental disorders
> **Excludes1**   borderline intellectual functioning, IQ above 70 to 84 (R41.83)

F70   **Mild intellectual disabilities**
IQ level 50-55 to approximately 70
Mild mental subnormality

F71   **Moderate intellectual disabilities**
IQ level 35-40 to 50-55
Moderate mental subnormality

F72   **Severe intellectual disabilities**
IQ 20-25 to 35-40
Severe mental subnormality

F73   **Profound intellectual disabilities**
IQ level below 20-25
Profound mental subnormality

● **F78**   **Other intellectual disabilities**

● **F78.A**   **Other genetic related intellectual disabilities**

F78.A1   **SYNGAP1-related intellectual disability**
Code also, if applicable, any associated:
autism spectrum disorder (F84.0)
autistic disorder (F84.0)
encephalopathy (G93.4-)
epilepsy and recurrent seizures (G40.-)
other pervasive developmental disorders (F84.8)
pervasive developmental disorder, NOS (F84.9)

F78.A9   **Other genetic related intellectual disability**
Code also, if applicable, any associated disorders

F79   **Unspecified intellectual disabilities**
Mental deficiency NOS
Mental subnormality NOS

PERVASIVE AND SPECIFIC DEVELOPMENTAL DISORDERS (F80-F89)

● **F80**   **Specific developmental disorders of speech and language**

F80.0   **Phonological disorder**
Communication disorder of unknown cause, characterized by failure to use age-appropriate sounds
Dyslalia
Functional speech articulation disorder
Lalling
Lisping
Phonological developmental disorder
Speech articulation developmental disorder
Speech-sound disorder
> **Excludes1**   speech articulation impairment due to aphasia NOS (R47.01)
> speech articulation impairment due to apraxia (R48.2)

> **Excludes2**   speech articulation impairment due to hearing loss (F80.4)
> speech articulation impairment due to intellectual disabilities (F70-F79)
> speech articulation impairment with expressive language developmental disorder (F80.1)
> speech articulation impairment with mixed receptive expressive language developmental disorder (F80.2)

▶ New   ▦ Revised   ~~deleted~~ Deleted   Excludes 1   Excludes 2   Includes   Use additional   Code first   Code also   Key words

   OGCR Official Guidelines   X Assign placeholder X   ● Use Additional Character(s)   ▶ Manifestation Code   🔖 Hierarchical Condition Category   **Coding Clinic**

F80.1   **Expressive language disorder**
Developmental dysphasia or aphasia, expressive type
> **Excludes1**   mixed receptive-expressive language disorder (F80.2)
> dysphasia and aphasia NOS (R47.-)
> **Excludes2**   acquired aphasia with epilepsy [Landau-Kleffner] (G40.80-)
> intellectual disabilities (F70-F79)
> pervasive developmental disorders (F84.-)
> selective mutism (F94.0)

F80.2   **Mixed receptive-expressive language disorder**
Developmental dysphasia or aphasia, receptive type
Developmental Wernicke's aphasia
> **Excludes1**   central auditory processing disorder (H93.25)
> dysphasia or aphasia NOS (R47.-)
> expressive language disorder (F80.1)
> expressive type dysphasia or aphasia (F80.1)
> word deafness (H93.25)
> **Excludes2**   acquired aphasia with epilepsy [Landau-Kleffner] (G40.80-)
> intellectual disabilities (F70-F79)
> pervasive developmental disorders (F84.-)
> selective mutism (F94.0)

F80.4   **Speech and language development delay due to hearing loss**
Code also type of hearing loss (H90.-, H91.-)

● **F80.8**   **Other developmental disorders of speech or language**

F80.81   **Childhood onset fluency disorder**
Cluttering NOS
Stuttering NOS
> **Excludes1**   adult onset fluency disorder (F98.5)
> fluency disorder in conditions classified elsewhere (R47.82)
> fluency disorder (stuttering) following cerebrovascular disease (I69. with final characters -23)

F80.82   **Social pragmatic communication disorder**
> **Excludes1**   Asperger's syndrome (F84.5)
> autistic disorder (F84.0)
> Coding Clinic: 2016, Q4, P16

F80.89   **Other developmental disorders of speech and language**
Coding Clinic: 2017, Q1, P27

F80.9   **Developmental disorder of speech and language, unspecified**
Communication disorder NOS
Language disorder NOS

● **F81**   **Specific developmental disorders of scholastic skills**

F81.0   **Specific reading disorder**
'Backward reading'
Developmental dyslexia
Specific learning disorder, with impairment in reading
Specific reading retardation
> **Excludes1**   alexia NOS (R48.0)
> dyslexia NOS (R48.0)

F81.2   **Mathematics disorder**
Developmental acalculia
Developmental arithmetical disorder
Developmental Gerstmann's syndrome
Specific learning disorder, with impairment in mathematics
> **Excludes1**   acalculia NOS (R48.8)
> **Excludes2**   arithmetical difficulties associated with a reading disorder (F81.0)
> arithmetical difficulties associated with a spelling disorder (F81.81)
> arithmetical difficulties due to inadequate teaching (Z55.8)

● **F81.8**   **Other developmental disorders of scholastic skills**

F81.81   **Disorder of written expression**
Specific learning disorder, with impairment in written expression
Specific spelling disorder

F81.89   **Other developmental disorders of scholastic skills**

F81.9   **Developmental disorder of scholastic skills, unspecified**
Knowledge acquisition disability NOS
Learning disability NOS
Learning disorder NOS
Coding Clinic: 2022, Q4, P41

F82   **Specific developmental disorder of motor function**
Clumsy child syndrome
Developmental coordination disorder
Developmental dyspraxia
> **Excludes1**   abnormalities of gait and mobility (R26.-)
> lack of coordination (R27.-)
> **Excludes2**   lack of coordination secondary to intellectual disabilities (F70-F79)

● **F84**   **Pervasive developmental disorders**
Code also any associated medical condition and intellectual disabilities

F84.0   **Autistic disorder**
Autism spectrum disorder
Infantile autism
Infantile psychosis
Kanner's syndrome
> **Excludes1**   Asperger's syndrome (F84.5)
> Coding Clinic: 2022, Q4, P41; 2017, Q1, P27

F84.2   **Rett's syndrome**
Neurodevelopmental disorder
> **Excludes1**   Asperger's syndrome (F84.5)
> Autistic disorder (F84.0)
> other childhood disintegrative disorder (F84.3)

F84.3   **Other childhood disintegrative disorder**   P
Dementia infantilis
At least two years of normal development followed by significant loss of language abilities, social skills, bowel/bladder control, motor skills
Disintegrative psychosis
Heller's syndrome
At least two years of normal development followed by significant loss of language abilities, social skills, bowel/bladder control, motor skills
Symbiotic psychosis
Abnormal relationship to mothering figure, characterized by intense separation anxiety, severe regression, giving up of useful speech, and autism
Use additional code to identify any associated neurological condition.
> **Excludes1**   Asperger's syndrome (F84.5)
> Autistic disorder (F84.0)
> Rett's syndrome (F84.2)

F84.5   **Asperger's syndrome**
Developmental disorder
Asperger's disorder
Autistic psychopathy
Schizoid disorder of childhood

F84.8   **Other pervasive developmental disorders**
Overactive disorder associated with intellectual disabilities and stereotyped movements

F84.9   **Pervasive developmental disorder, unspecified**
Atypical autism

F88   **Other disorders of psychological development**
Developmental agnosia
Global developmental delay
Other specified neurodevelopmental disorder

F89   **Unspecified disorder of psychological development**
Developmental disorder NOS
Neurodevelopmental disorder NOS

CHAPTER 5 (F01-F99)

BEHAVIORAL AND EMOTIONAL DISORDERS WITH ONSET USUALLY OCCURRING IN CHILDHOOD AND ADOLESCENCE (F90-F98)

Note: Codes within categories F90-F98 may be used regardless of the age of a patient. These disorders generally have onset within the childhood or adolescent years, but may continue throughout life or not be diagnosed until adulthood.

● **F90 Attention-deficit hyperactivity disorders**
Attention deficit disorder with hyperactivity=ADHD

Includes attention deficit disorder with hyperactivity
attention deficit syndrome with hyperactivity

Excludes2 anxiety disorders (F40.-, F41.-)
mood [affective] disorders (F30-F39)
pervasive developmental disorders (F84.-)
schizophrenia (F20.-)

F90.0 Attention-deficit hyperactivity disorder, predominantly inattentive type
Attention-deficit/hyperactivity disorder, predominantly inattentive presentation

F90.1 Attention-deficit hyperactivity disorder, predominantly hyperactive type
Attention-deficit/hyperactivity disorder, predominantly hyperactive impulsive presentation

F90.2 Attention-deficit hyperactivity disorder, combined type
Attention-deficit/hyperactivity disorder, combined presentation

F90.8 Attention-deficit hyperactivity disorder, other type

F90.9 Attention-deficit hyperactivity disorder, unspecified type
Attention-deficit hyperactivity disorder of childhood or adolescence NOS
Attention-deficit hyperactivity disorder NOS

● **F91 Conduct disorders**
Childhood/adolescence disruptive behavior disorder

Excludes1 antisocial behavior (Z72.81-)
antisocial personality disorder (F60.2)

Excludes2 conduct problems associated with attention-deficit hyperactivity disorder (F90.-)
mood [affective] disorders (F30-F39)
pervasive developmental disorders (F84.-)
schizophrenia (F20.-)

F91.0 Conduct disorder confined to family context

F91.1 Conduct disorder, childhood-onset type
Unsocialized conduct disorder
Conduct disorder, solitary aggressive type
Unsocialized aggressive disorder

F91.2 Conduct disorder, adolescent-onset type
Socialized conduct disorder
Conduct disorder, group type

F91.3 Oppositional defiant disorder

F91.8 Other conduct disorders
Other specified conduct disorder
Other specified disruptive disorder

F91.9 Conduct disorder, unspecified
Behavioral disorder NOS
Conduct disorder NOS
Disruptive behavior disorder NOS
Disruptive disorder NOS

● **F93 Emotional disorders with onset specific to childhood**

F93.0 Separation anxiety disorder of childhood
Excludes2 mood [affective] disorders (F30-F39)
nonpsychotic mental disorders (F40-F48)
phobic anxiety disorder of childhood (F40.8)
social phobia (F40.1)

F93.8 Other childhood emotional disorders
Identity disorder
Excludes2 gender identity disorder of childhood (F64.2)

F93.9 Childhood emotional disorder, unspecified

Item 5–2 Enuresis: Bed wetting by children at night. Causes can be either psychological or medical (diabetes, urinary tract infections, or abnormalities). **Encopresis:** Overflow incontinence of bowels sometimes resulting from chronic constipation or fecal impaction. Check the documentation for additional diagnoses.

● **F94 Disorders of social functioning with onset specific to childhood and adolescence**

F94.0 Selective mutism
Elective mutism
Excludes2 pervasive developmental disorders (F84.-)
schizophrenia (F20.-)
specific developmental disorders of speech and language (F80.-)
transient mutism as part of separation anxiety in young children (F93.0)

F94.1 Reactive attachment disorder of childhood
Use additional code to identify any associated failure to thrive or growth retardation
Excludes1 disinhibited attachment disorder of childhood (F94.2)
normal variation in pattern of selective attachment
Excludes2 Asperger's syndrome (F84.5)
maltreatment syndromes (T74.-)
sexual or physical abuse in childhood, resulting in psychosocial problems (Z62.81-)

F94.2 Disinhibited attachment disorder of childhood
Affectionless psychopathy
Institutional syndrome
Excludes1 reactive attachment disorder of childhood (F94.1)
Excludes2 Asperger's syndrome (F84.5)
attention-deficit hyperactivity disorders (F90.-)
hospitalism in children (F43.2-)

F94.8 Other childhood disorders of social functioning

F94.9 Childhood disorder of social functioning, unspecified

● **F95 Tic disorder**
Involuntary twitch

F95.0 Transient tic disorder
Provisional tic disorder

F95.1 Chronic motor or vocal tic disorder

F95.2 Tourette's disorder
Combined vocal and multiple motor tic disorder [de la Tourette]
Tourette's syndrome

F95.8 Other tic disorders

F95.9 Tic disorder, unspecified
Tic NOS

● **F98 Other behavioral and emotional disorders with onset usually occurring in childhood and adolescence**
Excludes2 breath-holding spells (R06.89)
gender identity disorder of childhood (F64.2)
Kleine-Levin syndrome (G47.13)
obsessive-compulsive disorder (F42.3-)
sleep disorders not due to a substance or known physiological condition (F51.-)

F98.0 Enuresis not due to a substance or known physiological condition
Enuresis: Urinary incontinence
Enuresis (primary) (secondary) of nonorganic origin
Functional enuresis
Psychogenic enuresis
Urinary incontinence of nonorganic origin
Excludes1 enuresis NOS (R32)

▶ New   ⇒ Revised   ~~deleted~~ Deleted   Excludes 1   Excludes 2   Includes   Use additional   Code first   Code also   Key words

OGCR Official Guidelines   X Assign placeholder X   ● Use Additional Character(s)   ⫶ Manifestation Code   🦉 Hierarchical Condition Category   **Coding Clinic**

F98.1   **Encopresis not due to a substance or known**
            physiological condition
            Encopresis: Fecal incontinence
            Functional encopresis
            Incontinence of feces of nonorganic origin
            Psychogenic encopresis

            Use additional code to identify the cause of any
            coexisting constipation.

            Excludes1   encopresis NOS (R15.-)

●**F98.2**   **Other feeding disorders of infancy and childhood**

            Excludes2   anorexia nervosa and other eating
                            disorders (F50.-)
                            feeding difficulties (R63.3-)
                            feeding problems of newborn (P92.-)
                            pica of infancy or childhood (F98.3)

   F98.21   **Rumination disorder of infancy and childhood**
               ▶Rumination disorder of infancy and childhood,
                in remission

               ▶ **Excludes1**   rumination disorder in adults
                                (F50.84)

   F98.29   **Other feeding disorders of infancy and early**
               childhood

F98.3   **Pica of infancy and childhood**
            Craving and eating substances such as paint, clay, or dirt to
            replace a nutritional deficit in the body.
            ▶Pica in infancy or childhood, in remission

            ▶ **Excludes1**   pica in adults (F50.83)

F98.4   **Stereotyped movement disorders**
            Stereotype/habit disorder

            Excludes1   abnormal involuntary movements (R25.-)

            Excludes2   compulsions in obsessive-compulsive
                            disorder (F42.-)
                            hair plucking (F63.3)
                            movement disorders of organic origin
                            (G20-G25)
                            nail-biting (F98.8)
                            nose-picking (F98.8)
                            stereotypies that are part of a broader
                            psychiatric condition (F01-F95)
                            thumb-sucking (F98.8)
                            tic disorders (F95.-)
                            trichotillomania (F63.3)

F98.5   **Adult onset fluency disorder**

            Excludes1   childhood onset fluency disorder (F80.81)
                            dysphasia (R47.02)
                            fluency disorder in conditions
                            classified elsewhere (R47.82)
                            fluency disorder (stuttering) following
                            cerebrovascular disease (I69. with
                            final characters -23)
                            tic disorders (F95.-)

F98.8   **Other specified behavioral and emotional disorders with**
            onset usually occurring in childhood and adolescence
            Excessive masturbation
            Nail-biting
            Nose-picking
            Thumb-sucking

F98.9   **Unspecified behavioral and emotional disorders with**
            onset usually occurring in childhood and adolescence

UNSPECIFIED MENTAL DISORDER (F99)

F99   **Mental disorder, not otherwise specified**
          Mental illness NOS

          Excludes1   unspecified mental disorder due to known
                          physiological condition (F09)

CHAPTER 6

DISEASES OF THE NERVOUS SYSTEM
(G00-G99)

OGCR Chapter-Specific Coding Guidelines

6. Chapter 6: Diseases of the Nervous System (G00-G99)

a. Dominant/nondominant side

Codes from category G81, Hemiplegia and hemiparesis, and subcategories, G83.1, Monoplegia of lower limb, G83.2, Monoplegia of upper limb, and G83.3, Monoplegia, unspecified, identify whether the dominant or nondominant side is affected. Should the affected side be documented, but not specified as dominant or nondominant, and the classification system does not indicate a default, code selection is as follows:

- For ambidextrous patients, the default should be dominant.
- If the left side is affected, the default is nondominant.
- If the right side is affected, the default is dominant.

b. Pain - Category G89

1) General coding information

Codes in category G89, Pain, not elsewhere classified, may be used in conjunction with codes from other categories and chapters to provide more detail about acute or chronic pain and neoplasm-related pain, unless otherwise indicated below.

If the pain is not specified as acute or chronic, post-thoracotomy, postprocedural, or neoplasm-related, do not assign codes from category G89.

A code from category G89 should not be assigned if the underlying (definitive) diagnosis is known, unless the reason for the encounter is pain control/management and not management of the underlying condition.

When an admission or encounter is for a procedure aimed at treating the underlying condition (e.g., spinal fusion, kyphoplasty), a code for the underlying condition (e.g., vertebral fracture, spinal stenosis) should be assigned as the principal diagnosis. No code from category G89 should be assigned.

(a) Category G89 Codes as Principal or First-Listed Diagnosis

Category G89 codes are acceptable as principal diagnosis or the first-listed code:

- When pain control or pain management is the reason for the admission/encounter (e.g., a patient with displaced intervertebral disc, nerve impingement and severe back pain presents for injection of steroid into the spinal canal). The underlying cause of the pain should be reported as an additional diagnosis, if known.
- When a patient is admitted for the insertion of a neurostimulator for pain control, assign the appropriate pain code as the principal or first-listed diagnosis. When an admission or encounter is for a procedure aimed at treating the underlying condition and a neurostimulator is inserted for pain control during the same admission/encounter, a code for the underlying condition should be assigned as the principal diagnosis and the appropriate pain code should be assigned as a secondary diagnosis.

(b) Use of Category G89 Codes in Conjunction with Site Specific Pain Codes

(i) Assigning Category G89 and Site-Specific Pain Codes

Codes from category G89 may be used in conjunction with codes that identify the site of pain (including codes from Chapter 18) if the category G89 code provides additional information. For example, if the code describes the site of the pain, but does not fully describe whether the pain is acute or chronic, then both codes should be assigned.

(ii) Sequencing of Category G89 Codes with Site-Specific Pain Codes

The sequencing of category G89 codes with site-specific pain codes (including Chapter 18 codes), is dependent on the circumstances of the encounter/admission as follows:

- If the encounter is for pain control or pain management, assign the code from category G89 followed by the code identifying the specific site of pain (e.g., encounter for pain management for acute neck pain from trauma is assigned code G89.11, Acute pain due to trauma, followed by code M54.2, Cervicalgia, to identify the site of pain).
- If the encounter is for any other reason except pain control or pain management, and a related definitive diagnosis has not been established (confirmed) by the provider, assign the code for the specific site of pain first, followed by the appropriate code from category G89.

2) Pain due to devices, implants and grafts

See Section I.C.19. Pain due to medical devices

3) Postoperative Pain

The provider's documentation should be used to guide the coding of postoperative pain, as well as *Section III. Reporting Additional Diagnoses* and *Section IV. Diagnostic Coding and Reporting in the Outpatient Setting.*

The default for post-thoracotomy and other postoperative pain not specified as acute or chronic is the code for the acute form.

Routine or expected postoperative pain immediately after surgery should not be coded.

(a) Postoperative pain not associated with specific postoperative complication

Postoperative pain not associated with a specific postoperative complication is assigned to the appropriate postoperative pain code in category G89.

(b) Postoperative pain associated with specific postoperative complication

Postoperative pain associated with a specific postoperative complication (such as painful wire sutures) is assigned to the appropriate code(s) found in Chapter 19, Injury, poisoning, and certain other consequences of external causes. If appropriate, use additional code(s) from category G89 to identify acute or chronic pain (G89.18 or G89.28).

4) Chronic pain

Chronic pain is classified to subcategory G89.2. There is no time frame defining when pain becomes chronic pain. The provider's documentation should be used to guide use of these codes.

5) Neoplasm Related Pain

Code G89.3 is assigned to pain documented as being related, associated or due to cancer, primary or secondary malignancy, or tumor. This code is assigned regardless of whether the pain is acute or chronic.

This code may be assigned as the principal or first-listed code when the stated reason for the admission/encounter is documented as pain control/pain management. The underlying neoplasm should be reported as an additional diagnosis.

When the reason for the admission/encounter is management of the neoplasm and the pain associated with the neoplasm is also documented, code G89.3 may be assigned as an additional diagnosis. It is not necessary to assign an additional code for the site of the pain.

See Section I.C.2 for instructions on the sequencing of neoplasms for all other stated reasons for the admission/encounter (except for pain control/pain management).

6) Chronic pain syndrome

Central pain syndrome (G89.0) and chronic pain syndrome (G89.4) are different than the term "chronic pain," and therefore codes should only be used when the provider has specifically documented this condition.

See Section I.C.5. Pain disorders related to psychological factors

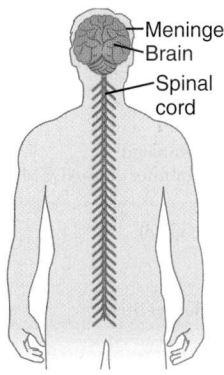

Meninges
Brain
Spinal cord

Figure 6-1   The brain and spinal cord make up the central nervous system.

Item 6-1   The two major classifications of the nervous system are the peripheral nervous system and the central nervous system (CNS). The central nervous system is composed of the brain and the spinal cord. The peripheral nervous system is composed of the parasympathetic and sympathetic systems. **Encephalitis** is the swelling of the brain. **Meningitis** is swelling of the covering of the brain, the meninges. Types and causes of brain infections are:

Type	Cause
purulent	bacterial
aseptic/abacterial	viral
chronic meningitis	mycobacterial and fungal

CHAPTER 6

DISEASES OF THE NERVOUS SYSTEM (G00-G99)

Excludes2	certain conditions originating in the perinatal period (P04-P96)
	certain infectious and parasitic diseases (A00-B99)
	complications of pregnancy, childbirth and the puerperium (O00-O9A)
	congenital malformations, deformations, and chromosomal abnormalities (Q00-Q99)
	endocrine, nutritional and metabolic diseases (E00-E88)
	injury, poisoning and certain other consequences of external causes (S00-T88)
	neoplasms (C00-D49)
	symptoms, signs and abnormal clinical and laboratory findings, not elsewhere classified (R00-R94)

This chapter contains the following blocks:

G00-G09	Inflammatory diseases of the central nervous system
G10-G14	Systemic atrophies primarily affecting the central nervous system
G20-G26	Extrapyramidal and movement disorders
G30-G32	Other degenerative diseases of the nervous system
G35-G37	Demyelinating diseases of the central nervous system
G40-G47	Episodic and paroxysmal disorders
G50-G59	Nerve, nerve root and plexus disorders
G60-G65	Polyneuropathies and other disorders of the peripheral nervous system
G70-G73	Diseases of myoneural junction and muscle
G80-G83	Cerebral palsy and other paralytic syndromes
G89-G99	Other disorders of the nervous system

INFLAMMATORY DISEASES OF THE CENTRAL NERVOUS SYSTEM (G00-G09)

● **G00**   **Bacterial meningitis, not elsewhere classified**
An infection of the cerebrospinal fluid surrounding the spinal cord and brain.

Includes	bacterial arachnoiditis
	bacterial leptomeningitis
	bacterial meningitis
	bacterial pachymeningitis

Excludes1	bacterial meningoencephalitis (G04.2)
	bacterial meningomyelitis (G04.2)

G00.0   Hemophilus meningitis
Meningitis due to Hemophilus influenzae

G00.1   Pneumococcal meningitis
Meningitis due to Streptococcal pneumoniae

G00.2   Streptococcal meningitis
Use additional code to further identify organism (B95.0-B95.5)

G00.3   Staphylococcal meningitis
Use additional code to further identify organism (B95.61-B95.8)

G00.8   Other bacterial meningitis
Meningitis due to Escherichia coli
Meningitis due to Friedländer bacillus
Meningitis due to Klebsiella
Use additional code to further identify organism (B96.-)

G00.9   Bacterial meningitis, unspecified
Meningitis due to gram-negative bacteria, unspecified
Purulent meningitis NOS
Pyogenic meningitis NOS
Suppurative meningitis NOS

▷ **G01**   *Meningitis in bacterial diseases classified elsewhere*
Code first underlying disease

Excludes1	meningitis (in):
	gonococcal (A54.81)
	leptospirosis (A27.81)
	listeriosis (A32.11)
	Lyme disease (A69.21)
	meningococcal (A39.0)
	neurosyphilis (A52.13)
	tuberculosis (A17.0)
	meningoencephalitis and meningomyelitis in bacterial diseases classified elsewhere (G05)

▷ **G02**   *Meningitis in other infectious and parasitic diseases classified elsewhere*
Code first underlying disease, such as:
African trypanosomiasis (B56.-)
poliovirus infection (A80.-)

Excludes1	candidal meningitis (B37.5)
	coccidioidomycosis meningitis (B38.4)
	cryptococcal meningitis (B45.1)
	herpesviral [herpes simplex] meningitis (B00.3)
	infectious mononucleosis complicated by meningitis (B27.- with fourth character 2)
	measles complicated by meningitis (B05.1)
	meningoencephalitis and meningomyelitis in other infectious and parasitic diseases classified elsewhere (G05)
	mumps meningitis (B26.1)
	rubella meningitis (B06.02)
	varicella [chickenpox] meningitis (B01.0)
	zoster meningitis (B02.1)

CHAPTER 6 (G00-G99)

CHAPTER 6 (G00-G99)

● **G03**   **Meningitis due to other and unspecified causes**
- **Includes**   arachnoiditis NOS
  - leptomeningitis NOS
  - meningitis NOS
  - pachymeningitis NOS
- **Excludes1**   meningoencephalitis (G04.-)
  - meningomyelitis (G04.-)

G03.0   **Nonpyogenic meningitis**
- Aseptic meningitis
- Nonbacterial meningitis

G03.1   **Chronic meningitis**

G03.2   **Benign recurrent meningitis [Mollaret]**

G03.8   **Meningitis due to other specified causes**

G03.9   **Meningitis, unspecified**
- Arachnoiditis (spinal) NOS

● **G04**   **Encephalitis, myelitis and encephalomyelitis**
- **Includes**   acute ascending myelitis
  - meningoencephalitis
  - meningomyelitis
- **Excludes1**   encephalopathy NOS (G93.40)
  - other noninfectious acute disseminated encephalomyelitis (noninfectious ADEM) (G04.81)
- **Excludes2**   acute transverse myelitis (G37.3)
  - alcoholic encephalopathy (G31.2)
  - multiple sclerosis (G35)
  - myalgic encephalomyelitis (G93.32)
  - subacute necrotizing myelitis (G37.4)
  - toxic encephalitis (G92.8)
  - toxic encephalopathy (G92.8)

● **G04.0**   **Acute disseminated encephalitis and encephalomyelitis (ADEM)**
- **Excludes1**   acute necrotizing hemorrhagic encephalopathy (G04.3-)

G04.00   **Acute disseminated encephalitis and encephalomyelitis, unspecified**

▷ **G04.01**   *Postinfectious acute disseminated encephalitis and encephalomyelitis (postinfectious ADEM)*
- **Excludes1**   post chickenpox encephalitis (B01.1)
  - post measles encephalitis (B05.0)
  - post measles myelitis (B05.1)

G04.02   **Postimmunization acute disseminated encephalitis, myelitis and encephalomyelitis**
- Encephalitis, post immunization
- Encephalomyelitis, post immunization
- Use additional code to identify the vaccine (T50.A-, T50.B-, T50.Z-)

G04.1   **Tropical spastic paraplegia** 🦠

G04.2   **Bacterial meningoencephalitis and meningomyelitis, not elsewhere classified**

● **G04.3**   **Acute necrotizing hemorrhagic encephalopathy**
- *Sudden and severe CNS disease with pathology of hemorrhages and necrosis of white matter*
- **Excludes1**   acute disseminated encephalitis and encephalomyelitis (G04.0-)

G04.30   **Acute necrotizing hemorrhagic encephalopathy, unspecified**

G04.31   **Postinfectious acute necrotizing hemorrhagic encephalopathy**

G04.32   **Postimmunization acute necrotizing hemorrhagic encephalopathy**
- Use additional code to identify vaccine (T50.A-, T50.B-, T50.Z-)

G04.39   **Other acute necrotizing hemorrhagic encephalopathy**
- Code also underlying etiology, if applicable

● **G04.8**   **Other encephalitis, myelitis and encephalomyelitis**
- Code also any associated seizure (G40.-, R56.9)

G04.81   **Other encephalitis and encephalomyelitis**
- Noninfectious acute disseminated encephalomyelitis (noninfectious ADEM)

G04.82   **Acute flaccid myelitis**
- **Excludes1**   transverse myelitis (G37.3)

G04.89   **Other myelitis** 🦠
- Coding Clinic: 2020, Q1, P14

● **G04.9**   **Encephalitis, myelitis and encephalomyelitis, unspecified**

G04.90   **Encephalitis and encephalomyelitis, unspecified**
- Ventriculitis (cerebral) NOS

G04.91   **Myelitis, unspecified** 🦠

● **G05**   **Encephalitis, myelitis and encephalomyelitis in diseases classified elsewhere**
- *Code first underlying disease, such as:*
  - congenital toxoplasmosis encephalitis, myelitis and encephalomyelitis (P37.1)
  - cytomegaloviral encephalitis, myelitis and encephalomyelitis (B25.8)
  - encephalitis, myelitis and encephalomyelitis (in) systemic lupus erythematosus (M32.19)
  - eosinophilic meningoencephalitis (B83.2)
  - human immunodeficiency virus [HIV] disease (B20)
  - poliovirus (A80.-)
  - suppurative otitis media (H66.01-H66.4)
  - systemic lupus erythematosus (M32.19)
  - trichinellosis (B75)
- **Excludes1**   adenoviral encephalitis, myelitis and encephalomyelitis (A85.1)
  - encephalitis, myelitis and encephalomyelitis (in) measles (B05.0)
  - enteroviral encephalitis, myelitis and encephalomyelitis (A85.0)
  - herpesviral [herpes simplex] encephalitis, myelitis and encephalomyelitis (B00.4)
  - listerial encephalitis, myelitis and encephalomyelitis (A32.12)
  - meningococcal encephalitis, myelitis and encephalomyelitis (A39.81)
  - mumps encephalitis, myelitis and encephalomyelitis (B26.2)
  - postchickenpox encephalitis, myelitis and encephalomyelitis (B01.1-)
  - rubella encephalitis, myelitis and encephalomyelitis (B06.01)
  - toxoplasmosis encephalitis, myelitis and encephalomyelitis (B58.2)
  - zoster encephalitis, myelitis and encephalomyelitis (B02.0)

▷ **G05.3**   *Encephalitis and encephalomyelitis in diseases classified elsewhere*
- Meningoencephalitis in diseases classified elsewhere
- *Code first underlying disease*

▷ **G05.4**   *Myelitis in diseases classified elsewhere* 🦠
- Meningomyelitis in diseases classified elsewhere

● **G06**   **Intracranial and intraspinal abscess and granuloma**
- *An accumulation of pus in either the brain or spinal cord*
- Use additional code (B95-B97) to identify infectious agent.

G06.0   **Intracranial abscess and granuloma**
- Brain [any part] abscess (embolic)
- Cerebellar abscess (embolic)
- Cerebral abscess (embolic)
- Intracranial epidural abscess or granuloma
- Intracranial extradural abscess or granuloma
- Intracranial subdural abscess or granuloma
- Otogenic abscess (embolic)
- **Excludes1**   tuberculous intracranial abscess and granuloma (A17.81)

▷ New   ⇒ Revised   ~~deleted~~ Deleted   Excludes 1   Excludes 2   Includes   Use additional   Code first   Code also   Key words
OGCR Official Guidelines   X Assign placeholder X   ● Use Additional Character(s)   ▷ Manifestation Code   🦠 Hierarchical Condition Category   Coding Clinic

G06.1   **Intraspinal abscess and granuloma**
Abscess (embolic) of spinal cord [any part]
Intraspinal epidural abscess or granuloma
Intraspinal extradural abscess or granuloma
Intraspinal subdural abscess or granuloma
> **Excludes1**   tuberculous intraspinal abscess and
> granuloma (A17.81)

G06.2   **Extradural and subdural abscess, unspecified**

G07   *Intracranial and intraspinal abscess and granuloma in diseases classified elsewhere*
Code first underlying disease, such as:
schistosomiasis granuloma of brain (B65.-)
> **Excludes1**   abscess of brain:
> amebic (A06.6)
> chromomycotic (B43.1)
> gonococcal (A54.82)
> tuberculous (A17.81)
> tuberculoma of meninges (A17.1)

G08   **Intracranial and intraspinal phlebitis and thrombophlebitis**
Septic embolism of intracranial or intraspinal venous sinuses and veins
Septic endophlebitis of intracranial or intraspinal venous sinuses and veins
Septic phlebitis of intracranial or intraspinal venous sinuses and veins
Septic thrombophlebitis of intracranial or intraspinal venous sinuses and veins
Septic thrombosis of intracranial or intraspinal venous sinuses and veins
> **Excludes1**   intracranial phlebitis and thrombophlebitis
> complicating:
> abortion, ectopic or molar pregnancy
> (O00-O07, O08.7)
> pregnancy, childbirth and the puerperium
> (O22.5, O87.3)
> nonpyogenic intracranial phlebitis and
> thrombophlebitis (I67.6)
> **Excludes2**   intracranial phlebitis and thrombophlebitis
> complicating nonpyogenic intraspinal
> phlebitis and thrombophlebitis (G95.1)

G09   **Sequelae of inflammatory diseases of central nervous system**
Note: Category G09 is to be used to indicate conditions
whose primary classification is to G00-G08 as the cause of
sequelae, themselves classifiable elsewhere. The 'sequelae'
include conditions specified as residuals.
*Code first condition resulting from (sequela) of inflammatory diseases
of central nervous system*

SYSTEMIC ATROPHIES PRIMARILY AFFECTING THE CENTRAL NERVOUS SYSTEM (G10-G14)

G10   **Huntington's disease** 🔎
*Genetic disease with degeneration of cells of the nervous system,
including brain*
Huntington's chorea
Huntington's dementia
Use Additional code, if applicable, to identify:
dementia with anxiety (F02.84, F02.A4, F02.B4, F02.C4)
dementia with behavioral disturbance (F02.81-, F02.A1-, F02.
B1-, F02.C1-)
dementia with mood disturbance (F02.83, F02.A3, F02.B3,
F02.C3)
dementia with psychotic disturbance (F02.82, F02.A2, F02.
B2, F02.C2)
dementia without behavioral disturbance (F02.80, F02.A0,
F02.B0, F02.C0)
mild neurocognitive disorder due to known physiological
condition (F06.7-)

● G11   **Hereditary ataxia**
Genetic neurological disorder affecting coordination
> **Excludes2**   cerebral palsy (G80.-)
> hereditary and idiopathic neuropathy (G60.-)
> metabolic disorders (E70-E88)

G11.0   Congenital nonprogressive ataxia 🔎
● G11.1   Early-onset cerebellar ataxia 🔎
    G11.10   **Early-onset cerebellar ataxia, unspecified**
    G11.11   **Friedreich ataxia**
Autosomal recessive Friedreich ataxia
Friedreich ataxia with retained reflexes
    G11.19   **Other early-onset cerebellar ataxia**
Early-onset cerebellar ataxia with essential
tremor
Early-onset cerebellar ataxia with myoclonus
[Hunt's ataxia]
Early-onset cerebellar ataxia with retained
tendon reflexes
X-linked recessive spinocerebellar ataxia
G11.2   Late-onset cerebellar ataxia 🔎   A
G11.3   Cerebellar ataxia with defective DNA repair 🔎
Ataxia telangiectasia [Louis-Bar]
> **Excludes2**   Cockayne's syndrome (Q87.19)
> other disorders of purine and pyrimidine
> metabolism (E79.-)
> xeroderma pigmentosum (Q82.1)
G11.4   Hereditary spastic paraplegia 🔎
G11.5   **Hypomyelination - hypogonadotropic hypogonadism - hypodontia**
4H syndrome
Pol III-related leukodystrophy
G11.6   **Leukodystrophy with vanishing white matter disease**
G11.8   Other hereditary ataxias 🔎
G11.9   Hereditary ataxia, unspecified 🔎
Hereditary cerebellar ataxia NOS
Hereditary cerebellar degeneration
Hereditary cerebellar disease
Hereditary cerebellar syndrome

● G12   **Spinal muscular atrophy and related syndromes**
G12.0   Infantile spinal muscular atrophy, type I [Werdnig-Hoffman] 🔎
G12.1   Other inherited spinal muscular atrophy 🔎
Adult form spinal muscular atrophy
Childhood form, type II spinal muscular atrophy
Distal spinal muscular atrophy
Juvenile form, type III spinal muscular atrophy
[Kugelberg-Welander]
Progressive bulbar palsy of childhood [Fazio-Londe]
Scapuloperoneal form spinal muscular atrophy
● G12.2   Motor neuron disease
*Progressive disease of motor neurons that carry impulses to
muscles to move*
    G12.20   **Motor neuron disease, unspecified** 🔎
    G12.21   Amyotrophic lateral sclerosis 🔎   A
Lou Gehrig's disease (ALS)
    G12.22   Progressive bulbar palsy 🔎
    G12.23   Primary lateral sclerosis 🔎
    G12.24   Familial motor neuron disease 🔎
    G12.25   Progressive spinal muscle atrophy 🔎
    G12.29   Other motor neuron disease 🔎
G12.8   Other spinal muscular atrophies and related syndromes 🔎
G12.9   Spinal muscular atrophy, unspecified 🔎

CHAPTER 6 (G00-G99)

Item 6–2 Huntington's chorea is an inherited degenerative disorder of
the central nervous system and is characterized by ceaseless, jerky movements
and progressive cognitive and behavioral deterioration.

● **G13** **Systemic atrophies primarily affecting central nervous system in diseases classified elsewhere**

▶ *G13.0* *Paraneoplastic neuromyopathy and neuropathy* 🐾
　　Carcinomatous neuromyopathy
　　Sensorial paraneoplastic neuropathy [Denny Brown]
　　Code first underlying neoplasm (C00-D49)

▶ *G13.1* *Other systemic atrophy primarily affecting central nervous system in neoplastic disease* 🐾
　　Paraneoplastic limbic encephalopathy
　　Code first underlying neoplasm (C00-D49)

▶ *G13.2* *Systemic atrophy primarily affecting the central nervous system in myxedema*
　　Code first underlying disease, such as:
　　　hypothyroidism (E03.-)
　　　myxedematous congenital iodine deficiency (E00.1)

▶ *G13.8* *Systemic atrophy primarily affecting central nervous system in other diseases classified elsewhere*
　　Code first underlying disease

G14 **Postpolio syndrome**
　| **Includes** | Postpolio myelitic syndrome |
　| **Excludes1** | sequelae of poliomyelitis (B91) |

EXTRAPYRAMIDAL AND MOVEMENT DISORDERS (G20-G26)

● **G20** **Parkinson's disease** 🐾
　Progressive disease of the nervous system that affects muscle coordination
　Hemiparkinsonism
　Idiopathic Parkinsonism or Parkinson's disease
　Paralysis agitans
　Parkinsonism or Parkinson's disease NOS
　Primary Parkinsonism or Parkinson's disease
　Use additional code, if applicable, to identify:
　　dementia with anxiety (F02.84, F02.A4, F02.B4, F02.C4)
　　dementia with behavioral disturbance (F02.81-, F02.A1-, F02.B1-, F02.C1-)
　　dementia with mood disturbance (F02.83, F02.A3, F02.B3, F02.C3)
　　dementia with psychotic disturbance (F02.82, F02.A2, F02.B2, F02.C2)
　　dementia without behavioral disturbance (F02.80, F02.A0, F02.B0, F02.C0)
　　mild neurocognitive disorder due to known physiological condition (F06.7-)
　Coding Clinic: 2017, Q2, P7-8; 2016, Q2, P7

● **G20.A** **Parkinson's disease without dyskinesia**
　　G20.A1 **Parkinson's disease without dyskinesia, without mention of fluctuations**
　　　Parkinson's disease NOS
　　　Parkinson's disease without dyskinesia, without mention of OFF episodes

　　G20.A2 **Parkinson's disease without dyskinesia, with fluctuations**
　　　Parkinson's disease without dyskinesia, with OFF episodes
　　　Coding Clinic: 2023, Q4, P17

● **G20.B** **Parkinson's disease with dyskinesia**
　　| **Excludes1** | drug induced dystonia (G24.0-) |
　　G20.B1 **Parkinson's disease with dyskinesia, without mention of fluctuations**
　　　Parkinson's disease with dyskinesia, without mention of OFF episodes
　　　Coding Clinic: 2023, Q4, P16

　　G20.B2 **Parkinson's disease with dyskinesia, with fluctuations**
　　　Parkinson's disease with dyskinesia, with OFF episodes
　　　Coding Clinic: 2023, Q4, P17

● **G20.C** **Parkinsonism, unspecified**
　　Parkinsonism, NOS
Excludes1	Parkinson's disease NOS (G20.A1)
	Parkinson's disease with dyskinesia (G20.B-)
	Parkinson's disease without dyskinesia (G20.A-)
	secondary parkinsonism (G20.-)

● **G21** **Secondary parkinsonism**
　Symptoms of Parkinson's caused by medicines, illness, or other nervous system disorder
Excludes1	~~dementia with Parkinsonism (G31.83)~~
	Huntington's disease (G10)
	▶neurocognitive disorder with Lewy bodies (G31.83)
	Shy-Drager syndrome (G90.3)
	syphilitic Parkinsonism (A52.19)

　G21.0 **Malignant neuroleptic syndrome**
　　Use additional code for adverse effect, if applicable, to identify drug (T43.3X5, T43.4X5, T43.505, T43.595)
　　| **Excludes1** | neuroleptic induced parkinsonism (G21.11) |

● **G21.1** **Other drug-induced secondary parkinsonism**
　　G21.11 **Neuroleptic induced parkinsonism** 🐾
　　　Use additional code for adverse effect, if applicable, to identify drug (T43.3X5, T43.4X5, T43.505, T43.595)
　　　| **Excludes1** | malignant neuroleptic syndrome (G21.0) |

　　G21.19 **Other drug induced secondary parkinsonism** 🐾
　　　Other medication-induced parkinsonism
　　　Use additional code for adverse effect, if applicable, to identify drug (T36-T50 with fifth or sixth character 5)

　G21.2 **Secondary parkinsonism due to other external agents** 🐾
　　Code first (T51-T65) to identify external agent

　G21.3 **Postencephalitic parkinsonism** 🐾
　G21.4 **Vascular parkinsonism** 🐾
　G21.8 **Other secondary parkinsonism** 🐾
　G21.9 **Secondary parkinsonism, unspecified** 🐾

● **G23** **Other degenerative diseases of basal ganglia**
　| **Excludes2** | multi-system degeneration of the autonomic nervous system (G90.3) |

　G23.0 **Hallervorden-Spatz disease** 🐾
　　Pigmentary pallidal degeneration

　G23.1 **Progressive supranuclear ophthalmoplegia [Steele-Richardson-Olszewski]** 🐾
　　Progressive supranuclear palsy

　G23.2 **Striatonigral degeneration** 🐾

　G23.3 **Hypomyelination with atrophy of the basal ganglia and cerebellum**
　　H-ABC

　G23.8 **Other specified degenerative diseases of basal ganglia** 🐾
　　Calcification of basal ganglia

　G23.9 **Degenerative disease of basal ganglia, unspecified** 🐾

● **G24** **Dystonia**
　Involuntary movements
　| **Includes** | dyskinesia |
　| **Excludes2** | athetoid cerebral palsy (G80.3) |

● **G24.0** **Drug induced dystonia**
　　Use additional code for adverse effect, if applicable, to identify drug (T36-T50 with fifth or sixth character 5)
　　G24.01 **Drug induced subacute dyskinesia**
　　　Drug induced blepharospasm
　　　Drug induced orofacial dyskinesia
　　　Neuroleptic induced tardive dyskinesia
　　　Tardive dyskinesia

　　G24.02 **Drug induced acute dystonia**
　　　Acute dystonic reaction to drugs
　　　Neuroleptic induced acute dystonia

　　G24.09 **Other drug induced dystonia**

　G24.1 **Genetic torsion dystonia**
　　Dystonia deformans progressiva
　　Dystonia musculorum deformans
　　Familial torsion dystonia
　　Idiopathic familial dystonia
　　Idiopathic (torsion) dystonia NOS
　　(Schwalbe-) Ziehen-Oppenheim disease

▶ New　　⇒ Revised　　~~deleted~~ Deleted　　Excludes 1　　Excludes 2　　Includes　　Use additional　　Code first　　Code also　　Key words

OGCR Official Guidelines　　X Assign placeholder X　　● Use Additional Character(s)　　▶ Manifestation Code　　🐾 Hierarchical Condition Category　　Coding Clinic

G24.2   **Idiopathic nonfamilial dystonia**

G24.3   **Spasmodic torticollis**
Head tilts toward one side and chin is elevated and turned toward opposite side (wry neck)

> **Excludes1**   congenital torticollis (Q68.0)
> hysterical torticollis (F44.4)
> ocular torticollis (R29.891)
> psychogenic torticollis (F45.8)
> torticollis NOS (M43.6)
> traumatic recurrent torticollis (S13.4)

G24.4   **Idiopathic orofacial dystonia**
Orofacial dyskinesia

> **Excludes1**   drug induced orofacial dyskinesia (G24.01)

G24.5   **Blepharospasm**
Tonic spasm of orbicularis oculi muscle, producing closure of eyelids

> **Excludes1**   drug induced blepharospasm (G24.01)

G24.8   **Other dystonia**
Acquired torsion dystonia NOS

G24.9   **Dystonia, unspecified**
Dyskinesia NOS

● **G25**   **Other extrapyramidal and movement disorders**
Extrapyramidal: Other than pyramidal tracts

> **Excludes2**   sleep related movement disorders (G47.6-)

G25.0   **Essential tremor**
Familial tremor

> **Excludes1**   tremor NOS (R25.1)

G25.1   **Drug-induced tremor**
Use additional code for adverse effect, if applicable, to identify drug (T36-T50 with fifth or sixth character 5)

G25.2   **Other specified forms of tremor**
Intention tremor

G25.3   **Myoclonus**
Shocklike contractions muscle(s)
Drug-induced myoclonus
Palatal myoclonus
Use additional code for adverse effect, if applicable, to identify drug (T36-T50 with fifth or sixth character 5)

> **Excludes1**   facial myokymia (G51.4)
> myoclonic epilepsy (G40.-)

G25.4   **Drug-induced chorea**
Use additional code for adverse effect, if applicable, to identify drug (T36-T50 with fifth or sixth character 5)

G25.5   **Other chorea**
Continual, involuntary, jerky, movements
Chorea NOS

> **Excludes1**   chorea NOS with heart involvement (I02.0)
> Huntington's chorea (G10)
> rheumatic chorea (I02.-)
> Sydenham's chorea (I02.-)

● G25.6   **Drug induced tics and other tics of organic origin**

G25.61   **Drug induced tics**
Use additional code for adverse effect, if applicable, to identify drug (T36-T50 with fifth or sixth character 5)

G25.69   **Other tics of organic origin**

> **Excludes1**   habit spasm (F95.9)
> tic NOS (F95.9)
> Tourette's syndrome (F95.2)

● G25.7   **Other and unspecified drug induced movement disorders**
Use additional code for adverse effect, if applicable, to identify drug (T36-T50 with fifth or sixth character 5)

G25.70   **Drug induced movement disorder, unspecified**

G25.71   **Drug induced akathisia**
Drug induced acathisia
Neuroleptic induced acute akathisia
Tardive akathisia

G25.79   **Other drug induced movement disorders**

● G25.8   **Other specified extrapyramidal and movement disorders**

G25.81   **Restless legs syndrome**

G25.82   **Stiff-man syndrome**

G25.83   **Benign shuddering attacks**

G25.89   **Other specified extrapyramidal and movement disorders**

G25.9   **Extrapyramidal and movement disorder, unspecified**

▷ **G26**   *Extrapyramidal and movement disorders in diseases classified elsewhere*
Code first underlying disease

OTHER DEGENERATIVE DISEASES OF THE NERVOUS SYSTEM (G30-G32)

● **G30**   **Alzheimer's disease**
Progressive central neurodegenerative disorder

> **Includes**   Alzheimer's dementia senile and presenile forms

Use additional code, if applicable, to identify:
   delirium, if applicable (F05)
   dementia with anxiety (F02.84, F02.A4, F02.B4, F02.C4)
   dementia with behavioral disturbance (F02.81-, F02.A1-, F02.B1-, F02.C1-)
   dementia with mood disturbance (F02.83, F02.A3, F02.B3, F02.C3)
   dementia with psychotic disturbance (F02.82, F02.A2, F02.B2, F02.C2)
   dementia without behavioral disturbance (F02.80, F02.A0, F02.B0, F02.C0)
   mild neurocognitive disorder due to known physiological condition (F06.7-)

> **Excludes1**   senile degeneration of brain NEC (G31.1)
> senile dementia NOS (F03.-)
> senility NOS (R41.81)

G30.0   **Alzheimer's disease with early onset**

G30.1   **Alzheimer's disease with late onset**   **A**
Coding Clinic: 2022, Q4, P15

G30.8   **Other Alzheimer's disease**

G30.9   **Alzheimer's disease, unspecified**
Coding Clinic: 2017, Q1, P43; 2016, Q2, P6; 2012, Q4, P95

● **G31**   **Other degenerative diseases of nervous system, not elsewhere classified**
Use additional
   code, if applicable, for codes G31.0-G31.83, G31.85-G31.9, to identify:
   dementia with behavioral disturbance (F02.81-, F02.A1-, F02.B1-, F02.C1-)
   dementia with mood disturbance (F02.83, F02.A3, F02.B3, F02.C3)
   dementia with psychotic disturbance (F02.82, F02.A2, F02.B2, F02.C2)
   dementia without behavioral disturbance (F02.80, F02.A0, F02.B0, F02.C0)
   mild neurocognitive disorder due to known physiological condition (F06.7-)

> **Excludes2**   Reye's syndrome (G93.7)

● G31.0   **Frontotemporal dementia**

G31.01   **Pick's disease**
Primary progressive aphasia
Progressive isolated aphasia

G31.09   **Other frontotemporal neurocognitive disorder**
Frontal dementia
Use Additional code, if applicable, to identify mild neurocognitive disorders due to known physiological condition (F06.7-)

G31.1   Senile degeneration of brain, not elsewhere classified
> Excludes1   Alzheimer's disease (G30.-)
>   senility NOS (R41.81)

G31.2   Degeneration of nervous system due to alcohol
Alcoholic cerebellar ataxia
Alcoholic cerebellar degeneration
Alcoholic cerebral degeneration
Alcoholic encephalopathy
Dysfunction of the autonomic nervous system due to alcohol
Code also associated alcoholism (F10.-)

● **G31.8   Other specified degenerative diseases of nervous system**

G31.80   Leukodystrophy, unspecified

G31.81   Alpers' disease
Rare neuronal degeneration of cerebral cortex disease of young children
Grey-matter degeneration
Coding Clinic: 2017, Q2, P7

G31.82   Leigh's disease
Rare neurometabolic disorder that affects central nervous system
Subacute necrotizing encephalopathy

G31.83   Neurocognitive disorder with Lewy bodies
Closely allied to Parkinson's Disease
Lewy body dementia
Lewy body disease
Use Additional code, if applicable, to identify mild neurocognitive disorders due to known physiological condition (F06.7-)
Coding Clinic: 2017, Q2, P7; 2016, Q4, P141

G31.84   Mild cognitive impairment of uncertain or unknown etiology
Mild cognitive disorder NOS
Mild neurocognitive disorder of uncertain or unknown etiology
Use Additional code to identify presence of:
alcohol abuse and dependence (F10.-)
exposure to environmental tobacco smoke (Z77.22)
history of tobacco dependence (Z87.891)
hypertension (I10-I1A)
occupational exposure to environmental tobacco smoke (Z57.31)
tobacco dependence (F17.-)
tobacco use (Z72.0)
> Excludes1   age related cognitive decline (R41.81)
>   altered mental status (R41.82)
>   cerebral degeneration (G31.9)
>   cerebrovascular diseases (I60-I69)
>   change in mental status (R41.82)
>   cognitive deficits following (sequelae of) cerebral hemorrhage or infarction (I69.01-, I69.11-, I69.21-, I69.31-, I69.81-, I69.91-)
>   cognitive impairment due to intracranial or head injury (S06.-)
>   dementia (F01.-, F02.-, F03.-)
>   mild neurocognitive disorder due to a known physiological condition (F06.7-)
>   neurologic neglect syndrome (R41.4)
>   personality change, nonpsychotic (F68.8)
Coding Clinic: 2021, Q3, P3

G31.85   Corticobasal degeneration

G31.86   Alexander disease

G31.89   Other specified degenerative diseases of nervous system

G31.9   Degenerative disease of nervous system, unspecified
Coding Clinic: 2021, Q3, P3

● **G32   Other degenerative disorders of nervous system in diseases classified elsewhere**

▷ *G32.0   Subacute combined degeneration of spinal cord in diseases classified elsewhere* 🦠
Dana-Putnam syndrome
Sclerosis of spinal cord (combined) (dorsolateral) (posterolateral)
Code first underlying disease, such as:
other dietary vitamin B12 deficiency anemia
pernicious (D51.0)
vitamin B12 deficiency anemia, unspecified (D51.8)
> Excludes1   syphilitic combined degeneration of spinal cord (A52.11)

● **G32.8   Other specified degenerative disorders of nervous system in diseases classified elsewhere**
Code first underlying disease, such as:
amyloidosis cerebral degeneration (E85.-)
cerebral degeneration (due to) hypothyroidism (E00.0-E03.9)
cerebral degeneration (due to) neoplasm (C00-D49)
cerebral degeneration (due to) vitamin B deficiency, except thiamine (E52-E53.-)
> Excludes1   superior hemorrhagic polioencephalitis [Wernicke's encephalopathy] (E51.2)

▷ *G32.81   Cerebellar ataxia in diseases classified elsewhere* 🦠
Code first underlying disease, such as:
celiac disease (with gluten ataxia) (K90.0)
cerebellar ataxia (in) neoplastic disease (paraneoplastic cerebellar degeneration) (C00-D49)
non-celiac gluten ataxia (M35.9)
> Excludes1   systemic atrophy primarily affecting the central nervous system in alcoholic cerebellar ataxia (G31.2)
>   systemic atrophy primarily affecting the central nervous system in myxedema (G13.2)

▷ *G32.89   Other specified degenerative disorders of nervous system in diseases classified elsewhere*
Degenerative encephalopathy in diseases classified elsewhere

DEMYELINATING DISEASES OF THE CENTRAL NERVOUS SYSTEM (G35-G37)

G35   Multiple sclerosis 🦠
Destruction of central nervous system; four types: relapsing remitting, secondary progressive, primary progressive, and progressive relapsing
Disseminated multiple sclerosis
Generalized multiple sclerosis
Multiple sclerosis NOS
Multiple sclerosis of brain stem
Multiple sclerosis of cord
Coding Clinic: 2021, Q1, P7

● **G36   Other acute disseminated demyelination**
> Excludes1   postinfectious encephalitis and encephalomyelitis NOS (G04.01)

G36.0   Neuromyelitis optica [Devic] 🦠
Inflammatory disorder in which immune system attacks optic nerves and spinal cord producing inflammation of optic nerve (optic neuritis) and spinal cord (myelitis)
Demyelination in optic neuritis
> Excludes1   optic neuritis NOS (H46)

G36.1   Acute and subacute hemorrhagic leukoencephalitis [Hurst] 🦠

Item 6–3   **Multiple sclerosis** (MS) is a nervous system disease affecting the brain and spinal cord by damaging the myelin sheath surrounding and protecting nerve cells. The damage slows down/blocks messages between the brain and body. Symptoms are visual disturbances, muscle weakness, coordination and balance issues, numbness, prickling, thinking and memory problems. The cause is unknown, though it is thought that it may be an autoimmune disease. It affects women more than men, between 20 and 40 years of age. MS can be mild, but it may cause the loss of ability to write, walk, and speak. There is no cure, but medication may slow or control symptoms.

G36.8   **Other specified acute disseminated demyelination** 🦟

G36.9   **Acute disseminated demyelination, unspecified** 🦟

● G37   **Other demyelinating diseases of central nervous system**
Destruction of central nervous system

    G37.0   **Diffuse sclerosis of central nervous system** 🦟
       Periaxial encephalitis
       Schilder's disease
       Excludes1   X linked adrenoleukodystrophy (E71.52-)

    G37.1   **Central demyelination of corpus callosum** 🦟

    G37.2   **Central pontine myelinolysis** 🦟
       Coding Clinic: 2022, Q2, P11

    G37.3   **Acute transverse myelitis in demyelinating disease of central nervous system** 🦟
       Acute transverse myelitis NOS
       Acute transverse myelopathy
       Excludes1   acute flaccid myelitis (G04.82)
                  multiple sclerosis (G35)
                  neuromyelitis optica [Devic] (G36.0)

    G37.4   **Subacute necrotizing myelitis of central nervous system** 🦟

    G37.5   **Concentric sclerosis [Baló] of central nervous system** 🦟

● G37.8   **Other specified demyelinating diseases of central nervous system** 🦟

      G37.81   **Myelin oligodendrocyte glycoprotein antibody disease**
          MOG antibody disease
          Code also associated manifestations, if known, such as:
          noninfectious acute disseminated encephalomyelitis (G04.81)
          neuromyelitis optica (G36.0)

      G37.89   **Other specified demyelinating diseases of central nervous system**

    G37.9   **Demyelinating disease of central nervous system, unspecified** 🦟

EPISODIC AND PAROXYSMAL DISORDERS (G40-G47)

● G40   **Epilepsy and recurrent seizures**
     Note: The following terms are to be considered equivalent to intractable: pharmacoresistant (pharmacologically resistant), treatment resistant, refractory (medically) and poorly controlled

     Excludes1   conversion disorder with seizures (F44.5)
               convulsions NOS (R56.9)
               post traumatic seizures (R56.1)
               seizure (convulsive) NOS (R56.9)
               seizure of newborn (P90)

     Excludes2   hippocampal sclerosis (G93.81)
               mesial temporal sclerosis (G93.81)
               temporal sclerosis (G93.81)
               Todd's paralysis (G83.84)

● G40.0   **Localization-related (focal) (partial) idiopathic epilepsy and epileptic syndromes with seizures of localized onset**
      Benign childhood epilepsy with centrotemporal EEG spikes
      Childhood epilepsy with occipital EEG paroxysms
      Excludes1   adult onset localization-related epilepsy (G40.1-, G40.2-)

● G40.00   **Localization-related (focal) (partial) idiopathic epilepsy and epileptic syndromes with seizures of localized onset, not intractable**
      Localization-related (focal) (partial) idiopathic epilepsy and epileptic syndromes with seizures of localized onset without intractability

      G40.001   **Localization-related (focal) (partial) idiopathic epilepsy and epileptic syndromes with seizures of localized onset, not intractable, with status epilepticus** 🦟

      G40.009   **Localization-related (focal) (partial) idiopathic epilepsy and epileptic syndromes with seizures of localized onset, not intractable, without status epilepticus** 🦟
          Localization-related (focal) (partial) idiopathic epilepsy and epileptic syndromes with seizures of localized onset NOS

● G40.01   **Localization-related (focal) (partial) idiopathic epilepsy and epileptic syndromes with seizures of localized onset, intractable**

      G40.011   **Localization-related (focal) (partial) idiopathic epilepsy and epileptic syndromes with seizures of localized onset, intractable, with status epilepticus** 🦟

      G40.019   **Localization-related (focal) (partial) idiopathic epilepsy and epileptic syndromes with seizures of localized onset, intractable, without status epilepticus** 🦟

● G40.1   **Localization-related (focal) (partial) symptomatic epilepsy and epileptic syndromes with simple partial seizures**
      Attacks without alteration of consciousness
      Epilepsia partialis continua [Kozhevnikof]
      Simple partial seizures developing into secondarily generalized seizures

● G40.10   **Localization-related (focal) (partial) symptomatic epilepsy and epileptic syndromes with simple partial seizures, not intractable**
      Localization-related (focal) (partial) symptomatic epilepsy and epileptic syndromes with simple partial seizures without intractability

      G40.101   **Localization-related (focal) (partial) symptomatic epilepsy and epileptic syndromes with simple partial seizures, not intractable, with status epilepticus** 🦟

      G40.109   **Localization-related (focal) (partial) symptomatic epilepsy and epileptic syndromes with simple partial seizures, not intractable, without status epilepticus** 🦟
          Localization-related (focal) (partial) symptomatic epilepsy and epileptic syndromes with simple partial seizures NOS
          Coding Clinic: 2023, Q3, P4

● G40.11   **Localization-related (focal) (partial) symptomatic epilepsy and epileptic syndromes with simple partial seizures, intractable**

      G40.111   **Localization-related (focal) (partial) symptomatic epilepsy and epileptic syndromes with simple partial seizures, intractable, with status epilepticus** 🦟

      G40.119   **Localization-related (focal) (partial) symptomatic epilepsy and epileptic syndromes with simple partial seizures, intractable, without status epilepticus** 🦟

● **G40.2** **Localization-related (focal) (partial) symptomatic epilepsy and epileptic syndromes with complex partial seizures**
     Attacks with alteration of consciousness, often with automatisms
     Complex partial seizures developing into secondarily generalized seizures

     ● **G40.20** **Localization-related (focal) (partial) symptomatic epilepsy and epileptic syndromes with complex partial seizures, not intractable**
         Localization-related (focal) (partial) symptomatic epilepsy and epileptic syndromes with complex partial seizures without intractability

         G40.201 **Localization-related (focal) (partial) symptomatic epilepsy and epileptic syndromes with complex partial seizures, not intractable, with status epilepticus** 🦠

         G40.209 **Localization-related (focal) (partial) symptomatic epilepsy and epileptic syndromes with complex partial seizures, not intractable, without status epilepticus** 🦠
           Localization-related (focal) (partial) symptomatic epilepsy and epileptic syndromes with complex partial seizures NOS

     ● **G40.21** **Localization-related (focal) (partial) symptomatic epilepsy and epileptic syndromes with complex partial seizures, intractable**

         G40.211 **Localization-related (focal) (partial) symptomatic epilepsy and epileptic syndromes with complex partial seizures, intractable, with status epilepticus** 🦠

         G40.219 **Localization-related (focal) (partial) symptomatic epilepsy and epileptic syndromes with complex partial seizures, intractable, without status epilepticus** 🦠

● **G40.3** **Generalized idiopathic epilepsy and epileptic syndromes**
     Code also MERRF syndrome, if applicable (E88.42)

     ● **G40.30** **Generalized idiopathic epilepsy and epileptic syndromes, not intractable**
         Generalized idiopathic epilepsy and epileptic syndromes without intractability

         G40.301 **Generalized idiopathic epilepsy and epileptic syndromes, not intractable, with status epilepticus** 🦠

         G40.309 **Generalized idiopathic epilepsy and epileptic syndromes, not intractable, without status epilepticus** 🦠
           Generalized idiopathic epilepsy and epileptic syndromes NOS

     ● **G40.31** **Generalized idiopathic epilepsy and epileptic syndromes, intractable**

         G40.311 **Generalized idiopathic epilepsy and epileptic syndromes, intractable, with status epilepticus** 🦠

         G40.319 **Generalized idiopathic epilepsy and epileptic syndromes, intractable, without status epilepticus** 🦠

● **G40.4** **Other generalized epilepsy and epileptic syndromes**
     Epilepsy with grand mal seizures on awakening
     Epilepsy with myoclonic absences
     Epilepsy with myoclonic-astatic seizures
     Grand mal seizure NOS
     Nonspecific atonic epileptic seizures
     Nonspecific clonic epileptic seizures
     Nonspecific myoclonic epileptic seizures
     Nonspecific tonic epileptic seizures
     Nonspecific tonic-clonic epileptic seizures
     Symptomatic early myoclonic encephalopathy

     ● **G40.40** **Other generalized epilepsy and epileptic syndromes, not intractable**
         Other generalized epilepsy and epileptic syndromes without intractability
         Other generalized epilepsy and epileptic syndromes NOS

         G40.401 **Other generalized epilepsy and epileptic syndromes, not intractable, with status epilepticus** 🦠

         G40.409 **Other generalized epilepsy and epileptic syndromes, not intractable, without status epilepticus** 🦠

     ● **G40.41** **Other generalized epilepsy and epileptic syndromes, intractable**

         G40.411 **Other generalized epilepsy and epileptic syndromes, intractable, with status epilepticus** 🦠

         G40.419 **Other generalized epilepsy and epileptic syndromes, intractable, without status epilepticus** 🦠

     G40.42 **Cyclin-Dependent Kinase-Like 5 Deficiency Disorder**
         CDKL5
         Use additional code, if known, to identify associated manifestations, such as:
         cortical blindness (H47.61-)
         global developmental delay (F88)

● **G40.5** **Epileptic seizures related to external causes**
     Epileptic seizures related to alcohol
     Epileptic seizures related to drugs
     Epileptic seizures related to hormonal changes
     Epileptic seizures related to sleep deprivation
     Epileptic seizures related to stress
     Code also, if applicable, associated epilepsy and recurrent seizures (G40.-)
     Use additional code for adverse effect, if applicable, to identify drug (T36-T50 with fifth or sixth character 5)

     ● **G40.50** **Epileptic seizures related to external causes, not intractable**

         G40.501 **Epileptic seizures related to external causes, not intractable, with status epilepticus** 🦠

         G40.509 **Epileptic seizures related to external causes, not intractable, without status epilepticus** 🦠
           Epileptic seizures related to external causes, NOS

● **G40.8** **Other epilepsy and recurrent seizures**
     Epilepsies and epileptic syndromes undetermined as to whether they are focal or generalized
     Landau-Kleffner syndrome

     ● **G40.80** **Other epilepsy**

         G40.801 **Other epilepsy, not intractable, with status epilepticus** 🦠
           Other epilepsy without intractability with status epilepticus

         G40.802 **Other epilepsy, not intractable, without status epilepticus** 🦠
           Other epilepsy NOS
           Other epilepsy without intractability without status epilepticus

         G40.803 **Other epilepsy, intractable, with status epilepticus** 🦠

         G40.804 **Other epilepsy, intractable, without status epilepticus** 🦠

     ● **G40.81** **Lennox-Gastaut syndrome**

         G40.811 **Lennox-Gastaut syndrome, not intractable, with status epilepticus** 🦠

         G40.812 **Lennox-Gastaut syndrome, not intractable, without status epilepticus** 🦠

CHAPTER 6 (G00-G99)

▶ New   ⇒ Revised   ~~deleted~~ Deleted   Excludes 1   Excludes 2   Includes   Use additional   Code first   Code also   Key words

OGCR Official Guidelines   X Assign placeholder X   ● Use Additional Character(s)   ▶ Manifestation Code   🦠 Hierarchical Condition Category   **Coding Clinic**

        G40.813   Lennox-Gastaut syndrome, intractable, with status epilepticus 🦟

        G40.814   Lennox-Gastaut syndrome, intractable, without status epilepticus 🦟

● **G40.82**   Epileptic spasms
         Infantile spasms
         Salaam attacks
         West's syndrome

        G40.821   Epileptic spasms, not intractable, with status epilepticus 🦟

        G40.822   Epileptic spasms, not intractable, without status epilepticus 🦟

        G40.823   Epileptic spasms, intractable, with status epilepticus 🦟

        G40.824   Epileptic spasms, intractable, without status e pilepticus 🦟

● **G40.83**   Dravet syndrome
         Polymorphic epilepsy in infancy (PMEI)
         Severe myoclonic epilepsy in infancy (SMEI)

        G40.833   Dravet syndrome, intractable, with status epilepticus

        G40.834   Dravet syndrome, intractable, without status epilepticus
                 Dravet syndrome NOS

▶● **G40.84**   KCNQ2-related epilepsy

   ▶ **G40.841**   KCNQ2-related epilepsy, not intractable, with status epilepticus

   ▶ **G40.842**   KCNQ2-related epilepsy, not intractable, without status epilepticus
               ▶KCNQ2-related epilepsy NOS

   ▶ **G40.843**   KCNQ2-related epilepsy, intractable, with status epilepticus

   ▶ **G40.844**   KCNQ2-related epilepsy, intractable, without status epilepticus

  G40.89   Other seizures 🦟

         Excludes1   post traumatic seizures (R56.1)
                       recurrent seizures NOS (G40.909)
                       seizure NOS (R56.9)

● **G40.9**   Epilepsy, unspecified

  ● **G40.90**   Epilepsy, unspecified, not intractable
         Epilepsy, unspecified, without intractability

        G40.901   Epilepsy, unspecified, not intractable, with status epilepticus 🦟

        G40.909   Epilepsy, unspecified, not intractable, without status epilepticus 🦟
                 Epilepsy NOS
                 Epileptic convulsions NOS
                 Epileptic fits NOS
                 Epileptic seizures NOS
                 Recurrent seizures NOS
                 Seizure disorder NOS
                 Coding Clinic: 2024, Q2, P9; 2021, Q2, P3

  ● **G40.91**   Epilepsy, unspecified, intractable
         Intractable seizure disorder NOS

        G40.911   Epilepsy, unspecified, intractable, with status epilepticus 🦟

        G40.919   Epilepsy, unspecified, intractable, without status epilepticus 🦟

● **G40.A**   Absence epileptic syndrome
         Childhood absence epilepsy [pyknolepsy]
         Juvenile absence epilepsy
         Absence epileptic syndrome, NOS

  ● **G40.A0**   Absence epileptic syndrome, not intractable

        G40.A01   Absence epileptic syndrome, not intractable, with status epilepticus 🦟

        G40.A09   Absence epileptic syndrome, not intractable, without status epilepticus 🦟

● **G40.A1**   Absence epileptic syndrome, intractable

        G40.A11   Absence epileptic syndrome, intractable, with status epilepticus 🦟

        G40.A19   Absence epileptic syndrome, intractable, without status epilepticus 🦟

● **G40.B**   Juvenile myoclonic epilepsy [impulsive petit mal]

  ● **G40.B0**   Juvenile myoclonic epilepsy, not intractable

        G40.B01   Juvenile myoclonic epilepsy, not intractable, with status epilepticus 🦟

        G40.B09   Juvenile myoclonic epilepsy, not intractable, without status epilepticus 🦟

  ● **G40.B1**   Juvenile myoclonic epilepsy, intractable

        G40.B11   Juvenile myoclonic epilepsy, intractable, with status epilepticus 🦟

        G40.B19   Juvenile myoclonic epilepsy, intractable, without status epilepticus 🦟

● **G40.C**   Lafora progressive myoclonus epilepsy
         Lafora body disease
         Code also, if applicable, associated conditions such as dementia (F02.8-)

  ● **G40.C0**   Lafora progressive myoclonus epilepsy, not intractable

        G40.C01   Lafora progressive myoclonus epilepsy, not intractable, with status epilepticus

        G40.C09   Lafora progressive myoclonus epilepsy, not intractable, without status epilepticus
                 Lafora progressive myoclonus epilepsy NOS

  ● **G40.C1**   Lafora progressive myoclonus epilepsy, intractable

        G40.C11   Lafora progressive myoclonus epilepsy, intractable, with status epilepticus

        G40.C19   Lafora progressive myoclonus epilepsy, intractable, without status epilepticus

● **G43**   Migraine

         Note: The following terms are to be considered equivalent to intractable: pharmacoresistant (pharmacologically resistant), treatment resistant, refractory (medically) and poorly controlled

         Use additional code for adverse effect, if applicable, to identify drug (T36-T50 with fifth or sixth character 5)

         Excludes1   headache NOS (R51.9)
                       lower half migraine (G44.00)

         Excludes2   headache syndromes (G44.-)

● **G43.0**   Migraine without aura
         Neurological disorder, generally recurring headaches without early symptom (aura)
         Common migraine

         Excludes1   chronic migraine without aura (G43.7-)

  ● **G43.00**   Migraine without aura, not intractable
         Neurological disorder, generally recurring headaches without early symptom (aura); resistant to cure, relief, or control
         Migraine without aura without mention of refractory migraine

        G43.001   Migraine without aura, not intractable, with status migrainosus

        G43.009   Migraine without aura, not intractable, without status migrainosus
                 Migraine without aura NOS

CHAPTER 6 (G00-G99)

Item 6–4 Migraine headache is described as an intense pulsing or throbbing pain in one area of the head. It can be accompanied by extreme sensitivity to light (photophobic) and sound and is three times more common in women than in men. Symptoms include nausea and vomiting. Research indicates migraine headaches are caused by inherited abnormalities in genes that control the activities of certain cell populations in the brain.

● **G43.01   Migraine without aura, intractable**
>   *Intractable migraine: Not easily cured or managed;*
>   *relentless pain from a migraine*
>   Migraine without aura with refractory migraine

    G43.011   Migraine without aura, intractable,
    with status migrainosus

    G43.019   Migraine without aura, intractable,
    without status migrainosus

● **G43.1   Migraine with aura**
>   Basilar migraine
>   Classical migraine
>   Migraine equivalents
>   Migraine preceded or accompanied by transient focal
>   neurological phenomena
>   Migraine triggered seizures
>   Migraine with acute-onset aura
>   Migraine with aura without headache (migraine
>   equivalents)
>   Migraine with prolonged aura
>   Migraine with typical aura
>   Retinal migraine
>   Code also any associated seizure (G40.-, R56.9)
>   chronic migraine with aura (G43.E-)
>   **Excludes1**   persistent migraine aura (G43.5-, G43.6-)

● **G43.10   Migraine with aura, not intractable**
>   Migraine with aura without mention of
>   refractory migraine

    G43.101   Migraine with aura, not intractable,
    with status migrainosus

    G43.109   Migraine with aura, not intractable,
    without status migrainosus
>   Migraine with aura NOS

● **G43.11   Migraine with aura, intractable**
>   Migraine with aura with refractory migraine

    G43.111   Migraine with aura, intractable, with
    status migrainosus

    G43.119   Migraine with aura, intractable,
    without status migrainosus

● **G43.4   Hemiplegic migraine**
>   *Inherited migraine disorder causing temporary paralysis of*
>   *one side of body followed by severe headache and nausea*
>   Familial migraine
>   Sporadic migraine

● **G43.40   Hemiplegic migraine, not intractable**
>   Hemiplegic migraine without refractory
>   migraine

    G43.401   Hemiplegic migraine, not intractable,
    with status migrainosus

    G43.409   Hemiplegic migraine, not intractable,
    without status migrainosus
>   Hemiplegic migraine NOS

● **G43.41   Hemiplegic migraine, intractable**
>   Hemiplegic migraine with refractory migraine

    G43.411   Hemiplegic migraine, intractable,
    with status migrainosus

    G43.419   Hemiplegic migraine, intractable,
    without status migrainosus

● **G43.5   Persistent migraine aura without cerebral infarction**

● **G43.50   Persistent migraine aura without cerebral**
infarction, not intractable
>   Persistent migraine aura without cerebral
>   infarction, without refractory migraine

    G43.501   Persistent migraine aura without
    cerebral infarction, not intractable,
    with status migrainosus

    G43.509   Persistent migraine aura without
    cerebral infarction, not intractable,
    without status migrainosus
>   Persistent migraine aura NOS

● **G43.51   Persistent migraine aura without cerebral**
infarction, intractable
>   Persistent migraine aura without cerebral
>   infarction, with refractory migraine

    G43.511   Persistent migraine aura without
    cerebral infarction, intractable, with
    status migrainosus

    G43.519   Persistent migraine aura without
    cerebral infarction, intractable,
    without status migrainosus

● **G43.6   Persistent migraine aura with cerebral infarction**
>   *Visual, motor, or psychic disturbances, paresthesias, and*
>   *related neurologic abnormalities accompanying*
>   *migraine*
>   Code also the type of cerebral infarction (I63.-)

● **G43.60   Persistent migraine aura with cerebral**
infarction, not intractable
>   Persistent migraine aura with cerebral
>   infarction, without refractory migraine

    G43.601   Persistent migraine aura with cerebral
    infarction, not intractable, with status
    migrainosus

    G43.609   Persistent migraine aura with cerebral
    infarction, not intractable, without
    status migrainosus

● **G43.61   Persistent migraine aura with cerebral**
infarction, intractable
>   Persistent migraine aura with cerebral
>   infarction, with refractory migraine

    G43.611   Persistent migraine aura with cerebral
    infarction, intractable, with status
    migrainosus

    G43.619   Persistent migraine aura with cerebral
    infarction, intractable, without status
    migrainosus

● **G43.7   Chronic migraine without aura**
>   Transformed migraine
>   **Excludes1**   migraine without aura (G43.0-)

● **G43.70   Chronic migraine without aura, not intractable**
>   Chronic migraine without aura, without
>   refractory migraine

    G43.701   Chronic migraine without aura, not
    intractable, with status migrainosus

    G43.709   Chronic migraine without aura,
    not intractable, without status
    migrainosus
>   Chronic migraine without aura NOS

● **G43.71   Chronic migraine without aura, intractable**
>   Chronic migraine without aura, with refractory
>   migraine

    G43.711   Chronic migraine without aura,
    intractable, with status migrainosus

    G43.719   Chronic migraine without aura,
    intractable, without status
    migrainosus

● **G43.8   Other migraine**

● **G43.80   Other migraine, not intractable**
>   Other migraine, without refractory migraine

    G43.801   Other migraine, not intractable, with
    status migrainosus

    G43.809   Other migraine, not intractable,
    without status migrainosus

● **G43.81   Other migraine, intractable**
>   Other migraine, with refractory migraine

    G43.811   Other migraine, intractable, with
    status migrainosus

    G43.819   Other migraine, intractable, without
    status migrainosus

▶ New   ⇒ Revised   ~~deleted~~ Deleted   Excludes 1   Excludes 2   Includes   Use additional   Code first   Code also   Key words

OGCR Official Guidelines   X Assign placeholder X   ● Use Additional Character(s)   ▶ Manifestation Code   🦟 Hierarchical Condition Category   **Coding Clinic**

● **G43.82   Menstrual migraine, not intractable**
Menstrual headache, not intractable
Menstrual migraine, without refractory migraine
Menstrually related migraine, not intractable
Pre-menstrual headache, not intractable
Pre-menstrual migraine, not intractable
Pure menstrual migraine, not intractable

Code also associated premenstrual tension
syndrome (N94.3)

  G43.821   Menstrual migraine, not intractable, with status migrainosus ♀

  G43.829   Menstrual migraine, not intractable, without status migrainosus ♀
Menstrual migraine NOS

● **G43.83   Menstrual migraine, intractable**
Menstrual headache, intractable
Menstrual migraine, with refractory migraine
Menstrually related migraine, intractable
Pre-menstrual headache, intractable
Pre-menstrual migraine, intractable
Pure menstrual migraine, intractable

Code also associated premenstrual tension
syndrome (N94.3)

  G43.831   Menstrual migraine, intractable, with status migrainosus ♀

  G43.839   Menstrual migraine, intractable, without status migrainosus ♀

● **G43.9   Migraine, unspecified**
  ● **G43.90   Migraine, unspecified, not intractable**
Migraine, unspecified, without refractory
migraine

  G43.901   Migraine, unspecified, not intractable, with status migrainosus
Status migrainosus NOS

  G43.909   Migraine, unspecified, not intractable, without status migrainosus
Migraine NOS

  ● **G43.91   Migraine, unspecified, intractable**
Migraine, unspecified, with refractory
migraine

  G43.911   Migraine, unspecified, intractable, with status migrainosus

  G43.919   Migraine, unspecified, intractable, without status migrainosus

● **G43.A   Cyclical vomiting**
  Excludes1   cyclical vomiting syndrome unrelated to migraine (R11.15)

  G43.A0   Cyclical vomiting, in migraine, not intractable
Cyclical vomiting, without refractory migraine

  G43.A1   Cyclical vomiting, in migraine, intractable
Cyclical vomiting, with refractory migraine

● **G43.B   Ophthalmoplegic migraine**
  G43.B0   Ophthalmoplegic migraine, not intractable
Ophthalmoplegic migraine, without refractory
migraine

  G43.B1   Ophthalmoplegic migraine, intractable
Ophthalmoplegic migraine, with refractory
migraine

● **G43.C   Periodic headache syndromes in child or adult**
  G43.C0   Periodic headache syndromes in child or adult, not intractable
Periodic headache syndromes in child or adult,
without refractory migraine

  G43.C1   Periodic headache syndromes in child or adult, intractable
Periodic headache syndromes in child or adult,
with refractory migraine

● **G43.D   Abdominal migraine**
  G43.D0   Abdominal migraine, not intractable
Abdominal migraine, without refractory
migraine

  G43.D1   Abdominal migraine, intractable
Abdominal migraine, with refractory migraine

● **G43.E   Chronic migraine with aura**
  Excludes1   migraine with aura (G43.1-)
  ● **G43.E0   Chronic migraine with aura, not intractable**
Chronic migraine with aura, without refractory
migraine

  G43.E01   Chronic migraine with aura, not intractable, with status migrainosus

  G43.E09   Chronic migraine with aura, not intractable, without status migrainosus
Chronic migraine with aura NOS

  ● **G43.E1   Chronic migraine with aura, intractable**
Chronic migraine with aura, with refractory
migraine

  G43.E11   Chronic migraine with aura, intractable, with status migrainosus

  G43.E19   Chronic migraine with aura, intractable, without status migrainosus

● **G44   Other headache syndromes**
  Excludes1   headache NOS (R51.9)
  Excludes2   atypical facial pain (G50.1)
               headache due to lumbar puncture (G97.1)
               migraines (G43.-)
               trigeminal neuralgia (G50.0)

  ● **G44.0   Cluster headaches and other trigeminal autonomic cephalgias (TAC)**
    ● **G44.00   Cluster headache syndrome, unspecified**
Ciliary neuralgia
Cluster headache NOS
Histamine cephalgia
Lower half migraine
Migrainous neuralgia

  G44.001   Cluster headache syndrome, unspecified, intractable

  G44.009   Cluster headache syndrome, unspecified, not intractable
Cluster headache syndrome NOS

  ● **G44.01   Episodic cluster headache**
  G44.011   Episodic cluster headache, intractable
  G44.019   Episodic cluster headache, not intractable
Episodic cluster headache NOS

  ● **G44.02   Chronic cluster headache**
  G44.021   Chronic cluster headache, intractable
  G44.029   Chronic cluster headache, not intractable
Chronic cluster headache NOS

  ● **G44.03   Episodic paroxysmal hemicrania**
Paroxysmal hemicrania NOS
  G44.031   Episodic paroxysmal hemicrania, intractable
  G44.039   Episodic paroxysmal hemicrania, not intractable
Episodic paroxysmal hemicrania
NOS

  ● **G44.04   Chronic paroxysmal hemicrania**
Unilateral headache
  G44.041   Chronic paroxysmal hemicrania, intractable
  G44.049   Chronic paroxysmal hemicrania, not intractable
Chronic paroxysmal hemicrania NOS

  ● **G44.05   Short lasting unilateral neuralgiform headache with conjunctival injection and tearing (SUNCT)**
  G44.051   Short lasting unilateral neuralgiform headache with conjunctival injection and tearing (SUNCT), intractable

CHAPTER 6 (G00-G99)

G44.059   **Short lasting unilateral neuralgiform headache with conjunctival injection and tearing (SUNCT), not intractable**
    Short lasting unilateral neuralgiform headache with conjunctival injection and tearing (SUNCT) NOS

● **G44.09**   **Other trigeminal autonomic cephalgias (TAC)**
    Cluster headaches

    G44.091   **Other trigeminal autonomic cephalgias (TAC), intractable**

    G44.099   **Other trigeminal autonomic cephalgias (TAC), not intractable**

G44.1   **Vascular headache, not elsewhere classified**
    Excludes2   cluster headache (G44.0)
              complicated headache syndromes (G44.5-)
              drug-induced headache (G44.4-)
              migraine (G43.-)
              other specified headache syndromes (G44.8-)
              post-traumatic headache (G44.3-)
              tension-type headache (G44.2-)

● **G44.2**   **Tension-type headache**
  ● **G44.20**   **Tension-type headache, unspecified**
    G44.201   **Tension-type headache, unspecified, intractable**
    G44.209   **Tension-type headache, unspecified, not intractable**
        Tension headache NOS

  ● **G44.21**   **Episodic tension-type headache**
    G44.211   **Episodic tension-type headache, intractable**
    G44.219   **Episodic tension-type headache, not intractable**
        Episodic tension-type headache NOS

  ● **G44.22**   **Chronic tension-type headache**
    G44.221   **Chronic tension-type headache, intractable**
    G44.229   **Chronic tension-type headache, not intractable**
        Chronic tension-type headache NOS

● **G44.3**   **Post-traumatic headache**
  ● **G44.30**   **Post-traumatic headache, unspecified**
    G44.301   **Post-traumatic headache, unspecified, intractable**
    G44.309   **Post-traumatic headache, unspecified, not intractable**
        Post-traumatic headache NOS

  ● **G44.31**   **Acute post-traumatic headache**
    G44.311   **Acute post-traumatic headache, intractable**
    G44.319   **Acute post-traumatic headache, not intractable**
        Acute post-traumatic headache NOS

  ● **G44.32**   **Chronic post-traumatic headache**
    G44.321   **Chronic post-traumatic headache, intractable**
    G44.329   **Chronic post-traumatic headache, not intractable**
        Chronic post-traumatic headache NOS

● **G44.4**   **Drug-induced headache, not elsewhere classified**
    Medication overuse headache
    Use additional code for adverse effect, if applicable, to identify drug (T36-T50 with fifth or sixth character 5)

    G44.40   **Drug-induced headache, not elsewhere classified, not intractable**
    G44.41   **Drug-induced headache, not elsewhere classified, intractable**

● **G44.5**   **Complicated headache syndromes**
    G44.51   **Hemicrania continua**
        Persistent unilateral headache
    G44.52   **New daily persistent headache (NDPH)**
    G44.53   **Primary thunderclap headache**
    G44.59   **Other complicated headache syndrome**

● **G44.8**   **Other specified headache syndromes**
    Excludes2   headache with orthostatic or positional component, not elsewhere classified (R51.0)

    G44.81   **Hypnic headache**
        Benign primary headaches
    G44.82   **Headache associated with sexual activity**
        Orgasmic headache
        Preorgasmic headache
    G44.83   **Primary cough headache**
    G44.84   **Primary exertional headache**
    G44.85   **Primary stabbing headache**
    G44.86   **Cervicogenic headache**
        Code also associated cervical spinal condition, if known
        Coding Clinic: 2021, Q4, P12
    G44.89   **Other headache syndrome**

● **G45**   **Transient cerebral ischemic attacks and related syndromes**
    Excludes1   neonatal cerebral ischemia (P91.0)
              transient retinal artery occlusion (H34.0-)
    Coding Clinic: 2023, Q1, P37; 2018, Q2, P9

  G45.0   **Vertebro-basilar artery syndrome**
  G45.1   **Carotid artery syndrome (hemispheric)**
  G45.2   **Multiple and bilateral precerebral artery syndromes**
  G45.3   **Amaurosis fugax**
    Transient visual loss in one eye
  G45.4   **Transient global amnesia**
    Episode of short-term memory loss, nonrecurrent, lasting few hours
    Excludes1   amnesia NOS (R41.3)
  G45.8   **Other transient cerebral ischemic attacks and related syndromes**
  G45.9   **Transient cerebral ischemic attack, unspecified**
    Spasm of cerebral artery
    TIA
    Transient cerebral ischemia NOS

● **G46**   **Vascular syndromes of brain in cerebrovascular diseases**
    Code first underlying cerebrovascular disease (I60-I69)
  G46.0   **Middle cerebral artery syndrome**
  G46.1   **Anterior cerebral artery syndrome**
  G46.2   **Posterior cerebral artery syndrome**
  G46.3   **Brain stem stroke syndrome**
    Benedikt syndrome
    Claude syndrome
    Foville syndrome
    Millard-Gubler syndrome
    Wallenberg syndrome
    Weber syndrome
  G46.4   **Cerebellar stroke syndrome**
  G46.5   **Pure motor lacunar syndrome**
    Occlusion of single deep penetrating artery
  G46.6   **Pure sensory lacunar syndrome**
  G46.7   **Other lacunar syndromes**
  G46.8   **Other vascular syndromes of brain in cerebrovascular diseases**

● **G47**   **Sleep disorders**
    Excludes2   nightmares (F51.5)
              nonorganic sleep disorders (F51.-)
              sleep terrors (F51.4)
              sleepwalking (F51.3)

CHAPTER 6 (G00-G99)

▶ New   ⇒ Revised   ~~deleted~~ Deleted   Excludes 1   Excludes 2   Includes   Use additional   Code first   Code also   Key words
OGCR Official Guidelines   X Assign placeholder X   ● Use Additional Character(s)   ▌ Manifestation Code   Hierarchical Condition Category   Coding Clinic

● G47.0 **Insomnia**
     Excludes2   alcohol related insomnia (F10.182,
                   F10.282, F10.982)
               drug-related insomnia (F11.182, F11.282,
                   F11.982, F13.182, F13.282, F13.982,
                   F14.182, F14.282, F14.982, F15.182,
                   F15.282, F15.982, F19.182, F19.282,
                   F19.982)
               idiopathic insomnia (F51.01)
               insomnia due to a mental disorder
                   (F51.05)
               insomnia not due to a substance or known
                   physiological condition (F51.0-)
               nonorganic insomnia (F51.0-)
               primary insomnia (F51.01)
               sleep apnea (G47.3-)

    G47.00 **Insomnia, unspecified**
        Insomnia NOS

    G47.01 **Insomnia due to medical condition**
        Code also associated medical condition

    G47.09 **Other insomnia**

● G47.1 **Hypersomnia**
     Excludes2   alcohol-related hypersomnia (F10.182,
                   F10.282, F10.982)
               drug-related hypersomnia (F11.182,
                   F11.282, F11.982, F13.182, F13.282,
                   F13.982, F14.182, F14.282, F14.982,
                   F15.182, F15.282, F15.982, F19.182,
                   F19.282, F19.982)
               hypersomnia due to a mental disorder
                   (F51.13)
               hypersomnia not due to a substance or
                   known physiological condition (F51.1-)
               primary hypersomnia (F51.11)
               sleep apnea (G47.3-)

    G47.10 **Hypersomnia, unspecified**
        Hypersomnia NOS

    G47.11 **Idiopathic hypersomnia with long sleep time**
        Idiopathic hypersomnia NOS

    G47.12 **Idiopathic hypersomnia without long sleep time**

    G47.13 **Recurrent hypersomnia**
        Kleine-Levin syndrome
        Menstrual related hypersomnia

    G47.14 **Hypersomnia due to medical condition**
        Code also associated medical condition

    G47.19 **Other hypersomnia**

● G47.2 **Circadian rhythm sleep disorders**
        Disorders of the sleep wake schedule
        Inversion of nyctohemeral rhythm
        Inversion of sleep rhythm

    G47.20 **Circadian rhythm sleep disorder, unspecified
             type**
        Sleep wake schedule disorder NOS

    G47.21 **Circadian rhythm sleep disorder, delayed sleep
             phase type**
        Delayed sleep phase syndrome

    G47.22 **Circadian rhythm sleep disorder, advanced
             sleep phase type**

    G47.23 **Circadian rhythm sleep disorder, irregular sleep
             wake type**
        Irregular sleep-wake pattern

    G47.24 **Circadian rhythm sleep disorder, free running
             type**
        Circadian rhythm sleep disorder, non-24-hour
            sleep-wake type

    G47.25 **Circadian rhythm sleep disorder, jet lag type**

    G47.26 **Circadian rhythm sleep disorder, shift work
             type**

   ▷ *G47.27 Circadian rhythm sleep disorder in conditions
           classified elsewhere*
        Code first underlying condition

    G47.29 **Other circadian rhythm sleep disorder**

● G47.3 **Sleep apnea**
    *Characterized by episodes in which breathing stops during
    sleep*
    Code also any associated underlying condition
     Excludes1   apnea NOS (R06.81)
                   Cheyne-Stokes breathing (R06.3)
                   pickwickian syndrome (E66.2)
                   sleep apnea of newborn (P28.3-)

    G47.30 **Sleep apnea, unspecified**
        Sleep apnea NOS

    G47.31 **Primary central sleep apnea**
        Idiopathic central sleep apnea

    G47.32 **High altitude periodic breathing**

    G47.33 **Obstructive sleep apnea (adult) (pediatric)**
        Obstructive sleep apnea hypopnea
         Excludes1   obstructive sleep apnea of
                      newborn (P28.3-)

    G47.34 **Idiopathic sleep related nonobstructive alveolar
             hypoventilation**
        Sleep related hypoxia

    G47.35 **Congenital central alveolar hypoventilation
             syndrome**

   ▷ *G47.36 Sleep related hypoventilation in conditions
           classified elsewhere*
        Sleep related hypoxemia in conditions
            classified elsewhere
        Code first underlying condition

   ▷ *G47.37 Central sleep apnea in conditions classified
           elsewhere*
        Code first underlying condition

    G47.39 **Other sleep apnea**

● G47.4 **Narcolepsy and cataplexy**
    *Cataplexy is a disorder evidenced by seizures including
    minor slacking of the facial muscles to complete
    collapse and often affects people who have **narcolepsy**,
    a disorder in which there is great difficulty remaining
    awake during the daytime.*

● G47.41 **Narcolepsy**
        G47.411 **Narcolepsy with cataplexy**
        G47.419 **Narcolepsy without cataplexy**
               Narcolepsy NOS

● G47.42 **Narcolepsy in conditions classified elsewhere**
        Code first underlying condition
   ▷ *G47.421 Narcolepsy in conditions classified
               elsewhere with cataplexy*
   ▷ *G47.429 Narcolepsy in conditions classified
               elsewhere without cataplexy*

● G47.5 **Parasomnia**
     Excludes1   alcohol induced parasomnia (F10.182,
                   F10.282, F10.982)
               drug induced parasomnia (F11.182,
                   F11.282, F11.982, F13.182, F13.282,
                   F13.982, F14.182, F14.282, F14.982,
                   F15.182, F15.282, F15.982, F19.182,
                   F19.282, F19.982)
               parasomnia not due to a substance or
                   known physiological condition (F51.8)

    G47.50 **Parasomnia, unspecified**
        Parasomnia NOS

    G47.51 **Confusional arousals**

    G47.52 **REM sleep behavior disorder**

    G47.53 **Recurrent isolated sleep paralysis**

   ▷ *G47.54 Parasomnia in conditions classified elsewhere*
        Code first underlying condition

    G47.59 **Other parasomnia**

● G47.6 **Sleep related movement disorders**
     Excludes2   restless legs syndrome (G25.81)

    G47.61 **Periodic limb movement disorder**

    G47.62 **Sleep related leg cramps**

CHAPTER 6 (G00–G99)

G47.63   **Sleep related bruxism**
   Excludes1 psychogenic bruxism (F45.8)
   Coding Clinic: 2016, Q4, P118

G47.69   **Other sleep related movement disorders**

G47.8   **Other sleep disorders**
  Other specified sleep-wake disorder

G47.9   **Sleep disorder, unspecified**
  Sleep disorder NOS
  Unspecified sleep-wake disorder

★ **(See Plate 6 of the Anatomy Illustrations.)**

NERVE, NERVE ROOT AND PLEXUS DISORDERS (G50-G59)

Excludes1 current traumatic nerve, nerve root and plexus
     disorders - see Injury, nerve by body region
    neuralgia NOS (M79.2)
    neuritis NOS (M79.2)
    peripheral neuritis in pregnancy (O26.82-)
    radiculitis NOS (M54.1-)

● **G50** **Disorders of trigeminal nerve**
  Includes disorders of 5th cranial nerve

G50.0 **Trigeminal neuralgia**
  Syndrome of paroxysmal facial pain
  Tic douloureux

G50.1 **Atypical facial pain**

G50.8 **Other disorders of trigeminal nerve**

G50.9 **Disorder of trigeminal nerve, unspecified**

● **G51** **Facial nerve disorders**
  Includes disorders of 7th cranial nerve

G51.0 **Bell's palsy**
  Facial palsy

G51.1 **Geniculate ganglionitis**
  Rare disorder with symptoms of severe pain deep in ear,
   spreading to ear canal, outer ear, mastoid or eye regions
   Excludes1 postherpetic geniculate ganglionitis
       (B02.21)

G51.2 **Melkersson's syndrome**
  Melkersson-Rosenthal syndrome

● G51.3 **Clonic hemifacial spasm**

  G51.31 **Clonic hemifacial spasm, right**

  G51.32 **Clonic hemifacial spasm, left**
    Coding Clinic: 2018, Q4, P10

  G51.33 **Clonic hemifacial spasm, bilateral**

  G51.39 **Clonic hemifacial spasm, unspecified**

G51.4 **Facial myokymia**
  Involuntary facial muscle movement

G51.8 **Other disorders of facial nerve**

G51.9 **Disorder of facial nerve, unspecified**

● **G52** **Disorders of other cranial nerves**
  Excludes2 disorders of acoustic [8th] nerve (H93.3)
     disorders of optic [2nd] nerve (H46, H47.0)
     paralytic strabismus due to nerve palsy
      (H49.0-H49.2)

G52.0 **Disorders of olfactory nerve**
  Disorders of 1st cranial nerve

G52.1 **Disorders of glossopharyngeal nerve**
  Disorder of 9th cranial nerve
  Glossopharyngeal neuralgia

G52.2 **Disorders of vagus nerve**
  Disorders of pneumogastric [10th] nerve

G52.3 **Disorders of hypoglossal nerve**
  Disorders of 12th cranial nerve

G52.7 **Disorders of multiple cranial nerves**
  Polyneuritis cranialis

G52.8 **Disorders of other specified cranial nerves**

G52.9 **Cranial nerve disorder, unspecified**

Item 6-5 Trigeminal neuralgia, tic douloureux, is a pain syndrome diagnosed from the patient's history alone. The condition is characterized by pain and a brief facial spasm or tic. Pain is unilateral and follows the sensory distribution of cranial nerve V, typically radiating to the maxillary (V2) or mandibular (V3) area.

Item 6-6 The most common facial nerve disorder is **Bell's Palsy,** which occurs suddenly and results in facial drooping unilaterally. This disorder is the result of a reaction to a virus that causes the facial nerve in the ear to swell, resulting in pressure in the bony canal.

▶ G53 *Cranial nerve disorders in diseases classified elsewhere*
  Code first underlying disease, such as:
   neoplasm (C00-D49)
   Excludes1 multiple cranial nerve palsy in sarcoidosis (D86.82)
      multiple cranial nerve palsy in syphilis (A52.15)
      postherpetic geniculate ganglionitis (B02.21)
      postherpetic trigeminal neuralgia (B02.22)

● G54 **Nerve root and plexus disorders**
  Raiculopathy (nerve root disorder) caused by pressure on nerve root,
   most common cause is herniation of intervertebral disk. Plexus
   disorders (plexopathies) are due to compression or injury.
   Excludes1 current traumatic nerve root and plexus disorders
      - see nerve injury by body region
     intervertebral disc disorders (M50-M51)
     neuralgia or neuritis NOS (M79.2)
     neuritis or radiculitis brachial NOS (M54.13)
     neuritis or radiculitis lumbar NOS (M54.16)
     neuritis or radiculitis lumbosacral NOS (M54.17)
     neuritis or radiculitis thoracic NOS (M54.14)
     radiculitis NOS (M54.10)
     radiculopathy NOS (M54.10)
     spondylosis (M47.-)

G54.0 **Brachial plexus disorders**
  Thoracic outlet syndrome
  Coding Clinic: 2023, Q2, P8

G54.1 **Lumbosacral plexus disorders**

G54.2 **Cervical root disorders, not elsewhere classified**

G54.3 **Thoracic root disorders, not elsewhere classified**

G54.4 **Lumbosacral root disorders, not elsewhere classified**

G54.5 **Neuralgic amyotrophy**
  Parsonage-Aldren-Turner syndrome
  Shoulder-girdle neuritis
   Excludes1 neuralgic amyotrophy in diabetes
       mellitus (E08-E13 with .44)

G54.6 **Phantom limb syndrome with pain** 🅗
  Sensations (cramping, itching) in a limb that no longer exists

G54.7 **Phantom limb syndrome without pain** 🅗
  Phantom limb syndrome NOS

G54.8 **Other nerve root and plexus disorders**

G54.9 **Nerve root and plexus disorder, unspecified**

▶ G55 *Nerve root and plexus compressions in diseases classified elsewhere*
  Code first underlying disease, such as:
   neoplasm (C00-D49)
   Excludes1 nerve root compression (due to) (in) ankylosing
      spondylitis (M45.-)
     nerve root compression (due to) (in)dorsopathies
      (M53.-, M54.-)
     nerve root compression (due to) (in)intervertebral
      disc disorders (M50.1-, M51.1-)
     nerve root compression (due to) (in)
      spondylopathies (M46.-, M48.-)
     nerve root compression (due to) (in) spondylosis
      (M47.0-, M47.2-)

★ **(See Plates 472 and 473 on pages 56 and 57.)**

● **G56　Mononeuropathies of upper limb**

　　Excludes1　current traumatic nerve disorder - see nerve injury by body region

● **G56.0　Carpal tunnel syndrome**

　　G56.00　Carpal tunnel syndrome, unspecified upper limb

　　G56.01　Carpal tunnel syndrome, right upper limb

　　G56.02　Carpal tunnel syndrome, left upper limb

　　G56.03　Carpal tunnel syndrome, bilateral upper limbs
　　　　　　Coding Clinic: 2016, Q4, P17

● **G56.1　Other lesions of median nerve**

　　G56.10　Other lesions of median nerve, unspecified side

　　G56.11　Other lesions of median nerve, right upper limb

　　G56.12　Other lesions of median nerve, left upper limb

　　G56.13　Other lesions of median nerve, bilateral upper limbs
　　　　　　Coding Clinic: 2016, Q4, P17

● **G56.2　Lesion of ulnar nerve**
　　　　　Tardy ulnar nerve palsy

　　G56.20　Lesion of ulnar nerve, unspecified upper limb

　　G56.21　Lesion of ulnar nerve, right upper limb

　　G56.22　Lesion of ulnar nerve, left upper limb

　　G56.23　Lesion of ulnar nerve, bilateral upper limbs
　　　　　　Coding Clinic: 2016, Q4, P17

● **G56.3　Lesion of radial nerve**

　　G56.30　Lesion of radial nerve, unspecified upper limb

　　G56.31　Lesion of radial nerve, right upper limb

　　G56.32　Lesion of radial nerve, left upper limb

　　G56.33　Lesion of radial nerve, bilateral upper limbs
　　　　　　Coding Clinic: 2016, Q4, P17

● **G56.4　Causalgia of upper limb**
　　　　　Intense burning pain and sensitivity to slight touch
　　　　　Complex regional pain syndrome II of upper limb

　　Excludes1　complex regional pain syndrome I of lower limb (G90.52-)
　　　　　　complex regional pain syndrome I of upper limb (G90.51-)
　　　　　　complex regional pain syndrome II of lower limb (G57.7-)
　　　　　　reflex sympathetic dystrophy of lower limb (G90.52-)
　　　　　　reflex sympathetic dystrophy (G90.51-)

　　G56.40　Causalgia of unspecified upper limb

　　G56.41　Causalgia of right upper limb

　　G56.42　Causalgia of left upper limb

　　G56.43　Causalgia of bilateral upper limbs
　　　　　　Coding Clinic: 2016, Q4, P17

● **G56.8　Other specified mononeuropathies of upper limb**
　　　　　Disease of a single nerve
　　　　　Interdigital neuroma of upper limb

　　G56.80　Other specified mononeuropathies of unspecified upper limb

　　G56.81　Other specified mononeuropathies of right upper limb

　　G56.82　Other specified mononeuropathies of left upper limb

　　G56.83　Other specified mononeuropathies of bilateral upper limbs
　　　　　　Coding Clinic: 2016, Q4, P17

● **G56.9　Unspecified mononeuropathy of upper limb**
　　　　　Disease of a single nerve

　　G56.90　Unspecified mononeuropathy of unspecified upper limb

　　G56.91　Unspecified mononeuropathy of right upper limb

　　G56.92　Unspecified mononeuropathy of left upper limb

　　G56.93　Unspecified mononeuropathy of bilateral upper limbs
　　　　　　Coding Clinic: 2016, Q4, P17

● **G57　Mononeuropathies of lower limb**

　　Excludes1　current traumatic nerve disorder - see nerve injury by body region

★ **(See Plates 544 and 545 on pages 58 and 59.)**

● **G57.0　Lesion of sciatic nerve**

　　Excludes1　sciatica NOS (M54.3-)

　　Excludes2　sciatica attributed to intervertebral disc disorder (M51.1.-)

　　G57.00　Lesion of sciatic nerve, unspecified lower limb

　　G57.01　Lesion of sciatic nerve, right lower limb

　　G57.02　Lesion of sciatic nerve, left lower limb

　　G57.03　Lesion of sciatic nerve, bilateral lower limbs
　　　　　　Coding Clinic: 2016, Q4, P1

● **G57.1　Meralgia paresthetica**
　　　　　Numbness or pain in outer thigh caused by injury to nerve
　　　　　Lateral cutaneous nerve of thigh syndrome

　　G57.10　Meralgia paresthetica, unspecified lower limb

　　G57.11　Meralgia paresthetica, right lower limb

　　G57.12　Meralgia paresthetica, left lower limb

　　G57.13　Meralgia paresthetica, bilateral lower limbs
　　　　　　Coding Clinic: 2016, Q4, P1

● **G57.2　Lesion of femoral nerve**

　　G57.20　Lesion of femoral nerve, unspecified lower limb

　　G57.21　Lesion of femoral nerve, right lower limb

　　G57.22　Lesion of femoral nerve, left lower limb

　　G57.23　Lesion of femoral nerve, bilateral lower limbs
　　　　　　Coding Clinic: 2016, Q4, P1

● **G57.3　Lesion of lateral popliteal nerve**
　　　　　Peroneal nerve palsy

　　G57.30　Lesion of lateral popliteal nerve, unspecified lower limb

　　G57.31　Lesion of lateral popliteal nerve, right lower limb

　　G57.32　Lesion of lateral popliteal nerve, left lower limb

　　G57.33　Lesion of lateral popliteal nerve, bilateral lower limbs
　　　　　　Coding Clinic: 2016, Q4, P1

● **G57.4　Lesion of medial popliteal nerve**

　　G57.40　Lesion of medial popliteal nerve, unspecified lower limb

　　G57.41　Lesion of medial popliteal nerve, right lower limb

　　G57.42　Lesion of medial popliteal nerve, left lower limb

　　G57.43　Lesion of medial popliteal nerve, bilateral lower limbs
　　　　　　Coding Clinic: 2016, Q4, P1

● **G57.5　Tarsal tunnel syndrome**

　　G57.50　Tarsal tunnel syndrome, unspecified lower limb

　　G57.51　Tarsal tunnel syndrome, right lower limb

　　G57.52　Tarsal tunnel syndrome, left lower limb

　　G57.53　Tarsal tunnel syndrome, bilateral lower limbs
　　　　　　Coding Clinic: 2016, Q4, P1

● **G57.6　Lesion of plantar nerve**
　　　　　Morton's metatarsalgia

　　G57.60　Lesion of plantar nerve, unspecified lower limb

　　G57.61　Lesion of plantar nerve, right lower limb

　　G57.62　Lesion of plantar nerve, left lower limb

　　G57.63　Lesion of plantar nerve, bilateral lower limbs
　　　　　　Coding Clinic: 2016, Q4, P1

CHAPTER 6 (G00-G99)

CHAPTER 6 (G00–G99)

- **G57.7 Causalgia of lower limb**
    Complex regional pain syndrome II of lower limb
    Excludes1   complex regional pain syndrome I of lower limb (G90.52-)
    complex regional pain syndrome I of upper limb (G90.51-)
    complex regional pain syndrome II of upper limb (G56.4-)
    reflex sympathetic dystrophy of lower limb (G90.52-)
    reflex sympathetic dystrophy of upper limb (G90.51-)

    G57.70   **Causalgia of unspecified lower limb**
    G57.71   **Causalgia of right lower limb**
    G57.72   **Causalgia of left lower limb**
    G57.73   **Causalgia of bilateral lower limbs**
         Coding Clinic: 2016, Q4, P1

- **G57.8 Other specified mononeuropathies of lower limb**
    Interdigital neuroma of lower limb

    G57.80   **Other specified mononeuropathies of unspecified lower limb**
    G57.81   **Other specified mononeuropathies of right lower limb**
    G57.82   **Other specified mononeuropathies of left lower limb**
    G57.83   **Other specified mononeuropathies of bilateral lower limbs**
         Coding Clinic: 2016, Q4, P17

- **G57.9 Unspecified mononeuropathy of lower limb**

    G57.90   **Unspecified mononeuropathy of unspecified lower limb**
    G57.91   **Unspecified mononeuropathy of right lower limb**
    G57.92   **Unspecified mononeuropathy of left lower limb**
    G57.93   **Unspecified mononeuropathy of bilateral lower limbs**
         Coding Clinic: 2016, Q4, P17

- **G58 Other mononeuropathies**
    G58.0   **Intercostal neuropathy**
    G58.7   **Mononeuritis multiplex**
    G58.8   **Other specified mononeuropathies**
    G58.9   **Mononeuropathy, unspecified**

▶ *G59*   *Mononeuropathy in diseases classified elsewhere*
    Code first underlying disease
    Excludes1   diabetic mononeuropathy (E08-E13 with .41)
    syphilitic nerve paralysis (A52.19)
    syphilitic neuritis (A52.15)
    tuberculous mononeuropathy (A17.83)

POLYNEUROPATHIES AND OTHER DISORDERS OF THE PERIPHERAL NERVOUS SYSTEM (G60-G65)

Excludes1   neuralgia NOS (M79.2)
neuritis NOS (M79.2)
peripheral neuritis in pregnancy (O26.82-)
radiculitis NOS (M54.10)

- **G60 Hereditary and idiopathic neuropathy**
    G60.0 Hereditary motor and sensory neuropathy
    Charcot-Marie-Tooth disease
    Déjerine-Sottas disease
    Hereditary motor and sensory neuropathy, types I-IV
    Hypertrophic neuropathy of infancy
    Peroneal muscular atrophy (axonal type) (hypertrophic type)
    Roussy-Lévy syndrome

    G60.1 Refsum's disease
    Genetic disorder affecting fatty acid metabolism
    Infantile Refsum disease

    G60.2 Neuropathy in association with hereditary ataxia
    G60.3 Idiopathic progressive neuropathy

- **G60.8 Other hereditary and idiopathic neuropathies**
    Dominantly inherited sensory neuropathy
    Morvan's disease
    Nelaton's syndrome
    Recessively inherited sensory neuropathy

    G60.9 Hereditary and idiopathic neuropathy, unspecified

- **G61 Inflammatory polyneuropathy**
    G61.0 Guillain-Barré syndrome 🔖 Ⓔ PDX 93
    Autoimmune disease affecting peripheral nervous system
    Acute (post-)infective polyneuritis
    Miller Fisher Syndrome

    G61.1 Serum neuropathy 🔖
    Use additional code for adverse effect, if applicable, to identify serum (T50.-)

- **G61.8 Other inflammatory polyneuropathies**
    G61.81   **Chronic inflammatory demyelinating polyneuritis** 🔖
    G61.82   **Multifocal motor neuropathy** 🔖
    MMN
    G61.89   **Other inflammatory polyneuropathies** 🔖

    G61.9 Inflammatory polyneuropathy, unspecified 🔖

- **G62 Other and unspecified polyneuropathies**
    G62.0 Drug-induced polyneuropathy 🔖
    Use additional code for adverse effect, if applicable, to identify drug (T36-T50 with fifth or sixth character 5)

    G62.1 Alcoholic polyneuropathy 🔖
    Malfunction of many peripheral nerves throughout the body
    Coding Clinic: 2019, Q3, P8

    G62.2 Polyneuropathy due to other toxic agents 🔖
    Code first (T51-T65) to identify toxic agent

Figure 6-2 Actions of parasympathetic and sympathetic nerves. (From Chabner: The Language of Medicine, ed 9, St. Louis, Saunders, 2011)

Item 6–7 The **peripheral nervous system** consists of 31 pairs of spinal nerves, 12 pairs of cranial nerves, and the autonomic nerves, which are divided into the parasympathetic and sympathetic nerves. The cranial nerves are: olfactory (I), optic (II), oculomotor (III), trochlear (IV), trigeminal (V), abducens (VI), facial (VII), vestibulocochlear (VIII), glossopharyngeal (IX), vagus (X), accessory (XI), and hypoglossal (XII).

▶ New   ⇒ Revised   ~~deleted~~ Deleted   Excludes 1   Excludes 2   Includes   Use additional   Code first   Code also   Key words

OGCR Official Guidelines   X Assign placeholder X   ● Use Additional Character(s)   ▶ Manifestation Code   🔖 Hierarchical Condition Category   Coding Clinic

● G62.8   **Other specified polyneuropathies**
     G62.81   **Critical illness polyneuropathy** 🔍
         Acute motor neuropathy
     G62.82   **Radiation-induced polyneuropathy** 🔍
         Use additional external cause code (W88-W90, X39.0-) to identify cause
         Coding Clinic: 2016, Q4, P18
     G62.89   **Other specified polyneuropathies**
         Coding Clinic: 2016, Q2, P11
   G62.9   **Polyneuropathy, unspecified**
     Neuropathy NOS

▷ *G63*   *Polyneuropathy in diseases classified elsewhere* 🔍
     Code first underlying disease, such as:
       amyloidosis (E85.-)
       endocrine disease, except diabetes (E00-E07, E15-E16, E20-E34)
       metabolic diseases (E70-E88)
       neoplasm (C00-D49)
       nutritional deficiency (E40-E64)
     Excludes1   polyneuropathy (in):
         diabetes mellitus (E08-E13 with .42)
         diphtheria (A36.83)
         infectious mononucleosis complicated by polyneuropathy (B27.0-B27.9 with fifth character 1)
         Lyme disease (A69.22)
         mumps (B26.84)
         postherpetic (B02.23)
         rheumatoid arthritis (M05.5-)
         scleroderma (M34.83)
         systemic lupus erythematosus (M32.19)
     Coding Clinic: 2023, Q3, P19-20; 2021, Q1, P7; 2012, Q4, P100

  G64   **Other disorders of peripheral nervous system**
     Disorder of peripheral nervous system NOS

● **G65**   **Sequelae of inflammatory and toxic polyneuropathies**
     Code first condition resulting from (sequela) of inflammatory and toxic polyneuropathies
   G65.0   **Sequelae of Guillain-Barré syndrome** 🔍
   G65.1   **Sequelae of other inflammatory polyneuropathy** 🔍
   G65.2   **Sequelae of toxic polyneuropathy** 🔍

DISEASES OF MYONEURAL JUNCTION AND MUSCLE (G70-G73)

● **G70**   **Myasthenia gravis and other myoneural disorders**
     Excludes1   botulism (A05.1, A48.51-A48.52)
         transient neonatal myasthenia gravis (P94.0)

● **G70.0**   **Myasthenia gravis**
     Acquired and results in fatigable muscle weakness exacerbated by activity and improved with rest
     G70.00   **Myasthenia gravis without (acute) exacerbation** 🔍
         Myasthenia gravis NOS
         Coding Clinic: 2022, Q3, P16
     G70.01   **Myasthenia gravis with (acute) exacerbation** 🔍
         Myasthenia gravis in crisis
   G70.1   **Toxic myoneural disorders** 🔍
     Dysfunction at junction of muscle and motor nerve (myoneural junction)
     Code first (T51-T65) to identify toxic agent
   G70.2   **Congenital and developmental myasthenia** 🔍
● **G70.8**   **Other specified myoneural disorders**
     G70.80   **Lambert-Eaton syndrome, unspecified** 🔍
         Lambert-Eaton syndrome NOS
     ▷ *G70.81*   *Lambert-Eaton syndrome in disease classified elsewhere* 🔍
         Code first underlying disease
         Excludes1   Lambert-Eaton syndrome in neoplastic disease (G73.1)
     G70.89   **Other specified myoneural disorders** 🔍
   G70.9   **Myoneural disorder, unspecified** 🔍

● **G71**   **Primary disorders of muscles**
     Excludes2   arthrogryposis multiplex congenita (Q74.3)
         metabolic disorders (E70-E88)
         myositis (M60.-)
● **G71.0**   **Muscular dystrophy** 🔍
     G71.00   **Muscular dystrophy, unspecified** 🔍
     G71.01   **Duchenne or Becker muscular dystrophy** 🔍
         Autosomal recessive, childhood type, muscular dystrophy resembling Duchenne or Becker muscular dystrophy
         Benign [Becker] muscular dystrophy
         Severe [Duchenne] muscular dystrophy
     G71.02   **Facioscapulohumeral muscular dystrophy** 🔍
         Scapulohumeral muscular dystrophy
         Coding Clinic: 2018, Q4, P12
●   **G71.03**   **Limb girdle muscular dystrophies**
       G71.031   **Autosomal dominant limb girdle muscular dystrophy**
         LGMD D4 calpain-3-related
         LGMD D5 collagen 6-related
         Limb girdle muscular dystrophy type 1
       G71.032   **Autosomal recessive limb girdle muscular dystrophy due to calpain-3 dysfunction**
         Limb girdle muscular dystrophy type 2A
         LGMD R1 calpain-3-related
         Primary calpainopathy
       G71.033   **Limb girdle muscular dystrophy due to dysferlin dysfunction**
         Dysferlinopathy
         LGMD R2 dysferlin-related
         Limb girdle muscular dystrophy type 2B
         Miyoshi Myopathy type 1
●   **G71.034**   **Limb girdle muscular dystrophy due to sarcoglycan dysfunction**
       G71.0340   **Limb girdle muscular dystrophy due to sarcoglycan dysfunction, unspecified**
         Sarcoglycanopathy, NOS
       G71.0341   **Limb girdle muscular dystrophy due to alpha sarcoglycan dysfunction**
         Alpha sarcoglycanopathy
         Limb-girdle muscular dystrophy due to alpha-sarcoglycan deficiency
         Limb girdle muscular dystrophy type 2D
       G71.0342   **Limb girdle muscular dystrophy due to beta sarcoglycan dysfunction**
         Beta sarcoglycanopathy
         Limb girdle muscular dystrophy due to beta-sarcoglycan deficiency
         Limb girdle muscular dystrophy type 2E
       G71.0349   **Limb girdle muscular dystrophy due to other sarcoglycan dysfunction**
         Delta sarcoglycanopathy
         Delta-sarcoglycan-related LGMD R6
         Gamma sarcoglycanopathy
         Gamma-sarcoglycan-related LGMD R5
         Limb girdle muscular dystrophy type 2C
         Limb girdle muscular dystrophy type 2F

CHAPTER 6 (G00-G99)

Item 6–8 Muscular dystrophies (MD) are a group of rare inherited muscle diseases. Voluntary muscles become progressively weaker. In the late stages of MD, fat and connective tissue replace muscle fibers. In some types of muscular dystrophy, heart muscles, other involuntary muscles, and other organs are affected. **Myopathies** is a general term for neuromuscular diseases in which the muscle fibers dysfunction for any one of many reasons, resulting in muscular weakness.

G71.035 **Limb girdle muscular dystrophy due to anoctamin-5 dysfunction**
Anoctamin-5-related LGMD R12
Anoctaminopathy
Autosomal recessive limb girdle muscular dystrophy type 2L
Miyoshi myopathy type 3

G71.038 **Other limb girdle muscular dystrophy**
LGMD R9 FKRP-related
LGMD R22 collagen 6-related
Limb girdle muscular dystrophy due to fukutin related protein dysfunction
Limb girdle muscular dystrophy type 2I
Other autosomal recessive limb girdle muscular dystrophy

G71.039 **Limb girdle muscular dystrophy, unspecified**

G71.09 **Other specified muscular dystrophies**
Benign scapuloperoneal muscular dystrophy with early contractures [Emery-Dreifuss]
Congenital muscular dystrophy NOS
Congenital muscular dystrophy with specific morphological abnormalities of the muscle fiber
Distal muscular dystrophy
Ocular muscular dystrophy
Oculopharyngeal muscular dystrophy
Scapuloperoneal muscular dystrophy

● G71.1 **Myotonic disorders**
Inherited disorder that affects muscles tone

G71.11 **Myotonic muscular dystrophy**
Dystrophia myotonica [Steinert]
Myotonia atrophica
Myotonic dystrophy
Proximal myotonic myopathy (PROMM)
Steinert disease

G71.12 **Myotonia congenita**
Acetazolamide responsive myotonia congenita
Dominant myotonia congenita [Thomsen disease]
Myotonia levior
Recessive myotonia congenita [Becker disease]

G71.13 **Myotonic chondrodystrophy**
Chondrodystrophic myotonia
Congenital myotonic chondrodystrophy
Schwartz-Jampel disease

G71.14 **Drug induced myotonia**
Use additional code for adverse effect, if applicable, to identify drug (T36-T50 with fifth or sixth character 5)

G71.19 **Other specified myotonic disorders**
Myotonia fluctuans
Myotonia permanens
Neuromyotonia [Isaacs]
Paramyotonia congenita (of von Eulenburg)
Pseudomyotonia
Symptomatic myotonia

● G71.2 **Congenital myopathies**
Excludes2 arthrogryposis multiplex congenita (Q74.3)

G71.20 **Congenital myopathy, unspecified**
G71.21 **Nemaline myopathy**

● G71.22 **Centronuclear myopathy**
G71.220 **X-linked myotubular myopathy**
Myotubular (centronuclear) myopathy

G71.228 **Other centronuclear myopathy**
Autosomal centronuclear myopathy
Autosomal dominant centronuclear myopathy
Autosomal recessive centronuclear myopathy
Centronuclear myopathy, NOS

G71.29 **Other congenital myopathy**
Central core disease
Minicore disease
Multicore disease
Multiminicore disease

G71.3 **Mitochondrial myopathy, not elsewhere classified**
Myopathies associated with increased number of enlarged, often abnormal, mitochondria in muscle fibers
Excludes1 Kearns-Sayre syndrome (H49.81)
Leber's disease (H47.21)
Leigh's encephalopathy (G31.82)
mitochondrial metabolism disorders (E88.4.-)
Reye's syndrome (G93.7)

G71.8 **Other primary disorders of muscles**
G71.9 **Primary disorder of muscle, unspecified**
Hereditary myopathy NOS

● G72 **Other and unspecified myopathies**
Excludes1 arthrogryposis multiplex congenita (Q74.3)
dermatopolymyositis (M33.-)
ischemic infarction of muscle (M62.2-)
myositis (M60.-)
polymyositis (M33.2.-)

G72.0 **Drug-induced myopathy**
Use additional code for adverse effect, if applicable, to identify drug (T36-T50 with fifth or sixth character 5)

G72.1 **Alcoholic myopathy**
Use additional code to identify alcoholism (F10.-)

G72.2 **Myopathy due to other toxic agents**
Code first (T51-T65) to identify toxic agent

G72.3 **Periodic paralysis**
Familial periodic paralysis
Hyperkalemic periodic paralysis (familial)
Hypokalemic periodic paralysis (familial)
Myotonic periodic paralysis (familial)
Normokalemic paralysis (familial)
Potassium sensitive periodic paralysis
Excludes1 paramyotonia congenita (of von Eulenburg) (G71.19)

● G72.4 **Inflammatory and immune myopathies, not elsewhere classified**
G72.41 **Inclusion body myositis [IBM]**
G72.49 **Other inflammatory and immune myopathies, not elsewhere classified**
Inflammatory myopathy NOS

● G72.8 **Other specified myopathies**
G72.81 **Critical illness myopathy**
Acute necrotizing myopathy
Acute quadriplegic myopathy
Intensive care (ICU) myopathy
Myopathy of critical illness

G72.89 **Other specified myopathies**
G72.9 **Myopathy, unspecified**

● **G73** **Disorders of myoneural junction and muscle in diseases classified elsewhere**

▶ *G73.1* *Lambert-Eaton syndrome in neoplastic disease* 🐾

Rare autoimmune disorder affecting calcium channels of nerve-muscle (neuromuscular) junction

Code first underlying neoplasm (C00-D49)

Excludes1   Lambert-Eaton syndrome not associated with neoplasm (G70.80-G70.81)

▶ *G73.3* *Myasthenic syndromes in other diseases classified elsewhere* 🐾

Code first underlying disease, such as:
     neoplasm (C00-D49)
     thyrotoxicosis (E05.-)

▶ *G73.7* *Myopathy in diseases classified elsewhere*

Code first underlying disease, such as:
     glycogen storage disease (E74.0-)
     hyperparathyroidism (E21.0, E21.3)
     hypoparathyroidism (E20.-)
     lipid storage disorders (E75.-)

Excludes1   myopathy in:
     rheumatoid arthritis (M05.32)
     sarcoidosis (D86.87)
     scleroderma (M34.82)
     Sjögren syndrome (M35.03)
     systemic lupus erythematosus (M32.19)

CEREBRAL PALSY AND OTHER PARALYTIC SYNDROMES (G80-G83)

● **G80** **Cerebral palsy**

Excludes1   hereditary spastic paraplegia (G11.4)

G80.0 **Spastic quadriplegic cerebral palsy** 🐾
     Congenital spastic paralysis (cerebral)

G80.1 **Spastic diplegic cerebral palsy** 🐾
     Spastic cerebral palsy NOS

G80.2 **Spastic hemiplegic cerebral palsy** 🐾

G80.3 **Athetoid cerebral palsy** 🐾
     Result of damage to cerebellum or basal ganglia responsible for processing neuromuscular signals
     Double athetosis (syndrome)
     Dyskinetic cerebral palsy
     Dystonic cerebral palsy
     Vogt disease

G80.4 **Ataxic cerebral palsy** 🐾
     Poor muscle tone and coordination

G80.8 **Other cerebral palsy** 🐾
     Mixed cerebral palsy syndromes

G80.9 **Cerebral palsy, unspecified** 🐾
     Cerebral palsy NOS

OGCR Section I.C.6.a.

Dominant/nondominant side

Codes from category G81, Hemiplegia and hemiparesis, and subcategories, G83.1, Monoplegia of lower limb, G83.2, Monoplegia of upper limb, and G83.3, Monoplegia, unspecified, identify whether the dominant and nondominant side is affected. Should the affected side be documented, but not specified as dominant or nondominant, and the classification system does not indicate a default, code selection is as follows:

- For ambidextrous patients, the default should be dominant.
- If the left side is affected, the default is nondominant.
- If the right side is affected, the default is dominant.

Item 6–9   **Hemiplegia** is complete paralysis of one side of the body—arm, leg, and trunk. **Hemiparesis** is a generalized weakness or incomplete paralysis of one side of the body. If most activities (eating, writing) are performed with the right hand, the right is the dominant side, and the left is the nondominant side. **Quadriplegia,** also called tetraplegia, is the complete paralysis of all four limbs. **Quadriparesis** is the incomplete paralysis of all four limbs. Nerve damage in C1–C4 is associated with lower limb paralysis, and C5–C7 damage is associated with upper limb paralysis. **Diplegia** is the paralysis of the upper limbs. **Monoplegia** is the complete paralysis of one limb.

● **G81** **Hemiplegia and hemiparesis**

Note: This category is to be used only when hemiplegia (complete)(incomplete) is reported without further specification, or is stated to be old or longstanding but of unspecified cause. The category is also for use in multiple coding to identify these types of hemiplegia resulting from any cause.

Excludes1   congenital cerebral palsy (G80.-)
     hemiplegia and hemiparesis due to sequela of cerebrovascular disease (I69.05-, I69.15-, I69.25-, I69.35-, I69.85-, I69.95-)

Coding Clinic: 2012, Q4, P106

● **G81.0** **Flaccid hemiplegia**
     Paralysis of half of body with loss of tone of muscles of paralyzed part and absence of tendon reflexes

     G81.00 **Flaccid hemiplegia affecting unspecified side** 🐾
     G81.01 **Flaccid hemiplegia affecting right dominant side** 🐾
     G81.02 **Flaccid hemiplegia affecting left dominant side** 🐾
     G81.03 **Flaccid hemiplegia affecting right nondominant side** 🐾
     G81.04 **Flaccid hemiplegia affecting left nondominant side** 🐾

● **G81.1** **Spastic hemiplegia**
     Paralysis of half of body with spasticity of muscles of paralyzed part and increased tendon reflexes

     G81.10 **Spastic hemiplegia affecting unspecified side** 🐾
     G81.11 **Spastic hemiplegia affecting right dominant side** 🐾
     G81.12 **Spastic hemiplegia affecting left dominant side** 🐾
     G81.13 **Spastic hemiplegia affecting right nondominant side** 🐾
     G81.14 **Spastic hemiplegia affecting left nondominant side** 🐾

● **G81.9** **Hemiplegia, unspecified**

     G81.90 **Hemiplegia, unspecified affecting unspecified side** 🐾
     G81.91 **Hemiplegia, unspecified affecting right dominant side** 🐾
     G81.92 **Hemiplegia, unspecified affecting left dominant side** 🐾
     G81.93 **Hemiplegia, unspecified affecting right nondominant side** 🐾
     G81.94 **Hemiplegia, unspecified affecting left nondominant side** 🐾
     Coding Clinic: 2015, Q1, P26

● **G82** **Paraplegia (paraparesis) and quadriplegia (quadriparesis)**

Note: This category is to be used only when the listed conditions are reported without further specification, or are stated to be old or longstanding but of unspecified cause. The category is also for use in multiple coding to identify these conditions resulting from any cause.

Excludes1   congenital cerebral palsy (G80.-)
     functional quadriplegia (R53.2)
     hysterical paralysis (F44.4)

● **G82.2** **Paraplegia**
     Paralysis of both lower limbs NOS
     Paraparesis (lower) NOS
     Paraplegia (lower) NOS

     G82.20 **Paraplegia, unspecified** 🐾
          Coding Clinic: 2017, Q3, P3
     G82.21 **Paraplegia, complete** 🐾
     G82.22 **Paraplegia, incomplete** 🐾

● **G82.5** **Quadriplegia**
     Paralysis of all limbs; AKA tetraplegia

     G82.50 **Quadriplegia, unspecified** 🐾
     G82.51 **Quadriplegia, C1-C4 complete** 🐾
     G82.52 **Quadriplegia, C1-C4 incomplete** 🐾
          Coding Clinic: 2024, Q2, P23
     G82.53 **Quadriplegia, C5-C7 complete** 🐾
     G82.54 **Quadriplegia, C5-C7 incomplete** 🐾

CHAPTER 6 (G00-G99)

● **G83** **Other paralytic syndromes**

> **Note:** This category is to be used only when the listed conditions are reported without further specification, or are stated to be old or longstanding but of unspecified cause. The category is also for use in multiple coding to identify these conditions resulting from any cause.

> **Includes**   paralysis (complete) (incomplete), except as in G80-G82

G83.0   **Diplegia of upper limbs** 🐾
> *Paralysis affecting limbs on both sides; AKA bilateral paralysis*
> Diplegia (upper)
> Paralysis of both upper limbs

● **G83.1**   **Monoplegia of lower limb**
> *Paralysis of limb on one side*
> Paralysis of lower limb

> **Excludes1**   monoplegia of lower limbs due to sequela of cerebrovascular disease (I69.04-, I69.14-, I69.24-, I69.34-, I69.84-, I69.94-)

> Coding Clinic: 2012, Q4, P106

G83.10   **Monoplegia of lower limb affecting unspecified side** 🐾

G83.11   **Monoplegia of lower limb affecting right dominant side** 🐾

G83.12   **Monoplegia of lower limb affecting left dominant side** 🐾

G83.13   **Monoplegia of lower limb affecting right nondominant side** 🐾

G83.14   **Monoplegia of lower limb affecting left nondominant side** 🐾

● **G83.2**   **Monoplegia of upper limb**
> Paralysis of upper limb

> **Excludes1**   monoplegia of upper limbs due to sequela of cerebrovascular disease (I69.03-, I69.13-, I69.23-, I69.33-, I69.83-, I69.93-)

> Coding Clinic: 2012, Q4, P106

G83.20   **Monoplegia of upper limb affecting unspecified side** 🐾

G83.21   **Monoplegia of upper limb affecting right dominant side** 🐾

G83.22   **Monoplegia of upper limb affecting left dominant side** 🐾

G83.23   **Monoplegia of upper limb affecting right nondominant side** 🐾

G83.24   **Monoplegia of upper limb affecting left nondominant side** 🐾

● **G83.3**   **Monoplegia, unspecified**
> Coding Clinic: 2012, Q4, P106

G83.30   **Monoplegia, unspecified affecting unspecified side** 🐾

G83.31   **Monoplegia, unspecified affecting right dominant side** 🐾

G83.32   **Monoplegia, unspecified affecting left dominant side** 🐾

G83.33   **Monoplegia, unspecified affecting right nondominant side** 🐾

G83.34   **Monoplegia, unspecified affecting left nondominant side** 🐾

G83.4   **Cauda equina syndrome** 🐾
> *Aching pain due to compression of spinal nerve roots*
> Neurogenic bladder due to cauda equina syndrome

> **Excludes1**   cord bladder NOS (G95.89)
> neurogenic bladder NOS (N31.9)
> Coding Clinic: 2024, Q1, P18

G83.5   **Locked-in state** 🐾
> Coding Clinic: 2022, Q2, P11

● **G83.8**   **Other specified paralytic syndromes**

> **Excludes1**   paralytic syndromes due to current spinal cord injury-code to spinal cord injury (S14, S24, S34)

G83.81   **Brown-Séquard syndrome** 🐾

G83.82   **Anterior cord syndrome** 🐾

G83.83   **Posterior cord syndrome** 🐾

G83.84   **Todd's paralysis (postepileptic)** 🐾

G83.89   **Other specified paralytic syndromes** 🐾

G83.9   **Paralytic syndrome, unspecified** 🐾

OTHER DISORDERS OF THE NERVOUS SYSTEM (G89-G99)

● **G89**   **Pain, not elsewhere classified**

> Code also related psychological factors associated with pain (F45.42)

> **Excludes1**   generalized pain NOS (R52)
> pain disorders exclusively related to psychological factors (F45.41)
> pain NOS (R52)

> **Excludes2**   atypical face pain (G50.1)
> headache syndromes (G44.-)
> localized pain, unspecified type - code to pain by site, such as:
>   abdomen pain (R10.-)
>   back pain (M54.9)
>   breast pain (N64.4)
>   chest pain (R07.1-R07.9)
>   ear pain (H92.0-)
>   eye pain (H57.1)
>   headache (R51.9)
>   joint pain (M25.5-)
>   limb pain (M79.6-)
>   lumbar region pain (M54.5-)
>   painful urination (R30.9)
>   pelvic and perineal pain (R10.2)
>   shoulder pain (M25.51-)
>   spine pain (M54.-)
>   throat pain (R07.0)
>   tongue pain (K14.6)
>   tooth pain (K08.8)
> renal colic (N23)
> migraines (G43.-)
> myalgia (M79.1-)
> pain from prosthetic devices, implants, and grafts (T82.84, T83.84, T84.84, T85.84-)
> phantom limb syndrome with pain (G54.6)
> vulvar vestibulitis (N94.810)
> vulvodynia (N94.81-)

G89.0   **Central pain syndrome**
> *Neurological condition causing intractable pain resulting from damage to CNS*
> Déjérine-Roussy syndrome
> Myelopathic pain syndrome
> Thalamic pain syndrome (hyperesthetic)

● **G89.1**   **Acute pain, not elsewhere classified**

G89.11   **Acute pain due to trauma**

G89.12   **Acute post-thoracotomy pain**
> Post-thoracotomy pain NOS

G89.18   **Other acute postprocedural pain**
> Postoperative pain NOS
> Postprocedural pain NOS

● **G89.2**   **Chronic pain, not elsewhere classified**

> **Excludes1**   causalgia, lower limb (G57.7-)
> causalgia, upper limb (G56.4-)
> central pain syndrome (G89.0)
> chronic pain syndrome (G89.4)
> complex regional pain syndrome II, lower limb (G57.7-)
> complex regional pain syndrome II, upper limb (G56.4-)
> neoplasm related chronic pain (G89.3)
> reflex sympathetic dystrophy (G90.5-)

G89.21   Chronic pain due to trauma

G89.22   Chronic post-thoracotomy pain

G89.28   Other chronic postprocedural pain
         Other chronic postoperative pain

G89.29   Other chronic pain
         Coding Clinic: 2023, Q3, P17

G89.3   Neoplasm related pain (acute) (chronic)
        Cancer associated pain
        Pain due to malignancy (primary) (secondary)
        Tumor associated pain

G89.4   Chronic pain syndrome
        Chronic pain associated with significant psychosocial
        dysfunction

● G90   Disorders of autonomic nervous system
        | Excludes1 | dysfunction of the autonomic nervous system due to alcohol (G31.2) |

● G90.0   Idiopathic peripheral autonomic neuropathy

        G90.01   Carotid sinus syncope
                 Carotid sinus syndrome

        G90.09   Other idiopathic peripheral autonomic
                 neuropathy
                 Idiopathic peripheral autonomic neuropathy
                 NOS

G90.1   Familial dysautonomia [Riley-Day] 🔖
        Inherited disorder that affects nerve function

G90.2   Horner's syndrome
        Due to damage of the sympathetic nervous system
        Bernard(-Horner) syndrome
        Cervical sympathetic dystrophy or paralysis

G90.3   Multi-system degeneration of the autonomic nervous
        system 🔖
        Neurogenic orthostatic hypotension [Shy-Drager]
        | Excludes1 | orthostatic hypotension NOS (I95.1) |

G90.4   Autonomic dysreflexia
        Syndrome resulting from lesions of spinal cord
        Use additional code to identify the cause, such as:
            fecal impaction (K56.41)
            pressure ulcer (pressure area) (L89.-)
            urinary tract infection (N39.0)

● G90.5   Complex regional pain syndrome I (CRPS I)
        Reflex sympathetic dystrophy
        | Excludes1 | causalgia of lower limb (G57.7-) |
        | | causalgia of upper limb (G56.4-) |
        | | complex regional pain syndrome II of lower limb (G57.7-) |
        | | complex regional pain syndrome II of upper limb (G56.4-) |

        G90.50   Complex regional pain syndrome I, unspecified

        ● G90.51   Complex regional pain syndrome I of upper
                   limb

                 G90.511   Complex regional pain syndrome I of
                           right upper limb

                 G90.512   Complex regional pain syndrome I of
                           left upper limb

                 G90.513   Complex regional pain syndrome I of
                           upper limb, bilateral

                 G90.519   Complex regional pain
                           syndrome I of unspecified
                           upper limb

        ● G90.52   Complex regional pain syndrome I of lower
                   limb

                 G90.521   Complex regional pain syndrome I of
                           right lower limb

                 G90.522   Complex regional pain syndrome I of
                           left lower limb

                 G90.523   Complex regional pain syndrome I of
                           lower limb, bilateral

                 G90.529   Complex regional pain
                           syndrome I of unspecified
                           lower limb

        G90.59   Complex regional pain syndrome I of other
                 specified site

G90.8   Other disorders of autonomic nervous system
        Coding Clinic: 2023, Q2, P9

        ▷ G90.81   Serotonin syndrome
                 ▷ Serotonin toxicity
                 ▷ *Code first poisoning due to drug or toxin, such as:*
                     ▷ linezolid (T36.8X- with sixth character 1-4)
                     ▷ monoamine oxidase inhibitors (T43.1X with
                        sixth character 1-4)
                     ▷ selective serotonin and norepinephrine
                        reuptake inhibitors [SSNRI] (T43.21with
                        sixth character 1-4)
                     ▷ selective serotonin reuptake inhibitors [SSRI]
                        (T43.22 with sixth character 1-4)
                 ▷ Use Additional code for adverse effect, if
                    applicable, to identify drug, such as:
                     ▷ linezolid (T36.8X5)
                     ▷ monoamine oxidase inhibitors (T43.1X5)
                     ▷ selective serotonin and norepinephrine
                        reuptake inhibitors [SSNRI](T43.215)
                     ▷ selective serotonin reuptake inhibitors [SSRI]
                        (T43.225)
                 ▷ Use Additional code, if applicable, to identify:
                     ▷ disseminated intravascular coagulation (D65)
                     ▷ hypertensive crisis (I16.-)
                     ▷ metabolic acidosis (E87.2-)
                     ▷ shock, not elsewhere classified (R57.-)
                     ▷ toxic encephalopathy (G92.-)
                     ▷ ventricular tachycardia (I47.2-)

        ▷ G90.89   Other disorders of autonomic nervous system

G90.9   Disorder of the autonomic nervous system, unspecified

G90.A   Postural orthostatic tachycardia syndrome [POTS]
        Chronic orthostatic intolerance
        Postural tachycardia syndrome
        Coding Clinic: 2022, Q4, P20

G90.B   LMNB1-related autosomal dominant leukodystrophy

● G91   Hydrocephalus
        Dilatation of cerebral ventricles, accompanied by accumulation of
        cerebrospinal fluid
        | Includes | acquired hydrocephalus |
        | Excludes1 | Arnold-Chiari syndrome with hydrocephalus (Q07.-) |
        | | congenital hydrocephalus (Q03.-) |
        | | spina bifida with hydrocephalus (Q05.-) |

G91.0   Communicating hydrocephalus
        Secondary normal pressure hydrocephalus

G91.1   Obstructive hydrocephalus

G91.2   (Idiopathic) normal pressure
        hydrocephalus
        Normal pressure hydrocephalus NOS

G91.3   Post-traumatic hydrocephalus, unspecified

▷ *G91.4   Hydrocephalus in diseases classified elsewhere*
        Code first underlying condition, such as:
            congenital syphilis (A50.4-)
            neoplasm (C00-D49)
            plasminogen deficiency (E88.02)
        | Excludes1 | hydrocephalus due to congenital toxoplasmosis (P37.1) |

G91.8   Other hydrocephalus

G91.9   Hydrocephalus, unspecified

G92   Toxic encephalopathy

- ● **G92.0   Immune effector cell-associated neurotoxicity syndrome**

    Code first underlying cause such as:
    complications of immune effector cellular therapy (T80.82)

    Code also, if applicable, associated signs and symptoms, such as:
    cerebral edema (G93.6)
    unspecified convulsions (R56.9)

    G92.00   Immune effector cell-associated neurotoxicity syndrome, grade unspecified
    ICANS, grade unspecified

    G92.01   Immune effector cell-associated neurotoxicity syndrome, grade 1
    ICANS, grade 1

    G92.02   Immune effector cell-associated neurotoxicity syndrome, grade 2
    ICANS, grade 2

    G92.03   Immune effector cell-associated neurotoxicity syndrome, grade 3
    ICANS, grade 3

    G92.04   Immune effector cell-associated neurotoxicity syndrome, grade 4
    ICANS, grade 4

    G92.05   Immune effector cell-associated neurotoxicity syndrome, grade 5
    ICANS, grade 5

- **G92.8   Other toxic encephalopathy**
    Toxic encephalitis
    Toxic metabolic encephalopathy

    Code first poisoning due to drug or toxin, if applicable, (T36-T65 with fifth or sixth character 1-4)

    Use Additional code for adverse effect, if applicable, to identify drug (T36-T50 with fifth or sixth character 5)
    Coding Clinic: 2024, Q2, P15; 2022, Q1, P53

- **G92.9   Unspecified toxic encephalopathy**
    Code first poisoning due to drug or toxin, if applicable, (T36-T65 with fifth or sixth character 1-4)

    Use Additional code for adverse effect, if applicable, to identify drug (T36-T50 with fifth or sixth character 5)

    Disorder or disease of brain caused by chemicals
    Coding Clinic: 2021, Q1, P13; 2017, Q1, P39-40

- ● **G93   Other disorders of brain**

    G93.0   Cerebral cysts
    Arachnoid cyst
    Porencephalic cyst, acquired
    Excludes1   acquired periventricular cysts of newborn (P91.1)
    congenital cerebral cysts (Q04.6)

    G93.1   Anoxic brain damage, not elsewhere classified 🍫
    Permanent brain damage by lack of oxygen perfusion through brain tissues.
    Excludes1   cerebral anoxia due to anesthesia during labor and delivery (O74.3)
    cerebral anoxia due to anesthesia during the puerperium (O89.2)
    neonatal anoxia (P84)

    G93.2   Benign intracranial hypertension
    Pseudotumor
    Excludes1   hypertensive encephalopathy (I67.4)
    obstructive hydrocephalus (G91.1)

- ● **G93.3   Postviral and related fatigue syndromes**
    Excludes1   chronic fatigue NOS (R53.82)

    Use Additional code, if applicable, for post COVID-19 condition, unspecified (U09.9)
    Excludes1   neurasthenia (F48.8)

    G93.31   Postviral fatigue syndrome

    G93.32   Myalgic encephalomyelitis/chronic fatigue syndrome
    Chronic fatigue syndrome
    ME/CFS
    Myalgic encephalomyelitis

    G93.39   Other post infection and related fatigue syndromes

- ● **G93.4   Other and unspecified encephalopathy**
    Excludes2   alcoholic encephalopathy (G31.2)
    encephalopathy in diseases classified elsewhere (G94)
    hypertensive encephalopathy (I67.4)
    Coding Clinic: 2024, Q2, P15; 2017, Q2, P9

    G93.40   Encephalopathy, unspecified

    G93.41   Metabolic encephalopathy
    Septic encephalopathy
    Coding Clinic: 2024, Q2, P15; 2017, Q2, P8; 2016, Q3, P42; 2015, Q3, P21

    G93.42   Megalencephalic leukoencephalopathy with subcortical cysts

    G93.43   Leukoencephalopathy with calcifications and cysts

    G93.44   Adult-onset leukodystrophy with axonal spheroids
    Adult-onset leukoencephalopathy with axonal spheroids and pigmented glia

    G93.45   Developmental and epileptic encephalopathy
    ▶ Early infantile epileptic encephalopathy
    ▶ Code also if applicable, associated disorders such as:
    ▶ developmental disorders of scholastic skills (F81.-)
    ▶ developmental disorder of speech and language (F80.-)
    ▶ epilepsy, by specific type (G40.-)
    ▶ intellectual disabilities (F70-F79)
    ▶ other neurodevelopmental disorder (F88)
    ▶ pervasive developmental disorders (F84.-)

    G93.49   Other encephalopathy
    Encephalopathy NEC
    Coding Clinic: 2021, Q2, P3; 2018, Q4, P16; 2018, Q2, P22; 2017, Q2, P9

    G93.5   Compression of brain 🍫
    Arnold-Chiari type 1 compression of brain
    Compression of brain (stem)
    Herniation of brain (stem)
    Excludes1   traumatic compression of brain (S06.A-)

    G93.6   Cerebral edema 🍫
    Excludes1   cerebral edema due to birth injury (P11.0)
    traumatic cerebral edema (S06.1-)
    Coding Clinic: 2022, Q3, P9,11

    G93.7   Reye's syndrome   P
    Life-threatening neurological condition, usually follows viral illness
    Code first (poisoning due to salicylates, if applicable (T39.0-, with sixth character 1-4)

    Use additional code for adverse effect due to salicylates, if applicable (T39.0-, with sixth character 5)

- ● **G93.8   Other specified disorders of brain**
    G93.81   Temporal sclerosis
    Hippocampal sclerosis
    Mesial temporal sclerosis

    G93.82   Brain death

    G93.89   Other specified disorders of brain
    Postradiation encephalopathy
    Coding Clinic: 2024, Q2, P15,16; 2019, Q3, P9; 2016, Q4, P7

    G93.9   Disorder of brain, unspecified

▶ New   ⇒ Revised   ~~deleted~~ Deleted   Excludes 1   Excludes 2   Includes   Use additional   Code first   Code also   Key words
OGCR Official Guidelines   X Assign placeholder X   ● Use Additional Character(s)   ▶ Manifestation Code   🍫 Hierarchical Condition Category   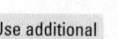 Coding Clinic

G94   *Other disorders of brain in diseases classified elsewhere*
> *Code first underlying disease*
> **Excludes1**   encephalopathy in congenital syphilis (A50.49)
> encephalopathy in influenza (J09.X9, J10.81, J11.81)
> encephalopathy in syphilis (A52.19)
> hydrocephalus in diseases classified elsewhere (G91.4)
> **Coding Clinic: 2018, Q2, P22; 2017, Q2, P8**

G95   **Other and unspecified diseases of spinal cord**
> **Excludes2**   myelitis (G04.-)

   G95.0   **Syringomyelia and syringobulbia** 🔲

G95.1   **Vascular myelopathies**
> **Excludes2**   intraspinal phlebitis and thrombophlebitis, except non-pyogenic (G08)

   G95.11   **Acute infarction of spinal cord (embolic) (nonembolic)** 🔲
> Anoxia of spinal cord
> Arterial thrombosis of spinal cord

   G95.19   **Other vascular myelopathies** 🔲
> Edema of spinal cord
> Hematomyelia
> Nonpyogenic intraspinal phlebitis and thrombophlebitis
> Subacute necrotic myelopathy
> **Coding Clinic: 2023, Q3, P21**

G95.2   **Other and unspecified cord compression**

   G95.20   Unspecified cord compression 🔲

   G95.29   Other cord compression 🔲

G95.8   **Other specified diseases of spinal cord**
> **Excludes1**   neurogenic bladder NOS (N31.9)
> neurogenic bladder due to cauda equina syndrome (G83.4)
> neuromuscular dysfunction of bladder without spinal cord lesion (N31.-)

   G95.81   **Conus medullaris syndrome** 🔲
> *Damage to gray matter and/or nerve roots in lower end of spinal cord*

   G95.89   **Other specified diseases of spinal cord** 🔲
> Cord bladder NOS
> Drug-induced myelopathy
> Radiation-induced myelopathy
> **Excludes1**   myelopathy NOS (G95.9)

   G95.9   **Disease of spinal cord, unspecified** 🔲
> Myelopathy NOS

G96   **Other disorders of central nervous system**

   G96.0   **Cerebrospinal fluid leak**
> Code also if applicable:
> intracranial hypotension (G96.81-)
> **Excludes1**   cerebrospinal fluid leak from spinal puncture (G97.0)
> **Coding Clinic: 2018, Q2, P13**

   G96.00   **Cerebrospinal fluid leak, unspecified**
> Code also if applicable:
> head injury (S00-S09)

   G96.01   **Cranial cerebrospinal fluid leak, spontaneous**
> Otorrhea due to spontaneous cerebrospinal fluid CSF leak
> Rhinorrhea due to spontaneous cerebrospinal fluid CSF leak
> Spontaneous cerebrospinal fluid leak from skull base

   G96.02   **Spinal cerebrospinal fluid leak, spontaneous**
> Spontaneous cerebrospinal fluid leak from spine

   G96.08   **Other cranial cerebrospinal fluid leak**
> Postoperative cranial cerebrospinal fluid leak
> Traumatic cranial cerebrospinal fluid leak
> Code also if applicable:
> head injury (S00-S09)

   G96.09   **Other spinal cerebrospinal fluid leak**
> Other spinal CSF leak
> Postoperative spinal cerebrospinal fluid leak
> Traumatic spinal cerebrospinal fluid leak
> Code also if applicable:
> head injury (S00-S09)
> **Coding Clinic: 2022, Q3, P24**

G96.1   **Disorders of meninges, not elsewhere classified**

   G96.11   **Dural tear**
> Code also intracranial hypotension, if applicable (G96.81-)
> **Excludes1**   accidental puncture or laceration of dura during a procedure (G97.41)

   G96.12   **Meningeal adhesions (cerebral) (spinal)**

   G96.19   **Other disorders of meninges, not elsewhere classified**

      G96.191   **Perineural cyst**
> Cervical nerve root cyst
> Lumbar nerve root cyst
> Sacral nerve root cyst
> Tarlov cyst
> Thoracic nerve root cyst

      G96.198   **Other disorders of meninges, not elsewhere classified**

G96.8   **Other specified disorders of central nervous system**

   G96.81   **Intracranial hypotension**
> Code also any associated diagnoses, such as:
> Brachial amyotrophy (G54.5)
> Cerebrospinal fluid leak from spine (G96.02)
> Cranial nerve disorders in diseases classified elsewhere (G53)
> Nerve root and compressions in diseases classified elsewhere (G55)
> Nonpyogenic thrombosis of intracranial venous system (I67.6)
> Nontraumatic intracerebral hemorrhage (I61.-)
> Nontraumatic subdural hemorrhage (I62.0-)
> Other and unspecified cord compression (G95.2-)
> Other secondary parkinsonism (G21.8)
> Reversible cerebrovascular vasoconstriction syndrome (I67.841)
> Spinal cord herniation (G95.89)
> Stroke (I63.-)
> Syringomyelia (G95.0)

      G96.810   **Intracranial hypotension, unspecified**

      G96.811   **Intracranial hypotension, spontaneous**

      G96.819   **Other intracranial hypotension**

   G96.89   **Other specified disorders of central nervous system**

   G96.9   **Disorder of central nervous system, unspecified**

G97   **Intraoperative and postprocedural complications and disorders of nervous system, not elsewhere classified**
> **Excludes2**   intraoperative and postprocedural cerebrovascular infarction (I97.81-, I97.82-)
> **Coding Clinic: 2016, Q4, P9**

   G97.0   **Cerebrospinal fluid leak from spinal puncture**
> Code also any associated diagnoses or complications, such as:
> intracranial hypotension following a procedure (G97.83-G97.84)

G97.1 **Other reaction to spinal and lumbar puncture**
Headache due to lumbar puncture
Other reaction to spinal dural puncture
Code also, if applicable, any associated headache with orthostatic component (R51.0)

G97.2 **Intracranial hypotension following ventricular shunting**
Code also any associated diagnoses or complications

● G97.3 **Intraoperative hemorrhage and hematoma of a nervous system organ or structure complicating a procedure**
Excludes1 intraoperative hemorrhage and hematoma of a nervous system organ or structure due to accidental puncture and laceration during a procedure (G97.4-)

    G97.31 **Intraoperative hemorrhage and hematoma of a nervous system organ or structure complicating a nervous system procedure**

    G97.32 **Intraoperative hemorrhage and hematoma of a nervous system organ or structure complicating other procedure**

● G97.4 **Accidental puncture and laceration of a nervous system organ or structure during a procedure**

    G97.41 **Accidental puncture or laceration of dura during a procedure**
Incidental (inadvertent) durotomy
Code also any associated diagnoses or complications
Coding Clinic: 2024, Q1, P21

    G97.48 **Accidental puncture and laceration of other nervous system organ or structure during a nervous system procedure**

    G97.49 **Accidental puncture and laceration of other nervous system organ or structure during other procedure**

● G97.5 **Postprocedural hemorrhage of a nervous system organ or structure following a procedure**

    G97.51 **Postprocedural hemorrhage of a nervous system organ or structure following a nervous system procedure**

    G97.52 **Postprocedural hemorrhage of a nervous system organ or structure following other procedure**

● G97.6 **Postprocedural hematoma and seroma of a nervous system organ or structure following a procedure**

    G97.61 **Postprocedural hematoma of a nervous system organ or structure following a nervous system procedure**

    G97.62 **Postprocedural hematoma of a nervous system organ or structure following other procedure**

    G97.63 **Postprocedural seroma of a nervous system organ or structure following a nervous system procedure**

    G97.64 **Postprocedural seroma of a nervous system organ or structure following other procedure**

● G97.8 **Other intraoperative and postprocedural complications and disorders of nervous system**
Use additional code to further specify disorder

    G97.81 **Other intraoperative complications of nervous system**

    G97.82 **Other postprocedural complications and disorders of nervous system**
Coding Clinic: 2022, Q1, P35

    G97.83 **Intracranial hypotension following lumbar cerebrospinal fluid shunting**
Code also any associated diagnoses or complications

    G97.84 **Intracranial hypotension following other procedure**
Code also, if applicable:
accidental puncture or laceration of dura during a procedure (G97.41)
cerebrospinal fluid leak from spinal puncture (G97.0)

● G98 **Other disorders of nervous system not elsewhere classified**
Includes nervous system disorder NOS

  G98.0 **Neurogenic arthritis, not elsewhere classified**
Nonsyphilitic neurogenic arthropathy NEC
Nonsyphilitic neurogenic spondylopathy NEC
Excludes1 spondylopathy (in):
syringomyelia and syringobulbia (G95.0)
tabes dorsalis (A52.11)

  G98.8 **Other disorders of nervous system**
Nervous system disorder NOS

● G99 **Other disorders of nervous system in diseases classified elsewhere**

  ▷ *G99.0 Autonomic neuropathy in diseases classified elsewhere*
Code first underlying disease, such as:
amyloidosis (E85.-)
gout (M1A.-, M10.-)
hyperthyroidism (E05.-)
Excludes1 diabetic autonomic neuropathy (E08-E13 with .43)

  ▷ *G99.2 Myelopathy in diseases classified elsewhere* 🦠
Code first underlying disease, such as:
neoplasm (C00-D49)
Excludes1 myelopathy in:
intervertebral disease (M50.0-, M51.0-)
spondylosis (M47.0-, M47.1-)

  ▷ *G99.8 Other specified disorders of nervous system in diseases classified elsewhere*
Code first underlying disorder, such as:
amyloidosis (E85.-)
avitaminosis (E56.-)
Excludes1 nervous system involvement in:
cysticercosis (B69.0)
rubella (B06.0-)
syphilis (A52.1-)

772
▶ New ⇛ Revised ~~deleted~~ Deleted Excludes 1 Excludes 2 Includes Use additional Code first Code also Key words
OGCR Official Guidelines X Assign placeholder X ● Use Additional Character(s) ▷ Manifestation Code 🦠 Hierarchical Condition Category Coding Clinic

CHAPTER 7

DISEASES OF THE EYE AND ADNEXA
(H00-H59)

OGCR Chapter-Specific Coding Guidelines

7. Chapter 7: Diseases of the Eye and Adnexa (H00-H59)

a. Glaucoma

1) **Assigning Glaucoma Codes**

Assign as many codes from category H40, Glaucoma, as needed to identify the type of glaucoma, the affected eye, and the glaucoma stage.

2) **Bilateral glaucoma with same type and stage**

When a patient has bilateral glaucoma and both eyes are documented as being the same type and stage, and there is a code for bilateral glaucoma, report only the code for the type of glaucoma, bilateral, with the seventh character for the stage.

When a patient has bilateral glaucoma and both eyes are documented as being the same type and stage, and the classification does not provide a code for bilateral glaucoma (i.e., subcategories H40.10, H40.11, and H40.20) report only one code for the type of glaucoma with the appropriate seventh character for the stage.

3) **Bilateral glaucoma stage with different types or stages**

When a patient has bilateral glaucoma and each eye is documented as having a different type or stage, and the classification distinguishes laterality, assign the appropriate code for each eye rather than the code for bilateral glaucoma.

When a patient has bilateral glaucoma and each eye is documented as having a different type, and the classification does not distinguish laterality (i.e., subcategories H40.10, H40.11 and H40.20), assign one code for each type of glaucoma with the appropriate seventh character for the stage.

When a patient has bilateral glaucoma and each eye is documented as having the same type, but different stage, and the classification does not distinguish laterality (i.e., subcategories H40.10, H40.11, and H40.20), assign a code for the type of glaucoma for each eye with the seventh character for the specific glaucoma stage documented for each eye.

4) **Patient admitted with glaucoma and stage evolves during the admission**

If a patient is admitted with glaucoma and the stage progresses during the admission, assign the code for highest stage documented.

5) **Indeterminate stage glaucoma**

Assignment of the seventh character "4" for "indeterminate stage" should be based on the clinical documentation. The seventh character "4" is used for glaucomas whose stage cannot be clinically determined. This seventh character should not be confused with the seventh character "0", unspecified, which should be assigned when there is no documentation regarding the stage of the glaucoma.

b. Blindness

If "blindness" or "low vision" of both eyes is documented but the visual impairment category is not documented, assign code H54.3, Unqualified visual loss, both eyes. If "blindness" or "low vision" in one eye is documented but the visual impairment category is not documented, assign a code from H54.6-, Unqualified visual loss, one eye. If "blindness" or "visual loss" is documented without any information about whether one or both eyes are affected, assign code H54.7, Unspecified visual loss.

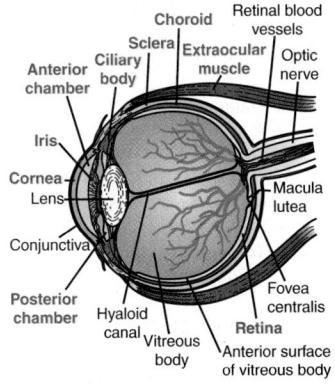

Figure 7-1 Eye and ocular adnexa. (From Buck CJ: Step-by-Step Medical Coding, ed 2016, St. Louis, Elsevier, 2016)

★**(See Plate 15 of the Anatomy Illustrations.)**

CHAPTER 7

DISEASES OF THE EYE AND ADNEXA
(H00-H59)

Note: Use an external cause code following the code for the eye condition, if applicable, to identify the cause of the eye condition

Excludes2 certain conditions originating in the perinatal period (P04-P96)

certain infectious and parasitic diseases (A00-B99)

complications of pregnancy, childbirth and the puerperium (O00-O9A)

congenital malformations, deformations, and chromosomal abnormalities (Q00-Q99)

diabetes mellitus related eye conditions (E09.3-, E10.3-, E11.3-, E13.3-)

endocrine, nutritional and metabolic diseases (E00-E88)

injury (trauma) of eye and orbit (S05.-)

injury, poisoning and certain other consequences of external causes (S00-T88)

neoplasms (C00-D49)

symptoms, signs and abnormal clinical and laboratory findings, not elsewhere classified (R00-R94)

syphilis related eye disorders (A50.01, A50.3-, A51.43, A52.71)

This chapter contains the following blocks:

H00-H05	Disorders of eyelid, lacrimal system and orbit
H10-H11	Disorders of conjunctiva
H15-H22	Disorders of sclera, cornea, iris and ciliary body
H25-H28	Disorders of lens
H30-H36	Disorders of choroid and retina
H40-H42	Glaucoma
H43-H44	Disorders of vitreous body and globe
H46-H47	Disorders of optic nerve and visual pathways
H49-H52	Disorders of ocular muscles, binocular movement, accommodation and refraction
H53-H54	Visual disturbances and blindness
H55-H57	Other disorders of eye and adnexa
H59	Intraoperative and postprocedural complications and disorders of eye and adnexa, not elsewhere classified

DISORDERS OF EYELID, LACRIMAL SYSTEM AND ORBIT (H00-H05)

Excludes2   open wound of eyelid (S01.1-)
superficial injury of eyelid (S00.1-, S00.2-)

● **H00   Hordeolum and chalazion**
Hordeolum: inflammatory staphylococcal infection of sebaceous
glands of eyelids; AKA stye. Chalazion: eyelid mass

● **H00.0   Hordeolum (externum) (internum) of eyelid**
Bacterial infection (staphylococcus) of the sebaceous gland of
the eyelid (stye)

● **H00.01   Hordeolum externum**
Hordeolum NOS
Stye

     H00.011   Hordeolum externum right upper eyelid

     H00.012   Hordeolum externum right lower eyelid

     H00.013   Hordeolum externum right eye, unspecified eyelid

     H00.014   Hordeolum externum left upper eyelid

     H00.015   Hordeolum externum left lower eyelid

     H00.016   Hordeolum externum left eye, unspecified eyelid

     H00.019   Hordeolum externum unspecified eye, unspecified eyelid

● **H00.02   Hordeolum internum**
Infection of meibomian gland

     H00.021   Hordeolum internum right upper eyelid

     H00.022   Hordeolum internum right lower eyelid

     H00.023   Hordeolum internum right eye, unspecified eyelid

     H00.024   Hordeolum internum left upper eyelid

     H00.025   Hordeolum internum left lower eyelid

     H00.026   Hordeolum internum left eye, unspecified eyelid

     H00.029   Hordeolum internum unspecified eye, unspecified eyelid

● **H00.03   Abscess of eyelid**
Furuncle of eyelid

     H00.031   Abscess of right upper eyelid

     H00.032   Abscess of right lower eyelid

     H00.033   Abscess of eyelid right eye, unspecified eyelid

     H00.034   Abscess of left upper eyelid

     H00.035   Abscess of left lower eyelid

     H00.036   Abscess of eyelid left eye, unspecified eyelid

     H00.039   Abscess of eyelid unspecified eye, unspecified eyelid

● **H00.1   Chalazion**
Often caused by accumulation of meibomian gland secretions
resulting from a blockage of duct.
Meibomian (gland) cyst

Excludes2   infected meibomian gland (H00.02-)

     H00.11   Chalazion right upper eyelid

     H00.12   Chalazion right lower eyelid

     H00.13   Chalazion right eye, unspecified eyelid

     H00.14   Chalazion left upper eyelid

     H00.15   Chalazion left lower eyelid

     H00.16   Chalazion left eye, unspecified eyelid

     H00.19   Chalazion unspecified eye, unspecified eyelid

● **H01   Other inflammation of eyelid**

● **H01.0   Blepharitis**
Inflammation of eyelids

Excludes1   blepharoconjunctivitis (H10.5-)

● **H01.00   Unspecified blepharitis**

     H01.001   Unspecified blepharitis right upper eyelid

     H01.002   Unspecified blepharitis right lower eyelid

     H01.003   Unspecified blepharitis right eye, unspecified eyelid

     H01.004   Unspecified blepharitis left upper eyelid

     H01.005   Unspecified blepharitis left lower eyelid

     H01.006   Unspecified blepharitis left eye, unspecified eyelid

     H01.009   Unspecified blepharitis unspecified eye, unspecified eyelid

     H01.00A   Unspecified blepharitis right eye, upper and lower eyelids

     H01.00B   Unspecified blepharitis left eye, upper and lower eyelids

● **H01.01   Ulcerative blepharitis**

     H01.011   Ulcerative blepharitis right upper eyelid

     H01.012   Ulcerative blepharitis right lower eyelid

     H01.013   Ulcerative blepharitis right eye, unspecified eyelid

     H01.014   Ulcerative blepharitis left upper eyelid

     H01.015   Ulcerative blepharitis left lower eyelid

     H01.016   Ulcerative blepharitis left eye, unspecified eyelid

     H01.019   Ulcerative blepharitis unspecified eye, unspecified eyelid

     H01.01A   Ulcerative blepharitis right eye, upper and lower eyelids

     H01.01B   Ulcerative blepharitis left eye, upper and lower eyelids

● **H01.02   Squamous blepharitis**

     H01.021   Squamous blepharitis right upper eyelid

     H01.022   Squamous blepharitis right lower eyelid

     H01.023   Squamous blepharitis right eye, unspecified eyelid

     H01.024   Squamous blepharitis left upper eyelid

     H01.025   Squamous blepharitis left lower eyelid

     H01.026   Squamous blepharitis left eye, unspecified eyelid

     H01.029   Squamous blepharitis unspecified eye, unspecified eyelid

     H01.02A   Squamous blepharitis right eye, upper and lower eyelids

     H01.02B   Squamous blepharitis left eye, upper and lower eyelids

● **H01.1   Noninfectious dermatoses of eyelid**

● **H01.11   Allergic dermatitis of eyelid**
Contact dermatitis of eyelid

     H01.111   Allergic dermatitis of right upper eyelid

     H01.112   Allergic dermatitis of right lower eyelid

     H01.113   Allergic dermatitis of right eye, unspecified eyelid

▶ New   ⇒ Revised   ~~deleted~~ Deleted   Excludes 1   Excludes 2   Includes   Use additional   Code first   Code also   Key words

OGCR Official Guidelines   X Assign placeholder X   ● Use Additional Character(s)   ▶ Manifestation Code   🏥 Hierarchical Condition Category   **Coding Clinic**

H01.114 Allergic dermatitis of left upper eyelid

H01.115 Allergic dermatitis of left lower eyelid

H01.116 Allergic dermatitis of left eye, unspecified eyelid

H01.119 Allergic dermatitis of unspecified eye, unspecified eyelid

● H01.12 Discoid lupus erythematosus of eyelid

H01.121 Discoid lupus erythematosus of right upper eyelid

H01.122 Discoid lupus erythematosus of right lower eyelid

H01.123 Discoid lupus erythematosus of right eye, unspecified eyelid

H01.124 Discoid lupus erythematosus of left upper eyelid

H01.125 Discoid lupus erythematosus of left lower eyelid

H01.126 Discoid lupus erythematosus of left eye, unspecified eyelid

H01.129 Discoid lupus erythematosus of unspecified eye, unspecified eyelid

● H01.13 Eczematous dermatitis of eyelid

H01.131 Eczematous dermatitis of right upper eyelid

H01.132 Eczematous dermatitis of right lower eyelid

H01.133 Eczematous dermatitis of right eye, unspecified eyelid

H01.134 Eczematous dermatitis of left upper eyelid

H01.135 Eczematous dermatitis of left lower eyelid

H01.136 Eczematous dermatitis of left eye, unspecified eyelid

H01.139 Eczematous dermatitis of unspecified eye, unspecified eyelid

● H01.14 Xeroderma of eyelid
Abnormally dry

H01.141 Xeroderma of right upper eyelid

H01.142 Xeroderma of right lower eyelid

H01.143 Xeroderma of right eye, unspecified eyelid

H01.144 Xeroderma of left upper eyelid

H01.145 Xeroderma of left lower eyelid

H01.146 Xeroderma of left eye, unspecified eyelid

H01.149 Xeroderma of unspecified eye, unspecified eyelid

H01.8 Other specified inflammations of eyelid

H01.9 Unspecified inflammation of eyelid
Inflammation of eyelid NOS

● H02 Other disorders of eyelid
Turning inward (inversion) of eyelid margin and ingrowing eyelashes

Excludes1 congenital malformations of eyelid (Q10.0-Q10.3)

● H02.0 Entropion and trichiasis of eyelid

● H02.00 Unspecified entropion of eyelid

H02.001 Unspecified entropion of right upper eyelid

H02.002 Unspecified entropion of right lower eyelid

H02.003 Unspecified entropion of right eye, unspecified eyelid

H02.004 Unspecified entropion of left upper eyelid

H02.005 Unspecified entropion of left lower eyelid

Figure 7-2 Right lower eyelid entropion. Note the inward rotation of the tarsal plate about the horizontal axis and the resultant contact between the mucocutaneous junction and ocular surface. (From Glynn M, Drake WM, Hutchison R: Hutchison's Clinical Methods: An Integrated Approach to Clinical Practice, Edinburgh, Saunders/Elsevier, 2012)

H02.006 Unspecified entropion of left eye, unspecified eyelid

H02.009 Unspecified entropion of unspecified eye, unspecified eyelid

● H02.01 Cicatricial entropion of eyelid
Scar

H02.011 Cicatricial entropion of right upper eyelid

H02.012 Cicatricial entropion of right lower eyelid

H02.013 Cicatricial entropion of right eye, unspecified eyelid

H02.014 Cicatricial entropion of left upper eyelid

H02.015 Cicatricial entropion of left lower eyelid

H02.016 Cicatricial entropion of left eye, unspecified eyelid

H02.019 Cicatricial entropion of unspecified eye, unspecified eyelid

● H02.02 Mechanical entropion of eyelid
Turning inward (inversion) of eyelid margin due to lack of support

H02.021 Mechanical entropion of right upper eyelid

H02.022 Mechanical entropion of right lower eyelid

H02.023 Mechanical entropion of right eye, unspecified eyelid

H02.024 Mechanical entropion of left upper eyelid

H02.025 Mechanical entropion of left lower eyelid

H02.026 Mechanical entropion of left eye, unspecified eyelid

H02.029 Mechanical entropion of unspecified eye, unspecified eyelid

● H02.03 Senile entropion of eyelid
Turning inward (inversion) of eyelid margin due to aging

H02.031 Senile entropion of right upper eyelid A

H02.032 Senile entropion of right lower eyelid A

H02.033 Senile entropion of right eye, unspecified eyelid A

H02.034 Senile entropion of left upper eyelid A

H02.035 Senile entropion of left lower eyelid A

H02.036 Senile entropion of left eye, unspecified eyelid A

H02.039 Senile entropion of unspecified eye, unspecified eyelid A

● H02.04 Spastic entropion of eyelid
Turning inward (inversion) of eyelid margin caused by spasm of muscle

H02.041 Spastic entropion of right upper eyelid

H02.042 Spastic entropion of right lower eyelid

H02.043 Spastic entropion of right eye, unspecified eyelid

CHAPTER 7 (H00-H59)

H02.044   Spastic entropion of left upper eyelid

H02.045   Spastic entropion of left lower eyelid

H02.046   Spastic entropion of left eye, unspecified eyelid

H02.049   Spastic entropion of unspecified eye, unspecified eyelid

● **H02.05**   Trichiasis without entropion
Ingrowing hairs of eyelashes

H02.051   Trichiasis without entropion right upper eyelid

H02.052   Trichiasis without entropion right lower eyelid

H02.053   Trichiasis without entropion right eye, unspecified eyelid

H02.054   Trichiasis without entropion left upper eyelid

H02.055   Trichiasis without entropion left lower eyelid

H02.056   Trichiasis without entropion left eye, unspecified eyelid

H02.059   Trichiasis without entropion unspecified eye, unspecified eyelid

● **H02.1**   Ectropion of eyelid
Eversion (pulling away) of eyelid

● **H02.10**   Unspecified ectropion of eyelid

H02.101   Unspecified ectropion of right upper eyelid

H02.102   Unspecified ectropion of right lower eyelid

H02.103   Unspecified ectropion of right eye, unspecified eyelid

H02.104   Unspecified ectropion of left upper eyelid

H02.105   Unspecified ectropion of left lower eyelid

H02.106   Unspecified ectropion of left eye, unspecified eyelid

H02.109   Unspecified ectropion of unspecified eye, unspecified eyelid

● **H02.11**   Cicatricial ectropion of eyelid
Pulling of eyelid down and away from eye due to scar or tightening

H02.111   Cicatricial ectropion of right upper eyelid

H02.112   Cicatricial ectropion of right lower eyelid

H02.113   Cicatricial ectropion of right eye, unspecified eyelid

H02.114   Cicatricial ectropion of left upper eyelid

H02.115   Cicatricial ectropion of left lower eyelid

H02.116   Cicatricial ectropion of left eye, unspecified eyelid

H02.119   Cicatricial ectropion of unspecified eye, unspecified eyelid

● **H02.12**   Mechanical ectropion of eyelid
Eversion (pulling away) of eyelid due to lack of support

H02.121   Mechanical ectropion of right upper eyelid

H02.122   Mechanical ectropion of right lower eyelid

H02.123   Mechanical ectropion of right eye, unspecified eyelid

H02.124   Mechanical ectropion of left upper eyelid

H02.125   Mechanical ectropion of left lower eyelid

H02.126   Mechanical ectropion of left eye, unspecified eyelid

H02.129   Mechanical ectropion of unspecified eye, unspecified eyelid

● **H02.13**   Senile ectropion of eyelid
Eversion (pulling away) of eyelid due to age

H02.131   Senile ectropion of right upper eyelid   A

H02.132   Senile ectropion of right lower eyelid   A

H02.133   Senile ectropion of right eye, unspecified eyelid   A

H02.134   Senile ectropion of left upper eyelid A

H02.135   Senile ectropion of left lower eyelid A

H02.136   Senile ectropion of left eye, unspecified eyelid   A

H02.139   Senile ectropion of unspecified eye, unspecified eyelid   A

● **H02.14**   Spastic ectropion of eyelid
Eversion (pulling away) of eyelid due to tonic muscle spasm

H02.141   Spastic ectropion of right upper eyelid

H02.142   Spastic ectropion of right lower eyelid

H02.143   Spastic ectropion of right eye, unspecified eyelid

H02.144   Spastic ectropion of left upper eyelid

H02.145   Spastic ectropion of left lower eyelid

H02.146   Spastic ectropion of left eye, unspecified eyelid

H02.149   Spastic ectropion of unspecified eye, unspecified eyelid

● **H02.15**   Paralytic ectropion of eyelid

H02.151   Paralytic ectropion of right upper eyelid

H02.152   Paralytic ectropion of right lower eyelid

H02.153   Paralytic ectropion of right eye, unspecified eyelid

H02.154   Paralytic ectropion of left upper eyelid

H02.155   Paralytic ectropion of left lower eyelid

H02.156   Paralytic ectropion of left eye, unspecified eyelid

H02.159   Paralytic ectropion of unspecified eye, unspecified eyelid

● **H02.2**   Lagophthalmos
Condition in which eye cannot completely close

● **H02.20**   Unspecified lagophthalmos

H02.201   Unspecified lagophthalmos right upper eyelid

H02.202   Unspecified lagophthalmos right lower eyelid

H02.203   Unspecified lagophthalmos right eye, unspecified eyelid

H02.204   Unspecified lagophthalmos left upper eyelid

H02.205   Unspecified lagophthalmos left lower eyelid

H02.206   Unspecified lagophthalmos left eye, unspecified eyelid

H02.209   Unspecified lagophthalmos unspecified eye, unspecified eyelid

H02.20A   Unspecified lagophthalmos right eye, upper and lower eyelids

H02.20B   Unspecified lagophthalmos left eye, upper and lower eyelids

H02.20C   Unspecified lagophthalmos, bilateral, upper and lower eyelids

CHAPTER 7 (H00–H59)

● **H02.21**   Cicatricial lagophthalmos
Upper or lower eyelid does not close due to scar or tightening

H02.211   Cicatricial lagophthalmos right upper eyelid

H02.212   Cicatricial lagophthalmos right lower eyelid

H02.213   Cicatricial lagophthalmos right eye, unspecified eyelid

H02.214   Cicatricial lagophthalmos left upper eyelid

H02.215   Cicatricial lagophthalmos left lower eyelid

H02.216   Cicatricial lagophthalmos left eye, unspecified eyelid

H02.219   Cicatricial lagophthalmos unspecified eye, unspecified eyelid

H02.21A   Cicatricial lagophthalmos right eye, upper and lower eyelids

H02.21B   Cicatricial lagophthalmos left eye, upper and lower eyelids

H02.21C   Cicatricial lagophthalmos, bilateral, upper and lower eyelids

● **H02.22**   Mechanical lagophthalmos
Inability to close lids due to structural disorder

H02.221   Mechanical lagophthalmos right upper eyelid

H02.222   Mechanical lagophthalmos right lower eyelid

H02.223   Mechanical lagophthalmos right eye, unspecified eyelid

H02.224   Mechanical lagophthalmos left upper eyelid

H02.225   Mechanical lagophthalmos left lower eyelid

H02.226   Mechanical lagophthalmos left eye, unspecified eyelid

H02.229   Mechanical lagophthalmos unspecified eye, unspecified eyelid

H02.22A   Mechanical lagophthalmos right eye, upper and lower eyelids

H02.22B   Mechanical lagophthalmos left eye, upper and lower eyelids

H02.22C   Mechanical lagophthalmos, bilateral, upper and lower eyelids

● **H02.23**   Paralytic lagophthalmos
Eyelids do not close due to paralysis

H02.231   Paralytic lagophthalmos right upper eyelid

H02.232   Paralytic lagophthalmos right lower eyelid

H02.233   Paralytic lagophthalmos right eye, unspecified eyelid

H02.234   Paralytic lagophthalmos left upper eyelid

H02.235   Paralytic lagophthalmos left lower eyelid

H02.236   Paralytic lagophthalmos left eye, unspecified eyelid

H02.239   Paralytic lagophthalmos unspecified eye, unspecified eyelid

H02.23A   Paralytic lagophthalmos right eye, upper and lower eyelids

H02.23B   Paralytic lagophthalmos left eye, upper and lower eyelids

H02.23C   Paralytic lagophthalmos, bilateral, upper and lower eyelids

Figure 7-3   Ptosis of eyelid. (From Kanski JJ: Clinical Diagnosis in Ophthalmology, London, Elsevier Mosby, 2006)

Item 7-1   Ptosis of eyelid is drooping of the upper eyelid over the pupil when the eyes are fully opened resulting from nerve or muscle damage, which may require surgical correction.

★ **(See Plate 17 of the Anatomy Illustrations.)**

● **H02.3**   Blepharochalasis
Relaxation of skin of eyelid, due to atrophy of intercellular tissue
Pseudoptosis

H02.30   Blepharochalasis unspecified eye, unspecified eyelid

H02.31   Blepharochalasis right upper eyelid

H02.32   Blepharochalasis right lower eyelid

H02.33   Blepharochalasis right eye, unspecified eyelid

H02.34   Blepharochalasis left upper eyelid

H02.35   Blepharochalasis left lower eyelid

H02.36   Blepharochalasis left eye, unspecified eyelid

● **H02.4**   Ptosis of eyelid
Falling forward, drooping, sagging of eyelid

● **H02.40**   Unspecified ptosis of eyelid

H02.401   Unspecified ptosis of right eyelid

H02.402   Unspecified ptosis of left eyelid

H02.403   Unspecified ptosis of bilateral eyelids

H02.409   Unspecified ptosis of unspecified eyelid

● **H02.41**   Mechanical ptosis of eyelid

H02.411   Mechanical ptosis of right eyelid

H02.412   Mechanical ptosis of left eyelid

H02.413   Mechanical ptosis of bilateral eyelids

H02.419   Mechanical ptosis of unspecified eyelid

● **H02.42**   Myogenic ptosis of eyelid

H02.421   Myogenic ptosis of right eyelid

H02.422   Myogenic ptosis of left eyelid

H02.423   Myogenic ptosis of bilateral eyelids

H02.429   Myogenic ptosis of unspecified eyelid

● **H02.43**   Paralytic ptosis of eyelid
Neurogenic ptosis of eyelid

H02.431   Paralytic ptosis of right eyelid

H02.432   Paralytic ptosis of left eyelid

H02.433   Paralytic ptosis of bilateral eyelids

H02.439   Paralytic ptosis unspecified eyelid

● **H02.5**   Other disorders affecting eyelid function

Excludes2   blepharospasm (G24.5)
organic tic (G25.69)
psychogenic tic (F95.-)

● **H02.51**   Abnormal innervation syndrome

H02.511   Abnormal innervation syndrome right upper eyelid

H02.512   Abnormal innervation syndrome right lower eyelid

H02.513   Abnormal innervation syndrome right eye, unspecified eyelid

H02.514   Abnormal innervation syndrome left upper eyelid

H02.515   Abnormal innervation syndrome left lower eyelid

H02.516   Abnormal innervation syndrome left eye, unspecified eyelid

H02.519   Abnormal innervation syndrome unspecified eye, unspecified eyelid

CHAPTER 7 (H00-H59)

● **H02.52 Blepharophimosis**
  Drooping of eyelid with reduced lid size
  Ankyloblepharon
  - H02.521 Blepharophimosis right upper eyelid
  - H02.522 Blepharophimosis right lower eyelid
  - H02.523 Blepharophimosis right eye, unspecified eyelid
  - H02.524 Blepharophimosis left upper eyelid
  - H02.525 Blepharophimosis left lower eyelid
  - H02.526 Blepharophimosis left eye, unspecified eyelid
  - H02.529 Blepharophimosis unspecified eye, unspecified lid

● **H02.53 Eyelid retraction**
  Eyelid lag
  - H02.531 Eyelid retraction right upper eyelid
  - H02.532 Eyelid retraction right lower eyelid
  - H02.533 Eyelid retraction right eye, unspecified eyelid
  - H02.534 Eyelid retraction left upper eyelid
  - H02.535 Eyelid retraction left lower eyelid
  - H02.536 Eyelid retraction left eye, unspecified eyelid
  - H02.539 Eyelid retraction unspecified eye, unspecified lid

H02.59 Other disorders affecting eyelid function
  Deficient blink reflex
  Sensory disorders

● **H02.6 Xanthelasma of eyelid**
  Yellow-to-orange patches or pimples clustered together on eyelid
  - H02.60 Xanthelasma of unspecified eye, unspecified eyelid
  - H02.61 Xanthelasma of right upper eyelid
  - H02.62 Xanthelasma of right lower eyelid
  - H02.63 Xanthelasma of right eye, unspecified eyelid
  - H02.64 Xanthelasma of left upper eyelid
  - H02.65 Xanthelasma of left lower eyelid
  - H02.66 Xanthelasma of left eye, unspecified eyelid

● **H02.7 Other and unspecified degenerative disorders of eyelid and periocular area**
  H02.70 Unspecified degenerative disorders of eyelid and periocular area
  ● **H02.71 Chloasma of eyelid and periocular area**
    Dyspigmentation of eyelid
    Hyperpigmentation of eyelid
    - H02.711 Chloasma of right upper eyelid and periocular area
    - H02.712 Chloasma of right lower eyelid and periocular area
    - H02.713 Chloasma of right eye, unspecified eyelid and periocular area
    - H02.714 Chloasma of left upper eyelid and periocular area
    - H02.715 Chloasma of left lower eyelid and periocular area
    - H02.716 Chloasma of left eye, unspecified eyelid and periocular area
    - H02.719 Chloasma of unspecified eye, unspecified eyelid and periocular area
  ● **H02.72 Madarosis of eyelid and periocular area**
    Loss of eyelashes and/or eyebrows
    Hypotrichosis of eyelid
    - H02.721 Madarosis of right upper eyelid and periocular area
    - H02.722 Madarosis of right lower eyelid and periocular area
    - H02.723 Madarosis of right eye, unspecified eyelid and periocular area

- H02.724 Madarosis of left upper eyelid and periocular area
- H02.725 Madarosis of left lower eyelid and periocular area
- H02.726 Madarosis of left eye, unspecified eyelid and periocular area
- H02.729 Madarosis of unspecified eye, unspecified eyelid and periocular area

● **H02.73 Vitiligo of eyelid and periocular area**
  Skin pigmentation disease characterized by white patches
  Hypopigmentation of eyelid
  - H02.731 Vitiligo of right upper eyelid and periocular area
  - H02.732 Vitiligo of right lower eyelid and periocular area
  - H02.733 Vitiligo of right eye, unspecified eyelid and periocular area
  - H02.734 Vitiligo of left upper eyelid and periocular area
  - H02.735 Vitiligo of left lower eyelid and periocular area
  - H02.736 Vitiligo of left eye, unspecified eyelid and periocular area
  - H02.739 Vitiligo of unspecified eye, unspecified eyelid and periocular area

H02.79 Other degenerative disorders of eyelid and periocular area

● **H02.8 Other specified disorders of eyelid**
  ● **H02.81 Retained foreign body in eyelid**
    Use additional code to identify the type of retained foreign body (Z18.-)
    Excludes1 laceration of eyelid with foreign body (S01.12-)
      retained intraocular foreign body (H44.6-, H44.7-)
      superficial foreign body of eyelid and periocular area (S00.25-)
    - H02.811 Retained foreign body in right upper eyelid
    - H02.812 Retained foreign body in right lower eyelid
    - H02.813 Retained foreign body in right eye, unspecified eyelid
    - H02.814 Retained foreign body in left upper eyelid
    - H02.815 Retained foreign body in left lower eyelid
    - H02.816 Retained foreign body in left eye, unspecified eyelid
    - H02.819 Retained foreign body in unspecified eye, unspecified eyelid
  ● **H02.82 Cysts of eyelid**
    Sebaceous cyst of eyelid
    - H02.821 Cysts of right upper eyelid
    - H02.822 Cysts of right lower eyelid
    - H02.823 Cysts of right eye, unspecified eyelid
    - H02.824 Cysts of left upper eyelid
    - H02.825 Cysts of left lower eyelid
    - H02.826 Cysts of left eye, unspecified eyelid
    - H02.829 Cysts of unspecified eye, unspecified eyelid
  ● **H02.83 Dermatochalasis of eyelid**
    Skin is inelastic and hangs loosely in folds
    - H02.831 Dermatochalasis of right upper eyelid
    - H02.832 Dermatochalasis of right lower eyelid
    - H02.833 Dermatochalasis of right eye, unspecified eyelid
    - H02.834 Dermatochalasis of left upper eyelid

H02.835   Dermatochalasis of left lower eyelid

H02.836   Dermatochalasis of left eye, unspecified eyelid

H02.839   Dermatochalasis of unspecified eye, unspecified eyelid

● H02.84   Edema of eyelid
           Hyperemia of eyelid

H02.841   Edema of right upper eyelid

H02.842   Edema of right lower eyelid

H02.843   Edema of right eye, unspecified eyelid

H02.844   Edema of left upper eyelid

H02.845   Edema of left lower eyelid

H02.846   Edema of left eye, unspecified eyelid

H02.849   Edema of unspecified eye, unspecified eyelid

● H02.85   Elephantiasis of eyelid
           *Massive secondary lymphedema with hypertrophy
           of skin and subcutaneous tissues
           (pachyderma)*

H02.851   Elephantiasis of right upper eyelid

H02.852   Elephantiasis of right lower eyelid

H02.853   Elephantiasis of right eye, unspecified eyelid

H02.854   Elephantiasis of left upper eyelid

H02.855   Elephantiasis of left lower eyelid

H02.856   Elephantiasis of left eye, unspecified eyelid

H02.859   Elephantiasis of unspecified eye, unspecified eyelid

● H02.86   Hypertrichosis of eyelid
           Excessive growth of hair

H02.861   Hypertrichosis of right upper eyelid

H02.862   Hypertrichosis of right lower eyelid

H02.863   Hypertrichosis of right eye, unspecified eyelid

H02.864   Hypertrichosis of left upper eyelid

H02.865   Hypertrichosis of left lower eyelid

H02.866   Hypertrichosis of left eye, unspecified eyelid

H02.869   Hypertrichosis of unspecified eye, unspecified eyelid

● H02.87   Vascular anomalies of eyelid

H02.871   Vascular anomalies of right upper eyelid

H02.872   Vascular anomalies of right lower eyelid

H02.873   Vascular anomalies of right eye, unspecified eyelid

H02.874   Vascular anomalies of left upper eyelid

H02.875   Vascular anomalies of left lower eyelid

H02.876   Vascular anomalies of left eye, unspecified eyelid

H02.879   Vascular anomalies of unspecified eye, unspecified eyelid

● H02.88   Meibomian gland dysfunction of eyelid

H02.881   Meibomian gland dysfunction right upper eyelid

H02.882   Meibomian gland dysfunction right lower eyelid

H02.883   Meibomian gland dysfunction of right eye, unspecified eyelid

H02.884   Meibomian gland dysfunction left upper eyelid

H02.885   Meibomian gland dysfunction left lower eyelid

H02.886   Meibomian gland dysfunction of left eye, unspecified eyelid

H02.889   Meibomian gland dysfunction of unspecified eye, unspecified eyelid

H02.88A   Meibomian gland dysfunction right eye, upper and lower eyelids

H02.88B   Meibomian gland dysfunction left eye, upper and lower eyelids

H02.89   Other specified disorders of eyelid
          Hemorrhage of eyelid

H02.9   Unspecified disorder of eyelid
         Disorder of eyelid NOS

● H04   Disorders of lacrimal system
    Excludes1   congenital malformations of lacrimal system
                 (Q10.4-Q10.6)

● H04.0   Dacryoadenitis
          Inflammation of lacrimal gland

● H04.00   Unspecified dacryoadenitis

H04.001   Unspecified dacryoadenitis, right lacrimal gland

H04.002   Unspecified dacryoadenitis, left lacrimal gland

H04.003   Unspecified dacryoadenitis, bilateral lacrimal glands

H04.009   Unspecified dacryoadenitis, unspecified lacrimal gland

● H04.01   Acute dacryoadenitis

H04.011   Acute dacryoadenitis, right lacrimal gland

H04.012   Acute dacryoadenitis, left lacrimal gland

H04.013   Acute dacryoadenitis, bilateral lacrimal glands

H04.019   Acute dacryoadenitis, unspecified lacrimal gland

★ **(See Plate 19 of the Anatomy Illustrations.)**

● H04.02   Chronic dacryoadenitis

H04.021   Chronic dacryoadenitis, right lacrimal gland

H04.022   Chronic dacryoadenitis, left lacrimal gland

H04.023   Chronic dacryoadenitis, bilateral lacrimal gland

H04.029   Chronic dacryoadenitis, unspecified lacrimal gland

● H04.03   Chronic enlargement of lacrimal gland

H04.031   Chronic enlargement of right lacrimal gland

H04.032   Chronic enlargement of left lacrimal gland

H04.033   Chronic enlargement of bilateral lacrimal glands

H04.039   Chronic enlargement of unspecified lacrimal gland

● H04.1   Other disorders of lacrimal gland

● H04.11   Dacryops
           Watery eye or distention of lacrimal duct due to fluid

H04.111   Dacryops of right lacrimal gland

H04.112   Dacryops of left lacrimal gland

H04.113   Dacryops of bilateral lacrimal glands

H04.119   Dacryops of unspecified lacrimal gland

Figure 7-4   Lacrimal apparatus. (From Buck CJ: Step-by-Step Medical Coding, 2016, St. Louis, Elsevier, 2016)

CHAPTER 7 (H00-H59)

● **H04.12**   **Dry eye syndrome**
     Tear film insufficiency, NOS

     H04.121   Dry eye syndrome of right lacrimal gland

     H04.122   Dry eye syndrome of left lacrimal gland

     H04.123   Dry eye syndrome of bilateral lacrimal glands

     H04.129   Dry eye syndrome of unspecified lacrimal gland

● **H04.13**   **Lacrimal cyst**
     Lacrimal cystic degeneration

     H04.131   Lacrimal cyst right lacrimal gland

     H04.132   Lacrimal cyst left lacrimal gland

     H04.133   Lacrimal cyst bilateral lacrimal glands

     H04.139   Lacrimal cyst unspecified lacrimal gland

● **H04.14**   **Primary lacrimal gland atrophy**

     H04.141   Primary lacrimal gland atrophy, right lacrimal gland

     H04.142   Primary lacrimal gland atrophy, left lacrimal gland

     H04.143   Primary lacrimal gland atrophy, bilateral lacrimal glands

     H04.149   Primary lacrimal gland atrophy, unspecified lacrimal gland

● **H04.15**   **Secondary lacrimal gland atrophy**

     H04.151   Secondary lacrimal gland atrophy, right lacrimal gland

     H04.152   Secondary lacrimal gland atrophy, left lacrimal gland

     H04.153   Secondary lacrimal gland atrophy, bilateral lacrimal glands

     H04.159   Secondary lacrimal gland atrophy, unspecified lacrimal gland

● **H04.16**   **Lacrimal gland dislocation**

     H04.161   Lacrimal gland dislocation, right lacrimal gland

     H04.162   Lacrimal gland dislocation, left lacrimal gland

     H04.163   Lacrimal gland dislocation, bilateral lacrimal glands

     H04.169   Lacrimal gland dislocation, unspecified lacrimal gland

     H04.19   Other specified disorders of lacrimal gland

● **H04.2**   **Epiphora**
     Overflow of tears due to stricture of lacrimal passages; AKA lacrimation

● **H04.20**   **Unspecified epiphora**

     H04.201   Unspecified epiphora, right side

     H04.202   Unspecified epiphora, left side

     H04.203   Unspecified epiphora, bilateral

     H04.209   Unspecified epiphora, unspecified side

● **H04.21**   **Epiphora due to excess lacrimation**

     H04.211   Epiphora due to excess lacrimation, right lacrimal gland

     H04.212   Epiphora due to excess lacrimation, left lacrimal gland

     H04.213   Epiphora due to excess lacrimation, bilateral lacrimal glands

     H04.219   Epiphora due to excess lacrimation, unspecified lacrimal gland

● **H04.22**   **Epiphora due to insufficient drainage**

     H04.221   Epiphora due to insufficient drainage, right side

     H04.222   Epiphora due to insufficient drainage, left side

     H04.223   Epiphora due to insufficient drainage, bilateral

     H04.229   Epiphora due to insufficient drainage, unspecified side

● **H04.3**   **Acute and unspecified inflammation of lacrimal passages**

     Excludes1   neonatal dacryocystitis (P39.1)

● **H04.30**   **Unspecified dacryocystitis**

     H04.301   Unspecified dacryocystitis of right lacrimal passage

     H04.302   Unspecified dacryocystitis of left lacrimal passage

     H04.303   Unspecified dacryocystitis of bilateral lacrimal passages

     H04.309   Unspecified dacryocystitis of unspecified lacrimal passage

● **H04.31**   **Phlegmonous dacryocystitis**
     Cellulitis of lacrimal sac

     H04.311   Phlegmonous dacryocystitis of right lacrimal passage

     H04.312   Phlegmonous dacryocystitis of left lacrimal passage

     H04.313   Phlegmonous dacryocystitis of bilateral lacrimal passages

     H04.319   Phlegmonous dacryocystitis of unspecified lacrimal passage

● **H04.32**   **Acute dacryocystitis**
     Acute dacryopericystitis

     H04.321   Acute dacryocystitis of right lacrimal passage

     H04.322   Acute dacryocystitis of left lacrimal passage

     H04.323   Acute dacryocystitis of bilateral lacrimal passages

     H04.329   Acute dacryocystitis of unspecified lacrimal passage

● **H04.33**   **Acute lacrimal canaliculitis**

     H04.331   Acute lacrimal canaliculitis of right lacrimal passage

     H04.332   Acute lacrimal canaliculitis of left lacrimal passage

     H04.333   Acute lacrimal canaliculitis of bilateral lacrimal passages

     H04.339   Acute lacrimal canaliculitis of unspecified lacrimal passage

● **H04.4**   **Chronic inflammation of lacrimal passages**

● **H04.41**   **Chronic dacryocystitis**
     Inflammation of lacrimal sac

     H04.411   Chronic dacryocystitis of right lacrimal passage

     H04.412   Chronic dacryocystitis of left lacrimal passage

     H04.413   Chronic dacryocystitis of bilateral lacrimal passages

     H04.419   Chronic dacryocystitis of unspecified lacrimal passage

● **H04.42**   **Chronic lacrimal canaliculitis**
     Inflammation of lacrimal ducts

     H04.421   Chronic lacrimal canaliculitis of right lacrimal passage

     H04.422   Chronic lacrimal canaliculitis of left lacrimal passage

     H04.423   Chronic lacrimal canaliculitis of bilateral lacrimal passages

     H04.429   Chronic lacrimal canaliculitis of unspecified lacrimal passage

● **H04.43**   **Chronic lacrimal mucocele**
     Accumulation of mucous secretion

     H04.431   Chronic lacrimal mucocele of right lacrimal passage

     H04.432   Chronic lacrimal mucocele of left lacrimal passage

     H04.433   Chronic lacrimal mucocele of bilateral lacrimal passages

     H04.439   Chronic lacrimal mucocele of unspecified lacrimal passage

▶ New   ⇒ Revised   ~~deleted~~ Deleted   Excludes 1   Excludes 2   Includes   Use additional   Code first   Code also   Key words

OGCR Official Guidelines   X Assign placeholder X   ● Use Additional Character(s)   ▶ Manifestation Code   🗘 Hierarchical Condition Category   **Coding Clinic**

- **H04.5   Stenosis and insufficiency of lacrimal passages**
  - **H04.51   Dacryolith**
    Concretion in lacrimal sac/duct; AKA lacrimal calculus
    - H04.511   Dacryolith of right lacrimal passage
    - H04.512   Dacryolith of left lacrimal passage
    - H04.513   Dacryolith of bilateral lacrimal passages
    - H04.519   Dacryolith of unspecified lacrimal passage
  - **H04.52   Eversion of lacrimal punctum**
    Turning out of lacrimal drainage opening
    - H04.521   Eversion of right lacrimal punctum
    - H04.522   Eversion of left lacrimal punctum
    - H04.523   Eversion of bilateral lacrimal punctum
    - H04.529   Eversion of unspecified lacrimal punctum
  - **H04.53   Neonatal obstruction of nasolacrimal duct**
    Excludes1   congenital stenosis and stricture of lacrimal duct (Q10.5)
    - H04.531   Neonatal obstruction of right nasolacrimal duct   N
    - H04.532   Neonatal obstruction of left nasolacrimal duct   N
    - H04.533   Neonatal obstruction of bilateral nasolacrimal duct   N
    - H04.539   Neonatal obstruction of unspecified nasolacrimal duct   N
  - **H04.54   Stenosis of lacrimal canaliculi**
    - H04.541   Stenosis of right lacrimal canaliculi
    - H04.542   Stenosis of left lacrimal canaliculi
    - H04.543   Stenosis of bilateral lacrimal canaliculi
    - H04.549   Stenosis of unspecified lacrimal canaliculi
  - **H04.55   Acquired stenosis of nasolacrimal duct**
    - H04.551   Acquired stenosis of right nasolacrimal duct
    - H04.552   Acquired stenosis of left nasolacrimal duct
    - H04.553   Acquired stenosis of bilateral nasolacrimal duct
    - H04.559   Acquired stenosis of unspecified nasolacrimal duct
  - **H04.56   Stenosis of lacrimal punctum**
    - H04.561   Stenosis of right lacrimal punctum
    - H04.562   Stenosis of left lacrimal punctum
    - H04.563   Stenosis of bilateral lacrimal punctum
    - H04.569   Stenosis of unspecified lacrimal punctum
  - **H04.57   Stenosis of lacrimal sac**
    - H04.571   Stenosis of right lacrimal sac
    - H04.572   Stenosis of left lacrimal sac
    - H04.573   Stenosis of bilateral lacrimal sac
    - H04.579   Stenosis of unspecified lacrimal sac
- **H04.6   Other changes of lacrimal passages**
  - **H04.61   Lacrimal fistula**
    - H04.611   Lacrimal fistula right lacrimal passage
    - H04.612   Lacrimal fistula left lacrimal passage
    - H04.613   Lacrimal fistula bilateral lacrimal passages
    - H04.619   Lacrimal fistula unspecified lacrimal passage
  - H04.69   Other changes of lacrimal passages

- **H04.8   Other disorders of lacrimal system**
  - **H04.81   Granuloma of lacrimal passages**
    Inflammatory response due to infectious or noninfectious agents
    - H04.811   Granuloma of right lacrimal passage
    - H04.812   Granuloma of left lacrimal passage
    - H04.813   Granuloma of bilateral lacrimal passages
    - H04.819   Granuloma of unspecified lacrimal passage
  - H04.89   Other disorders of lacrimal system
  - H04.9   Disorder of lacrimal system, unspecified
- **H05   Disorders of orbit**
  Excludes1   congenital malformation of orbit (Q10.7)
  - **H05.0   Acute inflammation of orbit**
    - H05.00   Unspecified acute inflammation of orbit
    - **H05.01   Cellulitis of orbit**
      Infection of soft tissue of orbit
      Abscess of orbit
      - H05.011   Cellulitis of right orbit
      - H05.012   Cellulitis of left orbit
      - H05.013   Cellulitis of bilateral orbits
      - H05.019   Cellulitis of unspecified orbit
    - **H05.02   Osteomyelitis of orbit**
      Infection of boney orbit of eye
      - H05.021   Osteomyelitis of right orbit
      - H05.022   Osteomyelitis of left orbit
      - H05.023   Osteomyelitis of bilateral orbits
      - H05.029   Osteomyelitis of unspecified orbit
    - **H05.03   Periostitis of orbit**
      Inflammation of periosteum (membrane covering bone surface)
      - H05.031   Periostitis of right orbit
      - H05.032   Periostitis of left orbit
      - H05.033   Periostitis of bilateral orbits
      - H05.039   Periostitis of unspecified orbit
    - **H05.04   Tenonitis of orbit**
      Inflammation of tenon capsule (space enclosing fascia of Tenon between eyeball and fat of orbit)
      - H05.041   Tenonitis of right orbit
      - H05.042   Tenonitis of left orbit
      - H05.043   Tenonitis of bilateral orbits
      - H05.049   Tenonitis of unspecified orbit
  - **H05.1   Chronic inflammatory disorders of orbit**
    - H05.10   Unspecified chronic inflammatory disorders of orbit
    - **H05.11   Granuloma of orbit**
      Pseudotumor (inflammatory) of orbit
      - H05.111   Granuloma of right orbit
      - H05.112   Granuloma of left orbit
      - H05.113   Granuloma of bilateral orbits
      - H05.119   Granuloma of unspecified orbit
    - **H05.12   Orbital myositis**
      Inflammation of extraocular muscles of orbit
      - H05.121   Orbital myositis, right orbit
      - H05.122   Orbital myositis, left orbit
      - H05.123   Orbital myositis, bilateral
      - H05.129   Orbital myositis, unspecified orbit

CHAPTER 7 (H00-H59)

Figure 7-5 Exophthalmos. (From Black JM, Hokanson JH: Medical-Surgical Nursing: Clinical Management for Positive Outcomes, St. Louis, Saunders Elsevier, 2009)

● H05.2   **Exophthalmic conditions**
  Bulging eyes
  H05.20   Unspecified exophthalmos
● H05.21   **Displacement (lateral) of globe**
  H05.211   Displacement (lateral) of globe, right eye
  H05.212   Displacement (lateral) of globe, left eye
  H05.213   Displacement (lateral) of globe, bilateral
  H05.219   Displacement (lateral) of globe, unspecified eye
● H05.22   **Edema of orbit**
  Orbital congestion
  H05.221   Edema of right orbit
  H05.222   Edema of left orbit
  H05.223   Edema of bilateral orbit
  H05.229   Edema of unspecified orbit
● H05.23   **Hemorrhage of orbit**
  H05.231   Hemorrhage of right orbit
  H05.232   Hemorrhage of left orbit
  H05.233   Hemorrhage of bilateral orbit
  H05.239   Hemorrhage of unspecified orbit
● H05.24   **Constant exophthalmos**
  Constant bulging eyes, often symptom of Graves disease
  H05.241   Constant exophthalmos, right eye
  H05.242   Constant exophthalmos, left eye
  H05.243   Constant exophthalmos, bilateral
  H05.249   Constant exophthalmos, unspecified eye
● H05.25   **Intermittent exophthalmos**
  Intermittent bulging eye occurring with bending forward or sharp turning of head
  H05.251   Intermittent exophthalmos, right eye
  H05.252   Intermittent exophthalmos, left eye
  H05.253   Intermittent exophthalmos, bilateral
  H05.259   Intermittent exophthalmos, unspecified eye
● H05.26   **Pulsating exophthalmos**
  Bulging eyes with pulsation and bruit, often due to aneurysm pushing eye forward
  H05.261   Pulsating exophthalmos, right eye
  H05.262   Pulsating exophthalmos, left eye
  H05.263   Pulsating exophthalmos, bilateral
  H05.269   Pulsating exophthalmos, unspecified eye

● H05.3   **Deformity of orbit**
  Excludes1   congenital deformity of orbit (Q10.7)
                  hypertelorism (Q75.2)
  H05.30   Unspecified deformity of orbit
● H05.31   **Atrophy of orbit**
  H05.311   Atrophy of right orbit
  H05.312   Atrophy of left orbit
  H05.313   Atrophy of bilateral orbit
  H05.319   Atrophy of unspecified orbit
● H05.32   **Deformity of orbit due to bone disease**
  Code also associated bone disease
  H05.321   Deformity of right orbit due to bone disease
  H05.322   Deformity of left orbit due to bone disease
  H05.323   Deformity of bilateral orbits due to bone disease
  H05.329   Deformity of unspecified orbit due to bone disease
● H05.33   **Deformity of orbit due to trauma or surgery**
  H05.331   Deformity of right orbit due to trauma or surgery
  H05.332   Deformity of left orbit due to trauma or surgery
  H05.333   Deformity of bilateral orbits due to trauma or surgery
  H05.339   Deformity of unspecified orbit due to trauma or surgery
● H05.34   **Enlargement of orbit**
  H05.341   Enlargement of right orbit
  H05.342   Enlargement of left orbit
  H05.343   Enlargement of bilateral orbits
  H05.349   Enlargement of unspecified orbit
● H05.35   **Exostosis of orbit**
  H05.351   Exostosis of right orbit
  H05.352   Exostosis of left orbit
  H05.353   Exostosis of bilateral orbits
  H05.359   Exostosis of unspecified orbit
● H05.4   **Enophthalmos**
  Recessed eyeball into orbit
● H05.40   **Unspecified enophthalmos**
  H05.401   Unspecified enophthalmos, right eye
  H05.402   Unspecified enophthalmos, left eye
  H05.403   Unspecified enophthalmos, bilateral
  H05.409   Unspecified enophthalmos, unspecified eye
● H05.41   **Enophthalmos due to atrophy of orbital tissue**
  H05.411   Enophthalmos due to atrophy of orbital tissue, right eye
  H05.412   Enophthalmos due to atrophy of orbital tissue, left eye
  H05.413   Enophthalmos due to atrophy of orbital tissue, bilateral
  H05.419   Enophthalmos due to atrophy of orbital tissue, unspecified eye
● H05.42   **Enophthalmos due to trauma or surgery**
  H05.421   Enophthalmos due to trauma or surgery, right eye
  H05.422   Enophthalmos due to trauma or surgery, left eye
  H05.423   Enophthalmos due to trauma or surgery, bilateral
  H05.429   Enophthalmos due to trauma or surgery, unspecified eye

▶ New   ⟜ Revised   ~~deleted~~ Deleted   Excludes 1   Excludes 2   Includes   Use additional   Code first   Code also   Key words
OGCR Official Guidelines   X Assign placeholder X   ● Use Additional Character(s)   ▶ Manifestation Code   ✎ Hierarchical Condition Category   Coding Clinic

CHAPTER 7 (H00-H59)

● **H05.5**   **Retained (old) foreign body following penetrating wound of orbit**
    Retrobulbar foreign body
    Use additional code to identify the type of retained foreign body (Z18.-)
    Excludes1   current penetrating wound of orbit (S05.4-)
    Excludes2   retained foreign body of eyelid (H02.81-)
          retained intraocular foreign body (H44.6-, H44.7-)

   H05.50   Retained (old) foreign body following penetrating wound of unspecified orbit
   H05.51   Retained (old) foreign body following penetrating wound of right orbit
   H05.52   Retained (old) foreign body following penetrating wound of left orbit
   H05.53   Retained (old) foreign body following penetrating wound of bilateral orbits

● **H05.8**   **Other disorders of orbit**
 ● H05.81   Cyst of orbit
      Encephalocele of orbit
     H05.811   Cyst of right orbit
     H05.812   Cyst of left orbit
     H05.813   Cyst of bilateral orbits
     H05.819   Cyst of unspecified orbit
 ● H05.82   Myopathy of extraocular muscles
      Weakness of muscles of eye
     H05.821   Myopathy of extraocular muscles, right orbit
     H05.822   Myopathy of extraocular muscles, left orbit
     H05.823   Myopathy of extraocular muscles, bilateral
     H05.829   Myopathy of extraocular muscles, unspecified orbit
   H05.89   Other disorders of orbit
  H05.9   Unspecified disorder of orbit

DISORDERS OF CONJUNCTIVA (H10-H11)

★ **(See Plate 18 of the Anatomy Illustrations.)**

● **H10**   **Conjunctivitis**
   Inflammation of membrane of the inside of the eyelid or on surface of eye (conjunctiva)
   Excludes1   keratoconjunctivitis (H16.2-)
 ● **H10.0**   **Mucopurulent conjunctivitis**
  ● H10.01   Acute follicular conjunctivitis
     H10.011   Acute follicular conjunctivitis, right eye
     H10.012   Acute follicular conjunctivitis, left eye
     H10.013   Acute follicular conjunctivitis, bilateral
     H10.019   Acute follicular conjunctivitis, unspecified eye
  ● H10.02   Other mucopurulent conjunctivitis
     H10.021   Other mucopurulent conjunctivitis, right eye
     H10.022   Other mucopurulent conjunctivitis, left eye
     H10.023   Other mucopurulent conjunctivitis, bilateral
     H10.029   Other mucopurulent conjunctivitis, unspecified eye
 ● **H10.1**   **Acute atopic conjunctivitis**
     Acute papillary conjunctivitis
   H10.10   Acute atopic conjunctivitis, unspecified eye
   H10.11   Acute atopic conjunctivitis, right eye
   H10.12   Acute atopic conjunctivitis, left eye
   H10.13   Acute atopic conjunctivitis, bilateral

● **H10.2**   **Other acute conjunctivitis**
 ● H10.21   Acute toxic conjunctivitis
     Acute chemical conjunctivitis
     Code first (T51-T65) to identify chemical and intent
     Excludes1   burn and corrosion of eye and adnexa (T26.-)
     H10.211   Acute toxic conjunctivitis, right eye
     H10.212   Acute toxic conjunctivitis, left eye
     H10.213   Acute toxic conjunctivitis, bilateral
     H10.219   Acute toxic conjunctivitis, unspecified eye
 ● H10.22   Pseudomembranous conjunctivitis
     H10.221   Pseudomembranous conjunctivitis, right eye
     H10.222   Pseudomembranous conjunctivitis, left eye
     H10.223   Pseudomembranous conjunctivitis, bilateral
     H10.229   Pseudomembranous conjunctivitis, unspecified eye
 ● H10.23   Serous conjunctivitis, except viral
     Excludes1   viral conjunctivitis (B30.-)
     H10.231   Serous conjunctivitis, except viral, right eye
     H10.232   Serous conjunctivitis, except viral, left eye
     H10.233   Serous conjunctivitis, except viral, bilateral
     H10.239   Serous conjunctivitis, except viral, unspecified eye
 ● **H10.3**   **Unspecified acute conjunctivitis**
     Excludes1   ophthalmia neonatorum NOS (P39.1)
   H10.30   Unspecified acute conjunctivitis, unspecified eye
   H10.31   Unspecified acute conjunctivitis, right eye
   H10.32   Unspecified acute conjunctivitis, left eye
   H10.33   Unspecified acute conjunctivitis, bilateral
 ● **H10.4**   **Chronic conjunctivitis**
  ● H10.40   Unspecified chronic conjunctivitis
     H10.401   Unspecified chronic conjunctivitis, right eye
     H10.402   Unspecified chronic conjunctivitis, left eye
     H10.403   Unspecified chronic conjunctivitis, bilateral
     H10.409   Unspecified chronic conjunctivitis, unspecified eye
  ● H10.41   Chronic giant papillary conjunctivitis
     Inflammation of membrane of the inside of the eyelid or on surface of eye often associated with contact lens wear
     H10.411   Chronic giant papillary conjunctivitis, right eye
     H10.412   Chronic giant papillary conjunctivitis, left eye
     H10.413   Chronic giant papillary conjunctivitis, bilateral
     H10.419   Chronic giant papillary conjunctivitis, unspecified eye
  ● H10.42   Simple chronic conjunctivitis
     H10.421   Simple chronic conjunctivitis, right eye
     H10.422   Simple chronic conjunctivitis, left eye
     H10.423   Simple chronic conjunctivitis, bilateral
     H10.429   Simple chronic conjunctivitis, unspecified eye

CHAPTER 7 (H00-H59)

● **H10.43** Chronic follicular conjunctivitis
Inflammation of membrane of the inside of the eyelid or on surface of eye due to topical medications or infection

H10.431 Chronic follicular conjunctivitis, **right eye**

H10.432 Chronic follicular conjunctivitis, **left eye**

H10.433 Chronic follicular conjunctivitis, **bilateral**

H10.439 Chronic follicular conjunctivitis, **unspecified eye**

H10.44 Vernal conjunctivitis
Affecting children, especially boys in which there are flattened papules with thick, gelatinous exudate on conjunctivae on inside of upper lid

Excludes1 vernal keratoconjunctivitis with limbar and corneal involvement (H16.26-)

H10.45 Other chronic allergic conjunctivitis

● **H10.5** Blepharoconjunctivitis
Inflammation of eyelids and conjunctiva

● **H10.50** Unspecified blepharoconjunctivitis

H10.501 Unspecified blepharoconjunctivitis, **right eye**

H10.502 Unspecified blepharoconjunctivitis, **left eye**

H10.503 Unspecified blepharoconjunctivitis, **bilateral**

H10.509 Unspecified blepharoconjunctivitis, **unspecified eye**

● **H10.51** Ligneous conjunctivitis
Code also underlying condition if known, such as:
plasminogen deficiency (E88.02)

H10.511 Ligneous conjunctivitis, **right eye**

H10.512 Ligneous conjunctivitis, **left eye**

H10.513 Ligneous conjunctivitis, **bilateral**

H10.519 Ligneous conjunctivitis, **unspecified eye**

● **H10.52** Angular blepharoconjunctivitis

H10.521 Angular blepharoconjunctivitis, **right eye**

H10.522 Angular blepharoconjunctivitis, **left eye**

H10.523 Angular blepharoconjunctivitis, **bilateral**

H10.529 Angular blepharoconjunctivitis, **unspecified eye**

● **H10.53** Contact blepharoconjunctivitis

H10.531 Contact blepharoconjunctivitis, **right eye**

H10.532 Contact blepharoconjunctivitis, **left eye**

H10.533 Contact blepharoconjunctivitis, **bilateral**

H10.539 Contact blepharoconjunctivitis, **unspecified eye**

● **H10.8** Other conjunctivitis

● **H10.81** Pingueculitis
Inflammation of a yellow, raised thickening on the white of the eye associated with chronic dry eyes

Excludes1 pinguecula (H11.15-)

H10.811 Pingueculitis, **right eye**

H10.812 Pingueculitis, **left eye**

H10.813 Pingueculitis, **bilateral**

H10.819 Pingueculitis, **unspecified eye**

● **H10.82** Rosacea conjunctivitis
Code first underlying rosacea dermatitis (L71.-)

H10.821 Rosacea conjunctivitis, **right eye**

H10.822 Rosacea conjunctivitis, **left eye**

H10.823 Rosacea conjunctivitis, **bilateral**
Coding Clinic: 2018, Q4, P15

H10.829 Rosacea conjunctivitis, **unspecified eye**

H10.89 Other conjunctivitis

H10.9 Unspecified conjunctivitis

● **H11** Other disorders of conjunctiva

Excludes1 keratoconjunctivitis (H16.2-)

● **H11.0** Pterygium of eye

Excludes1 pseudopterygium (H11.81-)

● **H11.00** Unspecified pterygium of eye

H11.001 Unspecified pterygium of **right eye**

H11.002 Unspecified pterygium of **left eye**

H11.003 Unspecified pterygium of eye, **bilateral**

H11.009 Unspecified pterygium of **unspecified eye**

● **H11.01** Amyloid pterygium

H11.011 Amyloid pterygium of **right eye**

H11.012 Amyloid pterygium of **left eye**

H11.013 Amyloid pterygium of eye, **bilateral**

H11.019 Amyloid pterygium of **unspecified eye**

● **H11.02** Central pterygium of eye

H11.021 Central pterygium of **right eye**

H11.022 Central pterygium of **left eye**

H11.023 Central pterygium of eye, **bilateral**

H11.029 Central pterygium of **unspecified eye**

● **H11.03** Double pterygium of eye

H11.031 Double pterygium of **right eye**

H11.032 Double pterygium of **left eye**

H11.033 Double pterygium of eye, **bilateral**

H11.039 Double pterygium of **unspecified eye**

● **H11.04** Peripheral pterygium of eye, **stationary**

H11.041 Peripheral pterygium, stationary, **right eye**

H11.042 Peripheral pterygium, stationary, **left eye**

H11.043 Peripheral pterygium, stationary, **bilateral**

H11.049 Peripheral pterygium, stationary, **unspecified eye**

● **H11.05** Peripheral pterygium of eye, **progressive**

H11.051 Peripheral pterygium, progressive, **right eye**

H11.052 Peripheral pterygium, progressive, **left eye**

H11.053 Peripheral pterygium, progressive, **bilateral**

H11.059 Peripheral pterygium, progressive, **unspecified eye**

● **H11.06** Recurrent pterygium of eye

H11.061 Recurrent pterygium of **right eye**

H11.062 Recurrent pterygium of **left eye**

H11.063 Recurrent pterygium of eye, **bilateral**

H11.069 Recurrent pterygium of **unspecified eye**

Figure 7-6 Double pterygium. Note both nasal and temporal pterygia in a 57-year-old farmer. (From Brightbill FS, McDonnell PJ: Corneal Surgery: Theory, Technique and Tissue, S.l., Mosby Elsevier, 2009)

Item 7-2 Pterygium is Greek for batlike. The condition is characterized by a membrane that extends from the limbus to the center of the cornea and resembles a wing.

▶ New   ▭ Revised   ~~deleted~~ Deleted   Excludes 1   Excludes 2   Includes   Use additional   Code first   Code also   Key words

OGCR Official Guidelines   X Assign placeholder X   ● Use Additional Character(s)   ▷ Manifestation Code   🦰 Hierarchical Condition Category   **Coding Clinic**

● H11.1   **Conjunctival degenerations and deposits**
    Excludes2   pseudopterygium (H11.81)
   H11.10   Unspecified conjunctival degenerations
● H11.11   Conjunctival deposits
     H11.111   Conjunctival deposits, right eye
     H11.112   Conjunctival deposits, left eye
     H11.113   Conjunctival deposits, bilateral
     H11.119   Conjunctival deposits, unspecified eye
● H11.12   Conjunctival concretions
     White to yellow nodules within or beneath conjunctiva
     H11.121   Conjunctival concretions, right eye
     H11.122   Conjunctival concretions, left eye
     H11.123   Conjunctival concretions, bilateral
     H11.129   Conjunctival concretions, unspecified eye
● H11.13   Conjunctival pigmentations
     Conjunctival argyrosis [argyria]
     H11.131   Conjunctival pigmentations, right eye
     H11.132   Conjunctival pigmentations, left eye
     H11.133   Conjunctival pigmentations, bilateral
     H11.139   Conjunctival pigmentations, unspecified eye
● H11.14   Conjunctival xerosis, unspecified
     Excludes1   xerosis of conjunctiva due to vitamin A deficiency (E50.0, E50.1)
     H11.141   Conjunctival xerosis, unspecified, right eye
     H11.142   Conjunctival xerosis, unspecified, left eye
     H11.143   Conjunctival xerosis, unspecified, bilateral
     H11.149   Conjunctival xerosis, unspecified, unspecified eye
● H11.15   Pinguecula
     Yellowish spot near sclerocorneal junction, usually on nasal side; associated with aging
     Excludes1   pingueculitis (H10.81-)
     H11.151   Pinguecula, right eye
     H11.152   Pinguecula, left eye
     H11.153   Pinguecula, bilateral
     H11.159   Pinguecula, unspecified eye
● H11.2   Conjunctival scars
● H11.21   Conjunctival adhesions and strands (localized)
     H11.211   Conjunctival adhesions and strands (localized), right eye
     H11.212   Conjunctival adhesions and strands (localized), left eye
     H11.213   Conjunctival adhesions and strands (localized), bilateral
     H11.219   Conjunctival adhesions and strands (localized), unspecified eye
● H11.22   Conjunctival granuloma
     H11.221   Conjunctival granuloma, right eye
     H11.222   Conjunctival granuloma, left eye
     H11.223   Conjunctival granuloma, bilateral
     H11.229   Conjunctival granuloma, unspecified
● H11.23   Symblepharon
     Adhesion between tarsal conjunctiva and bulbar conjunctiva
     H11.231   Symblepharon, right eye
     H11.232   Symblepharon, left eye
     H11.233   Symblepharon, bilateral
     H11.239   Symblepharon, unspecified eye

● H11.24   Scarring of conjunctiva
     H11.241   Scarring of conjunctiva, right eye
     H11.242   Scarring of conjunctiva, left eye
     H11.243   Scarring of conjunctiva, bilateral
     H11.249   Scarring of conjunctiva, unspecified eye
● H11.3   Conjunctival hemorrhage
     Subconjunctival hemorrhage
   H11.30   Conjunctival hemorrhage, unspecified eye
   H11.31   Conjunctival hemorrhage, right eye
   H11.32   Conjunctival hemorrhage, left eye
   H11.33   Conjunctival hemorrhage, bilateral
● H11.4   Other conjunctival vascular disorders and cysts
● H11.41   Vascular abnormalities of conjunctiva
     Conjunctival aneurysm
     H11.411   Vascular abnormalities of conjunctiva, right eye
     H11.412   Vascular abnormalities of conjunctiva, left eye
     H11.413   Vascular abnormalities of conjunctiva, bilateral
     H11.419   Vascular abnormalities of conjunctiva, unspecified eye
● H11.42   Conjunctival edema
     H11.421   Conjunctival edema, right eye
     H11.422   Conjunctival edema, left eye
     H11.423   Conjunctival edema, bilateral
     H11.429   Conjunctival edema, unspecified eye
● H11.43   Conjunctival hyperemia
     H11.431   Conjunctival hyperemia, right eye
     H11.432   Conjunctival hyperemia, left eye
     H11.433   Conjunctival hyperemia, bilateral
     H11.439   Conjunctival hyperemia, unspecified eye
● H11.44   Conjunctival cysts
     H11.441   Conjunctival cysts, right eye
     H11.442   Conjunctival cysts, left eye
     H11.443   Conjunctival cysts, bilateral
     H11.449   Conjunctival cysts, unspecified eye
● H11.8   Other specified disorders of conjunctiva
● H11.81   Pseudopterygium of conjunctiva
     Conjunctival scar attached to cornea
     H11.811   Pseudopterygium of conjunctiva, right eye
     H11.812   Pseudopterygium of conjunctiva, left eye
     H11.813   Pseudopterygium of conjunctiva, bilateral
     H11.819   Pseudopterygium of conjunctiva, unspecified eye
● H11.82   Conjunctivochalasis
     Conjunctiva bulges over eyelid margin or covers lower punctum
     H11.821   Conjunctivochalasis, right eye
     H11.822   Conjunctivochalasis, left eye
     H11.823   Conjunctivochalasis, bilateral
     H11.829   Conjunctivochalasis, unspecified eye
   H11.89   Other specified disorders of conjunctiva
  H11.9   Unspecified disorder of conjunctiva

CHAPTER 7 (H00-H59)

DISORDERS OF SCLERA, CORNEA, IRIS AND CILIARY BODY (H15-H22)

- ● H15   **Disorders of sclera**
  - ● H15.0   Scleritis
    - *Inflammation of the white (sclera and episclera) of the eye.*
    - ● H15.00   Unspecified scleritis
      - H15.001   Unspecified scleritis, right eye
      - H15.002   Unspecified scleritis, left eye
      - H15.003   Unspecified scleritis, bilateral
      - H15.009   Unspecified scleritis, unspecified eye
    - ● H15.01   Anterior scleritis
      - H15.011   Anterior scleritis, right eye
      - H15.012   Anterior scleritis, left eye
      - H15.013   Anterior scleritis, bilateral
      - H15.019   Anterior scleritis, unspecified eye
    - ● H15.02   Brawny scleritis
      - *Swelling around the cornea that is gelantinous in appearance*
      - H15.021   Brawny scleritis, right eye
      - H15.022   Brawny scleritis, left eye
      - H15.023   Brawny scleritis, bilateral
      - H15.029   Brawny scleritis, unspecified eye
    - ● H15.03   Posterior scleritis
      - Sclerotenonitis
      - H15.031   Posterior scleritis, right eye
      - H15.032   Posterior scleritis, left eye
      - H15.033   Posterior scleritis, bilateral
      - H15.039   Posterior scleritis, unspecified eye
    - ● H15.04   Scleritis with corneal involvement
      - H15.041   Scleritis with corneal involvement, right eye
      - H15.042   Scleritis with corneal involvement, left eye
      - H15.043   Scleritis with corneal involvement, bilateral
      - H15.049   Scleritis with corneal involvement, unspecified eye
    - ● H15.05   Scleromalacia perforans
      - *Necrotic without inflammation; usually associated with rheumatoid arthritis*
      - H15.051   Scleromalacia perforans, right eye
      - H15.052   Scleromalacia perforans, left eye
      - H15.053   Scleromalacia perforans, bilateral
      - H15.059   Scleromalacia perforans, unspecified eye
    - ● H15.09   Other scleritis
      - Scleral abscess
      - H15.091   Other scleritis, right eye
      - H15.092   Other scleritis, left eye
      - H15.093   Other scleritis, bilateral
      - H15.099   Other scleritis, unspecified eye
  - ● H15.1   Episcleritis
    - *Inflammation of the white (sclera and episclera) of the eye.*
    - ● H15.10   Unspecified episcleritis
      - H15.101   Unspecified episcleritis, right eye
      - H15.102   Unspecified episcleritis, left eye
      - H15.103   Unspecified episcleritis, bilateral
      - H15.109   Unspecified episcleritis, unspecified eye
    - ● H15.11   Episcleritis periodica fugax
      - *Transient, recurrent inflammation of portion of episclera (connective tissue on the surface of the sclera)*
      - H15.111   Episcleritis periodica fugax, right eye
      - H15.112   Episcleritis periodica fugax, left eye
      - H15.113   Episcleritis periodica fugax, bilateral
      - H15.119   Episcleritis periodica fugax, unspecified eye

- ● H15.12   Nodular episcleritis
    - *Characterized by tender, localized, moveable nodule within inflamed area*
    - H15.121   Nodular episcleritis, right eye
    - H15.122   Nodular episcleritis, left eye
    - H15.123   Nodular episcleritis, bilateral
    - H15.129   Nodular episcleritis, unspecified eye
  - ● H15.8   Other disorders of sclera
    - **Excludes2**   blue sclera (Q13.5)
      - degenerative myopia (H44.2-)
    - ● H15.81   Equatorial staphyloma
      - H15.811   Equatorial staphyloma, right eye
      - H15.812   Equatorial staphyloma, left eye
      - H15.813   Equatorial staphyloma, bilateral
      - H15.819   Equatorial staphyloma, unspecified eye
    - ● H15.82   Localized anterior staphyloma
      - H15.821   Localized anterior staphyloma, right eye
      - H15.822   Localized anterior staphyloma, left eye
      - H15.823   Localized anterior staphyloma, bilateral
      - H15.829   Localized anterior staphyloma, unspecified eye
    - ● H15.83   Staphyloma posticum
      - H15.831   Staphyloma posticum, right eye
      - H15.832   Staphyloma posticum, left eye
      - H15.833   Staphyloma posticum, bilateral
      - H15.839   Staphyloma posticum, unspecified eye
    - ● H15.84   Scleral ectasia
      - H15.841   Scleral ectasia, right eye
      - H15.842   Scleral ectasia, left eye
      - H15.843   Scleral ectasia, bilateral
      - H15.849   Scleral ectasia, unspecified eye
    - ● H15.85   Ring staphyloma
      - H15.851   Ring staphyloma, right eye
      - H15.852   Ring staphyloma, left eye
      - H15.853   Ring staphyloma, bilateral
      - H15.859   Ring staphyloma, unspecified eye
    - H15.89   Other disorders of sclera
  - H15.9   Unspecified disorder of sclera

- ● H16   **Keratitis**
  - ● H16.0   Corneal ulcer
    - ● H16.00   Unspecified corneal ulcer
      - H16.001   Unspecified corneal ulcer, right eye
      - H16.002   Unspecified corneal ulcer, left eye
      - H16.003   Unspecified corneal ulcer, bilateral
      - H16.009   Unspecified corneal ulcer, unspecified eye
    - ● H16.01   Central corneal ulcer
      - H16.011   Central corneal ulcer, right eye
      - H16.012   Central corneal ulcer, left eye
      - H16.013   Central corneal ulcer, bilateral
      - H16.019   Central corneal ulcer, unspecified eye
    - ● H16.02   Ring corneal ulcer
      - H16.021   Ring corneal ulcer, right eye
      - H16.022   Ring corneal ulcer, left eye
      - H16.023   Ring corneal ulcer, bilateral
      - H16.029   Ring corneal ulcer, unspecified eye
    - ● H16.03   Corneal ulcer with hypopyon
      - H16.031   Corneal ulcer with hypopyon, right eye
      - H16.032   Corneal ulcer with hypopyon, left eye
      - H16.033   Corneal ulcer with hypopyon, bilateral
      - H16.039   Corneal ulcer with hypopyon, unspecified eye

▶ New   ⇒ Revised   ~~deleted~~ Deleted   Excludes 1   Excludes 2   Includes   Use additional   Code first   Code also   Key words

OGCR Official Guidelines   X Assign placeholder X   ● Use Additional Character(s)   ▶ Manifestation Code   🦚 Hierarchical Condition Category   Coding Clinic

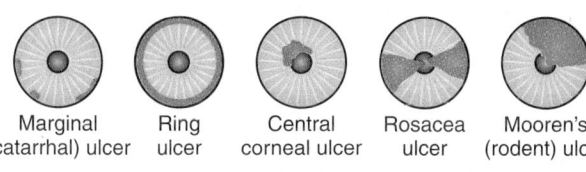

Figure 7-7 Corneal ulcers: marginal, ring, central corneal, rosacea, and Mooren's.

Item 7–3 An infected ulcer is usually called a **serpiginous** or **hypopyon** ulcer, which is a pus sac in the anterior chamber of the eye. **Marginal** ulcers are usually asymptomatic, not primary, and are often superficial and simple. More severe marginal ulcers spread to form a ring ulcer. **Ring** ulcers can extend around the entire corneal periphery. **Central corneal** ulcers develop when there is an abrasion to the epithelium and an infection develops in the eroded area. The **pyocyaneal** ulcer is the most serious corneal infection, which, if left untreated, can lead to loss of the eye.

● H16.04   Marginal corneal ulcer
    H16.041   Marginal corneal ulcer, right eye
    H16.042   Marginal corneal ulcer, left eye
    H16.043   Marginal corneal ulcer, bilateral
    H16.049   Marginal corneal ulcer, unspecified eye

● H16.05   Mooren's corneal ulcer
    H16.051   Mooren's corneal ulcer, right eye
    H16.052   Mooren's corneal ulcer, left eye
    H16.053   Mooren's corneal ulcer, bilateral
    H16.059   Mooren's corneal ulcer, unspecified eye

● H16.06   Mycotic corneal ulcer
    H16.061   Mycotic corneal ulcer, right eye
    H16.062   Mycotic corneal ulcer, left eye
    H16.063   Mycotic corneal ulcer, bilateral
    H16.069   Mycotic corneal ulcer, unspecified eye

● H16.07   Perforated corneal ulcer
    H16.071   Perforated corneal ulcer, right eye
    H16.072   Perforated corneal ulcer, left eye
    H16.073   Perforated corneal ulcer, bilateral
    H16.079   Perforated corneal ulcer, unspecified eye

● H16.1   Other and unspecified superficial keratitis without conjunctivitis
  ● H16.10   Unspecified superficial keratitis
    H16.101   Unspecified superficial keratitis, right eye
    H16.102   Unspecified superficial keratitis, left eye
    H16.103   Unspecified superficial keratitis, bilateral
    H16.109   Unspecified superficial keratitis, unspecified eye

  ● H16.11   Macular keratitis
    Areolar keratitis
    Nummular keratitis
    Stellate keratitis
    Striate keratitis
    H16.111   Macular keratitis, right eye
    H16.112   Macular keratitis, left eye
    H16.113   Macular keratitis, bilateral
    H16.119   Macular keratitis, unspecified eye

  ● H16.12   Filamentary keratitis
    H16.121   Filamentary keratitis, right eye
    H16.122   Filamentary keratitis, left eye
    H16.123   Filamentary keratitis, bilateral
    H16.129   Filamentary keratitis, unspecified eye

● H16.13   Photokeratitis
    Snow blindness
    Welders' keratitis
    H16.131   Photokeratitis, right eye
    H16.132   Photokeratitis, left eye
    H16.133   Photokeratitis, bilateral
    H16.139   Photokeratitis, unspecified eye

● H16.14   Punctate keratitis
    H16.141   Punctate keratitis, right eye
    H16.142   Punctate keratitis, left eye
    H16.143   Punctate keratitis, bilateral
    H16.149   Punctate keratitis, unspecified eye

● H16.2   Keratoconjunctivitis
  ● H16.20   Unspecified keratoconjunctivitis
    Superficial keratitis with conjunctivitis NOS
    H16.201   Unspecified keratoconjunctivitis, right eye
    H16.202   Unspecified keratoconjunctivitis, left eye
    H16.203   Unspecified keratoconjunctivitis, bilateral
    H16.209   Unspecified keratoconjunctivitis, unspecified eye

  ● H16.21   Exposure keratoconjunctivitis
    H16.211   Exposure keratoconjunctivitis, right eye
    H16.212   Exposure keratoconjunctivitis, left eye
    H16.213   Exposure keratoconjunctivitis, bilateral
    H16.219   Exposure keratoconjunctivitis, unspecified eye

  ● H16.22   Keratoconjunctivitis sicca, not specified as Sjögren's
    Excludes1   Sjogren's syndrome (M35.01)
    H16.221   Keratoconjunctivitis sicca, not specified as Sjögren's, right eye
    H16.222   Keratoconjunctivitis sicca, not specified as Sjögren's, left eye
    H16.223   Keratoconjunctivitis sicca, not specified as Sjögren's, bilateral
    H16.229   Keratoconjunctivitis sicca, not specified as Sjögren's, unspecified eye

  ● H16.23   Neurotrophic keratoconjunctivitis
    H16.231   Neurotrophic keratoconjunctivitis, right eye
    H16.232   Neurotrophic keratoconjunctivitis, left eye
    H16.233   Neurotrophic keratoconjunctivitis, bilateral
    H16.239   Neurotrophic keratoconjunctivitis, unspecified eye

  ● H16.24   Ophthalmia nodosa
    H16.241   Ophthalmia nodosa, right eye
    H16.242   Ophthalmia nodosa, left eye
    H16.243   Ophthalmia nodosa, bilateral
    H16.249   Ophthalmia nodosa, unspecified eye

  ● H16.25   Phlyctenular keratoconjunctivitis
    H16.251   Phlyctenular keratoconjunctivitis, right eye
    H16.252   Phlyctenular keratoconjunctivitis, left eye
    H16.253   Phlyctenular keratoconjunctivitis, bilateral
    H16.259   Phlyctenular keratoconjunctivitis, unspecified eye

CHAPTER 7 (H00-H59)

CHAPTER 7 (H00-H59)

● H16.26   Vernal keratoconjunctivitis, with limbar and corneal involvement

      Excludes1   vernal conjunctivitis without limbar and corneal involvement (H10.44)

    H16.261   Vernal keratoconjunctivitis, with limbar and corneal involvement, right eye

    H16.262   Vernal keratoconjunctivitis, with limbar and corneal involvement, left eye

    H16.263   Vernal keratoconjunctivitis, with limbar and corneal involvement, bilateral

    H16.269   Vernal keratoconjunctivitis, with limbar and corneal involvement, unspecified eye

● H16.29   Other keratoconjunctivitis

    H16.291   Other keratoconjunctivitis, right eye

    H16.292   Other keratoconjunctivitis, left eye

    H16.293   Other keratoconjunctivitis, bilateral

    H16.299   Other keratoconjunctivitis, unspecified eye

● H16.3   Interstitial and deep keratitis

 ● H16.30   Unspecified interstitial keratitis

    H16.301   Unspecified interstitial keratitis, right eye

    H16.302   Unspecified interstitial keratitis, left eye

    H16.303   Unspecified interstitial keratitis, bilateral

    H16.309   Unspecified interstitial keratitis, unspecified eye

 ● H16.31   Corneal abscess

    H16.311   Corneal abscess, right eye

    H16.312   Corneal abscess, left eye

    H16.313   Corneal abscess, bilateral

    H16.319   Corneal abscess, unspecified eye

 ● H16.32   Diffuse interstitial keratitis
      Cogan's syndrome

    H16.321   Diffuse interstitial keratitis, right eye

    H16.322   Diffuse interstitial keratitis, left eye

    H16.323   Diffuse interstitial keratitis, bilateral

    H16.329   Diffuse interstitial keratitis, unspecified eye

 ● H16.33   Sclerosing keratitis

    H16.331   Sclerosing keratitis, right eye

    H16.332   Sclerosing keratitis, left eye

    H16.333   Sclerosing keratitis, bilateral

    H16.339   Sclerosing keratitis, unspecified eye

 ● H16.39   Other interstitial and deep keratitis

    H16.391   Other interstitial and deep keratitis, right eye

    H16.392   Other interstitial and deep keratitis, left eye

    H16.393   Other interstitial and deep keratitis, bilateral

    H16.399   Other interstitial and deep keratitis, unspecified eye

● H16.4   Corneal neovascularization

 ● H16.40   Unspecified corneal neovascularization

    H16.401   Unspecified corneal neovascularization, right eye

    H16.402   Unspecified corneal neovascularization, left eye

    H16.403   Unspecified corneal neovascularization, bilateral

    H16.409   Unspecified corneal neovascularization, unspecified

 ● H16.41   Ghost vessels (corneal)

    H16.411   Ghost vessels (corneal), right eye

    H16.412   Ghost vessels (corneal), left eye

    H16.413   Ghost vessels (corneal), bilateral

    H16.419   Ghost vessels (corneal), unspecified eye

 ● H16.42   Pannus (corneal)

    H16.421   Pannus (corneal), right eye

    H16.422   Pannus (corneal), left eye

    H16.423   Pannus (corneal), bilateral

    H16.429   Pannus (corneal), unspecified eye

 ● H16.43   Localized vascularization of cornea

    H16.431   Localized vascularization of cornea, right eye

    H16.432   Localized vascularization of cornea, left eye

    H16.433   Localized vascularization of cornea, bilateral

    H16.439   Localized vascularization of cornea, unspecified eye

 ● H16.44   Deep vascularization of cornea

    H16.441   Deep vascularization of cornea, right eye

    H16.442   Deep vascularization of cornea, left eye

    H16.443   Deep vascularization of cornea, bilateral

    H16.449   Deep vascularization of cornea, unspecified eye

   H16.8   Other keratitis

   H16.9   Unspecified keratitis

● H17   Corneal scars and opacities

 ● H17.0   Adherent leukoma

    H17.00   Adherent leukoma, unspecified eye

    H17.01   Adherent leukoma, right eye

    H17.02   Adherent leukoma, left eye

    H17.03   Adherent leukoma, bilateral

 ● H17.1   Central corneal opacity

    H17.10   Central corneal opacity, unspecified eye

    H17.11   Central corneal opacity, right eye

    H17.12   Central corneal opacity, left eye

    H17.13   Central corneal opacity, bilateral

 ● H17.8   Other corneal scars and opacities

  ● H17.81   Minor opacity of cornea
      Corneal nebula

    H17.811   Minor opacity of cornea, right eye

    H17.812   Minor opacity of cornea, left eye

    H17.813   Minor opacity of cornea, bilateral

    H17.819   Minor opacity of cornea, unspecified eye

  ● H17.82   Peripheral opacity of cornea

    H17.821   Peripheral opacity of cornea, right eye

    H17.822   Peripheral opacity of cornea, left eye

    H17.823   Peripheral opacity of cornea, bilateral

    H17.829   Peripheral opacity of cornea, unspecified eye

    H17.89   Other corneal scars and opacities

   H17.9   Unspecified corneal scar and opacity

● H18   Other disorders of cornea

 ● H18.0   Corneal pigmentations and deposits

  ● H18.00   Unspecified corneal deposit

    H18.001   Unspecified corneal deposit, right eye

    H18.002   Unspecified corneal deposit, left eye

    H18.003   Unspecified corneal deposit, bilateral

    H18.009   Unspecified corneal deposit, unspecified eye

▶ New   ⇒ Revised   ~~deleted~~ Deleted   Excludes 1   Excludes 2   Includes   Use additional   Code first   Code also   Key words

OGCR Official Guidelines   X Assign placeholder X   ● Use Additional Character(s)   ▶ Manifestation Code   🗝 Hierarchical Condition Category   Coding Clinic

● H18.01   Anterior corneal pigmentations
     Staehli's line
     H18.011   Anterior corneal pigmentations, right eye
     H18.012   Anterior corneal pigmentations, left eye
     H18.013   Anterior corneal pigmentations, bilateral
     H18.019   Anterior corneal pigmentations, unspecified eye

● H18.02   Argentous corneal deposits
     H18.021   Argentous corneal deposits, right eye
     H18.022   Argentous corneal deposits, left eye
     H18.023   Argentous corneal deposits, bilateral
     H18.029   Argentous corneal deposits, unspecified eye

● H18.03   Corneal deposits in metabolic disorders
     Code also associated metabolic disorder
     H18.031   Corneal deposits in metabolic disorders, right eye
     H18.032   Corneal deposits in metabolic disorders, left eye
     H18.033   Corneal deposits in metabolic disorders, bilateral
     H18.039   Corneal deposits in metabolic disorders, unspecified eye

● H18.04   Kayser-Fleischer ring
     Code also associated Wilson's disease (E83.01)
     H18.041   Kayser-Fleischer ring, right eye
     H18.042   Kayser-Fleischer ring, left eye
     H18.043   Kayser-Fleischer ring, bilateral
     H18.049   Kayser-Fleischer ring, unspecified eye

● H18.05   Posterior corneal pigmentations
     Krukenberg's spindle
     H18.051   Posterior corneal pigmentations, right eye
     H18.052   Posterior corneal pigmentations, left eye
     H18.053   Posterior corneal pigmentations, bilateral
     H18.059   Posterior corneal pigmentations, unspecified eye

● H18.06   Stromal corneal pigmentations
     Hematocornea
     H18.061   Stromal corneal pigmentations, right eye
     H18.062   Stromal corneal pigmentations, left eye
     H18.063   Stromal corneal pigmentations, bilateral
     H18.069   Stromal corneal pigmentations, unspecified eye

● H18.1   Bullous keratopathy
     H18.10   Bullous keratopathy, unspecified eye
     H18.11   Bullous keratopathy, right eye
     H18.12   Bullous keratopathy, left eye
     H18.13   Bullous keratopathy, bilateral

● H18.2   Other and unspecified corneal edema
     H18.20   Unspecified corneal edema
     ● H18.21   Corneal edema secondary to contact lens
         Excludes2   other corneal disorders due to contact lens (H18.82-)
     H18.211   Corneal edema secondary to contact lens, right eye
     H18.212   Corneal edema secondary to contact lens, left eye
     H18.213   Corneal edema secondary to contact lens, bilateral
     H18.219   Corneal edema secondary to contact lens, unspecified eye

● H18.22   Idiopathic corneal edema
     H18.221   Idiopathic corneal edema, right eye
     H18.222   Idiopathic corneal edema, left eye
     H18.223   Idiopathic corneal edema, bilateral
     H18.229   Idiopathic corneal edema, unspecified eye

● H18.23   Secondary corneal edema
     H18.231   Secondary corneal edema, right eye
     H18.232   Secondary corneal edema, left eye
     H18.233   Secondary corneal edema, bilateral
     H18.239   Secondary corneal edema, unspecified eye

● H18.3   Changes of corneal membranes
     H18.30   Unspecified corneal membrane change
     ● H18.31   Folds and rupture in Bowman's membrane
     H18.311   Folds and rupture in Bowman's membrane, right eye
     H18.312   Folds and rupture in Bowman's membrane, left eye
     H18.313   Folds and rupture in Bowman's membrane, bilateral
     H18.319   Folds and rupture in Bowman's membrane, unspecified eye

● H18.32   Folds in Descemet's membrane
     H18.321   Folds in Descemet's membrane, right eye
     H18.322   Folds in Descemet's membrane, left eye
     H18.323   Folds in Descemet's membrane, bilateral
     H18.329   Folds in Descemet's membrane, unspecified eye

● H18.33   Rupture in Descemet's membrane
     H18.331   Rupture in Descemet's membrane, right eye
     H18.332   Rupture in Descemet's membrane, left eye
     H18.333   Rupture in Descemet's membrane, bilateral
     H18.339   Rupture in Descemet's membrane, unspecified eye

● H18.4   Corneal degeneration
     Excludes1   Mooren's ulcer (H16.0-)
         recurrent erosion of cornea (H18.83-)
     H18.40   Unspecified corneal degeneration
     ● H18.41   Arcus senilis
     Senile corneal changes
     H18.411   Arcus senilis, right eye
     H18.412   Arcus senilis, left eye
     H18.413   Arcus senilis, bilateral
     H18.419   Arcus senilis, unspecified eye

● H18.42   Band keratopathy
     H18.421   Band keratopathy, right eye
     H18.422   Band keratopathy, left eye
     H18.423   Band keratopathy, bilateral
     H18.429   Band keratopathy, unspecified eye
     H18.43   Other calcerous corneal degeneration

● H18.44   Keratomalacia
     Excludes1   keratomalacia due to vitamin A deficiency (E50.4)
     H18.441   Keratomalacia, right eye
     H18.442   Keratomalacia, left eye
     H18.443   Keratomalacia, bilateral
     H18.449   Keratomalacia, unspecified eye

CHAPTER 7 (H00-H59)

● H18.45   Nodular corneal degeneration
     H18.451   Nodular corneal degeneration, right eye
     H18.452   Nodular corneal degeneration, left eye
     H18.453   Nodular corneal degeneration, bilateral
     H18.459   Nodular corneal degeneration, unspecified eye
● H18.46   Peripheral corneal degeneration
     H18.461   Peripheral corneal degeneration, right eye
     H18.462   Peripheral corneal degeneration, left eye
     H18.463   Peripheral corneal degeneration, bilateral
     H18.469   Peripheral corneal degeneration, unspecified eye
   H18.49   Other corneal degeneration
● H18.5   Hereditary corneal dystrophies
   ● H18.50   Unspecified hereditary corneal dystrophies
     H18.501   Unspecified hereditary corneal dystrophies, right eye
     H18.502   Unspecified hereditary corneal dystrophies, left eye
     H18.503   Unspecified hereditary corneal dystrophies, bilateral
     H18.509   Unspecified hereditary corneal dystrophies, unspecified eye
   ● H18.51   Endothelial corneal dystrophy
     Fuchs' dystrophy
     H18.511   Endothelial corneal dystrophy, right eye
     H18.512   Endothelial corneal dystrophy, left eye
     H18.513   Endothelial corneal dystrophy, bilateral
     H18.519   Endothelial corneal dystrophy, unspecified eye
   ● H18.52   Epithelial (juvenile) corneal dystrophy
     H18.521   Epithelial (juvenile) corneal dystrophy, right eye
     H18.522   Epithelial (juvenile) corneal dystrophy, left eye
     H18.523   Epithelial (juvenile) corneal dystrophy, bilateral
     H18.529   Epithelial (juvenile) corneal dystrophy, unspecified eye
   ● H18.53   Granular corneal dystrophy
     H18.531   Granular corneal dystrophy, right eye
     H18.532   Granular corneal dystrophy, left eye
     H18.533   Granular corneal dystrophy, bilateral
     H18.539   Granular corneal dystrophy, unspecified eye
   ● H18.54   Lattice corneal dystrophy
     H18.541   Lattice corneal dystrophy, right eye
     H18.542   Lattice corneal dystrophy, left eye
     H18.543   Lattice corneal dystrophy, bilateral
     H18.549   Lattice corneal dystrophy, unspecified eye
   ● H18.55   Macular corneal dystrophy
     H18.551   Macular corneal dystrophy, right eye
     H18.552   Macular corneal dystrophy, left eye
     H18.553   Macular corneal dystrophy, bilateral
     H18.559   Macular corneal dystrophy, unspecified eye

● H18.59   Other hereditary corneal dystrophies
     H18.591   Other hereditary corneal dystrophies, right eye
     H18.592   Other hereditary corneal dystrophies, left eye
     H18.593   Other hereditary corneal dystrophies, bilateral
     H18.599   Other hereditary corneal dystrophies, unspecified eye
● H18.6   Keratoconus
   ● H18.60   Keratoconus, unspecified
     H18.601   Keratoconus, unspecified, right eye
     H18.602   Keratoconus, unspecified, left eye
     H18.603   Keratoconus, unspecified, bilateral
     H18.609   Keratoconus, unspecified, unspecified eye
   ● H18.61   Keratoconus, stable
     H18.611   Keratoconus, stable, right eye
     H18.612   Keratoconus, stable, left eye
     H18.613   Keratoconus, stable, bilateral
     H18.619   Keratoconus, stable, unspecified eye
   ● H18.62   Keratoconus, unstable
     Acute hydrops
     H18.621   Keratoconus, unstable, right eye
     H18.622   Keratoconus, unstable, left eye
     H18.623   Keratoconus, unstable, bilateral
     H18.629   Keratoconus, unstable, unspecified eye
● H18.7   Other and unspecified corneal deformities
     Excludes 1   congenital malformations of cornea (Q13.3-Q13.4)
   H18.70   Unspecified corneal deformity
   ● H18.71   Corneal ectasia
     H18.711   Corneal ectasia, right eye
     H18.712   Corneal ectasia, left eye
     H18.713   Corneal ectasia, bilateral
     H18.719   Corneal ectasia, unspecified eye
   ● H18.72   Corneal staphyloma
     H18.721   Corneal staphyloma, right eye
     H18.722   Corneal staphyloma, left eye
     H18.723   Corneal staphyloma, bilateral
     H18.729   Corneal staphyloma, unspecified eye
   ● H18.73   Descemetocele
     H18.731   Descemetocele, right eye
     H18.732   Descemetocele, left eye
     H18.733   Descemetocele, bilateral
     H18.739   Descemetocele, unspecified eye
   ● H18.79   Other corneal deformities
     H18.791   Other corneal deformities, right eye
     H18.792   Other corneal deformities, left eye
     H18.793   Other corneal deformities, bilateral
     H18.799   Other corneal deformities, unspecified eye

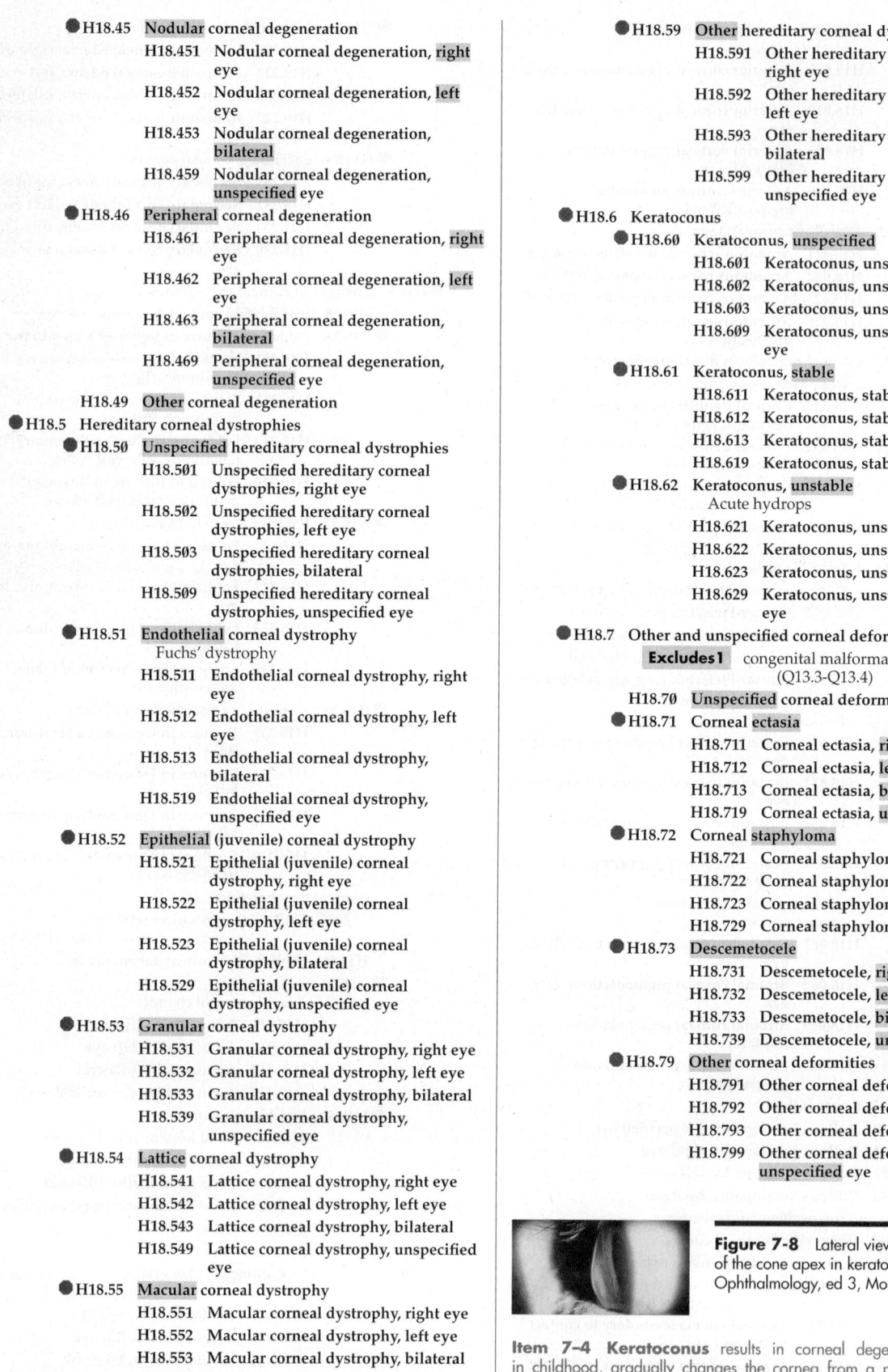

Figure 7-8 Lateral view of the displacement of the cone apex in keratoconus. (From Yanoff: Ophthalmology, ed 3, Mosby, Inc., 2008)

Item 7-4 Keratoconus results in corneal degeneration that begins in childhood, gradually changes the cornea from a round to cone shape, decreasing visual acuity. Treatment includes contact lenses. In severe cases the need for corneal transplant may be the treatment of choice; however, newer technologies may use high-frequency radio energy to shrink the edges of the cornea, pulling the central area back to a more normal shape. It can help delay or avoid the need for a corneal transplantation.

▶ New   ⇒ Revised   ~~deleted~~ Deleted   Excludes 1   Excludes 2   Includes   Use additional   Code first   Code also   Key words
OGCR Official Guidelines   X Assign placeholder X   ● Use Additional Character(s)   ▶ Manifestation Code   ⬚ Hierarchical Condition Category   **Coding Clinic**

● H18.8   Other specified disorders of cornea
   ● H18.81   Anesthesia and hypoesthesia of cornea
      H18.811   Anesthesia and hypoesthesia of cornea, right eye
      H18.812   Anesthesia and hypoesthesia of cornea, left eye
      H18.813   Anesthesia and hypoesthesia of cornea, bilateral
      H18.819   Anesthesia and hypoesthesia of cornea, unspecified eye
   ● H18.82   Corneal disorder due to contact lens
      Excludes2   corneal edema due to contact lens (H18.21-)
      H18.821   Corneal disorder due to contact lens, right eye
      H18.822   Corneal disorder due to contact lens, left eye
      H18.823   Corneal disorder due to contact lens, bilateral
      H18.829   Corneal disorder due to contact lens, unspecified eye
   ● H18.83   Recurrent erosion of cornea
      H18.831   Recurrent erosion of cornea, right eye
      H18.832   Recurrent erosion of cornea, left eye
      H18.833   Recurrent erosion of cornea, bilateral
      H18.839   Recurrent erosion of cornea, unspecified eye
   ● H18.89   Other specified disorders of cornea
      H18.891   Other specified disorders of cornea, right eye
      H18.892   Other specified disorders of cornea, left eye
      H18.893   Other specified disorders of cornea, bilateral
      H18.899   Other specified disorders of cornea, unspecified eye
   H18.9   Unspecified disorder of cornea

● H20   Iridocyclitis
   ● H20.0   Acute and subacute iridocyclitis
      Acute anterior uveitis
      Acute cyclitis
      Acute iritis
      Subacute anterior uveitis
      Subacute cyclitis
      Subacute iritis
      Excludes1   iridocyclitis, iritis, uveitis (due to) (in) diabetes mellitus (E08-E13 with .39)
         iridocyclitis, iritis, uveitis (due to) (in) diphtheria (A36.89)
         iridocyclitis, iritis, uveitis (due to) (in) gonococcal (A54.32)
         iridocyclitis, iritis, uveitis (due to) (in) herpes (simplex) (B00.51)
         iridocyclitis, iritis, uveitis (due to) (in) herpes zoster (B02.32)
         iridocyclitis, iritis, uveitis (due to) (in) late congenital syphilis (A50.39)
         iridocyclitis, iritis, uveitis (due to) (in) late syphilis (A52.71)
         iridocyclitis, iritis, uveitis (due to) (in) sarcoidosis (D86.83)
         iridocyclitis, iritis, uveitis (due to) (in) syphilis (A51.43)
         iridocyclitis, iritis, uveitis (due to) (in) toxoplasmosis (B58.09)
         iridocyclitis, iritis, uveitis (due to) (in) tuberculosis (A18.54)
      H20.00   Unspecified acute and subacute iridocyclitis

● H20.01   Primary iridocyclitis
      H20.011   Primary iridocyclitis, right eye
      H20.012   Primary iridocyclitis, left eye
      H20.013   Primary iridocyclitis, bilateral
      H20.019   Primary iridocyclitis, unspecified eye
● H20.02   Recurrent acute iridocyclitis
      H20.021   Recurrent acute iridocyclitis, right eye
      H20.022   Recurrent acute iridocyclitis, left eye
      H20.023   Recurrent acute iridocyclitis, bilateral
      H20.029   Recurrent acute iridocyclitis, unspecified eye
● H20.03   Secondary infectious iridocyclitis
      H20.031   Secondary infectious iridocyclitis, right eye
      H20.032   Secondary infectious iridocyclitis, left eye
      H20.033   Secondary infectious iridocyclitis, bilateral
      H20.039   Secondary infectious iridocyclitis, unspecified eye
● H20.04   Secondary noninfectious iridocyclitis
      H20.041   Secondary noninfectious iridocyclitis, right eye
      H20.042   Secondary noninfectious iridocyclitis, left eye
      H20.043   Secondary noninfectious iridocyclitis, bilateral
      H20.049   Secondary noninfectious iridocyclitis, unspecified eye
● H20.05   Hypopyon
      H20.051   Hypopyon, right eye
      H20.052   Hypopyon, left eye
      H20.053   Hypopyon, bilateral
      H20.059   Hypopyon, unspecified eye
● H20.1   Chronic iridocyclitis
      Use additional code for any associated cataract (H26.21-)
      Excludes2   posterior cyclitis (H30.2-)
      H20.10   Chronic iridocyclitis, unspecified eye
      H20.11   Chronic iridocyclitis, right eye
      H20.12   Chronic iridocyclitis, left eye
      H20.13   Chronic iridocyclitis, bilateral
● H20.2   Lens-induced iridocyclitis
      H20.20   Lens-induced iridocyclitis, unspecified eye
      H20.21   Lens-induced iridocyclitis, right eye
      H20.22   Lens-induced iridocyclitis, left eye
      H20.23   Lens-induced iridocyclitis, bilateral
● H20.8   Other iridocyclitis
      Excludes2   glaucomatocyclitis crises (H40.4-)
         posterior cyclitis (H30.2-)
         sympathetic uveitis (H44.13-)
● H20.81   Fuchs' heterochromic cyclitis
      H20.811   Fuchs' heterochromic cyclitis, right eye
      H20.812   Fuchs' heterochromic cyclitis, left eye
      H20.813   Fuchs' heterochromic cyclitis, bilateral
      H20.819   Fuchs' heterochromic cyclitis, unspecified eye
● H20.82   Vogt-Koyanagi syndrome
      H20.821   Vogt-Koyanagi syndrome, right eye
      H20.822   Vogt-Koyanagi syndrome, left eye

CHAPTER 7 (H00-H59)

H20.823 Vogt-Koyanagi syndrome, bilateral
H20.829 Vogt-Koyanagi syndrome, unspecified eye

H20.9 **Unspecified iridocyclitis**
Uveitis NOS

● H21 **Other disorders of iris and ciliary body**
Excludes2 sympathetic uveitis (H44.1-)
● H21.0 **Hyphema**
Excludes1 traumatic hyphema (S05.1-)
H21.00 Hyphema, unspecified eye
H21.01 Hyphema, right eye
H21.02 Hyphema, left eye
H21.03 Hyphema, bilateral
● H21.1 **Other vascular disorders of iris and ciliary body**
Neovascularization of iris or ciliary body
Rubeosis iridis
Rubeosis of iris
● H21.1X **Other vascular disorders of iris and ciliary body**
H21.1X1 Other vascular disorders of iris and ciliary body, right eye
H21.1X2 Other vascular disorders of iris and ciliary body, left eye
H21.1X3 Other vascular disorders of iris and ciliary body, bilateral
H21.1X9 Other vascular disorders of iris and ciliary body, unspecified eye
● H21.2 **Degeneration of iris and ciliary body**
● H21.21 Degeneration of chamber angle
H21.211 Degeneration of chamber angle, right eye
H21.212 Degeneration of chamber angle, left eye
H21.213 Degeneration of chamber angle, bilateral
H21.219 Degeneration of chamber angle, unspecified eye
● H21.22 Degeneration of ciliary body
H21.221 Degeneration of ciliary body, right eye
H21.222 Degeneration of ciliary body, left eye
H21.223 Degeneration of ciliary body, bilateral
H21.229 Degeneration of ciliary body, unspecified eye
● H21.23 Degeneration of iris (pigmentary)
Translucency of iris
H21.231 Degeneration of iris (pigmentary), right eye
H21.232 Degeneration of iris (pigmentary), left eye
H21.233 Degeneration of iris (pigmentary), bilateral
H21.239 Degeneration of iris (pigmentary), unspecified eye
● H21.24 Degeneration of pupillary margin
H21.241 Degeneration of pupillary margin, right eye
H21.242 Degeneration of pupillary margin, left eye
H21.243 Degeneration of pupillary margin, bilateral
H21.249 Degeneration of pupillary margin, unspecified eye
● H21.25 Iridoschisis
H21.251 Iridoschisis, right eye
H21.252 Iridoschisis, left eye

H21.253 Iridoschisis, bilateral
H21.259 Iridoschisis, unspecified eye
● H21.26 Iris atrophy (essential) (progressive)
H21.261 Iris atrophy (essential) (progressive), right eye
H21.262 Iris atrophy (essential) (progressive), left eye
H21.263 Iris atrophy (essential) (progressive), bilateral
H21.269 Iris atrophy (essential) (progressive), unspecified eye
● H21.27 Miotic pupillary cyst
H21.271 Miotic pupillary cyst, right eye
H21.272 Miotic pupillary cyst, left eye
H21.273 Miotic pupillary cyst, bilateral
H21.279 Miotic pupillary cyst, unspecified eye
H21.29 **Other iris atrophy**
● H21.3 **Cyst of iris, ciliary body and anterior chamber**
Excludes2 miotic pupillary cyst (H21.27-)
● H21.30 Idiopathic cysts of iris, ciliary body or anterior chamber
Cyst of iris, ciliary body or anterior chamber NOS
H21.301 Idiopathic cysts of iris, ciliary body or anterior chamber, right eye
H21.302 Idiopathic cysts of iris, ciliary body or anterior chamber, left eye
H21.303 Idiopathic cysts of iris, ciliary body or anterior chamber, bilateral
H21.309 Idiopathic cysts of iris, ciliary body or anterior chamber, unspecified eye
● H21.31 Exudative cysts of iris or anterior chamber
H21.311 Exudative cysts of iris or anterior chamber, right eye
H21.312 Exudative cysts of iris or anterior chamber, left eye
H21.313 Exudative cysts of iris or anterior chamber, bilateral
H21.319 Exudative cysts of iris or anterior chamber, unspecified eye
● H21.32 Implantation cysts of iris, ciliary body or anterior chamber
H21.321 Implantation cysts of iris, ciliary body or anterior chamber, right eye
H21.322 Implantation cysts of iris, ciliary body or anterior chamber, left eye
H21.323 Implantation cysts of iris, ciliary body or anterior chamber, bilateral
H21.329 Implantation cysts of iris, ciliary body or anterior chamber, unspecified eye
● H21.33 Parasitic cyst of iris, ciliary body or anterior chamber
H21.331 Parasitic cyst of iris, ciliary body or anterior chamber, right eye
H21.332 Parasitic cyst of iris, ciliary body or anterior chamber, left eye
H21.333 Parasitic cyst of iris, ciliary body or anterior chamber, bilateral
H21.339 Parasitic cyst of iris, ciliary body or anterior chamber, unspecified eye
● H21.34 Primary cyst of pars plana
H21.341 Primary cyst of pars plana, right eye
H21.342 Primary cyst of pars plana, left eye

▶ New   ⇒ Revised   ~~deleted~~ Deleted   Excludes 1   Excludes 2   Includes   Use additional   Code first   Code also   Key words
OGCR Official Guidelines   X Assign placeholder X   ● Use Additional Character(s)   ▷ Manifestation Code   🐾 Hierarchical Condition Category   Coding Clinic

H21.343   Primary cyst of pars plana, bilateral
H21.349   Primary cyst of pars plana, unspecified eye
● H21.35   Exudative cyst of pars plana
H21.351   Exudative cyst of pars plana, right eye
H21.352   Exudative cyst of pars plana, left eye
H21.353   Exudative cyst of pars plana, bilateral
H21.359   Exudative cyst of pars plana, unspecified eye
● H21.4   **Pupillary membranes**
Iris bombé
Pupillary occlusion
Pupillary seclusion
Excludes1   congenital pupillary membranes (Q13.8)
H21.40   Pupillary membranes, unspecified eye
H21.41   Pupillary membranes, right eye
H21.42   Pupillary membranes, left eye
H21.43   Pupillary membranes, bilateral
● H21.5   **Other and unspecified adhesions and disruptions of iris and ciliary body**
Excludes1   corectopia (Q13.2)
● H21.50   **Unspecified adhesions of iris**
Synechia (iris) NOS
H21.501   Unspecified adhesions of iris, right eye
H21.502   Unspecified adhesions of iris, left eye
H21.503   Unspecified adhesions of iris, bilateral
H21.509   Unspecified adhesions of iris and ciliary body, unspecified eye
● H21.51   Anterior synechiae (iris)
H21.511   Anterior synechiae (iris), right eye
H21.512   Anterior synechiae (iris), left eye
H21.513   Anterior synechiae (iris), bilateral
H21.519   Anterior synechiae (iris), unspecified eye
● H21.52   Goniosynechiae
H21.521   Goniosynechiae, right eye
H21.522   Goniosynechiae, left eye
H21.523   Goniosynechiae, bilateral
H21.529   Goniosynechiae, unspecified eye
● H21.53   Iridodialysis
H21.531   Iridodialysis, right eye
H21.532   Iridodialysis, left eye
H21.533   Iridodialysis, bilateral
H21.539   Iridodialysis, unspecified eye
● H21.54   Posterior synechiae (iris)
H21.541   Posterior synechiae (iris), right eye
H21.542   Posterior synechiae (iris), left eye
H21.543   Posterior synechiae (iris), bilateral
H21.549   Posterior synechiae (iris), unspecified eye
● H21.55   Recession of chamber angle
H21.551   Recession of chamber angle, right eye
H21.552   Recession of chamber angle, left eye
H21.553   Recession of chamber angle, bilateral
H21.559   Recession of chamber angle, unspecified eye
● H21.56   Pupillary abnormalities
Deformed pupil
Ectopic pupil
Rupture of sphincter, pupil
Excludes1   congenital deformity of pupil (Q13.2-)

H21.561   Pupillary abnormality, right eye
H21.562   Pupillary abnormality, left eye
H21.563   Pupillary abnormality, bilateral
H21.569   Pupillary abnormality, unspecified eye
● H21.8   **Other specified disorders of iris and ciliary body**
H21.81   Floppy iris syndrome
Intraoperative floppy iris syndrome (IFIS)
Use additional code for adverse effect, if applicable, to identify drug (T36-T50 with fifth or sixth character 5)
H21.82   Plateau iris syndrome (post-iridectomy) (postprocedural)
H21.89   Other specified disorders of iris and ciliary body
H21.9   **Unspecified disorder of iris and ciliary body**

▷ **H22**   *Disorders of iris and ciliary body in diseases classified elsewhere*
Code first underlying disease, such as:
gout (M1A.-, M10.-)
leprosy (A30.-)
parasitic disease (B89)

DISORDERS OF LENS (H25-H28)

● **H25**   **Age-related cataract**
Senile cataract
Excludes2   capsular glaucoma with pseudoexfoliation of lens (H40.1-)
● H25.0   **Age-related incipient cataract**
● H25.01   Cortical age-related cataract
H25.011   Cortical age-related cataract, right eye   A
H25.012   Cortical age-related cataract, left eye   A
H25.013   Cortical age-related cataract, bilateral   A
H25.019   Cortical age-related cataract, unspecified eye   A
● H25.03   Anterior subcapsular polar age-related cataract
H25.031   Anterior subcapsular polar age-related cataract, right eye   A
H25.032   Anterior subcapsular polar age-related cataract, left eye   A
H25.033   Anterior subcapsular polar age-related cataract, bilateral   A
H25.039   Anterior subcapsular polar age-related cataract, unspecified eye   A

Figure 7-9 Age-related cataract.
Nuclear sclerosis and cortical lens opacities are present. (From Ignatavicius DD, Workman ML: Medical-Surgical Nursing: Patient-Centered Collaborative Care, St. Louis, MO, Saunders/Elsevier, 2010)

Item 7-5 Senile cataracts are linked to the aging process. The most common area for the formation of a cataract is the cortical area of the lens. **Polar cataracts** can be either anterior or posterior. **Anterior polar cataracts** are more common and are small, white, capsular cataracts located on the anterior portion of the lens. **Total cataracts,** also called **complete** or **mature,** cause an opacity of all fibers of the lens. **Hypermature** describes a mature cataract with a swollen, milky cortex that covers the entire lens. **Immature,** also called **incipient,** cataracts have a clear cortex and are only slightly opaque. Treatment for all cataracts is the removal of the lens.

CHAPTER 7 (H00-H59)

CHAPTER 7 (H00-H59)

● H25.04 **Posterior subcapsular polar** age-related cataract

  H25.041 Posterior subcapsular polar age-related cataract, **right eye**   A

  H25.042 Posterior subcapsular polar age-related cataract, **left eye**   A

  H25.043 Posterior subcapsular polar age-related cataract, **bilateral**   A

  H25.049 Posterior subcapsular polar age-related cataract, **unspecified eye** A

● H25.09 Other age-related incipient cataract
  Coronary age-related cataract
  Punctate age-related cataract
  Water clefts

  H25.091 Other age-related incipient cataract, **right eye**   A

  H25.092 Other age-related incipient cataract, **left eye**   A

  H25.093 Other age-related incipient cataract, **bilateral**   A

  H25.099 Other age-related incipient cataract, **unspecified eye**   A

● H25.1 Age-related **nuclear** cataract
  Cataracta brunescens
  Nuclear sclerosis cataract

  H25.10 Age-related nuclear cataract, **unspecified eye**   A

  H25.11 Age-related nuclear cataract, **right eye**   A
          Coding Clinic: 2019, Q2, P30

  H25.12 Age-related nuclear cataract, **left eye**   A
          Coding Clinic: 2016, Q1, P33

  H25.13 Age-related nuclear cataract, **bilateral**   A
          Coding Clinic: 2016, Q1, P32

● H25.2 Age-related cataract, **morgagnian type**
  Age-related hypermature cataract

  H25.20 Age-related cataract, morgagnian type, **unspecified** eye   A

  H25.21 Age-related cataract, morgagnian type, **right eye**   A

  H25.22 Age-related cataract, morgagnian type, **left eye** A

  H25.23 Age-related cataract, morgagnian type, **bilateral**   A

● H25.8 Other age-related cataract

  ● H25.81 **Combined forms** of age-related cataract

    H25.811 Combined forms of age-related cataract, **right eye**   A

    H25.812 Combined forms of age-related cataract, **left eye**   A

    H25.813 Combined forms of age-related cataract, **bilateral**   A
             Coding Clinic: 2019, Q2, P30

    H25.819 Combined forms of age-related cataract, **unspecified eye** A

  H25.89 Other age-related cataract   A

  H25.9 **Unspecified** age-related cataract   A

● H26 Other cataract

  Excludes1 congenital cataract (Q12.0)

  ● H26.0 Infantile and juvenile cataract

    ● H26.00 **Unspecified** infantile and juvenile cataract

      H26.001 Unspecified infantile and juvenile cataract, **right eye**   P

      H26.002 Unspecified infantile and juvenile cataract, **left eye**   P

      H26.003 Unspecified infantile and juvenile cataract, **bilateral**   P

      H26.009 Unspecified infantile and juvenile cataract, **unspecified eye** P

  ● H26.01 Infantile and juvenile **cortical, lamellar, or zonular** cataract

    H26.011 Infantile and juvenile cortical, lamellar, or zonular cataract, **right eye**   P

    H26.012 Infantile and juvenile cortical, lamellar, or zonular cataract, **left eye** P

    H26.013 Infantile and juvenile cortical, lamellar, or zonular cataract, **bilateral**   P

    H26.019 Infantile and juvenile cortical, lamellar, or zonular cataract, **unspecified** eye P

  ● H26.03 Infantile and juvenile **nuclear** cataract

    H26.031 Infantile and juvenile nuclear cataract, **right eye**   P

    H26.032 Infantile and juvenile nuclear cataract, **left eye**   P

    H26.033 Infantile and juvenile nuclear cataract, **bilateral**   P

    H26.039 Infantile and juvenile nuclear cataract, **unspecified eye** P

  ● H26.04 Anterior subcapsular polar infantile and juvenile cataract

    H26.041 Anterior subcapsular polar infantile and juvenile cataract, **right eye**   P

    H26.042 Anterior subcapsular polar infantile and juvenile cataract, **left eye**   P

    H26.043 Anterior subcapsular polar infantile and juvenile cataract, **bilateral**   P

    H26.049 Anterior subcapsular polar infantile and juvenile cataract, **unspecified** eye P

  ● H26.05 **Posterior subcapsular polar** infantile and juvenile cataract

    H26.051 Posterior subcapsular polar infantile and juvenile cataract, **right eye**   P

    H26.052 Posterior subcapsular polar infantile and juvenile cataract, **left eye**   P

    H26.053 Posterior subcapsular polar infantile and juvenile cataract, **bilateral**   P

    H26.059 Posterior subcapsular polar infantile and juvenile cataract, **unspecified** eye P

  ● H26.06 **Combined forms** of infantile and juvenile cataract

    H26.061 Combined forms of infantile and juvenile cataract, **right eye**   P

    H26.062 Combined forms of infantile and juvenile cataract, **left eye**   P

    H26.063 Combined forms of infantile and juvenile cataract **bilateral**   P

    H26.069 Combined forms of infantile and juvenile cataract, **unspecified eye** P

  H26.09 Other infantile and juvenile cataract   P

● H26.1 Traumatic cataract

  Use additional code (Chapter 20) to identify external cause

  ● H26.10 **Unspecified** traumatic cataract

    H26.101 Unspecified traumatic cataract, **right eye**

    H26.102 Unspecified traumatic cataract, **left eye**

    H26.103 Unspecified traumatic cataract, **bilateral**

    H26.109 Unspecified traumatic cataract, **unspecified eye**

▶ New   ⇒ Revised   ~~deleted~~ Deleted   Excludes 1   Excludes 2   Includes   Use additional   Code first   Code also   Key words

OGCR Official Guidelines   X Assign placeholder X   ● Use Additional Character(s)   ▶ Manifestation Code   🅗 Hierarchical Condition Category   Coding Clinic

● H26.11   Localized traumatic opacities
    H26.111   Localized traumatic opacities, right eye
    H26.112   Localized traumatic opacities, left eye
    H26.113   Localized traumatic opacities, bilateral
    H26.119   Localized traumatic opacities, unspecified eye
● H26.12   Partially resolved traumatic cataract
    H26.121   Partially resolved traumatic cataract, right eye
    H26.122   Partially resolved traumatic cataract, left eye
    H26.123   Partially resolved traumatic cataract, bilateral
    H26.129   Partially resolved traumatic cataract, unspecified eye
● H26.13   Total traumatic cataract
    H26.131   Total traumatic cataract, right eye
    H26.132   Total traumatic cataract, left eye
    H26.133   Total traumatic cataract, bilateral
    H26.139   Total traumatic cataract, unspecified eye

● H26.2   Complicated cataract
    H26.20   Unspecified complicated cataract
      Cataracta complicata NOS
● H26.21   Cataract with neovascularization
      Code also, if applicable, associated condition, such as:
        chronic iridocyclitis (H20.1-)
    H26.211   Cataract with neovascularization, right eye
    H26.212   Cataract with neovascularization, left eye
    H26.213   Cataract with neovascularization, bilateral
    H26.219   Cataract with neovascularization, unspecified eye
● H26.22   Cataract secondary to ocular disorders (degenerative) (inflammatory)
      Code also associated ocular disorder
    H26.221   Cataract secondary to ocular disorders (degenerative) (inflammatory), right eye
    H26.222   Cataract secondary to ocular disorders (degenerative) (inflammatory), left eye
    H26.223   Cataract secondary to ocular disorders (degenerative) (inflammatory), bilateral
    H26.229   Cataract secondary to ocular disorders (degenerative) (inflammatory), unspecified eye
● H26.23   Glaucomatous flecks (subcapsular)
      Code first underlying glaucoma (H40-H42)
    H26.231   Glaucomatous flecks (subcapsular), right eye
    H26.232   Glaucomatous flecks (subcapsular), left eye
    H26.233   Glaucomatous flecks (subcapsular), bilateral
    H26.239   Glaucomatous flecks (subcapsular), unspecified eye
● H26.3   Drug-induced cataract
      Toxic cataract
      Use additional code for adverse effect, if applicable, to identify drug (T36-T50 with fifth or sixth character 5)
    H26.30   Drug-induced cataract, unspecified eye

    H26.31   Drug-induced cataract, right eye
    H26.32   Drug-induced cataract, left eye
    H26.33   Drug-induced cataract, bilateral
● H26.4   Secondary cataract
      Coding Clinic: 2018, Q2, P14
    H26.40   Unspecified secondary cataract
● H26.41   Soemmering's ring
    H26.411   Soemmering's ring, right eye
    H26.412   Soemmering's ring, left eye
    H26.413   Soemmering's ring, bilateral
    H26.419   Soemmering's ring, unspecified eye
● H26.49   Other secondary cataract
    H26.491   Other secondary cataract, right eye
    H26.492   Other secondary cataract, left eye
      Coding Clinic: 2018, Q2, P13
    H26.493   Other secondary cataract, bilateral
    H26.499   Other secondary cataract, unspecified eye
    H26.8   Other specified cataract
    H26.9   Unspecified cataract

● H27   Other disorders of lens
    Excludes1   congenital lens malformations (Q12.-)
        mechanical complications of intraocular lens implant (T85.2)
        pseudophakia (Z96.1)
● H27.0   Aphakia
      Acquired absence of lens
      Acquired aphakia
      Aphakia due to trauma
    Excludes1   cataract extraction status (Z98.4-)
        congenital absence of lens (Q12.3)
        congenital aphakia (Q12.3)
    H27.00   Aphakia, unspecified eye
    H27.01   Aphakia, right eye
    H27.02   Aphakia, left eye
    H27.03   Aphakia, bilateral
● H27.1   Dislocation of lens
    H27.10   Unspecified dislocation of lens
● H27.11   Subluxation of lens
    H27.111   Subluxation of lens, right eye
    H27.112   Subluxation of lens, left eye
    H27.113   Subluxation of lens, bilateral
    H27.119   Subluxation of lens, unspecified eye
● H27.12   Anterior dislocation of lens
    H27.121   Anterior dislocation of lens, right eye
    H27.122   Anterior dislocation of lens, left eye
    H27.123   Anterior dislocation of lens, bilateral
    H27.129   Anterior dislocation of lens, unspecified eye
● H27.13   Posterior dislocation of lens
    H27.131   Posterior dislocation of lens, right eye
    H27.132   Posterior dislocation of lens, left eye
    H27.133   Posterior dislocation of lens, bilateral
    H27.139   Posterior dislocation of lens, unspecified eye
    H27.8   Other specified disorders of lens
    H27.9   Unspecified disorder of lens

▸ H28   *Cataract in diseases classified elsewhere*
      Code first underlying disease, such as:
        hypoparathyroidism (E20.-)
        myotonia (G71.1-)
        myxedema (E03.-)
        protein-calorie malnutrition (E40-E46)
    Excludes1   cataract in diabetes mellitus (E08.36, E09.36, E10.36, E11.36, E13.36)

CHAPTER 7 (H00-H59)

DISORDERS OF CHOROID AND RETINA (H30-H36)

★ **(See Plate 16 of the Anatomy Illustrations.)**

● H30   Chorioretinal inflammation
  ● **H30.0**   **Focal chorioretinal inflammation**
      Focal chorioretinitis
      Focal choroiditis
      Focal retinitis
      Focal retinochoroiditis

    ● **H30.00**   Unspecified focal chorioretinal inflammation
        Focal chorioretinitis NOS
        Focal choroiditis NOS
        Focal retinitis NOS
        Focal retinochoroiditis NOS

      H30.001   Unspecified focal chorioretinal inflammation, right eye
      H30.002   Unspecified focal chorioretinal inflammation, left eye
      H30.003   Unspecified focal chorioretinal inflammation, bilateral
      H30.009   Unspecified focal chorioretinal inflammation, unspecified eye

    ● **H30.01**   Focal chorioretinal inflammation, juxtapapillary
      H30.011   Focal chorioretinal inflammation, juxtapapillary, right eye
      H30.012   Focal chorioretinal inflammation, juxtapapillary, left eye
      H30.013   Focal chorioretinal inflammation, juxtapapillary, bilateral
      H30.019   Focal chorioretinal inflammation, juxtapapillary, unspecified eye

    ● **H30.02**   Focal chorioretinal inflammation of posterior pole
      H30.021   Focal chorioretinal inflammation of posterior pole, right eye
      H30.022   Focal chorioretinal inflammation of posterior pole, left eye
      H30.023   Focal chorioretinal inflammation of posterior pole, bilateral
      H30.029   Focal chorioretinal inflammation of posterior pole, unspecified eye

    ● **H30.03**   Focal chorioretinal inflammation, peripheral
      H30.031   Focal chorioretinal inflammation, peripheral, right eye
      H30.032   Focal chorioretinal inflammation, peripheral, left eye
      H30.033   Focal chorioretinal inflammation, peripheral, bilateral
      H30.039   Focal chorioretinal inflammation, peripheral, unspecified eye

    ● **H30.04**   Focal chorioretinal inflammation, macular or paramacular
      H30.041   Focal chorioretinal inflammation, macular or paramacular, right eye
      H30.042   Focal chorioretinal inflammation, macular or paramacular, left eye
      H30.043   Focal chorioretinal inflammation, macular or paramacular, bilateral
      H30.049   Focal chorioretinal inflammation, macular or paramacular, unspecified eye

  ● **H30.1**   **Disseminated chorioretinal inflammation**
      Disseminated chorioretinitis
      Disseminated choroiditis
      Disseminated retinitis
      Disseminated retinochoroiditis
    Excludes2   exudative retinopathy (H35.02-)

  ● **H30.10**   Unspecified disseminated chorioretinal inflammation
      Disseminated chorioretinitis NOS
      Disseminated choroiditis NOS
      Disseminated retinitis NOS
      Disseminated retinochoroiditis NOS

      H30.101   Unspecified disseminated chorioretinal inflammation, right eye
      H30.102   Unspecified disseminated chorioretinal inflammation, left eye
      H30.103   Unspecified disseminated chorioretinal inflammation, bilateral
      H30.109   Unspecified disseminated chorioretinal inflammation, unspecified eye

  ● **H30.11**   Disseminated chorioretinal inflammation of posterior pole
      H30.111   Disseminated chorioretinal inflammation of posterior pole, right eye
      H30.112   Disseminated chorioretinal inflammation of posterior pole, left eye
      H30.113   Disseminated chorioretinal inflammation of posterior pole, bilateral
      H30.119   Disseminated chorioretinal inflammation of posterior pole, unspecified eye

  ● **H30.12**   Disseminated chorioretinal inflammation, peripheral
      H30.121   Disseminated chorioretinal inflammation, peripheral right eye
      H30.122   Disseminated chorioretinal inflammation, peripheral, left eye
      H30.123   Disseminated chorioretinal inflammation, peripheral, bilateral
      H30.129   Disseminated chorioretinal inflammation, peripheral, unspecified eye

  ● **H30.13**   Disseminated chorioretinal inflammation, generalized
      H30.131   Disseminated chorioretinal inflammation, generalized, right eye
      H30.132   Disseminated chorioretinal inflammation, generalized, left eye
      H30.133   Disseminated chorioretinal inflammation, generalized, bilateral
      H30.139   Disseminated chorioretinal inflammation, generalized, unspecified eye

  ● **H30.14**   Acute posterior multifocal placoid pigment epitheliopathy
      H30.141   Acute posterior multifocal placoid pigment epitheliopathy, right eye
      H30.142   Acute posterior multifocal placoid pigment epitheliopathy, left eye
      H30.143   Acute posterior multifocal placoid pigment epitheliopathy, bilateral
      H30.149   Acute posterior multifocal placoid pigment epitheliopathy, unspecified eye

  ● **H30.2**   **Posterior cyclitis**
      Pars planitis
    H30.20   Posterior cyclitis, unspecified eye
    H30.21   Posterior cyclitis, right eye
    H30.22   Posterior cyclitis, left eye
    H30.23   Posterior cyclitis, bilateral

▶ New   ⇒ Revised   ~~deleted~~ Deleted   Excludes 1   Excludes 2   Includes   Use additional   Code first   Code also   Key words
OGCR Official Guidelines   X Assign placeholder X   ● Use Additional Character(s)   ▸ Manifestation Code   🏥 Hierarchical Condition Category   Coding Clinic

● **H30.8   Other chorioretinal inflammations**
  ● **H30.81   Harada's disease**
       H30.811   Harada's disease, right eye
       H30.812   Harada's disease, left eye
       H30.813   Harada's disease, bilateral
       H30.819   Harada's disease, unspecified eye
  ● **H30.89   Other chorioretinal inflammations**
       H30.891   Other chorioretinal inflammations, right eye
       H30.892   Other chorioretinal inflammations, left eye
       H30.893   Other chorioretinal inflammations, bilateral
       H30.899   Other chorioretinal inflammations, unspecified eye
● **H30.9   Unspecified chorioretinal inflammation**
       Chorioretinitis NOS
       Choroiditis NOS
       Neuroretinitis NOS
       Retinitis NOS
       Retinochoroiditis NOS
      H30.90   Unspecified chorioretinal inflammation, unspecified eye
      H30.91   Unspecified chorioretinal inflammation, right eye
      H30.92   Unspecified chorioretinal inflammation, left eye
      H30.93   Unspecified chorioretinal inflammation, bilateral

● **H31   Other disorders of choroid**
  ● **H31.0   Chorioretinal scars**
       Excludes2   postsurgical chorioretinal scars (H59.81-)
    ● **H31.00   Unspecified chorioretinal scars**
       H31.001   Unspecified chorioretinal scars, right eye
       H31.002   Unspecified chorioretinal scars, left eye
       H31.003   Unspecified chorioretinal scars, bilateral
       H31.009   Unspecified chorioretinal scars, unspecified eye
    ● **H31.01   Macula scars of posterior pole (postinflammatory) (post-traumatic)**
       Excludes1   postprocedural chorioretinal scar (H59.81-)
       H31.011   Macula scars of posterior pole (postinflammatory) (post-traumatic), right eye
       H31.012   Macula scars of posterior pole (postinflammatory) (post-traumatic), left eye
       H31.013   Macula scars of posterior pole (postinflammatory) (post-traumatic), bilateral
       H31.019   Macula scars of posterior pole (postinflammatory) (post-traumatic), unspecified eye
    ● **H31.02   Solar retinopathy**
       H31.021   Solar retinopathy, right eye
       H31.022   Solar retinopathy, left eye
       H31.023   Solar retinopathy, bilateral
       H31.029   Solar retinopathy, unspecified eye
    ● **H31.09   Other chorioretinal scars**
       H31.091   Other chorioretinal scars, right eye
       H31.092   Other chorioretinal scars, left eye
       H31.093   Other chorioretinal scars, bilateral
       H31.099   Other chorioretinal scars, unspecified eye

● **H31.1   Choroidal degeneration**
       Excludes2   angioid streaks of macula (H35.33)
  ● **H31.10   Unspecified choroidal degeneration**
       Choroidal sclerosis NOS
       H31.101   Choroidal degeneration, unspecified, right eye
       H31.102   Choroidal degeneration, unspecified, left eye
       H31.103   Choroidal degeneration, unspecified, bilateral
       H31.109   Choroidal degeneration, unspecified, unspecified eye
  ● **H31.11   Age-related choroidal atrophy**
       H31.111   Age-related choroidal atrophy, right eye   **A**
       H31.112   Age-related choroidal atrophy, left eye   **A**
       H31.113   Age-related choroidal atrophy, bilateral   **A**
       H31.119   Age-related choroidal atrophy, unspecified eye   **A**
  ● **H31.12   Diffuse secondary atrophy of choroid**
       H31.121   Diffuse secondary atrophy of choroid, right eye
       H31.122   Diffuse secondary atrophy of choroid, left eye
       H31.123   Diffuse secondary atrophy of choroid, bilateral
       H31.129   Diffuse secondary atrophy of choroid, unspecified eye

● **H31.2   Hereditary choroidal dystrophy**
       Excludes2   hyperornithinemia (E72.4)
                   ornithinemia (E72.4)
      H31.20   Hereditary choroidal dystrophy, unspecified
      H31.21   Choroideremia
      H31.22   Choroidal dystrophy (central areolar) (generalized) (peripapillary)
      H31.23   Gyrate atrophy, choroid
      H31.29   Other hereditary choroidal dystrophy
● **H31.3   Choroidal hemorrhage and rupture**
  ● **H31.30   Unspecified choroidal hemorrhage**
       H31.301   Unspecified choroidal hemorrhage, right eye
       H31.302   Unspecified choroidal hemorrhage, left eye
       H31.303   Unspecified choroidal hemorrhage, bilateral
       H31.309   Unspecified choroidal hemorrhage, unspecified eye
  ● **H31.31   Expulsive choroidal hemorrhage**
       H31.311   Expulsive choroidal hemorrhage, right eye
       H31.312   Expulsive choroidal hemorrhage, left eye
       H31.313   Expulsive choroidal hemorrhage, bilateral
       H31.319   Expulsive choroidal hemorrhage, unspecified eye
  ● **H31.32   Choroidal rupture**
       H31.321   Choroidal rupture, right eye
       H31.322   Choroidal rupture, left eye
       H31.323   Choroidal rupture, bilateral
       H31.329   Choroidal rupture, unspecified eye

CHAPTER 7 (H00-H59)

CHAPTER 7 (H00-H59)

- H31.4 Choroidal detachment
    - H31.40 Unspecified choroidal detachment
        - H31.401 Unspecified choroidal detachment, right eye
        - H31.402 Unspecified choroidal detachment, left eye
        - H31.403 Unspecified choroidal detachment, bilateral
        - H31.409 Unspecified choroidal detachment, unspecified eye
    - H31.41 Hemorrhagic choroidal detachment
        - H31.411 Hemorrhagic choroidal detachment, right eye
        - H31.412 Hemorrhagic choroidal detachment, left eye
        - H31.413 Hemorrhagic choroidal detachment, bilateral
        - H31.419 Hemorrhagic choroidal detachment, unspecified eye
    - H31.42 Serous choroidal detachment
        - H31.421 Serous choroidal detachment, right eye
        - H31.422 Serous choroidal detachment, left eye
        - H31.423 Serous choroidal detachment, bilateral
        - H31.429 Serous choroidal detachment, unspecified eye
    - H31.8 Other specified disorders of choroid
    - H31.9 Unspecified disorder of choroid

- H32 *Chorioretinal disorders in diseases classified elsewhere*
    - *Code first* underlying disease, such as:
        - congenital toxoplasmosis (P37.1)
        - histoplasmosis (B39.-)
        - leprosy (A30.-)
    - **Excludes1** chorioretinitis (in):
        - toxoplasmosis (acquired) (B58.01)
        - tuberculosis (A18.53)

- H33 Retinal detachments and breaks
    - **Excludes1** detachment of retinal pigment epithelium (H35.72-, H35.73-)
    - H33.0 Retinal detachment with retinal break
        - Rhegmatogenous retinal detachment
        - **Excludes1** serous retinal detachment (without retinal break) (H33.2-)
        - H33.00 Unspecified retinal detachment with retinal break
            - H33.001 Unspecified retinal detachment with retinal break, right eye
            - H33.002 Unspecified retinal detachment with retinal break, left eye
            - H33.003 Unspecified retinal detachment with retinal break, bilateral
            - H33.009 Unspecified retinal detachment with retinal break, unspecified eye
        - H33.01 Retinal detachment with single break
            - H33.011 Retinal detachment with single break, right eye
            - H33.012 Retinal detachment with single break, left eye
            - H33.013 Retinal detachment with single break, bilateral
            - H33.019 Retinal detachment with single break, unspecified eye

NON-RHEGMATOGENOUS RETINAL DETACHMENT

VITREOUS DETACHMENT

RHEGMATOGENOUS RETINAL DETACHMENT

Figure 7-10 Retinal detachment. (From Kumar: Robbins and Cotran: Pathologic Basis of Disease, ed 7, Saunders, 2005)

Item 7-6 Retinal detachments and defects are conditions of the eye in which the retina separates from the underlying tissue. Initial detachment may be localized, requiring rapid treatment (medical emergency) to avoid the entire retina from detaching, which leads to vision loss and blindness.

- H33.02 Retinal detachment with multiple breaks
    - H33.021 Retinal detachment with multiple breaks, right eye
    - H33.022 Retinal detachment with multiple breaks, left eye
    - H33.023 Retinal detachment with multiple breaks, bilateral
    - H33.029 Retinal detachment with multiple breaks, unspecified eye
- H33.03 Retinal detachment with giant retinal tear
    - H33.031 Retinal detachment with giant retinal tear, right eye
    - H33.032 Retinal detachment with giant retinal tear, left eye
    - H33.033 Retinal detachment with giant retinal tear, bilateral
    - H33.039 Retinal detachment with giant retinal tear, unspecified eye
- H33.04 Retinal detachment with retinal dialysis
    - H33.041 Retinal detachment with retinal dialysis, right eye
    - H33.042 Retinal detachment with retinal dialysis, left eye
    - H33.043 Retinal detachment with retinal dialysis, bilateral
    - H33.049 Retinal detachment with retinal dialysis, unspecified eye

● **H33.05** Total retinal detachment
　　　H33.051 Total retinal detachment, right eye
　　　H33.052 Total retinal detachment, left eye
　　　H33.053 Total retinal detachment, bilateral
　　　H33.059 Total retinal detachment, unspecified eye

● **H33.1** Retinoschisis and retinal cysts
　　Excludes1 congenital retinoschisis (Q14.1)
　　　　　　　microcystoid degeneration of retina (H35.42-)

● **H33.10** Unspecified retinoschisis
　　　H33.101 Unspecified retinoschisis, right eye
　　　H33.102 Unspecified retinoschisis, left eye
　　　H33.103 Unspecified retinoschisis, bilateral
　　　H33.109 Unspecified retinoschisis, unspecified eye

● **H33.11** Cyst of ora serrata
　　　H33.111 Cyst of ora serrata, right eye
　　　H33.112 Cyst of ora serrata, left eye
　　　H33.113 Cyst of ora serrata, bilateral
　　　H33.119 Cyst of ora serrata, unspecified eye

● **H33.12** Parasitic cyst of retina
　　　H33.121 Parasitic cyst of retina, right eye
　　　H33.122 Parasitic cyst of retina, left eye
　　　H33.123 Parasitic cyst of retina, bilateral
　　　H33.129 Parasitic cyst of retina, unspecified eye

● **H33.19** Other retinoschisis and retinal cysts
　　　Pseudocyst of retina
　　　H33.191 Other retinoschisis and retinal cysts, right eye
　　　H33.192 Other retinoschisis and retinal cysts, left eye
　　　H33.193 Other retinoschisis and retinal cysts, bilateral
　　　H33.199 Other retinoschisis and retinal cysts, unspecified eye

● **H33.2** Serous retinal detachment
　　　Retinal detachment NOS
　　　Retinal detachment without retinal break
　　Excludes1 central serous chorioretinopathy (H35.71-)
　　　H33.20 Serous retinal detachment, unspecified eye
　　　H33.21 Serous retinal detachment, right eye
　　　H33.22 Serous retinal detachment, left eye
　　　H33.23 Serous retinal detachment, bilateral

● **H33.3** Retinal breaks without detachment
　　Excludes1 chorioretinal scars after surgery for detachment (H59.81-)
　　　　　　　peripheral retinal degeneration without break (H35.4-)

● **H33.30** Unspecified retinal break
　　　H33.301 Unspecified retinal break, right eye
　　　H33.302 Unspecified retinal break, left eye
　　　H33.303 Unspecified retinal break, bilateral
　　　H33.309 Unspecified retinal break, unspecified eye

● **H33.31** Horseshoe tear of retina without detachment
　　　Operculum of retina without detachment
　　　H33.311 Horseshoe tear of retina without detachment, right eye
　　　H33.312 Horseshoe tear of retina without detachment, left eye
　　　H33.313 Horseshoe tear of retina without detachment, bilateral

　　　H33.319 Horseshoe tear of retina without detachment, unspecified eye

● **H33.32** Round hole of retina without detachment
　　　H33.321 Round hole, right eye
　　　H33.322 Round hole, left eye
　　　H33.323 Round hole, bilateral
　　　H33.329 Round hole, unspecified eye

● **H33.33** Multiple defects of retina without detachment
　　　H33.331 Multiple defects of retina without detachment, right eye
　　　H33.332 Multiple defects of retina without detachment, left eye
　　　H33.333 Multiple defects of retina without detachment, bilateral
　　　H33.339 Multiple defects of retina without detachment, unspecified eye

● **H33.4** Traction detachment of retina
　　　Proliferative vitreo-retinopathy with retinal detachment
　　　H33.40 Traction detachment of retina, unspecified eye
　　　H33.41 Traction detachment of retina, right eye
　　　H33.42 Traction detachment of retina, left eye
　　　H33.43 Traction detachment of retina, bilateral

　　H33.8 Other retinal detachments

● **H34** Retinal vascular occlusions
　　　Blockage in vessel of the retina
　　Excludes1 amaurosis fugax (G45.3)

● **H34.0** Transient retinal artery occlusion
　　　H34.00 Transient retinal artery occlusion, unspecified eye
　　　H34.01 Transient retinal artery occlusion, right eye
　　　H34.02 Transient retinal artery occlusion, left eye
　　　H34.03 Transient retinal artery occlusion, bilateral

● **H34.1** Central retinal artery occlusion
　　　H34.10 Central retinal artery occlusion, unspecified eye
　　　H34.11 Central retinal artery occlusion, right eye
　　　H34.12 Central retinal artery occlusion, left eye
　　　H34.13 Central retinal artery occlusion, bilateral

● **H34.2** Other retinal artery occlusions

● **H34.21** Partial retinal artery occlusion
　　　Hollenhorst's plaque
　　　Retinal microembolism
　　　H34.211 Partial retinal artery occlusion, right eye
　　　H34.212 Partial retinal artery occlusion, left eye
　　　H34.213 Partial retinal artery occlusion, bilateral
　　　H34.219 Partial retinal artery occlusion, unspecified eye

● **H34.23** Retinal artery branch occlusion
　　　H34.231 Retinal artery branch occlusion, right eye
　　　H34.232 Retinal artery branch occlusion, left eye
　　　H34.233 Retinal artery branch occlusion, bilateral
　　　H34.239 Retinal artery branch occlusion, unspecified eye

CHAPTER 7 (H00-H59)

● H34.8   Other retinal vascular occlusions
          Coding Clinic: 2016, Q4, P19
   ● H34.81   Central retinal vein occlusion
              One of the following 7th characters is to
              be assigned to codes in subcategory
              H34.81 to designate the severity of the
              occlusion:

              | 0 | with macular edema |
              | 1 | with retinal neovascularization |
              | 2 | stable |
              | | Old central retinal vein occlusion |

       ● H34.811   Central retinal vein occlusion, right
                   eye
       ● H34.812   Central retinal vein occlusion, left eye
       ● H34.813   Central retinal vein occlusion,
                   bilateral
       ● H34.819   Central retinal vein occlusion,
                   unspecified eye
   ● H34.82   Venous engorgement
              Incipient retinal vein occlusion
              Partial retinal vein occlusion
         H34.821   Venous engorgement, right eye
         H34.822   Venous engorgement, left eye
         H34.823   Venous engorgement, bilateral
         H34.829   Venous engorgement, unspecified eye
   ● H34.83   Tributary (branch) retinal vein occlusion
              One of the following 7th characters is to
              be assigned to codes in subcategory
              H34.83 to designate the severity of the
              occlusion:

              | 0 | with macular edema |
              | 1 | with retinal neovascularization |
              | 2 | stable |
              | | Old tributary (branch) retinal vein occlusion |

       ● H34.831   Tributary (branch) retinal vein
                   occlusion, right eye
       ● H34.832   Tributary (branch) retinal vein
                   occlusion, left eye
       ● H34.833   Tributary (branch) retinal vein
                   occlusion, bilateral
       ● H34.839   Tributary (branch) retinal vein
                   occlusion, unspecified eye
   H34.9   Unspecified retinal vascular occlusion

● H35   Other retinal disorders
    Excludes2   diabetic retinal disorders (E08.311-E08.359,
                E09.311-E09.359, E10.311-E10.359,
                E11.311-E11.359, E13.311-E13.359)
  ● H35.0   Background retinopathy and retinal vascular changes
            Code also any associated hypertension (I10)
            OGCR Section I. C.9.a.5.

            Hypertensive Retinopathy
            Subcategory H35.0, Background retinopathy and
            retinal vascular changes, should be used with a
            code from category I10–I15, Hypertensive disease to
            include the systemic hypertension. The sequencing is
            based on the reason for the encounter.

       H35.00   Unspecified background retinopathy
   ● H35.01   Changes in retinal vascular appearance
              Retinal vascular sheathing
         H35.011   Changes in retinal vascular
                   appearance, right eye
         H35.012   Changes in retinal vascular
                   appearance, left eye

         H35.013   Changes in retinal vascular
                   appearance, bilateral
         H35.019   Changes in retinal vascular
                   appearance, unspecified eye
   ● H35.02   Exudative retinopathy
              Coats retinopathy
         H35.021   Exudative retinopathy, right eye
         H35.022   Exudative retinopathy, left eye
         H35.023   Exudative retinopathy, bilateral
         H35.029   Exudative retinopathy, unspecified
                   eye
   ● H35.03   Hypertensive retinopathy
         H35.031   Hypertensive retinopathy, right eye
         H35.032   Hypertensive retinopathy, left eye
         H35.033   Hypertensive retinopathy, bilateral
         H35.039   Hypertensive retinopathy, unspecified
                   eye
   ● H35.04   Retinal micro-aneurysms, unspecified
         H35.041   Retinal micro-aneurysms,
                   unspecified, right eye
         H35.042   Retinal micro-aneurysms,
                   unspecified, left eye
         H35.043   Retinal micro-aneurysms,
                   unspecified, bilateral
         H35.049   Retinal micro-aneurysms,
                   unspecified, unspecified eye
   ● H35.05   Retinal neovascularization, unspecified
         H35.051   Retinal neovascularization,
                   unspecified, right eye
         H35.052   Retinal neovascularization,
                   unspecified, left eye
         H35.053   Retinal neovascularization,
                   unspecified, bilateral
         H35.059   Retinal neovascularization,
                   unspecified, unspecified eye
   ● H35.06   Retinal vasculitis
              Eales disease
              Retinal perivasculitis
         H35.061   Retinal vasculitis, right eye
         H35.062   Retinal vasculitis, left eye
         H35.063   Retinal vasculitis, bilateral
         H35.069   Retinal vasculitis, unspecified eye
   ● H35.07   Retinal telangiectasis
         H35.071   Retinal telangiectasis, right eye
         H35.072   Retinal telangiectasis, left eye
         H35.073   Retinal telangiectasis, bilateral
         H35.079   Retinal telangiectasis, unspecified eye
   H35.09   Other intraretinal microvascular abnormalities
            Retinal varices
  ● H35.1   Retinopathy of prematurity
   ● H35.10   Retinopathy of prematurity, unspecified
              Retinopathy of prematurity NOS
         H35.101   Retinopathy of prematurity,
                   unspecified, right eye
         H35.102   Retinopathy of prematurity,
                   unspecified, left eye
         H35.103   Retinopathy of prematurity,
                   unspecified, bilateral
         H35.109   Retinopathy of prematurity,
                   unspecified, unspecified eye
   ● H35.11   Retinopathy of prematurity, stage 0
         H35.111   Retinopathy of prematurity, stage 0,
                   right eye
         H35.112   Retinopathy of prematurity, stage 0,
                   left eye

H35.113   Retinopathy of prematurity, stage 0, bilateral

H35.119   Retinopathy of prematurity, stage 0, unspecified eye

● H35.12   Retinopathy of prematurity, stage 1

H35.121   Retinopathy of prematurity, stage 1, right eye

H35.122   Retinopathy of prematurity, stage 1, left eye

H35.123   Retinopathy of prematurity, stage 1, bilateral

H35.129   Retinopathy of prematurity, stage 1, unspecified eye

● H35.13   Retinopathy of prematurity, stage 2

H35.131   Retinopathy of prematurity, stage 2, right eye

H35.132   Retinopathy of prematurity, stage 2, left eye

H35.133   Retinopathy of prematurity, stage 2, bilateral

H35.139   Retinopathy of prematurity, stage 2, unspecified eye

● H35.14   Retinopathy of prematurity, stage 3

H35.141   Retinopathy of prematurity, stage 3, right eye

H35.142   Retinopathy of prematurity, stage 3, left eye

H35.143   Retinopathy of prematurity, stage 3, bilateral

H35.149   Retinopathy of prematurity, stage 3, unspecified eye

● H35.15   Retinopathy of prematurity, stage 4

H35.151   Retinopathy of prematurity, stage 4, right eye

H35.152   Retinopathy of prematurity, stage 4, left eye

H35.153   Retinopathy of prematurity, stage 4, bilateral

H35.159   Retinopathy of prematurity, stage 4, unspecified eye

● H35.16   Retinopathy of prematurity, stage 5

H35.161   Retinopathy of prematurity, stage 5, right eye

H35.162   Retinopathy of prematurity, stage 5, left eye

H35.163   Retinopathy of prematurity, stage 5, bilateral

H35.169   Retinopathy of prematurity, stage 5, unspecified eye

● H35.17   Retrolental fibroplasia

H35.171   Retrolental fibroplasia, right eye

H35.172   Retrolental fibroplasia, left eye

H35.173   Retrolental fibroplasia, bilateral

H35.179   Retrolental fibroplasia, unspecified eye

● H35.2   Other non-diabetic proliferative retinopathy

Proliferative vitreo-retinopathy

Excludes1   proliferative vitreo-retinopathy with retinal detachment (H33.4-)

Thaslassemia proliferative retinopathy

Excludes2   proliferative sickle-cell retinopathy (H36.82-)

H35.20   Other non-diabetic proliferative retinopathy, unspecified eye

H35.21   Other non-diabetic proliferative retinopathy, right eye

H35.22   Other non-diabetic proliferative retinopathy, left eye

H35.23   Other non-diabetic proliferative retinopathy, bilateral

● H35.3   Degeneration of macula and posterior pole

H35.30   Unspecified macular degeneration   A

Age-related macular degeneration

● H35.31   Nonexudative age-related macular degeneration

Atrophic age-related macular degeneration

Dry age-related macular degeneration

One of the following 7th characters is to be assigned to codes in subcategory H35.31 to designate the stage of the disease:

> 0   stage unspecified
> 1   early dry stage
> 2   intermediate dry stage
> 3   advanced atrophic without subfoveal involvement
>   advanced dry stage
> 4   advanced atrophic with subfoveal involvement

● H35.311   Nonexudative age-related macular degeneration, right eye   A

Coding Clinic: 2016, Q4, P20-21

● H35.312   Nonexudative age-related macular degeneration, left eye   A

Coding Clinic: 2016, Q4, P20-21

● H35.313   Nonexudative age-related macular degeneration, bilateral   A

Coding Clinic: 2016, Q4, P20

● H35.319   Nonexudative age-related macular degeneration, unspecified eye   A

Coding Clinic: 2016, Q4, P20

● H35.32   Exudative age-related macular degeneration

Wet age-related macular degeneration

One of the following 7th characters is to be assigned to codes in subcategory H35.32 to designate the stage of the disease:

> 0   stage unspecified
> 1   with active choroidal neovascularization
> 2   with inactive choroidal neovascularization
>   with involuted or regressed neovascularization
> 3   with inactive scar

Coding Clinic: 2016, Q4, P20

● H35.321   Exudative age-related macular degeneration, right eye 🔁   A

● H35.322   Exudative age-related macular degeneration, left eye 🔁   A

● H35.323   Exudative age-related macular degeneration, bilateral 🔁   A

● H35.329   Exudative age-related macular degeneration, unspecified eye 🔁   A

H35.33   Angioid streaks of macula

● H35.34   Macular cyst, hole, or pseudohole

H35.341   Macular cyst, hole, or pseudohole, right eye

H35.342   Macular cyst, hole, or pseudohole, left eye

H35.343   Macular cyst, hole, or pseudohole, bilateral

H35.349   Macular cyst, hole, or pseudohole, unspecified eye

CHAPTER 7 (H00-H59)

Item 7-7 Macular degeneration is typically age-related, chronic, and is evidenced by deterioration of the macula (the part of the retina that provides for central field vision), resulting in blurred vision or a blind spot in the center of visual field while not affecting peripheral vision.

● H35.35   Cystoid macular degeneration

> Excludes1   cystoid macular edema following cataract surgery (H59.03-)

    H35.351   Cystoid macular degeneration, right eye

    H35.352   Cystoid macular degeneration, left eye

    H35.353   Cystoid macular degeneration, bilateral

    H35.359   Cystoid macular degeneration, unspecified eye

● H35.36   Drusen (degenerative) of macula

    H35.361   Drusen (degenerative) of macula, right eye
> Coding Clinic: 2016, Q4, P21

    H35.362   Drusen (degenerative) of macula, left eye
> Coding Clinic: 2016, Q4, P21

    H35.363   Drusen (degenerative) of macula, bilateral
> Coding Clinic: 2017, Q1, P51

    H35.369   Drusen (degenerative) of macula, unspecified eye

● H35.37   Puckering of macula

    H35.371   Puckering of macula, right eye

    H35.372   Puckering of macula, left eye

    H35.373   Puckering of macula, bilateral

    H35.379   Puckering of macula, unspecified eye

● H35.38   Toxic maculopathy

> *Code first poisoning due to drug or toxin, if applicable (T36-T65 with fifth or sixth character 1-4)*
>
> Use additional code for adverse effect, if applicable, to identify drug (T36-T50 with fifth or sixth character 5)

    H35.381   Toxic maculopathy, right eye

    H35.382   Toxic maculopathy, left eye

    H35.383   Toxic maculopathy, bilateral

    H35.389   Toxic maculopathy, unspecified eye

● H35.4   Peripheral retinal degeneration

> Excludes1   hereditary retinal degeneration (dystrophy) (H35.5-)
> peripheral retinal degeneration with retinal break (H33.3-)

    H35.40   Unspecified peripheral retinal degeneration

●   H35.41   Lattice degeneration of retina
              Palisade degeneration of retina

    H35.411   Lattice degeneration of retina, right eye

    H35.412   Lattice degeneration of retina, left eye

    H35.413   Lattice degeneration of retina, bilateral

    H35.419   Lattice degeneration of retina, unspecified eye

●   H35.42   Microcystoid degeneration of retina

    H35.421   Microcystoid degeneration of retina, right eye

    H35.422   Microcystoid degeneration of retina, left eye

    H35.423   Microcystoid degeneration of retina, bilateral

    H35.429   Microcystoid degeneration of retina, unspecified eye

● H35.43   Paving stone degeneration of retina

    H35.431   Paving stone degeneration of retina, right eye

    H35.432   Paving stone degeneration of retina, left eye

    H35.433   Paving stone degeneration of retina, bilateral

    H35.439   Paving stone degeneration of retina, unspecified eye

● H35.44   Age-related reticular degeneration of retina

    H35.441   Age-related reticular degeneration of retina, right eye   A

    H35.442   Age-related reticular degeneration of retina, left eye   A

    H35.443   Age-related reticular degeneration of retina, bilateral   A

    H35.449   Age-related reticular degeneration of retina, unspecified eye   A

● H35.45   Secondary pigmentary degeneration

    H35.451   Secondary pigmentary degeneration, right eye

    H35.452   Secondary pigmentary degeneration, left eye

    H35.453   Secondary pigmentary degeneration, bilateral

    H35.459   Secondary pigmentary degeneration, unspecified eye

● H35.46   Secondary vitreoretinal degeneration

    H35.461   Secondary vitreoretinal degeneration, right eye

    H35.462   Secondary vitreoretinal degeneration, left eye

    H35.463   Secondary vitreoretinal degeneration, bilateral

    H35.469   Secondary vitreoretinal degeneration, unspecified eye

● H35.5   Hereditary retinal dystrophy

> Excludes1   dystrophies primarily involving Bruch's membrane (H31.1-)

    H35.50   Unspecified hereditary retinal dystrophy

    H35.51   Vitreoretinal dystrophy

    H35.52   Pigmentary retinal dystrophy
             Albipunctate retinal dystrophy
             Retinitis pigmentosa
             Tapetoretinal dystrophy

    H35.53   Other dystrophies primarily involving the sensory retina
             Stargardt's disease

    H35.54   Dystrophies primarily involving the retinal pigment epithelium
             Vitelliform retinal dystrophy

● H35.6   Retinal hemorrhage

    H35.60   Retinal hemorrhage, unspecified eye

    H35.61   Retinal hemorrhage, right eye

    H35.62   Retinal hemorrhage, left eye

    H35.63   Retinal hemorrhage, bilateral

● H35.7   Separation of retinal layers

> Excludes1   retinal detachment (serous) (H33.2-)
> rhegmatogenous retinal detachment (H33.0-)

    H35.70   Unspecified separation of retinal layers

● H35.71   Central serous chorioretinopathy

    H35.711   Central serous chorioretinopathy, right eye

    H35.712   Central serous chorioretinopathy, left eye

    H35.713   Central serous chorioretinopathy, bilateral

    H35.719   Central serous chorioretinopathy, unspecified eye

▶ New   ⇒ Revised   ~~deleted~~ Deleted   Excludes 1   Excludes 2   Includes   Use additional   Code first   Code also   Key words

802   OGCR Official Guidelines   X Assign placeholder X   ● Use Additional Character(s)   ▶ Manifestation Code   HCC Hierarchical Condition Category   Coding Clinic

● **H35.72** **Serous** detachment of retinal pigment epithelium

    H35.721 Serous detachment of retinal pigment epithelium, **right eye**

    H35.722 Serous detachment of retinal pigment epithelium, **left eye**

    H35.723 Serous detachment of retinal pigment epithelium, **bilateral**

    H35.729 Serous detachment of retinal pigment epithelium, **unspecified** eye

● **H35.73** **Hemorrhagic** detachment of retinal pigment epithelium

    H35.731 Hemorrhagic detachment of retinal pigment epithelium, **right** eye

    H35.732 Hemorrhagic detachment of retinal pigment epithelium, **left** eye

    H35.733 Hemorrhagic detachment of retinal pigment epithelium, **bilateral**

    H35.739 Hemorrhagic detachment of retinal pigment epithelium, **unspecified** eye

● **H35.8** Other specified retinal disorders

    Excludes2 retinal hemorrhage (H35.6-)

  H35.81 Retinal **edema**

      Retinal cotton wool spots

  H35.82 Retinal **ischemia**

  H35.89 **Other** specified retinal disorders

  H35.9 **Unspecified** retinal disorder

◗ *H36* *Retinal disorders in diseases classified elsewhere*

    Code first underlying disease, such as:
      lipid storage disorders (E75.-)
      sickle-cell disorders (D57.-)

    Excludes1 arteriosclerotic retinopathy (H35.0-)
        diabetic retinopathy (E08.3-, E09.3-, E10.3-, E11.3-, E13.3-)

● **H36.8** Other retinal disorders in diseases classified elsewhere

  ● **H36.81** Nonproliferative sickle-cell retinopathy

    H36.811 Nonproliferative sickle-cell retinopathy, **right eye**

    H36.812 Nonproliferative sickle-cell retinopathy, **left eye**

    H36.813 Nonproliferative sickle-cell retinopathy, **bilateral**

    H36.819 Nonproliferative sickle-cell retinopathy, **unspecified eye**

  ● **H36.82** Proliferative sickle-cell retinopathy

    H36.821 Proliferative sickle-cell retinopathy, **right eye**

    H36.822 Proliferative sickle-cell retinopathy, **left eye**

    H36.823 Proliferative sickle-cell retinopathy, **bilateral**

    H36.829 Proliferative sickle-cell retinopathy, **unspecified eye**

  ● **H36.89** Other retinal disorders in diseases classified elsewhere

      Retinal dystrophy in lipid storage disorders

GLAUCOMA (H40-H42)

● **H40** Glaucoma

    Intraocular pressure (IOP) that is too high results from too much aqueous humor and because of excess production or inadequate drainage, optic nerve damage and vision loss may occur.

    Excludes1 absolute glaucoma (H44.51-)
        congenital glaucoma (Q15.0)
        traumatic glaucoma due to birth injury (P15.3)

● **H40.0** Glaucoma **suspect**

  ● **H40.00** Preglaucoma, **unspecified**

    H40.001 Preglaucoma, unspecified, **right eye**

    H40.002 Preglaucoma, unspecified, **left eye**

    H40.003 Preglaucoma, unspecified, **bilateral**

    H40.009 Preglaucoma, unspecified, **unspecified** eye

  ● **H40.01** **Open angle** with borderline findings, **low risk**

      Open angle, low risk

    H40.011 Open angle with borderline findings, low risk, **right eye**

    H40.012 Open angle with borderline findings, low risk, **left eye**

    H40.013 Open angle with borderline findings, low risk, **bilateral**

    H40.019 Open angle with borderline findings, low risk, **unspecified eye**

  ● **H40.02** **Open angle** with borderline findings, **high risk**

      Open angle, high risk

    H40.021 Open angle with borderline findings, high risk, **right eye**

    H40.022 Open angle with borderline findings, high risk, **left eye**

    H40.023 Open angle with borderline findings, high risk, **bilateral**

    H40.029 Open angle with borderline findings, high risk, **unspecified eye**

  ● **H40.03** **Anatomical narrow** angle

      Primary angle closure suspect

    H40.031 Anatomical narrow angle, **right eye**

    H40.032 Anatomical narrow angle, **left eye**

    H40.033 Anatomical narrow angle, **bilateral**

    H40.039 Anatomical narrow angle, **unspecified** eye

  ● **H40.04** **Steroid responder**

    H40.041 Steroid responder, **right eye**

    H40.042 Steroid responder, **left eye**

    H40.043 Steroid responder, **bilateral**

    H40.049 Steroid responder, **unspecified eye**

  ● **H40.05** Ocular **hypertension**

    H40.051 Ocular hypertension, **right eye**

    H40.052 Ocular hypertension, **left eye**

    H40.053 Ocular hypertension, **bilateral**

    H40.059 Ocular hypertension, **unspecified** eye

  ● **H40.06** Primary angle closure **without glaucoma damage**

    H40.061 Primary angle closure without glaucoma damage, **right eye**

    H40.062 Primary angle closure without glaucoma damage, **left eye**

    H40.063 Primary angle closure without glaucoma damage, **bilateral**

    H40.069 Primary angle closure without glaucoma damage, **unspecified** eye

CHAPTER 7 (H00-H59)

● **H40.1   Open-angle glaucoma**

X● **H40.10   Unspecified open-angle glaucoma**

One of the following 7th characters is to be assigned to code H40.10 to designate the stage of glaucoma

0	stage unspecified
1	mild stage
2	moderate stage
3	severe stage
4	indeterminate stage

● **H40.11   Primary open-angle glaucoma**

Chronic simple glaucoma

One of the following 7th characters is to be assigned to each code in subcategory H40.11 to designate the stage of glaucoma

0	stage unspecified
1	mild stage
2	moderate stage
3	severe stage
4	indeterminate stage

Coding Clinic: 2016, Q4, P22

● **H40.111   Primary open-angle glaucoma, right eye**

Coding Clinic: 2019, Q2, P31

● **H40.112   Primary open-angle glaucoma, left eye**

● **H40.113   Primary open-angle glaucoma, bilateral**

● **H40.119   Primary open-angle glaucoma, unspecified eye**

● **H40.12   Low-tension glaucoma**

One of the following 7th characters is to be assigned to each code in subcategory H40.12 to designate the stage of glaucoma

0	stage unspecified
1	mild stage
2	moderate stage
3	severe stage
4	indeterminate stage

● **H40.121   Low-tension glaucoma, right eye**

● **H40.122   Low-tension glaucoma, left eye**

● **H40.123   Low-tension glaucoma, bilateral**

● **H40.129   Low-tension glaucoma, unspecified eye**

● **H40.13   Pigmentary glaucoma**

One of the following 7th characters is to be assigned to each code in subcategory H40.13 to designate the stage of glaucoma

0	stage unspecified
1	mild stage
2	moderate stage
3	severe stage
4	indeterminate stage

● **H40.131   Pigmentary glaucoma, right eye**

● **H40.132   Pigmentary glaucoma, left eye**

● **H40.133   Pigmentary glaucoma, bilateral**

● **H40.139   Pigmentary glaucoma, unspecified eye**

● **H40.14   Capsular glaucoma with pseudoexfoliation of lens**

One of the following 7th characters is to be assigned to each code in subcategory H40.14 to designate the stage of glaucoma

0	stage unspecified
1	mild stage
2	moderate stage
3	severe stage
4	indeterminate stage

● **H40.141   Capsular glaucoma with pseudoexfoliation of lens, right eye**

● **H40.142   Capsular glaucoma with pseudoexfoliation of lens, left eye**

● **H40.143   Capsular glaucoma with pseudoexfoliation of lens, bilateral**

● **H40.149   Capsular glaucoma with pseudoexfoliation of lens, unspecified eye**

● **H40.15   Residual stage of open-angle glaucoma**

H40.151   Residual stage of open-angle glaucoma, right eye

H40.152   Residual stage of open-angle glaucoma, left eye

H40.153   Residual stage of open-angle glaucoma, bilateral

H40.159   Residual stage of open-angle glaucoma, unspecified eye

● **H40.2   Primary angle-closure glaucoma**

Excludes1   aqueous misdirection (H40.83-)
malignant glaucoma (H40.83-)

X● **H40.20   Unspecified primary angle-closure glaucoma**

One of the following 7th characters is to be assigned to code H40.20 to designate the stage of glaucoma

0	stage unspecified
1	mild stage
2	moderate stage
3	severe stage
4	indeterminate stage

● **H40.21   Acute angle-closure glaucoma**

Acute angle-closure glaucoma attack
Acute angle-closure glaucoma crisis

H40.211   Acute angle-closure glaucoma, right eye

H40.212   Acute angle-closure glaucoma, left eye

H40.213   Acute angle-closure glaucoma, bilateral

H40.219   Acute angle-closure glaucoma, unspecified eye

● **H40.22   Chronic angle-closure glaucoma**

Chronic primary angle closure glaucoma

One of the following 7th characters is to be assigned to each code in subcategory H40.22 to designate the stage of glaucoma

0	stage unspecified
1	mild stage
2	moderate stage
3	severe stage
4	indeterminate stage

● **H40.221   Chronic angle-closure glaucoma, right eye**

● **H40.222   Chronic angle-closure glaucoma, left eye**

▶ New   ⇒ Revised   ~~deleted~~ Deleted   Excludes 1   Excludes 2   Includes   Use additional   Code first   Code also   Key words

804   OGCR Official Guidelines   X Assign placeholder X   ● Use Additional Character(s)   ▌ Manifestation Code   🔖 Hierarchical Condition Category   Coding Clinic

● H40.223   Chronic angle-closure glaucoma, bilateral
● H40.229   Chronic angle-closure glaucoma, unspecified eye
● H40.23   Intermittent angle-closure glaucoma
   H40.231   Intermittent angle-closure glaucoma, right eye
   H40.232   Intermittent angle-closure glaucoma, left eye
   H40.233   Intermittent angle-closure glaucoma, bilateral
   H40.239   Intermittent angle-closure glaucoma, unspecified eye
● H40.24   Residual stage of angle-closure glaucoma
   H40.241   Residual stage of angle-closure glaucoma, right eye
   H40.242   Residual stage of angle-closure glaucoma, left eye
   H40.243   Residual stage of angle-closure glaucoma, bilateral
   H40.249   Residual stage of angle-closure glaucoma, unspecified eye

● **H40.3   Glaucoma secondary to eye trauma**
Code also underlying condition
One of the following 7th characters is to be assigned to each code in subcategory H40.3 to designate the stage of glaucoma

0	stage unspecified
1	mild stage
2	moderate stage
3	severe stage
4	indeterminate stage

X ● H40.30   Glaucoma secondary to eye trauma, unspecified eye
X ● H40.31   Glaucoma secondary to eye trauma, right eye
X ● H40.32   Glaucoma secondary to eye trauma, left eye
X ● H40.33   Glaucoma secondary to eye trauma, bilateral

● **H40.4   Glaucoma secondary to eye inflammation**
Code also underlying condition
One of the following 7th characters is to be assigned to each code in subcategory H40.4 to designate the stage of glaucoma

0	stage unspecified
1	mild stage
2	moderate stage
3	severe stage
4	indeterminate stage

X ● H40.40   Glaucoma secondary to eye inflammation, unspecified eye
X ● H40.41   Glaucoma secondary to eye inflammation, right eye
X ● H40.42   Glaucoma secondary to eye inflammation, left eye
X ● H40.43   Glaucoma secondary to eye inflammation, bilateral

● **H40.5   Glaucoma secondary to other eye disorders**
Code also underlying eye disorder
One of the following 7th characters is to be assigned to each code in subcategory H40.5 to designate the stage of glaucoma

0	stage unspecified
1	mild stage
2	moderate stage
3	severe stage
4	indeterminate stage

X ● H40.50   Glaucoma secondary to other eye disorders, unspecified eye
X ● H40.51   Glaucoma secondary to other eye disorders, right eye
X ● H40.52   Glaucoma secondary to other eye disorders, left eye
X ● H40.53   Glaucoma secondary to other eye disorders, bilateral

● **H40.6   Glaucoma secondary to drugs**
Use additional code for adverse effect, if applicable, to identify drug (T36-T50 with fifth or sixth character 5)
One of the following 7th characters is to be assigned to each code in subcategory H40.6 to designate the stage of glaucoma

0	stage unspecified
1	mild stage
2	moderate stage
3	severe stage
4	indeterminate stage

X ● H40.60   Glaucoma secondary to drugs, unspecified eye
X ● H40.61   Glaucoma secondary to drugs, right eye
X ● H40.62   Glaucoma secondary to drugs, left eye
X ● H40.63   Glaucoma secondary to drugs, bilateral

● **H40.8   Other glaucoma**
● H40.81   Glaucoma with increased episcleral venous pressure
   H40.811   Glaucoma with increased episcleral venous pressure, right eye
   H40.812   Glaucoma with increased episcleral venous pressure, left eye
   H40.813   Glaucoma with increased episcleral venous pressure, bilateral
   H40.819   Glaucoma with increased episcleral venous pressure, unspecified eye
● H40.82   Hypersecretion glaucoma
   H40.821   Hypersecretion glaucoma, right eye
   H40.822   Hypersecretion glaucoma, left eye
   H40.823   Hypersecretion glaucoma, bilateral
   H40.829   Hypersecretion glaucoma, unspecified eye
● H40.83   Aqueous misdirection
Malignant glaucoma
   H40.831   Aqueous misdirection, right eye
   H40.832   Aqueous misdirection, left eye
   H40.833   Aqueous misdirection, bilateral
   H40.839   Aqueous misdirection, unspecified eye
   H40.89   Other specified glaucoma
H40.9   Unspecified glaucoma

▶ *H42   Glaucoma in diseases classified elsewhere*
Code first underlying condition, such as:
amyloidosis (E85.-)
aniridia (Q13.1)
glaucoma (in) diabetes mellitus (E08.39, E09.39, E10.39, E11.39, E13.39)
Lowe's syndrome (E72.03)
Reiger anomaly (Q13.81)
specified metabolic disorder (E70-E88)

Excludes1   glaucoma (in) onchocerciasis (B73.02)
glaucoma (in) syphilis (A52.71)
glaucoma (in) tuberculous (A18.59)

DISORDERS OF VITREOUS BODY AND GLOBE (H43-H44)

● **H43   Disorders of vitreous body**

  ● **H43.0   Vitreous prolapse**

    Excludes1   vitreous syndrome following cataract surgery (H59.0-)

           traumatic vitreous prolapse (S05.2-)

     H43.00   Vitreous prolapse, unspecified eye

     H43.01   Vitreous prolapse, right eye

     H43.02   Vitreous prolapse, left eye

     H43.03   Vitreous prolapse, bilateral

  ● **H43.1   Vitreous hemorrhage**

     H43.10   Vitreous hemorrhage, unspecified eye 🐾

     H43.11   Vitreous hemorrhage, right eye 🐾

     H43.12   Vitreous hemorrhage, left eye 🐾

     H43.13   Vitreous hemorrhage, bilateral 🐾

  ● **H43.2   Crystalline deposits in vitreous body**

     H43.20   Crystalline deposits in vitreous body, unspecified eye

     H43.21   Crystalline deposits in vitreous body, right eye

     H43.22   Crystalline deposits in vitreous body, left eye

     H43.23   Crystalline deposits in vitreous body, bilateral

  ● **H43.3   Other vitreous opacities**

    ● **H43.31   Vitreous membranes and strands**

       H43.311   Vitreous membranes and strands, right eye

       H43.312   Vitreous membranes and strands, left eye

       H43.313   Vitreous membranes and strands, bilateral

       H43.319   Vitreous membranes and strands, unspecified eye

    ● **H43.39   Other vitreous opacities**

       Vitreous floaters

         Small clumps of cells that float in the vitreous of the eye, appearing as black specks or dots in the field of vision and common in the aging eye.

       H43.391   Other vitreous opacities, right eye

       H43.392   Other vitreous opacities, left eye

       H43.393   Other vitreous opacities, bilateral

       H43.399   Other vitreous opacities, unspecified eye

  ● **H43.8   Other disorders of vitreous body**

    Excludes1   proliferative vitreo-retinopathy with retinal detachment (H33.4)

    Excludes2   vitreous abscess (H44.02-)

    ● **H43.81   Vitreous degeneration**

       Vitreous detachment

       H43.811   Vitreous degeneration, right eye

       H43.812   Vitreous degeneration, left eye

       H43.813   Vitreous degeneration, bilateral

       H43.819   Vitreous degeneration, unspecified eye

    ● **H43.82   Vitreomacular adhesion**

       Vitreomacular traction

       H43.821   Vitreomacular adhesion, right eye   A

       H43.822   Vitreomacular adhesion, left eye   A

       H43.823   Vitreomacular adhesion, bilateral   A

       H43.829   Vitreomacular adhesion, unspecified eye   A

     H43.89   Other disorders of vitreous body

   H43.9   Unspecified disorder of vitreous body

● **H44   Disorders of globe**

  Includes   disorders affecting multiple structures of eye

  ● **H44.0   Purulent endophthalmitis**

     Use additional code to identify organism

    Excludes1   bleb associated endophthalmitis (H59.4-)

    ● **H44.00   Unspecified purulent endophthalmitis**

       H44.001   Unspecified purulent endophthalmitis, right eye

       H44.002   Unspecified purulent endophthalmitis, left eye

       H44.003   Unspecified purulent endophthalmitis, bilateral

       H44.009   Unspecified purulent endophthalmitis, unspecified eye

    ● **H44.01   Panophthalmitis (acute)**

       H44.011   Panophthalmitis (acute), right eye

       H44.012   Panophthalmitis (acute), left eye

       H44.013   Panophthalmitis (acute), bilateral

       H44.019   Panophthalmitis (acute), unspecified eye

    ● **H44.02   Vitreous abscess (chronic)**

       H44.021   Vitreous abscess (chronic), right eye

       H44.022   Vitreous abscess (chronic), left eye

       H44.023   Vitreous abscess (chronic), bilateral

       H44.029   Vitreous abscess (chronic), unspecified eye

  ● **H44.1   Other endophthalmitis**

    Excludes1   bleb associated endophthalmitis (H59.4-)

    Excludes2   ophthalmia nodosa (H16.2-)

    ● **H44.11   Panuveitis**

       H44.111   Panuveitis, right eye

       H44.112   Panuveitis, left eye

       H44.113   Panuveitis, bilateral

       H44.119   Panuveitis, unspecified eye

    ● **H44.12   Parasitic endophthalmitis, unspecified**   Ⓔⓧ DX 792

       H44.121   Parasitic endophthalmitis, unspecified, right eye

       H44.122   Parasitic endophthalmitis, unspecified, left eye

       H44.123   Parasitic endophthalmitis, unspecified, bilateral

       H44.129   Parasitic endophthalmitis, unspecified, unspecified eye

    ● **H44.13   Sympathetic uveitis**

       H44.131   Sympathetic uveitis, right eye

       H44.132   Sympathetic uveitis, left eye

       H44.133   Sympathetic uveitis, bilateral

       H44.139   Sympathetic uveitis, unspecified eye

     H44.19   Other endophthalmitis

  ● **H44.2   Degenerative myopia**

     Malignant myopia

     H44.20   Degenerative myopia, unspecified eye

     H44.21   Degenerative myopia, right eye

     H44.22   Degenerative myopia, left eye

     H44.23   Degenerative myopia, bilateral

    ● **H44.2A   Degenerative myopia with choroidal neovascularization**

       Use Additional code for any associated choroid disorders (H31.-)

       H44.2A1   Degenerative myopia with choroidal neovascularization, right eye

       H44.2A2   Degenerative myopia with choroidal neovascularization, left eye

---

▶ New   ⇒ Revised   ~~deleted~~ Deleted   Excludes 1   Excludes 2   Includes   Use additional   Code first   Code also   Key words

OGCR Official Guidelines   X Assign placeholder X   ● Use Additional Character(s)   ▶ Manifestation Code   🐾 Hierarchical Condition Category   Coding Clinic

         H44.2A3   Degenerative myopia with choroidal neovascularization, bilateral

         H44.2A9   Degenerative myopia with choroidal neovascularization, unspecified eye

● H44.2B   Degenerative myopia with macular hole

         H44.2B1   Degenerative myopia with macular hole, right eye

         H44.2B2   Degenerative myopia with macular hole, left eye

         H44.2B3   Degenerative myopia with macular hole, bilateral

         H44.2B9   Degenerative myopia with macular hole, unspecified eye

● H44.2C   Degenerative myopia with retinal detachment

         Use Additional code to identify the retinal detachment (H33.-)

         H44.2C1   Degenerative myopia with retinal detachment, right eye

         H44.2C2   Degenerative myopia with retinal detachment, left eye

         H44.2C3   Degenerative myopia with retinal detachment, bilateral

         H44.2C9   Degenerative myopia with retinal detachment, unspecified eye

● H44.2D   Degenerative myopia with foveoschisis

         H44.2D1   Degenerative myopia with foveoschisis, right eye

         H44.2D2   Degenerative myopia with foveoschisis, left eye

         H44.2D3   Degenerative myopia with foveoschisis, bilateral

         H44.2D9   Degenerative myopia with foveoschisis, unspecified eye

● H44.2E   Degenerative myopia with other maculopathy

         H44.2E1   Degenerative myopia with other maculopathy, right eye

         H44.2E2   Degenerative myopia with other maculopathy, left eye

         H44.2E3   Degenerative myopia with other maculopathy, bilateral

         H44.2E9   Degenerative myopia with other maculopathy, unspecified eye

● H44.3   Other and unspecified degenerative disorders of globe

     H44.30   Unspecified degenerative disorder of globe

● H44.31   Chalcosis

         H44.311   Chalcosis, right eye

         H44.312   Chalcosis, left eye

         H44.313   Chalcosis, bilateral

         H44.319   Chalcosis, unspecified eye

● H44.32   Siderosis of eye

         H44.321   Siderosis of eye, right eye

         H44.322   Siderosis of eye, left eye

         H44.323   Siderosis of eye, bilateral

         H44.329   Siderosis of eye, unspecified eye

● H44.39   Other degenerative disorders of globe

         H44.391   Other degenerative disorders of globe, right eye

         H44.392   Other degenerative disorders of globe, left eye

         H44.393   Other degenerative disorders of globe, bilateral

         H44.399   Other degenerative disorders of globe, unspecified eye

● H44.4   Hypotony of eye

     H44.40   Unspecified hypotony of eye

● H44.41   Flat anterior chamber hypotony of eye

         H44.411   Flat anterior chamber hypotony of right eye

         H44.412   Flat anterior chamber hypotony of left eye

         H44.413   Flat anterior chamber hypotony of eye, bilateral

         H44.419   Flat anterior chamber hypotony of unspecified eye

● H44.42   Hypotony of eye due to ocular fistula

         H44.421   Hypotony of right eye due to ocular fistula

         H44.422   Hypotony of left eye due to ocular fistula

         H44.423   Hypotony of eye due to ocular fistula, bilateral

         H44.429   Hypotony of unspecified eye due to ocular fistula

● H44.43   Hypotony of eye due to other ocular disorders

         H44.431   Hypotony of eye due to other ocular disorders, right eye

         H44.432   Hypotony of eye due to other ocular disorders, left eye

         H44.433   Hypotony of eye due to other ocular disorders, bilateral

         H44.439   Hypotony of eye due to other ocular disorders, unspecified eye

● H44.44   Primary hypotony of eye

         H44.441   Primary hypotony of right eye

         H44.442   Primary hypotony of left eye

         H44.443   Primary hypotony of eye, bilateral

         H44.449   Primary hypotony of unspecified eye

● H44.5   Degenerated conditions of globe

     H44.50   Unspecified degenerated conditions of globe

● H44.51   Absolute glaucoma

         H44.511   Absolute glaucoma, right eye

         H44.512   Absolute glaucoma, left eye

         H44.513   Absolute glaucoma, bilateral

         H44.519   Absolute glaucoma, unspecified eye

● H44.52   Atrophy of globe

         Phthisis bulbi

         H44.521   Atrophy of globe, right eye

         H44.522   Atrophy of globe, left eye

         H44.523   Atrophy of globe, bilateral

         H44.529   Atrophy of globe, unspecified eye

● H44.53   Leucocoria

         H44.531   Leucocoria, right eye

         H44.532   Leucocoria, left eye

         H44.533   Leucocoria, bilateral

         H44.539   Leucocoria, unspecified eye

● H44.6   Retained (old) intraocular foreign body, magnetic

         Use additional code to identify magnetic foreign body (Z18.11)

         Excludes 1   current intraocular foreign body (S05.-)

         Excludes 2   retained foreign body in eyelid (H02.81-)
                 retained (old) foreign body following penetrating wound of orbit (H05.5-)
                 retained (old) intraocular foreign body, nonmagnetic (H44.7-)

CHAPTER 7 (H00-H59)

CHAPTER 7 (H00-H59)

● **H44.60** Unspecified retained (old) intraocular foreign body, magnetic

     H44.601 Unspecified retained (old) intraocular foreign body, magnetic, right eye

     H44.602 Unspecified retained (old) intraocular foreign body, magnetic, left eye

     H44.603 Unspecified retained (old) intraocular foreign body, magnetic, bilateral

     H44.609 Unspecified retained (old) intraocular foreign body, magnetic, unspecified eye

● **H44.61** Retained (old) magnetic foreign body in anterior chamber

     H44.611 Retained (old) magnetic foreign body in anterior chamber, right eye

     H44.612 Retained (old) magnetic foreign body in anterior chamber, left eye

     H44.613 Retained (old) magnetic foreign body in anterior chamber, bilateral

     H44.619 Retained (old) magnetic foreign body in anterior chamber, unspecified eye

● **H44.62** Retained (old) magnetic foreign body in iris or ciliary body

     H44.621 Retained (old) magnetic foreign body in iris or ciliary body, right eye

     H44.622 Retained (old) magnetic foreign body in iris or ciliary body, left eye

     H44.623 Retained (old) magnetic foreign body in iris or ciliary body, bilateral

     H44.629 Retained (old) magnetic foreign body in iris or ciliary body, unspecified eye

● **H44.63** Retained (old) magnetic foreign body in lens

     H44.631 Retained (old) magnetic foreign body in lens, right eye

     H44.632 Retained (old) magnetic foreign body in lens, left eye

     H44.633 Retained (old) magnetic foreign body in lens, bilateral

     H44.639 Retained (old) magnetic foreign body in lens, unspecified eye

● **H44.64** Retained (old) magnetic foreign body in posterior wall of globe

     H44.641 Retained (old) magnetic foreign body in posterior wall of globe, right eye

     H44.642 Retained (old) magnetic foreign body in posterior wall of globe, left eye

     H44.643 Retained (old) magnetic foreign body in posterior wall of globe, bilateral

     H44.649 Retained (old) magnetic foreign body in posterior wall of globe, unspecified eye

● **H44.65** Retained (old) magnetic foreign body in vitreous body

     H44.651 Retained (old) magnetic foreign body in vitreous body, right eye

     H44.652 Retained (old) magnetic foreign body in vitreous body, left eye

     H44.653 Retained (old) magnetic foreign body in vitreous body, bilateral

     H44.659 Retained (old) magnetic foreign body in vitreous body, unspecified eye

● **H44.69** Retained (old) intraocular foreign body, magnetic, in other or multiple sites

     H44.691 Retained (old) intraocular foreign body, magnetic, in other or multiple sites, right eye

     H44.692 Retained (old) intraocular foreign body, magnetic, in other or multiple sites, left eye

     H44.693 Retained (old) intraocular foreign body, magnetic, in other or multiple sites, bilateral

     H44.699 Retained (old) intraocular foreign body, magnetic, in other or multiple sites, unspecified eye

● **H44.7** Retained (old) intraocular foreign body, nonmagnetic

     Use additional code to identify nonmagnetic foreign body (Z18.01-Z18.10, Z18.12, Z18.2-Z18.9)

     Excludes1   current intraocular foreign body (S05.-)

     Excludes2   retained foreign body in eyelid (H02.81-)
retained (old) foreign body following penetrating wound of orbit (H05.5-)
retained (old) intraocular foreign body, magnetic (H44.6-)

● **H44.70** Unspecified retained (old) intraocular foreign body, nonmagnetic

     H44.701 Unspecified retained (old) intraocular foreign body, nonmagnetic, right eye

     H44.702 Unspecified retained (old) intraocular foreign body, nonmagnetic, left eye

     H44.703 Unspecified retained (old) intraocular foreign body, nonmagnetic, bilateral

     H44.709 Unspecified retained (old) intraocular foreign body, nonmagnetic, unspecified eye

         Retained (old) intraocular foreign body NOS

● **H44.71** Retained (nonmagnetic) (old) foreign body in anterior chamber

     H44.711 Retained (nonmagnetic) (old) foreign body in anterior chamber, right eye

     H44.712 Retained (nonmagnetic) (old) foreign body in anterior chamber, left eye

     H44.713 Retained (nonmagnetic) (old) foreign body in anterior chamber, bilateral

     H44.719 Retained (nonmagnetic) (old) foreign body in anterior chamber, unspecified eye

● **H44.72** Retained (nonmagnetic) (old) foreign body in iris or ciliary body

     H44.721 Retained (nonmagnetic) (old) foreign body in iris or ciliary body, right eye

     H44.722 Retained (nonmagnetic) (old) foreign body in iris or ciliary body, left eye

     H44.723 Retained (nonmagnetic) (old) foreign body in iris or ciliary body, bilateral

     H44.729 Retained (nonmagnetic) (old) foreign body in iris or ciliary body, unspecified eye

● **H44.73** Retained (nonmagnetic) (old) foreign body in lens

     H44.731 Retained (nonmagnetic) (old) foreign body in lens, right eye

     H44.732 Retained (nonmagnetic) (old) foreign body in lens, left eye

     H44.733 Retained (nonmagnetic) (old) foreign body in lens, bilateral

     H44.739 Retained (nonmagnetic) (old) foreign body in lens, unspecified eye

● **H44.74** Retained (nonmagnetic) (old) foreign body in posterior wall of globe
    H44.741 Retained (nonmagnetic) (old) foreign body in posterior wall of globe, right eye
    H44.742 Retained (nonmagnetic) (old) foreign body in posterior wall of globe, left eye
    H44.743 Retained (nonmagnetic) (old) foreign body in posterior wall of globe, bilateral
    H44.749 Retained (nonmagnetic) (old) foreign body in posterior wall of globe, unspecified eye
● **H44.75** Retained (nonmagnetic) (old) foreign body in vitreous body
    H44.751 Retained (nonmagnetic) (old) foreign body in vitreous body, right eye
    H44.752 Retained (nonmagnetic) (old) foreign body in vitreous body, left eye
    H44.753 Retained (nonmagnetic) (old) foreign body in vitreous body, bilateral
    H44.759 Retained (nonmagnetic) (old) foreign body in vitreous body, unspecified eye
● **H44.79** Retained (old) intraocular foreign body, nonmagnetic, in other or multiple sites
    H44.791 Retained (old) intraocular foreign body, nonmagnetic, in other or multiple sites, right eye
    H44.792 Retained (old) intraocular foreign body, nonmagnetic, in other or multiple sites, left eye
    H44.793 Retained (old) intraocular foreign body, nonmagnetic, in other or multiple sites, bilateral
    H44.799 Retained (old) intraocular foreign body, nonmagnetic, in other or multiple sites, unspecified eye
● **H44.8** Other disorders of globe
   ● **H44.81** Hemophthalmos
    H44.811 Hemophthalmos, right eye
    H44.812 Hemophthalmos, left eye
    H44.813 Hemophthalmos, bilateral
    H44.819 Hemophthalmos, unspecified eye
   ● **H44.82** Luxation of globe
    H44.821 Luxation of globe, right eye
    H44.822 Luxation of globe, left eye
    H44.823 Luxation of globe, bilateral
    H44.829 Luxation of globe, unspecified eye
    H44.89 Other disorders of globe
  H44.9 Unspecified disorder of globe

★ **(See Plate 7 of the Anatomy Illustrations.)**

DISORDERS OF OPTIC NERVE AND VISUAL PATHWAYS (H46-H47)

● **H46** Optic neuritis
   Excludes2 ischemic optic neuropathy (H47.01-)
      neuromyelitis optica [Devic] (G36.0)
  ● **H46.0** Optic papillitis
    H46.00 Optic papillitis, unspecified eye
    H46.01 Optic papillitis, right eye
    H46.02 Optic papillitis, left eye
    H46.03 Optic papillitis, bilateral

● **H46.1** Retrobulbar neuritis
   Retrobulbar neuritis NOS
   Excludes1 syphilitic retrobulbar neuritis (A52.15)
    H46.10 Retrobulbar neuritis, unspecified eye
    H46.11 Retrobulbar neuritis, right eye
    H46.12 Retrobulbar neuritis, left eye
    H46.13 Retrobulbar neuritis, bilateral
  H46.2 Nutritional optic neuropathy
  H46.3 Toxic optic neuropathy
    Code first (T51-T65) to identify cause
  H46.8 Other optic neuritis
  H46.9 Unspecified optic neuritis
    Coding Clinic: 2023, Q3, P19

● **H47** Other disorders of optic [2nd] nerve and visual pathways
  ● **H47.0** Disorders of optic nerve, not elsewhere classified
   ● **H47.01** Ischemic optic neuropathy
    H47.011 Ischemic optic neuropathy, right eye
    H47.012 Ischemic optic neuropathy, left eye
    H47.013 Ischemic optic neuropathy, bilateral
    H47.019 Ischemic optic neuropathy, unspecified eye
   ● **H47.02** Hemorrhage in optic nerve sheath
    H47.021 Hemorrhage in optic nerve sheath, right eye
    H47.022 Hemorrhage in optic nerve sheath, left eye
    H47.023 Hemorrhage in optic nerve sheath, bilateral
    H47.029 Hemorrhage in optic nerve sheath, unspecified eye
   ● **H47.03** Optic nerve hypoplasia
    H47.031 Optic nerve hypoplasia, right eye
    H47.032 Optic nerve hypoplasia, left eye
    H47.033 Optic nerve hypoplasia, bilateral
    H47.039 Optic nerve hypoplasia, unspecified eye
   ● **H47.09** Other disorders of optic nerve, not elsewhere classified
    Compression of optic nerve
    H47.091 Other disorders of optic nerve, not elsewhere classified, right eye
    H47.092 Other disorders of optic nerve, not elsewhere classified, left eye
    H47.093 Other disorders of optic nerve, not elsewhere classified, bilateral
    H47.099 Other disorders of optic nerve, not elsewhere classified, unspecified eye
  ● **H47.1** Papilledema
    H47.10 Unspecified papilledema
    H47.11 Papilledema associated with increased intracranial pressure
    H47.12 Papilledema associated with decreased ocular pressure
    H47.13 Papilledema associated with retinal disorder
   ● **H47.14** Foster-Kennedy syndrome
    H47.141 Foster-Kennedy syndrome, right eye
    H47.142 Foster-Kennedy syndrome, left eye
    H47.143 Foster-Kennedy syndrome, bilateral
    H47.149 Foster-Kennedy syndrome, unspecified eye

CHAPTER 7 (H00-H59)

Figure 7-11   Stages of papilledema according to the Frisén grading scale. **A,** Very eary papilledema (Frisén stage 1). **B,** Early papilledema (Frisén stage 2). **C,** Moderate papilledema (Frisén stage 3). **D,** Marked papilledema (Frisén stage 4). **E,** Severe papilledema. (From Youmans JR, Winn HR: Youmans Neurological Surgery, Philadelphia, PA, Elsevier/Saunders, 2011)

Item 7-8   Papilledema is swelling of the optic disc caused by increased intracranial pressure. It is most often bilateral and occurs quickly (hours) or over weeks of time. It is a common symptom of a brain tumor. The term should not be used to describe optic disc swelling with underlying infectious, infiltrative, or inflammatory etiologies.

● **H47.2**   Optic atrophy
     H47.20   Unspecified optic atrophy
     ● H47.21   Primary optic atrophy
         H47.211   Primary optic atrophy, right eye
         H47.212   Primary optic atrophy, left eye
         H47.213   Primary optic atrophy, bilateral
         H47.219   Primary optic atrophy, unspecified eye
     H47.22   Hereditary optic atrophy
         Leber's optic atrophy
     ● H47.23   Glaucomatous optic atrophy
         H47.231   Glaucomatous optic atrophy, right eye
         H47.232   Glaucomatous optic atrophy, left eye
         H47.233   Glaucomatous optic atrophy, bilateral
         H47.239   Glaucomatous optic atrophy, unspecified eye
     ● H47.29   Other optic atrophy
         Temporal pallor of optic disc
         H47.291   Other optic atrophy, right eye
         H47.292   Other optic atrophy, left eye
         H47.293   Other optic atrophy, bilateral
         H47.299   Other optic atrophy, unspecified eye
● **H47.3**   Other disorders of optic disc
     ● H47.31   Coloboma of optic disc
         H47.311   Coloboma of optic disc, right eye
         H47.312   Coloboma of optic disc, left eye
         H47.313   Coloboma of optic disc, bilateral
         H47.319   Coloboma of optic disc, unspecified eye
     ● H47.32   Drusen of optic disc
         H47.321   Drusen of optic disc, right eye
         H47.322   Drusen of optic disc, left eye
         H47.323   Drusen of optic disc, bilateral
         H47.329   Drusen of optic disc, unspecified eye
     ● H47.33   Pseudopapilledema of optic disc
         H47.331   Pseudopapilledema of optic disc, right eye
         H47.332   Pseudopapilledema of optic disc, left eye
         H47.333   Pseudopapilledema of optic disc, bilateral
         H47.339   Pseudopapilledema of optic disc, unspecified eye

     ● H47.39   Other disorders of optic disc
         H47.391   Other disorders of optic disc, right eye
         H47.392   Other disorders of optic disc, left eye
         H47.393   Other disorders of optic disc, bilateral
         H47.399   Other disorders of optic disc, unspecified eye
● **H47.4**   Disorders of optic chiasm
     Code also underlying condition
     H47.41   Disorders of optic chiasm in (due to) inflammatory disorders
     H47.42   Disorders of optic chiasm in (due to) neoplasm
     H47.43   Disorders of optic chiasm in (due to) vascular disorders
     H47.49   Disorders of optic chiasm in (due to) other disorders
● **H47.5**   Disorders of other visual pathways
     Disorders of optic tracts, geniculate nuclei and optic radiations
     Code also underlying condition
     ● H47.51   Disorders of visual pathways in (due to) inflammatory disorders
         H47.511   Disorders of visual pathways in (due to) inflammatory disorders, right side
         H47.512   Disorders of visual pathways in (due to) inflammatory disorders, left side
         H47.519   Disorders of visual pathways in (due to) inflammatory disorders, unspecified side
     ● H47.52   Disorders of visual pathways in (due to) neoplasm
         H47.521   Disorders of visual pathways in (due to) neoplasm, right side
         H47.522   Disorders of visual pathways in (due to) neoplasm, left side
         H47.529   Disorders of visual pathways in (due to) neoplasm, unspecified side
     ● H47.53   Disorders of visual pathways in (due to) vascular disorders
         H47.531   Disorders of visual pathways in (due to) vascular disorders, right side
         H47.532   Disorders of visual pathways in (due to) vascular disorders, left side
         H47.539   Disorders of visual pathways in (due to) vascular disorders, unspecified side
● **H47.6**   Disorders of visual cortex
     Code also underlying condition
     Excludes1   injury to visual cortex S04.04-
     ● H47.61   Cortical blindness
         H47.611   Cortical blindness, right side of brain
         H47.612   Cortical blindness, left side of brain
         H47.619   Cortical blindness, unspecified side of brain
     ● H47.62   Disorders of visual cortex in (due to) inflammatory disorders
         H47.621   Disorders of visual cortex in (due to) inflammatory disorders, right side of brain
         H47.622   Disorders of visual cortex in (due to) inflammatory disorders, left side of brain
         H47.629   Disorders of visual cortex in (due to) inflammatory disorders, unspecified side of brain
     ● H47.63   Disorders of visual cortex in (due to) neoplasm
         H47.631   Disorders of visual cortex in (due to) neoplasm, right side of brain

▶ New   ⟹ Revised   ~~deleted~~ Deleted   Excludes 1   Excludes 2   Includes   Use additional   Code first   Code also   Key words
OGCR Official Guidelines   X Assign placeholder X   ● Use Additional Character(s)   ▶ Manifestation Code   🗞 Hierarchical Condition Category   Coding Clinic

H47.632 Disorders of visual cortex in (due to) neoplasm, left side of brain

H47.639 Disorders of visual cortex in (due to) neoplasm, unspecified side of brain

● H47.64 Disorders of visual cortex in (due to) vascular disorders

H47.641 Disorders of visual cortex in (due to) vascular disorders, right side of brain

H47.642 Disorders of visual cortex in (due to) vascular disorders, left side of brain

H47.649 Disorders of visual cortex in (due to) vascular disorders, unspecified side of brain

H47.9 Unspecified disorder of visual pathways

DISORDERS OF OCULAR MUSCLES, BINOCULAR MOVEMENT, ACCOMMODATION AND REFRACTION (H49-H52)

Excludes2 nystagmus and other irregular eye movements (H55)

● H49 Paralytic strabismus

Excludes2 internal ophthalmoplegia (H52.51-)
internuclear ophthalmoplegia (H51.2-)
progressive supranuclear ophthalmoplegia (G23.1)

● H49.0 Third [oculomotor] nerve palsy

H49.00 Third [oculomotor] nerve palsy, unspecified eye
H49.01 Third [oculomotor] nerve palsy, right eye
H49.02 Third [oculomotor] nerve palsy, left eye
H49.03 Third [oculomotor] nerve palsy, bilateral

● H49.1 Fourth [trochlear] nerve palsy

H49.10 Fourth [trochlear] nerve palsy, unspecified eye
H49.11 Fourth [trochlear] nerve palsy, right eye
H49.12 Fourth [trochlear] nerve palsy, left eye
H49.13 Fourth [trochlear] nerve palsy, bilateral

● H49.2 Sixth [abducent] nerve palsy

H49.20 Sixth [abducent] nerve palsy, unspecified eye
H49.21 Sixth [abducent] nerve palsy, right eye
H49.22 Sixth [abducent] nerve palsy, left eye
H49.23 Sixth [abducent] nerve palsy, bilateral

● H49.3 Total (external) ophthalmoplegia

H49.30 Total (external) ophthalmoplegia, unspecified eye
H49.31 Total (external) ophthalmoplegia, right eye
H49.32 Total (external) ophthalmoplegia, left eye
H49.33 Total (external) ophthalmoplegia, bilateral

● H49.4 Progressive external ophthalmoplegia

Excludes1 Kearns-Sayre syndrome (H49.81-)

H49.40 Progressive external ophthalmoplegia, unspecified eye
H49.41 Progressive external ophthalmoplegia, right eye
H49.42 Progressive external ophthalmoplegia, left eye
H49.43 Progressive external ophthalmoplegia, bilateral

● H49.8 Other paralytic strabismus

● H49.81 Kearns-Sayre syndrome

Progressive external ophthalmoplegia with pigmentary retinopathy

Code also, if applicable, other manifestations, such as:
heart block (I45.9)

H49.811 Kearns-Sayre syndrome, right eye 🔖
H49.812 Kearns-Sayre syndrome, left eye 🔖
H49.813 Kearns-Sayre syndrome, bilateral 🔖
H49.819 Kearns-Sayre syndrome, unspecified eye 🔖

● H49.88 Other paralytic strabismus

External ophthalmoplegia NOS

H49.881 Other paralytic strabismus, right eye
H49.882 Other paralytic strabismus, left eye
H49.883 Other paralytic strabismus, bilateral
H49.889 Other paralytic strabismus, unspecified eye

H49.9 Unspecified paralytic strabismus

● H50 Other strabismus

● H50.0 Esotropia

Convergent concomitant strabismus

Excludes1 intermittent esotropia (H50.31-, H50.32)

H50.00 Unspecified esotropia

● H50.01 Monocular esotropia

H50.011 Monocular esotropia, right eye
H50.012 Monocular esotropia, left eye

● H50.02 Monocular esotropia with A pattern

H50.021 Monocular esotropia with A pattern, right eye
H50.022 Monocular esotropia with A pattern, left eye

● H50.03 Monocular esotropia with V pattern

H50.031 Monocular esotropia with V pattern, right eye
H50.032 Monocular esotropia with V pattern, left eye

● H50.04 Monocular esotropia with other noncomitancies

H50.041 Monocular esotropia with other noncomitancies, right eye
H50.042 Monocular esotropia with other noncomitancies, left eye

H50.05 Alternating esotropia
H50.06 Alternating esotropia with A pattern
H50.07 Alternating esotropia with V pattern
H50.08 Alternating esotropia with other noncomitancies

● H50.1 Exotropia

Misalignment in which one eye deviates outward (away from nose) while the other fixates normally
Divergent concomitant strabismus

Excludes1 intermittent exotropia (H50.33-, H50.34)

H50.10 Unspecified exotropia

● H50.11 Monocular exotropia

H50.111 Monocular exotropia, right eye
H50.112 Monocular exotropia, left eye

Item 7-9 Strabismus or esotropia (crossed eyes) is a condition of the extraocular eye muscles, resulting in an inability of the eyes to focus and also affects depth perception.

Figure 7-12 A. Image of strabismus. **B.** Exotropia. (**A** from Yanoff: Ophthalmology, ed 3, Mosby, Inc., 2008. **B** from Zitelli BJ, Davis HW, Pediatric Physical Diagnosis: Atlas of Pediatric Physical Diagnosis, Philadelphia, Elsevier Saunders, 2012)

CHAPTER 7 (H00-H59)

H50.12 Monocular exotropia with A pattern
  H50.121 Monocular exotropia with A pattern, right eye
  H50.122 Monocular exotropia with A pattern, left eye
H50.13 Monocular exotropia with V pattern
  H50.131 Monocular exotropia with V pattern, right eye
  H50.132 Monocular exotropia with V pattern, left eye
H50.14 Monocular exotropia with other noncomitancies
  H50.141 Monocular exotropia with other noncomitancies, right eye
  H50.142 Monocular exotropia with other noncomitancies, left eye
H50.15 Alternating exotropia
H50.16 Alternating exotropia with A pattern
H50.17 Alternating exotropia with V pattern
H50.18 Alternating exotropia with other noncomitancies
H50.2 Vertical strabismus
  Hypertropia
  H50.21 Vertical strabismus, right eye
  H50.22 Vertical strabismus, left eye
H50.3 Intermittent heterotropia
  Displacement of an organ or part of an organ from its normal position
  H50.30 Unspecified intermittent heterotropia
  H50.31 Intermittent monocular esotropia
    H50.311 Intermittent monocular esotropia, right eye
    H50.312 Intermittent monocular esotropia, left eye
  H50.32 Intermittent alternating esotropia
  H50.33 Intermittent monocular exotropia
    H50.331 Intermittent monocular exotropia, right eye
    H50.332 Intermittent monocular exotropia, left eye
  H50.34 Intermittent alternating exotropia
H50.4 Other and unspecified heterotropia
  H50.40 Unspecified heterotropia
  H50.41 Cyclotropia
    H50.411 Cyclotropia, right eye
    H50.412 Cyclotropia, left eye
  H50.42 Monofixation syndrome
  H50.43 Accommodative component in esotropia
H50.5 Heterophoria
  One or both eyes wander away from the position where both eyes are looking together in the same direction
  H50.50 Unspecified heterophoria
  H50.51 Esophoria
    Eye deviates inward (toward the nose)
  H50.52 Exophoria
    Eye deviates outward (toward the ear)
  H50.53 Vertical heterophoria
  H50.54 Cyclophoria
  H50.55 Alternating heterophoria
H50.6 Mechanical strabismus
  H50.60 Mechanical strabismus, unspecified
  H50.61 Brown's sheath syndrome
    H50.611 Brown's sheath syndrome, right eye
    H50.612 Brown's sheath syndrome, left eye
  H50.62 Inferior oblique muscle entrapment
    H50.621 Inferior oblique muscle entrapment, right eye
    H50.622 Inferior oblique muscle entrapment, left eye

    H50.629 Inferior oblique muscle entrapment, unspecified eye
  H50.63 Inferior rectus muscle entrapment
    H50.631 Inferior rectus muscle entrapment, right eye
    H50.632 Inferior rectus muscle entrapment, left eye
    H50.639 Inferior rectus muscle entrapment, unspecified eye
  H50.64 Lateral rectus muscle entrapment
    H50.641 Lateral rectus muscle entrapment, right eye
    H50.642 Lateral rectus muscle entrapment, left eye
    H50.649 Lateral rectus muscle entrapment, unspecified eye
  H50.65 Medial rectus muscle entrapment
    H50.651 Medial rectus muscle entrapment, right eye
    H50.652 Medial rectus muscle entrapment, left eye
    H50.659 Medial rectus muscle entrapment, unspecified eye
  H50.66 Superior oblique muscle entrapment
    H50.661 Superior oblique muscle entrapment, right eye
    H50.662 Superior oblique muscle entrapment, left eye
    H50.669 Superior oblique muscle entrapment, unspecified eye
  H50.67 Superior rectus muscle entrapment
    H50.671 Superior rectus muscle entrapment, right eye
    H50.672 Superior rectus muscle entrapment, left eye
    H50.679 Superior rectus muscle entrapment, unspecified eye
  H50.68 Extraocular muscle entrapment, unspecified
    H50.681 Extraocular muscle entrapment, unspecified, right eye
    H50.682 Extraocular muscle entrapment, unspecified, left eye
    H50.689 Extraocular muscle entrapment, unspecified, unspecified eye
  H50.69 Other mechanical strabismus
    Strabismus due to adhesions
    Traumatic limitation of duction of eye muscle
H50.8 Other specified strabismus
  H50.81 Duane's syndrome
    H50.811 Duane's syndrome, right eye
    H50.812 Duane's syndrome, left eye
  H50.89 Other specified strabismus
H50.9 Unspecified strabismus

H51 Other disorders of binocular movement
  H51.0 Palsy (spasm) of conjugate gaze
  H51.1 Convergence insufficiency and excess
    H51.11 Convergence insufficiency
    H51.12 Convergence excess
  H51.2 Internuclear ophthalmoplegia
    H51.20 Internuclear ophthalmoplegia, unspecified eye
    H51.21 Internuclear ophthalmoplegia, right eye
    H51.22 Internuclear ophthalmoplegia, left eye
    H51.23 Internuclear ophthalmoplegia, bilateral
  H51.8 Other specified disorders of binocular movement
  H51.9 Unspecified disorder of binocular movement

Item 7-10 Disorders of refraction: **Hypermetropia,** or farsightedness, means focus at a distance is adequate but not on close objects. **Myopia** is near-sightedness or short-sightedness and means the focus on nearby objects is clear but distant objects appear blurred. **Astigmatism** is warping of the curvature of the cornea so light rays entering do not meet a single focal point, resulting in a distorted image. **Anisometropia** is unequal refractive power in which one eye may be myopic (near-sighted) and the other hyperopic (far-sighted). **Presbyopia** is the loss of focus on near objects, which occurs with age because the lens loses elasticity.

- H52   Disorders of refraction and accommodation
  - H52.0   Hypermetropia
    - H52.00   Hypermetropia, unspecified eye
    - H52.01   Hypermetropia, right eye
    - H52.02   Hypermetropia, left eye
    - H52.03   Hypermetropia, bilateral
  - H52.1   Myopia
    - **Excludes1**   degenerative myopia (H44.2-)
    - H52.10   Myopia, unspecified eye
    - H52.11   Myopia, right eye
    - H52.12   Myopia, left eye
    - H52.13   Myopia, bilateral
  - H52.2   Astigmatism
    - H52.20   Unspecified astigmatism
      - H52.201   Unspecified astigmatism, right eye
      - H52.202   Unspecified astigmatism, left eye
      - H52.203   Unspecified astigmatism, bilateral
      - H52.209   Unspecified astigmatism, unspecified eye
    - H52.21   Irregular astigmatism
      - H52.211   Irregular astigmatism, right eye
      - H52.212   Irregular astigmatism, left eye
      - H52.213   Irregular astigmatism, bilateral
      - H52.219   Irregular astigmatism, unspecified eye
    - H52.22   Regular astigmatism
      - H52.221   Regular astigmatism, right eye
      - H52.222   Regular astigmatism, left eye
      - H52.223   Regular astigmatism, bilateral
      - H52.229   Regular astigmatism, unspecified eye
  - H52.3   Anisometropia and aniseikonia
    - H52.31   Anisometropia
    - H52.32   Aniseikonia
  - H52.4   Presbyopia
  - H52.5   Disorders of accommodation
    - H52.51   Internal ophthalmoplegia (complete) (total)
      - H52.511   Internal ophthalmoplegia (complete) (total), right eye
      - H52.512   Internal ophthalmoplegia (complete) (total), left eye
      - H52.513   Internal ophthalmoplegia (complete) (total), bilateral
      - H52.519   Internal ophthalmoplegia (complete) (total), unspecified eye
    - H52.52   Paresis of accommodation
      - H52.521   Paresis of accommodation, right eye
      - H52.522   Paresis of accommodation, left eye
      - H52.523   Paresis of accommodation, bilateral
      - H52.529   Paresis of accommodation, unspecified eye
    - H52.53   Spasm of accommodation
      - H52.531   Spasm of accommodation, right eye
      - H52.532   Spasm of accommodation, left eye
      - H52.533   Spasm of accommodation, bilateral
      - H52.539   Spasm of accommodation, unspecified eye
  - H52.6   Other disorders of refraction
  - H52.7   Unspecified disorder of refraction

VISUAL DISTURBANCES AND BLINDNESS (H53-H54)

- H53   Visual disturbances
  - H53.0   Amblyopia ex anopsia
    - **Excludes1**   amblyopia due to vitamin A deficiency (E50.5)
    - H53.00   Unspecified amblyopia
      - H53.001   Unspecified amblyopia, right eye
      - H53.002   Unspecified amblyopia, left eye
      - H53.003   Unspecified amblyopia, bilateral
      - H53.009   Unspecified amblyopia, unspecified eye
    - H53.01   Deprivation amblyopia
      - H53.011   Deprivation amblyopia, right eye
      - H53.012   Deprivation amblyopia, left eye
      - H53.013   Deprivation amblyopia, bilateral
      - H53.019   Deprivation amblyopia, unspecified eye
    - H53.02   Refractive amblyopia
      - H53.021   Refractive amblyopia, right eye
      - H53.022   Refractive amblyopia, left eye
      - H53.023   Refractive amblyopia, bilateral
      - H53.029   Refractive amblyopia, unspecified eye
    - H53.03   Strabismic amblyopia
      - **Excludes1**   strabismus (H50.-)
      - H53.031   Strabismic amblyopia, right eye
      - H53.032   Strabismic amblyopia, left eye
      - H53.033   Strabismic amblyopia, bilateral
      - H53.039   Strabismic amblyopia, unspecified eye
    - H53.04   Amblyopia suspect
      - Coding Clinic: 2016, Q4, P22
      - H53.041   Amblyopia suspect, right eye
      - H53.042   Amblyopia suspect, left eye
      - H53.043   Amblyopia suspect, bilateral
      - H53.049   Amblyopia suspect, unspecified eye
  - H53.1   Subjective visual disturbances
    - **Excludes1**   subjective visual disturbances due to vitamin A deficiency (E50.5)
      visual hallucinations (R44.1)
    - H53.10   Unspecified subjective visual disturbances
    - H53.11   Day blindness
      Hemeralopia
    - H53.12   Transient visual loss
      Scintillating scotoma
      - **Excludes1**   amaurosis fugax (G45.3-)
        transient retinal artery occlusion (H34.0-)
      - Coding Clinic: 2022, Q1, P30
      - H53.121   Transient visual loss, right eye
      - H53.122   Transient visual loss, left eye
      - H53.123   Transient visual loss, bilateral
      - H53.129   Transient visual loss, unspecified eye
    - H53.13   Sudden visual loss
      - H53.131   Sudden visual loss, right eye
      - H53.132   Sudden visual loss, left eye
      - H53.133   Sudden visual loss, bilateral
      - H53.139   Sudden visual loss, unspecified eye
    - H53.14   Visual discomfort
      Asthenopia
      Photophobia
      - H53.141   Visual discomfort, right eye
      - H53.142   Visual discomfort, left eye
      - H53.143   Visual discomfort, bilateral
      - H53.149   Visual discomfort, unspecified

N Newborn Age: 0   **P** Pediatric Age: 0-17   **M** Maternity DX: 9-64   **A** Adult Age: 15-124

H53.15   Visual distortions of shape and size
Metamorphopsia

H53.16   Psychophysical visual disturbances

H53.19   Other subjective visual disturbances
Visual halos
Coding Clinic: 2022, Q1, P30

H53.2   **Diplopia**
Double vision
Coding Clinic: 2022, Q3, P10

● **H53.3**   **Other and unspecified disorders of binocular vision**

H53.30   Unspecified disorder of binocular vision

H53.31   Abnormal retinal correspondence

H53.32   Fusion with defective stereopsis

H53.33   Simultaneous visual perception without fusion

H53.34   Suppression of binocular vision

● **H53.4**   **Visual field defects**

H53.40   Unspecified visual field defects

● **H53.41**   Scotoma involving central area
Central scotoma

     H53.411   Scotoma involving central area, right eye

     H53.412   Scotoma involving central area, left eye

     H53.413   Scotoma involving central area, bilateral

     H53.419   Scotoma involving central area, unspecified eye

● **H53.42**   Scotoma of blind spot area
Enlarged blind spot

     H53.421   Scotoma of blind spot area, right eye

     H53.422   Scotoma of blind spot area, left eye

     H53.423   Scotoma of blind spot area, bilateral

     H53.429   Scotoma of blind spot area, unspecified eye

● **H53.43**   Sector or arcuate defects
Arcuate scotoma
Bjerrum scotoma

     H53.431   Sector or arcuate defects, right eye

     H53.432   Sector or arcuate defects, left eye

     H53.433   Sector or arcuate defects, bilateral

     H53.439   Sector or arcuate defects, unspecified eye

● **H53.45**   Other localized visual field defect
Peripheral visual field defect
Ring scotoma NOS
Scotoma NOS

     H53.451   Other localized visual field defect, right eye

     H53.452   Other localized visual field defect, left eye

     H53.453   Other localized visual field defect, bilateral

     H53.459   Other localized visual field defect, unspecified eye

● **H53.46**   Homonymous bilateral field defects
Homonymous hemianopia
Homonymous hemianopsia
Quadrant anopia
Quadrant anopsia

     H53.461   Homonymous bilateral field defects, right side

     H53.462   Homonymous bilateral field defects, left side

     H53.469   Homonymous bilateral field defects, unspecified side
Homonymous bilateral field defects NOS

H53.47   Heteronymous bilateral field defects
Heteronymous hemianop(s)ia

● **H53.48**   Generalized contraction of visual field

     H53.481   Generalized contraction of visual field, right eye

     H53.482   Generalized contraction of visual field, left eye

     H53.483   Generalized contraction of visual field, bilateral

     H53.489   Generalized contraction of visual field, unspecified eye

● **H53.5**   **Color vision deficiencies**
Color blindness

   Excludes2   day blindness (H53.11)

H53.50   Unspecified color vision deficiencies
Color blindness NOS

H53.51   Achromatopsia

H53.52   Acquired color vision deficiency

H53.53   Deuteranomaly
Deuteranopia

H53.54   Protanomaly
Protanopia

H53.55   Tritanomaly
Tritanopia

H53.59   Other color vision deficiencies

● **H53.6**   **Night blindness**

   Excludes1   night blindness due to vitamin A deficiency (E50.5)

H53.60   Unspecified night blindness

H53.61   Abnormal dark adaptation curve

H53.62   Acquired night blindness

H53.63   Congenital night blindness

H53.69   Other night blindness

● **H53.7**   **Vision sensitivity deficiencies**

H53.71   Glare sensitivity

H53.72   Impaired contrast sensitivity

H53.8   **Other visual disturbances**

H53.9   **Unspecified visual disturbance**

● **H54**   **Blindness and low vision**

Note: For definition of visual impairment categories see table below.

Code first any associated underlying cause of the blindness

   Excludes1   amaurosis fugax (G45.3)

● **H54.0**   **Blindness, both eyes**
Visual impairment categories 3, 4, 5 in both eyes.

   ● **H54.0X**   Blindness, both eyes, different category levels

     H54.0X3   Blindness right eye, category 3

       H54.0X33   Blindness right eye category 3, blindness left eye category 3

       H54.0X34   Blindness right eye category 3, blindness left eye category 4

       H54.0X35   Blindness right eye category 3, blindness left eye category 5

     ● **H54.0X4**   Blindness right eye, category 4

       H54.0X43   Blindness right eye category 4, blindness left eye category 3

       H54.0X44   Blindness right eye category 4, blindness left eye category 4

       H54.0X45   Blindness right eye category 4, blindness left eye category 5

▶ New   ⇒ Revised   ~~deleted~~ Deleted   Excludes 1   Excludes 2   Includes   Use additional   Code first   Code also   Key words
OGCR Official Guidelines   X Assign placeholder X   ● Use Additional Character(s)   ▶ Manifestation Code   🔖 Hierarchical Condition Category   Coding Clinic

● **H54.0X5**   Blindness right eye, category 5

     H54.0X53   Blindness right eye category 5, blindness left eye category 3

     H54.0X54   Blindness right eye category 5, blindness left eye category 4

     H54.0X55   Blindness right eye category 5, blindness left eye category 5

● **H54.1**   **Blindness, one eye, low vision other eye**
Visual impairment categories 3, 4, 5 in one eye, with categories 1 or 2 in the other eye.

   H54.10   Blindness, one eye, low vision other eye, unspecified eyes

● **H54.11**   Blindness, right eye, low vision left eye

   ● **H54.113**   Blindness right eye category 3, low vision left eye

     H54.1131   Blindness right eye category 3, low vision left eye category 1

     H54.1132   Blindness right eye category 3, low vision left eye category 2

   ● **H54.114**   Blindness right eye category 4, low vision left eye

     H54.1141   Blindness right eye category 4, low vision left eye category 1

     H54.1142   Blindness right eye category 4, low vision left eye category 2

   ● **H54.115**   Blindness right eye category 5, low vision left eye

     H54.1151   Blindness right eye category 5, low vision left eye category 1

     H54.1152   Blindness right eye category 5, low vision left eye category 2

● **H54.12**   Blindness, left eye, low vision right eye

   ● **H54.121**   Low vision right eye category 1, blindness left eye

     H54.1213   Low vision right eye category 1, blindness left eye category 3

     H54.1214   Low vision right eye category 1, blindness left eye category 4

     H54.1215   Low vision right eye category 1, blindness left eye category 5

   ● **H54.122**   Low vision right eye category 2, blindness left eye

     H54.1223   Low vision right eye category 2, blindness left eye category 3

     H54.1224   Low vision right eye category 2, blindness left eye category 4

     H54.1225   Low vision right eye category 2, blindness left eye category 5

● **H54.2**   **Low vision, both eyes**
Visual impairment categories 1 or 2 in both eyes.

   ● **H54.2X**   Low vision, both eyes, different category levels

     ● **H54.2X1**   Low vision, right eye, category 1

       H54.2X11   Low vision right eye category 1, low vision left eye category 1

       H54.2X12   Low vision right eye category 1, low vision left eye category 2

     ● **H54.2X2**   Low vision, right eye, category 2

       H54.2X21   Low vision right eye category 2, low vision left eye category 1

       H54.2X22   Low vision right eye category 2, low vision left eye category 2

  H54.3   **Unqualified visual loss, both eyes**
Visual impairment category 9 in both eyes.

● **H54.4**   **Blindness, one eye**
Visual impairment categories 3, 4, 5 in one eye [normal vision in other eye]

   H54.40   Blindness, one eye, unspecified eye

● **H54.41**   Blindness, right eye, normal vision left eye

   ● **H54.413**   Blindness, right eye, category 3

     H54.413A   Blindness right eye category 3, normal vision left eye

   ● **H54.414**   Blindness, right eye, category 4

     H54.414A   Blindness right eye category 4, normal vision left eye

   ● **H54.415**   Blindness, right eye, category 5

     H54.415A   Blindness right eye category 5, normal vision left eye

● **H54.42**   Blindness, left eye, normal vision right eye

   ● **H54.42A**   Blindness, left eye, category 3-5

     H54.42A3   Blindness left eye category 3, normal vision right eye

     H54.42A4   Blindness left eye category 4, normal vision right eye

     H54.42A5   Blindness left eye category 5, normal vision right eye

● **H54.5**   **Low vision, one eye**
Visual impairment categories 1 or 2 in one eye [normal vision in other eye].

   H54.50   Low vision, one eye, unspecified eye

● **H54.51**   Low vision, right eye, normal vision left eye

   ● **H54.511**   Low vision, right eye, category 1

     H54.511A   Low vision right eye category 1, normal vision left eye

   ● **H54.512**   Low vision, right eye, category 2

     H54.512A   Low vision right eye category 2, normal vision left eye

● **H54.52**   Low vision, left eye, normal vision right eye

   ● **H54.52A**   Low vision, left eye, category 1-2

     H54.52A1   Low vision left eye category 1, normal vision right eye

     H54.52A2   Low vision left eye category 2, normal vision right eye

● **H54.6**   **Unqualified visual loss, one eye**
Visual impairment category 9 in one eye [normal vision in other eye].

   H54.60   Unqualified visual loss, one eye, unspecified

   H54.61   Unqualified visual loss, right eye, normal vision left eye

   H54.62   Unqualified visual loss, left eye, normal vision right eye

OGCR Section I.C.7.b.

Blindness
If "blindness" or "low vision" of both eyes is documented but the visual impairment category is not documented, assign code H54.3, Unqualified visual loss, both eyes. If "blindness" or "low vision" in one eye is documented but the visual impairment category is not documented, assign a code from H54.6-, Unqualified visual loss, one eye. If "blindness" or "visual loss" is documented without any information about whether one or both eyes are affected, assign code H54.7, Unspecified visual loss.

H54.7 Unspecified visual loss
Visual impairment category 9 NOS

H54.8 Legal blindness, as defined in USA
Blindness NOS according to USA definition
Excludes1 legal blindness with specification of impairment level (H54.0-H54.7)

Note: The table below gives a classification of severity of visual impairment recommended by a WHO Study Group on the Prevention of Blindness, Geneva, 6-10 November 1972.

The term "low vision" in category H54 comprises categories 1 and 2 of the table, the term "blindness" categories 3, 4, and 5, and the term "unqualified visual loss" category 9.

If the extent of the visual field is taken into account, patients with a field no greater than 10 but greater than 5 around central fixation should be placed in category 3 and patients with a field no greater than 5 around central fixation should be placed in category 4, even if the central acuity is not impaired.

(Document 508 compliance requires all cells in the following table to be filled.)

Category of visual impairment	Visual acuity with best possible correction	
	Maximum less than:	Minimum equal to or better than:
—	6/18	6/60
3/10 (0.3)	1/10 (0.1)	—
20/70	20/200	—
—	6/60	3/60
1/10 (0.1)	1/20 (0.05)	—
20/200	20/400	—
—	3/60	1/60 (finger counting at one meter)
1/20 (0.05)	1/50 (0.02)	—
20/400	5/300 (20/1200)	—
—	1/60 (finger counting at one meter)	Light perception
1/50 (0.02)	—	—
5/300	—	—
—	No light perception	—
—	Undetermined or unspecified	—

OTHER DISORDERS OF EYE AND ADNEXA (H55–H57)

H55 Nystagmus and other irregular eye movements
H55.0 Nystagmus
Rapid, involuntary movements of the eyes in the horizontal or vertical direction
H55.00 Unspecified nystagmus
H55.01 Congenital nystagmus
H55.02 Latent nystagmus
H55.03 Visual deprivation nystagmus
H55.04 Dissociated nystagmus
H55.09 Other forms of nystagmus
H55.8 Other irregular eye movements
H55.81 Deficient saccadic eye movements
H55.82 Deficient smooth pursuit eye movements
H55.89 Other irregular eye movements

H57 Other disorders of eye and adnexa
H57.0 Anomalies of pupillary function
H57.00 Unspecified anomaly of pupillary function
H57.01 Argyll Robertson pupil, atypical
Excludes1 syphilitic Argyll Robertson pupil (A52.19)
H57.02 Anisocoria
H57.03 Miosis
H57.04 Mydriasis
H57.05 Tonic pupil
H57.051 Tonic pupil, right eye
H57.052 Tonic pupil, left eye
H57.053 Tonic pupil, bilateral
H57.059 Tonic pupil, unspecified eye
H57.09 Other anomalies of pupillary function
H57.1 Ocular pain
H57.10 Ocular pain, unspecified eye
H57.11 Ocular pain, right eye
H57.12 Ocular pain, left eye
H57.13 Ocular pain, bilateral
H57.8 Other specified disorders of eye and adnexa
H57.81 Brow ptosis
H57.811 Brow ptosis, right
H57.812 Brow ptosis, left
H57.813 Brow ptosis, bilateral
H57.819 Brow ptosis, unspecified
H57.89 Other specified disorders of eye and adnexa
H57.8A Foreign body sensation eye (ocular)
H57.8A1 Foreign body sensation, right eye
H57.8A2 Foreign body sensation, left eye
H57.8A3 Foreign body sensation, bilateral eyes
H57.8A9 Foreign body sensation, unspecified eye
H57.9 Unspecified disorder of eye and adnexa

INTRAOPERATIVE AND POSTPROCEDURAL COMPLICATIONS AND DISORDERS OF EYE AND ADNEXA, NOT ELSEWHERE CLASSIFIED (H59)

H59 Intraoperative and postprocedural complications and disorders of eye and adnexa, not elsewhere classified
Excludes1 mechanical complication of intraocular lens (T85.2)
mechanical complication of other ocular prosthetic devices, implants and grafts (T85.3)
pseudophakia (Z96.1)
secondary cataracts (H26.4-)

▶ New   ⇒ Revised   ~~deleted~~ Deleted   Excludes 1   Excludes 2   Includes   Use additional   Code first   Code also   Key words
OGCR Official Guidelines   X Assign placeholder X   ● Use Additional Character(s)   ▷ Manifestation Code   Hierarchical Condition Category   Coding Clinic

● H59.0   Disorders of the eye following cataract surgery

  ● H59.01   Keratopathy (bullous aphakic) following cataract surgery
        Vitreal corneal syndrome
        Vitreous (touch) syndrome

     H59.011   Keratopathy (bullous aphakic) following cataract surgery, right eye

     H59.012   Keratopathy (bullous aphakic) following cataract surgery, left eye

     H59.013   Keratopathy (bullous aphakic) following cataract surgery, bilateral

     H59.019   Keratopathy (bullous aphakic) following cataract surgery, unspecified eye

  ● H59.02   Cataract (lens) fragments in eye following cataract surgery

     H59.021   Cataract (lens) fragments in eye following cataract surgery, right eye

     H59.022   Cataract (lens) fragments in eye following cataract surgery, left eye

     H59.023   Cataract (lens) fragments in eye following cataract surgery, bilateral

     H59.029   Cataract (lens) fragments in eye following cataract surgery, unspecified eye

  ● H59.03   Cystoid macular edema following cataract surgery

     H59.031   Cystoid macular edema following cataract surgery, right eye

     H59.032   Cystoid macular edema following cataract surgery, left eye

     H59.033   Cystoid macular edema following cataract surgery, bilateral

     H59.039   Cystoid macular edema following cataract surgery, unspecified eye

  ● H59.09   Other disorders of the eye following cataract surgery

     H59.091   Other disorders of the right eye following cataract surgery

     H59.092   Other disorders of the left eye following cataract surgery

     H59.093   Other disorders of the eye following cataract surgery, bilateral

     H59.099   Other disorders of unspecified eye following cataract surgery

● H59.1   Intraoperative hemorrhage and hematoma of eye and adnexa complicating a procedure

     Excludes1   intraoperative hemorrhage and hematoma of eye and adnexa due to accidental puncture or laceration during a procedure (H59.2-)

  ● H59.11   Intraoperative hemorrhage and hematoma of eye and adnexa complicating an ophthalmic procedure

     H59.111   Intraoperative hemorrhage and hematoma of right eye and adnexa complicating an ophthalmic procedure

     H59.112   Intraoperative hemorrhage and hematoma of left eye and adnexa complicating an ophthalmic procedure

     H59.113   Intraoperative hemorrhage and hematoma of eye and adnexa complicating an ophthalmic procedure, bilateral

     H59.119   Intraoperative hemorrhage and hematoma of unspecified eye and adnexa complicating an ophthalmic procedure

  ● H59.12   Intraoperative hemorrhage and hematoma of eye and adnexa complicating other procedure

     H59.121   Intraoperative hemorrhage and hematoma of right eye and adnexa complicating other procedure

     H59.122   Intraoperative hemorrhage and hematoma of left eye and adnexa complicating other procedure

     H59.123   Intraoperative hemorrhage and hematoma of eye and adnexa complicating other procedure, bilateral

     H59.129   Intraoperative hemorrhage and hematoma of unspecified eye and adnexa complicating other procedure

● H59.2   Accidental puncture and laceration of eye and adnexa during a procedure

  ● H59.21   Accidental puncture and laceration of eye and adnexa during an ophthalmic procedure

     H59.211   Accidental puncture and laceration of right eye and adnexa during an ophthalmic procedure

     H59.212   Accidental puncture and laceration of left eye and adnexa during an ophthalmic procedure

     H59.213   Accidental puncture and laceration of eye and adnexa during an ophthalmic procedure, bilateral

     H59.219   Accidental puncture and laceration of unspecified eye and adnexa during an ophthalmic procedure

  ● H59.22   Accidental puncture and laceration of eye and adnexa during other procedure

     H59.221   Accidental puncture and laceration of right eye and adnexa during other procedure

     H59.222   Accidental puncture and laceration of left eye and adnexa during other procedure

     H59.223   Accidental puncture and laceration of eye and adnexa during other procedure, bilateral

     H59.229   Accidental puncture and laceration of unspecified eye and adnexa during other procedure

● H59.3   Postprocedural hemorrhage, hematoma, and seroma of eye and adnexa following other procedure
     Coding Clinic: 2016, Q4, P10

  ● H59.31   Postprocedural hemorrhage of eye and adnexa following an ophthalmic procedure

     H59.311   Postprocedural hemorrhage of right eye and adnexa following an ophthalmic procedure

     H59.312   Postprocedural hemorrhage of left eye and adnexa following an ophthalmic procedure

     H59.313   Postprocedural hemorrhage of eye and adnexa following an ophthalmic procedure, bilateral

     H59.319   Postprocedural hemorrhage of unspecified eye and adnexa following an ophthalmic procedure

  ● H59.32   Postprocedural hemorrhage of eye and adnexa following other procedure

     H59.321   Postprocedural hemorrhage of right eye and adnexa following other procedure

     H59.322   Postprocedural hemorrhage of left eye and adnexa following other procedure

H59.323   Postprocedural hemorrhage of eye and adnexa following other procedure, bilateral

H59.329   Postprocedural hemorrhage of unspecified eye and adnexa following other procedure

● H59.33   Postprocedural hematoma of eye and adnexa following an ophthalmic procedure

H59.331   Postprocedural hematoma of right eye and adnexa following an ophthalmic procedure

H59.332   Postprocedural hematoma of left eye and adnexa following an ophthalmic procedure

H59.333   Postprocedural hematoma of eye and adnexa following an ophthalmic procedure, bilateral

H59.339   Postprocedural hematoma of unspecified eye and adnexa following an ophthalmic procedure

● H59.34   Postprocedural hematoma of eye and adnexa following other procedure

H59.341   Postprocedural hematoma of right eye and adnexa following other procedure

H59.342   Postprocedural hematoma of left eye and adnexa following other procedure

H59.343   Postprocedural hematoma of eye and adnexa following other procedure, bilateral

H59.349   Postprocedural hematoma of unspecified eye and adnexa following other procedure

● H59.35   Postprocedural seroma of eye and adnexa following an ophthalmic procedure

H59.351   Postprocedural seroma of right eye and adnexa following an ophthalmic procedure

H59.352   Postprocedural seroma of left eye and adnexa following an ophthalmic procedure

H59.353   Postprocedural seroma of eye and adnexa following an ophthalmic procedure, bilateral

H59.359   Postprocedural seroma of unspecified eye and adnexa following an ophthalmic procedure

● H59.36   Postprocedural seroma of eye and adnexa following other procedure

H59.361   Postprocedural seroma of right eye and adnexa following other procedure

H59.362   Postprocedural seroma of left eye and adnexa following other procedure

H59.363   Postprocedural seroma of eye and adnexa following other procedure, bilateral

H59.369   Postprocedural seroma of unspecified eye and adnexa following other procedure

● H59.4   Inflammation (infection) of postprocedural bleb
Postprocedural blebitis

Excludes1   filtering (vitreous) bleb after glaucoma surgery status (Z98.83)

H59.40   Inflammation (infection) of postprocedural bleb, unspecified

H59.41   Inflammation (infection) of postprocedural bleb, stage 1

H59.42   Inflammation (infection) of postprocedural bleb, stage 2

H59.43   Inflammation (infection) of postprocedural bleb, stage 3
Bleb endophthalmitis

● H59.8   Other intraoperative and postprocedural complications and disorders of eye and adnexa, not elsewhere classified

● H59.81   Chorioretinal scars after surgery for detachment

H59.811   Chorioretinal scars after surgery for detachment, right eye

H59.812   Chorioretinal scars after surgery for detachment, left eye

H59.813   Chorioretinal scars after surgery for detachment, bilateral

H59.819   Chorioretinal scars after surgery for detachment, unspecified eye

H59.88   Other intraoperative complications of eye and adnexa, not elsewhere classified

H59.89   Other postprocedural complications and disorders of eye and adnexa, not elsewhere classified

▶ New   ⇒ Revised   ~~deleted~~ Deleted   Excludes 1   Excludes 2   Includes   Use additional   Code first   Code also   Key words
OGCR Official Guidelines   X Assign placeholder X   ● Use Additional Character(s)   ▶ Manifestation Code   🐾 Hierarchical Condition Category   Coding Clinic

CHAPTER 8

DISEASES OF THE EAR AND MASTOID PROCESS (H60-H95)

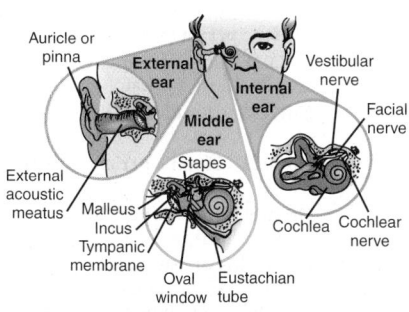

Figure 8-1 Auditory system. (From Buck CJ: Step-by-Step Medical Coding, ed 2016, St. Louis, Elsevier, 2016)

★**(See Plate 20 of the Anatomy Illustrations.)**

CHAPTER 8

DISEASES OF THE EAR AND MASTOID PROCESS (H60-H95)

Note: Use an external cause code following the code for the ear condition, if applicable, to identify the cause of the ear condition

Excludes2   certain conditions originating in the perinatal period (P04-P96)
certain infectious and parasitic diseases (A00-B99)
complications of pregnancy, childbirth and the puerperium (O00-O9A)
congenital malformations, deformations and chromosomal abnormalities (Q00-Q99)
endocrine, nutritional and metabolic diseases (E00-E88)
injury, poisoning and certain other consequences of external causes (S00-T88)
neoplasms (C00-D49)
symptoms, signs and abnormal clinical and laboratory findings, not elsewhere classified (R00-R94)

This chapter contains the following blocks:

H60-H62	Diseases of external ear
H65-H75	Diseases of middle ear and mastoid
H80-H83	Diseases of inner ear
H90-H94	Other disorders of ear
H95	Intraoperative and postprocedural complications and disorders of ear and mastoid process, not elsewhere classified

DISEASES OF EXTERNAL EAR (H60-H62)

● **H60**   Otitis externa
   ● **H60.0**   Abscess of external ear
     Boil of external ear
     Carbuncle of auricle or external auditory canal
     Furuncle of external ear
     H60.00   Abscess of external ear, unspecified ear
     H60.01   Abscess of right external ear
     H60.02   Abscess of left external ear
     H60.03   Abscess of external ear, bilateral

● **H60.1**   Cellulitis of external ear
     Cellulitis of auricle
     Cellulitis of external auditory canal
     H60.10   Cellulitis of external ear, unspecified ear
     H60.11   Cellulitis of right external ear
     H60.12   Cellulitis of left external ear
     H60.13   Cellulitis of external ear, bilateral
● **H60.2**   Malignant otitis externa
     H60.20   Malignant otitis externa, unspecified ear
     H60.21   Malignant otitis externa, right ear
     H60.22   Malignant otitis externa, left ear
     H60.23   Malignant otitis externa, bilateral
● **H60.3**   Other infective otitis externa
   ● **H60.31**   Diffuse otitis externa
     H60.311   Diffuse otitis externa, right ear
     H60.312   Diffuse otitis externa, left ear
     H60.313   Diffuse otitis externa, bilateral
     H60.319   Diffuse otitis externa, unspecified ear
   ● **H60.32**   Hemorrhagic otitis externa
     H60.321   Hemorrhagic otitis externa, right ear
     H60.322   Hemorrhagic otitis externa, left ear
     H60.323   Hemorrhagic otitis externa, bilateral
     H60.329   Hemorrhagic otitis externa, unspecified ear
   ● **H60.33**   Swimmer's ear
     H60.331   Swimmer's ear, right ear
     H60.332   Swimmer's ear, left ear
     H60.333   Swimmer's ear, bilateral
     H60.339   Swimmer's ear, unspecified ear
   ● **H60.39**   Other infective otitis externa
     H60.391   Other infective otitis externa, right ear
     H60.392   Other infective otitis externa, left ear
     H60.393   Other infective otitis externa, bilateral
     H60.399   Other infective otitis externa, unspecified ear
● **H60.4**   Cholesteatoma of external ear
     Keratosis obturans of external ear (canal)
     Excludes2   cholesteatoma of middle ear (H71.-)
      recurrent cholesteatoma of postmastoidectomy cavity (H95.0-)
     H60.40   Cholesteatoma of external ear, unspecified ear
     H60.41   Cholesteatoma of right external ear
     H60.42   Cholesteatoma of left external ear
     H60.43   Cholesteatoma of external ear, bilateral
● **H60.5**   Acute noninfective otitis externa
   ● **H60.50**   Unspecified acute noninfective otitis externa
     Acute otitis externa NOS
     H60.501   Unspecified acute noninfective otitis externa, right ear
     H60.502   Unspecified acute noninfective otitis externa, left ear
     H60.503   Unspecified acute noninfective otitis externa, bilateral
     H60.509   Unspecified acute noninfective otitis externa, unspecified ear
   ● **H60.51**   Acute actinic otitis externa
     H60.511   Acute actinic otitis externa, right ear
     H60.512   Acute actinic otitis externa, left ear
     H60.513   Acute actinic otitis externa, bilateral
     H60.519   Acute actinic otitis externa, unspecified ear

CHAPTER 8 (H60–H95)

- **H60.52** Acute chemical otitis externa
  - H60.521 Acute chemical otitis externa, right ear
  - H60.522 Acute chemical otitis externa, left ear
  - H60.523 Acute chemical otitis externa, bilateral
  - H60.529 Acute chemical otitis externa, unspecified ear
- **H60.53** Acute contact otitis externa
  - H60.531 Acute contact otitis externa, right ear
  - H60.532 Acute contact otitis externa, left ear
  - H60.533 Acute contact otitis externa, bilateral
  - H60.539 Acute contact otitis externa, unspecified ear
- **H60.54** Acute eczematoid otitis externa
  - H60.541 Acute eczematoid otitis externa, right ear
  - H60.542 Acute eczematoid otitis externa, left ear
  - H60.543 Acute eczematoid otitis externa, bilateral
  - H60.549 Acute eczematoid otitis externa, unspecified ear
- **H60.55** Acute reactive otitis externa
  - H60.551 Acute reactive otitis externa, right ear
  - H60.552 Acute reactive otitis externa, left ear
  - H60.553 Acute reactive otitis externa, bilateral
  - H60.559 Acute reactive otitis externa, unspecified ear
- **H60.59** Other noninfective acute otitis externa
  - H60.591 Other noninfective acute otitis externa, right ear
  - H60.592 Other noninfective acute otitis externa, left ear
  - H60.593 Other noninfective acute otitis externa, bilateral
  - H60.599 Other noninfective acute otitis externa, unspecified ear
- **H60.6** Unspecified chronic otitis externa
  - H60.60 Unspecified chronic otitis externa, unspecified ear
  - H60.61 Unspecified chronic otitis externa, right ear
  - H60.62 Unspecified chronic otitis externa, left ear
  - H60.63 Unspecified chronic otitis externa, bilateral
- **H60.8** Other otitis externa
  - **H60.8X** Other otitis externa
    - H60.8X1 Other otitis externa, right ear
    - H60.8X2 Other otitis externa, left ear
    - H60.8X3 Other otitis externa, bilateral
    - H60.8X9 Other otitis externa, unspecified ear
- **H60.9** Unspecified otitis externa
  - H60.90 Unspecified otitis externa, unspecified ear
  - H60.91 Unspecified otitis externa, right ear
  - H60.92 Unspecified otitis externa, left ear
  - H60.93 Unspecified otitis externa, bilateral
- **H61** Other disorders of external ear
  - **H61.0** Chondritis and perichondritis of external ear
    Chondrodermatitis nodularis chronica helicis
    Perichondritis of auricle
    Perichondritis of pinna
    - **H61.00** Unspecified perichondritis of external ear
      - H61.001 Unspecified perichondritis of right external ear
      - H61.002 Unspecified perichondritis of left external ear
      - H61.003 Unspecified perichondritis of external ear, bilateral
      - H61.009 Unspecified perichondritis of external ear, unspecified ear

- **H61.01** Acute perichondritis of external ear
  - H61.011 Acute perichondritis of right external ear
  - H61.012 Acute perichondritis of left external ear
  - H61.013 Acute perichondritis of external ear, bilateral
  - H61.019 Acute perichondritis of external ear, unspecified ear
- **H61.02** Chronic perichondritis of external ear
  - H61.021 Chronic perichondritis of right external ear
  - H61.022 Chronic perichondritis of left external ear
  - H61.023 Chronic perichondritis of external ear, bilateral
  - H61.029 Chronic perichondritis of external ear, unspecified ear
- **H61.03** Chondritis of external ear
  Chondritis of auricle
  Chondritis of pinna
  - H61.031 Chondritis of right external ear
  - H61.032 Chondritis of left external ear
    Coding Clinic: 2015, Q1, P18
  - H61.033 Chondritis of external ear, bilateral
  - H61.039 Chondritis of external ear, unspecified ear
- **H61.1** Noninfective disorders of pinna
  - **Excludes2** cauliflower ear (M95.1-)
    gouty tophi of ear (M1A.-)
  - **H61.10** Unspecified noninfective disorders of pinna
    Disorder of pinna NOS
    - H61.101 Unspecified noninfective disorders of pinna, right ear
    - H61.102 Unspecified noninfective disorders of pinna, left ear
    - H61.103 Unspecified noninfective disorders of pinna, bilateral
    - H61.109 Unspecified noninfective disorders of pinna, unspecified ear
  - **H61.11** Acquired deformity of pinna
    Acquired deformity of auricle
    - **Excludes2** cauliflower ear (M95.1-)
    - H61.111 Acquired deformity of pinna, right ear
    - H61.112 Acquired deformity of pinna, left ear
    - H61.113 Acquired deformity of pinna, bilateral
    - H61.119 Acquired deformity of pinna, unspecified ear
  - **H61.12** Hematoma of pinna
    Hematoma of auricle
    - H61.121 Hematoma of pinna, right ear
    - H61.122 Hematoma of pinna, left ear
    - H61.123 Hematoma of pinna, bilateral
    - H61.129 Hematoma of pinna, unspecified ear
  - **H61.19** Other noninfective disorders of pinna
    - H61.191 Noninfective disorders of pinna, right ear
    - H61.192 Noninfective disorders of pinna, left ear
    - H61.193 Noninfective disorders of pinna, bilateral
    - H61.199 Noninfective disorders of pinna, unspecified ear

▶ New   ⇒ Revised   ~~deleted~~ Deleted   Excludes 1   Excludes 2   Includes   Use additional   Code first   Code also   Key words
OGCR Official Guidelines   X Assign placeholder X   ● Use Additional Character(s)   ▶ Manifestation Code   🏷 Hierarchical Condition Category   Coding Clinic

● **H61.2 Impacted cerumen**
Wax in ear

   H61.20   Impacted cerumen, unspecified ear

   H61.21   Impacted cerumen, right ear

   H61.22   Impacted cerumen, left ear

   H61.23   Impacted cerumen, bilateral

● **H61.3 Acquired stenosis of external ear canal**
Collapse of external ear canal

   Excludes1   postprocedural stenosis of external ear canal (H95.81-)

  ● H61.30   **Acquired stenosis of external ear canal, unspecified**

     H61.301   Acquired stenosis of right external ear canal, unspecified

     H61.302   Acquired stenosis of left external ear canal, unspecified

     H61.303   Acquired stenosis of external ear canal, unspecified, bilateral

     H61.309   Acquired stenosis of external ear canal, unspecified, unspecified ear

  ● H61.31   **Acquired stenosis of external ear canal secondary to trauma**

     H61.311   Acquired stenosis of right external ear canal secondary to trauma

     H61.312   Acquired stenosis of left external ear canal secondary to trauma

     H61.313   Acquired stenosis of external ear canal secondary to trauma, bilateral

     H61.319   Acquired stenosis of external ear canal secondary to trauma, unspecified ear

  ● H61.32   **Acquired stenosis of external ear canal secondary to inflammation and infection**

     H61.321   Acquired stenosis of right external ear canal secondary to inflammation and infection

     H61.322   Acquired stenosis of left external ear canal secondary to inflammation and infection

     H61.323   Acquired stenosis of external ear canal secondary to inflammation and infection, bilateral

     H61.329   Acquired stenosis of external ear canal secondary to inflammation and infection, unspecified ear

  ● H61.39   **Other acquired stenosis of external ear canal**

     H61.391   Other acquired stenosis of right external ear canal

     H61.392   Other acquired stenosis of left external ear canal

     H61.393   Other acquired stenosis of external ear canal, bilateral

     H61.399   Other acquired stenosis of external ear canal, unspecified ear

● **H61.8 Other specified disorders of external ear**

  ● H61.81   **Exostosis of external canal**

     H61.811   Exostosis of right external canal

     H61.812   Exostosis of left external canal

     H61.813   Exostosis of external canal, bilateral

     H61.819   Exostosis of external canal, unspecified ear

  ● H61.89   **Other specified disorders of external ear**

     H61.891   Other specified disorders of right external ear

     H61.892   Other specified disorders of left external ear

     H61.893   Other specified disorders of external ear, bilateral

     H61.899   Other specified disorders of external ear, unspecified ear

● **H61.9 Disorder of external ear, unspecified**

   H61.90   Disorder of external ear, unspecified, unspecified ear

   H61.91   Disorder of right external ear, unspecified

   H61.92   Disorder of left external ear, unspecified

   H61.93   Disorder of external ear, unspecified, bilateral

● **H62 Disorders of external ear in diseases classified elsewhere**

  ● **H62.4 Otitis externa in other diseases classified elsewhere**

    Code first underlying disease, such as:
    erysipelas (A46)
    impetigo (L01.0-)

    Excludes1   otitis externa (in):
               candidiasis (B37.84)
               herpes viral [herpes simplex] (B00.1)
               herpes zoster (B02.8)

    H62.40   *Otitis externa in other diseases classified elsewhere, unspecified ear*

    H62.41   *Otitis externa in other diseases classified elsewhere, right ear*

    H62.42   *Otitis externa in other diseases classified elsewhere, left ear*

    H62.43   *Otitis externa in other diseases classified elsewhere, bilateral*

  ● **H62.8 Other disorders of external ear in diseases classified elsewhere**

    Code first underlying disease, such as:
    gout (M1A.-, M10.-)

   ● H62.8X   **Other disorders of external ear in diseases classified elsewhere**

     H62.8X1   *Other disorders of right external ear in diseases classified elsewhere*

     H62.8X2   *Other disorders of left external ear in diseases classified elsewhere*

     H62.8X3   *Other disorders of external ear in diseases classified elsewhere, bilateral*

     H62.8X9   *Other disorders of external ear in diseases classified elsewhere, unspecified ear*

DISEASES OF MIDDLE EAR AND MASTOID (H65-H75)

★ **(See Plate 21 of the Anatomy Illustrations.)**

● **H65 Nonsuppurative otitis media**
Bacterial or viral infection or inflammation of the middle ear; may result in fluid accumulation with pain and temporary hearing loss.

   Includes   nonsuppurative otitis media with myringitis

   Use additional code for any associated perforated tympanic membrane (H72.-)

   Use additional code to identify:
   exposure to environmental tobacco smoke (Z77.22)
   exposure to tobacco smoke in the perinatal period (P96.81)
   history of tobacco dependence (Z87.891)
   infectious agent (B95-B97)
   occupational exposure to environmental tobacco smoke (Z57.31)
   tobacco dependence (F17.-)
   tobacco use (Z72.0)

  ● **H65.0 Acute serous otitis media**
    Acute and subacute secretory otitis

   H65.00   Acute serous otitis media, unspecified ear

   H65.01   Acute serous otitis media, right ear

   H65.02   Acute serous otitis media, left ear

   H65.03   Acute serous otitis media, bilateral

   H65.04   Acute serous otitis media, recurrent, right ear

   H65.05   Acute serous otitis media, recurrent, left ear

   H65.06   Acute serous otitis media, recurrent, bilateral

   H65.07   Acute serous otitis media, recurrent, unspecified ear

● **H65.1**   **Other acute nonsuppurative otitis media**
> **Excludes1**   otitic barotrauma (T70.0)
>   otitis media (acute) NOS (H66.9)

  ● **H65.11**   **Acute and subacute allergic otitis media (mucoid) (sanguinous) (serous)**

      H65.111   Acute and subacute allergic otitis media (mucoid) (sanguinous) (serous), **right ear**

      H65.112   Acute and subacute allergic otitis media (mucoid) (sanguinous) (serous), **left ear**

      H65.113   Acute and subacute allergic otitis media (mucoid) (sanguinous) (serous), **bilateral**

      H65.114   Acute and subacute allergic otitis media (mucoid) (sanguinous) (serous), **recurrent, right ear**

      H65.115   Acute and subacute allergic otitis media (mucoid) (sanguinous) (serous), **recurrent, left ear**

      H65.116   Acute and subacute allergic otitis media (mucoid) (sanguinous) (serous), **recurrent, bilateral**

      H65.117   Acute and subacute allergic otitis media (mucoid) (sanguinous) (serous), **recurrent, unspecified ear**

      H65.119   Acute and subacute allergic otitis media (mucoid) (sanguinous) (serous), **unspecified ear**

  ● **H65.19**   **Other acute** nonsuppurative otitis media
> Acute and subacute mucoid otitis media
> Acute and subacute nonsuppurative otitis media NOS
> Acute and subacute sanguinous otitis media
> Acute and subacute seromucinous otitis media

      H65.191   Other acute nonsuppurative otitis media, **right ear**

      H65.192   Other acute nonsuppurative otitis media, **left ear**

      H65.193   Other acute nonsuppurative otitis media, **bilateral**

      H65.194   Other acute nonsuppurative otitis media, **recurrent, right ear**

      H65.195   Other acute nonsuppurative otitis media, **recurrent, left ear**

      H65.196   Other acute nonsuppurative otitis media, **recurrent, bilateral**

      H65.197   Other acute nonsuppurative otitis media **recurrent, unspecified ear**

      H65.199   Other acute nonsuppurative otitis media, **unspecified ear**

● **H65.2**   **Chronic serous otitis media**
> Chronic tubotympanal catarrh

  H65.20   **Chronic serous otitis media, unspecified ear**

  H65.21   **Chronic serous otitis media, right ear**

  H65.22   **Chronic serous otitis media, left ear**

  H65.23   **Chronic serous otitis media, bilateral**

● **H65.3**   **Chronic mucoid otitis media**
> Chronic mucinous otitis media
> Chronic secretory otitis media
> Chronic transudative otitis media
> Glue ear

> **Excludes1**   adhesive middle ear disease (H74.1)

  H65.30   **Chronic mucoid otitis media, unspecified ear**

  H65.31   **Chronic mucoid otitis media, right ear**

  H65.32   **Chronic mucoid otitis media, left ear**

  H65.33   **Chronic mucoid otitis media, bilateral**

● **H65.4**   **Other chronic nonsuppurative otitis media**

  ● **H65.41**   **Chronic allergic otitis media**

      H65.411   Chronic allergic otitis media, **right ear**

      H65.412   Chronic allergic otitis media, **left ear**

      H65.413   Chronic allergic otitis media, **bilateral**

      H65.419   Chronic allergic otitis media, **unspecified ear**

  ● **H65.49**   **Other chronic nonsuppurative otitis media**
> Chronic exudative otitis media
> Chronic nonsuppurative otitis media NOS
> Chronic otitis media with effusion (nonpurulent)
> Chronic seromucinous otitis media

      H65.491   Other chronic nonsuppurative otitis media, **right ear**

      H65.492   Other chronic nonsuppurative otitis media, **left ear**

      H65.493   Other chronic nonsuppurative otitis media, **bilateral**

      H65.499   Other chronic nonsuppurative otitis media, **unspecified ear**

● **H65.9**   **Unspecified nonsuppurative otitis media**
> Allergic otitis media NOS
> Catarrhal otitis media NOS
> Exudative otitis media NOS
> Mucoid otitis media NOS
> Otitis media with effusion (nonpurulent) NOS
> Secretory otitis media NOS
> Seromucinous otitis media NOS
> Serous otitis media NOS
> Transudative otitis media NOS

  H65.90   **Unspecified nonsuppurative otitis media, unspecified ear**

  H65.91   **Unspecified nonsuppurative otitis media, right ear**

  H65.92   **Unspecified nonsuppurative otitis media, left ear**

  H65.93   **Unspecified nonsuppurative otitis media, bilateral**

● **H66**   **Suppurative and unspecified otitis media**
> *Suppurative: Discharging pus*
> **Includes**   suppurative and unspecified otitis media with myringitis

> Use additional code to identify:
>   exposure to environmental tobacco smoke (Z77.22)
>   exposure to tobacco smoke in the perinatal period (P96.81)
>   history of tobacco dependence (Z87.891)
>   occupational exposure to environmental tobacco smoke (Z57.31)
>   tobacco dependence (F17.-)
>   tobacco use (Z72.0)

  ● **H66.0**   **Acute suppurative otitis media**

    ● **H66.00**   **Acute suppurative otitis media without spontaneous rupture of ear drum**

      H66.001   Acute suppurative otitis media without spontaneous rupture of ear drum, **right ear**
>   Coding Clinic: 2016, Q1, P34

      H66.002   Acute suppurative otitis media without spontaneous rupture of ear drum, **left ear**

      H66.003   Acute suppurative otitis media without spontaneous rupture of ear drum, **bilateral**

      H66.004   Acute suppurative otitis media without spontaneous rupture of ear drum, **recurrent, right ear**

      H66.005   Acute suppurative otitis media without spontaneous rupture of ear drum, **recurrent, left ear**

      H66.006   Acute suppurative otitis media without spontaneous rupture of ear drum, **recurrent, bilateral**

      H66.007   Acute suppurative otitis media without spontaneous rupture of ear drum, **recurrent, unspecified ear**

      H66.009   Acute suppurative otitis media without spontaneous rupture of ear drum, **unspecified ear**

- **H66.01** Acute suppurative otitis media with spontaneous rupture of ear drum
  - H66.011 Acute suppurative otitis media with spontaneous rupture of ear drum, right ear
  - H66.012 Acute suppurative otitis media with spontaneous rupture of ear drum, left ear
  - H66.013 Acute suppurative otitis media with spontaneous rupture of ear drum, bilateral
  - H66.014 Acute suppurative otitis media with spontaneous rupture of ear drum, recurrent, right ear
  - H66.015 Acute suppurative otitis media with spontaneous rupture of ear drum, recurrent, left ear
  - H66.016 Acute suppurative otitis media with spontaneous rupture of ear drum, recurrent, bilateral
  - H66.017 Acute suppurative otitis media with spontaneous rupture of ear drum, recurrent, unspecified ear
  - H66.019 Acute suppurative otitis media with spontaneous rupture of ear drum, unspecified ear
- **H66.1** Chronic tubotympanic suppurative otitis media
  Benign chronic suppurative otitis media
  Chronic tubotympanic disease
  Use additional code for any associated perforated tympanic membrane (H72.-)
  - H66.10 Chronic tubotympanic suppurative otitis media, unspecified
  - H66.11 Chronic tubotympanic suppurative otitis media, right ear
  - H66.12 Chronic tubotympanic suppurative otitis media, left ear
  - H66.13 Chronic tubotympanic suppurative otitis media, bilateral
- **H66.2** Chronic atticoantral suppurative otitis media
  Chronic atticoantral disease
  Use additional code for any associated perforated tympanic membrane (H72.-)
  - H66.20 Chronic atticoantral suppurative otitis media, unspecified ear
  - H66.21 Chronic atticoantral suppurative otitis media, right ear
  - H66.22 Chronic atticoantral suppurative otitis media, left ear
  - H66.23 Chronic atticoantral suppurative otitis media, bilateral
- **H66.3** Other chronic suppurative otitis media
  Chronic suppurative otitis media NOS
  Use additional code for any associated perforated tympanic membrane (H72.-)
  Excludes1 tuberculous otitis media (A18.6)
- **H66.3X** Other chronic suppurative otitis media
  - H66.3X1 Other chronic suppurative otitis media, right ear
  - H66.3X2 Other chronic suppurative otitis media, left ear
  - H66.3X3 Other chronic suppurative otitis media, bilateral
  - H66.3X9 Other chronic suppurative otitis media, unspecified ear

- **H66.4** Suppurative otitis media, unspecified
  Purulent otitis media NOS
  Use additional code for any associated perforated tympanic membrane (H72.-)
  - H66.40 Suppurative otitis media, unspecified, unspecified ear
  - H66.41 Suppurative otitis media, unspecified, right ear
  - H66.42 Suppurative otitis media, unspecified, left ear
  - H66.43 Suppurative otitis media, unspecified, bilateral
- **H66.9** Otitis media, unspecified
  Otitis media NOS
  Acute otitis media NOS
  Chronic otitis media NOS
  Use additional code for any associated perforated tympanic membrane (H72.-)
  - H66.90 Otitis media, unspecified, unspecified ear
  - H66.91 Otitis media, unspecified, right ear
  - H66.92 Otitis media, unspecified, left ear
  - H66.93 Otitis media, unspecified, bilateral
- **H67** Otitis media in diseases classified elsewhere
  Code first underlying disease, such as:
  plasminogen deficiency (E88.02)
  viral disease NEC (B00-B34)
  Use additional code for any associated perforated tympanic membrane (H72.-)
  Excludes1 otitis media in:
  influenza (J09.X9, J10.83, J11.83)
  measles (B05.3)
  scarlet fever (A38.0)
  tuberculosis (A18.6)
  - *H67.1* Otitis media in diseases classified elsewhere, right ear
  - *H67.2* Otitis media in diseases classified elsewhere, left ear
  - *H67.3* Otitis media in diseases classified elsewhere, bilateral
  - *H67.9* Otitis media in diseases classified elsewhere, unspecified ear
- **H68** Eustachian salpingitis and obstruction
  - **H68.0** Eustachian salpingitis
    - **H68.00** Unspecified Eustachian salpingitis
      - H68.001 Unspecified Eustachian salpingitis, right ear
      - H68.002 Unspecified Eustachian salpingitis, left ear
      - H68.003 Unspecified Eustachian salpingitis, bilateral
      - H68.009 Unspecified Eustachian salpingitis, unspecified ear
    - **H68.01** Acute Eustachian salpingitis
      - H68.011 Acute Eustachian salpingitis, right ear
      - H68.012 Acute Eustachian salpingitis, left ear
      - H68.013 Acute Eustachian salpingitis, bilateral
      - H68.019 Acute Eustachian salpingitis, unspecified ear
    - **H68.02** Chronic Eustachian salpingitis
      - H68.021 Chronic Eustachian salpingitis, right ear
      - H68.022 Chronic Eustachian salpingitis, left ear
      - H68.023 Chronic Eustachian salpingitis, bilateral
      - H68.029 Chronic Eustachian salpingitis, unspecified ear

CHAPTER 8 (H60-H95)

CHAPTER 8 (H60-H95)

- **H68.1   Obstruction of Eustachian tube**
  Stenosis of Eustachian tube
  Stricture of Eustachian tube
  - **H68.10   Unspecified obstruction of Eustachian tube**
    - H68.101   Unspecified obstruction of Eustachian tube, right ear
    - H68.102   Unspecified obstruction of Eustachian tube, left ear
    - H68.103   Unspecified obstruction of Eustachian tube, bilateral
    - H68.109   Unspecified obstruction of Eustachian tube, unspecified ear
  - **H68.11   Osseous obstruction of Eustachian tube**
    - H68.111   Osseous obstruction of Eustachian tube, right ear
    - H68.112   Osseous obstruction of Eustachian tube, left ear
    - H68.113   Osseous obstruction of Eustachian tube, bilateral
    - H68.119   Osseous obstruction of Eustachian tube, unspecified ear
  - **H68.12   Intrinsic cartilagenous obstruction of Eustachian tube**
    - H68.121   Intrinsic cartilagenous obstruction of Eustachian tube, right ear
    - H68.122   Intrinsic cartilagenous obstruction of Eustachian tube, left ear
    - H68.123   Intrinsic cartilagenous obstruction of Eustachian tube, bilateral
    - H68.129   Intrinsic cartilagenous obstruction of Eustachian tube, unspecified ear
  - **H68.13   Extrinsic cartilagenous obstruction of Eustachian tube**
    Compression of Eustachian tube
    - H68.131   Extrinsic cartilagenous obstruction of Eustachian tube, right ear
    - H68.132   Extrinsic cartilagenous obstruction of Eustachian tube, left ear
    - H68.133   Extrinsic cartilagenous obstruction of Eustachian tube, bilateral
    - H68.139   Extrinsic cartilagenous obstruction of Eustachian tube, unspecified ear
- **H69   Other and unspecified disorders of Eustachian tube**
  - **H69.0   Patulous Eustachian tube**
    - H69.00   Patulous Eustachian tube, unspecified ear
    - H69.01   Patulous Eustachian tube, right ear
    - H69.02   Patulous Eustachian tube, left ear
    - H69.03   Patulous Eustachian tube, bilateral
  - **H69.8   Other specified disorders of Eustachian tube**
    - H69.80   Other specified disorders of Eustachian tube, unspecified ear
    - H69.81   Other specified disorders of Eustachian tube, right ear
    - H69.82   Other specified disorders of Eustachian tube, left ear
    - H69.83   Other specified disorders of Eustachian tube, bilateral
  - **H69.9   Unspecified Eustachian tube disorder**
    - H69.90   Unspecified Eustachian tube disorder, unspecified ear
    - H69.91   Unspecified Eustachian tube disorder, right ear
    - H69.92   Unspecified Eustachian tube disorder, left ear
    - H69.93   Unspecified Eustachian tube disorder, bilateral

- **H70   Mastoiditis and related conditions**
  - **H70.0   Acute mastoiditis**
    Abscess of mastoid
    Empyema of mastoid
    - **H70.00   Acute mastoiditis without complications**
      - H70.001   Acute mastoiditis without complications, right ear
      - H70.002   Acute mastoiditis without complications, left ear
      - H70.003   Acute mastoiditis without complications, bilateral
      - H70.009   Acute mastoiditis without complications, unspecified ear
    - **H70.01   Subperiosteal abscess of mastoid**
      - H70.011   Subperiosteal abscess of mastoid, right ear
      - H70.012   Subperiosteal abscess of mastoid, left ear
      - H70.013   Subperiosteal abscess of mastoid, bilateral
      - H70.019   Subperiosteal abscess of mastoid, unspecified ear
    - **H70.09   Acute mastoiditis with other complications**
      - H70.091   Acute mastoiditis with other complications, right ear
      - H70.092   Acute mastoiditis with other complications, left ear
      - H70.093   Acute mastoiditis with other complications, bilateral
      - H70.099   Acute mastoiditis with other complications, unspecified ear
  - **H70.1   Chronic mastoiditis**
    Caries of mastoid
    Fistula of mastoid
    > **Excludes1**   tuberculous mastoiditis (A18.03)
    - H70.10   Chronic mastoiditis, unspecified ear
    - H70.11   Chronic mastoiditis, right ear
    - H70.12   Chronic mastoiditis, left ear
    - H70.13   Chronic mastoiditis, bilateral
  - **H70.2   Petrositis**
    Inflammation of petrous bone
    - **H70.20   Unspecified petrositis**
      - H70.201   Unspecified petrositis, right ear
      - H70.202   Unspecified petrositis, left ear
      - H70.203   Unspecified petrositis, bilateral
      - H70.209   Unspecified petrositis, unspecified ear
    - **H70.21   Acute petrositis**
      - H70.211   Acute petrositis, right ear
      - H70.212   Acute petrositis, left ear
      - H70.213   Acute petrositis, bilateral
      - H70.219   Acute petrositis, unspecified ear
    - **H70.22   Chronic petrositis**
      - H70.221   Chronic petrositis, right ear
      - H70.222   Chronic petrositis, left ear
      - H70.223   Chronic petrositis, bilateral
      - H70.229   Chronic petrositis, unspecified ear

Item 8-1   Mastoiditis is an infection of the portion of the temporal bone of the skull that is behind the ear (mastoid process) caused by an untreated otitis media, leading to an infection of the surrounding structures which may include the brain.

▶ New   ⇒ Revised   ~~deleted~~ Deleted   Excludes 1   Excludes 2   Includes   Use additional   Code first   Code also   Key words

824   OGCR Official Guidelines   X Assign placeholder X   ● Use Additional Character(s)   ▶ Manifestation Code   🗞 Hierarchical Condition Category   **Coding Clinic**

● H70.8 **Other mastoiditis and related conditions**
   Excludes1 preauricular sinus and cyst (Q18.1)
                  sinus, fistula, and cyst of branchial cleft
                  (Q18.0)
   ● H70.81 Postauricular fistula
      H70.811 Postauricular fistula, right ear
      H70.812 Postauricular fistula, left ear
      H70.813 Postauricular fistula, bilateral
      H70.819 Postauricular fistula, unspecified ear
   ● H70.89 Other mastoiditis and related conditions
      H70.891 Other mastoiditis and related
               conditions, right ear
      H70.892 Other mastoiditis and related
               conditions, left ear
      H70.893 Other mastoiditis and related
               conditions, bilateral
      H70.899 Other mastoiditis and related
               conditions, unspecified ear
● H70.9 **Unspecified mastoiditis**
   H70.90 Unspecified mastoiditis, unspecified ear
   H70.91 Unspecified mastoiditis, right ear
   H70.92 Unspecified mastoiditis, left ear
   H70.93 Unspecified mastoiditis, bilateral

● H71 **Cholesteatoma of middle ear**
   Excludes2 cholesteatoma of external ear (H60.4-)
                  recurrent cholesteatoma of postmastoidectomy
                  cavity (H95.0-)
● H71.0 **Cholesteatoma of attic**
   H71.00 Cholesteatoma of attic, unspecified ear
   H71.01 Cholesteatoma of attic, right ear
   H71.02 Cholesteatoma of attic, left ear
           Coding Clinic: 2021, Q3, P9
   H71.03 Cholesteatoma of attic, bilateral
● H71.1 **Cholesteatoma of tympanum**
   H71.10 Cholesteatoma of tympanum, unspecified ear
   H71.11 Cholesteatoma of tympanum, right ear
   H71.12 Cholesteatoma of tympanum, left ear
   H71.13 Cholesteatoma of tympanum, bilateral
● H71.2 **Cholesteatoma of mastoid**
   H71.20 Cholesteatoma of mastoid, unspecified ear
   H71.21 Cholesteatoma of mastoid, right ear
   H71.22 Cholesteatoma of mastoid, left ear
           Coding Clinic: 2021, Q3, P9
   H71.23 Cholesteatoma of mastoid, bilateral
● H71.3 **Diffuse cholesteatosis**
           Coding Clinic: 2021, Q3, P9
   H71.30 Diffuse cholesteatosis, unspecified ear
   H71.31 Diffuse cholesteatosis, right ear
   H71.32 Diffuse cholesteatosis, left ear
   H71.33 Diffuse cholesteatosis, bilateral
● H71.9 **Unspecified cholesteatoma**
   H71.90 Unspecified cholesteatoma, unspecified ear
   H71.91 Unspecified cholesteatoma, right ear
   H71.92 Unspecified cholesteatoma, left ear
   H71.93 Unspecified cholesteatoma, bilateral

★ **(See Plate 22 of the Anatomy Illustrations.)**

● H72 **Perforation of tympanic membrane**
   Hole or rupture in ear drum
   Includes persistent post-traumatic perforation of ear drum
                 postinflammatory perforation of ear drum
   Code first any associated otitis media (H65.-, H66.1-, H66.2-,
   H66.3-, H66.4-, H66.9-, H67.-)
   Excludes1 acute suppurative otitis media with rupture of
                  the tympanic membrane (H66.01-)
                  traumatic rupture of ear drum (S09.2-)
● H72.0 **Central perforation of tympanic membrane**
   H72.00 Central perforation of tympanic membrane,
           unspecified ear
   H72.01 Central perforation of tympanic membrane,
           right ear
   H72.02 Central perforation of tympanic membrane, left
           ear
   H72.03 Central perforation of tympanic membrane,
           bilateral
● H72.1 **Attic perforation of tympanic membrane**
   Perforation of pars flaccida
   H72.10 Attic perforation of tympanic membrane,
           unspecified ear
   H72.11 Attic perforation of tympanic membrane, right
           ear
   H72.12 Attic perforation of tympanic membrane, left
           ear
   H72.13 Attic perforation of tympanic membrane,
           bilateral
● H72.2 **Other marginal perforations of tympanic membrane**
   ● H72.2X Other marginal perforations of tympanic
             membrane
      H72.2X1 Other marginal perforations of
               tympanic membrane, right ear
      H72.2X2 Other marginal perforations of
               tympanic membrane, left ear
      H72.2X3 Other marginal perforations of
               tympanic membrane, bilateral
      H72.2X9 Other marginal perforations of
               tympanic membrane, unspecified ear
● H72.8 **Other perforations of tympanic membrane**
   ● H72.81 Multiple perforations of tympanic membrane
      H72.811 Multiple perforations of tympanic
               membrane, right ear
      H72.812 Multiple perforations of tympanic
               membrane, left ear
      H72.813 Multiple perforations of tympanic
               membrane, bilateral
      H72.819 Multiple perforations of tympanic
               membrane, unspecified ear
   ● H72.82 Total perforations of tympanic membrane
      H72.821 Total perforations of tympanic
               membrane, right ear
      H72.822 Total perforations of tympanic
               membrane, left ear
      H72.823 Total perforations of tympanic
               membrane, bilateral
      H72.829 Total perforations of tympanic
               membrane, unspecified ear
● H72.9 **Unspecified perforation of tympanic membrane**
   H72.90 Unspecified perforation of tympanic
           membrane, unspecified ear
   H72.91 Unspecified perforation of tympanic
           membrane, right ear
   H72.92 Unspecified perforation of tympanic
           membrane, left ear
   H72.93 Unspecified perforation of tympanic
           membrane, bilateral

CHAPTER 8 (H60-H95)

● H73   Other disorders of tympanic membrane
   ● H73.0   Acute myringitis
     Excludes1   acute myringitis with otitis media (H65, H66)
     ● H73.00   Unspecified acute myringitis
       Acute tympanitis NOS
       H73.001   Acute myringitis, right ear
       H73.002   Acute myringitis, left ear
       H73.003   Acute myringitis, bilateral
       H73.009   Acute myringitis, unspecified ear
     ● H73.01   Bullous myringitis
       H73.011   Bullous myringitis, right ear
       H73.012   Bullous myringitis, left ear
       H73.013   Bullous myringitis, bilateral
       H73.019   Bullous myringitis, unspecified ear
     ● H73.09   Other acute myringitis
       H73.091   Other acute myringitis, right ear
       H73.092   Other acute myringitis, left ear
       H73.093   Other acute myringitis, bilateral
       H73.099   Other acute myringitis, unspecified ear
   ● H73.1   Chronic myringitis
     Chronic tympanitis
     Excludes1   chronic myringitis with otitis media (H65, H66)
     H73.10   Chronic myringitis, unspecified ear
     H73.11   Chronic myringitis, right ear
     H73.12   Chronic myringitis, left ear
     H73.13   Chronic myringitis, bilateral
   ● H73.2   Unspecified myringitis
     H73.20   Unspecified myringitis, unspecified ear
     H73.21   Unspecified myringitis, right ear
     H73.22   Unspecified myringitis, left ear
     H73.23   Unspecified myringitis, bilateral
   ● H73.8   Other specified disorders of tympanic membrane
     ● H73.81   Atrophic flaccid tympanic membrane
       H73.811   Atrophic flaccid tympanic membrane, right ear
       H73.812   Atrophic flaccid tympanic membrane, left ear
       H73.813   Atrophic flaccid tympanic membrane, bilateral
       H73.819   Atrophic flaccid tympanic membrane, unspecified ear
     ● H73.82   Atrophic nonflaccid tympanic membrane
       H73.821   Atrophic nonflaccid tympanic membrane, right ear
       H73.822   Atrophic nonflaccid tympanic membrane, left ear
       H73.823   Atrophic nonflaccid tympanic membrane, bilateral
       H73.829   Atrophic nonflaccid tympanic membrane, unspecified ear
     ● H73.89   Other specified disorders of tympanic membrane
       H73.891   Other specified disorders of tympanic membrane, right ear
       H73.892   Other specified disorders of tympanic membrane, left ear
       H73.893   Other specified disorders of tympanic membrane, bilateral
       H73.899   Other specified disorders of tympanic membrane, unspecified ear

● H73.9   Unspecified disorder of tympanic membrane
   H73.90   Unspecified disorder of tympanic membrane, unspecified ear
   H73.91   Unspecified disorder of tympanic membrane, right ear
   H73.92   Unspecified disorder of tympanic membrane, left ear
   H73.93   Unspecified disorder of tympanic membrane, bilateral
● H74   Other disorders of middle ear mastoid
   Excludes2   mastoiditis (H70.-)
   ● H74.0   Tympanosclerosis
     H74.01   Tympanosclerosis, right ear
     H74.02   Tympanosclerosis, left ear
     H74.03   Tympanosclerosis, bilateral
     H74.09   Tympanosclerosis, unspecified ear
   ● H74.1   Adhesive middle ear disease
     Adhesive otitis
     Excludes1   glue ear (H65.3-)
     H74.11   Adhesive right middle ear disease
     H74.12   Adhesive left middle ear disease
     H74.13   Adhesive middle ear disease, bilateral
     H74.19   Adhesive middle ear disease, unspecified ear
   ● H74.2   Discontinuity and dislocation of ear ossicles
     H74.20   Discontinuity and dislocation of ear ossicles, unspecified ear
     H74.21   Discontinuity and dislocation of right ear ossicles
     H74.22   Discontinuity and dislocation of left ear ossicles
     H74.23   Discontinuity and dislocation of ear ossicles, bilateral
   ● H74.3   Other acquired abnormalities of ear ossicles
     ● H74.31   Ankylosis of ear ossicles
       H74.311   Ankylosis of ear ossicles, right ear
       H74.312   Ankylosis of ear ossicles, left ear
       H74.313   Ankylosis of ear ossicles, bilateral
       H74.319   Ankylosis of ear ossicles, unspecified ear
     ● H74.32   Partial loss of ear ossicles
       H74.321   Partial loss of ear ossicles, right ear
       H74.322   Partial loss of ear ossicles, left ear
       H74.323   Partial loss of ear ossicles, bilateral
       H74.329   Partial loss of ear ossicles, unspecified ear
     ● H74.39   Other acquired abnormalities of ear ossicles
       H74.391   Other acquired abnormalities of right ear ossicles
       H74.392   Other acquired abnormalities of left ear ossicles
       H74.393   Other acquired abnormalities of ear ossicles, bilateral
       H74.399   Other acquired abnormalities of ear ossicles, unspecified ear
   ● H74.4   Polyp of middle ear
     H74.40   Polyp of middle ear, unspecified ear
     H74.41   Polyp of right middle ear
     H74.42   Polyp of left middle ear
     H74.43   Polyp of middle ear, bilateral

▶ New   ⟹ Revised   ~~deleted~~ Deleted   Excludes 1   Excludes 2   Includes   Use additional   Code first   Code also   Key words
OGCR Official Guidelines   X Assign placeholder X   ● Use Additional Character(s)   ▶ Manifestation Code   🔖 Hierarchical Condition Category   Coding Clinic

● H74.8　Other specified disorders of middle ear and mastoid
　　● H74.8X　Other specified disorders of middle ear and mastoid
　　　　H74.8X1　Other specified disorders of right middle ear and mastoid
　　　　H74.8X2　Other specified disorders of left middle ear and mastoid
　　　　H74.8X3　Other specified disorders of middle ear and mastoid, bilateral
　　　　H74.8X9　Other specified disorders of middle ear and mastoid, unspecified ear
● H74.9　Unspecified disorder of middle ear and mastoid
　　H74.90　Unspecified disorder of middle ear and mastoid, unspecified ear
　　H74.91　Unspecified disorder of right middle ear and mastoid
　　H74.92　Unspecified disorder of left middle ear and mastoid
　　H74.93　Unspecified disorder of middle ear and mastoid, bilateral

● H75　Other disorders of middle ear and mastoid in diseases classified elsewhere
　　Code first underlying disease
● H75.0　Mastoiditis in infectious and parasitic diseases classified elsewhere
　　　Excludes1　mastoiditis (in):
　　　　　　　　　syphilis (A52.77)
　　　　　　　　　tuberculosis (A18.03)
　　▷ *H75.00　Mastoiditis in infectious and parasitic diseases classified elsewhere, unspecified ear*
　　▷ *H75.01　Mastoiditis in infectious and parasitic diseases classified elsewhere, right ear*
　　▷ *H75.02　Mastoiditis in infectious and parasitic diseases classified elsewhere, left ear*
　　▷ *H75.03　Mastoiditis in infectious and parasitic diseases classified elsewhere, bilateral*
● H75.8　Other specified disorders of middle ear and mastoid in diseases classified elsewhere
　　▷ *H75.80　Other specified disorders of middle ear and mastoid in diseases classified elsewhere, unspecified ear*
　　▷ *H75.81　Other specified disorders of right middle ear and mastoid in diseases classified elsewhere*
　　▷ *H75.82　Other specified disorders of left middle ear and mastoid in diseases classified elsewhere*
　　▷ *H75.83　Other specified disorders of middle ear and mastoid in diseases classified elsewhere, bilateral*

DISEASES OF INNER EAR (H80-H83)

★ **(See Plate 23 of the Anatomy Illustrations.)**

● H80　Otosclerosis
　　Inherited middle ear spongelike bone growth causing hearing loss
　　　Includes　Otospongiosis
● H80.0　Otosclerosis involving oval window, nonobliterative
　　H80.00　Otosclerosis involving oval window, nonobliterative, unspecified ear
　　H80.01　Otosclerosis involving oval window, nonobliterative, right ear
　　H80.02　Otosclerosis involving oval window, nonobliterative, left ear
　　H80.03　Otosclerosis involving oval window, nonobliterative, bilateral

● H80.1　Otosclerosis involving oval window, obliterative
　　H80.10　Otosclerosis involving oval window, obliterative, unspecified ear
　　H80.11　Otosclerosis involving oval window, obliterative, right ear
　　H80.12　Otosclerosis involving oval window, obliterative, left ear
　　H80.13　Otosclerosis involving oval window, obliterative, bilateral
● H80.2　Cochlear otosclerosis
　　　Otosclerosis involving otic capsule
　　　Otosclerosis involving round window
　　H80.20　Cochlear otosclerosis, unspecified ear
　　H80.21　Cochlear otosclerosis, right ear
　　H80.22　Cochlear otosclerosis, left ear
　　H80.23　Cochlear otosclerosis, bilateral
● H80.8　Other otosclerosis
　　H80.80　Other otosclerosis, unspecified ear
　　H80.81　Other otosclerosis, right ear
　　H80.82　Other otosclerosis, left ear
　　H80.83　Other otosclerosis, bilateral
● H80.9　Unspecified otosclerosis
　　H80.90　Unspecified otosclerosis, unspecified ear
　　H80.91　Unspecified otosclerosis, right ear
　　H80.92　Unspecified otosclerosis, left ear
　　H80.93　Unspecified otosclerosis, bilateral

● H81　Disorders of vestibular function
　　　Excludes1　epidemic vertigo (A88.1)
　　　　　　　　　vertigo NOS (R42)
● H81.0　Ménière's disease
　　　Vestibular disorder that produces recurring symptoms including severe and intermittent hearing loss including the feeling of ear pressure or pain
　　　Labyrinthine hydrops
　　　Ménière's syndrome or vertigo
　　H81.01　Ménière's disease, right ear
　　H81.02　Ménière's disease, left ear
　　H81.03　Ménière's disease, bilateral
　　H81.09　Ménière's disease, unspecified ear
● H81.1　Benign paroxysmal vertigo
　　H81.10　Benign paroxysmal vertigo, unspecified ear
　　H81.11　Benign paroxysmal vertigo, right ear
　　H81.12　Benign paroxysmal vertigo, left ear
　　H81.13　Benign paroxysmal vertigo, bilateral
● H81.2　Vestibular neuronitis
　　H81.20　Vestibular neuronitis, unspecified ear
　　H81.21　Vestibular neuronitis, right ear
　　H81.22　Vestibular neuronitis, left ear
　　H81.23　Vestibular neuronitis, bilateral
● H81.3　Other peripheral vertigo
　　● H81.31　Aural vertigo
　　　　H81.311　Aural vertigo, right ear
　　　　H81.312　Aural vertigo, left ear
　　　　H81.313　Aural vertigo, bilateral
　　　　H81.319　Aural vertigo, unspecified ear
　　● H81.39　Other peripheral vertigo
　　　　　Lermoyez' syndrome
　　　　　Otogenic vertigo
　　　　　Peripheral vertigo NOS
　　　　H81.391　Other peripheral vertigo, right ear
　　　　H81.392　Other peripheral vertigo, left ear
　　　　H81.393　Other peripheral vertigo, bilateral
　　　　H81.399　Other peripheral vertigo, unspecified ear
● H81.4　Vertigo of central origin
　　　Central positional nystagmus

● **H81.8   Other disorders of vestibular function**
  ● **H81.8X   Other disorders of vestibular function**
    H81.8X1   Other disorders of vestibular function, right ear
    H81.8X2   Other disorders of vestibular function, left ear
    H81.8X3   Other disorders of vestibular function, bilateral
    H81.8X9   Other disorders of vestibular function, unspecified ear
        Coding Clinic: 2022, Q2, P12

● **H81.9   Unspecified disorder of vestibular function**
    Vertiginous syndrome NOS
    H81.90   Unspecified disorder of vestibular function, unspecified ear
    H81.91   Unspecified disorder of vestibular function, right ear
    H81.92   Unspecified disorder of vestibular function, left ear
    H81.93   Unspecified disorder of vestibular function, bilateral

● **H82   Vertiginous syndromes in diseases classified elsewhere**
    Code first underlying disease
    Excludes1   epidemic vertigo (A88.1)
  ▷ *H82.1   Vertiginous syndromes in diseases classified elsewhere, right ear*
  ▷ *H82.2   Vertiginous syndromes in diseases classified elsewhere, left ear*
  ▷ *H82.3   Vertiginous syndromes in diseases classified elsewhere, bilateral*
  ▷ *H82.9   Vertiginous syndromes in diseases classified elsewhere, unspecified ear*

● **H83   Other diseases of inner ear**
  ● **H83.0   Labyrinthitis**
    Balance disorder that follows URI or head injury
    H83.01   Labyrinthitis, right ear
    H83.02   Labyrinthitis, left ear
    H83.03   Labyrinthitis, bilateral
    H83.09   Labyrinthitis, unspecified ear
  ● **H83.1   Labyrinthine fistula**
    H83.11   Labyrinthine fistula, right ear
    H83.12   Labyrinthine fistula, left ear
    H83.13   Labyrinthine fistula, bilateral
    H83.19   Labyrinthine fistula, unspecified ear
  ● **H83.2   Labyrinthine dysfunction**
    Labyrinthine hypersensitivity
    Labyrinthine hypofunction
    Labyrinthine loss of function
    ● **H83.2X   Labyrinthine dysfunction**
      H83.2X1   Labyrinthine dysfunction, right ear
      H83.2X2   Labyrinthine dysfunction, left ear
      H83.2X3   Labyrinthine dysfunction, bilateral
      H83.2X9   Labyrinthine dysfunction, unspecified ear
  ● **H83.3   Noise effects on inner ear**
    Acoustic trauma of inner ear
    Noise-induced hearing loss of inner ear
    ● **H83.3X   Noise effects on inner ear**
      H83.3X1   Noise effects on right inner ear
      H83.3X2   Noise effects on left inner ear
      H83.3X3   Noise effects on inner ear, bilateral
      H83.3X9   Noise effects on inner ear, unspecified ear

● **H83.8   Other specified diseases of inner ear**
  ● **H83.8X   Other specified diseases of inner ear**
    H83.8X1   Other specified diseases of right inner ear
    H83.8X2   Other specified diseases of left inner ear
    H83.8X3   Other specified diseases of inner ear, bilateral
    H83.8X9   Other specified diseases of inner ear, unspecified ear
● **H83.9   Unspecified disease of inner ear**
    H83.90   Unspecified disease of inner ear, unspecified ear
    H83.91   Unspecified disease of right inner ear
    H83.92   Unspecified disease of left inner ear
    H83.93   Unspecified disease of inner ear, bilateral

OTHER DISORDERS OF EAR (H90-H94)

● **H90   Conductive and sensorineural hearing loss**
    Excludes1   deaf nonspeaking NEC (H91.3)
        deafness NOS (H91.9-)
        hearing loss NOS (H91.9-)
        noise-induced hearing loss (H83.3-)
        ototoxic hearing loss (H91.0-)
        sudden (idiopathic) hearing loss (H91.2-)
  H90.0   Conductive hearing loss, bilateral
  ● **H90.1   Conductive hearing loss, unilateral with unrestricted hearing on the contralateral side**
    H90.11   Conductive hearing loss, unilateral, right ear, with unrestricted hearing on the contralateral side
    H90.12   Conductive hearing loss, unilateral, left ear, with unrestricted hearing on the contralateral side
  H90.2   Conductive hearing loss, unspecified
    Conductive deafness NOS
  H90.3   Sensorineural hearing loss, bilateral
  ● **H90.4   Sensorineural hearing loss, unilateral with unrestricted hearing on the contralateral side**
    H90.41   Sensorineural hearing loss, unilateral, right ear, with unrestricted hearing on the contralateral side
    H90.42   Sensorineural hearing loss, unilateral, left ear, with unrestricted hearing on the contralateral side
  H90.5   Unspecified sensorineural hearing loss
    Central hearing loss NOS
    Congenital deafness NOS
    Neural hearing loss NOS
    Perceptive hearing loss NOS
    Sensorineural deafness NOS
    Sensory hearing loss NOS
    Excludes1   abnormal auditory perception (H93.2-)
        psychogenic deafness (F44.6)
  H90.6   Mixed conductive and sensorineural hearing loss, bilateral
    Coding Clinic: 2015, Q2, P7
  ● **H90.7   Mixed conductive and sensorineural hearing loss, unilateral with unrestricted hearing on the contralateral side**
    H90.71   Mixed conductive and sensorineural hearing loss, unilateral, right ear, with unrestricted hearing on the contralateral side
    H90.72   Mixed conductive and sensorineural hearing loss, unilateral, left ear, with unrestricted hearing on the contralateral side
  H90.8   Mixed conductive and sensorineural hearing loss, unspecified

▶ New   ⇒ Revised   ~~deleted~~ Deleted   Excludes 1   Excludes 2   Includes   Use additional   Code first   Code also   Key words
OGCR Official Guidelines   X Assign placeholder X   ● Use Additional Character(s)   ▷ Manifestation Code   🔒 Hierarchical Condition Category   Coding Clinic

● **H90.A** Conductive and sensorineural hearing loss with restricted hearing on the contralateral side
Coding Clinic: 2016, Q4, P23-24

  ● **H90.A1** Conductive hearing loss, unilateral, with restricted hearing on the contralateral side

     H90.A11 Conductive hearing loss, unilateral, right ear with restricted hearing on the contralateral side

     H90.A12 Conductive hearing loss, unilateral, left ear with restricted hearing on the contralateral side
Coding Clinic: 2016, Q4, P25

  ● **H90.A2** Sensorineural hearing loss, unilateral, with restricted hearing on the contralateral side

     H90.A21 Sensorineural hearing loss, unilateral, right ear, with restricted hearing on the contralateral side

     H90.A22 Sensorineural hearing loss, unilateral, left ear, with restricted hearing on the contralateral side

  ● **H90.A3** Mixed conductive and sensorineural hearing loss, unilateral with restricted hearing on the contralateral side

     H90.A31 Mixed conductive and sensorineural hearing loss, unilateral, right ear with restricted hearing on the contralateral side

     H90.A32 Mixed conductive and sensorineural hearing loss, unilateral, left ear with restricted hearing on the contralateral side

● **H91** Other and unspecified hearing loss
     Excludes1   abnormal auditory perception (H93.2-)
                     hearing loss as classified in H90.-
                       impacted cerumen (H61.2-)
                       noise-induced hearing loss (H83.3-)
                       psychogenic deafness (F44.6)
                       transient ischemic deafness (H93.01-)

  ● **H91.0** Ototoxic hearing loss
     Code first poisoning due to drug or toxin, if applicable (T36-T65 with fifth or sixth character 1-4)
     Use additional code for adverse effect, if applicable, to identify drug (T36-T50 with fifth or sixth character 5)

     H91.01 Ototoxic hearing loss, right ear
     H91.02 Ototoxic hearing loss, left ear
     H91.03 Ototoxic hearing loss, bilateral
     H91.09 Ototoxic hearing loss, unspecified ear

  ● **H91.1** Presbycusis
     Presbyacusia
     H91.10 Presbycusis, unspecified ear
     H91.11 Presbycusis, right ear
     H91.12 Presbycusis, left ear
     H91.13 Presbycusis, bilateral

  ● **H91.2** Sudden idiopathic hearing loss
     Sudden hearing loss NOS
     H91.20 Sudden idiopathic hearing loss, unspecified ear
     H91.21 Sudden idiopathic hearing loss, right ear
     H91.22 Sudden idiopathic hearing loss, left ear
     H91.23 Sudden idiopathic hearing loss, bilateral

  H91.3 Deaf nonspeaking, not elsewhere classified

  ● **H91.8** Other specified hearing loss
    ● **H91.8X** Other specified hearing loss
       H91.8X1 Other specified hearing loss, right ear
       H91.8X2 Other specified hearing loss, left ear
       H91.8X3 Other specified hearing loss, bilateral
       H91.8X9 Other specified hearing loss, unspecified ear

● **H91.9** Unspecified hearing loss
     Deafness NOS
     High frequency deafness
     Low frequency deafness
   H91.90 Unspecified hearing loss, unspecified ear
   H91.91 Unspecified hearing loss, right ear
   H91.92 Unspecified hearing loss, left ear
   H91.93 Unspecified hearing loss, bilateral

● **H92** Otalgia and effusion of ear
  ● **H92.0** Otalgia
     H92.01 Otalgia, right ear
     H92.02 Otalgia, left ear
     H92.03 Otalgia, bilateral
     H92.09 Otalgia, unspecified ear

  ● **H92.1** Otorrhea
     Excludes1   leakage of cerebrospinal fluid through ear (G96.0)
     H92.10 Otorrhea, unspecified ear
     H92.11 Otorrhea, right ear
     H92.12 Otorrhea, left ear
     H92.13 Otorrhea, bilateral

  ● **H92.2** Otorrhagia
     Excludes1   traumatic otorrhagia - code to injury
     H92.20 Otorrhagia, unspecified ear
     H92.21 Otorrhagia, right ear
     H92.22 Otorrhagia, left ear
     H92.23 Otorrhagia, bilateral

● **H93** Other disorders of ear, not elsewhere classified
  ● **H93.0** Degenerative and vascular disorders of ear
     Excludes1   presbycusis (H91.1)
    ● **H93.01** Transient ischemic deafness
       H93.011 Transient ischemic deafness, right ear
       H93.012 Transient ischemic deafness, left ear
       H93.013 Transient ischemic deafness, bilateral
       H93.019 Transient ischemic deafness, unspecified ear

    ● **H93.09** Unspecified degenerative and vascular disorders of ear
       H93.091 Unspecified degenerative and vascular disorders of right ear
       H93.092 Unspecified degenerative and vascular disorders of left ear
       H93.093 Unspecified degenerative and vascular disorders of ear, bilateral
       H93.099 Unspecified degenerative and vascular disorders of unspecified ear

  ● **H93.1** Tinnitus
     Perception of sound (ringing, buzzing, humming, whistling tunes, or singing)
     H93.11 Tinnitus, right ear
     H93.12 Tinnitus, left ear
     H93.13 Tinnitus, bilateral
     H93.19 Tinnitus, unspecified ear

  ● **H93.A** Pulsatile tinnitus
     Coding Clinic: 2016, Q4, P25
     H93.A1 Pulsatile tinnitus, right ear
        Coding Clinic: 2023, Q2, P19; 2016, Q4, P26
     H93.A2 Pulsatile tinnitus, left ear
     H93.A3 Pulsatile tinnitus, bilateral
     H93.A9 Pulsatile tinnitus, unspecified ear

CHAPTER 8 (H60-H95)

● H93.2   Other abnormal auditory perceptions
　　　　Excludes2　auditory hallucinations (R44.0)
　　● H93.21　Auditory recruitment
　　　　　H93.211　Auditory recruitment, right ear
　　　　　H93.212　Auditory recruitment, left ear
　　　　　H93.213　Auditory recruitment, bilateral
　　　　　H93.219　Auditory recruitment, unspecified ear
　　● H93.22　Diplacusis
　　　　　H93.221　Diplacusis, right ear
　　　　　H93.222　Diplacusis, left ear
　　　　　H93.223　Diplacusis, bilateral
　　　　　H93.229　Diplacusis, unspecified ear
　　● H93.23　Hyperacusis
　　　　　H93.231　Hyperacusis, right ear
　　　　　H93.232　Hyperacusis, left ear
　　　　　H93.233　Hyperacusis, bilateral
　　　　　H93.239　Hyperacusis, unspecified ear
　　● H93.24　Temporary auditory threshold shift
　　　　　H93.241　Temporary auditory threshold shift, right ear
　　　　　H93.242　Temporary auditory threshold shift, left ear
　　　　　H93.243　Temporary auditory threshold shift, bilateral
　　　　　H93.249　Temporary auditory threshold shift, unspecified ear
　　　H93.25　Central auditory processing disorder
　　　　　Congenital auditory imperception
　　　　　Word deafness
　　　　　Excludes1　mixed receptive-expressive language disorder (F80.2)
　　● H93.29　Other abnormal auditory perceptions
　　　　　H93.291　Other abnormal auditory perceptions, right ear
　　　　　H93.292　Other abnormal auditory perceptions, left ear
　　　　　H93.293　Other abnormal auditory perceptions, bilateral
　　　　　H93.299　Other abnormal auditory perceptions, unspecified ear
● H93.3   Disorders of acoustic nerve
　　　Disorder of 8th cranial nerve
　　　Excludes1　acoustic neuroma (D33.3)
　　　　　　　　syphilitic acoustic neuritis (A52.15)
　　● H93.3X　Disorders of acoustic nerve
　　　　　H93.3X1　Disorders of right acoustic nerve
　　　　　H93.3X2　Disorders of left acoustic nerve
　　　　　H93.3X3　Disorders of bilateral acoustic nerves
　　　　　H93.3X9　Disorders of unspecified acoustic nerve
● H93.8   Other specified disorders of ear
　　● H93.8X　Other specified disorders of ear
　　　　　H93.8X1　Other specified disorders of right ear
　　　　　H93.8X2　Other specified disorders of left ear
　　　　　H93.8X3　Other specified disorders of ear, bilateral
　　　　　H93.8X9　Other specified disorders of ear, unspecified ear
● H93.9   Unspecified disorder of ear
　　　H93.90　Unspecified disorder of ear, unspecified ear
　　　H93.91　Unspecified disorder of right ear
　　　H93.92　Unspecified disorder of left ear
　　　H93.93　Unspecified disorder of ear, bilateral

● H94   Other disorders of ear in diseases classified elsewhere
　● H94.0　Acoustic neuritis in infectious and parasitic diseases classified elsewhere
　　　Code first underlying disease, such as:
　　　　parasitic disease (B65-B89)
　　　Excludes1　acoustic neuritis (in):
　　　　　　herpes zoster (B02.29)
　　　　　　syphilis (A52.15)
　　▷ *H94.00　Acoustic neuritis in infectious and parasitic diseases classified elsewhere, unspecified ear*
　　▷ *H94.01　Acoustic neuritis in infectious and parasitic diseases classified elsewhere, right ear*
　　▷ *H94.02　Acoustic neuritis in infectious and parasitic diseases classified elsewhere, left ear*
　　▷ *H94.03　Acoustic neuritis in infectious and parasitic diseases classified elsewhere, bilateral*
　● H94.8　Other specified disorders of ear in diseases classified elsewhere
　　　Code first underlying disease, such as:
　　　　congenital syphilis (A50.0)
　　　Excludes1　aural myiasis (B87.4)
　　　　　　syphilitic labyrinthitis (A52.79)
　　▷ *H94.80　Other specified disorders of ear in diseases classified elsewhere, unspecified ear*
　　▷ *H94.81　Other specified disorders of right ear in diseases classified elsewhere*
　　▷ *H94.82　Other specified disorders of left ear in diseases classified elsewhere*
　　▷ *H94.83　Other specified disorders of ear in diseases classified elsewhere, bilateral*

INTRAOPERATIVE AND POSTPROCEDURAL COMPLICATIONS AND DISORDERS OF EAR AND MASTOID PROCESS, NOT ELSEWHERE CLASSIFIED (H95)

● H95   Intraoperative and postprocedural complications and disorders of ear and mastoid process, not elsewhere classified
　　Coding Clinic: 2016, Q4, P10
　● H95.0　Recurrent cholesteatoma of postmastoidectomy cavity
　　　H95.00　Recurrent cholesteatoma of postmastoidectomy cavity, unspecified ear
　　　H95.01　Recurrent cholesteatoma of postmastoidectomy cavity, right ear
　　　H95.02　Recurrent cholesteatoma of postmastoidectomy cavity, left ear
　　　H95.03　Recurrent cholesteatoma of postmastoidectomy cavity, bilateral ears
　● H95.1　Other disorders of ear and mastoid process following mastoidectomy
　　● H95.11　Chronic inflammation of postmastoidectomy cavity
　　　　　H95.111　Chronic inflammation of postmastoidectomy cavity, right ear
　　　　　H95.112　Chronic inflammation of postmastoidectomy cavity, left ear
　　　　　H95.113　Chronic inflammation of postmastoidectomy cavity, bilateral ears
　　　　　H95.119　Chronic inflammation of postmastoidectomy cavity, unspecified ear
　　● H95.12　Granulation of postmastoidectomy cavity
　　　　　H95.121　Granulation of postmastoidectomy cavity, right ear
　　　　　H95.122　Granulation of postmastoidectomy cavity, left ear
　　　　　H95.123　Granulation of postmastoidectomy cavity, bilateral ears
　　　　　H95.129　Granulation of postmastoidectomy cavity, unspecified ear

● H95.13   Mucosal cyst of postmastoidectomy cavity
    H95.131   Mucosal cyst of postmastoidectomy cavity, **right** ear
    H95.132   Mucosal cyst of postmastoidectomy cavity, **left** ear
    H95.133   Mucosal cyst of postmastoidectomy cavity, **bilateral ears**
    H95.139   Mucosal cyst of postmastoidectomy cavity, **unspecified** ear

● H95.19   Other disorders following mastoidectomy
    H95.191   Other disorders following mastoidectomy, **right** ear
    H95.192   Other disorders following mastoidectomy, **left** ear
    H95.193   Other disorders following mastoidectomy, **bilateral ears**
    H95.199   Other disorders following mastoidectomy, **unspecified** ear

● H95.2   Intraoperative **hemorrhage and hematoma** of ear and mastoid process complicating a procedure

    Excludes1   intraoperative hemorrhage and hematoma of ear and mastoid process due to accidental puncture or laceration during a procedure (H95.3-)

    H95.21   Intraoperative hemorrhage and hematoma of ear and mastoid process complicating a procedure on the **ear and mastoid process**
    H95.22   Intraoperative hemorrhage and hematoma of ear and mastoid process complicating **other procedure**

● H95.3   **Accidental puncture and laceration** of ear and mastoid process during a procedure
    H95.31   Accidental puncture and laceration of the ear and mastoid process during a procedure on the **ear and mastoid process**
    H95.32   Accidental puncture and laceration of the ear and mastoid process during **other procedure**

● H95.4   Postprocedural **hemorrhage** of ear and mastoid process following a procedure
    H95.41   Postprocedural hemorrhage of ear and mastoid process following a procedure on the **ear and mastoid process**
    H95.42   Postprocedural hemorrhage of ear and mastoid process following **other procedure**

● H95.5   Postprocedural **hematoma and seroma** of ear and mastoid process following a procedure
    H95.51   Postprocedural **hematoma** of ear and mastoid process following a procedure on the **ear and mastoid process**
    H95.52   Postprocedural **hematoma** of ear and mastoid process following **other procedure**
    H95.53   Postprocedural **seroma** of ear and mastoid process following a procedure on the **ear and mastoid process**
    H95.54   Postprocedural **seroma** of ear and mastoid process following **other procedure**

● H95.8   Other intraoperative and postprocedural complications and disorders of the ear and mastoid process, not elsewhere classified

    Excludes2   postprocedural complications and disorders following mastoidectomy (H95.0-, H95.1-)

  ● H95.81   Postprocedural **stenosis** of external ear canal
    H95.811   Postprocedural stenosis of **right** external ear canal
    H95.812   Postprocedural stenosis of **left** external ear canal
    H95.813   Postprocedural stenosis of external ear canal, **bilateral**
    H95.819   Postprocedural stenosis of **unspecified** external ear canal

    H95.88   Other **intraoperative** complications and disorders of the ear and mastoid process, not elsewhere classified
        Use additional code, if applicable, to further specify disorder

    H95.89   Other **postprocedural** complications and disorders of the ear and mastoid process, not elsewhere classified
        Use additional code, if applicable, to further specify disorder

CHAPTER 8 (H60–H95)

CHAPTER 9

DISEASES OF THE CIRCULATORY SYSTEM
(I00-I99)

OGCR Chapter-Specific Coding Guidelines

9. **Chapter 9: Diseases of the Circulatory System (I00-I99)**
    a. **Hypertension**
    The classification presumes a causal relationship between hypertension and heart involvement and between hypertension and kidney involvement, as the two conditions are linked by the term "with" in the Alphabetic Index. These conditions should be coded as related even in the absence of provider documentation explicitly linking them, unless the documentation clearly states the conditions are unrelated.

    For hypertension and conditions not specifically linked by relational terms such as "with," "associated with" or "due to" in the classification, provider documentation must link the conditions in order to code them as related.

    1) **Hypertension with Heart Disease**
    Hypertension with heart conditions classified to I50.- or I51.4-I51.7, I51.89, I51.9, are assigned to, a code from category I11, Hypertensive heart disease. Use additional code(s) from category I50, Heart failure, to identify the type(s) of heart failure in those patients with heart failure.

    The same heart conditions (I50.-, I51.4-I51.7, I51.89, I51.9) with hypertension, are coded separately if the provider has documented they are unrelated to the hypertension. Sequence according to the circumstances of the admission/encounter.

    2) **Hypertensive Chronic Kidney Disease**
    Assign codes from category I12, Hypertensive chronic kidney disease, when both hypertension and a condition classifiable to category N18, Chronic kidney disease (CKD), are present. CKD should not be coded as hypertension if the provider indicates the CKD is not related to the hypertension.

    The appropriate code from category N18 should be used as a secondary code with a code from category I12 to identify the stage of chronic kidney disease.
    See Section I.C.14. Chronic kidney disease.
    If a patient has hypertensive chronic kidney disease and acute renal failure, an additional code for the acute renal failure is required.

    3) **Hypertensive Heart and Chronic Kidney Disease**
    Assign codes from combination category I13, Hypertensive heart and chronic kidney disease, when there is hypertension with both heart and kidney involvement. If heart failure is present, assign an additional code from category I50 to identify the type of heart failure.

    The appropriate code from category N18, Chronic kidney disease, should be used as a secondary code with a code from category I13 to identify the stage of chronic kidney disease.
    See Section I.C.14. Chronic kidney disease.
    The codes in category I13, Hypertensive heart and chronic kidney disease, are combination codes that include hypertension, heart disease and chronic kidney disease. The Includes note at I13 specifies that the conditions included at I11 and I12 are included together in I13. If a patient has hypertension, heart disease and chronic kidney disease then a code from I13 should be used, not individual codes for hypertension, heart disease and chronic kidney disease, or codes from I11 or I12.

    For patients with both acute renal failure and chronic kidney disease an additional code for acute renal failure is required.

    4) **Hypertensive Cerebrovascular Disease**
    For hypertensive cerebrovascular disease, first assign the appropriate code from categories I60-I69, followed by the appropriate hypertension code.

    5) **Hypertensive Retinopathy**
    Subcategory H35.0, Background retinopathy and retinal vascular changes, should be used with a code from category I10 – I15, Hypertensive disease to include the systemic hypertension. The sequencing is based on the reason for the encounter.

    6) **Hypertension, Secondary**
    Secondary hypertension is due to an underlying condition. Two codes are required: one to identify the underlying etiology and one from category I15 to identify the hypertension. Sequencing of codes is determined by the reason for admission/encounter.

    7) **Hypertension, Transient**
    Assign code R03.0, Elevated blood pressure reading without diagnosis of hypertension, unless patient has an established diagnosis of hypertension. Assign code O13.-, Gestational [pregnancy-induced] hypertension without significant proteinuria, or O14.-, Pre-eclampsia, for transient hypertension of pregnancy.

    8) **Hypertension, Controlled**
    This diagnostic statement usually refers to an existing state of hypertension under control by therapy. Assign the appropriate code from categories I10-I15, Hypertensive diseases.

    9) **Hypertension, Uncontrolled**
    Uncontrolled hypertension may refer to untreated hypertension or hypertension not responding to current therapeutic regimen. In either case, assign the appropriate code from categories I10-I15, Hypertensive diseases.

    10) **Hypertensive Crisis**
    Assign a code from category I16, Hypertensive crisis, for documented hypertensive urgency, hypertensive emergency or unspecified hypertensive crisis. Code also any identified hypertensive disease (I10-I15). The sequencing is based on the reason for the encounter.

    11) **Pulmonary Hypertension**
    Pulmonary hypertension is classified to category I27, Other pulmonary heart diseases. For secondary pulmonary hypertension (I27.1, I27.2-), code also any associated conditions or adverse effects of drugs or toxins. The sequencing is based on the reason for the encounter, except for adverse effects of drugs.
    See Section I.C.19.e Adverse Effects, Poisoning, Underdosing and Toxic Effects.

    b. **Atherosclerotic Coronary Artery Disease and Angina**
    ICD-10-CM has combination codes for atherosclerotic heart disease with angina pectoris. The subcategories for these codes are I25.11, Atherosclerotic heart disease of native coronary artery with angina pectoris and I25.7, Atherosclerosis of coronary artery bypass graft(s) and coronary artery of transplanted heart with angina pectoris.

    When using one of these combination codes it is not necessary to use an additional code for angina pectoris. A causal relationship can be assumed in a patient with both atherosclerosis and angina pectoris, unless the documentation indicates the angina is due to something other than the atherosclerosis.

    If a patient with coronary artery disease is admitted due to an acute myocardial infarction (AMI), the AMI should be sequenced before the coronary artery disease.
    See Section I.C.9. Acute myocardial infarction (AMI).

    c. **Intraoperative and Postprocedural Cerebrovascular Accident**
    Medical record documentation should clearly specify the cause-and-effect relationship between the medical intervention and the cerebrovascular accident in order to assign a code for intraoperative or postprocedural cerebrovascular accident.

    Proper code assignment depends on whether it was an infarction or hemorrhage and whether it occurred intraoperatively or postoperatively. If it was a cerebral hemorrhage, code assignment depends on the type of procedure performed.

    d. **Sequelae of Cerebrovascular Disease**
    1) **Category I69, Sequelae of Cerebrovascular disease**
    Category I69 is used to indicate conditions classifiable to categories I60-I67 as the causes of sequela (neurologic deficits), themselves classified elsewhere. These "late effects" include neurologic deficits that persist after initial onset of conditions classifiable to categories I60-I67. The neurologic deficits caused by cerebrovascular disease may be present from the onset or may arise at any time after the onset of the condition classifiable to categories I60-I67.

    Codes from category I69, Sequelae of cerebrovascular disease, that specify hemiplegia, hemiparesis and monoplegia identify whether the dominant or nondominant side is affected. Should the affected side be documented, but not specified as dominant or nondominant, and the classification system does not indicate a default, code selection is as follows:
    • For ambidextrous patients, the default should be dominant.
    • If the left side is affected, the default is nondominant.
    • If the right side is affected, the default is dominant.

    2) **Codes from category I69 with codes from I60-I67**
    Codes from category I69 may be assigned on a health care record with codes from I60-I67, if the patient has a current cerebrovascular disease and deficits from an old cerebrovascular disease.

3) Codes from category I69 and Personal history of transient ischemic attack (TIA) and cerebral infarction (Z86.73)

Codes from category I69 should not be assigned if the patient does not have neurologic deficits.

See Section I.C.21. 4. History (of) for use of personal history codes.

e. **Acute myocardial infarction (AMI)**

1) **Type 1 ST elevation myocardial infarction (STEMI) and non-ST elevation myocardial infarction (NSTEMI)**

The ICD-10-CM codes for acute type 1 myocardial infarction (AMI) identify the site, such as anterolateral wall or true posterior wall. Subcategories I21.0-I21.2 and code I21.3 are used for type 1 ST elevation myocardial infarction (STEMI). Code I21.4, non-ST elevation (NSTEMI) myocardial infarction, is used for type 1 non-ST elevation myocardial infarction (NSTEMI) and nontransmural MIs.

If a type 1 NSTEMI evolves to STEMI, assign the STEMI code. If a type 1 STEMI converts to NSTEMI due to thrombolytic therapy, it is still coded as STEMI.

For encounters occurring while the myocardial infarction is equal to, or less than, four weeks old, including transfers to another acute setting or a postacute setting, and the myocardial infarction meets the definition for "other diagnoses" (see Section III, Reporting Additional Diagnoses), codes from category I21 may continue to be reported. For encounters after the 4-week time frame and the patient is still receiving care related to the myocardial infarction, the appropriate aftercare code should be assigned, rather than a code from category I21. For old or healed myocardial infarctions not requiring further care, code I25.2, Old myocardial infarction, may be assigned.

2) **Acute myocardial infarction, unspecified**

Code I21.9, Acute myocardial infarction, unspecified, is the default for unspecified acute myocardial infarction or unspecified type. If only type 1 STEMI or transmural MI without the site is documented, assign code I21.3, ST elevation (STEMI) myocardial infarction of unspecified site.

3) **AMI documented as nontransmural or subendocardial but site provided**

If an AMI is documented as nontransmural or subendocardial, but the site is provided, it is still coded as a subendocardial AMI.

See Section I.C.21.3 for information on coding status post administration of tPA in a different facility within the last 24 hours.

4) **Subsequent acute myocardial infarction**

A code from category I22, Subsequent ST elevation (STEMI) and non-ST elevation (NSTEMI) myocardial infarction, is to be used when a patient who has suffered a type 1 or unspecified AMI has a new AMI within the 4-week time frame of the initial AMI. A code from category I22 must be used in conjunction with a code from category I21. The sequencing of the I22 and I21 codes depends on the circumstances of the encounter.

Do not assign code I22 for subsequent myocardial infarctions other than type 1 or unspecified. For subsequent type 2 AMI assign only code I21.A1. For subsequent type 4 or type 5 AMI, assign only code I21.A9.

If a subsequent myocardial infarction of one type occurs within 4 weeks of a myocardial infarction of a different type, assign the appropriate codes from category I21 to identify each type. Do not assign a code from I22. Codes from category I22 should only be assigned if both the initial and subsequent myocardial infarctions are type 1 or unspecified.

5) **Other Types of Myocardial Infarction**

The ICD-10-CM provides codes for different types of myocardial infarction. Type 1 myocardial infarctions are assigned to codes I21.0-I21.4 and I21.9.

Type 2 myocardial infarction, and myocardial infarction due to demand ischemia or secondary to ischemic balance, is assigned to code I21.A1, Myocardial infarction type 2 with a code for the underlying cause. Do not assign code I24.8, Other forms of acute ischemic heart disease for the demand ischemia. Sequencing of type 2 AMI or the underlying cause is dependent on the circumstances of admission. When a type 2 AMI code is described as NSTEMI or STEMI, only assign code I21.A1. Codes I21.01-I21.4 should only be assigned for type 1 AMIs.

Acute myocardial infarctions type 3, 4a, 4b, 4c, and 5 are assigned to code I21.A9, Other myocardial infarction type.

The "Code also" and "Code first" notes should be followed related to complications, and for coding of postprocedural myocardial infarctions during or following cardiac surgery.

Figure 9-1 Cardiovascular valves.

Item 9–1 Rheumatic fever is the inflammation of the valve(s) of the heart, usually the mitral or aortic, which leads to valve damage. Rheumatic heart inflammations are usually **pericarditis** (sac surrounding heart), **endocarditis** (heart cavity), or **myocarditis** (heart muscle).

CHAPTER 9

DISEASES OF THE CIRCULATORY SYSTEM (I00-I99)

Excludes2   certain conditions originating in the perinatal period (P04-P96)
certain infectious and parasitic diseases (A00-B99)
complications of pregnancy, childbirth and the puerperium (O00-O9A)
congenital malformations, deformations, and chromosomal abnormalities (Q00-Q99)
endocrine, nutritional and metabolic diseases (E00-E88)
injury, poisoning and certain other consequences of external causes (S00-T88)
neoplasms (C00-D49)
symptoms, signs and abnormal clinical and laboratory findings, not elsewhere classified (R00-R94)
systemic connective tissue disorders (M30-M36)
transient cerebral ischemic attacks and related syndromes (G45.-)

This chapter contains the following blocks:

I00-I02	Acute rheumatic fever
I05-I09	Chronic rheumatic heart diseases
I10-I1A	Hypertensive diseases
I20-I25	Ischemic heart diseases
I26-I28	Pulmonary heart disease and diseases of pulmonary circulation
I30-I5A	Other forms of heart disease
I60-I69	Cerebrovascular diseases
I70-I79	Diseases of arteries, arterioles and capillaries
I80-I89	Diseases of veins, lymphatic vessels and lymph nodes, not elsewhere classified
I95-I99	Other and unspecified disorders of the circulatory system

ACUTE RHEUMATIC FEVER (I00-I02)

I00   **Rheumatic fever without heart involvement**

     Includes   arthritis, rheumatic, acute or subacute

     Excludes1   rheumatic fever with heart involvement (I01.0-I01.9)

● **I01**   **Rheumatic fever with heart involvement**

     Excludes1   chronic diseases of rheumatic origin (I05-I09) unless rheumatic fever is also present or there is evidence of reactivation or activity of the rheumatic process.

   I01.0   **Acute rheumatic pericarditis**
       Any condition in I00 with pericarditis
       Rheumatic pericarditis (acute)

     Excludes1   acute pericarditis not specified as rheumatic (I30.-)

   I01.1   **Acute rheumatic endocarditis**
       Any condition in I00 with endocarditis or valvulitis
       Acute rheumatic valvulitis

Item 9–2 Rheumatic chorea, also called Sydenham's, juvenile, minor, simple, or St. Vitus' dance, is a major symptom of rheumatic fever and is characterized by ceaseless, involuntary, jerky, purposeless movements.

I01.2   **Acute rheumatic myocarditis**
Any condition in I00 with myocarditis

I01.8   **Other acute rheumatic heart disease**
Any condition in I00 with other or multiple types of heart involvement
Acute rheumatic pancarditis

I01.9   **Acute rheumatic heart disease, unspecified**
Any condition in I00 with unspecified type of heart involvement
Rheumatic carditis, acute
Rheumatic heart disease, active or acute

● **I02**   **Rheumatic chorea**
     Includes   Sydenham's chorea
     Excludes1   chorea NOS (G25.5)
                    Huntington's chorea (G10)

I02.0   **Rheumatic chorea with heart involvement**
Chorea NOS with heart involvement
Rheumatic chorea with heart involvement of any type classifiable under I01.-

I02.9   **Rheumatic chorea without heart involvement**
Rheumatic chorea NOS

CHRONIC RHEUMATIC HEART DISEASES (I05-I09)

● **I05**   **Rheumatic mitral valve diseases**
     Includes   conditions classifiable to both I05.0 and I05.2-I05.9, whether specified as rheumatic or not
     Excludes1   mitral valve disease specified as nonrheumatic (I34.-)
                    mitral valve disease with aortic and/or tricuspid valve involvement (I08.-)

I05.0   **Rheumatic mitral stenosis**
Mitral (valve) obstruction (rheumatic)

I05.1   **Rheumatic mitral insufficiency**
Rheumatic mitral incompetence
Rheumatic mitral regurgitation
     Excludes1   mitral insufficiency not specified as rheumatic (I34.0)

I05.2   **Rheumatic mitral stenosis with insufficiency**
Rheumatic mitral stenosis with incompetence or regurgitation

I05.8   **Other rheumatic mitral valve diseases**
Rheumatic mitral (valve) failure

I05.9   **Rheumatic mitral valve disease, unspecified**
Rheumatic mitral (valve) disorder (chronic) NOS

● **I06**   **Rheumatic aortic valve diseases**
     Excludes1   aortic valve disease not specified as rheumatic (I35.-)
                    aortic valve disease with mitral and/or tricuspid valve involvement (I08.-)

I06.0   **Rheumatic aortic stenosis**
Rheumatic aortic (valve) obstruction

I06.1   **Rheumatic aortic insufficiency**
Rheumatic aortic incompetence
Rheumatic aortic regurgitation

I06.2   **Rheumatic aortic stenosis with insufficiency**
Rheumatic aortic stenosis with incompetence or regurgitation

★ **(See Plate 33 of the Anatomy Illustrations.)**

Item 9–4 Aortic stenosis is the narrowing of the aortic valve located between the left ventricle and the aorta. **Aortic insufficiency** is the improper closure of the aortic valve, which may lead to enlargement (hypertrophy) of the left ventricle.

I06.8   **Other rheumatic aortic valve diseases**

I06.9   **Rheumatic aortic valve disease, unspecified**
Rheumatic aortic (valve) disease NOS

● **I07**   **Rheumatic tricuspid valve diseases**
     Includes   rheumatic tricuspid valve diseases specified as rheumatic or unspecified
     ~~Excludes1   tricuspid valve disease specified as nonrheumatic (I36.-)~~
                 ~~tricuspid valve disease with aortic and/or mitral valve involvement (I08.-)~~
     ▶ **Excludes2**   tricuspid valve disease specified as
         ▶ nonrheumatic (I36.-)
         ▶ tricuspid valve disease with aortic and/or mitral valve involvement (I08.-)

I07.0   **Rheumatic tricuspid stenosis**
Tricuspid (valve) stenosis (rheumatic)

I07.1   **Rheumatic tricuspid insufficiency**
Tricuspid (valve) insufficiency (rheumatic)

I07.2   **Rheumatic tricuspid stenosis and insufficiency**

I07.8   **Other rheumatic tricuspid valve diseases**

I07.9   **Rheumatic tricuspid valve disease, unspecified**
Rheumatic tricuspid valve disorder NOS

● **I08**   **Multiple valve diseases**
     Includes   multiple valve diseases specified as rheumatic or unspecified
     Excludes1   endocarditis, valve unspecified (I38)
                    multiple valve disease specified a nonrheumatic (I34.-, I35.-, I36.-, I37.-, I38.-, Q22.-, Q23.-, Q24.8-)
                    rheumatic valve disease NOS (I09.1)
     Coding Clinic: 2019, Q2, P5

I08.0   **Rheumatic disorders of both mitral and aortic valves**
Involvement of both mitral and aortic valves specified as rheumatic or unspecified
Coding Clinic: 2019, Q2, P5

I08.1   **Rheumatic disorders of both mitral and tricuspid valves**

I08.2   **Rheumatic disorders of both aortic and tricuspid valves**

I08.3   **Combined rheumatic disorders of mitral, aortic and tricuspid valves**

I08.8   **Other rheumatic multiple valve diseases**

I08.9   **Rheumatic multiple valve disease, unspecified**

● **I09**   **Other rheumatic heart diseases**
I09.0   **Rheumatic myocarditis**
     Excludes1   myocarditis not specified as rheumatic (I51.4)

I09.1   **Rheumatic diseases of endocardium, valve unspecified**
Rheumatic endocarditis (chronic)
Rheumatic valvulitis (chronic)
     Excludes1   endocarditis, valve unspecified (I38)

I09.2   **Chronic rheumatic pericarditis**
Adherent pericardium, rheumatic
Chronic rheumatic mediastinopericarditis
Chronic rheumatic myopericarditis
     Excludes1   chronic pericarditis not specified as rheumatic (I31.-)

● **I09.8**   **Other specified rheumatic heart diseases**
     I09.81   **Rheumatic heart failure** 🐾
           Use additional code to identify type of heart failure (I50.-)
     I09.89   **Other specified rheumatic heart diseases**
           Rheumatic disease of pulmonary valve

I09.9   **Rheumatic heart disease, unspecified**
Rheumatic carditis
     Excludes1   rheumatoid carditis (M05.31)

Item 9–3 Mitral stenosis is the narrowing of the mitral valve separating the left atrium from the left ventricle. **Mitral insufficiency** is the improper closure of the mitral valve, which may lead to enlargement (hypertrophy) of the left atrium.

▶ New   ⇒ Revised   ~~deleted~~ Deleted   Excludes 1   Excludes 2   Includes   Use additional   Code first   Code also   Key words
OGCR Official Guidelines   X Assign placeholder X   ● Use Additional Character(s)   ▶ Manifestation Code   🐾 Hierarchical Condition Category   Coding Clinic

Item 9-5 Hypertension is caused by high arterial blood pressure in the arteries. **Essential, primary,** or **idiopathic** hypertension occurs without identifiable organic cause. **Secondary** hypertension is that which has an organic cause. **Malignant** hypertension is severely elevated blood pressure. **Benign** hypertension is mildly elevated blood pressure.

HYPERTENSIVE DISEASES (I10-I16)

Use additional code to identify:
    exposure to environmental tobacco smoke (Z77.22)
    history of tobacco dependence (Z87.891)
    occupational exposure to environmental tobacco
        smoke (Z57.31)
    tobacco dependence (F17.-)
    tobacco use (Z72.0)

Excludes1	neonatal hypertension (P29.2) primary pulmonary hypertension (I27.0)
Excludes2	hypertensive disease complicating pregnancy, childbirth and the puerperium (O10-O11, O13-O16)

I10   Essential (primary) hypertension

Includes	high blood pressure hypertension (arterial) (benign) (essential) (malignant) (primary) (systemic)
Excludes1	hypertensive disease complicating pregnancy, childbirth and the puerperium (O10-O11, O13-O16)
Excludes2	essential (primary) hypertension involving vessels of brain (I60-I69) essential (primary) hypertension involving vessels of eye (H35.0-)

Coding Clinic: 2023, Q4, P24-25,42

●I11   Hypertensive heart disease

Includes	any condition in I50.- or I51.4-I51.7, I51.89, I51.9 due to hypertension

I11.0   Hypertensive heart disease with heart failure 🔊
    Hypertensive heart failure
    Use additional code to identify type of heart failure (I50.-)
    Coding Clinic: 2017, Q1, P47

I11.9   Hypertensive heart disease without heart failure
    Hypertensive heart disease NOS

OGCR Section I.C.9.a.2.

Hypertensive Chronic Kidney Disease
Assign codes from category I12, Hypertensive chronic kidney disease, when both hypertension and a condition classifiable to category N18, Chronic kidney disease (CKD), are present. CKD should not be coded as hypertension if the physician has specifically documented a different cause.

The appropriate code from category N18 should be used as a secondary code with a code from category I12 to identify the stage of chronic kidney disease.
See Section I.C.14. Chronic kidney disease.

If a patient has hypertensive chronic kidney disease and acute renal failure, an additional code for the acute renal failure is required.

●I12   Hypertensive chronic kidney disease

Includes	any condition in N18 and N26 - due to hypertension arteriosclerosis of kidney arteriosclerotic nephritis (chronic) (interstitial) hypertensive nephropathy nephrosclerosis
Excludes1	hypertension due to kidney disease (I15.0, I15.1) renovascular hypertension (I15.0) secondary hypertension (I15.-)
Excludes2	acute kidney failure (N17.-)

Coding Clinic: 2018, Q4, P89; 2016, Q4, P123

I12.0   Hypertensive chronic kidney disease with stage 5 chronic kidney disease or end stage renal disease 🔊
    Use additional code to identify the stage of chronic kidney disease (N18.5, N18.6)
    Coding Clinic: 2016, Q3, P23

I12.9   Hypertensive chronic kidney disease with stage 1 through stage 4 chronic kidney disease, or unspecified chronic kidney disease
    Hypertensive chronic kidney disease NOS
    Hypertensive renal disease NOS
    Use additional code to identify the stage of chronic kidney disease (N18.1-N18.4, N18.9)
    Coding Clinic: 2022, Q4, P6; 2018, Q4, P88

OGCR Section I.c.9.a.3.

Hypertensive Heart and Chronic Kidney Disease
Assign codes from combination category I13, Hypertensive heart and chronic kidney disease, when **there is hypertension with both heart and kidney involvement.** If heart failure is present, assign an additional code from category I50 to identify the type of heart failure.

The appropriate code from category N18, Chronic kidney disease, should be used as a secondary code with a code from category I13 to identify the stage of chronic kidney disease.
See Section I.C.14. Chronic kidney disease.

The codes in category I13, Hypertensive heart and chronic kidney disease, are combination codes that include hypertension, heart disease and chronic kidney disease. The Includes note at I13 specifies that the conditions included at I11 and I12 are included together in I13. If a patient has hypertension, heart disease and chronic kidney disease then a code from I13 should be used, not individual codes for hypertension, heart disease and chronic kidney disease, or codes from I11 or I12.

For patients with both acute renal failure and chronic kidney disease an additional code for acute renal failure is required.

●I13   Hypertensive heart and chronic kidney disease

Includes	any condition in I11.- with any condition in I12.- cardiorenal disease cardiovascular renal disease

Coding Clinic: 2022, Q4, P6

I13.0   Hypertensive heart and chronic kidney disease with heart failure and stage 1 through stage 4 chronic kidney disease, or unspecified chronic kidney disease 🔊
    Use additional code to identify type of heart failure (I50.-)
    Use additional code to identify stage of chronic kidney disease (N18.1-N18.4, N18.9)

●I13.1   Hypertensive heart and chronic kidney disease without heart failure

I13.10   Hypertensive heart and chronic kidney disease without heart failure, with stage 1 through stage 4 chronic kidney disease, or unspecified chronic kidney disease
    Hypertensive heart disease and hypertensive chronic kidney disease NOS
    Use additional code to identify the stage of chronic kidney disease (N18.1-N18.4, N18.9)

I13.11   Hypertensive heart and chronic kidney disease without heart failure, with stage 5 chronic kidney disease, or end stage renal disease 🔊
    Use additional code to identify the stage of chronic kidney disease (N18.5, N18.6)

I13.2   Hypertensive heart and chronic kidney disease with heart failure and with stage 5 chronic kidney disease, or end stage renal disease 🔊
    Use additional code to identify type of heart failure (I50.-)
    Use additional code to identify the stage of chronic kidney disease (N18.5, N18.6)

OGCR Section I.9.a.6.

Hypertension, Secondary
Secondary hypertension is due to an underlying condition.
Two codes are required: one to identify the underlying
etiology and one from category I15 to identify the
hypertension. Sequencing of codes is determined by the
reason for admission/encounter.

● **I15** **Secondary hypertension**

Code also underlying condition

Excludes1 postprocedural hypertension (I97.3)

Excludes2 secondary hypertension involving vessels of
brain (I60-I69)
secondary hypertension involving vessels of eye
(H35.0-)

I15.0 **Renovascular hypertension**

I15.1 **Hypertension secondary to other renal disorders**
Coding Clinic: 2016, Q3, P23

I15.2 **Hypertension secondary to endocrine disorders**
Coding Clinic: 2023, Q2, P16-17

I15.8 **Other secondary hypertension**

I15.9 **Secondary hypertension, unspecified**

● **I16** **Hypertensive crisis**

Code also any identified hypertensive disease (I10-I15, I1A)
Coding Clinic: 2016, Q4, P26-27, 123

I16.0 **Hypertensive urgency** (Ex) No exclusions

I16.1 **Hypertensive emergency**
Coding Clinic: 2023, Q4, P25

▶ Use Additional code, if applicable, to identify specific organ
dysfunction, such as:
▶ acute kidney injury (N17.-)
▶ acute myocardial infarction (I21.-)
▶ acute pulmonary edema (left and/or right ventricular
failure) (J81.0, I50.-)
▶ aortic dissection (I71.0-)
▶ cerebral hemorrhage (I60.-. I61.-, I62.-)
▶ cerebral infarction (I63.-)
▶ eclampsia (O15.-)
▶ hypertensive encephalopathy (I67.4)
▶ seizure (R56.9)

I16.9 **Hypertensive crisis, unspecified** , I1A Other hypertension

● **I1A** **Other hypertension**

I1A.0 **Resistant hypertension**
Apparent treatment resistant hypertension
Treatment resistant hypertension
True resistant hypertension

*Code first specific type of existing hypertension, if known,
such as:*
essential hypertension (I10)
secondary hypertension (I15.-)
Coding Clinic: 2023, Q4, P24-25

ISCHEMIC HEART DISEASES (I20-I25)

Code also the presence of hypertension (I10-I1A)

● **I20** **Angina pectoris**

*Chest pain/discomfort due to lack of oxygen to the heart muscle.
Principal symptom of myocardial infarction.*

Use additional code to identify:
exposure to environmental tobacco smoke (Z77.22)
history of tobacco dependence (Z87.891)
occupational exposure to environmental tobacco smoke (Z57.31)
tobacco dependence (F17.-)
tobacco use (Z72.0)

Excludes1 angina pectoris with atherosclerotic heart disease
of native coronary arteries (I25.1-)
atherosclerosis of coronary artery bypass graft(s)
and coronary artery of transplanted heart
with angina pectoris (I25.7-)
postinfarction angina (I23.7)

I20.0 **Unstable angina** 🏷️
Accelerated angina
Crescendo angina
De novo effort angina
Intermediate coronary syndrome
Preinfarction syndrome
Worsening effort angina

I20.1 **Angina pectoris with documented spasm** 🏷️
Angiospastic angina
Prinzmetal angina
Spasm-induced angina
Variant angina

I20.2 **Refractory angina pectoris**

● **I20.8** **Other forms of angina pectoris** 🏷️
Use additional code(s) for symptoms associated with
angina equivalent

I20.81 **Angina pectoris with coronary microvascular
dysfunction**
Angina pectoris with coronary microvascular
disease

I20.89 **Other forms of angina pectoris**
Angina equivalent
Angina of effort
Coronary slow flow syndrome
Stable angina
Stenocardia

I20.9 **Angina pectoris, unspecified** 🏷️
Angina NOS
Anginal syndrome
Cardiac angina
Ischemic chest pain

● **I21** **Acute myocardial infarction**

Includes cardiac infarction
coronary (artery) embolism
coronary (artery) occlusion
coronary (artery) rupture
coronary (artery) thrombosis
infarction of heart, myocardium, or ventricle
myocardial infarction specified as acute or with a
stated duration of 4 weeks (28 days) or less
from onset

Use additional code, if applicable, to identify:
exposure to environmental tobacco smoke (Z77.22)
history of tobacco dependence (Z87.891)
occupational exposure to environmental tobacco smoke (Z57.31)
status post administration of tPA (rtPA) in a different facility
within the last 24 hours prior to admission to current
facility (Z92.82)
tobacco dependence (F17.-)
tobacco use (Z72.0)

Excludes2 old myocardial infarction (I25.2)
postmyocardial infarction syndrome (I24.1)
subsequent type 1 myocardial infarction (I22.-)
Coding Clinic: 2016, Q4, P140; 2013, Q1, P25-26; 2012, Q4, P103

● **I21.0** **ST elevation (STEMI) myocardial infarction of anterior
wall**
Type 1 ST elevation myocardial infarction of anterior wall
Coding Clinic: 2013, Q1, P26

I21.01 **ST elevation (STEMI) myocardial
infarction involving left main coronary
artery** 🏷️

I21.02 **ST elevation (STEMI) myocardial infarction
involving left anterior descending coronary
artery** 🏷️
ST elevation (STEMI) myocardial infarction
involving diagonal coronary artery
Coding Clinic: 2013, Q1, P26

I21.09   **ST elevation (STEMI) myocardial infarction involving other coronary artery of anterior wall** 🐾
    Acute transmural myocardial infarction of anterior wall
    Anteroapical transmural (Q wave) infarction (acute)
    Anterolateral transmural (Q wave) infarction (acute)
    Anteroseptal transmural (Q wave) infarction (acute)
    Transmural (Q wave) infarction (acute) (of) anterior (wall) NOS
    Coding Clinic: 2012, Q4, P102, 104

● **I21.1**   **ST elevation (STEMI) myocardial infarction of inferior wall**
    Type 1 ST elevation myocardial infarction of inferior wall
    Coding Clinic: 2013, Q1, P26

I21.11   **ST elevation (STEMI) myocardial infarction involving right coronary artery** 🐾
    Inferoposterior transmural (Q wave) infarction (acute)

I21.19   **ST elevation (STEMI) myocardial infarction involving other coronary artery of inferior wall** 🐾
    Acute transmural myocardial infarction of inferior wall
    Inferolateral transmural (Q wave) infarction (acute)
    Transmural (Q wave) infarction (acute) (of) diaphragmatic wall
    Transmural (Q wave) infarction (acute) (of) inferior (wall) NOS

    Excludes2   ST elevation (STEMI) myocardial infarction involving left circumflex coronary artery (I21.21)

    Coding Clinic: 2012, Q4, P97

● **I21.2**   **ST elevation (STEMI) myocardial infarction of other sites**
    Type 1 ST elevation myocardial infarction of other sites
    Coding Clinic: 2013, Q1, P26

I21.21   **ST elevation (STEMI) myocardial infarction involving left circumflex coronary artery** 🐾
    ST elevation (STEMI) myocardial infarction involving oblique marginal coronary artery

I21.29   **ST elevation (STEMI) myocardial infarction involving other sites** 🐾
    Acute transmural myocardial infarction of other sites
    Apical-lateral transmural (Q wave) infarction (acute)
    Basal-lateral transmural (Q wave) infarction (acute)
    High lateral transmural (Q wave) infarction (acute)
    Lateral (wall) NOS transmural (Q wave) infarction (acute)
    Posterior (true) transmural (Q wave) infarction (acute)
    Posterobasal transmural (Q wave) infarction (acute)
    Posterolateral transmural (Q wave) infarction (acute)
    Posteroseptal transmural (Q wave) infarction (acute)
    Septal transmural (Q wave) infarction (acute) NOS

OGCR Section I.c.9.e.2.
Acute myocardial infarction, unspecified
Code I21.9, Acute myocardial infarction, unspecified, is the default for unspecified acute myocardial infarction or unspecified type. If only type 1 STEMI or transmural MI without the site is documented, assign I21.3, ST elevation (STEMI) myocardial infarction of unspecified site.

I21.3   **ST elevation (STEMI) myocardial infarction of unspecified site** 🐾
    Acute transmural myocardial infarction of unspecified site
    Transmural (Q wave) myocardial infarction NOS
    Type 1 ST elevation myocardial infarction of unspecified site
    Coding Clinic: 2013, Q1, P26

I21.4   **Non-ST elevation (NSTEMI) myocardial infarction** 🐾
    Acute subendocardial myocardial infarction
    Non-Q wave myocardial infarction NOS
    Nontransmural myocardial infarction NOS
    Type 1 non-ST elevation myocardial infarction
    Coding Clinic: 2024, Q1, P28; 2023, Q2, P29; 2021, Q3, P7; 2017, Q1, P44; 2015, Q2, P16; 2013, Q1, P26

I21.9   **Acute myocardial infarction, unspecified** 🐾
    Myocardial infarction (acute) NOS

● **I21.A**   **Other type of myocardial infarction**

I21.A1   **Myocardial infarction type 2** 🐾
    Myocardial infarction due to demand ischemia
    Myocardial infarction secondary to ischemic imbalance

    ➠ *Code first, if applicable, the underlying cause, such as:*
    anemia (D50.0-D64.9)
    chronic obstructive pulmonary disease (J44.-)
    paroxysmal tachycardia (I47.0-I47.9)
    shock (R57.0-R57.9)
    Coding Clinic: 2017, Q4, P13-14

I21.A9   **Other myocardial infarction type** 🐾
    Myocardial infarction associated with revascularization procedure
    Myocardial infarction type 3
    Myocardial infarction type 4a
    Myocardial infarction type 4b
    Myocardial infarction type 4c
    Myocardial infarction type 5

    Code first, if applicable, postprocedural myocardial infarction following cardiac surgery (I97.190), or postprocedural myocardial infarction during cardiac surgery (I97.790)

    Code also complication, if known and applicable, such as:
    (acute) stent occlusion (T82.897-)
    (acute) stent stenosis (T82.857-)
    (acute) stent thrombosis (T82.865-)
    cardiac arrest due to underlying cardiac condition (I46.2)
    complication of percutaneous coronary intervention (PCI) (I97.89)
    occlusion of coronary artery bypass graft (T82.218-)
    Coding Clinic: 2021, Q3, P6-7; 2019, Q2, P32-33

I21.B   **Myocardial infarction with coronary microvascular dysfunction**
    Myocardial infarction with coronary microvascular disease
    Myocardial infarction with nonobstructive coronary arteries
    [MINOCA] with microvascular disease

● I22   Subsequent ST elevation (STEMI) and non-ST elevation (NSTEMI) myocardial infarction

> **Includes**   acute myocardial infarction occurring within four weeks (28 days) of a previous acute myocardial infarction, regardless of site
> cardiac infarction
> coronary (artery) embolism
> coronary (artery) occlusion
> coronary (artery) rupture
> coronary (artery) thrombosis
> infarction of heart, myocardium, or ventricle
> recurrent myocardial infarction
> reinfarction of myocardium
> rupture of heart, myocardium, or ventricle
> subsequent type 1 myocardial infarction

> **Excludes1**   subsequent myocardial infarction, type 2 (I21.A1)
> subsequent myocardial infarction of other type (type 3) (type 4) (type 5) (I21.A9)

> Use additional code, if applicable, to identify:
> exposure to environmental tobacco smoke (Z77.22)
> history of tobacco dependence (Z87.891)
> occupational exposure to environmental tobacco smoke (Z57.31)
> status post administration of tPA (rtPA) in a different facility within the last 24 hours prior to admission to current facility (Z92.82)
> tobacco dependence (F17.-)
> tobacco use (Z72.0)
> Coding Clinic: 2017, Q4, P14; 2013, Q1, P25; 2012, Q4, P103

I22.0   Subsequent ST elevation (STEMI) myocardial infarction of anterior wall 🗝
> Subsequent acute transmural myocardial infarction of anterior wall
> Subsequent transmural (Q wave) infarction (acute)(of) anterior (wall) NOS
> Subsequent anteroapical transmural (Q wave) infarction (acute)
> Subsequent anterolateral transmural (Q wave) infarction (acute)
> Subsequent anteroseptal transmural (Q wave) infarction (acute)

I22.1   Subsequent ST elevation (STEMI) myocardial infarction of inferior wall 🗝
> Subsequent acute transmural myocardial infarction of inferior wall
> Subsequent transmural (Q wave) infarction (acute)(of) diaphragmatic wall
> Subsequent transmural (Q wave) infarction (acute)(of) inferior (wall) NOS
> Subsequent inferolateral transmural (Q wave) infarction (acute)
> Subsequent inferoposterior transmural (Q wave) infarction (acute)
> Coding Clinic: 2012, Q4, P97, 102, 104

I22.2   Subsequent non-ST elevation (NSTEMI) myocardial infarction 🗝
> Subsequent acute subendocardial myocardial infarction
> Subsequent non-Q wave myocardial infarction NOS
> Subsequent nontransmural myocardial infarction NOS

I22.8   Subsequent ST elevation (STEMI) myocardial infarction of other sites 🗝
> Subsequent acute transmural myocardial infarction of other sites
> Subsequent apical-lateral transmural (Q wave) myocardial infarction (acute)
> Subsequent basal-lateral transmural (Q wave) myocardial infarction (acute)
> Subsequent high lateral transmural (Q wave) myocardial infarction (acute)
> Subsequent transmural (Q wave) myocardial infarction (acute)(of) lateral (wall) NOS
> Subsequent posterior (true) transmural (Q wave) myocardial infarction (acute)
> Subsequent posterobasal transmural (Q wave) myocardial infarction (acute)
> Subsequent posterolateral transmural (Q wave) myocardial infarction (acute)
> Subsequent posteroseptal transmural (Q wave) myocardial infarction (acute)
> Subsequent septal NOS transmural (Q wave) myocardial infarction (acute)

I22.9   Subsequent ST elevation (STEMI) myocardial infarction of unspecified site 🗝
> Subsequent acute myocardial infarction of unspecified site
> Subsequent myocardial infarction (acute) NOS

● I23   Certain current complications following ST elevation (STEMI) and non-ST elevation (NSTEMI) myocardial infarction (within the 28 day period)
> Coding Clinic: 2017, Q2, P11

I23.0   Hemopericardium as current complication following acute myocardial infarction 🗝   A
> **Excludes1**   hemopericardium not specified as current complication following acute myocardial infarction (I31.2)

I23.1   Atrial septal defect as current complication following acute myocardial infarction 🗝   A
> **Excludes1**   acquired atrial septal defect not specified as current complication following acute myocardial infarction (I51.0)

I23.2   Ventricular septal defect as current complication following acute myocardial infarction 🗝   A
> **Excludes1**   acquired ventricular septal defect not specified as current complication following acute myocardial infarction (I51.0)

I23.3   Rupture of cardiac wall without hemopericardium as current complication following acute myocardial infarction 🗝   A
> Coding Clinic: 2017, Q2, P11

I23.4   Rupture of chordae tendineae as current complication following acute myocardial infarction 🗝
> **Excludes1**   rupture of chordae tendineae not specified as current complication following acute myocardial infarction (I51.1)

I23.5   Rupture of papillary muscle as current complication following acute myocardial infarction 🗝
> **Excludes1**   rupture of papillary muscle not specified as current complication following acute myocardial infarction (I51.2)

Item 9–6   Classification is based on the location of the atherosclerosis. **"Of native coronary artery"** indicates the atherosclerosis is within an original heart artery. **"Of autologous vein bypass graft"** indicates that the atherosclerosis is within a vein graft that was taken from within the patient. **"Of nonautologous biological bypass graft"** indicates the atherosclerosis is within a vessel grafted from other than the patient. **"Of artery bypass graft"** indicates the atherosclerosis is within an artery that was grafted from within the patient.

▶ New   ▥ Revised   ~~deleted~~ Deleted   Excludes 1   Excludes 2   Includes   Use additional   Code first   Code also   Key words
OGCR Official Guidelines   X Assign placeholder X   ● Use Additional Character(s)   ▶ Manifestation Code   🗝 Hierarchical Condition Category   Coding Clinic

I23.6 **Thrombosis of atrium, auricular appendage, and ventricle as current complications following acute myocardial infarction** 🔖 A

    Excludes1 thrombosis of atrium, auricular appendage, and ventricle not specified as current complication following acute myocardial infarction (I51.3)

I23.7 **Postinfarction angina** 🔖 A
    Coding Clinic: 2015, Q2, P16-17

I23.8 **Other current complications following acute myocardial infarction** 🔖 A

● I24 **Other acute ischemic heart diseases**
    Excludes1 angina pectoris (I20.-)
        transient myocardial ischemia in newborn (P29.4)
    Excludes2 non-ischemic myocardial injury (I5A)

I24.0 **Acute coronary thrombosis not resulting in myocardial infarction** 🔖
    Acute coronary (artery) (vein) embolism not resulting in myocardial infarction
    Acute coronary (artery) (vein) occlusion not resulting in myocardial infarction
    Acute coronary (artery) (vein) thromboembolism not resulting in myocardial infarction
    Excludes1 atherosclerotic heart disease (I25.1-)
    Coding Clinic: 2013, Q1, P24

I24.1 **Dressler's syndrome** 🔖
    Postmyocardial infarction syndrome
    Excludes1 postinfarction angina (I23.7)

● I24.8 **Other forms of acute ischemic heart disease** 🔖
    Excludes1 myocardial infarction due to demand ischemia (I21.A1)
    Coding Clinic: 2017, Q4, P13

    I24.81 **Acute coronary microvascular dysfunction**
        Acute (presentation of) coronary microvascular disease

    I24.89 **Other forms of acute ischemic heart disease**

I24.9 **Acute ischemic heart disease, unspecified** 🔖
    Excludes1 ischemic heart disease (chronic) NOS (I25.9)

● I25 **Chronic ischemic heart disease**
    Excludes2 non-ischemic myocardial injury (I5A)

    Use additional code to identify:
    chronic total occlusion of coronary artery (I25.82)
    exposure to environmental tobacco smoke (Z77.22)
    history of tobacco dependence (Z87.891)
    occupational exposure to environmental tobacco smoke (Z57.31)
    tobacco dependence (F17.-)
    tobacco use (Z72.0)

⭐ **(See Plates 218 and 219 on pages 74 and 75.)**

● I25.1 **Atherosclerotic heart disease of native coronary artery**
    Disease in which fatty deposits form on the walls of arteries
    Atherosclerotic cardiovascular disease
    Coronary (artery) atheroma
    Coronary (artery) atherosclerosis
    Coronary (artery) disease
    Coronary (artery) sclerosis
    Use additional code, if applicable, to identify:
    coronary atherosclerosis due to calcified coronary lesion (I25.84)
    coronary atherosclerosis due to lipid rich plaque (I25.83)
    Excludes2 atheroembolism (I75.-)
        atherosclerosis of coronary artery bypass graft(s) and transplanted heart (I25.7-)

    I25.10 **Atherosclerotic heart disease of native coronary artery without angina pectoris** A
        Atherosclerotic heart disease NOS
        Coding Clinic: 2024, Q1, P28; 2021, Q3, P6-7; 2015, Q2, P17; 2012, Q4, P92

OGCR See Section I.9.b.

Atherosclerotic Coronary Artery Disease and Angina

ICD-10-CM has combination codes for atherosclerotic heart disease with angina pectoris. The subcategories for these codes are I25.11, Atherosclerotic heart disease of native coronary artery with angina pectoris and I25.7, Atherosclerosis of coronary artery bypass graft(s) and coronary artery of transplanted heart with angina pectoris.

When using one of these combination codes it is not necessary to use an additional code for angina pectoris. A causal relationship can be assumed in a patient with both atherosclerosis and angina pectoris, unless the documentation indicates the angina is due to something other than the atherosclerosis.

If a patient with coronary artery disease is admitted due to an acute myocardial infarction (AMI), the AMI should be sequenced before the coronary artery disease.

See Section I.C.9. Acute myocardial infarction (AMI).

● I25.11 **Atherosclerotic heart disease of native coronary artery with angina pectoris**

    I25.110 **Atherosclerotic heart disease of native coronary artery with unstable angina pectoris** 🔖 A
        Excludes1 unstable angina without atherosclerotic heart disease (I20.0)

    I25.111 **Atherosclerotic heart disease of native coronary artery with angina pectoris with documented spasm** 🔖 A
        Excludes1 angina pectoris with documented spasm without atherosclerotic heart disease (I20.1)

    I25.112 **Atherosclerotic heart disease of native coronary artery with refractory angina pectoris** A

    I25.118 **Atherosclerotic heart disease of native coronary artery with other forms of angina pectoris** 🔖 A
        Excludes1 other forms of angina pectoris without atherosclerotic heart disease (I20.8-)
        Coding Clinic: 2015, Q2, P16-17

    I25.119 **Atherosclerotic heart disease of native coronary artery with unspecified angina pectoris** 🔖 A
        Atherosclerotic heart disease with angina NOS
        Atherosclerotic heart disease with ischemic chest pain
        Excludes1 unspecified angina pectoris without atherosclerotic heart disease (I20.9)

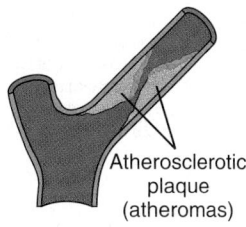

Figure 9-2 Atherosclerotic plaque.

Atherosclerotic plaque (atheromas)

CHAPTER 9 (I00-I99)

CHAPTER 9 (I00-I99)

I25.2   **Old myocardial infarction**
Healed myocardial infarction
Past myocardial infarction diagnosed by ECG or other investigation, but currently presenting no symptoms

I25.3   **Aneurysm of heart**
Mural aneurysm
Ventricular aneurysm

● **I25.4**   **Coronary artery aneurysm and dissection**

    I25.41   **Coronary artery aneurysm**
        Coronary arteriovenous fistula, acquired
        Excludes1   congenital coronary (artery) aneurysm (Q24.5)

    I25.42   **Coronary artery dissection**

I25.5   **Ischemic cardiomyopathy**
    Excludes2   coronary atherosclerosis (I25.1-, I25.7-)
    Coding Clinic: 2022, Q3, P18

I25.6   **Silent myocardial ischemia**

● **I25.7**   **Atherosclerosis of coronary artery bypass graft(s) and coronary artery of transplanted heart with angina pectoris**
Use additional code, if applicable, to identify:
    coronary atherosclerosis due to calcified coronary lesion (I25.84)
    coronary atherosclerosis due to lipid rich plaque (I25.83)
    Excludes1   atherosclerosis of bypass graft(s) of transplanted heart without angina pectoris (I25.812)
        atherosclerosis of coronary artery bypass graft(s) without angina pectoris (I25.810)
        atherosclerosis of native coronary artery of transplanted heart without angina pectoris (I25.811)

  ● **I25.70**   **Atherosclerosis of coronary artery bypass graft(s), unspecified, with angina pectoris**

    I25.700   **Atherosclerosis of coronary artery bypass graft(s), unspecified, with unstable angina pectoris** A
        Excludes1   unstable angina pectoris without atherosclerosis of coronary artery bypass graft (I20.0)

    I25.701   **Atherosclerosis of coronary artery bypass graft(s), unspecified, with angina pectoris with documented spasm** A
        Excludes1   angina pectoris with documented spasm without atherosclerosis of coronary artery bypass graft (I20.1)

    I25.702   **Atherosclerosis of coronary artery bypass graft(s), unspecified, with refractory angina pectoris** A
        Coding Clinic: 2022, Q4, P22

    I25.708   **Atherosclerosis of coronary artery bypass graft(s), unspecified, with other forms of angina pectoris** A
        Excludes1   other forms of angina pectoris without atherosclerosis of coronary artery bypass graft (I20.8-)

    I25.709   **Atherosclerosis of coronary artery bypass graft(s), unspecified, with unspecified angina pectoris** A
        Excludes1   unspecified angina pectoris without atherosclerosis of coronary artery bypass graft (I20.9)

  ● **I25.71**   **Atherosclerosis of autologous vein coronary artery bypass graft(s) with angina pectoris**

    I25.710   **Atherosclerosis of autologous vein coronary artery bypass graft(s) with unstable angina pectoris** A
        Excludes1   unstable angina without atherosclerosis of autologous vein coronary artery bypass graft(s) (I20.0)
        Excludes2   embolism or thrombus of coronary artery bypass graft(s) (T82.8-)

    I25.711   **Atherosclerosis of autologous vein coronary artery bypass graft(s) with angina pectoris with documented spasm** A
        Excludes1   angina pectoris with documented spasm without atherosclerosis of autologous vein coronary artery bypass graft(s) (I20.1)

    I25.712   **Atherosclerosis of autologous vein coronary artery bypass graft(s) with refractory angina pectoris** A

    I25.718   **Atherosclerosis of autologous vein coronary artery bypass graft(s) with other forms of angina pectoris** A
        Excludes1   other forms of angina pectoris without atherosclerosis of autologous vein coronary artery bypass graft(s) (I20.8-)

    I25.719   **Atherosclerosis of autologous vein coronary artery bypass graft(s) with unspecified angina pectoris** A
        Excludes1   unspecified angina pectoris without atherosclerosis of autologous vein coronary artery bypass graft(s) (I20.9)

  ● **I25.72**   **Atherosclerosis of autologous artery coronary artery bypass graft(s) with angina pectoris**
Atherosclerosis of internal mammary artery graft with angina pectoris

    I25.720   **Atherosclerosis of autologous artery coronary artery bypass graft(s) with unstable angina pectoris** A
        Excludes1   unstable angina without atherosclerosis of autologous artery coronary artery bypass graft(s) (I20.0)

▶ New   ⇒ Revised   ~~deleted~~ Deleted   Excludes 1   Excludes 2   Includes   Use additional   Code first   Code also   Key words
OGCR Official Guidelines   X Assign placeholder X   ● Use Additional Character(s)   ▶ Manifestation Code   🐾 Hierarchical Condition Category   **Coding Clinic**

I25.721   Atherosclerosis of autologous artery coronary artery bypass graft(s) with angina pectoris with documented spasm 🔖   A

     Excludes1   angina pectoris with documented spasm without atherosclerosis of autologous artery coronary artery bypass graft(s) (I20.1)

I25.722   Atherosclerosis of autologous artery coronary artery bypass graft(s) with refractory angina pectoris   A

I25.728   Atherosclerosis of autologous artery coronary artery bypass graft(s) with other forms of angina pectoris 🔖   A

     Excludes1   other forms of angina pectoris without atherosclerosis of autologous artery coronary artery bypass graft(s) (I20.8-)

I25.729   Atherosclerosis of autologous artery coronary artery bypass graft(s) with unspecified angina pectoris 🔖   A

     Excludes1   unspecified angina pectoris without atherosclerosis of autologous artery coronary artery bypass graft(s) (I20.9)

● I25.73   Atherosclerosis of nonautologous biological coronary artery bypass graft(s) with angina pectoris

I25.730   Atherosclerosis of nonautologous biological coronary artery bypass graft(s) with unstable angina pectoris 🔖   A

     Excludes1   unstable angina without atherosclerosis of nonautologous biological coronary artery bypass graft(s) (I20.0)

I25.731   Atherosclerosis of nonautologous biological coronary artery bypass graft(s) with angina pectoris with documented spasm 🔖   A

     Excludes1   angina pectoris with documented spasm without atherosclerosis of nonautologous biological coronary artery bypass graft(s) (I20.1)

I25.732   Atherosclerosis of nonautologous biological coronary artery bypass graft(s)with refractory angina pectoris   A

I25.738   Atherosclerosis of nonautologous biological coronary artery bypass graft(s) with other forms of angina pectoris 🔖   A

     Excludes1   other forms of angina pectoris without atherosclerosis of nonautologous biological coronary artery bypass graft(s) (I20.8-)

I25.739   Atherosclerosis of nonautologous biological coronary artery bypass graft(s) with unspecified angina pectoris 🔖   A

     Excludes1   unspecified angina pectoris without atherosclerosis of nonautologous biological coronary artery bypass graft(s) (I20.9)

● I25.75   Atherosclerosis of native coronary artery of transplanted heart with angina pectoris

     Excludes1   atherosclerosis of native coronary artery of transplanted heart without angina pectoris (I25.811)

I25.750   Atherosclerosis of native coronary artery of transplanted heart with unstable angina 🔖

I25.751   Atherosclerosis of native coronary artery of transplanted heart with angina pectoris with documented spasm 🔖

I25.752   Atherosclerosis of native coronary artery of transplanted heart with refractory angina pectoris   A

I25.758   Atherosclerosis of native coronary artery of transplanted heart with other forms of angina pectoris 🔖

I25.759   Atherosclerosis of native coronary artery of transplanted heart with unspecified angina pectoris 🔖

● I25.76   Atherosclerosis of bypass graft of coronary artery of transplanted heart with angina pectoris

     Excludes1   atherosclerosis of bypass graft of coronary artery of transplanted heart without angina pectoris (I25.812)

I25.760   Atherosclerosis of bypass graft of coronary artery of transplanted heart with unstable angina 🔖   A

I25.761   Atherosclerosis of bypass graft of coronary artery of transplanted heart with angina pectoris with documented spasm 🔖   A

I25.762   Atherosclerosis of bypass graft of coronary artery of transplanted heart with refractory angina pectoris   A

I25.768   Atherosclerosis of bypass graft of coronary artery of transplanted heart with other forms of angina pectoris 🔖   A

I25.769   Atherosclerosis of bypass graft of coronary artery of transplanted heart with unspecified angina pectoris 🔖   A

CHAPTER 9 (I00-I99)

● **I25.79** **Atherosclerosis of other coronary artery bypass graft(s) with angina pectoris**   A

    I25.790 **Atherosclerosis of other coronary artery bypass graft(s) with unstable angina pectoris** 🦠

          Excludes1   unstable angina without atherosclerosis of other coronary artery bypass graft(s) (I20.0)

    I25.791 **Atherosclerosis of other coronary artery bypass graft(s) with angina pectoris with documented spasm** 🦠   A

          Excludes1   angina pectoris with documented spasm without atherosclerosis of other coronary artery bypass graft(s) (I20.1)

    I25.792 **Atherosclerosis of other coronary artery bypass graft(s) with refractory angina pectoris**   A

    I25.798 **Atherosclerosis of other coronary artery bypass graft(s) with other forms of angina pectoris** 🦠   A

          Excludes1   other forms of angina pectoris without atherosclerosis of other coronary artery bypass graft(s) (I20.8-)

    I25.799 **Atherosclerosis of other coronary artery bypass graft(s) with unspecified angina pectoris** 🦠   A

          Excludes1   unspecified angina pectoris without atherosclerosis of other coronary artery bypass graft(s) (I20.9)

● **I25.8** **Other forms of chronic ischemic heart disease**

  ● **I25.81** **Atherosclerosis of other coronary vessels without angina pectoris**

     Use additional code, if applicable, to identify:
     coronary atherosclerosis due to calcified coronary lesion (I25.84)
     coronary atherosclerosis due to lipid rich plaque (I25.83)

      Excludes2   atherosclerotic heart disease of native coronary artery without angina pectoris (I25.10)

    I25.810 **Atherosclerosis of coronary artery bypass graft(s) without angina pectoris**   A
        Atherosclerosis of coronary artery bypass graft NOS

          Excludes1   atherosclerosis of coronary bypass graft(s) with angina pectoris (I25.70- -I25.73-, I25.79-)

        Coding Clinic: 2016, Q4, P86

    I25.811 **Atherosclerosis of native coronary artery of transplanted heart without angina pectoris**
        Atherosclerosis of native coronary artery of transplanted heart NOS

          Excludes1   atherosclerosis of native coronary artery of transplanted heart with angina pectoris (I25.75-)

    I25.812 **Atherosclerosis of bypass graft of coronary artery of transplanted heart without angina pectoris**   A
        Atherosclerosis of bypass graft of transplanted heart NOS

          Excludes1   atherosclerosis of bypass graft of transplanted heart with angina pectoris (I25.76)

  I25.82 **Chronic total occlusion of coronary artery**
     Complete occlusion of coronary artery
     Total occlusion of coronary artery

     Code first coronary atherosclerosis (I25.1-, I25.7-, I25.81-)

      Excludes1   acute coronary occlusion with myocardial infarction (I21.0-I21.B, I22.-)
           acute coronary occlusion without myocardial infarction (I24.0)

  I25.83 **Coronary atherosclerosis due to lipid rich plaque**   A

     Code first coronary atherosclerosis (I25.1-, I25.7-, I25.81-)

  I25.84 **Coronary atherosclerosis due to calcified coronary lesion**
     Coronary atherosclerosis due to severely calcified coronary lesion

     Code first coronary atherosclerosis (I25.1-, I25.7-, I25.81-)

  I25.85 **Chronic coronary microvascular dysfunction**
     Chronic (presentation of) coronary microvascular disease
     Coronary microvascular dysfunction NOS

  I25.89 **Other forms of chronic ischemic heart disease**

 I25.9 **Chronic ischemic heart disease, unspecified**
     Ischemic heart disease (chronic) NOS

PULMONARY HEART DISEASE AND DISEASES OF PULMONARY CIRCULATION (I26-I28)

● **I26** **Pulmonary embolism**

  Includes   cor pulmonale without embolism (I27.81)
         pulmonary (acute)(artery)(vein) infarction
         pulmonary (acute)(artery)(vein) thromboembolism
         pulmonary (acute)(artery)(vein) thrombosis

  Excludes2   chronic pulmonary embolism (I27.82)
         personal history of pulmonary embolism (Z86.711)
         pulmonary embolism due to trauma (T79.0, T79.1)
         pulmonary embolism due to complications of surgical and medical care (T80.0, T81.7-, T82.8-)
         pulmonary embolism complicating abortion, ectopic or molar pregnancy (O00-O07, O08.2)
         pulmonary embolism complicating pregnancy, childbirth and the puerperium (O88.-)
         septic (non-pulmonary) arterial embolism (I76)

  Coding Clinic: 2021, Q2, P10

Item 9–7 Pulmonary heart disease or **cor pulmonale** is right ventricle hypertrophy or RVH as a result of a respiratory disorder increasing back flow pressure to the right ventricle. Left untreated, cor pulmonale leads to right-heart failure and death.

CHAPTER 9 (I00-I99)

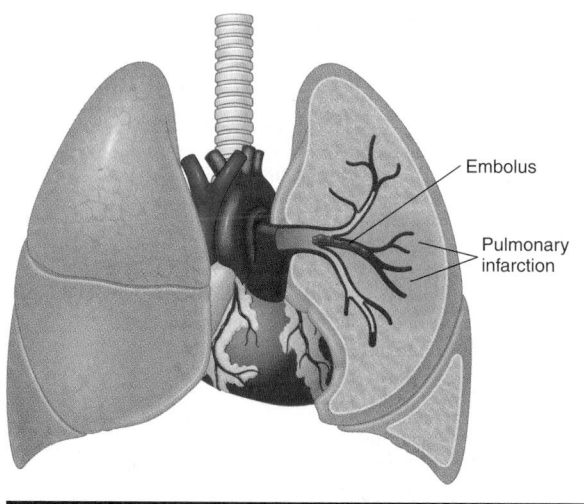

Figure 9-3 Pulmonary embolism. (From Chabner: The Language of Medicine, ed 8, St. Louis, Saunders, 2007)

● **I26.0** **Pulmonary embolism with acute cor pulmonale**

I26.01 **Septic pulmonary embolism with acute cor pulmonale** 🔊

  Code first underlying infection

I26.02 **Saddle embolus of pulmonary artery with acute cor pulmonale** 🔊

  ▶ **I26.03** **Cement embolism of pulmonary artery with acute cor pulmonale**

    ▶ *Code first complication of other artery following a procedure (T81.718)*

  ▶**I26.04** **Fat embolism of pulmonary artery with acute cor pulmonale**

    ▶ *Code first, if applicable:*
    complication of other artery following a procedure (T81.718)
    ▶*traumatic fat embolism (T79.1)*

I26.09 **Other pulmonary embolism with acute cor pulmonale** 🔊

  Acute cor pulmonale NOS
  ▶Other thrombotic pulmonary embolism with acute cor pulmonale

● **I26.9** **Pulmonary embolism without acute cor pulmonale**

I26.90 **Septic pulmonary embolism without acute cor pulmonale** 🔊

  Code first underlying infection

I26.92 **Saddle embolus of pulmonary artery without acute cor pulmonale** 🔊

◗**I26.93** **Single subsegmental thrombotic pulmonary embolism without acute cor pulmonale** 🔊

  Subsegmental pulmonary embolism NOS

◗**I26.94** **Multiple subsegmental thrombotic pulmonary emboli without acute cor pulmonale** 🔊
  Coding Clinic: 2022, Q2, P13; 2021, Q2, P10

  ▶ **I26.95** **Cement embolism of pulmonary artery without acute cor pulmonale**

    ▶ *Code first complication of other artery following a procedure (T81.718)*

  ▶**I26.96** **Fat embolism of pulmonary artery without acute cor pulmonale**

    ▶ *Code first, if applicable:*
    complication of other artery following a procedure (T81.718)
    ▶*traumatic fat embolism (T79.1)*

I26.99 **Other pulmonary embolism without acute cor pulmonale** 🔊

  Acute pulmonary embolism NOS
  ▶Other thrombotic pulmonary embolism with acute cor pulmonale
  Pulmonary embolism NOS
  Coding Clinic: 2022, Q2, P13; 2019, Q2, P22-23

● **I27** **Other pulmonary heart diseases**

I27.0 **Primary pulmonary hypertension** 🔊

  Heritable pulmonary arterial hypertension
  Idiopathic pulmonary arterial hypertension
  Primary group 1 pulmonary hypertension
  Primary pulmonary arterial hypertension

  Excludes1 persistent pulmonary hypertension of newborn (P29.30)
  pulmonary hypertension NOS (I27.20)
  secondary pulmonary arterial hypertension (I27.21)
  secondary pulmonary hypertension (I27.29)

I27.1 **Kyphoscoliotic heart disease** 🔊

● **I27.2** **Other secondary pulmonary hypertension**

  Code also associated underlying condition

  Excludes1 Eisenmenger's syndrome (I27.83)
  Coding Clinic: 2016, Q2, P8

I27.20 **Pulmonary hypertension, unspecified** 🔊

  Pulmonary hypertension NOS

I27.21 **Secondary pulmonary arterial hypertension** 🔊

  (Associated) (drug-induced) (toxin-induced) pulmonary arterial hypertension NOS
  (Associated) (drug-induced) (toxin-induced) (secondary) group 1 pulmonary hypertension

  Code also associated conditions if applicable, or adverse effects of drugs or toxins, such as:
  adverse effect of appetite depressants (T50.5X5)
  congenital heart disease (Q20-Q28)
  human immunodeficiency virus [HIV] disease (B20)
  polymyositis (M33.2-)
  portal hypertension (K76.6)
  rheumatoid arthritis (M05.-)
  schistosomiasis (B65.-)
  Sjögren syndrome (M35.0-)
  systemic sclerosis (M34.-)

I27.22 **Pulmonary hypertension due to left heart disease** 🔊

  Group 2 pulmonary hypertension

  Code also associated left heart disease, if known, such as:
  multiple valve disease (I08.-)
  rheumatic mitral valve diseases (I05.-)
  rheumatic aortic valve diseases (I06.-)

I27.23 **Pulmonary hypertension due to lung diseases and hypoxia** 🔊

  Group 3 pulmonary hypertension

  Code also associated lung disease, if known, such as:
  bronchiectasis (J47.-)
  cystic fibrosis with pulmonary manifestations (E84.0)
  interstitial lung disease (J84.-)
  pleural effusion (J90)
  sleep apnea (G47.3-)

I27.24 **Chronic thromboembolic pulmonary hypertension** 🔊

  Group 4 pulmonary hypertension

  Code also associated pulmonary embolism, if applicable (I26.-, I27.82)

CHAPTER 9 (I00–I99)

I27.29 Other secondary pulmonary hypertension 🅗
Group 5 pulmonary hypertension
Pulmonary hypertension with unclear multifactorial mechanisms
Pulmonary hypertension due to hematologic disorders
Pulmonary hypertension due to metabolic disorders
Pulmonary hypertension due to other systemic disorders
Code also other associated disorders, if known, such as:
chronic myeloid leukemia (C92.10-C92.22)
essential thrombocythemia (D47.3)
Gaucher disease (E75.22)
hypertensive chronic kidney disease with end stage renal disease (I12.0, I13.11,I13.2)
hyperthyroidism (E05.-)
hypothyroidism (E00-E03)
polycythemia vera (D45)
sarcoidosis (D86.-)

● **I27.8 Other specified pulmonary heart diseases**
I27.81 Cor pulmonale (chronic) 🅗
Cor pulmonale NOS
Code also, if applicable, right heart failure (I50.81-)
Excludes1   acute cor pulmonale (I26.0-)

I27.82 Chronic pulmonary embolism 🅗
Use additional code, if applicable, for associated long-term (current) use of anticoagulants (Z79.01)
Excludes1   personal history of pulmonary embolism (Z86.711)
Coding Clinic: 2021, Q2, P10

I27.83 Eisenmenger's syndrome 🅗
Eisenmenger's complex
(Irreversible) Eisenmenger's disease
Pulmonary hypertension with right to left shunt related to congenital heart disease
Code also underlying heart defect, if known, such as:
atrial septal defect (Q21.1-)
Eisenmenger's defect (Q21.8)
patent ductus arteriosus (Q25.0)
ventricular septal defect (Q21.0)

I27.89 Other specified pulmonary heart diseases 🅗

I27.9 Pulmonary heart disease, unspecified 🅗
Chronic cardiopulmonary disease

● **I28 Other diseases of pulmonary vessels**
I28.0 Arteriovenous fistula of pulmonary vessels 🅗
Excludes1   congenital arteriovenous fistula (Q25.72)

I28.1 Aneurysm of pulmonary artery 🅗
Excludes1   congenital aneurysm (Q25.79)
congenital arteriovenous aneurysm (Q25.72)

I28.8 Other diseases of pulmonary vessels 🅗
Pulmonary arteritis
Pulmonary endarteritis
Rupture of pulmonary vessels
Stenosis of pulmonary vessels
Stricture of pulmonary vessels

I28.9 Disease of pulmonary vessels, unspecified 🅗

OTHER FORMS OF HEART DISEASE (I30-I5A)

● **I30 Acute pericarditis**
Inflammation of pericardium (sac surrounding the heart) caused by an infection
Includes   acute mediastinopericarditis
acute myopericarditis
acute pericardial effusion
acute pleuropericarditis
acute pneumopericarditis
Excludes1   Dressler's syndrome (I24.1)
rheumatic pericarditis (acute) (I01.0)
➡ viral pericarditis due to Coxsackie virus (B33.23)

I30.0 Acute nonspecific idiopathic pericarditis

I30.1 Infective pericarditis
Pneumococcal pericarditis
Pneumopyopericardium
Purulent pericarditis
Pyopericarditis
Pyopericardium
Pyopneumopericardium
Staphylococcal pericarditis
Streptococcal pericarditis
Suppurative pericarditis
Viral pericarditis
Use additional code (B95-B97) to identify infectious agent

I30.8 Other forms of acute pericarditis

I30.9 Acute pericarditis, unspecified

● **I31 Other diseases of pericardium**
Excludes1   diseases of pericardium specified as rheumatic (I09.2)
postcardiotomy syndrome (I97.0)
traumatic injury to pericardium (S26.-)

I31.0 Chronic adhesive pericarditis
Accretio cordis
Adherent pericardium
Adhesive mediastinopericarditis

I31.1 Chronic constrictive pericarditis
Concretio cordis
Pericardial calcification

I31.2 Hemopericardium, not elsewhere classified
Excludes1   hemopericardium as current complication following acute myocardial infarction (I23.0)

● **I31.3 Pericardial effusion (noninflammatory)**
Excludes1   acute pericardial effusion (I30.9)
Coding Clinic: 2019, Q1, P16

I31.31 Malignant pericardial effusion in diseases classified elsewhere
Code first underlying neoplasm (C00-D49)
Coding Clinic: 2022, Q4, P24

I31.39 Other pericardial effusion (noninflammatory)
Chylopericardium

I31.4 Cardiac tamponade
Code first underlying cause

I31.8 Other specified diseases of pericardium
Epicardial plaques
Focal pericardial adhesions

I31.9 Disease of pericardium, unspecified
Pericarditis (chronic) NOS

▷ **I32 Pericarditis in diseases classified elsewhere**
Code first underlying disease
Excludes1   pericarditis (in):
coxsackie (virus) (B33.23)
gonococcal (A54.83)
meningococcal (A39.53)
rheumatoid (arthritis) (M05.31)
syphilitic (A52.06)
systemic lupus erythematosus (M32.12)
tuberculosis (A18.84)

▶ New   ⇒ Revised   ~~deleted~~ Deleted   Excludes 1   Excludes 2   Includes   Use additional   Code first   Code also   Key words
OGCR Official Guidelines   X Assign placeholder X   ● Use Additional Character(s)   ▷ Manifestation Code   🅗 Hierarchical Condition Category   Coding Clinic

● **I33**　**Acute and subacute endocarditis**
Inflammation/infection of lining of heart, affecting heart valves including
replacement valves and is usually caused by a bacterial infection
　　　Excludes1　acute rheumatic endocarditis (I01.1)
　　　　　　　　　endocarditis NOS (I38)

　　I33.0　**Acute and subacute infective endocarditis**
　　　　　Bacterial endocarditis (acute) (subacute)
　　　　　Infective endocarditis (acute) (subacute) NOS
　　　　　Endocarditis lenta (acute) (subacute)
　　　　　Malignant endocarditis (acute) (subacute)
　　　　　Purulent endocarditis (acute) (subacute)
　　　　　Septic endocarditis (acute) (subacute)
　　　　　Ulcerative endocarditis (acute) (subacute)
　　　　　Vegetative endocarditis (acute) (subacute)
　　　　　Use additional code (B95-B97) to identify infectious
　　　　　　agent

　　I33.9　**Acute and subacute endocarditis, unspecified**
　　　　　Acute endocarditis NOS
　　　　　Acute myoendocarditis NOS
　　　　　Acute periendocarditis NOS
　　　　　Subacute endocarditis NOS
　　　　　Subacute myoendocarditis NOS
　　　　　Subacute periendocarditis NOS

● **I34**　**Nonrheumatic mitral valve disorders**
　　Code also, if applicable:
　　nonrheumatic mitral (valve) annulus calcification (I34.81)
　　　Excludes1　mitral valve disease (I05.9)
　　　　　　　　　mitral valve failure (I05.8)
　　　　　　　　　mitral valve stenosis (I05.0)
　　　　　　　　　mitral valve disorder of unspecified cause with
　　　　　　　　　　diseases of aortic and/or tricuspid valve(s)
　　　　　　　　　　(I08.-)
　　　　　　　　　mitral valve disorder of unspecified cause with
　　　　　　　　　　mitral stenosis or obstruction (I05.0)
　　　　　　　　　mitral valve disorder specified as congenital
　　　　　　　　　　(Q23.2, Q23.9)
　　　　　　　　　mitral valve disorder specified as rheumatic
　　　　　　　　　　(I05.-)

　　I34.0　**Nonrheumatic mitral (valve) insufficiency**
　　　　　Nonrheumatic mitral (valve) incompetence NOS
　　　　　Nonrheumatic mitral (valve) regurgitation NOS

　　I34.1　**Nonrheumatic mitral (valve) prolapse**
　　　　　Floppy nonrheumatic mitral valve syndrome
　　　　　　Excludes1　Marfan's syndrome (Q87.4-)

　　I34.2　**Nonrheumatic mitral (valve) stenosis**
　　　　　Code also, if applicable:
　　　　　nonrheumatic mitral (valve) annulus calcification
　　　　　　(I34.81)

● **I34.8**　**Other nonrheumatic mitral valve disorders**
　　　I34.81　**Nonrheumatic mitral (valve) annulus**
　　　　　　calcification
　　　　　　Nonrheumatic mitral (valve) annular
　　　　　　　calcification
　　　　　　Mitral (valve) annulus calcification NOS
　　　　　　Code also, if applicable:
　　　　　　　nonrheumatic mitral (valve) insufficiency
　　　　　　　　(I34.0)
　　　　　　　nonrheumatic mitral (valve) stenosis (I34.2)
　　　I34.89　**Other nonrheumatic mitral valve disorders**
　　I34.9　**Nonrheumatic mitral valve disorder, unspecified**

● **I35**　**Nonrheumatic aortic valve disorders**
　　　~~**Excludes1**~~　~~aortic valve disorder of unspecified cause but~~
　　　　　　　　　~~with diseases of mitral and/or tricuspid~~
　　　　　　　　　~~valve(s) (I08.-)~~
　　　　　　　　~~aortic valve disorder specified as congenital~~
　　　　　　　　　~~(Q23.0, Q23.1)~~
　　　　　　　　~~aortic valve disorder specified as rheumatic (I06.-)~~
　　　　　　　　~~hypertrophic subaortic stenosis~~
　　Code also, if applicable, bicuspid aortic valve (Q23.81)
　　▶**Excludes2**　aortic valve disorder of unspecified cause but
　　　　　　　　　with diseases of mitral and/or tricuspid
　　　　　　　　　valve(s) (I08.-)
　　　　　　　▶aortic valve disorder specified as congenital
　　　　　　　　　(Q23.0, Q23.1)
　　　　　　　▶aortic valve disorder specified as rheumatic (I06.-)
　　　　　　　▶hypertrophic subaortic stenosis (I42.1)

　　I35.0　**Nonrheumatic aortic (valve) stenosis**
　　I35.1　**Nonrheumatic aortic (valve) insufficiency**
　　　　　Nonrheumatic aortic (valve) incompetence NOS
　　　　　Nonrheumatic aortic (valve) regurgitation NOS
　　I35.2　**Nonrheumatic aortic (valve) stenosis with insufficiency**
　　I35.8　**Other nonrheumatic aortic valve disorders**
　　I35.9　**Nonrheumatic aortic valve disorder, unspecified**

● **I36**　**Nonrheumatic tricuspid valve disorders**
　　　Excludes1　tricuspid valve disorders of unspecified cause
　　　　　　　　　(I07.-)
　　　　　　　　tricuspid valve disorders specified as congenital
　　　　　　　　　(Q22.4, Q22.8, Q22.9)
　　　　　　　　tricuspid valve disorders specified as rheumatic
　　　　　　　　　(I07.-)
　　　　　　　　tricuspid valve disorders with aortic and/or
　　　　　　　　　mitral valve involvement (I08.-)

　　I36.0　**Nonrheumatic tricuspid (valve) stenosis**
　　I36.1　**Nonrheumatic tricuspid (valve) insufficiency**
　　　　　Nonrheumatic tricuspid (valve) incompetence
　　　　　Nonrheumatic tricuspid (valve) regurgitation
　　I36.2　**Nonrheumatic tricuspid (valve) stenosis with**
　　　　　　insufficiency
　　I36.8　**Other nonrheumatic tricuspid valve disorders**
　　I36.9　**Nonrheumatic tricuspid valve disorder, unspecified**

● **I37**　**Nonrheumatic pulmonary valve disorders**
　　　Excludes1　pulmonary valve disorder specified as congenital
　　　　　　　　　(Q22.1, Q22.2, Q22.3)
　　　　　　　　pulmonary valve disorder specified as rheumatic
　　　　　　　　　(I09.89)

　　I37.0　**Nonrheumatic pulmonary valve stenosis**
　　I37.1　**Nonrheumatic pulmonary valve insufficiency**
　　　　　Nonrheumatic pulmonary valve incompetence
　　　　　Nonrheumatic pulmonary valve regurgitation
　　I37.2　**Nonrheumatic pulmonary valve stenosis with**
　　　　　　insufficiency
　　I37.8　**Other nonrheumatic pulmonary valve disorders**
　　I37.9　**Nonrheumatic pulmonary valve disorder, unspecified**
　　I38　**Endocarditis, valve unspecified**
　　　Includes　endocarditis (chronic) NOS
　　　　　　　valvular incompetence NOS
　　　　　　　valvular insufficiency NOS
　　　　　　　valvular regurgitation NOS
　　　　　　　valvular stenosis NOS
　　　　　　　valvulitis (chronic) NOS

　　　Excludes1　congenital insufficiency of cardiac valve NOS (Q24.8)
　　　　　　　　congenital stenosis of cardiac valve NOS (Q24.8)
　　　　　　　　endocardial fibroelastosis (I42.4)
　　　　　　　　endocarditis specified as rheumatic (I09.1)

CHAPTER 9 (I00-I99)

CHAPTER 9 (I00-I99)

▶ **I39** *Endocarditis and heart valve disorders in diseases classified elsewhere*

> *Code first underlying disease, such as:*
> Q fever (A78)

> **Excludes1**   endocardial involvement in:
> candidiasis (B37.6)
> gonococcal infection (A54.83)
> Libman-Sacks disease (M32.11)
> listerosis (A32.82)
> meningococcal infection (A39.51)
> rheumatoid arthritis (M05.31)
> syphilis (A52.03)
> tuberculosis (A18.84)
> typhoid fever (A01.02)

● **I40** **Acute myocarditis**

> *Inflammation of heart muscle due to infection (viral/bacterial)*

> **Includes**   subacute myocarditis
> **Excludes1**   acute rheumatic myocarditis (I01.2)

I40.0   **Infective myocarditis**
> Septic myocarditis
> Use additional code (B95-B97) to identify infectious agent

I40.1   **Isolated myocarditis**
> Fiedler's myocarditis
> Giant cell myocarditis
> Idiopathic myocarditis

I40.8   **Other acute myocarditis**

I40.9   **Acute myocarditis, unspecified**

▶ **I41** *Myocarditis in diseases classified elsewhere*

> *Code first underlying disease, such as:*
> typhus (A75.0-A75.9)

> **Excludes1**   myocarditis (in):
> Chagas' disease (chronic) (B57.2)
> acute (B57.0)
> coxsackie (virus) infection (B33.22)
> diphtheritic (A36.81)
> gonococcal (A54.83)
> influenzal (J09.X9, J10.82, J11.82)
> meningococcal (A39.52)
> mumps (B26.82)
> rheumatoid arthritis (M05.31)
> sarcoid (D86.85)
> syphilis (A52.06)
> toxoplasmosis (B58.81)
> tuberculous (A18.84)

● **I42** **Cardiomyopathy**

> *Disease of the heart muscle resulting in an abnormally enlarged, weakened, thickened, and/or stiffened muscles*

> **Includes**   myocardiopathy

> *Code first pre-existing cardiomyopathy complicating pregnancy and puerperium (O99.4)*

> **Excludes2**   ischemic cardiomyopathy (I25.5)
> peripartum cardiomyopathy (O90.3)
> ventricular hypertrophy (I51.7)

I42.0   **Dilated cardiomyopathy** 🐾
> Congestive cardiomyopathy

I42.1   **Obstructive hypertrophic cardiomyopathy** 🐾
> Hypertrophic subaortic stenosis (idiopathic)

I42.2   **Other hypertrophic cardiomyopathy** 🐾
> Nonobstructive hypertrophic cardiomyopathy

I42.3   **Endomyocardial (eosinophilic) disease** 🐾
> Endomyocardial (tropical) fibrosis
> Löffler's endocarditis

I42.4   **Endocardial fibroelastosis** 🐾
> Congenital cardiomyopathy
> Elastomyofibrosis

I42.5   **Other restrictive cardiomyopathy** 🐾
> Constrictive cardiomyopathy NOS

I42.6   **Alcoholic cardiomyopathy** 🐾
> Code also presence of alcoholism (F10.-)

I42.7   **Cardiomyopathy due to drug and external agent** 🐾
> *Code first poisoning due to drug or toxin, if applicable (T36-T65 with fifth or sixth character 1-4)*
> Use additional code for adverse effect, if applicable, to identify drug (T36-T50 with fifth or sixth character 5)
> **Coding Clinic: 2021, Q3, P8**

I42.8   **Other cardiomyopathies** 🐾

I42.9   **Cardiomyopathy, unspecified** 🐾
> Cardiomyopathy (primary) (secondary) NOS

▶ **I43** *Cardiomyopathy in diseases classified elsewhere* 🐾

> *Code first underlying disease, such as:*
> amyloidosis (E85.-)
> glycogen storage disease (E74.0-)
> gout (M10.0-)
> thyrotoxicosis (E05.0-E05.9-)

> **Excludes1**   cardiomyopathy (in):
> coxsackie (virus) (B33.24)
> diphtheria (A36.81)
> sarcoidosis (D86.85)
> tuberculosis (A18.84)
> **Coding Clinic: 2024, Q2, P9**

● **I44** **Atrioventricular and left bundle-branch block**

> *Conduction problem resulting in arrhythmias/dysrhythmias due to a lack of electrical impulses being transmitted normally through the heart*

I44.0   **Atrioventricular block, first degree**

I44.1   **Atrioventricular block, second degree**
> Atrioventricular block, type I and II
> Möbitz block, type I and II
> Second degree block, type I and II
> Wenckebach's block

I44.2   **Atrioventricular block, complete** 🐾
> Complete heart block NOS
> Third degree block
> **Coding Clinic: 2019, Q2, P4**

● **I44.3**   **Other and unspecified atrioventricular block**
> Atrioventricular block NOS

> **I44.30**   **Unspecified atrioventricular block**
> **I44.39**   **Other atrioventricular block**

I44.4   **Left anterior fascicular block**

I44.5   **Left posterior fascicular block**

● **I44.6**   **Other and unspecified fascicular block**

> **I44.60**   **Unspecified fascicular block**
> Left bundle-branch hemiblock NOS
> **I44.69**   **Other fascicular block**

I44.7   **Left bundle-branch block, unspecified**

● **I45** **Other conduction disorders**

I45.0   **Right fascicular block**

● **I45.1**   **Other and unspecified right bundle-branch block**

> **I45.10**   **Unspecified right bundle-branch block**
> Right bundle-branch block NOS
> **I45.19**   **Other right bundle-branch block**

I45.2   **Bifascicular block**

I45.3   **Trifascicular block**

I45.4   **Nonspecific intraventricular block**
> Bundle-branch block NOS

I45.5   **Other specified heart block**
> Sinoatrial block
> Sinoauricular block
> **Excludes1**   heart block NOS (I45.9)

I45.6   **Pre-excitation syndrome**
> Accelerated atrioventricular conduction
> Accessory atrioventricular conduction
> Anomalous atrioventricular excitation
> Lown-Ganong-Levine syndrome
> Pre-excitation atrioventricular conduction
> Wolff-Parkinson-White syndrome

● **I45.8**   **Other specified conduction disorders**

     I45.81   Long QT syndrome

     I45.89   Other specified conduction disorders

         Atrioventricular [AV] dissociation

         Interference dissociation

         Isorhythmic dissociation

         Nonparoxysmal AV nodal tachycardia

         Coding Clinic: 2013, Q2, P32

   I45.9   **Conduction disorder, unspecified**

         Heart block NOS

         Stokes-Adams syndrome

● **I46**   **Cardiac arrest**

     Excludes2   cardiogenic shock (R57.0)

   I46.2   **Cardiac arrest due to underlying cardiac condition** 🔖

         Code first underlying cardiac condition

         Coding Clinic: 2024, Q1, P27

   I46.8   **Cardiac arrest due to other underlying condition** 🔖

         Code first underlying condition

   I46.9   **Cardiac arrest, cause unspecified** 🔖

● **I47**   **Paroxysmal tachycardia**

     Code first tachycardia complicating:

         abortion or ectopic or molar pregnancy (O00-O07, O08.8)

         obstetric surgery and procedures (O75.4)

     Excludes1   tachycardia NOS (R00.0)

         sinoauricular tachycardia NOS (R00.0)

         sinus [sinusal] tachycardia NOS (R00.0)

   I47.0   **Re-entry ventricular arrhythmia** 🔖

● **I47.1**   **Supraventricular tachycardia** 🔖

     I47.10   Supraventricular tachycardia, unspecified

     I47.11   Inappropriate sinus tachycardia, so stated

         IST

     I47.19   Other supraventricular tachycardia

         Atrial (paroxysmal) tachycardia

         Atrioventricular [AV] (paroxysmal) tachycardia

         Atrioventricular re-entrant (nodal) tachycardia [AVNRT] [AVRT]

         Junctional (paroxysmal) tachycardia

         Nodal (paroxysmal) tachycardia

● **I47.2**   **Ventricular tachycardia** 🔖

     I47.20   Ventricular tachycardia, unspecified

     I47.21   Torsades de pointes

         Code also, if applicable, long QT syndrome (I45.81)

         Use Additional code for adverse effect, if applicable, to identify drug (T36-T50 with fifth or sixth character 5)

         Coding Clinic: 2022, Q4, P24

     I47.29   Other ventricular tachycardia

         Coding Clinic: 2021, Q3, P12; 2013, Q3, P23

   I47.9   **Paroxysmal tachycardia, unspecified** 🔖

         Bouveret (-Hoffman) syndrome

● **I48**   **Atrial fibrillation and flutter**

     Most common abnormal heart rhythm (arrhythmia) presenting as irregular, rapid beating (tachycardia) of the heart's upper chamber.

   I48.0   **Paroxysmal atrial fibrillation** 🔖

● **I48.1**   **Persistent atrial fibrillation** 🔖

     Rapid contractions of the upper heart chamber

     Excludes1   Permanent atrial fibrillation (I48.21)

     Coding Clinic: 2019, Q2, P3-4

     I48.11   Longstanding persistent atrial fibrillation

     I48.19   Other persistent atrial fibrillation

         Chronic persistent atrial fibrillation

         Persistent atrial fibrillation, NOS

● **I48.2**   **Chronic atrial fibrillation** 🔖

     Coding Clinic: 2019, Q2, P3

     I48.20   Chronic atrial fibrillation, unspecified

         Excludes1   Chronic persistent atrial fibrillation (I48.19)

     I48.21   Permanent atrial fibrillation

   I48.3   **Typical atrial flutter** 🔖

         Type I atrial flutter

   I48.4   **Atypical atrial flutter** 🔖

         Type II atrial flutter

● **I48.9**   **Unspecified atrial fibrillation and atrial flutter**

     I48.91   Unspecified atrial fibrillation 🔖

     I48.92   Unspecified atrial flutter 🔖

● **I49**   **Other cardiac arrhythmias**

     Code first cardiac arrhythmia complicating:

         abortion or ectopic or molar pregnancy (O00-O07, O08.8)

         obstetric surgery and procedures (O75.4)

     ~~Excludes1~~   ~~neonatal dysrhythmia (P29.1-)~~

         ~~sinoatrial bradycardia (R00.1)~~

         ~~sinus bradycardia (R00.1)~~

         ~~vagal bradycardia (R00.1)~~

     Excludes2   bradycardia NOS (R00.1)

         ▶neonatal dysrhythmia (P29.1-)

         ▶sinoatrial bradycardia (R00.1)

         ▶sinus bradycardia (R00.1)

         ▶vagal bradycardia (R00.1)

● **I49.0**   **Ventricular fibrillation and flutter**

     I49.01   Ventricular fibrillation 🔖

         MCC: If patient discharged alive

     I49.02   Ventricular flutter 🔖

   I49.1   **Atrial premature depolarization**

         Atrial premature beats

   I49.2   **Junctional premature depolarization** 🔖

   I49.3   **Ventricular premature depolarization**

● **I49.4**   **Other and unspecified premature depolarization**

     I49.40   Unspecified premature depolarization

         Premature beats NOS

     I49.49   Other premature depolarization

         Ectopic beats

         Extrasystoles

         Extrasystolic arrhythmias

         Premature contractions

   I49.5   **Sick sinus syndrome** 🔖

         Tachycardia-bradycardia syndrome

         Coding Clinic: 2019, Q1, P33

   I49.8   **Other specified cardiac arrhythmias**

         Brugada syndrome

         Coronary sinus rhythm disorder

         Ectopic rhythm disorder

         Nodal rhythm disorder

   I49.9   **Cardiac arrhythmia, unspecified**

         Arrhythmia (cardiac) NOS

● **I50**   **Heart failure**

     Code first heart failure complicating abortion or ectopic or molar pregnancy (O00-O07, O08.8)

         heart failure due to hypertension (I11.0)

         heart failure due to hypertension with chronic kidney disease (I13.-)

         heart failure following surgery (I97.13-)

         obstetric surgery and procedures (O75.4)

         rheumatic heart failure (I09.81)

     Excludes2   cardiac arrest (I46.-)

         neonatal cardiac failure (P29.0)

     Coding Clinic: 2017, Q1, P47; 2016, Q4, P122-123, Q1, P38; 2015, Q2, P15

Item 9–8 Congestive heart failure (CHF) is a condition in which the left ventricle of the heart cannot pump enough blood to the body. The blood flow from the heart slows or returns to the heart from the venous system (back flow) resulting in congestion (fluid accumulation) particularly in the abdomen. Most commonly, fluid collects in the lungs and results in shortness of breath, especially when in a reclining position.

I50.1   **Left ventricular failure, unspecified** 🐾
       Cardiac asthma
       Edema of lung with heart disease NOS
       Edema of lung with heart failure
       Left heart failure
       Pulmonary edema with heart disease NOS
       Pulmonary edema with heart failure

       Excludes1   edema of lung without heart disease or heart failure (J81.-)
                pulmonary edema without heart disease or failure (J81.-)

● **I50.2**   **Systolic (congestive) heart failure**
       Heart failure with reduced ejection fraction [HFrEF]
       Systolic left ventricular heart failure

       Code also end stage heart failure, if applicable (I50.84)

       Excludes1   combined systolic (congestive) and diastolic (congestive) heart failure (I50.4-)

   I50.20   **Unspecified systolic (congestive) heart failure** 🐾

   I50.21   **Acute systolic (congestive) heart failure** 🐾
       Presenting a short and relatively severe episode

   I50.22   **Chronic systolic (congestive) heart failure** 🐾
       Long-lasting, presenting over time

   I50.23   **Acute on chronic systolic (congestive) heart failure** 🐾
       Combination code. What was a chronic condition now has an acute exacerbation (to make more severe).
       Coding Clinic: 2013, Q2, P33

● **I50.3**   **Diastolic (congestive) heart failure**
       Diastolic left ventricular heart failure
       Heart failure with normal ejection fraction
       Heart failure with preserved ejection fraction [HFpEF]

       Code also end stage heart failure, if applicable (I50.84)

       Excludes1   combined systolic (congestive) and diastolic (congestive) heart failure (I50.4-)

   I50.30   **Unspecified diastolic (congestive) heart failure** 🐾

   I50.31   **Acute diastolic (congestive) heart failure** 🐾
       Coding Clinic: 2017, Q1, P46

   I50.32   **Chronic diastolic (congestive) heart failure** 🐾
       Coding Clinic: 2023, Q3, P14

   I50.33   **Acute on chronic diastolic (congestive) heart failure** 🐾
       Coding Clinic: 2024, Q2, P10

● **I50.4**   **Combined systolic (congestive) and diastolic (congestive) heart failure**
       Combined systolic and diastolic left ventricular heart failure
       Heart failure with reduced ejection fraction and diastolic dysfunction

       Code also end stage heart failure, if applicable (I50.84)

   I50.40   **Unspecified combined systolic (congestive) and diastolic (congestive) heart failure** 🐾

   I50.41   **Acute combined systolic (congestive) and diastolic (congestive) heart failure** 🐾

   I50.42   **Chronic combined systolic (congestive) and diastolic (congestive) heart failure** 🐾

   I50.43   **Acute on chronic combined systolic (congestive) and diastolic (congestive) heart failure** 🐾

● **I50.8**   **Other heart failure**

   ● **I50.81**   **Right heart failure**
       Right ventricular failure

     I50.810   **Right heart failure, unspecified** 🐾
       Right heart failure without mention of left heart failure
       Right ventricular failure NOS

     I50.811   **Acute right heart failure** 🐾
       Acute isolated right heart failure
       Acute (isolated) right ventricular failure

     I50.812   **Chronic right heart failure** 🐾
       Chronic isolated right heart failure
       Chronic (isolated) right ventricular failure

     I50.813   **Acute on chronic right heart failure** 🐾
       Acute on chronic isolated right heart failure
       Acute on chronic (isolated) right ventricular failure
       Acute decompensation of chronic (isolated) right ventricular failure
       Acute exacerbation of chronic (isolated) right ventricular failure
       Coding Clinic: 2023, Q3, P14

     I50.814   **Right heart failure due to left heart failure** 🐾
       Right ventricular failure secondary to left ventricular failure
       Code also the type of left ventricular failure, if known (I50.2-I50.43)

       Excludes1   Right heart failure with but not due to left heart failure (I50.82)

   I50.82   **Biventricular heart failure** 🐾
       Code also the type of left ventricular failure as systolic, diastolic, or combined, if known (I50.2-I50.43)

   I50.83   **High output heart failure** 🐾

   I50.84   **End stage heart failure** 🐾
       Stage D heart failure
       Code also the type of heart failure as systolic, diastolic, or combined, if known (I50.2-I50.43)
       Coding Clinic: 2022, Q3, P17

   I50.89   **Other heart failure** 🐾

I50.9   **Heart failure, unspecified** 🐾
       Cardiac, heart or myocardial failure NOS
       Congestive heart disease
       Congestive heart failure NOS

       Excludes2   fluid overload unrelated to congestive heart failure (E87.70)

       Coding Clinic: 2017, Q1, P45-46; 2015, Q2, P15; 2012, Q4, P92

● **I51**   **Complications and ill-defined descriptions of heart disease**

       Excludes1   any condition in I51.4-I51.9 due to hypertension (I11.-)
                any condition in I51.4-I51.9 due to hypertension and chronic kidney disease (I13.-)
                heart disease specified as rheumatic (I00-I09)

▶ New   ⇒ Revised   ~~deleted~~ Deleted   Excludes 1   Excludes 2   Includes   Use additional   Code first   Code also   Key words

OGCR Official Guidelines   X Assign placeholder X   ● Use Additional Character(s)   ▶ Manifestation Code   🐾 Hierarchical Condition Category   Coding Clinic

I51.0   **Cardiac septal defect, acquired**   **A**
     Acquired septal atrial defect (old)
     Acquired septal auricular defect (old)
     Acquired septal ventricular defect (old)
     Excludes1   cardiac septal defect as current complication following acute myocardial infarction (I23.1, I23.2)

I51.1   **Rupture of chordae tendineae, not elsewhere classified** 🔖
     Excludes1   rupture of chordae tendineae as current complication following acute myocardial infarction (I23.4)

I51.2   **Rupture of papillary muscle, not elsewhere classified** 🔖
     Excludes1   rupture of papillary muscle as current complication following acute myocardial infarction (I23.5)

I51.3   **Intracardiac thrombosis, not elsewhere classified**
     Apical thrombosis (old)
     Atrial thrombosis (old)
     Auricular thrombosis (old)
     Mural thrombosis (old)
     Ventricular thrombosis (old)
     Excludes1   intracardiac thrombosis as current complication following acute myocardial infarction (I23.6)
     Coding Clinic: 2013, Q1, P24

I51.4   **Myocarditis, unspecified** 🔖
     Chronic (interstitial) myocarditis
     Myocardial fibrosis
     Myocarditis NOS
     Excludes1   acute or subacute myocarditis (I40.-)
     Coding Clinic: 2016, Q4, P122

I51.5   **Myocardial degeneration** 🔖
     Fatty degeneration of heart or myocardium
     Myocardial disease
     Senile degeneration of heart or myocardium
     Coding Clinic: 2016, Q4, P122

I51.7   **Cardiomegaly**
     Cardiac dilatation
     Cardiac hypertrophy
     Ventricular dilatation
     Coding Clinic: 2016, Q4, P122

● **I51.8**   **Other ill-defined heart diseases**
     Coding Clinic: 2016, Q4, P122
     I51.81   **Takotsubo syndrome**
         Reversible left ventricular dysfunction following sudden emotional stress
         Stress induced cardiomyopathy
         Takotsubo cardiomyopathy
         Transient left ventricular apical ballooning syndrome
     I51.89   **Other ill-defined heart diseases**
         Carditis (acute)(chronic)
         Pancarditis (acute)(chronic)
         Coding Clinic: 2019, Q2, P6

I51.9   **Heart disease, unspecified**
     Coding Clinic: 2016, Q4, P122

▷ **I52**   *Other heart disorders in diseases classified elsewhere*
     Code first underlying disease, such as:
     congenital syphilis (A50.5)
     mucopolysaccharidosis (E76.3)
     schistosomiasis (B65.0-B65.9)
     Excludes1   heart disease (in):
         gonococcal infection (A54.83)
         meningococcal infection (A39.50)
         rheumatoid arthritis (M05.31)
         syphilis (A52.06)

CEREBROVASCULAR DISEASES (I60-I69)

Use additional code to identify presence of:
     alcohol abuse and dependence (F10.-)
     exposure to environmental tobacco smoke (Z77.22)
     history of tobacco dependence (Z87.891)
     hypertension (I10-I1A)
     occupational exposure to environmental tobacco smoke (Z57.31)
     tobacco dependence (F17.-)
     tobacco use (Z72.0)
     Excludes1   traumatic intracranial hemorrhage (S06.-)
     Coding Clinic: 2015, Q4, P40

I5A   **Non-ischemic myocardial injury (non-traumatic)**
     Acute (non-ischemic) myocardial injury
     Chronic (non-ischemic) myocardial injury
     Unspecified (non-ischemic) myocardial injury
     Code first the underlying cause, if known and applicable, such as:
         acute kidney failure (N17.-)
         acute myocarditis (I40.-)
         cardiomyopathy (I42.-)
         chronic kidney disease (CKD) (N18.-)
         heart failure (I50.-)
         hypertensive urgency (I16.0)
         nonrheumatic aortic valve disorders (I35.-)
         paroxysmal tachycardia (I47.-)
         pulmonary embolism (I26.-)
         pulmonary hypertension (I27.0, I27.2-)
         sepsis (A41.-)
         takotsubo syndrome (I51.81)
     Use additional code, if known, to indicate National Institutes of Health Stroke Scale (NIHSS) score (R29.7-)
     Excludes1   acute myocardial infarction (I21.-)
               injury of heart (S26.-)
     Excludes2   other acute ischemic heart diseases (I24.-)
     Coding Clinic: 2021, Q4, P15

● **I60**   **Nontraumatic subarachnoid hemorrhage**
     Excludes1   syphilitic ruptured cerebral aneurysm (A52.05)
     Excludes2   sequelae of subarachnoid hemorrhage (I69.0-)
     ● **I60.0**   **Nontraumatic subarachnoid hemorrhage from carotid siphon and bifurcation**
         I60.00   **Nontraumatic subarachnoid hemorrhage from unspecified carotid siphon and bifurcation** 🔖
         I60.01   **Nontraumatic subarachnoid hemorrhage from right carotid siphon and bifurcation** 🔖
         I60.02   **Nontraumatic subarachnoid hemorrhage from left carotid siphon and bifurcation** 🔖
     ● **I60.1**   **Nontraumatic subarachnoid hemorrhage from middle cerebral artery**
         I60.10   **Nontraumatic subarachnoid hemorrhage from unspecified middle cerebral artery** 🔖
         I60.11   **Nontraumatic subarachnoid hemorrhage from right middle cerebral artery** 🔖
         I60.12   **Nontraumatic subarachnoid hemorrhage from left middle cerebral artery** 🔖
     I60.2   **Nontraumatic subarachnoid hemorrhage from anterior communicating artery** 🔖
     ● **I60.3**   **Nontraumatic subarachnoid hemorrhage from posterior communicating artery**
         I60.30   **Nontraumatic subarachnoid hemorrhage from unspecified posterior communicating artery** 🔖
         I60.31   **Nontraumatic subarachnoid hemorrhage from right posterior communicating artery** 🔖
         I60.32   **Nontraumatic subarachnoid hemorrhage from left posterior communicating artery** 🔖
     I60.4   **Nontraumatic subarachnoid hemorrhage from basilar artery** 🔖

- **I60.5** Nontraumatic subarachnoid hemorrhage from vertebral artery
  - **I60.50** Nontraumatic subarachnoid hemorrhage from unspecified vertebral artery 🐾
  - **I60.51** Nontraumatic subarachnoid hemorrhage from right vertebral artery 🐾
  - **I60.52** Nontraumatic subarachnoid hemorrhage from left vertebral artery 🐾
- **I60.6** Nontraumatic subarachnoid hemorrhage from other intracranial arteries 🐾
- **I60.7** Nontraumatic subarachnoid hemorrhage from unspecified intracranial artery 🐾
  - Ruptured (congenital) berry aneurysm
  - Ruptured (congenital) cerebral aneurysm
  - Subarachnoid hemorrhage (nontraumatic) from cerebral artery NOS
  - Subarachnoid hemorrhage (nontraumatic) from communicating artery NOS
    - **Excludes1** berry aneurysm, nonruptured (I67.1)
- **I60.8** Other nontraumatic subarachnoid hemorrhage 🐾
  - Meningeal hemorrhage
  - Rupture of cerebral arteriovenous malformation
- **I60.9** Nontraumatic subarachnoid hemorrhage, unspecified 🐾

- **I61** Nontraumatic intracerebral hemorrhage
  - Use Additional code, if known, to indicate National Institutes of Health Stroke Scale (NIHSS) score (R29.7-)
  - **Excludes2** sequelae of intracerebral hemorrhage (I69.1-)
  - Coding Clinic: 2017, Q2, P10
  - **I61.0** Nontraumatic intracerebral hemorrhage in hemisphere, subcortical 🐾
    - Deep intracerebral hemorrhage (nontraumatic)
    - Coding Clinic: 2016, Q4, P27
  - **I61.1** Nontraumatic intracerebral hemorrhage in hemisphere, cortical 🐾
    - Cerebral lobe hemorrhage (nontraumatic)
    - Superficial intracerebral hemorrhage (nontraumatic)
    - Coding Clinic: 2016, Q4, P28
  - **I61.2** Nontraumatic intracerebral hemorrhage in hemisphere, unspecified 🐾
  - **I61.3** Nontraumatic intracerebral hemorrhage in brain stem 🐾
    - Coding Clinic: 2023, Q4, P42
  - **I61.4** Nontraumatic intracerebral hemorrhage in cerebellum 🐾
  - **I61.5** Nontraumatic intracerebral hemorrhage, intraventricular 🐾
  - **I61.6** Nontraumatic intracerebral hemorrhage, multiple localized 🐾
  - **I61.8** Other nontraumatic intracerebral hemorrhage 🐾
    - Coding Clinic: 2024, Q2, P25
  - **I61.9** Nontraumatic intracerebral hemorrhage, unspecified 🐾
    - Coding Clinic: 2022, Q3, P9-10

- **I62** Other and unspecified nontraumatic intracranial hemorrhage
  - Use Additional code, if known, to indicate National Institutes of Health Stroke Scale (NIHSS) score (R29.7-)
  - **Excludes2** sequelae of intracranial hemorrhage (I69.2)
  - **I62.0** Nontraumatic subdural hemorrhage
    - **I62.00** Nontraumatic subdural hemorrhage, unspecified 🐾
    - **I62.01** Nontraumatic acute subdural hemorrhage 🐾
    - **I62.02** Nontraumatic subacute subdural hemorrhage 🐾
    - **I62.03** Nontraumatic chronic subdural hemorrhage 🐾
  - **I62.1** Nontraumatic extradural hemorrhage 🐾
    - Nontraumatic epidural hemorrhage
    - Coding Clinic: 2023, Q3, P22
  - **I62.9** Nontraumatic intracranial hemorrhage, unspecified 🐾

★ **(See Plate 31 of the Anatomy Illustrations.)**

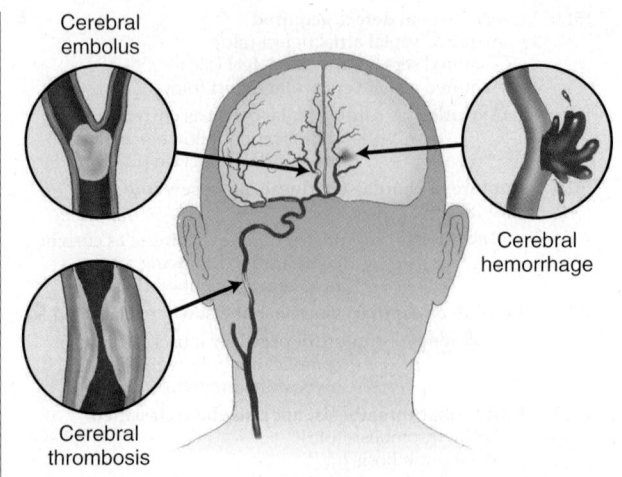

Figure 9-4 Events causing a stroke. (From Shiland: Mastering Healthcare Terminology, ed 1, St. Louis, Mosby, 2003)

- **I63** Cerebral infarction
  - **Excludes1** neonatal cerebral infarction (P91.82-)
  - **Excludes2** chronic, without residual deficits (sequelae) (Z86.73)
  - **Includes** occlusion and stenosis of cerebral and precerebral arteries, resulting in cerebral infarction
  - Use additional code, if applicable, to identify status post administration of tPA (rtPA) in a different facility within the last 24 hours prior to admission to current facility (Z92.82)
  - Use additional code, if known, to indicate National Institutes of Health Stroke Scale (NIHSS) score (R29.7-)
  - **Excludes2** sequelae of cerebral infarction (I69.3-)
  - Coding Clinic: 2016, Q4, P28, 61, 127
  - **I63.0** Cerebral infarction due to thrombosis of precerebral arteries
    - **I63.00** Cerebral infarction due to thrombosis of unspecified precerebral artery 🐾
    - **I63.01** Cerebral infarction due to thrombosis of vertebral artery
      - **I63.011** Cerebral infarction due to thrombosis of right vertebral artery 🐾
      - **I63.012** Cerebral infarction due to thrombosis of left vertebral artery 🐾
      - **I63.013** Cerebral infarction due to thrombosis of bilateral vertebral arteries 🐾
      - **I63.019** Cerebral infarction due to thrombosis of unspecified vertebral artery 🐾
    - **I63.02** Cerebral infarction due to thrombosis of basilar artery 🐾
    - **I63.03** Cerebral infarction due to thrombosis of carotid artery
      - **I63.031** Cerebral infarction due to thrombosis of right carotid artery 🐾
      - **I63.032** Cerebral infarction due to thrombosis of left carotid artery 🐾
      - **I63.033** Cerebral infarction due to thrombosis of bilateral carotid arteries 🐾
      - **I63.039** Cerebral infarction due to thrombosis of unspecified carotid artery 🐾
    - **I63.09** Cerebral infarction due to thrombosis of other precerebral artery 🐾

▶ New ⇒ Revised ~~deleted~~ Deleted | Excludes 1 | Excludes 2 | Includes | Use additional | Code first | Code also | Key words

OGCR Official Guidelines   X Assign placeholder X   ● Use Additional Character(s)   ▶ Manifestation Code   🐾 Hierarchical Condition Category   Coding Clinic

- I63.1   Cerebral infarction due to embolism of precerebral arteries
  - I63.10   Cerebral infarction due to embolism of unspecified precerebral artery 🔍
  - ● I63.11   Cerebral infarction due to embolism of vertebral artery
    - I63.111   Cerebral infarction due to embolism of right vertebral artery 🔍
    - I63.112   Cerebral infarction due to embolism of left vertebral artery 🔍
    - I63.113   Cerebral infarction due to embolism of bilateral vertebral arteries 🔍
    - I63.119   Cerebral infarction due to embolism of unspecified vertebral artery 🔍
  - I63.12   Cerebral infarction due to embolism of basilar artery 🔍
  - ● I63.13   Cerebral infarction due to embolism of carotid artery
    - I63.131   Cerebral infarction due to embolism of right carotid artery 🔍
    - I63.132   Cerebral infarction due to embolism of left carotid artery 🔍
    - I63.133   Cerebral infarction due to embolism of bilateral carotid arteries 🔍
    - I63.139   Cerebral infarction due to embolism of unspecified carotid artery 🔍
  - I63.19   Cerebral infarction due to embolism of other precerebral artery 🔍
- ● I63.2   Cerebral infarction due to unspecified occlusion or stenosis of precerebral arteries
  - I63.20   Cerebral infarction due to unspecified occlusion or stenosis of unspecified precerebral arteries 🔍
  - ● I63.21   Cerebral infarction due to unspecified occlusion or stenosis of vertebral arteries
    - I63.211   Cerebral infarction due to unspecified occlusion or stenosis of right vertebral artery 🔍
    - I63.212   Cerebral infarction due to unspecified occlusion or stenosis of left vertebral artery 🔍
    - I63.213   Cerebral infarction due to unspecified occlusion or stenosis of bilateral vertebral arteries 🔍
    - I63.219   Cerebral infarction due to unspecified occlusion or stenosis of unspecified vertebral artery 🔍
  - I63.22   Cerebral infarction due to unspecified occlusion or stenosis of basilar artery 🔍
  - ● I63.23   Cerebral infarction due to unspecified occlusion or stenosis of carotid arteries
    - I63.231   Cerebral infarction due to unspecified occlusion or stenosis of right carotid arteries 🔍
    - I63.232   Cerebral infarction due to unspecified occlusion or stenosis of left carotid arteries 🔍
    - I63.233   Cerebral infarction due to unspecified occlusion or stenosis of bilateral carotid arteries 🔍
    - I63.239   Cerebral infarction due to unspecified occlusion or stenosis of unspecified carotid artery 🔍
  - I63.29   Cerebral infarction due to unspecified occlusion or stenosis of other precerebral arteries 🔍
- ● I63.3   Cerebral infarction due to thrombosis of cerebral arteries
  - I63.30   Cerebral infarction due to thrombosis of unspecified cerebral artery 🔍
  - ● I63.31   Cerebral infarction due to thrombosis of middle cerebral artery

- I63.311   Cerebral infarction due to thrombosis of right middle cerebral artery 🔍
- I63.312   Cerebral infarction due to thrombosis of left middle cerebral artery 🔍
- I63.313   Cerebral infarction due to thrombosis of bilateral middle cerebral arteries 🔍
- I63.319   Cerebral infarction due to thrombosis of unspecified middle cerebral artery 🔍
- ● I63.32   Cerebral infarction due to thrombosis of anterior cerebral artery
  - I63.321   Cerebral infarction due to thrombosis of right anterior cerebral artery 🔍
  - I63.322   Cerebral infarction due to thrombosis of left anterior cerebral artery 🔍
  - I63.323   Cerebral infarction due to thrombosis of bilateral anterior cerebral arteries 🔍
  - I63.329   Cerebral infarction due to thrombosis of unspecified anterior cerebral artery 🔍
- ● I63.33   Cerebral infarction due to thrombosis of posterior cerebral artery
  - I63.331   Cerebral infarction due to thrombosis of right posterior cerebral artery 🔍
  - I63.332   Cerebral infarction due to thrombosis of left posterior cerebral artery 🔍
  - I63.333   Cerebral infarction due to thrombosis of bilateral posterior cerebral arteries 🔍
  - I63.339   Cerebral infarction due to thrombosis of unspecified posterior cerebral artery 🔍
- ● I63.34   Cerebral infarction due to thrombosis of cerebellar artery
  - I63.341   Cerebral infarction due to thrombosis of right cerebellar artery 🔍
  - I63.342   Cerebral infarction due to thrombosis of left cerebellar artery 🔍
  - I63.343   Cerebral infarction due to thrombosis of bilateral cerebellar arteries 🔍
  - I63.349   Cerebral infarction due to thrombosis of unspecified cerebellar artery 🔍
- I63.39   Cerebral infarction due to thrombosis of other cerebral artery 🔍
- ● I63.4   Cerebral infarction due to embolism of cerebral arteries
  - I63.40   Cerebral infarction due to embolism of unspecified cerebral artery 🔍
  - ● I63.41   Cerebral infarction due to embolism of middle cerebral artery
    - I63.411   Cerebral infarction due to embolism of right middle cerebral artery 🔍
    - I63.412   Cerebral infarction due to embolism of left middle cerebral artery 🔍
    - I63.413   Cerebral infarction due to embolism of bilateral middle cerebral arteries 🔍
    - I63.419   Cerebral infarction due to embolism of unspecified middle cerebral artery 🔍
  - ● I63.42   Cerebral infarction due to embolism of anterior cerebral artery
    - I63.421   Cerebral infarction due to embolism of right anterior cerebral artery 🔍
    - I63.422   Cerebral infarction due to embolism of left anterior cerebral artery 🔍
    - I63.423   Cerebral infarction due to embolism of bilateral anterior cerebral arteries 🔍
    - I63.429   Cerebral infarction due to embolism of unspecified anterior cerebral artery 🔍

- ● **I63.43** Cerebral infarction due to embolism of posterior cerebral artery
  - **I63.431** Cerebral infarction due to embolism of right posterior cerebral artery 🗇
  - **I63.432** Cerebral infarction due to embolism of left posterior cerebral artery 🗇
  - **I63.433** Cerebral infarction due to embolism of bilateral posterior cerebral arteries 🗇
  - **I63.439** Cerebral infarction due to embolism of unspecified posterior cerebral artery 🗇
- ● **I63.44** Cerebral infarction due to embolism of cerebellar artery
  - **I63.441** Cerebral infarction due to embolism of right cerebellar artery 🗇
  - **I63.442** Cerebral infarction due to embolism of left cerebellar artery 🗇
  - **I63.443** Cerebral infarction due to embolism of bilateral cerebellar arteries 🗇
  - **I63.449** Cerebral infarction due to embolism of unspecified cerebellar artery 🗇
  - **I63.49** Cerebral infarction due to embolism of other cerebral artery 🗇
- ● **I63.5** Cerebral infarction due to unspecified occlusion or stenosis of cerebral arteries
  - **I63.50** Cerebral infarction due to unspecified occlusion or stenosis of unspecified cerebral artery 🗇
  - ● **I63.51** Cerebral infarction due to unspecified occlusion or stenosis of middle cerebral artery
    - **I63.511** Cerebral infarction due to unspecified occlusion or stenosis of right middle cerebral artery 🗇
    - **I63.512** Cerebral infarction due to unspecified occlusion or stenosis of left middle cerebral artery 🗇
    - **I63.513** Cerebral infarction due to unspecified occlusion or stenosis of bilateral middle cerebral arteries 🗇
    - **I63.519** Cerebral infarction due to unspecified occlusion or stenosis of unspecified middle cerebral artery 🗇
  - ● **I63.52** Cerebral infarction due to unspecified occlusion or stenosis of anterior cerebral artery
    - **I63.521** Cerebral infarction due to unspecified occlusion or stenosis of right anterior cerebral artery 🗇
    - **I63.522** Cerebral infarction due to unspecified occlusion or stenosis of left anterior cerebral artery 🗇
    - **I63.523** Cerebral infarction due to unspecified occlusion or stenosis of bilateral anterior cerebral arteries 🗇
    - **I63.529** Cerebral infarction due to unspecified occlusion or stenosis of unspecified anterior cerebral artery 🗇
  - ● **I63.53** Cerebral infarction due to unspecified occlusion or stenosis of posterior cerebral artery
    - **I63.531** Cerebral infarction due to unspecified occlusion or stenosis of right posterior cerebral artery 🗇
    - **I63.532** Cerebral infarction due to unspecified occlusion or stenosis of left posterior cerebral artery 🗇
      Coding Clinic: 2024, Q1, P32; 2017, Q2, P10
    - **I63.533** Cerebral infarction due to unspecified occlusion or stenosis of bilateral posterior cerebral arteries 🗇
    - **I63.539** Cerebral infarction due to unspecified occlusion or stenosis of unspecified posterior cerebral artery 🗇

- ● **I63.54** Cerebral infarction due to unspecified occlusion or stenosis of cerebellar artery
  - **I63.541** Cerebral infarction due to unspecified occlusion or stenosis of right cerebellar artery 🗇
  - **I63.542** Cerebral infarction due to unspecified occlusion or stenosis of left cerebellar artery 🗇
  - **I63.543** Cerebral infarction due to unspecified occlusion or stenosis of bilateral cerebellar arteries 🗇
  - **I63.549** Cerebral infarction due to unspecified occlusion or stenosis of unspecified cerebellar artery 🗇
  - **I63.59** Cerebral infarction due to unspecified occlusion or stenosis of other cerebral artery 🗇
- **I63.6** Cerebral infarction due to cerebral venous thrombosis, nonpyogenic 🗇
- ● **I63.8** Other cerebral infarction 🗇
  - **I63.81** Other cerebral infarction due to occlusion or stenosis of small artery 🗇
    Lacunar infarction
    Coding Clinic: 2018, Q4, P16
  - **I63.89** Other cerebral infarction 🗇
    Coding Clinic: 2024, Q1, P26, 32; 2022, Q1, P25; 2017, Q2, P9
- **I63.9** Cerebral infarction, unspecified 🗇
  Stroke NOS
  Excludes2 transient cerebral ischemic attacks and related syndromes (G45.-)
  Coding Clinic: 2016, Q4, P62; 2015, Q1, P26
- ● **I65** Occlusion and stenosis of precerebral arteries, not resulting in cerebral infarction
  Includes embolism of precerebral artery
  narrowing of precerebral artery
  obstruction (complete) (partial) of precerebral artery
  thrombosis of precerebral artery
  Excludes1 insufficiency, NOS, of precerebral artery (G45.-)
  insufficiency of precerebral arteries causing cerebral infarction (I63.0-I63.2)
  - ● **I65.0** Occlusion and stenosis of vertebral artery
    - **I65.01** Occlusion and stenosis of right vertebral artery
    - **I65.02** Occlusion and stenosis of left vertebral artery
    - **I65.03** Occlusion and stenosis of bilateral vertebral arteries
    - **I65.09** Occlusion and stenosis of unspecified vertebral artery
  - **I65.1** Occlusion and stenosis of basilar artery
  - ● **I65.2** Occlusion and stenosis of carotid artery
    - **I65.21** Occlusion and stenosis of right carotid artery
    - **I65.22** Occlusion and stenosis of left carotid artery
    - **I65.23** Occlusion and stenosis of bilateral carotid arteries
      Coding Clinic: 2021, Q1, P4
    - **I65.29** Occlusion and stenosis of unspecified carotid artery
  - **I65.8** Occlusion and stenosis of other precerebral arteries
  - **I65.9** Occlusion and stenosis of unspecified precerebral artery
    Occlusion and stenosis of precerebral artery NOS
- ● **I66** Occlusion and stenosis of cerebral arteries, not resulting in cerebral infarction
  Includes embolism of cerebral artery
  narrowing of cerebral artery
  obstruction (complete) (partial) of cerebral artery
  thrombosis of cerebral artery
  Excludes1 occlusion and stenosis of cerebral artery causing cerebral infarction (I63.3-I63.5)

● **I66.0** **Occlusion and stenosis of middle cerebral artery**
　　I66.01 Occlusion and stenosis of right middle cerebral artery
　　I66.02 Occlusion and stenosis of left middle cerebral artery
　　I66.03 Occlusion and stenosis of bilateral middle cerebral arteries
　　I66.09 Occlusion and stenosis of unspecified middle cerebral artery

● **I66.1** **Occlusion and stenosis of anterior cerebral artery**
　　I66.11 Occlusion and stenosis of right anterior cerebral artery
　　I66.12 Occlusion and stenosis of left anterior cerebral artery
　　I66.13 Occlusion and stenosis of bilateral anterior cerebral arteries
　　I66.19 Occlusion and stenosis of unspecified anterior cerebral artery

● **I66.2** **Occlusion and stenosis of posterior cerebral artery**
　　I66.21 Occlusion and stenosis of right posterior cerebral artery
　　I66.22 Occlusion and stenosis of left posterior cerebral artery
　　I66.23 Occlusion and stenosis of bilateral posterior cerebral arteries
　　I66.29 Occlusion and stenosis of unspecified posterior cerebral artery

I66.3 **Occlusion and stenosis of cerebellar arteries**

I66.8 **Occlusion and stenosis of other cerebral arteries**
　　Occlusion and stenosis of perforating arteries

I66.9 **Occlusion and stenosis of unspecified cerebral artery**

● **I67** **Other cerebrovascular diseases**
　　Excludes1 Occlusion and stenosis of cerebral artery causing cerebral infarction (I63.3-I63.5-)
　　　　Occlusion and stenosis of precerebral artery causing cerebral infarction (I63.2-)
　　Excludes2 sequelae of the listed conditions (I69.8)

I67.0 **Dissection of cerebral arteries, nonruptured** 🔒
　　Excludes1 ruptured cerebral arteries (I60.7)
　　Coding Clinic: 2021, Q3, P5

I67.1 **Cerebral aneurysm, nonruptured**
　　Cerebral aneurysm NOS
　　Cerebral arteriovenous fistula, acquired
　　Internal carotid artery aneurysm, intracranial portion
　　Internal carotid artery aneurysm, NOS
　　Excludes1 congenital cerebral aneurysm, nonruptured (Q28.-)
　　　　ruptured cerebral aneurysm (I60.7)

I67.2 **Cerebral atherosclerosis**　　　　　　　A
　　Atheroma of cerebral and precerebral arteries

I67.3 **Progressive vascular leukoencephalopathy**
　　Binswanger's disease

I67.4 **Hypertensive encephalopathy**
　　Code also, if applicable, associated hypertensive conditions such as:
　　　　essential (primary) hypertension (I10)
　　　　hypertensive chronic kidney disease (I12.-)
　　　　hypertensive heart and chronic kidney disease (I13.-)
　　　　hypertensive heart disease (I11.-)
　　Excludes2 insufficiency, NOS, of precerebral arteries (G45.2)
　　Coding Clinic: 2023, Q4, P25

I67.5 **Moyamoya disease**

I67.6 **Nonpyogenic thrombosis of intracranial venous system**
　　Nonpyogenic thrombosis of cerebral vein
　　Nonpyogenic thrombosis of intracranial venous sinus
　　Excludes1 nonpyogenic thrombosis of intracranial venous system causing infarction (I63.6)

I67.7 **Cerebral arteritis, not elsewhere classified**
　　Granulomatous angiitis of the nervous system
　　Excludes1 allergic granulomatous angiitis (M30.1)

● **I67.8** **Other specified cerebrovascular diseases**
　　I67.81 **Acute cerebrovascular insufficiency**
　　　　Acute cerebrovascular insufficiency unspecified as to location or reversibility
　　I67.82 **Cerebral ischemia**
　　　　Chronic cerebral ischemia
　　I67.83 **Posterior reversible encephalopathy syndrome**
　　　　PRES
　　● **I67.84** **Cerebral vasospasm and vasoconstriction**
　　　　I67.841 **Reversible cerebrovascular vasoconstriction syndrome**
　　　　　　Call-Fleming syndrome
　　　　　　Code first underlying condition, if applicable, such as eclampsia (O15.00-O15.9)
　　　　I67.848 **Other cerebrovascular vasospasm and vasoconstriction**
　　● **I67.85** **Hereditary cerebrovascular diseases**
　　　　I67.850 **Cerebral autosomal dominant arteriopathy with subcortical infarcts and leukoencephalopathy**
　　　　　　CADASIL
　　　　　　Code also any associated diagnoses, such as:
　　　　　　　　epilepsy (G40.-), stroke (I63.-)
　　　　　　　　vascular dementia (F01.-)
　　　　I67.858 **Other hereditary cerebrovascular disease**
　　I67.89 **Other cerebrovascular disease**
　　　　Coding Clinic: 2023, Q2, P19

I67.9 **Cerebrovascular disease, unspecified**

● **I68** **Cerebrovascular disorders in diseases classified elsewhere**
　▷ **I68.0** *Cerebral amyloid angiopathy*
　　　Code first underlying amyloidosis (E85.-)
　▷ **I68.2** *Cerebral arteritis in other diseases classified elsewhere*
　　　Code first underlying disease
　　Excludes1 cerebral arteritis (in):
　　　　listerosis (A32.89)
　　　　systemic lupus erythematosus (M32.19)
　　　　syphilis (A52.04)
　　　　tuberculosis (A18.89)
　▷ **I68.8** *Other cerebrovascular disorders in diseases classified elsewhere*
　　　Code first underlying disease
　　Excludes1 syphilitic cerebral aneurysm (A52.05)

CHAPTER 9 (I00-I99)

OGCR Section I.c.9.d.

Sequelae of Cerebrovascular Disease

1) Category I69, Sequelae of Cerebrovascular disease
Category I69 is used to indicate conditions classifiable to categories I6Ø-I67 as the causes of sequela (neurologic deficits), themselves classified elsewhere. These "late effects" include neurologic deficits that persist after initial onset of conditions classifiable to categories I6Ø-I67. The neurologic deficits caused by cerebrovascular disease may be present from the onset of may arise at any time after the onset of the condition classifiable to categories I6Ø-I67.

Codes from category I69, Sequelae of cerebrovascular disease, that specify hemiplegia, hemiparesis and monoplegia identify whether the dominant or nondominant side is affected. Should the affected side be documented, but not specified as dominant or nondominant, and the classification system does not indicate a default, code selection is as follows:

For ambidextrous patients, the default should be dominant.
If the left side is affected, the default is nondominant.
If the right side is affected, the default is dominant.

2) Codes from category I69 with codes from I6Ø-I67
Codes from category I69 may be assigned on a health care record with codes from I6Ø-I67, if the patient has a current cerebrovascular disease and deficits from an old cerebrovascular disease.

● **I69**   **Sequelae** of cerebrovascular disease

    Note: Category I69 is to be used to indicate conditions in I6Ø-I67 as the cause of sequelae. The 'sequelae' include conditions specified as such or as residuals which may occur at any time after the onset of the causal condition.

    Excludes1   personal history of cerebral infarction without residual deficit (Z86.73)
          personal history of prolonged reversible ischemic neurologic deficit (PRIND) (Z86.73)
          personal history of reversible ischemic neurologcial deficit (RIND) (Z86.73)
          sequelae of traumatic intracranial injury (SØ6.-)

    Coding Clinic: 2016, Q4, P28; 2015, Q4, P40; 2012, Q4, P107

● **I69.Ø**   **Sequelae** of nontraumatic subarachnoid hemorrhage

    I69.ØØ   **Unspecified** sequelae of nontraumatic subarachnoid hemorrhage

    ● **I69.Ø1**   **Cognitive deficits** following nontraumatic subarachnoid hemorrhage

        I69.Ø1Ø   **Attention and concentration** deficit following nontraumatic subarachnoid hemorrhage

        I69.Ø11   **Memory** deficit following nontraumatic subarachnoid hemorrhage

        I69.Ø12   **Visuospatial** deficit and spatial neglect following nontraumatic subarachnoid hemorrhage

        I69.Ø13   **Psychomotor** deficit following nontraumatic subarachnoid hemorrhage

        I69.Ø14   **Frontal lobe and executive function** deficit following nontraumatic subarachnoid hemorrhage

        I69.Ø15   **Cognitive social or emotional** deficit following nontraumatic subarachnoid hemorrhage

        I69.Ø18   **Other symptoms and signs** involving cognitive functions following nontraumatic subarachnoid hemorrhage

        I69.Ø19   **Unspecified** symptoms and signs involving cognitive functions following nontraumatic subarachnoid hemorrhage

● **I69.Ø2**   **Speech and language deficits** following nontraumatic subarachnoid hemorrhage

    I69.Ø2Ø   **Aphasia** following nontraumatic subarachnoid hemorrhage

    I69.Ø21   **Dysphasia** following nontraumatic subarachnoid hemorrhage

    I69.Ø22   **Dysarthria** following nontraumatic subarachnoid hemorrhage

    I69.Ø23   **Fluency disorder** following nontraumatic subarachnoid hemorrhage
         Stuttering following nontraumatic subarachnoid hemorrhage

    I69.Ø28   **Other speech and language deficits** following nontraumatic subarachnoid hemorrhage

● **I69.Ø3**   **Monoplegia of upper limb** following nontraumatic subarachnoid hemorrhage

    I69.Ø31   Monoplegia of upper limb following nontraumatic subarachnoid hemorrhage affecting **right dominant side** 🏥

    I69.Ø32   Monoplegia of upper limb following nontraumatic subarachnoid hemorrhage affecting **left dominant side** 🏥

    I69.Ø33   Monoplegia of upper limb following nontraumatic subarachnoid hemorrhage affecting **right non-dominant side** 🏥

    I69.Ø34   Monoplegia of upper limb following nontraumatic subarachnoid hemorrhage affecting **left non-dominant side** 🏥

    I69.Ø39   Monoplegia of upper limb following nontraumatic subarachnoid hemorrhage affecting **unspecified side** 🏥

● **I69.Ø4**   **Monoplegia of lower limb** following nontraumatic subarachnoid hemorrhage

    I69.Ø41   Monoplegia of lower limb following nontraumatic subarachnoid hemorrhage affecting **right dominant side** 🏥

    I69.Ø42   Monoplegia of lower limb following nontraumatic subarachnoid hemorrhage affecting **left dominant side** 🏥

    I69.Ø43   Monoplegia of lower limb following nontraumatic subarachnoid hemorrhage affecting **right non-dominant side** 🏥

    I69.Ø44   Monoplegia of lower limb following nontraumatic subarachnoid hemorrhage affecting **left non-dominant side** 🏥

    I69.Ø49   Monoplegia of lower limb following nontraumatic subarachnoid hemorrhage affecting **unspecified side** 🏥

● **I69.Ø5**   **Hemiplegia and hemiparesis** following nontraumatic subarachnoid hemorrhage

    I69.Ø51   Hemiplegia and hemiparesis following nontraumatic subarachnoid hemorrhage affecting **right dominant side** 🏥

    I69.Ø52   Hemiplegia and hemiparesis following nontraumatic subarachnoid hemorrhage affecting **left dominant side** 🏥

    I69.Ø53   Hemiplegia and hemiparesis following nontraumatic subarachnoid hemorrhage affecting **right non-dominant side** 🏥

▶ New   ⇏ Revised   ~~deleted~~ Deleted   Excludes 1   Excludes 2   Includes   Use additional   Code first   Code also   Key words

OGCR Official Guidelines   X Assign placeholder X   ● Use Additional Character(s)   ▌ Manifestation Code   🏥 Hierarchical Condition Category   Coding Clinic

I69.054   **Hemiplegia and hemiparesis following nontraumatic subarachnoid hemorrhage affecting left non-dominant side** 🔎

I69.059   **Hemiplegia and hemiparesis following nontraumatic subarachnoid hemorrhage affecting unspecified side** 🔎

● I69.06   **Other paralytic syndrome following nontraumatic subarachnoid hemorrhage**

    Use additional code to identify type of paralytic syndrome, such as:
      locked-in state (G83.5)
      quadriplegia (G82.5-)

    Excludes1 hemiplegia/hemiparesis following nontraumatic subarachnoid hemorrhage (I69.05-)
                monoplegia of lower limb following nontraumatic subarachnoid hemorrhage (I69.04-)
                monoplegia of upper limb following nontraumatic subarachnoid hemorrhage (I69.03-)

I69.061   **Other paralytic syndrome following nontraumatic subarachnoid hemorrhage affecting right dominant side** 🔎

I69.062   **Other paralytic syndrome following nontraumatic subarachnoid hemorrhage affecting left dominant side** 🔎

I69.063   **Other paralytic syndrome following nontraumatic subarachnoid hemorrhage affecting right non-dominant side** 🔎

I69.064   **Other paralytic syndrome following nontraumatic subarachnoid hemorrhage affecting left non-dominant side** 🔎

I69.065   **Other paralytic syndrome following nontraumatic subarachnoid hemorrhage, bilateral** 🔎

I69.069   **Other paralytic syndrome following nontraumatic subarachnoid hemorrhage affecting unspecified side** 🔎

● I69.09   **Other sequelae of nontraumatic subarachnoid hemorrhage**

I69.090   **Apraxia following nontraumatic subarachnoid hemorrhage**

I69.091   **Dysphagia following nontraumatic subarachnoid hemorrhage**

    Use additional code to identify the type of dysphagia, if known (R13.11-R13.19)

I69.092   **Facial weakness following nontraumatic subarachnoid hemorrhage**

    Facial droop following nontraumatic subarachnoid hemorrhage

I69.093   **Ataxia following nontraumatic subarachnoid hemorrhage**

I69.098   **Other sequelae following nontraumatic subarachnoid hemorrhage**

    Alterations of sensation following nontraumatic subarachnoid hemorrhage
    Disturbance of vision following nontraumatic subarachnoid hemorrhage
    Use additional code to identify the sequelae

● I69.1   **Sequelae of nontraumatic intracerebral hemorrhage**

I69.10   **Unspecified sequelae of nontraumatic intracerebral hemorrhage**

● I69.11   **Cognitive deficits following nontraumatic intracerebral hemorrhage**

I69.110   **Attention and concentration deficit following nontraumatic intracerebral hemorrhage**

I69.111   **Memory deficit following nontraumatic intracerebral hemorrhage**

I69.112   **Visuospatial deficit and spatial neglect following nontraumatic intracerebral hemorrhage**

I69.113   **Psychomotor deficit following nontraumatic intracerebral hemorrhage**

I69.114   **Frontal lobe and executive function deficit following nontraumatic intracerebral hemorrhage**

I69.115   **Cognitive social or emotional deficit following nontraumatic intracerebral hemorrhage**

I69.118   **Other symptoms and signs involving cognitive functions following nontraumatic intracerebral hemorrhage**

I69.119   **Unspecified symptoms and signs involving cognitive functions following nontraumatic intracerebral hemorrhage**

● I69.12   **Speech and language deficits following nontraumatic intracerebral hemorrhage**

I69.120   **Aphasia following nontraumatic intracerebral hemorrhage**

I69.121   **Dysphasia following nontraumatic intracerebral hemorrhage**

I69.122   **Dysarthria following nontraumatic intracerebral hemorrhage**

I69.123   **Fluency disorder following nontraumatic intracerebral hemorrhage**

    Stuttering following nontraumatic intracerebral hemorrhage

I69.128   **Other speech and language deficits following nontraumatic intracerebral hemorrhage**

● I69.13   **Monoplegia of upper limb following nontraumatic intracerebral hemorrhage**

I69.131   **Monoplegia of upper limb following nontraumatic intracerebral hemorrhage affecting right dominant side** 🔎

I69.132   **Monoplegia of upper limb following nontraumatic intracerebral hemorrhage affecting left dominant side** 🔎

I69.133   **Monoplegia of upper limb following nontraumatic intracerebral hemorrhage affecting right non-dominant side** 🔎

I69.134   **Monoplegia of upper limb following nontraumatic intracerebral hemorrhage affecting left non-dominant side** 🔎

I69.139   **Monoplegia of upper limb following nontraumatic intracerebral hemorrhage affecting unspecified side** 🔎

CHAPTER 9 (I00–I99)

● **I69.14**   **Monoplegia of lower limb following** nontraumatic intracerebral hemorrhage

     I69.141   Monoplegia of lower limb following nontraumatic intracerebral hemorrhage affecting right dominant side 🐾

     I69.142   Monoplegia of lower limb following nontraumatic intracerebral hemorrhage affecting left dominant side 🐾

     I69.143   Monoplegia of lower limb following nontraumatic intracerebral hemorrhage affecting right non-dominant side 🐾

     I69.144   Monoplegia of lower limb following nontraumatic intracerebral hemorrhage affecting left non-dominant side 🐾

     I69.149   Monoplegia of lower limb following nontraumatic intracerebral hemorrhage affecting unspecified side 🐾

● **I69.15**   **Hemiplegia and hemiparesis** following nontraumatic intracerebral hemorrhage

     I69.151   Hemiplegia and hemiparesis following nontraumatic intracerebral hemorrhage affecting right dominant side 🐾

     I69.152   Hemiplegia and hemiparesis following nontraumatic intracerebral hemorrhage affecting left dominant side 🐾

     I69.153   Hemiplegia and hemiparesis following nontraumatic intracerebral hemorrhage affecting right non-dominant side 🐾

     I69.154   Hemiplegia and hemiparesis following nontraumatic intracerebral hemorrhage affecting left non-dominant side 🐾

     I69.159   Hemiplegia and hemiparesis following nontraumatic intracerebral hemorrhage affecting unspecified side 🐾

● **I69.16**   **Other paralytic syndrome** following nontraumatic intracerebral hemorrhage

     Use additional code to identify type of paralytic syndrome, such as:
     locked-in state (G83.5)
     quadriplegia (G82.5-)

     Excludes1   hemiplegia/hemiparesis following nontraumatic intracerebral hemorrhage (I69.15-)
             monoplegia of lower limb following nontraumatic intracerebral hemorrhage (I69.14-)
             monoplegia of upper limb following nontraumatic intracerebral hemorrhage (I69.13-)

     I69.161   Other paralytic syndrome following nontraumatic intracerebral hemorrhage affecting right dominant side 🐾

     I69.162   Other paralytic syndrome following nontraumatic intracerebral hemorrhage affecting left dominant side 🐾

     I69.163   Other paralytic syndrome following nontraumatic intracerebral hemorrhage affecting right non-dominant side 🐾

     I69.164   Other paralytic syndrome following nontraumatic intracerebral hemorrhage affecting left non-dominant side 🐾

     I69.165   Other paralytic syndrome following nontraumatic intracerebral hemorrhage, bilateral 🐾

     I69.169   Other paralytic syndrome following nontraumatic intracerebral hemorrhage affecting unspecified side 🐾

● **I69.19**   **Other sequelae of nontraumatic intracerebral hemorrhage**

     I69.190   Apraxia following nontraumatic intracerebral hemorrhage

     I69.191   Dysphagia following nontraumatic intracerebral hemorrhage
         Use additional code to identify the type of dysphagia, if known (R13.11-R13.19)

     I69.192   Facial weakness following nontraumatic intracerebral hemorrhage
         Facial droop following nontraumatic intracerebral hemorrhage

     I69.193   Ataxia following nontraumatic intracerebral hemorrhage

     I69.198   Other sequelae of nontraumatic intracerebral hemorrhage
         Alteration of sensations following nontraumatic intracerebral hemorrhage
         Disturbance of vision following nontraumatic intracerebral hemorrhage
         Use additional code to identify the sequelae

● **I69.2**   **Sequelae of other nontraumatic intracranial hemorrhage**

     I69.20   Unspecified sequelae of other nontraumatic intracranial hemorrhage

●   I69.21   **Cognitive deficits** following other nontraumatic intracranial hemorrhage

     I69.210   **Attention and concentration** deficit following other nontraumatic intracranial hemorrhage

     I69.211   **Memory** deficit following other nontraumatic intracranial hemorrhage

     I69.212   **Visuospatial deficit and spatial neglect** following other nontraumatic intracranial hemorrhage

     I69.213   **Psychomotor** deficit following other nontraumatic intracranial hemorrhage

     I69.214   **Frontal lobe and executive function** deficit following other nontraumatic intracranial hemorrhage

     I69.215   **Cognitive social or emotional** deficit following other nontraumatic intracranial hemorrhage

     I69.218   **Other symptoms and signs involving cognitive functions** following other nontraumatic intracranial hemorrhage

     I69.219   **Unspecified** symptoms and signs involving cognitive functions following other nontraumatic intracranial hemorrhage

●   I69.22   **Speech and language deficits** following other nontraumatic intracranial hemorrhage

     I69.220   Aphasia following other nontraumatic intracranial hemorrhage

     I69.221   Dysphasia following other nontraumatic intracranial hemorrhage

     I69.222   Dysarthria following other nontraumatic intracranial hemorrhage

▶ New   ⇒ Revised   ~~deleted~~ Deleted   Excludes 1   Excludes 2   Includes   Use additional   Code first   Code also   Key words

856   OGCR Official Guidelines   X Assign placeholder X   ● Use Additional Character(s)   ▷ Manifestation Code   🐾 Hierarchical Condition Category   **Coding Clinic**

I69.223   **Fluency disorder** following other nontraumatic intracranial hemorrhage
     Stuttering following other nontraumatic intracranial hemorrhage

I69.228   **Other speech and language deficits** following other nontraumatic intracranial hemorrhage

● **I69.23**   **Monoplegia of upper limb** following other nontraumatic intracranial hemorrhage

I69.231   Monoplegia of upper limb following other nontraumatic intracranial hemorrhage affecting right dominant side 🔁

I69.232   Monoplegia of upper limb following other nontraumatic intracranial hemorrhage affecting left dominant side 🔁

I69.233   Monoplegia of upper limb following other nontraumatic intracranial hemorrhage affecting right non-dominant side 🔁

I69.234   Monoplegia of upper limb following other nontraumatic intracranial hemorrhage affecting left non-dominant side 🔁

I69.239   Monoplegia of upper limb following other nontraumatic intracranial hemorrhage affecting unspecified side 🔁

● **I69.24**   **Monoplegia of lower limb** following other nontraumatic intracranial hemorrhage

I69.241   Monoplegia of lower limb following other nontraumatic intracranial hemorrhage affecting right dominant side 🔁

I69.242   Monoplegia of lower limb following other nontraumatic intracranial hemorrhage affecting left dominant side 🔁

I69.243   Monoplegia of lower limb following other nontraumatic intracranial hemorrhage affecting right non-dominant side 🔁

I69.244   Monoplegia of lower limb following other nontraumatic intracranial hemorrhage affecting left non-dominant side 🔁

I69.249   Monoplegia of lower limb following other nontraumatic intracranial hemorrhage affecting unspecified side 🔁

● **I69.25**   **Hemiplegia and hemiparesis** following other nontraumatic intracranial hemorrhage

I69.251   Hemiplegia and hemiparesis following other nontraumatic intracranial hemorrhage affecting right dominant side 🔁

I69.252   Hemiplegia and hemiparesis following other nontraumatic intracranial hemorrhage affecting left dominant side 🔁

I69.253   Hemiplegia and hemiparesis following other nontraumatic intracranial hemorrhage affecting right non-dominant side 🔁

I69.254   Hemiplegia and hemiparesis following other nontraumatic intracranial hemorrhage affecting left non-dominant side 🔁

I69.259   Hemiplegia and hemiparesis following other nontraumatic intracranial hemorrhage affecting unspecified side 🔁

● **I69.26**   **Other paralytic syndrome** following other nontraumatic intracranial hemorrhage

     Use additional code to identify type of paralytic syndrome, such as:
     locked-in state (G83.5)
     quadriplegia (G82.5-)

     Excludes1   hemiplegia/hemiparesis following other nontraumatic intracranial hemorrhage (I69.25-)
         monoplegia of lower limb following other nontraumatic intracranial hemorrhage (I69.24-)
         monoplegia of upper limb following other nontraumatic intracranial hemorrhage (I69.23-)

I69.261   Other paralytic syndrome following other nontraumatic intracranial hemorrhage affecting right dominant side 🔁

I69.262   Other paralytic syndrome following other nontraumatic intracranial hemorrhage affecting left dominant side 🔁

I69.263   Other paralytic syndrome following other nontraumatic intracranial hemorrhage affecting right non-dominant side 🔁

I69.264   Other paralytic syndrome following other nontraumatic intracranial hemorrhage affecting left non-dominant side 🔁

I69.265   Other paralytic syndrome following other nontraumatic intracranial hemorrhage, bilateral 🔁

I69.269   Other paralytic syndrome following other nontraumatic intracranial hemorrhage affecting unspecified side 🔁

● **I69.29**   **Other sequelae of other nontraumatic intracranial hemorrhage**

I69.290   **Apraxia** following other nontraumatic intracranial hemorrhage

I69.291   **Dysphagia** following other nontraumatic intracranial hemorrhage
     Use additional code to identify the type of dysphagia, if known (R13.11-R13.19)

I69.292   **Facial weakness** following other nontraumatic intracranial hemorrhage
     Facial droop following other nontraumatic intracranial hemorrhage

I69.293   **Ataxia** following other nontraumatic intracranial hemorrhage

I69.298   **Other sequelae** of other nontraumatic intracranial hemorrhage
     Alteration of sensation following other nontraumatic intracranial hemorrhage
     Disturbance of vision following other nontraumatic intracranial hemorrhage
     Use additional code to identify the sequelae

CHAPTER 9 (I00-I99)

● **I69.3**   **Sequelae of cerebral infarction**
Sequelae of stroke NOS
Coding Clinic: 2012, Q4, P92, 95

    I69.30   Unspecified sequelae of cerebral infarction

●   **I69.31**   Cognitive deficits following cerebral infarction

        I69.310   Attention and concentration deficit following cerebral infarction

        I69.311   Memory deficit following cerebral infarction

        I69.312   Visuospatial deficit and spatial neglect following cerebral infarction

        I69.313   Psychomotor deficit following cerebral infarction

        I69.314   Frontal lobe and executive function deficit following cerebral infarction

        I69.315   Cognitive social or emotional deficit following cerebral infarction

        I69.318   Other symptoms and signs involving cognitive functions following cerebral infarction

        I69.319   Unspecified symptoms and signs involving cognitive functions following cerebral infarction

●   **I69.32**   Speech and language deficits following cerebral infarction

        I69.320   Aphasia following cerebral infarction

        I69.321   Dysphasia following cerebral infarction
Coding Clinic: 2012, Q4, P91

        I69.322   Dysarthria following cerebral infarction
           Excludes2   transient ischemic attack (TIA) (G45.9)

        I69.323   Fluency disorder following cerebral infarction
Stuttering following cerebral infarction

        I69.328   Other speech and language deficits following cerebral infarction

●   **I69.33**   Monoplegia of upper limb following cerebral infarction
Coding Clinic: 2017, Q1, P47

        I69.331   Monoplegia of upper limb following cerebral infarction affecting right dominant side 🦠

        I69.332   Monoplegia of upper limb following cerebral infarction affecting left dominant side 🦠

        I69.333   Monoplegia of upper limb following cerebral infarction affecting right non-dominant side 🦠

        I69.334   Monoplegia of upper limb following cerebral infarction affecting left non-dominant side 🦠

        I69.339   Monoplegia of upper limb following cerebral infarction affecting unspecified side 🦠

●   **I69.34**   Monoplegia of lower limb following cerebral infarction
Coding Clinic: 2017, Q1, P47

        I69.341   Monoplegia of lower limb following cerebral infarction affecting right dominant side 🦠

        I69.342   Monoplegia of lower limb following cerebral infarction affecting left dominant side 🦠

        I69.343   Monoplegia of lower limb following cerebral infarction affecting right non-dominant side 🦠

        I69.344   Monoplegia of lower limb following cerebral infarction affecting left non-dominant side 🦠

        I69.349   Monoplegia of lower limb following cerebral infarction affecting unspecified side 🦠

●   **I69.35**   Hemiplegia and hemiparesis following cerebral infarction

        I69.351   Hemiplegia and hemiparesis following cerebral infarction affecting right dominant side 🦠
           Excludes2   transient ischemic attack (TIA) (G45.9)
        Coding Clinic: 2015, Q1, P25

        I69.352   Hemiplegia and hemiparesis following cerebral infarction affecting left dominant side 🦠

        I69.353   Hemiplegia and hemiparesis following cerebral infarction affecting right non-dominant side 🦠

        I69.354   Hemiplegia and hemiparesis following cerebral infarction affecting left non-dominant side 🦠
        Coding Clinic: 2012, Q4, P91

        I69.359   Hemiplegia and hemiparesis following cerebral infarction affecting unspecified side 🦠

●   **I69.36**   Other paralytic syndrome following cerebral infarction
Use additional code to identify type of paralytic syndrome, such as:
locked-in state (G83.5)
quadriplegia (G82.5-)
    Excludes1   hemiplegia/hemiparesis following cerebral infarction (I69.35-)
monoplegia of lower limb following cerebral infarction (I69.34-)
monoplegia of upper limb following cerebral infarction (I69.33-)

        I69.361   Other paralytic syndrome following cerebral infarction affecting right dominant side 🦠

        I69.362   Other paralytic syndrome following cerebral infarction affecting left dominant side 🦠

        I69.363   Other paralytic syndrome following cerebral infarction affecting right non-dominant side 🦠

        I69.364   Other paralytic syndrome following cerebral infarction affecting left non-dominant side 🦠

        I69.365   Other paralytic syndrome following cerebral infarction, bilateral 🦠

        I69.369   Other paralytic syndrome following cerebral infarction affecting unspecified side 🦠

●   **I69.39**   Other sequelae of cerebral infarction

        I69.390   Apraxia following cerebral infarction

        I69.391   Dysphagia following cerebral infarction
Use additional code to identify the type of dysphagia, if known (R13.11-R13.19)

        I69.392   Facial weakness following cerebral infarction
Facial droop following cerebral infarction
Coding Clinic: 2024, Q2, P13

▶ New   ⇨ Revised   ~~deleted~~ Deleted   Excludes 1   Excludes 2   Includes   Use additional   Code first   Code also   Key words
OGCR Official Guidelines   X Assign placeholder X   ● Use Additional Character(s)   ▶ Manifestation Code   🦠 Hierarchical Condition Category   Coding Clinic

I69.393   **Ataxia** following cerebral infarction

I69.398   **Other** sequelae of cerebral infarction

     Alteration of sensation following cerebral infarction

     Disturbance of vision following cerebral infarction

     Use additional code to identify the sequelae

     Coding Clinic: 2024, Q2, P13

● **I69.8**   **Sequelae** of other cerebrovascular diseases

    Excludes1   sequelae of traumatic intracranial injury (S06.-)

   I69.80   **Unspecified** sequelae of other cerebrovascular disease

● I69.81   **Cognitive deficits** following other cerebrovascular disease

    I69.810   **Attention and concentration** deficit following other cerebrovascular disease

    I69.811   **Memory** deficit following other cerebrovascular disease

    I69.812   **Visuospatial** deficit and spatial neglect following other cerebrovascular disease

    I69.813   **Psychomotor** deficit following other cerebrovascular disease

    I69.814   **Frontal lobe and executive function** deficit following other cerebrovascular disease

    I69.815   **Cognitive social or emotional** deficit following other cerebrovascular disease

    I69.818   **Other** symptoms and signs involving cognitive functions following other cerebrovascular disease

    I69.819   **Unspecified** symptoms and signs involving cognitive functions following other cerebrovascular disease

● I69.82   **Speech and language** deficits following other cerebrovascular disease

    I69.820   **Aphasia** following other cerebrovascular disease

    I69.821   **Dysphasia** following other cerebrovascular disease

    I69.822   **Dysarthria** following other cerebrovascular disease

    I69.823   **Fluency** disorder following other cerebrovascular disease

     Stuttering following other cerebrovascular disease

    I69.828   **Other** speech and language deficits following other cerebrovascular disease

     Coding Clinic: 2019, Q3, P9

● I69.83   **Monoplegia of upper limb** following other cerebrovascular disease

    I69.831   Monoplegia of upper limb following other cerebrovascular disease affecting **right dominant side** 🔖

    I69.832   Monoplegia of upper limb following other cerebrovascular disease affecting **left dominant side** 🔖

    I69.833   Monoplegia of upper limb following other cerebrovascular disease affecting **right non-dominant side** 🔖

    I69.834   Monoplegia of upper limb following other cerebrovascular disease affecting **left non-dominant side** 🔖

    I69.839   Monoplegia of upper limb following other cerebrovascular disease affecting **unspecified side** 🔖

● I69.84   **Monoplegia of lower limb** following other cerebrovascular disease

    I69.841   Monoplegia of lower limb following other cerebrovascular disease affecting **right dominant side** 🔖

    I69.842   Monoplegia of lower limb following other cerebrovascular disease affecting **left dominant side** 🔖

    I69.843   Monoplegia of lower limb following other cerebrovascular disease affecting **right non-dominant side** 🔖

    I69.844   Monoplegia of lower limb following other cerebrovascular disease affecting **left non-dominant side** 🔖

    I69.849   Monoplegia of lower limb following other cerebrovascular disease affecting **unspecified** side 🔖

● I69.85   **Hemiplegia and hemiparesis** following other cerebrovascular disease

    I69.851   Hemiplegia and hemiparesis following other cerebrovascular disease affecting **right dominant side** 🔖

    I69.852   Hemiplegia and hemiparesis following other cerebrovascular disease affecting **left dominant side** 🔖

    I69.853   Hemiplegia and hemiparesis following other cerebrovascular disease affecting **right non-dominant side** 🔖

    I69.854   Hemiplegia and hemiparesis following other cerebrovascular disease affecting **left non-dominant side** 🔖

    I69.859   Hemiplegia and hemiparesis following other cerebrovascular disease affecting **unspecified** side 🔖

● I69.86   **Other paralytic syndrome** following other cerebrovascular disease

     Use additional code to identify type of paralytic syndrome, such as: locked-in state (G83.5) quadriplegia (G82.5-)

    Excludes1   hemiplegia/hemiparesis following other cerebrovascular disease (I69.85-)

       monoplegia of lower limb following other cerebrovascular disease (I69.84-)

       monoplegia of upper limb following other cerebrovascular disease (I69.83-)

    I69.861   Other paralytic syndrome following other cerebrovascular disease affecting **right dominant side** 🔖

    I69.862   Other paralytic syndrome following other cerebrovascular disease affecting **left dominant side** 🔖

    I69.863   Other paralytic syndrome following other cerebrovascular disease affecting **right non-dominant side** 🔖

    I69.864   Other paralytic syndrome following other cerebrovascular disease affecting **left non-dominant side** 🔖

    I69.865   Other paralytic syndrome following other cerebrovascular disease, **bilateral** 🔖

    I69.869   Other paralytic syndrome following other cerebrovascular disease affecting **unspecified** side 🔖

● **I69.89 Other sequelae of other cerebrovascular disease**

    I69.890 Apraxia following other cerebrovascular disease

    I69.891 Dysphagia following other cerebrovascular disease
        Use additional code to identify the type of dysphagia, if known (R13.11-R13.19)

    I69.892 Facial weakness following other cerebrovascular disease
        Facial droop following other cerebrovascular disease

    I69.893 Ataxia following other cerebrovascular disease

    I69.898 Other sequelae of other cerebrovascular disease
        Alteration of sensation following other cerebrovascular disease
        Disturbance of vision following other cerebrovascular disease
        Use additional code to identify the sequelae

● **I69.9 Sequelae of unspecified cerebrovascular diseases**
    Excludes1 sequelae of stroke (I69.3)
        sequelae of traumatic intracranial injury (S06.-)

  I69.90 Unspecified sequelae of unspecified cerebrovascular disease

● **I69.91 Cognitive deficits following unspecified cerebrovascular disease**

    I69.910 Attention and concentration deficit following unspecified cerebrovascular disease

    I69.911 Memory deficit following unspecified cerebrovascular disease

    I69.912 Visuospatial deficit and spatial neglect following unspecified cerebrovascular disease

    I69.913 Psychomotor deficit following unspecified cerebrovascular disease

    I69.914 Frontal lobe and executive function deficit following unspecified cerebrovascular disease

    I69.915 Cognitive social or emotional deficit following unspecified cerebrovascular disease

    I69.918 Other symptoms and signs involving cognitive functions following unspecified cerebrovascular disease

    I69.919 Unspecified symptoms and signs involving cognitive functions following unspecified cerebrovascular disease

● **I69.92 Speech and language deficits following unspecified cerebrovascular disease**

    I69.920 Aphasia following unspecified cerebrovascular disease

    I69.921 Dysphasia following unspecified cerebrovascular disease

    I69.922 Dysarthria following unspecified cerebrovascular disease

    I69.923 Fluency disorder following unspecified cerebrovascular disease
        Stuttering following unspecified cerebrovascular disease

    I69.928 Other speech and language deficits following unspecified cerebrovascular disease

● **I69.93 Monoplegia of upper limb following unspecified cerebrovascular disease**

    I69.931 Monoplegia of upper limb following unspecified cerebrovascular disease affecting right dominant side 🐾

    I69.932 Monoplegia of upper limb following unspecified cerebrovascular disease affecting left dominant side 🐾

    I69.933 Monoplegia of upper limb following unspecified cerebrovascular disease affecting right non-dominant side 🐾

    I69.934 Monoplegia of upper limb following unspecified cerebrovascular disease affecting left non-dominant side 🐾

    I69.939 Monoplegia of upper limb following unspecified cerebrovascular disease affecting unspecified side 🐾

● **I69.94 Monoplegia of lower limb following unspecified cerebrovascular disease**

    I69.941 Monoplegia of lower limb following unspecified cerebrovascular disease affecting right dominant side 🐾

    I69.942 Monoplegia of lower limb following unspecified cerebrovascular disease affecting left dominant side 🐾

    I69.943 Monoplegia of lower limb following unspecified cerebrovascular disease affecting right non-dominant side 🐾

    I69.944 Monoplegia of lower limb following unspecified cerebrovascular disease affecting left non-dominant side 🐾

    I69.949 Monoplegia of lower limb following unspecified cerebrovascular disease affecting unspecified side 🐾

● **I69.95 Hemiplegia and hemiparesis following unspecified cerebrovascular disease**

    I69.951 Hemiplegia and hemiparesis following unspecified cerebrovascular disease affecting right dominant side 🐾

    I69.952 Hemiplegia and hemiparesis following unspecified cerebrovascular disease affecting left dominant side 🐾

    I69.953 Hemiplegia and hemiparesis following unspecified cerebrovascular disease affecting right non-dominant side 🐾

    I69.954 Hemiplegia and hemiparesis following unspecified cerebrovascular disease affecting left non-dominant side 🐾

    I69.959 Hemiplegia and hemiparesis following unspecified cerebrovascular disease affecting unspecified side 🐾

● **I69.96 Other paralytic syndrome following unspecified cerebrovascular disease**
    Use additional code to identify type of paralytic syndrome, such as:
    locked-in state (G83.5)
    quadriplegia (G82.5-)
    Excludes1 hemiplegia/hemiparesis following unspecified cerebrovascular disease (I69.95-)
        monoplegia of lower limb following unspecified cerebrovascular disease (I69.94-)
        monoplegia of upper limb following unspecified cerebrovascular disease (I69.93-)

    I69.961 Other paralytic syndrome following unspecified cerebrovascular disease affecting right dominant side 🐾

    I69.962 Other paralytic syndrome following unspecified cerebrovascular disease affecting left dominant side 🐾

▶ New   ⇒ Revised   ~~deleted~~ Deleted   Excludes 1   Excludes 2   Includes   Use additional   Code first   Code also   Key words

OGCR Official Guidelines   X Assign placeholder X   ● Use Additional Character(s)   ▷ Manifestation Code   🐾 Hierarchical Condition Category   Coding Clinic

I69.963   Other paralytic syndrome following unspecified cerebrovascular disease affecting right non-dominant side 🦟

I69.964   Other paralytic syndrome following unspecified cerebrovascular disease affecting left non-dominant side 🦟

I69.965   Other paralytic syndrome following unspecified cerebrovascular disease, bilateral 🦟

I69.969   Other paralytic syndrome following unspecified cerebrovascular disease affecting unspecified side 🦟

● **I69.99**   Other sequelae of unspecified cerebrovascular disease

I69.990   Apraxia following unspecified cerebrovascular disease

I69.991   Dysphagia following unspecified cerebrovascular disease

     Use additional code to identify the type of dysphagia, if known (R13.11-R13.19)

I69.992   Facial weakness following unspecified cerebrovascular disease

     Facial droop following unspecified cerebrovascular disease

I69.993   Ataxia following unspecified cerebrovascular disease

I69.998   Other sequelae following unspecified cerebrovascular disease

     Alteration in sensation following unspecified cerebrovascular disease

     Disturbance of vision following unspecified cerebrovascular disease

     Use additional code to identify the sequelae

DISEASES OF ARTERIES, ARTERIOLES AND CAPILLARIES (I70-I79)

● **I70**   **Atherosclerosis**

   Includes   arteriolosclerosis
                arterial degeneration
                arteriosclerosis
                arteriosclerotic vascular disease
                arteriovascular degeneration
                atheroma
                endarteritis deformans or obliterans
                senile arteritis
                senile endarteritis
                vascular degeneration

Use additional code to identify:
   exposure to environmental tobacco smoke (Z77.22)
   history of tobacco dependence (Z87.891)
   occupational exposure to environmental tobacco smoke (Z57.31)
   tobacco dependence (F17.-)
   tobacco use (Z72.0)

   Excludes2   arteriosclerotic cardiovascular disease (I25.1-)
                arteriosclerotic heart disease (I25.1-)
                atheroembolism (I75.-)
                cerebral atherosclerosis (I67.2)
                coronary atherosclerosis (I25.1-)
                mesenteric atherosclerosis (K55.1)
                precerebral atherosclerosis (I67.2)
                primary pulmonary atherosclerosis (I27.0)

I70.0   Atherosclerosis of aorta 🦟   A

I70.1   Atherosclerosis of renal artery 🦟   A
     Goldblatt's kidney
     Excludes2   atherosclerosis of renal arterioles (I12.-)

★ **(See Plates 500, 501, and 502 on pages 60 – 62.)**

● **I70.2**   Atherosclerosis of native arteries of the extremities
     Mönckeberg's (medial) sclerosis
     Use additional code, if applicable, to identify chronic total occlusion of artery of extremity (I70.92)
     Excludes2   atherosclerosis of bypass graft of extremities (I70.30-I70.79)

● **I70.20**   Unspecified atherosclerosis of native arteries of extremities

I70.201   Unspecified atherosclerosis of native arteries of extremities, right leg 🦟   A

I70.202   Unspecified atherosclerosis of native arteries of extremities, left leg 🦟   A

I70.203   Unspecified atherosclerosis of native arteries of extremities, bilateral legs 🦟   A

I70.208   Unspecified atherosclerosis of native arteries of extremities, other extremity 🦟   A

I70.209   Unspecified atherosclerosis of native arteries of extremities, unspecified extremity 🦟   A

● **I70.21**   Atherosclerosis of native arteries of extremities with intermittent claudication

I70.211   Atherosclerosis of native arteries of extremities with intermittent claudication, right leg 🦟   A

I70.212   Atherosclerosis of native arteries of extremities with intermittent claudication, left leg 🦟   A

I70.213   Atherosclerosis of native arteries of extremities with intermittent claudication, bilateral legs 🦟   A

I70.218   Atherosclerosis of native arteries of extremities with intermittent claudication, other extremity 🦟   A

I70.219   Atherosclerosis of native arteries of extremities with intermittent claudication, unspecified extremity 🦟   A

● **I70.22**   Atherosclerosis of native arteries of extremities with rest pain

   Includes   any condition classifiable to I70.21-
                chronic limb-threatening ischemia NOS of native arteries of extremities
                chronic limb-threatening ischemia of native arteries of extremities with rest pain
                critical limb ischemia NOS of native arteries of extremities
                critical limb ischemia of native arteries of extremities with rest pain

I70.221   Atherosclerosis of native arteries of extremities with rest pain, right leg 🦟   A

I70.222   Atherosclerosis of native arteries of extremities with rest pain, left leg 🦟 A

I70.223   Atherosclerosis of native arteries of extremities with rest pain, bilateral legs 🦟   A

I70.228   Atherosclerosis of native arteries of extremities with rest pain, other extremity 🦟   A

I70.229   Atherosclerosis of native arteries of extremities with rest pain, unspecified extremity 🦟   A

CHAPTER 9 (I00-I99)

CHAPTER 9 (I00-I99)

● **I70.23** Atherosclerosis of native arteries of right leg with ulceration

    Includes   any condition classifiable to I70.211 and I70.221
                  chronic limb-threatening ischemia of native arteries of right leg with ulceration
                  critical limb ischemia of native arteries of right leg with ulceration

    Use additional code to identify severity of ulcer (L97.-)

    I70.231 Atherosclerosis of native arteries of right leg with ulceration of thigh 🔖 A

    I70.232 Atherosclerosis of native arteries of right leg with ulceration of calf 🔖 A

    I70.233 Atherosclerosis of native arteries of right leg with ulceration of ankle 🔖 A

    I70.234 Atherosclerosis of native arteries of right leg with ulceration of heel and midfoot 🔖 A

         Atherosclerosis of native arteries of right leg with ulceration of plantar surface of midfoot

    I70.235 Atherosclerosis of native arteries of right leg with ulceration of other part of foot 🔖 A

         Atherosclerosis of native arteries of right leg extremities with ulceration of toe

    I70.238 Atherosclerosis of native arteries of right leg with ulceration of other part of lower leg 🔖 A

    I70.239 Atherosclerosis of native arteries of right leg with ulceration of unspecified site 🔖 A

● **I70.24** Atherosclerosis of native arteries of left leg with ulceration

    Includes   any condition classifiable to I70.212 and I70.222
                  chronic limb-threatening ischemia of native arteries of left leg with ulceration
                  critical limb ischemia of native arteries of left leg with ulceration

    Use additional code to identify severity of ulcer (L97.-)

    I70.241 Atherosclerosis of native arteries of left leg with ulceration of thigh 🔖 A

    I70.242 Atherosclerosis of native arteries of left leg with ulceration of calf 🔖 A

    I70.243 Atherosclerosis of native arteries of left leg with ulceration of ankle 🔖 A

    I70.244 Atherosclerosis of native arteries of left leg with ulceration of heel and midfoot 🔖 A

         Atherosclerosis of native arteries of left leg with ulceration of plantar surface of midfoot

    I70.245 Atherosclerosis of native arteries of left leg with ulceration of other part of foot 🔖 A

         Atherosclerosis of native arteries of left leg extremities with ulceration of toe

    I70.248 Atherosclerosis of native arteries of left leg with ulceration of other part of lower leg 🔖 A

    I70.249 Atherosclerosis of native arteries of left leg with ulceration of unspecified site 🔖 A

I70.25 Atherosclerosis of native arteries of other extremities with ulceration 🔖 A

    Includes   any condition classifiable to I70.218 and I70.228

    Use additional code to identify the severity of the ulcer (L98.49-)

● **I70.26** Atherosclerosis of native arteries of extremities with gangrene

    Includes   any condition classifiable to I70.21-, I70.22-, I70.23-, I70.24-, and I70.25-
                  chronic limb-threatening ischemia of native arteries of extremities with gangrene
                  critical limb ischemia of native arteries of extremities with gangrene

    Use additional code to identify the severity of any ulcer (L97.-, L98.49-), if applicable

    I70.261 Atherosclerosis of native arteries of extremities with gangrene, right leg A

    I70.262 Atherosclerosis of native arteries of extremities with gangrene, left leg 🔖 A

    I70.263 Atherosclerosis of native arteries of extremities with gangrene, bilateral legs 🔖 A

    I70.268 Atherosclerosis of native arteries of extremities with gangrene, other extremity 🔖 A

    I70.269 Atherosclerosis of native arteries of extremities with gangrene, unspecified extremity 🔖 A

● **I70.29** Other atherosclerosis of native arteries of extremities

    I70.291 Other atherosclerosis of native arteries of extremities, right leg 🔖 A

    I70.292 Other atherosclerosis of native arteries of extremities, left leg 🔖 A

    I70.293 Other atherosclerosis of native arteries of extremities, bilateral legs 🔖 A

    I70.298 Other atherosclerosis of native arteries of extremities, other extremity 🔖 A

    I70.299 Other atherosclerosis of native arteries of extremities, unspecified extremity 🔖 A

● **I70.3** Atherosclerosis of unspecified type of bypass graft(s) of the extremities

    Use additional code, if applicable, to identify chronic total occlusion of artery of extremity (I70.92)

    Excludes1   embolism or thrombus of bypass graft(s) of extremities (T82.8-)

● **I70.30** Unspecified atherosclerosis of unspecified type of bypass graft(s) of the extremities

    I70.301 Unspecified atherosclerosis of unspecified type of bypass graft(s) of the extremities, right leg 🔖 A

    I70.302 Unspecified atherosclerosis of unspecified type of bypass graft(s) of the extremities, left leg 🔖 A

    I70.303 Unspecified atherosclerosis of unspecified type of bypass graft(s) of the extremities, bilateral legs 🔖 A

    I70.308 Unspecified atherosclerosis of unspecified type of bypass graft(s) of the extremities, other extremity 🔖 A

    I70.309 Unspecified atherosclerosis of unspecified type of bypass graft(s) of the extremities, unspecified extremity 🔖 A

▶ New   ⟹ Revised   ~~deleted~~ Deleted   Excludes 1   Excludes 2   Includes   Use additional   Code first   Code also   Key words

OGCR Official Guidelines   X Assign placeholder X   ● Use Additional Character(s)   ▶ Manifestation Code   🔖 Hierarchical Condition Category   **Coding Clinic**

● **I70.31** **Atherosclerosis of unspecified type of bypass graft(s) of the extremities with intermittent claudication**

     I70.311   Atherosclerosis of unspecified type of bypass graft(s) of the extremities with intermittent claudication, right leg 🔳A

     I70.312   Atherosclerosis of unspecified type of bypass graft(s) of the extremities with intermittent claudication, left leg 🔳 A

     I70.313   Atherosclerosis of unspecified type of bypass graft(s) of the extremities with intermittent claudication, bilateral legs 🔳   A

     I70.318   Atherosclerosis of unspecified type of bypass graft(s) of the extremities with intermittent claudication, other extremity 🔳   A

     I70.319   Atherosclerosis of unspecified type of bypass graft(s) of the extremities with intermittent claudication, unspecified extremity 🔳   A

● **I70.32** **Atherosclerosis of unspecified type of bypass graft(s) of the extremities with rest pain**

     Includes   any condition classifiable to I70.31-
        chronic limb-threatening ischemia NOS of unspecified type of bypass graft(s) of the extremities
        chronic limb-threatening ischemia of unspecified type of bypass graft(s) of the extremities with rest pain, right leg
        critical limb ischemia NOS of unspecified type of bypass graft(s) of the extremities
        critical limb ischemia of unspecified type of bypass graft(s) of the extremities with rest pain

     I70.321   Atherosclerosis of unspecified type of bypass graft(s) of the extremities with rest pain, right leg 🔳   A

     I70.322   Atherosclerosis of unspecified type of bypass graft(s) of the extremities with rest pain, left leg 🔳   A

     I70.323   Atherosclerosis of unspecified type of bypass graft(s) of the extremities with rest pain, bilateral legs 🔳   A

     I70.328   Atherosclerosis of unspecified type of bypass graft(s) of the extremities with rest pain, other extremity 🔳   A

     I70.329   Atherosclerosis of unspecified type of bypass graft(s) of the extremities with rest pain, unspecified extremity 🔳   A

● **I70.33** **Atherosclerosis of unspecified type of bypass graft(s) of the right leg with ulceration**

     Includes   any condition classifiable to I70.311 and I70.321
        chronic limb-threatening ischemia of unspecified type of bypass graft(s) of the right leg with ulceration
        critical limb ischemia of unspecified type of bypass graft(s) of the right leg with ulceration

     Use additional code to identify severity of ulcer (L97.-)

     I70.331   Atherosclerosis of unspecified type of bypass graft(s) of the right leg with ulceration of thigh 🔳   A

     I70.332   Atherosclerosis of unspecified type of bypass graft(s) of the right leg with ulceration of calf 🔳   A

     I70.333   Atherosclerosis of unspecified type of bypass graft(s) of the right leg with ulceration of ankle 🔳   A

     I70.334   Atherosclerosis of unspecified type of bypass graft(s) of the right leg with ulceration of heel and midfoot 🔳   A
        Atherosclerosis of unspecified type of bypass graft(s) of right leg with ulceration of plantar surface of midfoot

     I70.335   Atherosclerosis of unspecified type of bypass graft(s) of the right leg with ulceration of other part of foot 🔳   A
        Atherosclerosis of unspecified type of bypass graft(s) of the right leg with ulceration of toe

     I70.338   Atherosclerosis of unspecified type of bypass graft(s) of the right leg with ulceration of other part of lower leg 🔳   A

     I70.339   Atherosclerosis of unspecified type of bypass graft(s) of the right leg with ulceration of unspecified site 🔳   A

● **I70.34** **Atherosclerosis of unspecified type of bypass graft(s) of the left leg with ulceration**

     Includes   any condition classifiable to I70.312 and I70.322
        chronic limb-threatening ischemia of unspecified type of bypass graft(s) of the left leg with ulceration
        critical limb ischemia of unspecified type of bypass graft(s) of the left leg with ulceration

     Use additional code to identify severity of ulcer (L97.-)

     I70.341   Atherosclerosis of unspecified type of bypass graft(s) of the left leg with ulceration of thigh 🔳   A

     I70.342   Atherosclerosis of unspecified type of bypass graft(s) of the left leg with ulceration of calf 🔳   A

     I70.343   Atherosclerosis of unspecified type of bypass graft(s) of the left leg with ulceration of ankle 🔳   A

     I70.344   Atherosclerosis of unspecified type of bypass graft(s) of the left leg with ulceration of heel and midfoot 🔳   A
        Atherosclerosis of unspecified type of bypass graft(s) of left leg with ulceration of plantar surface of midfoot

     I70.345   Atherosclerosis of unspecified type of bypass graft(s) of the left leg with ulceration of other part of foot 🔳   A
        Atherosclerosis of unspecified type of bypass graft(s) of the left leg with ulceration of toe

     I70.348   Atherosclerosis of unspecified type of bypass graft(s) of the left leg with ulceration of other part of lower leg 🔳   A

     I70.349   Atherosclerosis of unspecified type of bypass graft(s) of the left leg with ulceration of unspecified site 🔳   A

I70.35   Atherosclerosis of unspecified type of bypass graft(s) of other extremity with ulceration 🦠 A

     Includes   any condition classifiable to I70.318 and I70.328

     Use additional code to identify severity of ulcer (L98.49-)

● I70.36   Atherosclerosis of unspecified type of bypass graft(s) of the extremities with gangrene

     Includes   any condition classifiable to I70.31-, I70.32-, I70.33-, I70.34-, I70.35

           chronic limb-threatening ischemia of unspecified type of bypass graft(s) of the extremities with gangrene

           critical limb ischemia of unspecified type of bypass graft(s) of the extremities with gangrene

     Use additional code to identify the severity of any ulcer (L97.-, L98.49-), if applicable

     I70.361   Atherosclerosis of unspecified type of bypass graft(s) of the extremities with gangrene, right leg 🦠   A

     I70.362   Atherosclerosis of unspecified type of bypass graft(s) of the extremities with gangrene, left leg 🦠   A

     I70.363   Atherosclerosis of unspecified type of bypass graft(s) of the extremities with gangrene, bilateral legs 🦠   A

     I70.368   Atherosclerosis of unspecified type of bypass graft(s) of the extremities with gangrene, other extremity 🦠   A

     I70.369   Atherosclerosis of unspecified type of bypass graft(s) of the extremities with gangrene, unspecified extremity 🦠   A

● I70.39   Other atherosclerosis of unspecified type of bypass graft(s) of the extremities

     I70.391   Other atherosclerosis of unspecified type of bypass graft(s) of the extremities, right leg 🦠   A

     I70.392   Other atherosclerosis of unspecified type of bypass graft(s) of the extremities, left leg 🦠   A

     I70.393   Other atherosclerosis of unspecified type of bypass graft(s) of the extremities, bilateral legs 🦠   A

     I70.398   Other atherosclerosis of unspecified type of bypass graft(s) of the extremities, other extremity 🦠   A

     I70.399   Other atherosclerosis of unspecified type of bypass graft(s) of the extremities, unspecified extremity 🦠 A

● I70.4   Atherosclerosis of autologous vein bypass graft(s) of the extremities

     Use additional code, if applicable, to identify chronic total occlusion of artery of extremity (I70.92)

● I70.40   Unspecified atherosclerosis of autologous vein bypass graft(s) of the extremities

     I70.401   Unspecified atherosclerosis of autologous vein bypass graft(s) of the extremities, right leg 🦠   A

     I70.402   Unspecified atherosclerosis of autologous vein bypass graft(s) of the extremities, left leg 🦠   A

     I70.403   Unspecified atherosclerosis of autologous vein bypass graft(s) of the extremities, bilateral legs 🦠   A

     I70.408   Unspecified atherosclerosis of autologous vein bypass graft(s) of the extremities, other extremity 🦠   A

     I70.409   Unspecified atherosclerosis of autologous vein bypass graft(s) of the extremities, unspecified extremity 🦠 A

● I70.41   Atherosclerosis of autologous vein bypass graft(s) of the extremities with intermittent claudication

     I70.411   Atherosclerosis of autologous vein bypass graft(s) of the extremities with intermittent claudication, right leg 🦠 A

     I70.412   Atherosclerosis of autologous vein bypass graft(s) of the extremities with intermittent claudication, left leg 🦠   A

     I70.413   Atherosclerosis of autologous vein bypass graft(s) of the extremities with intermittent claudication, bilateral legs 🦠   A

     I70.418   Atherosclerosis of autologous vein bypass graft(s) of the extremities with intermittent claudication, other extremity 🦠   A

     I70.419   Atherosclerosis of autologous vein bypass graft(s) of the extremities with intermittent claudication, unspecified extremity 🦠   A

● I70.42   Atherosclerosis of autologous vein bypass graft(s) of the extremities with rest pain

     Includes   any condition classifiable to I70.41-

           chronic limb-threatening ischemia NOS of autologous vein bypass graft(s) of the extremities

           chronic limb-threatening ischemia of autologous vein bypass graft(s) of the extremities with rest pain

           critical limb ischemia NOS of autologous vein bypass graft(s) of the extremities

           critical limb ischemia of autologous vein bypass graft(s) of the extremities with rest pain

     I70.421   Atherosclerosis of autologous vein bypass graft(s) of the extremities with rest pain, right leg 🦠   A

     I70.422   Atherosclerosis of autologous vein bypass graft(s) of the extremities with rest pain, left leg 🦠   A

     I70.423   Atherosclerosis of autologous vein bypass graft(s) of the extremities with rest pain, bilateral legs 🦠   A

     I70.428   Atherosclerosis of autologous vein bypass graft(s) of the extremities with rest pain, other extremity 🦠   A

     I70.429   Atherosclerosis of autologous vein bypass graft(s) of the extremities with rest pain, unspecified extremity 🦠   A

● I70.43   Atherosclerosis of autologous vein bypass graft(s) of the right leg with ulceration

     Includes   any condition classifiable to I70.411 and I70.421

           chronic limb-threatening ischemia of autologous vein bypass graft(s) of the right leg with ulceration

           critical limb ischemia of autologous vein bypass graft(s) of the right leg with ulceration

     Use additional code to identify severity of ulcer (L97.-)

     I70.431   Atherosclerosis of autologous vein bypass graft(s) of the right leg with ulceration of thigh 🦠   A

I70.432   Atherosclerosis of autologous vein bypass graft(s) of the right leg with ulceration of calf 🔹   A

I70.433   Atherosclerosis of autologous vein bypass graft(s) of the right leg with ulceration of ankle 🔹   A

I70.434   Atherosclerosis of autologous vein bypass graft(s) of the right leg with ulceration of heel and midfoot 🔹   A
> Atherosclerosis of autologous vein bypass graft(s) of right leg with ulceration of plantar surface of midfoot

I70.435   Atherosclerosis of autologous vein bypass graft(s) of the right leg with ulceration of other part of foot 🔹   A
> Atherosclerosis of autologous vein bypass graft(s) of right leg with ulceration of toe

I70.438   Atherosclerosis of autologous vein bypass graft(s) of the right leg with ulceration of other part of lower leg 🔹   A

I70.439   Atherosclerosis of autologous vein bypass graft(s) of the right leg with ulceration of unspecified site 🔹   A

● I70.44   Atherosclerosis of autologous vein bypass graft(s) of the left leg with ulceration
> **Includes**   any condition classifiable to I70.412 and I70.422
> chronic limb-threatening ischemia of autologous vein bypass graft(s) of the left leg with ulceration
> critical limb ischemia of autologous vein bypass graft(s) of the left leg with ulceration

Use additional code to identify severity of ulcer (L97.-)

I70.441   Atherosclerosis of autologous vein bypass graft(s) of the left leg with ulceration of thigh 🔹   A

I70.442   Atherosclerosis of autologous vein bypass graft(s) of the left leg with ulceration of calf 🔹   A

I70.443   Atherosclerosis of autologous vein bypass graft(s) of the left leg with ulceration of ankle 🔹   A

I70.444   Atherosclerosis of autologous vein bypass graft(s) of the left leg with ulceration of heel and midfoot 🔹   A
> Atherosclerosis of autologous vein bypass graft(s) of left leg with ulceration of plantar surface of midfoot

I70.445   Atherosclerosis of autologous vein bypass graft(s) of the left leg with ulceration of other part of foot 🔹   A
> Atherosclerosis of autologous vein bypass graft(s) of left leg with ulceration of toe

I70.448   Atherosclerosis of autologous vein bypass graft(s) of the left leg with ulceration of other part of lower leg 🔹   A

I70.449   Atherosclerosis of autologous vein bypass graft(s) of the left leg with ulceration of unspecified site 🔹   A

I70.45   Atherosclerosis of autologous vein bypass graft(s) of other extremity with ulceration 🔹   A
> **Includes**   any condition classifiable to I70.418, I70.428, and I70.438

Use additional code to identify severity of ulcer (L98.49-)

● I70.46   Atherosclerosis of autologous vein bypass graft(s) of the extremities with gangrene
> **Includes**   any condition classifiable to I70.41-, I70.42-, and I70.43-, I70.44-, I70.45
> chronic limb-threatening ischemia of autologous vein bypass graft(s) of the extremities with gangrene
> critical limb ischemia of autologous vein bypass graft(s) of the extremities with gangrene

Use additional code to identify the severity of any ulcer (L97.-, L98.49-), if applicable

I70.461   Atherosclerosis of autologous vein bypass graft(s) of the extremities with gangrene, right leg   A

I70.462   Atherosclerosis of autologous vein bypass graft(s) of the extremities with gangrene, left leg 🔹   A

I70.463   Atherosclerosis of autologous vein bypass graft(s) of the extremities with gangrene, bilateral legs 🔹   A

I70.468   Atherosclerosis of autologous vein bypass graft(s) of the extremities with gangrene, other extremity 🔹   A

I70.469   Atherosclerosis of autologous vein bypass graft(s) of the extremities with gangrene, unspecified extremity 🔹   A

● I70.49   Other atherosclerosis of autologous vein bypass graft(s) of the extremities

I70.491   Other atherosclerosis of autologous vein bypass graft(s) of the extremities, right leg 🔹   A

I70.492   Other atherosclerosis of autologous vein bypass graft(s) of the extremities, left leg 🔹   A

I70.493   Other atherosclerosis of autologous vein bypass graft(s) of the extremities, bilateral legs 🔹   A

I70.498   Other atherosclerosis of autologous vein bypass graft(s) of the extremities, other extremity 🔹   A

I70.499   Other atherosclerosis of autologous vein bypass graft(s) of the extremities, unspecified extremity 🔹   A

● I70.5   Atherosclerosis of nonautologous biological bypass graft(s) of the extremities
Use additional code, if applicable, to identify chronic total occlusion of artery of extremity (I70.92)

● I70.50   Unspecified atherosclerosis of nonautologous biological bypass graft(s) of the extremities

I70.501   Unspecified atherosclerosis of nonautologous biological bypass graft(s) of the extremities, right leg 🔹   A

I70.502   Unspecified atherosclerosis of nonautologous biological bypass graft(s) of the extremities, left leg 🔹 A

I70.503   Unspecified atherosclerosis of nonautologous biological bypass graft(s) of the extremities, bilateral legs 🔹   A

CHAPTER 9 (I00–I99)

CHAPTER 9 (I00-I99)

I70.508   Unspecified atherosclerosis of nonautologous biological bypass graft(s) of the extremities, other extremity 🐾   A

I70.509   Unspecified atherosclerosis of nonautologous biological bypass graft(s) of the extremities, unspecified extremity 🐾   A

● I70.51   Atherosclerosis of nonautologous biological bypass graft(s) of the extremities intermittent claudication

I70.511   Atherosclerosis of nonautologous biological bypass graft(s) of the extremities with intermittent claudication, right leg 🐾   A

I70.512   Atherosclerosis of nonautologous biological bypass graft(s) of the extremities with intermittent claudication, left leg 🐾   A

I70.513   Atherosclerosis of nonautologous biological bypass graft(s) of the extremities with intermittent claudication, bilateral legs 🐾   A

I70.518   Atherosclerosis of nonautologous biological bypass graft(s) of the extremities with intermittent claudication, other extremity 🐾   A

I70.519   Atherosclerosis of nonautologous biological bypass graft(s) of the extremities with intermittent claudication, unspecified extremity 🐾 A

● I70.52   Atherosclerosis of nonautologous biological bypass graft(s) of the extremities with rest pain

Includes   any condition classifiable to I70.51-
chronic limb-threatening ischemia NOS of nonautologous biological bypass graft(s) of the extremities
chronic limb-threatening ischemia of nonautologous biological bypass graft(s) of the extremities with rest pain
critical limb ischemia NOS of nonautologous biological bypass graft(s) of the extremities
critical limb ischemia of nonautologous biological bypass graft(s) of the extremities with rest pain

I70.521   Atherosclerosis of nonautologous biological bypass graft(s) of the extremities with rest pain, right leg 🐾   A

I70.522   Atherosclerosis of nonautologous biological bypass graft(s) of the extremities with rest pain, left leg 🐾 A

I70.523   Atherosclerosis of nonautologous biological bypass graft(s) of the extremities with rest pain, bilateral legs 🐾   A

I70.528   Atherosclerosis of nonautologous biological bypass graft(s) of the extremities with rest pain, other extremity 🐾   A

I70.529   Atherosclerosis of nonautologous biological bypass graft(s) of the extremities with rest pain, unspecified extremity 🐾   A

● I70.53   Atherosclerosis of nonautologous biological bypass graft(s) of the right leg with ulceration

Includes   any condition classifiable to I70.511 and I70.521
chronic limb-threatening ischemia of nonautologous biological bypass graft(s) of the right leg with ulceration
critical limb ischemia of nonautologous biological bypass graft(s) of the right leg with ulceration

Use additional code to identify severity of ulcer (L97.-)

I70.531   Atherosclerosis of nonautologous biological bypass graft(s) of the right leg with ulceration of thigh 🐾 A

I70.532   Atherosclerosis of nonautologous biological bypass graft(s) of the right leg with ulceration of calf 🐾 A

I70.533   Atherosclerosis of nonautologous biological bypass graft(s) of the right leg with ulceration of ankle 🐾 A

I70.534   Atherosclerosis of nonautologous biological bypass graft(s) of the right leg with ulceration of heel and midfoot 🐾   A
Atherosclerosis of nonautologous biological bypass graft(s) of right leg with ulceration of plantar surface of midfoot

I70.535   Atherosclerosis of nonautologous biological bypass graft(s) of the right leg with ulceration of other part of foot 🐾   A
Atherosclerosis of nonautologous biological bypass graft(s) of the right leg with ulceration of toe

I70.538   Atherosclerosis of nonautologous biological bypass graft(s) of the right leg with ulceration of other part of lower leg 🐾   A

I70.539   Atherosclerosis of nonautologous biological bypass graft(s) of the right leg with ulceration of unspecified site 🐾   A

● I70.54   Atherosclerosis of nonautologous biological bypass graft(s) of the left leg with ulceration

Includes   any condition classifiable to I70.512 and I70.522
chronic limb-threatening ischemia of nonautologous biological bypass graft(s) of the left leg with ulceration
critical limb ischemia of nonautologous biological bypass graft(s) of the left leg with ulceration

Use additional code to identify severity of ulcer (L97.-)

I70.541   Atherosclerosis of nonautologous biological bypass graft(s) of the left leg with ulceration of thigh 🐾   A

I70.542   Atherosclerosis of nonautologous biological bypass graft(s) of the left leg with ulceration of calf 🐾   A

I70.543   Atherosclerosis of nonautologous biological bypass graft(s) of the left leg with ulceration of ankle 🐾   A

▶ New   ⇒ Revised   ~~deleted~~ Deleted   Excludes 1   Excludes 2   Includes   Use additional   Code first   Code also   Key words

OGCR Official Guidelines   X Assign placeholder X   ● Use Additional Character(s)   ▶ Manifestation Code   🐾 Hierarchical Condition Category   **Coding Clinic**

I70.544   Atherosclerosis of nonautologous biological bypass graft(s) of the left leg with ulceration of heel and midfoot 🔖   A
  Atherosclerosis of nonautologous biological bypass graft(s) of left leg with ulceration of plantar surface of midfoot

I70.545   Atherosclerosis of nonautologous biological bypass graft(s) of the left leg with ulceration of other part of foot 🔖   A
  Atherosclerosis of nonautologous biological bypass graft(s) of the left leg with ulceration of toe

I70.548   Atherosclerosis of nonautologous biological bypass graft(s) of the left leg with ulceration of other part of lower leg 🔖   A

I70.549   Atherosclerosis of nonautologous biological bypass graft(s) of the left leg with ulceration of unspecified site 🔖   A

I70.55   Atherosclerosis of nonautologous biological bypass graft(s) of other extremity with ulceration 🔖   A
 Includes any condition classifiable to I70.518, I70.528, and I70.538
 Use additional code to identify severity of ulcer (L98.49)

● I70.56   Atherosclerosis of nonautologous biological bypass graft(s) of the extremities with gangrene
 Includes any condition classifiable to I70.51-, I70.52-, and I70.53-, I70.54-, I70.55
  chronic limb-threatening ischemia of nonautologous biological bypass graft(s) of the extremities with gangrene
  critical limb ischemia of nonautologous biological bypass graft(s) of the extremities with gangrene
 Use additional code to identify the severity of any ulcer (L97.-, L98.49-), if applicable

I70.561   Atherosclerosis of nonautologous biological bypass graft(s) of the extremities with gangrene, right leg 🔖   A

I70.562   Atherosclerosis of nonautologous biological bypass graft(s) of the extremities with gangrene, left leg 🔖   A

I70.563   Atherosclerosis of nonautologous biological bypass graft(s) of the extremities with gangrene, bilateral legs 🔖   A

I70.568   Atherosclerosis of nonautologous biological bypass graft(s) of the extremities with gangrene, other extremity 🔖   A

I70.569   Atherosclerosis of nonautologous biological bypass graft(s) of the extremities with gangrene, unspecified extremity 🔖   A

● I70.59   Other atherosclerosis of nonautologous biological bypass graft(s) of the extremities

I70.591   Other atherosclerosis of nonautologous biological bypass graft(s) of the extremities, right leg 🔖   A

I70.592   Other atherosclerosis of nonautologous biological bypass graft(s) of the extremities, left leg 🔖   A

I70.593   Other atherosclerosis of nonautologous biological bypass graft(s) of the extremities, bilateral legs 🔖   A

I70.598   Other atherosclerosis of nonautologous biological bypass graft(s) of the extremities, other extremity 🔖   A

I70.599   Other atherosclerosis of nonautologous biological bypass graft(s) of the extremities, unspecified extremity 🔖   A

● I70.6   Atherosclerosis of nonbiological bypass graft(s) of the extremities
 Use additional code, if applicable, to identify chronic total occlusion of artery of extremity (I70.92)

● I70.60   Unspecified atherosclerosis of nonbiological bypass graft(s) of the extremities

I70.601   Unspecified atherosclerosis of nonbiological bypass graft(s) of the extremities, right leg 🔖   A

I70.602   Unspecified atherosclerosis of nonbiological bypass graft(s) of the extremities, left leg 🔖   A

I70.603   Unspecified atherosclerosis of nonbiological bypass graft(s) of the extremities, bilateral legs 🔖   A

I70.608   Unspecified atherosclerosis of nonbiological bypass graft(s) of the extremities, other extremity 🔖   A

I70.609   Unspecified atherosclerosis of nonbiological bypass graft(s) of the extremities, unspecified extremity 🔖   A

● I70.61   Atherosclerosis of nonbiological bypass graft(s) of the extremities with intermittent claudication

I70.611   Atherosclerosis of nonbiological bypass graft(s) of the extremities with intermittent claudication, right leg 🔖   A

I70.612   Atherosclerosis of nonbiological bypass graft(s) of the extremities with intermittent claudication, left leg 🔖   A

I70.613   Atherosclerosis of nonbiological bypass graft(s) of the extremities with intermittent claudication, bilateral legs 🔖   A

I70.618   Atherosclerosis of nonbiological bypass graft(s) of the extremities with intermittent claudication, other extremity 🔖   A

I70.619   Atherosclerosis of nonbiological bypass graft(s) of the extremities with intermittent claudication, unspecified extremity 🔖   A

● I70.62   Atherosclerosis of nonbiological bypass graft(s) of the extremities with rest pain
 Includes any condition classifiable to I70.61-
  chronic limb-threatening ischemia NOS of nonbiological bypass graft(s) of the extremities
  chronic limb-threatening ischemia of nonbiological bypass graft(s) of the extremities with rest pain
  critical limb ischemia NOS of nonbiological bypass graft(s) of the extremities
  critical limb ischemia of nonbiological bypass graft(s) of the extremities with rest pain

I70.621   Atherosclerosis of nonbiological bypass graft(s) of the extremities with rest pain, right leg 🔖   A

I70.622   Atherosclerosis of nonbiological bypass graft(s) of the extremities with rest pain, left leg 🔖   A

CHAPTER 9 (I00-I99)

I70.623   Atherosclerosis of nonbiological bypass graft(s) of the extremities with rest pain, bilateral legs 🦠   A

I70.628   Atherosclerosis of nonbiological bypass graft(s) of the extremities with rest pain, other extremity 🦠   A

I70.629   Atherosclerosis of nonbiological bypass graft(s) of the extremities with rest pain, unspecified extremity 🦠   A

● **I70.63**   Atherosclerosis of nonbiological bypass graft(s) of the right leg with ulceration

    Includes   any condition classifiable to I70.611 and I70.621
          chronic limb-threatening ischemia of nonbiological bypass graft(s) of the right leg with ulceration
          critical limb ischemia of nonbiological bypass graft(s) of the right leg with ulceration

    Use additional code to identify severity of ulcer (L97.-)

I70.631   Atherosclerosis of nonbiological bypass graft(s) of the right leg with ulceration of thigh 🦠   A

I70.632   Atherosclerosis of nonbiological bypass graft(s) of the right leg with ulceration of calf 🦠   A

I70.633   Atherosclerosis of nonbiological bypass graft(s) of the right leg with ulceration of ankle 🦠   A

I70.634   Atherosclerosis of nonbiological bypass graft(s) of the right leg with ulceration of heel and midfoot 🦠   A
      Atherosclerosis of nonbiological bypass graft(s) of right leg with ulceration of plantar surface of midfoot

I70.635   Atherosclerosis of nonbiological bypass graft(s) of the right leg with ulceration of other part of foot 🦠   A
      Atherosclerosis of nonbiological bypass graft(s) of the right leg with ulceration of toe

I70.638   Atherosclerosis of nonbiological bypass graft(s) of the right leg with ulceration of other part of lower leg 🦠   A

I70.639   Atherosclerosis of nonbiological bypass graft(s) of the right leg with ulceration of unspecified site 🦠   A

● **I70.64**   Atherosclerosis of nonbiological bypass graft(s) of the left leg with ulceration

    Includes   any condition classifiable to I70.612 and I70.622
          chronic limb-threatening ischemia of nonbiological bypass graft(s) of the left leg with ulceration
          critical limb ischemia of nonbiological bypass graft(s) of the left leg with ulceration

    Use additional code to identify severity of ulcer (L97.-)

I70.641   Atherosclerosis of nonbiological bypass graft(s) of the left leg with ulceration of thigh 🦠   A

I70.642   Atherosclerosis of nonbiological bypass graft(s) of the left leg with ulceration of calf 🦠   A

I70.643   Atherosclerosis of nonbiological bypass graft(s) of the left leg with ulceration of ankle 🦠   A

I70.644   Atherosclerosis of nonbiological bypass graft(s) of the left leg with ulceration of heel and midfoot 🦠   A
      Atherosclerosis of nonbiological bypass graft(s) of left leg with ulceration of plantar surface of midfoot

I70.645   Atherosclerosis of nonbiological bypass graft(s) of the left leg with ulceration of other part of foot 🦠   A
      Atherosclerosis of nonbiological bypass graft(s) of the left leg with ulceration of toe

I70.648   Atherosclerosis of nonbiological bypass graft(s) of the left leg with ulceration of other part of lower leg 🦠   A

I70.649   Atherosclerosis of nonbiological bypass graft(s) of the left leg with ulceration of unspecified site 🦠   A

I70.65   Atherosclerosis of nonbiological bypass graft(s) of other extremity with ulceration 🦠

    Includes   any condition classifiable to I70.618 and I70.628

    Use additional code to identify severity of ulcer (L98.49-)

● **I70.66**   Atherosclerosis of nonbiological bypass graft(s) of the extremities with gangrene

    Includes   any condition classifiable to I70.61-, I70.62-, I70.63-, I70.64-, I70.65
          chronic limb-threatening ischemia of nonbiological bypass graft(s) of the extremities with gangrene
          critical limb ischemia of nonbiological bypass graft(s) of the extremities with gangrene

    Use additional code to identify the severity of any ulcer (L97.-, L98.49-), if applicable

I70.661   Atherosclerosis of nonbiological bypass graft(s) of the extremities with gangrene, right leg 🦠   A

I70.662   Atherosclerosis of nonbiological bypass graft(s) of the extremities with gangrene, left leg 🦠   A

I70.663   Atherosclerosis of nonbiological bypass graft(s) of the extremities with gangrene, bilateral legs 🦠   A

I70.668   Atherosclerosis of nonbiological bypass graft(s) of the extremities with gangrene, other extremity 🦠   A

I70.669   Atherosclerosis of nonbiological bypass graft(s) of the extremities with gangrene, unspecified extremity 🦠   A

● **I70.69**   Other atherosclerosis of nonbiological bypass graft(s) of the extremities

I70.691   Other atherosclerosis of nonbiological bypass graft(s) of the extremities, right leg 🦠   A

I70.692   Other atherosclerosis of nonbiological bypass graft(s) of the extremities, left leg 🦠   A

I70.693   Other atherosclerosis of nonbiological bypass graft(s) of the extremities, bilateral legs 🦠   A

▶ New   ⇒ Revised   ~~deleted~~ Deleted   Excludes 1   Excludes 2   Includes   Use additional   Code first   Code also   Key words

OGCR Official Guidelines   X Assign placeholder X   ● Use Additional Character(s)   ▶ Manifestation Code   🦠 Hierarchical Condition Category   Coding Clinic

I70.698   Other atherosclerosis of nonbiological bypass graft(s) of the extremities, other extremity 🦴   A

I70.699   Other atherosclerosis of nonbiological bypass graft(s) of the extremities, unspecified extremity 🦴   A

● **I70.7**   Atherosclerosis of other type of bypass graft(s) of the extremities

> Use additional code, if applicable, to identify chronic total occlusion of artery of extremity (I70.92)

● **I70.70**   Unspecified atherosclerosis of other type of bypass graft(s) of the extremities

I70.701   Unspecified atherosclerosis of other type of bypass graft(s) of the extremities, right leg 🦴   A

I70.702   Unspecified atherosclerosis of other type of bypass graft(s) of the extremities, left leg 🦴   A

I70.703   Unspecified atherosclerosis of other type of bypass graft(s) of the extremities, bilateral legs 🦴   A

I70.708   Unspecified atherosclerosis of other type of bypass graft(s) of the extremities, other extremity 🦴   A

I70.709   Unspecified atherosclerosis of other type of bypass graft(s) of the extremities, unspecified extremity 🦴 A

● **I70.71**   Atherosclerosis of other type of bypass graft(s) of the extremities with intermittent claudication

I70.711   Atherosclerosis of other type of bypass graft(s) of the extremities with intermittent claudication, right leg 🦴A

I70.712   Atherosclerosis of other type of bypass graft(s) of the extremities with intermittent claudication, left leg 🦴   A

I70.713   Atherosclerosis of other type of bypass graft(s) of the extremities with intermittent claudication, bilateral legs 🦴   A

I70.718   Atherosclerosis of other type of bypass graft(s) of the extremities with intermittent claudication, other extremity 🦴   A

I70.719   Atherosclerosis of other type of bypass graft(s) of the extremities with intermittent claudication, unspecified extremity 🦴   A

● **I70.72**   Atherosclerosis of other type of bypass graft(s) of the extremities with rest pain

> **Includes**   any condition classifiable to I70.71-
> chronic limb-threatening ischemia NOS of other type of bypass graft(s) of the extremities
> chronic limb-threatening ischemia of other type of bypass graft(s) of the extremities with rest pain
> critical limb ischemia NOS of other type of bypass graft(s) of the extremities
> critical limb ischemia of other type of bypass graft(s) of the extremities with rest pain

I70.721   Atherosclerosis of other type of bypass graft(s) of the extremities with rest pain, right leg 🦴   A

I70.722   Atherosclerosis of other type of bypass graft(s) of the extremities with rest pain, left leg 🦴   A

I70.723   Atherosclerosis of other type of bypass graft(s) of the extremities with rest pain, bilateral legs 🦴   A

I70.728   Atherosclerosis of other type of bypass graft(s) of the extremities with rest pain, other extremity 🦴   A

I70.729   Atherosclerosis of other type of bypass graft(s) of the extremities with rest pain, unspecified extremity 🦴   A

● **I70.73**   Atherosclerosis of other type of bypass graft(s) of the right leg with ulceration

> **Includes**   any condition classifiable to I70.711 and I70.721
> chronic limb-threatening ischemia of other type of bypass graft(s) of the right leg with ulceration
> critical limb ischemia of other type of bypass graft(s) of the right leg with ulceration

> Use additional code to identify severity of ulcer (L97.-)

I70.731   Atherosclerosis of other type of bypass graft(s) of the right leg with ulceration of thigh 🦴   A

I70.732   Atherosclerosis of other type of bypass graft(s) of the right leg with ulceration of calf 🦴   A

I70.733   Atherosclerosis of other type of bypass graft(s) of the right leg with ulceration of ankle 🦴   A

I70.734   Atherosclerosis of other type of bypass graft(s) of the right leg with ulceration of heel and midfoot 🦴   A
> Atherosclerosis of other type of bypass graft(s) of right leg with ulceration of plantar surface of midfoot

I70.735   Atherosclerosis of other type of bypass graft(s) of the right leg with ulceration of other part of foot 🦴   A
> Atherosclerosis of other type of bypass graft(s) of right leg with ulceration of toe

I70.738   Atherosclerosis of other type of bypass graft(s) of the right leg with ulceration of other part of lower leg 🦴   A

I70.739   Atherosclerosis of other type of bypass graft(s) of the right leg with ulceration of unspecified site 🦴   A

● **I70.74**   Atherosclerosis of other type of bypass graft(s) of the left leg with ulceration

> **Includes**   any condition classifiable to I70.712 and I70.722
> chronic limb-threatening ischemia of other type of bypass graft(s) of the left leg with ulceration
> critical limb ischemia of other type of bypass graft(s) of the left leg with ulceration

> Use additional code to identify severity of ulcer (L97.-)

I70.741   Atherosclerosis of other type of bypass graft(s) of the left leg with ulceration of thigh 🦴   A

I70.742   Atherosclerosis of other type of bypass graft(s) of the left leg with ulceration of calf 🦴   A

I70.743   Atherosclerosis of other type of bypass graft(s) of the left leg with ulceration of ankle 🦴   A

CHAPTER 9 (I00-I99)

I70.744   **Atherosclerosis of other type of bypass graft(s) of the left leg with ulceration of heel and midfoot** 🅡   A
Atherosclerosis of other type of bypass graft(s) of left leg with ulceration of plantar surface of midfoot

I70.745   **Atherosclerosis of other type of bypass graft(s) of the left leg with ulceration of other part of foot** 🅡   A
Atherosclerosis of other type of bypass graft(s) of left leg with ulceration of toe

I70.748   **Atherosclerosis of other type of bypass graft(s) of the left leg with ulceration of other part of lower leg** 🅡   A

I70.749   **Atherosclerosis of other type of bypass graft(s) of the left leg with ulceration of unspecified site** 🅡   A

I70.75   **Atherosclerosis of other type of bypass graft(s) of other extremity with ulceration** 🅡   A
Includes   any condition classifiable to I70.718 and I70.728
Use additional code to identify severity of ulcer (L98.49)

●**I70.76**   **Atherosclerosis of other type of bypass graft(s) of the extremities with gangrene**
Includes   any condition classifiable to I70.71-, I70.72-, I70.73-, I70.74-, I70.75
chronic limb-threatening ischemia of other type of bypass graft(s) of the extremities with gangrene
critical limb ischemia of other type of bypass graft(s) of the extremities with gangrene
Use additional code to identify the severity of any ulcer (L97.-, L98.49-), if applicable

I70.761   **Atherosclerosis of other type of bypass graft(s) of the extremities with gangrene, right leg** 🅡   A

I70.762   **Atherosclerosis of other type of bypass graft(s) of the extremities with gangrene, left leg** 🅡   A

I70.763   **Atherosclerosis of other type of bypass graft(s) of the extremities with gangrene, bilateral legs** 🅡   A

I70.768   **Atherosclerosis of other type of bypass graft(s) of the extremities with gangrene, other extremity** 🅡   A

I70.769   **Atherosclerosis of other type of bypass graft(s) of the extremities with gangrene, unspecified extremity** 🅡   A

●**I70.79**   **Other atherosclerosis of other type of bypass graft(s) of the extremities**

I70.791   **Other atherosclerosis of other type of bypass graft(s) of the extremities, right leg** 🅡   A

I70.792   **Other atherosclerosis of other type of bypass graft(s) of the extremities, left leg** 🅡   A

I70.793   **Other atherosclerosis of other type of bypass graft(s) of the extremities, bilateral legs** 🅡   A

I70.798   **Other atherosclerosis of other type of bypass graft(s) of the extremities, other extremity** 🅡   A

I70.799   **Other atherosclerosis of other type of bypass graft(s) of the extremities, unspecified extremity** 🅡   A

I70.8   **Atherosclerosis of other arteries**   A

●**I70.9**   **Other and unspecified atherosclerosis**

I70.90   **Unspecified atherosclerosis**   A

I70.91   **Generalized atherosclerosis**   A

I70.92   **Chronic total occlusion of artery of the extremities** 🅡   A
Complete occlusion of artery of the extremities
Total occlusion of artery of the extremities
Code first atherosclerosis of arteries of the extremities (I70.2-, I70.3-, I70.4-, I70.5-, I70.6-, I70.7-)

●**I71**   **Aortic aneurysm and dissection**
Code first, if applicable:
syphilitic aortic aneurysm (A52.01)
traumatic aortic aneurysm (S25.09, S35.09)

●**I71.0**   **Dissection of aorta**

I71.00   **Dissection of unspecified site of aorta** 🅡

●**I71.01**   **Dissection of thoracic aorta** 🅡

I71.010   **Dissection of ascending aorta**
Coding Clinic: 2024, Q2, P17

I71.011   **Dissection of aortic arch**
Coding Clinic: 2024, Q2, P17

I71.012   **Dissection of descending thoracic aorta**
Coding Clinic: 2024, Q2, P17

I71.019   **Dissection of thoracic aorta, unspecified**

I71.02   **Dissection of abdominal aorta** 🅡

I71.03   **Dissection of thoracoabdominal aorta** 🅡

●**I71.1**   **Thoracic aortic aneurysm, ruptured** 🅡

I71.10   **Thoracic aortic aneurysm, ruptured, unspecified**

I71.11   **Aneurysm of the ascending aorta, ruptured**

I71.12   **Aneurysm of the aortic arch, ruptured**

I71.13   **Aneurysm of the descending thoracic aorta, ruptured**

●**I71.2**   **Thoracic aortic aneurysm, without rupture** 🅡

I71.20   **Thoracic aortic aneurysm, without rupture, unspecified**

I71.21   **Aneurysm of the ascending aorta, without rupture**

I71.22   **Aneurysm of the aortic arch, without rupture**

I71.23   **Aneurysm of the descending thoracic aorta, without rupture**

●**I71.3**   **Abdominal aortic aneurysm, ruptured** 🅡

I71.30   **Abdominal aortic aneurysm, ruptured, unspecified**

I71.31   **Pararenal abdominal aortic aneurysm, ruptured**

I71.32   **Juxtarenal abdominal aortic aneurysm, ruptured**

I71.33   **Infrarenal abdominal aortic aneurysm, ruptured**

●**I71.4**   **Abdominal aortic aneurysm, without rupture** 🅡

I71.40   **Abdominal aortic aneurysm, without rupture, unspecified**

I71.41   **Pararenal abdominal aortic aneurysm, without rupture**
Coding Clinic: 2024, Q2, P16

I71.42   **Juxtarenal abdominal aortic aneurysm, without rupture**

I71.43   **Infrarenal abdominal aortic aneurysm, without rupture**

●**I71.5**   **Thoracoabdominal aortic aneurysm, ruptured** 🅡

I71.50   **Thoracoabdominal aortic aneurysm, ruptured, unspecified**

I71.51   **Supraceliac aneurysm of the thoracoabdominal aorta, ruptured**

I71.52   **Paravisceral aneurysm of the thoracoabdominal aorta, ruptured**

▶ New   ⇒ Revised   ~~deleted~~ Deleted | Excludes 1 | | Excludes 2 | | Includes | | Use additional | | Code first | | Code also | | Key words |

OGCR Official Guidelines   X Assign placeholder X   ● Use Additional Character(s)   ▸ Manifestation Code   🅡 Hierarchical Condition Category   Coding Clinic

●I71.6   **Thoracoabdominal** aortic aneurysm, without rupture 🔖

     I71.60   Thoracoabdominal aortic aneurysm, without rupture, unspecified

     I71.61   Supraceliac aneurysm of the thoracoabdominal aorta, without rupture

     I71.62   Paravisceral aneurysm of the thoracoabdominal aorta, without rupture

I71.8   Aortic aneurysm of unspecified site, ruptured 🔖
     Rupture of aorta NOS

I71.9   Aortic aneurysm of unspecified site, without rupture 🔖
     Aneurysm of aorta
     Dilatation of aorta
     Hyaline necrosis of aorta

●I72   **Other aneurysm**

     Includes   aneurysm (cirsoid) (false) (ruptured)

     Excludes2   acquired aneurysm (I77.0)
                  aneurysm (of) aorta (I71.-)
                  aneurysm (of) arteriovenous NOS (Q27.3-)
                  carotid artery dissection (I77.71)
                  cerebral (nonruptured) aneurysm (I67.1)
                  coronary aneurysm (I25.4)
                  coronary artery dissection (I25.42)
                  dissection of artery NEC (I77.79)
                  dissection of precerebral artery, congenital (nonruptured) (Q28.1)
                  heart aneurysm (I25.3)
                  iliac artery dissection (I77.72)
                  precerebral artery, congential (nonruptured) (Q28.1)
                  pulmonary artery aneurysm (I28.1)
                  renal artery dissection (I77.73)
                  retinal aneurysm (H35.0)
                  ruptured cerebral aneurysm (I60.7)
                  varicose aneurysm (I77.0)
                  vertebral artery dissection (I77.74)

I72.0   Aneurysm of carotid artery 🔖
     Aneurysm of common carotid artery
     Aneurysm of external carotid artery
     Aneurysm of internal carotid artery, extracranial portion

     Excludes1   aneurysm of internal carotid artery, intracranial portion (I67.1)
                  aneurysm of internal carotid artery NOS (I67.1)

I72.1   Aneurysm of artery of upper extremity 🔖

I72.2   Aneurysm of renal artery 🔖

I72.3   Aneurysm of iliac artery 🔖

I72.4   Aneurysm of artery of lower extremity 🔖
     Coding Clinic: 2019, Q2, P22

Figure 9-5   Raynaud's syndrome. (From Hallett: Comprehensive Vascular and Endovascular Surgery, ed 2, Philadelphia, Mosby Ltd., 2010)

Item 9–9   An **embolus** is a mass of undissolved matter present in the blood that is transported by the blood current. A **thrombus** is a blood clot that occludes or shuts off a vessel. When a thrombus is dislodged, it becomes an embolus.

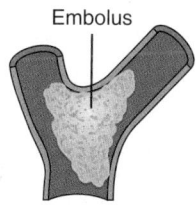

Embolus

Figure 9-6   An arterial embolus.

I72.5   Aneurysm of other precerebral arteries 🔖
     Aneurysm of basilar artery (trunk)

     Excludes2   aneurysm of carotid artery (I72.0)
                  aneurysm of vertebral artery (I72.6)
                  dissection of carotid artery (I77.71)
                  dissection of other precerebral arteries (I77.75)
                  dissection of vertebral artery (I77.74)
     Coding Clinic 2016, Q4, P28

I72.6   Aneurysm of vertebral artery 🔖
     Excludes2   dissection of vertebral artery (I77.74)
     Coding Clinic 2016, Q4, P28

I72.8   Aneurysm of other specified arteries 🔖

I72.9   Aneurysm of unspecified site 🔖

●I73   **Other peripheral vascular diseases**

     Excludes2   chilblains (T69.1)
                  frostbite (T33-T34)
                  immersion hand or foot (T69.0-)
                  spasm of cerebral artery (G45.9)
     Coding Clinic: 2018, Q4, P87-88

●I73.0   **Raynaud's syndrome**
     Diminishing oxygen supply to fingers, toes, nose, and ears when exposed to temperature changes or stress
     Raynaud's disease
     Raynaud's phenomenon (secondary)

     I73.00   Raynaud's syndrome without gangrene

     I73.01   Raynaud's syndrome with gangrene 🔖

I73.1   Thromboangiitis obliterans [Buerger's disease] 🔖
     Inflammatory occlusive disease resulting in poor circulation to the legs, feet, and sometimes the hands due to progressive inflammatory narrowing and eventually obliteration of the small arteries

●I73.8   **Other specified peripheral vascular diseases**

     Excludes1   diabetic (peripheral) angiopathy (E08-E13 with .51-.52)

     I73.81   Erythromelalgia 🔖

     I73.89   Other specified peripheral vascular diseases 🔖
           Acrocyanosis
           Erythrocyanosis
           Simple acroparesthesia [Schultze's type]
           Vasomotor acroparesthesia [Nothnagel's type]

I73.9   Peripheral vascular disease, unspecified 🔖
     Intermittent claudication
     Peripheral angiopathy NOS
     Spasm of artery

     Excludes1   atherosclerosis of the extremities (I70.2—I70.7-)
     Coding Clinic: 2018, Q4, P87

● **I74   Arterial embolism and thrombosis**

> **Includes**   embolic infarction
> embolic occlusion
> thrombotic infarction
> thrombotic occlusion

> *Code first* embolism and thrombosis complicating abortion or ectopic or molar pregnancy (O00-O07, O08.2)
> embolism and thrombosis complicating pregnancy, childbirth and the puerperium (O88.-)

> **Excludes2**   atheroembolism (I75.-)
> basilar embolism and thrombosis (I63.0-I63.2, I65.1)
> carotid embolism and thrombosis (I63.0-I63.2, I65.2)
> cerebral embolism and thrombosis (I63.3-I63.5, I66.-)
> coronary embolism and thrombosis (I21-I25)
> mesenteric embolism and thrombosis (K55.0-)
> ophthalmic embolism and thrombosis (H34.-)
> precerebral embolism and thrombosis NOS (I63.0-I63.2, I65.9)
> pulmonary embolism and thrombosis (I26.-)
> renal embolism and thrombosis (N28.0)
> retinal embolism and thrombosis (H34.-)
> septic embolism and thrombosis (I76)
> vertebral embolism and thrombosis (I63.0-I63.2, I65.0)

> Coding Clinic: 2023, Q2, P7

● **I74.0   Embolism and thrombosis of abdominal aorta**

    I74.01   Saddle embolus of abdominal aorta 🅠

    I74.09   Other arterial embolism and thrombosis of abdominal aorta 🅠
> Aortic bifurcation syndrome
> Aortoiliac obstruction
> Leriche's syndrome

● **I74.1   Embolism and thrombosis of other and unspecified parts of aorta**

    I74.10   Embolism and thrombosis of unspecified parts of aorta 🅠

    I74.11   Embolism and thrombosis of thoracic aorta 🅠

    I74.19   Embolism and thrombosis of other parts of aorta 🅠

I74.2   Embolism and thrombosis of arteries of the upper extremities 🅠

I74.3   Embolism and thrombosis of arteries of the lower extremities 🅠

I74.4   Embolism and thrombosis of arteries of extremities, unspecified 🅠
> Peripheral arteria l embolism NOS

I74.5   Embolism and thrombosis of iliac artery 🅠
> Coding Clinic: 2023, Q2, P7

I74.8   Embolism and thrombosis of other arteries 🅠

I74.9   Embolism and thrombosis of unspecified artery 🅠

● **I75   Atheroembolism**

> **Includes**   atherothrombotic microembolism
> cholesterol embolism

● **I75.0   Atheroembolism of extremities**

    ● **I75.01**   Atheroembolism of upper extremity

      I75.011   Atheroembolism of right upper extremity 🅠

      I75.012   Atheroembolism of left upper extremity 🅠

      I75.013   Atheroembolism of bilateral upper extremities 🅠

      I75.019   Atheroembolism of unspecified upper extremity 🅠

    ● **I75.02**   Atheroembolism of lower extremity

      I75.021   Atheroembolism of right lower extremity 🅠

      I75.022   Atheroembolism of left lower extremity 🅠

      I75.023   Atheroembolism of bilateral lower extremities 🅠

      I75.029   Atheroembolism of unspecified lower extremity 🅠

● **I75.8   Atheroembolism of other sites**

    I75.81   Atheroembolism of kidney 🅠
> Use additional code for any associated acute kidney failure and chronic kidney disease (N17.-, N18.-)

    I75.89   Atheroembolism of other site 🅠

I76   Septic arterial embolism 🅠

> *Code first* underlying infection, such as:
> infective endocarditis (I33.0)
> lung abscess (J85.-)

> Use additional code to identify the site of the embolism (I74.-)

> **Excludes2**   septic pulmonary embolism (I26.01, I26.90)

● **I77   Other disorders of arteries and arterioles**

> **Excludes2**   collagen (vascular) diseases (M30-M36)
> hypersensitivity angiitis (M31.0)
> pulmonary artery (I28.-)

I77.0   Arteriovenous fistula, acquired 🅠
> Aneurysmal varix
> Arteriovenous aneurysm, acquired

> **Excludes1**   arteriovenous aneurysm NOS (Q27.3-)
> presence of arteriovenous shunt (fistula) for dialysis (Z99.2)
> traumatic - see injury of blood vessel by body region

> **Excludes2**   cerebral (I67.1)
> coronary (I25.4)

I77.1   Stricture of artery 🅠
> Narrowing of artery
> Coding Clinic: 2021, Q3, P13

I77.2   Rupture of artery 🅠
> Erosion of artery
> Fistula of artery
> Ulcer of artery

> **Excludes1**   traumatic rupture of artery - see injury of blood vessel by body region

I77.3   Arterial fibromuscular dysplasia 🅠
> Fibromuscular hyperplasia (of) carotid artery
> Fibromuscular hyperplasia (of) renal artery

I77.4   Celiac artery compression syndrome 🅠
> Coding Clinic: 2021, Q3, P12-13

I77.5   Necrosis of artery 🅠

I77.6   Arteritis, unspecified 🅠
> Aortitis NOS
> Endarteritis NOS

> **Excludes1**   arteritis or endarteritis:
> aortic arch (M31.4)
> cerebral NEC (I67.7)
> coronary (I25.89)
> deformans (I70.-)
> giant cell (M31.5, M31.6)
> obliterans (I70.-)
> senile (I70.-)

● **I77.7   Other arterial dissection**

> **Excludes2**   dissection of aorta (I71.0-)
> dissection of coronary artery (I25.42)

    I77.70   Dissection of unspecified artery 🅠
> Coding Clinic 2016, Q4, P28

    I77.71   Dissection of carotid artery 🅠

    I77.72   Dissection of iliac artery 🅠

    I77.73   Dissection of renal artery 🅠

    I77.74   Dissection of vertebral artery 🅠

> **Excludes2**   aneurysm of vertebral artery (I72.6)

> Coding Clinic 2024, Q1, P26

▶ New   ⟹ Revised   ~~deleted~~ Deleted   Excludes 1   Excludes 2   Includes   Use additional   Code first   Code also   Key words

OGCR Official Guidelines   X Assign placeholder X   ● Use Additional Character(s)   ▌ Manifestation Code   🅠 Hierarchical Condition Category   **Coding Clinic**

I77.75 **Dissection of other precerebral arteries** 🔎
Dissection of basilar artery (trunk)
Excludes2   aneurysm of carotid artery (I72.0)
aneurysm of other precerebral arteries (I72.5)
aneurysm of vertebral artery (I72.6)
dissection of carotid artery (I77.71)
dissection of vertebral artery (I77.74)
Coding Clinic 2016, Q4, P28

I77.76 **Dissection of artery of upper extremity** 🔎
Coding Clinic 2016, Q4, P28

I77.77 **Dissection of artery of lower extremity** 🔎
Coding Clinic 2016, Q4, P28

I77.79 **Dissection of other specified artery** 🔎
Coding Clinic 2016, Q4, P28

I77.8 **Other specified disorders of arteries and arterioles**

I77.81 **Aortic ectasia**
Ectasis aorta
Excludes1   aortic aneurysm and dissection (I71.-)

I77.810 **Thoracic aortic ectasia** 🔎

I77.811 **Abdominal aortic ectasia** 🔎

I77.812 **Thoracoabdominal aortic ectasia** 🔎

I77.819 **Aortic ectasia, unspecified site** 🔎

I77.82 **Antineutrophilic cytoplasmic antibody [ANCA] vasculitis**
ANCA associated vasculitis
ANCA positive vasculitis
Excludes2   eosinophilic granulomatosis with polyangiitis (M30.1)
granulomatosis with polyangiitis (M31.3-)
microscopic polyangiitis (M31.7)

I77.89 **Other specified disorders of arteries and arterioles** 🔎
Coding Clinic 2021, Q1, P23

I77.9 **Disorder of arteries and arterioles, unspecified** 🔎
Coding Clinic 2021, Q1, P4

● I78 **Diseases of capillaries**

I78.0 **Hereditary hemorrhagic telangiectasia** 🔎
Rendu-Osler-Weber disease

I78.1 **Nevus, non-neoplastic**
Araneus nevus   Spider nevus
Senile nevus   Stellar nevus
Excludes1   nevus NOS (D22.-)
vascular NOS (Q82.5)
Excludes2   blue nevus (D22.-)
flammeus nevus (Q82.5)
hairy nevus (D22.-)
melanocytic nevus (D22.-)
pigmented nevus (D22.-)
portwine nevus (Q82.5)
sanguineous nevus (Q82.5)
strawberry nevus (Q82.5)
verrucous nevus (Q82.5)
Coding Clinic: 2019, Q1, P21

I78.8 **Other diseases of capillaries**

I78.9 **Disease of capillaries, unspecified**

● I79 **Disorders of arteries, arterioles and capillaries in diseases classified elsewhere**

▶ I79.0 *Aneurysm of aorta in diseases classified elsewhere* 🔎
Code first underlying disease
Excludes1   syphilitic aneurysm (A52.01)

▶ I79.1 *Aortitis in diseases classified elsewhere* 🔎
Code first underlying disease
Excludes1   syphilitic aortitis (A52.02)

▶ I79.8 *Other disorders of arteries, arterioles and capillaries in diseases classified elsewhere* 🔎
Code first underlying disease, such as:
amyloidosis (E85.-)
Excludes1   diabetic (peripheral) angiopathy (E08-E13 with .51-.52)
syphilitic endarteritis (A52.09)
tuberculous endarteritis (A18.89)

DISEASES OF VEINS, LYMPHATIC VESSELS AND LYMPH NODES, NOT ELSEWHERE CLASSIFIED (I80-I89)

● I80 **Phlebitis and thrombophlebitis**
Inflammation of a vein with infiltration of walls (phlebitis)
Includes   endophlebitis
inflammation, vein
periphlebitis
suppurative phlebitis
Code first phlebitis and thrombophlebitis complicating abortion, ectopic or molar pregnancy (O00-O07, O08.7)
phlebitis and thrombophlebitis complicating pregnancy, childbirth and the puerperium (O22.-, O87.-)
Excludes1   venous embolism and thrombosis of lower extremities (I82.4-, I82.5-, I82.81-)

● I80.0 **Phlebitis and thrombophlebitis of superficial vessels of lower extremities**
Phlebitis and thrombophlebitis of femoropopliteal vein

I80.00 **Phlebitis and thrombophlebitis of superficial vessels of unspecified lower extremity**

I80.01 **Phlebitis and thrombophlebitis of superficial vessels of right lower extremity**

I80.02 **Phlebitis and thrombophlebitis of superficial vessels of left lower extremity**

I80.03 **Phlebitis and thrombophlebitis of superficial vessels of lower extremities, bilateral**

● I80.1 **Phlebitis and thrombophlebitis of femoral vein**
Phlebitis and thrombophlebitis of common femoral vein
Phlebitis and thrombophlebitis of deep femoral vein

I80.10 **Phlebitis and thrombophlebitis of unspecified femoral vein** 🔎

I80.11 **Phlebitis and thrombophlebitis of right femoral vein** 🔎

I80.12 **Phlebitis and thrombophlebitis of left femoral vein** 🔎

I80.13 **Phlebitis and thrombophlebitis of femoral vein, bilateral** 🔎

● I80.2 **Phlebitis and thrombophlebitis of other and unspecified deep vessels of lower extremities**

● I80.20 **Phlebitis and thrombophlebitis of unspecified deep vessels of lower extremities**

I80.201 **Phlebitis and thrombophlebitis of unspecified deep vessels of right lower extremity** 🔎

I80.202 **Phlebitis and thrombophlebitis of unspecified deep vessels of left lower extremity** 🔎

I80.203 **Phlebitis and thrombophlebitis of unspecified deep vessels of lower extremities, bilateral** 🔎

I80.209 **Phlebitis and thrombophlebitis of unspecified deep vessels of unspecified lower extremity** 🔎

● I80.21 **Phlebitis and thrombophlebitis of iliac vein**
Phlebitis and thrombophlebitis of common iliac vein
Phlebitis and thrombophlebitis of external iliac vein
Phlebitis and thrombophlebitis of internal iliac vein

I80.211 **Phlebitis and thrombophlebitis of right iliac vein** 🔎

I80.212 **Phlebitis and thrombophlebitis of left iliac vein** 🔎

I80.213   Phlebitis and thrombophlebitis of iliac vein, bilateral 🦠

I80.219   Phlebitis and thrombophlebitis of unspecified iliac vein 🦠

⬤ **I80.22   Phlebitis and thrombophlebitis of popliteal vein**

I80.221   Phlebitis and thrombophlebitis of right popliteal vein 🦠

I80.222   Phlebitis and thrombophlebitis of left popliteal vein 🦠

I80.223   Phlebitis and thrombophlebitis of popliteal vein, bilateral 🦠

I80.229   Phlebitis and thrombophlebitis of unspecified popliteal vein 🦠

⬤ **I80.23   Phlebitis and thrombophlebitis of tibial vein**
Phlebitis and thrombophlebitis of anterior tibial vein
Phlebitis and thrombophlebitis of posterior tibial vein

I80.231   Phlebitis and thrombophlebitis of right tibial vein 🦠

I80.232   Phlebitis and thrombophlebitis of left tibial vein 🦠

I80.233   Phlebitis and thrombophlebitis of tibial vein, bilateral 🦠

I80.239   Phlebitis and thrombophlebitis of unspecified tibial vein 🦠

⬤ **I80.24   Phlebitis and thrombophlebitis of peroneal vein**

I80.241   Phlebitis and thrombophlebitis of right peroneal vein

I80.242   Phlebitis and thrombophlebitis of left peroneal vein

I80.243   Phlebitis and thrombophlebitis of peroneal vein, bilateral

I80.249   Phlebitis and thrombophlebitis of unspecified peroneal vein

⬤ **I80.25   Phlebitis and thrombophlebitis of calf muscular vein**
Phlebitis and thrombophlebitis of calf muscular vein, NOS
Phlebitis and thrombophlebitis of gastrocnemial vein
Phlebitis and thrombophlebitis of soleal vein

I80.251   Phlebitis and thrombophlebitis of right calf muscular vein

I80.252   Phlebitis and thrombophlebitis of left calf muscular vein

I80.253   Phlebitis and thrombophlebitis of calf muscular vein, bilateral

I80.259   Phlebitis and thrombophlebitis of unspecified calf muscular vein

⬤ **I80.29   Phlebitis and thrombophlebitis of other deep vessels of lower extremities**

I80.291   Phlebitis and thrombophlebitis of other deep vessels of right lower extremity 🦠

I80.292   Phlebitis and thrombophlebitis of other deep vessels of left lower extremity 🦠

I80.293   Phlebitis and thrombophlebitis of other deep vessels of lower extremity, bilateral 🦠

I80.299   Phlebitis and thrombophlebitis of other deep vessels of unspecified lower extremity 🦠

I80.3   Phlebitis and thrombophlebitis of lower extremities, unspecified

I80.8   Phlebitis and thrombophlebitis of other sites

I80.9   Phlebitis and thrombophlebitis of unspecified site

I81   Portal vein thrombosis
Portal (vein) obstruction

Excludes2   hepatic vein thrombosis (I82.0)
phlebitis of portal vein (K75.1)

Coding Clinic: 2019, Q4, P68

⬤ **I82   Other venous embolism and thrombosis**
Code first venous embolism and thrombosis complicating:
abortion, ectopic or molar pregnancy (O00-O07, O08.7)
pregnancy, childbirth and the puerperium (O22.-, O87.-)

Excludes2   venous embolism and thrombosis (of):
cerebral (I63.6, I67.6)
coronary (I21-I25)
intracranial and intraspinal, septic or NOS (G08)
intracranial, nonpyogenic (I67.6)
intraspinal, nonpyogenic (G95.1)
mesenteric (K55.0-)
portal (I81)
pulmonary (I26.-)

I82.0   Budd-Chiari syndrome 🦠
Hepatic vein thrombosis

I82.1   Thrombophlebitis migrans
"White leg" is the other term to describe a migrating thrombus.

⬤ **I82.2   Embolism and thrombosis of vena cava and other thoracic veins**

⬤ **I82.21   Embolism and thrombosis of superior vena cava**

I82.210   Acute embolism and thrombosis of superior vena cava 🦠
Embolism and thrombosis of superior vena cava NOS

I82.211   Chronic embolism and thrombosis of superior vena cava 🦠

⬤ **I82.22   Embolism and thrombosis of inferior vena cava**

I82.220   Acute embolism and thrombosis of inferior vena cava 🦠
Embolism and thrombosis of inferior vena cava NOS

I82.221   Chronic embolism and thrombosis of inferior vena cava 🦠

⬤ **I82.29   Embolism and thrombosis of other thoracic veins**
Embolism and thrombosis of brachiocephalic (innominate) vein

I82.290   Acute embolism and thrombosis of other thoracic veins 🦠

I82.291   Chronic embolism and thrombosis of other thoracic veins 🦠

I82.3   Embolism and thrombosis of renal vein 🦠

⬤ **I82.4   Acute embolism and thrombosis of deep veins of lower extremity**

I82.40   Acute embolism and thrombosis of unspecified deep veins of lower extremity
Deep vein thrombosis NOS
DVT NOS

Excludes1   acute embolism and thrombosis of unspecified deep veins of distal lower extremity (I82.4Z-)
acute embolism and thrombosis of unspecified deep veins of proximal lower extremity (I82.4Y-)

I82.401   Acute embolism and thrombosis of unspecified deep veins of right lower extremity 🦠

I82.402   Acute embolism and thrombosis of unspecified deep veins of left lower extremity 🦠

▶ New   ➡ Revised   ~~deleted~~ Deleted   Excludes 1   Excludes 2   Includes   Use additional   Code first   Code also   Key words
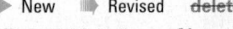 OGCR Official Guidelines   X Assign placeholder X   ⬤ Use Additional Character(s)   ▶ Manifestation Code   🦠 Hierarchical Condition Category   Coding Clinic

CHAPTER 9 (I00-I99)

　　　I82.403　Acute embolism and thrombosis of unspecified deep veins of lower extremity, bilateral 🦠

　　　I82.409　Acute embolism and thrombosis of unspecified deep veins of unspecified lower extremity 🦠

● I82.41　Acute embolism and thrombosis of femoral vein
　　　Acute embolism and thrombosis of common femoral vein
　　　Acute embolism and thrombosis of deep femoral vein

　　　I82.411　Acute embolism and thrombosis of right femoral vein 🦠

　　　I82.412　Acute embolism and thrombosis of left femoral vein 🦠
　　　　　　　　Coding Clinic: 2023, Q3, P12

　　　I82.413　Acute embolism and thrombosis of femoral vein, bilateral 🦠

　　　I82.419　Acute embolism and thrombosis of unspecified femoral vein 🦠

● I82.42　Acute embolism and thrombosis of iliac vein
　　　Acute embolism and thrombosis of common iliac vein
　　　Acute embolism and thrombosis of external iliac vein
　　　Acute embolism and thrombosis of internal iliac vein

　　　I82.421　Acute embolism and thrombosis of right iliac vein 🦠

　　　I82.422　Acute embolism and thrombosis of left iliac vein 🦠

　　　I82.423　Acute embolism and thrombosis of iliac vein, bilateral 🦠

　　　I82.429　Acute embolism and thrombosis of unspecified iliac vein 🦠

● I82.43　Acute embolism and thrombosis of popliteal vein

　　　I82.431　Acute embolism and thrombosis of right popliteal vein 🦠

　　　I82.432　Acute embolism and thrombosis of left popliteal vein 🦠

　　　I82.433　Acute embolism and thrombosis of popliteal vein, bilateral 🦠

　　　I82.439　Acute embolism and thrombosis of unspecified popliteal vein 🦠

● I82.44　Acute embolism and thrombosis of tibial vein
　　　Acute embolism and thrombosis of anterior tibial vein
　　　Acute embolism and thrombosis of posterior tibial vein

　　　I82.441　Acute embolism and thrombosis of right tibial vein 🦠

　　　I82.442　Acute embolism and thrombosis of left tibial vein 🦠

　　　I82.443　Acute embolism and thrombosis of tibial vein, bilateral 🦠

　　　I82.449　Acute embolism and thrombosis of unspecified tibial vein 🦠

● I82.45　Acute embolism and thrombosis of peroneal vein

　　　I82.451　Acute embolism and thrombosis of right peroneal vein

　　　I82.452　Acute embolism and thrombosis of left peroneal vein

　　　I82.453　Acute embolism and thrombosis of peroneal vein, bilateral

　　　I82.459　Acute embolism and thrombosis of unspecified peroneal vein

● I82.46　Acute embolism and thrombosis of calf muscular vein
　　　Acute embolism and thrombosis of calf muscular vein, NOS
　　　Acute embolism and thrombosis of gastrocnemial vein
　　　Acute embolism and thrombosis of soleal vein

　　　I82.461　Acute embolism and thrombosis of right calf muscular vein

　　　I82.462　Acute embolism and thrombosis of left calf muscular vein

　　　I82.463　Acute embolism and thrombosis of calf muscular vein, bilateral

　　　I82.469　Acute embolism and thrombosis of unspecified calf muscular vein

● I82.49　Acute embolism and thrombosis of other specified deep vein of lower extremity

　　　I82.491　Acute embolism and thrombosis of other specified deep vein of right lower extremity 🦠

　　　I82.492　Acute embolism and thrombosis of other specified deep vein of left lower extremity 🦠

　　　I82.493　Acute embolism and thrombosis of other specified deep vein of lower extremity, bilateral 🦠

　　　I82.499　Acute embolism and thrombosis of other specified deep vein of unspecified lower extremity 🦠

● I82.4Y　Acute embolism and thrombosis of unspecified deep veins of proximal lower extremity
　　　Acute embolism and thrombosis of deep vein of thigh NOS
　　　Acute embolism and thrombosis of deep vein of upper leg NOS

　　　I82.4Y1　Acute embolism and thrombosis of unspecified deep veins of right proximal lower extremity 🦠

　　　I82.4Y2　Acute embolism and thrombosis of unspecified deep veins of left proximal lower extremity 🦠

　　　I82.4Y3　Acute embolism and thrombosis of unspecified deep veins of proximal lower extremity, bilateral 🦠

　　　I82.4Y9　Acute embolism and thrombosis of unspecified deep veins of unspecified proximal lower extremity 🦠

● I82.4Z　Acute embolism and thrombosis of unspecified deep veins of distal lower extremity
　　　Acute embolism and thrombosis of deep vein of calf NOS
　　　Acute embolism and thrombosis of deep vein of lower leg NOS

　　　I82.4Z1　Acute embolism and thrombosis of unspecified deep veins of right distal lower extremity 🦠

　　　I82.4Z2　Acute embolism and thrombosis of unspecified deep veins of left distal lower extremity 🦠

　　　I82.4Z3　Acute embolism and thrombosis of unspecified deep veins of distal lower extremity, bilateral 🦠

　　　I82.4Z9　Acute embolism and thrombosis of unspecified deep veins of unspecified distal lower extremity 🦠

CHAPTER 9 (I00–I99)

- **I82.5** **Chronic embolism and thrombosis of deep veins of lower extremity**

  Use additional code, if applicable, for associated long-term (current) use of anticoagulants (Z79.01)

  Excludes1 personal history of venous embolism and thrombosis (Z86.718)

  - **I82.50** Chronic embolism and thrombosis of unspecified deep veins of lower extremity

    Excludes1 chronic embolism and thrombosis of unspecified deep veins of distal lower extremity (I82.5Z-)
    chronic embolism and thrombosis of unspecified deep veins of proximal lower extremity (I82.5Y-)

    - I82.501 Chronic embolism and thrombosis of unspecified deep veins of right lower extremity
    - I82.502 Chronic embolism and thrombosis of unspecified deep veins of left lower extremity
    - I82.503 Chronic embolism and thrombosis of unspecified deep veins of lower extremity, bilateral
    - I82.509 Chronic embolism and thrombosis of unspecified deep veins of unspecified lower extremity

  - **I82.51** Chronic embolism and thrombosis of femoral vein

    Chronic embolism and thrombosis of common femoral vein
    Chronic embolism and thrombosis of deep femoral vein

    - I82.511 Chronic embolism and thrombosis of right femoral vein
    - I82.512 Chronic embolism and thrombosis of left femoral vein
    - I82.513 Chronic embolism and thrombosis of femoral vein, bilateral
    - I82.519 Chronic embolism and thrombosis of unspecified femoral vein

  - **I82.52** Chronic embolism and thrombosis of iliac vein

    Chronic embolism and thrombosis of common iliac vein
    Chronic embolism and thrombosis of external iliac vein
    Chronic embolism and thrombosis of internal iliac vein

    - I82.521 Chronic embolism and thrombosis of right iliac vein
    - I82.522 Chronic embolism and thrombosis of left iliac vein
    - I82.523 Chronic embolism and thrombosis of iliac vein, bilateral
    - I82.529 Chronic embolism and thrombosis of unspecified iliac vein

  - **I82.53** Chronic embolism and thrombosis of popliteal vein
    - I82.531 Chronic embolism and thrombosis of right popliteal vein
    - I82.532 Chronic embolism and thrombosis of left popliteal vein
    - I82.533 Chronic embolism and thrombosis of popliteal vein, bilateral
    - I82.539 Chronic embolism and thrombosis of unspecified popliteal vein

  - **I82.54** Chronic embolism and thrombosis of tibial vein

    Chronic embolism and thrombosis of anterior tibial vein
    Chronic embolism and thrombosis of posterior tibial vein

    - I82.541 Chronic embolism and thrombosis of right tibial vein
    - I82.542 Chronic embolism and thrombosis of left tibial vein
    - I82.543 Chronic embolism and thrombosis of tibial vein, bilateral
    - I82.549 Chronic embolism and thrombosis of unspecified tibial vein

  - **I82.55** Chronic embolism and thrombosis of peroneal vein
    - I82.551 Chronic embolism and thrombosis of right peroneal vein
    - I82.552 Chronic embolism and thrombosis of left peroneal vein
    - I82.553 Chronic embolism and thrombosis of peroneal vein, bilateral
    - I82.559 Chronic embolism and thrombosis of unspecified peroneal vein

  - **I82.56** Chronic embolism and thrombosis of calf muscular vein

    Chronic embolism and thrombosis of calf muscular vein NOS
    Chronic embolism and thrombosis of gastrocnemial vein
    Chronic embolism and thrombosis of soleal vein

    - I82.561 Chronic embolism and thrombosis of right calf muscular vein
    - I82.562 Chronic embolism and thrombosis of left calf muscular vein
    - I82.563 Chronic embolism and thrombosis of calf muscular vein, bilateral
    - I82.569 Chronic embolism and thrombosis of unspecified calf muscular vein

  - **I82.59** Chronic embolism and thrombosis of other specified deep vein of lower extremity
    - I82.591 Chronic embolism and thrombosis of other specified deep vein of right lower extremity
    - I82.592 Chronic embolism and thrombosis of other specified deep vein of left lower extremity
    - I82.593 Chronic embolism and thrombosis of other specified deep vein of lower extremity, bilateral
    - I82.599 Chronic embolism and thrombosis of other specified deep vein of unspecified lower extremity

Item 9-10 Varicose/Varicosities (varix = singular, varices = plural): Enlarged, engorged, tortuous, twisted vascular vessels (veins, arteries, lymphatics). As such, the condition can present in various parts of the body, although the most familiar locations are the lower extremities. A common complication of varices is thrombophlebitis. Varicosities of the anus and rectum are called hemorrhoids.

Figure 9-7 Varicose veins of the legs. (Getty Image)

● **I82.5Y** Chronic embolism and thrombosis of unspecified deep veins of proximal lower extremity

Chronic embolism and thrombosis of deep veins of thigh NOS

Chronic embolism and thrombosis of deep veins of upper leg NOS

I82.5Y1 Chronic embolism and thrombosis of unspecified deep veins of right proximal lower extremity 🔗

I82.5Y2 Chronic embolism and thrombosis of unspecified deep veins of left proximal lower extremity 🔗

I82.5Y3 Chronic embolism and thrombosis of unspecified deep veins of proximal lower extremity, bilateral 🔗

I82.5Y9 Chronic embolism and thrombosis of unspecified deep veins of unspecified proximal lower extremity 🔗

● **I82.5Z** Chronic embolism and thrombosis of unspecified deep veins of distal lower extremity

Chronic embolism and thrombosis of deep veins of calf NOS

Chronic embolism and thrombosis of deep veins of lower leg NOS

I82.5Z1 Chronic embolism and thrombosis of unspecified deep veins of right distal lower extremity 🔗

I82.5Z2 Chronic embolism and thrombosis of unspecified deep veins of left distal lower extremity 🔗

I82.5Z3 Chronic embolism and thrombosis of unspecified deep veins of distal lower extremity, bilateral 🔗

I82.5Z9 Chronic embolism and thrombosis of unspecified deep veins of unspecified distal lower extremity 🔗

● **I82.6** Acute embolism and thrombosis of veins of upper extremity

● **I82.60** Acute embolism and thrombosis of unspecified veins of upper extremity

I82.601 Acute embolism and thrombosis of unspecified veins of right upper extremity

I82.602 Acute embolism and thrombosis of unspecified veins of left upper extremity

I82.603 Acute embolism and thrombosis of unspecified veins of upper extremity, bilateral

I82.609 Acute embolism and thrombosis of unspecified veins of unspecified upper extremity

● **I82.61** Acute embolism and thrombosis of superficial veins of upper extremity

Acute embolism and thrombosis of antecubital vein

Acute embolism and thrombosis of basilic vein

Acute embolism and thrombosis of cephalic vein

I82.611 Acute embolism and thrombosis of superficial veins of right upper extremity

I82.612 Acute embolism and thrombosis of superficial veins of left upper extremity

I82.613 Acute embolism and thrombosis of superficial veins of upper extremity, bilateral

I82.619 Acute embolism and thrombosis of superficial veins of unspecified upper extremity

● **I82.62** Acute embolism and thrombosis of deep veins of upper extremity

Acute embolism and thrombosis of brachial vein

Acute embolism and thrombosis of radial vein

Acute embolism and thrombosis of ulnar vein

I82.621 Acute embolism and thrombosis of deep veins of right upper extremity 🔗

I82.622 Acute embolism and thrombosis of deep veins of left upper extremity 🔗

I82.623 Acute embolism and thrombosis of deep veins of upper extremity, bilateral 🔗

I82.629 Acute embolism and thrombosis of deep veins of unspecified upper extremity 🔗

● **I82.7** Chronic embolism and thrombosis of veins of upper extremity

Use additional code, if applicable, for associated long-term (current) use of anticoagulants (Z79.01)

Excludes1 personal history of venous embolism and thrombosis (Z86.718)

● **I82.70** Chronic embolism and thrombosis of unspecified veins of upper extremity

I82.701 Chronic embolism and thrombosis of unspecified veins of right upper extremity

I82.702 Chronic embolism and thrombosis of unspecified veins of left upper extremity

I82.703 Chronic embolism and thrombosis of unspecified veins of upper extremity, bilateral

I82.709 Chronic embolism and thrombosis of unspecified veins of unspecified upper extremity

● **I82.71** Chronic embolism and thrombosis of superficial veins of upper extremity

Chronic embolism and thrombosis of antecubital vein

Chronic embolism and thrombosis of basilic vein

Chronic embolism and thrombosis of cephalic vein

I82.711 Chronic embolism and thrombosis of superficial veins of right upper extremity

I82.712 Chronic embolism and thrombosis of superficial veins of left upper extremity

I82.713 Chronic embolism and thrombosis of superficial veins of upper extremity, bilateral

I82.719 Chronic embolism and thrombosis of superficial veins of unspecified upper extremity

● **I82.72** Chronic embolism and thrombosis of deep veins of upper extremity

Chronic embolism and thrombosis of brachial vein

Chronic embolism and thrombosis of radial vein

Chronic embolism and thrombosis of ulnar vein

I82.721 Chronic embolism and thrombosis of deep veins of right upper extremity 🔗

I82.722 Chronic embolism and thrombosis of deep veins of left upper extremity 🔗

I82.723 Chronic embolism and thrombosis of deep veins of upper extremity, bilateral 🔗

I82.729 Chronic embolism and thrombosis of deep veins of unspecified upper extremity 🔗

● **I82.8** Embolism and thrombosis of other specified veins

> Use additional code, if applicable, for associated long-term (current) use of anticoagulants (Z79.01)

●● **I82.81** Embolism and thrombosis of superficial veins of lower extremities

> Embolism and thrombosis of saphenous vein (greater) (lesser)

- **I82.811** Embolism and thrombosis of superficial veins of right lower extremity
- **I82.812** Embolism and thrombosis of superficial veins of left lower extremity
- **I82.813** Embolism and thrombosis of superficial veins of lower extremities, bilateral
- **I82.819** Embolism and thrombosis of superficial veins of unspecified lower extremity

●● **I82.89** Embolism and thrombosis of other specified veins

- **I82.890** Acute embolism and thrombosis of other specified veins
- **I82.891** Chronic embolism and thrombosis of other specified veins

● **I82.9** Embolism and thrombosis of unspecified vein

- **I82.90** Acute embolism and thrombosis of unspecified vein
  > Embolism of vein NOS
  > Thrombosis (vein) NOS
- **I82.91** Chronic embolism and thrombosis of unspecified vein

● **I82.A** Embolism and thrombosis of axillary vein

●● **I82.A1** Acute embolism and thrombosis of axillary vein

- **I82.A11** Acute embolism and thrombosis of right axillary vein 🐾
- **I82.A12** Acute embolism and thrombosis of left axillary vein 🐾
- **I82.A13** Acute embolism and thrombosis of axillary vein, bilateral 🐾
- **I82.A19** Acute embolism and thrombosis of unspecified axillary vein 🐾

●● **I82.A2** Chronic embolism and thrombosis of axillary vein

- **I82.A21** Chronic embolism and thrombosis of right axillary vein 🐾
- **I82.A22** Chronic embolism and thrombosis of left axillary vein 🐾
- **I82.A23** Chronic embolism and thrombosis of axillary vein, bilateral 🐾
- **I82.A29** Chronic embolism and thrombosis of unspecified axillary vein 🐾

● **I82.B** Embolism and thrombosis of subclavian vein

●● **I82.B1** Acute embolism and thrombosis of subclavian vein

- **I82.B11** Acute embolism and thrombosis of right subclavian vein 🐾
- **I82.B12** Acute embolism and thrombosis of left subclavian vein 🐾
- **I82.B13** Acute embolism and thrombosis of subclavian vein, bilateral 🐾
- **I82.B19** Acute embolism and thrombosis of unspecified subclavian vein 🐾

●● **I82.B2** Chronic embolism and thrombosis of subclavian vein

- **I82.B21** Chronic embolism and thrombosis of right subclavian vein 🐾
- **I82.B22** Chronic embolism and thrombosis of left subclavian vein 🐾
- **I82.B23** Chronic embolism and thrombosis of subclavian vein, bilateral 🐾
- **I82.B29** Chronic embolism and thrombosis of unspecified subclavian vein 🐾

● **I82.C** Embolism and thrombosis of internal jugular vein

●● **I82.C1** Acute embolism and thrombosis of internal jugular vein

- **I82.C11** Acute embolism and thrombosis of right internal jugular vein 🐾
- **I82.C12** Acute embolism and thrombosis of left internal jugular vein 🐾
- **I82.C13** Acute embolism and thrombosis of internal jugular vein, bilateral 🐾
- **I82.C19** Acute embolism and thrombosis of unspecified internal jugular vein 🐾

●● **I82.C2** Chronic embolism and thrombosis of internal jugular vein

- **I82.C21** Chronic embolism and thrombosis of right internal jugular vein 🐾
- **I82.C22** Chronic embolism and thrombosis of left internal jugular vein 🐾
- **I82.C23** Chronic embolism and thrombosis of internal jugular vein, bilateral 🐾
- **I82.C29** Chronic embolism and thrombosis of unspecified internal jugular vein 🐾

● **I83** Varicose veins of lower extremities

> **Excludes2** varicose veins complicating pregnancy (O22.0-)
> varicose veins complicating the puerperium (O87.4)

● **I83.0** Varicose veins of lower extremities with ulcer

> Use additional code to identify severity of ulcer (L97.-)

●● **I83.00** Varicose veins of unspecified lower extremity with ulcer

- **I83.001** Varicose veins of unspecified lower extremity with ulcer of thigh 🐾   A
- **I83.002** Varicose veins of unspecified lower extremity with ulcer of calf 🐾   A
- **I83.003** Varicose veins of unspecified lower extremity with ulcer of ankle 🐾   A
- **I83.004** Varicose veins of unspecified lower extremity with ulcer of heel and midfoot 🐾   A
  > Varicose veins of unspecified lower extremity with ulcer of plantar surface of midfoot
- **I83.005** Varicose veins of unspecified lower extremity with ulcer other part of foot 🐾   A
  > Varicose veins of unspecified lower extremity with ulcer of toe
- **I83.008** Varicose veins of unspecified lower extremity with ulcer other part of lower leg 🐾   A
- **I83.009** Varicose veins of unspecified lower extremity with ulcer of unspecified site 🐾   A

●● **I83.01** Varicose veins of right lower extremity with ulcer

- **I83.011** Varicose veins of right lower extremity with ulcer of thigh 🐾   A
- **I83.012** Varicose veins of right lower extremity with ulcer of calf 🐾   A
- **I83.013** Varicose veins of right lower extremity with ulcer of ankle 🐾   A
- **I83.014** Varicose veins of right lower extremity with ulcer of heel and midfoot 🐾   A
  > Varicose veins of right lower extremity with ulcer of plantar surface of midfoot

▶ New   ⇒ Revised   ~~deleted~~ Deleted   Excludes 1   Excludes 2   Includes   Use additional   Code first   Code also   Key words
OGCR Official Guidelines   X Assign placeholder X   ● Use Additional Character(s)   ▶ Manifestation Code   🐾 Hierarchical Condition Category   Coding Clinic

I83.015   Varicose veins of right lower extremity with ulcer other part of foot 🔍   A
        Varicose veins of right lower extremity with ulcer of toe

I83.018   Varicose veins of right lower extremity with ulcer other part of lower leg 🔍   A

I83.019   Varicose veins of right lower extremity with ulcer of unspecified site 🔍   A

● I83.02   Varicose veins of left lower extremity with ulcer

I83.021   Varicose veins of left lower extremity with ulcer of thigh 🔍   A

I83.022   Varicose veins of left lower extremity with ulcer of calf 🔍   A

I83.023   Varicose veins of left lower extremity with ulcer of ankle 🔍   A

I83.024   Varicose veins of left lower extremity with ulcer of heel and midfoot 🔍   A
        Varicose veins of left lower extremity with ulcer of plantar surface of midfoot

I83.025   Varicose veins of left lower extremity with ulcer other part of foot 🔍   A
        Varicose veins of left lower extremity with ulcer of toe

I83.028   Varicose veins of left lower extremity with ulcer other part of lower leg 🔍   A

I83.029   Varicose veins of left lower extremity with ulcer of unspecified site 🔍   A

● I83.1   Varicose veins of lower extremities with inflammation

I83.10   Varicose veins of unspecified lower extremity with inflammation   A

I83.11   Varicose veins of right lower extremity with inflammation   A

I83.12   Varicose veins of left lower extremity with inflammation   A

● I83.2   Varicose veins of lower extremities with both ulcer and inflammation
    Use additional code to identify severity of ulcer (L97.-)

● I83.20   Varicose veins of unspecified lower extremity with both ulcer and inflammation

I83.201   Varicose veins of unspecified lower extremity with both ulcer of thigh and inflammation 🔍   A

I83.202   Varicose veins of unspecified lower extremity with both ulcer of calf and inflammation 🔍   A

I83.203   Varicose veins of unspecified lower extremity with both ulcer of ankle and inflammation 🔍   A

I83.204   Varicose veins of unspecified lower extremity with both ulcer of heel and midfoot and inflammation 🔍   A
        Varicose veins of unspecified lower extremity with both ulcer of plantar surface of midfoot and inflammation

I83.205   Varicose veins of unspecified lower extremity with both ulcer other part of foot and inflammation 🔍   A
        Varicose veins of unspecified lower extremity with both ulcer of toe and inflammation

I83.208   Varicose veins of unspecified lower extremity with both ulcer of other part of lower extremity and inflammation 🔍   A

I83.209   Varicose veins of unspecified lower extremity with both ulcer of unspecified site and inflammation 🔍   A

● I83.21   Varicose veins of right lower extremity with both ulcer and inflammation

I83.211   Varicose veins of right lower extremity with both ulcer of thigh and inflammation 🔍   A

I83.212   Varicose veins of right lower extremity with both ulcer of calf and inflammation 🔍   A

I83.213   Varicose veins of right lower extremity with both ulcer of ankle and inflammation 🔍   A

I83.214   Varicose veins of right lower extremity with both ulcer of heel and midfoot and inflammation 🔍   A
        Varicose veins of right lower extremity with both ulcer of plantar surface of midfoot and inflammation

I83.215   Varicose veins of right lower extremity with both ulcer other part of foot and inflammation 🔍   A
        Varicose veins of right lower extremity with both ulcer of toe and inflammation

I83.218   Varicose veins of right lower extremity with both ulcer of other part of lower extremity and inflammation 🔍   A

I83.219   Varicose veins of right lower extremity with both ulcer of unspecified site and inflammation 🔍 A

● I83.22   Varicose veins of left lower extremity with both ulcer and inflammation

I83.221   Varicose veins of left lower extremity with both ulcer of thigh and inflammation 🔍   A

I83.222   Varicose veins of left lower extremity with both ulcer of calf and inflammation 🔍   A

I83.223   Varicose veins of left lower extremity with both ulcer of ankle and inflammation 🔍   A

I83.224   Varicose veins of left lower extremity with both ulcer of heel and midfoot and inflammation 🔍   A
        Varicose veins of left lower extremity with both ulcer of plantar surface of midfoot and inflammation

I83.225   Varicose veins of left lower extremity with both ulcer other part of foot and inflammation 🔍   A
        Varicose veins of left lower extremity with both ulcer of toe and inflammation

I83.228   Varicose veins of left lower extremity with both ulcer of other part of lower extremity and inflammation 🔍   A

I83.229   Varicose veins of left lower extremity with both ulcer of unspecified site and inflammation 🔍   A

● I83.8   Varicose veins of lower extremities with other complications

● I83.81   Varicose veins of lower extremities with pain

I83.811   Varicose veins of right lower extremity with pain   A

I83.812   Varicose veins of left lower extremity with pain   A

I83.813   Varicose veins of bilateral lower extremities with pain   A

I83.819   Varicose veins of unspecified lower extremity with pain   A

● I83.89   **Varicose veins of lower extremities with other complications**
Varicose veins of lower extremities with edema
Varicose veins of lower extremities with swelling

     I83.891   **Varicose veins of right lower extremity with other complications**   A

     I83.892   **Varicose veins of left lower extremity with other complications**   A

     I83.893   **Varicose veins of bilateral lower extremities with other complications** A

     I83.899   **Varicose veins of unspecified lower extremity with other complications**   A

● I83.9   **Asymptomatic varicose veins of lower extremities**
Phlebectasia of lower extremities
Varicose veins of lower extremities
Varix of lower extremities

     I83.90   **Asymptomatic varicose veins of unspecified lower extremity**   A
Varicose veins NOS

     I83.91   **Asymptomatic varicose veins of right lower extremity**   A

     I83.92   **Asymptomatic varicose veins of left lower extremity**   A

     I83.93   **Asymptomatic varicose veins of bilateral lower extremities**   A

● **I85**   **Esophageal varices**
Use additional code to identify:
alcohol abuse and dependence (F10.-)

● **I85.0**   **Esophageal varices**
Idiopathic esophageal varices
Primary esophageal varices

     I85.00   **Esophageal varices without bleeding** 🔲
Esophageal varices NOS

     I85.01   **Esophageal varices with bleeding** 🔲

● **I85.1**   **Secondary esophageal varices**
Esophageal varices secondary to alcoholic liver disease
Esophageal varices secondary to cirrhosis of liver
Esophageal varices secondary to schistosomiasis
Esophageal varices secondary to toxic liver disease
Code first underlying disease

     I85.10   **Secondary esophageal varices without bleeding** 🔲

     I85.11   **Secondary esophageal varices with bleeding** 🔲

● **I86**   **Varicose veins of other sites**
   Excludes1   varicose veins of unspecified site (I83.9-)
   Excludes2   retinal varices (H35.0-)

I86.0   **Sublingual varices**

I86.1   **Scrotal varices**
Varicocele

I86.2   **Pelvic varices**

I86.3   **Vulval varices**
   Excludes1   vulval varices complicating childbirth and the puerperium (O87.8)
           vulval varices complicating pregnancy (O22.1-)

I86.4   **Gastric varices**

I86.8   **Varicose veins of other specified sites**   A
Varicose ulcer of nasal septum

● **I87**   **Other disorders of veins**

● **I87.0**   **Postthrombotic syndrome**
Chronic venous hypertension due to deep vein thrombosis
Postphlebitic syndrome
   Excludes1   chronic venous hypertension without deep vein thrombosis (I87.3-)

   ● I87.00   **Postthrombotic syndrome without complications**
Asymptomatic Postthrombotic syndrome

     I87.001   **Postthrombotic syndrome without complications of right lower extremity**

     I87.002   **Postthrombotic syndrome without complications of left lower extremity**

     I87.003   **Postthrombotic syndrome without complications of bilateral lower extremity**

     I87.009   **Postthrombotic syndrome without complications of unspecified extremity**
Postthrombotic syndrome NOS

   ● I87.01   **Postthrombotic syndrome with ulcer**
Use additional code to specify site and severity of ulcer (L97.-)

     I87.011   **Postthrombotic syndrome with ulcer of right lower extremity** 🔲

     I87.012   **Postthrombotic syndrome with ulcer of left lower extremity** 🔲

     I87.013   **Postthrombotic syndrome with ulcer of bilateral lower extremity** 🔲

     I87.019   **Postthrombotic syndrome with ulcer of unspecified lower extremity** 🔲

   ● I87.02   **Postthrombotic syndrome with inflammation**

     I87.021   **Postthrombotic syndrome with inflammation of right lower extremity**

     I87.022   **Postthrombotic syndrome with inflammation of left lower extremity**

     I87.023   **Postthrombotic syndrome with inflammation of bilateral lower extremity**

     I87.029   **Postthrombotic syndrome with inflammation of unspecified lower extremity**

   ● I87.03   **Postthrombotic syndrome with ulcer and inflammation**
Use additional code to specify site and severity of ulcer (L97.-)

     I87.031   **Postthrombotic syndrome with ulcer and inflammation of right lower extremity** 🔲

     I87.032   **Postthrombotic syndrome with ulcer and inflammation of left lower extremity** 🔲

     I87.033   **Postthrombotic syndrome with ulcer and inflammation of bilateral lower extremity** 🔲

     I87.039   **Postthrombotic syndrome with ulcer and inflammation of unspecified lower extremity** 🔲

   ● I87.09   **Postthrombotic syndrome with other complications**

     I87.091   **Postthrombotic syndrome with other complications of right lower extremity**

     I87.092   **Postthrombotic syndrome with other complications of left lower extremity**

     I87.093   **Postthrombotic syndrome with other complications of bilateral lower extremity**

     I87.099   **Postthrombotic syndrome with other complications of unspecified lower extremity**

I87.1   **Compression of vein**
Stricture of vein
Vena cava syndrome (inferior) (superior)
   Excludes2   compression of pulmonary vein (I28.8)
   Coding Clinic: 2023, Q2, P8

▶ New   ➡ Revised   ~~deleted~~ Deleted   Excludes 1   Excludes 2   Includes   Use additional   Code first   Code also   Key words
OGCR Official Guidelines   X Assign placeholder X   ● Use Additional Character(s)   ▷ Manifestation Code   🔲 Hierarchical Condition Category   **Coding Clinic**

I87.2 Venous insufficiency (chronic) (peripheral)
Stasis dermatitis

> Code also, if applicable, associated hypertensive conditions such as:
> essential (primary) hypertension (I10)
> hypertensive chronic kidney disease (I12.-)
> hypertensive heart and chronic kidney disease (I13.-)
> hypertensive heart disease (I11.-)

> Use Additional code, if applicable, to specify site and severity of ulcer (L97.-)

> **Excludes1**   stasis dermatitis with varicose veins of lower extremities (I83.1-, I83.2-)

> Coding Clinic: 2024, Q1, P16

● **I87.3 Chronic venous hypertension (idiopathic)**
Stasis edema

> **Excludes1**   chronic venous hypertension due to deep vein thrombosis (I87.0-)
> varicose veins of lower extremities (I83.-)

● **I87.30 Chronic venous hypertension (idiopathic) without complications**
Asymptomatic chronic venous hypertension (idiopathic)

     I87.301 Chronic venous hypertension (idiopathic) without complications of right lower extremity

     I87.302 Chronic venous hypertension (idiopathic) without complications of left lower extremity

     I87.303 Chronic venous hypertension (idiopathic) without complications of bilateral lower extremity

     I87.309 Chronic venous hypertension (idiopathic) without complications of unspecified lower extremity
Chronic venous hypertension NOS

● **I87.31 Chronic venous hypertension (idiopathic) with ulcer**

> Use additional code to specify site and severity of ulcer (L97.-)

     I87.311 Chronic venous hypertension (idiopathic) with ulcer of right lower extremity 🔗

     I87.312 Chronic venous hypertension (idiopathic) with ulcer of left lower extremity 🔗

     I87.313 Chronic venous hypertension (idiopathic) with ulcer of bilateral lower extremity 🔗

     I87.319 Chronic venous hypertension (idiopathic) with ulcer of unspecified lower extremity 🔗

● **I87.32 Chronic venous hypertension (idiopathic) with inflammation**

     I87.321 Chronic venous hypertension (idiopathic) with inflammation of right lower extremity

     I87.322 Chronic venous hypertension (idiopathic) with inflammation of left lower extremity

     I87.323 Chronic venous hypertension (idiopathic) with inflammation of bilateral lower extremity

     I87.329 Chronic venous hypertension (idiopathic) with inflammation of unspecified lower extremity

● **I87.33 Chronic venous hypertension (idiopathic) with ulcer and inflammation**

> Use additional code to specify site and severity of ulcer (L97.-)

     I87.331 Chronic venous hypertension (idiopathic) with ulcer and inflammation of right lower extremity 🔗

     I87.332 Chronic venous hypertension (idiopathic) with ulcer and inflammation of left lower extremity 🔗

     I87.333 Chronic venous hypertension (idiopathic) with ulcer and inflammation of bilateral lower extremity 🔗

     I87.339 Chronic venous hypertension (idiopathic) with ulcer and inflammation of unspecified lower extremity 🔗

● **I87.39 Chronic venous hypertension (idiopathic) with other complications**

     I87.391 Chronic venous hypertension (idiopathic) with other complications of right lower extremity

     I87.392 Chronic venous hypertension (idiopathic) with other complications of left lower extremity

     I87.393 Chronic venous hypertension (idiopathic) with other complications of bilateral lower extremity

     I87.399 Chronic venous hypertension (idiopathic) with other complications of unspecified lower extremity

I87.8 Other specified disorders of veins
Phlebosclerosis
Venofibrosis

I87.9 Disorder of vein, unspecified

● **I88 Nonspecific lymphadenitis**

> **Excludes1**   acute lymphadenitis, except mesenteric (L04.-)
> enlarged lymph nodes NOS (R59.-)
> human immunodeficiency virus [HIV] disease resulting in generalized lymphadenopathy (B20)

I88.0 Nonspecific mesenteric lymphadenitis
Mesenteric lymphadenitis (acute)(chronic)

I88.1 Chronic lymphadenitis, except mesenteric
Adenitis
Lymphadenitis

I88.8 Other nonspecific lymphadenitis

I88.9 Nonspecific lymphadenitis, unspecified
Lymphadenitis NOS

● **I89 Other noninfective disorders of lymphatic vessels and lymph nodes**

> **Excludes1**   chylocele, tunica vaginalis (nonfilarial) NOS (N50.89)
> enlarged lymph nodes NOS (R59.-)
> filarial chylocele (B74.-)
> hereditary lymphedema (Q82.0)

I89.0 Lymphedema, not elsewhere classified
Elephantiasis (nonfilarial) NOS
Lymphangiectasis
Obliteration, lymphatic vessel
Praecox lymphedema
Secondary lymphedema

> **Excludes1**   postmastectomy lymphedema (I97.2)
> Coding Clinic: 2024, Q1, P17

I89.1 Lymphangitis
Chronic lymphangitis
Lymphangitis NOS
Subacute lymphangitis

> **Excludes1**   acute lymphangitis (L03.-)

I89.8   **Other specified noninfective disorders of lymphatic vessels and lymph nodes**
Chylocele (nonfilarial)
Chylous ascites
Chylous cyst
Lipomelanotic reticulosis
Lymph node or vessel fistula
Lymph node or vessel infarction
Lymph node or vessel rupture

I89.9   **Noninfective disorder of lymphatic vessels and lymph nodes, unspecified**
Disease of lymphatic vessels NOS

OTHER AND UNSPECIFIED DISORDERS OF THE CIRCULATORY SYSTEM (I95-I99)

● **I95**   **Hypotension**
Subnormal arterial blood pressure
   Excludes1   cardiovascular collapse (R57.9)
                maternal hypotension syndrome (O26.5-)
                nonspecific low blood pressure reading NOS (R03.1)

  I95.0   **Idiopathic hypotension**

  I95.1   **Orthostatic hypotension**
Hypotension, postural
Moving from a sitting or reclining position to a standing position precipitates a sudden drop in blood pressure (hypotension).
   Excludes1   neurogenic orthostatic hypotension [Shy-Drager] (G90.3)
                orthostatic hypotension due to drugs (I95.2)
   Coding Clinic: 2023, Q2, P9

  I95.2   **Hypotension due to drugs**
Orthostatic hypotension due to drugs
Use additional code for adverse effect, if applicable, to identify drug (T36-T50 with fifth or sixth character 5)

  I95.3   **Hypotension of hemodialysis**
Intra-dialytic hypotension

 ● **I95.8**   **Other hypotension**
  I95.81   Postprocedural hypotension
  I95.89   Other hypotension
        Chronic hypotension

  I95.9   **Hypotension, unspecified**

I96   **Gangrene, not elsewhere classified** 🗲
Gangrenous cellulitis
   Excludes1   gangrene in atherosclerosis of native arteries of the extremities (I70.26)
                gangrene of certain specified sites - *see* Alphabetical Index
                gangrene in hernia (K40.1, K40.4, K41.1, K41.4, K42.1, K43.1-, K44.1, K45.1, K46.1)
                gangrene in other peripheral vascular diseases (I73.-)
                gas gangrene (A48.0)
                pyoderma gangrenosum (L88)
   Excludes2   gangrene in diabetes mellitus (E08-E13 with .52)
   Coding Clinic: 2018, Q4, P87; 2017, Q3, P6; 2013, Q2, P35

● **I97**   **Intraoperative and postprocedural complications and disorders of circulatory system, not elsewhere classified**
   Excludes2   postprocedural shock (T81.1-)
   Coding Clinic: 2019, Q2, P22

  I97.0   **Postcardiotomy syndrome**

 ● **I97.1**   **Other postprocedural cardiac functional disturbances**
   Excludes2   acute pulmonary insufficiency following thoracic surgery (J95.1)
                intraoperative cardiac functional disturbances (I97.7-)

   ● **I97.11**   Postprocedural cardiac insufficiency
     I97.110   Postprocedural cardiac insufficiency following cardiac surgery
     I97.111   Postprocedural cardiac insufficiency following other surgery

   ● **I97.12**   Postprocedural cardiac arrest
     I97.120   Postprocedural cardiac arrest following cardiac surgery
     I97.121   Postprocedural cardiac arrest following other surgery

   ● **I97.13**   Postprocedural heart failure
     Use additional code to identify the heart failure (I50.-)
     I97.130   Postprocedural heart failure following cardiac surgery
     I97.131   Postprocedural heart failure following other surgery

   ● **I97.19**   Other postprocedural cardiac functional disturbances
     Use additional code, if applicable, to further specify disorder
     I97.190   Other postprocedural cardiac functional disturbances following cardiac surgery
        Use Additional code, if applicable, for type 4 or type 5 myocardial infarction, to further specify disorder
        Coding Clinic: 2019, Q2, P32-33
     I97.191   Other postprocedural cardiac functional disturbances following other surgery

  I97.2   **Postmastectomy lymphedema syndrome**   A
Elephantiasis due to mastectomy
Obliteration of lymphatic vessels

  I97.3   **Postprocedural hypertension**

 ● **I97.4**   **Intraoperative hemorrhage and hematoma of a circulatory system organ or structure complicating a procedure**
   Excludes1   intraoperative hemorrhage and hematoma of a circulatory system organ or structure due to accidental puncture and laceration during a procedure (I97.5-)
   Excludes2   intraoperative cerebrovascular hemorrhage complicating a procedure (G97.3-)

   ● **I97.41**   Intraoperative hemorrhage and hematoma of a circulatory system organ or structure complicating a circulatory system procedure
     I97.410   Intraoperative hemorrhage and hematoma of a circulatory system organ or structure complicating a cardiac catheterization
     I97.411   Intraoperative hemorrhage and hematoma of a circulatory system organ or structure complicating a cardiac bypass
     I97.418   Intraoperative hemorrhage and hematoma of a circulatory system organ or structure complicating other circulatory system procedure

   I97.42   Intraoperative hemorrhage and hematoma of a circulatory system organ or structure complicating other procedure
     Coding Clinic: 2020, Q1, P20; 2016, Q4, P100

 ● **I97.5**   **Accidental puncture and laceration of a circulatory system organ or structure during a procedure**
   Excludes2   accidental puncture and laceration of brain during a procedure (G97.4-)

   I97.51   Accidental puncture and laceration of a circulatory system organ or structure during a circulatory system procedure
     Coding Clinic: 2019, Q2, P24

   I97.52   Accidental puncture and laceration of a circulatory system organ or structure during other procedure

---

▶ New   ⇒ Revised   ~~deleted~~ Deleted   Excludes 1   Excludes 2   Includes   Use additional   Code first   Code also   Key words

OGCR Official Guidelines   X Assign placeholder X   ● Use Additional Character(s)   ▷ Manifestation Code   🗲 Hierarchical Condition Category   Coding Clinic

● **I97.6** **Postprocedural hemorrhage, hematoma and seroma of a circulatory system organ or structure following a procedure**

     Excludes2   postprocedural cerebrovascular hemorrhage complicating a procedure (G97.5-)

     Coding Clinic: 2016, Q4, P10

   ● **I97.61** Postprocedural hemorrhage of a circulatory system organ or structure following a circulatory system procedure

     I97.610   Postprocedural hemorrhage of a circulatory system organ or structure following a cardiac catheterization

     I97.611   Postprocedural hemorrhage of a circulatory system organ or structure following cardiac bypass

     I97.618   Postprocedural hemorrhage of a circulatory system organ or structure following other circulatory system procedure

   ● **I97.62** Postprocedural hemorrhage, hematoma and seroma of a circulatory system organ or structure following other procedure

     I97.620   Postprocedural hemorrhage of a circulatory system organ or structure following other procedure

     I97.621   Postprocedural hematoma of a circulatory system organ or structure following other procedure

     I97.622   Postprocedural seroma of a circulatory system organ or structure following other procedure

   ● **I97.63** Postprocedural hematoma of a circulatory system organ or structure following a circulatory system procedure

     I97.630   Postprocedural hematoma of a circulatory system organ or structure following a cardiac catheterization

     I97.631   Postprocedural hematoma of a circulatory system organ or structure following cardiac bypass

     I97.638   Postprocedural hematoma of a circulatory system organ or structure following other circulatory system procedure

   ● **I97.64** Postprocedural seroma of a circulatory system organ or structure following a circulatory system procedure

     I97.640   Postprocedural seroma of a circulatory system organ or structure following a cardiac catheterization

     I97.641   Postprocedural seroma of a circulatory system organ or structure following cardiac bypass

     I97.648   Postprocedural seroma of a circulatory system organ or structure following other circulatory system procedure

● **I97.7** **Intraoperative cardiac functional disturbances**

     Excludes2   acute pulmonary insufficiency following thoracic surgery (J95.1)
        postprocedural cardiac functional disturbances (I97.1-)

   ● **I97.71** Intraoperative cardiac arrest

     I97.710   Intraoperative cardiac arrest during cardiac surgery

     I97.711   Intraoperative cardiac arrest during other surgery

   ● **I97.79** Other intraoperative cardiac functional disturbances

     Use additional code, if applicable, to further specify disorder

     I97.790   Other intraoperative cardiac functional disturbances during cardiac surgery

     I97.791   Other intraoperative cardiac functional disturbances during other surgery

● **I97.8** **Other intraoperative and postprocedural complications and disorders of the circulatory system, not elsewhere classified**

     Use additional code, if applicable, to further specify disorder

   ● **I97.81** Intraoperative cerebrovascular infarction

     I97.810   Intraoperative cerebrovascular infarction during cardiac surgery 🔒

     I97.811   Intraoperative cerebrovascular infarction during other surgery 🔒

   ● **I97.82** Postprocedural cerebrovascular infarction

     I97.820   Postprocedural cerebrovascular infarction following cardiac surgery 🔒

     I97.821   Postprocedural cerebrovascular infarction following other surgery 🔒

     I97.88   Other intraoperative complications of the circulatory system, not elsewhere classified

     I97.89   Other postprocedural complications and disorders of the circulatory system, not elsewhere classified

       Coding Clinic: 2024, Q1, P26; 2019, Q2, P32-33

● **I99** **Other and unspecified disorders of circulatory system**

   I99.8   Other disorder of circulatory system

   I99.9   Unspecified disorder of circulatory system

CHAPTER 10

DISEASES OF THE RESPIRATORY SYSTEM
(J00-J99)

OGCR Chapter-Specific Coding Guidelines

10. **Chapter 10: Diseases of the Respiratory System (J00-J99)**

a. **Chronic Obstructive Pulmonary Disease [COPD] and Asthma**

1) **Acute exacerbation of chronic obstructive bronchitis and asthma**

The codes in categories J44 and J45 distinguish between uncomplicated cases and those in acute exacerbation. An acute exacerbation is a worsening or a decompensation of a chronic condition. An acute exacerbation is not equivalent to an infection superimposed on a chronic condition, though an exacerbation may be triggered by an infection.

b. **Acute Respiratory Failure**

1) **Acute respiratory failure as principal diagnosis**

A code from subcategory J96.0, Acute respiratory failure, or subcategory J96.2, Acute and chronic respiratory failure, may be assigned as a principal diagnosis when it is the condition established after study to be chiefly responsible for occasioning the admission to the hospital, and the selection is supported by the Alphabetic Index and Tabular List. However, chapter-specific coding guidelines (such as obstetrics, poisoning, HIV, newborn) that provide sequencing direction take precedence.

2) **Acute respiratory failure as secondary diagnosis**

Respiratory failure may be listed as a secondary diagnosis if it occurs after admission, or if it is present on admission, but does not meet the definition of principal diagnosis.

3) **Sequencing of acute respiratory failure and another acute condition**

When a patient is admitted with respiratory failure and another acute condition (e.g., myocardial infarction, cerebrovascular accident, aspiration pneumonia), the principal diagnosis will not be the same in every situation. This applies whether the other acute condition is a respiratory or nonrespiratory condition. Selection of the principal diagnosis will be dependent on the circumstances of admission. If both the respiratory failure and the other acute condition are equally responsible for occasioning the admission to the hospital, and there are no chapter-specific sequencing rules, the guideline regarding two or more diagnoses that equally meet the definition for principal diagnosis *(Section II, C.)* may be applied in these situations.

If the documentation is not clear as to whether acute respiratory failure and another condition are equally responsible for occasioning the admission, query the provider for clarification.

c. **Influenza due to certain identified influenza viruses**

Code only confirmed cases of influenza due to certain identified influenza viruses (category J09), and due to other identified influenza virus (category J10). This is an exception to the hospital inpatient guideline Section II, H. (Uncertain Diagnosis).

In this context, "confirmation" does not require documentation of positive laboratory testing specific for avian or other novel influenza A or other identified influenza virus. However, coding should be based on the provider's diagnostic statement that the patient has avian influenza, or other novel influenza A, for category J09, or has another particular identified strain of influenza, such as H1N1 or H3N2, but not identified as novel or variant, for category J10.

If the provider records "suspected" or "possible" or "probable" avian influenza, or novel influenza, or other identified influenza, then the appropriate influenza code from category J11, Influenza due to unidentified influenza virus, should be assigned. A code from category J09, Influenza due to certain identified influenza viruses, should not be assigned nor should a code from category J10, Influenza due to other identified influenza virus.

d. **Ventilator associated Pneumonia**

1) **Documentation of Ventilator associated Pneumonia**

As with all procedural or postprocedural complications, code assignment is based on the provider's documentation of the relationship between the condition and the procedure.

Code J95.851, Ventilator associated pneumonia, should be assigned only when the provider has documented ventilator associated pneumonia (VAP). An additional code to identify the organism (e.g., Pseudomonas aeruginosa, code B96.5) should also be assigned. Do not assign an additional code from categories J12-J18 to identify the type of pneumonia.

Code J95.851 should not be assigned for cases where the patient has pneumonia and is on a mechanical ventilator and the provider has not specifically stated that the pneumonia is ventilator associated pneumonia. If the documentation is unclear as to whether the patient has a pneumonia that is a complication attributable to the mechanical ventilator, query the provider.

2) **Ventilator associated Pneumonia Develops after Admission**

A patient may be admitted with one type of pneumonia (e.g., code J13, Pneumonia due to Streptococcus pneumonia) and subsequently develop VAP. In this instance, the principal diagnosis would be the appropriate code from categories J12-J18 for the pneumonia diagnosed at the time of admission. Code J95.851, Ventilator associated pneumonia, would be assigned as an additional diagnosis when the provider has also documented the presence of ventilator associated pneumonia.

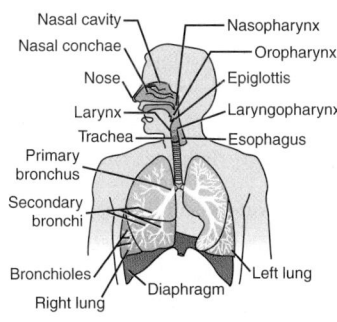

Figure 10-1 Respiratory system. (From Buck CJ: Step-by-Step Medical Coding, ed 2016, St. Louis, Elsevier, 2016)

Figure 10-2 Paranasal sinuses. (From Buck CJ: Step-by-Step Medical Coding, ed 2016, St. Louis, Elsevier, 2016)

Item 10–1 Pharyngitis is painful inflammation of the pharynx (sore throat). Ninety percent of the infections are caused by a virus with the remaining being bacterial and rarely a fungus (candidiasis). Other irritants such as pollutants, chemicals, or smoke may cause similar symptoms.

CHAPTER 10

DISEASES OF THE RESPIRATORY SYSTEM (J00-J99)

Note: When a respiratory condition is described as occurring in more than one site and is not specifically indexed, it should be classified to the lower anatomic site (e.g., tracheobronchitis to bronchitis in J40).

Use additional code, where applicable, to identify:
exposure to environmental tobacco smoke (Z77.22)
exposure to tobacco smoke in the perinatal period (P96.81)
history of tobacco dependence (Z87.891)
occupational exposure to environmental tobacco smoke (Z57.31)
tobacco dependence (F17.-)
tobacco use (Z72.0)

Excludes2   certain conditions originating in the perinatal period (P04-P96)
certain infectious and parasitic diseases (A00-B99)
complications of pregnancy, childbirth and the puerperium (O00-O99A)
congenital malformations, deformations and chromosomal abnormalities (Q00-Q99)
endocrine, nutritional and metabolic diseases (E00-E88)
injury, poisoning and certain other consequences of external causes (S00-T88)
neoplasms (C00-D49)
smoke inhalation (T59.81-)
symptoms, signs and abnormal clinical and laboratory findings, not elsewhere classified (R00-R94)

This chapter contains the following blocks:

J00-J06	Acute upper respiratory infections
J09-J18	Influenza and pneumonia
J20-J22	Other acute lower respiratory infections
J30-J39	Other diseases of upper respiratory tract
J40-J4A	Chronic lower respiratory diseases
J60-J70	Lung diseases due to external agents
J80-J84	Other respiratory diseases principally affecting the interstitium
J85-J86	Suppurative and necrotic conditions of the lower respiratory tract
J90-J94	Other diseases of the pleura
J95	Intraoperative and postprocedural complications and disorders of respiratory system, not elsewhere classified
J96-J99	Other diseases of the respiratory system

ACUTE UPPER RESPIRATORY INFECTIONS (J00-J06)

Use Additional code, if applicable, to identify resistance to antimicrobial drugs (Z16.-)

Excludes1   chronic obstructive pulmonary disease with acute lower respiratory infection (J44.0)

J00   Acute nasopharyngitis [common cold]
Acute rhinitis
Coryza (acute)
Infective nasopharyngitis NOS
Infective rhinitis
Nasal catarrh, acute
Nasopharyngitis NOS

Excludes1   acute pharyngitis (J02.-)
acute sore throat NOS (J02.9)
influenza virus with other respiratory manifestations (J09.X2, J10.1, J11.1)
pharyngitis NOS (J02.9)
rhinitis NOS (J31.0)
sore throat NOS (J02.9)

Excludes2   allergic rhinitis (J30.1-J30.9)
chronic pharyngitis (J31.2)
chronic rhinitis (J31.0)
chronic sore throat (J31.2)
nasopharyngitis, chronic (J31.1)
vasomotor rhinitis (J30.0)

★**(See Plate 27 of the Anatomy Illustrations.)**

●**J01   Acute sinusitis**
Includes   acute abscess of sinus
acute empyema of sinus
acute infection of sinus
acute inflammation of sinus
acute suppuration of sinus

Use additional code (B95-B97) to identify infectious agent.
Excludes1   sinusitis NOS (J32.9)
Excludes2   chronic sinusitis (J32.0-J32.8)

●**J01.0   Acute maxillary sinusitis**
Acute antritis
J01.00   Acute maxillary sinusitis, unspecified
J01.01   Acute recurrent maxillary sinusitis

●**J01.1   Acute frontal sinusitis**
J01.10   Acute frontal sinusitis, unspecified
J01.11   Acute recurrent frontal sinusitis

●**J01.2   Acute ethmoidal sinusitis**
J01.20   Acute ethmoidal sinusitis, unspecified
J01.21   Acute recurrent ethmoidal sinusitis

●**J01.3   Acute sphenoidal sinusitis**
J01.30   Acute sphenoidal sinusitis, unspecified
J01.31   Acute recurrent sphenoidal sinusitis

●**J01.4   Acute pansinusitis**
J01.40   Acute pansinusitis, unspecified
J01.41   Acute recurrent pansinusitis

CHAPTER 10 (J00-J99)

- **J01.8** **Other acute sinusitis**
  - **J01.80** **Other acute sinusitis**
    - Acute sinusitis involving more than one sinus but not pansinusitis
  - **J01.81** **Other acute recurrent sinusitis**
    - Acute recurrent sinusitis involving more than one sinus but not pansinusitis
- **J01.9** **Acute sinusitis, unspecified**
  - **J01.90** **Acute sinusitis, unspecified**
  - **J01.91** **Acute recurrent sinusitis, unspecified**
- **J02** **Acute pharyngitis**
  - **Includes** acute sore throat
  - **Excludes1** acute laryngopharyngitis (J06.0)
    - peritonsillar abscess (J36)
    - pharyngeal abscess (J39.1)
    - retropharyngeal abscess (J39.0)
  - **Excludes2** chronic pharyngitis (J31.2)
  - **J02.0** **Streptococcal pharyngitis**
    - Septic pharyngitis
    - Streptococcal sore throat
    - **Excludes2** scarlet fever (A38.-)
  - **J02.8** **Acute pharyngitis due to other specified organisms**
    - Use additional code (B95-B97) to identify infectious agent
    - **Excludes1** pharyngitis due to coxsackie virus (B08.5)
      - pharyngitis due to gonococcus (A54.5)
      - acute pharyngitis due to herpes [simplex] virus (B00.2)
      - acute pharyngitis due to infectious mononucleosis (B27.-)
      - enteroviral vesicular pharyngitis (B08.5)
  - **J02.9** **Acute pharyngitis, unspecified**
    - Gangrenous pharyngitis (acute)
    - Infective pharyngitis (acute) NOS
    - Pharyngitis (acute) NOS
    - Sore throat (acute) NOS
    - Suppurative pharyngitis (acute)
    - Ulcerative pharyngitis (acute)
    - **Excludes1** influenza virus with other respiratory manifestations (J09.X2, J10.1, J11.1)
- **J03** **Acute tonsillitis**
  - *Inflammation of pharyngeal tonsils caused by virus or bacteria*
  - **Excludes1** acute sore throat (J02.-)
    - hypertrophy of tonsils (J35.1)
    - peritonsillar abscess (J36)
    - sore throat NOS (J02.9)
    - streptococcal sore throat (J02.0)
  - **Excludes2** chronic tonsillitis (J35.0)
  - **J03.0** **Streptococcal tonsillitis**
    - **J03.00** **Acute streptococcal tonsillitis, unspecified**
    - **J03.01** **Acute recurrent streptococcal tonsillitis**
  - **J03.8** **Acute tonsillitis due to other specified organisms**
    - Use additional code (B95-B97) to identify infectious agent.
    - **Excludes1** diphtheritic tonsillitis (A36.0)
      - herpesviral pharyngotonsillitis (B00.2)
      - streptococcal tonsillitis (J03.0)
      - tuberculous tonsillitis (A15.8)
      - Vincent's tonsillitis (A69.1)
    - **J03.80** **Acute tonsillitis due to other specified organisms**
    - **J03.81** **Acute recurrent tonsillitis due to other specified organisms**
- **J03.9** **Acute tonsillitis, unspecified**
  - Follicular tonsillitis (acute)
  - Gangrenous tonsillitis (acute)
  - Infective tonsillitis (acute)
  - Tonsillitis (acute) NOS
  - Ulcerative tonsillitis (acute)
  - **Excludes1** influenza virus with other respiratory manifestations (J09.X2, J10.1, J11.1)
  - **J03.90** **Acute tonsillitis, unspecified**
  - **J03.91** **Acute recurrent tonsillitis, unspecified**
- **J04** **Acute laryngitis and tracheitis**
  - Use additional code (B95-B97) to identify infectious agent.
  - Code also influenza, if present, such as:
    - influenza due to identified novel influenza A virus with other respiratory manifestations (J09.X2)
    - influenza due to other identified influenza virus with other respiratory manifestations (J10.1)
    - influenza due to unidentified influenza virus with other respiratory manifestations (J11.1)
  - **Excludes1** acute obstructive laryngitis [croup] and epiglottitis (J05.-)
  - **Excludes2** laryngismus (stridulus) (J38.5)
  - **J04.0** **Acute laryngitis**
    - Edematous laryngitis (acute)
    - Laryngitis (acute) NOS
    - Subglottic laryngitis (acute)
    - Suppurative laryngitis (acute)
    - Ulcerative laryngitis (acute)
    - **Excludes1** acute obstructive laryngitis (J05.0)
    - **Excludes2** chronic laryngitis (J37.0)
  - **J04.1** **Acute tracheitis**
    - Acute viral tracheitis
    - Catarrhal tracheitis (acute)
    - Tracheitis (acute) NOS
    - **Excludes2** chronic tracheitis (J42)
    - **J04.10** **Acute tracheitis without obstruction**
    - **J04.11** **Acute tracheitis with obstruction**
  - **J04.2** **Acute laryngotracheitis**
    - Laryngotracheitis NOS
    - Tracheitis (acute) with laryngitis (acute)
    - **Excludes1** acute obstructive laryngotracheitis (J05.0)
    - **Excludes2** chronic laryngotracheitis (J37.1)
  - **J04.3** **Supraglottitis, unspecified**
    - **J04.30** **Supraglottitis, unspecified, without obstruction**
    - **J04.31** **Supraglottitis, unspecified, with obstruction**
- **J05** **Acute obstructive laryngitis [croup] and epiglottitis**
  - Use additional code (B95-B97) to identify infectious agent.
  - Code also influenza, if present, such as:
    - influenza due to identified novel influenza A virus with other respiratory manifestations (J09.X2)
    - influenza due to other identified influenza virus with other respiratory manifestations (J10.1)
    - influenza due to unidentified influenza virus with other respiratory manifestations (J11.1)
  - **J05.0** **Acute obstructive laryngitis [croup]**
    - Obstructive laryngitis (acute) NOS
    - Obstructive laryngotracheitis NOS
  - **J05.1** **Acute epiglottitis**
    - **Excludes2** epiglottitis, chronic (J37.0)
    - **J05.10** **Acute epiglottitis without obstruction**
      - Epiglottitis NOS
    - **J05.11** **Acute epiglottitis with obstruction**
- **J06** **Acute upper respiratory infections of multiple and unspecified sites**
  - **Excludes1** acute respiratory infection NOS (J22)
    - influenza virus with other respiratory manifestations (J09.X2, J10.1, J11.1)
    - streptococcal pharyngitis (J02.0)
  - **Coding Clinic: 2020, Q1, P22**

Item 10–2 **Laryngitis** is an inflammation of the larynx (voice box) resulting in hoarse voice or the complete loss of the voice. **Tracheitis** is an inflammation of the trachea (often following a URI) commonly caused by *staphylococcus aureus* resulting in inspiratory stridor (crowing sound on inspiration) and a crouplike cough.

▶ New   ⇒ Revised   ~~deleted~~ Deleted   Excludes 1   Excludes 2   Includes   Use additional   Code first   Code also   Key words
OGCR Official Guidelines   X Assign placeholder X   ● Use Additional Character(s)   ⫸ Manifestation Code   🏷 Hierarchical Condition Category   Coding Clinic

J06.0　**Acute laryngopharyngitis**

J06.9　**Acute upper respiratory infection, unspecified**
　　　Upper respiratory disease, acute
　　　Upper respiratory infection NOS

　　　Use additional code (B95-B97) to identify infectious
　　　　agent, if known, such as:
　　　　respiratory syncytial virus (RSV) (B97.4)

INFLUENZA AND PNEUMONIA (J09-J18)

Excludes2　allergic or eosinophilic pneumonia (J82)
　　　　　aspiration pneumonia NOS (J69.0)
　　　　　meconium pneumonia (P24.01)
　　　　　neonatal aspiration pneumonia (P24.-)
　　　　　pneumonia due to solids and liquids (J69.-)
　　　　　congenital pneumonia (P23.9)
　　　　　lipid pneumonia (J69.1)
　　　　　rheumatic pneumonia (I00)
　　　　　ventilator associated pneumonia (J95.851)
Coding Clinic: 2020, Q1, P22

● **J09**　**Influenza due to certain identified influenza viruses**
　　　Excludes1　influenza A/H1N1 (J10.-)
　　　　　　influenza due to other influenza viruses (J10.-)
　　　　　　influenza due to unidentified influenza virus
　　　　　　　(J11.-)
　　　　　　seasonal influenza due to other identified
　　　　　　　influenza virus (J10.-)
　　　　　　seasonal influenza due to unidentified influenza
　　　　　　　virus (J11.-)

● **J09.X**　**Influenza due to identified novel influenza A virus**
　　　　Avian influenza
　　　　Bird influenza
　　　　Influenza A/H5N1
　　　　Influenza of other animal origin, not bird or swine
　　　　Swine influenza virus (viruses that normally cause
　　　　　infections in pigs)
　　　　Coding Clinic: 2016, Q3, P11

　　J09.X1　**Influenza due to identified novel influenza A
　　　　　virus with pneumonia**
　　　　　　Code also , if applicable, associated:
　　　　　　　lung abscess (J85.1)
　　　　　　　other specified type of pneumonia

　　J09.X2　**Influenza due to identified novel influenza A
　　　　　virus with other respiratory manifestations**
　　　　　　Influenza due to identified novel influenza A
　　　　　　　virus NOS
　　　　　　Influenza due to identified novel influenza A
　　　　　　　virus with laryngitis
　　　　　　Influenza due to identified novel influenza A
　　　　　　　virus with pharyngitis
　　　　　　Influenza due to identified novel influenza A
　　　　　　　virus with upper respiratory symptoms
　　　　　　Use additional code, if applicable, for
　　　　　　　associated:
　　　　　　　pleural effusion (J91.8)
　　　　　　　sinusitis (J01.-)

　　J09.X3　**Influenza due to identified novel influenza A
　　　　　virus with gastrointestinal manifestations**
　　　　　　Influenza due to identified novel influenza A
　　　　　　　virus gastroenteritis
　　　　　　Excludes1　'intestinal flu' [viral
　　　　　　　　gastroenteritis] (A08.-)

　　J09.X9　**Influenza due to identified novel influenza A
　　　　　virus with other manifestations**
　　　　　　Influenza due to identified novel influenza A
　　　　　　　virus with encephalopathy
　　　　　　Influenza due to identified novel influenza A
　　　　　　　virus with myocarditis
　　　　　　Influenza due to identified novel influenza A
　　　　　　　virus with otitis media
　　　　　　Use additional code to identify manifestation

● **J10**　**Influenza due to other identified influenza virus**
　　　Includes　influenza A (non-novel)
　　　　　　influenza B
　　　　　　influenza C
　　　Excludes1　influenza due to avian influenza virus (J09.X-)
　　　　　　influenza due to swine flu (J09.X-)
　　　　　　influenza due to unidentified influenza virus
　　　　　　　(J11.-)

● **J10.0**　**Influenza due to other identified influenza virus with
　　　pneumonia**
　　　　Code also associated lung abscess, if applicable (J85.1)

　　J10.00　**Influenza due to other identified influenza
　　　　　virus with unspecified type of
　　　　　pneumonia**

　　J10.01　**Influenza due to other identified influenza virus
　　　　　with the same other identified influenza virus
　　　　　pneumonia**

　　J10.08　**Influenza due to other identified influenza virus
　　　　　with other specified pneumonia**
　　　　　　Code also other specified type of pneumonia
　　　　　　Coding Clinic: 2017, Q4, P96

　　J10.1　**Influenza due to other identified influenza virus with
　　　　other respiratory manifestations**
　　　　　Influenza due to other identified influenza virus NOS
　　　　　Influenza due to other identified influenza virus with
　　　　　　laryngitis
　　　　　Influenza due to other identified influenza virus with
　　　　　　pharyngitis
　　　　　Influenza due to other identified influenza virus with
　　　　　　upper respiratory symptoms
　　　　　Use additional code for associated pleural effusion, if
　　　　　　applicable (J91.8)
　　　　　Use additional code for associated sinusitis, if
　　　　　　applicable (J01.-)
　　　　　Coding Clinic: 2016, Q3, P11

　　J10.2　**Influenza due to other identified influenza virus with
　　　　gastrointestinal manifestations**
　　　　　Influenza due to other identified influenza virus
　　　　　　gastroenteritis
　　　　　Excludes1　'intestinal flu' [viral gastroenteritis]
　　　　　　　(A08.-)

● **J10.8**　**Influenza due to other identified influenza virus with
　　　other manifestations**

　　J10.81　**Influenza due to other identified influenza virus
　　　　　with encephalopathy**

　　J10.82　**Influenza due to other identified influenza virus
　　　　　with myocarditis**

　　J10.83　**Influenza due to other identified influenza virus
　　　　　with otitis media**
　　　　　　Use additional code for any associated
　　　　　　　perforated tympanic membrane (H72.-)

　　J10.89　**Influenza due to other identified influenza virus
　　　　　with other manifestations**
　　　　　　Use additional codes to identify the
　　　　　　　manifestations

● **J11**　**Influenza due to unidentified influenza virus**

● **J11.0**　**Influenza due to unidentified influenza virus with
　　　pneumonia**
　　　　Code also associated lung abscess, if applicable (J85.1)

　　J11.00　**Influenza due to unidentified influenza virus
　　　　　with unspecified type of pneumonia**
　　　　　　Influenza with pneumonia NOS
　　　　　　Coding Clinic: 2016, Q3, P12

　　J11.08　**Influenza due to unidentified influenza virus
　　　　　with specified pneumonia**
　　　　　　Code also other specified type of pneumonia

J11.1   **Influenza due to unidentified influenza virus with other respiratory manifestations**
Influenza NOS
Influenzal laryngitis NOS
Influenzal pharyngitis NOS
Influenza with upper respiratory symptoms NOS
Use additional code for associated pleural effusion, if applicable (J91.8)
Use additional code for associated sinusitis, if applicable (J01.-)

J11.2   **Influenza due to unidentified influenza virus with gastrointestinal manifestations**
Influenza gastroenteritis NOS
Excludes1   'intestinal flu' [viral gastroenteritis] (A08.-)

● **J11.8**   **Influenza due to unidentified influenza virus with other manifestations**
    J11.81   **Influenza due to unidentified influenza virus with encephalopathy**
Influenzal encephalopathy NOS
    J11.82   **Influenza due to unidentified influenza virus with myocarditis**
Influenzal myocarditis NOS
    J11.83   **Influenza due to unidentified influenza virus with otitis media**
Influenzal otitis media NOS
Use additional code for any associated perforated tympanic membrane (H72.-)
    J11.89   **Influenza due to unidentified influenza virus with other manifestations**
Use additional codes to identify the manifestations

● **J12**   **Viral pneumonia, not elsewhere classified**
Includes   bronchopneumonia due to viruses other than influenza viruses
Code first associated influenza, if applicable (J09.X1, J10.0-, J11.0-)
Code also associated abscess, if applicable (J85.1)
~~**Excludes1** aspiration pneumonia due to anesthesia during labor and delivery (O74.0)~~
~~aspiration pneumonia due to anesthesia during pregnancy (O29)~~
~~aspiration pneumonia due to anesthesia during puerperium (O89.0)~~
~~aspiration pneumonia due to solids and liquids (J69.-)~~
~~aspiration pneumonia NOS (J69.0)~~
~~congenital pneumonia (P23.0)~~
~~congenital rubella pneumonitis (P35.0)~~
~~interstitial pneumonia NOS (J84.9)~~
~~lipid pneumonia (J69.1)~~
~~neonatal aspiration pneumonia (P24.-)~~

▶ **Excludes2**   aspiration pneumonia due to anesthesia during labor and delivery (O74.0)
▶ aspiration pneumonia due to anesthesia during pregnancy (O29)
▶ aspiration pneumonia due to anesthesia during puerperium (O89.0)
▶ aspiration pneumonia due to solids and liquids (J69.-)
▶ aspiration pneumonia NOS (J69.0)
▶ congenital pneumonia (P23.0)
▶ congenital rubella pneumonitis (P35.0)
▶ interstitial pneumonia NOS (J84.9)
▶ lipid pneumonia (J69.1)
▶ neonatal aspiration pneumonia (P24.-)
Coding Clinic: 2021, Q1, P34

J12.0   **Adenoviral pneumonia**
J12.1   **Respiratory syncytial virus pneumonia**
RSV pneumonia
J12.2   **Parainfluenza virus pneumonia**
J12.3   **Human metapneumovirus pneumonia**
● **J12.8**   **Other viral pneumonia**
    J12.81   **Pneumonia due to SARS-associated coronavirus**
Severe acute respiratory syndrome NOS
    J12.82   **Pneumonia due to coronavirus disease 2019** (Ex)
No exclusions
Pneumonia due to 2019 novel coronavirus (SARS-CoV-2)
Pneumonia due to COVID-19
Code first COVID-19 (U07.1)
Coding Clinic: 2021, Q1, P33-34, 42, 47, 49
    J12.89   **Other viral pneumonia**
Coding Clinic: 2021, Q1, P33-34
J12.9   **Viral pneumonia, unspecified**

J13   **Pneumonia due to Streptococcus pneumoniae** 🐾
Bronchopneumonia due to S. pneumoniae
⇒*Code first, if applicable, associated influenza, if applicable (J09.X1, J10.0-, J11.0-)*
Code also, ~~associated abscess, if applicable (J85.1)~~
▶ if applicable, any associated condition such as:
▶ abscess (J85.1)
▶ aspiration pneumonia (J69.-)
Excludes1   congenital pneumonia due to S. pneumoniae (P23.6)
lobar pneumonia, unspecified organism (J18.1)
pneumonia due to other streptococci (J15.3-J15.4)

J14   **Pneumonia due to Hemophilus influenzae** 🐾
Bronchopneumonia due to H. influenzae
⇒*Code first, if applicable, associated influenza, if applicable (J09.X1, J10.0-, J11.0-)*
Code also, ~~associated abscess, if applicable (J85.1)~~
▶ if applicable, any associated condition such as:
▶ abscess (J85.1)
▶ aspiration pneumonia (J69.-)
Excludes1   congenital pneumonia due to H. influenzae (P23.6)

● **J15**   **Bacterial pneumonia, not elsewhere classified**
Includes   bronchopneumonia due to bacteria other than S. pneumoniae and H. influenzae
⇒*Code first, if applicable, associated influenza, if applicable (J09.X1, J10.0-, J11.0-)*
Code also, ~~associated abscess, if applicable (J85.1)~~
▶ if applicable, any associated condition such as:
▶ abscess (J85.1)
▶ aspiration pneumonia (J69.-)
Excludes1   chlamydial pneumonia (J16.0)
congenital pneumonia (P23.-)
Legionnaires' disease (A48.1)
spirochetal pneumonia (A69.8)
J15.0   **Pneumonia due to Klebsiella pneumoniae** 🐾
J15.1   **Pneumonia due to Pseudomonas** 🐾
● **J15.2**   **Pneumonia due to staphylococcus**
    J15.20   **Pneumonia due to staphylococcus, unspecified** 🐾
    ● **J15.21**   **Pneumonia due to staphylococcus aureus**
        J15.211   **Pneumonia due to Methicillin susceptible Staphylococcus aureus** 🐾
MSSA pneumonia
Pneumonia due to Staphylococcus aureus NOS
        J15.212   **Pneumonia due to Methicillin resistant Staphylococcus aureus** 🐾
    J15.29   **Pneumonia due to other staphylococcus** 🐾
J15.3   **Pneumonia due to streptococcus, group B** 🐾

Item 10–3 Pneumonia is an infection of the lungs, caused by a variety of microorganisms, including viruses, most commonly the Streptococcus pneumoniae (pneumococcus) bacteria, fungi, and parasites. Pneumonia occurs when the immune system is weakened, often by a URI or influenza.

▶ New   ⇒ Revised   ~~deleted~~ Deleted   Excludes 1   Excludes 2   Includes   Use additional   Code first   Code also   Key words

888   OGCR Official Guidelines   X Assign placeholder X   ● Use Additional Character(s)   ▷ Manifestation Code   🐾 Hierarchical Condition Category   Coding Clinic

J15.4   Pneumonia due to other streptococci 🦠

     Excludes1   pneumonia due to streptococcus, group B (J15.3)
                       pneumonia due to Streptococcus pneumoniae (J13)

J15.5   Pneumonia due to Escherichia coli 🦠

J15.6   Pneumonia due to other Gram-negative bacteria 🦠

J15.61   Pneumonia due to Acinetobacter baumannii

J15.69   Pneumonia due to other Gram-negative bacteria
         Pneumonia due to other aerobic Gram-negative bacteria
         Pneumonia due to Serratia marcescens

J15.7   Pneumonia due to Mycoplasma pneumoniae

J15.8   Pneumonia due to other specified bacteria 🦠

J15.9   Unspecified bacterial pneumonia
         Pneumonia due to gram-positive bacteria
         Coding Clinic: 2017, Q4, P96

● **J16**   Pneumonia due to other infectious organisms, not elsewhere classified

     ▰ *Code first, if applicable, associated influenza, if applicable (J09.X1, J10.0-, J11.0-)*

     ▶ Code also, ~~associated abscess, if applicable (J85.1)~~
       ▶ if applicable, any associated condition such as:
         ▶ abscess (J85.1)
         ▶ aspiration pneumonia (J69.-)

     Excludes1   congenital pneumonia (P23.-)
                       ornithosis (A70)
                       pneumocystosis (B59)
                       pneumonia NOS (J18.9)

J16.0   Chlamydial pneumonia

J16.8   Pneumonia due to other specified infectious organisms

▰ *J17*   *Pneumonia in diseases classified elsewhere*

     Code first underlying disease, such as:
         Q fever (A78)
         rheumatic fever (I00)
         schistosomiasis (B65.0-B65.9)

     ▶ Code also, if applicable, any associated condition such as:
       ▶ abscess (J85.1)
       ▶ aspiration pneumonia (J69.-)

     Excludes1   candidial pneumonia (B37.1)
                       chlamydial pneumonia (J16.0)
                       gonorrheal pneumonia (A54.84)
                       histoplasmosis pneumonia (B39.0-B39.2)
                       measles pneumonia (B05.2)
                       nocardiosis pneumonia (A43.0)
                       pneumocystosis (B59)
                       pneumonia due to Pneumocystis carinii (B59)
                       pneumonia due to Pneumocystis jiroveci (B59)
                       pneumonia in actinomycosis (A42.0)
                       pneumonia in anthrax (A22.1)
                       pneumonia in ascariasis (B77.81)
                       pneumonia in aspergillosis (B44.0-B44.1)
                       pneumonia in coccidioidomycosis (B38.0-B38.2)
                       pneumonia in cytomegalovirus disease (B25.0)
                       pneumonia in toxoplasmosis (B58.3)
                       rubella pneumonia (B06.81)
                       salmonella pneumonia (A02.22)
                       spirochetal infection NEC with pneumonia (A69.8)
                       tularemia pneumonia (A21.2)
                       typhoid fever with pneumonia (A01.03)
                       varicella pneumonia (B01.2)
                       whooping cough with pneumonia (A37 with fifth-character 1)

● **J18**   Pneumonia, unspecified organism

     ▰ *Code first, if applicable, associated influenza, if applicable (J09.X1, J10.0-, J11.0-)*

     ▶ Code also, if applicable, any associated condition such as:
       ▶ aspiration pneumonia (J69.-)

     Excludes1   congenital pneumonia (P23.0)
                       drug-induced interstitial lung disorder (J70.2-J70.4)
                       interstitial pneumonia NOS (J84.9)
                       neonatal aspiration pneumonia (P24.-)
                       pneumonitis due to fumes and vapors (J68.0)
                       usual interstitial pneumonia (J84.178)

     ▶ **Excludes2**   abscess of lung with pneumonia (J85.1)
                       ▶ aspiration pneumonia due to anesthesia during labor and delivery (O74.0)
                       ▶ aspiration pneumonia due to anesthesia during pregnancy (O29)
                       ▶ aspiration pneumonia due to anesthesia during puerperium (O89.0)
                       ▶ aspiration pneumonia due to solids and liquids (J69.-)
                       ▶ aspiration pneumonia NOS (J69.0)
                       ▶ lipid pneumonia (J69.1)
                       ▶ pneumonitis due to external agents (J67-J70)

J18.0   Bronchopneumonia, unspecified organism

     Excludes1   hypostatic bronchopneumonia (J18.2)
                       lipid pneumonia (J69.1)

     ▰ **Excludes2**   acute bronchiolitis (J21.-)
                       chronic bronchiolitis (J44.89)
                       ▶ other specified chronic obstructive pulmonary disease (J44.89)

J18.1   Lobar pneumonia, unspecified organism 🦠
         Coding Clinic: 2016, Q3, P15

J18.2   Hypostatic pneumonia, unspecified organism
         Hypostatic bronchopneumonia
         Passive pneumonia

J18.8   Other pneumonia, unspecified organism

J18.9   Pneumonia, unspecified organism
         Coding Clinic: Q3, P15; 2019, Q2, P28; Q1, P36; 2016, Q3, P15; 2012, Q4, P94

OTHER ACUTE LOWER RESPIRATORY INFECTIONS (J20-J22)

     Excludes2   chronic obstructive pulmonary disease with acute lower respiratory infection (J44.0)

● **J20**   Acute bronchitis
     Inflammation/irritation of the bronchial tubes lasting 2-3 weeks, most commonly caused by a virus

     Includes   acute and subacute bronchitis (with) bronchospasm
                       acute and subacute bronchitis (with) tracheitis
                       acute and subacute bronchitis (with) tracheobronchitis, acute
                       acute and subacute fibrinous bronchitis
                       acute and subacute membranous bronchitis
                       acute and subacute purulent bronchitis
                       acute and subacute septic bronchitis

     Excludes1   bronchitis NOS (J40)
                       tracheobronchitis NOS (J40)

     Excludes2   acute bronchitis with bronchiectasis (J47.0)
                       acute bronchitis with chronic obstructive asthma (J44.0)
                       acute bronchitis with chronic obstructive pulmonary disease (J44.0)
                       allergic bronchitis NOS (J45.909-)
                       bronchitis due to chemicals, fumes and vapors (J68.0)
                       chronic bronchitis NOS (J42)
                       chronic mucopurulent bronchitis (J41.1)
                       chronic obstructive bronchitis (J44.-)
                       chronic obstructive tracheobronchitis (J44.-)
                       chronic simple bronchitis (J41.0)
                       chronic tracheobronchitis (J42)

J20.0   Acute bronchitis due to Mycoplasma pneumoniae

J20.1   Acute bronchitis due to Hemophilus influenzae

J20.2   Acute bronchitis due to streptococcus

J20.3 Acute bronchitis due to coxsackievirus

J20.4 Acute bronchitis due to parainfluenza virus

J20.5 Acute bronchitis due to respiratory syncytial virus
Acute bronchitis due to RSV

J20.6 Acute bronchitis due to rhinovirus
Coding Clinic: 2016, Q3, P10

J20.7 Acute bronchitis due to echovirus

J20.8 Acute bronchitis due to other specified organisms
Coding Clinic: 2016, Q3, P11

J20.9 Acute bronchitis, unspecified
Coding Clinic: 2019, Q1, P35; 2016, Q3, P16

● **J21** Acute bronchiolitis
Bronchiolitis obliterans with organizing pneumonia (BOOP)
inflammation of bronchioles and surrounding tissue in lung

  Includes acute bronchiolitis with bronchospasm

  Excludes2 respiratory bronchiolitis interstitial lung disease
(J84.115)

J21.0 Acute bronchiolitis due to respiratory syncytial virus
Acute bronchitis due to RSV

J21.1 Acute bronchiolitis due to human metapneumovirus

J21.8 Acute bronchiolitis due to other specified organisms

J21.9 Acute bronchiolitis, unspecified
Bronchiolitis (acute)

  Excludes1 chronic bronchiolitis (J44.89)

J22 Unspecified acute lower respiratory infection
Acute (lower) respiratory (tract) infection NOS

  Excludes1 upper respiratory infection (acute) (J06.9)

Coding Clinic: 2020, Q1, P22-23

OTHER DISEASES OF UPPER RESPIRATORY TRACT (J30-J39)

● **J30** Vasomotor and allergic rhinitis

  Includes spasmodic rhinorrhea

  Excludes1 allergic rhinitis with asthma (bronchial) (J45.909)
rhinitis NOS (J31.0)

J30.0 Vasomotor rhinitis

J30.1 Allergic rhinitis due to pollen
Allergy NOS due to pollen
Hay fever
Pollinosis

J30.2 Other seasonal allergic rhinitis

J30.5 Allergic rhinitis due to food

● **J30.8** Other allergic rhinitis

  J30.81 Allergic rhinitis due to animal (cat) (dog) hair
and dander

  J30.89 Other allergic rhinitis
Perennial allergic rhinitis

J30.9 Allergic rhinitis, unspecified

● **J31** Chronic rhinitis, nasopharyngitis and pharyngitis

J31.0 Chronic rhinitis
Atrophic rhinitis (chronic)
Granulomatous rhinitis (chronic)
Hypertrophic rhinitis (chronic)
Obstructive rhinitis (chronic)
Ozena
Purulent rhinitis (chronic)
Rhinitis (chronic) NOS
Ulcerative rhinitis (chronic)

  Excludes1 allergic rhinitis (J30.1-J30.9)
vasomotor rhinitis (J30.0)

J31.1 Chronic nasopharyngitis

  Excludes2 acute nasopharyngitis (J00)

J31.2 Chronic pharyngitis
Chronic sore throat
Atrophic pharyngitis (chronic)
Granular pharyngitis (chronic)
Hypertrophic pharyngitis (chronic)

  Excludes2 acute pharyngitis (J02.9)

● **J32** Chronic sinusitis

  Includes sinus abscess
sinus empyema
sinus infection
sinus suppuration

  Excludes2 acute sinusitis (J01.-)

J32.0 Chronic maxillary sinusitis
Antritis (chronic)
Maxillary sinusitis NOS

J32.1 Chronic frontal sinusitis
Frontal sinusitis NOS

J32.2 Chronic ethmoidal sinusitis
Ethmoidal sinusitis NOS

  Excludes1 Woakes' ethmoiditis (J33.1)

J32.3 Chronic sphenoidal sinusitis
Sphenoidal sinusitis NOS

J32.4 Chronic pansinusitis
Pansinusitis NOS

J32.8 Other chronic sinusitis
Sinusitis (chronic) involving more than one sinus but
not pansinusitis

J32.9 Chronic sinusitis, unspecified
Sinusitis (chronic) NOS

● **J33** Nasal polyp

  Excludes1 adenomatous polyps (D14.0)

J33.0 Polyp of nasal cavity
Choanal polyp
Nasopharyngeal polyp

J33.1 Polypoid sinus degeneration
Woakes' syndrome or ethmoiditis

J33.8 Other polyp of sinus
Accessory polyp of sinus
Ethmoidal polyp of sinus
Maxillary polyp of sinus
Sphenoidal polyp of sinus

J33.9 Nasal polyp, unspecified

● **J34** Other and unspecified disorders of nose and nasal sinuses

  Excludes2 varicose ulcer of nasal septum (I86.8)

J34.0 Abscess, furuncle and carbuncle of nose
Cellulitis of nose
Necrosis of nose
Ulceration of nose

J34.1 Cyst and mucocele of nose and nasal sinus

J34.2 Deviated nasal septum
Deflection or deviation of septum (nasal) (acquired)

  Excludes1 congenital deviated nasal septum (Q67.4)

J34.3 Hypertrophy of nasal turbinates

Deviated
septal
cartilage

Figure 10-3 Deviated nasal septum.

Item 10–4 Nasal polyps are an abnormal growth of tissue (tumor) projecting from a mucous membrane and attached to the surface by a narrow elongated stalk (pedunculated). Nasal polyps usually originate in the ethmoid sinus but also may occur in the maxillary sinus. Symptoms are nasal block, sinusitis, anosmia, and secondary infections.

Item 10–5 A **deviated nasal septum** is the displacement of the septal cartilage that separates the nares. This displacement causes obstructed air flow through the nasal passages. A child can be born with this displacement (congenital), or the condition may be acquired through trauma, such as a sports injury. Symptoms include nasal block, sinusitis, and related secondary infections. Septoplasty is surgical repair of this condition.

▶ New   ⇒ Revised   ~~deleted~~ Deleted   Excludes 1   Excludes 2   Includes   Use additional   Code first   Code also   Key words
OGCR Official Guidelines   X Assign placeholder X   ● Use Additional Character(s)   ▶ Manifestation Code   🍊 Hierarchical Condition Category   Coding Clinic

● **J34.8**   **Other specified disorders of nose and nasal sinuses**

     J34.81   **Nasal mucositis (ulcerative)**

         Code also type of associated therapy, such as:
           antineoplastic and immunosuppressive
           drugs (T45.1X-)
           radiological procedure and radiotherapy
           (Y84.2)

         Excludes2   gastrointestinal mucositis
                 (ulcerative) (K92.81)
                 mucositis (ulcerative) of vagina
                 and vulva (N76.81)
                 oral mucositis (ulcerative) (K12.3-)

▶● **J34.82**   **Nasal valve collapse**
         ▶Nasal valve compromise
         ▶Nasal valve stenosis
         ▶ *Code first underlying cause, such as:*
           deviated nasal septum (J34.2)

▶● **J34.820**   **Internal nasal valve collapse**
     ▶**J34.8200** **Internal nasal valve collapse,**
                 unspecified
         ▶**J34.8201**   **Internal nasal valve**
                 collapse, static
             ▶Narrowing of the
                septum, head of the
                inferior turbinate
                and the upper
                lateral cartilage
         ▶**J34.8202**   **Internal nasal valve**
                 collapse, dynamic
             ▶Collapse or falling of the
                upper, middle
                sidewall of the nose
                on inspiration

▶● **J34.821**   **External nasal valve collapse**
         J34.8210   **External nasal valve**
                 collapse, unspecified
         J34.8211   **External nasal valve**
                 collapse, static
             ▶Fixed narrowing of the
                caudal septum,
                lower lateral
                cartilage, alar rim
                and nasal sill
         J34.8212   **External nasal valve**
                 collapse, dynamic
             ▶Collapse or falling of the
                lower sidewall or
                nostril of the nose
                on inspiration
         ▶**J34.829**   **Nasal valve collapse, unspecified**
            ▶Nasal valve collapse, NOS

     J34.89   **Other specified disorders of nose and nasal**
            sinuses
         Perforation of nasal septum NOS
         Rhinolith

     J34.9   **Unspecified disorder of nose and nasal sinuses**

● **J35**   **Chronic diseases of tonsils and adenoids**

   ● **J35.0**   **Chronic tonsillitis and adenoiditis**

         Excludes2   acute tonsillitis (J03.-)

     J35.01   **Chronic tonsillitis**

     J35.02   **Chronic adenoiditis**

     J35.03   **Chronic tonsillitis and adenoiditis**

     J35.1   **Hypertrophy of tonsils**
         Enlargement of tonsils

         Excludes1   hypertrophy of tonsils with tonsillitis
                 (J35.0-)

     J35.2   **Hypertrophy of adenoids**
         Enlargement of adenoids

         Excludes1   hypertrophy of adenoids with adenoiditis
                 (J35.0-)

     J35.3   **Hypertrophy of tonsils with hypertrophy of adenoids**

         Excludes1   hypertrophy of tonsils and adenoids with
                 tonsillitis and adenoiditis (J35.03)

     J35.8   **Other chronic diseases of tonsils and adenoids**
         Adenoid vegetations
         Amygdalolith
         Calculus, tonsil
         Cicatrix of tonsil (and adenoid)
         Tonsillar tag
         Ulcer of tonsil

     J35.9   **Chronic disease of tonsils and adenoids, unspecified**
         Disease (chronic) of tonsils and adenoids NOS

● **J36**   **Peritonsillar abscess**

     Includes   abscess of tonsil
                peritonsillar cellulitis
                quinsy

     Use additional code (B95-B97) to identify infectious agent.

     Excludes1   acute tonsillitis (J03.-)
                chronic tonsillitis (J35.0)
                retropharyngeal abscess (J39.0)
                tonsillitis NOS (J03.9-)

● **J37**   **Chronic laryngitis and laryngotracheitis**
     Use additional code to identify:
         exposure to environmental tobacco smoke (Z77.22)
         exposure to tobacco smoke in the perinatal period (P96.81)
         history of tobacco dependence (Z87.891)
         infectious agent (B95-B97)
         occupational exposure to environmental tobacco smoke (Z57.31)
         tobacco dependence (F17.-)
         tobacco use (Z72.0)

     J37.0   **Chronic laryngitis**
         Catarrhal laryngitis
         Hypertrophic laryngitis
         Sicca laryngitis

         Excludes2   acute laryngitis (J04.0)
                 obstructive (acute) laryngitis (J05.0)

     J37.1   **Chronic laryngotracheitis**
         Laryngitis, chronic, with tracheitis (chronic)
         Tracheitis, chronic, with laryngitis

         Excludes1   chronic tracheitis (J42)

         Excludes2   acute laryngotracheitis (J04.2)
                 acute tracheitis (J04.1)

● **J38**   **Diseases of vocal cords and larynx, not elsewhere classified**

     Excludes1   congenital laryngeal stridor (P28.89)
                obstructive laryngitis (acute) (J05.0)
                postprocedural subglottic stenosis (J95.5)
                stridor (R06.1)
                ulcerative laryngitis (J04.0)

   ● **J38.0**   **Paralysis of vocal cords and larynx**
         Laryngoplegia
         Paralysis of glottis

     J38.00   **Paralysis of vocal cords and larynx, unspecified**

     J38.01   **Paralysis of vocal cords and larynx, unilateral**

     J38.02   **Paralysis of vocal cords and larynx, bilateral**

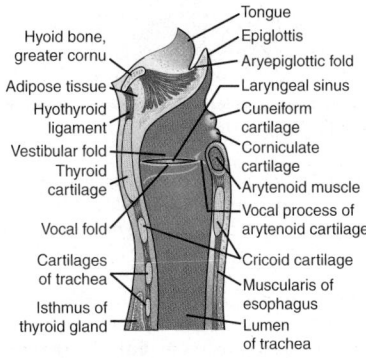

Figure 10-4   Coronal section of the larynx.

Item 10–6   The **larynx** extends from the tongue to the trachea and is divided into an upper and lower portion separated by folds. The framework of the larynx is cartilage composed of the single cricoid, thyroid, and epiglottic cartilages, and the paired arytenoid, cuneiform, and corniculate cartilages.

J38.1   **Polyp of vocal cord and larynx**
> **Excludes1**   adenomatous polyps (D14.1)

J38.2   **Nodules of vocal cords**
Chorditis (fibrinous)(nodosa)(tuberosa)
Singer's nodes
Teacher's nodes

J38.3   **Other diseases of vocal cords**
Abscess of vocal cords
Cellulitis of vocal cords
Granuloma of vocal cords
Leukokeratosis of vocal cords
Leukoplakia of vocal cords

J38.4   **Edema of larynx**
Edema (of) glottis
Subglottic edema
Supraglottic edema
> **Excludes1**   acute obstructive laryngitis [croup] (J05.0)
> edematous laryngitis (J04.0)

J38.5   **Laryngeal spasm**
Laryngismus (stridulus)

J38.6   **Stenosis of larynx**

J38.7   **Other diseases of larynx**
Abscess of larynx
Cellulitis of larynx
Disease of larynx NOS
Necrosis of larynx
Pachyderma of larynx
Perichondritis of larynx
Ulcer of larynx

● **J39**   **Other diseases of upper respiratory tract**
> **Excludes1**   acute respiratory infection NOS (J22)
> acute upper respiratory infection (J06.9)
> upper respiratory inflammation due to chemicals, gases, fumes or vapors (J68.2)

J39.0   **Retropharyngeal and parapharyngeal abscess**
Peripharyngeal abscess
> **Excludes1**   peritonsillar abscess (J36)

J39.1   **Other abscess of pharynx**
Cellulitis of pharynx
Nasopharyngeal abscess

J39.2   **Other diseases of pharynx**
Cyst of pharynx
Edema of pharynx
> **Excludes2**   chronic pharyngitis (J31.2)
> ulcerative pharyngitis (J02.9)

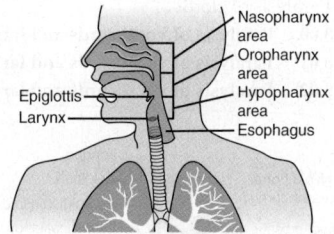

Figure 10-5   The pharynx.

Item 10–7   The **pharynx** is the passage for both food and air between the mouth and the esophagus and is divided into three areas: nasopharynx, oropharynx, and hypopharynx. The hypopharynx branches into the esophagus and the voice box.

Item 10–8   **Chronic bronchitis** is usually defined as being present in any patient who has persistent cough with sputum production for at least three months in at least two consecutive years. **Simple chronic bronchitis** is marked by a productive cough but no pathological airflow obstruction. **Chronic obstructive pulmonary disease (COPD)** is a group of conditions—bronchitis, emphysema, asthma, bronchiectasis, allergic alveolitis—marked by dyspnea. **Catarrhal** bronchitis is an acute form of bronchitis marked by profuse mucus and pus production (**mucopurulent** discharge). **Croupous** bronchitis, also known as pseudomembranous, fibrinous, plastic, exudative, or membranous, is marked by a violent cough and dyspnea.

J39.3   **Upper respiratory tract hypersensitivity reaction, site unspecified**
> **Excludes1**   hypersensitivity reaction of upper respiratory tract, such as:
> extrinsic allergic alveolitis (J67.9)
> pneumoconiosis (J60-J67.9)

J39.8   **Other specified diseases of upper respiratory tract**
Coding Clinic: 2023, Q1, P30

J39.9   **Disease of upper respiratory tract, unspecified**

CHRONIC LOWER RESPIRATORY DISEASES (J40-J4A)

> **Excludes1**   bronchitis due to chemicals, gases, fumes and vapors (J68.0)
> **Excludes2**   cystic fibrosis (E84.-)

J40   **Bronchitis, not specified as acute or chronic**
Bronchitis NOS
Catarrhal bronchitis
Bronchitis with tracheitis NOS
Tracheobronchitis NOS
Use additional code to identify:
exposure to environmental tobacco smoke (Z77.22)
exposure to tobacco smoke in the perinatal period (P96.81)
history of tobacco dependence (Z87.891)
occupational exposure to environmental tobacco smoke (Z57.31)
tobacco dependence (F17.-)
tobacco use (Z72.0)
> **Excludes1**   acute bronchitis (J20.-)
> allergic bronchitis NOS (J45.909-)
> asthmatic bronchitis NOS (J45.9-)
> bronchitis due to chemicals, gases, fumes and vapors (J68.0)

● **J41**   **Simple and mucopurulent chronic bronchitis**
Use additional code to identify:
exposure to environmental tobacco smoke (Z77.22)
exposure to tobacco smoke in the perinatal period (P96.81)
history of tobacco dependence (Z87.891)
occupational exposure to environmental tobacco smoke (Z57.31)
tobacco dependence (F17.-)
tobacco use (Z72.0)
> **Excludes2**   chronic bronchitis NOS (J42)
> chronic obstructive bronchitis (J44.-)

J41.0   **Simple chronic bronchitis** 🐄

J41.1   **Mucopurulent chronic bronchitis** 🐄

J41.8   **Mixed simple and mucopurulent chronic bronchitis** 🐄

J42   **Unspecified chronic bronchitis** 🐄
Chronic bronchitis NOS
Chronic tracheitis
Chronic tracheobronchitis
Use additional code to identify:
exposure to environmental tobacco smoke (Z77.22)
exposure to tobacco smoke in the perinatal period (P96.81)
history of tobacco dependence (Z87.891)
occupational exposure to environmental tobacco smoke (Z57.31)
tobacco dependence (F17.-)
tobacco use (Z72.0)
> **Excludes1**   bronchiolitis obliterans and bronchiolitis obliterans syndrome (J44.81)
> chronic asthmatic bronchitis (J44.-)
> chronic bronchitis with airways obstruction (J44.-)
> chronic emphysematous bronchitis (J44.-)
> chronic obstructive pulmonary disease NOS (J44.9)
> simple and mucopurulent chronic bronchitis (J41.-)

● **J43**   **Emphysema**
> **Excludes1**   compensatory emphysema (J98.3)
> emphysema due to inhalation of chemicals, gases, fumes or vapors (J68.4)
> interstitial emphysema (J98.2)
> mediastinal emphysema (J98.2)
> neonatal interstitial emphysema (P25.0)
> surgical (subcutaneous) emphysema (T81.82)
> **Excludes2**   emphysema with chronic (obstructive) bronchitis (J44.-)
> emphysematous (obstructive) bronchitis (J44.-)
> traumatic subcutaneous emphysema (T79.7)
Coding Clinic: 2024, Q2, P4

▶ New   ⇛ Revised   ~~deleted~~ Deleted   Excludes 1   Excludes 2   Includes   Use additional   Code first   Code also   Key words

OGCR Official Guidelines   X Assign placeholder X   ● Use Additional Character(s)   ▶ Manifestation Code   🐄 Hierarchical Condition Category   Coding Clinic

Figure 10-6   Emphysema. (From Shiland, BJ: Medical Terminology & Anatomy for ICD-10 Coding, ed 2, Mosby, 2015)

J43.0   **Unilateral pulmonary emphysema [MacLeod's syndrome]**
  Swyer-James syndrome
  Unilateral emphysema
  Unilateral hyperlucent lung
  Unilateral pulmonary artery functional hypoplasia
  Unilateral transparency of lung

J43.1   **Panlobular emphysema**
  Panacinar emphysema

J43.2   **Centrilobular emphysema**

J43.8   **Other emphysema**

J43.9   **Emphysema, unspecified**
  Bullous emphysema (lung)(pulmonary)
  Emphysema (lung)(pulmonary) NOS
  Emphysematous bleb
  Vesicular emphysema (lung)(pulmonary)
  Coding Clinic: 2024, Q2, P4, 5; 2019, Q1, P35-37; 2017, Q4, P97-98

● **J44**   **Other chronic obstructive pulmonary disease**
  Includes   asthma with chronic obstructive pulmonary disease
    chronic asthmatic (obstructive) bronchitis
    chronic bronchitis with airway obstruction
    chronic bronchitis with emphysema
    chronic emphysematous bronchitis
    chronic obstructive asthma
    chronic obstructive bronchitis
    chronic obstructive tracheobronchitis
  Code also type of asthma, if applicable (J45.-)
  Excludes1   chronic bronchitis NOS (J42)
    chronic simple and mucopurulent bronchitis (J41.-)
    chronic tracheitis (J42)
    chronic tracheobronchitis (J42)
  Excludes2   bronchiectasis (J47.-)
    emphysema without chronic bronchitis (J43.-)
  Coding Clinic: 2024, Q2, P3-6; 2019, Q1, P34-36; 2017, Q4, P97; 2017, Q1, P25; 2016, Q3, P16

J44.0   **Chronic obstructive pulmonary disease with (acute) lower respiratory infection**
  Code also to identify the infection
  Coding Clinic: 2024, Q2, P6; 2019, Q1, P35-36; 2017, Q4, P96; 2017, Q2, P30, Q1, P24-25; 2016, Q3, P15-16

J44.1   **Chronic obstructive pulmonary disease with (acute) exacerbation**
  Decompensated COPD
  Decompensated COPD with (acute) exacerbation
  Excludes2   chronic obstructive pulmonary disease [COPD] with acute bronchitis (J44.0)
    lung diseases due to external agents (J60-J70)
  Coding Clinic: 2024, Q2, P6; 2019, Q1, P34-35; 2017, Q4, P96; 2017, Q1, P26; 2016, Q3, P15-16, Q1, P36

● **J44.8**   **Other specified chronic obstructive pulmonary disease**
  J44.81   **Bronchiolitis obliterans and bronchiolitis obliterans syndrome**
    Obliterative bronchiolitis
    Code first, if applicable:
      complication of bone marrow transplant (T86.09)
      complication of stem cell transplant (T86.5)
      heart-lung transplant rejection (T86.31)
      lung transplant rejection (T86.810)
      other complications of heart-lung transplant (T86.39)
      other complications of lung transplant (T86.818)
    Code also, if applicable, associated conditions, such as:
      chronic graft-versus-host disease (D89.811)
      chronic lung allograft dysfunction (J4A.-)
      chronic respiratory conditions due to chemicals, gases, fumes and vapors (J68.4)
  J44.89   **Other specified chronic obstructive pulmonary disease**
    Chronic asthmatic (obstructive) bronchitis
    Chronic emphysematous bronchitis
    Coding Clinic: 2024, Q2, P3

J44.9   **Chronic obstructive pulmonary disease, unspecified**
  Chronic obstructive airway disease NOS
  Chronic obstructive lung disease NOS
  Excludes2   lung diseases due to external agents (J60-J70)
  Coding Clinic: 2024, Q2, P3, 4, 6; 2019, Q1, P36; 2017, Q4, P96-97; 2017, Q1, P24-25; 2016, Q1, P37

● **J45**   **Asthma**
  Allergic (predominantly) asthma
  Allergic bronchitis NOS
  Allergic rhinitis with asthma
  Atopic asthma
  Extrinsic allergic asthma
  Hay fever with asthma
  Idiosyncratic asthma
  Intrinsic nonallergic asthma
  Nonallergic asthma
  Use additional code to identify:
    eosinophilic asthma (J82.83)
    exposure to environmental tobacco smoke (Z77.22)
    exposure to tobacco smoke in the perinatal period (P96.81)
    history of tobacco dependence (Z87.891)
    occupational exposure to environmental tobacco smoke (Z57.31)
    tobacco dependence (F17.-)
    tobacco use (Z72.0)
  Excludes1   detergent asthma (J69.8)
    miner's asthma (J60)
    wheezing NOS (R06.2)
    wood asthma (J67.8)
  Excludes2   asthma with chronic obstructive pulmonary disease (J44.89)
    chronic asthmatic (obstructive) bronchitis (J44.89)
    chronic obstructive asthma (J44.89)
    other specified chronic obstructive pulmonary disease (J44.89)
  Coding Clinic: 2024, Q2, P3; 2019, Q1, P37; 2017, Q1, P25

● **J45.2**   **Mild intermittent asthma**
  J45.20   **Mild intermittent asthma, uncomplicated**
    Mild intermittent asthma NOS
  J45.21   **Mild intermittent asthma with (acute) exacerbation**
  J45.22   **Mild intermittent asthma with status asthmaticus**

Item 10-9 **Asthma** is a bronchial condition marked by airway obstruction, hyper-responsiveness, and inflammation. **Extrinsic** asthma, also known as allergic asthma, is characterized by the same symptoms that occur with exposure to allergens and is divided into the following types: **atopic, occupational,** and **allergic bronchopulmonary aspergillosis. Intrinsic** asthma occurs in patients who have no history of allergy or sensitivities to allergens and is divided into the following types: **nonreaginic** and **pharmacologic. Status asthmaticus** is the most severe form of asthma attack and can last for days or weeks.

Figure 10-7 Factors causing expiratory obstruction in asthma. **A.** Cross section of a bronchiole occluded by muscle spasm, swollen mucosa, and mucus. **B.** Longitudinal section of an obstructed bronchiole. **C.** Cross section of a clear bronchiole. (From Shiland: Mastering Healthcare Terminology, ed 1, St. Louis, Mosby, 2003)

● **J45.3 Mild persistent asthma**
   J45.30 Mild persistent asthma, uncomplicated
     Mild persistent asthma NOS
   J45.31 Mild persistent asthma with (acute) exacerbation
     Coding Clinic: 2016, Q1, P35
   J45.32 Mild persistent asthma with status asthmaticus
● **J45.4 Moderate persistent asthma**
   J45.40 Moderate persistent asthma, uncomplicated
     Moderate persistent asthma NOS
   J45.41 Moderate persistent asthma with (acute) exacerbation
     Coding Clinic: 2017, Q1, P26
   J45.42 Moderate persistent asthma with status asthmaticus
● **J45.5 Severe persistent asthma**
   J45.50 Severe persistent asthma, uncomplicated
     Severe persistent asthma NOS
   J45.51 Severe persistent asthma with (acute) exacerbation
   J45.52 Severe persistent asthma with status asthmaticus
● **J45.9 Other and unspecified asthma**
   ● **J45.90 Unspecified asthma**
     Asthmatic bronchitis NOS
     Childhood asthma NOS
     Late onset asthma
     J45.901 Unspecified asthma with (acute) exacerbation
      Coding Clinic: 2017, Q4, P96
     J45.902 Unspecified asthma with status asthmaticus

     J45.909 Unspecified asthma, uncomplicated
      Asthma NOS
      Excludes2 lung diseases due to external agents (J60-J70)
      Coding Clinic: 2024, Q2, P3; 2023, Q1, P17; 2017, Q4, P96; 2017, Q1, P25
   ● **J45.99 Other asthma**
     J45.990 Exercise induced bronchospasm
     J45.991 Cough variant asthma
     J45.998 Other asthma

● **J47 Bronchiectasis**
   Includes bronchiolectasis
   Use additional code to identify:
     exposure to environmental tobacco smoke (Z77.22)
     exposure to tobacco smoke in the perinatal period (P96.81)
     history of tobacco dependence (Z87.891)
     occupational exposure to environmental tobacco smoke (Z57.31)
     tobacco dependence (F17.-)
     tobacco use (Z72.0)
   Excludes1 congenital bronchiectasis (Q33.4)
     tuberculous bronchiectasis (current disease) (A15.0)
   Coding Clinic: 2024, Q2, P5,6
   J47.0 Bronchiectasis with acute lower respiratory infection
     Bronchiectasis with acute bronchitis
     Code also to identify infection, if applicable
   J47.1 Bronchiectasis with (acute) exacerbation
     Coding Clinic: 2021, Q1, P24
   J47.9 Bronchiectasis, uncomplicated
     Bronchiectasis NOS
     Coding Clinic: 2024, Q2, P5,6

LUNG DISEASES DUE TO EXTERNAL AGENTS (J60-J70)

   Excludes2 asthma (J45.-)
     malignant neoplasm of bronchus and lung (C34.-)

● **J4A Chronic lung allograft dysfunction**
   Code first, if applicable:
     heart-lung transplant rejection (T86.31)
     lung transplant rejection (T86.810)
     other complications of heart-lung transplant (T86.39)
     other complications of lung transplant (T86.818)
   Code also, if applicable, bronchiolitis obliterans syndrome (J44.81)
   J4A.0 Restrictive allograft syndrome
     Code also, if applicable, for mixed chronic lung allograft dysfunction, bronchiolitis obliterans syndrome (J44.81)
   J4A.8 Other chronic lung allograft dysfunction
   J4A.9 Chronic lung allograft dysfunction, unspecified

J60 Coalworker's pneumoconiosis   A
   Anthracosilicosis
   Anthracosis
   Black lung disease
   Coalworker's lung
   Excludes1 coalworker pneumoconiosis with tuberculosis, any type in A15 (J65)

J61 Pneumoconiosis due to asbestos and other mineral fibers   A
   Asbestosis
   Excludes1 pleural plaque with asbestosis (J92.0)
     pneumoconiosis with tuberculosis, any type in A15 (J65)

● **J62 Pneumoconiosis due to dust containing silica**
   Includes silicotic fibrosis (massive) of lung
   Excludes1 pneumoconiosis with tuberculosis, any type in A15 (J65)
   J62.0 Pneumoconiosis due to talc dust
   J62.8 Pneumoconiosis due to other dust containing silica
     Silicosis NOS

▶ New   ⇒ Revised   ~~deleted~~ Deleted   Excludes 1   Excludes 2   Includes   Use additional   Code first   Code also   Key words
OGCR Official Guidelines   X Assign placeholder X   ● Use Additional Character(s)   ▶ Manifestation Code   🐾 Hierarchical Condition Category   Coding Clinic

Figure 10-8 Progressive massive fibrosis superimposed on coal workers' pneumoconiosis. The large, blackened scars are located principally in the upper lobe. (From Frazier MS, Drzymkowski JW: Essentials of Human Diseases and Conditions, St. Louis, MO, Saunders, 2004)

Item 10–10   Pneumoconiosis refers to a lung condition resulting from exposure to inorganic or organic airborne particles, such as coal dust or moldy hay, as well as chemical fumes and vapors, such as insecticides. In this condition, the lungs retain the airborne particles.

● **J63   Pneumoconiosis due to other inorganic dusts**

> **Excludes1**   pneumoconiosis with tuberculosis, any type in A15 (J65)
>
> Coding Clinic: 2019, Q3, P8

   J63.0   Aluminosis (of lung) 🔖

   J63.1   Bauxite fibrosis (of lung) 🔖

   J63.2   Berylliosis 🔖

   J63.3   Graphite fibrosis (of lung) 🔖

   J63.4   Siderosis 🔖
> Coding Clinic: 2019, Q3, P8

   J63.5   Stannosis 🔖

   J63.6   Pneumoconiosis due to other specified inorganic dusts 🔖

  J64   Unspecified pneumoconiosis 🔖

> **Excludes1**   pneumonoconiosis with tuberculosis, any type in A15 (J65)

  J65   Pneumoconiosis associated with tuberculosis 🔖
> Any condition in J60-J64 with tuberculosis, any type in A15
> Silicotuberculosis

● **J66   Airway disease due to specific organic dust**

> **Excludes2**   allergic alveolitis (J67.-)
> asbestosis (J61)
> bagassosis (J67.1)
> farmer's lung (J67.0)
> hypersensitivity pneumonitis due to organic dust (J67.-)
> reactive airways dysfunction syndrome (J68.3)

   J66.0   Byssinosis 🔖
> Airway disease due to cotton dust

   J66.1   Flax-dressers' disease 🔖

   J66.2   Cannabinosis 🔖

   J66.8   Airway disease due to other specific organic dusts 🔖

● **J67   Hypersensitivity pneumonitis due to organic dust**

> **Includes**   allergic alveolitis and pneumonitis due to inhaled organic dust and particles of fungal, actinomycetic or other origin
>
> **Excludes1**   pneumonitis due to inhalation of chemicals, gases, fumes or vapors (J68.0)

   J67.0   Farmer's lung 🔖
> Harvester's lung
> Haymaker's lung
> Moldy hay disease

   J67.1   Bagassosis 🔖
> Bagasse disease
> Bagasse pneumonitis

   J67.2   Bird fancier's lung 🔖
> Budgerigar fancier's disease or lung
> Pigeon fancier's disease or lung

   J67.3   Suberosis 🔖
> Corkhandler's disease or lung
> Corkworker's disease or lung

   J67.4   Maltworker's lung 🔖
> Alveolitis due to Aspergillus clavatus

   J67.5   Mushroom-worker's lung 🔖

   J67.6   Maple-bark-stripper's lung 🔖
> Alveolitis due to Cryptostroma corticale
> Cryptostromosis

   J67.7   Air conditioner and humidifier lung 🔖
> Allergic alveolitis due to fungal, thermophilic actinomycetes and other organisms growing in ventilation [air conditioning] systems

   J67.8   Hypersensitivity pneumonitis due to other organic dusts 🔖
> Cheese-washer's lung
> Coffee-worker's lung
> Fish-meal worker's lung
> Furrier's lung
> Sequoiosis

   J67.9   Hypersensitivity pneumonitis due to unspecified organic dust 🔖
> Allergic alveolitis (extrinsic) NOS
> Hypersensitivity pneumonitis NOS

● **J68   Respiratory conditions due to inhalation of chemicals, gases, fumes and vapors**

> *Code first (T51-T65) to identify cause*
> Use additional code to identify associated respiratory conditions, such as:
> acute respiratory failure (J96.0-)

   J68.0   Bronchitis and pneumonitis due to chemicals, gases, fumes and vapors 🔖
> Chemical bronchitis (acute)
> Coding Clinic: 2019, Q2, P31-32

   J68.1   Pulmonary edema due to chemicals, gases, fumes and vapors 🔖
> Chemical pulmonary edema (acute) (chronic)
> > **Excludes1**   pulmonary edema (acute) (chronic) NOS (J81.-)

   J68.2   Upper respiratory inflammation due to chemicals, gases, fumes and vapors, not elsewhere classified 🔖

   J68.3   Other acute and subacute respiratory conditions due to chemicals, gases, fumes and vapors 🔖
> Reactive airways dysfunction syndrome

   J68.4   Chronic respiratory conditions due to chemicals, gases, fumes and vapors 🔖

> Code also, if applicable, chronic conditions, such as:
> emphysema (J43.-)
> obliterative bronchiolitis (J44.81)
> pulmonary fibrosis (J84.10)
> > **Excludes1**   chronic pulmonary edema due to chemicals, gases, fumes and vapors (J68.1)

   J68.8   Other respiratory conditions due to chemicals, gases, fumes and vapors 🔖

   J68.9   Unspecified respiratory condition due to chemicals, gases, fumes and vapors 🔖

● **J69   Pneumonitis due to solids and liquids**

▶ Code also, if applicable, other types of pneumonias

> **Excludes1**   neonatal aspiration syndromes (P24.-)
> postprocedural pneumonitis (J95.4)

   J69.0   Pneumonitis due to inhalation of food and vomit 🔖
> Aspiration pneumonia NOS
> Aspiration pneumonia (due to) food (regurgitated)
> Aspiration pneumonia (due to) gastric secretions
> Aspiration pneumonia (due to) milk
> Aspiration pneumonia (due to) vomit
>
> Code also any associated foreign body in respiratory tract (T17.-)
> > **Excludes1**   chemical pneumonitis due to anesthesia (J95.4)
> > obstetric aspiration pneumonitis (O74.0)
> Coding Clinic: 2021, Q1, P34; 2019, Q2, P7, 31-32; 2017, Q1, P24

   J69.1   Pneumonitis due to inhalation of oils and essences 🔖
> Exogenous lipoid pneumonia
> Lipid pneumonia NOS
>
> *Code first (T51-T65) to identify substance*
> > **Excludes1**   endogenous lipoid pneumonia (J84.89)

CHAPTER 10 (J00-J99)

CHAPTER 10 (J00-J99)

J69.8 **Pneumonitis due to inhalation of other solids and liquids** 🐾
     Pneumonitis due to aspiration of blood
     Pneumonitis due to aspiration of detergent
     Code first (T51-T65) to identify substance

● **J70** **Respiratory conditions due to other external agents**

   J70.0 **Acute pulmonary manifestations due to radiation** 🐾
     Radiation pneumonitis
     Use additional code (W88-W90, X39.0-) to identify the external cause

   J70.1 **Chronic and other pulmonary manifestations due to radiation** 🐾
     Fibrosis of lung following radiation
     Use additional code (W88-W90, X39.0-) to identify the external cause

   J70.2 **Acute drug-induced interstitial lung disorders** 🐾
     Use additional code for adverse effect, if applicable, to identify drug (T36-T50 with fifth or sixth character 5)
     Excludes1   interstitial pneumonia NOS (J84.9)
                  lymphoid interstitial pneumonia (J84.2)
     Coding Clinic: 2019, Q2, P28

   J70.3 **Chronic drug-induced interstitial lung disorders** 🐾
     Use additional code for adverse effect, if applicable, to identify drug (T36-T50 with fifth or sixth character 5)
     Excludes1   interstitial pneumonia NOS (J84.9)
                  lymphoid interstitial pneumonia (J84.2)

   J70.4 **Drug-induced interstitial lung disorders, unspecified** 🐾
     Use additional code for adverse effect, if applicable, to identify drug (T36-T50 with fifth or sixth character 5)
     Excludes1   interstitial pneumonia NOS (J84.9)
                  lymphoid interstitial pneumonia (J84.2)
     Coding Clinic: 2019, Q2, P28

   J70.5 **Respiratory conditions due to smoke inhalation** 🐾
     Code first smoke inhalation (T59.81-)
     Excludes2   smoke inhalation due to chemicals, gases, fumes and vapors (J68.9)

   J70.8 **Respiratory conditions due to other specified external agents** 🐾
     Code first (T51-T65) to identify the external agent

   J70.9 **Respiratory conditions due to unspecified external agent** 🐾
     Code first (T51-T65) to identify the external agent

OTHER RESPIRATORY DISEASES PRINCIPALLY AFFECTING THE INTERSTITIUM (J80-J84)

J80 **Acute respiratory distress syndrome** 🐾
     Acute respiratory distress syndrome in adult or child
     Adult hyaline membrane disease
     Excludes1   respiratory distress syndrome in newborn (perinatal) (P22.0)
     Coding Clinic: 2017, Q1, P26-27

● **J81** **Pulmonary edema**
     Use additional code to identify:
       exposure to environmental tobacco smoke (Z77.22)
       history of tobacco dependence (Z87.891)
       occupational exposure to environmental tobacco smoke (Z57.31)
       tobacco dependence (F17.-)
       tobacco use (Z72.0)
     Excludes1   chemical (acute) pulmonary edema (J68.1)
                  hypostatic pneumonia (J18.2)
                  passive pneumonia (J18.2)
                  pulmonary edema due to external agents (J60-J70)
                  pulmonary edema with heart disease NOS (I50.1)
                  pulmonary edema with heart failure (I50.1)

   J81.0 **Acute pulmonary edema** 🐾
     Acute edema of lung
     Coding Clinic: 2023, Q1, P25; 2017, Q1, P26

Figure 10-9   Bullous emphysema with large subpleural bullae *(upper left)*. (From Kumar: Robbins and Cotran: Pathologic Basis of Disease, ed 8, Saunders, An Imprint of Elsevier, 2009)

   J81.1 **Chronic pulmonary edema**
     Pulmonary congestion (chronic) (passive)
     Pulmonary edema NOS

J82 **Pulmonary eosinophilia, not elsewhere classified** 🐾
     Excludes2   pulmonary eosinophilia due to aspergillosis (B44.-)
                  pulmonary eosinophilia due to drugs (J70.2-J70.4)
                  pulmonary eosinophilia due to specified parasitic infection (B50-B83)
                  pulmonary eosinophilia due to systemic connective tissue disorders (M30-M36)
                  pulmonary infiltrate NOS (R91.8)

   ● **J82.8** **Pulmonary eosinophilia, not elsewhere classified**

     J82.81 **Chronic eosinophilic pneumonia**
       Eosinophilic pneumonia, NOS

     J82.82 **Acute eosinophilic pneumonia**

     J82.83 **Eosinophilic asthma**
       Code first asthma, by type, such as:
         mild intermittent asthma (J45.2-)
         mild persistent asthma (J45.3-)
         moderate persistent asthma (J45.4-)
         severe persistent asthma (J45.5-)

     J82.89 **Other pulmonary eosinophilia, not elsewhere classified**
       Allergic pneumonia
       Löffler's pneumonia
       Tropical (pulmonary) eosinophilia NOS

● **J84** **Other interstitial pulmonary diseases**
     Excludes1   drug-induced interstitial lung disorders (J70.2-J70.4)
                  interstitial emphysema (J98.2)
     Excludes2   lung diseases due to external agents (J60-J70)
     Coding Clinic: 2019, Q2, P28

   ● **J84.0** **Alveolar and parieto-alveolar conditions**

     J84.01 **Alveolar proteinosis** 🐾

     J84.02 **Pulmonary alveolar microlithiasis** 🐾

     ▷ **J84.03** *Idiopathic pulmonary hemosiderosis* 🐾
       Essential brown induration of lung
       Code first underlying disease, such as:
         disorders of iron metabolism (E83.1-)
       ▶ Code also, if applicable, associated condition
       Excludes1   acute idiopathic pulmonary hemorrhage in infants [AIPHI] (R04.81)

     J84.09 **Other alveolar and parieto-alveolar conditions** 🐾

   ● **J84.1** **Other interstitial pulmonary diseases with fibrosis**
     Excludes1   pulmonary fibrosis (chronic) due to inhalation of chemicals, gases, fumes or vapors (J68.4)
                  pulmonary fibrosis (chronic) following radiation (J70.1)

     J84.10 **Pulmonary fibrosis, unspecified** 🐾
       Capillary fibrosis of lung
       Cirrhosis of lung (chronic) NOS
       Fibrosis of lung (atrophic) (chronic) (confluent) (massive) (perialveolar) (peribronchial) NOS
       Induration of lung (chronic) NOS
       Postinflammatory pulmonary fibrosis
       Coding Clinic: 2024, Q2, P20

▶ New   ⇒ Revised   ~~deleted~~ Deleted   Excludes 1   Excludes 2   Includes   Use additional   Code first   Code also   Key words
OGCR Official Guidelines   X Assign placeholder X   ● Use Additional Character(s)   ▷ Manifestation Code   🐾 Hierarchical Condition Category   Coding Clinic

● J84.11　**Idiopathic interstitial pneumonia**
　　　　Excludes1　lymphoid interstitial pneumonia (J84.2)
　　　　　　　　　　pneumocystis pneumonia (B59)

　　J84.111　**Idiopathic interstitial pneumonia, not otherwise specified** 🔊

　　J84.112　**Idiopathic pulmonary fibrosis** 🔊
　　　　　　Cryptogenic fibrosing alveolitis
　　　　　　Idiopathic fibrosing alveolitis

　　J84.113　**Idiopathic non-specific interstitial pneumonitis** 🔊
　　　　　　Excludes1　non-specific interstitial pneumonia NOS, or due to known underlying cause (J84.89)

　　J84.114　**Acute interstitial pneumonitis** 🔊
　　　　　　Hamman-Rich syndrome
　　　　　　Excludes1　pneumocystis pneumonia (B59)

　　J84.115　**Respiratory bronchiolitis interstitial lung disease** 🔊

　　J84.116　**Cryptogenic organizing pneumonia** 🔊
　　　　　　Excludes1　organizing pneumonia NOS, or due to known underlying cause (J84.89)

　　J84.117　**Desquamative interstitial pneumonia** 🔊

◐ J84.17　*Other interstitial pulmonary diseases with fibrosis in diseases classified elsewhere* 🔊

　▷ J84.170　*Interstitial lung disease with progressive fibrotic phenotype in diseases classified elsewhere*
　　　　　　Progressive fibrotic interstitial lung disease
　　　　　　Code first underlying disease, such as:
　　　　　　　lung diseases due to external agents (J60-J70)
　　　　　　　rheumatoid arthritis (M05.00-M06.9)
　　　　　　　sarcoidosis (D86.-)
　　　　　　　systemic connective tissue disorders (M30-M36)

　▷ J84.178　*Other interstitial pulmonary diseases with fibrosis in diseases classified elsewhere*
　　　　　　Interstitial pneumonia (nonspecific) (usual) due to collagen vascular disease
　　　　　　Interstitial pneumonia (nonspecific) (usual) in diseases classified elsewhere
　　　　　　Organizing pneumonia due to collagen vascular disease
　　　　　　Organizing pneumonia in diseases classified elsewhere
　　　　　　Code first underlying disease, such as:
　　　　　　　progressive systemic sclerosis (M34.0)
　　　　　　　rheumatoid arthritis (M05.00-M06.9)
　　　　　　　systemic lupus erythematosis (M32.0-M32.9)

J84.2　**Lymphoid interstitial pneumonia** 🔊
　　　　Lymphoid interstitial pneumonitis

● J84.8　**Other specified interstitial pulmonary diseases**
　　　　Excludes1　exogenous lipoid pneumonia (J69.1)
　　　　　　　　　　unspecified lipoid pneumonia (J69.1)

　　J84.81　**Lymphangioleiomyomatosis** 🔊
　　　　　　Lymphangiomyomatosis

　　J84.82　**Adult pulmonary Langerhans cell histiocytosis** 🔊　　　　　　　　A
　　　　　　Adult PLCH

　　J84.83　**Surfactant mutations of the lung** 🔊

● J84.84　**Other interstitial lung diseases of childhood**

　　J84.841　**Neuroendocrine cell hyperplasia of infancy** 🔊

　　J84.842　**Pulmonary interstitial glycogenosis** 🔊

　　J84.843　**Alveolar capillary dysplasia with vein misalignment** 🔊

　　J84.848　**Other interstitial lung diseases of childhood** 🔊

　　J84.89　**Other specified interstitial pulmonary diseases** 🔊
　　　　　　Endogenous lipoid pneumonia
　　　　　　Interstitial pneumonitis
　　　　　　Non-specific interstitial pneumonitis NOS
　　　　　　Organizing pneumonia NOS
　　　　　　Code first, if applicable:
　　　　　　　poisoning due to drug or toxin (T51-T65 with fifth or sixth character to indicate intent), for toxic pneumonopathy underlying cause of pneumonopathy, if known
　　　　　　Use additional code, for adverse effect, to identify drug (T36-T50 with fifth or sixth character 5), if drug-induced
　　　　　　Excludes1　cryptogenic organizing pneumonia (J84.116)
　　　　　　　　　　idiopathic non-specific interstitial pneumonitis (J84.113)
　　　　　　　　　　lipoid pneumonia, exogenous or unspecified (J69.1)
　　　　　　　　　　lymphoid interstitial pneumonia (J84.2)

　　　　　　Coding Clinic: 2021, Q4, P106-107; 2021, Q1, P48; 2019, Q2, P28

J84.9　**Interstitial pulmonary disease, unspecified** 🔊
　　　　Interstitial pneumonia NOS

SUPPURATIVE AND NECROTIC CONDITIONS OF THE LOWER RESPIRATORY TRACT (J85-J86)

● J85　**Abscess of lung and mediastinum**
　　　　Use additional code (B95-B97) to identify infectious agent.

J85.0　**Gangrene and necrosis of lung** 🔊

J85.1　**Abscess of lung with pneumonia** 🔊
　　　　Code also the type of pneumonia

J85.2　**Abscess of lung without pneumonia** 🔊
　　　　Abscess of lung NOS

J85.3　**Abscess of mediastinum** 🔊

● J86　**Pyothorax**
　　▷Code also, if applicable, disruption of internal operation (surgical) wound (T81.32-)
　　　Use additional code (B95-B97) to identify infectious agent.
　　　Excludes1　abscess of lung (J85.-)
　　　　　　　　pyothorax due to tuberculosis (A15.6)

J86.0　**Pyothorax with fistula** 🔊
　　　　Bronchocutaneous fistula
　　　　Bronchopleural fistula
　　　　Hepatopleural fistula
　　　　Mediastinal fistula
　　　　Pleural fistula
　　　　Thoracic fistula
　　　　Any condition classifiable to J86.9 with fistula

J86.9　**Pyothorax without fistula** 🔊
　　　　Abscess of pleura
　　　　Abscess of thorax
　　　　Empyema (chest) (lung) (pleura)
　　　　Fibrinopurulent pleurisy
　　　　Purulent pleurisy
　　　　Pyopneumothorax
　　　　Septic pleurisy
　　　　Seropurulent pleurisy
　　　　Suppurative pleurisy

CHAPTER 10 (J00-J99)

OTHER DISEASES OF THE PLEURA (J90-J94)

J90   **Pleural effusion, not elsewhere classified**
Encysted pleurisy
Pleural effusion NOS
Pleurisy with effusion (exudative) (serous)
Excludes1   chylous (pleural) effusion (J94.0)
malignant pleural effusion (J91.0))
pleurisy NOS (R09.1)
tuberculous pleural effusion (A15.6)
Coding Clinic: 2015, Q2, P16

● **J91**   **Pleural effusion in conditions classified elsewhere**
Excludes2   pleural effusion in heart failure (I50.-)
pleural effusion in systemic lupus erythematosus (M32.13)

▷ *J91.0*   *Malignant pleural effusion*
Code first underlying neoplasm (C00-D49)
Coding Clinic: 2024, Q2, P11,12; 2022, Q3, P14-15

▷ *J91.8*   *Pleural effusion in other conditions classified elsewhere*
Code first underlying disease, such as:
filariasis (B74.0-B74.9)
influenza (J09.X2, J10.1, J11.1)
Coding Clinic: 2015, Q2, P16

● **J92**   **Pleural plaque**
Includes   pleural thickening
J92.0   **Pleural plaque with presence of asbestos**
J92.9   **Pleural plaque without asbestos**
Pleural plaque NOS

● **J93**   **Pneumothorax and air leak**
Collapsed lung
Excludes1   congenital or perinatal pneumothorax (P25.1)
postprocedural air leak (J95.812)
postprocedural pneumothorax (J95.811)
traumatic pneumothorax (S27.0)
tuberculous (current disease) pneumothorax (A15.-)
pyopneumothorax (J86.-)

J93.0   **Spontaneous tension pneumothorax**
Tension pneumothorax (most serious type) occurs when air (positive pressure) collects in the pleural space

● **J93.1**   **Other spontaneous pneumothorax**
J93.11   **Primary spontaneous pneumothorax**
J93.12   **Secondary spontaneous pneumothorax**
Code first underlying condition, such as:
catamenial pneumothorax due to endometriosis (N80.B-)
cystic fibrosis (E84.-)
eosinophilic pneumonia (J82)
lymphangioleiomyomatosis (J84.81)
malignant neoplasm of bronchus and lung (C34.-)
Marfan syndrome (Q87.4-)
pneumonia due to Pneumocystis carinii (B59)
secondary malignant neoplasm of lung (C78.0-)
spontaneous rupture of the esophagus (K22.3)

● **J93.8**   **Other pneumothorax and air leak**
J93.81   **Chronic pneumothorax**
J93.82   **Other air leak**
Persistent air leak
J93.83   **Other pneumothorax**
Acute pneumothorax
Spontaneous pneumothorax NOS

J93.9   **Pneumothorax, unspecified**
Pneumothorax NOS

● **J94**   **Other pleural conditions**
Excludes1   pleurisy NOS (R09.1)
traumatic hemopneumothorax (S27.2)
traumatic hemothorax (S27.1)
tuberculous pleural conditions (current disease) (A15.-)

J94.0   **Chylous effusion**
Chyliform effusion

J94.1   **Fibrothorax**

J94.2   **Hemothorax**
Hemopneumothorax

J94.8   **Other specified pleural conditions**
Hydropneumothorax
Hydrothorax
Coding Clinic: 2021, Q1, P49

J94.9   **Pleural condition, unspecified**

INTRAOPERATIVE AND POSTPROCEDURAL COMPLICATIONS AND DISORDERS OF RESPIRATORY SYSTEM, NOT ELSEWHERE CLASSIFIED (J95)

● **J95**   **Intraoperative and postprocedural complications and disorders of respiratory system, not elsewhere classified**
Excludes2   aspiration pneumonia (J69.-)
emphysema (subcutaneous) resulting from a procedure (T81.82)
hypostatic pneumonia (J18.2)
pulmonary manifestations due to radiation (J70.0- J70.1)

● **J95.0**   **Tracheostomy complications**
J95.00   **Unspecified tracheostomy complication** 🦝
J95.01   **Hemorrhage from tracheostomy stoma** 🦝
J95.02   **Infection of tracheostomy stoma** 🦝
Use additional code to identify type of infection, such as:
cellulitis of neck (L03.221)
sepsis (A40, A41.-)
J95.03   **Malfunction of tracheostomy stoma** 🦝
Mechanical complication of tracheostomy stoma
Obstruction of tracheostomy airway
Tracheal stenosis due to tracheostomy
J95.04   **Tracheo-esophageal fistula following tracheostomy** 🦝
J95.09   **Other tracheostomy complication** 🦝

J95.1   **Acute pulmonary insufficiency following thoracic surgery** 🦝
Excludes2   functional disturbances following cardiac surgery (I97.0, I97.1-)

J95.2   **Acute pulmonary insufficiency following nonthoracic surgery** 🦝
Excludes2   functional disturbances following cardiac surgery (I97.0, I97.1-)

J95.3   **Chronic pulmonary insufficiency following surgery** 🦝
Excludes2   functional disturbances following cardiac surgery (I97.0, I97.1-)

J95.4   **Chemical pneumonitis due to anesthesia**
Mendelson's syndrome
Postprocedural aspiration pneumonia
Use additional code for adverse effect, if applicable, to identify drug (T41.- with fifth or sixth character 5)
Excludes1   aspiration pneumonitis due to anesthesia complicating labor and delivery (O74.0)
aspiration pneumonitis due to anesthesia complicating pregnancy (O29)
aspiration pneumonitis due to anesthesia complicating the puerperium (O89.01)

J95.5   **Postprocedural subglottic stenosis**

Item 10-11 Empyema is a condition in which pus accumulates in a body cavity. Empyema **with fistula** occurs when the pus passes from one cavity to another organ or structure.

▶ New   ⇒ Revised   ~~deleted~~ Deleted   Excludes 1   Excludes 2   Includes   Use additional   Code first   Code also   Key words
OGCR Official Guidelines   X Assign placeholder X   ● Use Additional Character(s)   ▷ Manifestation Code   🦝 Hierarchical Condition Category   Coding Clinic

● **J95.6**   **Intraoperative hemorrhage and hematoma** of a respiratory system organ or structure complicating a procedure

> **Excludes1**   intraoperative hemorrhage and hematoma of a respiratory system organ or structure due to accidental puncture and laceration during procedure (J95.7-)

     J95.61   Intraoperative hemorrhage and hematoma of a respiratory system organ or structure complicating a respiratory system procedure

     J95.62   Intraoperative hemorrhage and hematoma of a respiratory system organ or structure complicating other procedure

● **J95.7**   **Accidental puncture and laceration** of a respiratory system organ or structure during a procedure

> **Excludes2**   postprocedural pneumothorax (J95.811)

     J95.71   Accidental puncture and laceration of a respiratory system organ or structure during a respiratory system procedure

     J95.72   Accidental puncture and laceration of a respiratory system organ or structure during other procedure

● **J95.8**   **Other intraoperative and postprocedural complications** and disorders of respiratory system, not elsewhere classified

> Coding Clinic: 2016, Q4, P10

● **J95.81**   **Postprocedural** pneumothorax and air leak

     J95.811   Postprocedural pneumothorax

> Coding Clinic: 2021, Q1, P49

     J95.812   Postprocedural air leak

● **J95.82**   **Postprocedural respiratory failure**

> **Excludes1**   Respiratory failure in other conditions (J96.-)

     J95.821   **Acute postprocedural respiratory failure** 🔖

> Postprocedural respiratory failure NOS

     J95.822   **Acute and chronic** postprocedural respiratory failure 🔖

● **J95.83**   **Postprocedural hemorrhage** of a respiratory system organ or structure following a procedure

     J95.830   Postprocedural hemorrhage of a respiratory system organ or structure following a respiratory system procedure

     J95.831   Postprocedural hemorrhage of a respiratory system organ or structure following other procedure

> Coding Clinic: 2023, Q2, P28

     J95.84   Transfusion-related acute lung injury (TRALI)

● **J95.85**   **Complication of respirator [ventilator]**

     J95.850   **Mechanical complication of respirator** 🔖

> **Excludes1**   encounter for respirator [ventilator] dependence during power failure (Z99.12)

     J95.851   **Ventilator associated pneumonia** 🔖

> Ventilator associated pneumonitis
>
> Use additional code to identify the organism, if known (B95.-, B96.-, B97.-)
>
> **Excludes1**   ventilator lung in newborn (P27.8)
>
> Coding Clinic: 2017, Q1, P25

     J95.859   **Other complication of respirator [ventilator]** 🔖

> Coding Clinic: 2021, Q1, P49

● **J95.86**   **Postprocedural hematoma and seroma** of a respiratory system organ or structure following a procedure

     J95.860   Postprocedural hematoma of a respiratory system organ or structure following a respiratory system procedure

     J95.861   Postprocedural hematoma of a respiratory system organ or structure following other procedure

     J95.862   Postprocedural seroma of a respiratory system organ or structure following a respiratory system procedure

     J95.863   Postprocedural seroma of a respiratory system organ or structure following other procedure

     J95.87   Transfusion-associated dyspnea (TAD)

> **Excludes1**   transfusion associated circulatory overload (TACO) (E87.71)
> transfusion-related acute lung injury (TRALI) (J95.84)

     J95.88   Other intraoperative complications of respiratory system, not elsewhere classified

     J95.89   Other postprocedural complications and disorders of respiratory system, not elsewhere classified

> Use additional code to identify disorder, such as:
> aspiration pneumonia (J69.-)
> bacterial or viral pneumonia (J12-J18)
>
> **Excludes2**   acute pulmonary insufficiency following thoracic surgery (J95.1)
> postprocedural subglottic stenosis (J95.5)

OTHER DISEASES OF THE RESPIRATORY SYSTEM (J96-J99)

● **J96**   **Respiratory failure, not elsewhere classified**

> **Excludes1**   acute respiratory distress syndrome (J80)
> cardiorespiratory failure (R09.2)
> newborn respiratory distress syndrome (P22.0)
> postprocedural respiratory failure (J95.82-)
> respiratory arrest (R09.2)
> respiratory arrest of newborn (P28.81)
> respiratory failure of newborn (P28.5)

● **J96.0**   **Acute respiratory failure**

     J96.00   Acute respiratory failure, unspecified whether with hypoxia or hypercapnia 🔖

> Coding Clinic: 2016, Q3, P14

     J96.01   Acute respiratory failure with hypoxia 🔖

> Coding Clinic: 2024, Q2, P11

     J96.02   Acute respiratory failure with hypercapnia 🔖

> Acute respiratory acidosis

● **J96.1**   **Chronic respiratory failure**

     J96.10   Chronic respiratory failure, unspecified whether with hypoxia or hypercapnia 🔖

> Coding Clinic: 2021, Q4, P105-106; 2021, Q1, P46; 2016, Q1, P38; 2015, Q1, P21

     J96.11   Chronic respiratory failure with hypoxia 🔖

     J96.12   Chronic respiratory failure with hypercapnia 🔖

> Chronic respiratory acidosis

● **J96.2**   **Acute and chronic respiratory failure**

> Acute on chronic respiratory failure

     J96.20   Acute and chronic respiratory failure, unspecified whether with hypoxia or hypercapnia 🔖

     J96.21   Acute and chronic respiratory failure with hypoxia 🔖

     J96.22   Acute and chronic respiratory failure with hypercapnia 🔖

● **J96.9**   **Respiratory failure, unspecified**
     J96.90   **Respiratory failure, unspecified, unspecified whether with hypoxia or hypercapnia** 🐾
         Coding Clinic: 2021, Q1, P44
     J96.91   **Respiratory failure, unspecified with hypoxia** 🐾
     J96.92   **Respiratory failure, unspecified with hypercapnia** 🐾

● **J98**   **Other respiratory disorders**
   Use additional code to identify:
     exposure to environmental tobacco smoke (Z77.22)
     exposure to tobacco smoke in the perinatal period (P96.81)
     history of tobacco dependence (Z87.891)
     occupational exposure to environmental tobacco smoke (Z57.31)
     tobacco dependence (F17.-)
     tobacco use (Z72.0)
   Excludes1   newborn apnea (P28.4-)
             newborn sleep apnea (P28.3-)
   Excludes2   apnea NOS (R06.81)
             sleep apnea (G47.3-)

● **J98.0**   **Diseases of bronchus, not elsewhere classified**
     J98.01   **Acute bronchospasm**
       Excludes1   acute bronchiolitis with bronchospasm (J21.-)
                acute bronchitis with bronchospasm (J20.-)
                asthma (J45.-)
                exercise induced bronchospasm (J45.990)
     J98.09   **Other diseases of bronchus, not elsewhere classified**
       Broncholithiasis
       Calcification of bronchus
       Stenosis of bronchus
       Tracheobronchial collapse
       Tracheobronchial dyskinesia
       Ulcer of bronchus
       Coding Clinic: 2022, Q3, P8

● **J98.1**   **Pulmonary collapse**
   Excludes1   therapeutic collapse of lung status (Z98.3)
     J98.11   **Atelectasis**
       Excludes1   newborn atelectasis
                tuberculous atelectasis (current disease) (A15)
     J98.19   **Other pulmonary collapse**
   J98.2   **Interstitial emphysema** 🐾
     Mediastinal emphysema
     Excludes1   emphysema NOS (J43.9)
             emphysema in newborn (P25.0)
             surgical emphysema (subcutaneous) (T81.82)
             traumatic subcutaneous emphysema (T79.7)

J98.3   **Compensatory emphysema** 🐾
J98.4   **Other disorders of lung**
   Calcification of lung
   Cystic lung disease (acquired)
   Lung disease NOS
   Pulmolithiasis
   Excludes1   acute interstitial pneumonitis (J84.114)
            pulmonary insufficiency following surgery (J95.1-J95.2)
   Coding Clinic: 2024, Q2, P20, 21

● **J98.5**   **Diseases of mediastinum, not elsewhere classified**
   Excludes2   abscess of mediastinum (J85.3)
   Coding Clinic: 2016, Q4, P29
     J98.51   **Mediastinitis**
       Code first underlying condition, if applicable, such as postoperative mediastinitis (T81.-)
     J98.59   **Other diseases of mediastinum, not elsewhere classified**
       Fibrosis of mediastinum
       Hernia of mediastinum
       Retraction of mediastinum
J98.6   **Disorders of diaphragm**
   Diaphragmatitis
   Paralysis of diaphragm
   Relaxation of diaphragm
   Excludes1   congenital malformation of diaphragm NEC (Q79.1)
            congenital diaphragmatic hernia (Q79.0)
   Excludes2   diaphragmatic hernia (K44.-)
J98.8   **Other specified respiratory disorders**
J98.9   **Respiratory disorder, unspecified**
   Respiratory disease (chronic) NOS

▷ **J99**   *Respiratory disorders in diseases classified elsewhere* 🐾
   Code first underlying disease, such as:
     amyloidosis (E85.-)
     ankylosing spondylitis (M45.-)
     congenital syphilis (A50.-)
     cryoglobulinemia (D89.1)
     early congenital syphilis (A50.-)
     plasminogen deficiency (E88.02)
     schistosomiasis (B65.0-B65.9)
   Excludes1   respiratory disorders in:
       amebiasis (A06.5)
       blastomycosis (B40.0-B40.2)
       candidiasis (B37.1)
       coccidioidomycosis (B38.0-B38.2)
       cystic fibrosis with pulmonary manifestations (E84.0)
       dermatomyositis (M33.01, M33.11)
       histoplasmosis (B39.0-B39.2)
       late syphilis (A52.72, A52.73)
       polymyositis (M33.21)
       Sjögren syndrome (M35.02)
       systemic lupus erythematosus (M32.13)
       systemic sclerosis (M34.81)
       Wegener's granulomatosis (M31.30-M31.31)

CHAPTER 11

DISEASES OF THE DIGESTIVE SYSTEM (K00-K95)

OGCR Chapter-Specific Coding Guidelines

11. Chapter 11: Diseases of the Digestive System (K00-K95)
Reserved for future guideline expansion

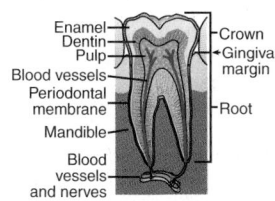

Figure 11-1 Anatomy of a tooth.

Item 11-1 **Anodontia** is the congenital absence of teeth. **Hypodontia** is partial anodontia. **Oligodontia** is the congenital absence of some teeth, whereas **supernumerary** is having more teeth than the normal number. **Mesiodens** are small extra teeth that often appear in pairs, although single small teeth are not uncommon.

CHAPTER 11

DISEASES OF THE DIGESTIVE SYSTEM (K00-K95)

Excludes2   certain conditions originating in the perinatal period (P04-P96)
certain infectious and parasitic diseases (A00-B99)
complications of pregnancy, childbirth and the puerperium (O00-O9A)
congenital malformations, deformations and chromosomal abnormalities (Q00-Q99)
endocrine, nutritional and metabolic diseases (E00-E88)
injury, poisoning and certain other consequences of external causes (S00-T88)
neoplasms (C00-D49)
symptoms, signs and abnormal clinical and laboratory findings, not elsewhere classified (R00-R94)

This chapter contains the following blocks:

K00-K14	Diseases of oral cavity and salivary glands
K20-K31	Diseases of esophagus, stomach and duodenum
K35-K38	Diseases of appendix
K40-K46	Hernia
K50-K52	Noninfective enteritis and colitis
K55-K64	Other diseases of intestines
K65-K68	Diseases of peritoneum and retroperitoneum
K70-K77	Diseases of liver
K80-K87	Disorders of gallbladder, biliary tract and pancreas
K90-K95	Other diseases of the digestive system

DISEASES OF ORAL CAVITY AND SALIVARY GLANDS (K00-K14)

● **K00** **Disorders of tooth development and eruption**
    Excludes2 embedded and impacted teeth (K01.-)

  K00.0 **Anodontia**
      Hypodontia
      Oligodontia
      Excludes1 acquired absence of teeth (K08.1-)

  K00.1 **Supernumerary teeth**
      Distomolar
      Fourth molar
      Mesiodens
      Paramolar
      Supplementary teeth
      Excludes2 supernumerary roots (K00.2)

  K00.2 **Abnormalities of size and form of teeth**
      Concrescence of teeth
      Fusion of teeth
      Gemination of teeth
      Dens evaginatus
      Dens in dente
      Dens invaginatus
      Enamel pearls
      Macrodontia
      Microdontia
      Peg-shaped [conical] teeth
      Supernumerary roots
      Taurodontism
      Tuberculum paramolare
      Excludes1 abnormalities of teeth due to congenital syphilis (A50.5)
              tuberculum Carabelli, which is regarded as a normal variation and should not be coded

  K00.3 **Mottled teeth**
      Dental fluorosis
      Mottling of enamel
      Nonfluoride enamel opacities
      Excludes2 deposits [accretions] on teeth (K03.6)

  K00.4 **Disturbances in tooth formation**
      Aplasia and hypoplasia of cementum
      Dilaceration of tooth
      Enamel hypoplasia (neonatal) (postnatal) (prenatal)
      Regional odontodysplasia
      Turner's tooth
      Excludes1 Hutchinson's teeth and mulberry molars in congenital syphilis (A50.5)
      Excludes2 mottled teeth (K00.3)

  K00.5 **Hereditary disturbances in tooth structure, not elsewhere classified**
      Amelogenesis imperfecta
      Dentinogenesis imperfecta
      Odontogenesis imperfecta
      Dentinal dysplasia
      Shell teeth

  K00.6 **Disturbances in tooth eruption**
      Dentia praecox
      Natal tooth
      Neonatal tooth
      Premature eruption of tooth
      Premature shedding of primary [deciduous] tooth
      Prenatal teeth
      Retained [persistent] primary tooth
      Excludes2 embedded and impacted teeth (K01.-)

  K00.7 **Teething syndrome**

  K00.8 **Other disorders of tooth development**
      Color changes during tooth formation
      Intrinsic staining of teeth NOS
      Excludes2 posteruptive color changes (K03.7)

  K00.9 **Disorder of tooth development, unspecified**
      Disorder of odontogenesis NOS

● **K01** **Embedded and impacted teeth**
    Excludes1 abnormal position of fully erupted teeth (M26.3-)

  K01.0 **Embedded teeth**

  K01.1 **Impacted teeth**

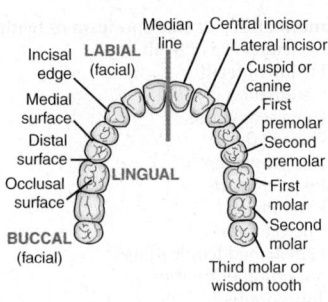

Figure 11-2 The permanent teeth within the dental arch.

Item 11–2 Each dental arch (jaw) normally contains 16 teeth. Tooth decay or **dental caries** is a disease of the enamel, dentin, and cementum of the tooth and can result in a cavity.

● **K02** **Dental caries**

    Includes caries of dentine
         dental cavities
         early childhood caries
         pre-eruptive caries
         recurrent caries (dentino enamel junction)
           (enamel) (to the pulp)
         tooth decay

    K02.3 **Arrested dental caries**
        Arrested coronal and root caries

  ● **K02.5** **Dental caries on pit and fissure surface**
        Dental caries on chewing surface of tooth

        K02.51 **Dental caries on pit and fissure surface limited to enamel**
            White spot lesions [initial caries] on pit and fissure surface of tooth

        K02.52 **Dental caries on pit and fissure surface penetrating into dentin**
            Primary dental caries, cervical origin

        K02.53 **Dental caries on pit and fissure surface penetrating into pulp**

  ● **K02.6** **Dental caries on smooth surface**

        K02.61 **Dental caries on smooth surface limited to enamel**
            White spot lesions [initial caries] on smooth surface of tooth

        K02.62 **Dental caries on smooth surface penetrating into dentin**

        K02.63 **Dental caries on smooth surface penetrating into pulp**

    K02.7 **Dental root caries**

    K02.9 **Dental caries, unspecified**

● **K03** **Other diseases of hard tissues of teeth**

    Excludes2 bruxism (F45.8)
           dental caries (K02.-)
           teeth-grinding NOS (F45.8)

    K03.0 **Excessive attrition of teeth**
        Approximal wear of teeth
        Occlusal wear of teeth

    K03.1 **Abrasion of teeth**
        Dentifrice abrasion of teeth
        Habitual abrasion of teeth
        Occupational abrasion of teeth
        Ritual abrasion of teeth
        Traditional abrasion of teeth
        Wedge defect NOS

    K03.2 **Erosion of teeth**
        Erosion of teeth due to diet
        Erosion of teeth due to drugs and medicaments
        Erosion of teeth due to persistent vomiting
        Erosion of teeth NOS
        Idiopathic erosion of teeth
        Occupational erosion of teeth

    K03.3 **Pathological resorption of teeth**
        Internal granuloma of pulp
        Resorption of teeth (external)

    K03.4 **Hypercementosis**
        Cementation hyperplasia

    K03.5 **Ankylosis of teeth**

    K03.6 **Deposits [accretions] on teeth**
        Betel deposits [accretions] on teeth
        Black deposits [accretions] on teeth
        Extrinsic staining of teeth NOS
        Green deposits [accretions] on teeth
        Materia alba deposits [accretions] on teeth
        Orange deposits [accretions] on teeth
        Staining of teeth NOS
        Subgingival dental calculus
        Supragingival dental calculus
        Tobacco deposits [accretions] on teeth

    K03.7 **Posteruptive color changes of dental hard tissues**
        Excludes2 deposits [accretions] on teeth (K03.6)

  ● **K03.8** **Other specified diseases of hard tissues of teeth**

        K03.81 **Cracked tooth**
            Excludes1 asymptomatic craze lines in enamel - omit code
                broken or fractured tooth due to trauma (S02.5)

        K03.89 **Other specified diseases of hard tissues of teeth**

    K03.9 **Disease of hard tissues of teeth, unspecified**

K04 **Diseases of pulp and periapical tissues**
    Coding Clinic: 2016, Q4, P29

  ● **K04.0** **Pulpitis**
        Acute pulpitis
        Chronic (hyperplastic) (ulcerative) pulpitis

        K04.01 **Reversible pulpitis**

        K04.02 **Irreversible pulpitis**

    K04.1 **Necrosis of pulp**
        Pulpal gangrene

    K04.2 **Pulp degeneration**
        Denticles
        Pulpal calcifications
        Pulpal stones

    K04.3 **Abnormal hard tissue formation in pulp**
        Secondary or irregular dentine

    K04.4 **Acute apical periodontitis of pulpal origin**
        Acute apical periodontitis NOS
        Excludes1 acute periodontitis (K05.2-)

    K04.5 **Chronic apical periodontitis**
        Apical or periapical granuloma
        Apical periodontitis NOS
        Excludes1 chronic periodontitis (K05.3-)

    K04.6 **Periapical abscess with sinus**
        Dental abscess with sinus
        Dentoalveolar abscess with sinus

    K04.7 **Periapical abscess without sinus**
        Dental abscess without sinus
        Dentoalveolar abscess without sinus

    K04.8 **Radicular cyst**
        Apical (periodontal) cyst
        Periapical cyst
        Residual radicular cyst
        Excludes2 lateral periodontal cyst (K09.0)

  ● **K04.9** **Other and unspecified diseases of pulp and periapical tissues**

        K04.90 **Unspecified diseases of pulp and periapical tissues**

        K04.99 **Other diseases of pulp and periapical tissues**

Item 11–3 **Acute gingivitis,** also known as orilitis or ulitis, is the short-term, severe inflammation of the gums (gingiva) caused by bacteria. **Chronic gingivitis** is persistent inflammation of the gums. When the gingivitis moves into the periodontium it is called periodontitis, also known as paradentitis.

▶ New　⇒ Revised　d̶e̶l̶e̶t̶e̶d̶ Deleted　Excludes 1　Excludes 2　Includes　Use additional　Code first　Code also　Key words

OGCR Official Guidelines　X Assign placeholder X　● Use Additional Character(s)　) Manifestation Code　🝏 Hierarchical Condition Category　Coding Clinic

902

● **K05** **Gingivitis and periodontal diseases**
   Use additional code to identify:
      alcohol abuse and dependence (F10.-)
      exposure to environmental tobacco smoke (Z77.22)
      exposure to tobacco smoke in the perinatal period (P96.81)
      history of tobacco dependence (Z87.891)
      occupational exposure to environmental tobacco smoke
         (Z57.31)
      tobacco dependence (F17.-)
      tobacco use (Z72.0)
   Coding Clinic: 2016, Q4, P29

● **K05.0** **Acute gingivitis**
   Excludes1 acute necrotizing ulcerative gingivitis
                     (A69.1)
                  herpesviral [herpes simplex]
                     gingivostomatitis (B00.2)

   K05.00 **Acute gingivitis, plaque induced**
              Acute gingivitis NOS
              Plaque induced gingival disease

   K05.01 **Acute gingivitis, non-plaque induced**

● **K05.1** **Chronic gingivitis**
      Desquamative gingivitis (chronic)
      Gingivitis (chronic) NOS
      Hyperplastic gingivitis (chronic)
      Pregnancy associated gingivitis
      Simple marginal gingivitis (chronic)
      Ulcerative gingivitis (chronic)
      *Code first, if applicable, diseases of the digestive system
         complicating pregnancy (O99.61-)*

   K05.10 **Chronic gingivitis, plaque induced**
              Chronic gingivitis NOS
              Gingivitis NOS

   K05.11 **Chronic gingivitis, non-plaque induced**

● **K05.2** **Aggressive periodontitis**
      Acute pericoronitis
      Excludes1 acute apical periodontitis (K04.4)
                     periapical abscess (K04.7)
                     periapical abscess with sinus (K04.6)

   K05.20 **Aggressive periodontitis, unspecified**

● **K05.21** **Aggressive periodontitis, localized**
              Periodontal abscess

      K05.211 **Aggressive periodontitis, localized,
                   slight**

      K05.212 **Aggressive periodontitis, localized,
                   moderate**

      K05.213 **Aggressive periodontitis, localized,
                   severe**

      K05.219 **Aggressive periodontitis, localized,
                   unspecified severity**

● **K05.22** **Aggressive periodontitis, generalized**

      K05.221 **Aggressive periodontitis, generalized,
                   slight**

      K05.222 **Aggressive periodontitis, generalized,
                   moderate**

      K05.223 **Aggressive periodontitis, generalized,
                   severe**

      K05.229 **Aggressive periodontitis, generalized,
                   unspecified severity**

● **K05.3** **Chronic periodontitis**
      Chronic pericoronitis
      Complex periodontitis
      Periodontitis NOS
      Simplex periodontitis
      Excludes1 chronic apical periodontitis (K04.5)

   K05.30 **Chronic periodontitis, unspecified**

● **K05.31** **Chronic periodontitis, localized**

      K05.311 **Chronic periodontitis, localized,
                   slight**

      K05.312 **Chronic periodontitis, localized,
                   moderate**

      K05.313 **Chronic periodontitis, localized,
                   severe**

      K05.319 **Chronic periodontitis, localized,
                   unspecified severity**

● **K05.32** **Chronic periodontitis, generalized**

      K05.321 **Chronic periodontitis, generalized,
                   slight**

      K05.322 **Chronic periodontitis, generalized,
                   moderate**

      K05.323 **Chronic periodontitis, generalized,
                   severe**

      K05.329 **Chronic periodontitis, generalized,
                   unspecified severity**

   K05.4 **Periodontosis**
      Juvenile periodontosis

   K05.5 **Other periodontal diseases**
      Combined periodontic-endodontic lesion
      Narrow gingival width (of periodontal soft tissue)
      Excludes2 leukoplakia of gingiva (K13.21)

   K05.6 **Periodontal disease, unspecified**

● **K06** **Other disorders of gingiva and edentulous alveolar ridge**
      Excludes2 acute gingivitis (K05.0)
                     atrophy of edentulous alveolar ridge (K08.2)
                     chronic gingivitis (K05.1)
                     gingivitis NOS (K05.1)
      Coding Clinic: 2016, Q4, P29

● **K06.0** **Gingival recession**
      Gingival recession (postinfective) (postprocedural)

   ● **K06.01** **Gingival recession, localized**

      K06.010 **Localized gingival recession,
                   unspecified**
                      Localized gingival recession, NOS

      K06.011 **Localized gingival recession, minimal**

      K06.012 **Localized gingival recession,
                   moderate**

      K06.013 **Localized gingival recession, severe**

   ● **K06.02** **Gingival recession, generalized**

      K06.020 **Generalized gingival recession,
                   unspecified**
                      Generalized gingival recession, NOS

      K06.021 **Generalized gingival recession,
                   minimal**

      K06.022 **Generalized gingival recession,
                   moderate**

      K06.023 **Generalized gingival recession,
                   severe**

   K06.1 **Gingival enlargement**
      Gingival fibromatosis

   K06.2 **Gingival and edentulous alveolar ridge lesions
              associated with trauma**
      Irritative hyperplasia of edentulous ridge [denture
         hyperplasia]
      Use additional code (Chapter 20) to identify external
         cause or denture status (Z97.2)

   K06.3 **Horizontal alveolar bone loss**

   K06.8 **Other specified disorders of gingiva and edentulous
              alveolar ridge**
      Fibrous epulis
      Flabby alveolar ridge
      Giant cell epulis
      Peripheral giant cell granuloma of gingiva
      Pyogenic granuloma of gingiva
      Vertical ridge deficiency
      Excludes2 gingival cyst (K09.0)

   K06.9 **Disorder of gingiva and edentulous alveolar ridge,
              unspecified**

CHAPTER 11 (K00-K95)

● **K08 Other disorders of teeth and supporting structures**

  Excludes2   dentofacial anomalies [including malocclusion] (M26.-)
          disorders of jaw (M27.-)

  Coding Clinic: 2016, Q4, P29

  K08.0 Exfoliation of teeth due to systemic causes
    Code also underlying systemic condition

● **K08.1 Complete loss of teeth**
    Acquired loss of teeth, complete

    Excludes1   congenital absence of teeth (K00.0)
          exfoliation of teeth due to systemic causes (K08.0)
          partial loss of teeth (K08.4-)

  ● **K08.10 Complete loss of teeth, unspecified cause**
    K08.101 Complete loss of teeth, unspecified cause, class I
    K08.102 Complete loss of teeth, unspecified cause, class II
    K08.103 Complete loss of teeth, unspecified cause, class III
    K08.104 Complete loss of teeth, unspecified cause, class IV
    K08.109 Complete loss of teeth, unspecified cause, unspecified class
      Edentulism NOS

  ● **K08.11 Complete loss of teeth due to trauma**
    K08.111 Complete loss of teeth due to trauma, class I
    K08.112 Complete loss of teeth due to trauma, class II
    K08.113 Complete loss of teeth due to trauma, class III
    K08.114 Complete loss of teeth due to trauma, class IV
    K08.119 Complete loss of teeth due to trauma, unspecified class

  ● **K08.12 Complete loss of teeth due to periodontal diseases**
    K08.121 Complete loss of teeth due to periodontal diseases, class I
    K08.122 Complete loss of teeth due to periodontal diseases, class II
    K08.123 Complete loss of teeth due to periodontal diseases, class III
    K08.124 Complete loss of teeth due to periodontal diseases, class IV
    K08.129 Complete loss of teeth due to periodontal diseases, unspecified class

  ● **K08.13 Complete loss of teeth due to caries**
    K08.131 Complete loss of teeth due to caries, class I
    K08.132 Complete loss of teeth due to caries, class II
    K08.133 Complete loss of teeth due to caries, class III
    K08.134 Complete loss of teeth due to caries, class IV
    K08.139 Complete loss of teeth due to caries, unspecified class

  ● **K08.19 Complete loss of teeth due to other specified cause**
    K08.191 Complete loss of teeth due to other specified cause, class I
    K08.192 Complete loss of teeth due to other specified cause, class II
    K08.193 Complete loss of teeth due to other specified cause, class III
    K08.194 Complete loss of teeth due to other specified cause, class IV
    K08.199 Complete loss of teeth due to other specified cause, unspecified class

● **K08.2 Atrophy of edentulous alveolar ridge**
  K08.20 Unspecified atrophy of edentulous alveolar ridge
    Atrophy of the mandible NOS
    Atrophy of the maxilla NOS
  K08.21 Minimal atrophy of the mandible
    Minimal atrophy of the edentulous mandible
  K08.22 Moderate atrophy of the mandible
    Moderate atrophy of the edentulous mandible
  K08.23 Severe atrophy of the mandible
    Severe atrophy of the edentulous mandible
  K08.24 Minimal atrophy of maxilla
    Minimal atrophy of the edentulous maxilla
  K08.25 Moderate atrophy of the maxilla
    Moderate atrophy of the edentulous maxilla
  K08.26 Severe atrophy of the maxilla
    Severe atrophy of the edentulous maxilla

● **K08.3 Retained dental root**

● **K08.4 Partial loss of teeth**
  Acquired loss of teeth, partial

  Excludes1   complete loss of teeth (K08.1-)
      congenital absence of teeth (K00.0)

  Excludes2   exfoliation of teeth due to systemic causes (K08.0)

  ● **K08.40 Partial loss of teeth, unspecified cause**
    K08.401 Partial loss of teeth, unspecified cause, class I
    K08.402 Partial loss of teeth, unspecified cause, class II
    K08.403 Partial loss of teeth, unspecified cause, class III
    K08.404 Partial loss of teeth, unspecified cause, class IV
    K08.409 Partial loss of teeth, unspecified cause, unspecified class
      Tooth extraction status NOS

  ● **K08.41 Partial loss of teeth due to trauma**
    K08.411 Partial loss of teeth due to trauma, class I
    K08.412 Partial loss of teeth due to trauma, class II
    K08.413 Partial loss of teeth due to trauma, class III
    K08.414 Partial loss of teeth due to trauma, class IV
    K08.419 Partial loss of teeth due to trauma, unspecified class

  ● **K08.42 Partial loss of teeth due to periodontal diseases**
    K08.421 Partial loss of teeth due to periodontal diseases, class I
    K08.422 Partial loss of teeth due to periodontal diseases, class II
    K08.423 Partial loss of teeth due to periodontal diseases, class III
    K08.424 Partial loss of teeth due to periodontal diseases, class IV
    K08.429 Partial loss of teeth due to periodontal diseases, unspecified class

  ● **K08.43 Partial loss of teeth due to caries**
    K08.431 Partial loss of teeth due to caries, class I
    K08.432 Partial loss of teeth due to caries, class II
    K08.433 Partial loss of teeth due to caries, class III

K08.434 **Partial loss of teeth due to caries, class IV**

K08.439 **Partial loss of teeth due to caries, unspecified class**

● K08.49 Partial loss of teeth due to other specified cause

K08.491 **Partial loss of teeth due to other specified cause, class I**

K08.492 **Partial loss of teeth due to other specified cause, class II**

K08.493 **Partial loss of teeth due to other specified cause, class III**

K08.494 **Partial loss of teeth due to other specified cause, class IV**

K08.499 **Partial loss of teeth due to other specified cause, unspecified class**

● K08.5 **Unsatisfactory restoration of tooth**
Defective bridge, crown, filling
Defective dental restoration

Excludes1 dental restoration status (Z98.811)

Excludes2 endosseous dental implant failure (M27.6-)
unsatisfactory endodontic treatment (M27.5-)

K08.50 **Unsatisfactory restoration of tooth, unspecified**
Defective dental restoration NOS

K08.51 **Open restoration margins of tooth**
Dental restoration failure of marginal integrity
Open margin on tooth restoration
Poor gingival margin to tooth restoration

K08.52 **Unrepairable overhanging of dental restorative materials**
Overhanging of tooth restoration

● K08.53 **Fractured dental restorative material**

Excludes1 cracked tooth (K03.81)
traumatic fracture of tooth (S02.5)

K08.530 **Fractured dental restorative material without loss of material**

K08.531 **Fractured dental restorative material with loss of material**

K08.539 **Fractured dental restorative material, unspecified**

K08.54 **Contour of existing restoration of tooth biologically incompatible with oral health**
Dental restoration failure of periodontal anatomical integrity
Unacceptable contours of existing restoration of tooth
Unacceptable morphology of existing restoration of tooth

K08.55 **Allergy to existing dental restorative material**
Use additional code to identify the specific type of allergy

K08.56 **Poor aesthetic of existing restoration of tooth**
Dental restoration aesthetically inadequate or displeasing

K08.59 **Other unsatisfactory restoration of tooth**
Other defective dental restoration

● K08.8 **Other specified disorders of teeth and supporting structures**

K08.81 **Primary occlusal trauma**

K08.82 **Secondary occlusal trauma**

K08.89 **Other specified disorders of teeth and supporting structures**
Enlargement of alveolar ridge NOS
Insufficient anatomic crown height
Insufficient clinical crown length
Irregular alveolar process
Toothache NOS

K08.9 **Disorder of teeth and supporting structures, unspecified**

Item 11–4 Atrophy is wasting away of a tissue or organ, whereas **hypertrophy** is overdevelopment or enlargement of a tissue or organ. **Sialoadenitis** is salivary gland inflammation. **Parotitis** is the inflammation of the parotid gland. In the epidemic form, parotitis is also known as mumps. **Sialolithiasis** is the formation of calculus within a salivary gland. **Mucocele** is a polyp composed of mucus.

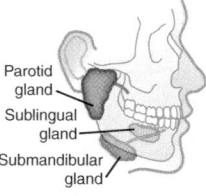

Figure 11-3 Major salivary glands.

Parotid gland
Sublingual gland
Submandibular gland

● K09 **Cysts of oral region, not elsewhere classified**

Includes lesions showing histological features both of aneurysmal cyst and of another fibro-osseous lesion

Excludes2 cysts of jaw (M27.0-, M27.4-)
radicular cyst (K04.8)

K09.0 **Developmental odontogenic cysts**
Dentigerous cyst
Eruption cyst
Follicular cyst
Gingival cyst
Lateral periodontal cyst
Primordial cyst

Excludes2 keratocysts (D16.4, D16.5)
odontogenic keratocystic tumors (D16.4, D16.5)

K09.1 **Developmental (nonodontogenic) cysts of oral region**
Cyst (of) incisive canal
Cyst (of) palatine of papilla
Globulomaxillary cyst
Median palatal cyst
Nasoalveolar cyst
Nasolabial cyst
Nasopalatine duct cyst

K09.8 **Other cysts of oral region, not elsewhere classified**
Dermoid cyst
Epidermoid cyst
Lymphoepithelial cyst
Epstein's pearl

K09.9 **Cyst of oral region, unspecified**

★ **(See Plate 28 of the Anatomy Illustrations.)**

● K11 **Diseases of salivary glands**
Use additional code to identify:
alcohol abuse and dependence (F10.-)
exposure to environmental tobacco smoke (Z77.22)
exposure to tobacco smoke in the perinatal period (P96.81)
history of tobacco dependence (Z87.891)
occupational exposure to environmental tobacco smoke (Z57.31)
tobacco dependence (F17.-)
tobacco use (Z72.0)

K11.0 **Atrophy of salivary gland**

K11.1 **Hypertrophy of salivary gland**

● K11.2 **Sialoadenitis**
Parotitis

Excludes1 epidemic parotitis (B26.-)
mumps (B26.-)
uveoparotid fever [Heerfordt] (D86.89)

K11.20 **Sialoadenitis, unspecified**

K11.21 **Acute sialoadenitis**

Excludes1 acute recurrent sialoadenitis (K11.22)

K11.22 **Acute recurrent sialoadenitis**

K11.23 **Chronic sialoadenitis**

K11.3 **Abscess of salivary gland**

CHAPTER 11 (K00-K95)

K11.4   **Fistula of salivary gland**
> **Excludes1**   congenital fistula of salivary gland (Q38.4)

K11.5   **Sialolithiasis**
> Calculus of salivary gland or duct
> Stone of salivary gland or duct

K11.6   **Mucocele of salivary gland**
> Mucous extravasation cyst of salivary gland
> Mucous retention cyst of salivary gland
> Ranula

K11.7   **Disturbances of salivary secretion**
> Hypoptyalism
> Ptyalism
> Xerostomia
> **Excludes2**   dry mouth NOS (R68.2)

K11.8   **Other diseases of salivary glands**
> Benign lymphoepithelial lesion of salivary gland
> Mikulicz' disease
> Necrotizing sialometaplasia
> Sialectasia
> Stenosis of salivary duct
> Stricture of salivary duct
> **Excludes1**   Sjögren syndrome (M35.0-)

K11.9   **Disease of salivary gland, unspecified**
> Sialoadenopathy NOS

● **K12**   **Stomatitis and related lesions**
> Use additional code to identify:
>   alcohol abuse and dependence (F10.-)
>   exposure to environmental tobacco smoke (Z77.22)
>   exposure to tobacco smoke in the perinatal period (P96.81)
>   history of tobacco dependence (Z87.891)
>   occupational exposure to environmental tobacco smoke (Z57.31)
>   tobacco dependence (F17.-)
>   tobacco use (Z72.0)
> **Excludes1**   cancrum oris (A69.0)
>   cheilitis (K13.0)
>   gangrenous stomatitis (A69.0)
>   herpesviral [herpes simplex] gingivostomatitis (B00.2)
>   noma (A69.0)

K12.0   **Recurrent oral aphthae**
> Aphthous stomatitis (major) (minor)
> Bednar's aphthae
> Periadenitis mucosa necrotica recurrens
> Recurrent aphthous ulcer
> Stomatitis herpetiformis

K12.1   **Other forms of stomatitis**
> Stomatitis NOS
> Denture stomatitis
> Ulcerative stomatitis
> Vesicular stomatitis
> **Excludes1**   acute necrotizing ulcerative stomatitis (A69.1)
>   Vincent's stomatitis (A69.1)

K12.2   **Cellulitis and abscess of mouth**
> Cellulitis of mouth (floor)
> Submandibular abscess
> **Excludes2**   abscess of salivary gland (K11.3)
>   abscess of tongue (K14.0)
>   periapical abscess (K04.6-K04.7)
>   periodontal abscess (K05.21)
>   peritonsillar abscess (J36)

● **K12.3**   **Oral mucositis (ulcerative)**
> Mucositis (oral) (oropharyneal)
> **Excludes2**   gastrointestinal mucositis (ulcerative) (K92.81)
>   mucositis (ulcerative) of vagina and vulva (N76.81)
>   nasal mucositis (ulcerative) (J34.81)

     K12.30   **Oral mucositis (ulcerative), unspecified**

     K12.31   **Oral mucositis (ulcerative) due to antineoplastic therapy**
> Use additional code for adverse effect, if applicable, to identify antineoplastic and immunosuppressive drugs (T45.1X5)
> Use additional code for other antineoplastic therapy, such as:
>   radiological procedure and radiotherapy (Y84.2)

     K12.32   **Oral mucositis (ulcerative) due to other drugs**
> Use additional code for adverse effect, if applicable, to identify drug (T36-T50 with fifth or sixth character 5)

     K12.33   **Oral mucositis (ulcerative) due to radiation**
> Use additional external cause code (W88-W90, X39.0-) to identify cause

     K12.39   **Other oral mucositis (ulcerative)**
> Viral oral mucositis (ulcerative)

● **K13**   **Other diseases of lip and oral mucosa**
> **Includes**   epithelial disturbances of tongue
> Use additional code to identify:
>   alcohol abuse and dependence (F10.-)
>   exposure to environmental tobacco smoke (Z77.22)
>   exposure to tobacco smoke in the perinatal period (P96.81)
>   history of tobacco dependence (Z87.891)
>   occupational exposure to environmental tobacco smoke (Z57.31)
>   tobacco dependence (F17.-)
>   tobacco use (Z72.0)
> **Excludes2**   certain disorders of gingiva and edentulous alveolar ridge (K05-K06)
>   cysts of oral region (K09.-)
>   diseases of tongue (K14.-)
>   stomatitis and related lesions (K12.-)

K13.0   **Diseases of lips**

Abscess of lips	Exfoliative cheilitis
Angular cheilitis	Fistula of lips
Cellulitis of lips	Glandular cheilitis
Cheilitis NOS	Hypertrophy of lips
Cheilodynia	Perlèche NEC
Cheilosis	

> **Excludes1**   ariboflavinosis (E53.0)
>   cheilitis due to radiation-related disorders (L55-L59)
>   congenital fistula of lips (Q38.0)
>   congenital hypertrophy of lips (Q18.6)
>   Perlèche due to candidiasis (B37.83)
>   Perlèche due to riboflavin deficiency (E53.0)

K13.1   **Cheek and lip biting**

● **K13.2**   **Leukoplakia and other disturbances of oral epithelium, including tongue**
> **Excludes1**   carcinoma in situ of oral epithelium (D00.0-)
>   hairy leukoplakia (K13.3)

     K13.21   **Leukoplakia of oral mucosa, including tongue**
> *Considered precancerous and evidenced by thickened white patches of epithelium on mucous membranes*
> Leukokeratosis of oral mucosa
> Leukoplakia of gingiva, lips, tongue
> **Excludes1**   hairy leukoplakia (K13.3)
>   leukokeratosis nicotina palati (K13.24)

Figure 11-4   Oral leukoplakia and associated. (From Swartz MH: Textbook of Physical Diagnosis: History and Examination, Philadelphia, PA, Saunders/Elsevier, 2010)

Item 11-5   **Stomatitis** is the inflammation of the oral mucosa. **Mucositis** is the inflammation of the mucous membranes lining the digestive tract from the mouth to the anus. It is a common side effect of chemotherapy and of radiotherapy that involves any part of the digestive tract.

▶ New   ◀ Revised   ~~deleted~~ Deleted   Excludes 1   Excludes 2   Includes   Use additional   Code first   Code also   Key words

906

OGCR Official Guidelines   X Assign placeholder X   ● Use Additional Character(s)   ▷ Manifestation Code   🔖 Hierarchical Condition Category   Coding Clinic

K13.22 **Minimal keratinized** residual ridge mucosa
    Minimal keratinization of alveolar ridge
    mucosa

K13.23 **Excessive keratinized** residual ridge mucosa
    Excessive keratinization of alveolar ridge
    mucosa

K13.24 **Leukokeratosis nicotina palati**
    Smoker's palate

K13.29 **Other** disturbances of oral epithelium,
including tongue
    Erythroplakia of mouth or tongue
    Focal epithelial hyperplasia of mouth or tongue
    Leukoedema of mouth or tongue
    Other oral epithelium disturbances

K13.3 **Hairy leukoplakia**

K13.4 **Granuloma and granuloma-like lesions of oral mucosa**
    Eosinophilic granuloma
    Granuloma pyogenicum
    Verrucous xanthoma

K13.5 **Oral submucous fibrosis**
    Submucous fibrosis of tongue

K13.6 **Irritative hyperplasia of oral mucosa**
    Excludes2 irritative hyperplasia of edentulous ridge
    [denture hyperplasia] (K06.2)

● K13.7 **Other and unspecified lesions of oral mucosa**
    K13.70 **Unspecified** lesions of oral mucosa
    K13.79 **Other lesions of oral mucosa**
        Focal oral mucinosis
    Coding Clinic: 2022, Q2, P8

★ **(See Plate 26 of the Anatomy Illustrations.)**

● K14 **Diseases of tongue**
    Use additional code to identify:
        alcohol abuse and dependence (F10.-)
        exposure to environmental tobacco smoke (Z77.22)
        history of tobacco dependence (Z87.891)
        occupational exposure to environmental tobacco smoke
        (Z57.31)
        tobacco dependence (F17.-)
        tobacco use (Z72.0)
    Excludes2 erythroplakia (K13.29)
         focal epithelial hyperplasia (K13.29)
         leukoedema of tongue (K13.29)
         leukoplakia of tongue (K13.21)
         hairy leukoplakia (K13.3)
         macroglossia (congenital) (Q38.2)
         submucous fibrosis of tongue (K13.5)

K14.0 **Glossitis**
    Abscess of tongue
    Ulceration (traumatic) of tongue
    Excludes1 atrophic glossitis (K14.4)

K14.1 **Geographic tongue**
    Benign migratory glossitis
    Glossitis areata exfoliativa

K14.2 **Median rhomboid glossitis**

K14.3 **Hypertrophy of tongue papillae**
    Black hairy tongue
    Coated tongue
    Hypertrophy of foliate papillae
    Lingua villosa nigra

K14.4 **Atrophy of tongue papillae**
    Atrophic glossitis

K14.5 **Plicated tongue**
    Fissured tongue   Scrotal tongue
    Furrowed tongue
    Excludes1 fissured tongue, congenital (Q38.3)

K14.6 **Glossodynia**
    Glossopyrosis   Painful tongue

K14.8 **Other diseases of tongue**
    Atrophy of tongue   Glossocele
    Crenated tongue   Glossoptosis
    Enlargement of tongue Hypertrophy of tongue

K14.9 **Disease of tongue, unspecified**
    Glossopathy NOS

DISEASES OF ESOPHAGUS, STOMACH AND DUODENUM (K20-K31)

    Excludes2 hiatus hernia (K44.-)

● K20 **Esophagitis**
    Use additional code to identify:
        alcohol abuse and dependence (F10.-)
    Excludes1 erosion of esophagus (K22.1-)
         esophagitis with gastro-esophageal reflux disease
         (K21.0-)
         reflux esophagitis (K21.0-)
         ulcerative esophagitis (K22.1-)
    Excludes2 eosinophilic gastritis or gastroenteritis (K52.81)
    Coding Clinic: 2023, Q1, P20

K20.0 **Eosinophilic esophagitis**

● K20.8 **Other esophagitis**
    K20.80 **Other esophagitis without bleeding**
        Abscess of esophagus
        Other esophagitis NOS
    K20.81 **Other esophagitis with bleeding**

● K20.9 **Esophagitis, unspecified**
    K20.90 **Esophagitis, unspecified without bleeding**
        Esophagitis NOS
    K20.91 **Esophagitis, unspecified with bleeding**

● K21 **Gastro-esophageal reflux disease**
    Excludes1 newborn esophageal reflux (P78.83)

● K21.0 **Gastro-esophageal reflux disease with esophagitis**
    K21.00 **Gastro-esophageal reflux disease with
esophagitis, without bleeding**
        Reflux esophagitis
    K21.01 **Gastro-esophageal reflux disease with
esophagitis, with bleeding**

K21.9 **Gastro-esophageal reflux disease without esophagitis**
    Esophageal reflux NOS
    Coding Clinic: 2016, Q1, P18

● K22 **Other diseases of esophagus**
    Excludes2 esophageal varices (I85.-)
    K22.0 **Achalasia of cardia**
        Achalasia NOS
        Cardiospasm
        Excludes1 congenital cardiospasm (Q39.5)

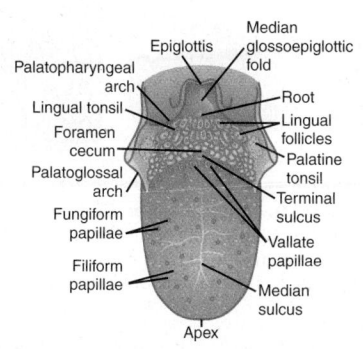

Figure 11-5 Structure of the tongue.

CHAPTER 11 (K00-K95)

● **K22.1**   **Ulcer of esophagus**
     Barrett's ulcer
     Erosion of esophagus
     Fungal ulcer of esophagus
     Peptic ulcer of esophagus
     Ulcer of esophagus due to ingestion of chemicals
     Ulcer of esophagus due to ingestion of drugs and
       medicaments
     Ulcerative esophagitis
     Code first poisoning due to drug or toxin, if applicable
       (T36-T65 with fifth or sixth character 1-4)
     Use additional code for adverse effect, if applicable, to
       identify drug (T36-T50 with fifth or sixth character 5)
     Excludes1   Barrett's esophagus (K22.87-)
   K22.10   **Ulcer of esophagus without bleeding**
       Ulcer of esophagus NOS
   K22.11   **Ulcer of esophagus with bleeding**
       Excludes2   bleeding esophageal varices
          (I85.01, I85.11)
       Coding Clinic: 2023, Q1, P20

● **K22.2**   **Esophageal obstruction**
     Compression of esophagus
     Constriction of esophagus
     Stenosis of esophagus
     Stricture of esophagus
     Excludes1   congenital stenosis or stricture of
          esophagus (Q39.3)
     Coding Clinic: 2024, Q2, P26

● **K22.3**   **Perforation of esophagus**
     Rupture of esophagus
     Excludes1   traumatic perforation of (thoracic)
          esophagus (S27.8-)

● **K22.4**   **Dyskinesia of esophagus**
     Difficulty in moving
     Corkscrew esophagus
     Diffuse esophageal spasm
     Spasm of esophagus
     Excludes1   cardiospasm (K22.0)

● **K22.5**   **Diverticulum of esophagus, acquired**
     Esophageal pouch, acquired
     Excludes1   diverticulum of esophagus (congenital)
          (Q39.6)

● **K22.6**   **Gastro-esophageal laceration-hemorrhage syndrome**
     Mallory-Weiss syndrome

Item 11–6   **Esophageal reflux** is the return flow of the contents of the stomach to the esophagus and is referred to as GERD and/or "heartburn." **Gastroesophageal reflux** is the return flow of the contents of the stomach and duodenum to the esophagus. **Esophageal leukoplakia** are white areas on the mucous membrane of the esophagus for which no specific cause can be identified.

Figure 11-6   The esophagus is the muscular tube that connects the pharynx and the stomach. The 10-inch (25 cm) long esophagus is divided into three parts: **cervical, thoracic,** and **abdominal.**

CERVICAL ESOPHAGUS
Left subclavian artery
First rib
Arch of aorta
Diaphragm
THORACIC ESOPHAGUS
ABDOMINAL ESOPHAGUS
Stomach

Item 11–7   **Achalasia** is a condition in which the smooth muscle fibers of the esophagus do not relax. Most frequently, this condition occurs at the esophagogastric sphincter. **Cardiospasm,** also known as **megaesophagus,** is achalasia of the thoracic esophagus.

● **K22.7**   **Barrett's esophagus**
     Barrett's disease
     Barrett's syndrome
     Excludes1   Barrett's ulcer (K22.1)
          malignant neoplasm of esophagus (C15.-)
   K22.70   **Barrett's esophagus without dysplasia**
       Barrett's esophagus NOS
● **K22.71**   **Barrett's esophagus with dysplasia**
     K22.710   **Barrett's esophagus with low grade**
       dysplasia
     K22.711   **Barrett's esophagus with high grade**
       dysplasia
     K22.719   **Barrett's esophagus with dysplasia,**
       unspecified

● **K22.8**   **Other specified diseases of esophagus**
   K22.81   **Esophageal polyp**
     Excludes1   benign neoplasm of esophagus (D13.0)
   K22.82 Esophagogastric junction polyp
     Excludes1   benign neoplasm of stomach (D13.1)
   K22.89   **Other specified disease of esophagus**
       Hemorrhage of esophagus NOS
     Excludes2   esophageal varices (I85.-)
          Paterson-Kelly syndrome (D50.1)
     Coding Clinic: 2024, Q2, P26; 2020, Q1, P16

   K22.9   **Disease of esophagus, unspecified**

▷ **K23**   *Disorders of esophagus in diseases classified elsewhere*
     Code first underlying disease, such as:
       congenital syphilis (A50.5)
     Excludes1   late syphilis (A52.79)
          megaesophagus due to Chagas' disease (B57.31)
          tuberculosis (A18.83)

● **K25**   **Gastric ulcer**
     Includes   erosion (acute) of stomach
       pylorus ulcer (peptic)
       stomach ulcer (peptic)
     Use additional code to identify:
       alcohol abuse and dependence (F10.-)
     Excludes1   acute gastritis (K29.0-)
          peptic ulcer NOS (K27.-)

   K25.0   **Acute gastric ulcer with hemorrhage**
       Coding Clinic: 2023, Q1, P16
   K25.1   **Acute gastric ulcer with perforation** 🏥
   K25.2   **Acute gastric ulcer with both hemorrhage and perforation** 🏥
   K25.3   **Acute gastric ulcer without hemorrhage or perforation**
   K25.4   **Chronic or unspecified gastric ulcer with hemorrhage**
       Coding Clinic: 2017, Q3, P27
   K25.5   **Chronic or unspecified gastric ulcer with perforation** 🏥
   K25.6   **Chronic or unspecified gastric ulcer with both hemorrhage and perforation** 🏥

A   B   C

Figure 11-7   **A.** Ulcer. **B.** Perforated ulcer. **C.** Laparoscopic view of a perforated duodenal ulcer *(arrow)* with fibrinous exudate on the adjacent peritoneum. (**C** from Feldman: Sleisenger & Fordtran's Gastrointestinal and Liver Disease, ed 8, Saunders, An Imprint of Elsevier, 2006)

Item 11–8   **Gastric ulcers** are lesions of the stomach that result in the death of the tissue and a defect of the surface. **Perforated ulcers** are those in which the lesion penetrates the gastric wall, leaving a hole. **Peptic ulcers** are lesions of the stomach or the duodenum. **Peptic** refers to the gastric juice, pepsin.

▶ New   ⇒ Revised   ~~deleted~~ Deleted   Excludes 1   Excludes 2   Includes   Use additional   Code first   Code also   Key words
OGCR Official Guidelines   X Assign placeholder X   ● Use Additional Character(s)   ▷ Manifestation Code   🏥 Hierarchical Condition Category   *Coding Clinic*

K25.7   Chronic gastric ulcer without hemorrhage or perforation

K25.9   Gastric ulcer, unspecified as acute or chronic, without hemorrhage or perforation
         Coding Clinic: 2021, Q1, P12

● **K26**   Duodenal ulcer

     Includes   erosion (acute) of duodenum
              duodenum ulcer (peptic)
              postpyloric ulcer (peptic)

     Use additional code to identify:
         alcohol abuse and dependence (F10.-)

     Excludes1   peptic ulcer NOS (K27.-)

K26.0   Acute duodenal ulcer with hemorrhage

K26.1   Acute duodenal ulcer with perforation 🦕

K26.2   Acute duodenal ulcer with both hemorrhage and perforation 🦕

K26.3   Acute duodenal ulcer without hemorrhage or perforation

K26.4   Chronic or unspecified duodenal ulcer with hemorrhage
         Coding Clinic: 2016, Q1, P14

K26.5   Chronic or unspecified duodenal ulcer with perforation 🦕

K26.6   Chronic or unspecified duodenal ulcer with both hemorrhage and perforation 🦕

K26.7   Chronic duodenal ulcer without hemorrhage or perforation
         Coding Clinic: 2023, Q2, P11

K26.9   Duodenal ulcer, unspecified as acute or chronic, without hemorrhage or perforation

● **K27**   Peptic ulcer, site unspecified

     Includes   gastroduodenal ulcer NOS
              peptic ulcer NOS

     Use additional code to identify:
         alcohol abuse and dependence (F10.-)

     Excludes1   peptic ulcer of newborn (P78.82)

K27.0   Acute peptic ulcer, site unspecified, with hemorrhage

K27.1   Acute peptic ulcer, site unspecified, with perforation 🦕

K27.2   Acute peptic ulcer, site unspecified, with both hemorrhage and perforation 🦕

K27.3   Acute peptic ulcer, site unspecified, without hemorrhage or perforation

K27.4   Chronic or unspecified peptic ulcer, site unspecified, with hemorrhage

K27.5   Chronic or unspecified peptic ulcer, site unspecified, with perforation 🦕

K27.6   Chronic or unspecified peptic ulcer, site unspecified, with both hemorrhage and perforation 🦕

K27.7   Chronic peptic ulcer, site unspecified, without hemorrhage or perforation

K27.9   Peptic ulcer, site unspecified, unspecified as acute or chronic, without hemorrhage or perforation

● **K28**   Gastrojejunal ulcer

     Includes   anastomotic ulcer (peptic) or erosion
              gastrocolic ulcer (peptic) or erosion
              gastrointestinal ulcer (peptic) or erosion
              gastrojejunal ulcer (peptic) or erosion
              jejunal ulcer (peptic) or erosion
              marginal ulcer (peptic) or erosion
              stomal ulcer (peptic) or erosion

     Use additional code to identify:
         alcohol abuse and dependence (F10.-)

     Excludes1   primary ulcer of small intestine (K63.3)

K28.0   Acute gastrojejunal ulcer with hemorrhage

K28.1   Acute gastrojejunal ulcer with perforation 🦕

K28.2   Acute gastrojejunal ulcer with both hemorrhage and perforation 🦕

K28.3   Acute gastrojejunal ulcer without hemorrhage or perforation

K28.4   Chronic or unspecified gastrojejunal ulcer with hemorrhage
         Coding Clinic: 2023, Q3, P10

K28.5   Chronic or unspecified gastrojejunal ulcer with perforation 🦕

K28.6   Chronic or unspecified gastrojejunal ulcer with both hemorrhage and perforation 🦕

K28.7   Chronic gastrojejunal ulcer without hemorrhage or perforation

K28.9   Gastrojejunal ulcer, unspecified as acute or chronic, without hemorrhage or perforation

● **K29**   Gastritis and duodenitis

     Excludes1   eosinophilic gastritis or gastroenteritis (K52.81)
              Zollinger-Ellison syndrome (E16.4)

● **K29.0**   Acute gastritis

       Use additional code to identify:
           alcohol abuse and dependence (F10.-)

       Excludes1   erosion (acute) of stomach (K25.-)

       K29.00   Acute gastritis without bleeding

       K29.01   Acute gastritis with bleeding

● **K29.2**   Alcoholic gastritis

       Use additional code to identify:
           alcohol abuse and dependence (F10.-)

       K29.20   Alcoholic gastritis without bleeding

       K29.21   Alcoholic gastritis with bleeding

● **K29.3**   Chronic superficial gastritis

       K29.30   Chronic superficial gastritis without bleeding

       K29.31   Chronic superficial gastritis with bleeding

● **K29.4**   Chronic atrophic gastritis
         Gastric atrophy

       K29.40   Chronic atrophic gastritis without bleeding

       K29.41   Chronic atrophic gastritis with bleeding

● **K29.5**   Unspecified chronic gastritis
         Chronic antral gastritis
         Chronic fundal gastritis

       K29.50   Unspecified chronic gastritis without bleeding

       K29.51   Unspecified chronic gastritis with bleeding

● **K29.6**   Other gastritis
         Giant hypertrophic gastritis
         Granulomatous gastritis
         Ménétrier's disease

       K29.60   Other gastritis without bleeding

       K29.61   Other gastritis with bleeding

● **K29.7**   Gastritis, unspecified

       K29.70   Gastritis, unspecified, without bleeding

       K29.71   Gastritis, unspecified, with bleeding

● **K29.8**   Duodenitis

       K29.80   Duodenitis without bleeding

       K29.81   Duodenitis with bleeding

● **K29.9**   Gastroduodenitis, unspecified

       K29.90   Gastroduodenitis, unspecified, without bleeding

       K29.91   Gastroduodenitis, unspecified, with bleeding

K30   Functional dyspepsia
       Indigestion

     Excludes1   dyspepsia NOS (R10.13)
              heartburn (R12)
              nervous dyspepsia (F45.8)
              neurotic dyspepsia (F45.8)
              psychogenic dyspepsia (F45.8)

Item 11-9 Gastritis is a severe inflammation of the stomach. **Atrophic gastritis** is a chronic inflammation of the stomach that results in destruction of the cells of the mucosa of the stomach. Duodenitis is an inflammation of the duodenum, the first section of the small intestine.

CHAPTER 11 (K00-K95)

Item 11–10 Achlorhydria, also known as gastric anacidity, is the absence of gastric acid.

● **K31 Other diseases of stomach and duodenum**
    Includes   functional disorders of stomach
      Excludes2   diabetic gastroparesis (E08.43, E09.43, E10.43,
                  E11.43, E13.43)
                  diverticulum of duodenum (K57.00-K57.13)

  K31.0 Acute dilatation of stomach
      Acute distention of stomach

  K31.1 Adult hypertrophic pyloric stenosis   A
      Pyloric stenosis NOS
       Excludes1   congenital or infantile pyloric stenosis
                  (Q40.0)
       Coding Clinic: 2023, Q3, P12

  K31.2 Hourglass stricture and stenosis of stomach
       Excludes1   congenital hourglass stomach (Q40.2)
                  hourglass contraction of stomach (K31.89)

  K31.3 Pylorospasm, not elsewhere classified
       Excludes1   congenital or infantile pylorospasm (Q40.0)
                  neurotic pylorospasm (F45.8)
                  psychogenic pylorospasm (F45.8)

  K31.4 Gastric diverticulum
       Excludes1   congenital diverticulum of stomach (Q40.2)

  K31.5 Obstruction of duodenum
      Constriction of duodenum
      Duodenal ileus (chronic)
      Stenosis of duodenum
        Narrowing
      Stricture of duodenum
        Narrowing
      Volvulus of duodenum
        Twisting/knotting
       Excludes1   congenital stenosis of duodenum (Q41.0)

  K31.6 Fistula of stomach and duodenum
      Gastrocolic fistula
      Gastrojejunocolic fistula
   ▶ Code also, if applicable, disruption of internal operation
      (surgical) wound (T81.32-)

  K31.7 Polyp of stomach and duodenum
       Excludes1   adenomatous polyp of stomach (D13.1)
       Coding Clinic: 2020, Q1, P16

● **K31.8 Other specified diseases of stomach and duodenum**
    ● **K31.81 Angiodysplasia of stomach and duodenum**
        **K31.811 Angiodysplasia of stomach and
                duodenum with bleeding**
                Coding Clinic: 2023, Q1, P16
        **K31.819 Angiodysplasia of stomach and
                duodenum without bleeding**
                Angiodysplasia of stomach and
                duodenum NOS
    **K31.82 Dieulafoy lesion (hemorrhagic) of stomach and
          duodenum**
        Excludes2   Dieulafoy lesion of intestine
                  (K63.81)
    K31.83 Achlorhydria
    K31.84 Gastroparesis
        Gastroparalysis
        Code first underlying disease, if known, such as:
          anorexia nervosa (F50.0-)
          diabetes mellitus (E08.43, E09.43, E10.43,
             E11.43, E13.43)
          scleroderma (M34.-)
    K31.89 Other diseases of stomach and duodenum
        Coding Clinic: 2024, Q2, P26; 2020, Q1, P16; 2017, Q1, P28

  K31.9 Disease of stomach and duodenum, unspecified

● **K31.A Gastric intestinal metaplasia**
    K31.A0 Gastric intestinal metaplasia, unspecified
        Gastric intestinal metaplasia indefinite for dysplasia
        Gastric intestinal metaplasia NOS
    ● **K31.A1 Gastric intestinal metaplasia without dysplasia**

    K31.A11 Gastric intestinal metaplasia without
            dysplasia, involving the antrum
    K31.A12 Gastric intestinal metaplasia without
            dysplasia, involving the body(corpus)
    K31.A13 Gastric intestinal metaplasia without
            dysplasia, involving the fundus
            involving the cardia
    K31.A14 Gastric intestinal metaplasia without
            dysplasia, involving the cardia
    K31.A15 Gastric intestinal metaplasia without
            dysplasia, involving multiple sites
    K31.A19 Gastric intestinal metaplasia without
            dysplasia, unspecified site

● **K31.A2 Gastric intestinal metaplasia with dysplasia**
    K31.A21 Gastric intestinal metaplasia with low
            grade dysplasia
    K31.A22 Gastric intestinal metaplasia with
            high grade dysplasia
    K31.A29 Gastric intestinal metaplasia with
            dysplasia, unspecified

DISEASES OF APPENDIX (K35-K38)

● **K35 Acute appendicitis**
  ● **K35.2 Acute appendicitis with generalized peritonitis**
    ● **K35.20 Acute appendicitis with generalized
         peritonitis, without abscess (Acute)
         appendicitis with generalized
         peritonitis NOS**
         Coding Clinic: 2018, Q4, P18
         K35.200 **Acute appendicitis with
              generalized peritonitis,
              without perforation or
              abscess**
              (Acute) appendicitis with
                generalized peritonitis
                without rupture or
                perforation of
                appendix NOS
         K35.201 **Acute appendicitis with
              generalized peritonitis,
              with perforation, without
              abscess**
              Appendicitis (acute) with
                generalized (diffuse)
                peritonitis following
                rupture or perforation
                of appendix NOS
        K35.209 Acute appendicitis with generalized
            peritonitis, without abscess,
            unspecified as to perforation
             (Acute) appendicitis with
              generalized peritonitis NOS
  ● **K35.21 Acute appendicitis with generalized peritonitis,
         with abscess**
        K35.210 Acute appendicitis with generalized
            peritonitis, without perforation, with
            abscess
            (Acute) appendicitis with
              generalized peritonitis without
              rupture or perforation of
              appendix, with abscess
        K35.211 Acute appendicitis with generalized
            peritonitis, with perforation and
            abscess
            Appendicitis (acute) with
              generalized (diffuse) peritonitis
              following rupture or
              perforation of appendix, with
              abscess
        K35.219 Acute appendicitis with generalized
            peritonitis, with abscess, unspecified
            as to perforation
            (Acute) appendicitis with
              generalized peritonitis and
              abscess NOS

▶ New   ⇒ Revised   ~~deleted~~ Deleted   Excludes 1   Excludes 2   Includes   Use additional   Code first   Code also   Key words

910   OGCR Official Guidelines   X Assign placeholder X   ● Use Additional Character(s)   ▶ Manifestation Code   ⬥ Hierarchical Condition Category   Coding Clinic

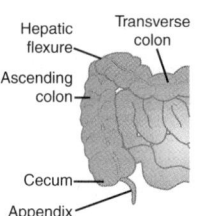

Figure 11-8 Acute appendicitis is the inflammation of the appendix, usually associated with obstruction. Most often this is a disease of adolescents and young adults.

● K35.3   Acute appendicitis with localized peritonitis

    K35.30   **Acute appendicitis with localized peritonitis, without perforation or gangrene**
       Acute appendicitis with localized peritonitis NOS

    K35.31   **Acute appendicitis with localized peritonitis and gangrene, without perforation**

    K35.32   **Acute appendicitis with perforation, localized peritonitis, and gangrene, without abscess**
       (Acute) appendicitis with perforation NOS
       Perforated appendix NOS
       Ruptured appendix (with localized peritonitis) NOS
       Coding Clinic: 2020, Q1, P16; 2018, Q4, P18

    K35.33   **Acute appendicitis with perforation, localized peritonitis, and gangrene, with abscess**
       (Acute) appendicitis with (peritoneal) abscess NOS
       Ruptured appendix with localized peritonitis and abscess

● K35.8   **Other and unspecified acute appendicitis**

    K35.80   Unspecified acute appendicitis
       Acute appendicitis NOS
       Acute appendicitis without (localized) (generalized) peritonitis

    ● K35.89   Other acute appendicitis

       K35.890   **Other acute appendicitis without perforation or gangrene**

       K35.891   **Other acute appendicitis without perforation, with gangrene**
         (Acute) appendicitis with gangrene NOS

K36   **Other appendicitis**
    Chronic appendicitis
    Recurrent appendicitis

K37   Unspecified appendicitis

    Excludes1   unspecified appendicitis with peritonitis (K35.2-, K35.3)

● K38   **Other diseases of appendix**

    K38.0   **Hyperplasia of appendix**

    K38.1   **Appendicular concretions**
       Fecalith of appendix
       Stercolith of appendix

    K38.2   **Diverticulum of appendix**

    K38.3   **Fistula of appendix**

    K38.8   **Other specified diseases of appendix**
       Intussusception of appendix

    K38.9   **Disease of appendix, unspecified**

HERNIA (K40-K46)

Note: Hernia with both gangrene and obstruction is classified to hernia with gangrene.

    Includes   acquired hernia
       congenital [except diaphragmatic or hiatus] hernia
       recurrent hernia

● K40   **Inguinal hernia**

    Includes   bubonocele
       direct inguinal hernia
       double inguinal hernia
       indirect inguinal hernia
       inguinal hernia NOS
       oblique inguinal hernia
       scrotal hernia

Item 11-11 Hernias of the groin are the most common type, accounting for 80 percent of all hernias. There are two major types of inguinal hernias: indirect (oblique) affecting men only and direct. **Indirect inguinal hernias** result when the intestines emerge through the abdominal wall in an indirect fashion through the inguinal canal. **Direct inguinal hernias** penetrate through the abdominal wall in a direct fashion. **Femoral hernias** occur at the femoral ring where the femoral vessels enter the thigh and is most common in women. An abdominal wall hernia is also called a ventral or epigastric hernia and occurs in both sexes. Classification is based on location of the hernia and whether there is obstruction or gangrene.

    Ventral, epigastric, or incisional hernia occurs on the abdominal surface caused by musculature weakness or a tear at a previous surgical site and is evidenced by a bulge that changes in size, becoming larger with exertion. An **incarcerated** hernia is one in which the intestines become trapped in the hernia. A **strangulated** hernia is one in which the blood supply to the intestines is lost. **Hiatal hernia** occurs when a loop of the stomach protrudes upward through the small opening in the diaphragm through which the esophagus passes, leaving the abdominal cavity and entering the chest. It occurs in both sexes.

Figure 11-9 Inguinal hernias are those that are located in the inguinal or iliac areas of the abdomen.

● K40.0   Bilateral inguinal hernia, with obstruction, without gangrene
       Inguinal hernia (bilateral) causing obstruction without gangrene
       Incarcerated inguinal hernia (bilateral) without gangrene
       Irreducible inguinal hernia (bilateral) without gangrene
       Strangulated inguinal hernia (bilateral) without gangrene

    K40.00   **Bilateral inguinal hernia, with obstruction, without gangrene, not specified as recurrent**
       Bilateral inguinal hernia, with obstruction, without gangrene NOS

    K40.01   **Bilateral inguinal hernia, with obstruction, without gangrene, recurrent**

● K40.1   Bilateral inguinal hernia, with gangrene

    K40.10   **Bilateral inguinal hernia, with gangrene, not specified as recurrent**
       Bilateral inguinal hernia, with gangrene NOS

    K40.11   **Bilateral inguinal hernia, with gangrene, recurrent**

● K40.2   Bilateral inguinal hernia, without obstruction or gangrene

    K40.20   **Bilateral inguinal hernia, without obstruction or gangrene, not specified as recurrent**
       Bilateral inguinal hernia NOS

    K40.21   **Bilateral inguinal hernia, without obstruction or gangrene, recurrent**

● K40.3   Unilateral inguinal hernia, with obstruction, without gangrene
       Inguinal hernia (unilateral) causing obstruction without gangrene
       Incarcerated inguinal hernia (unilateral) without gangrene
       Irreducible inguinal hernia (unilateral) without gangrene
       Strangulated inguinal hernia (unilateral) without gangrene

    K40.30   **Unilateral inguinal hernia, with obstruction, without gangrene, not specified as recurrent**
       Inguinal hernia, with obstruction NOS
       Unilateral inguinal hernia, with obstruction, without gangrene NOS

    K40.31   **Unilateral inguinal hernia, with obstruction, without gangrene, recurrent**

CHAPTER 11 (K00-K95)

CHAPTER 11 (K00-K95)

● **K40.4**   **Unilateral inguinal hernia, with gangrene**

     K40.40   **Unilateral inguinal hernia, with gangrene, not specified as recurrent**
         Inguinal hernia with gangrene NOS
         Unilateral inguinal hernia with gangrene NOS

     K40.41   **Unilateral inguinal hernia, with gangrene, recurrent**

● **K40.9**   **Unilateral inguinal hernia, without obstruction or gangrene**

     K40.90   **Unilateral inguinal hernia, without obstruction or gangrene, not specified as recurrent**
         Inguinal hernia NOS
         Unilateral inguinal hernia NOS
         Coding Clinic: 2021, Q3, P31

     K40.91   **Unilateral inguinal hernia, without obstruction or gangrene, recurrent**
         Coding Clinic: 2021, Q3, P31

● **K41**   **Femoral hernia**

● **K41.0**   **Bilateral femoral hernia, with obstruction, without gangrene**
     Femoral hernia (bilateral) causing obstruction, without gangrene
     Incarcerated femoral hernia (bilateral), without gangrene
     Irreducible femoral hernia (bilateral), without gangrene
     Strangulated femoral hernia (bilateral), without gangrene

     K41.00   **Bilateral femoral hernia, with obstruction, without gangrene, not specified as recurrent**
         Bilateral femoral hernia, with obstruction, without gangrene NOS

     K41.01   **Bilateral femoral hernia, with obstruction, without gangrene, recurrent**

● **K41.1**   **Bilateral femoral hernia, with gangrene**

     K41.10   **Bilateral femoral hernia, with gangrene, not specified as recurrent**
         Bilateral femoral hernia, with gangrene NOS

     K41.11   **Bilateral femoral hernia, with gangrene, recurrent**

● **K41.2**   **Bilateral femoral hernia, without obstruction or gangrene**

     K41.20   **Bilateral femoral hernia, without obstruction or gangrene, not specified as recurrent**
         Bilateral femoral hernia NOS

     K41.21   **Bilateral femoral hernia, without obstruction or gangrene, recurrent**

● **K41.3**   **Unilateral femoral hernia, with obstruction, without gangrene**
     Femoral hernia (unilateral) causing obstruction, without gangrene
     Incarcerated femoral hernia (unilateral), without gangrene
     Irreducible femoral hernia (unilateral), without gangrene
     Strangulated femoral hernia (unilateral), without gangrene

     K41.30   **Unilateral femoral hernia, with obstruction, without gangrene, not specified as recurrent**
         Femoral hernia, with obstruction NOS
         Unilateral femoral hernia, with obstruction NOS

     K41.31   **Unilateral femoral hernia, with obstruction, without gangrene, recurrent**
         Coding Clinic: 2021, Q3, P30

● **K41.4**   **Unilateral femoral hernia, with gangrene**

     K41.40   **Unilateral femoral hernia, with gangrene, not specified as recurrent**
         Femoral hernia, with gangrene NOS
         Unilateral femoral hernia, with gangrene NOS

     K41.41   **Unilateral femoral hernia, with gangrene, recurrent**

● **K41.9**   **Unilateral femoral hernia, without obstruction or gangrene**

     K41.90   **Unilateral femoral hernia, without obstruction or gangrene, not specified as recurrent**
         Femoral hernia NOS
         Unilateral femoral hernia NOS
         Coding Clinic: 2021, Q3, P30-31

     K41.91   **Unilateral femoral hernia, without obstruction or gangrene, recurrent**

● **K42**   **Umbilical hernia**

   Includes   paraumbilical hernia
   Excludes1   omphalocele (Q79.2)

   K42.0   **Umbilical hernia with obstruction, without gangrene**
     Umbilical hernia causing obstruction, without gangrene
     Incarcerated umbilical hernia, without gangrene
     Irreducible umbilical hernia, without gangrene
     Strangulated umbilical hernia, without gangrene

   K42.1   **Umbilical hernia with gangrene**
     Gangrenous umbilical hernia

   K42.9   **Umbilical hernia without obstruction or gangrene**
     Umbilical hernia NOS

● **K43**   **Ventral hernia**

   K43.0   **Incisional hernia with obstruction, without gangrene**
     Incisional hernia causing obstruction, without gangrene
     Incarcerated incisional hernia, without gangrene
     Irreducible incisional hernia, without gangrene
     Strangulated incisional hernia, without gangrene

   K43.1   **Incisional hernia with gangrene**
     Gangrenous incisional hernia

   K43.2   **Incisional hernia without obstruction or gangrene**
     Incisional hernia NOS

   K43.3   **Parastomal hernia with obstruction, without gangrene**
     Incarcerated parastomal hernia, without gangrene
     Irreducible parastomal hernia, without gangrene
     Parastomal hernia causing obstruction, without gangrene
     Strangulated parastomal hernia, without gangrene

   K43.4   **Parastomal hernia with gangrene**
     Gangrenous parastomal hernia

   K43.5   **Parastomal hernia without obstruction or gangrene**
     Parastomal hernia NOS

   K43.6   **Other and unspecified ventral hernia with obstruction, without gangrene**
     Epigastric hernia causing obstruction, without gangrene
     Hypogastric hernia causing obstruction, without gangrene
     Incarcerated epigastric hernia without gangrene
     Incarcerated hypogastric hernia without gangrene
     Incarcerated midline hernia without gangrene
     Incarcerated spigelian hernia without gangrene
     Incarcerated subxiphoid hernia without gangrene
     Irreducible epigastric hernia without gangrene
     Irreducible hypogastric hernia without gangrene
     Irreducible midline hernia without gangrene
     Irreducible spigelian hernia without gangrene
     Irreducible subxiphoid hernia without gangrene
     Midline hernia causing obstruction, without gangrene
     Spigelian hernia causing obstruction, without gangrene
     Strangulated epigastric hernia without gangrene
     Strangulated hypogastric hernia without gangrene
     Strangulated midline hernia without gangrene
     Strangulated spigelian hernia without gangrene
     Strangulated subxiphoid hernia without gangrene
     Subxiphoid hernia causing obstruction, without gangrene

   K43.7   **Other and unspecified ventral hernia with gangrene**
     Any condition listed under K43.6 specified as gangrenous

   K43.9   **Ventral hernia without obstruction or gangrene**
     Epigastric hernia
     Ventral hernia NOS

▶ New   ⇒ Revised   ~~deleted~~ Deleted   Excludes 1   Excludes 2   Includes   Use additional   Code first   Code also   Key words

OGCR Official Guidelines   X Assign placeholder X   ● Use Additional Character(s)   ▶ Manifestation Code   🔖 Hierarchical Condition Category   **Coding Clinic**

Item 11–12 Crohn's disease, also known as **regional enteritis,** is a chronic inflammatory disease of the intestines. Classification is based on location in the small (duodenum, ileum, jejunum) or large (cecum, colon, rectum, anal canal) intestine.

● **K44 Diaphragmatic hernia**
  Includes   hiatus hernia (esophageal) (sliding)
       paraesophageal hernia
  Excludes1   congenital diaphragmatic hernia (Q79.0)
       congenital hiatus hernia (Q40.1)

  K44.0 Diaphragmatic hernia with obstruction, without gangrene
     Diaphragmatic hernia causing obstruction
     Incarcerated diaphragmatic hernia
     Irreducible diaphragmatic hernia
     Strangulated diaphragmatic hernia
     Coding Clinic: 2022, Q2, P14

  K44.1 Diaphragmatic hernia with gangrene
     Gangrenous diaphragmatic hernia

  K44.9 Diaphragmatic hernia without obstruction or gangrene
     Diaphragmatic hernia NOS
     Coding Clinic: 2017, Q1, P7

● **K45 Other abdominal hernia**
  Includes   abdominal hernia, specified site NEC
       lumbar hernia
       obturator hernia
       pudendal hernia
       retroperitoneal hernia
       sciatic hernia

  K45.0 Other specified abdominal hernia with obstruction, without gangrene
     Other specified abdominal hernia causing obstruction
     Other specified incarcerated abdominal hernia
     Other specified irreducible abdominal hernia
     Other specified strangulated abdominal hernia

  K45.1 Other specified abdominal hernia with gangrene
     Any condition listed under K45 specified as gangrenous
     Coding Clinic: 2024, Q2, P22, 23

  K45.8 Other specified abdominal hernia without obstruction or gangrene

● **K46 Unspecified abdominal hernia**
  Includes   enterocele
       epiplocele
       hernia NOS
       interstitial hernia
       intestinal hernia
       intra-abdominal hernia
  Excludes1   vaginal enterocele (N81.5)

  K46.0 Unspecified abdominal hernia with obstruction, without gangrene , 1091
     Unspecified abdominal hernia causing obstruction
     Unspecified incarcerated abdominal hernia
     Unspecified irreducible abdominal hernia
     Unspecified strangulated abdominal hernia

  K46.1 Unspecified abdominal hernia with gangrene
     Any condition listed under K46 specified as gangrenous

  K46.9 Unspecified abdominal hernia without obstruction or gangrene
     Abdominal hernia NOS

⭑ **(See Plate 32 of the Anatomy Illustrations.)**

NONINFECTIVE ENTERITIS AND COLITIS (K50-K52)
  Includes   noninfective inflammatory bowel disease
  Excludes1   irritable bowel syndrome (K58.-)
       megacolon (K59.3-)

● **K50 Crohn's disease [regional enteritis]**
  Includes   granulomatous enteritis
  Use additional code to identify manifestations, such as:
  pyoderma gangrenosum (L88)
▶Use Additional code to identify any associated fistulas, if applicable:
   ▶anal fistula (K60.3-)
   ▶anorectal fistula (K60.5-)
   ▶rectal fistula (K60.4-)
  Excludes1   ulcerative colitis (K51.-)

● **K50.0 Crohn's disease of small intestine**
     Crohn's disease [regional enteritis] of duodenum
     Crohn's disease [regional enteritis] of ileum
     Crohn's disease [regional enteritis] of jejunum
     Regional ileitis
     Terminal ileitis
    Excludes1   Crohn's disease of both small and large intestine (K50.8-)

  K50.00 Crohn's disease of small intestine without complications 🔗

● **K50.01 Crohn's disease of small intestine with complications**
    K50.011 Crohn's disease of small intestine with rectal bleeding 🔗
    K50.012 Crohn's disease of small intestine with intestinal obstruction 🔗
    K50.013 Crohn's disease of small intestine with fistula 🔗
    K50.014 Crohn's disease of small intestine with abscess 🔗
       Coding Clinic: 2012, Q4, P104
    K50.018 Crohn's disease of small intestine with other complication 🔗
    K50.019 Crohn's disease of small intestine with unspecified complications 🔗

● **K50.1 Crohn's disease of large intestine**
     Crohn's disease [regional enteritis] of colon
     Crohn's disease [regional enteritis] of large bowel
     Crohn's disease [regional enteritis] of rectum
     Granulomatous colitis
     Regional colitis
    Excludes1   Crohn's disease of both small and large intestine (K50.8)

  K50.10 Crohn's disease of large intestine without complications 🔗

● **K50.11 Crohn's disease of large intestine with complications**
    K50.111 Crohn's disease of large intestine with rectal bleeding 🔗
    K50.112 Crohn's disease of large intestine with intestinal obstruction 🔗
    K50.113 Crohn's disease of large intestine with fistula 🔗
    K50.114 Crohn's disease of large intestine with abscess 🔗
       Coding Clinic: 2012, Q4, P104

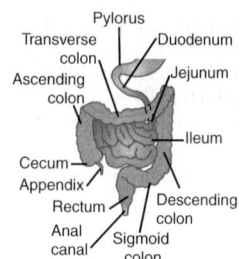

Figure 11-10 Small and large intestines.

CHAPTER 11 (K00-K95)

K50.118   Crohn's disease of large intestine with other complication 🖫

K50.119   Crohn's disease of large intestine with unspecified complications 🖫

● **K50.8**   Crohn's disease of both small and large intestine

    K50.80   Crohn's disease of both small and large intestine without complications 🖫

● **K50.81**   Crohn's disease of both small and large intestine with complications

      K50.811   Crohn's disease of both small and large intestine with rectal bleeding 🖫

      K50.812   Crohn's disease of both small and large intestine with intestinal obstruction 🖫

      K50.813   Crohn's disease of both small and large intestine with fistula 🖫

      K50.814   Crohn's disease of both small and large intestine with abscess 🖫
        Coding Clinic: 2012, Q4, P104

      K50.818   Crohn's disease of both small and large intestine with other complication 🖫

      K50.819   Crohn's disease of both small and large intestine with unspecified complications 🖫

● **K50.9**   Crohn's disease, unspecified

    K50.90   Crohn's disease, unspecified, without complications 🖫
      Crohn's disease NOS
      Regional enteritis NOS

● **K50.91**   Crohn's disease, unspecified, with complications

      K50.911   Crohn's disease, unspecified, with rectal bleeding 🖫

      K50.912   Crohn's disease, unspecified, with intestinal obstruction 🖫

      K50.913   Crohn's disease, unspecified, with fistula 🖫

      K50.914   Crohn's disease, unspecified, with abscess 🖫
        Coding Clinic: 2012, Q4, P104

      K50.918   Crohn's disease, unspecified, with other complication 🖫

      K50.919   Crohn's disease, unspecified, with unspecified complications 🖫

● **K51**   Ulcerative colitis
   Use additional code to identify manifestations, such as: pyoderma gangrenosum (L88)
  ▶ Use Additional code to identify any associated fistulas, if applicable:
    ▶ anal fistula (K60.3-)
    ▶ anorectal fistula (K60.5-)
    ▶ rectal fistula (K60.4-)
   Excludes1   Crohn's disease [regional enteritis] (K50.-)

● **K51.0**   Ulcerative (chronic) pancolitis
    Backwash ileitis

    K51.00   Ulcerative (chronic) pancolitis without complications 🖫
      Ulcerative (chronic) pancolitis NOS

● **K51.01**   Ulcerative (chronic) pancolitis with complications

      K51.011   Ulcerative (chronic) pancolitis with rectal bleeding 🖫

      K51.012   Ulcerative (chronic) pancolitis with intestinal obstruction 🖫

      K51.013   Ulcerative (chronic) pancolitis with fistula 🖫

      K51.014   Ulcerative (chronic) pancolitis with abscess 🖫

Item 11-13 Ulcerative colitis attacks the colonic mucosa and forms abscesses. The disease involves the intestines. Classification is based on the location:
- Enterocolitis: large and small intestine
- Ileocolitis: ileum and colon
- Proctitis: rectum
- Proctosigmoiditis: sigmoid colon and rectum

      K51.018   Ulcerative (chronic) pancolitis with other complication 🖫

      K51.019   Ulcerative (chronic) pancolitis with unspecified complications 🖫

● **K51.2**   Ulcerative (chronic) proctitis

    K51.20   Ulcerative (chronic) proctitis without complications 🖫
      Ulcerative (chronic) proctitis NOS

● **K51.21**   Ulcerative (chronic) proctitis with complications

      K51.211   Ulcerative (chronic) proctitis with rectal bleeding 🖫

      K51.212   Ulcerative (chronic) proctitis with intestinal obstruction 🖫

      K51.213   Ulcerative (chronic) proctitis with fistula 🖫

      K51.214   Ulcerative (chronic) proctitis with abscess 🖫

      K51.218   Ulcerative (chronic) proctitis with other complication 🖫

      K51.219   Ulcerative (chronic) proctitis with unspecified complications 🖫

● **K51.3**   Ulcerative (chronic) rectosigmoiditis

    K51.30   Ulcerative (chronic) rectosigmoiditis without complications 🖫
      Ulcerative (chronic) rectosigmoiditis NOS

● **K51.31**   Ulcerative (chronic) rectosigmoiditis with complications

      K51.311   Ulcerative (chronic) rectosigmoiditis with rectal bleeding 🖫

      K51.312   Ulcerative (chronic) rectosigmoiditis with intestinal obstruction 🖫

      K51.313   Ulcerative (chronic) rectosigmoiditis with fistula 🖫

      K51.314   Ulcerative (chronic) rectosigmoiditis with abscess 🖫

      K51.318   Ulcerative (chronic) rectosigmoiditis with other complication 🖫

      K51.319   Ulcerative (chronic) rectosigmoiditis with unspecified complications 🖫

● **K51.4**   Inflammatory polyps of colon

    Excludes2   adenomatous polyp of colon (D12.6)
        polyposis of colon (D12.6)
        polyps of colon NOS (K63.5)

    K51.40   Inflammatory polyps of colon without complications 🖫
      Inflammatory polyps of colon NOS

● **K51.41**   Inflammatory polyps of colon with complications

      K51.411   Inflammatory polyps of colon with rectal bleeding 🖫

      K51.412   Inflammatory polyps of colon with intestinal obstruction 🖫

      K51.413   Inflammatory polyps of colon with fistula 🖫

      K51.414   Inflammatory polyps of colon with abscess 🖫

      K51.418   Inflammatory polyps of colon with other complication 🖫

      K51.419   Inflammatory polyps of colon with unspecified complications 🖫

▶ New   ⇒ Revised   ~~deleted~~ Deleted   Excludes 1   Excludes 2   Includes   Use additional   Code first   Code also   Key words
OGCR Official Guidelines   X Assign placeholder X   ● Use Additional Character(s)   ▌ Manifestation Code   🖫 Hierarchical Condition Category   Coding Clinic

● K51.5   **Left sided colitis**
Left hemicolitis
  K51.50   **Left sided colitis without complications** 🔗
Left sided colitis NOS
● K51.51   **Left sided colitis with complications**
    K51.511   **Left sided colitis with rectal bleeding** 🔗
    K51.512   **Left sided colitis with intestinal obstruction** 🔗
    K51.513   **Left sided colitis with fistula** 🔗
    K51.514   **Left sided colitis with abscess** 🔗
    K51.518   **Left sided colitis with other complication** 🔗
    K51.519   **Left sided colitis with unspecified complications** 🔗
● K51.8   **Other ulcerative colitis**
  K51.80   **Other ulcerative colitis without complications** 🔗
● K51.81   **Other ulcerative colitis with complications**
    K51.811   **Other ulcerative colitis with rectal bleeding** 🔗
    K51.812   **Other ulcerative colitis with intestinal obstruction** 🔗
    K51.813   **Other ulcerative colitis with fistula** 🔗
    K51.814   **Other ulcerative colitis with abscess** 🔗
    K51.818   **Other ulcerative colitis with other complication** 🔗
    K51.819   **Other ulcerative colitis with unspecified complications** 🔗
● K51.9   **Ulcerative colitis, unspecified**
  K51.90   **Ulcerative colitis, unspecified, without complications** 🔗
● K51.91   **Ulcerative colitis, unspecified, with complications**
    K51.911   **Ulcerative colitis, unspecified with rectal bleeding** 🔗
    K51.912   **Ulcerative colitis, unspecified with intestinal obstruction** 🔗
    K51.913   **Ulcerative colitis, unspecified with fistula** 🔗
    K51.914   **Ulcerative colitis, unspecified with abscess** 🔗
    K51.918   **Ulcerative colitis, unspecified with other complication** 🔗
    K51.919   **Ulcerative colitis, unspecified with unspecified complications** 🔗
● K52   **Other and unspecified noninfective gastroenteritis and colitis**
  K52.0   **Gastroenteritis and colitis due to radiation**
  K52.1   **Toxic gastroenteritis and colitis**
Drug-induced gastroenteritis and colitis
Code first (T51-T65) to identify toxic agent
Use additional code for adverse effect, if applicable, to identify drug (T36-T50 with fifth or sixth character 5)
Coding Clinic: 2019, Q1, P17
● K52.2   **Allergic and dietetic gastroenteritis and colitis**
Food hypersensitivity gastroenteritis or colitis
Use additional code to identify type of food allergy (Z91.01-, Z91.02-)
    Excludes2   allergic eosinophilic colitis (K52.82)
allergic eosinophilic esophagitis (K20.0)
allergic eosinophilic gastritis (K52.81)
allergic eosinophilic gastroenteritis (K52.81)
Coding Clinic: 2016, Q4, P30-31
  K52.21   **Food protein-induced enterocolitis syndrome**
FPIES
Use additional code for hypovolemic shock, if present (R57.1)
  K52.22   **Food protein-induced enteropathy**

  K52.29   **Other allergic and dietetic gastroenteritis and colitis**
Allergic proctocolitis
Food hypersensitivity gastroenteritis or colitis
Food-induced eosinophilic proctocolitis
Food protein-induced proctocolitis
Immediate gastrointestinal hypersensitivity
Milk protein-induced proctocolitis
  K52.3   **Indeterminate colitis**
Colonic inflammatory bowel disease unclassified (IBDU)
    Excludes1   unspecified colitis (K52.9)
● K52.8   **Other specified noninfective gastroenteritis and colitis**
  K52.81   **Eosinophilic gastritis or gastroenteritis**
Eosinophilic enteritis
    Excludes2   eosinophilic esophagitis (K20.0)
  K52.82   **Eosinophilic colitis**
    Excludes2   allergic proctocolitis (K52.29)
food-induced eosinophilic proctocolitis (K52.29)
food protein-induced enterocolitis syndrome (FPIES) (K52.21)
food protein-induced proctocolitis (K52.29)
milk protein-induced proctocolitis (K52.29)
● K52.83   **Microscopic colitis**
Coding Clinic: 2016, Q4, P30-31
    K52.831   **Collagenous colitis**
    K52.832   **Lymphocytic colitis**
    K52.838   **Other microscopic colitis**
    K52.839   **Microscopic colitis, unspecified**
  K52.89   **Other specified noninfective gastroenteritis and colitis**
Coding Clinic: 2019, Q1, P21
  K52.9   **Noninfective gastroenteritis and colitis, unspecified**
Colitis NOS   Ileitis NOS
Enteritis NOS   Jejunitis NOS
Gastroenteritis NOS   Sigmoiditis NOS
    Excludes1   diarrhea NOS (R19.7)
functional diarrhea (K59.1)
infectious gastroenteritis and colitis NOS (A09)
neonatal diarrhea (noninfective) (P78.3)
psychogenic diarrhea (F45.8)
Coding Clinic: 2021, Q3, P3-4

OTHER DISEASES OF INTESTINES (K55-K64)

● K55   **Vascular disorders of intestine**
    Excludes1   necrotizing enterocolitis of newborn (P77.-)
    Excludes2   angioectasia (angiodysplasia) duodenum (K31.81)
● K55.0   **Acute vascular disorders of intestine**
Infarction of appendices epiploicae
Mesenteric (artery) (vein) embolism
Mesenteric (artery) (vein) infarction
Mesenteric (artery) (vein) thrombosis
Coding Clinic: 2019, Q4, P68
● K55.01   **Acute (reversible) ischemia of small intestine**
Coding Clinic: 2016, Q4, P32
    K55.011   **Focal (segmental) acute (reversible) ischemia of small intestine** 🔗
    K55.012   **Diffuse acute (reversible) ischemia of small intestine** 🔗
    K55.019   **Acute (reversible) ischemia of small intestine, extent unspecified** 🔗
● K55.02   **Acute infarction of small intestine**
Gangrene of small intestine
Necrosis of small intestine
Coding Clinic: 2016, Q4, P32
    K55.021   **Focal (segmental) acute infarction of small intestine** 🔗
    K55.022   **Diffuse acute infarction of small intestine** 🔗
    K55.029   **Acute infarction of small intestine, extent unspecified** 🔗

● **K55.03**   Acute (reversible) ischemia of large intestine
Acute fulminant ischemic colitis
Subacute ischemic colitis
Coding Clinic: 2016, Q4, P32

   K55.031   Focal (segmental) acute (reversible) ischemia of large intestine 🔖

   K55.032   Diffuse acute (reversible) ischemia of large intestine 🔖

   K55.039   Acute (reversible) ischemia of large intestine, extent unspecified 🔖
Coding Clinic: 2019, Q4, P68

● **K55.04**   Acute infarction of large intestine
Gangrene of large intestine
Necrosis of large intestine
Coding Clinic: 2016, Q4, P32

   K55.041   Focal (segmental) acute infarction of large intestine 🔖

   K55.042   Diffuse acute infarction of large intestine 🔖

   K55.049   Acute infarction of large intestine, extent unspecified 🔖

● **K55.05**   Acute (reversible) ischemia of intestine, part unspecified

   K55.051   Focal (segmental) acute (reversible) ischemia of intestine, part unspecified 🔖

   K55.052   Diffuse acute (reversible) ischemia of intestine, part unspecified 🔖

   K55.059   Acute (reversible) ischemia of intestine, part and extent unspecified 🔖

● **K55.06**   Acute infarction of intestine, part unspecified
Acute intestinal infarction
Gangrene of intestine
Necrosis of intestine

   K55.061   Focal (segmental) acute infarction of intestine, part unspecified 🔖

   K55.062   Diffuse acute infarction of intestine, part unspecified 🔖

   K55.069   Acute infarction of intestine, part and extent unspecified 🔖

K55.1   Chronic vascular disorders of intestine 🔖
Chronic ischemic colitis
Chronic ischemic enteritis
Chronic ischemic enterocolitis
Ischemic stricture of intestine
Mesenteric atherosclerosis
Mesenteric vascular insufficiency

● **K55.2**   Angiodysplasia of colon

   K55.20   Angiodysplasia of colon without hemorrhage

   K55.21   Angiodysplasia of colon with hemorrhage

● **K55.3**   Necrotizing enterocolitis

   Excludes1   necrotizing enterocolitis of newborn (P77.-)

   Excludes2   necrotizing enterocolitis due to Clostridium difficile (A04.7-)

   K55.30   Necrotizing enterocolitis, unspecified 🔖
Necrotizing enterocolitis, NOS

   K55.31   Stage 1 necrotizing enterocolitis 🔖
Necrotizing enterocolitis without pneumatosis, without perforation
Coding Clinic: 2016, Q4, P32

   K55.32   Stage 2 necrotizing enterocolitis 🔖
Necrotizing enterocolitis with pneumatosis, without perforation
Coding Clinic: 2016, Q4, P32

   K55.33   Stage 3 necrotizing enterocolitis 🔖
Necrotizing enterocolitis with perforation
Necrotizing enterocolitis with pneumatosis and perforation
Coding Clinic: 2016, Q4, P32

K55.8   Other vascular disorders of intestine 🔖

K55.9   Vascular disorder of intestine, unspecified 🔖
Ischemic colitis
Ischemic enteritis
Ischemic enterocolitis

● **K56**   Paralytic ileus and intestinal obstruction without hernia

   Excludes1   congenital stricture or stenosis of intestine (Q41-Q42)
cystic fibrosis with meconium ileus (E84.11)
ischemic stricture of intestine (K55.1)
meconium ileus NOS (P76.0)
neonatal intestinal obstructions classifiable to P76.-
obstruction of duodenum (K31.5)
postprocedural intestinal obstruction (K91.3-)

   Excludes2   stenosis of anus or rectum (K62.4)

K56.0   Paralytic ileus 🔖
Paralysis of bowel
Paralysis of colon
Paralysis of intestine

   Excludes1   gallstone ileus (K56.3)
ileus NOS (K56.7)
obstructive ileus NOS (K56.69-)

K56.1   Intussusception 🔖
Intussusception or invagination of bowel
Intussusception or invagination of colon
Intussusception or invagination of intestine
Intussusception or invagination of rectum

   Excludes2   intussusception of appendix (K38.8)
Coding Clinic: 2023, Q3, P12

K56.2   Volvulus 🔖
Strangulation of colon or intestine
Torsion of colon or intestine
Twist of colon or intestine

   Excludes2   volvulus of duodenum (K31.5)
Coding Clinic: 2024, Q2, P22

K56.3   Gallstone ileus 🔖
Obstruction of intestine by gallstone

● **K56.4**   Other impaction of intestine

   K56.41   Fecal impaction 🔖

    Excludes2   incomplete defecation (R15.0)
Coding Clinic: 2024, Q2, P6

   K56.49   Other impaction of intestine 🔖

● **K56.5**   Intestinal adhesions [bands] with obstruction (postinfection)
Abdominal hernia due to adhesions with obstruction
Peritoneal adhesions [bands] with intestinal obstruction (postinfection)

   K56.50   Intestinal adhesions [bands], unspecified as to partial versus complete obstruction 🔖
Intestinal adhesions with obstruction NOS

   K56.51   Intestinal adhesions [bands], with partial obstruction 🔖
Intestinal adhesions with incomplete obstruction

   K56.52   Intestinal adhesions [bands] with complete obstruction 🔖

● **K56.6**   Other and unspecified intestinal obstruction

   ● **K56.60**   Unspecified intestinal obstruction
Coding Clinic: 2017, Q2, P12

    K56.600   Partial intestinal obstruction, unspecified as to cause 🔖
Incomplete intestinal obstruction, NOS

▶ New   ⇒ Revised   ~~deleted~~ Deleted   Excludes 1   Excludes 2   Includes   Use additional   Code first   Code also   Key words
OGCR Official Guidelines   X Assign placeholder X   ● Use Additional Character(s)   ▷ Manifestation Code   🔖 Hierarchical Condition Category   Coding Clinic

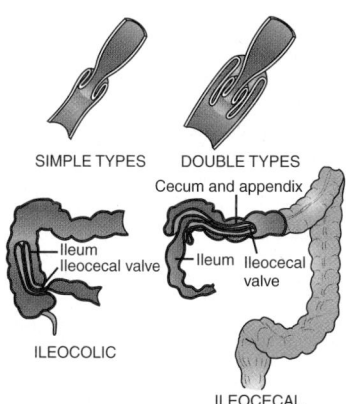

Figure 11-11   Types of intussusception.

Item 11–14   Intussusception is the prolapse (telescoping) of a part of the intestine into another adjacent part of the intestine. Intussusception may be enteric (ileoileal, jejunoileal, jejunojejunal), colic (colocolic), or intracolic (ileocecal, ileocolic).

Item 11–15   Volvulus is the twisting of a segment of the intestine, resulting in obstruction. Paralytic ileus is paralysis of the intestine. It need not be a complete paralysis, but it must prohibit the passage of food through the intestine and lead to intestinal blockage. It is a common aftermath of some types of surgery.

     K56.601   **Complete intestinal obstruction, unspecified as to cause** 🔁

     K56.609   **Unspecified intestinal obstruction, unspecified as to partial versus complete obstruction** 🔁
         Intestinal obstruction NOS

● K56.69   **Other intestinal obstruction**
     Enterostenosis NOS
     Obstructive ileus NOS
     Occlusion of colon or intestine NOS
     Stenosis of colon or intestine NOS
     Stricture of colon or intestine NOS
     Coding Clinic: 2017, Q2, P12

     K56.690   **Other partial intestinal obstruction** 🔁
         Other incomplete intestinal obstruction

     K56.691   **Other complete intestinal obstruction** 🔁

     K56.699   **Other intestinal obstruction unspecified as to partial versus complete obstruction** 🔁
         Other intestinal obstruction, NEC
         Coding Clinic: 2023, Q3, P11

K56.7   **Ileus, unspecified** 🔁

     Excludes1   obstructive ileus (K56.69-)

     Excludes2   intestinal obstruction with hernia (K40-K46)
     Coding Clinic: 2017, Q1, P41

● K57   **Diverticular disease of intestine**
     Code also if applicable peritonitis K65.-

     Excludes1   congenital diverticulum of intestine (Q43.8)
               Meckel's diverticulum (Q43.0)

     Excludes2   diverticulum of appendix (K38.2)
     Coding Clinic: 2022, Q1, P26

● K57.0   **Diverticulitis of small intestine with perforation and abscess**

     Excludes1   diverticulitis of both small and large intestine with perforation and abscess (K57.4-)

     K57.00   **Diverticulitis of small intestine with perforation and abscess without bleeding**

     K57.01   **Diverticulitis of small intestine with perforation and abscess with bleeding**

Figure 11-12   Diverticulosis. (From Shiland: Mastering Healthcare Terminology, ed 4, St. Louis, Mosby, 2012)

Item 11–16   Diverticula of the intestines are acquired herniations of the mucosa. Diverticulum (singular): Pocket or pouch that bulges outward through a weak spot (herniation) in the colon. Diverticula (plural). **Diverticulosis** is the condition of having diverticula. **Diverticulitis** is inflammation of these pouches or herniations. Classification is based on location (small intestine or colon) and whether it occurs with or without hemorrhage.

● K57.1   **Diverticular disease of small intestine without perforation or abscess**

     Excludes1   diverticular disease of both small and large intestine without perforation or abscess (K57.5-)

     K57.10   **Diverticulosis of small intestine without perforation or abscess without bleeding**
         Diverticular disease of small intestine NOS

     K57.11   **Diverticulosis of small intestine without perforation or abscess with bleeding**

     K57.12   **Diverticulitis of small intestine without perforation or abscess without bleeding**

     K57.13   **Diverticulitis of small intestine without perforation or abscess with bleeding**

● K57.2   **Diverticulitis of large intestine with perforation and abscess**

     Excludes1   diverticulitis of both small and large intestine with perforation and abscess (K57.4-)
     Coding Clinic: 2022, Q1, P27

     K57.20   **Diverticulitis of large intestine with perforation and abscess without bleeding**
         Coding Clinic: 2022, Q1, P26

     K57.21   **Diverticulitis of large intestine with perforation and abscess with bleeding**

● K57.3   **Diverticular disease of large intestine without perforation or abscess**

     Excludes1   diverticular disease of both small and large intestine without perforation or abscess (K57.5-)

     K57.30   **Diverticulosis of large intestine without perforation or abscess without bleeding**
         Diverticular disease of colon NOS

     K57.31   **Diverticulosis of large intestine without perforation or abscess with bleeding**

     K57.32   **Diverticulitis of large intestine without perforation or abscess without bleeding**

     K57.33   **Diverticulitis of large intestine without perforation or abscess with bleeding**

● K57.4   **Diverticulitis of both small and large intestine with perforation and abscess**

     K57.40   **Diverticulitis of both small and large intestine with perforation and abscess without bleeding**

     K57.41   **Diverticulitis of both small and large intestine with perforation and abscess with bleeding**

● **K57.5** **Diverticular disease of both small and large intestine without perforation or abscess**

    K57.50 **Diverticulosis of both small and large intestine without perforation or abscess without bleeding**
        Diverticular disease of both small and large intestine NOS

    K57.51 **Diverticulosis of both small and large intestine without perforation or abscess with bleeding**

    K57.52 **Diverticulitis of both small and large intestine without perforation or abscess without bleeding**

    K57.53 **Diverticulitis of both small and large intestine without perforation or abscess with bleeding**

● **K57.8** **Diverticulitis of intestine, part unspecified, with perforation and abscess**

    K57.80 **Diverticulitis of intestine, part unspecified, with perforation and abscess without bleeding**

    K57.81 **Diverticulitis of intestine, part unspecified, with perforation and abscess with bleeding**

● **K57.9** **Diverticular disease of intestine, part unspecified, without perforation or abscess**

    K57.90 **Diverticulosis of intestine, part unspecified, without perforation or abscess without bleeding**
        Diverticular disease of intestine NOS
        Coding Clinic: 2021, Q1, P12

    K57.91 **Diverticulosis of intestine, part unspecified, without perforation or abscess with bleeding**

    K57.92 **Diverticulitis of intestine, part unspecified, without perforation or abscess without bleeding**

    K57.93 **Diverticulitis of intestine, part unspecified, without perforation or abscess with bleeding**

● **K58** **Irritable bowel syndrome**

    Includes   irritable colon
                spastic colon

    K58.0 **Irritable bowel syndrome with diarrhea**

    K58.1 **Irritable bowel syndrome with constipation**
        Coding Clinic: 2016, Q4, P32

    K58.2 **Mixed irritable bowel syndrome**
        Coding Clinic: 2016, Q4, P32

    K58.8 **Other irritable bowel syndrome**
        Coding Clinic: 2016, Q4, P32

    K58.9 **Irritable bowel syndrome without diarrhea**
        ⇒Irritable bowel syndrome, unspecified

● **K59** **Other functional intestinal disorders**

    Excludes1   change in bowel habit NOS (R19.4)
                intestinal malabsorption (K90.-)
                psychogenic intestinal disorders (F45.8)

    Excludes2   functional disorders of stomach (K31.-)

● **K59.0** **Constipation**

    Excludes2   incomplete defecation (R15.0)
        Coding Clinic: 2024, Q2, P6

    K59.00 **Constipation, unspecified**

    K59.01 **Slow transit constipation**

    K59.02 **Outlet dysfunction constipation**
        Coding Clinic: 2023, Q1, P24

    K59.03 **Drug induced constipation**
        Use additional code for adverse effect, if applicable, to identify drug (T36-T50 with fifth or sixth character 5)
        Coding Clinic: 2016, Q4, P33

    K59.04 **Chronic idiopathic constipation**
        Functional constipation
        Coding Clinic: 2016, Q4, P33

    K59.09 **Other constipation**
        Chronic constipation

K59.1 **Functional diarrhea**

    Excludes1   diarrhea NOS (R19.7)
                irritable bowel syndrome with diarrhea (K58.0)

K59.2 **Neurogenic bowel, not elsewhere classified**

● **K59.3** **Megacolon, not elsewhere classified**
    Dilatation of colon
    Code first, if applicable (T51-T65) to identify toxic agent

    Excludes1   congenital megacolon (aganglionic) (Q43.1)
                megacolon (due to) (in) Chagas' disease (B57.32)
                megacolon (due to) (in) Clostridium difficile (A04.7-)
                megacolon (due to) (in) Hirschsprung's disease (Q43.1)
    Coding Clinic: 2016, Q4, P33

    K59.31 **Toxic megacolon** 🅗🅒

    K59.39 **Other megacolon**
        Megacolon NOS

K59.4 **Anal spasm**
    Proctalgia fugax

● **K59.8** **Other specified functional intestinal disorders**

    K59.81 Ogilvie syndrome
        Acute colonic pseudo-obstruction (ACPO)

    K59.89 Other specified functional intestinal disorders
        Atony of colon
        Pseudo-obstruction (acute) (chronic) of intestine

K59.9 **Functional intestinal disorder, unspecified**

● **K60** **Fissure and fistula of anal and rectal regions**

    Excludes1   fissure and fistula of anal and rectal regions with abscess or cellulitis (K61.-)
         ▶abscess or cellulitis off anal and rectal regions (K61.-)

    Excludes2   anal sphincter tear (healed) (nontraumatic) (old) (K62.81)

K60.0 **Acute anal fissure**

K60.1 **Chronic anal fissure**

K60.2 **Anal fissure, unspecified**

K60.3 **Anal fistula**
    ▶*Code first, if applicable:*
        ▶Crohn's disease (K50.-)
        ▶ulcerative colitis (K51.-)

    Excludes1   congenital fistula (Q43.6)

   ▶ **K60.30** **Anal fistula, unspecified**
        ▶Anal fistula NOS

   ▶● **K60.31** **Anal fistula, simple**
        ▶Low intersphincteric anal fistula
        ▶Superficial anal fistula

     ▶ **K60.311** **Anal fistula, simple, initial**
        ▶Anal fistula, simple, new

     ▶ **K60.312** **Anal fistula, simple, persistent**
        ▶Anal fistula, simple, chronic

     ▶ **K60.313** **Anal fistula, simple, recurrent**
        ▶Anal fistula simple, occurring following complete healing

     ▶ **K60.319** **Anal fistula, simple, unspecified**

   ▶● **K60.32** **Anal fistula, complex**
        ▶Extrasphincteric anal fistula
        ▶High intersphincteric anal fistula
        ▶Suprasphincteric anal fistula
        ▶Transsphincteric anal fistula

        ▶Code also, if applicable:
        ▶perianal abscess (K61.0)
        ▶rectovaginal fistula (N82.3)
        ▶stenosis of anus and rectum (K62.4)

     ▶ **K60.321** **Anal fistula, complex, initial**
        ▶Anal fistula, complex, new

▶ New   ⇒ Revised   ~~deleted~~ Deleted   Excludes 1   Excludes 2   Includes   Use additional   Code first   Code also   Key words
OGCR Official Guidelines   X Assign placeholder X   ● Use Additional Character(s)   ▶ Manifestation Code   🅗🅒 Hierarchical Condition Category   Coding Clinic

▶ **K60.322**   **Anal fistula, complex, persistent**
   ▶ Anal fistula, complex, chronic

▶ **K60.323**   **Anal fistula, complex, recurrent**
   ▶ Anal fistula complex, occurring following complete healing

▶ **K60.329**   **Anal fistula, complex, unspecified**

K60.4   **Rectal fistula**
Fistula of rectum to skin
▶ *Code first, if applicable:*
 ▶ Crohn's disease (K50.-)
 ▶ ulcerative colitis (K51.-)
Excludes1   congenital fistula (Q43.6)
      rectovaginal fistula (N82.3)
      vesicorectal fistula (N32.1)

▶ **K60.40**   **Rectal fistula, unspecified**
   ▶ Rectal fistula NOS

▶● **K60.41**   **Rectal fistula, simple**
   ▶ Low intersphincteric rectal fistula
   ▶ Superficial rectal fistula

   ▶ **K60.411**   **Rectal fistula, simple, initial**
     ▶ Rectal, fistula, simple, new

   ▶ **K60.412**   **Rectal fistula, simple, persistent**
     ▶ Rectal fistula, simple, chronic

   ▶ **K60.413**   **Rectal fistula, simple, recurrent**
     ▶ Rectal fistula simple, occurring following complete healing

   ▶ **K60.419**   **Rectal fistula, simple, unspecified**

▶● **K60.42**   **Rectal fistula, complex**
   ▶ Extrasphincteric rectal fistula
   ▶ High intersphincteric rectal fistula
   ▶ Suprasphincteric rectal fistula
   ▶ Transsphincteric rectal fistula
   ▶ *Code also, if applicable:*
     ▶ perianal abscess (K61.0)
     ▶ rectovaginal fistula (N82.3)
     ▶ stenosis of anus and rectum (K62.4)

   ▶ **K60.421**   **Rectal fistula, complex, initial**
     ▶ Rectal fistula, complex, new

   ▶ **K60.422**   **Rectal fistula, complex, persistent**
     ▶ Rectal fistula, complex, chronic

   ▶ **K60.423**   **Rectal fistula, complex, recurrent**
     ▶ Rectal fistula complex occurring following complete healing

   ▶ **K60.429**   **Rectal fistula, complex, unspecified**

K60.5   **Anorectal fistula**
▶ *Code first, if applicable:*
 ▶ Crohn's disease (K50.-)
 ▶ ulcerative colitis (K51.-)
Excludes1   congenital fistula (Q43.6)

▶ **K60.50**   **Anorectal fistula, unspecified**
   ▶ Anorectal fistula NOS

▶ **K60.51**   **Anorectal fistula, simple**
   ▶ Low intersphincteric anorectal fistula
   ▶ Superficial anorectal fistula

   ▶ **K60.511**   **Anorectal fistula, simple, initial**
     ▶ Anorectal fistula, simple, new

   ▶ **K60.512**   **Anorectal fistula, simple, persistent**
     ▶ Anorectal fistula, simple, chronic

   ▶ **K60.513**   **Anorectal fistula, simple, recurrent**
     ▶ Anorectal fistula simple, occurring following complete healing

   ▶ **K60.519**   **Anorectal fistula, simple, unspecified**

▶ **K60.52**   **Anorectal fistula, complex**
   ▶ Extrasphincteric anorectal fistula
   ▶ High intersphincteric anorectal fistula
   ▶ Suprasphincteric anorectal fistula
   ▶ Transsphincteric anorectal fistula
   ▶ *Code also, if applicable:*
     ▶ perianal abscess (K61.0)
     ▶ rectovaginal fistula (N82.3)
     ▶ stenosis of anus and rectum (K62.4)

▶ **K60.521**   **Anorectal fistula, complex, initial**
   ▶ Anorectal fistula, complex, new

▶ **K60.522**   **Anorectal fistula, complex, persistent**
   ▶ Anorectal fistula, complex, chronic

▶ **K60.523**   **Anorectal fistula, complex, recurrent**
   ▶ Anorectal fistula complex, occurring following complete healing

▶ **K60.529**   **Anorectal fistula, complex, unspecified**

● **K61**   **Abscess of anal and rectal regions**
Includes   abscess of anal and rectal regions
      cellulitis of anal and rectal regions

K61.0   **Anal abscess**
Perianal abscess
Excludes2   intrasphincteric abscess (K61.4)

K61.1   **Rectal abscess**
Perirectal abscess
Excludes1   ischiorectal abscess (K61.39)
Coding Clinic: 2012, Q4, P104

K61.2   **Anorectal abscess**

K61.3   **Ischiorectal abscess**
    K61.31   **Horseshoe abscess**
    K61.39   **Other ischiorectal abscess**
      Abscess of ischiorectal fossa
      Ischiorectal abscess, NOS

K61.4   **Intrasphincteric abscess**
Intersphincteric abscess

K61.5   **Supralevator abscess**

● **K62**   **Other diseases of anus and rectum**
Includes   anal canal
Excludes2   colostomy and enterostomy malfunction (K94.0-, K91.4-)
      fecal incontinence (R15.-)
      hemorrhoids (K64.-)

K62.0   **Anal polyp**
Coding Clinic: 2018, Q1, P7

K62.1   **Rectal polyp**
Excludes1   adenomatous polyp (D12.8)
Coding Clinic: 2018, Q1, P7

K62.2   **Anal prolapse**
Prolapse of anal canal

K62.3   **Rectal prolapse**
Prolapse of rectal mucosa

K62.4   **Stenosis of anus and rectum**
Stricture of anus (sphincter)
Coding Clinic: 2019, Q2, P13

K62.5   **Hemorrhage of anus and rectum**
Excludes1   gastrointestinal bleeding NOS (K92.2)
      melena (K92.1)
      neonatal rectal hemorrhage (P54.2)

K62.6   **Ulcer of anus and rectum**
Solitary ulcer of anus and rectum
Stercoral ulcer of anus and rectum
Excludes1   fissure and fistula of anus and rectum (K60.-)
      ulcerative colitis (K51.-)

K62.7   **Radiation proctitis**
Use additional code to identify the type of radiation (W88.-) or radiation therapy (Y84.2)
Coding Clinic: 2019, Q1, P21

Item 11–17 A **fissure** is a groove in the surface, whereas a **fistula** is an abnormal passage. An **abscess** is an accumulation of pus in a tissue cavity resulting from a bacterial or parasitic infection.

CHAPTER 11 (K00-K95)

CHAPTER 11 (K00-K95)

● **K62.8**   **Other specified diseases of anus and rectum**
>   **Excludes2**   ulcerative proctitis (K51.2)

   K62.81   **Anal sphincter tear (healed) (nontraumatic) (old)**
      Tear of anus, nontraumatic
      Use additional code for any associated fecal incontinence (R15.-)
>   **Excludes2**   anal fissure (K60.-)
>   anal sphincter tear (healed) (old) complicating delivery (O34.7-)
>   traumatic tear of anal sphincter (S31.831)

   K62.82   **Dysplasia of anus**
      Anal intraepithelial neoplasia I and II (AIN I and II) (histologically confirmed)
      Dysplasia of anus NOS
      Mild and moderate dysplasia of anus (histologically confirmed)
>   **Excludes1**   abnormal results from anal cytologic examination without histologic confirmation (R85.61-)
>   anal intraepithelial neoplasia III (D01.3)
>   carcinoma in situ of anus (D01.3)
>   HGSIL of anus (R85.613)
>   severe dysplasia of anus (D01.3)

   K62.89   **Other specified diseases of anus and rectum**
      Proctitis NOS
      Use additional code for any associated fecal incontinence (R15.-)

  K62.9   **Disease of anus and rectum, unspecified**

● **K63**   **Other diseases of intestine**

  K63.0   **Abscess of intestine**
>   **Excludes1**   abscess of intestine with Crohn's disease (K50.014, K50.114, K50.814, K50.914)
>   abscess of intestine with diverticular disease (K57.0, K57.2, K57.4, K57.8)
>   abscess of intestine with ulcerative colitis (K51.014, K51.214, K51.314, K51.414, K51.514, K51.814, K51.914)
>   **Excludes2**   abscess of anal and rectal regions (K61.-)
>   abscess of appendix (K35.3-)

  K63.1   **Perforation of intestine (nontraumatic)** 🕸
      Perforation (nontraumatic) of rectum
>   **Excludes1**   perforation (nontraumatic) of duodenum (K26.-)
>   perforation (nontraumatic) of intestine with diverticular disease (K57.0, K57.2, K57.4, K57.8)
>   **Excludes2**   perforation (nontraumatic) of appendix (K35.2-, K35.3)

  K63.2   **Fistula of intestine**
▶   Code also, if applicable, disruption of internal operation (surgical) wound (T81.32-)
>   **Excludes1**   fistula of duodenum (K31.6)
>   fistula of intestine with Crohn's disease (K50.013, K50.113, K50.813, K50.913)
>   fistula of intestine with ulcerative colitis (K51.013, K51.213, K51.313, K51.413, K51.513, K51.813, K51.913)
>   **Excludes2**   fistula of anal and rectal regions (K60.-)
>   fistula of appendix (K38.3)
>   intestinal-genital fistula, female (N82.2-N82.4)
>   vesicointestinal fistula (N32.1)

Coding Clinic: 2017, Q3, P4

  K63.3   **Ulcer of intestine**
      Primary ulcer of small intestine
>   **Excludes1**   duodenal ulcer (K26.-)
>   gastrointestinal ulcer (K28.-)
>   gastrojejunal ulcer (K28.-)
>   jejunal ulcer (K28.-)
>   peptic ulcer, site unspecified (K27.-)
>   ulcer of intestine with perforation (K63.1)
>   ulcer of anus or rectum (K62.6)
>   ulcerative colitis (K51.-)

  K63.4   **Enteroptosis**
  K63.5   **Polyp of colon**
>   **Excludes2**   adenomatous polyp of colon (D12.-)
>   inflammatory polyp of colon (K51.4-)
>   polyposis of colon (D12.6)

Coding Clinic: 2019, Q1, P33; 2017, Q1, P15-16; 2015, Q2, P14

● **K63.8**   **Other specified diseases of intestine**
   K63.81   **Dieulafoy lesion of intestine**
>   **Excludes2**   Dieulafoy lesion of stomach and duodenum (K31.82)

   ● **K63.82**   **Intestinal microbial overgrowth**
     ● **K63.821**   **Small intestinal bacterial overgrowth**
       K63.8211   **Small intestinal bacterial overgrowth, hydrogen-subtype**
       K63.8212   **Small intestinal bacterial overgrowth, hydrogen sulfide-subtype**
       K63.8219   **Small intestinal bacterial overgrowth, unspecified**
     K63.822   **Small intestinal fungal overgrowth**
     K63.829   **Intestinal methanogen overgrowth, unspecified**

   K63.89   **Other specified diseases of intestine**
Coding Clinic: 2013, Q2, P31

  K63.9   **Disease of intestine, unspecified**

● **K64**   **Hemorrhoids and perianal venous thrombosis**
>   **Includes**   piles
>   **Excludes1**   hemorrhoids complicating childbirth and the puerperium (O87.2)
>   hemorrhoids complicating pregnancy (O22.4)

  K64.0   **First degree hemorrhoids**
      Grade/stage I hemorrhoids
      Hemorrhoids (bleeding) without prolapse outside of anal canal

  K64.1   **Second degree hemorrhoids**
      Grade/stage II hemorrhoids
      Hemorrhoids (bleeding) that prolapse with straining, but retract spontaneously

  K64.2   **Third degree hemorrhoids**
      Grade/stage III hemorrhoids
      Hemorrhoids (bleeding) that prolapse with straining and require manual replacement back inside anal canal

  K64.3   **Fourth degree hemorrhoids**
      Grade/stage IV hemorrhoids
      Hemorrhoids (bleeding) with prolapsed tissue that cannot be manually replaced

  K64.4   **Residual hemorrhoidal skin tags**
      External hemorrhoids, NOS
      Skin tags of anus

  K64.5   **Perianal venous thrombosis**
      External hemorrhoids with thrombosis
      Perianal hematoma
      Thrombosed hemorrhoids NOS

  K64.8   **Other hemorrhoids**
      Internal hemorrhoids, without mention of degree
      Prolapsed hemorrhoids, degree not specified

  K64.9   **Unspecified hemorrhoids**
      Hemorrhoids (bleeding) NOS
      Hemorrhoids (bleeding) without mention of degree

▶ New   ⇒ Revised   ~~deleted~~ Deleted   Excludes 1   Excludes 2   Includes   Use additional   Code first   Code also   Key words

920   OGCR Official Guidelines   X Assign placeholder X   ● Use Additional Character(s)   ▮ Manifestation Code   🕸 Hierarchical Condition Category   Coding Clinic

DISEASES OF PERITONEUM AND RETROPERITONEUM (K65-K68)

● **K65**   **Peritonitis**

Use additional code (B95-B97), to identify infectious agent, if known

Code also if applicable diverticular disease of intestine (K57.-)

> **Excludes1**   acute appendicitis with generalized peritonitis (K35.2-)
> aseptic peritonitis (T81.6)
> benign paroxysmal peritonitis (E85.0)
> chemical peritonitis (T81.6)
> gonococcal peritonitis (A54.85)
> neonatal peritonitis (P78.0-P78.1)
> pelvic peritonitis, female (N73.3-N73.5)
> periodic familial peritonitis (E85.0)
> peritonitis due to talc or other foreign substance (T81.6)
> peritonitis in chlamydia (A74.81)
> peritonitis in diphtheria (A36.89)
> peritonitis in syphilis (late) (A52.74)
> peritonitis in tuberculosis (A18.31)
> peritonitis with or following abortion or ectopic or molar pregnancy (O00-O07, O08.0)
> peritonitis with or following appendicitis (K35.-)
> puerperal peritonitis (O85)
> retroperitoneal infections (K68.-)

Coding Clinic: 2022, Q1, P26

K65.0   **Generalized (acute) peritonitis** 🔗
Pelvic peritonitis (acute), male
Subphrenic peritonitis (acute)
Suppurative peritonitis (acute)

K65.1   **Peritoneal abscess** 🔗
Abdominopelvic abscess
Abscess (of) omentum
Abscess (of) peritoneum
Mesenteric abscess
Retrocecal abscess
Subdiaphragmatic abscess
Subhepatic abscess
Subphrenic abscess
Coding Clinic: 2024, Q1, P20; 2022, Q1, P26; 2019, Q1, P15

K65.2   **Spontaneous bacterial peritonitis** 🔗
> **Excludes1**   bacterial peritonitis NOS (K65.9)

K65.3   **Choleperitonitis** 🔗
Peritonitis due to bile

K65.4   **Sclerosing mesenteritis** 🔗
Fat necrosis of peritoneum
(Idiopathic) sclerosing mesenteric fibrosis
Mesenteric lipodystrophy
Mesenteric panniculitis
Retractile mesenteritis

K65.8   **Other peritonitis** 🔗
Chronic proliferative peritonitis
Peritonitis due to urine

K65.9   **Peritonitis, unspecified** 🔗
Bacterial peritonitis NOS
Coding Clinic: 2013, Q2, P31

● **K66**   **Other disorders of peritoneum**
> **Excludes2**   ascites (R18.-)
> peritoneal effusion (chronic) (R18.8)

K66.0   **Peritoneal adhesions (postprocedural) (postinfection)**
Adhesions (of) abdominal (wall)
Adhesions (of) diaphragm
Adhesions (of) intestine
Adhesions (of) male pelvis
Adhesions (of) omentum
Adhesions (of) stomach
Adhesive bands
Mesenteric adhesions

> ~~**Excludes1** female pelvic adhesions [bands] (N73.6)~~
> ~~peritoneal adhesions with intestinal~~
> ~~obstruction (K56.5-)~~

> ▷ **Excludes2**   female pelvic adhesions [bands] (N73.6)
> ▷ female pelvic postprocedural adhesions (N99.4)

Item 11-18   **Peritonitis** is an inflammation of the lining (peritoneum) of the abdominal cavity and surface of the intestines.

Item 11-19   **Retroperitoneal infections** occur between the posterior parietal peritoneum and posterior abdominal wall where the kidneys, adrenal glands, ureters, duodenum, ascending colon, descending colon, pancreas, and the large vessels and nerves are located.

K66.1   **Hemoperitoneum**
Peritoneal hematoma
Peritoneal hemorrhage
> **Excludes1**   traumatic hemoperitoneum (S36.8-)
> **Excludes2**   retroperitoneal hematoma (K68.3)
> retroperitoneal hemorrhage (K68.3)
Coding Clinic: 2022, Q1, P22-23

K66.8   **Other specified disorders of peritoneum**

K66.9   **Disorder of peritoneum, unspecified**

▷ **K67**   *Disorders of peritoneum in infectious diseases classified elsewhere* 🔗
> *Code first underlying disease, such as:*
> congenital syphilis (A50.0)
> helminthiasis (B65.0-B83.9)
> **Excludes1**   peritonitis in chlamydia (A74.81)
> peritonitis in diphtheria (A36.89)
> peritonitis in gonococcal (A54.85)
> peritonitis in syphilis (late) (A52.74)
> peritonitis in tuberculosis (A18.31)

● **K68**   **Disorders of retroperitoneum**
● **K68.1**   **Retroperitoneal abscess**
     K68.11   **Postprocedural retroperitoneal abscess**
> **Excludes2**   infection following procedure (T81.44)

     K68.12   **Psoas muscle abscess** 🔗

     K68.19   **Other retroperitoneal abscess** 🔗
Coding Clinic: 2019, Q1, P15

K68.2   **Retroperitoneal fibrosis**
Code also, if applicable, associated obstruction of ureter (N13.5)

K68.3   **Retroperitoneal hematoma**
Retroperitoneal hemorrhage

K68.9   **Other disorders of retroperitoneum**

DISEASES OF LIVER (K70-K77)

> **Excludes1**   jaundice NOS (R17)
> **Excludes2**   hemochromatosis (E83.11-)
> Reye's syndrome (G93.7)
> viral hepatitis (B15-B19)
> Wilson's disease (E83.01)

● **K70**   **Alcoholic liver disease**
Use additional code to identify:
alcohol abuse and dependence (F10.-)

K70.0   **Alcoholic fatty liver**   A

● **K70.1**   **Alcoholic hepatitis**
     K70.10   **Alcoholic hepatitis without ascites**   A
     K70.11   **Alcoholic hepatitis with ascites**   A

K70.2   **Alcoholic fibrosis and sclerosis of liver**   A

● **K70.3**   **Alcoholic cirrhosis of liver**
Alcoholic cirrhosis NOS
     K70.30   **Alcoholic cirrhosis of liver without ascites** 🔗   A
     K70.31   **Alcoholic cirrhosis of liver with ascites** 🔗   A
         Coding Clinic: 2018, Q1, P5

● **K70.4**   **Alcoholic hepatic failure**
Acute alcoholic hepatic failure
Alcoholic hepatic failure NOS
Chronic alcoholic hepatic failure
Subacute alcoholic hepatic failure

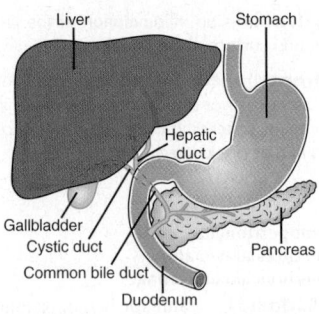

Figure 11-13   Liver and bile ducts.

Item 11–20 Cirrhosis is the progressive fibrosis of the liver resulting in loss of liver function. The main causes of cirrhosis of the liver are alcohol abuse, chronic hepatitis (inflammation of the liver), biliary disease, and excessive amounts of iron. **Alcoholic cirrhosis of the liver** is also called portal, Laënnec's, or fatty nutritional cirrhosis.

            K70.40   Alcoholic hepatic failure without coma   A
            K70.41   Alcoholic hepatic failure with coma   A
    K70.9   Alcoholic liver disease, unspecified   A

● **K71**   **Toxic liver disease**
     Includes   drug-induced idiosyncratic (unpredictable) liver disease
               drug-induced toxic (predictable) liver disease
     Code first poisoning due to drug or toxin, if applicable (T36-T65 with fifth or sixth character 1-4)
     Use additional code for adverse effect, if applicable, to identify drug (T36-T50 with fifth or sixth character 5)
     Excludes2   alcoholic liver disease (K70.-)
                 Budd-Chiari syndrome (I82.0)
   K71.0   **Toxic liver disease with cholestasis**
        Cholestasis with hepatocyte injury
        'Pure' cholestasis
 ● **K71.1**   **Toxic liver disease with hepatic necrosis**
        Hepatic failure (acute) (chronic) due to drugs
      K71.10   Toxic liver disease with hepatic necrosis, without coma
      K71.11   Toxic liver disease with hepatic necrosis, with coma
   K71.2   Toxic liver disease with acute hepatitis
   K71.3   Toxic liver disease with chronic persistent hepatitis
   K71.4   Toxic liver disease with chronic lobular hepatitis
 ● **K71.5**   **Toxic liver disease with chronic active hepatitis**
        Toxic liver disease with lupoid hepatitis
      K71.50   Toxic liver disease with chronic active hepatitis without ascites
      K71.51   Toxic liver disease with chronic active hepatitis with ascites
          Coding Clinic: 2018, Q1, P4
   K71.6   Toxic liver disease with hepatitis, not elsewhere classified
   K71.7   Toxic liver disease with fibrosis and cirrhosis of liver
   K71.8   Toxic liver disease with other disorders of liver
        Toxic liver disease with focal nodular hyperplasia
        Toxic liver disease with hepatic granulomas
        Toxic liver disease with peliosis hepatis
        Toxic liver disease with veno-occlusive disease of liver
        Coding Clinic: 2024, Q1, P25
   K71.9   Toxic liver disease, unspecified

● **K72**   **Hepatic failure, not elsewhere classified**
     Includes   fulminant hepatitis NEC, with hepatic failure
               liver (cell) necrosis with hepatic failure
               malignant hepatitis NEC, with hepatic failure
               yellow liver atrophy or dystrophy
     Excludes1   alcoholic hepatic failure (K70.4)
               hepatic failure with toxic liver disease (K71.1-)
               icterus of newborn (P55-P59)
               postprocedural hepatic failure (K91.82)
     Excludes2   hepatic failure complicating abortion or ectopic or molar pregnancy (O00-O07, O08.8)
               hepatic failure complicating pregnancy, childbirth and the puerperium (O26.6-)
               viral hepatitis with hepatic coma (B15-B19)
 ● **K72.0**   **Acute and subacute hepatic failure**
        Acute non-viral hepatitis NOS
        Coding Clinic: 2015, Q2, P17
      K72.00   Acute and subacute hepatic failure without coma
          Coding Clinic: 2021, Q1, P13; 2015, Q2, P17
      K72.01   Acute and subacute hepatic failure with coma
 ● **K72.1**   **Chronic hepatic failure**
        End stage liver disease
      K72.10   Chronic hepatic failure without coma
          Coding Clinic: 2021, Q1, P13; 2017, Q1, P41
      K72.11   Chronic hepatic failure with coma
          Coding Clinic: 2020, Q1, P15
 ● **K72.9**   **Hepatic failure, unspecified**
      K72.90   Hepatic failure, unspecified without coma
          Coding Clinic: 2022, Q1, P53; 2018, Q4, P21
      K72.91   Hepatic failure, unspecified with coma
        Hepatic coma NOS
        Coding Clinic: 2016, Q2, P35

● **K73**   **Chronic hepatitis, not elsewhere classified**
     Excludes1   alcoholic hepatitis (chronic) (K70.1-)
               drug-induced hepatitis (chronic) (K71.-)
               granulomatous hepatitis (chronic) NEC (K75.3)
               reactive, nonspecific hepatitis (chronic) (K75.2)
               viral hepatitis (chronic) (B15-B19)
   K73.0   Chronic persistent hepatitis, not elsewhere classified
   K73.1   Chronic lobular hepatitis, not elsewhere classified
   K73.2   Chronic active hepatitis, not elsewhere classified
   K73.8   Other chronic hepatitis, not elsewhere classified
   K73.9   Chronic hepatitis, unspecified

● **K74**   **Fibrosis and cirrhosis of liver**
     Code also, if applicable, viral hepatitis (acute) (chronic) (B15-B19)
     Excludes1   alcoholic cirrhosis (of liver) (K70.3)
               alcoholic fibrosis of liver (K70.2)
               cardiac sclerosis of liver (K76.1)
               cirrhosis (of liver) with toxic liver disease (K71.7)
               congenital cirrhosis (of liver) (P78.81)
               pigmentary cirrhosis (of liver) (E83.110)
 ● **K74.0**   **Hepatic fibrosis**
        Code first underlying liver disease, such as:
          nonalcoholic steatohepatitis (NASH) (K75.81)
      K74.00   Hepatic fibrosis, unspecified
      K74.01   Hepatic fibrosis, early fibrosis
         Hepatic fibrosis, stage F1 or stage F2
      K74.02   Hepatic fibrosis, advanced fibrosis
         Hepatic fibrosis, stage F3
         Excludes1   cirrhosis of liver (K74.6-)
                 hepatic fibrosis, stage F4 (K74.6-)
   K74.1   Hepatic sclerosis
   K74.2   Hepatic fibrosis with hepatic sclerosis

▶ New   ⇒ Revised   ~~deleted~~ Deleted   Excludes 1   Excludes 2   Includes   Use additional   Code first   Code also   Key words
OGCR Official Guidelines   X Assign placeholder X   ● Use Additional Character(s)   ▶ Manifestation Code   Hierarchical Condition Category   Coding Clinic

K74.3   **Primary biliary cirrhosis** 🔗
> Chronic nonsuppurative destructive cholangitis
> Primary biliary cholangitis
> **Excludes2**   primary sclerosing cholangitis (K83.01)

K74.4   **Secondary biliary cirrhosis** 🔗

K74.5   **Biliary cirrhosis, unspecified** 🔗

● K74.6   **Other and unspecified cirrhosis of liver**
> K74.60   **Unspecified cirrhosis of liver** 🔗
> > Cirrhosis (of liver) NOS
> > **Coding Clinic: 2018, Q1, P4**

> K74.69   **Other cirrhosis of liver** 🔗
> > Cryptogenic cirrhosis (of liver)
> > Macronodular cirrhosis (of liver)
> > Micronodular cirrhosis (of liver)
> > Mixed type cirrhosis (of liver)
> > Portal cirrhosis (of liver)
> > Postnecrotic cirrhosis (of liver)

● **K75**   **Other inflammatory liver diseases**
> **Excludes2**   toxic liver disease (K71.-)

K75.0   **Abscess of liver**
> Cholangitic hepatic abscess
> Hematogenous hepatic abscess
> Hepatic abscess NOS
> Lymphogenic hepatic abscess
> Pylephlebitic hepatic abscess
> **Excludes1**   amebic liver abscess (A06.4)
> > cholangitis without liver abscess (K83.09)
> > pylephlebitis without liver abscess (K75.1)
> **Excludes2**   acute or subacute hepatitis NOS (B17.9)
> > acute or subacute non-viral hepatitis (K72.0)
> > chronic hepatitis NEC (K73.8)

K75.1   **Phlebitis of portal vein**
> Pylephlebitis
> **Excludes1**   pylephlebitic liver abscess (K75.0)

K75.2   **Nonspecific reactive hepatitis**
> **Excludes1**   acute or subacute hepatitis (K72.0-)
> > chronic hepatitis NEC (K73.-)
> > viral hepatitis (B15-B19)

K75.3   **Granulomatous hepatitis, not elsewhere classified**
> **Excludes1**   acute or subacute hepatitis (K72.0-)
> > chronic hepatitis NEC (K73.-)
> > viral hepatitis (B15-B19)

K75.4   **Autoimmune hepatitis** 🔗
> Lupoid hepatitis NEC

● K75.8   **Other specified inflammatory liver diseases**
> K75.81   **Nonalcoholic steatohepatitis (NASH)**
> > Use additional code, if applicable, hepatic fibrosis (K74.0-)

> K75.89   **Other specified inflammatory liver diseases**

K75.9   **Inflammatory liver disease, unspecified**
> Hepatitis NOS
> **Excludes1**   acute or subacute hepatitis (K72.0-)
> > chronic hepatitis NEC (K73.-)
> > viral hepatitis (B15-B19)
> **Coding Clinic: 2015, Q2, P17**

● **K76**   **Other diseases of liver**
> **Excludes2**   alcoholic liver disease (K70.-)
> > amyloid degeneration of liver (E85.-)
> > cystic disease of liver (congenital) (Q44.6)
> > hepatic vein thrombosis (I82.0)
> > hepatomegaly NOS (R16.0)
> > pigmentary cirrhosis (of liver) (E83.110)
> > portal vein thrombosis (I81)
> > toxic liver disease (K71.-)

K76.0   **Fatty (change of) liver, not elsewhere classified**
> Nonalcoholic fatty liver disease (NAFLD)
> **Excludes1**   nonalcoholic steatohepatitis (NASH) (K75.81)

K76.1   **Chronic passive congestion of liver**
> Cardiac cirrhosis
> Cardiac sclerosis

K76.2   **Central hemorrhagic necrosis of liver**
> **Excludes1**   liver necrosis with hepatic failure (K72.-)

K76.3   **Infarction of liver**

K76.4   **Peliosis hepatis**
> Hepatic angiomatosis

K76.5   **Hepatic veno-occlusive disease**
> **Excludes1**   Budd-Chiari syndrome (I82.0)

K76.6   **Portal hypertension** 🔗
> Use additional code for any associated complications, such as:
> > portal hypertensive gastropathy (K31.89)
> **Coding Clinic: 2020, Q1, P15**

K76.7   **Hepatorenal syndrome** 🔗
> **Excludes1**   hepatorenal syndrome following labor and delivery (O90.41)
> > postprocedural hepatorenal syndrome (K91.83)

● K76.8   **Other specified diseases of liver**
> K76.81   **Hepatopulmonary syndrome** 🔗
> > *Code first underlying liver disease, such as:*
> > alcoholic cirrhosis of liver (K70.3-)
> > cirrhosis of liver without mention of alcohol (K74.6-)

> K76.82   **Hepatic encephalopathy**
> > Hepatic encephalopathy, NOS
> > Hepatic encephalopathy without coma
> > Hepatocerebral intoxication
> > Portal-systemic encephalopathy
> > Code also underlying liver disease, such as:
> > > acute and subacute hepatic failure without coma (K72.00)
> > > alcoholic hepatic failure without coma (K70.40)
> > > chronic hepatic failure without coma (K72.10)
> > > hepatic failure with toxic liver disease without coma (K71.10)
> > > hepatic failure without coma (K72.90)
> > > icterus of newborn (P55-P59)
> > > postprocedural hepatic failure (K91.82)
> > > viral hepatitis without hepatic coma (B15.9, B16.1, B16.9, B17.10, B19.10, B19.20, B19.9)
> > **Excludes1**   acute and subacute hepatic failure with coma (K72.01)
> > > alcoholic hepatic failure with coma (K70.41)
> > > chronic hepatic failure with coma (K72.11)
> > > hepatic failure with coma (K72.91)

> K76.89   **Other specified diseases of liver**
> > Cyst (simple) of liver
> > Focal nodular hyperplasia of liver
> > Hepatoptosis

K76.9   **Liver disease, unspecified**

▶ **K77**   *Liver disorders in diseases classified elsewhere*   (Ex) No exclusions
> *Code first underlying disease, such as:*
> amyloidosis (E85.-)
> congenital syphilis (A50.0, A50.5)
> congenital toxoplasmosis (P37.1)
> infectious mononucleosis with liver disease (B27.0-B27.9 with fifth character 9)
> schistosomiasis (B65.0-B65.9)
> **Excludes1**   alcoholic hepatitis (K70.1-)
> > alcoholic liver disease (K70.-)
> > cytomegaloviral hepatitis (B25.1)
> > herpesviral [herpes simplex] hepatitis (B00.81)
> > mumps hepatitis (B26.81)
> > sarcoidosis with liver disease (D86.89)
> > secondary syphilis with liver disease (A51.45)
> > syphilis (late) with liver disease (A52.74)
> > toxoplasmosis (acquired) hepatitis (B58.1)
> > tuberculosis with liver disease (A18.83)

CHAPTER 11 (K00-K95)

DISORDERS OF GALLBLADDER, BILIARY TRACT AND PANCREAS (K80–K87)

● **K80   Cholelithiasis**
  Presence or formation of gallstones
  Excludes1   retained cholelithiasis following cholecystectomy
            (K91.86)

● **K80.0   Calculus of gallbladder with acute cholecystitis**
  Any condition listed in K80.2 with acute cholecystitis

  Use additional code if applicable for associated
      gangrene of gallbladder (K82.A1), or perforation of
      gallbladder (K82.A2)
  *Check documentation for acute/chronic gallbladder/common
      bile duct either with or without obstruction.*

  **K80.00   Calculus of gallbladder with acute cholecystitis
            without obstruction**
            Coding Clinic: 2023, Q2, P12; 2018, Q4, P20

  **K80.01   Calculus of gallbladder with acute cholecystitis
            with obstruction**

● **K80.1   Calculus of gallbladder with other
          cholecystitis**

  Use additional code if applicable for associated
      gangrene of gallbladder (K82.A1), or perforation of
      gallbladder (K82.A2)

  **K80.10   Calculus of gallbladder with chronic
            cholecystitis without obstruction**
            Cholelithiasis with cholecystitis NOS

  **K80.11   Calculus of gallbladder with chronic
            cholecystitis with obstruction**

  **K80.12   Calculus of gallbladder with acute and chronic
            cholecystitis without obstruction**

  **K80.13   Calculus of gallbladder with acute and chronic
            cholecystitis with obstruction**

  **K80.18   Calculus of gallbladder with other cholecystitis
            without obstruction**

  **K80.19   Calculus of gallbladder with other cholecystitis
            with obstruction**

● **K80.2   Calculus of gallbladder without cholecystitis**
  Cholecystolithiasis without cholecystitis
  Cholelithiasis (without cholecystitis)
  Colic (recurrent) of gallbladder (without cholecystitis)
  Gallstone (impacted) of cystic duct (without
      cholecystitis)
  Gallstone (impacted) of gallbladder (without
      cholecystitis)

  **K80.20   Calculus of gallbladder without cholecystitis
            without obstruction**

  **K80.21   Calculus of gallbladder without cholecystitis
            with obstruction**

● **K80.3   Calculus of bile duct with cholangitis**
  Any condition listed in K80.5 with cholangitis

  **K80.30   Calculus of bile duct with cholangitis,
            unspecified, without obstruction**

  **K80.31   Calculus of bile duct with cholangitis,
            unspecified, with obstruction**

  **K80.32   Calculus of bile duct with acute cholangitis
            without obstruction**

  **K80.33   Calculus of bile duct with acute cholangitis
            with obstruction**

  **K80.34   Calculus of bile duct with chronic cholangitis
            without obstruction**

  **K80.35   Calculus of bile duct with chronic cholangitis
            with obstruction**

  **K80.36   Calculus of bile duct with acute and chronic
            cholangitis without obstruction**

  **K80.37   Calculus of bile duct with acute and chronic
            cholangitis with obstruction**

● **K80.4   Calculus of bile duct with cholecystitis**
  Any condition listed in K80.5 with cholecystitis (with
      cholangitis)

  Code also, if applicable, fistula of bile duct (K83.3)

  Use additional code if applicable for associated
      gangrene of gallbladder (K82.A1), or perforation of
      gallbladder (K82.A2)

  **K80.40   Calculus of bile duct with cholecystitis,
            unspecified, without obstruction**

  **K80.41   Calculus of bile duct with cholecystitis,
            unspecified, with obstruction**
            Coding Clinic: 2019, Q1, P18

  **K80.42   Calculus of bile duct with acute cholecystitis
            without obstruction**

  **K80.43   Calculus of bile duct with acute cholecystitis
            with obstruction**

  **K80.44   Calculus of bile duct with chronic cholecystitis
            without obstruction**

  **K80.45   Calculus of bile duct with chronic cholecystitis
            with obstruction**

  **K80.46   Calculus of bile duct with acute and chronic
            cholecystitis without obstruction**

  **K80.47   Calculus of bile duct with acute and chronic
            cholecystitis with obstruction**

● **K80.5   Calculus of bile duct without cholangitis or cholecystitis**
  Choledocholithiasis (without cholangitis or cholecystitis)
  Gallstone (impacted) of bile duct NOS (without
      cholangitis or cholecystitis)
  Gallstone (impacted) of common duct (without
      cholangitis or cholecystitis)
  Gallstone (impacted) of hepatic duct (without cholangitis
      or cholecystitis)
  Hepatic cholelithiasis (without cholangitis or cholecystitis)
  Hepatic colic (recurrent) (without cholangitis or
      cholecystitis)

  **K80.50   Calculus of bile duct without cholangitis or
            cholecystitis without obstruction**

  **K80.51   Calculus of bile duct without cholangitis or
            cholecystitis with obstruction**

● **K80.6   Calculus of gallbladder and bile duct with cholecystitis**
  Use additional code if applicable for associated
      gangrene of gallbladder (K82.A1), or perforation of
      gallbladder (K82.A2)

  **K80.60   Calculus of gallbladder and bile duct with
            cholecystitis, unspecified, without obstruction**

  **K80.61   Calculus of gallbladder and bile duct with
            cholecystitis, unspecified, with obstruction**

  **K80.62   Calculus of gallbladder and bile duct
            with acute cholecystitis without obstruction**

  **K80.63   Calculus of gallbladder and bile duct with
            acute cholecystitis with obstruction**

  **K80.64   Calculus of gallbladder and bile duct with
            chronic cholecystitis without obstruction**

  **K80.65   Calculus of gallbladder and bile duct with
            chronic cholecystitis with obstruction**

  **K80.66   Calculus of gallbladder and bile duct with
            acute and chronic cholecystitis without
            obstruction**

  **K80.67   Calculus of gallbladder and bile duct with
            acute and chronic cholecystitis with obstruction**

● **K80.7   Calculus of gallbladder and bile duct without
          cholecystitis**

  **K80.70   Calculus of gallbladder and bile duct without
            cholecystitis without obstruction**

  **K80.71   Calculus of gallbladder and bile duct without
            cholecystitis with obstruction**

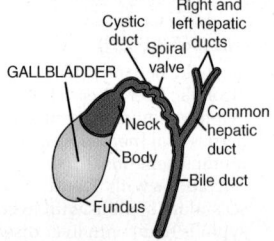

Figure 11-14   Gallbladder and bile ducts.

▶ New   ⇒ Revised   ~~deleted~~ Deleted   Excludes 1   Excludes 2   Includes   Use additional   Code first   Code also   Key words

OGCR Official Guidelines   X Assign placeholder X   ● Use Additional Character(s)   ⟩ Manifestation Code   🗪 Hierarchical Condition Category   Coding Clinic

● **K80.8**   **Other cholelithiasis**

     K80.80   Other cholelithiasis without obstruction

     K80.81   Other cholelithiasis with obstruction

● **K81**   **Cholecystitis**

Chronic or acute inflammation of the gallbladder

Use additional code if applicable for associated gangrene of gallbladder (K82.A1), or perforation of gallbladder (K82.A2)

     Excludes1   cholecystitis with cholelithiasis (K80.-)

     K81.0   **Acute cholecystitis**

         Abscess of gallbladder
         Angiocholecystitis
         Emphysematous (acute) cholecystitis
         Empyema of gallbladder
         Gangrene of gallbladder
         Gangrenous cholecystitis
         Suppurative cholecystitis

     K81.1   **Chronic cholecystitis**

     K81.2   **Acute cholecystitis with chronic cholecystitis**

     K81.9   **Cholecystitis, unspecified**

● **K82**   **Other diseases of gallbladder**

     Excludes1   nonvisualization of gallbladder (R93.2)
                 postcholecystectomy syndrome (K91.5)

     K82.0   **Obstruction of gallbladder**

         Occlusion of cystic duct or gallbladder without cholelithiasis
         Stenosis of cystic duct or gallbladder without cholelithiasis
         Stricture of cystic duct or gallbladder without cholelithiasis

         Excludes1   obstruction of gallbladder with cholelithiasis (K80.-)

     K82.1   **Hydrops of gallbladder**

         Mucocele of gallbladder

     K82.2   **Perforation of gallbladder**

         Rupture of cystic duct or gallbladder

         Excludes1   Perforation of gallbladder in cholecystitis (K82.A2)

     K82.3   **Fistula of gallbladder**

         Cholecystocolic fistula
         Cholecystoduodenal fistula
         Coding Clinic: 2019, Q1, P18

     K82.4   **Cholesterolosis of gallbladder**

         Strawberry gallbladder

         Excludes1   cholesterolosis of gallbladder with cholecystitis (K81.-)
                 cholesterolosis of gallbladder with cholelithiasis (K80.-)

     K82.8   **Other specified diseases of gallbladder**

         Adhesions of cystic duct or gallbladder
         Atrophy of cystic duct or gallbladder
         Cyst of cystic duct or gallbladder
         Dyskinesia of cystic duct or gallbladder
         Hypertrophy of cystic duct or gallbladder
         Nonfunctioning of cystic duct or gallbladder
         Ulcer of cystic duct or gallbladder

     K82.9   **Disease of gallbladder, unspecified**

● **K82.A**   **Disorders of gallbladder in diseases classified elsewhere**

Code first the type of cholecystitis (K81.-), or cholelithiasis with cholecystitis (K80.00-K80.19, K80.40-K80.47, K80.60-K80.67)

     ◗ **K82.A1**   *Gangrene of gallbladder in cholecystitis*
                 Coding Clinic: 2018, Q4, P20

     ● **K82.A2**   **Perforation of gallbladder in cholecystitis**
                 Coding Clinic: 2018, Q4, P20

● **K83**   **Other diseases of biliary tract**

     Excludes1   postcholecystectomy syndrome (K91.5)

     Excludes2   conditions involving the gallbladder (K81-K82)
                 conditions involving the cystic duct (K81-K82)

● **K83.0**   **Cholangitis**

     Excludes1   cholangitic liver abscess (K75.0)
                 cholangitis with choledocholithiasis (K80.3-, K80.4-)

     Excludes2   chronic nonsuppurative destructive cholangitis (K74.3)
                 primary biliary cholangitis (K74.3)
                 primary biliary cirrhosis (K74.3)

     K83.01   **Primary sclerosing cholangitis**
             Coding Clinic: 2018, Q4, P21

     K83.09   **Other cholangitis**
             Ascending cholangitis
             Cholangitis NOS
             Primary cholangitis
             Recurrent cholangitis
             Sclerosing cholangitis
             Secondary cholangitis
             Stenosing cholangitis
             Suppurative cholangitis

     K83.1   **Obstruction of bile duct**

         Occlusion of bile duct without cholelithiasis
         Stenosis of bile duct without cholelithiasis
         Stricture of bile duct without cholelithiasis

         Excludes1   congenital obstruction of bile duct (Q44.3)
                 obstruction of bile duct with cholelithiasis (K80.-)

         Coding Clinic: 2023, Q1, P27; 2016, Q1, P18

     K83.2   **Perforation of bile duct**
         Rupture of bile duct

     K83.3   **Fistula of bile duct**
         Choledochoduodenal fistula

     K83.4   **Spasm of sphincter of Oddi**

     K83.5   **Biliary cyst**

     K83.8   **Other specified diseases of biliary tract**
         Adhesions of biliary tract
         Atrophy of biliary tract
         Hypertrophy of biliary tract
         Ulcer of biliary tract

     K83.9   **Disease of biliary tract, unspecified**

● **K85**   **Acute pancreatitis**

Inflammatory process in which pancreatic enzymes autodigest the gland

     Includes   acute (recurrent) pancreatitis
               subacute pancreatitis

Coding Clinic: 2016, Q4, P34

● **K85.0**   **Idiopathic acute pancreatitis**

     K85.00   **Idiopathic acute pancreatitis without necrosis or infection**

     K85.01   **Idiopathic acute pancreatitis with uninfected necrosis**

     K85.02   **Idiopathic acute pancreatitis with infected necrosis**

● **K85.1**   **Biliary acute pancreatitis**

     Gallstone pancreatitis

     K85.10   **Biliary acute pancreatitis without necrosis or infection**
            Coding Clinic: 2023, Q2, P12

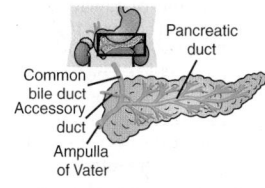

Figure 11-15   Pancreatic ductal system.

CHAPTER 11 (K00-K95)

K85.11 Biliary acute pancreatitis with uninfected necrosis

K85.12 Biliary acute pancreatitis with infected necrosis

● **K85.2 Alcohol induced acute pancreatitis**
> **Excludes2** alcohol induced chronic pancreatitis (K86.0)

K85.20 Alcohol induced acute pancreatitis without necrosis or infection
Coding Clinic: 2020, Q1, P9

K85.21 Alcohol induced acute pancreatitis with uninfected necrosis

K85.22 Alcohol induced acute pancreatitis with infected necrosis

● **K85.3 Drug induced acute pancreatitis**
> Use additional code for adverse effect, if applicable, to identify drug (T36-T50 with fifth or sixth character 5)
> Use additional code to identify drug abuse and dependence (F11.-F17.-)

K85.30 Drug induced acute pancreatitis without necrosis or infection

K85.31 Drug induced acute pancreatitis with uninfected necrosis

K85.32 Drug induced acute pancreatitis with infected necrosis

● **K85.8 Other acute pancreatitis**

K85.80 Other acute pancreatitis without necrosis or infection

K85.81 Other acute pancreatitis with uninfected necrosis

K85.82 Other acute pancreatitis with infected necrosis

● **K85.9 Acute pancreatitis, unspecified**
Pancreatitis NOS

K85.90 Acute pancreatitis without necrosis or infection, unspecified

K85.91 Acute pancreatitis with uninfected necrosis, unspecified

K85.92 Acute pancreatitis with infected necrosis, unspecified

● **K86 Other diseases of pancreas**
> **Excludes2** fibrocystic disease of pancreas (E84.-)
> islet cell tumor (of pancreas) (D13.7)
> pancreatic steatorrhea (K90.3)

K86.0 Alcohol-induced chronic pancreatitis 🅗
> Use additional code to identify:
> alcohol abuse and dependence (F10.-)
> Code also exocrine pancreatic insufficiency (K86.81)
> **Excludes2** alcohol induced acute pancreatitis (K85.2-)

K86.1 Other chronic pancreatitis 🅗
Chronic pancreatitis NOS
Infectious chronic pancreatitis
Recurrent chronic pancreatitis
Relapsing chronic pancreatitis
> Code also exocrine pancreatic insufficiency (K86.81)

K86.2 Cyst of pancreas

K86.3 Pseudocyst of pancreas

● **K86.8 Other specified diseases of pancreas**
Coding Clinic: 2016, Q4, P34

K86.81 Exocrine pancreatic insufficiency

K86.89 Other specified diseases of pancreas
Aseptic pancreatic necrosis, unrelated to acute pancreatitis
Atrophy of pancreas
Calculus of pancreas
Cirrhosis of pancreas
Fibrosis of pancreas
Pancreatic fat necrosis, unrelated to acute pancreatitis
Pancreatic infantilism
Pancreatic necrosis NOS, unrelated to acute pancreatitis

K86.9 Disease of pancreas, unspecified

▷ **K87 Disorders of gallbladder, biliary tract and pancreas in diseases classified elsewhere**
> *Code first underlying disease*
> **Excludes1** cytomegaloviral pancreatitis (B25.2)
> mumps pancreatitis (B26.3)
> syphilitic gallbladder (A52.74)
> syphilitic pancreas (A52.74)
> tuberculosis of gallbladder (A18.83)
> tuberculosis of pancreas (A18.83)

OTHER DISEASES OF THE DIGESTIVE SYSTEM (K90-K95)

● **K90 Intestinal malabsorption**
> **Excludes1** intestinal malabsorption following gastrointestinal surgery (K91.2)

K90.0 Celiac disease
Celiac disease with steatorrhea
Celiac gluten-sensitive enteropathy
Nontropical sprue
> Use additional code for associated disorders including:
> dermatitis herpetiformis (L13.0)
> gluten ataxia (G32.81)
> Code also exocrine pancreatic insufficiency (K86.81)

K90.1 Tropical sprue
Sprue NOS
Tropical steatorrhea

K90.2 Blind loop syndrome, not elsewhere classified
Blind loop syndrome NOS
> **Excludes1** congenital blind loop syndrome (Q43.8)
> postsurgical blind loop syndrome (K91.2)

K90.3 Pancreatic steatorrhea

● **K90.4 Other malabsorption due to intolerance**
> **Excludes2** celiac gluten-sensitive enteropathy (K90.0)
> lactose intolerance (E73.-)
Coding Clinic: 2016, Q4, P35-36

K90.41 Non-celiac gluten sensitivity
Gluten sensitivity NOS
Non-celiac gluten sensitive enteropathy

K90.49 Malabsorption due to intolerance, not elsewhere classified
Malabsorption due to intolerance to carbohydrate
Malabsorption due to intolerance to fat
Malabsorption due to intolerance to protein
Malabsorption due to intolerance to starch

● **K90.8 Other intestinal malabsorption**

K90.81 Whipple's disease

● K90.82 Short bowel syndrome
Short gut syndrome

K90.821 Short bowel syndrome with colon in continuity
Short bowel syndrome with colonic continuity
Coding Clinic: 2023, Q4, P32

K90.822 Short bowel syndrome without colon in continuity
Short bowel syndrome without colonic continuity
Coding Clinic: 2023, Q4, P33

K90.829 Short bowel syndrome, unspecified

K90.83 Intestinal failure

K90.89 Other intestinal malabsorption

K90.9 Intestinal malabsorption, unspecified
Coding Clinic: 2017, Q4, P108-109

● **K91 Intraoperative and postprocedural complications and disorders of digestive system, not elsewhere classified**
> **Excludes2** complications of artificial opening of digestive system (K94.-)
> complications of bariatric procedures (K95.-)
> gastrojejunal ulcer (K28.-)
> postprocedural (radiation) retroperitoneal abscess (K68.11)
> radiation colitis (K52.0)
> radiation gastroenteritis (K52.0)
> radiation proctitis (K62.7)
Coding Clinic: 2016, Q4, P10

CHAPTER 11 (K00-K95)

▶ New ⇒ Revised ~~deleted~~ Deleted Excludes 1 Excludes 2 Includes Use additional Code first Code also Key words
OGCR Official Guidelines X Assign placeholder X ● Use Additional Character(s) ▷ Manifestation Code 🅗 Hierarchical Condition Category Coding Clinic

K91.0 Vomiting following gastrointestinal surgery

K91.1 Postgastric surgery syndromes
Dumping syndrome
Postgastrectomy syndrome
Postvagotomy syndrome

K91.2 Postsurgical malabsorption, not elsewhere classified
Postsurgical blind loop syndrome
> **Excludes1** malabsorption osteomalacia in adults (M83.2)
> malabsorption osteoporosis, postsurgical (M80.8-, M81.8)

● **K91.3 Postprocedural intestinal obstruction**
Coding Clinic: 2017, Q1, P40-41

   K91.30 Postprocedural intestinal obstruction, unspecified as to partial versus complete
Postprocedural intestinal obstruction NOS

   K91.31 Postprocedural partial intestinal obstruction
Postprocedural incomplete intestinal obstruction

   K91.32 Postprocedural complete intestinal obstruction

K91.5 Postcholecystectomy syndrome

● **K91.6 Intraoperative hemorrhage and hematoma of a digestive system organ or structure complicating a procedure**
> **Excludes1** intraoperative hemorrhage and hematoma of a digestive system organ or structure due to accidental puncture and laceration during a procedure (K91.7-)

   K91.61 Intraoperative hemorrhage and hematoma of a digestive system organ or structure complicating a digestive system procedure
Coding Clinic: 2020, Q1, P20

   K91.62 Intraoperative hemorrhage and hematoma of a digestive system organ or structure complicating other procedure

● **K91.7 Accidental puncture and laceration of a digestive system organ or structure during a procedure**

   K91.71 Accidental puncture and laceration of a digestive system organ or structure during a digestive system procedure
Coding Clinic: 2022, Q1, P51-52; 2021, Q2, P12

   K91.72 Accidental puncture and laceration of a digestive system organ or structure during other procedure
Coding Clinic: 2022, Q1, P51; 2019, Q2, P24

● **K91.8 Other intraoperative and postprocedural complications and disorders of digestive system**

   K91.81 Other intraoperative complications of digestive system

   K91.82 Postprocedural hepatic failure

   K91.83 Postprocedural hepatorenal syndrome

●   **K91.84 Postprocedural hemorrhage of a digestive system organ or structure following a procedure**

     K91.840 Postprocedural hemorrhage of a digestive system organ or structure following a digestive system procedure
Coding Clinic: 2016, Q1, P15

     K91.841 Postprocedural hemorrhage of a digestive system organ or structure following other procedure

●   **K91.85 Complications of intestinal pouch**

     K91.850 Pouchitis 🦠
Inflammation of internal ileoanal pouch

     K91.858 Other complications of intestinal pouch 🦠
Coding Clinic: 2019, Q2, P13

   K91.86 Retained cholelithiasis following cholecystectomy

●   **K91.87 Postprocedural hematoma and seroma of a digestive system organ or structure following a procedure**

     K91.870 Postprocedural hematoma of a digestive system organ or structure following a digestive system procedure
Coding Clinic: 2022, Q1, P24

     K91.871 Postprocedural hematoma of a digestive system organ or structure following other procedure

     K91.872 Postprocedural seroma of a digestive system organ or structure following a digestive system procedure

     K91.873 Postprocedural seroma of a digestive system organ or structure following other procedure

   K91.89 Other postprocedural complications and disorders of digestive system
Use additional code, if applicable, to further specify disorder
> **Excludes2** postprocedural retroperitoneal abscess (K68.11)
Coding Clinic: 2017, Q1, P41

● **K92 Other diseases of digestive system**
> **Excludes1** neonatal gastrointestinal hemorrhage (P54.0-P54.3)

K92.0 Hematemesis

K92.1 Melena
> **Excludes1** occult blood in feces (R19.5)

K92.2 Gastrointestinal hemorrhage, unspecified
Gastric hemorrhage NOS
Intestinal hemorrhage NOS
> **Excludes1** acute hemorrhagic gastritis (K29.01)
> hemorrhage of anus and rectum (K62.5)
> angiodysplasia of stomach with hemorrhage (K31.811)
> diverticular disease with hemorrhage (K57.-)
> gastritis and duodenitis with hemorrhage (K29.-)
> peptic ulcer with hemorrhage (K25-K28)
Coding Clinic: 2021, Q1, P12

● **K92.8 Other specified diseases of the digestive system**

   K92.81 Gastrointestinal mucositis (ulcerative)
Code also type of associated therapy, such as:
antineoplastic and immunosuppressive drugs (T45.1X-)
radiological procedure and radiotherapy (Y84.2)
> **Excludes2** mucositis (ulcerative) of vagina and vulva (N76.81)
> nasal mucositis (ulcerative) (J34.81)
> oral mucositis (ulcerative) (K12.3-)

   K92.89 Other specified diseases of the digestive system

K92.9 Disease of digestive system, unspecified

● **K94 Complications of artificial openings of the digestive system**

●   **K94.0 Colostomy complications**

   K94.00 Colostomy complication, unspecified 🦠

   K94.01 Colostomy hemorrhage 🦠

   K94.02 Colostomy infection 🦠
Use additional code to specify type of infection, such as:
cellulitis of abdominal wall (L03.311)
sepsis (A40.-, A41.-)

   K94.03 Colostomy malfunction 🦠
Mechanical complication of colostomy

   K94.09 Other complications of colostomy 🦠

●   **K94.1 Enterostomy complications**

   K94.10 Enterostomy complication, unspecified 🦠

   K94.11 Enterostomy hemorrhage 🦠

   K94.12 Enterostomy infection 🦠
Use additional code to specify type of infection, such as:
cellulitis of abdominal wall (L03.311)
sepsis (A40.-, A41.-)

   K94.13 Enterostomy malfunction 🦠
Mechanical complication of enterostomy
Coding Clinic: 2021, Q4, P18

   K94.19 Other complications of enterostomy 🦠

● **K94.2   Gastrostomy complications**
      K94.20   Gastrostomy complication, unspecified 🐾
      K94.21   Gastrostomy hemorrhage 🐾
      K94.22   Gastrostomy infection 🐾
           Use additional code to specify type of
              infection, such as:
                cellulitis of abdominal wall (L03.311)
                sepsis (A40.-, A41.-)
      K94.23   Gastrostomy malfunction 🐾
           Mechanical complication of gastrostomy
      K94.29   Other complications of gastrostomy 🐾
● **K94.3 Esophagostomy complications**
      K94.30   Esophagostomy complications, unspecified 🐾
      K94.31   Esophagostomy hemorrhage 🐾
      K94.32   Esophagostomy infection 🐾
           Use additional code to identify the infection
      K94.33   Esophagostomy malfunction 🐾
           Mechanical complication of esophagostomy
      K94.39   Other complications of esophagostomy 🐾

● **K95   Complications of bariatric procedures**
  ● **K95.0   Complications of gastric band procedure**
      K95.01   Infection due to gastric band procedure
           Use additional code to specify type of infection
              or organism, such as:
                bacterial and viral infectious agents (B95.-,
                  B96.-)
                cellulitis of abdominal wall (L03.311)
                sepsis (A40.-, A41.-)
      K95.09   Other complications of gastric band procedure
           Use additional code, if applicable, to further
              specify complication
  ● **K95.8   Complications of other bariatric procedure**
        Excludes1   complications of gastric band surgery
                  (K95.0-)
      K95.81   Infection due to other bariatric procedure
           Use additional code to specify type of infection
              or organism, such as:
                bacterial and viral infectious agents (B95.-,
                  B96.-)
                cellulitis of abdominal wall (L03.311)
                sepsis (A40.-, A41.-)
      **K95.89   Other complications of other bariatric
              procedure**
           Use additional code, if applicable, to further
              specify complication

CHAPTER 11 (K00-K95)

▶ New   ➡ Revised   ~~deleted~~ Deleted   Excludes 1   Excludes 2   Includes   Use additional   Code first   Code also   Key words
OGCR Official Guidelines   X Assign placeholder X   ● Use Additional Character(s)   ▶ Manifestation Code   🐾 Hierarchical Condition Category   Coding Clinic

CHAPTER 12

DISEASES OF THE SKIN AND SUBCUTANEOUS TISSUE (L00-L99)

12. Chapter 12: Diseases of the Skin and Subcutaneous Tissue (L00-L99)

a. Pressure ulcer stage codes

1) **Pressure ulcer stages**
Codes from category L89, Pressure ulcer, identify the site of the pressure ulcer as well as the stage of the ulcer.
   The ICD-10-CM classifies pressure ulcer stages based on severity, which is designated by stages 1-4, unspecified stage and unstageable.
   Assign as many codes from category L89 as needed to identify all the pressure ulcers the patient has, if applicable.
   See Section I.B.14 for pressure ulcer stage documentation by clinicians other than patient's provider.

2) **Unstageable pressure ulcers**
Assignment of the code for unstageable pressure ulcer (L89.--0) should be based on the clinical documentation. These codes are used for pressure ulcers whose stage cannot be clinically determined (e.g., the ulcer is covered by eschar or has been treated with a skin or muscle graft) and pressure ulcers that are documented as deep tissue injury but not documented as due to trauma. This code should not be confused with the codes for unspecified stage (L89.--9). When there is no documentation regarding the stage of the pressure ulcer, assign the appropriate code for unspecified stage (L89.--9).

3) **Documented pressure ulcer stage**
Assignment of the pressure ulcer stage code should be guided by clinical documentation of the stage or documentation of the terms found in the Alphabetic Index. For clinical terms describing the stage that are not found in the Alphabetic Index, and there is no documentation of the stage, the provider should be queried.

4) **Patients admitted with pressure ulcers documented as healed**
No code is assigned if the documentation states that the pressure ulcer is completely healed.

5) **Patients admitted with pressure ulcers documented as healing**
Pressure ulcers described as healing should be assigned the appropriate pressure ulcer stage code based on the documentation in the medical record. If the documentation does not provide information about the stage of the healing pressure ulcer, assign the appropriate code for unspecified stage.
   If the documentation is unclear as to whether the patient has a current (new) pressure ulcer or if the patient is being treated for a healing pressure ulcer, query the provider.
   For ulcers that were present on admission but healed at the time of discharge, assign the code for the site and stage of the pressure ulcer at the time of admission.

6) **Patient admitted with pressure ulcer evolving into another stage during the admission**
If a patient is admitted to an inpatient hospital with a pressure ulcer at one stage and it progresses to a higher stage, two separate codes should be assigned: one code for the site and stage of the ulcer on admission and a second code for the same ulcer site and the highest stage reported during the stay.

b. Non-Pressure Chronic Ulcers

1) **Patients admitted with non-pressure ulcers documented as healed**
No code is assigned if the documentation states that the non-pressure ulcer is completely healed.

2) **Patients admitted with non-pressure ulcers documented as healing**
Non-pressure ulcers described as healing should be assigned the appropriate non-pressure ulcer code based on the documentation in the medical record. If the documentation does not provide information about the severity of the healing non-pressure ulcer, assign the appropriate code for unspecified severity.
   If the documentation is unclear as to whether the patient has a current (new) non-pressure ulcer or if the patient is being treated for a healing non-pressure ulcer, query the provider.
   For ulcers that were present on admission but healed at the time of discharge, assign the code for the site and severity of the non-pressure ulcer at the time of admission.

3) **Patient admitted with non-pressure ulcer that progresses to another severity level during the admission**
If a patient is admitted to an inpatient hospital with a non-pressure ulcer at one severity level and it progresses to a higher severity level, two separate codes should be assigned: one code for the site and severity level of the ulcer on admission and a second code for the same ulcer site and the highest severity level reported during the stay.
   See Section I.B.14 for pressure ulcer stage documentation by clinicians other than patient's provider.

Figure 12-1 Furuncle, also known as a boil, is a staphylococcal infection. The organism enters the body through a hair follicle and so furuncles usually appear in hairy areas of the body. A cluster of furuncles is known as a carbuncle and involves infection into the deep subcutaneous fascia. These usually appear on the back and neck. (**B** from Habif TP, Binnick AN, Meyerson LB: Clinical Dermatology: A Color Guide to Diagnosis and Therapy, S.l., Mosby Elsevier, 2010)

CHAPTER 12

DISEASES OF THE SKIN AND SUBCUTANEOUS TISSUE (L00-L99)

Excludes2   certain conditions originating in the perinatal period (P04-P96)
certain infectious and parasitic diseases (A00-B99)
complications of pregnancy, childbirth and the puerperium (O00-O9A)
congenital malformations, deformations, and chromosomal abnormalities (Q00-Q99)
endocrine, nutritional and metabolic diseases (E00-E88)
lipomelanotic reticulosis (I89.8)
neoplasms (C00-D49)
symptoms, signs and abnormal clinical and laboratory findings, not elsewhere classified (R00-R94)
systemic connective tissue disorders (M30-M36)
viral warts (B07.-)

This chapter contains the following blocks:

L00-L08	Infections of the skin and subcutaneous tissue
L10-L14	Bullous disorders
L20-L30	Dermatitis and eczema
L40-L45	Papulosquamous disorders
L49-L54	Urticaria and erythema
L55-L59	Radiation-related disorders of the skin and subcutaneous tissue
L60-L75	Disorders of skin appendages
L76	Intraoperative and postprocedural complications of skin and subcutaneous tissue
L80-L99	Other disorders of the skin and subcutaneous tissue

INFECTIONS OF THE SKIN AND SUBCUTANEOUS TISSUE (L00-L08)

Use additional code (B95-B97) to identify infectious agent.

Excludes2   hordeolum (H00.0)
infective dermatitis (L30.3)
local infections of skin classified in Chapter 1
lupus panniculitis (L93.2)
panniculitis NOS (M79.3)
panniculitis of neck and back (M54.0-)
Perlèche NOS (K13.0)
Perlèche due to candidiasis (B37.0)
Perlèche due to riboflavin deficiency (E53.0)
pyogenic granuloma (L98.0)
relapsing panniculitis [Weber-Christian] (M35.6)
viral warts (B07.-)
zoster (B02.-)

Figure 12-2 Impetigo. A thick, honey-yellow adherent crust covers the entire eroded surface. (From James WD, Elston DM, Berger TG, Andrews GC: Andrews' Diseases of the Skin: Clinical Dermatology, London, Saunders/Elsevier, 2011)

CHAPTER 12 (L00-L99)

L00   Staphylococcal scalded skin syndrome
     Ritter's disease
     Use additional code to identify percentage of skin exfoliation (L49.-)
     Excludes1   bullous impetigo (L01.03)
                     pemphigus neonatorum (L01.03)
                     toxic epidermal necrolysis [Lyell] (L51.2)

● L01   Impetigo
     Contagious skin infection caused by a streptococcus or staphylococcus aureus, common skin infections among children
     Excludes1   impetigo herpetiformis (L40.1)
     ● L01.0   Impetigo
              Impetigo contagiosa
              Impetigo vulgaris
         L01.00   Impetigo, unspecified
                  Impetigo NOS
         L01.01   Non-bullous impetigo
         L01.02   Bockhart's impetigo
                  Impetigo follicularis
                  Perifolliculitis NOS
                  Superficial pustular perifolliculitis
         L01.03   Bullous impetigo
                  Impetigo neonatorum
                  Pemphigus neonatorum
                  Neonate = newborn
         L01.09   Other impetigo
                  Ulcerative impetigo
     L01.1   Impetiginization of other dermatoses

● L02   Cutaneous abscess, furuncle and carbuncle
     Use additional code to identify organism (B95-B96)
     Excludes2   abscess of anus and rectal regions (K61.-)
                     abscess of female genital organs (external) (N76.4)
                     abscess of male genital organs (external) (N48.2, N49.-)
     ● L02.0   Cutaneous abscess, furuncle and carbuncle of face
         Excludes2   abscess of ear, external (H60.0)
                     abscess of eyelid (H00.0)
                     abscess of head [any part, except face] (L02.8)
                     abscess of lacrimal gland (H04.0)
                     abscess of lacrimal passages (H04.3)
                     abscess of mouth (K12.2)
                     abscess of nose (J34.0)
                     abscess of orbit (H05.0)
                     submandibular abscess (K12.2)
         L02.01   Cutaneous abscess of face
         L02.02   Furuncle of face
                  Boil of face
                  Folliculitis of face
         L02.03   Carbuncle of face
     ● L02.1   Cutaneous abscess, furuncle and carbuncle of neck
         L02.11   Cutaneous abscess of neck
         L02.12   Furuncle of neck
                  Boil of neck
                  Folliculitis of neck
         L02.13   Carbuncle of neck

● L02.2   Cutaneous abscess, furuncle and carbuncle of trunk
     Excludes1   non-newborn omphalitis (L08.82)
                     omphalitis of newborn (P38.-)
     Excludes2   abscess of breast (N61.1)
                     abscess of buttocks (L02.3)
                     abscess of female external genital organs (N76.4)
                     abscess of male external genital organs (N48.2, N49.-)
                     abscess of hip (L02.4)
     ● L02.21   Cutaneous abscess of trunk
         L02.211   Cutaneous abscess of abdominal wall
         L02.212   Cutaneous abscess of back [any part, except buttock]
         L02.213   Cutaneous abscess of chest wall
         L02.214   Cutaneous abscess of groin
         L02.215   Cutaneous abscess of perineum
         L02.216   Cutaneous abscess of umbilicus
         L02.219   Cutaneous abscess of trunk, unspecified
     ● L02.22   Furuncle of trunk
             Boil of trunk
             Folliculitis of trunk
         L02.221   Furuncle of abdominal wall
         L02.222   Furuncle of back [any part, except buttock]
         L02.223   Furuncle of chest wall
         L02.224   Furuncle of groin
         L02.225   Furuncle of perineum
         L02.226   Furuncle of umbilicus
         L02.229   Furuncle of trunk, unspecified
     ● L02.23   Carbuncle of trunk
         L02.231   Carbuncle of abdominal wall
         L02.232   Carbuncle of back [any part, except buttock]
         L02.233   Carbuncle of chest wall
         L02.234   Carbuncle of groin
         L02.235   Carbuncle of perineum
         L02.236   Carbuncle of umbilicus
         L02.239   Carbuncle of trunk, unspecified

● L02.3   Cutaneous abscess, furuncle and carbuncle of buttock
     Excludes1   pilonidal cyst with abscess (L05.01)
     L02.31   Cutaneous abscess of buttock
             Cutaneous abscess of gluteal region
     L02.32   Furuncle of buttock
             Boil of buttock
             Folliculitis of buttock
             Furuncle of gluteal region
     L02.33   Carbuncle of buttock
             Carbuncle of gluteal region

● L02.4   Cutaneous abscess, furuncle and carbuncle of limb
     Excludes2   Cutaneous abscess, furuncle and carbuncle of groin (L02.214, L02.224, L02.234)
                   Cutaneous abscess, furuncle and carbuncle of hand (L02.5-)
                   Cutaneous abscess, furuncle and carbuncle of foot (L02.6-)
     ● L02.41   Cutaneous abscess of limb
         L02.411   Cutaneous abscess of right axilla
         L02.412   Cutaneous abscess of left axilla
         L02.413   Cutaneous abscess of right upper limb
         L02.414   Cutaneous abscess of left upper limb
         L02.415   Cutaneous abscess of right lower limb
         L02.416   Cutaneous abscess of left lower limb
         L02.419   Cutaneous abscess of limb, unspecified

▶ New   ⇒ Revised   ~~deleted~~ Deleted   Excludes 1   Excludes 2   Includes   Use additional   Code first   Code also   Key words

OGCR Official Guidelines   X Assign placeholder X   ● Use Additional Character(s)   ▶ Manifestation Code   ⚕ Hierarchical Condition Category   **Coding Clinic**

● **L02.42** Furuncle of limb
      Boil of limb
      Folliculitis of limb
    L02.421 Furuncle of right axilla
    L02.422 Furuncle of left axilla
    L02.423 Furuncle of right upper limb
    L02.424 Furuncle of left upper limb
    L02.425 Furuncle of right lower limb
    L02.426 Furuncle of left lower limb
    L02.429 Furuncle of limb, unspecified
● **L02.43** Carbuncle of limb
    L02.431 Carbuncle of right axilla
    L02.432 Carbuncle of left axilla
    L02.433 Carbuncle of right upper limb
    L02.434 Carbuncle of left upper limb
    L02.435 Carbuncle of right lower limb
    L02.436 Carbuncle of left lower limb
    L02.439 Carbuncle of limb, unspecified
● **L02.5** Cutaneous abscess, furuncle and carbuncle of hand
  ● **L02.51** Cutaneous abscess of hand
      L02.511 Cutaneous abscess of right hand
      L02.512 Cutaneous abscess of left hand
      L02.519 Cutaneous abscess of unspecified hand
  ● **L02.52** Furuncle hand
        Boil of hand
        Folliculitis of hand
      L02.521 Furuncle right hand
      L02.522 Furuncle left hand
      L02.529 Furuncle unspecified hand
  ● **L02.53** Carbuncle of hand
      L02.531 Carbuncle of right hand
      L02.532 Carbuncle of left hand
      L02.539 Carbuncle of unspecified hand
● **L02.6** Cutaneous abscess, furuncle and carbuncle of foot
  ● **L02.61** Cutaneous abscess of foot
      L02.611 Cutaneous abscess of right foot
      L02.612 Cutaneous abscess of left foot
      L02.619 Cutaneous abscess of unspecified foot
  ● **L02.62** Furuncle of foot
        Boil of foot
        Folliculitis of foot
      L02.621 Furuncle of right foot
      L02.622 Furuncle of left foot
      L02.629 Furuncle of unspecified foot
  ● **L02.63** Carbuncle of foot
      L02.631 Carbuncle of right foot
      L02.632 Carbuncle of left foot
      L02.639 Carbuncle of unspecified foot
● **L02.8** Cutaneous abscess, furuncle and carbuncle of other sites
  ● **L02.81** Cutaneous abscess of other sites
      L02.811 Cutaneous abscess of head [any part, except face]
      L02.818 Cutaneous abscess of other sites
  ● **L02.82** Furuncle of other sites
        Boil of other sites
        Folliculitis of other sites
      L02.821 Furuncle of head [any part, except face]
      L02.828 Furuncle of other sites

● **L02.83** Carbuncle of other sites
      L02.831 Carbuncle of head [any part, except face]
      L02.838 Carbuncle of other sites
● **L02.9** Cutaneous abscess, furuncle and carbuncle, unspecified
    L02.91 Cutaneous abscess, unspecified
    L02.92 Furuncle, unspecified
        Boil NOS
        Furunculosis NOS
    L02.93 Carbuncle, unspecified
● **L03** Cellulitis and acute lymphangitis
    Excludes2 cellulitis of anal and rectal region (K61.-)
        cellulitis of external auditory canal (H60.1)
        cellulitis of eyelid (H00.0)
        cellulitis of female external genital organs (N76.4)
        cellulitis of lacrimal apparatus (H04.3)
        cellulitis of male external genital organs (N48.2, N49.-)
        cellulitis of mouth (K12.2)
        cellulitis of nose (J34.0)
        eosinophilic cellulitis [Wells] (L98.3)
        febrile neutrophilic dermatosis [Sweet] (L98.2)
        lymphangitis (chronic) (subacute) (I89.1)
● **L03.0** Cellulitis and acute lymphangitis of finger and toe
      Infection of nail
      Onychia
      Paronychia
      Perionychia
  ● **L03.01** Cellulitis of finger
        Felon
        Whitlow
        Excludes1 herpetic whitlow (B00.89)
      L03.011 Cellulitis of right finger
      L03.012 Cellulitis of left finger
      L03.019 Cellulitis of unspecified finger
  ● **L03.02** Acute lymphangitis of finger
        Hangnail with lymphangitis of finger
      L03.021 Acute lymphangitis of right finger
      L03.022 Acute lymphangitis of left finger
      L03.029 Acute lymphangitis of unspecified finger
  ● **L03.03** Cellulitis of toe
      L03.031 Cellulitis of right toe
      L03.032 Cellulitis of left toe
      L03.039 Cellulitis of unspecified toe
  ● **L03.04** Acute lymphangitis of toe
        Hangnail with lymphangitis of toe
      L03.041 Acute lymphangitis of right toe
      L03.042 Acute lymphangitis of left toe
      L03.049 Acute lymphangitis of unspecified toe
● **L03.1** Cellulitis and acute lymphangitis of other parts of limb
  ● **L03.11** Cellulitis of other parts of limb
        Excludes2 cellulitis of fingers (L03.01-)
            cellulitis of toes (L03.03-)
            groin (L03.314)
      L03.111 Cellulitis of right axilla
      L03.112 Cellulitis of left axilla
      L03.113 Cellulitis of right upper limb
      L03.114 Cellulitis of left upper limb
            Coding Clinic: 2019, Q1, P13
      L03.115 Cellulitis of right lower limb
      L03.116 Cellulitis of left lower limb
      L03.119 Cellulitis of unspecified part of limb

Item 12-1 Onychia is an inflammation of the tissue surrounding the nail with pus accumulation and loss of the nail, resulting from microscopic pathogens entering through small wounds. **Paronychia** is a nail disease also known as felon or whitlow and is a bacterial or fungal infection.

Item 12-2 Cellulitis is an acute spreading bacterial infection below the surface of the skin characterized by redness (erythema), warmth, swelling, pain, fever, chills, and enlarged lymph nodes ("swollen glands").

CHAPTER 12 (L00-L99)

CHAPTER 12 (L00-L99)

● **L03.12**   Acute lymphangitis of other parts of limb

     Excludes2   acute lymphangitis of fingers (L03.2-)

                acute lymphangitis of toes (L03.04-)

                acute lymphangitis of groin (L03.324)

   L03.121   Acute lymphangitis of right axilla

   L03.122   Acute lymphangitis of left axilla

   L03.123   Acute lymphangitis of right upper limb

   L03.124   Acute lymphangitis of left upper limb

   L03.125   Acute lymphangitis of right lower limb

   L03.126   Acute lymphangitis of left lower limb

   L03.129   Acute lymphangitis of unspecified part of limb

● **L03.2**   Cellulitis and acute lymphangitis of face and neck

   ● **L03.21**   Cellulitis and acute lymphangitis of face

     L03.211   Cellulitis of face

         Excludes2   abscess of orbit (H05.01-)

                cellulitis of ear (H60.1-)

                cellulitis of eyelid (H00.0-)

                cellulitis of head (L03.81)

                cellulitis of lacrimal apparatus (H04.3)

                cellulitis of lip (K13.0)

                cellulitis of mouth (K12.2)

                cellulitis of nose (internal) (J34.0)

                cellulitis of orbit (H05.01-)

                cellulitis of scalp (L03.81)

     L03.212   Acute lymphangitis of face

     L03.213   Periorbital cellulitis

         Preseptal cellulitis

         Coding Clinic: 2016, Q4, P36

   ● **L03.22**   Cellulitis and acute lymphangitis of neck

     L03.221   Cellulitis of neck

     L03.222   Acute lymphangitis of neck

● **L03.3**   Cellulitis and acute lymphangitis of trunk

   ● **L03.31**   Cellulitis of trunk

         Excludes2   cellulitis of anal and rectal regions (K61.-)

                cellulitis of breast NOS (N61.0)

                cellulitis of female external genital organs (N76.4)

                cellulitis of male external genital organs (N48.2, N49.-)

                omphalitis of newborn (P38.-)

                puerperal cellulitis of breast (O91.2)

     L03.311   Cellulitis of abdominal wall

         Excludes2   cellulitis of umbilicus (L03.316)

                cellulitis of groin (L03.314)

     L03.312   Cellulitis of back [any part except buttock]

     L03.313   Cellulitis of chest wall

     L03.314   Cellulitis of groin

     L03.315   Cellulitis of perineum

     L03.316   Cellulitis of umbilicus

     L03.317   Cellulitis of buttock

     L03.319   Cellulitis of trunk, unspecified

   ● **L03.32**   Acute lymphangitis of trunk

     L03.321   Acute lymphangitis of abdominal wall

     L03.322   Acute lymphangitis of back [any part except buttock]

     L03.323   Acute lymphangitis of chest wall

     L03.324   Acute lymphangitis of groin

     L03.325   Acute lymphangitis of perineum

     L03.326   Acute lymphangitis of umbilicus

     L03.327   Acute lymphangitis of buttock

     L03.329   Acute lymphangitis of trunk, unspecified

● **L03.8**   Cellulitis and acute lymphangitis of other sites

   ● **L03.81**   Cellulitis of other sites

     L03.811   Cellulitis of head [any part, except face]

         Cellulitis of scalp

         Excludes2   cellulitis of face (L03.211)

     L03.818   Cellulitis of other sites

   ● **L03.89**   Acute lymphangitis of other sites

     L03.891   Acute lymphangitis of head [any part, except face]

     L03.898   Acute lymphangitis of other sites

● **L03.9**   Cellulitis and acute lymphangitis, unspecified

   L03.90   Cellulitis, unspecified

   L03.91   Acute lymphangitis, unspecified

     Excludes1   lymphangitis NOS (I89.1)

● **L04**   **Acute lymphadenitis**

   Short-term inflammation of lymph nodes which can be regionalized to involve a given area of the lymph system or systemic involving much of the body

   Includes   abscess (acute) of lymph nodes, except mesenteric

              acute lymphadenitis, except mesenteric

   Excludes1   chronic or subacute lymphadenitis, except mesenteric (I88.1)

              enlarged lymph nodes (R59.-)

              human immunodeficiency virus [HIV] disease resulting in generalized lymphadenopathy (B20)

              lymphadenitis NOS (I88.9)

              nonspecific mesenteric lymphadenitis (I88.0)

   L04.0   Acute lymphadenitis of face, head and neck

   L04.1   Acute lymphadenitis of trunk

   L04.2   Acute lymphadenitis of upper limb

     Acute lymphadenitis of axilla

     Acute lymphadenitis of shoulder

   L04.3   Acute lymphadenitis of lower limb

     Acute lymphadenitis of hip

     Excludes2   acute lymphadenitis of groin (L04.1)

   L04.8   Acute lymphadenitis of other sites

   L04.9   Acute lymphadenitis, unspecified

● **L05**   **Pilonidal cyst and sinus**

   ● **L05.0**   Pilonidal cyst and sinus with abscess

     L05.01   Pilonidal cyst with abscess

         Pilonidal abscess

         Pilonidal dimple with abscess

         Postanal dimple with abscess

         Excludes2   congenital sacral dimple (Q82.6)

                parasacral dimple (Q82.6)

     L05.02   Pilonidal sinus with abscess

         Coccygeal fistula with abscess

         Coccygeal sinus with abscess

         Pilonidal fistula with abscess

Item 12–3   **Abscess** is a localized collection of pus in tissues or organs and is a sign of infection, resulting in swelling and inflammation.

▶ New   ⇒ Revised   ~~deleted~~ Deleted   Excludes 1   Excludes 2   Includes   Use additional   Code first   Code also   Key words

OGCR Official Guidelines   X Assign placeholder X   ● Use Additional Character(s)   ▶ Manifestation Code   🅗 Hierarchical Condition Category   Coding Clinic

Item 12–4 Pilonidal cyst, also called a coccygeal cyst, is the result of a disorder called pilonidal disease. The cyst usually contains hair and pus.

● **L05.9   Pilonidal cyst and sinus without abscess**

     L05.91   Pilonidal cyst without abscess
         Pilonidal dimple
         Postanal dimple
         Pilonidal cyst NOS

         Excludes2   congenital sacral dimple (Q82.6)
                       parasacral dimple (Q82.6)

     L05.92   Pilonidal sinus without abscess
         Coccygeal fistula
         Coccygeal sinus without abscess
         Pilonidal fistula

● **L08   Other local infections of skin and subcutaneous tissue**

     L08.0   Pyoderma
         Dermatitis gangrenosa
         Purulent dermatitis
         Septic dermatitis
         Suppurative dermatitis

         Excludes1   pyoderma gangrenosum (L88)
                       pyoderma vegetans (L08.81)

     L08.1   Erythrasma

●   **L08.8   Other specified local infections of the skin and subcutaneous tissue**

     L08.81   Pyoderma vegetans

         Excludes1   pyoderma gangrenosum (L88)
                       pyoderma NOS (L08.0)

     L08.82   Omphalitis not of newborn

         Excludes1   omphalitis of newborn (P38.-)

     L08.89   Other specified local infections of the skin and subcutaneous tissue

     L08.9   Local infection of the skin and subcutaneous tissue, unspecified

BULLOUS DISORDERS (L10-L14)

Excludes1   benign familial pemphigus [Hailey-Hailey] (Q82.8)
                 staphylococcal scalded skin syndrome (L00)
                 toxic epidermal necrolysis [Lyell] (L51.2)

● **L10   Pemphigus**

     Excludes1   pemphigus neonatorum (L01.03)

     L10.0   Pemphigus vulgaris
     L10.1   Pemphigus vegetans
     L10.2   Pemphigus foliaceous
     L10.3   Brazilian pemphigus [fogo selvagem]
     L10.4   Pemphigus erythematosus
         Senear-Usher syndrome
     L10.5   Drug-induced pemphigus

         Use additional code for adverse effect, if applicable, to identify drug (T36-T50 with fifth or sixth character 5)

●   **L10.8   Other pemphigus**
     L10.81   Paraneoplastic pemphigus
     L10.89   Other pemphigus
     L10.9   Pemphigus, unspecified

tem 12–5 Dermatitis herpetiformis, also known as Duhring's disease, is a systemic disease characterized by small blisters (3 to 5 mm) and occasionally large bullae (> 5 mm).

Figure 12-3   Dermatitis herpetiformis. (From Terhorst D: BASICS Dermatologie, München, Elsevier, Urban & Fischer, 2011)

● **L11   Other acantholytic disorders**

     L11.0   Acquired keratosis follicularis

         Excludes1   keratosis follicularis (congenital) [Darier-White] (Q82.8)

     L11.1   Transient acantholytic dermatosis [Grover]
     L11.8   Other specified acantholytic disorders
     L11.9   Acantholytic disorder, unspecified

● **L12   Pemphigoid**

     Excludes1   herpes gestationis (O26.4-)
                 impetigo herpetiformis (L40.1)

     L12.0   Bullous pemphigoid
     L12.1   Cicatricial pemphigoid
         Benign mucous membrane pemphigoid

     L12.2   Chronic bullous disease of childhood   P
         Juvenile dermatitis herpetiformis

●   **L12.3   Acquired epidermolysis bullosa**

         Excludes1   epidermolysis bullosa (congenital) (Q81.-)

     L12.30   Acquired epidermolysis bullosa, unspecified 🔗
     L12.31   Epidermolysis bullosa due to drug 🔗

         Use additional code for adverse effect, if applicable, to identify drug (T36-T50 with fifth or sixth character 5)

     L12.35   Other acquired epidermolysis bullosa 🔗
     L12.8   Other pemphigoid
     L12.9   Pemphigoid, unspecified

● **L13   Other bullous disorders**

     L13.0   Dermatitis herpetiformis
         Duhring's disease
         Hydroa herpetiformis

         Excludes1   juvenile dermatitis herpetiformis (L12.2)
                       senile dermatitis herpetiformis (L12.0)

     L13.1   Subcorneal pustular dermatitis
         Sneddon-Wilkinson disease

     L13.8   Other specified bullous disorders
     L13.9   Bullous disorder, unspecified

▷ *L14   Bullous disorders in diseases classified elsewhere*
     Code first underlying disease

DERMATITIS AND ECZEMA (L20-L30)

Note: In this block the terms dermatitis and eczema are used synonymously and interchangeably.

     Excludes2   chronic (childhood) granulomatous disease (D71)
                 dermatitis gangrenosa (L08.0)
                 dermatitis herpetiformis (L13.0)
                 dry skin dermatitis (L85.3)
                 factitial dermatitis (L98.1)
                 perioral dermatitis (L71.0)
                 radiation-related disorders of the skin and subcutaneous tissue (L55-L59)
                 stasis dermatitis (I87.2)

● **L20   Atopic dermatitis**

     L20.0   Besnier's prurigo

●   **L20.8   Other atopic dermatitis**

         Excludes2   circumscribed neurodermatitis (L28.0)

     L20.81   Atopic neurodermatitis
         Diffuse neurodermatitis
     L20.82   Flexural eczema
     L20.83   Infantile (acute) (chronic) eczema   P
     L20.84   Intrinsic (allergic) eczema
     L20.89   Other atopic dermatitis
     L20.9   Atopic dermatitis, unspecified

Item 12–6 Seborrheic dermatitis is characterized by greasy, scaly, red patches and is associated with oily skin and scalp.

Figure 12-4　Seborrheic dermatitis. (Getty Image)

● **L21 Seborrheic dermatitis**

　　　Excludes2　infective dermatitis (L30.3)
　　　　　　　　　　seborrheic keratosis (L82.-)

　　L21.0 Seborrhea capitis
　　　　Cradle cap
　　　　Coding Clinic: 2018, Q1, P6

　　L21.1 Seborrheic infantile dermatitis　　　　　　　P

　　L21.8 Other seborrheic dermatitis

　　L21.9 Seborrheic dermatitis, unspecified
　　　　Seborrhea NOS

L22 Diaper dermatitis
　　　Diaper erythema
　　　Diaper rash
　　　Psoriasiform diaper rash
　　　Coding Clinic: 2021, Q4, P18

● **L23 Allergic contact dermatitis**

　　　Excludes1　allergy NOS (T78.40)
　　　　　　　　　　contact dermatitis NOS (L25.9)
　　　　　　　　　　dermatitis NOS (L30.9)

　　　Excludes2　dermatitis due to substances taken internally (L27.-)
　　　　　　　　　　dermatitis of eyelid (H01.1-)
　　　　　　　　　　diaper dermatitis (L22)
　　　　　　　　　　eczema of external ear (H60.5-)
　　　　　　　　　　irritant contact dermatitis (L24.-)
　　　　　　　　　　perioral dermatitis (L71.0)
　　　　　　　　　　radiation-related disorders of the skin and
　　　　　　　　　　　　subcutaneous tissue (L55-L59)

　　L23.0 Allergic contact dermatitis due to metals
　　　　Allergic contact dermatitis due to chromium
　　　　Allergic contact dermatitis due to nickel

　　L23.1 Allergic contact dermatitis due to adhesives

　　L23.2 Allergic contact dermatitis due to cosmetics

　　L23.3 Allergic contact dermatitis due to drugs in contact with skin

　　　　Use additional code for adverse effect, if applicable, to
　　　　　　identify drug (T36-T50 with fifth or sixth character 5)

　　　　Excludes2　dermatitis due to ingested drugs and
　　　　　　　　　　　medicaments (L27.0-L27.1)

　　L23.4 Allergic contact dermatitis due to dyes

　　L23.5 Allergic contact dermatitis due to other chemical products
　　　　Allergic contact dermatitis due to cement
　　　　Allergic contact dermatitis due to insecticide
　　　　Allergic contact dermatitis due to plastic
　　　　Allergic contact dermatitis due to rubber

Item 12–7 Atopic dermatitis, also known as atopic eczema, infantile eczema, disseminated neuro dermatitis, flexural eczema, and *prurigo diathesique* (Besnier), is characterized by intense itching and is often hereditary.

Figure 12-5　Atopic dermatitis. (From Chabner D-E: The Language of Medicine, St. Louis, MO, Saunders/Elsevier, 2007)

L23.6 Allergic contact dermatitis due to food in contact with the skin
　　　Excludes2　dermatitis due to ingested food (L27.2)

L23.7 Allergic contact dermatitis due to plants, except food
　　　Excludes2　allergy NOS due to pollen (J30.1)

● **L23.8 Allergic contact dermatitis due to other agents**

　　L23.81　Allergic contact dermatitis due to animal (cat) (dog) dander
　　　　Allergic contact dermatitis due to animal (cat) (dog) hair

　　L23.89　Allergic contact dermatitis due to other agents

L23.9 Allergic contact dermatitis, unspecified cause
　　　Allergic contact eczema NOS

● **L24 Irritant contact dermatitis**

　　　Excludes1　allergy NOS (T78.40)
　　　　　　　　　　contact dermatitis NOS (L25.9)
　　　　　　　　　　dermatitis NOS (L30.9)

　　　Excludes2　allergic contact dermatitis (L23.-)
　　　　　　　　　　dermatitis due to substances taken internally (L27.-)
　　　　　　　　　　dermatitis of eyelid (H01.1-)
　　　　　　　　　　diaper dermatitis (L22)
　　　　　　　　　　eczema of external ear (H60.5-)
　　　　　　　　　　perioral dermatitis (L71.0)
　　　　　　　　　　radiation-related disorders of the skin and
　　　　　　　　　　　　subcutaneous tissue (L55-L59)

　　L24.0 Irritant contact dermatitis due to detergents

　　L24.1 Irritant contact dermatitis due to oils and greases

　　L24.2 Irritant contact dermatitis due to solvents
　　　　Irritant contact dermatitis due to chlorocompound
　　　　Irritant contact dermatitis due to cyclohexane
　　　　Irritant contact dermatitis due to ester
　　　　Irritant contact dermatitis due to glycol
　　　　Irritant contact dermatitis due to hydrocarbon
　　　　Irritant contact dermatitis due to ketone

　　L24.3 Irritant contact dermatitis due to cosmetics

　　L24.4 Irritant contact dermatitis due to drugs in contact with skin

　　　　Use additional code for adverse effect, if applicable,
　　　　　　to identify drug (T36-T50 with fifth or sixth
　　　　　　character 5)

　　L24.5 Irritant contact dermatitis due to other chemical products
　　　　Irritant contact dermatitis due to cement
　　　　Irritant contact dermatitis due to insecticide
　　　　Irritant contact dermatitis due to plastic
　　　　Irritant contact dermatitis due to rubber

　　L24.6 Irritant contact dermatitis due to food in contact with skin
　　　Excludes2　dermatitis due to ingested food (L27.2)

　　L24.7 Irritant contact dermatitis due to plants, except food
　　　Excludes2　allergy NOS to pollen (J30.1)

● **L24.8 Irritant contact dermatitis due to other agents**

　　L24.81　Irritant contact dermatitis due to metals
　　　　Irritant contact dermatitis due to chromium
　　　　Irritant contact dermatitis due to nickel

　　L24.89　Irritant contact dermatitis due to other agents
　　　　Irritant contact dermatitis due to dyes

　　L24.9 Irritant contact dermatitis, unspecified cause
　　　Irritant contact eczema NOS

● **L24.A Irritant contact dermatitis due to friction or contact with body fluids**
　　　Excludes1　virritant contact dermatitis related to
　　　　　　　　　　stoma or fistula (L24.B-)
　　　Excludes2　erythema intertrigo (L30.4)

　　L24.A0 Irritant contact dermatitis due to friction or contact with body fluids, unspecified

　　L24.A1 Irritant contact dermatitis due to saliva

　　L24.A2 Irritant contact dermatitis due to fecal, urinary or dual incontinence
　　　Excludes1　diaper dermatitis (L22)
　　　　　　Coding Clinic: 2021, Q4, P18

▶ New　⇥ Revised　~~deleted~~ Deleted　Excludes 1　Excludes 2　Includes　Use additional　Code first　Code also　Key words

OGCR Official Guidelines　X Assign placeholder X　● Use Additional Character(s)　▶ Manifestation Code　🔖 Hierarchical Condition Category　Coding Clinic

L24.A9 **Irritant contact dermatitis due friction or contact with other specified body fluids**
Irritant contact dermatitis related to endotracheal tube
Wound fluids, exudate

● **L24.B Irritant contact dermatitis related to stoma or fistula**
Use additional code to identify any artificial opening status (Z93.-), if applicable, for contact dermatitis related to stoma secretions

L24.B0 **Irritant contact dermatitis related to unspecified stoma or fistula**
Irritant contact dermatitis related to fistula NOS
Irritant contact dermatitis related to stoma NOS

L24.B1 **Irritant contact dermatitis related to digestive stoma or fistula**
Irritant contact dermatitis related to gastrostomy
Irritant contact dermatitis related to jejunostomy
Irritant contact dermatitis related to saliva or spit fistula

L24.B2 **Irritant contact dermatitis related to respiratory stoma or fistula**
Irritant contact dermatitis related to tracheostomy

L24.B3 **Irritant contact dermatitis related to fecal or urinary stoma or fistula**
Irritant contact dermatitis related to colostomy
Irritant contact dermatitis related to enterocutaneous fistula
Irritant contact dermatitis related to ileostomy
Coding Clinic: 2021, Q4, P17,19

● **L25 Unspecified contact dermatitis**
Excludes1 allergic contact dermatitis (L23.-)
allergy NOS (T78.40)
dermatitis NOS (L30.9)
irritant contact dermatitis (L24.-)
Excludes2 dermatitis due to ingested substances (L27.-)
dermatitis of eyelid (H01.1-)
eczema of external ear (H60.5-)
perioral dermatitis (L71.0)
radiation-related disorders of the skin and subcutaneous tissue (L55-L59)

L25.0 **Unspecified contact dermatitis due to cosmetics**
L25.1 **Unspecified contact dermatitis due to drugs in contact with skin**
Use additional code for adverse effect, if applicable, to identify drug (T36-T50 with fifth or sixth character 5)
Excludes2 dermatitis due to ingested drugs and medicaments (L27.0-L27.1)
L25.2 **Unspecified contact dermatitis due to dyes**
L25.3 **Unspecified contact dermatitis due to other chemical products**
Unspecified contact dermatitis due to cement
Unspecified contact dermatitis due to insecticide
L25.4 **Unspecified contact dermatitis due to food in contact with skin**
Excludes2 dermatitis due to ingested food (L27.2)
L25.5 **Unspecified contact dermatitis due to plants, except food**
Excludes1 nettle rash (L50.9)
Excludes2 allergy NOS due to pollen (J30.1)
L25.8 **Unspecified contact dermatitis due to other agents**
L25.9 **Unspecified contact dermatitis, unspecified cause**
Contact dermatitis (occupational) NOS
Contact eczema (occupational) NOS

● **L26 Exfoliative dermatitis**
Hebra's pityriasis
Excludes1 Ritter's disease (L00)

● **L27 Dermatitis due to substances taken internally**
Excludes1 allergy NOS (T78.40)
Excludes2 adverse food reaction, except dermatitis (T78.0-T78.1)
contact dermatitis (L23-L25)
drug photoallergic response (L56.1)
drug phototoxic response (L56.0)
urticaria (L50.-)

L27.0 **Generalized skin eruption due to drugs and medicaments taken internally**
Use additional code for adverse effect, if applicable, to identify drug (T36-T50 with fifth or sixth character 5)

L27.1 **Localized skin eruption due to drugs and medicaments taken internally**
Use additional code for adverse effect, if applicable, to identify drug (T36-T50 with fifth or sixth character 5)

L27.2 **Dermatitis due to ingested food**
Excludes2 dermatitis due to food in contact with skin (L23.6, L24.6, L25.4)

L27.8 **Dermatitis due to other substances taken internally**
L27.9 **Dermatitis due to unspecified substance taken internally**

● **L28 Lichen simplex chronicus and prurigo**
L28.0 **Lichen simplex chronicus**
Circumscribed neurodermatitis
Lichen NOS
L28.1 **Prurigo nodularis**
L28.2 **Other prurigo**
Prurigo NOS   Prurigo mitis
Prurigo Hebra   Urticaria papulosa

● **L29 Pruritus**
Excludes1 neurotic excoriation (L98.1)
psychogenic pruritus (F45.8)
L29.0 **Pruritus ani**
L29.1 **Pruritus scroti**
L29.2 **Pruritus vulvae**
L29.3 **Anogenital pruritus, unspecified**
L29.8 **Other pruritus**
▶ L29.81 **Cholestatic pruritus**
▶ Code also, if applicable, type of liver disease
▶ Use Additional code for adverse effect, if applicable, to identify drug (T36-T50 with fifth or sixth character 5)
▶ L29.89 **Other pruritus**
L29.9 **Pruritus, unspecified**
Itch NOS

● **L30 Other and unspecified dermatitis**
Excludes2 contact dermatitis (L23-L25)
dry skin dermatitis (L85.3)
small plaque parapsoriasis (L41.3)
stasis dermatitis (I87.2)
L30.0 **Nummular dermatitis**
L30.1 **Dyshidrosis [pompholyx]**
L30.2 **Cutaneous autosensitization**
Candidid [levurid]   Eczematid
Dermatophytid
L30.3 **Infective dermatitis**
Infectious eczematoid dermatitis
L30.4 **Erythema intertrigo**
L30.5 **Pityriasis alba**
Coding Clinic: 2018, Q1, P6
L30.8 **Other specified dermatitis**
L30.9 **Dermatitis, unspecified**
Eczema NOS

PAPULOSQUAMOUS DISORDERS (L40-L45)

- **L40**   **Psoriasis**
  - **L40.0**   **Psoriasis vulgaris**
    - Nummular psoriasis   Plaque psoriasis
  - **L40.1**   **Generalized pustular psoriasis**
    - Impetigo herpetiformis   Von Zumbusch's disease
  - **L40.2**   **Acrodermatitis continua**
  - **L40.3**   **Pustulosis palmaris et plantaris**
  - **L40.4**   **Guttate psoriasis**
  - ● **L40.5**   **Arthropathic psoriasis**
    - **L40.50**   Arthropathic psoriasis, unspecified 🐾
    - **L40.51**   Distal interphalangeal psoriatic arthropathy 🐾
    - **L40.52**   Psoriatic arthritis mutilans 🐾
    - **L40.53**   Psoriatic spondylitis 🐾
    - **L40.54**   Psoriatic juvenile arthropathy 🐾
    - **L40.59**   Other psoriatic arthropathy 🐾
  - **L40.8**   **Other psoriasis**
    - Flexural psoriasis
  - **L40.9**   **Psoriasis, unspecified**

- **L41**   **Parapsoriasis**
  - **Excludes1**   poikiloderma vasculare atrophicans (L94.5)
  - **L41.0**   **Pityriasis lichenoides et varioliformis acuta**
    - Mucha-Habermann disease
  - **L41.1**   **Pityriasis lichenoides chronica**
  - **L41.3**   **Small plaque parapsoriasis**
  - **L41.4**   **Large plaque parapsoriasis**
  - **L41.5**   **Retiform parapsoriasis**
  - **L41.8**   **Other parapsoriasis**
  - **L41.9**   **Parapsoriasis, unspecified**

- L42   **Pityriasis rosea**

- **L43**   **Lichen planus**
  - ⇒ **Excludes1**   lichen planopilaris (L66.1-)
  - **L43.0**   **Hypertrophic lichen planus**
  - **L43.1**   **Bullous lichen planus**
  - **L43.2**   **Lichenoid drug reaction**
    - Use additional code for adverse effect, if applicable, to identify drug (T36-T50 with fifth or sixth character 5)
  - **L43.3**   **Subacute (active) lichen planus**
    - Lichen planus tropicus
  - **L43.8**   **Other lichen planus**
  - **L43.9**   **Lichen planus, unspecified**

- **L44**   **Other papulosquamous disorders**
  - **L44.0**   **Pityriasis rubra pilaris**
  - **L44.1**   **Lichen nitidus**
  - **L44.2**   **Lichen striatus**
  - **L44.3**   **Lichen ruber moniliformis**
  - **L44.4**   **Infantile papular acrodermatitis [Gianotti-Crosti]**   P
  - **L44.8**   **Other specified papulosquamous disorders**
  - **L44.9**   **Papulosquamous disorder, unspecified**

- ▶ *L45*   *Papulosquamous disorders in diseases classified elsewhere*
  - *Code first underlying disease*

URTICARIA AND ERYTHEMA (L49-L54)

- **Excludes1**   Lyme disease (A69.2-)
  - rosacea (L71.-)

- ● **L49**   **Exfoliation due to erythematous conditions according to extent of body surface involved**
  - *Code first erythematous condition causing exfoliation, such as:*
    - Ritter's disease (L00)
    - (Staphylococcal) scalded skin syndrome (L00)
    - Stevens-Johnson syndrome (L51.1)
    - Stevens-Johnson syndrome-toxic epidermal necrolysis overlap syndrome (L51.3)
    - Toxic epidermal necrolysis (L51.2)
  - **L49.0**   **Exfoliation due to erythematous condition involving less than 10 percent of body surface**
    - Exfoliation due to erythematous condition NOS
  - **L49.1**   **Exfoliation due to erythematous condition involving 10-19 percent of body surface**
  - **L49.2**   **Exfoliation due to erythematous condition involving 20-29 percent of body surface**
  - **L49.3**   **Exfoliation due to erythematous condition involving 30-39 percent of body surface** (Ex) No exclusions
  - **L49.4**   **Exfoliation due to erythematous condition involving 40-49 percent of body surface** (Ex) No exclusions
  - **L49.5**   **Exfoliation due to erythematous condition involving 50-59 percent of body surface** (Ex) No exclusions
  - **L49.6**   **Exfoliation due to erythematous condition involving 60-69 percent of body surface** (Ex) No exclusions
  - **L49.7**   **Exfoliation due to erythematous condition involving 70-79 percent of body surface** (Ex) No exclusions
  - **L49.8**   **Exfoliation due to erythematous condition involving 80-89 percent of body surface** (Ex) No exclusions
  - **L49.9**   **Exfoliation due to erythematous condition involving 90 or more percent of body surface** (Ex) No exclusions

- ● **L50**   **Urticaria**
  - **Excludes1**   allergic contact dermatitis (L23.-)
    - angioneurotic edema (T78.3)
    - giant urticaria (T78.3)
    - hereditary angio-edema (D84.1)
    - Quincke's edema (T78.3)
    - serum urticaria (T80.6-)
    - solar urticaria (L56.3)
    - urticaria neonatorum (P83.8)
    - urticaria papulosa (L28.2)
    - urticaria pigmentosa (D47.01)
  - **L50.0**   **Allergic urticaria**
  - **L50.1**   **Idiopathic urticaria**
  - **L50.2**   **Urticaria due to cold and heat**
    - **Excludes2**   familial cold urticaria (M04.2)
  - **L50.3**   **Dermatographic urticaria**
  - **L50.4**   **Vibratory urticaria**
  - **L50.5**   **Cholinergic urticaria**
  - **L50.6**   **Contact urticaria**

Figure 12-6   Erythematous plaques with silvery scales in a patient with psoriasis. (Getty Image)

Item 12–8 Psoriasis is a chronic, recurrent inflammatory skin disease characterized by small patches covered with thick, silvery scales. **Parapsoriasis** is a treatment-resistant erythroderma. **Pityriasis rosea** is characterized by a herald patch that is a single large lesion and that usually appears on the trunk and is followed by scattered, smaller lesions.

▶ New   ⇒ Revised   ~~deleted~~ Deleted   Excludes 1   Excludes 2   Includes   Use additional   Code first   Code also   Key words

OGCR Official Guidelines   X Assign placeholder X   ● Use Additional Character(s)   ▶ Manifestation Code   🐾 Hierarchical Condition Category   Coding Clinic

Figure 12-7 Urticaria (hives). *(Courtesy of David Effron, MD.)* (Getty Image)

Item 12–9 Urticaria is a vascular reaction in which wheals surrounded by a red halo appear and cause severe itching. The causes of urticaria or hives are extensive and varied (e.g., food, heat, cold, drugs, stress, infections).

L50.8 Other urticaria
 Chronic urticaria
 Recurrent periodic urticaria

L50.9 Urticaria, unspecified

● **L51 Erythema multiforme**
 Use additional code for adverse effect, if applicable, to identify drug (T36-T50 with fifth or sixth character 5)
 Use additional code to identify associated manifestations, such as:
 arthropathy associated with dermatological disorders (M14.8-)
 conjunctival edema (H11.42)
 conjunctivitis (H10.22-)
 corneal scars and opacities (H17.-)
 corneal ulcer (H16.0-)
 edema of eyelid (H02.84-)
 inflammation of eyelid (H01.8)
 keratoconjunctivitis sicca (H16.22-)
 mechanical lagophthalmos (H02.22-)
 stomatitis (K12.-)
 symblepharon (H11.23-)
 Use additional code to identify percentage of skin exfoliation (L49.-)

 Excludes1 staphylococcal scalded skin syndrome (L00)
 Ritter's disease (L00)

L51.0 Nonbullous erythema multiforme
L51.1 Stevens-Johnson syndrome 🔖
L51.2 Toxic epidermal necrolysis [Lyell] 🔖
L51.3 Stevens-Johnson syndrome-toxic epidermal necrolysis overlap syndrome 🔖
 SJS-TEN overlap syndrome
L51.8 Other erythema multiforme
L51.9 Erythema multiforme, unspecified
 Erythema iris
 Erythema multiforme major NOS
 Erythema multiforme minor NOS
 Herpes iris

L52 Erythema nodosum
 Excludes1 tuberculous erythema nodosum (A18.4)

● **L53 Other erythematous conditions**
 Excludes1 erythema ab igne (L59.0)
 erythema due to external agents in contact with skin (L23-L25)
 erythema intertrigo (L30.4)

L53.0 Toxic erythema
 Code first poisoning due to drug or toxin, if applicable (T36-T65 with fifth or sixth character 1-4)
 Use additional code for adverse effect, if applicable, to identify drug (T36-T50 with fifth or sixth character 5)
 Excludes1 neonatal erythema toxicum (P83.1)
L53.1 Erythema annulare centrifugum
L53.2 Erythema marginatum
L53.3 Other chronic figurate erythema
L53.8 Other specified erythematous conditions
L53.9 Erythematous condition, unspecified
 Erythema NOS
 Erythroderma NOS

◗ *L54 Erythema in diseases classified elsewhere*
 Code first underlying disease

RADIATION-RELATED DISORDERS OF THE SKIN AND SUBCUTANEOUS TISSUE (L55-L59)

● **L55 Sunburn**
L55.0 Sunburn of first degree
L55.1 Sunburn of second degree
L55.2 Sunburn of third degree
L55.9 Sunburn, unspecified

● **L56 Other acute skin changes due to ultraviolet radiation**
 Use additional code to identify the source of the ultraviolet radiation (W89, X32)
L56.0 Drug phototoxic response
 Use additional code for adverse effect, if applicable, to identify drug (T36-T50 with fifth or sixth character 5)
L56.1 Drug photoallergic response
 Use additional code for adverse effect, if applicable, to identify drug (T36-T50 with fifth or sixth character 5)
L56.2 Photocontact dermatitis [berloque dermatitis]
L56.3 Solar urticaria
L56.4 Polymorphous light eruption
L56.5 Disseminated superficial actinic porokeratosis (DSAP)
L56.8 Other specified acute skin changes due to ultraviolet radiation
L56.9 Acute skin change due to ultraviolet radiation, unspecified

● **L57 Skin changes due to chronic exposure to nonionizing radiation**
 Use additional code to identify the source of the ultraviolet radiation (W89), or other nonionizing radiation (W90)
L57.0 Actinic keratosis
 Keratosis NOS   Solar keratosis
 Senile keratosis
L57.1 Actinic reticuloid
L57.2 Cutis rhomboidalis nuchae
L57.3 Poikiloderma of Civatte
L57.4 Cutis laxa senilis
 Elastosis senilis
L57.5 Actinic granuloma
L57.8 Other skin changes due to chronic exposure to nonionizing radiation
 Farmer's skin   Solar dermatitis
 Sailor's skin
L57.9 Skin changes due to chronic exposure to nonionizing radiation, unspecified

● **L58 Radiodermatitis**
 Use additional code to identify the source of the radiation (W88, W90)
L58.0 Acute radiodermatitis
L58.1 Chronic radiodermatitis
L58.9 Radiodermatitis, unspecified

● **L59 Other disorders of skin and subcutaneous tissue related to radiation**
L59.0 Erythema ab igne [dermatitis ab igne]
L59.8 Other specified disorders of the skin and subcutaneous tissue related to radiation
 Coding Clinic: 2017, Q1, P34
L59.9 Disorder of the skin and subcutaneous tissue related to radiation, unspecified

---

N Newborn Age: 0   P Pediatric Age: 0–17   M Maternity DX: 9–64   A Adult Age: 15–124

CHAPTER 12 (L00-L99)

CHAPTER 12 (L00–L99)

DISORDERS OF SKIN APPENDAGES (L60-L75)

Excludes1   congenital malformations of integument (Q84.-)

● **L60**   **Nail disorders**

    Excludes2   clubbing of nails (R68.3)
                onychia and paronychia (L03.0-)

    L60.0   **Ingrowing nail**

    L60.1   **Onycholysis**

    L60.2   **Onychogryphosis**

    L60.3   **Nail dystrophy**

    L60.4   **Beau's lines**

    L60.5   **Yellow nail syndrome**

    L60.8   **Other nail disorders**

    L60.9   **Nail disorder, unspecified**

▷ **L62**   *Nail disorders in diseases classified elsewhere*

    Code first underlying disease, such as:
        pachydermoperiostosis (M89.4-)

● **L63**   **Alopecia areata**

    L63.0   **Alopecia (capitis) totalis**

    L63.1   **Alopecia universalis**

    L63.2   **Ophiasis**

    L63.8   **Other alopecia areata**

    L63.9   **Alopecia areata, unspecified**

● **L64**   **Androgenic alopecia**

    Includes   male-pattern baldness

    L64.0   **Drug-induced androgenic alopecia**

        Use additional code for adverse effect, if applicable, to identify drug (T36-T50 with fifth or sixth character 5)

    L64.8   **Other androgenic alopecia**

    L64.9   **Androgenic alopecia, unspecified**

● **L65**   **Other nonscarring hair loss**

    Use additional code for adverse effect, if applicable, to identify drug (T36-T50 with fifth or sixth character 5)

    Excludes1   trichotillomania (F63.3)

    L65.0   **Telogen effluvium**

    L65.1   **Anagen effluvium**

    L65.2   **Alopecia mucinosa**

    L65.8   **Other specified nonscarring hair loss**

    L65.9   **Nonscarring hair loss, unspecified**
          Alopecia NOS

● **L66**   **Cicatricial alopecia [scarring hair loss]**

    L66.0   **Pseudopelade**

    L66.1   **Lichen planopilaris**
         ~~Follicular lichen planus~~

    ▷L66.10   **Lichen planopilaris, unspecified**

    ▷L66.11   **Classic lichen planopilaris**
             ▷Follicular lichen planus

    ▷L66.12   **Frontal fibrosing alopecia**
             ▷FFA

    ▷L66.19   **Other lichen planopilaris**
             ▷Lassueur Graham-Little Piccardi syndrome

    L66.2   **Folliculitis decalvans**

    L66.3   **Perifolliculitis capitis abscedens**

    L66.4   **Folliculitis ulerythematosa reticulata**

    L66.8   **Other cicatricial alopecia**
         Coding Clinic: 2015, Q1, P19

    ▷L66.81   **Central centrifugal cicatricial alopecia**
             ▷AddCCCA

    ▷L66.89   **Other cicatricial alopecia**

    L66.9   **Cicatricial alopecia, unspecified**

Item 12-10 **Alopecia** is lack of hair and takes many forms. The most common is male pattern alopecia, also known as **androgenetic alopecia. Telogen effluvium** is early and excessive loss of hair resulting from a trauma to the hair follicle (fever, drugs, surgery, etc.).

Figure 12-8   Male pattern alopecia.

● **L67**   **Hair color and hair shaft abnormalities**

    Excludes1   monilethrix (Q84.1)
              pili annulati (Q84.1)
              telogen effluvium (L65.0)

    L67.0   **Trichorrhexis nodosa**

    L67.1   **Variations in hair color**
         Canities
         Greyness, hair (premature)
         Heterochromia of hair
         Poliosis circumscripta, acquired
         Poliosis NOS

    L67.8   **Other hair color and hair shaft abnormalities**
         Fragilitas crinium

    L67.9   **Hair color and hair shaft abnormality, unspecified**

● **L68**   **Hypertrichosis**

    Includes   excess hair

    Excludes1   congenital hypertrichosis (Q84.2)
              persistent lanugo (Q84.2)

    L68.0   **Hirsutism**
         Excessive growth of hair

    L68.1   **Acquired hypertrichosis lanuginosa**

    L68.2   **Localized hypertrichosis**

    L68.3   **Polytrichia**

    L68.8   **Other hypertrichosis**

    L68.9   **Hypertrichosis, unspecified**

● **L70**   **Acne**

    Excludes2   acne keloid (L73.0)

    L70.0   **Acne vulgaris**

    L70.1   **Acne conglobata**

    L70.2   **Acne varioliformis**
         Acne necrotica miliaris

    L70.3   **Acne tropica**

    L70.4   **Infantile acne**   P

    L70.5   **Acné excoriée**
         Acné excoriée des jeunes filles
         Picker's acne

    L70.8   **Other acne**

    L70.9   **Acne, unspecified**

● **L71**   **Rosacea**

    Use additional code for adverse effect, if applicable, to identify drug (T36-T50 with fifth or sixth character 5)

    L71.0   **Perioral dermatitis**

    L71.1   **Rhinophyma**

    L71.8   **Other rosacea**
         Coding Clinic: 2018, Q4, P15

    L71.9   **Rosacea, unspecified**

▷ New   ⇒ Revised   ~~deleted~~ Deleted   Excludes 1   Excludes 2   Includes   Use additional   Code first   Code also   Key words

938   OGCR Official Guidelines   X Assign placeholder X   ● Use Additional Character(s)   ▷ Manifestation Code   🔖 Hierarchical Condition Category   Coding Clinic

● **L72** Follicular cysts of skin and subcutaneous tissue
   L72.0 Epidermal cyst
●   **L72.1** Pilar and trichodermal cyst
     L72.11 Pilar cyst
     L72.12 Trichodermal cyst
        Trichilemmal (proliferating) cyst
   L72.3 Sebaceous cyst
     Excludes2 pilar cyst (L72.11)
        trichilemmal (proliferating) cyst (L72.12)
   L72.2 Steatocystoma multiplex
   L72.8 Other follicular cysts of the skin and subcutaneous tissue
   L72.9 Follicular cyst of the skin and subcutaneous tissue, unspecified

● **L73** Other follicular disorders
   L73.0 Acne keloid
   L73.1 Pseudofolliculitis barbae
   L73.2 Hidradenitis suppurativa
   L73.8 Other specified follicular disorders
     Sycosis barbae
   L73.9 Follicular disorder, unspecified

● **L74** Eccrine sweat disorders
   Excludes2 generalized hyperhidrosis (R61)
   L74.0 Miliaria rubra
   L74.1 Miliaria crystallina
   L74.2 Miliaria profunda
     Miliaria tropicalis
   L74.3 Miliaria, unspecified
   L74.4 Anhidrosis
     Hypohidrosis
●   **L74.5** Focal hyperhidrosis
●   **L74.51** Primary focal hyperhidrosis
      L74.510 Primary focal hyperhidrosis, axilla
      L74.511 Primary focal hyperhidrosis, face
      L74.512 Primary focal hyperhidrosis, palms
      L74.513 Primary focal hyperhidrosis, soles
      L74.519 Primary focal hyperhidrosis, unspecified
     L74.52 Secondary focal hyperhidrosis
       Frey's syndrome
   L74.8 Other eccrine sweat disorders
   L74.9 Eccrine sweat disorder, unspecified
     Sweat gland disorder NOS

● **L75** Apocrine sweat disorders
   Excludes1 dyshidrosis (L30.1)
     hidradenitis suppurativa (L73.2)
   L75.0 Bromhidrosis
   L75.1 Chromhidrosis
   L75.2 Apocrine miliaria
     Fox-Fordyce disease
   L75.8 Other apocrine sweat disorders
   L75.9 Apocrine sweat disorder, unspecified
     Intraoperative and postprocedural complications of skin and subcutaneous tissue (L76)

INTRAOPERATIVE AND POSTPROCEDURAL COMPLICATIONS OF SKIN AND SUBCUTANEOUS TISSUE (L76)

● **L76** Intraoperative and postprocedural complications of skin and subcutaneous tissue
   Coding Clinic: 2016, Q4, P10
●   **L76.0** Intraoperative hemorrhage and hematoma of skin and subcutaneous tissue complicating a procedure
     Excludes1 intraoperative hemorrhage and hematoma of skin and subcutaneous tissue due to accidental puncture and laceration during a procedure (L76.1-)

     L76.01 Intraoperative hemorrhage and hematoma of skin and subcutaneous tissue complicating a dermatologic procedure
     L76.02 Intraoperative hemorrhage and hematoma of skin and subcutaneous tissue complicating other procedure
●   **L76.1** Accidental puncture and laceration of skin and subcutaneous tissue during a procedure
     L76.11 Accidental puncture and laceration of skin and subcutaneous tissue during a dermatologic procedure
     L76.12 Accidental puncture and laceration of skin and subcutaneous tissue during other procedure
●   **L76.2** Postprocedural hemorrhage of skin and subcutaneous tissue following a procedure
     L76.21 Postprocedural hemorrhage of skin and subcutaneous tissue following a dermatologic procedure
     L76.22 Postprocedural hemorrhage of skin and subcutaneous tissue following other procedure
●   **L76.3** Postprocedural hematoma and seroma of skin and subcutaneous tissue following a procedure
     L76.31 Postprocedural hematoma of skin and subcutaneous tissue following a dermatologic procedure
     L76.32 Postprocedural hematoma of skin and subcutaneous tissue following other procedure
     L76.33 Postprocedural seroma of skin and subcutaneous tissue following a dermatologic procedure
     L76.34 Postprocedural seroma of skin and subcutaneous tissue following other procedure
●   **L76.8** Other intraoperative and postprocedural complications of skin and subcutaneous tissue
     Use additional code, if applicable, to further specify disorder
     L76.81 Other intraoperative complications of skin and subcutaneous tissue
     L76.82 Other postprocedural complications of skin and subcutaneous tissue
      Coding Clinic: 2017, Q3, P6

OTHER DISORDERS OF THE SKIN AND SUBCUTANEOUS TISSUE (L80-L99)

  L80 Vitiligo
   Excludes2 vitiligo of eyelids (H02.73-)
     vitiligo of vulva (N90.89)

● **L81** Other disorders of pigmentation
   Excludes1 birthmark NOS (Q82.5)
     Peutz-Jeghers syndrome (Q85.89)
   Excludes2 nevus - see Alphabetical Index
   L81.0 Postinflammatory hyperpigmentation
   L81.1 Chloasma
   L81.2 Freckles
   L81.3 Café au lait spots
   L81.4 Other melanin hyperpigmentation
     Lentigo
   L81.5 Leukoderma, not elsewhere classified
   L81.6 Other disorders of diminished melanin formation
   L81.7 Pigmented purpuric dermatosis
     Angioma serpiginosum
   L81.8 Other specified disorders of pigmentation
     Iron pigmentation
     Tattoo pigmentation
   L81.9 Disorder of pigmentation, unspecified

CHAPTER 12 (L00-L99)

● **L82 Seborrheic keratosis**

    Includes basal cell papilloma
                  dermatosis papulosa nigra
                  Leser-Trélat disease

    Excludes2 seborrheic dermatitis (L21.-)

   L82.0 Inflamed seborrheic keratosis
        Coding Clinic: 2023, Q2, P12; 2021, Q3, P11

   L82.1 Other seborrheic keratosis
        Seborrheic keratosis NOS

L83 Acanthosis nigricans
    Confluent and reticulated papillomatosis

L84 Corns and callosities
    Callus
    Clavus

● **L85 Other epidermal thickening**

    Excludes2 hypertrophic disorders of the skin (L91.-)

   L85.0 Acquired ichthyosis
        Excludes1 congenital ichthyosis (Q80.-)

   L85.1 Acquired keratosis [keratoderma] palmaris et plantaris
        Excludes1 inherited keratosis palmaris et plantaris (Q82.8)

   L85.2 Keratosis punctata (palmaris et plantaris)

   L85.3 Xerosis cutis
        Dry skin dermatitis

   L85.8 Other specified epidermal thickening
        Cutaneous horn

   L85.9 Epidermal thickening, unspecified

▷ *L86 Keratoderma in diseases classified elsewhere*
    Firm horny papules that have a cobblestone appearance
     Code first underlying disease, such as:
      Reiter's disease (M02.3-)
     Excludes1 gonococcal keratoderma (A54.89)
             gonococcal keratosis (A54.89)
             keratoderma due to vitamin A deficiency (E50.8)
             keratosis due to vitamin A deficiency (E50.8)
             xeroderma due to vitamin A deficiency (E50.8)

● **L87 Transepidermal elimination disorders**

    Excludes1 granuloma annulare (perforating) (L92.0)

   L87.0 Keratosis follicularis et parafollicularis in cutem penetrans
        Kyrle disease
        Hyperkeratosis follicularis penetrans

   L87.1 Reactive perforating collagenosis

   L87.2 Elastosis perforans serpiginosa

   L87.8 Other transepidermal elimination disorders

   L87.9 Transepidermal elimination disorder, unspecified

L88 Pyoderma gangrenosum
    Phagedenic pyoderma
    Excludes1 dermatitis gangrenosa (L08.0)

OGCR Section I.B.14.

General Coding Guidelines

Documentation for BMI, *Depth of* Non-pressure ulcers, Pressure Ulcer Stages, **Coma Scale,** and *NIH Stroke Scale*

For the Body Mass Index (BMI), depth of non-pressure chronic ulcers, pressure ulcer stage, **coma scale,** and NIH stroke scale (NIHSS) codes, code assignment may be based on medical record documentation from clinicians who are not the patient's provider (i.e., physician or other qualified healthcare practitioner legally accountable for establishing the patient's diagnosis), since this information is typically documented by other clinicians involved in the care of the patient (e.g., a dietitian often documents the BMI, a nurse often documents the pressure ulcer stages, **and an emergency medical technician often documents the coma scale**). However, the associated diagnosis (such as overweight, obesity, **acute stroke,** or pressure ulcer) must be documented by the patient's provider. If there is conflicting medical record documentation, either from the same clinician or different clinicians, the patient's attending provider should be queried for clarification. The BMI, **coma scale,** and NHSS codes should only be reported as secondary diagnoses.

● **L89 Pressure ulcer**

    Includes bed sore   pressure area
             decubitus ulcer   pressure sore
             plaster ulcer

   Code first any associated gangrene (I96)

    Excludes2 decubitus (trophic) ulcer of cervix (uteri) (N86)
             diabetic ulcers (E08.621, E08.622, E09.621, E09.622, E10.621, E10.622, E11.621, E11.622, E13.621, E13.622)
             non-pressure chronic ulcer of skin (L97.-)
             skin infections (L00-L08)
             varicose ulcer (I83.0, I83.2)
     Coding Clinic: 2019, Q4, P11; 2018, Q2, P22; 2016, Q4, P124

  ● **L89.0 Pressure ulcer of elbow**

    ● **L89.00 Pressure ulcer of unspecified elbow**

       L89.000 Pressure ulcer of unspecified elbow, unstageable 🔖

       L89.001 Pressure ulcer of unspecified elbow, stage 1
           Healing pressure ulcer of unspecified elbow, stage 1
           Pressure pre-ulcer skin changes limited to persistent focal edema, unspecified elbow

       L89.002 Pressure ulcer of unspecified elbow, stage 2
           Healing pressure ulcer of unspecified elbow, stage 2
           Pressure ulcer with abrasion, blister, partial thickness skin loss involving epidermis and/or dermis, unspecified elbow

       L89.003 Pressure ulcer of unspecified elbow, stage 3 🔖
           Healing pressure ulcer of unspecified elbow, stage 3
           Pressure ulcer with full thickness skin loss involving damage or necrosis of subcutaneous tissue, unspecified elbow

       L89.004 Pressure ulcer of unspecified elbow, stage 4 🔖
           Healing pressure ulcer of unspecified elbow, stage 4
           Pressure ulcer with necrosis of soft tissues through to underlying muscle, tendon, or bone, unspecified elbow

       L89.006 Pressure-induced deep tissue damage of unspecified elbow

---

▶ New ➡ Revised ~~deleted~~ Deleted Excludes 1 Excludes 2 Includes Use additional Code first Code also Key words

OGCR Official Guidelines X Assign placeholder X ● Use Additional Character(s) ▶ Manifestation Code 🔖 Hierarchical Condition Category Coding Clinic

L89.009   **Pressure ulcer of unspecified elbow, unspecified stage**
        Healing pressure ulcer of elbow NOS
        Healing pressure ulcer of unspecified elbow, unspecified stage

●**L89.01** **Pressure ulcer of right elbow**
    L89.010   **Pressure ulcer of right elbow, unstageable** 🔖
    L89.011   **Pressure ulcer of right elbow, stage 1**
        Healing pressure ulcer of right elbow, stage 1
        Pressure pre-ulcer skin changes limited to persistent focal edema, right elbow
    L89.012   **Pressure ulcer of right elbow, stage 2**
        Healing pressure ulcer of right elbow, stage 2
        Pressure ulcer with abrasion, blister, partial thickness skin loss involving epidermis and/or dermis, right elbow
    L89.013   **Pressure ulcer of right elbow, stage 3** 🔖
        Healing pressure ulcer of right elbow, stage 3
        Pressure ulcer with full thickness skin loss involving damage or necrosis of subcutaneous tissue, right elbow

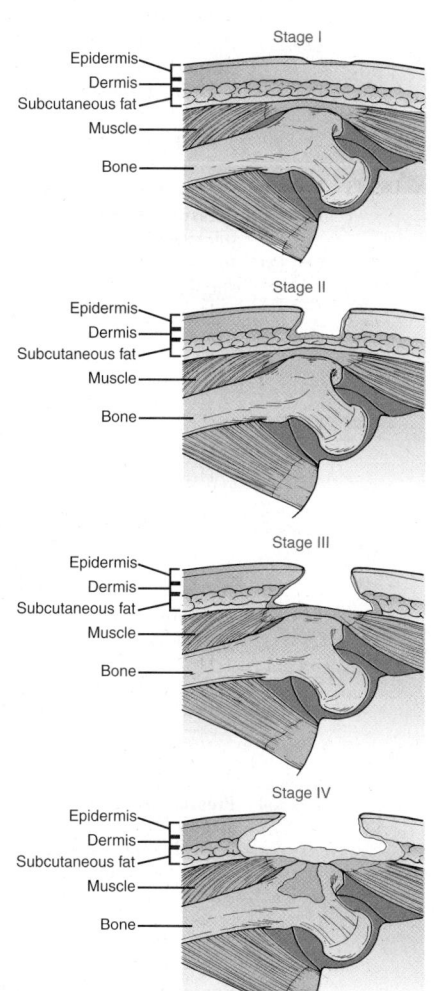

Epidermis — Dermis — Subcutaneous fat — Muscle — Bone
Stage I

Epidermis — Dermis — Subcutaneous fat — Muscle — Bone
Stage II

Epidermis — Dermis — Subcutaneous fat — Muscle — Bone
Stage III

Epidermis — Dermis — Subcutaneous fat — Muscle — Bone
Stage IV

Figure 12-9 Stage I, II, III, and IV of pressure ulcers.

L89.014   **Pressure ulcer of right elbow, stage 4** 🔖
        Healing pressure ulcer of right elbow, stage 4
        Pressure ulcer with necrosis of soft tissues through to underlying muscle, tendon, or bone, right elbow
L89.016   **Pressure-induced deep tissue damage of right elbow**
L89.019   **Pressure ulcer of right elbow, unspecified stage**
        Healing pressure ulcer of right elbow NOS

●**L89.02** **Pressure ulcer of left elbow**
    L89.020   **Pressure ulcer of left elbow, unstageable** 🔖
    L89.021   **Pressure ulcer of left elbow, stage 1**
        Healing pressure ulcer of left elbow, stage 1
        Pressure pre-ulcer skin changes limited to persistent focal edema, left elbow
    L89.022   **Pressure ulcer of left elbow, stage 2**
        Healing pressure ulcer of left elbow, stage 2
        Pressure ulcer with abrasion, blister, partial thickness skin loss involving epidermis and/or dermis, left elbow
    L89.023   **Pressure ulcer of left elbow, stage 3** 🔖
        Healing pressure ulcer of left elbow, stage 3
        Pressure ulcer with full thickness skin loss involving damage or necrosis of subcutaneous tissue, left elbow
    L89.024   **Pressure ulcer of left elbow, stage 4** 🔖
        Healing pressure ulcer of left elbow, stage 4
        Pressure ulcer with necrosis of soft tissues through to underlying muscle, tendon, or bone, left elbow
    L89.026   **Pressure-induced deep tissue damage of left elbow**
    L89.029   **Pressure ulcer of left elbow, unspecified stage**
        Healing pressure ulcer of left elbow NOS

●**L89.1** **Pressure ulcer of back**
  ●**L89.10** **Pressure ulcer of unspecified part of back**
    L89.100   **Pressure ulcer of unspecified part of back, unstageable** 🔖
    L89.101   **Pressure ulcer of unspecified part of back, stage 1**
        Healing pressure ulcer of unspecified part of back, stage 1
        Pressure pre-ulcer skin changes limited to persistent focal edema, unspecified part of back
    L89.102   **Pressure ulcer of unspecified part of back, stage 2**
        Healing pressure ulcer of unspecified part of back, stage 2
        Pressure ulcer with abrasion, blister, partial thickness skin loss involving epidermis and/or dermis, unspecified part of back

L89.103 Pressure ulcer of unspecified part of back, stage 3 🦠
    Healing pressure ulcer of unspecified part of back, stage 3
    Pressure ulcer with full thickness skin loss involving damage or necrosis of subcutaneous tissue, unspecified part of back

L89.104 Pressure ulcer of unspecified part of back, stage 4 🦠
    Healing pressure ulcer of unspecified part of back, stage 4
    Pressure ulcer with necrosis of soft tissues through to underlying muscle, tendon, or bone, unspecified part of back

L89.106 Pressure-induced deep tissue damage of unspecified part of back

L89.109 Pressure ulcer of unspecified part of back, unspecified stage
    Healing pressure ulcer of unspecified part of back NOS
    Healing pressure ulcer of unspecified part of back, unspecified stage

● **L89.11** Pressure ulcer of right upper back
    Pressure ulcer of right shoulder blade

L89.110 Pressure ulcer of right upper back, unstageable 🦠

L89.111 Pressure ulcer of right upper back, stage 1
    Healing pressure ulcer of right upper back, stage 1
    Pressure pre-ulcer skin changes limited to persistent focal edema, right upper back

L89.112 Pressure ulcer of right upper back, stage 2
    Healing pressure ulcer of right upper back, stage 2
    Pressure ulcer with abrasion, blister, partial thickness skin loss involving epidermis and/or dermis, right upper back

L89.113 Pressure ulcer of right upper back, stage 3 🦠
    Healing pressure ulcer of right upper back, stage 3
    Pressure ulcer with full thickness skin loss involving damage or necrosis of subcutaneous tissue, right upper back

L89.114 Pressure ulcer of right upper back, stage 4 🦠
    Healing pressure ulcer of right upper back, stage 4
    Pressure ulcer with necrosis of soft tissues through to underlying muscle, tendon, or bone, right upper back

L89.116 Pressure-induced deep tissue damage of right upper back

L89.119 Pressure ulcer of right upper back, unspecified stage
    Healing pressure ulcer of right upper back NOS
    Healing pressure ulcer of right upper back, unspecified stage

● **L89.12** Pressure ulcer of left upper back
    Pressure ulcer of left shoulder blade

L89.120 Pressure ulcer of left upper back, unstageable 🦠

L89.121 Pressure ulcer of left upper back, stage 1
    Healing pressure ulcer of left upper back, stage 1
    Pressure pre-ulcer skin changes limited to persistent focal edema, left upper back

L89.122 Pressure ulcer of left upper back, stage 2
    Healing pressure ulcer of left upper back, stage 2
    Pressure ulcer with abrasion, blister, partial thickness skin loss involving epidermis and/or dermis, left upper back

L89.123 Pressure ulcer of left upper back, stage 3 🦠
    Healing pressure ulcer of left upper back, stage 3
    Pressure ulcer with full thickness skin loss involving damage or necrosis of subcutaneous tissue, left upper back

L89.124 Pressure ulcer of left upper back, stage 4 🦠
    Healing pressure ulcer of left upper back, stage 4
    Pressure ulcer with necrosis of soft tissues through to underlying muscle, tendon, or bone, left upper back

L89.126 Pressure-induced deep tissue damage of left upper back

L89.129 Pressure ulcer of left upper back, unspecified stage
    Healing pressure ulcer of left upper back NOS
    Healing pressure ulcer of left upper back, unspecified stage

● **L89.13** Pressure ulcer of right lower back

L89.130 Pressure ulcer of right lower back, unstageable 🦠

L89.131 Pressure ulcer of right lower back, stage 1
    Healing pressure ulcer of right lower back, stage 1
    Pressure pre-ulcer skin changes limited to persistent focal edema, right lower back

L89.132 Pressure ulcer of right lower back, stage 2
    Healing pressure ulcer of right lower back, stage 2
    Pressure ulcer with abrasion, blister, partial thickness skin loss involving epidermis and/or dermis, right lower back

L89.133 Pressure ulcer of right lower back, stage 3 🦠
    Healing pressure ulcer of right lower back, stage 3
    Pressure ulcer with full thickness skin loss involving damage or necrosis of subcutaneous tissue, right lower back

L89.134 Pressure ulcer of right lower back, stage 4 🦠
    Healing pressure ulcer of right lower back, stage 4
    Pressure ulcer with necrosis of soft tissues through to underlying muscle, tendon, or bone, right lower back

L89.136 Pressure-induced deep tissue damage of right lower back

L89.139   **Pressure ulcer of right lower back, unspecified stage**
    Healing pressure ulcer of right lower back NOS
    Healing pressure ulcer of right lower back, unspecified stage

● **L89.14   Pressure ulcer of left lower back**

L89.140   **Pressure ulcer of left lower back, unstageable** 🔖

L89.141   **Pressure ulcer of left lower back, stage 1**
    Healing pressure ulcer of left lower back, stage 1
    Pressure pre-ulcer skin changes limited to persistent focal edema, left lower back

L89.142   **Pressure ulcer of left lower back, stage 2**
    Healing pressure ulcer of left lower back, stage 2
    Pressure ulcer with abrasion, blister, partial thickness skin loss involving epidermis and/or dermis, left lower back

L89.143   **Pressure ulcer of left lower back, stage 3** 🔖
    Healing pressure ulcer of left lower back, stage 3
    Pressure ulcer with full thickness skin loss involving damage or necrosis of subcutaneous tissue, left lower back

L89.144   **Pressure ulcer of left lower back, stage 4** 🔖
    Healing pressure ulcer of left lower back, stage 4
    Pressure ulcer with necrosis of soft tissues through to underlying muscle, tendon, or bone, left lower back

L89.146   **Pressure-induced deep tissue damage of left lower back**

L89.149   **Pressure ulcer of left lower back, unspecified stage**
    Healing pressure ulcer of left lower back NOS
    Healing pressure ulcer of left lower back, unspecified stage

● **L89.15   Pressure ulcer of sacral region**
    Pressure ulcer of coccyx
    Pressure ulcer of tailbone
    Coding Clinic: 2021, Q3, P10

L89.150   **Pressure ulcer of sacral region, unstageable** 🔖

L89.151   **Pressure ulcer of sacral region, stage 1**
    Healing pressure ulcer of sacral region, stage 1
    Pressure pre-ulcer skin changes limited to persistent focal edema, sacral region

L89.152   **Pressure ulcer of sacral region, stage 2**
    Healing pressure ulcer of sacral region, stage 2
    Pressure ulcer with abrasion, blister, partial thickness skin loss involving epidermis and/or dermis, sacral region

L89.153   **Pressure ulcer of sacral region, stage 3** 🔖
    Healing pressure ulcer of sacral region, stage 3
    Pressure ulcer with full thickness skin loss involving damage or necrosis of subcutaneous tissue, sacral region
    Coding Clinic: 2021, Q3, P10

L89.154   **Pressure ulcer of sacral region, stage 4** 🔖
    Healing pressure ulcer of sacral region, stage 4
    Pressure ulcer with necrosis of soft tissues through to underlying muscle, tendon, or bone, sacral region
    Coding Clinic: 2022, Q2, P9; 2021, Q1, P24

L89.156   **Pressure-induced deep tissue damage of sacral region**

L89.159   **Pressure ulcer of sacral region, unspecified stage**
    Healing pressure ulcer of sacral region NOS
    Healing pressure ulcer of sacral region, unspecified stage

● **L89.2   Pressure ulcer of hip**

 ● **L89.20   Pressure ulcer of unspecified hip**

L89.200   **Pressure ulcer of unspecified hip, unstageable** 🔖

L89.201   **Pressure ulcer of unspecified hip, stage 1**
    Healing pressure ulcer of unspecified hip back, stage 1
    Pressure pre-ulcer skin changes limited to persistent focal edema, unspecified hip

L89.202   **Pressure ulcer of unspecified hip, stage 2**
    Healing pressure ulcer of unspecified hip, stage 2
    Pressure ulcer with abrasion, blister, partial thickness skin loss involving epidermis and/or dermis, unspecified hip

L89.203   **Pressure ulcer of unspecified hip, stage 3** 🔖
    Healing pressure ulcer of unspecified hip, stage 3
    Pressure ulcer with full thickness skin loss involving damage or necrosis of subcutaneous tissue, unspecified hip

L89.204   **Pressure ulcer of unspecified hip, stage 4** 🔖
    Healing pressure ulcer of unspecified hip, stage 4
    Pressure ulcer with necrosis of soft tissues through to underlying muscle, tendon, or bone, unspecified hip

L89.206   **Pressure-induced deep tissue damage of unspecified hip**

L89.209   **Pressure ulcer of unspecified hip, unspecified stage**
    Healing pressure ulcer of unspecified hip NOS
    Healing pressure ulcer of unspecified hip, unspecified stage

 ● **L89.21   Pressure ulcer of right hip**

L89.210   **Pressure ulcer of right hip, unstageable** 🔖

L89.211   **Pressure ulcer of right hip, stage 1**
    Healing pressure ulcer of right hip back, stage 1
    Pressure pre-ulcer skin changes limited to persistent focal edema, right hip

CHAPTER 12 (L00-L99)

L89.212   Pressure ulcer of right hip, stage 2
Healing pressure ulcer of right hip, stage 2
Pressure ulcer with abrasion, blister, partial thickness skin loss involving epidermis and/or dermis, right hip

L89.213   Pressure ulcer of right hip, stage 3 🝰
Healing pressure ulcer of right hip, stage 3
Pressure ulcer with full thickness skin loss involving damage or necrosis of subcutaneous tissue, right hip

L89.214   Pressure ulcer of right hip, stage 4 🝰
Healing pressure ulcer of right hip, stage 4
Pressure ulcer with necrosis of soft tissues through to underlying muscle, tendon, or bone, right hip

L89.216   Pressure-induced deep tissue damage of right hip

L89.219   Pressure ulcer of right hip, unspecified stage
Healing pressure ulcer of right hip NOS
Healing pressure ulcer of right hip, unspecified stage

● **L89.22   Pressure ulcer of left hip**

L89.220   Pressure ulcer of left hip, unstageable 🝰

L89.221   Pressure ulcer of left hip, stage 1
Healing pressure ulcer of left hip back, stage 1
Pressure pre-ulcer skin changes limited to persistent focal edema, left hip

L89.222   Pressure ulcer of left hip, stage 2
Healing pressure ulcer of left hip, stage 2
Pressure ulcer with abrasion, blister, partial thickness skin loss involving epidermis and/or dermis, left hip

L89.223   Pressure ulcer of left hip, stage 3 🝰
Healing pressure ulcer of left hip, stage 3
Pressure ulcer with full thickness skin loss involving damage or necrosis of subcutaneous tissue, left hip

L89.224   Pressure ulcer of left hip, stage 4 🝰
Healing pressure ulcer of left hip, stage 4
Pressure ulcer with necrosis of soft tissues through to underlying muscle, tendon, or bone, left hip

L89.226   Pressure-induced deep tissue damage of left hip

L89.229   Pressure ulcer of left hip, unspecified stage
Healing pressure ulcer of left hip NOS
Healing pressure ulcer of left hip, unspecified stage

● **L89.3   Pressure ulcer of buttock**

● **L89.30   Pressure ulcer of unspecified buttock**

L89.300   Pressure ulcer of unspecified buttock, unstageable 🝰

L89.301   Pressure ulcer of unspecified buttock, stage 1
Healing pressure ulcer of unspecified buttock, stage 1
Pressure pre-ulcer skin changes limited to persistent focal edema, unspecified buttock

L89.302   Pressure ulcer of unspecified buttock, stage 2
Healing pressure ulcer of unspecified buttock, stage 2
Pressure ulcer with abrasion, blister, partial thickness skin loss involving epidermis and/or dermis, unspecified buttock

L89.303   Pressure ulcer of unspecified buttock, stage 3 🝰
Healing pressure ulcer of unspecified buttock, stage 3
Pressure ulcer with full thickness skin loss involving damage or necrosis of subcutaneous tissue, unspecified buttock

L89.304   Pressure ulcer of unspecified buttock, stage 4 🝰
Healing pressure ulcer of unspecified buttock, stage 4
Pressure ulcer with necrosis of soft tissues through to underlying muscle, tendon, or bone, unspecified buttock

L89.306   Pressure-induced deep tissue damage of unspecified buttock

L89.309   Pressure ulcer of unspecified buttock, unspecified stage
Healing pressure ulcer of unspecified buttock NOS
Healing pressure ulcer of unspecified buttock, unspecified stage

● **L89.31   Pressure ulcer of right buttock**

L89.310   Pressure ulcer of right buttock, unstageable 🝰

L89.311   Pressure ulcer of right buttock, stage 1
Healing pressure ulcer of right buttock, stage 1
Pressure pre-ulcer skin changes limited to persistent focal edema, right buttock

L89.312   Pressure ulcer of right buttock, stage 2
Healing pressure ulcer of right buttock, stage 2
Pressure ulcer with abrasion, blister, partial thickness skin loss involving epidermis and/or dermis, right buttock

L89.313   Pressure ulcer of right buttock, stage 3 🝰
Healing pressure ulcer of right buttock, stage 3
Pressure ulcer with full thickness skin loss involving damage or necrosis of subcutaneous tissue, right buttock

▶ New   ⇒ Revised   ~~deleted~~ Deleted   Excludes 1   Excludes 2   Includes   Use additional   Code first   Code also   Key words
OGCR Official Guidelines   X Assign placeholder X   ● Use Additional Character(s)   ▶ Manifestation Code   🝰 Hierarchical Condition Category   Coding Clinic

L89.314   **Pressure ulcer of right buttock, stage 4** 🔍
> Healing pressure ulcer of right buttock, stage 4
> Pressure ulcer with necrosis of soft tissues through to underlying muscle, tendon, or bone, right buttock

L89.316 **Pressure-induced deep tissue damage of right buttock**

L89.319   **Pressure ulcer of right buttock, unspecified stage**
> Healing pressure ulcer of right buttock NOS
> Healing pressure ulcer of right buttock, unspecified stage

● **L89.32**   **Pressure ulcer of left buttock**

L89.320   **Pressure ulcer of left buttock, unstageable** 🔍

L89.321   **Pressure ulcer of left buttock, stage 1**
> Healing pressure ulcer of left buttock, stage 1
> Pressure pre-ulcer skin changes limited to persistent focal edema, left buttock

L89.322   **Pressure ulcer of left buttock, stage 2**
> Healing pressure ulcer of left buttock, stage 2
> Pressure ulcer with abrasion, blister, partial thickness skin loss involving epidermis and/or dermis, left buttock

L89.323   **Pressure ulcer of left buttock, stage 3** 🔍
> Healing pressure ulcer of left buttock, stage 3
> Pressure ulcer with full thickness skin loss involving damage or necrosis of subcutaneous tissue, left buttock

L89.324   **Pressure ulcer of left buttock, stage 4** 🔍
> Healing pressure ulcer of left buttock, stage 4
> Pressure ulcer with necrosis of soft tissues through to underlying muscle, tendon, or bone, left buttock

L89.326   **Pressure-induced deep tissue damage of left buttock**

L89.329   **Pressure ulcer of left buttock, unspecified stage**
> Healing pressure ulcer of left buttock NOS
> Healing pressure ulcer of left buttock, unspecified stage

● **L89.4**   **Pressure ulcer of contiguous site of back, buttock and hip**

L89.40   **Pressure ulcer of contiguous site of back, buttock and hip, unspecified stage**
> Healing pressure ulcer of contiguous site of back, buttock and hip NOS
> Healing pressure ulcer of contiguous site of back, buttock and hip, unspecified stage

L89.41   **Pressure ulcer of contiguous site of back, buttock and hip, stage 1**
> Healing pressure ulcer of contiguous site of back, buttock and hip, stage 1
> Pressure pre-ulcer skin changes limited to persistent focal edema, contiguous site of back, buttock and hip

L89.42   **Pressure ulcer of contiguous site of back, buttock and hip, stage 2**
> Healing pressure ulcer of contiguous site of back, buttock and hip, stage 2
> Pressure ulcer with abrasion, blister, partial thickness skin loss involving epidermis and/or dermis, contiguous site of back, buttock and hip

L89.43   **Pressure ulcer of contiguous site of back, buttock and hip, stage 3** 🔍
> Healing pressure ulcer of contiguous site of back, buttock and hip, stage 3
> Pressure ulcer with full thickness skin loss involving damage or necrosis of subcutaneous tissue, contiguous site of back, buttock and hip

L89.44   **Pressure ulcer of contiguous site of back, buttock and hip, stage 4** 🔍
> Healing pressure ulcer of contiguous site of back, buttock and hip, stage 4
> Pressure ulcer with necrosis of soft tissues through to underlying muscle, tendon, or bone, contiguous site of back, buttock and hip

L89.45   **Pressure ulcer of contiguous site of back, buttock and hip, unstageable** 🔍

L89.46   **Pressure-induced deep tissue damage of contiguous site of back, buttock and hip**

● **L89.5**   **Pressure ulcer of ankle**

  ● **L89.50**   **Pressure ulcer of unspecified ankle**

L89.500   **Pressure ulcer of unspecified ankle, unstageable** 🔍

L89.501   **Pressure ulcer of unspecified ankle, stage 1**
> Healing pressure ulcer of unspecified ankle, stage 1
> Pressure pre-ulcer skin changes limited to persistent focal edema, unspecified ankle

L89.502   **Pressure ulcer of unspecified ankle, stage 2**
> Healing pressure ulcer of unspecified ankle, stage 2
> Pressure ulcer with abrasion, blister, partial thickness skin loss involving epidermis and/or dermis, unspecified ankle

L89.503   **Pressure ulcer of unspecified ankle, stage 3** 🔍
> Healing pressure ulcer of unspecified ankle, stage 3
> Pressure ulcer with full thickness skin loss involving damage or necrosis of subcutaneous tissue, unspecified ankle

L89.504   **Pressure ulcer of unspecified ankle, stage 4** 🔍
> Healing pressure ulcer of unspecified ankle, stage 4
> Pressure ulcer with necrosis of soft tissues through to underlying muscle, tendon, or bone, unspecified ankle

L89.506   **Pressure-induced deep tissue damage of unspecified ankle**

L89.509   **Pressure ulcer of unspecified ankle, unspecified stage**
> Healing pressure ulcer of unspecified ankle NOS
> Healing pressure ulcer of unspecified ankle, unspecified stage

ICD-10-CM

- L89.51 Pressure ulcer of right ankle
- L89.510 Pressure ulcer of right ankle, unstageable
- L89.511 Pressure ulcer of right ankle, stage 1
  - Healing pressure ulcer of right ankle, stage 1
  - Pressure pre-ulcer skin changes limited to persistent focal edema, right ankle
- L89.512 Pressure ulcer of right ankle, stage 2
  - Healing pressure ulcer of right ankle, stage 2
  - Pressure ulcer with abrasion, blister, partial thickness skin loss involving epidermis and/or dermis, right ankle
- L89.513 Pressure ulcer of right ankle, stage 3
  - Healing pressure ulcer of right ankle, stage 3
  - Pressure ulcer with full thickness skin loss involving damage or necrosis of subcutaneous tissue, right ankle
- L89.514 Pressure ulcer of right ankle, stage 4
  - Healing pressure ulcer of right ankle, stage 4
  - Pressure ulcer with necrosis of soft tissues through to underlying muscle, tendon, or bone, right ankle
- L89.516 Pressure-induced deep tissue damage of right ankle
- L89.519 Pressure ulcer of right ankle, unspecified stage
  - Healing pressure ulcer of right ankle NOS
  - Healing pressure ulcer of right ankle, unspecified stage
- L89.52 Pressure ulcer of left ankle
- L89.520 Pressure ulcer of left ankle, unstageable
- L89.521 Pressure ulcer of left ankle, stage 1
  - Healing pressure ulcer of left ankle, stage 1
  - Pressure pre-ulcer skin changes limited to persistent focal edema, left ankle
- L89.522 Pressure ulcer of left ankle, stage 2
  - Healing pressure ulcer of left ankle, stage 2
  - Pressure ulcer with abrasion, blister, partial thickness skin loss involving epidermis and/or dermis, left ankle
- L89.523 Pressure ulcer of left ankle, stage 3
  - Healing pressure ulcer of left ankle, stage 3
  - Pressure ulcer with full thickness skin loss involving damage or necrosis of subcutaneous tissue, left ankle
- L89.524 Pressure ulcer of left ankle, stage 4
  - Healing pressure ulcer of left ankle, stage 4
  - Pressure ulcer with necrosis of soft tissues through to underlying muscle, tendon, or bone, left ankle
- L89.526 Pressure-induced deep tissue damage of left ankle

- L89.529 Pressure ulcer of left ankle, unspecified stage
  - Healing pressure ulcer of left ankle NOS
  - Healing pressure ulcer of left ankle, unspecified stage
- L89.6 Pressure ulcer of heel
- L89.60 Pressure ulcer of unspecified heel
- L89.600 Pressure ulcer of unspecified heel, unstageable
- L89.601 Pressure ulcer of unspecified heel, stage 1
  - Healing pressure ulcer of unspecified heel, stage 1
  - Pressure pre-ulcer skin changes limited to persistent focal edema, unspecified heel
- L89.602 Pressure ulcer of unspecified heel, stage 2
  - Healing pressure ulcer of unspecified heel, stage 2
  - Pressure ulcer with abrasion, blister, partial thickness skin loss involving epidermis and/or dermis, unspecified heel
- L89.603 Pressure ulcer of unspecified heel, stage 3
  - Healing pressure ulcer of unspecified heel, stage 3
  - Pressure ulcer with full thickness skin loss involving damage or necrosis of subcutaneous tissue, unspecified heel
- L89.604 Pressure ulcer of unspecified heel, stage 4
  - Healing pressure ulcer of unspecified heel, stage 4
  - Pressure ulcer with necrosis of soft tissues through to underlying muscle, tendon, or bone, unspecified heel
- L89.606 Pressure-induced deep tissue damage of unspecified heel
- L89.609 Pressure ulcer of unspecified heel, unspecified stage
  - Healing pressure ulcer of unspecified heel NOS
  - Healing pressure ulcer of unspecified heel, unspecified stage
- L89.61 Pressure ulcer of right heel
- L89.610 Pressure ulcer of right heel, unstageable
- L89.611 Pressure ulcer of right heel, stage 1
  - Healing pressure ulcer of right heel, stage 1
  - Pressure pre-ulcer skin changes limited to persistent focal edema, right heel
- L89.612 Pressure ulcer of right heel, stage 2
  - Healing pressure ulcer of right heel, stage 2
  - Pressure ulcer with abrasion, blister, partial thickness skin loss involving epidermis and/or dermis, right heel
- L89.613 Pressure ulcer of right heel, stage 3
  - Healing pressure ulcer of right heel, stage 3
  - Pressure ulcer with full thickness skin loss involving damage or necrosis of subcutaneous tissue, right heel

946

L89.614   **Pressure ulcer of right heel, stage 4** 🔖
            Healing pressure ulcer of right heel,
                stage 4
            Pressure ulcer with necrosis of soft
                tissues through to underlying
                muscle, tendon, or bone, right
                heel

L89.616   **Pressure-induced deep tissue damage
            of right heel**

L89.619   **Pressure ulcer of right heel,
            unspecified stage**
            Healing pressure ulcer of right heel
                NOS
            Healing pressure ulcer of right heel,
                unspecified stage

● **L89.62 Pressure ulcer of left heel**

L89.620   **Pressure ulcer of left heel,
            unstageable** 🔖

L89.621   **Pressure ulcer of left heel, stage 1**
            Healing pressure ulcer of left heel,
                stage 1
            Pressure pre-ulcer skin changes
                limited to persistent focal
                edema, left heel

L89.622   **Pressure ulcer of left heel, stage 2**
            Healing pressure ulcer of left heel,
                stage 2
            Pressure ulcer with abrasion, blister,
                partial thickness skin loss
                involving epidermis and/or
                dermis, left heel
            Coding Clinic: 2016, Q4, P142

L89.623   **Pressure ulcer of left heel, stage 3** 🔖
            Healing pressure ulcer of left heel,
                stage 3
            Pressure ulcer with full thickness
                skin loss involving damage or
                necrosis of subcutaneous tissue,
                left heel
            Coding Clinic: 2016, Q4, P142

L89.624   **Pressure ulcer of left heel, stage 4** 🔖
            Healing pressure ulcer of left heel,
                stage 4
            Pressure ulcer with necrosis of soft
                tissues through to underlying
                muscle, tendon, or bone, left
                heel

L89.626   **Pressure-induced deep tissue damage
            of left heel**

L89.629   **Pressure ulcer of left heel, unspecified
            stage**
            Healing pressure ulcer of left heel
                NOS
            Healing pressure ulcer of left heel,
                unspecified stage

● **L89.8 Pressure ulcer of other site**

● **L89.81 Pressure ulcer of head**
            Pressure ulcer of face

L89.810   **Pressure ulcer of head, unstageable** 🔖

L89.811   **Pressure ulcer of head, stage 1**
            Healing pressure ulcer of head,
                stage 1
            Pressure pre-ulcer skin changes
                limited to persistent focal
                edema, head

L89.812   **Pressure ulcer of head, stage 2**
            Healing pressure ulcer of head,
                stage 2
            Pressure ulcer with abrasion, blister,
                partial thickness skin loss
                involving epidermis and/or
                dermis, head

L89.813   **Pressure ulcer of head, stage 3** 🔖
            Healing pressure ulcer of head,
                stage 3
            Pressure ulcer with full thickness
                skin loss involving damage or
                necrosis of subcutaneous tissue,
                head

L89.814   **Pressure ulcer of head, stage 4** 🔖
            Healing pressure ulcer of head,
                stage 4
            Pressure ulcer with necrosis of soft
                tissues through to underlying
                muscle, tendon, or bone, head

L89.816   **Pressure-induced deep tissue damage
            of head**

L89.819   **Pressure ulcer of head, unspecified
            stage**
            Healing pressure ulcer of head NOS
            Healing pressure ulcer of head,
                unspecified stage

● **L89.89 Pressure ulcer of other site**

L89.890   **Pressure ulcer of other site,
            unstageable** 🔖

L89.891   **Pressure ulcer of other site, stage 1**
            Healing pressure ulcer of other site,
                stage 1
            Pressure pre-ulcer skin changes
                limited to persistent focal
                edema, other site

L89.892   **Pressure ulcer of other site, stage 2**
            Healing pressure ulcer of other site,
                stage 2
            Pressure ulcer with abrasion, blister,
                partial thickness skin loss
                involving epidermis and/or
                dermis, other site

L89.893   **Pressure ulcer of other site, stage 3** 🔖
            Healing pressure ulcer of other site,
                stage 3
            Pressure ulcer with full thickness
                skin loss involving damage or
                necrosis of subcutaneous tissue,
                other site

L89.894   **Pressure ulcer of other site, stage 4** 🔖
            Healing pressure ulcer of other site,
                stage 4
            Pressure ulcer with necrosis of soft
                tissues through to underlying
                muscle, tendon, or bone, other
                site

L89.899   **Pressure ulcer of other site,
            unspecified stage**
            Healing pressure ulcer of other site
                NOS
            Healing pressure ulcer of other site,
                unspecified stage

● **L89.9 Pressure ulcer of unspecified site**

L89.90   **Pressure ulcer of unspecified site, unspecified
            stage**
            Healing pressure ulcer of unspecified site NOS
            Healing pressure ulcer of unspecified site,
                unspecified stage

L89.91   **Pressure ulcer of unspecified site, stage 1**
            Healing pressure ulcer of unspecified site,
                stage 1
            Pressure pre-ulcer skin changes limited to
                persistent focal edema, unspecified site

L89.92   **Pressure ulcer of unspecified site, stage 2**
            Healing pressure ulcer of unspecified site,
                stage 2
            Pressure ulcer with abrasion, blister, partial
                thickness skin loss involving epidermis
                and/or dermis, unspecified site

CHAPTER 12 (L00–L99)

Item 12–11 Scleroderma means hard skin. It is a group of diseases that causes abnormal growth of connective tissues that support the skin and organs. There are two types: localized scleroderma affecting the skin and systemic scleroderma affecting blood vessels and internal organs and the skin.

L89.93   **Pressure ulcer of unspecified site, stage 3** 🐾
       Healing pressure ulcer of unspecified site, stage 3
       Pressure ulcer with full thickness skin loss involving damage or necrosis of subcutaneous tissue, unspecified site

L89.94   **Pressure ulcer of unspecified site, stage 4** 🐾
       Healing pressure ulcer of unspecified site, stage 4
       Pressure ulcer with necrosis of soft tissues through to underlying muscle, tendon, or bone, unspecified site

L89.95   **Pressure ulcer of unspecified site, unstageable** 🐾

L89.96   **Pressure-induced deep tissue damage of unspecified site**

● **L90**   **Atrophic disorders of skin**

L90.0   **Lichen sclerosus et atrophicus**
       Excludes2   lichen sclerosus of external female genital organs (N90.4)
                   lichen sclerosus of external male genital organs (N48.0)

L90.1   **Anetoderma of Schweninger-Buzzi**

L90.2   **Anetoderma of Jadassohn-Pellizzari**

L90.3   **Atrophoderma of Pasini and Pierini**

L90.4   **Acrodermatitis chronica atrophicans**

L90.5   **Scar conditions and fibrosis of skin**
       Adherent scar (skin)
       Cicatrix
       Disfigurement of skin due to scar
       Fibrosis of skin NOS
       Scar NOS
       Excludes2   hypertrophic scar (L91.0)
                   keloid scar (L91.0)
       Coding Clinic: 2016, Q2, P5; 2015, Q1, P19

L90.6   **Striae atrophicae**

L90.8   **Other atrophic disorders of skin**

L90.9   **Atrophic disorder of skin, unspecified**

● **L91**   **Hypertrophic disorders of skin**

L91.0   **Keloid scar**
       Hypertrophic scar
       Keloid
       Excludes2   acne keloid (L73.0)
                   scar NOS (L90.5)

L91.8   **Other hypertrophic disorders of the skin**

L91.9   **Hypertrophic disorder of the skin, unspecified**

● **L92**   **Granulomatous disorders of skin and subcutaneous tissue**
       Excludes2   actinic granuloma (L57.5)

L92.0   **Granuloma annulare**
       Perforating granuloma annulare

L92.1   **Necrobiosis lipoidica, not elsewhere classified**
       Excludes1   necrobiosis lipoidica associated with diabetes mellitus (E08-E13 with .620)

L92.2   **Granuloma faciale [eosinophilic granuloma of skin]**

L92.3   **Foreign body granuloma of the skin and subcutaneous tissue**
       Use additional code to identify the type of retained foreign body (Z18.-)

L92.8   **Other granulomatous disorders of the skin and subcutaneous tissue**

L92.9   **Granulomatous disorder of the skin and subcutaneous tissue, unspecified**
       Excludes2   umbilical granuloma (P83.81)

● **L93**   **Lupus erythematosus**
       Use additional code for adverse effect, if applicable, to identify drug (T36-T50 with fifth or sixth character 5)
       Excludes1   lupus exedens (A18.4)
                   lupus vulgaris (A18.4)
                   scleroderma (M34.-)
                   systemic lupus erythematosus (M32.-)

L93.0   **Discoid lupus erythematosus**
       Lupus erythematosus NOS

L93.1   **Subacute cutaneous lupus erythematosus**

L93.2   **Other local lupus erythematosus**
       Lupus erythematosus profundus
       Lupus panniculitis

● **L94**   **Other localized connective tissue disorders**
       Excludes1   systemic connective tissue disorders (M30-M36)

L94.0   **Localized scleroderma [morphea]**
       Circumscribed scleroderma

L94.1   **Linear scleroderma**
       En coup de sabre lesion

L94.2   **Calcinosis cutis**

L94.3   **Sclerodactyly**

L94.4   **Gottron's papules**

L94.5   **Poikiloderma vasculare atrophicans**

L94.6   **Ainhum**

L94.8   **Other specified localized connective tissue disorders**

L94.9   **Localized connective tissue disorder, unspecified**

● **L95**   **Vasculitis limited to skin, not elsewhere classified**
       Excludes1   angioma serpiginosum (L81.7)
                   Henoch(-Schönlein) purpura (D69.0)
                   hypersensitivity angiitis (M31.0)
                   lupus panniculitis (L93.2)
                   panniculitis NOS (M79.3)
                   panniculitis of neck and back (M54.0-)
                   polyarteritis nodosa (M30.0)
                   relapsing panniculitis (M35.6)
                   rheumatoid vasculitis (M05.2)
                   serum sickness (T80.6-)
                   urticaria (L50.-)
                   Wegener's granulomatosis (M31.3-)

L95.0   **Livedoid vasculitis**
       Atrophie blanche (en plaque)

L95.1   **Erythema elevatum diutinum**

L95.8   **Other vasculitis limited to the skin**

L95.9   **Vasculitis limited to the skin, unspecified**

● **L97**   **Non-pressure chronic ulcer of lower limb, not elsewhere classified**
       Includes   chronic ulcer of skin of lower limb NOS
                 non-healing ulcer of skin
                 non-infected sinus of skin
                 trophic ulcer NOS
                 tropical ulcer NOS
                 ulcer of skin of lower limb NOS

       Code first any associated underlying condition, such as:
       any associated gangrene (I96)
       atherosclerosis of the lower extremities (I70.23-, I70.24-, I70.33-, I70.34-, I70.43-, I70.44-, I70.53-, I70.54-, I70.63-, I70.64-, I70.73-, I70.74-)
       chronic venous hypertension (I87.31-, I87.33-)
       diabetic ulcers (E08.621, E08.622, E09.621, E09.622, E10.621, E10.622, E11.621, E11.622, E13.621, E13.622)
       postphlebitic syndrome (I87.01-, I87.03-)
       postthrombotic syndrome (I87.01-, I87.03-)
       varicose ulcer (I83.0-, I83.2-)
       Excludes2   pressure ulcer (pressure area) (L89.-)
                   skin infections (L00-L08)
                   specific infections classified to A00-B99

▶ New   ⇒ Revised   ~~deleted~~ Deleted   Excludes 1   Excludes 2   Includes   Use additional   Code first   Code also   Key words

OGCR Official Guidelines   **X** Assign placeholder X   ● Use Additional Character(s)   ▶ Manifestation Code   🐾 Hierarchical Condition Category   **Coding Clinic**

● **L97.1**   Non-pressure chronic ulcer of thigh

  ● **L97.10**   Non-pressure chronic ulcer of unspecified thigh

     L97.101   Non-pressure chronic ulcer of unspecified thigh limited to breakdown of skin 🔖

     L97.102   Non-pressure chronic ulcer of unspecified thigh with fat layer exposed 🔖

     L97.103   Non-pressure chronic ulcer of unspecified thigh with necrosis of muscle 🔖

     L97.104   Non-pressure chronic ulcer of unspecified thigh with necrosis of bone 🔖

     L97.105   Non-pressure chronic ulcer of unspecified thigh with muscle involvement without evidence of necrosis 🔖

     L97.106   Non-pressure chronic ulcer of unspecified thigh with bone involvement without evidence of necrosis 🔖

     L97.108   Non-pressure chronic ulcer of unspecified thigh with other specified severity 🔖

     L97.109   Non-pressure chronic ulcer of unspecified thigh with unspecified severity 🔖

  ● **L97.11**   Non-pressure chronic ulcer of right thigh

     L97.111   Non-pressure chronic ulcer of right thigh limited to breakdown of skin 🔖

     L97.112   Non-pressure chronic ulcer of right thigh with fat layer exposed 🔖

     L97.113   Non-pressure chronic ulcer of right thigh with necrosis of muscle 🔖

     L97.114   Non-pressure chronic ulcer of right thigh with necrosis of bone 🔖

     L97.115   Non-pressure chronic ulcer of right thigh with muscle involvement without evidence of necrosis 🔖

     L97.116   Non-pressure chronic ulcer of right thigh with bone involvement without evidence of necrosis 🔖

     L97.118   Non-pressure chronic ulcer of right thigh with other specified severity 🔖

     L97.119   Non-pressure chronic ulcer of right thigh with unspecified severity 🔖

  ● **L97.12**   Non-pressure chronic ulcer of left thigh

     L97.121   Non-pressure chronic ulcer of left thigh limited to breakdown of skin 🔖

     L97.122   Non-pressure chronic ulcer of left thigh with fat layer exposed 🔖

     L97.123   Non-pressure chronic ulcer of left thigh with necrosis of muscle 🔖

     L97.124   Non-pressure chronic ulcer of left thigh with necrosis of bone 🔖

     L97.125   Non-pressure chronic ulcer of left thigh with muscle involvement without evidence of necrosis 🔖

     L97.126   Non-pressure chronic ulcer of left thigh with bone involvement without evidence of necrosis 🔖

     L97.128   Non-pressure chronic ulcer of left thigh with other specified severity 🔖

     L97.129   Non-pressure chronic ulcer of left thigh with unspecified severity 🔖

● **L97.2**   Non-pressure chronic ulcer of calf

  ● **L97.20**   Non-pressure chronic ulcer of unspecified calf

     L97.201   Non-pressure chronic ulcer of unspecified calf limited to breakdown of skin 🔖

     L97.202   Non-pressure chronic ulcer of unspecified calf with fat layer exposed 🔖

     L97.203   Non-pressure chronic ulcer of unspecified calf with necrosis of muscle 🔖

     L97.204   Non-pressure chronic ulcer of unspecified calf with necrosis of bone 🔖

     L97.205   Non-pressure chronic ulcer of unspecified calf with muscle involvement without evidence of necrosis 🔖

     L97.206   Non-pressure chronic ulcer of unspecified calf with bone involvement without evidence of necrosis 🔖

     L97.208   Non-pressure chronic ulcer of unspecified calf with other specified severity 🔖

     L97.209   Non-pressure chronic ulcer of unspecified calf with unspecified severity 🔖

  ● **L97.21**   Non-pressure chronic ulcer of right calf

     L97.211   Non-pressure chronic ulcer of right calf limited to breakdown of skin 🔖

     L97.212   Non-pressure chronic ulcer of right calf with fat layer exposed 🔖

     L97.213   Non-pressure chronic ulcer of right calf with necrosis of muscle 🔖

     L97.214   Non-pressure chronic ulcer of right calf with necrosis of bone 🔖

     L97.215   Non-pressure chronic ulcer of right calf with muscle involvement without evidence of necrosis 🔖

     L97.216   Non-pressure chronic ulcer of right calf with bone involvement without evidence of necrosis 🔖

     L97.218   Non-pressure chronic ulcer of right calf with other specified severity 🔖

     L97.219   Non-pressure chronic ulcer of right calf with unspecified severity 🔖

       Coding Clinic: 2024, Q1, P16

  ● **L97.22**   Non-pressure chronic ulcer of left calf

     L97.221   Non-pressure chronic ulcer of left calf limited to breakdown of skin 🔖

     L97.222   Non-pressure chronic ulcer of left calf with fat layer exposed 🔖

     L97.223   Non-pressure chronic ulcer of left calf with necrosis of muscle 🔖

     L97.224   Non-pressure chronic ulcer of left calf with necrosis of bone 🔖

     L97.225   Non-pressure chronic ulcer of left calf with muscle involvement without evidence of necrosis 🔖

     L97.226   Non-pressure chronic ulcer of left calf with bone involvement without evidence of necrosis 🔖

     L97.228   Non-pressure chronic ulcer of left calf with other specified severity 🔖

     L97.229   Non-pressure chronic ulcer of left calf with unspecified severity 🔖

CHAPTER 12 (L00-L99)

● **L97.3**   Non-pressure chronic ulcer of ankle
  ● **L97.30**   Non-pressure chronic ulcer of unspecified ankle

     L97.301   Non-pressure chronic ulcer of unspecified ankle limited to breakdown of skin 🐾

     L97.302   Non-pressure chronic ulcer of unspecified ankle with fat layer exposed 🐾

     L97.303   Non-pressure chronic ulcer of unspecified ankle with necrosis of muscle 🐾

     L97.304   Non-pressure chronic ulcer of unspecified ankle with necrosis of bone 🐾

     L97.305   Non-pressure chronic ulcer of unspecified ankle with muscle involvement without evidence of necrosis 🐾

     L97.306   Non-pressure chronic ulcer of unspecified ankle with bone involvement without evidence of necrosis 🐾

     L97.308   Non-pressure chronic ulcer of unspecified ankle with other specified severity 🐾

     L97.309   Non-pressure chronic ulcer of unspecified ankle with unspecified severity 🐾

  ● **L97.31**   Non-pressure chronic ulcer of right ankle

     L97.311   Non-pressure chronic ulcer of right ankle limited to breakdown of skin 🐾

     L97.312   Non-pressure chronic ulcer of right ankle with fat layer exposed 🐾

     L97.313   Non-pressure chronic ulcer of right ankle with necrosis of muscle 🐾

     L97.314   Non-pressure chronic ulcer of right ankle with necrosis of bone 🐾

     L97.315   Non-pressure chronic ulcer of right ankle with muscle involvement without evidence of necrosis 🐾
             Coding Clinic: 2017, Q4, P17

     L97.316   Non-pressure chronic ulcer of right ankle with bone involvement without evidence of necrosis 🐾

     L97.318   Non-pressure chronic ulcer of right ankle with other specified severity 🐾

     L97.319   Non-pressure chronic ulcer of right ankle with unspecified severity 🐾

  ● **L97.32**   Non-pressure chronic ulcer of left ankle

     L97.321   Non-pressure chronic ulcer of left ankle limited to breakdown of skin 🐾

     L97.322   Non-pressure chronic ulcer of left ankle with fat layer exposed 🐾
             Coding Clinic: 2021, Q1, P8

     L97.323   Non-pressure chronic ulcer of left ankle with necrosis of muscle 🐾

     L97.324   Non-pressure chronic ulcer of left ankle with necrosis of bone 🐾

     L97.325   Non-pressure chronic ulcer of left ankle with muscle involvement without evidence of necrosis 🐾

     L97.326   Non-pressure chronic ulcer of left ankle with bone involvement without evidence of necrosis 🐾

     L97.328   Non-pressure chronic ulcer of left ankle with other specified severity 🐾

     L97.329   Non-pressure chronic ulcer of left ankle with unspecified severity 🐾

● **L97.4**   Non-pressure chronic ulcer of heel and midfoot
    Non-pressure chronic ulcer of plantar surface of midfoot
  ● **L97.40**   Non-pressure chronic ulcer of unspecified heel and midfoot

     L97.401   Non-pressure chronic ulcer of unspecified heel and midfoot limited to breakdown of skin 🐾

     L97.402   Non-pressure chronic ulcer of unspecified heel and midfoot with fat layer exposed 🐾

     L97.403   Non-pressure chronic ulcer of unspecified heel and midfoot with necrosis of muscle 🐾

     L97.404   Non-pressure chronic ulcer of unspecified heel and midfoot with necrosis of bone 🐾

     L97.405   Non-pressure chronic ulcer of unspecified heel and midfoot with muscle involvement without evidence of necrosis 🐾

     L97.406   Non-pressure chronic ulcer of unspecified heel and midfoot with bone involvement without evidence of necrosis 🐾

     L97.408   Non-pressure chronic ulcer of unspecified heel and midfoot with other specified severity 🐾

     L97.409   Non-pressure chronic ulcer of unspecified heel and midfoot with unspecified severity 🐾

  ● **L97.41**   Non-pressure chronic ulcer of right heel and midfoot

     L97.411   Non-pressure chronic ulcer of right heel and midfoot limited to breakdown of skin 🐾

     L97.412   Non-pressure chronic ulcer of right heel and midfoot with fat layer exposed 🐾

     L97.413   Non-pressure chronic ulcer of right heel and midfoot with necrosis of muscle 🐾

     L97.414   Non-pressure chronic ulcer of right heel and midfoot with necrosis of bone 🐾

     L97.415   Non-pressure chronic ulcer of right heel and midfoot with muscle involvement without evidence of necrosis 🐾

     L97.416   Non-pressure chronic ulcer of right heel and midfoot with bone involvement without evidence of necrosis 🐾

     L97.418   Non-pressure chronic ulcer of right heel and midfoot with other specified severity 🐾

     L97.419   Non-pressure chronic ulcer of right heel and midfoot with unspecified severity 🐾

  ● **L97.42**   Non-pressure chronic ulcer of left heel and midfoot

     L97.421   Non-pressure chronic ulcer of left heel and midfoot limited to breakdown of skin 🐾
             Coding Clinic: 2016, Q1, P13

     L97.422   Non-pressure chronic ulcer of left heel and midfoot with fat layer exposed 🐾

     L97.423   Non-pressure chronic ulcer of left heel and midfoot with necrosis of muscle 🐾

     L97.424   Non-pressure chronic ulcer of left heel and midfoot with necrosis of bone 🐾

▶ New   ⇒ Revised   ~~deleted~~ Deleted   Excludes 1   Excludes 2   Includes   Use additional   Code first   Code also   Key words

OGCR Official Guidelines   X Assign placeholder X   ● Use Additional Character(s)   ▶ Manifestation Code   🐾 Hierarchical Condition Category   Coding Clinic

L97.425   Non-pressure chronic ulcer of left heel and midfoot with muscle involvement without evidence of necrosis 🔎

L97.426   Non-pressure chronic ulcer of left heel and midfoot with bone involvement without evidence of necrosis 🔎

L97.428   Non-pressure chronic ulcer of left heel and midfoot with other specified severity 🔎

L97.429   Non-pressure chronic ulcer of left heel and midfoot with unspecified severity 🔎

● **L97.5**   Non-pressure chronic ulcer of other part of foot
     Non-pressure chronic ulcer of toe

   ● **L97.50**   Non-pressure chronic ulcer of other part of unspecified foot

L97.501   Non-pressure chronic ulcer of other part of unspecified foot limited to breakdown of skin 🔎

L97.502   Non-pressure chronic ulcer of other part of unspecified foot with fat layer exposed 🔎

L97.503   Non-pressure chronic ulcer of other part of unspecified foot with necrosis of muscle 🔎

L97.504   Non-pressure chronic ulcer of other part of unspecified foot with necrosis of bone 🔎

L97.505   Non-pressure chronic ulcer of other part of unspecified foot with muscle involvement without evidence of necrosis 🔎

L97.506   Non-pressure chronic ulcer of other part of unspecified foot with bone involvement without evidence of necrosis 🔎

L97.508   Non-pressure chronic ulcer of other part of unspecified foot with other specified severity 🔎

L97.509   Non-pressure chronic ulcer of other part of unspecified foot with unspecified severity 🔎

   ● **L97.51**   Non-pressure chronic ulcer of other part of right foot

L97.511   Non-pressure chronic ulcer of other part of right foot limited to breakdown of skin 🔎
     Coding Clinic: 2020, Q1, P12

L97.512   Non-pressure chronic ulcer of other part of right foot with fat layer exposed 🔎

L97.513   Non-pressure chronic ulcer of other part of right foot with necrosis of muscle 🔎

L97.514   Non-pressure chronic ulcer of other part of right foot with necrosis of bone 🔎

L97.515   Non-pressure chronic ulcer of other part of right foot with muscle involvement without evidence of necrosis 🔎

L97.516   Non-pressure chronic ulcer of other part of right foot with bone involvement without evidence of necrosis 🔎

L97.518   Non-pressure chronic ulcer of other part of right foot with other specified severity 🔎

L97.519   Non-pressure chronic ulcer of other part of right foot with unspecified severity 🔎

● **L97.52**   Non-pressure chronic ulcer of other part of left foot

L97.521   Non-pressure chronic ulcer of other part of left foot limited to breakdown of skin 🔎

L97.522   Non-pressure chronic ulcer of other part of left foot with fat layer exposed 🔎

L97.523   Non-pressure chronic ulcer of other part of left foot with necrosis of muscle 🔎

L97.524   Non-pressure chronic ulcer of other part of left foot with necrosis of bone 🔎

L97.525   Non-pressure chronic ulcer of other part of left foot with muscle involvement without evidence of necrosis 🔎

L97.526   Non-pressure chronic ulcer of other part of left foot with bone involvement without evidence of necrosis 🔎

L97.528   Non-pressure chronic ulcer of other part of left foot with other specified severity 🔎

L97.529   Non-pressure chronic ulcer of other part of left foot with unspecified severity 🔎

● **L97.8**   Non-pressure chronic ulcer of other part of lower leg

   ● **L97.80**   Non-pressure chronic ulcer of other part of unspecified lower leg

L97.801   Non-pressure chronic ulcer of other part of unspecified lower leg limited to breakdown of skin 🔎

L97.802   Non-pressure chronic ulcer of other part of unspecified lower leg with fat layer exposed 🔎

L97.803   Non-pressure chronic ulcer of other part of unspecified lower leg with necrosis of muscle 🔎

L97.804   Non-pressure chronic ulcer of other part of unspecified lower leg with necrosis of bone 🔎

L97.805   Non-pressure chronic ulcer of other part of unspecified lower leg with muscle involvement without evidence of necrosis 🔎

L97.806   Non-pressure chronic ulcer of other part of unspecified lower leg with bone involvement without evidence of necrosis 🔎

L97.808   Non-pressure chronic ulcer of other part of unspecified lower leg with other specified severity 🔎

L97.809   Non-pressure chronic ulcer of other part of unspecified lower leg with unspecified severity 🔎

   ● **L97.81**   Non-pressure chronic ulcer of other part of right lower leg

L97.811   Non-pressure chronic ulcer of other part of right lower leg limited to breakdown of skin 🔎

L97.812   Non-pressure chronic ulcer of other part of right lower leg with fat layer exposed 🔎

L97.813   Non-pressure chronic ulcer of other part of right lower leg with necrosis of muscle 🔎

L97.814   Non-pressure chronic ulcer of other part of right lower leg with necrosis of bone 🔎

CHAPTER 12 (L00-L99)

L97.815 Non-pressure chronic ulcer of other part of right lower leg with muscle involvement without evidence of necrosis 🦠

L97.816 Non-pressure chronic ulcer of other part of right lower leg with bone involvement without evidence of necrosis 🦠

L97.818 Non-pressure chronic ulcer of other part of right lower leg with other specified severity 🦠

L97.819 Non-pressure chronic ulcer of other part of right lower leg with unspecified severity 🦠

● **L97.82** Non-pressure chronic ulcer of other part of left lower leg

L97.821 Non-pressure chronic ulcer of other part of left lower leg limited to breakdown of skin 🦠

L97.822 Non-pressure chronic ulcer of other part of left lower leg with fat layer exposed 🦠

L97.823 Non-pressure chronic ulcer of other part of left lower leg with necrosis of muscle 🦠

L97.824 Non-pressure chronic ulcer of other part of left lower leg with necrosis of bone 🦠

L97.825 Non-pressure chronic ulcer of other part of left lower leg with muscle involvement without evidence of necrosis 🦠

L97.826 Non-pressure chronic ulcer of other part of left lower leg with bone involvement without evidence of necrosis 🦠

L97.828 Non-pressure chronic ulcer of other part of left lower leg with other specified severity 🦠

L97.829 Non-pressure chronic ulcer of other part of left lower leg with unspecified severity 🦠

● **L97.9** Non-pressure chronic ulcer of unspecified part of lower leg

● **L97.90** Non-pressure chronic ulcer of unspecified part of unspecified lower leg

L97.901 Non-pressure chronic ulcer of unspecified part of unspecified lower leg limited to breakdown of skin 🦠

L97.902 Non-pressure chronic ulcer of unspecified part of unspecified lower leg with fat layer exposed 🦠

L97.903 Non-pressure chronic ulcer of unspecified part of unspecified lower leg with necrosis of muscle 🦠

L97.904 Non-pressure chronic ulcer of unspecified part of unspecified lower leg with necrosis of bone 🦠

L97.905 Non-pressure chronic ulcer of unspecified part of unspecified lower leg with muscle involvement without evidence of necrosis 🦠

L97.906 Non-pressure chronic ulcer of unspecified part of unspecified lower leg with bone involvement without evidence of necrosis 🦠

L97.908 Non-pressure chronic ulcer of unspecified part of unspecified lower leg with other specified severity 🦠

L97.909 Non-pressure chronic ulcer of unspecified part of unspecified lower leg with unspecified severity 🦠

● **L97.91** Non-pressure chronic ulcer of unspecified part of right lower leg

L97.911 Non-pressure chronic ulcer of unspecified part of right lower leg limited to breakdown of skin 🦠

L97.912 Non-pressure chronic ulcer of unspecified part of right lower leg with fat layer exposed 🦠

L97.913 Non-pressure chronic ulcer of unspecified part of right lower leg with necrosis of muscle 🦠

L97.914 Non-pressure chronic ulcer of unspecified part of right lower leg with necrosis of bone 🦠

L97.915 Non-pressure chronic ulcer of unspecified part of right lower leg with muscle involvement without evidence of necrosis 🦠

L97.916 Non-pressure chronic ulcer of unspecified part of right lower leg with bone involvement without evidence of necrosis 🦠

L97.918 Non-pressure chronic ulcer of unspecified part of right lower leg with other specified severity 🦠

L97.919 Non-pressure chronic ulcer of unspecified part of right lower leg with unspecified severity 🦠

● **L97.92** Non-pressure chronic ulcer of unspecified part of left lower leg

L97.921 Non-pressure chronic ulcer of unspecified part of left lower leg limited to breakdown of skin 🦠

L97.922 Non-pressure chronic ulcer of unspecified part of left lower leg with fat layer exposed 🦠

L97.923 Non-pressure chronic ulcer of unspecified part of left lower leg with necrosis of muscle 🦠

L97.924 Non-pressure chronic ulcer of unspecified part of left lower leg with necrosis of bone 🦠

L97.925 Non-pressure chronic ulcer of unspecified part of left lower leg with muscle involvement without evidence of necrosis 🦠

L97.926 Non-pressure chronic ulcer of unspecified part of left lower leg with bone involvement without evidence of necrosis 🦠

L97.928 Non-pressure chronic ulcer of unspecified part of left lower leg with other specified severity 🦠

L97.929 Non-pressure chronic ulcer of unspecified part of left lower leg with unspecified severity 🦠

● **L98** Other disorders of skin and subcutaneous tissue, not elsewhere classified

L98.0 Pyogenic granuloma

Excludes2 pyogenic granuloma of gingiva (K06.8)
pyogenic granuloma of maxillary alveolar ridge (K04.5)
pyogenic granuloma of oral mucosa (K13.4)

L98.1 Factitial dermatitis
Neurotic excoriation

Excludes1 Excoriation (skin-picking) disorder (F42.4)

Coding Clinic: 2016, Q4, P15

L98.2 Febrile neutrophilic dermatosis [Sweet]

L98.3 Eosinophilic cellulitis [Wells]

▶ New ⇒ Revised ~~deleted~~ Deleted Excludes 1 Excludes 2 Includes Use additional Code first Code also Key words
OGCR Official Guidelines X Assign placeholder X ● Use Additional Character(s) ▷ Manifestation Code 🦠 Hierarchical Condition Category Coding Clinic

● **L98.4 Non-pressure chronic ulcer of skin, not elsewhere classified**
    Chronic ulcer of skin NOS
    Tropical ulcer NOS
    Ulcer of skin NOS
    Excludes2   pressure ulcer (pressure area) (L89.-)
                  gangrene (I96)
                  skin infections (L00-L08)
                  specific infections classified to A00-B99
                  ulcer of lower limb NEC (L97.-)
                  varicose ulcer (I83.0-I83.93)

● **L98.41 Non-pressure chronic ulcer of buttock**

    L98.411 Non-pressure chronic ulcer of buttock limited to breakdown of skin

    L98.412 Non-pressure chronic ulcer of buttock with fat layer exposed

    L98.413 Non-pressure chronic ulcer of buttock with necrosis of muscle

    L98.414 Non-pressure chronic ulcer of buttock with necrosis of bone

    L98.415 Non-pressure chronic ulcer of buttock with muscle involvement without evidence of necrosis

    L98.416 Non-pressure chronic ulcer of buttock with bone involvement without evidence of necrosis

    L98.418 Non-pressure chronic ulcer of buttock with other specified severity

    L98.419 Non-pressure chronic ulcer of buttock with unspecified severity

● **L98.42 Non-pressure chronic ulcer of back**

    L98.421 Non-pressure chronic ulcer of back limited to breakdown of skin

    L98.422 Non-pressure chronic ulcer of back with fat layer exposed

    L98.423 Non-pressure chronic ulcer of back with necrosis of muscle

    L98.424 Non-pressure chronic ulcer of back with necrosis of bone

    L98.425 Non-pressure chronic ulcer of back with muscle involvement without evidence of necrosis

    L98.426 Non-pressure chronic ulcer of back with bone involvement without evidence of necrosis

    L98.428 Non-pressure chronic ulcer of back with other specified severity

    L98.429 Non-pressure chronic ulcer of back with unspecified severity

● **L98.49 Non-pressure chronic ulcer of skin of other sites**
    Non-pressure chronic ulcer of skin NOS

    L98.491 Non-pressure chronic ulcer of skin of other sites limited to breakdown of skin

    L98.492 Non-pressure chronic ulcer of skin of other sites with fat layer exposed

    L98.493 Non-pressure chronic ulcer of skin of other sites with necrosis of muscle

    L98.494 Non-pressure chronic ulcer of skin of other sites with necrosis of bone

    L98.495 Non-pressure chronic ulcer of skin of other sites with muscle involvement without evidence of necrosis

    L98.496 Non-pressure chronic ulcer of skin of other sites with bone involvement without evidence of necrosis

    L98.498 Non-pressure chronic ulcer of skin of other sites with other specified severity

    L98.499 Non-pressure chronic ulcer of skin of other sites with unspecified severity

L98.5 Mucinosis of the skin
    Focal mucinosis
    Lichen myxedematosus
    Reticular erythematous mucinosis
    Excludes1 focal oral mucinosis (K13.79)
                 myxedema (E03.9)

L98.6 Other infiltrative disorders of the skin and subcutaneous tissue
    Excludes1 hyalinosis cutis et mucosae (E78.89)

L98.7 Excessive and redundant skin and subcutaneous tissue
    Loose or sagging skin following bariatric surgery weight loss
    Loose or sagging skin following dietary weight loss
    Loose or sagging skin, NOS
    Excludes2 acquired excess or redundant skin of eyelid (H02.3-)
                 congenital excess or redundant skin of eyelid (Q10.3)
                 skin changes due to chronic exposure to nonionizing radiation (L57.-)
    Coding Clinic: 2022, Q3, P11; 2016, Q4, P36

L98.8 Other specified disorders of the skin and subcutaneous tissue
    Coding Clinic: 2013, Q2, P32

L98.9 Disorder of the skin and subcutaneous tissue, unspecified

▸ *L99* *Other disorders of skin and subcutaneous tissue in diseases classified elsewhere*
    Code first underlying disease, such as:
    amyloidosis (E85.-)
    Excludes1 skin disorders in diabetes (E08-E13 with .62-)
                 skin disorders in gonorrhea (A54.89)
                 skin disorders in syphilis (A51.31, A52.79)

CHAPTER 12 (L00-L99)

CHAPTER 13

DISEASES OF THE MUSCULOSKELETAL SYSTEM AND CONNECTIVE TISSUE (M00-M99)

OGCR Chapter-Specific Coding Guidelines

13. Chapter 13: Diseases of the Musculoskeletal System and Connective Tissue (M00-M99)

a. Site and laterality

Most of the codes within Chapter 13 have site and laterality designations. The site represents the bone, joint or the muscle involved. For some conditions where more than one bone, joint or muscle is usually involved, such as osteoarthritis, there is a "multiple sites" code available. For categories where no multiple site code is provided and more than one bone, joint or muscle is involved, multiple codes should be used to indicate the different sites involved.

1) Bone versus joint

For certain conditions, the bone may be affected at the upper or lower end (e.g., avascular necrosis of bone, M87, Osteoporosis, M80, M81). Though the portion of the bone affected may be at the joint, the site designation will be the bone, not the joint.

b. Acute traumatic versus chronic or recurrent musculoskeletal conditions

Many musculoskeletal conditions are a result of previous injury or trauma to a site, or are recurrent conditions. Bone, joint or muscle conditions that are the result of a healed injury are usually found in Chapter 13. Recurrent bone, joint or muscle conditions are also usually found in Chapter 13. Any current, acute injury should be coded to the appropriate injury code from Chapter 19. Chronic or recurrent conditions should generally be coded with a code from Chapter 13. If it is difficult to determine from the documentation in the record which code is best to describe a condition, query the provider.

c. Coding of Pathologic Fractures

7th character A is for use as long as the patient is receiving active treatment for the fracture. While the patient may be seen by a new or different provider over the course of treatment for a pathological fracture, assignment of the 7th character is based on whether the patient is undergoing active treatment and not whether the provider is seeing the patient for the first time.

7th character, D is to be used for encounters after the patient has completed active treatment for the fracture and is receiving routine care for the fracture during the healing or recovery phase. The other 7th characters, listed under each subcategory in the Tabular List, are to be used for subsequent encounters for treatment of problems associated with the healing, such as malunions, nonunions, and sequelae.

Care for complications of surgical treatment for fracture repairs during the healing or recovery phase should be coded with the appropriate complication codes.

See Section I.C.19. Coding of traumatic fractures.

d. Osteoporosis

Osteoporosis is a systemic condition, meaning that all bones of the musculoskeletal system are affected. Therefore, site is not a component of the codes under category M81, Osteoporosis without current pathological fracture. The site codes under category M80, Osteoporosis with current pathological fracture, identify the site of the fracture, not the osteoporosis.

1) Osteoporosis without pathological fracture

Category M81, Osteoporosis without current pathological fracture, is for use for patients with osteoporosis who do not currently have a pathologic fracture due to the osteoporosis, even if they have had a fracture in the past. For patients with a history of osteoporosis fractures, status code Z87.310, Personal history of (healed) osteoporosis fracture, should follow the code from M81.

2) Osteoporosis with current pathological fracture

Category M80, Osteoporosis with current pathological fracture, is for patients who have a current pathologic fracture at the time of an encounter. The codes under M80 identify the site of the fracture. A code from category M80, not a traumatic fracture code, should be used for any patient with known osteoporosis who suffers a fracture, even if the patient had a minor fall or trauma, if that fall or trauma would not usually break a normal, healthy bone.

CHAPTER 13

DISEASES OF THE MUSCULOSKELETAL SYSTEM AND CONNECTIVE TISSUE (M00-M99)

Note: Use an external cause code following the code for the musculoskeletal condition, if applicable, to identify the cause of the musculoskeletal condition

Excludes2   arthropathic psoriasis (L40.5-)
certain conditions originating in the perinatal period (P04-P96)
certain infectious and parasitic diseases (A00-B99)
compartment syndrome (traumatic) (T79.A-)
complications of pregnancy, childbirth and the puerperium (O00-O9A)
congenital malformations, deformations, and chromosomal abnormalities (Q00-Q99)
endocrine, nutritional and metabolic diseases (E00-E88)
injury, poisoning and certain other consequences of external causes (S00-T88)
neoplasms (C00-D49)
symptoms, signs and abnormal clinical and laboratory findings, not elsewhere classified (R00-R94)

This chapter contains the following blocks:

M00-M02	Infectious arthropathies
M04	Autoinflammatory syndromes
M05-M14	Inflammatory polyarthropathies
M15-M19	Osteoarthritis
M20-M25	Other joint disorders
M26-M27	Dentofacial anomalies [including malocclusion] and other disorders of jaw
M30-M36	Systemic connective tissue disorders
M40-M43	Deforming dorsopathies
M45-M49	Spondylopathies
M50-M54	Other dorsopathies
M60-M63	Disorders of muscles
M65-M67	Disorders of synovium and tendon
M70-M79	Other soft tissue disorders
M80-M85	Disorders of bone density and structure
M86-M90	Other osteopathies
M91-M94	Chondropathies
M95	Other disorders of the musculoskeletal system and connective tissue
M96	Intraoperative and postprocedural complications and disorders of musculoskeletal system, not elsewhere classified
M97	Periprosthetic fracture around internal prosthetic joint
M99	Biomechanical lesions, not elsewhere classified

Coding Clinic: 2016, Q4, P124

ARTHROPATHIES (M00-M25)

Includes   Disorders affecting predominantly peripheral (limb) joints

INFECTIOUS ARTHROPATHIES (M00-M02)

Note: This block comprises arthropathies due to microbiological agents.

Distinction is made between the following types of etiological relationship:

a) direct infection of joint, where organisms invade synovial tissue and microbial antigen is present in the joint;

b) indirect infection, which may be of two types: a reactive arthropathy, where microbial infection of the body is established but neither organisms nor antigens can be identified in the joint, and a postinfective arthropathy, where microbial antigen is present but recovery of an organism is inconstant and evidence of local multiplication is lacking.

▶ New   ◆ Revised   ~~deleted~~ Deleted   Excludes 1   Excludes 2   Includes   Use additional   Code first   Code also   Key words

OGCR Official Guidelines   X Assign placeholder X   ● Use Additional Character(s)   ▶ Manifestation Code   ⚙ Hierarchical Condition Category   Coding Clinic

● **M00**   Pyogenic arthritis
     Excludes2   infection and inflammatory reaction due to
              internal joint prosthesis (T84.5-)

● **M00.0**   Staphylococcal arthritis and polyarthritis
       Use additional code (B95.61-B95.8) to identify bacterial
         agent
     M00.00   Staphylococcal arthritis, unspecified joint 🦠
   ● **M00.01**   Staphylococcal arthritis, shoulder
       M00.011   Staphylococcal arthritis, right
             shoulder 🦠
       M00.012   Staphylococcal arthritis, left
             shoulder 🦠
       M00.019   Staphylococcal arthritis, unspecified
             shoulder 🦠
   ● **M00.02**   Staphylococcal arthritis, elbow
       M00.021   Staphylococcal arthritis, right
             elbow 🦠
       M00.022   Staphylococcal arthritis, left elbow 🦠
       M00.029   Staphylococcal arthritis, unspecified
             elbow 🦠
   ● **M00.03**   Staphylococcal arthritis, wrist
       Staphylococcal arthritis of carpal bones
       M00.031   Staphylococcal arthritis, right wrist 🦠
       M00.032   Staphylococcal arthritis, left wrist 🦠
       M00.039   Staphylococcal arthritis, unspecified
             wrist 🦠
   ● **M00.04**   Staphylococcal arthritis, hand
       Staphylococcal arthritis of metacarpus and
         phalanges
       M00.041   Staphylococcal arthritis, right hand 🦠
       M00.042   Staphylococcal arthritis, left hand 🦠
       M00.049   Staphylococcal arthritis, unspecified
             hand 🦠
   ● **M00.05**   Staphylococcal arthritis, hip
       M00.051   Staphylococcal arthritis, right hip 🦠
       M00.052   Staphylococcal arthritis, left hip 🦠
       M00.059   Staphylococcal arthritis, unspecified
             hip 🦠
   ● **M00.06**   Staphylococcal arthritis, knee
       M00.061   Staphylococcal arthritis, right knee 🦠
       M00.062   Staphylococcal arthritis, left knee 🦠
       M00.069   Staphylococcal arthritis, unspecified
             knee 🦠
   ● **M00.07**   Staphylococcal arthritis, ankle and foot
       Staphylococcal arthritis, tarsus, metatarsus and
         phalanges
       M00.071   Staphylococcal arthritis, right ankle
             and foot 🦠
       M00.072   Staphylococcal arthritis, left ankle
             and foot 🦠
       M00.079   Staphylococcal arthritis, unspecified
             ankle and foot 🦠
     M00.08   Staphylococcal arthritis, vertebrae 🦠
     M00.09   Staphylococcal polyarthritis 🦠
● **M00.1**   Pneumococcal arthritis and polyarthritis
     M00.10   Pneumococcal arthritis, unspecified joint 🦠
   ● **M00.11**   Pneumococcal arthritis, shoulder
       M00.111   Pneumococcal arthritis, right
             shoulder 🦠
       M00.112   Pneumococcal arthritis, left
             shoulder 🦠
       M00.119   Pneumococcal arthritis, unspecified
             shoulder 🦠

● **M00.12**   Pneumococcal arthritis, elbow
       M00.121   Pneumococcal arthritis, right
             elbow 🦠
       M00.122   Pneumococcal arthritis, left elbow 🦠
       M00.129   Pneumococcal arthritis, unspecified
             elbow 🦠
● **M00.13**   Pneumococcal arthritis, wrist
       Pneumococcal arthritis of carpal bones
       M00.131   Pneumococcal arthritis, right wrist 🦠
       M00.132   Pneumococcal arthritis, left wrist 🦠
       M00.139   Pneumococcal arthritis, unspecified
             wrist 🦠
● **M00.14**   Pneumococcal arthritis, hand
       Pneumococcal arthritis of metacarpus and
         phalanges
       M00.141   Pneumococcal arthritis, right hand 🦠
       M00.142   Pneumococcal arthritis, left hand 🦠
       M00.149   Pneumococcal arthritis, unspecified
             hand 🦠
● **M00.15**   Pneumococcal arthritis, hip
       M00.151   Pneumococcal arthritis, right hip 🦠
       M00.152   Pneumococcal arthritis, left hip 🦠
       M00.159   Pneumococcal arthritis, unspecified
             hip 🦠
● **M00.16**   Pneumococcal arthritis, knee
       M00.161   Pneumococcal arthritis, right knee 🦠
       M00.162   Pneumococcal arthritis, left knee 🦠
       M00.169   Pneumococcal arthritis, unspecified
             knee 🦠
● **M00.17**   Pneumococcal arthritis, ankle and foot
       Pneumococcal arthritis, tarsus, metatarsus and
         phalanges
       M00.171   Pneumococcal arthritis, right ankle
             and foot 🦠
       M00.172   Pneumococcal arthritis, left ankle and
             foot 🦠
       M00.179   Pneumococcal arthritis, unspecified
             ankle and foot 🦠
     M00.18   Pneumococcal arthritis, vertebrae 🦠
     M00.19   Pneumococcal polyarthritis 🦠
● **M00.2**   Other streptococcal arthritis and polyarthritis
       Use additional code (B95.0-B95.2, B95.4-B95.5) to
         identify bacterial agent
     M00.20   Other streptococcal arthritis, unspecified
            joint 🦠
   ● **M00.21**   Other streptococcal arthritis, shoulder
       M00.211   Other streptococcal arthritis, right
             shoulder 🦠
       M00.212   Other streptococcal arthritis, left
             shoulder 🦠
       M00.219   Other streptococcal arthritis,
             unspecified shoulder 🦠
   ● **M00.22**   Other streptococcal arthritis, elbow
       M00.221   Other streptococcal arthritis, right
             elbow 🦠
       M00.222   Other streptococcal arthritis, left
             elbow 🦠
       M00.229   Other streptococcal arthritis,
             unspecified elbow 🦠
   ● **M00.23**   Other streptococcal arthritis, wrist
       Other streptococcal arthritis of carpal bones
       M00.231   Other streptococcal arthritis, right
             wrist 🦠
       M00.232   Other streptococcal arthritis, left
             wrist 🦠
       M00.239   Other streptococcal arthritis,
             unspecified wrist 🦠

CHAPTER 13 (M00-M99)

- M00.24 **Other streptococcal arthritis, hand**
  Other streptococcal arthritis metacarpus and phalanges
  - M00.241 **Other streptococcal arthritis, right hand** 🦠
  - M00.242 **Other streptococcal arthritis, left hand** 🦠
  - M00.249 **Other streptococcal arthritis, unspecified hand** 🦠
- M00.25 **Other streptococcal arthritis, hip**
  - M00.251 **Other streptococcal arthritis, right hip** 🦠
  - M00.252 **Other streptococcal arthritis, left hip** 🦠
  - M00.259 **Other streptococcal arthritis, unspecified hip** 🦠
- M00.26 **Other streptococcal arthritis, knee**
  - M00.261 **Other streptococcal arthritis, right knee** 🦠
  - M00.262 **Other streptococcal arthritis, left knee** 🦠
  - M00.269 **Other streptococcal arthritis, unspecified knee** 🦠
- M00.27 **Other streptococcal arthritis, ankle and foot**
  Other streptococcal arthritis, tarsus, metatarsus and phalanges
  - M00.271 **Other streptococcal arthritis, right ankle and foot** 🦠
  - M00.272 **Other streptococcal arthritis, left ankle and foot** 🦠
  - M00.279 **Other streptococcal arthritis, unspecified ankle and foot** 🦠
  - M00.28 **Other streptococcal arthritis, vertebrae** 🦠
  - M00.29 **Other streptococcal polyarthritis** 🦠
- M00.8 **Arthritis and polyarthritis due to other bacteria**
  Use additional code (B96) to identify bacteria
  - M00.80 **Arthritis due to other bacteria, unspecified joint** 🦠
  - M00.81 **Arthritis due to other bacteria, shoulder**
    - M00.811 **Arthritis due to other bacteria, right shoulder** 🦠
    - M00.812 **Arthritis due to other bacteria, left shoulder** 🦠
    - M00.819 **Arthritis due to other bacteria, unspecified shoulder** 🦠
  - M00.82 **Arthritis due to other bacteria, elbow**
    - M00.821 **Arthritis due to other bacteria, right elbow** 🦠
    - M00.822 **Arthritis due to other bacteria, left elbow** 🦠
    - M00.829 **Arthritis due to other bacteria, unspecified elbow** 🦠
  - M00.83 **Arthritis due to other bacteria, wrist**
    Arthritis due to other bacteria, carpal bones
    - M00.831 **Arthritis due to other bacteria, right wrist** 🦠
    - M00.832 **Arthritis due to other bacteria, left wrist** 🦠
    - M00.839 **Arthritis due to other bacteria, unspecified wrist** 🦠
  - M00.84 **Arthritis due to other bacteria, hand**
    Arthritis due to other bacteria, metacarpus and phalanges
    - M00.841 **Arthritis due to other bacteria, right hand** 🦠
    - M00.842 **Arthritis due to other bacteria, left hand** 🦠
    - M00.849 **Arthritis due to other bacteria, unspecified hand** 🦠

- M00.85 **Arthritis due to other bacteria, hip**
  - M00.851 **Arthritis due to other bacteria, right hip** 🦠
  - M00.852 **Arthritis due to other bacteria, left hip** 🦠
  - M00.859 **Arthritis due to other bacteria, unspecified hip** 🦠
- M00.86 **Arthritis due to other bacteria, knee**
  - M00.861 **Arthritis due to other bacteria, right knee** 🦠
  - M00.862 **Arthritis due to other bacteria, left knee** 🦠
    Coding Clinic: 2019, Q3, P16
  - M00.869 **Arthritis due to other bacteria, unspecified knee** 🦠
- M00.87 **Arthritis due to other bacteria, ankle and foot**
  Arthritis due to other bacteria, tarsus, metatarsus, and phalanges
  - M00.871 **Arthritis due to other bacteria, right ankle and foot** 🦠
  - M00.872 **Arthritis due to other bacteria, left ankle and foot** 🦠
  - M00.879 **Arthritis due to other bacteria, unspecified ankle and foot** 🦠
  - M00.88 **Arthritis due to other bacteria, vertebrae** 🦠
  - M00.89 **Polyarthritis due to other bacteria** 🦠
- M00.9 **Pyogenic arthritis, unspecified** 🦠
  Infective arthritis NOS

- M01 **Direct infections of joint in infectious and parasitic diseases classified elsewhere**
  Code first underlying disease, such as:
  leprosy [Hansen's disease] (A30.-)
  mycoses (B35-B49)
  O'nyong-nyong fever (A92.1)
  paratyphoid fever (A01.1-A01.4)
  Excludes1 arthropathy in Lyme disease (A69.23)
  gonococcal arthritis (A54.42)
  meningococcal arthritis (A39.83)
  mumps arthritis (B26.85)
  postinfective arthropathy (M02.-)
  postmeningococcal arthritis (A39.84)
  reactive arthritis (M02.3)
  rubella arthritis (B06.82)
  sarcoidosis arthritis (D86.86)
  typhoid fever arthritis (A01.04)
  tuberculosis arthritis (A18.01-A18.02)
  - M01.X **Direct infection of joint in infectious and parasitic diseases classified elsewhere**
    - *M01.X0 Direct infection of unspecified joint in infectious and parasitic diseases classified elsewhere* 🦠
    - M01.X1 **Direct infection of shoulder joint in infectious and parasitic diseases classified elsewhere**
      - *M01.X11 Direct infection of right shoulder in infectious and parasitic diseases classified elsewhere* 🦠
      - *M01.X12 Direct infection of left shoulder in infectious and parasitic diseases classified elsewhere* 🦠
      - *M01.X19 Direct infection of unspecified shoulder in infectious and parasitic diseases classified elsewhere* 🦠
    - M01.X2 **Direct infection of elbow in infectious and parasitic diseases classified elsewhere**
      - *M01.X21 Direct infection of right elbow in infectious and parasitic diseases classified elsewhere* 🦠
      - *M01.X22 Direct infection of left elbow in infectious and parasitic diseases classified elsewhere* 🦠
      - *M01.X29 Direct infection of unspecified elbow in infectious and parasitic diseases classified elsewhere* 🦠

● **M01.X3**   Direct infection of wrist in infectious and parasitic diseases classified elsewhere
> Direct infection of carpal bones in infectious and parasitic diseases classified elsewhere

    ▸ *M01.X31*   *Direct infection of right wrist in infectious and parasitic diseases classified elsewhere* 🔄

    ▸ *M01.X32*   *Direct infection of left wrist in infectious and parasitic diseases classified elsewhere* 🔄

    ▸ *M01.X39*   *Direct infection of unspecified wrist in infectious and parasitic diseases classified elsewhere* 🔄

● **M01.X4**   Direct infection of hand in infectious and parasitic diseases classified elsewhere
> Direct infection of metacarpus and phalanges in infectious and parasitic diseases classified elsewhere

    ▸ *M01.X41*   *Direct infection of right hand in infectious and parasitic diseases classified elsewhere* 🔄

    ▸ *M01.X42*   *Direct infection of left hand in infectious and parasitic diseases classified elsewhere* 🔄

    ▸ *M01.X49*   *Direct infection of unspecified hand in infectious and parasitic diseases classified elsewhere* 🔄

● **M01.X5**   Direct infection of hip in infectious and parasitic diseases classified elsewhere

    ▸ *M01.X51*   *Direct infection of right hip in infectious and parasitic diseases classified elsewhere* 🔄

    ▸ *M01.X52*   *Direct infection of left hip in infectious and parasitic diseases classified elsewhere* 🔄

    ▸ *M01.X59*   *Direct infection of unspecified hip in infectious and parasitic diseases classified elsewhere* 🔄

● **M01.X6**   Direct infection of knee in infectious and parasitic diseases classified elsewhere

    ▸ *M01.X61*   *Direct infection of right knee in infectious and parasitic diseases classified elsewhere* 🔄

    ▸ *M01.X62*   *Direct infection of left knee in infectious and parasitic diseases classified elsewhere* 🔄

    ▸ *M01.X69*   *Direct infection of unspecified knee in infectious and parasitic diseases classified elsewhere* 🔄

● **M01.X7**   Direct infection of ankle and foot in infectious and parasitic diseases classified elsewhere
> Direct infection of tarsus, metatarsus and phalanges in infectious and parasitic diseases classified elsewhere

    ▸ *M01.X71*   *Direct infection of right ankle and foot in infectious and parasitic diseases classified elsewhere* 🔄

    ▸ *M01.X72*   *Direct infection of left ankle and foot in infectious and parasitic diseases classified elsewhere* 🔄

    ▸ *M01.X79*   *Direct infection of unspecified ankle and foot in infectious and parasitic diseases classified elsewhere* 🔄

▸ *M01.X8*   *Direct infection of vertebrae in infectious and parasitic diseases classified elsewhere* 🔄

▸ *M01.X9*   *Direct infection of multiple joints in infectious and parasitic diseases classified elsewhere* 🔄

● **M02**   Postinfective and reactive arthropathies
> *Code first* underlying disease, such as:
> congenital syphilis [Clutton's joints] (A50.5)
> enteritis due to Yersinia enterocolitica (A04.6)
> infective endocarditis (I33.0)
> viral hepatitis (B15-B19)

    Excludes1   Behçet's disease (M35.2)
                direct infections of joint in infectious and parasitic diseases classified elsewhere (M01.-)
                postmeningococcal arthritis (A39.84)
                mumps arthritis (B26.85)
                rubella arthritis (B06.82)
                syphilis arthritis (late) (A52.77)
                rheumatic fever (I00)
                tabetic arthropathy [Charcôt's] (A52.16)

● **M02.0**   Arthropathy following intestinal bypass

    M02.00   Arthropathy following intestinal bypass, unspecified site

    ● **M02.01**   Arthropathy following intestinal bypass, shoulder

       M02.011   Arthropathy following intestinal bypass, right shoulder

       M02.012   Arthropathy following intestinal bypass, left shoulder

       M02.019   Arthropathy following intestinal bypass, unspecified shoulder

    ● **M02.02**   Arthropathy following intestinal bypass, elbow

       M02.021   Arthropathy following intestinal bypass, right elbow

       M02.022   Arthropathy following intestinal bypass, left elbow

       M02.029   Arthropathy following intestinal bypass, unspecified elbow

    ● **M02.03**   Arthropathy following intestinal bypass, wrist
> Arthropathy following intestinal bypass, carpal bones

       M02.031   Arthropathy following intestinal bypass, right wrist

       M02.032   Arthropathy following intestinal bypass, left wrist

       M02.039   Arthropathy following intestinal bypass, unspecified wrist

    ● **M02.04**   Arthropathy following intestinal bypass, hand
> Arthropathy following intestinal bypass, metacarpals and phalanges

       M02.041   Arthropathy following intestinal bypass, right hand

       M02.042   Arthropathy following intestinal bypass, left hand

       M02.049   Arthropathy following intestinal bypass, unspecified hand

    ● **M02.05**   Arthropathy following intestinal bypass, hip

       M02.051   Arthropathy following intestinal bypass, right hip

       M02.052   Arthropathy following intestinal bypass, left hip

       M02.059   Arthropathy following intestinal bypass, unspecified hip

    ● **M02.06**   Arthropathy following intestinal bypass, knee

       M02.061   Arthropathy following intestinal bypass, right knee

       M02.062   Arthropathy following intestinal bypass, left knee

       M02.069   Arthropathy following intestinal bypass, unspecified knee

    ● **M02.07**   Arthropathy following intestinal bypass, ankle and foot
> Arthropathy following intestinal bypass, tarsus, metatarsus and phalanges

       M02.071   Arthropathy following intestinal bypass, right ankle and foot

M02.072 Arthropathy following intestinal bypass, left ankle and foot

M02.079 Arthropathy following intestinal bypass, unspecified ankle and foot

M02.08 Arthropathy following intestinal bypass, vertebrae

M02.09 Arthropathy following intestinal bypass, multiple sites

● M02.1 Postdysenteric arthropathy

M02.10 Postdysenteric arthropathy, unspecified site 🐾

● M02.11 Postdysenteric arthropathy, shoulder

M02.111 Postdysenteric arthropathy, right shoulder 🐾

M02.112 Postdysenteric arthropathy, left shoulder 🐾

M02.119 Postdysenteric arthropathy, unspecified shoulder 🐾

● M02.12 Postdysenteric arthropathy, elbow

M02.121 Postdysenteric arthropathy, right elbow 🐾

M02.122 Postdysenteric arthropathy, left elbow 🐾

M02.129 Postdysenteric arthropathy, unspecified elbow 🐾

● M02.13 Postdysenteric arthropathy, wrist
Postdysenteric arthropathy, carpal bones

M02.131 Postdysenteric arthropathy, right wrist 🐾

M02.132 Postdysenteric arthropathy, left wrist 🐾

M02.139 Postdysenteric arthropathy, unspecified wrist 🐾

● M02.14 Postdysenteric arthropathy, hand
Postdysenteric arthropathy, metacarpus and phalanges

M02.141 Postdysenteric arthropathy, right hand 🐾

M02.142 Postdysenteric arthropathy, left hand 🐾

M02.149 Postdysenteric arthropathy, unspecified hand 🐾

● M02.15 Postdysenteric arthropathy, hip

M02.151 Postdysenteric arthropathy, right hip 🐾

M02.152 Postdysenteric arthropathy, left hip 🐾

M02.159 Postdysenteric arthropathy, unspecified hip 🐾

● M02.16 Postdysenteric arthropathy, knee

M02.161 Postdysenteric arthropathy, right knee 🐾

M02.162 Postdysenteric arthropathy, left knee 🐾

M02.169 Postdysenteric arthropathy, unspecified knee 🐾

● M02.17 Postdysenteric arthropathy, ankle and foot
Postdysenteric arthropathy, tarsus, metatarsus and phalanges

M02.171 Postdysenteric arthropathy, right ankle and foot 🐾

M02.172 Postdysenteric arthropathy, left ankle and foot 🐾

M02.179 Postdysenteric arthropathy, unspecified ankle and foot 🐾

M02.18 Postdysenteric arthropathy, vertebrae 🐾

M02.19 Postdysenteric arthropathy, multiple sites 🐾

● M02.2 Postimmunization arthropathy

M02.20 Postimmunization arthropathy, unspecified site

● M02.21 Postimmunization arthropathy, shoulder

M02.211 Postimmunization arthropathy, right shoulder

M02.212 Postimmunization arthropathy, left shoulder

M02.219 Postimmunization arthropathy, unspecified shoulder

● M02.22 Postimmunization arthropathy, elbow

M02.221 Postimmunization arthropathy, right elbow

M02.222 Postimmunization arthropathy, left elbow

M02.229 Postimmunization arthropathy, unspecified elbow

● M02.23 Postimmunization arthropathy, wrist
Postimmunization arthropathy, carpal bones

M02.231 Postimmunization arthropathy, right wrist

M02.232 Postimmunization arthropathy, left wrist

M02.239 Postimmunization arthropathy, unspecified wrist

● M02.24 Postimmunization arthropathy, hand
Postimmunization arthropathy, metacarpus and phalanges

M02.241 Postimmunization arthropathy, right hand

M02.242 Postimmunization arthropathy, left hand

M02.249 Postimmunization arthropathy, unspecified hand

● M02.25 Postimmunization arthropathy, hip

M02.251 Postimmunization arthropathy, right hip

M02.252 Postimmunization arthropathy, left hip

M02.259 Postimmunization arthropathy, unspecified hip

● M02.26 Postimmunization arthropathy, knee

M02.261 Postimmunization arthropathy, right knee

M02.262 Postimmunization arthropathy, left knee

M02.269 Postimmunization arthropathy, unspecified knee

● M02.27 Postimmunization arthropathy, ankle and foot
Postimmunization arthropathy, tarsus, metatarsus and phalanges

M02.271 Postimmunization arthropathy, right ankle and foot

M02.272 Postimmunization arthropathy, left ankle and foot

M02.279 Postimmunization arthropathy, unspecified ankle and foot

M02.28 Postimmunization arthropathy, vertebrae

M02.29 Postimmunization arthropathy, multiple sites

● M02.3 Reiter's disease
Reactive arthritis

M02.30 Reiter's disease, unspecified site 🐾

● M02.31 Reiter's disease, shoulder

M02.311 Reiter's disease, right shoulder 🐾

M02.312 Reiter's disease, left shoulder 🐾

M02.319 Reiter's disease, unspecified shoulder 🐾

● M02.32 Reiter's disease, elbow

M02.321 Reiter's disease, right elbow 🐾

M02.322 Reiter's disease, left elbow 🐾

M02.329 Reiter's disease, unspecified elbow 🐾

● M02.33   Reiter's disease, wrist
      Reiter's disease, carpal bones
    M02.331   Reiter's disease, right wrist 🦿
    M02.332   Reiter's disease, left wrist 🦿
    M02.339   Reiter's disease, unspecified wrist 🦿
● M02.34   Reiter's disease, hand
      Reiter's disease, metacarpus and phalanges
    M02.341   Reiter's disease, right hand 🦿
    M02.342   Reiter's disease, left hand 🦿
    M02.349   Reiter's disease, unspecified hand 🦿
● M02.35   Reiter's disease, hip
    M02.351   Reiter's disease, right hip 🦿
    M02.352   Reiter's disease, left hip 🦿
    M02.359   Reiter's disease, unspecified hip 🦿
● M02.36   Reiter's disease, knee
    M02.361   Reiter's disease, right knee 🦿
    M02.362   Reiter's disease, left knee 🦿
    M02.369   Reiter's disease, unspecified knee 🦿
● M02.37   Reiter's disease, ankle and foot
      Reiter's disease, tarsus, metatarsus and
        phalanges
    M02.371   Reiter's disease, right ankle and
          foot 🦿
    M02.372   Reiter's disease, left ankle and foot 🦿
    M02.379   Reiter's disease, unspecified ankle
          and foot 🦿
  M02.38   Reiter's disease, vertebrae 🦿
  M02.39   Reiter's disease, multiple sites 🦿
● M02.8   Other reactive arthropathies
  ▸ *M02.80   Other reactive arthropathies, unspecified site* 🦿
  ● M02.81   Other reactive arthropathies, shoulder
    ▸ *M02.811   Other reactive arthropathies, right*
        shoulder 🦿
    ▸ *M02.812   Other reactive arthropathies, left*
        shoulder 🦿
    ▸ *M02.819   Other reactive arthropathies,*
        unspecified shoulder 🦿
  ● M02.82   Other reactive arthropathies, elbow
    ▸ *M02.821   Other reactive arthropathies, right*
        elbow 🦿
    ▸ *M02.822   Other reactive arthropathies, left*
        elbow 🦿
    ▸ *M02.829   Other reactive arthropathies,*
        unspecified elbow 🦿
  ● M02.83   Other reactive arthropathies, wrist
      Other reactive arthropathies, carpal bones
    ▸ *M02.831   Other reactive arthropathies, right*
        wrist 🦿
    ▸ *M02.832   Other reactive arthropathies, left*
        wrist 🦿
    ▸ *M02.839   Other reactive arthropathies,*
        unspecified wrist 🦿
  ● M02.84   Other reactive arthropathies, hand
      Other reactive arthropathies, metacarpus and
        phalanges
    ▸ *M02.841   Other reactive arthropathies, right*
        hand 🦿
    ▸ *M02.842   Other reactive arthropathies, left*
        hand 🦿
    ▸ *M02.849   Other reactive arthropathies,*
        unspecified hand 🦿
  ● M02.85   Other reactive arthropathies, hip
    ▸ *M02.851   Other reactive arthropathies, right*
        hip 🦿
    ▸ *M02.852   Other reactive arthropathies, left*
        hip 🦿
    ▸ *M02.859   Other reactive arthropathies,*
        unspecified hip 🦿

● M02.86   Other reactive arthropathies, knee
    ▸ *M02.861   Other reactive arthropathies, right*
        knee 🦿
    ▸ *M02.862   Other reactive arthropathies, left*
        knee 🦿
    ▸ *M02.869   Other reactive arthropathies,*
        unspecified knee 🦿
● M02.87   Other reactive arthropathies, ankle and foot
      Other reactive arthropathies, tarsus,
        metatarsus and phalanges
    ▸ *M02.871   Other reactive arthropathies, right*
        ankle and foot 🦿
    ▸ *M02.872   Other reactive arthropathies, left ankle*
        and foot 🦿
    ▸ *M02.879   Other reactive arthropathies,*
        unspecified ankle and foot 🦿
  ▸ *M02.88   Other reactive arthropathies, vertebrae* 🦿
  ▸ *M02.89   Other reactive arthropathies, multiple sites* 🦿
▸ *M02.9   Reactive arthropathy, unspecified* 🦿

AUTOINFLAMMATORY SYNDROMES (M04)

● M04   Autoinflammatory syndromes
   Excludes2   Crohn's disease (K50.-)
   Coding Clinic: 2016, Q4, P37
  M04.1   Periodic fever syndromes 🦿
      Familial Mediterranean fever
      Hyperimmunoglobin D syndrome
      Mevalonate kinase deficiency
      Tumor necrosis factor receptor associated periodic
        syndrome [TRAPS]
  M04.2   Cryopyrin-associated periodic syndromes 🦿
      Chronic infantile neurological, cutaneous and articular
        syndrome [CINCA]
      Familial cold autoinflammatory syndrome
      Familial cold urticaria
      Muckle-Wells syndrome
      Neonatal onset multisystemic inflammatory disorder
        [NOMID]
  M04.8   Other autoinflammatory syndromes 🦿
      Blau syndrome
      Deficiency of interleukin 1 receptor antagonist [DIRA]
      Majeed syndrome
      Periodic fever, aphthous stomatitis, pharyngitis, and
        adenopathy syndrome [PFAPA]
      Pyogenic arthritis, pyoderma gangrenosum, and acne
        syndrome [PAPA]
  M04.9   Autoinflammatory syndrome, unspecified 🦿

INFLAMMATORY POLYARTHROPATHIES (M05-M14)

● M05   Rheumatoid arthritis with rheumatoid factor
   Excludes1   rheumatic fever (I00)
               juvenile rheumatoid arthritis (M08.-)
               rheumatoid arthritis of spine (M45.-)
  ● M05.0   Felty's syndrome
      Rheumatoid arthritis with splenoadenomegaly and
        leukopenia
    M05.00   Felty's syndrome, unspecified site 🦿
  ● M05.01   Felty's syndrome, shoulder
      M05.011   Felty's syndrome, right shoulder 🦿
      M05.012   Felty's syndrome, left shoulder 🦿
      M05.019   Felty's syndrome, unspecified
          shoulder 🦿

Item 13-1   Rheumatoid arthritis (RA) is a chronic systemic inflammatory autoimmune disease of undetermined etiology involving primarily the synovial membranes and articular structures of multiple joints. It can also affect other organs, including the eyes, blood vessels, heart, and lungs. The disease is often progressive. In late stages, deformity, ankylosis, and other **inflammatory polyarthropathies** develop.

CHAPTER 13 (M00-M99)

● M05.02   Felty's syndrome, elbow
　　　M05.021   Felty's syndrome, right elbow 🐾
　　　M05.022   Felty's syndrome, left elbow 🐾
　　　M05.029   Felty's syndrome, unspecified elbow 🐾
● M05.03   Felty's syndrome, wrist
　　　　　Felty's syndrome, carpal bones
　　　M05.031   Felty's syndrome, right wrist 🐾
　　　M05.032   Felty's syndrome, left wrist 🐾
　　　M05.039   Felty's syndrome, unspecified wrist 🐾
● M05.04   Felty's syndrome, hand
　　　　　Felty's syndrome, metacarpus and phalanges
　　　M05.041   Felty's syndrome, right hand 🐾
　　　M05.042   Felty's syndrome, left hand 🐾
　　　M05.049   Felty's syndrome, unspecified hand 🐾
● M05.05   Felty's syndrome, hip
　　　M05.051   Felty's syndrome, right hip 🐾
　　　M05.052   Felty's syndrome, left hip 🐾
　　　M05.059   Felty's syndrome, unspecified hip 🐾
● M05.06   Felty's syndrome, knee
　　　M05.061   Felty's syndrome, right knee 🐾
　　　M05.062   Felty's syndrome, left knee 🐾
　　　M05.069   Felty's syndrome, unspecified knee 🐾
● M05.07   Felty's syndrome, ankle and foot
　　　　　Felty's syndrome, tarsus, metatarsus and
　　　　　　phalanges
　　　M05.071   Felty's syndrome, right ankle and
　　　　　　foot 🐾
　　　M05.072   Felty's syndrome, left ankle and foot 🐾
　　　M05.079   Felty's syndrome, unspecified ankle
　　　　　　and foot 🐾
　　　M05.09   Felty's syndrome, multiple sites 🐾
● M05.1   Rheumatoid lung disease with rheumatoid arthritis
　　　M05.10   Rheumatoid lung disease with rheumatoid
　　　　　arthritis of unspecified site 🐾
● M05.11   Rheumatoid lung disease with rheumatoid
　　　arthritis of shoulder
　　　M05.111   Rheumatoid lung disease with
　　　　　rheumatoid arthritis of right
　　　　　shoulder 🐾
　　　M05.112   Rheumatoid lung disease with
　　　　　rheumatoid arthritis of left shoulder 🐾
　　　M05.119   Rheumatoid lung disease with
　　　　　rheumatoid arthritis of unspecified
　　　　　shoulder 🐾
● M05.12   Rheumatoid lung disease with rheumatoid
　　　arthritis of elbow
　　　M05.121   Rheumatoid lung disease with
　　　　　rheumatoid arthritis of right elbow 🐾
　　　M05.122   Rheumatoid lung disease with
　　　　　rheumatoid arthritis of left elbow 🐾
　　　M05.129   Rheumatoid lung disease with
　　　　　rheumatoid arthritis of unspecified
　　　　　elbow 🐾
● M05.13   Rheumatoid lung disease with rheumatoid
　　　arthritis of wrist
　　　　　Rheumatoid lung disease with rheumatoid
　　　　　　arthritis, carpal bones
　　　M05.131   Rheumatoid lung disease with
　　　　　rheumatoid arthritis of right wrist 🐾
　　　M05.132   Rheumatoid lung disease with
　　　　　rheumatoid arthritis of left wrist 🐾
　　　M05.139   Rheumatoid lung disease with
　　　　　rheumatoid arthritis of unspecified
　　　　　wrist 🐾

● M05.14   Rheumatoid lung disease with rheumatoid
　　　arthritis of hand
　　　　　Rheumatoid lung disease with rheumatoid
　　　　　　arthritis, metacarpus and phalanges
　　　M05.141   Rheumatoid lung disease with
　　　　　rheumatoid arthritis of right hand 🐾
　　　M05.142   Rheumatoid lung disease with
　　　　　rheumatoid arthritis of left hand 🐾
　　　M05.149   Rheumatoid lung disease with
　　　　　rheumatoid arthritis of unspecified
　　　　　hand 🐾
● M05.15   Rheumatoid lung disease with rheumatoid
　　　arthritis of hip
　　　M05.151   Rheumatoid lung disease with
　　　　　rheumatoid arthritis of right hip 🐾
　　　M05.152   Rheumatoid lung disease with
　　　　　rheumatoid arthritis of left hip 🐾
　　　M05.159   Rheumatoid lung disease with
　　　　　rheumatoid arthritis of unspecified
　　　　　hip 🐾
● M05.16   Rheumatoid lung disease with rheumatoid
　　　arthritis of knee
　　　M05.161   Rheumatoid lung disease with
　　　　　rheumatoid arthritis of right knee 🐾
　　　M05.162   Rheumatoid lung disease with
　　　　　rheumatoid arthritis of left knee 🐾
　　　M05.169   Rheumatoid lung disease with
　　　　　rheumatoid arthritis of unspecified
　　　　　knee 🐾
● M05.17   Rheumatoid lung disease with rheumatoid
　　　arthritis of ankle and foot
　　　　　Rheumatoid lung disease with rheumatoid
　　　　　　arthritis, tarsus, metatarsus and phalanges
　　　M05.171   Rheumatoid lung disease with
　　　　　rheumatoid arthritis of right ankle
　　　　　and foot 🐾
　　　M05.172   Rheumatoid lung disease with
　　　　　rheumatoid arthritis of left ankle and
　　　　　foot 🐾
　　　M05.179   Rheumatoid lung disease with
　　　　　rheumatoid arthritis of unspecified
　　　　　ankle and foot 🐾
　　　M05.19   Rheumatoid lung disease with rheumatoid
　　　　　arthritis of multiple sites 🐾
● M05.2   Rheumatoid vasculitis with rheumatoid arthritis
　　　M05.20   Rheumatoid vasculitis with rheumatoid
　　　　　arthritis of unspecified site 🐾
● M05.21   Rheumatoid vasculitis with rheumatoid
　　　arthritis of shoulder
　　　M05.211   Rheumatoid vasculitis with
　　　　　rheumatoid arthritis of right
　　　　　shoulder 🐾
　　　M05.212   Rheumatoid vasculitis with
　　　　　rheumatoid arthritis of left
　　　　　shoulder 🐾
　　　M05.219   Rheumatoid vasculitis with
　　　　　rheumatoid arthritis of unspecified
　　　　　shoulder 🐾
● M05.22   Rheumatoid vasculitis with rheumatoid
　　　arthritis of elbow
　　　M05.221   Rheumatoid vasculitis with
　　　　　rheumatoid arthritis of right elbow 🐾
　　　M05.222   Rheumatoid vasculitis with
　　　　　rheumatoid arthritis of left elbow 🐾
　　　M05.229   Rheumatoid vasculitis with
　　　　　rheumatoid arthritis of unspecified
　　　　　elbow 🐾

● M05.23 Rheumatoid vasculitis with rheumatoid arthritis of wrist
    Rheumatoid vasculitis with rheumatoid arthritis, carpal bones

  M05.231 Rheumatoid vasculitis with rheumatoid arthritis of right wrist 🐾

  M05.232 Rheumatoid vasculitis with rheumatoid arthritis of left wrist 🐾

  M05.239 Rheumatoid vasculitis with rheumatoid arthritis of unspecified wrist 🐾

● M05.24 Rheumatoid vasculitis with rheumatoid arthritis of hand
    Rheumatoid vasculitis with rheumatoid arthritis, metacarpus and phalanges

  M05.241 Rheumatoid vasculitis with rheumatoid arthritis of right hand 🐾

  M05.242 Rheumatoid vasculitis with rheumatoid arthritis of left hand 🐾

  M05.249 Rheumatoid vasculitis with rheumatoid arthritis of unspecified hand 🐾

● M05.25 Rheumatoid vasculitis with rheumatoid arthritis of hip

  M05.251 Rheumatoid vasculitis with rheumatoid arthritis of right hip 🐾

  M05.252 Rheumatoid vasculitis with rheumatoid arthritis of left hip 🐾

  M05.259 Rheumatoid vasculitis with rheumatoid arthritis of unspecified hip 🐾

● M05.26 Rheumatoid vasculitis with rheumatoid arthritis of knee

  M05.261 Rheumatoid vasculitis with rheumatoid arthritis of right knee 🐾

  M05.262 Rheumatoid vasculitis with rheumatoid arthritis of left knee 🐾

  M05.269 Rheumatoid vasculitis with rheumatoid arthritis of unspecified knee 🐾

● M05.27 Rheumatoid vasculitis with rheumatoid arthritis of ankle and foot
    Rheumatoid vasculitis with rheumatoid arthritis, tarsus, metatarsus and phalanges

  M05.271 Rheumatoid vasculitis with rheumatoid arthritis of right ankle and foot 🐾

  M05.272 Rheumatoid vasculitis with rheumatoid arthritis of left ankle and foot 🐾

  M05.279 Rheumatoid vasculitis with rheumatoid arthritis of unspecified ankle and foot 🐾

  M05.29 Rheumatoid vasculitis with rheumatoid arthritis of multiple sites 🐾

● M05.3 Rheumatoid heart disease with rheumatoid arthritis
  Rheumatoid carditis
  Rheumatoid endocarditis
  Rheumatoid myocarditis
  Rheumatoid pericarditis

  M05.30 Rheumatoid heart disease with rheumatoid arthritis of unspecified site 🐾

● M05.31 Rheumatoid heart disease with rheumatoid arthritis of shoulder

  M05.311 Rheumatoid heart disease with rheumatoid arthritis of right shoulder 🐾

  M05.312 Rheumatoid heart disease with rheumatoid arthritis of left shoulder 🐾

  M05.319 Rheumatoid heart disease with rheumatoid arthritis of unspecified shoulder 🐾

● M05.32 Rheumatoid heart disease with rheumatoid arthritis of elbow

  M05.321 Rheumatoid heart disease with rheumatoid arthritis of right elbow 🐾

  M05.322 Rheumatoid heart disease with rheumatoid arthritis of left elbow 🐾

  M05.329 Rheumatoid heart disease with rheumatoid arthritis of unspecified elbow 🐾

● M05.33 Rheumatoid heart disease with rheumatoid arthritis of wrist
    Rheumatoid heart disease with rheumatoid arthritis, carpal bones

  M05.331 Rheumatoid heart disease with rheumatoid arthritis of right wrist 🐾

  M05.332 Rheumatoid heart disease with rheumatoid arthritis of left wrist 🐾

  M05.339 Rheumatoid heart disease with rheumatoid arthritis of unspecified wrist 🐾

● M05.34 Rheumatoid heart disease with rheumatoid arthritis of hand
    Rheumatoid heart disease with rheumatoid arthritis, metacarpus and phalanges

  M05.341 Rheumatoid heart disease with rheumatoid arthritis of right hand 🐾

  M05.342 Rheumatoid heart disease with rheumatoid arthritis of left hand 🐾

  M05.349 Rheumatoid heart disease with rheumatoid arthritis of unspecified hand 🐾

● M05.35 Rheumatoid heart disease with rheumatoid arthritis of hip

  M05.351 Rheumatoid heart disease with rheumatoid arthritis of right hip 🐾

  M05.352 Rheumatoid heart disease with rheumatoid arthritis of left hip 🐾

  M05.359 Rheumatoid heart disease with rheumatoid arthritis of unspecified hip 🐾

● M05.36 Rheumatoid heart disease with rheumatoid arthritis of knee

  M05.361 Rheumatoid heart disease with rheumatoid arthritis of right knee 🐾

  M05.362 Rheumatoid heart disease with rheumatoid arthritis of left knee 🐾

  M05.369 Rheumatoid heart disease with rheumatoid arthritis of unspecified knee 🐾

● M05.37 Rheumatoid heart disease with rheumatoid arthritis of ankle and foot
    Rheumatoid heart disease with rheumatoid arthritis, tarsus, metatarsus and phalanges

  M05.371 Rheumatoid heart disease with rheumatoid arthritis of right ankle and foot 🐾

  M05.372 Rheumatoid heart disease with rheumatoid arthritis of left ankle and foot 🐾

  M05.379 Rheumatoid heart disease with rheumatoid arthritis of unspecified ankle and foot 🐾

  M05.39 Rheumatoid heart disease with rheumatoid arthritis of multiple sites 🐾

● M05.4 Rheumatoid myopathy with rheumatoid arthritis

  M05.40 Rheumatoid myopathy with rheumatoid arthritis of unspecified site 🐾

● M05.41 Rheumatoid myopathy with rheumatoid arthritis of shoulder

  M05.411 Rheumatoid myopathy with rheumatoid arthritis of right shoulder 🐾

CHAPTER 13 (M00-M99)

M05.412   Rheumatoid myopathy with rheumatoid arthritis of left shoulder 🐾

M05.419   Rheumatoid myopathy with rheumatoid arthritis of unspecified shoulder 🐾

● M05.42   Rheumatoid myopathy with rheumatoid arthritis of elbow

M05.421   Rheumatoid myopathy with rheumatoid arthritis of right elbow 🐾

M05.422   Rheumatoid myopathy with rheumatoid arthritis of left elbow 🐾

M05.429   Rheumatoid myopathy with rheumatoid arthritis of unspecified elbow 🐾

● M05.43   Rheumatoid myopathy with rheumatoid arthritis of wrist
Rheumatoid myopathy with rheumatoid arthritis, carpal bones

M05.431   Rheumatoid myopathy with rheumatoid arthritis of right wrist 🐾

M05.432   Rheumatoid myopathy with rheumatoid arthritis of left wrist 🐾

M05.439   Rheumatoid myopathy with rheumatoid arthritis of unspecified wrist 🐾

● M05.44   Rheumatoid myopathy with rheumatoid arthritis of hand
Rheumatoid myopathy with rheumatoid arthritis, metacarpus and phalanges

M05.441   Rheumatoid myopathy with rheumatoid arthritis of right hand 🐾

M05.442   Rheumatoid myopathy with rheumatoid arthritis of left hand 🐾

M05.449   Rheumatoid myopathy with rheumatoid arthritis of unspecified hand 🐾

● M05.45   Rheumatoid myopathy with rheumatoid arthritis of hip

M05.451   Rheumatoid myopathy with rheumatoid arthritis of right hip 🐾

M05.452   Rheumatoid myopathy with rheumatoid arthritis of left hip 🐾

M05.459   Rheumatoid myopathy with rheumatoid arthritis of unspecified hip 🐾

● M05.46   Rheumatoid myopathy with rheumatoid arthritis of knee

M05.461   Rheumatoid myopathy with rheumatoid arthritis of right knee 🐾

M05.462   Rheumatoid myopathy with rheumatoid arthritis of left knee 🐾

M05.469   Rheumatoid myopathy with rheumatoid arthritis of unspecified knee 🐾

● M05.47   Rheumatoid myopathy with rheumatoid arthritis of ankle and foot
Rheumatoid myopathy with rheumatoid arthritis, tarsus, metatarsus and phalanges

M05.471   Rheumatoid myopathy with rheumatoid arthritis of right ankle and foot 🐾

M05.472   Rheumatoid myopathy with rheumatoid arthritis of left ankle and foot 🐾

M05.479   Rheumatoid myopathy with rheumatoid arthritis of unspecified ankle and foot 🐾

M05.49   Rheumatoid myopathy with rheumatoid arthritis of multiple sites 🐾

● M05.5   Rheumatoid polyneuropathy with rheumatoid arthritis

M05.50   Rheumatoid polyneuropathy with rheumatoid arthritis of unspecified site 🐾

● M05.51   Rheumatoid polyneuropathy with rheumatoid arthritis of shoulder

M05.511   Rheumatoid polyneuropathy with rheumatoid arthritis of right shoulder 🐾

M05.512   Rheumatoid polyneuropathy with rheumatoid arthritis of left shoulder 🐾

M05.519   Rheumatoid polyneuropathy with rheumatoid arthritis of unspecified shoulder 🐾

● M05.52   Rheumatoid polyneuropathy with rheumatoid arthritis of elbow

M05.521   Rheumatoid polyneuropathy with rheumatoid arthritis of right elbow 🐾

M05.522   Rheumatoid polyneuropathy with rheumatoid arthritis of left elbow 🐾

M05.529   Rheumatoid polyneuropathy with rheumatoid arthritis of unspecified elbow 🐾

● M05.53   Rheumatoid polyneuropathy with rheumatoid arthritis of wrist
Rheumatoid polyneuropathy with rheumatoid arthritis, carpal bones

M05.531   Rheumatoid polyneuropathy with rheumatoid arthritis of right wrist 🐾

M05.532   Rheumatoid polyneuropathy with rheumatoid arthritis of left wrist 🐾

M05.539   Rheumatoid polyneuropathy with rheumatoid arthritis of unspecified wrist 🐾

● M05.54   Rheumatoid polyneuropathy with rheumatoid arthritis of hand
Rheumatoid polyneuropathy with rheumatoid arthritis, metacarpus and phalanges

M05.541   Rheumatoid polyneuropathy with rheumatoid arthritis of right hand 🐾

M05.542   Rheumatoid polyneuropathy with rheumatoid arthritis of left hand 🐾

M05.549   Rheumatoid polyneuropathy with rheumatoid arthritis of unspecified hand 🐾

● M05.55   Rheumatoid polyneuropathy with rheumatoid arthritis of hip

M05.551   Rheumatoid polyneuropathy with rheumatoid arthritis of right hip 🐾

M05.552   Rheumatoid polyneuropathy with rheumatoid arthritis of left hip 🐾

M05.559   Rheumatoid polyneuropathy with rheumatoid arthritis of unspecified hip 🐾

● M05.56   Rheumatoid polyneuropathy with rheumatoid arthritis of knee

M05.561   Rheumatoid polyneuropathy with rheumatoid arthritis of right knee 🐾

M05.562   Rheumatoid polyneuropathy with rheumatoid arthritis of left knee 🐾

M05.569   Rheumatoid polyneuropathy with rheumatoid arthritis of unspecified knee 🐾

● M05.57   Rheumatoid polyneuropathy with rheumatoid arthritis of ankle and foot
Rheumatoid polyneuropathy with rheumatoid arthritis, tarsus, metatarsus and phalanges

M05.571   Rheumatoid polyneuropathy with rheumatoid arthritis of right ankle and foot

▶ New   ⇒ Revised   deleted Deleted   Excludes 1   Excludes 2   Includes   Use additional   Code first   Code also   Key words
OGCR Official Guidelines   X Assign placeholder X   ● Use Additional Character(s)   ▶ Manifestation Code   🐾 Hierarchical Condition Category   Coding Clinic

M05.572 Rheumatoid polyneuropathy with rheumatoid arthritis of left ankle and foot 🔄

M05.579 Rheumatoid polyneuropathy with rheumatoid arthritis of unspecified ankle and foot 🔄

M05.59 Rheumatoid polyneuropathy with rheumatoid arthritis of multiple sites 🔄

● M05.6 Rheumatoid arthritis with involvement of other organs and systems

M05.60 Rheumatoid arthritis of unspecified site with involvement of other organs and systems 🔄

● M05.61 Rheumatoid arthritis of shoulder with involvement of other organs and systems

M05.611 Rheumatoid arthritis of right shoulder with involvement of other organs and systems 🔄

M05.612 Rheumatoid arthritis of left shoulder with involvement of other organs and systems 🔄

M05.619 Rheumatoid arthritis of unspecified shoulder with involvement of other organs and systems 🔄

● M05.62 Rheumatoid arthritis of elbow with involvement of other organs and systems

M05.621 Rheumatoid arthritis of right elbow with involvement of other organs and systems 🔄

M05.622 Rheumatoid arthritis of left elbow with involvement of other organs and systems 🔄

M05.629 Rheumatoid arthritis of unspecified elbow with involvement of other organs and systems 🔄

● M05.63 Rheumatoid arthritis of wrist with involvement of other organs and systems
Rheumatoid arthritis of carpal bones with involvement of other organs and systems

M05.631 Rheumatoid arthritis of right wrist with involvement of other organs and systems 🔄

M05.632 Rheumatoid arthritis of left wrist with involvement of other organs and systems 🔄

M05.639 Rheumatoid arthritis of unspecified wrist with involvement of other organs and systems 🔄

● M05.64 Rheumatoid arthritis of hand with involvement of other organs and systems
Rheumatoid arthritis of metacarpus and phalanges with involvement of other organs and systems

M05.641 Rheumatoid arthritis of right hand with involvement of other organs and systems 🔄

M05.642 Rheumatoid arthritis of left hand with involvement of other organs and systems 🔄

M05.649 Rheumatoid arthritis of unspecified hand with involvement of other organs and systems 🔄

● M05.65 Rheumatoid arthritis of hip with involvement of other organs and systems

M05.651 Rheumatoid arthritis of right hip with involvement of other organs and systems 🔄

M05.652 Rheumatoid arthritis of left hip with involvement of other organs and systems 🔄

M05.659 Rheumatoid arthritis of unspecified hip with involvement of other organs and systems 🔄

● M05.66 Rheumatoid arthritis of knee with involvement of other organs and systems

M05.661 Rheumatoid arthritis of right knee with involvement of other organs and systems 🔄

M05.662 Rheumatoid arthritis of left knee with involvement of other organs and systems 🔄

M05.669 Rheumatoid arthritis of unspecified knee with involvement of other organs and systems 🔄

● M05.67 Rheumatoid arthritis of ankle and foot with involvement of other organs and systems
Rheumatoid arthritis of tarsus, metatarsus and phalanges with involvement of other organs and systems

M05.671 Rheumatoid arthritis of right ankle and foot with involvement of other organs and systems 🔄

M05.672 Rheumatoid arthritis of left ankle and foot with involvement of other organs and systems 🔄

M05.679 Rheumatoid arthritis of unspecified ankle and foot with involvement of other organs and systems 🔄

M05.69 Rheumatoid arthritis of multiple sites with involvement of other organs and systems 🔄

● M05.7 Rheumatoid arthritis with rheumatoid factor without organ or systems involvement

M05.70 Rheumatoid arthritis with rheumatoid factor of unspecified site without organ or systems involvement 🔄

● M05.71 Rheumatoid arthritis with rheumatoid factor of shoulder without organ or systems involvement

M05.711 Rheumatoid arthritis with rheumatoid factor of right shoulder without organ or systems involvement 🔄

M05.712 Rheumatoid arthritis with rheumatoid factor of left shoulder without organ or systems involvement 🔄

M05.719 Rheumatoid arthritis with rheumatoid factor of unspecified shoulder without organ or systems involvement 🔄

● M05.72 Rheumatoid arthritis with rheumatoid factor of elbow without organ or systems involvement

M05.721 Rheumatoid arthritis with rheumatoid factor of right elbow without organ or systems involvement 🔄

M05.722 Rheumatoid arthritis with rheumatoid factor of left elbow without organ or systems involvement 🔄

M05.729 Rheumatoid arthritis with rheumatoid factor of unspecified elbow without organ or systems involvement 🔄

● M05.73 Rheumatoid arthritis with rheumatoid factor of wrist without organ or systems involvement

M05.731 Rheumatoid arthritis with rheumatoid factor of right wrist without organ or systems involvement 🔄

M05.732 Rheumatoid arthritis with rheumatoid factor of left wrist without organ or systems involvement 🔄

M05.739 Rheumatoid arthritis with rheumatoid factor of unspecified wrist without organ or systems involvement 🔄

● M05.74 Rheumatoid arthritis with rheumatoid factor of hand without organ or systems involvement

    M05.741 Rheumatoid arthritis with rheumatoid factor of right hand without organ or systems involvement 🐾

    M05.742 Rheumatoid arthritis with rheumatoid factor of left hand without organ or systems involvement 🐾

    M05.749 Rheumatoid arthritis with rheumatoid factor of unspecified hand without organ or systems involvement 🐾

● M05.75 Rheumatoid arthritis with rheumatoid factor of hip without organ or systems involvement

    M05.751 Rheumatoid arthritis with rheumatoid factor of right hip without organ or systems involvement 🐾

    M05.752 Rheumatoid arthritis with rheumatoid factor of left hip without organ or systems involvement 🐾

    M05.759 Rheumatoid arthritis with rheumatoid factor of unspecified hip without organ or systems involvement 🐾

● M05.76 Rheumatoid arthritis with rheumatoid factor of knee without organ or systems involvement

    M05.761 Rheumatoid arthritis with rheumatoid factor of right knee without organ or systems involvement 🐾

    M05.762 Rheumatoid arthritis with rheumatoid factor of left knee without organ or systems involvement 🐾

    M05.769 Rheumatoid arthritis with rheumatoid factor of unspecified knee without organ or systems involvement 🐾

● M05.77 Rheumatoid arthritis with rheumatoid factor of ankle and foot without organ or systems involvement

    M05.771 Rheumatoid arthritis with rheumatoid factor of right ankle and foot without organ or systems involvement 🐾

    M05.772 Rheumatoid arthritis with rheumatoid factor of left ankle and foot without organ or systems involvement 🐾

    M05.779 Rheumatoid arthritis with rheumatoid factor of unspecified ankle and foot without organ or systems involvement 🐾

M05.79 Rheumatoid arthritis with rheumatoid factor of multiple sites without organ or systems involvement 🐾

M05.7A Rheumatoid arthritis with rheumatoid factor of other specified site without organ or systems involvement

● M05.8 Other rheumatoid arthritis with rheumatoid factor

    M05.80 Other rheumatoid arthritis with rheumatoid factor of unspecified site 🐾

● M05.81 Other rheumatoid arthritis with rheumatoid factor of shoulder

    M05.811 Other rheumatoid arthritis with rheumatoid factor of right shoulder 🐾

    M05.812 Other rheumatoid arthritis with rheumatoid factor of left shoulder 🐾

    M05.819 Other rheumatoid arthritis with rheumatoid factor of unspecified shoulder 🐾

● M05.82 Other rheumatoid arthritis with rheumatoid factor of elbow

    M05.821 Other rheumatoid arthritis with rheumatoid factor of right elbow 🐾

    M05.822 Other rheumatoid arthritis with rheumatoid factor of left elbow 🐾

    M05.829 Other rheumatoid arthritis with rheumatoid factor of unspecified elbow 🐾

● M05.83 Other rheumatoid arthritis with rheumatoid factor of wrist

    M05.831 Other rheumatoid arthritis with rheumatoid factor of right wrist 🐾

    M05.832 Other rheumatoid arthritis with rheumatoid factor of left wrist 🐾

    M05.839 Other rheumatoid arthritis with rheumatoid factor of unspecified wrist 🐾

● M05.84 Other rheumatoid arthritis with rheumatoid factor of hand

    M05.841 Other rheumatoid arthritis with rheumatoid factor of right hand 🐾

    M05.842 Other rheumatoid arthritis with rheumatoid factor of left hand 🐾

    M05.849 Other rheumatoid arthritis with rheumatoid factor of unspecified hand 🐾

● M05.85 Other rheumatoid arthritis with rheumatoid factor of hip

    M05.851 Other rheumatoid arthritis with rheumatoid factor of right hip 🐾

    M05.852 Other rheumatoid arthritis with rheumatoid factor of left hip 🐾

    M05.859 Other rheumatoid arthritis with rheumatoid factor of unspecified hip 🐾

● M05.86 Other rheumatoid arthritis with rheumatoid factor of knee

    M05.861 Other rheumatoid arthritis with rheumatoid factor of right knee 🐾

    M05.862 Other rheumatoid arthritis with rheumatoid factor of left knee 🐾

    M05.869 Other rheumatoid arthritis with rheumatoid factor of unspecified knee 🐾

● M05.87 Other rheumatoid arthritis with rheumatoid factor of ankle and foot

    M05.871 Other rheumatoid arthritis with rheumatoid factor of right ankle and foot 🐾

    M05.872 Other rheumatoid arthritis with rheumatoid factor of left ankle and foot 🐾

    M05.879 Other rheumatoid arthritis with rheumatoid factor of unspecified ankle and foot 🐾

M05.89 Other rheumatoid arthritis with rheumatoid factor of multiple sites 🐾

M05.8A Other rheumatoid arthritis with rheumatoid factor of other specified site

M05.9 Rheumatoid arthritis with rheumatoid factor, unspecified 🐾

● M06 Other rheumatoid arthritis
Coding Clinic: 2024, Q1, P17

  ● M06.0 Rheumatoid arthritis without rheumatoid factor

    M06.00 Rheumatoid arthritis without rheumatoid factor, unspecified site 🐾

  ● M06.01 Rheumatoid arthritis without rheumatoid factor, shoulder

    M06.011 Rheumatoid arthritis without rheumatoid factor, right shoulder 🐾

▶ New ⟹ Revised ~~deleted~~ Deleted Excludes 1 Excludes 2 Includes Use additional Code first Code also Key words

OGCR Official Guidelines X Assign placeholder X ● Use Additional Character(s) ▷ Manifestation Code 🐾 Hierarchical Condition Category Coding Clinic

M06.012   Rheumatoid arthritis without rheumatoid factor, left shoulder ✺

M06.019   Rheumatoid arthritis without rheumatoid factor, unspecified shoulder ✺

● M06.02   Rheumatoid arthritis without rheumatoid factor, elbow

    M06.021   Rheumatoid arthritis without rheumatoid factor, right elbow ✺

    M06.022   Rheumatoid arthritis without rheumatoid factor, left elbow ✺

    M06.029   Rheumatoid arthritis without rheumatoid factor, unspecified elbow ✺

● M06.03   Rheumatoid arthritis without rheumatoid factor, wrist

    M06.031   Rheumatoid arthritis without rheumatoid factor, right wrist ✺

    M06.032   Rheumatoid arthritis without rheumatoid factor, left wrist ✺

    M06.039   Rheumatoid arthritis without rheumatoid factor, unspecified wrist ✺

● M06.04   Rheumatoid arthritis without rheumatoid factor, hand

    M06.041   Rheumatoid arthritis without rheumatoid factor, right hand ✺

    M06.042   Rheumatoid arthritis without rheumatoid factor, left hand ✺

    M06.049   Rheumatoid arthritis without rheumatoid factor, unspecified hand ✺

● M06.05   Rheumatoid arthritis without rheumatoid factor, hip

    M06.051   Rheumatoid arthritis without rheumatoid factor, right hip ✺

    M06.052   Rheumatoid arthritis without rheumatoid factor, left hip ✺

    M06.059   Rheumatoid arthritis without rheumatoid factor, unspecified hip ✺

● M06.06   Rheumatoid arthritis without rheumatoid factor, knee

    M06.061   Rheumatoid arthritis without rheumatoid factor, right knee ✺

    M06.062   Rheumatoid arthritis without rheumatoid factor, left knee ✺

    M06.069   Rheumatoid arthritis without rheumatoid factor, unspecified knee ✺

● M06.07   Rheumatoid arthritis without rheumatoid factor, ankle and foot

    M06.071   Rheumatoid arthritis without rheumatoid factor, right ankle and foot ✺

    M06.072   Rheumatoid arthritis without rheumatoid factor, left ankle and foot ✺

    M06.079   Rheumatoid arthritis without rheumatoid factor, unspecified ankle and foot ✺

M06.08   Rheumatoid arthritis without rheumatoid factor, vertebrae ✺

M06.09   Rheumatoid arthritis without rheumatoid factor, multiple sites ✺

M06.0A   Rheumatoid arthritis without rheumatoid factor, other specified site

M06.1   **Adult-onset Still's disease** ✺   A

    Excludes1   Still's disease NOS (M08.2-)

● M06.2   **Rheumatoid bursitis**

    M06.20   Rheumatoid bursitis, unspecified site ✺

● M06.21   Rheumatoid bursitis, shoulder

    M06.211   Rheumatoid bursitis, right shoulder ✺

    M06.212   Rheumatoid bursitis, left shoulder ✺

    M06.219   Rheumatoid bursitis, unspecified shoulder ✺

● M06.22   Rheumatoid bursitis, elbow

    M06.221   Rheumatoid bursitis, right elbow ✺

    M06.222   Rheumatoid bursitis, left elbow ✺

    M06.229   Rheumatoid bursitis, unspecified elbow ✺

● M06.23   Rheumatoid bursitis, wrist

    M06.231   Rheumatoid bursitis, right wrist ✺

    M06.232   Rheumatoid bursitis, left wrist ✺

    M06.239   Rheumatoid bursitis, unspecified wrist ✺

● M06.24   Rheumatoid bursitis, hand

    M06.241   Rheumatoid bursitis, right hand ✺

    M06.242   Rheumatoid bursitis, left hand ✺

    M06.249   Rheumatoid bursitis, unspecified hand ✺

● M06.25   Rheumatoid bursitis, hip

    M06.251   Rheumatoid bursitis, right hip ✺

    M06.252   Rheumatoid bursitis, left hip ✺

    M06.259   Rheumatoid bursitis, unspecified hip ✺

● M06.26   Rheumatoid bursitis, knee

    M06.261   Rheumatoid bursitis, right knee ✺

    M06.262   Rheumatoid bursitis, left knee ✺

    M06.269   Rheumatoid bursitis, unspecified knee ✺

● M06.27   Rheumatoid bursitis, ankle and foot

    M06.271   Rheumatoid bursitis, right ankle and foot ✺

    M06.272   Rheumatoid bursitis, left ankle and foot ✺

    M06.279   Rheumatoid bursitis, unspecified ankle and foot ✺

    M06.28   Rheumatoid bursitis, vertebrae ✺

    M06.29   Rheumatoid bursitis, multiple sites ✺

● M06.3   **Rheumatoid nodule**

    M06.30   Rheumatoid nodule, unspecified site ✺

● M06.31   Rheumatoid nodule, shoulder

    M06.311   Rheumatoid nodule, right shoulder ✺

    M06.312   Rheumatoid nodule, left shoulder ✺

    M06.319   Rheumatoid nodule, unspecified shoulder ✺

● M06.32   Rheumatoid nodule, elbow

    M06.321   Rheumatoid nodule, right elbow ✺

    M06.322   Rheumatoid nodule, left elbow ✺

    M06.329   Rheumatoid nodule, unspecified elbow ✺

● M06.33   Rheumatoid nodule, wrist

    M06.331   Rheumatoid nodule, right wrist ✺

    M06.332   Rheumatoid nodule, left wrist ✺

    M06.339   Rheumatoid nodule, unspecified wrist ✺

● M06.34   Rheumatoid nodule, hand

    M06.341   Rheumatoid nodule, right hand ✺

    M06.342   Rheumatoid nodule, left hand ✺

    M06.349   Rheumatoid nodule, unspecified hand ✺

CHAPTER 13 (M00-M99)

● M06.35 Rheumatoid nodule, hip
    M06.351 Rheumatoid nodule, right hip 🦥
    M06.352 Rheumatoid nodule, left hip 🦥
    M06.359 Rheumatoid nodule, unspecified hip 🦥
● M06.36 Rheumatoid nodule, knee
    M06.361 Rheumatoid nodule, right knee 🦥
    M06.362 Rheumatoid nodule, left knee 🦥
    M06.369 Rheumatoid nodule, unspecified knee 🦥
● M06.37 Rheumatoid nodule, ankle and foot
    M06.371 Rheumatoid nodule, right ankle and foot 🦥
    M06.372 Rheumatoid nodule, left ankle and foot 🦥
    M06.379 Rheumatoid nodule, unspecified ankle and foot 🦥
M06.38 Rheumatoid nodule, vertebrae 🦥
M06.39 Rheumatoid nodule, multiple sites 🦥
M06.4 Inflammatory polyarthropathy 🦥
    Excludes1   polyarthritis NOS (M13.0)
    Coding Clinic: 2024, Q1, P17
● M06.8 Other specified rheumatoid arthritis
    M06.80 Other specified rheumatoid arthritis, unspecified site 🦥
● M06.81 Other specified rheumatoid arthritis, shoulder
    M06.811 Other specified rheumatoid arthritis, right shoulder 🦥
    M06.812 Other specified rheumatoid arthritis, left shoulder 🦥
    M06.819 Other specified rheumatoid arthritis, unspecified shoulder 🦥
● M06.82 Other specified rheumatoid arthritis, elbow
    M06.821 Other specified rheumatoid arthritis, right elbow 🦥
    M06.822 Other specified rheumatoid arthritis, left elbow 🦥
    M06.829 Other specified rheumatoid arthritis, unspecified elbow 🦥
● M06.83 Other specified rheumatoid arthritis, wrist
    M06.831 Other specified rheumatoid arthritis, right wrist 🦥
    M06.832 Other specified rheumatoid arthritis, left wrist 🦥
    M06.839 Other specified rheumatoid arthritis, unspecified wrist 🦥
● M06.84 Other specified rheumatoid arthritis, hand
    M06.841 Other specified rheumatoid arthritis, right hand 🦥
    M06.842 Other specified rheumatoid arthritis, left hand 🦥
    M06.849 Other specified rheumatoid arthritis, unspecified hand 🦥
● M06.85 Other specified rheumatoid arthritis, hip
    M06.851 Other specified rheumatoid arthritis, right hip 🦥
    M06.852 Other specified rheumatoid arthritis, left hip 🦥
    M06.859 Other specified rheumatoid arthritis, unspecified hip 🦥
● M06.86 Other specified rheumatoid arthritis, knee
    M06.861 Other specified rheumatoid arthritis, right knee 🦥
    M06.862 Other specified rheumatoid arthritis, left knee 🦥
    M06.869 Other specified rheumatoid arthritis, unspecified knee 🦥

● M06.87 Other specified rheumatoid arthritis, ankle and foot
    M06.871 Other specified rheumatoid arthritis, right ankle and foot 🦥
    M06.872 Other specified rheumatoid arthritis, left ankle and foot 🦥
    M06.879 Other specified rheumatoid arthritis, unspecified ankle and foot 🦥
M06.88 Other specified rheumatoid arthritis, vertebrae 🦥
M06.89 Other specified rheumatoid arthritis, multiple sites 🦥
M06.8A Other specified rheumatoid arthritis, other specified site
M06.9 Rheumatoid arthritis, unspecified 🦥
    Coding Clinic: 2024, Q1, P17
● M07 Enteropathic arthropathies
    Code also associated enteropathy, such as:
    regional enteritis [Crohn's disease] (K50.-)
    ulcerative colitis (K51.-)
    Excludes1   psoriatic arthropathies (L40.5-)
● M07.6 Enteropathic arthropathies
    M07.60 Enteropathic arthropathies, unspecified site
● M07.61 Enteropathic arthropathies, shoulder
    M07.611 Enteropathic arthropathies, right shoulder
    M07.612 Enteropathic arthropathies, left shoulder
    M07.619 Enteropathic arthropathies, unspecified shoulder
● M07.62 Enteropathic arthropathies, elbow
    M07.621 Enteropathic arthropathies, right elbow
    M07.622 Enteropathic arthropathies, left elbow
    M07.629 Enteropathic arthropathies, unspecified elbow
● M07.63 Enteropathic arthropathies, wrist
    M07.631 Enteropathic arthropathies, right wrist
    M07.632 Enteropathic arthropathies, left wrist
    M07.639 Enteropathic arthropathies, unspecified wrist
● M07.64 Enteropathic arthropathies, hand
    M07.641 Enteropathic arthropathies, right hand
    M07.642 Enteropathic arthropathies, left hand
    M07.649 Enteropathic arthropathies, unspecified hand
● M07.65 Enteropathic arthropathies, hip
    M07.651 Enteropathic arthropathies, right hip
    M07.652 Enteropathic arthropathies, left hip
    M07.659 Enteropathic arthropathies, unspecified hip
● M07.66 Enteropathic arthropathies, knee
    M07.661 Enteropathic arthropathies, right knee
    M07.662 Enteropathic arthropathies, left knee
    M07.669 Enteropathic arthropathies, unspecified knee
● M07.67 Enteropathic arthropathies, ankle and foot
    M07.671 Enteropathic arthropathies, right ankle and foot
    M07.672 Enteropathic arthropathies, left ankle and foot
    M07.679 Enteropathic arthropathies, unspecified ankle and foot
M07.68 Enteropathic arthropathies, vertebrae
M07.69 Enteropathic arthropathies, multiple sites

▶ New ⇒ Revised ~~deleted~~ Deleted Excludes 1 Excludes 2 Includes Use additional Code first Code also Key words
OGCR Official Guidelines X Assign placeholder X ● Use Additional Character(s) ▷ Manifestation Code 🦥 Hierarchical Condition Category Coding Clinic

● **M08   Juvenile arthritis**

> Code also any associated underlying condition, such as:
> regional enteritis [Crohn's disease] (K50.-)
> ulcerative colitis (K51.-)
>
> **Excludes1**   arthropathy in Whipple's disease (M14.8)
> Felty's syndrome (M05.0)
> juvenile dermatomyositis (M33.0-)
> psoriatic juvenile arthropathy (L40.54)

● **M08.0   Unspecified juvenile rheumatoid arthritis**

> Juvenile rheumatoid arthritis with or without rheumatoid factor

   M08.00   Unspecified juvenile rheumatoid arthritis of unspecified site 🔍

●   **M08.01**   Unspecified juvenile rheumatoid arthritis, shoulder

     M08.011   Unspecified juvenile rheumatoid arthritis, right shoulder 🔍

     M08.012   Unspecified juvenile rheumatoid arthritis, left shoulder 🔍

     M08.019   Unspecified juvenile rheumatoid arthritis, unspecified shoulder 🔍

●   **M08.02**   Unspecified juvenile rheumatoid arthritis of elbow

     M08.021   Unspecified juvenile rheumatoid arthritis, right elbow 🔍

     M08.022   Unspecified juvenile rheumatoid arthritis, left elbow 🔍

     M08.029   Unspecified juvenile rheumatoid arthritis, unspecified elbow 🔍

●   **M08.03**   Unspecified juvenile rheumatoid arthritis, wrist

     M08.031   Unspecified juvenile rheumatoid arthritis, right wrist 🔍

     M08.032   Unspecified juvenile rheumatoid arthritis, left wrist 🔍

     M08.039   Unspecified juvenile rheumatoid arthritis, unspecified wrist 🔍

●   **M08.04**   Unspecified juvenile rheumatoid arthritis, hand

     M08.041   Unspecified juvenile rheumatoid arthritis, right hand 🔍

     M08.042   Unspecified juvenile rheumatoid arthritis, left hand 🔍

     M08.049   Unspecified juvenile rheumatoid arthritis, unspecified hand 🔍

●   **M08.05**   Unspecified juvenile rheumatoid arthritis, hip

     M08.051   Unspecified juvenile rheumatoid arthritis, right hip 🔍

     M08.052   Unspecified juvenile rheumatoid arthritis, left hip 🔍

     M08.059   Unspecified juvenile rheumatoid arthritis, unspecified hip 🔍

●   **M08.06**   Unspecified juvenile rheumatoid arthritis, knee

     M08.061   Unspecified juvenile rheumatoid arthritis, right knee 🔍

     M08.062   Unspecified juvenile rheumatoid arthritis, left knee 🔍

     M08.069   Unspecified juvenile rheumatoid arthritis, unspecified knee 🔍

●   **M08.07**   Unspecified juvenile rheumatoid arthritis, ankle and foot

     M08.071   Unspecified juvenile rheumatoid arthritis, right ankle and foot 🔍

     M08.072   Unspecified juvenile rheumatoid arthritis, left ankle and foot 🔍

     M08.079   Unspecified juvenile rheumatoid arthritis, unspecified ankle and foot 🔍

   M08.08   Unspecified juvenile rheumatoid arthritis, vertebrae 🔍

   M08.09   Unspecified juvenile rheumatoid arthritis, multiple sites 🔍

   M08.0A   Unspecified juvenile rheumatoid arthritis, other specified site

● **M08.1   Juvenile ankylosing spondylitis** 🔍

> **Excludes1**   ankylosing spondylitis in adults (M45.0-)

● **M08.2   Juvenile rheumatoid arthritis with systemic onset**

> Still's disease NOS
>
> **Excludes1**   adult-onset Still's disease (M06.1-)

   M08.20   Juvenile rheumatoid arthritis with systemic onset, unspecified site 🔍

●   **M08.21**   Juvenile rheumatoid arthritis with systemic onset, shoulder

     M08.211   Juvenile rheumatoid arthritis with systemic onset, right shoulder 🔍

     M08.212   Juvenile rheumatoid arthritis with systemic onset, left shoulder 🔍

     M08.219   Juvenile rheumatoid arthritis with systemic onset, unspecified shoulder 🔍

●   **M08.22**   Juvenile rheumatoid arthritis with systemic onset, elbow

     M08.221   Juvenile rheumatoid arthritis with systemic onset, right elbow 🔍

     M08.222   Juvenile rheumatoid arthritis with systemic onset, left elbow 🔍

     M08.229   Juvenile rheumatoid arthritis with systemic onset, unspecified elbow 🔍

●   **M08.23**   Juvenile rheumatoid arthritis with systemic onset, wrist

     M08.231   Juvenile rheumatoid arthritis with systemic onset, right wrist 🔍

     M08.232   Juvenile rheumatoid arthritis with systemic onset, left wrist 🔍

     M08.239   Juvenile rheumatoid arthritis with systemic onset, unspecified wrist 🔍

●   **M08.24**   Juvenile rheumatoid arthritis with systemic onset, hand

     M08.241   Juvenile rheumatoid arthritis with systemic onset, right hand 🔍

     M08.242   Juvenile rheumatoid arthritis with systemic onset, left hand 🔍

     M08.249   Juvenile rheumatoid arthritis with systemic onset, unspecified hand 🔍

●   **M08.25**   Juvenile rheumatoid arthritis with systemic onset, hip

     M08.251   Juvenile rheumatoid arthritis with systemic onset, right hip 🔍

     M08.252   Juvenile rheumatoid arthritis with systemic onset, left hip 🔍

     M08.259   Juvenile rheumatoid arthritis with systemic onset, unspecified hip 🔍

●   **M08.26**   Juvenile rheumatoid arthritis with systemic onset, knee

     M08.261   Juvenile rheumatoid arthritis with systemic onset, right knee 🔍

     M08.262   Juvenile rheumatoid arthritis with systemic onset, left knee 🔍

     M08.269   Juvenile rheumatoid arthritis with systemic onset, unspecified knee 🔍

●   **M08.27**   Juvenile rheumatoid arthritis with systemic onset, ankle and foot

     M08.271   Juvenile rheumatoid arthritis with systemic onset, right ankle and foot 🔍

     M08.272   Juvenile rheumatoid arthritis with systemic onset, left ankle and foot 🔍

     M08.279   Juvenile rheumatoid arthritis with systemic onset, unspecified ankle and foot 🔍

CHAPTER 13 (M00-M99)

- **M08.28**   Juvenile rheumatoid arthritis with systemic onset, vertebrae 🐾
- **M08.29**   Juvenile rheumatoid arthritis with systemic onset, multiple sites 🐾
- **M08.2A**   Juvenile rheumatoid arthritis with systemic onset, other specified site
- **M08.3**   Juvenile rheumatoid polyarthritis (seronegative)
- ● **M08.4**   Pauciarticular juvenile rheumatoid arthritis
  - **M08.40**   Pauciarticular juvenile rheumatoid arthritis, unspecified site 🐾
  - ● **M08.41**   Pauciarticular juvenile rheumatoid arthritis, shoulder
    - **M08.411**   Pauciarticular juvenile rheumatoid arthritis, right shoulder 🐾
    - **M08.412**   Pauciarticular juvenile rheumatoid arthritis, left shoulder 🐾
    - **M08.419**   Pauciarticular juvenile rheumatoid arthritis, unspecified shoulder 🐾
  - ● **M08.42**   Pauciarticular juvenile rheumatoid arthritis, elbow
    - **M08.421**   Pauciarticular juvenile rheumatoid arthritis, right elbow 🐾
    - **M08.422**   Pauciarticular juvenile rheumatoid arthritis, left elbow 🐾
    - **M08.429**   Pauciarticular juvenile rheumatoid arthritis, unspecified elbow 🐾
  - ● **M08.43**   Pauciarticular juvenile rheumatoid arthritis, wrist
    - **M08.431**   Pauciarticular juvenile rheumatoid arthritis, right wrist 🐾
    - **M08.432**   Pauciarticular juvenile rheumatoid arthritis, left wrist 🐾
    - **M08.439**   Pauciarticular juvenile rheumatoid arthritis, unspecified wrist 🐾
  - ● **M08.44**   Pauciarticular juvenile rheumatoid arthritis, hand
    - **M08.441**   Pauciarticular juvenile rheumatoid arthritis, right hand 🐾
    - **M08.442**   Pauciarticular juvenile rheumatoid arthritis, left hand 🐾
    - **M08.449**   Pauciarticular juvenile rheumatoid arthritis, unspecified hand 🐾
  - ● **M08.45**   Pauciarticular juvenile rheumatoid arthritis, hip
    - **M08.451**   Pauciarticular juvenile rheumatoid arthritis, right hip 🐾
    - **M08.452**   Pauciarticular juvenile rheumatoid arthritis, left hip 🐾
    - **M08.459**   Pauciarticular juvenile rheumatoid arthritis, unspecified hip 🐾
  - ● **M08.46**   Pauciarticular juvenile rheumatoid arthritis, knee
    - **M08.461**   Pauciarticular juvenile rheumatoid arthritis, right knee 🐾
    - **M08.462**   Pauciarticular juvenile rheumatoid arthritis, left knee 🐾
    - **M08.469**   Pauciarticular juvenile rheumatoid arthritis, unspecified knee 🐾
  - ● **M08.47**   Pauciarticular juvenile rheumatoid arthritis, ankle and foot
    - **M08.471**   Pauciarticular juvenile rheumatoid arthritis, right ankle and foot 🐾
    - **M08.472**   Pauciarticular juvenile rheumatoid arthritis, left ankle and foot 🐾
    - **M08.479**   Pauciarticular juvenile rheumatoid arthritis, unspecified ankle and foot 🐾
  - **M08.48**   Pauciarticular juvenile rheumatoid arthritis, vertebrae 🐾
  - **M08.4A**   Pauciarticular juvenile rheumatoid arthritis, other specified site

- ● **M08.8**   Other juvenile arthritis
  - **M08.80**   Other juvenile arthritis, unspecified site 🐾
  - ● **M08.81**   Other juvenile arthritis, shoulder
    - **M08.811**   Other juvenile arthritis, right shoulder 🐾
    - **M08.812**   Other juvenile arthritis, left shoulder 🐾
    - **M08.819**   Other juvenile arthritis, unspecified shoulder 🐾
  - ● **M08.82**   Other juvenile arthritis, elbow
    - **M08.821**   Other juvenile arthritis, right elbow 🐾
    - **M08.822**   Other juvenile arthritis, left elbow 🐾
    - **M08.829**   Other juvenile arthritis, unspecified elbow 🐾
  - ● **M08.83**   Other juvenile arthritis, wrist
    - **M08.831**   Other juvenile arthritis, right wrist 🐾
    - **M08.832**   Other juvenile arthritis, left wrist 🐾
    - **M08.839**   Other juvenile arthritis, unspecified wrist 🐾
  - ● **M08.84**   Other juvenile arthritis, hand
    - **M08.841**   Other juvenile arthritis, right hand 🐾
    - **M08.842**   Other juvenile arthritis, left hand 🐾
    - **M08.849**   Other juvenile arthritis, unspecified hand 🐾
  - ● **M08.85**   Other juvenile arthritis, hip
    - **M08.851**   Other juvenile arthritis, right hip 🐾
    - **M08.852**   Other juvenile arthritis, left hip 🐾
    - **M08.859**   Other juvenile arthritis, unspecified hip 🐾
  - ● **M08.86**   Other juvenile arthritis, knee
    - **M08.861**   Other juvenile arthritis, right knee 🐾
    - **M08.862**   Other juvenile arthritis, left knee 🐾
    - **M08.869**   Other juvenile arthritis, unspecified knee 🐾
  - ● **M08.87**   Other juvenile arthritis, ankle and foot
    - **M08.871**   Other juvenile arthritis, right ankle and foot 🐾
    - **M08.872**   Other juvenile arthritis, left ankle and foot 🐾
    - **M08.879**   Other juvenile arthritis, unspecified ankle and foot 🐾
  - **M08.88**   Other juvenile arthritis, other specified site 🐾
    Other juvenile arthritis, vertebrae
  - **M08.89**   Other juvenile arthritis, multiple sites 🐾
- ● **M08.9**   Juvenile arthritis, unspecified

  Excludes1   juvenile rheumatoid arthritis, unspecified (M08.0-)

  - **M08.90**   Juvenile arthritis, unspecified, unspecified site 🐾
  - ● **M08.91**   Juvenile arthritis, unspecified, shoulder
    - **M08.911**   Juvenile arthritis, unspecified, right shoulder 🐾
    - **M08.912**   Juvenile arthritis, unspecified, left shoulder 🐾
    - **M08.919**   Juvenile arthritis, unspecified, unspecified shoulder 🐾
  - ● **M08.92**   Juvenile arthritis, unspecified, elbow
    - **M08.921**   Juvenile arthritis, unspecified, right elbow 🐾
    - **M08.922**   Juvenile arthritis, unspecified, left elbow 🐾
    - **M08.929**   Juvenile arthritis, unspecified, unspecified elbow 🐾

▶ New   ⇒ Revised   ~~deleted~~ Deleted   Excludes 1   Excludes 2   Includes   Use additional   Code first   Code also   Key words

OGCR Official Guidelines   X Assign placeholder X   ● Use Additional Character(s)   ▶ Manifestation Code   🐾 Hierarchical Condition Category   **Coding Clinic**

- M08.93 Juvenile arthritis, unspecified, wrist
  - M08.931 Juvenile arthritis, unspecified, right wrist 🔁
  - M08.932 Juvenile arthritis, unspecified, left wrist 🔁
  - M08.939 Juvenile arthritis, unspecified, unspecified wrist 🔁
- M08.94 Juvenile arthritis, unspecified, hand
  - M08.941 Juvenile arthritis, unspecified, right hand 🔁
  - M08.942 Juvenile arthritis, unspecified, left hand 🔁
  - M08.949 Juvenile arthritis, unspecified, unspecified hand 🔁
- M08.95 Juvenile arthritis, unspecified, hip
  - M08.951 Juvenile arthritis, unspecified, right hip 🔁
  - M08.952 Juvenile arthritis, unspecified, left hip 🔁
  - M08.959 Juvenile arthritis, unspecified, unspecified hip 🔁
- M08.96 Juvenile arthritis, unspecified, knee
  - M08.961 Juvenile arthritis, unspecified, right knee 🔁
  - M08.962 Juvenile arthritis, unspecified, left knee 🔁
  - M08.969 Juvenile arthritis, unspecified, unspecified knee 🔁
- M08.97 Juvenile arthritis, unspecified, ankle and foot
  - M08.971 Juvenile arthritis, unspecified, right ankle and foot 🔁
  - M08.972 Juvenile arthritis, unspecified, left ankle and foot 🔁
  - M08.979 Juvenile arthritis, unspecified, unspecified ankle and foot 🔁
  - M08.98 Juvenile arthritis, unspecified, vertebrae 🔁
  - M08.99 Juvenile arthritis, unspecified, multiple sites 🔁
  - M08.9A Juvenile arthritis, unspecified, other specified site

- **M1A Chronic gout**

  Use additional code to identify:
       Autonomic neuropathy in diseases classified elsewhere (G99.0)
       Calculus of urinary tract in diseases classified elsewhere (N22)
       Cardiomyopathy in diseases classified elsewhere (I43)
       Disorders of external ear in diseases classified elsewhere (H61.1-, H62.8-)
       Disorders of iris and ciliary body in diseases classified elsewhere (H22)
       Glomerular disorders in diseases classified elsewhere (N08)

  Excludes1   gout NOS (M10.-)

  Excludes2   acute gout (M10.-)

  The appropriate 7th character is to be added to each code from category M1A

0	without tophus (tophi)
1	with tophus (tophi)

  - **M1A.0 Idiopathic chronic gout**
    Chronic gouty bursitis
    Primary chronic gout
    - X● M1A.00 Idiopathic chronic gout, unspecified site
    - M1A.01 Idiopathic chronic gout, shoulder
      - M1A.011 Idiopathic chronic gout, right shoulder
      - M1A.012 Idiopathic chronic gout, left shoulder
      - M1A.019 Idiopathic chronic gout, unspecified shoulder

  - M1A.02 Idiopathic chronic gout, elbow
    - M1A.021 Idiopathic chronic gout, right elbow
    - M1A.022 Idiopathic chronic gout, left elbow
    - M1A.029 Idiopathic chronic gout, unspecified elbow
  - M1A.03 Idiopathic chronic gout, wrist
    - M1A.031 Idiopathic chronic gout, right wrist
    - M1A.032 Idiopathic chronic gout, left wrist
    - M1A.039 Idiopathic chronic gout, unspecified wrist
  - M1A.04 Idiopathic chronic gout, hand
    - M1A.041 Idiopathic chronic gout, right hand
    - M1A.042 Idiopathic chronic gout, left hand
    - M1A.049 Idiopathic chronic gout, unspecified hand
  - M1A.05 Idiopathic chronic gout, hip
    - M1A.051 Idiopathic chronic gout, right hip
    - M1A.052 Idiopathic chronic gout, left hip
    - M1A.059 Idiopathic chronic gout, unspecified hip
  - M1A.06 Idiopathic chronic gout, knee
    - M1A.061 Idiopathic chronic gout, right knee
    - M1A.062 Idiopathic chronic gout, left knee
    - M1A.069 Idiopathic chronic gout, unspecified knee
  - M1A.07 Idiopathic chronic gout, ankle and foot
    - M1A.071 Idiopathic chronic gout, right ankle and foot
    - M1A.072 Idiopathic chronic gout, left ankle and foot
    - M1A.079 Idiopathic chronic gout, unspecified ankle and foot
  - X● M1A.08 Idiopathic chronic gout, vertebrae
  - X● M1A.09 Idiopathic chronic gout, multiple sites
- **M1A.1 Lead-induced chronic gout**
    Code first toxic effects of lead and its compounds (T56.0-)
    - X● M1A.10 Lead-induced chronic gout, unspecified site
    - M1A.11 Lead-induced chronic gout, shoulder
      - M1A.111 Lead-induced chronic gout, right shoulder
      - M1A.112 Lead-induced chronic gout, left shoulder
      - M1A.119 Lead-induced chronic gout, unspecified shoulder
    - M1A.12 Lead-induced chronic gout, elbow
      - M1A.121 Lead-induced chronic gout, right elbow
      - M1A.122 Lead-induced chronic gout, left elbow
      - M1A.129 Lead-induced chronic gout, unspecified elbow
    - M1A.13 Lead-induced chronic gout, wrist
      - M1A.131 Lead-induced chronic gout, right wrist
      - M1A.132 Lead-induced chronic gout, left wrist
      - M1A.139 Lead-induced chronic gout, unspecified wrist
    - M1A.14 Lead-induced chronic gout, hand
      - M1A.141 Lead-induced chronic gout, right hand
      - M1A.142 Lead-induced chronic gout, left hand
      - M1A.149 Lead-induced chronic gout, unspecified hand
    - M1A.15 Lead-induced chronic gout, hip
      - M1A.151 Lead-induced chronic gout, right hip
      - M1A.152 Lead-induced chronic gout, left hip
      - M1A.159 Lead-induced chronic gout, unspecified hip

CHAPTER 13 (M00-M99)

- ● M1A.16 Lead-induced chronic gout, knee
  - ● M1A.161 Lead-induced chronic gout, right knee
  - ● M1A.162 Lead-induced chronic gout, left knee
  - ● M1A.169 Lead-induced chronic gout, unspecified knee
- ● M1A.17 Lead-induced chronic gout, ankle and foot
  - ● M1A.171 Lead-induced chronic gout, right ankle and foot
  - ● M1A.172 Lead-induced chronic gout, left ankle and foot
  - ● M1A.179 Lead-induced chronic gout, unspecified ankle and foot
- X ● M1A.18 Lead-induced chronic gout, vertebrae
- X ● M1A.19 Lead-induced chronic gout, multiple sites
- ● M1A.2 Drug-induced chronic gout

  Use additional code for adverse effect, if applicable, to identify drug (T36-T50 with fifth or sixth character 5)

- X ● M1A.20 Drug-induced chronic gout, unspecified site
- ● M1A.21 Drug-induced chronic gout, shoulder
  - ● M1A.211 Drug-induced chronic gout, right shoulder
  - ● M1A.212 Drug-induced chronic gout, left shoulder
  - ● M1A.219 Drug-induced chronic gout, unspecified shoulder
- ● M1A.22 Drug-induced chronic gout, elbow
  - ● M1A.221 Drug-induced chronic gout, right elbow
  - ● M1A.222 Drug-induced chronic gout, left elbow
  - ● M1A.229 Drug-induced chronic gout, unspecified elbow
- ● M1A.23 Drug-induced chronic gout, wrist
  - ● M1A.231 Drug-induced chronic gout, right wrist
  - ● M1A.232 Drug-induced chronic gout, left wrist
  - ● M1A.239 Drug-induced chronic gout, unspecified wrist
- ● M1A.24 Drug-induced chronic gout, hand
  - ● M1A.241 Drug-induced chronic gout, right hand
  - ● M1A.242 Drug-induced chronic gout, left hand
  - ● M1A.249 Drug-induced chronic gout, unspecified hand
- ● M1A.25 Drug-induced chronic gout, hip
  - ● M1A.251 Drug-induced chronic gout, right hip
  - ● M1A.252 Drug-induced chronic gout, left hip
  - ● M1A.259 Drug-induced chronic gout, unspecified hip
- ● M1A.26 Drug-induced chronic gout, knee
  - ● M1A.261 Drug-induced chronic gout, right knee
  - ● M1A.262 Drug-induced chronic gout, left knee
  - ● M1A.269 Drug-induced chronic gout, unspecified knee
- ● M1A.27 Drug-induced chronic gout, ankle and foot
  - ● M1A.271 Drug-induced chronic gout, right ankle and foot
  - ● M1A.272 Drug-induced chronic gout, left ankle and foot
  - ● M1A.279 Drug-induced chronic gout, unspecified ankle and foot
- X ● M1A.28 Drug-induced chronic gout, vertebrae
- X ● M1A.29 Drug-induced chronic gout, multiple sites

- ● M1A.3 Chronic gout due to renal impairment

  Code first associated renal disease

- X ● M1A.30 Chronic gout due to renal impairment, unspecified site
- ● M1A.31 Chronic gout due to renal impairment, shoulder
  - ● M1A.311 Chronic gout due to renal impairment, right shoulder
  - ● M1A.312 Chronic gout due to renal impairment, left shoulder
  - ● M1A.319 Chronic gout due to renal impairment, unspecified shoulder
- ● M1A.32 Chronic gout due to renal impairment, elbow
  - ● M1A.321 Chronic gout due to renal impairment, right elbow
  - ● M1A.322 Chronic gout due to renal impairment, left elbow
  - ● M1A.329 Chronic gout due to renal impairment, unspecified elbow
- ● M1A.33 Chronic gout due to renal impairment, wrist
  - ● M1A.331 Chronic gout due to renal impairment, right wrist
  - ● M1A.332 Chronic gout due to renal impairment, left wrist
  - ● M1A.339 Chronic gout due to renal impairment, unspecified wrist
- ● M1A.34 Chronic gout due to renal impairment, hand
  - ● M1A.341 Chronic gout due to renal impairment, right hand
  - ● M1A.342 Chronic gout due to renal impairment, left hand
  - ● M1A.349 Chronic gout due to renal impairment, unspecified hand
- ● M1A.35 Chronic gout due to renal impairment, hip
  - ● M1A.351 Chronic gout due to renal impairment, right hip
  - ● M1A.352 Chronic gout due to renal impairment, left hip
  - ● M1A.359 Chronic gout due to renal impairment, unspecified hip
- ● M1A.36 Chronic gout due to renal impairment, knee
  - ● M1A.361 Chronic gout due to renal impairment, right knee
  - ● M1A.362 Chronic gout due to renal impairment, left knee
  - ● M1A.369 Chronic gout due to renal impairment, unspecified knee
- ● M1A.37 Chronic gout due to renal impairment, ankle and foot
  - ● M1A.371 Chronic gout due to renal impairment, right ankle and foot
  - ● M1A.372 Chronic gout due to renal impairment, left ankle and foot
  - ● M1A.379 Chronic gout due to renal impairment, unspecified ankle and foot
- X ● M1A.38 Chronic gout due to renal impairment, vertebrae
- X ● M1A.39 Chronic gout due to renal impairment, multiple sites
- ● M1A.4 Other secondary chronic gout

  Code first associated condition

- X ● M1A.40 Other secondary chronic gout, unspecified site
- ● M1A.41 Other secondary chronic gout, shoulder
  - ● M1A.411 Other secondary chronic gout, right shoulder
  - ● M1A.412 Other secondary chronic gout, left shoulder
  - ● M1A.419 Other secondary chronic gout, unspecified shoulder

▶ New   ⇨ Revised   ~~deleted~~ Deleted   Excludes 1   Excludes 2   Includes   Use additional   Code first   Code also   Key words

OGCR Official Guidelines   X Assign placeholder X   ● Use Additional Character(s)   ▶ Manifestation Code   🔗 Hierarchical Condition Category   Coding Clinic

- M1A.42 Other secondary chronic gout, elbow
  - M1A.421 Other secondary chronic gout, right elbow
  - M1A.422 Other secondary chronic gout, left elbow
  - M1A.429 Other secondary chronic gout, unspecified elbow
- M1A.43 Other secondary chronic gout, wrist
  - M1A.431 Other secondary chronic gout, right wrist
  - M1A.432 Other secondary chronic gout, left wrist
  - M1A.439 Other secondary chronic gout, unspecified wrist
- M1A.44 Other secondary chronic gout, hand
  - M1A.441 Other secondary chronic gout, right hand
  - M1A.442 Other secondary chronic gout, left hand
  - M1A.449 Other secondary chronic gout, unspecified hand
- M1A.45 Other secondary chronic gout, hip
  - M1A.451 Other secondary chronic gout, right hip
  - M1A.452 Other secondary chronic gout, left hip
  - M1A.459 Other secondary chronic gout, unspecified hip
- M1A.46 Other secondary chronic gout, knee
  - M1A.461 Other secondary chronic gout, right knee
  - M1A.462 Other secondary chronic gout, left knee
  - M1A.469 Other secondary chronic gout, unspecified knee
- M1A.47 Other secondary chronic gout, ankle and foot
  - M1A.471 Other secondary chronic gout, right ankle and foot
  - M1A.472 Other secondary chronic gout, left ankle and foot
  - M1A.479 Other secondary chronic gout, unspecified ankle and foot
- X ● M1A.48 Other secondary chronic gout, vertebrae
- X ● M1A.49 Other secondary chronic gout, multiple sites
- X ● M1A.9 Chronic gout, unspecified

- M10   **Gout**

  Accumulation of uric acid that results in swollen, red, hot, painful, stiff joints

  Acute gout
  Gout attack
  Gout flare
  Podagra

  Use additional code to identify:
      Autonomic neuropathy in diseases classified elsewhere (G99.0)
      Calculus of urinary tract in diseases classified elsewhere (N22)
      Cardiomyopathy in diseases classified elsewhere (I43)
      Disorders of external ear in diseases classified elsewhere (H61.1-, H62.8-)
      Disorders of iris and ciliary body in diseases classified elsewhere (H22)
      Glomerular disorders in diseases classified elsewhere (N08)

  Excludes2   chronic gout (M1A.-)

  - M10.0   **Idiopathic gout**
    Gouty bursitis
    Primary gout
    - M10.00 Idiopathic gout, unspecified site
    - M10.01 Idiopathic gout, shoulder
      - M10.011 Idiopathic gout, right shoulder
      - M10.012 Idiopathic gout, left shoulder
      - M10.019 Idiopathic gout, unspecified shoulder

- M10.02 Idiopathic gout, elbow
  - M10.021 Idiopathic gout, right elbow
  - M10.022 Idiopathic gout, left elbow
  - M10.029 Idiopathic gout, unspecified elbow
- M10.03 Idiopathic gout, wrist
  - M10.031 Idiopathic gout, right wrist
  - M10.032 Idiopathic gout, left wrist
  - M10.039 Idiopathic gout, unspecified wrist
- M10.04 Idiopathic gout, hand
  - M10.041 Idiopathic gout, right hand
  - M10.042 Idiopathic gout, left hand
  - M10.049 Idiopathic gout, unspecified hand
- M10.05 Idiopathic gout, hip
  - M10.051 Idiopathic gout, right hip
  - M10.052 Idiopathic gout, left hip
  - M10.059 Idiopathic gout, unspecified hip
- M10.06 Idiopathic gout, knee
  - M10.061 Idiopathic gout, right knee
  - M10.062 Idiopathic gout, left knee
  - M10.069 Idiopathic gout, unspecified knee
- M10.07 Idiopathic gout, ankle and foot
  - M10.071 Idiopathic gout, right ankle and foot
  - M10.072 Idiopathic gout, left ankle and foot
  - M10.079 Idiopathic gout, unspecified ankle and foot
- M10.08 Idiopathic gout, vertebrae
- M10.09 Idiopathic gout, multiple sites
- M10.1   **Lead-induced gout**

  Code first toxic effects of lead and its compounds (T56.0-)
  - M10.10 Lead-induced gout, unspecified site
  - M10.11 Lead-induced gout, shoulder
    - M10.111 Lead-induced gout, right shoulder
    - M10.112 Lead-induced gout, left shoulder
    - M10.119 Lead-induced gout, unspecified shoulder
  - M10.12 Lead-induced gout, elbow
    - M10.121 Lead-induced gout, right elbow
    - M10.122 Lead-induced gout, left elbow
    - M10.129 Lead-induced gout, unspecified elbow
  - M10.13 Lead-induced gout, wrist
    - M10.131 Lead-induced gout, right wrist
    - M10.132 Lead-induced gout, left wrist
    - M10.139 Lead-induced gout, unspecified wrist
  - M10.14 Lead-induced gout, hand
    - M10.141 Lead-induced gout, right hand
    - M10.142 Lead-induced gout, left hand
    - M10.149 Lead-induced gout, unspecified hand
  - M10.15 Lead-induced gout, hip
    - M10.151 Lead-induced gout, right hip
    - M10.152 Lead-induced gout, left hip
    - M10.159 Lead-induced gout, unspecified hip
  - M10.16 Lead-induced gout, knee
    - M10.161 Lead-induced gout, right knee
    - M10.162 Lead-induced gout, left knee
    - M10.169 Lead-induced gout, unspecified knee
  - M10.17 Lead-induced gout, ankle and foot
    - M10.171 Lead-induced gout, right ankle and foot
    - M10.172 Lead-induced gout, left ankle and foot
    - M10.179 Lead-induced gout, unspecified ankle and foot
  - M10.18 Lead-induced gout, vertebrae
  - M10.19 Lead-induced gout, multiple sites

CHAPTER 13 (M00-M99)

● **M10.2 Drug-induced gout**
   Use additional code for adverse effect, if applicable, to identify drug (T36-T50 with fifth or sixth character 5)
   M10.20 Drug-induced gout, unspecified site
● **M10.21** Drug-induced gout, shoulder
   M10.211 Drug-induced gout, right shoulder
   M10.212 Drug-induced gout, left shoulder
   M10.219 Drug-induced gout, unspecified shoulder
● **M10.22** Drug-induced gout, elbow
   M10.221 Drug-induced gout, right elbow
   M10.222 Drug-induced gout, left elbow
   M10.229 Drug-induced gout, unspecified elbow
● **M10.23** Drug-induced gout, wrist
   M10.231 Drug-induced gout, right wrist
   M10.232 Drug-induced gout, left wrist
   M10.239 Drug-induced gout, unspecified wrist
● **M10.24** Drug-induced gout, hand
   M10.241 Drug-induced gout, right hand
   M10.242 Drug-induced gout, left hand
   M10.249 Drug-induced gout, unspecified hand
● **M10.25** Drug-induced gout, hip
   M10.251 Drug-induced gout, right hip
   M10.252 Drug-induced gout, left hip
   M10.259 Drug-induced gout, unspecified hip
● **M10.26** Drug-induced gout, knee
   M10.261 Drug-induced gout, right knee
   M10.262 Drug-induced gout, left knee
   M10.269 Drug-induced gout, unspecified knee
● **M10.27** Drug-induced gout, ankle and foot
   M10.271 Drug-induced gout, right ankle and foot
   M10.272 Drug-induced gout, left ankle and foot
   M10.279 Drug-induced gout, unspecified ankle and foot
   M10.28 Drug-induced gout, vertebrae
   M10.29 Drug-induced gout, multiple sites
● **M10.3 Gout due to renal impairment**
   Code also associated renal disease
   M10.30 Gout due to renal impairment, unspecified site
● **M10.31** Gout due to renal impairment, shoulder
   M10.311 Gout due to renal impairment, right shoulder
   M10.312 Gout due to renal impairment, left shoulder
   M10.319 Gout due to renal impairment, unspecified shoulder
● **M10.32** Gout due to renal impairment, elbow
   M10.321 Gout due to renal impairment, right elbow
   M10.322 Gout due to renal impairment, left elbow
   M10.329 Gout due to renal impairment, unspecified elbow
● **M10.33** Gout due to renal impairment, wrist
   M10.331 Gout due to renal impairment, right wrist
   M10.332 Gout due to renal impairment, left wrist
   M10.339 Gout due to renal impairment, unspecified wrist

● **M10.34** Gout due to renal impairment, hand
   M10.341 Gout due to renal impairment, right hand
   M10.342 Gout due to renal impairment, left hand
   M10.349 Gout due to renal impairment, unspecified hand
● **M10.35** Gout due to renal impairment, hip
   M10.351 Gout due to renal impairment, right hip
   M10.352 Gout due to renal impairment, left hip
   M10.359 Gout due to renal impairment, unspecified hip
● **M10.36** Gout due to renal impairment, knee
   M10.361 Gout due to renal impairment, right knee
   M10.362 Gout due to renal impairment, left knee
   M10.369 Gout due to renal impairment, unspecified knee
● **M10.37** Gout due to renal impairment, ankle and foot
   M10.371 Gout due to renal impairment, right ankle and foot
   M10.372 Gout due to renal impairment, left ankle and foot
   M10.379 Gout due to renal impairment, unspecified ankle and foot
   M10.38 Gout due to renal impairment, vertebrae
   M10.39 Gout due to renal impairment, multiple sites
● **M10.4 Other secondary gout**
   Code first associated condition
   M10.40 Other secondary gout, unspecified site
● **M10.41** Other secondary gout, shoulder
   M10.411 Other secondary gout, right shoulder
   M10.412 Other secondary gout, left shoulder
   M10.419 Other secondary gout, unspecified shoulder
● **M10.42** Other secondary gout, elbow
   M10.421 Other secondary gout, right elbow
   M10.422 Other secondary gout, left elbow
   M10.429 Other secondary gout, unspecified elbow
● **M10.43** Other secondary gout, wrist
   M10.431 Other secondary gout, right wrist
   M10.432 Other secondary gout, left wrist
   M10.439 Other secondary gout, unspecified wrist
● **M10.44** Other secondary gout, hand
   M10.441 Other secondary gout, right hand
   M10.442 Other secondary gout, left hand
   M10.449 Other secondary gout, unspecified hand
● **M10.45** Other secondary gout, hip
   M10.451 Other secondary gout, right hip
   M10.452 Other secondary gout, left hip
   M10.459 Other secondary gout, unspecified hip
● **M10.46** Other secondary gout, knee
   M10.461 Other secondary gout, right knee
   M10.462 Other secondary gout, left knee
   M10.469 Other secondary gout, unspecified knee

● M10.47   Other secondary gout, ankle and foot
    M10.471   Other secondary gout, right ankle and foot
    M10.472   Other secondary gout, left ankle and foot
    M10.479   Other secondary gout, unspecified ankle and foot
  M10.48   Other secondary gout, vertebrae
  M10.49   Other secondary gout, multiple sites
M10.9   Gout, unspecified
    Gout NOS

● M11   Other crystal arthropathies
  ● M11.0   Hydroxyapatite deposition disease
    M11.00   Hydroxyapatite deposition disease, unspecified site
    ● M11.01   Hydroxyapatite deposition disease, shoulder
      M11.011   Hydroxyapatite deposition disease, right shoulder
      M11.012   Hydroxyapatite deposition disease, left shoulder
      M11.019   Hydroxyapatite deposition disease, unspecified shoulder
    ● M11.02   Hydroxyapatite deposition disease, elbow
      M11.021   Hydroxyapatite deposition disease, right elbow
      M11.022   Hydroxyapatite deposition disease, left elbow
      M11.029   Hydroxyapatite deposition disease, unspecified elbow
    ● M11.03   Hydroxyapatite deposition disease, wrist
      M11.031   Hydroxyapatite deposition disease, right wrist
      M11.032   Hydroxyapatite deposition disease, left wrist
      M11.039   Hydroxyapatite deposition disease, unspecified wrist
    ● M11.04   Hydroxyapatite deposition disease, hand
      M11.041   Hydroxyapatite deposition disease, right hand
      M11.042   Hydroxyapatite deposition disease, left hand
      M11.049   Hydroxyapatite deposition disease, unspecified hand
    ● M11.05   Hydroxyapatite deposition disease, hip
      M11.051   Hydroxyapatite deposition disease, right hip
      M11.052   Hydroxyapatite deposition disease, left hip
      M11.059   Hydroxyapatite deposition disease, unspecified hip
    ● M11.06   Hydroxyapatite deposition disease, knee
      M11.061   Hydroxyapatite deposition disease, right knee
      M11.062   Hydroxyapatite deposition disease, left knee
      M11.069   Hydroxyapatite deposition disease, unspecified knee
    ● M11.07   Hydroxyapatite deposition disease, ankle and foot
      M11.071   Hydroxyapatite deposition disease, right ankle and foot
      M11.072   Hydroxyapatite deposition disease, left ankle and foot
      M11.079   Hydroxyapatite deposition disease, unspecified ankle and foot
    M11.08   Hydroxyapatite deposition disease, vertebrae
    M11.09   Hydroxyapatite deposition disease, multiple sites

  ● M11.1   Familial chondrocalcinosis
    M11.10   Familial chondrocalcinosis, unspecified site
    ● M11.11   Familial chondrocalcinosis, shoulder
      M11.111   Familial chondrocalcinosis, right shoulder
      M11.112   Familial chondrocalcinosis, left shoulder
      M11.119   Familial chondrocalcinosis, unspecified shoulder
    ● M11.12   Familial chondrocalcinosis, elbow
      M11.121   Familial chondrocalcinosis, right elbow
      M11.122   Familial chondrocalcinosis, left elbow
      M11.129   Familial chondrocalcinosis, unspecified elbow
    ● M11.13   Familial chondrocalcinosis, wrist
      M11.131   Familial chondrocalcinosis, right wrist
      M11.132   Familial chondrocalcinosis, left wrist
      M11.139   Familial chondrocalcinosis, unspecified wrist
    ● M11.14   Familial chondrocalcinosis, hand
      M11.141   Familial chondrocalcinosis, right hand
      M11.142   Familial chondrocalcinosis, left hand
      M11.149   Familial chondrocalcinosis, unspecified hand
    ● M11.15   Familial chondrocalcinosis, hip
      M11.151   Familial chondrocalcinosis, right hip
      M11.152   Familial chondrocalcinosis, left hip
      M11.159   Familial chondrocalcinosis, unspecified hip
    ● M11.16   Familial chondrocalcinosis, knee
      M11.161   Familial chondrocalcinosis, right knee
      M11.162   Familial chondrocalcinosis, left knee
      M11.169   Familial chondrocalcinosis, unspecified knee
    ● M11.17   Familial chondrocalcinosis, ankle and foot
      M11.171   Familial chondrocalcinosis, right ankle and foot
      M11.172   Familial chondrocalcinosis, left ankle and foot
      M11.179   Familial chondrocalcinosis, unspecified ankle and foot
    M11.18   Familial chondrocalcinosis, vertebrae
    M11.19   Familial chondrocalcinosis, multiple sites
  ● M11.2   Other chondrocalcinosis
    Chondrocalcinosis NOS
    M11.20   Other chondrocalcinosis, unspecified site
    ● M11.21   Other chondrocalcinosis, shoulder
      M11.211   Other chondrocalcinosis, right shoulder
      M11.212   Other chondrocalcinosis, left shoulder
      M11.219   Other chondrocalcinosis, unspecified shoulder
    ● M11.22   Other chondrocalcinosis, elbow
      M11.221   Other chondrocalcinosis, right elbow
      M11.222   Other chondrocalcinosis, left elbow
      M11.229   Other chondrocalcinosis, unspecified elbow
    ● M11.23   Other chondrocalcinosis, wrist
      M11.231   Other chondrocalcinosis, right wrist
      M11.232   Other chondrocalcinosis, left wrist
      M11.239   Other chondrocalcinosis, unspecified wrist

CHAPTER 13 (M00-M99)

CHAPTER 13 (M00-M99)

● M11.24 Other chondrocalcinosis, hand
　　　　M11.241 Other chondrocalcinosis, right hand
　　　　M11.242 Other chondrocalcinosis, left hand
　　　　M11.249 Other chondrocalcinosis, unspecified hand
● M11.25 Other chondrocalcinosis, hip
　　　　M11.251 Other chondrocalcinosis, right hip
　　　　M11.252 Other chondrocalcinosis, left hip
　　　　M11.259 Other chondrocalcinosis, unspecified hip
● M11.26 Other chondrocalcinosis, knee
　　　　M11.261 Other chondrocalcinosis, right knee
　　　　M11.262 Other chondrocalcinosis, left knee
　　　　M11.269 Other chondrocalcinosis, unspecified knee
● M11.27 Other chondrocalcinosis, ankle and foot
　　　　M11.271 Other chondrocalcinosis, right ankle and foot
　　　　M11.272 Other chondrocalcinosis, left ankle and foot
　　　　M11.279 Other chondrocalcinosis, unspecified ankle and foot
　　M11.28 Other chondrocalcinosis, vertebrae
　　M11.29 Other chondrocalcinosis, multiple sites
● M11.8 Other specified crystal arthropathies
　　M11.80 Other specified crystal arthropathies, unspecified site
● M11.81 Other specified crystal arthropathies, shoulder
　　　　M11.811 Other specified crystal arthropathies, right shoulder
　　　　M11.812 Other specified crystal arthropathies, left shoulder
　　　　M11.819 Other specified crystal arthropathies, unspecified shoulder
● M11.82 Other specified crystal arthropathies, elbow
　　　　M11.821 Other specified crystal arthropathies, right elbow
　　　　M11.822 Other specified crystal arthropathies, left elbow
　　　　M11.829 Other specified crystal arthropathies, unspecified elbow
● M11.83 Other specified crystal arthropathies, wrist
　　　　M11.831 Other specified crystal arthropathies, right wrist
　　　　M11.832 Other specified crystal arthropathies, left wrist
　　　　M11.839 Other specified crystal arthropathies, unspecified wrist
● M11.84 Other specified crystal arthropathies, hand
　　　　M11.841 Other specified crystal arthropathies, right hand
　　　　M11.842 Other specified crystal arthropathies, left hand
　　　　M11.849 Other specified crystal arthropathies, unspecified hand
● M11.85 Other specified crystal arthropathies, hip
　　　　M11.851 Other specified crystal arthropathies, right hip
　　　　M11.852 Other specified crystal arthropathies, left hip
　　　　M11.859 Other specified crystal arthropathies, unspecified hip
● M11.86 Other specified crystal arthropathies, knee
　　　　M11.861 Other specified crystal arthropathies, right knee
　　　　M11.862 Other specified crystal arthropathies, left knee
　　　　M11.869 Other specified crystal arthropathies, unspecified knee

● M11.87 Other specified crystal arthropathies, ankle and foot
　　　　M11.871 Other specified crystal arthropathies, right ankle and foot
　　　　M11.872 Other specified crystal arthropathies, left ankle and foot
　　　　M11.879 Other specified crystal arthropathies, unspecified ankle and foot
　　M11.88 Other specified crystal arthropathies, vertebrae
　　M11.89 Other specified crystal arthropathies, multiple sites
　　M11.9 Crystal arthropathy, unspecified

● M12 Other and unspecified arthropathy
　　Excludes1 arthrosis (M15-M19)
　　　　　　 cricoarytenoid arthropathy (J38.7)
● M12.0 Chronic postrheumatic arthropathy [Jaccoud]
　　M12.00 Chronic postrheumatic arthropathy [Jaccoud], unspecified site 🔾
● M12.01 Chronic postrheumatic arthropathy [Jaccoud], shoulder
　　　　M12.011 Chronic postrheumatic arthropathy [Jaccoud], right shoulder 🔾
　　　　M12.012 Chronic postrheumatic arthropathy [Jaccoud], left shoulder 🔾
　　　　M12.019 Chronic postrheumatic arthropathy [Jaccoud], unspecified shoulder 🔾
● M12.02 Chronic postrheumatic arthropathy [Jaccoud], elbow
　　　　M12.021 Chronic postrheumatic arthropathy [Jaccoud], right elbow 🔾
　　　　M12.022 Chronic postrheumatic arthropathy [Jaccoud], left elbow 🔾
　　　　M12.029 Chronic postrheumatic arthropathy [Jaccoud], unspecified elbow 🔾
● M12.03 Chronic postrheumatic arthropathy [Jaccoud], wrist
　　　　M12.031 Chronic postrheumatic arthropathy [Jaccoud], right wrist 🔾
　　　　M12.032 Chronic postrheumatic arthropathy [Jaccoud], left wrist 🔾
　　　　M12.039 Chronic postrheumatic arthropathy [Jaccoud], unspecified wrist 🔾
● M12.04 Chronic postrheumatic arthropathy [Jaccoud], hand
　　　　M12.041 Chronic postrheumatic arthropathy [Jaccoud], right hand 🔾
　　　　M12.042 Chronic postrheumatic arthropathy [Jaccoud], left hand 🔾
　　　　M12.049 Chronic postrheumatic arthropathy [Jaccoud], unspecified hand 🔾
● M12.05 Chronic postrheumatic arthropathy [Jaccoud], hip
　　　　M12.051 Chronic postrheumatic arthropathy [Jaccoud], right hip 🔾
　　　　M12.052 Chronic postrheumatic arthropathy [Jaccoud], left hip 🔾
　　　　M12.059 Chronic postrheumatic arthropathy [Jaccoud], unspecified hip 🔾
● M12.06 Chronic postrheumatic arthropathy [Jaccoud], knee
　　　　M12.061 Chronic postrheumatic arthropathy [Jaccoud], right knee 🔾
　　　　M12.062 Chronic postrheumatic arthropathy [Jaccoud], left knee 🔾
　　　　M12.069 Chronic postrheumatic arthropathy [Jaccoud], unspecified knee 🔾

▶ New　　⇒ Revised　　~~deleted~~ Deleted　　Excludes 1　　Excludes 2　　Includes　　Use additional　　Code first　　Code also　　Key words
OGCR Official Guidelines　　X Assign placeholder X　　● Use Additional Character(s)　　▷ Manifestation Code　　🔾 Hierarchical Condition Category　　Coding Clinic

● M12.07   Chronic postrheumatic arthropathy [Jaccoud], ankle and foot

     M12.071   Chronic postrheumatic arthropathy [Jaccoud], right ankle and foot 🔗

     M12.072   Chronic postrheumatic arthropathy [Jaccoud], left ankle and foot 🔗

     M12.079   Chronic postrheumatic arthropathy [Jaccoud], unspecified ankle and foot 🔗

   M12.08   Chronic postrheumatic arthropathy [Jaccoud], other specified site 🔗

       Chronic postrheumatic arthropathy [Jaccoud], vertebrae

   M12.09   Chronic postrheumatic arthropathy [Jaccoud], multiple sites 🔗

● M12.1   **Kaschin-Beck disease**

     Osteochondroarthrosis deformans endemica

   M12.10   Kaschin-Beck disease, unspecified site

● M12.11   Kaschin-Beck disease, shoulder

     M12.111   Kaschin-Beck disease, right shoulder

     M12.112   Kaschin-Beck disease, left shoulder

     M12.119   Kaschin-Beck disease, unspecified shoulder

● M12.12   Kaschin-Beck disease, elbow

     M12.121   Kaschin-Beck disease, right elbow

     M12.122   Kaschin-Beck disease, left elbow

     M12.129   Kaschin-Beck disease, unspecified elbow

● M12.13   Kaschin-Beck disease, wrist

     M12.131   Kaschin-Beck disease, right wrist

     M12.132   Kaschin-Beck disease, left wrist

     M12.139   Kaschin-Beck disease, unspecified wrist

● M12.14   Kaschin-Beck disease, hand

     M12.141   Kaschin-Beck disease, right hand

     M12.142   Kaschin-Beck disease, left hand

     M12.149   Kaschin-Beck disease, unspecified hand

● M12.15   Kaschin-Beck disease, hip

     M12.151   Kaschin-Beck disease, right hip

     M12.152   Kaschin-Beck disease, left hip

     M12.159   Kaschin-Beck disease, unspecified hip

● M12.16   Kaschin-Beck disease, knee

     M12.161   Kaschin-Beck disease, right knee

     M12.162   Kaschin-Beck disease, left knee

     M12.169   Kaschin-Beck disease, unspecified knee

● M12.17   Kaschin-Beck disease, ankle and foot

     M12.171   Kaschin-Beck disease, right ankle and foot

     M12.172   Kaschin-Beck disease, left ankle and foot

     M12.179   Kaschin-Beck disease, unspecified ankle and foot

   M12.18   Kaschin-Beck disease, vertebrae

   M12.19   Kaschin-Beck disease, multiple sites

● M12.2   **Villonodular synovitis (pigmented)**

   M12.20   Villonodular synovitis (pigmented), unspecified site

● M12.21   Villonodular synovitis (pigmented), shoulder

     M12.211   Villonodular synovitis (pigmented), right shoulder

     M12.212   Villonodular synovitis (pigmented), left shoulder

     M12.219   Villonodular synovitis (pigmented), unspecified shoulder

● M12.22   Villonodular synovitis (pigmented), elbow

     M12.221   Villonodular synovitis (pigmented), right elbow

     M12.222   Villonodular synovitis (pigmented), left elbow

     M12.229   Villonodular synovitis (pigmented), unspecified elbow

● M12.23   Villonodular synovitis (pigmented), wrist

     M12.231   Villonodular synovitis (pigmented), right wrist

     M12.232   Villonodular synovitis (pigmented), left wrist

     M12.239   Villonodular synovitis (pigmented), unspecified wrist

● M12.24   Villonodular synovitis (pigmented), hand

     M12.241   Villonodular synovitis (pigmented), right hand

     M12.242   Villonodular synovitis (pigmented), left hand

     M12.249   Villonodular synovitis (pigmented), unspecified hand

● M12.25   Villonodular synovitis (pigmented), hip

     M12.251   Villonodular synovitis (pigmented), right hip

     M12.252   Villonodular synovitis (pigmented), left hip

     M12.259   Villonodular synovitis (pigmented), unspecified hip

● M12.26   Villonodular synovitis (pigmented), knee

     M12.261   Villonodular synovitis (pigmented), right knee

     M12.262   Villonodular synovitis (pigmented), left knee

     M12.269   Villonodular synovitis (pigmented), unspecified knee

● M12.27   Villonodular synovitis (pigmented), ankle and foot

     M12.271   Villonodular synovitis (pigmented), right ankle and foot

     M12.272   Villonodular synovitis (pigmented), left ankle and foot

     M12.279   Villonodular synovitis (pigmented), unspecified ankle and foot

   M12.28   Villonodular synovitis (pigmented), other specified site

       Villonodular synovitis (pigmented), vertebrae

   M12.29   Villonodular synovitis (pigmented), multiple sites

● M12.3   **Palindromic rheumatism**

   M12.30   Palindromic rheumatism, unspecified site

● M12.31   Palindromic rheumatism, shoulder

     M12.311   Palindromic rheumatism, right shoulder

     M12.312   Palindromic rheumatism, left shoulder

     M12.319   Palindromic rheumatism, unspecified shoulder

● M12.32   Palindromic rheumatism, elbow

     M12.321   Palindromic rheumatism, right elbow

     M12.322   Palindromic rheumatism, left elbow

     M12.329   Palindromic rheumatism, unspecified elbow

● M12.33   Palindromic rheumatism, wrist

     M12.331   Palindromic rheumatism, right wrist

     M12.332   Palindromic rheumatism, left wrist

     M12.339   Palindromic rheumatism, unspecified wrist

CHAPTER 13 (M00-M99)

- M12.34 Palindromic rheumatism, hand
  - M12.341 Palindromic rheumatism, right hand
  - M12.342 Palindromic rheumatism, left hand
  - M12.349 Palindromic rheumatism, unspecified hand
- M12.35 Palindromic rheumatism, hip
  - M12.351 Palindromic rheumatism, right hip
  - M12.352 Palindromic rheumatism, left hip
  - M12.359 Palindromic rheumatism, unspecified hip
- M12.36 Palindromic rheumatism, knee
  - M12.361 Palindromic rheumatism, right knee
  - M12.362 Palindromic rheumatism, left knee
  - M12.369 Palindromic rheumatism, unspecified knee
- M12.37 Palindromic rheumatism, ankle and foot
  - M12.371 Palindromic rheumatism, right ankle and foot
  - M12.372 Palindromic rheumatism, left ankle and foot
  - M12.379 Palindromic rheumatism, unspecified ankle and foot
- M12.38 Palindromic rheumatism, other specified site
  - Palindromic rheumatism, vertebrae
- M12.39 Palindromic rheumatism, multiple sites
- M12.4 Intermittent hydrarthrosis
  - M12.40 Intermittent hydrarthrosis, unspecified site
  - M12.41 Intermittent hydrarthrosis, shoulder
    - M12.411 Intermittent hydrarthrosis, right shoulder
    - M12.412 Intermittent hydrarthrosis, left shoulder
    - M12.419 Intermittent hydrarthrosis, unspecified shoulder
  - M12.42 Intermittent hydrarthrosis, elbow
    - M12.421 Intermittent hydrarthrosis, right elbow
    - M12.422 Intermittent hydrarthrosis, left elbow
    - M12.429 Intermittent hydrarthrosis, unspecified elbow
  - M12.43 Intermittent hydrarthrosis, wrist
    - M12.431 Intermittent hydrarthrosis, right wrist
    - M12.432 Intermittent hydrarthrosis, left wrist
    - M12.439 Intermittent hydrarthrosis, unspecified wrist
  - M12.44 Intermittent hydrarthrosis, hand
    - M12.441 Intermittent hydrarthrosis, right hand
    - M12.442 Intermittent hydrarthrosis, left hand
    - M12.449 Intermittent hydrarthrosis, unspecified hand
  - M12.45 Intermittent hydrarthrosis, hip
    - M12.451 Intermittent hydrarthrosis, right hip
    - M12.452 Intermittent hydrarthrosis, left hip
    - M12.459 Intermittent hydrarthrosis, unspecified hip
  - M12.46 Intermittent hydrarthrosis, knee
    - M12.461 Intermittent hydrarthrosis, right knee
    - M12.462 Intermittent hydrarthrosis, left knee
    - M12.469 Intermittent hydrarthrosis, unspecified knee
  - M12.47 Intermittent hydrarthrosis, ankle and foot
    - M12.471 Intermittent hydrarthrosis, right ankle and foot
    - M12.472 Intermittent hydrarthrosis, left ankle and foot
    - M12.479 Intermittent hydrarthrosis, unspecified ankle and foot

- M12.48 Intermittent hydrarthrosis, other site
- M12.49 Intermittent hydrarthrosis, multiple sites
- M12.5 Traumatic arthropathy
  - **Excludes1** current injury-see Alphabetic Index
    post-traumatic osteoarthritis of first carpometacarpal joint (M18.2-M18.3)
    post-traumatic osteoarthritis of hip (M16.4-M16.5)
    post-traumatic osteoarthritis of knee (M17.2-M17.3)
    post-traumatic osteoarthritis NOS (M19.1-)
    post-traumatic osteoarthritis of other single joints (M19.1-)
  - M12.50 Traumatic arthropathy, unspecified site
  - M12.51 Traumatic arthropathy, shoulder
    - M12.511 Traumatic arthropathy, right shoulder
    - M12.512 Traumatic arthropathy, left shoulder
    - M12.519 Traumatic arthropathy, unspecified shoulder
  - M12.52 Traumatic arthropathy, elbow
    - M12.521 Traumatic arthropathy, right elbow
    - M12.522 Traumatic arthropathy, left elbow
    - M12.529 Traumatic arthropathy, unspecified elbow
  - M12.53 Traumatic arthropathy, wrist
    - M12.531 Traumatic arthropathy, right wrist
    - M12.532 Traumatic arthropathy, left wrist
    - M12.539 Traumatic arthropathy, unspecified wrist
  - M12.54 Traumatic arthropathy, hand
    - M12.541 Traumatic arthropathy, right hand
    - M12.542 Traumatic arthropathy, left hand
    - M12.549 Traumatic arthropathy, unspecified hand
  - M12.55 Traumatic arthropathy, hip
    - M12.551 Traumatic arthropathy, right hip
    - M12.552 Traumatic arthropathy, left hip
      Coding Clinic: 2015, Q1, P17
    - M12.559 Traumatic arthropathy, unspecified hip
  - M12.56 Traumatic arthropathy, knee
    - M12.561 Traumatic arthropathy, right knee
    - M12.562 Traumatic arthropathy, left knee
    - M12.569 Traumatic arthropathy, unspecified knee
  - M12.57 Traumatic arthropathy, ankle and foot
    - M12.571 Traumatic arthropathy, right ankle and foot
    - M12.572 Traumatic arthropathy, left ankle and foot
    - M12.579 Traumatic arthropathy, unspecified ankle and foot
  - M12.58 Traumatic arthropathy, other specified site
    - Traumatic arthropathy, vertebrae
  - M12.59 Traumatic arthropathy, multiple sites
- M12.8 Other specific arthropathies, not elsewhere classified
  - Transient arthropathy
  - M12.80 Other specific arthropathies, not elsewhere classified, unspecified site
  - M12.81 Other specific arthropathies, not elsewhere classified, shoulder
    - M12.811 Other specific arthropathies, not elsewhere classified, right shoulder
    - M12.812 Other specific arthropathies, not elsewhere classified, left shoulder
    - M12.819 Other specific arthropathies, not elsewhere classified, unspecified shoulder

▶ New   ⇒ Revised   ~~deleted~~ Deleted   Excludes 1   Excludes 2   Includes   Use additional   Code first   Code also   Key words

OGCR Official Guidelines   X Assign placeholder X   ● Use Additional Character(s)   ▷ Manifestation Code   ℞ Hierarchical Condition Category   Coding Clinic

●M12.82 Other specific arthropathies, not elsewhere classified, elbow
  M12.821 Other specific arthropathies, not elsewhere classified, right elbow
  M12.822 Other specific arthropathies, not elsewhere classified, left elbow
  M12.829 Other specific arthropathies, not elsewhere classified, unspecified elbow
●M12.83 Other specific arthropathies, not elsewhere classified, wrist
  M12.831 Other specific arthropathies, not elsewhere classified, right wrist
  M12.832 Other specific arthropathies, not elsewhere classified, left wrist
  M12.839 Other specific arthropathies, not elsewhere classified, unspecified wrist
●M12.84 Other specific arthropathies, not elsewhere classified, hand
  M12.841 Other specific arthropathies, not elsewhere classified, right hand
  M12.842 Other specific arthropathies, not elsewhere classified, left hand
  M12.849 Other specific arthropathies, not elsewhere classified, unspecified hand
●M12.85 Other specific arthropathies, not elsewhere classified, hip
  M12.851 Other specific arthropathies, not elsewhere classified, right hip
  M12.852 Other specific arthropathies, not elsewhere classified, left hip
  M12.859 Other specific arthropathies, not elsewhere classified, unspecified hip
●M12.86 Other specific arthropathies, not elsewhere classified, knee
  M12.861 Other specific arthropathies, not elsewhere classified, right knee
  M12.862 Other specific arthropathies, not elsewhere classified, left knee
  M12.869 Other specific arthropathies, not elsewhere classified, unspecified knee
●M12.87 Other specific arthropathies, not elsewhere classified, ankle and foot
  M12.871 Other specific arthropathies, not elsewhere classified, right ankle and foot
  M12.872 Other specific arthropathies, not elsewhere classified, left ankle and foot
  M12.879 Other specific arthropathies, not elsewhere classified, unspecified ankle and foot
  M12.88 Other specific arthropathies, not elsewhere classified, other specified site
    Other specific arthropathies, not elsewhere classified, vertebrae
  M12.89 Other specific arthropathies, not elsewhere classified, multiple sites
M12.9 Arthropathy, unspecified

●M13 Other arthritis
  Excludes1 arthrosis (M15-M19)
            osteoarthritis (M15-M19)
  M13.0 Polyarthritis, unspecified
●M13.1 Monoarthritis, not elsewhere classified
  M13.10 Monoarthritis, not elsewhere classified, unspecified site

●M13.11 Monoarthritis, not elsewhere classified, shoulder
  M13.111 Monoarthritis, not elsewhere classified, right shoulder
  M13.112 Monoarthritis, not elsewhere classified, left shoulder
  M13.119 Monoarthritis, not elsewhere classified, unspecified shoulder
●M13.12 Monoarthritis, not elsewhere classified, elbow
  M13.121 Monoarthritis, not elsewhere classified, right elbow
  M13.122 Monoarthritis, not elsewhere classified, left elbow
  M13.129 Monoarthritis, not elsewhere classified, unspecified elbow
●M13.13 Monoarthritis, not elsewhere classified, wrist
  M13.131 Monoarthritis, not elsewhere classified, right wrist
  M13.132 Monoarthritis, not elsewhere classified, left wrist
  M13.139 Monoarthritis, not elsewhere classified, unspecified wrist
●M13.14 Monoarthritis, not elsewhere classified, hand
  M13.141 Monoarthritis, not elsewhere classified, right hand
  M13.142 Monoarthritis, not elsewhere classified, left hand
  M13.149 Monoarthritis, not elsewhere classified, unspecified hand
●M13.15 Monoarthritis, not elsewhere classified, hip
  M13.151 Monoarthritis, not elsewhere classified, right hip
  M13.152 Monoarthritis, not elsewhere classified, left hip
  M13.159 Monoarthritis, not elsewhere classified, unspecified hip
●M13.16 Monoarthritis, not elsewhere classified, knee
  M13.161 Monoarthritis, not elsewhere classified, right knee
  M13.162 Monoarthritis, not elsewhere classified, left knee
  M13.169 Monoarthritis, not elsewhere classified, unspecified knee
●M13.17 Monoarthritis, not elsewhere classified, ankle and foot
  M13.171 Monoarthritis, not elsewhere classified, right ankle and foot
  M13.172 Monoarthritis, not elsewhere classified, left ankle and foot
  M13.179 Monoarthritis, not elsewhere classified, unspecified ankle and foot
●M13.8 Other specified arthritis
    Allergic arthritis
    Excludes1 osteoarthritis (M15-M19)
  M13.80 Other specified arthritis, unspecified site
●M13.81 Other specified arthritis, shoulder
  M13.811 Other specified arthritis, right shoulder
  M13.812 Other specified arthritis, left shoulder
  M13.819 Other specified arthritis, unspecified shoulder
●M13.82 Other specified arthritis, elbow
  M13.821 Other specified arthritis, right elbow
  M13.822 Other specified arthritis, left elbow
  M13.829 Other specified arthritis, unspecified elbow

● M13.83 Other specified arthritis, wrist
   M13.831 Other specified arthritis, right wrist
   M13.832 Other specified arthritis, left wrist
   M13.839 Other specified arthritis, unspecified wrist
● M13.84 Other specified arthritis, hand
   M13.841 Other specified arthritis, right hand
   M13.842 Other specified arthritis, left hand
   M13.849 Other specified arthritis, unspecified hand
● M13.85 Other specified arthritis, hip
   M13.851 Other specified arthritis, right hip
   M13.852 Other specified arthritis, left hip
   M13.859 Other specified arthritis, unspecified hip
● M13.86 Other specified arthritis, knee
   M13.861 Other specified arthritis, right knee
   M13.862 Other specified arthritis, left knee
   M13.869 Other specified arthritis, unspecified knee
● M13.87 Other specified arthritis, ankle and foot
   M13.871 Other specified arthritis, right ankle and foot
   M13.872 Other specified arthritis, left ankle and foot
   M13.879 Other specified arthritis, unspecified ankle and foot
  M13.88 Other specified arthritis, other site
  M13.89 Other specified arthritis, multiple sites
● M14 Arthropathies in other diseases classified elsewhere
  Excludes1 arthropathy in:
    diabetes mellitus (E08-E13 with .61-)
    hematological disorders (M36.2-M36.3)
    hypersensitivity reactions (M36.4)
    neoplastic disease (M36.1)
    neurosyphillis (A52.16)
    sarcoidosis (D86.86)
   enteropathic arthropathies (M07.0-)
   juvenile psoriatic arthropathy (L40.54)
   lipoid dermatoarthritis (E78.81)
● M14.6 Charcôt's joint
  Neuropathic arthropathy
  Excludes1 Charcôt's joint in diabetes mellitus (E08-E13 with .610)
     Charcôt's joint in tabes dorsalis (A52.16)
  M14.60 Charcôt's joint, unspecified site
● M14.61 Charcôt's joint, shoulder
   M14.611 Charcôt's joint, right shoulder
   M14.612 Charcôt's joint, left shoulder
   M14.619 Charcôt's joint, unspecified shoulder
● M14.62 Charcôt's joint, elbow
   M14.621 Charcôt's joint, right elbow
   M14.622 Charcôt's joint, left elbow
   M14.629 Charcôt's joint, unspecified elbow
● M14.63 Charcôt's joint, wrist
   M14.631 Charcôt's joint, right wrist
   M14.632 Charcôt's joint, left wrist
   M14.639 Charcôt's joint, unspecified wrist
● M14.64 Charcôt's joint, hand
   M14.641 Charcôt's joint, right hand
   M14.642 Charcôt's joint, left hand
   M14.649 Charcôt's joint, unspecified hand
● M14.65 Charcôt's joint, hip
   M14.651 Charcôt's joint, right hip
   M14.652 Charcôt's joint, left hip
   M14.659 Charcôt's joint, unspecified hip

● M14.66 Charcôt's joint, knee
   M14.661 Charcôt's joint, right knee
   M14.662 Charcôt's joint, left knee
   M14.669 Charcôt's joint, unspecified knee
● M14.67 Charcôt's joint, ankle and foot
   M14.671 Charcôt's joint, right ankle and foot
   M14.672 Charcôt's joint, left ankle and foot
   M14.679 Charcôt's joint, unspecified ankle and foot
  M14.68 Charcôt's joint, vertebrae
  M14.69 Charcôt's joint, multiple sites
● M14.8 Arthropathies in other specified diseases classified elsewhere
  Code first underlying disease, such as:
    amyloidosis (E85.-)
    erythema multiforme (L51.-)
    erythema nodosum (L52)
    hemochromatosis (E83.11-)
    hyperparathyroidism (E21.-)
    hypothyroidism (E00-E03)
    sickle-cell disorders (D57.-)
    thyrotoxicosis [hyperthyroidism] (E05.-)
    Whipple's disease (K90.81)
  ▶ *M14.80 Arthropathies in other specified diseases classified elsewhere, unspecified site*
● *M14.81 Arthropathies in other specified diseases classified elsewhere, shoulder*
  ▶ *M14.811 Arthropathies in other specified diseases classified elsewhere, right shoulder*
  ▶ *M14.812 Arthropathies in other specified diseases classified elsewhere, left shoulder*
  ▶ *M14.819 Arthropathies in other specified diseases classified elsewhere, unspecified shoulder*
● *M14.82 Arthropathies in other specified diseases classified elsewhere, elbow*
  ▶ *M14.821 Arthropathies in other specified diseases classified elsewhere, right elbow*
  ▶ *M14.822 Arthropathies in other specified diseases classified elsewhere, left elbow*
  ▶ *M14.829 Arthropathies in other specified diseases classified elsewhere, unspecified elbow*
● *M14.83 Arthropathies in other specified diseases classified elsewhere, wrist*
  ▶ *M14.831 Arthropathies in other specified diseases classified elsewhere, right wrist*
  ▶ *M14.832 Arthropathies in other specified diseases classified elsewhere, left wrist*
  ▶ *M14.839 Arthropathies in other specified diseases classified elsewhere, unspecified wrist*
● *M14.84 Arthropathies in other specified diseases classified elsewhere, hand*
  ▶ *M14.841 Arthropathies in other specified diseases classified elsewhere, right hand*
  ▶ *M14.842 Arthropathies in other specified diseases classified elsewhere, left hand*
  ▶ *M14.849 Arthropathies in other specified diseases classified elsewhere, unspecified hand*

▶ New   ⟹ Revised   ~~deleted~~ Deleted   Excludes 1   Excludes 2   Includes   Use additional   Code first   Code also   Key words
OGCR Official Guidelines   X Assign placeholder X   ● Use Additional Character(s)   ▶ Manifestation Code   🝔 Hierarchical Condition Category   Coding Clinic

● M14.85 Arthropathies in other specified diseases classified elsewhere, hip
- ▷ *M14.851 Arthropathies in other specified diseases classified elsewhere, right hip*
- ▷ *M14.852 Arthropathies in other specified diseases classified elsewhere, left hip*
- ▷ *M14.859 Arthropathies in other specified diseases classified elsewhere, unspecified hip*

● M14.86 Arthropathies in other specified diseases classified elsewhere, knee
- ▷ *M14.861 Arthropathies in other specified diseases classified elsewhere, right knee*
- ▷ *M14.862 Arthropathies in other specified diseases classified elsewhere, left knee*
- ▷ *M14.869 Arthropathies in other specified diseases classified elsewhere, unspecified knee*

● M14.87 Arthropathies in other specified diseases classified elsewhere, ankle and foot
- ▷ *M14.871 Arthropathies in other specified diseases classified elsewhere, right ankle and foot*
- ▷ *M14.872 Arthropathies in other specified diseases classified elsewhere, left ankle and foot*
- ▷ *M14.879 Arthropathies in other specified diseases classified elsewhere, unspecified ankle and foot*

- ▷ *M14.88 Arthropathies in other specified diseases classified elsewhere, vertebrae*
- ▷ *M14.89 Arthropathies in other specified diseases classified elsewhere, multiple sites*

OSTEOARTHRITIS (M15-M19)

Osteoarthritis is the most common degenerative joint disease and form of arthritis that breaks down the cartilage causing pain, swelling, and reduced motion in the joints.

    Excludes2   osteoarthritis of spine (M47.-)

● M15 Polyosteoarthritis
    Includes   arthritis of multiple sites
    Excludes1 bilateral involvement of single joint (M16-M19)

M15.0 Primary generalized (osteo)arthritis

M15.1 Heberden's nodes (with arthropathy)
    Interphalangeal distal osteoarthritis

M15.2 Bouchard's nodes (with arthropathy)
    Juxtaphalangeal distal osteoarthritis

M15.3 Secondary multiple arthritis
    Post-traumatic polyosteoarthritis

M15.4 Erosive (osteo)arthritis

M15.8 Other polyosteoarthritis

M15.9 Polyosteoarthritis, unspecified
    Generalized osteoarthritis NOS

● M16 Osteoarthritis of hip

M16.0 Bilateral primary osteoarthritis of hip
    Coding Clinic: 2018, Q2, P15; 2016, Q4, P146

● M16.1 Unilateral primary osteoarthritis of hip
    Primary osteoarthritis of hip NOS

    M16.10 Unilateral primary osteoarthritis, unspecified hip

    M16.11 Unilateral primary osteoarthritis, right hip

    M16.12 Unilateral primary osteoarthritis, left hip

M16.2 Bilateral osteoarthritis resulting from hip dysplasia

● M16.3 Unilateral osteoarthritis resulting from hip dysplasia
    Dysplastic osteoarthritis of hip NOS

    M16.30 Unilateral osteoarthritis resulting from hip dysplasia, unspecified hip

    M16.31 Unilateral osteoarthritis resulting from hip dysplasia, right hip

    M16.32 Unilateral osteoarthritis resulting from hip dysplasia, left hip

M16.4 Bilateral post-traumatic osteoarthritis of hip

● M16.5 Unilateral post-traumatic osteoarthritis of hip
    Post-traumatic osteoarthritis of hip NOS

    M16.50 Unilateral post-traumatic osteoarthritis, unspecified hip

    M16.51 Unilateral post-traumatic osteoarthritis, right hip

    M16.52 Unilateral post-traumatic osteoarthritis, left hip

M16.6 Other bilateral secondary osteoarthritis of hip

M16.7 Other unilateral secondary osteoarthritis of hip
    Secondary osteoarthritis of hip NOS

M16.9 Osteoarthritis of hip, unspecified

● M17 Osteoarthritis of knee

M17.0 Bilateral primary osteoarthritis of knee

● M17.1 Unilateral primary osteoarthritis of knee
    Primary osteoarthritis of knee NOS

    M17.10 Unilateral primary osteoarthritis, unspecified knee
        Coding Clinic: 2016, Q4, P147

    M17.11 Unilateral primary osteoarthritis, right knee

    M17.12 Unilateral primary osteoarthritis, left knee
        Coding Clinic: 2016, Q4, P146

M17.2 Bilateral post-traumatic osteoarthritis of knee

● M17.3 Unilateral post-traumatic osteoarthritis of knee
    Post-traumatic osteoarthritis of knee NOS

    M17.30 Unilateral post-traumatic osteoarthritis, unspecified knee

    M17.31 Unilateral post-traumatic osteoarthritis, right knee

    M17.32 Unilateral post-traumatic osteoarthritis, left knee

M17.4 Other bilateral secondary osteoarthritis of knee

M17.5 Other unilateral secondary osteoarthritis of knee
    Secondary osteoarthritis of knee NOS

M17.9 Osteoarthritis of knee, unspecified
    Coding Clinic: 2016, Q4, P146

● M18 Osteoarthritis of first carpometacarpal joint

M18.0 Bilateral primary osteoarthritis of first carpometacarpal joints

● M18.1 Unilateral primary osteoarthritis of first carpometacarpal joint
    Primary osteoarthritis of first carpometacarpal joint NOS

    M18.10 Unilateral primary osteoarthritis of first carpometacarpal joint, unspecified hand

    M18.11 Unilateral primary osteoarthritis of first carpometacarpal joint, right hand

    M18.12 Unilateral primary osteoarthritis of first carpometacarpal joint, left hand

M18.2 Bilateral post-traumatic osteoarthritis of first carpometacarpal joints

● M18.3 Unilateral post-traumatic osteoarthritis of first carpometacarpal joint
    Post-traumatic osteoarthritis of first carpometacarpal joint NOS

    M18.30 Unilateral post-traumatic osteoarthritis of first carpometacarpal joint, unspecified hand

    M18.31 Unilateral post-traumatic osteoarthritis of first carpometacarpal joint, right hand

    M18.32 Unilateral post-traumatic osteoarthritis of first carpometacarpal joint, left hand

CHAPTER 13 (M00-M99)

M18.4 Other bilateral secondary osteoarthritis of first carpometacarpal joints

● **M18.5 Other unilateral secondary osteoarthritis of first carpometacarpal joint**
     Secondary osteoarthritis of first carpometacarpal joint NOS

     M18.50 Other unilateral secondary osteoarthritis of first carpometacarpal joint, unspecified hand

     M18.51 Other unilateral secondary osteoarthritis of first carpometacarpal joint, right hand

     M18.52 Other unilateral secondary osteoarthritis of first carpometacarpal joint, left hand

M18.9 Osteoarthritis of first carpometacarpal joint, unspecified

● **M19 Other and unspecified osteoarthritis**

     Excludes1 polyarthritis (M15.-)

     Excludes2 arthrosis of spine (M47.-)
                   hallux rigidus (M20.2)
                   osteoarthritis of spine (M47.-)

● **M19.0 Primary osteoarthritis of other joints**

     ● **M19.01 Primary osteoarthritis, shoulder**

         M19.011 Primary osteoarthritis, right shoulder
            Coding Clinic: 2016, Q4, P145

         M19.012 Primary osteoarthritis, left shoulder

         M19.019 Primary osteoarthritis, unspecified shoulder

     ● **M19.02 Primary osteoarthritis, elbow**

         M19.021 Primary osteoarthritis, right elbow

         M19.022 Primary osteoarthritis, left elbow

         M19.029 Primary osteoarthritis, unspecified elbow

     ● **M19.03 Primary osteoarthritis, wrist**

         M19.031 Primary osteoarthritis, right wrist

         M19.032 Primary osteoarthritis, left wrist

         M19.039 Primary osteoarthritis, unspecified wrist

     ● **M19.04 Primary osteoarthritis, hand**

         Excludes2 primary osteoarthritis of first carpometacarpal joint (M18.0-, M18.1-)

         M19.041 Primary osteoarthritis, right hand

         M19.042 Primary osteoarthritis, left hand

         M19.049 Primary osteoarthritis, unspecified hand

     ● **M19.07 Primary osteoarthritis ankle and foot**

         M19.071 Primary osteoarthritis, right ankle and foot

         M19.072 Primary osteoarthritis, left ankle and foot

         M19.079 Primary osteoarthritis, unspecified ankle and foot

     M19.09 Primary osteoarthritis, other specified site

● **M19.1 Post-traumatic osteoarthritis of other joints**

     ● **M19.11 Post-traumatic osteoarthritis, shoulder**

         M19.111 Post-traumatic osteoarthritis, right shoulder

         M19.112 Post-traumatic osteoarthritis, left shoulder

         M19.119 Post-traumatic osteoarthritis, unspecified shoulder

     ● **M19.12 Post-traumatic osteoarthritis, elbow**

         M19.121 Post-traumatic osteoarthritis, right elbow

         M19.122 Post-traumatic osteoarthritis, left elbow

         M19.129 Post-traumatic osteoarthritis, unspecified elbow

● **M19.13 Post-traumatic osteoarthritis, wrist**

     M19.131 Post-traumatic osteoarthritis, right wrist

     M19.132 Post-traumatic osteoarthritis, left wrist

     M19.139 Post-traumatic osteoarthritis, unspecified wrist

● **M19.14 Post-traumatic osteoarthritis, hand**

     Excludes2 post-traumatic osteoarthritis of first carpometacarpal joint (M18.2-, M18.3-)

     M19.141 Post-traumatic osteoarthritis, right hand

     M19.142 Post-traumatic osteoarthritis, left hand

     M19.149 Post-traumatic osteoarthritis, unspecified hand

● **M19.17 Post-traumatic osteoarthritis, ankle and foot**

     M19.171 Post-traumatic osteoarthritis, right ankle and foot

     M19.172 Post-traumatic osteoarthritis, left ankle and foot

     M19.179 Post-traumatic osteoarthritis, unspecified ankle and foot

     M19.19 Post-traumatic osteoarthritis, other specified site

● **M19.2 Secondary osteoarthritis of other joints**

     ● **M19.21 Secondary osteoarthritis, shoulder**

         M19.211 Secondary osteoarthritis, right shoulder

         M19.212 Secondary osteoarthritis, left shoulder

         M19.219 Secondary osteoarthritis, unspecified shoulder

     ● **M19.22 Secondary osteoarthritis, elbow**

         M19.221 Secondary osteoarthritis, right elbow

         M19.222 Secondary osteoarthritis, left elbow

         M19.229 Secondary osteoarthritis, unspecified elbow

     ● **M19.23 Secondary osteoarthritis, wrist**

         M19.231 Secondary osteoarthritis, right wrist

         M19.232 Secondary osteoarthritis, left wrist

         M19.239 Secondary osteoarthritis, unspecified wrist

     ● **M19.24 Secondary osteoarthritis, hand**

         M19.241 Secondary osteoarthritis, right hand

         M19.242 Secondary osteoarthritis, left hand

         M19.249 Secondary osteoarthritis, unspecified hand

     ● **M19.27 Secondary osteoarthritis, ankle and foot**

         M19.271 Secondary osteoarthritis, right ankle and foot

         M19.272 Secondary osteoarthritis, left ankle and foot

         M19.279 Secondary osteoarthritis, unspecified ankle and foot

     M19.29 Secondary osteoarthritis, other specified site

● **M19.9 Osteoarthritis, unspecified site**

     M19.90 Unspecified osteoarthritis, unspecified site
         Arthrosis NOS
         Arthritis NOS
         Osteoarthritis NOS
         Coding Clinic: 2016, Q4, P147

     M19.91 Primary osteoarthritis, unspecified site
         Primary osteoarthritis NOS

     M19.92 Post-traumatic osteoarthritis, unspecified site
         Post-traumatic osteoarthritis NOS

     M19.93 Secondary osteoarthritis, unspecified site
         Secondary osteoarthritis NOS

▶ New   ⇒ Revised   ~~deleted~~ Deleted   Excludes 1   Excludes 2   Includes   Use additional   Code first   Code also   Key words

OGCR Official Guidelines   X Assign placeholder X   ● Use Additional Character(s)   ▶ Manifestation Code   🔖 Hierarchical Condition Category   Coding Clinic

OTHER JOINT DISORDERS (M20-M25)

Excludes2   joints of the spine (M40-M54)

● **M20** **Acquired deformities of fingers and toes**
   Excludes1   acquired absence of fingers and toes (Z89.-)
           congenital absence of fingers and toes (Q71.3-, Q72.3-)
           congenital deformities and malformations of fingers and toes (Q66.-, Q68-Q70, Q74.-)

● **M20.0** **Deformity of finger(s)**
   Excludes1   clubbing of fingers (R68.3)
           palmar fascial fibromatosis [Dupuytren] (M72.0)
           trigger finger (M65.3)

● **M20.00** **Unspecified deformity of finger(s)**
   M20.001 Unspecified deformity of right finger(s)
   M20.002 Unspecified deformity of left finger(s)
   M20.009 Unspecified deformity of unspecified finger(s)

● **M20.01** **Mallet finger**
   M20.011 Mallet finger of right finger(s)
   M20.012 Mallet finger of left finger(s)
   M20.019 Mallet finger of unspecified finger(s)

● **M20.02** **Boutonnière deformity**
   M20.021 Boutonnière deformity of right finger(s)
   M20.022 Boutonnière deformity of left finger(s)
   M20.029 Boutonnière deformity of unspecified finger(s)

● **M20.03** **Swan-neck deformity**
   M20.031 Swan-neck deformity of right finger(s)
   M20.032 Swan-neck deformity of left finger(s)
   M20.039 Swan-neck deformity of unspecified finger(s)

● **M20.09** **Other deformity of finger(s)**
   M20.091 Other deformity of right finger(s)
   M20.092 Other deformity of left finger(s)
   M20.099 Other deformity of finger(s), unspecified finger(s)

● **M20.1** **Hallux valgus (acquired)**
   Excludes2   bunion (M21.6-)
   Coding Clinic: 2016, Q4, P38
   M20.10 Hallux valgus (acquired), unspecified foot
   M20.11 Hallux valgus (acquired), right foot
   M20.12 Hallux valgus (acquired), left foot

● **M20.2** **Hallux rigidus**
   M20.20 Hallux rigidus, unspecified foot
   M20.21 Hallux rigidus, right foot
   M20.22 Hallux rigidus, left foot

● **M20.3** **Hallux varus (acquired)**
   M20.30 Hallux varus (acquired), unspecified foot
   M20.31 Hallux varus (acquired), right foot
   M20.32 Hallux varus (acquired), left foot

● **M20.4** **Other hammer toe(s) (acquired)**
   M20.40 Other hammer toe(s) (acquired), unspecified foot
   M20.41 Other hammer toe(s) (acquired), right foot
   M20.42 Other hammer toe(s) (acquired), left foot

Figure 13-1   Hallux valgus.

Item 13-2 Hallux valgus is a sometimes painful structural deformity caused by an inflammation of the bursal sac at the base of the metatarsophalangeal joint (big toe). **Hallus varus** is a deviation of the great toe to the inner side of the foot or away from the next toe.

● **M20.5** **Other deformities of toe(s) (acquired)**
   ● **M20.5X** **Other deformities of toe(s) (acquired)**
       M20.5X1 Other deformities of toe(s) (acquired), right foot
       M20.5X2 Other deformities of toe(s) (acquired), left foot
       M20.5X9 Other deformities of toe(s) (acquired), unspecified foot

● **M20.6** **Acquired deformities of toe(s), unspecified**
   M20.60 Acquired deformities of toe(s), unspecified, unspecified foot
   M20.61 Acquired deformities of toe(s), unspecified, right foot
   M20.62 Acquired deformities of toe(s), unspecified, left foot

● **M21** **Other acquired deformities of limbs**
   Excludes1   acquired absence of limb (Z89.-)
           congenital absence of limbs (Q71-Q73)
           congenital deformities and malformations of limbs (Q65-Q66, Q68-Q74)
   Excludes2   acquired deformities of fingers or toes (M20.-)
           coxa plana (M91.2)

● **M21.0** **Valgus deformity, not elsewhere classified**
   Excludes1   metatarsus valgus (Q66.6)
           talipes calcaneovalgus (Q66.4-)
   M21.00 Valgus deformity, not elsewhere classified, unspecified site

● **M21.02** **Valgus deformity, not elsewhere classified, elbow**
       Cubitus valgus
       M21.021 Valgus deformity, not elsewhere classified, right elbow
       M21.022 Valgus deformity, not elsewhere classified, left elbow
       M21.029 Valgus deformity, not elsewhere classified, unspecified elbow

Item 13-3 Cubitus valgus is a deformity of the elbow resulting in an increased carrying angle in which the arm extends at the side and the palm faces forward, which results in the forearm and hand extended at greater than 15 degrees.

Item 13-4 Cubitus varus is a deformity of the elbow resulting in the arm extended at the side and the palm facing forward so that the forearm and hand are held at less than 5 degrees, decreasing the carrying angle.

CHAPTER 13 (M00-M99)

CHAPTER 13 (M00-M99)

● M21.05 Valgus deformity, not elsewhere classified, hip
    M21.051 Valgus deformity, not elsewhere classified, right hip
    M21.052 Valgus deformity, not elsewhere classified, left hip
    M21.059 Valgus deformity, not elsewhere classified, unspecified hip
● M21.06 Valgus deformity, not elsewhere classified, knee
      Genu valgum
      Knock knee
    M21.061 Valgus deformity, not elsewhere classified, right knee
    M21.062 Valgus deformity, not elsewhere classified, left knee
    M21.069 Valgus deformity, not elsewhere classified, unspecified knee
● M21.07 Valgus deformity, not elsewhere classified, ankle
    M21.071 Valgus deformity, not elsewhere classified, right ankle
    M21.072 Valgus deformity, not elsewhere classified, left ankle
    M21.079 Valgus deformity, not elsewhere classified, unspecified ankle
● M21.1 Varus deformity, not elsewhere classified
    Excludes1   metatarsus varus (Q66.22-)
                  tibia vara (M92.51-)
   M21.10 Varus deformity, not elsewhere classified, unspecified site
● M21.12 Varus deformity, not elsewhere classified, elbow
      Cubitus varus, elbow
    M21.121 Varus deformity, not elsewhere classified, right elbow
    M21.122 Varus deformity, not elsewhere classified, left elbow
    M21.129 Varus deformity, not elsewhere classified, unspecified elbow
● M21.15 Varus deformity, not elsewhere classified, hip
    M21.151 Varus deformity, not elsewhere classified, right hip
    M21.152 Varus deformity, not elsewhere classified, left hip
    M21.159 Varus deformity, not elsewhere classified, unspecified
● M21.16 Varus deformity, not elsewhere classified, knee
      Bow leg
      Genu varum
    M21.161 Varus deformity, not elsewhere classified, right knee
    M21.162 Varus deformity, not elsewhere classified, left knee
    M21.169 Varus deformity, not elsewhere classified, unspecified knee
● M21.17 Varus deformity, not elsewhere classified, ankle
    M21.171 Varus deformity, not elsewhere classified, right ankle
    M21.172 Varus deformity, not elsewhere classified, left ankle
    M21.179 Varus deformity, not elsewhere classified, unspecified ankle
● M21.2 Flexion deformity
   M21.20 Flexion deformity, unspecified site
● M21.21 Flexion deformity, shoulder
    M21.211 Flexion deformity, right shoulder
    M21.212 Flexion deformity, left shoulder
    M21.219 Flexion deformity, unspecified shoulder

● M21.22 Flexion deformity, elbow
    M21.221 Flexion deformity, right elbow
    M21.222 Flexion deformity, left elbow
    M21.229 Flexion deformity, unspecified elbow
● M21.23 Flexion deformity, wrist
    M21.231 Flexion deformity, right wrist
    M21.232 Flexion deformity, left wrist
    M21.239 Flexion deformity, unspecified wrist
● M21.24 Flexion deformity, finger joints
    M21.241 Flexion deformity, right finger joints
    M21.242 Flexion deformity, left finger joints
    M21.249 Flexion deformity, unspecified finger joints
● M21.25 Flexion deformity, hip
    M21.251 Flexion deformity, right hip
    M21.252 Flexion deformity, left hip
    M21.259 Flexion deformity, unspecified hip
● M21.26 Flexion deformity, knee
    M21.261 Flexion deformity, right knee
    M21.262 Flexion deformity, left knee
    M21.269 Flexion deformity, unspecified knee
● M21.27 Flexion deformity, ankle and toes
    M21.271 Flexion deformity, right ankle and toes
    M21.272 Flexion deformity, left ankle and toes
    M21.279 Flexion deformity, unspecified ankle and toes
● M21.3 Wrist or foot drop (acquired)
   ● M21.33 Wrist drop (acquired)
    M21.331 Wrist drop, right wrist
    M21.332 Wrist drop, left wrist
    M21.339 Wrist drop, unspecified wrist
   ● M21.37 Foot drop (acquired)
    M21.371 Foot drop, right foot
    M21.372 Foot drop, left foot
    M21.379 Foot drop, unspecified foot
● M21.4 Flat foot [pes planus] (acquired)
    Excludes1   congenital pes planus (Q66.5-)
   M21.40 Flat foot [pes planus] (acquired), unspecified foot
   M21.41 Flat foot [pes planus] (acquired), right foot
   M21.42 Flat foot [pes planus] (acquired), left foot
● M21.5 Acquired clawhand, clubhand, clawfoot and clubfoot
    Excludes1   clubfoot, not specified as acquired (Q66.89)
   ● M21.51 Acquired clawhand
    M21.511 Acquired clawhand, right hand
    M21.512 Acquired clawhand, left hand
    M21.519 Acquired clawhand, unspecified hand
   ● M21.52 Acquired clubhand
    M21.521 Acquired clubhand, right hand
    M21.522 Acquired clubhand, left hand
    M21.529 Acquired clubhand, unspecified hand
   ● M21.53 Acquired clawfoot
    M21.531 Acquired clawfoot, right foot
    M21.532 Acquired clawfoot, left foot
    M21.539 Acquired clawfoot, unspecified foot
   ● M21.54 Acquired clubfoot
    M21.541 Acquired clubfoot, right foot
    M21.542 Acquired clubfoot, left foot
    M21.549 Acquired clubfoot, unspecified foot

▶ New   ⇒ Revised   ~~deleted~~ Deleted   Excludes 1   Excludes 2   Includes   Use additional   Code first   Code also   Key words

OGCR Official Guidelines   X Assign placeholder X   ● Use Additional Character(s)   ▌ Manifestation Code   🅗 Hierarchical Condition Category   **Coding Clinic**

● **M21.6**   **Other acquired deformities of foot**
     Excludes2   deformities of toe (acquired)
                (M20.1-M20.6-)
   ● **M21.61**   **Bunion**
         Coding Clinic: 2016, Q4, P38
       M21.611   Bunion of right foot
       M21.612   Bunion of left foot
       M21.619   Bunion of unspecified foot
   ● **M21.62**   **Bunionette**
         Coding Clinic: 2016, Q4, P38
       M21.621   Bunionette of right foot
       M21.622   Bunionette of left foot
       M21.629   Bunionette of unspecified foot
   ● **M21.6X**   **Other acquired deformities of foot**
       M21.6X1   Other acquired deformities of right foot
         Coding Clinic: 2023, Q3, P21
       M21.6X2   Other acquired deformities of left foot
       M21.6X9   Other acquired deformities of unspecified foot
● **M21.7**   **Unequal limb length (acquired)**
     Note: The site used should correspond to the shorter limb.
     M21.70   Unequal limb length (acquired), unspecified site
   ● **M21.72**   **Unequal limb length (acquired), humerus**
       M21.721   Unequal limb length (acquired), right humerus
       M21.722   Unequal limb length (acquired), left humerus
       M21.729   Unequal limb length (acquired), unspecified humerus
   ● **M21.73**   **Unequal limb length (acquired), ulna and radius**
       M21.731   Unequal limb length (acquired), right ulna
       M21.732   Unequal limb length (acquired), left ulna
       M21.733   Unequal limb length (acquired), right radius
       M21.734   Unequal limb length (acquired), left radius
       M21.739   Unequal limb length (acquired), unspecified ulna and radius
   ● **M21.75**   **Unequal limb length (acquired), femur**
       M21.751   Unequal limb length (acquired), right femur
       M21.752   Unequal limb length (acquired), left femur
       M21.759   Unequal limb length (acquired), unspecified femur
   ● **M21.76**   **Unequal limb length (acquired), tibia and fibula**
       M21.761   Unequal limb length (acquired), right tibia
       M21.762   Unequal limb length (acquired), left tibia
       M21.763   Unequal limb length (acquired), right fibula
       M21.764   Unequal limb length (acquired), left fibula
       M21.769   Unequal limb length (acquired), unspecified tibia and fibula
● **M21.8**   **Other specified acquired deformities of limbs**
     Excludes2   coxa plana (M91.2)
     M21.80   Other specified acquired deformities of unspecified limb

● **M21.82**   **Other specified acquired deformities of upper arm**
     M21.821   Other specified acquired deformities of right upper arm
     M21.822   Other specified acquired deformities of left upper arm
     M21.829   Other specified acquired deformities of unspecified upper arm
● **M21.83**   **Other specified acquired deformities of forearm**
     M21.831   Other specified acquired deformities of right forearm
     M21.832   Other specified acquired deformities of left forearm
     M21.839   Other specified acquired deformities of unspecified forearm
● **M21.85**   **Other specified acquired deformities of thigh**
     M21.851   Other specified acquired deformities of right thigh
     M21.852   Other specified acquired deformities of left thigh
     M21.859   Other specified acquired deformities of unspecified thigh
● **M21.86**   **Other specified acquired deformities of lower leg**
     M21.861   Other specified acquired deformities of right lower leg
     M21.862   Other specified acquired deformities of left lower leg
     M21.869   Other specified acquired deformities of unspecified lower leg
● **M21.9**   **Unspecified acquired deformity of limb and hand**
     M21.90   Unspecified acquired deformity of unspecified limb
● **M21.92**   **Unspecified acquired deformity of upper arm**
     M21.921   Unspecified acquired deformity of right upper arm
     M21.922   Unspecified acquired deformity of left upper arm
     M21.929   Unspecified acquired deformity of unspecified upper arm
● **M21.93**   **Unspecified acquired deformity of forearm**
     M21.931   Unspecified acquired deformity of right forearm
     M21.932   Unspecified acquired deformity of left forearm
     M21.939   Unspecified acquired deformity of unspecified forearm
● **M21.94**   **Unspecified acquired deformity of hand**
     M21.941   Unspecified acquired deformity of hand, right hand
     M21.942   Unspecified acquired deformity of hand, left hand
     M21.949   Unspecified acquired deformity of hand, unspecified hand
● **M21.95**   **Unspecified acquired deformity of thigh**
     M21.951   Unspecified acquired deformity of right thigh
     M21.952   Unspecified acquired deformity of left thigh
     M21.959   Unspecified acquired deformity of unspecified thigh
● **M21.96**   **Unspecified acquired deformity of lower leg**
     M21.961   Unspecified acquired deformity of right lower leg
     M21.962   Unspecified acquired deformity of left lower leg
     M21.969   Unspecified acquired deformity of unspecified lower leg

CHAPTER 13 (M00-M99)

● **M22   Disorder of patella**
    Excludes2   traumatic dislocation of patella (S83.0-)
  ● **M22.0   Recurrent dislocation of patella**
      M22.00   Recurrent dislocation of patella, unspecified knee
      M22.01   Recurrent dislocation of patella, right knee
      M22.02   Recurrent dislocation of patella, left knee
  ● **M22.1   Recurrent subluxation of patella**
      Incomplete dislocation of patella
      M22.10   Recurrent subluxation of patella, unspecified knee
      M22.11   Recurrent subluxation of patella, right knee
      M22.12   Recurrent subluxation of patella, left knee
  ● **M22.2   Patellofemoral disorders**
    ● **M22.2X   Patellofemoral disorders**
      M22.2X1   Patellofemoral disorders, right knee
      M22.2X2   Patellofemoral disorders, left knee
      M22.2X9   Patellofemoral disorders, unspecified knee
  ● **M22.3   Other derangements of patella**
    ● **M22.3X   Other derangements of patella**
      M22.3X1   Other derangements of patella, right knee
      M22.3X2   Other derangements of patella, left knee
      M22.3X9   Other derangements of patella, unspecified knee
  ● **M22.4   Chondromalacia patellae**
      M22.40   Chondromalacia patellae, unspecified knee
      M22.41   Chondromalacia patellae, right knee
      M22.42   Chondromalacia patellae, left knee
  ● **M22.8   Other disorders of patella**
    ● **M22.8X   Other disorders of patella**
      M22.8X1   Other disorders of patella, right knee
      M22.8X2   Other disorders of patella, left knee
      M22.8X9   Other disorders of patella, unspecified knee
  ● **M22.9   Unspecified disorder of patella**
      M22.90   Unspecified disorder of patella, unspecified knee
      M22.91   Unspecified disorder of patella, right knee
      M22.92   Unspecified disorder of patella, left knee

● **M23   Internal derangement of knee**
    Excludes1   ankylosis (M24.66)
                  deformity of knee (M21.-)
                  osteochondritis dissecans (M93.2)
    Excludes2   current injury - see injury of knee and lower leg (S80-S89)
                  recurrent dislocation or subluxation of joints (M24.4)
                  recurrent dislocation or subluxation of patella (M22.0-M22.1)
    Coding Clinic: 2019, Q2, P26
  ● **M23.0   Cystic meniscus**
    ● **M23.00   Cystic meniscus, unspecified meniscus**
      Cystic meniscus, unspecified lateral meniscus
      Cystic meniscus, unspecified medial meniscus
      M23.000   Cystic meniscus, unspecified lateral meniscus, right knee
      M23.001   Cystic meniscus, unspecified lateral meniscus, left knee
      M23.002   Cystic meniscus, unspecified lateral meniscus, unspecified knee
      M23.003   Cystic meniscus, unspecified medial meniscus, right knee
      M23.004   Cystic meniscus, unspecified medial meniscus, left knee

      M23.005   Cystic meniscus, unspecified medial meniscus, unspecified knee
      M23.006   Cystic meniscus, unspecified meniscus, right knee
      M23.007   Cystic meniscus, unspecified meniscus, left knee
      M23.009   Cystic meniscus, unspecified meniscus, unspecified knee
  ● **M23.01   Cystic meniscus, anterior horn of medial meniscus**
      M23.011   Cystic meniscus, anterior horn of medial meniscus, right knee
      M23.012   Cystic meniscus, anterior horn of medial meniscus, left knee
      M23.019   Cystic meniscus, anterior horn of medial meniscus, unspecified knee
  ● **M23.02   Cystic meniscus, posterior horn of medial meniscus**
      M23.021   Cystic meniscus, posterior horn of medial meniscus, right knee
      M23.022   Cystic meniscus, posterior horn of medial meniscus, left knee
      M23.029   Cystic meniscus, posterior horn of medial meniscus, unspecified knee
  ● **M23.03   Cystic meniscus, other medial meniscus**
      M23.031   Cystic meniscus, other medial meniscus, right knee
      M23.032   Cystic meniscus, other medial meniscus, left knee
      M23.039   Cystic meniscus, other medial meniscus, unspecified knee
  ● **M23.04   Cystic meniscus, anterior horn of lateral meniscus**
      M23.041   Cystic meniscus, anterior horn of lateral meniscus, right knee
      M23.042   Cystic meniscus, anterior horn of lateral meniscus, left knee
      M23.049   Cystic meniscus, anterior horn of lateral meniscus, unspecified knee
  ● **M23.05   Cystic meniscus, posterior horn of lateral meniscus**
      M23.051   Cystic meniscus, posterior horn of lateral meniscus, right knee
      M23.052   Cystic meniscus, posterior horn of lateral meniscus, left knee
      M23.059   Cystic meniscus, posterior horn of lateral meniscus, unspecified knee
  ● **M23.06   Cystic meniscus, other lateral meniscus**
      M23.061   Cystic meniscus, other lateral meniscus, right knee
      M23.062   Cystic meniscus, other lateral meniscus, left knee
      M23.069   Cystic meniscus, other lateral meniscus, unspecified knee

★**(See Plate 34 of the Anatomy Illustrations.)**

  ● **M23.2   Derangement of meniscus due to old tear or injury**
      Old bucket-handle tear
    ● **M23.20   Derangement of unspecified meniscus due to old tear or injury**
      Derangement of unspecified lateral meniscus due to old tear or injury
      Derangement of unspecified medial meniscus due to old tear or injury
      M23.200   Derangement of unspecified lateral meniscus due to old tear or injury, right knee
      M23.201   Derangement of unspecified lateral meniscus due to old tear or injury, left knee

▶ New   ⇒ Revised   ~~deleted~~ Deleted   Excludes 1   Excludes 2   Includes   Use additional   Code first   Code also   Key words
OGCR Official Guidelines   **X** Assign placeholder X   ● Use Additional Character(s)   ▌ Manifestation Code   🏷 Hierarchical Condition Category   **Coding Clinic**

M23.202   Derangement of unspecified lateral meniscus due to old tear or injury, unspecified knee

M23.203   Derangement of unspecified medial meniscus due to old tear or injury, right knee

M23.204   Derangement of unspecified medial meniscus due to old tear or injury, left knee

M23.205   Derangement of unspecified medial meniscus due to old tear or injury, unspecified knee

M23.206   Derangement of unspecified meniscus due to old tear or injury, right knee

M23.207   Derangement of unspecified meniscus due to old tear or injury, left knee

M23.209   Derangement of unspecified meniscus due to old tear or injury, unspecified knee

● M23.21   Derangement of anterior horn of medial meniscus due to old tear or injury

M23.211   Derangement of anterior horn of medial meniscus due to old tear or injury, right knee

M23.212   Derangement of anterior horn of medial meniscus due to old tear or injury, left knee

M23.219   Derangement of anterior horn of medial meniscus due to old tear or injury, unspecified knee

● M23.22   Derangement of posterior horn of medial meniscus due to old tear or injury

M23.221   Derangement of posterior horn of medial meniscus due to old tear or injury, right knee

M23.222   Derangement of posterior horn of medial meniscus due to old tear or injury, left knee

M23.229   Derangement of posterior horn of medial meniscus due to old tear or injury, unspecified knee

● M23.23   Derangement of other medial meniscus due to old tear or injury

M23.231   Derangement of other medial meniscus due to old tear or injury, right knee

M23.232   Derangement of other medial meniscus due to old tear or injury, left knee

M23.239   Derangement of other medial meniscus due to old tear or injury, unspecified knee

● M23.24   Derangement of anterior horn of lateral meniscus due to old tear or injury

M23.241   Derangement of anterior horn of lateral meniscus due to old tear or injury, right knee

M23.242   Derangement of anterior horn of lateral meniscus due to old tear or injury, left knee

M23.249   Derangement of anterior horn of lateral meniscus due to old tear or injury, unspecified knee

● M23.25   Derangement of posterior horn of lateral meniscus due to old tear or injury

M23.251   Derangement of posterior horn of lateral meniscus due to old tear or injury, right knee

M23.252   Derangement of posterior horn of lateral meniscus due to old tear or injury, left knee

M23.259   Derangement of posterior horn of lateral meniscus due to old tear or injury, unspecified knee

● M23.26   Derangement of other lateral meniscus due to old tear or injury

M23.261   Derangement of other lateral meniscus due to old tear or injury, right knee

M23.262   Derangement of other lateral meniscus due to old tear or injury, left knee

M23.269   Derangement of other lateral meniscus due to old tear or injury, unspecified knee

● M23.3   **Other meniscus derangements**
Degenerate meniscus
Detached meniscus
Retained meniscus

● M23.30   Other meniscus derangements, unspecified meniscus
Other meniscus derangements, unspecified lateral meniscus
Other meniscus derangements, unspecified medial meniscus

M23.300   Other meniscus derangements, unspecified lateral meniscus, right knee

M23.301   Other meniscus derangements, unspecified lateral meniscus, left knee

M23.302   Other meniscus derangements, unspecified lateral meniscus, unspecified knee

M23.303   Other meniscus derangements, unspecified medial meniscus, right knee

M23.304   Other meniscus derangements, unspecified medial meniscus, left knee

M23.305   Other meniscus derangements, unspecified medial meniscus, unspecified knee

M23.306   Other meniscus derangements, unspecified meniscus, right knee

M23.307   Other meniscus derangements, unspecified meniscus, left knee

M23.309   Other meniscus derangements, unspecified meniscus, unspecified knee

● M23.31   Other meniscus derangements, anterior horn of medial meniscus

M23.311   Other meniscus derangements, anterior horn of medial meniscus, right knee

M23.312   Other meniscus derangements, anterior horn of medial meniscus, left knee

M23.319   Other meniscus derangements, anterior horn of medial meniscus, unspecified knee

● M23.32   Other meniscus derangements, posterior horn of medial meniscus

M23.321   Other meniscus derangements, posterior horn of medial meniscus, right knee

M23.322   Other meniscus derangements, posterior horn of medial meniscus, left knee

M23.329   Other meniscus derangements, posterior horn of medial meniscus, unspecified knee

CHAPTER 13 (M00-M99)

● M23.33 Other meniscus derangements, other medial meniscus
      M23.331 Other meniscus derangements, other medial meniscus, right knee
      M23.332 Other meniscus derangements, other medial meniscus, left knee
      M23.339 Other meniscus derangements, other medial meniscus, unspecified knee
● M23.34 Other meniscus derangements, anterior horn of lateral meniscus
      M23.341 Other meniscus derangements, anterior horn of lateral meniscus, right knee
      M23.342 Other meniscus derangements, anterior horn of lateral meniscus, left knee
      M23.349 Other meniscus derangements, anterior horn of lateral meniscus, unspecified knee
● M23.35 Other meniscus derangements, posterior horn of lateral meniscus
      M23.351 Other meniscus derangements, posterior horn of lateral meniscus, right knee
      M23.352 Other meniscus derangements, posterior horn of lateral meniscus, left knee
      M23.359 Other meniscus derangements, posterior horn of lateral meniscus, unspecified knee
● M23.36 Other meniscus derangements, other lateral meniscus
      M23.361 Other meniscus derangements, other lateral meniscus, right knee
      M23.362 Other meniscus derangements, other lateral meniscus, left knee
      M23.369 Other meniscus derangements, other lateral meniscus, unspecified knee
● M23.4 Loose body in knee
      M23.40 Loose body in knee, unspecified knee
      M23.41 Loose body in knee, right knee
      M23.42 Loose body in knee, left knee
● M23.5 Chronic instability of knee
      M23.50 Chronic instability of knee, unspecified knee
      M23.51 Chronic instability of knee, right knee
      M23.52 Chronic instability of knee, left knee
● M23.6 Other spontaneous disruption of ligament(s) of knee
   ● M23.60 Other spontaneous disruption of unspecified ligament of knee
         M23.601 Other spontaneous disruption of unspecified ligament of right knee
         M23.602 Other spontaneous disruption of unspecified ligament of left knee
         M23.609 Other spontaneous disruption of unspecified ligament of unspecified knee
   ● M23.61 Other spontaneous disruption of anterior cruciate ligament of knee
         M23.611 Other spontaneous disruption of anterior cruciate ligament of right knee
         M23.612 Other spontaneous disruption of anterior cruciate ligament of left knee
         M23.619 Other spontaneous disruption of anterior cruciate ligament of unspecified knee
   ● M23.62 Other spontaneous disruption of posterior cruciate ligament of knee
         M23.621 Other spontaneous disruption of posterior cruciate ligament of right knee

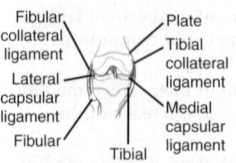

Figure 13-2 Collateral and cruciate ligament of knee. (From DeLee: DeLee and Drez's Orthopaedic Sports Medicine, ed 3, Saunders, 2009)

         M23.622 Other spontaneous disruption of posterior cruciate ligament of left knee
         M23.629 Other spontaneous disruption of posterior cruciate ligament of unspecified knee
   ● M23.63 Other spontaneous disruption of medial collateral ligament of knee
         M23.631 Other spontaneous disruption of medial collateral ligament of right knee
         M23.632 Other spontaneous disruption of medial collateral ligament of left knee
         M23.639 Other spontaneous disruption of medial collateral ligament of unspecified knee
   ● M23.64 Other spontaneous disruption of lateral collateral ligament of knee
         M23.641 Other spontaneous disruption of lateral collateral ligament of right knee
         M23.642 Other spontaneous disruption of lateral collateral ligament of left knee
         M23.649 Other spontaneous disruption of lateral collateral ligament of unspecified knee
   ● M23.67 Other spontaneous disruption of capsular ligament of knee
         M23.671 Other spontaneous disruption of capsular ligament of right knee
         M23.672 Other spontaneous disruption of capsular ligament of left knee
         M23.679 Other spontaneous disruption of capsular ligament of unspecified knee
● M23.8 Other internal derangements of knee
      Laxity of ligament of knee
      Snapping knee
   ● M23.8X Other internal derangements of knee
         M23.8X1 Other internal derangements of right knee
         M23.8X2 Other internal derangements of left knee
         M23.8X9 Other internal derangements of unspecified knee
● M23.9 Unspecified internal derangement of knee
      M23.90 Unspecified internal derangement of unspecified knee
      M23.91 Unspecified internal derangement of right knee
      M23.92 Unspecified internal derangement of left knee
● M24 Other specific joint derangements
   Excludes1 current injury - see injury of joint by body region
   Excludes2 ganglion (M67.4)
                  snapping knee (M23.8-)
                  temporomandibular joint disorders (M26.6-)
● M24.0 Loose body in joint
   Excludes2 loose body in knee (M23.4)
      M24.00 Loose body in unspecified joint
   ● M24.01 Loose body in shoulder
         M24.011 Loose body in right shoulder
         M24.012 Loose body in left shoulder
         M24.019 Loose body in unspecified shoulder

▶ New   ⇒ Revised   ~~deleted~~ Deleted   Excludes 1   Excludes 2   Includes   Use additional   Code first   Code also   Key words
OGCR Official Guidelines   X Assign placeholder X   ● Use Additional Character(s)   ▶ Manifestation Code   🐾 Hierarchical Condition Category   Coding Clinic

● M24.02 Loose body in elbow
  M24.021 Loose body in right elbow
  M24.022 Loose body in left elbow
  M24.029 Loose body in unspecified elbow
● M24.03 Loose body in wrist
  M24.031 Loose body in right wrist
  M24.032 Loose body in left wrist
  M24.039 Loose body in unspecified wrist
● M24.04 Loose body in finger joints
  M24.041 Loose body in right finger joint(s)
  M24.042 Loose body in left finger joint(s)
  M24.049 Loose body in unspecified finger joint(s)
● M24.05 Loose body in hip
  M24.051 Loose body in right hip
  M24.052 Loose body in left hip
  M24.059 Loose body in unspecified hip
● M24.07 Loose body in ankle and toe joints
  M24.071 Loose body in right ankle
  M24.072 Loose body in left ankle
  M24.073 Loose body in unspecified ankle
  M24.074 Loose body in right toe joint(s)
  M24.075 Loose body in left toe joint(s)
  M24.076 Loose body in unspecified toe joints
  M24.08 Loose body, other site
● M24.1 Other articular cartilage disorders
  Excludes2 chondrocalcinosis (M11.1-, M11.2-)
              internal derangement of knee (M23.-)
              metastatic calcification (E83.59)
              ochronosis (E70.29)
  M24.10 Other articular cartilage disorders, unspecified site
● M24.11 Other articular cartilage disorders, shoulder
  M24.111 Other articular cartilage disorders, right shoulder
  M24.112 Other articular cartilage disorders, left shoulder
  M24.119 Other articular cartilage disorders, unspecified shoulder
● M24.12 Other articular cartilage disorders, elbow
  M24.121 Other articular cartilage disorders, right elbow
  M24.122 Other articular cartilage disorders, left elbow
  M24.129 Other articular cartilage disorders, unspecified elbow
● M24.13 Other articular cartilage disorders, wrist
  M24.131 Other articular cartilage disorders, right wrist
  M24.132 Other articular cartilage disorders, left wrist
  M24.139 Other articular cartilage disorders, unspecified wrist
● M24.14 Other articular cartilage disorders, hand
  M24.141 Other articular cartilage disorders, right hand
  M24.142 Other articular cartilage disorders, left hand
  M24.149 Other articular cartilage disorders, unspecified hand
● M24.15 Other articular cartilage disorders, hip
  M24.151 Other articular cartilage disorders, right hip
  M24.152 Other articular cartilage disorders, left hip
  M24.159 Other articular cartilage disorders, unspecified hip

● M24.17 Other articular cartilage disorders, ankle and foot
  M24.171 Other articular cartilage disorders, right ankle
  M24.172 Other articular cartilage disorders, left ankle
  M24.173 Other articular cartilage disorders, unspecified ankle
  M24.174 Other articular cartilage disorders, right foot
  M24.175 Other articular cartilage disorders, left foot
  M24.176 Other articular cartilage disorders, unspecified foot
  M24.19 Other articular cartilage disorders, other specified site
● M24.2 Disorder of ligament
  Instability secondary to old ligament injury
  Ligamentous laxity NOS
  Excludes1 familial ligamentous laxity (M35.7)
  Excludes2 internal derangement of knee (M23.5-M23.8X9)
  M24.20 Disorder of ligament, unspecified site
● M24.21 Disorder of ligament, shoulder
  M24.211 Disorder of ligament, right shoulder
  M24.212 Disorder of ligament, left shoulder
  M24.219 Disorder of ligament, unspecified shoulder
● M24.22 Disorder of ligament, elbow
  M24.221 Disorder of ligament, right elbow
  M24.222 Disorder of ligament, left elbow
  M24.229 Disorder of ligament, unspecified elbow
● M24.23 Disorder of ligament, wrist
  M24.231 Disorder of ligament, right wrist
  M24.232 Disorder of ligament, left wrist
  M24.239 Disorder of ligament, unspecified wrist
● M24.24 Disorder of ligament, hand
  M24.241 Disorder of ligament, right hand
  M24.242 Disorder of ligament, left hand
  M24.249 Disorder of ligament, unspecified hand
● M24.25 Disorder of ligament, hip
  M24.251 Disorder of ligament, right hip
  M24.252 Disorder of ligament, left hip
  M24.259 Disorder of ligament, unspecified hip
● M24.27 Disorder of ligament, ankle and foot
  M24.271 Disorder of ligament, right ankle
  M24.272 Disorder of ligament, left ankle
  M24.273 Disorder of ligament, unspecified ankle
  M24.274 Disorder of ligament, right foot
  M24.275 Disorder of ligament, left foot
  M24.276 Disorder of ligament, unspecified foot
  M24.28 Disorder of ligament, vertebrae
      Coding Clinic: 2023, Q2, P13-14
  M24.29 Disorder of ligament, other specified site
● M24.3 Pathological dislocation of joint, not elsewhere classified
  Excludes1 congenital dislocation or displacement of joint - see congenital malformations and deformations of the musculoskeletal system (Q65-Q79)
              current injury - see injury of joints and ligaments by body region
              recurrent dislocation of joint (M24.4-)
  M24.30 Pathological dislocation of unspecified joint, not elsewhere classified

● M24.31 Pathological dislocation of shoulder, not elsewhere classified
 M24.311 Pathological dislocation of right shoulder, not elsewhere classified
 M24.312 Pathological dislocation of left shoulder, not elsewhere classified
 M24.319 Pathological dislocation of unspecified shoulder, not elsewhere classified

● M24.32 Pathological dislocation of elbow, not elsewhere classified
 M24.321 Pathological dislocation of right elbow, not elsewhere classified
 M24.322 Pathological dislocation of left elbow, not elsewhere classified
 M24.329 Pathological dislocation of unspecified elbow, not elsewhere classified

● M24.33 Pathological dislocation of wrist, not elsewhere classified
 M24.331 Pathological dislocation of right wrist, not elsewhere classified
 M24.332 Pathological dislocation of left wrist, not elsewhere classified
 M24.339 Pathological dislocation of unspecified wrist, not elsewhere classified

● M24.34 Pathological dislocation of hand, not elsewhere classified
 M24.341 Pathological dislocation of right hand, not elsewhere classified
 M24.342 Pathological dislocation of left hand, not elsewhere classified
 M24.349 Pathological dislocation of unspecified hand, not elsewhere classified

● M24.35 Pathological dislocation of hip, not elsewhere classified
 M24.351 Pathological dislocation of right hip, not elsewhere classified
   Coding Clinic: 2022, Q1, P32
 M24.352 Pathological dislocation of left hip, not elsewhere classified
   Coding Clinic: 2022, Q1, P32
 M24.359 Pathological dislocation of unspecified hip, not elsewhere classified

● M24.36 Pathological dislocation of knee, not elsewhere classified
 M24.361 Pathological dislocation of right knee, not elsewhere classified
 M24.362 Pathological dislocation of left knee, not elsewhere classified
 M24.369 Pathological dislocation of unspecified knee, not elsewhere classified

● M24.37 Pathological dislocation of ankle and foot, not elsewhere classified
 M24.371 Pathological dislocation of right ankle, not elsewhere classified
 M24.372 Pathological dislocation of left ankle, not elsewhere classified
 M24.373 Pathological dislocation of unspecified ankle, not elsewhere classified
 M24.374 Pathological dislocation of right foot, not elsewhere classified
 M24.375 Pathological dislocation of left foot, not elsewhere classified

 M24.376 Pathological dislocation of unspecified foot, not elsewhere classified
 M24.39 Pathological dislocation of other specified joint, not elsewhere classified

● M24.4 Recurrent dislocation of joint
   Recurrent subluxation of joint
   Excludes2 recurrent dislocation of patella (M22.0-M22.1)
        recurrent vertebral dislocation (M43.3-, M43.4, M43.5-)
 M24.40 Recurrent dislocation, unspecified joint
● M24.41 Recurrent dislocation, shoulder
 M24.411 Recurrent dislocation, right shoulder
 M24.412 Recurrent dislocation, left shoulder
 M24.419 Recurrent dislocation, unspecified shoulder
● M24.42 Recurrent dislocation, elbow
 M24.421 Recurrent dislocation, right elbow
 M24.422 Recurrent dislocation, left elbow
 M24.429 Recurrent dislocation, unspecified elbow
● M24.43 Recurrent dislocation, wrist
 M24.431 Recurrent dislocation, right wrist
 M24.432 Recurrent dislocation, left wrist
 M24.439 Recurrent dislocation, unspecified wrist
● M24.44 Recurrent dislocation, hand and finger(s)
 M24.441 Recurrent dislocation, right hand
 M24.442 Recurrent dislocation, left hand
 M24.443 Recurrent dislocation, unspecified hand
 M24.444 Recurrent dislocation, right finger
 M24.445 Recurrent dislocation, left finger
 M24.446 Recurrent dislocation, unspecified finger
● M24.45 Recurrent dislocation, hip
 M24.451 Recurrent dislocation, right hip
 M24.452 Recurrent dislocation, left hip
 M24.459 Recurrent dislocation, unspecified hip
● M24.46 Recurrent dislocation, knee
 M24.461 Recurrent dislocation, right knee
 M24.462 Recurrent dislocation, left knee
 M24.469 Recurrent dislocation, unspecified knee
● M24.47 Recurrent dislocation, ankle, foot and toes
 M24.471 Recurrent dislocation, right ankle
 M24.472 Recurrent dislocation, left ankle
 M24.473 Recurrent dislocation, unspecified ankle
 M24.474 Recurrent dislocation, right foot
 M24.475 Recurrent dislocation, left foot
 M24.476 Recurrent dislocation, unspecified foot
 M24.477 Recurrent dislocation, right toe(s)
 M24.478 Recurrent dislocation, left toe(s)
 M24.479 Recurrent dislocation, unspecified toe(s)
 M24.49 Recurrent dislocation, other specified joint
● M24.5 Contracture of joint
   Excludes1 contracture of muscle without contracture of joint (M62.4-)
        contracture of tendon (sheath) without contracture of joint (M62.4-)
        Dupuytren's contracture (M72.0)
   Excludes2 acquired deformities of limbs (M20-M21)
 M24.50 Contracture, unspecified joint

▶ New ⇒ Revised ~~deleted~~ Deleted Excludes 1 Excludes 2 Includes Use additional Code first Code also Key words
OGCR Official Guidelines X Assign placeholder X ● Use Additional Character(s) ▶ Manifestation Code 🦢 Hierarchical Condition Category Coding Clinic

● M24.51 Contracture, shoulder
    M24.511 Contracture, right shoulder
    M24.512 Contracture, left shoulder
    M24.519 Contracture, unspecified shoulder
● M24.52 Contracture, elbow
    M24.521 Contracture, right elbow
    M24.522 Contracture, left elbow
    M24.529 Contracture, unspecified elbow
● M24.53 Contracture, wrist
    M24.531 Contracture, right wrist
    M24.532 Contracture, left wrist
    M24.539 Contracture, unspecified wrist
● M24.54 Contracture, hand
    M24.541 Contracture, right hand
    M24.542 Contracture, left hand
    M24.549 Contracture, unspecified hand
● M24.55 Contracture, hip
    M24.551 Contracture, right hip
      Coding Clinic: 2016, Q2, P6
    M24.552 Contracture, left hip
      Coding Clinic: 2016, Q2, P6
    M24.559 Contracture, unspecified hip
● M24.56 Contracture, knee
    M24.561 Contracture, right knee
      Coding Clinic: 2016, Q2, P6
    M24.562 Contracture, left knee
      Coding Clinic: 2016, Q2, P6
    M24.569 Contracture, unspecified knee
● M24.57 Contracture, ankle and foot
    M24.571 Contracture, right ankle
    M24.572 Contracture, left ankle
    M24.573 Contracture, unspecified ankle
    M24.574 Contracture, right foot
    M24.575 Contracture, left foot
    M24.576 Contracture, unspecified foot
  M24.59 Contracture, other specified joint
● M24.6 Ankylosis of joint
    Excludes1 stiffness of joint without ankylosis (M25.6-)
    Excludes2 spine (M43.2-)
  M24.60 Ankylosis, unspecified joint
● M24.61 Ankylosis, shoulder
    M24.611 Ankylosis, right shoulder
    M24.612 Ankylosis, left shoulder
    M24.619 Ankylosis, unspecified shoulder
● M24.62 Ankylosis, elbow
    M24.621 Ankylosis, right elbow
    M24.622 Ankylosis, left elbow
    M24.629 Ankylosis, unspecified elbow
● M24.63 Ankylosis, wrist
    M24.631 Ankylosis, right wrist
    M24.632 Ankylosis, left wrist
    M24.639 Ankylosis, unspecified wrist
● M24.64 Ankylosis, hand
    M24.641 Ankylosis, right hand
    M24.642 Ankylosis, left hand
    M24.649 Ankylosis, unspecified hand
● M24.65 Ankylosis, hip
    M24.651 Ankylosis, right hip
    M24.652 Ankylosis, left hip
    M24.659 Ankylosis, unspecified hip

● M24.66 Ankylosis, knee
    M24.661 Ankylosis, right knee
    M24.662 Ankylosis, left knee
    M24.669 Ankylosis, unspecified knee
● M24.67 Ankylosis, ankle and foot
    M24.671 Ankylosis, right ankle
    M24.672 Ankylosis, left ankle
    M24.673 Ankylosis, unspecified ankle
    M24.674 Ankylosis, right foot
    M24.675 Ankylosis, left foot
    M24.676 Ankylosis, unspecified foot
  M24.69 Ankylosis, other specified joint
M24.7 Protrusio acetabuli
● M24.8 Other specific joint derangements, not elsewhere classified
    Excludes2 iliotibial band syndrome (M76.3)
  M24.80 Other specific joint derangements of unspecified joint, not elsewhere classified
● M24.81 Other specific joint derangements of shoulder, not elsewhere classified
    M24.811 Other specific joint derangements of right shoulder, not elsewhere classified
    M24.812 Other specific joint derangements of left shoulder, not elsewhere classified
    M24.819 Other specific joint derangements of unspecified shoulder, not elsewhere classified
● M24.82 Other specific joint derangements of elbow, not elsewhere classified
    M24.821 Other specific joint derangements of right elbow, not elsewhere classified
    M24.822 Other specific joint derangements of left elbow, not elsewhere classified
    M24.829 Other specific joint derangements of unspecified elbow, not elsewhere classified
● M24.83 Other specific joint derangements of wrist, not elsewhere classified
    M24.831 Other specific joint derangements of right wrist, not elsewhere classified
    M24.832 Other specific joint derangements of left wrist, not elsewhere classified
    M24.839 Other specific joint derangements of unspecified wrist, not elsewhere classified
● M24.84 Other specific joint derangements of hand, not elsewhere classified
    M24.841 Other specific joint derangements of right hand, not elsewhere classified
    M24.842 Other specific joint derangements of left hand, not elsewhere classified
    M24.849 Other specific joint derangements of unspecified hand, not elsewhere classified
● M24.85 Other specific joint derangements of hip, not elsewhere classified
    Irritable hip
    M24.851 Other specific joint derangements of right hip, not elsewhere classified
    M24.852 Other specific joint derangements of left hip, not elsewhere classified
    M24.859 Other specific joint derangements of unspecified hip, not elsewhere classified

CHAPTER 13 (M00-M99)

Item 13–5 Ankylosis or arthrokleisis is a consolidation of a joint due to disease, injury, or surgical procedure. Spondylosis is the degeneration of the vertebral processes and formation of osteophytes and commonly occurs with age. **Spondylitis** or ankylosing spondylitis is a type of arthritis that affects the spine or backbone, causing back pain and stiffness.

CHAPTER 13 (M00-M99)

● M24.87   Other specific joint derangements of ankle and foot, not elsewhere classified
     M24.871   Other specific joint derangements of right ankle, not elsewhere classified
     M24.872   Other specific joint derangements of left ankle, not elsewhere classified
     M24.873   Other specific joint derangements of unspecified ankle, not elsewhere classified
     M24.874   Other specific joint derangements of right foot, not elsewhere classified
     M24.875   Other specific joint derangements left foot, not elsewhere classified
     M24.876   Other specific joint derangements of unspecified foot, not elsewhere classified
   M24.89   Other specific joint derangement of other specified joint, not elsewhere classified
   M24.9   Joint derangement, unspecified

● M25   Other joint disorder, not elsewhere classified
   Excludes2   abnormality of gait and mobility (R26.-)
               acquired deformities of limb (M20-M21)
               calcification of bursa (M71.4-)
               calcification of shoulder (joint) (M75.3)
               calcification of tendon (M65.2-)
               difficulty in walking (R26.2)
               temporomandibular joint disorder (M26.6-)

● M25.0   Hemarthrosis
   Excludes1   current injury - see injury of joint by body region
               hemophilic arthropathy (M36.2)
   M25.00   Hemarthrosis, unspecified joint
● M25.01   Hemarthrosis, shoulder
     M25.011   Hemarthrosis, right shoulder
     M25.012   Hemarthrosis, left shoulder
     M25.019   Hemarthrosis, unspecified shoulder
● M25.02   Hemarthrosis, elbow
     M25.021   Hemarthrosis, right elbow
     M25.022   Hemarthrosis, left elbow
     M25.029   Hemarthrosis, unspecified elbow
● M25.03   Hemarthrosis, wrist
     M25.031   Hemarthrosis, right wrist
     M25.032   Hemarthrosis, left wrist
     M25.039   Hemarthrosis, unspecified wrist
● M25.04   Hemarthrosis, hand
     M25.041   Hemarthrosis, right hand
     M25.042   Hemarthrosis, left hand
     M25.049   Hemarthrosis, unspecified hand
● M25.05   Hemarthrosis, hip
     M25.051   Hemarthrosis, right hip
     M25.052   Hemarthrosis, left hip
     M25.059   Hemarthrosis, unspecified hip
● M25.06   Hemarthrosis, knee
     M25.061   Hemarthrosis, right knee
     M25.062   Hemarthrosis, left knee
     M25.069   Hemarthrosis, unspecified knee
● M25.07   Hemarthrosis, ankle and foot
     M25.071   Hemarthrosis, right ankle
     M25.072   Hemarthrosis, left ankle
     M25.073   Hemarthrosis, unspecified ankle
     M25.074   Hemarthrosis, right foot
     M25.075   Hemarthrosis, left foot
     M25.076   Hemarthrosis, unspecified foot
   M25.08   Hemarthrosis, other specified site
            Hemarthrosis, vertebrae

● M25.1   Fistula of joint
   M25.10   Fistula, unspecified joint
● M25.11   Fistula, shoulder
     M25.111   Fistula, right shoulder
     M25.112   Fistula, left shoulder
     M25.119   Fistula, unspecified shoulder
● M25.12   Fistula, elbow
     M25.121   Fistula, right elbow
     M25.122   Fistula, left elbow
     M25.129   Fistula, unspecified elbow
● M25.13   Fistula, wrist
     M25.131   Fistula, right wrist
     M25.132   Fistula, left wrist
     M25.139   Fistula, unspecified wrist
● M25.14   Fistula, hand
     M25.141   Fistula, right hand
     M25.142   Fistula, left hand
     M25.149   Fistula, unspecified hand
● M25.15   Fistula, hip
     M25.151   Fistula, right hip
     M25.152   Fistula, left hip
     M25.159   Fistula, unspecified hip
● M25.16   Fistula, knee
     M25.161   Fistula, right knee
     M25.162   Fistula, left knee
     M25.169   Fistula, unspecified knee
● M25.17   Fistula, ankle and foot
     M25.171   Fistula, right ankle
     M25.172   Fistula, left ankle
     M25.173   Fistula, unspecified ankle
     M25.174   Fistula, right foot
     M25.175   Fistula, left foot
     M25.176   Fistula, unspecified foot
   M25.18   Fistula, other specified site
            Fistula, vertebrae

● M25.2   Flail joint
   M25.20   Flail joint, unspecified joint
● M25.21   Flail joint, shoulder
     M25.211   Flail joint, right shoulder
     M25.212   Flail joint, left shoulder
     M25.219   Flail joint, unspecified shoulder
● M25.22   Flail joint, elbow
     M25.221   Flail joint, right elbow
     M25.222   Flail joint, left elbow
     M25.229   Flail joint, unspecified elbow
● M25.23   Flail joint, wrist
     M25.231   Flail joint, right wrist
     M25.232   Flail joint, left wrist
     M25.239   Flail joint, unspecified wrist
● M25.24   Flail joint, hand
     M25.241   Flail joint, right hand
     M25.242   Flail joint, left hand
     M25.249   Flail joint, unspecified hand
● M25.25   Flail joint, hip
     M25.251   Flail joint, right hip
     M25.252   Flail joint, left hip
     M25.259   Flail joint, unspecified hip
● M25.26   Flail joint, knee
     M25.261   Flail joint, right knee
     M25.262   Flail joint, left knee
     M25.269   Flail joint, unspecified knee

▶ New   ⇒ Revised   ~~deleted~~ Deleted   Excludes 1   Excludes 2   Includes   Use additional   Code first   Code also   Key words

OGCR Official Guidelines   X Assign placeholder X   ● Use Additional Character(s)   ▶ Manifestation Code   🅗 Hierarchical Condition Category   Coding Clinic

● M25.27 Flail joint, ankle and foot
    M25.271 Flail joint, right ankle and foot
    M25.272 Flail joint, left ankle and foot
    M25.279 Flail joint, unspecified ankle and foot
  M25.28 Flail joint, other site
● M25.3 Other instability of joint
    Excludes1 instability of joint secondary to old
            ligament injury (M24.2-)
            instability of joint secondary to removal
            of joint prosthesis (M96.8-)
    Excludes2 spinal instabilities (M53.2-)
  M25.30 Other instability, unspecified joint
● M25.31 Other instability, shoulder
    M25.311 Other instability, right shoulder
    M25.312 Other instability, left shoulder
    M25.319 Other instability, unspecified
           shoulder
● M25.32 Other instability, elbow
    M25.321 Other instability, right elbow
    M25.322 Other instability, left elbow
    M25.329 Other instability, unspecified elbow
● M25.33 Other instability, wrist
    M25.331 Other instability, right wrist
    M25.332 Other instability, left wrist
    M25.339 Other instability, unspecified wrist
● M25.34 Other instability, hand
    M25.341 Other instability, right hand
    M25.342 Other instability, left hand
    M25.349 Other instability, unspecified hand
● M25.35 Other instability, hip
    M25.351 Other instability, right hip
    M25.352 Other instability, left hip
    M25.359 Other instability, unspecified hip
● M25.36 Other instability, knee
    M25.361 Other instability, right knee
    M25.362 Other instability, left knee
    M25.369 Other instability, unspecified knee
● M25.37 Other instability, ankle and foot
    M25.371 Other instability, right ankle
    M25.372 Other instability, left ankle
    M25.373 Other instability, unspecified ankle
    M25.374 Other instability, right foot
    M25.375 Other instability, left foot
    M25.376 Other instability, unspecified foot
  M25.39 Other instability of joint
● M25.4 Effusion of joint
    Excludes1 hydrarthrosis in yaws (A66.6)
            intermittent hydrarthrosis (M12.4-)
            other infective (teno)synovitis (M65.1-)
  M25.40 Effusion, unspecified joint
● M25.41 Effusion, shoulder
    M25.411 Effusion, right shoulder
    M25.412 Effusion, left shoulder
    M25.419 Effusion, unspecified shoulder
● M25.42 Effusion, elbow
    M25.421 Effusion, right elbow
    M25.422 Effusion, left elbow
    M25.429 Effusion, unspecified elbow
● M25.43 Effusion, wrist
    M25.431 Effusion, right wrist
    M25.432 Effusion, left wrist
    M25.439 Effusion, unspecified wrist

● M25.44 Effusion, hand
    M25.441 Effusion, right hand
    M25.442 Effusion, left hand
    M25.449 Effusion, unspecified hand
● M25.45 Effusion, hip
    M25.451 Effusion, right hip
    M25.452 Effusion, left hip
    M25.459 Effusion, unspecified hip
● M25.46 Effusion, knee
    M25.461 Effusion, right knee
    M25.462 Effusion, left knee
    M25.469 Effusion, unspecified knee
● M25.47 Effusion, ankle and foot
    M25.471 Effusion, right ankle
    M25.472 Effusion, left ankle
    M25.473 Effusion, unspecified ankle
    M25.474 Effusion, right foot
    M25.475 Effusion, left foot
    M25.476 Effusion, unspecified foot
  M25.48 Effusion, other site
● M25.5 Pain in joint
    Excludes2 pain in hand (M79.64-)
            pain in fingers (M79.64-)
            pain in foot (M79.67-)
            pain in limb (M79.6-)
            pain in toes (M79.67-)
  M25.50 Pain in unspecified joint
● M25.51 Pain in shoulder
    M25.511 Pain in right shoulder
    M25.512 Pain in left shoulder
    M25.519 Pain in unspecified shoulder
● M25.52 Pain in elbow
    M25.521 Pain in right elbow
    M25.522 Pain in left elbow
    M25.529 Pain in unspecified elbow
● M25.53 Pain in wrist
    M25.531 Pain in right wrist
    M25.532 Pain in left wrist
    M25.539 Pain in unspecified wrist
● M25.54 Pain in joints of hand
    Coding Clinic: 2016, Q4, P38
    M25.541 Pain in joints of right hand
    M25.542 Pain in joints of left hand
    M25.549 Pain in joints of unspecified hand
            Pain in joints of hand NOS
● M25.55 Pain in hip
    M25.551 Pain in right hip
    M25.552 Pain in left hip
    M25.559 Pain in unspecified hip
● M25.56 Pain in knee
    M25.561 Pain in right knee
    M25.562 Pain in left knee
    M25.569 Pain in unspecified knee
● M25.57 Pain in ankle and joints of foot
    M25.571 Pain in right ankle and joints of right
            foot
    M25.572 Pain in left ankle and joints of left
            foot
    M25.579 Pain in unspecified ankle and joints
            of unspecified foot
  M25.59 Pain in other specified joint

●M25.6 **Stiffness of joint, not elsewhere classified**
   Excludes1   ankylosis of joint (M24.6-)
               contracture of joint (M24.5-)
   M25.60 Stiffness of unspecified joint, not elsewhere classified
   ●M25.61 Stiffness of shoulder, not elsewhere classified
      M25.611 Stiffness of right shoulder, not elsewhere classified
      M25.612 Stiffness of left shoulder, not elsewhere classified
      M25.619 Stiffness of unspecified shoulder, not elsewhere classified
   ●M25.62 Stiffness of elbow, not elsewhere classified
      M25.621 Stiffness of right elbow, not elsewhere classified
      M25.622 Stiffness of left elbow, not elsewhere classified
      M25.629 Stiffness of unspecified elbow, not elsewhere classified
   ●M25.63 Stiffness of wrist, not elsewhere classified
      M25.631 Stiffness of right wrist, not elsewhere classified
      M25.632 Stiffness of left wrist, not elsewhere classified
      M25.639 Stiffness of unspecified wrist, not elsewhere classified
   ●M25.64 Stiffness of hand, not elsewhere classified
      M25.641 Stiffness of right hand, not elsewhere classified
      M25.642 Stiffness of left hand, not elsewhere classified
      M25.649 Stiffness of unspecified hand, not elsewhere classified
   ●M25.65 Stiffness of hip, not elsewhere classified
      M25.651 Stiffness of right hip, not elsewhere classified
      M25.652 Stiffness of left hip, not elsewhere classified
      M25.659 Stiffness of unspecified hip, not elsewhere classified
   ●M25.66 Stiffness of knee, not elsewhere classified
      M25.661 Stiffness of right knee, not elsewhere classified
      M25.662 Stiffness of left knee, not elsewhere classified
      M25.669 Stiffness of unspecified knee, not elsewhere classified
   ●M25.67 Stiffness of ankle and foot, not elsewhere classified
      M25.671 Stiffness of right ankle, not elsewhere classified
      M25.672 Stiffness of left ankle, not elsewhere classified
      M25.673 Stiffness of unspecified ankle, not elsewhere classified
      M25.674 Stiffness of right foot, not elsewhere classified
      M25.675 Stiffness of left foot, not elsewhere classified
      M25.676 Stiffness of unspecified foot, not elsewhere classified
   M25.69 Stiffness of other specified joint, not elsewhere classified
●M25.7 **Osteophyte**
   M25.70 Osteophyte, unspecified joint
   ●M25.71 Osteophyte, shoulder
      M25.711 Osteophyte, right shoulder
      M25.712 Osteophyte, left shoulder
      M25.719 Osteophyte, unspecified shoulder
   ●M25.72 Osteophyte, elbow
      M25.721 Osteophyte, right elbow
      M25.722 Osteophyte, left elbow
      M25.729 Osteophyte, unspecified elbow
   ●M25.73 Osteophyte, wrist
      M25.731 Osteophyte, right wrist
      M25.732 Osteophyte, left wrist
      M25.739 Osteophyte, unspecified wrist
   ●M25.74 Osteophyte, hand
      M25.741 Osteophyte, right hand
      M25.742 Osteophyte, left hand
      M25.749 Osteophyte, unspecified hand
   ●M25.75 Osteophyte, hip
      M25.751 Osteophyte, right hip
      M25.752 Osteophyte, left hip
      M25.759 Osteophyte, unspecified hip
   ●M25.76 Osteophyte, knee
      M25.761 Osteophyte, right knee
      M25.762 Osteophyte, left knee
      M25.769 Osteophyte, unspecified knee
   ●M25.77 Osteophyte, ankle and foot
      M25.771 Osteophyte, right ankle
      M25.772 Osteophyte, left ankle
      M25.773 Osteophyte, unspecified ankle
      M25.774 Osteophyte, right foot
      M25.775 Osteophyte, left foot
      M25.776 Osteophyte, unspecified foot
   M25.78 Osteophyte, vertebrae
●M25.8 **Other specified joint disorders**
   M25.80 Other specified joint disorders, unspecified joint
   ●M25.81 Other specified joint disorders, shoulder
            Coding Clinic: 2022, Q3, P18
      M25.811 Other specified joint disorders, right shoulder
      M25.812 Other specified joint disorders, left shoulder
               Coding Clinic: 2022, Q3, P18
      M25.819 Other specified joint disorders, unspecified shoulder
   ●M25.82 Other specified joint disorders, elbow
      M25.821 Other specified joint disorders, right elbow
      M25.822 Other specified joint disorders, left elbow
      M25.829 Other specified joint disorders, unspecified elbow
   ●M25.83 Other specified joint disorders, wrist
      M25.831 Other specified joint disorders, right wrist
      M25.832 Other specified joint disorders, left wrist
      M25.839 Other specified joint disorders, unspecified wrist
   ●M25.84 Other specified joint disorders, hand
      M25.841 Other specified joint disorders, right hand
      M25.842 Other specified joint disorders, left hand
      M25.849 Other specified joint disorders, unspecified hand
   ●M25.85 Other specified joint disorders, hip
      M25.851 Other specified joint disorders, right hip
      M25.852 Other specified joint disorders, left hip
      M25.859 Other specified joint disorders, unspecified hip

▶ New   ⇒ Revised   ~~deleted~~ Deleted   Excludes 1   Excludes 2   Includes   Use additional   Code first   Code also   Key words
OGCR Official Guidelines   X Assign placeholder X   ● Use Additional Character(s)   ▷ Manifestation Code   �hb Hierarchical Condition Category   Coding Clinic

● M25.86 Other specified joint disorders, knee
    M25.861 Other specified joint disorders, right knee
    M25.862 Other specified joint disorders, left knee
    M25.869 Other specified joint disorders, unspecified knee
● M25.87 Other specified joint disorders, ankle and foot
    M25.871 Other specified joint disorders, right ankle and foot
    M25.872 Other specified joint disorders, left ankle and foot
    M25.879 Other specified joint disorders, unspecified ankle and foot
M25.9 Joint disorder, unspecified

DENTOFACIAL ANOMALIES [INCLUDING MALOCCLUSION] AND OTHER DISORDERS OF JAW (M26-M27)

Excludes1 hemifacial atrophy or hypertrophy (Q67.4)
    unilateral condylar hyperplasia or hypoplasia (M27.8)

● M26 Dentofacial anomalies [including malocclusion]
● M26.0 Major anomalies of jaw size
    Excludes1 acromegaly (E22.0)
        Robin's syndrome (Q87.0)
    M26.00 Unspecified anomaly of jaw size
    M26.01 Maxillary hyperplasia
    M26.02 Maxillary hypoplasia
    M26.03 Mandibular hyperplasia
    M26.04 Mandibular hypoplasia
    M26.05 Macrogenia
    M26.06 Microgenia
    M26.07 Excessive tuberosity of jaw
        Entire maxillary tuberosity
    M26.09 Other specified anomalies of jaw size
● M26.1 Anomalies of jaw-cranial base relationship
    M26.10 Unspecified anomaly of jaw-cranial base relationship
    M26.11 Maxillary asymmetry
    M26.12 Other jaw asymmetry
    M26.19 Other specified anomalies of jaw-cranial base relationship
        Coding Clinic: 2020, Q1, P21
● M26.2 Anomalies of dental arch relationship
    M26.20 Unspecified anomaly of dental arch relationship
  ● M26.21 Malocclusion, Angle's class
    M26.211 Malocclusion, Angle's class I
        Neutro-occlusion
    M26.212 Malocclusion, Angle's class II
        Disto-occlusion Division I
        Disto-occlusion Division II
    M26.213 Malocclusion, Angle's class III
        Mesio-occlusion
    M26.219 Malocclusion, Angle's class, unspecified

Figure 13-3 Dentofacial malocclusion.

Item 13–6 Hyperplasia is a condition of overdevelopment, whereas **hypoplasia** is a condition of underdevelopment. **Macrogenia** is overdevelopment of the chin, whereas **microgenia** is underdevelopment of the chin.

● M26.22 Open occlusal relationship
    M26.220 Open anterior occlusal relationship
        Anterior open bite
    M26.221 Open posterior occlusal relationship
        Posterior open bite
M26.23 Excessive horizontal overlap
    Excessive horizontal overjet
M26.24 Reverse articulation
    Crossbite (anterior) (posterior)
M26.25 Anomalies of interarch distance
M26.29 Other anomalies of dental arch relationship
    Midline deviation of dental arch
    Overbite (excessive) deep
    Overbite (excessive) horizontal
    Overbite (excessive) vertical
    Posterior lingual occlusion of mandibular teeth
● M26.3 Anomalies of tooth position of fully erupted tooth or teeth
    Excludes2 embedded and impacted teeth (K01.-)
    M26.30 Unspecified anomaly of tooth position of fully erupted tooth or teeth
        Abnormal spacing of fully erupted tooth or teeth NOS
        Displacement of fully erupted tooth or teeth NOS
        Transposition of fully erupted tooth or teeth NOS
    M26.31 Crowding of fully erupted teeth
    M26.32 Excessive spacing of fully erupted teeth
        Diastema of fully erupted tooth or teeth NOS
    M26.33 Horizontal displacement of fully erupted tooth or teeth
        Tipped tooth or teeth
        Tipping of fully erupted tooth
    M26.34 Vertical displacement of fully erupted tooth or teeth
        Extruded tooth
        Infraeruption of tooth or teeth
        Supraeruption of tooth or teeth
    M26.35 Rotation of fully erupted tooth or teeth
    M26.36 Insufficient interocclusal distance of fully erupted teeth (ridge)
        Lack of adequate intermaxillary vertical dimension of fully erupted teeth
    M26.37 Excessive interocclusal distance of fully erupted teeth
        Excessive intermaxillary vertical dimension of fully erupted teeth
        Loss of occlusal vertical dimension of fully erupted teeth
    M26.39 Other anomalies of tooth position of fully erupted tooth or teeth
M26.4 Malocclusion, unspecified
● M26.5 Dentofacial functional abnormalities
    Excludes1 bruxism (F45.8)
        teeth-grinding NOS (F45.8)
    M26.50 Dentofacial functional abnormalities, unspecified
    M26.51 Abnormal jaw closure
    M26.52 Limited mandibular range of motion
    M26.53 Deviation in opening and closing of the mandible
    M26.54 Insufficient anterior guidance
        Insufficient anterior occlusal guidance
    M26.55 Centric occlusion maximum intercuspation discrepancy
        Excludes1 centric occlusion NOS (M26.59)
    M26.56 Non-working side interference
        Balancing side interference

CHAPTER 13 (M00-M99)

M26.57   Lack of posterior occlusal support

M26.59   Other dentofacial functional abnormalities
Centric occlusion (of teeth) NOS
Malocclusion due to abnormal swallowing
Malocclusion due to mouth breathing
Malocclusion due to tongue, lip or finger habits

● M26.6   **Temporomandibular joint disorders**

      Excludes2   current temporomandibular joint dislocation (S03.0)
                   current temporomandibular joint sprain (S03.4)

      Coding Clinic: 2016, Q4, P38-39

   ● M26.60   Temporomandibular joint disorder, unspecified

      M26.601   **Right** temporomandibular joint disorder, unspecified

      M26.602   **Left** temporomandibular joint disorder, unspecified

      M26.603   **Bilateral** temporomandibular joint disorder, unspecified

      M26.609   **Unspecified** temporomandibular joint disorder, unspecified side
Temporomandibular joint disorder NOS

   ● M26.61   **Adhesions and ankylosis of temporomandibular joint**

      M26.611   Adhesions and ankylosis of **right** temporomandibular joint

      M26.612   Adhesions and ankylosis of **left** temporomandibular joint

      M26.613   Adhesions and ankylosis of **bilateral** temporomandibular joint

      M26.619   Adhesions and ankylosis of temporomandibular joint, **unspecified** side

   ● M26.62   **Arthralgia of temporomandibular joint**

      M26.621   Arthralgia of **right** temporomandibular joint

      M26.622   Arthralgia of **left** temporomandibular joint

      M26.623   Arthralgia of **bilateral** temporomandibular joint

      M26.629   Arthralgia of temporomandibular joint, **unspecified** side

   ● M26.63   **Articular disc disorder of temporomandibular joint**

      M26.631   Articular disc disorder of **right** temporomandibular joint

      M26.632   Articular disc disorder of **left** temporomandibular joint

      M26.633   Articular disc disorder of **bilateral** temporomandibular joint

      M26.639   Articular disc disorder of temporomandibular joint, **unspecified** side

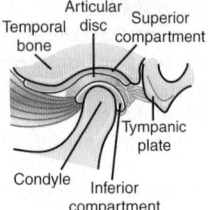

Figure 13-4   Temporomandibular joint.

Item 13-7 Dysfunction of the temporomandibular joint is termed **temporomandibular joint (TMJ) syndrome** and is characterized by pain and tenderness/spasm of the muscles of mastication, joint noise, and in the later stages, limited mandibular movement.

● M26.64   Arthritis of temporomandibular joint

      M26.641   Arthritis of right temporomandibular joint

      M26.642   Arthritis of left temporomandibular joint

      M26.643   Arthritis of bilateral temporomandibular joint

      M26.649   Arthritis of unspecified temporomandibular joint

● M26.65   Arthropathy of temporomandibular joint

      M26.651   Arthropathy of right temporomandibular joint

      M26.652   Arthropathy of left temporomandibular joint

      M26.653   Arthropathy of bilateral temporomandibular joint

      M26.659   Arthropathy of unspecified temporomandibular joint

   M26.69   **Other** specified disorders of temporomandibular joint

● M26.7   Dental alveolar anomalies

   M26.70   **Unspecified** alveolar anomaly

   M26.71   Alveolar **maxillary hyperplasia**

   M26.72   Alveolar **mandibular hyperplasia**

   M26.73   Alveolar **maxillary hypoplasia**

   M26.74   Alveolar **mandibular hypoplasia**

   M26.79   **Other** specified alveolar anomalies

● M26.8   Other dentofacial anomalies

   M26.81   **Anterior soft tissue impingement**
Anterior soft tissue impingement on teeth

   M26.82   **Posterior soft tissue impingement**
Posterior soft tissue impingement on teeth

   M26.89   **Other** dentofacial anomalies

M26.9   Dentofacial anomaly, **unspecified**

● M27   **Other diseases of jaws**

M27.0   Developmental disorders of jaws
Latent bone cyst of jaw
Stafne's cyst
Torus mandibularis
Torus palatinus

M27.1   Giant cell granuloma, central
Giant cell granuloma NOS

      Excludes1   peripheral giant cell granuloma (K06.8)

M27.2   Inflammatory conditions of jaws
Osteitis of jaw(s)
Osteomyelitis (neonatal) jaw(s)
Osteoradionecrosis jaw(s)
Periostitis jaw(s)
Sequestrum of jaw bone
Use additional code (W88-W90, X39.0) to identify radiation, if radiation-induced

      Excludes2   osteonecrosis of jaw due to drug (M87.180)

M27.3   Alveolitis of jaws
Alveolar osteitis
Dry socket

● M27.4   Other and unspecified cysts of jaw

      Excludes1   cysts of oral region (K09.-)
                latent bone cyst of jaw (M27.0)
                Stafne's cyst (M27.0)

   M27.40   **Unspecified** cyst of jaw
Cyst of jaw NOS

   M27.49   **Other** cysts of jaw
Aneurysmal cyst of jaw
Hemorrhagic cyst of jaw
Traumatic cyst of jaw

● M27.5   Periradicular pathology associated with previous endodontic treatment

   M27.51   Perforation of root canal space due to endodontic treatment

   M27.52   Endodontic overfill

▶ New   ⇒ Revised   ~~deleted~~ Deleted   Excludes 1   Excludes 2   Includes   Use additional   Code first   Code also   Key words

994   OGCR Official Guidelines   X Assign placeholder X   ● Use Additional Character(s)   ▶ Manifestation Code   Ⓗ Hierarchical Condition Category   Coding Clinic

M27.53   **Endodontic underfill**

M27.59   **Other periradicular pathology associated with previous endodontic treatment**

● M27.6   **Endosseous dental implant failure**

M27.61   Osseointegration **failure of dental implant**
Hemorrhagic complications of dental implant placement
Iatrogenic osseointegration failure of dental implant
Osseointegration failure of dental implant due to complications of systemic disease
Osseointegration failure of dental implant due to poor bone quality
Pre-integration failure of dental implant NOS
Pre-osseointegration failure of dental implant

M27.62   Post-osseointegration biological **failure of dental implant**
Failure of dental implant due to lack of attached gingiva
Failure of dental implant due to occlusal trauma (caused by poor prosthetic design)
Failure of dental implant due to parafunctional habits
Failure of dental implant due to periodontal infection (peri–implantitis)
Failure of dental implant due to poor oral hygiene
Iatrogenic post-osseointegration failure of dental implant
Post-osseointegration failure of dental implant due to complications of systemic disease

M27.63   Post-osseointegration mechanical **failure of dental implant**
Failure of dental prosthesis causing loss of dental implant
Fracture of dental implant
Excludes2   cracked tooth (K03.81)
fractured dental restorative material with loss of material (K08.531)
fractured dental restorative material without loss of material (K08.530)
fractured tooth (S02.5)

M27.69   **Other endosseous dental implant failure**
Dental implant failure NOS

M27.8   **Other specified diseases of jaws**
Cherubism
Exostosis
Fibrous dysplasia
Unilateral condylar hyperplasia
Unilateral condylar hypoplasia
Excludes1   jaw pain (R68.84)

M27.9   **Disease of jaws, unspecified**

SYSTEMIC CONNECTIVE TISSUE DISORDERS (M30-M36)

Includes   autoimmune disease NOS
collagen (vascular) disease NOS
systemic autoimmune disease
systemic collagen (vascular) disease

Excludes1   autoimmune disease, single organ or single cell-type - code to relevant condition category

● M30   **Polyarteritis nodosa and related conditions**
Excludes1   microscopic polyarteritis (M31.7)

M30.0   **Polyarteritis nodosa** 🔎

M30.1   **Polyarteritis with lung involvement [Churg-Strauss]** 🔎
Allergic granulomatous angiitis
Eosinophilic granulomatosis with polyangiitis [EGPA]
Coding Clinic: 2021, Q1, P23

M30.2   **Juvenile polyarteritis** 🔎

M30.3   **Mucocutaneous lymph node syndrome [Kawasaki]** 🔎

M30.8   **Other conditions related to polyarteritis nodosa** 🔎
Polyangiitis overlap syndrome

● M31   **Other necrotizing vasculopathies**

M31.0   **Hypersensitivity angiitis** 🔎
Goodpasture's syndrome

● M31.1   **Thrombotic microangiopathy** 🔎

M31.10   **Thrombotic microangiopathy, unspecified**

M31.11   **Hematopoietic stem cell transplantation-associated thrombotic microangiopathy [HSCT-TMA]**
Transplant-associated thrombotic microangiopathy [TA-TMA]
Code first if applicable:
complications of bone marrow transplant (T86.0-)
complications of stem cell transplant (T86.5)
Use Additional code to identify specific organ dysfunction, such as:
acute kidney failure (N17.-)
acute respiratory distress syndrome (J80)
capillary leak syndrome (I78.8)
diffuse alveolar hemorrhage (R04.89)
encephalopathy (metabolic) (septic) (G93.41)
fluid overload, unspecified (E87.70)
graft versus host disease (D89.81-)
hemolytic uremic syndrome (D59.3-)
hepatic failure (K72.-)
hepatic veno-occlusive disease (K76.5)
idiopathic interstitial pneumonia (J84.11-)
sinusoidal obstruction syndrome (K76.5)

M31.19   **Other thrombotic microangiopathy**
Thrombotic thrombocytopenic purpura

M31.2   **Lethal midline granuloma** 🔎

● M31.3   **Wegener's granulomatosis**
Granulomatosis with polyangiitis
Necrotizing respiratory granulomatosis
Coding Clinic: 2021, Q1, P23

M31.30   **Wegener's granulomatosis without renal involvement** 🔎
Wegener's granulomatosis NOS
Coding Clinic: 2021, Q2, P10

M31.31   **Wegener's granulomatosis with renal involvement** 🔎

M31.4   **Aortic arch syndrome [Takayasu]** 🔎

M31.5   **Giant cell arteritis with polymyalgia rheumatica** 🔎

M31.6   **Other giant cell arteritis** 🔎

M31.7   **Microscopic polyangiitis** 🔎
Microscopic polyarteritis
Excludes1   polyarteritis nodosa (M30.0)
Coding Clinic: 2021, Q1, P23

M31.8   **Other specified necrotizing vasculopathies** 🔎
Hypocomplementemic vasculitis
Septic vasculitis

M31.9   **Necrotizing vasculopathy, unspecified** 🔎

● M32   **Systemic lupus erythematosus (SLE)**
Autoimmune inflammatory connective tissue disease of unknown cause that occurs most often in women
Excludes1   lupus erythematosus (discoid) (NOS) (L93.0)

M32.0   **Drug-induced systemic lupus erythematosus** 🔎
Use additional code for adverse effect, if applicable, to identify drug (T36-T50 with fifth or sixth character 5)

● M32.1   **Systemic lupus erythematosus with organ or system involvement**

M32.10   **Systemic lupus erythematosus, organ or system involvement unspecified** 🔎

M32.11   **Endocarditis in systemic lupus erythematosus** 🔎
Libman-Sacks disease

CHAPTER 13 (M00-M99)

M32.12 Pericarditis in systemic lupus erythematosus 🐾
Lupus pericarditis

M32.13 Lung involvement in systemic lupus erythematosus 🐾
Pleural effusion due to systemic lupus erythematosus

M32.14 Glomerular disease in systemic lupus erythematosus 🐾
Lupus renal disease NOS

M32.15 Tubulo-interstitial nephropathy in systemic lupus erythematosus 🐾

M32.19 Other organ or system involvement in systemic lupus erythematosus 🐾
Use additional code(s) to identify organ or system involvement, such as encephalitis (G05.3)

M32.8 Other forms of systemic lupus erythematosus 🐾

M32.9 Systemic lupus erythematosus, unspecified 🐾
SLE NOS
Systemic lupus erythematosus NOS
Systemic lupus erythematosus without organ involvement

● **M33 Dermatopolymyositis**

● **M33.0 Juvenile dermatomyositis**

M33.00 Juvenile dermatomyositis, organ involvement unspecified 🐾

M33.01 Juvenile dermatomyositis with respiratory involvement 🐾

M33.02 Juvenile dermatomyositis with myopathy 🐾

M33.03 Juvenile dermatomyositis without myopathy 🐾

M33.09 Juvenile dermatomyositis with other organ involvement 🐾

● **M33.1 Other dermatomyositis**
Adult dermatomyositis

M33.10 Other dermatomyositis, organ involvement unspecified 🐾

M33.11 Other dermatomyositis with respiratory involvement 🐾

M33.12 Other dermatomyositis with myopathy 🐾

M33.13 Other dermatomyositis without myopathy 🐾
Dermatomyositis NOS

M33.19 Other dermatomyositis with other organ involvement 🐾

● **M33.2 Polymyositis**

M33.20 Polymyositis, organ involvement unspecified 🐾

M33.21 Polymyositis with respiratory involvement 🐾

M33.22 Polymyositis with myopathy 🐾

M33.29 Polymyositis with other organ involvement 🐾

● **M33.9 Dermatopolymyositis, unspecified**

M33.90 Dermatopolymyositis, unspecified, organ involvement unspecified 🐾

M33.91 Dermatopolymyositis, unspecified with respiratory involvement 🐾

M33.92 Dermatopolymyositis, unspecified with myopathy 🐾

M33.93 Dermatopolymyositis, unspecified without myopathy 🐾

M33.99 Dermatopolymyositis, unspecified with other organ involvement 🐾

● **M34 Systemic sclerosis [scleroderma]**

Excludes1   circumscribed scleroderma (L94.0)
neonatal scleroderma (P83.88)

M34.0 Progressive systemic sclerosis 🐾

M34.1 CR(E)ST syndrome 🐾
Combination of calcinosis, Raynaud's phenomenon, esophageal dysfunction, sclerodactyly, telangiectasia

Item 13–8 Polymyalgia rheumatica is a syndrome characterized by aching and morning stiffness and is related to aging and hereditary predisposition.

M34.2 Systemic sclerosis induced by drug and chemical 🐾
Code first poisoning due to drug or toxin, if applicable (T36-T65 with fifth or sixth character 1-4)
Use additional code for adverse effect, if applicable, to identify drug (T36-T50 with fifth or sixth character 5)

● **M34.8 Other forms of systemic sclerosis**

M34.81 Systemic sclerosis with lung involvement 🐾
Code also if applicable:
other interstitial pulmonary diseases (J84.89)
secondary pulmonary arterial hypertension (I27.21)

M34.82 Systemic sclerosis with myopathy 🐾

M34.83 Systemic sclerosis with polyneuropathy 🐾

M34.89 Other systemic sclerosis 🐾

M34.9 Systemic sclerosis, unspecified 🐾

● **M35 Other systemic involvement of connective tissue**

Excludes1   reactive perforating collagenosis (L87.1)

● **M35.0 Sjögren syndrome**
Sicca syndrome
Use Additional code to identify associated manifestations

Excludes1   dry mouth, unspecified (R68.2)

M35.00 Sjögren syndrome, unspecified 🐾

M35.01 Sjögren syndrome with keratoconjunctivitis 🐾

M35.02 Sjögren syndrome with lung involvement 🐾

M35.03 Sjögren syndrome with myopathy 🐾

M35.04 Sjögren syndrome with tubulo-interstitial nephropathy 🐾
Renal tubular acidosis in sicca syndrome

M35.05 Sjögren syndrome with inflammatory arthritis

M35.06 Sjögren syndrome with peripheral nervous system involvement

M35.07 Sjögren syndrome with central nervous system involvement

M35.08 Sjögren syndrome with gastrointestinal involvement

M35.09 Sjögren syndrome with other organ involvement 🐾

M35.0A Sjögren syndrome with glomerular disease

M35.0B Sjögren syndrome with vasculitis

M35.0C Sjögren syndrome with dental involvement

M35.1 Other overlap syndromes 🐾
Mixed connective tissue disease

Excludes1   polyangiitis overlap syndrome (M30.8)

M35.2 Behçet's disease 🐾

M35.3 Polymyalgia rheumatica 🐾

Excludes1   polymyalgia rheumatica with giant cell arteritis (M31.5)

M35.4 Diffuse (eosinophilic) fasciitis

M35.5 Multifocal fibrosclerosis 🐾

M35.6 Relapsing panniculitis [Weber-Christian]

Excludes1   lupus panniculitis (L93.2)
panniculitis NOS (M79.3-)

M35.7 Hypermobility syndrome
Familial ligamentous laxity

Excludes1   ligamentous laxity, NOS (M24.2-)

Excludes2   Ehlers-Danlos syndromes (Q79.6-)

▶ New   ⇒ Revised   ~~deleted~~ Deleted   Excludes 1   Excludes 2   Includes   Use additional   Code first   Code also   Key words

OGCR Official Guidelines   X Assign placeholder X   ● Use Additional Character(s)   ▶ Manifestation Code   🐾 Hierarchical Condition Category   Coding Clinic

● **M35.8** **Other specified systemic involvement of connective tissue** 🔍
   Coding Clinic: 2021, Q4, P102; 2021, Q1, P36

   M35.81 Multisystem inflammatory syndrome
       MIS-A
       MIS-C
       Multisystem inflammatory syndrome in adults
       Multisystem inflammatory syndrome in children
       Pediatric inflammatory multisystem syndrome
       PIMS

       Code first, if applicable, COVID-19 (U07.1)

       Code also any associated complications such as:
           acute hepatic failure (K72.0-)
           acute kidney failure (N17.-)
           acute myocarditis (I40.-)
           acute respiratory distress syndrome (J80)
           cardiac arrhythmia (I47-I49.-)
           pneumonia due to COVID-19 (J12.82)
           severe sepsis (R65.2-)
           viral cardiomyopathy (B33.24)
           viral pericarditis (B33.23)

       Use additional code, if applicable, for:
           exposure to COVID-19 or SARS-C
               personal history of COVID-19 (Z86.16)
           post COVID-19 condition (U09.9)
       Coding Clinic: 2021, Q4, P102; 2021, Q1, P36, 42

   M35.89 Other specified systemic involvement of connective tissue

M35.9 Systemic involvement of connective tissue, unspecified 🔍
       Autoimmune disease (systemic) NOS
       Collagen (vascular) disease NOS

● **M36** **Systemic disorders of connective tissue in diseases classified elsewhere**
   Excludes2 arthropathies in diseases classified elsewhere (M14.-)

▹ **M36.0** *Dermato(poly)myositis in neoplastic disease* 🔍
       Code first underlying neoplasm (C00-D49)

▹ **M36.1** *Arthropathy in neoplastic disease*
       Code first underlying neoplasm, such as:
           leukemia (C91-C95)
           malignant histiocytosis (C96.A)
           multiple myeloma (C90.0)

▹ **M36.2** *Hemophilic arthropathy*
       Hemarthrosis in hemophilic arthropathy
       Code first underlying disease, such as:
           factor VIII deficiency (D66)
           with vascular defect (D68.0-)
           factor IX deficiency (D67)
           hemophilia (classical) (D66)
           hemophilia B (D67)
           hemophilia C (D68.1)

▹ **M36.3** *Arthropathy in other blood disorders*
▹ **M36.4** *Arthropathy in hypersensitivity reactions classified elsewhere*
       Code first underlying disease, such as:
           Henoch (-Schönlein) purpura (D69.0)
           serum sickness (T80.6-)

▹ **M36.8** *Systemic disorders of connective tissue in other diseases classified elsewhere* 🔍
       Code first underlying disease, such as:
           alkaptonuria (E70.29)
           hypogammaglobulinemia (D80.-)
           ochronosis (E70.29)

DORSOPATHIES (M40-M54)

DEFORMING DORSOPATHIES (M40-M43)

● **M40** **Kyphosis and lordosis**
   Excludes1 congenital kyphosis and lordosis (Q76.4)
                  kyphoscoliosis (M41.-)
                  postprocedural kyphosis and lordosis (M96.-)
   Code first underlying disease

● **M40.0** **Postural kyphosis**
   Excludes1 osteochondrosis of spine (M42.-)
   M40.00 Postural kyphosis, site unspecified
   M40.03 Postural kyphosis, cervicothoracic region
   M40.04 Postural kyphosis, thoracic region
   M40.05 Postural kyphosis, thoracolumbar region

● **M40.1 Other secondary kyphosis**
   M40.10 Other secondary kyphosis, site unspecified
   M40.12 Other secondary kyphosis, cervical region
   M40.13 Other secondary kyphosis, cervicothoracic region
   M40.14 Other secondary kyphosis, thoracic region
   M40.15 Other secondary kyphosis, thoracolumbar region

● **M40.2 Other and unspecified kyphosis**
   ● **M40.20 Unspecified kyphosis**
       M40.202 Unspecified kyphosis, cervical region
       M40.203 Unspecified kyphosis, cervicothoracic region
       M40.204 Unspecified kyphosis, thoracic region
       M40.205 Unspecified kyphosis, thoracolumbar region
       M40.209 Unspecified kyphosis, site unspecified
   ● **M40.29 Other kyphosis**
       M40.292 Other kyphosis, cervical region
       M40.293 Other kyphosis, cervicothoracic region
       M40.294 Other kyphosis, thoracic region
       M40.295 Other kyphosis, thoracolumbar region
       M40.299 Other kyphosis, site unspecified

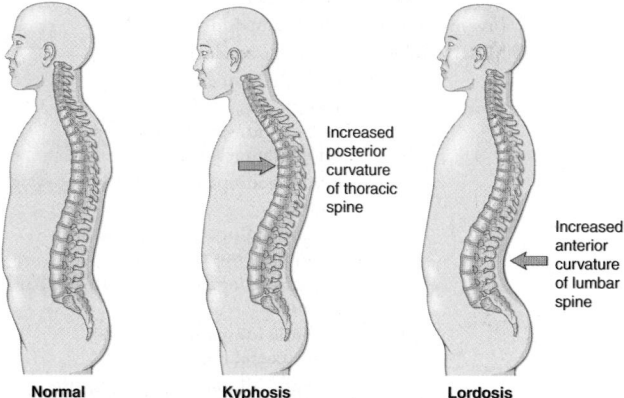

Increased posterior curvature of thoracic spine

Increased anterior curvature of lumbar spine

Normal   Kyphosis   Lordosis

Figure 13-5 Kyphosis, Lordosis, Scoliosis. (From Chabner: The Language of Medicine, ed 8, St. Louis, Saunders, 2007)

Item 13–9 **Kyphosis** is an abnormal curvature of the spine. **Senile kyphosis** is a result of disc degeneration causing ossification (turning to bone). **Adolescent** or **juvenile** kyphosis is also known as **Scheuermann's disease,** a condition in which the discs of the lower thoracic spine herniate, causing the disc space to narrow and the spine to tilt forward. This condition is attributed to poor posture. **Lordosis or swayback** is an abnormal curvature of the spine resulting in an inward curve of the lumbar spine just above the buttocks. **Scoliosis** causes a sideways curve to the spine. The curves are S- or C-shaped, and it is most commonly acquired in late childhood and early teen years, when growth is fast.

CHAPTER 13 (M00-M99)

CHAPTER 13 (M00-M99)

- **M40.3 Flatback syndrome**
  - M40.30 Flatback syndrome, site unspecified
  - M40.35 Flatback syndrome, thoracolumbar region
  - M40.36 Flatback syndrome, lumbar region
  - M40.37 Flatback syndrome, lumbosacral region
- **M40.4 Postural lordosis**
  - *Abnormal increase in the normal curvature of the lumbar spine (sway back)*
  - Acquired lordosis
  - M40.40 Postural lordosis, site unspecified
  - M40.45 Postural lordosis, thoracolumbar region
  - M40.46 Postural lordosis, lumbar region
  - M40.47 Postural lordosis, lumbosacral region
- **M40.5 Lordosis, unspecified**
  - M40.50 Lordosis, unspecified, site unspecified
  - M40.55 Lordosis, unspecified, thoracolumbar region
  - M40.56 Lordosis, unspecified, lumbar region
  - M40.57 Lordosis, unspecified, lumbosacral region

- **M41 Scoliosis**
  - **Includes** kyphoscoliosis
  - **Excludes1** congenital scoliosis NOS (Q67.5)
    congenital scoliosis due to bony malformation (Q76.3)
    postural congenital scoliosis (Q67.5)
    kyphoscoliotic heart disease (I27.1)
  - **Excludes2** postprocedural scoliosis (M96.89)
    postradiation scoliosis (M96.5)
  - **M41.0 Infantile idiopathic scoliosis**
    - M41.00 Infantile idiopathic scoliosis, site unspecified
    - M41.02 Infantile idiopathic scoliosis, cervical region
    - M41.03 Infantile idiopathic scoliosis, cervicothoracic region
    - M41.04 Infantile idiopathic scoliosis, thoracic region
    - M41.05 Infantile idiopathic scoliosis, thoracolumbar region
    - M41.06 Infantile idiopathic scoliosis, lumbar region
    - M41.07 Infantile idiopathic scoliosis, lumbosacral region
    - M41.08 Infantile idiopathic scoliosis, sacral and sacrococcygeal region
  - **M41.1 Juvenile and adolescent idiopathic scoliosis**
    - **M41.11 Juvenile idiopathic scoliosis**
      - M41.112 Juvenile idiopathic scoliosis, cervical region
      - M41.113 Juvenile idiopathic scoliosis, cervicothoracic region
      - M41.114 Juvenile idiopathic scoliosis, thoracic region
      - M41.115 Juvenile idiopathic scoliosis, thoracolumbar region
      - M41.116 Juvenile idiopathic scoliosis, lumbar region
      - M41.117 Juvenile idiopathic scoliosis, lumbosacral region
      - M41.119 Juvenile idiopathic scoliosis, site unspecified
    - **M41.12 Adolescent idiopathic scoliosis**
      - M41.122 Adolescent idiopathic scoliosis, cervical region
      - M41.123 Adolescent idiopathic scoliosis, cervicothoracic region
      - M41.124 Adolescent idiopathic scoliosis, thoracic region
      - M41.125 Adolescent idiopathic scoliosis, thoracolumbar region
        - Coding Clinic: 2024, Q1, P23
      - M41.126 Adolescent idiopathic scoliosis, lumbar region

- M41.127 Adolescent idiopathic scoliosis, lumbosacral region
- M41.129 Adolescent idiopathic scoliosis, site unspecified
- **M41.2 Other idiopathic scoliosis**
  - M41.20 Other idiopathic scoliosis, site unspecified
  - M41.22 Other idiopathic scoliosis, cervical region
  - M41.23 Other idiopathic scoliosis, cervicothoracic region
  - M41.24 Other idiopathic scoliosis, thoracic region
  - M41.25 Other idiopathic scoliosis, thoracolumbar region
  - M41.26 Other idiopathic scoliosis, lumbar region
  - M41.27 Other idiopathic scoliosis, lumbosacral region
- **M41.3 Thoracogenic scoliosis**
  - M41.30 Thoracogenic scoliosis, site unspecified
  - M41.34 Thoracogenic scoliosis, thoracic region
  - M41.35 Thoracogenic scoliosis, thoracolumbar region
- **M41.4 Neuromuscular scoliosis**
  - Scoliosis secondary to cerebral palsy, Friedreich's ataxia, poliomyelitis and other neuromuscular disorders
  - Code also underlying condition
  - M41.40 Neuromuscular scoliosis, site unspecified
  - M41.41 Neuromuscular scoliosis, occipito-atlanto-axial region
  - M41.42 Neuromuscular scoliosis, cervical region
  - M41.43 Neuromuscular scoliosis, cervicothoracic region
  - M41.44 Neuromuscular scoliosis, thoracic region
  - M41.45 Neuromuscular scoliosis, thoracolumbar region
  - M41.46 Neuromuscular scoliosis, lumbar region
  - M41.47 Neuromuscular scoliosis, lumbosacral region
- **M41.5 Other secondary scoliosis**
  - Coding Clinic: 2019, Q1, P19
  - *Code first underlying disease*
  - M41.50 Other secondary scoliosis, site unspecified
  - M41.52 Other secondary scoliosis, cervical region
  - M41.53 Other secondary scoliosis, cervicothoracic region
  - M41.54 Other secondary scoliosis, thoracic region
  - M41.55 Other secondary scoliosis, thoracolumbar region
  - M41.56 Other secondary scoliosis, lumbar region
  - M41.57 Other secondary scoliosis, lumbosacral region
- **M41.8 Other forms of scoliosis**
  - Coding Clinic: 2022, Q1, P30
  - M41.80 Other forms of scoliosis, site unspecified
  - M41.82 Other forms of scoliosis, cervical region
  - M41.83 Other forms of scoliosis, cervicothoracic region
  - M41.84 Other forms of scoliosis, thoracic region
  - M41.85 Other forms of scoliosis, thoracolumbar region
  - M41.86 Other forms of scoliosis, lumbar region
  - M41.87 Other forms of scoliosis, lumbosacral region
  - M41.9 Scoliosis, unspecified
    - Coding Clinic: 2022, Q1, P30
- **M42 Spinal osteochondrosis**
  - **M42.0 Juvenile osteochondrosis of spine**
    - Calvé's disease
    - Scheuermann's disease
    - **Excludes1** postural kyphosis (M40.0)
    - M42.00 Juvenile osteochondrosis of spine, site unspecified
    - M42.01 Juvenile osteochondrosis of spine, occipito-atlanto-axial region
    - M42.02 Juvenile osteochondrosis of spine, cervical region
    - M42.03 Juvenile osteochondrosis of spine, cervicothoracic region
    - M42.04 Juvenile osteochondrosis of spine, thoracic region

▶ New   ⇒ Revised   ~~deleted~~ Deleted   Excludes 1   Excludes 2   Includes   Use additional   Code first   Code also   Key words

OGCR Official Guidelines   X Assign placeholder X   ● Use Additional Character(s)   ▶ Manifestation Code   ⚑ Hierarchical Condition Category   Coding Clinic

M42.05 **Juvenile osteochondrosis of spine, thoracolumbar region**

M42.06 **Juvenile osteochondrosis of spine, lumbar region**

M42.07 **Juvenile osteochondrosis of spine, lumbosacral region**

M42.08 **Juvenile osteochondrosis of spine, sacral and sacrococcygeal region**

M42.09 **Juvenile osteochondrosis of spine, multiple sites in spine**

● **M42.1 Adult osteochondrosis of spine**

M42.10 **Adult osteochondrosis of spine, site unspecified**   A

M42.11 **Adult osteochondrosis of spine, occipitoatlanto-axial region**   A

M42.12 **Adult osteochondrosis of spine, cervical region**   A

M42.13 **Adult osteochondrosis of spine, cervicothoracic region**   A

M42.14 **Adult osteochondrosis of spine, thoracic region**   A

M42.15 **Adult osteochondrosis of spine, thoracolumbar region**   A

M42.16 **Adult osteochondrosis of spine, lumbar region**   A

M42.17 **Adult osteochondrosis of spine, lumbosacral region**   A

M42.18 **Adult osteochondrosis of spine, sacral and sacrococcygeal region**   A

M42.19 **Adult osteochondrosis of spine, multiple sites in spine**   A

M42.9 **Spinal osteochondrosis, unspecified**

● **M43 Other deforming dorsopathies**

  Excludes1   congenital spondylolysis and spondylolisthesis (Q76.2)
      hemivertebra (Q76.3-Q76.4)
      Klippel-Feil syndrome (Q76.1)
      lumbarization and sacralization (Q76.4)
      platyspondylisis (Q76.4)
      spina bifida occulta (Q76.0)
      spinal curvature in osteoporosis (M80.-)
      spinal curvature in Paget's disease of bone [osteitis deformans] (M88.-)

● **M43.0 Spondylolysis**

  Excludes1   congenital spondylolysis (Q76.2)
      spondylolisthesis (M43.1)
  Coding Clinic: 2023, Q3, P20

M43.00 **Spondylolysis, site unspecified**
M43.01 **Spondylolysis, occipito-atlanto-axial region**
M43.02 **Spondylolysis, cervical region**
M43.03 **Spondylolysis, cervicothoracic region**
M43.04 **Spondylolysis, thoracic region**
M43.05 **Spondylolysis, thoracolumbar region**
M43.06 **Spondylolysis, lumbar region**
M43.07 **Spondylolysis, lumbosacral region**
M43.08 **Spondylolysis, sacral and sacrococcygeal region**
M43.09 **Spondylolysis, multiple sites in spine**

● **M43.1 Spondylolisthesis**

  Excludes1   acute traumatic of lumbosacral region (S33.1)
      acute traumatic of sites other than lumbosacral - code to Fracture, vertebra, by region
      congenital spondylolisthesis (Q76.2)
  Coding Clinic: 2023, Q3, P20

M43.10 **Spondylolisthesis, site unspecified**
M43.11 **Spondylolisthesis, occipito-atlanto-axial region**
M43.12 **Spondylolisthesis, cervical region**
M43.13 **Spondylolisthesis, cervicothoracic region**
M43.14 **Spondylolisthesis, thoracic region**

M43.15 **Spondylolisthesis, thoracolumbar region**
M43.16 **Spondylolisthesis, lumbar region**
  Coding Clinic: 2024, Q1, P18
M43.17 **Spondylolisthesis, lumbosacral region**
  Coding Clinic: 2023, Q3, P20
M43.18 **Spondylolisthesis, sacral and sacrococcygeal region**
M43.19 **Spondylolisthesis, multiple sites in spine**

● **M43.2 Fusion of spine**

Ankylosis of spinal joint

  Excludes1   ankylosing spondylitis (M45.0-)
      congenital fusion of spine (Q76.4)

  Excludes2   arthrodesis status (Z98.1)
      pseudoarthrosis after fusion or arthrodesis (M96.0)

M43.20 **Fusion of spine, site unspecified**
M43.21 **Fusion of spine, occipito-atlanto-axial region**
M43.22 **Fusion of spine, cervical region**
M43.23 **Fusion of spine, cervicothoracic region**
M43.24 **Fusion of spine, thoracic region**
M43.25 **Fusion of spine, thoracolumbar region**
M43.26 **Fusion of spine, lumbar region**
M43.27 **Fusion of spine, lumbosacral region**
M43.28 **Fusion of spine, sacral and sacrococcygeal region**

M43.3 **Recurrent atlantoaxial dislocation with myelopathy**
M43.4 **Other recurrent atlantoaxial dislocation**

● **M43.5 Other recurrent vertebral dislocation**

  Excludes1   biomechanical lesions NEC (M99.-)

● **M43.5X Other recurrent vertebral dislocation**

M43.5X2 **Other recurrent vertebral dislocation, cervical region**
M43.5X3 **Other recurrent vertebral dislocation, cervicothoracic region**
M43.5X4 **Other recurrent vertebral dislocation, thoracic region**
M43.5X5 **Other recurrent vertebral dislocation, thoracolumbar region**
M43.5X6 **Other recurrent vertebral dislocation, lumbar region**
M43.5X7 **Other recurrent vertebral dislocation, lumbosacral region**
M43.5X8 **Other recurrent vertebral dislocation, sacral and sacrococcygeal region**
M43.5X9 **Other recurrent vertebral dislocation, site unspecified**

M43.6 **Torticollis**

  Excludes1   congenital (sternomastoid) torticollis (Q68.0)
      current injury - see Injury, of spine, by body region ocular torticollis (R29.891)
      psychogenic torticollis (F45.8)
      spasmodic torticollis (G24.3)
      torticollis due to birth injury (P15.2)

● **M43.8 Other specified deforming dorsopathies**

  Excludes2   kyphosis and lordosis (M40.-)
      scoliosis (M41.-)

● **M43.8X Other specified deforming dorsopathies**

M43.8X1 **Other specified deforming dorsopathies, occipito-atlanto-axial region**
M43.8X2 **Other specified deforming dorsopathies, cervical region**
M43.8X3 **Other specified deforming dorsopathies, cervicothoracic region**
M43.8X4 **Other specified deforming dorsopathies, thoracic region**
M43.8X5 **Other specified deforming dorsopathies, thoracolumbar region**
M43.8X6 **Other specified deforming dorsopathies, lumbar region**
M43.8X7 **Other specified deforming dorsopathies, lumbosacral region**

Item 13-10 Spondylolisthesis is a condition caused by the slipping forward of one disc over another.

CHAPTER 13 (M00-M99)

CHAPTER 13 (M00-M99)

M43.8X8   Other specified deforming dorsopathies, sacral and sacrococcygeal region

M43.8X9   Other specified deforming dorsopathies, site unspecified

M43.9   Deforming dorsopathy, unspecified
Curvature of spine NOS

SPONDYLOPATHIES (M45-M49)

● M45   Ankylosing spondylitis
Rheumatoid arthritis of spine

Excludes1   arthropathy in Reiter's disease (M02.3-)
juvenile (ankylosing) spondylitis (M08.1)

Excludes2   Behçet's disease (M35.2)

M45.0   Ankylosing spondylitis of multiple sites in spine 🔴

M45.1   Ankylosing spondylitis of occipito-atlanto-axial region 🔴

M45.2   Ankylosing spondylitis of cervical region 🔴

M45.3   Ankylosing spondylitis of cervicothoracic region 🔴

M45.4   Ankylosing spondylitis of thoracic region 🔴

M45.5   Ankylosing spondylitis of thoracolumbar region 🔴

M45.6   Ankylosing spondylitis lumbar region 🔴

M45.7   Ankylosing spondylitis of lumbosacral region 🔴

M45.8   Ankylosing spondylitis sacral and sacrococcygeal region 🔴

M45.9   Ankylosing spondylitis of unspecified sites in spine 🔴

● M45.A   Non-radiographic axial spondyloarthritis

M45.A0   Non-radiographic axial spondyloarthritis of unspecified sites in spine

M45.A1   Non-radiographic axial spondyloarthritis of occipito-atlanto-axial region

M45.A2   Non-radiographic axial spondyloarthritis of cervical region

M45.A3   Non-radiographic axial spondyloarthritis of cervicothoracic region

M45.A4   Non-radiographic axial spondyloarthritis of thoracic region

M45.A5   Non-radiographic axial spondyloarthritis of thoracolumbar region

M45.A6   Non-radiographic axial spondyloarthritis of lumbar region

M45.A7   Non-radiographic axial spondyloarthritis of lumbosacral region

M45.A8   Non-radiographic axial spondyloarthritis of sacral and sacrococcygeal region

M45.AB   Non-radiographic axial spondyloarthritis of multiple sites in spine

● M46   Other inflammatory spondylopathies

● M46.0   Spinal enthesopathy
Disorder of ligamentous or muscular attachments of spine

M46.00   Spinal enthesopathy, site unspecified 🔴

M46.01   Spinal enthesopathy, occipito-atlanto-axial region 🔴

M46.02   Spinal enthesopathy, cervical region 🔴

M46.03   Spinal enthesopathy, cervicothoracic region 🔴

M46.04   Spinal enthesopathy, thoracic region 🔴

M46.05   Spinal enthesopathy, thoracolumbar region 🔴

M46.06   Spinal enthesopathy, lumbar region 🔴

M46.07   Spinal enthesopathy, lumbosacral region 🔴

M46.08   Spinal enthesopathy, sacral and sacrococcygeal region 🔴

M46.09   Spinal enthesopathy, multiple sites in spine 🔴

M46.1   Sacroiliitis, not elsewhere classified 🔴

● M46.2   Osteomyelitis of vertebra

M46.20   Osteomyelitis of vertebra, site unspecified 🔴

M46.21   Osteomyelitis of vertebra, occipito-atlanto-axial region 🔴

M46.22   Osteomyelitis of vertebra, cervical region 🔴

M46.23   Osteomyelitis of vertebra, cervicothoracic region 🔴

M46.24   Osteomyelitis of vertebra, thoracic region 🔴

M46.25   Osteomyelitis of vertebra, thoracolumbar region 🔴

M46.26   Osteomyelitis of vertebra, lumbar region 🔴

M46.27   Osteomyelitis of vertebra, lumbosacral region 🔴

M46.28   Osteomyelitis of vertebra, sacral and sacrococcygeal region 🔴

● M46.3   Infection of intervertebral disc (pyogenic)
Use additional code (B95-B97) to identify infectious agent

M46.30   Infection of intervertebral disc (pyogenic), site unspecified 🔴

M46.31   Infection of intervertebral disc (pyogenic), occipito-atlanto-axial region 🔴

M46.32   Infection of intervertebral disc (pyogenic), cervical region 🔴

M46.33   Infection of intervertebral disc (pyogenic), cervicothoracic region 🔴

M46.34   Infection of intervertebral disc (pyogenic), thoracic region 🔴

M46.35   Infection of intervertebral disc (pyogenic), thoracolumbar region 🔴

M46.36   Infection of intervertebral disc (pyogenic), lumbar region 🔴

M46.37   Infection of intervertebral disc (pyogenic), lumbosacral region 🔴

M46.38   Infection of intervertebral disc (pyogenic), sacral and sacrococcygeal region 🔴

M46.39   Infection of intervertebral disc (pyogenic), multiple sites in spine 🔴

● M46.4   Discitis, unspecified

M46.40   Discitis, unspecified, site unspecified

M46.41   Discitis, unspecified, occipito-atlanto-axial region

M46.42   Discitis, unspecified, cervical region

M46.43   Discitis, unspecified, cervicothoracic region

M46.44   Discitis, unspecified, thoracic region

M46.45   Discitis, unspecified, thoracolumbar region

M46.46   Discitis, unspecified, lumbar region

M46.47   Discitis, unspecified, lumbosacral region

M46.48   Discitis, unspecified, sacral and sacrococcygeal region

M46.49   Discitis, unspecified, multiple sites in spine

● M46.5   Other infective spondylopathies

M46.50   Other infective spondylopathies, site unspecified 🔴

M46.51   Other infective spondylopathies, occipitoatlanto-axial region 🔴

M46.52   Other infective spondylopathies, cervical region 🔴

M46.53   Other infective spondylopathies, cervicothoracic region 🔴

M46.54   Other infective spondylopathies, thoracic region 🔴

M46.55   Other infective spondylopathies, thoracolumbar region 🔴

M46.56   Other infective spondylopathies, lumbar region 🔴

M46.57   Other infective spondylopathies, lumbosacral region 🔴

M46.58   Other infective spondylopathies, sacral and sacrococcygeal region 🔴

M46.59   Other infective spondylopathies, multiple sites in spine 🔴

● M46.8   Other specified inflammatory spondylopathies

M46.80   Other specified inflammatory spondylopathies, site unspecified 🔴

M46.81   Other specified inflammatory spondylopathies, occipito-atlanto-axial region 🔴

▶ New   ⇒ Revised   ~~deleted~~ Deleted   Excludes 1   Excludes 2   Includes   Use additional   Code first   Code also   Key words

1000   OGCR Official Guidelines   X Assign placeholder X   ● Use Additional Character(s)   ▷ Manifestation Code   🔴 Hierarchical Condition Category   Coding Clinic

M46.82   Other specified inflammatory spondylopathies, cervical region 🔒

M46.83   Other specified inflammatory spondylopathies, cervicothoracic region 🔒

M46.84   Other specified inflammatory spondylopathies, thoracic region 🔒

M46.85   Other specified inflammatory spondylopathies, thoracolumbar region 🔒

M46.86   Other specified inflammatory spondylopathies, lumbar region 🔒

M46.87   Other specified inflammatory spondylopathies, lumbosacral region 🔒

M46.88   Other specified inflammatory spondylopathies, sacral and sacrococcygeal region 🔒

M46.89   Other specified inflammatory spondylopathies, multiple sites in spine 🔒

● M46.9   Unspecified inflammatory spondylopathy

M46.90   Unspecified inflammatory spondylopathy, site unspecified 🔒

M46.91   Unspecified inflammatory spondylopathy, occipito-atlanto-axial region 🔒

M46.92   Unspecified inflammatory spondylopathy, cervical region 🔒
     Coding Clinic: 2019, Q3, P10

M46.93   Unspecified inflammatory spondylopathy, cervicothoracic region 🔒

M46.94   Unspecified inflammatory spondylopathy, thoracic region 🔒

M46.95   Unspecified inflammatory spondylopathy, thoracolumbar region 🔒

M46.96   Unspecified inflammatory spondylopathy, lumbar region 🔒

M46.97   Unspecified inflammatory spondylopathy, lumbosacral region 🔒

M46.98   Unspecified inflammatory spondylopathy, sacral and sacrococcygeal region 🔒

M46.99   Unspecified inflammatory spondylopathy, multiple sites in spine 🔒

● M47   Spondylosis

Includes   arthrosis or osteoarthritis of spine
degeneration of facet joints

● M47.0   Anterior spinal and vertebral artery compression syndromes
     Coding Clinic: 2019, Q3, P10

● M47.01   Anterior spinal artery compression syndromes

M47.011   Anterior spinal artery compression syndromes, occipito-atlanto-axial region

M47.012   Anterior spinal artery compression syndromes, cervical region
     Coding Clinic: 2023, Q1, P37

M47.013   Anterior spinal artery compression syndromes, cervicothoracic region

M47.014   Anterior spinal artery compression syndromes, thoracic region

M47.015   Anterior spinal artery compression syndromes, thoracolumbar region

M47.016   Anterior spinal artery compression syndromes, lumbar region

M47.019   Anterior spinal artery compression syndromes, site unspecified

● M47.02   Vertebral artery compression syndromes

M47.021   Vertebral artery compression syndromes, occipito-atlanto-axial region

M47.022   Vertebral artery compression syndromes, cervical region
     Coding Clinic: 2023, Q1, P37

M47.029   Vertebral artery compression syndromes, site unspecified

● M47.1   Other spondylosis with myelopathy
Spondylogenic compression of spinal cord
Excludes1   vertebral subluxation (M43.3-M43.5X9)

M47.10   Other spondylosis with myelopathy, site unspecified

M47.11   Other spondylosis with myelopathy, occipito-atlanto-axial region

M47.12   Other spondylosis with myelopathy, cervical region
     Coding Clinic: 2020, Q1, P17

M47.13   Other spondylosis with myelopathy, cervicothoracic region

M47.14   Other spondylosis with myelopathy, thoracic region

M47.15   Other spondylosis with myelopathy, thoracolumbar region

M47.16   Other spondylosis with myelopathy, lumbar region

● M47.2   Other spondylosis with radiculopathy

M47.20   Other spondylosis with radiculopathy, site unspecified

M47.21   Other spondylosis with radiculopathy, occipito-atlanto-axial region

M47.22   Other spondylosis with radiculopathy, cervical region
     Coding Clinic: 2020, Q1, P17

M47.23   Other spondylosis with radiculopathy, cervicothoracic region

M47.24   Other spondylosis with radiculopathy, thoracic region

M47.25   Other spondylosis with radiculopathy, thoracolumbar region

M47.26   Other spondylosis with radiculopathy, lumbar region

M47.27   Other spondylosis with radiculopathy, lumbosacral region

M47.28   Other spondylosis with radiculopathy, sacral and sacrococcygeal region

● M47.8   Other spondylosis

● M47.81   Spondylosis without myelopathy or radiculopathy

M47.811   Spondylosis without myelopathy or radiculopathy, occipito-atlanto-axial region

M47.812   Spondylosis without myelopathy or radiculopathy, cervical region
     Coding Clinic: 2019, Q3, P10-11; 2018, Q2, P15

M47.813   Spondylosis without myelopathy or radiculopathy, cervicothoracic region

M47.814   Spondylosis without myelopathy or radiculopathy, thoracic region

M47.815   Spondylosis without myelopathy or radiculopathy, thoracolumbar region

M47.816   Spondylosis without myelopathy or radiculopathy, lumbar region

M47.817   Spondylosis without myelopathy or radiculopathy, lumbosacral region

M47.818   Spondylosis without myelopathy or radiculopathy, sacral and sacrococcygeal region

M47.819   Spondylosis without myelopathy or radiculopathy, site unspecified

● M47.89   Other spondylosis

M47.891   Other spondylosis, occipito-atlanto-axial region

M47.892   Other spondylosis, cervical region

M47.893   Other spondylosis, cervicothoracic region

M47.894   Other spondylosis, thoracic region

CHAPTER 13 (M00-M99)

        M47.895   Other spondylosis, thoracolumbar region

        M47.896   Other spondylosis, lumbar region

        M47.897   Other spondylosis, lumbosacral region

        M47.898   Other spondylosis, sacral and sacrococcygeal region

        M47.899   Other spondylosis, site unspecified

    M47.9   Spondylosis, unspecified

● **M48   Other spondylopathies**

  ● **M48.0   Spinal stenosis**
        Caudal stenosis

    M48.00   Spinal stenosis, site unspecified

    M48.01   Spinal stenosis, occipito-atlanto-axial region

    M48.02   Spinal stenosis, cervical region
        Coding Clinic: 2020, Q1, P17

    M48.03   Spinal stenosis, cervicothoracic region

    M48.04   Spinal stenosis, thoracic region

    M48.05   Spinal stenosis, thoracolumbar region

  ● M48.06   Spinal stenosis, lumbar region
        Coding Clinic: 2017, Q3, P24

        M48.061   Spinal stenosis, lumbar region without neurogenic claudication
            Spinal stenosis, lumbar region NOS

        M48.062   Spinal stenosis, lumbar region with neurogenic claudication
            Coding Clinic: 2017, Q4, P19

    M48.07   Spinal stenosis, lumbosacral region

    M48.08   Spinal stenosis, sacral and sacrococcygeal region

  ● **M48.1   Ankylosing hyperostosis [Forestier]**
        Diffuse idiopathic skeletal hyperostosis [DISH]

    M48.10   Ankylosing hyperostosis [Forestier], site unspecified

    M48.11   Ankylosing hyperostosis [Forestier], occipito-atlanto-axial region

    M48.12   Ankylosing hyperostosis [Forestier], cervical region

    M48.13   Ankylosing hyperostosis [Forestier], cervicothoracic region

    M48.14   Ankylosing hyperostosis [Forestier], thoracic region

    M48.15   Ankylosing hyperostosis [Forestier], thoracolumbar region

    M48.16   Ankylosing hyperostosis [Forestier], lumbar region

    M48.17   Ankylosing hyperostosis [Forestier], lumbosacral region

    M48.18   Ankylosing hyperostosis [Forestier], sacral and sacrococcygeal region

    M48.19   Ankylosing hyperostosis [Forestier], multiple sites in spine

  ● **M48.2   Kissing spine**

    M48.20   Kissing spine, site unspecified

    M48.21   Kissing spine, occipito-atlanto-axial region

    M48.22   Kissing spine, cervical region

    M48.23   Kissing spine, cervicothoracic region

    M48.24   Kissing spine, thoracic region

    M48.25   Kissing spine, thoracolumbar region

    M48.26   Kissing spine, lumbar region

    M48.27   Kissing spine, lumbosacral region

  ● **M48.3   Traumatic spondylopathy**

    M48.30   Traumatic spondylopathy, site unspecified

    M48.31   Traumatic spondylopathy, occipito-atlanto-axial region

    M48.32   Traumatic spondylopathy, cervical region

    M48.33   Traumatic spondylopathy, cervicothoracic region

    M48.34   Traumatic spondylopathy, thoracic region

    M48.35   Traumatic spondylopathy, thoracolumbar region

    M48.36   Traumatic spondylopathy, lumbar region

    M48.37   Traumatic spondylopathy, lumbosacral region

    M48.38   Traumatic spondylopathy, sacral and sacrococcygeal region

● **M48.4   Fatigue fracture of vertebra**
    Stress fracture of vertebra

> **Excludes1**   pathological fracture NOS (M84.4-)
> pathological fracture of vertebra due to neoplasm (M84.58)
> pathological fracture of vertebra due to other diagnosis (M84.68)
> pathological fracture of vertebra due to osteoporosis (M80.-)
> traumatic fracture of vertebrae (S12.0-S12.3-, S22.0-, S32.0-)

The appropriate 7th character is to be added to each code from subcategory M48.4:

> A   initial encounter for fracture
> D   subsequent encounter for fracture with routine healing
> G   subsequent encounter for fracture with delayed healing
> S   sequela of fracture

  X● M48.40   Fatigue fracture of vertebra, site unspecified

  X● M48.41   Fatigue fracture of vertebra, occipitoatlanto-axial region

  X● M48.42   Fatigue fracture of vertebra, cervical region

  X● M48.43   Fatigue fracture of vertebra, cervicothoracic region

  X● M48.44   Fatigue fracture of vertebra, thoracic region

  X● M48.45   Fatigue fracture of vertebra, thoracolumbar region

  X● M48.46   Fatigue fracture of vertebra, lumbar region

  X● M48.47   Fatigue fracture of vertebra, lumbosacral region

  X● M48.48   Fatigue fracture of vertebra, sacral and sacrococcygeal region

● **M48.5   Collapsed vertebra, not elsewhere classified**
    Collapsed vertebra NOS
    Compression fracture of vertebra NOS
    Wedging of vertebra NOS

> **Excludes1**   current injury - see Injury of spine, by body region
> fatigue fracture of vertebra (M48.4)
> pathological fracture of vertebra due to neoplasm (M84.58)
> pathological fracture of vertebra due to other diagnosis (M84.68)
> pathological fracture of vertebra due to osteoporosis (M80.-)
> pathological fracture NOS (M84.4-)
> stress fracture of vertebra (M48.4-)
> traumatic fracture of vertebra (S12.-, S22.-, S32.-)

The appropriate 7th character is to be added to each code from subcategory M48.5:

> A   initial encounter for fracture
> D   subsequent encounter for fracture with routine healing
> G   subsequent encounter for fracture with delayed healing
> S   sequela of fracture

  X● M48.50   Collapsed vertebra, not elsewhere classified, site unspecified A 🐾

  X● M48.51   Collapsed vertebra, not elsewhere classified, occipito-atlanto-axial region A 🐾

▶ New   ⇒ Revised   ~~deleted~~ Deleted   Excludes 1   Excludes 2   Includes   Use additional   Code first   Code also   Key words

OGCR Official Guidelines   X Assign placeholder X   ● Use Additional Character(s)   ▶ Manifestation Code   🐾 Hierarchical Condition Category   Coding Clinic

X ● M48.52 **Collapsed vertebra, not elsewhere classified, cervical region** A 🔖

X ● M48.53 **Collapsed vertebra, not elsewhere classified, cervicothoracic region** A 🔖

X ● M48.54 **Collapsed vertebra, not elsewhere classified, thoracic region** A 🔖

X ● M48.55 **Collapsed vertebra, not elsewhere classified, thoracolumbar region** A 🔖

X ● M48.56 **Collapsed vertebra, not elsewhere classified, lumbar region** A 🔖

X ● M48.57 **Collapsed vertebra, not elsewhere classified, lumbosacral region** A 🔖

X ● M48.58 **Collapsed vertebra, not elsewhere classified, sacral and sacrococcygeal region** A 🔖

● M48.8 **Other specified spondylopathies**
Ossification of posterior longitudinal ligament

● M48.8X **Other specified spondylopathies**

M48.8X1 **Other specified spondylopathies, occipito-atlanto-axial region** 🔖

M48.8X2 **Other specified spondylopathies, cervical region** 🔖

M48.8X3 **Other specified spondylopathies, cervicothoracic region** 🔖

M48.8X4 **Other specified spondylopathies, thoracic region** 🔖

M48.8X5 **Other specified spondylopathies, thoracolumbar region** 🔖

M48.8X6 **Other specified spondylopathies, lumbar region** 🔖

M48.8X7 **Other specified spondylopathies, lumbosacral region** 🔖

M48.8X8 **Other specified spondylopathies, sacral and sacrococcygeal region** 🔖

M48.8X9 **Other specified spondylopathies, site unspecified** 🔖

M48.9 **Spondylopathy, unspecified**

● M49 **Spondylopathies in diseases classified elsewhere**

Includes curvature of spine in diseases classified elsewhere
deformity of spine in diseases classified elsewhere
kyphosis in diseases classified elsewhere
scoliosis in diseases classified elsewhere
spondylopathy in diseases classified elsewhere

Code first underlying disease, such as:
brucellosis (A23.-)
Charcot-Marie-Tooth disease (G60.0)
enterobacterial infections (A01-A04)
osteitis fibrosa cystica (E21.0)

Excludes1 curvature of spine in tuberculosis [Pott's] (A18.01)
enteropathic arthropathies (M07.-)
gonococcal spondylitis (A54.41)
neuropathic [tabes dorsalis] spondylitis (A52.11)
neuropathic spondylopathy in syringomyelia (G95.0)
neuropathic spondylopathy in tabes dorsalis (A52.11)
nonsyphilitic neuropathic spondylopathy NEC (G98.0)
spondylitis in syphilis (acquired) (A52.77)
tuberculous spondylitis (A18.01)
typhoid fever spondylitis (A01.05)

● M49.8 **Spondylopathy in diseases classified elsewhere**

❯ *M49.80 Spondylopathy in diseases classified elsewhere, site unspecified* 🔖

❯ *M49.81 Spondylopathy in diseases classified elsewhere, occipito-atlanto-axial region* 🔖

❯ *M49.82 Spondylopathy in diseases classified elsewhere, cervical region* 🔖

❯ *M49.83 Spondylopathy in diseases classified elsewhere, cervicothoracic region* 🔖

❯ *M49.84 Spondylopathy in diseases classified elsewhere, thoracic region* 🔖

❯ *M49.85 Spondylopathy in diseases classified elsewhere, thoracolumbar region* 🔖

❯ *M49.86 Spondylopathy in diseases classified elsewhere, lumbar region* 🔖

❯ *M49.87 Spondylopathy in diseases classified elsewhere, lumbosacral region* 🔖

❯ *M49.88 Spondylopathy in diseases classified elsewhere, sacral and sacrococcygeal region* 🔖

❯ *M49.89 Spondylopathy in diseases classified elsewhere, multiple sites in spine* 🔖

OTHER DORSOPATHIES (M50-M54)

Excludes1 current injury - see injury of spine by body region
discitis NOS (M46.4-)

● M50 **Cervical disc disorders**

Includes cervicothoracic disc disorders with cervicalgia
cervicothoracic disc disorders
Coding Clinic: 2016, Q1, P17

● M50.0 **Cervical disc disorder with myelopathy**

M50.00 **Cervical disc disorder with myelopathy, unspecified cervical region**

M50.01 **Cervical disc disorder with myelopathy, high cervical region**
C2-C3 disc disorder with myelopathy
C3-C4 disc disorder with myelopathy
Coding Clinic: 2016, Q1, P17

● M50.02 **Cervical disc disorder with myelopathy, mid-cervical region**
Coding Clinic: 2016, Q4, P39-40

M50.020 **Cervical disc disorder with myelopathy, mid-cervical region, unspecified level**

M50.021 **Cervical disc disorder at C4-C5 level with myelopathy**
C4-C5 disc disorder with myelopathy

M50.022 **Cervical disc disorder at C5-C6 level with myelopathy**
C5-C6 disc disorder with myelopathy

M50.023 **Cervical disc disorder at C6-C7 level with myelopathy**
C6-C7 disc disorder with myelopathy

M50.03 **Cervical disc disorder with myelopathy, cervicothoracic region**
C7-T1 disc disorder with myelopathy

● M50.1 **Cervical disc disorder with radiculopathy**

Excludes2 brachial radiculitis NOS (M54.13)

M50.10 **Cervical disc disorder with radiculopathy, unspecified cervical region**

M50.11 **Cervical disc disorder with radiculopathy, high cervical region**
C2-C3 disc disorder with radiculopathy
C3 radiculopathy due to disc disorder
C3-C4 disc disorder with radiculopathy
C4 radiculopathy due to disc disorder

● M50.12 **Cervical disc disorder with radiculopathy, mid-cervical region**
Coding Clinic: 2016, Q4, P39-40

M50.120 **Mid-cervical disc disorder, unspecified level**

M50.121 **Cervical disc disorder at C4-C5 level with radiculopathy**
C4-C5 disc disorder with radiculopathy
C5 radiculopathy due to disc disorder

M50.122 **Cervical disc disorder at C5-C6 level with radiculopathy**
  C5-C6 disc disorder with radiculopathy
  C6 radiculopathy due to disc disorder

M50.123 **Cervical disc disorder at C6-C7 level with radiculopathy**
  C6-C7 disc disorder with radiculopathy
  C7 radiculopathy due to disc disorder

M50.13 **Cervical disc disorder with radiculopathy, cervicothoracic region**
  C7-T1 disc disorder with radiculopathy
  C8 radiculopathy due to disc disorder

● M50.2 **Other cervical disc displacement**
  Coding Clinic: 2016, Q4, P40

M50.20 **Other cervical disc displacement, unspecified cervical region**

M50.21 **Other cervical disc displacement, high cervical region**
  Other C2-C3 cervical disc displacement
  Other C3-C4 cervical disc displacement
  Coding Clinic: 2021, Q4, P12

● M50.22 **Other cervical disc displacement, mid-cervical region**

M50.220 **Other cervical disc displacement, mid-cervical region, unspecified level**

M50.221 **Other cervical disc displacement at C4-C5 level**
  Other C4-C5 cervical disc displacement

M50.222 **Other cervical disc displacement at C5-C6 level**
  Other C5-C6 cervical disc displacement

M50.223 **Other cervical disc displacement at C6-C7 level**
  Other C6-C7 cervical disc displacement

M50.23 **Other cervical disc displacement, cervicothoracic region**
  Other C7-T1 cervical disc displacement

● M50.3 **Other cervical disc degeneration**
  Coding Clinic: 2016, Q4, P40

M50.30 **Other cervical disc degeneration, unspecified cervical region**

M50.31 **Other cervical disc degeneration, high cervical region**
  Other C2-C3 cervical disc degeneration
  Other C3-C4 cervical disc degeneration

● M50.32 **Other cervical disc degeneration, mid-cervical region**

M50.320 **Other cervical disc degeneration, mid-cervical region, unspecified level**

M50.321 **Other cervical disc degeneration at C4-C5 level**
  Other C4-C5 cervical disc degeneration

M50.322 **Other cervical disc degeneration at C5-C6 level**
  Other C5-C6 cervical disc degeneration

M50.323 **Other cervical disc degeneration at C6-C7 level**
  Other C6-C7 cervical disc degeneration

M50.33 **Other cervical disc degeneration, cervicothoracic region**
  Other C7-T1 cervical disc degeneration

● M50.8 **Other cervical disc disorders**
  Coding Clinic: 2016, Q4, P40

M50.80 **Other cervical disc disorders, unspecified cervical region**

M50.81 **Other cervical disc disorders, high cervical region**
  Other C2-C3 cervical disc disorders
  Other C3-C4 cervical disc disorders

● M50.82 **Other cervical disc disorders, mid-cervical region**

M50.820 **Other cervical disc disorders, mid-cervical region, unspecified level**

M50.821 **Other cervical disc disorders at C4-C5 level**
  Other C4-C5 cervical disc disorders

M50.822 **Other cervical disc disorders at C5-C6 level**
  Other C5-C6 cervical disc disorders

M50.823 **Other cervical disc disorders at C6-C7 level**
  Other C6-C7 cervical disc disorders

M50.83 **Other cervical disc disorders, cervicothoracic region**
  Other C7-T1 cervical disc disorders

● M50.9 **Cervical disc disorder, unspecified**
  Coding Clinic: 2016, Q4, P40

M50.90 **Cervical disc disorder, unspecified, unspecified cervical region**

M50.91 **Cervical disc disorder, unspecified, high cervical region**
  C2-C3 cervical disc disorder, unspecified
  C3-C4 cervical disc disorder, unspecified

● M50.92 **Cervical disc disorder, unspecified, mid-cervical region**

M50.920 **Unspecified cervical disc disorder, mid-cervical region, unspecified level**

M50.921 **Unspecified cervical disc disorder at C4-C5 level**
  Unspecified C4-C5 cervical disc disorder

M50.922 **Unspecified cervical disc disorder at C5-C6 level**
  Unspecified C5-C6 cervical disc disorder

M50.923 **Unspecified cervical disc disorder at C6-C7 level**
  Unspecified C6-C7 cervical disc disorder

M50.93 **Cervical disc disorder, unspecified, cervicothoracic region**
  C7-T1 cervical disc disorder, unspecified

● M51 **Thoracic, thoracolumbar, and lumbosacral intervertebral disc disorders**

  Excludes2 cervical and cervicothoracic disc disorders (M50.-)
  sacral and sacrococcygeal disorders (M53.3)

● M51.0 **Thoracic, thoracolumbar and lumbosacral intervertebral disc disorders with myelopathy**

M51.04 **Intervertebral disc disorders with myelopathy, thoracic region**

M51.05 **Intervertebral disc disorders with myelopathy, thoracolumbar region**

M51.06 **Intervertebral disc disorders with myelopathy, lumbar region**

● **M51.1** **Thoracic, thoracolumbar and lumbosacral intervertebral disc disorders with radiculopathy**
Sciatica due to intervertebral disc disorder

     Excludes1   lumbar radiculitis NOS (M54.16)
                sciatica NOS (M54.3)

     M51.14 **Intervertebral disc disorders with radiculopathy, thoracic region**

     M51.15 **Intervertebral disc disorders with radiculopathy, thoracolumbar region**

     M51.16 **Intervertebral disc disorders with radiculopathy, lumbar region**

     M51.17 **Intervertebral disc disorders with radiculopathy, lumbosacral region**

● **M51.2** **Other thoracic, thoracolumbar and lumbosacral intervertebral disc displacement**
Lumbago due to displacement of intervertebral disc

     M51.24 **Other intervertebral disc displacement, thoracic region**

     M51.25 **Other intervertebral disc displacement, thoracolumbar region**

     M51.26 **Other intervertebral disc displacement, lumbar region**

     M51.27 **Other intervertebral disc displacement, lumbosacral region**

● **M51.3** **Other thoracic, thoracolumbar and lumbosacral intervertebral disc degeneration**
     Coding Clinic: 2013, Q3, P22

     M51.34 **Other intervertebral disc degeneration, thoracic region**

     M51.35 **Other intervertebral disc degeneration, thoracolumbar region**

     M51.36 **Other intervertebral disc degeneration, lumbar region**
         Coding Clinic: 2018, Q2, P15

         ▶**M51.360** **Other intervertebral disc degeneration, lumbar region with discogenic back pain only**
             ▶Other intervertebral disc degeneration, lumbar region with axial back pain only

         ▶**M51.361** **Other intervertebral disc degeneration, lumbar region with lower extremity pain only**
             ▶Other intervertebral disc degeneration, lumbar region with leg pain only
             ▶Other intervertebral disc degeneration, lumbar region with referred sclerotomal pain only

         ▶**M51.362** **Other intervertebral disc degeneration, lumbar region with discogenicback pain and lower extremity pain**
             ▶Other intervertebral disc degeneration, lumbar region with discogenic back pain and leg pain
             ▶Other intervertebral disc degeneration, lumbar region with axial back pain and referred sclerotomal pain

         ▶**M51.369** **Other intervertebral disc degeneration, lumbar region without mention of lumbar back pain or lower extremity pain**
             ▶Other intervertebral disc degeneration, lumbar region without mention of lumbar back pain or leg pain
             ▶Other intervertebral disc degeneration, lumbar region, NOS

     M51.37 **Other intervertebral disc degeneration, lumbosacral region**
         Coding Clinic: 2022, Q1, P26

         ▶**M51.370** **Other intervertebral disc degeneration, lumbosacral region with discogenic back pain only**
             ▶Other intervertebral disc degeneration, lumbosacral region with axial back pain only

         ▶**M51.371** **Other intervertebral disc degeneration, lumbosacral region with lower extremity pain only**
             ▶Other intervertebral disc degeneration, lumbosacral region with leg pain only
             ▶Other intervertebral disc degeneration, lumbosacral region with referred sclerotomal pain only

         ▶**M51.372** **Other intervertebral disc degeneration, lumbosacral region with discogenic back pain and lower extremity pain**
             ▶Other intervertebral disc degeneration, lumbosacral region with discogenic backpain and leg pain
             ▶Other intervertebral disc degeneration, lumbosacral region with axial back pain and referred sclerotomal pain

         ▶**M51.379** **Other intervertebral disc degeneration, lumbosacral region without mention of lumbar back pain or lower extremity pain**
             ▶Other intervertebral disc degeneration, lumbosacral region without mention of lumbar back pain or leg pain
             ▶Other intervertebral disc degeneration, lumbosacral region, NOS

● **M51.4** **Schmorl's nodes**

     M51.44 **Schmorl's nodes, thoracic region**

     M51.45 **Schmorl's nodes, thoracolumbar region**

     M51.46 **Schmorl's nodes, lumbar region**

     M51.47 **Schmorl's nodes, lumbosacral region**

● **M51.8** **Other thoracic, thoracolumbar and lumbosacral intervertebral disc disorders**

     M51.84 **Other intervertebral disc disorders, thoracic region**

     M51.85 **Other intervertebral disc disorders, thoracolumbar region**

     M51.86 **Other intervertebral disc disorders, lumbar region**

     M51.87 **Other intervertebral disc disorders, lumbosacral region**

     M51.9 **Unspecified thoracic, thoracolumbar and lumbosacral intervertebral disc disorder**

● **M51.A** **Other lumbar and lumbosacral annulus fibrosus disc defects**

     M51.A0 **Intervertebral annulus fibrosus defect, lumbar region, unspecified size**
         Code first, if applicable, lumbar disc herniation (M51.06, M51.16, M51.26)

     M51.A1 **Intervertebral annulus fibrosus defect, small, lumbar region**
         Code first, if applicable, lumbar disc herniation (M51.06, M51.16, M51.26)

     M51.A2 **Intervertebral annulus fibrosus defect, large, lumbar region**
         Code first, if applicable, lumbar disc herniation (M51.06, M51.16, M51.26)

CHAPTER 13 (M00-M99)

M51.A3   Intervertebral annulus fibrosus defect, lumbosacral region, unspecified size

     Code first, if applicable, lumbosacral disc herniation (M51.17, M51.27)

M51.A4   Intervertebral annulus fibrosus defect, small, lumbosacral region

     Code first, if applicable, lumbosacral disc herniation (M51.17, M51.27)

M51.A5   Intervertebral annulus fibrosus defect, large, lumbosacral region

     Code first, if applicable, lumbosacral disc herniation (M51.17, M51.27)

● **M53   Other and unspecified dorsopathies, not elsewhere classified**

   M53.0   Cervicocranial syndrome
     Posterior cervical sympathetic syndrome

   M53.1   Cervicobrachial syndrome
     Excludes2   cervical disc disorder (M50.-)
               thoracic outlet syndrome (G54.0)

  ● **M53.2   Spinal instabilities**

   ● **M53.2X   Spinal instabilities**

     M53.2X1   Spinal instabilities, occipito-atlanto-axial region

     M53.2X2   Spinal instabilities, cervical region

     M53.2X3   Spinal instabilities, cervicothoracic region

     M53.2X4   Spinal instabilities, thoracic region

     M53.2X5   Spinal instabilities, thoracolumbar region

     M53.2X6   Spinal instabilities, lumbar region

     M53.2X7   Spinal instabilities, lumbosacral region

     M53.2X8   Spinal instabilities, sacral and sacrococcygeal region

     M53.2X9   Spinal instabilities, site unspecified

   M53.3   Sacrococcygeal disorders, not elsewhere classified
     Coccygodynia

  ● **M53.8   Other specified dorsopathies**

     M53.80   Other specified dorsopathies, site unspecified

     M53.81   Other specified dorsopathies, occipito-atlanto-axial region

     M53.82   Other specified dorsopathies, cervical region

     M53.83   Other specified dorsopathies, cervicothoracic region

     M53.84   Other specified dorsopathies, thoracic region

     M53.85   Other specified dorsopathies, thoracolumbar region

     M53.86   Other specified dorsopathies, lumbar region

     M53.87   Other specified dorsopathies, lumbosacral region

     M53.88   Other specified dorsopathies, sacral and sacrococcygeal region

   M53.9   Dorsopathy, unspecified

● **M54   Dorsalgia**
   Excludes1   psychogenic dorsalgia (F45.41)

  ● **M54.0   Panniculitis affecting regions of neck and back**
     Excludes1   lupus panniculitis (L93.2)
               panniculitis NOS (M79.3)
               relapsing [Weber-Christian] panniculitis (M35.6)

     M54.00   Panniculitis affecting regions of neck and back, site unspecified

     M54.01   Panniculitis affecting regions of neck and back, occipito-atlanto-axial region

     M54.02   Panniculitis affecting regions of neck and back, cervical region

     M54.03   Panniculitis affecting regions of neck and back, cervicothoracic region

     M54.04   Panniculitis affecting regions of neck and back, thoracic region

     M54.05   Panniculitis affecting regions of neck and back, thoracolumbar region

     M54.06   Panniculitis affecting regions of neck and back, lumbar region

     M54.07   Panniculitis affecting regions of neck and back, lumbosacral region

     M54.08   Panniculitis affecting regions of neck and back, sacral and sacrococcygeal region

     M54.09   Panniculitis affecting regions, neck and back, multiple sites in spine

  ● **M54.1   Radiculopathy**
     Brachial neuritis or radiculitis NOS
     Lumbar neuritis or radiculitis NOS
     Lumbosacral neuritis or radiculitis NOS
     Thoracic neuritis or radiculitis NOS
     Radiculitis NOS

     Excludes1   neuralgia and neuritis NOS (M79.2)
               radiculopathy with cervical disc disorder (M50.1)
               radiculopathy with lumbar and other intervertebral disc disorder (M51.1-)
               radiculopathy with spondylosis (M47.2-)

     M54.10   Radiculopathy, site unspecified

     M54.11   Radiculopathy, occipito-atlanto-axial region

     M54.12   Radiculopathy, cervical region

     M54.13   Radiculopathy, cervicothoracic region

     M54.14   Radiculopathy, thoracic region

     M54.15   Radiculopathy, thoracolumbar region

     M54.16   Radiculopathy, lumbar region

     M54.17   Radiculopathy, lumbosacral region

     M54.18   Radiculopathy, sacral and sacrococcygeal region

   M54.2   Cervicalgia
     Excludes1   cervicalgia due to intervertebral cervical disc disorder (M50.-)

  ● **M54.3   Sciatica**
     ▶ **Excludes1**   intervertebral disc degeneration, lumbar region with lower extremity pain only (M51.361)
            ▶ intervertebral disc degeneration, lumbosacral region with lower extremity pain only (M51.371)
            lesion of sciatic nerve (G57.0)
            sciatica due to intervertebral disc disorder (M51.1-)
            sciatica with lumbago (M54.4-)

     M54.30   Sciatica, unspecified side

     M54.31   Sciatica, right side

     M54.32   Sciatica, left side

  ● **M54.4   Lumbago with sciatica**
     ▶ **Excludes1**   intervertebral disc degeneration, lumbar region with discogenic back pain and lower extremity pain (M51.362)
            ▶ intervertebral disc degeneration, lumbosacral region with discogenic back pain and lower extremity pain (M51.372)
            lumbago with sciatica due to intervertebral disc disorder (M51.1-)

     M54.40   Lumbago with sciatica, unspecified side

     M54.41   Lumbago with sciatica, right side

     M54.42   Lumbago with sciatica, left side
       Coding Clinic: 2016, Q2, P7

▶ New   ⇒ Revised   ~~deleted~~ Deleted   Excludes 1   Excludes 2   Includes   Use additional   Code first   Code also   Key words

OGCR Official Guidelines   X Assign placeholder X   ● Use Additional Character(s)   ▶ Manifestation Code   🔖 Hierarchical Condition Category   Coding Clinic

● M54.5 **Low back pain**
  ▶ **Excludes1**   intervertebral disc degeneration, lumbar
                  region with discogenic back pain
                  only (M51.360)
              ▶ intervertebral disc degeneration,
                  lumbosacral region with discogenic
                  back pain only (M51.370)
                low back strain (S39.012)
                lumbago due to intervertebral disc
                  displacement (M51.2-)
                lumbago with sciatica (M54.4-)

  M54.50 **Low back pain, unspecified**
          Loin pain
          Lumbago NOS
  M54.51 **Vertebrogenic low back pain**
          Low back vertebral endplate pain
          Coding Clinic: 2021, Q4, P22
  M54.59 **Other low back pain**
● M54.6 **Pain in thoracic spine**
      Excludes1   pain in thoracic spine due to
                  intervertebral disc disorder (M51.)
● M54.8 **Other dorsalgia**
      Excludes1   dorsalgia in thoracic region (M54.6)
                  low back pain (M54.5-)
  M54.81 **Occipital neuralgia**
  M54.89 **Other dorsalgia**
● M54.9 **Dorsalgia, unspecified**
          Backache NOS
          Back pain NOS

SOFT TISSUE DISORDERS (M60-M79)

DISORDERS OF MUSCLES (M60-M63)

  Excludes1   dermatopolymyositis (M33.-)
              muscular dystrophies and myopathies (G71-G72)
              myopathy in amyloidosis (E85.-)
              myopathy in polyarteritis nodosa (M30.0)
              myopathy in rheumatoid arthritis (M05.32)
              myopathy in scleroderma (M34.-)
              myopathy in Sjögren's syndrome (M35.03)
              myopathy in systemic lupus erythematosus (M32.-)

● M60 **Myositis**
      Excludes2   inclusion body myositis [IBM] (G72.41)
● M60.0 **Infective myositis**
          Tropical pyomyositis
          Use additional code (B95-B97) to identify infectious
              agent
  ● M60.00 **Infective myositis, unspecified site**
      M60.000 **Infective myositis, unspecified right
               arm**
                Infective myositis, right upper limb
                  NOS
      M60.001 **Infective myositis, unspecified left
               arm**
                Infective myositis, left upper limb
                  NOS
      M60.002 **Infective myositis, unspecified arm**
                Infective myositis, upper limb NOS
      M60.003 **Infective myositis, unspecified right
               leg**
                Infective myositis, right lower limb
                  NOS
      M60.004 **Infective myositis, unspecified left leg**
                Infective myositis, left lower limb
                  NOS
      M60.005 **Infective myositis, unspecified leg**
                Infective myositis, lower limb NOS
      M60.009 **Infective myositis, unspecified site**

● M60.01 **Infective myositis, shoulder**
      M60.011 Infective myositis, **right shoulder**
      M60.012 Infective myositis, **left shoulder**
      M60.019 Infective myositis, **unspecified
               shoulder**
● M60.02 **Infective myositis, upper arm**
      M60.021 Infective myositis, **right upper arm**
      M60.022 Infective myositis, **left upper arm**
      M60.029 Infective myositis, **unspecified upper
               arm**
● M60.03 **Infective myositis, forearm**
      M60.031 Infective myositis, **right forearm**
      M60.032 Infective myositis, **left forearm**
      M60.039 Infective myositis, **unspecified
               forearm**
● M60.04 **Infective myositis, hand and fingers**
      M60.041 Infective myositis, **right hand**
      M60.042 Infective myositis, **left hand**
      M60.043 Infective myositis, **unspecified hand**
      M60.044 Infective myositis, **right finger(s)**
      M60.045 Infective myositis, **left finger(s)**
      M60.046 Infective myositis, **unspecified
               finger(s)**
● M60.05 **Infective myositis, thigh**
      M60.051 Infective myositis, **right thigh**
      M60.052 Infective myositis, **left thigh**
      M60.059 Infective myositis, **unspecified thigh**
● M60.06 **Infective myositis, lower leg**
      M60.061 Infective myositis, **right lower leg**
      M60.062 Infective myositis, **left lower leg**
      M60.069 Infective myositis, **unspecified lower
               leg**
● M60.07 **Infective myositis, ankle, foot and toes**
      M60.070 Infective myositis, **right ankle**
      M60.071 Infective myositis, **left ankle**
      M60.072 Infective myositis, **unspecified ankle**
      M60.073 Infective myositis, **right foot**
      M60.074 Infective myositis, **left foot**
      M60.075 Infective myositis, **unspecified foot**
      M60.076 Infective myositis, **right toe(s)**
      M60.077 Infective myositis, **left toe(s)**
      M60.078 Infective myositis, **unspecified toe(s)**
  M60.08 Infective myositis, **other site**
  M60.09 Infective myositis, **multiple sites**
● M60.1 **Interstitial myositis**
  M60.10 Interstitial myositis of **unspecified site**
● M60.11 **Interstitial myositis, shoulder**
      M60.111 Interstitial myositis, **right shoulder**
      M60.112 Interstitial myositis, **left shoulder**
      M60.119 Interstitial myositis, **unspecified
               shoulder**
● M60.12 **Interstitial myositis, upper arm**
      M60.121 Interstitial myositis, **right upper arm**
      M60.122 Interstitial myositis, **left upper arm**
      M60.129 Interstitial myositis, **unspecified
               upper arm**
● M60.13 **Interstitial myositis, forearm**
      M60.131 Interstitial myositis, **right forearm**
      M60.132 Interstitial myositis, **left forearm**
      M60.139 Interstitial myositis, **unspecified
               forearm**
● M60.14 **Interstitial myositis, hand**
      M60.141 Interstitial myositis, **right hand**
      M60.142 Interstitial myositis, **left hand**
      M60.149 Interstitial myositis, **unspecified hand**

● M60.15 Interstitial myositis, thigh
   M60.151 Interstitial myositis, right thigh
   M60.152 Interstitial myositis, left thigh
   M60.159 Interstitial myositis, unspecified thigh
● M60.16 Interstitial myositis, lower leg
   M60.161 Interstitial myositis, right lower leg
   M60.162 Interstitial myositis, left lower leg
   M60.169 Interstitial myositis, unspecified lower leg
● M60.17 Interstitial myositis, ankle and foot
   M60.171 Interstitial myositis, right ankle and foot
   M60.172 Interstitial myositis, left ankle and foot
   M60.179 Interstitial myositis, unspecified ankle and foot
  M60.18 Interstitial myositis, other site
  M60.19 Interstitial myositis, multiple sites
● M60.2 Foreign body granuloma of soft tissue, not elsewhere classified
   Use additional code to identify the type of retained foreign body (Z18.-)
   Excludes1 foreign body granuloma of skin and subcutaneous tissue (L92.3)
  M60.20 Foreign body granuloma of soft tissue, not elsewhere classified, unspecified site
● M60.21 Foreign body granuloma of soft tissue, not elsewhere classified, shoulder
   M60.211 Foreign body granuloma of soft tissue, not elsewhere classified, right shoulder
   M60.212 Foreign body granuloma of soft tissue, not elsewhere classified, left shoulder
   M60.219 Foreign body granuloma of soft tissue, not elsewhere classified, unspecified shoulder
● M60.22 Foreign body granuloma of soft tissue, not elsewhere classified, upper arm
   M60.221 Foreign body granuloma of soft tissue, not elsewhere classified, right upper arm
   M60.222 Foreign body granuloma of soft tissue, not elsewhere classified, left upper arm
   M60.229 Foreign body granuloma of soft tissue, not elsewhere classified, unspecified upper arm
● M60.23 Foreign body granuloma of soft tissue, not elsewhere classified, forearm
   M60.231 Foreign body granuloma of soft tissue, not elsewhere classified, right forearm
   M60.232 Foreign body granuloma of soft tissue, not elsewhere classified, left forearm
   M60.239 Foreign body granuloma of soft tissue, not elsewhere classified, unspecified forearm
● M60.24 Foreign body granuloma of soft tissue, not elsewhere classified, hand
   M60.241 Foreign body granuloma of soft tissue, not elsewhere classified, right hand
   M60.242 Foreign body granuloma of soft tissue, not elsewhere classified, left hand
   M60.249 Foreign body granuloma of soft tissue, not elsewhere classified, unspecified hand

● M60.25 Foreign body granuloma of soft tissue, not elsewhere classified, thigh
   M60.251 Foreign body granuloma of soft tissue, not elsewhere classified, right thigh
   M60.252 Foreign body granuloma of soft tissue, not elsewhere classified, left thigh
   M60.259 Foreign body granuloma of soft tissue, not elsewhere classified, unspecified thigh
● M60.26 Foreign body granuloma of soft tissue, not elsewhere classified, lower leg
   M60.261 Foreign body granuloma of soft tissue, not elsewhere classified, right lower leg
   M60.262 Foreign body granuloma of soft tissue, not elsewhere classified, left lower leg
   M60.269 Foreign body granuloma of soft tissue, not elsewhere classified, unspecified lower leg
● M60.27 Foreign body granuloma of soft tissue, not elsewhere classified, ankle and foot
   M60.271 Foreign body granuloma of soft tissue, not elsewhere classified, right ankle and foot
   M60.272 Foreign body granuloma of soft tissue, not elsewhere classified, left ankle and foot
   M60.279 Foreign body granuloma of soft tissue, not elsewhere classified, unspecified ankle and foot
  M60.28 Foreign body granuloma of soft tissue, not elsewhere classified, other site
● M60.8 Other myositis
  M60.80 Other myositis, unspecified site
● M60.81 Other myositis shoulder
   M60.811 Other myositis, right shoulder
   M60.812 Other myositis, left shoulder
   M60.819 Other myositis, unspecified shoulder
● M60.82 Other myositis, upper arm
   M60.821 Other myositis, right upper arm
   M60.822 Other myositis, left upper arm
   M60.829 Other myositis, unspecified upper arm
● M60.83 Other myositis, forearm
   M60.831 Other myositis, right forearm
   M60.832 Other myositis, left forearm
   M60.839 Other myositis, unspecified forearm
● M60.84 Other myositis, hand
   M60.841 Other myositis, right hand
   M60.842 Other myositis, left hand
   M60.849 Other myositis, unspecified hand
● M60.85 Other myositis, thigh
   M60.851 Other myositis, right thigh
   M60.852 Other myositis, left thigh
   M60.859 Other myositis, unspecified thigh
● M60.86 Other myositis, lower leg
   M60.861 Other myositis, right lower leg
   M60.862 Other myositis, left lower leg
   M60.869 Other myositis, unspecified lower leg
● M60.87 Other myositis, ankle and foot
   M60.871 Other myositis, right ankle and foot
   M60.872 Other myositis, left ankle and foot
   M60.879 Other myositis, unspecified ankle and foot
  M60.88 Other myositis, other site
  M60.89 Other myositis, multiple sites
M60.9 Myositis, unspecified

▶ New ⇒ Revised ~~deleted~~ Deleted Excludes 1 Excludes 2 Includes Use additional Code first Code also Key words
OGCR Official Guidelines X Assign placeholder X ● Use Additional Character(s) ▶ Manifestation Code 🐾 Hierarchical Condition Category **Coding Clinic**

● **M61   Calcification and ossification of muscle**
   ● **M61.0   Myositis ossificans traumatica**
       M61.00   Myositis ossificans traumatica, unspecified site
     ● M61.01   Myositis ossificans traumatica, shoulder
          M61.011   Myositis ossificans traumatica, right shoulder
          M61.012   Myositis ossificans traumatica, left shoulder
          M61.019   Myositis ossificans traumatica, unspecified shoulder
     ● M61.02   Myositis ossificans traumatica, upper arm
          M61.021   Myositis ossificans traumatica, right upper arm
          M61.022   Myositis ossificans traumatica, left upper arm
          M61.029   Myositis ossificans traumatica, unspecified upper arm
     ● M61.03   Myositis ossificans traumatica, forearm
          M61.031   Myositis ossificans traumatica, right forearm
          M61.032   Myositis ossificans traumatica, left forearm
          M61.039   Myositis ossificans traumatica, unspecified forearm
     ● M61.04   Myositis ossificans traumatica, hand
          M61.041   Myositis ossificans traumatica, right hand
          M61.042   Myositis ossificans traumatica, left hand
          M61.049   Myositis ossificans traumatica, unspecified hand
     ● M61.05   Myositis ossificans traumatica, thigh
          M61.051   Myositis ossificans traumatica, right thigh
          M61.052   Myositis ossificans traumatica, left thigh
          M61.059   Myositis ossificans traumatica, unspecified thigh
     ● M61.06   Myositis ossificans traumatica, lower leg
          M61.061   Myositis ossificans traumatica, right lower leg
          M61.062   Myositis ossificans traumatica, left lower leg
          M61.069   Myositis ossificans traumatica, unspecified lower leg
     ● M61.07   Myositis ossificans traumatica, ankle and foot
          M61.071   Myositis ossificans traumatica, right ankle and foot
          M61.072   Myositis ossificans traumatica, left ankle and foot
          M61.079   Myositis ossificans traumatica, unspecified ankle and foot
       M61.08   Myositis ossificans traumatica, other site
       M61.09   Myositis ossificans traumatica, multiple sites
   ● **M61.1   Myositis ossificans progressiva**
       Fibrodysplasia ossificans progressiva
       M61.10   Myositis ossificans progressiva, unspecified site
     ● M61.11   Myositis ossificans progressiva, shoulder
          M61.111   Myositis ossificans progressiva, right shoulder
          M61.112   Myositis ossificans progressiva, left shoulder
          M61.119   Myositis ossificans progressiva, unspecified shoulder

   ● M61.12   Myositis ossificans progressiva, upper arm
          M61.121   Myositis ossificans progressiva, right upper arm
          M61.122   Myositis ossificans progressiva, left upper arm
          M61.129   Myositis ossificans progressiva, unspecified arm
   ● M61.13   Myositis ossificans progressiva, forearm
          M61.131   Myositis ossificans progressiva, right forearm
          M61.132   Myositis ossificans progressiva, left forearm
          M61.139   Myositis ossificans progressiva, unspecified forearm
   ● M61.14   Myositis ossificans progressiva, hand and finger(s)
          M61.141   Myositis ossificans progressiva, right hand
          M61.142   Myositis ossificans progressiva, left hand
          M61.143   Myositis ossificans progressiva, unspecified hand
          M61.144   Myositis ossificans progressiva, right finger(s)
          M61.145   Myositis ossificans progressiva, left finger(s)
          M61.146   Myositis ossificans progressiva, unspecified finger(s)
   ● M61.15   Myositis ossificans progressiva, thigh
          M61.151   Myositis ossificans progressiva, right thigh
          M61.152   Myositis ossificans progressiva, left thigh
          M61.159   Myositis ossificans progressiva, unspecified thigh
   ● M61.16   Myositis ossificans progressiva, lower leg
          M61.161   Myositis ossificans progressiva, right lower leg
          M61.162   Myositis ossificans progressiva, left lower leg
          M61.169   Myositis ossificans progressiva, unspecified lower leg
   ● M61.17   Myositis ossificans progressiva, ankle, foot and toe(s)
          M61.171   Myositis ossificans progressiva, right ankle
          M61.172   Myositis ossificans progressiva, left ankle
          M61.173   Myositis ossificans progressiva, unspecified ankle
          M61.174   Myositis ossificans progressiva, right foot
          M61.175   Myositis ossificans progressiva, left foot
          M61.176   Myositis ossificans progressiva, unspecified foot
          M61.177   Myositis ossificans progressiva, right toe(s)
          M61.178   Myositis ossificans progressiva, left toe(s)
          M61.179   Myositis ossificans progressiva, unspecified toe(s)
       M61.18   Myositis ossificans progressiva, other site
       M61.19   Myositis ossificans progressiva, multiple sites

CHAPTER 13 (M00-M99)

● **M61.2 Paralytic calcification and ossification of muscle**
Myositis ossificans associated with quadriplegia or paraplegia

    M61.20 Paralytic calcification and ossification of muscle, unspecified site

    ● **M61.21** Paralytic calcification and ossification of muscle, shoulder

        M61.211 Paralytic calcification and ossification of muscle, right shoulder

        M61.212 Paralytic calcification and ossification of muscle, left shoulder

        M61.219 Paralytic calcification and ossification of muscle, unspecified shoulder

    ● **M61.22** Paralytic calcification and ossification of muscle, upper arm

        M61.221 Paralytic calcification and ossification of muscle, right upper arm

        M61.222 Paralytic calcification and ossification of muscle, left upper arm

        M61.229 Paralytic calcification and ossification of muscle, unspecified upper arm

    ● **M61.23** Paralytic calcification and ossification of muscle, forearm

        M61.231 Paralytic calcification and ossification of muscle, right forearm

        M61.232 Paralytic calcification and ossification of muscle, left forearm

        M61.239 Paralytic calcification and ossification of muscle, unspecified forearm

    ● **M61.24** Paralytic calcification and ossification of muscle, hand

        M61.241 Paralytic calcification and ossification of muscle, right hand

        M61.242 Paralytic calcification and ossification of muscle, left hand

        M61.249 Paralytic calcification and ossification of muscle, unspecified hand

    ● **M61.25** Paralytic calcification and ossification of muscle, thigh

        M61.251 Paralytic calcification and ossification of muscle, right thigh

        M61.252 Paralytic calcification and ossification of muscle, left thigh

        M61.259 Paralytic calcification and ossification of muscle, unspecified thigh

    ● **M61.26** Paralytic calcification and ossification of muscle, lower leg

        M61.261 Paralytic calcification and ossification of muscle, right lower leg

        M61.262 Paralytic calcification and ossification of muscle, left lower leg

        M61.269 Paralytic calcification and ossification of muscle, unspecified lower leg

    ● **M61.27** Paralytic calcification and ossification of muscle, ankle and foot

        M61.271 Paralytic calcification and ossification of muscle, right ankle and foot

        M61.272 Paralytic calcification and ossification of muscle, left ankle and foot

        M61.279 Paralytic calcification and ossification of muscle, unspecified ankle and foot

    M61.28 Paralytic calcification and ossification of muscle, other site

    M61.29 Paralytic calcification and ossification of muscle, multiple sites

● **M61.3 Calcification and ossification of muscles associated with burns**
Myositis ossificans associated with burns

    M61.30 Calcification and ossification of muscles associated with burns, unspecified site

    ● **M61.31** Calcification and ossification of muscles associated with burns, shoulder

        M61.311 Calcification and ossification of muscles associated with burns, right shoulder

        M61.312 Calcification and ossification of muscles associated with burns, left shoulder

        M61.319 Calcification and ossification of muscles associated with burns, unspecified shoulder

    ● **M61.32** Calcification and ossification of muscles associated with burns, upper arm

        M61.321 Calcification and ossification of muscles associated with burns, right upper arm

        M61.322 Calcification and ossification of muscles associated with burns, left upper arm

        M61.329 Calcification and ossification of muscles associated with burns, unspecified upper arm

    ● **M61.33** Calcification and ossification of muscles associated with burns, forearm

        M61.331 Calcification and ossification of muscles associated with burns, right forearm

        M61.332 Calcification and ossification of muscles associated with burns, left forearm

        M61.339 Calcification and ossification of muscles associated with burns, unspecified forearm

    ● **M61.34** Calcification and ossification of muscles associated with burns, hand

        M61.341 Calcification and ossification of muscles associated with burns, right hand

        M61.342 Calcification and ossification of muscles associated with burns, left hand

        M61.349 Calcification and ossification of muscles associated with burns, unspecified hand

    ● **M61.35** Calcification and ossification of muscles associated with burns, thigh

        M61.351 Calcification and ossification of muscles associated with burns, right thigh

        M61.352 Calcification and ossification of muscles associated with burns, left thigh

        M61.359 Calcification and ossification of muscles associated with burns, unspecified thigh

    ● **M61.36** Calcification and ossification of muscles associated with burns, lower leg

        M61.361 Calcification and ossification of muscles associated with burns, right lower leg

        M61.362 Calcification and ossification of muscles associated with burns, left lower leg

        M61.369 Calcification and ossification of muscles associated with burns, unspecified lower leg

    ● **M61.37** Calcification and ossification of muscles associated with burns, ankle and foot

        M61.371 Calcification and ossification of muscles associated with burns, right ankle and foot

M61.372 Calcification and ossification of muscles associated with burns, left ankle and foot

M61.379 Calcification and ossification of muscles associated with burns, unspecified ankle and foot

M61.38 Calcification and ossification of muscles associated with burns, other site

M61.39 Calcification and ossification of muscles associated with burns, multiple sites

● M61.4 Other calcification of muscle

> Excludes1   calcific tendinitis NOS (M65.2-)
> calcific tendinitis of shoulder (M75.3)

M61.40 Other calcification of muscle, unspecified site

● M61.41 Other calcification of muscle, shoulder

M61.411 Other calcification of muscle, right shoulder

M61.412 Other calcification of muscle, left shoulder

M61.419 Other calcification of muscle, unspecified shoulder

● M61.42 Other calcification of muscle, upper arm

M61.421 Other calcification of muscle, right upper arm

M61.422 Other calcification of muscle, left upper arm

M61.429 Other calcification of muscle, unspecified upper arm

● M61.43 Other calcification of muscle, forearm

M61.431 Other calcification of muscle, right forearm

M61.432 Other calcification of muscle, left forearm

M61.439 Other calcification of muscle, unspecified forearm

● M61.44 Other calcification of muscle, hand

M61.441 Other calcification of muscle, right hand

M61.442 Other calcification of muscle, left hand

M61.449 Other calcification of muscle, unspecified hand

● M61.45 Other calcification of muscle, thigh

M61.451 Other calcification of muscle, right thigh

M61.452 Other calcification of muscle, left thigh

M61.459 Other calcification of muscle, unspecified thigh

● M61.46 Other calcification of muscle, lower leg

M61.461 Other calcification of muscle, right lower leg

M61.462 Other calcification of muscle, left lower leg

M61.469 Other calcification of muscle, unspecified lower leg

● M61.47 Other calcification of muscle, ankle and foot

M61.471 Other calcification of muscle, right ankle and foot

M61.472 Other calcification of muscle, left ankle and foot

M61.479 Other calcification of muscle, unspecified ankle and foot

M61.48 Other calcification of muscle, other site

M61.49 Other calcification of muscle, multiple sites

● M61.5 Other ossification of muscle

M61.50 Other ossification of muscle, unspecified site

● M61.51 Other ossification of muscle, shoulder

M61.511 Other ossification of muscle, right shoulder

M61.512 Other ossification of muscle, left shoulder

M61.519 Other ossification of muscle, unspecified shoulder

● M61.52 Other ossification of muscle, upper arm

M61.521 Other ossification of muscle, right upper arm

M61.522 Other ossification of muscle, left upper arm

M61.529 Other ossification of muscle, unspecified upper arm

● M61.53 Other ossification of muscle, forearm

M61.531 Other ossification of muscle, right forearm

M61.532 Other ossification of muscle, left forearm

M61.539 Other ossification of muscle, unspecified forearm

● M61.54 Other ossification of muscle, hand

M61.541 Other ossification of muscle, right hand

M61.542 Other ossification of muscle, left hand

M61.549 Other ossification of muscle, unspecified hand

● M61.55 Other ossification of muscle, thigh

M61.551 Other ossification of muscle, right thigh

M61.552 Other ossification of muscle, left thigh

M61.559 Other ossification of muscle, unspecified thigh

● M61.56 Other ossification of muscle, lower leg

M61.561 Other ossification of muscle, right lower leg

M61.562 Other ossification of muscle, left lower leg

M61.569 Other ossification of muscle, unspecified lower leg

● M61.57 Other ossification of muscle, ankle and foot

M61.571 Other ossification of muscle, right ankle and foot

M61.572 Other ossification of muscle, left ankle and foot

M61.579 Other ossification of muscle, unspecified ankle and foot

M61.58 Other ossification of muscle, other site

M61.59 Other ossification of muscle, multiple sites

M61.9 Calcification and ossification of muscle, unspecified

● M62 Other disorders of muscle

> Excludes1   alcoholic myopathy (G72.1)
> cramp and spasm (R25.2)
> drug-induced myopathy (G72.0)
> myalgia (M79.1-)
> stiff-man syndrome (G25.82)

> Excludes2   nontraumatic hematoma of muscle (M79.81)

● M62.0 Separation of muscle (nontraumatic)
Diastasis of muscle

> Excludes1   diastasis recti complicating pregnancy, labor and delivery (O71.8)
> traumatic separation of muscle - see strain of muscle by body region

M62.00 Separation of muscle (nontraumatic), unspecified site

● M62.01 Separation of muscle (nontraumatic), shoulder

    M62.011   Separation of muscle (nontraumatic), right shoulder

    M62.012   Separation of muscle (nontraumatic), left shoulder

    M62.019   Separation of muscle (nontraumatic), unspecified shoulder

● M62.02   Separation of muscle (nontraumatic), upper arm

    M62.021   Separation of muscle (nontraumatic), right upper arm

    M62.022   Separation of muscle (nontraumatic), left upper arm

    M62.029   Separation of muscle (nontraumatic), unspecified upper arm

● M62.03   Separation of muscle (nontraumatic), forearm

    M62.031   Separation of muscle (nontraumatic), right forearm

    M62.032   Separation of muscle (nontraumatic), left forearm

    M62.039   Separation of muscle (nontraumatic), unspecified forearm

● M62.04   Separation of muscle (nontraumatic), hand

    M62.041   Separation of muscle (nontraumatic), right hand

    M62.042   Separation of muscle (nontraumatic), left hand

    M62.049   Separation of muscle (nontraumatic), unspecified hand

● M62.05   Separation of muscle (nontraumatic), thigh

    M62.051   Separation of muscle (nontraumatic), right thigh

    M62.052   Separation of muscle (nontraumatic), left thigh

    M62.059   Separation of muscle (nontraumatic), unspecified thigh

● M62.06   Separation of muscle (nontraumatic), lower leg

    M62.061   Separation of muscle (nontraumatic), right lower leg

    M62.062   Separation of muscle (nontraumatic), left lower leg

    M62.069   Separation of muscle (nontraumatic), unspecified lower leg

● M62.07   Separation of muscle (nontraumatic), ankle and foot

    M62.071   Separation of muscle (nontraumatic), right ankle and foot

    M62.072   Separation of muscle (nontraumatic), left ankle and foot

    M62.079   Separation of muscle (nontraumatic), unspecified ankle and foot

M62.08   Separation of muscle (nontraumatic), other site

● M62.1   Other rupture of muscle (nontraumatic)

    Excludes1   traumatic rupture of muscle - see strain of muscle by body region

    Excludes2   rupture of tendon (M66.-)

M62.10   Other rupture of muscle (nontraumatic), unspecified site

● M62.11   Other rupture of muscle (nontraumatic), shoulder

    M62.111   Other rupture of muscle (nontraumatic), right shoulder

    M62.112   Other rupture of muscle (nontraumatic), left shoulder

    M62.119   Other rupture of muscle (nontraumatic), unspecified shoulder

● M62.12   Other rupture of muscle (nontraumatic), upper arm

    M62.121   Other rupture of muscle (nontraumatic), right upper arm

    M62.122   Other rupture of muscle (nontraumatic), left upper arm

    M62.129   Other rupture of muscle (nontraumatic), unspecified upper arm

● M62.13   Other rupture of muscle (nontraumatic), forearm

    M62.131   Other rupture of muscle (nontraumatic), right forearm

    M62.132   Other rupture of muscle (nontraumatic), left forearm

    M62.139   Other rupture of muscle (nontraumatic), unspecified forearm

● M62.14   Other rupture of muscle (nontraumatic), hand

    M62.141   Other rupture of muscle (nontraumatic), right hand

    M62.142   Other rupture of muscle (nontraumatic), left hand

    M62.149   Other rupture of muscle (nontraumatic), unspecified hand

● M62.15   Other rupture of muscle (nontraumatic), thigh

    M62.151   Other rupture of muscle (nontraumatic), right thigh

    M62.152   Other rupture of muscle (nontraumatic), left thigh

    M62.159   Other rupture of muscle (nontraumatic), unspecified thigh

● M62.16   Other rupture of muscle (nontraumatic), lower leg

    M62.161   Other rupture of muscle (nontraumatic), right lower leg

    M62.162   Other rupture of muscle (nontraumatic), left lower leg

    M62.169   Other rupture of muscle (nontraumatic), unspecified lower leg

● M62.17   Other rupture of muscle (nontraumatic), ankle and foot

    M62.171   Other rupture of muscle (nontraumatic), right ankle and foot

    M62.172   Other rupture of muscle (nontraumatic), left ankle and foot

    M62.179   Other rupture of muscle (nontraumatic), unspecified ankle and foot

M62.18   Other rupture of muscle (nontraumatic), other site

● M62.2   Nontraumatic ischemic infarction of muscle

    Excludes1   compartment syndrome (traumatic) (T79.A-)
          nontraumatic compartment syndrome (M79.A-)
          traumatic ischemia of muscle (T79.6)
          rhabdomyolysis (M62.82)
          Volkmann's ischemic contracture (T79.6)

M62.20   Nontraumatic ischemic infarction of muscle, unspecified site

● M62.21   Nontraumatic ischemic infarction of muscle, shoulder

    M62.211   Nontraumatic ischemic infarction of muscle, right shoulder

    M62.212   Nontraumatic ischemic infarction of muscle, left shoulder

    M62.219   Nontraumatic ischemic infarction of muscle, unspecified shoulder

● M62.22   Nontraumatic ischemic infarction of muscle, upper arm

    M62.221   Nontraumatic ischemic infarction of muscle, right upper arm

    M62.222   Nontraumatic ischemic infarction of muscle, left upper arm

    M62.229   Nontraumatic ischemic infarction of muscle, unspecified upper arm

▶ New   ⇒ Revised   ~~deleted~~ Deleted   Excludes 1   Excludes 2   Includes   Use additional   Code first   Code also   Key words

OGCR Official Guidelines   X Assign placeholder X   ● Use Additional Character(s)   ▶ Manifestation Code   🏷 Hierarchical Condition Category   Coding Clinic

● **M62.23**   Nontraumatic ischemic infarction of muscle, forearm

     M62.231   Nontraumatic ischemic infarction of muscle, right forearm

     M62.232   Nontraumatic ischemic infarction of muscle, left forearm

     M62.239   Nontraumatic ischemic infarction of muscle, unspecified forearm

● **M62.24**   Nontraumatic ischemic infarction of muscle, hand

     M62.241   Nontraumatic ischemic infarction of muscle, right hand

     M62.242   Nontraumatic ischemic infarction of muscle, left hand

     M62.249   Nontraumatic ischemic infarction of muscle, unspecified hand

● **M62.25**   Nontraumatic ischemic infarction of muscle, thigh

     M62.251   Nontraumatic ischemic infarction of muscle, right thigh

     M62.252   Nontraumatic ischemic infarction of muscle, left thigh

     M62.259   Nontraumatic ischemic infarction of muscle, unspecified thigh

● **M62.26**   Nontraumatic ischemic infarction of muscle, lower leg

     M62.261   Nontraumatic ischemic infarction of muscle, right lower leg

     M62.262   Nontraumatic ischemic infarction of muscle, left lower leg

     M62.269   Nontraumatic ischemic infarction of muscle, unspecified lower leg

● **M62.27**   Nontraumatic ischemic infarction of muscle, ankle and foot

     M62.271   Nontraumatic ischemic infarction of muscle, right ankle and foot

     M62.272   Nontraumatic ischemic infarction of muscle, left ankle and foot

     M62.279   Nontraumatic ischemic infarction of muscle, unspecified ankle and foot

   M62.28   Nontraumatic ischemic infarction of muscle, other site

   M62.3   Immobility syndrome (paraplegic)

   M62.4   Contracture of muscle

     Contracture of tendon (sheath)

     Excludes1   contracture of joint (M24.5-)

   M62.40   Contracture of muscle, unspecified site

● **M62.41**   Contracture of muscle, shoulder

     M62.411   Contracture of muscle, right shoulder

     M62.412   Contracture of muscle, left shoulder

     M62.419   Contracture of muscle, unspecified shoulder

● **M62.42**   Contracture of muscle, upper arm

     M62.421   Contracture of muscle, right upper arm

     M62.422   Contracture of muscle, left upper arm

     M62.429   Contracture of muscle, unspecified upper arm

● **M62.43**   Contracture of muscle, forearm

     M62.431   Contracture of muscle, right forearm

     M62.432   Contracture of muscle, left forearm

     M62.439   Contracture of muscle, unspecified forearm

● **M62.44**   Contracture of muscle, hand

     M62.441   Contracture of muscle, right hand

     M62.442   Contracture of muscle, left hand

     M62.449   Contracture of muscle, unspecified hand

● **M62.45**   Contracture of muscle, thigh

     M62.451   Contracture of muscle, right thigh

     M62.452   Contracture of muscle, left thigh

     M62.459   Contracture of muscle, unspecified thigh

● **M62.46**   Contracture of muscle, lower leg

     M62.461   Contracture of muscle, right lower leg

     M62.462   Contracture of muscle, left lower leg
       Coding Clinic: 2023, Q2, P14

     M62.469   Contracture of muscle, unspecified lower leg

● **M62.47**   Contracture of muscle, ankle and foot

     M62.471   Contracture of muscle, right ankle and foot

     M62.472   Contracture of muscle, left ankle and foot

     M62.479   Contracture of muscle, unspecified ankle and foot

   M62.48   Contracture of muscle, other site

   M62.49   Contracture of muscle, multiple sites

● **M62.5**   Muscle wasting and atrophy, not elsewhere classified

     Disuse atrophy NEC

     Excludes1   neuralgic amyotrophy (G54.5)
                 progressive muscular atrophy (G12.21)
                 sarcopenia (M62.84)

     Excludes2   pelvic muscle wasting (N81.84)

   M62.50   Muscle wasting and atrophy, not elsewhere classified, unspecified site

● **M62.51**   Muscle wasting and atrophy, not elsewhere classified, shoulder

     M62.511   Muscle wasting and atrophy, not elsewhere classified, right shoulder

     M62.512   Muscle wasting and atrophy, not elsewhere classified, left shoulder

     M62.519   Muscle wasting and atrophy, not elsewhere classified, unspecified shoulder

● **M62.52**   Muscle wasting and atrophy, not elsewhere classified, upper arm

     M62.521   Muscle wasting and atrophy, not elsewhere classified, right upper arm

     M62.522   Muscle wasting and atrophy, not elsewhere classified, left upper arm

     M62.529   Muscle wasting and atrophy, not elsewhere classified, unspecified upper arm

● **M62.53**   Muscle wasting and atrophy, not elsewhere classified, forearm

     M62.531   Muscle wasting and atrophy, not elsewhere classified, right forearm

     M62.532   Muscle wasting and atrophy, not elsewhere classified, left forearm

     M62.539   Muscle wasting and atrophy, not elsewhere classified, unspecified forearm

● **M62.54**   Muscle wasting and atrophy, not elsewhere classified, hand

     M62.541   Muscle wasting and atrophy, not elsewhere classified, right hand

     M62.542   Muscle wasting and atrophy, not elsewhere classified, left hand

     M62.549   Muscle wasting and atrophy, not elsewhere classified, unspecified hand

● **M62.55**   Muscle wasting and atrophy, not elsewhere classified, thigh

     M62.551   Muscle wasting and atrophy, not elsewhere classified, right thigh

     M62.552   Muscle wasting and atrophy, not elsewhere classified, left thigh

CHAPTER 13 (M00-M99)

M62.559 Muscle wasting and atrophy, not elsewhere classified, unspecified thigh

● M62.56 Muscle wasting and atrophy, not elsewhere classified, lower leg

M62.561 Muscle wasting and atrophy, not elsewhere classified, right lower leg

M62.562 Muscle wasting and atrophy, not elsewhere classified, left lower leg

M62.569 Muscle wasting and atrophy, not elsewhere classified, unspecified lower leg

● M62.57 Muscle wasting and atrophy, not elsewhere classified, ankle and foot

M62.571 Muscle wasting and atrophy, not elsewhere classified, right ankle and foot

M62.572 Muscle wasting and atrophy, not elsewhere classified, left ankle and foot

M62.579 Muscle wasting and atrophy, not elsewhere classified, unspecified ankle and foot

M62.58 Muscle wasting and atrophy, not elsewhere classified, other site

M62.59 Muscle wasting and atrophy, not elsewhere classified, multiple sites

● M62.5A Muscle wasting and atrophy, not elsewhere classified, back

M62.5A0 Muscle wasting and atrophy, not elsewhere classified, back, cervical

M62.5A1 Muscle wasting and atrophy, not elsewhere classified, back, thoracic

M62.5A2 Muscle wasting and atrophy, not elsewhere classified, back, lumbosacral

M62.5A9 Muscle wasting and atrophy, not elsewhere classified, back, unspecified level

● M62.8 Other specified disorders of muscle

Excludes2 nontraumatic hematoma of muscle (M79.81)

M62.81 Muscle weakness (generalized)

Excludes1 muscle weakness in sarcopenia (M62.84)

M62.82 Rhabdomyolysis

Excludes1 traumatic rhabdomyolysis (T79.6)

Coding Clinic: 2019, Q2, P12

● M62.83 Muscle spasm

M62.830 Muscle spasm of back

M62.831 Muscle spasm of calf
Charley-horse

M62.838 Other muscle spasm

M62.84 Sarcopenia
Age-related sarcopenia

Code first underlying disease, if applicable, such as:
disorders of myoneural junction and muscle disease in diseases classified elsewhere (G73.-)
other and unspecified myopathies (G72.-)
primary disorders of muscles (G71.-)

Coding Clinic: 2016, Q4, P41

▷ M62.85 Dyfunction of the multifidus muscles, lumbar region

M62.89 Other specified disorders of muscle
Muscle (sheath) hernia

M62.9 Disorder of muscle, unspecified

● M63 Disorders of muscle in diseases classified elsewhere

Code first underlying disease, such as:
leprosy (A30.-)
neoplasm (C49.-, C79.89, D21.-, D48.1-)
schistosomiasis (B65.-)
trichinellosis (B75)

Excludes1 myopathy in cysticercosis (B69.81)
myopathy in endocrine diseases (G73.7)
myopathy in metabolic diseases (G73.7)
myopathy in sarcoidosis (D86.87)
myopathy in secondary syphilis (A51.49)
myopathy in syphilis (late) (A52.78)
myopathy in toxoplasmosis (B58.82)
myopathy in tuberculosis (A18.09)

● M63.8 Disorders of muscle in diseases classified elsewhere

▷ M63.80 Disorders of muscle in diseases classified elsewhere, unspecified site

● M63.81 Disorders of muscle in diseases classified elsewhere, shoulder

▷ M63.811 Disorders of muscle in diseases classified elsewhere, right shoulder

▷ M63.812 Disorders of muscle in diseases classified elsewhere, left shoulder

▷ M63.819 Disorders of muscle in diseases classified elsewhere, unspecified shoulder

● M63.82 Disorders of muscle in diseases classified elsewhere, upper arm

▷ M63.821 Disorders of muscle in diseases classified elsewhere, right upper arm

▷ M63.822 Disorders of muscle in diseases classified elsewhere, left upper arm

▷ M63.829 Disorders of muscle in diseases classified elsewhere, unspecified upper arm

● M63.83 Disorders of muscle in diseases classified elsewhere, forearm

▷ M63.831 Disorders of muscle in diseases classified elsewhere, right forearm

▷ M63.832 Disorders of muscle in diseases classified elsewhere, left forearm

▷ M63.839 Disorders of muscle in diseases classified elsewhere, unspecified forearm

● M63.84 Disorders of muscle in diseases classified elsewhere, hand

▷ M63.841 Disorders of muscle in diseases classified elsewhere, right hand

▷ M63.842 Disorders of muscle in diseases classified elsewhere, left hand

▷ M63.849 Disorders of muscle in diseases classified elsewhere, unspecified hand

● M63.85 Disorders of muscle in diseases classified elsewhere, thigh

▷ M63.851 Disorders of muscle in diseases classified elsewhere, right thigh

▷ M63.852 Disorders of muscle in diseases classified elsewhere, left thigh

▷ M63.859 Disorders of muscle in diseases classified elsewhere, unspecified thigh

● M63.86 Disorders of muscle in diseases classified elsewhere, lower leg

▷ M63.861 Disorders of muscle in diseases classified elsewhere, right lower leg

▷ M63.862 Disorders of muscle in diseases classified elsewhere, left lower leg

▷ M63.869 Disorders of muscle in diseases classified elsewhere, unspecified lower leg

● **M63.87** **Disorders of muscle in diseases classified elsewhere, ankle and foot**
  ▷ *M63.871* *Disorders of muscle in diseases classified elsewhere, right ankle and foot*
  ▷ *M63.872* *Disorders of muscle in diseases classified elsewhere, left ankle and foot*
  ▷ *M63.879* *Disorders of muscle in diseases classified elsewhere, unspecified ankle and foot*
  ▷ *M63.88* *Disorders of muscle in diseases classified elsewhere, other site*
  ▷ *M63.89* *Disorders of muscle in diseases classified elsewhere, multiple sites*

DISORDERS OF SYNOVIUM AND TENDON (M65-M67)

● **M65** **Synovitis and tenosynovitis**
  Excludes1　chronic crepitant synovitis of hand and wrist (M70.0-)
  　　　　　current injury - see injury of ligament or tendon by body region
  　　　　　soft tissue disorders related to use, overuse and pressure (M70.-)
  ● **M65.0** **Abscess of tendon sheath**
  　　　Use additional code (B95-B96) to identify bacterial agent
  　　M65.00 Abscess of tendon sheath, unspecified site
  ● **M65.01** Abscess of tendon sheath, shoulder
  　　　M65.011 Abscess of tendon sheath, right shoulder
  　　　M65.012 Abscess of tendon sheath, left shoulder
  　　　M65.019 Abscess of tendon sheath, unspecified shoulder
  ● **M65.02** Abscess of tendon sheath, upper arm
  　　　M65.021 Abscess of tendon sheath, right upper arm
  　　　M65.022 Abscess of tendon sheath, left upper arm
  　　　M65.029 Abscess of tendon sheath, unspecified upper arm
  ● **M65.03** Abscess of tendon sheath, forearm
  　　　M65.031 Abscess of tendon sheath, right forearm
  　　　M65.032 Abscess of tendon sheath, left forearm
  　　　M65.039 Abscess of tendon sheath, unspecified forearm
  ● **M65.04** Abscess of tendon sheath, hand
  　　　M65.041 Abscess of tendon sheath, right hand
  　　　M65.042 Abscess of tendon sheath, left hand
  　　　M65.049 Abscess of tendon sheath, unspecified hand
  ● **M65.05** Abscess of tendon sheath, thigh
  　　　M65.051 Abscess of tendon sheath, right thigh
  　　　M65.052 Abscess of tendon sheath, left thigh
  　　　M65.059 Abscess of tendon sheath, unspecified thigh

● **M65.06** Abscess of tendon sheath, lower leg
  　　　M65.061 Abscess of tendon sheath, right lower leg
  　　　M65.062 Abscess of tendon sheath, left lower leg
  　　　M65.069 Abscess of tendon sheath, unspecified lower leg
● **M65.07** Abscess of tendon sheath, ankle and foot
  　　　M65.071 Abscess of tendon sheath, right ankle and foot
  　　　M65.072 Abscess of tendon sheath, left ankle and foot
  　　　M65.079 Abscess of tendon sheath, unspecified ankle and foot
  　　M65.08 Abscess of tendon sheath, other site
● **M65.1** Other infective (teno)synovitis
  　　M65.10 Other infective (teno)synovitis, unspecified site
● **M65.11** Other infective (teno)synovitis, shoulder
  　　　M65.111 Other infective (teno)synovitis, right shoulder
  　　　M65.112 Other infective (teno)synovitis, left shoulder
  　　　M65.119 Other infective (teno)synovitis, unspecified shoulder
● **M65.12** Other infective (teno)synovitis, elbow
  　　　M65.121 Other infective (teno)synovitis, right elbow
  　　　M65.122 Other infective (teno)synovitis, left elbow
  　　　M65.129 Other infective (teno)synovitis, unspecified elbow
● **M65.13** Other infective (teno)synovitis, wrist
  　　　M65.131 Other infective (teno)synovitis, right wrist
  　　　M65.132 Other infective (teno)synovitis, left wrist
  　　　M65.139 Other infective (teno)synovitis, unspecified wrist
● **M65.14** Other infective (teno)synovitis, hand
  　　　M65.141 Other infective (teno)synovitis, right hand
  　　　M65.142 Other infective (teno)synovitis, left hand
  　　　M65.149 Other infective (teno)synovitis, unspecified hand
● **M65.15** Other infective (teno)synovitis, hip
  　　　M65.151 Other infective (teno)synovitis, right hip
  　　　M65.152 Other infective (teno)synovitis, left hip
  　　　M65.159 Other infective (teno)synovitis, unspecified hip
● **M65.16** Other infective (teno)synovitis, knee
  　　　M65.161 Other infective (teno)synovitis, right knee
  　　　M65.162 Other infective (teno)synovitis, left knee
  　　　M65.169 Other infective (teno)synovitis, unspecified knee
● **M65.17** Other infective (teno)synovitis, ankle and foot
  　　　M65.171 Other infective (teno)synovitis, right ankle and foot
  　　　M65.172 Other infective (teno)synovitis, left ankle and foot
  　　　M65.179 Other infective (teno)synovitis, unspecified ankle and foot
  　　M65.18 Other infective (teno)synovitis, other site
  　　M65.19 Other infective (teno)synovitis, multiple sites

Item 13-11 Synovitis is an inflammation of a synovial membrane resulting in pain on motion and is characterized by fluctuating swelling due to effusion in a synovial sac. **Tenosynovitis** is an inflammation of a tendon sheath and occurs most commonly in the wrists, hands, and feet. Bursitis is inflammation of a bursa (fluid-filled sac) caused by repetitive use, trauma, infection, or systemic inflammatory disease. Bursae act as protectors and facilitate movement between bones and overlapping muscles (deep bursae) or between bones and tendons/skin (superficial bursae).

CHAPTER 13 (M00-M99)

● M65.2 Calcific tendinitis
    Excludes1   tendinitis as classified in M75-M77
            calcified tendinitis of shoulder (M75.3)
    M65.20 Calcific tendinitis, unspecified site
● M65.22 Calcific tendinitis, upper arm
    M65.221 Calcific tendinitis, right upper arm
    M65.222 Calcific tendinitis, left upper arm
    M65.229 Calcific tendinitis, unspecified upper arm
● M65.23 Calcific tendinitis, forearm
    M65.231 Calcific tendinitis, right forearm
    M65.232 Calcific tendinitis, left forearm
    M65.239 Calcific tendinitis, unspecified forearm
● M65.24 Calcific tendinitis, hand
    M65.241 Calcific tendinitis, right hand
    M65.242 Calcific tendinitis, left hand
    M65.249 Calcific tendinitis, unspecified hand
● M65.25 Calcific tendinitis, thigh
    M65.251 Calcific tendinitis, right thigh
    M65.252 Calcific tendinitis, left thigh
    M65.259 Calcific tendinitis, unspecified thigh
● M65.26 Calcific tendinitis, lower leg
    M65.261 Calcific tendinitis, right lower leg
    M65.262 Calcific tendinitis, left lower leg
    M65.269 Calcific tendinitis, unspecified lower leg
● M65.27 Calcific tendinitis, ankle and foot
    M65.271 Calcific tendinitis, right ankle and foot
    M65.272 Calcific tendinitis, left ankle and foot
    M65.279 Calcific tendinitis, unspecified ankle and foot
    M65.28 Calcific tendinitis, other site
    M65.29 Calcific tendinitis, multiple sites
● M65.3 Trigger finger
    Nodular tendinous disease
    M65.30 Trigger finger, unspecified finger
● M65.31 Trigger thumb
    M65.311 Trigger thumb, right thumb
    M65.312 Trigger thumb, left thumb
    M65.319 Trigger thumb, unspecified thumb
● M65.32 Trigger finger, index finger
    M65.321 Trigger finger, right index finger
    M65.322 Trigger finger, left index finger
    M65.329 Trigger finger, unspecified index finger
● M65.33 Trigger finger, middle finger
    M65.331 Trigger finger, right middle finger
    M65.332 Trigger finger, left middle finger
    M65.339 Trigger finger, unspecified middle finger
● M65.34 Trigger finger, ring finger
    M65.341 Trigger finger, right ring finger
    M65.342 Trigger finger, left ring finger
    M65.349 Trigger finger, unspecified ring finger
● M65.35 Trigger finger, little finger
    M65.351 Trigger finger, right little finger
    M65.352 Trigger finger, left little finger
    M65.359 Trigger finger, unspecified little finger
M65.4 Radial styloid tenosynovitis [de Quervain]

● M65.8 Other synovitis and tenosynovitis
    M65.80 Other synovitis and tenosynovitis, unspecified site
● M65.81 Other synovitis and tenosynovitis, shoulder
    M65.811 Other synovitis and tenosynovitis, right shoulder
    M65.812 Other synovitis and tenosynovitis, left shoulder
    M65.819 Other synovitis and tenosynovitis, unspecified shoulder
● M65.82 Other synovitis and tenosynovitis, upper arm
    M65.821 Other synovitis and tenosynovitis, right upper arm
    M65.822 Other synovitis and tenosynovitis, left upper arm
    M65.829 Other synovitis and tenosynovitis, unspecified upper arm
● M65.83 Other synovitis and tenosynovitis, forearm
    M65.831 Other synovitis and tenosynovitis, right forearm
    M65.832 Other synovitis and tenosynovitis, left forearm
    M65.839 Other synovitis and tenosynovitis, unspecified forearm
● M65.84 Other synovitis and tenosynovitis, hand
    M65.841 Other synovitis and tenosynovitis, right hand
    M65.842 Other synovitis and tenosynovitis, left hand
    M65.849 Other synovitis and tenosynovitis, unspecified hand
● M65.85 Other synovitis and tenosynovitis, thigh
    M65.851 Other synovitis and tenosynovitis, right thigh
    M65.852 Other synovitis and tenosynovitis, left thigh
    M65.859 Other synovitis and tenosynovitis, unspecified thigh
● M65.86 Other synovitis and tenosynovitis, lower leg
    M65.861 Other synovitis and tenosynovitis, right lower leg
    M65.862 Other synovitis and tenosynovitis, left lower leg
    M65.869 Other synovitis and tenosynovitis, unspecified lower leg
● M65.87 Other synovitis and tenosynovitis, ankle and foot
    M65.871 Other synovitis and tenosynovitis, right ankle and foot
    M65.872 Other synovitis and tenosynovitis, left ankle and foot
    M65.879 Other synovitis and tenosynovitis, unspecified ankle and foot
    M65.88 Other synovitis and tenosynovitis, other site
    M65.89 Other synovitis and tenosynovitis, multiple sites
M65.9 Synovitis and tenosynovitis, unspecified
  ▶M65.90 Unspecified synovitis and tenosynovitis, unspecified site
  ▶● M65.91 Unspecified synovitis and tenosynovitis, shoulder
    ▶M65.911 Unspecified synovitis and tenosynovitis, right shoulder
    ▶M65.912 Unspecified synovitis and tenosynovitis, left shoulder
    ▶M65.919 Unspecified synovitis and tenosynovitis, unspecified shoulder

▶ New   ➡ Revised   ~~deleted~~ Deleted   Excludes 1   Excludes 2   Includes   Use additional   Code first   Code also   Key words
OGCR Official Guidelines   **X** Assign placeholder X   ● Use Additional Character(s)   ▶ Manifestation Code   🏥 Hierarchical Condition Category   **Coding Clinic**

▷ ● M65.92 Unspecified synovitis and tenosynovitis, upper arm
    ▷ M65.921 Unspecified synovitis and tenosynovitis, right upper arm
    ▷ M65.922 Unspecified synovitis and tenosynovitis, left upper arm
    ▷ M65.929 Unspecified synovitis and tenosynovitis, unspecified upper arm
▷ ● M65.93 Unspecified synovitis and tenosynovitis, forearm
    ▷ M65.931 Unspecified synovitis and tenosynovitis, right forearm
    ▷ M65.932 Unspecified synovitis and tenosynovitis, left forearm
    ▷ M65.939 Unspecified synovitis and tenosynovitis, unspecified forearm
▷ ● M65.94 Unspecified synovitis and tenosynovitis, hand
    ▷ M65.941 Unspecified synovitis and tenosynovitis, right hand
    ▷ M65.942 Unspecified synovitis and tenosynovitis, left hand
    ▷ M65.949 Unspecified synovitis and tenosynovitis, unspecified hand
▷ ● M65.95 Unspecified synovitis and tenosynovitis, thigh
    ▷ M65.951 Unspecified synovitis and tenosynovitis, right thigh
    ▷ M65.952 Unspecified synovitis and tenosynovitis, left thigh
    ▷ M65.959 Unspecified synovitis and tenosynovitis, unspecified thigh
▷ ● M65.96 Unspecified synovitis and tenosynovitis, lower leg
    ▷ M65.961 Unspecified synovitis and tenosynovitis, right lower leg
    ▷ M65.962 Unspecified synovitis and tenosynovitis, left lower leg
    ▷ M65.969 Unspecified synovitis and tenosynovitis, unspecified lower leg
▷ ● M65.97 Unspecified synovitis and tenosynovitis, ankle and foot
    ▷ M65.971 Unspecified synovitis and tenosynovitis, right ankle and foot
    ▷ M65.972 Unspecified synovitis and tenosynovitis, left ankle and foot
    ▷ M65.979 Unspecified synovitis and tenosynovitis, unspecified ankle and foot
  ▷ M65.98 Unspecified synovitis and tenosynovitis, other site
  ▷ M65.99 Unspecified synovitis and tenosynovitis, multiple sites

● M66 Spontaneous rupture of synovium and tendon

Includes	rupture that occurs when a normal force is applied to tissues that are inferred to have less than normal strength
Excludes2	rotator cuff syndrome (M75.1-)
	rupture where an abnormal force is applied to normal tissue - see injury of tendon by body region

  M66.0 Rupture of popliteal cyst
● M66.1 Rupture of synovium
    Rupture of synovial cyst
    Excludes2 rupture of popliteal cyst (M66.0)
    M66.10 Rupture of synovium, unspecified joint
  ● M66.11 Rupture of synovium, shoulder
    M66.111 Rupture of synovium, right shoulder
    M66.112 Rupture of synovium, left shoulder
    M66.119 Rupture of synovium, unspecified shoulder

● M66.12 Rupture of synovium, elbow
    M66.121 Rupture of synovium, right elbow
    M66.122 Rupture of synovium, left elbow
    M66.129 Rupture of synovium, unspecified elbow
● M66.13 Rupture of synovium, wrist
    M66.131 Rupture of synovium, right wrist
    M66.132 Rupture of synovium, left wrist
    M66.139 Rupture of synovium, unspecified wrist
● M66.14 Rupture of synovium, hand and fingers
    M66.141 Rupture of synovium, right hand
    M66.142 Rupture of synovium, left hand
    M66.143 Rupture of synovium, unspecified hand
    M66.144 Rupture of synovium, right finger(s)
    M66.145 Rupture of synovium, left finger(s)
    M66.146 Rupture of synovium, unspecified finger(s)
● M66.15 Rupture of synovium, hip
    M66.151 Rupture of synovium, right hip
    M66.152 Rupture of synovium, left hip
    M66.159 Rupture of synovium, unspecified hip
● M66.17 Rupture of synovium, ankle, foot and toes
    M66.171 Rupture of synovium, right ankle
    M66.172 Rupture of synovium, left ankle
    M66.173 Rupture of synovium, unspecified ankle
    M66.174 Rupture of synovium, right foot
    M66.175 Rupture of synovium, left foot
    M66.176 Rupture of synovium, unspecified foot
    M66.177 Rupture of synovium, right toe(s)
    M66.178 Rupture of synovium, left toe(s)
    M66.179 Rupture of synovium, unspecified toe(s)
  M66.18 Rupture of synovium, other site
● M66.2 Spontaneous rupture of extensor tendons
  M66.20 Spontaneous rupture of extensor tendons, unspecified site
  ● M66.21 Spontaneous rupture of extensor tendons, shoulder
    M66.211 Spontaneous rupture of extensor tendons, right shoulder
    M66.212 Spontaneous rupture of extensor tendons, left shoulder
    M66.219 Spontaneous rupture of extensor tendons, unspecified shoulder
  ● M66.22 Spontaneous rupture of extensor tendons, upper arm
    M66.221 Spontaneous rupture of extensor tendons, right upper arm
    M66.222 Spontaneous rupture of extensor tendons, left upper arm
    M66.229 Spontaneous rupture of extensor tendons, unspecified upper arm
  ● M66.23 Spontaneous rupture of extensor tendons, forearm
    M66.231 Spontaneous rupture of extensor tendons, right forearm
    M66.232 Spontaneous rupture of extensor tendons, left forearm
    M66.239 Spontaneous rupture of extensor tendons, unspecified forearm

CHAPTER 13 (M00-M99)

● M66.24 Spontaneous rupture of extensor tendons, hand

   M66.241 Spontaneous rupture of extensor tendons, right hand

   M66.242 Spontaneous rupture of extensor tendons, left hand

   M66.249 Spontaneous rupture of extensor tendons, unspecified hand

● M66.25 Spontaneous rupture of extensor tendons, thigh

   M66.251 Spontaneous rupture of extensor tendons, right thigh

   M66.252 Spontaneous rupture of extensor tendons, left thigh

   M66.259 Spontaneous rupture of extensor tendons, unspecified thigh

● M66.26 Spontaneous rupture of extensor tendons, lower leg

   M66.261 Spontaneous rupture of extensor tendons, right lower leg

   M66.262 Spontaneous rupture of extensor tendons, left lower leg

   M66.269 Spontaneous rupture of extensor tendons, unspecified lower leg

● M66.27 Spontaneous rupture of extensor tendons, ankle and foot

   M66.271 Spontaneous rupture of extensor tendons, right ankle and foot

   M66.272 Spontaneous rupture of extensor tendons, left ankle and foot

   M66.279 Spontaneous rupture of extensor tendons, unspecified ankle and foot

  M66.28 Spontaneous rupture of extensor tendons, other site

  M66.29 Spontaneous rupture of extensor tendons, multiple sites

● M66.3 Spontaneous rupture of flexor tendons

  M66.30 Spontaneous rupture of flexor tendons, unspecified site

● M66.31 Spontaneous rupture of flexor tendons, shoulder

   M66.311 Spontaneous rupture of flexor tendons, right shoulder

   M66.312 Spontaneous rupture of flexor tendons, left shoulder

   M66.319 Spontaneous rupture of flexor tendons, unspecified shoulder

● M66.32 Spontaneous rupture of flexor tendons, upper arm

   M66.321 Spontaneous rupture of flexor tendons, right upper arm

   M66.322 Spontaneous rupture of flexor tendons, left upper arm

   M66.329 Spontaneous rupture of flexor tendons, unspecified upper arm

● M66.33 Spontaneous rupture of flexor tendons, forearm

   M66.331 Spontaneous rupture of flexor tendons, right forearm

   M66.332 Spontaneous rupture of flexor tendons, left forearm

   M66.339 Spontaneous rupture of flexor tendons, unspecified forearm

● M66.34 Spontaneous rupture of flexor tendons, hand

   M66.341 Spontaneous rupture of flexor tendons, right hand

   M66.342 Spontaneous rupture of flexor tendons, left hand

   M66.349 Spontaneous rupture of flexor tendons, unspecified hand

● M66.35 Spontaneous rupture of flexor tendons, thigh

   M66.351 Spontaneous rupture of flexor tendons, right thigh

   M66.352 Spontaneous rupture of flexor tendons, left thigh

   M66.359 Spontaneous rupture of flexor tendons, unspecified thigh

● M66.36 Spontaneous rupture of flexor tendons, lower leg

   M66.361 Spontaneous rupture of flexor tendons, right lower leg

   M66.362 Spontaneous rupture of flexor tendons, left lower leg

   M66.369 Spontaneous rupture of flexor tendons, unspecified lower leg

● M66.37 Spontaneous rupture of flexor tendons, ankle and foot

   M66.371 Spontaneous rupture of flexor tendons, right ankle and foot

   M66.372 Spontaneous rupture of flexor tendons, left ankle and foot

   M66.379 Spontaneous rupture of flexor tendons, unspecified ankle and foot

  M66.38 Spontaneous rupture of flexor tendons, other site

  M66.39 Spontaneous rupture of flexor tendons, multiple sites

● M66.8 Spontaneous rupture of other tendons

  M66.80 Spontaneous rupture of other tendons, unspecified site

● M66.81 Spontaneous rupture of other tendons, shoulder

   M66.811 Spontaneous rupture of other tendons, right shoulder

   M66.812 Spontaneous rupture of other tendons, left shoulder

   M66.819 Spontaneous rupture of other tendons, unspecified shoulder

● M66.82 Spontaneous rupture of other tendons, upper arm

   M66.821 Spontaneous rupture of other tendons, right upper arm

   M66.822 Spontaneous rupture of other tendons, left upper arm

   M66.829 Spontaneous rupture of other tendons, unspecified upper arm

● M66.83 Spontaneous rupture of other tendons, forearm

   M66.831 Spontaneous rupture of other tendons, right forearm

   M66.832 Spontaneous rupture of other tendons, left forearm

   M66.839 Spontaneous rupture of other tendons, unspecified forearm

● M66.84 Spontaneous rupture of other tendons, hand

   M66.841 Spontaneous rupture of other tendons, right hand

   M66.842 Spontaneous rupture of other tendons, left hand

   M66.849 Spontaneous rupture of other tendons, unspecified hand

● M66.85 Spontaneous rupture of other tendons, thigh

   M66.851 Spontaneous rupture of other tendons, right thigh

   M66.852 Spontaneous rupture of other tendons, left thigh

   M66.859 Spontaneous rupture of other tendons, unspecified thigh

● M66.86 Spontaneous rupture of other tendons, lower leg

   M66.861 Spontaneous rupture of other tendons, right lower leg

   M66.862 Spontaneous rupture of other tendons, left lower leg

   M66.869 Spontaneous rupture of other tendons, unspecified lower leg

● **M66.87** Spontaneous rupture of other tendons, ankle and foot

     M66.871 Spontaneous rupture of other tendons, right ankle and foot

     M66.872 Spontaneous rupture of other tendons, left ankle and foot

     M66.879 Spontaneous rupture of other tendons, unspecified ankle and foot

   M66.88 Spontaneous rupture of other tendons, other sites

   M66.89 Spontaneous rupture of other tendons, multiple sites

M66.9 Spontaneous rupture of unspecified tendon

     Rupture at musculotendinous junction, nontraumatic

● **M67** **Other disorders of synovium and tendon**

   Excludes1   palmar fascial fibromatosis [Dupuytren] (M72.0)
               tendinitis NOS (M77.9-)
               xanthomatosis localized to tendons (E78.2)

● **M67.0** Short Achilles tendon (acquired)

   M67.00 Short Achilles tendon (acquired), unspecified ankle

   M67.01 Short Achilles tendon (acquired), right ankle

   M67.02 Short Achilles tendon (acquired), left ankle

● **M67.2** Synovial hypertrophy, not elsewhere classified

     Excludes1   villonodular synovitis (pigmented) (M12.2-)

   M67.20 Synovial hypertrophy, not elsewhere classified, unspecified site

● **M67.21** Synovial hypertrophy, not elsewhere classified, shoulder

     M67.211 Synovial hypertrophy, not elsewhere classified, right shoulder

     M67.212 Synovial hypertrophy, not elsewhere classified, left shoulder

     M67.219 Synovial hypertrophy, not elsewhere classified, unspecified shoulder

● **M67.22** Synovial hypertrophy, not elsewhere classified, upper arm

     M67.221 Synovial hypertrophy, not elsewhere classified, right upper arm

     M67.222 Synovial hypertrophy, not elsewhere classified, left upper arm

     M67.229 Synovial hypertrophy, not elsewhere classified, unspecified upper arm

● **M67.23** Synovial hypertrophy, not elsewhere classified, forearm

     M67.231 Synovial hypertrophy, not elsewhere classified, right forearm

     M67.232 Synovial hypertrophy, not elsewhere classified, left forearm

     M67.239 Synovial hypertrophy, not elsewhere classified, unspecified forearm

● **M67.24** Synovial hypertrophy, not elsewhere classified, hand

     M67.241 Synovial hypertrophy, not elsewhere classified, right hand

     M67.242 Synovial hypertrophy, not elsewhere classified, left hand

     M67.249 Synovial hypertrophy, not elsewhere classified, unspecified hand

● **M67.25** Synovial hypertrophy, not elsewhere classified, thigh

     M67.251 Synovial hypertrophy, not elsewhere classified, right thigh

     M67.252 Synovial hypertrophy, not elsewhere classified, left thigh

     M67.259 Synovial hypertrophy, not elsewhere classified, unspecified thigh

● **M67.26** Synovial hypertrophy, not elsewhere classified, lower leg

     M67.261 Synovial hypertrophy, not elsewhere classified, right lower leg

     M67.262 Synovial hypertrophy, not elsewhere classified, left lower leg

     M67.269 Synovial hypertrophy, not elsewhere classified, unspecified lower leg

● **M67.27** Synovial hypertrophy, not elsewhere classified, ankle and foot

     M67.271 Synovial hypertrophy, not elsewhere classified, right ankle and foot

     M67.272 Synovial hypertrophy, not elsewhere classified, left ankle and foot

     M67.279 Synovial hypertrophy, not elsewhere classified, unspecified ankle and foot

   M67.28 Synovial hypertrophy, not elsewhere classified, other site

   M67.29 Synovial hypertrophy, not elsewhere classified, multiple sites

● **M67.3** Transient synovitis

     Toxic synovitis

     Excludes1   palindromic rheumatism (M12.3-)

   M67.30 Transient synovitis, unspecified site

● **M67.31** Transient synovitis, shoulder

     M67.311 Transient synovitis, right shoulder

     M67.312 Transient synovitis, left shoulder

     M67.319 Transient synovitis, unspecified shoulder

● **M67.32** Transient synovitis, elbow

     M67.321 Transient synovitis, right elbow

     M67.322 Transient synovitis, left elbow

     M67.329 Transient synovitis, unspecified elbow

● **M67.33** Transient synovitis, wrist

     M67.331 Transient synovitis, right wrist

     M67.332 Transient synovitis, left wrist

     M67.339 Transient synovitis, unspecified wrist

● **M67.34** Transient synovitis, hand

     M67.341 Transient synovitis, right hand

     M67.342 Transient synovitis, left hand

     M67.349 Transient synovitis, unspecified hand

● **M67.35** Transient synovitis, hip

     M67.351 Transient synovitis, right hip

     M67.352 Transient synovitis, left hip

     M67.359 Transient synovitis, unspecified hip

● **M67.36** Transient synovitis, knee

     M67.361 Transient synovitis, right knee

     M67.362 Transient synovitis, left knee

     M67.369 Transient synovitis, unspecified knee

● **M67.37** Transient synovitis, ankle and foot

     M67.371 Transient synovitis, right ankle and foot

     M67.372 Transient synovitis, left ankle and foot

     M67.379 Transient synovitis, unspecified ankle and foot

   M67.38 Transient synovitis, other site

   M67.39 Transient synovitis, multiple sites

● **M67.4** Ganglion

     Ganglion of joint or tendon (sheath)

     Excludes1   ganglion in yaws (A66.6)

     Excludes2   cyst of bursa (M71.2-M71.3)
               cyst of synovium (M71.2-M71.3)

   M67.40 Ganglion, unspecified site

● **M67.41** Ganglion, shoulder

     M67.411 Ganglion, right shoulder

     M67.412 Ganglion, left shoulder

     M67.419 Ganglion, unspecified shoulder

CHAPTER 13 (M00-M99)

- M67.42 **Ganglion, elbow**
  - M67.421 Ganglion, right elbow
  - M67.422 Ganglion, left elbow
  - M67.429 Ganglion, unspecified elbow
- M67.43 **Ganglion, wrist**
  - M67.431 Ganglion, right wrist
  - M67.432 Ganglion, left wrist
  - M67.439 Ganglion, unspecified wrist
- M67.44 **Ganglion, hand**
  - M67.441 Ganglion, right hand
  - M67.442 Ganglion, left hand
  - M67.449 Ganglion, unspecified hand
- M67.45 **Ganglion, hip**
  - M67.451 Ganglion, right hip
  - M67.452 Ganglion, left hip
  - M67.459 Ganglion, unspecified hip
- M67.46 **Ganglion, knee**
  - M67.461 Ganglion, right knee
  - M67.462 Ganglion, left knee
  - M67.469 Ganglion, unspecified knee
- M67.47 **Ganglion, ankle and foot**
  - M67.471 Ganglion, right ankle and foot
  - M67.472 Ganglion, left ankle and foot
  - M67.479 Ganglion, unspecified ankle and foot
- M67.48 Ganglion, other site
- M67.49 Ganglion, multiple sites
- M67.5 **Plica syndrome**
  Plica knee
  - M67.50 Plica syndrome, unspecified knee
  - M67.51 Plica syndrome, right knee
  - M67.52 Plica syndrome, left knee
- M67.8 **Other specified disorders of synovium and tendon**
  - M67.80 Other specified disorders of synovium and tendon, unspecified site
  - M67.81 Other specified disorders of synovium and tendon, shoulder
    - M67.811 Other specified disorders of synovium, right shoulder
    - M67.812 Other specified disorders of synovium, left shoulder
    - M67.813 Other specified disorders of tendon, right shoulder
    - M67.814 Other specified disorders of tendon, left shoulder
    - M67.819 Other specified disorders of synovium and tendon, unspecified shoulder
  - M67.82 Other specified disorders of synovium and tendon, elbow
    - M67.821 Other specified disorders of synovium, right elbow
    - M67.822 Other specified disorders of synovium, left elbow
    - M67.823 Other specified disorders of tendon, right elbow
    - M67.824 Other specified disorders of tendon, left elbow
    - M67.829 Other specified disorders of synovium and tendon, unspecified elbow
  - M67.83 Other specified disorders of synovium and tendon, wrist
    - M67.831 Other specified disorders of synovium, right wrist
    - M67.832 Other specified disorders of synovium, left wrist
    - M67.833 Other specified disorders of tendon, right wrist

- M67.834 Other specified disorders of tendon, left wrist
- M67.839 Other specified disorders of synovium and tendon, unspecified wrist
- M67.84 Other specified disorders of synovium and tendon, hand
  - M67.841 Other specified disorders of synovium, right hand
  - M67.842 Other specified disorders of synovium, left hand
  - M67.843 Other specified disorders of tendon, right hand
  - M67.844 Other specified disorders of tendon, left hand
  - M67.849 Other specified disorders of synovium and tendon, unspecified hand
- M67.85 Other specified disorders of synovium and tendon, hip
  - M67.851 Other specified disorders of synovium, right hip
  - M67.852 Other specified disorders of synovium, left hip
  - M67.853 Other specified disorders of tendon, right hip
  - M67.854 Other specified disorders of tendon, left hip
  - M67.859 Other specified disorders of synovium and tendon, unspecified hip
- M67.86 Other specified disorders of synovium and tendon, knee
  - M67.861 Other specified disorders of synovium, right knee
  - M67.862 Other specified disorders of synovium, left knee
  - M67.863 Other specified disorders of tendon, right knee
  - M67.864 Other specified disorders of tendon, left knee
  - M67.869 Other specified disorders of synovium and tendon, unspecified knee
- M67.87 Other specified disorders of synovium and tendon, ankle and foot
  - M67.871 Other specified disorders of synovium, right ankle and foot
  - M67.872 Other specified disorders of synovium, left ankle and foot
  - M67.873 Other specified disorders of tendon, right ankle and foot
  - M67.874 Other specified disorders of tendon, left ankle and foot
  - M67.879 Other specified disorders of synovium and tendon, unspecified ankle and foot
- M67.88 Other specified disorders of synovium and tendon, other site
- M67.89 Other specified disorders of synovium and tendon, multiple sites
- M67.9 **Unspecified disorder of synovium and tendon**
  - M67.90 Unspecified disorder of synovium and tendon, unspecified site
  - M67.91 Unspecified disorder of synovium and tendon, shoulder
    - M67.911 Unspecified disorder of synovium and tendon, right shoulder
    - M67.912 Unspecified disorder of synovium and tendon, left shoulder
    - M67.919 Unspecified disorder of synovium and tendon, unspecified shoulder

CHAPTER 13 (M00-M99)

- **M67.92** Unspecified disorder of synovium and tendon, upper arm
  - M67.921 Unspecified disorder of synovium and tendon, right upper arm
  - M67.922 Unspecified disorder of synovium and tendon, left upper arm
  - M67.929 Unspecified disorder of synovium and tendon, unspecified upper arm
- **M67.93** Unspecified disorder of synovium and tendon, forearm
  - M67.931 Unspecified disorder of synovium and tendon, right forearm
  - M67.932 Unspecified disorder of synovium and tendon, left forearm
  - M67.939 Unspecified disorder of synovium and tendon, unspecified forearm
- **M67.94** Unspecified disorder of synovium and tendon, hand
  - M67.941 Unspecified disorder of synovium and tendon, right hand
  - M67.942 Unspecified disorder of synovium and tendon, left hand
  - M67.949 Unspecified disorder of synovium and tendon, unspecified hand
- **M67.95** Unspecified disorder of synovium and tendon, thigh
  - M67.951 Unspecified disorder of synovium and tendon, right thigh
  - M67.952 Unspecified disorder of synovium and tendon, left thigh
  - M67.959 Unspecified disorder of synovium and tendon, unspecified thigh
- **M67.96** Unspecified disorder of synovium and tendon, lower leg
  - M67.961 Unspecified disorder of synovium and tendon, right lower leg
  - M67.962 Unspecified disorder of synovium and tendon, left lower leg
  - M67.969 Unspecified disorder of synovium and tendon, unspecified lower leg
- **M67.97** Unspecified disorder of synovium and tendon, ankle and foot
  - M67.971 Unspecified disorder of synovium and tendon, right ankle and foot
  - M67.972 Unspecified disorder of synovium and tendon, left ankle and foot
  - M67.979 Unspecified disorder of synovium and tendon, unspecified ankle and foot
  - M67.98 Unspecified disorder of synovium and tendon, other site
  - M67.99 Unspecified disorder of synovium and tendon, multiple sites

OTHER SOFT TISSUE DISORDERS (M70-M79)

- **M70** Soft tissue disorders related to use, overuse and pressure
  - **Includes** soft tissue disorders of occupational origin
  - Use additional external cause code to identify activity causing disorder (Y93.-)
  - **Excludes1** bursitis NOS (M71.9-)
  - **Excludes2** bursitis of shoulder (M75.5)
    - enthesopathies (M76-M77)
    - pressure ulcer (pressure area) (L89.-)
- **M70.0** Crepitant synovitis (acute) (chronic) of hand and wrist
  - **M70.03** Crepitant synovitis (acute) (chronic), wrist
    - M70.031 Crepitant synovitis (acute) (chronic), right wrist
    - M70.032 Crepitant synovitis (acute) (chronic), left wrist
    - M70.039 Crepitant synovitis (acute) (chronic), unspecified wrist

- **M70.04** Crepitant synovitis (acute) (chronic), hand
  - M70.041 Crepitant synovitis (acute) (chronic), right hand
  - M70.042 Crepitant synovitis (acute) (chronic), left hand
  - M70.049 Crepitant synovitis (acute) (chronic), unspecified hand
- **M70.1** Bursitis of hand
  - M70.10 Bursitis, unspecified hand
  - M70.11 Bursitis, right hand
  - M70.12 Bursitis, left hand
- **M70.2** Olecranon bursitis
  - M70.20 Olecranon bursitis, unspecified elbow
  - M70.21 Olecranon bursitis, right elbow
  - M70.22 Olecranon bursitis, left elbow
- **M70.3** Other bursitis of elbow
  - M70.30 Other bursitis of elbow, unspecified elbow
  - M70.31 Other bursitis of elbow, right elbow
  - M70.32 Other bursitis of elbow, left elbow
- **M70.4** Prepatellar bursitis
  - M70.40 Prepatellar bursitis, unspecified knee
  - M70.41 Prepatellar bursitis, right knee
  - M70.42 Prepatellar bursitis, left knee
- **M70.5** Other bursitis of knee
  - M70.50 Other bursitis of knee, unspecified knee
  - M70.51 Other bursitis of knee, right knee
  - M70.52 Other bursitis of knee, left knee
- **M70.6** Trochanteric bursitis
  - Trochanteric tendinitis
  - M70.60 Trochanteric bursitis, unspecified hip
  - M70.61 Trochanteric bursitis, right hip
  - M70.62 Trochanteric bursitis, left hip
- **M70.7** Other bursitis of hip
  - Ischial bursitis
  - M70.70 Other bursitis of hip, unspecified hip
  - M70.71 Other bursitis of hip, right hip
  - M70.72 Other bursitis of hip, left hip
- **M70.8** Other soft tissue disorders related to use, overuse and pressure
  - M70.80 Other soft tissue disorders related to use, overuse and pressure of unspecified site
  - **M70.81** Other soft tissue disorders related to use, overuse and pressure of shoulder
    - M70.811 Other soft tissue disorders related to use, overuse and pressure, right shoulder
    - M70.812 Other soft tissue disorders related to use, overuse and pressure, left shoulder
    - M70.819 Other soft tissue disorders related to use, overuse and pressure, unspecified shoulder
  - **M70.82** Other soft tissue disorders related to use, overuse and pressure of upper arm
    - M70.821 Other soft tissue disorders related to use, overuse and pressure, right upper arm
    - M70.822 Other soft tissue disorders related to use, overuse and pressure, left upper arm
    - M70.829 Other soft tissue disorders related to use, overuse and pressure, unspecified upper arms
  - **M70.83** Other soft tissue disorders related to use, overuse and pressure of forearm
    - M70.831 Other soft tissue disorders related to use, overuse and pressure, right forearm

CHAPTER 13 (M00–M99)

M70.832   Other soft tissue disorders related to use, overuse and pressure, **left forearm**

M70.839   Other soft tissue disorders related to use, overuse and pressure, **unspecified forearm**

● M70.84   Other soft tissue disorders related to use, overuse and pressure of **hand**

M70.841   Other soft tissue disorders related to use, overuse and pressure, **right hand**

M70.842   Other soft tissue disorders related to use, overuse and pressure, **left hand**

M70.849   Other soft tissue disorders related to use, overuse and pressure, **unspecified hand**

● M70.85   Other soft tissue disorders related to use, overuse and pressure of **thigh**

M70.851   Other soft tissue disorders related to use, overuse and pressure, **right thigh**

M70.852   Other soft tissue disorders related to use, overuse and pressure, **left thigh**

M70.859   Other soft tissue disorders related to use, overuse and pressure, **unspecified thigh**

● M70.86   Other soft tissue disorders related to use, overuse and pressure **lower leg**

M70.861   Other soft tissue disorders related to use, overuse and pressure, **right lower leg**

M70.862   Other soft tissue disorders related to use, overuse and pressure, **left lower leg**

M70.869   Other soft tissue disorders related to use, overuse and pressure, **unspecified leg**

● M70.87   Other soft tissue disorders related to use, overuse and pressure of **ankle and foot**

M70.871   Other soft tissue disorders related to use, overuse and pressure, **right ankle and foot**

M70.872   Other soft tissue disorders related to use, overuse and pressure, **left ankle and foot**

M70.879   Other soft tissue disorders related to use, overuse and pressure, **unspecified ankle and foot**

M70.88   Other soft tissue disorders related to use, overuse and pressure **other site**

M70.89   Other soft tissue disorders related to use, overuse and pressure **multiple sites**

● M70.9   **Unspecified** soft tissue disorder related to use, overuse and pressure

M70.90   Unspecified soft tissue disorder related to use, overuse and pressure of **unspecified site**

● M70.91   Unspecified soft tissue disorder related to use, overuse and pressure of **shoulder**

M70.911   Unspecified soft tissue disorder related to use, overuse and pressure, **right shoulder**

M70.912   Unspecified soft tissue disorder related to use, overuse and pressure, **left shoulder**

M70.919   Unspecified soft tissue disorder related to use, overuse and pressure, **unspecified shoulder**

● M70.92   Unspecified soft tissue disorder related to use, overuse and pressure of **upper arm**

M70.921   Unspecified soft tissue disorder related to use, overuse and pressure, **right upper arm**

M70.922   Unspecified soft tissue disorder related to use, overuse and pressure, **left upper arm**

M70.929   Unspecified soft tissue disorder related to use, overuse and pressure, **unspecified upper arm**

● M70.93   Unspecified soft tissue disorder related to use, overuse and pressure of **forearm**

M70.931   Unspecified soft tissue disorder related to use, overuse and pressure, **right forearm**

M70.932   Unspecified soft tissue disorder related to use, overuse and pressure, **left forearm**

M70.939   Unspecified soft tissue disorder related to use, overuse and pressure, **unspecified forearm**

● M70.94   Unspecified soft tissue disorder related to use, overuse and pressure of **hand**

M70.941   Unspecified soft tissue disorder related to use, overuse and pressure, **right hand**

M70.942   Unspecified soft tissue disorder related to use, overuse and pressure, **left hand**

M70.949   Unspecified soft tissue disorder related to use, overuse and pressure, **unspecified hand**

● M70.95   Unspecified soft tissue disorder related to use, overuse and pressure of **thigh**

M70.951   Unspecified soft tissue disorder related to use, overuse and pressure, **right thigh**

M70.952   Unspecified soft tissue disorder related to use, overuse and pressure, **left thigh**

M70.959   Unspecified soft tissue disorder related to use, overuse and pressure, **unspecified thigh**

● M70.96   Unspecified soft tissue disorder related to use, overuse and pressure **lower leg**

M70.961   Unspecified soft tissue disorder related to use, overuse and pressure, **right lower leg**

M70.962   Unspecified soft tissue disorder related to use, overuse and pressure, **left lower leg**

M70.969   Unspecified soft tissue disorder related to use, overuse and pressure, **unspecified lower leg**

● M70.97   Unspecified soft tissue disorder related to use, overuse and pressure of **ankle and foot**

M70.971   Unspecified soft tissue disorder related to use, overuse and pressure, **right ankle and foot**

M70.972   Unspecified soft tissue disorder related to use, overuse and pressure, **left ankle and foot**

M70.979   Unspecified soft tissue disorder related to use, overuse and pressure, **unspecified ankle and foot**

M70.98   Unspecified soft tissue disorder related to use, overuse and pressure **other**

M70.99   Unspecified soft tissue disorder related to use, overuse and pressure **multiple sites**

● M71   Other bursopathies

Excludes1   bunion (M20.1)
bursitis related to use, overuse or pressure (M70.-)
enthesopathies (M76-M77)

● M71.0   Abscess of bursa

Use additional code (B95.-, B96.-) to identify causative organism

M71.00   Abscess of bursa, **unspecified** site

▶ New   ⇒ Revised   ~~deleted~~ Deleted   Excludes 1   Excludes 2   Includes   Use additional   Code first   Code also   Key words
OGCR Official Guidelines   X Assign placeholder X   ● Use Additional Character(s)   ▷ Manifestation Code   ⬙ Hierarchical Condition Category   Coding Clinic

● M71.01 Abscess of bursa, shoulder
     M71.011 Abscess of bursa, right shoulder
     M71.012 Abscess of bursa, left shoulder
     M71.019 Abscess of bursa, unspecified shoulder
● M71.02 Abscess of bursa, elbow
     M71.021 Abscess of bursa, right elbow
     M71.022 Abscess of bursa, left elbow
     M71.029 Abscess of bursa, unspecified elbow
● M71.03 Abscess of bursa, wrist
     M71.031 Abscess of bursa, right wrist
     M71.032 Abscess of bursa, left wrist
     M71.039 Abscess of bursa, unspecified wrist
● M71.04 Abscess of bursa, hand
     M71.041 Abscess of bursa, right hand
     M71.042 Abscess of bursa, left hand
     M71.049 Abscess of bursa, unspecified hand
● M71.05 Abscess of bursa, hip
     M71.051 Abscess of bursa, right hip
     M71.052 Abscess of bursa, left hip
     M71.059 Abscess of bursa, unspecified hip
● M71.06 Abscess of bursa, knee
     M71.061 Abscess of bursa, right knee
     M71.062 Abscess of bursa, left knee
     M71.069 Abscess of bursa, unspecified knee
● M71.07 Abscess of bursa, ankle and foot
     M71.071 Abscess of bursa, right ankle and foot
     M71.072 Abscess of bursa, left ankle and foot
     M71.079 Abscess of bursa, unspecified ankle and foot
     M71.08 Abscess of bursa, other site
     M71.09 Abscess of bursa, multiple sites
● M71.1 Other infective bursitis
     Use additional code (B95.-, B96.-) to identify causative organism
     M71.10 Other infective bursitis, unspecified site
● M71.11 Other infective bursitis, shoulder
     M71.111 Other infective bursitis, right shoulder
     M71.112 Other infective bursitis, left shoulder
     M71.119 Other infective bursitis, unspecified shoulder
● M71.12 Other infective bursitis, elbow
     M71.121 Other infective bursitis, right elbow
     M71.122 Other infective bursitis, left elbow
     M71.129 Other infective bursitis, unspecified elbow
● M71.13 Other infective bursitis, wrist
     M71.131 Other infective bursitis, right wrist
     M71.132 Other infective bursitis, left wrist
     M71.139 Other infective bursitis, unspecified wrist
● M71.14 Other infective bursitis, hand
     M71.141 Other infective bursitis, right hand
     M71.142 Other infective bursitis, left hand
     M71.149 Other infective bursitis, unspecified hand
● M71.15 Other infective bursitis, hip
     M71.151 Other infective bursitis, right hip
     M71.152 Other infective bursitis, left hip
     M71.159 Other infective bursitis, unspecified hip

● M71.16 Other infective bursitis, knee
     M71.161 Other infective bursitis, right knee
     M71.162 Other infective bursitis, left knee
     M71.169 Other infective bursitis, unspecified knee
● M71.17 Other infective bursitis, ankle and foot
     M71.171 Other infective bursitis, right ankle and foot
     M71.172 Other infective bursitis, left ankle and foot
     M71.179 Other infective bursitis, unspecified ankle and foot
     M71.18 Other infective bursitis, other site
     M71.19 Other infective bursitis, multiple sites
● M71.2 Synovial cyst of popliteal space [Baker]
     Popliteal space = popliteal cavity, popliteal fossa. Depression in the posterior aspect of the knee (behind the knee).
     Excludes1 synovial cyst of popliteal space with rupture (M66.0)
     M71.20 Synovial cyst of popliteal space [Baker], unspecified knee
     M71.21 Synovial cyst of popliteal space [Baker], right knee
     M71.22 Synovial cyst of popliteal space [Baker], left knee
● M71.3 Other bursal cyst
     Synovial cyst NOS
     Excludes1 synovial cyst with rupture (M66.1-)
     M71.30 Other bursal cyst, unspecified site
● M71.31 Other bursal cyst, shoulder
     M71.311 Other bursal cyst, right shoulder
     M71.312 Other bursal cyst, left shoulder
     M71.319 Other bursal cyst, unspecified shoulder
● M71.32 Other bursal cyst, elbow
     M71.321 Other bursal cyst, right elbow
     M71.322 Other bursal cyst, left elbow
     M71.329 Other bursal cyst, unspecified elbow
● M71.33 Other bursal cyst, wrist
     M71.331 Other bursal cyst, right wrist
     M71.332 Other bursal cyst, left wrist
     M71.339 Other bursal cyst, unspecified wrist
● M71.34 Other bursal cyst, hand
     M71.341 Other bursal cyst, right hand
     M71.342 Other bursal cyst, left hand
     M71.349 Other bursal cyst, unspecified hand
● M71.35 Other bursal cyst, hip
     M71.351 Other bursal cyst, right hip
     M71.352 Other bursal cyst, left hip
     M71.359 Other bursal cyst, unspecified hip
● M71.37 Other bursal cyst, ankle and foot
     M71.371 Other bursal cyst, right ankle and foot
     M71.372 Other bursal cyst, left ankle and foot
     M71.379 Other bursal cyst, unspecified ankle and foot
     M71.38 Other bursal cyst, other site
     M71.39 Other bursal cyst, multiple sites
● M71.4 Calcium deposit in bursa
     Excludes2 calcium deposit in bursa of shoulder (M75.3)
     M71.40 Calcium deposit in bursa, unspecified site
● M71.42 Calcium deposit in bursa, elbow
     M71.421 Calcium deposit in bursa, right elbow
     M71.422 Calcium deposit in bursa, left elbow
     M71.429 Calcium deposit in bursa, unspecified elbow

CHAPTER 13 (M00-M99)

● M71.43 Calcium deposit in bursa, wrist
 M71.431 Calcium deposit in bursa, right wrist
 M71.432 Calcium deposit in bursa, left wrist
 M71.439 Calcium deposit in bursa, unspecified wrist
● M71.44 Calcium deposit in bursa, hand
 M71.441 Calcium deposit in bursa, right hand
 M71.442 Calcium deposit in bursa, left hand
 M71.449 Calcium deposit in bursa, unspecified hand
● M71.45 Calcium deposit in bursa, hip
 M71.451 Calcium deposit in bursa, right hip
 M71.452 Calcium deposit in bursa, left hip
 M71.459 Calcium deposit in bursa, unspecified hip
● M71.46 Calcium deposit in bursa, knee
 M71.461 Calcium deposit in bursa, right knee
 M71.462 Calcium deposit in bursa, left knee
 M71.469 Calcium deposit in bursa, unspecified knee
● M71.47 Calcium deposit in bursa, ankle and foot
 M71.471 Calcium deposit in bursa, right ankle and foot
 M71.472 Calcium deposit in bursa, left ankle and foot
 M71.479 Calcium deposit in bursa, unspecified ankle and foot
 M71.48 Calcium deposit in bursa, other site
 M71.49 Calcium deposit in bursa, multiple sites
● M71.5 Other bursitis, not elsewhere classified

Excludes1 bursitis NOS (M71.9-)
Excludes2 bursitis of shoulder (M75.5)
bursitis of tibial collateral [Pellegrini-Stieda] (M76.4-)

 M71.50 Other bursitis, not elsewhere classified, unspecified site
● M71.52 Other bursitis, not elsewhere classified, elbow
 M71.521 Other bursitis, not elsewhere classified, right elbow
 M71.522 Other bursitis, not elsewhere classified, left elbow
 M71.529 Other bursitis, not elsewhere classified, unspecified elbow
● M71.53 Other bursitis, not elsewhere classified, wrist
 M71.531 Other bursitis, not elsewhere classified, right wrist
 M71.532 Other bursitis, not elsewhere classified, left wrist
 M71.539 Other bursitis, not elsewhere classified, unspecified wrist
● M71.54 Other bursitis, not elsewhere classified, hand
 M71.541 Other bursitis, not elsewhere classified, right hand
 M71.542 Other bursitis, not elsewhere classified, left hand
 M71.549 Other bursitis, not elsewhere classified, unspecified hand
● M71.55 Other bursitis, not elsewhere classified, hip
 M71.551 Other bursitis, not elsewhere classified, right hip
 M71.552 Other bursitis, not elsewhere classified, left hip
 M71.559 Other bursitis, not elsewhere classified, unspecified hip
● M71.56 Other bursitis, not elsewhere classified, knee
 M71.561 Other bursitis, not elsewhere classified, right knee

 M71.562 Other bursitis, not elsewhere classified, left knee
 M71.569 Other bursitis, not elsewhere classified, unspecified knee
● M71.57 Other bursitis, not elsewhere classified, ankle and foot
 M71.571 Other bursitis, not elsewhere classified, right ankle and foot
 M71.572 Other bursitis, not elsewhere classified, left ankle and foot
 M71.579 Other bursitis, not elsewhere classified, unspecified ankle and foot
 M71.58 Other bursitis, not elsewhere classified, other site
● M71.8 Other specified bursopathies
 M71.80 Other specified bursopathies, unspecified site
● M71.81 Other specified bursopathies, shoulder
 M71.811 Other specified bursopathies, right shoulder
 M71.812 Other specified bursopathies, left shoulder
 M71.819 Other specified bursopathies, unspecified shoulder
● M71.82 Other specified bursopathies, elbow
 M71.821 Other specified bursopathies, right elbow
 M71.822 Other specified bursopathies, left elbow
 M71.829 Other specified bursopathies, unspecified elbow
● M71.83 Other specified bursopathies, wrist
 M71.831 Other specified bursopathies, right wrist
 M71.832 Other specified bursopathies, left wrist
 M71.839 Other specified bursopathies, unspecified wrist
● M71.84 Other specified bursopathies, hand
 M71.841 Other specified bursopathies, right hand
 M71.842 Other specified bursopathies, left hand
 M71.849 Other specified bursopathies, unspecified hand
● M71.85 Other specified bursopathies, hip
 M71.851 Other specified bursopathies, right hip
 M71.852 Other specified bursopathies, left hip
 M71.859 Other specified bursopathies, unspecified hip
● M71.86 Other specified bursopathies, knee
 M71.861 Other specified bursopathies, right knee
 M71.862 Other specified bursopathies, left knee
 M71.869 Other specified bursopathies, unspecified knee
● M71.87 Other specified bursopathies, ankle and foot
 M71.871 Other specified bursopathies, right ankle and foot
 M71.872 Other specified bursopathies, left ankle and foot
 M71.879 Other specified bursopathies, unspecified ankle and foot
 M71.88 Other specified bursopathies, other site
 M71.89 Other specified bursopathies, multiple sites
M71.9 Bursopathy, unspecified
Bursitis NOS

▶ New ⟹ Revised ~~deleted~~ Deleted Excludes 1 Excludes 2 Includes Use additional Code first Code also Key words
OGCR Official Guidelines X Assign placeholder X ● Use Additional Character(s) ▶ Manifestation Code 🔖 Hierarchical Condition Category **Coding Clinic**

● M72 **Fibroblastic disorders**

> **Excludes2**   retroperitoneal fibromatosis (D48.3)

M72.0 **Palmar fascial fibromatosis [Dupuytren]**   **A**

M72.1 **Knuckle pads**

M72.2 **Plantar fascial fibromatosis**
   Plantar fasciitis

M72.4 **Pseudosarcomatous fibromatosis**
   Nodular fasciitis

M72.6 **Necrotizing fasciitis** 🦠
   Use additional code (B95.-, B96.-) to identify causative
   organism

M72.8 **Other fibroblastic disorders**
   Abscess of fascia
   Fasciitis NEC
   Other infective fasciitis
   Use additional code to (B95.-, B96.-) identify causative
   organism

> **Excludes1**   diffuse (eosinophilic) fasciitis (M35.4)
>   necrotizing fasciitis (M72.6)
>   nodular fasciitis (M72.4)
>   perirenal fasciitis NOS (N13.5)
>   perirenal fasciitis with infection (N13.6)
>   plantar fasciitis (M72.2)

M72.9 **Fibroblastic disorder, unspecified**
   Fasciitis NOS
   Fibromatosis NOS

● M75 **Shoulder lesions**

> **Excludes2**   shoulder-hand syndrome (M89.0-)

● M75.0 **Adhesive capsulitis of shoulder**
   Frozen shoulder
   Periarthritis of shoulder

   M75.00 **Adhesive capsulitis of unspecified shoulder**
   M75.01 **Adhesive capsulitis of right shoulder**
   M75.02 **Adhesive capsulitis of left shoulder**
      Coding Clinic: 2015, Q2, P23

● M75.1 **Rotator cuff tear or rupture, not specified as traumatic**
   Rotator cuff syndrome
   Supraspinatus syndrome
   Supraspinatus tear or rupture, not specified as
      traumatic

> **Excludes1**   tear of rotator cuff, traumatic (S46.01-)
> *Gradual onset due to repetitive stress to rotator cuff*

   ● M75.10 **Unspecified rotator cuff tear or rupture, not specified as traumatic**
      M75.100 **Unspecified rotator cuff tear or rupture of unspecified shoulder, not specified as traumatic**
      M75.101 **Unspecified rotator cuff tear or rupture of right shoulder, not specified as traumatic**
      M75.102 **Unspecified rotator cuff tear or rupture of left shoulder, not specified as traumatic**

   ● M75.11 **Incomplete rotator cuff tear or rupture not specified as traumatic**
      M75.110 **Incomplete rotator cuff tear or rupture of unspecified shoulder, not specified as traumatic**
      M75.111 **Incomplete rotator cuff tear or rupture of right shoulder, not specified as traumatic**
      M75.112 **Incomplete rotator cuff tear or rupture of left shoulder, not specified as traumatic**

   ● M75.12 **Complete rotator cuff tear or rupture not specified as traumatic**
      M75.120 **Complete rotator cuff tear or rupture of unspecified shoulder, not specified as traumatic**

M75.121 **Complete rotator cuff tear or rupture of right shoulder, not specified as traumatic**

M75.122 **Complete rotator cuff tear or rupture of left shoulder, not specified as traumatic**

● M75.2 **Bicipital tendinitis**
   M75.20 **Bicipital tendinitis, unspecified shoulder**
   M75.21 **Bicipital tendinitis, right shoulder**
   M75.22 **Bicipital tendinitis, left shoulder**

● M75.3 **Calcific tendinitis of shoulder**
   Calcified bursa of shoulder
   M75.30 **Calcific tendinitis of unspecified shoulder**
   M75.31 **Calcific tendinitis of right shoulder**
   M75.32 **Calcific tendinitis of left shoulder**

● M75.4 **Impingement syndrome of shoulder**
   M75.40 **Impingement syndrome of unspecified shoulder**
      Coding Clinic: 2022, Q3, P18-19
   M75.41 **Impingement syndrome of right shoulder**
   M75.42 **Impingement syndrome of left shoulder**

● M75.5 **Bursitis of shoulder**
   M75.50 **Bursitis of unspecified shoulder**
   M75.51 **Bursitis of right shoulder**
   M75.52 **Bursitis of left shoulder**

● M75.8 **Other shoulder lesions**
   M75.80 **Other shoulder lesions, unspecified shoulder**
   M75.81 **Other shoulder lesions, right shoulder**
   M75.82 **Other shoulder lesions, left shoulder**

● M75.9 **Shoulder lesion, unspecified**
   M75.90 **Shoulder lesion, unspecified, unspecified shoulder**
   M75.91 **Shoulder lesion, unspecified, right shoulder**
   M75.92 **Shoulder lesion, unspecified, left shoulder**

● M76 **Enthesopathies, lower limb, excluding foot**

> **Excludes2**   bursitis due to use, overuse and pressure (M70.-)
>   enthesopathies of ankle and foot (M77.5-)

● M76.0 **Gluteal tendinitis**
   M76.00 **Gluteal tendinitis, unspecified hip**
   M76.01 **Gluteal tendinitis, right hip**
   M76.02 **Gluteal tendinitis, left hip**

● M76.1 **Psoas tendinitis**
   M76.10 **Psoas tendinitis, unspecified hip**
   M76.11 **Psoas tendinitis, right hip**
   M76.12 **Psoas tendinitis, left hip**

● M76.2 **Iliac crest spur**
   M76.20 **Iliac crest spur, unspecified hip**
   M76.21 **Iliac crest spur, right hip**
   M76.22 **Iliac crest spur, left hip**

● M76.3 **Iliotibial band syndrome**
   M76.30 **Iliotibial band syndrome, unspecified leg**
   M76.31 **Iliotibial band syndrome, right leg**
   M76.32 **Iliotibial band syndrome, left leg**

● M76.4 **Tibial collateral bursitis [Pellegrini-Stieda]**
   M76.40 **Tibial collateral bursitis [Pellegrini-Stieda], unspecified leg**
   M76.41 **Tibial collateral bursitis [Pellegrini-Stieda], right leg**
   M76.42 **Tibial collateral bursitis [Pellegrini-Stieda], left leg**

● M76.5 **Patellar tendinitis**
   M76.50 **Patellar tendinitis, unspecified knee**
   M76.51 **Patellar tendinitis, right knee**
   M76.52 **Patellar tendinitis, left knee**

CHAPTER 13 (M00-M99)

● **M76.6**   Achilles tendinitis
     Achilles bursitis
     M76.60   Achilles tendinitis, unspecified leg
     M76.61   Achilles tendinitis, right leg
     M76.62   Achilles tendinitis, left leg

● **M76.7**   Peroneal tendinitis
     M76.70   Peroneal tendinitis, unspecified leg
     M76.71   Peroneal tendinitis, right leg
     M76.72   Peroneal tendinitis, left leg

● **M76.8**   Other specified enthesopathies of lower limb, excluding foot
     ● M76.81   Anterior tibial syndrome
       M76.811   Anterior tibial syndrome, right leg
       M76.812   Anterior tibial syndrome, left leg
       M76.819   Anterior tibial syndrome, unspecified leg
     ● M76.82   Posterior tibial tendinitis
       M76.821   Posterior tibial tendinitis, right leg
       M76.822   Posterior tibial tendinitis, left leg
       M76.829   Posterior tibial tendinitis, unspecified leg
     ● M76.89   Other specified enthesopathies of lower limb, excluding foot
       M76.891   Other specified enthesopathies of right lower limb, excluding foot
       M76.892   Other specified enthesopathies of left lower limb, excluding foot
       M76.899   Other specified enthesopathies of unspecified lower limb, excluding foot

M76.9   Unspecified enthesopathy, lower limb, excluding foot

● **M77**   Other enthesopathies
     Excludes1   bursitis NOS (M71.9-)
     Excludes2   bursitis due to use, overuse and pressure (M70.-)
              osteophyte (M25.7)
              spinal enthesopathy (M46.0-)

● **M77.0**   Medial epicondylitis
     M77.00   Medial epicondylitis, unspecified elbow
     M77.01   Medial epicondylitis, right elbow
     M77.02   Medial epicondylitis, left elbow

● **M77.1**   Lateral epicondylitis
     Tennis elbow
     M77.10   Lateral epicondylitis, unspecified elbow
     M77.11   Lateral epicondylitis, right elbow
     M77.12   Lateral epicondylitis, left elbow

● **M77.2**   Periarthritis of wrist
     M77.20   Periarthritis, unspecified wrist
     M77.21   Periarthritis, right wrist
     M77.22   Periarthritis, left wrist

● **M77.3**   Calcaneal spur
     M77.30   Calcaneal spur, unspecified foot
     M77.31   Calcaneal spur, right foot
     M77.32   Calcaneal spur, left foot

● **M77.4**   Metatarsalgia
     Excludes1   Morton's metatarsalgia (G57.6)
     M77.40   Metatarsalgia, unspecified foot
     M77.41   Metatarsalgia, right foot
     M77.42   Metatarsalgia, left foot

● **M77.5**   Other enthesopathy of foot and ankle
     M77.50   Other enthesopathy of unspecified foot and ankle
     M77.51   Other enthesopathy of right foot and ankle
     M77.52   Other enthesopathy of left foot and ankle

M77.8   Other enthesopathies, not elsewhere classified

M77.9   Enthesopathy, unspecified

     Bone spur NOS
     Capsulitis NOS
     Periarthritis NOS
     Tendinitis NOS

● **M79**   Other and unspecified soft tissue disorders, not elsewhere classified
     Excludes1   psychogenic rheumatism (F45.8)
              soft tissue pain, psychogenic (F45.41)

M79.0   Rheumatism, unspecified
     Excludes1   fibromyalgia (M79.7)
              palindromic rheumatism (M12.3-)

● **M79.1**   Myalgia
     Myofascial pain syndrome
     M79.10   Myalgia, unspecified site
     M79.11   Myalgia of mastication muscle
     M79.12   Myalgia of auxiliary muscles, head and neck
     M79.18   Myalgia, other site
       Excludes1   fibromyalgia (M79.7)
                myositis (M60.-)

M79.2   Neuralgia and neuritis, unspecified
     Excludes1   brachial radiculitis NOS (M54.1)
              lumbosacral radiculitis NOS (M54.1)
              mononeuropathies (G56-G58)
              radiculitis NOS (M54.1)
              sciatica (M54.3-M54.4)

M79.3   Panniculitis, unspecified
     Excludes1   lupus panniculitis (L93.2)
              neck and back panniculitis (M54.0-)
              relapsing [Weber-Christian] panniculitis (M35.6)

     Coding Clinic: 2024, Q1, P16

M79.4   Hypertrophy of (infrapatellar) fat pad

M79.5   Residual foreign body in soft tissue
     Excludes1   foreign body granuloma of skin and subcutaneous tissue (L92.3)
              foreign body granuloma of soft tissue (M60.2-)

● **M79.6**   Pain in limb, hand, foot, fingers and toes
     Excludes2   pain in joint (M25.5-)
     ● M79.60   Pain in limb, unspecified
       M79.601   Pain in right arm
           Pain in right upper limb NOS
       M79.602   Pain in left arm
           Pain in left upper limb NOS
       M79.603   Pain in arm, unspecified
           Pain in upper limb NOS
       M79.604   Pain in right leg
           Pain in right lower limb NOS
       M79.605   Pain in left leg
           Pain in left lower limb NOS
       M79.606   Pain in leg, unspecified
           Pain in lower limb NOS
       M79.609   Pain in unspecified limb
           Pain in limb NOS
     ● M79.62   Pain in upper arm
       Pain in axillary region
       M79.621   Pain in right upper arm
       M79.622   Pain in left upper arm
       M79.629   Pain in unspecified upper arm
     ● M79.63   Pain in forearm
       M79.631   Pain in right forearm
       M79.632   Pain in left forearm
       M79.639   Pain in unspecified forearm

▶ New   ⇒ Revised   ~~deleted~~ Deleted   Excludes 1   Excludes 2   Includes   Use additional   Code first   Code also   Key words

OGCR Official Guidelines   X Assign placeholder X   ● Use Additional Character(s)   ▶ Manifestation Code   🅗 Hierarchical Condition Category   Coding Clinic

● M79.64 Pain in hand and fingers
    M79.641 Pain in right hand
    M79.642 Pain in left hand
    M79.643 Pain in unspecified hand
    M79.644 Pain in right finger(s)
    M79.645 Pain in left finger(s)
    M79.646 Pain in unspecified finger(s)
● M79.65 Pain in thigh
    M79.651 Pain in right thigh
    M79.652 Pain in left thigh
    M79.659 Pain in unspecified thigh
● M79.66 Pain in lower leg
    M79.661 Pain in right lower leg
    M79.662 Pain in left lower leg
    M79.669 Pain in unspecified lower leg
● M79.67 Pain in foot and toes
    M79.671 Pain in right foot
    M79.672 Pain in left foot
    M79.673 Pain in unspecified foot
    M79.674 Pain in right toe(s)
    M79.675 Pain in left toe(s)
    M79.676 Pain in unspecified toe(s)

M79.7 **Fibromyalgia**
    Fibromyositis
    Fibrositis
    Myofibrositis

● M79.A **Nontraumatic compartment syndrome**
    Code first, if applicable, associated postprocedural complication
    Excludes1 compartment syndrome NOS (T79.A-)
               fibromyalgia (M79.7) nontraumatic
                 ischemic infarction of muscle (M62.2-)
               traumatic compartment syndrome (T79.A-)

  ● M79.A1 **Nontraumatic compartment syndrome of upper extremity**
    Nontraumatic compartment syndrome of shoulder, arm, forearm, wrist, hand, and fingers
    M79.A11 **Nontraumatic compartment syndrome of right upper extremity**
    M79.A12 **Nontraumatic compartment syndrome of left upper extremity**
    M79.A19 **Nontraumatic compartment syndrome of unspecified upper extremity**

  ● M79.A2 **Nontraumatic compartment syndrome of lower extremity**
    Nontraumatic compartment syndrome of hip, buttock, thigh, leg, foot, and toes
    M79.A21 **Nontraumatic compartment syndrome of right lower extremity**
    M79.A22 **Nontraumatic compartment syndrome of left lower extremity**
    M79.A29 **Nontraumatic compartment syndrome of unspecified lower extremity**
    M79.A3 **Nontraumatic compartment syndrome of abdomen**
    M79.A9 **Nontraumatic compartment syndrome of other sites**

● M79.8 **Other specified soft tissue disorders**
    M79.81 **Nontraumatic hematoma of soft tissue**
        Nontraumatic hematoma of muscle
        Nontraumatic seroma of muscle and soft tissue
    M79.89 **Other specified soft tissue disorders**
        Polyalgia

M79.9 **Soft tissue disorder, unspecified**

OGCR See Section I.C., Chapter 13.d.

Osteoporosis

Osteoporosis is a systemic condition, meaning that all bones of the musculoskeletal system are affected. Therefore, site is not a component of the codes under category M81, Osteoporosis without current pathological fracture. The site codes under category M80, Osteoporosis with current pathological fracture, identify the site of the fracture, not the osteoporosis.

1) Osteoporosis without pathological fracture

Category M81, Osteoporosis without current pathological fracture, is for use for patients with osteoporosis who do not currently have a pathologic fracture due to the osteoporosis, even if they have had a fracture in the past. For patients with a history of osteoporosis fractures, status code Z87.310, Personal history of (healed) osteoporosis fracture, should follow the code from M81.

2) Osteoporosis with current pathological fracture

Category M80, Osteoporosis with current pathological fracture, is for patients who have a current pathologic fracture at the time of an encounter. The codes under M80 identify the site of the fracture. A code from category M80, not a traumatic fracture code, should be used for any patient with known osteoporosis who suffers a fracture, even if the patient had a minor fall or trauma, if that fall or trauma would not usually break a normal, healthy bone.

OSTEOPATHIES AND CHONDROPATHIES (M80-M94)

DISORDERS OF BONE DENSITY AND STRUCTURE (M80-M85)

M80 **Osteoporosis with current pathological fracture**
    Excessive skeletal fragility (porous bone) resulting in bone fractures
    Includes osteoporosis with current fragility fracture
    Use additional code to identify major osseous defect, if applicable (M89.7-)
    Excludes1 collapsed vertebra NOS (M48.5)
               pathological fracture NOS (M84.4)
               wedging of vertebra NOS (M48.5)
    Excludes2 personal history of (healed) osteoporosis fracture (Z87.310)
    Coding Clinic: 2018, Q2, P12

The appropriate 7th character is to be added to each code from category M80:

A	initial encounter for fracture *All encounters involving diagnosis and treatment*
D	subsequent encounter for fracture with routine healing
G	subsequent encounter for fracture with delayed healing *Encounters for attention to casting or fixation devices, medication, and follow-up visits during the healing phase*
K	subsequent encounter for fracture with nonunion *Total failure of fracture healing*
P	subsequent encounter for fracture with malunion *Fracture ends do not heal together correctly.*
S	sequela

● M80.0 **Age-related osteoporosis with current pathological fracture**
    Involutional osteoporosis with current pathological fracture
    Osteoporosis NOS with current pathological fracture
    Postmenopausal osteoporosis with current pathological fracture
    Senile osteoporosis with current pathological fracture
  X ● M80.00 **Age-related osteoporosis with current pathological fracture, unspecified site** A
  ● M80.01 **Age-related osteoporosis with current pathological fracture, shoulder**
    ● M80.011 **Age-related osteoporosis with current pathological fracture, right shoulder** A
    ● M80.012 **Age-related osteoporosis with current pathological fracture, left shoulder** A

● **M80.019** Age-related osteoporosis with current pathological fracture, unspecified shoulder   A

● **M80.02** Age-related osteoporosis with current pathological fracture, humerus

  ● **M80.021** Age-related osteoporosis with current pathological fracture, right humerus   A

  ● **M80.022** Age-related osteoporosis with current pathological fracture, left humerus   A

  ● **M80.029** Age-related osteoporosis with current pathological fracture, unspecified humerus   A

● **M80.03** Age-related osteoporosis with current pathological fracture, forearm
  Age-related osteoporosis with current pathological fracture of wrist

  ● **M80.031** Age-related osteoporosis with current pathological fracture, right forearm   A

  ● **M80.032** Age-related osteoporosis with current pathological fracture, left forearm   A

  ● **M80.039** Age-related osteoporosis with current pathological fracture, unspecified forearm   A

● **M80.04** Age-related osteoporosis with current pathological fracture, hand

  ● **M80.041** Age-related osteoporosis with current pathological fracture, right hand   A

  ● **M80.042** Age-related osteoporosis with current pathological fracture, left hand   A

  ● **M80.049** Age-related osteoporosis with current pathological fracture, unspecified hand   A

● **M80.05** Age-related osteoporosis with current pathological fracture, femur
  Age-related osteoporosis with current pathological fracture of hip

  ● **M80.051** Age-related osteoporosis with current pathological fracture, right femur A 🐾   A

  ● **M80.052** Age-related osteoporosis with current pathological fracture, left femur A 🐾 A
  Coding Clinic: 2018, Q2, P12

  ● **M80.059** Age-related osteoporosis with current pathological fracture, unspecified femur A 🐾   A

● **M80.06** Age-related osteoporosis with current pathological fracture, lower leg

  ● **M80.061** Age-related osteoporosis with current pathological fracture, right lower leg A

  ● **M80.062** Age-related osteoporosis with current pathological fracture, left lower leg A

  ● **M80.069** Age-related osteoporosis with current pathological fracture, unspecified lower leg   A

● **M80.07** Age-related osteoporosis with current pathological fracture, ankle and foot

  ● **M80.071** Age-related osteoporosis with current pathological fracture, right ankle and foot   A

  ● **M80.072** Age-related osteoporosis with current pathological fracture, left ankle and foot   A

  ● **M80.079** Age-related osteoporosis with current pathological fracture, unspecified ankle and foot   A

X ● **M80.08** Age-related osteoporosis with current pathological fracture, vertebra(e) A 🐾   A

● **M80.0A** Age-related osteoporosis with current pathological fracture, other site   A

● **M80.0B** Age-related osteoporosis with current pathological fracture, pelvis

  M80.0B1 Age-related osteoporosis with current pathological fracture, right pelvis

  M80.0B2 Age-related osteoporosis with current pathological fracture, left pelvis

  M80.0B9 Age-related osteoporosis with current pathological fracture, unspecified pelvis

● **M80.8** Other osteoporosis with current pathological fracture
  Drug-induced osteoporosis with current pathological fracture
  Idiopathic osteoporosis with current pathological fracture
  Osteoporosis of disuse with current pathological fracture
  Postoophorectomy osteoporosis with current pathological fracture
  Postsurgical malabsorption osteoporosis with current pathological fracture
  Post-traumatic osteoporosis with current pathological fracture
  Use additional code for adverse effect, if applicable, to identify drug (T36-T50 with fifth or sixth character 5)

X ● **M80.80** Other osteoporosis with current pathological fracture, unspecified site   A

● **M80.81** Other osteoporosis with pathological fracture, shoulder

  ● **M80.811** Other osteoporosis with current pathological fracture, right shoulder

  ● **M80.812** Other osteoporosis with current pathological fracture, left shoulder

  ● **M80.819** Other osteoporosis with current pathological fracture, unspecified shoulder

● **M80.82** Other osteoporosis with current pathological fracture, humerus

  ● **M80.821** Other osteoporosis with current pathological fracture, right humerus

  ● **M80.822** Other osteoporosis with current pathological fracture, left humerus

  ● **M80.829** Other osteoporosis with current pathological fracture, unspecified humerus

● **M80.83** Other osteoporosis with current pathological fracture, forearm
  Other osteoporosis with current pathological fracture of wrist

  ● **M80.831** Other osteoporosis with current pathological fracture, right forearm

  ● **M80.832** Other osteoporosis with current pathological fracture, left forearm

  ● **M80.839** Other osteoporosis with current pathological fracture, unspecified forearm

● **M80.84** Other osteoporosis with current pathological fracture, hand

  ● **M80.841** Other osteoporosis with current pathological fracture, right hand

  ● **M80.842** Other osteoporosis with current pathological fracture, left hand

  ● **M80.849** Other osteoporosis with current pathological fracture, unspecified hand

▶ New   ➡ Revised   ~~deleted~~ Deleted   Excludes 1   Excludes 2   Includes   Use additional   Code first   Code also   Key words
OGCR Official Guidelines   X Assign placeholder X   ● Use Additional Character(s)   ▶ Manifestation Code   🐾 Hierarchical Condition Category   Coding Clinic

● **M80.85　Other osteoporosis with current pathological fracture, femur**
　　　　Other osteoporosis with current pathological fracture of hip

　　● **M80.851　Other osteoporosis with current pathological fracture, right femur A** 🔗

　　● **M80.852　Other osteoporosis with current pathological fracture, left femur A** 🔗

　　● **M80.859　Other osteoporosis with current pathological fracture, unspecified femur A** 🔗

● **M80.86　Other osteoporosis with current pathological fracture, lower leg**

　　● **M80.861　Other osteoporosis with current pathological fracture, right lower leg**

　　● **M80.862　Other osteoporosis with current pathological fracture, left lower leg**

　　● **M80.869　Other osteoporosis with current pathological fracture, unspecified lower leg**

● **M80.87　Other osteoporosis with current pathological fracture, ankle and foot**

　　● **M80.871　Other osteoporosis with current pathological fracture, right ankle and foot**

　　● **M80.872　Other osteoporosis with current pathological fracture, left ankle and foot**

　　● **M80.879　Other osteoporosis with current pathological fracture, unspecified ankle and foot**

X ● **M80.88　Other osteoporosis with current pathological fracture, vertebra(e) A** 🔗

　M80.8A　Other osteoporosis with current pathological fracture, other site

● **M80.8B　Other osteoporosis with current pathological fracture, pelvis**

　　　M80.8B1　Other osteoporosis with current pathological fracture, right pelvis

　　　M80.8B2　Other osteoporosis with current pathological fracture, left pelvis

　　　M80.8B9　Other osteoporosis with current pathological fracture, unspecified pelvis

● **M81　Osteoporosis without current pathological fracture**
　　Use additional code to identify:
　　major osseous defect, if applicable (M89.7-)
　　personal history of (healed) osteoporosis fracture, if applicable (Z87.310)

　　Excludes1　osteoporosis with current pathological fracture (M80.-)
　　　　　　　　Sudeck's atrophy (M89.0)

　M81.0　Age-related osteoporosis without current pathological fracture　　　　　　　　　　　　A
　　　Involutional osteoporosis without current pathological fracture
　　　Osteoporosis NOS
　　　Postmenopausal osteoporosis without current pathological fracture
　　　Senile osteoporosis without current pathological fracture

　M81.6　Localized osteoporosis [Lequesne]
　　　Excludes1　Sudeck's atrophy (M89.0)

● **M81.8　Other osteoporosis without current pathological fracture**
　　Drug-induced osteoporosis without current pathological fracture
　　Idiopathic osteoporosis without current pathological fracture
　　Osteoporosis of disuse without current pathological fracture
　　Postoophorectomy osteoporosis without current pathological fracture
　　Postsurgical malabsorption osteoporosis without current pathological fracture
　　Post-traumatic osteoporosis without current pathological fracture

　　Use additional code for adverse effect, if applicable, to identify drug (T36-T50 with fifth or sixth character 5)

● **M83　Adult osteomalacia**
　　Excludes2　infantile and juvenile osteomalacia (E55.0)
　　　　　　　　renal osteodystrophy (N25.0)
　　　　　　　　rickets (active) (E55.0)
　　　　　　　　rickets (active) sequelae (E64.3)
　　　　　　　　vitamin D-resistant osteomalacia (E83.31)
　　　　　　　　vitamin D-resistant rickets (active) (E83.31)

　M83.0　Puerperal osteomalacia　　　　　　　　　　　M
　M83.1　Senile osteomalacia　　　　　　　　　　　　A
　M83.2　Adult osteomalacia due to malabsorption　　A
　　　Postsurgical malabsorption osteomalacia in adults
　M83.3　Adult osteomalacia due to malnutrition　　A
　M83.4　Aluminum bone disease
　M83.5　Other drug-induced osteomalacia in adults　A
　　　Use additional code for adverse effect, if applicable, to identify drug (T36-T50 with fifth or sixth character 5)
　M83.8　Other adult osteomalacia　　　　　　　　　A
　M83.9　Adult osteomalacia, unspecified　　　　　　A

● **M84　Disorder of continuity of bone**
　　Excludes2　traumatic fracture of bone-see fracture, by site

● **M84.3　Stress fracture**
　　Fatigue fracture
　　March fracture
　　Stress fracture NOS
　　Stress reaction
　　Use additional external cause code(s) to identify the cause of the stress fracture
　　Excludes1　pathological fracture NOS (M84.4.-)
　　　　　　　　pathological fracture due to osteoporosis (M80.-)
　　　　　　　　traumatic fracture (S12.-, S22.-, S32.-, S42.-, S52.-, S62.-, S72.-, S82.-, S92.-)
　　Excludes2　personal history of (healed) stress (fatigue) fracture (Z87.312)
　　　　　　　　stress fracture of vertebra (M48.4-)
　　The appropriate 7th character is to be added to each code from subcategory M84.3:

　　┌───┐
　　│ A　initial encounter for fracture　　　　　　　│
　　│ D　subsequent encounter for fracture with routine healing │
　　│ G　subsequent encounter for fracture with delayed healing │
　　│ K　subsequent encounter for fracture with nonunion │
　　│ P　subsequent encounter for fracture with malunion │
　　│ S　sequela　　　　　　　　　　　　　　　　　　│
　　└───┘

X ● **M84.30　Stress fracture, unspecified site**
● **M84.31　Stress fracture, shoulder**
　　● **M84.311　Stress fracture, right shoulder**
　　● **M84.312　Stress fracture, left shoulder**
　　● **M84.319　Stress fracture, unspecified shoulder**
● **M84.32　Stress fracture, humerus**
　　● **M84.321　Stress fracture, right humerus**
　　● **M84.322　Stress fracture, left humerus**
　　● **M84.329　Stress fracture, unspecified humerus**

CHAPTER 13 (M00-M99)

CHAPTER 13 (M00-M99)

● M84.33 Stress fracture, ulna and radius
- ● M84.331 Stress fracture, right ulna
- ● M84.332 Stress fracture, left ulna
- ● M84.333 Stress fracture, right radius
- ● M84.334 Stress fracture, left radius
- ● M84.339 Stress fracture, unspecified ulna and radius

● M84.34 Stress fracture, hand and fingers
- ● M84.341 Stress fracture, right hand
- ● M84.342 Stress fracture, left hand
- ● M84.343 Stress fracture, unspecified hand
- ● M84.344 Stress fracture, right finger(s)
- ● M84.345 Stress fracture, left finger(s)
- ● M84.346 Stress fracture, unspecified finger(s)

● M84.35 Stress fracture, pelvis and femur
Stress fracture, hip
- ● M84.350 Stress fracture, pelvis
- ● M84.351 Stress fracture, right femur
- ● M84.352 Stress fracture, left femur
- ● M84.353 Stress fracture, unspecified femur
- ● M84.359 Stress fracture, hip, unspecified

● M84.36 Stress fracture, tibia and fibula
- ● M84.361 Stress fracture, right tibia
- ● M84.362 Stress fracture, left tibia
- ● M84.363 Stress fracture, right fibula
- ● M84.364 Stress fracture, left fibula
- ● M84.369 Stress fracture, unspecified tibia and fibula

● M84.37 Stress fracture, ankle, foot and toes
- ● M84.371 Stress fracture, right ankle
- ● M84.372 Stress fracture, left ankle
- ● M84.373 Stress fracture, unspecified ankle
- ● M84.374 Stress fracture, right foot
- ● M84.375 Stress fracture, left foot
- ● M84.376 Stress fracture, unspecified foot
- ● M84.377 Stress fracture, right toe(s)
- ● M84.378 Stress fracture, left toe(s)
- ● M84.379 Stress fracture, unspecified toe(s)

X ● M84.38 Stress fracture, other site
> **Excludes2** stress fracture of vertebra (M48.4-)

● M84.4 Pathological fracture, not elsewhere classified
Chronic fracture
Pathological fracture NOS
> **Excludes1** collapsed vertebra NEC (M48.5)
> pathological fracture in neoplastic disease (M84.5-)
> pathological fracture in osteoporosis (M80.-)
> pathological fracture in other disease (M84.6-)
> stress fracture (M84.3-)
> traumatic fracture (S12.-, S22.-, S32.-, S42.-, S52.-, S62.-, S72.-, S82.-, S92.-)

> **Excludes2** personal history of (healed) pathological fracture (Z87.311)

The appropriate 7th character is to be added to each code from subcategory M84.4:

A	initial encounter for fracture
D	subsequent encounter for fracture with routine healing
G	subsequent encounter for fracture with delayed healing
K	subsequent encounter for fracture with nonunion
P	subsequent encounter for fracture with malunion
S	sequela

X ● M84.40 Pathological fracture, unspecified site
● M84.41 Pathological fracture, shoulder
- ● M84.411 Pathological fracture, right shoulder
- ● M84.412 Pathological fracture, left shoulder
- ● M84.419 Pathological fracture, unspecified shoulder

● M84.42 Pathological fracture, humerus
- ● M84.421 Pathological fracture, right humerus
- ● M84.422 Pathological fracture, left humerus
- ● M84.429 Pathological fracture, unspecified humerus

● M84.43 Pathological fracture, ulna and radius
- ● M84.431 Pathological fracture, right ulna
- ● M84.432 Pathological fracture, left ulna
- ● M84.433 Pathological fracture, right radius
- ● M84.434 Pathological fracture, left radius
- ● M84.439 Pathological fracture, unspecified ulna and radius

● M84.44 Pathological fracture, hand and fingers
- ● M84.441 Pathological fracture, right hand
- ● M84.442 Pathological fracture, left hand
- ● M84.443 Pathological fracture, unspecified hand
- ● M84.444 Pathological fracture, right finger(s)
- ● M84.445 Pathological fracture, left finger(s)
- ● M84.446 Pathological fracture, unspecified finger(s)

● M84.45 Pathological fracture, femur and pelvis
- ● M84.451 Pathological fracture, right femur A
- ● M84.452 Pathological fracture, left femur A
- ● M84.453 Pathological fracture, unspecified femur A
- ● M84.454 Pathological fracture, pelvis A
  Coding Clinic: 2016, Q4, P43
- ● M84.459 Pathological fracture, hip, unspecified A

● M84.46 Pathological fracture, tibia and fibula
- ● M84.461 Pathological fracture, right tibia
- ● M84.462 Pathological fracture, left tibia
- ● M84.463 Pathological fracture, right fibula
- ● M84.464 Pathological fracture, left fibula
- ● M84.469 Pathological fracture, unspecified tibia and fibula

● M84.47 Pathological fracture, ankle, foot and toes
- ● M84.471 Pathological fracture, right ankle
- ● M84.472 Pathological fracture, left ankle
- ● M84.473 Pathological fracture, unspecified ankle
- ● M84.474 Pathological fracture, right foot
- ● M84.475 Pathological fracture, left foot
- ● M84.476 Pathological fracture, unspecified foot
- ● M84.477 Pathological fracture, right toe(s)
- ● M84.478 Pathological fracture, left toe(s)
- ● M84.479 Pathological fracture, unspecified toe(s)

X ● M84.48 Pathological fracture, other site

New | Revised | deleted Deleted | Excludes 1 | Excludes 2 | Includes | Use additional | Code first | Code also | Key words
OGCR Official Guidelines | X Assign placeholder X | ● Use Additional Character(s) | Manifestation Code | Hierarchical Condition Category | Coding Clinic

● **M84.5 Pathological fracture in neoplastic disease**

Code also underlying neoplasm

The appropriate 7th character is to be added to each code from subcategory M84.5:

A	initial encounter for fracture
D	subsequent encounter for fracture with routine healing
G	subsequent encounter for fracture with delayed healing
K	subsequent encounter for fracture with nonunion
P	subsequent encounter for fracture with malunion
S	sequela

X ● **M84.50** Pathological fracture in neoplastic disease, unspecified site

● **M84.51** Pathological fracture in neoplastic disease, shoulder

  ● **M84.511** Pathological fracture in neoplastic disease, right shoulder

  ● **M84.512** Pathological fracture in neoplastic disease, left shoulder

  ● **M84.519** Pathological fracture in neoplastic disease, unspecified shoulder

● **M84.52** Pathological fracture in neoplastic disease, humerus

  ● **M84.521** Pathological fracture in neoplastic disease, right humerus

  ● **M84.522** Pathological fracture in neoplastic disease, left humerus

  ● **M84.529** Pathological fracture in neoplastic disease, unspecified humerus

● **M84.53** Pathological fracture in neoplastic disease, ulna and radius

  ● **M84.531** Pathological fracture in neoplastic disease, right ulna

  ● **M84.532** Pathological fracture in neoplastic disease, left ulna

  ● **M84.533** Pathological fracture in neoplastic disease, right radius

  ● **M84.534** Pathological fracture in neoplastic disease, left radius

  ● **M84.539** Pathological fracture in neoplastic disease, unspecified ulna and radius

● **M84.54** Pathological fracture in neoplastic disease, hand

  ● **M84.541** Pathological fracture in neoplastic disease, right hand

  ● **M84.542** Pathological fracture in neoplastic disease, left hand

  ● **M84.549** Pathological fracture in neoplastic disease, unspecified hand

● **M84.55** Pathological fracture in neoplastic disease, pelvis and femur

  ● **M84.550** Pathological fracture in neoplastic disease, pelvis

  ● **M84.551** Pathological fracture in neoplastic disease, right femur A

  ● **M84.552** Pathological fracture in neoplastic disease, left femur A

  ● **M84.553** Pathological fracture in neoplastic disease, unspecified femur A

  ● **M84.559** Pathological fracture in neoplastic disease, hip, unspecified A

● **M84.56** Pathological fracture in neoplastic disease, tibia and fibula

  ● **M84.561** Pathological fracture in neoplastic disease, right tibia

  ● **M84.562** Pathological fracture in neoplastic disease, left tibia

  ● **M84.563** Pathological fracture in neoplastic disease, right fibula

  ● **M84.564** Pathological fracture in neoplastic disease, left fibula

  ● **M84.569** Pathological fracture in neoplastic disease, unspecified tibia and fibula

● **M84.57** Pathological fracture in neoplastic disease, ankle and foot

  ● **M84.571** Pathological fracture in neoplastic disease, right ankle

  ● **M84.572** Pathological fracture in neoplastic disease, left ankle

  ● **M84.573** Pathological fracture in neoplastic disease, unspecified ankle

  ● **M84.574** Pathological fracture in neoplastic disease, right foot

  ● **M84.575** Pathological fracture in neoplastic disease, left foot

  ● **M84.576** Pathological fracture in neoplastic disease, unspecified foot

X ● **M84.58** Pathological fracture in neoplastic disease, other specified site

Pathological fracture in neoplastic disease, vertebrae

● **M84.6 Pathological fracture in other disease**

Code also underlying condition

Excludes1 pathological fracture in osteoporosis (M80.-)

The appropriate 7th character is to be added to each code from subcategory M84.6:

A	initial encounter for fracture
D	subsequent encounter for fracture with routine healing
G	subsequent encounter for fracture with delayed healing
K	subsequent encounter for fracture with nonunion
P	subsequent encounter for fracture with malunion
S	sequela

X ● **M84.60** Pathological fracture in other disease, unspecified site

● **M84.61** Pathological fracture in other disease, shoulder

  ● **M84.611** Pathological fracture in other disease, right shoulder

  ● **M84.612** Pathological fracture in other disease, left shoulder

  ● **M84.619** Pathological fracture in other disease, unspecified shoulder

CHAPTER 13 (M00-M99)

CHAPTER 13 (M00-M99)

- M84.62   Pathological fracture in other disease, humerus
  - M84.621   Pathological fracture in other disease, right humerus
  - M84.622   Pathological fracture in other disease, left humerus
  - M84.629   Pathological fracture in other disease, unspecified humerus
- M84.63   Pathological fracture in other disease, ulna and radius
  - M84.631   Pathological fracture in other disease, right ulna
  - M84.632   Pathological fracture in other disease, left ulna
  - M84.633   Pathological fracture in other disease, right radius
  - M84.634   Pathological fracture in other disease, left radius
  - M84.639   Pathological fracture in other disease, unspecified ulna and radius
- M84.64   Pathological fracture in other disease, hand
  - M84.641   Pathological fracture in other disease, right hand
  - M84.642   Pathological fracture in other disease, left hand
  - M84.649   Pathological fracture in other disease, unspecified hand
- M84.65   Pathological fracture in other disease, pelvis and femur
  - M84.650   Pathological fracture in other disease, pelvis
  - M84.651   Pathological fracture in other disease, right femur A 🦠
  - M84.652   Pathological fracture in other disease, left femur A 🦠
  - M84.653   Pathological fracture in other disease, unspecified femur A 🦠
  - M84.659   Pathological fracture in other disease, hip, unspecified A 🦠
- M84.66   Pathological fracture in other disease, tibia and fibula
  - M84.661   Pathological fracture in other disease, right tibia
  - M84.662   Pathological fracture in other disease, left tibia
  - M84.663   Pathological fracture in other disease, right fibula
  - M84.664   Pathological fracture in other disease, left fibula
  - M84.669   Pathological fracture in other disease, unspecified tibia and fibula
- M84.67   Pathological fracture in other disease, ankle and foot
  - M84.671   Pathological fracture in other disease, right ankle
  - M84.672   Pathological fracture in other disease, left ankle
  - M84.673   Pathological fracture in other disease, unspecified ankle
  - M84.674   Pathological fracture in other disease, right foot
  - M84.675   Pathological fracture in other disease, left foot
  - M84.676   Pathological fracture in other disease, unspecified foot
- X ● M84.68   Pathological fracture in other disease, other site

- M84.7   Nontraumatic fracture, not elsewhere classified
  - M84.75   Atypical femoral fracture

    The appropriate 7th character is to be added to each code from M84.75:

A	initial encounter for fracture
D	subsequent encounter for fracture with routine healing
G	subsequent encounter for fracture with delayed healing
K	subsequent encounter for fracture with nonunion
P	subsequent encounter for fracture with malunion
S	sequela

    Coding Clinic: 2016, Q4, P41
    - M84.750   Atypical femoral fracture, unspecified
    - M84.751   Incomplete atypical femoral fracture, right leg
    - M84.752   Incomplete atypical femoral fracture, left leg
    - M84.753   Incomplete atypical femoral fracture, unspecified leg
    - M84.754   Complete transverse atypical femoral fracture, right leg A 🦠
    - M84.755   Complete transverse atypical femoral fracture, left leg A 🦠
    - M84.756   Complete transverse atypical femoral fracture, unspecified leg A 🦠
    - M84.757   Complete oblique atypical femoral fracture, right leg A 🦠
    - M84.758   Complete oblique atypical femoral fracture, left leg A 🦠
    - M84.759   Complete oblique atypical femoral fracture, unspecified leg A 🦠
- M84.8   Other disorders of continuity of bone
  - M84.80   Other disorders of continuity of bone, unspecified site
  - M84.81   Other disorders of continuity of bone, shoulder
    - M84.811   Other disorders of continuity of bone, right shoulder
    - M84.812   Other disorders of continuity of bone, left shoulder
    - M84.819   Other disorders of continuity of bone, unspecified shoulder
  - M84.82   Other disorders of continuity of bone, humerus
    - M84.821   Other disorders of continuity of bone, right humerus
    - M84.822   Other disorders of continuity of bone, left humerus
    - M84.829   Other disorders of continuity of bone, unspecified humerus
  - M84.83   Other disorders of continuity of bone, ulna and radius
    - M84.831   Other disorders of continuity of bone, right ulna
    - M84.832   Other disorders of continuity of bone, left ulna
    - M84.833   Other disorders of continuity of bone, right radius
    - M84.834   Other disorders of continuity of bone, left radius
    - M84.839   Other disorders of continuity of bone, unspecified ulna and radius
  - M84.84   Other disorders of continuity of bone, hand
    - M84.841   Other disorders of continuity of bone, right hand
    - M84.842   Other disorders of continuity of bone, left hand

M84.849   Other disorders of continuity of bone, unspecified hand

● M84.85   Other disorders of continuity of bone, pelvic region and thigh

     M84.851   Other disorders of continuity of bone, right pelvic region and thigh

     M84.852   Other disorders of continuity of bone, left pelvic region and thigh

     M84.859   Other disorders of continuity of bone, unspecified pelvic region and thigh

● M84.86   Other disorders of continuity of bone, tibia and fibula

     M84.861   Other disorders of continuity of bone, right tibia

     M84.862   Other disorders of continuity of bone, left tibia

     M84.863   Other disorders of continuity of bone, right fibula

     M84.864   Other disorders of continuity of bone, left fibula

     M84.869   Other disorders of continuity of bone, unspecified tibia and fibula

● M84.87   Other disorders of continuity of bone, ankle and foot

     M84.871   Other disorders of continuity of bone, right ankle and foot

     M84.872   Other disorders of continuity of bone, left ankle and foot

     M84.879   Other disorders of continuity of bone, unspecified ankle and foot

M84.88   Other disorders of continuity of bone, other site

M84.9   Disorder of continuity of bone, unspecified

● M85   Other disorders of bone density and structure

     Excludes1   osteogenesis imperfecta (Q78.0)
                 osteopetrosis (Q78.2)
                 osteopoikilosis (Q78.8)
                 polyostotic fibrous dysplasia (Q78.1)

● M85.0   Fibrous dysplasia (monostotic)

     Excludes2   fibrous dysplasia of jaw (M27.8)

     M85.00   Fibrous dysplasia (monostotic), unspecified site

● M85.01   Fibrous dysplasia (monostotic), shoulder

     M85.011   Fibrous dysplasia (monostotic), right shoulder

     M85.012   Fibrous dysplasia (monostotic), left shoulder

     M85.019   Fibrous dysplasia (monostotic), unspecified shoulder

● M85.02   Fibrous dysplasia (monostotic), upper arm

     M85.021   Fibrous dysplasia (monostotic), right upper arm

     M85.022   Fibrous dysplasia (monostotic), left upper arm

     M85.029   Fibrous dysplasia (monostotic), unspecified upper arm

● M85.03   Fibrous dysplasia (monostotic), forearm

     M85.031   Fibrous dysplasia (monostotic), right forearm

     M85.032   Fibrous dysplasia (monostotic), left forearm

     M85.039   Fibrous dysplasia (monostotic), unspecified forearm

● M85.04   Fibrous dysplasia (monostotic), hand

     M85.041   Fibrous dysplasia (monostotic), right hand

     M85.042   Fibrous dysplasia (monostotic), left hand

     M85.049   Fibrous dysplasia (monostotic), unspecified hand

● M85.05   Fibrous dysplasia (monostotic), thigh

     M85.051   Fibrous dysplasia (monostotic), right thigh

     M85.052   Fibrous dysplasia (monostotic), left thigh

     M85.059   Fibrous dysplasia (monostotic), unspecified thigh

● M85.06   Fibrous dysplasia (monostotic), lower leg

     M85.061   Fibrous dysplasia (monostotic), right lower leg

     M85.062   Fibrous dysplasia (monostotic), left lower leg

     M85.069   Fibrous dysplasia (monostotic), unspecified lower leg

● M85.07   Fibrous dysplasia (monostotic), ankle and foot

     M85.071   Fibrous dysplasia (monostotic), right ankle and foot

     M85.072   Fibrous dysplasia (monostotic), left ankle and foot

     M85.079   Fibrous dysplasia (monostotic), unspecified ankle and foot

M85.08   Fibrous dysplasia (monostotic), other site

M85.09   Fibrous dysplasia (monostotic), multiple sites

● M85.1   Skeletal fluorosis

     M85.10   Skeletal fluorosis, unspecified site

● M85.11   Skeletal fluorosis, shoulder

     M85.111   Skeletal fluorosis, right shoulder

     M85.112   Skeletal fluorosis, left shoulder

     M85.119   Skeletal fluorosis, unspecified shoulder

● M85.12   Skeletal fluorosis, upper arm

     M85.121   Skeletal fluorosis, right upper arm

     M85.122   Skeletal fluorosis, left upper arm

     M85.129   Skeletal fluorosis, unspecified upper arm

● M85.13   Skeletal fluorosis, forearm

     M85.131   Skeletal fluorosis, right forearm

     M85.132   Skeletal fluorosis, left forearm

     M85.139   Skeletal fluorosis, unspecified forearm

● M85.14   Skeletal fluorosis, hand

     M85.141   Skeletal fluorosis, right hand

     M85.142   Skeletal fluorosis, left hand

     M85.149   Skeletal fluorosis, unspecified hand

● M85.15   Skeletal fluorosis, thigh

     M85.151   Skeletal fluorosis, right thigh

     M85.152   Skeletal fluorosis, left thigh

     M85.159   Skeletal fluorosis, unspecified thigh

● M85.16   Skeletal fluorosis, lower leg

     M85.161   Skeletal fluorosis, right lower leg

     M85.162   Skeletal fluorosis, left lower leg

     M85.169   Skeletal fluorosis, unspecified lower leg

● M85.17   Skeletal fluorosis, ankle and foot

     M85.171   Skeletal fluorosis, right ankle and foot

     M85.172   Skeletal fluorosis, left ankle and foot

     M85.179   Skeletal fluorosis, unspecified ankle and foot

M85.18   Skeletal fluorosis, other site

M85.19   Skeletal fluorosis, multiple sites

M85.2   Hyperostosis of skull

● M85.3   Osteitis condensans

     M85.30   Osteitis condensans, unspecified site

● M85.31   Osteitis condensans, shoulder

     M85.311   Osteitis condensans, right shoulder

     M85.312   Osteitis condensans, left shoulder

     M85.319   Osteitis condensans, unspecified shoulder

● M85.32   Osteitis condensans, upper arm
     M85.321   Osteitis condensans, right upper arm
     M85.322   Osteitis condensans, left upper arm
     M85.329   Osteitis condensans, unspecified upper arm

● M85.33   Osteitis condensans, forearm
     M85.331   Osteitis condensans, right forearm
     M85.332   Osteitis condensans, left forearm
     M85.339   Osteitis condensans, unspecified forearm

● M85.34   Osteitis condensans, hand
     M85.341   Osteitis condensans, right hand
     M85.342   Osteitis condensans, left hand
     M85.349   Osteitis condensans, unspecified hand

● M85.35   Osteitis condensans, thigh
     M85.351   Osteitis condensans, right thigh
     M85.352   Osteitis condensans, left thigh
     M85.359   Osteitis condensans, unspecified thigh

● M85.36   Osteitis condensans, lower leg
     M85.361   Osteitis condensans, right lower leg
     M85.362   Osteitis condensans, left lower leg
     M85.369   Osteitis condensans, unspecified lower leg

● M85.37   Osteitis condensans, ankle and foot
     M85.371   Osteitis condensans, right ankle and foot
     M85.372   Osteitis condensans, left ankle and foot
     M85.379   Osteitis condensans, unspecified ankle and foot

   M85.38   Osteitis condensans, other site
   M85.39   Osteitis condensans, multiple sites

● M85.4   Solitary bone cyst
    Excludes2   solitary cyst of jaw (M27.4)
   M85.40   Solitary bone cyst, unspecified site

● M85.41   Solitary bone cyst, shoulder
     M85.411   Solitary bone cyst, right shoulder
     M85.412   Solitary bone cyst, left shoulder
     M85.419   Solitary bone cyst, unspecified shoulder

● M85.42   Solitary bone cyst, humerus
     M85.421   Solitary bone cyst, right humerus
     M85.422   Solitary bone cyst, left humerus
     M85.429   Solitary bone cyst, unspecified humerus

● M85.43   Solitary bone cyst, ulna and radius
     M85.431   Solitary bone cyst, right ulna and radius
     M85.432   Solitary bone cyst, left ulna and radius
     M85.439   Solitary bone cyst, unspecified ulna and radius

● M85.44   Solitary bone cyst, hand
     M85.441   Solitary bone cyst, right hand
     M85.442   Solitary bone cyst, left hand
     M85.449   Solitary bone cyst, unspecified hand

● M85.45   Solitary bone cyst, pelvis
     M85.451   Solitary bone cyst, right pelvis
     M85.452   Solitary bone cyst, left pelvis
     M85.459   Solitary bone cyst, unspecified pelvis

● M85.46   Solitary bone cyst, tibia and fibula
     M85.461   Solitary bone cyst, right tibia and fibula
     M85.462   Solitary bone cyst, left tibia and fibula

     M85.469   Solitary bone cyst, unspecified tibia and fibula

● M85.47   Solitary bone cyst, ankle and foot
     M85.471   Solitary bone cyst, right ankle and foot
     M85.472   Solitary bone cyst, left ankle and foot
     M85.479   Solitary bone cyst, unspecified ankle and foot

   M85.48   Solitary bone cyst, other site

● M85.5   Aneurysmal bone cyst
    Excludes2   aneurysmal cyst of jaw (M27.4)
   M85.50   Aneurysmal bone cyst, unspecified site

● M85.51   Aneurysmal bone cyst, shoulder
     M85.511   Aneurysmal bone cyst, right shoulder
     M85.512   Aneurysmal bone cyst, left shoulder
     M85.519   Aneurysmal bone cyst, unspecified shoulder

● M85.52   Aneurysmal bone cyst, upper arm
     M85.521   Aneurysmal bone cyst, right upper arm
     M85.522   Aneurysmal bone cyst, left upper arm
     M85.529   Aneurysmal bone cyst, unspecified upper arm

● M85.53   Aneurysmal bone cyst, forearm
     M85.531   Aneurysmal bone cyst, right forearm
     M85.532   Aneurysmal bone cyst, left forearm
     M85.539   Aneurysmal bone cyst, unspecified forearm

● M85.54   Aneurysmal bone cyst, hand
     M85.541   Aneurysmal bone cyst, right hand
     M85.542   Aneurysmal bone cyst, left hand
     M85.549   Aneurysmal bone cyst, unspecified hand

● M85.55   Aneurysmal bone cyst, thigh
     M85.551   Aneurysmal bone cyst, right thigh
     M85.552   Aneurysmal bone cyst, left thigh
     M85.559   Aneurysmal bone cyst, unspecified thigh

● M85.56   Aneurysmal bone cyst, lower leg
     M85.561   Aneurysmal bone cyst, right lower leg
     M85.562   Aneurysmal bone cyst, left lower leg
     M85.569   Aneurysmal bone cyst, unspecified lower leg

● M85.57   Aneurysmal bone cyst, ankle and foot
     M85.571   Aneurysmal bone cyst, right ankle and foot
     M85.572   Aneurysmal bone cyst, left ankle and foot
     M85.579   Aneurysmal bone cyst, unspecified ankle and foot

   M85.58   Aneurysmal bone cyst, other site
   M85.59   Aneurysmal bone cyst, multiple sites

● M85.6   Other cyst of bone
    Excludes1   cyst of jaw NEC (M27.4)
               osteitis fibrosa cystica generalisata [von Recklinghausen's disease of bone] (E21.Ø)
   M85.60   Other cyst of bone, unspecified site

● M85.61   Other cyst of bone, shoulder
     M85.611   Other cyst of bone, right shoulder
     M85.612   Other cyst of bone, left shoulder
     M85.619   Other cyst of bone, unspecified shoulder

● M85.62   Other cyst of bone, upper arm
     M85.621   Other cyst of bone, right upper arm
     M85.622   Other cyst of bone, left upper arm
     M85.629   Other cyst of bone, unspecified upper arm

● **M85.63**   Other cyst of bone, forearm
   M85.631   Other cyst of bone, right forearm
   M85.632   Other cyst of bone, left forearm
   M85.639   Other cyst of bone, unspecified forearm
● **M85.64**   Other cyst of bone, hand
   M85.641   Other cyst of bone, right hand
   M85.642   Other cyst of bone, left hand
   M85.649   Other cyst of bone, unspecified hand
● **M85.65**   Other cyst of bone, thigh
   M85.651   Other cyst of bone, right thigh
   M85.652   Other cyst of bone, left thigh
   M85.659   Other cyst of bone, unspecified thigh
● **M85.66**   Other cyst of bone, lower leg
   M85.661   Other cyst of bone, right lower leg
   M85.662   Other cyst of bone, left lower leg
   M85.669   Other cyst of bone, unspecified lower leg
● **M85.67**   Other cyst of bone, ankle and foot
   M85.671   Other cyst of bone, right ankle and foot
   M85.672   Other cyst of bone, left ankle and foot
   M85.679   Other cyst of bone, unspecified ankle and foot
  M85.68   Other cyst of bone, other site
  M85.69   Other cyst of bone, multiple sites
● **M85.8**   Other specified disorders of bone density and structure
   Hyperostosis of bones, except skull
   Osteosclerosis, acquired
   Excludes1   diffuse idiopathic skeletal hyperostosis [DISH] (M48.1)
    osteosclerosis congenita (Q77.4)
    osteosclerosis fragilitas (generalista) (Q78.2)
    osteosclerosis myelofibrosis (D75.81)
  M85.80   Other specified disorders of bone density and structure, unspecified site
● **M85.81**   Other specified disorders of bone density and structure, shoulder
   M85.811   Other specified disorders of bone density and structure, right shoulder
   M85.812   Other specified disorders of bone density and structure, left shoulder
   M85.819   Other specified disorders of bone density and structure, unspecified shoulder
● **M85.82**   Other specified disorders of bone density and structure, upper arm
   M85.821   Other specified disorders of bone density and structure, right upper arm
   M85.822   Other specified disorders of bone density and structure, left upper arm
   M85.829   Other specified disorders of bone density and structure, unspecified upper arm
● **M85.83**   Other specified disorders of bone density and structure, forearm
   M85.831   Other specified disorders of bone density and structure, right forearm
   M85.832   Other specified disorders of bone density and structure, left forearm
   M85.839   Other specified disorders of bone density and structure, unspecified forearm
● **M85.84**   Other specified disorders of bone density and structure, hand
   M85.841   Other specified disorders of bone density and structure, right hand
   M85.842   Other specified disorders of bone density and structure, left hand

   M85.849   Other specified disorders of bone density and structure, unspecified hand
● **M85.85**   Other specified disorders of bone density and structure, thigh
   M85.851   Other specified disorders of bone density and structure, right thigh
   M85.852   Other specified disorders of bone density and structure, left thigh
   M85.859   Other specified disorders of bone density and structure, unspecified thigh
● **M85.86**   Other specified disorders of bone density and structure, lower leg
   M85.861   Other specified disorders of bone density and structure, right lower leg
   M85.862   Other specified disorders of bone density and structure, left lower leg
   M85.869   Other specified disorders of bone density and structure, unspecified lower leg
● **M85.87**   Other specified disorders of bone density and structure, ankle and foot
   M85.871   Other specified disorders of bone density and structure, right ankle and foot
   M85.872   Other specified disorders of bone density and structure, left ankle and foot
   M85.879   Other specified disorders of bone density and structure, unspecified ankle and foot
  M85.88   Other specified disorders of bone density and structure, other site
  M85.89   Other specified disorders of bone density and structure, multiple sites
  M85.9   Disorder of bone density and structure, unspecified
   Coding Clinic: 2021, Q3, P11

OTHER OSTEOPATHIES (M86-M90)

  Excludes1   postprocedural osteopathies (M96.-)

● **M86**   **Osteomyelitis**
   Use additional code (B95-B97) to identify infectious agent
   Use additional code to identify major osseous defect, if applicable (M89.7-)
   Excludes1   osteomyelitis due to:
    echinococcus (B67.2)
    gonococcus (A54.43)
    salmonella (A02.24)
   Excludes2   ostemyelitis of:
    orbit (H05.0-)
    petrous bone (H70.2-)
    vertebra (M46.2-)
● **M86.0**   Acute hematogenous osteomyelitis
   M86.00   Acute hematogenous osteomyelitis, unspecified site
 ● M86.01   Acute hematogenous osteomyelitis, shoulder
    M86.011   Acute hematogenous osteomyelitis, right shoulder
    M86.012   Acute hematogenous osteomyelitis, left shoulder
    M86.019   Acute hematogenous osteomyelitis, unspecified shoulder
 ● M86.02   Acute hematogenous osteomyelitis, humerus
    M86.021   Acute hematogenous osteomyelitis, right humerus
    M86.022   Acute hematogenous osteomyelitis, left humerus
    M86.029   Acute hematogenous osteomyelitis, unspecified humerus

CHAPTER 13 (M00-M99)

Figure 13-6   Osteomyelitis of the spine. A lateral view of the lower thoracic spine demonstrates destruction of the disk space *(arrow)* as well as destruction of the adjoining vertebral bodies. (From Mettler: Essentials of Radiology, ed 2, Saunders, An Imprint of Elsevier, 2005)

Item 13–12 Osteomyelitis is an inflammation of the bone. **Acute osteomyelitis** is a rapidly destructive, pus-producing infection capable of causing severe bone destruction. **Chronic osteomyelitis** can remain long after the initial acute episode has passed and may lead to a recurrence of the acute phase. **Brodie's abscess** is an encapsulated focal abscess that must be surgically drained. **Periostitis** is an inflammation of the periosteum, a dense membrane composed of fibrous connective tissue that closely wraps all bone, except those with articulating surfaces in joints, which are covered by synovial membranes.

- M86.03   Acute hematogenous osteomyelitis, radius and ulna
    - M86.031   Acute hematogenous osteomyelitis, right radius and ulna
    - M86.032   Acute hematogenous osteomyelitis, left radius and ulna
    - M86.039   Acute hematogenous osteomyelitis, unspecified radius and ulna
- M86.04   Acute hematogenous osteomyelitis, hand
    - M86.041   Acute hematogenous osteomyelitis, right hand
    - M86.042   Acute hematogenous osteomyelitis, left hand
    - M86.049   Acute hematogenous osteomyelitis, unspecified hand
- M86.05   Acute hematogenous osteomyelitis, femur
    - M86.051   Acute hematogenous osteomyelitis, right femur
    - M86.052   Acute hematogenous osteomyelitis, left femur
    - M86.059   Acute hematogenous osteomyelitis, unspecified femur
- M86.06   Acute hematogenous osteomyelitis, tibia and fibula
    - M86.061   Acute hematogenous osteomyelitis, right tibia and fibula
    - M86.062   Acute hematogenous osteomyelitis, left tibia and fibula
    - M86.069   Acute hematogenous osteomyelitis, unspecified tibia and fibula
- M86.07   Acute hematogenous osteomyelitis, ankle and foot
    - M86.071   Acute hematogenous osteomyelitis, right ankle and foot
    - M86.072   Acute hematogenous osteomyelitis, left ankle and foot
    - M86.079   Acute hematogenous osteomyelitis, unspecified ankle and foot
    - M86.08   Acute hematogenous osteomyelitis, other sites
    - M86.09   Acute hematogenous osteomyelitis, multiple sites
- M86.1   Other acute osteomyelitis
    - M86.10   Other acute osteomyelitis, unspecified site
- M86.11   Other acute osteomyelitis, shoulder
    - M86.111   Other acute osteomyelitis, right shoulder
    - M86.112   Other acute osteomyelitis, left shoulder

- M86.119   Other acute osteomyelitis, unspecified shoulder
- M86.12   Other acute osteomyelitis, humerus
    - M86.121   Other acute osteomyelitis, right humerus
    - M86.122   Other acute osteomyelitis, left humerus
    - M86.129   Other acute osteomyelitis, unspecified humerus
- M86.13   Other acute osteomyelitis, radius and ulna
    - M86.131   Other acute osteomyelitis, right radius and ulna
    - M86.132   Other acute osteomyelitis, left radius and ulna
    - M86.139   Other acute osteomyelitis, unspecified radius and ulna
- M86.14   Other acute osteomyelitis, hand
    - M86.141   Other acute osteomyelitis, right hand
    - M86.142   Other acute osteomyelitis, left hand
    - M86.149   Other acute osteomyelitis, unspecified hand
- M86.15   Other acute osteomyelitis, femur
    - M86.151   Other acute osteomyelitis, right femur
    - M86.152   Other acute osteomyelitis, left femur
    - M86.159   Other acute osteomyelitis, unspecified femur
- M86.16   Other acute osteomyelitis, tibia and fibula
    - M86.161   Other acute osteomyelitis, right tibia and fibula
    - M86.162   Other acute osteomyelitis, left tibia and fibula
    - M86.169   Other acute osteomyelitis, unspecified tibia and fibula
- M86.17   Other acute osteomyelitis, ankle and foot
    - M86.171   Other acute osteomyelitis, right ankle and foot
        - Coding Clinic: 2020, Q1, P12
    - M86.172   Other acute osteomyelitis, left ankle and foot
    - M86.179   Other acute osteomyelitis, unspecified ankle and foot
    - M86.18   Other acute osteomyelitis, other site
    - M86.19   Other acute osteomyelitis, multiple sites
- M86.2   Subacute osteomyelitis
    - M86.20   Subacute osteomyelitis, unspecified site
- M86.21   Subacute osteomyelitis, shoulder
    - M86.211   Subacute osteomyelitis, right shoulder
    - M86.212   Subacute osteomyelitis, left shoulder
    - M86.219   Subacute osteomyelitis, unspecified shoulder
- M86.22   Subacute osteomyelitis, humerus
    - M86.221   Subacute osteomyelitis, right humerus
    - M86.222   Subacute osteomyelitis, left humerus
    - M86.229   Subacute osteomyelitis, unspecified humerus
- M86.23   Subacute osteomyelitis, radius and ulna
    - M86.231   Subacute osteomyelitis, right radius and ulna
    - M86.232   Subacute osteomyelitis, left radius and ulna
    - M86.239   Subacute osteomyelitis, unspecified radius and ulna

▶ New   ⇒ Revised   ~~deleted~~ Deleted   Excludes 1   Excludes 2   Includes   Use additional   Code first   Code also   Key words
OGCR Official Guidelines   X Assign placeholder X   ● Use Additional Character(s)   ▸ Manifestation Code   🐾 Hierarchical Condition Category   Coding Clinic

● **M86.24** Subacute osteomyelitis, hand
     M86.241 Subacute osteomyelitis, right hand 🔖
     M86.242 Subacute osteomyelitis, left hand 🔖
     M86.249 Subacute osteomyelitis, unspecified hand 🔖

● **M86.25** Subacute osteomyelitis, femur
     M86.251 Subacute osteomyelitis, right femur 🔖
     M86.252 Subacute osteomyelitis, left femur 🔖
     M86.259 Subacute osteomyelitis, unspecified femur 🔖

● **M86.26** Subacute osteomyelitis, tibia and fibula
     M86.261 Subacute osteomyelitis, right tibia and fibula 🔖
     M86.262 Subacute osteomyelitis, left tibia and fibula 🔖
     M86.269 Subacute osteomyelitis, unspecified tibia and fibula 🔖

● **M86.27** Subacute osteomyelitis, ankle and foot
     M86.271 Subacute osteomyelitis, right ankle and foot 🔖
     M86.272 Subacute osteomyelitis, left ankle and foot 🔖
     M86.279 Subacute osteomyelitis, unspecified ankle and foot 🔖

M86.28 Subacute osteomyelitis, other site 🔖
M86.29 Subacute osteomyelitis, multiple sites 🔖

● **M86.3** Chronic multifocal osteomyelitis
     M86.30 Chronic multifocal osteomyelitis, unspecified site 🔖

● **M86.31** Chronic multifocal osteomyelitis, shoulder
     M86.311 Chronic multifocal osteomyelitis, right shoulder 🔖
     M86.312 Chronic multifocal osteomyelitis, left shoulder 🔖
     M86.319 Chronic multifocal osteomyelitis, unspecified shoulder 🔖

● **M86.32** Chronic multifocal osteomyelitis, humerus
     M86.321 Chronic multifocal osteomyelitis, right humerus 🔖
     M86.322 Chronic multifocal osteomyelitis, left humerus 🔖
     M86.329 Chronic multifocal osteomyelitis, unspecified humerus 🔖

● **M86.33** Chronic multifocal osteomyelitis, radius and ulna
     M86.331 Chronic multifocal osteomyelitis, right radius and ulna 🔖
     M86.332 Chronic multifocal osteomyelitis, left radius and ulna 🔖
     M86.339 Chronic multifocal osteomyelitis, unspecified radius and ulna 🔖

● **M86.34** Chronic multifocal osteomyelitis, hand
     M86.341 Chronic multifocal osteomyelitis, right hand 🔖
     M86.342 Chronic multifocal osteomyelitis, left hand 🔖
     M86.349 Chronic multifocal osteomyelitis, unspecified hand 🔖

● **M86.35** Chronic multifocal osteomyelitis, femur
     M86.351 Chronic multifocal osteomyelitis, right femur 🔖
     M86.352 Chronic multifocal osteomyelitis, left femur 🔖
     M86.359 Chronic multifocal osteomyelitis, unspecified femur 🔖

● **M86.36** Chronic multifocal osteomyelitis, tibia and fibula
     M86.361 Chronic multifocal osteomyelitis, right tibia and fibula 🔖
     M86.362 Chronic multifocal osteomyelitis, left tibia and fibula 🔖
     M86.369 Chronic multifocal osteomyelitis, unspecified tibia and fibula 🔖

● **M86.37** Chronic multifocal osteomyelitis, ankle and foot
     M86.371 Chronic multifocal osteomyelitis, right ankle and foot 🔖
     M86.372 Chronic multifocal osteomyelitis, left ankle and foot 🔖
     M86.379 Chronic multifocal osteomyelitis, unspecified ankle and foot 🔖

M86.38 Chronic multifocal osteomyelitis, other site 🔖
M86.39 Chronic multifocal osteomyelitis, multiple sites 🔖

● **M86.4** Chronic osteomyelitis with draining sinus
     M86.40 Chronic osteomyelitis with draining sinus, unspecified site 🔖

● **M86.41** Chronic osteomyelitis with draining sinus, shoulder
     M86.411 Chronic osteomyelitis with draining sinus, right shoulder 🔖
     M86.412 Chronic osteomyelitis with draining sinus, left shoulder 🔖
     M86.419 Chronic osteomyelitis with draining sinus, unspecified shoulder 🔖

● **M86.42** Chronic osteomyelitis with draining sinus, humerus
     M86.421 Chronic osteomyelitis with draining sinus, right humerus 🔖
     M86.422 Chronic osteomyelitis with draining sinus, left humerus 🔖
     M86.429 Chronic osteomyelitis with draining sinus, unspecified humerus 🔖

● **M86.43** Chronic osteomyelitis with draining sinus, radius and ulna
     M86.431 Chronic osteomyelitis with draining sinus, right radius and ulna 🔖
     M86.432 Chronic osteomyelitis with draining sinus, left radius and ulna 🔖
     M86.439 Chronic osteomyelitis with draining sinus, unspecified radius and ulna 🔖

● **M86.44** Chronic osteomyelitis with draining sinus, hand
     M86.441 Chronic osteomyelitis with draining sinus, right hand 🔖
     M86.442 Chronic osteomyelitis with draining sinus, left hand 🔖
     M86.449 Chronic osteomyelitis with draining sinus, unspecified hand 🔖

● **M86.45** Chronic osteomyelitis with draining sinus, femur
     M86.451 Chronic osteomyelitis with draining sinus, right femur 🔖
     M86.452 Chronic osteomyelitis with draining sinus, left femur 🔖
     M86.459 Chronic osteomyelitis with draining sinus, unspecified femur 🔖

● **M86.46** Chronic osteomyelitis with draining sinus, tibia and fibula
     M86.461 Chronic osteomyelitis with draining sinus, right tibia and fibula 🔖
     M86.462 Chronic osteomyelitis with draining sinus, left tibia and fibula 🔖
     M86.469 Chronic osteomyelitis with draining sinus, unspecified tibia and fibula 🔖

CHAPTER 13 (M00-M99)

● M86.47   Chronic osteomyelitis with draining sinus, ankle and foot

    M86.471   Chronic osteomyelitis with draining sinus, right ankle and foot 🐾

    M86.472   Chronic osteomyelitis with draining sinus, left ankle and foot 🐾

    M86.479   Chronic osteomyelitis with draining sinus, unspecified ankle and foot 🐾

M86.48   Chronic osteomyelitis with draining sinus, other site 🐾

M86.49   Chronic osteomyelitis with draining sinus, multiple sites 🐾

● M86.5   Other chronic hematogenous osteomyelitis

    M86.50   Other chronic hematogenous osteomyelitis, unspecified site 🐾

● M86.51   Other chronic hematogenous osteomyelitis, shoulder

    M86.511   Other chronic hematogenous osteomyelitis, right shoulder 🐾

    M86.512   Other chronic hematogenous osteomyelitis, left shoulder 🐾

    M86.519   Other chronic hematogenous osteomyelitis, unspecified shoulder 🐾

● M86.52   Other chronic hematogenous osteomyelitis, humerus

    M86.521   Other chronic hematogenous osteomyelitis, right humerus 🐾

    M86.522   Other chronic hematogenous osteomyelitis, left humerus 🐾

    M86.529   Other chronic hematogenous osteomyelitis, unspecified humerus 🐾

● M86.53   Other chronic hematogenous osteomyelitis, radius and ulna

    M86.531   Other chronic hematogenous osteomyelitis, right radius and ulna 🐾

    M86.532   Other chronic hematogenous osteomyelitis, left radius and ulna 🐾

    M86.539   Other chronic hematogenous osteomyelitis, unspecified radius and ulna 🐾

● M86.54   Other chronic hematogenous osteomyelitis, hand

    M86.541   Other chronic hematogenous osteomyelitis, right hand 🐾

    M86.542   Other chronic hematogenous osteomyelitis, left hand 🐾

    M86.549   Other chronic hematogenous osteomyelitis, unspecified hand 🐾

● M86.55   Other chronic hematogenous osteomyelitis, femur

    M86.551   Other chronic hematogenous osteomyelitis, right femur 🐾

    M86.552   Other chronic hematogenous osteomyelitis, left femur 🐾

    M86.559   Other chronic hematogenous osteomyelitis, unspecified femur 🐾

● M86.56   Other chronic hematogenous osteomyelitis, tibia and fibula

    M86.561   Other chronic hematogenous osteomyelitis, right tibia and fibula 🐾

    M86.562   Other chronic hematogenous osteomyelitis, left tibia and fibula 🐾

    M86.569   Other chronic hematogenous osteomyelitis, unspecified tibia and fibula 🐾

● M86.57   Other chronic hematogenous osteomyelitis, ankle and foot

    M86.571   Other chronic hematogenous osteomyelitis, right ankle and foot 🐾

    M86.572   Other chronic hematogenous osteomyelitis, left ankle and foot 🐾

    M86.579   Other chronic hematogenous osteomyelitis, unspecified ankle and foot 🐾

M86.58   Other chronic hematogenous osteomyelitis, other site 🐾

M86.59   Other chronic hematogenous osteomyelitis, multiple sites 🐾

● M86.6   Other chronic osteomyelitis

    M86.60   Other chronic osteomyelitis, unspecified site 🐾

● M86.61   Other chronic osteomyelitis, shoulder

    M86.611   Other chronic osteomyelitis, right shoulder 🐾

    M86.612   Other chronic osteomyelitis, left shoulder 🐾

    M86.619   Other chronic osteomyelitis, unspecified shoulder 🐾

● M86.62   Other chronic osteomyelitis, humerus

    M86.621   Other chronic osteomyelitis, right humerus 🐾

    M86.622   Other chronic osteomyelitis, left humerus 🐾

    M86.629   Other chronic osteomyelitis, unspecified humerus 🐾

● M86.63   Other chronic osteomyelitis, radius and ulna

    M86.631   Other chronic osteomyelitis, right radius and ulna 🐾

    M86.632   Other chronic osteomyelitis, left radius and ulna 🐾

    M86.639   Other chronic osteomyelitis, unspecified radius and ulna 🐾

● M86.64   Other chronic osteomyelitis, hand

    M86.641   Other chronic osteomyelitis, right hand 🐾

    M86.642   Other chronic osteomyelitis, left hand 🐾

    M86.649   Other chronic osteomyelitis, unspecified hand 🐾

● M86.65   Other chronic osteomyelitis, thigh

    M86.651   Other chronic osteomyelitis, right thigh 🐾

    M86.652   Other chronic osteomyelitis, left thigh 🐾

    M86.659   Other chronic osteomyelitis, unspecified thigh 🐾

● M86.66   Other chronic osteomyelitis, tibia and fibula

    M86.661   Other chronic osteomyelitis, right tibia and fibula 🐾

    M86.662   Other chronic osteomyelitis, left tibia and fibula 🐾

    M86.669   Other chronic osteomyelitis, unspecified tibia and fibula 🐾

● M86.67   Other chronic osteomyelitis, ankle and foot

    M86.671   Other chronic osteomyelitis, right ankle and foot 🐾
         Coding Clinic: 2016, Q1, P13

    M86.672   Other chronic osteomyelitis, left ankle and foot 🐾

    M86.679   Other chronic osteomyelitis, unspecified ankle and foot 🐾

M86.68   Other chronic osteomyelitis, other site 🐾

M86.69   Other chronic osteomyelitis, multiple sites 🐾

▶ New   ⇒ Revised   ~~deleted~~ Deleted   Excludes 1   Excludes 2   Includes   Use additional   Code first   Code also   Key words

OGCR Official Guidelines   X Assign placeholder X   ● Use Additional Character(s)   ▶ Manifestation Code   🐾 Hierarchical Condition Category   *Coding Clinic*

● M86.8 **Other osteomyelitis**
　　Brodie's abscess
　　● M86.8X **Other osteomyelitis**
　　　　M86.8X0 Other osteomyelitis, multiple sites 🔍
　　　　M86.8X1 Other osteomyelitis, shoulder 🔍
　　　　M86.8X2 Other osteomyelitis, upper arm 🔍
　　　　M86.8X3 Other osteomyelitis, forearm 🔍
　　　　M86.8X4 Other osteomyelitis, hand 🔍
　　　　M86.8X5 Other osteomyelitis, thigh 🔍
　　　　M86.8X6 Other osteomyelitis, lower leg 🔍
　　　　M86.8X7 Other osteomyelitis, ankle and foot 🔍
　　　　M86.8X8 Other osteomyelitis, other site 🔍
　　　　　　Coding Clinic: 2022, Q1, P31
　　　　M86.8X9 Other osteomyelitis, unspecified sites 🔍
● M86.9 **Osteomyelitis, unspecified** 🔍
　　Infection of bone NOS
　　Periostitis without osteomyelitis

● M87 **Osteonecrosis**
　　Includes　avascular necrosis of bone
　　Use additional code to identify major osseous defect, if applicable (M89.7-)
　　Excludes1　juvenile osteonecrosis (M91-M92)
　　　　osteochondropathies (M90-M93)

● M87.0 **Idiopathic aseptic necrosis of bone**
　　M87.00 Idiopathic aseptic necrosis of unspecified bone 🔍
　　● M87.01 Idiopathic aseptic necrosis of shoulder
　　　　Idiopathic aseptic necrosis of clavicle and scapula
　　　　M87.011 Idiopathic aseptic necrosis of right shoulder 🔍
　　　　M87.012 Idiopathic aseptic necrosis of left shoulder 🔍
　　　　M87.019 Idiopathic aseptic necrosis of unspecified shoulder 🔍
　　● M87.02 Idiopathic aseptic necrosis of humerus
　　　　M87.021 Idiopathic aseptic necrosis of right humerus 🔍
　　　　M87.022 Idiopathic aseptic necrosis of left humerus 🔍
　　　　M87.029 Idiopathic aseptic necrosis of unspecified humerus 🔍
　　● M87.03 Idiopathic aseptic necrosis of radius, ulna and carpus
　　　　M87.031 Idiopathic aseptic necrosis of right radius 🔍
　　　　M87.032 Idiopathic aseptic necrosis of left radius 🔍
　　　　M87.033 Idiopathic aseptic necrosis of unspecified radius 🔍
　　　　M87.034 Idiopathic aseptic necrosis of right ulna 🔍
　　　　M87.035 Idiopathic aseptic necrosis of left ulna 🔍
　　　　M87.036 Idiopathic aseptic necrosis of unspecified ulna 🔍
　　　　M87.037 Idiopathic aseptic necrosis of right carpus 🔍
　　　　M87.038 Idiopathic aseptic necrosis of left carpus 🔍
　　　　M87.039 Idiopathic aseptic necrosis of unspecified carpus 🔍

● M87.04 **Idiopathic aseptic necrosis of hand and fingers**
　　Idiopathic aseptic necrosis of metacarpals and phalanges of hands
　　M87.041 Idiopathic aseptic necrosis of right hand 🔍
　　M87.042 Idiopathic aseptic necrosis of left hand 🔍
　　M87.043 Idiopathic aseptic necrosis of unspecified hand 🔍
　　M87.044 Idiopathic aseptic necrosis of right finger(s) 🔍
　　M87.045 Idiopathic aseptic necrosis of left finger(s) 🔍
　　M87.046 Idiopathic aseptic necrosis of unspecified finger(s) 🔍
● M87.05 **Idiopathic aseptic necrosis of pelvis and femur**
　　M87.050 Idiopathic aseptic necrosis of pelvis 🔍
　　M87.051 Idiopathic aseptic necrosis of right femur 🔍
　　M87.052 Idiopathic aseptic necrosis of left femur 🔍
　　M87.059 Idiopathic aseptic necrosis of unspecified femur 🔍
　　　　Idiopathic aseptic necrosis of hip NOS
● M87.06 **Idiopathic aseptic necrosis of tibia and fibula**
　　M87.061 Idiopathic aseptic necrosis of right tibia 🔍
　　M87.062 Idiopathic aseptic necrosis of left tibia 🔍
　　M87.063 Idiopathic aseptic necrosis of unspecified tibia 🔍
　　M87.064 Idiopathic aseptic necrosis of right fibula 🔍
　　M87.065 Idiopathic aseptic necrosis of left fibula 🔍
　　M87.066 Idiopathic aseptic necrosis of unspecified fibula 🔍
● M87.07 **Idiopathic aseptic necrosis of ankle, foot and toes**
　　Idiopathic aseptic necrosis of metatarsus, tarsus, and phalanges of toes
　　M87.071 Idiopathic aseptic necrosis of right ankle 🔍
　　M87.072 Idiopathic aseptic necrosis of left ankle 🔍
　　M87.073 Idiopathic aseptic necrosis of unspecified ankle 🔍
　　M87.074 Idiopathic aseptic necrosis of right foot 🔍
　　M87.075 Idiopathic aseptic necrosis of left foot 🔍
　　M87.076 Idiopathic aseptic necrosis of unspecified foot 🔍
　　M87.077 Idiopathic aseptic necrosis of right toe(s) 🔍
　　M87.078 Idiopathic aseptic necrosis of left toe(s) 🔍
　　M87.079 Idiopathic aseptic necrosis of unspecified toe(s) 🔍
　　M87.08 Idiopathic aseptic necrosis of bone, other site 🔍
　　M87.09 Idiopathic aseptic necrosis of bone, multiple sites 🔍

CHAPTER 13 (M00-M99)

● M87.1 **Osteonecrosis due to drugs**

Use additional code for adverse effect, if applicable, to identify drug (T36-T50 with fifth or sixth character 5)

M87.10 Osteonecrosis due to drugs, unspecified bone 🐾

● M87.11 Osteonecrosis due to drugs, shoulder

    M87.111 Osteonecrosis due to drugs, right shoulder 🐾

    M87.112 Osteonecrosis due to drugs, left shoulder 🐾

    M87.119 Osteonecrosis due to drugs, unspecified shoulder 🐾

● M87.12 Osteonecrosis due to drugs, humerus

    M87.121 Osteonecrosis due to drugs, right humerus 🐾

    M87.122 Osteonecrosis due to drugs, left humerus 🐾

    M87.129 Osteonecrosis due to drugs, unspecified humerus 🐾

● M87.13 Osteonecrosis due to drugs of radius, ulna and carpus

    M87.131 Osteonecrosis due to drugs of right radius 🐾

    M87.132 Osteonecrosis due to drugs of left radius 🐾

    M87.133 Osteonecrosis due to drugs of unspecified radius 🐾

    M87.134 Osteonecrosis due to drugs of right ulna 🐾

    M87.135 Osteonecrosis due to drugs of left ulna 🐾

    M87.136 Osteonecrosis due to drugs of unspecified ulna 🐾

    M87.137 Osteonecrosis due to drugs of right carpus 🐾

    M87.138 Osteonecrosis due to drugs of left carpus 🐾

    M87.139 Osteonecrosis due to drugs of unspecified carpus 🐾

● M87.14 Osteonecrosis due to drugs, hand and fingers

    M87.141 Osteonecrosis due to drugs, right hand 🐾

    M87.142 Osteonecrosis due to drugs, left hand 🐾

    M87.143 Osteonecrosis due to drugs, unspecified hand 🐾

    M87.144 Osteonecrosis due to drugs, right finger(s) 🐾

    M87.145 Osteonecrosis due to drugs, left finger(s) 🐾

    M87.146 Osteonecrosis due to drugs, unspecified finger(s) 🐾

● M87.15 Osteonecrosis due to drugs, pelvis and femur

    M87.150 Osteonecrosis due to drugs, pelvis 🐾

    M87.151 Osteonecrosis due to drugs, right femur 🐾

    M87.152 Osteonecrosis due to drugs, left femur 🐾

    M87.159 Osteonecrosis due to drugs, unspecified femur 🐾

● M87.16 Osteonecrosis due to drugs, tibia and fibula

    M87.161 Osteonecrosis due to drugs, right tibia 🐾

    M87.162 Osteonecrosis due to drugs, left tibia 🐾

    M87.163 Osteonecrosis due to drugs, unspecified tibia 🐾

    M87.164 Osteonecrosis due to drugs, right fibula 🐾

    M87.165 Osteonecrosis due to drugs, left fibula 🐾

    M87.166 Osteonecrosis due to drugs, unspecified fibula 🐾

● M87.17 Osteonecrosis due to drugs, ankle, foot and toes

    M87.171 Osteonecrosis due to drugs, right ankle 🐾

    M87.172 Osteonecrosis due to drugs, left ankle 🐾

    M87.173 Osteonecrosis due to drugs, unspecified ankle 🐾

    M87.174 Osteonecrosis due to drugs, right foot 🐾

    M87.175 Osteonecrosis due to drugs, left foot 🐾

    M87.176 Osteonecrosis due to drugs, unspecified foot 🐾

    M87.177 Osteonecrosis due to drugs, right toe(s) 🐾

    M87.178 Osteonecrosis due to drugs, left toe(s) 🐾

    M87.179 Osteonecrosis due to drugs, unspecified toe(s) 🐾

● M87.18 Osteonecrosis due to drugs, other site

    M87.180 Osteonecrosis due to drugs, jaw 🐾

    M87.188 Osteonecrosis due to drugs, other site 🐾

    M87.19 Osteonecrosis due to drugs, multiple sites 🐾

● M87.2 **Osteonecrosis due to previous trauma**

M87.20 Osteonecrosis due to previous trauma, unspecified bone 🐾

● M87.21 Osteonecrosis due to previous trauma, shoulder

    M87.211 Osteonecrosis due to previous trauma, right shoulder 🐾

    M87.212 Osteonecrosis due to previous trauma, left shoulder 🐾

    M87.219 Osteonecrosis due to previous trauma, unspecified shoulder 🐾

● M87.22 Osteonecrosis due to previous trauma, humerus

    M87.221 Osteonecrosis due to previous trauma, right humerus 🐾

    M87.222 Osteonecrosis due to previous trauma, left humerus 🐾

    M87.229 Osteonecrosis due to previous trauma, unspecified humerus 🐾

● M87.23 Osteonecrosis due to previous trauma of radius, ulna and carpus

    M87.231 Osteonecrosis due to previous trauma of right radius 🐾

    M87.232 Osteonecrosis due to previous trauma of left radius 🐾

    M87.233 Osteonecrosis due to previous trauma of unspecified radius 🐾

    M87.234 Osteonecrosis due to previous trauma of right ulna 🐾

    M87.235 Osteonecrosis due to previous trauma of left ulna 🐾

    M87.236 Osteonecrosis due to previous trauma of unspecified ulna 🐾

    M87.237 Osteonecrosis due to previous trauma of right carpus 🐾

    M87.238 Osteonecrosis due to previous trauma of left carpus 🐾

    M87.239 Osteonecrosis due to previous trauma of unspecified carpus 🐾

▶ New   ➡ Revised   ~~deleted~~ Deleted   Excludes 1   Excludes 2   Includes   Use additional   Code first   Code also   Key words

OGCR Official Guidelines   X Assign placeholder X   ● Use Additional Character(s)   ▶ Manifestation Code   🐾 Hierarchical Condition Category   Coding Clinic

● M87.24 Osteonecrosis due to previous trauma, hand and fingers

     M87.241 Osteonecrosis due to previous trauma, right hand 🐾

     M87.242 Osteonecrosis due to previous trauma, left hand 🐾

     M87.243 Osteonecrosis due to previous trauma, unspecified hand 🐾

     M87.244 Osteonecrosis due to previous trauma, right finger(s) 🐾

     M87.245 Osteonecrosis due to previous trauma, left finger(s) 🐾

     M87.246 Osteonecrosis due to previous trauma, unspecified finger(s) 🐾

● M87.25 Osteonecrosis due to previous trauma, pelvis and femur

     M87.250 Osteonecrosis due to previous trauma, pelvis 🐾

     M87.251 Osteonecrosis due to previous trauma, right femur 🐾

     M87.252 Osteonecrosis due to previous trauma, left femur 🐾

     M87.256 Osteonecrosis due to previous trauma, unspecified femur 🐾

● M87.26 Osteonecrosis due to previous trauma, tibia and fibula

     M87.261 Osteonecrosis due to previous trauma, right tibia 🐾

     M87.262 Osteonecrosis due to previous trauma, left tibia 🐾

     M87.263 Osteonecrosis due to previous trauma, unspecified tibia 🐾

     M87.264 Osteonecrosis due to previous trauma, right fibula 🐾

     M87.265 Osteonecrosis due to previous trauma, left fibula 🐾

     M87.266 Osteonecrosis due to previous trauma, unspecified fibula 🐾

● M87.27 Osteonecrosis due to previous trauma, ankle, foot and toes

     M87.271 Osteonecrosis due to previous trauma, right ankle 🐾

     M87.272 Osteonecrosis due to previous trauma, left ankle 🐾

     M87.273 Osteonecrosis due to previous trauma, unspecified ankle 🐾

     M87.274 Osteonecrosis due to previous trauma, right foot 🐾

     M87.275 Osteonecrosis due to previous trauma, left foot 🐾

     M87.276 Osteonecrosis due to previous trauma, unspecified foot 🐾

     M87.277 Osteonecrosis due to previous trauma, right toe(s) 🐾

     M87.278 Osteonecrosis due to previous trauma, left toe(s) 🐾

     M87.279 Osteonecrosis due to previous trauma, unspecified toe(s) 🐾

   M87.28 Osteonecrosis due to previous trauma, other site 🐾

   M87.29 Osteonecrosis due to previous trauma, multiple sites 🐾

● M87.3 Other secondary osteonecrosis

   M87.30 Other secondary osteonecrosis, unspecified bone 🐾

● M87.31 Other secondary osteonecrosis, shoulder

     M87.311 Other secondary osteonecrosis, right shoulder 🐾

     M87.312 Other secondary osteonecrosis, left shoulder 🐾

     M87.319 Other secondary osteonecrosis, unspecified shoulder 🐾

● M87.32 Other secondary osteonecrosis, humerus

     M87.321 Other secondary osteonecrosis, right humerus 🐾

     M87.322 Other secondary osteonecrosis, left humerus 🐾

     M87.329 Other secondary osteonecrosis, unspecified humerus 🐾

● M87.33 Other secondary osteonecrosis of radius, ulna and carpus

     M87.331 Other secondary osteonecrosis of right radius 🐾

     M87.332 Other secondary osteonecrosis of left radius 🐾

     M87.333 Other secondary osteonecrosis of unspecified radius 🐾

     M87.334 Other secondary osteonecrosis of right ulna 🐾

     M87.335 Other secondary osteonecrosis of left ulna 🐾

     M87.336 Other secondary osteonecrosis of unspecified ulna 🐾

     M87.337 Other secondary osteonecrosis of right carpus 🐾

     M87.338 Other secondary osteonecrosis of left carpus 🐾

     M87.339 Other secondary osteonecrosis of unspecified carpus 🐾

● M87.34 Other secondary osteonecrosis, hand and fingers

     M87.341 Other secondary osteonecrosis, right hand 🐾

     M87.342 Other secondary osteonecrosis, left hand 🐾

     M87.343 Other secondary osteonecrosis, unspecified hand 🐾

     M87.344 Other secondary osteonecrosis, right finger(s) 🐾

     M87.345 Other secondary osteonecrosis, left finger(s) 🐾

     M87.346 Other secondary osteonecrosis, unspecified finger(s) 🐾

● M87.35 Other secondary osteonecrosis, pelvis and femur

     M87.350 Other secondary osteonecrosis, pelvis 🐾

     M87.351 Other secondary osteonecrosis, right femur 🐾

     M87.352 Other secondary osteonecrosis, left femur 🐾

     M87.353 Other secondary osteonecrosis, unspecified femur 🐾

● M87.36 Other secondary osteonecrosis, tibia and fibula

     M87.361 Other secondary osteonecrosis, right tibia 🐾

     M87.362 Other secondary osteonecrosis, left tibia 🐾

     M87.363 Other secondary osteonecrosis, unspecified tibia 🐾

     M87.364 Other secondary osteonecrosis, right fibula 🐾

     M87.365 Other secondary osteonecrosis, left fibula 🐾

     M87.366 Other secondary osteonecrosis, unspecified fibula 🐾

CHAPTER 13 (M00-M99)

- M87.37   Other secondary osteonecrosis, ankle and foot
  - M87.371   Other secondary osteonecrosis, right ankle 🔖
  - M87.372   Other secondary osteonecrosis, left ankle 🔖
  - M87.373   Other secondary osteonecrosis, unspecified ankle 🔖
  - M87.374   Other secondary osteonecrosis, right foot 🔖
  - M87.375   Other secondary osteonecrosis, left foot 🔖
  - M87.376   Other secondary osteonecrosis, unspecified foot 🔖
  - M87.377   Other secondary osteonecrosis, right toe(s) 🔖
  - M87.378   Other secondary osteonecrosis, left toe(s) 🔖
  - M87.379   Other secondary osteonecrosis, unspecified toe(s) 🔖
- M87.38   Other secondary osteonecrosis, other site 🔖
- M87.39   Other secondary osteonecrosis, multiple sites 🔖

- M87.8   **Other osteonecrosis**
  - M87.80   Other osteonecrosis, unspecified bone 🔖
  - M87.81   Other osteonecrosis, shoulder
    - M87.811   Other osteonecrosis, right shoulder 🔖
    - M87.812   Other osteonecrosis, left shoulder 🔖
    - M87.819   Other osteonecrosis, unspecified shoulder 🔖
  - M87.82   Other osteonecrosis, humerus
    - M87.821   Other osteonecrosis, right humerus 🔖
    - M87.822   Other osteonecrosis, left humerus 🔖
    - M87.829   Other osteonecrosis, unspecified humerus 🔖
  - M87.83   Other osteonecrosis of radius, ulna and carpus
    - M87.831   Other osteonecrosis of right radius 🔖
    - M87.832   Other osteonecrosis of left radius 🔖
    - M87.833   Other osteonecrosis of unspecified radius 🔖
    - M87.834   Other osteonecrosis of right ulna 🔖
    - M87.835   Other osteonecrosis of left ulna 🔖
    - M87.836   Other osteonecrosis of unspecified ulna 🔖
    - M87.837   Other osteonecrosis of right carpus 🔖
    - M87.838   Other osteonecrosis of left carpus 🔖
    - M87.839   Other osteonecrosis of unspecified carpus 🔖
  - M87.84   Other osteonecrosis, hand and fingers
    - M87.841   Other osteonecrosis, right hand 🔖
    - M87.842   Other osteonecrosis, left hand 🔖
    - M87.843   Other osteonecrosis, unspecified hand 🔖
    - M87.844   Other osteonecrosis, right finger(s) 🔖
    - M87.845   Other osteonecrosis, left finger(s) 🔖
    - M87.849   Other osteonecrosis, unspecified finger(s) 🔖
  - M87.85   Other osteonecrosis, pelvis and femur
    - M87.850   Other osteonecrosis, pelvis 🔖
    - M87.851   Other osteonecrosis, right femur 🔖
    - M87.852   Other osteonecrosis, left femur 🔖
    - M87.859   Other osteonecrosis, unspecified femur 🔖
  - M87.86   Other osteonecrosis, tibia and fibula
    - M87.861   Other osteonecrosis, right tibia 🔖
    - M87.862   Other osteonecrosis, left tibia 🔖

- M87.863   Other osteonecrosis, unspecified tibia 🔖
- M87.864   Other osteonecrosis, right fibula 🔖
- M87.865   Other osteonecrosis, left fibula 🔖
- M87.869   Other osteonecrosis, unspecified fibula 🔖
- M87.87   Other osteonecrosis, ankle, foot and toes
  - M87.871   Other osteonecrosis, right ankle 🔖
  - M87.872   Other osteonecrosis, left ankle 🔖
  - M87.873   Other osteonecrosis, unspecified ankle 🔖
  - M87.874   Other osteonecrosis, right foot 🔖
  - M87.875   Other osteonecrosis, left foot 🔖
  - M87.876   Other osteonecrosis, unspecified foot 🔖
  - M87.877   Other osteonecrosis, right toe(s) 🔖
  - M87.878   Other osteonecrosis, left toe(s) 🔖
  - M87.879   Other osteonecrosis, unspecified toe(s) 🔖
- M87.88   Other osteonecrosis, other site 🔖
- M87.89   Other osteonecrosis, multiple sites 🔖
- M87.9   **Osteonecrosis, unspecified** 🔖
  Necrosis of bone NOS

- M88   **Osteitis deformans [Paget's disease of bone]**
  Chronic disorder that results in enlarged and deformed bones. The excessive breakdown and formation of bone tissue causes bones to weaken and results in bone pain, arthritis, deformities, and fractures.

  Excludes1   osteitis deformans in neoplastic disease (M90.6)

  - M88.0   **Osteitis deformans of skull**
  - M88.1   **Osteitis deformans of vertebrae**
  - M88.8   **Osteitis deformans of other bones**
    - M88.81   Osteitis deformans of shoulder
      - M88.811   Osteitis deformans of right shoulder
      - M88.812   Osteitis deformans of left shoulder
      - M88.819   Osteitis deformans of unspecified shoulder
    - M88.82   Osteitis deformans of upper arm
      - M88.821   Osteitis deformans of right upper arm
      - M88.822   Osteitis deformans of left upper arm
      - M88.829   Osteitis deformans of unspecified upper arm
    - M88.83   Osteitis deformans of forearm
      - M88.831   Osteitis deformans of right forearm
      - M88.832   Osteitis deformans of left forearm
      - M88.839   Osteitis deformans of unspecified forearm
    - M88.84   Osteitis deformans of hand
      - M88.841   Osteitis deformans of right hand
      - M88.842   Osteitis deformans of left hand
      - M88.849   Osteitis deformans of unspecified hand
    - M88.85   Osteitis deformans of thigh
      - M88.851   Osteitis deformans of right thigh
      - M88.852   Osteitis deformans of left thigh
      - M88.859   Osteitis deformans of unspecified thigh
    - M88.86   Osteitis deformans of lower leg
      - M88.861   Osteitis deformans of right lower leg
      - M88.862   Osteitis deformans of left lower leg
      - M88.869   Osteitis deformans of unspecified lower leg
    - M88.87   Osteitis deformans of ankle and foot
      - M88.871   Osteitis deformans of right ankle and foot

▶ New   ⇒ Revised   ~~deleted~~ Deleted   Excludes 1   Excludes 2   Includes   Use additional   Code first   Code also   Key words

OGCR Official Guidelines   X Assign placeholder X   ● Use Additional Character(s)   ▶ Manifestation Code   🔖 Hierarchical Condition Category   Coding Clinic

M88.872 Osteitis deformans of left ankle and foot

M88.879 Osteitis deformans of unspecified ankle and foot

M88.88 Osteitis deformans of other bones

　　　　Excludes2　osteitis deformans of skull (M88.0)

　　　　　　　　　　osteitis deformans of vertebrae (M88.1)

M88.89 Osteitis deformans of multiple sites

M88.9 Osteitis deformans of unspecified bone

● M89 Other disorders of bone

　● M89.0 Algoneurodystrophy

　　　　Shoulder-hand syndrome
　　　　Sudeck's atrophy

　　　　Excludes1　causalgia, lower limb (G57.7-)

　　　　　　　　　　causalgia, upper limb (G56.4-)

　　　　　　　　　　complex regional pain syndrome II, lower limb (G57.7-)

　　　　　　　　　　complex regional pain syndrome II, upper limb (G56.4-)

　　　　　　　　　　reflex sympathetic dystrophy (G90.5-)

　　　M89.00 Algoneurodystrophy, unspecified site

　● M89.01 Algoneurodystrophy, shoulder

　　　M89.011 Algoneurodystrophy, right shoulder

　　　M89.012 Algoneurodystrophy, left shoulder

　　　M89.019 Algoneurodystrophy, unspecified shoulder

　● M89.02 Algoneurodystrophy, upper arm

　　　M89.021 Algoneurodystrophy, right upper arm

　　　M89.022 Algoneurodystrophy, left upper arm

　　　M89.029 Algoneurodystrophy, unspecified upper arm

　● M89.03 Algoneurodystrophy, forearm

　　　M89.031 Algoneurodystrophy, right forearm

　　　M89.032 Algoneurodystrophy, left forearm

　　　M89.039 Algoneurodystrophy, unspecified forearm

　● M89.04 Algoneurodystrophy, hand

　　　M89.041 Algoneurodystrophy, right hand

　　　M89.042 Algoneurodystrophy, left hand

　　　M89.049 Algoneurodystrophy, unspecified hand

　● M89.05 Algoneurodystrophy, thigh

　　　M89.051 Algoneurodystrophy, right thigh

　　　M89.052 Algoneurodystrophy, left thigh

　　　M89.059 Algoneurodystrophy, unspecified thigh

　● M89.06 Algoneurodystrophy, lower leg

　　　M89.061 Algoneurodystrophy, right lower leg

　　　M89.062 Algoneurodystrophy, left lower leg

　　　M89.069 Algoneurodystrophy, unspecified lower leg

　● M89.07 Algoneurodystrophy, ankle and foot

　　　M89.071 Algoneurodystrophy, right ankle and foot

　　　M89.072 Algoneurodystrophy, left ankle and foot

　　　M89.079 Algoneurodystrophy, unspecified ankle and foot

　　M89.08 Algoneurodystrophy, other site

　　M89.09 Algoneurodystrophy, multiple sites

● M89.1 Physeal arrest

　　Arrest of growth plate
　　Epiphyseal arrest
　　Growth plate arrest

● M89.12 Physeal arrest, humerus

　　M89.121 Complete physeal arrest, right proximal humerus

　　M89.122 Complete physeal arrest, left proximal humerus

　　M89.123 Partial physeal arrest, right proximal humerus

　　M89.124 Partial physeal arrest, left proximal humerus

　　M89.125 Complete physeal arrest, right distal humerus

　　M89.126 Complete physeal arrest, left distal humerus

　　M89.127 Partial physeal arrest, right distal humerus

　　M89.128 Partial physeal arrest, left distal humerus

　　M89.129 Physeal arrest, humerus, unspecified

● M89.13 Physeal arrest, forearm

　　M89.131 Complete physeal arrest, right distal radius

　　M89.132 Complete physeal arrest, left distal radius

　　M89.133 Partial physeal arrest, right distal radius

　　M89.134 Partial physeal arrest, left distal radius

　　M89.138 Other physeal arrest of forearm

　　M89.139 Physeal arrest, forearm, unspecified

● M89.15 Physeal arrest, femur

　　M89.151 Complete physeal arrest, right proximal femur

　　M89.152 Complete physeal arrest, left proximal femur

　　M89.153 Partial physeal arrest, right proximal femur

　　M89.154 Partial physeal arrest, left proximal femur

　　M89.155 Complete physeal arrest, right distal femur

　　M89.156 Complete physeal arrest, left distal femur

　　M89.157 Partial physeal arrest, right distal femur

　　M89.158 Partial physeal arrest, left distal femur

　　M89.159 Physeal arrest, femur, unspecified

● M89.16 Physeal arrest, lower leg

　　M89.160 Complete physeal arrest, right proximal tibia

　　M89.161 Complete physeal arrest, left proximal tibia

　　M89.162 Partial physeal arrest, right proximal tibia

　　M89.163 Partial physeal arrest, left proximal tibia

　　M89.164 Complete physeal arrest, right distal tibia

　　M89.165 Complete physeal arrest, left distal tibia

　　M89.166 Partial physeal arrest, right distal tibia

　　M89.167 Partial physeal arrest, left distal tibia

　　M89.168 Other physeal arrest of lower leg

　　M89.169 Physeal arrest, lower leg, unspecified

　M89.18 Physeal arrest, other site

CHAPTER 13 (M00-M99)

● **M89.2 Other disorders of bone development and growth**

   M89.20 Other disorders of bone development and growth, unspecified site

   ● M89.21 Other disorders of bone development and growth, shoulder

      M89.211 Other disorders of bone development and growth, right shoulder

      M89.212 Other disorders of bone development and growth, left shoulder

      M89.219 Other disorders of bone development and growth, unspecified shoulder

   ● M89.22 Other disorders of bone development and growth, humerus

      M89.221 Other disorders of bone development and growth, right humerus

      M89.222 Other disorders of bone development and growth, left humerus

      M89.229 Other disorders of bone development and growth, unspecified humerus

   ● M89.23 Other disorders of bone development and growth, ulna and radius

      M89.231 Other disorders of bone development and growth, right ulna

      M89.232 Other disorders of bone development and growth, left ulna

      M89.233 Other disorders of bone development and growth, right radius

      M89.234 Other disorders of bone development and growth, left radius

      M89.239 Other disorders of bone development and growth, unspecified ulna and radius

   ● M89.24 Other disorders of bone development and growth, hand

      M89.241 Other disorders of bone development and growth, right hand

      M89.242 Other disorders of bone development and growth, left hand

      M89.249 Other disorders of bone development and growth, unspecified hand

   ● M89.25 Other disorders of bone development and growth, femur

      M89.251 Other disorders of bone development and growth, right femur

      M89.252 Other disorders of bone development and growth, left femur

      M89.259 Other disorders of bone development and growth, unspecified femur

   ● M89.26 Other disorders of bone development and growth, tibia and fibula

      M89.261 Other disorders of bone development and growth, right tibia

      M89.262 Other disorders of bone development and growth, left tibia

      M89.263 Other disorders of bone development and growth, right fibula

      M89.264 Other disorders of bone development and growth, left fibula

      M89.269 Other disorders of bone development and growth, unspecified lower leg

   ● M89.27 Other disorders of bone development and growth, ankle and foot

      M89.271 Other disorders of bone development and growth, right ankle and foot

      M89.272 Other disorders of bone development and growth, left ankle and foot

      M89.279 Other disorders of bone development and growth, unspecified ankle and foot

   M89.28 Other disorders of bone development and growth, other site

   M89.29 Other disorders of bone development and growth, multiple sites

● **M89.3 Hypertrophy of bone**

   M89.30 Hypertrophy of bone, unspecified site

   ● M89.31 Hypertrophy of bone, shoulder

      M89.311 Hypertrophy of bone, right shoulder

      M89.312 Hypertrophy of bone, left shoulder

      M89.319 Hypertrophy of bone, unspecified shoulder

   ● M89.32 Hypertrophy of bone, humerus

      M89.321 Hypertrophy of bone, right humerus

      M89.322 Hypertrophy of bone, left humerus

      M89.329 Hypertrophy of bone, unspecified humerus

   ● M89.33 Hypertrophy of bone, ulna and radius

      M89.331 Hypertrophy of bone, right ulna

      M89.332 Hypertrophy of bone, left ulna

      M89.333 Hypertrophy of bone, right radius

      M89.334 Hypertrophy of bone, left radius

      M89.339 Hypertrophy of bone, unspecified ulna and radius

   ● M89.34 Hypertrophy of bone, hand

      M89.341 Hypertrophy of bone, right hand

      M89.342 Hypertrophy of bone, left hand

      M89.349 Hypertrophy of bone, unspecified hand

   ● M89.35 Hypertrophy of bone, femur

      M89.351 Hypertrophy of bone, right femur

      M89.352 Hypertrophy of bone, left femur

      M89.359 Hypertrophy of bone, unspecified femur

   ● M89.36 Hypertrophy of bone, tibia and fibula

      M89.361 Hypertrophy of bone, right tibia

      M89.362 Hypertrophy of bone, left tibia

      M89.363 Hypertrophy of bone, right fibula

      M89.364 Hypertrophy of bone, left fibula

      M89.369 Hypertrophy of bone, unspecified tibia and fibula

   ● M89.37 Hypertrophy of bone, ankle and foot

      M89.371 Hypertrophy of bone, right ankle and foot

      M89.372 Hypertrophy of bone, left ankle and foot

      M89.379 Hypertrophy of bone, unspecified ankle and foot

   M89.38 Hypertrophy of bone, other site

   M89.39 Hypertrophy of bone, multiple sites

● **M89.4 Other hypertrophic osteoarthropathy**
   Marie-Bamberger disease
   Pachydermoperiostosis

   M89.40 Other hypertrophic osteoarthropathy, unspecified site

   ● M89.41 Other hypertrophic osteoarthropathy, shoulder

      M89.411 Other hypertrophic osteoarthropathy, right shoulder

      M89.412 Other hypertrophic osteoarthropathy, left shoulder

      M89.419 Other hypertrophic osteoarthropathy, unspecified shoulder

   ● M89.42 Other hypertrophic osteoarthropathy, upper arm

      M89.421 Other hypertrophic osteoarthropathy, right upper arm

      M89.422 Other hypertrophic osteoarthropathy, left upper arm

▶ New ⇒ Revised ~~deleted~~ Deleted | Excludes 1 | Excludes 2 | Includes | Use additional | Code first | Code also | Key words

OGCR Official Guidelines X Assign placeholder X ● Use Additional Character(s) ▶ Manifestation Code 🔖 Hierarchical Condition Category Coding Clinic

● M89.429 Other hypertrophic osteoarthropathy, unspecified upper arm
● **M89.43** Other hypertrophic osteoarthropathy, forearm
    M89.431 Other hypertrophic osteoarthropathy, right forearm
    M89.432 Other hypertrophic osteoarthropathy, left forearm
    M89.439 Other hypertrophic osteoarthropathy, unspecified forearm
● **M89.44** Other hypertrophic osteoarthropathy, hand
    M89.441 Other hypertrophic osteoarthropathy, right hand
    M89.442 Other hypertrophic osteoarthropathy, left hand
    M89.449 Other hypertrophic osteoarthropathy, unspecified hand
● **M89.45** Other hypertrophic osteoarthropathy, thigh
    M89.451 Other hypertrophic osteoarthropathy, right thigh
    M89.452 Other hypertrophic osteoarthropathy, left thigh
    M89.459 Other hypertrophic osteoarthropathy, unspecified thigh
● **M89.46** Other hypertrophic osteoarthropathy, lower leg
    M89.461 Other hypertrophic osteoarthropathy, right lower leg
    M89.462 Other hypertrophic osteoarthropathy, left lower leg
    M89.469 Other hypertrophic osteoarthropathy, unspecified lower leg
● **M89.47** Other hypertrophic osteoarthropathy, ankle and foot
    M89.471 Other hypertrophic osteoarthropathy, right ankle and foot
    M89.472 Other hypertrophic osteoarthropathy, left ankle and foot
    M89.479 Other hypertrophic osteoarthropathy, unspecified ankle and foot
  M89.48 Other hypertrophic osteoarthropathy, other site
  M89.49 Other hypertrophic osteoarthropathy, multiple sites
● **M89.5** Osteolysis
    Use additional code to identify major osseous defect, if applicable (M89.7-)
    Excludes2 periprosthetic osteolysis of internal prosthetic joint (T84.05-)
  M89.50 Osteolysis, unspecified site
● **M89.51** Osteolysis, shoulder
    M89.511 Osteolysis, right shoulder
    M89.512 Osteolysis, left shoulder
    M89.519 Osteolysis, unspecified shoulder
● **M89.52** Osteolysis, upper arm
    M89.521 Osteolysis, right upper arm
    M89.522 Osteolysis, left upper arm
    M89.529 Osteolysis, unspecified upper arm
● **M89.53** Osteolysis, forearm
    M89.531 Osteolysis, right forearm
    M89.532 Osteolysis, left forearm
    M89.539 Osteolysis, unspecified forearm
● **M89.54** Osteolysis, hand
    M89.541 Osteolysis, right hand
    M89.542 Osteolysis, left hand
    M89.549 Osteolysis, unspecified hand
● **M89.55** Osteolysis, thigh
    M89.551 Osteolysis, right thigh
    M89.552 Osteolysis, left thigh
    M89.559 Osteolysis, unspecified thigh

● **M89.56** Osteolysis, lower leg
    M89.561 Osteolysis, right lower leg
    M89.562 Osteolysis, left lower leg
    M89.569 Osteolysis, unspecified lower leg
● **M89.57** Osteolysis, ankle and foot
    M89.571 Osteolysis, right ankle and foot
    M89.572 Osteolysis, left ankle and foot
    M89.579 Osteolysis, unspecified ankle and foot
  M89.58 Osteolysis, other site
  M89.59 Osteolysis, multiple sites
● **M89.6** Osteopathy after poliomyelitis
    Use additional code (B91) to identify previous poliomyelitis
    Excludes1 postpolio syndrome (G14)
  M89.60 Osteopathy after poliomyelitis, unspecified site 🦴
● **M89.61** Osteopathy after poliomyelitis, shoulder
    M89.611 Osteopathy after poliomyelitis, right shoulder 🦴
    M89.612 Osteopathy after poliomyelitis, left shoulder 🦴
    M89.619 Osteopathy after poliomyelitis, unspecified shoulder 🦴
● **M89.62** Osteopathy after poliomyelitis, upper arm
    M89.621 Osteopathy after poliomyelitis, right upper arm 🦴
    M89.622 Osteopathy after poliomyelitis, left upper arm 🦴
    M89.629 Osteopathy after poliomyelitis, unspecified upper arm 🦴
● **M89.63** Osteopathy after poliomyelitis, forearm
    M89.631 Osteopathy after poliomyelitis, right forearm 🦴
    M89.632 Osteopathy after poliomyelitis, left forearm 🦴
    M89.639 Osteopathy after poliomyelitis, unspecified forearm 🦴
● **M89.64** Osteopathy after poliomyelitis, hand
    M89.641 Osteopathy after poliomyelitis, right hand 🦴
    M89.642 Osteopathy after poliomyelitis, left hand 🦴
    M89.649 Osteopathy after poliomyelitis, unspecified hand 🦴
● **M89.65** Osteopathy after poliomyelitis, thigh
    M89.651 Osteopathy after poliomyelitis, right thigh 🦴
    M89.652 Osteopathy after poliomyelitis, left thigh 🦴
    M89.659 Osteopathy after poliomyelitis, unspecified thigh 🦴
● **M89.66** Osteopathy after poliomyelitis, lower leg
    M89.661 Osteopathy after poliomyelitis, right lower leg 🦴
    M89.662 Osteopathy after poliomyelitis, left lower leg 🦴
    M89.669 Osteopathy after poliomyelitis, unspecified lower leg 🦴
● **M89.67** Osteopathy after poliomyelitis, ankle and foot
    M89.671 Osteopathy after poliomyelitis, right ankle and foot 🦴
    M89.672 Osteopathy after poliomyelitis, left ankle and foot 🦴
    M89.679 Osteopathy after poliomyelitis, unspecified ankle and foot 🦴
  M89.68 Osteopathy after poliomyelitis, other site 🦴
  M89.69 Osteopathy after poliomyelitis, multiple sites 🦴

● **M89.7   Major osseous defect**
  Code first underlying disease, if known, such as:
    aseptic necrosis of bone (M87.-)
    malignant neoplasm of bone (C40.-)
    osteolysis (M89.5-)
    osteomyelitis (M86.-)
    osteonecrosis (M87.-)
    osteoporosis (M80.-, M81.-)
    periprosthetic osteolysis (T84.05-)

  M89.70   Major osseous defect, unspecified site

● **M89.71   Major osseous defect, shoulder region**
    Major osseous defect clavicle or scapula
    M89.711   Major osseous defect, right shoulder region
    M89.712   Major osseous defect, left shoulder region
    M89.719   Major osseous defect, unspecified shoulder region

● **M89.72   Major osseous defect, humerus**
    M89.721   Major osseous defect, right humerus
    M89.722   Major osseous defect, left humerus
    M89.729   Major osseous defect, unspecified humerus

● **M89.73   Major osseous defect, forearm**
    Major osseous defect of radius and ulna
    M89.731   Major osseous defect, right forearm
    M89.732   Major osseous defect, left forearm
    M89.739   Major osseous defect, unspecified forearm

● **M89.74   Major osseous defect, hand**
    Major osseous defect of carpus, fingers, metacarpus
    M89.741   Major osseous defect, right hand
    M89.742   Major osseous defect, left hand
    M89.749   Major osseous defect, unspecified hand

● **M89.75   Major osseous defect, pelvic region and thigh**
    Major osseous defect of femur and pelvis
    M89.751   Major osseous defect, right pelvic region and thigh
    M89.752   Major osseous defect, left pelvic region and thigh
    M89.759   Major osseous defect, unspecified pelvic region and thigh

● **M89.76   Major osseous defect, lower leg**
    Major osseous defect of fibula and tibia
    M89.761   Major osseous defect, right lower leg
    M89.762   Major osseous defect, left lower leg
    M89.769   Major osseous defect, unspecified lower leg

● **M89.77   Major osseous defect, ankle and foot**
    Major osseous defect of metatarsus, tarsus, toes
    M89.771   Major osseous defect, right ankle and foot
    M89.772   Major osseous defect, left ankle and foot
    M89.779   Major osseous defect, unspecified ankle and foot

  M89.78   Major osseous defect, other site
  M89.79   Major osseous defect, multiple sites

● **M89.8   Other specified disorders of bone**
    Infantile cortical hyperostoses
    Post-traumatic subperiosteal ossification
    Coding Clinic: 2022, Q2, P10

● **M89.8X   Other specified disorders of bone**
    M89.8X0   Other specified disorders of bone, multiple sites
    M89.8X1   Other specified disorders of bone, shoulder

    M89.8X2   Other specified disorders of bone, upper arm
    M89.8X3   Other specified disorders of bone, forearm
      Coding Clinic: 2019, Q3, P10
    M89.8X4   Other specified disorders of bone, hand
    M89.8X5   Other specified disorders of bone, thigh
    M89.8X6   Other specified disorders of bone, lower leg
    M89.8X7   Other specified disorders of bone, ankle and foot
    M89.8X8   Other specified disorders of bone, other site
      Coding Clinic: 2023, Q2, P19
    M89.8X9   Other specified disorders of bone, unspecified site

  M89.9   Disorder of bone, unspecified

● **M90   Osteopathies in diseases classified elsewhere**
  Excludes1   osteochondritis, osteomyelitis, and osteopathy (in):
      cryptococcosis (B45.3)
      diabetes mellitus (E08-E13 with .69-)
      gonococcal (A54.43)
      neurogenic syphilis (A52.11)
      renal osteodystrophy (N25.0)
      salmonellosis (A02.24)
      secondary syphilis (A51.46)
      syphilis (late) (A52.77)

● **M90.5   Osteonecrosis in diseases classified elsewhere**
    Code first underlying disease, such as:
      caisson disease (T70.3)
      hemoglobinopathy (D50-D64)

  ▸ *M90.50   Osteonecrosis in diseases classified elsewhere, unspecified site* 🐾

● *M90.51   Osteonecrosis in diseases classified elsewhere, shoulder*
    ▸ *M90.511   Osteonecrosis in diseases classified elsewhere, right shoulder* 🐾
    ▸ *M90.512   Osteonecrosis in diseases classified elsewhere, left shoulder* 🐾
    ▸ *M90.519   Osteonecrosis in diseases classified elsewhere, unspecified shoulder* 🐾

● *M90.52   Osteonecrosis in diseases classified elsewhere, upper arm*
    ▸ *M90.521   Osteonecrosis in diseases classified elsewhere, right upper arm* 🐾
    ▸ *M90.522   Osteonecrosis in diseases classified elsewhere, left upper arm* 🐾
    ▸ *M90.529   Osteonecrosis in diseases classified elsewhere, unspecified upper arm* 🐾

● *M90.53   Osteonecrosis in diseases classified elsewhere, forearm*
    ▸ *M90.531   Osteonecrosis in diseases classified elsewhere, right forearm* 🐾
    ▸ *M90.532   Osteonecrosis in diseases classified elsewhere, left forearm* 🐾
    ▸ *M90.539   Osteonecrosis in diseases classified elsewhere, unspecified forearm* 🐾

● *M90.54   Osteonecrosis in diseases classified elsewhere, hand*
    ▸ *M90.541   Osteonecrosis in diseases classified elsewhere, right hand* 🐾
    ▸ *M90.542   Osteonecrosis in diseases classified elsewhere, left hand* 🐾
    ▸ *M90.549   Osteonecrosis in diseases classified elsewhere, unspecified hand* 🐾

▸ New   ⇒ Revised   ~~deleted~~ Deleted   Excludes 1   Excludes 2   Includes   Use additional   Code first   Code also   Key words

OGCR Official Guidelines   X Assign placeholder X   ● Use Additional Character(s)   ▸ Manifestation Code   🐾 Hierarchical Condition Category   Coding Clinic

- **M90.55** Osteonecrosis in diseases classified elsewhere, thigh
  - *M90.551* *Osteonecrosis in diseases classified elsewhere, right thigh* 🔗
  - *M90.552* *Osteonecrosis in diseases classified elsewhere, left thigh* 🔗
  - *M90.559* *Osteonecrosis in diseases classified elsewhere, unspecified thigh* 🔗
- **M90.56** Osteonecrosis in diseases classified elsewhere, lower leg
  - *M90.561* *Osteonecrosis in diseases classified elsewhere, right lower leg* 🔗
  - *M90.562* *Osteonecrosis in diseases classified elsewhere, left lower leg* 🔗
  - *M90.569* *Osteonecrosis in diseases classified elsewhere, unspecified lower leg* 🔗
- **M90.57** Osteonecrosis in diseases classified elsewhere, ankle and foot
  - *M90.571* *Osteonecrosis in diseases classified elsewhere, right ankle and foot* 🔗
  - *M90.572* *Osteonecrosis in diseases classified elsewhere, left ankle and foot* 🔗
  - *M90.579* *Osteonecrosis in diseases classified elsewhere, unspecified ankle and foot* 🔗
  - *M90.58* *Osteonecrosis in diseases classified elsewhere, other site* 🔗
  - *M90.59* *Osteonecrosis in diseases classified elsewhere, multiple sites* 🔗
- **M90.6** Osteitis deformans in neoplastic diseases
  Osteitis deformans in malignant neoplasm of bone
  Code first the neoplasm (C40.-, C41.-)
  > **Excludes1**   osteitis deformans [Paget's disease of bone] (M88.-)
  - *M90.60* *Osteitis deformans in neoplastic diseases, unspecified site*
- **M90.61** Osteitis deformans in neoplastic diseases, shoulder
  - *M90.611* *Osteitis deformans in neoplastic diseases, right shoulder*
  - *M90.612* *Osteitis deformans in neoplastic diseases, left shoulder*
  - *M90.619* *Osteitis deformans in neoplastic diseases, unspecified shoulder*
- **M90.62** Osteitis deformans in neoplastic diseases, upper arm
  - *M90.621* *Osteitis deformans in neoplastic diseases, right upper arm*
  - *M90.622* *Osteitis deformans in neoplastic diseases, left upper arm*
  - *M90.629* *Osteitis deformans in neoplastic diseases, unspecified upper arm*
- **M90.63** Osteitis deformans in neoplastic diseases, forearm
  - *M90.631* *Osteitis deformans in neoplastic diseases, right forearm*
  - *M90.632* *Osteitis deformans in neoplastic diseases, left forearm*
  - *M90.639* *Osteitis deformans in neoplastic diseases, unspecified forearm*
- **M90.64** Osteitis deformans in neoplastic diseases, hand
  - *M90.641* *Osteitis deformans in neoplastic diseases, right hand*
  - *M90.642* *Osteitis deformans in neoplastic diseases, left hand*
  - *M90.649* *Osteitis deformans in neoplastic diseases, unspecified hand*
- **M90.65** Osteitis deformans in neoplastic diseases, thigh
  - *M90.651* *Osteitis deformans in neoplastic diseases, right thigh*

  - *M90.652* *Osteitis deformans in neoplastic diseases, left thigh*
  - *M90.659* *Osteitis deformans in neoplastic diseases, unspecified thigh*
- **M90.66** Osteitis deformans in neoplastic diseases, lower leg
  - *M90.661* *Osteitis deformans in neoplastic diseases, right lower leg*
  - *M90.662* *Osteitis deformans in neoplastic diseases, left lower leg*
  - *M90.669* *Osteitis deformans in neoplastic diseases, unspecified lower leg*
- **M90.67** Osteitis deformans in neoplastic diseases, ankle and foot
  - *M90.671* *Osteitis deformans in neoplastic diseases, right ankle and foot*
  - *M90.672* *Osteitis deformans in neoplastic diseases, left ankle and foot*
  - *M90.679* *Osteitis deformans in neoplastic diseases, unspecified ankle and foot*
  - *M90.68* *Osteitis deformans in neoplastic diseases, other site*
  - *M90.69* *Osteitis deformans in neoplastic diseases, multiple sites*
- **M90.8** Osteopathy in diseases classified elsewhere
  Code first underlying disease, such as:
    rickets (E55.0)
    vitamin-D-resistant rickets (E83.31)
  - *M90.80* *Osteopathy in diseases classified elsewhere, unspecified site*
- **M90.81** Osteopathy in diseases classified elsewhere, shoulder
  - *M90.811* *Osteopathy in diseases classified elsewhere, right shoulder*
  - *M90.812* *Osteopathy in diseases classified elsewhere, left shoulder*
  - *M90.819* *Osteopathy in diseases classified elsewhere, unspecified shoulder*
- **M90.82** Osteopathy in diseases classified elsewhere, upper arm
  - *M90.821* *Osteopathy in diseases classified elsewhere, right upper arm*
  - *M90.822* *Osteopathy in diseases classified elsewhere, left upper arm*
  - *M90.829* *Osteopathy in diseases classified elsewhere, unspecified upper arm*
- **M90.83** Osteopathy in diseases classified elsewhere, forearm
  - *M90.831* *Osteopathy in diseases classified elsewhere, right forearm*
  - *M90.832* *Osteopathy in diseases classified elsewhere, left forearm*
  - *M90.839* *Osteopathy in diseases classified elsewhere, unspecified forearm*
- **M90.84** Osteopathy in diseases classified elsewhere, hand
  - *M90.841* *Osteopathy in diseases classified elsewhere, right hand*
  - *M90.842* *Osteopathy in diseases classified elsewhere, left hand*
  - *M90.849* *Osteopathy in diseases classified elsewhere, unspecified hand*
- **M90.85** Osteopathy in diseases classified elsewhere, thigh
  - *M90.851* *Osteopathy in diseases classified elsewhere, right thigh*
  - *M90.852* *Osteopathy in diseases classified elsewhere, left thigh*
  - *M90.859* *Osteopathy in diseases classified elsewhere, unspecified thigh*

CHAPTER 13 (M00-M99)

● M90.86 **Osteopathy in diseases classified elsewhere, lower leg**
  ▸ *M90.861 Osteopathy in diseases classified elsewhere, right lower leg*
  ▸ *M90.862 Osteopathy in diseases classified elsewhere, left lower leg*
  ▸ *M90.869 Osteopathy in diseases classified elsewhere, unspecified lower leg*
● M90.87 **Osteopathy in diseases classified elsewhere, ankle and foot**
  ▸ *M90.871 Osteopathy in diseases classified elsewhere, right ankle and foot*
  ▸ *M90.872 Osteopathy in diseases classified elsewhere, left ankle and foot*
  ▸ *M90.879 Osteopathy in diseases classified elsewhere, unspecified ankle and foot*
  ▸ *M90.88 Osteopathy in diseases classified elsewhere, other site*
  ▸ *M90.89 Osteopathy in diseases classified elsewhere, multiple sites*

CHONDROPATHIES (M91-M94)

Excludes1 postprocedural chondropathies (M96.-)

● M91 Juvenile osteochondrosis of hip and pelvis
  Excludes1 slipped upper femoral epiphysis (nontraumatic) (M93.0-)

M91.0 **Juvenile osteochondrosis of pelvis**
  Osteochondrosis (juvenile) of acetabulum
  Osteochondrosis (juvenile) of iliac crest [Buchanan]
  Osteochondrosis (juvenile) of ischiopubic synchondrosis [van Neck]
  Osteochondrosis (juvenile) of symphysis pubis [Pierson]
● M91.1 **Juvenile osteochondrosis of head of femur [Legg-Calvé-Perthes]**
  M91.10 Juvenile osteochondrosis of head of femur [Legg-Calvé-Perthes], unspecified leg
  M91.11 Juvenile osteochondrosis of head of femur [Legg-Calvé-Perthes], right leg
  M91.12 Juvenile osteochondrosis of head of femur [Legg-Calvé-Perthes], left leg
● M91.2 **Coxa plana**
  Hip deformity due to previous juvenile osteochondrosis
  M91.20 Coxa plana, unspecified hip
  M91.21 Coxa plana, right hip
  M91.22 Coxa plana, left hip
● M91.3 **Pseudocoxalgia**
  M91.30 Pseudocoxalgia, unspecified hip
  M91.31 Pseudocoxalgia, right hip
  M91.32 Pseudocoxalgia, left hip
● M91.4 **Coxa magna**
  M91.40 Coxa magna, unspecified hip
  M91.41 Coxa magna, right hip
  M91.42 Coxa magna, left hip
● M91.8 **Other juvenile osteochondrosis of hip and pelvis**
  Juvenile osteochondrosis after reduction of congenital dislocation of hip
  M91.80 Other juvenile osteochondrosis of hip and pelvis, unspecified leg
  M91.81 Other juvenile osteochondrosis of hip and pelvis, right leg
  M91.82 Other juvenile osteochondrosis of hip and pelvis, left leg
● M91.9 **Juvenile osteochondrosis of hip and pelvis, unspecified**
  M91.90 Juvenile osteochondrosis of hip and pelvis, unspecified, unspecified leg
  M91.91 Juvenile osteochondrosis of hip and pelvis, unspecified, right leg
  M91.92 Juvenile osteochondrosis of hip and pelvis, unspecified, left leg

● M92 Other juvenile osteochondrosis
● M92.0 **Juvenile osteochondrosis of humerus**
  Osteochondrosis (juvenile) of capitulum of humerus [Panner]
  Osteochondrosis (juvenile) of head of humerus [Haas]
  M92.00 Juvenile osteochondrosis of humerus, unspecified arm
  M92.01 Juvenile osteochondrosis of humerus, right arm
  M92.02 Juvenile osteochondrosis of humerus, left arm
● M92.1 **Juvenile osteochondrosis of radius and ulna**
  Osteochondrosis (juvenile) of lower ulna [Burns]
  Osteochondrosis (juvenile) of radial head [Brailsford]
  M92.10 Juvenile osteochondrosis of radius and ulna, unspecified arm
  M92.11 Juvenile osteochondrosis of radius and ulna, right arm
  M92.12 Juvenile osteochondrosis of radius and ulna, left arm
● M92.2 **Juvenile osteochondrosis, hand**
  ● M92.20 Unspecified juvenile osteochondrosis, hand
    M92.201 Unspecified juvenile osteochondrosis, right hand
    M92.202 Unspecified juvenile osteochondrosis, left hand
    M92.209 Unspecified juvenile osteochondrosis, unspecified hand
  ● M92.21 Osteochondrosis (juvenile) of carpal lunate [Kienböck]
    M92.211 Osteochondrosis (juvenile) of carpal lunate [Kienböck], right hand
    M92.212 Osteochondrosis (juvenile) of carpal lunate [Kienböck], left hand
    M92.219 Osteochondrosis (juvenile) of carpal lunate [Kienböck], unspecified hand
  ● M92.22 Osteochondrosis (juvenile) of metacarpal heads [Mauclaire]
    M92.221 Osteochondrosis (juvenile) of metacarpal heads [Mauclaire], right hand
    M92.222 Osteochondrosis (juvenile) of metacarpal heads [Mauclaire], left hand
    M92.229 Osteochondrosis (juvenile) of metacarpal heads [Mauclaire], unspecified hand
  ● M92.29 Other juvenile osteochondrosis, hand
    M92.291 Other juvenile osteochondrosis, right hand
    M92.292 Other juvenile osteochondrosis, left hand
    M92.299 Other juvenile osteochondrosis, unspecified hand
● M92.3 Other juvenile osteochondrosis, upper limb
  M92.30 Other juvenile osteochondrosis, unspecified upper limb
  M92.31 Other juvenile osteochondrosis, right upper limb
  M92.32 Other juvenile osteochondrosis, left upper limb
● M92.4 Juvenile osteochondrosis of patella
  Osteochondrosis (juvenile) of primary patellar center [Köhler]
  Osteochondrosis (juvenile) of secondary patellar center [Sinding Larsen]
  M92.40 Juvenile osteochondrosis of patella, unspecified knee
  M92.41 Juvenile osteochondrosis of patella, right knee
  M92.42 Juvenile osteochondrosis of patella, left knee
● M92.5 Juvenile osteochondrosis of tibia and fibula

CHAPTER 13 (M00-M99)

▸ New ⇒ Revised deleted Deleted Excludes 1 Excludes 2 Includes Use additional Code first Code also Key words
OGCR Official Guidelines X Assign placeholder X ● Use Additional Character(s) ▸ Manifestation Code Hierarchical Condition Category Coding Clinic

● M92.50   Unspecified juvenile osteochondrosis of tibia and fibula

     M92.501   Unspecified juvenile osteochondrosis, right leg

     M92.502   Unspecified juvenile osteochondrosis, left leg

     M92.503   Unspecified juvenile osteochondrosis, bilateral leg

     M92.509   Unspecified juvenile osteochondrosis, unspecified leg

● M92.51   Juvenile osteochondrosis of proximal tibia
     Blount disease
     Tibia vara

     M92.511   Juvenile osteochondrosis of proximal tibia, right leg

     M92.512   Juvenile osteochondrosis of proximal tibia, left leg

     M92.513   Juvenile osteochondrosis of proximal tibia, bilateral

     M92.519   Juvenile osteochondrosis of proximal tibia, unspecified leg

● M92.52   Juvenile osteochondrosis of tibia tubercle
     Osgood-Schlatter disease

     M92.521   Juvenile osteochondrosis of tibia tubercle, right leg

     M92.522   Juvenile osteochondrosis of tibia tubercle, left leg

     M92.523   Juvenile osteochondrosis of tibia tubercle, bilateral

     M92.529   Juvenile osteochondrosis of tibia tubercle, unspecified leg

  M92.59   Other juvenile osteochondrosis of tibia and fibula

     M92.591   Other juvenile osteochondrosis of tibia and fibula, right leg

     M92.592   Other juvenile osteochondrosis of tibia and fibula, left leg

     M92.593   Other juvenile osteochondrosis of tibia and fibula, bilateral

     M92.599   Other juvenile osteochondrosis of tibia and fibula, unspecified leg

● M92.6   Juvenile osteochondrosis of tarsus
     Osteochondrosis (juvenile) of calcaneum [Sever]
     Osteochondrosis (juvenile) of os tibiale externum [Haglund]
     Osteochondrosis (juvenile) of talus [Diaz]
     Osteochondrosis (juvenile) of tarsal navicular [Köhler]

     M92.60   Juvenile osteochondrosis of tarsus, unspecified ankle

     M92.61   Juvenile osteochondrosis of tarsus, right ankle

     M92.62   Juvenile osteochondrosis of tarsus, left ankle

● M92.7   Juvenile osteochondrosis of metatarsus
     Osteochondrosis (juvenile) of fifth metatarsus [Iselin]
     Osteochondrosis (juvenile) of second metatarsus [Freiberg]

     M92.70   Juvenile osteochondrosis of metatarsus, unspecified foot

     M92.71   Juvenile osteochondrosis of metatarsus, right foot

     M92.72   Juvenile osteochondrosis of metatarsus, left foot

  M92.8   Other specified juvenile osteochondrosis
     ~~Calcaneal apophysitis~~

  M92.9   Juvenile osteochondrosis, unspecified
     Juvenile apophysitis NOS
     Juvenile epiphysitis NOS
     Juvenile osteochondritis NOS
     Juvenile osteochondrosis NOS

● M93   Other osteochondropathies
    Excludes2   osteochondrosis of spine (M42.-)

● M93.0   Slipped upper femoral epiphysis (nontraumatic)
     Slipped capital femoral epiphysis (SCFE)
     Slipped upper femoral epiphysis (SUFE)
    Use additional code for associated chondrolysis (M94.3)

● M93.00   Unspecified slipped upper femoral epiphysis (nontraumatic)

     M93.001   Unspecified slipped upper femoral epiphysis (nontraumatic), right hip

     M93.002   Unspecified slipped upper femoral epiphysis (nontraumatic), left hip

     M93.003   Unspecified slipped upper femoral epiphysis (nontraumatic), unspecified hip

     M93.004   Unspecified slipped upper femoral epiphysis (nontraumatic), bilateral hips

● M93.01   Acute slipped upper femoral epiphysis, stable (nontraumatic)

     M93.011   Acute slipped upper femoral epiphysis, stable (nontraumatic), right hip

     M93.012   Acute slipped upper femoral epiphysis, stable (nontraumatic), left hip

     M93.013   Acute slipped upper femoral epiphysis, stable (nontraumatic), unspecified hip

     M93.014   Acute slipped upper femoral epiphysis, stable (nontraumatic), bilateral hips

● M93.02   Chronic slipped upper femoral epiphysis, stable (nontraumatic)

     M93.021   Chronic slipped upper femoral epiphysis, stable (nontraumatic), right hip

     M93.022   Chronic slipped upper femoral epiphysis, stable (nontraumatic), left hip

     M93.023   Chronic slipped upper femoral epiphysis, stable (nontraumatic), unspecified hip

     M93.024   Chronic slipped upper femoral epiphysis, stable (nontraumatic), bilateral hips

● M93.03   Acute on chronic slipped upper femoral epiphysis, stable (nontraumatic)

     M93.031   Acute on chronic slipped upper femoral epiphysis, stable (nontraumatic), right hip

     M93.032   Acute on chronic slipped upper femoral epiphysis, stable (nontraumatic), left hip

     M93.033   Acute on chronic slipped upper femoral epiphysis, stable (nontraumatic), unspecified hip

     M93.034   Acute on chronic slipped upper femoral epiphysis, stable (nontraumatic), bilateral hips

● M93.04   Acute slipped upper femoral epiphysis, unstable (nontraumatic)

     M93.041   Acute slipped upper femoral epiphysis, unstable (nontraumatic), right hip

     M93.042   Acute slipped upper femoral epiphysis, unstable (nontraumatic), left hip

M93.043 Acute slipped upper femoral epiphysis, unstable (nontraumatic), unspecified hip

M93.044 Acute slipped upper femoral epiphysis, unstable (nontraumatic), bilateral hips

● M93.05 Acute on chronic slipped upper femoral epiphysis, unstable (nontraumatic)

M93.051 Acute on chronic slipped upper femoral epiphysis, unstable (nontraumatic), right hip

M93.052 Acute on chronic slipped upper femoral epiphysis, unstable (nontraumatic), left hip

M93.053 Acute on chronic slipped upper femoral epiphysis, unstable (nontraumatic), unspecified hip

M93.054 Acute on chronic slipped upper femoral epiphysis, unstable (nontraumatic), bilateral hips

● M93.06 Acute slipped upper femoral epiphysis, unspecified stability (nontraumatic)

M93.061 Acute slipped upper femoral epiphysis, unspecified stability (nontraumatic), right hip

M93.062 Acute slipped upper femoral epiphysis, unspecified stability (nontraumatic), left hip

M93.063 Acute slipped upper femoral epiphysis, unspecified stability (nontraumatic), unspecified hip

M93.064 Acute slipped upper femoral epiphysis, unspecified stability (nontraumatic), bilateral hips

● M93.07 Acute on chronic slipped upper femoral epiphysis, unspecified stability (nontraumatic)

M93.071 Acute on chronic slipped upper femoral epiphysis, unspecified stability (nontraumatic), right hip

M93.072 Acute on chronic slipped upper femoral epiphysis, unspecified stability (nontraumatic), left hip

M93.073 Acute on chronic slipped upper femoral epiphysis, unspecified stability (nontraumatic), unspecified hip

M93.074 Acute on chronic slipped upper femoral epiphysis, unspecified stability (nontraumatic), bilateral hips

M93.1 Kienböck's disease of adults   A
Adult osteochondrosis of carpal lunates

● M93.2 Osteochondritis dissecans

M93.20 Osteochondritis dissecans of unspecified site

● M93.21 Osteochondritis dissecans of shoulder

M93.211 Osteochondritis dissecans, right shoulder

M93.212 Osteochondritis dissecans, left shoulder

M93.219 Osteochondritis dissecans, unspecified shoulder

● M93.22 Osteochondritis dissecans of elbow

M93.221 Osteochondritis dissecans, right elbow

M93.222 Osteochondritis dissecans, left elbow

M93.229 Osteochondritis dissecans, unspecified elbow

● M93.23 Osteochondritis dissecans of wrist

M93.231 Osteochondritis dissecans, right wrist

M93.232 Osteochondritis dissecans, left wrist

M93.239 Osteochondritis dissecans, unspecified wrist

● M93.24 Osteochondritis dissecans of joints of hand

M93.241 Osteochondritis dissecans, joints of right hand

M93.242 Osteochondritis dissecans, joints of left hand

M93.249 Osteochondritis dissecans, joints of unspecified hand

● M93.25 Osteochondritis dissecans of hip

M93.251 Osteochondritis dissecans, right hip

M93.252 Osteochondritis dissecans, left hip

M93.259 Osteochondritis dissecans, unspecified hip

● M93.26 Osteochondritis dissecans knee

M93.261 Osteochondritis dissecans, right knee

M93.262 Osteochondritis dissecans, left knee

M93.269 Osteochondritis dissecans, unspecified knee

● M93.27 Osteochondritis dissecans of ankle and joints of foot

M93.271 Osteochondritis dissecans, right ankle and joints of right foot

M93.272 Osteochondritis dissecans, left ankle and joints of left foot

M93.279 Osteochondritis dissecans, unspecified ankle and joints of foot

M93.28 Osteochondritis dissecans other site

M93.29 Osteochondritis dissecans multiple sites

● M93.8 Other specified osteochondropathies

M93.80 Other specified osteochondropathies of unspecified site

● M93.81 Other specified osteochondropathies of shoulder

M93.811 Other specified osteochondropathies, right shoulder

M93.812 Other specified osteochondropathies, left shoulder

M93.819 Other specified osteochondropathies, unspecified shoulder

● M93.82 Other specified osteochondropathies of upper arm

M93.821 Other specified osteochondropathies, right upper arm

M93.822 Other specified osteochondropathies, left upper arm

M93.829 Other specified osteochondropathies, unspecified upper arm

● M93.83 Other specified osteochondropathies of forearm

M93.831 Other specified osteochondropathies, right forearm

M93.832 Other specified osteochondropathies, left forearm

M93.839 Other specified osteochondropathies, unspecified forearm

● M93.84 Other specified osteochondropathies of hand

M93.841 Other specified osteochondropathies, right hand

M93.842 Other specified osteochondropathies, left hand

M93.849 Other specified osteochondropathies, unspecified hand

● M93.85 Other specified osteochondropathies of thigh

M93.851 Other specified osteochondropathies, right thigh

M93.852 Other specified osteochondropathies, left thigh

M93.859 Other specified osteochondropathies, unspecified thigh

● M93.86   Other specified osteochondropathies lower leg
      M93.861   Other specified osteochondropathies, right lower leg
      M93.862   Other specified osteochondropathies, left lower leg
      M93.869   Other specified osteochondropathies, unspecified lower leg
● M93.87   Other specified osteochondropathies of ankle and foot
      M93.871   Other specified osteochondropathies, right ankle and foot
      M93.872   Other specified osteochondropathies, left ankle and foot
      M93.879   Other specified osteochondropathies, unspecified ankle and foot
   M93.88   Other specified osteochondropathies other
   M93.89   Other specified osteochondropathies multiple sites
M93.9   Osteochondropathy, unspecified
      Apophysitis NOS
      Epiphysitis NOS
      Osteochondritis NOS
      Osteochondrosis NOS
   M93.90   Osteochondropathy, unspecified of unspecified site
● M93.91   Osteochondropathy, unspecified of shoulder
      M93.911   Osteochondropathy, unspecified, right shoulder
      M93.912   Osteochondropathy, unspecified, left shoulder
      M93.919   Osteochondropathy, unspecified, unspecified shoulder
● M93.92   Osteochondropathy, unspecified of upper arm
      M93.921   Osteochondropathy, unspecified, right upper arm
      M93.922   Osteochondropathy, unspecified, left upper arm
      M93.929   Osteochondropathy, unspecified, unspecified upper arm
● M93.93   Osteochondropathy, unspecified of forearm
      M93.931   Osteochondropathy, unspecified, right forearm
      M93.932   Osteochondropathy, unspecified, left forearm
      M93.939   Osteochondropathy, unspecified, unspecified forearm
● M93.94   Osteochondropathy, unspecified of hand
      M93.941   Osteochondropathy, unspecified, right hand
      M93.942   Osteochondropathy, unspecified, left hand
      M93.949   Osteochondropathy, unspecified, unspecified hand
● M93.95   Osteochondropathy, unspecified of thigh
      M93.951   Osteochondropathy, unspecified, right thigh
      M93.952   Osteochondropathy, unspecified, left thigh
      M93.959   Osteochondropathy, unspecified, unspecified thigh
● M93.96   Osteochondropathy, unspecified lower leg
      M93.961   Osteochondropathy, unspecified, right lower leg
      M93.962   Osteochondropathy, unspecified, left lower leg
      M93.969   Osteochondropathy, unspecified, unspecified lower leg

● M93.97   Osteochondropathy, unspecified of ankle and foot
      M93.971   Osteochondropathy, unspecified, right ankle and foot
      M93.972   Osteochondropathy, unspecified, left ankle and foot
      M93.979   Osteochondropathy, unspecified, unspecified ankle and foot
   M93.98   Osteochondropathy, unspecified other
   M93.99   Osteochondropathy, unspecified multiple sites
● M94   Other disorders of cartilage
   M94.0   Chondrocostal junction syndrome [Tietze]
      Costochondritis
   M94.1   Relapsing polychondritis
● M94.2   Chondromalacia
      Excludes1   chondromalacia patellae (M22.4)
   M94.20   Chondromalacia, unspecified site
● M94.21   Chondromalacia, shoulder
      M94.211   Chondromalacia, right shoulder
      M94.212   Chondromalacia, left shoulder
      M94.219   Chondromalacia, unspecified shoulder
● M94.22   Chondromalacia, elbow
      M94.221   Chondromalacia, right elbow
      M94.222   Chondromalacia, left elbow
      M94.229   Chondromalacia, unspecified elbow
● M94.23   Chondromalacia, wrist
      M94.231   Chondromalacia, right wrist
      M94.232   Chondromalacia, left wrist
      M94.239   Chondromalacia, unspecified wrist
● M94.24   Chondromalacia, joints of hand
      M94.241   Chondromalacia, joints of right hand
      M94.242   Chondromalacia, joints of left hand
      M94.249   Chondromalacia, joints of unspecified hand
● M94.25   Chondromalacia, hip
      M94.251   Chondromalacia, right hip
      M94.252   Chondromalacia, left hip
      M94.259   Chondromalacia, unspecified hip
● M94.26   Chondromalacia, knee
      M94.261   Chondromalacia, right knee
      M94.262   Chondromalacia, left knee
      M94.269   Chondromalacia, unspecified knee
● M94.27   Chondromalacia, ankle and joints of foot
      M94.271   Chondromalacia, right ankle and joints of right foot
      M94.272   Chondromalacia, left ankle and joints of left foot
      M94.279   Chondromalacia, unspecified ankle and joints of foot
   M94.28   Chondromalacia, other site
   M94.29   Chondromalacia, multiple sites
● M94.3   Chondrolysis
      Code first any associated slipped upper femoral epiphysis (nontraumatic) (M93.0-)
● M94.35   Chondrolysis, hip
      M94.351   Chondrolysis, right hip
      M94.352   Chondrolysis, left hip
      M94.359   Chondrolysis, unspecified hip
● M94.8   Other specified disorders of cartilage
● M94.8X   Other specified disorders of cartilage
      M94.8X0   Other specified disorders of cartilage, multiple sites
      M94.8X1   Other specified disorders of cartilage, shoulder
      M94.8X2   Other specified disorders of cartilage, upper arm

M94.8X3 Other specified disorders of cartilage, forearm

M94.8X4 Other specified disorders of cartilage, hand

M94.8X5 Other specified disorders of cartilage, thigh

M94.8X6 Other specified disorders of cartilage, lower leg

M94.8X7 Other specified disorders of cartilage, ankle and foot

M94.8X8 Other specified disorders of cartilage, other site

M94.8X9 Other specified disorders of cartilage, unspecified sites

M94.9 Disorder of cartilage, unspecified

OTHER DISORDERS OF THE MUSCULOSKELETAL SYSTEM AND CONNECTIVE TISSUE (M95)

● M95 Other acquired deformities of musculoskeletal system and connective tissue

Excludes2 acquired absence of limbs and organs (Z89-Z90)
acquired deformities of limbs (M20-M21)
congenital malformations and deformations of the musculoskeletal system (Q65-Q79)
deforming dorsopathies (M40-M43)
dentofacial anomalies [including malocclusion] (M26.-)
postprocedural musculoskeletal disorders (M96.-)

M95.0 Acquired deformity of nose
Excludes2 deviated nasal septum (J34.2)

● M95.1 Cauliflower ear
Excludes2 other acquired deformities of ear (H61.1)

M95.10 Cauliflower ear, unspecified ear
M95.11 Cauliflower ear, right ear
M95.12 Cauliflower ear, left ear

M95.2 Other acquired deformity of head
Coding Clinic: 2023, Q1, P31

M95.3 Acquired deformity of neck

M95.4 Acquired deformity of chest and rib
Coding Clinic: 2022, Q2, P14

M95.5 Acquired deformity of pelvis
Excludes1 maternal care for known or suspected disproportion (O33.-)

M95.8 Other specified acquired deformities of musculoskeletal system

M95.9 Acquired deformity of musculoskeletal system, unspecified

INTRAOPERATIVE AND POSTPROCEDURAL COMPLICATIONS AND DISORDERS OF MUSCULOSKELETAL SYSTEM, NOT ELSEWHERE CLASSIFIED (M96)

● M96 Intraoperative and postprocedural complications and disorders of musculoskeletal system, not elsewhere classified

Excludes2 arthropathy following intestinal bypass (M02.0-)
complications of internal orthopedic prosthetic devices, implants and grafts (T84.-)
disorders associated with osteoporosis (M80)
periprosthetic fracture around internal prosthetic joint (M97.-)
presence of functional implants and other devices (Z96-Z97)

M96.0 Pseudarthrosis after fusion or arthrodesis

M96.1 Postlaminectomy syndrome, not elsewhere classified
Coding Clinic: 2024, Q1, P18

M96.2 Postradiation kyphosis

M96.3 Postlaminectomy kyphosis

M96.4 Postsurgical lordosis

M96.5 Postradiation scoliosis

● M96.6 Fracture of bone following insertion of orthopedic implant, joint prosthesis, or bone plate
Intraoperative fracture of bone during insertion of orthopedic implant, joint prosthesis, or bone plate
Excludes2 complication of internal orthopedic devices, implants or grafts (T84.-)

● M96.62 Fracture of humerus following insertion of orthopedic implant, joint prosthesis, or bone plate

M96.621 Fracture of humerus following insertion of orthopedic implant, joint prosthesis, or bone plate, right arm 🐾

M96.622 Fracture of humerus following insertion of orthopedic implant, joint prosthesis, or bone plate, left arm 🐾

M96.629 Fracture of humerus following insertion of orthopedic implant, joint prosthesis, or bone plate, unspecified arm 🐾

● M96.63 Fracture of radius or ulna following insertion of orthopedic implant, joint prosthesis, or bone plate

M96.631 Fracture of radius or ulna following insertion of orthopedic implant, joint prosthesis, or bone plate, right arm 🐾

M96.632 Fracture of radius or ulna following insertion of orthopedic implant, joint prosthesis, or bone plate, left arm 🐾

M96.639 Fracture of radius or ulna following insertion of orthopedic implant, joint prosthesis, or bone plate, unspecified arm 🐾

M96.65 Fracture of pelvis following insertion of orthopedic implant, joint prosthesis, or bone plate 🐾

● M96.66 Fracture of femur following insertion of orthopedic implant, joint prosthesis, or bone plate

M96.661 Fracture of femur following insertion of orthopedic implant, joint prosthesis, or bone plate, right leg 🐾

M96.662 Fracture of femur following insertion of orthopedic implant, joint prosthesis, or bone plate, left leg 🐾

M96.669 Fracture of femur following insertion of orthopedic implant, joint prosthesis, or bone plate, unspecified leg 🐾

● M96.67 Fracture of tibia or fibula following insertion of orthopedic implant, joint prosthesis, or bone plate

M96.671 Fracture of tibia or fibula following insertion of orthopedic implant, joint prosthesis, or bone plate, right leg 🐾

M96.672 Fracture of tibia or fibula following insertion of orthopedic implant, joint prosthesis, or bone plate, left leg 🐾

M96.679 Fracture of tibia or fibula following insertion of orthopedic implant, joint prosthesis, or bone plate, unspecified leg 🐾

M96.69 Fracture of other bone following insertion of orthopedic implant, joint prosthesis, or bone plate 🐾

● M96.8 Other intraoperative and postprocedural complications and disorders of musculoskeletal system, not elsewhere classified
Coding Clinic: 2016, Q4, P10

● **M96.81** **Intraoperative hemorrhage and hematoma of a musculoskeletal structure complicating a procedure**

    Excludes1   intraoperative hemorrhage and hematoma of a musculoskeletal structure due to accidental puncture and laceration during a procedure (M96.82-)

    M96.810   Intraoperative hemorrhage and hematoma of a musculoskeletal structure complicating a musculoskeletal system procedure

    M96.811   Intraoperative hemorrhage and hematoma of a musculoskeletal structure complicating other procedure

● **M96.82** **Accidental puncture and laceration of a musculoskeletal structure during a procedure**

    M96.820   Accidental puncture and laceration of a musculoskeletal structure during a musculoskeletal system procedure

    M96.821   Accidental puncture and laceration of a musculoskeletal structure during other procedure

● **M96.83** **Postprocedural hemorrhage of a musculoskeletal structure following a procedure**

    M96.830   Postprocedural hemorrhage of a musculoskeletal structure following a musculoskeletal system procedure

    M96.831   Postprocedural hemorrhage of a musculoskeletal structure following other procedure

● **M96.84** **Postprocedural hematoma and seroma of a musculoskeletal structure following a procedure**

    M96.840   Postprocedural hematoma of a musculoskeletal structure following a musculoskeletal system procedure

    M96.841   Postprocedural hematoma of a musculoskeletal structure following other procedure
        Coding Clinic: 2016, Q4, P10

    M96.842   Postprocedural seroma of a musculoskeletal structure following a musculoskeletal system procedure

    M96.843   Postprocedural seroma of a musculoskeletal structure following other procedure
        Coding Clinic: 2023, Q2, P13

    M96.89 **Other intraoperative and postprocedural complications and disorders of the musculoskeletal system**

        Instability of joint secondary to removal of joint prosthesis

        Use additional code, if applicable, to further specify disorder
        Coding Clinic: 2 2024, Q1, P18, 23; 023, Q2, P14; 2022, Q2, P14; 2021, Q1, P5

● **M96.A** **Fracture of ribs, sternum and thorax associated with compression of the chest and cardiopulmonary resuscitation**

    M96.A1 **Fracture of sternum associated with chest compression and cardiopulmonary resuscitation**

        Fracture of xiphoid process associated with chest compression and cardiopulmonary resuscitation

    M96.A2 **Fracture of one rib associated with chest compression and cardiopulmonary resuscitation**

    M96.A3 **Multiple fractures of ribs associated with chest compression and cardiopulmonary resuscitation**
        Coding Clinic: 2022, Q4, P32-33

    M96.A4 **Flail chest associated with chest compression and cardiopulmonary resuscitation**

    M96.A9 **Other fracture associated with chest compression and cardiopulmonary resuscitation**

PERIPROSTHETIC FRACTURE AROUND INTERNAL PROSTHETIC JOINT (M97)

● **M97** **Periprosthetic fracture around internal prosthetic joint**

    Code first if known, the specific type and cause of fracture, such as traumatic or pathological

    Excludes2   fracture of bone following insertion of orthopedic implant, joint prosthesis or bone plate (M96.6-)
        breakage (fracture) of prosthetic joint (T84.01-)
    Coding Clinic: 2016, Q4, P42

    The appropriate 7th character is to be added to each code from category M97:

A	initial encounter
D	subsequent encounter
S	sequela

● **M97.0** **Periprosthetic fracture around internal prosthetic hip joint**

    X● **M97.01**   Periprosthetic fracture around internal prosthetic right hip joint ✺
        Coding Clinic: 2016, Q4, P43

    X● **M97.02**   Periprosthetic fracture around internal prosthetic left hip joint ✺

● **M97.1** **Periprosthetic fracture around internal prosthetic knee joint**

    X● **M97.11**   Periprosthetic fracture around internal prosthetic right knee joint

    X● **M97.12**   Periprosthetic fracture around internal prosthetic left knee joint

● **M97.2** **Periprosthetic fracture around internal prosthetic ankle joint**

    X● **M97.21**   Periprosthetic fracture around internal prosthetic right ankle joint

    X● **M97.22**   Periprosthetic fracture around internal prosthetic left ankle joint

● **M97.3** **Periprosthetic fracture around internal prosthetic shoulder joint**

    X● **M97.31**   Periprosthetic fracture around internal prosthetic right shoulder joint

    X● **M97.32**   Periprosthetic fracture around internal prosthetic left shoulder joint

● **M97.4** **Periprosthetic fracture around internal prosthetic elbow joint**

    X● **M97.41**   Periprosthetic fracture around internal prosthetic right elbow joint

    X● **M97.42**   Periprosthetic fracture around internal prosthetic left elbow joint

X● **M97.8** **Periprosthetic fracture around other internal prosthetic joint**

    Periprosthetic fracture around internal prosthetic finger joint

    Periprosthetic fracture around internal prosthetic spinal joint

    Periprosthetic fracture around internal prosthetic toe joint

    Periprosthetic fracture around internal prosthetic wrist joint

    Use additional code to identify the joint (Z96.6-)

X● **M97.9** **Periprosthetic fracture around unspecified internal prosthetic joint**

BIOMECHANICAL LESIONS, NOT ELSEWHERE CLASSIFIED (M99)

● **M99   Biomechanical lesions, not elsewhere classified**

> **Note:** This category should not be used if the condition can be classified elsewhere.

  ● **M99.0   Segmental and somatic dysfunction**

    M99.00   Segmental and somatic dysfunction of head region

    M99.01   Segmental and somatic dysfunction of cervical region

    M99.02   Segmental and somatic dysfunction of thoracic region

    M99.03   Segmental and somatic dysfunction of lumbar region

    M99.04   Segmental and somatic dysfunction of sacral region

    M99.05   Segmental and somatic dysfunction of pelvic region

    M99.06   Segmental and somatic dysfunction of lower extremity

    M99.07   Segmental and somatic dysfunction of upper extremity

    M99.08   Segmental and somatic dysfunction of rib cage

    M99.09   Segmental and somatic dysfunction of abdomen and other regions

  ● **M99.1   Subluxation complex (vertebral)**

    M99.10   Subluxation complex (vertebral) of head region

    M99.11   Subluxation complex (vertebral) of cervical region

    M99.12   Subluxation complex (vertebral) of thoracic region

    M99.13   Subluxation complex (vertebral) of lumbar region

    M99.14   Subluxation complex (vertebral) of sacral region

    M99.15   Subluxation complex (vertebral) of pelvic region

    M99.16   Subluxation complex (vertebral) of lower extremity

    M99.17   Subluxation complex (vertebral) of upper extremity

    M99.18   Subluxation complex (vertebral) of rib cage

    M99.19   Subluxation complex (vertebral) of abdomen and other regions

  ● **M99.2   Subluxation stenosis of neural canal**

    M99.20   Subluxation stenosis of neural canal of head region

    M99.21   Subluxation stenosis of neural canal of cervical region

    M99.22   Subluxation stenosis of neural canal of thoracic region

    M99.23   Subluxation stenosis of neural canal of lumbar region

    M99.24   Subluxation stenosis of neural canal of sacral region

    M99.25   Subluxation stenosis of neural canal of pelvic region

    M99.26   Subluxation stenosis of neural canal of lower extremity

    M99.27   Subluxation stenosis of neural canal of upper extremity

    M99.28   Subluxation stenosis of neural canal of rib cage

    M99.29   Subluxation stenosis of neural canal of abdomen and other regions

  ● **M99.3   Osseous stenosis of neural canal**

    M99.30   Osseous stenosis of neural canal of head region

    M99.31   Osseous stenosis of neural canal of cervical region

    M99.32   Osseous stenosis of neural canal of thoracic region

    M99.33   Osseous stenosis of neural canal of lumbar region

    M99.34   Osseous stenosis of neural canal of sacral region

    M99.35   Osseous stenosis of neural canal of pelvic region

    M99.36   Osseous stenosis of neural canal of lower extremity

    M99.37   Osseous stenosis of neural canal of upper extremity

    M99.38   Osseous stenosis of neural canal of rib cage

    M99.39   Osseous stenosis of neural canal of abdomen and other regions

  ● **M99.4   Connective tissue stenosis of neural canal**

    M99.40   Connective tissue stenosis of neural canal of head region

    M99.41   Connective tissue stenosis of neural canal of cervical region

    M99.42   Connective tissue stenosis of neural canal of thoracic region

    M99.43   Connective tissue stenosis of neural canal of lumbar region

    M99.44   Connective tissue stenosis of neural canal of sacral region

    M99.45   Connective tissue stenosis of neural canal of pelvic region

    M99.46   Connective tissue stenosis of neural canal of lower extremity

    M99.47   Connective tissue stenosis of neural canal of upper extremity

    M99.48   Connective tissue stenosis of neural canal of rib cage

    M99.49   Connective tissue stenosis of neural canal of abdomen and other regions

  ● **M99.5   Intervertebral disc stenosis of neural canal**

    M99.50   Intervertebral disc stenosis of neural canal of head region

    M99.51   Intervertebral disc stenosis of neural canal of cervical region

    M99.52   Intervertebral disc stenosis of neural canal of thoracic region

    M99.53   Intervertebral disc stenosis of neural canal of lumbar region

    M99.54   Intervertebral disc stenosis of neural canal of sacral region

    M99.55   Intervertebral disc stenosis of neural canal of pelvic region

    M99.56   Intervertebral disc stenosis of neural canal of lower extremity

    M99.57   Intervertebral disc stenosis of neural canal of upper extremity

    M99.58   Intervertebral disc stenosis of neural canal of rib cage

    M99.59   Intervertebral disc stenosis of neural canal of abdomen and other regions

  ● **M99.6   Osseous and subluxation stenosis of intervertebral foramina**

    M99.60   Osseous and subluxation stenosis of intervertebral foramina of head region

    M99.61   Osseous and subluxation stenosis of intervertebral foramina of cervical region

    M99.62   Osseous and subluxation stenosis of intervertebral foramina of thoracic region

    M99.63   Osseous and subluxation stenosis of intervertebral foramina of lumbar region

    M99.64   Osseous and subluxation stenosis of intervertebral foramina of sacral region

    M99.65   Osseous and subluxation stenosis of intervertebral foramina of pelvic region

    M99.66   Osseous and subluxation stenosis of intervertebral foramina of lower extremity

▶ New   ⇛ Revised   ~~deleted~~ Deleted   Excludes 1   Excludes 2   Includes   Use additional   Code first   Code also   Key words

OGCR Official Guidelines   X Assign placeholder X   ● Use Additional Character(s)   ▹ Manifestation Code   Hierarchical Condition Category   Coding Clinic

M99.67   Osseous and subluxation stenosis of intervertebral foramina of upper extremity

M99.68   Osseous and subluxation stenosis of intervertebral foramina of rib cage

M99.69   Osseous and subluxation stenosis of intervertebral foramina of abdomen and other regions

● M99.7   Connective tissue and disc stenosis of intervertebral foramina

M99.70   Connective tissue and disc stenosis of intervertebral foramina of head region

M99.71   Connective tissue and disc stenosis of intervertebral foramina of cervical region

M99.72   Connective tissue and disc stenosis of intervertebral foramina of thoracic region

M99.73   Connective tissue and disc stenosis of intervertebral foramina of lumbar region

M99.74   Connective tissue and disc stenosis of intervertebral foramina of sacral region

M99.75   Connective tissue and disc stenosis of intervertebral foramina of pelvic region

M99.76   Connective tissue and disc stenosis of intervertebral foramina of lower extremity

M99.77   Connective tissue and disc stenosis of intervertebral foramina of upper extremity

M99.78   Connective tissue and disc stenosis of intervertebral foramina of rib cage

M99.79   Connective tissue and disc stenosis of intervertebral foramina of abdomen and other regions

● M99.8   Other biomechanical lesions

M99.80   Other biomechanical lesions of head region

M99.81   Other biomechanical lesions of cervical region

M99.82   Other biomechanical lesions of thoracic region

M99.83   Other biomechanical lesions of lumbar region

M99.84   Other biomechanical lesions of sacral region

M99.85   Other biomechanical lesions of pelvic region

M99.86   Other biomechanical lesions of lower extremity

M99.87   Other biomechanical lesions of upper extremity

M99.88   Other biomechanical lesions of rib cage

M99.89   Other biomechanical lesions of abdomen and other regions

M99.9   Biomechanical lesion, unspecified

CHAPTER 14

DISEASES OF THE GENITOURINARY SYSTEM (N00-N99)

OGCR Chapter-Specific Coding Guidelines

14. Chapter 14: Diseases of Genitourinary System (N00-N99)

a. Chronic kidney disease

1) Stages of chronic kidney disease (CKD)

The ICD-10-CM classifies CKD based on severity. The severity of CKD is designated by stages 1-5. Stage 2, code N18.2, equates to mild CKD; stage 3, code N18.3, equates to moderate CKD; and stage 4, code N18.4, equates to severe CKD. Code N18.6, End stage renal disease (ESRD), is assigned when the provider has documented end-stage-renal disease (ESRD).

    If both a stage of CKD and ESRD are documented, assign code N18.6 only.

2) Chronic kidney disease and kidney transplant status

Patients who have undergone kidney transplant may still have some form of chronic kidney disease CKD because the kidney transplant may not fully restore kidney function. Therefore, the presence of CKD alone does not constitute a transplant complication. Assign the appropriate N18 code for the patient's stage of CKD and code Z94.0, Kidney transplant status. If a transplant complication such as failure or rejection or other transplant complication is documented, see Section I.C.19.g for information on coding complications of a kidney transplant. If the documentation is unclear as to whether the patient has a complication of the transplant, query the provider.

3) Chronic kidney disease with other conditions

Patients with CKD may also suffer from other serious conditions, most commonly diabetes mellitus and hypertension. The sequencing of the CKD code in relationship to codes for other contributing conditions is based on the conventions in the Tabular List.

See I.C.9. Hypertensive chronic kidney disease.

See I.C.19. Chronic kidney disease and kidney transplant complications.

Item 14–1 Nephritis (inflammation) or **nephropathy** (disease) **with lesion of proliferative glomerulonephritis** results from a streptococcal infection.

    Nephritis (inflammation) or **nephropathy** (disease) **with lesion of membranous glomerulonephritis** is characterized by deposits along the epithelial side of the basement membrane.

    Nephritis (inflammation) or **nephropathy** (disease) **with lesion of membranoproliferative glomerulonephritis** is characterized by alterations in the basement membranes of the kidney and the glomerular cells.

    Nephritis (inflammation) or **nephropathy** (disease) **with lesion of rapidly progressive glomerulonephritis** is characterized by rapid and progressive decline in renal function.

    Nephritis (inflammation) or **nephropathy** (disease) **with lesion of renal cortical necrosis** is characterized by death of the cortical tissues.

    Nephritis (inflammation) or **nephropathy** (disease) **with lesion of renal medullary necrosis** is characterized by death of the tissues that collect urine.

Figure 14-1 Kidneys within the urinary system.

Item 14–2 Glomerulonephritis is nephritis accompanied by inflammation of the glomeruli of the kidney, resulting in the degeneration of the glomeruli and the nephrons.

    Acute glomerulonephritis primarily affects children and young adults and is usually a result of a streptococcal infection.

    Proliferative glomerulonephritis is the acute form of the disease resulting from a streptococcal infection.

    Rapidly progressive glomerulonephritis, also known as **crescentic** or **malignant glomerulonephritis**, is the acute form of the disease, which leads quickly to rapid and progressive decline in renal function.

CHAPTER 14

DISEASES OF THE GENITOURINARY SYSTEM (N00-N99)

Excludes2   certain conditions originating in the perinatal period (P04-P96)

certain infectious and parasitic diseases (A00-B99)

complications of pregnancy, childbirth and the puerperium (O00-O9A)

congenital malformations, deformations and chromosomal abnormalities (Q00-Q99)

endocrine, nutritional and metabolic diseases (E00-E88)

injury, poisoning and certain other consequences of external causes (S00-T88)

neoplasms (C00-D49)

symptoms, signs and abnormal clinical and laboratory findings, not elsewhere classified (R00-R94)

This chapter contains the following blocks:

N00-N08	Glomerular diseases
N10-N16	Renal tubulo-interstitial diseases
N17-N19	Acute kidney failure and chronic kidney disease
N20-N23	Urolithiasis
N25-N29	Other disorders of kidney and ureter
N30-N39	Other diseases of the urinary system
N40-N53	Diseases of male genital organs
N60-N65	Disorders of breast
N70-N77	Inflammatory diseases of female pelvic organs
N80-N98	Noninflammatory disorders of female genital tract
N99	Intraoperative and postprocedural complications and disorders of genitourinary system, not elsewhere classified

GLOMERULAR DISEASES (N00-N08)

Code also any associated kidney failure (N17-N19)

Excludes1   hypertensive chronic kidney disease (I12.-)

● **N00** **Acute nephritic syndrome**

    Includes   acute glomerular disease
                  acute glomerulonephritis
                  acute nephritis

    Excludes1   acute tubulo-interstitial nephritis (N10)
                  nephritic syndrome NOS (N05.-)

  N00.0 **Acute nephritic syndrome with minor glomerular abnormality**

        Acute nephritic syndrome with minimal change lesion

  N00.1 **Acute nephritic syndrome with focal and segmental glomerular lesions**

        Acute nephritic syndrome with focal and segmental hyalinosis

        Acute nephritic syndrome with focal and segmental sclerosis

        Acute nephritic syndrome with focal glomerulonephritis

  N00.2 **Acute nephritic syndrome with diffuse membranous glomerulonephritis**

  N00.3 **Acute nephritic syndrome with diffuse mesangial proliferative glomerulonephritis**

▶ New   ⇒ Revised   deleted Deleted   Excludes 1   Excludes 2   Includes   Use additional   Code first   Code also   Key words

OGCR Official Guidelines   X Assign placeholder X   ● Use Additional Character(s)   ▶ Manifestation Code   🔖 Hierarchical Condition Category   Coding Clinic

N00.4 **Acute nephritic syndrome with** diffuse endocapillary proliferative glomerulonephritis

N00.5 **Acute nephritic syndrome with** diffuse mesangiocapillary glomerulonephritis
>   Acute nephritic syndrome with membranoproliferative glomerulonephritis, types 1 and 3, or NOS
>
>   **Excludes1** Acute nephritic syndrome with C3 glomerulonephritis (N00.A)
>   Acute nephritic syndrome with C3 glomerulopathy (N00.A)

N00.6 **Acute nephritic syndrome with** dense deposit disease
>   Acute nephritic syndrome with C3 glomerulopathy with dense deposit disease
>   Acute nephritic syndrome with membranoproliferative glomerulonephritis, type 2

N00.7 **Acute nephritic syndrome with** diffuse crescentic glomerulonephritis
>   Acute nephritic syndrome with extracapillary glomerulonephritis

N00.8 **Acute nephritic syndrome with** other morphologic changes
>   Acute nephritic syndrome with proliferative glomerulonephritis NOS

N00.9 **Acute nephritic syndrome with** unspecified morphologic changes

N00.A **Acute nephritic syndrome with C3 glomerulonephritis**
>   Acute nephritic syndrome with C3 glomerulopathy, NOS
>
>   **Excludes1** Acute nephritic syndrome (with C3 glomerulopathy) with dense deposit disease (N00.6)

● **N01 Rapidly progressive nephritic syndrome**
>   **Includes** rapidly progressive glomerular disease
>   rapidly progressive glomerulonephritis
>   rapidly progressive nephritis
>
>   **Excludes1** nephritic syndrome NOS (N05.-)

N01.0 **Rapidly progressive nephritic syndrome with** minor glomerular abnormality
>   Rapidly progressive nephritic syndrome with minimal change lesion

N01.1 **Rapidly progressive nephritic syndrome with** focal and segmental glomerular lesions
>   Rapidly progressive nephritic syndrome with focal and segmental hyalinosis
>   Rapidly progressive nephritic syndrome with focal and segmental sclerosis
>   Rapidly progressive nephritic syndrome with focal glomerulonephritis

N01.2 **Rapidly progressive nephritic syndrome with** diffuse membranous glomerulonephritis

N01.3 **Rapidly progressive nephritic syndrome with** diffuse mesangial proliferative glomerulonephritis

N01.4 **Rapidly progressive nephritic syndrome with** diffuse endocapillary proliferative glomerulonephritis

N01.5 **Rapidly progressive nephritic syndrome with** diffuse mesangiocapillary glomerulonephritis
>   Rapidly progressive nephritic syndrome with membranoproliferative glomerulonephritis, types 1 and 3, or NOS
>
>   **Excludes1** Rapidly progressive nephritic syndrome with C3 glomerulonephritis (N01.A)
>   Rapidly progressive nephritic syndrome with C3 glomerulopathy (N01.A)

N01.6 **Rapidly progressive nephritic syndrome with** dense deposit disease
>   Rapidly progressive nephritic syndrome with C3 glomerulopathy with dense deposit disease
>   Rapidly progressive nephritic syndrome with membranoproliferative glomerulonephritis, type 2

N01.7 **Rapidly progressive nephritic syndrome with** diffuse crescentic glomerulonephritis
>   Rapidly progressive nephritic syndrome with extracapillary glomerulonephritis

N01.8 **Rapidly progressive nephritic syndrome with** other morphologic changes
>   Rapidly progressive nephritic syndrome with proliferative glomerulonephritis NOS

N01.9 **Rapidly progressive nephritic syndrome with** unspecified morphologic changes

N01.A **Rapidly progressive nephritic syndrome with C3 glomerulonephritis**
>   Rapidly progressive nephritic syndrome with C3 glomerulopathy, NOS
>
>   **Excludes1** Rapidly progressive nephritic syndrome (with C3 glomerulopathy) with dense deposit disease (N01.6)

● **N02 Recurrent and persistent hematuria**
>   **Excludes1** acute cystitis with hematuria (N30.01)
>   hematuria NOS (R31.9)
>   hematuria not associated with specified morphologic lesions (R31.-)

N02.0 **Recurrent and persistent hematuria with** minor glomerular abnormality
>   Recurrent and persistent hematuria with minimal change lesion

N02.1 **Recurrent and persistent hematuria with** focal and segmental glomerular lesions
>   Recurrent and persistent hematuria with focal and segmental hyalinosis
>   Recurrent and persistent hematuria with focal and segmental sclerosis
>   Recurrent and persistent hematuria with focal glomerulonephritis

N02.2 **Recurrent and persistent hematuria with** diffuse membranous glomerulonephritis

N02.3 **Recurrent and persistent hematuria with** diffuse mesangial proliferative glomerulonephritis

N02.4 **Recurrent and persistent hematuria with** diffuse endocapillary proliferative glomerulonephritis

N02.5 **Recurrent and persistent hematuria with** diffuse mesangiocapillary glomerulonephritis
>   Recurrent and persistent hematuria with membranoproliferative glomerulonephritis, types 1 and 3, or NOS
>
>   **Excludes1** Recurrent and persistent hematuria with C3 glomerulonephritis (N02.A)
>   Recurrent and persistent hematuria with C3 glomerulopathy (N02.A)

N02.6 **Recurrent and persistent hematuria with** dense deposit disease
>   Recurrent and persistent hematuria with C3 glomerulopathy with dense deposit disease
>   Recurrent and persistent hematuria with membranoproliferative glomerulonephritis, type 2

N02.7 **Recurrent and persistent hematuria with** diffuse crescentic glomerulonephritis
>   Recurrent and persistent hematuria with extracapillary glomerulonephritis

N02.8 **Recurrent and persistent hematuria with** other morphologic changes
>   Recurrent and persistent hematuria with proliferative glomerulonephritis NOS

N02.9 **Recurrent and persistent hematuria with** unspecified morphologic changes
>   Coding Clinic: 2017, Q2, P5

CHAPTER 14 (N00-N99)

N02.A   Recurrent and persistent hematuria with C3 glomerulonephritis

Recurrent and persistent hematuria with C3 glomerulopathy

> **Excludes1**   Recurrent and persistent hematuria (with C3 glomerulopathy) with dense deposit disease (N02.6)

● **N02.B   Recurrent and persistent immunoglobulin A nephropathy**

N02.B1   Recurrent and persistent immunoglobulin A nephropathy with glomerular lesion

N02.B2   Recurrent and persistent immunoglobulin A nephropathy with focal and segmental glomerular lesion

> Recurrent and persistent immunoglobulin A nephropathy with focal and segmental hyalinosis or sclerosis

N02.B3   Recurrent and persistent immunoglobulin A nephropathy with diffuse membranoproliferative glomerulonephritis

N02.B4   Recurrent and persistent immunoglobulin A nephropathy with diffuse membranous glomerulonephritis

N02.B5   Recurrent and persistent immunoglobulin A nephropathy with diffuse mesangial proliferative glomerulonephritis

N02.B6   Recurrent and persistent immunoglobulin A nephropathy with diffuse mesangiocapillary glomerulonephritis

N02.B9   Other recurrent and persistent immunoglobulin A nephropathy

● **N03   Chronic nephritic syndrome**

> **Includes**   chronic glomerular disease
> chronic glomerulonephritis
> chronic nephritis

> **Excludes1**   chronic tubulo-interstitial nephritis (N11.-)
> diffuse sclerosing glomerulonephritis (N05.8-)
> nephritic syndrome NOS (N05.-)

N03.0   Chronic nephritic syndrome with minor glomerular abnormality

> Chronic nephritic syndrome with minimal change lesion

N03.1   Chronic nephritic syndrome with focal and segmental glomerular lesions

> Chronic nephritic syndrome with focal and segmental hyalinosis
> Chronic nephritic syndrome with focal and segmental sclerosis
> Chronic nephritic syndrome with focal glomerulonephritis

N03.2   Chronic nephritic syndrome with diffuse membranous glomerulonephritis

N03.3   Chronic nephritic syndrome with diffuse mesangial proliferative glomerulonephritis

N03.4   Chronic nephritic syndrome with diffuse endocapillary proliferative glomerulonephritis

N03.5   Chronic nephritic syndrome with diffuse mesangiocapillary glomerulonephritis

> Chronic nephritic syndrome with membranoproliferative glomerulonephritis, types 1 and 3, or NOS

> **Excludes1**   Chronic nephritic syndrome with C3 glomerulonephritis (N03.A)
> Chronic nephritic syndrome with C3 glomerulopathy (N03.A)

N03.6   Chronic nephritic syndrome with dense deposit disease

> Chronic nephritic syndrome with C3 glomerulopathy with dense deposit disease
> Chronic nephritic syndrome with membranoproliferative glomerulonephritis, type 2

N03.7   Chronic nephritic syndrome with diffuse crescentic glomerulonephritis

> Chronic nephritic syndrome with extracapillary glomerulonephritis

N03.8   Chronic nephritic syndrome with other morphologic changes

> Chronic nephritic syndrome with proliferative glomerulonephritis NOS

N03.9   Chronic nephritic syndrome with unspecified morphologic changes

N03.A   Chronic nephritic syndrome with C3 glomerulonephritis

> Chronic nephritic syndrome with C3 glomerulopathy

> **Excludes1**   Chronic nephritic syndrome (with C3 glomerulopathy) with dense deposit disease (N03.6)

● **N04   Nephrotic syndrome**

> **Includes**   congenital nephrotic syndrome
> lipoid nephrosis

N04.0   Nephrotic syndrome with minor glomerular abnormality

> Nephrotic syndrome with minimal change lesion

N04.1   Nephrotic syndrome with focal and segmental glomerular lesions

> Nephrotic syndrome with focal and segmental hyalinosis
> Nephrotic syndrome with focal and segmental sclerosis
> Nephrotic syndrome with focal glomerulonephritis

● **N04.2   Nephrotic syndrome with diffuse membranous glomerulonephritis**

N04.20   Nephrotic syndrome with diffuse membranous glomerulonephritis, unspecified

> Membranous nephropathy NOS with nephrotic syndrome

N04.21   Primary membranous nephropathy with nephrotic syndrome

> Idiopathic membranous nephropathy with nephrotic syndrome

N04.22   Secondary membranous nephropathy with nephrotic syndrome

> *Code first, if applicable, other disease or disorder or poisoning causing membranous nephropathy*

> Use Additional code, if applicable, for adverse effect of drug causing membranous nephropathy

N04.29   Other nephrotic syndrome with diffuse membranous glomerulonephritis

N04.3   Nephrotic syndrome with diffuse mesangial proliferative glomerulonephritis

N04.4   Nephrotic syndrome with diffuse endocapillary proliferative glomerulonephritis

N04.5   Nephrotic syndrome with diffuse mesangiocapillary glomerulonephritis

> Nephrotic syndrome with membranoproliferative glomerulonephritis, types 1 and 3, or NOS

> **Excludes1**   Nephrotic syndrome with C3 glomerulonephritis (N04.A)
> Nephrotic syndrome with C3 glomerulopathy (N04.A)

Item 14–3 Chronic glomerulonephritis (GN) persists over a period of years, with remissions and exacerbation.

Chronic GN with lesion of proliferative glomerulonephritis results from a streptococcal infection.

Chronic GN with lesion of membranous glomerulonephritis, also known as membranous nephropathy, is characterized by deposits along the epithelial side of the basement membrane.

Chronic GN with lesion of membrano-proliferative glomerulonephritis (MPGN) is a group of disorders characterized by alterations in the basement membranes of the kidney and the glomerular cells.

Chronic GN with lesion of rapidly progressive glomerulonephritis is characterized by necrosis, endothelial proliferation, and mesangial proliferation. The condition is marked by rapid and progressive decline in renal function.

▶ New   ⟹ Revised   ~~deleted~~ Deleted   Excludes 1   Excludes 2   Includes   Use additional   Code first   Code also   Key words

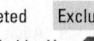 OGCR Official Guidelines   X Assign placeholder X   ● Use Additional Character(s)   ▶ Manifestation Code   🅗 Hierarchical Condition Category   **Coding Clinic**

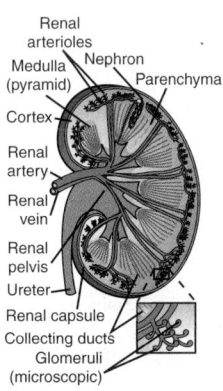

Renal
arterioles
Medulla   Nephron
(pyramid)   Parenchyma
Cortex
Renal
artery
Renal
vein
Renal
pelvis
Ureter
Renal capsule
Collecting ducts
Glomeruli
(microscopic)

Figure 14-2 Kidney cross section.

Item 14–4 Nephrotic syndrome (NS) is marked by massive proteinuria (protein in the urine) and water retention. Patients with NS are particularly vulnerable to staphylococcal and pneumococcal infections. NS with lesion of proliferative glomerulonephritis results from a streptococcal infection. NS with lesion of membranous glomerulonephritis results in thickening of the capillary walls. NS with lesion of minimal change glomerulonephritis is usually a benign disorder that occurs mostly in children and requires electron microscopy (biopsy) to verify changes in the glomeruli.

N04.6   **Nephrotic syndrome with** dense deposit disease
      Nephrotic syndrome with C3 glomerulopathy with dense deposit disease
      Nephrotic syndrome with membranoproliferative glomerulonephritis, type 2

N04.7   **Nephrotic syndrome with** diffuse crescentic glomerulonephritis
      Nephrotic syndrome with extracapillary glomerulonephritis

N04.8   **Nephrotic syndrome with** other morphologic changes
      Nephrotic syndrome with proliferative glomerulonephritis NOS

N04.9   **Nephrotic syndrome with** unspecified morphologic changes

N04.A   **Nephrotic syndrome with** C3 glomerulonephritis
      Nephrotic syndrome with C3 glomerulopathy
      Excludes1   Nephrotic syndrome (with C3 glomerulopathy) with dense deposit disease (N04.6)

● N05   **Unspecified nephritic syndrome**
      Includes   glomerular disease NOS
              glomerulonephritis NOS
              nephritis NOS
              nephropathy NOS and renal disease NOS with morphological lesion specified in .0-.8

      Excludes1   nephropathy NOS with no stated morphological lesion (N28.9)
              renal disease NOS with no stated morphological lesion (N28.9)
              tubulo-interstitial nephritis NOS (N12)

N05.0   **Unspecified nephritic syndrome with** minor glomerular abnormality
      Unspecified nephritic syndrome with minimal change lesion

N05.1   **Unspecified nephritic syndrome with focal and** segmental glomerular lesions
      Unspecified nephritic syndrome with focal and segmental hyalinosis
      Unspecified nephritic syndrome with focal and segmental sclerosis
      Unspecified nephritic syndrome with focal glomerulonephritis

N05.2   **Unspecified nephritic syndrome with** diffuse membranous glomerulonephritis

N05.3   **Unspecified nephritic syndrome with** diffuse mesangial proliferative glomerulonephritis

N05.4   **Unspecified nephritic syndrome with** diffuse endocapillary proliferative glomerulonephritis

N05.5   **Unspecified nephritic syndrome with** diffuse mesangiocapillary glomerulonephritis
      Unspecified nephritic syndrome with membranoproliferative glomerulonephritis, types 1 and 3, or NOS
      Excludes1   Unspecified nephritic syndrome with C3 glomerulonephritis (N05.A)
              Unspecified nephritic syndrome with C3 glomerulopathy (N05.A)

N05.6   **Unspecified nephritic syndrome with** dense deposit disease
      Unspecified nephritic syndrome with C3 glomerulopathy with dense deposit disease
      Unspecified nephritic syndrome with membranoproliferative glomerulonephritis, type 2

N05.7   **Unspecified nephritic syndrome with** diffuse crescentic glomerulonephritis
      Unspecified nephritic syndrome with extracapillary glomerulonephritis

N05.8   **Unspecified nephritic syndrome with** other morphologic changes
      Unspecified nephritic syndrome with proliferative glomerulonephritis NOS

N05.9   **Unspecified nephritic syndrome with** unspecified morphologic changes

N05.A   **Unspecified nephritic syndrome with** C3 glomerulonephritis
      Unspecified nephritic syndrome with C3 glomerulopathy
      Excludes1   Unspecified nephritic syndrome (with C3 glomerulopathy) with dense deposit disease(N05.6)

● N06   **Isolated proteinuria with specified morphological lesion**
      Excludes1   proteinuria not associated with specific morphologic lesions (R80.0)

N06.0   **Isolated proteinuria with** minor glomerular abnormality
      Isolated proteinuria with minimal change lesion

N06.1   **Isolated proteinuria with** focal and segmental glomerular lesions
      Isolated proteinuria with focal and segmental hyalinosis
      Isolated proteinuria with focal and segmental sclerosis
      Isolated proteinuria with focal glomerulonephritis

N06.2   **Isolated proteinuria with** diffuse membranous glomerulonephritis

  ● N06.20   **Isolated proteinuria with diffuse membranous glomerulonephritis, unspecified**
      Membranous nephropathy, NOS
      Excludes1   membranous nephropathy NOS with nephrotic syndrome (N04.20)

  N06.21   **Primary membranous nephropathy with isolated proteinuria**
      Idiopathic membranous nephropathy (with isolated proteinuria)
      Primary membranous nephropathy, NOS
      Excludes1   primary membranous nephropathy with nephrotic syndrome (N04.21)

  N06.22   **Secondary membranous nephropathy with isolated proteinuria**
      Secondary membranous nephropathy, NOS
      Code first, if applicable, other disease or disorder or poisoning causing membranous nephropathy
      Use Additional code, if applicable, for adverse effect of drug causing membranous nephropathy
      Excludes1   secondary membranous nephropathy with nephrotic syndrome (N04.22)

  N06.29   **Other isolated proteinuria with diffuse membranous glomerulonephritis**

CHAPTER 14 (N00-N99)

N06.3 **Isolated proteinuria with diffuse mesangial proliferative glomerulonephritis**

N06.4 **Isolated proteinuria with diffuse endocapillary proliferative glomerulonephritis**

N06.5 **Isolated proteinuria with diffuse mesangiocapillary glomerulonephritis**
Isolated proteinuria with membranoproliferative glomerulonephritis, types 1 and 3, or NOS

> **Excludes1**   Isolated proteinuria with C3 glomerulonephritis (N06.A)
> Isolated proteinuria with C3 glomerulopathy (N06.A)

N06.6 **Isolated proteinuria with dense deposit disease**
Isolated proteinuria with C3 glomerulopathy with dense deposit disease
Isolated proteinuria with membranoproliferative glomerulonephritis, type 2

N06.7 **Isolated proteinuria with diffuse crescentic glomerulonephritis**
Isolated proteinuria with extracapillary glomerulonephritis

N06.8 **Isolated proteinuria with other morphologic lesion**
Isolated proteinuria with proliferative glomerulonephritis NOS

N06.9 **Isolated proteinuria with unspecified morphologic lesion**

N06.A **Isolated proteinuria with C3 glomerulonephritis**
Isolated proteinuria with C3 glomerulopathy

> **Excludes1**   Isolated proteinuria (with C3 glomerulopathy) with dense deposit disease (N06.6)

● **N07** **Hereditary nephropathy, not elsewhere classified**

> **Excludes2**   Alport's syndrome (Q87.81-)
> hereditary amyloid nephropathy (E85.-)
> nail patella syndrome (Q87.2)
> non-neuropathic heredofamilial amyloidosis (E85.-)

N07.0 **Hereditary nephropathy, not elsewhere classified with minor glomerular abnormality**
Hereditary nephropathy, not elsewhere classified with minimal change lesion

N07.1 **Hereditary nephropathy, not elsewhere classified with focal and segmental glomerular lesions**
Hereditary nephropathy, not elsewhere classified with focal and segmental hyalinosis
Hereditary nephropathy, not elsewhere classified with focal and segmental sclerosis
Hereditary nephropathy, not elsewhere classified with focal glomerulonephritis

N07.2 **Hereditary nephropathy, not elsewhere classified with diffuse membranous glomerulonephritis**

N07.3 **Hereditary nephropathy, not elsewhere classified with diffuse mesangial proliferative glomerulonephritis**

N07.4 **Hereditary nephropathy, not elsewhere classified with diffuse endocapillary proliferative glomerulonephritis**

N07.5 **Hereditary nephropathy, not elsewhere classified with diffuse mesangiocapillary glomerulonephritis**
Hereditary nephropathy, not elsewhere classified with membranoproliferative glomerulonephritis, types 1 and 3, or NOS

> **Excludes1**   Hereditary nephropathy, not elsewhere classified with C3 glomerulonephritis (N07.A)
> Hereditary nephropathy, not elsewhere classified with C3 glomerulopathy (N07.A)

N07.6 **Hereditary nephropathy, not elsewhere classified with dense deposit disease**
Hereditary nephropathy, not elsewhere classified with C3 glomerulopathy with dense deposit disease
Hereditary nephropathy, not elsewhere classified with membranoproliferative glomerulonephritis, type 2

N07.7 **Hereditary nephropathy, not elsewhere classified with diffuse crescentic glomerulonephritis**
Hereditary nephropathy, not elsewhere classified with extracapillary glomerulonephritis

N07.8 **Hereditary nephropathy, not elsewhere classified with other morphologic lesions**
Hereditary nephropathy, not elsewhere classified with proliferative glomerulonephritis NOS

N07.9 **Hereditary nephropathy, not elsewhere classified with unspecified morphologic lesions**

N07.A **Hereditary nephropathy, not elsewhere classified with C3 glomerulonephritis**
Hereditary nephropathy, not elsewhere classified with C3 glomerulopathy

> **Excludes1**   Hereditary nephropathy, not elsewhere classified (with C3 glomerulopathy) with dense deposit disease (N07.6)

▷ *N08* *Glomerular disorders in diseases classified elsewhere*
Glomerulonephritis
Nephritis
Nephropathy

> *Code first underlying disease, such as:*
> amyloidosis (E85.-)
> congenital syphilis (A50.5)
> cryoglobulinemia (D89.1)
> disseminated intravascular coagulation (D65)
> gout (M1A.-, M10.-)
> microscopic polyangiitis (M31.7)
> multiple myeloma (C90.0-)
> sepsis (A40.0-A41.9)
> sickle-cell disease (D57.0-D57.8)

> **Excludes1**   glomerulonephritis, nephritis and nephropathy (in):
> antiglomerular basement membrane disease (M31.0)
> diabetes (E08-E13 with .21)
> gonococcal (A54.21)
> Goodpasture's syndrome (M31.0)
> hemolytic-uremic syndrome (D59.3)
> lupus (M32.14)
> mumps (B26.83)
> syphilis (A52.75)
> systemic lupus erythematosus (M32.14)
> Wegener's granulomatosis (M31.31)
> pyelonephritis in diseases classified elsewhere (N16)
> renal tubulo-interstitial disorders classified elsewhere (N16)

RENAL TUBULO-INTERSTITIAL DISEASES (N10-N16)

> **Includes**   pyelonephritis
> **Excludes1**   pyeloureteritis cystica (N28.85)

N10 **Acute pyelonephritis**
Acute infectious interstitial nephritis
Acute pyelitis
Acute tubulo-interstitial nephritis
Hemoglobin nephrosis
Myoglobin nephrosis
Use additional code (B95-B97), to identify infectious agent
Coding Clinic: 2019, Q3, P13-14

● **N11** **Chronic tubulo-interstitial nephritis**

> **Includes**   chronic infectious interstitial nephritis
> chronic pyelitis
> chronic pyelonephritis

Use additional code (B95-B97), to identify infectious agent

Figure 14-3 Acute pyelonephritis. Cortical surface exhibits grayish white areas of inflammation and abscess formation. (From Frazier MS, Drzymkowski JW: Essentials of Human Diseases and Conditions, St. Louis, Saunders/Elsevier, 2009)

Item 14–5 Pyelonephritis is an infection of the kidneys and ureters and may be chronic or acute in one or both kidneys.

N11.0   Nonobstructive reflux-associated chronic pyelonephritis
   Pyelonephritis (chronic) associated with (vesicoureteral) reflux
   | Excludes1 | vesicoureteral reflux NOS (N13.70) |

N11.1   Chronic obstructive pyelonephritis
   Pyelonephritis (chronic) associated with anomaly of pelviureteric junction
   Pyelonephritis (chronic) associated with anomaly of pyeloureteric junction
   Pyelonephritis (chronic) associated with crossing of vessel
   Pyelonephritis (chronic) associated with kinking of ureter
   Pyelonephritis (chronic) associated with obstruction of ureter
   Pyelonephritis (chronic) associated with stricture of pelviureteric junction
   Pyelonephritis (chronic) associated with stricture of ureter
   | Excludes1 | calculous pyelonephritis (N20.9) |
   | | obstructive uropathy (N13.-) |

N11.8   Other chronic tubulo-interstitial nephritis
   Nonobstructive chronic pyelonephritis NOS

N11.9   Chronic tubulo-interstitial nephritis, unspecified
   Chronic interstitial nephritis NOS
   Chronic pyelitis NOS
   Chronic pyelonephritis NOS

N12   Tubulo-interstitial nephritis, not specified as acute or chronic
   Interstitial nephritis NOS
   Pyelitis NOS
   Pyelonephritis NOS
   | Excludes1 | calculous pyelonephritis (N20.9) |

●**N13   Obstructive and reflux uropathy**
Excludes2	calculus of kidney and ureter without hydronephrosis (N20.-)
	congenital obstructive defects of renal pelvis and ureter (Q62.0-Q62.3)
	hydronephrosis with ureteropelvic junction obstruction (Q62.11)
	obstructive pyelonephritis (N11.1)

N13.0   Hydronephrosis with ureteropelvic junction obstruction
   Hydronephrosis due to acquired occlusion of ureteropelvic junction
   | Excludes2 | Hydronephrosis with ureteropelvic junction obstruction due to calculus (N13.2) |
   Coding Clinic: 2016, Q4, P43

N13.1   Hydronephrosis with ureteral stricture, not elsewhere classified
   | Excludes1 | hydronephrosis with ureteral stricture with infection (N13.6) |

N13.2   Hydronephrosis with renal and ureteral calculous obstruction
   | Excludes1 | hydronephrosis with renal and ureteral calculous obstruction with infection (N13.6) |

Figure 14-4 Hydronephrosis of the kidney, with marked dilatation of pelvis and calyces and thinning of renal parenchyma. (From Kumar: Robbins and Cotran: Pathologic Basis of Disease, ed 8, Saunders, An Imprint of Elsevier, 2009)

●**N13.3   Other and unspecified hydronephrosis**
   | Excludes1 | hydronephrosis with infection (N13.6) |
   N13.30   Unspecified hydronephrosis
   N13.39   Other hydronephrosis

N13.4   Hydroureter
Excludes1	congenital hydroureter (Q62.3-)
	hydroureter with infection (N13.6)
	vesicoureteral-reflux with hydroureter (N13.73-)

N13.5   Crossing vessel and stricture of ureter without hydronephrosis
   Kinking and stricture of ureter without hydronephrosis
   | Excludes1 | crossing vessel and stricture of ureter without hydronephrosis with infection (N13.6) |
   Coding Clinic: 2016, Q4, P43

N13.6   Pyonephrosis
   Conditions in N13.0-N13.5 with infection
   Obstructive uropathy with infection
   Use additional code (B95-B97), to identify infectious agent
   Coding Clinic: 2018, Q2, P21

●**N13.7   Vesicoureteral-reflux**
   | Excludes1 | reflux-associated pyelonephritis (N11.0) |
   N13.70   Vesicoureteral-reflux, unspecified
   Occurs when urine flows from bladder back into ureters
   Vesicoureteral-reflux NOS
   N13.71   Vesicoureteral-reflux without reflux nephropathy
   ●**N13.72   Vesicoureteral-reflux with reflux nephropathy without hydroureter**
   N13.721   Vesicoureteral-reflux with reflux nephropathy without hydroureter, unilateral
   N13.722   Vesicoureteral-reflux with reflux nephropathy without hydroureter, bilateral
   N13.729   Vesicoureteral-reflux with reflux nephropathy without hydroureter, unspecified
   ●**N13.73   Vesicoureteral-reflux with reflux nephropathy with hydroureter**
   N13.731   Vesicoureteral-reflux with reflux nephropathy with hydroureter, unilateral
   N13.732   Vesicoureteral-reflux with reflux nephropathy with hydroureter, bilateral
   N13.739   Vesicoureteral-reflux with reflux nephropathy with hydroureter, unspecified

N13.8   Other obstructive and reflux uropathy
   Urinary tract obstruction due to specified cause
   Code first, if applicable, any causal condition first, such as:
   enlarged prostate (N40.1)

N13.9   Obstructive and reflux uropathy, unspecified
   Urinary tract obstruction NOS

CHAPTER 14 (N00-N99)

● **N14 Drug- and heavy-metal-induced tubulo-interstitial and tubular conditions**

Code first poisoning due to drug or toxin, if applicable (T36-T65 with fifth or sixth character 1-4)

Use additional code for adverse effect, if applicable, to identify drug (T36-T50 with fifth or sixth character 5)

N14.0 Analgesic nephropathy

● **N14.1 Nephropathy induced by other drugs, medicaments and biological substances**
Coding Clinic: 2021, Q3, P9-10

　N14.11 Contrast-induced nephropathy
　　Contrast medium, radiography nephropathy
　　Excludes2 acute kidney failure (N17.-)
　Coding Clinic: 2022, Q4, P33

　N14.19 Nephropathy induced by other drugs, medicaments and biological substances

N14.2 Nephropathy induced by unspecified drug, medicament or biological substance

N14.3 Nephropathy induced by heavy metals

N14.4 Toxic nephropathy, not elsewhere classified

● **N15 Other renal tubulo-interstitial diseases**

N15.0 Balkan nephropathy
　Balkan endemic nephropathy

N15.1 Renal and perinephric abscess

N15.8 Other specified renal tubulo-interstitial diseases

N15.9 Renal tubulo-interstitial disease, unspecified
　Infection of kidney NOS
　Excludes1 urinary tract infection NOS (N39.0)

▷ *N16 Renal tubulo-interstitial disorders in diseases classified elsewhere*
　Pyelonephritis
　Tubulo-interstitial nephritis
　Code first underlying disease, such as:
　　brucellosis (A23.0-A23.9)
　　cryoglobulinemia (D89.1)
　　glycogen storage disease (E74.0-)
　　leukemia (C91-C95)
　　lymphoma (C81.0-C85.9, C96.0-C96.9)
　　multiple myeloma (C90.0-)
　　sepsis (A40.0-A41.9)
　　Wilson's disease (E83.01)
　　Excludes1 diphtheritic pyelonephritis and tubulo-interstitial nephritis (A36.84)
　　　pyelonephritis and tubulo-interstitial nephritis in candidiasis (B37.49)
　　　pyelonephritis and tubulo-interstitial nephritis in cystinosis (E72.04)
　　　pyelonephritis and tubulo-interstitial nephritis in salmonella infection (A02.25)
　　　pyelonephritis and tubulo-interstitial nephritis in sarcoidosis (D86.84)
　　　pyelonephritis and tubulo-interstitial nephritis in Sjögren syndrome (M35.04)
　　　pyelonephritis and tubulo-interstitial nephritis in systemic lupus erythematosus (M32.15)
　　　pyelonephritis and tubulo-interstitial nephritis in toxoplasmosis (B58.83)
　　　renal tubular degeneration in diabetes (E08-E13 with .29)
　　　syphilitic pyelonephritis and tubulo-interstitial nephritis (A52.75)

ACUTE KIDNEY FAILURE AND CHRONIC KIDNEY DISEASE (N17-N19)

Excludes2 congenital renal failure (P96.0)
　drug- and heavy-metal-induced tubulo-interstitial and tubular conditions (N14.-)
　extrarenal uremia (R39.2)
　hemolytic-uremic syndrome (D59.3-)
　hepatorenal syndrome (K76.7)
　postpartum hepatorenal syndrome (O90.41)
　posttraumatic renal failure (T79.5)
　prerenal uremia (R39.2)
　renal failure complicating abortion or ectopic or molar pregnancy (O00-O07, O08.4)
　renal failure following labor and delivery (O90.41)
　renal failure postprocedural (N99.0)

● **N17 Acute kidney failure**
Code also associated underlying condition
Excludes1 posttraumatic renal failure (T79.5)

N17.0 Acute kidney failure with tubular necrosis 🐾
　Acute tubular necrosis
　Renal tubular necrosis
　Tubular necrosis NOS
　Coding Clinic: 2022, Q4, P33 ; 2021, Q3, P10

N17.1 Acute kidney failure with acute cortical necrosis 🐾
　Acute cortical necrosis
　Cortical necrosis NOS
　Renal cortical necrosis

N17.2 Acute kidney failure with medullary necrosis 🐾
　Medullary [papillary] necrosis NOS
　Acute medullary [papillary] necrosis
　Renal medullary [papillary] necrosis

N17.8 Other acute kidney failure 🐾

N17.9 Acute kidney failure, unspecified 🐾
　Acute kidney injury (nontraumatic)
　Excludes2 traumatic kidney injury (S37.0-)
　Coding Clinic: 2023, Q3, P5; 2019, Q2, P7,25

● **N18 Chronic kidney disease (CKD)**
Code first any associated:
　diabetic chronic kidney disease (E08.22, E09.22, E10.22, E11.22, E13.22)
　hypertensive chronic kidney disease (I12.-, I13.-)
Use additional code to identify kidney transplant status, if applicable, (Z94.0)
Coding Clinic: 2018, Q4, P89; 2016, Q4, P123

N18.1 Chronic kidney disease, stage 1

N18.2 Chronic kidney disease, stage 2 (mild)

● **N18.3 Chronic kidney disease, stage 3 (moderate)**
Coding Clinic: 2022, Q4, P6

　N18.30 Chronic kidney disease, stage 3 unspecified
　N18.31 Chronic kidney disease, stage 3a
　N18.32 Chronic kidney disease, stage 3b

N18.4 Chronic kidney disease, stage 4 (severe) 🐾
Coding Clinic: 2023, Q1, P18; 2022, Q4, P14; 2013, Q1, P24

N18.5 Chronic kidney disease, stage 5 🐾
　Excludes1 chronic kidney disease, stage 5 requiring chronic dialysis (N18.6)

N18.6 End stage renal disease 🐾
　Chronic kidney disease requiring chronic dialysis
　Use additional code to identify dialysis status (Z99.2)
　Coding Clinic: 2022, Q3, P16; 2016, Q3, P23, Q1, P13

Item 14-6 Decreased blood flow is the usual cause of **acute renal failure** that offers a good prognosis for recovery.
Chronic renal failure is usually the result of long-standing kidney disease and is a very serious condition that generally results in death.

▷ New   ⇒ Revised   ~~deleted~~ Deleted   Excludes 1   Excludes 2   Includes   Use additional   Code first   Code also   Key words
OGCR Official Guidelines   X Assign placeholder X   ● Use Additional Character(s)   ▷ Manifestation Code   🐾 Hierarchical Condition Category   Coding Clinic

CHAPTER 14 (N00-N99)

Multiple calculi

Figure 14-5   Multiple urinary calculi.

N18.9   Chronic kidney disease, unspecified
    Chronic renal disease
    Chronic renal failure NOS
    Chronic renal insufficiency
    Chronic uremia NOS
    Diffuse sclerosing glomerulonephritis NOS
    Coding Clinic: 2018, Q4, P88

N19   Unspecified kidney failure
    Uremia NOS
    Excludes1   acute kidney failure (N17.-)
               chronic kidney disease (N18.-)
               chronic uremia (N18.9)
               extrarenal uremia (R39.2)
               prerenal uremia (R39.2)
               renal insufficiency (acute) (N28.9)
               uremia of newborn (P96.0)

UROLITHIASIS (N20-N23)

N20   Calculus of kidney and ureter
    Calculous pyelonephritis
    Excludes1   nephrocalcinosis (E83.59)
               that with hydronephrosis (N13.2)
    Coding Clinic: 2019, Q3, P14

   N20.0   Calculus of kidney
       Nephrolithiasis NOS   Staghorn calculus
       Renal calculus   Stone in kidney
       Renal stone
       Coding Clinic: 2019, Q3, P13; 2017, Q1, P5

   N20.1   Calculus of ureter
       Calculus of the ureteropelvic junction
       Ureteric stone
       Coding Clinic: 2016, Q3, P24

   N20.2   Calculus of kidney with calculus of ureter
   N20.9   Urinary calculus, unspecified

N21   Calculus of lower urinary tract
    Includes   calculus of lower urinary tract with cystitis and urethritis

   N21.0   Calculus in bladder
       Calculus in diverticulum of bladder
       Urinary bladder stone
       Excludes2   staghorn calculus (N20.0)
       Coding Clinic: 2015, Q2, P9

   N21.1   Calculus in urethra
       Excludes2   calculus of prostate (N42.0)

   N21.8   Other lower urinary tract calculus
   N21.9   Calculus of lower urinary tract, unspecified
       Excludes1   calculus of urinary tract NOS (N20.9)

N22   Calculus of urinary tract in diseases classified elsewhere
    Code first underlying disease, such as:
      gout (M1A.-, M10.-)
      schistosomiasis (B65.0-B65.9)

N23   Unspecified renal colic

OTHER DISORDERS OF KIDNEY AND URETER (N25-N29)
    Excludes2   disorders of kidney and ureter with urolithiasis (N20-N23)

N25   Disorders resulting from impaired renal tubular function
   N25.0   Renal osteodystrophy
       Azotemic osteodystrophy
       Phosphate-losing tubular disorders
       Renal rickets
       Renal short stature
       Excludes2   metabolic disorders classifiable to E70-E88

   N25.1   Nephrogenic diabetes insipidus
       Excludes1   diabetes insipidus NOS (E23.2)

   N25.8   Other disorders resulting from impaired renal tubular function
     N25.81   Secondary hyperparathyroidism of renal origin
         Excludes1   secondary hyperparathyroidism, non-renal (E21.1)
         Excludes2   metabolic disorders classifiable to E70-E88

     N25.89   Other disorders resulting from impaired renal tubular function
         Hypokalemic nephropathy
         Lightwood-Albright syndrome
         Renal tubular acidosis NOS

   N25.9   Disorder resulting from impaired renal tubular function, unspecified

N26   Unspecified contracted kidney
    Excludes1   contracted kidney due to hypertension (I12.-)
             diffuse sclerosing glomerulonephritis (N05.8.-)
             hypertensive nephrosclerosis (arteriolar) (arteriosclerotic) (I12.-)
             small kidney of unknown cause (N27.-)

   N26.1   Atrophy of kidney (terminal)
   N26.2   Page kidney
   N26.9   Renal sclerosis, unspecified

N27   Small kidney of unknown cause
    Includes   oligonephronia
   N27.0   Small kidney, unilateral
   N27.1   Small kidney, bilateral
   N27.9   Small kidney, unspecified

N28   Other disorders of kidney and ureter, not elsewhere classified
   N28.0   Ischemia and infarction of kidney
       Renal artery embolism
       Renal artery obstruction
       Renal artery occlusion
       Renal artery thrombosis
       Renal infarct
       Excludes1   atherosclerosis of renal artery (extrarenal part) (I70.1)
             congenital stenosis of renal artery (Q27.1)
             Goldblatt's kidney (I70.1)

   N28.1   Cyst of kidney, acquired
       Cyst (multiple) (solitary) of kidney, (acquired)
       Excludes1   cystic kidney disease (congenital) (Q61.-)

   N28.8   Other specified disorders of kidney and ureter
       Excludes1   hydroureter (N13.4)
             ureteric stricture with hydronephrosis (N13.1)
             ureteric stricture without hydronephrosis (N13.5)

     N28.81   Hypertrophy of kidney
     N28.82   Megaloureter
     N28.83   Nephroptosis
     N28.84   Pyelitis cystica

N28.85   **Pyeloureteritis cystica**

N28.86   **Ureteritis cystica**

N28.89   **Other specified disorders of kidney and ureter**
Coding Clinic: 2023, Q3, P5

N28.9   **Disorder of kidney and ureter, unspecified**
Nephropathy NOS
Renal disease (acute) NOS
Renal insufficiency (acute)

> **Excludes1**   chronic renal insufficiency (N18.9)
> unspecified nephritic syndrome (N05.-)

Coding Clinic: 2016, Q1, P13

▷ N29   *Other disorders of kidney and ureter in diseases classified elsewhere*

Code first underlying disease, such as:
amyloidosis (E85.-)
nephrocalcinosis (E83.59)
schistosomiasis (B65.0-B65.9)

> **Excludes1**   disorders of kidney and ureter in:
> cystinosis (E72.0)
> gonorrhea (A54.21)
> syphilis (A52.75)
> tuberculosis (A18.11)

OTHER DISEASES OF THE URINARY SYSTEM (N30-N39)

> **Excludes2**   urinary infection (complicating):
> abortion or ectopic or molar pregnancy
> (O00-O07, O08.8)
> pregnancy, childbirth and the puerperium
> (O23.-, O75.3, O86.2-)

● N30   **Cystitis**
Infection of bladder and irritation in lower urinary tract
Use additional code to identify infectious agent (B95-B97)

> **Excludes1**   prostatocystitis (N41.3)

● N30.0   **Acute cystitis**

> **Excludes1**   irradiation cystitis (N30.4-)
> trigonitis (N30.3-)

N30.00   **Acute cystitis without hematuria**

N30.01   **Acute cystitis with hematuria**

● N30.1   **Interstitial cystitis (chronic)**
Ongoing infection of kidney glomeruli and tubules

N30.10   **Interstitial cystitis (chronic) without hematuria**

N30.11   **Interstitial cystitis (chronic) with hematuria**

● N30.2   **Other chronic cystitis**

N30.20   **Other chronic cystitis without hematuria**

N30.21   **Other chronic cystitis with hematuria**

● N30.3   **Trigonitis**
Inflammation of triangular area of bladder (where the ureters and urethra come together)
Urethrotrigonitis

N30.30   **Trigonitis without hematuria**

N30.31   **Trigonitis with hematuria**

● N30.4   **Irradiation cystitis**

N30.40   **Irradiation cystitis without hematuria**

N30.41   **Irradiation cystitis with hematuria**

● N30.8   **Other cystitis**
Abscess of bladder

N30.80   **Other cystitis without hematuria**

N30.81   **Other cystitis with hematuria**

● N30.9   **Cystitis, unspecified**

N30.90   **Cystitis, unspecified without hematuria**

N30.91   **Cystitis, unspecified with hematuria**

● N31   **Neuromuscular dysfunction of bladder, not elsewhere classified**
Use additional code to identify any associated urinary incontinence (N39.3-N39.4-)

> **Excludes1**   cord bladder NOS (G95.89)
> neurogenic bladder due to cauda equina
> syndrome (G83.4)
> neuromuscular dysfunction due to spinal cord
> lesion (G95.89)

N31.0   **Uninhibited neuropathic bladder, not elsewhere classified**

N31.1   **Reflex neuropathic bladder, not elsewhere classified**

N31.2   **Flaccid neuropathic bladder, not elsewhere classified**
Atonic (motor) (sensory) neuropathic bladder
Diminished tone of bladder muscle
Autonomous neuropathic bladder
Nonreflex neuropathic bladder

N31.8   **Other neuromuscular dysfunction of bladder**

N31.9   **Neuromuscular dysfunction of bladder, unspecified**
Neurogenic bladder dysfunction NOS

● N32   **Other disorders of bladder**

> **Excludes2**   calculus of bladder (N21.0)
> cystocele (N81.1-)
> hernia or prolapse of bladder, female (N81.1-)

N32.0   **Bladder-neck obstruction**
Bladder-neck stenosis (acquired)

> **Excludes1**   congenital bladder-neck obstruction
> (Q64.3-)

N32.1   **Vesicointestinal fistula**
Vesicorectal fistula

N32.2   **Vesical fistula, not elsewhere classified**

> **Excludes1**   fistula between bladder and female
> genital tract (N82.0-N82.1)

N32.3   **Diverticulum of bladder**
Formation of sac from a herniation of wall of bladder

> **Excludes1**   congenital diverticulum of bladder (Q64.6)
> diverticulitis of bladder (N30.8-)

● N32.8   **Other specified disorders of bladder**

N32.81   **Overactive bladder**
Detrusor muscle hyperactivity

> **Excludes1**   frequent urination due to
> specified bladder condition-
> code to condition

N32.89   **Other specified disorders of bladder**
Bladder hemorrhage
Bladder hypertrophy
Calcified bladder
Contracted bladder

N32.9   **Bladder disorder, unspecified**

▷ N33   *Bladder disorders in diseases classified elsewhere*
Code first underlying disease, such as:
schistosomiasis (B65.0-B65.9)

> **Excludes1**   bladder disorder in syphilis (A52.76)
> bladder disorder in tuberculosis (A18.12)
> candidal cystitis (B37.41)
> chlamydial cystitis(A56.01)
> cystitis in gonorrhea (A54.01)
> cystitis in neurogenic bladder (N31.-)
> diphtheritic cystitis (A36.85)
> syphilitic cystitis (A52.76)
> trichomonal cystitis (A59.03)

● N34   **Urethritis and urethral syndrome**
Use additional code (B95-B97), to identify infectious agent

> **Excludes2**   Reiter's disease (M02.3-)
> urethritis in diseases with a predominantly sexual
> mode of transmission (A50-A64)
> urethrotrigonitis (N30.3-)

N34.0   **Urethral abscess**
Abscess (of) Cowper's gland
Abscess (of) Littré's gland
Abscess (of) urethral (gland)
Periurethral abscess

> **Excludes1**   urethral caruncle (N36.2)

N34.1   **Nonspecific urethritis**
Nongonococcal urethritis
Nonvenereal urethritis

N34.2   **Other urethritis**
Inflammation of urethra
Meatitis, urethral
Postmenopausal urethritis
Ulcer of urethra (meatus)
Urethritis NOS

N34.3   **Urethral syndrome, unspecified**

- ● N35   Urethral stricture
  Narrowing of lumen of urethra caused by scarring due to infection or injury
  Excludes1   congenital urethral stricture (Q64.3-)
  postprocedural urethral stricture (N99.1-)
  - ● N35.0   Post-traumatic urethral stricture
    Urethral stricture due to injury
    Excludes1   postprocedural urethral stricture (N99.1-)
    - ● N35.01   Post-traumatic urethral stricture, male
      - N35.010   Post-traumatic urethral stricture, male, meatal
      - N35.011   Post-traumatic bulbous urethral stricture
      - N35.012   Post-traumatic membranous urethral stricture
      - N35.013   Post-traumatic anterior urethral stricture
      - N35.014   Post-traumatic urethral stricture, male, unspecified
      - N35.016   Post-traumatic urethral stricture, male, overlapping sites
    - ● N35.02   Post-traumatic urethral stricture, female
      - N35.021   Urethral stricture due to childbirth
      - N35.028   Other post-traumatic urethral stricture, female
  - ● N35.1   Postinfective urethral stricture, not elsewhere classified
    Excludes1   urethral stricture associated with schistosomiasis (B65.-, N29)
    gonococcal urethral stricture (A54.01)
    syphilitic urethral stricture (A52.76)
    - ● N35.11   Postinfective urethral stricture, not elsewhere classified, male
      - N35.111   Postinfective urethral stricture, not elsewhere classified, male, meatal
      - N35.112   Postinfective bulbous urethral stricture, not elsewhere classified, male
      - N35.113   Postinfective membranous urethral stricture, not elsewhere classified, male
      - N35.114   Postinfective anterior urethral stricture, not elsewhere classified, male
      - N35.116   Postinfective urethral stricture, not elsewhere classified, male, overlapping sites
      - N35.119   Postinfective urethral stricture, not elsewhere classified, male, unspecified
    - N35.12   Postinfective urethral stricture, not elsewhere classified, female
  - ● N35.8   Other urethral stricture
    Excludes1   postprocedural urethral stricture (N99.1-)
    - ● N35.81   Other urethral stricture, male
      - N35.811   Other urethral stricture, male, meatal
      - N35.812   Other bulbous urethral stricture, male
      - N35.813   Other membranous urethral stricture, male
      - N35.814   Other anterior urethral stricture, male
      - N35.816   Other urethral stricture, male, overlapping sites
      - N35.819   Other urethral stricture, male, unspecified site
    - N35.82   Other urethral stricture, female
  - ● N35.9   Urethral stricture, unspecified
    - ● N35.91   Urethral stricture, unspecified, male
      - N35.911   Unspecified urethral stricture, male, meatal
      - N35.912   Unspecified bulbous urethral stricture, male
      - N35.913   Unspecified membranous urethral stricture, male

-      N35.914   Unspecified anterior urethral stricture, male
-      N35.916   Unspecified urethral stricture, male, overlapping sites
-      N35.919   Unspecified urethral stricture, male, unspecified site
  Pinhole meatus NOS
  Urethral stricture NOS
  - N35.92   Unspecified urethral stricture, female

- ● N36   Other disorders of urethra
  - N36.0   Urethral fistula
    Urethroperineal fistula
    Urethrorectal fistula
    Urinary fistula NOS
    Excludes1   urethroscrotal fistula (N50.89)
    urethrovaginal fistula (N82.1)
    urethrovesicovaginal fistula (N82.1)
  - N36.1   Urethral diverticulum
  - N36.2   Urethral caruncle
  - ● N36.4   Urethral functional and muscular disorders
    Use additional code to identify associated urinary stress incontinence (N39.3)
    - N36.41   Hypermobility of urethra
    - N36.42   Intrinsic sphincter deficiency (ISD)
    - N36.43   Combined hypermobility of urethra and intrinsic sphincter deficiency
    - N36.44   Muscular disorders of urethra
      Bladder sphincter dyssynergy
  - N36.5   Urethral false passage
  - N36.8   Other specified disorders of urethra
    Excludes1   congenital urethrocele (Q64.7)
    female urethrocele (N81.0)
    Coding Clinic: 2022, Q2, P7
  - N36.9   Urethral disorder, unspecified

- ▷ N37   *Urethral disorders in diseases classified elsewhere*
  Code first underlying disease
  Excludes1   urethritis (in):
  candidal infection (B37.41)
  chlamydial (A56.01)
  gonorrhea (A54.01)
  syphilis (A52.76)
  trichomonal infection (A59.03)
  tuberculosis (A18.13)

- ● N39   Other disorders of urinary system
  Excludes2   hematuria NOS (R31.-)
  recurrent or persistent hematuria (N02.-)
  recurrent or persistent hematuria with specified morphological lesion (N02.-)
  proteinuria NOS (R80.-)
  - N39.0   Urinary tract infection, site not specified
    Use additional code (B95-B97), to identify infectious agent
    Excludes1   candidiasis of urinary tract (B37.4-)
    neonatal urinary tract infection (P39.3)
    ▷ pyonephrosis (N13.6)
    pyuria (R82.81)
    urinary tract infection of specified site, such as:
    cystitis (N30.-)
    urethritis (N34.-)
    Coding Clinic: 2018, Q2, P22; Q1, P16; 2012, Q4, P94
  - N39.3   Stress incontinence (female) (male)
    Code also any associated overactive bladder (N32.81)
    Excludes1   mixed incontinence (N39.46)
    Coding Clinic: 2021, Q4, P18

CHAPTER 14 (N00-N99)

● **N39.4** **Other specified urinary incontinence**
Code also any associated overactive bladder (N32.81)
> **Excludes1** enuresis NOS (R32)
> functional urinary incontinence (R39.81)
> urinary incontinence associated with cognitive impairment (R39.81)
> urinary incontinence NOS (R32)
> urinary incontinence of nonorganic origin (F98.0)

     N39.41 **Urge incontinence**
> **Excludes1** mixed incontinence (N39.46)

     N39.42 **Incontinence without sensory awareness**
Insensible (urinary) incontinence

     N39.43 **Post-void dribbling**

     N39.44 **Nocturnal enuresis**
> **Excludes2** nocturnal polyuria (R35.81)

     N39.45 **Continuous leakage**

     N39.46 **Mixed incontinence**
Urge and stress incontinence

     ● **N39.49** **Other specified urinary incontinence**
        N39.490 **Overflow incontinence**
        N39.491 **Coital incontinence**
          Coding Clinic: 2016, Q4, P44

        N39.492 **Postural (urinary) incontinence**
          Coding Clinic: 2016, Q4, P44

        N39.498 **Other specified urinary incontinence**
Reflex incontinence
Total incontinence

N39.8 **Other specified disorders of urinary system**

N39.9 **Disorder of urinary system, unspecified**

DISEASES OF MALE GENITAL ORGANS (N40-N53)

★ **(See Plate 5 of the Anatomy Illustrations.)**

● **N40** **Benign prostatic hyperplasia**
> **Includes** adenofibromatous hypertrophy of prostate
> benign hypertrophy of the prostate
> *Enlargement of prostate gland usually occurring with age and causing obstructed urine flow*
> benign prostatic hypertrophy
> BPH
> enlarged prostate
> nodular prostate
> polyp of prostate

> **Excludes1** benign neoplasms of prostate (adenoma, benign) (fibroadenoma) (fibroma) (myoma) (D29.1)
> malignant neoplasm of prostate (C61)

     N40.0 **Benign prostatic hyperplasia without lower urinary tract symptoms** A
Enlarged prostate without LUTS
Enlarged prostate NOS

     N40.1 **Benign prostatic hyperplasia with lower urinary tract symptoms** A
Enlarged prostate with LUTS
Use additional code for associated symptoms, when specified:
incomplete bladder emptying (R39.14)
nocturia (R35.1)
straining on urination (R39.16)
urinary frequency (R35.0)
urinary hesitancy (R39.11)
urinary incontinence (N39.4-)
urinary obstruction (N13.8)
urinary retention (R33.8)
urinary urgency (R39.15)
weak urinary stream (R39.12)
Coding Clinic: 2018, Q4, P55

     N40.2 **Nodular prostate without lower urinary tract symptoms** A
Nodular prostate without LUTS

     N40.3 **Nodular prostate with lower urinary tract symptoms** A
Use additional code for associated symptoms, when specified:
incomplete bladder emptying (R39.14)
nocturia (R35.1)
straining on urination (R39.16)
urinary frequency (R35.0)
urinary hesitancy (R39.11)
urinary incontinence (N39.4-)
urinary obstruction (N13.8)
urinary retention (R33.8)
urinary urgency (R39.15)
weak urinary stream (R39.12)

● **N41** **Inflammatory diseases of prostate**
Use additional code (B95-B97), to identify infectious agent

     N41.0 **Acute prostatitis** A
        Coding Clinic: 2024, Q1, P16

     N41.1 **Chronic prostatitis** A

     N41.2 **Abscess of prostate** A

     N41.3 **Prostatocystitis** A
        Coding Clinic: 2024, Q1, P16

     N41.4 **Granulomatous prostatitis** A

     N41.8 **Other inflammatory diseases of prostate** A

     N41.9 **Inflammatory disease of prostate, unspecified** A
Prostatitis NOS

● **N42** **Other and unspecified disorders of prostate**
     N42.0 **Calculus of prostate** A
Prostatic stone

     N42.1 **Congestion and hemorrhage of prostate** A
> **Excludes1** enlarged prostate (N40.-)
> hematuria (R31.-)
> hyperplasia of prostate (N40.-)
> inflammatory diseases of prostate (N41.-)

     ● **N42.3** **Dysplasia of prostate**
        Coding Clinic: 2016, Q4, P44
        N42.30 **Unspecified dysplasia of prostate**
        N42.31 **Prostatic intraepithelial neoplasia**
PIN
Prostatic intraepithelial neoplasia I (PIN I)
Prostatic intraepithelial neoplasia II (PIN II)
> **Excludes1** prostatic intraepithelial neoplasia III (PIN III) (D07.5)

        N42.32 **Atypical small acinar proliferation of prostate**
        N42.39 **Other dysplasia of prostate**

     ● **N42.8** **Other specified disorders of prostate**
        N42.81 **Prostatodynia syndrome** A
Painful prostate syndrome
        N42.82 **Prostatosis syndrome** A
        N42.83 **Cyst of prostate** A
        N42.89 **Other specified disorders of prostate** A

     N42.9 **Disorder of prostate, unspecified** A

Figure 14-6 Benign prostatic hyperplasia. (From Shiland: Mastering Healthcare Terminology, ed 3, St. Louis, Mosby, 2010)

▶ New   ⇒ Revised   ~~deleted~~ Deleted   Excludes 1   Excludes 2   Includes   Use additional   Code first   Code also   Key words

OGCR Official Guidelines   X Assign placeholder X   ● Use Additional Character(s)   ▶ Manifestation Code   Ⓗ Hierarchical Condition Category   Coding Clinic

Item 14-7　Hydrocele is a sac of fluid accumulating in the testes membrane.

Blood
vessels
Vas
deferens
Epididymis
Testis
A
Hydrocele

Figure 14-7　A. Hydrocele. **B.** Newborn with large right hydrocele. (**B** from Nelson WE, Kliegman R: Nelson Textbook of Pediatrics, Philadelphia, Saunders Elsevier, 2011)

● N43　**Hydrocele and spermatocele**

　　Includes　　hydrocele of spermatic cord, testis or tunica vaginalis

　　Excludes1　congenital hydrocele (P83.5)

　　N43.0　**Encysted hydrocele**

　　N43.1　**Infected hydrocele**

　　　　　　Use additional code (B95-B97), to identify infectious agent

　　N43.2　**Other hydrocele**

　　N43.3　**Hydrocele, unspecified**

　● N43.4　**Spermatocele of epididymis**
　　　　　　Spermatic cyst

　　　　N43.40　**Spermatocele of epididymis, unspecified**

　　　　N43.41　**Spermatocele of epididymis, single**

　　　　N43.42　**Spermatocele of epididymis, multiple**

● N44　**Noninflammatory disorders of testis**

　● N44.0　**Torsion of testis**

　　　　N44.00　**Torsion of testis, unspecified**

　　　　N44.01　**Extravaginal torsion of spermatic cord**

　　　　N44.02　**Intravaginal torsion of spermatic cord**
　　　　　　　　Torsion of spermatic cord NOS

　　　　N44.03　**Torsion of appendix testis**

　　　　N44.04　**Torsion of appendix epididymis**

　　N44.1　**Cyst of tunica albuginea testis**

　　N44.2　**Benign cyst of testis**

　　N44.8　**Other noninflammatory disorders of the testis**

● N45　**Orchitis and epididymitis**
　　　Orchitis is inflammation of one or both of the testes as a result of mumps or other infection, trauma, or metastasis. Epididymitis is inflammation of the tubular structure that connects the testicle with the vas deferens.

　　　Use additional code (B95-B97), to identify infectious agent

　　N45.1　**Epididymitis**

　　N45.2　**Orchitis**

　　N45.3　**Epididymo-orchitis**

　　N45.4　**Abscess of epididymis or testis**

● N46　**Male infertility**

　　Excludes1　vasectomy status (Z98.52)

　● N46.0　**Azoospermia**
　　　　　　Absolute male infertility
　　　　　　Male infertility due to germinal (cell) aplasia
　　　　　　Male infertility due to spermatogenic arrest (complete)

　　　　N46.01　**Organic azoospermia**　　　　　　　　A
　　　　　　　　Azoospermia NOS

　　● N46.02　**Azoospermia due to extratesticular causes**
　　　　　　　　Code also associated cause

　　　　　N46.021　**Azoospermia due to drug therapy**　A

　　　　　N46.022　**Azoospermia due to infection**　　　A

　　　　　N46.023　**Azoospermia due to obstruction of efferent ducts**　　　　　　　　　　　　A

Item 14-8 Male infertility is the inability of the female sex partner to conceive after one year of unprotected intercourse.
　　Azoospermia is no sperm ejaculated and **oligospermia** is few sperm ejaculated—both resulting in infertility. Extratesticular causes such as injury, infections, radiation, and chemotherapy may also cause male infertility.

　　　　　N46.024　**Azoospermia due to radiation**　　A

　　　　　N46.025　**Azoospermia due to systemic disease**　　　　　　　　　　　　　　A

　　　　　N46.029　**Azoospermia due to other extratesticular causes**　　　　　　　A

　● N46.1　**Oligospermia**
　　　　　　Male infertility due to germinal cell desquamation
　　　　　　Male infertility due to hypospermatogenesis
　　　　　　Male infertility due to incomplete spermatogenic arrest

　　　　N46.11　**Organic oligospermia**　　　　　　　　A
　　　　　　　　Oligospermia NOS

　　● N46.12　**Oligospermia due to extratesticular causes**
　　　　　　　　Code also associated cause

　　　　　N46.121　**Oligospermia due to drug therapy**　A

　　　　　N46.122　**Oligospermia due to infection**　　A

　　　　　N46.123　**Oligospermia due to obstruction of efferent ducts**　　　　　　　　A

　　　　　N46.124　**Oligospermia due to radiation**　A

　　　　　N46.125　**Oligospermia due to systemic disease**　　　　　　　　　　　　　　A

　　　　　N46.129　**Oligospermia due to other extratesticular causes**　　　　　　　A

　　N46.8　**Other male infertility**　　　　　　　　　A

　　N46.9　**Male infertility, unspecified**　　　　　　A

● N47　**Disorders of prepuce**

　　N47.0　**Adherent prepuce, newborn**　　　　　　N

　　N47.1　**Phimosis**

　　N47.2　**Paraphimosis**

　　N47.3　**Deficient foreskin**

　　N47.4　**Benign cyst of prepuce**

　　N47.5　**Adhesions of prepuce and glans penis**

　　N47.6　**Balanoposthitis**
　　　　　　Use additional code (B95-B97), to identify infectious agent
　　　　　　Excludes1　balanitis (N48.1)

　　N47.7　**Other inflammatory diseases of prepuce**
　　　　　　Use additional code (B95-B97), to identify infectious agent

　　N47.8　**Other disorders of prepuce**

● N48　**Other disorders of penis**

　　N48.0　**Leukoplakia of penis**
　　　　　　Balanitis xerotica obliterans
　　　　　　Kraurosis of penis
　　　　　　Lichen sclerosus of external male genital organs
　　　　　　Excludes1　carcinoma in situ of penis (D07.4)

　　N48.1　**Balanitis**
　　　　　　Use additional code (B95-B97), to identify infectious agent
　　　　　　Excludes1　amebic balanitis (A06.8)
　　　　　　　　　　　　　balanitis xerotica obliterans (N48.0)
　　　　　　　　　　　　　candidal balanitis (B37.42)
　　　　　　　　　　　　　gonococcal balanitis (A54.23)
　　　　　　　　　　　　　herpesviral [herpes simplex] balanitis (A60.01)

CHAPTER 14 (N00-N99)

Item 14–9 Seminal vesiculitis is an inflammation of the seminal vesicle. **Spermatocele** is a benign cystic accumulation of sperm arising from the head of the epididymis. **Torsion of the testis** is a medical emergency occurring most commonly in boys 7 to 12 years of age and results from a congenital abnormality of the covering of the testis allowing the testis to twist within its sac and cutting off the blood supply to the testis.

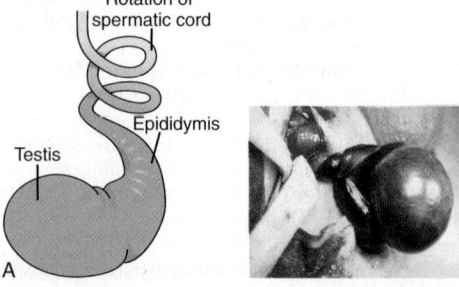

Figure 14-8 A. Torsion of testis. **B.** Torsion of the testis. (**B** from Kliegman R, Nelson WE: Nelson Textbook of Pediatrics, Philadelphia, Saunders, 2007)

● **N48.2 Other inflammatory disorders of penis**
Use additional code (B95-B97), to identify infectious agent
   Excludes1 balanitis (N48.1)
              balanitis xerotica obliterans (N48.0)
              balanoposthitis (N47.6)
   N48.21 **Abscess of corpus cavernosum and penis**
   N48.22 **Cellulitis of corpus cavernosum and penis**
   N48.29 **Other inflammatory disorders of penis**
● **N48.3 Priapism**
Painful erection
Code first underlying cause
   N48.30 **Priapism, unspecified**
   N48.31 **Priapism due to trauma**
  ▸N48.32 *Priapism due to disease classified elsewhere*
   N48.33 **Priapism, drug-induced**
   N48.39 **Other priapism**
  N48.5 **Ulcer of penis**
  N48.6 **Induration penis plastica**
Peyronie's disease
Plastic induration of penis
● **N48.8 Other specified disorders of penis**
   N48.81 **Thrombosis of superficial vein of penis**
   N48.82 **Acquired torsion of penis**
       Acquired torsion of penis NOS
       Excludes1 congenital torsion of penis (Q55.63)
   N48.83 **Acquired buried penis**
       Excludes1 congenital hidden penis (Q55.64)
   N48.89 **Other specified disorders of penis**
  N48.9 **Disorder of penis, unspecified**

● **N49 Inflammatory disorders of male genital organs, not elsewhere classified**
Use additional code (B95-B97), to identify infectious agent
   Excludes1 inflammation of penis (N48.1, N48.2-)
           orchitis and epididymitis (N45.-)
  N49.0 **Inflammatory disorders of seminal vesicle**
Vesiculitis NOS
  N49.1 **Inflammatory disorders of spermatic cord, tunica vaginalis and vas deferens**
Vasitis
  N49.2 **Inflammatory disorders of scrotum**
  N49.3 **Fournier gangrene**

N49.8 **Inflammatory disorders of other specified male genital organs**
Inflammation of multiple sites in male genital organs
N49.9 **Inflammatory disorder of unspecified male genital organ**
Abscess of unspecified male genital organ
Boil of unspecified male genital organ
Carbuncle of unspecified male genital organ
Cellulitis of unspecified male genital organ

● N50 **Other and unspecified disorders of male genital organs**
   Excludes2 torsion of testis (N44.0-)
N50.0 **Atrophy of testis**
N50.1 **Vascular disorders of male genital organs**
Hematocele, NOS, of male genital organs
Hemorrhage of male genital organs
Thrombosis of male genital organs
N50.3 **Cyst of epididymis**
● N50.8 **Other specified disorders of male genital organs**
Coding Clinic: 2016, Q4, P45
  ● N50.81 **Testicular pain**
     N50.811 **Right testicular pain**
     N50.812 **Left testicular pain**
     N50.819 **Testicular pain, unspecified**
  N50.82 **Scrotal pain**
  N50.89 **Other specified disorders of the male genital organs**
Atrophy of scrotum, seminal vesicle, spermatic cord, tunica vaginalis and vas deferens
Chylocele, tunica vaginalis (nonfilarial) NOS
Edema of scrotum, seminal vesicle, spermatic cord, tunica vaginalis and vas deferens
Hypertrophy of scrotum, seminal vesicle, spermatic cord, tunica vaginalis and vas deferens
Stricture of spermatic cord, tunica vaginalis, and vas deferens
Ulcer of scrotum, seminal vesicle, spermatic cord, testis, tunica vaginalis and vas deferens
Urethroscrotal fistula
N50.9 **Disorder of male genital organs, unspecified**

▸ N51 *Disorders of male genital organs in diseases classified elsewhere*
Code first underlying disease, such as:
filariasis (B74.0-B74.9)
   Excludes1 amebic balanitis (A06.8)
         candidal balanitis (B37.42)
         gonococcal balanitis (A54.23)
         gonococcal prostatitis (A54.22)
         herpesviral [herpes simplex] balanitis (A60.01)
         trichomonal prostatitis (A59.02)
         tuberculous prostatitis (A18.14)

● N52 **Male erectile dysfunction**
   Excludes1 psychogenic impotence (F52.21)
● N52.0 **Vasculogenic erectile dysfunction**
  N52.01 **Erectile dysfunction due to arterial insufficiency**   A
  N52.02 **Corporo-venous occlusive erectile dysfunction** A
  N52.03 **Combined arterial insufficiency and corporo-venous occlusive erectile dysfunction**   A
▸ N52.1 *Erectile dysfunction due to diseases classified elsewhere* A
Code first underlying disease
N52.2 **Drug-induced erectile dysfunction**   A
● N52.3 **Postprocedural erectile dysfunction**
  N52.31 **Erectile dysfunction following radical prostatectomy**   A
  N52.32 **Erectile dysfunction following radical cystectomy**   A
  N52.33 **Erectile dysfunction following urethral surgery**   A
  N52.34 **Erectile dysfunction following simple prostatectomy**   A

▸ New   ⇒ Revised   ~~deleted~~ Deleted   Excludes 1   Excludes 2   Includes   Use additional   Code first   Code also   Key words
OGCR Official Guidelines   X Assign placeholder X   ● Use Additional Character(s)   ▸ Manifestation Code   Hierarchical Condition Category   Coding Clinic

N52.35　Erectile dysfunction following radiation therapy　A
　　Coding Clinic: 2016, Q4, P45

N52.36　Erectile dysfunction following interstitial seed therapy　A
　　Coding Clinic: 2016, Q4, P45

N52.37　Erectile dysfunction following prostate ablative therapy　A
　　Erectile dysfunction following cryotherapy
　　Erectile dysfunction following other prostate ablative therapies
　　Erectile dysfunction following ultrasound ablative therapies
　　Coding Clinic: 2016, Q4, P45

N52.39　Other and unspecified postprocedural erectile dysfunction　A

N52.8　Other male erectile dysfunction　A

N52.9　Male erectile dysfunction, unspecified　A
　　Impotence NOS

● N53　Other male sexual dysfunction
　　Excludes1　psychogenic sexual dysfunction (F52.-)
● N53.1　Ejaculatory dysfunction
　　Excludes1　premature ejaculation (F52.4)
　　N53.11　Retarded ejaculation
　　N53.12　Painful ejaculation
　　N53.13　Anejaculatory orgasm
　　N53.14　Retrograde ejaculation
　　N53.19　Other ejaculatory dysfunction
　　　　Ejaculatory dysfunction NOS
　N53.8　Other male sexual dysfunction
　N53.9　Unspecified male sexual dysfunction

DISORDERS OF BREAST (N60-N65)
　Excludes1　disorders of breast associated with childbirth (O91-O92)

● N60　Benign mammary dysplasia
　Benign lumpiness of breast
　　Includes　fibrocystic mastopathy
● N60.0　Solitary cyst of breast
　　Cyst of breast
　　N60.01　Solitary cyst of right breast
　　N60.02　Solitary cyst of left breast
　　N60.09　Solitary cyst of unspecified breast
● N60.1　Diffuse cystic mastopathy
　　Cystic breast
　　Fibrocystic disease of breast
　　Excludes1　diffuse cystic mastopathy with epithelial proliferation (N60.3-)
　　N60.11　Diffuse cystic mastopathy of right breast　A
　　N60.12　Diffuse cystic mastopathy of left breast　A
　　N60.19　Diffuse cystic mastopathy of unspecified breast　A
● N60.2　Fibroadenosis of breast
　　Adenofibrosis of breast
　　Excludes2　fibroadenoma of breast (D24.-)
　　N60.21　Fibroadenosis of right breast
　　N60.22　Fibroadenosis of left breast
　　N60.29　Fibroadenosis of unspecified breast
● N60.3　Fibrosclerosis of breast
　　Cystic mastopathy with epithelial proliferation
　　N60.31　Fibrosclerosis of right breast
　　N60.32　Fibrosclerosis of left breast
　　N60.39　Fibrosclerosis of unspecified breast
● N60.4　Mammary duct ectasia
　　N60.41　Mammary duct ectasia of right breast
　　N60.42　Mammary duct ectasia of left breast
　　N60.49　Mammary duct ectasia of unspecified breast

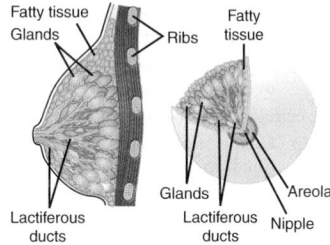

Figure 14-9　Breast.

● N60.8　Other benign mammary dysplasias
　　N60.81　Other benign mammary dysplasias of right breast
　　N60.82　Other benign mammary dysplasias of left breast
　　N60.89　Other benign mammary dysplasias of unspecified breast
● N60.9　Unspecified benign mammary dysplasia
　　N60.91　Unspecified benign mammary dysplasia of right breast
　　N60.92　Unspecified benign mammary dysplasia of left breast
　　N60.99　Unspecified benign mammary dysplasia of unspecified breast

● N61　Inflammatory disorders of breast
　　Excludes1　inflammatory carcinoma of breast (C50.9)
　　　inflammatory disorder of breast associated with childbirth (O91.-)
　　　neonatal infective mastitis (P39.0)
　　　thrombophlebitis of breast [Mondor's disease] (I80.8)
　N61.0　Mastitis without abscess
　　Infective mastitis (acute) (nonpuerperal) (subacute)
　　Mastitis (acute) (nonpuerperal) (subacute) NOS
　　Cellulitis (acute) (nonpuerperal) (subacute) of breast NOS
　　Cellulitis (acute) (nonpuerperal) (subacute) of nipple NOS
　N61.1　Abscess of the breast and nipple
　　Abscess (acute) (chronic) (nonpuerperal) of areola
　　Abscess (acute) (chronic) (nonpuerperal) of breast
　　Carbuncle of breast
　　Mastitis with abscess
● N61.2　Granulomatous mastitis
　　N61.20　Granulomatous mastitis, unspecified breast
　　N61.21　Granulomatous mastitis, right breast
　　N61.22　Granulomatous mastitis, left breast
　　N61.23　Granulomatous mastitis, bilateral breast

N62　Hypertrophy of breast
　　Gynecomastia
　　Hypertrophy of breast NOS
　　Massive pubertal hypertrophy of breast
　　Excludes1　breast engorgement of newborn (P83.4)
　　　disproportion of reconstructed breast (N65.1)

● N63　Unspecified lump in breast
　　Nodule(s) NOS in breast
　　N63.0　Unspecified lump in unspecified breast
● N63.1　Unspecified lump in the right breast
　　N63.10　Unspecified lump in the right breast, unspecified quadrant
　　　Coding Clinic: 2022, Q3, P8
　　N63.11　Unspecified lump in the right breast, upper outer quadrant
　　　Coding Clinic: 2017, Q4, P19
　　N63.12　Unspecified lump in the right breast, upper inner quadrant
　　N63.13　Unspecified lump in the right breast, lower outer quadrant

CHAPTER 14 (N00-N99)

N63.14 Unspecified lump in the right breast, lower inner quadrant

N63.15 Unspecified lump in the right breast, overlapping quadrants

● **N63.2** Unspecified lump in the left breast

N63.20 Unspecified lump in the left breast, unspecified quadrant

N63.21 Unspecified lump in the left breast, upper outer quadrant

N63.22 Unspecified lump in the left breast, upper inner quadrant

N63.23 Unspecified lump in the left breast, lower outer quadrant

N63.24 Unspecified lump in the left breast, lower inner quadrant

N63.25 Unspecified lump in the left breast, overlapping quadrants

● **N63.3** Unspecified lump in axillary tail

N63.31 Unspecified lump in axillary tail of the right breast

N63.32 Unspecified lump in axillary tail of the left breast

● **N63.4** Unspecified lump in breast, subareolar

N63.41 Unspecified lump in right breast, subareolar

N63.42 Unspecified lump in left breast, subareolar

● **N64** Other disorders of breast

> **Excludes2** mechanical complication of breast prosthesis and implant (T85.4-)

N64.0 Fissure and fistula of nipple

N64.1 Fat necrosis of breast
Fat necrosis (segmental) of breast
Code first breast necrosis due to breast graft (T85.898)

N64.2 Atrophy of breast

N64.3 Galactorrhea not associated with childbirth
Excessive or spontaneous flow of milk

N64.4 Mastodynia

● **N64.5** Other signs and symptoms in breast

> **Excludes2** abnormal findings on diagnostic imaging of breast (R92.-)

N64.51 Induration of breast

N64.52 Nipple discharge

> **Excludes1** abnormal findings in nipple discharge (R89.-)

N64.53 Retraction of nipple

N64.59 Other signs and symptoms in breast

● **N64.8** Other specified disorders of breast

N64.81 Ptosis of breast   A

> **Excludes1** ptosis of native breast in relation to reconstructed breast (N65.1)

N64.82 Hypoplasia of breast   A
Micromastia

> **Excludes1** congenital absence of breast (Q83.0)
>
> hypoplasia of native breast in relation to reconstructed breast (N65.1)

N64.89 Other specified disorders of breast
Galactocele
Subinvolution of breast (postlactational)
Coding Clinic: 2019, Q1, P32; 2018, Q1, P4

N64.9 Disorder of breast, unspecified
Coding Clinic: 2018, Q1, P4

● **N65** Deformity and disproportion of reconstructed breast

N65.0 Deformity of reconstructed breast   A
Contour irregularity in reconstructed breast
Excess tissue in reconstructed breast
Misshapen reconstructed breast

N65.1 Disproportion of reconstructed breast   A
Breast asymmetry between native breast and reconstructed breast
Disproportion between native breast and reconstructed breast

INFLAMMATORY DISEASES OF FEMALE PELVIC ORGANS (N70-N77)

> **Excludes1** inflammatory diseases of female pelvic organs complicating:
> abortion or ectopic or molar pregnancy (O00-O07, O08.0)
> pregnancy, childbirth and the puerperium (O23.-, O75.3, O85, O86.-)

★ **(See Plate 35 of the Anatomy Illustrations.)**

● **N70** Salpingitis and oophoritis
Oophoritis = inflammation of ovary
Salpingitis = inflammation of falloplan tube

> **Includes** abscess (of) fallopian tube
> abscess (of) ovary
> pyosalpinx
> salpingo-oophoritis
> tubo-ovarian abscess
> tubo-ovarian inflammatory disease

Use additional code (B95-B97), to identify infectious agent

> **Excludes1** gonococcal infection (A54.24)
> tuberculous infection (A18.17)

● **N70.0** Acute salpingitis and oophoritis

N70.01 Acute salpingitis

N70.02 Acute oophoritis

N70.03 Acute salpingitis and oophoritis

● **N70.1** Chronic salpingitis and oophoritis
Hydrosalpinx

N70.11 Chronic salpingitis

N70.12 Chronic oophoritis

N70.13 Chronic salpingitis and oophoritis

● **N70.9** Salpingitis and oophoritis, unspecified

N70.91 Salpingitis, unspecified

N70.92 Oophoritis, unspecified

N70.93 Salpingitis and oophoritis, unspecified

● **N71** Inflammatory disease of uterus, except cervix

> **Includes** endo (myo) metritis
> metritis
> myometritis
> pyometra
> uterine abscess

Use additional code (B95-B97), to identify infectious agent

> **Excludes1** hyperplastic endometritis (N85.0-)
> infection of uterus following delivery (O85, O86.-)

N71.0 Acute inflammatory disease of uterus

N71.1 Chronic inflammatory disease of uterus

N71.9 Inflammatory disease of uterus, unspecified

N72 Inflammatory disease of cervix uteri

> **Includes** cervicitis (with or without erosion or ectropion)
> endocervicitis (with or without erosion or ectropion)
> exocervicitis (with or without erosion or ectropion)

Use additional code (B95-B97), to identify infectious agent

> **Excludes1** erosion and ectropion of cervix without cervicitis (N86)

● **N73** Other female pelvic inflammatory diseases

Use additional code (B95-B97), to identify infectious agent

N73.0 Acute parametritis and pelvic cellulitis
Abscess of broad ligament
Abscess of parametrium
Pelvic cellulitis, female

▶ New ⇒ Revised ~~deleted~~ Deleted Excludes 1 Excludes 2 Includes Use additional Code first Code also Key words

OGCR Official Guidelines X Assign placeholder X ● Use Additional Character(s) ▶ Manifestation Code 🐱 Hierarchical Condition Category Coding Clinic

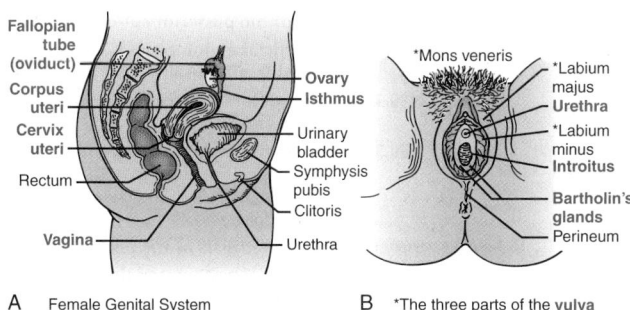

A   Female Genital System   B   *The three parts of the **vulva***

Figure 14-10   A. Female genital system. **B.** External female genital system. (From Buck CJ: Step-by-Step Medical Coding, ed 2016, St. Louis, Elsevier, 2016)

Item 14–10 Salpingitis is an infection of one or both fallopian tubes. **Oophoritis** is an infection of one or both ovaries.

N73.1   **Chronic parametritis and pelvic cellulitis**
Any condition in N73.0 specified as chronic
> **Excludes1**   tuberculous parametritis and pelvic cellultis (A18.17)

N73.2   **Unspecified parametritis and pelvic cellulitis**
Any condition in N73.0 unspecified whether acute or chronic

N73.3   **Female acute pelvic peritonitis**

N73.4   **Female chronic pelvic peritonitis**
> **Excludes1**   tuberculous pelvic (female) peritonitis (A18.17)

N73.5   **Female pelvic peritonitis, unspecified**

N73.6   **Female pelvic peritoneal adhesions (postinfective)**
> **Excludes2**   postprocedural pelvic peritoneal adhesions (N99.4)

N73.8   **Other specified female pelvic inflammatory diseases**

N73.9   **Female pelvic inflammatory disease, unspecified**
Female pelvic infection or inflammation NOS

⟩ **N74**   *Female pelvic inflammatory disorders in diseases classified elsewhere*
> *Code first underlying disease*
> **Excludes1**   chlamydial cervicitis (A56.02)
> chlamydial pelvic inflammatory disease (A56.11)
> gonococcal cervicitis (A54.03)
> gonococcal pelvic inflammatory disease (A54.24)
> herpesviral [herpes simplex] cervicitis (A60.03)
> herpesviral [herpes simplex] pelvic inflammatory disease (A60.09)
> syphilitic cervicitis (A52.76)
> syphilitic pelvic inflammatory disease (A52.76)
> trichomonal cervicitis (A59.09)
> tuberculous cervicitis (A18.16)
> tuberculous pelvic inflammatory disease (A18.17)

● **N75**   **Diseases of Bartholin's gland**

N75.0   **Cyst of Bartholin's gland**
> *Cysts filled with liquid or semisolid material*

N75.1   **Abscess of Bartholin's gland**
> *Localized collection of pus*

N75.8   **Other diseases of Bartholin's gland**
Bartholinitis

N75.9   **Disease of Bartholin's gland, unspecified**

● **N76**   **Other inflammation of vagina and vulva**
Use additional code (B95-B97), to identify infectious agent
> **Excludes2**   senile (atrophic) vaginitis (N95.2)
> vulvar vestibulitis (N94.810)

N76.0   **Acute vaginitis**
Acute vulvovaginitis
Vaginitis NOS
Vulvovaginitis NOS

N76.1   **Subacute and chronic vaginitis**
Chronic vulvovaginitis
Subacute vulvovaginitis

N76.2   **Acute vulvitis**
Vulvitis NOS

N76.3   **Subacute and chronic vulvitis**

N76.4   **Abscess of vulva**
Furuncle of vulva

N76.5   **Ulceration of vagina**

N76.6   **Ulceration of vulva**

● N76.8   **Other specified inflammation of vagina and vulva**

N76.81   **Mucositis (ulcerative) of vagina and vulva**
> Code also type of associated therapy, such as:
> antineoplastic and immunosuppressive drugs (T45.1X-)
> radiological procedure and radiotherapy (Y84.2)
> **Excludes2**   gastrointestinal mucositis (ulcerative) (K92.81)
> nasal mucositis (ulcerative) (J34.81)
> oral mucositis (ulcerative) (K12.3-)

N76.82   **Fournier disease of vagina and vulva**
Fournier gangrene of vagina and vulva
> Code also, if applicable, diabetes mellitus (E08-E13 with .9)
> **Excludes1**   gangrene in diabetes mellitus (E08-E13 with .52)

N76.89   **Other specified inflammation of vagina and vulva**

● **N77**   **Vulvovaginal ulceration and inflammation in diseases classified elsewhere**

⟩ **N77.0**   *Ulceration of vulva in diseases classified elsewhere*
> *Code first underlying disease, such as:*
> Behçet's disease (M35.2)
> **Excludes1**   ulceration of vulva in gonococcal infection (A54.02)
> ulceration of vulva in herpesviral [herpes simplex] infection (A60.04)
> ulceration of vulva in syphilis (A51.0)
> ulceration of vulva in tuberculosis (A18.18)

⟩ **N77.1**   *Vaginitis, vulvitis and vulvovaginitis in diseases classified elsewhere*
> *Code first underlying disease, such as:*
> pinworm (B80)
> **Excludes1**   candidial vulvovaginitis (B37.3-)
> chlamydial vulvovaginitis (A56.02)
> gonococcal vulvovaginitis (A54.02)
> herpesviral [herpes simplex] vulvovaginitis (A60.04)
> trichomonal vulvovaginitis (A59.01)
> tuberculous vulvovaginitis (A18.18)
> vulvovaginitis in early syphilis (A51.0)
> vulvovaginitis in late syphilis (A52.76)

NONINFLAMMATORY DISORDERS OF FEMALE GENITAL TRACT (N80-N98)

● **N80**   **Endometriosis**

● **N80.0**   **Endometriosis of uterus**
Endometriosis of the cervix
> **Excludes1**   stromal endometriosis (D39.0)

N80.00   **Endometriosis of the uterus, unspecified**

N80.01   **Superficial endometriosis of the uterus**

N80.02   **Deep endometriosis of the uterus**
Deep retrocervical endometriosis

N80.03   **Adenomyosis of the uterus**
Adenomyosis NOS

● **N80.1**   **Endometriosis of ovary**

● N80.10   **Endometriosis of ovary, unspecified depth**

N80.101   **Endometriosis of right ovary, unspecified depth**

N80.102   **Endometriosis of left ovary, unspecified depth**

N80.103 Endometriosis of bilateral ovaries, unspecified depth

N80.109 Endometriosis of ovary, unspecified side, unspecified depth
Endometriosis of ovary NOS

● N80.11 Superficial endometriosis of the ovary

N80.111 Superficial endometriosis of right ovary
Coding Clinic: 2022, Q4, P36

N80.112 Superficial endometriosis of left ovary

N80.113 Superficial endometriosis of bilateral ovaries

N80.119 Superficial endometriosis of ovary, unspecified ovary

● N80.12 Deep endometriosis of ovary
Deep ovarian endometriosis
Endometrioma

N80.121 Deep endometriosis of right ovary

N80.122 Deep endometriosis of left ovary

N80.123 Deep endometriosis of bilateral ovaries

N80.129 Deep endometriosis of ovary, unspecified ovary

● N80.2 Endometriosis of fallopian tube

● N80.20 Endometriosis of fallopian tube, unspecified depth

N80.201 Endometriosis of right fallopian tube, unspecified depth

N80.202 Endometriosis of left fallopian tube, unspecified depth

N80.203 Endometriosis of bilateral fallopian tubes, unspecified depth

N80.209 Endometriosis of unspecified fallopian tube, unspecified depth
Endometriosis fallopian tube NOS

● N80.21 Superficial endometriosis of fallopian tube

N80.211 Superficial endometriosis of right fallopian tube

N80.212 Superficial endometriosis of left fallopian tube

N80.213 Superficial endometriosis of bilateral fallopian tubes

N80.219 Superficial endometriosis of unspecified fallopian tube

● N80.22 Deep endometriosis of the fallopian tube
Deep endometriosis involving muscular wall of fallopian tube

N80.221 Deep endometriosis of right fallopian tube

N80.222 Deep endometriosis of left fallopian tube

N80.223 Deep endometriosis of bilateral fallopian tubes

N80.229 Deep endometriosis of unspecified fallopian tube

● N80.3 Endometriosis of pelvic peritoneum

N80.30 Endometriosis of pelvic peritoneum, unspecified
Endometriosis of the retroperitoneum NOS

● N80.31 Endometriosis of the anterior cul-de-sac

N80.311 Superficial endometriosis of the anterior cul-de-sac

N80.312 Deep endometriosis of the anterior cul-de-sac

N80.319 Endometriosis of the anterior cul-de-sac, unspecified depth
Endometriosis of the anterior cul-de-sac NOS

● N80.32 Endometriosis of the posterior cul-de-sac

N80.321 Superficial endometriosis of the posterior cul-de-sac

N80.322 Deep endometriosis of the posterior cul-de-sac

N80.329 Endometriosis of the posterior cul-de-sac, unspecified depth
Endometriosis of the posterior cul-de-sac NOS

● N80.33 Superficial endometriosis of the pelvic sidewall

N80.331 Superficial endometriosis of the right pelvic sidewall

N80.332 Superficial endometriosis of the left pelvic sidewall

N80.333 Superficial endometriosis of bilateral pelvic sidewall

N80.339 Superficial endometriosis of pelvic sidewall, unspecified side

● N80.34 Deep endometriosis of the pelvic sidewall

N80.341 Deep endometriosis of the right pelvic sidewall

N80.342 Deep endometriosis of the left pelvic sidewall

N80.343 Deep endometriosis of the bilateral pelvic sidewall

N80.349 Deep endometriosis of the pelvic sidewall, unspecified side
Coding Clinic: 2022, Q4, P36

● N80.35 Endometriosis of the pelvic sidewall, unspecified depth

N80.351 Endometriosis of the right pelvic sidewall, unspecified depth

N80.352 Endometriosis of the left pelvic sidewall, unspecified depth

N80.353 Endometriosis of bilateral pelvic sidewall, unspecified depth

N80.359 Endometriosis of pelvic sidewall, unspecified side, unspecified depth
Endometriosis of the pelvic sidewall NOS

● N80.36 Superficial endometriosis of the pelvic brim

N80.361 Superficial endometriosis of the right pelvic brim

N80.362 Superficial endometriosis of the left pelvic brim

N80.363 Superficial endometriosis of bilateral pelvic brim

N80.369 Superficial endometriosis of the pelvic brim, unspecified side

● N80.37 Deep endometriosis of the pelvic brim

N80.371 Deep endometriosis of the right pelvic brim

N80.372 Deep endometriosis of the left pelvic brim

N80.373 Deep endometriosis of bilateral pelvic brim

N80.379 Deep endometriosis of the pelvic brim, unspecified side

● N80.38 Endometriosis of the pelvic brim, unspecified depth

N80.381 Endometriosis of the right pelvic brim, unspecified depth

N80.382 Endometriosis of the left pelvic brim, unspecified depth

N80.383 Endometriosis of bilateral pelvic brim, unspecified depth

N80.389 Endometriosis of the pelvic brim, unspecified side, unspecified depth
Endometriosis of the pelvic brim NOS

▶ New   ⇒ Revised   ~~deleted~~ Deleted   Excludes 1   Excludes 2   Includes   Use additional   Code first   Code also   Key words
OGCR Official Guidelines   X Assign placeholder X   ● Use Additional Character(s)   ▶ Manifestation Code   🝑 Hierarchical Condition Category   Coding Clinic

● N80.39 Endometriosis of other pelvic peritoneum

    N80.391 Superficial endometriosis of the pelvic peritoneum, other specified sites

    N80.392 Deep endometriosis of the pelvic peritoneum, other specified sites

    N80.399 Endometriosis of the pelvic peritoneum, other specified sites, unspecified depth

● N80.3A Superficial endometriosis of the uterosacral ligament(s)

    N80.3A1 Superficial endometriosis of the right uterosacral ligament

    N80.3A2 Superficial endometriosis of the left uterosacral ligament

    N80.3A3 Superficial endometriosis of the bilateral uterosacral ligament(s)

    N80.3A9 Superficial endometriosis of the uterosacral ligament(s), unspecified side

● N80.3B Deep endometriosis of the uterosacral ligament(s)

    N80.3B1 Deep endometriosis of the right uterosacral ligament

    N80.3B2 Deep endometriosis of the left uterosacral ligament

    N80.3B3 Deep endometriosis of bilateral uterosacral ligament(s)

    N80.3B9 Deep endometriosis of the uterosacral ligament(s), unspecified side

● N80.3C Endometriosis of the uterosacral ligament(s), unspecified depth

    N80.3C1 Endometriosis of the right uterosacral ligament, unspecified depth

    N80.3C2 Endometriosis of the left uterosacral ligament, unspecified depth

    N80.3C3 Endometriosis of bilateral uterosacral ligament(s), unspecified depth

    N80.3C9 Endometriosis of the uterosacral ligament(s), unspecified side, unspecified depth
        Endometriosis of the uterosacral ligament(s) NOS

● N80.4 Endometriosis of rectovaginal septum and vagina

    N80.40 Endometriosis of rectovaginal septum, unspecified involvement of vagina
        Endometriosis of the rectovaginal septum, NOS

    N80.41 Endometriosis of rectovaginal septum without involvement of vagina

    N80.42 Endometriosis of rectovaginal septum with involvement of vagina

● N80.5 Endometriosis of intestine

    N80.50 Endometriosis of intestine, unspecified

  ● N80.51 Endometriosis of the rectum

    N80.511 Superficial endometriosis of the rectum

    N80.512 Deep endometriosis of the rectum
        Deep endometriosis of the rectum, multifocal

    N80.519 Endometriosis of the rectum, unspecified depth
        Endometriosis of the rectum NOS

  ● N80.52 Endometriosis of the sigmoid colon

    N80.521 Superficial endometriosis of the sigmoid colon

    N80.522 Deep endometriosis of the sigmoid colon

    N80.529 Endometriosis of the sigmoid colon, unspecified depth
        Endometriosis of the sigmoid colon NOS

● N80.53 Endometriosis of the cecum

    N80.531 Superficial endometriosis of the cecum

    N80.532 Deep endometriosis of the cecum

    N80.539 Endometriosis of the cecum, unspecified depth
        Endometriosis of the cecum NOS

● N80.54 Endometriosis of the appendix

    N80.541 Superficial endometriosis of the appendix

    N80.542 Deep endometriosis of the appendix

    N80.549 Endometriosis of the appendix, unspecified depth
        Endometriosis of the appendix NOS

● N80.55 Endometriosis of other parts of the colon
    Endometriosis of descending colon
    Endometriosis of transverse colon

    N80.551 Superficial endometriosis of other parts of the colon

    N80.552 Deep endometriosis of other parts of the colon

    N80.559 Endometriosis of other parts of the colon, unspecified depth
        Endometriosis of colon NOS

N80.6 Endometriosis in cutaneous scar

N80.8 Other endometriosis
    Endometriosis of other sites

N80.9 Endometriosis, unspecified

● N80.A Endometriosis of bladder and ureters

    N80.A0 Endometriosis of bladder, unspecified depth
        Endometriosis of bladder NOS

    N80.A1 Superficial endometriosis of bladder

    N80.A2 Deep endometriosis of bladder

  ● N80.A4 Superficial endometriosis of ureter
    Extrinsic endometriosis of ureter

    Code also, if applicable, obstructive and reflux uropathy (N13.-)

    N80.A41 Superficial endometriosis of right ureter

    N80.A42 Superficial endometriosis of left ureter

    N80.A43 Superficial endometriosis of bilateral ureters

    N80.A49 Superficial endometriosis of unspecified ureter

  ● N80.A5 Deep endometriosis of ureter
    Intrinsic endometriosis of ureter

    Code also, if applicable, obstructive and reflux uropathy (N13.-)

    N80.A51 Deep endometriosis of right ureter

    N80.A52 Deep endometriosis of left ureter

    N80.A53 Deep endometriosis of bilateral ureters

    N80.A59 Deep endometriosis of unspecified ureter

  ● N80.A6 Endometriosis of ureter, unspecified depth

    Code also, if applicable, obstructive and reflux uropathy (N13.-)

    N80.A61 Endometriosis of right ureter, unspecified depth

    N80.A62 Endometriosis of left ureter, unspecified depth

    N80.A63 Endometriosis of bilateral ureters, unspecified depth

    N80.A69 Endometriosis of unspecified ureter, unspecified depth

Item 14–11 **Endometriosis** is a condition for which no clear cause has been identified. Endometrial tissue is expelled from the uterus into the abdominal cavity and can implant onto a variety of organs. Classification is based on the site of implant of the endometrial tissue.

- ● **N80.B** **Endometriosis of cardiothoracic space**
      Endometriosis of thorax
      Code also, if applicable:
         catamenial hemothorax (J94.2)
         catamenial pneumothorax (J93.12)
   - **N80.B1** **Endometriosis of pleura**
   - **N80.B2** **Endometriosis of lung**
   - ● **N80.B3** **Endometriosis of diaphragm**
      - **N80.B31** **Superficial endometriosis of diaphragm**
      - **N80.B32** **Deep endometriosis of diaphragm**
      - **N80.B39** **Endometriosis of diaphragm, unspecified depth**
            Endometriosis of the diaphragm NOS
   - **N80.B4** **Endometriosis of the pericardial space**
   - **N80.B5** **Endometriosis of the mediastinal space**
   - **N80.B6** **Endometriosis of cardiothoracic space**
- **N80.C** **Endometriosis of the abdomen**
   - **N80.C0** **Endometriosis of the abdomen, unspecified**
         Endometriosis of the abdomen NOS
   - ● **N80.C1** **Endometriosis of the anterior abdominal wall**
      - **N80.C10** **Endometriosis of the anterior abdominal wall, subcutaneous tissue**
      - **N80.C11** **Endometriosis of the anterior abdominal wall, fascia and muscular layers**
      - **N80.C19** **Endometriosis of the anterior abdominal wall, unspecified depth**
            Endometriosis of the anterior abdominal wall NOS
   - **N80.C2** **Endometriosis of the umbilicus**
   - **N80.C3** **Endometriosis of the inguinal canal**
   - **N80.C4** **Endometriosis of extra-pelvic abdominal peritoneum**
   - **N80.C9** **Endometriosis of other site of abdomen**
- ● **N80.D** **Endometriosis of the pelvic nerves**
      Endometriosis of the nerves of the retroperitoneum
   - **N80.D0** **Endometriosis of the pelvic nerves, unspecified**
         Endometriosis of nerve of the retroperitoneum, NOS
   - **N80.D1** **Endometriosis of the sacral splanchnic nerves**
         Endometriosis of the pelvic splanchnic nerves
   - **N80.D2** **Endometriosis of the sacral nerve roots**
   - **N80.D3** **Endometriosis of the obturator nerve**
   - **N80.D4** **Endometriosis of the sciatic nerve**
   - **N80.D5** **Endometriosis of the pudendal nerve**
   - **N80.D6** **Endometriosis of the femoral nerve**
   - **N80.D9** **Endometriosis of other pelvic nerve**
         Endometriosis of the other nerves of the retroperitoneum

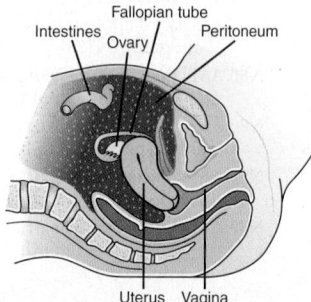

Figure 14-11 Sites of potential endometrial implants.

Figure 14-12 Three stages of uterine prolapse. **A.** Uterus is prolapsed. **B.** Vagina and uterus are prolapsed (incomplete uterovaginal prolapse). **C.** Vagina and uterus are completely prolapsed and are exposed through the external genitalia (complete uterovaginal prolapse).

- ● **N81** **Female genital prolapse**
      Excludes1 genital prolapse complicating pregnancy, labor or delivery (O34.5-)
            prolapse and hernia of ovary and fallopian tube (N83.4-)
            prolapse of vaginal vault after hysterectomy (N99.3)
   - **N81.0** **Urethrocele**
         Excludes1 urethrocele with cystocele (N81.1-)
               urethrocele with prolapse of uterus (N81.2-N81.4)
   - ● **N81.1** **Cystocele**
         Cystocele with urethrocele
         Cystourethrocele
         Excludes1 cystocele with prolapse of uterus (N81.2-N81.4)
      - **N81.10** **Cystocele, unspecified**
            Prolapse of (anterior) vaginal wall NOS
      - **N81.11** **Cystocele, midline**
      - **N81.12** **Cystocele, lateral**
            Paravaginal cystocele
   - **N81.2** **Incomplete uterovaginal prolapse**
         First degree uterine prolapse
         Prolapse of cervix NOS
         Second degree uterine prolapse
         Excludes1 cervical stump prolapse (N81.85)
   - **N81.3** **Complete uterovaginal prolapse**
         Procidentia (uteri) NOS
         Third degree uterine prolapse
   - **N81.4** **Uterovaginal prolapse, unspecified**
         Prolapse of uterus NOS
   - **N81.5** **Vaginal enterocele**
         Excludes1 enterocele with prolapse of uterus (N81.2-N81.4)
   - **N81.6** **Rectocele**
         Prolapse of posterior vaginal wall
         Use additional code for any associated fecal incontinence, if applicable (R15.-)
         Excludes1 rectocele with prolapse of uterus (N81.2-N81.4)
         Excludes2 perineocele (N81.81)
               rectal prolapse (K62.3)
   - ● **N81.8** **Other female genital prolapse**
      - **N81.81** **Perineocele**
      - **N81.82** **Incompetence or weakening of pubocervical tissue**
      - **N81.83** **Incompetence or weakening of rectovaginal tissue**
      - **N81.84** **Pelvic muscle wasting**
            Disuse atrophy of pelvic muscles and anal sphincter
      - **N81.85** **Cervical stump prolapse**
      - **N81.89** **Other female genital prolapse**
            Deficient perineum
            Old laceration of muscles of pelvic floor
   - **N81.9** **Female genital prolapse, unspecified**

▶ New   ⇒ Revised   ~~deleted~~ Deleted   Excludes 1   Excludes 2   Includes   Use additional   Code first   Code also   Key words

OGCR Official Guidelines   X Assign placeholder X   ● Use Additional Character(s)   ▶ Manifestation Code   🔖 Hierarchical Condition Category   Coding Clinic

● N82 Fistulae involving female genital tract
   Excludes1 vesicointestinal fistulae (N32.1)

   N82.0 **Vesicovaginal fistula**

   N82.1 Other female urinary-genital tract fistulae
      Cervicovesical fistula
      Ureterovaginal fistula
      Urethrovaginal fistula
      Uteroureteric fistula
      Uterovesical fistula
      Coding Clinic: 2017, Q3, P4

   N82.2 Fistula of vagina to small intestine

   N82.3 Fistula of vagina to large intestine
      Rectovaginal fistula

   N82.4 Other female intestinal-genital tract fistulae
      Intestinouterine fistula

   N82.5 Female genital tract-skin fistulae
      Uterus to abdominal wall fistula
      Vaginoperineal fistula

   N82.8 Other female genital tract fistulae

   N82.9 Female genital tract fistula, unspecified

● N83 Noninflammatory disorders of ovary, fallopian tube and broad ligament
   Excludes2 hydrosalpinx (N70.1-)

● N83.0 Follicular cyst of ovary
      Cyst of graafian follicle
      Hemorrhagic follicular cyst (of ovary)
      Coding Clinic: 2016, Q4, P46

      N83.00 Follicular cyst of ovary, unspecified side

      N83.01 Follicular cyst of right ovary

      N83.02 Follicular cyst of left ovary

● N83.1 Corpus luteum cyst
      Hemorrhagic corpus luteum cyst
      Coding Clinic: 2016, Q4, P46

      N83.10 Corpus luteum cyst of ovary, unspecified side

      N83.11 Corpus luteum cyst of right ovary

      N83.12 Corpus luteum cyst of left ovary
         Coding Clinic: 2022, Q1, P23

● N83.2 Other and unspecified ovarian cysts
      Excludes1 developmental ovarian cyst (Q50.1)
         neoplastic ovarian cyst (D27.-)
         polycystic ovarian syndrome (E28.2)
         Stein-Leventhal syndrome (E28.2)
      Coding Clinic: 2016, Q4, P46

   ● N83.20 Unspecified ovarian cysts
         Coding Clinic: 2022, Q1, P23

         N83.201 Unspecified ovarian cyst, right side

         N83.202 Unspecified ovarian cyst, left side
            Coding Clinic: 2022, Q1, P23

         N83.209 Unspecified ovarian cyst, unspecified side
            Ovarian cyst, NOS

   ● N83.29 Other ovarian cysts
         Retention cyst of ovary
         Simple cyst of ovary

         N83.291 Other ovarian cyst, right side

         N83.292 Other ovarian cyst, left side

         N83.299 Other ovarian cyst, unspecified side

● N83.3 Acquired atrophy of ovary and fallopian tube
      Coding Clinic: 2016, Q4, P46

   ● N83.31 Acquired atrophy of ovary

         N83.311 Acquired atrophy of right ovary

         N83.312 Acquired atrophy of left ovary

         N83.319 Acquired atrophy of ovary, unspecified side
            Acquired atrophy of ovary, NOS

   ● N83.32 Acquired atrophy of fallopian tube

         N83.321 Acquired atrophy of right fallopian tube

         N83.322 Acquired atrophy of left fallopian tube

         N83.329 Acquired atrophy of fallopian tube, unspecified side
            Acquired atrophy of fallopian tube, NOS

   ● N83.33 Acquired atrophy of ovary and fallopian tube

         N83.331 Acquired atrophy of right ovary and fallopian tube

         N83.332 Acquired atrophy of left ovary and fallopian tube

         N83.339 Acquired atrophy of ovary and fallopian tube, unspecified side
            Acquired atrophy of ovary and fallopian tube, NOS

● N83.4 Prolapse and hernia of ovary and fallopian tube
      Coding Clinic: 2016, Q4, P46

      N83.40 Prolapse and hernia of ovary and fallopian tube, unspecified side
         Prolapse and hernia of ovary and fallopian tube, NOS

      N83.41 Prolapse and hernia of right ovary and fallopian tube

      N83.42 Prolapse and hernia of left ovary and fallopian tube

● N83.5 Torsion of ovary, ovarian pedicle and fallopian tube
      Torsion of accessory tube
      Coding Clinic: 2016, Q4, P46

   ● N83.51 Torsion of ovary and ovarian pedicle

         N83.511 Torsion of right ovary and ovarian pedicle

         N83.512 Torsion of left ovary and ovarian pedicle

         N83.519 Torsion of ovary and ovarian pedicle, unspecified side
            Torsion of ovary and ovarian pedicle, NOS

   ● N83.52 Torsion of fallopian tube
         Torsion of hydatid of Morgagni

         N83.521 Torsion of right fallopian tube

         N83.522 Torsion of left fallopian tube

         N83.529 Torsion of fallopian tube, unspecified side
            Torsion of fallopian tube, NOS

      N83.53 Torsion of ovary, ovarian pedicle and fallopian tube

   N83.6 Hematosalpinx
      Excludes1 hematosalpinx (with) (in):
         hematocolpos (N89.7)
         hematometra (N85.7)
         tubal pregnancy (O00.1-)

   N83.7 Hematoma of broad ligament

   N83.8 Other noninflammatory disorders of ovary, fallopian tube and broad ligament
      Broad ligament laceration syndrome [Allen-Masters]

   N83.9 Noninflammatory disorder of ovary, fallopian tube and broad ligament, unspecified

● N84 Polyp of female genital tract
   Excludes1 adenomatous polyp (D28.-)
      placental polyp (O90.89)

   N84.0 Polyp of corpus uteri
      Polyp of endometrium
      Polyp of uterus NOS
      Excludes1 polypoid endometrial hyperplasia (N85.0-)

   N84.1 Polyp of cervix uteri
      Mucous polyp of cervix

   N84.2 Polyp of vagina

   N84.3 Polyp of vulva
      Polyp of labia

   N84.8 Polyp of other parts of female genital tract

   N84.9 Polyp of female genital tract, unspecified

CHAPTER 14 (N00–N99)

● **N85   Other noninflammatory disorders of uterus, except cervix**

    Excludes1   endometriosis (N80.-)

           inflammatory diseases of uterus (N71.-)

           noninflammatory disorders of cervix, except

              malposition (N86-N88)

           polyp of corpus uteri (N84.0)

           uterine prolapse (N81.-)

  ● **N85.0   Endometrial hyperplasia**

      N85.00   Endometrial hyperplasia, unspecified

          Hyperplasia (adenomatous) (cystic)

            (glandular) of endometrium

          Hyperplastic endometritis

      N85.01   Benign endometrial hyperplasia

          Endometrial hyperplasia (complex) (simple)

            without atypia

      N85.02   Endometrial intraepithelial neoplasia [EIN]

          Endometrial hyperplasia with atypia

          Excludes1   malignant neoplasm of

                endometrium (with

                endometrial intraepithelial

                neoplasia [EIN]) (C54.1)

  N85.2   Hypertrophy of uterus

      Bulky or enlarged uterus

      Excludes1   puerperal hypertrophy of uterus (O90.89)

  N85.3   Subinvolution of uterus

      Excludes1   puerperal subinvolution of uterus

                (O90.89)

  N85.4   Malposition of uterus

      Anteversion of uterus

      Retroflexion of uterus

      Retroversion of uterus

      Excludes1   malposition of uterus complicating

                pregnancy, labor or delivery (O34.5-,

                O65.5)

  N85.5   Inversion of uterus

      Excludes1   current obstetric trauma (O71.2)

                postpartum inversion of uterus (O71.2)

  N85.6   Intrauterine synechiae

  N85.7   Hematometra

      Hematosalpinx with hematometra

      Excludes1   hematometra with hematocolpos (N89.7)

  N85.8   Other specified noninflammatory disorders of uterus

      Atrophy of uterus, acquired

      Fibrosis of uterus NOS

  N85.9   Noninflammatory disorder of uterus, unspecified

      Disorder of uterus NOS

  N85.A   Isthmocele

      Isthmocele (non-pregnant state)

      Code also any associated conditions such as:

          abnormal uterine and vaginal bleeding, unspecified

            (N93.9)

          female infertility of uterine origin (N97.2)

          pelvic and perineal pain (R10.2)

      Excludes1   maternal care for cesarean scar defect

                (isthmocele) (O34.22)

          Coding Clinic: 2022, Q4, P37

● **N86   Erosion and ectropion of cervix uteri**

    Decubitus (trophic) ulcer of cervix

    Eversion of cervix

    Excludes1   erosion and ectropion of cervix with cervicitis

              (N72)

● **N87   Dysplasia of cervix uteri**

    Excludes1   abnormal results from cervical cytologic

              examination without histologic confirmation

              (R87.61-)

           carcinoma in situ of cervix uteri (D06.-)

           cervical intraepithelial neoplasia III [CIN III]

             (D06.-)

           HGSIL of cervix (R87.613)

           severe dysplasia of cervix uteri (D06.-)

  N87.0   Mild cervical dysplasia

      Cervical intraepithelial neoplasia I [CIN I]

  N87.1   Moderate cervical dysplasia

      Cervical intraepithelial neoplasia II [CIN II]

  N87.9   Dysplasia of cervix uteri, unspecified

      Anaplasia of cervix

      Cervical atypism

      Cervical dysplasia NOS

● **N88   Other noninflammatory disorders of cervix uteri**

    Excludes2   inflammatory disease of cervix (N72)

              polyp of cervix (N84.1)

  N88.0   Leukoplakia of cervix uteri

  N88.1   Old laceration of cervix uteri

      Adhesions of cervix

      Excludes1   current obstetric trauma (O71.3)

  N88.2   Stricture and stenosis of cervix uteri

      Excludes1   stricture and stenosis of cervix uteri

                complicating labor (O65.5)

  N88.3   Incompetence of cervix uteri

      Investigation and management of (suspected) cervical

         incompetence in a nonpregnant woman

      Excludes1   cervical incompetence complicating

                pregnancy (O34.3-)

  N88.4   Hypertrophic elongation of cervix uteri

  N88.8   Other specified noninflammatory disorders of cervix uteri

      Excludes1   current obstetric trauma (O71.3)

  N88.9   Noninflammatory disorder of cervix uteri, unspecified

● **N89   Other noninflammatory disorders of vagina**

    Excludes1   abnormal results from vaginal cytologic

              examination without histologic confirmation

              (R87.62-)

           carcinoma in situ of vagina (D07.2)

           HGSIL of vagina (R87.623)

           inflammation of vagina (N76.-)

           senile (atrophic) vaginitis (N95.2)

           severe dysplasia of vagina (D07.2)

           trichomonal leukorrhea (A59.00)

           vaginal intraepithelial neoplasia [VAIN], grade

             III (D07.2)

  N89.0   Mild vaginal dysplasia

      Vaginal intraepithelial neoplasia [VAIN], grade I

  N89.1   Moderate vaginal dysplasia

      Vaginal intraepithelial neoplasia [VAIN], grade II

  N89.3   Dysplasia of vagina, unspecified

  N89.4   Leukoplakia of vagina

  N89.5   Stricture and atresia of vagina

      Vaginal adhesions   Vaginal stenosis

      Excludes1   congenital atresia or stricture (Q52.4)

                postprocedural adhesions of vagina

                (N99.2)

  N89.6   Tight hymenal ring

      Rigid hymen   Tight introitus

      Excludes1   imperforate hymen (Q52.3)

  N89.7   Hematocolpos

      Hematocolpos with hematometra or hematosalpinx

      Coding Clinic: 2016, Q4, P59

  N89.8   Other specified noninflammatory disorders of vagina

      Leukorrhea NOS

      Old vaginal laceration

      Pessary ulcer of vagina

      Excludes1   current obstetric trauma (O70.-, O71.4,

                O71.7-O71.8)

                old laceration involving muscles of pelvic

                floor (N81.8)

  N89.9   Noninflammatory disorder of vagina, unspecified

▶ New   ⇒ Revised   ~~deleted~~ Deleted   Excludes 1   Excludes 2   Includes   Use additional   Code first   Code also   Key words

OGCR Official Guidelines   X Assign placeholder X   ● Use Additional Character(s)   ▷ Manifestation Code   Hierarchical Condition Category   Coding Clinic

● **N90**   **Other noninflammatory disorders of vulva and perineum**
     Excludes1   anogenital (venereal) warts (A63.0)
                 carcinoma in situ of vulva (D07.1)
                 condyloma acuminatum (A63.0)
                 current obstetric trauma (O70.-, O71.7-O71.8)
                 inflammation of vulva (N76.-)
                 severe dysplasia of vulva (D07.1)
                 vulvar intraepithelial neoplasm III [VIN III]
                   (D07.1)

     N90.0   **Mild vulvar dysplasia**
           Vulvar intraepithelial neoplasia [VIN], grade I

     N90.1   **Moderate vulvar dysplasia**
           Vulvar intraepithelial neoplasia [VIN], grade II

     N90.3   **Dysplasia of vulva, unspecified**

     N90.4   **Leukoplakia of vulva**
           Dystrophy of vulva
           Kraurosis of vulva
           Lichen sclerosus of external female genital organs

     N90.5   **Atrophy of vulva**
           Stenosis of vulva

●   **N90.6**   **Hypertrophy of vulva**
           Coding Clinic: 2016, Q4, P46

         N90.60   **Unspecified hypertrophy of vulva**
                Unspecified hypertrophy of labia

         N90.61   **Childhood asymmetric labium majus enlargement**
                CALME

         N90.69   **Other specified hypertrophy of vulva**
                Other specified hypertrophy of labia

     N90.7   **Vulvar cyst**

●   **N90.8**   **Other specified noninflammatory disorders of vulva and perineum**

●   **N90.81**   **Female genital mutilation status**
                Female genital cutting status

            N90.810   **Female genital mutilation status, unspecified**
                   Female genital cutting status, unspecified
                   Female genital mutilation status NOS

            N90.811   **Female genital mutilation Type I status**
                   Clitorectomy status
                   Female genital cutting Type I status

            N90.812   **Female genital mutilation Type II status**
                   Clitorectomy with excision of labia minora status
                   Female genital cutting Type II status

            N90.813   **Female genital mutilation Type III status**
                   Female genital cutting Type III status
                   Infibulation status

            N90.818   **Other female genital mutilation status**
                   Female genital cutting Type IV status
                   Female genital mutilation Type IV status
                   Other female genital cutting status

         N90.89   **Other specified noninflammatory disorders of vulva and perineum**
                Adhesions of vulva
                Hypertrophy of clitoris

     N90.9   **Noninflammatory disorder of vulva and perineum, unspecified**

● **N91**   **Absent, scanty and rare menstruation**
     Excludes1   ovarian dysfunction (E28.-)

     N91.0   **Primary amenorrhea**

     N91.1   **Secondary amenorrhea**

     N91.2   **Amenorrhea, unspecified**

     N91.3   **Primary oligomenorrhea**

     N91.4   **Secondary oligomenorrhea**

     N91.5   **Oligomenorrhea, unspecified**
           Hypomenorrhea NOS

● **N92**   **Excessive, frequent and irregular menstruation**
     Excludes1   postmenopausal bleeding (N95.0)
                 precocious puberty (menstruation) (E30.1)

     N92.0   **Excessive and frequent menstruation with regular cycle**
           Heavy periods NOS   Polymenorrhea
           Menorrhagia NOS

     N92.1   **Excessive and frequent menstruation with irregular cycle**
           Irregular intermenstrual bleeding
           Irregular, shortened intervals between menstrual bleeding
           Menometrorrhagia
           Metrorrhagia

     N92.2   **Excessive menstruation at puberty**   P
           Excessive bleeding associated with onset of menstrual periods
           Pubertal menorrhagia
           Puberty bleeding

     N92.3   **Ovulation bleeding**
           Regular intermenstrual bleeding

     N92.4   **Excessive bleeding in the premenopausal period**
           Climacteric menorrhagia or metrorrhagia
           Menopausal menorrhagia or metrorrhagia
           Perimenopausal bleeding
           Perimenopausal menorrhagia or metrorrhagia
           Preclimacteric menorrhagia or metrorrhagia
           Premenopausal menorrhagia or metrorrhagia

     N92.5   **Other specified irregular menstruation**

     N92.6   **Irregular menstruation, unspecified**
           Irregular bleeding NOS
           Irregular periods NOS
         Excludes1   irregular menstruation with:
                     lengthened intervals or scanty bleeding (N91.3-N91.5)
                     shortened intervals or excessive bleeding (N92.1)

● **N93**   **Other abnormal uterine and vaginal bleeding**
     Excludes1   neonatal vaginal hemorrhage (P54.6)
                 precocious puberty (menstruation) (E30.1)
                 pseudomenses (P54.6)

     N93.0   **Postcoital and contact bleeding**

     N93.1   **Pre-pubertal vaginal bleeding**
           Coding Clinic: 2016, Q4, P47

     N93.8   **Other specified abnormal uterine and vaginal bleeding**
           Dysfunctional or functional uterine or vaginal bleeding NOS

     N93.9   **Abnormal uterine and vaginal bleeding, unspecified**

● **N94**   **Pain and other conditions associated with female genital organs and menstrual cycle**

     N94.0   **Mittelschmerz**
           Ovulation pain

●   **N94.1**   **Dyspareunia**
           Painful intercourse/coitus
         Excludes1   psychogenic dyspareunia (F52.6)
         Coding Clinic: 2016, Q4, P47

         N94.10   **Unspecified dyspareunia**

         N94.11   **Superficial (introital) dyspareunia**

         N94.12   **Deep dyspareunia**

         N94.19   **Other specified dyspareunia**

     N94.2   **Vaginismus**
           Vagina tightness
         Excludes1   psychogenic vaginismus (F52.5)

CHAPTER 14 (N00–N99)

N94.3 **Premenstrual tension syndrome**
AKA: PMS
Code also associated menstrual migraine (G43.82-, G43.83-)
> **Excludes1** Premenstrual dysphoric disorder (F32.81)
> Coding Clinic: 2016, Q4, P14

N94.4 **Primary dysmenorrhea**
Lifelong painful menstruation

N94.5 **Secondary dysmenorrhea**
Later onset of painful menstruation

N94.6 **Dysmenorrhea, unspecified**
> **Excludes1** psychogenic dysmenorrhea (F45.8)

● **N94.8** **Other specified conditions associated with female genital organs and menstrual cycle**
  ● **N94.81** **Vulvodynia**
     N94.810 **Vulvar vestibulitis**
     N94.818 **Other vulvodynia**
     N94.819 **Vulvodynia, unspecified**
       Vulvodynia NOS
   N94.89 **Other specified conditions associated with female genital organs and menstrual cycle**

N94.9 **Unspecified condition associated with female genital organs and menstrual cycle**

● **N95** **Menopausal and other perimenopausal disorders**
Menopausal and other perimenopausal disorders due to naturally occurring (age-related) menopause and perimenopause
> **Excludes1** excessive bleeding in the premenopausal period (N92.4)
> menopausal and perimenopausal disorders due to artificial or premature menopause (E89.4-, E28.31-)
> premature menopause (E28.31-)
> **Excludes2** postmenopausal osteoporosis (M81.0-)
> postmenopausal osteoporosis with current pathological fracture (M80.0-)
> postmenopausal urethritis (N34.2)

N95.0 **Postmenopausal bleeding**

N95.1 **Menopausal and female climacteric states**
Symptoms such as flushing, sleeplessness, headache, lack of concentration, associated with natural (age-related) menopause
Use additional code for associated symptoms
> **Excludes1** asymptomatic menopausal state (Z78.0)
> symptoms associated with artificial menopause (E89.41)
> symptoms associated with premature menopause (E28.310)

N95.2 **Postmenopausal atrophic vaginitis**
Senile (atrophic) vaginitis

N95.8 **Other specified menopausal and perimenopausal disorders**

N95.9 **Unspecified menopausal and perimenopausal disorder**

N96 **Recurrent pregnancy loss**
Investigation or care in a nonpregnant woman with history of recurrent pregnancy loss
> **Excludes1** recurrent pregnancy loss with current pregnancy (O26.2-)

● **N97** **Female infertility**
> **Includes** inability to achieve a pregnancy
> sterility, female NOS
> **Excludes2** female infertility associated with:
> hypopituitarism (E23.0)
> Stein-Leventhal syndrome (E28.2)
> incompetence of cervix uteri (N88.3)
> Coding Clinic: 2022, Q2, P16

N97.0 **Female infertility associated with anovulation**
> Coding Clinic: 2022, Q2, P16

N97.1 **Female infertility of tubal origin**
Female infertility associated with congenital anomaly of tube
Female infertility due to tubal block
Female infertility due to tubal occlusion
Female infertility due to tubal stenosis

N97.2 **Female infertility of uterine origin**
Female infertility associated with congenital anomaly of uterus
Female infertility due to nonimplantation of ovum

N97.8 **Female infertility of other origin**

N97.9 **Female infertility, unspecified**

● **N98** **Complications associated with artificial fertilization**
N98.0 **Infection associated with artificial insemination**
N98.1 **Hyperstimulation of ovaries**
Hyperstimulation of ovaries NOS
Hyperstimulation of ovaries associated with induced ovulation
N98.2 **Complications of attempted introduction of fertilized ovum following in vitro fertilization**
N98.3 **Complications of attempted introduction of embryo in embryo transfer**
N98.8 **Other complications associated with artificial fertilization**
N98.9 **Complication associated with artificial fertilization, unspecified**

INTRAOPERATIVE AND POSTPROCEDURAL COMPLICATIONS AND DISORDERS OF GENITOURINARY SYSTEM, NOT ELSEWHERE CLASSIFIED (N99)

● **N99** **Intraoperative and postprocedural complications and disorders of genitourinary system, not elsewhere classified**
> **Excludes2** irradiation cystitis (N30.4-)
> postoophorectomy osteoporosis with current pathological fracture (M80.8-)
> postoophorectomy osteoporosis without current pathological fracture (M81.8)

N99.0 **Postprocedural (acute) (chronic) kidney failure**
Use additional code to type of kidney disease

● **N99.1** **Postprocedural urethral stricture**
Postcatheterization urethral stricture
  ● **N99.11** **Postprocedural urethral stricture, male**
     N99.110 **Postprocedural urethral stricture, male, meatal**
     N99.111 **Postprocedural bulbous urethral stricture, male**
     N99.112 **Postprocedural membranous urethral stricture, male**
     N99.113 **Postprocedural anterior bulbous urethral stricture, male**
       Coding Clinic: 2016, Q4, P48
     N99.114 **Postprocedural urethral stricture, male, unspecified**
     N99.115 **Postprocedural fossa navicularis urethral stricture**
       Coding Clinic: 2016, Q4, P47
     N99.116 **Postprocedural urethral stricture, male, overlapping sites**
   N99.12 **Postprocedural urethral stricture, female**

N99.2 **Postprocedural adhesions of vagina**
N99.3 **Prolapse of vaginal vault after hysterectomy**
N99.4 **Postprocedural pelvic peritoneal adhesions**
> **Excludes2** pelvic peritoneal adhesions NOS (N73.6)
> postinfective pelvic peritoneal adhesions (N73.6)

▶ New   ⇒ Revised   ~~deleted~~ Deleted   Excludes 1   Excludes 2   Includes   Use additional   Code first   Code also   Key words
OGCR Official Guidelines   X Assign placeholder X   ● Use Additional Character(s)   ▶ Manifestation Code   🔒 Hierarchical Condition Category   Coding Clinic

● N99.5   **Complications of stoma of urinary tract**
     Excludes2   mechanical complication of urinary catheter (T83.0-)

   ● N99.51   Complication of cystostomy
     N99.510   Cystostomy hemorrhage 🔏
     N99.511   Cystostomy infection 🔏
     N99.512   Cystostomy malfunction 🔏
     N99.518   Other cystostomy complication 🔏

   ● N99.52   Complication of incontinent external stoma of urinary tract
     N99.520   Hemorrhage of incontinent external stoma of urinary tract 🔏
     N99.521   Infection of incontinent external stoma of urinary tract 🔏
         Coding Clinic: 2016, Q4, P48
     N99.522   Malfunction of incontinent external stoma of urinary tract 🔏
     N99.523   Herniation of incontinent stoma of urinary tract 🔏
         Coding Clinic: 2016, Q4, P48
     N99.524   Stenosis of incontinent stoma of urinary tract 🔏
         Coding Clinic: 2016, Q4, P48
     N99.528   Other complication of incontinent external stoma of urinary tract 🔏

   ● N99.53   Complication of continent stoma of urinary tract
     N99.530   Hemorrhage of continent stoma of urinary tract 🔏
     N99.531   Infection of continent stoma of urinary tract 🔏
     N99.532   Malfunction of continent stoma of urinary tract 🔏
     N99.533   Herniation of continent stoma of urinary tract 🔏
         Coding Clinic: 2016, Q4, P48
     N99.534   Stenosis of continent stoma of urinary tract 🔏
         Coding Clinic: 2016, Q4, P48
     N99.538   Other complication of continent stoma of urinary tract 🔏

● N99.6   **Intraoperative hemorrhage and hematoma of a genitourinary system organ or structure complicating a procedure**
     Excludes1   intraoperative hemorrhage and hematoma of a genitourinary system organ or structure due to accidental puncture or laceration during a procedure (N99.7-)

   N99.61   Intraoperative hemorrhage and hematoma of a genitourinary system organ or structure complicating a genitourinary system procedure
   N99.62   Intraoperative hemorrhage and hematoma of a genitourinary system organ or structure complicating other procedure

● N99.7   **Accidental puncture and laceration of a genitourinary system organ or structure during a procedure**
   N99.71   Accidental puncture and laceration of a genitourinary system organ or structure during a genitourinary system procedure
   N99.72   Accidental puncture and laceration of a genitourinary system organ or structure during other procedure

● N99.8   **Other intraoperative and postprocedural complications and disorders of genitourinary system**
     Coding Clinic: 2016, Q4, P10

   N99.81   Other intraoperative complications of genitourinary system
   ● N99.82   Postprocedural hemorrhage of a genitourinary system organ or structure following a procedure
     N99.820   Postprocedural hemorrhage of a genitourinary system organ or structure following a genitourinary system procedure
     N99.821   Postprocedural hemorrhage of a genitourinary system organ or structure following other procedure

   N99.83   Residual ovary syndrome
   ● N99.84   Postprocedural hematoma and seroma of a genitourinary system organ or structure following a procedure
     N99.840   Postprocedural hematoma of a genitourinary system organ or structure following a genitourinary system procedure
     N99.841   Postprocedural hematoma of a genitourinary system organ or structure following other procedure
     N99.842   Postprocedural seroma of a genitourinary system organ or structure following a genitourinary system procedure
     N99.843   Postprocedural seroma of a genitourinary system organ or structure following other procedure

   N99.85   Post endometrial ablation syndrome
     Coding Clinic: 2019, Q4, P12
   N99.89   Other postprocedural complications and disorders of genitourinary system

CHAPTER 14 (N00-N99)

CHAPTER 15

PREGNANCY, CHILDBIRTH, AND THE PUERPERIUM (O00-O9A)

OGCR Chapter-Specific Coding Guidelines

15. **Chapter 15: Pregnancy, Childbirth, and the Puerperium (O00-O9A)**

a. General Rules for Obstetric Cases

1) Codes from Chapter 15 and sequencing priority
Obstetric cases require codes from Chapter 15, codes in the range O00-O9A, Pregnancy, Childbirth, and the Puerperium. Chapter 15 codes have sequencing priority over codes from other chapters. Additional codes from other chapters may be used in conjunction with Chapter 15 codes to further specify conditions. Should the provider document that the pregnancy is incidental to the encounter, then code Z33.1, Pregnant state, incidental, should be used in place of any Chapter 15 codes. It is the provider's responsibility to state that the condition being treated is not affecting the pregnancy.

2) Chapter 15 codes used only on the maternal record
Chapter 15 codes are to be used only on the maternal record, never on the record of the newborn.

3) Final character for trimester
The majority of codes in Chapter 15 have a final character indicating the trimester of pregnancy. The timeframes for the trimesters are indicated at the beginning of the chapter. If trimester is not a component of a code it is because the condition always occurs in a specific trimester, or the concept of trimester of pregnancy is not applicable. Certain codes have characters for only certain trimesters because the condition does not occur in all trimesters, but it may occur in more than just one.

Assignment of the final character for trimester should be based on the provider's documentation of the trimester (or number of weeks) for the current admission/encounter. This applies to the assignment of trimester for pre-existing conditions as well as those that develop during or are due to the pregnancy. The provider's documentation of the number of weeks may be used to assign the appropriate code identifying the trimester.

Whenever delivery occurs during the current admission, and there is an "in childbirth" option for the obstetric complication being coded, the "in childbirth" code should be assigned.

4) Selection of trimester for inpatient admissions that encompass more than one trimester
In instances when a patient is admitted to a hospital for complications of pregnancy during one trimester and remains in the hospital into a subsequent trimester, the trimester character for the antepartum complication code should be assigned on the basis of the trimester when the complication developed, not the trimester of the discharge. If the condition developed prior to the current admission/encounter or represents a pre-existing condition, the trimester character for the trimester at the time of the admission/encounter should be assigned.

5) Unspecified trimester
Each category that includes codes for trimester has a code for "unspecified trimester." The "unspecified trimester" code should rarely be used, such as when the documentation in the record is insufficient to determine the trimester and it is not possible to obtain clarification.

6) 7th character for Fetus Identification
Where applicable, a 7th character is to be assigned for certain categories (O31, O32, O33.3 - O33.6, O35, O36, O40, O41, O60.1, O60.2, O64, and O69) to identify the fetus for which the complication code applies.

Assign 7th character "0":
• For single gestations
• When the documentation in the record is insufficient to determine the fetus affected and it is not possible to obtain clarification.
• When it is not possible to clinically determine which fetus is affected.

b. Selection of OB Principal or First-listed Diagnosis

1) Routine outpatient prenatal visits
For routine outpatient prenatal visits when no complications are present, a code from category Z34, Encounter for supervision of normal pregnancy, should be used as the first-listed diagnosis. These codes should not be used in conjunction with Chapter 15 codes.

2) Supervision of High-Risk Pregnancy
Codes from category O09, Supervision of high-risk pregnancy, are intended for use only during the prenatal period. For complications during the labor or delivery episode as a result of a high-risk pregnancy, assign the applicable complication codes from Chapter 15. If there are no complications during the labor or delivery episode, assign code O80, Encounter for full-term uncomplicated delivery.

For routine prenatal outpatient visits for patients with high-risk pregnancies, a code from category O09, Supervision of high-risk pregnancy, should be used as the first-listed diagnosis. Secondary Chapter 15 codes may be used in conjunction with these codes if appropriate.

3) Episodes when no delivery occurs
In episodes when no delivery occurs, the principal diagnosis should correspond to the principal complication of the pregnancy which necessitated the encounter. Should more than one complication exist, all of which are treated or monitored, any of the complications codes may be sequenced first.

4) When a delivery occurs
When an obstetric patient is admitted and delivers during that admission, the condition that prompted the admission should be sequenced as the principal diagnosis. If multiple conditions prompted the admission, sequence the one most related to the delivery as the principal diagnosis. A code for any complication of the delivery should be assigned as an additional diagnosis. In cases of cesarean delivery, if the patient was admitted with a condition that resulted in the performance of a cesarean procedure, that condition should be selected as the principal diagnosis. If the reason for the admission was unrelated to the condition resulting in the cesarean delivery, the condition related to the reason for the admission should be selected as the principal diagnosis.

5) Outcome of delivery
A code from category Z37, Outcome of delivery, should be included on every maternal record when a delivery has occurred. These codes are not to be used on subsequent records or on the newborn record.

c. Pre-existing conditions versus conditions due to the pregnancy
Certain categories in Chapter 15 distinguish between conditions of the mother that existed prior to pregnancy (pre-existing) and those that are a direct result of pregnancy. When assigning codes from Chapter 15, it is important to assess if a condition was pre-existing prior to pregnancy or developed during or due to the pregnancy in order to assign the correct code.

Categories that do not distinguish between pre-existing and pregnancy-related conditions may be used for either. It is acceptable to use codes specifically for the puerperium with codes complicating pregnancy and childbirth if a condition arises postpartum during the delivery encounter.

d. Pre-existing hypertension in pregnancy
Category O10, Pre-existing hypertension complicating pregnancy, childbirth and the puerperium, includes codes for hypertensive heart and hypertensive chronic kidney disease. When assigning one of the O10 codes that includes hypertensive heart disease or hypertensive chronic kidney disease, it is necessary to add a secondary code from the appropriate hypertension category to specify the type of heart failure or chronic kidney disease.
See Section I.C.9. Hypertension.

e. Fetal Conditions Affecting the Management of the Mother

1) Codes from categories O35 and O36
Codes from categories O35, Maternal care for known or suspected fetal abnormality and damage, and O36, Maternal care for other fetal problems, are assigned only when the fetal condition is actually responsible for modifying the management of the mother, i.e., by requiring diagnostic studies, additional observation, special care, or termination of pregnancy. The fact that the fetal condition exists does not justify assigning a code from this series to the mother's record.

2) In utero surgery
In cases when surgery is performed on the fetus, a diagnosis code from category O35, Maternal care for known or suspected fetal abnormality and damage, should be assigned identifying the fetal condition. Assign the appropriate procedure code for the procedure performed.

No code from Chapter 16, the perinatal codes, should be used on the mother's record to identify fetal conditions. Surgery performed in utero on a fetus is still to be coded as an obstetric encounter.

f. HIV Infection in Pregnancy, Childbirth, and the Puerperium
During pregnancy, childbirth or the puerperium, a patient admitted because of an HIV-related illness should receive a principal diagnosis from subcategory O98.7-, Human immunodeficiency [HIV] disease complicating pregnancy, childbirth and the puerperium, followed by the code(s) for the HIV-related illness(es).

Patients with asymptomatic HIV infection status admitted during pregnancy, childbirth, or the puerperium should receive codes of O98.7- and Z21, Asymptomatic human immunodeficiency virus [HIV] infection status.

g. Diabetes mellitus in pregnancy
Diabetes mellitus is a significant complicating factor in pregnancy. Pregnant women who are diabetic should be assigned a code from category O24, Diabetes mellitus in pregnancy, childbirth, and the puerperium, first, followed by the appropriate diabetes code(s) (E08-E13) from Chapter 4.

h. **Long-term use of insulin and oral hypoglycemics**
See Section I.C.4.a.3 for information on the long-term use of insulin and oral hypoglycemic.

i. **Gestational (pregnancy induced) diabetes**
Gestational (pregnancy induced) diabetes can occur during the second and third trimester of pregnancy in women who were not diabetic prior to pregnancy. Gestational diabetes can cause complications in the pregnancy similar to those of pre-existing diabetes mellitus. It also puts the woman at greater risk of developing diabetes after the pregnancy. Codes for gestational diabetes are in subcategory O24.4, Gestational diabetes mellitus. No other code from category O24, Diabetes mellitus in pregnancy, childbirth, and the puerperium, should be used with a code from O24.4.

The codes under subcategory O24.4 include diet controlled, insulin controlled, and controlled by oral hypoglycemic drugs. If a patient with gestational diabetes is treated with both diet and insulin, only the code for insulin-controlled is required. If a patient with gestational diabetes is treated with both diet and oral hypoglycemic medications, only the code for "controlled by oral hypoglycemic drugs" is required. Code Z79.4, Long-term (current) use of insulin or code Z79.84, Long-term (current) use of oral hypoglycemic drugs, should not be assigned with codes from subcategory O24.4.

An abnormal glucose tolerance in pregnancy is assigned a code from subcategory O99.81, Abnormal glucose complicating pregnancy, childbirth, and the puerperium.

j. **Sepsis and septic shock complicating abortion, pregnancy, childbirth and the puerperium**
When assigning a Chapter 15 code for sepsis complicating abortion, pregnancy, childbirth, and the puerperium, a code for the specific type of infection should be assigned as an additional diagnosis. If severe sepsis is present, a code from subcategory R65.2, Severe sepsis, and code(s) for associated organ dysfunction(s) should also be assigned as additional diagnoses.

k. **Puerperal sepsis**
Code O85, Puerperal sepsis, should be assigned with a secondary code to identify the causal organism (e.g., for a bacterial infection, assign a code from category B95-B96, Bacterial infections in conditions classified elsewhere). A code from category A40, Streptococcal sepsis, or A41, Other sepsis, should not be used for puerperal sepsis. If applicable, use additional codes to identify severe sepsis (R65.2-) and any associated acute organ dysfunction.

l. **Alcohol, tobacco and drug use during pregnancy, childbirth and the puerperium**
1) **Alcohol use during pregnancy, childbirth and the puerperium**
Codes under subcategory O99.31, Alcohol use complicating pregnancy, childbirth, and the puerperium, should be assigned for any pregnancy case when a mother uses alcohol during the pregnancy or postpartum. A secondary code from category F10, Alcohol-related disorders, should also be assigned to identify manifestations of the alcohol use.

2) **Tobacco use during pregnancy, childbirth, and the puerperium**
Codes under subcategory O99.33, Smoking (tobacco) complicating pregnancy, childbirth, and the puerperium, should be assigned for any pregnancy case when a mother uses any type of tobacco product during the pregnancy or postpartum. A secondary code from category F17, Nicotine dependence, should also be assigned to identify the type of nicotine dependence.

3) **Drug use during pregnancy, childbirth and the puerperium**
Codes under subcategory O99.32, Drug use complicating pregnancy, childbirth, and the puerperium, should be assigned for any pregnancy case when a mother uses drugs during the pregnancy or postpartum. This can involve illegal drugs, or inappropriate use or abuse of prescription drugs. Secondary code(s) from categories F11-F16 and F18-F19 should also be assigned to identify manifestations of the drug use.

m. **Poisoning, toxic effects, adverse effects and underdosing in a pregnant patient**
A code from subcategory O9A.2, Injury, poisoning and certain other consequences of external causes complicating pregnancy, childbirth, and the puerperium, should be sequenced first, followed by the appropriate injury, poisoning, toxic effect, adverse effect or underdosing code, and then the additional code(s) that specifies the condition caused by the poisoning, toxic effect, adverse effect or underdosing.
See Section I.C.19. Adverse effects, poisoning, underdosing and toxic effects.

n. **Normal Delivery, Code O80**
1) **Encounter for full-term uncomplicated delivery**
Code O80 should be assigned when a woman is admitted for a full-term normal delivery and delivers a single, healthy infant without any complications antepartum, during the delivery, or postpartum during the delivery episode. Code O80 is always a principal diagnosis. It is not to be used if any other code from Chapter 15 is needed to describe a current complication of the antenatal, delivery, or perinatal period. Additional codes from other chapters may be used with code O80 if they are not related to or are in any way complicating the pregnancy.

2) **Uncomplicated delivery with resolved antepartum complication**
Code O80 may be used if the patient had a complication at some point during the pregnancy, but the complication is not present at the time of the admission for delivery.

3) **Outcome of delivery for O80**
Z37.0, Single live birth, is the only outcome of delivery code appropriate for use with O80.

o. **The Peripartum and Postpartum Periods**
1) **Peripartum and Postpartum periods**
The postpartum period begins immediately after delivery and continues for six weeks following delivery. The peripartum period is defined as the last month of pregnancy to five months postpartum.

2) **Peripartum and postpartum complication**
A postpartum complication is any complication occurring within the six-week period.

3) **Pregnancy-related complications after 6 week period**
Chapter 15 codes may also be used to describe pregnancy-related complications after the peripartum or postpartum period if the provider documents that a condition is pregnancy related.

4) **Admission for routine postpartum care following delivery outside hospital**
When the mother delivers outside the hospital prior to admission and is admitted for routine postpartum care and no complications are noted, code Z39.0, Encounter for care and examination of mother immediately after delivery, should be assigned as the principal diagnosis.

5) **Pregnancy associated cardiomyopathy**
Pregnancy associated cardiomyopathy, code O90.3, is unique in that it may be diagnosed in the third trimester of pregnancy but may continue to progress months after delivery. For this reason, it is referred to as peripartum cardiomyopathy. Code O90.3 is only for use when the cardiomyopathy develops as a result of pregnancy in a woman who did not have pre-existing heart disease.

p. **Code O94, Sequelae of complication of pregnancy, childbirth, and the puerperium**
1) **Code O94**
Code O94, Sequelae of complication of pregnancy, childbirth, and the puerperium, is for use in those cases when an initial complication of a pregnancy develops a sequelae requiring care or treatment at a future date.

2) **After the initial postpartum period**
This code may be used at any time after the initial postpartum period.

3) **Sequencing of Code O94**
This code, like all sequela codes, is to be sequenced following the code describing the sequelae of the complication.

q. **Termination of Pregnancy and Spontaneous abortions**
1) **Abortion with Liveborn Fetus**
When an attempted termination of pregnancy results in a liveborn fetus assign code Z33.2, Encounter for elective termination of pregnancy and a code from category Z37, Outcome of Delivery.

2) **Retained Products of Conception following an abortion**
Subsequent encounters for retained products of conception following a spontaneous abortion or elective termination of pregnancy, without complications are assigned O03.4, Incomplete spontaneous, abortion without complication, or codes O07.4, Failed attempted termination of pregnancy without complication. This advice is appropriate even when the patient was discharged previously with a discharge diagnosis of complete abortion. If the patient has a specific complication associated with the spontaneous abortion or elective termination of pregnancy in addition to retained products of conception, assign the appropriate complication in category O03 or O07 instead of code O03.4 or O07.4

3) **Complications leading to abortion**
Codes from Chapter 15 may be used as additional codes to identify any documented complications of the pregnancy in conjunction with codes in categories in O04, O07 and O08.

r. **Abuse in a pregnant patient**
For suspected or confirmed cases of abuse of a pregnant patient, a code(s) from subcategories O9A.3, Physical abuse complicating pregnancy, childbirth, and the puerperium, O9A.4, Sexual abuse complicating pregnancy, childbirth, and the puerperium, and O9A.5, Psychological abuse complicating pregnancy, childbirth, and the puerperium, should be sequenced first, followed by the appropriate codes (if applicable) to identify any associated current injury due to physical abuse, sexual abuse, and the perpetrator of abuse.
See Section I.C.19. Adult and child abuse, neglect and other maltreatment.

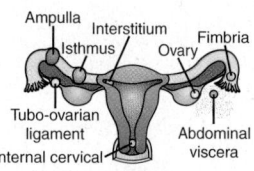

Figure 15-1   Implantation sites of ectopic pregnancy.

Item 15–1   Ectopic pregnancy most often occurs in the fallopian tube. Pregnancy outside the uterus may end in a lifethreatening rupture.

⭐ **(See Plate 4 of the Anatomy Illustrations.)**

CHAPTER 15

PREGNANCY, CHILDBIRTH, AND THE PUERPERIUM (O00–O9A)

Note: CODES FROM THIS CHAPTER ARE FOR USE ONLY ON MATERNAL RECORDS, NEVER ON NEWBORN RECORDS

Codes from this chapter are for use for conditions related to or aggravated by the pregnancy, childbirth, or by the puerperium (maternal causes or obstetric causes)

Trimesters are counted from the first day of the last menstrual period. They are defined as follows:

1st trimester - less than 14 weeks 0 days

2nd trimester - 14 weeks 0 days to less than 28 weeks 0 days

3rd trimester - 28 weeks 0 days until delivery

Use additional code , if applicable, from category Z3A, Weeks of gestation, to identify the specific week of the pregnancy, if known.

Excludes1   supervision of normal pregnancy (Z34.-)

Excludes2   mental and behavioral disorders associated with the puerperium (F53.-)
         obstetrical tetanus (A34)
         postpartum necrosis of pituitary gland (E23.0)
         puerperal osteomalacia (M83.0)

This chapter contains the following blocks:

O00–O08	Pregnancy with abortive outcome
O09	Supervision of high risk pregnancy
O10–O16	Edema, proteinuria and hypertensive disorders in pregnancy, childbirth and the puerperium
O20–O29	Other maternal disorders predominantly related to pregnancy
O30–O48	Maternal care related to the fetus and amniotic cavity and possible delivery problems
O60–O77	Complications of labor and delivery
O80, O82	Encounter for delivery
O85–O92	Complications predominantly related to the puerperium
O94–O9A	Other obstetric conditions, not elsewhere classified

PREGNANCY WITH ABORTIVE OUTCOME (O00–O08)

Excludes1   continuing pregnancy in multiple gestation after abortion of one fetus or more (O31.1-, O31.3-)

Coding Clinic: 2016, Q4, P130

● O00   **Ectopic pregnancy**

Includes   ruptured ectopic pregnancy

Use additional code from category O08 to identify any associated complication

● O00.0   **Abdominal pregnancy**

Excludes1   maternal care for viable fetus in abdominal pregnancy (O36.7-)

Coding Clinic: 2016, Q4, P49

     O00.00   **Abdominal pregnancy without intrauterine pregnancy**   M
         Abdominal pregnancy NOS

     O00.01   **Abdominal pregnancy with intrauterine pregnancy**   M

● O00.1   **Tubal pregnancy**
     Fallopian pregnancy
     Rupture of (fallopian) tube due to pregnancy
     Tubal abortion

Coding Clinic: 2016, Q4, P49

   ● O00.10   **Tubal pregnancy without intrauterine pregnancy**
         Tubal pregnancy NOS

         O00.101   **Right tubal pregnancy without intrauterine pregnancy**   M

         O00.102   **Left tubal pregnancy without intrauterine pregnancy**   M

         O00.109   **Unspecified tubal pregnancy without intrauterine pregnancy**   M

   ● O00.11   **Tubal pregnancy with intrauterine pregnancy**

         O00.111   **Right tubal pregnancy with intrauterine pregnancy**   M

         O00.112   **Left tubal pregnancy with intrauterine pregnancy**   M

         O00.119   **Unspecified tubal pregnancy with intrauterine pregnancy**   M

● O00.2   **Ovarian pregnancy**

Coding Clinic: 2016, Q4, P49

   ● O00.20   **Ovarian pregnancy without intrauterine pregnancy**
         Ovarian pregnancy NOS

         O00.201   **Right ovarian pregnancy without intrauterine pregnancy**   M

         O00.202   **Left ovarian pregnancy without intrauterine pregnancy**   M

         O00.209   **Unspecified ovarian pregnancy without intrauterine pregnancy**   M

   ● O00.21   **Ovarian pregnancy with intrauterine pregnancy**

         O00.211   **Right ovarian pregnancy with intrauterine pregnancy**   M

         O00.212   **Left ovarian pregnancy with intrauterine pregnancy**   M

         O00.219   **Unspecified ovarian pregnancy with intrauterine pregnancy**   M

● O00.8   **Other ectopic pregnancy**
     Cervical pregnancy
     Cornual pregnancy
     Intraligamentous pregnancy
     Mural pregnancy

Coding Clinic: 2016, Q4, P49

     O00.80   **Other ectopic pregnancy without intrauterine pregnancy**   M
         Other ectopic pregnancy NOS

     O00.81   **Other ectopic pregnancy with intrauterine pregnancy**   M

▶ New   ⇒ Revised   ~~deleted~~ Deleted   Excludes 1   Excludes 2   Includes   Use additional   Code first   Code also   Key words

OGCR Official Guidelines   X Assign placeholder X   ● Use Additional Character(s)   ▶ Manifestation Code   🏥 Hierarchical Condition Category   **Coding Clinic**

● **O00.9**   **Ectopic pregnancy, unspecified**
     Coding Clinic: 2016, Q4, P49

     O00.90   **Unspecified ectopic pregnancy without intrauterine pregnancy**   M
          Ectopic pregnancy NOS

     O00.91   **Unspecified ectopic pregnancy with intrauterine pregnancy**   M

● **O01**   **Hydatidiform mole**
     Use additional code from category O08 to identify any associated complication

     Excludes1   chorioadenoma (destruens) (D39.2)
                 malignant hydatidiform mole (D39.2)

     O01.0   **Classical hydatidiform mole**   M
         Complete hydatidiform mole

     O01.1   **Incomplete and partial hydatidiform mole**   M

     O01.9   **Hydatidiform mole, unspecified**   M
         Trophoblastic disease NOS
         Vesicular mole NOS

● **O02**   **Other abnormal products of conception**
     Use additional code from category O08 to identify any associated complication

     Excludes1   papyraceous fetus (O31.0-)

     O02.0   **Blighted ovum and nonhydatidiform mole**   M
         Carneous mole   Molar pregnancy NEC
         Fleshy mole   Pathological ovum
         Intrauterine mole NOS

     O02.1   **Missed abortion**   M
         Early fetal death, before completion of 20 weeks of gestation, with retention of dead fetus

         Excludes1   failed induced abortion (O07.-)
                    fetal death (intrauterine) (late) (O36.4)
                    missed abortion with blighted ovum (O02.0)
                    missed abortion with hydatidiform mole (O01.-)
                    missed abortion with nonhydatidiform (O02.0)
                    missed abortion with other abnormal products of conception (O02.8-)
                    missed delivery (O36.4)
                    stillbirth (P95)
         Coding Clinic: 2022, Q2, P3-4; 2019, Q3, P12

● **O02.8**   **Other specified abnormal products of conception**
         Excludes1   abnormal products of conception with blighted ovum (O02.0)
                    abnormal products of conception with hydatidiform mole (O01.-)
                    abnormal products of conception with nonhydatidiform mole (O02.0)

     O02.81   **Inappropriate change in quantitative human chorionic gonadotropin (hCG) in early pregnancy**   M
         Biochemical pregnancy
         Chemical pregnancy
         Inappropriate level of quantitative human chorionic gonadotropin (hCG) for gestational age in early pregnancy

     O02.89   **Other abnormal products of conception**   M

     O02.9   **Abnormal product of conception, unspecified**   M

● **O03**   **Spontaneous abortion**
     Coding Clinic: 2023, Q1, P17
     Note: Incomplete abortion includes retained products of conception following spontaneous abortion.
     Includes   miscarriage

     O03.0   **Genital tract and pelvic infection following incomplete spontaneous abortion**   M
         Endometritis following incomplete spontaneous abortion
         Oophoritis following incomplete spontaneous abortion
         Parametritis following incomplete spontaneous abortion
         Pelvic peritonitis following incomplete spontaneous abortion
         Salpingitis following incomplete spontaneous abortion
         Salpingo-oophoritis following incomplete spontaneous abortion

         Excludes1   sepsis following incomplete spontaneous abortion (O03.37)
                    urinary tract infection following incomplete spontaneous abortion (O03.38)

     O03.1   **Delayed or excessive hemorrhage following incomplete spontaneous abortion**   M
         Afibrinogenemia following incomplete spontaneous abortion
         Defibrination syndrome following incomplete spontaneous abortion
         Hemolysis following incomplete spontaneous abortion
         Intravascular coagulation following incomplete spontaneous abortion

     O03.2   **Embolism following incomplete spontaneous abortion**   M
         Air embolism following incomplete spontaneous abortion
         Amniotic fluid embolism following incomplete spontaneous abortion
         Blood-clot embolism following incomplete spontaneous abortion
         Embolism NOS following incomplete spontaneous abortion
         Fat embolism following incomplete spontaneous abortion
         Pulmonary embolism following incomplete spontaneous abortion
         Pyemic embolism following incomplete spontaneous abortion
         Septic or septicopyemic embolism following incomplete spontaneous abortion
         Soap embolism following incomplete spontaneous abortion

     ● **O03.3**   **Other and unspecified complications following incomplete spontaneous abortion**

     O03.30   **Unspecified complication following incomplete spontaneous abortion**   M

     O03.31   **Shock following incomplete spontaneous abortion**   M
         Circulatory collapse following incomplete spontaneous abortion
         Shock (postprocedural) following incomplete spontaneous abortion

         Excludes1   shock due to infection following incomplete spontaneous abortion (O03.37)

     O03.32   **Renal failure following incomplete spontaneous abortion**   M
         Kidney failure (acute) following incomplete spontaneous abortion
         Oliguria following incomplete spontaneous abortion
         Renal shutdown following incomplete spontaneous abortion
         Renal tubular necrosis following incomplete spontaneous abortion
         Uremia following incomplete spontaneous abortion

Item 15–2 A **hydatidiform** mole is an overproduction of placental tissue. The tumor secretes a hormone, chorionic gonadotropic hormone (CGH), that indicates a positive pregnancy test. There is no viable fetus. More than 80% of hydatidiform moles are noncancerous.

O03.33   **Metabolic disorder following incomplete spontaneous abortion**   M

O03.34   **Damage to pelvic organs following incomplete spontaneous abortion**   M

Laceration, perforation, tear or chemical damage of bladder following incomplete spontaneous abortion

Laceration, perforation, tear or chemical damage of bowel following incomplete spontaneous abortion

Laceration, perforation, tear or chemical damage of broad ligament following incomplete spontaneous abortion

Laceration, perforation, tear or chemical damage of cervix following incomplete spontaneous abortion

Laceration, perforation, tear or chemical damage of periurethral tissue following incomplete spontaneous abortion

Laceration, perforation, tear or chemical damage of uterus following incomplete spontaneous abortion

Laceration, perforation, tear or chemical damage of vagina following incomplete spontaneous abortion

O03.35   **Other venous complications following incomplete spontaneous abortion**   M

O03.36   **Cardiac arrest following incomplete spontaneous abortion**   M

O03.37   **Sepsis following incomplete spontaneous abortion**   M

Use additional code to identify infectious agent (B95-B97)

Use additional code to identify severe sepsis, if applicable (R65.2-)

Excludes1   septic or septicopyemic embolism following incomplete spontaneous abortion (O03.2)

O03.38   **Urinary tract infection following incomplete spontaneous abortion**   M

Cystitis following incomplete spontaneous abortion

O03.39   **Incomplete spontaneous abortion with other complications**   M

O03.4   **Incomplete spontaneous abortion without complication**   M

Coding Clinic: 2023, Q1, P17

O03.5   **Genital tract and pelvic infection following complete or unspecified spontaneous abortion**   M

Endometritis following complete or unspecified spontaneous abortion

Oophoritis following complete or unspecified spontaneous abortion

Parametritis following complete or unspecified spontaneous abortion

Pelvic peritonitis following complete or unspecified spontaneous abortion

Salpingitis following complete or unspecified spontaneous abortion

Salpingo-oophoritis following complete or unspecified spontaneous abortion

Excludes1   sepsis following complete or unspecified spontaneous abortion (O03.87)

urinary tract infection following complete or unspecified spontaneous abortion (O03.88)

O03.6   **Delayed or excessive hemorrhage following complete or unspecified spontaneous abortion**   M

Afibrinogenemia following complete or unspecified spontaneous abortion

Defibrination syndrome following complete or unspecified spontaneous abortion

Hemolysis following complete or unspecified spontaneous abortion

Intravascular coagulation following complete or unspecified spontaneous abortion

Coding Clinic: 2022, Q1, P19

O03.7   **Embolism following complete or unspecified spontaneous abortion**   M

Air embolism following complete or unspecified spontaneous abortion

Amniotic fluid embolism following complete or unspecified spontaneous abortion

Blood-clot embolism following complete or unspecified spontaneous abortion

Embolism NOS following complete or unspecified spontaneous abortion

Fat embolism following complete or unspecified spontaneous abortion

Pulmonary embolism following complete or unspecified spontaneous abortion

Pyemic embolism following complete or unspecified spontaneous abortion

Septic or septicopyemic embolism following complete or unspecified spontaneous abortion

Soap embolism following complete or unspecified spontaneous abortion

● O03.8   **Other and unspecified complications following complete or unspecified spontaneous abortion**

O03.80   **Unspecified complication following complete or unspecified spontaneous abortion**   M

O03.81   **Shock following complete or unspecified spontaneous abortion**   M

Circulatory collapse following complete or unspecified spontaneous abortion

Shock (postprocedural) following complete or unspecified spontaneous abortion

Excludes1   shock due to infection following complete or unspecified spontaneous abortion (O03.87)

O03.82   **Renal failure following complete or unspecified spontaneous abortion**   M

Kidney failure (acute) following complete or unspecified spontaneous abortion

Oliguria following complete or unspecified spontaneous abortion

Renal shutdown following complete or unspecified spontaneous abortion

Renal tubular necrosis following complete or unspecified spontaneous abortion

Uremia following complete or unspecified spontaneous abortion

O03.83   **Metabolic disorder following complete or unspecified spontaneous abortion**   M

O03.84   **Damage to pelvic organs following complete or unspecified spontaneous abortion**   M

Laceration, perforation, tear or chemical damage of bladder following complete or unspecified spontaneous abortion

Laceration, perforation, tear or chemical damage of bowel following complete or unspecified spontaneous abortion

Laceration, perforation, tear or chemical damage of broad ligament following complete or unspecified spontaneous abortion

Laceration, perforation, tear or chemical damage of cervix following complete or unspecified spontaneous abortion

Laceration, perforation, tear or chemical damage of periurethral tissue following complete or unspecified spontaneous abortion

Laceration, perforation, tear or chemical damage of uterus following complete or unspecified spontaneous abortion

Laceration, perforation, tear or chemical damage of vagina following complete or unspecified spontaneous abortion

▶ New   ⇒ Revised   ~~deleted~~ Deleted   Excludes 1   Excludes 2   Includes   Use additional   Code first   Code also   Key words

OGCR Official Guidelines   X Assign placeholder X   ● Use Additional Character(s)   ▷ Manifestation Code   🄷 Hierarchical Condition Category   Coding Clinic

O03.85   **Other venous complications following complete or unspecified spontaneous abortion**   M

O03.86   **Cardiac arrest following complete or unspecified spontaneous abortion**   M

O03.87   **Sepsis following complete or unspecified spontaneous abortion**   M

    Use additional code to identify infectious agent (B95-B97)

    Use additional code to identify severe sepsis, if applicable (R65.2-)

    Excludes1   septic or septicopyemic embolism following complete or unspecified spontaneous abortion (O03.7)

O03.88   **Urinary tract infection following complete or unspecified spontaneous abortion**   M

    Cystitis following complete or unspecified spontaneous abortion

O03.89   **Complete or unspecified spontaneous abortion with other complications**   M

O03.9   **Complete or unspecified spontaneous abortion without complication**   M

    Miscarriage NOS

    Spontaneous abortion NOS

● **O04**   **Complications following (induced) termination of pregnancy**

    Includes   complications following (induced) termination of pregnancy

    Excludes2   encounter for elective termination of pregnancy, uncomplicated (Z33.2)

          failed attempted termination of pregnancy (O07.-)

    Coding Clinic: 2023, Q2, P15-16; 2023, Q1, P17

O04.5   **Genital tract and pelvic infection following (induced) termination of pregnancy**   M

    Endometritis following (induced) termination of pregnancy

    Oophoritis following (induced) termination of pregnancy

    Parametritis following (induced) termination of pregnancy

    Pelvic peritonitis following (induced) termination of pregnancy

    Salpingitis following (induced) termination of pregnancy

    Salpingo-oophoritis following (induced) termination of pregnancy

    Excludes1   sepsis following (induced) termination of pregnancy (O04.87)

          urinary tract infection following (induced) termination of pregnancy (O04.88)

O04.6   **Delayed or excessive hemorrhage following (induced) termination of pregnancy**   M

    Afibrinogenemia following (induced) termination of pregnancy

    Defibrination syndrome following (induced) termination of pregnancy

    Hemolysis following (induced) termination of pregnancy

    Intravascular coagulation following (induced) termination of pregnancy

    Coding Clinic: 2023, Q2, P15-16; 2019, Q3, P12

O04.7   **Embolism following (induced) termination of pregnancy**   M

    Air embolism following (induced) termination of pregnancy

    Amniotic fluid embolism following (induced) termination of pregnancy

    Blood-clot embolism following (induced) termination of pregnancy

    Embolism NOS following (induced) termination of pregnancy

    Fat embolism following (induced) termination of pregnancy

    Pulmonary embolism following (induced) termination of pregnancy

    Pyemic embolism following (induced) termination of pregnancy

    Septic or septicopyemic embolism following (induced) termination of pregnancy

    Soap embolism following (induced) termination of pregnancy

● **O04.8**   **(Induced) termination of pregnancy with other and unspecified complications**

O04.80   **(Induced) termination of pregnancy with unspecified complications**   M

O04.81   **Shock following (induced) termination of pregnancy**   M

    Circulatory collapse following (induced) termination of pregnancy

    Shock (postprocedural) following (induced) termination of pregnancy

    Excludes1   shock due to infection following (induced) termination of pregnancy (O04.87)

O04.82   **Renal failure following (induced) termination of pregnancy**   M

    Kidney failure (acute) following (induced) termination of pregnancy

    Oliguria following (induced) termination of pregnancy

    Renal shutdown following (induced) termination of pregnancy

    Renal tubular necrosis following (induced) termination of pregnancy

    Uremia following (induced) termination of pregnancy

O04.83   **Metabolic disorder following (induced) termination of pregnancy**   M

O04.84   **Damage to pelvic organs following (induced) termination of pregnancy**   M

    Laceration, perforation, tear or chemical damage of bladder following (induced) termination of pregnancy

    Laceration, perforation, tear or chemical damage of bowel following (induced) termination of pregnancy

    Laceration, perforation, tear or chemical damage of broad ligament following (induced) termination of pregnancy

    Laceration, perforation, tear or chemical damage of cervix following (induced) termination of pregnancy

    Laceration, perforation, tear or chemical damage of periurethral tissue following (induced) termination of pregnancy

    Laceration, perforation, tear or chemical damage of uterus following (induced) termination of pregnancy

    Laceration, perforation, tear or chemical damage of vagina following (induced) termination of pregnancy

O04.85   **Other venous complications following (induced) termination of pregnancy**   M

O04.86   **Cardiac arrest following (induced) termination of pregnancy**   M

O04.87   **Sepsis following (induced) termination of pregnancy**   M

Use additional code to identify infectious agent (B95-B97)

Use additional code to identify severe sepsis, if applicable (R65.2-)

Excludes1   septic or septicopyemic embolism following (induced) termination of pregnancy (O04.7)

O04.88   **Urinary tract infection following (induced) termination of pregnancy**   M

Cystitis following (induced) termination of pregnancy

O04.89   **(Induced) termination of pregnancy with other complications**   M

● **O07**   **Failed attempted termination of pregnancy**

Includes   failure of attempted induction of termination of pregnancy
incomplete elective abortion

Excludes1   incomplete spontaneous abortion (O03.0-)

Coding Clinic: 2023, Q1, P17

O07.0   **Genital tract and pelvic infection following failed attempted termination of pregnancy**   M

Endometritis following failed attempted termination of pregnancy

Oophoritis following failed attempted termination of pregnancy

Parametritis following failed attempted termination of pregnancy

Pelvic peritonitis following failed attempted termination of pregnancy

Salpingitis following failed attempted termination of pregnancy

Salpingo-oophoritis following failed attempted termination of pregnancy

Excludes1   sepsis following failed attempted termination of pregnancy (O07.37)
urinary tract infection following failed attempted termination of pregnancy (O07.38)

O07.1   **Delayed or excessive hemorrhage following failed attempted termination of pregnancy**   M

Afibrinogenemia following failed attempted termination of pregnancy

Defibrination syndrome following failed attempted termination of pregnancy

Hemolysis following failed attempted termination of pregnancy

Intravascular coagulation following failed attempted termination of pregnancy

O07.2   **Embolism following failed attempted termination of pregnancy**   M

Air embolism following failed attempted termination of pregnancy

Amniotic fluid embolism following failed attempted termination of pregnancy

Blood-clot embolism following failed attempted termination of pregnancy

Embolism NOS following failed attempted termination of pregnancy

Fat embolism following failed attempted termination of pregnancy

Pulmonary embolism following failed attempted termination of pregnancy

Pyemic embolism following failed attempted termination of pregnancy

Septic or septicopyemic embolism following failed attempted termination of pregnancy

Soap embolism following failed attempted termination of pregnancy

● **O07.3**   **Failed attempted termination of pregnancy with other and unspecified complications**

O07.30   **Failed attempted termination of pregnancy with unspecified complications**   M

O07.31   **Shock following failed attempted termination of pregnancy**   M

Circulatory collapse following failed attempted termination of pregnancy

Shock (postprocedural) following failed attempted termination of pregnancy

Excludes1   shock due to infection following failed attempted termination of pregnancy (O07.37)

O07.32   **Renal failure following failed attempted termination of pregnancy**   M

Kidney failure (acute) following failed attempted termination of pregnancy

Oliguria following failed attempted termination of pregnancy

Renal shutdown following failed attempted termination of pregnancy

Renal tubular necrosis following failed attempted termination of pregnancy

Uremia following failed attempted termination of pregnancy

O07.33   **Metabolic disorder following failed attempted termination of pregnancy**   M

O07.34   **Damage to pelvic organs following failed attempted termination of pregnancy**   M

Laceration, perforation, tear or chemical damage of bladder following failed attempted termination of pregnancy

Laceration, perforation, tear or chemical damage of bowel following failed attempted termination of pregnancy

Laceration, perforation, tear or chemical damage of broad ligament following failed attempted termination of pregnancy

Laceration, perforation, tear or chemical damage of cervix following failed attempted termination of pregnancy

Laceration, perforation, tear or chemical damage of periurethral tissue following failed attempted termination of pregnancy

Laceration, perforation, tear or chemical damage of uterus following failed attempted termination of pregnancy

Laceration, perforation, tear or chemical damage of vagina following failed attempted termination of pregnancy

O07.35   **Other venous complications following failed attempted termination of pregnancy**   M

O07.36   **Cardiac arrest following failed attempted termination of pregnancy**   M

O07.37   **Sepsis following failed attempted termination of pregnancy**   M

Use additional code (B95-B97), to identify infectious agent

Use additional code (R65.2-) to identify severe sepsis, if applicable

Excludes1   septic or septicopyemic embolism following failed attempted termination of pregnancy (O07.2)

O07.38   **Urinary tract infection following failed attempted termination of pregnancy**   M

Cystitis following failed attempted termination of pregnancy

O07.39   **Failed attempted termination of pregnancy with other complications**   M

O07.4   **Failed attempted termination of pregnancy without complication**   M

▶ New   ⇒ Revised   ~~deleted~~ Deleted   Excludes 1   Excludes 2   Includes   Use additional   Code first   Code also   Key words

OGCR Official Guidelines   X Assign placeholder X   ● Use Additional Character(s)   ▶ Manifestation Code   🏷 Hierarchical Condition Category   Coding Clinic

● O08 **Complications following ectopic and molar**
       pregnancy
       This category is for use with categories O00-O02 to identify any
       associated complications.
       Coding Clinic: 2023, Q1, P17

   O08.0 **Genital tract and pelvic infection** following ectopic and
          molar pregnancy   M
          Endometritis following ectopic and molar pregnancy
          Oophoritis following ectopic and molar pregnancy
          Parametritis following ectopic and molar pregnancy
          Pelvic peritonitis following ectopic and molar
            pregnancy
          Salpingitis following ectopic and molar pregnancy
          Salpingo-oophoritis following ectopic and molar
            pregnancy
          Excludes1   sepsis following ectopic and molar
                          pregnancy (O08.82)
                          urinary tract infection (O08.83)

   O08.1 **Delayed or excessive hemorrhage** following ectopic and
          molar pregnancy   M
          Afibrinogenemia following ectopic and molar
            pregnancy
          Defibrination syndrome following ectopic and molar
            pregnancy
          Hemolysis following ectopic and molar pregnancy
          Intravascular coagulation following ectopic and molar
            pregnancy
          Excludes1   delayed or excessive hemorrhage due to
                          incomplete abortion (O03.1)

   O08.2 **Embolism following ectopic and molar pregnancy**   M
          Air embolism following ectopic and molar pregnancy
          Amniotic fluid embolism following ectopic and molar
            pregnancy
          Blood-clot embolism following ectopic and molar
            pregnancy
          Embolism NOS following ectopic and molar pregnancy
          Fat embolism following ectopic and molar pregnancy
          Pulmonary embolism following ectopic and molar
            pregnancy
          Pyemic embolism following ectopic and molar pregnancy
          Septic or septicopyemic embolism following ectopic
            and molar pregnancy
          Soap embolism following ectopic and molar pregnancy

   O08.3 **Shock following ectopic and molar pregnancy**   M
          Circulatory collapse following ectopic and molar
            pregnancy
          Shock (postprocedural) following ectopic and molar
            pregnancy
          Excludes1   shock due to infection following ectopic
                          and molar pregnancy (O08.82)

   O08.4 **Renal failure** following ectopic and molar
          pregnancy   M
          Kidney failure (acute) following ectopic and molar
            pregnancy
          Oliguria following ectopic and molar pregnancy
          Renal shutdown following ectopic and molar
            pregnancy
          Renal tubular necrosis following ectopic and molar
            pregnancy
          Uremia following ectopic and molar pregnancy

   O08.5 **Metabolic disorders following an ectopic and molar**
          pregnancy   M

   O08.6 **Damage to pelvic organs** and tissues following an
          ectopic and molar pregnancy   M
          Laceration, perforation, tear or chemical damage of
            bladder following an ectopic and molar pregnancy
          Laceration, perforation, tear or chemical damage of bowel
            following an ectopic and molar pregnancy
          Laceration, perforation, tear or chemical damage of broad
            ligament following an ectopic and molar pregnancy
          Laceration, perforation, tear or chemical damage of cervix
            following an ectopic and molar pregnancy
          Laceration, perforation, tear or chemical damage of
            periurethral tissue following an ectopic and molar
            pregnancy
          Laceration, perforation, tear or chemical damage of uterus
            following an ectopic and molar pregnancy
          Laceration, perforation, tear or chemical damage of
            vagina following an ectopic and molar pregnancy

   O08.7 **Other venous complications** following an ectopic and
          molar pregnancy   M

● O08.8 **Other complications** following an ectopic and molar
          pregnancy

   O08.81 **Cardiac arrest** following an ectopic and molar
           pregnancy   M

   O08.82 **Sepsis** following ectopic and molar
           pregnancy   M
           Use additional code (B95-B97), to identify
             infectious agent
           Use additional code (R65.2-) to identify severe
             sepsis, if applicable
           Excludes1   septic or septicopyemic
                           embolism following ectopic
                           and molar pregnancy
                           (O08.2)

   O08.83 **Urinary tract** infection following an ectopic and
           molar pregnancy   M
           Cystitis following an ectopic and molar
             pregnancy

   O08.89 **Other** complications following an ectopic and
           molar pregnancy   M

   O08.9 **Unspecified** complication following an ectopic and
          molar pregnancy   M

SUPERVISION OF HIGH RISK PREGNANCY (O09)

● O09 **Supervision of high risk pregnancy**
       Coding Clinic: 2016, Q4, P125, 150

   ● O09.0 **Supervision of pregnancy with history of infertility**

      O09.00 **Supervision of pregnancy with history of**
              infertility, unspecified trimester   M

      O09.01 **Supervision of pregnancy with history of**
              infertility, first trimester   M

      O09.02 **Supervision of pregnancy with history of**
              infertility, second trimester   M

      O09.03 **Supervision of pregnancy with history of**
              infertility, third trimester   M

   ● O09.1 **Supervision of pregnancy with history of ectopic**
            pregnancy
            Coding Clinic: 2016, Q4, P49-50

      O09.10 **Supervision of pregnancy with history of**
              ectopic pregnancy, unspecified trimester   M

      O09.11 **Supervision of pregnancy with history**
              of ectopic pregnancy, first trimester   M

      O09.12 **Supervision of pregnancy with history**
              of ectopic pregnancy, second trimester   M

      O09.13 **Supervision of pregnancy with history**
              of ectopic pregnancy, third trimester   M

● **O09.A Supervision of pregnancy with history of molar pregnancy**
Coding Clinic: 2016, Q4, P50

  O09.A0 Supervision of pregnancy with history of molar pregnancy, unspecified trimester   M

  O09.A1 Supervision of pregnancy with history of molar pregnancy, first trimester   M

  O09.A2 Supervision of pregnancy with history of molar pregnancy, second trimester   M

  O09.A3 Supervision of pregnancy with history of molar pregnancy, third trimester   M

● **O09.2 Supervision of pregnancy with other poor reproductive or obstetric history**

  Excludes2 pregnancy care for patient with history of recurrent pregnancy loss (O26.2-)

 ● **O09.21 Supervision of pregnancy with history of pre-term labor**

  O09.211 Supervision of pregnancy with history of pre-term labor, first trimester   M

  O09.212 Supervision of pregnancy with history of pre-term labor, second trimester   M

  O09.213 Supervision of pregnancy with history of pre-term labor, third trimester   M

  O09.219 Supervision of pregnancy with history of pre-term labor, unspecified trimester   M

 ● **O09.29 Supervision of pregnancy with other poor reproductive or obstetric history**
  Supervision of pregnancy with history of neonatal death
  Supervision of pregnancy with history of stillbirth

  O09.291 Supervision of pregnancy with other poor reproductive or obstetric history, first trimester   M

  O09.292 Supervision of pregnancy with other poor reproductive or obstetric history, second trimester   M

  O09.293 Supervision of pregnancy with other poor reproductive or obstetric history, third trimester   M

  O09.299 Supervision of pregnancy with other poor reproductive or obstetric history, unspecified trimester   M

● **O09.3 Supervision of pregnancy with insufficient antenatal care**
  Supervision of concealed pregnancy
  Supervision of hidden pregnancy

  O09.30 Supervision of pregnancy with insufficient antenatal care, unspecified trimester   M

  O09.31 Supervision of pregnancy with insufficient antenatal care, first trimester   M

  O09.32 Supervision of pregnancy with insufficient antenatal care, second trimester   M

  O09.33 Supervision of pregnancy with insufficient antenatal care, third trimester   M

● **O09.4 Supervision of pregnancy with grand multiparity**

  O09.40 Supervision of pregnancy with grand multiparity, unspecified trimester   M

  O09.41 Supervision of pregnancy with grand multiparity, first trimester   M

  O09.42 Supervision of pregnancy with grand multiparity, second trimester   M

  O09.43 Supervision of pregnancy with grand multiparity, third trimester   M

● **O09.5 Supervision of elderly primigravida and multigravida**
Pregnancy for a female 35 years and older at expected date of delivery

 ● **O09.51 Supervision of elderly primigravida**

  O09.511 Supervision of elderly primigravida, first trimester   M

  O09.512 Supervision of elderly primigravida, second trimester   M

  O09.513 Supervision of elderly primigravida, third trimester   M

  O09.519 Supervision of elderly primigravida, unspecified trimester   M

 ● **O09.52 Supervision of elderly multigravida**

  O09.521 Supervision of elderly multigravida, first trimester   M

  O09.522 Supervision of elderly multigravida, second trimester   M

  O09.523 Supervision of elderly multigravida, third trimester   M
Coding Clinic: 2016, Q4, P150

  O09.529 Supervision of elderly multigravida, unspecified trimester   M

● **O09.6 Supervision of young primigravida and multigravida**
Supervision of pregnancy for a female less than 16 years old at expected date of delivery

 ● **O09.61 Supervision of young primigravida**

  O09.611 Supervision of young primigravida, first trimester   M

  O09.612 Supervision of young primigravida, second trimester   M

  O09.613 Supervision of young primigravida, third trimester   M

  O09.619 Supervision of young primigravida, unspecified trimester   M

 ● **O09.62 Supervision of young multigravida**

  O09.621 Supervision of young multigravida, first trimester   M

  O09.622 Supervision of young multigravida, second trimester   M

  O09.623 Supervision of young multigravida, third trimester   M

  O09.629 Supervision of young multigravida, unspecified trimester   M

● **O09.7 Supervision of high risk pregnancy due to social problems**

  O09.70 Supervision of high risk pregnancy due to social problems, unspecified trimester   M

  O09.71 Supervision of high risk pregnancy due to social problems, first trimester   M

  O09.72 Supervision of high risk pregnancy due to social problems, second trimester   M

  O09.73 Supervision of high risk pregnancy due to social problems, third trimester   M

● **O09.8 Supervision of other high risk pregnancies**

 ● **O09.81 Supervision of pregnancy resulting from assisted reproductive technology**
  Supervision of pregnancy resulting from in-vitro fertilization

  Excludes2 gestational carrier status (Z33.3)

  O09.811 Supervision of pregnancy resulting from assisted reproductive technology, first trimester   M

  O09.812 Supervision of pregnancy resulting from assisted reproductive technology, second trimester   M

▶ New   ⇒ Revised   ~~deleted~~ Deleted   Excludes 1   Excludes 2   Includes   Use additional   Code first   Code also   Key words
OGCR Official Guidelines   X Assign placeholder X   ● Use Additional Character(s)   ▷ Manifestation Code   Hierarchical Condition Category   Coding Clinic

O09.813 Supervision of pregnancy resulting from assisted reproductive technology, third trimester M

O09.819 Supervision of pregnancy resulting from assisted reproductive technology, unspecified trimester M

● O09.82 Supervision of pregnancy with history of in utero procedure during previous pregnancy

O09.821 Supervision of pregnancy with history of in utero procedure during previous pregnancy, first trimester M

O09.822 Supervision of pregnancy with history of in utero procedure during previous pregnancy, second trimester M

O09.823 Supervision of pregnancy with history of in utero procedure during previous pregnancy, third trimester M

O09.829 Supervision of pregnancy with history of in utero procedure during previous pregnancy, unspecified trimester M

Excludes1 supervision of pregnancy affected by in utero procedure during current pregnancy (O35.7)

● O09.89 Supervision of other high risk pregnancies

O09.891 Supervision of other high risk pregnancies, first trimester M

O09.892 Supervision of other high risk pregnancies, second trimester M

O09.893 Supervision of other high risk pregnancies, third trimester M

O09.899 Supervision of other high risk pregnancies, unspecified trimester M

● O09.9 Supervision of high risk pregnancy, unspecified

O09.90 Supervision of high risk pregnancy, unspecified, unspecified trimester M

O09.91 Supervision of high risk pregnancy, unspecified, first trimester M

O09.92 Supervision of high risk pregnancy, unspecified, second trimester M

O09.93 Supervision of high risk pregnancy, unspecified, third trimester M

EDEMA, PROTEINURIA AND HYPERTENSIVE DISORDERS IN PREGNANCY, CHILDBIRTH AND THE PUERPERIUM (O10-O16)

● O10 Pre-existing hypertension complicating pregnancy, childbirth and the puerperium

Includes pre-existing hypertension with pre-existing proteinuria complicating pregnancy, childbirth and the puerperium

Excludes2 pre-existing hypertension with superimposed pre-eclampsia complicating pregnancy, childbirth and the puerperium (O11.-)

Coding Clinic: 2016, Q4, P50

● O10.0 Pre-existing essential hypertension complicating pregnancy, childbirth and the puerperium
Any condition in I10 specified as a reason for obstetric care during pregnancy, childbirth or the puerperium

● O10.01 Pre-existing essential hypertension complicating pregnancy

O10.011 Pre-existing essential hypertension complicating pregnancy, first trimester M

O10.012 Pre-existing essential hypertension complicating pregnancy, second trimester M

O10.013 Pre-existing essential hypertension complicating pregnancy, third trimester M

O10.019 Pre-existing essential hypertension complicating pregnancy, unspecified trimester M

O10.02 Pre-existing essential hypertension complicating childbirth M

O10.03 Pre-existing essential hypertension complicating the puerperium M

● O10.1 Pre-existing hypertensive heart disease complicating pregnancy, childbirth and the puerperium
Any condition in I11 specified as a reason for obstetric care during pregnancy, childbirth or the puerperium
Use additional code from I11 to identify the type of hypertensive heart disease

● O10.11 Pre-existing hypertensive heart disease complicating pregnancy

O10.111 Pre-existing hypertensive heart disease complicating pregnancy, first trimester M

O10.112 Pre-existing hypertensive heart disease complicating pregnancy, second trimester M

O10.113 Pre-existing hypertensive heart disease complicating pregnancy, third trimester M

O10.119 Pre-existing hypertensive heart disease complicating pregnancy, unspecified trimester M

O10.12 Pre-existing hypertensive heart disease complicating childbirth M

O10.13 Pre-existing hypertensive heart disease complicating the puerperium M

● O10.2 Pre-existing hypertensive chronic kidney disease complicating pregnancy, childbirth and the puerperium
Any condition in I12 specified as a reason for obstetric care during pregnancy, childbirth or the puerperium
Use additional code from I12 to identify the type of hypertensive chronic kidney disease

● O10.21 Pre-existing hypertensive chronic kidney disease complicating pregnancy

O10.211 Pre-existing hypertensive chronic kidney disease complicating pregnancy, first trimester M

O10.212 Pre-existing hypertensive chronic kidney disease complicating pregnancy, second trimester M

O10.213 Pre-existing hypertensive chronic kidney disease complicating pregnancy, third trimester M

O10.219 Pre-existing hypertensive chronic kidney disease complicating pregnancy, unspecified trimester M

O10.22 Pre-existing hypertensive chronic kidney disease complicating childbirth M

O10.23 Pre-existing hypertensive chronic kidney disease complicating the puerperium M

● **O10.3 Pre-existing hypertensive heart and chronic kidney disease complicating pregnancy, childbirth and the puerperium**

> Any condition in I13 specified as a reason for obstetric care during pregnancy, childbirth or the puerperium
>
> Use additional code from I13 to identify the type of hypertensive heart and chronic kidney disease

● **O10.31 Pre-existing hypertensive heart and chronic kidney disease complicating pregnancy**

     O10.311 Pre-existing hypertensive heart and chronic kidney disease complicating pregnancy, first trimester   M

     O10.312 Pre-existing hypertensive heart and chronic kidney disease complicating pregnancy, second trimester   M

     O10.313 Pre-existing hypertensive heart and chronic kidney disease complicating pregnancy, third trimester   M

     O10.319 Pre-existing hypertensive heart and chronic kidney disease complicating pregnancy, unspecified trimester   M

   O10.32 Pre-existing hypertensive heart and chronic kidney disease complicating childbirth   M

   O10.33 Pre-existing hypertensive heart and chronic kidney disease complicating the puerperium   M

● **O10.4 Pre-existing secondary hypertension complicating pregnancy, childbirth and the puerperium**

> Any condition in I15 specified as a reason for obstetric care during pregnancy, childbirth or the puerperium
>
> Use additional code from I15 to identify the type of secondary hypertension

● **O10.41 Pre-existing secondary hypertension complicating pregnancy**

     O10.411 Pre-existing secondary hypertension complicating pregnancy, first trimester   M

     O10.412 Pre-existing secondary hypertension complicating pregnancy, second trimester   M

     O10.413 Pre-existing secondary hypertension complicating pregnancy, third trimester   M

     O10.419 Pre-existing secondary hypertension complicating pregnancy, unspecified trimester   M

   O10.42 Pre-existing secondary hypertension complicating childbirth   M

   O10.43 Pre-existing secondary hypertension complicating the puerperium   M

● **O10.9 Unspecified pre-existing hypertension complicating pregnancy, childbirth and the puerperium**

● **O10.91 Unspecified pre-existing hypertension complicating pregnancy**

     O10.911 Unspecified pre-existing hypertension complicating pregnancy, first trimester   M

     O10.912 Unspecified pre-existing hypertension complicating pregnancy, second trimester   M

     O10.913 Unspecified pre-existing hypertension complicating pregnancy, third trimester   M

     O10.919 Unspecified pre-existing hypertension complicating pregnancy, unspecified trimester   M

   O10.92 Unspecified pre-existing hypertension complicating childbirth   M

   O10.93 Unspecified pre-existing hypertension complicating the puerperium   M

● **O11 Pre-existing hypertension with pre-eclampsia**

> **Includes**   conditions in O10 complicated by pre-eclampsia pre-eclampsia superimposed pre-existing hypertension
>
> Use additional code from O10 to identify the type of hypertension
>
> Coding Clinic: 2016, Q4, P50

   O11.1 Pre-existing hypertension with pre-eclampsia, first trimester   M

   O11.2 Pre-existing hypertension with pre-eclampsia, second trimester   M

   O11.3 Pre-existing hypertension with pre-eclampsia, third trimester   M

   O11.4 Pre-existing hypertension with pre-eclampsia, complicating childbirth   M

   O11.5 Pre-existing hypertension with pre-eclampsia, complicating the puerperium   M

   O11.9 Pre-existing hypertension with pre-eclampsia, unspecified trimester   M

● **O12 Gestational [pregnancy-induced] edema and proteinuria without hypertension**

> Coding Clinic: 2016, Q4, P50

● **O12.0 Gestational edema**

     O12.00 Gestational edema, unspecified trimester   M

     O12.01 Gestational edema, first trimester   M

     O12.02 Gestational edema, second trimester   M

     O12.03 Gestational edema, third trimester   M

     O12.04 Gestational edema, complicating childbirth   M

     O12.05 Gestational edema, complicating the puerperium   M

● **O12.1 Gestational proteinuria**

     O12.10 Gestational proteinuria, unspecified trimester   M

     O12.11 Gestational proteinuria, first trimester   M

     O12.12 Gestational proteinuria, second trimester   M

     O12.13 Gestational proteinuria, third trimester   M

     O12.14 Gestational proteinuria, complicating childbirth   M

     O12.15 Gestational proteinuria, complicating the puerperium   M

● **O12.2 Gestational edema with proteinuria**

     O12.20 Gestational edema with proteinuria, unspecified trimester   M

     O12.21 Gestational edema with proteinuria, first trimester   M

     O12.22 Gestational edema with proteinuria, second trimester   M

     O12.23 Gestational edema with proteinuria, third trimester   M

     O12.24 Gestational edema with proteinuria, complicating childbirth   M

     O12.25 Gestational edema with proteinuria, complicating the puerperium   M

● **O13 Gestational [pregnancy-induced] hypertension without significant proteinuria**

> **Includes**   gestational hypertension NOS transient hypertension of pregnancy
>
> Coding Clinic: 2016, Q4, P50

   O13.1 Gestational [pregnancy-induced] hypertension without significant proteinuria, first trimester   M

   O13.2 Gestational [pregnancy-induced] hypertension without significant proteinuria, second trimester   M

   O13.3 Gestational [pregnancy-induced] hypertension without significant proteinuria, third trimester   M

   O13.4 Gestational [pregnancy-induced] hypertension without significant proteinuria, complicating childbirth   M

   O13.5 Gestational [pregnancy-induced] hypertension without significant proteinuria, complicating the puerperium   M

   O13.9 Gestational [pregnancy-induced] hypertension without significant proteinuria, unspecified trimester   M

▶ New   ⇒ Revised   ~~deleted~~ Deleted   Excludes 1   Excludes 2   Includes   Use additional   Code first   Code also   Key words

OGCR Official Guidelines   X Assign placeholder X   ● Use Additional Character(s)   ▶ Manifestation Code   🦪 Hierarchical Condition Category   Coding Clinic

● **O14** **Pre-eclampsia**

    Excludes1   pre-existing hypertension with pre-eclampsia (O11)

    Coding Clinic: 2016, Q4, P50

  ● **O14.0** Mild to moderate pre-eclampsia

      O14.00   Mild to moderate pre-eclampsia, unspecified trimester   **M**

      O14.02   Mild to moderate pre-eclampsia, second trimester   **M**

      O14.03   Mild to moderate pre-eclampsia, third trimester   **M**

      O14.04   Mild to moderate pre-eclampsia, complicating childbirth
          Coding Clinic: 2019, Q2, P8   **M**

      O14.05   Mild to moderate pre-eclampsia, complicating the puerperium   **M**

  ● **O14.1** Severe pre-eclampsia

      Excludes1   HELLP syndrome (O14.2-)

      H=hemolysis, EL=elevated liver enzymes, LP=low platelet count

      Coding Clinic: 2019, Q3, P12

      O14.10   Severe pre-eclampsia, unspecified trimester   **M**

      O14.12   Severe pre-eclampsia, second trimester   **M**

      O14.13   Severe pre-eclampsia, third trimester   **M**

      O14.14   Severe pre-eclampsia complicating childbirth   **M**

      O14.15   Severe pre-eclampsia, complicating the puerperium   **M**

  ● **O14.2** HELLP syndrome

      Severe pre-eclampsia with hemolysis, elevated liver enzymes and low platelet count (HELLP)

      O14.20   HELLP syndrome (HELLP), unspecified trimester   **M**

      O14.22   HELLP syndrome (HELLP), second trimester   **M**

      O14.23   HELLP syndrome (HELLP), third trimester   **M**

      O14.24   HELLP syndrome, complicating childbirth   **M**

      O14.25   HELLP syndrome, complicating the puerperium   **M**

  ● **O14.9** Unspecified pre-eclampsia

      O14.90   Unspecified pre-eclampsia, unspecified trimester   **M**

      O14.92   Unspecified pre-eclampsia, second trimester   **M**

      O14.93   Unspecified pre-eclampsia, third trimester   **M**

      O14.94   Unspecified pre-eclampsia, complicating childbirth   **M**

      O14.95   Unspecified pre-eclampsia, complicating the puerperium   **M**

● **O15** **Eclampsia**

    Includes   convulsions following conditions in O10-O14 and O16

  ● **O15.0** Eclampsia complicating pregnancy
      Coding Clinic: 2016, Q4, P50

      O15.00   Eclampsia complicating pregnancy, unspecified trimester   **M**

      O15.02   Eclampsia complicating pregnancy, second trimester   **M**

      O15.03   Eclampsia complicating pregnancy, third trimester   **M**

    O15.1   Eclampsia complicating labor   **M**

    O15.2   Eclampsia complicating the puerperium   **M**

    O15.9   Eclampsia, unspecified as to time period   **M**
      Eclampsia NOS

● **O16** **Unspecified maternal hypertension**
    Coding Clinic: 2016, Q4, P50

    O16.1   Unspecified maternal hypertension, first trimester   **M**

    O16.2   Unspecified maternal hypertension, second trimester   **M**

    O16.3   Unspecified maternal hypertension, third trimester   **M**

    O16.4   Unspecified maternal hypertension, complicating childbirth   **M**

    O16.5   Unspecified maternal hypertension, complicating the puerperium   **M**

    O16.9   Unspecified maternal hypertension, unspecified trimester   **M**

OTHER MATERNAL DISORDERS PREDOMINANTLY RELATED TO PREGNANCY (O20-O29)

    Excludes2   maternal care related to the fetus and amniotic cavity and possible delivery problems (O30-O48)

             maternal diseases classifiable elsewhere but complicating pregnancy, labor and delivery, and the puerperium (O98-O99)

● **O20** **Hemorrhage in early pregnancy**

    Includes   hemorrhage before completion of 20 weeks gestation

    Excludes1   pregnancy with abortive outcome (O00-O08)

    O20.0   Threatened abortion   **M**
      Hemorrhage specified as due to threatened abortion

    O20.8   Other hemorrhage in early pregnancy   **M**
      Coding Clinic: 2023, Q3, P18

    O20.9   Hemorrhage in early pregnancy, unspecified   **M**

● **O21** **Excessive vomiting in pregnancy**

    O21.0   Mild hyperemesis gravidarum   **M**
      Hyperemesis gravidarum, mild or unspecified, starting before the end of the 20th week of gestation

    O21.1   Hyperemesis gravidarum with metabolic disturbance   **M**
      Hyperemesis gravidarum, starting before the end of the 20th week of gestation, with metabolic disturbance such as carbohydrate depletion
      Hyperemesis gravidarum, starting before the end of the 20th week of gestation, with metabolic disturbance such as dehydration
      Hyperemesis gravidarum, starting before the end of the 20th week of gestation, with metabolic disturbance such as electrolyte imbalance

    O21.2   Late vomiting of pregnancy   **M**
      Excessive vomiting starting after 20 completed weeks of gestation

    O21.8   Other vomiting complicating pregnancy   **M**
      Vomiting due to diseases classified elsewhere, complicating pregnancy
      Use additional code, to identify cause

    O21.9   Vomiting of pregnancy, unspecified   **M**

● **O22** **Venous complications and hemorrhoids in pregnancy**

    Excludes1   venous complications of:
          abortion NOS (O03.9)
          ectopic or molar pregnancy (O08.7)
          failed attempted abortion (O07.35)
          induced abortion (O04.85)
          spontaneous abortion (O03.89)

    Excludes2   obstetric pulmonary embolism (O88.-)
          venous complications and hemorrhoids of childbirth and the puerperium (O87.-)

● **O22.0   Varicose veins of lower extremity in pregnancy**
Varicose veins NOS in pregnancy

     O22.00   Varicose veins of lower extremity in pregnancy, unspecified trimester   M

     O22.01   Varicose veins of lower extremity in pregnancy, first trimester   M

     O22.02   Varicose veins of lower extremity in pregnancy, second trimester   M

     O22.03   Varicose veins of lower extremity in pregnancy, third trimester   M

● **O22.1   Genital varices in pregnancy**
Perineal varices in pregnancy
Vaginal varices in pregnancy
Vulval varices in pregnancy

     O22.10   Genital varices in pregnancy, unspecified trimester   M

     O22.11   Genital varices in pregnancy, first trimester   M

     O22.12   Genital varices in pregnancy, second trimester   M

     O22.13   Genital varices in pregnancy, third trimester   M

● **O22.2   Superficial thrombophlebitis in pregnancy**
Phlebitis in pregnancy NOS
Thrombophlebitis of legs in pregnancy
Thrombosis in pregnancy NOS

Use additional code to identify the superficial thrombophlebitis (I80.0-)

     O22.20   Superficial thrombophlebitis in pregnancy, unspecified trimester   M

     O22.21   Superficial thrombophlebitis in pregnancy, first trimester   M

     O22.22   Superficial thrombophlebitis in pregnancy, second trimester   M

     O22.23   Superficial thrombophlebitis in pregnancy, third trimester   M

● **O22.3   Deep phlebothrombosis in pregnancy**
Deep vein thrombosis, antepartum

Use additional code to identify the deep vein thrombosis (I82.4-, I82.5-, I82.62-, I82.72-)

Use additional code, if applicable, for associated long-term (current) use of anticoagulants (Z79.01)

     O22.30   Deep phlebothrombosis in pregnancy, unspecified trimester   M

     O22.31   Deep phlebothrombosis in pregnancy, first trimester   M

     O22.32   Deep phlebothrombosis in pregnancy, second trimester   M

     O22.33   Deep phlebothrombosis in pregnancy, third trimester   M

● **O22.4   Hemorrhoids in pregnancy**

     O22.40   Hemorrhoids in pregnancy, unspecified trimester   M

     O22.41   Hemorrhoids in pregnancy, first trimester   M

     O22.42   Hemorrhoids in pregnancy, second trimester   M

     O22.43   Hemorrhoids in pregnancy, third trimester   M

● **O22.5   Cerebral venous thrombosis in pregnancy**
Cerebrovenous sinus thrombosis in pregnancy

     O22.50   Cerebral venous thrombosis in pregnancy, unspecified trimester   M

     O22.51   Cerebral venous thrombosis in pregnancy, first trimester   M

     O22.52   Cerebral venous thrombosis in pregnancy, second trimester   M

     O22.53   Cerebral venous thrombosis in pregnancy, third trimester   M

● **O22.8   Other venous complications in pregnancy**

     ● **O22.8X   Other venous complications in pregnancy**

         O22.8X1   Other venous complications in pregnancy, first trimester   M

         O22.8X2   Other venous complications in pregnancy, second trimester   M

         O22.8X3   Other venous complications in pregnancy, third trimester   M

         O22.8X9   Other venous complications in pregnancy, unspecified trimester   M

● **O22.9   Venous complication in pregnancy, unspecified**
Gestational phlebitis NOS
Gestational phlebopathy NOS
Gestational thrombosis NOS

     O22.90   Venous complication in pregnancy, unspecified, unspecified trimester   M

     O22.91   Venous complication in pregnancy, unspecified, first trimester   M

     O22.92   Venous complication in pregnancy, unspecified, second trimester   M

     O22.93   Venous complication in pregnancy, unspecified, third trimester   M

● **O23   Infections of genitourinary tract in pregnancy**

Use additional code to identify organism (B95.-, B96.-)

Excludes2   gonococcal infections complicating pregnancy, childbirth and the puerperium (O98.2)
infections with a predominantly sexual mode of transmission NOS complicating pregnancy, childbirth and the puerperium (O98.3)
syphilis complicating pregnancy, childbirth and the puerperium (O98.1)
tuberculosis of genitourinary system complicating pregnancy, childbirth and the puerperium (O98.0)
venereal disease NOS complicating pregnancy, childbirth and the puerperium (O98.3)

● **O23.0   Infections of kidney in pregnancy**
Pyelonephritis in pregnancy

     O23.00   Infections of kidney in pregnancy, unspecified trimester   M

     O23.01   Infections of kidney in pregnancy, first trimester   M

     O23.02   Infections of kidney in pregnancy, second trimester   M

     O23.03   Infections of kidney in pregnancy, third trimester   M

● **O23.1   Infections of bladder in pregnancy**

     O23.10   Infections of bladder in pregnancy, unspecified trimester   M

     O23.11   Infections of bladder in pregnancy, first trimester   M

     O23.12   Infections of bladder in pregnancy, second trimester   M

     O23.13   Infections of bladder in pregnancy, third trimester   M

● **O23.2   Infections of urethra in pregnancy**

     O23.20   Infections of urethra in pregnancy, unspecified trimester   M

     O23.21   Infections of urethra in pregnancy, first trimester   M

     O23.22   Infections of urethra in pregnancy, second trimester   M

     O23.23   Infections of urethra in pregnancy, third trimester   M

● O23.3   Infections of other parts of urinary tract in pregnancy

    O23.30   Infections of other parts of urinary tract in pregnancy, unspecified trimester   **M**

    O23.31   Infections of other parts of urinary tract in pregnancy, first trimester   **M**

    O23.32   Infections of other parts of urinary tract in pregnancy, second trimester   **M**

    O23.33   Infections of other parts of urinary tract in pregnancy, third trimester   **M**

● O23.4   Unspecified infection of urinary tract in pregnancy

    O23.40   Unspecified infection of urinary tract in pregnancy, unspecified trimester   **M**

    O23.41   Unspecified infection of urinary tract in pregnancy, first trimester   **M**

    O23.42   Unspecified infection of urinary tract in pregnancy, second trimester   **M**

    O23.43   Unspecified infection of urinary tract in pregnancy, third trimester   **M**

● O23.5   Infections of the genital tract in pregnancy

   ● O23.51   Infection of cervix in pregnancy

       O23.511   Infections of cervix in pregnancy, first trimester   **M**

       O23.512   Infections of cervix in pregnancy, second trimester   **M**

       O23.513   Infections of cervix in pregnancy, third trimester   **M**

       O23.519   Infections of cervix in pregnancy, unspecified trimester   **M**

   ● O23.52   Salpingo-oophoritis in pregnancy

       Oophoritis = inflammation of ovary
       Salpingitis = inflammation of fallopian tube
       Oophoritis in pregnancy
       Salpingitis in pregnancy

       O23.521   Salpingo-oophoritis in pregnancy, first trimester   **M**

       O23.522   Salpingo-oophoritis in pregnancy, second trimester   **M**

       O23.523   Salpingo-oophoritis in pregnancy, third trimester   **M**

       O23.529   Salpingo-oophoritis in pregnancy, unspecified trimester   **M**

   ● O23.59   Infection of other part of genital tract in pregnancy
       Coding Clinic: 2022, Q1, P20

       O23.591   Infection of other part of genital tract in pregnancy, first trimester   **M**

       O23.592   Infection of other part of genital tract in pregnancy, second trimester   **M**

       O23.593   Infection of other part of genital tract in pregnancy, third trimester   **M**
       Coding Clinic: 2022, Q1, P20

       O23.599   Infection of other part of genital tract in pregnancy, unspecified trimester   **M**

● O23.9   Unspecified genitourinary tract infection in pregnancy
    Genitourinary tract infection in pregnancy NOS

    O23.90   Unspecified genitourinary tract infection in pregnancy, unspecified trimester   **M**

    O23.91   Unspecified genitourinary tract infection in pregnancy, first trimester   **M**

    O23.92   Unspecified genitourinary tract infection in pregnancy, second trimester   **M**

    O23.93   Unspecified genitourinary tract infection in pregnancy, third trimester   **M**

OGCR   Section I.C.15.g.

Diabetes mellitus in pregnancy
Diabetes mellitus is a significant complicating factor in pregnancy. Pregnant women who are diabetic should be assigned a code from category O24, Diabetes mellitus in pregnancy, childbirth, and the puerperium, first, followed by the appropriate diabetes code(s) (E08-E13) from Chapter 4.

● O24   Diabetes mellitus in pregnancy, childbirth, and the puerperium

   ● O24.0   Pre-existing type 1 diabetes mellitus, in pregnancy, childbirth and the puerperium
      Juvenile onset diabetes mellitus, in pregnancy, childbirth and the puerperium
      Ketosis-prone diabetes mellitus in pregnancy, childbirth and the puerperium
      Use additional code from category E10 to further identify any manifestations

     ● O24.01   Pre-existing type 1 diabetes mellitus, in pregnancy

        O24.011   Pre-existing type 1 diabetes mellitus, in pregnancy, first trimester   **M**

        O24.012   Pre-existing type 1 diabetes mellitus, in pregnancy, second trimester   **M**

        O24.013   Pre-existing type 1 diabetes mellitus, in pregnancy, third trimester   **M**

        O24.019   Pre-existing type 1 diabetes mellitus, in pregnancy, unspecified trimester   **M**

     O24.02   Pre-existing type 1 diabetes mellitus, in childbirth   **M**

     O24.03   Pre-existing type 1 diabetes mellitus, in the puerperium   **M**

   ● O24.1   Pre-existing type 2 diabetes mellitus, in pregnancy, childbirth and the puerperium
      Insulin-resistant diabetes mellitus in pregnancy, childbirth and the puerperium
      Use additional code (for):
       from category E11 to further identify any manifestations
       long-term (current) use of insulin (Z79.4)
      ▶ Use additional injectable non-insulin antidiabetic drugs (Z79.85)

     ● O24.11   Pre-existing type 2 diabetes mellitus, in pregnancy

        O24.111   Pre-existing type 2 diabetes mellitus, in pregnancy, first trimester   **M**

        O24.112   Pre-existing type 2 diabetes mellitus, in pregnancy, second trimester   **M**

        O24.113   Pre-existing type 2 diabetes mellitus, in pregnancy, third trimester   **M**

        O24.119   Pre-existing type 2 diabetes mellitus, in pregnancy, unspecified trimester   **M**

     O24.12   Pre-existing type 2 diabetes mellitus, in childbirth   **M**

     O24.13   Pre-existing type 2 diabetes mellitus, in the puerperium   **M**

   ● O24.3   Unspecified pre-existing diabetes mellitus in pregnancy, childbirth and the puerperium
      Use additional code (for):
       from category E11 to further identify any manifestation
       long-term (current) use of insulin (Z79.4)
      ▶ Use additional injectable non-insulin antidiabetic drugs (Z79.85)

     ● O24.31   Unspecified pre-existing diabetes mellitus in pregnancy

        O24.311   Unspecified pre-existing diabetes mellitus in pregnancy, first trimester   **M**

        O24.312   Unspecified pre-existing diabetes mellitus in pregnancy, second trimester   **M**

O24.313   Unspecified pre-existing diabetes
mellitus in pregnancy, **third
trimester**   M

O24.319   Unspecified pre-existing diabetes
mellitus in pregnancy, **unspecified
trimester**   M

O24.32   Unspecified pre-existing diabetes mellitus in
childbirth   M

O24.33   Unspecified pre-existing diabetes mellitus in
the puerperium   M

● O24.4   **Gestational diabetes mellitus**
Diabetes mellitus arising in pregnancy
Gestational diabetes mellitus NOS
Coding Clinic: 2016, Q4, P50, 126

● O24.41   Gestational diabetes mellitus in **pregnancy**

O24.410   Gestational diabetes mellitus in
pregnancy, **diet controlled**   M

O24.414   Gestational diabetes mellitus in
pregnancy, **insulin controlled**   M

O24.415   Gestational diabetes mellitus
in pregnancy, **controlled by oral
hypoglycemic drugs**   M
Gestational diabetes mellitus in
pregnancy, controlled by oral
antidiabetic drugs
Coding Clinic: 2016, Q4, P50

O24.419   Gestational diabetes mellitus in
pregnancy, **unspecified control**   M
Coding Clinic: 2015, Q4, P34

● O24.42   Gestational diabetes mellitus in **childbirth**

O24.420   Gestational diabetes mellitus in
childbirth, **diet controlled**   M

O24.424   Gestational diabetes mellitus in
childbirth, **insulin controlled**   M

O24.425   Gestational diabetes mellitus
in childbirth, **controlled by oral
hypoglycemic drugs**   M
Gestational diabetes mellitus in
childbirth, controlled by oral
antidiabetic drugs
Coding Clinic: 2016, Q4, P50

O24.429   Gestational diabetes mellitus in
childbirth, **unspecified control**   M

OGCR Section I.C.15.i.

Gestational (pregnancy induced) diabetes
Gestational (pregnancy induced) diabetes can occur during the second
and third trimester of pregnancy in women who were not diabetic
prior to pregnancy. Gestational diabetes can cause complications
in the pregnancy similar to those of pre-existing diabetes mellitus.
It also puts the woman at greater risk of developing diabetes after
the pregnancy. Codes for gestational diabetes are in subcategory
O24.4, Gestational diabetes mellitus. No other code from category
O24, Diabetes mellitus in pregnancy, childbirth, and the puerperium,
should be used with a code from O24.4

The codes under subcategory O24.4 include diet controlled, insulin
controlled, **and controlled by oral hypoglycemic drugs.** If a patient
with gestational diabetes is treated with both diet and insulin,
only the code for insulin-controlled is required. **If a patient with
gestational diabetes is treated with both diet and oral hypoglycemic
medications, only the code for "controlled by oral hypoglycemic
drugs" is required.** Code Z79.4, Long-term (current) use of insulin **or
code Z79.84, Long-term (current) use of oral hypoglycemic drugs,**
should not be assigned with codes from subcategory O24.4.

An abnormal glucose tolerance in pregnancy is assigned a code from
subcategory O99.81, Abnormal glucose complicating pregnancy,
childbirth, and the puerperium.

● O24.43   Gestational diabetes mellitus in the **puerperium**

O24.430   Gestational diabetes mellitus in the
puerperium, **diet controlled**   M

O24.434   Gestational diabetes mellitus in the
puerperium, **insulin controlled**   M

O24.435   Gestational diabetes mellitus in
puerperium, **controlled by oral
hypoglycemic drugs**   M
Gestational diabetes mellitus in
puerperium, controlled by oral
antidiabetic drugs
Coding Clinic: 2016, Q4, P50

O24.439   Gestational diabetes mellitus in the
puerperium, **unspecified control**   M

● O24.8   **Other pre-existing diabetes mellitus in pregnancy,
childbirth, and the puerperium**
Use additional code (for):
from categories E08, E09 and E13 to further identify
any manifestation
long-term (current) use of insulin (Z79.4)
▶ Use additional injectable non-insulin antidiabetic drugs
(Z79.85)

● O24.81   Other pre-existing diabetes mellitus in
pregnancy

O24.811   Other pre-existing diabetes mellitus
in pregnancy, **first trimester**   M

O24.812   Other pre-existing diabetes mellitus
in pregnancy, **second trimester**   M

O24.813   Other pre-existing diabetes mellitus
in pregnancy, **third trimester**   M

O24.819   Other pre-existing diabetes mellitus
in pregnancy, **unspecified trimester**   M

O24.82   Other pre-existing diabetes mellitus in
childbirth   M

O24.83   Other pre-existing diabetes mellitus in the
puerperium   M

● O24.9   **Unspecified diabetes mellitus in pregnancy, childbirth
and the puerperium**
⟹ Use additional code (for):
▶ from categories E08, E09 and E13 to further
identify any manifestation
▶ injectable non-insulin antidiabetic drugs
(Z79.85)
▶ long-term (current) use of insulin (Z79.4)
*Unknown whether patient was diabetic before pregnancy
occurred*

● O24.91   Unspecified diabetes mellitus in **pregnancy**

O24.911   Unspecified diabetes mellitus in
pregnancy, **first trimester**   M

O24.912   Unspecified diabetes mellitus in
pregnancy, **second trimester**   M

O24.913   Unspecified diabetes mellitus in
pregnancy, **third trimester**   M

O24.919   Unspecified diabetes mellitus in
pregnancy, **unspecified trimester**   M

O24.92   Unspecified diabetes mellitus in **childbirth**   M

O24.93   Unspecified diabetes mellitus in the
puerperium   M

● O25   **Malnutrition** in pregnancy, childbirth and the puerperium

● O25.1   Malnutrition in **pregnancy**

O25.10   Malnutrition in pregnancy, **unspecified
trimester**   M

O25.11   Malnutrition in pregnancy, **first trimester**   M

O25.12   Malnutrition in pregnancy, **second trimester**   M

O25.13   Malnutrition in pregnancy, **third trimester**   M

O25.2   Malnutrition in **childbirth**   M

O25.3   Malnutrition in the **puerperium**   M

● O26   **Maternal care for other conditions predominantly related to
pregnancy**

● O26.0   **Excessive weight gain in pregnancy**
Excludes2   gestational edema (O12.0, O12.2)

O26.00   Excessive weight gain in pregnancy, **unspecified
trimester**   M

O26.01   Excessive weight gain in pregnancy, **first
trimester**   M

O26.02   Excessive weight gain in pregnancy, second
          trimester   M
O26.03   Excessive weight gain in pregnancy, third
          trimester   M
● O26.1   Low weight gain in pregnancy
O26.10   Low weight gain in pregnancy, unspecified
          trimester   M
O26.11   Low weight gain in pregnancy, first trimester   M
O26.12   Low weight gain in pregnancy, second
          trimester   M
O26.13   Low weight gain in pregnancy, third
          trimester   M
● O26.2   Pregnancy care for patient with recurrent pregnancy loss
O26.20   Pregnancy care for patient with recurrent
          pregnancy loss, unspecified trimester   M
O26.21   Pregnancy care for patient with recurrent
          pregnancy loss, first trimester   M
O26.22   Pregnancy care for patient with recurrent
          pregnancy loss, second trimester   M
O26.23   Pregnancy care for patient with recurrent
          pregnancy loss, third trimester   M
● O26.3   Retained intrauterine contraceptive device in pregnancy
O26.30   Retained intrauterine contraceptive device in
          pregnancy, unspecified trimester   M
O26.31   Retained intrauterine contraceptive device in
          pregnancy, first trimester   M
O26.32   Retained intrauterine contraceptive device in
          pregnancy, second trimester   M
O26.33   Retained intrauterine contraceptive device in
          pregnancy, third trimester   M
● O26.4   Herpes gestationis
O26.40   Herpes gestationis, unspecified trimester   M
O26.41   Herpes gestationis, first trimester   M
O26.42   Herpes gestationis, second trimester   M
O26.43   Herpes gestationis, third trimester   M
● O26.5   Maternal hypotension syndrome
          Supine hypotensive syndrome
O26.50   Maternal hypotension syndrome, unspecified
          trimester   M
O26.51   Maternal hypotension syndrome, first
          trimester   M
O26.52   Maternal hypotension syndrome, second
          trimester   M
O26.53   Maternal hypotension syndrome, third
          trimester   M
● O26.6   Liver and biliary tract disorders in pregnancy, childbirth
          and the puerperium
          Use additional code to identify the specific disorder
          Excludes2 hepatorenal syndrome following labor
                         and delivery (O90.41)
● O26.61 Liver and biliary tract disorders in
          pregnancy
O26.611   Liver and biliary tract disorders
          in pregnancy, first trimester   M
O26.612   Liver and biliary tract disorders
          in pregnancy, second trimester   M
O26.613   Liver and biliary tract disorders
          in pregnancy, third trimester   M
O26.619   Liver and biliary tract disorders in
          pregnancy, unspecified trimester   M
O26.62   Liver and biliary tract disorders in childbirth   M
          Coding Clinic: 2023, Q1, P26-27
O26.63   Liver and biliary tract disorders in the
          puerperium   M
● O26.64 Intrahepatic cholestasis of pregnancy
O26.641   Intrahepatic cholestasis of pregnancy,
          first trimester   M
O26.642   Intrahepatic cholestasis of pregnancy,
          second trimester   M

O26.643   Intrahepatic cholestasis of pregnancy,
          third trimester   M
O26.649   Intrahepatic cholestasis of pregnancy,
          unspecified trimester   M
● O26.7   Subluxation of symphysis (pubis) in pregnancy,
          childbirth and the puerperium
          Excludes1 traumatic separation of symphysis
                         (pubis) during childbirth (O71.6)
● O26.71 Subluxation of symphysis (pubis) in pregnancy
O26.711   Subluxation of symphysis (pubis) in
          pregnancy, first trimester   M
O26.712   Subluxation of symphysis (pubis) in
          pregnancy, second trimester   M
O26.713   Subluxation of symphysis (pubis) in
          pregnancy, third trimester   M
O26.719   Subluxation of symphysis (pubis) in
          pregnancy, unspecified trimester   M
O26.72   Subluxation of symphysis (pubis) in
          childbirth   M
O26.73   Subluxation of symphysis (pubis) in the
          puerperium   M
● O26.8   Other specified pregnancy related conditions
● O26.81 Pregnancy related exhaustion and fatigue
O26.811   Pregnancy related exhaustion and
          fatigue, first trimester   M
O26.812   Pregnancy related exhaustion and
          fatigue, second trimester   M
O26.813   Pregnancy related exhaustion and
          fatigue, third trimester   M
O26.819   Pregnancy related exhaustion and
          fatigue, unspecified trimester   M
● O26.82 Pregnancy related peripheral neuritis
O26.821   Pregnancy related peripheral neuritis,
          first trimester   M
O26.822   Pregnancy related peripheral neuritis,
          second trimester   M
O26.823   Pregnancy related peripheral neuritis,
          third trimester   M
O26.829   Pregnancy related peripheral neuritis,
          unspecified trimester   M
● O26.83 Pregnancy related renal disease
          Use additional code to identify the specific
          disorder
O26.831   Pregnancy related renal disease, first
          trimester   M
O26.832   Pregnancy related renal disease,
          second trimester   M
O26.833   Pregnancy related renal disease, third
          trimester   M
O26.839   Pregnancy related renal disease,
          unspecified trimester   M
● O26.84 Uterine size-date discrepancy complicating
          pregnancy
          Excludes1 encounter for suspected problem
                         with fetal growth ruled out
                         (Z03.74)
O26.841   Uterine size-date discrepancy, first
          trimester   M
O26.842   Uterine size-date discrepancy, second
          trimester   M
O26.843   Uterine size-date discrepancy, third
          trimester   M
O26.849   Uterine size-date discrepancy,
          unspecified trimester   M
● O26.85 Spotting complicating pregnancy
O26.851   Spotting complicating pregnancy, first
          trimester   M
O26.852   Spotting complicating pregnancy,
          second trimester   M

O26.853　Spotting complicating pregnancy, third trimester　M

O26.859　Spotting complicating pregnancy, unspecified trimester　M

O26.86　Pruritic urticarial papules and plaques of pregnancy (PUPPP)　M
Polymorphic eruption of pregnancy

● O26.87　Cervical shortening

Excludes1　encounter for suspected cervical shortening ruled out (Z03.75)

O26.872　Cervical shortening, second trimester　M

O26.873　Cervical shortening, third trimester　M

O26.879　Cervical shortening, unspecified trimester　M

● O26.89　Other specified pregnancy related conditions
Use Additional code, if applicable, to identify specific condition such as insulin resistance(E88.81-)

O26.891　Other specified pregnancy related conditions, first trimester　M

O26.892　Other specified pregnancy related conditions, second trimester　M

O26.893　Other specified pregnancy related conditions, third trimester　M
Coding Clinic: 2015, Q3, P40

O26.899　Other specified pregnancy related conditions, unspecified trimester　M

● O26.9　Pregnancy related conditions, unspecified

O26.90　Pregnancy related conditions, unspecified, unspecified trimester　M

O26.91　Pregnancy related conditions, unspecified, first trimester　M

O26.92　Pregnancy related conditions, unspecified, second trimester　M

O26.93　Pregnancy related conditions, unspecified, third trimester　M

● O28　Abnormal findings on antenatal screening of mother

Excludes1　diagnostic findings classified elsewhere - see Alphabetical Index

O28.0　Abnormal hematological finding on antenatal screening of mother　M

O28.1　Abnormal biochemical finding on antenatal screening of mother　M

O28.2　Abnormal cytological finding on antenatal screening of mother　M

O28.3　Abnormal ultrasonic finding on antenatal screening of mother　M
Coding Clinic: 2016, Q4, P5

O28.4　Abnormal radiological finding on antenatal screening of mother　M

O28.5　Abnormal chromosomal and genetic finding on antenatal screening of mother

O28.8　Other abnormal findings on antenatal screening of mother　M

O28.9　Unspecified abnormal findings on antenatal screening of mother　M

● O29　Complications of anesthesia during pregnancy

Includes　maternal complications arising from the administration of a general, regional or local anesthetic, analgesic or other sedation during pregnancy

Use additional code, if necessary, to identify the complication

Excludes2　complications of anesthesia during labor and delivery (O74.-)
complications of anesthesia during the puerperium (O89.-)

● O29.0　Pulmonary complications of anesthesia during pregnancy

● O29.01　Aspiration pneumonitis due to anesthesia during pregnancy
Inhalation of stomach contents or secretions NOS due to anesthesia during pregnancy
Mendelson's syndrome due to anesthesia during pregnancy

O29.011　Aspiration pneumonitis due to anesthesia during pregnancy, first trimester　M

O29.012　Aspiration pneumonitis due to anesthesia during pregnancy, second trimester　M

O29.013　Aspiration pneumonitis due to anesthesia during pregnancy, third trimester　M

O29.019　Aspiration pneumonitis due to anesthesia during pregnancy, unspecified trimester　M

● O29.02　Pressure collapse of lung due to anesthesia during pregnancy

O29.021　Pressure collapse of lung due to anesthesia during pregnancy, first trimester　M

O29.022　Pressure collapse of lung due to anesthesia during pregnancy, second trimester　M

O29.023　Pressure collapse of lung due to anesthesia during pregnancy, third trimester　M

O29.029　Pressure collapse of lung due to anesthesia during pregnancy, unspecified trimester　M

● O29.09　Other pulmonary complications of anesthesia during pregnancy

O29.091　Other pulmonary complications of anesthesia during pregnancy, first trimester　M

O29.092　Other pulmonary complications of anesthesia during pregnancy, second trimester　M

O29.093　Other pulmonary complications of anesthesia during pregnancy, third trimester　M

O29.099　Other pulmonary complications of anesthesia during pregnancy, unspecified trimester　M

● O29.1　Cardiac complications of anesthesia during pregnancy

● O29.11　Cardiac arrest due to anesthesia during pregnancy

O29.111　Cardiac arrest due to anesthesia during pregnancy, first trimester　M

O29.112　Cardiac arrest due to anesthesia during pregnancy, second trimester　M

O29.113　Cardiac arrest due to anesthesia during pregnancy, third trimester　M

O29.119　Cardiac arrest due to anesthesia during pregnancy, unspecified trimester　M

● O29.12　Cardiac failure due to anesthesia during pregnancy

O29.121　Cardiac failure due to anesthesia during pregnancy, first trimester　M

O29.122　Cardiac failure due to anesthesia during pregnancy, second trimester　M

O29.123　Cardiac failure due to anesthesia during pregnancy, third trimester　M

O29.129　Cardiac failure due to anesthesia during pregnancy, unspecified trimester　M

● O29.19   Other cardiac complications of anesthesia during pregnancy
    O29.191   Other cardiac complications of anesthesia during pregnancy, first trimester   M
    O29.192   Other cardiac complications of anesthesia during pregnancy, second trimester   M
    O29.193   Other cardiac complications of anesthesia during pregnancy, third trimester   M
    O29.199   Other cardiac complications of anesthesia during pregnancy, unspecified trimester   M

● O29.2   Central nervous system complications of anesthesia during pregnancy
   ● O29.21   Cerebral anoxia due to anesthesia during pregnancy
    O29.211   Cerebral anoxia due to anesthesia during pregnancy, first trimester   M
    O29.212   Cerebral anoxia due to anesthesia during pregnancy, second trimester   M
    O29.213   Cerebral anoxia due to anesthesia during pregnancy, third trimester   M
    O29.219   Cerebral anoxia due to anesthesia during pregnancy, unspecified trimester   M
   ● O29.29   Other central nervous system complications of anesthesia during pregnancy
    O29.291   Other central nervous system complications of anesthesia during pregnancy, first trimester   M
    O29.292   Other central nervous system complications of anesthesia during pregnancy, second trimester   M
    O29.293   Other central nervous system complications of anesthesia during pregnancy, third trimester   M
    O29.299   Other central nervous system complications of anesthesia during pregnancy, unspecified trimester   M

● O29.3   Toxic reaction to local anesthesia during pregnancy
   ● O29.3X   Toxic reaction to local anesthesia during pregnancy
    O29.3X1   Toxic reaction to local anesthesia during pregnancy, first trimester   M
    O29.3X2   Toxic reaction to local anesthesia during pregnancy, second trimester   M
    O29.3X3   Toxic reaction to local anesthesia during pregnancy, third trimester   M
    O29.3X9   Toxic reaction to local anesthesia during pregnancy, unspecified trimester   M

● O29.4   Spinal and epidural anesthesia induced headache during pregnancy
    O29.40   Spinal and epidural anesthesia induced headache during pregnancy, unspecified trimester   M
    O29.41   Spinal and epidural anesthesia induced headache during pregnancy, first trimester   M
    O29.42   Spinal and epidural anesthesia induced headache during pregnancy, second trimester   M
    O29.43   Spinal and epidural anesthesia induced headache during pregnancy, third trimester   M

● O29.5   Other complications of spinal and epidural anesthesia during pregnancy
   ● O29.5X   Other complications of spinal and epidural anesthesia during pregnancy
    O29.5X1   Other complications of spinal and epidural anesthesia during pregnancy, first trimester   M
    O29.5X2   Other complications of spinal and epidural anesthesia during pregnancy, second trimester   M
    O29.5X3   Other complications of spinal and epidural anesthesia during pregnancy, third trimester   M
    O29.5X9   Other complications of spinal and epidural anesthesia during pregnancy, unspecified trimester   M

● O29.6   Failed or difficult intubation for anesthesia during pregnancy
    O29.60   Failed or difficult intubation for anesthesia during pregnancy, unspecified trimester   M
    O29.61   Failed or difficult intubation for anesthesia during pregnancy, first trimester   M
    O29.62   Failed or difficult intubation for anesthesia during pregnancy, second trimester   M
    O29.63   Failed or difficult intubation for anesthesia during pregnancy, third trimester   M

● O29.8   Other complications of anesthesia during pregnancy
   ● O29.8X   Other complications of anesthesia during pregnancy
    O29.8X1   Other complications of anesthesia during pregnancy, first trimester   M
    O29.8X2   Other complications of anesthesia during pregnancy, second trimester   M
    O29.8X3   Other complications of anesthesia during pregnancy, third trimester   M
    O29.8X9   Other complications of anesthesia during pregnancy, unspecified trimester   M

● O29.9   Unspecified complication of anesthesia during pregnancy
    O29.90   Unspecified complication of anesthesia during pregnancy, unspecified trimester   M
    O29.91   Unspecified complication of anesthesia during pregnancy, first trimester   M
    O29.92   Unspecified complication of anesthesia during pregnancy, second trimester   M
    O29.93   Unspecified complication of anesthesia during pregnancy, third trimester   M

MATERNAL CARE RELATED TO THE FETUS AND AMNIOTIC CAVITY AND POSSIBLE DELIVERY PROBLEMS (O30-O48)

● O30   Multiple gestation
   Code also any complications specific to multiple gestation
   Coding Clinic: 2016, Q4, P51
   ● O30.0   Twin pregnancy
    ● O30.00   Twin pregnancy, unspecified number of placenta and unspecified number of amniotic sacs
     O30.001   Twin pregnancy, unspecified number of placenta and unspecified number of amniotic sacs, first trimester   M
     O30.002   Twin pregnancy, unspecified number of placenta and unspecified number of amniotic sacs, second trimester   M
     O30.003   Twin pregnancy, unspecified number of placenta and unspecified number of amniotic sacs, third trimester   M
     O30.009   Twin pregnancy, unspecified number of placenta and unspecified number of amniotic sacs, unspecified trimester   M
    ● O30.01   Twin pregnancy, monochorionic/monoamniotic
     Twin pregnancy, one placenta, one amniotic sac
     Excludes1   conjoined twins (O30.02-)
     O30.011   Twin pregnancy, monochorionic/monoamniotic, first trimester   M
     O30.012   Twin pregnancy, monochorionic/monoamniotic, second trimester   M

CHAPTER 15 (O00-O9A)

O30.013   Twin pregnancy, monochorionic/monoamniotic, third trimester   M

O30.019   Twin pregnancy, monochorionic/monoamniotic, unspecified trimester   M

● O30.02   Conjoined twin pregnancy

O30.021   Conjoined twin pregnancy, first trimester   M

O30.022   Conjoined twin pregnancy, second trimester   M

O30.023   Conjoined twin pregnancy, third trimester   M

O30.029   Conjoined twin pregnancy, unspecified trimester   M

● O30.03   Twin pregnancy, monochorionic/diamniotic
Twin pregnancy, one placenta, two amniotic sacs

O30.031   Twin pregnancy, monochorionic/diamniotic, first trimester   M

O30.032   Twin pregnancy, monochorionic/diamniotic, second trimester   M

O30.033   Twin pregnancy, monochorionic/diamniotic, third trimester   M

O30.039   Twin pregnancy, monochorionic/diamniotic, unspecified trimester   M

● O30.04   Twin pregnancy, dichorionic/diamniotic
Twin pregnancy, two placentae, two amniotic sacs

O30.041   Twin pregnancy, dichorionic/diamniotic, first trimester   M

O30.042   Twin pregnancy, dichorionic/diamniotic, second trimester   M

O30.043   Twin pregnancy, dichorionic/diamniotic, third trimester   M

O30.049   Twin pregnancy, dichorionic/diamniotic, unspecified trimester   M

● O30.09   Twin pregnancy, unable to determine number of placenta and number of amniotic sacs

O30.091   Twin pregnancy, unable to determine number of placenta and number of amniotic sacs, first trimester   M

O30.092   Twin pregnancy, unable to determine number of placenta and number of amniotic sacs, second trimester   M

O30.093   Twin pregnancy, unable to determine number of placenta and number of amniotic sacs, third trimester   M

O30.099   Twin pregnancy, unable to determine number of placenta and number of amniotic sacs, unspecified trimester   M

● O30.1   Triplet pregnancy

● O30.10   Triplet pregnancy, unspecified number of placenta and unspecified number of amniotic sacs

O30.101   Triplet pregnancy, unspecified number of placenta and unspecified number of amniotic sacs, first trimester   M

O30.102   Triplet pregnancy, unspecified number of placenta and unspecified number of amniotic sacs, second trimester   M

O30.103   Triplet pregnancy, unspecified number of placenta and unspecified number of amniotic sacs, third trimester   M
Coding Clinic: 2016, Q2, P8

O30.109   Triplet pregnancy, unspecified number of placenta and unspecified number of amniotic sacs, unspecified trimester

● O30.11   Triplet pregnancy with two or more monochorionic fetuses

O30.111   Triplet pregnancy with two or more monochorionic fetuses, first trimester   M

O30.112   Triplet pregnancy with two or more monochorionic fetuses, second trimester   M

O30.113   Triplet pregnancy with two or more monochorionic fetuses, third trimester   M

O30.119   Triplet pregnancy with two or more monochorionic fetuses, unspecified trimester   M

● O30.12   Triplet pregnancy with two or more monoamniotic fetuses

O30.121   Triplet pregnancy with two or more monoamniotic fetuses, first trimester   M

O30.122   Triplet pregnancy with two or more monoamniotic fetuses, second trimester   M

O30.123   Triplet pregnancy with two or more monoamniotic fetuses, third trimester   M

O30.129   Triplet pregnancy with two or more monoamniotic fetuses, unspecified trimester   M

● O30.13   Triplet pregnancy, trichorionic/triamniotic

O30.131   Triplet pregnancy, trichorionic/triamniotic, first trimester   M

O30.132   Triplet pregnancy, trichorionic/triamniotic, second trimester   M

O30.133   Triplet pregnancy, trichorionic/triamniotic, third trimester   M

O30.139   Triplet pregnancy, trichorionic/triamniotic, unspecified trimester   M

● O30.19   Triplet pregnancy, unable to determine number of placenta and number of amniotic sacs

O30.191   Triplet pregnancy, unable to determine number of placenta and number of amniotic sacs, first trimester   M

O30.192   Triplet pregnancy, unable to determine number of placenta and number of amniotic sacs, second trimester   M

O30.193   Triplet pregnancy, unable to determine number of placenta and number of amniotic sacs, third trimester   M

O30.199   Triplet pregnancy, unable to determine number of placenta and number of amniotic sacs, unspecified trimester   M

● O30.2   Quadruplet pregnancy

● O30.20   Quadruplet pregnancy, unspecified number of placenta and unspecified number of amniotic sacs

O30.201   Quadruplet pregnancy, unspecified number of placenta and unspecified number of amniotic sacs, first trimester   M

O30.202   Quadruplet pregnancy, unspecified number of placenta and unspecified number of amniotic sacs, second trimester   M

O30.203   Quadruplet pregnancy, unspecified number of placenta and unspecified number of amniotic sacs, third trimester   M

O30.209   Quadruplet pregnancy, unspecified number of placenta and unspecified number of amniotic sacs, unspecified trimester   M

● O30.21   Quadruplet pregnancy with two or more monochorionic fetuses

  O30.211   Quadruplet pregnancy with two or more monochorionic fetuses, first trimester   M

  O30.212   Quadruplet pregnancy with two or more monochorionic fetuses, second trimester   M

  O30.213   Quadruplet pregnancy with two or more monochorionic fetuses, third trimester   M

  O30.219   Quadruplet pregnancy with two or more monochorionic fetuses, unspecified trimester   M

● O30.22   Quadruplet pregnancy with two or more monoamniotic fetuses

  O30.221   Quadruplet pregnancy with two or more monoamniotic fetuses, first trimester   M

  O30.222   Quadruplet pregnancy with two or more monoamniotic fetuses, second trimester   M

  O30.223   Quadruplet pregnancy with two or more monoamniotic fetuses, third trimester   M

  O30.229   Quadruplet pregnancy with two or more monoamniotic fetuses, unspecified trimester   M

● O30.23   Quadruplet pregnancy, quadrachorionic/quadra-amniotic

  O30.231   Quadruplet pregnancy, quadrachorionic/quadra-amniotic, first trimester   M

  O30.232   Quadruplet pregnancy, quadrachorionic/quadra-amniotic, second trimester   M

  O30.233   Quadruplet pregnancy, quadrachorionic/quadra-amniotic, third trimester   M

  O30.239   Quadruplet pregnancy, quadrachorionic/quadra-amniotic, unspecifiedtrimester   M

● O30.29   Quadruplet pregnancy, unable to determine number of placenta and number of amniotic sacs

  O30.291   Quadruplet pregnancy, unable to determine number of placenta and number of amniotic sacs, first trimester   M

  O30.292   Quadruplet pregnancy, unable to determine number of placenta and number of amniotic sacs, second trimester   M

  O30.293   Quadruplet pregnancy, unable to determine number of placenta and number of amniotic sacs, third trimester   M

  O30.299   Quadruplet pregnancy, unable to determine number of placenta and number of amniotic sacs, unspecified trimester   M

● O30.8   Other specified multiple gestation
Multiple gestation pregnancy greater then quadruplets

● O30.80   Other specified multiple gestation, unspecified number of placenta and unspecified number of amniotic sacs

  O30.801   Other specified multiple gestation, unspecified number of placenta and unspecified number of amniotic sacs, first trimester   M

  O30.802   Other specified multiple gestation, unspecified number of placenta and unspecified number of amniotic sacs, second trimester   M

  O30.803   Other specified multiple gestation, unspecified number of placenta and unspecified number of amniotic sacs, third trimester   M

  O30.809   Other specified multiple gestation, unspecified number of placenta and unspecified number of amniotic sacs, unspecified trimester   M

● O30.81   Other specified multiple gestation with two or more monochorionic fetuses

  O30.811   Other specified multiple gestation with two or more monochorionic fetuses, first trimester   M

  O30.812   Other specified multiple gestation with two or more monochorionic fetuses, second trimester   M

  O30.813   Other specified multiple gestation with two or more monochorionic fetuses, third trimester   M

  O30.819   Other specified multiple gestation with two or more monochorionic fetuses, unspecified trimester   M

● O30.82   Other specified multiple gestation with two or more monoamniotic fetuses

  O30.821   Other specified multiple gestation with two or more monoamniotic fetuses, first trimester   M

  O30.822   Other specified multiple gestation with two or more monoamniotic fetuses, second trimester   M

  O30.823   Other specified multiple gestation with two or more monoamniotic fetuses, third trimester   M

  O30.829   Other specified multiple gestation with two or more monoamniotic fetuses, unspecified trimester   M

● O30.83   Other specified multiple gestation, number of chorions and amnions are both equalto the number of fetuses
Pentachorionic, penta-amniotic pregnancy (quintuplets)
Hexachorionic, hexa-amniotic pregnancy (sextuplets)
Heptachorionic, hepta-amniotic pregnancy (septuplets)

  O30.831   Other specified multiple gestation, number of chorions and amnions are both equal to the number of fetuses, first trimester   M

  O30.832   Other specified multiple gestation, number of chorions and amnions are both equal to the number of fetuses, second trimester   M

  O30.833   Other specified multiple gestation, number of chorions and amnions are both equal to the number of fetuses, third trimester   M

  O30.839   Other specified multiple gestation, number of chorions and amnions are both equal to the number of fetuses, unspecified trimester   M

● O30.89   Other specified multiple gestation, unable to determine number of placenta and number of amniotic sacs

     O30.891   Other specified multiple gestation, unable to determine number of placenta and number of amniotic sacs, first trimester   M

     O30.892   Other specified multiple gestation, unable to determine number of placenta and number of amniotic sacs, second trimester   M

     O30.893   Other specified multiple gestation, unable to determine number of placenta and number of amniotic sacs, third trimester   M

     O30.899   Other specified multiple gestation, unable to determine number of placenta and number of amniotic sacs, unspecified trimester   M

● O30.9   Multiple gestation, unspecified
     Multiple pregnancy NOS

     O30.90   Multiple gestation, unspecified, unspecified trimester   M

     O30.91   Multiple gestation, unspecified, first trimester   M

     O30.92   Multiple gestation, unspecified, second trimester   M

     O30.93   Multiple gestation, unspecified, third trimester   M

● **O31**   **Complications specific to multiple gestation**

Excludes2   delayed delivery of second twin, triplet, etc. (O63.2)
     malpresentation of one fetus or more (O32.9)
     placental transfusion syndromes (O43.0-)

Coding Clinic: 2012, Q4, P107

One of the following 7th characters is to be assigned to each code under category O31. 7th character 0 is for single gestations and multiple gestations where the fetus is unspecified. 7th characters 1 through 9 are for cases of multiple gestations to identify the fetus for which the code applies. The appropriate code from category O30, Multiple gestation, must also be assigned when assigning a code from category O31 that has a 7th character of 1 through 9.

0	not applicable or unspecified
1	fetus 1
2	fetus 2
3	fetus 3
4	fetus 4
5	fetus 5
9	other fetus

● O31.0   Papyraceous fetus
     Fetus compressus

X ● O31.00   Papyraceous fetus, unspecified trimester   M

X ● O31.01   Papyraceous fetus, first trimester   M

X ● O31.02   Papyraceous fetus, second trimester   M

X ● O31.03   Papyraceous fetus, third trimester   M

● O31.1   Continuing pregnancy after spontaneous abortion of one fetus or more

X ● O31.10   Continuing pregnancy after spontaneous abortion of one fetus or more, unspecified trimester   M

X ● O31.11   Continuing pregnancy after spontaneous abortion of one fetus or more, first trimester   M

X ● O31.12   Continuing pregnancy after spontaneous abortion of one fetus or more, second trimester   M

X ● O31.13   Continuing pregnancy after spontaneous abortion of one fetus or more, third trimester   M

● O31.2   Continuing pregnancy after intrauterine death of one fetus or more

X ● O31.20   Continuing pregnancy after intrauterine death of one fetus or more, unspecified trimester   M

X ● O31.21   Continuing pregnancy after intrauterine death of one fetus or more, first trimester   M

X ● O31.22   Continuing pregnancy after intrauterine death of one fetus or more, second trimester   M

X ● O31.23   Continuing pregnancy after intrauterine death of one fetus or more, third trimester   M

● O31.3   Continuing pregnancy after elective fetal reduction of one fetus or more
     Continuing pregnancy after selective termination of one fetus or more

X ● O31.30   Continuing pregnancy after elective fetal reduction of one fetus or more, unspecified trimester   M

X ● O31.31   Continuing pregnancy after elective fetal reduction of one fetus or more, first trimester   M

X ● O31.32   Continuing pregnancy after elective fetal reduction of one fetus or more, second trimester   M

X ● O31.33   Continuing pregnancy after elective fetal reduction of one fetus or more, third trimester   M

● O31.8   Other complications specific to multiple gestation

● O31.8X   Other complications specific to multiple gestation

● O31.8X1   Other complications specific to multiple gestation, first trimester   M

● O31.8X2   Other complications specific to multiple gestation, second trimester   M

● O31.8X3   Other complications specific to multiple gestation, third trimester   M

● O31.8X9   Other complications specific to multiple gestation, unspecified trimester   M

● **O32**   **Maternal care for malpresentation of fetus**

Includes   the listed conditions as a reason for observation, hospitalization or other obstetric care of the mother, or for cesarean delivery before onset of labor

Excludes1   malpresentation of fetus with obstructed labor (O64.-)

Coding Clinic: 2012, Q4, P107

One of the following 7th characters is to be assigned to each code under category O32. 7th character 0 is for single gestations and multiple gestations where the fetus is unspecified. 7th characters 1 through 9 are for cases of multiple gestations to identify the fetus for which the code applies. The appropriate code from category O30, Multiple gestation, must also be assigned when assigning a code from category O32 that has a 7th character of 1 through 9.

0	not applicable or unspecified
1	fetus 1
2	fetus 2
3	fetus 3
4	fetus 4
5	fetus 5
9	other fetus

X ● O32.0   Maternal care for unstable lie   M

X ● O32.1   Maternal care for breech presentation   M
     Maternal care for buttocks presentation
     Maternal care for complete breech
     Maternal care for frank breech

     Excludes1   footling presentation (O32.8)
            incomplete breech (O32.8)

X ● O32.2   Maternal care for transverse and oblique lie   M
     Maternal care for oblique presentation
     Maternal care for transverse presentation

▶ New   ⇒ Revised   ~~deleted~~ Deleted   Excludes 1   Excludes 2   Includes   Use additional   Code first   Code also   Key words

OGCR Official Guidelines   X Assign placeholder X   ● Use Additional Character(s)   ▌ Manifestation Code   🦋 Hierarchical Condition Category   Coding Clinic

X● **O32.3** **Maternal care for face, brow and chin presentation** M

X● **O32.4** **Maternal care for high head at term** M
Maternal care for failure of head to enter pelvic brim

X● **O32.6** **Maternal care for compound presentation** M

X● **O32.8** **Maternal care for other malpresentation of fetus** M
Maternal care for footling presentation
Maternal care for incomplete breech

X● **O32.9** **Maternal care for malpresentation of fetus, unspecified** M

● **O33** **Maternal care for disproportion**
Includes the listed conditions as a reason for observation, hospitalization or other obstetric care of the mother, or for cesarean delivery before onset of labor

Excludes1 disproportion with obstructed labor (O65-O66)

O33.0 **Maternal care for disproportion due to deformity of maternal pelvic bones** M
Maternal care for disproportion due to pelvic deformity causing disproportion NOS

O33.1 **Maternal care for disproportion due to generally contracted pelvis** M
Maternal care for disproportion due to contracted pelvis NOS causing disproportion

O33.2 **Maternal care for disproportion due to inlet contraction of pelvis** M
Maternal care for disproportion due to inlet contraction (pelvis) causing disproportion

X● **O33.3** **Maternal care for disproportion due to outlet contraction of pelvis** M
Maternal care for disproportion due to mid-cavity contraction (pelvis)
Maternal care for disproportion due to outlet contraction (pelvis)
One of the following 7th characters is to be assigned to code O33.3. 7th character Ø is for single gestations and multiple gestations where the fetus is unspecified. 7th characters 1 through 9 are for cases of multiple gestations to identify the fetus for which the code applies. The appropriate code from category O30, Multiple gestation, must also be assigned when assigning code O33.3 with a 7th character of 1 through 9.

Ø	not applicable or unspecified
1	fetus 1
2	fetus 2
3	fetus 3
4	fetus 4
5	fetus 5
9	other fetus

X● **O33.4** **Maternal care for disproportion of mixed maternal and fetal origin** M
One of the following 7th characters is to be assigned to code O33.4. 7th character Ø is for single gestations and multiple gestations where the fetus is unspecified. 7th characters 1 through 9 are for cases of multiple gestations to identify the fetus for which the code applies. The appropriate code from category O30, Multiple gestation, must also be assigned when assigning code O33.4 with a 7th character of 1 through 9.

Ø	not applicable or unspecified
1	fetus 1
2	fetus 2
3	fetus 3
4	fetus 4
5	fetus 5
9	other fetus

X● **O33.5** **Maternal care for disproportion due to unusually large fetus** M
Maternal care for disproportion due to disproportion of fetal origin with normally formed fetus
Maternal care for disproportion due to fetal disproportion NOS
One of the following 7th characters is to be assigned to code O33.5. 7th character Ø is for single gestations and multiple gestations where the fetus is unspecified. 7th characters 1 through 9 are for cases of multiple gestations to identify the fetus for which the code applies. The appropriate code from category O30, Multiple gestation, must also be assigned when assigning code O33.5 with a 7th character of 1 through 9.

Ø	not applicable or unspecified
1	fetus 1
2	fetus 2
3	fetus 3
4	fetus 4
5	fetus 5
9	other fetus

X● **O33.6** **Maternal care for disproportion due to hydrocephalic fetus** M
One of the following 7th characters is to be assigned to code O33.6. 7th character Ø is for single gestations and multiple gestations where the fetus is unspecified. 7th characters 1 through 9 are for cases of multiple gestations to identify the fetus for which the code applies. The appropriate code from category O30, Multiple gestation, must also be assigned when assigning code O33.6 with a 7th character of 1 through 9.

Ø	not applicable or unspecified
1	fetus 1
2	fetus 2
3	fetus 3
4	fetus 4
5	fetus 5
9	other fetus

X● **O33.7** **Maternal care for disproportion due to other fetal deformities** M
Maternal care for disproportion due to fetal ascites
Maternal care for disproportion due to fetal hydrops
Maternal care for disproportion due to fetal meningomyelocele
Maternal care for disproportion due to fetal sacral teratoma
Maternal care for disproportion due to fetal tumor

Excludes1 obstructed labor due to other fetal deformities (O66.3)

Coding Clinic: 2016, Q4, P51

One of the following 7th characters is to be assigned to code O33.7. 7th character Ø is for single gestations and multiple gestations where the fetus is unspecified. 7th characters 1 through 9 are for cases of multiple gestations to identify the fetus for which the code applies. The appropriate code from category O30, Multiple gestation, must also be assigned when assigning code O33.7 with a 7th character of 1 through 9.

Ø	not applicable or unspecified
1	fetus 1
2	fetus 2
3	fetus 3
4	fetus 4
5	fetus 5
9	other fetus

O33.8 **Maternal care for disproportion of other origin** M

O33.9 **Maternal care for disproportion, unspecified** M
Maternal care for disproportion due to cephalopelvic disproportion NOS
Maternal care for disproportion due to fetopelvic disproportion NOS

● **O34**   **Maternal care for abnormality of pelvic organs**

     Includes   the listed conditions as a reason for hospitalization or other obstetric care of the mother, or for cesarean delivery before onset of labor

     Code first any associated obstructed labor (O65.5)

     Use additional code for specific condition

● **O34.0**   **Maternal care for congenital malformation of uterus**
     Maternal care for double uterus
     Maternal care for uterus bicornis

     O34.00   Maternal care for unspecified congenital malformation of uterus, unspecified trimester   M

     O34.01   Maternal care for unspecified congenital malformation of uterus, first trimester   M

     O34.02   Maternal care for unspecified congenital malformation of uterus, second trimester   M

     O34.03   Maternal care for unspecified congenital malformation of uterus, third trimester   M

● **O34.1**   **Maternal care for benign tumor of corpus uteri**

     Excludes2   maternal care for benign tumor of cervix (O34.4-)
                   maternal care for malignant neoplasm of uterus (O9A.1-)

     O34.10   Maternal care for benign tumor of corpus uteri, unspecified trimester   M

     O34.11   Maternal care for benign tumor of corpus uteri, first trimester   M

     O34.12   Maternal care for benign tumor of corpus uteri, second trimester   M

     O34.13   Maternal care for benign tumor of corpus uteri, third trimester   M

● **O34.2**   **Maternal care due to uterine scar from previous surgery**
     Coding Clinic: 2016, Q4, P76

     ● **O34.21**   Maternal care for scar from previous cesarean delivery
         Coding Clinic: 2016, Q4, P51

         O34.211   Maternal care for low transverse scar from previous cesarean delivery   M

         O34.212   Maternal care for vertical scar from previous cesarean delivery   M
                 Maternal care for classical scar from previous cesarean delivery

         O34.218   Maternal care for other type scar from previous cesarean delivery   M
                 Mid-transverse T incision

         O34.219   Maternal care for unspecified type scar from previous cesarean delivery   M

     O34.22   Maternal care for cesarean scar defect (isthmocele)   M

     O34.29   Maternal care due to uterine scar from other previous surgery   M
             Maternal care due to uterine scar from other transmural uterine incision

● **O34.3**   **Maternal care for cervical incompetence**
     Maternal care for cerclage with or without cervical incompetence
     Maternal care for Shirodkar suture with or without cervical incompetence

     O34.30   Maternal care for cervical incompetence, unspecified trimester   M

     O34.31   Maternal care for cervical incompetence, first trimester   M

     O34.32   Maternal care for cervical incompetence, second trimester   M

     O34.33   Maternal care for cervical incompetence, third trimester   M

● **O34.4**   **Maternal care for other abnormalities of cervix**

     O34.40   Maternal care for other abnormalities of cervix, unspecified trimester   M

     O34.41   Maternal care for other abnormalities of cervix, first trimester   M

     O34.42   Maternal care for other abnormalities of cervix, second trimester   M

     O34.43   Maternal care for other abnormalities of cervix, third trimester   M

● **O34.5**   **Maternal care for other abnormalities of gravid uterus**

     ● **O34.51**   Maternal care for incarceration of gravid uterus

         O34.511   Maternal care for incarceration of gravid uterus, first trimester   M

         O34.512   Maternal care for incarceration of gravid uterus, second trimester   M

         O34.513   Maternal care for incarceration of gravid uterus, third trimester   M

         O34.519   Maternal care for incarceration of gravid uterus, unspecified trimester   M

     ● **O34.52**   Maternal care for prolapse of gravid uterus

         O34.521   Maternal care for prolapse of gravid uterus, first trimester   M

         O34.522   Maternal care for prolapse of gravid uterus, second trimester   M

         O34.523   Maternal care for prolapse of gravid uterus, third trimester   M

         O34.529   Maternal care for prolapse of gravid uterus, unspecified trimester   M

     ● **O34.53**   Maternal care for retroversion of gravid uterus

         O34.531   Maternal care for retroversion of gravid uterus, first trimester   M

         O34.532   Maternal care for retroversion of gravid uterus, second trimester   M

         O34.533   Maternal care for retroversion of gravid uterus, third trimester   M

         O34.539   Maternal care for retroversion of gravid uterus, unspecified trimester   M

     ● **O34.59**   Maternal care for other abnormalities of gravid uterus

         O34.591   Maternal care for other abnormalities of gravid uterus, first trimester   M

         O34.592   Maternal care for other abnormalities of gravid uterus, second trimester   M

         O34.593   Maternal care for other abnormalities of gravid uterus, third trimester   M

         O34.599   Maternal care for other abnormalities of gravid uterus, unspecified trimester   M

● **O34.6**   **Maternal care for abnormality of vagina**

     Excludes2   maternal care for vaginal varices in pregnancy (O22.1-)

     O34.60   Maternal care for abnormality of vagina, unspecified trimester   M

     O34.61   Maternal care for abnormality of vagina, first trimester   M

     O34.62   Maternal care for abnormality of vagina, second trimester   M

     O34.63   Maternal care for abnormality of vagina, third trimester   M

● **O34.7**   **Maternal care for abnormality of vulva and perineum**

     Excludes2   maternal care for perineal and vulval varices in pregnancy (O22.1-)

     O34.70   Maternal care for abnormality of vulva and perineum, unspecified trimester   M

     O34.71   Maternal care for abnormality of vulva and perineum, first trimester   M

     O34.72   Maternal care for abnormality of vulva and perineum, second trimester   M

     O34.73   Maternal care for abnormality of vulva and perineum, third trimester   M

● **O34.8**   **Maternal care for other abnormalities of pelvic organs**

     O34.80   Maternal care for other abnormalities of pelvic organs, unspecified trimester   M

     O34.81   Maternal care for other abnormalities of pelvic organs, first trimester   M

O34.82   Maternal care for other abnormalities of pelvic organs, second trimester   M

O34.83   Maternal care for other abnormalities of pelvic organs, third trimester   M

● O34.9   Maternal care for abnormality of pelvic organ, unspecified

O34.90   Maternal care for abnormality of pelvic organ, unspecified, unspecified trimester   M

O34.91   Maternal care for abnormality of pelvic organ, unspecified, first trimester   M

O34.92   Maternal care for abnormality of pelvic organ, unspecified, second trimester   M

O34.93   Maternal care for abnormality of pelvic organ, unspecified, third trimester   M

● O35   Maternal care for known or suspected fetal abnormality and damage

Includes   the listed conditions in the fetus as a reason for hospitalization or other obstetric care to the mother, or for termination of pregnancy

Code also any associated maternal condition

Excludes1   encounter for suspected maternal and fetal conditions ruled out (Z03.7-)

One of the following 7th characters is to be assigned to each code under category O35. 7th character 0 is for single gestations and multiple gestations where the fetus is unspecified. 7th characters 1 through 9 are for cases of multiple gestations to identify the fetus for which the code applies. The appropriate code from category O30, Multiple gestation, must also be assigned when assigning a code from category O35 that has a 7th character of 1 through 9.

0	not applicable or unspecified
1	fetus 1
2	fetus 2
3	fetus 3
4	fetus 4
5	fetus 5
9	other fetus

X ● O35.0   Maternal care for (suspected) central nervous system malformation in fetus   M

Excludes2   chromosomal abnormality in fetus (O35.1-)

X ● O35.00   Maternal care for (suspected) central nervous system malformation or damage in fetus, unspecified   M

X ● O35.01   Maternal care for (suspected) central nervous system malformation or damage in fetus, agenesis of the corpus callosum   M

X ● O35.02   Maternal care for (suspected) central nervous system malformation or damage in fetus, anencephaly   M

X ● O35.03   Maternal care for (suspected) central nervous system malformation or damage in fetus, choroid plexus cysts   M

X ● O35.04   Maternal care for (suspected) central nervous system malformation or damage in fetus, encephalocele   M

X ● O35.05   Maternal care for (suspected) central nervous system malformation or damage in fetus, holoprosencephaly   M

X ● O35.06   Maternal care for (suspected) central nervous system malformation or damage in fetus, hydrocephaly   M

     Maternal care for fetal hydrocephalus

X ● O35.07   Maternal care for (suspected) central nervous system malformation or damage in fetus, microcephaly   M

X ● O35.08   Maternal care for (suspected) central nervous system malformation or damage in fetus, spina bifida   M

X ● O35.09   Maternal care for (suspected) other central nervous system malformation or damage in Fetus   M

X ● O35.1   Maternal care for (suspected) chromosomal abnormality in fetus   M

X ● O35.10   Maternal care for (suspected) chromosomal abnormality in fetus, unspecified   M

X ● O35.11   Maternal care for (suspected) chromosomal abnormality in fetus, Trisomy 13   M

X ● O35.12   Maternal care for (suspected) chromosomal abnormality in fetus, Trisomy 18   M

X ● O35.13   Maternal care for (suspected) chromosomal abnormality in fetus, Trisomy 21   M

X ● O35.14   Maternal care for (suspected) chromosomal abnormality in fetus, Turner Syndrome   M

X ● O35.15   Maternal care for (suspected) chromosomal abnormality in fetus, sex chromosome Abnormality   M

X ● O35.19   Maternal care for (suspected) chromosomal abnormality in fetus, other chromosomal abnormality   M

X ● O35.2   Maternal care for (suspected) hereditary disease in fetus   M

Excludes2   chromosomal abnormality in fetus (O35.1-)

X ● O35.3   Maternal care for (suspected) damage to fetus from viral disease in mother   M

     Maternal care for damage to fetus from maternal cytomegalovirus infection

     Maternal care for damage to fetus from maternal rubella

     Coding Clinic: 2016, Q4, P6

X ● O35.4   Maternal care for (suspected) damage to fetus from alcohol   M

X ● O35.5   Maternal care for (suspected) damage to fetus by drugs   M

     Maternal care for damage to fetus from drug addiction

X ● O35.6   Maternal care for (suspected) damage to fetus by radiation   M

X ● O35.7   Maternal care for (suspected) damage to fetus by other medical procedures   M

     Maternal care for damage to fetus by amniocentesis

     Maternal care for damage to fetus by biopsy procedures

     Maternal care for damage to fetus by hematological investigation

     Maternal care for damage to fetus by intrauterine contraceptive device

     Maternal care for damage to fetus by intrauterine surgery

X ● O35.8   Maternal care for other (suspected) fetal abnormality and damage   M

     Maternal care for damage to fetus from maternal listeriosis

     Maternal care for damage to fetus from maternal toxoplasmosis

X ● O35.9   Maternal care for (suspected) fetal abnormality and damage, unspecified   M

X ● O35.A   Maternal care for other (suspected) fetal abnormality and damage, fetal facial anomalies   M

X ● O35.B   Maternal care for other (suspected) fetal abnormality and damage, fetal cardiac anomalies   M

X ● O35.C   Maternal care for other (suspected) fetal abnormality and damage, fetal pulmonary anomalies   M

X ● O35.D   Maternal care for other (suspected) fetal abnormality and damage, fetal gastrointestinal anomalies   M

X ● O35.E   Maternal care for other (suspected) fetal abnormality and damage, fetal genitourinary anomalies   M

X ● O35.F   Maternal care for other (suspected) fetal abnormality and damage, fetal musculoskeletal anomalies of trunk   M

Excludes2   maternal care for other (suspected) fetal abnormality and damage, fetal lower extremities anomalies (O35.H)

     maternal care for other (suspected) fetal abnormality and damage, fetal upper extremities anomalies (O35.G)

X ● O35.G   Maternal care for other (suspected) fetal abnormality and damage, fetal upper extremities anomalies   M

X ● O35.H   Maternal care for other (suspected) fetal abnormality and damage, fetal lower extremities Anomalies   M

CHAPTER 15 (O00-O9A)

CHAPTER 15 (O00-O9A)

OGCR Section I.C.15.e.1.

Fetal Conditions Affecting the Management of the Mother
1) Code from categories O35 and O36
Codes from categories O35, Maternal care for known or suspected fetal abnormality and damage, and O36, Maternal care for other fetal problems, are assigned only when the fetal condition is actually responsible for modifying the management of the mother, i.e., by requiring diagnostic studies, additional observation, special care, or termination of pregnancy. The fact that the fetal condition exists does not justify assigning a code from this series to the mother's record.
2) In utero surgery
In cases when surgery is performed on the fetus, a diagnosis code from category O35, Maternal care for known or suspected fetal abnormality and damage, should be assigned identifying the fetal condition. Assign the appropriate procedure code for the procedure performed.
No code from Chapter 16, the perinatal codes, should be used on the mother's record to identify fetal conditions. Surgery performed in utero on a fetus is still to be coded as an obstetric encounter.

● **O36**   **Maternal care for other fetal problems**

     Includes   the listed conditions in the fetus as a reason for hospitalization or other obstetric care of the mother, or for termination of pregnancy

     Excludes1   encounter for suspected maternal and fetal conditions ruled out (Z03.7-)
                   placental transfusion syndromes (O43.0-)

     Excludes2   labor and delivery complicated by fetal stress (O77.-)

     One of the following 7th characters is to be assigned to each code under category O36. 7th character 0 is for single gestations and multiple gestations where the fetus is unspecified. 7th characters 1 through 9 are for cases of multiple gestations to identify the fetus for which the code applies. The appropriate code from category O30, Multiple gestation, must also be assigned when assigning a code from category O36 that has a 7th character of 1 through 9.

0	not applicable or unspecified
1	fetus 1
2	fetus 2
3	fetus 3
4	fetus 4
5	fetus 5
9	other fetus

Coding Clinic: 2015, Q3, P40

● **O36.0**   **Maternal care for rhesus isoimmunization**
     Maternal care for Rh incompatibility (with hydrops fetalis)

     ● **O36.01**   **Maternal care for anti-D [Rh] antibodies**

         ● **O36.011**   **Maternal care for anti-D [Rh] antibodies, first trimester**   M

         ● **O36.012**   **Maternal care for anti-D [Rh] antibodies, second trimester**   M

         ● **O36.013**   **Maternal care for anti-D [Rh] antibodies, third trimester**   M

         ● **O36.019**   **Maternal care for anti-D [Rh] antibodies, unspecified trimester**   M

     ● **O36.09**   **Maternal care for other rhesus isoimmunization**

         ● **O36.091**   **Maternal care for other rhesus isoimmunization, first trimester**

         ● **O36.092**   **Maternal care for other rhesus isoimmunization, second trimester**   M

         ● **O36.093**   **Maternal care for other rhesus isoimmunization, third trimester**   M
             Coding Clinic: 2015, Q3, P40

         ● **O36.099**   **Maternal care for other rhesus isoimmunization, unspecified trimester**   M

● **O36.1**   **Maternal care for other isoimmunization**
     Maternal care for ABO isoimmunization

     ● **O36.11**   **Maternal care for Anti-A sensitization**
         Maternal care for isoimmunization NOS (with hydrops fetalis)

         ● **O36.111**   **Maternal care for Anti-A sensitization, first trimester**   M

         ● **O36.112**   **Maternal care for Anti-A sensitization, second trimester**   M

         ● **O36.113**   **Maternal care for Anti-A sensitization, third trimester**   M

         ● **O36.119**   **Maternal care for Anti-A sensitization, unspecified trimester**   M

     ● **O36.19**   **Maternal care for other isoimmunization**
         Maternal care for Anti-B sensitization

         ● **O36.191**   **Maternal care for other isoimmunization, first trimester**   M

         ● **O36.192**   **Maternal care for other isoimmunization, second trimester**   M

         ● **O36.193**   **Maternal care for other isoimmunization, third trimester**   M

         ● **O36.199**   **Maternal care for other isoimmunization, unspecified trimester**   M

● **O36.2**   **Maternal care for hydrops fetalis**
     Maternal care for hydrops fetalis NOS
     Maternal care for hydrops fetalis not associated with isoimmunization

     Excludes1   hydrops fetalis associated with ABO isoimmunization (O36.1-)
                  hydrops fetalis associated with rhesus isoimmunization (O36.0-)

     ● **O36.20**   **Maternal care for hydrops fetalis, unspecified trimester**   M

     ● **O36.21**   **Maternal care for hydrops fetalis, first trimester**   M

     ● **O36.22**   **Maternal care for hydrops fetalis, second trimester**   M

     ● **O36.23**   **Maternal care for hydrops fetalis, third trimester**   M

● **O36.4**   **Maternal care for intrauterine death**   M
     Maternal care for intrauterine fetal death NOS
     Maternal care for intrauterine fetal death after completion of 20 weeks of gestation
     Maternal care for late fetal death
     Maternal care for missed delivery

     Excludes1   missed abortion (O02.1)
                  stillbirth (P95)
     Coding Clinic: 2022, Q2, P3-4

● **O36.5**   **Maternal care for known or suspected poor fetal growth**

     ● **O36.51**   **Maternal care for known or suspected placental insufficiency**

         ● **O36.511**   **Maternal care for known or suspected placental insufficiency, first trimester**   M

         ● **O36.512**   **Maternal care for known or suspected placental insufficiency, second trimester**   M

         ● **O36.513**   **Maternal care for known or suspected placental insufficiency, third trimester**   M

         ● **O36.519**   **Maternal care for known or suspected placental insufficiency, unspecified trimester**   M

     ● **O36.59**   **Maternal care for other known or suspected poor fetal growth**
         Maternal care for known or suspected light-for-dates NOS
         Maternal care for known or suspected small-for-dates NOS

         ● **O36.591**   **Maternal care for other known or suspected poor fetal growth, first trimester**   M

▶ New   ⇒ Revised   ~~deleted~~ Deleted   Excludes 1   Excludes 2   Includes   Use additional   Code first   Code also   Key words

OGCR Official Guidelines   X Assign placeholder X   ▶ Use Additional Character(s)   ▶ Manifestation Code   🔶 Hierarchical Condition Category   Coding Clinic

● O36.592   Maternal care for other known or suspected poor fetal growth, second trimester   M

● O36.593   Maternal care for other known or suspected poor fetal growth, third trimester   M

● O36.599   Maternal care for other known or suspected poor fetal growth, unspecified trimester   M

● O36.6   Maternal care for excessive fetal growth
     Maternal care for known or suspected large-for-dates

X ● O36.60   Maternal care for excessive fetal growth, unspecified trimester   M

X ● O36.61   Maternal care for excessive fetal growth, first trimester   M

X ● O36.62   Maternal care for excessive fetal growth, second trimester   M

X ● O36.63   Maternal care for excessive fetal growth, third trimester   M

● O36.7   Maternal care for viable fetus in abdominal pregnancy

X ● O36.70   Maternal care for viable fetus in abdominal pregnancy, unspecified trimester   M

X ● O36.71   Maternal care for viable fetus in abdominal pregnancy, first trimester   M

X ● O36.72   Maternal care for viable fetus in abdominal pregnancy, second trimester   M

X ● O36.73   Maternal care for viable fetus in abdominal pregnancy, third trimester   M

● O36.8   Maternal care for other specified fetal problems

X ● O36.80   Pregnancy with inconclusive fetal viability   M
     Encounter to determine fetal viability of pregnancy
     Coding Clinic: 2019, Q2, P29

● O36.81   Decreased fetal movements

● O36.812   Decreased fetal movements, second trimester   M

● O36.813   Decreased fetal movements, third trimester   M

● O36.819   Decreased fetal movements, unspecified trimester   M

● O36.82   Fetal anemia and thrombocytopenia

● O36.821   Fetal anemia and thrombocytopenia, first trimester   M

● O36.822   Fetal anemia and thrombocytopenia, second trimester   M

● O36.823   Fetal anemia and thrombocytopenia, third trimester   M

● O36.829   Fetal anemia and thrombocytopenia, unspecified trimester   M

● O36.83   Maternal care for abnormalities of the fetal heart rate or rhythm
     Maternal care for depressed fetal heart rate tones
     Maternal care for fetal bradycardia
     Maternal care for fetal heart rate abnormal variability
     Maternal care for fetal heart rate decelerations
     Maternal care for fetal heart rate irregularity
     Maternal care for fetal tachycardia
     Maternal care for non-reassuring fetal heart rate or rhythm

● O36.831   Maternal care for abnormalities of the fetal heart rate or rhythm, first trimester   M

● O36.832   Maternal care for abnormalities of the fetal heart rate or rhythm, second trimester   M

● O36.833   Maternal care for abnormalities of the fetal heart rate or rhythm, third trimester   M

● O36.839   Maternal care for abnormalities of the fetal heart rate or rhythm, unspecified trimester   M

● O36.89   Maternal care for other specified fetal problems

● O36.891   Maternal care for other specified fetal problems, first trimester   M

● O36.892   Maternal care for other specified fetal problems, second trimester   M

● O36.893   Maternal care for other specified fetal problems, third trimester   M

● O36.899   Maternal care for other specified fetal problems, unspecified trimester   M

● O36.9   Maternal care for fetal problem, unspecified

X ● O36.90   Maternal care for fetal problem, unspecified, unspecified trimester   M

X ● O36.91   Maternal care for fetal problem, unspecified, first trimester   M

X ● O36.92   Maternal care for fetal problem, unspecified, second trimester   M

X ● O36.93   Maternal care for fetal problem, unspecified, third trimester   M

● O40   Polyhydramnios
     Overabundance of amniotic fluid
     Includes   hydramnios
     Excludes1   encounter for suspected maternal and fetal conditions ruled out (Z03.7-)

One of the following 7th characters is to be assigned to each code under category O40. 7th character Ø is for single gestations and multiple gestations where the fetus is unspecified. 7th characters 1 through 9 are for cases of multiple gestations to identify the fetus for which the code applies. The appropriate code from category O30, Multiple gestation, must also be assigned when assigning a code from category O40 that has a 7th character of 1 through 9.

Ø	not applicable or unspecified
1	fetus 1
2	fetus 2
3	fetus 3
4	fetus 4
5	fetus 5
9	other fetus

X ● O40.1   Polyhydramnios, first trimester   M

X ● O40.2   Polyhydramnios, second trimester   M

X ● O40.3   Polyhydramnios, third trimester   M

X ● O40.9   Polyhydramnios, unspecified trimester   M

● O41   Other disorders of amniotic fluid and membranes
     Excludes1   encounter for suspected maternal and fetal conditions ruled out (Z03.7-)

One of the following 7th characters is to be assigned to each code under category O41. 7th character Ø is for single gestations and multiple gestations where the fetus is unspecified. 7th characters 1 through 9 are for cases of multiple gestations to identify the fetus for which the code applies. The appropriate code from category O30, Multiple gestation, must also be assigned when assigning a code from category O41 that has a 7th character of 1 through 9.

Ø	not applicable or unspecified
1	fetus 1
2	fetus 2
3	fetus 3
4	fetus 4
5	fetus 5
9	other fetus

● O41.0   Oligohydramnios
     Scant volume of amniotic fluid
     Oligohydramnios without rupture of membranes

X ● O41.00   Oligohydramnios, unspecified trimester   M

X ● O41.01   Oligohydramnios, first trimester   M

X ● O41.02   Oligohydramnios, second trimester   M

X ● O41.03   Oligohydramnios, third trimester   M

CHAPTER 15 (OØØ–O9A)

CHAPTER 15 (O00-O9A)

● O41.1   Infection of amniotic sac and membranes
   ● O41.10   Infection of amniotic sac and membranes, unspecified
      ● O41.101   Infection of amniotic sac and membranes, unspecified, first trimester   M
      ● O41.102   Infection of amniotic sac and membranes, unspecified, second trimester   M
      ● O41.103   Infection of amniotic sac and membranes, unspecified, third trimester   M
      ● O41.109   Infection of amniotic sac and membranes, unspecified, unspecified trimester   M
   ● O41.12   Chorioamnionitis
      Coding Clinic: 2019, Q2, P34-35
      ● O41.121   Chorioamnionitis, first trimester   M
      ● O41.122   Chorioamnionitis, second trimester   M
      ● O41.123   Chorioamnionitis, third trimester   M
      ● O41.129   Chorioamnionitis, unspecified trimester   M
   ● O41.14   Placentitis
      ● O41.141   Placentitis, first trimester   M
      ● O41.142   Placentitis, second trimester   M
      ● O41.143   Placentitis, third trimester   M
      ● O41.149   Placentitis, unspecified trimester   M
● O41.8   Other specified disorders of amniotic fluid and membranes
   ● O41.8X   Other specified disorders of amniotic fluid and membranes
      ● O41.8X1   Other specified disorders of amniotic fluid and membranes, first trimester M
      ● O41.8X2   Other specified disorders of amniotic fluid and membranes, second trimester   M
      ● O41.8X3   Other specified disorders of amniotic fluid and membranes, third trimester   M
         Coding Clinic: 2024, Q1, P14
      ● O41.8X9   Other specified disorders of amniotic fluid and membranes, unspecified trimester   M
● O41.9   Disorder of amniotic fluid and membranes, unspecified
   X ● O41.90   Disorder of amniotic fluid and membranes, unspecified, unspecified trimester   M
   X ● O41.91   Disorder of amniotic fluid and membranes, unspecified, first trimester   M
   X ● O41.92   Disorder of amniotic fluid and membranes, unspecified, second trimester   M
   X ● O41.93   Disorder of amniotic fluid and membranes, unspecified, third trimester   M

● O42   Premature rupture of membranes
   Coding Clinic: 2023, Q3, P17
  ● O42.0   Premature rupture of membranes, onset of labor within 24 hours of rupture
   O42.00   Premature rupture of membranes, onset of labor within 24 hours of rupture, unspecified weeks of gestation   M
   ● O42.01   Preterm premature rupture of membranes, onset of labor within 24 hours of rupture
      Premature rupture of membranes before 37 completed weeks of gestation
      O42.011   Preterm premature rupture of membranes, onset of labor within 24 hours of rupture, first trimester   M
      O42.012   Preterm premature rupture of membranes, onset of labor within 24 hours of rupture, second trimester   M

      O42.013   Preterm premature rupture of membranes, onset of labor within 24 hours of rupture, third trimester   M
      O42.019   Preterm premature rupture of membranes, onset of labor within 24 hours of rupture, unspecified trimester   M
   O42.02   Full-term premature rupture of membranes, onset of labor within 24 hours of rupture   M
      Premature rupture of membranes at or after 37 completed weeks of gestation, onset of labor within 24 hours of rupture
● O42.1   Premature rupture of membranes, onset of labor more than 24 hours following rupture
   O42.10   Premature rupture of membranes, onset of labor more than 24 hours following rupture, unspecified weeks of gestation   M
  ● O42.11   Preterm premature rupture of membranes, onset of labor more than 24 hours following rupture
      Premature rupture of membranes before 37 completed weeks of gestation
      O42.111   Preterm premature rupture of membranes, onset of labor more than 24 hours following rupture, first trimester   M
      O42.112   Preterm premature rupture of membranes, onset of labor more than 24 hours following rupture, second trimester   M
      O42.113   Preterm premature rupture of membranes, onset of labor more than 24 hours following rupture, third trimester   M
      O42.119   Preterm premature rupture of membranes, onset of labor more than 24 hours following rupture, unspecified trimester   M
   O42.12   Full-term premature rupture of membranes, onset of labor more than 24 hours following rupture   M
      Premature rupture of membranes at or after 37 completed weeks of gestation, onset of labor more than 24 hours following rupture
● O42.9   Premature rupture of membranes, unspecified as to length of time between rupture and onset of labor
   O42.90   Premature rupture of membranes, unspecified as to length of time between rupture and onset of labor, unspecified weeks of gestation   M
  ● O42.91   Preterm premature rupture of membranes, unspecified as to length of time between rupture and onset of labor
      Premature rupture of membranes before 37 completed weeks of gestation
      O42.911   Preterm premature rupture of membranes, unspecified as to length of time between rupture and onset of labor, first trimester   M
      O42.912   Preterm premature rupture of membranes, unspecified as to length of time between rupture and onset of labor, second trimester   M
      O42.913   Preterm premature rupture of membranes, unspecified as to length of time between rupture and onset of labor, third trimester   M
      O42.919   Preterm premature rupture of membranes, unspecified as to length of time between rupture and onset of labor, unspecified trimester   M

▶ New   ⇒ Revised   ~~deleted~~ Deleted   Excludes 1   Excludes 2   Includes   Use additional   Code first   Code also   Key words

OGCR Official Guidelines   X Assign placeholder X   ● Use Additional Character(s)   ▶ Manifestation Code   ⊕ Hierarchical Condition Category   Coding Clinic

O42.92 **Full-term premature rupture of membranes, unspecified as to length of time between rupture and onset of labor**   M

     Premature rupture of membranes at or after 37 completed weeks of gestation, unspecified as to length of time between rupture and onset of labor

● O43   **Placental disorders**

     Excludes2   maternal care for poor fetal growth due to placental insufficiency (O36.5-)

          placenta previa (O44.-)

          placental polyp (O90.89)

          placentitis (O41.14-)

          premature separation of placenta [abruptio placentae] (O45.-)

● O43.0   **Placental transfusion syndromes**

   ● O43.01   **Fetomaternal placental transfusion syndrome**

        Maternofetal placental transfusion syndrome

     O43.011   Fetomaternal placental transfusion syndrome, first trimester   M

     O43.012   Fetomaternal placental transfusion syndrome, second trimester   M

     O43.013   Fetomaternal placental transfusion syndrome, third trimester   M

     O43.019   Fetomaternal placental transfusion syndrome, unspecified trimester   M

   ● O43.02   **Fetus-to-fetus placental transfusion syndrome**

     O43.021   Fetus-to-fetus placental transfusion syndrome, first trimester   M

     O43.022   Fetus-to-fetus placental transfusion syndrome, second trimester   M

     O43.023   Fetus-to-fetus placental transfusion syndrome, third trimester   M

     O43.029   Fetus-to-fetus placental transfusion syndrome, unspecified trimester   M

● O43.1   **Malformation of placenta**

   ● O43.10   **Malformation of placenta, unspecified**

        Abnormal placenta NOS

     O43.101   Malformation of placenta, unspecified, first trimester   M

     O43.102   Malformation of placenta, unspecified, second trimester   M

     O43.103   Malformation of placenta, unspecified, third trimester   M

     O43.109   Malformation of placenta, unspecified, unspecified trimester   M

   ● O43.11   **Circumvallate placenta**

     O43.111   Circumvallate placenta, first trimester   M

     O43.112   Circumvallate placenta, second trimester   M

     O43.113   Circumvallate placenta, third trimester   M

     O43.119   Circumvallate placenta, unspecified trimester   M

   ● O43.12   **Velamentous insertion of umbilical cord**

     O43.121   Velamentous insertion of umbilical cord, first trimester   M

     O43.122   Velamentous insertion of umbilical cord, second trimester   M

     O43.123   Velamentous insertion of umbilical cord, third trimester   M

     O43.129   Velamentous insertion of umbilical cord, unspecified trimester   M

   ● O43.19   **Other malformation of placenta**

     O43.191   Other malformation of placenta, first trimester   M

     O43.192   Other malformation of placenta, second trimester   M

     O43.193   Other malformation of placenta, third trimester   M

     O43.199   Other malformation of placenta, unspecified trimester   M

● O43.2   **Morbidly adherent placenta**

     Code also associated third stage postpartum hemorrhage, if applicable (O72.0)

     Excludes1   retained placenta (O73.-)

   ● O43.21   **Placenta accreta**

     O43.211   Placenta accreta, first trimester   M

     O43.212   Placenta accreta, second trimester   M

     O43.213   Placenta accreta, third trimester   M

     O43.219   Placenta accreta, unspecified trimester   M

   ● O43.22   **Placenta increta**

     O43.221   Placenta increta, first trimester   M

     O43.222   Placenta increta, second trimester   M

        Coding Clinic: 2022, Q1, P21

     O43.223   Placenta increta, third trimester   M

     O43.229   Placenta increta, unspecified trimester   M

   ● O43.23   **Placenta percreta**

     O43.231   Placenta percreta, first trimester   M

     O43.232   Placenta percreta, second trimester   M

     O43.233   Placenta percreta, third trimester   M

     O43.239   Placenta percreta, unspecified trimester   M

● O43.8   **Other placental disorders**

   ● O43.81   **Placental infarction**

     O43.811   Placental infarction, first trimester   M

     O43.812   Placental infarction, second trimester   M

     O43.813   Placental infarction, third trimester   M

     O43.819   Placental infarction, unspecified trimester   M

   ● O43.89   **Other placental disorders**

        Placental dysfunction

     O43.891   Other placental disorders, first trimester   M

     O43.892   Other placental disorders, second trimester   M

     O43.893   Other placental disorders, third trimester   M

     O43.899   Other placental disorders, unspecified trimester   M

● O43.9   **Unspecified placental disorder**

     O43.90   Unspecified placental disorder, unspecified trimester   M

     O43.91   Unspecified placental disorder, first trimester   M

     O43.92   Unspecified placental disorder, second trimester   M

     O43.93   Unspecified placental disorder, third trimester   M

Figure 15-2   A. Marginal placento previa. **B.** Partial placenta previa. **C.** Total placento previa.

Item 15–3   Placenta previa is a condition in which the opening of the cervix is obstructed by the displaced placenta. The three types, marginal, partial, and total, are varying degrees of placenta displacement. Placenta abruption is the premature breaking away of the placenta from the site of the uterine implant before the delivery of the fetus.

CHAPTER 15 (O00-O9A)

CHAPTER 15 (O00-O9A)

● O44   Placenta previa

     Coding Clinic: 2016, Q4, P52

● O44.0   Complete placenta previa NOS or without hemorrhage

     Placenta previa NOS

     O44.00   Complete placenta previa NOS or without hemorrhage, unspecified trimester   M

     O44.01   Complete placenta previa NOS or without hemorrhage, first trimester   M

     O44.02   Complete placenta previa NOS or without hemorrhage, second trimester   M

     O44.03   Complete placenta previa NOS or without hemorrhage, third trimester   M

● O44.1   Complete placenta previa with hemorrhage

     Excludes1   labor and delivery complicated by hemorrhage from vasa previa (O69.4)

     O44.10   Complete placenta previa with hemorrhage, unspecified trimester   M

     O44.11   Complete placenta previa with hemorrhage, first trimester   M

     O44.12   Complete placenta previa with hemorrhage, second trimester   M

     O44.13   Complete placenta previa with hemorrhage, third trimester   M

● O44.2   Partial placenta previa without hemorrhage

     Marginal placenta previa, NOS or without hemorrhage

     O44.20   Partial placenta previa NOS or without hemorrhage, unspecified trimester   M

     O44.21   Partial placenta previa NOS or without hemorrhage, first trimester   M

     O44.22   Partial placenta previa NOS or without hemorrhage, second trimester   M

     O44.23   Partial placenta previa NOS or without hemorrhage, third trimester   M

● O44.3   Partial placenta previa with hemorrhage

     Marginal placenta previa with hemorrhage

     O44.30   Partial placenta previa with hemorrhage, unspecified trimester   M

     O44.31   Partial placenta previa with hemorrhage, first trimester   M

     O44.32   Partial placenta previa with hemorrhage, second trimester   M

     O44.33   Partial placenta previa with hemorrhage, third trimester   M

● O44.4   Low lying placenta NOS or without hemorrhage

     Low implantation of placenta NOS or without hemorrhage

     O44.40   Low lying placenta NOS or without hemorrhage, unspecified trimester   M

     O44.41   Low lying placenta NOS or without hemorrhage, first trimester   M

     O44.42   Low lying placenta NOS or without hemorrhage, second trimester   M

     O44.43   Low lying placenta NOS or without hemorrhage, third trimester   M

● O44.5   Low lying placenta with hemorrhage

     Low implantation of placenta with hemorrhage

Figure 15-3 Abruptio placentae is classified according to the grade of separation of the placenta from the uterine wall. **A.** Mild separation in which hemorrhage is internal. **B.** Moderate separation in which there is external hemorrhage. **C.** Severe separation in which there is external hemorrhage and extreme separation.

     O44.50   Low lying placenta with hemorrhage, unspecified trimester   M

     O44.51   Low lying placenta with hemorrhage, first trimester   M

     O44.52   Low lying placenta with hemorrhage, second trimester   M

     O44.53   Low lying placenta with hemorrhage, third trimester   M

● O45   Premature separation of placenta [abruptio placentae]

● O45.0   Premature separation of placenta with coagulation defect

● O45.00   Premature separation of placenta with coagulation defect, unspecified

     O45.001   Premature separation of placenta with coagulation defect, unspecified, first trimester   M

     O45.002   Premature separation of placenta with coagulation defect, unspecified, second trimester   M

     O45.003   Premature separation of placenta with coagulation defect, unspecified, third trimester   M

     O45.009   Premature separation of placenta with coagulation defect, unspecified, unspecified trimester   M

● O45.01   Premature separation of placenta with afibrinogenemia

     Premature separation of placenta with hypofibrinogenemia

     O45.011   Premature separation of placenta with afibrinogenemia, first trimester   M

     O45.012   Premature separation of placenta with afibrinogenemia, second trimester   M

     O45.013   Premature separation of placenta with afibrinogenemia, third trimester   M

     O45.019   Premature separation of placenta with afibrinogenemia, unspecified trimester   M

● O45.02   Premature separation of placenta with disseminated intravascular coagulation

     O45.021   Premature separation of placenta with disseminated intravascular coagulation, first trimester   M

     O45.022   Premature separation of placenta with disseminated intravascular coagulation, second trimester   M

     O45.023   Premature separation of placenta with disseminated intravascular coagulation, third trimester   M

     O45.029   Premature separation of placenta with disseminated intravascular coagulation, unspecified trimester   M

● O45.09   Premature separation of placenta with other coagulation defect

     O45.091   Premature separation of placenta with other coagulation defect, first trimester   M

     O45.092   Premature separation of placenta with other coagulation defect, second trimester   M

     O45.093   Premature separation of placenta with other coagulation defect, third trimester   M

     O45.099   Premature separation of placenta with other coagulation defect, unspecified trimester   M

● O45.8   Other premature separation of placenta

● O45.8X   Other premature separation of placenta

     O45.8X1   Other premature separation of placenta, first trimester   M

     O45.8X2   Other premature separation of placenta, second trimester   M

▶ New   ⟹ Revised   ~~deleted~~ Deleted   Excludes 1   Excludes 2   Includes   Use additional   Code first   Code also   Key words

OGCR Official Guidelines   X Assign placeholder X   ● Use Additional Character(s)   ▷ Manifestation Code   🗱 Hierarchical Condition Category   Coding Clinic

      O45.8X3   Other premature separation of placenta, third trimester   **M**

      O45.8X9   Other premature separation of placenta, unspecified trimester   **M**

● **O45.9**   Premature separation of placenta, unspecified
     Abruptio placentae NOS

      O45.90   Premature separation of placenta, unspecified, unspecified trimester   **M**

      O45.91   Premature separation of placenta, unspecified, first trimester   **M**

      O45.92   Premature separation of placenta, unspecified, second trimester   **M**

      O45.93   Premature separation of placenta, unspecified, third trimester   **M**

● **O46**   Antepartum hemorrhage, not elsewhere classified

     Excludes1   hemorrhage in early pregnancy (O20.-)
                intrapartum hemorrhage NEC (O67.-)
                placenta previa (O44.-)
                premature separation of placenta [abruptio placentae] (O45.-)

● **O46.0**   Antepartum hemorrhage with coagulation defect

  ● **O46.00**   Antepartum hemorrhage with coagulation defect, unspecified

      O46.001   Antepartum hemorrhage with coagulation defect, unspecified, first trimester   **M**

      O46.002   Antepartum hemorrhage with coagulation defect, unspecified, second trimester   **M**

      O46.003   Antepartum hemorrhage with coagulation defect, unspecified, third trimester   **M**

      O46.009   Antepartum hemorrhage with coagulation defect, unspecified, unspecified trimester   **M**

  ● **O46.01**   Antepartum hemorrhage with afibrinogenemia
       Antepartum hemorrhage with hypofibrinogenemia

      O46.011   Antepartum hemorrhage with afibrinogenemia, first trimester   **M**

      O46.012   Antepartum hemorrhage with afibrinogenemia, second trimester   **M**

      O46.013   Antepartum hemorrhage with afibrinogenemia, third trimester   **M**

      O46.019   Antepartum hemorrhage with afibrinogenemia, unspecified trimester   **M**

  ● **O46.02**   Antepartum hemorrhage with disseminated intravascular coagulation

      O46.021   Antepartum hemorrhage with disseminated intravascular coagulation, first trimester   **M**

      O46.022   Antepartum hemorrhage with disseminated intravascular coagulation, second trimester   **M**

      O46.023   Antepartum hemorrhage with disseminated intravascular coagulation, third trimester   **M**

      O46.029   Antepartum hemorrhage with disseminated intravascular coagulation, unspecified trimester   **M**

  ● **O46.09**   Antepartum hemorrhage with other coagulation defect

      O46.091   Antepartum hemorrhage with other coagulation defect, first trimester   **M**

      O46.092   Antepartum hemorrhage with other coagulation defect, second trimester   **M**

      O46.093   Antepartum hemorrhage with other coagulation defect, third trimester   **M**

      O46.099   Antepartum hemorrhage with other coagulation defect, unspecified trimester   **M**

● **O46.8**   Other antepartum hemorrhage

  ● **O46.8x**   Other antepartum hemorrhage

      O46.8x1   Other antepartum hemorrhage, first trimester   **M**

      O46.8x2   Other antepartum hemorrhage, second trimester   **M**

      O46.8x3   Other antepartum hemorrhage, third trimester   **M**

      O46.8x9   Other antepartum hemorrhage, unspecified trimester   **M**

● **O46.9**   Antepartum hemorrhage, unspecified

      O46.90   Antepartum hemorrhage, unspecified, unspecified trimester   **M**

      O46.91   Antepartum hemorrhage, unspecified, first trimester   **M**

      O46.92   Antepartum hemorrhage, unspecified, second trimester   **M**

      O46.93   Antepartum hemorrhage, unspecified, third trimester   **M**

● **O47**   False labor

     Includes   Braxton Hicks contractions
                threatened labor

     Excludes1   preterm labor (O60.-)

● **O47.0**   False labor before 37 completed weeks of gestation

      O47.00   False labor before 37 completed weeks of gestation, unspecified trimester   **M**

      O47.02   False labor before 37 completed weeks of gestation, second trimester   **M**

      O47.03   False labor before 37 completed weeks of gestation, third trimester   **M**

    O47.1   False labor at or after 37 completed weeks of gestation   **M**
        Coding Clinic: 2021, Q1, P10

    O47.9   False labor, unspecified   **M**

● **O48**   Late pregnancy

    O48.0   Post-term pregnancy   **M**
        Pregnancy over 40 completed weeks to 42 completed weeks gestation
        Coding Clinic: 2022, Q2 P3-4

    O48.1   Prolonged pregnancy   **M**
        Pregnancy which has advanced beyond 42 completed weeks gestation
        Coding Clinic: 2022, Q2 P3-4

COMPLICATIONS OF LABOR AND DELIVERY (O60-O77)

● **O60**   Preterm labor

     Includes   onset (spontaneous) of labor before 37 completed weeks of gestation

     Excludes1   false labor (O47.0-)
                threatened labor NOS (O47.0-)

● **O60.0**   Preterm labor without delivery

      O60.00   Preterm labor without delivery, unspecified trimester   **M**

      O60.02   Preterm labor without delivery, second trimester   **M**

      O60.03   Preterm labor without delivery, third trimester   **M**

● **O60.1 Preterm labor with preterm delivery**

One of the following 7th characters is to be assigned to each code under subcategory O60.1. 7th character 0 is for single gestations and multiple gestations where the fetus is unspecified. 7th characters 1 through 9 are for cases of multiple gestations to identify the fetus for which the code applies. The appropriate code from category O30, Multiple gestation, must also be assigned when assigning a code from subcategory O60.1 that has a 7th character of 1 through 9.

0	not applicable or unspecified
1	fetus 1
2	fetus 2
3	fetus 3
4	fetus 4
5	fetus 5
9	other fetus

Coding Clinic: 2016, Q2, P11

X● **O60.10 Preterm labor with preterm delivery, unspecified trimester** M
Preterm labor with delivery NOS

X● **O60.12 Preterm labor second trimester with preterm delivery second trimester** M

X● **O60.13 Preterm labor second trimester with preterm delivery third trimester** M

X● **O60.14 Preterm labor third trimester with preterm delivery third trimester** M
Coding Clinic: 2016, Q2, P10

● **O60.2 Term delivery with preterm labor**

One of the following 7th characters is to be assigned to each code under subcategory O60.2. 7th character 0 is for single gestations and multiple gestations where the fetus is unspecified. 7th characters 1 through 9 are for cases of multiple gestations to identify the fetus for which the code applies. The appropriate code from category O30, Multiple gestation, must also be assigned when assigning a code from subcategory O60.2 that has a 7th character of 1 through 9.

0	not applicable or unspecified
1	fetus 1
2	fetus 2
3	fetus 3
4	fetus 4
5	fetus 5
9	other fetus

X● **O60.20 Term delivery with preterm labor, unspecified trimester** M

X● **O60.22 Term delivery with preterm labor, second trimester** M

X● **O60.23 Term delivery with preterm labor, third trimester** M

● **O61 Failed induction of labor**

O61.0 Failed medical induction of labor M
Failed induction (of labor) by oxytocin
Failed induction (of labor) by prostaglandins

O61.1 Failed instrumental induction of labor M
Failed mechanical induction (of labor)
Failed surgical induction (of labor)

O61.8 Other failed induction of labor M

O61.9 Failed induction of labor, unspecified M

● **O62 Abnormalities of forces of labor**

O62.0 Primary inadequate contractions M
Failure of cervical dilatation
Primary hypotonic uterine dysfunction
Uterine inertia during latent phase of labor
Coding Clinic: 2024, Q1, P13

O62.1 Secondary uterine inertia M
Arrested active phase of labor
Secondary hypotonic uterine dysfunction

O62.2 Other uterine inertia M
Atony of uterus without hemorrhage
Atony of uterus NOS
Desultory labor
Hypotonic uterine dysfunction NOS
Irregular labor
Poor contractions
Slow slope active phase of labor
Uterine inertia NOS

Excludes1 atony of uterus with hemorrhage (postpartum) (O72.1)
postpartum atony of uterus without hemorrhage (O75.89)

O62.3 Precipitate labor M

O62.4 Hypertonic, incoordinate, and prolonged uterine contractions M
Cervical spasm
Contraction ring dystocia
Dyscoordinate labor
Hour-glass contraction of uterus
Hypertonic uterine dysfunction
Incoordinate uterine action
Tetanic contractions
Uterine dystocia NOS
Uterine spasm

Excludes1 dystocia (fetal) (maternal) NOS (O66.9)

O62.8 Other abnormalities of forces of labor M

O62.9 Abnormality of forces of labor, unspecified M

● **O63 Long labor**

O63.0 Prolonged first stage (of labor) M

O63.1 Prolonged second stage (of labor) M

O63.2 Delayed delivery of second twin, triplet, etc. M

O63.9 Long labor, unspecified M
Prolonged labor NOS

● **O64 Obstructed labor due to malposition and malpresentation of fetus**

One of the following 7th characters is to be assigned to each code under category O64. 7th character 0 is for single gestations and multiple gestations where the fetus is unspecified. 7th characters 1 through 9 are for cases of multiple gestations to identify the fetus for which the code applies. The appropriate code from category O30, Multiple gestation, must also be assigned when assigning a code from category O64 that has a 7th character of 1 through 9.

0	not applicable or unspecified
1	fetus 1
2	fetus 2
3	fetus 3
4	fetus 4
5	fetus 5
9	other fetus

X● **O64.0 Obstructed labor due to incomplete rotation of fetal head** M
Deep transverse arrest
Obstructed labor due to persistent occipitoiliac (position)
Obstructed labor due to persistent occipitoposterior (position)
Obstructed labor due to persistent occipitosacral (position)
Obstructed labor due to persistent occipitotransverse (position)

X● **O64.1 Obstructed labor due to breech presentation** M
Obstructed labor due to buttocks presentation
Obstructed labor due to complete breech presentation
Obstructed labor due to frank breech presentation

X● **O64.2 Obstructed labor due to face presentation** M
Obstructed labor due to chin presentation

X● **O64.3 Obstructed labor due to brow presentation** M

▶ New   ⇒ Revised   ~~deleted~~ Deleted   Excludes 1   Excludes 2   Includes   Use additional   Code first   Code also   Key words

OGCR Official Guidelines   X Assign placeholder X   ● Use Additional Character(s)   ▷ Manifestation Code   ⌘ Hierarchical Condition Category   Coding Clinic

Figure 15-5 Hydrocephalic fetus causing disproportion.

Figure 15-4 Five types of malposition and malpresentation of the fetus: **A.** Breech. **B.** Vertex. **C.** Face. **D.** Brow. **E.** Shoulder.

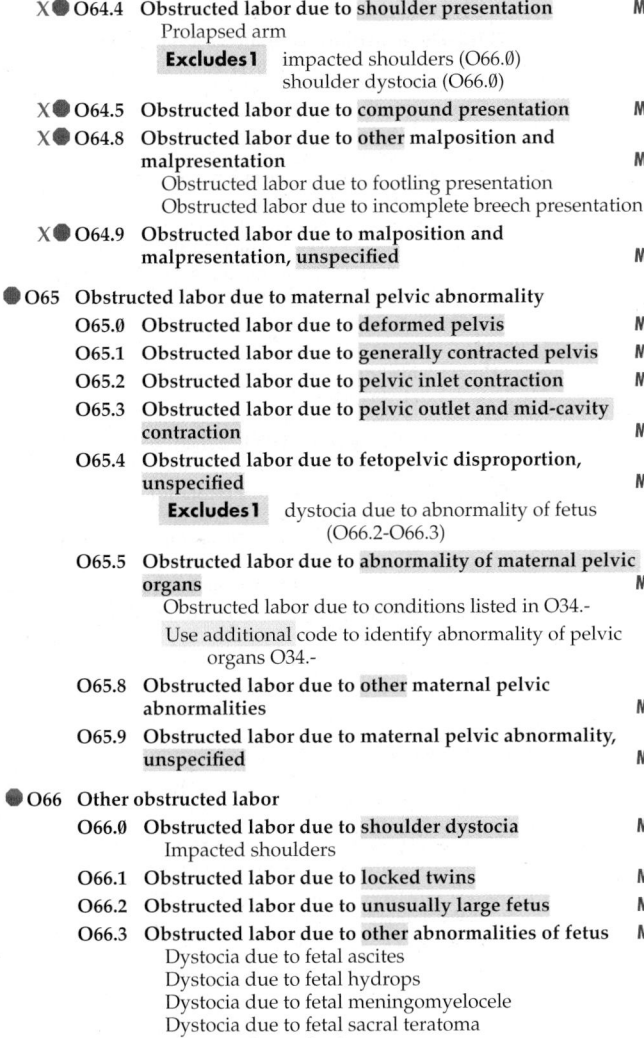

X ● **O64.4**   **Obstructed labor due to shoulder presentation**   M
Prolapsed arm

     Excludes 1   impacted shoulders (O66.0)
                  shoulder dystocia (O66.0)

X ● **O64.5**   **Obstructed labor due to compound presentation**   M

X ● **O64.8**   **Obstructed labor due to other malposition and malpresentation**   M
Obstructed labor due to footling presentation
Obstructed labor due to incomplete breech presentation

X ● **O64.9**   **Obstructed labor due to malposition and malpresentation, unspecified**   M

● **O65**   **Obstructed labor due to maternal pelvic abnormality**

   O65.0   **Obstructed labor due to deformed pelvis**   M

   O65.1   **Obstructed labor due to generally contracted pelvis**   M

   O65.2   **Obstructed labor due to pelvic inlet contraction**   M

   O65.3   **Obstructed labor due to pelvic outlet and mid-cavity contraction**   M

   O65.4   **Obstructed labor due to fetopelvic disproportion, unspecified**   M

     Excludes 1   dystocia due to abnormality of fetus (O66.2-O66.3)

   O65.5   **Obstructed labor due to abnormality of maternal pelvic organs**   M
Obstructed labor due to conditions listed in O34.-
Use additional code to identify abnormality of pelvic organs O34.-

   O65.8   **Obstructed labor due to other maternal pelvic abnormalities**   M

   O65.9   **Obstructed labor due to maternal pelvic abnormality, unspecified**   M

● **O66**   **Other obstructed labor**

   O66.0   **Obstructed labor due to shoulder dystocia**   M
Impacted shoulders

   O66.1   **Obstructed labor due to locked twins**   M

   O66.2   **Obstructed labor due to unusually large fetus**   M

   O66.3   **Obstructed labor due to other abnormalities of fetus**   M
Dystocia due to fetal ascites
Dystocia due to fetal hydrops
Dystocia due to fetal meningomyelocele
Dystocia due to fetal sacral teratoma
Dystocia due to fetal tumor
Dystocia due to hydrocephalic fetus
Use additional code to identify cause of obstruction

● **O66.4**   **Failed trial of labor**

   O66.40   **Failed trial of labor, unspecified**   M

   O66.41   **Failed attempted vaginal birth after previous cesarean delivery**   M
Code first rupture of uterus, if applicable (O71.0-, O71.1)

   O66.5   **Attempted application of vacuum extractor and forceps**   M
Attempted application of vacuum or forceps, with subsequent delivery by forceps or cesarean delivery

   O66.6   **Obstructed labor due to other multiple fetuses**   M

   O66.8   **Other specified obstructed labor**   M
Use additional code to identify cause of obstruction

   O66.9   **Obstructed labor, unspecified**   M
Dystocia NOS
Fetal dystocia NOS
Maternal dystocia NOS

● **O67**   **Labor and delivery complicated by intrapartum hemorrhage, not elsewhere classified**

     Excludes 1   antepartum hemorrhage NEC (O46.-)
                placenta previa (O44.-)
                premature separation of placenta [abruptio placentae] (O45.-)

     Excludes 2   postpartum hemorrhage (O72.-)

   O67.0   **Intrapartum hemorrhage with coagulation defect**   M
Intrapartum hemorrhage (excessive) associated with afibrinogenemia
Intrapartum hemorrhage (excessive) associated with disseminated intravascular coagulation
Intrapartum hemorrhage (excessive) associated with hyperfibrinolysis
Intrapartum hemorrhage (excessive) associated with hypofibrinogenemia

   O67.8   **Other intrapartum hemorrhage**   M
Excessive intrapartum hemorrhage

   O67.9   **Intrapartum hemorrhage, unspecified**   M

● **O68**   **Labor and delivery complicated by abnormality of fetal acid-base balance**   M
Fetal acidemia complicating labor and delivery
Fetal acidosis complicating labor and delivery
Fetal alkalosis complicating labor and delivery
Fetal metabolic acidemia complicating labor and delivery

     Excludes 1   fetal stress NOS (O77.9)
                labor and delivery complicated by electrocardiographic evidence of fetal stress (O77.8)
                labor and delivery complicated by ultrasonic evidence of fetal stress (O77.8)

     Excludes 2   abnormality in fetal heart rate or rhythm (O76)
                labor and delivery complicated by meconium in amniotic fluid (O77.0)

CHAPTER 15 (O00-O9A)

● O69   **Labor and delivery complicated by** umbilical cord complications

One of the following 7th characters is to be assigned to each code under category O69. 7th character Ø is for single gestations and multiple gestations where the fetus is unspecified. 7th characters 1 through 9 are for cases of multiple gestations to identify the fetus for which the code applies. The appropriate code from category O30, Multiple gestation, must also be assigned when assigning a code from category O69 that has a 7th character of 1 through 9.

Ø	not applicable or unspecified
1	fetus 1
2	fetus 2
3	fetus 3
4	fetus 4
5	fetus 5
9	other fetus

X ● O69.0   **Labor and delivery complicated by** prolapse of cord   M

X ● O69.1   **Labor and delivery complicated by** cord around neck, with compression   M

> **Excludes1**   labor and delivery complicated by cord around neck, without compression (O69.81)

X ● O69.2   **Labor and delivery complicated by** other cord entanglement, with compression   M

Labor and delivery complicated by compression of cord NOS

Labor and delivery complicated by entanglement of cords of twins in monoamniotic sac

Labor and delivery complicated by knot in cord

> **Excludes1**   labor and delivery complicated by other cord entanglement, without compression (O69.82)

X ● O69.3   **Labor and delivery complicated by** short cord   M

X ● O69.4   **Labor and delivery complicated by** vasa previa   M

Labor and delivery complicated by hemorrhage from vasa previa

X ● O69.5   **Labor and delivery complicated by** vascular lesion of cord   M

Labor and delivery complicated by cord bruising

Labor and delivery complicated by cord hematoma

Labor and delivery complicated by thrombosis of umbilical vessels

● O69.8   **Labor and delivery complicated by** other cord complications

X ● O69.81   **Labor and delivery complicated by** cord around neck, without compression   M

X ● O69.82   **Labor and delivery complicated by** other cord entanglement, without compression   M

X ● O69.89   **Labor and delivery complicated by** other cord complications   M

Coding Clinic: 2023, Q2, P29

X ● O69.9   **Labor and delivery complicated by** cord complication, unspecified   M

● O70   **Perineal laceration during delivery**

> **Includes**   episiotomy extended by laceration
> **Excludes1**   obstetric high vaginal laceration alone (O71.4)

O70.0   **First degree perineal laceration during delivery**   M

Perineal laceration, rupture or tear involving fourchette during delivery

Perineal laceration, rupture or tear involving labia during delivery

Perineal laceration, rupture or tear involving skin during delivery

Perineal laceration, rupture or tear involving vagina during delivery

Perineal laceration, rupture or tear involving vulva during delivery

Slight perineal laceration, rupture or tear during delivery

Figure 15-6   Perineal lacerations: **A.** First-degree is laceration of superficial tissues. **B.** Second-degree is limited to the pelvic floor and may involve the perineal or vaginal muscles. **C.** Third-degree involves the anal sphincter. **D.** Fourth-degree involves anal or rectal mucosa.

O70.1   **Second degree perineal laceration during delivery**   M

Perineal laceration, rupture or tear during delivery as in O70.0, also involving pelvic floor

Perineal laceration, rupture or tear during delivery as in O70.0, also involving perineal muscles

Perineal laceration, rupture or tear during delivery as in O70.0, also involving vaginal muscles

> **Excludes1**   perineal laceration involving anal sphincter (O70.2)

Coding Clinic: 2016, Q4, P53; Q2, P34

● O70.2   **Third degree perineal laceration during delivery**

Perineal laceration, rupture or tear during delivery as in O70.1, also involving anal sphincter

Perineal laceration, rupture or tear during delivery as in O70.1, also involving rectovaginal septum

Perineal laceration, rupture or tear during delivery as in O70.1, also involving sphincter NOS

> **Excludes1**   anal sphincter tear during delivery without third degree perineal laceration (O70.4)
> perineal laceration involving anal or rectal mucosa (O70.3)

O70.20   **Third degree perineal laceration during delivery, unspecified**   M

O70.21   **Third degree perineal laceration during delivery, IIIa**   M

Third degree perineal laceration during delivery with less than 50% of external anal sphincter (EAS) thickness torn

O70.22   **Third degree perineal laceration during delivery, IIIb**   M

Third degree perineal laceration during delivery with more than 50% external anal sphincter (EAS) thickness torn

O70.23   **Third degree perineal laceration during delivery, IIIc**   M

Third degree perineal laceration during delivery with both external anal sphincter (EAS) and internal anal sphincter (IAS) torn

O70.3   **Fourth degree perineal laceration during delivery**   M

Perineal laceration, rupture or tear during delivery as in O70.2, also involving anal mucosa

Perineal laceration, rupture or tear during delivery as in O70.2, also involving rectal mucosa

O70.4   **Anal sphincter tear complicating delivery, not associated with third degree laceration**   M

> **Excludes1**   anal sphincter tear with third degree perineal laceration (O70.2)

O70.9   **Perineal laceration during delivery, unspecified**   M

● **O71   Other obstetric trauma**
   Includes   obstetric damage from instruments
● **O71.0   Rupture of uterus (spontaneous) before onset of labor**
   Excludes1   disruption of (current) cesarean delivery wound (O90.0)
   laceration of uterus, NEC (O71.81)
   O71.00   Rupture of uterus before onset of labor, unspecified trimester   M
   O71.02   Rupture of uterus before onset of labor, second trimester   M
   O71.03   Rupture of uterus before onset of labor, third trimester   M
   O71.1   Rupture of uterus during labor   M
   Rupture of uterus not stated as occurring before onset of labor
   Excludes1   disruption of cesarean delivery wound (O90.0)
   laceration of uterus, NEC (O71.81)
   O71.2   Postpartum inversion of uterus   M
   O71.3   Obstetric laceration of cervix   M
   Annular detachment of cervix
   O71.4   Obstetric high vaginal laceration alone   M
   Laceration of vaginal wall without perineal laceration
   Excludes1   obstetric high vaginal laceration with perineal laceration (O70.-)
   O71.5   Other obstetric injury to pelvic organs   M
   Obstetric injury to bladder
   Obstetric injury to urethra
   Excludes2   obstetric periurethral trauma (O71.82)
   O71.6   Obstetric damage to pelvic joints and ligaments   M
   Obstetric avulsion of inner symphyseal cartilage
   Obstetric damage to coccyx
   Obstetric traumatic separation of symphysis (pubis)
   O71.7   Obstetric hematoma of pelvis   M
   Obstetric hematoma of perineum
   Obstetric hematoma of vagina
   Obstetric hematoma of vulva
● **O71.8   Other specified obstetric trauma**
   O71.81   Laceration of uterus, not elsewhere classified   M
   O71.82   Other specified trauma to perineum and vulva   M
   Obstetric periurethral trauma
   O71.89   Other specified obstetric trauma   M
   O71.9   Obstetric trauma, unspecified   M
● **O72   Postpartum hemorrhage**
   Includes   hemorrhage after delivery of fetus or infant
   O72.0   Third-stage hemorrhage   M
   Hemorrhage associated with retained, trapped or adherent placenta
   Retained placenta NOS
   Code also type of adherent placenta (O43.2-)
   O72.1   Other immediate postpartum hemorrhage   M
   Hemorrhage following delivery of placenta
   Postpartum hemorrhage (atonic) NOS
   Uterine atony with hemorrhage
   Excludes1   uterine atony NOS (O62.2)
   uterine atony without hemorrhage (O62.2)
   postpartum atony of uterus without hemorrhage (O75.89)
   Coding Clinic: 2023, Q2, P15

   O72.2   Delayed and secondary postpartum hemorrhage   M
   Hemorrhage associated with retained portions of placenta or membranes after the first 24 hours following delivery of placenta
   Retained products of conception NOS, following delivery
   O72.3   Postpartum coagulation defects   M
   Postpartum afibrinogenemia
   Postpartum fibrinolysis
● **O73   Retained placenta and membranes, without hemorrhage**
   Excludes1   placenta accreta (O43.21-)
   placenta increta (O43.22-)
   placenta percreta (O43.23-)
   O73.0   Retained placenta without hemorrhage   M
   Adherent placenta, without hemorrhage
   Trapped placenta without hemorrhage
   O73.1   Retained portions of placenta and membranes, without hemorrhage   M
   Retained products of conception following delivery, without hemorrhage
● **O74   Complications of anesthesia during labor and delivery**
   Includes   maternal complications arising from the administration of a general, regional or local anesthetic, analgesic or other sedation during labor and delivery
   Use additional code, if applicable, to identify specific complication
   O74.0   Aspiration pneumonitis due to anesthesia during labor and delivery   M
   Inhalation of stomach contents or secretions NOS due to anesthesia during labor and delivery
   Mendelson's syndrome due to anesthesia during labor and delivery
   O74.1   Other pulmonary complications of anesthesia during labor and delivery   M
   O74.2   Cardiac complications of anesthesia during labor and delivery   M
   O74.3   Central nervous system complications of anesthesia during labor and delivery   M
   O74.4   Toxic reaction to local anesthesia during labor and delivery   M
   O74.5   Spinal and epidural anesthesia-induced headache during labor and delivery   M
   O74.6   Other complications of spinal and epidural anesthesia during labor and delivery   M
   O74.7   Failed or difficult intubation for anesthesia during labor and delivery   M
   O74.8   Other complications of anesthesia during labor and delivery   M
   O74.9   Complication of anesthesia during labor and delivery, unspecified   M
● **O75   Other complications of labor and delivery, not elsewhere classified**
   Excludes2   puerperal (postpartum) infection (O86.-)
   puerperal (postpartum) sepsis (O85)
   O75.0   Maternal distress during labor and delivery   M
   O75.1   Shock during or following labor and delivery   M
   Obstetric shock following labor and delivery
   O75.2   Pyrexia during labor, not elsewhere classified   M
   O75.3   Other infection during labor   M
   Sepsis during labor
   Use additional code (B95-B97), to identify infectious agent

Figure 15-7 The four stages of normal delivery: **I.** Lightening, which occurs 2 to 4 weeks before birth, at which time the fetus turns with head toward the vagina. **II.** Regular contractions begin, the amniotic sac ruptures, and dilation is complete. **III.** Delivery of the head and rotation. **IV.** Expulsion of placenta.

O75.4 Other complications of obstetric surgery and procedures   M
     Cardiac arrest following obstetric surgery or procedures
     Cardiac failure following obstetric surgery or procedures
     Cerebral anoxia following obstetric surgery or procedures
     Pulmonary edema following obstetric surgery or procedures
     Use additional code to identify specific complication
     Excludes2   complications of anesthesia during labor and delivery (O74.-)
                  disruption of obstetrical (surgical) wound (O90.0-O90.1)
                  hematoma of obstetrical (surgical) wound (O90.2)
                  infection of obstetrical (surgical) wound (O86.0-)

O75.5 Delayed delivery after artificial rupture of membranes   M
● **O75.8 Other specified complications of labor and delivery**
     O75.81 Maternal exhaustion complicating labor and delivery   M
     O75.82 Onset (spontaneous) of labor after 37 completed weeks of gestation but before 39 completed weeks gestation, with delivery by (planned) cesarean section   M
          Delivery by (planned) cesarean section occurring after 37 completed weeks of gestation but before 39 completed weeks gestation due to (spontaneous) onset of labor
          Code first to specify reason for planned cesarean section such as:
          cephalopelvic disproportion (normally formed fetus) (O33.9)
          previous cesarean delivery (O34.21-)
          Coding Clinic: 2022, Q2, P3-4
     O75.89 Other specified complications of labor and delivery   M
O75.9 Complication of labor and delivery, unspecified   M

O76 Abnormality in fetal heart rate and rhythm complicating labor and delivery   M
     Depressed fetal heart rate tones complicating labor and delivery
     Fetal bradycardia complicating labor and delivery
     Fetal heart rate decelerations complicating labor and delivery
     Fetal heart rate irregularity complicating labor and delivery
     Fetal heart rate abnormal variability complicating labor and delivery
     Fetal tachycardia complicating labor and delivery
     Non-reassuring fetal heart rate or rhythm complicating labor and delivery
     Excludes1   fetal stress NOS (O77.9)
               labor and delivery complicated by electrocardiographic evidence of fetal stress (O77.8)
               labor and delivery complicated by ultrasonic evidence of fetal stress (O77.8)
     Excludes2   fetal metabolic acidemia (O68)
               other fetal stress (O77.0-O77.1)

● **O77 Other fetal stress complicating labor and delivery**
     O77.0 Labor and delivery complicated by meconium in amniotic fluid   M
          Coding Clinic: 2022, Q2, P16-17
     O77.1 Fetal stress in labor or delivery due to drug administration   M
     O77.8 Labor and delivery complicated by other evidence of fetal stress   M
          Labor and delivery complicated by electrocardiographic evidence of fetal stress
          Labor and delivery complicated by ultrasonic evidence of fetal stress
          Excludes1   abnormality of fetal acid-base balance (O68)
                      abnormality in fetal heart rate or rhythm (O76)
                      fetal metabolic acidemia (O68)
     O77.9 Labor and delivery complicated by fetal stress, unspecified   M
          Excludes1   abnormality of fetal acid-base balance (O68)
                      abnormality in fetal heart rate or rhythm (O76)
                      fetal metabolic acidemia (O68)

OGCR Section I.C., Chapter 15.n.

Normal Delivery, Code O80

1) Encounter for full-term uncomplicated delivery

Code O80 should be assigned when a woman is admitted for a full-term normal delivery and delivers a single, healthy infant without any complications antepartum, during the delivery, or postpartum during the delivery episode. Code O80 is always a principal diagnosis. It is not to be used if any other code from Chapter 15 is needed to describe a current complication of the antenatal, delivery, or perinatal period. Additional codes from other chapters may be used with code O80 if they are not related to or are in any way complicating the pregnancy.

2) Uncomplicated delivery with resolved antepartum complication

Code O80 may be used if the patient had a complication at some point during the pregnancy, but the complication is not present at the time of the admission for delivery.

3) Outcome of delivery for O80

Z37.0, Single live brith, is the only outcome of delivery code appropriate for use with O80.

ENCOUNTER FOR DELIVERY (O80-O82)

O80 Encounter for full-term uncomplicated delivery   M
     Delivery requiring minimal or no assistance, with or without episiotomy, without fetal manipulation [e.g., rotation version] or instrumentation [forceps] of a spontaneous, cephalic, vaginal, full-term, single, live-born infant. This code is for use as a single diagnosis code and is not to be used with any other code from Chapter 15.
     Use additional code to indicate outcome of delivery (Z37.0)
     Coding Clinic: 2016, Q4, P124, 150

O82 Encounter for cesarean delivery without indication   M
     Use additional code to indicate outcome of delivery (Z37.0)

▶ New   ⇒ Revised   ~~deleted~~ Deleted   Excludes 1   Excludes 2   Includes   Use additional   Code first   Code also   Key words
OGCR Official Guidelines   X Assign placeholder X   ● Use Additional Character(s)   ▶ Manifestation Code   Hierarchical Condition Category   Coding Clinic

COMPLICATIONS PREDOMINANTLY RELATED TO THE PUERPERIUM (O85-O92)

Excludes2   mental and behavioral disorders associated with the puerperium (F53.-)
obstetrical tetanus (A34)
puerperal osteomalacia (M83.0)

O85 Puerperal sepsis   M
Postpartum sepsis
Puerperal peritonitis
Puerperal pyemia
Use additional code (B95-B97), to identify infectious agent
Use additional code (R65.2-) to identify severe sepsis, if applicable

Excludes1   fever of unknown origin following delivery (O86.4)
~~genital tract infection following delivery (O86.1-)~~
obstetric pyemic and septic embolism (O88.3-)
puerperal septic thrombophlebitis (O86.81)
~~urinary tract infection following delivery (O86.2-)~~

 ▶ **Excludes2**   genital tract infection following delivery (O86.1-)

                ▶sepsis during labor (O75.3)
                ▶urinary tract infection following delivery (O86.2-)

Coding Clinic: 2022, Q2, P5; 2018, Q4, P23

● O86 Other puerperal infections
Use additional code (B95-B97), to identify infectious agent

Excludes2   infection during labor (O75.3)
obstetrical tetanus (A34)

● O86.0 Infection of obstetric surgical wound
Infected cesarean delivery wound following delivery
Infected perineal repair following delivery

Excludes1   complications of procedures, not elsewhere classified (T81.44)
postprocedural fever NOS (R50.82)
postprocedural retroperitoneal abscess (K68.11)

O86.00 **Infection of obstetric surgical wound, unspecified**   M

O86.01 **Infection of obstetric surgical wound, superficial incisional site**   M
Subcutaneous abscess following an obstetrical procedure
Stitch abscess following an obstetrical procedure

O86.02 **Infection of obstetric surgical wound, deep incisional site**   M
Intramuscular abscess following an obstetrical procedure
Sub-fascial abscess following an obstetrical procedure
Coding Clinic: 2018, Q4, P23

O86.03 **Infection of obstetric surgical wound, organ and space site**   M
Intraabdominal abscess following an obstetrical procedure
Subphrenic abscess following an obstetrical procedure

O86.04 **Sepsis following an obstetrical procedure**   M
Use additional code to identify the sepsis

O86.09 **Infection of obstetric surgical wound, other surgical site**   M

● O86.1 Other infection of genital tract following delivery

O86.11 **Cervicitis following delivery**   M
O86.12 **Endometritis following delivery**   M
O86.13 **Vaginitis following delivery**   M
O86.19 **Other infection of genital tract following delivery**   M

● O86.2 Urinary tract infection following delivery

O86.20 **Urinary tract infection following delivery, unspecified**   M
Puerperal urinary tract infection NOS
Coding Clinic: 2022, Q2, P5

O86.21 **Infection of kidney following delivery**   M

O86.22 **Infection of bladder following delivery**   M
Infection of urethra following delivery

O86.29 **Other urinary tract infection following delivery**   M

O86.4 Pyrexia of unknown origin following delivery   M
Puerperal infection NOS following delivery
Puerperal pyrexia NOS following delivery

Excludes2   pyrexia during labor (O75.2)

● O86.8 Other specified puerperal infections
O86.81 **Puerperal septic thrombophlebitis**   M
O86.89 **Other specified puerperal infections**   M

● O87 Venous complications and hemorrhoids in the puerperium

Includes   venous complications in labor, delivery and the puerperium

Excludes2   obstetric embolism (O88.-)
puerperal septic thrombophlebitis (O86.81)
venous complications in pregnancy (O22.-)

O87.0 Superficial thrombophlebitis in the puerperium   M
Puerperal phlebitis NOS
Puerperal thrombosis NOS
Use additional code, if applicable, to identify the superficial vein thrombosis, such as thrombosis of superficial vessels of lower extremities (I80.0-)

O87.1 Deep phlebothrombosis in the puerperium   M
Deep vein thrombosis, postpartum
Pelvic thrombophlebitis, postpartum
Use additional code to identify the deep vein thrombosis (I82.4-, I82.5-, I82.62-, I82.72-)
Use additional code, if applicable, for associated long-term (current) use of anticoagulants (Z79.01)

O87.2 Hemorrhoids in the puerperium   M

O87.3 Cerebral venous thrombosis in the puerperium   M
Cerebrovenous sinus thrombosis in the puerperium

O87.4 Varicose veins of lower extremity in the puerperium   M

O87.8 Other venous complications in the puerperium   M
Genital varices in the puerperium

O87.9 Venous complication in the puerperium, unspecified   M
Puerperal phlebopathy NOS

O88 Obstetric embolism

Excludes1   embolism complicating abortion NOS (O03.2)
embolism complicating ectopic or molar pregnancy (O08.2)
embolism complicating failed attempted abortion (O07.2)
embolism complicating induced abortion (O04.7)
embolism complicating spontaneous abortion (O03.2, O03.7)

● O88.0 Obstetric air embolism
● O88.01 Obstetric air embolism in pregnancy

O88.011 **Air embolism in pregnancy, first trimester**   M

O88.012 **Air embolism in pregnancy, second trimester**   M

O88.013 **Air embolism in pregnancy, third trimester**   M

O88.019 **Air embolism in pregnancy, unspecified trimester**   M

O88.02 **Air embolism in childbirth**   M

O88.03 **Air embolism in the puerperium**   M

● **O88.1 Amniotic fluid embolism**
    Anaphylactoid syndrome in pregnancy

  ● **O88.11 Amniotic fluid embolism in pregnancy**

      O88.111 Amniotic fluid embolism in pregnancy, first trimester   M

      O88.112 Amniotic fluid embolism in pregnancy, second trimester   M

      O88.113 Amniotic fluid embolism in pregnancy, third trimester   M

      O88.119 Amniotic fluid embolism in pregnancy, unspecified trimester   M

    O88.12 Amniotic fluid embolism in childbirth   M

    O88.13 Amniotic fluid embolism in the puerperium   M

● **O88.2 Obstetric thromboembolism**

  ● **O88.21 Thromboembolism in pregnancy**
      Obstetric (pulmonary) embolism NOS

      O88.211 Thromboembolism in pregnancy, first trimester   M

      O88.212 Thromboembolism in pregnancy, second trimester   M

      O88.213 Thromboembolism in pregnancy, third trimester   M

      O88.219 Thromboembolism in pregnancy, unspecified trimester   M

    O88.22 Thromboembolism in childbirth   M

    O88.23 Thromboembolism in the puerperium   M
      Puerperal (pulmonary) embolism NOS

● **O88.3 Obstetric pyemic and septic embolism**

  ● **O88.31 Pyemic and septic embolism in pregnancy**

      O88.311 Pyemic and septic embolism in pregnancy, first trimester   M

      O88.312 Pyemic and septic embolism in pregnancy, second trimester   M

      O88.313 Pyemic and septic embolism in pregnancy, third trimester   M

      O88.319 Pyemic and septic embolism in pregnancy, unspecified trimester   M

    O88.32 Pyemic and septic embolism in childbirth   M

    O88.33 Pyemic and septic embolism in the puerperium   M

● **O88.8 Other obstetric embolism**
    Obstetric fat embolism

  ● **O88.81 Other embolism in pregnancy**

      O88.811 Other embolism in pregnancy, first trimester   M

      O88.812 Other embolism in pregnancy, second trimester   M

      O88.813 Other embolism in pregnancy, third trimester   M

      O88.819 Other embolism in pregnancy, unspecified trimester   M

    O88.82 Other embolism in childbirth   M

    O88.83 Other embolism in the puerperium   M

● **O89 Complications of anesthesia during the puerperium**

  Includes   maternal complications arising from the administration of a general, regional or local anesthetic, analgesic or other sedation during the puerperium

  Use additional code, if applicable, to identify specific complication

● **O89.0 Pulmonary complications of anesthesia during the puerperium**

  O89.01 Aspiration pneumonitis due to anesthesia during the puerperium   M
    Inhalation of stomach contents or secretions NOS due to anesthesia during the puerperium
    Mendelson's syndrome due to anesthesia during the puerperium

  O89.09 Other pulmonary complications of anesthesia during the puerperium   M

O89.1 Cardiac complications of anesthesia during the puerperium   M

O89.2 Central nervous system complications of anesthesia during the puerperium   M

O89.3 Toxic reaction to local anesthesia during the puerperium   M

O89.4 Spinal and epidural anesthesia-induced headache during the puerperium   M

O89.5 Other complications of spinal and epidural anesthesia during the puerperium   M

O89.6 Failed or difficult intubation for anesthesia during the puerperium   M

O89.8 Other complications of anesthesia during the puerperium   M

O89.9 Complication of anesthesia during the puerperium, unspecified   M

● **O90 Complications of the puerperium, not elsewhere classified**

O90.0 Disruption of cesarean delivery wound   M
    Dehiscence of cesarean delivery wound

    Excludes1   rupture of uterus (spontaneous) before onset of labor (O71.0-)
             rupture of uterus during labor (O71.1)

O90.1 Disruption of perineal obstetric wound
    Disruption of wound of episiotomy
    Disruption of wound of perineal laceration
    Secondary perineal tear

O90.2 Hematoma of obstetric wound   M

O90.3 Peripartum cardiomyopathy   M
    Conditions in I42.- arising during pregnancy and the puerperium

    Excludes1   pre-existing heart disease complicating pregnancy and the puerperium (O99.4-)

  Coding Clinic: 2022, Q3, P16-18

● **O90.4 Postpartum acute kidney failure**   M

    Excludes1   non-anuria and oliguria (R34)

  O90.41 Hepatorenal syndrome following labor and delivery   M

  O90.49 Other postpartum acute kidney failure   M
    Postpartum acute kidney failure
    Puerperal anuria
    Puerperal oliguria

O90.5 Postpartum thyroiditis   M

O90.6 Postpartum mood disturbance   M
    Postpartum blues   Postpartum sadness
    Postpartum dysphoria

    Excludes1   postpartum depression (F53.0)
             puerperal psychosis (F53.1)

● **O90.8 Other complications of the puerperium, not elsewhere classified**

  O90.81 Anemia of the puerperium   M
    Postpartum anemia NOS

      Excludes1   pre-existing anemia complicating the puerperium (O99.03)

  O90.89 Other complications of the puerperium, not elsewhere classified   M
    Placental polyp

O90.9 Complication of the puerperium, unspecified   M

● **O91 Infections of breast associated with pregnancy, the puerperium and lactation**

  Use additional code to identify infection

● **O91.0 Infection of nipple associated with pregnancy, the puerperium and lactation**

  ● **O91.01 Infection of nipple associated with pregnancy**
    Gestational abscess of nipple

    O91.011 Infection of nipple associated with pregnancy, first trimester   M

    O91.012 Infection of nipple associated with pregnancy, second trimester   M

▶ New   ⇒ Revised   ~~deleted~~ Deleted   Excludes 1   Excludes 2   Includes   Use additional   Code first   Code also   Key words

OGCR Official Guidelines   X Assign placeholder X   ● Use Additional Character(s)   ▶ Manifestation Code   ⬡ Hierarchical Condition Category   Coding Clinic

O91.013   Infection of nipple associated with pregnancy, third trimester   M

O91.019   Infection of nipple associated with pregnancy, unspecified trimester   M

O91.02   Infection of nipple associated with the puerperium   M
Puerperal abscess of nipple

O91.03   Infection of nipple associated with lactation   M
Abscess of nipple associated with lactation

● O91.1   Abscess of breast associated with pregnancy, the puerperium and lactation

   ● O91.11   Abscess of breast associated with pregnancy
Gestational mammary abscess
Gestational purulent mastitis
Gestational subareolar abscess

O91.111   Abscess of breast associated with pregnancy, first trimester   M

O91.112   Abscess of breast associated with pregnancy, second trimester   M

O91.113   Abscess of breast associated with pregnancy, third trimester   M

O91.119   Abscess of breast associated with pregnancy, unspecified trimester   M

O91.12   Abscess of breast associated with the puerperium   M
Puerperal mammary abscess
Puerperal purulent mastitis
Puerperal subareolar abscess

O91.13   Abscess of breast associated with lactation   M
Mammary abscess associated with lactation
Purulent mastitis associated with lactation
Subareolar abscess associated with lactation

● O91.2   Nonpurulent mastitis associated with pregnancy, the puerperium and lactation

   ● O91.21   Nonpurulent mastitis associated with pregnancy
Gestational interstitial mastitis
Gestational lymphangitis of breast
Gestational mastitis NOS
Gestational parenchymatous mastitis

O91.211   Nonpurulent mastitis associated with pregnancy, first trimester   M

O91.212   Nonpurulent mastitis associated with pregnancy, second trimester   M

O91.213   Nonpurulent mastitis associated with pregnancy, third trimester   M

O91.219   Nonpurulent mastitis associated with pregnancy, unspecified trimester   M

O91.22   Nonpurulent mastitis associated with the puerperium   M
Puerperal interstitial mastitis
Puerperal lymphangitis of breast
Puerperal mastitis NOS
Puerperal parenchymatous mastitis

O91.23   Nonpurulent mastitis associated with lactation   M
Interstitial mastitis associated with lactation
Lymphangitis of breast associated with lactation
Mastitis NOS associated with lactation
Parenchymatous mastitis associated with lactation

● O92   Other disorders of breast and disorders of lactation associated with pregnancy and the puerperium

   ● O92.0   Retracted nipple associated with pregnancy, the puerperium, and lactation

     ● O92.01   Retracted nipple associated with pregnancy

O92.011   Retracted nipple associated with pregnancy, first trimester   M

O92.012   Retracted nipple associated with pregnancy, second trimester   M

O92.013   Retracted nipple associated with pregnancy, third trimester   M

O92.019   Retracted nipple associated with pregnancy, unspecified trimester   M

O92.02   Retracted nipple associated with the puerperium   M

O92.03   Retracted nipple associated with lactation   M

● O92.1   Cracked nipple associated with pregnancy, the puerperium, and lactation
Fissure of nipple, gestational or puerperal

   ● O92.11   Cracked nipple associated with pregnancy

O92.111   Cracked nipple associated with pregnancy, first trimester   M

O92.112   Cracked nipple associated with pregnancy, second trimester   M

O92.113   Cracked nipple associated with pregnancy, third trimester   M

O92.119   Cracked nipple associated with pregnancy, unspecified trimester   M

O92.12   Cracked nipple associated with the puerperium   M

O92.13   Cracked nipple associated with lactation   M

● O92.2   Other and unspecified disorders of breast associated with pregnancy and the puerperium

O92.20   Unspecified disorder of breast associated with pregnancy and the puerperium   M

O92.29   Other disorders of breast associated with pregnancy and the puerperium   M

O92.3   Agalactia   M
Primary agalactia

   Excludes1   elective agalactia (O92.5)
secondary agalactia (O92.5)
therapeutic agalactia (O92.5)

O92.4   Hypogalactia   M

O92.5   Suppressed lactation   M
Elective agalactia   Therapeutic agalactia
Secondary agalactia

   Excludes1   primary agalactia (O92.3)

O92.6   Galactorrhea   M

● O92.7   Other and unspecified disorders of lactation

O92.70   Unspecified disorders of lactation   M

O92.79   Other disorders of lactation   M
Puerperal galactocele

OTHER OBSTETRIC CONDITIONS, NOT ELSEWHERE CLASSIFIED (O94-O9A)

O94   Sequelae of complication of pregnancy, childbirth, and the puerperium   M

Note: This category is to be used to indicate conditions in O00-O77.-, O85-O94 and O98-O9A.- as the cause of late effects. The "sequelae" include conditions specified as such, or as late effects, which may occur at any time after the puerperium.

Code first condition resulting from (sequela) of complication of pregnancy, childbirth, and the puerperium
Coding Clinic: 2022, Q3, P17-18

O98   Maternal infectious and parasitic diseases classifiable elsewhere but complicating pregnancy, childbirth and the puerperium

   Includes   the listed conditions when complicating the pregnant state, when aggravated by the pregnancy, or as a reason for obstetric care

Use additional code (Chapter 1), to identify specific infectious or parasitic disease

   Excludes2   herpes gestationis (O26.4-)
infectious carrier state (O99.82-, O99.83-)
obstetrical tetanus (A34)
puerperal infection (O86.-)
puerperal sepsis (O85)
when the reason for maternal care is that the disease is known or suspected to have affected the fetus (O35-O36)

- O98.0 **Tuberculosis** complicating pregnancy, childbirth and the puerperium
  Conditions in A15-A19
  - O98.01 Tuberculosis complicating **pregnancy**
    - O98.011 Tuberculosis complicating pregnancy, **first trimester** M
    - O98.012 Tuberculosis complicating pregnancy, **second trimester** M
    - O98.013 Tuberculosis complicating pregnancy, **third trimester** M
    - O98.019 Tuberculosis complicating pregnancy, **unspecified trimester** M
  - O98.02 Tuberculosis complicating **childbirth** M
  - O98.03 Tuberculosis complicating the **puerperium** M
- O98.1 **Syphilis** complicating pregnancy, childbirth and the puerperium
  Conditions in A50-A53
  - O98.11 Syphilis complicating **pregnancy**
    - O98.111 Syphilis complicating pregnancy, **first trimester** M
    - O98.112 Syphilis complicating pregnancy, **second trimester** M
    - O98.113 Syphilis complicating pregnancy, **third trimester** M
    - O98.119 Syphilis complicating pregnancy, **unspecified trimester** M
  - O98.12 Syphilis complicating **childbirth** M
  - O98.13 Syphilis complicating the **puerperium** M
- O98.2 **Gonorrhea** complicating pregnancy, childbirth and the puerperium
  Conditions in A54.-
  - O98.21 Gonorrhea complicating **pregnancy**
    - O98.211 Gonorrhea complicating pregnancy, **first trimester** M
    - O98.212 Gonorrhea complicating pregnancy, **second trimester** M
    - O98.213 Gonorrhea complicating pregnancy, **third trimester** M
    - O98.219 Gonorrhea complicating pregnancy, **unspecified trimester** M
  - O98.22 Gonorrhea complicating **childbirth** M
  - O98.23 Gonorrhea complicating the **puerperium** M
- O98.3 **Other infections with a predominantly sexual mode of transmission** complicating pregnancy, childbirth and the puerperium
  Conditions in A55-A64
  - O98.31 Other infections with a predominantly sexual mode of transmission complicating **pregnancy**
    - O98.311 Other infections with a predominantly sexual mode of transmission complicating pregnancy, **first trimester** M
    - O98.312 Other infections with a predominantly sexual mode of transmission complicating pregnancy, **second trimester** M
    - O98.313 Other infections with a predominantly sexual mode of transmission complicating pregnancy, **third trimester** M
    - O98.319 Other infections with a predominantly sexual mode of transmission complicating pregnancy, **unspecified trimester** M
  - O98.32 Other infections with a predominantly sexual mode of transmission complicating childbirth M
    Coding Clinic: 2020, Q1, P20

- O98.33 Other infections with a predominantly sexual mode of transmission complicating the **puerperium** M
- O98.4 **Viral hepatitis** complicating pregnancy, childbirth and the puerperium
  Conditions in B15-B19
  - O98.41 Viral hepatitis complicating **pregnancy**
    - O98.411 Viral hepatitis complicating pregnancy, **first trimester** M
    - O98.412 Viral hepatitis complicating pregnancy, **second trimester** M
    - O98.413 Viral hepatitis complicating pregnancy, **third trimester** M
    - O98.419 Viral hepatitis complicating pregnancy, **unspecified trimester** M
  - O98.42 Viral hepatitis complicating **childbirth** M
  - O98.43 Viral hepatitis complicating the **puerperium** M
- O98.5 **Other viral diseases** complicating pregnancy, childbirth and the puerperium
  Conditions in A80-B09, B25-B34, R87.81-, R87.82-
  Excludes:1 human immunodeficiency virus [HIV] disease complicating pregnancy, childbirth and the puerperium (O98.7-)
  - O98.51 Other viral diseases complicating **pregnancy**
    - O98.511 Other viral diseases complicating pregnancy, **first trimester** M
    - O98.512 Other viral diseases complicating pregnancy, **second trimester** M
      Coding Clinic: 2016, Q4, P5-6
    - O98.513 Other viral diseases complicating pregnancy, **third trimester** M
      Coding Clinic: 2016, Q4, P6
    - O98.519 Other viral diseases complicating pregnancy, **unspecified trimester** M
  - O98.52 Other viral diseases complicating **childbirth** M
  - O98.53 Other viral diseases complicating the **puerperium** M
- O98.6 **Protozoal diseases** complicating pregnancy, childbirth and the puerperium
  Conditions in B50-B64
  - O98.61 Protozoal diseases complicating **pregnancy**
    - O98.611 Protozoal diseases complicating pregnancy, **first trimester** M
    - O98.612 Protozoal diseases complicating pregnancy, **second trimester** M
    - O98.613 Protozoal diseases complicating pregnancy, **third trimester** M
    - O98.619 Protozoal diseases complicating pregnancy, **unspecified trimester** M
  - O98.62 Protozoal diseases complicating **childbirth** M
  - O98.63 Protozoal diseases complicating the **puerperium** M
- O98.7 **Human immunodeficiency virus [HIV] disease** complicating pregnancy, childbirth and the puerperium
  Use additional code to identify the type of HIV disease:
    Acquired immune deficiency syndrome (AIDS) (B20)
    Asymptomatic HIV status (Z21)
    HIV positive NOS (Z21)
    Symptomatic HIV disease (B20)

● **O98.71 Human immunodeficiency virus [HIV] disease complicating pregnancy**

    O98.711 Human immunodeficiency virus [HIV] disease complicating pregnancy, first trimester   M

    O98.712 Human immunodeficiency virus [HIV] disease complicating pregnancy, second trimester   M

    O98.713 Human immunodeficiency virus [HIV] disease complicating pregnancy, third trimester   M

    O98.719 Human immunodeficiency virus [HIV] disease complicating pregnancy, unspecified trimester   M

  O98.72 Human immunodeficiency virus [HIV] disease complicating childbirth   M

  O98.73 Human immunodeficiency virus [HIV] disease complicating the puerperium   M

● **O98.8 Other maternal infectious and parasitic diseases complicating pregnancy, childbirth and the puerperium**

  ● **O98.81 Other maternal infectious and parasitic diseases complicating pregnancy**

    O98.811 Other maternal infectious and parasitic diseases complicating pregnancy, first trimester   M

    O98.812 Other maternal infectious and parasitic diseases complicating pregnancy, second trimester   M

    O98.813 Other maternal infectious and parasitic diseases complicating pregnancy, third trimester   M

    O98.819 Other maternal infectious and parasitic diseases complicating pregnancy, unspecified trimester   M

  O98.82 Other maternal infectious and parasitic diseases complicating childbirth   M
    Coding Clinic: 2020, Q1, P10

  O98.83 Other maternal infectious and parasitic diseases complicating the puerperium   M
    Coding Clinic: 2022, Q2, P5

● **O98.9 Unspecified maternal infectious and parasitic disease complicating pregnancy, childbirth and the puerperium**

  ● **O98.91 Unspecified maternal infectious and parasitic disease complicating pregnancy**

    O98.911 Unspecified maternal infectious and parasitic disease complicating pregnancy, first trimester   M

    O98.912 Unspecified maternal infectious and parasitic disease complicating pregnancy, second trimester   M

    O98.913 Unspecified maternal infectious and parasitic disease complicating pregnancy, third trimester   M

    O98.919 Unspecified maternal infectious and parasitic disease complicating pregnancy, unspecified trimester   M

  O98.92 Unspecified maternal infectious and parasitic disease complicating childbirth   M

  O98.93 Unspecified maternal infectious and parasitic disease complicating the puerperium   M

● **O99 Other maternal diseases classifiable elsewhere but complicating pregnancy, childbirth and the puerperium**

  Includes: conditions which complicate the pregnant state, are aggravated by the pregnancy or are a main reason for obstetric care

  Use additional code to identify specific condition

  Excludes2 when the reason for maternal care is that the condition is known or suspected to have affected the fetus (O35-O36)

  Coding Clinic: 2018, Q4, P8-9

  ● **O99.0 Anemia complicating pregnancy, childbirth and the puerperium**
    Conditions in D50-D64

    Excludes1 anemia arising in the puerperium (O90.81) postpartum anemia NOS (O90.81)

    ● **O99.01 Anemia complicating pregnancy**

      O99.011 Anemia complicating pregnancy, first trimester   M

      O99.012 Anemia complicating pregnancy, second trimester   M

      O99.013 Anemia complicating pregnancy, third trimester   M

      O99.019 Anemia complicating pregnancy, unspecified trimester   M

    O99.02 Anemia complicating childbirth   M

    O99.03 Anemia complicating the puerperium   M

      Excludes1 postpartum anemia not preexisting prior to delivery (O90.81)

  ● **O99.1 Other diseases of the blood and blood-forming organs and certain disorders involving the immune mechanism complicating pregnancy, childbirth and the puerperium**
    Conditions in D65-D89

    Excludes1 hemorrhage with coagulation defects (O45.-, O46.0-, O67.0, O72.3)

    ● **O99.11 Other diseases of the blood and blood-forming organs and certain disorders involving the immune mechanism complicating pregnancy**

      O99.111 Other diseases of the blood and blood-forming organs and certain disorders involving the immune mechanism complicating pregnancy, first trimester   M

      O99.112 Other diseases of the blood and blood-forming organs and certain disorders involving the immune mechanism complicating pregnancy, second trimester   M

      O99.113 Other diseases of the blood and blood-forming organs and certain disorders involving the immune mechanism complicating pregnancy, third trimester   M

      O99.119 Other diseases of the blood and blood-forming organs and certain disorders involving the immune mechanism complicating pregnancy, unspecified trimester   M

CHAPTER 15 (O00-O9A)

CHAPTER 15 (O00-O9A)

O99.12   Other diseases of the blood and blood-forming organs and certain disorders involving the immune mechanism complicating childbirth   M

O99.13   Other diseases of the blood and blood-forming organs and certain disorders involving the immune mechanism complicating the puerperium   M

● O99.2   Endocrine, nutritional and metabolic diseases complicating pregnancy, childbirth and the puerperium
Conditions in E00-E89

Excludes2   diabetes mellitus (O24.-)
malnutrition (O25.-)
postpartum thyroiditis (O90.5)

● O99.21   Obesity complicating pregnancy, childbirth, and the puerperium
Use additional code to identify the type of obesity (E66.-)

O99.210   Obesity complicating pregnancy, unspecified trimester   M

O99.211   Obesity complicating pregnancy, first trimester   M

O99.212   Obesity complicating pregnancy, second trimester   M

O99.213   Obesity complicating pregnancy, third trimester   M

O99.214   Obesity complicating childbirth   M
Coding Clinic: 2021, Q2, P10-11; 2018, Q4, P80

O99.215   Obesity complicating the puerperium   M

● O99.28   Other endocrine, nutritional and metabolic diseases complicating pregnancy, childbirth and the puerperium

O99.280   Endocrine, nutritional and metabolic diseases complicating pregnancy, unspecified trimester   M

O99.281   Endocrine, nutritional and metabolic diseases complicating pregnancy, first trimester   M

O99.282   Endocrine, nutritional and metabolic diseases complicating pregnancy, second trimester   M

O99.283   Endocrine, nutritional and metabolic diseases complicating pregnancy, third trimester   M

O99.284   Endocrine, nutritional and metabolic diseases complicating childbirth   M

O99.285   Endocrine, nutritional and metabolic diseases complicating the puerperium   M
Coding Clinic: 2021, Q1, P9

● O99.3   Mental disorders and diseases of the nervous system complicating pregnancy, childbirth and the puerperium

● O99.31   Alcohol use complicating pregnancy, childbirth, and the puerperium
Use additional code(s) from F10 to identify manifestations of the alcohol use

O99.310   Alcohol use complicating pregnancy, unspecified trimester   M

O99.311   Alcohol use complicating pregnancy, first trimester   M

O99.312   Alcohol use complicating pregnancy, second trimester   M

O99.313   Alcohol use complicating pregnancy, third trimester   M

O99.314   Alcohol use complicating childbirth   M

O99.315   Alcohol use complicating the puerperium   M

● O99.32   Drug use complicating pregnancy, childbirth, and the puerperium
Use additional code(s) from F11-F16 and F18-F19 to identify manifestations of the drug use

O99.320   Drug use complicating pregnancy, unspecified trimester   M

O99.321   Drug use complicating pregnancy, first trimester   M

O99.322   Drug use complicating pregnancy, second trimester   M

O99.323   Drug use complicating pregnancy, third trimester   M

O99.324   Drug use complicating childbirth   M

O99.325   Drug use complicating the puerperium   M

● O99.33   Tobacco use disorder complicating pregnancy, childbirth, and the puerperium
Smoking complicating pregnancy, childbirth, and the puerperium
Use additional code from category F17 to identify type of tobacco nicotine dependence

O99.330   Smoking (tobacco) complicating pregnancy, unspecified trimester   M

O99.331   Smoking (tobacco) complicating pregnancy, first trimester   M

O99.332   Smoking (tobacco) complicating pregnancy, second trimester   M

O99.333   Smoking (tobacco) complicating pregnancy, third trimester   M

O99.334   Smoking (tobacco) complicating childbirth   M

O99.335   Smoking (tobacco) complicating the puerperium   M

● O99.34   Other mental disorders complicating pregnancy, childbirth, and the puerperium
Conditions in F01-F09, F20-F52 and F54-F99

Excludes2   postpartum mood disturbance (O90.6)
postnatal psychosis (F53.1)
puerperal psychosis (F53.1)
Coding Clinic: 2018, Q4, P9

O99.340   Other mental disorders complicating pregnancy, unspecified trimester   M

O99.341   Other mental disorders complicating pregnancy, first trimester   M

O99.342   Other mental disorders complicating pregnancy, second trimester   M

O99.343   Other mental disorders complicating pregnancy, third trimester   M

O99.344   Other mental disorders complicating childbirth   M

O99.345   Other mental disorders complicating the puerperium   M
Coding Clinic: 2018, Q4, P8-9

● O99.35   Diseases of the nervous system complicating pregnancy, childbirth, and the puerperium
Conditions in G00-G99

Excludes2   pregnancy related peripheral neuritis (O26.8-)

O99.350   Diseases of the nervous system complicating pregnancy, unspecified trimester   M

O99.351   Diseases of the nervous system complicating pregnancy, first trimester   M

O99.352   Diseases of the nervous system complicating pregnancy, second trimester   M

▶ New   ⇒ Revised   ~~deleted~~ Deleted   Excludes 1   Excludes 2   Includes   Use additional   Code first   Code also   Key words
OGCR Official Guidelines   X Assign placeholder X   ● Use Additional Character(s)   ▶ Manifestation Code   🏥 Hierarchical Condition Category   **Coding Clinic**

       O99.353   Diseases of the nervous system complicating pregnancy, third trimester   M

       O99.354   Diseases of the nervous system complicating childbirth   M

       O99.355   Diseases of the nervous system complicating the puerperium   M

● O99.4   **Diseases of the circulatory system** complicating pregnancy, childbirth and the puerperium
     Conditions in I00-I99

     Excludes1   peripartum cardiomyopathy (O90.3)

     Excludes2   hypertensive disorders (O10-O16)
       obstetric embolism (O88.-)
       venous complications and cerebrovenous sinus thrombosis in labor, childbirth and the puerperium (O87.-)
       venous complications and cerebrovenous sinus thrombosis in pregnancy (O22.-)

   ● O99.41   Diseases of the circulatory system complicating pregnancy
       Coding Clinic: 2016, Q2, P8

       O99.411   Diseases of the circulatory system complicating pregnancy, first trimester   M

       O99.412   Diseases of the circulatory system complicating pregnancy, second trimester   M

       O99.413   Diseases of the circulatory system complicating pregnancy, third trimester   M

       O99.419   Diseases of the circulatory system complicating pregnancy, unspecified trimester   M

   O99.42   Diseases of the circulatory system complicating childbirth   M

   O99.43   Diseases of the circulatory system complicating the puerperium   M

● O99.5   **Diseases of the respiratory system** complicating pregnancy, childbirth and the puerperium
     Conditions in J00-J99

   ● O99.51   Diseases of the respiratory system complicating pregnancy

       O99.511   Diseases of the respiratory system complicating pregnancy, first trimester   M

       O99.512   Diseases of the respiratory system complicating pregnancy, second trimester   M

       O99.513   Diseases of the respiratory system complicating pregnancy, third trimester   M

       O99.519   Diseases of the respiratory system complicating pregnancy, unspecified trimester   M

   O99.52   Diseases of the respiratory system complicating childbirth   M

   O99.53   Diseases of the respiratory system complicating the puerperium   M

● O99.6   **Diseases of the digestive system** complicating pregnancy, childbirth and the puerperium
     Conditions in K00-K93

     Excludes2   hemorrhoids in pregnancy (O22.4-)
       liver and biliary tract disorders in pregnancy, childbirth and the puerperium (O26.6-)

● O99.61   Diseases of the digestive system complicating pregnancy

       O99.611   Diseases of the digestive system complicating pregnancy, first trimester   M

       O99.612   Diseases of the digestive system complicating pregnancy, second trimester   M

       O99.613   Diseases of the digestive system complicating pregnancy, third trimester   M

       O99.619   Diseases of the digestive system complicating pregnancy, unspecified trimester   M

   O99.62   Diseases of the digestive system complicating childbirth   M

   O99.63   Diseases of the digestive system complicating the puerperium   M

● O99.7   **Diseases of the skin and subcutaneous tissue** complicating pregnancy, childbirth and the puerperium
     Conditions in L00-L99

     Excludes2   herpes gestationis (O26.4)
       pruritic urticarial papules and plaques of pregnancy (PUPPP) (O26.86)

● O99.71   Diseases of the skin and subcutaneous tissue complicating pregnancy

       O99.711   Diseases of the skin and subcutaneous tissue complicating pregnancy, first trimester   M

       O99.712   Diseases of the skin and subcutaneous tissue complicating pregnancy, second trimester   M

       O99.713   Diseases of the skin and subcutaneous tissue complicating pregnancy, third trimester   M

       O99.719   Diseases of the skin and subcutaneous tissue complicating pregnancy, unspecified trimester   M

   O99.72   Diseases of the skin and subcutaneous tissue complicating childbirth   M

   O99.73   Diseases of the skin and subcutaneous tissue complicating the puerperium   M

● O99.8   **Other specified diseases and conditions** complicating pregnancy, childbirth and the puerperium
     Conditions in D00-D48, H00-H95, M00-N99, and Q00-Q99

     Use additional code to identify condition

     Excludes2   genitourinary infections in pregnancy (O23.-)
       infection of genitourinary tract following delivery (O86.1-O86.4)
       malignant neoplasm complicating pregnancy, childbirth and the puerperium (O9A.1-)
       maternal care for known or suspected abnormality of maternal pelvic organs (O34.-)
       postpartum acute kidney failure (O90.49)
       traumatic injuries in pregnancy (O9A.2-)

● O99.81   Abnormal glucose complicating pregnancy, childbirth and the puerperium

     Excludes1   gestational diabetes (O24.4-)

       O99.810   Abnormal glucose complicating pregnancy   M

       O99.814   Abnormal glucose complicating childbirth   M

       O99.815   Abnormal glucose complicating the puerperium   M

CHAPTER 15 (O00-O9A)

CHAPTER 15 (O00-O9A)

● O99.82   **Streptococcus B carrier state** complicating pregnancy, childbirth and the puerperium

    Excludes1   Carrier of streptococcus group B (GBS) in a nonpregnant woman (Z22.330)

  O99.820   Streptococcus B carrier state complicating pregnancy   M

  O99.824   Streptococcus B carrier state complicating childbirth   M
         Coding Clinic: 2019, Q2, P9

  O99.825   Streptococcus B carrier state complicating the puerperium   M

● O99.83   **Other infection carrier state** complicating pregnancy, childbirth and the puerperium

     Use additional code to identify the carrier state (Z22.-)

  O99.830   Other infection carrier state complicating pregnancy   M

  O99.834   Other infection carrier state complicating childbirth   M

  O99.835   Other infection carrier state complicating the puerperium   M

● O99.84   **Bariatric surgery status** complicating pregnancy, childbirth and the puerperium

     Gastric banding status complicating pregnancy, childbirth and the puerperium
     Gastric bypass status for obesity complicating pregnancy, childbirth and the puerperium
     Obesity surgery status complicating pregnancy, childbirth and the puerperium

  O99.840   Bariatric surgery status complicating pregnancy, unspecified trimester   M

  O99.841   Bariatric surgery status complicating pregnancy, first trimester   M

  O99.842   Bariatric surgery status complicating pregnancy, second trimester   M

  O99.843   Bariatric surgery status complicating pregnancy, third trimester   M

  O99.844   Bariatric surgery status complicating childbirth   M

  O99.845   Bariatric surgery status complicating the puerperium   M

● O99.89   **Other specified diseases and conditions** complicating pregnancy, childbirth and the puerperium   M

  O99.891   Other specified diseases and conditions complicating pregnancy   M

  O99.892   Other specified diseases and conditions complicating childbirth   M
         Coding Clinic: 2023, Q3, P17

  O99.893   Other specified diseases and conditions complicating puerperium   M

OGCR   Section I.C.2.l.3.

Malignant neoplasm in a pregnant patient

When a pregnant woman has a malignant neoplasm, a code from subcategory O9A.1-, Malignant neoplasm complicating pregnancy, childbirth, and the puerperium, should be sequenced first, followed by the appropriate code from Chapter 2 to indicate the type of neoplasm.

● O9A   **Maternal malignant neoplasms, traumatic injuries and abuse classifiable elsewhere but complicating pregnancy, childbirth and the puerperium**

● O9A.1   **Malignant neoplasm complicating pregnancy, childbirth and the puerperium**

     Conditions in C00-C96

     Use additional code to identify neoplasm

    Excludes2   maternal care for benign tumor of corpus uteri (O34.1-)
             maternal care for benign tumor of cervix (O34.4-)

● O9A.11   Malignant neoplasm complicating pregnancy

  O9A.111   Malignant neoplasm complicating pregnancy, first trimester   M

  O9A.112   Malignant neoplasm complicating pregnancy, second trimester   M

  O9A.113   Malignant neoplasm complicating pregnancy, third trimester   M

  O9A.119   Malignant neoplasm complicating pregnancy, unspecified trimester   M

  O9A.12   Malignant neoplasm complicating childbirth   M

  O9A.13   Malignant neoplasm complicating the puerperium   M
         Coding Clinic: 2015, Q3, P19

● O9A.2   **Injury, poisoning and certain other consequences of external causes** complicating pregnancy, childbirth and the puerperium

     Conditions in S00-T88, except T74 and T76

     Use additional code(s) to identify the injury or poisoning

    Excludes2   physical, sexual and psychological abuse complicating pregnancy, childbirth and the puerperium (O9A.3-, O9A.4-, O9A.5-)

● O9A.21   Injury, poisoning and certain other consequences of external causes complicating pregnancy

  O9A.211   Injury, poisoning and certain other consequences of external causes complicating pregnancy, first trimester   M

  O9A.212   Injury, poisoning and certain other consequences of external causes complicating pregnancy, second trimester   M

  O9A.213   Injury, poisoning and certain other consequences of external causes complicating pregnancy, third trimester   M

  O9A.219   Injury, poisoning and certain other consequences of external causes complicating pregnancy, unspecified trimester   M

  O9A.22   Injury, poisoning and certain other consequences of external causes complicating childbirth   M

  O9A.23   Injury, poisoning and certain other consequences of external causes complicating the puerperium   M

● O9A.3   **Physical abuse** complicating pregnancy, childbirth and the puerperium

     Conditions in T74.11 or T76.11

     Use additional code (if applicable):
       to identify any associated current injury due to physical abuse
       to identify the perpetrator of abuse (Y07.-)

    Excludes2   sexual abuse complicating pregnancy, childbirth and the puerperium (O9A.4)

● O9A.31   Physical abuse complicating pregnancy

  O9A.311   Physical abuse complicating pregnancy, first trimester   M

  O9A.312   Physical abuse complicating pregnancy, second trimester   M

  O9A.313   Physical abuse complicating pregnancy, third trimester   M

  O9A.319   Physical abuse complicating pregnancy, unspecified trimester   M

  O9A.32   Physical abuse complicating childbirth   M

  O9A.33   Physical abuse complicating the puerperium   M

▶ New   ⇛ Revised   ~~deleted~~ Deleted   Excludes 1   Excludes 2   Includes   Use additional   Code first   Code also   Key words

OGCR Official Guidelines   X Assign placeholder X   ● Use Additional Character(s)   ◗ Manifestation Code   🦉 Hierarchical Condition Category   **Coding Clinic**

● O9A.4   **Sexual abuse complicating pregnancy, childbirth and the puerperium**

Conditions in T74.21 or T76.21

Use additional code (if applicable):

to identify any associated current injury due to sexual abuse

to identify the perpetrator of abuse (Y07.-)

● O9A.41   Sexual abuse complicating pregnancy

     O9A.411   Sexual abuse complicating pregnancy, first trimester   **M**

     O9A.412   Sexual abuse complicating pregnancy, second trimester   **M**

     O9A.413   Sexual abuse complicating pregnancy, third trimester   **M**

     O9A.419   Sexual abuse complicating pregnancy, unspecified trimester   **M**

   O9A.42   Sexual abuse complicating childbirth   **M**

   O9A.43   Sexual abuse complicating the puerperium   **M**

● O9A.5   **Psychological abuse complicating pregnancy, childbirth and the puerperium**

Conditions in T74.31 or T76.31

Use additional code to identify the perpetrator of abuse (Y07.-)

● O9A.51   Psychological abuse complicating pregnancy

     O9A.511   Psychological abuse complicating pregnancy, first trimester   **M**

     O9A.512   Psychological abuse complicating pregnancy, second trimester   **M**

     O9A.513   Psychological abuse complicating pregnancy, third trimester   **M**

     O9A.519   Psychological abuse complicating pregnancy, unspecified trimester   **M**

   O9A.52   Psychological abuse complicating childbirth   **M**

   O9A.53   Psychological abuse complicating the puerperium   **M**

CHAPTER 16

CERTAIN CONDITIONS ORIGINATING IN THE PERINATAL PERIOD (P00-P96)

OGCR Chapter-Specific Coding Guidelines

16. **Chapter 16: Certain Conditions Originating in the Perinatal Period (P00-P96)**
For coding and reporting purposes the perinatal period is defined as before birth through the 28th day following birth. The following guidelines are provided for reporting purposes

a. General Perinatal Rules

1) Use of Chapter 16 Codes
Codes in this chapter are never for use on the maternal record. Codes from Chapter 15, the obstetric chapter, are never permitted on the newborn record. Chapter 16 codes may be used throughout the life of the patient if the condition is still present.

2) Principal Diagnosis for Birth Record
When coding the birth episode in a newborn record, assign a code from category Z38, Liveborn infants according to place of birth and type of delivery, as the principal diagnosis. A code from category Z38 is assigned only once, to a newborn at the time of birth. If a newborn is transferred to another institution, a code from category Z38 should not be used at the receiving hospital.
A code from category Z38 is used only on the newborn record, not on the mother's record.

3) Use of Codes from other Chapters with Codes from Chapter 16
Codes from other chapters may be used with codes from chapter 16 if the codes from the other chapters provide more specific detail. Codes for signs and symptoms may be assigned when a definitive diagnosis has not been established. If the reason for the encounter is a perinatal condition, the code from Chapter 16 should be sequenced first.

4) Use of Chapter 16 Codes after the Perinatal Period
Should a condition originate in the perinatal period, and continue throughout the life of the patient, the perinatal code should continue to be used regardless of the patient's age.

5) Birth process or community acquired conditions
If a newborn has a condition that may be either due to the birth process or community acquired and the documentation does not indicate which it is, the default is due to the birth process and the code from Chapter 16 should be used. If the condition is community-acquired, a code from Chapter 16 should not be assigned.

6) Code all clinically significant conditions
All clinically significant conditions noted on routine newborn examination should be coded. A condition is clinically significant if it requires:
- clinical evaluation; or
- therapeutic treatment; or
- diagnostic procedures; or
- extended length of hospital stay; or
- increased nursing care and/or monitoring; or
- has implications for future health care needs

Note: The perinatal guidelines listed above are the same as the general coding guidelines for "additional diagnoses", except for the final point regarding implications for future health care needs. Codes should be assigned for conditions that have been specified by the provider as having implications for future health care needs.

b. Observation and Evaluation of Newborns for Suspected Conditions Not Found

1) Use of Z05 codes
Assign a code from category Z05, Observation and evaluation of newborns and infants for suspected conditions ruled out, to identify those instances when a healthy newborn is evaluated for a suspected condition that is determined after study not to be present. Do not use a code from category Z05 when the patient has identified signs or symptoms of a suspected problem; in such cases code the sign or symptom.

2) Z05 on Other than the Birth Record
A code from category Z05 may also be assigned as a principal or first-listed code for readmissions or encounters when the code from category Z38 code no longer applies. Codes from category Z05 are for use only for healthy newborns and infants for which no condition after study is found to be present.

3) Z05 on a birth record
A code from category Z05 is to be used as a secondary code after the code from category Z38, Liveborn infants according to place of birth and type of delivery.

c. Coding Additional Perinatal Diagnoses

1) Assigning codes for conditions that require treatment
Assign codes for conditions that require treatment or further investigation, prolong the length of stay, or require resource utilization.

2) Codes for conditions specified as having implications for future health care needs
Assign codes for conditions that have been specified by the provider as having implications for future health care needs.
Note: This guideline should not be used for adult patients.

d. Prematurity and Fetal Growth Retardation
Providers utilize different criteria in determining prematurity. A code for prematurity should not be assigned unless it is documented. Assignment of codes in categories P05, Disorders of newborn related to slow fetal growth and fetal malnutrition, and P07, Disorders of newborn related to short gestation and low birth weight, not elsewhere classified, should be based on the recorded birth weight and estimated gestational age.
When both birth weight and gestational age are available, two codes from category P07 should be assigned, with the code for birth weight sequenced before the code for gestational age.

e. Low birth weight and immaturity status
Codes from category P07, Disorders of newborn related to short gestation and low birth weight, not elsewhere classified, are for use for a child or adult who was premature or had a low birth weight as a newborn and this is affecting the patient's current health status.
See Section I.C.21. Factors influencing health status and contact with health services, Status.

f. Bacterial Sepsis of Newborn
Category P36, Bacterial sepsis of newborn, includes congenital sepsis. If a perinate is documented as having sepsis without documentation of congenital or community acquired, the default is congenital and a code from category P36 should be assigned. If the P36 code includes the causal organism, an additional code from category B95, Streptococcus, Staphylococcus, and Enterococcus as the cause of diseases classified elsewhere, or B96, Other bacterial agents as the cause of diseases classified elsewhere, should not be assigned. If the P36 code does not include the causal organism, assign an additional code from category B96. If applicable, use additional codes to identify severe sepsis (R65.2-) and any associated acute organ dysfunction.

g. Stillbirth
Code P95, Stillbirth, is only for use in institutions that maintain separate records for stillbirths. No other code should be used with P95. Code P95 should not be used on the mother's record.

CHAPTER 16

CERTAIN CONDITIONS ORIGINATING IN THE PERINATAL PERIOD (P00-P96)

Note: Codes from this chapter are for use on newborn records only, never on maternal records.

> **Includes**   conditions that have their origin in the fetal or perinatal period (before birth through the first 28 days after birth) even if morbidity occurs later

> **Excludes2**   congenital malformations, deformations and chromosomal abnormalities (Q00-Q99)
> endocrine, nutritional and metabolic diseases (E00-E88)
> injury, poisoning and certain other consequences of external causes (S00-T88)
> neoplasms (C00-D49)
> tetanus neonatorum (A33)

This chapter contains the following blocks:

P00-P04	Newborn affected by maternal factors and by complications of pregnancy, labor, and delivery
P05-P08	Disorders of newborns related to length of gestation and fetal growth
P09	Abnormal findings on neonatal screening
P10-P15	Birth trauma
P19-P29	Respiratory and cardiovascular disorders specific to the perinatal period
P35-P39	Infections specific to the perinatal period
P50-P61	Hemorrhagic and hematological disorders of newborn
P70-P74	Transitory endocrine and metabolic disorders specific to newborn
P76-P78	Digestive system disorders of newborn
P80-P83	Conditions involving the integument and temperature regulation of newborn
P84	Other problems with newborn
P90-P96	Other disorders originating in the perinatal period

NEWBORN AFFECTED BY MATERNAL FACTORS AND BY COMPLICATIONS OF PREGNANCY, LABOR, AND DELIVERY (P00–P04)

Note: These codes are for use when the listed maternal conditions are specified as the cause of confirmed morbidity or potential morbidity which have their origin in the perinatal period (before birth through the first 28 days after birth).

● **P00**   **Newborn affected by maternal conditions that may be unrelated to present pregnancy**

Code first any current condition in newborn

> **Excludes2**   encounter for observation of newborn for suspected diseases and conditions ruled out (Z05.-)
> newborn affected by maternal complications of pregnancy (P01.-)
> newborn affected by maternal endocrine and metabolic disorders (P70–P74)
> newborn affected by noxious substances transmitted via placenta or breast milk (P04.-)

Coding Clinic: 2016, Q4, P54

P00.0   **Newborn affected by maternal hypertensive disorders**
Newborn affected by maternal conditions classifiable to O10-O11, O13-O16

P00.1   **Newborn affected by maternal renal and urinary tract diseases**
Newborn affected by maternal conditions classifiable to N00-N39

P00.2   **Newborn affected by maternal infectious and parasitic diseases**
Newborn affected by maternal infectious disease classifiable to A00-B99, J09 and J10

> **Excludes1**   maternal genital tract or other localized infections (P00.8)

> **Excludes2**   infections specific to the perinatal period (P35-P39)
> newborn affected by (positive) maternal group B streptococcus (GBS) colonization (P00.82)

Coding Clinic: 2019, Q2, P10; 2015, Q3, P21

P00.3   **Newborn affected by other maternal circulatory and respiratory diseases**
Newborn affected by maternal conditions classifiable to I00-I99, J00-J99, Q20-Q34 and not included in P00.0, P00.2

P00.4   **Newborn affected by maternal nutritional disorders**
Newborn affected by maternal disorders classifiable to E40-E64
Maternal malnutrition NOS

P00.5   **Newborn affected by maternal injury**
Newborn affected by maternal conditions classifiable to O9A.2-

P00.6   **Newborn affected by surgical procedure on mother**
Newborn affected by amniocentesis

> **Excludes1**   Cesarean delivery for present delivery (P03.4)
> damage to placenta from amniocentesis, cesarean delivery or surgical induction (P02.1)
> previous surgery to uterus or pelvic organs (P03.89)

> **Excludes2**   newborn affected by complication of (fetal) intrauterine procedure (P96.5)

P00.7   **Newborn affected by other medical procedures on mother, not elsewhere classified**
Newborn affected by radiation to mother

> **Excludes1**   damage to placenta from amniocentesis, cesarean delivery or surgical induction (P02.1)
> newborn affected by other complications of labor and delivery (P03.-)

● **P00.8**   **Newborn affected by other maternal conditions**

P00.81   **Newborn affected by periodontal disease in mother**

P00.82   **Newborn affected by (positive) maternal group B streptococcus (GBS) colonization**
Contact with positive maternal group B streptococcus
Coding Clinic: 2021, Q4, P23

P00.89   **Newborn affected by other maternal conditions**
Newborn affected by conditions classifiable to T80-T88
Newborn affected by maternal genital tract or other localized infections
Newborn affected by maternal systemic lupus erythematosus
Use additional code to identify infectious agent, if known

> **Excludes2**   newborn affected by positive maternal group B streptococcus (GBS) colonization (P00.82)

Coding Clinic: 2019, Q2, P9

P00.9   **Newborn affected by unspecified maternal condition**

● **P01**   **Newborn affected by maternal complications of pregnancy**

Code first any current condition in newborn

> **Excludes2**   encounter for observation of newborn for suspected diseases and conditions ruled out (Z05.-)

Coding Clinic: 2016, Q4, P54

P01.0   **Newborn affected by incompetent cervix**

P01.1   **Newborn affected by premature rupture of membranes**

CHAPTER 16 (P00-P96)

P01.2   Newborn affected by oligohydramnios

> **Excludes1**   oligohydramnios due to premature rupture of membranes (P01.1)

P01.3   Newborn affected by polyhydramnios
Excess of amniotic fluid, usually > 2000 mL
Newborn affected by hydramnios

P01.4   Newborn affected by ectopic pregnancy
Newborn affected by abdominal pregnancy

P01.5   Newborn affected by multiple pregnancy
Newborn affected by triplet (pregnancy)
Newborn affected by twin (pregnancy)

P01.6   Newborn affected by maternal death

P01.7   Newborn affected by malpresentation before labor
Newborn affected by breech presentation before labor
Newborn affected by external version before labor
Newborn affected by face presentation before labor
Newborn affected by transverse lie before labor
Newborn affected by unstable lie before labor

P01.8   Newborn affected by other maternal complications of pregnancy

P01.9   Newborn affected by maternal complication of pregnancy, unspecified

● **P02   Newborn affected by complications of placenta, cord and membranes**

Code first any current condition in newborn

> **Excludes2**   encounter for observation of newborn for suspected diseases and conditions ruled out (Z05.-)

Coding Clinic: 2016, Q4, P54

P02.0   Newborn affected by placenta previa

P02.1   Newborn affected by other forms of placental separation and hemorrhage
Newborn affected by abruptio placenta
Newborn affected by accidental hemorrhage
Newborn affected by antepartum hemorrhage
Newborn affected by damage to placenta from amniocentesis, cesarean delivery or surgical induction
Newborn affected by maternal blood loss
Newborn affected by premature separation of placenta

● **P02.2   Newborn affected by other and unspecified morphological and functional abnormalities of placenta**

P02.20   Newborn affected by unspecified morphological and functional abnormalities of placenta

P02.29   Newborn affected by other morphological and functional abnormalities of placenta
Newborn affected by placental dysfunction
Newborn affected by placental infarction
Newborn affected by placental insufficiency

P02.3   Newborn affected by placental transfusion syndromes
Newborn affected by placental and cord abnormalities resulting in twin-to-twin or other transplacental transfusion

P02.4   Newborn affected by prolapsed cord

P02.5   Newborn affected by other compression of umbilical cord
Newborn affected by umbilical cord (tightly) around neck
Newborn affected by entanglement of umbilical cord
Newborn affected by knot in umbilical cord
Coding Clinic: 2022, Q1, P22

● **P02.6   Newborn affected by other and unspecified conditions of umbilical cord**

P02.60   Newborn affected by unspecified conditions of umbilical cord

P02.69   Newborn affected by other conditions of umbilical cord
Newborn affected by short umbilical cord
Newborn affected by vasa previa

> **Excludes1**   newborn affected by single umbilical artery (Q27.0)

● **P02.7   Newborn affected by chorioamnionitis**
Inflammation of chorion and amnion

P02.70   Newborn affected by fetal inflammatory response syndrome 🔹
Newborn affected by FIRS

P02.78   Newborn affected by other conditions from chorioamnionitis
Newborn affected by amnionitis
Newborn affected by membranitis
Newborn affected by placentitis

P02.8   Newborn affected by other abnormalities of membranes

P02.9   Newborn affected by abnormality of membranes, unspecified

● **P03   Newborn affected by other complications of labor and delivery**

Code first any current condition in newborn

> **Excludes2**   encounter for observation of newborn for suspected diseases and conditions ruled out (Z05.-)

Coding Clinic: 2016, Q4, P54

P03.0   Newborn affected by breech delivery and extraction

P03.1   Newborn affected by other malpresentation, malposition and disproportion during labor and delivery
Newborn affected by contracted pelvis
Newborn affected by conditions classifiable to O64-O66
Newborn affected by persistent occipitoposterior
Newborn affected by transverse lie

P03.2   Newborn affected by forceps delivery

P03.3   Newborn affected by delivery by vacuum extractor [ventouse]

P03.4   Newborn affected by Cesarean delivery

P03.5   Newborn affected by precipitate delivery
Newborn affected by rapid second stage

P03.6   Newborn affected by abnormal uterine contractions
Newborn affected by conditions classifiable to O62.-, except O62.3
Newborn affected by hypertonic labor
Newborn affected by uterine inertia

● **P03.8   Newborn affected by other specified complications of labor and delivery**

● **P03.81   Newborn affected by abnormality in fetal (intrauterine) heart rate or rhythm**

> **Excludes1**   neonatal cardiac dysrhythmia (P29.1-)

P03.810   Newborn affected by abnormality in fetal (intrauterine) heart rate or rhythm before the onset of labor

P03.811   Newborn affected by abnormality in fetal (intrauterine) heart rate or rhythm during labor

P03.819   Newborn affected by abnormality in fetal (intrauterine) heart rate or rhythm, unspecified as to time of onset

P03.82   Meconium passage during delivery

> **Excludes1**   meconium aspiration (P24.00, P24.01)
> meconium staining (P96.83)

P03.89   Newborn affected by other specified complications of labor and delivery
Newborn affected by abnormality of maternal soft tissues
Newborn affected by conditions classifiable to O60-O75 and by procedures used in labor and delivery not included in P02.- and P03.0-P03.6
Newborn affected by induction of labor

P03.9   Newborn affected by complication of labor and delivery, unspecified

---

▶ New   ⟹ Revised   ~~deleted~~ Deleted   Excludes 1   Excludes 2   Includes   Use additional   Code first   Code also   Key words

OGCR Official Guidelines   X Assign placeholder X   ● Use Additional Character(s)   ▶ Manifestation Code   🔹 Hierarchical Condition Category   Coding Clinic

● **P04**   **Newborn affected by noxious substances transmitted via placenta or breast milk**

Code first any current condition in newborn, if applicable

    Includes   nonteratogenic effects of substances transmitted via placenta

    Excludes2   congenital malformations (Q00-Q99)
          encounter for observation of newborn for suspected diseases and conditions ruled out (Z05.-)
          neonatal jaundice from excessive hemolysis due to drugs or toxins transmitted from mother (P58.4)
          newborn in contact with and (suspected) exposures hazardous to health not transmitted via placenta or breast milk (Z77.-)

    Coding Clinic: 2016, Q4, P54

P04.0   **Newborn affected by maternal anesthesia and analgesia in pregnancy, labor and delivery**
     Newborn affected by reactions and intoxications from maternal opiates and tranquilizers administered for procedures during pregnancy or labor and delivery

     Excludes2   newborn affected by other maternal medication (P04.1-)

● **P04.1**   **Newborn affected by other maternal medication**
     Code first , if applicable, withdrawal symptoms from maternal use of drugs of addiction (P96.1)
     withdrawal symptoms from therapeutic use of drugs in newborn (P96.2)

     Excludes1   dysmorphism due to warfarin (Q86.2)
          fetal hydantoin syndrome (Q86.1)

     Excludes2   maternal anesthesia and analgesia in pregnancy, labor and delivery (P04.0)
          maternal use of drugs of addiction (P04.4-)

    P04.11   **Newborn affected by maternal antineoplastic chemotherapy**

    P04.12   **Newborn affected by maternal cytotoxic drugs**

    P04.13   **Newborn affected by maternal use of anticonvulsants**

    P04.14   **Newborn affected by maternal use of opiates**

    P04.15   **Newborn affected by maternal use of antidepressants**

    P04.16   **Newborn affected by maternal use of amphetamines**

    P04.17   **Newborn affected by maternal use of sedative-hypnotics**

    P04.1A   **Newborn affected by maternal use of anxiolytics**

    P04.18   **Newborn affected by other maternal medication**

    P04.19   **Newborn affected by maternal use of unspecified medication**
      Coding Clinic: 2016, Q4, P55

P04.2   **Newborn affected by maternal use of tobacco**
     Newborn affected by exposure in utero to tobacco smoke

     Excludes2   newborn exposure to environmental tobacco smoke (P96.81)

P04.3   **Newborn affected by maternal use of alcohol**

     Excludes1   fetal alcohol syndrome (Q86.0)

● **P04.4**   **Newborn affected by maternal use of drugs of addiction**

    P04.40   **Newborn affected by maternal use of unspecified drugs of addiction**

    P04.41   **Newborn affected by maternal use of cocaine**

    P04.42   **Newborn affected by maternal use of hallucinogens**

     Excludes2   newborn affected by other maternal medication (P04.1-)

P04.49   **Newborn affected by maternal use of other drugs of addiction**

     Excludes2   newborn affected by maternal anesthesia and analgesia (P04.0)
          withdrawal symptoms from maternal use of drugs of addiction (P96.1)

P04.5   **Newborn affected by maternal use of nutritional chemical substances**

P04.6   **Newborn affected by maternal exposure to environmental chemical substances**

● **P04.8**   **Newborn affected by other maternal noxious substances**

    P04.81   **Newborn affected by maternal use of cannabis**

    P04.89   **Newborn affected by other maternal noxious substances**

P04.9   **Newborn affected by maternal noxious substance, unspecified**

OGCR   Section I.C.16.d.

Prematurity and Fetal Growth Retardation

Providers utilize different criteria in determining prematurity. A code for prematurity should not be assigned unless it is documented. Assignment of codes in categories P05, Disorders of newborn related to slow fetal growth and fetal malnutrition, and P07, Disorders of newborn related to short gestation and low birth weight, not elsewhere classified, should be based on the recorded birth weight and estimated gestational age.

When both birth weight and gestational age are available, two codes from category P07 should be assigned, with the code for birth weight sequenced before the code for gestational age.

DISORDERS OF NEWBORN RELATED TO LENGTH OF GESTATION AND FETAL GROWTH (P05-P08)

● **P05**   **Disorders of newborn related to slow fetal growth and fetal malnutrition**
     Coding Clinic: 2016, Q4, P56

● **P05.0**   **Newborn light for gestational age**
     Newborn light-for-dates
     Weight below but length above 10th percentile for gestational age

    P05.00   **Newborn light for gestational age, unspecified weight**

    P05.01   **Newborn light for gestational age, less than 500 grams**

    P05.02   **Newborn light for gestational age, 500-749 grams**

    P05.03   **Newborn light for gestational age, 750-999 grams**

    P05.04   **Newborn light for gestational age, 1000-1249 grams**

    P05.05   **Newborn light for gestational age, 1250-1499 grams**

    P05.06   **Newborn light for gestational age, 1500-1749 grams**

    P05.07   **Newborn light for gestational age, 1750-1999 grams**

    P05.08   **Newborn light for gestational age, 2000-2499 grams**

    P05.09   **Newborn light for gestational age, 2500 grams and over**
      Newborn light for gestational age, other
      Coding Clinic: 2016, Q4, P55

CHAPTER 16 (P00-P96)

● **P05.1**   **Newborn small for gestational age**
Newborn small-and-light-for-dates
Newborn small-for-dates
Weight and length below 10th percentile for gestational age

     P05.10   **Newborn small for gestational age, unspecified weight**

     P05.11   **Newborn small for gestational age, less than 500 grams**

     P05.12   **Newborn small for gestational age, 500-749 grams**

     P05.13   **Newborn small for gestational age, 750-999 grams**

     P05.14   **Newborn small for gestational age, 1000-1249 grams**

     P05.15   **Newborn small for gestational age, 1250-1499 grams**

     P05.16   **Newborn small for gestational age, 1500-1749 grams**

     P05.17   **Newborn small for gestational age, 1750-1999 grams**

     P05.18   **Newborn small for gestational age, 2000-2499 grams**

     P05.19   **Newborn small for gestational age, other**
Newborn small for gestational age, 2500 grams and over
Coding Clinic: 2016, Q4, P55

P05.2   **Newborn affected by fetal (intrauterine) malnutrition not light or small for gestational age**
Infant, not light or small for gestational age, showing signs of fetal malnutrition, such as dry, peeling skin and loss of subcutaneous tissue

     Excludes1   newborn affected by fetal malnutrition with light for gestational age (P05.0-)
newborn affected by fetal malnutrition with small for gestational age (P05.1-)

P05.9   **Newborn affected by slow intrauterine growth, unspecified**
Newborn affected by fetal growth retardation NOS

● **P07**   **Disorders of newborn related to short gestation and low birth weight, not elsewhere classified**
Note: When both birth weight and gestational age of the newborn are available, both should be coded with birth weight sequenced before gestational age.

     Includes   the listed conditions, without further specification, as the cause of morbidity or additional care, in newborn

● **P07.0**   **Extremely low birth weight newborn**
Newborn birth weight 999 g. or less

     Excludes1   low birth weight due to slow fetal growth and fetal malnutrition (P05.-)

     P07.00   **Extremely low birth weight newborn, unspecified weight**

     P07.01   **Extremely low birth weight newborn, less than 500 grams**

     P07.02   **Extremely low birth weight newborn, 500-749 grams**

     P07.03   **Extremely low birth weight newborn, 750-999 grams**

● **P07.1**   **Other low birth weight newborn**
Newborn birth weight 1000-2499 g.

     Excludes1   low birth weight due to slow fetal growth and fetal malnutrition (P05.-)

     P07.10   **Other low birth weight newborn, unspecified weight**

     P07.14   **Other low birth weight newborn, 1000-1249 grams**

     P07.15   **Other low birth weight newborn, 1250-1499 grams**

     P07.16   **Other low birth weight newborn, 1500-1749 grams**

     P07.17   **Other low birth weight newborn, 1750-1999 grams**

     P07.18   **Other low birth weight newborn, 2000-2499 grams**

● **P07.2**   **Extreme immaturity of newborn**
Less than 28 completed weeks (less than 196 completed days) of gestation

     P07.20   **Extreme immaturity of newborn, unspecified weeks of gestation**
Gestational age less than 28 completed weeks NOS

     P07.21   **Extreme immaturity of newborn, gestational age less than 23 completed weeks**
Extreme immaturity of newborn, gestational age less than 23 weeks, 0 days

     P07.22   **Extreme immaturity of newborn, gestational age 23 completed weeks**
Extreme immaturity of newborn, gestational age 23 weeks, 0 days through 23 weeks, 6 days

     P07.23   **Extreme immaturity of newborn, gestational age 24 completed weeks**
Extreme immaturity of newborn, gestational age 24 weeks, 0 days through 24 weeks, 6 days

     P07.24   **Extreme immaturity of newborn, gestational age 25 completed weeks**
Extreme immaturity of newborn, gestational age 25 weeks, 0 days through 25 weeks, 6 days

     P07.25   **Extreme immaturity of newborn, gestational age 26 completed weeks**
Extreme immaturity of newborn, gestational age 26 weeks, 0 days through 26 weeks, 6 days

     P07.26   **Extreme immaturity of newborn, gestational age 27 completed weeks**
Extreme immaturity of newborn, gestational age 27 weeks, 0 days through 27 weeks, 6 days

● **P07.3**   **Preterm [premature] newborn [other]**
28 completed weeks or more but less than 37 completed weeks (196 completed days but less than 259 completed days) of gestation
Prematurity NOS

     P07.30   **Preterm newborn, unspecified weeks of gestation**

     P07.31   **Preterm newborn, gestational age 28 completed weeks**
Preterm newborn, gestational age 28 weeks, 0 days through 28 weeks, 6 days

     P07.32   **Preterm newborn, gestational age 29 completed weeks**
Preterm newborn, gestational age 29 weeks, 0 days through 29 weeks, 6 days

     P07.33   **Preterm newborn, gestational age 30 completed weeks**
Preterm newborn, gestational age 30 weeks, 0 days through 30 weeks, 6 days

     P07.34   **Preterm newborn, gestational age 31 completed weeks**
Preterm newborn, gestational age 31 weeks, 0 days through 31 weeks, 6 days

     P07.35   **Preterm newborn, gestational age 32 completed weeks**
Preterm newborn, gestational age 32 weeks, 0 days through 32 weeks, 6 days

     P07.36   **Preterm newborn, gestational age 33 completed weeks**
Preterm newborn, gestational age 33 weeks, 0 days through 33 weeks, 6 days

▶ New   ⇒ Revised   ~~deleted~~ Deleted   Excludes 1   Excludes 2   Includes   Use additional   Code first   Code also   Key words

OGCR Official Guidelines   X Assign placeholder X   ● Use Additional Character(s)   ▶ Manifestation Code   🔖 Hierarchical Condition Category   **Coding Clinic**

P07.37   **Preterm newborn, gestational age 34 completed weeks**
> Preterm newborn, gestational age 34 weeks, 0 days through 34 weeks, 6 days
> *Coding Clinic: 2017, Q2, P7*

P07.38   **Preterm newborn, gestational age 35 completed weeks**
> Preterm newborn, gestational age 35 weeks, 0 days through 35 weeks, 6 days

P07.39   **Preterm newborn, gestational age 36 completed weeks**
> Preterm newborn, gestational age 36 weeks, 0 days through 36 weeks, 6 days
> *Coding Clinic: 2017, Q3, P26*

● **P08**   **Disorders of newborn related to long gestation and high birth weight**
> **Note:** When both birth weight and gestational age of the newborn are available, priority of assignment should be given to birth weight.
> **Includes**   the listed conditions, without further specification, as causes of morbidity or additional care, in newborn

P08.0   **Exceptionally large newborn baby**
> Usually implies a birth weight of 4500 g. or more
> **Excludes1**   syndrome of infant of diabetic mother (P70.1)
> syndrome of infant of mother with gestational diabetes (P70.0)

P08.1   **Other heavy for gestational age newborn**
> Other newborn heavy- or large-for-dates regardless of period of gestation
> Usually implies a birth weight of 4000 g. to 4499 g.
> **Excludes1**   newborn with a birth weight of 4500 or more (P08.0)
> syndrome of infant of diabetic mother (P70.1)
> syndrome of infant of mother with gestational diabetes (P70.0)

● **P08.2**   **Late newborn, not heavy for gestational age**

P08.21   **Post-term newborn**
> Newborn with gestation period over 40 completed weeks to 42 completed weeks

P08.22   **Prolonged gestation of newborn**
> Newborn with gestation period over 42 completed weeks (294 days or more), not heavy- or large-for-dates
> Postmaturity NOS

ABNORMAL FINDINGS ON NEONATAL SCREENING (P09)

● **P09**   **Abnormal findings on neonatal screening**
> Includes: Abnormal findings on state mandated newborn screens
> Failed newborn screening
> **Excludes2**   nonspecific serologic evidence of human immunodeficiency virus [HIV] (R75)

P09.1   **Abnormal findings on neonatal screening for inborn errors of metabolism**

P09.2   **Abnormal findings on neonatal screening for congenital endocrine disease**
> Abnormal findings on neonatal screening for congenital adrenal hyperplasia
> Abnormal findings on neonatal screening for hypothyroidism screen

P09.3   **Abnormal findings on neonatal screening for congenital hematologic disorders**
> Abnormal findings for hemoglobinopathy screening
> Abnormal findings on red cell membrane defects screen
> Abnormal findings on sickle cell screen

P09.4   **Abnormal findings on neonatal screening for cystic fibrosis**

P09.5   **Abnormal findings on neonatal screening for critical congenital heart disease**
> Neonatal congenital heart disease screening failure

P09.6   **Abnormal findings on neonatal screening for neonatal hearing loss**
> **Excludes2**   encounter for hearing examination following failed hearing screening (Z01.110)

P09.8   **Other abnormal findings on neonatal screening**

P09.9   **Abnormal findings on neonatal screening, unspecified**

BIRTH TRAUMA (P10-P15)

● **P10**   **Intracranial laceration and hemorrhage due to birth injury**
> **Excludes1**   intracranial hemorrhage of newborn NOS (P52.9)
> intracranial hemorrhage of newborn due to anoxia or hypoxia (P52.-)
> nontraumatic intracranial hemorrhage of newborn (P52.-)

P10.0   **Subdural hemorrhage due to birth injury**
> Subdural hematoma (localized) due to birth injury
> **Excludes1**   subdural hemorrhage accompanying tentorial tear (P10.4)

P10.1   **Cerebral hemorrhage due to birth injury**

P10.2   **Intraventricular hemorrhage due to birth injury**

P10.3   **Subarachnoid hemorrhage due to birth injury**

P10.4   **Tentorial tear due to birth injury**
> *Pertaining to tentorium of cerebellum (extension of dura mater that separates cerebellum from inferior portion of occipital lobes)*

P10.8   **Other intracranial lacerations and hemorrhages due to birth injury**

P10.9   **Unspecified intracranial laceration and hemorrhage due to birth injury**

● **P11**   **Other birth injuries to central nervous system**

P11.0   **Cerebral edema due to birth injury**

P11.1   **Other specified brain damage due to birth injury**

P11.2   **Unspecified brain damage due to birth injury**

P11.3   **Birth injury to facial nerve**
> Facial palsy due to birth injury

P11.4   **Birth injury to other cranial nerves**

P11.5   **Birth injury to spine and spinal cord**
> Fracture of spine due to birth injury

P11.9   **Birth injury to central nervous system, unspecified**

● **P12**   **Birth injury to scalp**

P12.0   **Cephalhematoma due to birth injury**

P12.1   **Chignon (from vacuum extraction) due to birth injury**

P12.2   **Epicranial subaponeurotic hemorrhage due to birth injury**
> Subgaleal hemorrhage

P12.3   **Bruising of scalp due to birth injury**

P12.4   **Injury of scalp of newborn due to monitoring equipment**
> Sampling incision of scalp of newborn
> Scalp clip (electrode) injury of newborn

● **P12.8**   **Other birth injuries to scalp**

P12.81   **Caput succedaneum**

P12.89   **Other birth injuries to scalp**

P12.9   **Birth injury to scalp, unspecified**

● **P13**   **Birth injury to skeleton**
> **Excludes2**   birth injury to spine (P11.5)

P13.0   **Fracture of skull due to birth injury**

P13.1   **Other birth injuries to skull**
> **Excludes1**   cephalhematoma (P12.0)

P13.2   **Birth injury to femur**

P13.3   **Birth injury to other long bones**

CHAPTER 16 (P00-P96)

Item 16-1 The **peripheral nervous system** consists of 31 pairs of spinal nerves, 12 pairs of cranial nerves, and the autonomic nerves, which are divided into the parasympathetic and sympathetic nerves. The cranial nerves are: olfactory (I), optic (II), oculomotor (III), trochlear (IV), trigeminal (V), abducens (VI), facial (VII), vestibulocochlear (VIII), glossopharyngeal (IX), vagus (X), accessory (XI), and hypoglossal (XII).

Central Nervous System
- Brain
- Spinal cord

Peripheral Nervous System
- Cranial nerves (12)
- Spinal nerves
  cervical (8)
  thoracic (12)
  lumbar (5)
  sacral (5)
  coccyx (1)

Figure 16-1 The central nervous system consists of the brain and spinal cord. The peripheral nervous system consists of nerves that lie outside the skull and spinal cord. (From Stoy: Mosby's EMT-Basic Textbook, ed 2, St. Louis, Mosby, 2007)

P13.4　**Fracture of clavicle due to birth injury**

P13.8　**Birth injuries to other parts of skeleton**

P13.9　**Birth injury to skeleton, unspecified**

● P14　**Birth injury to peripheral nervous system**

P14.0　**Erb's paralysis due to birth injury**

P14.1　**Klumpke's paralysis due to birth injury**

P14.2　**Phrenic nerve paralysis due to birth injury**

P14.3　**Other brachial plexus birth injuries**

P14.8　**Birth injuries to other parts of peripheral nervous system**

P14.9　**Birth injury to peripheral nervous system, unspecified**

● P15　**Other birth injuries**

P15.0　**Birth injury to liver**
Rupture of liver due to birth injury

P15.1　**Birth injury to spleen**
Rupture of spleen due to birth injury

P15.2　**Sternomastoid injury due to birth injury**

P15.3　**Birth injury to eye**
Subconjunctival hemorrhage due to birth injury
Traumatic glaucoma due to birth injury

P15.4　**Birth injury to face**
Facial congestion due to birth injury

P15.5　**Birth injury to external genitalia**

P15.6　**Subcutaneous fat necrosis due to birth injury**

P15.8　**Other specified birth injuries**

P15.9　**Birth injury, unspecified**

RESPIRATORY AND CARDIOVASCULAR DISORDERS SPECIFIC TO THE PERINATAL PERIOD (P19-P29)

● P19　**Metabolic acidemia in newborn**

Includes　metabolic acidemia in newborn

P19.0　**Metabolic acidemia in newborn first noted before onset of labor**

P19.1　**Metabolic acidemia in newborn first noted during labor**

P19.2　**Metabolic acidemia noted at birth**

P19.9　**Metabolic acidemia in newborn, unspecified**

● P22　**Respiratory distress of newborn**
Coding Clinic: 2019, Q2, P29

P22.0　**Respiratory distress syndrome of newborn**
Cardiorespiratory distress syndrome of newborn
Hyaline membrane disease
Idiopathic respiratory distress syndrome [IRDS or RDS] of newborn
Pulmonary hypoperfusion syndrome
Respiratory distress syndrome, type I

Excludes2　respiratory arrest of newborn (P28.81)
respiratory failure of newborn NOS (P28.5)

Coding Clinic: 2019, Q2, P29

P22.1　**Transient tachypnea of newborn**
Idiopathic tachypnea of newborn
Respiratory distress syndrome, type II
Wet lung syndrome

P22.8　**Other respiratory distress of newborn**

Excludes1　respiratory arrest of newborn (P28.81)
respiratory failure of newborn NOS (P28.5)

P22.9　**Respiratory distress of newborn, unspecified**

Excludes1　respiratory arrest of newborn (P28.81)
respiratory failure of newborn NOS (P28.5)

● P23　**Congenital pneumonia**

Includes　infective pneumonia acquired in utero or during birth

Excludes1　neonatal pneumonia resulting from aspiration (P24.-)

P23.0　**Congenital pneumonia due to viral agent**
Use additional code (B97) to identify organism

Excludes1　congenital rubella pneumonitis (P35.0)

P23.1　**Congenital pneumonia due to Chlamydia**

P23.2　**Congenital pneumonia due to staphylococcus**

P23.3　**Congenital pneumonia due to streptococcus, group B**

P23.4　**Congenital pneumonia due to Escherichia coli**

P23.5　**Congenital pneumonia due to Pseudomonas**

P23.6　**Congenital pneumonia due to other bacterial agents**
Congenital pneumonia due to Hemophilus influenzae
Congenital pneumonia due to Klebsiella pneumoniae
Congenital pneumonia due to Mycoplasma
Congenital pneumonia due to Streptococcus, except group B
Use additional code (B95-B96) to identify organism

P23.8　**Congenital pneumonia due to other organisms**

P23.9　**Congenital pneumonia, unspecified**

● P24　**Neonatal aspiration**

Includes　aspiration in utero and during delivery

● P24.0　**Meconium aspiration**

Excludes1　meconium passage (without aspiration) during delivery (P03.82)
meconium staining (P96.83)

P24.00　**Meconium aspiration without respiratory symptoms**
Meconium aspiration NOS

▶ New　⇒ Revised　~~deleted~~ Deleted　| Excludes 1 |　| Excludes 2 |　| Includes |　| Use additional |　| Code first |　| Code also |　| Key words |

OGCR Official Guidelines　X Assign placeholder X　● Use Additional Character(s)　▶ Manifestation Code　🔍 Hierarchical Condition Category　Coding Clinic

P24.01 Meconium aspiration with respiratory symptoms
  Meconium aspiration pneumonia
  Meconium aspiration pneumonitis
  Meconium aspiration syndrome NOS
  Use additional code to identify any secondary pulmonary hypertension, if applicable (I27.2-)

● **P24.1 Neonatal aspiration of (clear) amniotic fluid and mucus**
  Neonatal aspiration of liquor (amnii)

P24.10 Neonatal aspiration of (clear) amniotic fluid and mucus without respiratory symptoms
  Neonatal aspiration of amniotic fluid and mucus NOS

P24.11 Neonatal aspiration of (clear) amniotic fluid and mucus with respiratory symptoms
  Neonatal aspiration of amniotic fluid and mucus with pneumonia
  Neonatal aspiration of amniotic fluid and mucus with pneumonitis
  Use additional code to identify any secondary pulmonary hypertension, if applicable (I27.2-)

● **P24.2 Neonatal aspiration of blood**

P24.20 Neonatal aspiration of blood without respiratory symptoms
  Neonatal aspiration of blood NOS

P24.21 Neonatal aspiration of blood with respiratory symptoms
  Neonatal aspiration of blood with pneumonia
  Neonatal aspiration of blood with pneumonitis
  Use additional code to identify any secondary pulmonary hypertension, if applicable (I27.2-)

● **P24.3 Neonatal aspiration of milk and regurgitated food**
  Neonatal aspiration of stomach contents

P24.30 Neonatal aspiration of milk and regurgitated food without respiratory symptoms
  Neonatal aspiration of milk and regurgitated food NOS

P24.31 Neonatal aspiration of milk and regurgitated food with respiratory symptoms
  Neonatal aspiration of milk and regurgitated food with pneumonia
  Neonatal aspiration of milk and regurgitated food with pneumonitis
  Use additional code to identify any secondary pulmonary hypertension, if applicable (I27.2-)

● **P24.8 Other neonatal aspiration**

P24.80 Other neonatal aspiration without respiratory symptoms
  Neonatal aspiration NEC

P24.81 Other neonatal aspiration with respiratory symptoms
  Neonatal aspiration pneumonia NEC
  Neonatal aspiration with pneumonitis NEC
  Neonatal aspiration with pneumonia NOS
  Neonatal aspiration with pneumonitis NOS
  Use additional code to identify any secondary pulmonary hypertension, if applicable (I27.2-)

P24.9 Neonatal aspiration, unspecified

● **P25 Interstitial emphysema and related conditions originating in the perinatal period**

P25.0 Interstitial emphysema originating in the perinatal period

P25.1 Pneumothorax originating in the perinatal period

P25.2 Pneumomediastinum originating in the perinatal period

P25.3 Pneumopericardium originating in the perinatal period

P25.8 Other conditions related to interstitial emphysema originating in the perinatal period

● **P26 Pulmonary hemorrhage originating in the perinatal period**
  Excludes1   acute idiopathic hemorrhage in infants over 28 days old (R04.81)

P26.0 Tracheobronchial hemorrhage originating in the perinatal period

P26.1 Massive pulmonary hemorrhage originating in the perinatal period

P26.8 Other pulmonary hemorrhages originating in the perinatal period

P26.9 Unspecified pulmonary hemorrhage originating in the perinatal period

● **P27 Chronic respiratory disease originating in the perinatal period**
  Excludes2   respiratory distress of newborn (P22.0-P22.9)

P27.0 Wilson-Mikity syndrome
  Pulmonary dysmaturity

P27.1 Bronchopulmonary dysplasia originating in the perinatal period

P27.8 Other chronic respiratory diseases originating in the perinatal period
  Congenital pulmonary fibrosis
  Ventilator lung in newborn

P27.9 Unspecified chronic respiratory disease originating in the perinatal period

● **P28 Other respiratory conditions originating in the perinatal period**
  Code also, if applicable, congenital malformations of the respiratory system (Q30-Q34)

P28.0 Primary atelectasis of newborn
  Failure of lungs to expand properly at birth
  Primary failure to expand terminal respiratory units
  Pulmonary hypoplasia associated with short gestation
  Pulmonary immaturity NOS

● **P28.1 Other and unspecified atelectasis of newborn**

P28.10 Unspecified atelectasis of newborn
  Atelectasis of newborn NOS

P28.11 Resorption atelectasis without respiratory distress syndrome
  Excludes1   resorption atelectasis with respiratory distress syndrome (P22.0)

P28.19 Other atelectasis of newborn
  Partial atelectasis of newborn
  Secondary atelectasis of newborn

P28.2 Cyanotic attacks of newborn
  Excludes1   apnea of newborn (P28.3- - P28.4-)

● **P28.3 Primary sleep apnea of newborn**
  Sleep apnea of newborn NOS
  Excludes2   other apnea of newborn (P28.4-)

P28.30 Primary sleep apnea of newborn, unspecified
  Transient oxygen desaturation spells of newborn during sleep

P28.31 Primary central sleep apnea of newborn

P28.32 Primary obstructive sleep apnea of newborn

P28.33 Primary mixed sleep apnea of newborn

P28.39 Other primary sleep apnea of newborn

● **P28.4 Other apnea of newborn**
  Excludes2   primary sleep apnea of newborn (P28.3-)

P28.40 Unspecified apnea of newborn
  Apnea of newborn, NOS
  Transient oxygen desaturation spells of newborn

P28.41 Central neonatal apnea of newborn

P28.42 Obstructive apnea of newborn

P28.43 Mixed neonatal apnea of newborn

P28.49 Other apnea of newborn
  Apnea of prematurity

CHAPTER 16 (P00-P96)

P28.5   Respiratory failure of newborn
    Excludes2 respiratory arrest of newborn (P28.81)
      ➡respiratory distress of newborn (P22.0)
    Coding Clinic: 2019, Q2, P29

● **P28.8   Other specified respiratory conditions of newborn**
    P28.81   Respiratory arrest of newborn
      Coding Clinic: 2017, Q2, P6
    P28.89   Other specified respiratory conditions of newborn
      Congenital laryngeal stridor
      Sniffles in newborn
      Snuffles in newborn
      Excludes1 early congenital syphilitic rhinitis (A50.05)

P28.9   Respiratory condition of newborn, unspecified
    Respiratory depression in newborn
    Code also associated underlying condition

● **P29   Cardiovascular disorders originating in the perinatal period**
    Excludes2 congenital malformations of the circulatory system (Q20-Q28)

P29.0   Neonatal cardiac failure
● **P29.1   Neonatal cardiac dysrhythmia**
    P29.11   Neonatal tachycardia
    P29.12   Neonatal bradycardia
P29.2   Neonatal hypertension
● **P29.3   Persistent fetal circulation**
    P29.30   Pulmonary hypertension of newborn
      Persistent pulmonary hypertension of newborn
    P29.38   Other persistent fetal circulation
      Delayed closure of ductus arteriosus
P29.4   Transient myocardial ischemia in newborn
● **P29.8   Other cardiovascular disorders originating in the perinatal period**
    P29.81   Cardiac arrest of newborn
    P29.89   Other cardiovascular disorders originating in the perinatal period
P29.9   Cardiovascular disorder originating in the perinatal period, unspecified

INFECTIONS SPECIFIC TO THE PERINATAL PERIOD (P35-P39)

Infections acquired in utero, during birth via the umbilicus, or during the first 28 days after birth
    Excludes2 asymptomatic human immunodeficiency virus [HIV] infection status (Z21)
      congenital gonococcal infection (A54.-)
      congenital pneumonia (P23.-)
      congenital syphilis (A50.-)
      human immunodeficiency virus [HIV] disease (B20)
      infant botulism (A48.51)
      infectious diseases not specific to the perinatal period (A00-B99, J09, J10.-)
      intestinal infectious disease (A00-A09)
      laboratory evidence of human immunodeficiency virus [HIV] (R75)
      tetanus neonatorum (A33)

● **P35   Congenital viral diseases**
    Includes infections acquired in utero or during birth

P35.0   Congenital rubella syndrome
    Congenital rubella pneumonitis
P35.1   Congenital cytomegalovirus infection
    Viruses transmitted by multiple routes that cause mild/subclinical infection
P35.2   Congenital herpesviral [herpes simplex] infection
P35.3   Congenital viral hepatitis
P35.4   Congenital Zika virus disease
    Use additional code to identify manifestations of congenital Zika virus disease
    Coding Clinic: 2018, Q4, P26
P35.8   Other congenital viral diseases
    Congenital varicella [chickenpox]
    Coding Clinic: 2016, Q4, P7
P35.9   Congenital viral disease, unspecified

● **P36   Bacterial sepsis of newborn**
    Includes congenital sepsis
    Use additional code(s), if applicable, to identify severe sepsis (R65.2-) and associated acute organ dysfunction(s)

P36.0   Sepsis of newborn due to streptococcus, group B 🅗
● **P36.1   Sepsis of newborn due to other and unspecified streptococci**
    P36.10   Sepsis of newborn due to unspecified streptococci 🅗
    P36.19   Sepsis of newborn due to other streptococci 🅗
P36.2   Sepsis of newborn due to Staphylococcus aureus 🅗
● **P36.3   Sepsis of newborn due to other and unspecified staphylococci**
    P36.30   Sepsis of newborn due to unspecified staphylococci 🅗
    P36.39   Sepsis of newborn due to other staphylococci 🅗
P36.4   Sepsis of newborn due to Escherichia coli 🅗
P36.5   Sepsis of newborn due to anaerobes 🅗
P36.8   Other bacterial sepsis of newborn 🅗
    Use additional code from category B96 to identify organism
P36.9   Bacterial sepsis of newborn, unspecified 🅗

● **P37   Other congenital infectious and parasitic diseases**
    Excludes2 congenital syphilis (A50.-)
      infectious neonatal diarrhea (A00-A09)
      necrotizing enterocolitis in newborn (P77.-)
      noninfectious neonatal diarrhea (P78.3)
      ophthalmia neonatorum due to gonococcus (A54.31)
      tetanus neonatorum (A33)

P37.0   Congenital tuberculosis
P37.1   Congenital toxoplasmosis
    Parasitic infection, often causing mild flu-like illness
    Hydrocephalus due to congenital toxoplasmosis
P37.2   Neonatal (disseminated) listeriosis
    Acquired transplacentally or during/after parturition in which symptoms are those of sepsis
P37.3   Congenital falciparum malaria
P37.4   Other congenital malaria
P37.5   Neonatal candidiasis
P37.8   Other specified congenital infectious and parasitic diseases
P37.9   Congenital infectious or parasitic disease, unspecified

● **P38   Omphalitis of newborn**
    Inflammation of umbilicus
    Excludes1 omphalitis not of newborn (L08.82)
      tetanus omphalitis (A33)
      umbilical hemorrhage of newborn (P51.-)
P38.1   Omphalitis with mild hemorrhage
P38.9   Omphalitis without hemorrhage
    Omphalitis of newborn NOS

● **P39   Other infections specific to the perinatal period**
    Use additional code to identify organism or specific infection
P39.0   Neonatal infective mastitis
    Excludes1 breast engorgement of newborn (P83.4)
      noninfective mastitis of newborn (P83.4)
P39.1   Neonatal conjunctivitis and dacryocystitis
    Neonatal chlamydial conjunctivitis
    Ophthalmia neonatorum NOS
    Neonate = newborn
    Excludes1 gonococcal conjunctivitis (A54.31)
P39.2   Intra-amniotic infection affecting newborn, not elsewhere classified
P39.3   Neonatal urinary tract infection
P39.4   Neonatal skin infection
    Neonatal pyoderma
    Excludes1 pemphigus neonatorum (L00)
      staphylococcal scalded skin syndrome (L00)
P39.8   Other specified infections specific to the perinatal period
P39.9   Infection specific to the perinatal period, unspecified

▶ New ➡ Revised ~~deleted~~ Deleted Excludes 1 Excludes 2 Includes Use additional Code first Code also Key words
OGCR Official Guidelines X Assign placeholder X ● Use Additional Character(s) ▶ Manifestation Code 🅗 Hierarchical Condition Category Coding Clinic

HEMORRHAGIC AND HEMATOLOGICAL DISORDERS OF NEWBORN (P50-P61)

> **Excludes1**   congenital stenosis and stricture of bile ducts (Q44.3)
> Crigler-Najjar syndrome (E80.5)
> Dubin-Johnson syndrome (E80.6)
> Gilbert syndrome (E80.4)
> hereditary hemolytic anemias (D55-D58)

● **P50   Newborn affected by intrauterine (fetal) blood loss**

> **Excludes1**   congenital anemia from intrauterine (fetal) blood loss (P61.3)

P50.0   Newborn affected by intrauterine (fetal) blood loss from vasa previa

P50.1   Newborn affected by intrauterine (fetal) blood loss from ruptured cord

P50.2   Newborn affected by intrauterine (fetal) blood loss from placenta

P50.3   Newborn affected by hemorrhage into co-twin

P50.4   Newborn affected by hemorrhage into maternal circulation

P50.5   Newborn affected by intrauterine (fetal) blood loss from cut end of co-twin's cord

P50.8   Newborn affected by other intrauterine (fetal) blood loss

P50.9   Newborn affected by intrauterine (fetal) blood loss, unspecified
Newborn affected by fetal hemorrhage NOS

● **P51   Umbilical hemorrhage of newborn**

> **Excludes1**   omphalitis with mild hemorrhage (P38.1)
> umbilical hemorrhage from cut end of co-twins cord (P50.5)

P51.0   Massive umbilical hemorrhage of newborn

P51.8   Other umbilical hemorrhages of newborn
Slipped umbilical ligature NOS

P51.9   Umbilical hemorrhage of newborn, unspecified

● **P52   Intracranial nontraumatic hemorrhage of newborn**

> **Includes**   intracranial hemorrhage due to anoxia or hypoxia
> **Excludes1**   intracranial hemorrhage due to birth injury (P10.-)
> intracranial hemorrhage due to other injury (S06.-)

P52.0   Intraventricular (nontraumatic) hemorrhage, grade 1, of newborn
Subependymal hemorrhage (without intraventricular extension)
Bleeding into germinal matrix

P52.1   Intraventricular (nontraumatic) hemorrhage, grade 2, of newborn
Subependymal hemorrhage with intraventricular extension
Bleeding into ventricle

● **P52.2   Intraventricular (nontraumatic) hemorrhage, grade 3 and grade 4, of newborn**

P52.21   Intraventricular (nontraumatic) hemorrhage, grade 3, of newborn
Subependymal hemorrhage with intraventricular extension with enlargement of ventricle

P52.22   Intraventricular (nontraumatic) hemorrhage, grade 4, of newborn
Bleeding into cerebral cortex
Subependymal hemorrhage with intracerebral extension

P52.3   Unspecified intraventricular (nontraumatic) hemorrhage of newborn

P52.4   Intracerebral (nontraumatic) hemorrhage of newborn

P52.5   Subarachnoid (nontraumatic) hemorrhage of newborn

P52.6   Cerebellar (nontraumatic) and posterior fossa hemorrhage of newborn

P52.8   Other intracranial (nontraumatic) hemorrhages of newborn

P52.9   Intracranial (nontraumatic) hemorrhage of newborn, unspecified

P53   Hemorrhagic disease of newborn
Vitamin K deficiency of newborn

● **P54   Other neonatal hemorrhages**

> **Excludes1**   newborn affected by (intrauterine) blood loss (P50.-)
> pulmonary hemorrhage originating in the perinatal period (P26.-)

P54.0   Neonatal hematemesis
Vomiting of blood

> **Excludes1**   neonatal hematemesis due to swallowed maternal blood (P78.2)

P54.1   Neonatal melena
Dark-colored feces stained with blood pigments

> **Excludes1**   neonatal melena due to swallowed maternal blood (P78.2)

P54.2   Neonatal rectal hemorrhage

P54.3   Other neonatal gastrointestinal hemorrhage

P54.4   Neonatal adrenal hemorrhage

P54.5   Neonatal cutaneous hemorrhage
Neonatal bruising
Neonatal ecchymoses
Neonatal petechiae
Neonatal superficial hematomata

> **Excludes2**   bruising of scalp due to birth injury (P12.3)
> cephalhematoma due to birth injury (P12.0)

P54.6   Neonatal vaginal hemorrhage
Neonatal pseudomenses

P54.8   Other specified neonatal hemorrhages

P54.9   Neonatal hemorrhage, unspecified

● **P55   Hemolytic disease of newborn**
AKA erythroblastosis fetalis and is due to Rh isoimmunization, result of Rh blood factor incompatibilities between mother (Rh negative) and fetus (Rh positive)

P55.0   Rh isoimmunization of newborn

P55.1   ABO isoimmunization of newborn
Coding Clinic: 2015, Q3, P20

P55.8   Other hemolytic diseases of newborn

P55.9   Hemolytic disease of newborn, unspecified

● **P56   Hydrops fetalis due to hemolytic disease**
Caused by maternal sensitization to fetal blood group antigen

> **Excludes1**   hydrops fetalis NOS (P83.2)

P56.0   Hydrops fetalis due to isoimmunization

● **P56.9   Hydrops fetalis due to other and unspecified hemolytic disease**

P56.90   Hydrops fetalis due to unspecified hemolytic disease

P56.99   Hydrops fetalis due to other hemolytic disease

● **P57   Kernicterus**
High levels of bilirubin in blood, with severe neural symptoms

P57.0   Kernicterus due to isoimmunization

P57.8   Other specified kernicterus

> **Excludes1**   Crigler-Najjar syndrome (E80.5)

P57.9   Kernicterus, unspecified

● **P58   Neonatal jaundice due to other excessive hemolysis**

> **Excludes1**   jaundice due to isoimmunization (P55-P57)

P58.0   Neonatal jaundice due to bruising

P58.1   Neonatal jaundice due to bleeding

P58.2   Neonatal jaundice due to infection

P58.3   Neonatal jaundice due to polycythemia

CHAPTER 16 (P00-P96)

CHAPTER 16 (P00–P96)

● P58.4   Neonatal jaundice due to drugs or toxins transmitted from mother or given to newborn

Code first poisoning due to drug or toxin, if applicable (T36-T65 with fifth or sixth character 1-4)

Use additional code for adverse effect, if applicable, to identify drug (T36-T50 with fifth or sixth character 5)

   P58.41   Neonatal jaundice due to drugs or toxins transmitted from mother
   P58.42   Neonatal jaundice due to drugs or toxins given to newborn

P58.5   Neonatal jaundice due to swallowed maternal blood
P58.8   Neonatal jaundice due to other specified excessive hemolysis
P58.9   Neonatal jaundice due to excessive hemolysis, unspecified

● P59   Neonatal jaundice from other and unspecified causes

   Excludes1   jaundice due to inborn errors of metabolism (E70-E88)
                kernicterus (P57.-)

P59.0   Neonatal jaundice associated with preterm delivery
         Hyperbilirubinemia of prematurity
         Jaundice due to delayed conjugation associated with preterm delivery

P59.1   Inspissated bile syndrome
● P59.2   Neonatal jaundice from other and unspecified hepatocellular damage

      Excludes1   congenital viral hepatitis (P35.3)

   P59.20   Neonatal jaundice from unspecified hepatocellular damage
   P59.29   Neonatal jaundice from other hepatocellular damage
             Neonatal giant cell hepatitis
             Neonatal (idiopathic) hepatitis

P59.3   Neonatal jaundice from breast milk inhibitor
P59.8   Neonatal jaundice from other specified causes
P59.9   Neonatal jaundice, unspecified
         Neonatal physiological jaundice (intense)(prolonged) NOS
         Coding Clinic: 2015, Q3, P20

P60   Disseminated intravascular coagulation of newborn
       Defibrination syndrome of newborn

● P61   Other perinatal hematological disorders

   Excludes1   transient hypogammaglobulinemia of infancy (D80.7)

P61.0   Transient neonatal thrombocytopenia
         Lack of sufficient numbers of circulating throm bocytes (platelets)
         Neonatal thrombocytopenia due to exchange transfusion
         Neonatal thrombocytopenia due to idiopathic maternal thrombocytopenia
         Neonatal thrombocytopenia due to isoimmunization

P61.1   Polycythemia neonatorum
         Neonate = newborn

P61.2   Anemia of prematurity
P61.3   Congenital anemia from fetal blood loss
P61.4   Other congenital anemias, not elsewhere classified
         Congenital anemia NOS

P61.5   Transient neonatal neutropenia
         Low levels of granulocytic neutrophilic white blood cells

      Excludes1   congenital neutropenia (nontransient) (D70.0)

P61.6   Other transient neonatal disorders of coagulation
P61.8   Other specified perinatal hematological disorders
P61.9   Perinatal hematological disorder, unspecified

TRANSITORY ENDOCRINE AND METABOLIC DISORDERS SPECIFIC TO NEWBORN (P70-P74)

   Includes   transitory endocrine and metabolic disturbances caused by the infant's response to maternal endocrine and metabolic factors, or its adjustment to extrauterine environment

● P70   Transitory disorders of carbohydrate metabolism specific to newborn

P70.0   Syndrome of infant of mother with gestational diabetes
         Newborn (with hypoglycemia) affected by maternal gestational diabetes

      Excludes1   newborn (with hypoglycemia) affected by maternal (pre-existing) diabetes mellitus (P70.1)
                   syndrome of infant of a diabetic mother (P70.1)

P70.1   Syndrome of infant of a diabetic mother
         Newborn (with hypoglycemia) affected by maternal (pre-existing) diabetes mellitus

      Excludes1   newborn (with hypoglycemia) affected by maternal gestational diabetes (P70.0)
                   syndrome of infant of mother with gestational diabetes (P70.0)

P70.2   Neonatal diabetes mellitus
P70.3   Iatrogenic neonatal hypoglycemia
P70.4   Other neonatal hypoglycemia
         Transitory neonatal hypoglycemia
P70.8   Other transitory disorders of carbohydrate metabolism of newborn
P70.9   Transitory disorder of carbohydrate metabolism of newborn, unspecified

● P71   Transitory neonatal disorders of calcium and magnesium metabolism

P71.0   Cow's milk hypocalcemia in newborn
P71.1   Other neonatal hypocalcemia

      Excludes1   neonatal hypoparathyroidism (P71.4)

P71.2   Neonatal hypomagnesemia
P71.3   Neonatal tetany without calcium or magnesium deficiency
         Neonatal tetany NOS
P71.4   Transitory neonatal hypoparathyroidism
P71.8   Other transitory neonatal disorders of calcium and magnesium metabolism
         Coding Clinic: 2016, Q4, P55
P71.9   Transitory neonatal disorder of calcium and magnesium metabolism, unspecified

● P72   Other transitory neonatal endocrine disorders

   Excludes1   congenital hypothyroidism with or without goiter (E03.0-E03.1)
                dyshormogenetic goiter (E07.1)
                Pendred's syndrome (E07.1)

P72.0   Neonatal goiter, not elsewhere classified
         Transitory congenital goiter with normal functioning
P72.1   Transitory neonatal hyperthyroidism
         Neonatal thyrotoxicosis
P72.2   Other transitory neonatal disorders of thyroid function, not elsewhere classified
         Transitory neonatal hypothyroidism
P72.8   Other specified transitory neonatal endocrine disorders
P72.9   Transitory neonatal endocrine disorder, unspecified

● P74   Other transitory neonatal electrolyte and metabolic disturbances

P74.0   Late metabolic acidosis of newborn

      Excludes1   (fetal) metabolic acidosis of newborn (P19)

P74.1   Dehydration of newborn

▶ New   ⇒ Revised   ~~deleted~~ Deleted   Excludes 1   Excludes 2   Includes   Use additional   Code first   Code also   Key words

OGCR Official Guidelines   X Assign placeholder X   ● Use Additional Character(s)   ▶ Manifestation Code   🅗 Hierarchical Condition Category   Coding Clinic

● **P74.2** **Disturbances of sodium balance of newborn**
Coding Clinic: 2018, Q2, P6
     P74.21 Hypernatremia of newborn
     P74.22 Hyponatremia of newborn
● **P74.3** **Disturbances of potassium balance of newborn**
     P74.31 Hyperkalemia of newborn
     P74.32 Hypokalemia of newborn
● **P74.4** **Other transitory electrolyte disturbances of newborn**
     P74.41 **Alkalosis of newborn**
          Hyperbicarbonatemia
     ● **P74.42** **Disturbances of chlorine balance of newborn**
          P74.421 **Hyperchloremia of newborn**
              Hyperchloremic metabolic acidosis
                 Excludes2 late metabolic acidosis of the newborn (P74.0)
          P74.422 **Hypochloremia of newborn**
     P74.49 **Other transitory electrolyte disturbance of newborn**
● **P74.5** **Transitory tyrosinemia of newborn**
● **P74.6** **Transitory hyperammonemia of newborn**
● **P74.8** **Other transitory metabolic disturbances of newborn**
     Amino-acid metabolic disorders described as transitory
● **P74.9** **Transitory metabolic disturbance of newborn, unspecified**

DIGESTIVE SYSTEM DISORDERS OF NEWBORN (P76-P78)

● **P76** **Other intestinal obstruction of newborn**
     P76.0 **Meconium plug syndrome**
          Fetal stool obstruction in large intestine, present at birth; may be symptom of organic disease.
          Meconium ileus NOS
          Excludes1 meconium ileus in cystic fibrosis (E84.11)
     P76.1 **Transitory ileus of newborn**
          Temporary obstruction of ileus (small intestine)
          Excludes1 Hirschsprung's disease (Q43.1)
     P76.2 **Intestinal obstruction due to inspissated milk**
          Being thickened, dried, or made less fluid
     P76.8 **Other specified intestinal obstruction of newborn**
          Excludes1 intestinal obstruction classifiable to K56.-
     P76.9 **Intestinal obstruction of newborn, unspecified**
● **P77** **Necrotizing enterocolitis of newborn**
     P77.1 **Stage 1 necrotizing enterocolitis in newborn**
          Necrotizing enterocolitis without pneumatosis, without perforation
     P77.2 **Stage 2 necrotizing enterocolitis in newborn**
          Necrotizing enterocolitis with pneumatosis, without perforation
     P77.3 **Stage 3 necrotizing enterocolitis in newborn**
          Necrotizing enterocolitis with perforation
          Necrotizing enterocolitis with pneumatosis and perforation
     P77.9 **Necrotizing enterocolitis in newborn, unspecified**
          Necrotizing enterocolitis in newborn, NOS
● **P78** **Other perinatal digestive system disorders**
     Excludes1 cystic fibrosis (E84.0-E84.9)
          neonatal gastrointestinal hemorrhages (P54.0-P54.3)
     P78.0 **Perinatal intestinal perforation**
          Meconium peritonitis
     P78.1 **Other neonatal peritonitis**
          Neonatal peritonitis NOS
     P78.2 **Neonatal hematemesis and melena due to swallowed maternal blood**
     P78.3 **Noninfective neonatal diarrhea**
          Neonatal diarrhea NOS

● **P78.8** **Other specified perinatal digestive system disorders**
     P78.81 **Congenital cirrhosis (of liver)**
     P78.82 **Peptic ulcer of newborn**
     P78.83 **Newborn esophageal reflux**
          Neonatal esophageal reflux
     P78.84 **Gestational alloimmune liver disease**
          GALD
          Neonatal hemochromatosis
          Excludes1 hemochromatosis (E83.11-)
     P78.89 **Other specified perinatal digestive system disorders**
     P78.9 **Perinatal digestive system disorder, unspecified**

CONDITIONS INVOLVING THE INTEGUMENT AND TEMPERATURE REGULATION OF NEWBORN (P80-P83)

● **P80** **Hypothermia of newborn**
     P80.0 **Cold injury syndrome**
          Severe and usually chronic hypothermia associated with a pink flushed appearance, edema and neurological and biochemical abnormalities.
          Excludes1 mild hypothermia of newborn (P80.8)
     P80.8 **Other hypothermia of newborn**
          Mild hypothermia of newborn
     P80.9 **Hypothermia of newborn, unspecified**
● **P81** **Other disturbances of temperature regulation of newborn**
     P81.0 **Environmental hyperthermia of newborn**
     P81.8 **Other specified disturbances of temperature regulation of newborn**
     P81.9 **Disturbance of temperature regulation of newborn, unspecified**
          Fever of newborn NOS
● **P83** **Other conditions of integument specific to newborn**
     Excludes1 congenital malformations of skin and integument (Q80-Q84)
          hydrops fetalis due to hemolytic disease (P56.-)
          neonatal skin infection (P39.4)
          staphylococcal scalded skin syndrome (L00)
     Excludes2 cradle cap (L21.0)
          diaper [napkin] dermatitis (L22)
     P83.0 **Sclerema neonatorum**
          Neonate = newborn
     P83.1 **Neonatal erythema toxicum**
          Benign, generalized, transient pustules that become firm vesicles
     P83.2 **Hydrops fetalis not due to hemolytic disease**
          Severe, life-threatening problem of severe edema (swelling) as a result of too much fluid leaving blood and entering tissue
          Hydrops fetalis NOS
     ● **P83.3** **Other and unspecified edema specific to newborn**
          P83.30 **Unspecified edema specific to newborn**
          P83.39 **Other edema specific to newborn**
     P83.4 **Breast engorgement of newborn**
          Noninfective mastitis of newborn
     P83.5 **Congenital hydrocele**
     P83.6 **Umbilical polyp of newborn**
     ● **P83.8** **Other specified conditions of integument specific to newborn**
          P83.81 **Umbilical granuloma**
              Excludes2 Granulomatous disorder of the skin and subcutaneous tissue, unspecified (L92.9)
          P83.88 **Other specified conditions of integument specific to newborn**
              Bronze baby syndrome
              Neonatal scleroderma
              Urticaria neonatorum
     P83.9 **Condition of the integument specific to newborn, unspecified**

CHAPTER 16 (P00-P96)

OTHER PROBLEMS WITH NEWBORN (P84)

P84   Other problems with newborn
       Acidemia of newborn
       Acidosis of newborn
       Anoxia of newborn NOS
       Asphyxia of newborn NOS
       Hypercapnia of newborn
       Hypoxemia of newborn
       Hypoxia of newborn NOS
       Mixed metabolic and respiratory acidosis of newborn

> **Excludes1**   intracranial hemorrhage due to anoxia or hypoxia
>   (P52.-)
>   hypoxic ischemic encephalopathy [HIE] (P91.6-)
>   late metabolic acidosis of newborn (P74.0)

OTHER DISORDERS ORIGINATING IN THE PERINATAL PERIOD (P90-P96)

P90   Convulsions of newborn

> **Excludes1**   benign myoclonic epilepsy in infancy (G40.3-)
>   benign neonatal convulsions (familial) (G40.3-)

● P91   Other disturbances of cerebral status of newborn

    P91.0   Neonatal cerebral ischemia

    > **Excludes1**   Neonatal cerebral infarction (P91.82-)

    P91.1   Acquired periventricular cysts of newborn

    P91.2   Neonatal cerebral leukomalacia
             Degeneration of white matter adjacent to cerebral ventricles
             following cerebral hypoxia or brain ischemia in neonates
             Periventricular leukomalacia

    P91.3   Neonatal cerebral irritability

    P91.4   Neonatal cerebral depression

    P91.5   Neonatal coma

  ● P91.6   Hypoxic ischemic encephalopathy [HIE]

    > **Excludes1**   Neonatal cerebral depression (P91.4)
    >   Neonatal cerebral irritability (P91.3)
    >   Neonatal coma (P91.5)

       P91.60   Hypoxic ischemic encephalopathy [HIE],
                 unspecified

       P91.61   Mild hypoxic ischemic encephalopathy
                 [HIE]

       P91.62   Moderate hypoxic ischemic encephalopathy
                 [HIE]

       P91.63   Severe hypoxic ischemic encephalopathy [HIE]

  ● P91.8   Other specified disturbances of cerebral status of newborn

    ● P91.81   Neonatal encephalopathy

       ▷ *P91.811   Neonatal encephalopathy in diseases*
         classified elsewhere
             Code first underlying condition, if known,
                such as:
                congenital cirrhosis (of liver) (P78.81)
                intracranial nontraumatic
                   hemorrhage of newborn (P52.-)
                kernicterus (P57.-)

       P91.819   Neonatal encephalopathy, unspecified

    ● P91.82   Neonatal cerebral infarction
             Neonatal stroke
             Perinatal arterial ischemic stroke
             Perinatal cerebral infarction

       > **Excludes1**   cerebral infarction (I63.-)

       > **Excludes2**   intracranial hemorrhage of
       >   newborn (P52.-)

       P91.821   Neonatal cerebral infarction, right
                  side of brain

       P91.822   Neonatal cerebral infarction, left side
                  of brain

       P91.823   Neonatal cerebral infarction, bilateral

       P91.829   Neonatal cerebral infarction,
                  unspecified side

       P91.88   Other specified disturbances of cerebral status
                 of newborn

    P91.9   Disturbance of cerebral status of newborn, unspecified

● P92   Feeding problems of newborn

> **Excludes2**   feeding problems in child over 28 days old
>   (R63.3-)

Coding Clinic: 2017, Q1, P28; 2016, Q3, P19

  ● P92.0   Vomiting of newborn

    > **Excludes1**   vomiting of child over 28 days old (R11.-)

       P92.01   Bilious vomiting of newborn

       > **Excludes1**   bilious vomiting in child over
       >   28 days old (R11.14)

       P92.09   Other vomiting of newborn

       > **Excludes1**   regurgitation of food in newborn
       >   (P92.1)

    P92.1   Regurgitation and rumination of newborn

    P92.2   Slow feeding of newborn

    P92.3   Underfeeding of newborn

    P92.4   Overfeeding of newborn

    P92.5   Neonatal difficulty in feeding at breast
             Coding Clinic: 2017, Q1, P28; 2016, Q3, P19

    P92.6   Failure to thrive in newborn

       > **Excludes1**   failure to thrive in child over 28 days old
       >   (R62.51)

    P92.8   Other feeding problems of newborn

    P92.9   Feeding problem of newborn, unspecified

● P93   Reactions and intoxications due to drugs administered to
         newborn

> **Includes**   reactions and intoxications due to drugs
>   administered to fetus affecting newborn

> **Excludes1**   jaundice due to drugs or toxins transmitted from
>   mother or given to newborn (P58.4-)
>   reactions and intoxications from maternal
>   opiates, tranquilizers and other medication
>   (P04.0-P04.1, P04.4-)
>   withdrawal symptoms from maternal use of
>   drugs of addiction (P96.1)
>   withdrawal symptoms from therapeutic use of
>   drugs in newborn (P96.2)

    P93.0   Grey baby syndrome
             Grey syndrome from chloramphenicol administration
             in newborn

    P93.8   Other reactions and intoxications due to drugs
             administered to newborn
             Use additional code for adverse effect, if applicable,
                to identify drug (T36-T50 with fifth or sixth
                character 5)

● P94   Disorders of muscle tone of newborn

    P94.0   Transient neonatal myasthenia gravis

       > **Excludes1**   myasthenia gravis (G70.0)

    P94.1   Congenital hypertonia

    P94.2   Congenital hypotonia
             Floppy baby syndrome, unspecified

    P94.8   Other disorders of muscle tone of newborn

    P94.9   Disorder of muscle tone of newborn, unspecified

OGCR Section I.C.16.g.

Stillbirth
Code P95, Stillbirth, is only for use for institutions that maintain
separate records for stillbirths. No other code should be used with P95.
Code P95 should not be used on the mother's record.

P95   Stillbirth
       Deadborn fetus NOS
       Fetal death of unspecified cause
       Stillbirth NOS

> **Excludes1**   maternal care for intrauterine death (O36.4)
>   missed abortion (O02.1)
>   outcome of delivery, stillbirth (Z37.1, Z37.3,
>   Z37.4, Z37.7)

▷ New   ⇒ Revised   ~~deleted~~ Deleted   Excludes 1   Excludes 2   Includes   Use additional   Code first   Code also   Key words

OGCR Official Guidelines   X Assign placeholder X   ● Use Additional Character(s)   ▷ Manifestation Code   🗞 Hierarchical Condition Category   **Coding Clinic**

● **P96**   **Other conditions originating in the perinatal period**

     P96.0   **Congenital renal failure**
             Uremia of newborn

     P96.1   **Neonatal withdrawal symptoms from maternal use of drugs of addiction**
             Drug withdrawal syndrome in infant of dependent mother
             Neonatal abstinence syndrome

             Excludes1   reactions and intoxications from maternal opiates and tranquilizers administered during labor and delivery (P04.0)

     P96.2   **Withdrawal symptoms from therapeutic use of drugs in newborn**

     P96.3   **Wide cranial sutures of newborn**
             Neonatal craniotabes

     P96.5   **Complication to newborn due to (fetal) intrauterine procedure**

             Excludes2   newborn affected by amniocentesis (P00.6)

● **P96.8**   **Other specified conditions originating in the perinatal period**

     P96.81   **Exposure to (parental) (environmental) tobacco smoke in the perinatal period**

             Excludes2   newborn affected by in utero exposure to tobacco (P04.2)
                             exposure to environmental tobacco smoke after the perinatal period (Z77.22)

     P96.82   **Delayed separation of umbilical cord**

     P96.83   **Meconium staining**

             Excludes1   meconium aspiration (P24.00, P24.01)
                             meconium passage during delivery (P03.82)

     P96.89   **Other specified conditions originating in the perinatal period**
             Use additional code to specify condition

     P96.9   **Condition originating in the perinatal period, unspecified**
             Congenital debility NOS

CHAPTER 17

CONGENITAL MALFORMATIONS, DEFORMATIONS, AND CHROMOSOMAL ABNORMALITIES (Q00-Q99)

OGCR Chapter-Specific Coding Guidelines

17. Chapter 17: Congenital malformations, deformations, and chromosomal abnormalities (Q00-Q99)
Assign an appropriate code(s) from categories Q00-Q99, Congenital malformations, deformations, and chromosomal abnormalities when a malformation/deformation or chromosomal abnormality is documented. A malformation/deformation/ or chromosomal abnormality may be the principal/first-listed diagnosis on a record or a secondary diagnosis.
When a malformation/deformation/or chromosomal abnormality does not have a unique code assignment, assign additional code(s) for any manifestations that may be present.
When the code assignment specifically identifies the malformation/deformation/or chromosomal abnormality, manifestations that are an inherent component of the anomaly should not be coded separately. Additional codes should be assigned for manifestations that are not an inherent component.
Codes from Chapter 17 may be used throughout the life of the patient. If a congenital malformation or deformity has been corrected, a personal history code should be used to identify the history of the malformation or deformity. Although present at birth, malformation/deformation/or chromosomal abnormality may not be identified until later in life. Whenever the condition is diagnosed by the physician, it is appropriate to assign a code from codes Q00-Q99.
For the birth admission, the appropriate code from category Z38, Liveborn infants, according to place of birth and type of delivery, should be sequenced as the principal diagnosis, followed by any congenital anomaly codes, Q00-Q99.

CHAPTER 17

CONGENITAL MALFORMATIONS, DEFORMATIONS, AND CHROMOSOMAL ABNORMALITIES (Q00-Q99)

Note: Codes from this chapter are not for use on maternal records

Excludes2 inborn errors of metabolism (E70-E88)

This chapter contains the following blocks:

Q00-Q07	Congenital malformations of the nervous system
Q10-Q18	Congenital malformations of eye, ear, face and neck
Q20-Q28	Congenital malformations of the circulatory system
Q30-Q34	Congenital malformations of the respiratory system
Q35-Q37	Cleft lip and cleft palate
Q38-Q45	Other congenital malformations of the digestive system
Q50-Q56	Congenital malformations of genital organs
Q60-Q64	Congenital malformations of the urinary system
Q65-Q79	Congenital malformations and deformations of the musculoskeletal system
Q80-Q89	Other congenital malformations
Q90-Q99	Chromosomal abnormalities, not elsewhere classified

Figure 17-1 An infant with a large occipital encephalocele. The large skin-covered encephalocele is visible. (From Swaiman KF, Ashwal S, Ferriero DM: Pediatric Neurology: Principles and Practice, Philadelphia, Saunders, 2012)

CONGENITAL MALFORMATIONS OF THE NERVOUS SYSTEM (Q00–Q07)

● **Q00 Anencephaly and similar malformations**
    Q00.0 Anencephaly 🐾
        Absence of skull with cerebral hemispheres missing or reduced to small masses attached to base of cranium
        Acephaly
        Acrania
        Amyelencephaly
        Hemianencephaly
        Hemicephaly

    Q00.1 Craniorachischisis 🐾
        Developmental anomaly consisting of fissure of cranium and vertebral column

    Q00.2 Iniencephaly 🐾
        Developmental anomaly characterized by enlargement of foramen magnum and absence of laminae and spinous processes of cervical, dorsal

● **Q01 Encephalocele**
    Sac-like protrusions of brain and membranes visible through an opening in skull

Includes	Arnold-Chiari syndrome, type III
	encephalocystocele
	encephalomyelocele
	hydroencephalocele
	hydromeningocele, cranial
	meningocele, cerebral
	meningoencephalocele

Excludes1	Meckel-Gruber syndrome (Q61.9)

    Q01.0 Frontal encephalocele 🐾
    Q01.1 Nasofrontal encephalocele 🐾
    Q01.2 Occipital encephalocele 🐾
    Q01.8 Encephalocele of other sites 🐾
    Q01.9 Encephalocele, unspecified 🐾

Q02 Microcephaly 🐾
    Head size measures significantly below normal based on standardized charts

Includes	hydromicrocephaly
	micrencephalon

Code first, if applicable, congenital Zika virus disease

Excludes1	Meckel-Gruber syndrome (Q61.9)

Coding Clinic: 2018, Q4, P26; 2016, Q4, P7

● **Q03 Congenital hydrocephalus**
    Accumulation of cerebrospinal fluid in ventricles resulting in swelling and enlargement

Includes	hydrocephalus in newborn
Excludes1	Arnold-Chiari syndrome, type II (Q07.0-)
	acquired hydrocephalus (G91.-)
	hydrocephalus due to congenital toxoplasmosis (P37.1)
	hydrocephalus with spina bifida (Q05.0-Q05.4)

    Q03.0 Malformations of aqueduct of Sylvius 🐾
        Anomaly of aqueduct of Sylvius
        Obstruction of aqueduct of Sylvius, congenital
        Stenosis of aqueduct of Sylvius

    Q03.1 Atresia of foramina of Magendie and Luschka 🐾
        Dandy-Walker syndrome

    Q03.8 Other congenital hydrocephalus 🐾

    Q03.9 Congenital hydrocephalus, unspecified 🐾

● **Q04 Other congenital malformations of brain**

Excludes1	cyclopia (Q87.0)
	macrocephaly (Q75.3)

▶ New   ⬛ Revised   ~~deleted~~ Deleted   Excludes 1   Excludes 2   Includes   Use additional   Code first   Code also   Key words
OGCR Official Guidelines   X Assign placeholder X   ● Use Additional Character(s)   ▶ Manifestation Code   🐾 Hierarchical Condition Category   **Coding Clinic**

Q04.0 Congenital malformations of corpus callosum 🔍
Agenesis of corpus callosum

Q04.1 Arhinencephaly 🔍
Congenital absence of olfactory bulbs, tract, or nerves

Q04.2 Holoprosencephaly 🔍
Failure of cleavage of forebrain (prosencephalon) resulting in incomplete or absent cortical separation and deficits in midline facial development

Q04.3 Other reduction deformities of brain 🔍
Absence of part of brain
Agenesis of part of brain
Cerebral cortex are not fully formed, brain surface is smooth
Agyria
Aplasia of part of brain
Hydranencephaly
Hypoplasia of part of brain
Lissencephaly
Congenital malformation or absence of convolutions of cerebral cortex
Microgyria
Malformation of brain characterized by excessive number of small convolutions (gyri) on surface
Pachygyria
Reduction in number of sulci of cerebrum
> **Excludes1**   congenital malformations of corpus callosum (Q04.0)

Q04.4 Septo-optic dysplasia of brain 🔍

Q04.5 Megalencephaly 🔍
Abnormally large brain

Q04.6 Congenital cerebral cysts 🔍
Porencephaly   Schizencephaly
> **Excludes1**   acquired porencephalic cyst (G93.0)

Q04.8 Other specified congenital malformations of brain 🔍
Arnold-Chiari syndrome, type IV
Macrogyria

Q04.9 Congenital malformation of brain, unspecified 🔍
Congenital anomaly NOS of brain
Congenital deformity NOS of brain
Congenital disease or lesion NOS of brain
Multiple anomalies NOS of brain, congenital

● **Q05   Spina bifida**
Developmental anomaly characterized by defective closure of vertebral arch, through which spinal cord and meninges may protrude
> **Includes**   hydromeningocele (spinal)
> meningocele (spinal)
> meningomyelocele
> myelocele
> myelomeningocele
> rachischisis
> spina bifida (aperta)(cystica)
> syringomyelocele

Use additional code for any associated paraplegia (paraparesis) (G82.2-)
> **Excludes1**   Arnold-Chiari syndrome, type II (Q07.0-)
> spina bifida occulta (Q76.0)

Q05.0 Cervical spina bifida with hydrocephalus 🔍

Q05.1 Thoracic spina bifida with hydrocephalus 🔍
Dorsal spina bifida with hydrocephalus
Thoracolumbar spina bifida with hydrocephalus

Q05.2 Lumbar spina bifida with hydrocephalus 🔍
Lumbosacral spina bifida with hydrocephalus

Q05.3 Sacral spina bifida with hydrocephalus 🔍

Q05.4 Unspecified spina bifida with hydrocephalus 🔍

Q05.5 Cervical spina bifida without hydrocephalus 🔍

Q05.6 Thoracic spina bifida without hydrocephalus 🔍
Dorsal spina bifida NOS
Thoracolumbar spina bifida NOS

Q05.7 Lumbar spina bifida without hydrocephalus 🔍
Lumbosacral spina bifida NOS

Q05.8 Sacral spina bifida without hydrocephalus 🔍

Q05.9 Spina bifida, unspecified 🔍

● **Q06   Other congenital malformations of spinal cord**

Q06.0 Amyelia 🔍
Congenital absence of spinal cord

Q06.1 Hypoplasia and dysplasia of spinal cord 🔍
Underdevelopment of spinal cord
Atelomyelia
Congenitally incomplete development of spinal cord
Myelatelia
Myelodysplasia of spinal cord
Defective development of spinal cord, especially lower segments

Q06.2 Diastematomyelia 🔍
Congenital anomaly, associated with spina bifida, in which spinal cord is split into halves and surrounded by dural sac

Q06.3 Other congenital cauda equina malformations 🔍

Q06.4 Hydromyelia 🔍
Dilation of central canal of spinal cord with increased fluid accumulation
Hydrorachis

Q06.8 Other specified congenital malformations of spinal cord 🔍

Q06.9 Congenital malformation of spinal cord, unspecified 🔍
Congenital anomaly NOS of spinal cord
Congenital deformity NOS of spinal cord
Congenital disease or lesion NOS of spinal cord

● **Q07   Other congenital malformations of nervous system**
> **Excludes2**   congenital central alveolar hypoventilation syndrome (G47.35)
> familial dysautonomia [Riley-Day] (G90.1)
> neurofibromatosis (nonmalignant) (Q85.0-)

● **Q07.0 Arnold-Chiari syndrome**
Herniation of cerebellar tonsils and vermis through foramen magnum into spinal canal
Arnold-Chiari syndrome, type II
> **Excludes1**   Arnold-Chiari syndrome, type III (Q01.-)
> Arnold-Chiari syndrome, type IV (Q04.8)

Q07.00 Arnold-Chiari syndrome without spina bifida or hydrocephalus 🔍

Q07.01 Arnold-Chiari syndrome with spina bifida 🔍

Q07.02 Arnold-Chiari syndrome with hydrocephalus 🔍

Q07.03 Arnold-Chiari syndrome with spina bifida and hydrocephalus 🔍

Q07.8 Other specified congenital malformations of nervous system 🔍
Agenesis of nerve
Displacement of brachial plexus
Jaw-winking syndrome
Marcus Gunn's syndrome

Q07.9 Congenital malformation of nervous system, unspecified 🔍
Congenital anomaly NOS of nervous system
Congenital deformity NOS of nervous system
Congenital disease or lesion NOS of nervous system

CONGENITAL MALFORMATIONS OF EYE, EAR, FACE AND NECK (Q10-Q18)

> **Excludes2**   cleft lip and cleft palate (Q35-Q37)
> congenital malformation of cervical spine (Q05.0, Q05.5, Q67.5, Q76.0-Q76.4)
> congenital malformation of larynx (Q31.-)
> congenital malformation of lip NEC (Q38.0)
> congenital malformation of nose (Q30.-)
> congenital malformation of parathyroid gland (Q89.2)
> congenital malformation of thyroid gland (Q89.2)

● **Q10   Congenital malformations of eyelid, lacrimal apparatus and orbit**
> **Excludes1**   cryptophthalmos NOS (Q11.2)
> cryptophthalmos syndrome (Q87.0)

CHAPTER 17 (Q00-Q99)

Q10.0 Congenital ptosis
Prolapse or drooping of upper eyelid from paralysis of third nerve or from sympathetic innervations

Q10.1 Congenital ectropion
Outward turning of eyelid

Q10.2 Congenital entropion
Inward turning of eyelid

Q10.3 Other congenital malformations of eyelid
Ablepharon
Blepharophimosis, congenital
Coloboma of eyelid
Congenital absence or agenesis of cilia
Congenital absence or agenesis of eyelid
Congenital accessory eyelid
Congenital accessory eye muscle
Congenital malformation of eyelid NOS

Q10.4 Absence and agenesis of lacrimal apparatus
Congenital absence of punctum lacrimale

Q10.5 Congenital stenosis and stricture of lacrimal duct

Q10.6 Other congenital malformations of lacrimal apparatus
Congenital malformation of lacrimal apparatus NOS

Q10.7 Congenital malformation of orbit

● **Q11 Anophthalmos, microphthalmos and macrophthalmos**
Absence of eye and optic pit

Q11.0 Cystic eyeball

Q11.1 Other anophthalmos
Anophthalmos NOS
Agenesis of eye
Absence of eye
Aplasia of eye

Q11.2 Microphthalmos
Partial absence of eye and optic pit
Cryptophthalmos NOS
Dysplasia of eye
Hypoplasia of eye
Rudimentary eye
Excludes1 cryptophthalmos syndrome (Q87.0)

Q11.3 Macrophthalmos
Congenital enlargement of eyes
Excludes1 macrophthalmos in congenital glaucoma (Q15.0)

● **Q12 Congenital lens malformations**

Q12.0 Congenital cataract
Q12.1 Congenital displaced lens
Q12.2 Coloboma of lens
Q12.3 Congenital aphakia
Q12.4 Spherophakia
Smaller, more spherical optic lens than normal
Q12.8 Other congenital lens malformations
Microphakia
Q12.9 Congenital lens malformation, unspecified

● **Q13 Congenital malformations of anterior segment of eye**

Q13.0 Coloboma of iris
Coloboma NOS
Q13.1 Absence of iris
Aniridia
Use additional code for associated glaucoma (H42)
Q13.2 Other congenital malformations of iris
Anisocoria, congenital
Atresia of pupil
Congenital malformation of iris NOS
Corectopia
Q13.3 Congenital corneal opacity

Q13.4 Other congenital corneal malformations
Congenital malformation of cornea NOS
Microcornea
Peter's anomaly
Q13.5 Blue sclera
Condition of unusual blueness of sclera; not harmful
● **Q13.8 Other congenital malformations of anterior segment of eye**
▶ **Q13.81 Rieger anomaly**
▶Axenfeld-Rieger syndrome
▶Code also any other associated congenital malformations such as cardiac defects
Use additional code for associated glaucoma (H42)
Q13.89 Other congenital malformations of anterior segment of eye
Q13.9 Congenital malformation of anterior segment of eye, unspecified

● **Q14 Congenital malformations of posterior segment of eye**
Excludes2 optic nerve hypoplasia (H47.03-)
Q14.0 Congenital malformation of vitreous humor
Congenital vitreous opacity
Q14.1 Congenital malformation of retina
Congenital retinal aneurysm
Q14.2 Congenital malformation of optic disc
Coloboma of optic disc
Q14.3 Congenital malformation of choroid
Q14.8 Other congenital malformations of posterior segment of eye
Coloboma of the fundus
Q14.9 Congenital malformation of posterior segment of eye, unspecified

● **Q15 Other congenital malformations of eye**
Excludes1 congenital nystagmus (H55.01)
ocular albinism (E70.31-)
optic nerve hypoplasia (H47.03-)
retinitis pigmentosa (H35.52)
Q15.0 Congenital glaucoma
Axenfeld's anomaly
Buphthalmos
Congenital syndrome characterized by enlargement of the eye with symptoms of glaucoma.
Glaucoma of childhood
Glaucoma of newborn
Hydrophthalmos
Keratoglobus, congenital, with glaucoma
Macrocornea with glaucoma
Macrophthalmos in congenital glaucoma
Megalocornea with glaucoma
Q15.8 Other specified congenital malformations of eye
Q15.9 Congenital malformation of eye, unspecified
Congenital anomaly of eye
Congenital deformity of eye

● **Q16 Congenital malformations of ear causing impairment of hearing**
Excludes1 congenital deafness (H90.-)
Q16.0 Congenital absence of (ear) auricle
Q16.1 Congenital absence, atresia and stricture of auditory canal (external)
Congenital atresia or stricture of osseous meatus
Q16.2 Absence of eustachian tube
Q16.3 Congenital malformation of ear ossicles
Congenital fusion of ear ossicles
Q16.4 Other congenital malformations of middle ear
Congenital malformation of middle ear NOS
Q16.5 Congenital malformation of inner ear
Congenital anomaly of membranous labyrinth
Congenital anomaly of organ of Corti
Q16.9 Congenital malformation of ear causing impairment of hearing, unspecified
Congenital absence of ear NOS

Figure 17-2 Bilateral congenital **hydrophthalmia,** in which the eyes are very large in comparison to the other facial features due to glaucoma.

▶ New   ⇒ Revised   deleted Deleted   Excludes 1   Excludes 2   Includes   Use additional   Code first   Code also   Key words
OGCR Official Guidelines   X Assign placeholder X   ● Use Additional Character(s)   ▶ Manifestation Code   🗣 Hierarchical Condition Category   Coding Clinic

● **Q17 Other congenital malformations of ear**

    Excludes1   congenital malformations of ear with impairment
of hearing (Q16.0-Q16.9)

                  preauricular sinus (Q18.1)

    Q17.0 Accessory auricle
        Accessory tragus
        Polyotia
        Preauricular appendage or tag
        Supernumerary ear
        Supernumerary lobule

    Q17.1 Macrotia
        Enlarged ears

    Q17.2 Microtia
        An abnormally small or underdeveloped external ear

    Q17.3 Other misshapen ear
        Pointed ear

    Q17.4 Misplaced ear
        Low-set ears
        Excludes1   cervical auricle (Q18.2)

    Q17.5 Prominent ear
        Bat ear

    Q17.8 Other specified congenital malformations of ear
        Congenital absence of lobe of ear

    Q17.9 Congenital malformation of ear, unspecified
        Congenital anomaly of ear NOS

● **Q18 Other congenital malformations of face and neck**

    Excludes1   cleft lip and cleft palate (Q35-Q37)
                  conditions classified to Q67.0-Q67.4
                  congenital malformations of skull and face bones
(Q75.-)
                  cyclopia (Q87.0)
                  dentofacial anomalies [including malocclusion]
(M26.-)
                  malformation syndromes affecting facial
appearance (Q87.0)
                  persistent thyroglossal duct (Q89.2)

    Q18.0 Sinus, fistula and cyst of branchial cleft
        Branchial vestige
        *Branchial remnants (cysts, fistula, skin tags) that are
developmental anomalies*

    Q18.1 Preauricular sinus and cyst
        Fistula of auricle, congenital
        Cervicoaural fistula
        *Abnormal passage in neck originating from first branchial
cleft*

    Q18.2 Other branchial cleft malformations
        Branchial cleft malformation NOS
        Cervical auricle
        Otocephaly

    Q18.3 Webbing of neck
        Pterygium colli
        Thick fold of skin on side of neck

    Q18.4 Macrostomia
        *Results from failure of union of maxillary and mandibular
processes, results in abnormally large mouth*

    Q18.5 Microstomia

    Q18.6 Macrocheilia
        Excessive size of lips
        Hypertrophy of lip, congenital

    Q18.7 Microcheilia
        Abnormal smallness of lips

    Q18.8 Other specified congenital malformations of face and neck
        Medial cyst of face and neck
        Medial fistula of face and neck
        Medial sinus of face and neck

    Q18.9 Congenital malformation of face and neck, unspecified
        Congenital anomaly NOS of face and neck

CONGENITAL MALFORMATIONS OF THE CIRCULATORY SYSTEM (Q20-Q28)

● **Q20 Congenital malformations of cardiac chambers and connections**

    Excludes1   dextrocardia with situs inversus (Q89.3)
                  mirror-image atrial arrangement with situs
inversus (Q89.3)

    Q20.0 Common arterial trunk
        Persistent truncus arteriosus
        Excludes1   aortic septal defect (Q21.4)

    Q20.1 Double outlet right ventricle
        Taussig-Bing syndrome

    Q20.2 Double outlet left ventricle

    Q20.3 Discordant ventriculoarterial connection
        Dextrotransposition of aorta
        Transposition of great vessels (complete)

    Q20.4 Double inlet ventricle
        Common ventricle
        Cor triloculare biatriatum
        Single ventricle

    Q20.5 Discordant atrioventricular connection
        Corrected transposition
        Levotransposition
        Ventricular inversion

    Q20.6 Isomerism of atrial appendages
        Isomerism of atrial appendages with asplenia or
polysplenia

    Q20.8 Other congenital malformations of cardiac chambers and connections
        Cor binoculare

    Q20.9 Congenital malformation of cardiac chambers and connections, unspecified

● **Q21 Congenital malformations of cardiac septa**

    Excludes1   acquired cardiac septal defect (I51.0)

    Q21.0 Ventricular septal defect
        Roger's disease

    Q21.1 Atrial septal defect
        Excludes 2   ostium primum atrial septal defect
(type I) (Q21.20)

        Q21.10 Atrial septal defect, unspecified

        Q21.11 Secundum atrial septal defect
            Fenestrated atrial septum
            Patent or persistent ostium secundum defect
(type II)

        Q21.12 Patent foramen ovale
            Persistent foramen ovale

        Q21.13 Coronary sinus atrial septal defect
            Coronary sinus defect
            Unroofed coronary sinus

        Q21.14 Superior sinus venosus atrial septal defect
            Superior vena cava type atrial septal defect

        Q21.15 Inferior sinus venosus atrial septal defect
            Inferior vena cava type atrial septal defect

        Q21.16 Sinus venosus atrial septal defect, unspecified
            Sinus venosus defect, NOS

        Q21.19 Other specified atrial septal defect
            Common atrium
            Other specified atrial septal abnormality

    Q21.2 Atrioventricular septal defect
        Atrioventricular canal defect
        Endocardial cushion defect
        Ostium primum atrial septal defect (type I)

        Q21.20 Atrioventricular septal defect, unspecified as to partial or complete
            Atrioventricular canal, NOS
            Endocardial cushion defect NOS
            Ostium primum atrial septal defect (type I) NOS

CHAPTER 17 (Q00-Q99)

Q21.21　**Partial atrioventricular septal defect**
　　　Incomplete atrioventricular canal
　　　Incomplete atrioventricular septal defect
　　　Incomplete endocardial cushion defect
　　　Ostium primum atrial septal defect (type I)
　　　　with separate atrioventricular valves
　　　Partial atrioventricular canal
　　　Partial endocardial cushion defect

Q21.22　**Transitional atrioventricular septal defect**
　　　Intermediate atrioventricular canal
　　　Intermediate atrioventricular septal defect
　　　Intermediate endocardial cushion defect
　　　Ostium primum atrial septal defect (type I)
　　　　with separate atrioventricular valves and
　　　　a small or restrictive inlet VSD
　　　Transitional atrioventricular canal
　　　Transitional endocardial cushion defect

Q21.23　**Complete atrioventricular septal defect**
　　　Common atrioventricular canal
　　　Common atrioventricular septal defect
　　　Common endocardial cushion defect
　　　Ostium primum atrial septal defect (type I)
　　　　with common atrioventricular valve and a
　　　　moderate or larger inlet VSD

Q21.3　**Tetralogy of Fallot**
　　　Ventricular septal defect with pulmonary stenosis or
　　　atresia, dextroposition of aorta and hypertrophy of
　　　right ventricle.

Q21.4　**Aortopulmonary septal defect**
　　　Aortic septal defect
　　　Aortopulmonary window

Q21.8　**Other congenital malformations of cardiac septa**
　　　Eisenmenger's defect
　　　Pentalogy of Fallot
　　　Code also, if applicable:
　　　　Eisenmenger's complex (I27.83)
　　　　Eisenmenger's syndrome (I27.83)

Q21.9　**Congenital malformation of cardiac septum, unspecified**
　　　Septal (heart) defect NOS

● Q22　**Congenital malformations of pulmonary and tricuspid valves**

Q22.0　**Pulmonary valve atresia**

Q22.1　**Congenital pulmonary valve stenosis**

Q22.2　**Congenital pulmonary valve insufficiency**
　　　Congenital pulmonary valve regurgitation

Q22.3　**Other congenital malformations of pulmonary valve**
　　　Congenital malformation of pulmonary valve NOS
　　　Supernumerary cusps of pulmonary valve

Q22.4　**Congenital tricuspid stenosis**
　　　Congenital tricuspid atresia

Q22.5　**Ebstein's anomaly**
　　　Malformation of tricuspid valve

Q22.6　**Hypoplastic right heart syndrome**

Q22.8　**Other congenital malformations of tricuspid valve**

Q22.9　**Congenital malformation of tricuspid valve, unspecified**

● Q23　**Congenital malformations of aortic and mitral valves**

Q23.0　**Congenital stenosis of aortic valve**
　　　Congenital aortic atresia
　　　Congenital aortic stenosis NOS
　　　Excludes1　congenital stenosis of aortic valve in
　　　　　hypoplastic left heart syndrome
　　　　　(Q23.4)
　　　　congenital subaortic stenosis (Q24.4)
　　　　supravalvular aortic stenosis (congenital)
　　　　　(Q25.3)

Q23.1　**Congenital insufficiency of aortic valve**
　　　~~Bicuspid aortic valve~~
　　　Congenital aortic insufficiency

Q23.2　**Congenital mitral stenosis**
　　　Congenital mitral atresia

Q23.3　**Congenital mitral insufficiency**

Q23.4　**Hypoplastic left heart syndrome**

Q23.8　**Other congenital malformations of aortic and mitral valves**
▶ Q23.81　**Bicuspid aortic valve**
　　　▶Congenital bicuspid aortic valve
　　　▶Unicuspid (congenital) aortic valve (at birth)
　　　▶Code also, if applicable, acquired aortic valve
　　　　disorders, such as:
　　　　▶aortic (valve) insufficiency (nonrheumatic)
　　　　　(I35.1)
　　　　▶aortic (valve) stenosis (nonrheumatic) (I35.0)
　　　　▶aortic (valve) stenosis with insufficiency
　　　　　(nonrheumatic) (I35.2)
▶ Q23.82　**Congenital mitral valve cleft leaflet**
　　　▶Cleft mitral valve leaflet at birth
▶ Q23.88　**Other congenital malformations of aortic and mitral valves**

Q23.9　**Congenital malformation of aortic and mitral valves, unspecified**

● Q24　**Other congenital malformations of heart**
　　　Excludes1　endocardial fibroelastosis (I42.4)

Q24.0　**Dextrocardia**
　　　Heart is located in right hemithorax
　　　Excludes1　dextrocardia with situs inversus (Q89.3)
　　　　isomerism of atrial appendages (with
　　　　　asplenia or polysplenia) (Q20.6)
　　　　mirror-image atrial arrangement with
　　　　　situs inversus (Q89.3)

Q24.1　**Levocardia**
　　　Normal position of heart but related structures on wrong side

Q24.2　**Cor triatriatum**
　　　Congenital heart defect; left atrium is subdivided

Q24.3　**Pulmonary infundibular stenosis**
　　　Subvalvular pulmonic stenosis

Q24.4　**Congenital subaortic stenosis**

Q24.5　**Malformation of coronary vessels**
　　　Congenital coronary (artery) aneurysm

Q24.6　**Congenital heart block**

Q24.8　**Other specified congenital malformations of heart**
　　　Congenital diverticulum of left ventricle
　　　Congenital malformation of myocardium
　　　Congenital malformation of pericardium
　　　Malposition of heart
　　　Uhl's disease

Q24.9　**Congenital malformation of heart, unspecified**
　　　Congenital anomaly of heart
　　　Congenital disease of heart

● Q25　**Congenital malformations of great arteries**

Q25.0　**Patent ductus arteriosus**
　　　Fetal blood vessel connecting left pulmonary artery directly
　　　　to descending aorta
　　　Patent ductus Botallo
　　　Persistent ductus arteriosus

Q25.1　**Coarctation of aorta**
　　　Coarctation of aorta (preductal) (postductal)
　　　Stenosis of aorta
　　　Coding Clinic: 2016, Q4, P56-57

● Q25.2　**Atresia of aorta** (Ex) PDX 1536
　　　Coding Clinic: 2016, Q4, P56

Q25.21　**Interruption of aortic arch**
　　　Atresia of aortic arch

Q25.29　**Other atresia of aorta**
　　　Atresia of aorta

Q25.3　**Supravalvular aortic stenosis**
　　　Excludes1　congenital aortic stenosis NOS (Q23.0)
　　　　congenital stenosis of aortic valve (Q23.0)

● Q25.4　**Other congenital malformations of aorta**
　　　Excludes1　hypoplasia of aorta in hypoplastic left
　　　　　heart syndrome (Q23.4)
　　　Coding Clinic: 2016, Q4, P57

Q25.40　**Congenital malformation of aorta unspecified**

Q25.41　**Absence and aplasia of aorta**

Q25.42   **Hypoplasia of aorta**

Q25.43   **Congenital aneurysm of aorta**
    Congenital aneurysm of aortic root
    Congenital aneurysm of aortic sinus

Q25.44   **Congenital dilation of aorta**

Q25.45   **Double aortic arch**
    Vascular ring of aorta

Q25.46   **Tortuous aortic arch**
    Persistent convolutions of aortic arch

Q25.47   **Right aortic arch**
    Persistent right aortic arch

Q25.48   **Anomalous origin of subclavian artery**

Q25.49   **Other congenital malformations of aorta**
    Aortic arch
    Bovine arch

Q25.5   **Atresia of pulmonary artery**

Q25.6   **Stenosis of pulmonary artery**
    Supravalvular pulmonary stenosis

● Q25.7   **Other congenital malformations of pulmonary artery**

    Q25.71   **Coarctation of pulmonary artery**

    Q25.72   **Congenital pulmonary arteriovenous malformation**
       Congenital pulmonary arteriovenous aneurysm

    Q25.79   **Other congenital malformations of pulmonary artery**
       Aberrant pulmonary artery
       Agenesis of pulmonary artery
       Congenital aneurysm of pulmonary artery
       Congenital anomaly of pulmonary artery
       Hypoplasia of pulmonary artery

Q25.8   **Other congenital malformations of other great arteries**

Q25.9   **Congenital malformation of great arteries, unspecified**

● Q26   Congenital malformations of great veins

Q26.0   **Congenital stenosis of vena cava**
    Congenital stenosis of vena cava (inferior)(superior)

Q26.1   **Persistent left superior vena cava**

Q26.2   **Total anomalous pulmonary venous connection**
    Total anomalous pulmonary venous return [TAPVR], subdiaphragmatic
    Total anomalous pulmonary venous return [TAPVR], supradiaphragmatic

Q26.3   **Partial anomalous pulmonary venous connection**
    Partial anomalous pulmonary venous return

Q26.4   **Anomalous pulmonary venous connection, unspecified**

Q26.5   **Anomalous portal venous connection**

Q26.6   **Portal vein-hepatic artery fistula**

Q26.8   **Other congenital malformations of great veins**
    Absence of vena cava (inferior) (superior)
    Azygos continuation of inferior vena cava
    Persistent left posterior cardinal vein
    Scimitar syndrome

Q26.9   **Congenital malformation of great vein, unspecified**
    Congenital anomaly of vena cava (inferior) (superior) NOS

● Q27   Other congenital malformations of peripheral vascular system
    Excludes2   anomalies of cerebral and precerebral vessels (Q28.0-Q28.3)
           anomalies of coronary vessels (Q24.5)
           anomalies of pulmonary artery (Q25.5-Q25.7)
           congenital retinal aneurysm (Q14.1)
           hemangioma and lymphangioma (D18.-)

Q27.0   **Congenital absence and hypoplasia of umbilical artery**
    Single umbilical artery

Q27.1   **Congenital renal artery stenosis**

Q27.2   **Other congenital malformations of renal artery**
    Congenital malformation of renal artery NOS
    Multiple renal arteries

● Q27.3   **Arteriovenous malformation (peripheral)**
    Arteriovenous aneurysm
    Excludes1   acquired arteriovenous aneurysm (I77.0)
    Excludes2   arteriovenous malformation of cerebral vessels (Q28.2)
              arteriovenous malformation of precerebral vessels (Q28.0)

    Q27.30   **Arteriovenous malformation, site unspecified**

    Q27.31   **Arteriovenous malformation of vessel of upper limb**

    Q27.32   **Arteriovenous malformation of vessel of lower limb**

    Q27.33   **Arteriovenous malformation of digestive system vessel**

    Q27.34   **Arteriovenous malformation of renal vessel**

    Q27.39   **Arteriovenous malformation, other site**

Q27.4   **Congenital phlebectasia**

Q27.8   **Other specified congenital malformations of peripheral vascular system**
    Absence of peripheral vascular system
    Atresia of peripheral vascular system
    Congenital aneurysm (peripheral)
    Congenital stricture, artery
    Congenital varix
    Excludes1   arteriovenous malformation (Q27.3-)

Q27.9   **Congenital malformation of peripheral vascular system, unspecified**
    Anomaly of artery or vein NOS

● Q28   Other congenital malformations of circulatory system
    Excludes1   congenital aneurysm NOS (Q27.8)
           congenital coronary aneurysm (Q24.5)
           ruptured cerebral arteriovenous malformation (I60.8)
           ruptured malformation of precerebral vessels (I72.0)
    Excludes2   congenital peripheral aneurysm (Q27.8)
           congenital pulmonary aneurysm (Q25.79)
           congenital retinal aneurysm (Q14.1)

Q28.0   **Arteriovenous malformation of precerebral vessels**
    Congenital arteriovenous precerebral aneurysm (nonruptured)

Q28.1   **Other malformations of precerebral vessels**
    Congenital malformation of precerebral vessels NOS
    Congenital precerebral aneurysm (nonruptured)

Q28.2   **Arteriovenous malformation of cerebral vessels**
    Arteriovenous malformation of brain NOS
    Congenital arteriovenous cerebral aneurysm (nonruptured)

Q28.3   **Other malformations of cerebral vessels**
    Congenital cerebral aneurysm (nonruptured)
    Congenital malformation of cerebral vessels NOS
    Developmental venous anomaly

Q28.8   **Other specified congenital malformations of circulatory system**
    Congenital aneurysm, specified site NEC
    Spinal vessel anomaly

Q28.9   **Congenital malformation of circulatory system, unspecified**

CONGENITAL MALFORMATIONS OF THE RESPIRATORY SYSTEM (Q30-Q34)

● Q30   Congenital malformations of nose
    Excludes1   congenital deviation of nasal septum (Q67.4)

Q30.0   **Choanal atresia**
    Atresia of nares (anterior) (posterior)
    Congenital stenosis of nares (anterior) (posterior)

Q30.1   **Agenesis and underdevelopment of nose**
    Congenital absent of nose

Q30.2   **Fissured, notched and cleft** nose

Q30.3   **Congenital** perforated **nasal septum**

Q30.8   **Other congenital malformations of nose**
          Accessory nose
          Congenital anomaly of nasal sinus wall
          Coding Clinic: 2022, Q2, P17

Q30.9   **Congenital malformation of nose, unspecified**

● Q31   **Congenital malformations of larynx**
          Excludes1   congenital laryngeal stridor NOS (P28.89)

Q31.0   **Web of larynx**
          Glottic web of larynx
          Subglottic web of larynx
          Web of larynx NOS

Q31.1   **Congenital subglottic stenosis**

Q31.2   **Laryngeal hypoplasia**

Q31.3   **Laryngocele**

Q31.5   **Congenital laryngomalacia**

Q31.8   **Other congenital malformations of larynx**
          Absence of larynx
          Agenesis of larynx
          Atresia of larynx
          Congenital cleft thyroid cartilage
          Congenital fissure of epiglottis
          Congenital stenosis of larynx NEC
          Posterior cleft of cricoid cartilage

Q31.9   **Congenital malformation of larynx, unspecified**

● Q32   **Congenital malformations of trachea and bronchus**
          Excludes1   congenital bronchiectasis (Q33.4)

Q32.0   **Congenital tracheomalacia**

Q32.1   **Other congenital malformations of trachea**
          Atresia of trachea
          Congenital anomaly of tracheal cartilage
          Congenital dilatation of trachea
          Congenital malformation of trachea
          Congenital stenosis of trachea
          Congenital tracheocele

Q32.2   **Congenital bronchomalacia**

Q32.3   **Congenital stenosis of bronchus**

Q32.4   **Other congenital malformations of bronchus**
          Absence of bronchus
          Agenesis of bronchus
          Atresia of bronchus
          Congenital diverticulum of bronchus
          Congenital malformation of bronchus NOS

● Q33   **Congenital malformations of lung**

Q33.0   **Congenital cystic lung**
          Congenital cystic lung disease
          Congenital honeycomb lung
          Congenital polycystic lung disease
          Excludes1   cystic fibrosis (E84.0)
                          cystic lung disease, acquired or
                          unspecified (J98.4)

Q33.1   **Accessory lobe of lung**
          Azygos lobe (fissured), lung

Q33.2   **Sequestration of lung**

Q33.3   **Agenesis of lung**
          Congenital absence of lung (lobe)

Q33.4   **Congenital bronchiectasis**

Q33.5   **Ectopic tissue in lung**

Q33.6   **Congenital hypoplasia and dysplasia of lung**
          Excludes1   pulmonary hypoplasia associated with
                          short gestation (P28.0)

Q33.8   **Other congenital malformations of lung**

Q33.9   **Congenital malformation of lung, unspecified**

● Q34   Other congenital malformations of **respiratory system**
          Excludes2   congenital central alveolar hypoventilation
                          syndrome (G47.35)

Q34.0   **Anomaly of pleura**

Q34.1   **Congenital cyst of mediastinum**

Q34.8   **Other specified congenital malformations of respiratory
          system**
          Atresia of nasopharynx

Q34.9   **Congenital malformation of respiratory system,
          unspecified**
          Congenital absence of respiratory system
          Congenital anomaly of respiratory system NOS

CLEFT LIP AND CLEFT PALATE (Q35-Q37)

Use additional code to identify associated malformation of the
nose (Q30.2)

Excludes2   Robin's syndrome (Q87.0)

● Q35   Cleft palate
          Includes   fissure of palate
                         palatoschisis
          Excludes1   cleft palate with cleft lip (Q37.-)

Q35.1   **Cleft hard palate**

Q35.3   **Cleft soft palate**

Q35.5   **Cleft hard palate with cleft soft palate**

Q35.7   **Cleft uvula**

Q35.9   **Cleft palate, unspecified**
          Cleft palate NOS

● Q36   Cleft lip
          Includes   cheiloschisis
                         congenital fissure of lip
                         harelip
                         labium leporinum
          Excludes1   cleft lip with cleft palate (Q37.-)

Q36.0   **Cleft lip, bilateral**

Q36.1   **Cleft lip, median**

Q36.9   **Cleft lip, unilateral**
          Cleft lip NOS

● Q37   Cleft palate with cleft lip
          Includes   cheilopalatoschisis

Q37.0   **Cleft hard palate with bilateral cleft lip**

Q37.1   **Cleft hard palate with unilateral cleft lip**
          Cleft hard palate with cleft lip NOS

Q37.2   **Cleft soft palate with bilateral cleft lip**

Q37.3   **Cleft soft palate with unilateral cleft lip**
          Cleft soft palate with cleft lip NOS

Q37.4   **Cleft hard and soft palate with bilateral cleft lip**

Q37.5   **Cleft hard and soft palate with unilateral cleft lip**
          Cleft hard and soft palate with cleft lip NOS

Q37.8   **Unspecified cleft palate with bilateral cleft lip**

Q37.9   **Unspecified cleft palate with unilateral cleft lip**
          Cleft palate with cleft lip NOS

Figure 17-3   Cleft palate.

▶ New   ⇒ Revised   ~~deleted~~ Deleted   Excludes 1   Excludes 2   Includes   Use additional   Code first   Code also   Key words

OGCR Official Guidelines   X Assign placeholder X   ● Use Additional Character(s)   ▶ Manifestation Code   🐾 Hierarchical Condition Category   Coding Clinic

OTHER CONGENITAL MALFORMATIONS OF THE DIGESTIVE SYSTEM (Q38-Q45)

● **Q38 Other congenital malformations of tongue, mouth and pharynx**

> **Excludes1** dentofacial anomalies (M26.-)
> macrostomia (Q18.4)
> microstomia (Q18.5)

Q38.0 Congenital malformations of lips, not elsewhere classified
Congenital fistula of lip
Congenital malformation of lip NOS
Van der Woude's syndrome

> **Excludes1** cleft lip (Q36.-)
> cleft lip with cleft palate (Q37.-)
> macrocheilia (Q18.6)
> microcheilia (Q18.7)

Q38.1 Ankyloglossia
Restricted movement of tongue resulting in speech difficulty
Tongue tie

Q38.2 Macroglossia
Excessive size of tongue
Congenital hypertrophy of tongue

Q38.3 Other congenital malformations of tongue
Aglossia
Bifid tongue
Congenital adhesion of tongue
Congenital fissure of tongue
Congenital malformation of tongue NOS
Double tongue
Hypoglossia
Hypoplasia of tongue
Microglossia

Q38.4 Congenital malformations of salivary glands and ducts
Atresia of salivary glands and ducts
Congenital absence of salivary glands and ducts
Congenital accessory salivary glands and ducts
Congenital fistula of salivary gland

Q38.5 Congenital malformations of palate, not elsewhere classified
Congenital absence of uvula
Congenital malformation of palate NOS
Congenital high arched palate

> **Excludes1** cleft palate (Q35.-)
> cleft palate with cleft lip (Q37.-)

Q38.6 Other congenital malformations of mouth
Congenital malformation of mouth NOS

Q38.7 Congenital pharyngeal pouch
Congenital diverticulum of pharynx

> **Excludes1** pharyngeal pouch syndrome (D82.1)

Q38.8 Other congenital malformations of pharynx
Congenital malformation of pharynx NOS
Imperforate pharynx

● **Q39 Congenital malformations of esophagus**

Q39.0 Atresia of esophagus without fistula
Atresia of esophagus NOS

Q39.1 Atresia of esophagus with tracheo-esophageal fistula
Atresia of esophagus with broncho-esophageal fistula

Q39.2 Congenital tracheo-esophageal fistula without atresia
Congenital tracheo-esophageal fistula NOS

Q39.3 Congenital stenosis and stricture of esophagus

Q39.4 Esophageal web

Q39.5 Congenital dilatation of esophagus
Congenital cardiospasm

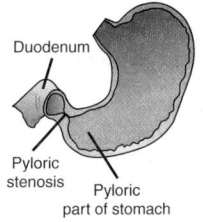
Duodenum
Pyloric stenosis
Pyloric part of stomach

Figure 17-4 Pyloric stenosis.

Q39.6 Congenital diverticulum of esophagus
Congenital esophageal pouch

Q39.8 Other congenital malformations of esophagus
Congenital absence of esophagus
Congenital displacement of esophagus
Congenital duplication of esophagus

Q39.9 Congenital malformation of esophagus, unspecified

● **Q40 Other congenital malformations of upper alimentary tract**

Q40.0 Congenital hypertrophic pyloric stenosis
Congenital or infantile constriction
Congenital or infantile hypertrophy
Congenital or infantile spasm
Congenital or infantile stenosis
Congenital or infantile stricture

Q40.1 Congenital hiatus hernia
Congenital displacement of cardia through esophageal hiatus

> **Excludes1** congenital diaphragmatic hernia (Q79.0)

Q40.2 Other specified congenital malformations of stomach
Congenital displacement of stomach
Congenital diverticulum of stomach
Congenital hourglass stomach
Congenital duplication of stomach
Megalogastria
Microgastria

Q40.3 Congenital malformation of stomach, unspecified

Q40.8 Other specified congenital malformations of upper alimentary tract

Q40.9 Congenital malformation of upper alimentary tract, unspecified
Congenital anomaly of upper alimentary tract
Congenital deformity of upper alimentary tract

● **Q41 Congenital absence, atresia and stenosis of small intestine**

> **Includes** congenital obstruction, occlusion or stricture of small intestine or intestine NOS

> **Excludes1** cystic fibrosis with intestinal manifestation (E84.11)
> meconium ileus NOS (without cystic fibrosis) (P76.0)

Q41.0 Congenital absence, atresia and stenosis of duodenum

Q41.1 Congenital absence, atresia and stenosis of jejunum
Apple peel syndrome
Imperforate jejunum

Q41.2 Congenital absence, atresia and stenosis of ileum

Q41.8 Congenital absence, atresia and stenosis of other specified parts of small intestine

Q41.9 Congenital absence, atresia and stenosis of small intestine, part unspecified
Congenital absence, atresia and stenosis of intestine NOS

● **Q42 Congenital absence, atresia and stenosis of large intestine**

> **Includes** congenital obstruction, occlusion and stricture of large intestine

Q42.0 Congenital absence, atresia and stenosis of rectum with fistula

Q42.1 Congenital absence, atresia and stenosis of rectum without fistula
Imperforate rectum

Q42.2 Congenital absence, atresia and stenosis of anus with fistula

Q42.3 Congenital absence, atresia and stenosis of anus without fistula
Imperforate anus

Q42.8 Congenital absence, atresia and stenosis of other parts of large intestine

Q42.9 Congenital absence, atresia and stenosis of large intestine, part unspecified

CHAPTER 17 (Q00-Q99)

CHAPTER 17 (Q00–Q99)

● **Q43**   **Other congenital malformations of intestine**

     Q43.0   **Meckel's diverticulum (displaced) (hypertrophic)**
         Congenital abnormality in which a pouch remains on the lower end of the small intestine
         Persistent omphalomesenteric duct
         Persistent vitelline duct

     Q43.1   **Hirschsprung's disease**
         Developmental disorder of enteric nervous system characterized by absence of ganglion cells in distal colon resulting in functional obstruction
         Aganglionosis
         Congenital (aganglionic) megacolon

     Q43.2   **Other congenital functional disorders of colon**
         Congenital dilatation of colon

     Q43.3   **Congenital malformations of intestinal fixation**
         Congenital omental, anomalous adhesions [bands]
         Congenital peritoneal adhesions [bands]
         Incomplete rotation of cecum and colon
         Insufficient rotation of cecum and colon
         Jackson's membrane
         Malrotation of colon
         Rotation failure of cecum and colon
         Universal mesentery

     Q43.4   **Duplication of intestine**

     Q43.5   **Ectopic anus**
         Anal opening in abnormal location

     Q43.6   **Congenital fistula of rectum and anus**
         Excludes1   congenital fistula of anus with absence, atresia and stenosis (Q42.2)
                 congenital fistula of rectum with absence, atresia and stenosis (Q42.0)
                 congenital rectovaginal fistula (Q52.2)
                 congenital urethrorectal fistula (Q64.73)
                 pilonidal fistula or sinus (L05.-)

     Q43.7   **Persistent cloaca**
         Malformation in which rectum, vagina, and urinary tract form one channel; AKA congenital cloaca
         Cloaca NOS

     Q43.8   **Other specified congenital malformations of intestine**
         Congenital blind loop syndrome
         Congenital diverticulitis, colon
         Congenital diverticulum, intestine
         Dolichocolon
         Megaloappendix
         Megaloduodenum
         Microcolon
         Transposition of appendix
         Transposition of colon
         Transposition of intestine

     Q43.9   **Congenital malformation of intestine, unspecified**

● **Q44**   **Congenital malformations of gallbladder, bile ducts and liver**

     Q44.0   **Agenesis, aplasia and hypoplasia of gallbladder**
         Congenital absence of gallbladder

     Q44.1   **Other congenital malformations of gallbladder**
         Congenital malformation of gallbladder NOS
         Intrahepatic gallbladder

     Q44.2   **Atresia of bile ducts**

     Q44.3   **Congenital stenosis and stricture of bile ducts**

     Q44.4   **Choledochal cyst**

     Q44.5   **Other congenital malformations of bile ducts**
         Accessory hepatic duct
         Biliary duct duplication
         Congenital malformation of bile duct NOS
         Cystic duct duplication

     Q44.6   **Cystic disease of liver**
         Fibrocystic disease of liver

● **Q44.7**   **Other congenital malformations of liver**
         Code also associated underlying condition

     Q44.70   **Other congenital malformation of liver, unspecified**
         Congenital malformation of liver, NOS

     Q44.71   **Alagille syndrome**
         Alagille-Watson syndrome

     Q44.79   **Other congenital malformations of liver**
         Accessory liver
         Congenital absence of liver
         Congenital hepatomegaly

● **Q45**   **Other congenital malformations of digestive system**
     Excludes2   congenital diaphragmatic hernia (Q79.0)
                 congenital hiatus hernia (Q40.1)

     Q45.0   **Agenesis, aplasia and hypoplasia of pancreas**
         Congenital absence of pancreas

     Q45.1   **Annular pancreas**

     Q45.2   **Congenital pancreatic cyst**

     Q45.3   **Other congenital malformations of pancreas and pancreatic duct**
         Accessory pancreas
         Congenital malformation of pancreas or pancreatic duct NOS
         Excludes1   congenital diabetes mellitus (E10.-)
                 cystic fibrosis (E84.0-E84.9)
                 fibrocystic disease of pancreas (E84.-)
                 neonatal diabetes mellitus (P70.2)

     Q45.8   **Other specified congenital malformations of digestive system**
         Absence (complete) (partial) of alimentary tract NOS
         Duplication of digestive system
         Malposition, congenital of digestive system

     Q45.9   **Congenital malformation of digestive system, unspecified**
         Congenital anomaly of digestive system
         Congenital deformity of digestive system

CONGENITAL MALFORMATIONS OF GENITAL ORGANS (Q50-Q56)

     Excludes1   androgen insensitivity syndrome (E34.5-)
                 syndromes associated with anomalies in the number and form of chromosomes (Q90-Q99)

● **Q50**   **Congenital malformations of ovaries, fallopian tubes and broad ligaments**

     ● **Q50.0**   **Congenital absence of ovary**
         Excludes1   Turner's syndrome (Q96.-)

     Q50.01   **Congenital absence of ovary, unilateral**

     Q50.02   **Congenital absence of ovary, bilateral**

     Q50.1   **Developmental ovarian cyst**

     Q50.2   **Congenital torsion of ovary**

     ● **Q50.3**   **Other congenital malformations of ovary**

     Q50.31   **Accessory ovary**

     Q50.32   **Ovarian streak**
         Inadequate ovaries with absent follicular and hormonal function
         46, XX with streak gonads

     Q50.39   **Other congenital malformation of ovary**
         Congenital malformation of ovary NOS

     Q50.4   **Embryonic cyst of fallopian tube**
         Fimbrial cyst

     Q50.5   **Embryonic cyst of broad ligament**
         Epoophoron cyst
         Parovarian cyst

     Q50.6   **Other congenital malformations of fallopian tube and broad ligament**
         Absence of fallopian tube and broad ligament
         Accessory fallopian tube and broad ligament
         Atresia of fallopian tube and broad ligament
         Congenital malformation of fallopian tube or broad ligament NOS

● Q51　Congenital malformations of uterus and cervix
　Q51.0　Agenesis and aplasia of uterus
　　　　　Congenital absence of uterus
● Q51.1　Doubling of uterus with doubling of cervix and vagina
　　Q51.10　Doubling of uterus with doubling of cervix and vagina without obstruction
　　　　　　Doubling of uterus with doubling of cervix and vagina NOS
　　Q51.11　Doubling of uterus with doubling of cervix and vagina with obstruction
● Q51.2　Other doubling of uterus
　　　　　Doubling of uterus NOS
　　　　　Septate uterus
　　Q51.21　Complete doubling of uterus
　　　　　　Complete septate uterus
　　Q51.22　Partial doubling of uterus
　　　　　　Partial septate uterus
　　Q51.28　Other and unspecified doubling of uterus
　　　　　　Septate uterus NOS
　Q51.3　Bicornate uterus
　　　　　Bicornate uterus, complete or partial
　　　　　Birth defect in which uterus has two separate "horns" that form top of uterus
　Q51.4　Unicornate uterus
　　　　　Unicornate uterus with or without a separate uterine horn
　　　　　Uterus with only one functioning horn
　　　　　Uterus with half being undeveloped
　Q51.5　Agenesis and aplasia of cervix
　　　　　Congenital absence of cervix
　Q51.6　Embryonic cyst of cervix
　Q51.7　Congenital fistulae between uterus and digestive and urinary tracts
● Q51.8　Other congenital malformations of uterus and cervix
　● Q51.81　Other congenital malformations of uterus
　　　Q51.810　Arcuate uterus
　　　　　　　Arcuatus uterus
　　　Q51.811　Hypoplasia of uterus
　　　Q51.818　Other congenital malformations of uterus
　　　　　　　Müllerian anomaly of uterus NEC
　● Q51.82　Other congenital malformations of cervix
　　　Q51.820　Cervical duplication
　　　Q51.821　Hypoplasia of cervix
　　　Q51.828　Other congenital malformations of cervix
　Q51.9　Congenital malformation of uterus and cervix, unspecified

● Q52　Other congenital malformations of female genitalia
　Q52.0　Congenital absence of vagina
　　　　　Vaginal agenesis, total or partial
● Q52.1　Doubling of vagina
　　Excludes1　doubling of vagina with doubling of uterus and cervix (Q51.1-)
　　Q52.10　Doubling of vagina, unspecified
　　　　　　Septate vagina NOS
　　Q52.11　Transverse vaginal septum
　● Q52.12　Longitudinal vaginal septum
　　　Coding Clinic: 2016, Q4, P58
　　　Q52.120　Longitudinal vaginal septum, nonobstructing
　　　Q52.121　Longitudinal vaginal septum, obstructing, right side
　　　Q52.122　Longitudinal vaginal septum, obstructing, left side
　　　Q52.123　Longitudinal vaginal septum, microperforate, right side

　　　Q52.124　Longitudinal vaginal septum, microperforate, left side
　　　　　　　Coding Clinic: 2016, Q4, P59
　　　Q52.129　Other and unspecified longitudinal vaginal septum
　Q52.2　Congenital rectovaginal fistula
　　　　Excludes1　cloaca (Q43.7)
　Q52.3　Imperforate hymen
　　　　　Membrane (hymen) completely closes vaginal orifice
　Q52.4　Other congenital malformations of vagina
　　　　　Canal of Nuck cyst, congenital
　　　　　Congenital malformation of vagina NOS
　　　　　Embryonic vaginal cyst
　　　　　Gartner's duct cyst
　　　　　Coding Clinic: 2022, Q2, P16
　Q52.5　Fusion of labia
　Q52.6　Congenital malformation of clitoris
● Q52.7　Other and unspecified congenital malformations of vulva
　　Q52.70　Unspecified congenital malformations of vulva
　　　　　　Congenital malformation of vulva NOS
　　Q52.71　Congenital absence of vulva
　　Q52.79　Other congenital malformations of vulva
　　　　　　Congenital cyst of vulva
　Q52.8　Other specified congenital malformations of female genitalia
　Q52.9　Congenital malformation of female genitalia, unspecified

● Q53　Undescended and ectopic testicle
　● Q53.0　Ectopic testis
　　　Q53.00　Ectopic testis, unspecified
　　　Q53.01　Ectopic testis, unilateral
　　　Q53.02　Ectopic testes, bilateral
　● Q53.1　Undescended testicle, unilateral
　　　Q53.10　Unspecified undescended testicle, unilateral
　　● Q53.11　Abdominal testis, unilateral
　　　　Q53.111　Unilateral intraabdominal testis
　　　　Q53.112　Unilateral inguinal testis
　　　Q53.12　Ectopic perineal testis, unilateral
　　　Q53.13　Unilateral high scrotal testis
　● Q53.2　Undescended testicle, bilateral
　　　Q53.20　Undescended testicle, unspecified, bilateral
　　● Q53.21　Abdominal testis, bilateral
　　　　Q53.211　Bilateral intraabdominal testes
　　　　Q53.212　Bilateral inguinal testes
　　　Q53.22　Ectopic perineal testis, bilateral
　　　Q53.23　Bilateral high scrotal testes
　Q53.9　Undescended testicle, unspecified
　　　　　Cryptorchism NOS

Item 17–1 Testes form in the abdomen of the male and only descend into the scrotum during normal embryonic development. "Ectopic" testes are out of their normal place or "retained" (left behind) in the abdomen. Crypto (hidden) orchism (testicle) is a major risk factor for testicular cancer.

ECTOPIC TESTES	CRYPTORCHID TESTES
Penile	Abdominal
Superficial inguinal	Inguinal
(most common)	Prepubic
Femoral	(most common)

Figure 17-5 Undescended testes and the positions of the testes in various types of cryptorchidism or abnormal paths of descent.

● **Q54   Hypospadias**
Birth defect of male; urethra opens in abnormal location on shaft
   Excludes1   epispadias (Q64.0)
   Q54.0   Hypospadias, balanic
      Hypospadias, coronal
      Hypospadias, glandular
   Q54.1   Hypospadias, penile
   Q54.2   Hypospadias, penoscrotal
   Q54.3   Hypospadias, perineal
   Q54.4   Congenital chordee
      Chordee without hypospadias
   Q54.8   Other hypospadias
      Hypospadias with intersex state
   Q54.9   Hypospadias, unspecified

● **Q55   Other congenital malformations of male genital organs**
   Excludes1   congenital hydrocele (P83.5)
                hypospadias (Q54.-)
   Q55.0   Absence and aplasia of testis
      Monorchism
   Q55.1   Hypoplasia of testis and scrotum
      Fusion of testes
● **Q55.2   Other and unspecified congenital malformations of testis and scrotum**
   Q55.20   Unspecified congenital malformations of testis and scrotum
      Congenital malformation of testis or scrotum NOS
   Q55.21   Polyorchism
      Developmental anomaly characterized by presence of more than two testes
   Q55.22   Retractile testis
   Q55.23   Scrotal transposition
   Q55.29   Other congenital malformations of testis and scrotum
   Q55.3   Atresia of vas deferens
      Code first any associated cystic fibrosis (E84.-)
   Q55.4   Other congenital malformations of vas deferens, epididymis, seminal vesicles and prostate
      Absence or aplasia of prostate
      Absence or aplasia of spermatic cord
      Congenital malformation of vas deferens, epididymis, seminal vesicles or prostate NOS
   Q55.5   Congenital absence and aplasia of penis
● **Q55.6   Other congenital malformations of penis**
   Q55.61   Curvature of penis (lateral)
   Q55.62   Hypoplasia of penis
      Underdevelopment penis
      Micropenis
   Q55.63   Congenital torsion of penis
      Excludes1   acquired torsion of penis (N48.82)
   Q55.64   Hidden penis
      Buried penis
      Concealed penis
      Excludes1   acquired buried penis (N48.83)
   Q55.69   Other congenital malformation of penis
      Congenital malformation of penis NOS
   Q55.7   Congenital vasocutaneous fistula
      Abnormal opening between vas deferens and skin
   Q55.8   Other specified congenital malformations of male genital organs
   Q55.9   Congenital malformation of male genital organ, unspecified
      Congenital anomaly of male genital organ
      Congenital deformity of male genital organ

● **Q56   Indeterminate sex and pseudohermaphroditism**
Internal reproductive organs are opposite external physical characteristics.
   Excludes1   46,XX true hermaphrodite (Q99.1)
                androgen insensitivity syndrome (E34.5-)
                chimera 46,XX/46,XY true hermaphrodite (Q99.0)
                female pseudohermaphroditism with adrenocortical disorder (E25.-)
                pseudohermaphroditism with specified chromosomal anomaly (Q96-Q99)
                pure gonadal dysgenesis (Q99.1)
   Q56.0   Hermaphroditism, not elsewhere classified
      Ovotestis
   Q56.1   Male pseudohermaphroditism, not elsewhere classified
      46, XY with streak gonads
      Male pseudohermaphroditism NOS
   Q56.2   Female pseudohermaphroditism, not elsewhere classified
      Female pseudohermaphroditism NOS
   Q56.3   Pseudohermaphroditism, unspecified
   Q56.4   Indeterminate sex, unspecified
      Ambiguous genitalia

CONGENITAL MALFORMATIONS OF THE URINARY SYSTEM (Q60-Q64)

● **Q60   Renal agenesis and other reduction defects of kidney**
   Includes   congenital absence of kidney
                congenital atrophy of kidney
                infantile atrophy of kidney
   Q60.0   Renal agenesis, unilateral
   Q60.1   Renal agenesis, bilateral
   Q60.2   Renal agenesis, unspecified
   Q60.3   Renal hypoplasia, unilateral
   Q60.4   Renal hypoplasia, bilateral
   Q60.5   Renal hypoplasia, unspecified
   Q60.6   Potter's syndrome

● **Q61   Cystic kidney disease**
Cysts that develop in failing kidney due to end-stage renal disease
   Excludes1   acquired cyst of kidney (N28.1)
                Potter's syndrome (Q60.6)
● **Q61.0   Congenital renal cyst**
   Q61.00   Congenital renal cyst, unspecified
      Cyst of kidney NOS (congenital)
   Q61.01   Congenital single renal cyst
   Q61.02   Congenital multiple renal cysts
● **Q61.1   Polycystic kidney, infantile type**
      Polycystic kidney, autosomal recessive
   Q61.11   Cystic dilatation of collecting ducts
   Q61.19   Other polycystic kidney, infantile type
   Q61.2   Polycystic kidney, adult type
      Polycystic kidney, autosomal dominant
   Q61.3   Polycystic kidney, unspecified
      Coding Clinic: 2016, Q3, P23
   Q61.4   Renal dysplasia
      Multicystic dysplastic kidney
      Multicystic kidney (development)
      Multicystic kidney disease
      Multicystic renal dysplasia
      Excludes1   polycystic kidney disease (Q61.11-Q61.3)
   Q61.5   Medullary cystic kidney
      Nephronophthisis
      Sponge kidney NOS
   Q61.8   Other cystic kidney diseases
      Fibrocystic kidney
      Fibrocystic renal degeneration or disease
   Q61.9   Cystic kidney disease, unspecified
      Meckel-Gruber syndrome

▶ New   ⇒ Revised   ~~deleted~~ Deleted   Excludes 1   Excludes 2   Includes   Use additional   Code first   Code also   Key words
OGCR Official Guidelines   X Assign placeholder X   ● Use Additional Character(s)   ▶ Manifestation Code   🐴 Hierarchical Condition Category   Coding Clinic

● Q62 Congenital obstructive defects of renal pelvis and congenital malformations of ureter

Q62.0 Congenital hydronephrosis

● Q62.1 Congenital occlusion of ureter
    Atresia and stenosis of ureter
    Q62.10 Congenital occlusion of ureter, unspecified
    Q62.11 Congenital occlusion of ureteropelvic junction
    Q62.12 Congenital occlusion of ureterovesical orifice

Q62.2 Congenital megaureter
    Congenital dilatation of ureter

● Q62.3 Other obstructive defects of renal pelvis and ureter
    Q62.31 Congenital ureterocele, orthotopic
    Q62.32 Cecoureterocele
        Ectopic ureterocele
    Q62.39 Other obstructive defects of renal pelvis and ureter
        Ureteropelvic junction obstruction NOS

Q62.4 Agenesis of ureter
    Congenital absence ureter

Q62.5 Duplication of ureter
    Accessory ureter
    Double ureter

● Q62.6 Malposition of ureter
    Q62.60 Malposition of ureter, unspecified
    Q62.61 Deviation of ureter
    Q62.62 Displacement of ureter
    Q62.63 Anomalous implantation of ureter
        Ectopia of ureter
        Ectopic ureter
    Q62.69 Other malposition of ureter

Q62.7 Congenital vesico-uretero-renal reflux

Q62.8 Other congenital malformations of ureter
    Anomaly of ureter NOS

● Q63 Other congenital malformations of kidney
    Excludes1 congenital nephrotic syndrome (N04.-)

Q63.0 Accessory kidney

Q63.1 Lobulated, fused and horseshoe kidney

Q63.2 Ectopic kidney
    Congenital displaced kidney
    Malrotation of kidney

Q63.3 Hyperplastic and giant kidney
    Compensatory hypertrophy of kidney

Q63.8 Other specified congenital malformations of kidney
    Congenital renal calculi

Q63.9 Congenital malformation of kidney, unspecified

● Q64 Other congenital malformations of urinary system

Q64.0 Epispadias
    Urethral opening somewhere on dorsum of penis
    Excludes1 hypospadias (Q54.-)

● Q64.1 Exstrophy of urinary bladder
    Bladder is exposed, inside out, and protrudes through abdominal wall
    Q64.10 Exstrophy of urinary bladder, unspecified
        Ectopia vesicae
    Q64.11 Supravesical fissure of urinary bladder
    Q64.12 Cloacal exstrophy of urinary bladder
    Q64.19 Other exstrophy of urinary bladder
        Extroversion of bladder

Q64.2 Congenital posterior urethral valves

● Q64.3 Other atresia and stenosis of urethra and bladder neck
    Q64.31 Congenital bladder neck obstruction
        Congenital obstruction of vesicourethral orifice
    Q64.32 Congenital stricture of urethra
    Q64.33 Congenital stricture of urinary meatus
    Q64.39 Other atresia and stenosis of urethra and bladder neck
        Atresia and stenosis of urethra and bladder neck NOS

Q64.4 Malformation of urachus
    Cyst of urachus
    Patent urachus
    Prolapse of urachus

Q64.5 Congenital absence of bladder and urethra

Q64.6 Congenital diverticulum of bladder

● Q64.7 Other and unspecified congenital malformations of bladder and urethra
    Excludes1 congenital prolapse of bladder (mucosa) (Q79.4)
    Q64.70 Unspecified congenital malformation of bladder and urethra
        Malformation of bladder or urethra NOS
    Q64.71 Congenital prolapse of urethra
    Q64.72 Congenital prolapse of urinary meatus
    Q64.73 Congenital urethrorectal fistula
    Q64.74 Double urethra
    Q64.75 Double urinary meatus
    Q64.79 Other congenital malformations of bladder and urethra

Q64.8 Other specified congenital malformations of urinary system

Q64.9 Congenital malformation of urinary system, unspecified
    Congenital anomaly NOS of urinary system
    Congenital deformity NOS of urinary system

CONGENITAL MALFORMATIONS AND DEFORMATIONS OF THE MUSCULOSKELETAL SYSTEM (Q65-Q79)

● Q65 Congenital deformities of hip
    Excludes1 clicking hip (R29.4)

● Q65.0 Congenital dislocation of hip, unilateral
    Q65.00 Congenital dislocation of unspecified hip, unilateral
    Q65.01 Congenital dislocation of right hip, unilateral
    Q65.02 Congenital dislocation of left hip, unilateral

Q65.1 Congenital dislocation of hip, bilateral

Q65.2 Congenital dislocation of hip, unspecified

● Q65.3 Congenital partial dislocation of hip, unilateral
    Q65.30 Congenital partial dislocation of unspecified hip, unilateral
    Q65.31 Congenital partial dislocation of right hip, unilateral
    Q65.32 Congenital partial dislocation of left hip, unilateral

Q65.4 Congenital partial dislocation of hip, bilateral

Q65.5 Congenital partial dislocation of hip, unspecified

Q65.6 Congenital unstable hip
    Congenital dislocatable hip

Item 17–2 Equinus foot is a term referring to the hoof of a horse. The deformity is usually congenital or spastic. **Talipes equinovarus** is referred to as clubfoot. The foot tends to be smaller than normal, with the heel pointing downward and the forefoot turning inward. The heel cord (Achilles tendon) is tight, causing the heel to be drawn up toward the leg.

Figure 17-6 Supination and cavus deformity of forefoot. (From Kliegman R, Nelson WE: Nelson Textbook of Pediatrics, Philadelphia, Saunders, 2007)

CHAPTER 17 (Q00-Q99)

CHAPTER 17 (Q00-Q99)

Figure 17-7   Talipes. (From Dorland: Dorland's Illustrated Medical Dictionary, ed 31, Saunders, 2007, p 1893)

● Q65.8   **Other congenital deformities of hip**
     Q65.81   Congenital coxa valga
     Q65.82   Congenital coxa vara
     Q65.89   Other specified congenital deformities of hip
         Anteversion of femoral neck
         Congenital acetabular dysplasia
   Q65.9   **Congenital deformity of hip, unspecified**

● Q66   **Congenital deformities of feet**
     Excludes1   reduction defects of feet (Q72.-)
               valgus deformities (acquired) (M21.0-)
               varus deformities (acquired) (M21.1-)

● Q66.0   **Congenital talipes equinovarus**
     Heel is turned inward from midline and foot is plantar flexed; AKA clubfoot
     Q66.00   Congenital talipes equinovarus, unspecified foot
     Q66.01   Congenital talipes equinovarus, right foot
     Q66.02   Congenital talipes equinovarus, left foot

● Q66.1   **Congenital talipes calcaneovarus**
     Deformity of foot in which heel is turned toward midline of body and anterior of foot is elevated
     Q66.10   Congenital talipes calcaneovarus, unspecified foot
     Q66.11   Congenital talipes calcaneovarus, right foot
     Q66.12   Congenital talipes calcaneovarus, left foot

● Q66.2   **Congenital metatarsus (primus) varus**
     Angulation of first metatarsal bone toward midline of body
     Coding Clinic: 2016, Q4, P59
     ● Q66.21   Congenital metatarsus primus varus
         Q66.211   Congenital metatarsus primus varus, right foot
         Q66.212   Congenital metatarsus primus varus, left foot
         Q66.219   Congenital metatarsus primus varus, unspecified foot
     ● Q66.22   Congenital metatarsus adductus
         Congenital metatarsus varus
         Q66.221   Congenital metatarsus adductus, right foot
         Q66.222   Congenital metatarsus adductus, left foot
         Q66.229   Congenital metatarsus adductus, unspecified foot

● Q66.3   **Other congenital varus deformities of feet**
     Hallux varus, congenital
     Q66.30   Other congenital varus deformities of feet, unspecified foot

     Q66.31   Other congenital varus deformities of feet, right foot
     Q66.32   Other congenital varus deformities of feet, left foot
● Q66.4   **Congenital talipes calcaneovalgus**
     Q66.40   Congenital talipes calcaneovalgus, unspecified foot
     Q66.41   Congenital talipes calcaneovalgus, right foot
     Q66.42   Congenital talipes calcaneovalgus, left foot
● Q66.5   **Congenital pes planus**
     Congenital flat foot
     Congenital rigid flat foot
     Congenital spastic (everted) flat foot
     Excludes1   pes planus, acquired (M21.4)
     Q66.50   Congenital pes planus, unspecified foot
     Q66.51   Congenital pes planus, right foot
     Q66.52   Congenital pes planus, left foot
   Q66.6   **Other congenital valgus deformities of feet**
     Inward angulation
     Congenital metatarsus valgus
● Q66.7   **Congenital pes cavus**
     Q66.70   Congenital pes cavus, unspecified foot
     Q66.71   Congenital pes cavus, right foot
     Q66.72   Congenital pes cavus, left foot
● Q66.8   **Other congenital deformities of feet**
     Q66.80   Congenital vertical talus deformity, unspecified foot
     Q66.81   Congenital vertical talus deformity, right foot
     Q66.82   Congenital vertical talus deformity, left foot
     Q66.89   Other specified congenital deformities of feet
         Congenital asymmetric talipes
         Congenital clubfoot NOS
         Congenital talipes NOS
         Congenital tarsal coalition
         Hammer toe, congenital
● Q66.9   **Congenital deformity of feet, unspecified**
     Q66.90   Congenital deformity of feet, unspecified, unspecified foot
     Q66.91   Congenital deformity of feet, unspecified, right foot
     Q66.92   Congenital deformity of feet, unspecified, left foot
● Q67   **Congenital musculoskeletal deformities of head, face, spine and chest**
     Excludes1   congenital malformation syndromes classified to Q87.-
               Potter's syndrome (Q60.6)
   Q67.0   **Congenital facial asymmetry**
   Q67.1   **Congenital compression facies**
   Q67.2   **Dolichocephaly**
     Long head dimension
     Excludes1   sagittal craniosynostosis (Q75.01)
   Q67.3   **Plagiocephaly**
     Asymmetric shape of head resulting from irregular closure of cranial sutures
     Excludes1   coronal craniosynostosis (Q75.02-)
               lambdoid craniosynostosis (Q75.04-)

Figure 17-8   Mild to moderate inbowing of the lower leg. (From Lissauer T, Clayden G: Illustrated Textbook of Paediatrics, Edinburgh, Mosby, 2011)

▶ New   ⇒ Revised   ~~deleted~~ Deleted   Excludes 1   Excludes 2   Includes   Use additional   Code first   Code also   Key words
OGCR Official Guidelines   X Assign placeholder X   ● Use Additional Character(s)   ▶ Manifestation Code   🔒 Hierarchical Condition Category   **Coding Clinic**

Q67.4 **Other congenital deformities of skull, face and jaw**
Congenital depressions in skull
Congenital hemifacial atrophy or hypertrophy
Deviation of nasal septum, congenital
Squashed or bent nose, congenital

> **Excludes1**   dentofacial anomalies [including malocclusion] (M26.-)
> syphilitic saddle nose (A50.5)

Q67.5 **Congenital deformity of spine**
Congenital postural scoliosis
Congenital scoliosis NOS

> **Excludes1**   infantile idiopathic scoliosis (M41.0)
> scoliosis due to congenital bony malformation (Q76.3)

Q67.6 **Pectus excavatum**
Congenital funnel chest
Funnel-shaped chest depression

Q67.7 **Pectus carinatum**
Congenital pigeon chest

Q67.8 **Other congenital deformities of chest**
Congenital deformity of chest wall NOS

● Q68 **Other congenital musculoskeletal deformities**

> **Excludes1**   reduction defects of limb(s) (Q71-Q73)
> **Excludes2**   congenital myotonic chondrodystrophy (G71.13)

Q68.0 **Congenital deformity of sternocleidomastoid muscle**
Congenital contracture of sternocleidomastoid (muscle)
Congenital (sternomastoid) torticollis
Sternomastoid tumor (congenital)

Q68.1 **Congenital deformity of finger(s) and hand**
Congenital clubfinger
Spade-like hand (congenital)

Q68.2 **Congenital deformity of knee**
Congenital dislocation of knee
Congenital genu recurvatum
Hyperextension of knee resulting from hypermobility

Q68.3 **Congenital bowing of femur**

> **Excludes1**   anteversion of femur (neck) (Q65.89)

Q68.4 **Congenital bowing of tibia and fibula**

Q68.5 **Congenital bowing of long bones of leg, unspecified**

Q68.6 **Discoid meniscus**

Q68.8 **Other specified congenital musculoskeletal deformities**
Congenital deformity of clavicle
Congenital deformity of elbow
Congenital deformity of forearm
Congenital deformity of scapula
Congenital deformity of wrist
Congenital dislocation of elbow
Congenital dislocation of shoulder
Congenital dislocation of wrist

● Q69 **Polydactyly**
AKA hyperdactyly, consists of supernumerary fingers or toes

Q69.0 **Accessory finger(s)**

Q69.1 **Accessory thumb(s)**

Q69.2 **Accessory toe(s)**
Accessory hallux

Q69.9 **Polydactyly, unspecified**
Supernumerary digit(s) NOS

Figure 17-9 Thumb and index finger. (From Chung K: Hand and Upper Extremity Reconstruction, 1e, Saunders, 2008)

● Q70 **Syndactyly**
Webbing between distal phalanges of adjacent digits

● Q70.0 **Fused fingers**
Complex syndactyly of fingers with synostosis

Q70.00   Fused fingers, unspecified hand
Q70.01   Fused fingers, right hand
Q70.02   Fused fingers, left hand
Q70.03   Fused fingers, bilateral

● Q70.1 **Webbed fingers**
Simple syndactyly of fingers without synostosis

Q70.10   Webbed fingers, unspecified hand
Q70.11   Webbed fingers, right hand
Q70.12   Webbed fingers, left hand
Q70.13   Webbed fingers, bilateral

● Q70.2 **Fused toes**
Complex syndactyly of toes with synostosis

Q70.20   Fused toes, unspecified foot
Q70.21   Fused toes, right foot
Q70.22   Fused toes, left foot
Q70.23   Fused toes, bilateral

● Q70.3 **Webbed toes**
Simple syndactyly of toes without synostosis

Q70.30   Webbed toes, unspecified foot
Q70.31   Webbed toes, right foot
Q70.32   Webbed toes, left foot
Q70.33   Webbed toes, bilateral

Q70.4 **Polysyndactyly, unspecified**

> **Excludes1**   specified syndactyly of hand and feet - code to specified conditions (Q70.0- -Q70.3-)

Extra and webbed digits

Q70.9 **Syndactyly, unspecified**
Symphalangy NOS

● Q71 **Reduction defects of upper limb**

● Q71.0 **Congenital complete absence of upper limb**

Q71.00   Congenital complete absence of unspecified upper limb
Q71.01   Congenital complete absence of right upper limb
Q71.02   Congenital complete absence of left upper limb
Q71.03   Congenital complete absence of upper limb, bilateral

● Q71.1 **Congenital absence of upper arm and forearm with hand present**

Q71.10   Congenital absence of unspecified upper arm and forearm with hand present
Q71.11   Congenital absence of right upper arm and forearm with hand present
Q71.12   Congenital absence of left upper arm and forearm with hand present
Q71.13   Congenital absence of upper arm and forearm with hand present, bilateral

● Q71.2 **Congenital absence of both forearm and hand**

Q71.20   Congenital absence of both forearm and hand, unspecified upper limb
Q71.21   Congenital absence of both forearm and hand, right upper limb
Q71.22   Congenital absence of both forearm and hand, left upper limb
Q71.23   Congenital absence of both forearm and hand, bilateral

● Q71.3 **Congenital absence of hand and finger**

Q71.30   Congenital absence of unspecified hand and finger
Q71.31   Congenital absence of right hand and finger
Q71.32   Congenital absence of left hand and finger
Q71.33   Congenital absence of hand and finger, bilateral

● **Q71.4** Longitudinal reduction defect of radius
Clubhand (congenital)
Radial clubhand

     Q71.40 Longitudinal reduction defect of unspecified radius

     Q71.41 Longitudinal reduction defect of right radius

     Q71.42 Longitudinal reduction defect of left radius

     Q71.43 Longitudinal reduction defect of radius, bilateral

● **Q71.5** Longitudinal reduction defect of ulna

     Q71.50 Longitudinal reduction defect of unspecified ulna

     Q71.51 Longitudinal reduction defect of right ulna

     Q71.52 Longitudinal reduction defect of left ulna

     Q71.53 Longitudinal reduction defect of ulna, bilateral

● **Q71.6** Lobster-claw hand

     Q71.60 Lobster-claw hand, unspecified hand

     Q71.61 Lobster-claw right hand

     Q71.62 Lobster-claw left hand

     Q71.63 Lobster-claw hand, bilateral

● **Q71.8** Other reduction defects of upper limb

     ● **Q71.81** Congenital shortening of upper limb

         Q71.811 Congenital shortening of right upper limb

         Q71.812 Congenital shortening of left upper limb

         Q71.813 Congenital shortening of upper limb, bilateral

         Q71.819 Congenital shortening of unspecified upper limb

     ● **Q71.89** Other reduction defects of upper limb

         Q71.891 Other reduction defects of right upper limb

         Q71.892 Other reduction defects of left upper limb

         Q71.893 Other reduction defects of upper limb, bilateral

         Q71.899 Other reduction defects of unspecified upper limb

● **Q71.9** Unspecified reduction defect of upper limb

     Q71.90 Unspecified reduction defect of unspecified upper limb

     Q71.91 Unspecified reduction defect of right upper limb

     Q71.92 Unspecified reduction defect of left upper limb

     Q71.93 Unspecified reduction defect of upper limb, bilateral

● **Q72** Reduction defects of lower limb

     ● **Q72.0** Congenital complete absence of lower limb

     Q72.00 Congenital complete absence of unspecified lower limb

     Q72.01 Congenital complete absence of right lower limb

     Q72.02 Congenital complete absence of left lower limb

     Q72.03 Congenital complete absence of lower limb, bilateral

     ● **Q72.1** Congenital absence of thigh and lower leg with foot present

     Q72.10 Congenital absence of unspecified thigh and lower leg with foot present

     Q72.11 Congenital absence of right thigh and lower leg with foot present

     Q72.12 Congenital absence of left thigh and lower leg with foot present

     Q72.13 Congenital absence of thigh and lower leg with foot present, bilateral

     ● **Q72.2** Congenital absence of both lower leg and foot

     Q72.20 Congenital absence of both lower leg and foot, unspecified lower limb

     Q72.21 Congenital absence of both lower leg and foot, right lower limb

     Q72.22 Congenital absence of both left lower leg and foot, left lower limb

     Q72.23 Congenital absence of both lower leg and foot, bilateral

● **Q72.3** Congenital absence of foot and toe(s)

     Q72.30 Congenital absence of unspecified foot and toe(s)

     Q72.31 Congenital absence of right foot and toe(s)

     Q72.32 Congenital absence of left foot and toe(s)

     Q72.33 Congenital absence of foot and toe(s), bilateral

● **Q72.4** Longitudinal reduction defect of femur
Proximal femoral focal deficiency

     Q72.40 Longitudinal reduction defect of unspecified femur

     Q72.41 Longitudinal reduction defect of right femur

     Q72.42 Longitudinal reduction defect of left femur

     Q72.43 Longitudinal reduction defect of femur, bilateral

● **Q72.5** Longitudinal reduction defect of tibia

     Q72.50 Longitudinal reduction defect of unspecified tibia

     Q72.51 Longitudinal reduction defect of right tibia

     Q72.52 Longitudinal reduction defect of left tibia

     Q72.53 Longitudinal reduction defect of tibia, bilateral

● **Q72.6** Longitudinal reduction defect of fibula

     Q72.60 Longitudinal reduction defect of unspecified fibula

     Q72.61 Longitudinal reduction defect of right fibula

     Q72.62 Longitudinal reduction defect of left fibula

     Q72.63 Longitudinal reduction defect of fibula, bilateral

● **Q72.7** Split foot

     Q72.70 Split foot, unspecified lower limb

     Q72.71 Split foot, right lower limb

     Q72.72 Split foot, left lower limb

     Q72.73 Split foot, bilateral

● **Q72.8** Other reduction defects of lower limb

     ● **Q72.81** Congenital shortening of lower limb

         Q72.811 Congenital shortening of right lower limb

         Q72.812 Congenital shortening of left lower limb

         Q72.813 Congenital shortening of lower limb, bilateral

         Q72.819 Congenital shortening of unspecified lower limb

     ● **Q72.89** Other reduction defects of lower limb

         Q72.891 Other reduction defects of right lower limb

         Q72.892 Other reduction defects of left lower limb

         Q72.893 Other reduction defects of lower limb, bilateral

         Q72.899 Other reduction defects of unspecified lower limb

● **Q72.9** Unspecified reduction defect of lower limb

     Q72.90 Unspecified reduction defect of unspecified lower limb

     Q72.91 Unspecified reduction defect of right lower limb

     Q72.92 Unspecified reduction defect of left lower limb

     Q72.93 Unspecified reduction defect of lower limb, bilateral

● **Q73** Reduction defects of unspecified limb

     Q73.0 Congenital absence of unspecified limb(s)
Amelia NOS

     Q73.1 Phocomelia, unspecified limb(s)
Phocomelia NOS
Absence/shortening of long bones primarily as a result of thalidomide

▶ New   ⇒ Revised   ~~deleted~~ Deleted   Excludes 1   Excludes 2   Includes   Use additional   Code first   Code also   Key words

OGCR Official Guidelines   X Assign placeholder X   ● Use Additional Character(s)   ▌ Manifestation Code   ✎ Hierarchical Condition Category   **Coding Clinic**

Figure 17-10 Generalized craniosynostosis without symptoms or signs of increased intracranial pressure. (From Goetz C: Textbook of Clinical Neurology, St. Louis, MO, Elsevier, 2007)

Item 17–3 **Anencephalus** is a congenital deformity of the cranial vault. **Craniosynostosis,** also known as craniostenosis and stenocephaly, signifies any form of congenital deformity of the skull that results from the premature closing of the sutures of the skull. **Iniencephaly** is a deformity in which the head and neck are flexed backward to a great extent and the head is very large in comparison to the shortened body.

Q73.8   **Other reduction defects of unspecified limb(s)**
        Longitudinal reduction deformity of unspecified limb(s)
        Ectromelia of limb NOS
            Gross hypoplasia or aplasia of one or more long bones of
            limb(s)
        Hemimelia of limb NOS
            Absence of one-half of long bone
        Reduction defect of limb NOS

● Q74   **Other congenital malformations of limb(s)**
        Excludes1   polydactyly (Q69.-)
                        reduction defect of limb (Q71-Q73)
                        syndactyly (Q70.-)

Q74.0   **Other congenital malformations of upper limb(s), including shoulder girdle**
        Accessory carpal bones
        Cleidocranial dysostosis
        Congenital pseudarthrosis of clavicle
        Macrodactylia (fingers)
        Madelung's deformity
        Radioulnar synostosis
        Sprengel's deformity
        Triphalangeal thumb

Q74.1   **Congenital malformation of knee**
        Congenital absence of patella
        Congenital dislocation of patella
        Congenital genu valgum
        Congenital genu varum
        Rudimentary patella
        Excludes1   congenital dislocation of knee (Q68.2)
                        congenital genu recurvatum (Q68.2)
                        nail patella syndrome (Q87.2)

Q74.2   **Other congenital malformations of lower limb(s), including pelvic girdle**
        Congenital fusion of sacroiliac joint
        Congenital malformation of ankle joint
        Congenital malformation of sacroiliac joint
        Excludes1   anteversion of femur (neck) (Q65.89)

Q74.3   **Arthrogryposis multiplex congenita**
Q74.8   **Other specified congenital malformations of limb(s)**
Q74.9   **Unspecified congenital malformation of limb(s)**
        Congenital anomaly of limb(s) NOS

● Q75   **Other congenital malformations of skull and face bones**
        Excludes1   congenital malformation of face NOS (Q18.-)
                        congenital malformation syndromes classified to
                            Q87.-
                        dentofacial anomalies [including malocclusion]
                            (M26.-)
                        musculoskeletal deformities of head and face
                            (Q67.0-Q67.4)
                        skull defects associated with congenital
                            anomalies of brain such as:
                        anencephaly (Q00.0)
                        encephalocele (Q01.-)
                        hydrocephalus (Q03.-)
                        microcephaly (Q02)

● Q75.0   **Craniosynostosis**
          Premature closure of sutures of skull
  ● Q75.00   **Craniosynostosis unspecified**
             Craniosynostosis NOS
        Q75.001   **Craniosynostosis unspecified, unilateral**
        Q75.002   **Craniosynostosis unspecified, bilateral**
        Q75.009   **Craniosynostosis unspecified**
                  Imperfect fusion of skull
  ● Q75.01   **Sagittal craniosynostosis**
             Non-deformational dolichocephaly
             Non-deformational scaphocephaly
             Excludes1   plagiocephaly (Q67.3)
  ● Q75.02   **Coronal craniosynostosis**
             Non-deformational anterior plagiocephaly
             Excludes1   dolichocephaly (Q67.2)
        Q75.021   **Coronal craniosynostosis unilateral**
                  Non-deformational anterior
                  plagiocephaly
        Q75.022   **Coronal craniosynostosis bilateral**
                  Non-deformational brachycephaly
        Q75.029   **Coronal craniosynostosis unspecified**
  ● Q75.03   **Metopic craniosynostosis**
             Trigonocephaly
  ● Q75.04   **Lambdoid craniosynostosis**
             Non-deformational posterior plagiocephaly
             Excludes1   dolichocephaly (Q67.2)
        Q75.041   **Lambdoid craniosynostosis, unilateral**
        Q75.042   **Lambdoid craniosynostosis, bilateral**
        Q75.049   **Lambdoid craniosynostosis, unspecified**
  ● Q75.05   **Multi-suture craniosynostosis**
        Q75.051   **Cloverleaf skull**
                  Kleeblattschaedel skull
        Q75.052   **Pansynostosis**
        Q75.058   **Other multi-suture craniosynostosis**
                  Excludes1   coronal
                                  craniosynostosis,
                                  bilateral
                                  (Q75.022)
                                  lambdoid
                                  craniosynostosis,
                                  bilateral
                                  (Q75.042)

      Q75.08   **Other single-suture craniosynostosis**

Q75.1   **Craniofacial dysostosis**
        Congenital deformity of head
        Crouzon's disease

Q75.2   **Hypertelorism**

Q75.3   **Macrocephaly**
        Unusually large size of head; AKA megalocephaly

Q75.4   **Mandibulofacial dysostosis**
        Franceschetti syndrome
        Treacher Collins syndrome

Q75.5   **Oculomandibular dysostosis**
        Ossification of occular and mandibular bones

Q75.8   **Other specified congenital malformations of skull and face bones**
        Absence of skull bone, congenital
        Congenital deformity of forehead
        Platybasia

Q75.9   **Congenital malformation of skull and face bones, unspecified**
        Congenital anomaly of face bones NOS
        Congenital anomaly of skull NOS

● Q76   **Congenital malformations of spine and bony thorax**
        Excludes1   congenital musculoskeletal deformities of spine
                        and chest (Q67.5-Q67.8)

Q76.0   **Spina bifida occulta**
        Excludes1   meningocele (spinal) (Q05.-)
                        spina bifida (aperta) (cystica) (Q05.-)

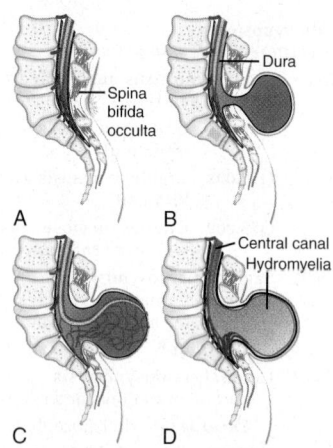

Figure 17-11 **A.** Spina bifida occulta. **B.** Meningocele.
C. Myelomeningocele. **D.** Myelocystocele (syringomyelocele)
or hydromyelia.

Item 17–4 **Spina bifida** is a midline spinal defect in which one or more vertebrae fail to fuse, leaving an opening in the vertebral canal. When the defect is not visible, it is called spina bifida occulta, and when it is visible, it is called spina bifida cystica.

Q76.1 **Klippel-Feil syndrome**
Cervical fusion syndrome

Q76.2 **Congenital spondylolisthesis**
Congenital spondylolysis
Excludes1 spondylolisthesis (acquired) (M43.1-)
spondylolysis (acquired) (M43.0-)

Q76.3 **Congenital scoliosis due to congenital bony malformation**
Hemivertebra fusion or failure of segmentation with scoliosis
Coding Clinic: 2022, Q4, P41

● **Q76.4** **Other congenital malformations of spine, not associated with scoliosis**

   ● **Q76.41** **Congenital kyphosis**
Abnormal increase in convexity curvature of thoracic spinal column; AKA humpback

      Q76.411 **Congenital kyphosis, occipito-atlanto-axial region**

      Q76.412 **Congenital kyphosis, cervical region**

      Q76.413 **Congenital kyphosis, cervicothoracic region**

      Q76.414 **Congenital kyphosis, thoracic region**

      Q76.415 **Congenital kyphosis, thoracolumbar region**

      Q76.419 **Congenital kyphosis, unspecified region**

   ● **Q76.42** **Congenital lordosis**
An abnormal increase in curvature of lumbar spine (sway back)

      Q76.425 **Congenital lordosis, thoracolumbar region**

      Q76.426 **Congenital lordosis, lumbar region**

      Q76.427 **Congenital lordosis, lumbosacral region**

      Q76.428 **Congenital lordosis, sacral and sacrococcygeal region**

      Q76.429 **Congenital lordosis, unspecified region**

Q76.49 **Other congenital malformations of spine, not associated with scoliosis**
Congenital absence of vertebra NOS
Congenital fusion of spine NOS
Congenital malformation of lumbosacral (joint) (region) NOS
Congenital malformation of spine NOS
Hemivertebra NOS
Malformation of spine NOS
Platyspondylisis NOS
Supernumerary vertebra NOS

Q76.5 **Cervical rib**
Supernumerary rib in cervical region

Q76.6 **Other congenital malformations of ribs**
Accessory rib
Congenital absence of rib
Congenital fusion of ribs
Congenital malformation of ribs NOS
Excludes1 short rib syndrome (Q77.2)

Q76.7 **Congenital malformation of sternum**
Congenital absence of sternum
Sternum bifidum

Q76.8 **Other congenital malformations of bony thorax**

Q76.9 **Congenital malformation of bony thorax, unspecified**

● **Q77** **Osteochondrodysplasia with defects of growth of tubular bones and spine**
Excludes1 mucopolysaccharidosis (E76.0-E76.3)
Excludes2 congenital myotonic chondrodystrophy (G71.13)

Q77.0 **Achondrogenesis**
Hypochondrogenesis

Q77.1 **Thanatophoric short stature**

Q77.2 **Short rib syndrome**
Asphyxiating thoracic dysplasia [Jeune]

Q77.3 **Chondrodysplasia punctata**
Benign cartilaginous neoplasms
Excludes1 rhizomelic chondrodysplasia punctata (E71.43)

Q77.4 **Achondroplasia**
Disturbance of epiphyseal chondroblastic growth and maturation, results in dwarfism
Hypochondroplasia
Osteosclerosis congenita

Q77.5 **Diastrophic dysplasia**

Q77.6 **Chondroectodermal dysplasia**
Defective development of skin, hair, teeth, with polydactyly and defect of cardiac septum
Ellis-van Creveld syndrome

Q77.7 **Spondyloepiphyseal dysplasia**

Q77.8 **Other osteochondrodysplasia with defects of growth of tubular bones and spine**

Q77.9 **Osteochondrodysplasia with defects of growth of tubular bones and spine, unspecified**

● **Q78** **Other osteochondrodysplasias**
Disorder of development of bone and cartilage; common cause of dwarfism
Excludes2 congenital myotonic chondrodystrophy (G71.13)

Q78.0 **Osteogenesis imperfecta**
Fragilitas ossium
Osteopsathyrosis

Q78.1 **Polyostotic fibrous dysplasia**
Albright(-McCune)(-Sternberg) syndrome

Q78.2 **Osteopetrosis**
Abnormally dense bone; AKA marble bones disease, ivory bones
Albers-Schönberg syndrome
Osteosclerosis NOS

Q78.3 **Progressive diaphyseal dysplasia**
Camurati-Engelmann syndrome

Q78.4 **Enchondromatosis**
Thinning of overlying cortex of bone and distorted length
Maffucci's syndrome
Ollier's disease

Q78.5 Metaphyseal dysplasia
Disturbance in enchondral bone growth, causing ends of shafts to remain larger than normal in circumference
Pyle's syndrome

Q78.6 Multiple congenital exostoses
Diaphyseal aclasis

Q78.8 Other specified osteochondrodysplasias
Osteopoikilosis

Q78.9 Osteochondrodysplasia, unspecified
Chondrodystrophy NOS
AKA skeletal dysplasia (dwarfism) caused by genetic mutations affecting hyaline cartilage capping long bones and vertebrae
Osteodystrophy NOS

● **Q79 Congenital malformations of musculoskeletal system, not elsewhere classified**
> **Excludes2** congenital (sternomastoid) torticollis (Q68.0)

Q79.0 Congenital diaphragmatic hernia
> **Excludes1** congenital hiatus hernia (Q40.1)

Q79.1 Other congenital malformations of diaphragm
Absence of diaphragm
Congenital malformation of diaphragm NOS
Eventration of diaphragm

Q79.2 Exomphalos
Abdominal hernia in which part of intestine protrudes at umbilicus; AKA exomphalos and exumbilication
Omphalocele
> **Excludes1** umbilical hernia (K42.-)

Q79.3 Gastroschisis
Congenital fissure of anterior abdominal wall often with protrusion of small/large intestine

Q79.4 Prune belly syndrome
Congenital prolapse of bladder mucosa
Eagle-Barrett syndrome

● **Q79.5 Other congenital malformations of abdominal wall**
> **Excludes1** umbilical hernia (K42.-)

Q79.51 Congenital hernia of bladder

Q79.59 Other congenital malformations of abdominal wall

● **Q79.6 Ehlers-Danlos syndromes**
Group of inherited disorders of connective tissue; AKA cutis hyperelastica

Q79.60 Ehlers-Danlos syndrome, unspecified

Q79.61 Classical Ehlers-Danlos syndrome
Classical EDS (cEDS)

Q79.62 Hypermobile Ehlers-Danlos syndrome
Hypermobile EDS (hEDS)

Q79.63 Vascular Ehlers-Danlos syndrome
Vascular EDS (vEDS)

Q79.69 Other Ehlers-Danlos syndromes

Q79.8 Other congenital malformations of musculoskeletal system
Absence of muscle
Absence of tendon
Accessory muscle
Amyotrophia congenita
Congenital constricting bands
Congenital shortening of tendon
Poland syndrome

Q79.9 Congenital malformation of musculoskeletal system, unspecified
Congenital anomaly of musculoskeletal system NOS
Congenital deformity of musculoskeletal system NOS

OTHER CONGENITAL MALFORMATIONS (Q80-Q89)

● **Q80 Congenital ichthyosis**
Characterized by increased keratinization, resulting in noninflammatory scaling of skin
> **Excludes1** Refsum's disease (G60.1)

Q80.0 Ichthyosis vulgaris

Q80.1 X-linked ichthyosis

Q80.2 Lamellar ichthyosis
Collodion baby

Q80.3 Congenital bullous ichthyosiform erythroderma

Q80.4 Harlequin fetus

Q80.8 Other congenital ichthyosis

Q80.9 Congenital ichthyosis, unspecified

● **Q81 Epidermolysis bullosa**
Loosening of epidermis

Q81.0 Epidermolysis bullosa simplex
> **Excludes1** Cockayne's syndrome (Q87.19)

Q81.1 Epidermolysis bullosa letalis
Herlitz' syndrome

Q81.2 Epidermolysis bullosa dystrophica

Q81.8 Other epidermolysis bullosa

Q81.9 Epidermolysis bullosa, unspecified

● **Q82 Other congenital malformations of skin**
> **Excludes1** acrodermatitis enteropathica (E83.2)
> congenital erythropoietic porphyria (E80.0)
> pilonidal cyst or sinus (L05.-)
> Sturge-Weber (-Dimitri) syndrome (Q85.89)

Q82.0 Hereditary lymphedema
Characterized by swelling of subcutaneous tissue caused by obstruction of lymphatic vessels and resulting edema of lymph fluid

Q82.1 Xeroderma pigmentosum
Extreme sensitivity to ultraviolet rays that most commonly affects the eyes and skin, but may also involve the nervous system

Q82.2 Congenital cutaneous mastocytosis
Characterized by infiltrates of mast cells in tissues/organs
Congenital diffuse cutaneous mastocytosis
Congenital maculopapular cutaneous mastocytosis
Congenital urticaria pigmentosa
> **Excludes1** cutaneous mastocytosis NOS (D47.01)
> diffuse cutaneous mastocytosis (with onset after newborn period) (D47.01)
> malignant mastocytosis (C96.2-)
> systemic mastocytosis (D47.02)
> urticaria pigmentosa (non-congenital) (with onset after newborn period) (D47.01)

Q82.3 Incontinentia pigmenti
Characterized by hypopigmented cutaneous in adults and early childhood

Q82.4 Ectodermal dysplasia (anhidrotic)
Absence/deficiency of tissues/structures, including teeth, hair, nails, and certain glands
> **Excludes1** Ellis-van Creveld syndrome (Q77.6)

Q82.5 Congenital non-neoplastic nevus
Birthmark NOS
Flammeus Nevus
Portwine Nevus
Sanguineous Nevus
Strawberry Nevus
Vascular Nevus NOS
Verrucous Nevus
> **Excludes2** Café au lait spots (L81.3)
> lentigo (L81.4)
> nevus NOS (D22.-)
> araneus nevus (I78.1)
> melanocytic nevus (D22.-)
> pigmented nevus (D22.-)
> spider nevus (I78.1)
> stellar nevus (I78.1)

Q82.6 Congenital sacral dimple
Parasacral dimple
> **Excludes2** pilonidal cyst with abscess (L05.01)
> pilonidal cyst without abscess (L05.91)
Coding Clinic: 2016, Q4, P60

CHAPTER 17 (Q00-Q99)

Q82.8   Other specified congenital malformations of skin
Abnormal palmar creases
Accessory skin tags
Benign familial pemphigus [Hailey-Hailey]
Congenital poikiloderma
Cutis laxa (hyperelastica)
Dermatoglyphic anomalies
Inherited keratosis palmaris et plantaris
Keratosis follicularis [Darier-White]
> **Excludes1**   Ehlers-Danlos syndromes (Q79.6-)
> Coding Clinic: 2016, Q1, P17

Q82.9   Congenital malformation of skin, unspecified

● **Q83   Congenital malformations of breast**
> **Excludes2**   absence of pectoral muscle (Q79.8)
> hypoplasia of breast (N64.82)
> micromastia (N64.82)

Q83.0   Congenital absence of breast with absent nipple

Q83.1   Accessory breast
Supernumerary breast

Q83.2   Absent nipple

Q83.3   Accessory nipple
Supernumerary nipple

Q83.8   Other congenital malformations of breast

Q83.9   Congenital malformation of breast, unspecified

● **Q84   Other congenital malformations of integument**

Q84.0   Congenital alopecia
Congenital atrichosis

Q84.1   Congenital morphological disturbances of hair, not elsewhere classified
Beaded hair
Monilethrix
Pili annulati
> **Excludes1**   Menkes' kinky hair syndrome (E83.09)

Q84.2   Other congenital malformations of hair
Congenital hypertrichosis
Congenital malformation of hair NOS
Persistent lanugo

Q84.3   Anonychia
Absence of nail
> **Excludes1**   nail patella syndrome (Q87.2)

Q84.4   Congenital leukonychia
Opaque, whitish discoloration of nails; AKA leukopathia unguium

Q84.5   Enlarged and hypertrophic nails
Congenital onychauxis
Pachyonychia

Q84.6   Other congenital malformations of nails
Congenital clubnail
Congenital koilonychia
Congenital malformation of nail NOS

Q84.8   Other specified congenital malformations of integument
Aplasia cutis congenita

Q84.9   Congenital malformation of integument, unspecified
Congenital anomaly of integument NOS
Congenital deformity of integument NOS

● **Q85   Phakomatoses, not elsewhere classified**
> **Excludes1**   ataxia telangiectasia [Louis-Bar] (G11.3)
> familial dysautonomia [Riley-Day] (G90.1)

● **Q85.0   Neurofibromatosis (nonmalignant)**
Developmental changes in nervous system and other structures, with formation of neurofibromas

Q85.00   Neurofibromatosis, unspecified 🅱

Q85.01   Neurofibromatosis, type 1 🅱
Von Recklinghausen disease

Q85.02   Neurofibromatosis, type 2 🅱
Acoustic neurofibromatosis

Q85.03   Schwannomatosis 🅱

Q85.09   Other neurofibromatosis 🅱

Q85.1   Tuberous sclerosis 🅱
Bourneville's disease
Epiloia

● **Q85.8   Other phakomatoses, not elsewhere classified** 🅱
> **Excludes1**   Meckel-Gruber syndrome (Q61.9)
> Coding Clinic: 2021, Q3, P12

Q85.81   PTEN hamartoma tumor syndrome
PHTS
PTEN related Cowden syndrome
> Code also, if applicable, genetic susceptibility to malignant neoplasm (Z15.0-)
> Coding Clinic: 2022, Q4, P41

Q85.82   Other Cowden syndrome

Q85.83   Von Hippel-Lindau syndrome
> Code also manifestations
> Coding Clinic: 2023, Q2, P16

Q85.89   Other phakomatoses, not elsewhere classified
Peutz-Jeghers syndrome
Sturge-Weber(-Dimitri) syndrome

Q85.9   Phakomatosis, unspecified 🅱
Hamartosis NOS

● **Q86   Congenital malformation syndromes due to known exogenous causes, not elsewhere classified**
> **Excludes2**   iodine-deficiency-related hypothyroidism (E00-E02)
> nonteratogenic effects of substances transmitted via placenta or breast milk (P04.-)

Q86.0   Fetal alcohol syndrome (dysmorphic)

Q86.1   Fetal hydantoin syndrome
Meadow's syndrome

Q86.2   Dysmorphism due to warfarin

Q86.8   Other congenital malformation syndromes due to known exogenous causes

● **Q87   Other specified congenital malformation syndromes affecting multiple systems**
> Use additional code(s) to identify all associated manifestations

Q87.0   Congenital malformation syndromes predominantly affecting facial appearance
Acrocephalopolysyndactyly
Acrocephalosyndactyly [Apert]
Cryptophthalmos syndrome
Cyclopia
Goldenhar syndrome
Moebius syndrome
Oro-facial-digital syndrome
Robin syndrome
Whistling face

● **Q87.1   Congenital malformation syndromes predominantly associated with short stature**

Q87.11   Prader-Willi syndrome

Q87.19   Other congenital malformation syndromes predominantly associated with short stature
Aarskog syndrome
Cockayne syndrome
De Lange syndrome
Dubowitz syndrome
Noonan syndrome
Robinow-Silverman-Smith syndrome
Russell-Silver syndrome
Seckel syndrome
> **Excludes1**   Ellis-van Creveld syndrome (Q77.6)
> Smith-Lemli-Opitz syndrome (E78.72)

Q87.2   Congenital malformation syndromes predominantly involving limbs
Holt-Oram syndrome
Klippel-Trenaunay-Weber syndrome
Nail patella syndrome
Rubinstein-Taybi syndrome
Sirenomelia syndrome
Thrombocytopenia with absent radius [TAR] syndrome
VATER syndrome

Q87.3 **Congenital malformation syndromes involving early overgrowth**
Beckwith-Wiedemann syndrome
Sotos' syndrome
Weaver syndrome

● **Q87.4** **Marfan's syndrome**

Q87.40 **Marfan's syndrome, unspecified**

● **Q87.41** **Marfan syndrome with cardiovascular manifestations**

Q87.410 **Marfan syndrome with aortic dilation**

Q87.418 **Marfan syndrome with other cardiovascular manifestations**

Q87.42 **Marfan syndrome with ocular manifestations**

Q87.43 **Marfan syndrome with skeletal manifestation**

Q87.5 **Other congenital malformation syndromes with other skeletal changes**

● **Q87.8** **Other specified congenital malformation syndromes, not elsewhere classified**

Excludes1 Zellweger syndrome (E71.510)

Q87.81 **Alport syndrome**
Progressive sensorineural hearing loss, progressive pyelonephritis or glomerulonephritis, and ocular defects
Use additional code to identify stage of chronic kidney disease (N18.1-N18.6)

Q87.82 **Arterial tortuosity syndrome**
Coding Clinic: 2016, Q4, P60-61

Q87.83 **Bardet-Biedl syndrome**

Q87.84 **Laurence-Moon syndrome**

Q87.85 **MED13L syndrome**
Asadollahi-Rauch syndrome
Mediator complex subunit 13L syndrome
Code also, if applicable, any associated manifestations such as:
autism spectrum disorder (F84.0-)
congenital malformations of cardiac septa (Q21.-)
epilepsy and recurrent seizures (G40.-)
intellectual disability (F70-F79)

▶ **Q87.86** **Kleefstra syndrome**

Q87.89 **Other specified congenital malformation syndromes, not elsewhere classified**

● **Q89** **Other congenital malformations, not elsewhere classified**

● **Q89.0** **Congenital absence and malformations of spleen**

Excludes1 isomerism of atrial appendages (with asplenia or polysplenia) (Q20.6)

Q89.01 **Asplenia (congenital)**

Q89.09 **Congenital malformations of spleen**
Congenital splenomegaly

Q89.1 **Congenital malformations of adrenal gland**

Excludes1 adrenogenital disorders (E25.-)
congenital adrenal hyperplasia (E25.0)

Q89.2 **Congenital malformations of other endocrine glands**
Congenital malformation of parathyroid or thyroid gland
Persistent thyroglossal duct
Thyroglossal cyst

Excludes1 congenital goiter (E03.0)
congenital hypothyroidism (E03.1)

Q89.3 **Situs inversus**
Lateral transposition of viscera of thorax and abdomen
Dextrocardia with situs inversus
Mirror-image atrial arrangement with situs inversus
Situs inversus or transversus abdominalis
Situs inversus or transversus thoracis
Transposition of abdominal viscera
Transposition of thoracic viscera

Excludes1 dextrocardia NOS (Q24.0)

Q89.4 **Conjoined twins**
Craniopagus
Dicephaly
Pygopagus
Thoracopagus

Q89.7 **Multiple congenital malformations, not elsewhere classified**
Multiple congenital anomalies NOS
Multiple congenital deformities NOS

Excludes1 congenital malformation syndromes affecting multiple systems (Q87.-)

Q89.8 **Other specified congenital malformations**
Use additional code(s) to identify all associated manifestations
Coding Clinic: 2021, Q3, P12

Q89.9 **Congenital malformation, unspecified**
Congenital anomaly NOS
Congenital deformity NOS

CHROMOSOMAL ABNORMALITIES, NOT ELSEWHERE CLASSIFIED (Q90-Q99)

Excludes2 mitochondrial metabolic disorders (E88.4-)

● **Q90** **Down syndrome**
Code also associated physical condition(s), such as atrioventricular septal defect (Q21.2-)
Use additional code(s) to identify any associated and degree of intellectual disabilities (F70-F79)

Q90.0 **Trisomy 21, nonmosaicism (meiotic nondisjunction)**
Trisomy 21, nondisjunction, accounts for 95% of Downs syndrome cases

Q90.1 **Trisomy 21, mosaicism (mitotic nondisjunction)**

Q90.2 **Trisomy 21, translocation**

Q90.9 **Down syndrome, unspecified**
Trisomy 21 NOS

● **Q91** **Trisomy 18 and Trisomy 13**

Q91.0 **Trisomy 18, nonmosaicism (meiotic nondisjunction)**

Q91.1 **Trisomy 18, mosaicism (mitotic nondisjunction)**

Q91.2 **Trisomy 18, translocation**

Q91.3 **Trisomy 18, unspecified**

Q91.4 **Trisomy 13, nonmosaicism (meiotic nondisjunction)**

Q91.5 **Trisomy 13, mosaicism (mitotic nondisjunction)**

Q91.6 **Trisomy 13, translocation**

Q91.7 **Trisomy 13, unspecified**

● **Q92** **Other trisomies and partial trisomies of the autosomes, not elsewhere classified**

Includes unbalanced translocations and insertions

Excludes1 trisomies of chromosomes 13, 18, 21 (Q90-Q91)

Q92.0 **Whole chromosome trisomy, nonmosaicism (meiotic nondisjunction)**

Q92.1 **Whole chromosome trisomy, mosaicism (mitotic nondisjunction)**

Q92.2 **Partial trisomy**
Less than whole arm duplicated
Whole arm or more duplicated

Excludes1 partial trisomy due to unbalanced translocation (Q92.5)

Q92.5 **Duplications with other complex rearrangements**
Partial trisomy due to unbalanced translocations
Code also any associated deletions due to unbalanced translocations, inversions and insertions (Q93.7)

● **Q92.6** **Marker chromosomes**
Trisomies due to dicentrics
Trisomies due to extra rings
Trisomies due to isochromosomes
Individual with marker heterochromatin

Q92.61 **Marker chromosomes in normal individual**

Q92.62 **Marker chromosomes in abnormal individual**

Q92.7 **Triploidy and polyploidy**

Q92.8 **Other specified trisomies and partial trisomies of autosomes**
Duplications identified by fluorescence in situ hybridization (FISH)
Duplications identified by in situ hybridization (ISH)
Duplications seen only at prometaphase

Q92.9 **Trisomy and partial trisomy of autosomes, unspecified**

● **Q93　Monosomies and deletions from the autosomes, not elsewhere classified**

Q93.0　Whole chromosome monosomy, nonmosaicism (meiotic nondisjunction)

Q93.1　Whole chromosome monosomy, mosaicism (mitotic nondisjunction)

Q93.2　Chromosome replaced with ring, dicentric or isochromosome

Q93.3　Deletion of short arm of chromosome 4
　　Wolff-Hirschorn syndrome

Q93.4　Deletion of short arm of chromosome 5
　　Cri-du-chat syndrome

● **Q93.5　Other deletions of part of a chromosome**

　　Q93.51　Angelman syndrome

　　Q93.52　Phelan-McDermid syndrome
　　　　22q13.3 deletion syndrome
　　　　Use additional code(s) to identify any associated conditions, such as:
　　　　　　autism spectrum disorder (F84.0)
　　　　　　degree of intellectual disabilities (F70-F79)
　　　　　　epilepsy and recurrent seizures (G40.-)
　　　　　　lymphedema (I89.0)

　　Q93.59　Other deletions of part of a chromosome

Q93.7　Deletions with other complex rearrangements
　　Deletions due to unbalanced translocations, inversions and insertions
　　Code also any associated duplications due to unbalanced translocations, inversions and insertions (Q92.5)

● **Q93.8　Other deletions from the autosomes**

　　Q93.81　Velo-cardio-facial syndrome
　　　　Deletion 22q11.2
　　　　Coding Clinic: 2019, Q3, P14

　　Q93.82　Williams syndrome

　　Q93.88　Other microdeletions Miller-Dieker syndrome
　　　　Smith-Magenis syndrome

　　Q93.89　Other deletions from the autosomes
　　　　Deletions identified by fluorescence in situ hybridization (FISH)
　　　　Deletions identified by in situ hybridization (ISH)
　　　　Deletions seen only at prometaphase

Q93.9　Deletion from autosomes, unspecified

● **Q95　Balanced rearrangements and structural markers, not elsewhere classified**

　　Includes　Robertsonian and balanced reciprocal translocations and insertions

Q95.0　Balanced translocation and insertion in normal individual

Q95.1　Chromosome inversion in normal individual

Q95.2　Balanced autosomal rearrangement in abnormal individual

Q95.3　Balanced sex/autosomal rearrangement in abnormal individual

Q95.5　Individual with autosomal fragile site

Q95.8　Other balanced rearrangements and structural markers

Q95.9　Balanced rearrangement and structural marker, unspecified

● **Q96　Turner's syndrome**
　Caused by missing or incomplete X chromosome affecting growth and sexual development

　　Excludes1　Noonan syndrome (Q87.19)

Q96.0　Karyotype 45, X

Q96.1　Karyotype 46, X iso (Xq)
　　Karyotype 46, isochromosome Xq

Q96.2　Karyotype 46, X with abnormal sex chromosome, except iso (Xq)
　　Karyotype 46, X with abnormal sex chromosome, except isochromosome Xq

Q96.3　Mosaicism, 45, X/46, XX or XY

Q96.4　Mosaicism, 45, X/other cell line(s) with abnormal sex chromosome

Q96.8　Other variants of Turner's syndrome

Q96.9　Turner's syndrome, unspecified

● **Q97　Other sex chromosome abnormalities, female phenotype, not elsewhere classified**

　　Excludes1　Turner's syndrome (Q96.-)

Q97.0　Karyotype 47, XXX

Q97.1　Female with more than three X chromosomes

Q97.2　Mosaicism, lines with various numbers of X chromosomes

Q97.3　Female with 46, XY karyotype

Q97.8　Other specified sex chromosome abnormalities, female phenotype

Q97.9　Sex chromosome abnormality, female phenotype, unspecified

● **Q98　Other sex chromosome abnormalities, male phenotype, not elsewhere classified**

Q98.0　Klinefelter syndrome karyotype 47, XXY

Q98.1　Klinefelter syndrome, male with more than two X chromosomes

Q98.3　Other male with 46, XX karyotype

Q98.4　Klinefelter syndrome, unspecified

Q98.5　Karyotype 47, XYY

Q98.6　Male with structurally abnormal sex chromosome

Q98.7　Male with sex chromosome mosaicism

Q98.8　Other specified sex chromosome abnormalities, male phenotype

Q98.9　Sex chromosome abnormality, male phenotype, unspecified

● **Q99　Other chromosome abnormalities, not elsewhere classified**

Q99.0　Chimera 46, XX/46, XY
　　Chimera 46, XX/46, XY true hermaphrodite

Q99.1　46, XX true hermaphrodite
　　46, XX with streak gonads
　　46, XY with streak gonads
　　Pure gonadal dysgenesis

Q99.2　Fragile X chromosome
　　Fragile X syndrome

Q99.8　Other specified chromosome abnormalities

Q99.9　Chromosomal abnormality, unspecified

CHAPTER 18

SYMPTOMS, SIGNS, AND ABNORMAL CLINICAL AND LABORATORY FINDINGS, NOT ELSEWHERE CLASSIFIED (R00-R99)

OGCR Chapter-Specific Coding Guidelines

18. **Chapter 18: Symptoms, signs, and abnormal clinical and laboratory findings, not elsewhere classified (R00-R99)**
Chapter 18 includes symptoms, signs, abnormal results of clinical or other investigative procedures, and ill-defined conditions regarding which no diagnosis classifiable elsewhere is recorded. Signs and symptoms that point to a specific diagnosis have been assigned to a category in other chapters of the classification.

a. Use of symptom codes
Codes that describe symptoms and signs are acceptable for reporting purposes when a related definitive diagnosis has not been established (confirmed) by the provider.

b. Use of a symptom code with a definitive diagnosis code
Codes for signs and symptoms may be reported in addition to a related definitive diagnosis when the sign or symptom is not routinely associated with that diagnosis, such as the various signs and symptoms associated with complex syndromes. The definitive diagnosis code should be sequenced before the symptom code.

Signs or symptoms that are associated routinely with a disease process should not be assigned as additional codes, unless otherwise instructed by the classification.

c. Combination codes that include symptoms
ICD-10-CM contains a number of combination codes that identify both the definitive diagnosis and common symptoms of that diagnosis. When using one of these combination codes, an additional code should not be assigned for the symptom.

d. Repeated falls
Code R29.6, Repeated falls, is for use for encounters when a patient has recently fallen and the reason for the fall is being investigated.

Code Z91.81, History of falling, is for use when a patient has fallen in the past and is at risk for future falls. When appropriate, both codes R29.6 and Z91.81 may be assigned together.

e. Coma scale
The coma scale codes (R40.2-) can be used in conjunction with traumatic brain injury codes, acute cerebrovascular disease or sequelae of cerebrovascular disease codes. These codes are primarily for use by trauma registries, but they may be used in any setting where this information is collected. The coma scale may also be used to assess the status of the central nervous system for other non-trauma conditions, such as monitoring patients in the intensive care unit regardless of medical condition. The coma scale codes should be sequenced after the diagnosis code(s).

These codes, one from each subcategory, are needed to complete the scale. The 7th character indicates when the scale was recorded. The 7th character should match for all three codes.

At a minimum, report the initial score documented on presentation at your facility. This may be a score from the emergency medicine technician (EMT) or in the emergency department. If desired, a facility may choose to capture multiple coma scale scores.

Assign code R40.24, Glasgow coma scale, total score, when only the total score is documented in the medical record and not the individual score(s).

Do not report codes for individual or total Glasgow coma scale scores for a patient with a medically induced coma or a sedated patient.

See Section I.B.14 for coma scale documentation by clinicians other than patient's provider.

f. Functional quadriplegia
GUIDELINE HAS BEEN DELETED EFFECTIVE OCTOBER 1, 2017

g. SIRS due to Non-Infectious Process
The systemic inflammatory response syndrome (SIRS) can develop as a result of certain non-infectious disease processes, such as trauma, malignant neoplasm, or pancreatitis. When SIRS is documented with a noninfectious condition, and no subsequent infection is documented, the code for the underlying condition, such as an injury, should be assigned, followed by code R65.10, Systemic inflammatory response syndrome (SIRS) of non-infectious origin without acute organ dysfunction, or code R65.11, Systemic inflammatory response syndrome (SIRS) of non-infectious origin with acute organ dysfunction. If an associated acute organ dysfunction is documented, the appropriate code(s) for the specific type of organ dysfunction(s) should be assigned in addition to code R65.11. If acute organ dysfunction is documented, but it cannot be determined if the acute organ dysfunction is associated with SIRS or due to another condition (e.g., directly due to the trauma), the provider should be queried.

h. Death NOS
Code R99, Ill-defined and unknown cause of mortality, is only for use in the very limited circumstance when a patient who has already died is brought into an emergency department or other healthcare facility and is pronounced dead upon arrival. It does not represent the discharge disposition of death.

i. NIHSS Stroke Scale
The NIH stroke scale (NIHSS) codes (R29.7- -) can be used in conjunction with acute stroke codes (I63) to identify the patient's neurological status and the severity of the stroke. The stroke scale codes should be sequenced after the acute stroke diagnosis code(s).

At a minimum, report the initial score documented. If desired, a facility may choose to capture multiple stroke scale scores.

See Section I.B.14 for NIHSS stroke scale documentation by clinicians other than patient's provider.

CHAPTER 18

SYMPTOMS, SIGNS, AND ABNORMAL CLINICAL AND LABORATORY FINDINGS, NOT ELSEWHERE CLASSIFIED (RØØ-R99)

Note: This chapter includes symptoms, signs, abnormal results of clinical or other investigative procedures, and ill-defined conditions regarding which no diagnosis classifiable elsewhere is recorded.

Signs and symptoms that point rather definitely to a given diagnosis have been assigned to a category in other chapters of the classification. In general, categories in this chapter include the less well-defined conditions and symptoms that, without the necessary study of the case to establish a final diagnosis, point perhaps equally to two or more diseases or to two or more systems of the body. Practically all categories in the chapter could be designated "not otherwise specified", "unknown etiology" or "transient". The Alphabetical Index should be consulted to determine which symptoms and signs are to be allocated here and which to other chapters. The residual subcategories, numbered .8, are generally provided for other relevant symptoms that cannot be allocated elsewhere in the classification.

The conditions and signs or symptoms included in categories RØØ-R94 consist of:
(a) cases for which no more specific diagnosis can be made even after all the facts bearing on the case have been investigated;
(b) signs or symptoms existing at the time of initial encounter that proved to be transient and whose causes could not be determined;
(c) provisional diagnosis in a patient who failed to return for further investigation or care;
(d) cases referred elsewhere for investigation or treatment before the diagnosis was made;
(e) cases in which a more precise diagnosis was not available for any other reason;
(f) certain symptoms, for which supplementary information is provided, that represent important problems in medical care in their own right.

> **Excludes2**   abnormal findings on antenatal screening of mother (O28.-)
> certain conditions originating in the perinatal period (PØ4-P96)
> signs and symptoms classified in the body system chapters
> signs and symptoms of breast (N63, N64.5)

This chapter contains the following blocks:

RØØ-RØ9	Symptoms and signs involving the circulatory and respiratory systems
R10-R19	Symptoms and signs involving the digestive system and abdomen
R20-R23	Symptoms and signs involving the skin and subcutaneous tissue
R25-R29	Symptoms and signs involving the nervous and musculoskeletal systems
R30-R39	Symptoms and signs involving the genitourinary system
R40-R46	Symptoms and signs involving cognition, perception, emotional state and behavior
R47-R49	Symptoms and signs involving speech and voice
R50-R69	General symptoms and signs
R70-R79	Abnormal findings on examination of blood, without diagnosis
R80-R82	Abnormal findings on examination of urine, without diagnosis
R83-R89	Abnormal findings on examination of other body fluids, substances and tissues, without diagnosis
R90-R94	Abnormal findings on diagnostic imaging and in function studies, without diagnosis
R97	Abnormal tumor markers
R99	Ill-defined and unknown cause of mortality

SYMPTOMS AND SIGNS INVOLVING THE CIRCULATORY AND RESPIRATORY SYSTEMS (RØØ-RØ9)

● **RØØ**   **Abnormalities of heart beat**

> **Excludes1**   abnormalities originating in the perinatal period (P29.1-)
> inappropriate sinus tachycardia, so stated (I47.11)

> **Excludes2**   specified arrhythmias (I47-I49)

RØØ.0   **Tachycardia, unspecified**
Rapid heart rate >100 beats
Rapid heart beat
Sinoauricular tachycardia NOS
Sinus [sinusal] tachycardia NOS

> **Excludes1**   neonatal tachycardia (P29.11)
> paroxysmal tachycardia (I47.-)

Coding Clinic: 2022, Q4, P47

RØØ.1   **Bradycardia, unspecified**
Slow heart rate, <60
Sinoatrial bradycardia
Sinus bradycardia
Slow heart beat
Vagal bradycardia

Use additional code for adverse effect, if applicable, to identify drug (T36-T50 with fifth or sixth character 5)

> **Excludes1**   neonatal bradycardia (P29.12)

RØØ.2   **Palpitations**
Awareness of heart beat

RØØ.8   **Other abnormalities of heart beat**

RØØ.9   **Unspecified abnormalities of heart beat**

▶ New   ⇒ Revised   ~~deleted~~ Deleted   Excludes 1   Excludes 2   Includes   Use additional   Code first   Code also   Key words
OGCR Official Guidelines   X Assign placeholder X   ● Use Additional Character(s)   ▶ Manifestation Code   🐾 Hierarchical Condition Category   Coding Clinic

● **R01**   **Cardiac murmurs and other cardiac sounds**

    Excludes1   cardiac murmurs and sounds originating in the perinatal period (P29.8)

   R01.0   **Benign and innocent cardiac murmurs**
        Functional cardiac murmur

   R01.1   **Cardiac murmur, unspecified**
        Cardiac bruit NOS
        Heart murmur NOS
        Systolic murmur NOS

   R01.2   **Other cardiac sounds**
        Cardiac dullness, increased or decreased
        Precordial friction

OGCR Section I.C.9.a.7.

Hypertension, Transient

Assign code R03.0, Elevated blood pressure reading without diagnosis of hypertension, unless patient has an established diagnosis of hypertension. Assign code O13.-, Gestational [pregnancy-induced] hypertension with significant proteinuria, or O14.-, Pre-eclampsia, for transient hypertension of pregnancy.

● **R03**   **Abnormal blood-pressure reading, without diagnosis**

   R03.0   **Elevated blood-pressure reading, without diagnosis of hypertension**
        Note: This category is to be used to record an episode of elevated blood pressure in a patient in whom no formal diagnosis of hypertension has been made, or as an isolated incidental finding.

   R03.1   **Nonspecific low blood-pressure reading**
      Excludes1   hypotension (I95.-)
           maternal hypotension syndrome (O26.5-)
           neurogenic orthostatic hypotension (G90.3)

● **R04**   **Hemorrhage from respiratory passages**

   R04.0   **Epistaxis**
        Hemorrhage from nose
        Nosebleed
        Coding Clinic: 2023, Q2, P28; 2018, Q4, P38

   R04.1   **Hemorrhage from throat**
      Excludes2   hemoptysis (R04.2)

   R04.2   **Hemoptysis**
        Blood-stained sputum
        Cough with hemorrhage

●   **R04.8**   **Hemorrhage from other sites in respiratory passages**

     R04.81   **Acute idiopathic pulmonary hemorrhage in infants**   P
           AIPHI
           Acute idiopathic hemorrhage in infants over 28 days old
        Excludes1   perinatal pulmonary hemorrhage (P26.-)
                von Willebrand's disease (D68.0-)

     R04.89   **Hemorrhage from other sites in respiratory passages**
           Pulmonary hemorrhage NOS

   R04.9   **Hemorrhage from respiratory passages, unspecified**

● **R05**   **Cough**

     Excludes1   paroxysmal cough due to Bordetella pertussis (A37.0-)
           smoker's cough (J41.0)

     Excludes2   cough with hemorrhage (R04.2))

   R05.1   **Acute cough**

   R05.2   **Subacute cough**

   R05.3   **Chronic cough**
        Persistent cough
        Refractory cough
        Unexplained cough

   R05.4   **Cough syncope**
        Code first syncope and collapse (R55)

   R05.8   **Other specified cough**

   R05.9   **Cough, unspecified**

● **R06**   **Abnormalities of breathing**

     Excludes1   acute respiratory distress syndrome (J80)
           respiratory arrest (R09.2)
           respiratory arrest of newborn (P28.81)
           respiratory distress syndrome of newborn (P22.-)
           respiratory failure (J96.-)
           respiratory failure of newborn (P28.5)

●   **R06.0**   **Dyspnea**
        Excludes1   tachypnea NOS (R06.82)
                transient tachypnea of newborn (P22.1)

     R06.00   **Dyspnea, unspecified**
           Coding Clinic: 2017, Q1, P26-27

     R06.01   **Orthopnea**

     R06.02   **Shortness of breath**

     R06.03   **Acute respiratory distress**

     R06.09   **Other forms of dyspnea**

   R06.1   **Stridor**
        Harsh, high-pitched breath sound
      Excludes1   congenital laryngeal stridor (P28.89)
           laryngismus (stridulus) (J38.5)

   R06.2   **Wheezing**
      Excludes1   Asthma (J45.-)
      Coding Clinic: 2016, Q2, P34

   R06.3   **Periodic breathing**
        Cheyne-Stokes breathing
        An abnormal pattern of breathing with gradually increasing and decreasing tidal volume with some periods of apnea

   R06.4   **Hyperventilation**
      Excludes1   psychogenic hyperventilation (F45.8)

   R06.5   **Mouth breathing**
      Excludes2   dry mouth NOS (R68.2)

   R06.6   **Hiccough**
      Excludes1   psychogenic hiccough (F45.8)

   R06.7   **Sneezing**

●   **R06.8**   **Other abnormalities of breathing**

     R06.81   **Apnea, not elsewhere classified**
           Apnea NOS
        Excludes1   apnea (of) newborn (P28.4-)
                sleep apnea (G47.3-)
                sleep apnea of newborn (primary) (P28.3-)

     R06.82   **Tachypnea, not elsewhere classified**
           Tachypnea NOS
        Excludes1   transitory tachypnea of newborn (P22.1)

     R06.83   **Snoring**

     R06.89   **Other abnormalities of breathing**
           Breath-holding (spells)
           Sighing

   R06.9   **Unspecified abnormalities of breathing**

● **R07**   **Pain in throat and chest**

     Excludes1   epidemic myalgia (B33.0)
     Excludes2   jaw pain R68.84
           pain in breast (N64.4)

   R07.0   **Pain in throat**
      Excludes1   chronic sore throat (J31.2)
           sore throat (acute) NOS (J02.9)
      Excludes2   dysphagia (R13.1-)
           pain in neck (M54.2)

   R07.1   **Chest pain on breathing**
        Painful respiration

   R07.2   **Precordial pain**

● **R07.8 Other chest pain**
    R07.81 Pleurodynia
        Pleurodynia NOS
        Excludes1 epidemic pleurodynia (B33.0)
    R07.82 Intercostal pain
    R07.89 Other chest pain
        Anterior chest-wall pain NOS
        Coding Clinic: 2021, Q1, P42
  R07.9 Chest pain, unspecified

● **R09 Other symptoms and signs involving the circulatory and respiratory system**
    Excludes1 acute respiratory distress syndrome (J80)
        respiratory arrest of newborn (P28.81)
        respiratory distress syndrome of newborn (P22.0)
        respiratory failure (J96.-)
        respiratory failure of newborn (P28.5)
● **R09.0 Asphyxia and hypoxemia**
    Excludes1 asphyxia due to carbon monoxide (T58.-)
        asphyxia due to foreign body in respiratory tract (T17.-)
        birth (intrauterine) asphyxia (P84)
        hyperventilation (R06.4)
        traumatic asphyxia (T71.-)
    Excludes2 hypercapnia (R06.89)
    R09.01 Asphyxia
    R09.02 Hypoxemia
        Coding Clinic: 2019, Q3, P15
  R09.1 Pleurisy
    Occurs when double membrane (pleura) lining chest cavity and lung surface becomes inflamed, causing sharp pain on inspiration/expiration
    Excludes1 pleurisy with effusion (J90)
  R09.2 Respiratory arrest 🦠
    Cardiorespiratory failure
    Excludes1 cardiac arrest (I46.-)
        respiratory arrest of newborn (P28.81)
        respiratory distress of newborn (P22.0)
        respiratory failure (J96.-)
        respiratory failure of newborn (P28.5)
        respiratory insufficiency (R06.89)
        respiratory insufficiency of newborn (P28.5)
  R09.3 Abnormal sputum
    Abnormal amount of sputum
    Abnormal color of sputum
    Abnormal odor of sputum
    Excessive sputum
    Excludes1 blood-stained sputum (R04.2)
● **R09.8 Other specified symptoms and signs involving the circulatory and respiratory systems**
    R09.81 Nasal congestion
    R09.82 Postnasal drip
    R09.89 Other specified symptoms and signs involving the circulatory and respiratory systems
        Bruit (arterial)
        Abnormal chest percussion
        Friction sounds in chest
        Chest tympany
        Choking sensation
        Rales
          Wet rattling, clicking, crackling sounds on auscultation
        Weak pulse
        Excludes2 foreign body in throat (T17.2-)
                  wheezing (R06.2)
        Coding Clinic: 2021, Q1, P42
● **R09.A Foreign body sensation of the circulatory and respiratory system**
    R09.A0 Foreign body sensation, unspecified
    R09.A1 Foreign body sensation, nose

    R09.A2 Foreign body sensation, throat
        Foreign body sensation globus
    R09.A9 Foreign body sensation, other site

SYMPTOMS AND SIGNS INVOLVING THE DIGESTIVE SYSTEM AND ABDOMEN (R10-R19)

Excludes2 congenital or infantile pylorospasm (Q40.0)
    gastrointestinal hemorrhage (K92.0-K92.2)
    intestinal obstruction (K56.-)
    newborn gastrointestinal hemorrhage (P54.0-P54.3)
    newborn intestinal obstruction (P76.-)
    pylorospasm (K31.3)
    signs and symptoms involving the urinary system (R30-R39)
    symptoms referable to female genital organs (N94.-)
    symptoms referable to male genital organs (N48-N50)

● **R10 Abdominal and pelvic pain**
    Excludes1 renal colic (N23)
    Excludes2 dorsalgia (M54.-)
        flatulence and related conditions (R14.-)
  R10.0 Acute abdomen
    Severe abdominal pain (generalized) (with abdominal rigidity)
    Excludes1 abdominal rigidity NOS (R19.3)
        generalized abdominal pain NOS (R10.84)
        localized abdominal pain (R10.1-R10.3-)
● **R10.1 Pain localized to upper abdomen**
    R10.10 Upper abdominal pain, unspecified
    R10.11 Right upper quadrant pain
    R10.12 Left upper quadrant pain
    R10.13 Epigastric pain
        Dyspepsia
        Excludes1 functional dyspepsia (K30)
  R10.2 Pelvic and perineal pain
    Excludes1 vulvodynia (N94.81)
● **R10.3 Pain localized to other parts of lower abdomen**
    R10.30 Lower abdominal pain, unspecified
    R10.31 Right lower quadrant pain
    R10.32 Left lower quadrant pain
    R10.33 Periumbilical pain
● **R10.8 Other abdominal pain**
  ● **R10.81 Abdominal tenderness**
    Abdominal tenderness NOS
    R10.811 Right upper quadrant abdominal tenderness
    R10.812 Left upper quadrant abdominal tenderness
    R10.813 Right lower quadrant abdominal tenderness
    R10.814 Left lower quadrant abdominal tenderness
    R10.815 Periumbilic abdominal tenderness
    R10.816 Epigastric abdominal tenderness
    R10.817 Generalized abdominal tenderness
    R10.819 Abdominal tenderness, unspecified site
  ● **R10.82 Rebound abdominal tenderness**
    R10.821 Right upper quadrant rebound abdominal tenderness
    R10.822 Left upper quadrant rebound abdominal tenderness
    R10.823 Right lower quadrant rebound abdominal tenderness
    R10.824 Left lower quadrant rebound abdominal tenderness
    R10.825 Periumbilic rebound abdominal tenderness

▶ New ⇒ Revised ~~deleted~~ Deleted Excludes 1 Excludes 2 Includes Use additional Code first Code also Key words

1162 OGCR Official Guidelines X Assign placeholder X ● Use Additional Character(s) ▷ Manifestation Code 🦠 Hierarchical Condition Category Coding Clinic

R10.826   **Epigastric rebound abdominal tenderness**

R10.827   **Generalized rebound abdominal tenderness**

R10.829   **Rebound abdominal tenderness, unspecified site**

R10.83   **Colic**   P
     Colic NOS
     Infantile colic
     Excludes1   colic in adult and child over 12 months old (R10.84)

R10.84   **Generalized abdominal pain**
     Excludes1   generalized abdominal pain associated with acute abdomen (R10.0)

R10.9   **Unspecified abdominal pain**

● **R11**   **Nausea and vomiting**
     Excludes1   cyclical vomiting associated with migraine (G43.A-)
         excessive vomiting in pregnancy (O21.-)
         hematemesis (K92.0)
         neonatal hematemesis (P54.0)
         newborn vomiting (P92.0-)
         psychogenic vomiting (F50.89)
         vomiting associated with bulimia nervosa (F50.2-)
         vomiting following gastrointestinal surgery (K91.0)
     Coding Clinic: 2017, Q1, P27

● R11.0   **Nausea**
     Nausea NOS
     Nausea without vomiting

● R11.1   **Vomiting**

R11.10   **Vomiting, unspecified**
     Vomiting NOS

R11.11   **Vomiting without nausea**

R11.12   **Projectile vomiting**

R11.13   **Vomiting of fecal matter**

R11.14   **Bilious vomiting**
     Bilious emesis

R11.15   **Cyclical vomiting syndrome unrelated to migraine**
     Cyclic vomiting syndrome NOS
     Persistent vomiting
     Excludes1   cyclical vomiting in migraine (G43.A-)
     Excludes2   bulimia nervosa (F50.20)
         diabetes mellitus due to underlying condition (E08.-)

R11.2   **Nausea with vomiting, unspecified**
     Persistent nausea with vomiting NOS
     Coding Clinic: 2020, Q1, P8

R12   **Heartburn**
     Excludes1   dyspepsia NOS (R10.13)
         functional dyspepsia (K30)

● **R13**   **Aphagia and dysphagia**

R13.0   **Aphagia**
     Inability to swallow
     Excludes1   psychogenic aphagia (F50.9)

● R13.1   **Dysphagia**
     Difficulty swallowing
     Code first, if applicable, dysphagia following cerebrovascular disease (I69. with final characters -91)
     Excludes1   psychogenic dysphagia (F45.8)

R13.10   **Dysphagia, unspecified**
     Difficulty in swallowing NOS

R13.11   **Dysphagia, oral phase**

R13.12   **Dysphagia, oropharyngeal phase**

R13.13   **Dysphagia, pharyngeal phase**

R13.14   **Dysphagia, pharyngoesophageal phase**

R13.19   **Other dysphagia**
     Cervical dysphagia
     Neurogenic dysphagia

● **R14**   **Flatulence and related conditions**
     Excludes1   psychogenic aerophagy (F45.8)

R14.0   **Abdominal distension (gaseous)**
     Bloating
     Tympanites (abdominal) (intestinal)

R14.1   **Gas pain**

R14.2   **Eructation**
     Belching air from stomach through mouth

R14.3   **Flatulence**

● **R15**   **Fecal incontinence**
     Includes   encopresis NOS
     Excludes1   fecal incontinence of nonorganic origin (F98.1)

R15.0   **Incomplete defecation**
     Excludes1   constipation (K59.0-)
         fecal impaction (K56.41)

R15.1   **Fecal smearing**
     Fecal soiling

R15.2   **Fecal urgency**

R15.9   **Full incontinence of feces**
     Fecal incontinence NOS

● **R16**   **Hepatomegaly and splenomegaly, not elsewhere classified**
     Enlargement of liver or spleen

R16.0   **Hepatomegaly, not elsewhere classified**
     Hepatomegaly NOS

R16.1   **Splenomegaly, not elsewhere classified**
     Splenomegaly NOS

R16.2   **Hepatomegaly with splenomegaly, not elsewhere classified**
     Hepatosplenomegaly NOS

R17   **Unspecified jaundice**
     Excludes1   neonatal jaundice (P55, P57-P59)

● **R18**   **Ascites**
     Includes   fluid in peritoneal cavity
     Excludes1   ascites in alcoholic cirrhosis (K70.31)
         ascites in alcoholic hepatitis (K70.11)
         ascites in toxic liver disease with chronic active hepatitis (K71.51)

R18.0   **Malignant ascites**
     Code first malignancy, such as:
         malignant neoplasm of ovary (C56.-)
         secondary malignant neoplasm of retroperitoneum and peritoneum (C78.6)

R18.8   **Other ascites**
     Ascites NOS
     Peritoneal effusion (chronic)
     Coding Clinic: 2018, Q1, P4

● **R19**   **Other symptoms and signs involving the digestive system and abdomen**
     Excludes1   acute abdomen (R10.0)

● R19.0   **Intra-abdominal and pelvic swelling, mass and lump**
     Excludes1   abdominal distension (gaseous) (R14.-)
         ascites (R18.-)

R19.00   **Intra-abdominal and pelvic swelling, mass and lump, unspecified site**

R19.01   **Right upper quadrant abdominal swelling, mass and lump**

R19.02   **Left upper quadrant abdominal swelling, mass and lump**

R19.03   **Right lower quadrant abdominal swelling, mass and lump**

R19.04   **Left lower quadrant abdominal swelling, mass and lump**

R19.05   **Periumbilic swelling, mass or lump**
     Diffuse or generalized umbilical swelling or mass

R19.06   **Epigastric swelling, mass or lump**

R19.07   **Generalized intra-abdominal and pelvic swelling, mass and lump**

CHAPTER 18 (R00-R99)

CHAPTER 18 (R00-R99)

Diffuse or generalized intra-abdominal swelling or mass NOS
Diffuse or generalized pelvic swelling or mass NOS

R19.09 **Other intra-abdominal and pelvic swelling, mass and lump**

● R19.1 **Abnormal bowel sounds**

R19.11 **Absent bowel sounds**

R19.12 **Hyperactive bowel sounds**

R19.15 **Other abnormal bowel sounds**
Abnormal bowel sounds NOS

R19.2 **Visible peristalsis**
Hyperperistalsis

● R19.3 **Abdominal rigidity**

Excludes1   abdominal rigidity with severe abdominal pain (R10.0)

R19.30 **Abdominal rigidity, unspecified site**

R19.31 **Right upper quadrant abdominal rigidity**

R19.32 **Left upper quadrant abdominal rigidity**

R19.33 **Right lower quadrant abdominal rigidity**

R19.34 **Left lower quadrant abdominal rigidity**

R19.35 **Periumbilic abdominal rigidity**

R19.36 **Epigastric abdominal rigidity**

R19.37 **Generalized abdominal rigidity**

R19.4 **Change in bowel habit**

Excludes1   constipation (K59.0-)
functional diarrhea (K59.1)

R19.5 **Other fecal abnormalities**
Abnormal stool color
Bulky stools
Mucus in stools
Occult blood in feces
Occult blood in stools

Excludes1   melena (K92.1)
neonatal melena (P54.1)
Coding Clinic: 2021, Q1, P10; 2019, Q1, P32

R19.6 **Halitosis**

R19.7 **Diarrhea, unspecified**
Diarrhea NOS

Excludes1   functional diarrhea (K59.1)
neonatal diarrhea (P78.3)
psychogenic diarrhea (F45.8)
Coding Clinic: 2021, Q3, P4

R19.8 **Other specified symptoms and signs involving the digestive system and abdomen**

SYMPTOMS AND SIGNS INVOLVING THE SKIN AND SUBCUTANEOUS TISSUE (R20-R23)

Excludes2   symptoms relating to breast (N64.4-N64.5)

● R20 **Disturbances of skin sensation**

Excludes1   dissociative anesthesia and sensory loss (F44.6)
psychogenic disturbances (F45.8)

R20.0 **Anesthesia of skin**
Loss of sensation

R20.1 **Hypoesthesia of skin**
Unpleasant abnormal sensation

R20.2 **Paresthesia of skin**
Abnormal touch sensation, including burning, prickling, often in absence of external stimulus
Formication   Tingling skin
Pins and needles

Excludes1   acroparesthesia (I73.8)

R20.3 **Hyperesthesia**

R20.8 **Other disturbances of skin sensation**

R20.9 **Unspecified disturbances of skin sensation**

R21 **Rash and other nonspecific skin eruption**

Includes   rash NOS

Excludes1   specified type of rash- code to condition
vesicular eruption (R23.8)

● R22 **Localized swelling, mass and lump of skin and subcutaneous tissue**

Includes   subcutaneous nodules (localized) (superficial)

Excludes1   abnormal findings on diagnostic imaging (R90-R93)
edema (R60.-)
enlarged lymph nodes (R59.-)
localized adiposity (E65)
swelling of joint (M25.4-)

R22.0 **Localized swelling, mass and lump, head**

R22.1 **Localized swelling, mass and lump, neck**

R22.2 **Localized swelling, mass and lump, trunk**

Excludes1   intra-abdominal or pelvic mass and lump (R19.0-)
intra-abdominal or pelvic swelling (R19.0-)

Excludes2   breast mass and lump (N63)
Coding Clinic: 2022, Q3, P8

● R22.3 **Localized swelling, mass and lump, upper limb**

R22.30 **Localized swelling, mass and lump, unspecified upper limb**

R22.31 **Localized swelling, mass and lump, right upper limb**

R22.32 **Localized swelling, mass and lump, left upper limb**

R22.33 **Localized swelling, mass and lump, upper limb, bilateral**

● R22.4 **Localized swelling, mass and lump, lower limb**

R22.40 **Localized swelling, mass and lump, unspecified lower limb**

R22.41 **Localized swelling, mass and lump, right lower limb**

R22.42 **Localized swelling, mass and lump, left lower limb**

R22.43 **Localized swelling, mass and lump, lower limb, bilateral**

R22.9 **Localized swelling, mass and lump, unspecified**

● R23 **Other skin changes**

R23.0 **Cyanosis**

Excludes1   acrocyanosis (I73.8)
cyanotic attacks of newborn (P28.2)

R23.1 **Pallor**
Clammy skin

R23.2 **Flushing**
Excessive blushing
Code first, if applicable, menopausal and female climacteric states (N95.1)

R23.3 **Spontaneous ecchymoses**
Small hemorrhagic spot of skin; AKA black and blue spot
Petechiae

Excludes1   ecchymoses of newborn (P54.5)
purpura (D69.-)

R23.4 **Changes in skin texture**
Desquamation of skin   Scaling of skin
Induration of skin

Excludes1   epidermal thickening NOS (L85.9)

R23.8 **Other skin changes**

R23.9 **Unspecified skin changes**

SYMPTOMS AND SIGNS INVOLVING THE NERVOUS AND MUSCULOSKELETAL SYSTEMS (R25-R29)

● R25 **Abnormal involuntary movements**

Excludes1   specific movement disorders (G20-G26)
stereotyped movement disorders (F98.4)
tic disorders (F95.-)

R25.0 **Abnormal head movements**

R25.1 **Tremor, unspecified**

Excludes1   chorea NOS (G25.5)
essential tremor (G25.0)
hysterical tremor (F44.4)
intention tremor (G25.2)

R25.2 **Cramp and spasm**

     Excludes2   carpopedal spasm (R29.0)
                   charley-horse (M62.831)
                   infantile spasms (G40.4-)
                   muscle spasm of back (M62.830)
                   muscle spasm of calf (M62.831)

R25.3 **Fasciculation**
     Twitching NOS

R25.8 **Other abnormal involuntary movements**

R25.9 **Unspecified abnormal involuntary movements**

● R26 **Abnormalities of gait and mobility**

     Excludes1   ataxia NOS (R27.0)
                   hereditary ataxia (G11.-)
                   locomotor (syphilitic) ataxia (A52.11)
                   immobility syndrome (paraplegic) (M62.3)

R26.0 **Ataxic gait**
     Staggering gait
     Coding Clinic: 2022, Q2, P12

R26.1 **Paralytic gait**
     Spastic gait

R26.2 **Difficulty in walking, not elsewhere classified**

     Excludes1   falling (R29.6)
                   unsteadiness on feet (R26.81)
     Coding Clinic: 2016, Q2, P7

● R26.8 **Other abnormalities of gait and mobility**

     R26.81   **Unsteadiness on feet**

     R26.89   **Other abnormalities of gait and mobility**

R26.9 **Unspecified abnormalities of gait and mobility**

● R27 **Other lack of coordination**

     Excludes1   ataxic gait (R26.0)
                   hereditary ataxia (G11.-)
                   vertigo NOS (R42)

R27.0 **Ataxia, unspecified**

     Excludes1   ataxia following cerebrovascular disease
                   (I69. with final characters -93)
     Coding Clinic: 2022, Q3, P10

R27.8 **Other lack of coordination**

R27.9 **Unspecified lack of coordination**

● R29 **Other symptoms and signs involving the nervous and musculoskeletal systems**

R29.0 **Tetany**
     Hyperexcitability of nerves and muscles characterized by spasm, twitching, and cramps
     Carpopedal spasm

     Excludes1   hysterical tetany (F44.5)
                   neonatal tetany (P71.3)
                   parathyroid tetany (E20.9)
                   post-thyroidectomy tetany (E89.2)

R29.1 **Meningismus**

R29.2 **Abnormal reflex**

     Excludes2   abnormal pupillary reflex (H57.0)
                   hyperactive gag reflex (J39.2)
                   vasovagal reaction or syncope (R55)

R29.3 **Abnormal posture**

R29.4 **Clicking hip**

     Excludes1   congenital deformities of hip (Q65.-)

R29.5 **Transient paralysis**
     Code first any associated spinal cord injury (S14.0, S14.1-, S24.0, S24.1-, S34.0-, S34.1-)

     Excludes1   transient ischemic attack (G45.9)

R29.6 **Repeated falls**
     Falling
     Tendency to fall

     Excludes2   at risk for falling (Z91.81)
                   history of falling (Z91.81)

OGCR Section I.C.18.d.

Repeated falls

Code R29.6, Repeated falls, is for use for encounters when a patient has recently fallen and the reason for the fall is being investigated.

Code Z91.81, History of falling, is for use when a patient has fallen in the past and is at risk for future falls. When appropriate, both codes R29.6 and Z91.81 may be assigned together.

Coding Clinic: 2016, Q2, P7

● R29.7 **National Institutes of Health Stroke Scale (NIHSS) score**
     Code first the type of cerebral infarction (I63.-)
     Coding Clinic: 2016, Q4, P61, 127

● R29.70   **NIHSS score 0-9**
     R29.700   **NIHSS score 0**
     R29.701   **NIHSS score 1**
     R29.702   **NIHSS score 2**
     R29.703   **NIHSS score 3**
     R29.704   **NIHSS score 4**
     R29.705   **NIHSS score 5**
     R29.706   **NIHSS score 6**
     R29.707   **NIHSS score 7**
     R29.708   **NIHSS score 8**
     R29.709   **NIHSS score 9**

● R29.71   **NIHSS score 10-19**
     R29.710   **NIHSS score 10**
     R29.711   **NIHSS score 11**
     R29.712   **NIHSS score 12**
     R29.713   **NIHSS score 13**
     R29.714   **NIHSS score 14**
     R29.715   **NIHSS score 15**
     R29.716   **NIHSS score 16**
     R29.717   **NIHSS score 17**
     R29.718   **NIHSS score 18**
     R29.719   **NIHSS score 19**

● R29.72   **NIHSS score 20-29**
     R29.720   **NIHSS score 20**
     R29.721   **NIHSS score 21**
     R29.722   **NIHSS score 22**
     R29.723   **NIHSS score 23**
     R29.724   **NIHSS score 24**
     R29.725   **NIHSS score 25**
     R29.726   **NIHSS score 26**
     R29.727   **NIHSS score 27**
     R29.728   **NIHSS score 28**
     R29.729   **NIHSS score 29**

OGCR Section I.C.18.i.

NIHSS Stroke Scale

The NIH stroke scale (NIHSS) codes (R29.7- -) can be used in conjunction with acute stroke codes (I63) to identify the patient's neurological status and the severity of the stroke. The stroke scale codes should be sequenced after the acute stroke diagnosis code(s).

At a minimum, report the initial score documented. If desired, a facility may choose to capture multiple stroke scale scores.

● R29.73   **NIHSS score 30-39**
     R29.730   **NIHSS score 30**
                 Coding Clinic: 2016, Q4, P62
     R29.731   **NIHSS score 31**
     R29.732   **NIHSS score 32**
     R29.733   **NIHSS score 33**
     R29.734   **NIHSS score 34**
     R29.735   **NIHSS score 35**
     R29.736   **NIHSS score 36**
     R29.737   **NIHSS score 37**
     R29.738   **NIHSS score 38**
     R29.739   **NIHSS score 39**

CHAPTER 18 (R00-R99)

● R29.74   **NIHSS score 40-42**
    R29.740   **NIHSS score 40**
    R29.741   **NIHSS score 41**
    R29.742   **NIHSS score 42**

● R29.8   **Other symptoms and signs involving the nervous and musculoskeletal systems**

   ● R29.81   **Other symptoms and signs involving the nervous system**

     R29.810   **Facial weakness**
       Facial droop

       Excludes1   Bell's palsy (G51.0)
         facial weakness following cerebrovascular disease (I69. with final characters -92)

       Coding Clinic: 2022, Q3, P9

     R29.818   **Other symptoms and signs involving the nervous system**

   ● R29.89   **Other symptoms and signs involving the musculoskeletal system**

       Excludes2   pain in limb (M79.6-)

     R29.890   **Loss of height**

       Excludes1   osteoporosis (M80-M81)

     R29.891   **Ocular torticollis**

       Excludes1   congenital (sterno-mastoid) torticollis Q68.0
         psychogenic torticollis (F45.8)
         spasmodic torticollis (G24.3)
         torticollis due to birth injury (P15.8)
         torticollis NOS M43.6

     R29.898   **Other symptoms and signs involving the musculoskeletal system**

● R29.9   **Unspecified symptoms and signs involving the nervous and musculoskeletal systems**

     R29.90   **Unspecified symptoms and signs involving the nervous system**

     R29.91   **Unspecified symptoms and signs involving the musculoskeletal system**

SYMPTOMS AND SIGNS INVOLVING THE GENITOURINARY SYSTEM (R30-R39)

● R30   **Pain associated with micturition**

   Excludes1   psychogenic pain associated with micturition (F45.8)

   R30.0   **Dysuria**
     Painful urination
     Strangury

   R30.1   **Vesical tenesmus**
     Straining to urinate, with sensation of a full bladder even when empty

   R30.9   **Painful micturition, unspecified**
     Painful urination NOS

● R31   **Hematuria**

   Excludes1   hematuria included with underlying conditions, such as:
     acute cystitis with hematuria (N30.01)
     recurrent and persistent hematuria in glomerular diseases (N02.-)

   R31.0   **Gross hematuria**
     Coding Clinic: 2017, Q1, P17

   R31.1   **Benign essential microscopic hematuria**

● R31.2   **Other microscopic hematuria**
     Coding Clinic: 2016, Q4, P62

     R31.21   **Asymptomatic microscopic hematuria**
       AMH

     R31.29   **Other microscopic hematuria**

   R31.9   **Hematuria, unspecified**
     Coding Clinic: 2017, Q1, P6

R32   **Unspecified urinary incontinence**
   Enuresis NOS

   Excludes1   functional urinary incontinence (R39.81)
     nonorganic enuresis (F98.0)
     stress incontinence and other specified urinary incontinence (N39.3-N39.4-)
     urinary incontinence associated with cognitive impairment (R39.81)
   Coding Clinic: 2021, Q4, P18

● R33   **Retention of urine**
   Excludes1   psychogenic retention of urine (F45.8)

   R33.0   **Drug induced retention of urine**
     Use additional code for adverse effect, if applicable, to identify drug (T36-T50 with fifth or sixth character 5)

   R33.8   **Other retention of urine**
     Code first, if applicable, any causal condition, such as:
     enlarged prostate (N40.1)
     Coding Clinic: 2018, Q4, P55

   R33.9   **Retention of urine, unspecified**

R34   **Anuria and oliguria**
   Excludes1   anuria and oliguria complicating abortion or ectopic or molar pregnancy (O00-O07, O08.4)
     anuria and oliguria complicating pregnancy (O26.83-)
     anuria and oliguria complicating the puerperium (O90.49)

● R35   **Polyuria**
   Passage of excessive volume of urine
   Code first, if applicable, any causal condition, such as:
   enlarged prostate (N40.1)
   Excludes1   psychogenic polyuria (F45.8)

   R35.0   **Frequency of micturition**
     Discharge or passage of urine; AKA uresis

   R35.1   **Nocturia**
     Urinary frequency at night

   ● R35.8   **Other polyuria**

     R35.81   **Nocturnal polyuria**
       Excludes2   nocturnal enuresis (N39.44)

     R35.89   **Other polyuria**
       Polyuria NOS

● R36   **Urethral discharge**

   R36.0   **Urethral discharge without blood**

   R36.1   **Hematospermia**
     Presence of blood in semen

   R36.9   **Urethral discharge, unspecified**
     Penile discharge NOS
     Urethrorrhea

R37   **Sexual dysfunction, unspecified**

● R39   **Other and unspecified symptoms and signs involving the genitourinary system**

   R39.0   **Extravasation of urine**
     Leakage, discharge

- **R39.1** **Other difficulties with micturition**
    Code first, if applicable, any causal condition, such as:
    enlarged prostate (N40.1)
    - R39.11 **Hesitancy of micturition**
    - R39.12 **Poor urinary stream**
        Weak urinary steam
    - R39.13 **Splitting of urinary stream**
    - R39.14 **Feeling of incomplete bladder emptying**
    - R39.15 **Urgency of urination**
        Excludes1 urge incontinence (N39.41, N39.46)
    - R39.16 **Straining to void**
    - **R39.19** **Other difficulties with micturition**
        Coding Clinic: 2016, Q4, P63
        - R39.191 **Need to immediately re-void**
        - R39.192 **Position dependent micturition**
        - R39.198 **Other difficulties with micturition**
- R39.2 **Extrarenal uremia**
    Prerenal uremia
    Excludes1 uremia NOS (N19)
- **R39.8** **Other symptoms and signs involving the genitourinary system**
    - R39.81 **Functional urinary incontinence**
        Urinary incontinence due to cognitive impairment, or severe physical disability or immobility
        Excludes1 stress incontinence and other specified urinary incontinence (N39.3-N39.4-) urinary incontinence NOS (R32)
    - R39.82 **Chronic bladder pain**
        Coding Clinic: 2016, Q4, P64
    - R39.83 **Unilateral non-palpable testicle**
    - R39.84 **Bilateral non-palpable testicles**
    - R39.89 **Other symptoms and signs involving the genitourinary system**
        Coding Clinic: 2016, Q4, P64
- R39.9 **Unspecified symptoms and signs involving the genitourinary system**

SYMPTOMS AND SIGNS INVOLVING COGNITION, PERCEPTION, EMOTIONAL STATE AND BEHAVIOR (R40-R46)

Excludes2 symptoms and signs constituting part of a pattern of mental disorder (F01-F99)
Coding Clinic: 2015, Q4, P40

- R40 **Somnolence, stupor and coma**
    Excludes1 neonatal coma (P91.5)
    somnolence, stupor and coma in diabetes (E08-E13)
    somnolence, stupor and coma in hepatic failure (K72.-)
    somnolence, stupor and coma in hypoglycemia (nondiabetic) (E15)
    - R40.0 **Somnolence**
        Drowsiness
        Excludes1 coma (R40.2-)
    - R40.1 **Stupor**
        Lowered level of consciousness
        Catatonic stupor
        Semicoma
        Excludes1 catatonic schizophrenia (F20.2)
        coma (R40.2-)
        depressive stupor (F31-F33)
        dissociative stupor (F44.2)
        manic stupor (F30.2)

- R40.2 **Coma**
    Code first any associated:
    fracture of skull (S02.-)
    intracranial injury (S06.-)
    Note: One code from each subcategory R40.21-R40-23 is required to complete the coma scale
    Coding Clinic: 2021, Q4, P112; 2016, Q4, P127
    - R40.20 **Unspecified coma**
        Coma NOS
        Unconsciousness NOS
        Coding Clinic: 2021, Q4, P112
    - R40.21 **Coma scale, eyes open**
        The following appropriate 7th character is to be added to subcategory R40.21-:

0	unspecified time
1	in the field [EMT or ambulance]
2	at arrival to emergency department
3	at hospital admission
4	24 hours or more after hospital admission

        Coding Clinic: 2021, Q4, P112; 2017, Q4, P25; 2015, Q2, P18
        - R40.211 **Coma scale, eyes open, never**
            Coma scale eye opening score of 1
        - R40.212 **Coma scale, eyes open, to pain**
            Coma scale eye opening score of 2
        - R40.213 **Coma scale, eyes open, to sound**
            Coma scale eye opening score of 3
        - R40.214 **Coma scale, eyes open, spontaneous**
            Coma scale eye opening score of 4
    - R40.22 **Coma scale, best verbal response**
        The following appropriate 7th character is to be added to subcategory R40.22-:

0	unspecified time
1	in the field [EMT or ambulance]
2	at arrival to emergency department
3	at hospital admission
4	24 hours or more after hospital admission

        Coding Clinic: 2021, Q4, P112; 2017, Q4, P25; 2015, Q2, P18
        - R40.221 **Coma scale, best verbal response, none**
            Coma scale verbal score of 1
        - R40.222 **Coma scale, best verbal response, incomprehensible words**
            Coma scale verbal score of 2
            Incomprehensible sounds (2-5 years of age)
            Moans/grunts to pain; restless (< 2 years old)

CHAPTER 18 (R00-R99)

● **R40.223**   **Coma scale, best verbal response, inappropriate words**
Coma scale verbal score of 3
Inappropriate crying or screaming (< 2 years of age)
Screaming (2-5 years of age)

● **R40.224**   **Coma scale, best verbal response, confused conversation**
Coma scale verbal score of 4
Inappropriate words (2-5 years of age)
Irritable cries (< 2 years of age)

● **R40.225**   **Coma scale, best verbal response, oriented**
Coma scale verbal score of 5
Cooing or babbling or crying appropriately (< 2 years of age)
Uses appropriate words (2- 5 years of age)

● **R40.23**   **Coma scale, best motor response**
The following appropriate 7th character is to be added to subcategory R40.23-:

0	unspecified time
1	in the field [EMT or ambulance]
2	at arrival to emergency department
3	at hospital admission
4	24 hours or more after hospital admission

Coding Clinic: 2017, Q4, P25; 2015, Q2, P18

● **R40.231**   **Coma scale, best motor response, none** 🐾
Coma scale motor score of 1

Glasgow Coma Scale

Eye Opening Response	
• Spontaneous--open with blinking at baseline	4 points
• To verbal stimuli, command, speech	3 points
• To pain only (not applied to face)	2 points
• No response	1 point
Verbal Response	
• Oriented	5 points
• Confused conversation, but able to answer questions	4 points
• Inappropriate words	3 points
• Incomprehensible speech	2 points
• No response	1 point
Motor Response	
• Obeys commands for movement	6 points
• Purposeful movement to painful stimulus	5 points
• Withdraws in response to pain	4 points
• Flexion in response to pain (decorticate posturing)	3 points
• Extension response in response to pain (decerebrate posturing)	2 points
• No response	1 point
Categorization:	
Coma: No eye opening, no ability to follow commands, no word verbalizations (3-8)	
Head Injury Classification:	
Severe Head Injury--GCS score of 8 or less	
Moderate Head Injury--GCS score of 9 to 12	
Mild head injury--GCS score of 13 to 15	
(Adapted from: Advanced Trauma Life Support: Course for Physicians, American College of Surgeons, 1993). http://www.bt.cdc.gov/masscasualtires/gscale.asp	

Figure 18-1

● **R40.232**   **Coma scale, best motor response, extension** 🐾
Abnormal extensor posturing to pain or noxious stimuli (< 2 years of age)
Coma scale motor score of 2
Extensor posturing to pain or noxious stimuli (2-5 years of age)

● **R40.233**   **Coma scale, best motor response, abnormal flexion**
Coma scale motor score of 3
Abnormal flexure posturing to pain or noxious stimuli (2-5 years of age)
Flexion/decorticate posturing (< 2 years of age)

● **R40.234**   **Coma scale, best motor response, flexion withdrawal** 🐾
Coma scale motor score of 4
Withdraws from pain or noxious stimuli (2-5 years of age)

● **R40.235**   **Coma scale, best motor response, localizes pain**
Coma scale motor score of 5
Localizes pain (2-5 years of age)
Withdraws to touch (< 2 years of age)

● **R40.236**   **Coma scale, best motor response, obeys commands**
Coma scale motor score of 6
Normal or spontaneous movement (< 2 years of age)
Obeys commands (2-5 years of age)

● **R40.24**   **Glasgow coma scale, total score**
Note: Assign a code from subcategory R40.24, when only the total coma score is documented
The following appropriate 7th character is to be added to subcategory R40.24-:

0	unspecified time
1	in the field [EMT or ambulance]
2	at arrival to emergency department
3	at hospital admission
4	24 hours or more after hospital admission

Coding Clinic: 2016, Q4, P64; 2015, Q2, P18

● **R40.241**   **Glasgow coma scale score 13-15**
● **R40.242**   **Glasgow coma scale score 9-12**
● **R40.243**   **Glasgow coma scale score 3-8** 🐾
● **R40.244**   **Other coma, without documented Glasgow coma scale score, or with partial score reported** 🐾

R40.2A   **Nontraumatic coma due to underlying condition**
Secondary coma
Code first underlying condition
Coding Clinic: 2023, Q4, P42

R40.3   **Persistent vegetative state** 🐾
R40.4   **Transient alteration of awareness**

● **R41**   **Other symptoms and signs involving cognitive functions and awareness**
Excludes1   dissociative [conversion] disorders (F44.-)
mild cognitive impairment, of uncertain or unknown etiology (G31.84)

R41.0   **Disorientation, unspecified**
Confusion NOS   Delirium NOS
▶ **Excludes1**   delirium due to known physiological condition (F05)
Coding Clinic: 2022, Q2, P11; 2019, Q2, P34; 2016, Q4, P71

R41.1   **Anterograde amnesia**
R41.2   **Retrograde amnesia**

▶ New   ⇒ Revised   ~~deleted~~ Deleted   Excludes 1   Excludes 2   Includes   Use additional   Code first   Code also   Key words
OGCR Official Guidelines   X Assign placeholder X   ● Use Additional Character(s)   ▶ Manifestation Code   🐾 Hierarchical Condition Category   Coding Clinic

R41.3 **Other amnesia**
    Amnesia NOS
    Memory loss NOS
    Excludes1 amnestic disorder due to known
                      physiologic condition (F04)
                    amnestic syndrome due to psychoactive
                      substance use (F10-F19 with 5th
                      character .6)
                    mild memory disturbance due to known
                      physiological condition (F06.8)
                    transient global amnesia (G45.4)

R41.4 **Neurologic neglect syndrome**
    Asomatognosia   Left-sided neglect
    Hemi-akinesia   Sensory neglect
    Hemi-inattention   Visuospatial neglect
    Hemispatial neglect
    Excludes1 visuospatial deficit (R41.842)

● **R41.8** **Other symptoms and signs involving cognitive
    functions and awareness**
    R41.81 **Age-related cognitive decline**   A
          Senility NOS
    R41.82 **Altered mental status, unspecified**
          Change in mental status NOS
          Excludes1 altered level of consciousness
                     (R40.-)
                  altered mental status due to
                     known condition - code to
                     condition
                  delirium NOS (R41.0)
          Coding Clinic: 2012, Q4, P98
    R41.83 **Borderline intellectual functioning**
          IQ level 71 to 84
          Excludes1 intellectual disabilities (F70-F79)
    ● **R41.84** **Other specified cognitive deficit**
          ▶ *Code first the underlying condition, if known, such*
            as:
          ▶ schizophrenia (F20.-)
          Excludes1 cognitive deficits as sequelae
                     of cerebrovascular disease
                     (I69.01-, I69.11-, I69.21-,
                     I69.31-, I69.81-, I69.91-)
        R41.840 **Attention and concentration deficit**
             Excludes1 attention-deficit
                     hyperactivity
                     disorders (F90.-)
        R41.841 **Cognitive communication deficit**
        R41.842 **Visuospatial deficit**
        R41.843 **Psychomotor deficit**
        R41.844 **Frontal lobe and executive function
            deficit**
    ▶ **R41.85** **Anosognosia**
    R41.89 **Other symptoms and signs involving cognitive
          functions and awareness**
          ~~Anosognosia~~

R41.9 **Unspecified symptoms and signs involving cognitive
    functions and awareness**
    Unspecified neurocognitive disorder

R42 **Dizziness and giddiness**
    Light-headedness
    Vertigo NOS
    Excludes1 vertiginous syndromes (H81.-)
                  vertigo from infrasound (T75.23)
    Coding Clinic: 2015, Q4, P40

● **R43** **Disturbances of smell and taste**
    R43.0 **Anosmia**
          *Absence of sense of smell; AKA anosphresia and olfactory
            anesthesia*
    R43.1 **Parosmia**
    R43.2 **Parageusia**
          *Perversion of sense of taste or bad taste in mouth; AKA
            dysgeusia*

R43.8 **Other disturbances of smell and taste**
    Mixed disturbance of smell and taste
R43.9 **Unspecified disturbances of smell and taste**

● **R44** **Other symptoms and signs involving general sensations and
    perceptions**
    Excludes1 alcoholic hallucinations (F10.151, F10.251, F10.951)
                hallucinations in drug psychosis (F11-F19 with
                    fifth to sixth characters 51)
                hallucinations in mood disorders with psychotic
                    symptoms (F30.2, F31.5, F32.3, F33.3)
                hallucinations in schizophrenia, schizotypal and
                    delusional disorders (F20-F29)
    Excludes2 disturbances of skin sensation (R20.-)
    R44.0 **Auditory hallucinations**
    R44.1 **Visual hallucinations**
    R44.2 **Other hallucinations**
    R44.3 **Hallucinations, unspecified**
          Coding Clinic: 2022, Q2, P11
    R44.8 **Other symptoms and signs involving general sensations
          and perceptions**
    R44.9 **Unspecified symptoms and signs involving general
          sensations and perceptions**

● **R45** **Symptoms and signs involving emotional state**
    R45.0 **Nervousness**
          Nervous tension
    R45.1 **Restlessness and agitation**
    R45.2 **Unhappiness**
    R45.3 **Demoralization and apathy**
          Excludes1 anhedonia (R45.84)
    R45.4 **Irritability and anger**
    R45.5 **Hostility**
    R45.6 **Violent behavior**
    R45.7 **State of emotional shock and stress, unspecified**
  ● **R45.8** **Other symptoms and signs involving emotional state**
        R45.81 **Low self-esteem**
        R45.82 **Worries**
        R45.83 **Excessive crying of child, adolescent or adult**
             Excludes1 excessive crying of infant (baby)
                     R68.11
        R45.84 **Anhedonia**
          Total loss of feeling of pleasure in pleasurable acts
      ● **R45.85** **Homicidal and suicidal ideations**
          Excludes1 suicide attempt (T14.91)
          R45.850 **Homicidal ideations**
          R45.851 **Suicidal ideations**
             Coding Clinic: 2022, Q1, P29
        R45.86 **Emotional lability**
        R45.87 **Impulsiveness**
        R45.88 **Nonsuicidal self-harm**
          Nonsuicidal self-injury
          Nonsuicidal self-mutilation
          Self-inflicted injury without suicidal intent
          Code also injury, if known
          Coding Clinic: 2021, Q4, P27
        R45.89 **Other symptoms and signs involving emotional
          state**
          Flat affect
          Loneliness

● **R46** **Symptoms and signs involving appearance and behavior**
    Excludes1 appearance and behavior in schizophrenia,
                schizotypal and delusional disorders
                (F20-F29)
             mental and behavioral disorders (F01-F99)
    R46.0 **Very low level of personal hygiene**
    R46.1 **Bizarre personal appearance**
    R46.2 **Strange and inexplicable behavior**
    R46.3 **Overactivity**
    R46.4 **Slowness and poor responsiveness**
          Excludes1 stupor (R40.1)

CHAPTER 18 (R00-R99)

R46.5   Suspiciousness and marked evasiveness

R46.6   Undue concern and preoccupation with stressful events

R46.7   Verbosity and circumstantial detail obscuring reason for contact

● R46.8   Other symptoms and signs involving appearance and behavior

     R46.81   Obsessive-compulsive behavior

         Excludes1   obsessive-compulsive disorder (F42.-)

     R46.89   Other symptoms and signs involving appearance and behavior

SYMPTOMS AND SIGNS INVOLVING SPEECH AND VOICE (R47-R49)

● R47   Speech disturbances, not elsewhere classified

     Excludes1   autism (F84.0)

         cluttering (F80.81)

         specific developmental disorders of speech and language (F80.-)

         stuttering (F80.81)

● R47.0   Dysphasia and aphasia

     R47.01   Aphasia

         Excludes1   aphasia following cerebrovascular disease (I69. with final characters -20)

         progressive isolated aphasia (G31.01)

         Coding Clinic: 2022, Q3, P9

     R47.02   Dysphasia

         Impairment in comprehension of speech, caused by left-sided brain damage

         Excludes1   dysphasia following cerebrovascular disease (I69. with final characters -21)

R47.1   Dysarthria and anarthria

     Motor speech disorder

     Excludes1   dysarthria following cerebrovascular disease (I69. with final characters -22)

     Coding Clinic: 2022, Q3, P9

● R47.8   Other speech disturbances

     Excludes1   dysarthria following cerebrovascular disease (I69. with final characters -28)

     R47.81   Slurred speech

     ▷ R47.82   *Fluency disorder in conditions classified elsewhere*

         Stuttering in conditions classified elsewhere

         Code first underlying disease or condition, such as: Parkinson's disease (G20.-)

         Excludes1   adult onset fluency disorder (F98.5)

         childhood onset fluency disorder (F80.81)

         fluency disorder (stuttering) following cerebrovascular disease (I69. with final characters -23)

     R47.89   Other speech disturbances

R47.9   Unspecified speech disturbances

● R48   Dyslexia and other symbolic dysfunctions, not elsewhere classified

     Excludes1   specific developmental disorders of scholastic skills (F81.-)

R48.0   Dyslexia and alexia

R48.1   Agnosia

     Loss of ability to recognize objects, persons, sounds, shapes, or smells

     Astereognosia (astereognosis)

     Autotopagnosia

     Excludes1   visual object agnosia (R48.3)

R48.2   Apraxia

     Loss of ability to execute or carry out learned purposeful movements

     Excludes1   apraxia following cerebrovascular disease (I69. with final characters -90)

R48.3   Visual agnosia

     Prosopagnosia

     Simultanagnosia (asimultagnosia)

R48.8   Other symbolic dysfunctions

     Acalculia

     Difficulty performing simple mathematical tasks resulting from neurological injury

     Agraphia

     Coding Clinic: 2017, Q1, P27

R48.9   Unspecified symbolic dysfunctions

● R49   Voice and resonance disorders

     Excludes1   psychogenic voice and resonance disorders (F44.4)

R49.0   Dysphonia

     Hoarseness

R49.1   Aphonia

     Loss of voice

● R49.2   Hypernasality and hyponasality

     R49.21   Hypernasality

     R49.22   Hyponasality

R49.8   Other voice and resonance disorders

R49.9   Unspecified voice and resonance disorder

     Change in voice NOS

     Resonance disorder NOS

GENERAL SYMPTOMS AND SIGNS (R50-R69)

● R50   Fever of other and unknown origin

     Excludes1   chills without fever (R68.83)

         febrile convulsions (R56.0-)

         fever of unknown origin during labor (O75.2)

         fever of unknown origin in newborn (P81.9)

         hypothermia due to illness (R68.0)

         malignant hyperthermia due to anesthesia (T88.3)

         puerperal pyrexia NOS (O86.4)

R50.2   Drug induced fever

     Use additional code for adverse effect, if applicable, to identify drug (T36-T50 with fifth or sixth character 5)

     Excludes1   postvaccination (postimmunization) fever (R50.83)

● R50.8   Other specified fever

     ▷ R50.81   *Fever presenting with conditions classified elsewhere*

         Code first underlying condition when associated fever is present, such as with:

         leukemia (C91-C95)

         neutropenia (D70.-)

         sickle-cell disease (D57.)

         Coding Clinic: 2023, Q4, P7; 2019, Q2, P25

     R50.82   Postprocedural fever

         Excludes1   postprocedural infection (T81.44)

         posttransfusion fever (R50.84)

         postvaccination (postimmunization) fever (R50.83)

     R50.83   Postvaccination fever

         Postimmunization fever

     R50.84   Febrile nonhemolytic transfusion reaction

         FNHTR

         Posttransfusion fever

▶ New   ⇒ Revised   ~~deleted~~ Deleted   Excludes 1   Excludes 2   Includes   Use additional   Code first   Code also   Key words

OGCR Official Guidelines   X Assign placeholder X   ● Use Additional Character(s)   ▷ Manifestation Code   🦺 Hierarchical Condition Category   Coding Clinic

R50.9   **Fever, unspecified**
     Fever NOS
     Fever of unknown origin [FUO]
     Fever with chills
     Fever with rigors
     Hyperpyrexia NOS
     Persistent fever
     Pyrexia NOS

●R51   Headache
     Excludes2   atypical face pain (G50.1)
               migraine and other headache syndromes
                  (G43-G44)
               trigeminal neuralgia (G50.0)

R51.0   **Headache with orthostatic component, not elsewhere classified**
     Headache with positional component, not elsewhere classified

R51.9   Headache, unspecified
     Facial pain NOS

R52   **Pain, unspecified**
     Acute pain NOS
     Generalized pain NOS
     Excludes1   acute and chronic pain, not elsewhere classified
               (G89.-)
               localized pain, unspecified type - code to pain by
                  site, such as:
                  abdomen pain (R10.-)
                  back pain (M54.9)
                  breast pain (N64.4)
                  chest pain (R07.1-R07.9)
                  ear pain (H92.0-)
                  eye pain (H57.1)
                  headache (R51.9)
                  joint pain (M25.5-)
                  limb pain (M79.6-)
                  lumbar region pain (M54.5-)
                  pelvic and perineal pain (R10.2)
                  shoulder pain (M25.51-)
                  spine pain (M54.-)
                  throat pain (R07.0)
                  tongue pain (K14.6)
                  tooth pain (K08.8)
                  renal colic (N23)
               pain disorders exclusively related to
                  psychological factors (F45.41)

●R53   Malaise and fatigue
R53.0   **Neoplastic (malignant) related fatigue**
     Code first associated neoplasm

R53.1   **Weakness**
     Asthenia NOS
     Excludes1   age-related weakness (R54)
               muscle weakness (generalized) (M62.81)
               sarcopenia (M62.84)
               senile asthenia (R54)
     Coding Clinic: 2021, Q4, P103; 2017, Q1, P7

R53.2   **Functional quadriplegia** 🔖
     Complete immobility due to severe physical disability
     or frailty
     Excludes1   frailty NOS (R54)
               hysterical paralysis (F44.4)
               immobility syndrome (M62.3)
               neurologic quadriplegia (G82.5-)
               quadriplegia (G82.50)
     Coding Clinic: 2022, Q4, P15; 2016, Q2, P6

●R53.8   Other malaise and fatigue
     Excludes1   combat exhaustion and fatigue (F43.0)
               congenital debility (P96.9)
               exhaustion and fatigue due to excessive
                  exertion (T73.3)
               exhaustion and fatigue due to exposure
                  (T73.2)
               exhaustion and fatigue due to heat (T67.-)
               exhaustion and fatigue due to pregnancy
                  (O26.8-)
               exhaustion and fatigue due to recurrent
                  depressive episode (F33)
               exhaustion and fatigue due to senile
                  debility (R54)

R53.81   **Other malaise**
     Chronic debility
     Debility NOS
     General physical deterioration
     Malaise NOS
     Nervous debility
     Excludes1   age-related physical debility
               (R54)
     Coding Clinic: 2021, Q1, P43

R53.82   **Chronic fatigue, unspecified**
     Excludes1   chronic fatigue syndrome
                  (G93.32)
                 myalgic encephalomyelitis
                  (G93.32)
                 other post infection and related
                  fatigue syndromes (G93.39)
                 postviral fatigue syndrome
                  (G93.31)

R53.83   **Other fatigue**
     Fatigue NOS   Lethargy
     Lack of energy   Tiredness
     Excludes2   exhaustion and fatigue due to
                  depressive episode (F32.-)
     Coding Clinic: 2017, Q1, P7

R54   **Age-related physical debility**   A
     Frailty   Senile asthenia
     Old age   Senile debility
     Senescence
     Excludes1   age-related cognitive decline (R41.81)
               sarcopenia (M62.84)
               senile psychosis (F03.-)
               senility NOS (R41.81)

R55   **Syncope and collapse**
     Blackout
     Fainting
     Vasovagal attack
     Excludes1   cardiogenic shock (R57.0)
               carotid sinus syncope (G90.01)
               heat syncope (T67.1)
               neurocirculatory asthenia (F45.8)
               neurogenic orthostatic hypotension (G90.3)
               orthostatic hypotension (I95.1)
               postprocedural shock (T81.1-)
               psychogenic syncope (F48.8)
               shock NOS (R57.9)
               shock complicating or following abortion or
                  ectopic or molar pregnancy (O00-O07, O08.3)
               shock complicating or following labor and
                  delivery (O75.1)
               Stokes-Adams attack (I45.9)
               unconsciousness NOS (R40.2-)

●R56   Convulsions, not elsewhere classified
     Excludes1   dissociative convulsions and seizures (F44.5)
               epileptic convulsions and seizures (G40.-)
               newborn convulsions and seizures (P90)

●R56.0   Febrile convulsions
R56.00   **Simple febrile convulsions** 🔖
     Febrile convulsion NOS
     Febrile seizure NOS

CHAPTER 18 (R00-R99)

R56.01 **Complex febrile convulsions** 🐾
 Atypical febrile seizure
 Complex febrile seizure
 Complicated febrile seizure
 Excludes1 status epilepticus (G40.901)

R56.1 **Post traumatic seizures** 🐾
 Excludes1 post traumatic epilepsy (G40.-)

R56.9 **Unspecified convulsions** 🐾
 Convulsion disorder Recurrent convulsions
 Fit NOS   Seizure(s) (convulsive) NOS
 Coding Clinic: 2022, Q4, P46; 2021, Q1, P3; 2019, Q4, P18

● **R57** **Shock, not elsewhere classified**
 Excludes1 anaphylactic shock NOS (T78.2)
  anaphylactic reaction or shock due to adverse
   food reaction (T78.0-)
  anaphylactic shock due to adverse effect of
   correct drug or medicament properly
   administered (T88.6)
  anaphylactic shock due to serum (T80.5-)
  electric shock (T75.4)
  obstetric shock (O75.1)
  postprocedural shock (T81.1-)
  psychic shock (F43.0)
  shock complicating or following ectopic or molar
   pregnancy (O00-O07, O08.3)
  shock due to anesthesia (T88.2)
  shock due to lightning (T75.01)
  traumatic shock (T79.4)
  toxic shock syndrome (A48.3)

R57.0 **Cardiogenic shock** 🐾
 Excludes2 septic shock (R65.21)

R57.1 **Hypovolemic shock** 🐾
 Decreased blood volume (loss)
 Coding Clinic: 2019, Q2, P7-8

R57.8 **Other shock** 🐾

R57.9 **Shock, unspecified** 🐾
 Failure of peripheral circulation NOS
 Resulting in significant blood pressure drop

R58 **Hemorrhage, not elsewhere classified**
 Hemorrhage NOS
 Excludes1 hemorrhage included with underlying
   conditions, such as:
   acute duodenal ulcer with hemorrhage (K26.0)
   acute gastritis with bleeding (K29.01)
   ulcerative enterocolitis with rectal bleeding
    (K51.01)

● **R59** **Enlarged lymph nodes**
 Includes swollen glands
 Excludes1 lymphadenitis NOS (I88.9)
  acute lymphadenitis (L04.-)
  chronic lymphadenitis (I88.1)
  mesenteric (acute) (chronic) lymphadenitis (I88.0)

R59.0 **Localized enlarged lymph nodes**

R59.1 **Generalized enlarged lymph nodes**
 Lymphadenopathy NOS

R59.9 **Enlarged lymph nodes, unspecified**

● **R60** **Edema, not elsewhere classified**
 Excludes1 angioneurotic edema (T78.3)
  ascites (R18.-)
  cerebral edema (G93.6)
  cerebral edema due to birth injury (P11.0)
  edema of larynx (J38.4)
  edema of nasopharynx (J39.2)
  edema of pharynx (J39.2)
  gestational edema (O12.0-)
  hereditary edema (Q82.0)
  hydrops fetalis NOS (P83.2)
  hydrothorax (J94.8)
  hydrops fetalis NOS (P83.2)
  newborn edema (P83.3)
  pulmonary edema (J81.-)

R60.0 **Localized edema**

R60.1 **Generalized edema**
 Excludes2 nutritional edema (E40-E46)

R60.9 **Edema, unspecified**
 Fluid retention NOS

R61 **Generalized hyperhidrosis**
 Excessive sweating
 Night sweats
 Secondary hyperhidrosis
 Code first, if applicable, menopausal and female climacteric states
  (N95.1)
 Excludes1 focal (primary) (secondary) hyperhidrosis
   (L74.5-)
  Frey's syndrome (L74.52)
  localized (primary) (secondary) hyperhidrosis
   (L74.5-)

● **R62** **Lack of expected normal physiological development in childhood and adults**
 Excludes1 delayed puberty (E30.0)
  gonadal dysgenesis (Q99.1)
  hypopituitarism (E23.0)

R62.0 **Delayed milestone in childhood**   P
 Delayed attainment of expected physiological
  developmental stage
 Late talker
 Late walker

● **R62.5** **Other and unspecified lack of expected normal physiological development in childhood**
 Excludes1 HIV disease resulting in failure to thrive
   (B20)
  physical retardation due to malnutrition
   (E45)

R62.50 **Unspecified lack of expected normal physiological development in childhood**
 Infantilism NOS

R62.51 **Failure to thrive (child)**   P
 Failure to gain weight
 Excludes1 failure to thrive in child under 28
   days old (P92.6)
 Coding Clinic: 2018, Q4, P82

R62.52 **Short stature (child)**
 Lack of growth   Short stature NOS
 Physical retardation
 Excludes1 short stature due to endocrine
   disorder (E34.3-)

R62.59 **Other lack of expected normal physiological development in childhood**

R62.7 **Adult failure to thrive**   A

● **R63** **Symptoms and signs concerning food and fluid intake**
 Excludes1 bulimia NOS (F50.2-)

R63.0 **Anorexia**
 Loss of appetite
 Excludes1 anorexia nervosa (F50.0-)
  loss of appetite of nonorganic origin
   (F50.89)

R63.1 **Polydipsia**
 Excessive thirst

R63.2 **Polyphagia**
 Excessive eating   Hyperalimentation NOS

● **R63.3** **Feeding difficulties**
 Excludes2 eating disorders (F50.-)
  feeding problems of newborn (P92.-)
  infant feeding disorder of nonorganic
   origin (F98.2-)

R63.30 **Feeding difficulties, unspecified**   P

▶ New ⬧ Revised ~~deleted~~ Deleted Excludes 1 Excludes 2 Includes Use additional Code first Code also Key words
OGCR Official Guidelines X Assign placeholder X ● Use Additional Character(s) ▶ Manifestation Code 🐾 Hierarchical Condition Category Coding Clinic

R63.31   **Pediatric feeding disorder, acute**
     Pediatric feeding dysfunction, acute
       Code also, if applicable, associated conditions
         such as:
       aspiration pneumonia (J69.0)
       dysphagia (R13.1-)
       gastro-esophageal reflux disease (K21.-)
       malnutrition (E40-E46)

R63.32   **Pediatric feeding disorder, chronic**   P
     Pediatric feeding dysfunction, chronic
       Code also, if applicable, associated conditions
         such as:
       aspiration pneumonia (J69.0)
       dysphagia (R13.1-)
       gastro-esophageal reflux disease (K21.-)
       malnutrition (E40-E46)

R63.39   **Other feeding difficulties**
     Feeding problem (elderly) (infant) NOS
     Picky eater
     Coding Clinic: 2017, Q1, P27; 2016, Q3, P19

R63.4   **Abnormal weight loss**

R63.5   **Abnormal weight gain**
     Excludes1   excessive weight gain in pregnancy
                (O26.0-)
                obesity (E66.-)

R63.6   **Underweight**
     Use additional code to identify body mass index (BMI),
       if known (Z68.-)
     Excludes1   abnormal weight loss (R63.4)
                anorexia nervosa (F50.0-)
                malnutrition (E40-E46)

R63.8   **Other symptoms and signs concerning food and fluid
intake**

R64   **Cachexia** 🔊
     Excludes1   abnormal weight loss (R63.4)
                cachexia due to underlying condition (E88.A)
                nutritional marasmus (E41)
     Coding Clinic: 2017, Q3, P25

● R65   **Symptoms and signs specifically associated with systemic
inflammation and infection**

   ● R65.1   **Systemic inflammatory response syndrome (SIRS) of
non-infectious origin**
       Code first underlying condition, such as:
         heatstroke (T67.0-)
         injury and trauma (S00-T88)
       Excludes1   sepsis - code to infection
                  severe sepsis (R65.2)
       Coding Clinic: 2019, Q2, P38

     R65.10   **Systemic inflammatory response syndrome
(SIRS) of non-infectious origin without acute
organ dysfunction** 🔊
         Systemic inflammatory response syndrome
           (SIRS) NOS
         Coding Clinic: 2019, Q2, P25, 38

     R65.11   **Systemic inflammatory response syndrome
(SIRS) of non-infectious origin with acute
organ dysfunction** 🔊
         Use additional code to identify specific acute
           organ dysfunction, such as:
         acute kidney failure (N17.-)
         acute respiratory failure (J96.0-)
         critical illness myopathy (G72.81)
         critical illness polyneuropathy (G62.81)
         disseminated intravascular coagulopathy
          [DIC] (D65)
         encephalopathy (metabolic) (septic) (G93.41)
         hepatic failure (K72.0-)

OGCR Section I.C.18.g.

SIRS due to Non-Infectious Process
The systemic inflammatory response syndrome (SIRS) can develop as a result of certain non-infectious disease processes, such as trauma, malignant neoplasm, or pancreatitis. When SIRS is documented with a noninfectious condition, and no subsequent infection is documented, the code for the underlying condition, such as an injury, should be assigned, followed by code R65.10, Systemic inflammatory response syndrome (SIRS) of non-infectious origin without acute organ dysfunction, or code R65.11, Systemic inflammatory response syndrome (SIRS) of non-infectious origin with acute organ dysfunction. If an associated acute organ dysfunction is documented, the appropriate code(s) for the specific type of organ dysfunction(s) should be assigned in addition to code R65.11. If acute organ dysfunction is documented, but it cannot be determined if the acute organ dysfunction is associated with SIRS or due to another condition (e.g., directly due to the trauma), the provider should be queried.

● R65.2   **Severe sepsis**
     Infection with associated acute organ dysfunction
     Sepsis with acute organ dysfunction
     Sepsis with multiple organ dysfunction
     Systemic inflammatory response syndrome due to
       infectious process with acute organ dysfunction
     Code first underlying infection, such as:
       infection following a procedure (T81.44)
       infections following infusion, transfusion and
         therapeutic injection (T80.2-)
       puerperal sepsis (O85)
       sepsis following complete or unspecified
         spontaneous abortion (O03.87)
       sepsis following ectopic and molar pregnancy
         (O08.82)
       sepsis following incomplete spontaneous abortion
         (O03.37)
       sepsis following (induced) termination of pregnancy
         (O04.87)
       sepsis NOS (A41.9)
     Use additional code to identify specific acute organ
       dysfunction, such as:
       acute kidney failure (N17.-)
       acute respiratory failure (J96.0-)
       critical illness myopathy (G72.81)
       critical illness polyneuropathy (G62.81)
       disseminated intravascular coagulopathy [DIC] (D65)
       encephalopathy (metabolic) (septic) (G93.41)
       hepatic failure (K72.0-)
     Coding Clinic: 2017, Q4, P99; 2016, Q3, P8

     R65.20   **Severe sepsis without septic shock** 🔊
         Severe sepsis NOS
         Coding Clinic: 2019, Q1, P14; 2018, Q4, P90; 2016, Q3, P14

     R65.21   **Severe sepsis with septic shock** 🔊

● R68   **Other general symptoms and signs**

     R68.0   **Hypothermia, not associated with low environmental
temperature**
       Excludes1   hypothermia NOS (accidental) (T68)
                  hypothermia due to anesthesia (T88.51)
                  hypothermia due to low environmental
                    temperature (T68)
                  newborn hypothermia (P80.-)

   ● R68.1   **Nonspecific symptoms peculiar to infancy**
       Excludes1   colic, infantile (R10.83)
                  neonatal cerebral irritability (P91.3)
                  teething syndrome (K00.7)

     R68.11   **Excessive crying of infant (baby)**   P
         Excludes1   excessive crying of child,
                    adolescent, or adult (R45.83)

     R68.12   **Fussy infant (baby)**   P
         Irritable infant

CHAPTER 18 (R00-R99)

R68.13 **Apparent life threatening event in infant (ALTE)** P
Apparent life threatening event in newborn
Brief resolved unexplained event (BRUE)
Code first confirmed diagnosis, if known
Use additional code(s) for associated signs
and symptoms if no confirmed diagnosis
established, or if signs and symptoms are
not associated routinely with confirmed
diagnosis, or provide additional
information for cause of ALTE

R68.19 **Other nonspecific symptoms peculiar to infancy**
P

R68.2 **Dry mouth, unspecified**

Excludes1 dry mouth due to dehydration (E86.0)
dry mouth due to Sjögren syndrome
(M35.0-)
~~salivary gland hyposecretion (K11.7)~~

▶ Excludes2 salivary gland hyposecretion (K11.7)

R68.3 **Clubbing of fingers**
Clubbing of nails

Excludes1 congenital clubfinger (Q68.1)

● R68.8 **Other general symptoms and signs**

R68.81 **Early satiety**

R68.82 **Decreased libido**   A
Decreased sexual desire

R68.83 **Chills (without fever)**
Chills NOS

Excludes1 chills with fever (R50.9)

R68.84 **Jaw pain**
Mandibular pain
Maxilla pain

Excludes1 temporomandibular joint
arthralgia (M26.62-)

R68.89 **Other general symptoms and signs**

R69 **Illness, unspecified**
Unknown and unspecified cases of morbidity

ABNORMAL FINDINGS ON EXAMINATION OF BLOOD, WITHOUT DIAGNOSIS (R70-R79)

Excludes2 abnormal findings on antenatal screening of
mother (O28.-)
abnormalities of lipids (E78.-)
abnormalities of platelets and thrombocytes
(D69.-)
abnormalities of white blood cells classified
elsewhere (D70-D72)
coagulation hemorrhagic disorders (D65-D68)
diagnostic abnormal findings classified
elsewhere —*see* Alphabetical Index
hemorrhagic and hematological disorders of
newborn (P50-P61)

● R70 **Elevated erythrocyte sedimentation rate and abnormality of
plasma viscosity**

R70.0 **Elevated erythrocyte sedimentation rate**

R70.1 **Abnormal plasma viscosity**

● R71 **Abnormality of red blood cells**

Excludes1 anemias (D50-D64)
anemia of premature infant (P61.2)
benign (familial) polycythemia (D75.0)
congenital anemias (P61.2-P61.4)
newborn anemia due to isoimmunization (P55.-)
polycythemia neonatorum (P61.1)
polycythemia NOS (D75.1)
polycythemia vera (D45)
secondary polycythemia (D75.1)

R71.0 **Precipitous drop in hematocrit**
Drop (precipitous) in hemoglobin
Drop in hematocrit
Blood volume that has decreased red blood cells

R71.8 **Other abnormality of red blood cells**
Abnormal red-cell morphology NOS
Abnormal red-cell volume NOS
Anisocytosis
Red blood cells of unequal size
Poikilocytosis
Red blood cells of abnormal shape

● R73 **Elevated blood glucose level**

Excludes1 diabetes mellitus (E08-E13)
diabetes mellitus in pregnancy, childbirth and the
puerperium (O24.-)
neonatal disorders (P70.0-P70.2)
postsurgical hypoinsulinemia (E89.1)

● R73.0 **Abnormal glucose**

Excludes1 abnormal glucose in pregnancy (O99.81-)
diabetes mellitus (E08-E13)
dysmetabolic syndrome X (E88.81-)
gestational diabetes (O24.4-)
glycosuria (R81)
hypoglycemia (E16.2)
▶type 1 diabetes mellitus, presymptomatic
(E10.A-)

R73.01 **Impaired fasting glucose**
Elevated fasting glucose

R73.02 **Impaired glucose tolerance (oral)**
Elevated glucose tolerance

R73.03 **Prediabetes**
Latent diabetes
Coding Clinic: 2016, Q4, P65

R73.09 **Other abnormal glucose**
Abnormal glucose NOS
Abnormal non-fasting glucose tolerance
Coding Clinic: 2016, Q4, P65

R73.9 **Hyperglycemia, unspecified**

● R74 **Abnormal serum enzyme levels**

● R74.0 **Nonspecific elevation of levels of transaminase and
lactic acid dehydrogenase [LDH]**

R74.01 **Elevation of levels of liver transaminase levels**
Elevation of levels of alanine transaminase
(ALT)
Elevation of levels of aspartate transaminase
(AST)

R74.02 **Elevation of levels of lactic acid dehydrogenase
[LDH]**

R74.8 **Abnormal levels of other serum enzymes**
Abnormal level of acid phosphatase
Abnormal level of alkaline phosphatase
Abnormal level of amylase
Abnormal level of lipase [triacylglycerol lipase]
Coding Clinic: 2019, Q2, P6

R74.9 **Abnormal serum enzyme level, unspecified**

R75 **Inconclusive laboratory evidence of human immunodeficiency
virus [HIV]**
Nonconclusive HIV-test finding in infants

Excludes1 asymptomatic human immunodeficiency virus
[HIV] infection status (Z21)
human immunodeficiency virus [HIV] disease
(B20)

▶ New   ⇒ Revised   ~~deleted~~ Deleted   Excludes 1   Excludes 2   Includes   Use additional   Code first   Code also   Key words
OGCR Official Guidelines   X Assign placeholder X   ● Use Additional Character(s)   ▶ Manifestation Code   🔒 Hierarchical Condition Category   Coding Clinic

● **R76   Other abnormal immunological findings in serum**

　R76.0   Raised antibody titer

　　Excludes1　isoimmunization in pregnancy
　　　　　　　　　(O36.0-O36.1)
　　　　　　　　isoimmunization affecting newborn (P55.-)
　　Coding Clinic: 2021, Q1, P7

● **R76.1   Nonspecific reaction to test for tuberculosis**

　**R76.11   Nonspecific reaction to tuberculin skin test
　　　　　　without active tuberculosis**
　　　　Abnormal result of Mantoux test
　　　　PPD positive
　　　　Tuberculin (skin test) positive
　　　　Tuberculin (skin test) reactor

　　　　Excludes1　nonspecific reaction to cell
　　　　　　　　　　mediated immunity
　　　　　　　　　　measurement of gamma
　　　　　　　　　　interferon antigen response
　　　　　　　　　　without active tuberculosis
　　　　　　　　　　(R76.12)

　**R76.12   Nonspecific reaction to cell mediated immunity
　　　　　　measurement of gamma interferon antigen
　　　　　　response without active tuberculosis**
　　　　Nonspecific reaction to QuantiFERON-TB test
　　　　　　(QFT) without active tuberculosis

　　　　Excludes1　nonspecific reaction to tuberculin
　　　　　　　　　　skin test without active
　　　　　　　　　　tuberculosis (R76.11)
　　　　　　　　　　positive tuberculin skin test
　　　　　　　　　　(R76.11)

　**R76.8   Other specified abnormal immunological findings in
　　　　　serum**
　　　　Raised level of immunoglobulins NOS
　　　　Coding Clinic: 2021, Q1, P7

　R76.9   Abnormal immunological finding in serum, unspecified

● **R77   Other abnormalities of plasma proteins**

　　Excludes1　disorders of plasma-protein metabolism (E88.0-)

　R77.0   Abnormality of albumin

　R77.1   Abnormality of globulin
　　　　Hyperglobulinemia NOS

　R77.2   Abnormality of alphafetoprotein

　R77.8   Other specified abnormalities of plasma proteins
　　　　Coding Clinic: 2019, Q2, P6

　R77.9   Abnormality of plasma protein, unspecified
　　　　Coding Clinic: 2019, Q2, P6

● **R78   Findings of drugs and other substances, not normally found in
　　　blood**

　　Use additional code to identify any retained foreign body, if
　　applicable (Z18.-)

　　Excludes2　mental or behavioral disorders due to
　　　　　　　　psychoactive substance use (F10-F19)

　R78.0   Finding of alcohol in blood
　　　　Use additional external cause code (Y90.-), for detail
　　　　　regarding alcohol level.

　R78.1   Finding of opiate drug in blood

　R78.2   Finding of cocaine in blood

　R78.3   Finding of hallucinogen in blood

　R78.4   Finding of other drugs of addictive potential in blood

　R78.5   Finding of other psychotropic drug in blood

　R78.6   Finding of steroid agent in blood

● **R78.7   Finding of abnormal level of heavy metals in blood**

　R78.71   Abnormal lead level in blood
　　　　Excludes1　lead poisoning (T56.0-)

　**R78.79   Finding of abnormal level of heavy metals in
　　　　　　blood**

● **R78.8   Finding of other specified substances, not normally
　　　　found in blood**

　R78.81   Bacteremia
　　　　Blood poisoning/bacteremia
　　　　Excludes1　sepsis-code to specified infection

　**R78.89   Finding of other specified substances, not
　　　　　　normally found in blood**
　　　　Finding of abnormal level of lithium in blood

　**R78.9   Finding of unspecified substance, not normally found in
　　　　　blood**

● **R79   Other abnormal findings of blood chemistry**

　　Use additional code to identify any retained foreign body, if
　　applicable (Z18.-)

　　Excludes1　asymptomatic hyperuricemia (E79.0)
　　　　　　　　hyperglycemia NOS (R73.9)
　　　　　　　　hypoglycemia NOS (E16.2)
　　　　　　　　neonatal hypoglycemia (P70.3-P70.4)
　　　　　　　　specific findings indicating disorder of amino-
　　　　　　　　　acid metabolism (E70-E72)
　　　　　　　　specific findings indicating disorder of
　　　　　　　　　carbohydrate metabolism (E73-E74)
　　　　　　　　specific findings indicating disorder of lipid
　　　　　　　　　metabolism (E75.-)

　R79.0   Abnormal level of blood mineral
　　　　Abnormal blood level of cobalt
　　　　Abnormal blood level of copper
　　　　Abnormal blood level of iron
　　　　Abnormal blood level of magnesium
　　　　Abnormal blood level of mineral NEC
　　　　Abnormal blood level of zinc

　　　　Excludes1　abnormal level of lithium (R78.89)
　　　　　　　　　　disorders of mineral metabolism (E83.-)
　　　　　　　　　　neonatal hypomagnesemia (P71.2)
　　　　　　　　　　nutritional mineral deficiency (E58-E61)

　R79.1   Abnormal coagulation profile
　　　　Abnormal or prolonged bleeding time
　　　　Abnormal or prolonged coagulation time
　　　　Abnormal or prolonged partial thromboplastin time [PTT]
　　　　Abnormal or prolonged prothrombin time [PT]
　　　　Low von Willebrand factor

　　　　Excludes1　coagulation defects (D68.-)

　　　　Excludes2　abnormality of fluid, electrolyte or acid-
　　　　　　　　　　base balance (E86-E87)

● **R79.8   Other specified abnormal findings of blood chemistry**

　R79.81   Abnormal blood-gas level

　R79.82   Elevated C-reactive protein (CRP)

　R79.83   Abnormal findings of blood amino-acid level
　　　　Homocysteinemia

　　　　Excludes1　disorders of amino-acid metabolism
　　　　　　　　　　(E70-E72)

　　　　Coding Clinic: 2021, Q4, P28

　**R79.89   Other specified abnormal findings of blood
　　　　　　chemistry**
　　　　Coding Clinic: 2019, Q2, P6

　R79.9   Abnormal finding of blood chemistry, unspecified

**ABNORMAL FINDINGS ON EXAMINATION OF URINE,
WITHOUT DIAGNOSIS (R80-R82)**

　Excludes1　abnormal findings on antenatal screening of
　　　　　　　　mother (O28.-)
　　　　　　　diagnostic abnormal findings classified elsewhere
　　　　　　　　- see Alphabetical Index
　　　　　　　specific findings indicating disorder of amino-
　　　　　　　　acid metabolism (E70-E72)
　　　　　　　specific findings indicating disorder of
　　　　　　　　carbohydrate metabolism (E73-E74)

CHAPTER 18 (R00-R99)

● R80   Proteinuria
        Excludes1   gestational proteinuria (O12.1-)
    R80.0   Isolated proteinuria
            Idiopathic proteinuria
            Excludes1   isolated proteinuria with specific
                        morphological lesion (N06.-)
    R80.1   Persistent proteinuria, unspecified
    R80.2   Orthostatic proteinuria, unspecified
            Postural proteinuria
    R80.3   Bence Jones proteinuria
    R80.8   Other proteinuria
    R80.9   Proteinuria, unspecified
            Albuminuria NOS

R81   Glycosuria
        Excludes1   renal glycosuria (E74.818)

● R82   Other and unspecified abnormal findings in urine
        Includes   chromoabnormalities in urine
        Use additional code to identify any retained foreign body, if
        applicable (Z18.-)
        Excludes2   hematuria (R31.-)
    R82.0   Chyluria
            White milky urine
            Excludes1   filarial chyluria (B74.-)
    R82.1   Myoglobinuria
            Presence of myoglobin (iron containing protein) in urine
    R82.2   Biliuria
            Presence of bile pigments/salts in urine
    R82.3   Hemoglobinuria
            Presence of hemoglobin in urine
            Excludes1   hemoglobinuria due to hemolysis from
                        external causes NEC (D59.6)
                        hemoglobinuria due to paroxysmal
                        nocturnal [Marchiafava-Micheli]
                        (D59.5)
    R82.4   Acetonuria
            Ketonuria
    R82.5   Elevated urine levels of drugs, medicaments and
            biological substances
            Elevated urine levels of catecholamines
            Elevated urine levels of indoleacetic acid
            Elevated urine levels of 17-ketosteroids
            Elevated urine levels of steroids
    R82.6   Abnormal urine levels of substances chiefly
            nonmedicinal as to source
            Abnormal urine level of heavy metals
● R82.7   Abnormal findings on microbiological examination of
          urine
            Excludes1   colonization status (Z22.-)
            Coding Clinic: 2016, Q4, P65
    R82.71 Bacteriuria
    R82.79 Other abnormal findings on microbiological
            examination of urine
                Positive culture findings of urine
● R82.8   Abnormal findings on cytological and histological
          examination of urine
    R82.81 Pyuria
            Sterile pyuria
            Coding Clinic: 2019, Q4, P16
    R82.89 Other abnormal findings on cytological and
            histological examination of urine
● R82.9   Other and unspecified abnormal findings in urine
    R82.90 Unspecified abnormal findings in urine
    R82.91 Other chromoabnormalities of urine
            Chromoconversion (dipstick)
            Idiopathic dipstick converts positive for blood
                with no cellular forms in sediment
            Excludes1   hemoglobinuria (R82.3)
                        myoglobinuria (R82.1)

    R82.99 Other abnormal findings in urine
        R82.991 Hypocitraturia
        R82.992 Hyperoxaluria
                Excludes1   Primary hyperoxaluria
                            (E72.53)
        R82.993 Hyperuricosuria
        R82.994 Hypercalciuria
                Idiopathic hypercalciuria
        R82.998 Other abnormal findings in urine
                Cells and casts in urine
                Crystalluria
                Melanuria

ABNORMAL FINDINGS ON EXAMINATION OF OTHER BODY FLUIDS, SUBSTANCES AND TISSUES, WITHOUT DIAGNOSIS (R83-R89)

        Excludes1   abnormal findings on antenatal screening of
                    mother (O28.-)
                    diagnostic abnormal findings classified elsewhere
                    - see Alphabetical Index
        Excludes2   abnormal findings on examination of blood,
                    without diagnosis (R70-R79)
                    abnormal findings on examination of urine,
                    without diagnosis (R80-R82)
                    abnormal tumor markers (R97.-)

● R83   Abnormal findings in cerebrospinal fluid
    R83.0   Abnormal level of enzymes in cerebrospinal fluid
    R83.1   Abnormal level of hormones in cerebrospinal fluid
    R83.2   Abnormal level of other drugs, medicaments and
            biological substances in cerebrospinal fluid
    R83.3   Abnormal level of substances chiefly nonmedicinal as to
            source in cerebrospinal fluid
    R83.4   Abnormal immunological findings in cerebrospinal
            fluid
    R83.5   Abnormal microbiological findings in cerebrospinal
            fluid
                Positive culture findings in cerebrospinal fluid
            Excludes1   colonization status (Z22.-)
    R83.6   Abnormal cytological findings in cerebrospinal fluid
    R83.8   Other abnormal findings in cerebrospinal fluid
                Abnormal chromosomal findings in cerebrospinal fluid
    R83.9   Unspecified abnormal finding in cerebrospinal fluid

● R84   Abnormal findings in specimens from respiratory organs and
        thorax
        Includes   abnormal findings in bronchial washings
                    abnormal findings in nasal secretions
                    abnormal findings in pleural fluid
                    abnormal findings in sputum
                    abnormal findings in throat scrapings
        Excludes1   blood-stained sputum (R04.2)
    R84.0   Abnormal level of enzymes in specimens from
            respiratory organs and thorax
    R84.1   Abnormal level of hormones in specimens from
            respiratory organs and thorax
    R84.2   Abnormal level of other drugs, medicaments and
            biological substances in specimens from respiratory
            organs and thorax
    R84.3   Abnormal level of substances chiefly nonmedicinal as to
            source in specimens from respiratory organs and thorax
    R84.4   Abnormal immunological findings in specimens from
            respiratory organs and thorax
    R84.5   Abnormal microbiological findings in specimens from
            respiratory organs and thorax
                Positive culture findings in specimens from respiratory
                organs and thorax
            Excludes1   colonization status (Z22.-)
    R84.6   Abnormal cytological findings in specimens from
            respiratory organs and thorax
    R84.7   Abnormal histological findings in specimens from
            respiratory organs and thorax

R84.8   Other abnormal findings in specimens from respiratory organs and thorax
> Abnormal chromosomal findings in specimens from respiratory organs and thorax

R84.9   Unspecified abnormal finding in specimens from respiratory organs and thorax

● R85   Abnormal findings in specimens from digestive organs and abdominal cavity

> **Includes**   abnormal findings in peritoneal fluid
> abnormal findings in saliva

> **Excludes 1**   cloudy peritoneal dialysis effluent (R88.0)
> fecal abnormalities (R19.5)

R85.0   Abnormal level of enzymes in specimens from digestive organs and abdominal cavity

R85.1   Abnormal level of hormones in specimens from digestive organs and abdominal cavity

R85.2   Abnormal level of other drugs, medicaments and biological substances in specimens from digestive organs and abdominal cavity

R85.3   Abnormal level of substances chiefly nonmedicinal as to source in specimens from digestive organs and abdominal cavity

R85.4   Abnormal immunological findings in specimens from digestive organs and abdominal cavity

R85.5   Abnormal microbiological findings in specimens from digestive organs and abdominal cavity
> Positive culture findings in specimens from digestive organs and abdominal cavity

> **Excludes 1**   colonization status (Z22.-)

● R85.6   Abnormal cytological findings in specimens from digestive organs and abdominal cavity

    ● R85.61   Abnormal cytologic smear of anus

> **Excludes 1**   abnormal cytological findings in specimens from other digestive organs and abdominal cavity (R85.69)
> carcinoma in situ of anus (histologically confirmed) (D01.3)
> anal intraepithelial neoplasia I [AIN I] (K62.82)
> anal intraepithelial neoplasia II [AIN II] (K62.82)
> anal intraepithelial neoplasia III [AIN III] (D01.3)
> dysplasia (mild) (moderate) of anus (histologically confirmed) (K62.82)
> severe dysplasia of anus (histologically confirmed) (D01.3)

> **Excludes 2**   anal high risk human papillomavirus (HPV) DNA test positive (R85.81)
> anal low risk human papillomavirus (HPV) DNA test positive (R85.82)

     R85.610   Atypical squamous cells of undetermined significance on cytologic smear of anus (ASC-US)

     R85.611   Atypical squamous cells cannot exclude high grade squamous intraepithelial lesion on cytologic smear of anus (ASC-H)

     R85.612   Low grade squamous intraepithelial lesion on cytologic smear of anus (LGSIL)

     R85.613   High grade squamous intraepithelial lesion on cytologic smear of anus (HGSIL)

     R85.614   Cytologic evidence of malignancy on smear of anus

     R85.615   Unsatisfactory cytologic smear of anus
> Inadequate sample of cytologic smear of anus

     R85.616   Satisfactory anal smear but lacking transformation zone

     R85.618   Other abnormal cytological findings on specimens from anus

     R85.619   Unspecified abnormal cytological findings in specimens from anus
> Abnormal anal cytology NOS
> Atypical glandular cells of anus NOS

    R85.69   Abnormal cytological findings in specimens from other digestive organs and abdominal cavity

R85.7   Abnormal histological findings in specimens from digestive organs and abdominal cavity

● R85.8   Other abnormal findings in specimens from digestive organs and abdominal cavity

    R85.81   Anal high risk human papillomavirus (HPV) DNA test positive

> **Excludes 1**   anogenital warts due to human papillomavirus (HPV) (A63.0)
> condyloma acuminatum (A63.0)

    R85.82   Anal low risk human papillomavirus (HPV) DNA test positive
> Use additional code for associated human papillomavirus (B97.7)

    R85.89   Other abnormal findings in specimens from digestive organs and abdominal cavity
> Abnormal chromosomal findings in specimens from digestive organs and abdominal cavity

R85.9   Unspecified abnormal finding in specimens from digestive organs and abdominal cavity

● R86   Abnormal findings in specimens from male genital organs

> **Includes**   abnormal findings in prostatic secretions
> abnormal findings in semen, seminal fluid
> abnormal spermatozoa

> **Excludes 1**   azoospermia (N46.0-)
> oligospermia (N46.1-)

R86.0   Abnormal level of enzymes in specimens from male genital organs

R86.1   Abnormal level of hormones in specimens from male genital organs

R86.2   Abnormal level of other drugs, medicaments and biological substances in specimens from male genital organs

R86.3   Abnormal level of substances chiefly nonmedicinal as to source in specimens from male genital organs

R86.4   Abnormal immunological findings in specimens from male genital organs

R86.5   Abnormal microbiological findings in specimens from male genital organs
> Positive culture findings in specimens from male genital organs

> **Excludes 1**   colonization status (Z22.-)

R86.6   Abnormal cytological findings in specimens from male genital organs

R86.7   Abnormal histological findings in specimens from male genital organs

R86.8   Other abnormal findings in specimens from male genital organs
> Abnormal chromosomal findings in specimens from male genital organs

R86.9   Unspecified abnormal finding in specimens from male genital organs

CHAPTER 18 (R00–R99)

● **R87** **Abnormal findings in specimens from female genital organs**

    Includes   abnormal findings in secretion and smears from cervix uteri

                    abnormal findings in secretion and smears from vagina

                    abnormal findings in secretion and smears from vulva

R87.0 **Abnormal level of enzymes in specimens from female genital organs**

R87.1 **Abnormal level of hormones in specimens from female genital organs**

R87.2 **Abnormal level of other drugs, medicaments and biological substances in specimens from female genital organs**

R87.3 **Abnormal level of substances chiefly nonmedicinal as to source in specimens from female genital organs**

R87.4 **Abnormal immunological findings in specimens from female genital organs**

R87.5 **Abnormal microbiological findings in specimens from female genital organs**

    Positive culture findings in specimens from female genital organs

    Excludes1   colonization status (Z22.-)

● **R87.6** **Abnormal cytological findings in specimens from female genital organs**

    ● **R87.61** **Abnormal cytological findings in specimens from cervix uteri**

        Excludes1   abnormal cytological findings in specimens from other female genital organs (R87.69)

                    abnormal cytological findings in specimens from vagina (R87.62-)

                    carcinoma in situ of cervix uteri (histologically confirmed) (D06.-)

                    cervical intraepithelial neoplasia I [CIN I] (N87.0)

                    cervical intraepithelial neoplasia II [CIN II] (N87.1)

                    cervical intraepithelial neoplasia III [CIN III] (D06.-)

                    dysplasia (mild) (moderate) of cervix uteri (histologically confirmed) (N87.-)

                    severe dysplasia of cervix uteri (histologically confirmed) (D06.-)

        Excludes2   cervical high risk human papillomavirus (HPV) DNA test positive (R87.810)

                    cervical low risk human papillomavirus (HPV) DNA test positive (R87.820)

        R87.610 **Atypical squamous cells of undetermined significance on cytologic smear of cervix (ASC-US)**

        R87.611 **Atypical squamous cells cannot exclude high grade squamous intraepithelial lesion on cytologic smear of cervix (ASC-H)**

        R87.612 **Low grade squamous intraepithelial lesion on cytologic smear of cervix (LGSIL)**

        R87.613 **High grade squamous intraepithelial lesion on cytologic smear of cervix (HGSIL)**

        R87.614 **Cytologic evidence of malignancy on smear of cervix**

        R87.615 **Unsatisfactory cytologic smear of cervix**

            Inadequate sample of cytologic smear of cervix

R87.616 **Satisfactory cervical smear but lacking transformation zone**

R87.618 **Other abnormal cytological findings on specimens from cervix uteri**

R87.619 **Unspecified abnormal cytological findings in specimens from cervix uteri**

    Abnormal cervical cytology NOS

    Abnormal Papanicolaou smear of cervix NOS

    Abnormal thin preparation smear of cervix NOS

    Atypical endocervical cells of cervix NOS

    Atypical endometrial cells of cervix NOS

    Atypical glandular cells of cervix NOS

● **R87.62** **Abnormal cytological findings in specimens from vagina**

    Use additional code to identify acquired absence of uterus and cervix, if applicable (Z90.71-)

    Excludes1   abnormal cytological findings in specimens from cervix uteri (R87.61-)

                    abnormal cytological findings in specimens from other female genital organs (R87.69)

                    carcinoma in situ of vagina (histologically confirmed) (D07.2)

                    vaginal intraepithelial neoplasia I [VAIN I] (N89.0)

                    vaginal intraepithelial neoplasia II [VAIN II] (N89.1)

                    vaginal intraepithelial neoplasia III [VAIN III] (D07.2)

                    dysplasia (mild) (moderate) of vagina (histologically confirmed) (N89.-)

                    severe dysplasia of vagina (histologically confirmed) (D07.2)

    Excludes2   vaginal high risk human papillomavirus (HPV) DNA test positive (R87.811)

                    vaginal low risk human papillomavirus (HPV) DNA test positive (R87.821)

    R87.620 **Atypical squamous cells of undetermined significance on cytologic smear of vagina (ASC-US)**

    R87.621 **Atypical squamous cells cannot exclude high grade squamous intraepithelial lesion on cytologic smear of vagina (ASC-H)**

    R87.622 **Low grade squamous intraepithelial lesion on cytologic smear of vagina (LGSIL)**

    R87.623 **High grade squamous intraepithelial lesion on cytologic smear of vagina (HGSIL)**

    R87.624 **Cytologic evidence of malignancy on smear of vagina**

    R87.625 **Unsatisfactory cytologic smear of vagina**

        Inadequate sample of cytologic smear of vagina

    R87.628 **Other abnormal cytological findings on specimens from vagina**

▶ New   ⇒ Revised   ~~deleted~~ Deleted   Excludes 1   Excludes 2   Includes   Use additional   Code first   Code also   Key words

OGCR Official Guidelines   X Assign placeholder X   ● Use Additional Character(s)   ⟩ Manifestation Code   🦠 Hierarchical Condition Category   Coding Clinic

R87.629 **Unspecified abnormal cytological findings in specimens from vagina**
Abnormal Papanicolaou smear of vagina NOS
Abnormal thin preparation smear of vagina NOS
Abnormal vaginal cytology NOS
Atypical endocervical cells of vagina NOS
Atypical endometrial cells of vagina NOS
Atypical glandular cells of vagina NOS

R87.69 **Abnormal cytological findings in specimens from other female genital organs**
Abnormal cytological findings in specimens from female genital organs NOS
 Excludes1 dysplasia of vulva (histologically confirmed) (N90.0-N90.3)

R87.7 **Abnormal histological findings in specimens from female genital organs**
 Excludes1 carcinoma in situ (histologically confirmed) of female genital organs (D06-D07.3)
    cervical intraepithelial neoplasia I [CIN I] (N87.0)
    cervical intraepithelial neoplasia II [CIN II] (N87.1)
    cervical intraepithelial neoplasia III [CIN III] (D06.-)
    dysplasia (mild) (moderate) of cervix uteri (histologically confirmed) (N87.-)
    dysplasia (mild) (moderate) of vagina (histologically confirmed) (N89.-)
    vaginal intraepithelial neoplasia I [VAIN I] (N89.0)
    vaginal intraepithelial neoplasia II [VAIN II] (N89.1)
    vaginal intraepithelial neoplasia III [VAIN III] (D07.2)
    severe dysplasia of cervix uteri (histologically confirmed) (D06.-)
    severe dysplasia of vagina (histologically confirmed) (D07.2)

● R87.8 **Other abnormal findings in specimens from female genital organs**

● R87.81 **High risk human papillomavirus (HPV) DNA test positive from female genital organs**
 Excludes1 anogenital warts due to human papillomavirus (HPV) (A63.0)
    condyloma acuminatum (A63.0)

R87.810 **Cervical high risk human papillomavirus (HPV) DNA test positive**

R87.811 **Vaginal high risk human papillomavirus (HPV) DNA test positive**

● R87.82 **Low risk human papillomavirus (HPV) DNA test positive from female genital organs**
Use additional code for associated human papillomavirus (B97.7)

R87.820 **Cervical low risk human papillomavirus (HPV) DNA test positive**

R87.821 **Vaginal low risk human papillomavirus (HPV) DNA test positive**

R87.89 **Other abnormal findings in specimens from female genital organs**
Abnormal chromosomal findings in specimens from female genital organs

R87.9 **Unspecified abnormal finding in specimens from female genital organs**

● R88 **Abnormal findings in other body fluids and substances**
R88.0 **Cloudy (hemodialysis) (peritoneal) dialysis effluent**
R88.8 **Abnormal findings in other body fluids and substances**

● R89 **Abnormal findings in specimens from other organs, systems and tissues**
 Includes abnormal findings in nipple discharge
    abnormal findings in synovial fluid
    abnormal findings in wound secretions

R89.0 **Abnormal level of enzymes in specimens from other organs, systems and tissues**

R89.1 **Abnormal level of hormones in specimens from other organs, systems and tissues**

R89.2 **Abnormal level of other drugs, medicaments and biological substances in specimens from other organs, systems and tissues**

R89.3 **Abnormal level of substances chiefly nonmedicinal as to source in specimens from other organs, systems and tissues**

R89.4 **Abnormal immunological findings in specimens from other organs, systems and tissues**

R89.5 **Abnormal microbiological findings in specimens from other organs, systems and tissues**
Positive culture findings in specimens from other organs, systems and tissues
 Excludes1 colonization status (Z22.-)

R89.6 **Abnormal cytological findings in specimens from other organs, systems and tissues**

R89.7 **Abnormal histological findings in specimens from other organs, systems and tissues**

R89.8 **Other abnormal findings in specimens from other organs, systems and tissues**
Abnormal chromosomal findings in specimens from other organs, systems and tissues

R89.9 **Unspecified abnormal finding in specimens from other organs, systems and tissues**

ABNORMAL FINDINGS ON DIAGNOSTIC IMAGING AND IN FUNCTION STUDIES, WITHOUT DIAGNOSIS (R90-R94)

 Includes nonspecific abnormal findings on diagnostic imaging by computerized axial tomography [CAT scan]
    nonspecific abnormal findings on diagnostic imaging by magnetic resonance imaging [MRI][NMR]
    nonspecific abnormal findings on diagnostic imaging by positron emission tomography [PET scan]
    nonspecific abnormal findings on diagnostic imaging by thermography
    nonspecific abnormal findings on diagnostic imaging by ultrasound [echogram]
    nonspecific abnormal findings on diagnostic imaging by X-ray examination
 Excludes1 abnormal findings on antenatal screening of mother (O28.-)
    diagnostic abnormal findings classified elsewhere - see Alphabetical Index

● R90 **Abnormal findings on diagnostic imaging of central nervous system**
R90.0 **Intracranial space-occupying lesion found on diagnostic imaging of central nervous system**

● R90.8 **Other abnormal findings on diagnostic imaging of central nervous system**
R90.81 **Abnormal echoencephalogram**
R90.82 **White matter disease, unspecified**
R90.89 **Other abnormal findings on diagnostic imaging of central nervous system**
Other cerebrovascular abnormality found on diagnostic imaging of central nervous system

● **R91 Abnormal findings on diagnostic imaging of lung**
  R91.1 Solitary pulmonary nodule
    Coin lesion lung
    Solitary pulmonary nodule, subsegmental branch of the bronchial tree
  R91.8 Other nonspecific abnormal finding of lung field
    Lung mass NOS found on diagnostic imaging of lung
    Pulmonary infiltrate NOS
    Shadow, lung

● **R92 Abnormal and inconclusive findings on diagnostic imaging of breast**
  R92.0 Mammographic microcalcification found on diagnostic imaging of breast
    Excludes2 mammographic calcification (calculus) found on diagnostic imaging of breast (R92.1)
  R92.1 Mammographic calcification found on diagnostic imaging of breast
    Mammographic calculus found on diagnostic imaging of breast
  R92.2 Inconclusive mammogram
    Inconclusive mammogram NEC
    Inconclusive mammography NEC
    Coding Clinic: 2015, Q1, P24
●   **R92.3 Mammographic density found on imaging of breast**
    Code also, if applicable, inconclusive mammogram (R92.2)
    R92.30 Dense breasts, unspecified
      Dense breasts NOS
      Low density
●   **R92.31 Mammographic fatty tissue density of breast**
      Breast Imaging Reporting and Data System (BI-RADS): A
      Breast Imaging Reporting and Data System (BI-RADS): 1
      R92.311 Mammographic fatty tissue density, right breast
      R92.312 Mammographic fatty tissue density, left breast
      R92.313 Mammographic fatty tissue density, bilateral breasts
●   **R92.32 Mammographic fibroglandular density of breast**
      Breast Imaging Reporting and Data System (BI-RADS): B
      Breast Imaging Reporting and Data System (BI-RADS): 2
      R92.321 Mammographic fibroglandular density, right breast
      R92.322 Mammographic fibroglandular density, left breast
      R92.323 Mammographic fibroglandular density, bilateral breasts
●   **R92.33 Mammographic heterogeneous density of breast**
      Breast Imaging Reporting and Data System (BI-RADS): C
      Breast Imaging Reporting and Data System (BI-RADS): 3
      R92.331 Mammographic heterogeneous density, right breast
      R92.332 Mammographic heterogeneous density, left breast
      R92.333 Mammographic heterogeneous density, bilateral breasts
      Coding Clinic: 2023, Q4, P44

●   **R92.34 Mammographic extreme density of breast**
      Breast Imaging Reporting and Data System (BI-RADS): D
      Breast Imaging Reporting and Data System (BI-RADS): 4
      R92.341 Mammographic extreme density, right breast
      R92.342 Mammographic extreme density, left breast
      R92.343 Mammographic extreme density, bilateral breasts
  R92.8 Other abnormal and inconclusive findings on diagnostic imaging of breast

● **R93 Abnormal findings on diagnostic imaging of other body structures**
  R93.0 Abnormal findings on diagnostic imaging of skull and head, not elsewhere classified
    Excludes1 intracranial space-occupying lesion found on diagnostic imaging (R90.0)
  R93.1 Abnormal findings on diagnostic imaging of heart and coronary circulation
    Abnormal echocardiogram NOS
    Abnormal heart shadow
  R93.2 Abnormal findings on diagnostic imaging of liver and biliary tract
    Nonvisualization of gallbladder
  R93.3 Abnormal findings on diagnostic imaging of other parts of digestive tract
●   **R93.4 Abnormal findings on diagnostic imaging of urinary organs**
    Excludes2 hypertrophy of kidney (N28.81)
    Coding Clinic: 2016, Q4, P66
    R93.41 Abnormal radiologic findings on diagnostic imaging of renal pelvis, ureter, or bladder
      Filling defect of bladder found on diagnostic imaging
      Filling defect of renal pelvis found on diagnostic imaging
      Filling defect of ureter found on diagnostic imaging
●   **R93.42 Abnormal radiologic findings on diagnostic imaging of kidney**
      R93.421 Abnormal radiologic findings on diagnostic imaging of right kidney
      R93.422 Abnormal radiologic findings on diagnostic imaging of left kidney
      R93.429 Abnormal radiologic findings on diagnostic imaging of unspecified kidney
    R93.49 Abnormal radiologic findings on diagnostic imaging of other urinary organs
  R93.5 Abnormal findings on diagnostic imaging of other abdominal regions, including retroperitoneum
  R93.6 Abnormal findings on diagnostic imaging of limbs
    Excludes2 abnormal finding in skin and subcutaneous tissue (R93.8-)
    Coding Clinic: 2020, Q1, P14
  R93.7 Abnormal findings on diagnostic imaging of other parts of musculoskeletal system
    Excludes2 abnormal findings on diagnostic imaging of skull (R93.0)

CHAPTER 18 (R00-R99)

▶ New ➡ Revised ~~deleted~~ Deleted | Excludes 1 | Excludes 2 | Includes | Use additional | Code first | Code also | Key words
OGCR Official Guidelines X Assign placeholder X ● Use Additional Character(s) ▶ Manifestation Code 🔑 Hierarchical Condition Category Coding Clinic

Figure 18-2 Cranial nerves. (From Patton and Thibodeau: Anatomy and physiology, ed 7, St. Louis, Mosby, 2009)

Trochlear nerve (IV)

Optic nerve (II)

Olfactory nerve (I)

Abducens nerve (VI)

Oculomotor nerve (III)

Trigeminal nerve (V)

Facial nerve (VII)

Vestibulocochlear nerve (VIII)

Glossopharyngeal nerve (IX)

Vagus nerve (X)

Accessory nerve (XI)

Hypoglossal nerve (XII)

● **R93.8** **Abnormal findings on diagnostic imaging of other specified body structures**

 ● **R93.81** **Abnormal radiologic findings on diagnostic imaging of testis**

  R93.811 **Abnormal radiologic findings on diagnostic imaging of right testicle**

  R93.812 **Abnormal radiologic findings on diagnostic imaging of left testicle**

  R93.813 **Abnormal radiologic findings on diagnostic imaging of testicles, bilateral**

  R93.819 **Abnormal radiologic findings on diagnostic imaging of unspecified testicle**

 R93.89 **Abnormal findings on diagnostic imaging of other specified body structures**
  Abnormal finding by radioisotope localization of placenta
  Abnormal radiological finding in skin and subcutaneous tissue
  Mediastinal shift

R93.9 **Diagnostic imaging inconclusive due to excess body fat of patient**

● **R94** **Abnormal results of function studies**

 Includes abnormal results of radionuclide [radioisotope] uptake studies
  abnormal results of scintigraphy

 ● **R94.0** **Abnormal results of function studies of central nervous system**

  R94.01 **Abnormal electroencephalogram [EEG]**

  R94.02 **Abnormal brain scan**

  R94.09 **Abnormal results of other function studies of central nervous system**

● **R94.1** **Abnormal results of function studies of peripheral nervous system and special senses**

 ● **R94.11** **Abnormal results of function studies of eye**

  R94.110 **Abnormal electro-oculogram [EOG]**

  R94.111 **Abnormal electroretinogram [ERG]**
   Abnormal retinal function study

  R94.112 **Abnormal visually evoked potential [VEP]**

  R94.113 **Abnormal oculomotor study**

  R94.118 **Abnormal results of other function studies of eye**

 ● **R94.12** **Abnormal results of function studies of ear and other special senses**

  R94.120 **Abnormal auditory function study**
   Coding Clinic: 2016, Q3, P17

  R94.121 **Abnormal vestibular function study**

  R94.128 **Abnormal results of other function studies of ear and other special senses**

 ● **R94.13** **Abnormal results of function studies of peripheral nervous system**

  R94.130 **Abnormal response to nerve stimulation, unspecified**

  R94.131 **Abnormal electromyogram [EMG]**

   Excludes1 electromyogram of eye (R94.113)

  R94.138 **Abnormal results of other function studies of peripheral nervous system**

Item 18-1 The **peripheral nervous system** consists of 31 pairs of spinal nerves, 12 pairs of cranial nerves, and the autonomic nerves, which are divided into the parasympathetic and sympathetic nerves. The cranial nerves are: olfactory (I), optic (II), oculomotor (III), trochlear (IV), trigeminal (V), abducens (VI), facial (VII), vestibulocochlear (VIII), glossopharyngeal (IX), vagus (X), accessory (XI), and hypoglossal (XII).

R94.2   **Abnormal results of pulmonary function studies**
  Reduced ventilatory capacity
  Reduced vital capacity

● R94.3   **Abnormal results of cardiovascular function studies**

  R94.30 **Abnormal result of cardiovascular function study, unspecified**

  R94.31 **Abnormal electrocardiogram [ECG] [EKG]**
    Excludes1 long QT syndrome (I45.81)

  R94.39 **Abnormal result of other cardiovascular function study**
    Abnormal electrophysiological intracardiac studies
    Abnormal phonocardiogram
    Abnormal vectorcardiogram
    Coding Clinic: 2023, Q1, P25

R94.4   **Abnormal results of kidney function studies**
  Abnormal renal function test

R94.5   **Abnormal results of liver function studies**

R94.6   **Abnormal results of thyroid function studies**

R94.7   **Abnormal results of other endocrine function studies**
  Excludes2 abnormal glucose (R73.0-)

R94.8   **Abnormal results of function studies of other organs and systems**
  Abnormal basal metabolic rate [BMR]
  Abnormal bladder function test
  Abnormal splenic function test

ABNORMAL TUMOR MARKERS (R97)

● R97 **Abnormal tumor markers**
  Elevated tumor associated antigens [TAA]
  Elevated tumor specific antigens [TSA]

  R97.0 **Elevated carcinoembryonic antigen [CEA]**

  R97.1 **Elevated cancer antigen 125 [CA 125]**

● R97.2 **Elevated prostate specific antigen [PSA]**
    Coding Clinic: 2016, Q4, P66

    R97.20 **Elevated prostate specific antigen [PSA]** A

    R97.21 **Rising PSA following treatment for malignant neoplasm of prostate** A
      Coding Clinic: 2023, Q2, P5

  R97.8 **Other abnormal tumor markers**

ILL-DEFINED AND UNKNOWN CAUSE OF MORTALITY (R99)

R99 **Ill-defined and unknown cause of mortality**
  Death (unexplained) NOS
  Unspecified cause of mortality

OGCR Section I.C.18.h.

 Death NOS

 Code R99, Ill-defined and unknown cause of mortality, is only for use in the very limited circumstance when a patient who has already died is brought into the emergency department or other healthcare facility and is pronounced dead upon arrival. It does not represent the discharge disposition of death.

▶ New ➡ Revised ~~deleted~~ Deleted Excludes 1 Excludes 2 Includes Use additional Code first Code also Key words
OGCR Official Guidelines X Assign placeholder X ● Use Additional Character(s) ▶ Manifestation Code Hierarchical Condition Category Coding Clinic

CHAPTER 19

INJURY, POISONING AND CERTAIN OTHER CONSEQUENCES OF EXTERNAL CAUSES (S00-T88)

OGCR Chapter-Specific Coding Guidelines

19. **Chapter 19: Injury, poisoning, and certain other consequences of external causes (S00-T88)**

    a. **Application of 7th Characters in Chapter 19**
    Most categories in Chapter 19 have a 7th character requirement for each applicable code. Most categories in this chapter have three 7th character values (with the exception of fractures): A, initial encounter, D, subsequent encounter and S, sequela. Categories for traumatic fractures have additional 7th character values. While the patient may be seen by a new or different provider over the course of treatment for an injury, assignment of the 7th character is based on whether the patient is undergoing active treatment and not whether the provider is seeing the patient for the first time.

    For complication codes, active treatment refers to treatment for the condition described by the code, even though it may be related to an earlier precipitating problem. For example, code T84.50XA, Infection and inflammatory reaction due to unspecified internal joint prosthesis, initial encounter, is used when active treatment is provided for the infection, even though the condition relates to the prosthetic device, implant or graft that was placed at a previous encounter.

    7th character "A", initial encounter is used for each encounter where the patient is receiving active treatment for the condition.

    7th character "D" subsequent encounter is used for encounters after the patient has completed active treatment of the condition and is receiving routine care for the condition during the healing or recovery phase.

    The aftercare Z codes should not be used for aftercare for conditions such as injuries or poisonings, where 7th characters are provided to identify subsequent care. For example, for aftercare of an injury, assign the acute injury code with the 7th character "D" (subsequent encounter).

    7th character "S", sequela, is for use for complications or conditions that arise as a direct result of a condition, such as scar formation after a burn. The scars are sequelae of the burn. When using 7th character "S", it is necessary to use both the injury code that precipitated the sequela and the code for the sequela itself. The "S" is added only to the injury code, not the sequela code. The 7th character "S" identifies the injury responsible for the sequela. The specific type of sequela (e.g. scar) is sequenced first, followed by the injury code.

    See Section I.B.10. Sequelae, (Late Effects).

    b. **Coding of Injuries**
    When coding injuries, assign separate codes for each injury unless a combination code is provided, in which case the combination code is assigned. Codes from category T07, Unspecified multiple injuries should not be assigned in the inpatient setting unless information for a more specific code is not available. Traumatic injury codes (S00-T14.9) are not to be used for normal, healing surgical wounds or to identify complications of surgical wounds.

    The code for the most serious injury, as determined by the provider and the focus of treatment, is sequenced first.

    1) **Superficial injuries**
    Superficial injuries such as abrasions or contusions are not coded when associated with more severe injuries of the same site.

    2) **Primary injury with damage to nerves/blood vessels**
    When a primary injury results in minor damage to peripheral nerves or blood vessels, the primary injury is sequenced first with additional code(s) for injuries to nerves and spinal cord (such as category S04), and/or injury to blood vessels (such as category S15). When the primary injury is to the blood vessels or nerves, that injury should be sequenced first.

    c. **Coding of Traumatic Fractures**
    The principles of multiple coding of injuries should be followed in coding fractures. Fractures of specified sites are coded individually by site in accordance with both the provisions within categories S02, S12, S22, S32, S42, S49, S52, S59, S62, S72, S79, S82, S89, S92 and the level of detail furnished by medical record content.

    A fracture not indicated as open or closed should be coded to closed. A fracture not indicated whether displaced or not displaced should be coded to displaced.

    More specific guidelines are as follows:

    1) **Initial vs. Subsequent Encounter for Fractures**
    Traumatic fractures are coded using the appropriate 7th character for initial encounter (A, B, C) for each encounter where the patient is receiving active treatment for the fracture. The appropriate 7th character for initial encounter should also be assigned for a patient who delayed seeking treatment for the fracture or nonunion.

    Fractures are coded using the appropriate 7th character for subsequent care for encounters after the patient has completed active treatment of the fracture and is receiving routine care for the fracture during the healing or recovery phase.

    Care for complications of surgical treatment for fracture repairs during the healing or recovery phase should be coded with the appropriate complication codes.

    Care of complications of fractures, such as malunion and nonunion, should be reported with the appropriate 7th character for subsequent care with nonunion (K, M, N,) or subsequent care with malunion (P, Q, R).

    Malunion/nonunion: The appropriate 7th character for initial encounter should also be assigned for a patient who delayed seeking treatment for the fracture or nonunion.

    The open fracture designations in the assignment of the 7th character for fractures of the forearm, femur and lower leg, including ankle are based on the Gustilo open fracture classification. When the Gustilo classification type is not specified for an open fracture, the 7th character for open fracture type I or II should be assigned (B, E, H, M, Q).

    A code from category M80, not a traumatic fracture code, should be used for any patient with known osteoporosis who suffers a fracture, even if the patient had a minor fall or trauma, if that fall or trauma would not usually break a normal, healthy bone.

    See Section I.C.13. Osteoporosis.

    The aftercare Z codes should not be used for aftercare for traumatic fractures. For aftercare of a traumatic fracture, assign the acute fracture code with the appropriate 7th character.

    2) **Multiple fractures sequencing**
    Multiple fractures are sequenced in accordance with the severity of the fracture.

    d. **Coding of Burns and Corrosions**
    The ICD-10-CM makes a distinction between burns and corrosions. The burn codes are for thermal burns, except sunburns, that come from a heat source, such as a fire or hot appliance. The burn codes are also for burns resulting from electricity and radiation. Corrosions are burns due to chemicals. The guidelines are the same for burns and corrosions.

    Current burns (T20-T25) are classified by depth, extent and by agent (X code). Burns are classified by depth as first degree (erythema), second degree (blistering), and third degree (full-thickness involvement). Burns of the eye and internal organs (T26-T28) are classified by site, but not by degree.

    1) **Sequencing of burn and related condition codes**
    Sequence first the code that reflects the highest degree of burn when more than one burn is present.

    a. When the reason for the admission or encounter is for treatment of external multiple burns, sequence first the code that reflects the burn of the highest degree.

    b. When a patient has both internal and external burns, the circumstances of admission govern the selection of the principal diagnosis or first-listed diagnosis.

    c. When a patient is admitted for burn injuries and other related conditions such as smoke inhalation and/or respiratory failure, the circumstances of admission govern the selection of the principal or first-listed diagnosis.

2) Burns of the same *anatomic* site

Classify burns of the same anatomic site and on the same side but of different degrees to the subcategory identifying the highest degree recorded in the diagnosis (e.g., for second- and third-degree burns of right thigh, assign only code T24.311-).

3) Non-healing burns

Non-healing burns are coded as acute burns.

Necrosis of burned skin should be coded as a non-healed burn.

4) Infected Burn

For any documented infected burn site, use an additional code for the infection.

5) Assign separate codes for each burn site

When coding burns, assign separate codes for each burn site. Category T30, Burn and corrosion, body region unspecified is extremely vague and should rarely be used.

Codes for burns of "multiple sites" should only be assigned when the medical record documentation does not specify the individual sites.

6) Burns and Corrosions Classified According to Extent of Body Surface Involved

Assign codes from category T31, Burns classified according to extent of body surface involved, or T32, Corrosions classified according to extent of body surface involved, when the site of the burn is not specified or when there is a need for additional data. It is advisable to use category T31 as additional coding when needed to provide data for evaluating burn mortality, such as that needed by burn units. It is also advisable to use category T31 as an additional code for reporting purposes when there is mention of a third-degree burn involving 20 percent or more of the body surface.

Categories T31 and T32 are based on the classic "rule of nines" in estimating body surface involved: head and neck are assigned nine percent, each arm nine percent, each leg 18 percent, the anterior trunk 18 percent, posterior trunk 18 percent, and genitalia one percent. Providers may change these percentage assignments where necessary to accommodate infants and children who have proportionately larger heads than adults, and patients who have large buttocks, thighs, or abdomen that involve burns.

7) Encounters for treatment of sequela of burns

Encounters for the treatment of the late effects of burns or corrosions (i.e., scars or joint contractures) should be coded with a burn or corrosion code with the 7th character "S" for sequela.

8) Sequelae with a late effect code and current burn

When appropriate, both a code for a current burn or corrosion with 7th character "A" or "D" and a burn or corrosion code with 7th character "S" may be assigned on the same record (when both a current burn and sequelae of an old burn exist). Burns and corrosions do not heal at the same rate and a current healing wound may still exist with sequela of a healed burn or corrosion.

See Section I.B.10. Sequela, (Late Effects).

9) Use of an external cause code with burns and corrosions

An external cause code should be used with burns and corrosions to identify the source and intent of the burn, as well as the place where it occurred.

e. Adverse Effects, Poisoning , Underdosing and Toxic Effects

Codes in categories T36-T65 are combination codes that include the substance that was taken as well as the intent. No additional external cause code is required for poisonings, toxic effects, adverse effects and underdosing codes.

1) Do not code directly from the Table of Drugs

Do not code directly from the Table of Drugs and Chemicals. Always refer back to the Tabular List.

2) Use as many codes as necessary to describe

Use as many codes as necessary to describe completely all drugs, medicinal or biological substances.

3) If the same code would describe the causative agent

If the same code would describe the causative agent for more than one adverse reaction, poisoning, toxic effect or underdosing, assign the code only once.

4) If two or more drugs, medicinal or biological substances

If two or more drugs, medicinal or biological substances are reported, code each individually unless a combination code is listed in the Table of Drugs and Chemicals.

5) The occurrence of drug toxicity is classified in ICD-10-CM as follows:

(a) Adverse Effect

When coding an adverse effect of a drug that has been correctly prescribed and properly administered, assign the appropriate code for the nature of the adverse effect followed by the appropriate code for the adverse effect of the drug (T36-T50). The code for the drug should have a 5th or 6th character "5" (for example T36.0X5-) Examples of the nature of an adverse effect are tachycardia, delirium, gastrointestinal hemorrhaging, vomiting, hypokalemia, hepatitis, renal failure, or respiratory failure.

(b) Poisoning

When coding a poisoning or reaction to the improper use of a medication (e.g., overdose, wrong substance given or taken in error, wrong route of administration), first assign the appropriate code from categories T36-T50. The poisoning codes have an associated intent as their 5th or 6th character (accidental, intentional self-harm, assault and undetermined). If the intent of the poisoning is unknown or unspecified, code the intent as accidental intent. The undetermined intent is only for use if the documentation in the record specifies that the intent cannot be determined. Use additional code(s) for all manifestations of poisonings.

If there is also a diagnosis of abuse or dependence of the substance, the abuse or dependence is assigned as an additional code.

Examples of poisoning include:

(i) Error was made in drug prescription
Errors made in drug prescription or in the administration of the drug by provider, nurse, patient, or other person.

(ii) Overdose of a drug intentionally taken If an overdose of a drug was intentionally taken or administered and resulted in drug toxicity, it would be coded as a poisoning.

(iii) Nonprescribed drug taken with correctly prescribed and properly administered drug. If a nonprescribed drug or medicinal agent was taken in combination with a correctly prescribed and properly administered drug, any drug toxicity or other reaction resulting from the interaction of the two drugs would be classified as a poisoning.

(iv) Interaction of drug(s) and alcohol. When a reaction results from the interaction of a drug(s) and alcohol, this would be classified as poisoning.

See Section I.C.4. if poisoning is the result of insulin pump malfunctions.

(c) Underdosing

Underdosing refers to taking less of a medication than is prescribed by a provider or a manufacturer's instruction. Discontinuing the use of a prescribed medication on the patient's own initiative (not directed by the patient's provider) is also classified as an underdosing. For underdosing, assign the code from categories T36-T50 (fifth or sixth character "6").

Codes for underdosing should never be assigned as principal or first-listed codes. If a patient has a relapse or exacerbation of the medical condition for which the drug is prescribed because of the reduction in dose, then the medical condition itself should be coded.

Noncompliance (Z91.12-, Z91.13- and Z91.14-) or complication of care (Y63.6-Y63.9) codes are to be used with an underdosing code to indicate intent, if known.

(d) Toxic Effects

When a harmful substance is ingested or comes in contact with a person, this is classified as a toxic effect. The toxic effect codes are in categories T51-T65.

Toxic effect codes have an associated intent: accidental, intentional self-harm, assault and undetermined.

f. Adult and child abuse, neglect and other maltreatment

Sequence first the appropriate code from categories T74 (Adult and child abuse, neglect and other maltreatment, confirmed) or T76 (Adult and child abuse, neglect and other maltreatment, suspected) for abuse, neglect and other maltreatment, followed by any accompanying mental health or injury code(s).

If the documentation in the medical record states abuse or neglect it is coded as confirmed (T74.-). It is coded as suspected if it is documented as suspected (T76.-).

For cases of confirmed abuse or neglect an external cause code from the assault section (X92-Y09) should be added to identify the cause of any physical injuries. A perpetrator code (Y07) should be added when the perpetrator of the abuse is known. For suspected cases of abuse or neglect, do not report external cause or perpetrator code.

If a suspected case of abuse, neglect or mistreatment is ruled out during an encounter code Z04.71, Encounter for examination and observation following alleged physical adult abuse, ruled out, or code Z04.72, Encounter for examination and observation following alleged child physical abuse, ruled out, should be used, not a code from T76.

If a suspected case of alleged rape or sexual abuse is ruled out during an encounter code Z04.41, Encounter for examination and observation following alleged adult rape or code Z04.42, Encounter for examination and observation following alleged child rape, should be used, not a code from T76.

If a suspected case of forced sexual exploitation or forced labor exploitation is ruled out during an encounter, code Z04.81, Encounter for examination and observation of victim following forced sexual exploitation, or code Z04.82, Encounter for examination and observation of victim following forced labor exploitation, should be used, not a code from T76.

See Section I.C.15. Abuse in a pregnant patient.

g. Complications of care

1) General guidelines for complications of care

(a) Documentation of complications of care

See Section I.B.16. for information on documentation of complications of care.

2) Pain due to medical devices

Pain associated with devices, implants or grafts left in a surgical site (for example painful hip prosthesis) is assigned to the appropriate code(s) found in Chapter 19, Injury, poisoning, and certain other consequences of external causes. Specific codes for pain due to medical devices are found in the T code section of the ICD-10-CM. Use additional code(s) from category G89 to identify acute or chronic pain due to presence of the device, implant or graft (G89.18 or G89.28).

3) Transplant complications

(a) Transplant complications other than kidney

Codes under category T86, Complications of transplanted organs and tissues, are for use for both complications and rejection of transplanted organs. A transplant complication code is only assigned if the complication affects the function of the transplanted organ. Two codes are required to fully describe a transplant complication: the appropriate code from category T86 and a secondary code that identifies the complication.

Pre-existing conditions or conditions that develop after the transplant are not coded as complications unless they affect the function of the transplanted organs.

See I.C.21. for transplant organ removal status.

See I.C.2. for malignant neoplasm associated with transplanted organ.

(b) Kidney transplant complications

Patients who have undergone kidney transplant may still have some form of chronic kidney disease (CKD) because the kidney transplant may not fully restore kidney function. Code T86.1- should be assigned for documented complications of a kidney transplant, such as transplant failure or rejection or other transplant complication. Code T86.1- should not be assigned for post kidney transplant patients who have chronic kidney (CKD) unless a transplant complication such as transplant failure or rejection is documented. If the documentation is unclear as to whether the patient has a complication of the transplant, query the provider.

Conditions that affect the function of the transplanted kidney, other than CKD, should be assigned a code from subcategory T86.1, Complications of transplanted organ, Kidney, and a secondary code that identifies the complication.

For patients with CKD following a kidney transplant, but who do not have a complication such as failure or rejection, *see Section I.C.14. Chronic kidney disease and kidney transplant status.*

4) Complication codes that include the external cause

As with certain other T codes, some of the complications of care codes have the external cause included in the code. The code includes the nature of the complication as well as the type of procedure that caused the complication. No external cause code indicating the type of procedure is necessary for these codes.

5) Complications of care codes within the body system chapters

Intraoperative and postprocedural complication codes are found within the body system chapters with codes specific to the organs and structures of that body system. These codes should be sequenced first, followed by a code(s) for the specific complication, if applicable.

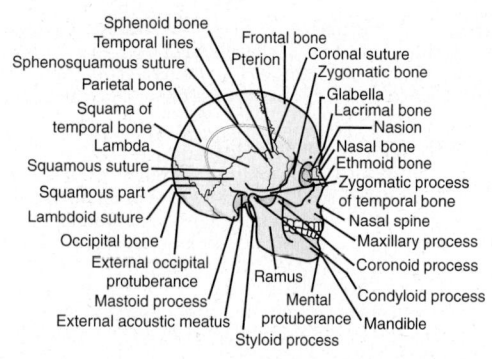

Figure 19-1 Lateral view of skull.

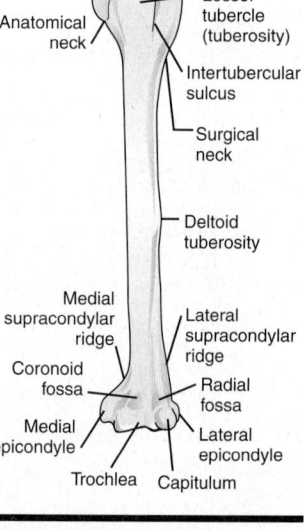

Figure 19-2 Frontal view of skull.

Figure 19-3 Anterior view of vertebral column.

Figure 19-4 Vertebra viewed from above.

Figure 19-5 Anterior view of rib cage.

Figure 19-6 Anterior aspect of left humerus.

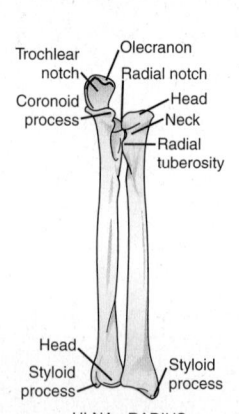

Figure 19-7 Anterior aspect of left radius and ulna.

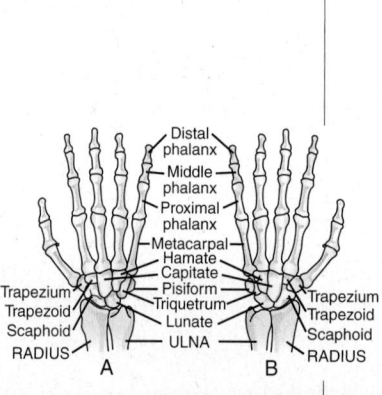

Figure 19-8 Right hand and wrist: **A.** Dorsal surface. **B.** Palmar surface.

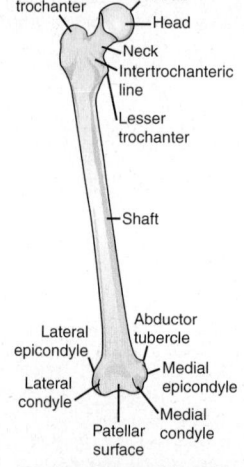

Figure 19-9 Anterior aspect of right femur.

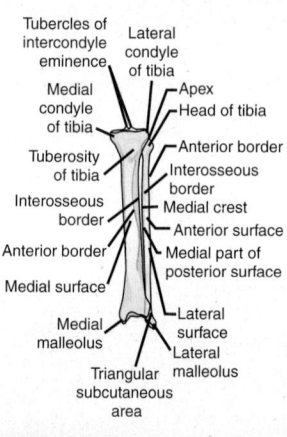

Figure 19-10 Anterior aspect of left tibia and fibula.

▶ New ⟾ Revised ~~deleted~~ Deleted Excludes 1 Excludes 2 Includes Use additional Code first Code also Key words

OGCR Official Guidelines X Assign placeholder X ● Use Additional Character(s) ▸ Manifestation Code Hierarchical Condition Category Coding Clinic

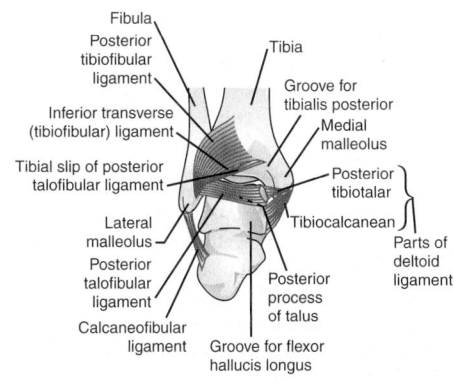

Figure 19-11 Posterior aspect of the left ankle joint.

Figure 19-12 Right foot viewed from above.

CHAPTER 19

INJURY, POISONING AND CERTAIN OTHER CONSEQUENCES OF EXTERNAL CAUSES (S00-T88)

Note: Use secondary code(s) from Chapter 20, External causes of morbidity, to indicate cause of injury. Codes within the T section that include the external cause do not require an additional external cause code.

Use additional code to identify any retained foreign body, if applicable (Z18.-)

Excludes1 birth trauma (P10-P15)
obstetric trauma (O70-O71)

Note: The chapter uses the S-section for coding different types of injuries related to single body regions and the T-section to cover injuries to unspecified body regions as well as poisoning and certain other consequences of external causes.

This chapter contains the following blocks:

S00-S09	Injuries to the head
S10-S19	Injuries to the neck
S20-S29	Injuries to the thorax
S30-S39	Injuries to the abdomen, lower back, lumbar spine, pelvis and external genitals
S40-S49	Injuries to the shoulder and upper arm
S50-S59	Injuries to the elbow and forearm
S60-S69	Injuries to the wrist, hand, and fingers
S70-S79	Injuries to the hip and thigh
S80-S89	Injuries to the knee and lower leg
S90-S99	Injuries to the ankle and foot

T07	Injuries involving multiple body regions
T14	Injury of unspecified body region
T15-T19	Effects of foreign body entering through natural orifice
T20-T25	Burns and corrosions of external body surface, specified by site
T26-T28	Burns and corrosions confined to eye and internal organs
T30-T32	Burns and corrosions of multiple and unspecified body regions
T33-T34	Frostbite
T36-T50	Poisoning by, adverse effect of and underdosing of drugs, medicaments and biological substances
T51-T65	Toxic effects of substances chiefly nonmedicinal as to source
T66-T78	Other and unspecified effects of external causes
T79	Certain early complications of trauma
T80-T88	Complications of surgical and medical care, not elsewhere classified

INJURIES TO THE HEAD (S00-S09)

Includes   injuries of ear
injuries of eye
injuries of face [any part]
injuries of gum
injuries of jaw
injuries of oral cavity
injuries of palate
injuries of periocular area
injuries of scalp
injuries of temporomandibular joint area
injuries of tongue
injuries of tooth

Code also for any associated infection

Excludes2 burns and corrosions (T20-T32)
effects of foreign body in ear (T16)
effects of foreign body in larynx (T17.3)
effects of foreign body in mouth NOS (T18.0)
effects of foreign body in nose (T17.0-T17.1)
effects of foreign body in pharynx (T17.2)
effects of foreign body on external eye (T15.-)
frostbite (T33-T34)
insect bite or sting, venomous (T63.4)

● S00 **Superficial injury of head**

Excludes1 diffuse cerebral contusion (S06.2-)
focal cerebral contusion (S06.3-)
injury of eye and orbit (S05.-)
open wound of head (S01.-)

The appropriate 7th character is to be added to each code from category S00

A	initial encounter
	All encounters involving diagnosis and treatment
D	subsequent encounter
	Encounters during the healing phase
S	sequela

● S00.0 **Superficial injury of scalp**
X ● S00.00 **Unspecified** superficial injury of scalp
X ● S00.01 **Abrasion** of scalp
X ● S00.02 **Blister (nonthermal)** of scalp
X ● S00.03 **Contusion** of scalp
Bruise of scalp
Hematoma of scalp
X ● S00.04 **External constriction** of part of scalp
X ● S00.05 **Superficial foreign body** of scalp
Splinter in the scalp
X ● S00.06 **Insect bite (nonvenomous)** of scalp
X ● S00.07 **Other** superficial bite of scalp
Excludes1 open bite of scalp (S01.05)

● **S00.1**   **Contusion of eyelid and periocular area**
Black eye
    Excludes2   contusion of eyeball and orbital tissues
(S05.1-)

X● **S00.10**   Contusion of unspecified eyelid and periocular area

X● **S00.11**   Contusion of right eyelid and periocular area

X● **S00.12**   Contusion of left eyelid and periocular area

● **S00.2**   **Other and unspecified superficial injuries of eyelid and periocular area**
    Excludes2   superficial injury of conjunctiva and cornea (S05.0-)

● **S00.20**   Unspecified superficial injury of eyelid and periocular area

   ● S00.201   Unspecified superficial injury of right eyelid and periocular area

   ● S00.202   Unspecified superficial injury of left eyelid and periocular area

   ● S00.209   Unspecified superficial injury of unspecified eyelid and periocular area

● **S00.21**   Abrasion of eyelid and periocular area

   ● S00.211   Abrasion of right eyelid and periocular area

   ● S00.212   Abrasion of left eyelid and periocular area

   ● S00.219   Abrasion of unspecified eyelid and periocular area

● **S00.22**   Blister (nonthermal) of eyelid and periocular area

   ● S00.221   Blister (nonthermal) of right eyelid and periocular area

   ● S00.222   Blister (nonthermal) of left eyelid and periocular area

   ● S00.229   Blister (nonthermal) of unspecified eyelid and periocular area

● **S00.24**   External constriction of eyelid and periocular area

   ● S00.241   External constriction of right eyelid and periocular area

   ● S00.242   External constriction of left eyelid and periocular area

   ● S00.249   External constriction of unspecified eyelid and periocular area

● **S00.25**   Superficial foreign body of eyelid and periocular area
Splinter of eyelid and periocular area
    Excludes2   retained foreign body in eyelid (H02.81-)

   ● S00.251   Superficial foreign body of right eyelid and periocular area

   ● S00.252   Superficial foreign body of left eyelid and periocular area

   ● S00.259   Superficial foreign body of unspecified eyelid and periocular area

● **S00.26**   Insect bite (nonvenomous) of eyelid and periocular area

   ● S00.261   Insect bite (nonvenomous) of right eyelid and periocular area

   ● S00.262   Insect bite (nonvenomous) of left eyelid and periocular area

   ● S00.269   Insect bite (nonvenomous) of unspecified eyelid and periocular area

● **S00.27**   Other superficial bite of eyelid and periocular area
    Excludes1   open bite of eyelid and periocular area (S01.15)

   ● S00.271   Other superficial bite of right eyelid and periocular area

   ● S00.272   Other superficial bite of left eyelid and periocular area

   ● S00.279   Other superficial bite of unspecified eyelid and periocular area

● **S00.3**   **Superficial injury of nose**

X● **S00.30**   Unspecified superficial injury of nose

X● **S00.31**   Abrasion of nose

X● **S00.32**   Blister (nonthermal) of nose

X● **S00.33**   Contusion of nose
Bruise of nose
Hematoma of nose

X● **S00.34**   External constriction of nose

X● **S00.35**   Superficial foreign body of nose
Splinter in the nose

X● **S00.36**   Insect bite (nonvenomous) of nose

X● **S00.37**   Other superficial bite of nose
    Excludes1   open bite of nose (S01.25)

● **S00.4**   **Superficial injury of ear**

● **S00.40**   Unspecified superficial injury of ear

   ● S00.401   Unspecified superficial injury of right ear

   ● S00.402   Unspecified superficial injury of left ear

   ● S00.409   Unspecified superficial injury of unspecified ear

● **S00.41**   Abrasion of ear

   ● S00.411   Abrasion of right ear

   ● S00.412   Abrasion of left ear

   ● S00.419   Abrasion of unspecified ear

● **S00.42**   Blister (nonthermal) of ear

   ● S00.421   Blister (nonthermal) of right ear

   ● S00.422   Blister (nonthermal) of left ear

   ● S00.429   Blister (nonthermal) of unspecified ear

● **S00.43**   Contusion of ear
Bruise of ear
Hematoma of ear

   ● S00.431   Contusion of right ear

   ● S00.432   Contusion of left ear

   ● S00.439   Contusion of unspecified ear

● **S00.44**   External constriction of ear

   ● S00.441   External constriction of right ear

   ● S00.442   External constriction of left ear

   ● S00.449   External constriction of unspecified ear

● **S00.45**   Superficial foreign body of ear
Splinter in the ear

   ● S00.451   Superficial foreign body of right ear

   ● S00.452   Superficial foreign body of left ear

   ● S00.459   Superficial foreign body of unspecified ear

● **S00.46**   Insect bite (nonvenomous) of ear

   ● S00.461   Insect bite (nonvenomous) of right ear

   ● S00.462   Insect bite (nonvenomous) of left ear

   ● S00.469   Insect bite (nonvenomous) of unspecified ear

● **S00.47** Other superficial bite of ear
　　Excludes1 open bite of ear (S01.35)
　　● **S00.471** Other superficial bite of right ear
　　● **S00.472** Other superficial bite of left ear
　　● **S00.479** Other superficial bite of unspecified ear
● **S00.5** Superficial injury of lip and oral cavity
　● **S00.50** Unspecified superficial injury of lip and oral cavity
　　● **S00.501** Unspecified superficial injury of lip
　　● **S00.502** Unspecified superficial injury of oral cavity
　● **S00.51** Abrasion of lip and oral cavity
　　● **S00.511** Abrasion of lip
　　● **S00.512** Abrasion of oral cavity
　● **S00.52** Blister (nonthermal) of lip and oral cavity
　　● **S00.521** Blister (nonthermal) of lip
　　● **S00.522** Blister (nonthermal) of oral cavity
　● **S00.53** Contusion of lip and oral cavity
　　● **S00.531** Contusion of lip
　　　Bruise of lip
　　　Hematoma of lip
　　● **S00.532** Contusion of oral cavity
　　　Bruise of oral cavity
　　　Hematoma of oral cavity
　● **S00.54** External constriction of lip and oral cavity
　　● **S00.541** External constriction of lip
　　● **S00.542** External constriction of oral cavity
　● **S00.55** Superficial foreign body of lip and oral cavity
　　● **S00.551** Superficial foreign body of lip
　　　Splinter of lip and oral cavity
　　● **S00.552** Superficial foreign body of oral cavity
　　　Splinter of lip and oral cavity
　● **S00.56** Insect bite (nonvenomous) of lip and oral cavity
　　● **S00.561** Insect bite (nonvenomous) of lip
　　● **S00.562** Insect bite (nonvenomous) of oral cavity
　● **S00.57** Other superficial bite of lip and oral cavity
　　● **S00.571** Other superficial bite of lip
　　　Excludes1 open bite of lip (S01.551)
　　● **S00.572** Other superficial bite of oral cavity
　　　Excludes1 open bite of oral cavity (S01.552)
● **S00.8** Superficial injury of other parts of head
　Superficial injuries of face [any part]
　X ● **S00.80** Unspecified superficial injury of other part of head
　X ● **S00.81** Abrasion of other part of head
　X ● **S00.82** Blister (nonthermal) of other part of head
　X ● **S00.83** Contusion of other part of head
　　Bruise of other part of head
　　Hematoma of other part of head
　X ● **S00.84** External constriction of other part of head
　X ● **S00.85** Superficial foreign body of other part of head
　　Splinter in other part of head
　X ● **S00.86** Insect bite (nonvenomous) of other part of head
　X ● **S00.87** Other superficial bite of other part of head
　　Excludes1 open bite of other part of head (S01.85)
● **S00.9** Superficial injury of unspecified part of head
　X ● **S00.90** Unspecified superficial injury of unspecified part of head
　X ● **S00.91** Abrasion of unspecified part of head
　X ● **S00.92** Blister (nonthermal) of unspecified part of head
　X ● **S00.93** Contusion of unspecified part of head
　　Bruise of head
　　Hematoma of head
　X ● **S00.94** External constriction of unspecified part of head

X ● **S00.95** Superficial foreign body of unspecified part of head
　Splinter of head
X ● **S00.96** Insect bite (nonvenomous) of unspecified part of head
X ● **S00.97** Other superficial bite of unspecified part of head
　　Excludes1 open bite of head (S01.95)

● **S01** Open wound of head
　Code also any associated:
　　injury of cranial nerve (S04.-)
　　injury of muscle and tendon of head (S09.1-)
　　intracranial injury (S06.-)
　　wound infection
　Excludes1 open skull fracture (S02.- with 7th character B)
　Excludes2 injury of eye and orbit (S05.-)
　　traumatic amputation of part of head (S08.-)
　The appropriate 7th character is to be added to each code from category S01

A	initial encounter
D	subsequent encounter
S	sequela

● **S01.0** Open wound of scalp
　　Excludes1 avulsion of scalp (S08.0-)
　X ● **S01.00** Unspecified open wound of scalp
　X ● **S01.01** Laceration without foreign body of scalp
　X ● **S01.02** Laceration with foreign body of scalp
　　Coding Clinic: 2015, Q1, P5-7
　X ● **S01.03** Puncture wound without foreign body of scalp
　X ● **S01.04** Puncture wound with foreign body of scalp
　X ● **S01.05** Open bite of scalp
　　Bite of scalp NOS
　　Excludes1 superficial bite of scalp (S00.06, S00.07-)
● **S01.1** Open wound of eyelid and periocular area
　Open wound of eyelid and periocular area with or without involvement of lacrimal passages
　● **S01.10** Unspecified open wound of eyelid and periocular area
　　● **S01.101** Unspecified open wound of right eyelid and periocular area
　　● **S01.102** Unspecified open wound of left eyelid and periocular area
　　● **S01.109** Unspecified open wound of unspecified eyelid and periocular area
　● **S01.11** Laceration without foreign body of eyelid and periocular area
　　● **S01.111** Laceration without foreign body of right eyelid and periocular area
　　● **S01.112** Laceration without foreign body of left eyelid and periocular area
　　● **S01.119** Laceration without foreign body of unspecified eyelid and periocular area
　● **S01.12** Laceration with foreign body of eyelid and periocular area
　　● **S01.121** Laceration with foreign body of right eyelid and periocular area
　　● **S01.122** Laceration with foreign body of left eyelid and periocular area
　　● **S01.129** Laceration with foreign body of unspecified eyelid and periocular area
　● **S01.13** Puncture wound without foreign body of eyelid and periocular area
　　● **S01.131** Puncture wound without foreign body of right eyelid and periocular area

CHAPTER 19 (S00–T88)

● S01.132   Puncture wound without foreign
             body of left eyelid and periocular area
● S01.139   Puncture wound without foreign
             body of unspecified eyelid and
             periocular area
● S01.14   Puncture wound with foreign body of eyelid
           and periocular area
   ● S01.141   Puncture wound with foreign body of
               right eyelid and periocular area
   ● S01.142   Puncture wound with foreign body of
               left eyelid and periocular area
   ● S01.149   Puncture wound with foreign body of
               unspecified eyelid and periocular area
● S01.15   Open bite of eyelid and periocular area
           Bite of eyelid and periocular area NOS
      Excludes1   superficial bite of eyelid and
                      periocular area (S00.26,
                      S00.27)
   ● S01.151   Open bite of right eyelid and
               periocular area
   ● S01.152   Open bite of left eyelid and
               periocular area
   ● S01.159   Open bite of unspecified eyelid and
               periocular area
● S01.2   Open wound of nose
   X ● S01.20   Unspecified open wound of nose
   X ● S01.21   Laceration without foreign body of nose
               Coding Clinic: 2015, Q1, P5-6
   X ● S01.22   Laceration with foreign body of nose
   X ● S01.23   Puncture wound without foreign body of nose
   X ● S01.24   Puncture wound with foreign body of nose
   X ● S01.25   Open bite of nose
               Bite of nose NOS
          Excludes1   superficial bite of nose (S00.36,
                          S00.37)
● S01.3   Open wound of ear
   ● S01.30   Unspecified open wound of ear
      ● S01.301   Unspecified open wound of right ear
      ● S01.302   Unspecified open wound of left ear
      ● S01.309   Unspecified open wound of
                  unspecified ear
   ● S01.31   Laceration without foreign body of ear
      ● S01.311   Laceration without foreign body of
                  right ear
      ● S01.312   Laceration without foreign body of
                  left ear
      ● S01.319   Laceration without foreign body of
                  unspecified ear
   ● S01.32   Laceration with foreign body of ear
      ● S01.321   Laceration with foreign body of right
                  ear
      ● S01.322   Laceration with foreign body of left
                  ear
      ● S01.329   Laceration with foreign body of
                  unspecified ear
   ● S01.33   Puncture wound without foreign body of ear
      ● S01.331   Puncture wound without foreign
                  body of right ear
      ● S01.332   Puncture wound without foreign
                  body of left ear
      ● S01.339   Puncture wound without foreign
                  body of unspecified ear
   ● S01.34   Puncture wound with foreign body of ear
      ● S01.341   Puncture wound with foreign body of
                  right ear
      ● S01.342   Puncture wound with foreign body of
                  left ear
      ● S01.349   Puncture wound with foreign body of
                  unspecified ear

● S01.35   Open bite of ear
           Bite of ear NOS
      Excludes1   superficial bite of ear (S00.46,
                      S00.47)
   ● S01.351   Open bite of right ear
   ● S01.352   Open bite of left ear
   ● S01.359   Open bite of unspecified ear
● S01.4   Open wound of cheek and temporomandibular area
   ● S01.40   Unspecified open wound of cheek and
              temporomandibular area
      ● S01.401   Unspecified open wound of right
                  cheek and temporomandibular area
      ● S01.402   Unspecified open wound of left cheek
                  and temporomandibular area
      ● S01.409   Unspecified open wound
                  of unspecified cheek and
                  temporomandibular area
   ● S01.41   Laceration without foreign body of cheek and
              temporomandibular area
      ● S01.411   Laceration without foreign body of
                  right cheek and temporomandibular
                  area
                  Coding Clinic: 2015, Q1, P5-7
      ● S01.412   Laceration without foreign body of
                  left cheek and temporomandibular
                  area
      ● S01.419   Laceration without foreign
                  body of unspecified cheek and
                  temporomandibular area
   ● S01.42   Laceration with foreign body of cheek and
              temporomandibular area
      ● S01.421   Laceration with foreign body of right
                  cheek and temporomandibular area
      ● S01.422   Laceration with foreign body of left
                  cheek and temporomandibular area
      ● S01.429   Laceration with foreign body
                  of unspecified cheek and
                  temporomandibular area
   ● S01.43   Puncture wound without foreign body of cheek
              and temporomandibular area
      ● S01.431   Puncture wound without
                  foreign body of right cheek and
                  temporomandibular area
      ● S01.432   Puncture wound without
                  foreign body of left cheek and
                  temporomandibular area
      ● S01.439   Puncture wound without foreign
                  body of unspecified cheek and
                  temporomandibular area
   ● S01.44   Puncture wound with foreign body of cheek
              and temporomandibular area
      ● S01.441   Puncture wound with foreign body of
                  right cheek and temporomandibular
                  area
      ● S01.442   Puncture wound with foreign body
                  of left cheek and temporomandibular
                  area
      ● S01.449   Puncture wound with foreign
                  body of unspecified cheek and
                  temporomandibular area
   ● S01.45   Open bite of cheek and temporomandibular
              area
              Bite of cheek and temporomandibular area NOS
         Excludes2   superficial bite of cheek and
                         temporomandibular area
                         (S00.86, S00.87)
      ● S01.451   Open bite of right cheek and
                  temporomandibular area
      ● S01.452   Open bite of left cheek and
                  temporomandibular area
      ● S01.459   Open bite of unspecified cheek and
                  temporomandibular area

▶ New   ⇒ Revised   ~~deleted~~ Deleted   Excludes 1   Excludes 2   Includes   Use additional   Code first   Code also   Key words
OGCR Official Guidelines   X Assign placeholder X   ● Use Additional Character(s)   ▶ Manifestation Code   🅗 Hierarchical Condition Category   Coding Clinic

● S01.5   Open wound of lip and oral cavity
  Excludes2   tooth dislocation (S03.2)
                   tooth fracture (S02.5)
  ● S01.50   Unspecified open wound of lip and oral cavity
    ● S01.501   Unspecified open wound of lip
    ● S01.502   Unspecified open wound of oral
                 cavity
  ● S01.51   Laceration of lip and oral cavity without foreign
              body
    ● S01.511   Laceration without foreign body of
                 lip
    ● S01.512   Laceration without foreign body of
                 oral cavity
  ● S01.52   Laceration of lip and oral cavity with foreign
              body
    ● S01.521   Laceration with foreign body of lip
    ● S01.522   Laceration with foreign body of oral
                 cavity
  ● S01.53   Puncture wound of lip and oral cavity without
              foreign body
    ● S01.531   Puncture wound without foreign
                 body of lip
    ● S01.532   Puncture wound without foreign
                 body of oral cavity
  ● S01.54   Puncture wound of lip and oral cavity with
              foreign body
    ● S01.541   Puncture wound with foreign body of
                 lip
    ● S01.542   Puncture wound with foreign body of
                 oral cavity
  ● S01.55   Open bite of lip and oral cavity
    ● S01.551   Open bite of lip
                 Bite of lip NOS
                 Excludes1   superficial bite of lip
                                  (S00.571)
    ● S01.552   Open bite of oral cavity
                 Bite of oral cavity NOS
                 Excludes1   superficial bite of oral
                                  cavity (S00.572)

● S01.8   Open wound of other parts of head
  X ● S01.80   Unspecified open wound of other part of head
  X ● S01.81   Laceration without foreign body of other part
                of head
  X ● S01.82   Laceration with foreign body of other part of
                head
  X ● S01.83   Puncture wound without foreign body of other
                part of head
  X ● S01.84   Puncture wound with foreign body of other
                part of head
  X ● S01.85   Open bite of other part of head
                Bite of other part of head NOS
                Excludes1   superficial bite of other part of
                                 head (S00.87)

● S01.9   Open wound of unspecified part of head
  X ● S01.90   Unspecified open wound of unspecified part of
                head
  X ● S01.91   Laceration without foreign body of unspecified
                part of head
  X ● S01.92   Laceration with foreign body of unspecified
                part of head
  X ● S01.93   Puncture wound without foreign body of
                unspecified part of head
  X ● S01.94   Puncture wound with foreign body of
                unspecified part of head
  X ● S01.95   Open bite of unspecified part of head
                Bite of head NOS
                Excludes1   superficial bite of head NOS
                                 (S00.97)

● S02   Fracture of skull and facial bones
  Note: A fracture not indicated as open or closed should be
             coded to closed
             The appropriate 7th character is to be added to each code
             from category S02

A	initial encounter for closed fracture
B	initial encounter for open fracture
D	subsequent encounter for fracture with routine healing
G	subsequent encounter for fracture with delayed healing
K	subsequent encounter for fracture with nonunion
S	sequela

  Code also any associated intracranial injury (S06.-)
  X ● S02.0   Fracture of vault of skull A, B, S 🐾
               Fracture of frontal bone
               Fracture of parietal bone
  ● S02.1   Fracture of base of skull
    Excludes2   lateral orbital wall (S02.84-)
                     medial orbital wall (S02.83-)
                     orbital floor (S02.3-)
    Coding Clinic: 2016, Q4, P66
    ● S02.10   Unspecified fracture of base of skull
      ● S02.101   Fracture of base of skull, right
                   side A, B, S 🐾
      ● S02.102   Fracture of base of skull, left
                   side A, B, S 🐾
      ● S02.109   Fracture of base of skull, unspecified
                   side A, B, S 🐾
    ● S02.11   Fracture of occiput
      ● S02.110   Type I occipital condyle fracture,
                   unspecified side A, B, S 🐾
      ● S02.111   Type II occipital condyle fracture,
                   unspecified side A, B, S 🐾
      ● S02.112   Type III occipital condyle fracture,
                   unspecified side A, B, S 🐾
      ● S02.113   Unspecified occipital condyle
                   fracture A, B, S 🐾
      ● S02.118   Other fracture of occiput, unspecified
                   side A, B, S 🐾
      ● S02.119   Unspecified fracture of
                   occiput A, B, S 🐾
      ● S02.11A   Type I occipital condyle fracture, right
                   side A, B, S 🐾
      ● S02.11B   Type I occipital condyle fracture, left
                   side A, B, S 🐾
      ● S02.11C   Type II occipital condyle fracture,
                   right side A, B, S 🐾
      ● S02.11D   Type II occipital condyle fracture, left
                   side A, B, S 🐾
      ● S02.11E   Type III occipital condyle fracture,
                   right side A, B, S 🐾
      ● S02.11F   Type III occipital condyle fracture,
                   left side A, B, S 🐾
      ● S02.11G   Other fracture of occiput, right side
                   A, B, S 🐾
      ● S02.11H   Other fracture of occiput, left side
                   A, B, S 🐾
    S02.12   Fracture of orbital roof
      S02.121   Fracture of orbital roof, right side
      S02.122   Fracture of orbital roof, left side
      S02.129   Fracture of orbital roof, unspecified
                 side

CHAPTER 19 (S00–T88)

X ● **S02.19** **Other fracture of base of skull** A, B, S 🦠
    Fracture of anterior fossa of base of skull
    Fracture of ethmoid sinus
    Fracture of frontal sinus
    Fracture of middle fossa of base of skull
    Fracture of posterior fossa of base of skull
    Fracture of sphenoid
    Fracture of temporal bone
    Coding Clinic: 2024, Q2, P15

X ● **S02.2** **Fracture of nasal bones**

● **S02.3** **Fracture of orbital floor**
    Fracture of inferior orbital wall
    Excludes1 orbit NOS (S02.85)
    Excludes2 lateral orbital wall (S02.84-)
             medial orbital wall (S02.83-)
             orbital roof (S02.1-)
    Coding Clinic: 2016, Q4, P66

   X ● **S02.30** **Fracture of orbital floor, unspecified side** A, B, S 🦠

   X ● **S02.31** **Fracture of orbital floor, right side** A, B, S 🦠

   X ● **S02.32** **Fracture of orbital floor, left side** A, B, S 🦠

● **S02.4** **Fracture of malar, maxillary and zygoma bones**
    Fracture of superior maxilla
    Fracture of upper jaw (bone)
    Fracture of zygomatic process of temporal bone
    Coding Clinic: 2016, Q4, P66

   ● **S02.40** **Fracture of malar, maxillary and zygoma bones, unspecified**
      ● **S02.400** **Malar fracture unspecified side** A, B, S 🦠
      ● **S02.401** **Maxillary fracture, unspecified side** A, B, S 🦠
      ● **S02.402** **Zygomatic fracture, unspecified side** A, B, S 🦠
      ● **S02.40A** **Malar fracture, right side** A, B, S 🦠
      ● **S02.40B** **Malar fracture, left side** A, B, S 🦠
      ● **S02.40C** **Maxillary fracture, right side** A, B, S 🦠
      ● **S02.40D** **Maxillary fracture, left side** A, B, S 🦠
      ● **S02.40E** **Zygomatic fracture, right side** A, B, S 🦠
      ● **S02.40F** **Zygomatic fracture, left side** A, B, S 🦠

   ● **S02.41** **LeFort fracture**
      ● **S02.411** **LeFort I fracture** A, B, S 🦠
      ● **S02.412** **LeFort II fracture** A, B, S 🦠
      ● **S02.413** **LeFort III fracture** A, B, S 🦠

   X ● **S02.42** **Fracture of alveolus of maxilla** A, B, S 🦠

X ● **S02.5** **Fracture of tooth (traumatic) Broken tooth**
    Excludes1 cracked tooth (nontraumatic) (K03.81)

● **S02.6** **Fracture of mandible**
    Fracture of lower jaw (bone)
    Coding Clinic: 2016, Q4, P66

   ● **S02.60** **Fracture of mandible of unspecified site**
      ● **S02.600** **Fracture of unspecified part of body of mandible, unspecified side** A, B, S 🦠
      ● **S02.601** **Fracture of unspecified part of body of right mandible** A, B, S 🦠
      ● **S02.602** **Fracture of unspecified part of body of left mandible** A, B, S 🦠
      ● **S02.609** **Fracture of mandible, unspecified** A, B, S 🦠

   ● **S02.61** **Fracture of condylar process of mandible**
      ● **S02.610** **Fracture of condylar process of mandible, unspecified side** A, B, S 🦠
      ● **S02.611** **Fracture of condylar process of right mandible** A, B, S 🦠
            Coding Clinic: 2021, Q1, P6
      ● **S02.612** **Fracture of condylar process of left mandible** A, B, S 🦠

● **S02.62** **Fracture of subcondylar process of mandible**
    ● **S02.620** **Fracture of subcondylar process of mandible, unspecified side** A, B, S 🦠
    ● **S02.621** **Fracture of subcondylar process of right mandible** A, B, S 🦠
    ● **S02.622** **Fracture of subcondylar process of left mandible** A, B, S 🦠

● **S02.63** **Fracture of coronoid process of mandible**
    ● **S02.630** **Fracture of coronoid process of mandible, unspecified side** A, B, S 🦠
    ● **S02.631** **Fracture of coronoid process of right mandible** A, B, S 🦠
    ● **S02.632** **Fracture of coronoid process of left mandible** A, B, S 🦠

● **S02.64** **Fracture of ramus of mandible**
    ● **S02.640** **Fracture of ramus of mandible, unspecified side** A, B, S 🦠
    ● **S02.641** **Fracture of ramus of right mandible** A, B, S 🦠
    ● **S02.642** **Fracture of ramus of left mandible** A, B, S 🦠

● **S02.65** **Fracture of angle of mandible**
    ● **S02.650** **Fracture of angle of mandible, unspecified side** A, B, S 🦠
    ● **S02.651** **Fracture of angle of right mandible** A, B, S 🦠
    ● **S02.652** **Fracture of angle of left mandible** A, B, S 🦠

X ● **S02.66** **Fracture of symphysis of mandible** A, B, S 🦠
    Coding Clinic: 2021, Q1, P6

● **S02.67** **Fracture of alveolus of mandible**
    ● **S02.670** **Fracture of alveolus of mandible, unspecified side** A, B, S 🦠
    ● **S02.671** **Fracture of alveolus of right mandible** A, B, S 🦠
    ● **S02.672** **Fracture of alveolus of left mandible** A, B, S 🦠

X ● **S02.69** **Fracture of mandible of other specified site** A, B, S 🦠

● **S02.8** **Fractures of other specified skull and facial bones**
    Fracture of palate
    Excludes2 lateral orbital wall (S02.84-)
             medial orbital wall (S02.83-)
    Coding Clinic: 2016, Q4, P66

   X ● **S02.80** **Fracture of other specified skull and facial bones, unspecified side** A, B, S 🦠

   X ● **S02.81** **Fracture of other specified skull and facial bones, right side** A, B, S 🦠

   X ● **S02.82** **Fracture of other specified skull and facial bones, left side** A, B, S 🦠

   ● **S02.83** **Fracture of medial orbital wall**
      Excludes2 orbital floor (S02.3-)
               orbital roof (S02.12-)
      S02.831 **Fracture of medial orbital wall, right side**
      S02.832 **Fracture of medial orbital wall, left side**
      S02.839 **Fracture of medial orbital wall, unspecified side**

   ● **S02.84** **Fracture of lateral orbital wall**
      Excludes2 orbital floor (S02.3-)
               orbital roof (S02.12-)
      S02.841 **Fracture of lateral orbital wall, right side**
      S02.842 **Fracture of lateral orbital wall, left side**
      S02.849 **Fracture of lateral orbital wall, unspecified side**

▶ New ⇒ Revised ~~deleted~~ Deleted Excludes 1 Excludes 2 Includes Use additional Code first Code also Key words

OGCR Official Guidelines X Assign placeholder X ● Use Additional Character(s) ▶ Manifestation Code 🦠 Hierarchical Condition Category Coding Clinic

Figure 19-13 Cranial nerves. (From Patton and Thibodeau: Anatomy and physiology, ed 7, St. Louis, Mosby, 2009)

Trochlear nerve (IV)

Olfactory nerve (I)

Optic nerve (II)

Abducens nerve (VI)

Oculomotor nerve (III)

Trigeminal nerve (V)

Facial nerve (VII)

Vestibulocochlear nerve (VIII)

Glossopharyngeal nerve (IX)

Vagus nerve (X)　Accessory nerve (XI)

Hypoglossal nerve (XII)

CHAPTER 19 (S00-T88)

S02.85 Fracture of orbit, unspecified
　Fracture of orbit NOS
　Fracture of orbit wall NOS
　Excludes1　lateral orbital wall (S02.84-)
　　　　　medial orbital wall (S02.83-)
　　　　　orbital floor (S02.3-)
　　　　　orbital roof (S02.12-)

● **S02.9　Fracture of unspecified skull and facial bones**
　X● **S02.91　Unspecified fracture of skull A, B, S** 🔗
　X● **S02.92　Unspecified fracture of facial bones A, B, S** 🔗

● **S03　Dislocation and sprain of joints and ligaments of head**
　Includes　avulsion of joint (capsule) or ligament of head
　　　　laceration of cartilage, joint (capsule) or ligament of head
　　　　sprain of cartilage, joint (capsule) or ligament of head
　　　　traumatic hemarthrosis of joint or ligament of head
　　　　traumatic rupture of joint or ligament of head
　　　　traumatic subluxation of joint or ligament of head
　　　　traumatic tear of joint or ligament of head

　Code also any associated open wound
　Excludes2　Strain of muscle or tendon of head (S09.1)
　The appropriate 7th character is to be added to each code from category S03

A	initial encounter
D	subsequent encounter
S	sequela

● **S03.0　Dislocation of jaw**
　Dislocation of jaw (cartilage) (meniscus)
　Dislocation of mandible
　Dislocation of temporomandibular (joint)
　Coding Clinic: 2016, Q4, P67
　X● **S03.00　Dislocation of jaw, unspecified side**
　X● **S03.01　Dislocation of jaw, right side**

X● **S03.02　Dislocation of jaw, left side**
X● **S03.03　Dislocation of jaw, bilateral side**
X● **S03.1　Dislocation of septal cartilage of nose**
X● **S03.2　Dislocation of tooth**
● **S03.4　Sprain of jaw**
　Sprain of temporomandibular (joint) (ligament)
　Coding Clinic: 2016, Q4, P67
　X● **S03.40　Sprain of jaw, unspecified side**
　X● **S03.41　Sprain of jaw, right side**
　X● **S03.42　Sprain of jaw, left side**
　X● **S03.43　Sprain of jaw, bilateral side**
X● **S03.8　Sprain of joints and ligaments of other parts of head**
X● **S03.9　Sprain of joints and ligaments of unspecified parts of head**

● **S04　Injury of cranial nerve**
　The selection of side should be based on the side of the body being affected
　Code first any associated intracranial injury (S06.-)
　Code also any associated:
　　open wound of head (S01.-)
　　skull fracture (S02.-)
　The appropriate 7th character is to be added to each code from category S04

A	initial encounter
D	subsequent encounter
S	sequela

● **S04.0　Injury of optic nerve and pathways**
　Use additional code to identify any visual field defect or blindness (H53.4-, H54.-)
　● **S04.01　Injury of optic nerve**
　　Injury of 2nd cranial nerve
　　● **S04.011　Injury of optic nerve, right eye**

● S04.012   Injury of optic nerve, left eye

● S04.019   Injury of optic nerve, unspecified eye
      Injury of optic nerve NOS

X ● S04.02   Injury of optic chiasm

● S04.03   Injury of optic tract and pathways
      Injury of optic radiation

     ● S04.031   Injury of optic tract and pathways, right side

     ● S04.032   Injury of optic tract and pathways, left side

     ● S04.039   Injury of optic tract and pathways, unspecified side
        Injury of optic tract and pathways NOS

● S04.04   Injury of visual cortex

     ● S04.041   Injury of visual cortex, right side

     ● S04.042   Injury of visual cortex, left side

     ● S04.049   Injury of visual cortex, unspecified side
        Injury of visual cortex NOS

● S04.1   Injury of oculomotor nerve
      Injury of 3rd cranial nerve

X ● S04.10   Injury of oculomotor nerve, unspecified side

X ● S04.11   Injury of oculomotor nerve, right side

X ● S04.12   Injury of oculomotor nerve, left side

● S04.2   Injury of trochlear nerve
      Injury of 4th cranial nerve

X ● S04.20   Injury of trochlear nerve, unspecified side

X ● S04.21   Injury of trochlear nerve, right side

X ● S04.22   Injury of trochlear nerve, left side

● S04.3   Injury of trigeminal nerve
      Injury of 5th cranial nerve

X ● S04.30   Injury of trigeminal nerve, unspecified side

X ● S04.31   Injury of trigeminal nerve, right side

X ● S04.32   Injury of trigeminal nerve, left side

● S04.4   Injury of abducent nerve
      Injury of 6th cranial nerve

X ● S04.40   Injury of abducent nerve, unspecified side

X ● S04.41   Injury of abducent nerve, right side

X ● S04.42   Injury of abducent nerve, left side

● S04.5   Injury of facial nerve
      Injury of 7th cranial nerve

X ● S04.50   Injury of facial nerve, unspecified side

X ● S04.51   Injury of facial nerve, right side

X ● S04.52   Injury of facial nerve, left side

● S04.6   Injury of acoustic nerve
      Injury of auditory nerve
      Injury of 8th cranial nerve

X ● S04.60   Injury of acoustic nerve, unspecified side

X ● S04.61   Injury of acoustic nerve, right side

X ● S04.62   Injury of acoustic nerve, left side

● S04.7   Injury of accessory nerve
      Injury of 11th cranial nerve

X ● S04.70   Injury of accessory nerve, unspecified side

X ● S04.71   Injury of accessory nerve, right side

X ● S04.72   Injury of accessory nerve, left side

● S04.8   Injury of other cranial nerves

● S04.81   Injury of olfactory [1st] nerve

     ● S04.811   Injury of olfactory [1st] nerve, right side

     ● S04.812   Injury of olfactory [1st] nerve, left side

     ● S04.819   Injury of olfactory [1st] nerve, unspecified side

● S04.89   Injury of other cranial nerves
      Injury of vagus [10th] nerve

     ● S04.891   Injury of other cranial nerves, right side

     ● S04.892   Injury of other cranial nerves, left side

     ● S04.899   Injury of other cranial nerves, unspecified side

X ● S04.9   Injury of unspecified cranial nerve

● S05   Injury of eye and orbit

    Includes   open wound of eye and orbit

    Excludes2   2nd cranial [optic] nerve injury (S04.0-)
        3rd cranial [oculomotor] nerve injury (S04.1-)
        open wound of eyelid and periocular area (S01.1-)
        orbital bone fracture (S02.1-, S02.3-, S02.8-)
        superficial injury of eyelid (S00.1-S00.2)

   The appropriate 7th character is to be added to each code from category S05

> A   initial encounter
> D   subsequent encounter
> S   sequela

● S05.0   Injury of conjunctiva and corneal abrasion without foreign body

    Excludes1   foreign body in conjunctival sac (T15.1)
        foreign body in cornea (T15.0)

X ● S05.00   Injury of conjunctiva and corneal abrasion without foreign body, unspecified eye

X ● S05.01   Injury of conjunctiva and corneal abrasion without foreign body, right eye

X ● S05.02   Injury of conjunctiva and corneal abrasion without foreign body, left eye

● S05.1   Contusion of eyeball and orbital tissues
      Traumatic hyphema

    Excludes2   black eye NOS (S00.1)
        contusion of eyelid and periocular area (S00.1)

X ● S05.10   Contusion of eyeball and orbital tissues, unspecified eye

X ● S05.11   Contusion of eyeball and orbital tissues, right eye

X ● S05.12   Contusion of eyeball and orbital tissues, left eye

● S05.2   Ocular laceration and rupture with prolapse or loss of intraocular tissue

X ● S05.20   Ocular laceration and rupture with prolapse or loss of intraocular tissue, unspecified eye

X ● S05.21   Ocular laceration and rupture with prolapse or loss of intraocular tissue, right eye

X ● S05.22   Ocular laceration and rupture with prolapse or loss of intraocular tissue, left eye

● S05.3   Ocular laceration without prolapse or loss of intraocular tissue
      Laceration of eye NOS

X ● S05.30   Ocular laceration without prolapse or loss of intraocular tissue, unspecified eye

X ● S05.31   Ocular laceration without prolapse or loss of intraocular tissue, right eye

X ● S05.32   Ocular laceration without prolapse or loss of intraocular tissue, left eye

● S05.4   Penetrating wound of orbit with or without foreign body

    Excludes2   retained (old) foreign body following penetrating wound in orbit (H05.5-)

X ● S05.40   Penetrating wound of orbit with or without foreign body, unspecified eye

X ● S05.41   Penetrating wound of orbit with or without foreign body, right eye

X ● S05.42   Penetrating wound of orbit with or without foreign body, left eye

● S05.5   Penetrating wound with foreign body of eyeball

    Excludes2   retained (old) intraocular foreign body (H44.6-, H44.7)

X ● S05.50   Penetrating wound with foreign body of unspecified eyeball

▶ New   ⇒ Revised   ~~deleted~~ Deleted   Excludes 1   Excludes 2   Includes   Use additional   Code first   Code also   Key words

OGCR Official Guidelines   X Assign placeholder X   ● Use Additional Character(s)   ▶ Manifestation Code   🝖 Hierarchical Condition Category   **Coding Clinic**

X ● **S05.51** Penetrating wound with foreign body of right eyeball

X ● **S05.52** Penetrating wound with foreign body of left eyeball

● **S05.6** Penetrating wound without foreign body of eyeball
Ocular penetration NOS

X ● **S05.60** Penetrating wound without foreign body of unspecified eyeball

X ● **S05.61** Penetrating wound without foreign body of right eyeball

X ● **S05.62** Penetrating wound without foreign body of left eyeball

● **S05.7** Avulsion of eye
Traumatic enucleation

X ● **S05.70** Avulsion of unspecified eye

X ● **S05.71** Avulsion of right eye

X ● **S05.72** Avulsion of left eye

● **S05.8** Other injuries of eye and orbit
Lacrimal duct injury

● **S05.8X** Other injuries of eye and orbit

● **S05.8X1** Other injuries of right eye and orbit

● **S05.8X2** Other injuries of left eye and orbit

● **S05.8X9** Other injuries of unspecified eye and orbit

● **S05.9** Unspecified injury of eye and orbit
Injury of eye NOS

X ● **S05.90** Unspecified injury of unspecified eye and orbit

X ● **S05.91** Unspecified injury of right eye and orbit

X ● **S05.92** Unspecified injury of left eye and orbit

● **S06** Intracranial injury

Includes   traumatic brain injury

Code also any associated:
open wound of head (S01.-)
skull fracture (S02.-)

Excludes1   head injury NOS (S09.90)

The appropriate 7th character is to be added to each code from category S06

A	initial encounter
D	subsequent encounter
S	sequela

Note: 7th characters D and S do not apply to codes in category S06 with 6th character 7 - death due to brain injury prior to regaining consciousness, or 8 - death due to other cause prior to regaining consciousness.
Coding Clinic: 2015, Q4, P40

● **S06.0** Concussion
Commotio cerebri

Excludes1   concussion with other intracranial injuries classified in subcategories S06.1- to S06.6- , and S06.81- to S06.82-, code to specified intracranial injury

Coding Clinic: 2016, Q4, P67

● **S06.0X** Concussion

● **S06.0X0** Concussion without loss of consciousness S 🐾

● **S06.0X1** Concussion with loss of consciousness of 30 minutes or less S 🐾
Concussion with brief loss of consciousness

● **S06.0X9** Concussion with loss of consciousness of unspecified duration S 🐾
Coding Clinic: 2016, Q4, P68

● **S06.0XA** Concussion with loss of consciousness status unknown
Concussion NOS

● **S06.1** Traumatic cerebral edema
Diffuse traumatic cerebral edema
Focal traumatic cerebral edema
Coding Clinic: 2016, Q4, P67

● **S06.1X** Traumatic cerebral edema

● **S06.1X0** Traumatic cerebral edema without loss of consciousness A, S 🐾
Coding Clinic: 2015, Q1, P12

● **S06.1X1** Traumatic cerebral edema with loss of consciousness of 30 minutes or less A, S 🐾
Traumatic cerebral edema with brief loss of consciousness

● **S06.1X2** Traumatic cerebral edema with loss of consciousness of 31 minutes to 59 minutes A, S 🐾

● **S06.1X3** Traumatic cerebral edema with loss of consciousness of 1 hour to 5 hours 59 minutes A, S 🐾

● **S06.1X4** Traumatic cerebral edema with loss of consciousness of 6 hours to 24 hours A, S 🐾

● **S06.1X5** Traumatic cerebral edema with loss of consciousness greater than 24 hours with return to pre-existing conscious level A, S 🐾

● **S06.1X6** Traumatic cerebral edema with loss of consciousness greater than 24 hours without return to pre-existing conscious level with patient surviving A, S 🐾

● **S06.1X7** Traumatic cerebral edema with loss of consciousness of any duration with death due to brain injury prior to regaining consciousness

● **S06.1X8** Traumatic cerebral edema with loss of consciousness of any duration with death due to other cause prior to regaining consciousness

● **S06.1X9** Traumatic cerebral edema with loss of consciousness of unspecified duration A, S 🐾

● **S06.1XA** Traumatic cerebral edema with loss of consciousness status unknown
Traumatic cerebral edema NOS

● **S06.2** Diffuse traumatic brain injury
Diffuse axonal brain injury

Excludes1   traumatic diffuse cerebral edema (S06.1X-)

Use Additional code, if applicable, for traumatic brain compression or herniation (S06.A-)

● **S06.2X** Diffuse traumatic brain injury

● **S06.2X0** Diffuse traumatic brain injury without loss of consciousness A, S 🐾

● **S06.2X1** Diffuse traumatic brain injury with loss of consciousness of 30 minutes or less A, S 🐾
Diffuse traumatic brain injury with brief loss of consciousness

● **S06.2X2** Diffuse traumatic brain injury with loss of consciousness of 31 minutes to 59 minutes A, S 🐾

● **S06.2X3** Diffuse traumatic brain injury with loss of consciousness of 1 hour to 5 hours 59 minutes A, S 🐾

● **S06.2X4** Diffuse traumatic brain injury with loss of consciousness of 6 hours to 24 hours A, S 🐾

● **S06.2X5** Diffuse traumatic brain injury with loss of consciousness greater than 24 hours with return to pre-existing conscious levels A, S 🐾

● S06.2X6 **Diffuse traumatic brain injury with loss of consciousness greater than 24 hours without return to pre-existing conscious level with patient surviving** A, S 🐾

● S06.2X7 **Diffuse traumatic brain injury with loss of consciousness of any duration with death due to brain injury prior to regaining consciousness**

● S06.2X8 **Diffuse traumatic brain injury with loss of consciousness of any duration with death due to other cause prior to regaining consciousness**

● S06.2X9 **Diffuse traumatic brain injury with loss of consciousness of unspecified duration** A, S 🐾
    Diffuse traumatic brain injury NOS

● S06.2XA **Diffuse traumatic brain injury with loss of consciousness status unknown**
    Diffuse traumatic brain injury NOS

● S06.3 **Focal traumatic brain injury**

Excludes2 any condition classifiable to S06.4-S06.6
    focal cerebral edema (S06.1)

Use Additional code, if applicable, for traumatic brain compression or herniation (S06.A-)

● S06.30 **Unspecified focal traumatic brain injury**

● S06.300 **Unspecified focal traumatic brain injury without loss of consciousness** A, S 🐾

● S06.301 **Unspecified focal traumatic brain injury with loss of consciousness of 30 minutes or less** A, S 🐾
    Unspecified focal traumatic brain injury with brief loss of consciousness

● S06.302 **Unspecified focal traumatic brain injury with loss of consciousness of 31 minutes to 59 minutes** A, S 🐾

● S06.303 **Unspecified focal traumatic brain injury with loss of consciousness of 1 hour to 5 hours 59 minutes** A, S 🐾

● S06.304 **Unspecified focal traumatic brain injury with loss of consciousness of 6 hours to 24 hours** A, S 🐾

● S06.305 **Unspecified focal traumatic brain injury with loss of consciousness greater than 24 hours with return to pre-existing conscious level** A, S 🐾

● S06.306 **Unspecified focal traumatic brain injury with loss of consciousness greater than 24 hours without return to pre-existing conscious level with patient surviving** A, S 🐾

● S06.307 **Unspecified focal traumatic brain injury with loss of consciousness of any duration with death due to brain injury prior to regaining consciousness**

● S06.308 **Unspecified focal traumatic brain injury with loss of consciousness of any duration with death due to other cause prior to regaining consciousness**

● S06.309 **Unspecified focal traumatic brain injury with loss of consciousness of unspecified duration** A, S 🐾

● S06.30A **Unspecified focal traumatic brain injury with loss of consciousness status unknown**
    Unspecified focal traumatic brain injury NOS

● S06.31 **Contusion and laceration of right cerebrum**

● S06.310 **Contusion and laceration of right cerebrum without loss of consciousness** A, S 🐾

● S06.311 **Contusion and laceration of right cerebrum with loss of consciousness of 30 minutes or less** A, S 🐾
    Contusion and laceration of right cerebrum with brief loss of consciousness

● S06.312 **Contusion and laceration of right cerebrum with loss of consciousness of 31 minutes to 59 minutes** A, S 🐾

● S06.313 **Contusion and laceration of right cerebrum with loss of consciousness of 1 hour to 5 hours 59 minutes** A, S 🐾

● S06.314 **Contusion and laceration of right cerebrum with loss of consciousness of 6 hours to 24 hours** A, S 🐾

● S06.315 **Contusion and laceration of right cerebrum with loss of consciousness greater than 24 hours with return to pre-existing conscious level** A, S 🐾

● S06.316 **Contusion and laceration of right cerebrum with loss of consciousness greater than 24 hours without return to pre-existing conscious level with patient surviving** A, S 🐾

● S06.317 **Contusion and laceration of right cerebrum with loss of consciousness of any duration with death due to brain injury prior to regaining consciousness**

● S06.318 **Contusion and laceration of right cerebrum with loss of consciousness of any duration with death due to other cause prior to regaining consciousness**

● S06.319 **Contusion and laceration of right cerebrum with loss of consciousness of unspecified duration** A, S 🐾

● S06.31A **Contusion and laceration of right cerebrum with loss of consciousness status unknown**
    Contusion and laceration of right cerebrum NOS

● S06.32 **Contusion and laceration of left cerebrum**

● S06.320 **Contusion and laceration of left cerebrum without loss of consciousness** A, S 🐾

● S06.321 **Contusion and laceration of left cerebrum with loss of consciousness of 30 minutes or less** A, S 🐾
    Contusion and laceration of left cerebrum with brief loss of consciousness

● S06.322 **Contusion and laceration of left cerebrum with loss of consciousness of 31 minutes to 59 minutes** A, S 🐾

● S06.323 **Contusion and laceration of left cerebrum with loss of consciousness of 1 hour to 5 hours 59 minutes** A, S 🐾

● S06.324 **Contusion and laceration of left cerebrum with loss of consciousness of 6 hours to 24 hours** A, S 🐾

● S06.325 **Contusion and laceration of left cerebrum with loss of consciousness greater than 24 hours with return to pre-existing conscious level** A, S 🐾

● S06.326   Contusion and laceration of left cerebrum with loss of consciousness greater than 24 hours without return to pre-existing conscious level with patient surviving A, S 🔁

● S06.327   Contusion and laceration of left cerebrum with loss of consciousness of any duration with death due to brain injury prior to regaining consciousness

● S06.328   Contusion and laceration of left cerebrum with loss of consciousness of any duration with death due to other cause prior to regaining consciousness

● S06.329   Contusion and laceration of left cerebrum with loss of consciousness of unspecified duration A, S 🔁

● S06.32A   Contusion and laceration of left cerebrum with loss of consciousness status unknown
            Contusion and laceration of left cerebrum NOS

● S06.33   Contusion and laceration of cerebrum, unspecified

● S06.330   Contusion and laceration of cerebrum, unspecified, without loss of consciousness A, S 🔁

● S06.331   Contusion and laceration of cerebrum, unspecified, with loss of consciousness of 30 minutes or less A, S 🔁
            Contusion and laceration of cerebrum, unspecified, with brief loss of consciousness

● S06.332   Contusion and laceration of cerebrum, unspecified, with loss of consciousness of 31 minutes to 59 minutes A, S 🔁

● S06.333   Contusion and laceration of cerebrum, unspecified, with loss of consciousness of 1 hour to 5 hours 59 minutes A, S 🔁

● S06.334   Contusion and laceration of cerebrum, unspecified, with loss of consciousness of 6 hours to 24 hours A, S 🔁

● S06.335   Contusion and laceration of cerebrum, unspecified, with loss of consciousness greater than 24 hours with return to pre-existing conscious level A, S 🔁

● S06.336   Contusion and laceration of cerebrum, unspecified, with loss of consciousness greater than 24 hours without return to pre-existing conscious level with patient surviving A, S 🔁

● S06.337   Contusion and laceration of cerebrum, unspecified, with loss of consciousness of any duration with death due to brain injury prior to regaining consciousness

● S06.338   Contusion and laceration of cerebrum, unspecified, with loss of consciousness of any duration with death due to other cause prior to regaining consciousness

● S06.339   Contusion and laceration of cerebrum, unspecified, with loss of consciousness of unspecified duration A, S 🔁

● S06.33A   Contusion and laceration of cerebrum, unspecified, with loss of consciousness status unknown
            Contusion and laceration of cerebrum NOS

● S06.34   Traumatic hemorrhage of right cerebrum
            Traumatic intracerebral hemorrhage and hematoma of right cerebrum

● S06.340   Traumatic hemorrhage of right cerebrum without loss of consciousness A, S 🔁
            Coding Clinic: 2015, Q1, P12

● S06.341   Traumatic hemorrhage of right cerebrum with loss of consciousness of 30 minutes or less A, S 🔁
            Traumatic hemorrhage of right cerebrum with brief loss of consciousness

● S06.342   Traumatic hemorrhage of right cerebrum with loss of consciousness of 31 minutes to 59 minutes A, S 🔁

● S06.343   Traumatic hemorrhage of right cerebrum with loss of consciousness of 1 hours to 5 hours 59 minutes A, S 🔁

● S06.344   Traumatic hemorrhage of right cerebrum with loss of consciousness of 6 hours to 24 hours A, S 🔁

● S06.345   Traumatic hemorrhage of right cerebrum with loss of consciousness greater than 24 hours with return to pre-existing conscious level A, S 🔁

● S06.346   Traumatic hemorrhage of right cerebrum with loss of consciousness greater than 24 hours without return to pre-existing conscious level with patient surviving A, S 🔁

● S06.347   Traumatic hemorrhage of right cerebrum with loss of consciousness of any duration with death due to brain injury prior to regaining consciousness

● S06.348   Traumatic hemorrhage of right cerebrum with loss of consciousness of any duration with death due to other cause prior to regaining consciousness

● S06.349   Traumatic hemorrhage of right cerebrum with loss of consciousness of unspecified duration A, S 🔁

● S06.34A   Traumatic hemorrhage of right cerebrum with loss of consciousness status unknown
            Traumatic hemorrhage of right cerebrum NOS

● S06.35   Traumatic hemorrhage of left cerebrum
            Traumatic intracerebral hemorrhage and hematoma of left cerebrum

● S06.350   Traumatic hemorrhage of left cerebrum without loss of consciousness A, S 🔁

● S06.351   Traumatic hemorrhage of left cerebrum with loss of consciousness of 30 minutes or less A, S 🔁
            Traumatic hemorrhage of left cerebrum with brief loss of consciousness

● S06.352   Traumatic hemorrhage of left cerebrum with loss of consciousness of 31 minutes to 59 minutes A, S 🔁

● S06.353   Traumatic hemorrhage of left cerebrum with loss of consciousness of 1 hours to 5 hours 59 minutes A, S 🔁

● S06.354   Traumatic hemorrhage of left cerebrum with loss of consciousness of 6 hours to 24 hours A, S 🔁

● S06.355   Traumatic hemorrhage of left cerebrum with loss of consciousness greater than 24 hours with return to pre-existing conscious level A, S 🐾

● S06.356   Traumatic hemorrhage of left cerebrum with loss of consciousness greater than 24 hours without return to pre-existing conscious level with patient surviving A, S 🐾

● S06.357   Traumatic hemorrhage of left cerebrum with loss of consciousness of any duration with death due to brain injury prior to regaining consciousness

● S06.358   Traumatic hemorrhage of left cerebrum with loss of consciousness of any duration with death due to other cause prior to regaining consciousness

● S06.359   Traumatic hemorrhage of left cerebrum with loss of consciousness of unspecified duration A, S 🐾

● S06.35A   Traumatic hemorrhage of left cerebrum with loss of consciousness status unknown
     Traumatic hemorrhage of left cerebrum NOS

● S06.36   Traumatic hemorrhage of cerebrum, unspecified
     Traumatic intracerebral hemorrhage and hematoma, unspecified

● S06.360   Traumatic hemorrhage of cerebrum, unspecified, without loss of consciousness A, S 🐾

● S06.361   Traumatic hemorrhage of cerebrum, unspecified, with loss of consciousness of 30 minutes or less A, S 🐾
     Traumatic hemorrhage of cerebrum, unspecified, with brief loss of consciousness

● S06.362   Traumatic hemorrhage of cerebrum, unspecified, with loss of consciousness of 31 minutes to 59 minutes A, S 🐾

● S06.363   Traumatic hemorrhage of cerebrum, unspecified, with loss of consciousness of 1 hours to 5 hours 59 minutes A, S 🐾

● S06.364   Traumatic hemorrhage of cerebrum, unspecified, with loss of consciousness of 6 hours to 24 hours A, S 🐾

● S06.365   Traumatic hemorrhage of cerebrum, unspecified, with loss of consciousness greater than 24 hours with return to pre-existing conscious level A, S 🐾

● S06.366   Traumatic hemorrhage of cerebrum, unspecified, with loss of consciousness greater than 24 hours without return to pre-existing conscious level with patient surviving A, S 🐾

● S06.367   Traumatic hemorrhage of cerebrum, unspecified, with loss of consciousness of any duration with death due to brain injury prior to regaining consciousness

● S06.368   Traumatic hemorrhage of cerebrum, unspecified, with loss of consciousness of any duration with death due to other cause prior to regaining consciousness

● S06.369   Traumatic hemorrhage of cerebrum, unspecified, with loss of consciousness of unspecified duration A, S 🐾

● S06.36A   Traumatic hemorrhage of cerebrum, unspecified, with loss of consciousness status unknown
     Traumatic hemorrhage of cerebrum NOS

● S06.37   Contusion, laceration, and hemorrhage of cerebellum

● S06.370   Contusion, laceration, and hemorrhage of cerebellum without loss of consciousness A, S 🐾

● S06.371   Contusion, laceration, and hemorrhage of cerebellum with loss of consciousness of 30 minutes or less A, S 🐾
     Contusion, laceration, and hemorrhage of cerebellum with brief loss of consciousness

● S06.372   Contusion, laceration, and hemorrhage of cerebellum with loss of consciousness of 31 minutes to 59 minutes A, S 🐾

● S06.373   Contusion, laceration, and hemorrhage of cerebellum with loss of consciousness of 1 hour to 5 hours 59 minutes A, S 🐾

● S06.374   Contusion, laceration, and hemorrhage of cerebellum with loss of consciousness of 6 hours to 24 hours A, S 🐾

● S06.375   Contusion, laceration, and hemorrhage of cerebellum with loss of consciousness greater than 24 hours with return to pre-existing conscious level A, S 🐾

● S06.376   Contusion, laceration, and hemorrhage of cerebellum with loss of consciousness greater than 24 hours without return to pre-existing conscious level with patient surviving A, S 🐾

● S06.377   Contusion, laceration, and hemorrhage of cerebellum with loss of consciousness of any duration with death due to brain injury prior to regaining consciousness

● S06.378   Contusion, laceration, and hemorrhage of cerebellum with loss of consciousness of any duration with death due to other cause prior to regaining consciousness

● S06.379   Contusion, laceration, and hemorrhage of cerebellum with loss of consciousness of unspecified duration A, S 🐾

● S06.37A   Contusion, laceration, and hemorrhage of cerebellum with loss of consciousness status unknown
     Contusion, laceration, and hemorrhage of cerebellum NOS

● S06.38   Contusion, laceration, and hemorrhage of brainstem

● S06.380   Contusion, laceration, and hemorrhage of brainstem without loss of consciousness A, S 🐾

● S06.381   Contusion, laceration, and hemorrhage of brainstem with loss of consciousness of 30 minutes or less A, S 🐾
     Contusion, laceration, and hemorrhage of brainstem with brief loss of consciousness

- ● S06.382 Contusion, laceration, and hemorrhage of brainstem with loss of consciousness of 31 minutes to 59 minutes A, S 🐾
- ● S06.383 Contusion, laceration, and hemorrhage of brainstem with loss of consciousness of 1 hour to 5 hours 59 minutes A, S 🐾
- ● S06.384 Contusion, laceration, and hemorrhage of brainstem with loss of consciousness of 6 hours to 24 hours A, S 🐾
- ● S06.385 Contusion, laceration, and hemorrhage of brainstem with loss of consciousness greater than 24 hours with return to pre-existing conscious level A, S 🐾
- ● S06.386 Contusion, laceration, and hemorrhage of brainstem with loss of consciousness greater than 24 hours without return to pre-existing conscious level with patient surviving A, S 🐾
- ● S06.387 Contusion, laceration, and hemorrhage of brainstem with loss of consciousness of any duration with death due to brain injury prior to regaining consciousness
- ● S06.388 Contusion, laceration, and hemorrhage of brainstem with loss of consciousness of any duration with death due to other cause prior to regaining consciousness
- ● S06.389 Contusion, laceration, and hemorrhage of brainstem with loss of consciousness of unspecified duration A, S 🐾
- ● S06.38A Contusion, laceration, and hemorrhage of brainstem with loss of consciousness status unknown
    Contusion, laceration, and hemorrhage of brainstem NOS

- ● S06.4 **Epidural hemorrhage**
    Situated outside dura mater
    Extradural hemorrhage NOS
    Intracranial hemorrhage due to trauma
    Extradural hemorrhage (traumatic)
  - ● S06.4X Epidural hemorrhage
    - ● S06.4X0 Epidural hemorrhage without loss of consciousness A, S 🐾
    - ● S06.4X1 Epidural hemorrhage with loss of consciousness of 30 minutes or less A, S 🐾
        Epidural hemorrhage with brief loss of consciousness
    - ● S06.4X2 Epidural hemorrhage with loss of consciousness of 31 minutes to 59 minutes A, S 🐾
    - ● S06.4X3 Epidural hemorrhage with loss of consciousness of 1 hour to 5 hours 59 minutes A, S 🐾
    - ● S06.4X4 Epidural hemorrhage with loss of consciousness of 6 hours to 24 hours A, S 🐾
    - ● S06.4X5 Epidural hemorrhage with loss of consciousness greater than 24 hours with return to pre-existing conscious level A, S 🐾
    - ● S06.4X6 Epidural hemorrhage with loss of consciousness greater than 24 hours without return to pre-existing conscious level with patient surviving A, S 🐾

- ● S06.4X7 Epidural hemorrhage with loss of consciousness of any duration with death due to brain injury prior to regaining consciousness
- ● S06.4X8 Epidural hemorrhage with loss of consciousness of any duration with death due to other causes prior to regaining consciousness
- ● S06.4X9 Epidural hemorrhage with loss of consciousness of unspecified duration A, S 🐾
- ● S06.4XA Epidural hemorrhage with loss of consciousness status unknown
    Epidural hemorrhage NOS

- ● S06.5 **Traumatic subdural hemorrhage**
    Use Additional code, if applicable, for traumatic brain compression or herniation (S06.A-)
    Coding Clinic: 2024, Q2, P15
  - ● S06.5X Traumatic subdural hemorrhage
    - ● S06.5X0 Traumatic subdural hemorrhage without loss of consciousness A, S 🐾
        Coding Clinic: 2021, Q1, P4; 2018, Q2, P13; 2015, Q3, P37
    - ● S06.5X1 Traumatic subdural hemorrhage with loss of consciousness of 30 minutes or less A, S 🐾
        Traumatic subdural hemorrhage with brief loss of consciousness
    - ● S06.5X2 Traumatic subdural hemorrhage with loss of consciousness of 31 minutes to 59 minutes A, S 🐾
    - ● S06.5X3 Traumatic subdural hemorrhage with loss of consciousness of 1 hour to 5 hours 59 minutes A, S 🐾
    - ● S06.5X4 Traumatic subdural hemorrhage with loss of consciousness of 6 hours to 24 hours A, S 🐾
    - ● S06.5X5 Traumatic subdural hemorrhage with loss of consciousness greater than 24 hours with return to pre-existing conscious level A, S 🐾
    - ● S06.5X6 Traumatic subdural hemorrhage with loss of consciousness greater than 24 hours without return to pre-existing conscious level with patient surviving A, S 🐾
        Coding Clinic: 2021, Q2, P5
    - ● S06.5X7 Traumatic subdural hemorrhage with loss of consciousness of any duration with death due to brain injury before regaining consciousness
    - ● S06.5X8 Traumatic subdural hemorrhage with loss of consciousness of any duration with death due to other cause before regaining consciousness
    - ● S06.5X9 Traumatic subdural hemorrhage with loss of consciousness of unspecified duration A, S 🐾
    - ● S06.5XA Traumatic subdural hemorrhage with loss of consciousness status unknown
        Traumatic subdural hemorrhage NOS
        Coding Clinic: 2022, Q4, P45

- ● S06.6 **Traumatic subarachnoid hemorrhage**
    Between arachnoid and pia mater
    Use Additional code, if applicable, for traumatic brain compression or herniation (S06.A-)
    Coding Clinic: 2016, Q4, P67
  - ● S06.6X Traumatic subarachnoid hemorrhage
    - ● S06.6X0 Traumatic subarachnoid hemorrhage without loss of consciousness A, S 🐾
        Coding Clinic: 2015, Q3, P37

CHAPTER 19 (S00-T88)

● S06.6X1   Traumatic subarachnoid hemorrhage with loss of consciousness of 30 minutes or less A, S 🐾
     Traumatic subarachnoid hemorrhage with brief loss of consciousness

● S06.6X2   Traumatic subarachnoid hemorrhage with loss of consciousness of 31 minutes to 59 minutes A, S 🐾

● S06.6X3   Traumatic subarachnoid hemorrhage with loss of consciousness of 1 hour to 5 hours 59 minutes A, S 🐾

● S06.6X4   Traumatic subarachnoid hemorrhage with loss of consciousness of 6 hours to 24 hours A, S 🐾

● S06.6X5   Traumatic subarachnoid hemorrhage with loss of consciousness greater than 24 hours with return to pre-existing conscious level A, S 🐾

● S06.6X6   Traumatic subarachnoid hemorrhage with loss of consciousness greater than 24 hours without return to pre-existing conscious level with patient surviving A, S 🐾
     Coding Clinic: 2021, Q2, P5

● S06.6X7   Traumatic subarachnoid hemorrhage with loss of consciousness of any duration with death due to brain injury prior to regaining consciousness

● S06.6X8   Traumatic subarachnoid hemorrhage with loss of consciousness of any duration with death due to other cause prior to regaining consciousness

● S06.6X9   Traumatic subarachnoid hemorrhage with loss of consciousness of unspecified duration A, S 🐾

● S06.6XA   Traumatic subarachnoid hemorrhage with loss of consciousness status unknown
     Traumatic subarachnoid hemorrhage NOS
     Coding Clinic: 2022, Q4, P45

● S06.8   Other specified intracranial injuries

● S06.81   Injury of right internal carotid artery, intracranial portion, not elsewhere classified
     Coding Clinic: 2016, Q4, P67

● S06.810   Injury of right internal carotid artery, intracranial portion, not elsewhere classified without loss of consciousness A, S 🐾

● S06.811   Injury of right internal carotid artery, intracranial portion, not elsewhere classified with loss of consciousness of 30 minutes or less A, S 🐾
     Injury of right internal carotid artery, intracranial portion, not elsewhere classified with brief loss of consciousness

● S06.812   Injury of right internal carotid artery, intracranial portion, not elsewhere classified with loss of consciousness of 31 minutes to 59 minutes A, S 🐾

● S06.813   Injury of right internal carotid artery, intracranial portion, not elsewhere classified with loss of consciousness of 1 hour to 5 hours 59 minutes A, S 🐾

● S06.814   Injury of right internal carotid artery, intracranial portion, not elsewhere classified with loss of consciousness of 6 hours to 24 hours A, S 🐾

● S06.815   Injury of right internal carotid artery, intracranial portion, not elsewhere classified with loss of consciousness greater than 24 hours with return to pre-existing conscious level A, S 🐾

● S06.816   Injury of right internal carotid artery, intracranial portion, not elsewhere classified with loss of consciousness greater than 24 hours without return to pre-existing conscious level with patient surviving A, S 🐾

● S06.817   Injury of right internal carotid artery, intracranial portion, not elsewhere classified with loss of consciousness of any duration with death due to brain injury prior to regaining consciousness

● S06.818   Injury of right internal carotid artery, intracranial portion, not elsewhere classified with loss of consciousness of any duration with death due to other cause prior to regaining consciousness

● S06.819   Injury of right internal carotid artery, intracranial portion, not elsewhere classified with loss of consciousness of unspecified duration A, S 🐾

● S06.81A   Injury of right internal carotid artery, intracranial portion, not elsewhere classified with loss of consciousness status unknown
     Injury of right internal carotid artery, intracranial portion, not elsewhere classified NOS

● S06.82   Injury of left internal carotid artery, intracranial portion, not elsewhere classified
     Coding Clinic: 2016, Q4, P67

● S06.820   Injury of left internal carotid artery, intracranial portion, not elsewhere classified without loss of consciousness A, S 🐾

● S06.821   Injury of left internal carotid artery, intracranial portion, not elsewhere classified with loss of consciousness of 30 minutes or less A, S 🐾
     Injury of left internal carotid artery, intracranial portion, not elsewhere classified with brief loss of consciousness

● S06.822   Injury of left internal carotid artery, intracranial portion, not elsewhere classified with loss of consciousness of 31 minutes to 59 minutes A, S 🐾

● S06.823   Injury of left internal carotid artery, intracranial portion, not elsewhere classified with loss of consciousness of 1 hour to 5 hours 59 minutes A, S 🐾

● S06.824   Injury of left internal carotid artery, intracranial portion, not elsewhere classified with loss of consciousness of 6 hours to 24 hours A, S 🐾

● S06.825   Injury of left internal carotid artery, intracranial portion, not elsewhere classified with loss of consciousness greater than 24 hours with return to pre-existing conscious level

● S06.826   Injury of left internal carotid artery, intracranial portion, not elsewhere classified with loss of consciousness greater than 24 hours without return to pre-existing conscious level with patient surviving A, S 🐾

● S06.827 Injury of left internal carotid artery, intracranial portion, not elsewhere classified with loss of consciousness of any duration with death due to brain injury prior to regaining consciousness

● S06.828 Injury of left internal carotid artery, intracranial portion, not elsewhere classified with loss of consciousness of any duration with death due to other cause prior to regaining consciousness

● S06.829 Injury of left internal carotid artery, intracranial portion, not elsewhere classified with loss of consciousness of unspecified duration A, S 🐾

● S06.82A Injury of left internal carotid artery, intracranial portion, not elsewhere classified with loss of consciousness status unknown

> Injury of left internal carotid artery, intracranial portion, not elsewhere classified NOS

● S06.89 Other specified intracranial injury

Excludes1 concussion (S06.0X-)

● S06.890 Other specified intracranial injury without loss of consciousness A, S 🐾

Coding Clinic: 2024, Q2, P16

● S06.891 Other specified intracranial injury with loss of consciousness of 30 minutes or less A, S 🐾

> Other specified intracranial injury with brief loss of consciousness

● S06.892 Other specified intracranial injury with loss of consciousness of 31 minutes to 59 minutes A, S 🐾

● S06.893 Other specified intracranial injury with loss of consciousness of 1 hour to 5 hours 59 minutes A, S 🐾

● S06.894 Other specified intracranial injury with loss of consciousness of 6 hours to 24 hours A, S 🐾

● S06.895 Other specified intracranial injury with loss of consciousness greater than 24 hours with return to pre-existing conscious level A, S 🐾

● S06.896 Other specified intracranial injury with loss of consciousness greater than 24 hours without return to pre-existing conscious level with patient surviving A, S 🐾

● S06.897 Other specified intracranial injury with loss of consciousness of any duration with death due to brain injury prior to regaining consciousness

● S06.898 Other specified intracranial injury with loss of consciousness of any duration with death due to other cause prior to regaining consciousness

● S06.899 Other specified intracranial injury with loss of consciousness of unspecified duration A, S 🐾

● S06.89A Other specified intracranial injury with loss of consciousness status unknown

● S06.8A Primary blast injury of brain, not elsewhere classified

Code also, if applicable, focal traumatic brain injury (S06.3-)

Excludes2 traumatic cerebral edema (S06.1)

● S06.8A0 Primary blast injury of brain, not elsewhere classified without loss of consciousness

● S06.8A1 Primary blast injury of brain, not elsewhere classified with loss of consciousness of 30 minutes or less

> Primary blast injury of brain, not elsewhere classified with brief loss of consciousness

● S06.8A2 Primary blast injury of brain, not elsewhere classified with loss of consciousness of 31 minutes to 59 minutes

● S06.8A3 Primary blast injury of brain, not elsewhere classified with loss of consciousness of 1 hour to 5 hours 59 minutes

● S06.8A4 Primary blast injury of brain, not elsewhere classified with loss of consciousness of 6 hours to 24 hours

● S06.8A5 Primary blast injury of brain, not elsewhere classified with loss of consciousness greater than 24 hours with return to pre-existing conscious level

● S06.8A6 Primary blast injury of brain, not elsewhere classified with loss of consciousness greater than 24 hours without return to pre-existing conscious level with patient surviving

● S06.8A7 Primary blast injury of brain, not elsewhere classified with loss of consciousness of any duration with death due to brain injury prior to regaining consciousness

● S06.8A8 Primary blast injury of brain, not elsewhere classified with loss of consciousness of any duration with death due to other cause prior to regaining consciousness

● S06.8AA Primary blast injury of brain, not elsewhere classified with loss of consciousness status unknown

> Primary blast injury of brain NOS

● S06.8A9 Primary blast injury of brain, not elsewhere classified with loss of consciousness of unspecified duration

● S06.9 Unspecified intracranial injury

> Brain injury NOS
> Head injury NOS with loss of consciousness
> Traumatic brain injury NOS

Excludes1 conditions classifiable to S06.0- to S06.8- code to specified intracranial injury head injury NOS (S09.90)

● S06.9X Unspecified intracranial injury

● S06.9X0 Unspecified intracranial injury without loss of consciousness A, S 🐾

● S06.9X1 Unspecified intracranial injury with loss of consciousness of 30 minutes or less A, S 🐾

> Unspecified intracranial injury with brief loss of consciousness

● S06.9X2 Unspecified intracranial injury with loss of consciousness of 31 minutes to 59 minutes A, S 🐾

CHAPTER 19 (S00–T88)

● **S06.9X3**   Unspecified intracranial injury with loss of consciousness of 1 hour to 5 hours 59 minutes A, S 🦠

● **S06.9X4**   Unspecified intracranial injury with loss of consciousness of 6 hours to 24 hours A, S 🦠

● **S06.9X5**   Unspecified intracranial injury with loss of consciousness greater than 24 hours with return to pre-existing conscious level A, S 🦠

● **S06.9X6**   Unspecified intracranial injury with loss of consciousness greater than 24 hours without return to pre-existing conscious level with patient surviving A, S 🦠

● **S06.9X7**   Unspecified intracranial injury with loss of consciousness of any duration with death due to brain injury prior to regaining consciousness

● **S06.9X8**   Unspecified intracranial injury with loss of consciousness of any duration with death due to other cause prior to regaining consciousness

● **S06.9X9**   Unspecified intracranial injury with loss of consciousness of unspecified duration A, S 🦠

● **S06.9XA**   Unspecified intracranial injury with loss of consciousness status unknown

● **S06.A**   **Traumatic brain compression and herniation**
Traumatic cerebral compression

Code first the underlying traumatic brain injury, such as:
diffuse traumatic brain injury (S06.2-)
focal traumatic brain injury (S06.3-)
traumatic subdural hemorrhage (S06.5-)
traumatic subarachnoid hemorrhage (S06.6-)

S06.A0   **Traumatic brain compression without herniation**
Traumatic brain compression NOS
Traumatic cerebral compression NOS

S06.A1   **Traumatic brain compression with herniation**
Traumatic brain herniation
Traumatic brainstem compression with herniation
Traumatic cerebellar compression with herniation
Traumatic cerebral compression with herniation

● **S07**   **Crushing injury of head**
Use additional code for all associated injuries, such as:
intracranial injuries (S06.-)
skull fractures (S02.-)

The appropriate 7th character is to be added to each code from category S07

A	initial encounter
D	subsequent encounter
S	sequela

X● **S07.0**   Crushing injury of face
X● **S07.1**   Crushing injury of skull
X● **S07.8**   Crushing injury of other parts of head
X● **S07.9**   Crushing injury of head, part unspecified

● **S08**   **Avulsion and traumatic amputation of part of head**
An amputation not identified as partial or complete should be coded to complete

The appropriate 7th character is to be added to each code from category S08

A	initial encounter
D	subsequent encounter
S	sequela

X● **S08.0**   Avulsion of scalp

● **S08.1**   Traumatic amputation of ear
  ● **S08.11**   Complete traumatic amputation of ear
    ● **S08.111**   Complete traumatic amputation of right ear
    ● **S08.112**   Complete traumatic amputation of left ear
    ● **S08.119**   Complete traumatic amputation of unspecified ear
  ● **S08.12**   Partial traumatic amputation of ear
    ● **S08.121**   Partial traumatic amputation of right ear
    ● **S08.122**   Partial traumatic amputation of left ear
    ● **S08.129**   Partial traumatic amputation of unspecified ear

● **S08.8**   Traumatic amputation of other parts of head
  ● **S08.81**   Traumatic amputation of nose
    ● **S08.811**   Complete traumatic amputation of nose
    ● **S08.812**   Partial traumatic amputation of nose
X● **S08.89**   Traumatic amputation of other parts of head

● **S09**   **Other and unspecified injuries of head**
The appropriate 7th character is to be added to each code from category S09

A	initial encounter
D	subsequent encounter
S	sequela

X● **S09.0**   **Injury of blood vessels of head, not elsewhere classified**
    Excludes1   injury of cerebral blood vessels (S06.-)
                 injury of precerebral blood vessels (S15.-)

● **S09.1**   **Injury of muscle and tendon of head**
Code also any associated open wound (S01.-)
    Excludes2   sprain to joints and ligament of head (S03.9)
X● **S09.10**   Unspecified injury of muscle and tendon of head
     Injury of muscle and tendon of head NOS
X● **S09.11**   Strain of muscle and tendon of head
X● **S09.12**   Laceration of muscle and tendon of head
X● **S09.19**   Other specified injury of muscle and tendon of head

● **S09.2**   **Traumatic rupture of ear drum**
    Excludes1   traumatic rupture of ear drum due to blast injury (S09.31-)
X● **S09.20**   Traumatic rupture of unspecified ear drum
X● **S09.21**   Traumatic rupture of right ear drum
X● **S09.22**   Traumatic rupture of left ear drum

● **S09.3**   **Other specified and unspecified injury of middle and inner ear**
    Excludes1   injury to ear NOS (S09.91-)
    Excludes2   injury to external ear (S00.4-, S01.3-, S08.1-)
● **S09.30**   Unspecified injury of middle and inner ear
  ● **S09.301**   Unspecified injury of right middle and inner ear
  ● **S09.302**   Unspecified injury of left middle and inner ear
  ● **S09.309**   Unspecified injury of unspecified middle and inner ear
● **S09.31**   Primary blast injury of ear
     Blast injury of ear NOS
  ● **S09.311**   Primary blast injury of right ear
  ● **S09.312**   Primary blast injury of left ear
  ● **S09.313**   Primary blast injury of ear, bilateral
  ● **S09.319**   Primary blast injury of unspecified ear
● **S09.39**   Other specified injury of middle and inner ear
     Secondary blast injury to ear

▶ New   ⇒ Revised   ~~deleted~~ Deleted   Excludes 1   Excludes 2   Includes   Use additional   Code first   Code also   Key words
OGCR Official Guidelines   X Assign placeholder X   ● Use Additional Character(s)   ▌ Manifestation Code   🦠 Hierarchical Condition Category   **Coding Clinic**

● S09.391   Other specified injury of right middle and inner ear

● S09.392   Other specified injury of left middle and inner ear

● S09.399   Other specified injury of unspecified middle and inner ear

X ● **S09.8**   Other specified injuries of head

● **S09.9**   Unspecified injury of face and head

   X ● **S09.90**   Unspecified injury of head
      Head injury NOS

     Excludes1   brain injury NOS (S06.9-)
            head injury NOS with loss of consciousness (S06.9-)
            intracranial injury NOS (S06.9-)

   X ● **S09.91**   Unspecified injury of ear
      Injury of ear NOS

   X ● **S09.92**   Unspecified injury of nose
      Injury of nose NOS

   X ● **S09.93**   Unspecified injury of face
      Injury of face NOS

INJURIES TO THE NECK (S10-S19)

Includes   injuries of nape
         injuries of supraclavicular region
         injuries of throat

Excludes2   burns and corrosions (T20-T32)
         effects of foreign body in esophagus (T18.1)
         effects of foreign body in larynx (T17.3)
         effects of foreign body in pharynx (T17.2)
         effects of foreign body in trachea (T17.4)
         frostbite (T33-T34)
         insect bite or sting, venomous (T63.4)

● **S10**   Superficial injury of neck

   The appropriate 7th character is to be added to each code from category S10

    A   initial encounter
    D   subsequent encounter
    S   sequela

   X ● **S10.0**   Contusion of throat
      Contusion of cervical esophagus
      Contusion of larynx
      Contusion of pharynx
      Contusion of trachea

● **S10.1**   Other and unspecified superficial injuries of throat

   X ● **S10.10**   Unspecified superficial injuries of throat

   X ● **S10.11**   Abrasion of throat

   X ● **S10.12**   Blister (nonthermal) of throat

   X ● **S10.14**   External constriction of part of throat

   X ● **S10.15**   Superficial foreign body of throat
      Splinter in the throat

   X ● **S10.16**   Insect bite (nonvenomous) of throat

   X ● **S10.17**   Other superficial bite of throat

     Excludes1   open bite of throat (S11.85)

● **S10.8**   Superficial injury of other specified parts of neck

   X ● **S10.80**   Unspecified superficial injury of other specified part of neck

   X ● **S10.81**   Abrasion of other specified part of neck

   X ● **S10.82**   Blister (nonthermal) of other specified part of neck

   X ● **S10.83**   Contusion of other specified part of neck

   X ● **S10.84**   External constriction of other specified part of neck

   X ● **S10.85**   Superficial foreign body of other specified part of neck
      Splinter in other part of neck

   X ● **S10.86**   Insect bite of other specified part of neck

   X ● **S10.87**   Other superficial bite of other specified part of neck

     Excludes1   open bite of other specified parts of neck (S11.85)

● **S10.9**   Superficial injury of unspecified part of neck

   X ● **S10.90**   Unspecified superficial injury of unspecified part of neck

   X ● **S10.91**   Abrasion of unspecified part of neck

   X ● **S10.92**   Blister (nonthermal) of unspecified part of neck

   X ● **S10.93**   Contusion of unspecified part of neck

   X ● **S10.94**   External constriction of unspecified part of neck

   X ● **S10.95**   Superficial foreign body of unspecified part of neck

   X ● **S10.96**   Insect bite of unspecified part of neck

   X ● **S10.97**   Other superficial bite of unspecified part of neck

● **S11**   Open wound of neck

   Code also any associated:
     spinal cord injury (S14.0, S14.1-)
     wound infection

     Excludes2   open fracture of vertebra (S12.- with 7th character B)

   The appropriate 7th character is to be added to each code from category S11

    A   initial encounter
    D   subsequent encounter
    S   sequela

● **S11.0**   Open wound of larynx and trachea

   ● **S11.01**   Open wound of larynx

     Excludes2   open wound of vocal cord (S11.03)

     ● S11.011   Laceration without foreign body of larynx

     ● S11.012   Laceration with foreign body of larynx

     ● S11.013   Puncture wound without foreign body of larynx

     ● S11.014   Puncture wound with foreign body of larynx

     ● S11.015   Open bite of larynx
        Bite of larynx NOS

     ● S11.019   Unspecified open wound of larynx

   ● **S11.02**   Open wound of trachea
      Open wound of cervical trachea
      Open wound of trachea NOS

     Excludes2   open wound of thoracic trachea (S27.5-)

     ● S11.021   Laceration without foreign body of trachea

     ● S11.022   Laceration with foreign body of trachea

     ● S11.023   Puncture wound without foreign body of trachea

     ● S11.024   Puncture wound with foreign body of trachea

     ● S11.025   Open bite of trachea
        Bite of trachea NOS

     ● S11.029   Unspecified open wound of trachea

   ● **S11.03**   Open wound of vocal cord

     ● S11.031   Laceration without foreign body of vocal cord

     ● S11.032   Laceration with foreign body of vocal cord

     ● S11.033   Puncture wound without foreign body of vocal cord

     ● S11.034   Puncture wound with foreign body of vocal cord

● **S11.035**   **Open bite of vocal cord**
     Bite of vocal cord NOS

● **S11.039**   **Unspecified open wound of vocal cord**

● **S11.1**   **Open wound of thyroid gland**

X● **S11.10**   **Unspecified open wound of thyroid gland**

X● **S11.11**   **Laceration without foreign body of thyroid gland**

X● **S11.12**   **Laceration with foreign body of thyroid gland**

X● **S11.13**   **Puncture wound without foreign body of thyroid gland**

X● **S11.14**   **Puncture wound with foreign body of thyroid gland**

X● **S11.15**   **Open bite of thyroid gland**
     Bite of thyroid gland NOS

● **S11.2**   **Open wound of pharynx and cervical esophagus**

     Excludes1   open wound of esophagus NOS (S27.8-)

X● **S11.20**   **Unspecified open wound of pharynx and cervical esophagus**

X● **S11.21**   **Laceration without foreign body of pharynx and cervical esophagus**

X● **S11.22**   **Laceration with foreign body of pharynx and cervical esophagus**

X● **S11.23**   **Puncture wound without foreign body of pharynx and cervical esophagus**

X● **S11.24**   **Puncture wound with foreign body of pharynx and cervical esophagus**

X● **S11.25**   **Open bite of pharynx and cervical esophagus**

     Bite of pharynx and cervical esophagus NOS

● **S11.8**   **Open wound of other specified parts of neck**

X● **S11.80**   **Unspecified open specified wound of other part of neck**

X● **S11.81**   **Laceration without foreign body of other specified part of neck**

X● **S11.82**   **Laceration with foreign body of other specified part of neck**

X● **S11.83**   **Puncture wound without foreign body of other specified part of neck**

X● **S11.84**   **Puncture wound with foreign body of other specified part of neck**

X● **S11.85**   **Open bite of other specified part of neck**
     Bite of other part of neck NOS

     Excludes1   superficial bite of other specified part of neck (S10.87)

X● **S11.89**   **Other open wound of other part of neck**

● **S11.9**   **Open wound of unspecified part of neck**

X● **S11.90**   **Unspecified open wound of unspecified part of neck**

X● **S11.91**   **Laceration without foreign body of unspecified part of neck**

X● **S11.92**   **Laceration with foreign body of unspecified part of neck**

X● **S11.93**   **Puncture wound without foreign body of unspecified part of neck**

X● **S11.94**   **Puncture wound with foreign body of unspecified part of neck**

X● **S11.95**   **Open bite of unspecified part of neck**
     Bite of neck NOS

     Excludes1   superficial bite of neck (S10.97)

● **S12**   **Fracture of cervical vertebra and other parts of neck**

     Note: A fracture not indicated as displaced or nondisplaced should be coded to displaced

     A fracture not indicated as open or closed should be coded to closed

     Includes   fracture of cervical neural arch
                  fracture of cervical spine
                  fracture of cervical spinous process
                  fracture of cervical transverse process
                  fracture of cervical vertebral arch
                  fracture of neck

     Code first any associated cervical spinal cord injury (S14.0, S14.1-)

     The appropriate 7th character is to be added to all codes from subcategories S12.0-S12.6

     A   initial encounter for closed fracture
     B   initial encounter for open fracture
     D   subsequent encounter for fracture with routine healing
     G   subsequent encounter for fracture with delayed healing
     K   subsequent encounter for fracture with nonunion
     S   sequela

● **S12.0**   **Fracture of first cervical vertebra**
     Atlas

   ● **S12.00**   **Unspecified fracture of first cervical vertebra**

     ● **S12.000**   **Unspecified displaced fracture of first cervical vertebra A, B** 🐾

     ● **S12.001**   **Unspecified nondisplaced fracture of first cervical vertebra A, B** 🐾

   X● **S12.01**   **Stable burst fracture of first cervical vertebra A, B** 🐾

   X● **S12.02**   **Unstable burst fracture of first cervical vertebra A, B** 🐾

   ● **S12.03**   **Posterior arch fracture of first cervical vertebra**

     ● **S12.030**   **Displaced posterior arch fracture of first cervical vertebra A, B** 🐾

     ● **S12.031**   **Nondisplaced posterior arch fracture of first cervical vertebra A, B** 🐾

   ● **S12.04**   **Lateral mass fracture of first cervical vertebra**

     ● **S12.040**   **Displaced lateral mass fracture of first cervical vertebra A, B** 🐾

     ● **S12.041**   **Nondisplaced lateral mass fracture of first cervical vertebra A, B** 🐾

   ● **S12.09**   **Other fracture of first cervical vertebra**

     ● **S12.090**   **Other displaced fracture of first cervical vertebra A, B** 🐾

     ● **S12.091**   **Other nondisplaced fracture of first cervical vertebra A, B** 🐾

● **S12.1**   **Fracture of second cervical vertebra**
     Axis

   ● **S12.10**   **Unspecified fracture of second cervical vertebra**

     ● **S12.100**   **Unspecified displaced fracture of second cervical vertebra A, B** 🐾
             Coding Clinic: 2024, Q2, P23

     ● **S12.101**   **Unspecified nondisplaced fracture of second cervical vertebra A, B** 🐾

   ● **S12.11**   **Type II dens fracture**

     ● **S12.110**   **Anterior displaced Type II dens fracture A, B** 🐾

     ● **S12.111**   **Posterior displaced Type II dens fracture A, B** 🐾

     ● **S12.112**   **Nondisplaced Type II dens fracture A, B** 🐾

   ● **S12.12**   **Other dens fracture**

     ● **S12.120**   **Other displaced dens fracture A, B** 🐾

     ● **S12.121**   **Other nondisplaced dens fracture A, B** 🐾

▶ New   ⇒ Revised   ~~deleted~~ Deleted   Excludes 1   Excludes 2   Includes   Use additional   Code first   Code also   Key words

OGCR Official Guidelines   X Assign placeholder X   ● Use Additional Character(s)   ▶ Manifestation Code   🐾 Hierarchical Condition Category   Coding Clinic

CHAPTER 19 (S00-T88)

● S12.13   Unspecified traumatic spondylolisthesis of second cervical vertebra
   ● S12.130   Unspecified traumatic displaced spondylolisthesis of second cervical vertebra A, B 🦴
   ● S12.131   Unspecified traumatic nondisplaced spondylolisthesis of second cervical vertebra A, B 🦴
X ● S12.14   Type III traumatic spondylolisthesis of second cervical vertebra A, B 🦴
● S12.15   Other traumatic spondylolisthesis of second cervical vertebra
   ● S12.150   Other traumatic displaced spondylolisthesis of second cervical vertebra A, B 🦴
   ● S12.151   Other traumatic nondisplaced spondylolisthesis of second cervical vertebra A, B 🦴
● S12.19   Other fracture of second cervical vertebra
   ● S12.190   Other displaced fracture of second cervical vertebra A, B 🦴
   ● S12.191   Other nondisplaced fracture of second cervical vertebra A, B 🦴
● S12.2   Fracture of third cervical vertebra
   ● S12.20   Unspecified fracture of third cervical vertebra
     ● S12.200   Unspecified displaced fracture of third cervical vertebra A, B 🦴
     ● S12.201   Unspecified nondisplaced fracture of third cervical vertebra A, B 🦴
   ● S12.23   Unspecified traumatic spondylolisthesis of third cervical vertebra
     ● S12.230   Unspecified traumatic displaced spondylolisthesis of third cervical vertebra A, B 🦴
     ● S12.231   Unspecified traumatic nondisplaced spondylolisthesis of third cervical vertebra A, B 🦴
X ● S12.24   Type III traumatic spondylolisthesis of third cervical vertebra A, B 🦴
   ● S12.25   Other traumatic spondylolisthesis of third cervical vertebra
     ● S12.250   Other traumatic displaced spondylolisthesis of third cervical vertebra A, B 🦴
     ● S12.251   Other traumatic nondisplaced spondylolisthesis of third cervical vertebra A, B 🦴
   ● S12.29   Other fracture of third cervical vertebra
     ● S12.290   Other displaced fracture of third cervical vertebra A, B 🦴
     ● S12.291   Other nondisplaced fracture of third cervical vertebra A, B 🦴
● S12.3   Fracture of fourth cervical vertebra
   ● S12.30   Unspecified fracture of fourth cervical vertebra
     ● S12.300   Unspecified displaced fracture of fourth cervical vertebra A, B 🦴
     ● S12.301   Unspecified nondisplaced fracture of fourth cervical vertebra A, B 🦴
   ● S12.33   Unspecified traumatic spondylolisthesis of fourth cervical vertebra
     ● S12.330   Unspecified traumatic displaced spondylolisthesis of fourth cervical vertebra A, B 🦴
     ● S12.331   Unspecified traumatic nondisplaced spondylolisthesis of fourth cervical vertebra A, B 🦴
X ● S12.34   Type III traumatic spondylolisthesis of fourth cervical vertebra A, B 🦴

● S12.35   Other traumatic spondylolisthesis of fourth cervical vertebra
   ● S12.350   Other traumatic displaced spondylolisthesis of fourth cervical vertebra A, B 🦴
   ● S12.351   Other traumatic nondisplaced spondylolisthesis of fourth cervical vertebra A, B 🦴
● S12.39   Other fracture of fourth cervical vertebra
   ● S12.390   Other displaced fracture of fourth cervical vertebra A, B 🦴
   ● S12.391   Other nondisplaced fracture of fourth cervical vertebra A, B 🦴
● S12.4   Fracture of fifth cervical vertebra
   ● S12.40   Unspecified fracture of fifth cervical vertebra
     ● S12.400   Unspecified displaced fracture of fifth cervical vertebra A, B 🦴
     ● S12.401   Unspecified nondisplaced fracture of fifth cervical vertebra A, B 🦴
   ● S12.43   Unspecified traumatic spondylolisthesis of fifth cervical vertebra
     ● S12.430   Unspecified traumatic displaced spondylolisthesis of fifth cervical vertebra A, B 🦴
     ● S12.431   Unspecified traumatic nondisplaced spondylolisthesis of fifth cervical vertebra A, B 🦴
X ● S12.44   Type III traumatic spondylolisthesis of fifth cervical vertebra A, B 🦴
   ● S12.45   Other traumatic spondylolisthesis of fifth cervical vertebra
     ● S12.450   Other traumatic displaced spondylolisthesis of fifth cervical vertebra A, B 🦴
     ● S12.451   Other traumatic nondisplaced spondylolisthesis of fifth cervical vertebra A, B 🦴
   ● S12.49   Other fracture of fifth cervical vertebra
     ● S12.490   Other displaced fracture of fifth cervical vertebra A, B 🦴
     ● S12.491   Other nondisplaced fracture of fifth cervical vertebra A, B 🦴
● S12.5   Fracture of sixth cervical vertebra
   ● S12.50   Unspecified fracture of sixth cervical vertebra
     ● S12.500   Unspecified displaced fracture of sixth cervical vertebra A, B 🦴
     ● S12.501   Unspecified nondisplaced fracture of sixth cervical vertebra A, B 🦴
   ● S12.53   Unspecified traumatic spondylolisthesis of sixth cervical vertebra
     ● S12.530   Unspecified traumatic displaced spondylolisthesis of sixth cervical vertebra A, B 🦴
     ● S12.531   Unspecified traumatic nondisplaced spondylolisthesis of sixth cervical vertebra A, B 🦴
X ● S12.54   Type III traumatic spondylolisthesis of sixth cervical vertebra A, B 🦴
   ● S12.55   Other traumatic spondylolisthesis of sixth cervical vertebra
     ● S12.550   Other traumatic displaced spondylolisthesis of sixth cervical vertebra A, B 🦴
     ● S12.551   Other traumatic nondisplaced spondylolisthesis of sixth cervical vertebra A, B 🦴
   ● S12.59   Other fracture of sixth cervical vertebra
     ● S12.590   Other displaced fracture of sixth cervical vertebra A, B 🦴
     ● S12.591   Other nondisplaced fracture of sixth cervical vertebra A, B 🦴

CHAPTER 19 (S00–T88)

CHAPTER 19 (S00-T88)

● **S12.6**   **Fracture of seventh cervical vertebra**
    S12.60   **Unspecified fracture of seventh cervical vertebra**
       ● **S12.600**   **Unspecified displaced fracture of seventh cervical vertebra** A, B 🦠
       ● **S12.601**   **Unspecified nondisplaced fracture of seventh cervical vertebra** A, B 🦠
    ● **S12.63**   **Unspecified traumatic spondylolisthesis of seventh cervical vertebra**
       ● **S12.630**   **Unspecified traumatic displaced spondylolisthesis of seventh cervical vertebra** A, B 🦠
       ● **S12.631**   **Unspecified traumatic nondisplaced spondylolisthesis of seventh cervical vertebra** A, B 🦠
X ● **S12.64**   **Type III traumatic spondylolisthesis of seventh cervical vertebra** A, B 🦠
    ● **S12.65**   **Other traumatic spondylolisthesis of seventh cervical vertebra**
       ● **S12.650**   **Other traumatic displaced spondylolisthesis of seventh cervical vertebra** A, B 🦠
       ● **S12.651**   **Other traumatic nondisplaced spondylolisthesis of seventh cervical vertebra** A, B 🦠
    ● **S12.69**   **Other fracture of seventh cervical vertebra**
       ● **S12.690**   **Other displaced fracture of seventh cervical vertebra** A, B 🦠
       ● **S12.691**   **Other nondisplaced fracture of seventh cervical vertebra** A, B 🦠

X ● **S12.8**   **Fracture of other parts of neck** A 🦠
    Hyoid bone   Thyroid cartilage
    Larynx   Trachea
    The appropriate 7th character is to be added to code S12.8

A	initial encounter
D	subsequent encounter
S	sequela

X ● **S12.9**   **Fracture of neck, unspecified** A 🦠
    Fracture of neck NOS
    Fracture of cervical spine NOS
    Fracture of cervical vertebra NOS
    The appropriate 7th character is to be added to code S12.9

A	initial encounter
D	subsequent encounter
S	sequela

● **S13**   **Dislocation and sprain of joints and ligaments at neck level**
    Includes   avulsion of joint or ligament at neck level
                   laceration of cartilage, joint or ligament at neck level
                   sprain of cartilage, joint or ligament at neck level
                   traumatic hemarthrosis of joint or ligament at neck level
                   traumatic rupture of joint or ligament at neck level
                   traumatic subluxation of joint or ligament at neck level
                   traumatic tear of joint or ligament at neck level
    Code also any associated open wound
    Excludes2   strain of muscle or tendon at neck level (S16.1)
    The appropriate 7th character is to be added to each code from category S13

A	initial encounter
D	subsequent encounter
S	sequela

X ● **S13.0**   **Traumatic rupture of cervical intervertebral disc**
    Excludes1   rupture or displacement (nontraumatic) of cervical intervertebral disc NOS (M50.-)

● **S13.1**   **Subluxation and dislocation of cervical vertebrae**
    Code also any associated:
       open wound of neck (S11.-)
       spinal cord injury (S14.1-)
    Excludes2   fracture of cervical vertebrae (S12.0-S12.3-)
    ● **S13.10**   **Subluxation and dislocation of unspecified cervical vertebrae**
       ● **S13.100**   **Subluxation of unspecified cervical vertebrae**
       ● **S13.101**   **Dislocation of unspecified cervical vertebrae**
    ● **S13.11**   **Subluxation and dislocation of C0/C1 cervical vertebrae**
       Subluxation and dislocation of atlantooccipital joint
       Subluxation and dislocation of atloidooccipital joint
       Subluxation and dislocation of occipitoatloid joint
       ● **S13.110**   **Subluxation of C0/C1 cervical vertebrae**
       ● **S13.111**   **Dislocation of C0/C1 cervical vertebrae**
    ● **S13.12**   **Subluxation and dislocation of C1/C2 cervical vertebrae**
       Subluxation and dislocation of atlantoaxial joint
       ● **S13.120**   **Subluxation of C1/C2 cervical vertebrae**
       ● **S13.121**   **Dislocation of C1/C2 cervical vertebrae**
    ● **S13.13**   **Subluxation and dislocation of C2/C3 cervical vertebrae**
       ● **S13.130**   **Subluxation of C2/C3 cervical vertebrae**
       ● **S13.131**   **Dislocation of C2/C3 cervical vertebrae**
    ● **S13.14**   **Subluxation and dislocation of C3/C4 cervical vertebrae**
       ● **S13.140**   **Subluxation of C3/C4 cervical vertebrae**
       ● **S13.141**   **Dislocation of C3/C4 cervical vertebrae**
    ● **S13.15**   **Subluxation and dislocation of C4/C5 cervical vertebrae**
       ● **S13.150**   **Subluxation of C4/C5 cervical vertebrae**
       ● **S13.151**   **Dislocation of C4/C5 cervical vertebrae**
    ● **S13.16**   **Subluxation and dislocation of C5/C6 cervical vertebrae**
       ● **S13.160**   **Subluxation of C5/C6 cervical vertebrae**
       ● **S13.161**   **Dislocation of C5/C6 cervical vertebrae**
    ● **S13.17**   **Subluxation and dislocation of C6/C7 cervical vertebrae**
       ● **S13.170**   **Subluxation of C6/C7 cervical vertebrae**
       ● **S13.171**   **Dislocation of C6/C7 cervical vertebrae**
    ● **S13.18**   **Subluxation and dislocation of C7/T1 cervical vertebrae**
       ● **S13.180**   **Subluxation of C7/T1 cervical vertebrae**
       ● **S13.181**   **Dislocation of C7/T1 cervical vertebrae**

▶ New   ⇒ Revised   ~~deleted~~ Deleted   Excludes 1   Excludes 2   Includes   Use additional   Code first   Code also   Key words

OGCR Official Guidelines   X Assign placeholder X   ● Use Additional Character(s)   ▶ Manifestation Code   🦠 Hierarchical Condition Category   Coding Clinic

● **S13.2**　Dislocation of other and unspecified parts of neck
　　X ● **S13.20**　Dislocation of unspecified parts of neck
　　X ● **S13.29**　Dislocation of other parts of neck
X ● **S13.4**　Sprain of ligaments of cervical spine
　　　　Sprain of anterior longitudinal (ligament), cervical
　　　　Sprain of atlanto-axial (joints)
　　　　Sprain of atlanto-occipital (joints)
　　　　Whiplash injury of cervical spine
X ● **S13.5**　Sprain of thyroid region
　　　　Sprain of cricoarytenoid (joint) (ligament)
　　　　Sprain of cricothyroid (joint) (ligament)
　　　　Sprain of thyroid cartilage
X ● **S13.8**　Sprain of joints and ligaments of other parts of neck
X ● **S13.9**　Sprain of joints and ligaments of unspecified parts of neck

● **S14**　Injury of nerves and spinal cord at neck level
　　　Note: Code to highest level of cervical cord injury
　　　　Code also any associated:
　　　　　fracture of cervical vertebra (S12.0--S12.6.-)
　　　　　open wound of neck (S11.-)
　　　　　transient paralysis (R29.5)
　　　　The appropriate 7th character is to be added to each code from category S14

A	initial encounter
D	subsequent encounter
S	sequela

X ● **S14.0**　Concussion and edema of cervical spinal cord A, D, S 🔗
　　　　Coding Clinic: 2024, Q2, P24
● **S14.1**　Other and unspecified injuries of cervical spinal cord
　　● **S14.10**　Unspecified injury of cervical spinal cord
　　　　● **S14.101**　Unspecified injury at C1 level of cervical spinal cord A, D, S 🔗
　　　　● **S14.102**　Unspecified injury at C2 level of cervical spinal cord A, D, S 🔗
　　　　● **S14.103**　Unspecified injury at C3 level of cervical spinal cord A, D, S 🔗
　　　　● **S14.104**　Unspecified injury at C4 level of cervical spinal cord A, D, S 🔗
　　　　● **S14.105**　Unspecified injury at C5 level of cervical spinal cord A, D, S 🔗
　　　　● **S14.106**　Unspecified injury at C6 level of cervical spinal cord A, D, S 🔗
　　　　● **S14.107**　Unspecified injury at C7 level of cervical spinal cord A, D, S 🔗
　　　　● **S14.108**　Unspecified injury at C8 level of cervical spinal cord A, D, S 🔗
　　　　● **S14.109**　Unspecified injury at unspecified level of cervical spinal cord A, D, S 🔗
　　　　　　　Injury of cervical spinal cord NOS
　　● **S14.11**　Complete lesion of cervical spinal cord
　　　　● **S14.111**　Complete lesion at C1 level of cervical spinal cord A, D, S 🔗
　　　　● **S14.112**　Complete lesion at C2 level of cervical spinal cord A, D, S 🔗
　　　　● **S14.113**　Complete lesion at C3 level of cervical spinal cord A, D, S 🔗
　　　　● **S14.114**　Complete lesion at C4 level of cervical spinal cord A, D, S 🔗
　　　　● **S14.115**　Complete lesion at C5 level of cervical spinal cord A, D, S 🔗
　　　　● **S14.116**　Complete lesion at C6 level of cervical spinal cord A, D, S 🔗
　　　　● **S14.117**　Complete lesion at C7 level of cervical spinal cord A, D, S 🔗
　　　　● **S14.118**　Complete lesion at C8 level of cervical spinal cord A, D, S 🔗
　　　　● **S14.119**　Complete lesion at unspecified level of cervical spinal cord A, D, S 🔗

● **S14.12**　Central cord syndrome of cervical spinal cord
　　● **S14.121**　Central cord syndrome at C1 level of cervical spinal cord A, D, S 🔗
　　● **S14.122**　Central cord syndrome at C2 level of cervical spinal cord A, D, S 🔗
　　● **S14.123**　Central cord syndrome at C3 level of cervical spinal cord A, D, S 🔗
　　　　　Coding Clinic: 2024, Q2, P23
　　● **S14.124**　Central cord syndrome at C4 level of cervical spinal cord A, D, S 🔗
　　● **S14.125**　Central cord syndrome at C5 level of cervical spinal cord A, D, S 🔗
　　● **S14.126**　Central cord syndrome at C6 level of cervical spinal cord A, D, S 🔗
　　● **S14.127**　Central cord syndrome at C7 level of cervical spinal cord A, D, S 🔗
　　● **S14.128**　Central cord syndrome at C8 level of cervical spinal cord A, D, S 🔗
　　● **S14.129**　Central cord syndrome at unspecified level of cervical spinal cord A, D, S 🔗
● **S14.13**　Anterior cord syndrome of cervical spinal cord
　　● **S14.131**　Anterior cord syndrome at C1 level of cervical spinal cord A, D, S 🔗
　　● **S14.132**　Anterior cord syndrome at C2 level of cervical spinal cord A, D, S 🔗
　　● **S14.133**　Anterior cord syndrome at C3 level of cervical spinal cord A, D, S 🔗
　　● **S14.134**　Anterior cord syndrome at C4 level of cervical spinal cord A, D, S 🔗
　　● **S14.135**　Anterior cord syndrome at C5 level of cervical spinal cord A, D, S 🔗
　　● **S14.136**　Anterior cord syndrome at C6 level of cervical spinal cord A, D, S 🔗
　　● **S14.137**　Anterior cord syndrome at C7 level of cervical spinal cord A, D, S 🔗
　　● **S14.138**　Anterior cord syndrome at C8 level of cervical spinal cord A, D, S 🔗
　　● **S14.139**　Anterior cord syndrome at unspecified level of cervical spinal cord A, D, S 🔗
● **S14.14**　Brown-Séquard syndrome of cervical spinal cord
　　● **S14.141**　Brown-Séquard syndrome at C1 level of cervical spinal cord A, D, S 🔗
　　● **S14.142**　Brown-Séquard syndrome at C2 level of cervical spinal cord A, D, S 🔗
　　● **S14.143**　Brown-Séquard syndrome at C3 level of cervical spinal cord A, D, S 🔗
　　● **S14.144**　Brown-Séquard syndrome at C4 level of cervical spinal cord A, D, S 🔗
　　● **S14.145**　Brown-Séquard syndrome at C5 level of cervical spinal cord A, D, S 🔗
　　● **S14.146**　Brown-Séquard syndrome at C6 level of cervical spinal cord A, D, S 🔗
　　● **S14.147**　Brown-Séquard syndrome at C7 level of cervical spinal cord A, D, S 🔗
　　● **S14.148**　Brown-Séquard syndrome at C8 level of cervical spinal cord A, D, S 🔗
　　● **S14.149**　Brown-Séquard syndrome at unspecified level of cervical spinal cord A, D, S 🔗
● **S14.15**　Other incomplete lesions of cervical spinal cord
　　　　Incomplete lesion of cervical spinal cord NOS
　　　　Posterior cord syndrome of cervical spinal cord
　　● **S14.151**　Other incomplete lesion at C1 level of cervical spinal cord A, D, S 🔗
　　● **S14.152**　Other incomplete lesion at C2 level of cervical spinal cord A, D, S 🔗
　　● **S14.153**　Other incomplete lesion at C3 level of cervical spinal cord A, D, S 🔗

● S14.154   Other incomplete lesion at C4 level of cervical spinal cord A, D, S 🐾

● S14.155   Other incomplete lesion at C5 level of cervical spinal cord A, D, S 🐾

● S14.156   Other incomplete lesion at C6 level of cervical spinal cord A, D, S 🐾

● S14.157   Other incomplete lesion at C7 level of cervical spinal cord A, D, S 🐾

● S14.158   Other incomplete lesion at C8 level of cervical spinal cord A, D, S 🐾

● S14.159   Other incomplete lesion at unspecified level of cervical spinal cord A, D, S 🐾

X● S14.2   Injury of nerve root of cervical spine

X● S14.3   Injury of brachial plexus

X● S14.4   Injury of peripheral nerves of neck

X● S14.5   Injury of cervical sympathetic nerves

X● S14.8   Injury of other specified nerves of neck

X● S14.9   Injury of unspecified nerves of neck

● S15   **Injury of blood vessels at neck level**

Code also any associated open wound (S11.-)

The appropriate 7th character is to be added to each code from category S15

A	initial encounter
D	subsequent encounter
S	sequela

● S15.0   **Injury of carotid artery of neck**

Injury of carotid artery (common) (external) (internal, extracranial portion)

Injury of carotid artery NOS

Excludes1   injury of internal carotid artery, intracranial portion (S06.8)

● S15.00   Unspecified injury of carotid artery

● S15.001   Unspecified injury of right carotid artery

● S15.002   Unspecified injury of left carotid artery

● S15.009   Unspecified injury of unspecified carotid artery

● S15.01   Minor laceration of carotid artery

Incomplete transection of carotid artery

Laceration of carotid artery NOS

Superficial laceration of carotid artery

● S15.011   Minor laceration of right carotid artery

● S15.012   Minor laceration of left carotid artery

● S15.019   Minor laceration of unspecified carotid artery

● S15.02   Major laceration of carotid artery

Complete transection of carotid artery

Traumatic rupture of carotid artery

● S15.021   Major laceration of right carotid artery

● S15.022   Major laceration of left carotid artery

● S15.029   Major laceration of unspecified carotid artery

● S15.09   Other specified injury of carotid artery

● S15.091   Other specified injury of right carotid artery

● S15.092   Other specified injury of left carotid artery

● S15.099   Other specified injury of unspecified carotid artery

● S15.1   **Injury of vertebral artery**

● S15.10   Unspecified injury of vertebral artery

● S15.101   Unspecified injury of right vertebral artery

● S15.102   Unspecified injury of left vertebral artery

● S15.109   Unspecified injury of unspecified vertebral artery

● S15.11   Minor laceration of vertebral artery

Incomplete transection of vertebral artery

Laceration of vertebral artery NOS

Superficial laceration of vertebral artery

● S15.111   Minor laceration of right vertebral artery

● S15.112   Minor laceration of left vertebral artery

● S15.119   Minor laceration of unspecified vertebral artery

● S15.12   Major laceration of vertebral artery

Complete transection of vertebral artery

Traumatic rupture of vertebral artery

● S15.121   Major laceration of right vertebral artery

● S15.122   Major laceration of left vertebral artery

● S15.129   Major laceration of unspecified vertebral artery

● S15.19   Other specified injury of vertebral artery

● S15.191   Other specified injury of right vertebral artery

● S15.192   Other specified injury of left vertebral artery

● S15.199   Other specified injury of unspecified vertebral artery

● S15.2   **Injury of external jugular vein**

● S15.20   Unspecified injury of external jugular vein

● S15.201   Unspecified injury of right external jugular vein

● S15.202   Unspecified injury of left external jugular vein

● S15.209   Unspecified injury of unspecified external jugular vein

● S15.21   Minor laceration of external jugular vein

Incomplete transection of external jugular vein

Laceration of external jugular vein NOS

Superficial laceration of external jugular vein

● S15.211   Minor laceration of right external jugular vein

● S15.212   Minor laceration of left external jugular vein

● S15.219   Minor laceration of unspecified external jugular vein

● S15.22   Major laceration of external jugular vein

Complete transection of external jugular vein

Traumatic rupture of external jugular vein

● S15.221   Major laceration of right external jugular vein

● S15.222   Major laceration of left external jugular vein

● S15.229   Major laceration of unspecified external jugular vein

● S15.29   Other specified injury of external jugular vein

● S15.291   Other specified injury of right external jugular vein

● S15.292   Other specified injury of left external jugular vein

● S15.299   Other specified injury of unspecified external jugular vein

● S15.3   **Injury of internal jugular vein**

● S15.30   Unspecified injury of internal jugular vein

● S15.301   Unspecified injury of right internal jugular vein

● S15.302   Unspecified injury of left internal jugular vein

● S15.309   Unspecified injury of unspecified internal jugular vein

▶ New   ⇨ Revised   ~~deleted~~ Deleted   Excludes 1   Excludes 2   Includes   Use additional   Code first   Code also   Key words

OGCR Official Guidelines   X Assign placeholder X   ● Use Additional Character(s)   ▸ Manifestation Code   🐾 Hierarchical Condition Category   Coding Clinic

- S15.31   Minor laceration of internal jugular vein
  - Incomplete transection of internal jugular vein
  - Laceration of internal jugular vein NOS
  - Superficial laceration of internal jugular vein
  - S15.311   Minor laceration of right internal jugular vein
  - S15.312   Minor laceration of left internal jugular vein
  - S15.319   Minor laceration of unspecified internal jugular vein
- S15.32   Major laceration of internal jugular vein
  - Complete transection of internal jugular vein
  - Traumatic rupture of internal jugular vein
  - S15.321   Major laceration of right internal jugular vein
  - S15.322   Major laceration of left internal jugular vein
  - S15.329   Major laceration of unspecified internal jugular vein
- S15.39   Other specified injury of internal jugular vein
  - S15.391   Other specified injury of right internal jugular vein
  - S15.392   Other specified injury of left internal jugular vein
  - S15.399   Other specified injury of unspecified internal jugular vein
- X⬤ S15.8   Injury of other specified blood vessels at neck level
- X⬤ S15.9   Injury of unspecified blood vessel at neck level

- ⬤ S16   Injury of muscle, fascia and tendon at neck level
  - Code also any associated open wound (S11.-)
  - **Excludes2**   sprain of joint or ligament at neck level (S13.9)
  - The appropriate 7th character is to be added to each code from category S16

A	initial encounter
D	subsequent encounter
S	sequela

  - X⬤ S16.1   Strain of muscle, fascia and tendon at neck level
  - X⬤ S16.2   Laceration of muscle, fascia and tendon at neck level
  - X⬤ S16.8   Other specified injury of muscle, fascia and tendon at neck level
  - X⬤ S16.9   Unspecified injury of muscle, fascia and tendon at neck level

- ⬤ S17   Crushing injury of neck
  - Use additional code for all associated injuries, such as:
    - injury of blood vessels (S15.-)
    - open wound of neck (S11.-)
    - spinal cord injury (S14.0, S14.1-)
    - vertebral fracture (S12.0--S12.3-)
  - The appropriate 7th character is to be added to each code from category S17

A	initial encounter
D	subsequent encounter
S	sequela

  - X⬤ S17.0   Crushing injury of larynx and trachea
  - X⬤ S17.8   Crushing injury of other specified parts of neck
  - X⬤ S17.9   Crushing injury of neck, part unspecified

- ⬤ S19   Other and unspecified injuries of neck
  - The appropriate 7th character is to be added to each code from category S19

A	initial encounter
D	subsequent encounter
S	sequela

  - ⬤ S19.8   Other specified injuries of neck
    - X⬤ S19.80   Other specified injuries of unspecified part of neck

- X⬤ S19.81   Other specified injuries of larynx
- X⬤ S19.82   Other specified injuries of cervical trachea
  - **Excludes2**   other specified injury of thoracic trachea (S27.5-)
- X⬤ S19.83   Other specified injuries of vocal cord
- X⬤ S19.84   Other specified injuries of thyroid gland
- X⬤ S19.85   Other specified injuries of pharynx and cervical esophagus
  - **Coding Clinic: 2022, Q1, P27**
- X⬤ S19.89   Other specified injuries of other specified part of neck
- X⬤ S19.9   Unspecified injury of neck

INJURIES TO THE THORAX (S20-S29)

Includes	injuries of breast
	injuries of chest (wall)
	injuries of interscapular area

Excludes2	burns and corrosions (T20-T32)
	effects of foreign body in bronchus (T17.5)
	effects of foreign body in esophagus (T18.1)
	effects of foreign body in lung (T17.8)
	effects of foreign body in trachea (T17.4)
	frostbite (T33-T34)
	injuries of axilla
	injuries of clavicle
	injuries of scapular region
	injuries of shoulder
	insect bite or sting, venomous (T63.4)

- ⬤ S20   Superficial injury of thorax
  - The appropriate 7th character is to be added to each code from category S20

A	initial encounter
D	subsequent encounter
S	sequela

  - ⬤ S20.0   Contusion of breast
    - X⬤ S20.00   Contusion of breast, unspecified breast
    - X⬤ S20.01   Contusion of right breast
    - X⬤ S20.02   Contusion of left breast
  - ⬤ S20.1   Other and unspecified superficial injuries of breast
    - ⬤ S20.10   Unspecified superficial injuries of breast
      - S20.101   Unspecified superficial injuries of breast, right breast
      - S20.102   Unspecified superficial injuries of breast, left breast
      - S20.109   Unspecified superficial injuries of breast, unspecified breast
    - ⬤ S20.11   Abrasion of breast
      - S20.111   Abrasion of breast, right breast
      - S20.112   Abrasion of breast, left breast
      - S20.119   Abrasion of breast, unspecified breast
    - ⬤ S20.12   Blister (nonthermal) of breast
      - S20.121   Blister (nonthermal) of breast, right breast
      - S20.122   Blister (nonthermal) of breast, left breast
      - S20.129   Blister (nonthermal) of breast, unspecified breast
    - ⬤ S20.14   External constriction of part of breast
      - S20.141   External constriction of part of breast, right breast
      - S20.142   External constriction of part of breast, left breast
      - S20.149   External constriction of part of breast, unspecified breast
    - ⬤ S20.15   Superficial foreign body of breast
      - Splinter in the breast
      - S20.151   Superficial foreign body of breast, right breast

CHAPTER 19 (S00-T88)

CHAPTER 19 (S00-T88)

● S20.152   Superficial foreign body of breast, left breast

● S20.159   Superficial foreign body of breast, unspecified breast

● S20.16   Insect bite (nonvenomous) of breast

   ● S20.161   Insect bite (nonvenomous) of breast, right breast

   ● S20.162   Insect bite (nonvenomous) of breast, left breast

   ● S20.169   Insect bite (nonvenomous) of breast, unspecified breast

● S20.17   Other superficial bite of breast

   Excludes1   open bite of breast (S21.05-)

   ● S20.171   Other superficial bite of breast, right breast

   ● S20.172   Other superficial bite of breast, left breast

   ● S20.179   Other superficial bite of breast, unspecified breast

● S20.2   Contusion of thorax

  X ● S20.20   Contusion of thorax, unspecified

  ● S20.21   Contusion of front wall of thorax

   ● S20.211   Contusion of right front wall of thorax

   ● S20.212   Contusion of left front wall of thorax

   S20.213   Contusion of bilateral front wall of thorax

   S20.214   Contusion of middle front wall of thorax

   ● S20.219   Contusion of unspecified front wall of thorax

  ● S20.22   Contusion of back wall of thorax

   ● S20.221   Contusion of right back wall of thorax

   ● S20.222   Contusion of left back wall of thorax

   S20.223   Contusion of bilateral back wall of thorax

   S20.224   Contusion of middle back wall of thorax

   ● S20.229   Contusion of unspecified back wall of thorax

● S20.3   Other and unspecified superficial injuries of front wall of thorax

  ● S20.30   Unspecified superficial injuries of front wall of thorax

   ● S20.301   Unspecified superficial injuries of right front wall of thorax

   ● S20.302   Unspecified superficial injuries of left front wall of thorax

   S20.303   Unspecified superficial injuries of bilateral front wall of thorax

   S20.304   Unspecified superficial injuries of middle front wall of thorax

   ● S20.309   Unspecified superficial injuries of unspecified front wall of thorax

  ● S20.31   Abrasion of front wall of thorax

   ● S20.311   Abrasion of right front wall of thorax

   ● S20.312   Abrasion of left front wall of thorax

   S20.313   Abrasion of bilateral front wall of thorax

   S20.314   Abrasion of middle front wall of thorax

   ● S20.319   Abrasion of unspecified front wall of thorax

  ● S20.32   Blister (nonthermal) of front wall of thorax

   ● S20.321   Blister (nonthermal) of right front wall of thorax

   ● S20.322   Blister (nonthermal) of left front wall of thorax

   S20.323   Blister (nonthermal) of bilateral front wall of thorax

   S20.324   Blister (nonthermal) of middle front wall of thorax

   ● S20.329   Blister (nonthermal) of unspecified front wall of thorax

● S20.34   External constriction of front wall of thorax

   ● S20.341   External constriction of right front wall of thorax

   ● S20.342   External constriction of left front wall of thorax

   S20.343   External constriction of bilateral front wall of thorax

   S20.344   External constriction of middle front wall of thorax

   ● S20.349   External constriction of unspecified front wall of thorax

● S20.35   Superficial foreign body of front wall of thorax

   Splinter in front wall of thorax

   ● S20.351   Superficial foreign body of right front wall of thorax

   ● S20.352   Superficial foreign body of left front wall of thorax

   S20.353   Superficial foreign body of bilateral front wall of thorax

   S20.354   Superficial foreign body of middle front wall of thorax

   ● S20.359   Superficial foreign body of unspecified front wall of thorax

● S20.36   Insect bite (nonvenomous) of front wall of thorax

   ● S20.361   Insect bite (nonvenomous) of right front wall of thorax

   ● S20.362   Insect bite (nonvenomous) of left front wall of thorax

   S20.363   Insect bite (nonvenomous) of bilateral front wall of thorax

   S20.364   Insect bite (nonvenomous) of middle front wall of thorax

   ● S20.369   Insect bite (nonvenomous) of unspecified front wall of thorax

● S20.37   Other superficial bite of front wall of thorax

   Excludes1   open bite of front wall of thorax (S21.14)

   ● S20.371   Other superficial bite of right front wall of thorax

   ● S20.372   Other superficial bite of left front wall of thorax

   S20.373   Other superficial bite of bilateral front wall of thorax

   S20.374   Other superficial bite of middle front wall of thorax

   ● S20.379   Other superficial bite of unspecified front wall of thorax

● S20.4   Other and unspecified superficial injuries of back wall of thorax

  ● S20.40   Unspecified superficial injuries of back wall of thorax

   ● S20.401   Unspecified superficial injuries of right back wall of thorax

   ● S20.402   Unspecified superficial injuries of left back wall of thorax

   ● S20.409   Unspecified superficial injuries of unspecified back wall of thorax

  ● S20.41   Abrasion of back wall of thorax

   ● S20.411   Abrasion of right back wall of thorax

   ● S20.412   Abrasion of left back wall of thorax

   ● S20.419   Abrasion of unspecified back wall of thorax

  ● S20.42   Blister (nonthermal) of back wall of thorax

   ● S20.421   Blister (nonthermal) of right back wall of thorax

---

▶ New   ⇒ Revised   ~~deleted~~ Deleted   Excludes 1   Excludes 2   Includes   Use additional   Code first   Code also   Key words

OGCR Official Guidelines   X Assign placeholder X   ● Use Additional Character(s)   ▶ Manifestation Code   🔖 Hierarchical Condition Category   **Coding Clinic**

● S20.422   Blister (nonthermal) of left back wall
             of thorax
● S20.429   Blister (nonthermal) of unspecified
             back wall of thorax
● S20.44   External constriction of back wall of thorax
   ● S20.441   External constriction of right back
                wall of thorax
   ● S20.442   External constriction of left back wall
                of thorax
   ● S20.449   External constriction of unspecified
                back wall of thorax
● S20.45   Superficial foreign body of back wall of thorax
             Splinter of back wall of thorax
   ● S20.451   Superficial foreign body of right back
                wall of thorax
   ● S20.452   Superficial foreign body of left back
                wall of thorax
   ● S20.459   Superficial foreign body of
                unspecified back wall of thorax
● S20.46   Insect bite (nonvenomous) of back wall of thorax
   ● S20.461   Insect bite (nonvenomous) of right
                back wall of thorax
   ● S20.462   Insect bite (nonvenomous) of left
                back wall of thorax
   ● S20.469   Insect bite (nonvenomous) of
                unspecified back wall of thorax
● S20.47   Other superficial bite of back wall of thorax
       Excludes1   open bite of back wall of thorax
                        (S21.24)
   ● S20.471   Other superficial bite of right back
                wall of thorax
   ● S20.472   Other superficial bite of left back wall
                of thorax
   ● S20.479   Other superficial bite of unspecified
                back wall of thorax
● S20.9   Superficial injury of unspecified parts of thorax
       Excludes1   contusion of thorax NOS (S20.20)
 X ● S20.90   Unspecified superficial injury of unspecified
              parts of thorax
              Superficial injury of thoracic wall NOS
 X ● S20.91   Abrasion of unspecified parts of thorax
 X ● S20.92   Blister (nonthermal) of unspecified parts of
              thorax
 X ● S20.94   External constriction of unspecified parts of
              thorax
 X ● S20.95   Superficial foreign body of unspecified parts of
              thorax
              Splinter in thorax NOS
 X ● S20.96   Insect bite (nonvenomous) of unspecified parts
              of thorax
 X ● S20.97   Other superficial bite of unspecified parts of
              thorax
          Excludes1   open bite of thorax NOS (S21.95)

● S21   Open wound of thorax
    Code also any associated injury such as:
        injury of heart (S26.-)
        injury of intrathoracic organs (S27.-)
        rib fracture (S22.3-, S22.4-)
        spinal cord injury (S24.0-, S24.1-)
        traumatic hemothorax (S27.1)
        traumatic hemopneumothorax (S27.3)
        traumatic pneumothorax (S27.0)
        wound infection
    Excludes1   traumatic amputation (partial) of thorax (S28.1)
    The appropriate 7th character is to be added to each code from
        category S21

A	initial encounter
D	subsequent encounter
S	sequela

Item 19–1 Pneumothorax is a collection of gas (positive air
pressure) in the pleural space, resulting in the lung collapsing. A **tension
pneumothorax** is life-threatening and is a result of air in the pleural space
causing a displacement in the mediastinal structures and cardiopulmonary
function compromise. A **traumatic pneumothorax** results from blunt or
penetrating injury that disrupts the parietal/visceral pleura. **Hemothorax** is
blood or bloody fluid in the pleural cavity as a result of traumatic blood vessel
rupture or inflammation of the lungs from pneumonia.

● S21.0   Open wound of breast
   ● S21.00   Unspecified open wound of breast
      ● S21.001   Unspecified open wound of right
                   breast
      ● S21.002   Unspecified open wound of left
                   breast
      ● S21.009   Unspecified open wound of
                   unspecified breast
   ● S21.01   Laceration without foreign body of breast
      ● S21.011   Laceration without foreign body of
                   right breast
      ● S21.012   Laceration without foreign body of
                   left breast
      ● S21.019   Laceration without foreign body of
                   unspecified breast
   ● S21.02   Laceration with foreign body of breast
      ● S21.021   Laceration with foreign body of right
                   breast
      ● S21.022   Laceration with foreign body of left
                   breast
      ● S21.029   Laceration with foreign body of
                   unspecified breast
   ● S21.03   Puncture wound without foreign body of breast
      ● S21.031   Puncture wound without foreign
                   body of right breast
      ● S21.032   Puncture wound without foreign
                   body of left breast
      ● S21.039   Puncture wound without foreign
                   body of unspecified breast
   ● S21.04   Puncture wound with foreign body of breast
      ● S21.041   Puncture wound with foreign body of
                   right breast
      ● S21.042   Puncture wound with foreign body of
                   left breast
      ● S21.049   Puncture wound with foreign body of
                   unspecified breast
   ● S21.05   Open bite of breast
                Bite of breast NOS
          Excludes1   superficial bite of breast (S20.17)
      ● S21.051   Open bite of right breast
      ● S21.052   Open bite of left breast
      ● S21.059   Open bite of unspecified breast
● S21.1   Open wound of front wall of thorax without penetration
           into thoracic cavity
           Open wound of chest without penetration into thoracic
               cavity
   ● S21.10   Unspecified open wound of front wall of thorax
               without penetration into thoracic cavity
      ● S21.101   Unspecified open wound of right
                   front wall of thorax without
                   penetration into thoracic cavity
      ● S21.102   Unspecified open wound of left front
                   wall of thorax without penetration
                   into thoracic cavity
      ● S21.109   Unspecified open wound of
                   unspecified front wall of thorax
                   without penetration into thoracic
                   cavity

CHAPTER 19 (S00–T88)

CHAPTER 19 (S00-T88)

● **S21.11**   **Laceration without foreign body of front wall of thorax without penetration into thoracic cavity**

  ● **S21.111**   Laceration without foreign body of right front wall of thorax without penetration into thoracic cavity

  ● **S21.112**   Laceration without foreign body of left front wall of thorax without penetration into thoracic cavity

  ● **S21.119**   Laceration without foreign body of unspecified front wall of thorax without penetration into thoracic cavity

● **S21.12**   **Laceration with foreign body of front wall of thorax without penetration into thoracic cavity**

  ● **S21.121**   Laceration with foreign body of right front wall of thorax without penetration into thoracic cavity

  ● **S21.122**   Laceration with foreign body of left front wall of thorax without penetration into thoracic cavity

  ● **S21.129**   Laceration with foreign body of unspecified front wall of thorax without penetration into thoracic cavity

● **S21.13**   **Puncture wound without foreign body of front wall of thorax without penetration into thoracic cavity**

  ● **S21.131**   Puncture wound without foreign body of right front wall of thorax without penetration into thoracic cavity

  ● **S21.132**   Puncture wound without foreign body of left front wall of thorax without penetration into thoracic cavity

  ● **S21.139**   Puncture wound without foreign body of unspecified front wall of thorax without penetration into thoracic cavity

● **S21.14**   **Puncture wound with foreign body of front wall of thorax without penetration into thoracic cavity**

  ● **S21.141**   Puncture wound with foreign body of right front wall of thorax without penetration into thoracic cavity

  ● **S21.142**   Puncture wound with foreign body of left front wall of thorax without penetration into thoracic cavity

  ● **S21.149**   Puncture wound with foreign body of unspecified front wall of thorax without penetration into thoracic cavity

● **S21.15**   **Open bite of front wall of thorax without penetration into thoracic cavity**
     Bite of front wall of thorax NOS

     Excludes1   superficial bite of front wall of thorax (S20.37)

  ● **S21.151**   Open bite of right front wall of thorax without penetration into thoracic cavity

  ● **S21.152**   Open bite of left front wall of thorax without penetration into thoracic cavity

  ● **S21.159**   Open bite of unspecified front wall of thorax without penetration into thoracic cavity

● **S21.2**   **Open wound of back wall of thorax without penetration into thoracic cavity**

  ● **S21.20**   **Unspecified open wound of back wall of thorax without penetration into thoracic cavity**

    ● **S21.201**   Unspecified open wound of right back wall of thorax without penetration into thoracic cavity

    ● **S21.202**   Unspecified open wound of left back wall of thorax without penetration into thoracic cavity

    ● **S21.209**   Unspecified open wound of unspecified back wall of thorax without penetration into thoracic cavity

  ● **S21.21**   **Laceration without foreign body of back wall of thorax without penetration into thoracic cavity**

    ● **S21.211**   Laceration without foreign body of right back wall of thorax without penetration into thoracic cavity

    ● **S21.212**   Laceration without foreign body of left back wall of thorax without penetration into thoracic cavity

    ● **S21.219**   Laceration without foreign body of unspecified back wall of thorax without penetration into thoracic cavity

  ● **S21.22**   **Laceration with foreign body of back wall of thorax without penetration into thoracic cavity**

    ● **S21.221**   Laceration with foreign body of right back wall of thorax without penetration into thoracic cavity

    ● **S21.222**   Laceration with foreign body of left back wall of thorax without penetration into thoracic cavity

    ● **S21.229**   Laceration with foreign body of unspecified back wall of thorax without penetration into thoracic cavity

  ● **S21.23**   **Puncture wound without foreign body of back wall of thorax without penetration into thoracic cavity**

    ● **S21.231**   Puncture wound without foreign body of right back wall of thorax without penetration into thoracic cavity

    ● **S21.232**   Puncture wound without foreign body of left back wall of thorax without penetration into thoracic cavity

    ● **S21.239**   Puncture wound without foreign body of unspecified back wall of thorax without penetration into thoracic cavity

  ● **S21.24**   **Puncture wound with foreign body of back wall of thorax without penetration into thoracic cavity**

    ● **S21.241**   Puncture wound with foreign body of right back wall of thorax without penetration into thoracic cavity

    ● **S21.242**   Puncture wound with foreign body of left back wall of thorax without penetration into thoracic cavity

    ● **S21.249**   Puncture wound with foreign body of unspecified back wall of thorax without penetration into thoracic cavity

  ● **S21.25**   **Open bite of back wall of thorax without penetration into thoracic cavity**
     Bite of back wall of thorax NOS

     Excludes1   superficial bite of back wall of thorax (S20.47)

    ● **S21.251**   Open bite of right back wall of thorax without penetration into thoracic cavity

● S21.252 Open bite of left back wall of thorax without penetration into thoracic cavity

● S21.259 Open bite of unspecified back wall of thorax without penetration into thoracic cavity

● S21.3 Open wound of front wall of thorax with penetration into thoracic cavity

Open wound of chest with penetration into thoracic cavity

● S21.30 Unspecified open wound of front wall of thorax with penetration into thoracic cavity

● S21.301 Unspecified open wound of right front wall of thorax with penetration into thoracic cavity

● S21.302 Unspecified open wound of left front wall of thorax with penetration into thoracic cavity

● S21.309 Unspecified open wound of unspecified front wall of thorax with penetration into thoracic cavity

● S21.31 Laceration without foreign body of front wall of thorax with penetration into thoracic cavity

● S21.311 Laceration without foreign body of right front wall of thorax with penetration into thoracic cavity

● S21.312 Laceration without foreign body of left front wall of thorax with penetration into thoracic cavity

● S21.319 Laceration without foreign body of unspecified front wall of thorax with penetration into thoracic cavity

● S21.32 Laceration with foreign body of front wall of thorax with penetration into thoracic cavity

● S21.321 Laceration with foreign body of right front wall of thorax with penetration into thoracic cavity

● S21.322 Laceration with foreign body of left front wall of thorax with penetration into thoracic cavity

● S21.329 Laceration with foreign body of unspecified front wall of thorax with penetration into thoracic cavity

● S21.33 Puncture wound without foreign body of front wall of thorax with penetration into thoracic cavity

● S21.331 Puncture wound without foreign body of right front wall of thorax with penetration into thoracic cavity

● S21.332 Puncture wound without foreign body of left front wall of thorax with penetration into thoracic cavity

● S21.339 Puncture wound without foreign body of unspecified front wall of thorax with penetration into thoracic cavity

● S21.34 Puncture wound with foreign body of front wall of thorax with penetration into thoracic cavity

● S21.341 Puncture wound with foreign body of right front wall of thorax with penetration into thoracic cavity

● S21.342 Puncture wound with foreign body of left front wall of thorax with penetration into thoracic cavity

● S21.349 Puncture wound with foreign body of unspecified front wall of thorax with penetration into thoracic cavity

● S21.35 Open bite of front wall of thorax with penetration into thoracic cavity

Excludes1   superficial bite of front wall of thorax (S20.37)

● S21.351 Open bite of right front wall of thorax with penetration into thoracic cavity

● S21.352 Open bite of left front wall of thorax with penetration into thoracic cavity

● S21.359 Open bite of unspecified front wall of thorax with penetration into thoracic cavity

● S21.4 Open wound of back wall of thorax with penetration into thoracic cavity

● S21.40 Unspecified open wound of back wall of thorax with penetration into thoracic cavity

● S21.401 Unspecified open wound of right back wall of thorax with penetration into thoracic cavity

● S21.402 Unspecified open wound of left back wall of thorax with penetration into thoracic cavity

● S21.409 Unspecified open wound of unspecified back wall of thorax with penetration into thoracic cavity

● S21.41 Laceration without foreign body of back wall of thorax with penetration into thoracic cavity

● S21.411 Laceration without foreign body of right back wall of thorax with penetration into thoracic cavity

● S21.412 Laceration without foreign body of left back wall of thorax with penetration into thoracic cavity

● S21.419 Laceration without foreign body of unspecified back wall of thorax with penetration into thoracic cavity

● S21.42 Laceration with foreign body of back wall of thorax with penetration into thoracic cavity

● S21.421 Laceration with foreign body of right back wall of thorax with penetration into thoracic cavity

● S21.422 Laceration with foreign body of left back wall of thorax with penetration into thoracic cavity

● S21.429 Laceration with foreign body of unspecified back wall of thorax with penetration into thoracic cavity

● S21.43 Puncture wound without foreign body of back wall of thorax with penetration into thoracic cavity

● S21.431 Puncture wound without foreign body of right back wall of thorax with penetration into thoracic cavity

● S21.432 Puncture wound without foreign body of left back wall of thorax with penetration into thoracic cavity

● S21.439 Puncture wound without foreign body of unspecified back wall of thorax with penetration into thoracic cavity

● S21.44 Puncture wound with foreign body of back wall of thorax with penetration into thoracic cavity

● S21.441 Puncture wound with foreign body of right back wall of thorax with penetration into thoracic cavity

● S21.442 Puncture wound with foreign body of left back wall of thorax with penetration into thoracic cavity

● S21.449 Puncture wound with foreign body of unspecified back wall of thorax with penetration into thoracic cavity

CHAPTER 19 (S00-T88)

● S21.45   **Open bite of back wall of thorax with penetration into thoracic cavity**
     Bite of back wall of thorax NOS

     Excludes1   superficial bite of back wall of thorax (S20.47)

   ● S21.451   Open bite of right back wall of thorax with penetration into thoracic cavity

   ● S21.452   Open bite of left back wall of thorax with penetration into thoracic cavity

   ● S21.459   Open bite of unspecified back wall of thorax with penetration into thoracic cavity

● S21.9   **Open wound of unspecified part of thorax**
     Open wound of thoracic wall NOS

   X ● S21.90   Unspecified open wound of unspecified part of thorax

   X ● S21.91   Laceration without foreign body of unspecified part of thorax

   X ● S21.92   Laceration with foreign body of unspecified part of thorax

   X ● S21.93   Puncture wound without foreign body of unspecified part of thorax

   X ● S21.94   Puncture wound with foreign body of unspecified part of thorax

   X ● S21.95   Open bite of unspecified part of thorax

     Excludes1   superficial bite of thorax (S20.97)

● S22   **Fracture of rib(s), sternum and thoracic spine**

   Note: A fracture not indicated as displaced or nondisplaced should be coded to displaced

     A fracture not indicated as open or closed should be coded to closed

   Includes   fracture of thoracic neural arch
         fracture of thoracic spinous process
         fracture of thoracic transverse process
         fracture of thoracic vertebra
         fracture of thoracic vertebral arch

➡ Code also, if applicable, any associated condition such as:
     injury of intrathoracic organ (S27.-)
     spinal cord injury (S24.0-, S24.1-)
   ▶ traumatic hemopneumothorax (S27.2)
   ▶ traumatic hemothorax (S27.1-)
   ▶ traumatic pneumothorax (S27.0)

   Excludes1   transection of thorax (S28.1)
   Excludes2   fracture of clavicle (S42.0-)
                 fracture of scapula (S42.1-)

   The appropriate 7th character is to be added to each code from category S22

A	initial encounter for closed fracture
B	initial encounter for open fracture
D	subsequent encounter for fracture with routine healing
G	subsequent encounter for fracture with delayed healing
K	subsequent encounter for fracture with nonunion
S	sequela

● S22.0   **Fracture of thoracic vertebra**

   ● S22.00   Fracture of unspecified thoracic vertebra

     ● S22.000   Wedge compression fracture of unspecified thoracic vertebra A, B 🐾

     ● S22.001   Stable burst fracture of unspecified thoracic vertebra A, B 🐾

     ● S22.002   Unstable burst fracture of unspecified thoracic vertebra A, B 🐾

     ● S22.008   Other fracture of unspecified thoracic vertebra A, B 🐾

     ● S22.009   Unspecified fracture of unspecified thoracic vertebra A, B 🐾

   ● S22.01   Fracture of first thoracic vertebra

     ● S22.010   Wedge compression fracture of first thoracic vertebra A, B 🐾

     ● S22.011   Stable burst fracture of first thoracic vertebra A, B 🐾

     ● S22.012   Unstable burst fracture of first thoracic vertebra A, B 🐾

     ● S22.018   Other fracture of first thoracic vertebra A, B 🐾

     ● S22.019   Unspecified fracture of first thoracic vertebra A, B 🐾

   ● S22.02   Fracture of second thoracic vertebra

     ● S22.020   Wedge compression fracture of second thoracic vertebra A, B 🐾

     ● S22.021   Stable burst fracture of second thoracic vertebra A, B 🐾

     ● S22.022   Unstable burst fracture of second thoracic vertebra A, B 🐾

     ● S22.028   Other fracture of second thoracic vertebra A, B 🐾

     ● S22.029   Unspecified fracture of second thoracic vertebra A, B 🐾

   ● S22.03   Fracture of third thoracic vertebra

     ● S22.030   Wedge compression fracture of third thoracic vertebra A, B 🐾

     ● S22.031   Stable burst fracture of third thoracic vertebra A, B 🐾

     ● S22.032   Unstable burst fracture of third thoracic vertebra A, B 🐾

     ● S22.038   Other fracture of third thoracic vertebra A, B 🐾

     ● S22.039   Unspecified fracture of third thoracic vertebra A, B 🐾

   ● S22.04   Fracture of fourth thoracic vertebra

     ● S22.040   Wedge compression fracture of fourth thoracic vertebra A, B 🐾

     ● S22.041   Stable burst fracture of fourth thoracic vertebra A, B 🐾

     ● S22.042   Unstable burst fracture of fourth thoracic vertebra A, B 🐾

     ● S22.048   Other fracture of fourth thoracic vertebra A, B 🐾

     ● S22.049   Unspecified fracture of fourth thoracic vertebra A, B 🐾

   ● S22.05   Fracture of T5-T6 vertebra

     ● S22.050   Wedge compression fracture of T5-T6 vertebra A, B 🐾

     ● S22.051   Stable burst fracture of T5-T6 vertebra A, B 🐾

     ● S22.052   Unstable burst fracture of T5-T6 vertebra A, B 🐾

     ● S22.058   Other fracture of T5-T6 vertebra A, B 🐾

     ● S22.059   Unspecified fracture of T5-T6 vertebra A, B 🐾

   ● S22.06   Fracture of T7-T8 vertebra

     ● S22.060   Wedge compression fracture of T7-T8 vertebra A, B 🐾

     ● S22.061   Stable burst fracture of T7-T8 vertebra A, B 🐾

     ● S22.062   Unstable burst fracture of T7-T8 vertebra A, B 🐾

     ● S22.068   Other fracture of T7-T8 thoracic vertebra A, B 🐾

     ● S22.069   Unspecified fracture of T7-T8 vertebra A, B 🐾

   ● S22.07   Fracture of T9-T10 vertebra

     ● S22.070   Wedge compression fracture of T9-T10 vertebra A, B 🐾

     ● S22.071   Stable burst fracture of T9-T10 vertebra A, B 🐾

     ● S22.072   Unstable burst fracture of T9-T10 vertebra A, B 🐾

     ● S22.078   Other fracture of T9-T10 vertebra A, B 🐾

● S22.079   Unspecified fracture of T9-T10 vertebra A, B 🔖

● S22.08   Fracture of T11-T12 vertebra

   ● S22.080   Wedge compression fracture of T11-T12 vertebra A, B 🔖

   ● S22.081   Stable burst fracture of T11-T12 vertebra A, B 🔖

   ● S22.082   Unstable burst fracture of T11-T12 vertebra A, B 🔖

   ● S22.088   Other fracture of T11-T12 vertebra A, B 🔖

   ● S22.089   Unspecified fracture of T11-T12 vertebra A, B 🔖

● S22.2   Fracture of sternum

  X● S22.20   Unspecified fracture of sternum

  X● S22.21   Fracture of manubrium

  X● S22.22   Fracture of body of sternum

  X● S22.23   Sternal manubrial dissociation

  X● S22.24   Fracture of xiphoid process

● S22.3 Fracture of one rib

  X● S22.31   Fracture of one rib, right side

  X● S22.32   Fracture of one rib, left side

  X● S22.39   Fracture of one rib, unspecified side

● S22.4   Multiple fractures of ribs

    Fractures of two or more ribs

    Excludes1   flail chest (S22.5-)

  X● S22.41   Multiple fractures of ribs, right side

  X● S22.42   Multiple fractures of ribs, left side

  X● S22.43   Multiple fractures of ribs, bilateral

  X● S22.49   Multiple fractures of ribs, unspecified side

X● S22.5   Flail chest

    Unstable chest due to sternum and/or rib fracture

X● S22.9   Fracture of bony thorax, part unspecified

● S23   Dislocation and sprain of joints and ligaments of thorax

  Includes   avulsion of joint or ligament of thorax
    laceration of cartilage, joint or ligament of thorax
    sprain of cartilage, joint or ligament of thorax
    traumatic hemarthrosis of joint or ligament of thorax
    traumatic rupture of joint or ligament of thorax
    traumatic subluxation of joint or ligament of thorax
    traumatic tear of joint or ligament of thorax

  Code also any associated: open wound

  Excludes2   dislocation, sprain of sternoclavicular joint (S43.2, S43.6)
    strain of muscle or tendon of thorax (S29.01-)

  The appropriate 7th character is to be added to each code from category S23

A	initial encounter
D	subsequent encounter
S	sequela

X● S23.0   Traumatic rupture of thoracic intervertebral disc

    Excludes1   rupture or displacement (nontraumatic) of thoracic intervertebral disc NOS (M51.- with fifth character 4)

● S23.1   Subluxation and dislocation of thoracic vertebra

    Code also any associated
      open wound of thorax (S21.-)
      spinal cord injury (S24.0-, S24.1-)

    Excludes2   fracture of thoracic vertebrae (S22.0-)

  ● S23.10   Subluxation and dislocation of unspecified thoracic vertebra

    ● S23.100   Subluxation of unspecified thoracic vertebra

    ● S23.101   Dislocation of unspecified thoracic vertebra

● S23.11   Subluxation and dislocation of T1/T2 thoracic vertebra

  ● S23.110   Subluxation of T1/T2 thoracic vertebra

  ● S23.111   Dislocation of T1/T2 thoracic vertebra

● S23.12   Subluxation and dislocation of T2/T3-T3/T4 thoracic vertebra

  ● S23.120   Subluxation of T2/T3 thoracic vertebra

  ● S23.121   Dislocation of T2/T3 thoracic vertebra

  ● S23.122   Subluxation of T3/T4 thoracic vertebra

  ● S23.123   Dislocation of T3/T4 thoracic vertebra

● S23.13   Subluxation and dislocation of T4/T5-T5/T6 thoracic vertebra

  ● S23.130   Subluxation of T4/T5 thoracic vertebra

  ● S23.131   Dislocation of T4/T5 thoracic vertebra

  ● S23.132   Subluxation of T5/T6 thoracic vertebra

  ● S23.133   Dislocation of T5/T6 thoracic vertebra

● S23.14   Subluxation and dislocation of T6/T7-T7/T8 thoracic vertebra

  ● S23.140   Subluxation of T6/T7 thoracic vertebra

  ● S23.141   Dislocation of T6/T7 thoracic vertebra

  ● S23.142   Subluxation of T7/T8 thoracic vertebra

  ● S23.143   Dislocation of T7/T8 thoracic vertebra

● S23.15   Subluxation and dislocation of T8/T9-T9/T10 thoracic vertebra

  ● S23.150   Subluxation of T8/T9 thoracic vertebra

  ● S23.151   Dislocation of T8/T9 thoracic vertebra

  ● S23.152   Subluxation of T9/T10 thoracic vertebra

  ● S23.153   Dislocation of T9/T10 thoracic vertebra

● S23.16   Subluxation and dislocation of T10/T11-T11/T12 thoracic vertebra

  ● S23.160   Subluxation of T10/T11 thoracic vertebra

  ● S23.161   Dislocation of T10/T11 thoracic vertebra

  ● S23.162   Subluxation of T11/T12 thoracic vertebra

  ● S23.163   Dislocation of T11/T12 thoracic vertebra

● S23.17   Subluxation and dislocation of T12/L1 thoracic vertebra

  ● S23.170   Subluxation of T12/L1 thoracic vertebra

  ● S23.171   Dislocation of T12/L1 thoracic vertebra

● S23.2   Dislocation of other and unspecified parts of thorax

  X● S23.20   Dislocation of unspecified part of thorax

  X● S23.29   Dislocation of other parts of thorax

X● S23.3   Sprain of ligaments of thoracic spine

● S23.4   Sprain of ribs and sternum

  X● S23.41   Sprain of ribs

  ● S23.42   Sprain of sternum

    ● S23.420   Sprain of sternoclavicular (joint) (ligament)

    ● S23.421   Sprain of chondrosternal joint

    ● S23.428   Other sprain of sternum

    ● S23.429   Unspecified sprain of sternum

X● S23.8   Sprain of other specified parts of thorax

X● S23.9   Sprain of unspecified parts of thorax

CHAPTER 19 (S00-T88)

● **S24**   **Injury of nerves and spinal cord at thorax level**

Note: Code to highest level of thoracic spinal cord injury.

Injuries to the spinal cord (S24.0 and S24.1) refer to the cord level and not bone level injury, and can affect nerve roots at and below the level given.

Code also any associated:
fracture of thoracic vertebra (S22.0-)
open wound of thorax (S21.-)
transient paralysis (R29.5)

Excludes2   injury of brachial plexus (S14.3)

The appropriate 7th character is to be added to each code from category S24

> A   initial encounter
> D   subsequent encounter
> S   sequela

X● **S24.0**   **Concussion and edema of** thoracic spinal cord A, D, S 🐾

● **S24.1**   **Other and unspecified injuries of thoracic spinal cord**

  ● **S24.10**   **Unspecified** injury of thoracic spinal cord

    ● **S24.101**   Unspecified injury at **T1 level of** thoracic spinal cord A, D, S 🐾

    ● **S24.102**   Unspecified injury at **T2-T6 level of** thoracic spinal cord A, D, S 🐾

    ● **S24.103**   Unspecified injury at **T7-T10 level of** thoracic spinal cord A, D, S 🐾

    ● **S24.104**   Unspecified injury at **T11-T12 level of** thoracic spinal cord A, D, S 🐾

    ● **S24.109**   Unspecified injury at **unspecified level** of thoracic spinal cord A, D, S 🐾
       Injury of thoracic spinal cord NOS

  ● **S24.11**   **Complete lesion of thoracic spinal cord**

    ● **S24.111**   Complete lesion at **T1 level of** thoracic spinal cord A, D, S 🐾

    ● **S24.112**   Complete lesion at **T2-T6 level of** thoracic spinal cord A, D, S 🐾

    ● **S24.113**   Complete lesion at **T7-T10 level of** thoracic spinal cord A, D, S 🐾

    ● **S24.114**   Complete lesion at **T11-T12 level of** thoracic spinal cord A, D, S 🐾

    ● **S24.119**   Complete lesion at **unspecified level** of thoracic spinal cord A, D, S 🐾

  ● **S24.13**   **Anterior cord syndrome** of thoracic spinal cord

    ● **S24.131**   Anterior cord syndrome at **T1 level of** thoracic spinal cord A, D, S 🐾

    ● **S24.132**   Anterior cord syndrome at **T2-T6 level** of thoracic spinal cord A, D, S 🐾

    ● **S24.133**   Anterior cord syndrome at **T7-T10 level** of thoracic spinal cord A, D, S 🐾

    ● **S24.134**   Anterior cord syndrome at **T11-T12 level** of thoracic spinal cord A, D, S 🐾

    ● **S24.139**   Anterior cord syndrome at **unspecified level** of thoracic spinal cord A, D, S 🐾

  ● **S24.14**   **Brown-Séquard syndrome** of thoracic spinal cord

    ● **S24.141**   Brown-Séquard syndrome at **T1 level** of thoracic spinal cord A, D, S 🐾

    ● **S24.142**   Brown-Séquard syndrome at **T2-T6 level** of thoracic spinal cord A, D, S 🐾

    ● **S24.143**   Brown-Séquard syndrome at **T7-T10 level** of thoracic spinal cord A, D, S 🐾

    ● **S24.144**   Brown-Séquard syndrome at **T11-T12 level** of thoracic spinal cord A, D, S 🐾

    ● **S24.149**   Brown-Séquard syndrome at **unspecified level** of thoracic spinal cord A, D, S 🐾

  ● **S24.15**   **Other incomplete lesions of thoracic spinal cord**
     Incomplete lesion of thoracic spinal cord NOS
     Posterior cord syndrome of thoracic spinal cord

    ● **S24.151**   Other incomplete lesion at **T1 level of** thoracic spinal cord A, D, S 🐾

    ● **S24.152**   Other incomplete lesion at **T2-T6 level** of thoracic spinal cord A, D, S 🐾

    ● **S24.153**   Other incomplete lesion at **T7-T10 level** of thoracic spinal cord A, D, S 🐾

    ● **S24.154**   Other incomplete lesion at **T11-T12 level** of thoracic spinal cord A, D, S 🐾

    ● **S24.159**   Other incomplete lesion at **unspecified level** of thoracic spinal cord A, D, S 🐾

X● **S24.2**   **Injury of nerve root of thoracic spine**

X● **S24.3**   **Injury of peripheral nerves of thorax**

X● **S24.4**   **Injury of thoracic sympathetic nervous system**
     Injury of cardiac plexus
     Injury of esophageal plexus
     Injury of pulmonary plexus
     Injury of stellate ganglion
     Injury of thoracic sympathetic ganglion

X● **S24.8**   **Injury of other specified nerves of thorax**

X● **S24.9**   **Injury of** unspecified **nerve of thorax**

● **S25**   **Injury of blood vessels of thorax**

The appropriate 7th character is to be added to each code from category S25

> A   initial encounter
> D   subsequent encounter
> S   sequela

Code also any associated open wound (S21.-)

● **S25.0**   **Injury of** thoracic aorta
     Injury of aorta NOS

  X● **S25.00**   **Unspecified** injury of thoracic aorta

  X● **S25.01**   **Minor laceration** of thoracic aorta
     Incomplete transection of thoracic aorta
     Laceration of thoracic aorta NOS
     Superficial laceration of thoracic aorta

  X● **S25.02**   **Major laceration** of thoracic aorta
     Complete transection of thoracic aorta
     Traumatic rupture of thoracic aorta

  X● **S25.09**   **Other specified injury of thoracic aorta**

● **S25.1**   **Injury of innominate or** subclavian **artery**

  ● **S25.10**   **Unspecified** injury of innominate or subclavian artery

    ● **S25.101**   Unspecified injury of **right** innominate or subclavian artery

    ● **S25.102**   Unspecified injury of **left** innominate or subclavian artery

    ● **S25.109**   Unspecified injury of **unspecified** innominate or subclavian artery

  ● **S25.11**   **Minor laceration** of innominate or subclavian artery
     Incomplete transection of innominate or subclavian artery
     Laceration of innominate or subclavian artery NOS
     Superficial laceration of innominate or subclavian artery

    ● **S25.111**   Minor laceration of **right** innominate or subclavian artery

    ● **S25.112**   Minor laceration of **left** innominate or subclavian artery

    ● **S25.119**   Minor laceration of **unspecified** innominate or subclavian artery

  ● **S25.12**   **Major laceration** of innominate or subclavian artery
     Complete transection of innominate or subclavian artery
     Traumatic rupture of innominate or subclavian artery

    ● **S25.121**   Major laceration of **right** innominate or subclavian artery

▶ New   ⇒ Revised   ~~deleted~~ Deleted   Excludes 1   Excludes 2   Includes   Use additional   Code first   Code also   Key words

OGCR Official Guidelines   X Assign placeholder X   ● Use Additional Character(s)   ▷ Manifestation Code   🐾 Hierarchical Condition Category   **Coding Clinic**

● S25.122   Major laceration of left innominate or subclavian artery

● S25.129   Major laceration of unspecified innominate or subclavian artery

● S25.19   Other specified injury of innominate or subclavian artery

  ● S25.191   Other specified injury of right innominate or subclavian artery

  ● S25.192   Other specified injury of left innominate or subclavian artery

  ● S25.199   Other specified injury of unspecified innominate or subclavian artery

● S25.2   Injury of superior vena cava

  Injury of vena cava NOS

X● S25.20   Unspecified injury of superior vena cava

X● S25.21   Minor laceration of superior vena cava

  Incomplete transection of superior vena cava

  Laceration of superior vena cava NOS

  Superficial laceration of superior vena cava

X● S25.22   Major laceration of superior vena cava

  Complete transection of superior vena cava

  Traumatic rupture of superior vena cava

X● S25.29   Other specified injury of superior vena cava

● S25.3   Injury of innominate or subclavian vein

● S25.30   Unspecified injury of innominate or subclavian vein

  ● S25.301   Unspecified injury of right innominate or subclavian vein

  ● S25.302   Unspecified injury of left innominate or subclavian vein

  ● S25.309   Unspecified injury of unspecified innominate or subclavian vein

● S25.31   Minor laceration of innominate or subclavian vein

  Incomplete transection of innominate or subclavian vein

  Laceration of innominate or subclavian vein NOS

  Superficial laceration of innominate or subclavian vein

  ● S25.311   Minor laceration of right innominate or subclavian vein

  ● S25.312   Minor laceration of left innominate or subclavian vein

  ● S25.319   Minor laceration of unspecified innominate or subclavian vein

● S25.32   Major laceration of innominate or subclavian vein

  Complete transection of innominate or subclavian vein

  Traumatic rupture of innominate or subclavian vein

  ● S25.321   Major laceration of right innominate or subclavian vein

  ● S25.322   Major laceration of left innominate or subclavian vein

  ● S25.329   Major laceration of unspecified innominate or subclavian vein

● S25.39   Other specified injury of innominate or subclavian vein

  ● S25.391   Other specified injury of right innominate or subclavian vein

  ● S25.392   Other specified injury of left innominate or subclavian vein

  ● S25.399   Other specified injury of unspecified innominate or subclavian vein

● S25.4   Injury of pulmonary blood vessels

● S25.40   Unspecified injury of pulmonary blood vessels

  ● S25.401   Unspecified injury of right pulmonary blood vessels

  ● S25.402   Unspecified injury of left pulmonary blood vessels

  ● S25.409   Unspecified injury of unspecified pulmonary blood vessels

● S25.41   Minor laceration of pulmonary blood vessels

  Incomplete transection of pulmonary blood vessels

  Laceration of pulmonary blood vessels NOS

  Superficial laceration of pulmonary blood vessels

  ● S25.411   Minor laceration of right pulmonary blood vessels

  ● S25.412   Minor laceration of left pulmonary blood vessels

  ● S25.419   Minor laceration of unspecified pulmonary blood vessels

● S25.42   Major laceration of pulmonary blood vessels

  Complete transection of pulmonary blood vessels

  Traumatic rupture of pulmonary blood vessels

  ● S25.421   Major laceration of right pulmonary blood vessels

  ● S25.422   Major laceration of left pulmonary blood vessels

  ● S25.429   Major laceration of unspecified pulmonary blood vessels

● S25.49   Other specified injury of pulmonary blood vessels

  ● S25.491   Other specified injury of right pulmonary blood vessels

  ● S25.492   Other specified injury of left pulmonary blood vessels

  ● S25.499   Other specified injury of unspecified pulmonary blood vessels

● S25.5   Injury of intercostal blood vessels

● S25.50   Unspecified injury of intercostal blood vessels

  ● S25.501   Unspecified injury of intercostal blood vessels, right side

  ● S25.502   Unspecified injury of intercostal blood vessels, left side

  ● S25.509   Unspecified injury of intercostal blood vessels, unspecified side

● S25.51   Laceration of intercostal blood vessels

  ● S25.511   Laceration of intercostal blood vessels, right side

  ● S25.512   Laceration of intercostal blood vessels, left side

  ● S25.519   Laceration of intercostal blood vessels, unspecified side

● S25.59   Other specified injury of intercostal blood vessels

  ● S25.591   Other specified injury of intercostal blood vessels, right side

  ● S25.592   Other specified injury of intercostal blood vessels, left side

  ● S25.599   Other specified injury of intercostal blood vessels, unspecified side

● S25.8   Injury of other blood vessels of thorax

  Injury of azygos vein

  Injury of mammary artery or vein

● S25.80   Unspecified injury of other blood vessels of thorax

  ● S25.801   Unspecified injury of other blood vessels of thorax, right side

  ● S25.802   Unspecified injury of other blood vessels of thorax, left side

  ● S25.809   Unspecified injury of other blood vessels of thorax, unspecified side

● S25.81   Laceration of other blood vessels of thorax

  ● S25.811   Laceration of other blood vessels of thorax, right side

  ● S25.812   Laceration of other blood vessels of thorax, left side

  ● S25.819   Laceration of other blood vessels of thorax, unspecified side

CHAPTER 19 (S00–T88)

Item 19–2 Pneumothorax is a collection of gas (positive air pressure) in the pleural space resulting in the lung collapsing. A **tension pneumothorax** is life-threatening and is a result of air in the pleural space causing a displacement in the mediastinal structures and cardiopulmonary function compromise. A **traumatic pneumothorax** results from blunt or penetrating injury that disrupts the parietal/visceral pleura. **Hemothorax** is blood or bloody fluid in the pleural cavity as a result of traumatic blood vessel rupture or inflammation of the lungs from pneumonia.

● S25.89   **Other specified injury of other blood vessels of thorax**

     ● S25.891   Other specified injury of other blood vessels of thorax, **right side**

     ● S25.892   Other specified injury of other blood vessels of thorax, **left side**

     ● S25.899   Other specified injury of other blood vessels of thorax, **unspecified side**

● S25.9   **Injury of unspecified blood vessel of thorax**

   X ● S25.90   Unspecified injury of unspecified blood vessel of thorax

   X ● S25.91   Laceration of unspecified blood vessel of thorax

   X ● S25.99   Other specified injury of unspecified blood vessel of thorax

● **S26   Injury of heart**

The appropriate 7th character is to be added to each code from category S26

A	initial encounter
D	subsequent encounter
S	sequela

Code also any associated:
   open wound of thorax (S21.-)
   traumatic hemopneumothorax (S27.2)
   traumatic hemothorax (S27.1)
   traumatic pneumothorax (S27.0)

● S26.0   **Injury of heart with hemopericardium**
     Hemopericardium: effusion of blood within pericardium

   X ● S26.00   Unspecified injury of heart with hemopericardium

   X ● S26.01   Contusion of heart with hemopericardium

   ● S26.02   Laceration of heart with hemopericardium

     ● S26.020   Mild laceration of heart with hemopericardium
       Laceration of heart without penetration of heart chamber

     ● S26.021   Moderate laceration of heart with hemopericardium
       Laceration of heart with penetration of heart chamber

     ● S26.022   Major laceration of heart with hemopericardium
       Laceration of heart with penetration of multiple heart chambers

   X ● S26.09   Other injury of heart with hemopericardium

● S26.1   **Injury of heart without hemopericardium**
     Hemopericardium: effusion of blood within pericardium

   X ● S26.10   Unspecified injury of heart without hemopericardium

   X ● S26.11   Contusion of heart without hemopericardium

   X ● S26.12   Laceration of heart without hemopericardium

   X ● S26.19   Other injury of heart without hemopericardium

● S26.9   **Injury of heart, unspecified with or without hemopericardium**
     Hemopericardium: effusion of blood within pericardium

   X ● S26.90   Unspecified injury of heart, unspecified with or without hemopericardium

   X ● S26.91   Contusion of heart, unspecified with or without hemopericardium

   X ● S26.92   **Laceration of heart, unspecified with or without hemopericardium**
     Laceration of heart NOS

   X ● S26.99   **Other injury of heart, unspecified with or without hemopericardium**

● **S27   Injury of other and unspecified intrathoracic organs**

Code also any associated open wound of thorax (S21.-)

Excludes2   injury of cervical esophagus (S10-S19)
       injury of trachea (cervical) (S10-S19)

The appropriate 7th character is to be added to each code from category S27

A	initial encounter
D	subsequent encounter
S	sequela

   X ● S27.0   **Traumatic pneumothorax**

     Excludes1   spontaneous pneumothorax (J93.-)

   X ● S27.1   **Traumatic hemothorax**

   X ● S27.2   **Traumatic hemopneumothorax**

   ● S27.3   **Other and unspecified injuries of lung**

     ● S27.30   Unspecified injury of lung

       ● S27.301   Unspecified injury of lung, **unilateral**

       ● S27.302   Unspecified injury of lung, **bilateral**

       ● S27.309   Unspecified injury of lung, **unspecified**

     ● S27.31   Primary blast injury of lung
       Blast injury of lung NOS

       ● S27.311   Primary blast injury of lung, **unilateral**

       ● S27.312   Primary blast injury of lung, **bilateral**

       ● S27.319   Primary blast injury of lung, **unspecified**

     ● S27.32   Contusion of lung

       ● S27.321   Contusion of lung, **unilateral**

       ● S27.322   Contusion of lung, **bilateral**

       ● S27.329   Contusion of lung, **unspecified**

     ● S27.33   Laceration of lung

       ● S27.331   Laceration of lung, **unilateral**

       ● S27.332   Laceration of lung, **bilateral**

       ● S27.339   Laceration of lung, **unspecified**

     ● S27.39   Other injuries of lung
       Secondary blast injury of lung

       ● S27.391   Other injuries of lung, **unilateral**

       ● S27.392   Other injuries of lung, **bilateral**

       ● S27.399   Other injuries of lung, **unspecified**

   ● S27.4   **Injury of bronchus**

     ● S27.40   Unspecified injury of bronchus

       ● S27.401   Unspecified injury of bronchus, **unilateral**

       ● S27.402   Unspecified injury of bronchus, **bilateral**

       ● S27.409   Unspecified injury of bronchus, **unspecified**

     ● S27.41   Primary blast injury of bronchus
       Blast injury of bronchus NOS

       ● S27.411   Primary blast injury of bronchus, **unilateral**

       ● S27.412   Primary blast injury of bronchus, **bilateral**

       ● S27.419   Primary blast injury of bronchus, **unspecified**

     ● S27.42   Contusion of bronchus

       ● S27.421   Contusion of bronchus, **unilateral**

       ● S27.422   Contusion of bronchus, **bilateral**

       ● S27.429   Contusion of bronchus, **unspecified**

▶ New   ⇒ Revised   ~~deleted~~ Deleted   Excludes 1   Excludes 2   Includes   Use additional   Code first   Code also   Key words

OGCR Official Guidelines   X Assign placeholder X   ● Use Additional Character(s)   ▶ Manifestation Code   ✿ Hierarchical Condition Category   **Coding Clinic**

● S27.43   Laceration of bronchus
     ● S27.431   Laceration of bronchus, unilateral
     ● S27.432   Laceration of bronchus, bilateral
     ● S27.439   Laceration of bronchus, unspecified
   ● S27.49   Other injury of bronchus
       Secondary blast injury of bronchus
     ● S27.491   Other injury of bronchus, unilateral
     ● S27.492   Other injury of bronchus, bilateral
     ● S27.499   Other injury of bronchus, unspecified
● S27.5   Injury of thoracic trachea
  X ● S27.50   Unspecified injury of thoracic trachea
  X ● S27.51   Primary blast injury of thoracic trachea
       Blast injury of thoracic trachea NOS
  X ● S27.52   Contusion of thoracic trachea
  X ● S27.53   Laceration of thoracic trachea
  X ● S27.59   Other injury of thoracic trachea
       Secondary blast injury of thoracic trachea
● S27.6   Injury of pleura
  X ● S27.60   Unspecified injury of pleura
  X ● S27.63   Laceration of pleura
  X ● S27.69   Other injury of pleura
● S27.8   Injury of other specified intrathoracic organs
   ● S27.80   Injury of diaphragm
     ● S27.802   Contusion of diaphragm
     ● S27.803   Laceration of diaphragm
     ● S27.808   Other injury of diaphragm
     ● S27.809   Unspecified injury of diaphragm
   ● S27.81   Injury of esophagus (thoracic part)
     ● S27.812   Contusion of esophagus (thoracic part)
     ● S27.813   Laceration of esophagus (thoracic part)
     ● S27.818   Other injury of esophagus (thoracic part)
     ● S27.819   Unspecified injury of esophagus (thoracic part)
   ● S27.89   Injury of other specified intrathoracic organs
       Injury of lymphatic thoracic duct
       Injury of thymus gland
     ● S27.892   Contusion of other specified intrathoracic organs
     ● S27.893   Laceration of other specified intrathoracic organs
     ● S27.898   Other injury of other specified intrathoracic organs
     ● S27.899   Unspecified injury of other specified intrathoracic organs
  X ● S27.9   Injury of unspecified intrathoracic organ

● S28   Crushing injury of thorax, and traumatic amputation of part of thorax

The appropriate 7th character is to be added to each code from category S28

A	initial encounter
D	subsequent encounter
S	sequela

  X ● S28.0   **Crushed chest**
       Use additional code for all associated injuries
       Excludes1   flail chest (S22.5)
  X ● S28.1   **Traumatic amputation (partial) of part of thorax, except breast**
   ● S28.2   **Traumatic amputation of breast**
     ● S28.21   **Complete traumatic amputation of breast**
       Traumatic amputation of breast NOS
       ● S28.211   **Complete traumatic amputation of right breast**

       ● S28.212   Complete traumatic amputation of left breast
       ● S28.219   Complete traumatic amputation of unspecified breast
     ● S28.22   Partial traumatic amputation of breast
       ● S28.221   Partial traumatic amputation of right breast
       ● S28.222   Partial traumatic amputation of left breast
       ● S28.229   Partial traumatic amputation of unspecified breast

● S29   Other and unspecified injuries of thorax

Code also any associated open wound (S21.-)

The appropriate 7th character is to be added to each code from category S29

A	initial encounter
D	subsequent encounter
S	sequela

   ● S29.0   Injury of muscle and tendon at thorax level
     ● S29.00   Unspecified injury of muscle and tendon of thorax
       ● S29.001   Unspecified injury of muscle and tendon of front wall of thorax
       ● S29.002   Unspecified injury of muscle and tendon of back wall of thorax
       ● S29.009   Unspecified injury of muscle and tendon of unspecified wall of thorax
     ● S29.01   Strain of muscle and tendon of thorax
       ● S29.011   Strain of muscle and tendon of front wall of thorax
       ● S29.012   Strain of muscle and tendon of back wall of thorax
       ● S29.019   Strain of muscle and tendon of unspecified wall of thorax
     ● S29.02   Laceration of muscle and tendon of thorax
       ● S29.021   Laceration of muscle and tendon of front wall of thorax
       ● S29.022   Laceration of muscle and tendon of back wall of thorax
       ● S29.029   Laceration of muscle and tendon of unspecified wall of thorax
     ● S29.09   Other injury of muscle and tendon of thorax
       ● S29.091   Other injury of muscle and tendon of front wall of thorax
       ● S29.092   Other injury of muscle and tendon of back wall of thorax
       ● S29.099   Other injury of muscle and tendon of unspecified wall of thorax
  X ● S29.8   Other specified injuries of thorax
  X ● S29.9   Unspecified injury of thorax

INJURIES TO THE ABDOMEN, LOWER BACK, LUMBAR SPINE PELVIS AND EXTERNAL GENITALS (S30-S39)

Includes	injuries to the abdominal wall
	injuries to the anus
	injuries to the buttock
	injuries to the external genitalia
	injuries to the flank
	injuries to the groin
Excludes2	burns and corrosions (T20-T32)
	effects of foreign body in anus and rectum (T18.5)
	effects of foreign body in genitourinary tract (T19.-)
	effects of foreign body in stomach, small intestine and colon (T18.2-T18.4)
	frostbite (T33-T34)
	insect bite or sting, venomous (T63.4)

CHAPTER 19 (S00-T88)

● **S30** **Superficial injury of abdomen, lower back, pelvis and external genitals**

Excludes2 superficial injury of hip (S70.-)

The appropriate 7th character is to be added to each code from category S30

A	initial encounter
D	subsequent encounter
S	sequela

X● **S30.0** Contusion of lower back and pelvis
         Contusion of buttock

X● **S30.1** Contusion of abdominal wall
         Contusion of flank
         Contusion of groin

● **S30.2** Contusion of external genital organs

  ● **S30.20** Contusion of unspecified external genital organ

    ● **S30.201** Contusion of unspecified external genital organ, male

    ● **S30.202** Contusion of unspecified external genital organ, female

  X● **S30.21** Contusion of penis

  X● **S30.22** Contusion of scrotum and testes

  X● **S30.23** Contusion of vagina and vulva

X● **S30.3** Contusion of anus

● **S30.8** Other superficial injuries of abdomen, lower back, pelvis and external genitals

  ● **S30.81** Abrasion of abdomen, lower back, pelvis and external genitals

    ● **S30.810** Abrasion of lower back and pelvis
    ● **S30.811** Abrasion of abdominal wall
    ● **S30.812** Abrasion of penis
    ● **S30.813** Abrasion of scrotum and testes
    ● **S30.814** Abrasion of vagina and vulva
    ● **S30.815** Abrasion of unspecified external genital organs, male
    ● **S30.816** Abrasion of unspecified external genital organs, female
    ● **S30.817** Abrasion of anus

  ● **S30.82** Blister (nonthermal) of abdomen, lower back, pelvis and external genitals

    ● **S30.820** Blister (nonthermal) of lower back and pelvis
    ● **S30.821** Blister (nonthermal) of abdominal wall
    ● **S30.822** Blister (nonthermal) of penis
    ● **S30.823** Blister (nonthermal) of scrotum and testes
    ● **S30.824** Blister (nonthermal) of vagina and vulva
    ● **S30.825** Blister (nonthermal) of unspecified external genital organs, male
    ● **S30.826** Blister (nonthermal) of unspecified external genital organs, female
    ● **S30.827** Blister (nonthermal) of anus

  ● **S30.84** External constriction of abdomen, lower back, pelvis and external genitals

    ● **S30.840** External constriction of lower back and pelvis
    ● **S30.841** External constriction of abdominal wall
    ● **S30.842** External constriction of penis
       Hair tourniquet syndrome of penis
       Use additional cause code to identify the constricting item (W49.0-)
    ● **S30.843** External constriction of scrotum and testes
    ● **S30.844** External constriction of vagina and vulva

● **S30.845** External constriction of unspecified external genital organs, male
● **S30.846** External constriction of unspecified external genital organs, female

● **S30.85** Superficial foreign body of abdomen, lower back, pelvis and external genitals
     Splinter in the abdomen, lower back, pelvis and external genitals

  ● **S30.850** Superficial foreign body of lower back and pelvis
  ● **S30.851** Superficial foreign body of abdominal wall
  ● **S30.852** Superficial foreign body of penis
  ● **S30.853** Superficial foreign body of scrotum and testes
  ● **S30.854** Superficial foreign body of vagina and vulva
  ● **S30.855** Superficial foreign body of unspecified external genital organs, male
  ● **S30.856** Superficial foreign body of unspecified external genital organs, female
  ● **S30.857** Superficial foreign body of anus

● **S30.86** Insect bite (nonvenomous) of abdomen, lower back, pelvis and external genitals

  ● **S30.860** Insect bite (nonvenomous) of lower back and pelvis
  ● **S30.861** Insect bite (nonvenomous) of abdominal wall
  ● **S30.862** Insect bite (nonvenomous) of penis
  ● **S30.863** Insect bite (nonvenomous) of scrotum and testes
  ● **S30.864** Insect bite (nonvenomous) of vagina and vulva
  ● **S30.865** Insect bite (nonvenomous) of unspecified external genital organs, male
  ● **S30.866** Insect bite (nonvenomous) of unspecified external genital organs, female
  ● **S30.867** Insect bite (nonvenomous) of anus

● **S30.87** Other superficial bite of abdomen, lower back, pelvis and external genitals

  Excludes1 open bite of abdomen, lower back, pelvis and external genitals (S31.05, S31.15, S31.25, S31.35, S31.45, S31.55)

  ● **S30.870** Other superficial bite of lower back and pelvis
  ● **S30.871** Other superficial bite of abdominal wall
  ● **S30.872** Other superficial bite of penis
  ● **S30.873** Other superficial bite of scrotum and testes
  ● **S30.874** Other superficial bite of vagina and vulva
  ● **S30.875** Other superficial bite of unspecified external genital organs, male
  ● **S30.876** Other superficial bite of unspecified external genital organs, female
  ● **S30.877** Other superficial bite of anus

● **S30.9** Unspecified superficial injury of abdomen, lower back, pelvis and external genitals

  X● **S30.91** Unspecified superficial injury of lower back and pelvis
  X● **S30.92** Unspecified superficial injury of abdominal wall
  X● **S30.93** Unspecified superficial injury of penis

▶ New   ⇒ Revised   ~~deleted~~ Deleted   Excludes 1   Excludes 2   Includes   Use additional   Code first   Code also   Key words
OGCR Official Guidelines   X Assign placeholder X   ● Use Additional Character(s)   ▶ Manifestation Code   🝾 Hierarchical Condition Category   **Coding Clinic**

X⬤ **S30.94** Unspecified superficial injury of scrotum and testes

X⬤ **S30.95** Unspecified superficial injury of vagina and vulva

X⬤ **S30.96** Unspecified superficial injury of unspecified external genital organs, male

X⬤ **S30.97** Unspecified superficial injury of unspecified external genital organs, female

X⬤ **S30.98** Unspecified superficial injury of anus

⬤ **S31** **Open wound of abdomen, lower back, pelvis and external genitals**

Code also any associated:
spinal cord injury (S24.0, S24.1-, S34.0-, S34.1-)
wound infection

Excludes1 traumatic amputation of part of abdomen, lower back and pelvis (S38.2-, S38.3)

Excludes2 open wound of hip (S71.00-S71.02)
open fracture of pelvis (S32.1--S32.9 with 7th character B)

The appropriate 7th character is to be added to each code from category S31

A	initial encounter
D	subsequent encounter
S	sequela

⬤ **S31.0** **Open wound of lower back and pelvis**

⬤ **S31.00** Unspecified open wound of lower back and pelvis

  ⬤ **S31.000** Unspecified open wound of lower back and pelvis without penetration into retroperitoneum
Unspecified open wound of lower back and pelvis NOS

  ⬤ **S31.001** Unspecified open wound of lower back and pelvis with penetration into retroperitoneum

⬤ **S31.01** Laceration without foreign body of lower back and pelvis

  ⬤ **S31.010** Laceration without foreign body of lower back and pelvis without penetration into retroperitoneum
Laceration without foreign body of lower back and pelvis NOS

  ⬤ **S31.011** Laceration without foreign body of lower back and pelvis with penetration into retroperitoneum

⬤ **S31.02** Laceration with foreign body of lower back and pelvis

  ⬤ **S31.020** Laceration with foreign body of lower back and pelvis without penetration into retroperitoneum
Laceration with foreign body of lower back and pelvis NOS

  ⬤ **S31.021** Laceration with foreign body of lower back and pelvis with penetration into retroperitoneum

⬤ **S31.03** Puncture wound without foreign body of lower back and pelvis

  ⬤ **S31.030** Puncture wound without foreign body of lower back and pelvis without penetration into retroperitoneum
Puncture wound without foreign body of lower back and pelvis NOS

  ⬤ **S31.031** Puncture wound without foreign body of lower back and pelvis with penetration into retroperitoneum

⬤ **S31.04** Puncture wound with foreign body of lower back and pelvis

  ⬤ **S31.040** Puncture wound with foreign body of lower back and pelvis without penetration into retroperitoneum
Puncture wound with foreign body of lower back and pelvis NOS

  ⬤ **S31.041** Puncture wound with foreign body of lower back and pelvis with penetration into retroperitoneum

⬤ **S31.05** Open bite of lower back and pelvis
Bite of lower back and pelvis NOS

Excludes1 superficial bite of lower back and pelvis (S30.860, S30.870)

  ⬤ **S31.050** Open bite of lower back and pelvis without penetration into retroperitoneum
Open bite of lower back and pelvis NOS

  ⬤ **S31.051** Open bite of lower back and pelvis with penetration into retroperitoneum

⬤ **S31.1** **Open wound of abdominal wall without penetration into peritoneal cavity**
Open wound of abdominal wall NOS

Excludes2 open wound of abdominal wall with penetration into peritoneal cavity (S31.6-)

⬤ **S31.10** Unspecified open wound of abdominal wall without penetration into peritoneal cavity

  ⬤ **S31.100** Unspecified open wound of abdominal wall, right upper quadrant without penetration into peritoneal cavity

  ⬤ **S31.101** Unspecified open wound of abdominal wall, left upper quadrant without penetration into peritoneal cavity

CHAPTER 19 (S00-T88)

CHAPTER 19 (S00-T88)

- S31.102 Unspecified open wound of abdominal wall, epigastric region without penetration into peritoneal cavity

- S31.103 Unspecified open wound of abdominal wall, right lower quadrant without penetration into peritoneal cavity

- S31.104 Unspecified open wound of abdominal wall, left lower quadrant without penetration into peritoneal cavity

- S31.105 Unspecified open wound of abdominal wall, periumbilic region without penetration into peritoneal cavity

- S31.109 Unspecified open wound of abdominal wall, unspecified quadrant without penetration into peritoneal cavity

    Unspecified open wound of abdominal wall NOS

- S31.11 Laceration without foreign body of abdominal wall without penetration into peritoneal cavity

    - S31.110 Laceration without foreign body of abdominal wall, right upper quadrant without penetration into peritoneal cavity

    - S31.111 Laceration without foreign body of abdominal wall, left upper quadrant without penetration into peritoneal cavity

    - S31.112 Laceration without foreign body of abdominal wall, epigastric region without penetration into peritoneal cavity

    - S31.113 Laceration without foreign body of abdominal wall, right lower quadrant without penetration into peritoneal cavity

    - S31.114 Laceration without foreign body of abdominal wall, left lower quadrant without penetration into peritoneal cavity

    - S31.115 Laceration without foreign body of abdominal wall, periumbilic region without penetration into peritoneal cavity

    - S31.119 Laceration without foreign body of abdominal wall, unspecified quadrant without penetration into peritoneal cavity

- S31.12 Laceration with foreign body of abdominal wall without penetration into peritoneal cavity

    - S31.120 Laceration of abdominal wall with foreign body, right upper quadrant without penetration into peritoneal cavity

    - S31.121 Laceration of abdominal wall with foreign body, left upper quadrant without penetration into peritoneal cavity

    - S31.122 Laceration of abdominal wall with foreign body, epigastric region without penetration into peritoneal cavity

    - S31.123 Laceration of abdominal wall with foreign body, right lower quadrant without penetration into peritoneal cavity

    - S31.124 Laceration of abdominal wall with foreign body, left lower quadrant without penetration into peritoneal cavity

- S31.125 Laceration of abdominal wall with foreign body, periumbilic region without penetration into peritoneal cavity

- S31.129 Laceration of abdominal wall with foreign body, unspecified quadrant without penetration into peritoneal cavity

- S31.13 Puncture wound of abdominal wall without foreign body without penetration into peritoneal cavity

    - S31.130 Puncture wound of abdominal wall without foreign body, right upper quadrant without penetration into peritoneal cavity

    - S31.131 Puncture wound of abdominal wall without foreign body, left upper quadrant without penetration into peritoneal cavity

    - S31.132 Puncture wound of abdominal wall without foreign body, epigastric region without penetration into peritoneal cavity

    - S31.133 Puncture wound of abdominal wall without foreign body, right lower quadrant without penetration into peritoneal cavity

    - S31.134 Puncture wound of abdominal wall without foreign body, left lower quadrant without penetration into peritoneal cavity

    - S31.135 Puncture wound of abdominal wall without foreign body, periumbilic region without penetration into peritoneal cavity

    - S31.139 Puncture wound of abdominal wall without foreign body, unspecified quadrant without penetration into peritoneal cavity

- S31.14 Puncture wound of abdominal wall with foreign body without penetration into peritoneal cavity

    - S31.140 Puncture wound of abdominal wall with foreign body, right upper quadrant without penetration into peritoneal cavity

    - S31.141 Puncture wound of abdominal wall with foreign body, left upper quadrant without penetration into peritoneal cavity

    - S31.142 Puncture wound of abdominal wall with foreign body, epigastric region without penetration into peritoneal cavity

    - S31.143 Puncture wound of abdominal wall with foreign body, right lower quadrant without penetration into peritoneal cavity

    - S31.144 Puncture wound of abdominal wall with foreign body, left lower quadrant without penetration into peritoneal cavity

    - S31.145 Puncture wound of abdominal wall with foreign body, periumbilic region without penetration into peritoneal cavity

    - S31.149 Puncture wound of abdominal wall with foreign body, unspecified quadrant without penetration into peritoneal cavity

▶ New   ⇨ Revised   ~~deleted~~ Deleted   Excludes 1   Excludes 2   Includes   Use additional   Code first   Code also   Key words
OGCR Official Guidelines   X Assign placeholder X   ● Use Additional Character(s)   ▶ Manifestation Code   🦘 Hierarchical Condition Category   **Coding Clinic**

● **S31.15**   **Open bite of abdominal wall without penetration into peritoneal cavity**
    Bite of abdominal wall NOS

    Excludes1   superficial bite of abdominal wall (S30.871)

   ● **S31.150**   Open bite of abdominal wall, right upper quadrant without penetration into peritoneal cavity

   ● **S31.151**   Open bite of abdominal wall, left upper quadrant without penetration into peritoneal cavity

   ● **S31.152**   Open bite of abdominal wall, epigastric region without penetration into peritoneal cavity

   ● **S31.153**   Open bite of abdominal wall, right lower quadrant without penetration into peritoneal cavity

   ● **S31.154**   Open bite of abdominal wall, left lower quadrant without penetration into peritoneal cavity

   ● **S31.155**   Open bite of abdominal wall, periumbilic region without penetration into peritoneal cavity

   ● **S31.159**   Open bite of abdominal wall, unspecified quadrant without penetration into peritoneal cavity

● **S31.2**   **Open wound of penis**

  X ● **S31.20**   Unspecified open wound of penis

  X ● **S31.21**   Laceration without foreign body of penis

  X ● **S31.22**   Laceration with foreign body of penis

  X ● **S31.23**   Puncture wound without foreign body of penis

  X ● **S31.24**   Puncture wound with foreign body of penis

  X ● **S31.25**   Open bite of penis
     Bite of penis NOS

     Excludes1   superficial bite of penis (S30.862, S30.872)

● **S31.3**   **Open wound of scrotum and testes**

  X ● **S31.30**   Unspecified open wound of scrotum and testes

  X ● **S31.31**   Laceration without foreign body of scrotum and testes

  X ● **S31.32**   Laceration with foreign body of scrotum and testes

  X ● **S31.33**   Puncture wound without foreign body of scrotum and testes

  X ● **S31.34**   Puncture wound with foreign body of scrotum and testes

  X ● **S31.35**   Open bite of scrotum and testes
     Bite of scrotum and testes NOS

     Excludes1   superficial bite of scrotum and testes (S30.863, S30.873)

● **S31.4**   **Open wound of vagina and vulva**

    Excludes1   injury to vagina and vulva during delivery (O70.-, O71.4)

  X ● **S31.40**   Unspecified open wound of vagina and vulva

  X ● **S31.41**   Laceration without foreign body of vagina and vulva

  X ● **S31.42**   Laceration with foreign body of vagina and vulva

  X ● **S31.43**   Puncture wound without foreign body of vagina and vulva

  X ● **S31.44**   Puncture wound with foreign body of vagina and vulva

  X ● **S31.45**   Open bite of vagina and vulva
     Bite of vagina and vulva NOS

     Excludes1   superficial bite of vagina and vulva (S30.864, S30.874)

● **S31.5**   **Open wound of unspecified external genital organs**

    Excludes1   traumatic amputation of external genital organs (S38.21, S38.22)

  ● **S31.50**   Unspecified open wound of unspecified external genital organs

   ● **S31.501**   Unspecified open wound of unspecified external genital organs, male

   ● **S31.502**   Unspecified open wound of unspecified external genital organs, female

  ● **S31.51**   Laceration without foreign body of unspecified external genital organs

   ● **S31.511**   Laceration without foreign body of unspecified external genital organs, male

   ● **S31.512**   Laceration without foreign body of unspecified external genital organs, female

  ● **S31.52**   Laceration with foreign body of unspecified external genital organs

   ● **S31.521**   Laceration with foreign body of unspecified external genital organs, male

   ● **S31.522**   Laceration with foreign body of unspecified external genital organs, female

  ● **S31.53**   Puncture wound without foreign body of unspecified external genital organs

   ● **S31.531**   Puncture wound without foreign body of unspecified external genital organs, male

   ● **S31.532**   Puncture wound without foreign body of unspecified external genital organs, female

  ● **S31.54**   Puncture wound with foreign body of unspecified external genital organs

   ● **S31.541**   Puncture wound with foreign body of unspecified external genital organs, male

   ● **S31.542**   Puncture wound with foreign body of unspecified external genital organs, female

  ● **S31.55**   Open bite of unspecified external genital organs
     Bite of unspecified external genital organs NOS

     Excludes1   superficial bite of unspecified external genital organs (S30.865, S30.866, S30.875, S30.876)

   ● **S31.551**   Open bite of unspecified external genital organs, male

   ● **S31.552**   Open bite of unspecified external genital organs, female

● **S31.6**   **Open wound of abdominal wall with penetration into peritoneal cavity**
    Coding Clinic: 2023, Q3, P9

  ● **S31.60**   Unspecified open wound of abdominal wall with penetration into peritoneal cavity

   ● **S31.600**   Unspecified open wound of abdominal wall, right upper quadrant with penetration into peritoneal cavity

   ● **S31.601**   Unspecified open wound of abdominal wall, left upper quadrant with penetration into peritoneal cavity

   ● **S31.602**   Unspecified open wound of abdominal wall, epigastric region with penetration into peritoneal cavity

● S31.603   Unspecified open wound of abdominal wall, right lower quadrant with penetration into peritoneal cavity

● S31.604   Unspecified open wound of abdominal wall, left lower quadrant with penetration into peritoneal cavity

● S31.605   Unspecified open wound of abdominal wall, periumbilic region with penetration into peritoneal cavity

● S31.609   Unspecified open wound of abdominal wall, unspecified quadrant with penetration into peritoneal cavity

● S31.61   Laceration without foreign body of abdominal wall with penetration into peritoneal cavity

● S31.610   Laceration without foreign body of abdominal wall, right upper quadrant with penetration into peritoneal cavity

● S31.611   Laceration without foreign body of abdominal wall, left upper quadrant with penetration into peritoneal cavity

● S31.612   Laceration without foreign body of abdominal wall, epigastric region with penetration into peritoneal cavity

● S31.613   Laceration without foreign body of abdominal wall, right lower quadrant with penetration into peritoneal cavity
     Coding Clinic: 2015, Q4, P37

● S31.614   Laceration without foreign body of abdominal wall, left lower quadrant with penetration into peritoneal cavity

● S31.615   Laceration without foreign body of abdominal wall, periumbilic region with penetration into peritoneal cavity

● S31.619   Laceration without foreign body of abdominal wall, unspecified quadrant with penetration into peritoneal cavity

● S31.62   Laceration with foreign body of abdominal wall with penetration into peritoneal cavity

● S31.620   Laceration with foreign body of abdominal wall, right upper quadrant with penetration into peritoneal cavity

● S31.621   Laceration with foreign body of abdominal wall, left upper quadrant with penetration into peritoneal cavity

● S31.622   Laceration with foreign body of abdominal wall, epigastric region with penetration into peritoneal cavity

● S31.623   Laceration with foreign body of abdominal wall, right lower quadrant with penetration into peritoneal cavity

● S31.624   Laceration with foreign body of abdominal wall, left lower quadrant with penetration into peritoneal cavity

● S31.625   Laceration with foreign body of abdominal wall, periumbilic region with penetration into peritoneal cavity

● S31.629   Laceration with foreign body of abdominal wall, unspecified quadrant with penetration into peritoneal cavity

● S31.63   Puncture wound without foreign body of abdominal wall with penetration into peritoneal cavity

● S31.630   Puncture wound without foreign body of abdominal wall, right upper quadrant with penetration into peritoneal cavity

● S31.631   Puncture wound without foreign body of abdominal wall, left upper quadrant with penetration into peritoneal cavity

● S31.632   Puncture wound without foreign body of abdominal wall, epigastric region with penetration into peritoneal cavity

● S31.633   Puncture wound without foreign body of abdominal wall, right lower quadrant with penetration into peritoneal cavity

● S31.634   Puncture wound without foreign body of abdominal wall, left lower quadrant with penetration into peritoneal cavity

● S31.635   Puncture wound without foreign body of abdominal wall, periumbilic region with penetration into peritoneal cavity

● S31.639   Puncture wound without foreign body of abdominal wall, unspecified quadrant with penetration into peritoneal cavity

● S31.64   Puncture wound with foreign body of abdominal wall with penetration into peritoneal cavity

● S31.640   Puncture wound with foreign body of abdominal wall, right upper quadrant with penetration into peritoneal cavity

● S31.641   Puncture wound with foreign body of abdominal wall, left upper quadrant with penetration into peritoneal cavity

● S31.642   Puncture wound with foreign body of abdominal wall, epigastric region with penetration into peritoneal cavity

● S31.643   Puncture wound with foreign body of abdominal wall, right lower quadrant with penetration into peritoneal cavity

● S31.644   Puncture wound with foreign body of abdominal wall, left lower quadrant with penetration into peritoneal cavity

● S31.645   Puncture wound with foreign body of abdominal wall, periumbilic region with penetration into peritoneal cavity

● S31.649   Puncture wound with foreign body of abdominal wall, unspecified quadrant with penetration into peritoneal cavity

CHAPTER 19 (S00-T88)

● **S31.65**   **Open bite** of abdominal wall with penetration into peritoneal cavity

> **Excludes1**   superficial bite of abdominal wall (S30.861, S30.871)

   ● **S31.650**   Open bite of abdominal wall, **right upper** quadrant with penetration into peritoneal cavity

   ● **S31.651**   Open bite of abdominal wall, **left upper** quadrant with penetration into peritoneal cavity

   ● **S31.652**   Open bite of abdominal wall, **epigastric region** with penetration into peritoneal cavity

   ● **S31.653**   Open bite of abdominal wall, **right lower** quadrant with penetration into peritoneal cavity

   ● **S31.654**   Open bite of abdominal wall, **left lower** quadrant with penetration into peritoneal cavity

   ● **S31.655**   Open bite of abdominal wall, **periumbilic region** with penetration into peritoneal cavity

   ● **S31.659**   Open bite of abdominal wall, **unspecified** quadrant with penetration into peritoneal cavity

● **S31.8**   **Open wound of** other parts of abdomen, lower back and pelvis

  ● **S31.80**   **Open wound of** unspecified buttock

   ● **S31.801**   **Laceration without foreign** body of unspecified buttock

   ● **S31.802**   **Laceration with foreign body of** unspecified buttock

   ● **S31.803**   **Puncture wound without foreign body of** unspecified buttock

   ● **S31.804**   **Puncture wound with foreign body of** unspecified buttock

   ● **S31.805**   **Open bite of** unspecified buttock

> Bite of buttock NOS
>
> **Excludes1**   superficial bite of buttock (S30.870)

   ● **S31.809**   **Unspecified** open wound of unspecified buttock

  ● **S31.81**   **Open wound of** right buttock

   ● **S31.811**   **Laceration without foreign** body of right buttock

   ● **S31.812**   **Laceration with foreign body of right** buttock

   ● **S31.813**   **Puncture wound without foreign body of** right buttock

   ● **S31.814**   **Puncture wound with foreign body of** right buttock

   ● **S31.815**   **Open bite of** right buttock

> Bite of right buttock NOS
>
> **Excludes1**   superficial bite of buttock (S30.870)

   ● **S31.819**   **Unspecified** open wound of right buttock

  ● **S31.82**   **Open wound of** left buttock

   ● **S31.821**   **Laceration without foreign body of** left buttock

   ● **S31.822**   **Laceration with foreign body of left** buttock

   ● **S31.823**   **Puncture wound without foreign body of** left buttock

   ● **S31.824**   **Puncture wound with foreign body of** left buttock

   ● **S31.825**   **Open bite of** left buttock

> Bite of left buttock NOS
>
> **Excludes1**   superficial bite of buttock (S30.870)

   ● **S31.829**   **Unspecified** open wound of left buttock

● **S31.83**   **Open wound of** anus

  ● **S31.831**   **Laceration without foreign body of** anus

  ● **S31.832**   **Laceration with foreign body of** anus

  ● **S31.833**   **Puncture wound without foreign body of** anus

  ● **S31.834**   **Puncture wound with foreign body of** anus

  ● **S31.835**   **Open bite** of anus

> Bite of anus NOS
>
> **Excludes1**   superficial bite of anus (S30.877)

  ● **S31.839**   **Unspecified open wound of anus**

● **S32**   **Fracture of lumbar spine and pelvis**

> **Note:** A fracture not indicated as displaced or nondisplaced should be coded to displaced
>
> A fracture not indicated as opened or closed should be coded to closed

> **Includes**   fracture of lumbosacral neural arch
> fracture of lumbosacral spinous process
> fracture of lumbosacral transverse process
> fracture of lumbosacral vertebra
> fracture of lumbosacral vertebral arch

Code first any associated spinal cord and spinal nerve injury (S34.-)

Excludes1   transection of abdomen (S38.3)

Excludes2   fracture of hip NOS (S72.0-)

The appropriate 7th character is to be added to each code from category S32

A	initial encounter for closed fracture
B	initial encounter for open fracture
D	subsequent encounter for fracture with routine healing
G	subsequent encounter for fracture with delayed healing
K	subsequent encounter for fracture with nonunion
S	sequela

● **S32.0**   **Fracture of** lumbar vertebra

> Fracture of lumbar spine NOS

  ● **S32.00**   **Fracture of** unspecified lumbar vertebra

   ● **S32.000**   **Wedge compression** fracture of unspecified lumbar vertebra A, B 🦴

   ● **S32.001**   **Stable burst** fracture of unspecified lumbar vertebra A, B 🦴

   ● **S32.002**   **Unstable burst** fracture of unspecified lumbar vertebra A, B 🦴

   ● **S32.008**   **Other** fracture of unspecified lumbar vertebra A, B 🦴

   ● **S32.009**   **Unspecified** fracture of unspecified lumbar vertebra A, B 🦴

  ● **S32.01**   **Fracture of** first lumbar vertebra

   ● **S32.010**   **Wedge compression** fracture of first lumbar vertebra A, B 🦴

   ● **S32.011**   **Stable burst** fracture of first lumbar vertebra A, B 🦴

   ● **S32.012**   **Unstable burst** fracture of first lumbar vertebra A, B 🦴

   ● **S32.018**   **Other** fracture of first lumbar vertebra A, B 🦴

   ● **S32.019**   **Unspecified** fracture of first lumbar vertebra A, B 🦴

  ● **S32.02**   **Fracture of** second lumbar vertebra

   ● **S32.020**   **Wedge compression** fracture of second lumbar vertebra A, B 🦴

   ● **S32.021**   **Stable burst** fracture of second lumbar vertebra A, B 🦴

● S32.022   Unstable burst fracture of second lumbar vertebra A, B 🦘

● S32.028   Other fracture of second lumbar vertebra A, B 🦘

● S32.029   Unspecified fracture of second lumbar vertebra A, B 🦘

● S32.03   Fracture of third lumbar vertebra

 ● S32.030   Wedge compression fracture of third lumbar vertebra A, B 🦘

 ● S32.031   Stable burst fracture of third lumbar vertebra A, B 🦘

 ● S32.032   Unstable burst fracture of third lumbar vertebra A, B 🦘

 ● S32.038   Other fracture of third lumbar vertebra A, B 🦘

 ● S32.039   Unspecified fracture of third lumbar vertebra A, B 🦘

● S32.04   Fracture of fourth lumbar vertebra

 ● S32.040   Wedge compression fracture of fourth lumbar vertebra A, B 🦘

 ● S32.041   Stable burst fracture of fourth lumbar vertebra A, B 🦘

 ● S32.042   Unstable burst fracture of fourth lumbar vertebra A, B 🦘

 ● S32.048   Other fracture of fourth lumbar vertebra A, B 🦘

 ● S32.049   Unspecified fracture of fourth lumbar vertebra A, B 🦘

● S32.05   Fracture of fifth lumbar vertebra

 ● S32.050   Wedge compression fracture of fifth lumbar vertebra A, B 🦘

 ● S32.051   Stable burst fracture of fifth lumbar vertebra A, B 🦘

 ● S32.052   Unstable burst fracture of fifth lumbar vertebra A, B 🦘

 ● S32.058   Other fracture of fifth lumbar vertebra A, B 🦘

 ● S32.059   Unspecified fracture of fifth lumbar vertebra A, B 🦘

● S32.1   Fracture of sacrum
For vertical fractures, code to most medial fracture extension
Use two codes if both a vertical and transverse fracture are present
Code also any associated fracture of pelvic ring (S32.8-)

X ● S32.10   Unspecified fracture of sacrum A, B 🦘

● S32.11   Zone I fracture of sacrum
Vertical sacral ala fracture of sacrum

 ● S32.110   Nondisplaced Zone I fracture of sacrum A, B 🦘

 ● S32.111   Minimally displaced Zone I fracture of sacrum A, B 🦘

 ● S32.112   Severely displaced Zone I fracture of sacrum A, B 🦘

 ● S32.119   Unspecified Zone I fracture of sacrum A, B 🦘

● S32.12   Zone II fracture of sacrum
Vertical foraminal region fracture of sacrum

 ● S32.120   Nondisplaced Zone II fracture of sacrum A, B 🦘

 ● S32.121   Minimally displaced Zone II fracture of sacrum A, B 🦘

 ● S32.122   Severely displaced Zone II fracture of sacrum A, B 🦘

 ● S32.129   Unspecified Zone II fracture of sacrum A, B 🦘

● S32.13   Zone III fracture of sacrum
Vertical fracture into spinal canal region of sacrum

 ● S32.130   Nondisplaced Zone III fracture of sacrum A, B 🦘

 ● S32.131   Minimally displaced Zone III fracture of sacrum A, B 🦘

 ● S32.132   Severely displaced Zone III fracture of sacrum A, B 🦘

 ● S32.139   Unspecified Zone III fracture of sacrum A, B 🦘

X ● S32.14   Type 1 fracture of sacrum A, B 🦘
Transverse flexion fracture of sacrum without displacement

X ● S32.15   Type 2 fracture of sacrum A, B 🦘
Transverse flexion fracture of sacrum with posterior displacement

X ● S32.16   Type 3 fracture of sacrum A, B 🦘
Transverse extension fracture of sacrum with anterior displacement

X ● S32.17   Type 4 fracture of sacrum A, B 🦘
Transverse segmental comminution of upper sacrum

X ● S32.19   Other fracture of sacrum A, B 🦘

X ● S32.2   Fracture of coccyx A, B 🦘

● S32.3   Fracture of ilium

 Excludes1   fracture of ilium with associated disruption of pelvic ring (S32.8-)

● S32.30   Unspecified fracture of ilium

 ● S32.301   Unspecified fracture of right ilium A, B 🦘

 ● S32.302   Unspecified fracture of left ilium A, B 🦘

 ● S32.309   Unspecified fracture of unspecified ilium A, B 🦘

● S32.31   Avulsion fracture of ilium

 ● S32.311   Displaced avulsion fracture of right ilium A, B 🦘

 ● S32.312   Displaced avulsion fracture of left ilium A, B 🦘

 ● S32.313   Displaced avulsion fracture of unspecified ilium A, B 🦘

 ● S32.314   Nondisplaced avulsion fracture of right ilium A, B 🦘

 ● S32.315   Nondisplaced avulsion fracture of left ilium A, B 🦘

 ● S32.316   Nondisplaced avulsion fracture of unspecified ilium A, B 🦘

● S32.39   Other fracture of ilium

 ● S32.391   Other fracture of right ilium A, B 🦘

 ● S32.392   Other fracture of left ilium A, B 🦘

 ● S32.399   Other fracture of unspecified ilium A, B 🦘

● S32.4   Fracture of acetabulum
Code also any associated fracture of pelvic ring (S32.8-)

● S32.40   Unspecified fracture of acetabulum

 ● S32.401   Unspecified fracture of right acetabulum A, B 🦘

 ● S32.402   Unspecified fracture of left acetabulum A, B 🦘

 ● S32.409   Unspecified fracture of unspecified acetabulum A, B 🦘

● S32.41   Fracture of anterior wall of acetabulum

 ● S32.411   Displaced fracture of anterior wall of right acetabulum A, B 🦘

 ● S32.412   Displaced fracture of anterior wall of left acetabulum A, B 🦘

 ● S32.413   Displaced fracture of anterior wall of unspecified acetabulum A, B 🦘

● S32.414   Nondisplaced fracture of anterior wall of right acetabulum A, B 🔒

● S32.415   Nondisplaced fracture of anterior wall of left acetabulum A, B 🔒

● S32.416   Nondisplaced fracture of anterior wall of unspecified acetabulum A, B 🔒

● S32.42   Fracture of posterior wall of acetabulum

● S32.421   Displaced fracture of posterior wall of right acetabulum A, B 🔒

● S32.422   Displaced fracture of posterior wall of left acetabulum A, B 🔒

● S32.423   Displaced fracture of posterior wall of unspecified acetabulum A, B 🔒

● S32.424   Nondisplaced fracture of posterior wall of right acetabulum A, B 🔒

● S32.425   Nondisplaced fracture of posterior wall of left acetabulum A, B 🔒

● S32.426   Nondisplaced fracture of posterior wall of unspecified acetabulum A, B 🔒

● S32.43   Fracture of anterior column [iliopubic] of acetabulum

● S32.431   Displaced fracture of anterior column [iliopubic] of right acetabulum A, B 🔒

● S32.432   Displaced fracture of anterior column [iliopubic] of left acetabulum A, B 🔒

● S32.433   Displaced fracture of anterior column [iliopubic] of unspecified acetabulum A, B 🔒

● S32.434   Nondisplaced fracture of anterior column [iliopubic] of right acetabulum A, B 🔒

● S32.435   Nondisplaced fracture of anterior column [iliopubic] of left acetabulum A, B 🔒

● S32.436   Nondisplaced fracture of anterior column [iliopubic] of unspecified acetabulum A, B 🔒

● S32.44   Fracture of posterior column [ilioischial] of acetabulum

● S32.441   Displaced fracture of posterior column [ilioischial] of right acetabulum A, B 🔒

● S32.442   Displaced fracture of posterior column [ilioischial] of left acetabulum A, B 🔒

● S32.443   Displaced fracture of posterior column [ilioischial] of unspecified acetabulum A, B 🔒

● S32.444   Nondisplaced fracture of posterior column [ilioischial] of right acetabulum A, B 🔒

● S32.445   Nondisplaced fracture of posterior column [ilioischial] of left acetabulum A, B 🔒

● S32.446   Nondisplaced fracture of posterior column [ilioischial] of unspecified acetabulum A, B 🔒

● S32.45   Transverse fracture of acetabulum

● S32.451   Displaced transverse fracture of right acetabulum A, B 🔒

● S32.452   Displaced transverse fracture of left acetabulum A, B 🔒

● S32.453   Displaced transverse fracture of unspecified acetabulum A, B 🔒

● S32.454   Nondisplaced transverse fracture of right acetabulum A, B 🔒

● S32.455   Nondisplaced transverse fracture of left acetabulum A, B 🔒

● S32.456   Nondisplaced transverse fracture of unspecified acetabulum A, B 🔒

● S32.46   Associated transverse-posterior fracture of acetabulum

● S32.461   Displaced associated transverse-posterior fracture of right acetabulum A, B 🔒

● S32.462   Displaced associated transverse-posterior fracture of left acetabulum A, B 🔒

● S32.463   Displaced associated transverse-posterior fracture of unspecified acetabulum A, B 🔒

● S32.464   Nondisplaced associated transverse-posterior fracture of right acetabulum A, B 🔒

● S32.465   Nondisplaced associated transverse-posterior fracture of left acetabulum A, B 🔒

● S32.466   Nondisplaced associated transverse-posterior fracture of unspecified acetabulum A, B 🔒

● S32.47   Fracture of medial wall of acetabulum

● S32.471   Displaced fracture of medial wall of right acetabulum A, B 🔒

● S32.472   Displaced fracture of medial wall of left acetabulum A, B 🔒

● S32.473   Displaced fracture of medial wall of unspecified acetabulum A, B 🔒

● S32.474   Nondisplaced fracture of medial wall of right acetabulum A, B 🔒

● S32.475   Nondisplaced fracture of medial wall of left acetabulum A, B 🔒

● S32.476   Nondisplaced fracture of medial wall of unspecified acetabulum A, B 🔒

● S32.48   Dome fracture of acetabulum

● S32.481   Displaced dome fracture of right acetabulum A, B 🔒

● S32.482   Displaced dome fracture of left acetabulum A, B 🔒

● S32.483   Displaced dome fracture of unspecified acetabulum A, B 🔒

● S32.484   Nondisplaced dome fracture of right acetabulum A, B 🔒

● S32.485   Nondisplaced dome fracture of left acetabulum A, B 🔒

● S32.486   Nondisplaced dome fracture of unspecified acetabulum A, B 🔒

● S32.49   Other fracture of acetabulum

● S32.491   Other fracture of right acetabulum A, B 🔒

● S32.492   Other fracture of left acetabulum A, B 🔒

● S32.499   Other fracture of unspecified acetabulum A, B 🔒

● S32.5   Fracture of pubis

    Excludes1   fracture of pubis with associated disruption of pelvic ring (S32.8-)

● S32.50   Unspecified fracture of pubis

● S32.501   Unspecified fracture of right pubis A, B 🔒

● S32.502   Unspecified fracture of left pubis A, B 🔒

● S32.509   Unspecified fracture of unspecified pubis A, B 🔒

S32.51   Fracture of superior rim of pubis
- ● **S32.511   Fracture of superior rim of right pubis**
  A, B 🐾
- ● **S32.512   Fracture of superior rim of left pubis**
  A, B 🐾
- ● **S32.519   Fracture of superior rim of unspecified pubis** A, B 🐾

S32.59   Other specified fracture of pubis
- ● **S32.591   Other specified fracture of right pubis**
  A, B 🐾
- ● **S32.592   Other specified fracture of left pubis**
  A, B 🐾
- ● **S32.599   Other specified fracture of unspecified pubis** A, B 🐾

● **S32.6   Fracture of ischium**
> **Excludes1**   fracture of ischium with associated disruption of pelvic ring (S32.8-)

- ● **S32.60   Unspecified fracture of ischium**
  - ● **S32.601   Unspecified fracture of right ischium** A, B 🐾
  - ● **S32.602   Unspecified fracture of left ischium** A, B 🐾
  - ● **S32.609   Unspecified fracture of unspecified ischium** A, B 🐾

- ● **S32.61   Avulsion fracture of ischium**
  - ● **S32.611   Displaced avulsion fracture of right ischium** A, B 🐾
  - ● **S32.612   Displaced avulsion fracture of left ischium** A, B 🐾
  - ● **S32.613   Displaced avulsion fracture of unspecified ischium** A, B 🐾
  - ● **S32.614   Nondisplaced avulsion fracture of right ischium** A, B 🐾
  - ● **S32.615   Nondisplaced avulsion fracture of left ischium** A, B 🐾
  - ● **S32.616   Nondisplaced avulsion fracture of unspecified ischium** A, B 🐾

- ● **S32.69   Other specified fracture of ischium**
  - ● **S32.691   Other specified fracture of right ischium** A, B 🐾
  - ● **S32.692   Other specified fracture of left ischium** A, B 🐾
  - ● **S32.699   Other specified fracture of unspecified ischium** A, B 🐾

● **S32.8   Fracture of other parts of pelvis**
> Code also any associated:
> fracture of acetabulum (S32.4-)
> sacral fracture (S32.1-)

- ● **S32.81   Multiple fractures of pelvis with disruption of pelvic ring**
  > Multiple pelvic fractures with disruption of pelvic circle
  - ● **S32.810   Multiple fractures of pelvis with stable disruption of pelvic ring** A, B 🐾
  - ● **S32.811   Multiple fractures of pelvis with unstable disruption of pelvic ring** A, B 🐾

- X ● **S32.82   Multiple fractures of pelvis without disruption of pelvic ring** A, B 🐾
  > Multiple pelvic fractures without disruption of pelvic circle

- X ● **S32.89   Fracture of other parts of pelvis** A, B 🐾

X ● **S32.9   Fracture of unspecified parts of lumbosacral spine and pelvis** A, B 🐾
> Fracture of lumbosacral spine NOS
> Fracture of pelvis NOS
> **Coding Clinic: 2012, Q4, P93**

● **S33   Dislocation and sprain of joints and ligaments of lumbar spine and pelvis**
> **Includes**   avulsion of joint or ligament of lumbar spine and pelvis
> laceration of cartilage, joint or ligament of lumbar spine and pelvis
> sprain of cartilage, joint or ligament of lumbar spine and pelvis
> traumatic hemarthrosis of joint or ligament of lumbar spine and pelvis
> traumatic rupture of joint or ligament of lumbar spine and pelvis
> traumatic subluxation of joint or ligament of lumbar spine and pelvis
> traumatic tear of joint or ligament of lumbar spine and pelvis

Code also any associated open wound
> **Excludes1**   nontraumatic rupture or displacement of lumbar intervertebral disc NOS (M51.-)
> obstetric damage to pelvic joints and ligaments (O71.6)

> **Excludes2**   dislocation and sprain of joints and ligaments of hip (S73.-)
> strain of muscle of lower back and pelvis (S39.01-)

The appropriate 7th character is to be added to each code from category S33

A	initial encounter
D	subsequent encounter
S	sequela

X ● **S33.0   Traumatic rupture of lumbar intervertebral disc**
> **Excludes1**   rupture or displacement (nontraumatic) of lumbar intervertebral disc NOS (M51.- with fifth character 6)

● **S33.1   Subluxation and dislocation of lumbar vertebra**
> Code also any associated:
> open wound of abdomen, lower back and pelvis (S31)
> spinal cord injury (S24.0, S24.1-, S34.0-, S34.1-)
> **Excludes2**   fracture of lumbar vertebrae (S32.0-)

- ● **S33.10   Subluxation and dislocation of unspecified lumbar vertebra**
  - ● **S33.100   Subluxation of unspecified lumbar vertebra**
  - ● **S33.101   Dislocation of unspecified lumbar vertebra**

- ● **S33.11   Subluxation and dislocation of L1/L2 lumbar vertebra**
  - ● **S33.110   Subluxation of L1/L2 lumbar vertebra**
  - ● **S33.111   Dislocation of L1/L2 lumbar vertebra**

- ● **S33.12   Subluxation and dislocation of L2/L3 lumbar vertebra**
  - ● **S33.120   Subluxation of L2/L3 lumbar vertebra**
  - ● **S33.121   Dislocation of L2/L3 lumbar vertebra**

- ● **S33.13   Subluxation and dislocation of L3/L4 lumbar vertebra**
  - ● **S33.130   Subluxation of L3/L4 lumbar vertebra**
  - ● **S33.131   Dislocation of L3/L4 lumbar vertebra**

- ● **S33.14   Subluxation and dislocation of L4/L5 lumbar vertebra**
  - ● **S33.140   Subluxation of L4/L5 lumbar vertebra**
  - ● **S33.141   Dislocation of L4/L5 lumbar vertebra**

X ● **S33.2   Dislocation of sacroiliac and sacrococcygeal joint**

● **S33.3   Dislocation of other and unspecified parts of lumbar spine and pelvis**
- X ● **S33.30   Dislocation of unspecified parts of lumbar spine and pelvis**
- X ● **S33.39   Dislocation of other parts of lumbar spine and pelvis**

X ● **S33.4   Traumatic rupture of symphysis pubis**

▶ New   ⇒ Revised   ~~deleted~~ Deleted   Excludes 1   Excludes 2   Includes   Use additional   Code first   Code also   Key words
OGCR Official Guidelines   X Assign placeholder X   ● Use Additional Character(s)   ▌ Manifestation Code   🐾 Hierarchical Condition Category   Coding Clinic

X● **S33.5**   Sprain of ligaments of lumbar spine
X● **S33.6**   Sprain of sacroiliac joint
X● **S33.8**   Sprain of other parts of lumbar spine and pelvis
X● **S33.9**   Sprain of unspecified parts of lumbar spine and pelvis

● **S34**   **Injury of lumbar and sacral spinal cord and nerves at abdomen, lower back and pelvis level**

> **Note:** Code to highest level of lumbar cord injury
>
> Injuries to the spinal cord (S34.0 and S34.1) refer to the cord level and not bone level injury, and can affect nerve roots at and below the level given.
>
> The appropriate 7th character is to be added to each code from category S34

> | | |
> |---|---|
> | A | initial encounter |
> | D | subsequent encounter |
> | S | sequela |

> Code also any associated:
> fracture of vertebra (S22.0-, S32.0-)
> open wound of abdomen, lower back and pelvis (S31.-)
> transient paralysis (R29.5)

● **S34.0**   **Concussion and edema of lumbar and sacral spinal cord**

X● **S34.01**   Concussion and edema of lumbar spinal cord A, D, S 🐾

X● **S34.02**   Concussion and edema of sacral spinal cord A, D, S 🐾
> Concussion and edema of conus medullaris

● **S34.1**   **Other and unspecified injury of lumbar and sacral spinal cord**

● **S34.10**   Unspecified injury to lumbar spinal cord

● **S34.101**   Unspecified injury to L_1 level of lumbar spinal cord A, D, S 🐾
> Unspecified injury to lumbar spinal cord level 1

● **S34.102**   Unspecified injury to L_2 level of lumbar spinal cord A, D, S 🐾
> Unspecified injury to lumbar spinal cord level 2

● **S34.103**   Unspecified injury to L_3 level of lumbar spinal cord A, D, S 🐾
> Unspecified injury to lumbar spinal cord level 3

● **S34.104**   Unspecified injury to L_4 level of lumbar spinal cord A, D, S 🐾
> Unspecified injury to lumbar spinal cord level 4

● **S34.105**   Unspecified injury to L_5 level of lumbar spinal cord A, D, S 🐾
> Unspecified injury to lumbar spinal cord level 5

● **S34.109**   Unspecified injury to unspecified level of lumbar spinal cord A, D, S 🐾

● **S34.11**   Complete lesion of lumbar spinal cord

● **S34.111**   Complete lesion of L_1 level of lumbar spinal cord A, D, S 🐾
> Complete lesion of lumbar spinal cord level 1

● **S34.112**   Complete lesion of L_2 level of lumbar spinal cord A, D, S 🐾
> Complete lesion of lumbar spinal cord level 2

● **S34.113**   Complete lesion of L_3 level of lumbar spinal cord A, D, S 🐾
> Complete lesion of lumbar spinal cord level 3

● **S34.114**   Complete lesion of L_4 level of lumbar spinal cord A, D, S 🐾
> Complete lesion of lumbar spinal cord level 4

● **S34.115**   Complete lesion of L_5 level of lumbar spinal cord A, D, S 🐾
> Complete lesion of lumbar spinal cord level 5

● **S34.119**   Complete lesion of unspecified level of lumbar spinal cord A, D, S 🐾

● **S34.12**   Incomplete lesion of lumbar spinal cord

● **S34.121**   Incomplete lesion of L_1 level of lumbar spinal cord A, D, S 🐾
> Incomplete lesion of lumbar spinal cord level 1

● **S34.122**   Incomplete lesion of L_2 level of lumbar spinal cord A, D, S 🐾
> Incomplete lesion of lumbar spinal cord level 2

● **S34.123**   Incomplete lesion of L_3 level of lumbar spinal cord A, D, S 🐾
> Incomplete lesion of lumbar spinal cord level 3

● **S34.124**   Incomplete lesion of L_4 level of lumbar spinal cord A, D, S 🐾
> Incomplete lesion of lumbar spinal cord level 4

● **S34.125**   Incomplete lesion of L_5 level of lumbar spinal cord A, D, S 🐾
> Incomplete lesion of lumbar spinal cord level 5

● **S34.129**   Incomplete lesion of unspecified level of lumbar spinal cord A, D, S 🐾

● **S34.13**   Other and unspecified injury to sacral spinal cord
> Other injury to conus medullaris

● **S34.131**   Complete lesion of sacral spinal cord A, D, S 🐾
> Complete lesion of conus medullaris

● **S34.132**   Incomplete lesion of sacral spinal cord A, D, S 🐾
> Incomplete lesion of conus medullaris

● **S34.139**   Unspecified injury to sacral spinal cord A, D, S 🐾
> Unspecified injury of conus medullaris

● **S34.2**   **Injury of nerve root of lumbar and sacral spine**

X● **S34.21**   Injury of nerve root of lumbar spine
X● **S34.22**   Injury of nerve root of sacral spine

X● **S34.3**   **Injury of cauda equina A, D, S 🐾**
X● **S34.4**   **Injury of lumbosacral plexus**
X● **S34.5**   **Injury of lumbar, sacral and pelvic sympathetic nerves**
> Injury of celiac ganglion or plexus
> Injury of hypogastric plexus
> Injury of mesenteric plexus (inferior) (superior)
> Injury of splanchnic nerve

X● **S34.6**   **Injury of peripheral nerve(s) at abdomen, lower back and pelvis level**
X● **S34.8**   **Injury of other nerves at abdomen, lower back and pelvis level**
X● **S34.9**   **Injury of unspecified nerves at abdomen, lower back and pelvis level**

● **S35**   **Injury of blood vessels at abdomen, lower back and pelvis level**

> The appropriate 7th character is to be added to each code from category S35

> | | |
> |---|---|
> | A | initial encounter |
> | D | subsequent encounter |
> | S | sequela |

> Code also any associated open wound (S31.-)

● **S35.0**   **Injury of abdominal aorta**

> **Excludes1**   injury of aorta NOS (S25.0)

X● **S35.00**   Unspecified injury of abdominal aorta
X● **S35.01**   Minor laceration of abdominal aorta
> Incomplete transection of abdominal aorta
> Laceration of abdominal aorta NOS
> Superficial laceration of abdominal aorta

X ● **S35.02** **Major laceration of abdominal aorta**
Complete transection of abdominal aorta
Traumatic rupture of abdominal aorta

X ● **S35.09** **Other injury of abdominal aorta**

● **S35.1** **Injury of inferior vena cava**
Injury of hepatic vein

Excludes1 injury of vena cava NOS (S25.2)

X ● **S35.10** **Unspecified injury of inferior vena cava**

X ● **S35.11** **Minor laceration of inferior vena cava**
Incomplete transection of inferior vena cava
Laceration of inferior vena cava NOS
Superficial laceration of inferior vena cava

X ● **S35.12** **Major laceration of inferior vena cava**
Complete transection of inferior vena cava
Traumatic rupture of inferior vena cava

X ● **S35.19** **Other injury of inferior vena cava**

● **S35.2** **Injury of celiac or mesenteric artery and branches**

● **S35.21** **Injury of celiac artery**

● **S35.211** **Minor laceration of celiac artery**
Incomplete transection of celiac artery
Laceration of celiac artery NOS
Superficial laceration of celiac artery

● **S35.212** **Major laceration of celiac artery**
Complete transection of celiac artery
Traumatic rupture of celiac artery

● **S35.218** **Other injury of celiac artery**

● **S35.219** **Unspecified injury of celiac artery**

● **S35.22** **Injury of superior mesenteric artery**

● **S35.221** **Minor laceration of superior mesenteric artery**
Incomplete transection of superior mesenteric artery
Laceration of superior mesenteric artery NOS
Superficial laceration of superior mesenteric artery

● **S35.222** **Major laceration of superior mesenteric artery**
Complete transection of superior mesenteric artery
Traumatic rupture of superior mesenteric artery

● **S35.228** **Other injury of superior mesenteric artery**

● **S35.229** **Unspecified injury of superior mesenteric artery**

● **S35.23** **Injury of inferior mesenteric artery**

● **S35.231** **Minor laceration of inferior mesenteric artery**
Incomplete transection of inferior mesenteric artery
Laceration of inferior mesenteric artery NOS
Superficial laceration of inferior mesenteric artery

● **S35.232** **Major laceration of inferior mesenteric artery**
Complete transection of inferior mesenteric artery
Traumatic rupture of inferior mesenteric artery

● **S35.238** **Other injury of inferior mesenteric artery**

● **S35.239** **Unspecified injury of inferior mesenteric artery**

● **S35.29** **Injury of branches of celiac and mesenteric artery**
Injury of gastric artery
Injury of gastroduodenal artery
Injury of hepatic artery
Injury of splenic artery

● **S35.291** **Minor laceration of branches of celiac and mesenteric artery**
Incomplete transection of branches of celiac and mesenteric artery
Laceration of branches of celiac and mesenteric artery NOS
Superficial laceration of branches of celiac and mesenteric artery

● **S35.292** **Major laceration of branches of celiac and mesenteric artery**
Complete transection of branches of celiac and mesenteric artery
Traumatic rupture of branches of celiac and mesenteric artery

● **S35.298** **Other injury of branches of celiac and mesenteric artery**

● **S35.299** **Unspecified injury of branches of celiac and mesenteric artery**

● **S35.3** **Injury of portal or splenic vein and branches**

● **S35.31** **Injury of portal vein**

● **S35.311** **Laceration of portal vein**

● **S35.318** **Other specified injury of portal vein**

● **S35.319** **Unspecified injury of portal vein**

● **S35.32** **Injury of splenic vein**

● **S35.321** **Laceration of splenic vein**

● **S35.328** **Other specified injury of splenic vein**

● **S35.329** **Unspecified injury of splenic vein**

● **S35.33** **Injury of superior mesenteric vein**

● **S35.331** **Laceration of superior mesenteric vein**

● **S35.338** **Other specified injury of superior mesenteric vein**

● **S35.339** **Unspecified injury of superior mesenteric vein**

● **S35.34** **Injury of inferior mesenteric vein**

● **S35.341** **Laceration of inferior mesenteric vein**

● **S35.348** **Other specified injury of inferior mesenteric vein**

● **S35.349** **Unspecified injury of inferior mesenteric vein**

● **S35.4** **Injury of renal blood vessels**

● **S35.40** **Unspecified injury of renal blood vessel**

● **S35.401** **Unspecified injury of right renal artery**

● **S35.402** **Unspecified injury of left renal artery**

● **S35.403** **Unspecified injury of unspecified renal artery**

● **S35.404** **Unspecified injury of right renal vein**

● **S35.405** **Unspecified injury of left renal vein**

● **S35.406** **Unspecified injury of unspecified renal vein**

● **S35.41** **Laceration of renal blood vessel**

● **S35.411** **Laceration of right renal artery**

● **S35.412** **Laceration of left renal artery**

● **S35.413** **Laceration of unspecified renal artery**

● **S35.414** **Laceration of right renal vein**

● **S35.415** **Laceration of left renal vein**

● **S35.416** **Laceration of unspecified renal vein**

CHAPTER 19 (S00-T88)

● S35.49 Other specified injury of renal blood vessel
  ● S35.491 Other specified injury of right renal artery
  ● S35.492 Other specified injury of left renal artery
  ● S35.493 Other specified injury of unspecified renal artery
  ● S35.494 Other specified injury of right renal vein
  ● S35.495 Other specified injury of left renal vein
  ● S35.496 Other specified injury of unspecified renal vein
● S35.5 Injury of iliac blood vessels
  X ● S35.50 Injury of unspecified iliac blood vessel(s)
  ● S35.51 Injury of iliac artery or vein
    Injury of hypogastric artery or vein
    ● S35.511 Injury of right iliac artery
    ● S35.512 Injury of left iliac artery
    ● S35.513 Injury of unspecified iliac artery
    ● S35.514 Injury of right iliac vein
    ● S35.515 Injury of left iliac vein
    ● S35.516 Injury of unspecified iliac vein
  ● S35.53 Injury of uterine artery or vein
    ● S35.531 Injury of right uterine artery
    ● S35.532 Injury of left uterine artery
    ● S35.533 Injury of unspecified uterine artery
    ● S35.534 Injury of right uterine vein
    ● S35.535 Injury of left uterine vein
    ● S35.536 Injury of unspecified uterine vein
  X ● S35.59 Injury of other iliac blood vessels
● S35.8 Injury of other blood vessels at abdomen, lower back and pelvis level
  Injury of ovarian artery or vein
  ● S35.8X Injury of other blood vessels at abdomen, lower back and pelvis level
    ● S35.8X1 Laceration of other blood vessels at abdomen, lower back and pelvis level
    ● S35.8X8 Other specified injury of other blood vessels at abdomen, lower back and pelvis level
    ● S35.8X9 Unspecified injury of other blood vessels at abdomen, lower back and pelvis level
● S35.9 Injury of unspecified blood vessel at abdomen, lower back and pelvis level
  X ● S35.90 Unspecified injury of unspecified blood vessel at abdomen, lower back and pelvis level
  X ● S35.91 Laceration of unspecified blood vessel at abdomen, lower back and pelvis level
  X ● S35.99 Other specified injury of unspecified blood vessel at abdomen, lower back and pelvis level

● S36 Injury of intra-abdominal organs
  The appropriate 7th character is to be added to each code from category S36

A	initial encounter
D	subsequent encounter
S	sequela

  Code also any associated open wound (S31.-)
● S36.0 Injury of spleen
  X ● S36.00 Unspecified injury of spleen
  ● S36.02 Contusion of spleen
    ● S36.020 Minor contusion of spleen
      Contusion of spleen less than 2 cm

● S36.021 Major contusion of spleen
    Contusion of spleen greater than 2 cm
● S36.029 Unspecified contusion of spleen
    Coding Clinic: 2015, Q2, P36, Q1, P11
● S36.03 Laceration of spleen
  ● S36.030 Superficial (capsular) laceration of spleen
    Laceration of spleen less than 1 cm
    Minor laceration of spleen
  ● S36.031 Moderate laceration of spleen
    Laceration of spleen 1 to 3 cm
    Coding Clinic: 2022, Q1, P23;
      2015, Q2, P36, Q1, P11
  ● S36.032 Major laceration of spleen
    Avulsion of spleen
    Laceration of spleen greater than 3 cm
    Massive laceration of spleen
    Multiple moderate lacerations of spleen
    Stellate laceration of spleen
  ● S36.039 Unspecified laceration of spleen
X ● S36.09 Other injury of spleen
● S36.1 Injury of liver and gallbladder and bile duct
  ● S36.11 Injury of liver
    Coding Clinic: 2024, Q1, P25
    ● S36.112 Contusion of liver
    ● S36.113 Laceration of liver, unspecified degree
    ● S36.114 Minor laceration of liver
      Laceration involving capsule only, or, without significant involvement of hepatic parenchyma [i.e., less than 1 cm deep]
    ● S36.115 Moderate laceration of liver
      Laceration involving parenchyma but without major disruption of parenchyma [i.e., less than 10 cm long and less than 3 cm deep]
    ● S36.116 Major laceration of liver
      Laceration with significant disruption of hepatic parenchyma [i.e., greater than 10 cm long and 3 cm deep]
      Multiple moderate lacerations, with or without hematoma
      Stellate laceration of liver
    ● S36.118 Other injury of liver
    ● S36.119 Unspecified injury of liver
      Coding Clinic: 2015, Q2, P17
  ● S36.12 Injury of gallbladder
    ● S36.122 Contusion of gallbladder
    ● S36.123 Laceration of gallbladder
    ● S36.128 Other injury of gallbladder
    ● S36.129 Unspecified injury of gallbladder
  X ● S36.13 Injury of bile duct
● S36.2 Injury of pancreas
  ● S36.20 Unspecified injury of pancreas
    ● S36.200 Unspecified injury of head of pancreas
    ● S36.201 Unspecified injury of body of pancreas
    ● S36.202 Unspecified injury of tail of pancreas
    ● S36.209 Unspecified injury of unspecified part of pancreas
  ● S36.22 Contusion of pancreas
    ● S36.220 Contusion of head of pancreas
    ● S36.221 Contusion of body of pancreas

CHAPTER 19 (S00-T88)

- S36.222   Contusion of tail of pancreas
- S36.229   Contusion of unspecified part of pancreas
- S36.23   Laceration of pancreas, unspecified degree
  - S36.230   Laceration of head of pancreas, unspecified degree
  - S36.231   Laceration of body of pancreas, unspecified degree
  - S36.232   Laceration of tail of pancreas, unspecified degree
  - S36.239   Laceration of unspecified part of pancreas, unspecified degree
- S36.24   Minor laceration of pancreas
  - S36.240   Minor laceration of head of pancreas
  - S36.241   Minor laceration of body of pancreas
  - S36.242   Minor laceration of tail of pancreas
  - S36.249   Minor laceration of unspecified part of pancreas
- S36.25   Moderate laceration of pancreas
  - S36.250   Moderate laceration of head of pancreas
  - S36.251   Moderate laceration of body of pancreas
  - S36.252   Moderate laceration of tail of pancreas
  - S36.259   Moderate laceration of unspecified part of pancreas
- S36.26   Major laceration of pancreas
  - S36.260   Major laceration of head of pancreas
  - S36.261   Major laceration of body of pancreas
  - S36.262   Major laceration of tail of pancreas
  - S36.269   Major laceration of unspecified part of pancreas
- S36.29   Other injury of pancreas
  - S36.290   Other injury of head of pancreas
  - S36.291   Other injury of body of pancreas
  - S36.292   Other injury of tail of pancreas
  - S36.299   Other injury of unspecified part of pancreas
- S36.3   Injury of stomach
  - X ● S36.30   Unspecified injury of stomach
  - X ● S36.32   Contusion of stomach
  - X ● S36.33   Laceration of stomach
  - X ● S36.39   Other injury of stomach
- S36.4   Injury of small intestine
  - S36.40   Unspecified injury of small intestine
    - S36.400   Unspecified injury of duodenum
    - S36.408   Unspecified injury of other part of small intestine
    - S36.409   Unspecified injury of unspecified part of small intestine
  - S36.41   Primary blast injury of small intestine
    Blast injury of small intestine NOS
    - S36.410   Primary blast injury of duodenum
    - S36.418   Primary blast injury of other part of small intestine
    - S36.419   Primary blast injury of unspecified part of small intestine
  - S36.42   Contusion of small intestine
    - S36.420   Contusion of duodenum
    - S36.428   Contusion of other part of small intestine
    - S36.429   Contusion of unspecified part of small intestine

- S36.43   Laceration of small intestine
  - S36.430   Laceration of duodenum
  - S36.438   Laceration of other part of small intestine
  - S36.439   Laceration of unspecified part of small intestine
- S36.49   Other injury of small intestine
  - S36.490   Other injury of duodenum
  - S36.498   Other injury of other part of small intestine
    Coding Clinic: 2023, Q3, P8-9
  - S36.499   Other injury of unspecified part of small intestine
- S36.5   Injury of colon
  Excludes2   injury of rectum (S36.6-)
  - S36.50   Unspecified injury of colon
    - S36.500   Unspecified injury of ascending [right] colon
    - S36.501   Unspecified injury of transverse colon
    - S36.502   Unspecified injury of descending [left] colon
    - S36.503   Unspecified injury of sigmoid colon
    - S36.508   Unspecified injury of other part of colon
    - S36.509   Unspecified injury of unspecified part of colon
  - S36.51   Primary blast injury of colon
    Blast injury of colon NOS
    - S36.510   Primary blast injury of ascending [right] colon
    - S36.511   Primary blast injury of transverse colon
    - S36.512   Primary blast injury of descending [left] colon
    - S36.513   Primary blast injury of sigmoid colon
    - S36.518   Primary blast injury of other part of colon
    - S36.519   Primary blast injury of unspecified part of colon
  - S36.52   Contusion of colon
    - S36.520   Contusion of ascending [right] colon
    - S36.521   Contusion of transverse colon
    - S36.522   Contusion of descending [left] colon
    - S36.523   Contusion of sigmoid colon
    - S36.528   Contusion of other part of colon
    - S36.529   Contusion of unspecified part of colon
  - S36.53   Laceration of colon
    - S36.530   Laceration of ascending [right] colon
    - S36.531   Laceration of transverse colon
    - S36.532   Laceration of descending [left] colon
    - S36.533   Laceration of sigmoid colon
    - S36.538   Laceration of other part of colon
    - S36.539   Laceration of unspecified part of colon
  - S36.59   Other injury of colon
    Secondary blast injury of colon
    - S36.590   Other injury of ascending [right] colon
      Coding Clinic: 2023, Q3, P8-9
    - S36.591   Other injury of transverse colon
    - S36.592   Other injury of descending [left] colon
    - S36.593   Other injury of sigmoid colon
    - S36.598   Other injury of other part of colon
    - S36.599   Other injury of unspecified part of colon

▶ New   ⇒ Revised   deleted Deleted   Excludes 1   Excludes 2   Includes   Use additional   Code first   Code also   Key words
OGCR Official Guidelines   X Assign placeholder X   ● Use Additional Character(s)   ▷ Manifestation Code   🔎 Hierarchical Condition Category   Coding Clinic

● **S36.6**   **Injury of rectum**
   X● **S36.60**   **Unspecified** injury of rectum
   X● **S36.61**   **Primary blast injury** of rectum
      Blast injury of rectum NOS
   X● **S36.62**   **Contusion** of rectum
   X● **S36.63**   **Laceration** of rectum
   X● **S36.69**   **Other injury** of rectum
      Secondary blast injury of rectum

● **S36.8**   **Injury of other intra-abdominal organs**
   X● **S36.81**   Injury of **peritoneum**
   ● **S36.89**   Injury of **other intra-abdominal organs**
      Injury of retroperitoneum
     ● **S36.892**   **Contusion** of other intra-abdominal organs
     ● **S36.893**   **Laceration** of other intra-abdominal organs
     ● **S36.898**   **Other injury** of other intra-abdominal organs
     ● **S36.899**   **Unspecified** injury of other intra-abdominal organs

● **S36.9**   **Injury of unspecified intra-abdominal organ**
   X● **S36.90**   **Unspecified** injury of unspecified intra-abdominal organ
   X● **S36.92**   **Contusion** of unspecified intra-abdominal organ
   X● **S36.93**   **Laceration** of unspecified intra-abdominal organ
   X● **S36.99**   **Other injury** of unspecified intra-abdominal organ

● **S37**   **Injury of urinary and pelvic organs**
   Code also any associated open wound (S31.-)

   Excludes1   obstetric trauma to pelvic organs (O71.-)
   Excludes2   injury of peritoneum (S36.81)
      injury of retroperitoneum (S36.89-)

   The appropriate 7th character is to be added to each code from category S37

A	initial encounter
D	subsequent encounter
S	sequela

● **S37.0**   **Injury of kidney**
   Excludes2   acute kidney injury (nontraumatic) (N17.9)
   ● **S37.00**   **Unspecified injury of kidney**
     ● **S37.001**   Unspecified injury of **right** kidney
     ● **S37.002**   Unspecified injury of **left** kidney
     ● **S37.009**   Unspecified injury of **unspecified** kidney
   ● **S37.01**   **Minor contusion of kidney**
      Contusion of kidney less than 2 cm
      Contusion of kidney NOS
     ● **S37.011**   Minor contusion of **right** kidney
     ● **S37.012**   Minor contusion of **left** kidney
     ● **S37.019**   Minor contusion of **unspecified** kidney
   ● **S37.02**   **Major contusion of kidney**
      Contusion of kidney greater than 2 cm
     ● **S37.021**   Major contusion of **right** kidney
     ● **S37.022**   Major contusion of **left** kidney
     ● **S37.029**   Major contusion of **unspecified** kidney
   ● **S37.03**   **Laceration of kidney, unspecified degree**
     ● **S37.031**   Laceration of **right** kidney, unspecified degree
     ● **S37.032**   Laceration of **left** kidney, unspecified degree
     ● **S37.039**   Laceration of **unspecified** kidney, unspecified degree

   ● **S37.04**   **Minor laceration of kidney**
      Laceration of kidney less than 1 cm
     ● **S37.041**   Minor laceration of **right** kidney
     ● **S37.042**   Minor laceration of **left** kidney
     ● **S37.049**   Minor laceration of **unspecified** kidney
   ● **S37.05**   **Moderate laceration of kidney**
      Laceration of kidney 1 to 3 cm
     ● **S37.051**   Moderate laceration of **right** kidney
     ● **S37.052**   Moderate laceration of **left** kidney
     ● **S37.059**   Moderate laceration of **unspecified** kidney
   ● **S37.06**   **Major laceration of kidney**
      Avulsion of kidney
      Laceration of kidney greater than 3 cm
      Massive laceration of kidney
      Multiple moderate lacerations of kidney
      Stellate laceration of kidney
     ● **S37.061**   Major laceration of **right** kidney
     ● **S37.062**   Major laceration of **left** kidney
     ● **S37.069**   Major laceration of **unspecified** kidney
   ● **S37.09**   **Other injury of kidney**
     ● **S37.091**   Other injury of **right** kidney
     ● **S37.092**   Other injury of **left** kidney
     ● **S37.099**   Other injury of **unspecified** kidney

● **S37.1**   **Injury of ureter**
   X● **S37.10**   **Unspecified** injury of ureter
   X● **S37.12**   **Contusion** of ureter
   X● **S37.13**   **Laceration** of ureter
   X● **S37.19**   **Other injury** of ureter

● **S37.2**   **Injury of bladder**
   X● **S37.20**   **Unspecified** injury of bladder
   X● **S37.22**   **Contusion** of bladder
   X● **S37.23**   **Laceration** of bladder
   X● **S37.29**   **Other injury** of bladder

● **S37.3**   **Injury of urethra**
   X● **S37.30**   **Unspecified** injury of urethra
   X● **S37.32**   **Contusion** of urethra
   X● **S37.33**   **Laceration** of urethra
   X● **S37.39**   **Other injury** of urethra

● **S37.4**   **Injury of ovary**
   ● **S37.40**   **Unspecified injury of ovary**
     ● **S37.401**   Unspecified injury of ovary, **unilateral**
     ● **S37.402**   Unspecified injury of ovary, **bilateral**
     ● **S37.409**   Unspecified injury of ovary, **unspecified**
   ● **S37.42**   **Contusion of ovary**
     ● **S37.421**   Contusion of ovary, **unilateral**
     ● **S37.422**   Contusion of ovary, **bilateral**
     ● **S37.429**   Contusion of ovary, **unspecified**
   ● **S37.43**   **Laceration of ovary**
     ● **S37.431**   Laceration of ovary, **unilateral**
     ● **S37.432**   Laceration of ovary, **bilateral**
     ● **S37.439**   Laceration of ovary, **unspecified**
   ● **S37.49**   **Other injury of ovary**
     ● **S37.491**   Other injury of ovary, **unilateral**
     ● **S37.492**   Other injury of ovary, **bilateral**
     ● **S37.499**   Other injury of ovary, **unspecified**

- S37.5　Injury of fallopian tube
  - S37.50　Unspecified injury of fallopian tube
    - S37.501　Unspecified injury of fallopian tube, unilateral
    - S37.502　Unspecified injury of fallopian tube, bilateral
    - S37.509　Unspecified injury of fallopian tube, unspecified
  - S37.51　Primary blast injury of fallopian tube
    Blast injury of fallopian tube NOS
    - S37.511　Primary blast injury of fallopian tube, unilateral
    - S37.512　Primary blast injury of fallopian tube, bilateral
    - S37.519　Primary blast injury of fallopian tube, unspecified
  - S37.52　Contusion of fallopian tube
    - S37.521　Contusion of fallopian tube, unilateral
    - S37.522　Contusion of fallopian tube, bilateral
    - S37.529　Contusion of fallopian tube, unspecified
  - S37.53　Laceration of fallopian tube
    - S37.531　Laceration of fallopian tube, unilateral
    - S37.532　Laceration of fallopian tube, bilateral
    - S37.539　Laceration of fallopian tube, unspecified
  - S37.59　Other injury of fallopian tube
    Secondary blast injury of fallopian tube
    - S37.591　Other injury of fallopian tube, unilateral
    - S37.592　Other injury of fallopian tube, bilateral
    - S37.599　Other injury of fallopian tube, unspecified
- S37.6　Injury of uterus
  - **Excludes1**　injury to gravid uterus (O9A.2-)
    injury to uterus during delivery (O71.-)
  - X S37.60　Unspecified injury of uterus
  - X S37.62　Contusion of uterus
  - X S37.63　Laceration of uterus
  - X S37.69　Other injury of uterus
- S37.8　Injury of other urinary and pelvic organs
  - S37.81　Injury of adrenal gland
    - S37.812　Contusion of adrenal gland
    - S37.813　Laceration of adrenal gland
    - S37.818　Other injury of adrenal gland
    - S37.819　Unspecified injury of adrenal gland
  - S37.82　Injury of prostate
    - S37.822　Contusion of prostate
    - S37.823　Laceration of prostate
    - S37.828　Other injury of prostate
    - S37.829　Unspecified injury of prostate
  - S37.89　Injury of other urinary and pelvic organ
    - S37.892　Contusion of other urinary and pelvic organ
    - S37.893　Laceration of other urinary and pelvic organ
    - S37.898　Other injury of other urinary and pelvic organ
    - S37.899　Unspecified injury of other urinary and pelvic organ

- S37.9　Injury of unspecified urinary and pelvic organ
  - X S37.90　Unspecified injury of unspecified urinary and pelvic organ
  - X S37.92　Contusion of unspecified urinary and pelvic organ
  - X S37.93　Laceration of unspecified urinary and pelvic organ
  - X S37.99　Other injury of unspecified urinary and pelvic organ
- S38　Crushing injury and traumatic amputation of abdomen, lower back, pelvis and external genitals
  An amputation not identified as partial or complete should be coded to complete
  The appropriate 7th character is to be added to each code from category S38

A	initial encounter
D	subsequent encounter
S	sequela

  - S38.0　Crushing injury of external genital organs
    Use additional code for any associated injuries
    - S38.00　Crushing injury of unspecified external genital organs
      - S38.001　Crushing injury of unspecified external genital organs, male
      - S38.002　Crushing injury of unspecified external genital organs, female
    - X S38.01　Crushing injury of penis
    - X S38.02　Crushing injury of scrotum and testis
    - X S38.03　Crushing injury of vulva
  - X S38.1　Crushing injury of abdomen, lower back, and pelvis
    Use additional code for all associated injuries, such as:
    fracture of thoracic or lumbar spine and pelvis (S22.0-, S32.-)
    injury to intra-abdominal organs (S36.-)
    injury to urinary and pelvic organs (S37.-)
    open wound of abdominal wall (S31.-)
    spinal cord injury (S34.0, S34.1-)
    - **Excludes2**　crushing injury of external genital organs (S38.0-)
  - S38.2　Traumatic amputation of external genital organs
    - S38.21　Traumatic amputation of female external genital organs
      Traumatic amputation of clitoris
      Traumatic amputation of labium (majus) (minus)
      Traumatic amputation of vulva
      - S38.211　Complete traumatic amputation of female external genital organs
      - S38.212　Partial traumatic amputation of female external genital organs
    - S38.22　Traumatic amputation of penis
      - S38.221　Complete traumatic amputation of penis
      - S38.222　Partial traumatic amputation of penis
    - S38.23　Traumatic amputation of scrotum and testis
      - S38.231　Complete traumatic amputation of scrotum and testis
      - S38.232　Partial traumatic amputation of scrotum and testis
  - X S38.3　Transection (partial) of abdomen

▶ New　⇒ Revised　deleted Deleted　Excludes 1　Excludes 2　Includes　Use additional　Code first　Code also　Key words
OGCR Official Guidelines　X Assign placeholder X　● Use Additional Character(s)　▷ Manifestation Code　🐄 Hierarchical Condition Category　Coding Clinic

● **S39   Other and unspecified injuries of abdomen, lower back, pelvis and external genitals**

Code also any associated open wound (S31.-)

    Excludes2   sprain of joints and ligaments of lumbar spine and pelvis (S33.-)

The appropriate 7th character is to be added to each code from category S39

> A   initial encounter
> D   subsequent encounter
> S   sequela

● **S39.0   Injury of muscle, fascia and tendon of abdomen, lower back and pelvis**

   ● **S39.00   Unspecified injury of muscle, fascia and tendon of abdomen, lower back and pelvis**

     ● **S39.001   Unspecified injury of muscle, fascia and tendon of abdomen**

     ● **S39.002   Unspecified injury of muscle, fascia and tendon of lower back**

     ● **S39.003   Unspecified injury of muscle, fascia and tendon of pelvis**

   ● **S39.01   Strain of muscle, fascia and tendon of abdomen, lower back and pelvis**

     ● **S39.011   Strain of muscle, fascia and tendon of abdomen**

     ● **S39.012   Strain of muscle, fascia and tendon of lower back**
        Coding Clinic: 2016, Q4, P74

     ● **S39.013   Strain of muscle, fascia and tendon of pelvis**

   ● **S39.02   Laceration of muscle, fascia and tendon of abdomen, lower back and pelvis**

     ● **S39.021   Laceration of muscle, fascia and tendon of abdomen**

     ● **S39.022   Laceration of muscle, fascia and tendon of lower back**

     ● **S39.023   Laceration of muscle, fascia and tendon of pelvis**

   ● **S39.09   Other injury of muscle, fascia and tendon of abdomen, lower back and pelvis**

     ● **S39.091   Other injury of muscle, fascia and tendon of abdomen**

     ● **S39.092   Other injury of muscle, fascia and tendon of lower back**

     ● **S39.093   Other injury of muscle, fascia and tendon of pelvis**

● **S39.8   Other specified injuries of abdomen, lower back, pelvis and external genitals**

   X ● **S39.81   Other specified injuries of abdomen**

   X ● **S39.82   Other specified injuries of lower back**

   X ● **S39.83   Other specified injuries of pelvis**

   ● **S39.84   Other specified injuries of external genitals**

     ● **S39.840   Fracture of corpus cavernosum penis**

     ● **S39.848   Other specified injuries of external genitals**

● **S39.9   Unspecified injury of abdomen, lower back, pelvis and external genitals**

   X ● **S39.91   Unspecified injury of abdomen**

   X ● **S39.92   Unspecified injury of lower back**

   X ● **S39.93   Unspecified injury of pelvis**

   X ● **S39.94   Unspecified injury of external genitals**

INJURIES TO THE SHOULDER AND UPPER ARM (S40-S49)

Includes	injuries of axilla injuries of scapular region
Excludes2	burns and corrosions (T20-T32)
	frostbite (T33-T34)
	injuries of elbow (S50-S59)
	insect bite or sting, venomous (T63.4)

● **S40   Superficial injury of shoulder and upper arm**

The appropriate 7th character is to be added to each code from category S40

> A   initial encounter
> D   subsequent encounter
> S   sequela

● **S40.0   Contusion of shoulder and upper arm**

   ● **S40.01   Contusion of shoulder**

     ● **S40.011   Contusion of right shoulder**

     ● **S40.012   Contusion of left shoulder**

     ● **S40.019   Contusion of unspecified shoulder**

   ● **S40.02   Contusion of upper arm**

     ● **S40.021   Contusion of right upper arm**

     ● **S40.022   Contusion of left upper arm**

     ● **S40.029   Contusion of unspecified upper arm**

● **S40.2   Other superficial injuries of shoulder**

   ● **S40.21   Abrasion of shoulder**

     ● **S40.211   Abrasion of right shoulder**

     ● **S40.212   Abrasion of left shoulder**

     ● **S40.219   Abrasion of unspecified shoulder**

   ● **S40.22   Blister (nonthermal) of shoulder**

     ● **S40.221   Blister (nonthermal) of right shoulder**

     ● **S40.222   Blister (nonthermal) of left shoulder**

     ● **S40.229   Blister (nonthermal) of unspecified shoulder**

   ● **S40.24   External constriction of shoulder**

     ● **S40.241   External constriction of right shoulder**

     ● **S40.242   External constriction of left shoulder**

     ● **S40.249   External constriction of unspecified shoulder**

   ● **S40.25   Superficial foreign body of shoulder**
      Splinter in the shoulder

     ● **S40.251   Superficial foreign body of right shoulder**

     ● **S40.252   Superficial foreign body of left shoulder**

     ● **S40.259   Superficial foreign body of unspecified shoulder**

   ● **S40.26   Insect bite (nonvenomous) of shoulder**

     ● **S40.261   Insect bite (nonvenomous) of right shoulder**

     ● **S40.262   Insect bite (nonvenomous) of left shoulder**

     ● **S40.269   Insect bite (nonvenomous) of unspecified shoulder**

   ● **S40.27   Other superficial bite of shoulder**

       Excludes1   open bite of shoulder (S41.05)

     ● **S40.271   Other superficial bite of right shoulder**

     ● **S40.272   Other superficial bite of left shoulder**

     ● **S40.279   Other superficial bite of unspecified shoulder**

● **S40.8   Other superficial injuries of upper arm**

   ● **S40.81   Abrasion of upper arm**

     ● **S40.811   Abrasion of right upper arm**

     ● **S40.812   Abrasion of left upper arm**

     ● **S40.819   Abrasion of unspecified upper arm**

CHAPTER 19 (S00-T88)

- S40.82   **Blister (nonthermal) of upper arm**
  - S40.821   Blister (nonthermal) of right upper arm
  - S40.822   Blister (nonthermal) of left upper arm
  - S40.829   Blister (nonthermal) of unspecified upper arm
- S40.84   **External constriction of upper arm**
  - S40.841   External constriction of right upper arm
  - S40.842   External constriction of left upper arm
  - S40.849   External constriction of unspecified upper arm
- S40.85   **Superficial foreign body of upper arm**
  Splinter in the upper arm
  - S40.851   Superficial foreign body of right upper arm
  - S40.852   Superficial foreign body of left upper arm
  - S40.859   Superficial foreign body of unspecified upper arm
- S40.86   **Insect bite (nonvenomous) of upper arm**
  - S40.861   Insect bite (nonvenomous) of right upper arm
  - S40.862   Insect bite (nonvenomous) of left upper arm
  - S40.869   Insect bite (nonvenomous) of unspecified upper arm
- S40.87   **Other superficial bite of upper arm**
  - **Excludes1**   open bite of upper arm (S41.14)
  - **Excludes2**   other superficial bite of shoulder (S40.27-)
  - S40.871   Other superficial bite of right upper arm
  - S40.872   Other superficial bite of left upper arm
  - S40.879   Other superficial bite of unspecified upper arm
- S40.9   **Unspecified superficial injury of shoulder and upper arm**
  - S40.91   **Unspecified superficial injury of shoulder**
    - S40.911   Unspecified superficial injury of right shoulder
    - S40.912   Unspecified superficial injury of left shoulder
    - S40.919   Unspecified superficial injury of unspecified shoulder
  - S40.92   **Unspecified superficial injury of upper arm**
    - S40.921   Unspecified superficial injury of right upper arm
    - S40.922   Unspecified superficial injury of left upper arm
    - S40.929   Unspecified superficial injury of unspecified upper arm

- S41   **Open wound of shoulder and upper arm**
  Code also any associated wound infection
  - **Excludes1**   traumatic amputation of shoulder and upper arm (S48.-)
  - **Excludes2**   open fracture of shoulder and upper arm (S42.- with 7th character B or C)

  The appropriate 7th character is to be added to each code from category S41

A	initial encounter
D	subsequent encounter
S	sequela

  - S41.0   **Open wound of shoulder**
    - S41.00   **Unspecified open wound of shoulder**
      - S41.001   Unspecified open wound of right shoulder
      - S41.002   Unspecified open wound of left shoulder
      - S41.009   Unspecified open wound of unspecified shoulder
    - S41.01   **Laceration without foreign body of shoulder**
      - S41.011   Laceration without foreign body of right shoulder
      - S41.012   Laceration without foreign body of left shoulder
      - S41.019   Laceration without foreign body of unspecified shoulder
    - S41.02   **Laceration with foreign body of shoulder**
      - S41.021   Laceration with foreign body of right shoulder
      - S41.022   Laceration with foreign body of left shoulder
      - S41.029   Laceration with foreign body of unspecified shoulder
    - S41.03   **Puncture wound without foreign body of shoulder**
      - S41.031   Puncture wound without foreign body of right shoulder
      - S41.032   Puncture wound without foreign body of left shoulder
      - S41.039   Puncture wound without foreign body of unspecified shoulder
    - S41.04   **Puncture wound with foreign body of shoulder**
      - S41.041   Puncture wound with foreign body of right shoulder
      - S41.042   Puncture wound with foreign body of left shoulder
      - S41.049   Puncture wound with foreign body of unspecified shoulder
    - S41.05   **Open bite of shoulder**
      Bite of shoulder NOS
      - **Excludes1**   superficial bite of shoulder (S40.27)
      - S41.051   Open bite of right shoulder
      - S41.052   Open bite of left shoulder
      - S41.059   Open bite of unspecified shoulder
  - S41.1   **Open wound of upper arm**
    - S41.10   **Unspecified open wound of upper arm**
      - S41.101   Unspecified open wound of right upper arm
      - S41.102   Unspecified open wound of left upper arm
      - S41.109   Unspecified open wound of unspecified upper arm
    - S41.11   **Laceration without foreign body of upper arm**
      - S41.111   Laceration without foreign body of right upper arm
      - S41.112   Laceration without foreign body of left upper arm
      - S41.119   Laceration without foreign body of unspecified upper arm
    - S41.12   **Laceration with foreign body of upper arm**
      - S41.121   Laceration with foreign body of right upper arm
      - S41.122   Laceration with foreign body of left upper arm
      - S41.129   Laceration with foreign body of unspecified upper arm
    - S41.13   **Puncture wound without foreign body of upper arm**
      - S41.131   Puncture wound without foreign body of right upper arm
      - S41.132   Puncture wound without foreign body of left upper arm
      - S41.139   Puncture wound without foreign body of unspecified upper arm

▶ New   ⇒ Revised   ~~deleted~~ Deleted   Excludes 1   Excludes 2   Includes   Use additional   Code first   Code also   Key words
OGCR Official Guidelines   X Assign placeholder X   ● Use Additional Character(s)   ▶ Manifestation Code   🔖 Hierarchical Condition Category   Coding Clinic

- S41.14   Puncture wound with foreign body of upper arm
  - S41.141   Puncture wound with foreign body of right upper arm
  - S41.142   Puncture wound with foreign body of left upper arm
  - S41.149   Puncture wound with foreign body of unspecified upper arm
- S41.15   Open bite of upper arm
  Bite of upper arm NOS
  > **Excludes1**   superficial bite of upper arm (S40.87)
  - S41.151   Open bite of right upper arm
  - S41.152   Open bite of left upper arm
  - S41.159   Open bite of unspecified upper arm

- S42   Fracture of shoulder and upper arm
  Note: A fracture not indicated as displaced or nondisplaced should be coded to displaced

  A fracture not indicated as open or closed should be coded to closed

  > **Excludes1**   periprosthetic fracture around internal prosthetic shoulder joint (M97.3)
  > traumatic amputation of shoulder and upper arm (S48.-)

  The appropriate 7th character is to be added to all codes from category S42

A	initial encounter for closed fracture
B	initial encounter for open fracture
D	subsequent encounter for fracture with routine healing
G	subsequent encounter for fracture with delayed healing
K	subsequent encounter for fracture with nonunion
P	subsequent encounter for fracture with malunion
S	sequela

- S42.0   Fracture of clavicle
  - S42.00   Fracture of unspecified part of clavicle
    - S42.001   Fracture of unspecified part of right clavicle
    - S42.002   Fracture of unspecified part of left clavicle
    - S42.009   Fracture of unspecified part of unspecified clavicle
      Coding Clinic: 2012, Q4, P3
  - S42.01   Fracture of sternal end of clavicle
    - S42.011   Anterior displaced fracture of sternal end of right clavicle
    - S42.012   Anterior displaced fracture of sternal end of left clavicle
    - S42.013   Anterior displaced fracture of sternal end of unspecified clavicle
      Displaced fracture of sternal end of clavicle NOS
    - S42.014   Posterior displaced fracture of sternal end of right clavicle
    - S42.015   Posterior displaced fracture of sternal end of left clavicle
    - S42.016   Posterior displaced fracture of sternal end of unspecified clavicle
    - S42.017   Nondisplaced fracture of sternal end of right clavicle
    - S42.018   Nondisplaced fracture of sternal end of left clavicle
    - S42.019   Nondisplaced fracture of sternal end of unspecified clavicle
  - S42.02   Fracture of shaft of clavicle
    - S42.021   Displaced fracture of shaft of right clavicle
    - S42.022   Displaced fracture of shaft of left clavicle
    - S42.023   Displaced fracture of shaft of unspecified clavicle
    - S42.024   Nondisplaced fracture of shaft of right clavicle
    - S42.025   Nondisplaced fracture of shaft of left clavicle
    - S42.026   Nondisplaced fracture of shaft of unspecified clavicle
  - S42.03   Fracture of lateral end of clavicle
    Fracture of acromial end of clavicle
    - S42.031   Displaced fracture of lateral end of right clavicle
    - S42.032   Displaced fracture of lateral end of left clavicle
    - S42.033   Displaced fracture of lateral end of unspecified clavicle
    - S42.034   Nondisplaced fracture of lateral end of right clavicle
    - S42.035   Nondisplaced fracture of lateral end of left clavicle
    - S42.036   Nondisplaced fracture of lateral end of unspecified clavicle
- S42.1   Fracture of scapula
  - S42.10   Fracture of unspecified part of scapula
    - S42.101   Fracture of unspecified part of scapula, right shoulder
    - S42.102   Fracture of unspecified part of scapula, left shoulder
    - S42.109   Fracture of unspecified part of scapula, unspecified shoulder
  - S42.11   Fracture of body of scapula
    - S42.111   Displaced fracture of body of scapula, right shoulder
    - S42.112   Displaced fracture of body of scapula, left shoulder
    - S42.113   Displaced fracture of body of scapula, unspecified shoulder
    - S42.114   Nondisplaced fracture of body of scapula, right shoulder
    - S42.115   Nondisplaced fracture of body of scapula, left shoulder
    - S42.116   Nondisplaced fracture of body of scapula, unspecified shoulder
  - S42.12   Fracture of acromial process
    - S42.121   Displaced fracture of acromial process, right shoulder
    - S42.122   Displaced fracture of acromial process, left shoulder
    - S42.123   Displaced fracture of acromial process, unspecified shoulder
    - S42.124   Nondisplaced fracture of acromial process, right shoulder
    - S42.125   Nondisplaced fracture of acromial process, left shoulder
    - S42.126   Nondisplaced fracture, of acromial process, unspecified shoulder
  - S42.13   Fracture of coracoid process
    - S42.131   Displaced fracture of coracoid process, right shoulder
    - S42.132   Displaced fracture of coracoid process, left shoulder
    - S42.133   Displaced fracture of coracoid process, unspecified shoulder
    - S42.134   Nondisplaced fracture of coracoid process, right shoulder
    - S42.135   Nondisplaced fracture of coracoid process, left shoulder
    - S42.136   Nondisplaced fracture of coracoid process, unspecified shoulder

CHAPTER 19 (S00-T88)

● S42.14   Fracture of glenoid cavity of scapula
- ● S42.141   Displaced fracture of glenoid cavity of scapula, right shoulder
- ● S42.142   Displaced fracture of glenoid cavity of scapula, left shoulder
- ● S42.143   Displaced fracture of glenoid cavity of scapula, unspecified shoulder
- ● S42.144   Nondisplaced fracture of glenoid cavity of scapula, right shoulder
- ● S42.145   Nondisplaced fracture of glenoid cavity of scapula, left shoulder
- ● S42.146   Nondisplaced fracture of glenoid cavity of scapula, unspecified shoulder

● S42.15   Fracture of neck of scapula
- ● S42.151   Displaced fracture of neck of scapula, right shoulder
- ● S42.152   Displaced fracture of neck of scapula, left shoulder
- ● S42.153   Displaced fracture of neck of scapula, unspecified shoulder
- ● S42.154   Nondisplaced fracture of neck of scapula, right shoulder
- ● S42.155   Nondisplaced fracture of neck of scapula, left shoulder
- ● S42.156   Nondisplaced fracture of neck of scapula, unspecified shoulder

● S42.19   Fracture of other part of scapula
- ● S42.191   Fracture of other part of scapula, right shoulder
- ● S42.192   Fracture of other part of scapula, left shoulder
- ● S42.199   Fracture of other part of scapula, unspecified shoulder

● S42.2   Fracture of upper end of humerus
   Fracture of proximal end of humerus
> **Excludes2**   fracture of shaft of humerus (S42.3-) physeal fracture of upper end of humerus (S49.0-)

● S42.20   Unspecified fracture of upper end of humerus
- ● S42.201   Unspecified fracture of upper end of right humerus
- ● S42.202   Unspecified fracture of upper end of left humerus
- ● S42.209   Unspecified fracture of upper end of unspecified humerus

● S42.21   Unspecified fracture of surgical neck of humerus
   Fracture of neck of humerus NOS
- ● S42.211   Unspecified displaced fracture of surgical neck of right humerus
- ● S42.212   Unspecified displaced fracture of surgical neck of left humerus
- ● S42.213   Unspecified displaced fracture of surgical neck of unspecified humerus
- ● S42.214   Unspecified nondisplaced fracture of surgical neck of right humerus
- ● S42.215   Unspecified nondisplaced fracture of surgical neck of left humerus
- ● S42.216   Unspecified nondisplaced fracture of surgical neck of unspecified humerus

● S42.22   2-part fracture of surgical neck of humerus
- ● S42.221   2-part displaced fracture of surgical neck of right humerus
- ● S42.222   2-part displaced fracture of surgical neck of left humerus
- ● S42.223   2-part displaced fracture of surgical neck of unspecified humerus
- ● S42.224   2-part nondisplaced fracture of surgical neck of right humerus

- ● S42.225   2-part nondisplaced fracture of surgical neck of left humerus
- ● S42.226   2-part nondisplaced fracture of surgical neck of unspecified humerus

● S42.23   3-part fracture of surgical neck of humerus
- ● S42.231   3-part fracture of surgical neck of right humerus
- ● S42.232   3-part fracture of surgical neck of left humerus
- ● S42.239   3-part fracture of surgical neck of unspecified humerus

● S42.24   4-part fracture of surgical neck of humerus
- ● S42.241   4-part fracture of surgical neck of right humerus
- ● S42.242   4-part fracture of surgical neck of left humerus
- ● S42.249   4-part fracture of surgical neck of unspecified humerus

● S42.25   Fracture of greater tuberosity of humerus
- ● S42.251   Displaced fracture of greater tuberosity of right humerus
- ● S42.252   Displaced fracture of greater tuberosity of left humerus
- ● S42.253   Displaced fracture of greater tuberosity of unspecified humerus
- ● S42.254   Nondisplaced fracture of greater tuberosity of right humerus
- ● S42.255   Nondisplaced fracture of greater tuberosity of left humerus
- ● S42.256   Nondisplaced fracture of greater tuberosity of unspecified humerus

● S42.26   Fracture of lesser tuberosity of humerus
- ● S42.261   Displaced fracture of lesser tuberosity of right humerus
- ● S42.262   Displaced fracture of lesser tuberosity of left humerus
- ● S42.263   Displaced fracture of lesser tuberosity of unspecified humerus
- ● S42.264   Nondisplaced fracture of lesser tuberosity of right humerus
- ● S42.265   Nondisplaced fracture of lesser tuberosity of left humerus
- ● S42.266   Nondisplaced fracture of lesser tuberosity of unspecified humerus

● S42.27   Torus fracture of upper end of humerus
   The appropriate 7th character is to be added to all codes in subcategory S42.27

> A   initial encounter for closed fracture
> D   subsequent encounter for fracture with routine healing
> G   subsequent encounter for fracture with delayed healing
> K   subsequent encounter for fracture with nonunion
> P   subsequent encounter for fracture with malunion
> S   sequela

- ● S42.271   Torus fracture of upper end of right humerus
- ● S42.272   Torus fracture of upper end of left humerus
- ● S42.279   Torus fracture of upper end of unspecified humerus

● S42.29   Other fracture of upper end of humerus
   Fracture of anatomical neck of humerus
   Fracture of articular head of humerus
- ● S42.291   Other displaced fracture of upper end of right humerus
- ● S42.292   Other displaced fracture of upper end of left humerus

▶ New   ⇒ Revised   ~~deleted~~ Deleted   Excludes 1   Excludes 2   Includes   Use additional   Code first   Code also   Key words
OGCR Official Guidelines   X Assign placeholder X   ● Use Additional Character(s)   ▶ Manifestation Code   Hierarchical Condition Category   **Coding Clinic**

Coding Clinic: 2024, Q2, P24

● S42.293　Other displaced fracture of upper end of unspecified humerus

● S42.294　Other nondisplaced fracture of upper end of right humerus

● S42.295　Other nondisplaced fracture of upper end of left humerus
Coding Clinic: 2019, Q1, P19

● S42.296　Other nondisplaced fracture of upper end of unspecified humerus

● S42.3　**Fracture of shaft of humerus**
　　Fracture of humerus NOS
　　Fracture of upper arm NOS

　　Excludes2　physeal fractures of upper end of humerus (S49.0-)
　　　　　　　physeal fractures of lower end of humerus (S49.1-)

● S42.30　Unspecified fracture of shaft of humerus

● S42.301　Unspecified fracture of shaft of humerus, right arm

● S42.302　Unspecified fracture of shaft of humerus, left arm

● S42.309　Unspecified fracture of shaft of humerus, unspecified arm

● S42.31　Greenstick fracture of shaft of humerus

　　The appropriate 7th character is to be added to all codes in subcategory S42.3

A	initial encounter for closed fracture
D	subsequent encounter for fracture with routine healing
G	subsequent encounter for fracture with delayed healing
K	subsequent encounter for fracture with nonunion
P	subsequent encounter for fracture with malunion
S	sequela

● S42.311　Greenstick fracture of shaft of humerus, right arm

● S42.312　Greenstick fracture of shaft of humerus, left arm

● S42.319　Greenstick fracture of shaft of humerus, unspecified arm

● S42.32　Transverse fracture of shaft of humerus

● S42.321　Displaced transverse fracture of shaft of humerus, right arm

● S42.322　Displaced transverse fracture of shaft of humerus, left arm

● S42.323　Displaced transverse fracture of shaft of humerus, unspecified arm

● S42.324　Nondisplaced transverse fracture of shaft of humerus, right arm

● S42.325　Nondisplaced transverse fracture of shaft of humerus, left arm

● S42.326　Nondisplaced transverse fracture of shaft of humerus, unspecified arm

● S42.33　Oblique fracture of shaft of humerus

● S42.331　Displaced oblique fracture of shaft of humerus, right arm

● S42.332　Displaced oblique fracture of shaft of humerus, left arm

● S42.333　Displaced oblique fracture of shaft of humerus, unspecified arm

● S42.334　Nondisplaced oblique fracture of shaft of humerus, right arm

● S42.335　Nondisplaced oblique fracture of shaft of humerus, left arm

● S42.336　Nondisplaced oblique fracture of shaft of humerus, unspecified arm

● S42.34　Spiral fracture of shaft of humerus

● S42.341　Displaced spiral fracture of shaft of humerus, right arm

● S42.342　Displaced spiral fracture of shaft of humerus, left arm

● S42.343　Displaced spiral fracture of shaft of humerus, unspecified arm

● S42.344　Nondisplaced spiral fracture of shaft of humerus, right arm

● S42.345　Nondisplaced spiral fracture of shaft of humerus, left arm

● S42.346　Nondisplaced spiral fracture of shaft of humerus, unspecified arm

● S42.35　Comminuted fracture of shaft of humerus

● S42.351　Displaced comminuted fracture of shaft of humerus, right arm

● S42.352　Displaced comminuted fracture of shaft of humerus, left arm

● S42.353　Displaced comminuted fracture of shaft of humerus, unspecified arm

● S42.354　Nondisplaced comminuted fracture of shaft of humerus, right arm

● S42.355　Nondisplaced comminuted fracture of shaft of humerus, left arm

● S42.356　Nondisplaced comminuted fracture of shaft of humerus, unspecified arm

● S42.36　Segmental fracture of shaft of humerus

● S42.361　Displaced segmental fracture of shaft of humerus, right arm

● S42.362　Displaced segmental fracture of shaft of humerus, left arm

● S42.363　Displaced segmental fracture of shaft of humerus, unspecified arm

● S42.364　Nondisplaced segmental fracture of shaft of humerus, right arm

● S42.365　Nondisplaced segmental fracture of shaft of humerus, left arm

● S42.366　Nondisplaced segmental fracture of shaft of humerus, unspecified arm

● S42.39　Other fracture of shaft of humerus

● S42.391　Other fracture of shaft of right humerus

● S42.392　Other fracture of shaft of left humerus

● S42.399　Other fracture of shaft of unspecified humerus

● S42.4　**Fracture of lower end of humerus**
　　Fracture of distal end of humerus

　　Excludes2　fracture of shaft of humerus (S42.3-)
　　　　　　　physeal fracture of lower end of humerus (S49.1-)

● S42.40　Unspecified fracture of lower end of humerus
　　Fracture of elbow NOS

● S42.401　Unspecified fracture of lower end of right humerus

● S42.402　Unspecified fracture of lower end of left humerus

● S42.409　Unspecified fracture of lower end of unspecified humerus

● S42.41　Simple supracondylar fracture without intercondylar fracture of humerus

● S42.411　Displaced simple supracondylar fracture without intercondylar fracture of right humerus

● S42.412　Displaced simple supracondylar fracture without intercondylar fracture of left humerus

● S42.413　Displaced simple supracondylar fracture without intercondylar fracture of unspecified humerus

CHAPTER 19 (S00-T88)

● S42.414   Nondisplaced simple supracondylar fracture without intercondylar fracture of right humerus

● S42.415   Nondisplaced simple supracondylar fracture without intercondylar fracture of left humerus

● S42.416   Nondisplaced simple supracondylar fracture without intercondylar fracture of unspecified humerus

● S42.42   Comminuted supracondylar fracture without intercondylar fracture of humerus

● S42.421   Displaced comminuted supracondylar fracture without intercondylar fracture of right humerus

● S42.422   Displaced comminuted supracondylar fracture without intercondylar fracture of left humerus

● S42.423   Displaced comminuted supracondylar fracture without intercondylar fracture of unspecified humerus

● S42.424   Nondisplaced comminuted supracondylar fracture without intercondylar fracture of right humerus

● S42.425   Nondisplaced comminuted supracondylar fracture without intercondylar fracture of left humerus

● S42.426   Nondisplaced comminuted supracondylar fracture without intercondylar fracture of unspecified humerus

● S42.43   Fracture (avulsion) of lateral epicondyle of humerus

● S42.431   Displaced fracture (avulsion) of lateral epicondyle of right humerus

● S42.432   Displaced fracture (avulsion) of lateral epicondyle of left humerus

● S42.433   Displaced fracture (avulsion) of lateral epicondyle of unspecified humerus

● S42.434   Nondisplaced fracture (avulsion) of lateral epicondyle of right humerus

● S42.435   Nondisplaced fracture (avulsion) of lateral epicondyle of left humerus

● S42.436   Nondisplaced fracture (avulsion) of lateral epicondyle of unspecified humerus

● S42.44   Fracture (avulsion) of medial epicondyle of humerus

● S42.441   Displaced fracture (avulsion) of medial epicondyle of right humerus

● S42.442   Displaced fracture (avulsion) of medial epicondyle of left humerus

● S42.443   Displaced fracture (avulsion) of medial epicondyle of unspecified humerus

● S42.444   Nondisplaced fracture (avulsion) of medial epicondyle of right humerus

● S42.445   Nondisplaced fracture (avulsion) of medial epicondyle of left humerus

● S42.446   Nondisplaced fracture (avulsion) of medial epicondyle of unspecified humerus

● S42.447   Incarcerated fracture (avulsion) of medial epicondyle of right humerus

● S42.448   Incarcerated fracture (avulsion) of medial epicondyle of left humerus

● S42.449   Incarcerated fracture (avulsion) of medial epicondyle of unspecified humerus

● S42.45   Fracture of lateral condyle of humerus
Fracture of capitellum of humerus

● S42.451   Displaced fracture of lateral condyle of right humerus

● S42.452   Displaced fracture of lateral condyle of left humerus

● S42.453   Displaced fracture of lateral condyle of unspecified humerus

● S42.454   Nondisplaced fracture of lateral condyle of right humerus

● S42.455   Nondisplaced fracture of lateral condyle of left humerus

● S42.456   Nondisplaced fracture of lateral condyle of unspecified humerus

● S42.46   Fracture of medial condyle of humerus
Trochlea fracture of humerus

● S42.461   Displaced fracture of medial condyle of right humerus

● S42.462   Displaced fracture of medial condyle of left humerus

● S42.463   Displaced fracture of medial condyle of unspecified humerus

● S42.464   Nondisplaced fracture of medial condyle of right humerus

● S42.465   Nondisplaced fracture of medial condyle of left humerus

● S42.466   Nondisplaced fracture of medial condyle of unspecified humerus

● S42.47   Transcondylar fracture of humerus

● S42.471   Displaced transcondylar fracture of right humerus

● S42.472   Displaced transcondylar fracture of left humerus

● S42.473   Displaced transcondylar fracture of unspecified humerus

● S42.474   Nondisplaced transcondylar fracture of right humerus

● S42.475   Nondisplaced transcondylar fracture of left humerus

● S42.476   Nondisplaced transcondylar fracture of unspecified humerus

● S42.48   Torus fracture of lower end of humerus

The appropriate 7th character is to be added to all codes in subcategory S42.48

A	initial encounter for closed fracture
D	subsequent encounter for fracture with routine healing
G	subsequent encounter for fracture with delayed healing
K	subsequent encounter for fracture with nonunion
P	subsequent encounter for fracture with malunion
S	sequela

● S42.481   Torus fracture of lower end of right humerus

● S42.482   Torus fracture of lower end of left humerus

● S42.489   Torus fracture of lower end of unspecified humerus

● S42.49   Other fracture of lower end of humerus

● S42.491   Other displaced fracture of lower end of right humerus

● S42.492   Other displaced fracture of lower end of left humerus

● S42.493   Other displaced fracture of lower end of unspecified humerus

● S42.494   Other nondisplaced fracture of lower end of right humerus

▶ New   ⇒ Revised   ~~deleted~~ Deleted   Excludes 1   Excludes 2   Includes   Use additional   Code first   Code also   Key words

OGCR Official Guidelines   X Assign placeholder X   ● Use Additional Character(s)   ▶ Manifestation Code   🔖 Hierarchical Condition Category   Coding Clinic

● S42.495   Other nondisplaced fracture of lower end of left humerus

● S42.496   Other nondisplaced fracture of lower end of unspecified humerus

● **S42.9**   **Fracture of shoulder girdle, part unspecified**
     Fracture of shoulder NOS

X ● S42.90   Fracture of unspecified shoulder girdle, part unspecified

X ● S42.91   Fracture of right shoulder girdle, part unspecified

X ● S42.92   Fracture of left shoulder girdle, part unspecified

● **S43**   **Dislocation and sprain of joints and ligaments of shoulder girdle**

> **Includes**   avulsion of joint or ligament of shoulder girdle
> laceration of cartilage, joint or ligament of shoulder girdle
> sprain of cartilage, joint or ligament of shoulder girdle
> traumatic hemarthrosis of joint or ligament of shoulder girdle
> traumatic rupture of joint or ligament of shoulder girdle
> traumatic subluxation of joint or ligament of shoulder girdle
> traumatic tear of joint or ligament of shoulder girdle

Code also any associated open wound

> **Excludes2**   strain of muscle, fascia and tendon of shoulder and upper arm (S46.-)

The appropriate 7th character is to be added to each code from category S43

> A   initial encounter
> D   subsequent encounter
> S   sequela

● **S43.0**   **Subluxation and dislocation of shoulder joint**
     Dislocation of glenohumeral joint
     Subluxation of glenohumeral joint

   ● S43.00   Unspecified subluxation and dislocation of shoulder joint
       Dislocation of humerus NOS
       Subluxation of humerus NOS

     ● S43.001   Unspecified subluxation of right shoulder joint

     ● S43.002   Unspecified subluxation of left shoulder joint

     ● S43.003   Unspecified subluxation of unspecified shoulder joint

     ● S43.004   Unspecified dislocation of right shoulder joint

     ● S43.005   Unspecified dislocation of left shoulder joint

     ● S43.006   Unspecified dislocation of unspecified shoulder joint

   ● S43.01   Anterior subluxation and dislocation of humerus

     ● S43.011   Anterior subluxation of right humerus

     ● S43.012   Anterior subluxation of left humerus

     ● S43.013   Anterior subluxation of unspecified humerus

     ● S43.014   Anterior dislocation of right humerus

     ● S43.015   Anterior dislocation of left humerus

     ● S43.016   Anterior dislocation of unspecified humerus

   ● S43.02   Posterior subluxation and dislocation of humerus

     ● S43.021   Posterior subluxation of right humerus

     ● S43.022   Posterior subluxation of left humerus

     ● S43.023   Posterior subluxation of unspecified humerus

     ● S43.024   Posterior dislocation of right humerus

     ● S43.025   Posterior dislocation of left humerus

     ● S43.026   Posterior dislocation of unspecified humerus

   ● S43.03   Inferior subluxation and dislocation of humerus

     ● S43.031   Inferior subluxation of right humerus

     ● S43.032   Inferior subluxation of left humerus

     ● S43.033   Inferior subluxation of unspecified humerus

     ● S43.034   Inferior dislocation of right humerus

     ● S43.035   Inferior dislocation of left humerus

     ● S43.036   Inferior dislocation of unspecified humerus

   ● S43.08   Other subluxation and dislocation of shoulder joint

     ● S43.081   Other subluxation of right shoulder joint

     ● S43.082   Other subluxation of left shoulder joint

     ● S43.083   Other subluxation of unspecified shoulder joint

     ● S43.084   Other dislocation of right shoulder joint

     ● S43.085   Other dislocation of left shoulder joint

     ● S43.086   Other dislocation of unspecified shoulder joint

● **S43.1**   **Subluxation and dislocation of acromioclavicular joint**

   ● S43.10   Unspecified dislocation of acromioclavicular joint

     ● S43.101   Unspecified dislocation of right acromioclavicular joint

     ● S43.102   Unspecified dislocation of left acromioclavicular joint

     ● S43.109   Unspecified dislocation of unspecified acromioclavicular joint

   ● S43.11   Subluxation of acromioclavicular joint

     ● S43.111   Subluxation of right acromioclavicular joint

     ● S43.112   Subluxation of left acromioclavicular joint

     ● S43.119   Subluxation of unspecified acromioclavicular joint

   ● S43.12   Dislocation of acromioclavicular joint, 100%-200% displacement

     ● S43.121   Dislocation of right acromioclavicular joint, 100%-200% displacement

     ● S43.122   Dislocation of left acromioclavicular joint, 100%-200% displacement

     ● S43.129   Dislocation of unspecified acromioclavicular joint, 100%-200% displacement

   ● S43.13   Dislocation of acromioclavicular joint, greater than 200% displacement

     ● S43.131   Dislocation of right acromioclavicular joint, greater than 200% displacement

     ● S43.132   Dislocation of left acromioclavicular joint, greater than 200% displacement

     ● S43.139   Dislocation of unspecified acromioclavicular joint, greater than 200% displacement

CHAPTER 19 (S00-T88)

- S43.14   Inferior dislocation of acromioclavicular joint
  - S43.141   Inferior dislocation of right acromioclavicular joint
  - S43.142   Inferior dislocation of left acromioclavicular joint
  - S43.149   Inferior dislocation of unspecified acromioclavicular joint
- S43.15   Posterior dislocation of acromioclavicular joint
  - S43.151   Posterior dislocation of right acromioclavicular joint
  - S43.152   Posterior dislocation of left acromioclavicular joint
  - S43.159   Posterior dislocation of unspecified acromioclavicular joint
- S43.2   Subluxation and dislocation of sternoclavicular joint
  - S43.20   Unspecified subluxation and dislocation of sternoclavicular joint
    - S43.201   Unspecified subluxation of right sternoclavicular joint
    - S43.202   Unspecified subluxation of left sternoclavicular joint
    - S43.203   Unspecified subluxation of unspecified sternoclavicular joint
    - S43.204   Unspecified dislocation of right sternoclavicular joint
    - S43.205   Unspecified dislocation of left sternoclavicular joint
    - S43.206   Unspecified dislocation of unspecified sternoclavicular joint
  - S43.21   Anterior subluxation and dislocation of sternoclavicular joint
    - S43.211   Anterior subluxation of right sternoclavicular joint
    - S43.212   Anterior subluxation of left sternoclavicular joint
    - S43.213   Anterior subluxation of unspecified sternoclavicular joint
    - S43.214   Anterior dislocation of right sternoclavicular joint
    - S43.215   Anterior dislocation of left sternoclavicular joint
    - S43.216   Anterior dislocation of unspecified sternoclavicular joint
  - S43.22   Posterior subluxation and dislocation of sternoclavicular joint
    - S43.221   Posterior subluxation of right sternoclavicular joint
    - S43.222   Posterior subluxation of left sternoclavicular joint
    - S43.223   Posterior subluxation of unspecified sternoclavicular joint
    - S43.224   Posterior dislocation of right sternoclavicular joint
    - S43.225   Posterior dislocation of left sternoclavicular joint
    - S43.226   Posterior dislocation of unspecified sternoclavicular joint
- S43.3   Subluxation and dislocation of other and unspecified parts of shoulder girdle
  - S43.30   Subluxation and dislocation of unspecified parts of shoulder girdle
    - Dislocation of shoulder girdle NOS
    - Subluxation of shoulder girdle NOS
    - S43.301   Subluxation of unspecified parts of right shoulder girdle
    - S43.302   Subluxation of unspecified parts of left shoulder girdle
    - S43.303   Subluxation of unspecified parts of unspecified shoulder girdle
    - S43.304   Dislocation of unspecified parts of right shoulder girdle

- S43.305   Dislocation of unspecified parts of left shoulder girdle
- S43.306   Dislocation of unspecified parts of unspecified shoulder girdle
- S43.31   Subluxation and dislocation of scapula
  - S43.311   Subluxation of right scapula
  - S43.312   Subluxation of left scapula
  - S43.313   Subluxation of unspecified scapula
  - S43.314   Dislocation of right scapula
  - S43.315   Dislocation of left scapula
  - S43.316   Dislocation of unspecified scapula
- S43.39   Subluxation and dislocation of other parts of shoulder girdle
  - S43.391   Subluxation of other parts of right shoulder girdle
  - S43.392   Subluxation of other parts of left shoulder girdle
  - S43.393   Subluxation of other parts of unspecified shoulder girdle
  - S43.394   Dislocation of other parts of right shoulder girdle
  - S43.395   Dislocation of other parts of left shoulder girdle
  - S43.396   Dislocation of other parts of unspecified shoulder girdle
- S43.4   Sprain of shoulder joint
  - S43.40   Unspecified sprain of shoulder joint
    - S43.401   Unspecified sprain of right shoulder joint
    - S43.402   Unspecified sprain of left shoulder joint
    - S43.409   Unspecified sprain of unspecified shoulder joint
  - S43.41   Sprain of coracohumeral (ligament)
    - S43.411   Sprain of right coracohumeral (ligament)
    - S43.412   Sprain of left coracohumeral (ligament)
    - S43.419   Sprain of unspecified coracohumeral (ligament)
  - S43.42   Sprain of rotator cuff capsule
    - *Encounters during the healing phase*
    - **Excludes1**   rotator cuff syndrome (complete) (incomplete), not specified as traumatic (M75.1-)
    - **Excludes2**   injury of tendon of rotator cuff (S46.0-)
    - S43.421   Sprain of right rotator cuff capsule
    - S43.422   Sprain of left rotator cuff capsule
    - S43.429   Sprain of unspecified rotator cuff capsule
  - S43.43   Superior glenoid labrum lesion
    - SLAP lesion
    - Coding Clinic: 2019, Q2, P27
    - S43.431   Superior glenoid labrum lesion of right shoulder
    - S43.432   Superior glenoid labrum lesion of left shoulder
      - Coding Clinic: 2024, Q2, P24
    - S43.439   Superior glenoid labrum lesion of unspecified shoulder
  - S43.49   Other sprain of shoulder joint
    - S43.491   Other sprain of right shoulder joint
    - S43.492   Other sprain of left shoulder joint
    - S43.499   Other sprain of unspecified shoulder joint

▶ New   ⇒ Revised   ~~deleted~~ Deleted   Excludes 1   Excludes 2   Includes   Use additional   Code first   Code also   Key words
OGCR Official Guidelines   X Assign placeholder X   ● Use Additional Character(s)   ▶ Manifestation Code   Hierarchical Condition Category   Coding Clinic

● **S43.5** Sprain of acromioclavicular joint
          Sprain of acromioclavicular ligament
    X ● **S43.50**   Sprain of unspecified acromioclavicular joint
    X ● **S43.51**   Sprain of right acromioclavicular joint
    X ● **S43.52**   Sprain of left acromioclavicular joint
● **S43.6** Sprain of sternoclavicular joint
    X ● **S43.60**   Sprain of unspecified sternoclavicular joint
    X ● **S43.61**   Sprain of right sternoclavicular joint
    X ● **S43.62**   Sprain of left sternoclavicular joint
● **S43.8** Sprain of other specified parts of shoulder girdle
    X ● **S43.80**   Sprain of other specified parts of unspecified shoulder girdle
    X ● **S43.81**   Sprain of other specified parts of right shoulder girdle
    X ● **S43.82**   Sprain of other specified parts of left shoulder girdle
● **S43.9** Sprain of unspecified parts of shoulder girdle
    X ● **S43.90**   Sprain of unspecified parts of unspecified shoulder girdle
                 Sprain of shoulder girdle NOS
    X ● **S43.91**   Sprain of unspecified parts of right shoulder girdle
    X ● **S43.92**   Sprain of unspecified parts of left shoulder girdle

● **S44** Injury of nerves at shoulder and upper arm level
       Code also any associated open wound (S41.-)
       Excludes2 injury of brachial plexus (S14.3-)
       The appropriate 7th character is to be added to each code from category S44

A	initial encounter
D	subsequent encounter
S	sequela

● **S44.0** Injury of ulnar nerve at upper arm level
         Excludes1 ulnar nerve NOS (S54.0)
    X ● **S44.00**   Injury of ulnar nerve at upper arm level, unspecified arm
    X ● **S44.01**   Injury of ulnar nerve at upper arm level, right arm
    X ● **S44.02**   Injury of ulnar nerve at upper arm level, left arm
● **S44.1** Injury of median nerve at upper arm level
         Excludes1 median nerve NOS (S54.1)
    X ● **S44.10**   Injury of median nerve at upper arm level, unspecified arm
    X ● **S44.11**   Injury of median nerve at upper arm level, right arm
    X ● **S44.12**   Injury of median nerve at upper arm level, left arm
● **S44.2** Injury of radial nerve at upper arm level
         Excludes1 radial nerve NOS (S54.2)
    X ● **S44.20**   Injury of radial nerve at upper arm level, unspecified arm
    X ● **S44.21**   Injury of radial nerve at upper arm level, right arm
    X ● **S44.22**   Injury of radial nerve at upper arm level, left arm
● **S44.3** Injury of axillary nerve
    X ● **S44.30**   Injury of axillary nerve, unspecified arm
    X ● **S44.31**   Injury of axillary nerve, right arm
    X ● **S44.32**   Injury of axillary nerve, left arm
● **S44.4** Injury of musculocutaneous nerve
    X ● **S44.40**   Injury of musculocutaneous nerve, unspecified arm
    X ● **S44.41**   Injury of musculocutaneous nerve, right arm
    X ● **S44.42**   Injury of musculocutaneous nerve, left arm

● **S44.5** Injury of cutaneous sensory nerve at shoulder and upper arm level
    X ● **S44.50**   Injury of cutaneous sensory nerve at shoulder and upper arm level, unspecified arm
    X ● **S44.51**   Injury of cutaneous sensory nerve at shoulder and upper arm level, right arm
    X ● **S44.52**   Injury of cutaneous sensory nerve at shoulder and upper arm level, left arm
● **S44.8** Injury of other nerves at shoulder and upper arm level
    ● **S44.8X** Injury of other nerves at shoulder and upper arm level
        ● **S44.8X1**   Injury of other nerves at shoulder and upper arm level, right arm
        ● **S44.8X2**   Injury of other nerves at shoulder and upper arm level, left arm
        ● **S44.8X9**   Injury of other nerves at shoulder and upper arm level, unspecified arm
● **S44.9** Injury of unspecified nerve at shoulder and upper arm level
    X ● **S44.90**   Injury of unspecified nerve at shoulder and upper arm level, unspecified arm
    X ● **S44.91**   Injury of unspecified nerve at shoulder and upper arm level, right arm
    X ● **S44.92**   Injury of unspecified nerve at shoulder and upper arm level, left arm

● **S45** Injury of blood vessels at shoulder and upper arm level
       Code also any associated open wound (S41.-)
       Excludes2 injury of subclavian artery (S25.1)
                     injury of subclavian vein (S25.3)
       The appropriate 7th character is to be added to each code from category S45

A	initial encounter
D	subsequent encounter
S	sequela

● **S45.0** Injury of axillary artery
    ● **S45.00** Unspecified injury of axillary artery
        ● **S45.001**   Unspecified injury of axillary artery, right side
        ● **S45.002**   Unspecified injury of axillary artery, left side
        ● **S45.009**   Unspecified injury of axillary artery, unspecified side
    ● **S45.01** Laceration of axillary artery
        ● **S45.011**   Laceration of axillary artery, right side
        ● **S45.012**   Laceration of axillary artery, left side
        ● **S45.019**   Laceration of axillary artery, unspecified side
    ● **S45.09** Other specified injury of axillary artery
        ● **S45.091**   Other specified injury of axillary artery, right side
        ● **S45.092**   Other specified injury of axillary artery, left side
        ● **S45.099**   Other specified injury of axillary artery, unspecified side
● **S45.1** Injury of brachial artery
    ● **S45.10** Unspecified injury of brachial artery
        ● **S45.101**   Unspecified injury of brachial artery, right side
        ● **S45.102**   Unspecified injury of brachial artery, left side
        ● **S45.109**   Unspecified injury of brachial artery, unspecified side
    ● **S45.11** Laceration of brachial artery
        ● **S45.111**   Laceration of brachial artery, right side
        ● **S45.112**   Laceration of brachial artery, left side
        ● **S45.119**   Laceration of brachial artery, unspecified side

- S45.19 Other specified injury of brachial artery
  - S45.191 Other specified injury of brachial artery, right side
  - S45.192 Other specified injury of brachial artery, left side
  - S45.199 Other specified injury of brachial artery, unspecified side
- S45.2 Injury of axillary or brachial vein
  - S45.20 Unspecified injury of axillary or brachial vein
    - S45.201 Unspecified injury of axillary or brachial vein, right side
    - S45.202 Unspecified injury of axillary or brachial vein, left side
    - S45.209 Unspecified injury of axillary or brachial vein, unspecified side
  - S45.21 Laceration of axillary or brachial vein
    - S45.211 Laceration of axillary or brachial vein, right side
    - S45.212 Laceration of axillary or brachial vein, left side
    - S45.219 Laceration of axillary or brachial vein, unspecified side
  - S45.29 Other specified injury of axillary or brachial vein
    - S45.291 Other specified injury of axillary or brachial vein, right side
    - S45.292 Other specified injury of axillary or brachial vein, left side
    - S45.299 Other specified injury of axillary or brachial vein, unspecified side
- S45.3 Injury of superficial vein at shoulder and upper arm level
  - S45.30 Unspecified injury of superficial vein at shoulder and upper arm level
    - S45.301 Unspecified injury of superficial vein at shoulder and upper arm level, right arm
    - S45.302 Unspecified injury of superficial vein at shoulder and upper arm level, left arm
    - S45.309 Unspecified injury of superficial vein at shoulder and upper arm level, unspecified arm
  - S45.31 Laceration of superficial vein at shoulder and upper arm level
    - S45.311 Laceration of superficial vein at shoulder and upper arm level, right arm
    - S45.312 Laceration of superficial vein at shoulder and upper arm level, left arm
    - S45.319 Laceration of superficial vein at shoulder and upper arm level, unspecified arm
  - S45.39 Other specified injury of superficial vein at shoulder and upper arm level
    - S45.391 Other specified injury of superficial vein at shoulder and upper arm level, right arm
    - S45.392 Other specified injury of superficial vein at shoulder and upper arm level, left arm
    - S45.399 Other specified injury of superficial vein at shoulder and upper arm level, unspecified arm

- S45.8 Injury of other specified blood vessels at shoulder and upper arm level
  - S45.80 Unspecified injury of other specified blood vessels at shoulder and upper arm level
    - S45.801 Unspecified injury of other specified blood vessels at shoulder and upper arm level, right arm
    - S45.802 Unspecified injury of other specified blood vessels at shoulder and upper arm level, left arm
    - S45.809 Unspecified injury of other specified blood vessels at shoulder and upper arm level, unspecified arm
  - S45.81 Laceration of other specified blood vessels at shoulder and upper arm level
    - S45.811 Laceration of other specified blood vessels at shoulder and upper arm level, right arm
    - S45.812 Laceration of other specified blood vessels at shoulder and upper arm level, left arm
    - S45.819 Laceration of other specified blood vessels at shoulder and upper arm level, unspecified arm
  - S45.89 Other specified injury of other specified blood vessels at shoulder and upper arm level
    - S45.891 Other specified injury of other specified blood vessels at shoulder and upper arm level, right arm
    - S45.892 Other specified injury of other specified blood vessels at shoulder and upper arm level, left arm
    - S45.899 Other specified injury of other specified blood vessels at shoulder and upper arm level, unspecified arm
- S45.9 Injury of unspecified blood vessel at shoulder and upper arm level
  - S45.90 Unspecified injury of unspecified blood vessel at shoulder and upper arm level
    - S45.901 Unspecified injury of unspecified blood vessel at shoulder and upper arm level, right arm
    - S45.902 Unspecified injury of unspecified blood vessel at shoulder and upper arm level, left arm
    - S45.909 Unspecified injury of unspecified blood vessel at shoulder and upper arm level, unspecified arm
  - S45.91 Laceration of unspecified blood vessel at shoulder and upper arm level
    - S45.911 Laceration of unspecified blood vessel at shoulder and upper arm level, right arm
    - S45.912 Laceration of unspecified blood vessel at shoulder and upper arm level, left arm
    - S45.919 Laceration of unspecified blood vessel at shoulder and upper arm level, unspecified arm
  - S45.99 Other specified injury of unspecified blood vessel at shoulder and upper arm level
    - S45.991 Other specified injury of unspecified blood vessel at shoulder and upper arm level, right arm
    - S45.992 Other specified injury of unspecified blood vessel at shoulder and upper arm level, left arm
    - S45.999 Other specified injury of unspecified blood vessel at shoulder and upper arm level, unspecified arm

CHAPTER 19 (S00-T88)

▶ New ⇒ Revised ~~deleted~~ Deleted Excludes 1 Excludes 2 Includes Use additional Code first Code also Key words

OGCR Official Guidelines X Assign placeholder X ● Use Additional Character(s) ⟩ Manifestation Code 🝳 Hierarchical Condition Category Coding Clinic

●S46   Injury of muscle, fascia and tendon at shoulder and upper arm level
> Code also any associated open wound (S41.-)
>> **Excludes2**   injury of muscle, fascia and tendon at elbow (S56.-)
>>   sprain of joints and ligaments of shoulder girdle (S43.9)
> The appropriate 7th character is to be added to each code from category S46

A	initial encounter
D	subsequent encounter
S	sequela

●S46.0   Injury of muscle(s) and tendon(s) of the rotator cuff of shoulder

    ●S46.00   Unspecified injury of muscle(s) and tendon(s) of the rotator cuff of shoulder

       ●S46.001   Unspecified injury of muscle(s) and tendon(s) of the rotator cuff of right shoulder

       ●S46.002   Unspecified injury of muscle(s) and tendon(s) of the rotator cuff of left shoulder

       ●S46.009   Unspecified injury of muscle(s) and tendon(s) of the rotator cuff of unspecified shoulder

    ●S46.01   Strain of muscle(s) and tendon(s) of the rotator cuff of shoulder
> *Acute onset due to trauma to rotator cuff muscle/tendon*

       ●S46.011   Strain of muscle(s) and tendon(s) of the rotator cuff of right shoulder

       ●S46.012   Strain of muscle(s) and tendon(s) of the rotator cuff of left shoulder

       ●S46.019   Strain of muscle(s) and tendon(s) of the rotator cuff of unspecified shoulder

    ●S46.02   Laceration of muscle(s) and tendon(s) of the rotator cuff of shoulder

       ●S46.021   Laceration of muscle(s) and tendon(s) of the rotator cuff of right shoulder

       ●S46.022   Laceration of muscle(s) and tendon(s) of the rotator cuff of left shoulder

       ●S46.029   Laceration of muscle(s) and tendon(s) of the rotator cuff of unspecified shoulder

    ●S46.09   Other injury of muscle(s) and tendon(s) of the rotator cuff of shoulder

       ●S46.091   Other injury of muscle(s) and tendon(s) of the rotator cuff of right shoulder

       ●S46.092   Other injury of muscle(s) and tendon(s) of the rotator cuff of left shoulder

       ●S46.099   Other injury of muscle(s) and tendon(s) of the rotator cuff of unspecified shoulder

●S46.1   Injury of muscle, fascia and tendon of long head of biceps

    ●S46.10   Unspecified injury of muscle, fascia and tendon of long head of biceps

       ●S46.101   Unspecified injury of muscle, fascia and tendon of long head of biceps, right arm

       ●S46.102   Unspecified injury of muscle, fascia and tendon of long head of biceps, left arm

       ●S46.109   Unspecified injury of muscle, fascia and tendon of long head of biceps, unspecified arm

    ●S46.11   Strain of muscle, fascia and tendon of long head of biceps
> **Coding Clinic: 2019, Q2, P27**

       ●S46.111   Strain of muscle, fascia and tendon of long head of biceps, right arm

       ●S46.112   Strain of muscle, fascia and tendon of long head of biceps, left arm

       ●S46.119   Strain of muscle, fascia and tendon of long head of biceps, unspecified arm

    ●S46.12   Laceration of muscle, fascia and tendon of long head of biceps

       ●S46.121   Laceration of muscle, fascia and tendon of long head of biceps, right arm

       ●S46.122   Laceration of muscle, fascia and tendon of long head of biceps, left arm

       ●S46.129   Laceration of muscle, fascia and tendon of long head of biceps, unspecified arm

    ●S46.19   Other injury of muscle, fascia and tendon of long head of biceps

       ●S46.191   Other injury of muscle, fascia and tendon of long head of biceps, right arm

       ●S46.192   Other injury of muscle, fascia and tendon of long head of biceps, left arm

       ●S46.199   Other injury of muscle, fascia and tendon of long head of biceps, unspecified arm

●S46.2   Injury of muscle, fascia and tendon of other parts of biceps

    ●S46.20   Unspecified injury of muscle, fascia and tendon of other parts of biceps

       ●S46.201   Unspecified injury of muscle, fascia and tendon of other parts of biceps, right arm

       ●S46.202   Unspecified injury of muscle, fascia and tendon of other parts of biceps, left arm

       ●S46.209   Unspecified injury of muscle, fascia and tendon of other parts of biceps, unspecified arm

    ●S46.21   Strain of muscle, fascia and tendon of other parts of biceps

       ●S46.211   Strain of muscle, fascia and tendon of other parts of biceps, right arm

       ●S46.212   Strain of muscle, fascia and tendon of other parts of biceps, left arm

       ●S46.219   Strain of muscle, fascia and tendon of other parts of biceps, unspecified arm

    ●S46.22   Laceration of muscle, fascia and tendon of other parts of biceps

       ●S46.221   Laceration of muscle, fascia and tendon of other parts of biceps, right arm

       ●S46.222   Laceration of muscle, fascia and tendon of other parts of biceps, left arm

       ●S46.229   Laceration of muscle, fascia and tendon of other parts of biceps, unspecified arm

    ●S46.29   Other injury of muscle, fascia and tendon of other parts of biceps

       ●S46.291   Other injury of muscle, fascia and tendon of other parts of biceps, right arm

       ●S46.292   Other injury of muscle, fascia and tendon of other parts of biceps, left arm

       ●S46.299   Other injury of muscle, fascia and tendon of other parts of biceps, unspecified arm

CHAPTER 19 (S00-T88)

- S46.3 Injury of muscle, fascia and tendon of triceps
  - S46.30 Unspecified injury of muscle, fascia and tendon of triceps
    - S46.301 Unspecified injury of muscle, fascia and tendon of triceps, right arm
    - S46.302 Unspecified injury of muscle, fascia and tendon of triceps, left arm
    - S46.309 Unspecified injury of muscle, fascia and tendon of triceps, unspecified arm
  - S46.31 Strain of muscle, fascia and tendon of triceps
    - S46.311 Strain of muscle, fascia and tendon of triceps, right arm
    - S46.312 Strain of muscle, fascia and tendon of triceps, left arm
    - S46.319 Strain of muscle, fascia and tendon of triceps, unspecified arm
  - S46.32 Laceration of muscle, fascia and tendon of triceps
    - S46.321 Laceration of muscle, fascia and tendon of triceps, right arm
    - S46.322 Laceration of muscle, fascia and tendon of triceps, left arm
    - S46.329 Laceration of muscle, fascia and tendon of triceps, unspecified arm
  - S46.39 Other injury of muscle, fascia and tendon of triceps
    - S46.391 Other injury of muscle, fascia and tendon of triceps, right arm
    - S46.392 Other injury of muscle, fascia and tendon of triceps, left arm
    - S46.399 Other injury of muscle, fascia and tendon of triceps, unspecified arm
- S46.8 Injury of other muscles, fascia and tendons at shoulder and upper arm level
  - S46.80 Unspecified injury of other muscles, fascia and tendons at shoulder and upper arm level
    - S46.801 Unspecified injury of other muscles, fascia and tendons at shoulder and upper arm level, right arm
    - S46.802 Unspecified injury of other muscles, fascia and tendons at shoulder and upper arm level, left arm
    - S46.809 Unspecified injury of other muscles, fascia and tendons at shoulder and upper arm level, unspecified arm
  - S46.81 Strain of other muscles, fascia and tendons at shoulder and upper arm level
    - S46.811 Strain of other muscles, fascia and tendons at shoulder and upper arm level, right arm
    - S46.812 Strain of other muscles, fascia and tendons at shoulder and upper arm level, left arm
    - S46.819 Strain of other muscles, fascia and tendons at shoulder and upper arm level, unspecified arm
  - S46.82 Laceration of other muscles, fascia and tendons at shoulder and upper arm level
    - S46.821 Laceration of other muscles, fascia and tendons at shoulder and upper arm level, right arm
    - S46.822 Laceration of other muscles, fascia and tendons at shoulder and upper arm level, left arm
    - S46.829 Laceration of other muscles, fascia and tendons at shoulder and upper arm level, unspecified arm

- S46.89 Other injury of other muscles, fascia and tendons at shoulder and upper arm level
  - S46.891 Other injury of other muscles, fascia and tendons at shoulder and upper arm level, right arm
  - S46.892 Other injury of other muscles, fascia and tendons at shoulder and upper arm level, left arm
  - S46.899 Other injury of other muscles, fascia and tendons at shoulder and upper arm level, unspecified arm
- S46.9 Injury of unspecified muscle, fascia and tendon at shoulder and upper arm level
  - S46.90 Unspecified injury of unspecified muscle, fascia and tendon at shoulder and upper arm level
    - S46.901 Unspecified injury of unspecified muscle, fascia and tendon at shoulder and upper arm level, right arm
    - S46.902 Unspecified injury of unspecified muscle, fascia and tendon at shoulder and upper arm level, left arm
    - S46.909 Unspecified injury of unspecified muscle, fascia and tendon at shoulder and upper arm level, unspecified arm
  - S46.91 Strain of unspecified muscle, fascia and tendon at shoulder and upper arm level
    - S46.911 Strain of unspecified muscle, fascia and tendon at shoulder and upper arm level, right arm
    - S46.912 Strain of unspecified muscle, fascia and tendon at shoulder and upper arm level, left arm
    - S46.919 Strain of unspecified muscle, fascia and tendon at shoulder and upper arm level, unspecified arm
  - S46.92 Laceration of unspecified muscle, fascia and tendon at shoulder and upper arm level
    - S46.921 Laceration of unspecified muscle, fascia and tendon at shoulder and upper arm level, right arm
    - S46.922 Laceration of unspecified muscle, fascia and tendon at shoulder and upper arm level, left arm
    - S46.929 Laceration of unspecified muscle, fascia and tendon at shoulder and upper arm level, unspecified arm
  - S46.99 Other injury of unspecified muscle, fascia and tendon at shoulder and upper arm level
    - S46.991 Other injury of unspecified muscle, fascia and tendon at shoulder and upper arm level, right arm
    - S46.992 Other injury of unspecified muscle, fascia and tendon at shoulder and upper arm level, left arm
    - S46.999 Other injury of unspecified muscle, fascia and tendon at shoulder and upper arm level, unspecified arm

▶ New   ⇒ Revised   ~~deleted~~ Deleted   Excludes 1   Excludes 2   Includes   Use additional   Code first   Code also   Key words

OGCR Official Guidelines   X Assign placeholder X   ● Use Additional Character(s)   ▶ Manifestation Code   🐾 Hierarchical Condition Category   Coding Clinic

● S47   **Crushing injury of shoulder and upper arm**
　　　　Use additional code for all associated injuries
　　　　Excludes2　crushing injury of elbow (S57.0-)
　　　　The appropriate 7th character is to be added to each code from
　　　　category S47

　　　　| A | initial encounter |
　　　　| D | subsequent encounter |
　　　　| S | sequela |

X ● **S47.1**　Crushing injury of right shoulder and upper arm
X ● **S47.2**　Crushing injury of left shoulder and upper arm
X ● **S47.9**　Crushing injury of shoulder and upper arm, unspecified
　　　　　　arm

● S48   **Traumatic amputation of shoulder and upper arm**
　　　　An amputation not identified as partial or complete should be
　　　　coded to complete
　　　　Excludes1　traumatic amputation at elbow level (S58.0)
　　　　The appropriate 7th character is to be added to each code from
　　　　category S48

　　　　| A | initial encounter |
　　　　| D | subsequent encounter |
　　　　| S | sequela |

● **S48.0**　**Traumatic amputation at shoulder joint**
　● **S48.01**　Complete traumatic amputation at shoulder
　　　　　　joint
　　● **S48.011**　Complete traumatic amputation at
　　　　　　　right shoulder joint A, S 🐾
　　● **S48.012**　Complete traumatic amputation at left
　　　　　　　shoulder joint A, S 🐾
　　● **S48.019**　Complete traumatic amputation at
　　　　　　　unspecified shoulder joint A, S 🐾
　● **S48.02**　Partial traumatic amputation at shoulder joint
　　● **S48.021**　Partial traumatic amputation at right
　　　　　　　shoulder joint A, S 🐾
　　● **S48.022**　Partial traumatic amputation at left
　　　　　　　shoulder joint A, S 🐾
　　● **S48.029**　Partial traumatic amputation at
　　　　　　　unspecified shoulder joint A, S 🐾
● **S48.1**　Traumatic amputation at level between shoulder and
　　　　elbow
　● **S48.11**　Complete traumatic amputation at level
　　　　　　between shoulder and elbow
　　● **S48.111**　Complete traumatic amputation at
　　　　　　　level between right shoulder and
　　　　　　　elbow A, S 🐾
　　● **S48.112**　Complete traumatic amputation at
　　　　　　　level between left shoulder and
　　　　　　　elbow A, S 🐾
　　● **S48.119**　Complete traumatic amputation at
　　　　　　　level between unspecified shoulder
　　　　　　　and elbow A, S 🐾
　● **S48.12**　Partial traumatic amputation at level between
　　　　　　shoulder and elbow
　　● **S48.121**　Partial traumatic amputation at level
　　　　　　　between right shoulder and elbow
　　　　　　　A, S 🐾
　　● **S48.122**　Partial traumatic amputation at level
　　　　　　　between left shoulder and elbow
　　　　　　　A, S 🐾
　　● **S48.129**　Partial traumatic amputation at level
　　　　　　　between unspecified shoulder and
　　　　　　　elbow A, S 🐾

● S48.9   **Traumatic amputation of shoulder and upper arm, level
　　　　unspecified**
　● **S48.91**　Complete traumatic amputation of shoulder
　　　　　　and upper arm, level unspecified
　　● **S48.911**　Complete traumatic amputation of
　　　　　　　right shoulder and upper arm, level
　　　　　　　unspecified A, S 🐾
　　● **S48.912**　Complete traumatic amputation of
　　　　　　　left shoulder and upper arm, level
　　　　　　　unspecified A, S 🐾
　　● **S48.919**　Complete traumatic amputation of
　　　　　　　unspecified shoulder and upper arm,
　　　　　　　level unspecified A, S 🐾
　● **S48.92**　Partial traumatic amputation of shoulder and
　　　　　　upper arm, level unspecified
　　● **S48.921**　Partial traumatic amputation of right
　　　　　　　shoulder and upper arm, level
　　　　　　　unspecified A, S 🐾
　　● **S48.922**　Partial traumatic amputation of left
　　　　　　　shoulder and upper arm, level
　　　　　　　unspecified A, S 🐾
　　● **S48.929**　Partial traumatic amputation of
　　　　　　　unspecified shoulder and upper
　　　　　　　arm, level unspecified A, S 🐾

● S49   **Other and unspecified injuries of shoulder and upper arm**
　　　　The appropriate 7th character is to be added to each code from
　　　　subcategories S49.0 and S49.1

　　　　| A | initial encounter for closed fracture |
　　　　| D | subsequent encounter for fracture with routine healing |
　　　　| G | subsequent encounter for fracture with delayed healing |
　　　　| K | subsequent encounter for fracture with nonunion |
　　　　| P | subsequent encounter for fracture with malunion |
　　　　| S | sequela |

● **S49.0**　Physeal fracture of upper end of humerus
　● **S49.00**　Unspecified physeal fracture of upper end of
　　　　　　humerus
　　● **S49.001**　Unspecified physeal fracture of upper
　　　　　　　end of humerus, right arm
　　● **S49.002**　Unspecified physeal fracture of upper
　　　　　　　end of humerus, left arm
　　● **S49.009**　Unspecified physeal fracture of upper
　　　　　　　end of humerus, unspecified arm
　● **S49.01**　Salter-Harris Type I physeal fracture of upper
　　　　　　end of humerus
　　● **S49.011**　Salter-Harris Type I physeal fracture
　　　　　　　of upper end of humerus, right arm
　　● **S49.012**　Salter-Harris Type I physeal fracture
　　　　　　　of upper end of humerus, left arm
　　● **S49.019**　Salter-Harris Type I physeal fracture
　　　　　　　of upper end of humerus, unspecified
　　　　　　　arm
　● **S49.02**　Salter-Harris Type II physeal fracture of upper
　　　　　　end of humerus
　　● **S49.021**　Salter-Harris Type II physeal fracture
　　　　　　　of upper end of humerus, right arm
　　● **S49.022**　Salter-Harris Type II physeal fracture
　　　　　　　of upper end of humerus, left arm
　　● **S49.029**　Salter-Harris Type II physeal fracture
　　　　　　　of upper end of humerus, unspecified
　　　　　　　arm
　● **S49.03**　Salter-Harris Type III physeal fracture of upper
　　　　　　end of humerus
　　● **S49.031**　Salter-Harris Type III physeal fracture
　　　　　　　of upper end of humerus, right arm
　　● **S49.032**　Salter-Harris Type III physeal fracture
　　　　　　　of upper end of humerus, left arm
　　● **S49.039**　Salter-Harris Type III physeal fracture
　　　　　　　of upper end of humerus, unspecified
　　　　　　　arm

CHAPTER 19 (S00–T88)

Item 19–3   SALTER-HARRIS TYPE 1: epiphysis is completely separated from end of bone, or metaphysic growth plate remains attached to epiphysis
  SALTER-HARRIS TYPE 2: epiphysis and growth plate are partially separated from metaphysis, which is cracked—most common type
  SALTER-HARRIS TYPE 3: fracture occurring through epiphysis and separates part of epiphysis and growth plate from metaphysis fracture, usually at distal end of tibia
  SALTER-HARRIS TYPE 4: fracture runs through epiphysis, across growth plate, into metaphysic, surgery is required to restore joint surface to normal and align growth plate

- ● S49.04   Salter-Harris Type IV physeal fracture of upper end of humerus
  - ● S49.041   Salter-Harris Type IV physeal fracture of upper end of humerus, **right** arm
  - ● S49.042   Salter-Harris Type IV physeal fracture of upper end of humerus, **left** arm
  - ● S49.049   Salter-Harris Type IV physeal fracture of upper end of humerus, **unspecified** arm
- ● S49.09   Other physeal fracture of upper end of humerus
  - ● S49.091   Other physeal fracture of upper end of humerus, **right** arm
  - ● S49.092   Other physeal fracture of upper end of humerus, **left** arm
  - ● S49.099   Other physeal fracture of upper end of humerus, **unspecified** arm
- ● S49.1   Physeal fracture of **lower** end of humerus
  - ● S49.10   Unspecified physeal fracture of lower end of humerus
    - ● S49.101   Unspecified physeal fracture of lower end of humerus, **right** arm
    - ● S49.102   Unspecified physeal fracture of lower end of humerus, **left** arm
    - ● S49.109   Unspecified physeal fracture of lower end of humerus, **unspecified** arm
  - ● S49.11   Salter-Harris Type I physeal fracture of lower end of humerus
    - ● S49.111   Salter-Harris Type I physeal fracture of lower end of humerus, **right** arm
    - ● S49.112   Salter-Harris Type I physeal fracture of lower end of humerus, **left** arm
    - ● S49.119   Salter-Harris Type I physeal fracture of lower end of humerus, **unspecified** arm
  - ● S49.12   Salter-Harris Type II physeal fracture of lower end of humerus
    - ● S49.121   Salter-Harris Type II physeal fracture of lower end of humerus, **right** arm
    - ● S49.122   Salter-Harris Type II physeal fracture of lower end of humerus, **left** arm
    - ● S49.129   Salter-Harris Type II physeal fracture of lower end of humerus, **unspecified** arm
  - ● S49.13   Salter-Harris Type III physeal fracture of lower end of humerus
    - ● S49.131   Salter-Harris Type III physeal fracture of lower end of humerus, **right** arm
    - ● S49.132   Salter-Harris Type III physeal fracture of lower end of humerus, **left** arm
    - ● S49.139   Salter-Harris Type III physeal fracture of lower end of humerus, **unspecified** arm

- ● S49.14   Salter-Harris Type IV physeal fracture of lower end of humerus
  - ● S49.141   Salter-Harris Type IV physeal fracture of lower end of humerus, **right** arm
  - ● S49.142   Salter-Harris Type IV physeal fracture of lower end of humerus, **left** arm
  - ● S49.149   Salter-Harris Type IV physeal fracture of lower end of humerus, **unspecified** arm
- ● S49.19   Other physeal fracture of lower end of humerus
  - ● S49.191   Other physeal fracture of lower end of humerus, **right** arm
  - ● S49.192   Other physeal fracture of lower end of humerus, **left** arm
  - ● S49.199   Other physeal fracture of lower end of humerus, **unspecified** arm
- ● S49.8   Other specified injuries of shoulder and upper arm
  The appropriate 7th character is to be added to each code in subcategory S49.8

A	initial encounter
D	subsequent encounter
S	sequela

  - X ● S49.80   Other specified injuries of shoulder and upper arm, **unspecified** arm
  - X ● S49.81   Other specified injuries of **right** shoulder and upper arm
  - X ● S49.82   Other specified injuries of **left** shoulder and upper arm
- ● S49.9   Unspecified injury of shoulder and upper arm
  The appropriate 7th character is to be added to each code in subcategory S49.9

A	initial encounter
D	subsequent encounter
S	sequela

  - X ● S49.90   Unspecified injury of shoulder and upper arm, **unspecified** arm
  - X ● S49.91   Unspecified injury of **right** shoulder and upper arm
  - X ● S49.92   Unspecified injury of **left** shoulder and upper arm

---

INJURIES TO THE ELBOW AND FOREARM (S50-S59)

Excludes2   burns and corrosions (T20-T32)
                frostbite (T33-T34)
                injuries of wrist and hand (S60-S69)
                insect bite or sting, venomous (T63.4)

- ● S50   Superficial injury of elbow and forearm
  Excludes2   superficial injury of wrist and hand (S60.-)
  The appropriate 7th character is to be added to each code from category S50

A	initial encounter
D	subsequent encounter
S	sequela

  - ● S50.0   Contusion of **elbow**
    - X ● S50.00   Contusion of **unspecified** elbow
    - X ● S50.01   Contusion of **right** elbow
    - X ● S50.02   Contusion of **left** elbow
  - ● S50.1   Contusion of **forearm**
    - X ● S50.10   Contusion of **unspecified** forearm
    - X ● S50.11   Contusion of **right** forearm
    - X ● S50.12   Contusion of **left** forearm

▶ New   ⇒ Revised   ~~deleted~~ Deleted   Excludes 1   Excludes 2   Includes   Use additional   Code first   Code also   Key words
OGCR Official Guidelines   X Assign placeholder X   ● Use Additional Character(s)   ▶ Manifestation Code   🦚 Hierarchical Condition Category   Coding Clinic

● **S50.3**   Other superficial injuries of elbow
   ● **S50.31**   Abrasion of elbow
     ● **S50.311**   Abrasion of right elbow
     ● **S50.312**   Abrasion of left elbow
     ● **S50.319**   Abrasion of unspecified elbow
   ● **S50.32**   Blister (nonthermal) of elbow
     ● **S50.321**   Blister (nonthermal) of right elbow
     ● **S50.322**   Blister (nonthermal) of left elbow
     ● **S50.329**   Blister (nonthermal) of unspecified elbow
   ● **S50.34**   External constriction of elbow
     ● **S50.341**   External constriction of right elbow
     ● **S50.342**   External constriction of left elbow
     ● **S50.349**   External constriction of unspecified elbow
   ● **S50.35**   Superficial foreign body of elbow
     Splinter in the elbow
     ● **S50.351**   Superficial foreign body of right elbow
     ● **S50.352**   Superficial foreign body of left elbow
     ● **S50.359**   Superficial foreign body of unspecified elbow
   ● **S50.36**   Insect bite (nonvenomous) of elbow
     ● **S50.361**   Insect bite (nonvenomous) of right elbow
     ● **S50.362**   Insect bite (nonvenomous) of left elbow
     ● **S50.369**   Insect bite (nonvenomous) of unspecified elbow
   ● **S50.37**   Other superficial bite of elbow
     Excludes1   open bite of elbow (S51.04)
     ● **S50.371**   Other superficial bite of right elbow
     ● **S50.372**   Other superficial bite of left elbow
     ● **S50.379**   Other superficial bite of unspecified elbow
● **S50.8**   Other superficial injuries of forearm
   ● **S50.81**   Abrasion of forearm
     ● **S50.811**   Abrasion of right forearm
     ● **S50.812**   Abrasion of left forearm
     ● **S50.819**   Abrasion of unspecified forearm
   ● **S50.82**   Blister (nonthermal) of forearm
     ● **S50.821**   Blister (nonthermal) of right forearm
     ● **S50.822**   Blister (nonthermal) of left forearm
     ● **S50.829**   Blister (nonthermal) of unspecified forearm
   ● **S50.84**   External constriction of forearm
     ● **S50.841**   External constriction of right forearm
     ● **S50.842**   External constriction of left forearm
     ● **S50.849**   External constriction of unspecified forearm
   ● **S50.85**   Superficial foreign body of forearm
     Splinter in the forearm
     ● **S50.851**   Superficial foreign body of right forearm
     ● **S50.852**   Superficial foreign body of left forearm
     ● **S50.859**   Superficial foreign body of unspecified forearm

● **S50.86**   Insect bite (nonvenomous) of forearm
     ● **S50.861**   Insect bite (nonvenomous) of right forearm
     ● **S50.862**   Insect bite (nonvenomous) of left forearm
     ● **S50.869**   Insect bite (nonvenomous) of unspecified forearm
   ● **S50.87**   Other superficial bite of forearm
     Excludes1   open bite of forearm (S51.84)
     ● **S50.871**   Other superficial bite of right forearm
     ● **S50.872**   Other superficial bite of left forearm
     ● **S50.879**   Other superficial bite of unspecified forearm
● **S50.9**   Unspecified superficial injury of elbow and forearm
   ● **S50.90**   Unspecified superficial injury of elbow
     ● **S50.901**   Unspecified superficial injury of right elbow
     ● **S50.902**   Unspecified superficial injury of left elbow
     ● **S50.909**   Unspecified superficial injury of unspecified elbow
   ● **S50.91**   Unspecified superficial injury of forearm
     ● **S50.911**   Unspecified superficial injury of right forearm
     ● **S50.912**   Unspecified superficial injury of left forearm
     ● **S50.919**   Unspecified superficial injury of unspecified forearm

● **S51**   Open wound of elbow and forearm
   Code also any associated wound infection
   Excludes1   open fracture of elbow and forearm (S52.- with open fracture 7th character)
           traumatic amputation of elbow and forearm (S58.-)
   Excludes2   open wound of wrist and hand (S61.-)
   The appropriate 7th character is to be added to each code from category S51

> A   initial encounter
> D   subsequent encounter
> S   sequela

   ● **S51.0**   Open wound of elbow
     ● **S51.00**   Unspecified open wound of elbow
       ● **S51.001**   Unspecified open wound of right elbow
         Coding Clinic: 2012, Q4, P108
       ● **S51.002**   Unspecified open wound of left elbow
       ● **S51.009**   Unspecified open wound of unspecified elbow
         Open wound of elbow NOS
     ● **S51.01**   Laceration without foreign body of elbow
       ● **S51.011**   Laceration without foreign body of right elbow
       ● **S51.012**   Laceration without foreign body of left elbow
       ● **S51.019**   Laceration without foreign body of unspecified elbow
     ● **S51.02**   Laceration with foreign body of elbow
       ● **S51.021**   Laceration with foreign body of right elbow
       ● **S51.022**   Laceration with foreign body of left elbow
       ● **S51.029**   Laceration with foreign body of unspecified elbow

● **S51.03**   **Puncture wound without foreign body of elbow**
    ● **S51.031**   **Puncture wound without foreign body of right elbow**
    ● **S51.032**   **Puncture wound without foreign body of left elbow**
    ● **S51.039**   **Puncture wound without foreign body of unspecified elbow**

● **S51.04**   **Puncture wound with foreign body of elbow**
    ● **S51.041**   **Puncture wound with foreign body of right elbow**
    ● **S51.042**   **Puncture wound with foreign body of left elbow**
    ● **S51.049**   **Puncture wound with foreign body of unspecified elbow**

● **S51.05**   **Open bite of elbow**
    Bite of elbow NOS
      Excludes1   superficial bite of elbow (S50.36, S50.37)
    ● **S51.051**   **Open bite, right elbow**
    ● **S51.052**   **Open bite, left elbow**
    ● **S51.059**   **Open bite, unspecified elbow**

● **S51.8**   **Open wound of forearm**
    Excludes2   open wound of elbow (S51.0-)

● **S51.80**   **Unspecified open wound of forearm**
    ● **S51.801**   **Unspecified open wound of right forearm**
    ● **S51.802**   **Unspecified open wound of left forearm**
    ● **S51.809**   **Unspecified open wound of unspecified forearm**
       Open wound of forearm NOS

● **S51.81**   **Laceration without foreign body of forearm**
    ● **S51.811**   **Laceration without foreign body of right forearm**
    ● **S51.812**   **Laceration without foreign body of left forearm**
    ● **S51.819**   **Laceration without foreign body of unspecified forearm**

● **S51.82**   **Laceration with foreign body of forearm**
    ● **S51.821**   **Laceration with foreign body of right forearm**
    ● **S51.822**   **Laceration with foreign body of left forearm**
    ● **S51.829**   **Laceration with foreign body of unspecified forearm**

● **S51.83**   **Puncture wound without foreign body of forearm**
    ● **S51.831**   **Puncture wound without foreign body of right forearm**
    ● **S51.832**   **Puncture wound without foreign body of left forearm**
    ● **S51.839**   **Puncture wound without foreign body of unspecified forearm**

● **S51.84**   **Puncture wound with foreign body of forearm**
    ● **S51.841**   **Puncture wound with foreign body of right forearm**
    ● **S51.842**   **Puncture wound with foreign body of left forearm**
    ● **S51.849**   **Puncture wound with foreign body of unspecified forearm**

● **S51.85**   **Open bite of forearm**
    Bite of forearm NOS
      Excludes1   superficial bite of forearm (S50.86, S50.87)
    ● **S51.851**   **Open bite of right forearm**
    ● **S51.852**   **Open bite of left forearm**
    ● **S51.859**   **Open bite of unspecified forearm**

● **S52**   **Fracture of forearm**
    Note: A fracture not identified as displaced or nondisplaced should be coded to displaced
      A fracture not designated as open or closed should be coded to closed
      The open fracture designations are based on the Gustilo open fracture classification
    Excludes1   traumatic amputation of forearm (S58.-)
    Excludes2   fracture at wrist and hand level (S62.-)
       periprosthetic fracture around internal prosthetic elbow joint (M97.4)

The appropriate 7th character is to be added to all codes from category S52

A	initial encounter for closed fracture
B	initial encounter for open fracture type I or II initial encounter for open fracture NOS
C	initial encounter for open fracture type IIIA, IIIB, or IIIC
D	subsequent encounter for closed fracture with routine healing
E	subsequent encounter for open fracture type I or II with routine healing
F	subsequent encounter for open fracture type IIIA, IIIB, or IIIC with routine healing
G	subsequent encounter for closed fracture with delayed healing
H	subsequent encounter for open fracture type I or II with delayed healing
J	subsequent encounter for open fracture type IIIA, IIIB, or IIIC with delayed healing
K	subsequent encounter for closed fracture with nonunion
M	subsequent encounter for open fracture type I or II with nonunion
N	subsequent encounter for open fracture type IIIA, IIIB, or IIIC with nonunion
P	subsequent encounter for closed fracture with malunion
Q	subsequent encounter for open fracture type I or II with malunion
R	subsequent encounter for open fracture type IIIA, IIIB, or IIIC with malunion
S	sequela

Coding Clinic: 2016, Q1, P33

● **S52.0**   **Fracture of upper end of ulna**
    Fracture of proximal end of ulna
    Excludes2   fracture of elbow NOS (S42.40-)
       fractures of shaft of ulna (S52.2-)

● **S52.00**   **Unspecified fracture of upper end of ulna**
    ● **S52.001**   **Unspecified fracture of upper end of right ulna**
    ● **S52.002**   **Unspecified fracture of upper end of left ulna**
    ● **S52.009**   **Unspecified fracture of upper end of unspecified ulna**

● **S52.01**   **Torus fracture of upper end of ulna**
    The appropriate 7th character is to be added to all codes in subcategory S52.01

A	initial encounter for closed fracture
D	subsequent encounter for fracture with routine healing
G	subsequent encounter for fracture with delayed healing
K	subsequent encounter for fracture with nonunion
P	subsequent encounter for fracture with malunion
S	sequela

▶ New   ⟰ Revised   ~~deleted~~ Deleted   Excludes 1   Excludes 2   Includes   Use additional   Code first   Code also   Key words

OGCR Official Guidelines   X Assign placeholder X   ● Use Additional Character(s)   ▶ Manifestation Code   🝔 Hierarchical Condition Category   **Coding Clinic**

● S52.011   Torus fracture of upper end of right ulna

● S52.012   Torus fracture of upper end of left ulna

● S52.019   Torus fracture of upper end of unspecified ulna

● S52.02   Fracture of olecranon process without intraarticular extension of ulna

　● S52.021   Displaced fracture of olecranon process without intraarticular extension of right ulna

　● S52.022   Displaced fracture of olecranon process without intraarticular extension of left ulna

　● S52.023   Displaced fracture of olecranon process without intraarticular extension of unspecified ulna

　● S52.024   Nondisplaced fracture of olecranon process without intraarticular extension of right ulna

　● S52.025   Nondisplaced fracture of olecranon process without intraarticular extension of left ulna

　● S52.026   Nondisplaced fracture of olecranon process without intraarticular extension of unspecified ulna

● S52.03   Fracture of olecranon process with intraarticular extension of ulna

　● S52.031   Displaced fracture of olecranon process with intraarticular extension of right ulna

　● S52.032   Displaced fracture of olecranon process with intraarticular extension of left ulna

　● S52.033   Displaced fracture of olecranon process with intraarticular extension of unspecified ulna

　● S52.034   Nondisplaced fracture of olecranon process with intraarticular extension of right ulna

　● S52.035   Nondisplaced fracture of olecranon process with intraarticular extension of left ulna

　● S52.036   Nondisplaced fracture of olecranon process with intraarticular extension of unspecified ulna

● S52.04   Fracture of coronoid process of ulna

　● S52.041   Displaced fracture of coronoid process of right ulna

　● S52.042   Displaced fracture of coronoid process of left ulna

　● S52.043   Displaced fracture of coronoid process of unspecified ulna

　● S52.044   Nondisplaced fracture of coronoid process of right ulna

　● S52.045   Nondisplaced fracture of coronoid process of left ulna

　● S52.046   Nondisplaced fracture of coronoid process of unspecified ulna

● S52.09   Other fracture of upper end of ulna

　● S52.091   Other fracture of upper end of right ulna

　● S52.092   Other fracture of upper end of left ulna

　● S52.099   Other fracture of upper end of unspecified ulna

● S52.1   Fracture of upper end of radius
Fracture of proximal end of radius

Excludes2　physeal fractures of upper end of radius (S59.2-)
　　　　　　　fracture of shaft of radius (S52.3-)

● S52.10   Unspecified fracture of upper end of radius

　● S52.101   Unspecified fracture of upper end of right radius

　● S52.102   Unspecified fracture of upper end of left radius

　● S52.109   Unspecified fracture of upper end of unspecified radius

● S52.11   Torus fracture of upper end of radius

The appropriate 7th character is to be added to all codes in subcategory S52.11

A	initial encounter for closed fracture
D	subsequent encounter for fracture with routine healing
G	subsequent encounter for fracture with delayed healing
K	subsequent encounter for fracture with nonunion
P	subsequent encounter for fracture with malunion
S	sequela

　● S52.111   Torus fracture of upper end of right radius

　● S52.112   Torus fracture of upper end of left radius

　● S52.119   Torus fracture of upper end of unspecified radius

● S52.12   Fracture of head of radius

　● S52.121   Displaced fracture of head of right radius

　● S52.122   Displaced fracture of head of left radius

　● S52.123   Displaced fracture of head of unspecified radius

　● S52.124   Nondisplaced fracture of head of right radius

　● S52.125   Nondisplaced fracture of head of left radius

　● S52.126   Nondisplaced fracture of head of unspecified radius

● S52.13   Fracture of neck of radius

　● S52.131   Displaced fracture of neck of right radius

　● S52.132   Displaced fracture of neck of left radius

　● S52.133   Displaced fracture of neck of unspecified radius

　● S52.134   Nondisplaced fracture of neck of right radius

　● S52.135   Nondisplaced fracture of neck of left radius

　● S52.136   Nondisplaced fracture of neck of unspecified radius

● S52.18   Other fracture of upper end of radius

　● S52.181   Other fracture of upper end of right radius

　● S52.182   Other fracture of upper end of left radius

　● S52.189   Other fracture of upper end of unspecified radius

- S52.2   Fracture of shaft of ulna
  - S52.20   Unspecified fracture of shaft of ulna
    Fracture of ulna NOS
    - S52.201   Unspecified fracture of shaft of right ulna
    - S52.202   Unspecified fracture of shaft of left ulna
    - S52.209   Unspecified fracture of shaft of unspecified ulna
  - S52.21   Greenstick fracture of shaft of ulna

    The appropriate 7th character is to be added to all codes in subcategory S52.21

A	initial encounter for closed fracture
D	subsequent encounter for fracture with routine healing
G	subsequent encounter for fracture with delayed healing
K	subsequent encounter for fracture with nonunion
P	subsequent encounter for fracture with malunion
S	sequela

    - S52.211   Greenstick fracture of shaft of right ulna
    - S52.212   Greenstick fracture of shaft of left ulna
    - S52.219   Greenstick fracture of shaft of unspecified ulna
  - S52.22   Transverse fracture of shaft of ulna
    - S52.221   Displaced transverse fracture of shaft of right ulna
    - S52.222   Displaced transverse fracture of shaft of left ulna
    - S52.223   Displaced transverse fracture of shaft of unspecified ulna
    - S52.224   Nondisplaced transverse fracture of shaft of right ulna
    - S52.225   Nondisplaced transverse fracture of shaft of left ulna
    - S52.226   Nondisplaced transverse fracture of shaft of unspecified ulna
  - S52.23   Oblique fracture of shaft of ulna
    - S52.231   Displaced oblique fracture of shaft of right ulna
    - S52.232   Displaced oblique fracture of shaft of left ulna
    - S52.233   Displaced oblique fracture of shaft of unspecified ulna
    - S52.234   Nondisplaced oblique fracture of shaft of right ulna
    - S52.235   Nondisplaced oblique fracture of shaft of left ulna
    - S52.236   Nondisplaced oblique fracture of shaft of unspecified ulna
  - S52.24   Spiral fracture of shaft of ulna
    - S52.241   Displaced spiral fracture of shaft of ulna, right arm
    - S52.242   Displaced spiral fracture of shaft of ulna, left arm
    - S52.243   Displaced spiral fracture of shaft of ulna, unspecified arm
    - S52.244   Nondisplaced spiral fracture of shaft of ulna, right arm
    - S52.245   Nondisplaced spiral fracture of shaft of ulna, left arm
    - S52.246   Nondisplaced spiral fracture of shaft of ulna, unspecified arm

- S52.25   Comminuted fracture of shaft of ulna
  - S52.251   Displaced comminuted fracture of shaft of ulna, right arm
  - S52.252   Displaced comminuted fracture of shaft of ulna, left arm
  - S52.253   Displaced comminuted fracture of shaft of ulna, unspecified arm
  - S52.254   Nondisplaced comminuted fracture of shaft of ulna, right arm
  - S52.255   Nondisplaced comminuted fracture of shaft of ulna, left arm
  - S52.256   Nondisplaced comminuted fracture of shaft of ulna, unspecified arm
- S52.26   Segmental fracture of shaft of ulna
  - S52.261   Displaced segmental fracture of shaft of ulna, right arm
  - S52.262   Displaced segmental fracture of shaft of ulna, left arm
  - S52.263   Displaced segmental fracture of shaft of ulna, unspecified arm
  - S52.264   Nondisplaced segmental fracture of shaft of ulna, right arm
  - S52.265   Nondisplaced segmental fracture of shaft of ulna, left arm
  - S52.266   Nondisplaced segmental fracture of shaft of ulna, unspecified arm
- S52.27   Monteggia's fracture of ulna
  Fracture of upper shaft of ulna with dislocation of radial head
  - S52.271   Monteggia's fracture of right ulna
  - S52.272   Monteggia's fracture of left ulna
  - S52.279   Monteggia's fracture of unspecified ulna
- S52.28   Bent bone of ulna
  - S52.281   Bent bone of right ulna
  - S52.282   Bent bone of left ulna
  - S52.283   Bent bone of unspecified ulna
- S52.29   Other fracture of shaft of ulna
  - S52.291   Other fracture of shaft of right ulna
  - S52.292   Other fracture of shaft of left ulna
  - S52.299   Other fracture of shaft of unspecified ulna
- S52.3   Fracture of shaft of radius
  - S52.30   Unspecified fracture of shaft of radius
    - S52.301   Unspecified fracture of shaft of right radius
    - S52.302   Unspecified fracture of shaft of left radius
    - S52.309   Unspecified fracture of shaft of unspecified radius
  - S52.31   Greenstick fracture of shaft of radius

    The appropriate 7th character is to be added to all codes in subcategory S52.31

A	initial encounter for closed fracture
D	subsequent encounter for fracture with routine healing
G	subsequent encounter for fracture with delayed healing
K	subsequent encounter for fracture with nonunion
P	subsequent encounter for fracture with malunion
S	sequela

    - S52.311   Greenstick fracture of shaft of radius, right arm

▶ New   ⇛ Revised   deleted Deleted   Excludes 1   Excludes 2   Includes   Use additional   Code first   Code also   Key words

OGCR Official Guidelines   X Assign placeholder X   ● Use Additional Character(s)   ▶ Manifestation Code   🆑 Hierarchical Condition Category   Coding Clinic

● S52.312   Greenstick fracture of shaft of radius, left arm
● S52.319   Greenstick fracture of shaft of radius, unspecified arm
● S52.32   Transverse fracture of shaft of radius
● S52.321   Displaced transverse fracture of shaft of right radius
● S52.322   Displaced transverse fracture of shaft of left radius
● S52.323   Displaced transverse fracture of shaft of unspecified radius
● S52.324   Nondisplaced transverse fracture of shaft of right radius
● S52.325   Nondisplaced transverse fracture of shaft of left radius
● S52.326   Nondisplaced transverse fracture of shaft of unspecified radius
● S52.33   Oblique fracture of shaft of radius
● S52.331   Displaced oblique fracture of shaft of right radius
● S52.332   Displaced oblique fracture of shaft of left radius
● S52.333   Displaced oblique fracture of shaft of unspecified radius
● S52.334   Nondisplaced oblique fracture of shaft of right radius
● S52.335   Nondisplaced oblique fracture of shaft of left radius
● S52.336   Nondisplaced oblique fracture of shaft of unspecified radius
● S52.34   Spiral fracture of shaft of radius
● S52.341   Displaced spiral fracture of shaft of radius, right arm
● S52.342   Displaced spiral fracture of shaft of radius, left arm
● S52.343   Displaced spiral fracture of shaft of radius, unspecified arm
● S52.344   Nondisplaced spiral fracture of shaft of radius, right arm
● S52.345   Nondisplaced spiral fracture of shaft of radius, left arm
● S52.346   Nondisplaced spiral fracture of shaft of radius, unspecified arm
● S52.35   Comminuted fracture of shaft of radius
● S52.351   Displaced comminuted fracture of shaft of radius, right arm
● S52.352   Displaced comminuted fracture of shaft of radius, left arm
● S52.353   Displaced comminuted fracture of shaft of radius, unspecified arm
● S52.354   Nondisplaced comminuted fracture of shaft of radius, right arm
● S52.355   Nondisplaced comminuted fracture of shaft of radius, left arm
● S52.356   Nondisplaced comminuted fracture of shaft of radius, unspecified arm
● S52.36   Segmental fracture of shaft of radius
● S52.361   Displaced segmental fracture of shaft of radius, right arm
● S52.362   Displaced segmental fracture of shaft of radius, left arm
● S52.363   Displaced segmental fracture of shaft of radius, unspecified arm
● S52.364   Nondisplaced segmental fracture of shaft of radius, right arm
● S52.365   Nondisplaced segmental fracture of shaft of radius, left arm
● S52.366   Nondisplaced segmental fracture of shaft of radius, unspecified arm

● S52.37   Galeazzi's fracture
        Fracture of lower shaft of radius with radioulnar joint dislocation
● S52.371   Galeazzi's fracture of right radius
● S52.372   Galeazzi's fracture of left radius
● S52.379   Galeazzi's fracture of unspecified radius
● S52.38   Bent bone of radius
● S52.381   Bent bone of right radius
● S52.382   Bent bone of left radius
● S52.389   Bent bone of unspecified radius
● S52.39   Other fracture of shaft of radius
● S52.391   Other fracture of shaft of radius, right arm
● S52.392   Other fracture of shaft of radius, left arm
● S52.399   Other fracture of shaft of radius, unspecified arm
● S52.5   Fracture of lower end of radius
        Fracture of distal end of radius
        Excludes2   physeal fractures of lower end of radius (S59.2-)
● S52.50   Unspecified fracture of the lower end of radius
● S52.501   Unspecified fracture of the lower end of right radius
● S52.502   Unspecified fracture of the lower end of left radius
● S52.509   Unspecified fracture of the lower end of unspecified radius
● S52.51   Fracture of radial styloid process
● S52.511   Displaced fracture of right radial styloid process
● S52.512   Displaced fracture of left radial styloid process
● S52.513   Displaced fracture of unspecified radial styloid process
● S52.514   Nondisplaced fracture of right radial styloid process
● S52.515   Nondisplaced fracture of left radial styloid process
● S52.516   Nondisplaced fracture of unspecified radial styloid process
● S52.52   Torus fracture of lower end of radius
        The appropriate 7th character is to be added to all codes in subcategory S52.52

A	initial encounter for closed fracture
D	subsequent encounter for fracture with routine healing
G	subsequent encounter for fracture with delayed healing
K	subsequent encounter for fracture with nonunion
P	subsequent encounter for fracture with malunion
S	sequela

● S52.521   Torus fracture of lower end of right radius
● S52.522   Torus fracture of lower end of left radius
● S52.529   Torus fracture of lower end of unspecified radius
● S52.53   Colles' fracture
● S52.531   Colles' fracture of right radius
● S52.532   Colles' fracture of left radius
        Coding Clinic: 2016, Q2, P5
● S52.539   Colles' fracture of unspecified radius

CHAPTER 19 (SØØ-T88)

● S52.54   **Smith's fracture**
- ● S52.541   Smith's fracture of right radius
- ● S52.542   Smith's fracture of left radius
- ● S52.549   Smith's fracture of unspecified radius

● S52.55   **Other extraarticular fracture of lower end of radius**
- ● S52.551   Other extraarticular fracture of lower end of right radius
- ● S52.552   Other extraarticular fracture of lower end of left radius
- ● S52.559   Other extraarticular fracture of lower end of unspecified radius
- ● S52.56   Barton's fracture
- ● S52.561   Barton's fracture of right radius
- ● S52.562   Barton's fracture of left radius
- ● S52.569   Barton's fracture of unspecified radius

● S52.57   **Other intraarticular fracture of lower end of radius**
- ● S52.571   Other intraarticular fracture of lower end of right radius
- ● S52.572   Other intraarticular fracture of lower end of left radius
- ● S52.579   Other intraarticular fracture of lower end of unspecified radius
- ● S52.59   Other fractures of lower end of radius
- ● S52.591   Other fractures of lower end of right radius
  > **Coding Clinic: 2019, Q3, P10**
- ● S52.592   Other fractures of lower end of left radius
- ● S52.599   Other fractures of lower end of unspecified radius
- ● S52.6   Fracture of lower end of ulna

● S52.60   **Unspecified fracture of lower end of ulna**
- ● S52.601   Unspecified fracture of lower end of right ulna
- ● S52.602   Unspecified fracture of lower end of left ulna
- ● S52.609   Unspecified fracture of lower end of unspecified ulna
- ● S52.61   Fracture of ulna styloid process
- ● S52.611   Displaced fracture of right ulna styloid process
- ● S52.612   Displaced fracture of left ulna styloid process
- ● S52.613   Displaced fracture of unspecified ulna styloid process
- ● S52.614   Nondisplaced fracture of right ulna styloid process
- ● S52.615   Nondisplaced fracture of left ulna styloid process
- ● S52.616   Nondisplaced fracture of unspecified ulna styloid process
- ● S52.62   Torus fracture of lower end of ulna

The appropriate 7th character is to be added to all codes in subcategory S52.62

A	initial encounter for closed fracture
D	subsequent encounter for fracture with routine healing
G	subsequent encounter for fracture with delayed healing
K	subsequent encounter for fracture with nonunion
P	subsequent encounter for fracture with malunion
S	sequela

- ● S52.621   Torus fracture of lower end of right ulna
- ● S52.622   Torus fracture of lower end of left ulna
- ● S52.629   Torus fracture of lower end of unspecified ulna
- ● S52.69   Other fracture of lower end of ulna
- ● S52.691   Other fracture of lower end of right ulna
  > **Coding Clinic: 2019, Q3, P10**
- ● S52.692   Other fracture of lower end of left ulna
- ● S52.699   Other fracture of lower end of unspecified ulna
- ● S52.9   Unspecified fracture of forearm

X ● S52.90   Unspecified fracture of unspecified forearm
X ● S52.91   Unspecified fracture of right forearm
X ● S52.92   Unspecified fracture of left forearm

● S53   **Dislocation and sprain of joints and ligaments of elbow**

Includes   avulsion of joint or ligament of elbow
laceration of cartilage, joint or ligament of elbow
sprain of cartilage, joint or ligament of elbow
traumatic hemarthrosis of joint or ligament of elbow
traumatic rupture of joint or ligament of elbow
traumatic subluxation of joint or ligament of elbow
traumatic tear of joint or ligament of elbow

Code also any associated open wound

Excludes2   strain of muscle, fascia and tendon at forearm level (S56.-)

The appropriate 7th character is to be added to each code from category S53

A	initial encounter
D	subsequent encounter
S	sequela

● S53.0   **Subluxation and dislocation of radial head**
Dislocation of radiohumeral joint
Subluxation of radiohumeral joint

Excludes1   Monteggia's fracture-dislocation (S52.27-)

- ● S53.00   Unspecified subluxation and dislocation of radial head
- ● S53.001   Unspecified subluxation of right radial head
- ● S53.002   Unspecified subluxation of left radial head
- ● S53.003   Unspecified subluxation of unspecified radial head
- ● S53.004   Unspecified dislocation of right radial head
- ● S53.005   Unspecified dislocation of left radial head
- ● S53.006   Unspecified dislocation of unspecified radial head

● S53.01   **Anterior subluxation and dislocation of radial head**
Anteriomedial subluxation and dislocation of radial head
- ● S53.011   Anterior subluxation of right radial head
- ● S53.012   Anterior subluxation of left radial head
- ● S53.013   Anterior subluxation of unspecified radial head
- ● S53.014   Anterior dislocation of right radial head
- ● S53.015   Anterior dislocation of left radial head
- ● S53.016   Anterior dislocation of unspecified radial head

● S53.02   Posterior subluxation and dislocation of radial head
   Posteriolateral subluxation and dislocation of radial head

 ● S53.021   Posterior subluxation of right radial head

 ● S53.022   Posterior subluxation of left radial head

 ● S53.023   Posterior subluxation of unspecified radial head

 ● S53.024   Posterior dislocation of right radial head

 ● S53.025   Posterior dislocation of left radial head

 ● S53.026   Posterior dislocation of unspecified radial head

● S53.03   Nursemaid's elbow

 ● S53.031   Nursemaid's elbow, right elbow
    Coding Clinic: 2015, Q1, P7-8

 ● S53.032   Nursemaid's elbow, left elbow

 ● S53.033   Nursemaid's elbow, unspecified elbow

● S53.09   Other subluxation and dislocation of radial head

 ● S53.091   Other subluxation of right radial head

 ● S53.092   Other subluxation of left radial head

 ● S53.093   Other subluxation of unspecified radial head

 ● S53.094   Other dislocation of right radial head

 ● S53.095   Other dislocation of left radial head

 ● S53.096   Other dislocation of unspecified radial head

● S53.1   Subluxation and dislocation of ulnohumeral joint
  Subluxation and dislocation of elbow NOS

  Excludes1 dislocation of radial head alone (S53.0-)

● S53.10   Unspecified subluxation and dislocation of ulnohumeral joint

 ● S53.101   Unspecified subluxation of right ulnohumeral joint

 ● S53.102   Unspecified subluxation of left ulnohumeral joint

 ● S53.103   Unspecified subluxation of unspecified ulnohumeral joint

 ● S53.104   Unspecified dislocation of right ulnohumeral joint

 ● S53.105   Unspecified dislocation of left ulnohumeral joint

 ● S53.106   Unspecified dislocation of unspecified ulnohumeral joint

● S53.11   Anterior subluxation and dislocation of ulnohumeral joint

 ● S53.111   Anterior subluxation of right ulnohumeral joint

 ● S53.112   Anterior subluxation of left ulnohumeral joint

 ● S53.113   Anterior subluxation of unspecified ulnohumeral joint

 ● S53.114   Anterior dislocation of right ulnohumeral joint
    Coding Clinic: 2012, Q4, P108

 ● S53.115   Anterior dislocation of left ulnohumeral joint

 ● S53.116   Anterior dislocation of unspecified ulnohumeral joint

● S53.12   Posterior subluxation and dislocation of ulnohumeral joint

 ● S53.121   Posterior subluxation of right ulnohumeral joint

 ● S53.122   Posterior subluxation of left ulnohumeral joint

 ● S53.123   Posterior subluxation of unspecified ulnohumeral joint

 ● S53.124   Posterior dislocation of right ulnohumeral joint

 ● S53.125   Posterior dislocation of left ulnohumeral joint

 ● S53.126   Posterior dislocation of unspecified ulnohumeral joint

● S53.13   Medial subluxation and dislocation of ulnohumeral joint

 ● S53.131   Medial subluxation of right ulnohumeral joint

 ● S53.132   Medial subluxation of left ulnohumeral joint

 ● S53.133   Medial subluxation of unspecified ulnohumeral joint

 ● S53.134   Medial dislocation of right ulnohumeral joint

 ● S53.135   Medial dislocation of left ulnohumeral joint

 ● S53.136   Medial dislocation of unspecified ulnohumeral joint

● S53.14   Lateral subluxation and dislocation of ulnohumeral joint

 ● S53.141   Lateral subluxation of right ulnohumeral joint

 ● S53.142   Lateral subluxation of left ulnohumeral joint

 ● S53.143   Lateral subluxation of unspecified ulnohumeral joint

 ● S53.144   Lateral dislocation of right ulnohumeral joint

 ● S53.145   Lateral dislocation of left ulnohumeral joint

 ● S53.146   Lateral dislocation of unspecified ulnohumeral joint

● S53.19   Other subluxation and dislocation of ulnohumeral joint

 ● S53.191   Other subluxation of right ulnohumeral joint

 ● S53.192   Other subluxation of left ulnohumeral joint

 ● S53.193   Other subluxation of unspecified ulnohumeral joint

 ● S53.194   Other dislocation of right ulnohumeral joint

 ● S53.195   Other dislocation of left ulnohumeral joint

 ● S53.196   Other dislocation of unspecified ulnohumeral joint

● S53.2   Traumatic rupture of radial collateral ligament

  Excludes1 sprain of radial collateral ligament NOS (S53.43-)

X ● S53.20   Traumatic rupture of unspecified radial collateral ligament

X ● S53.21   Traumatic rupture of right radial collateral ligament

X ● S53.22   Traumatic rupture of left radial collateral ligament

● S53.3   Traumatic rupture of ulnar collateral ligament

  Excludes1 sprain of ulnar collateral ligament (S53.44-)

X ● S53.30   Traumatic rupture of unspecified ulnar collateral ligament

X ● S53.31   Traumatic rupture of right ulnar collateral ligament

X ● S53.32   Traumatic rupture of left ulnar collateral ligament

CHAPTER 19 (S00-T88)

● **S53.4 Sprain of elbow**
> **Excludes2**   traumatic rupture of radial collateral ligament (S53.2-)
> traumatic rupture of ulnar collateral ligament (S53.3-)

   ● **S53.40 Unspecified sprain of elbow**
     ● **S53.401** Unspecified sprain of right elbow
     ● **S53.402** Unspecified sprain of left elbow
     ● **S53.409** Unspecified sprain of unspecified elbow
       Sprain of elbow NOS

   ● **S53.41 Radiohumeral (joint) sprain**
     ● **S53.411** Radiohumeral (joint) sprain of right elbow
     ● **S53.412** Radiohumeral (joint) sprain of left elbow
     ● **S53.419** Radiohumeral (joint) sprain of unspecified elbow

   ● **S53.42 Ulnohumeral (joint) sprain**
     ● **S53.421** Ulnohumeral (joint) sprain of right elbow
     ● **S53.422** Ulnohumeral (joint) sprain of left elbow
     ● **S53.429** Ulnohumeral (joint) sprain of unspecified elbow

   ● **S53.43 Radial collateral ligament sprain**
     ● **S53.431** Radial collateral ligament sprain of right elbow
     ● **S53.432** Radial collateral ligament sprain of left elbow
     ● **S53.439** Radial collateral ligament sprain of unspecified elbow

   ● **S53.44 Ulnar collateral ligament sprain**
     ● **S53.441** Ulnar collateral ligament sprain of right elbow
     ● **S53.442** Ulnar collateral ligament sprain of left elbow
     ● **S53.449** Ulnar collateral ligament sprain of unspecified elbow

   ● **S53.49 Other sprain of elbow**
     ● **S53.491** Other sprain of right elbow
     ● **S53.492** Other sprain of left elbow
     ● **S53.499** Other sprain of unspecified elbow

● **S54 Injury of nerves at forearm level**
> Code also any associated open wound (S51.-)
> **Excludes2**   injury of nerves at wrist and hand level (S64.-)

> The appropriate 7th character is to be added to each code from category S54

> | | |
> |---|---|
> | A | initial encounter |
> | D | subsequent encounter |
> | S | sequela |

● **S54.0 Injury of ulnar nerve at forearm level**
   Injury of ulnar nerve NOS
   X ● **S54.00** Injury of ulnar nerve at forearm level, unspecified arm
   X ● **S54.01** Injury of ulnar nerve at forearm level, right arm
   X ● **S54.02** Injury of ulnar nerve at forearm level, left arm

● **S54.1 Injury of median nerve at forearm level**
   Injury of median nerve NOS
   X ● **S54.10** Injury of median nerve at forearm level, unspecified arm
   X ● **S54.11** Injury of median nerve at forearm level, right arm
   X ● **S54.12** Injury of median nerve at forearm level, left arm

● **S54.2 Injury of radial nerve at forearm level**
   Injury of radial nerve NOS
   X ● **S54.20** Injury of radial nerve at forearm level, unspecified arm
   X ● **S54.21** Injury of radial nerve at forearm level, right arm
   X ● **S54.22** Injury of radial nerve at forearm level, left arm

● **S54.3 Injury of cutaneous sensory nerve at forearm level**
   X ● **S54.30** Injury of cutaneous sensory nerve at forearm level, unspecified arm
   X ● **S54.31** Injury of cutaneous sensory nerve at forearm level, right arm
   X ● **S54.32** Injury of cutaneous sensory nerve at forearm level, left arm

● **S54.8 Injury of other nerves at forearm level**
   ● **S54.8X** Injury of other nerves at forearm level
     ● **S54.8X1** Injury of other nerves at forearm level, right arm
     ● **S54.8X2** Injury of other nerves at forearm level, left arm
     ● **S54.8X9** Injury of other nerves at forearm level, unspecified arm

● **S54.9 Injury of unspecified nerve at forearm level**
   X ● **S54.90** Injury of unspecified nerve at forearm level, unspecified arm
   X ● **S54.91** Injury of unspecified nerve at forearm level, right arm
   X ● **S54.92** Injury of unspecified nerve at forearm level, left arm

● **S55 Injury of blood vessels at forearm level**
> Code also any associated open wound (S51.-)
> **Excludes2**   injury of blood vessels at wrist and hand level (S65.-)
> injury of brachial vessels (S45.1-S45.2)

> The appropriate 7th character is to be added to each code from category S55

> | | |
> |---|---|
> | A | initial encounter |
> | D | subsequent encounter |
> | S | sequela |

● **S55.0 Injury of ulnar artery at forearm level**
   ● **S55.00 Unspecified injury of ulnar artery at forearm level**
     ● **S55.001** Unspecified injury of ulnar artery at forearm level, right arm
     ● **S55.002** Unspecified injury of ulnar artery at forearm level, left arm
     ● **S55.009** Unspecified injury of ulnar artery at forearm level, unspecified arm

   ● **S55.01 Laceration of ulnar artery at forearm level**
     ● **S55.011** Laceration of ulnar artery at forearm level, right arm
     ● **S55.012** Laceration of ulnar artery at forearm level, left arm
     ● **S55.019** Laceration of ulnar artery at forearm level, unspecified arm

   ● **S55.09 Other specified injury of ulnar artery at forearm level**
     ● **S55.091** Other specified injury of ulnar artery at forearm level, right arm
     ● **S55.092** Other specified injury of ulnar artery at forearm level, left arm
     ● **S55.099** Other specified injury of ulnar artery at forearm level, unspecified arm

▶ New   ⇒ Revised   ~~deleted~~ Deleted   Excludes 1   Excludes 2   Includes   Use additional   Code first   Code also   Key words

OGCR Official Guidelines   X Assign placeholder X   ● Use Additional Character(s)   ▶ Manifestation Code   ℞ Hierarchical Condition Category   **Coding Clinic**

● S55.1   Injury of radial artery at forearm level
    ● S55.10   Unspecified injury of radial artery at forearm level
        ● S55.101   Unspecified injury of radial artery at forearm level, right arm
        ● S55.102   Unspecified injury of radial artery at forearm level, left arm
        ● S55.109   Unspecified injury of radial artery at forearm level, unspecified arm
    ● S55.11   Laceration of radial artery at forearm level
        ● S55.111   Laceration of radial artery at forearm level, right arm
        ● S55.112   Laceration of radial artery at forearm level, left arm
        ● S55.119   Laceration of radial artery at forearm level, unspecified arm
    ● S55.19   Other specified injury of radial artery at forearm level
        ● S55.191   Other specified injury of radial artery at forearm level, right arm
        ● S55.192   Other specified injury of radial artery at forearm level, left arm
        ● S55.199   Other specified injury of radial artery at forearm level, unspecified arm
● S55.2   Injury of vein at forearm level
    ● S55.20   Unspecified injury of vein at forearm level
        ● S55.201   Unspecified injury of vein at forearm level, right arm
        ● S55.202   Unspecified injury of vein at forearm level, left arm
        ● S55.209   Unspecified injury of vein at forearm level, unspecified arm
    ● S55.21   Laceration of vein at forearm level
        ● S55.211   Laceration of vein at forearm level, right arm
        ● S55.212   Laceration of vein at forearm level, left arm
        ● S55.219   Laceration of vein at forearm level, unspecified arm
    ● S55.29   Other specified injury of vein at forearm level
        ● S55.291   Other specified injury of vein at forearm level, right arm
        ● S55.292   Other specified injury of vein at forearm level, left arm
        ● S55.299   Other specified injury of vein at forearm level, unspecified arm
    ● S55.8   Injury of other blood vessels at forearm level
    ● S55.80   Unspecified injury of other blood vessels at forearm level
        ● S55.801   Unspecified injury of other blood vessels at forearm level, right arm
        ● S55.802   Unspecified injury of other blood vessels at forearm level, left arm
        ● S55.809   Unspecified injury of other blood vessels at forearm level, unspecified arm
    ● S55.81   Laceration of other blood vessels at forearm level
        ● S55.811   Laceration of other blood vessels at forearm level, right arm
        ● S55.812   Laceration of other blood vessels at forearm level, left arm
        ● S55.819   Laceration of other blood vessels at forearm level, unspecified arm

    ● S55.89   Other specified injury of other blood vessels at forearm level
        ● S55.891   Other specified injury of other blood vessels at forearm level, right arm
        ● S55.892   Other specified injury of other blood vessels at forearm level, left arm
        ● S55.899   Other specified injury of other blood vessels at forearm level, unspecified arm
● S55.9   Injury of unspecified blood vessel at forearm level
    ● S55.90   Unspecified injury of unspecified blood vessel at forearm level
        ● S55.901   Unspecified injury of unspecified blood vessel at forearm level, right arm
        ● S55.902   Unspecified injury of unspecified blood vessel at forearm level, left arm
        ● S55.909   Unspecified injury of unspecified blood vessel at forearm level, unspecified arm
    ● S55.91   Laceration of unspecified blood vessel at forearm level
        ● S55.911   Laceration of unspecified blood vessel at forearm level, right arm
        ● S55.912   Laceration of unspecified blood vessel at forearm level, left arm
        ● S55.919   Laceration of unspecified blood vessel at forearm level, unspecified arm
    ● S55.99   Other specified injury of unspecified blood vessel at forearm level
        ● S55.991   Other specified injury of unspecified blood vessel at forearm level, right arm
        ● S55.992   Other specified injury of unspecified blood vessel at forearm level, left arm
        ● S55.999   Other specified injury of unspecified blood vessel at forearm level, unspecified arm
● S56   Injury of muscle, fascia and tendon at forearm level
    Code also any associated open wound (S51.-)
    Excludes2   injury of muscle, fascia and tendon at or below wrist (S66.-)
                     sprain of joints and ligaments of elbow (S53.4-)
    The appropriate 7th character is to be added to each code from category S56

    | A | initial encounter |
    | D | subsequent encounter |
    | S | sequela |

    ● S56.0   Injury of flexor muscle, fascia and tendon of thumb at forearm level
        ● S56.00   Unspecified injury of flexor muscle, fascia and tendon of thumb at forearm level
            ● S56.001   Unspecified injury of flexor muscle, fascia and tendon of right thumb at forearm level
            ● S56.002   Unspecified injury of flexor muscle, fascia and tendon of left thumb at forearm level
            ● S56.009   Unspecified injury of flexor muscle, fascia and tendon of unspecified thumb at forearm level

CHAPTER 19 (S00-T88)

● S56.01   Strain of flexor muscle, fascia and tendon of thumb at forearm level
- ● S56.011   Strain of flexor muscle, fascia and tendon of right thumb at forearm level
- ● S56.012   Strain of flexor muscle, fascia and tendon of left thumb at forearm level
- ● S56.019   Strain of flexor muscle, fascia and tendon of unspecified thumb at forearm level

● S56.02   Laceration of flexor muscle, fascia and tendon of thumb at forearm level
- ● S56.021   Laceration of flexor muscle, fascia and tendon of right thumb at forearm level
- ● S56.022   Laceration of flexor muscle, fascia and tendon of left thumb at forearm level
- ● S56.029   Laceration of flexor muscle, fascia and tendon of unspecified thumb at forearm level

● S56.09   Other injury of flexor muscle, fascia and tendon of thumb at forearm level
- ● S56.091   Other injury of flexor muscle, fascia and tendon of right thumb at forearm level
- ● S56.092   Other injury of flexor muscle, fascia and tendon of left thumb at forearm level
- ● S56.099   Other injury of flexor muscle, fascia and tendon of unspecified thumb at forearm level

● S56.1   Injury of flexor muscle, fascia and tendon of other and unspecified finger at forearm level

● S56.10   Unspecified injury of flexor muscle, fascia and tendon of other and unspecified finger at forearm level
- ● S56.101   Unspecified injury of flexor muscle, fascia and tendon of right index finger at forearm level
- ● S56.102   Unspecified injury of flexor muscle, fascia and tendon of left index finger at forearm level
- ● S56.103   Unspecified injury of flexor muscle, fascia and tendon of right middle finger at forearm level
- ● S56.104   Unspecified injury of flexor muscle, fascia and tendon of left middle finger at forearm level
- ● S56.105   Unspecified injury of flexor muscle, fascia and tendon of right ring finger at forearm level
- ● S56.106   Unspecified injury of flexor muscle, fascia and tendon of left ring finger at forearm level
- ● S56.107   Unspecified injury of flexor muscle, fascia and tendon of right little finger at forearm level
- ● S56.108   Unspecified injury of flexor muscle, fascia and tendon of left little finger at forearm level
- ● S56.109   Unspecified injury of flexor muscle, fascia and tendon of unspecified finger at forearm level

● S56.11   Strain of flexor muscle, fascia and tendon of other and unspecified finger at forearm level
- ● S56.111   Strain of flexor muscle, fascia and tendon of right index finger at forearm level
- ● S56.112   Strain of flexor muscle, fascia and tendon of left index finger at forearm level

- ● S56.113   Strain of flexor muscle, fascia and tendon of right middle finger at forearm level
- ● S56.114   Strain of flexor muscle, fascia and tendon of left middle finger at forearm level
- ● S56.115   Strain of flexor muscle, fascia and tendon of right ring finger at forearm level
- ● S56.116   Strain of flexor muscle, fascia and tendon of left ring finger at forearm level
- ● S56.117   Strain of flexor muscle, fascia and tendon of right little finger at forearm level
- ● S56.118   Strain of flexor muscle, fascia and tendon of left little finger at forearm level
- ● S56.119   Strain of flexor muscle, fascia and tendon of finger of unspecified finger at forearm level

● S56.12   Laceration of flexor muscle, fascia and tendon of other and unspecified finger at forearm level
- ● S56.121   Laceration of flexor muscle, fascia and tendon of right index finger at forearm level
- ● S56.122   Laceration of flexor muscle, fascia and tendon of left index finger at forearm level
- ● S56.123   Laceration of flexor muscle, fascia and tendon of right middle finger at forearm level
- ● S56.124   Laceration of flexor muscle, fascia and tendon of left middle finger at forearm level
- ● S56.125   Laceration of flexor muscle, fascia and tendon of right ring finger at forearm level
- ● S56.126   Laceration of flexor muscle, fascia and tendon of left ring finger at forearm level
- ● S56.127   Laceration of flexor muscle, fascia and tendon of right little finger at forearm level
- ● S56.128   Laceration of flexor muscle, fascia and tendon of left little finger at forearm level
- ● S56.129   Laceration of flexor muscle, fascia and tendon of unspecified finger at forearm level

● S56.19   Other injury of flexor muscle, fascia and tendon of other and unspecified finger at forearm level
- ● S56.191   Other injury of flexor muscle, fascia and tendon of right index finger at forearm level
- ● S56.192   Other injury of flexor muscle, fascia and tendon of left index finger at forearm level
- ● S56.193   Other injury of flexor muscle, fascia and tendon of right middle finger at forearm level
- ● S56.194   Other injury of flexor muscle, fascia and tendon of left middle finger at forearm level
- ● S56.195   Other injury of flexor muscle, fascia and tendon of right ring finger at forearm level
- ● S56.196   Other injury of flexor muscle, fascia and tendon of left ring finger at forearm level

▶ New   ⇒ Revised   ~~deleted~~ Deleted   Excludes 1   Excludes 2   Includes   Use additional   Code first   Code also   Key words

OGCR Official Guidelines   X Assign placeholder X   ● Use Additional Character(s)   ▷ Manifestation Code   🔖 Hierarchical Condition Category   **Coding Clinic**

- S56.197   Other injury of flexor muscle, fascia and tendon of right little finger at forearm level
- S56.198   Other injury of flexor muscle, fascia and tendon of left little finger at forearm level
- S56.199   Other injury of flexor muscle, fascia and tendon of unspecified finger at forearm level
- S56.2   Injury of other flexor muscle, fascia and tendon at forearm level
  - S56.20   Unspecified injury of other flexor muscle, fascia and tendon at forearm level
    - S56.201   Unspecified injury of other flexor muscle, fascia and tendon at forearm level, right arm
    - S56.202   Unspecified injury of other flexor muscle, fascia and tendon at forearm level, left arm
    - S56.209   Unspecified injury of other flexor muscle, fascia and tendon at forearm level, unspecified arm
  - S56.21   Strain of other flexor muscle, fascia and tendon at forearm level
    - S56.211   Strain of other flexor muscle, fascia and tendon at forearm level, right arm
    - S56.212   Strain of other flexor muscle, fascia and tendon at forearm level, left arm
    - S56.219   Strain of other flexor muscle, fascia and tendon at forearm level, unspecified arm
  - S56.22   Laceration of other flexor muscle, fascia and tendon at forearm level
    - S56.221   Laceration of other flexor muscle, fascia and tendon at forearm level, right arm
    - S56.222   Laceration of other flexor muscle, fascia and tendon at forearm level, left arm
    - S56.229   Laceration of other flexor muscle, fascia and tendon at forearm level, unspecified arm
  - S56.29   Other injury of other flexor muscle, fascia and tendon at forearm level
    - S56.291   Other injury of other flexor muscle, fascia and tendon at forearm level, right arm
    - S56.292   Other injury of other flexor muscle, fascia and tendon at forearm level, left arm
    - S56.299   Other injury of other flexor muscle, fascia and tendon at forearm level, unspecified arm
- S56.3   Injury of extensor or abductor muscles, fascia and tendons of thumb at forearm level
  - S56.30   Unspecified injury of extensor or abductor muscles, fascia and tendons of thumb at forearm level
    - S56.301   Unspecified injury of extensor or abductor muscles, fascia and tendons of right thumb at forearm level
    - S56.302   Unspecified injury of extensor or abductor muscles, fascia and tendons of left thumb at forearm level
    - S56.309   Unspecified injury of extensor or abductor muscles, fascia and tendons of unspecified thumb at forearm level

- S56.31   Strain of extensor or abductor muscles, fascia and tendons of thumb at forearm level
  - S56.311   Strain of extensor or abductor muscles, fascia and tendons of right thumb at forearm level
  - S56.312   Strain of extensor or abductor muscles, fascia and tendons of left thumb at forearm level
  - S56.319   Strain of extensor or abductor muscles, fascia and tendons of unspecified thumb at forearm level
- S56.32   Laceration of extensor or abductor muscles, fascia and tendons of thumb at forearm level
  - S56.321   Laceration of extensor or abductor muscles, fascia and tendons of right thumb at forearm level
  - S56.322   Laceration of extensor or abductor muscles, fascia and tendons of left thumb at forearm level
  - S56.329   Laceration of extensor or abductor muscles, fascia and tendons of unspecified thumb at forearm level
  - S56.39   Other injury of extensor or abductor muscles, fascia and tendons of thumb at forearm level
  - S56.391   Other injury of extensor or abductor muscles, fascia and tendons of right thumb at forearm level
  - S56.392   Other injury of extensor or abductor muscles, fascia and tendons of left thumb at forearm level
  - S56.399   Other injury of extensor or abductor muscles, fascia and tendons of unspecified thumb at forearm level
- S56.4   Injury of extensor muscle, fascia and tendon of other and unspecified finger at forearm level
  - S56.40   Unspecified injury of extensor muscle, fascia and tendon of other and unspecified finger at forearm level
    - S56.401   Unspecified injury of extensor muscle, fascia and tendon of right index finger at forearm level
    - S56.402   Unspecified injury of extensor muscle, fascia and tendon of left index finger at forearm level
    - S56.403   Unspecified injury of extensor muscle, fascia and tendon of right middle finger at forearm level
    - S56.404   Unspecified injury of extensor muscle, fascia and tendon of left middle finger at forearm level
    - S56.405   Unspecified injury of extensor muscle, fascia and tendon of right ring finger at forearm level
    - S56.406   Unspecified injury of extensor muscle, fascia and tendon of left ring finger at forearm level
    - S56.407   Unspecified injury of extensor muscle, fascia and tendon of right little finger at forearm level
    - S56.408   Unspecified injury of extensor muscle, fascia and tendon of left little finger at forearm level
    - S56.409   Unspecified injury of extensor muscle, fascia and tendon of unspecified finger at forearm level

● S56.41   **Strain** of extensor muscle, fascia and tendon of other and unspecified finger at forearm level

    ● S56.411   Strain of extensor muscle, fascia and tendon of right index finger at forearm level

    ● S56.412   Strain of extensor muscle, fascia and tendon of left index finger at forearm level

    ● S56.413   Strain of extensor muscle, fascia and tendon of right middle finger at forearm level

    ● S56.414   Strain of extensor muscle, fascia and tendon of left middle finger at forearm level

    ● S56.415   Strain of extensor muscle, fascia and tendon of right ring finger at forearm level

    ● S56.416   Strain of extensor muscle, fascia and tendon of left ring finger at forearm level

    ● S56.417   Strain of extensor muscle, fascia and tendon of right little finger at forearm level

    ● S56.418   Strain of extensor muscle, fascia and tendon of left little finger at forearm level

    ● S56.419   Strain of extensor muscle, fascia and tendon of finger, unspecified finger at forearm level

● S56.42   **Laceration** of extensor muscle, fascia and tendon of other and unspecified finger at forearm level

    ● S56.421   Laceration of extensor muscle, fascia and tendon of right index finger at forearm level

    ● S56.422   Laceration of extensor muscle, fascia and tendon of left index finger at forearm level

    ● S56.423   Laceration of extensor muscle, fascia and tendon of right middle finger at forearm level

    ● S56.424   Laceration of extensor muscle, fascia and tendon of left middle finger at forearm level

    ● S56.425   Laceration of extensor muscle, fascia and tendon of right ring finger at forearm level

    ● S56.426   Laceration of extensor muscle, fascia and tendon of left ring finger at forearm level

    ● S56.427   Laceration of extensor muscle, fascia and tendon of right little finger at forearm level

    ● S56.428   Laceration of extensor muscle, fascia and tendon of left little finger at forearm level

    ● S56.429   Laceration of extensor muscle, fascia and tendon of unspecified finger at forearm level

● S56.49   Other injury of extensor muscle, fascia and tendon of other and unspecified finger at forearm level

    ● S56.491   Other injury of extensor muscle, fascia and tendon of right index finger at forearm level

    ● S56.492   Other injury of extensor muscle, fascia and tendon of left index finger at forearm level

● S56.493   Other injury of extensor muscle, fascia and tendon of right middle finger at forearm level

● S56.494   Other injury of extensor muscle, fascia and tendon of left middle finger at forearm level

● S56.495   Other injury of extensor muscle, fascia and tendon of right ring finger at forearm level

● S56.496   Other injury of extensor muscle, fascia and tendon of left ring finger at forearm level

● S56.497   Other injury of extensor muscle, fascia and tendon of right little finger at forearm level

● S56.498   Other injury of extensor muscle, fascia and tendon of left little finger at forearm level

● S56.499   Other injury of extensor muscle, fascia and tendon of unspecified finger at forearm level

● S56.5   Injury of other extensor muscle, fascia and tendon at forearm level

    ● S56.50   Unspecified injury of other extensor muscle, fascia and tendon at forearm level

        ● S56.501   Unspecified injury of other extensor muscle, fascia and tendon at forearm level, right arm

        ● S56.502   Unspecified injury of other extensor muscle, fascia and tendon at forearm level, left arm

        ● S56.509   Unspecified injury of other extensor muscle, fascia and tendon at forearm level, unspecified arm

    ● S56.51   Strain of other extensor muscle, fascia and tendon at forearm level

        ● S56.511   Strain of other extensor muscle, fascia and tendon at forearm level, right arm

        ● S56.512   Strain of other extensor muscle, fascia and tendon at forearm level, left arm

        ● S56.519   Strain of other extensor muscle, fascia and tendon at forearm level, unspecified arm

    ● S56.52   Laceration of other extensor muscle, fascia and tendon at forearm level

        ● S56.521   Laceration of other extensor muscle, fascia and tendon at forearm level, right arm

        ● S56.522   Laceration of other extensor muscle, fascia and tendon at forearm level, left arm

        ● S56.529   Laceration of other extensor muscle, fascia and tendon at forearm level, unspecified arm

    ● S56.59   Other injury of other extensor muscle, fascia and tendon at forearm level

        ● S56.591   Other injury of other extensor muscle, fascia and tendon at forearm level, right arm

        ● S56.592   Other injury of other extensor muscle, fascia and tendon at forearm level, left arm

        ● S56.599   Other injury of other extensor muscle, fascia and tendon at forearm level, unspecified arm

▶ New   ⟾ Revised   ~~deleted~~ Deleted   Excludes 1   Excludes 2   Includes   Use additional   Code first   Code also   Key words

OGCR Official Guidelines   X Assign placeholder X   ● Use Additional Character(s)   ▶ Manifestation Code   Hierarchical Condition Category   **Coding Clinic**

● S56.8   Injury of other muscles, fascia and tendons at forearm level
- ● S56.80   Unspecified injury of other muscles, fascia and tendons at forearm level
  - ● S56.801   Unspecified injury of other muscles, fascia and tendons at forearm level, right arm
  - ● S56.802   Unspecified injury of other muscles, fascia and tendons at forearm level, left arm
  - ● S56.809   Unspecified injury of other muscles, fascia and tendons at forearm level, unspecified arm
- ● S56.81   Strain of other muscles, fascia and tendons at forearm level
  - ● S56.811   Strain of other muscles, fascia and tendons at forearm level, right arm
  - ● S56.812   Strain of other muscles, fascia and tendons at forearm level, left arm
  - ● S56.819   Strain of other muscles, fascia and tendons at forearm level, unspecified arm
- ● S56.82   Laceration of other muscles, fascia and tendons at forearm level
  - ● S56.821   Laceration of other muscles, fascia and tendons at forearm level, right arm
  - ● S56.822   Laceration of other muscles, fascia and tendons at forearm level, left arm
  - ● S56.829   Laceration of other muscles, fascia and tendons at forearm level, unspecified arm
- ● S56.89   Other injury of other muscles, fascia and tendons at forearm level
  - ● S56.891   Other injury of other muscles, fascia and tendons at forearm level, right arm
  - ● S56.892   Other injury of other muscles, fascia and tendons at forearm level, left arm
  - ● S56.899   Other injury of other muscles, fascia and tendons at forearm level, unspecified arm

● S56.9   Injury of unspecified muscles, fascia and tendons at forearm level
- ● S56.90   Unspecified injury of unspecified muscles, fascia and tendons at forearm level
  - ● S56.901   Unspecified injury of unspecified muscles, fascia and tendons at forearm level, right arm
  - ● S56.902   Unspecified injury of unspecified muscles, fascia and tendons at forearm level, left arm
  - ● S56.909   Unspecified injury of unspecified muscles, fascia and tendons at forearm level, unspecified arm
- ● S56.91   Strain of unspecified muscles, fascia and tendons at forearm level
  - ● S56.911   Strain of unspecified muscles, fascia and tendons at forearm level, right arm
  - ● S56.912   Strain of unspecified muscles, fascia and tendons at forearm level, left arm
  - ● S56.919   Strain of unspecified muscles, fascia and tendons at forearm level, unspecified arm

● S56.92   Laceration of unspecified muscles, fascia and tendons at forearm level
- ● S56.921   Laceration of unspecified muscles, fascia and tendons at forearm level, right arm
- ● S56.922   Laceration of unspecified muscles, fascia and tendons at forearm level, left arm
- ● S56.929   Laceration of unspecified muscles, fascia and tendons at forearm level, unspecified arm

● S56.99   Other injury of unspecified muscles, fascia and tendons at forearm level
- ● S56.991   Other injury of unspecified muscles, fascia and tendons at forearm level, right arm
- ● S56.992   Other injury of unspecified muscles, fascia and tendons at forearm level, left arm
- ● S56.999   Other injury of unspecified muscles, fascia and tendons at forearm level, unspecified arm

● S57   Crushing injury of elbow and forearm

Use additional code(s) for all associated injuries

Excludes2   crushing injury of wrist and hand (S67.-)

The appropriate 7th character is to be added to each code from category S57

A	initial encounter
D	subsequent encounter
S	sequela

- ● S57.0   Crushing injury of elbow
  - X ● S57.00   Crushing injury of unspecified elbow
  - X ● S57.01   Crushing injury of right elbow
  - X ● S57.02   Crushing injury of left elbow
- ● S57.8   Crushing injury of forearm
  - X ● S57.80   Crushing injury of unspecified forearm
  - X ● S57.81   Crushing injury of right forearm
  - X ● S57.82   Crushing injury of left forearm

● S58   Traumatic amputation of elbow and forearm

An amputation not identified as partial or complete should be coded to complete

Excludes1   traumatic amputation of wrist and hand (S68.-)

The appropriate 7th character is to be added to each code from category S58

A	initial encounter
D	subsequent encounter
S	sequela

- ● S58.0   Traumatic amputation at elbow level
  - ● S58.01   Complete traumatic amputation at elbow level
    - ● S58.011   Complete traumatic amputation at elbow level, right arm A, S 🔖
    - ● S58.012   Complete traumatic amputation at elbow level, left arm A, S 🔖
    - ● S58.019   Complete traumatic amputation at elbow level, unspecified arm A, S 🔖
  - ● S58.02   Partial traumatic amputation at elbow level
    - ● S58.021   Partial traumatic amputation at elbow level, right arm A, S 🔖
    - ● S58.022   Partial traumatic amputation at elbow level, left arm A, S 🔖
    - ● S58.029   Partial traumatic amputation at elbow level, unspecified arm A, S 🔖

- S58.1 Traumatic amputation at level between elbow and wrist
  - S58.11 Complete traumatic amputation at level between elbow and wrist
    - S58.111 Complete traumatic amputation at level between elbow and wrist, right arm A, S 🐾
    - S58.112 Complete traumatic amputation at level between elbow and wrist, left arm A, S 🐾
    - S58.119 Complete traumatic amputation at level between elbow and wrist, unspecified arm A, S 🐾
  - S58.12 Partial traumatic amputation at level between elbow and wrist
    - S58.121 Partial traumatic amputation at level between elbow and wrist, right arm A, S 🐾
    - S58.122 Partial traumatic amputation at level between elbow and wrist, left arm A, S 🐾
    - S58.129 Partial traumatic amputation at level between elbow and wrist, unspecified arm A, S 🐾
- S58.9 Traumatic amputation of forearm, level unspecified
  - Excludes1 traumatic amputation of wrist (S68.-)
  - S58.91 Complete traumatic amputation of forearm, level unspecified
    - S58.911 Complete traumatic amputation of right forearm, level unspecified A, S 🐾
    - S58.912 Complete traumatic amputation of left forearm, level unspecified A, S 🐾
    - S58.919 Complete traumatic amputation of unspecified forearm, level unspecified A, S 🐾
  - S58.92 Partial traumatic amputation of forearm, level unspecified
    - S58.921 Partial traumatic amputation of right forearm, level unspecified A, S 🐾
    - S58.922 Partial traumatic amputation of left forearm, level unspecified A, S 🐾
    - S58.929 Partial traumatic amputation of unspecified forearm, level unspecified A, S 🐾
- S59 Other and unspecified injuries of elbow and forearm
  - Excludes2 other and unspecified injuries of wrist and hand (S69.-)

  The appropriate 7th character is to be added to each code from subcategories S59.0, S59.1, and S59.2

A	initial encounter for closed fracture
D	subsequent encounter for fracture with routine healing
G	subsequent encounter for fracture with delayed healing
K	subsequent encounter for fracture with nonunion
P	subsequent encounter for fracture with malunion
S	sequela

- S59.0 Physeal fracture of lower end of ulna
  - S59.00 Unspecified physeal fracture of lower end of ulna
    - S59.001 Unspecified physeal fracture of lower end of ulna, right arm
    - S59.002 Unspecified physeal fracture of lower end of ulna, left arm
    - S59.009 Unspecified physeal fracture of lower end of ulna, unspecified arm

Item 19-4 SALTER-HARRIS TYPE 1: epiphysis is completely separated from end of bone, or metaphysic growth plate remains attached to epiphysis
  SALTER-HARRIS TYPE 2: epiphysis and growth plate are partially separated from metaphysis, which is cracked—most common type
  SALTER-HARRIS TYPE 3: fracture occurring through epiphysis and separates part of epiphysis and growth plate from metaphysis fracture, usually at distal end of tibia
  SALTER-HARRIS TYPE 4: fracture runs through epiphysis, across growth plate, into metaphysic, surgery is required to restore joint surface to normal and align growth plate

  - S59.01 Salter-Harris Type I physeal fracture of lower end of ulna
    - S59.011 Salter-Harris Type I physeal fracture of lower end of ulna, right arm
    - S59.012 Salter-Harris Type I physeal fracture of lower end of ulna, left arm
    - S59.019 Salter-Harris Type I physeal fracture of lower end of ulna, unspecified arm
  - S59.02 Salter-Harris Type II physeal fracture of lower end of ulna
    - S59.021 Salter-Harris Type II physeal fracture of lower end of ulna, right arm
    - S59.022 Salter-Harris Type II physeal fracture of lower end of ulna, left arm
    - S59.029 Salter-Harris Type II physeal fracture of lower end of ulna, unspecified arm
  - S59.03 Salter-Harris Type III physeal fracture of lower end of ulna
    - S59.031 Salter-Harris Type III physeal fracture of lower end of ulna, right arm
    - S59.032 Salter-Harris Type III physeal fracture of lower end of ulna, left arm
    - S59.039 Salter-Harris Type III physeal fracture of lower end of ulna, unspecified arm
  - S59.04 Salter-Harris Type IV physeal fracture of lower end of ulna
    - S59.041 Salter-Harris Type IV physeal fracture of lower end of ulna, right arm
    - S59.042 Salter-Harris Type IV physeal fracture of lower end of ulna, left arm
    - S59.049 Salter-Harris Type IV physeal fracture of lower end of ulna, unspecified arm
  - S59.09 Other physeal fracture of lower end of ulna
    - S59.091 Other physeal fracture of lower end of ulna, right arm
    - S59.092 Other physeal fracture of lower end of ulna, left arm
    - S59.099 Other physeal fracture of lower end of ulna, unspecified arm
- S59.1 Physeal fracture of upper end of radius
  - S59.10 Unspecified physeal fracture of upper end of radius
    - S59.101 Unspecified physeal fracture of upper end of radius, right arm
    - S59.102 Unspecified physeal fracture of upper end of radius, left arm
    - S59.109 Unspecified physeal fracture of upper end of radius, unspecified arm
  - S59.11 Salter-Harris Type I physeal fracture of upper end of radius
    - S59.111 Salter-Harris Type I physeal fracture of upper end of radius, right arm
    - S59.112 Salter-Harris Type I physeal fracture of upper end of radius, left arm
    - S59.119 Salter-Harris Type I physeal fracture of upper end of radius, unspecified arm

CHAPTER 19 (S00-T88)

● S59.12   Salter-Harris Type II physeal fracture of upper end of radius
     ● S59.121   Salter-Harris Type II physeal fracture of upper end of radius, right arm
     ● S59.122   Salter-Harris Type II physeal fracture of upper end of radius, left arm
     ● S59.129   Salter-Harris Type II physeal fracture of upper end of radius, unspecified arm

● S59.13   Salter-Harris Type III physeal fracture of upper end of radius
     ● S59.131   Salter-Harris Type III physeal fracture of upper end of radius, right arm
     ● S59.132   Salter-Harris Type III physeal fracture of upper end of radius, left arm
     ● S59.139   Salter-Harris Type III physeal fracture of upper end of radius, unspecified arm

● S59.14   Salter-Harris Type IV physeal fracture of upper end of radius
     ● S59.141   Salter-Harris Type IV physeal fracture of upper end of radius, right arm
     ● S59.142   Salter-Harris Type IV physeal fracture of upper end of radius, left arm
     ● S59.149   Salter-Harris Type IV physeal fracture of upper end of radius, unspecified arm

● S59.19   Other physeal fracture of upper end of radius
     ● S59.191   Other physeal fracture of upper end of radius, right arm
     ● S59.192   Other physeal fracture of upper end of radius, left arm
     ● S59.199   Other physeal fracture of upper end of radius, unspecified arm

● S59.2   Physeal fracture of lower end of radius
     ● S59.20   Unspecified physeal fracture of lower end of radius
         ● S59.201   Unspecified physeal fracture of lower end of radius, right arm
         ● S59.202   Unspecified physeal fracture of lower end of radius, left arm
         ● S59.209   Unspecified physeal fracture of lower end of radius, unspecified arm
     ● S59.21   Salter-Harris Type I physeal fracture of lower end of radius
         ● S59.211   Salter-Harris Type I physeal fracture of lower end of radius, right arm
         ● S59.212   Salter-Harris Type I physeal fracture of lower end of radius, left arm
         ● S59.219   Salter-Harris Type I physeal fracture of lower end of radius, unspecified arm
     ● S59.22   Salter-Harris Type II physeal fracture of lower end of radius
         ● S59.221   Salter-Harris Type II physeal fracture of lower end of radius, right arm
         ● S59.222   Salter-Harris Type II physeal fracture of lower end of radius, left arm
         ● S59.229   Salter-Harris Type II physeal fracture of lower end of radius, unspecified arm

● S59.23   Salter-Harris Type III physeal fracture of lower end of radius
     ● S59.231   Salter-Harris Type III physeal fracture of lower end of radius, right arm
     ● S59.232   Salter-Harris Type III physeal fracture of lower end of radius, left arm
     ● S59.239   Salter-Harris Type III physeal fracture of lower end of radius, unspecified arm

● S59.24   Salter-Harris Type IV physeal fracture of lower end of radius
     ● S59.241   Salter-Harris Type IV physeal fracture of lower end of radius, right arm
     ● S59.242   Salter-Harris Type IV physeal fracture of lower end of radius, left arm
     ● S59.249   Salter-Harris Type IV physeal fracture of lower end of radius, unspecified arm

● S59.29   Other physeal fracture of lower end of radius
     ● S59.291   Other physeal fracture of lower end of radius, right arm
     ● S59.292   Other physeal fracture of lower end of radius, left arm
     ● S59.299   Other physeal fracture of lower end of radius, unspecified arm

● S59.8   Other specified injuries of elbow and forearm

The appropriate 7th character is to be added to each code in subcategory S59.8

A	initial encounter
D	subsequent encounter
S	sequela

     ● S59.80   Other specified injuries of elbow
         ● S59.801   Other specified injuries of right elbow
         ● S59.802   Other specified injuries of left elbow
         ● S59.809   Other specified injuries of unspecified elbow
     ● S59.81   Other specified injuries of forearm
         ● S59.811   Other specified injuries right forearm
         ● S59.812   Other specified injuries left forearm
         ● S59.819   Other specified injuries unspecified forearm

● S59.9   Unspecified injury of elbow and forearm

The appropriate 7th character is to be added to each code in subcategory S59.9

A	initial encounter
D	subsequent encounter
S	sequela

     ● S59.90   Unspecified injury of elbow
         ● S59.901   Unspecified injury of right elbow
         ● S59.902   Unspecified injury of left elbow
         ● S59.909   Unspecified injury of unspecified elbow
     ● S59.91   Unspecified injury of forearm
         ● S59.911   Unspecified injury of right forearm
         ● S59.912   Unspecified injury of left forearm
         ● S59.919   Unspecified injury of unspecified forearm

CHAPTER 19 (S00-T88)

INJURIES TO THE WRIST, HAND AND FINGERS (S60-S69)

Excludes2   burns and corrosions (T20-T32)
frostbite (T33-T34)
insect bite or sting, venomous (T63.4)

● S60   **Superficial injury of wrist, hand and fingers**

The appropriate 7th character is to be added to each code from category S60

A	initial encounter
D	subsequent encounter
S	sequela

● S60.0   **Contusion of finger without damage to nail**

     Excludes1   contusion involving nail (matrix) (S60.1)

X ● S60.00   Contusion of unspecified finger without damage to nail
         Contusion of finger(s) NOS

● S60.01   Contusion of thumb without damage to nail

   ● S60.011   Contusion of right thumb without damage to nail

   ● S60.012   Contusion of left thumb without damage to nail

   ● S60.019   Contusion of unspecified thumb without damage to nail

● S60.02   Contusion of index finger without damage to nail

   ● S60.021   Contusion of right index finger without damage to nail

   ● S60.022   Contusion of left index finger without damage to nail

   ● S60.029   Contusion of unspecified index finger without damage to nail

● S60.03   Contusion of middle finger without damage to nail

   ● S60.031   Contusion of right middle finger without damage to nail

   ● S60.032   Contusion of left middle finger without damage to nail

   ● S60.039   Contusion of unspecified middle finger without damage to nail

● S60.04   Contusion of ring finger without damage to nail

   ● S60.041   Contusion of right ring finger without damage to nail

   ● S60.042   Contusion of left ring finger without damage to nail

   ● S60.049   Contusion of unspecified ring finger without damage to nail

● S60.05   Contusion of little finger without damage to nail

   ● S60.051   Contusion of right little finger without damage to nail

   ● S60.052   Contusion of left little finger without damage to nail

   ● S60.059   Contusion of unspecified little finger without damage to nail

● S60.1   **Contusion of finger with damage to nail**

X ● S60.10   Contusion of unspecified finger with damage to nail

● S60.11   Contusion of thumb with damage to nail

   ● S60.111   Contusion of right thumb with damage to nail

   ● S60.112   Contusion of left thumb with damage to nail

   ● S60.119   Contusion of unspecified thumb with damage to nail

● S60.12   Contusion of index finger with damage to nail

   ● S60.121   Contusion of right index finger with damage to nail

   ● S60.122   Contusion of left index finger with damage to nail

   ● S60.129   Contusion of unspecified index finger with damage to nail

● S60.13   Contusion of middle finger with damage to nail

   ● S60.131   Contusion of right middle finger with damage to nail

   ● S60.132   Contusion of left middle finger with damage to nail

   ● S60.139   Contusion of unspecified middle finger with damage to nail

● S60.14   Contusion of ring finger with damage to nail

   ● S60.141   Contusion of right ring finger with damage to nail

   ● S60.142   Contusion of left ring finger with damage to nail

   ● S60.149   Contusion of unspecified ring finger with damage to nail

● S60.15   Contusion of little finger with damage to nail

   ● S60.151   Contusion of right little finger with damage to nail

   ● S60.152   Contusion of left little finger with damage to nail

   ● S60.159   Contusion of unspecified little finger with damage to nail

● S60.2   **Contusion of wrist and hand**

     Excludes2   contusion of fingers (S60.0-, S60.1-)

● S60.21   Contusion of wrist

   ● S60.211   Contusion of right wrist

   ● S60.212   Contusion of left wrist

   ● S60.219   Contusion of unspecified wrist

● S60.22   Contusion of hand

   ● S60.221   Contusion of right hand

   ● S60.222   Contusion of left hand

   ● S60.229   Contusion of unspecified hand

● S60.3   **Other superficial injuries of thumb**

● S60.31   Abrasion of thumb

   ● S60.311   Abrasion of right thumb

   ● S60.312   Abrasion of left thumb

   ● S60.319   Abrasion of unspecified thumb

● S60.32   Blister (nonthermal) of thumb

   ● S60.321   Blister (nonthermal) of right thumb

   ● S60.322   Blister (nonthermal) of left thumb

   ● S60.329   Blister (nonthermal) of unspecified thumb

● S60.34   External constriction of thumb
     Hair tourniquet syndrome of thumb
     Use additional cause code to identify the constricting item (W49.0-)

   ● S60.341   External constriction of right thumb

   ● S60.342   External constriction of left thumb

   ● S60.349   External constriction of unspecified thumb

● S60.35   Superficial foreign body of thumb
     Splinter in the thumb

   ● S60.351   Superficial foreign body of right thumb

   ● S60.352   Superficial foreign body of left thumb

   ● S60.359   Superficial foreign body of unspecified thumb

▶ New   ⇥ Revised   ~~deleted~~ Deleted   Excludes 1   Excludes 2   Includes   Use additional   Code first   Code also   Key words

OGCR Official Guidelines   X Assign placeholder X   ● Use Additional Character(s)   ▶ Manifestation Code   Hierarchical Condition Category   Coding Clinic

● S60.36　Insect bite (nonvenomous) of thumb
　● S60.361　Insect bite (nonvenomous) of right thumb
　● S60.362　Insect bite (nonvenomous) of left thumb
　● S60.369　Insect bite (nonvenomous) of unspecified thumb
● S60.37　Other superficial bite of thumb
　　Excludes1　open bite of thumb (S61.05-, S61.15-)
　● S60.371　Other superficial bite of right thumb
　● S60.372　Other superficial bite of left thumb
　● S60.379　Other superficial bite of unspecified thumb
● S60.39　Other superficial injuries of thumb
　● S60.391　Other superficial injuries of right thumb
　● S60.392　Other superficial injuries of left thumb
　● S60.399　Other superficial injuries of unspecified thumb
● S60.4　Other superficial injuries of other fingers
　● S60.41　Abrasion of fingers
　　● S60.410　Abrasion of right index finger
　　● S60.411　Abrasion of left index finger
　　● S60.412　Abrasion of right middle finger
　　● S60.413　Abrasion of left middle finger
　　● S60.414　Abrasion of right ring finger
　　● S60.415　Abrasion of left ring finger
　　● S60.416　Abrasion of right little finger
　　● S60.417　Abrasion of left little finger
　　● S60.418　Abrasion of other finger
　　　　Abrasion of specified finger with unspecified laterality
　　● S60.419　Abrasion of unspecified finger
　● S60.42　Blister (nonthermal) of fingers
　　● S60.420　Blister (nonthermal) of right index finger
　　● S60.421　Blister (nonthermal) of left index finger
　　● S60.422　Blister (nonthermal) of right middle finger
　　● S60.423　Blister (nonthermal) of left middle finger
　　● S60.424　Blister (nonthermal) of right ring finger
　　● S60.425　Blister (nonthermal) of left ring finger
　　● S60.426　Blister (nonthermal) of right little finger
　　● S60.427　Blister (nonthermal) of left little finger
　　● S60.428　Blister (nonthermal) of other finger
　　　　Blister (nonthermal) of specified finger with unspecified laterality
　　● S60.429　Blister (nonthermal) of unspecified finger
　● S60.44　External constriction of fingers
　　　Hair tourniquet syndrome of finger
　　　Use additional cause code to identify the constricting item (W49.0-)
　　● S60.440　External constriction of right index finger
　　● S60.441　External constriction of left index finger
　　● S60.442　External constriction of right middle finger

● S60.443　External constriction of left middle finger
● S60.444　External constriction of right ring finger
● S60.445　External constriction of left ring finger
● S60.446　External constriction of right little finger
● S60.447　External constriction of left little finger
● S60.448　External constriction of other finger
　　External constriction of specified finger with unspecified laterality
● S60.449　External constriction of unspecified finger
● S60.45　Superficial foreign body of fingers
　　Splinter in the finger(s)
　● S60.450　Superficial foreign body of right index finger
　● S60.451　Superficial foreign body of left index finger
　● S60.452　Superficial foreign body of right middle finger
　● S60.453　Superficial foreign body of left middle finger
　● S60.454　Superficial foreign body of right ring finger
　● S60.455　Superficial foreign body of left ring finger
　● S60.456　Superficial foreign body of right little finger
　● S60.457　Superficial foreign body of left little finger
　● S60.458　Superficial foreign body of other finger
　　　Superficial foreign body of specified finger with unspecified laterality
　● S60.459　Superficial foreign body of unspecified finger
● S60.46　Insect bite (nonvenomous) of fingers
　● S60.460　Insect bite (nonvenomous) of right index finger
　● S60.461　Insect bite (nonvenomous) of left index finger
　● S60.462　Insect bite (nonvenomous) of right middle finger
　● S60.463　Insect bite (nonvenomous) of left middle finger
　● S60.464　Insect bite (nonvenomous) of right ring finger
　● S60.465　Insect bite (nonvenomous) of left ring finger
　● S60.466　Insect bite (nonvenomous) of right little finger
　● S60.467　Insect bite (nonvenomous) of left little finger
　● S60.468　Insect bite (nonvenomous) of other finger
　　　Insect bite (nonvenomous) of specified finger with unspecified laterality
　● S60.469　Insect bite (nonvenomous) of unspecified finger
● S60.47　Other superficial bite of fingers
　　Excludes1　open bite of fingers (S61.25-, S61.35-)
　● S60.470　Other superficial bite of right index finger
　● S60.471　Other superficial bite of left index finger

CHAPTER 19 (S00-T88)

● S60.472   Other superficial bite of right middle finger
● S60.473   Other superficial bite of left middle finger
● S60.474   Other superficial bite of right ring finger
● S60.475   Other superficial bite of left ring finger
● S60.476   Other superficial bite of right little finger
● S60.477   Other superficial bite of left little finger
● S60.478   Other superficial bite of other finger
    Other superficial bite of specified finger with unspecified laterality
● S60.479   Other superficial bite of unspecified finger

● S60.5   Other superficial injuries of hand
   Excludes2   superficial injuries of fingers (S60.3-, S60.4-)
● S60.51   Abrasion of hand
 ● S60.511   Abrasion of right hand
 ● S60.512   Abrasion of left hand
 ● S60.519   Abrasion of unspecified hand
● S60.52   Blister (nonthermal) of hand
 ● S60.521   Blister (nonthermal) of right hand
 ● S60.522   Blister (nonthermal) of left hand
 ● S60.529   Blister (nonthermal) of unspecified hand
● S60.54   External constriction of hand
 ● S60.541   External constriction of right hand
 ● S60.542   External constriction of left hand
 ● S60.549   External constriction of unspecified hand
● S60.55   Superficial foreign body of hand
   Splinter in the hand
 ● S60.551   Superficial foreign body of right hand
 ● S60.552   Superficial foreign body of left hand
 ● S60.559   Superficial foreign body of unspecified hand
● S60.56   Insect bite (nonvenomous) of hand
 ● S60.561   Insect bite (nonvenomous) of right hand
 ● S60.562   Insect bite (nonvenomous) of left hand
 ● S60.569   Insect bite (nonvenomous) of unspecified hand
● S60.57   Other superficial bite of hand
   Excludes1   open bite of hand (S61.45-)
 ● S60.571   Other superficial bite of hand of right hand
 ● S60.572   Other superficial bite of hand of left hand
 ● S60.579   Other superficial bite of hand of unspecified hand
● S60.8   Other superficial injuries of wrist
● S60.81   Abrasion of wrist
 ● S60.811   Abrasion of right wrist
 ● S60.812   Abrasion of left wrist
 ● S60.819   Abrasion of unspecified wrist
● S60.82   Blister (nonthermal) of wrist
 ● S60.821   Blister (nonthermal) of right wrist
 ● S60.822   Blister (nonthermal) of left wrist
 ● S60.829   Blister (nonthermal) of unspecified wrist

● S60.84   External constriction of wrist
 ● S60.841   External constriction of right wrist
 ● S60.842   External constriction of left wrist
 ● S60.849   External constriction of unspecified wrist
● S60.85   Superficial foreign body of wrist
   Splinter in the wrist
 ● S60.851   Superficial foreign body of right wrist
 ● S60.852   Superficial foreign body of left wrist
 ● S60.859   Superficial foreign body of unspecified wrist
● S60.86   Insect bite (nonvenomous) of wrist
 ● S60.861   Insect bite (nonvenomous) of right wrist
 ● S60.862   Insect bite (nonvenomous) of left wrist
 ● S60.869   Insect bite (nonvenomous) of unspecified wrist
● S60.87   Other superficial bite of wrist
   Excludes1   open bite of wrist (S61.55)
 ● S60.871   Other superficial bite of right wrist
 ● S60.872   Other superficial bite of left wrist
 ● S60.879   Other superficial bite of unspecified wrist
● S60.9   Unspecified superficial injury of wrist, hand and fingers
● S60.91   Unspecified superficial injury of wrist
 ● S60.911   Unspecified superficial injury of right wrist
 ● S60.912   Unspecified superficial injury of left wrist
 ● S60.919   Unspecified superficial injury of unspecified wrist
● S60.92   Unspecified superficial injury of hand
 ● S60.921   Unspecified superficial injury of right hand
 ● S60.922   Unspecified superficial injury of left hand
 ● S60.929   Unspecified superficial injury of unspecified hand
● S60.93   Unspecified superficial injury of thumb
 ● S60.931   Unspecified superficial injury of right thumb
 ● S60.932   Unspecified superficial injury of left thumb
 ● S60.939   Unspecified superficial injury of unspecified thumb
● S60.94   Unspecified superficial injury of other fingers
 ● S60.940   Unspecified superficial injury of right index finger
 ● S60.941   Unspecified superficial injury of left index finger
 ● S60.942   Unspecified superficial injury of right middle finger
 ● S60.943   Unspecified superficial injury of left middle finger
 ● S60.944   Unspecified superficial injury of right ring finger
 ● S60.945   Unspecified superficial injury of left ring finger
 ● S60.946   Unspecified superficial injury of right little finger
 ● S60.947   Unspecified superficial injury of left little finger
 ● S60.948   Unspecified superficial injury of other finger
    Unspecified superficial injury of specified finger with unspecified laterality
 ● S60.949   Unspecified superficial injury of unspecified finger

- S61   Open wound of wrist, hand and fingers

    Code also any associated wound infection

    Excludes1   open fracture of wrist, hand and finger (S62.- with 7th character B)

                traumatic amputation of wrist and hand (S68.-)

    The appropriate 7th character is to be added to each code from category S61

A	initial encounter
D	subsequent encounter
S	sequela

    - S61.0   Open wound of thumb without damage to nail

        Excludes1   open wound of thumb with damage to nail (S61.1-)

        - S61.00   Unspecified open wound of thumb without damage to nail

            - S61.001   Unspecified open wound of right thumb without damage to nail
            - S61.002   Unspecified open wound of left thumb without damage to nail
            - S61.009   Unspecified open wound of unspecified thumb without damage to nail

        - S61.01   Laceration without foreign body of thumb without damage to nail

            - S61.011   Laceration without foreign body of right thumb without damage to nail
            - S61.012   Laceration without foreign body of left thumb without damage to nail
            - S61.019   Laceration without foreign body of unspecified thumb without damage to nail

        - S61.02   Laceration with foreign body of thumb without damage to nail

            - S61.021   Laceration with foreign body of right thumb without damage to nail
            - S61.022   Laceration with foreign body of left thumb without damage to nail
            - S61.029   Laceration with foreign body of unspecified thumb without damage to nail

        - S61.03   Puncture wound without foreign body of thumb without damage to nail

            - S61.031   Puncture wound without foreign body of right thumb without damage to nail
            - S61.032   Puncture wound without foreign body of left thumb without damage to nail
            - S61.039   Puncture wound without foreign body of unspecified thumb without damage to nail

        - S61.04   Puncture wound with foreign body of thumb without damage to nail

            - S61.041   Puncture wound with foreign body of right thumb without damage to nail
            - S61.042   Puncture wound with foreign body of left thumb without damage to nail
            - S61.049   Puncture wound with foreign body of unspecified thumb without damage to nail

        - S61.05   Open bite of thumb without damage to nail

            Bite of thumb NOS

            Excludes1   superficial bite of thumb (S60.36-, S60.37-)

            - S61.051   Open bite of right thumb without damage to nail
            - S61.052   Open bite of left thumb without damage to nail
            - S61.059   Open bite of unspecified thumb without damage to nail

    - S61.1   Open wound of thumb with damage to nail

        - S61.10   Unspecified open wound of thumb with damage to nail

            - S61.101   Unspecified open wound of right thumb with damage to nail
            - S61.102   Unspecified open wound of left thumb with damage to nail
            - S61.109   Unspecified open wound of unspecified thumb with damage to nail

        - S61.11   Laceration without foreign body of thumb with damage to nail

            - S61.111   Laceration without foreign body of right thumb with damage to nail
            - S61.112   Laceration without foreign body of left thumb with damage to nail
            - S61.119   Laceration without foreign body of unspecified thumb with damage to nail

        - S61.12   Laceration with foreign body of thumb with damage to nail

            - S61.121   Laceration with foreign body of right thumb with damage to nail
            - S61.122   Laceration with foreign body of left thumb with damage to nail
            - S61.129   Laceration with foreign body of unspecified thumb with damage to nail

        - S61.13   Puncture wound without foreign body of thumb with damage to nail

            - S61.131   Puncture wound without foreign body of right thumb with damage to nail
            - S61.132   Puncture wound without foreign body of left thumb with damage to nail
            - S61.139   Puncture wound without foreign body of unspecified thumb with damage to nail

        - S61.14   Puncture wound with foreign body of thumb with damage to nail

            - S61.141   Puncture wound with foreign body of right thumb with damage to nail
            - S61.142   Puncture wound with foreign body of left thumb with damage to nail
            - S61.149   Puncture wound with foreign body of unspecified thumb with damage to nail

        - S61.15   Open bite of thumb with damage to nail

            Bite of thumb with damage to nail NOS

            Excludes1   superficial bite of thumb (S60.36-, S60.37-)

            - S61.151   Open bite of right thumb with damage to nail
            - S61.152   Open bite of left thumb with damage to nail
            - S61.159   Open bite of unspecified thumb with damage to nail

    - S61.2   Open wound of other finger without damage to nail

        Excludes1   open wound of finger involving nail (matrix) (S61.3-)

        Excludes2   open wound of thumb without damage to nail (S61.0-)

        - S61.20   Unspecified open wound of other finger without damage to nail

            - S61.200   Unspecified open wound of right index finger without damage to nail
            - S61.201   Unspecified open wound of left index finger without damage to nail
            - S61.202   Unspecified open wound of right middle finger without damage to nail

CHAPTER 19 (S00-T88)

● S61.203   Unspecified open wound of left middle finger without damage to nail

● S61.204   Unspecified open wound of right ring finger without damage to nail

● S61.205   Unspecified open wound of left ring finger without damage to nail

● S61.206   Unspecified open wound of right little finger without damage to nail

● S61.207   Unspecified open wound of left little finger without damage to nail

● S61.208   Unspecified open wound of other finger without damage to nail
          Unspecified open wound of specified finger with unspecified laterality without damage to nail

● S61.209   Unspecified open wound of unspecified finger without damage to nail

● S61.21   Laceration without foreign body of finger without damage to nail

● S61.210   Laceration without foreign body of right index finger without damage to nail

● S61.211   Laceration without foreign body of left index finger without damage to nail

● S61.212   Laceration without foreign body of right middle finger without damage to nail

● S61.213   Laceration without foreign body of left middle finger without damage to nail

● S61.214   Laceration without foreign body of right ring finger without damage to nail

● S61.215   Laceration without foreign body of left ring finger without damage to nail

● S61.216   Laceration without foreign body of right little finger without damage to nail

● S61.217   Laceration without foreign body of left little finger without damage to nail

● S61.218   Laceration without foreign body of other finger without damage to nail
          Laceration without foreign body of specified finger with unspecified laterality without damage to nail

● S61.219   Laceration without foreign body of unspecified finger without damage to nail

● S61.22   Laceration with foreign body of finger without damage to nail

● S61.220   Laceration with foreign body of right index finger without damage to nail

● S61.221   Laceration with foreign body of left index finger without damage to nail

● S61.222   Laceration with foreign body of right middle finger without damage to nail

● S61.223   Laceration with foreign body of left middle finger without damage to nail

● S61.224   Laceration with foreign body of right ring finger without damage to nail

● S61.225   Laceration with foreign body of left ring finger without damage to nail

● S61.226   Laceration with foreign body of right little finger without damage to nail

● S61.227   Laceration with foreign body of left little finger without damage to nail

● S61.228   Laceration with foreign body of other finger without damage to nail
          Laceration with foreign body of specified finger with unspecified laterality without damage to nail

● S61.229   Laceration with foreign body of unspecified finger without damage to nail

● S61.23   Puncture wound without foreign body of finger without damage to nail

● S61.230   Puncture wound without foreign body of right index finger without damage to nail

● S61.231   Puncture wound without foreign body of left index finger without damage to nail

● S61.232   Puncture wound without foreign body of right middle finger without damage to nail

● S61.233   Puncture wound without foreign body of left middle finger without damage to nail

● S61.234   Puncture wound without foreign body of right ring finger without damage to nail

● S61.235   Puncture wound without foreign body of left ring finger without damage to nail

● S61.236   Puncture wound without foreign body of right little finger without damage to nail

● S61.237   Puncture wound without foreign body of left little finger without damage to nail

● S61.238   Puncture wound without foreign body of other finger without damage to nail
          Puncture wound without foreign body of specified finger with unspecified laterality without damage to nail

● S61.239   Puncture wound without foreign body of unspecified finger without damage to nail

● S61.24   Puncture wound with foreign body of finger without damage to nail

● S61.240   Puncture wound with foreign body of right index finger without damage to nail

● S61.241   Puncture wound with foreign body of left index finger without damage to nail

● S61.242   Puncture wound with foreign body of right middle finger without damage to nail

● S61.243   Puncture wound with foreign body of left middle finger without damage to nail

● S61.244   Puncture wound with foreign body of right ring finger without damage to nail

● S61.245   Puncture wound with foreign body of left ring finger without damage to nail

● S61.246   Puncture wound with foreign body of right little finger without damage to nail

● S61.247   Puncture wound with foreign body of left little finger without damage to nail

▶ New   ⇒ Revised   ~~deleted~~ Deleted   Excludes 1   Excludes 2   Includes   Use additional   Code first   Code also   Key words

OGCR Official Guidelines   X Assign placeholder X   ● Use Additional Character(s)   ▷ Manifestation Code   🝔 Hierarchical Condition Category   Coding Clinic

● S61.248   Puncture wound with foreign body of other finger without damage to nail
  Puncture wound with foreign body of specified finger with unspecified laterality without damage to nail

● S61.249   Puncture wound with foreign body of unspecified finger without damage to nail

● S61.25   Open bite of finger without damage to nail
  Bite of finger without damage to nail NOS

  Excludes1 superficial bite of finger (S60.46-, S60.47-)

 ● S61.250   Open bite of right index finger without damage to nail

 ● S61.251   Open bite of left index finger without damage to nail

 ● S61.252   Open bite of right middle finger without damage to nail

 ● S61.253   Open bite of left middle finger without damage to nail

 ● S61.254   Open bite of right ring finger without damage to nail

 ● S61.255   Open bite of left ring finger without damage to nail

 ● S61.256   Open bite of right little finger without damage to nail

 ● S61.257   Open bite of left little finger without damage to nail

 ● S61.258   Open bite of other finger without damage to nail
   Open bite of specified finger with unspecified laterality without damage to nail

 ● S61.259   Open bite of unspecified finger without damage to nail

● S61.3   Open wound of other finger with damage to nail

 ● S61.30   Unspecified open wound of finger with damage to nail

  ● S61.300   Unspecified open wound of right index finger with damage to nail

  ● S61.301   Unspecified open wound of left index finger with damage to nail

  ● S61.302   Unspecified open wound of right middle finger with damage to nail

  ● S61.303   Unspecified open wound of left middle finger with damage to nail

  ● S61.304   Unspecified open wound of right ring finger with damage to nail

  ● S61.305   Unspecified open wound of left ring finger with damage to nail

  ● S61.306   Unspecified open wound of right little finger with damage to nail

  ● S61.307   Unspecified open wound of left little finger with damage to nail

  ● S61.308   Unspecified open wound of other finger with damage to nail
   Unspecified open wound of specified finger with unspecified laterality with damage to nail

  ● S61.309   Unspecified open wound of unspecified finger with damage to nail

 ● S61.31   Laceration without foreign body of finger with damage to nail

  ● S61.310   Laceration without foreign body of right index finger with damage to nail

  ● S61.311   Laceration without foreign body of left index finger with damage to nail

● S61.312   Laceration without foreign body of right middle finger with damage to nail

● S61.313   Laceration without foreign body of left middle finger with damage to nail

● S61.314   Laceration without foreign body of right ring finger with damage to nail

● S61.315   Laceration without foreign body of left ring finger with damage to nail

● S61.316   Laceration without foreign body of right little finger with damage to nail

● S61.317   Laceration without foreign body of left little finger with damage to nail

● S61.318   Laceration without foreign body of other finger with damage to nail
  Laceration without foreign body of specified finger with unspecified laterality with damage to nail

● S61.319   Laceration without foreign body of unspecified finger with damage to nail

● S61.32   Laceration with foreign body of finger with damage to nail

 ● S61.320   Laceration with foreign body of right index finger with damage to nail

 ● S61.321   Laceration with foreign body of left index finger with damage to nail

 ● S61.322   Laceration with foreign body of right middle finger with damage to nail

 ● S61.323   Laceration with foreign body of left middle finger with damage to nail

 ● S61.324   Laceration with foreign body of right ring finger with damage to nail

 ● S61.325   Laceration with foreign body of left ring finger with damage to nail

 ● S61.326   Laceration with foreign body of right little finger with damage to nail

 ● S61.327   Laceration with foreign body of left little finger with damage to nail

 ● S61.328   Laceration with foreign body of other finger with damage to nail
   Laceration with foreign body of specified finger with unspecified laterality with damage to nail

 ● S61.329   Laceration with foreign body of unspecified finger with damage to nail

● S61.33   Puncture wound without foreign body of finger with damage to nail

 ● S61.330   Puncture wound without foreign body of right index finger with damage to nail

 ● S61.331   Puncture wound without foreign body of left index finger with damage to nail

 ● S61.332   Puncture wound without foreign body of right middle finger with damage to nail

 ● S61.333   Puncture wound without foreign body of left middle finger with damage to nail

 ● S61.334   Puncture wound without foreign body of right ring finger with damage to nail

 ● S61.335   Puncture wound without foreign body of left ring finger with damage to nail

 ● S61.336   Puncture wound without foreign body of right little finger with damage to nail

CHAPTER 19 (S00-T88)

● S61.337 Puncture wound without foreign body of **left little** finger with damage to nail

● S61.338 Puncture wound without foreign body of **other** finger with damage to nail
  Puncture wound without foreign body of specified finger with unspecified laterality with damage to nail

● S61.339 Puncture wound without foreign body of **unspecified** finger with damage to nail

● S61.34 Puncture wound with foreign body of finger with damage to nail

● S61.340 Puncture wound with foreign body of **right index** finger with damage to nail

● S61.341 Puncture wound with foreign body of **left index** finger with damage to nail

● S61.342 Puncture wound with foreign body of **right middle** finger with damage to nail

● S61.343 Puncture wound with foreign body of **left middle** finger with damage to nail

● S61.344 Puncture wound with foreign body of **right ring** finger with damage to nail

● S61.345 Puncture wound with foreign body of **left ring** finger with damage to nail

● S61.346 Puncture wound with foreign body of **right little** finger with damage to nail

● S61.347 Puncture wound with foreign body of **left little** finger with damage to nail

● S61.348 Puncture wound with foreign body of **other** finger with damage to nail
  Puncture wound with foreign body of specified finger with unspecified laterality with damage to nail

● S61.349 Puncture wound with foreign body of **unspecified** finger with damage to nail

● S61.35 Open bite of finger with damage to nail
  Bite of finger with damage to nail NOS
  Excludes1 superficial bite of finger (S60.46-, S60.47-)

● S61.350 Open bite of **right index** finger with damage to nail

● S61.351 Open bite of **left index** finger with damage to nail

● S61.352 Open bite of **right middle** finger with damage to nail

● S61.353 Open bite of **left middle** finger with damage to nail

● S61.354 Open bite of **right ring** finger with damage to nail

● S61.355 Open bite of **left ring** finger with damage to nail

● S61.356 Open bite of **right little** finger with damage to nail

● S61.357 Open bite of **left little** finger with damage to nail

● S61.358 Open bite of **other** finger with damage to nail
  Open bite of specified finger with unspecified laterality with damage to nail

● S61.359 Open bite of **unspecified** finger with damage to nail

● S61.4 Open wound of **hand**

● S61.40 Unspecified open wound of hand

● S61.401 Unspecified open wound of **right** hand

● S61.402 Unspecified open wound of **left** hand

● S61.409 Unspecified open wound of **unspecified** hand

● S61.41 Laceration without foreign body of hand

● S61.411 Laceration without foreign body of **right** hand

● S61.412 Laceration without foreign body of **left** hand

● S61.419 Laceration without foreign body of **unspecified** hand

● S61.42 Laceration with foreign body of hand

● S61.421 Laceration with foreign body of **right** hand

● S61.422 Laceration with foreign body of **left** hand

● S61.429 Laceration with foreign body of **unspecified** hand

● S61.43 Puncture wound without foreign body of hand

● S61.431 Puncture wound without foreign body of **right** hand

● S61.432 Puncture wound without foreign body of **left** hand

● S61.439 Puncture wound without foreign body of **unspecified** hand

● S61.44 Puncture wound with foreign body of hand

● S61.441 Puncture wound with foreign body of **right** hand

● S61.442 Puncture wound with foreign body of **left** hand

● S61.449 Puncture wound with foreign body of **unspecified** hand

● S61.45 Open bite of hand
  Bite of hand NOS
  Excludes1 superficial bite of hand (S60.56-, S60.57-)

● S61.451 Open bite of **right** hand

● S61.452 Open bite of **left** hand

● S61.459 Open bite of **unspecified** hand

● S61.5 Open wound of **wrist**

● S61.50 Unspecified open wound of wrist

● S61.501 Unspecified open wound of **right** wrist

● S61.502 Unspecified open wound of **left** wrist

● S61.509 Unspecified open wound of **unspecified** wrist

● S61.51 Laceration without foreign body of wrist

● S61.511 Laceration without foreign body of **right** wrist

● S61.512 Laceration without foreign body of **left** wrist

● S61.519 Laceration without foreign body of **unspecified** wrist

● S61.52 Laceration with foreign body of wrist

● S61.521 Laceration with foreign body of **right** wrist

● S61.522 Laceration with foreign body of **left** wrist

● S61.529 Laceration with foreign body of **unspecified** wrist

● S61.53 Puncture wound without foreign body of wrist

● S61.531 Puncture wound without foreign body of **right** wrist

● S61.532 Puncture wound without foreign body of **left** wrist

● S61.539 Puncture wound without foreign body of **unspecified** wrist

▶ New   ⇒ Revised   ~~deleted~~ Deleted   Excludes 1   Excludes 2   Includes   Use additional   Code first   Code also   Key words

OGCR Official Guidelines   X Assign placeholder X   ● Use Additional Character(s)   ▶ Manifestation Code   🔖 Hierarchical Condition Category   Coding Clinic

● S61.54　Puncture wound with foreign body of wrist
　　● S61.541　Puncture wound with foreign body of right wrist
　　● S61.542　Puncture wound with foreign body of left wrist
　　● S61.549　Puncture wound with foreign body of unspecified wrist
● S61.55　Open bite of wrist
　　　　　Bite of wrist NOS
　　　　Excludes1　superficial bite of wrist (S60.86-, S60.87-)
　　● S61.551　Open bite of right wrist
　　● S61.552　Open bite of left wrist
　　● S61.559　Open bite of unspecified wrist

● S62　Fracture at wrist and hand level
　　Note: A fracture not indicated as displaced or nondisplaced should be coded to displaced
　　A fracture not indicated as open or closed should be coded to closed
　　Excludes1　traumatic amputation of wrist and hand (S68.-)
　　Excludes2　fracture of distal parts of ulna and radius (S52.-)
　　The appropriate 7th character is to be added to each code from category S62

A	initial encounter for closed fracture
B	initial encounter for open fracture
D	subsequent encounter for fracture with routine healing
G	subsequent encounter for fracture with delayed healing
K	subsequent encounter for fracture with nonunion
P	subsequent encounter for fracture with malunion
S	sequela

● S62.0　Fracture of navicular [scaphoid] bone of wrist
　　●　　S62.00　Unspecified fracture of navicular [scaphoid] bone of wrist
　　　　● S62.001　Unspecified fracture of navicular [scaphoid] bone of right wrist
　　　　● S62.002　Unspecified fracture of navicular [scaphoid] bone of left wrist
　　　　　　　Coding Clinic: 2012, Q4, P106
　　　　● S62.009　Unspecified fracture of navicular [scaphoid] bone of unspecified wrist
　　● S62.01　Fracture of distal pole of navicular [scaphoid] bone of wrist
　　　　　　Fracture of volar tuberosity of navicular [scaphoid] bone of wrist
　　　　● S62.011　Displaced fracture of distal pole of navicular [scaphoid] bone of right wrist
　　　　● S62.012　Displaced fracture of distal pole of navicular [scaphoid] bone of left wrist
　　　　● S62.013　Displaced fracture of distal pole of navicular [scaphoid] bone of unspecified wrist
　　　　● S62.014　Nondisplaced fracture of distal pole of navicular [scaphoid] bone of right wrist
　　　　● S62.015　Nondisplaced fracture of distal pole of navicular [scaphoid] bone of left wrist
　　　　● S62.016　Nondisplaced fracture of distal pole of navicular [scaphoid] bone of unspecified wrist
　　● S62.02　Fracture of middle third of navicular [scaphoid] bone of wrist
　　　　● S62.021　Displaced fracture of middle third of navicular [scaphoid] bone of right wrist
　　　　● S62.022　Displaced fracture of middle third of navicular [scaphoid] bone of left wrist

● S62.023　Displaced fracture of middle third of navicular [scaphoid] bone of unspecified wrist
● S62.024　Nondisplaced fracture of middle third of navicular [scaphoid] bone of right wrist
● S62.025　Nondisplaced fracture of middle third of navicular [scaphoid] bone of left wrist
● S62.026　Nondisplaced fracture of middle third of navicular [scaphoid] bone of unspecified wrist
● S62.03　Fracture of proximal third of navicular [scaphoid] bone of wrist
　　● S62.031　Displaced fracture of proximal third of navicular [scaphoid] bone of right wrist
　　● S62.032　Displaced fracture of proximal third of navicular [scaphoid] bone of left wrist
　　● S62.033　Displaced fracture of proximal third of navicular [scaphoid] bone of unspecified wrist
　　● S62.034　Nondisplaced fracture of proximal third of navicular [scaphoid] bone of right wrist
　　● S62.035　Nondisplaced fracture of proximal third of navicular [scaphoid] bone of left wrist
　　● S62.036　Nondisplaced fracture of proximal third of navicular [scaphoid] bone of unspecified wrist
● S62.1　Fracture of other and unspecified carpal bone(s)
　　Excludes2　fracture of scaphoid of wrist (S62.0-)
● S62.10　Fracture of unspecified carpal bone
　　　　Fracture of wrist NOS
　　● S62.101　Fracture of unspecified carpal bone, right wrist
　　● S62.102　Fracture of unspecified carpal bone, left wrist
　　　　　Coding Clinic: 2012, Q4, P95
　　● S62.109　Fracture of unspecified carpal bone, unspecified wrist
● S62.11　Fracture of triquetrum [cuneiform] bone of wrist
　　● S62.111　Displaced fracture of triquetrum [cuneiform] bone, right wrist
　　● S62.112　Displaced fracture of triquetrum [cuneiform] bone, left wrist
　　● S62.113　Displaced fracture of triquetrum [cuneiform] bone, unspecified wrist
　　● S62.114　Nondisplaced fracture of triquetrum [cuneiform] bone, right wrist
　　● S62.115　Nondisplaced fracture of triquetrum [cuneiform] bone, left wrist
　　● S62.116　Nondisplaced fracture of triquetrum [cuneiform] bone, unspecified wrist
● S62.12　Fracture of lunate [semilunar]
　　● S62.121　Displaced fracture of lunate [semilunar], right wrist
　　● S62.122　Displaced fracture of lunate [semilunar], left wrist
　　● S62.123　Displaced fracture of lunate [semilunar], unspecified wrist
　　● S62.124　Nondisplaced fracture of lunate [semilunar], right wrist
　　● S62.125　Nondisplaced fracture of lunate [semilunar], left wrist
　　● S62.126　Nondisplaced fracture of lunate [semilunar], unspecified wrist

- S62.13   Fracture of capitate [os magnum] bone
  - S62.131   Displaced fracture of capitate [os magnum] bone, right wrist
  - S62.132   Displaced fracture of capitate [os magnum] bone, left wrist
  - S62.133   Displaced fracture of capitate [os magnum] bone, unspecified wrist
  - S62.134   Nondisplaced fracture of capitate [os magnum] bone, right wrist
  - S62.135   Nondisplaced fracture of capitate [os magnum] bone, left wrist
  - S62.136   Nondisplaced fracture of capitate [os magnum] bone, unspecified wrist
- S62.14   Fracture of body of hamate [unciform] bone
  Fracture of hamate [unciform] bone NOS
  - S62.141   Displaced fracture of body of hamate [unciform] bone, right wrist
  - S62.142   Displaced fracture of body of hamate [unciform] bone, left wrist
  - S62.143   Displaced fracture of body of hamate [unciform] bone, unspecified wrist
  - S62.144   Nondisplaced fracture of body of hamate [unciform] bone, right wrist
  - S62.145   Nondisplaced fracture of body of hamate [unciform] bone, left wrist
  - S62.146   Nondisplaced fracture of body of hamate [unciform] bone, unspecified wrist
- S62.15   Fracture of hook process of hamate [unciform] bone
  Fracture of unciform process of hamate [unciform] bone
  - S62.151   Displaced fracture of hook process of hamate [unciform] bone, right wrist
  - S62.152   Displaced fracture of hook process of hamate [unciform] bone, left wrist
  - S62.153   Displaced fracture of hook process of hamate [unciform] bone, unspecified wrist
  - S62.154   Nondisplaced fracture of hook process of hamate [unciform] bone, right wrist
  - S62.155   Nondisplaced fracture of hook process of hamate [unciform] bone, left wrist
  - S62.156   Nondisplaced fracture of hook process of hamate [unciform] bone, unspecified wrist
- S62.16   Fracture of pisiform
  - S62.161   Displaced fracture of pisiform, right wrist
  - S62.162   Displaced fracture of pisiform, left wrist
  - S62.163   Displaced fracture of pisiform, unspecified wrist
  - S62.164   Nondisplaced fracture of pisiform, right wrist
  - S62.165   Nondisplaced fracture of pisiform, left wrist
  - S62.166   Nondisplaced fracture of pisiform, unspecified wrist
- S62.17   Fracture of trapezium [larger multangular]
  - S62.171   Displaced fracture of trapezium [larger multangular], right wrist
  - S62.172   Displaced fracture of trapezium [larger multangular], left wrist
  - S62.173   Displaced fracture of trapezium [larger multangular], unspecified wrist
  - S62.174   Nondisplaced fracture of trapezium [larger multangular], right wrist
  - S62.175   Nondisplaced fracture of trapezium [larger multangular], left wrist
  - S62.176   Nondisplaced fracture of trapezium [larger multangular], unspecified wrist
- S62.18   Fracture of trapezoid [smaller multangular]
  - S62.181   Displaced fracture of trapezoid [smaller multangular], right wrist
  - S62.182   Displaced fracture of trapezoid [smaller multangular], left wrist
  - S62.183   Displaced fracture of trapezoid [smaller multangular], unspecified wrist
  - S62.184   Nondisplaced fracture of trapezoid [smaller multangular], right wrist
  - S62.185   Nondisplaced fracture of trapezoid [smaller multangular], left wrist
  - S62.186   Nondisplaced fracture of trapezoid [smaller multangular], unspecified wrist
- S62.2   Fracture of first metacarpal bone
  - S62.20   Unspecified fracture of first metacarpal bone
    - S62.201   Unspecified fracture of first metacarpal bone, right hand
    - S62.202   Unspecified fracture of first metacarpal bone, left hand
    - S62.209   Unspecified fracture of first metacarpal bone, unspecified hand
  - S62.21   Bennett's fracture
    - S62.211   Bennett's fracture, right hand
    - S62.212   Bennett's fracture, left hand
    - S62.213   Bennett's fracture, unspecified hand
  - S62.22   Rolando's fracture
    - S62.221   Displaced Rolando's fracture, right hand
    - S62.222   Displaced Rolando's fracture, left hand
    - S62.223   Displaced Rolando's fracture, unspecified hand
    - S62.224   Nondisplaced Rolando's fracture, right hand
    - S62.225   Nondisplaced Rolando's fracture, left hand
    - S62.226   Nondisplaced Rolando's fracture, unspecified hand
  - S62.23   Other fracture of base of first metacarpal bone
    - S62.231   Other displaced fracture of base of first metacarpal bone, right hand
    - S62.232   Other displaced fracture of base of first metacarpal bone, left hand
    - S62.233   Other displaced fracture of base of first metacarpal bone, unspecified hand
    - S62.234   Other nondisplaced fracture of base of first metacarpal bone, right hand
    - S62.235   Other nondisplaced fracture of base of first metacarpal bone, left hand
    - S62.236   Other nondisplaced fracture of base of first metacarpal bone, unspecified hand
  - S62.24   Fracture of shaft of first metacarpal bone
    - S62.241   Displaced fracture of shaft of first metacarpal bone, right hand
    - S62.242   Displaced fracture of shaft of first metacarpal bone, left hand
    - S62.243   Displaced fracture of shaft of first metacarpal bone, unspecified hand
    - S62.244   Nondisplaced fracture of shaft of first metacarpal bone, right hand

● S62.245   Nondisplaced fracture of shaft of first metacarpal bone, left hand

● S62.246   Nondisplaced fracture of shaft of first metacarpal bone, unspecified hand

● S62.25   Fracture of neck of first metacarpal bone

  ● S62.251   Displaced fracture of neck of first metacarpal bone, right hand

  ● S62.252   Displaced fracture of neck of first metacarpal bone, left hand

  ● S62.253   Displaced fracture of neck of first metacarpal bone, unspecified hand

  ● S62.254   Nondisplaced fracture of neck of first metacarpal bone, right hand

  ● S62.255   Nondisplaced fracture of neck of first metacarpal bone, left hand

  ● S62.256   Nondisplaced fracture of neck of first metacarpal bone, unspecified hand

● S62.29   Other fracture of first metacarpal bone

  ● S62.291   Other fracture of first metacarpal bone, right hand

  ● S62.292   Other fracture of first metacarpal bone, left hand

  ● S62.299   Other fracture of first metacarpal bone, unspecified hand

● S62.3   Fracture of other and unspecified metacarpal bone

    Excludes2   fracture of first metacarpal bone (S62.2-)

● S62.30   Unspecified fracture of other metacarpal bone

  ● S62.300   Unspecified fracture of second metacarpal bone, right hand

  ● S62.301   Unspecified fracture of second metacarpal bone, left hand

  ● S62.302   Unspecified fracture of third metacarpal bone, right hand

  ● S62.303   Unspecified fracture of third metacarpal bone, left hand

  ● S62.304   Unspecified fracture of fourth metacarpal bone, right hand

  ● S62.305   Unspecified fracture of fourth metacarpal bone, left hand

  ● S62.306   Unspecified fracture of fifth metacarpal bone, right hand

  ● S62.307   Unspecified fracture of fifth metacarpal bone, left hand

  ● S62.308   Unspecified fracture of other metacarpal bone

     Unspecified fracture of specified metacarpal bone with unspecified laterality

  ● S62.309   Unspecified fracture of unspecified metacarpal bone

● S62.31   Displaced fracture of base of other metacarpal bone

  ● S62.310   Displaced fracture of base of second metacarpal bone, right hand

  ● S62.311   Displaced fracture of base of second metacarpal bone, left hand

  ● S62.312   Displaced fracture of base of third metacarpal bone, right hand

  ● S62.313   Displaced fracture of base of third metacarpal bone, left hand

  ● S62.314   Displaced fracture of base of fourth metacarpal bone, right hand

  ● S62.315   Displaced fracture of base of fourth metacarpal bone, left hand

  ● S62.316   Displaced fracture of base of fifth metacarpal bone, right hand

  ● S62.317   Displaced fracture of base of fifth metacarpal bone, left hand

● S62.318   Displaced fracture of base of other metacarpal bone

    Displaced fracture of base of specified metacarpal bone with unspecified laterality

● S62.319   Displaced fracture of base of unspecified metacarpal bone

● S62.32   Displaced fracture of shaft of other metacarpal bone

  ● S62.320   Displaced fracture of shaft of second metacarpal bone, right hand

  ● S62.321   Displaced fracture of shaft of second metacarpal bone, left hand

  ● S62.322   Displaced fracture of shaft of third metacarpal bone, right hand

  ● S62.323   Displaced fracture of shaft of third metacarpal bone, left hand

  ● S62.324   Displaced fracture of shaft of fourth metacarpal bone, right hand

  ● S62.325   Displaced fracture of shaft of fourth metacarpal bone, left hand

  ● S62.326   Displaced fracture of shaft of fifth metacarpal bone, right hand

  ● S62.327   Displaced fracture of shaft of fifth metacarpal bone, left hand

  ● S62.328   Displaced fracture of shaft of other metacarpal bone

     Displaced fracture of shaft of specified metacarpal bone with unspecified laterality

  ● S62.329   Displaced fracture of shaft of unspecified metacarpal bone

● S62.33   Displaced fracture of neck of other metacarpal bone

  ● S62.330   Displaced fracture of neck of second metacarpal bone, right hand

  ● S62.331   Displaced fracture of neck of second metacarpal bone, left hand

  ● S62.332   Displaced fracture of neck of third metacarpal bone, right hand

  ● S62.333   Displaced fracture of neck of third metacarpal bone, left hand

  ● S62.334   Displaced fracture of neck of fourth metacarpal bone, right hand

  ● S62.335   Displaced fracture of neck of fourth metacarpal bone, left hand

  ● S62.336   Displaced fracture of neck of fifth metacarpal bone, right hand

  ● S62.337   Displaced fracture of neck of fifth metacarpal bone, left hand

  ● S62.338   Displaced fracture of neck of other metacarpal bone

     Displaced fracture of neck of specified metacarpal bone with unspecified laterality

  ● S62.339   Displaced fracture of neck of unspecified metacarpal bone

● S62.34   Nondisplaced fracture of base of other metacarpal bone

  ● S62.340   Nondisplaced fracture of base of second metacarpal bone, right hand

  ● S62.341   Nondisplaced fracture of base of second metacarpal bone, left hand

  ● S62.342   Nondisplaced fracture of base of third metacarpal bone, right hand

  ● S62.343   Nondisplaced fracture of base of third metacarpal bone, left hand

  ● S62.344   Nondisplaced fracture of base of fourth metacarpal bone, right hand

  ● S62.345   Nondisplaced fracture of base of fourth metacarpal bone, left hand

CHAPTER 19 (S00-T88)

● S62.346   Nondisplaced fracture of base of fifth metacarpal bone, right hand

● S62.347   Nondisplaced fracture of base of fifth metacarpal bone, left hand

● S62.348   Nondisplaced fracture of base of other metacarpal bone
       Nondisplaced fracture of base of specified metacarpal bone with unspecified laterality

● S62.349   Nondisplaced fracture of base of unspecified metacarpal bone

● S62.35   Nondisplaced fracture of shaft of other metacarpal bone

● S62.350   Nondisplaced fracture of shaft of second metacarpal bone, right hand

● S62.351   Nondisplaced fracture of shaft of second metacarpal bone, left hand

● S62.352   Nondisplaced fracture of shaft of third metacarpal bone, right hand

● S62.353   Nondisplaced fracture of shaft of third metacarpal bone, left hand

● S62.354   Nondisplaced fracture of shaft of fourth metacarpal bone, right hand

● S62.355   Nondisplaced fracture of shaft of fourth metacarpal bone, left hand

● S62.356   Nondisplaced fracture of shaft of fifth metacarpal bone, right hand

● S62.357   Nondisplaced fracture of shaft of fifth metacarpal bone, left hand

● S62.358   Nondisplaced fracture of shaft of other metacarpal bone
       Nondisplaced fracture of shaft of specified metacarpal bone with unspecified laterality

● S62.359   Nondisplaced fracture of shaft of unspecified metacarpal bone

● S62.36   Nondisplaced fracture of neck of other metacarpal bone

● S62.360   Nondisplaced fracture of neck of second metacarpal bone, right hand

● S62.361   Nondisplaced fracture of neck of second metacarpal bone, left hand

● S62.362   Nondisplaced fracture of neck of third metacarpal bone, right hand

● S62.363   Nondisplaced fracture of neck of third metacarpal bone, left hand

● S62.364   Nondisplaced fracture of neck of fourth metacarpal bone, right hand

● S62.365   Nondisplaced fracture of neck of fourth metacarpal bone, left hand

● S62.366   Nondisplaced fracture of neck of fifth metacarpal bone, right hand

● S62.367   Nondisplaced fracture of neck of fifth metacarpal bone, left hand

● S62.368   Nondisplaced fracture of neck of other metacarpal bone
       Nondisplaced fracture of neck of specified metacarpal bone with unspecified laterality

● S62.369   Nondisplaced fracture of neck of unspecified metacarpal bone

● S62.39   Other fracture of other metacarpal bone

● S62.390   Other fracture of second metacarpal bone, right hand

● S62.391   Other fracture of second metacarpal bone, left hand

● S62.392   Other fracture of third metacarpal bone, right hand

● S62.393   Other fracture of third metacarpal bone, left hand

● S62.394   Other fracture of fourth metacarpal bone, right hand

● S62.395   Other fracture of fourth metacarpal bone, left hand

● S62.396   Other fracture of fifth metacarpal bone, right hand

● S62.397   Other fracture of fifth metacarpal bone, left hand

● S62.398   Other fracture of other metacarpal bone
       Other fracture of specified metacarpal bone with unspecified laterality

● S62.399   Other fracture of unspecified metacarpal bone

● S62.5   Fracture of thumb

● S62.50   Fracture of unspecified phalanx of thumb

● S62.501   Fracture of unspecified phalanx of right thumb

● S62.502   Fracture of unspecified phalanx of left thumb

● S62.509   Fracture of unspecified phalanx of unspecified thumb

● S62.51   Fracture of proximal phalanx of thumb

● S62.511   Displaced fracture of proximal phalanx of right thumb

● S62.512   Displaced fracture of proximal phalanx of left thumb

● S62.513   Displaced fracture of proximal phalanx of unspecified thumb

● S62.514   Nondisplaced fracture of proximal phalanx of right thumb

● S62.515   Nondisplaced fracture of proximal phalanx of left thumb

● S62.516   Nondisplaced fracture of proximal phalanx of unspecified thumb

● S62.52   Fracture of distal phalanx of thumb

● S62.521   Displaced fracture of distal phalanx of right thumb

● S62.522   Displaced fracture of distal phalanx of left thumb

● S62.523   Displaced fracture of distal phalanx of unspecified thumb

● S62.524   Nondisplaced fracture of distal phalanx of right thumb

● S62.525   Nondisplaced fracture of distal phalanx of left thumb

● S62.526   Nondisplaced fracture of distal phalanx of unspecified thumb

● S62.6   Fracture of other and unspecified finger(s)
   Excludes2   fracture of thumb (S62.5-)

● S62.60   Fracture of unspecified phalanx of finger

● S62.600   Fracture of unspecified phalanx of right index finger

● S62.601   Fracture of unspecified phalanx of left index finger

● S62.602   Fracture of unspecified phalanx of right middle finger

● S62.603   Fracture of unspecified phalanx of left middle finger

● S62.604   Fracture of unspecified phalanx of right ring finger

● S62.605   Fracture of unspecified phalanx of left ring finger

● S62.606   Fracture of unspecified phalanx of right little finger

● S62.607   Fracture of unspecified phalanx of left little finger

● S62.608   Fracture of unspecified phalanx of other finger
       Fracture of unspecified phalanx of specified finger with unspecified laterality

▶ New   ⟹ Revised   ~~deleted~~ Deleted   Excludes 1   Excludes 2   Includes   Use additional   Code first   Code also   Key words

OGCR Official Guidelines   X Assign placeholder X   ● Use Additional Character(s)   ▶ Manifestation Code   🜂 Hierarchical Condition Category   Coding Clinic

● S62.609 Fracture of unspecified phalanx of unspecified finger

● S62.61 Displaced fracture of proximal phalanx of finger

● S62.610 Displaced fracture of proximal phalanx of right index finger

● S62.611 Displaced fracture of proximal phalanx of left index finger

● S62.612 Displaced fracture of proximal phalanx of right middle finger

● S62.613 Displaced fracture of proximal phalanx of left middle finger

● S62.614 Displaced fracture of proximal phalanx of right ring finger

● S62.615 Displaced fracture of proximal phalanx of left ring finger

● S62.616 Displaced fracture of proximal phalanx of right little finger

● S62.617 Displaced fracture of proximal phalanx of left little finger

● S62.618 Displaced fracture of proximal phalanx of other finger
   Displaced fracture of proximal phalanx of specified finger with unspecified laterality

● S62.619 Displaced fracture of proximal phalanx of unspecified finger

● S62.62 Displaced fracture of middle phalanx of finger

● S62.620 Displaced fracture of middle phalanx of right index finger

● S62.621 Displaced fracture of middle phalanx of left index finger

● S62.622 Displaced fracture of middle phalanx of right middle finger

● S62.623 Displaced fracture of middle phalanx of left middle finger

● S62.624 Displaced fracture of middle phalanx of right ring finger

● S62.625 Displaced fracture of middle phalanx of left ring finger

● S62.626 Displaced fracture of middle phalanx of right little finger

● S62.627 Displaced fracture of middle phalanx of left little finger

● S62.628 Displaced fracture of middle phalanx of other finger
   Displaced fracture of middle phalanx of specified finger with unspecified laterality

● S62.629 Displaced fracture of middle phalanx of unspecified finger

● S62.63 Displaced fracture of distal phalanx of finger

● S62.630 Displaced fracture of distal phalanx of right index finger

● S62.631 Displaced fracture of distal phalanx of left index finger

● S62.632 Displaced fracture of distal phalanx of right middle finger

● S62.633 Displaced fracture of distal phalanx of left middle finger

● S62.634 Displaced fracture of distal phalanx of right ring finger

● S62.635 Displaced fracture of distal phalanx of left ring finger

● S62.636 Displaced fracture of distal phalanx of right little finger

● S62.637 Displaced fracture of distal phalanx of left little finger

● S62.638 Displaced fracture of distal phalanx of other finger
   Displaced fracture of distal phalanx of specified finger with unspecified laterality

● S62.639 Displaced fracture of distal phalanx of unspecified finger

● S62.64 Nondisplaced fracture of proximal phalanx of finger

● S62.640 Nondisplaced fracture of proximal phalanx of right index finger

● S62.641 Nondisplaced fracture of proximal phalanx of left index finger

● S62.642 Nondisplaced fracture of proximal phalanx of right middle finger

● S62.643 Nondisplaced fracture of proximal phalanx of left middle finger

● S62.644 Nondisplaced fracture of proximal phalanx of right ring finger

● S62.645 Nondisplaced fracture of proximal phalanx of left ring finger

● S62.646 Nondisplaced fracture of proximal phalanx of right little finger

● S62.647 Nondisplaced fracture of proximal phalanx of left little finger

● S62.648 Nondisplaced fracture of proximal phalanx of other finger
   Nondisplaced fracture of proximal phalanx of specified finger with unspecified laterality

● S62.649 Nondisplaced fracture of proximal phalanx of unspecified finger

● S62.65 Nondisplaced fracture of middle phalanx of finger

● S62.650 Nondisplaced fracture of middle phalanx of right index finger

● S62.651 Nondisplaced fracture of middle phalanx of left index finger

● S62.652 Nondisplaced fracture of middle phalanx of right middle finger

● S62.653 Nondisplaced fracture of middle phalanx of left middle finger

● S62.654 Nondisplaced fracture of middle phalanx of right ring finger

● S62.655 Nondisplaced fracture of middle phalanx of left ring finger

● S62.656 Nondisplaced fracture of middle phalanx of right little finger

● S62.657 Nondisplaced fracture of middle phalanx of left little finger

● S62.658 Nondisplaced fracture of middle phalanx of other finger
   Nondisplaced fracture of middle phalanx of specified finger with unspecified laterality

● S62.659 Nondisplaced fracture of middle phalanx of unspecified finger

● S62.66 Nondisplaced fracture of distal phalanx of finger

● S62.660 Nondisplaced fracture of distal phalanx of right index finger

● S62.661 Nondisplaced fracture of distal phalanx of left index finger

● S62.662 Nondisplaced fracture of distal phalanx of right middle finger

● S62.663 Nondisplaced fracture of distal phalanx of left middle finger

● S62.664 Nondisplaced fracture of distal phalanx of right ring finger

● S62.665 Nondisplaced fracture of distal phalanx of left ring finger

CHAPTER 19 (S00-T88)

Figure 19-14 Dorsal dislocation of the distal phalanx of the index finger. (From Hardy M, Snaith B: Musculoskeletal Trauma: A Guide to Assessment and Diagnosis, 1e, Elsevier, 2011)

● S62.666   Nondisplaced fracture of distal phalanx of right little finger

● S62.667   Nondisplaced fracture of distal phalanx of left little finger

● S62.668   Nondisplaced fracture of distal phalanx of other finger
       Nondisplaced fracture of distal phalanx of specified finger with unspecified laterality

● S62.669   Nondisplaced fracture of distal phalanx of unspecified finger

● S62.9   Unspecified fracture of wrist and hand

X ● S62.90   Unspecified fracture of unspecified wrist and hand

X ● S62.91   Unspecified fracture of right wrist and hand

X ● S62.92   Unspecified fracture of left wrist and hand

● S63   **Dislocation and sprain of joints and ligaments at wrist and hand level**

     Includes   avulsion of joint or ligament at wrist and hand level
       laceration of cartilage, joint or ligament at wrist and hand level
       sprain of cartilage, joint or ligament at wrist and hand level
       traumatic hemarthrosis of joint or ligament at wrist and hand level
       traumatic rupture of joint or ligament at wrist and hand level
       traumatic subluxation of joint or ligament at wrist and hand level
       traumatic tear of joint or ligament at wrist and hand level

     Code also any associated open wound

     Excludes2   strain of muscle, fascia and tendon of wrist and hand (S66.-)

     The appropriate 7th character is to be added to each code from category S63

       A   initial encounter
       D   subsequent encounter
       S   sequela

● S63.0   **Subluxation and dislocation of wrist and hand joints**

● S63.00   **Unspecified subluxation and dislocation of wrist and hand**
       Dislocation of carpal bone NOS
       Dislocation of distal end of radius NOS
       Subluxation of carpal bone NOS
       Subluxation of distal end of radius NOS

● S63.001   Unspecified subluxation of right wrist and hand

● S63.002   Unspecified subluxation of left wrist and hand

● S63.003   Unspecified subluxation of unspecified wrist and hand

● S63.004   Unspecified dislocation of right wrist and hand

● S63.005   Unspecified dislocation of left wrist and hand

● S63.006   Unspecified dislocation of unspecified wrist and hand

● S63.01   Subluxation and dislocation of distal radioulnar joint

● S63.011   Subluxation of distal radioulnar joint of right wrist

● S63.012   Subluxation of distal radioulnar joint of left wrist

● S63.013   Subluxation of distal radioulnar joint of unspecified wrist

● S63.014   Dislocation of distal radioulnar joint of right wrist

● S63.015   Dislocation of distal radioulnar joint of left wrist

● S63.016   Dislocation of distal radioulnar joint of unspecified wrist

● S63.02   Subluxation and dislocation of radiocarpal joint

● S63.021   Subluxation of radiocarpal joint of right wrist

● S63.022   Subluxation of radiocarpal joint of left wrist

● S63.023   Subluxation of radiocarpal joint of unspecified wrist

● S63.024   Dislocation of radiocarpal joint of right wrist

● S63.025   Dislocation of radiocarpal joint of left wrist

● S63.026   Dislocation of radiocarpal joint of unspecified wrist

● S63.03   Subluxation and dislocation of midcarpal joint

● S63.031   Subluxation of midcarpal joint of right wrist

● S63.032   Subluxation of midcarpal joint of left wrist

● S63.033   Subluxation of midcarpal joint of unspecified wrist

● S63.034   Dislocation of midcarpal joint of right wrist

● S63.035   Dislocation of midcarpal joint of left wrist

● S63.036   Dislocation of midcarpal joint of unspecified wrist

● S63.04   Subluxation and dislocation of carpometacarpal joint of thumb

     Excludes2   interphalangeal subluxation and dislocation of thumb (S63.1-)

● S63.041   Subluxation of carpometacarpal joint of right thumb

● S63.042   Subluxation of carpometacarpal joint of left thumb

● S63.043   Subluxation of carpometacarpal joint of unspecified thumb

● S63.044   Dislocation of carpometacarpal joint of right thumb

CHAPTER 19 (S00-T88)

● S63.045　Dislocation of carpometacarpal joint of left thumb

● S63.046　Dislocation of carpometacarpal joint of unspecified thumb

● S63.05　Subluxation and dislocation of other carpometacarpal joint

　　　Excludes2　subluxation and dislocation of carpometacarpal joint of thumb (S63.04-)

● S63.051　Subluxation of other carpometacarpal joint of right hand

● S63.052　Subluxation of other carpometacarpal joint of left hand

● S63.053　Subluxation of other carpometacarpal joint of unspecified hand

● S63.054　Dislocation of other carpometacarpal joint of right hand

● S63.055　Dislocation of other carpometacarpal joint of left hand

● S63.056　Dislocation of other carpometacarpal joint of unspecified hand

● S63.06　Subluxation and dislocation of metacarpal (bone), proximal end

● S63.061　Subluxation of metacarpal (bone), proximal end of right hand

● S63.062　Subluxation of metacarpal (bone), proximal end of left hand

● S63.063　Subluxation of metacarpal (bone), proximal end of unspecified hand

● S63.064　Dislocation of metacarpal (bone), proximal end of right hand

● S63.065　Dislocation of metacarpal (bone), proximal end of left hand

● S63.066　Dislocation of metacarpal (bone), proximal end of unspecified hand

● S63.07　Subluxation and dislocation of distal end of ulna

● S63.071　Subluxation of distal end of right ulna

● S63.072　Subluxation of distal end of left ulna

● S63.073　Subluxation of distal end of unspecified ulna

● S63.074　Dislocation of distal end of right ulna

● S63.075　Dislocation of distal end of left ulna

● S63.076　Dislocation of distal end of unspecified ulna

● S63.09　Other subluxation and dislocation of wrist and hand

● S63.091　Other subluxation of right wrist and hand

● S63.092　Other subluxation of left wrist and hand

● S63.093　Other subluxation of unspecified wrist and hand

● S63.094　Other dislocation of right wrist and hand

● S63.095　Other dislocation of left wrist and hand

● S63.096　Other dislocation of unspecified wrist and hand

● S63.1　Subluxation and dislocation of thumb

● S63.10　Unspecified subluxation and dislocation of thumb

● S63.101　Unspecified subluxation of right thumb

● S63.102　Unspecified subluxation of left thumb

● S63.103　Unspecified subluxation of unspecified thumb

● S63.104　Unspecified dislocation of right thumb

● S63.105　Unspecified dislocation of left thumb

● S63.106　Unspecified dislocation of unspecified thumb

● S63.11　Subluxation and dislocation of metacarpophalangeal joint of thumb

● S63.111　Subluxation of metacarpophalangeal joint of right thumb

● S63.112　Subluxation of metacarpophalangeal joint of left thumb

● S63.113　Subluxation of metacarpophalangeal joint of unspecified thumb

● S63.114　Dislocation of metacarpophalangeal joint of right thumb

● S63.115　Dislocation of metacarpophalangeal joint of left thumb

● S63.116　Dislocation of metacarpophalangeal joint of unspecified thumb

● S63.12　Subluxation and dislocation of interphalangeal joint of thumb

● S63.121　Subluxation of interphalangeal joint of right thumb

● S63.122　Subluxation of interphalangeal joint of left thumb

● S63.123　Subluxation of interphalangeal joint of unspecified thumb

● S63.124　Dislocation of interphalangeal joint of right thumb

● S63.125　Dislocation of interphalangeal joint of left thumb

● S63.126　Dislocation of interphalangeal joint of unspecified thumb

● S63.2　Subluxation and dislocation of other finger(s)

　　　Excludes2　subluxation and dislocation of thumb (S63.1-)

● S63.20　Unspecified subluxation of other finger

● S63.200　Unspecified subluxation of right index finger

● S63.201　Unspecified subluxation of left index finger

● S63.202　Unspecified subluxation of right middle finger

● S63.203　Unspecified subluxation of left middle finger

● S63.204　Unspecified subluxation of right ring finger

● S63.205　Unspecified subluxation of left ring finger

● S63.206　Unspecified subluxation of right little finger

● S63.207　Unspecified subluxation of left little finger

● S63.208　Unspecified subluxation of other finger

　　　Unspecified subluxation of specified finger with unspecified laterality

● S63.209　Unspecified subluxation of unspecified finger

● S63.21　Subluxation of metacarpophalangeal joint of finger

● S63.210　Subluxation of metacarpophalangeal joint of right index finger

● S63.211　Subluxation of metacarpophalangeal joint of left index finger

● S63.212　Subluxation of metacarpophalangeal joint of right middle finger

● S63.213　Subluxation of metacarpophalangeal joint of left middle finger

● S63.214　Subluxation of metacarpophalangeal joint of right ring finger

- ● S63.215 Subluxation of metacarpophalangeal joint of left ring finger
- ● S63.216 Subluxation of metacarpophalangeal joint of right little finger
- ● S63.217 Subluxation of metacarpophalangeal joint of left little finger
- ● S63.218 Subluxation of metacarpophalangeal joint of other finger
  - Subluxation of metacarpophalangeal joint of specified finger with unspecified laterality
- ● S63.219 Subluxation of metacarpophalangeal joint of unspecified finger
- ● S63.22 Subluxation of unspecified interphalangeal joint of finger
  - ● S63.220 Subluxation of unspecified interphalangeal joint of right index finger
  - ● S63.221 Subluxation of unspecified interphalangeal joint of left index finger
  - ● S63.222 Subluxation of unspecified interphalangeal joint of right middle finger
  - ● S63.223 Subluxation of unspecified interphalangeal joint of left middle finger
  - ● S63.224 Subluxation of unspecified interphalangeal joint of right ring finger
  - ● S63.225 Subluxation of unspecified interphalangeal joint of left ring finger
  - ● S63.226 Subluxation of unspecified interphalangeal joint of right little finger
  - ● S63.227 Subluxation of unspecified interphalangeal joint of left little finger
  - ● S63.228 Subluxation of unspecified interphalangeal joint of other finger
    - Subluxation of unspecified interphalangeal joint of specified finger with unspecified laterality
  - ● S63.229 Subluxation of unspecified interphalangeal joint of unspecified finger
- ● S63.23 Subluxation of proximal interphalangeal joint of finger
  - ● S63.230 Subluxation of proximal interphalangeal joint of right index finger
  - ● S63.231 Subluxation of proximal interphalangeal joint of left index finger
  - ● S63.232 Subluxation of proximal interphalangeal joint of right middle finger
  - ● S63.233 Subluxation of proximal interphalangeal joint of left middle finger
  - ● S63.234 Subluxation of proximal interphalangeal joint of right ring finger
  - ● S63.235 Subluxation of proximal interphalangeal joint of left ring finger
  - ● S63.236 Subluxation of proximal interphalangeal joint of right little finger

- ● S63.237 Subluxation of proximal interphalangeal joint of left little finger
- ● S63.238 Subluxation of proximal interphalangeal joint of other finger
  - Subluxation of proximal interphalangeal joint of specified finger with unspecified laterality
- ● S63.239 Subluxation of proximal interphalangeal joint of unspecified finger
- ● S63.24 Subluxation of distal interphalangeal joint of finger
  - ● S63.240 Subluxation of distal interphalangeal joint of right index finger
  - ● S63.241 Subluxation of distal interphalangeal joint of left index finger
  - ● S63.242 Subluxation of distal interphalangeal joint of right middle finger
  - ● S63.243 Subluxation of distal interphalangeal joint of left middle finger
  - ● S63.244 Subluxation of distal interphalangeal joint of right ring finger
  - ● S63.245 Subluxation of distal interphalangeal joint of left ring finger
  - ● S63.246 Subluxation of distal interphalangeal joint of right little finger
  - ● S63.247 Subluxation of distal interphalangeal joint of left little finger
  - ● S63.248 Subluxation of distal interphalangeal joint of other finger
    - Subluxation of distal interphalangeal joint of specified finger with unspecified laterality
  - ● S63.249 Subluxation of distal interphalangeal joint of unspecified finger
- ● S63.25 Unspecified dislocation of other finger
  - ● S63.250 Unspecified dislocation of right index finger
  - ● S63.251 Unspecified dislocation of left index finger
  - ● S63.252 Unspecified dislocation of right middle finger
  - ● S63.253 Unspecified dislocation of left middle finger
  - ● S63.254 Unspecified dislocation of right ring finger
  - ● S63.255 Unspecified dislocation of left ring finger
  - ● S63.256 Unspecified dislocation of right little finger
  - ● S63.257 Unspecified dislocation of left little finger
  - ● S63.258 Unspecified dislocation of other finger
    - Unspecified dislocation of specified finger with unspecified laterality
  - ● S63.259 Unspecified dislocation of unspecified finger
    - Unspecified dislocation of unspecified finger with unspecified laterality
- ● S63.26 Dislocation of metacarpophalangeal joint of finger
  - ● S63.260 Dislocation of metacarpophalangeal joint of right index finger
  - ● S63.261 Dislocation of metacarpophalangeal joint of left index finger
  - ● S63.262 Dislocation of metacarpophalangeal joint of right middle finger

● S63.263   Dislocation of metacarpophalangeal joint of left middle finger

● S63.264   Dislocation of metacarpophalangeal joint of right ring finger

● S63.265   Dislocation of metacarpophalangeal joint of left ring finger

● S63.266   Dislocation of metacarpophalangeal joint of right little finger

● S63.267   Dislocation of metacarpophalangeal joint of left little finger

● S63.268   Dislocation of metacarpophalangeal joint of other finger

    Dislocation of metacarpophalangeal joint of specified finger with unspecified laterality

● S63.269   Dislocation of metacarpophalangeal joint of unspecified finger

● S63.27   Dislocation of unspecified interphalangeal joint of finger

● S63.270   Dislocation of unspecified interphalangeal joint of right index finger

● S63.271   Dislocation of unspecified interphalangeal joint of left index finger

● S63.272   Dislocation of unspecified interphalangeal joint of right middle finger

● S63.273   Dislocation of unspecified interphalangeal joint of left middle finger

● S63.274   Dislocation of unspecified interphalangeal joint of right ring finger

● S63.275   Dislocation of unspecified interphalangeal joint of left ring finger

● S63.276   Dislocation of unspecified interphalangeal joint of right little finger

● S63.277   Dislocation of unspecified interphalangeal joint of left little finger

● S63.278   Dislocation of unspecified interphalangeal joint of other finger

    Dislocation of unspecified interphalangeal joint of specified finger with unspecified laterality

● S63.279   Dislocation of unspecified interphalangeal joint of unspecified finger

    Dislocation of unspecified interphalangeal joint of unspecified finger without specified laterality

● S63.28   Dislocation of proximal interphalangeal joint of finger

● S63.280   Dislocation of proximal interphalangeal joint of right index finger

● S63.281   Dislocation of proximal interphalangeal joint of left index finger

● S63.282   Dislocation of proximal interphalangeal joint of right middle finger

● S63.283   Dislocation of proximal interphalangeal joint of left middle finger

● S63.284   Dislocation of proximal interphalangeal joint of right ring finger

● S63.285   Dislocation of proximal interphalangeal joint of left ring finger

● S63.286   Dislocation of proximal interphalangeal joint of right little finger

● S63.287   Dislocation of proximal interphalangeal joint of left little finger

● S63.288   Dislocation of proximal interphalangeal joint of other finger

    Dislocation of proximal interphalangeal joint of specified finger with unspecified laterality

● S63.289   Dislocation of proximal interphalangeal joint of unspecified finger

● S63.29   Dislocation of distal interphalangeal joint of finger

● S63.290   Dislocation of distal interphalangeal joint of right index finger

● S63.291   Dislocation of distal interphalangeal joint of left index finger

● S63.292   Dislocation of distal interphalangeal joint of right middle finger

● S63.293   Dislocation of distal interphalangeal joint of left middle finger

● S63.294   Dislocation of distal interphalangeal joint of right ring finger

● S63.295   Dislocation of distal interphalangeal joint of left ring finger

● S63.296   Dislocation of distal interphalangeal joint of right little finger

● S63.297   Dislocation of distal interphalangeal joint of left little finger

● S63.298   Dislocation of distal interphalangeal joint of other finger

    Dislocation of distal interphalangeal joint of specified finger with unspecified laterality

● S63.299   Dislocation of distal interphalangeal joint of unspecified finger

● S63.3   Traumatic rupture of ligament of wrist

● S63.30   Traumatic rupture of unspecified ligament of wrist

● S63.301   Traumatic rupture of unspecified ligament of right wrist

● S63.302   Traumatic rupture of unspecified ligament of left wrist

● S63.309   Traumatic rupture of unspecified ligament of unspecified wrist

● S63.31   Traumatic rupture of collateral ligament of wrist

● S63.311   Traumatic rupture of collateral ligament of right wrist

● S63.312   Traumatic rupture of collateral ligament of left wrist

● S63.319   Traumatic rupture of collateral ligament of unspecified wrist

● S63.32   Traumatic rupture of radiocarpal ligament

● S63.321   Traumatic rupture of right radiocarpal ligament

● S63.322   Traumatic rupture of left radiocarpal ligament

CHAPTER 19 (S00-T88)

● S63.329   Traumatic rupture of unspecified radiocarpal ligament

● S63.33   Traumatic rupture of ulnocarpal (palmar) ligament

  ● S63.331   Traumatic rupture of right ulnocarpal (palmar) ligament

  ● S63.332   Traumatic rupture of left ulnocarpal (palmar) ligament

  ● S63.339   Traumatic rupture of unspecified ulnocarpal (palmar) ligament

● S63.39   Traumatic rupture of other ligament of wrist

  ● S63.391   Traumatic rupture of other ligament of right wrist

  ● S63.392   Traumatic rupture of other ligament of left wrist

  ● S63.399   Traumatic rupture of other ligament of unspecified wrist

● S63.4   Traumatic rupture of ligament of finger at metacarpophalangeal and interphalangeal joint(s)

 ● S63.40   Traumatic rupture of unspecified ligament of finger at metacarpophalangeal and interphalangeal joint

  ● S63.400   Traumatic rupture of unspecified ligament of right index finger at metacarpophalangeal and interphalangeal joint

  ● S63.401   Traumatic rupture of unspecified ligament of left index finger at metacarpophalangeal and interphalangeal joint

  ● S63.402   Traumatic rupture of unspecified ligament of right middle finger at metacarpophalangeal and interphalangeal joint

  ● S63.403   Traumatic rupture of unspecified ligament of left middle finger at metacarpophalangeal and interphalangeal joint

  ● S63.404   Traumatic rupture of unspecified ligament of right ring finger at metacarpophalangeal and interphalangeal joint

  ● S63.405   Traumatic rupture of unspecified ligament of left ring finger at metacarpophalangeal and interphalangeal joint

  ● S63.406   Traumatic rupture of unspecified ligament of right little finger at metacarpophalangeal and interphalangeal joint

  ● S63.407   Traumatic rupture of unspecified ligament of left little finger at metacarpophalangeal and interphalangeal joint

  ● S63.408   Traumatic rupture of unspecified ligament of other finger at metacarpophalangeal and interphalangeal joint
          Traumatic rupture of unspecified ligament of specified finger with unspecified laterality at metacarpophalangeal and interphalangeal joint

  ● S63.409   Traumatic rupture of unspecified ligament of unspecified finger at metacarpophalangeal and interphalangeal joint

● S63.41   Traumatic rupture of collateral ligament of finger at metacarpophalangeal and interphalangeal joint

  ● S63.410   Traumatic rupture of collateral ligament of right index finger at metacarpophalangeal and interphalangeal joint

  ● S63.411   Traumatic rupture of collateral ligament of left index finger at metacarpophalangeal and interphalangeal joint

  ● S63.412   Traumatic rupture of collateral ligament of right middle finger at metacarpophalangeal and interphalangeal joint

  ● S63.413   Traumatic rupture of collateral ligament of left middle finger at metacarpophalangeal and interphalangeal joint

  ● S63.414   Traumatic rupture of collateral ligament of right ring finger at metacarpophalangeal and interphalangeal joint

  ● S63.415   Traumatic rupture of collateral ligament of left ring finger at metacarpophalangeal and interphalangeal joint

  ● S63.416   Traumatic rupture of collateral ligament of right little finger at metacarpophalangeal and interphalangeal joint

  ● S63.417   Traumatic rupture of collateral ligament of left little finger at metacarpophalangeal and interphalangeal joint

  ● S63.418   Traumatic rupture of collateral ligament of other finger at metacarpophalangeal and interphalangeal joint
          Traumatic rupture of collateral ligament of specified finger with unspecified laterality at metacarpophalangeal and interphalangeal joint

  ● S63.419   Traumatic rupture of collateral ligament of unspecified finger at metacarpophalangeal and interphalangeal joint

● S63.42   Traumatic rupture of palmar ligament of finger at metacarpophalangeal and interphalangeal joint

  ● S63.420   Traumatic rupture of palmar ligament of right index finger at metacarpophalangeal and interphalangeal joint

  ● S63.421   Traumatic rupture of palmar ligament of left index finger at metacarpophalangeal and interphalangeal joint

  ● S63.422   Traumatic rupture of palmar ligament of right middle finger at metacarpophalangeal and interphalangeal joint

  ● S63.423   Traumatic rupture of palmar ligament of left middle finger at metacarpophalangeal and interphalangeal joint

  ● S63.424   Traumatic rupture of palmar ligament of right ring finger at metacarpophalangeal and interphalangeal joint

▶ New   ⮕ Revised   ~~deleted~~ Deleted   Excludes 1   Excludes 2   Includes   Use additional   Code first   Code also   Key words
OGCR Official Guidelines   X Assign placeholder X   ● Use Additional Character(s)   ▶ Manifestation Code   Hierarchical Condition Category   **Coding Clinic**

● S63.425   Traumatic rupture of palmar ligament of left ring finger at metacarpophalangeal and interphalangeal joint

● S63.426   Traumatic rupture of palmar ligament of right little finger at metacarpophalangeal and interphalangeal joint

● S63.427   Traumatic rupture of palmar ligament of left little finger at metacarpophalangeal and interphalangeal joint

● S63.428   Traumatic rupture of palmar ligament of other finger at metacarpophalangeal and interphalangeal joint

     Traumatic rupture of palmar ligament of specified finger with unspecified laterality at metacarpophalangeal and interphalangeal joint

● S63.429   Traumatic rupture of palmar ligament of unspecified finger at metacarpophalangeal and interphalangeal joint

● S63.43   Traumatic rupture of volar plate of finger at metacarpophalangeal and interphalangeal joint

● S63.430   Traumatic rupture of volar plate of right index finger at metacarpophalangeal and interphalangeal joint

● S63.431   Traumatic rupture of volar plate of left index finger at metacarpophalangeal and interphalangeal joint

● S63.432   Traumatic rupture of volar plate of right middle finger at metacarpophalangeal and interphalangeal joint

● S63.433   Traumatic rupture of volar plate of left middle finger at metacarpophalangeal and interphalangeal joint

● S63.434   Traumatic rupture of volar plate of right ring finger at metacarpophalangeal and interphalangeal joint

● S63.435   Traumatic rupture of volar plate of left ring finger at metacarpophalangeal and interphalangeal joint

● S63.436   Traumatic rupture of volar plate of right little finger at metacarpophalangeal and interphalangeal joint

● S63.437   Traumatic rupture of volar plate of left little finger at metacarpophalangeal and interphalangeal joint

● S63.438   Traumatic rupture of volar plate of other finger at metacarpophalangeal and interphalangeal joint

     Traumatic rupture of volar plate of specified finger with unspecified laterality at metacarpophalangeal and interphalangeal joint

● S63.439   Traumatic rupture of volar plate of unspecified finger at metacarpophalangeal and interphalangeal joint

● S63.49   Traumatic rupture of other ligament of finger at metacarpophalangeal and interphalangeal joint

● S63.490   Traumatic rupture of other ligament of right index finger at metacarpophalangeal and interphalangeal joint

● S63.491   Traumatic rupture of other ligament of left index finger at metacarpophalangeal and interphalangeal joint

● S63.492   Traumatic rupture of other ligament of right middle finger at metacarpophalangeal and interphalangeal joint

● S63.493   Traumatic rupture of other ligament of left middle finger at metacarpophalangeal and interphalangeal joint

● S63.494   Traumatic rupture of other ligament of right ring finger at metacarpophalangeal and interphalangeal joint

● S63.495   Traumatic rupture of other ligament of left ring finger at metacarpophalangeal and interphalangeal joint

● S63.496   Traumatic rupture of other ligament of right little finger at metacarpophalangeal and interphalangeal joint

● S63.497   Traumatic rupture of other ligament of left little finger at metacarpophalangeal and interphalangeal joint

● S63.498   Traumatic rupture of other ligament of other finger at metacarpophalangeal and interphalangeal joint

     Traumatic rupture of ligament of specified finger with unspecified laterality at metacarpophalangeal and interphalangeal joint

● S63.499   Traumatic rupture of other ligament of unspecified finger at metacarpophalangeal and interphalangeal joint

● S63.5   Other and unspecified sprain of wrist

● S63.50   Unspecified sprain of wrist

● S63.501   Unspecified sprain of right wrist

● S63.502   Unspecified sprain of left wrist

● S63.509   Unspecified sprain of unspecified wrist

● S63.51   Sprain of carpal (joint)

● S63.511   Sprain of carpal joint of right wrist

● S63.512   Sprain of carpal joint of left wrist

● S63.519   Sprain of carpal joint of unspecified wrist

● S63.52   Sprain of radiocarpal joint

     Excludes1   traumatic rupture of radiocarpal ligament (S63.32-)

● S63.521   Sprain of radiocarpal joint of right wrist

● S63.522   Sprain of radiocarpal joint of left wrist

● S63.529   Sprain of radiocarpal joint of unspecified wrist

● S63.59   Other specified sprain of wrist

● S63.591   Other specified sprain of right wrist

● S63.592   Other specified sprain of left wrist

● S63.599   Other specified sprain of unspecified wrist

CHAPTER 19 (S00-T88)

● **S63.6**   Other and unspecified sprain of finger(s)
     Excludes1   traumatic rupture of ligament of finger at metacarpophalangeal and interphalangeal joint(s) (S63.4-)
   ● **S63.60**   Unspecified sprain of thumb
     ● S63.601   Unspecified sprain of right thumb
     ● S63.602   Unspecified sprain of left thumb
     ● S63.609   Unspecified sprain of unspecified thumb
   ● **S63.61**   Unspecified sprain of other and unspecified finger(s)
     ● S63.610   Unspecified sprain of right index finger
     ● S63.611   Unspecified sprain of left index finger
     ● S63.612   Unspecified sprain of right middle finger
     ● S63.613   Unspecified sprain of left middle finger
     ● S63.614   Unspecified sprain of right ring finger
     ● S63.615   Unspecified sprain of left ring finger
     ● S63.616   Unspecified sprain of right little finger
     ● S63.617   Unspecified sprain of left little finger
     ● S63.618   Unspecified sprain of other finger
        Unspecified sprain of specified finger with unspecified laterality
     ● S63.619   Unspecified sprain of unspecified finger
   ● **S63.62**   Sprain of interphalangeal joint of thumb
     ● S63.621   Sprain of interphalangeal joint of right thumb
     ● S63.622   Sprain of interphalangeal joint of left thumb
     ● S63.629   Sprain of interphalangeal joint of unspecified thumb
   ● **S63.63**   Sprain of interphalangeal joint of other and unspecified finger(s)
     ● S63.630   Sprain of interphalangeal joint of right index finger
     ● S63.631   Sprain of interphalangeal joint of left index finger
     ● S63.632   Sprain of interphalangeal joint of right middle finger
     ● S63.633   Sprain of interphalangeal joint of left middle finger
     ● S63.634   Sprain of interphalangeal joint of right ring finger
     ● S63.635   Sprain of interphalangeal joint of left ring finger
     ● S63.636   Sprain of interphalangeal joint of right little finger
     ● S63.637   Sprain of interphalangeal joint of left little finger
     ● S63.638   Sprain of interphalangeal joint of other finger
     ● S63.639   Sprain of interphalangeal joint of unspecified finger
   ● **S63.64**   Sprain of metacarpophalangeal joint of thumb
     ● S63.641   Sprain of metacarpophalangeal joint of right thumb
     ● S63.642   Sprain of metacarpophalangeal joint of left thumb
     ● S63.649   Sprain of metacarpophalangeal joint of unspecified thumb
   ● **S63.65**   Sprain of metacarpophalangeal joint of other and unspecified finger(s)
     ● S63.650   Sprain of metacarpophalangeal joint of right index finger

     ● S63.651   Sprain of metacarpophalangeal joint of left index finger
     ● S63.652   Sprain of metacarpophalangeal joint of right middle finger
     ● S63.653   Sprain of metacarpophalangeal joint of left middle finger
     ● S63.654   Sprain of metacarpophalangeal joint of right ring finger
     ● S63.655   Sprain of metacarpophalangeal joint of left ring finger
     ● S63.656   Sprain of metacarpophalangeal joint of right little finger
     ● S63.657   Sprain of metacarpophalangeal joint of left little finger
     ● S63.658   Sprain of metacarpophalangeal joint of other finger
        Sprain of metacarpophalangeal joint of specified finger with unspecified laterality
     ● S63.659   Sprain of metacarpophalangeal joint of unspecified finger
   ● **S63.68**   Other sprain of thumb
     ● S63.681   Other sprain of right thumb
     ● S63.682   Other sprain of left thumb
     ● S63.689   Other sprain of unspecified thumb
   ● **S63.69**   Other sprain of other and unspecified finger(s)
     ● S63.690   Other sprain of right index finger
     ● S63.691   Other sprain of left index finger
     ● S63.692   Other sprain of right middle finger
     ● S63.693   Other sprain of left middle finger
     ● S63.694   Other sprain of right ring finger
     ● S63.695   Other sprain of left ring finger
     ● S63.696   Other sprain of right little finger
     ● S63.697   Other sprain of left little finger
     ● S63.698   Other sprain of other finger
        Other sprain of specified finger with unspecified laterality
     ● S63.699   Other sprain of unspecified finger
● **S63.8**   Sprain of other part of wrist and hand
   ● **S63.8X**   Sprain of other part of wrist and hand
     ● S63.8X1   Sprain of other part of right wrist and hand
     ● S63.8X2   Sprain of other part of left wrist and hand
     ● S63.8X9   Sprain of other part of unspecified wrist and hand
● **S63.9**   Sprain of unspecified part of wrist and hand
   X ● **S63.90**   Sprain of unspecified part of unspecified wrist and hand
   X ● **S63.91**   Sprain of unspecified part of right wrist and hand
   X ● **S63.92**   Sprain of unspecified part of left wrist and hand

● **S64**   Injury of nerves at wrist and hand level
   The appropriate 7th character is to be added to each code from category S64

> A   initial encounter
> D   subsequent encounter
> S   sequela

   Code also any associated open wound (S61.-)
● **S64.0**   Injury of ulnar nerve at wrist and hand level
   X ● **S64.00**   Injury of ulnar nerve at wrist and hand level of unspecified arm
   X ● **S64.01**   Injury of ulnar nerve at wrist and hand level of right arm
   X ● **S64.02**   Injury of ulnar nerve at wrist and hand level of left arm

▶ New   ⟹ Revised   ~~deleted~~ Deleted   Excludes 1   Excludes 2   Includes   Use additional   Code first   Code also   Key words
OGCR Official Guidelines   X Assign placeholder X   ● Use Additional Character(s)   ▶ Manifestation Code   Hierarchical Condition Category   Coding Clinic

CHAPTER 19 (S00-T88)

● S64.1   Injury of median nerve at wrist and hand level
   X ● S64.10   Injury of median nerve at wrist and hand level of unspecified arm
   X ● S64.11   Injury of median nerve at wrist and hand level of right arm
   X ● S64.12   Injury of median nerve at wrist and hand level of left arm
● S64.2   Injury of radial nerve at wrist and hand level
   X ● S64.20   Injury of radial nerve at wrist and hand level of unspecified arm
   X ● S64.21   Injury of radial nerve at wrist and hand level of right arm
   X ● S64.22   Injury of radial nerve at wrist and hand level of left arm
● S64.3   Injury of digital nerve of thumb
   X ● S64.30   Injury of digital nerve of unspecified thumb
   X ● S64.31   Injury of digital nerve of right thumb
   X ● S64.32   Injury of digital nerve of left thumb
● S64.4   Injury of digital nerve of other and unspecified finger
   X ● S64.40   Injury of digital nerve of unspecified finger
   ● S64.49   Injury of digital nerve of other finger
     ● S64.490   Injury of digital nerve of right index finger
     ● S64.491   Injury of digital nerve of left index finger
     ● S64.492   Injury of digital nerve of right middle finger
     ● S64.493   Injury of digital nerve of left middle finger
     ● S64.494   Injury of digital nerve of right ring finger
     ● S64.495   Injury of digital nerve of left ring finger
     ● S64.496   Injury of digital nerve of right little finger
     ● S64.497   Injury of digital nerve of left little finger
     ● S64.498   Injury of digital nerve of other finger
       Injury of digital nerve of specified finger with unspecified laterality
● S64.8   Injury of other nerves at wrist and hand level
   ● S64.8X   Injury of other nerves at wrist and hand level
     ● S64.8X1   Injury of other nerves at wrist and hand level of right arm
     ● S64.8X2   Injury of other nerves at wrist and hand level of left arm
     ● S64.8X9   Injury of other nerves at wrist and hand level of unspecified arm
● S64.9   Injury of unspecified nerve at wrist and hand level
   X ● S64.90   Injury of unspecified nerve at wrist and hand level of unspecified arm
   X ● S64.91   Injury of unspecified nerve at wrist and hand level of right arm
   X ● S64.92   Injury of unspecified nerve at wrist and hand level of left arm

● S65   Injury of blood vessels at wrist and hand level
   The appropriate 7th character is to be added to each code from category S65

     | | |
     A   initial encounter
     D   subsequent encounter
     S   sequela

   Code also any associated open wound (S61.-)

● S65.0   Injury of ulnar artery at wrist and hand level
   ● S65.00   Unspecified injury of ulnar artery at wrist and hand level
     ● S65.001   Unspecified injury of ulnar artery at wrist and hand level of right arm
     ● S65.002   Unspecified injury of ulnar artery at wrist and hand level of left arm
     ● S65.009   Unspecified injury of ulnar artery at wrist and hand level of unspecified arm
   ● S65.01   Laceration of ulnar artery at wrist and hand level
     ● S65.011   Laceration of ulnar artery at wrist and hand level of right arm
     ● S65.012   Laceration of ulnar artery at wrist and hand level of left arm
     ● S65.019   Laceration of ulnar artery at wrist and hand level of unspecified arm
   ● S65.09   Other specified injury of ulnar artery at wrist and hand level
     ● S65.091   Other specified injury of ulnar artery at wrist and hand level of right arm
     ● S65.092   Other specified injury of ulnar artery at wrist and hand level of left arm
     ● S65.099   Other specified injury of ulnar artery at wrist and hand level of unspecified arm
● S65.1   Injury of radial artery at wrist and hand level
   ● S65.10   Unspecified injury of radial artery at wrist and hand level
     ● S65.101   Unspecified injury of radial artery at wrist and hand level of right arm
     ● S65.102   Unspecified injury of radial artery at wrist and hand level of left arm
     ● S65.109   Unspecified injury of radial artery at wrist and hand level of unspecified arm
   ● S65.11   Laceration of radial artery at wrist and hand level
     ● S65.111   Laceration of radial artery at wrist and hand level of right arm
     ● S65.112   Laceration of radial artery at wrist and hand level of left arm
     ● S65.119   Laceration of radial artery at wrist and hand level of unspecified arm
   ● S65.19   Other specified injury of radial artery at wrist and hand level
     ● S65.191   Other specified injury of radial artery at wrist and hand level of right arm
     ● S65.192   Other specified injury of radial artery at wrist and hand level of left arm
     ● S65.199   Other specified injury of radial artery at wrist and hand level of unspecified arm
● S65.2   Injury of superficial palmar arch
   ● S65.20   Unspecified injury of superficial palmar arch
     ● S65.201   Unspecified injury of superficial palmar arch of right hand
     ● S65.202   Unspecified injury of superficial palmar arch of left hand
     ● S65.209   Unspecified injury of superficial palmar arch of unspecified hand
   ● S65.21   Laceration of superficial palmar arch
     ● S65.211   Laceration of superficial palmar arch of right hand
     ● S65.212   Laceration of superficial palmar arch of left hand
     ● S65.219   Laceration of superficial palmar arch of unspecified hand

● S65.29   Other specified injury of superficial palmar arch
    ● S65.291   Other specified injury of superficial palmar arch of right hand
    ● S65.292   Other specified injury of superficial palmar arch of left hand
    ● S65.299   Other specified injury of superficial palmar arch of unspecified hand

● S65.3   Injury of deep palmar arch
   ● S65.30   Unspecified injury of deep palmar arch
    ● S65.301   Unspecified injury of deep palmar arch of right hand
    ● S65.302   Unspecified injury of deep palmar arch of left hand
    ● S65.309   Unspecified injury of deep palmar arch of unspecified hand
   ● S65.31   Laceration of deep palmar arch
    ● S65.311   Laceration of deep palmar arch of right hand
    ● S65.312   Laceration of deep palmar arch of left hand
    ● S65.319   Laceration of deep palmar arch of unspecified hand
   ● S65.39   Other specified injury of deep palmar arch
    ● S65.391   Other specified injury of deep palmar arch of right hand
    ● S65.392   Other specified injury of deep palmar arch of left hand
    ● S65.399   Other specified injury of deep palmar arch of unspecified hand

● S65.4   Injury of blood vessel of thumb
   ● S65.40   Unspecified injury of blood vessel of thumb
    ● S65.401   Unspecified injury of blood vessel of right thumb
    ● S65.402   Unspecified injury of blood vessel of left thumb
    ● S65.409   Unspecified injury of blood vessel of unspecified thumb
   ● S65.41   Laceration of blood vessel of thumb
    ● S65.411   Laceration of blood vessel of right thumb
    ● S65.412   Laceration of blood vessel of left thumb
    ● S65.419   Laceration of blood vessel of unspecified thumb
   ● S65.49   Other specified injury of blood vessel of thumb
    ● S65.491   Other specified injury of blood vessel of right thumb
    ● S65.492   Other specified injury of blood vessel of left thumb
    ● S65.499   Other specified injury of blood vessel of unspecified thumb

● S65.5   Injury of blood vessel of other and unspecified finger
   ● S65.50   Unspecified injury of blood vessel of other and unspecified finger
    ● S65.500   Unspecified injury of blood vessel of right index finger
    ● S65.501   Unspecified injury of blood vessel of left index finger
    ● S65.502   Unspecified injury of blood vessel of right middle finger
    ● S65.503   Unspecified injury of blood vessel of left middle finger
    ● S65.504   Unspecified injury of blood vessel of right ring finger
    ● S65.505   Unspecified injury of blood vessel of left ring finger
    ● S65.506   Unspecified injury of blood vessel of right little finger
    ● S65.507   Unspecified injury of blood vessel of left little finger
    ● S65.508   Unspecified injury of blood vessel of other finger
      Unspecified injury of blood vessel of specified finger with unspecified laterality
    ● S65.509   Unspecified injury of blood vessel of unspecified finger
   ● S65.51   Laceration of blood vessel of other and unspecified finger
    ● S65.510   Laceration of blood vessel of right index finger
    ● S65.511   Laceration of blood vessel of left index finger
    ● S65.512   Laceration of blood vessel of right middle finger
    ● S65.513   Laceration of blood vessel of left middle finger
    ● S65.514   Laceration of blood vessel of right ring finger
    ● S65.515   Laceration of blood vessel of left ring finger
    ● S65.516   Laceration of blood vessel of right little finger
    ● S65.517   Laceration of blood vessel of left little finger
    ● S65.518   Laceration of blood vessel of other finger
      Laceration of blood vessel of specified finger with unspecified laterality
    ● S65.519   Laceration of blood vessel of unspecified finger
   ● S65.59   Other specified injury of blood vessel of other and unspecified finger
    ● S65.590   Other specified injury of blood vessel of right index finger
    ● S65.591   Other specified injury of blood vessel of left index finger
    ● S65.592   Other specified injury of blood vessel of right middle finger
    ● S65.593   Other specified injury of blood vessel of left middle finger
    ● S65.594   Other specified injury of blood vessel of right ring finger
    ● S65.595   Other specified injury of blood vessel of left ring finger
    ● S65.596   Other specified injury of blood vessel of right little finger
    ● S65.597   Other specified injury of blood vessel of left little finger
    ● S65.598   Other specified injury of blood vessel of other finger
      Other specified injury of blood vessel of specified finger with unspecified laterality
    ● S65.599   Other specified injury of blood vessel of unspecified finger

● S65.8   Injury of other blood vessels at wrist and hand level
   ● S65.80   Unspecified injury of other blood vessels at wrist and hand level
    ● S65.801   Unspecified injury of other blood vessels at wrist and hand level of right arm
    ● S65.802   Unspecified injury of other blood vessels at wrist and hand level of left arm

● S65.809   Unspecified injury of other blood vessels at wrist and hand level of unspecified arm

● S65.81   Laceration of other blood vessels at wrist and hand level

  ● S65.811   Laceration of other blood vessels at wrist and hand level of right arm

  ● S65.812   Laceration of other blood vessels at wrist and hand level of left arm

  ● S65.819   Laceration of other blood vessels at wrist and hand level of unspecified arm

● S65.89   Other specified injury of other blood vessels at wrist and hand level

  ● S65.891   Other specified injury of other blood vessels at wrist and hand level of right arm

  ● S65.892   Other specified injury of other blood vessels at wrist and hand level of left arm

  ● S65.899   Other specified injury of other blood vessels at wrist and hand level of unspecified arm

● S65.9   Injury of unspecified blood vessel at wrist and hand level

 ● S65.90   Unspecified injury of unspecified blood vessel at wrist and hand level

  ● S65.901   Unspecified injury of unspecified blood vessel at wrist and hand level of right arm

  ● S65.902   Unspecified injury of unspecified blood vessel at wrist and hand level of left arm

  ● S65.909   Unspecified injury of unspecified blood vessel at wrist and hand level of unspecified arm

 ● S65.91   Laceration of unspecified blood vessel at wrist and hand level

  ● S65.911   Laceration of unspecified blood vessel at wrist and hand level of right arm

  ● S65.912   Laceration of unspecified blood vessel at wrist and hand level of left arm

  ● S65.919   Laceration of unspecified blood vessel at wrist and hand level of unspecified arm

 ● S65.99   Other specified injury of unspecified blood vessel at wrist and hand level

  ● S65.991   Other specified injury of unspecified blood vessel at wrist and hand of right arm

  ● S65.992   Other specified injury of unspecified blood vessel at wrist and hand of left arm

  ● S65.999   Other specified injury of unspecified blood vessel at wrist and hand of unspecified arm

● S66   Injury of muscle, fascia and tendon at wrist and hand level

Code also any associated open wound (S61.-)

Excludes2   sprain of joints and ligaments of wrist and hand (S63.-)

The appropriate 7th character is to be added to each code from category S66

A	initial encounter
D	subsequent encounter
S	sequela

● S66.0   Injury of long flexor muscle, fascia and tendon of thumb at wrist and hand level

● S66.00   Unspecified injury of long flexor muscle, fascia and tendon of thumb at wrist and hand level

  ● S66.001   Unspecified injury of long flexor muscle, fascia and tendon of right thumb at wrist and hand level

  ● S66.002   Unspecified injury of long flexor muscle, fascia and tendon of left thumb at wrist and hand level

  ● S66.009   Unspecified injury of long flexor muscle, fascia and tendon of unspecified thumb at wrist and hand level

● S66.01   Strain of long flexor muscle, fascia and tendon of thumb at wrist and hand level

  ● S66.011   Strain of long flexor muscle, fascia and tendon of right thumb at wrist and hand level

  ● S66.012   Strain of long flexor muscle, fascia and tendon of left thumb at wrist and hand level

  ● S66.019   Strain of long flexor muscle, fascia and tendon of unspecified thumb at wrist and hand level

● S66.02   Laceration of long flexor muscle, fascia and tendon of thumb at wrist and hand level

  ● S66.021   Laceration of long flexor muscle, fascia and tendon of right thumb at wrist and hand level

  ● S66.022   Laceration of long flexor muscle, fascia and tendon of left thumb at wrist and hand level

  ● S66.029   Laceration of long flexor muscle, fascia and tendon of unspecified thumb at wrist and hand level

● S66.09   Other specified injury of long flexor muscle, fascia and tendon of thumb at wrist and hand level

  ● S66.091   Other specified injury of long flexor muscle, fascia and tendon of right thumb at wrist and hand level

  ● S66.092   Other specified injury of long flexor muscle, fascia and tendon of left thumb at wrist and hand level

  ● S66.099   Other specified injury of long flexor muscle, fascia and tendon of unspecified thumb at wrist and hand level

● S66.1   Injury of flexor muscle, fascia and tendon of other and unspecified finger at wrist and hand level

Excludes2   injury of long flexor muscle, fascia and tendon of thumb at wrist and hand level (S66.0-)

● S66.10   Unspecified injury of flexor muscle, fascia and tendon of other and unspecified finger at wrist and hand level

  ● S66.100   Unspecified injury of flexor muscle, fascia and tendon of right index finger at wrist and hand level

  ● S66.101   Unspecified injury of flexor muscle, fascia and tendon of left index finger at wrist and hand level

  ● S66.102   Unspecified injury of flexor muscle, fascia and tendon of right middle finger at wrist and hand level

  ● S66.103   Unspecified injury of flexor muscle, fascia and tendon of left middle finger at wrist and hand level

  ● S66.104   Unspecified injury of flexor muscle, fascia and tendon of right ring finger at wrist and hand level

  ● S66.105   Unspecified injury of flexor muscle, fascia and tendon of left ring finger at wrist and hand level

CHAPTER 19 (S00-T88)

● S66.106   Unspecified injury of flexor muscle, fascia and tendon of right little finger at wrist and hand level

● S66.107   Unspecified injury of flexor muscle, fascia and tendon of left little finger at wrist and hand level

● S66.108   Unspecified injury of flexor muscle, fascia and tendon of other finger at wrist and hand level

      Unspecified injury of flexor muscle, fascia and tendon of specified finger with unspecified laterality at wrist and hand level

● S66.109   Unspecified injury of flexor muscle, fascia and tendon of unspecified finger at wrist and hand level

● S66.11   Strain of flexor muscle, fascia and tendon of other and unspecified finger at wrist and hand level

● S66.110   Strain of flexor muscle, fascia and tendon of right index finger at wrist and hand level

● S66.111   Strain of flexor muscle, fascia and tendon of left index finger at wrist and hand level

● S66.112   Strain of flexor muscle, fascia and tendon of right middle finger at wrist and hand level

● S66.113   Strain of flexor muscle, fascia and tendon of left middle finger at wrist and hand level

● S66.114   Strain of flexor muscle, fascia and tendon of right ring finger at wrist and hand level

● S66.115   Strain of flexor muscle, fascia and tendon of left ring finger at wrist and hand level

● S66.116   Strain of flexor muscle, fascia and tendon of right little finger at wrist and hand level

● S66.117   Strain of flexor muscle, fascia and tendon of left little finger at wrist and hand level

● S66.118   Strain of flexor muscle, fascia and tendon of other finger at wrist and hand level

      Strain of flexor muscle, fascia and tendon of specified finger with unspecified laterality at wrist and hand level

● S66.119   Strain of flexor muscle, fascia and tendon of unspecified finger at wrist and hand level

● S66.12   Laceration of flexor muscle, fascia and tendon of other and unspecified finger at wrist and hand level

● S66.120   Laceration of flexor muscle, fascia and tendon of right index finger at wrist and hand level

● S66.121   Laceration of flexor muscle, fascia and tendon of left index finger at wrist and hand level

● S66.122   Laceration of flexor muscle, fascia and tendon of right middle finger at wrist and hand level

● S66.123   Laceration of flexor muscle, fascia and tendon of left middle finger at wrist and hand level

● S66.124   Laceration of flexor muscle, fascia and tendon of right ring finger at wrist and hand level

● S66.125   Laceration of flexor muscle, fascia and tendon of left ring finger at wrist and hand level

● S66.126   Laceration of flexor muscle, fascia and tendon of right little finger at wrist and hand level

● S66.127   Laceration of flexor muscle, fascia and tendon of left little finger at wrist and hand level

● S66.128   Laceration of flexor muscle, fascia and tendon of other finger at wrist and hand level

      Laceration of flexor muscle, fascia and tendon of specified finger with unspecified laterality at wrist and hand level

● S66.129   Laceration of flexor muscle, fascia and tendon of unspecified finger at wrist and hand level

● S66.19   Other injury of flexor muscle, fascia and tendon of other and unspecified finger at wrist and hand level

● S66.190   Other injury of flexor muscle, fascia and tendon of right index finger at wrist and hand level

● S66.191   Other injury of flexor muscle, fascia and tendon of left index finger at wrist and hand level

● S66.192   Other injury of flexor muscle, fascia and tendon of right middle finger at wrist and hand level

● S66.193   Other injury of flexor muscle, fascia and tendon of left middle finger at wrist and hand level

● S66.194   Other injury of flexor muscle, fascia and tendon of right ring finger at wrist and hand level

● S66.195   Other injury of flexor muscle, fascia and tendon of left ring finger at wrist and hand level

● S66.196   Other injury of flexor muscle, fascia and tendon of right little finger at wrist and hand level

● S66.197   Other injury of flexor muscle, fascia and tendon of left little finger at wrist and hand level

● S66.198   Other injury of flexor muscle, fascia and tendon of other finger at wrist and hand level

      Other injury of flexor muscle, fascia and tendon of specified finger with unspecified laterality at wrist and hand level

● S66.199   Other injury of flexor muscle, fascia and tendon of unspecified finger at wrist and hand level

● S66.2   Injury of extensor muscle, fascia and tendon of thumb at wrist and hand level

● S66.20   Unspecified injury of extensor muscle, fascia and tendon of thumb at wrist and hand level

● S66.201   Unspecified injury of extensor muscle, fascia and tendon of right thumb at wrist and hand level

● S66.202   Unspecified injury of extensor muscle, fascia and tendon of left thumb at wrist and hand level

● S66.209   Unspecified injury of extensor muscle, fascia and tendon of unspecified thumb at wrist and hand level

● S66.21   Strain of extensor muscle, fascia and tendon of thumb at wrist and hand level

● S66.211   Strain of extensor muscle, fascia and tendon of right thumb at wrist and hand level

▶ New   ⇒ Revised   ~~deleted~~ Deleted   Excludes 1   Excludes 2   Includes   Use additional   Code first   Code also   Key words

OGCR Official Guidelines   X Assign placeholder X   ● Use Additional Character(s)   ▶ Manifestation Code   ℞ Hierarchical Condition Category   Coding Clinic

● **S66.212**   Strain of extensor muscle, fascia and tendon of left thumb at wrist and hand level

● **S66.219**   Strain of extensor muscle, fascia and tendon of unspecified thumb at wrist and hand level

● **S66.22**   Laceration of extensor muscle, fascia and tendon of thumb at wrist and hand level

    ● **S66.221**   Laceration of extensor muscle, fascia and tendon of right thumb at wrist and hand level

    ● **S66.222**   Laceration of extensor muscle, fascia and tendon of left thumb at wrist and hand level

    ● **S66.229**   Laceration of extensor muscle, fascia and tendon of unspecified thumb at wrist and hand level

● **S66.29**   Other specified injury of extensor muscle, fascia and tendon of thumb at wrist and hand level

    ● **S66.291**   Other specified injury of extensor muscle, fascia and tendon of right thumb at wrist and hand level

    ● **S66.292**   Other specified injury of extensor muscle, fascia and tendon of left thumb at wrist and hand level

    ● **S66.299**   Other specified injury of extensor muscle, fascia and tendon of unspecified thumb at wrist and hand level

● **S66.3**   Injury of extensor muscle, fascia and tendon of other and unspecified finger at wrist and hand level

      Excludes2   injury of extensor muscle, fascia and tendon of thumb at wrist and hand level (S66.2-)

   ● **S66.30**   Unspecified injury of extensor muscle, fascia and tendon of other and unspecified finger at wrist and hand level

    ● **S66.300**   Unspecified injury of extensor muscle, fascia and tendon of right index finger at wrist and hand level

    ● **S66.301**   Unspecified injury of extensor muscle, fascia and tendon of left index finger at wrist and hand level

    ● **S66.302**   Unspecified injury of extensor muscle, fascia and tendon of right middle finger at wrist and hand level

    ● **S66.303**   Unspecified injury of extensor muscle, fascia and tendon of left middle finger at wrist and hand level

    ● **S66.304**   Unspecified injury of extensor muscle, fascia and tendon of right ring finger at wrist and hand level

    ● **S66.305**   Unspecified injury of extensor muscle, fascia and tendon of left ring finger at wrist and hand level

    ● **S66.306**   Unspecified injury of extensor muscle, fascia and tendon of right little finger at wrist and hand level

    ● **S66.307**   Unspecified injury of extensor muscle, fascia and tendon of left little finger at wrist and hand level

    ● **S66.308**   Unspecified injury of extensor muscle, fascia and tendon of other finger at wrist and hand level

        Unspecified injury of extensor muscle, fascia and tendon of specified finger with unspecified laterality at wrist and hand level

    ● **S66.309**   Unspecified injury of extensor muscle, fascia and tendon of unspecified finger at wrist and hand level

● **S66.31**   Strain of extensor muscle, fascia and tendon of other and unspecified finger at wrist and hand level

    ● **S66.310**   Strain of extensor muscle, fascia and tendon of right index finger at wrist and hand level

    ● **S66.311**   Strain of extensor muscle, fascia and tendon of left index finger at wrist and hand level

    ● **S66.312**   Strain of extensor muscle, fascia and tendon of right middle finger at wrist and hand level

    ● **S66.313**   Strain of extensor muscle, fascia and tendon of left middle finger at wrist and hand level

    ● **S66.314**   Strain of extensor muscle, fascia and tendon of right ring finger at wrist and hand level

    ● **S66.315**   Strain of extensor muscle, fascia and tendon of left ring finger at wrist and hand level

    ● **S66.316**   Strain of extensor muscle, fascia and tendon of right little finger at wrist and hand level

    ● **S66.317**   Strain of extensor muscle, fascia and tendon of left little finger at wrist and hand level

    ● **S66.318**   Strain of extensor muscle, fascia and tendon of other finger at wrist and hand level

        Strain of extensor muscle, fascia and tendon of specified finger with unspecified laterality at wrist and hand level

    ● **S66.319**   Strain of extensor muscle, fascia and tendon of unspecified finger at wrist and hand level

● **S66.32**   Laceration of extensor muscle, fascia and tendon of other and unspecified finger at wrist and hand level

    ● **S66.320**   Laceration of extensor muscle, fascia and tendon of right index finger at wrist and hand level

    ● **S66.321**   Laceration of extensor muscle, fascia and tendon of left index finger at wrist and hand level

    ● **S66.322**   Laceration of extensor muscle, fascia and tendon of right middle finger at wrist and hand level

    ● **S66.323**   Laceration of extensor muscle, fascia and tendon of left middle finger at wrist and hand level

    ● **S66.324**   Laceration of extensor muscle, fascia and tendon of right ring finger at wrist and hand level

    ● **S66.325**   Laceration of extensor muscle, fascia and tendon of left ring finger at wrist and hand level

    ● **S66.326**   Laceration of extensor muscle, fascia and tendon of right little finger at wrist and hand level

    ● **S66.327**   Laceration of extensor muscle, fascia and tendon of left little finger at wrist and hand level

    ● **S66.328**   Laceration of extensor muscle, fascia and tendon of other finger at wrist and hand level

        Laceration of extensor muscle, fascia and tendon of specified finger with unspecified laterality at wrist and hand level

    ● **S66.329**   Laceration of extensor muscle, fascia and tendon of unspecified finger at wrist and hand level

CHAPTER 19 (S00-T88)

- ● S66.39   Other injury of extensor muscle, fascia and tendon of other and unspecified finger at wrist and hand level
  - ● S66.390   Other injury of extensor muscle, fascia and tendon of right index finger at wrist and hand level
  - ● S66.391   Other injury of extensor muscle, fascia and tendon of left index finger at wrist and hand level
  - ● S66.392   Other injury of extensor muscle, fascia and tendon of right middle finger at wrist and hand level
  - ● S66.393   Other injury of extensor muscle, fascia and tendon of left middle finger at wrist and hand level
  - ● S66.394   Other injury of extensor muscle, fascia and tendon of right ring finger at wrist and hand level
  - ● S66.395   Other injury of extensor muscle, fascia and tendon of left ring finger at wrist and hand level
  - ● S66.396   Other injury of extensor muscle, fascia and tendon of right little finger at wrist and hand level
  - ● S66.397   Other injury of extensor muscle, fascia and tendon of left little finger at wrist and hand level
  - ● S66.398   Other injury of extensor muscle, fascia and tendon of other finger at wrist and hand level

    Other injury of extensor muscle, fascia and tendon of specified finger with unspecified laterality at wrist and hand level
  - ● S66.399   Other injury of extensor muscle, fascia and tendon of unspecified finger at wrist and hand level
- ● S66.4   Injury of intrinsic muscle, fascia and tendon of thumb at wrist and hand level
  - ● S66.40   Unspecified injury of intrinsic muscle, fascia and tendon of thumb at wrist and hand level
    - ● S66.401   Unspecified injury of intrinsic muscle, fascia and tendon of right thumb at wrist and hand level
    - ● S66.402   Unspecified injury of intrinsic muscle, fascia and tendon of left thumb at wrist and hand level
    - ● S66.409   Unspecified injury of intrinsic muscle, fascia and tendon of unspecified thumb at wrist and hand level
  - ● S66.41   Strain of intrinsic muscle, fascia and tendon of thumb at wrist and hand level
    - ● S66.411   Strain of intrinsic muscle, fascia and tendon of right thumb at wrist and hand level
    - ● S66.412   Strain of intrinsic muscle, fascia and tendon of left thumb at wrist and hand level
    - ● S66.419   Strain of intrinsic muscle, fascia and tendon of unspecified thumb at wrist and hand level
  - ● S66.42   Laceration of intrinsic muscle, fascia and tendon of thumb at wrist and hand level
    - ● S66.421   Laceration of intrinsic muscle, fascia and tendon of right thumb at wrist and hand level
    - ● S66.422   Laceration of intrinsic muscle, fascia and tendon of left thumb at wrist and hand level

- ● S66.429   Laceration of intrinsic muscle, fascia and tendon of unspecified thumb at wrist and hand level
  - ● S66.49   Other specified injury of intrinsic muscle, fascia and tendon of thumb at wrist and hand level
    - ● S66.491   Other specified injury of intrinsic muscle, fascia and tendon of right thumb at wrist and hand level
    - ● S66.492   Other specified injury of intrinsic muscle, fascia and tendon of left thumb at wrist and hand level
    - ● S66.499   Other specified injury of intrinsic muscle, fascia and tendon of unspecified thumb at wrist and hand level
- ● S66.5   Injury of intrinsic muscle, fascia and tendon of other and unspecified finger at wrist and hand level

  Excludes2   injury of intrinsic muscle, fascia and tendon of thumb at wrist and hand level (S66.4-)
  - ● S66.50   Unspecified injury of intrinsic muscle, fascia and tendon of other and unspecified finger at wrist and hand level
    - ● S66.500   Unspecified injury of intrinsic muscle, fascia and tendon of right index finger at wrist and hand level
    - ● S66.501   Unspecified injury of intrinsic muscle, fascia and tendon of left index finger at wrist and hand level
    - ● S66.502   Unspecified injury of intrinsic muscle, fascia and tendon of right middle finger at wrist and hand level
    - ● S66.503   Unspecified injury of intrinsic muscle, fascia and tendon of left middle finger at wrist and hand level
    - ● S66.504   Unspecified injury of intrinsic muscle, fascia and tendon of right ring finger at wrist and hand level
    - ● S66.505   Unspecified injury of intrinsic muscle, fascia and tendon of left ring finger at wrist and hand level
    - ● S66.506   Unspecified injury of intrinsic muscle, fascia and tendon of right little finger at wrist and hand level
    - ● S66.507   Unspecified injury of intrinsic muscle, fascia and tendon of left little finger at wrist and hand level
    - ● S66.508   Unspecified injury of intrinsic muscle, fascia and tendon of other finger at wrist and hand level

      Unspecified injury of intrinsic muscle, fascia and tendon of specified finger with unspecified laterality at wrist and hand level
    - ● S66.509   Unspecified injury of intrinsic muscle, fascia and tendon of unspecified finger at wrist and hand level
  - ● S66.51   Strain of intrinsic muscle, fascia and tendon of other and unspecified finger at wrist and hand level
    - ● S66.510   Strain of intrinsic muscle, fascia and tendon of right index finger at wrist and hand level
    - ● S66.511   Strain of intrinsic muscle, fascia and tendon of left index finger at wrist and hand level
    - ● S66.512   Strain of intrinsic muscle, fascia and tendon of right middle finger at wrist and hand level

- ● S66.513   Strain of intrinsic muscle, fascia and tendon of left middle finger at wrist and hand level
- ● S66.514   Strain of intrinsic muscle, fascia and tendon of right ring finger at wrist and hand level
- ● S66.515   Strain of intrinsic muscle, fascia and tendon of left ring finger at wrist and hand level
- ● S66.516   Strain of intrinsic muscle, fascia and tendon of right little finger at wrist and hand level
- ● S66.517   Strain of intrinsic muscle, fascia and tendon of left little finger at wrist and hand level
- ● S66.518   Strain of intrinsic muscle, fascia and tendon of other finger at wrist and hand level

  Strain of intrinsic muscle, fascia and tendon of specified finger with unspecified laterality at wrist and hand level
- ● S66.519   Strain of intrinsic muscle, fascia and tendon of unspecified finger at wrist and hand level
- ● S66.52   Laceration of intrinsic muscle, fascia and tendon of other and unspecified finger at wrist and hand level
  - ● S66.520   Laceration of intrinsic muscle, fascia and tendon of right index finger at wrist and hand level
  - ● S66.521   Laceration of intrinsic muscle, fascia and tendon of left index finger at wrist and hand level
  - ● S66.522   Laceration of intrinsic muscle, fascia and tendon of right middle finger at wrist and hand level
  - ● S66.523   Laceration of intrinsic muscle, fascia and tendon of left middle finger at wrist and hand level
  - ● S66.524   Laceration of intrinsic muscle, fascia and tendon of right ring finger at wrist and hand level
  - ● S66.525   Laceration of intrinsic muscle, fascia and tendon of left ring finger at wrist and hand level
  - ● S66.526   Laceration of intrinsic muscle, fascia and tendon of right little finger at wrist and hand level
  - ● S66.527   Laceration of intrinsic muscle, fascia and tendon of left little finger at wrist and hand level
  - ● S66.528   Laceration of intrinsic muscle, fascia and tendon of other finger at wrist and hand level

    Laceration of intrinsic muscle, fascia and tendon of specified finger with unspecified laterality at wrist and hand level
  - ● S66.529   Laceration of intrinsic muscle, fascia and tendon of unspecified finger at wrist and hand level
- ● S66.59   Other injury of intrinsic muscle, fascia and tendon of other and unspecified finger at wrist and hand level
  - ● S66.590   Other injury of intrinsic muscle, fascia and tendon of right index finger at wrist and hand level
  - ● S66.591   Other injury of intrinsic muscle, fascia and tendon of left index finger at wrist and hand level

- ● S66.592   Other injury of intrinsic muscle, fascia and tendon of right middle finger at wrist and hand level
- ● S66.593   Other injury of intrinsic muscle, fascia and tendon of left middle finger at wrist and hand level
- ● S66.594   Other injury of intrinsic muscle, fascia and tendon of right ring finger at wrist and hand level
- ● S66.595   Other injury of intrinsic muscle, fascia and tendon of left ring finger at wrist and hand level
- ● S66.596   Other injury of intrinsic muscle, fascia and tendon of right little finger at wrist and hand level
- ● S66.597   Other injury of intrinsic muscle, fascia and tendon of left little finger at wrist and hand level
- ● S66.598   Other injury of intrinsic muscle, fascia and tendon of other finger at wrist and hand level

  Other injury of intrinsic muscle, fascia and tendon of specified finger with unspecified laterality at wrist and hand level
- ● S66.599   Other injury of intrinsic muscle, fascia and tendon of unspecified finger at wrist and hand level
- ● S66.8   Injury of other specified muscles, fascia and tendons at wrist and hand level
  - ● S66.80   Unspecified injury of other specified muscles, fascia and tendons at wrist and hand level
    - ● S66.801   Unspecified injury of other specified muscles, fascia and tendons at wrist and hand level, right hand
    - ● S66.802   Unspecified injury of other specified muscles, fascia and tendons at wrist and hand level, left hand
    - ● S66.809   Unspecified injury of other specified muscles, fascia and tendons at wrist and hand level, unspecified hand
  - ● S66.81   Strain of other specified muscles, fascia and tendons at wrist and hand level
    - ● S66.811   Strain of other specified muscles, fascia and tendons at wrist and hand level, right hand
    - ● S66.812   Strain of other specified muscles, fascia and tendons at wrist and hand level, left hand
    - ● S66.819   Strain of other specified muscles, fascia and tendons at wrist and hand level, unspecified hand
  - ● S66.82   Laceration of other specified muscles, fascia and tendons at wrist and hand level
    - ● S66.821   Laceration of other specified muscles, fascia and tendons at wrist and hand level, right hand
    - ● S66.822   Laceration of other specified muscles, fascia and tendons at wrist and hand level, left hand
    - ● S66.829   Laceration of other specified muscles, fascia and tendons at wrist and hand level, unspecified hand
  - ● S66.89   Other injury of other specified muscles, fascia and tendons at wrist and hand level
    - ● S66.891   Other injury of other specified muscles, fascia and tendons at wrist and hand level, right hand

CHAPTER 19 (S00-T88)

● S66.892   Other injury of other specified muscles, fascia and tendons at wrist and hand level, left hand

● S66.899   Other injury of other specified muscles, fascia and tendons at wrist and hand level, unspecified hand

● S66.9   Injury of unspecified muscle, fascia and tendon at wrist and hand level

   ● S66.90   Unspecified injury of unspecified muscle, fascia and tendon at wrist and hand level

     ● S66.901   Unspecified injury of unspecified muscle, fascia and tendon at wrist and hand level, right hand

     ● S66.902   Unspecified injury of unspecified muscle, fascia and tendon at wrist and hand level, left hand

     ● S66.909   Unspecified injury of unspecified muscle, fascia and tendon at wrist and hand level, unspecified hand

   ● S66.91   Strain of unspecified muscle, fascia and tendon at wrist and hand level

     ● S66.911   Strain of unspecified muscle, fascia and tendon at wrist and hand level, right hand

     ● S66.912   Strain of unspecified muscle, fascia and tendon at wrist and hand level, left hand

     ● S66.919   Strain of unspecified muscle, fascia and tendon at wrist and hand level, unspecified hand

   ● S66.92   Laceration of unspecified muscle, fascia and tendon at wrist and hand level

     ● S66.921   Laceration of unspecified muscle, fascia and tendon at wrist and hand level, right hand

     ● S66.922   Laceration of unspecified muscle, fascia and tendon at wrist and hand level, left hand

     ● S66.929   Laceration of unspecified muscle, fascia and tendon at wrist and hand level, unspecified hand

   ● S66.99   Other injury of unspecified muscle, fascia and tendon at wrist and hand level

     ● S66.991   Other injury of unspecified muscle, fascia and tendon at wrist and hand level, right hand

     ● S66.992   Other injury of unspecified muscle, fascia and tendon at wrist and hand level, left hand

     ● S66.999   Other injury of unspecified muscle, fascia and tendon at wrist and hand level, unspecified hand

● S67   Crushing injury of wrist, hand and fingers

   Use additional code for all associated injuries, such as:
     fracture of wrist and hand (S62.-)
     open wound of wrist and hand (S61.-)

   The appropriate 7th character is to be added to each code from category S67

A	initial encounter
D	subsequent encounter
S	sequela

   ● S67.0   Crushing injury of thumb

     X ● S67.00   Crushing injury of unspecified thumb
     X ● S67.01   Crushing injury of right thumb
     X ● S67.02   Crushing injury of left thumb

● S67.1   Crushing injury of other and unspecified finger(s)

   Excludes2   crushing injury of thumb (S67.0-)

   X ● S67.10   Crushing injury of unspecified finger(s)

   ● S67.19   Crushing injury of other finger(s)

     ● S67.190   Crushing injury of right index finger
     ● S67.191   Crushing injury of left index finger
     ● S67.192   Crushing injury of right middle finger
     ● S67.193   Crushing injury of left middle finger
     ● S67.194   Crushing injury of right ring finger
     ● S67.195   Crushing injury of left ring finger
     ● S67.196   Crushing injury of right little finger
     ● S67.197   Crushing injury of left little finger
     ● S67.198   Crushing injury of other finger
         Crushing injury of specified finger with unspecified laterality

● S67.2   Crushing injury of hand

   Excludes2   crushing injury of fingers (S67.1-)
         crushing injury of thumb (S67.0-)

   X ● S67.20   Crushing injury of unspecified hand
   X ● S67.21   Crushing injury of right hand
   X ● S67.22   Crushing injury of left hand

● S67.3   Crushing injury of wrist

   X ● S67.30   Crushing injury of unspecified wrist
   X ● S67.31   Crushing injury of right wrist
   X ● S67.32   Crushing injury of left wrist

● S67.4   Crushing injury of wrist and hand

   Excludes1   crushing injury of hand alone (S67.2-)
         crushing injury of wrist alone (S67.3-)

   Excludes2   crushing injury of fingers (S67.1-)
         crushing injury of thumb (S67.0-)

   X ● S67.40   Crushing injury of unspecified wrist and hand
   X ● S67.41   Crushing injury of right wrist and hand
   X ● S67.42   Crushing injury of left wrist and hand

● S67.9   Crushing injury of unspecified part(s) of wrist, hand and fingers

   X ● S67.90   Crushing injury of unspecified part(s) of unspecified wrist, hand and fingers
   X ● S67.91   Crushing injury of unspecified part(s) of right wrist, hand and fingers
   X ● S67.92   Crushing injury of unspecified part(s) of left wrist, hand and fingers

● S68   Traumatic amputation of wrist, hand and fingers

   An amputation not identified as partial or complete should be coded to complete

   The appropriate 7th character is to be added to each code from category S68

A	initial encounter
D	subsequent encounter
S	sequela

● S68.0   Traumatic metacarpophalangeal amputation of thumb
   Traumatic amputation of thumb NOS

   ● S68.01   Complete traumatic metacarpophalangeal amputation of thumb

     ● S68.011   Complete traumatic metacarpophalangeal amputation of right thumb S 🐾

     ● S68.012   Complete traumatic metacarpophalangeal amputation of left thumb S 🐾

     ● S68.019   Complete traumatic metacarpophalangeal amputation of unspecified thumb S 🐾

S68.02   **Partial** traumatic metacarpophalangeal amputation of thumb

- S68.021   Partial traumatic metacarpophalangeal amputation of **right thumb** S 🔖
- S68.022   Partial traumatic metacarpophalangeal amputation of **left thumb** S 🔖
- S68.029   Partial traumatic metacarpophalangeal amputation of **unspecified thumb** S 🔖

S68.1   Traumatic **metacarpophalangeal** amputation of other and unspecified **finger**

   Traumatic amputation of finger NOS

   Excludes2   traumatic metacarpophalangeal amputation of thumb (S68.0-)

- S68.11   **Complete** traumatic metacarpophalangeal amputation of other and unspecified finger

  - S68.110   Complete traumatic metacarpophalangeal amputation of **right index** finger S 🔖
  - S68.111   Complete traumatic metacarpophalangeal amputation of **left index** finger S 🔖
  - S68.112   Complete traumatic metacarpophalangeal amputation of **right middle** finger S 🔖
  - S68.113   Complete traumatic metacarpophalangeal amputation of **left middle** finger S 🔖
  - S68.114   Complete traumatic metacarpophalangeal amputation of **right ring** finger S 🔖
  - S68.115   Complete traumatic metacarpophalangeal amputation of **left ring** finger S 🔖
  - S68.116   Complete traumatic metacarpophalangeal amputation of **right little** finger S 🔖
  - S68.117   Complete traumatic metacarpophalangeal amputation of **left little** finger S 🔖
  - S68.118   Complete traumatic metacarpophalangeal amputation of **other** finger S 🔖

    Complete traumatic metacarpophalangeal amputation of specified finger with unspecified laterality

  - S68.119   Complete traumatic metacarpophalangeal amputation of **unspecified** finger S 🔖

- S68.12   **Partial** traumatic metacarpophalangeal amputation of other and unspecified finger

  - S68.120   Partial traumatic metacarpophalangeal amputation of **right index** finger S 🔖
  - S68.121   Partial traumatic metacarpophalangeal amputation of **left index** finger S 🔖
  - S68.122   Partial traumatic metacarpophalangeal amputation of **right middle** finger S 🔖
  - S68.123   Partial traumatic metacarpophalangeal amputation of **left middle** finger S 🔖
  - S68.124   Partial traumatic metacarpophalangeal amputation of **right ring** finger S 🔖
  - S68.125   Partial traumatic metacarpophalangeal amputation of **left ring** finger S 🔖

- S68.126   Partial traumatic metacarpophalangeal amputation of **right little** finger S 🔖
- S68.127   Partial traumatic metacarpophalangeal amputation of **left little** finger S 🔖
- S68.128   Partial traumatic metacarpophalangeal amputation of **other** finger S 🔖

  Partial traumatic metacarpophalangeal amputation of specified finger with unspecified laterality

- S68.129   Partial traumatic metacarpophalangeal amputation of **unspecified** finger S 🔖

S68.4   Traumatic amputation of **hand** at wrist level

   Traumatic amputation of hand NOS
   Traumatic amputation of wrist

- S68.41   **Complete** traumatic amputation of hand at wrist level

  - S68.411   Complete traumatic amputation of **right** hand at wrist level A, S 🔖
  - S68.412   Complete traumatic amputation of **left** hand at wrist level A, S 🔖
  - S68.419   Complete traumatic amputation of **unspecified** hand at wrist level A, S 🔖

- S68.42   **Partial** traumatic amputation of hand at wrist level

  - S68.421   Partial traumatic amputation of **right** hand at wrist level A, S 🔖
  - S68.422   Partial traumatic amputation of **left** hand at wrist level A, S 🔖
  - S68.429   Partial traumatic amputation of **unspecified** hand at wrist level A, S 🔖

S68.5   Traumatic **transphalangeal** amputation of **thumb**

   Traumatic interphalangeal joint amputation of thumb

- S68.51   **Complete** traumatic transphalangeal amputation of thumb

  - S68.511   Complete traumatic transphalangeal amputation of **right** thumb S 🔖
  - S68.512   Complete traumatic transphalangeal amputation of **left** thumb S 🔖
  - S68.519   Complete traumatic transphalangeal amputation of **unspecified** thumb S 🔖

- S68.52   **Partial** traumatic transphalangeal amputation of thumb

  - S68.521   Partial traumatic transphalangeal amputation of **right** thumb S 🔖
  - S68.522   Partial traumatic transphalangeal amputation of **left** thumb S 🔖
  - S68.529   Partial traumatic transphalangeal amputation of **unspecified** thumb S 🔖

S68.6   Traumatic **transphalangeal** amputation of other and unspecified **finger**

- S68.61   **Complete** traumatic transphalangeal amputation of other and unspecified finger(s)

  - S68.610   Complete traumatic transphalangeal amputation of **right index** finger S 🔖
  - S68.611   Complete traumatic transphalangeal amputation of **left index** finger S 🔖
  - S68.612   Complete traumatic transphalangeal amputation of **right middle** finger S 🔖
  - S68.613   Complete traumatic transphalangeal amputation of **left middle** finger S 🔖
  - S68.614   Complete traumatic transphalangeal amputation of **right ring** finger S 🔖
  - S68.615   Complete traumatic transphalangeal amputation of **left ring** finger S 🔖

● S68.616   Complete traumatic transphalangeal amputation of **right little finger** S 🐾

● S68.617   Complete traumatic transphalangeal amputation of **left little finger** S 🐾

● S68.618   Complete traumatic transphalangeal amputation of **other finger** S 🐾
    Complete traumatic transphalangeal amputation of specified finger with unspecified laterality

● S68.619   Complete traumatic transphalangeal amputation of **unspecified finger** S 🐾

● S68.62   Partial traumatic transphalangeal amputation of **other and unspecified finger**

  ● S68.620   Partial traumatic transphalangeal amputation of **right index finger** S 🐾

  ● S68.621   Partial traumatic transphalangeal amputation of **left index finger** S 🐾

  ● S68.622   Partial traumatic transphalangeal amputation of **right middle finger** S 🐾

  ● S68.623   Partial traumatic transphalangeal amputation of **left middle finger** S 🐾

  ● S68.624   Partial traumatic transphalangeal amputation of **right ring finger** S 🐾

  ● S68.625   Partial traumatic transphalangeal amputation of **left ring finger** S 🐾

  ● S68.626   Partial traumatic transphalangeal amputation of **right little finger** S 🐾

  ● S68.627   Partial traumatic transphalangeal amputation of **left little finger** S 🐾

  ● S68.628   Partial traumatic transphalangeal amputation of **other finger** S 🐾
    Partial traumatic transphalangeal amputation of specified finger with unspecified laterality

  ● S68.629   Partial traumatic transphalangeal amputation of **unspecified finger** S 🐾

● S68.7   Traumatic **transmetacarpal amputation of hand**

  ● S68.71   Complete traumatic transmetacarpal amputation of hand

    ● S68.711   Complete traumatic transmetacarpal amputation of **right hand** A, S 🐾

    ● S68.712   Complete traumatic transmetacarpal amputation of **left hand** A, S 🐾

    ● S68.719   Complete traumatic transmetacarpal amputation of **unspecified hand** A, S 🐾

  ● S68.72   Partial traumatic transmetacarpal amputation of hand

    ● S68.721   Partial traumatic transmetacarpal amputation of **right hand** A, S 🐾

    ● S68.722   Partial traumatic transmetacarpal amputation of **left hand** A, S 🐾

    ● S68.729   Partial traumatic transmetacarpal amputation of **unspecified hand** A, S 🐾

● S69   Other and unspecified injuries of wrist, hand and finger(s)
The appropriate 7th character is to be added to each code from category S69

A	initial encounter
D	subsequent encounter
S	sequela

● S69.8   **Other** specified injuries of wrist, hand and finger(s)

  X ● S69.80   Other specified injuries of **unspecified** wrist, hand and finger(s)

  X ● S69.81   Other specified injuries of **right** wrist, hand and finger(s)

  X ● S69.82   Other specified injuries of **left** wrist, hand and finger(s)

● S69.9   **Unspecified** injury of wrist, hand and finger(s)

  X ● S69.90   Unspecified injury of **unspecified** wrist, hand and finger(s)

  X ● S69.91   Unspecified injury of **right** wrist, hand and finger(s)

  X ● S69.92   Unspecified injury of **left** wrist, hand and finger(s)

INJURIES TO THE HIP AND THIGH (S70-S79)

Excludes2   burns and corrosions (T20-T32)
frostbite (T33-T34)
snake bite (T63.0-)
venomous insect bite or sting (T63.4-)

● S70   Superficial injury of hip and thigh
The appropriate 7th character is to be added to each code from category S70

A	initial encounter
D	subsequent encounter
S	sequela

● S70.0   Contusion of hip

  X ● S70.00   Contusion of **unspecified** hip

  X ● S70.01   Contusion of **right** hip

  X ● S70.02   Contusion of **left** hip

● S70.1   Contusion of **thigh**

  X ● S70.10   Contusion of **unspecified** thigh

  X ● S70.11   Contusion of **right** thigh

  X ● S70.12   Contusion of **left** thigh

● S70.2   Other superficial injuries of **hip**

  ● S70.21   **Abrasion** of hip

    ● S70.211   Abrasion, **right hip**

    ● S70.212   Abrasion, **left hip**

    ● S70.219   Abrasion, **unspecified** hip

  ● S70.22   **Blister** (nonthermal) of hip

    ● S70.221   Blister (nonthermal), **right hip**

    ● S70.222   Blister (nonthermal), **left hip**

    ● S70.229   Blister (nonthermal), **unspecified** hip

  ● S70.24   **External constriction** of hip

    ● S70.241   External constriction, **right hip**

    ● S70.242   External constriction, **left hip**

    ● S70.249   External constriction, **unspecified** hip

  ● S70.25   **Superficial foreign** body of hip
    Splinter in the hip

    ● S70.251   Superficial foreign body, **right hip**

    ● S70.252   Superficial foreign body, **left hip**

    ● S70.259   Superficial foreign body, **unspecified** hip

  ● S70.26   **Insect bite** (nonvenomous) of hip

    ● S70.261   Insect bite (nonvenomous), **right hip**

    ● S70.262   Insect bite (nonvenomous), **left hip**

    ● S70.269   Insect bite (nonvenomous), **unspecified** hip

  ● S70.27   **Other superficial bite** of hip
    Excludes1   open bite of hip (S71.05-)

    ● S70.271   Other superficial bite of hip, **right hip**

    ● S70.272   Other superficial bite of hip, **left hip**

    ● S70.279   Other superficial bite of hip, **unspecified** hip

● S70.3   Other superficial injuries of **thigh**

  ● S70.31   **Abrasion** of thigh

    ● S70.311   Abrasion, **right thigh**

    ● S70.312   Abrasion, **left thigh**

    ● S70.319   Abrasion, **unspecified** thigh

- **S70.32**   Blister (nonthermal) of thigh
  - **S70.321**   Blister (nonthermal), right thigh
  - **S70.322**   Blister (nonthermal), left thigh
  - **S70.329**   Blister (nonthermal), unspecified thigh
- **S70.34**   External constriction of thigh
  - **S70.341**   External constriction, right thigh
  - **S70.342**   External constriction, left thigh
  - **S70.349**   External constriction, unspecified thigh
- **S70.35**   Superficial foreign body of thigh
    Splinter in the thigh
  - **S70.351**   Superficial foreign body, right thigh
  - **S70.352**   Superficial foreign body, left thigh
  - **S70.359**   Superficial foreign body, unspecified thigh
- **S70.36**   Insect bite (nonvenomous) of thigh
  - **S70.361**   Insect bite (nonvenomous), right thigh
  - **S70.362**   Insect bite (nonvenomous), left thigh
  - **S70.369**   Insect bite (nonvenomous), unspecified thigh
- **S70.37**   Other superficial bite of thigh
    Excludes1   open bite of thigh (S71.15)
  - **S70.371**   Other superficial bite of right thigh
  - **S70.372**   Other superficial bite of left thigh
  - **S70.379**   Other superficial bite of unspecified thigh
- **S70.9**   Unspecified superficial injury of hip and thigh
  - **S70.91**   Unspecified superficial injury of hip
    - **S70.911**   Unspecified superficial injury of right hip
    - **S70.912**   Unspecified superficial injury of left hip
    - **S70.919**   Unspecified superficial injury of unspecified hip
  - **S70.92**   Unspecified superficial injury of thigh
    - **S70.921**   Unspecified superficial injury of right thigh
    - **S70.922**   Unspecified superficial injury of left thigh
    - **S70.929**   Unspecified superficial injury of unspecified thigh

- **S71**   Open wound of hip and thigh
    Code also any associated wound infection
    Excludes1   open fracture of hip and thigh (S72.-)
                   traumatic amputation of hip and thigh (S78.-)
    Excludes2   bite of venomous animal (T63.-)
                   open wound of ankle, foot and toes (S91.-)
                   open wound of knee and lower leg (S81.-)
    The appropriate 7th character is to be added to each code from category S71

    | A | initial encounter |
    | D | subsequent encounter |
    | S | sequela |

  - **S71.0**   Open wound of hip
    - **S71.00**   Unspecified open wound of hip
      - **S71.001**   Unspecified open wound, right hip
      - **S71.002**   Unspecified open wound, left hip
      - **S71.009**   Unspecified open wound, unspecified hip
    - **S71.01**   Laceration without foreign body of hip
      - **S71.011**   Laceration without foreign body, right hip

- **S71.012**   Laceration without foreign body, left hip
- **S71.019**   Laceration without foreign body, unspecified hip
- **S71.02**   Laceration with foreign body of hip
  - **S71.021**   Laceration with foreign body, right hip
  - **S71.022**   Laceration with foreign body, left hip
  - **S71.029**   Laceration with foreign body, unspecified hip
- **S71.03**   Puncture wound without foreign body of hip
  - **S71.031**   Puncture wound without foreign body, right hip
  - **S71.032**   Puncture wound without foreign body, left hip
  - **S71.039**   Puncture wound without foreign body, unspecified hip
- **S71.04**   Puncture wound with foreign body of hip
  - **S71.041**   Puncture wound with foreign body, right hip
  - **S71.042**   Puncture wound with foreign body, left hip
  - **S71.049**   Puncture wound with foreign body, unspecified hip
- **S71.05**   Open bite of hip
    Bite of hip NOS
    Excludes1   superficial bite of hip (S70.26, S70.27)
  - **S71.051**   Open bite, right hip
  - **S71.052**   Open bite, left hip
  - **S71.059**   Open bite, unspecified hip
- **S71.1**   Open wound of thigh
  - **S71.10**   Unspecified open wound of thigh
    - **S71.101**   Unspecified open wound, right thigh
    - **S71.102**   Unspecified open wound, left thigh
    - **S71.109**   Unspecified open wound, unspecified thigh
  - **S71.11**   Laceration without foreign body of thigh
    - **S71.111**   Laceration without foreign body, right thigh
    - **S71.112**   Laceration without foreign body, left thigh
    - **S71.119**   Laceration without foreign body, unspecified thigh
  - **S71.12**   Laceration with foreign body of thigh
    - **S71.121**   Laceration with foreign body, right thigh
    - **S71.122**   Laceration with foreign body, left thigh
    - **S71.129**   Laceration with foreign body, unspecified thigh
  - **S71.13**   Puncture wound without foreign body of thigh
    - **S71.131**   Puncture wound without foreign body, right thigh
    - **S71.132**   Puncture wound without foreign body, left thigh
        Coding Clinic: 2023, Q3, P12
    - **S71.139**   Puncture wound without foreign body, unspecified thigh
  - **S71.14**   Puncture wound with foreign body of thigh
    - **S71.141**   Puncture wound with foreign body, right thigh
    - **S71.142**   Puncture wound with foreign body, left thigh
    - **S71.149**   Puncture wound with foreign body, unspecified thigh

CHAPTER 19 (S00-T88)

● S71.15   **Open bite of thigh**
            Bite of thigh NOS
            Excludes1   superficial bite of thigh (S70.37-)
        ● S71.151   Open bite, **right thigh**
        ● S71.152   Open bite, **left thigh**
        ● S71.159   Open bite, **unspecified thigh**

● S72   **Fracture of femur**
        Note: A fracture not indicated as displaced or nondisplaced
               should be coded to displaced
               A fracture not indicated as open or closed should be coded
               to closed
               The open fracture designations are based on the Gustilo
               open fracture classification
        Excludes1   traumatic amputation of hip and thigh (S78.-)
        Excludes2   fracture of lower leg and ankle (S82.-)
                        fracture of foot (S92.-)
                        periprosthetic fracture of prosthetic implant of
                        hip (M97.0-)
        The appropriate 7th character is to be added to all codes from
            category S72

A	initial encounter for closed fracture
B	initial encounter for open fracture type I or II
	initial encounter for open fracture NOS
C	initial encounter for open fracture type IIIA, IIIB, or IIIC
D	subsequent encounter for closed fracture with routine healing
E	subsequent encounter for open fracture type I or II with routine healing
F	subsequent encounter for open fracture type IIIA, IIIB, or IIIC with routine healing
G	subsequent encounter for closed fracture with delayed healing
H	subsequent encounter for open fracture type I or II with delayed healing
J	subsequent encounter for open fracture type IIIA, IIIB, or IIIC with delayed healing
K	subsequent encounter for closed fracture with nonunion
M	subsequent encounter for open fracture type I or II with nonunion
N	subsequent encounter for open fracture type IIIA, IIIB, or IIIC with nonunion
P	subsequent encounter for closed fracture with malunion
Q	subsequent encounter for open fracture type I or II with malunion
R	subsequent encounter for open fracture type IIIA, IIIB, or IIIC with malunion
S	sequela

● S72.0   **Fracture of head and neck of femur**
            Excludes2   physeal fracture of lower end of femur
                            (S79.1-)
                            physeal fracture of upper end of femur (S79.0-)
        ● S72.00   **Fracture of unspecified part of neck of femur**
                    Fracture of hip NOS
                    Fracture of neck of femur NOS
                ● S72.001   **Fracture of unspecified part of neck of
                            right femur** A, B, C 🏥
                ● S72.002   **Fracture of unspecified part of neck of
                            left femur** A, B, C 🏥
                            Coding Clinic: 2015, Q4, P37, Q1, P17
                ● S72.009   **Fracture of unspecified part of neck of
                            unspecified femur** A, B, C 🏥
        ● S72.01   **Unspecified intracapsular fracture of femur**
                    Subcapital fracture of femur
                ● S72.011   **Unspecified intracapsular fracture of
                            right femur** A, B, C 🏥
                ● S72.012   **Unspecified intracapsular fracture of
                            left femur** A, B, C 🏥
                ● S72.019   **Unspecified intracapsular fracture of
                            unspecified femur** A, B, C 🏥
        ● S72.02   **Fracture of epiphysis (separation) (upper) of
                    femur**
                    Transepiphyseal fracture of femur
                    Fracture and separation across growth plate
                    Excludes1   capital femoral epiphyseal fracture
                                    (pediatric) of femur (S79.01-)
                                    Salter-Harris Type I physeal
                                    fracture of upper end of
                                    femur (S79.01-)
                ● S72.021   **Displaced fracture of epiphysis
                            (separation) (upper) of right femur**
                            A, B, C 🏥
                ● S72.022   **Displaced fracture of epiphysis
                            (separation) (upper) of left femur**
                            A, B, C 🏥
                ● S72.023   **Displaced fracture of epiphysis
                            (separation) (upper) of unspecified
                            femur** A, B, C 🏥
                ● S72.024   **Nondisplaced fracture of epiphysis
                            (separation) (upper) of right femur**
                            A, B, C 🏥
                ● S72.025   **Nondisplaced fracture of epiphysis
                            (separation) (upper) of left femur**
                            A, B, C 🏥
                ● S72.026   **Nondisplaced fracture of epiphysis
                            (separation) (upper) of unspecified
                            femur** A, B, C 🏥

▶ New   ⇒ Revised   ~~deleted~~ Deleted   Excludes 1   Excludes 2   Includes   Use additional   Code first   Code also   Key words
OGCR Official Guidelines   X Assign placeholder X   ● Use Additional Character(s)   ▶ Manifestation Code   🏥 Hierarchical Condition Category   Coding Clinic

● **S72.03**   **Midcervical** fracture of femur
Transcervical fracture of femur NOS

   ● **S72.031**   Displaced midcervical fracture of right femur A, B, C 🔖

   ● **S72.032**   Displaced midcervical fracture of left femur A, B, C 🔖

   ● **S72.033**   Displaced midcervical fracture of unspecified femur A, B, C 🔖

   ● **S72.034**   Nondisplaced midcervical fracture of right femur A, B, C 🔖

   ● **S72.035**   Nondisplaced midcervical fracture of left femur A, B, C 🔖

   ● **S72.036**   Nondisplaced midcervical fracture of unspecified femur A, B, C 🔖

● **S72.04**   Fracture of **base of neck** of femur
Cervicotrochanteric fracture of femur

   ● **S72.041**   Displaced fracture of base of neck of right femur A, B, C 🔖

   ● **S72.042**   Displaced fracture of base of neck of left femur A, B, C 🔖

   ● **S72.043**   Displaced fracture of base of neck of unspecified femur A, B, C 🔖

   ● **S72.044**   Nondisplaced fracture of base of neck of right femur A, B, C 🔖

   ● **S72.045**   Nondisplaced fracture of base of neck of left femur A, B, C 🔖

   ● **S72.046**   Nondisplaced fracture of base of neck of unspecified femur A, B, C 🔖

● **S72.05**   **Unspecified** fracture of head of femur
Fracture of head of femur NOS

   ● **S72.051**   Unspecified fracture of head of right femur A, B, C 🔖

   ● **S72.052**   Unspecified fracture of head of left femur A, B, C 🔖

   ● **S72.059**   Unspecified fracture of head of unspecified femur A, B, C 🔖

● **S72.06**   **Articular** fracture of head of femur

   ● **S72.061**   Displaced articular fracture of head of right femur A, B, C 🔖

   ● **S72.062**   Displaced articular fracture of head of left femur A, B, C 🔖

   ● **S72.063**   Displaced articular fracture of head of unspecified femur A, B, C 🔖

   ● **S72.064**   Nondisplaced articular fracture of head of right femur A, B, C 🔖

   ● **S72.065**   Nondisplaced articular fracture of head of left femur A, B, C 🔖

   ● **S72.066**   Nondisplaced articular fracture of head of unspecified femur A, B, C 🔖

● **S72.09**   **Other** fracture of **head and neck** of femur

   ● **S72.091**   Other fracture of head and neck of right femur A, B, C 🔖

   ● **S72.092**   Other fracture of head and neck of left femur A, B, C 🔖

   ● **S72.099**   Other fracture of head and neck of unspecified femur A, B, C 🔖

● **S72.1**   **Pertrochanteric** fracture
Fracture extending close to, but not into, joint

  ● **S72.10**   **Unspecified trochanteric** fracture of femur
Fracture of trochanter NOS

   ● **S72.101**   Unspecified trochanteric fracture of right femur A, B, C 🔖

   ● **S72.102**   Unspecified trochanteric fracture of left femur A, B, C 🔖

   ● **S72.109**   Unspecified trochanteric fracture of unspecified femur A, B, C 🔖

  ● **S72.11**   Fracture of **greater trochanter** of femur

   ● **S72.111**   Displaced fracture of greater trochanter of right femur A, B, C 🔖

   ● **S72.112**   Displaced fracture of greater trochanter of left femur A, B, C 🔖

   ● **S72.113**   Displaced fracture of greater trochanter of unspecified femur A, B, C 🔖

   ● **S72.114**   Nondisplaced fracture of greater trochanter of right femur A, B, C 🔖

   ● **S72.115**   Nondisplaced fracture of greater trochanter of left femur A, B, C 🔖

   ● **S72.116**   Nondisplaced fracture of greater trochanter of unspecified femur A, B, C 🔖

  ● **S72.12**   Fracture of **lesser trochanter** of femur

   ● **S72.121**   Displaced fracture of lesser trochanter of right femur A, B, C 🔖

   ● **S72.122**   Displaced fracture of lesser trochanter of left femur A, B, C 🔖

   ● **S72.123**   Displaced fracture of lesser trochanter of unspecified femur A, B, C 🔖

   ● **S72.124**   Nondisplaced fracture of lesser trochanter of right femur A, B, C 🔖

   ● **S72.125**   Nondisplaced fracture of lesser trochanter of left femur A, B, C 🔖

   ● **S72.126**   Nondisplaced fracture of lesser trochanter of unspecified femur A, B, C 🔖

  ● **S72.13**   **Apophyseal** fracture of femur
Pertaining to articulations between articular facets of adjacent vertebrae

    Excludes1   chronic (nontraumatic) slipped upper femoral epiphysis (M93.0-)

   ● **S72.131**   Displaced apophyseal fracture of right femur A, B, C 🔖

   ● **S72.132**   Displaced apophyseal fracture of left femur A, B, C 🔖

   ● **S72.133**   Displaced apophyseal fracture of unspecified femur A, B, C 🔖

   ● **S72.134**   Nondisplaced apophyseal fracture of right femur A, B, C 🔖

   ● **S72.135**   Nondisplaced apophyseal fracture of left femur A, B, C 🔖

   ● **S72.136**   Nondisplaced apophyseal fracture of unspecified femur A, B, C 🔖

  ● **S72.14**   **Intertrochanteric** fracture of femur

   ● **S72.141**   Displaced intertrochanteric fracture of right femur A, B, C 🔖
       Coding Clinic: 2016, Q3, P17

   ● **S72.142**   Displaced intertrochanteric fracture of left femur A, B, C 🔖

   ● **S72.143**   Displaced intertrochanteric fracture of unspecified femur A, B, C 🔖

   ● **S72.144**   Nondisplaced intertrochanteric fracture of right femur A, B, C 🔖

   ● **S72.145**   Nondisplaced intertrochanteric fracture of left femur A, B, C 🔖

   ● **S72.146**   Nondisplaced intertrochanteric fracture of unspecified femur A, B, C 🔖

● **S72.2**   **Subtrochanteric** fracture of femur
Subtrochanteric: inferior to trochanter

  X ● **S72.21**   Displaced subtrochanteric fracture of right femur A, B, C 🔖

  X ● **S72.22**   Displaced subtrochanteric fracture of left femur A, B, C 🔖

  X ● **S72.23**   Displaced subtrochanteric fracture of unspecified femur A, B, C 🔖

  X ● **S72.24**   Nondisplaced subtrochanteric fracture of right femur A, B, C 🔖

X ● S72.25   Nondisplaced subtrochanteric fracture of left femur A, B, C 🐾

X ● S72.26   Nondisplaced subtrochanteric fracture of unspecified femur A, B, C 🐾

● S72.3   Fracture of shaft of femur

  ● S72.30   Unspecified fracture of shaft of femur

    ● S72.301   Unspecified fracture of shaft of right femur A, B, C 🐾
      Coding Clinic: 2018, Q2, P12

    ● S72.302   Unspecified fracture of shaft of left femur A, B, C 🐾

    ● S72.309   Unspecified fracture of shaft of unspecified femur A, B, C 🐾

  ● S72.32   Transverse fracture of shaft of femur

    ● S72.321   Displaced transverse fracture of shaft of right femur A, B, C 🐾

    ● S72.322   Displaced transverse fracture of shaft of left femur A, B, C 🐾

    ● S72.323   Displaced transverse fracture of shaft of unspecified femur A, B, C 🐾

    ● S72.324   Nondisplaced transverse fracture of shaft of right femur A, B, C 🐾

    ● S72.325   Nondisplaced transverse fracture of shaft of left femur A, B, C 🐾

    ● S72.326   Nondisplaced transverse fracture of shaft of unspecified femur A, B, C 🐾

  ● S72.33   Oblique fracture of shaft of femur

    ● S72.331   Displaced oblique fracture of shaft of right femur A, B, C 🐾

    ● S72.332   Displaced oblique fracture of shaft of left femur A, B, C 🐾

    ● S72.333   Displaced oblique fracture of shaft of unspecified femur A, B, C 🐾

    ● S72.334   Nondisplaced oblique fracture of shaft of right femur A, B, C 🐾

    ● S72.335   Nondisplaced oblique fracture of shaft of left femur A, B, C 🐾

    ● S72.336   Nondisplaced oblique fracture of shaft of unspecified femur A, B, C 🐾

  ● S72.34   Spiral fracture of shaft of femur

    ● S72.341   Displaced spiral fracture of shaft of right femur A, B, C 🐾

    ● S72.342   Displaced spiral fracture of shaft of left femur A, B, C 🐾

    ● S72.343   Displaced spiral fracture of shaft of unspecified femur A, B, C 🐾

    ● S72.344   Nondisplaced spiral fracture of shaft of right femur A, B, C 🐾

    ● S72.345   Nondisplaced spiral fracture of shaft of left femur A, B, C 🐾

    ● S72.346   Nondisplaced spiral fracture of shaft of unspecified femur A, B, C 🐾

  ● S72.35   Comminuted fracture of shaft of femur

    ● S72.351   Displaced comminuted fracture of shaft of right femur A, B, C 🐾

    ● S72.352   Displaced comminuted fracture of shaft of left femur A, B, C 🐾

    ● S72.353   Displaced comminuted fracture of shaft of unspecified femur A, B, C 🐾

    ● S72.354   Nondisplaced comminuted fracture of shaft of right femur A, B, C 🐾

    ● S72.355   Nondisplaced comminuted fracture of shaft of left femur A, B, C 🐾

    ● S72.356   Nondisplaced comminuted fracture of shaft of unspecified femur A, B, C 🐾

  ● S72.36   Segmental fracture of shaft of femur

    ● S72.361   Displaced segmental fracture of shaft of right femur A, B, C 🐾

    ● S72.362   Displaced segmental fracture of shaft of left femur A, B, C 🐾

    ● S72.363   Displaced segmental fracture of shaft of unspecified femur A, B, C 🐾

    ● S72.364   Nondisplaced segmental fracture of shaft of right femur A, B, C 🐾

    ● S72.365   Nondisplaced segmental fracture of shaft of left femur A, B, C 🐾

    ● S72.366   Nondisplaced segmental fracture of shaft of unspecified femur A, B, C 🐾

  ● S72.39   Other fracture of shaft of femur

    ● S72.391   Other fracture of shaft of right femur A, B, C 🐾

    ● S72.392   Other fracture of shaft of left femur A, B, C 🐾

    ● S72.399   Other fracture of shaft of unspecified femur A, B, C 🐾

● S72.4   Fracture of lower end of femur
Fracture of distal end of femur

  Excludes2   fracture of shaft of femur (S72.3-)
    physeal fracture of lower end of femur (S79.1-)

  ● S72.40   Unspecified fracture of lower end of femur

    ● S72.401   Unspecified fracture of lower end of right femur A, B, C 🐾
      Coding Clinic: 2016, Q4, P43

    ● S72.402   Unspecified fracture of lower end of left femur A, B, C 🐾

    ● S72.409   Unspecified fracture of lower end of unspecified femur A, B, C 🐾

  ● S72.41   Unspecified condyle fracture of lower end of femur
Condyle fracture of femur NOS

    ● S72.411   Displaced unspecified condyle fracture of lower end of right femur A, B, C 🐾

    ● S72.412   Displaced unspecified condyle fracture of lower end of left femur A, B, C 🐾

    ● S72.413   Displaced unspecified condyle fracture of lower end of unspecified femur A, B, C 🐾

    ● S72.414   Nondisplaced unspecified condyle fracture of lower end of right femur A, B, C 🐾

    ● S72.415   Nondisplaced unspecified condyle fracture of lower end of left femur A, B, C 🐾

    ● S72.416   Nondisplaced unspecified condyle fracture of lower end of unspecified femur A, B, C 🐾

  ● S72.42   Fracture of lateral condyle of femur

    ● S72.421   Displaced fracture of lateral condyle of right femur A, B, C 🐾

    ● S72.422   Displaced fracture of lateral condyle of left femur A, B, C 🐾

    ● S72.423   Displaced fracture of lateral condyle of unspecified femur A, B, C 🐾

    ● S72.424   Nondisplaced fracture of lateral condyle of right femur A, B, C 🐾

    ● S72.425   Nondisplaced fracture of lateral condyle of left femur A, B, C 🐾

    ● S72.426   Nondisplaced fracture of lateral condyle of unspecified femur A, B, C 🐾

  ● S72.43   Fracture of medial condyle of femur

    ● S72.431   Displaced fracture of medial condyle of right femur A, B, C 🐾

    ● S72.432   Displaced fracture of medial condyle of left femur A, B, C 🐾

    ● S72.433   Displaced fracture of medial condyle of unspecified femur A, B, C 🐾

▶ New   ⇒ Revised   d̶e̶l̶e̶t̶e̶d̶ Deleted   Excludes 1   Excludes 2   Includes   Use additional   Code first   Code also   Key words
OGCR Official Guidelines   X Assign placeholder X   ● Use Additional Character(s)   ▷ Manifestation Code   🐾 Hierarchical Condition Category   Coding Clinic

CHAPTER 19 (S00-T88)

● S72.434   Nondisplaced fracture of medial condyle of **right** femur A, B, C 🦴

● S72.435   Nondisplaced fracture of medial condyle of **left** femur A, B, C 🦴

● S72.436   Nondisplaced fracture of medial condyle of **unspecified** femur A, B, C 🦴

● S72.44   Fracture of **lower epiphysis** (separation) of femur

> **Excludes1**   Salter-Harris Type I physeal fracture of lower end of femur (S79.11-)

● S72.441   **Displaced** fracture of lower epiphysis (separation) of **right** femur A, B, C 🦴

● S72.442   **Displaced** fracture of lower epiphysis (separation) of **left** femur A, B, C 🦴

● S72.443   **Displaced** fracture of lower epiphysis (separation) of **unspecified** femur A, B, C 🦴

● S72.444   **Nondisplaced** fracture of lower epiphysis (separation) of **right** femur A, B, C 🦴

● S72.445   **Nondisplaced** fracture of lower epiphysis (separation) of **left** femur A, B, C 🦴

● S72.446   **Nondisplaced** fracture of lower epiphysis (separation) of **unspecified** femur A, B, C 🦴

● S72.45   Supracondylar fracture **without intracondylar extension** of lower end of femur

> Supracondylar fracture of lower end of femur NOS

> **Excludes1**   supracondylar fracture with intracondylar extension of lower end of femur (S72.46-)

● S72.451   **Displaced** supracondylar fracture without intracondylar extension of lower end of **right** femur A, B, C 🦴

● S72.452   **Displaced** supracondylar fracture without intracondylar extension of lower end of **left** femur A, B, C 🦴

● S72.453   **Displaced** supracondylar fracture without intracondylar extension of lower end of **unspecified** femur A, B, C 🦴

● S72.454   **Nondisplaced** supracondylar fracture without intracondylar extension of lower end of **right** femur A, B, C 🦴

● S72.455   **Nondisplaced** supracondylar fracture without intracondylar extension of lower end of **left** femur A, B, C 🦴

● S72.456   **Nondisplaced** supracondylar fracture without intracondylar extension of lower end of **unspecified** femur A, B, C 🦴

● S72.46   Supracondylar fracture **with intracondylar** extension of lower end of femur

> **Excludes1**   supracondylar fracture without intracondylar extension of lower end of femur (S72.45-)

● S72.461   **Displaced** supracondylar fracture with intracondylar extension of lower end of **right** femur A, B, C 🦴

● S72.462   **Displaced** supracondylar fracture with intracondylar extension of lower end of **left** femur A, B, C 🦴

● S72.463   **Displaced** supracondylar fracture with intracondylar extension of lower end of **unspecified** femur A, B, C 🦴

● S72.464   **Nondisplaced** supracondylar fracture with intracondylar extension of lower end of **right** femur A, B, C 🦴

● S72.465   **Nondisplaced** supracondylar fracture with intracondylar extension of lower end of **left** femur A, B, C 🦴

● S72.466   **Nondisplaced** supracondylar fracture with intracondylar extension of lower end of **unspecified** femur A, B, C 🦴

● S72.47   Torus fracture of lower end of femur

> The appropriate 7th character is to be added to all codes in subcategory S72.47

A	initial encounter for closed fracture
D	subsequent encounter for fracture with routine healing
G	subsequent encounter for fracture with delayed healing
K	subsequent encounter for fracture with nonunion
P	subsequent encounter for fracture with malunion
S	sequela

● S72.471   Torus fracture of lower end of **right** femur A 🦴

● S72.472   Torus fracture of lower end of **left** femur A 🦴

● S72.479   Torus fracture of lower end of **unspecified** femur A 🦴

● S72.49   Other fracture of lower end of femur

● S72.491   Other fracture of lower end of **right** femur A, B, C 🦴

● S72.492   Other fracture of lower end of **left** femur A, B, C 🦴

● S72.499   Other fracture of lower end of **unspecified** femur A, B, C 🦴

● S72.8   Other fracture of femur

● S72.8X   Other fracture of femur

● S72.8X1   Other fracture of **right** femur A, B, C 🦴

● S72.8X2   Other fracture of **left** femur A, B, C 🦴

● S72.8X9   Other fracture of **unspecified** femur A, B, C 🦴

● S72.9   **Unspecified** fracture of femur

> Fracture of thigh NOS
> Fracture of upper leg NOS

> **Excludes1**   fracture of hip NOS (S72.00-, S72.01-)

X ● S72.90   Unspecified fracture of **unspecified** femur A, B, C 🦴

> **Coding Clinic: 2012, Q4, P94**

X ● S72.91   Unspecified fracture of **right** femur A, B, C 🦴

X ● S72.92   Unspecified fracture of **left** femur A, B, C 🦴

● S73   Dislocation and sprain of joint and ligaments of hip

> **Includes**   avulsion of joint or ligament of hip
> laceration of cartilage, joint or ligament of hip
> sprain of cartilage, joint or ligament of hip
> traumatic hemarthrosis of joint or ligament of hip
> traumatic rupture of joint or ligament of hip
> traumatic subluxation of joint or ligament of hip
> traumatic tear of joint or ligament of hip

> Code also any associated open wound

> **Excludes2**   strain of muscle, fascia and tendon of hip and thigh (S76.-)

> The appropriate 7th character is to be added to each code from category S73

A	initial encounter
D	subsequent encounter
S	sequela

● S73.0   Subluxation and dislocation of **hip**

> *Out of position*

> **Excludes2**   dislocation and subluxation of hip prosthesis (T84.020, T84.021)

CHAPTER 19 (S00-T88)

● **S73.00**   Unspecified subluxation and dislocation of hip
       Dislocation of hip NOS
       Subluxation of hip NOS
     ● **S73.001**   Unspecified subluxation of right hip A
     ● **S73.002**   Unspecified subluxation of left hip A
     ● **S73.003**   Unspecified subluxation of unspecified hip A
     ● **S73.004**   Unspecified dislocation of right hip A
     ● **S73.005**   Unspecified dislocation of left hip A
     ● **S73.006**   Unspecified dislocation of unspecified hip A

● **S73.01**   Posterior subluxation and dislocation of hip
     ● **S73.011**   Posterior subluxation of right hip A
     ● **S73.012**   Posterior subluxation of left hip A
     ● **S73.013**   Posterior subluxation of unspecified hip A
     ● **S73.014**   Posterior dislocation of right hip A
     ● **S73.015**   Posterior dislocation of left hip A
     ● **S73.016**   Posterior dislocation of unspecified hip A

● **S73.02**   Obturator subluxation and dislocation of hip
     ● **S73.021**   Obturator subluxation of right hip A
     ● **S73.022**   Obturator subluxation of left hip A
     ● **S73.023**   Obturator subluxation of unspecified hip A
     ● **S73.024**   Obturator dislocation of right hip A
     ● **S73.025**   Obturator dislocation of left hip A
     ● **S73.026**   Obturator dislocation of unspecified hip A

● **S73.03**   Other anterior subluxation and dislocation of hip
     ● **S73.031**   Other anterior subluxation of right hip A
     ● **S73.032**   Other anterior subluxation of left hip A
     ● **S73.033**   Other anterior subluxation of unspecified hip A
     ● **S73.034**   Other anterior dislocation of right hip A
     ● **S73.035**   Other anterior dislocation of left hip A
     ● **S73.036**   Other anterior dislocation of unspecified hip A

● **S73.04**   Central subluxation and dislocation of hip
     ● **S73.041**   Central subluxation of right hip A
     ● **S73.042**   Central subluxation of left hip A
     ● **S73.043**   Central subluxation of unspecified hip A
     ● **S73.044**   Central dislocation of right hip A
     ● **S73.045**   Central dislocation of left hip A
     ● **S73.046**   Central dislocation of unspecified hip A

● **S73.1**   Sprain of hip
   ● **S73.10**   Unspecified sprain of hip
     ● **S73.101**   Unspecified sprain of right hip
     ● **S73.102**   Unspecified sprain of left hip
     ● **S73.109**   Unspecified sprain of unspecified hip

   ● **S73.11**   Iliofemoral ligament sprain of hip
     ● **S73.111**   Iliofemoral ligament sprain of right hip
     ● **S73.112**   Iliofemoral ligament sprain of left hip
     ● **S73.119**   Iliofemoral ligament sprain of unspecified hip

   ● **S73.12**   Ischiocapsular (ligament) sprain of hip
     ● **S73.121**   Ischiocapsular ligament sprain of right hip
     ● **S73.122**   Ischiocapsular ligament sprain of left hip
     ● **S73.129**   Ischiocapsular ligament sprain of unspecified hip

   ● **S73.19**   Other sprain of hip
     ● **S73.191**   Other sprain of right hip
     ● **S73.192**   Other sprain of left hip
     ● **S73.199**   Other sprain of unspecified hip

● **S74**   Injury of nerves at hip and thigh level
     Code also any associated open wound (S71.-)
     Excludes2   injury of nerves at ankle and foot level (S94.-)
               injury of nerves at lower leg level (S84.-)
     The appropriate 7th character is to be added to each code from category S74

A	initial encounter
D	subsequent encounter
S	sequela

● **S74.0**   Injury of sciatic nerve at hip and thigh level
   X ● **S74.00**   Injury of sciatic nerve at hip and thigh level, unspecified leg
   X ● **S74.01**   Injury of sciatic nerve at hip and thigh level, right leg
   X ● **S74.02**   Injury of sciatic nerve at hip and thigh level, left leg

● **S74.1**   Injury of femoral nerve at hip and thigh level
   X ● **S74.10**   Injury of femoral nerve at hip and thigh level, unspecified leg
   X ● **S74.11**   Injury of femoral nerve at hip and thigh level, right leg
   X ● **S74.12**   Injury of femoral nerve at hip and thigh level, left leg

● **S74.2**   Injury of cutaneous sensory nerve at hip and thigh level
   X ● **S74.20**   Injury of cutaneous sensory nerve at hip and thigh level, unspecified leg
   X ● **S74.21**   Injury of cutaneous sensory nerve at hip and high level, right leg
   X ● **S74.22**   Injury of cutaneous sensory nerve at hip and thigh level, left leg

● **S74.8**   Injury of other nerves at hip and thigh level
   ● **S74.8X**   Injury of other nerves at hip and thigh level
     ● **S74.8X1**   Injury of other nerves at hip and thigh level, right leg
     ● **S74.8X2**   Injury of other nerves at hip and thigh level, left leg
     ● **S74.8X9**   Injury of other nerves at hip and thigh level, unspecified leg

● **S74.9**   Injury of unspecified nerve at hip and thigh level
   X ● **S74.90**   Injury of unspecified nerve at hip and thigh level, unspecified leg
   X ● **S74.91**   Injury of unspecified nerve at hip and thigh level, right leg
   X ● **S74.92**   Injury of unspecified nerve at hip and thigh level, left leg

▶ New   ⇒ Revised   ~~deleted~~ Deleted   Excludes 1   Excludes 2   Includes   Use additional   Code first   Code also   Key words
OGCR Official Guidelines   X Assign placeholder X   ● Use Additional Character(s)   ▶ Manifestation Code   🐾 Hierarchical Condition Category   **Coding Clinic**

● **S75**   **Injury of blood vessels at hip and thigh level**
     Code also any associated open wound (S71.-)
     Excludes2   injury of blood vessels at lower leg level (S85.-)
                      injury of popliteal artery (S85.0)
     The appropriate 7th character is to be added to each code from
        category S75

> A   initial encounter
> D   subsequent encounter
> S   sequela

● **S75.0**   **Injury of femoral artery**
   ● **S75.00**   **Unspecified** injury of femoral artery
      ● **S75.001**   Unspecified injury of femoral artery, **right leg**
      ● **S75.002**   Unspecified injury of femoral artery, **left leg**
      ● **S75.009**   Unspecified injury of femoral artery, **unspecified leg**
   ● **S75.01**   **Minor laceration** of femoral artery
        Incomplete transection of femoral artery
        Laceration of femoral artery NOS
        Superficial laceration of femoral artery
      ● **S75.011**   Minor laceration of femoral artery, **right leg**
      ● **S75.012**   Minor laceration of femoral artery, **left leg**
      ● **S75.019**   Minor laceration of femoral artery, **unspecified leg**
   ● **S75.02**   **Major laceration** of femoral artery
        Complete transection of femoral artery
        Traumatic rupture of femoral artery
      ● **S75.021**   Major laceration of femoral artery, **right leg**
      ● **S75.022**   Major laceration of femoral artery, **left leg**
              Coding Clinic: 2023, Q3, P12
      ● **S75.029**   Major laceration of femoral artery, **unspecified leg**
   ● **S75.09**   **Other** specified injury of femoral artery
      ● **S75.091**   Other specified injury of femoral artery, **right leg**
      ● **S75.092**   Other specified injury of femoral artery, **left leg**
      ● **S75.099**   Other specified injury of femoral artery, **unspecified leg**
● **S75.1**   **Injury of femoral vein at hip and thigh level**
   ● **S75.10**   **Unspecified** injury of femoral vein at hip and thigh level
      ● **S75.101**   Unspecified injury of femoral vein at hip and thigh level, **right leg**
      ● **S75.102**   Unspecified injury of femoral vein at hip and thigh level, **left leg**
      ● **S75.109**   Unspecified injury of femoral vein at hip and thigh level, **unspecified leg**
   ● **S75.11**   **Minor laceration** of femoral vein at hip and thigh level
        Incomplete transection of femoral vein at hip and thigh level
        Laceration of femoral vein at hip and thigh level NOS
        Superficial laceration of femoral vein at hip and thigh level
      ● **S75.111**   Minor laceration of femoral vein at hip and thigh level, **right leg**
      ● **S75.112**   Minor laceration of femoral vein at hip and thigh level, **left leg**
      ● **S75.119**   Minor laceration of femoral vein at hip and thigh level, **unspecified leg**

   ● **S75.12**   **Major laceration** of femoral vein at hip and thigh level
        Complete transection of femoral vein at hip and thigh level
        Traumatic rupture of femoral vein at hip and thigh level
      ● **S75.121**   Major laceration of femoral vein at hip and thigh level, **right leg**
      ● **S75.122**   Major laceration of femoral vein at hip and thigh level, **left leg**
              Coding Clinic: 2023, Q3, P12
      ● **S75.129**   Major laceration of femoral vein at hip and thigh level, **unspecified leg**
   ● **S75.19**   **Other** specified injury of femoral vein at hip and thigh level
      ● **S75.191**   Other specified injury of femoral vein at hip and thigh level, **right leg**
      ● **S75.192**   Other specified injury of femoral vein at hip and thigh level, **left leg**
      ● **S75.199**   Other specified injury of femoral vein at hip and thigh level, **unspecified leg**
● **S75.2**   **Injury of greater saphenous vein at hip and thigh level**
     Excludes1   greater saphenous vein NOS (S85.3)
   ● **S75.20**   **Unspecified** injury of greater saphenous vein at hip and thigh level
      ● **S75.201**   Unspecified injury of greater saphenous vein at hip and thigh level, **right leg**
      ● **S75.202**   Unspecified injury of greater saphenous vein at hip and thigh level, **left leg**
      ● **S75.209**   Unspecified injury of greater saphenous vein at hip and thigh level, **unspecified** leg
   ● **S75.21**   **Minor laceration** of greater saphenous vein at hip and thigh level
        Incomplete transection of greater saphenous vein at hip and thigh level
        Laceration of greater saphenous vein at hip and thigh level NOS
        Superficial laceration of greater saphenous vein at hip and thigh level
      ● **S75.211**   Minor laceration of greater saphenous vein at hip and thigh level, **right leg**
      ● **S75.212**   Minor laceration of greater saphenous vein at hip and thigh level, **left leg**
      ● **S75.219**   Minor laceration of greater saphenous vein at hip and thigh level, **unspecified** leg
   ● **S75.22**   **Major laceration** of greater saphenous vein at hip and thigh level
        Complete transection of greater saphenous vein at hip and thigh level
        Traumatic rupture of greater saphenous vein at hip and thigh level
      ● **S75.221**   Major laceration of greater saphenous vein at hip and thigh level, **right leg**
      ● **S75.222**   Major laceration of greater saphenous vein at hip and thigh level, **left leg**
      ● **S75.229**   Major laceration of greater saphenous vein at hip and thigh level, **unspecified** leg
   ● **S75.29**   **Other** specified injury of greater saphenous vein at hip and thigh level
      ● **S75.291**   Other specified injury of greater saphenous vein at hip and thigh level, **right** leg
      ● **S75.292**   Other specified injury of greater saphenous vein at hip and thigh level, **left** leg
      ● **S75.299**   Other specified injury of greater saphenous vein at hip and thigh level, **unspecified** leg

- ● S75.8   Injury of other blood vessels at hip and thigh level
  - ● S75.80   Unspecified injury of other blood vessels at hip and thigh level
    - ● S75.801   Unspecified injury of other blood vessels at hip and thigh level, right leg
    - ● S75.802   Unspecified injury of other blood vessels at hip and thigh level, left leg
    - ● S75.809   Unspecified injury of other blood vessels at hip and thigh level, unspecified leg
  - ● S75.81   Laceration of other blood vessels at hip and thigh level
    - ● S75.811   Laceration of other blood vessels at hip and thigh level, right leg
    - ● S75.812   Laceration of other blood vessels at hip and thigh level, left leg
    - ● S75.819   Laceration of other blood vessels at hip and thigh level, unspecified leg
  - ● S75.89   Other specified injury of other blood vessels at hip and thigh level
    - ● S75.891   Other specified injury of other blood vessels at hip and thigh level, right leg
    - ● S75.892   Other specified injury of other blood vessels at hip and thigh level, left leg
    - ● S75.899   Other specified injury of other blood vessels at hip and thigh level, unspecified leg
- ● S75.9   Injury of unspecified blood vessel at hip and thigh level
  - ● S75.90   Unspecified injury of unspecified blood vessel at hip and thigh level
    - ● S75.901   Unspecified injury of unspecified blood vessel at hip and thigh level, right leg
    - ● S75.902   Unspecified injury of unspecified blood vessel at hip and thigh level, left leg
    - ● S75.909   Unspecified injury of unspecified blood vessel at hip and thigh level, unspecified leg
  - ● S75.91   Laceration of unspecified blood vessel at hip and thigh level
    - ● S75.911   Laceration of unspecified blood vessel at hip and thigh level, right leg
    - ● S75.912   Laceration of unspecified blood vessel at hip and thigh level, left leg
    - ● S75.919   Laceration of unspecified blood vessel at hip and thigh level, unspecified leg
  - ● S75.99   Other specified injury of unspecified blood vessel at hip and thigh level
    - ● S75.991   Other specified injury of unspecified blood vessel at hip and thigh level, right leg
    - ● S75.992   Other specified injury of unspecified blood vessel at hip and thigh level, left leg
    - ● S75.999   Other specified injury of unspecified blood vessel at hip and thigh level, unspecified leg
- ● S76   Injury of muscle, fascia and tendon at hip and thigh level

  Code also any associated open wound (S71.-)

  Excludes2   injury of muscle, fascia and tendon at lower leg level (S86)

  sprain of joint and ligament of hip (S73.1)

  The appropriate 7th character is to be added to each code from category S76

A	initial encounter
D	subsequent encounter
S	sequela

- ● S76.0   Injury of muscle, fascia and tendon of hip
  - ● S76.00   Unspecified injury of muscle, fascia and tendon of hip
    - ● S76.001   Unspecified injury of muscle, fascia and tendon of right hip
    - ● S76.002   Unspecified injury of muscle, fascia and tendon of left hip
    - ● S76.009   Unspecified injury of muscle, fascia and tendon of unspecified hip
  - ● S76.01   Strain of muscle, fascia and tendon of hip
    - ● S76.011   Strain of muscle, fascia and tendon of right hip
    - ● S76.012   Strain of muscle, fascia and tendon of left hip
    - ● S76.019   Strain of muscle, fascia and tendon of unspecified hip
  - ● S76.02   Laceration of muscle, fascia and tendon of hip
    - ● S76.021   Laceration of muscle, fascia and tendon of right hip
    - ● S76.022   Laceration of muscle, fascia and tendon of left hip
    - ● S76.029   Laceration of muscle, fascia and tendon of unspecified hip
  - ● S76.09   Other specified injury of muscle, fascia and tendon of hip
    - ● S76.091   Other specified injury of muscle, fascia and tendon of right hip
    - ● S76.092   Other specified injury of muscle, fascia and tendon of left hip
    - ● S76.099   Other specified injury of muscle, fascia and tendon of unspecified hip
- ● S76.1   Injury of quadriceps muscle, fascia and tendon

  Injury of patellar ligament (tendon)
  - ● S76.10   Unspecified injury of quadriceps muscle, fascia and tendon
    - ● S76.101   Unspecified injury of right quadriceps muscle, fascia and tendon
    - ● S76.102   Unspecified injury of left quadriceps muscle, fascia and tendon
    - ● S76.109   Unspecified injury of unspecified quadriceps muscle, fascia and tendon
  - ● S76.11   Strain of quadriceps muscle, fascia and tendon
    - ● S76.111   Strain of right quadriceps muscle, fascia and tendon
    - ● S76.112   Strain of left quadriceps muscle, fascia and tendon
    - ● S76.119   Strain of unspecified quadriceps muscle, fascia and tendon
  - ● S76.12   Laceration of quadriceps muscle, fascia and tendon
    - ● S76.121   Laceration of right quadriceps muscle, fascia and tendon
    - ● S76.122   Laceration of left quadriceps muscle, fascia and tendon
    - ● S76.129   Laceration of unspecified quadriceps muscle, fascia and tendon
  - ● S76.19   Other specified injury of quadriceps muscle, fascia and tendon
    - ● S76.191   Other specified injury of right quadriceps muscle, fascia and tendon
    - ● S76.192   Other specified injury of left quadriceps muscle, fascia and tendon
    - ● S76.199   Other specified injury of unspecified quadriceps muscle, fascia and tendon
- ● S76.2   Injury of adductor muscle, fascia and tendon of thigh
  - ● S76.20   Unspecified injury of adductor muscle, fascia and tendon of thigh
    - ● S76.201   Unspecified injury of adductor muscle, fascia and tendon of right thigh

▶ New   ⟹ Revised   ~~deleted~~ Deleted   Excludes 1   Excludes 2   Includes   Use additional   Code first   Code also   Key words

OGCR Official Guidelines   X Assign placeholder X   ● Use Additional Character(s)   ▌ Manifestation Code   🝙 Hierarchical Condition Category   Coding Clinic

● S76.202   Unspecified injury of adductor muscle, fascia and tendon of left thigh

● S76.209   Unspecified injury of adductor muscle, fascia and tendon of unspecified thigh

● S76.21   Strain of adductor muscle, fascia and tendon of thigh

   ● S76.211   Strain of adductor muscle, fascia and tendon of right thigh

   ● S76.212   Strain of adductor muscle, fascia and tendon of left thigh

   ● S76.219   Strain of adductor muscle, fascia and tendon of unspecified thigh

● S76.22   Laceration of adductor muscle, fascia and tendon of thigh

   ● S76.221   Laceration of adductor muscle, fascia and tendon of right thigh

   ● S76.222   Laceration of adductor muscle, fascia and tendon of left thigh

   ● S76.229   Laceration of adductor muscle, fascia and tendon of unspecified thigh

● S76.29   Other injury of adductor muscle, fascia and tendon of thigh

   ● S76.291   Other injury of adductor muscle, fascia and tendon of right thigh

   ● S76.292   Other injury of adductor muscle, fascia and tendon of left thigh

   ● S76.299   Other injury of adductor muscle, fascia and tendon of unspecified thigh

● S76.3   Injury of muscle, fascia and tendon of the posterior muscle group at thigh level

 ● S76.30   Unspecified injury of muscle, fascia and tendon of the posterior muscle group at thigh level

   ● S76.301   Unspecified injury of muscle, fascia and tendon of the posterior muscle group at thigh level, right thigh

   ● S76.302   Unspecified injury of muscle, fascia and tendon of the posterior muscle group at thigh level, left thigh

   ● S76.309   Unspecified injury of muscle, fascia and tendon of the posterior muscle group at thigh level, unspecified thigh

 ● S76.31   Strain of muscle, fascia and tendon of the posterior muscle group at thigh level

   ● S76.311   Strain of muscle, fascia and tendon of the posterior muscle group at thigh level, right thigh

   ● S76.312   Strain of muscle, fascia and tendon of the posterior muscle group at thigh level, left thigh

   ● S76.319   Strain of muscle, fascia and tendon of the posterior muscle group at thigh level, unspecified thigh

 ● S76.32   Laceration of muscle, fascia and tendon of the posterior muscle group at thigh level

   ● S76.321   Laceration of muscle, fascia and tendon of the posterior muscle group at thigh level, right thigh

   ● S76.322   Laceration of muscle, fascia and tendon of the posterior muscle group at thigh level, left thigh

   ● S76.329   Laceration of muscle, fascia and tendon of the posterior muscle group at thigh level, unspecified thigh

 ● S76.39   Other specified injury of muscle, fascia and tendon of the posterior muscle group at thigh level

   ● S76.391   Other specified injury of muscle, fascia and tendon of the posterior muscle group at thigh level, right thigh

   ● S76.392   Other specified injury of muscle, fascia and tendon of the posterior muscle group at thigh level, left thigh

   ● S76.399   Other specified injury of muscle, fascia and tendon of the posterior muscle group at thigh level, unspecified thigh

● S76.8   Injury of other specified muscles, fascia and tendons at thigh level

 ● S76.80   Unspecified injury of other specified muscles, fascia and tendons at thigh level

   ● S76.801   Unspecified injury of other specified muscles, fascia and tendons at thigh level, right thigh

   ● S76.802   Unspecified injury of other specified muscles, fascia and tendons at thigh level, left thigh

   ● S76.809   Unspecified injury of other specified muscles, fascia and tendons at thigh level, unspecified thigh

 ● S76.81   Strain of other specified specified muscles, fascia and tendons at thigh level

   ● S76.811   Strain of other specified muscles, fascia and tendons at thigh level, right thigh

   ● S76.812   Strain of other specified muscles, fascia and tendons at thigh level, left thigh

   ● S76.819   Strain of other specified muscles, fascia and tendons at thigh level, unspecified thigh

 ● S76.82   Laceration of other specified muscles, fascia and tendons at thigh level

   ● S76.821   Laceration of other specified muscles, fascia and tendons at thigh level, right thigh

   ● S76.822   Laceration of other specified muscles, fascia and tendons at thigh level, left thigh

   ● S76.829   Laceration of other specified muscles, fascia and tendons at thigh level, unspecified thigh

 ● S76.89   Other injury of other specified muscles, fascia and tendons at thigh level

   ● S76.891   Other injury of other specified muscles, fascia and tendons at thigh level, right thigh

   ● S76.892   Other injury of other specified muscles, fascia and tendons at thigh level, left thigh

   ● S76.899   Other injury of other specified muscles, fascia and tendons at thigh level, unspecified thigh

● S76.9   Injury of unspecified muscles, fascia and tendons at thigh level

 ● S76.90   Unspecified injury of unspecified muscles, fascia and tendons at thigh level

   ● S76.901   Unspecified injury of unspecified muscles, fascia and tendons at thigh level, right thigh

   ● S76.902   Unspecified injury of unspecified muscles, fascia and tendons at thigh level, left thigh

   ● S76.909   Unspecified injury of unspecified muscles, fascia and tendons at thigh level, unspecified thigh

 ● S76.91   Strain of unspecified muscles, fascia and tendons at thigh level

CHAPTER 19 (S00-T88)

- **S76.911** Strain of unspecified muscles, fascia and tendons at thigh level, right thigh
- **S76.912** Strain of unspecified muscles, fascia and tendons at thigh level, left thigh
- **S76.919** Strain of unspecified muscles fascia and tendons at thigh level, unspecified thigh
- **S76.92** Laceration of unspecified muscles, fascia and tendons at thigh level
  - **S76.921** Laceration of unspecified muscles, fascia and tendons at thigh level, right thigh
  - **S76.922** Laceration of unspecified muscles, fascia and tendons at thigh level, left thigh
  - **S76.929** Laceration of unspecified muscles, fascia and tendons at thigh level, unspecified thigh
- **S76.99** Other specified injury of unspecified muscles, fascia and tendons at thigh level
  - **S76.991** Other specified injury of unspecified muscles, fascia and tendons at thigh level, right thigh
  - **S76.992** Other specified injury of unspecified muscles, fascia and tendons at thigh level, left thigh
  - **S76.999** Other specified injury of unspecified muscles, fascia and tendons at thigh level, unspecified thigh

- **S77 Crushing injury of hip and thigh**

  Use additional code(s) for all associated injuries

  Excludes2 crushing injury of ankle and foot (S97.-)
  crushing injury of lower leg (S87.-)

  The appropriate 7th character is to be added to each code from category S77

A	initial encounter
D	subsequent encounter
S	sequela

  - **S77.0** Crushing injury of hip
    - X **S77.00** Crushing injury of unspecified hip
    - X **S77.01** Crushing injury of right hip
    - X **S77.02** Crushing injury of left hip
  - **S77.1** Crushing injury of thigh
    - X **S77.10** Crushing injury of unspecified thigh
    - X **S77.11** Crushing injury of right thigh
    - X **S77.12** Crushing injury of left thigh
  - **S77.2** Crushing injury of hip with thigh
    - X **S77.20** Crushing injury of unspecified hip with thigh
    - X **S77.21** Crushing injury of right hip with thigh
    - X **S77.22** Crushing injury of left hip with thigh

- **S78 Traumatic amputation of hip and thigh**

  An amputation not identified as partial or complete should be coded to complete

  Excludes1 traumatic amputation of knee (S88.0-)

  The appropriate 7th character is to be added to each code from category S78

A	initial encounter
D	subsequent encounter
S	sequela

  - **S78.0** Traumatic amputation at hip joint
    - **S78.01** Complete traumatic amputation at hip joint
      - **S78.011** Complete traumatic amputation at right hip joint A, D, S
      - **S78.012** Complete traumatic amputation at left hip joint A, D, S
      - **S78.019** Complete traumatic amputation at unspecified hip joint A, D, S

- **S78.02** Partial traumatic amputation at hip joint
  - **S78.021** Partial traumatic amputation at right hip joint A, D, S
  - **S78.022** Partial traumatic amputation at left hip joint A, D, S
  - **S78.029** Partial traumatic amputation at unspecified hip joint A, D, S
- **S78.1** Traumatic amputation at level between hip and knee
  Excludes1 traumatic amputation of knee (S88.0-)
  - **S78.11** Complete traumatic amputation at level between hip and knee
    - **S78.111** Complete traumatic amputation at level between right hip and knee A, D, S
    - **S78.112** Complete traumatic amputation at level between left hip and knee A, D, S
    - **S78.119** Complete traumatic amputation at level between unspecified hip and knee A, D, S
  - **S78.12** Partial traumatic amputation at level between hip and knee
    - **S78.121** Partial traumatic amputation at level between right hip and knee A, D, S
    - **S78.122** Partial traumatic amputation at level between left hip and knee A, D, S
    - **S78.129** Partial traumatic amputation at level between unspecified hip and knee A, D, S
- **S78.9** Traumatic amputation of hip and thigh, level unspecified
  - **S78.91** Complete traumatic amputation of hip and thigh, level unspecified
    - **S78.911** Complete traumatic amputation of right hip and thigh, level unspecified A, D, S
    - **S78.912** Complete traumatic amputation of left hip and thigh, level unspecified A, D, S
    - **S78.919** Complete traumatic amputation of unspecified hip and thigh, level unspecified A, D, S
  - **S78.92** Partial traumatic amputation of hip and thigh, level unspecified
    - **S78.921** Partial traumatic amputation of right hip and thigh, level unspecified A, D, S
    - **S78.922** Partial traumatic amputation of left hip and thigh, level unspecified A, D, S
    - **S78.929** Partial traumatic amputation of unspecified hip and thigh, level unspecified A, D, S

- **S79 Other and unspecified injuries of hip and thigh**

  Note: A fracture not indicated as open or closed should be coded to closed

  The appropriate 7th character is to be added to each code from subcategories S79.0 and S79.1

A	initial encounter for closed fracture
D	subsequent encounter for fracture with routine healing
G	subsequent encounter for fracture with delayed healing
K	subsequent encounter for fracture with nonunion
P	subsequent encounter for fracture with malunion
S	sequela

  - **S79.0** Physeal fracture of upper end of femur
    Excludes1 apophyseal fracture of upper end of femur (S72.13-)
    nontraumatic slipped upper femoral epiphysis (M93.0-)

Item 19–5 SALTER-HARRIS TYPE 1: epiphysis is completely separated from end of bone, or metaphysic growth plate remains attached to epiphysis

SALTER-HARRIS TYPE 2: epiphysis and growth plate are partially separated from metaphysis, which is cracked—most common type

SALTER-HARRIS TYPE 3: fracture occurring through epiphysis and separates part of epiphysis and growth plate from metaphysis fracture, usually at distal end of tibia

SALTER-HARRIS TYPE 4: fracture runs through epiphysis, across growth plate, into metaphysic; surgery is required to restore joint surface to normal and align growth plate

- **S79.00** Unspecified physeal fracture of upper end of femur
  - **S79.001** Unspecified physeal fracture of upper end of right femur A 🦉
  - **S79.002** Unspecified physeal fracture of upper end of left femur A 🦉
  - **S79.009** Unspecified physeal fracture of upper end of unspecified femur A 🦉
- **S79.01** Salter-Harris Type I physeal fracture of upper end of femur

  Acute on chronic slipped capital femoral epiphysis (traumatic)

  Acute slipped capital femoral epiphysis (traumatic)

  Capital femoral epiphyseal fracture

  Excludes1 chronic slipped upper femoral epiphysis (nontraumatic) (M93.02-)

  - **S79.011** Salter-Harris Type I physeal fracture of upper end of right femur A 🦉
  - **S79.012** Salter-Harris Type I physeal fracture of upper end of left femur A 🦉
  - **S79.019** Salter-Harris Type I physeal fracture of upper end of unspecified femur A 🦉
- **S79.09** Other physeal fracture of upper end of femur
  - **S79.091** Other physeal fracture of upper end of right femur A 🦉
  - **S79.092** Other physeal fracture of upper end of left femur A 🦉
  - **S79.099** Other physeal fracture of upper end of unspecified femur A 🦉
- **S79.1** Physeal fracture of lower end of femur
  - **S79.10** Unspecified physeal fracture of lower end of femur
    - **S79.101** Unspecified physeal fracture of lower end of right femur A 🦉
    - **S79.102** Unspecified physeal fracture of lower end of left femur A 🦉
    - **S79.109** Unspecified physeal fracture of lower end of unspecified femur A 🦉
  - **S79.11** Salter-Harris Type I physeal fracture of lower end of femur
    - **S79.111** Salter-Harris Type I physeal fracture of lower end of right femur A 🦉
    - **S79.112** Salter-Harris Type I physeal fracture of lower end of left femur A 🦉
    - **S79.119** Salter-Harris Type I physeal fracture of lower end of unspecified femur A 🦉
  - **S79.12** Salter-Harris Type II physeal fracture of lower end of femur
    - **S79.121** Salter-Harris Type II physeal fracture of lower end of right femur A 🦉
    - **S79.122** Salter-Harris Type II physeal fracture of lower end of left femur A 🦉
    - **S79.129** Salter-Harris Type II physeal fracture of lower end of unspecified femur A 🦉
  - **S79.13** Salter-Harris Type III physeal fracture of lower end of femur
    - **S79.131** Salter-Harris Type III physeal fracture of lower end of right femur A 🦉
    - **S79.132** Salter-Harris Type III physeal fracture of lower end of left femur A 🦉
    - **S79.139** Salter-Harris Type III physeal fracture of lower end of unspecified femur A 🦉
  - **S79.14** Salter-Harris Type IV physeal fracture of lower end of femur
    - **S79.141** Salter-Harris Type IV physeal fracture of lower end of right femur A 🦉
    - **S79.142** Salter-Harris Type IV physeal fracture of lower end of left femur A 🦉
    - **S79.149** Salter-Harris Type IV physeal fracture of lower end of unspecified femur A 🦉
  - **S79.19** Other physeal fracture of lower end of femur
    - **S79.191** Other physeal fracture of lower end of right femur A 🦉
    - **S79.192** Other physeal fracture of lower end of left femur A 🦉
    - **S79.199** Other physeal fracture of lower end of unspecified femur A 🦉
- **S79.8 Other specified injuries of hip and thigh**

  The appropriate 7th character is to be added to each code in subcategory S79.8

A	initial encounter
D	subsequent encounter
S	sequela

  - **S79.81** Other specified injuries of hip
    - **S79.811** Other specified injuries of right hip
    - **S79.812** Other specified injuries of left hip
    - **S79.819** Other specified injuries of unspecified hip
  - **S79.82** Other specified injuries of thigh
    - **S79.821** Other specified injuries of right thigh
    - **S79.822** Other specified injuries of left thigh
    - **S79.829** Other specified injuries of unspecified thigh
- **S79.9** Unspecified injury of hip and thigh

  The appropriate 7th character is to be added to each code in subcategory S79.9

A	initial encounter
D	subsequent encounter
S	sequela

  - **S79.91** Unspecified injury of hip
    - **S79.911** Unspecified injury of right hip
    - **S79.912** Unspecified injury of left hip
    - **S79.919** Unspecified injury of unspecified hip
  - **S79.92** Unspecified injury of thigh
    - **S79.921** Unspecified injury of right thigh
    - **S79.922** Unspecified injury of left thigh
    - **S79.929** Unspecified injury of unspecified thigh

INJURIES TO THE KNEE AND LOWER LEG (S80-S89)

Excludes2   burns and corrosions (T20-T32)
frostbite (T33-T34)
injuries of ankle and foot, except fracture of ankle and malleolus (S90-S99)
insect bite or sting, venomous (T63.4)

● **S80**   **Superficial injury of knee and lower leg**

Excludes2   superficial injury of ankle and foot (S90.-)

The appropriate 7th character is to be added to each code from category S80

> A   initial encounter
> D   subsequent encounter
> S   sequela

● **S80.0**   **Contusion of knee**
   X ● **S80.00**   Contusion of unspecified knee
   X ● **S80.01**   Contusion of right knee
   X ● **S80.02**   Contusion of left knee
● **S80.1**   **Contusion of lower leg**
   X ● **S80.10**   Contusion of unspecified lower leg
   X ● **S80.11**   Contusion of right lower leg
   X ● **S80.12**   Contusion of left lower leg
● **S80.2**   **Other superficial injuries of knee**
   ● **S80.21**   **Abrasion of knee**
     ● **S80.211**   Abrasion, right knee
     ● **S80.212**   Abrasion, left knee
     ● **S80.219**   Abrasion, unspecified knee
   ● **S80.22**   **Blister (nonthermal) of knee**
     ● **S80.221**   Blister (nonthermal), right knee
     ● **S80.222**   Blister (nonthermal), left knee
     ● **S80.229**   Blister (nonthermal), unspecified knee
   ● **S80.24**   **External constriction of knee**
     ● **S80.241**   External constriction, right knee
     ● **S80.242**   External constriction, left knee
     ● **S80.249**   External constriction, unspecified knee
   ● **S80.25**   **Superficial foreign body of knee**
     Splinter in the knee
     ● **S80.251**   Superficial foreign body, right knee
     ● **S80.252**   Superficial foreign body, left knee
     ● **S80.259**   Superficial foreign body, unspecified knee
   ● **S80.26**   **Insect bite (nonvenomous) of knee**
     ● **S80.261**   Insect bite (nonvenomous), right knee
     ● **S80.262**   Insect bite (nonvenomous), left knee
     ● **S80.269**   Insect bite (nonvenomous), unspecified knee
   ● **S80.27**   **Other superficial bite of knee**
     Excludes1   open bite of knee (S81.05-)
     ● **S80.271**   Other superficial bite of right knee
     ● **S80.272**   Other superficial bite of left knee
     ● **S80.279**   Other superficial bite of unspecified knee
● **S80.8**   **Other superficial injuries of lower leg**
   ● **S80.81**   **Abrasion of lower leg**
     ● **S80.811**   Abrasion, right lower leg
     ● **S80.812**   Abrasion, left lower leg
     ● **S80.819**   Abrasion, unspecified lower leg
   ● **S80.82**   **Blister (nonthermal) of lower leg**
     ● **S80.821**   Blister (nonthermal), right lower leg
     ● **S80.822**   Blister (nonthermal), left lower leg
     ● **S80.829**   Blister (nonthermal), unspecified lower leg

● **S80.84**   **External constriction of lower leg**
   ● **S80.841**   External constriction, right lower leg
   ● **S80.842**   External constriction, left lower leg
   ● **S80.849**   External constriction, unspecified lower leg
● **S80.85**   **Superficial foreign body of lower leg**
   Splinter in the lower leg
   ● **S80.851**   Superficial foreign body, right lower leg
   ● **S80.852**   Superficial foreign body, left lower leg
   ● **S80.859**   Superficial foreign body, unspecified lower leg
● **S80.86**   **Insect bite (nonvenomous) of lower leg**
   ● **S80.861**   Insect bite (nonvenomous), right lower leg
   ● **S80.862**   Insect bite (nonvenomous), left lower leg
   ● **S80.869**   Insect bite (nonvenomous), unspecified lower leg
● **S80.87**   **Other superficial bite of lower leg**
   Excludes1   open bite of lower leg (S81.85-)
   ● **S80.871**   Other superficial bite, right lower leg
   ● **S80.872**   Other superficial bite, left lower leg
   ● **S80.879**   Other superficial bite, unspecified lower leg
● **S80.9**   **Unspecified superficial injury of knee and lower leg**
   ● **S80.91**   **Unspecified superficial injury of knee**
     ● **S80.911**   Unspecified superficial injury of right knee
     ● **S80.912**   Unspecified superficial injury of left knee
     ● **S80.919**   Unspecified superficial injury of unspecified knee
   ● **S80.92**   **Unspecified superficial injury of lower leg**
     ● **S80.921**   Unspecified superficial injury of right lower leg
     ● **S80.922**   Unspecified superficial injury of left lower leg
     ● **S80.929**   Unspecified superficial injury of unspecified lower leg

● **S81**   **Open wound of knee and lower leg**
Code also any associated wound infection
Excludes1   open fracture of knee and lower leg (S82.-)
traumatic amputation of lower leg (S88.-)
Excludes2   open wound of ankle and foot (S91.-)

The appropriate 7th character is to be added to each code from category S81

> A   initial encounter
> D   subsequent encounter
> S   sequela

● **S81.0**   **Open wound of knee**
   ● **S81.00**   **Unspecified open wound of knee**
     ● **S81.001**   Unspecified open wound, right knee
     ● **S81.002**   Unspecified open wound, left knee
     ● **S81.009**   Unspecified open wound, unspecified knee
   ● **S81.01**   **Laceration without foreign body of knee**
     ● **S81.011**   Laceration without foreign body, right knee
     ● **S81.012**   Laceration without foreign body, left knee
     ● **S81.019**   Laceration without foreign body, unspecified knee
   ● **S81.02**   **Laceration with foreign body of knee**
     ● **S81.021**   Laceration with foreign body, right knee

---

▶ New   ⇒ Revised   ~~deleted~~ Deleted   Excludes 1   Excludes 2   Includes   Use additional   Code first   Code also   Key words

OGCR Official Guidelines   X Assign placeholder X   ● Use Additional Character(s)   ▶ Manifestation Code   🐾 Hierarchical Condition Category   **Coding Clinic**

● S81.022 Laceration with foreign body, left knee

● S81.029 Laceration with foreign body, unspecified knee

● S81.03 Puncture wound without foreign body of knee

  ● S81.031 Puncture wound without foreign body, right knee

  ● S81.032 Puncture wound without foreign body, left knee

  ● S81.039 Puncture wound without foreign body, unspecified knee

● S81.04 Puncture wound with foreign body of knee

  ● S81.041 Puncture wound with foreign body, right knee

  ● S81.042 Puncture wound with foreign body, left knee

  ● S81.049 Puncture wound with foreign body, unspecified knee

● S81.05 Open bite of knee
    Bite of knee NOS

    Excludes1 superficial bite of knee (S80.27-)

  ● S81.051 Open bite, right knee
  ● S81.052 Open bite, left knee
  ● S81.059 Open bite, unspecified knee

● S81.8 Open wound of lower leg

  ● S81.80 Unspecified open wound of lower leg

    ● S81.801 Unspecified open wound, right lower leg

    ● S81.802 Unspecified open wound, left lower leg

    ● S81.809 Unspecified open wound, unspecified lower leg

  ● S81.81 Laceration without foreign body of lower leg

    ● S81.811 Laceration without foreign body, right lower leg

    ● S81.812 Laceration without foreign body, left lower leg

    ● S81.819 Laceration without foreign body, unspecified lower leg

  ● S81.82 Laceration with foreign body of lower leg

    ● S81.821 Laceration with foreign body, right lower leg

    ● S81.822 Laceration with foreign body, left lower leg

    ● S81.829 Laceration with foreign body, unspecified lower leg

  ● S81.83 Puncture wound without foreign body of lower leg

    ● S81.831 Puncture wound without foreign body, right lower leg

    ● S81.832 Puncture wound without foreign body, left lower leg

    ● S81.839 Puncture wound without foreign body, unspecified lower leg

  ● S81.84 Puncture wound with foreign body of lower leg

    ● S81.841 Puncture wound with foreign body, right lower leg
        Coding Clinic: 2016, Q3, P46

    ● S81.842 Puncture wound with foreign body, left lower leg

    ● S81.849 Puncture wound with foreign body, unspecified lower leg

  ● S81.85 Open bite of lower leg
      Bite of lower leg NOS

      Excludes1 superficial bite of lower leg (S80.86-, S80.87-)

    ● S81.851 Open bite, right lower leg
    ● S81.852 Open bite, left lower leg
    ● S81.859 Open bite, unspecified lower leg

● S82 Fracture of lower leg, including ankle
    Note: A fracture not indicated as displaced or nondisplaced should be coded to displaced

    A fracture not indicated as open or closed should be coded to closed

    The open fracture designations are based on the Gustilo open fracture classification

    Includes fracture of malleolus

    Excludes1 traumatic amputation of lower leg (S88.-)

    Excludes2 fracture of foot, except ankle (S92.-)
        periprosthetic fracture around internal prosthetic ankle joint (M97.2)
        periprosthetic fracture around internal of prosthetic implant of knee joint (M97.1-)

    The appropriate 7th character is to be added to all codes from category S82

A	initial encounter for closed fracture
B	initial encounter for open fracture type I or II initial encounter for open fracture NOS
C	initial encounter for open fracture type IIIA, IIIB, or IIIC
D	subsequent encounter for closed fracture with routine healing
E	subsequent encounter for open fracture type I or II with routine healing
F	subsequent encounter for open fracture type IIIA, IIIB, or IIIC with routine healing
G	subsequent encounter for closed fracture with delayed healing
H	subsequent encounter for open fracture type I or II with delayed healing
J	subsequent encounter for open fracture type IIIA, IIIB, or IIIC with delayed healing
K	subsequent encounter for closed fracture with nonunion
M	subsequent encounter for open fracture type I or II with nonunion
N	subsequent encounter for open fracture type IIIA, IIIB, or IIIC with nonunion
P	subsequent encounter for closed fracture with malunion
Q	subsequent encounter for open fracture type I or II with malunion
R	subsequent encounter for open fracture type IIIA, IIIB, or IIIC with malunion
S	sequela

● S82.0 Fracture of patella
    Knee cap

  ● S82.00 Unspecified fracture of patella

    ● S82.001 Unspecified fracture of right patella
    ● S82.002 Unspecified fracture of left patella
    ● S82.009 Unspecified fracture of unspecified patella

  ● S82.01 Osteochondral fracture of patella

    ● S82.011 Displaced osteochondral fracture of right patella

    ● S82.012 Displaced osteochondral fracture of left patella

    ● S82.013 Displaced osteochondral fracture of unspecified patella

    ● S82.014 Nondisplaced osteochondral fracture of right patella

    ● S82.015 Nondisplaced osteochondral fracture of left patella

    ● S82.016 Nondisplaced osteochondral fracture of unspecified patella

  ● S82.02 Longitudinal fracture of patella

    ● S82.021 Displaced longitudinal fracture of right patella

    ● S82.022 Displaced longitudinal fracture of left patella

● S82.023 Displaced longitudinal fracture of unspecified patella

● S82.024 Nondisplaced longitudinal fracture of right patella

● S82.025 Nondisplaced longitudinal fracture of left patella

● S82.026 Nondisplaced longitudinal fracture of unspecified patella

● S82.03 Transverse fracture of patella

● S82.031 Displaced transverse fracture of right patella

● S82.032 Displaced transverse fracture of left patella

● S82.033 Displaced transverse fracture of unspecified patella

● S82.034 Nondisplaced transverse fracture of right patella

● S82.035 Nondisplaced transverse fracture of left patella

● S82.036 Nondisplaced transverse fracture of unspecified patella

● S82.04 Comminuted fracture of patella

● S82.041 Displaced comminuted fracture of right patella

● S82.042 Displaced comminuted fracture of left patella

● S82.043 Displaced comminuted fracture of unspecified patella

● S82.044 Nondisplaced comminuted fracture of right patella

● S82.045 Nondisplaced comminuted fracture of left patella

● S82.046 Nondisplaced comminuted fracture of unspecified patella

● S82.09 Other fracture of patella

● S82.091 Other fracture of right patella

● S82.092 Other fracture of left patella

● S82.099 Other fracture of unspecified patella

● S82.1 Fracture of upper end of tibia
Fracture of proximal end of tibia

Excludes2 fracture of shaft of tibia (S82.2-)
physeal fracture of upper end of tibia (S89.0-)

● S82.10 Unspecified fracture of upper end of tibia

● S82.101 Unspecified fracture of upper end of right tibia

● S82.102 Unspecified fracture of upper end of left tibia

● S82.109 Unspecified fracture of upper end of unspecified tibia

● S82.11 Fracture of tibial spine

● S82.111 Displaced fracture of right tibial spine

● S82.112 Displaced fracture of left tibial spine

● S82.113 Displaced fracture of unspecified tibial spine

● S82.114 Nondisplaced fracture of right tibial spine

● S82.115 Nondisplaced fracture of left tibial spine

● S82.116 Nondisplaced fracture of unspecified tibial spine

● S82.12 Fracture of lateral condyle of tibia

● S82.121 Displaced fracture of lateral condyle of right tibia

● S82.122 Displaced fracture of lateral condyle of left tibia

● S82.123 Displaced fracture of lateral condyle of unspecified tibia

● S82.124 Nondisplaced fracture of lateral condyle of right tibia

● S82.125 Nondisplaced fracture of lateral condyle of left tibia

● S82.126 Nondisplaced fracture of lateral condyle of unspecified tibia

● S82.13 Fracture of medial condyle of tibia

● S82.131 Displaced fracture of medial condyle of right tibia

● S82.132 Displaced fracture of medial condyle of left tibia

● S82.133 Displaced fracture of medial condyle of unspecified tibia

● S82.134 Nondisplaced fracture of medial condyle of right tibia

● S82.135 Nondisplaced fracture of medial condyle of left tibia

● S82.136 Nondisplaced fracture of medial condyle of unspecified tibia

● S82.14 Bicondylar fracture of tibia
Fracture of tibial plateau NOS

● S82.141 Displaced bicondylar fracture of right tibia

● S82.142 Displaced bicondylar fracture of left tibia

● S82.143 Displaced bicondylar fracture of unspecified tibia

● S82.144 Nondisplaced bicondylar fracture of right tibia

● S82.145 Nondisplaced bicondylar fracture of left tibia

● S82.146 Nondisplaced bicondylar fracture of unspecified tibia

● S82.15 Fracture of tibial tuberosity

● S82.151 Displaced fracture of right tibial tuberosity

● S82.152 Displaced fracture of left tibial tuberosity

● S82.153 Displaced fracture of unspecified tibial tuberosity

● S82.154 Nondisplaced fracture of right tibial tuberosity

● S82.155 Nondisplaced fracture of left tibial tuberosity

● S82.156 Nondisplaced fracture of unspecified tibial tuberosity

● S82.16 Torus fracture of upper end of tibia

The appropriate 7th character is to be added to all codes in subcategory S82.16

A	initial encounter for closed fracture
D	subsequent encounter for fracture with routine healing
G	subsequent encounter for fracture with delayed healing
K	subsequent encounter for fracture with nonunion
P	subsequent encounter for fracture with malunion
S	sequela

● S82.161 Torus fracture of upper end of right tibia

● S82.162 Torus fracture of upper end of left tibia

● S82.169 Torus fracture of upper end of unspecified tibia

● S82.19 Other fracture of upper end of tibia

● S82.191 Other fracture of upper end of right tibia

▶ New   ⇒ Revised   ~~deleted~~ Deleted   Excludes 1   Excludes 2   Includes   Use additional   Code first   Code also   Key words

OGCR Official Guidelines   X Assign placeholder X   ● Use Additional Character(s)   ▷ Manifestation Code   🅗 Hierarchical Condition Category   **Coding Clinic**

- S82.192   Other fracture of upper end of left tibia
- S82.199   Other fracture of upper end of unspecified tibia
- S82.2   Fracture of shaft of tibia
  - S82.20   Unspecified fracture of shaft of tibia
    Fracture of tibia NOS
    - S82.201   Unspecified fracture of shaft of right tibia
    - S82.202   Unspecified fracture of shaft of left tibia
    - S82.209   Unspecified fracture of shaft of unspecified tibia
  - S82.22   Transverse fracture of shaft of tibia
    - S82.221   Displaced transverse fracture of shaft of right tibia
    - S82.222   Displaced transverse fracture of shaft of left tibia
    - S82.223   Displaced transverse fracture of shaft of unspecified tibia
    - S82.224   Nondisplaced transverse fracture of shaft of right tibia
    - S82.225   Nondisplaced transverse fracture of shaft of left tibia
    - S82.226   Nondisplaced transverse fracture of shaft of unspecified tibia
  - S82.23   Oblique fracture of shaft of tibia
    - S82.231   Displaced oblique fracture of shaft of right tibia
    - S82.232   Displaced oblique fracture of shaft of left tibia
    - S82.233   Displaced oblique fracture of shaft of unspecified tibia
    - S82.234   Nondisplaced oblique fracture of shaft of right tibia
      Coding Clinic: 2015, Q1, P9-10
    - S82.235   Nondisplaced oblique fracture of shaft of left tibia
    - S82.236   Nondisplaced oblique fracture of shaft of unspecified tibia
  - S82.24   Spiral fracture of shaft of tibia
    Toddler fracture
    - S82.241   Displaced spiral fracture of shaft of right tibia
    - S82.242   Displaced spiral fracture of shaft of left tibia
    - S82.243   Displaced spiral fracture of shaft of unspecified tibia
    - S82.244   Nondisplaced spiral fracture of shaft of right tibia
    - S82.245   Nondisplaced spiral fracture of shaft of left tibia
    - S82.246   Nondisplaced spiral fracture of shaft of unspecified tibia
  - S82.25   Comminuted fracture of shaft of tibia
    - S82.251   Displaced comminuted fracture of shaft of right tibia
      Coding Clinic: 2015, Q2, P6
    - S82.252   Displaced comminuted fracture of shaft of left tibia
    - S82.253   Displaced comminuted fracture of shaft of unspecified tibia
    - S82.254   Nondisplaced comminuted fracture of shaft of right tibia
    - S82.255   Nondisplaced comminuted fracture of shaft of left tibia
    - S82.256   Nondisplaced comminuted fracture of shaft of unspecified tibia

- S82.26   Segmental fracture of shaft of tibia
  - S82.261   Displaced segmental fracture of shaft of right tibia
  - S82.262   Displaced segmental fracture of shaft of left tibia
  - S82.263   Displaced segmental fracture of shaft of unspecified tibia
  - S82.264   Nondisplaced segmental fracture of shaft of right tibia
  - S82.265   Nondisplaced segmental fracture of shaft of left tibia
  - S82.266   Nondisplaced segmental fracture of shaft of unspecified tibia
- S82.29   Other fracture of shaft of tibia
  - S82.291   Other fracture of shaft of right tibia
  - S82.292   Other fracture of shaft of left tibia
  - S82.299   Other fracture of shaft of unspecified tibia
- S82.3   Fracture of lower end of tibia
  - **Excludes1**   bimalleolar fracture of lower leg (S82.84-)
    fracture of medial malleolus alone (S82.5-)
    Maisonneuve's fracture (S82.86-)
    pilon fracture of distal tibia (S82.87-)
    trimalleolar fractures of lower leg (S82.85-)
  - S82.30   Unspecified fracture of lower end of tibia
    - S82.301   Unspecified fracture of lower end of right tibia
    - S82.302   Unspecified fracture of lower end of left tibia
    - S82.309   Unspecified fracture of lower end of unspecified tibia
  - S82.31   Torus fracture of lower end of tibia

    The appropriate 7th character is to be added to all codes in subcategory S82.31

A	initial encounter for closed fracture
D	subsequent encounter for fracture with routine healing
G	subsequent encounter for fracture with delayed healing
K	subsequent encounter for fracture with nonunion
P	subsequent encounter for fracture with malunion
S	sequela

    - S82.311   Torus fracture of lower end of right tibia
    - S82.312   Torus fracture of lower end of left tibia
    - S82.319   Torus fracture of lower end of unspecified tibia
  - S82.39   Other fracture of lower end of tibia
    - S82.391   Other fracture of lower end of right tibia
    - S82.392   Other fracture of lower end of left tibia
      Coding Clinic: 2015, Q1, P25
    - S82.399   Other fracture of lower end of unspecified tibia
- S82.4   Fracture of shaft of fibula
  - **Excludes2**   fracture of lateral malleolus alone (S82.6-)
  - S82.40   Unspecified fracture of shaft of fibula
    - S82.401   Unspecified fracture of shaft of right fibula
    - S82.402   Unspecified fracture of shaft of left fibula
    - S82.409   Unspecified fracture of shaft of unspecified fibula

CHAPTER 19 (S00-T88)

- S82.42 **Transverse** fracture of shaft of fibula
  - S82.421 Displaced transverse fracture of shaft of **right** fibula
  - S82.422 Displaced transverse fracture of shaft of **left** fibula
  - S82.423 Displaced transverse fracture of shaft of **unspecified** fibula
  - S82.424 Nondisplaced transverse fracture of shaft of **right** fibula
  - S82.425 Nondisplaced transverse fracture of shaft of **left** fibula
  - S82.426 Nondisplaced transverse fracture of shaft of **unspecified** fibula
- S82.43 **Oblique** fracture of shaft of fibula
  - S82.431 Displaced oblique fracture of shaft of **right** fibula
  - S82.432 Displaced oblique fracture of shaft of **left** fibula
  - S82.433 Displaced oblique fracture of shaft of **unspecified** fibula
  - S82.434 Nondisplaced oblique fracture of shaft of **right** fibula
  - S82.435 Nondisplaced oblique fracture of shaft of **left** fibula
  - S82.436 Nondisplaced oblique fracture of shaft of **unspecified** fibula
- S82.44 **Spiral** fracture of shaft of fibula
  - S82.441 Displaced spiral fracture of shaft of **right** fibula
  - S82.442 Displaced spiral fracture of shaft of **left** fibula
  - S82.443 Displaced spiral fracture of shaft of **unspecified** fibula
  - S82.444 Nondisplaced spiral fracture of shaft of **right** fibula
  - S82.445 Nondisplaced spiral fracture of shaft of **left** fibula
  - S82.446 Nondisplaced spiral fracture of shaft of **unspecified** fibula
- S82.45 **Comminuted** fracture of shaft of fibula
  - S82.451 Displaced comminuted fracture of shaft of **right** fibula
  - S82.452 Displaced comminuted fracture of shaft of **left** fibula
  - S82.453 Displaced comminuted fracture of shaft of **unspecified** fibula
  - S82.454 Nondisplaced comminuted fracture of shaft of **right** fibula
  - S82.455 Nondisplaced comminuted fracture of shaft of **left** fibula
  - S82.456 Nondisplaced comminuted fracture of shaft of **unspecified** fibula
- S82.46 **Segmental** fracture of shaft of fibula
  - S82.461 Displaced segmental fracture of shaft of **right** fibula
  - S82.462 Displaced segmental fracture of shaft of **left** fibula
  - S82.463 Displaced segmental fracture of shaft of **unspecified** fibula
  - S82.464 Nondisplaced segmental fracture of shaft of **right** fibula
  - S82.465 Nondisplaced segmental fracture of shaft of **left** fibula
  - S82.466 Nondisplaced segmental fracture of shaft of **unspecified** fibula
- S82.49 **Other** fracture of shaft of fibula
  - S82.491 Other fracture of shaft of **right** fibula
  - S82.492 Other fracture of shaft of **left** fibula
  - S82.499 Other fracture of shaft of **unspecified** fibula

- S82.5 Fracture of **medial malleolus**
  - **Excludes1** pilon fracture of distal tibia (S82.87-)
    Salter-Harris type III of lower end of tibia (S89.13-)
    Salter-Harris type IV of lower end of tibia (S89.14-)
  - X● S82.51 Displaced fracture of medial malleolus of **right** tibia
  - X● S82.52 Displaced fracture of medial malleolus of **left** tibia
  - X● S82.53 Displaced fracture of medial malleolus of **unspecified** tibia
  - X● S82.54 Nondisplaced fracture of medial malleolus of **right** tibia
  - X● S82.55 Nondisplaced fracture of medial malleolus of **left** tibia
  - X● S82.56 Nondisplaced fracture of medial malleolus of **unspecified** tibia
- S82.6 Fracture of **lateral malleolus**
  - **Excludes1** pilon fracture of distal tibia (S82.87-)
  - X● S82.61 Displaced fracture of lateral malleolus of **right** fibula
  - X● S82.62 Displaced fracture of lateral malleolus of **left** fibula
  - X● S82.63 Displaced fracture of lateral malleolus of **unspecified** fibula
  - X● S82.64 Nondisplaced fracture of lateral malleolus of **right** fibula
  - X● S82.65 Nondisplaced fracture of lateral malleolus of **left** fibula
  - X● S82.66 Nondisplaced fracture of lateral malleolus of **unspecified** fibula
- S82.8 Other fractures of lower leg
  - S82.81 **Torus** fracture of **upper end** of fibula

    The appropriate 7th character is to be added to all codes in subcategory S82.81

A	initial encounter for closed fracture
D	subsequent encounter for fracture with routine healing
G	subsequent encounter for fracture with delayed healing
K	subsequent encounter for fracture with nonunion
P	subsequent encounter for fracture with malunion
S	sequela

    - S82.811 Torus fracture of upper end of **right** fibula
    - S82.812 Torus fracture of upper end of **left** fibula
    - S82.819 Torus fracture of upper end of **unspecified** fibula
  - S82.82 Torus fracture of **lower end** of fibula

    The appropriate 7th character is to be added to all codes in subcategory S82.82

A	initial encounter for closed fracture
D	subsequent encounter for fracture with routine healing
G	subsequent encounter for fracture with delayed healing
K	subsequent encounter for fracture with nonunion
P	subsequent encounter for fracture with malunion
S	sequela

    - S82.821 Torus fracture of lower end of **right** fibula
    - S82.822 Torus fracture of lower end of **left** fibula

▶ New ⇒ Revised ~~deleted~~ Deleted | Excludes 1 | Excludes 2 | Includes | Use additional | Code first | Code also | Key words

OGCR Official Guidelines X Assign placeholder X ● Use Additional Character(s) ▷ Manifestation Code ⬡ Hierarchical Condition Category **Coding Clinic**

● S82.829   Torus fracture of lower end of unspecified fibula

● S82.83   Other fracture of upper and lower end of fibula

● S82.831   Other fracture of upper and lower end of right fibula

● S82.832   Other fracture of upper and lower end of left fibula
Coding Clinic: 2015, Q1, P9-10

● S82.839   Other fracture of upper and lower end of unspecified fibula

● S82.84   Bimalleolar fracture of lower leg

● S82.841   Displaced bimalleolar fracture of right lower leg

● S82.842   Displaced bimalleolar fracture of left lower leg

● S82.843   Displaced bimalleolar fracture of unspecified lower leg

● S82.844   Nondisplaced bimalleolar fracture of right lower leg

● S82.845   Nondisplaced bimalleolar fracture of left lower leg

● S82.846   Nondisplaced bimalleolar fracture of unspecified lower leg

● S82.85   Trimalleolar fracture of lower leg

● S82.851   Displaced trimalleolar fracture of right lower leg

● S82.852   Displaced trimalleolar fracture of left lower leg

● S82.853   Displaced trimalleolar fracture of unspecified lower leg

● S82.854   Nondisplaced trimalleolar fracture of right lower leg

● S82.855   Nondisplaced trimalleolar fracture of left lower leg

● S82.856   Nondisplaced trimalleolar fracture of unspecified lower leg

● S82.86   Maisonneuve's fracture

● S82.861   Displaced Maisonneuve's fracture of right leg

● S82.862   Displaced Maisonneuve's fracture of left leg

● S82.863   Displaced Maisonneuve's fracture of unspecified leg

● S82.864   Nondisplaced Maisonneuve's fracture of right leg

● S82.865   Nondisplaced Maisonneuve's fracture of left leg

● S82.866   Nondisplaced Maisonneuve's fracture of unspecified leg

● S82.87   Pilon fracture of tibia

● S82.871   Displaced pilon fracture of right tibia
● S82.872   Displaced pilon fracture of left tibia
● S82.873   Displaced pilon fracture of unspecified tibia
● S82.874   Nondisplaced pilon fracture of right tibia
● S82.875   Nondisplaced pilon fracture of left tibia
● S82.876   Nondisplaced pilon fracture of unspecified tibia

● S82.89   Other fractures of lower leg
Fracture of ankle NOS

● S82.891   Other fracture of right lower leg
● S82.892   Other fracture of left lower leg
● S82.899   Other fracture of unspecified lower leg

● S82.9   Unspecified fracture of lower leg

X ● S82.90   Unspecified fracture of unspecified lower leg
X ● S82.91   Unspecified fracture of right lower leg
X ● S82.92   Unspecified fracture of left lower leg

● S83   Dislocation and sprain of joints and ligaments of knee

Includes   avulsion of joint or ligament of knee
laceration of cartilage, joint or ligament of knee
sprain of cartilage, joint or ligament of knee
traumatic hemarthrosis of joint or ligament of knee
traumatic rupture of joint or ligament of knee
traumatic subluxation of joint or ligament of knee
traumatic tear of joint or ligament of knee

Code also any associated open wound

Excludes2   derangement of patella (M22.0-M22.3)
injury of patellar ligament (tendon) (S76.1-)
internal derangement of knee (M23.-)
old dislocation of knee (M24.36)
pathological dislocation of knee (M24.36)
recurrent dislocation of knee (M22.0)
strain of muscle, fascia and tendon of lower leg (S86.-)

Coding Clinic: 2019, Q2, P26

The appropriate 7th character is to be added to each code from category S83

A	initial encounter
D	subsequent encounter
S	sequela

● S83.0   Subluxation and dislocation of patella

● S83.00   Unspecified subluxation and dislocation of patella

● S83.001   Unspecified subluxation of right patella
● S83.002   Unspecified subluxation of left patella
● S83.003   Unspecified subluxation of unspecified patella
● S83.004   Unspecified dislocation of right patella
● S83.005   Unspecified dislocation of left patella
● S83.006   Unspecified dislocation of unspecified patella

● S83.01   Lateral subluxation and dislocation of patella

● S83.011   Lateral subluxation of right patella
● S83.012   Lateral subluxation of left patella
● S83.013   Lateral subluxation of unspecified patella
● S83.014   Lateral dislocation of right patella
● S83.015   Lateral dislocation of left patella
● S83.016   Lateral dislocation of unspecified patella

● S83.09   Other subluxation and dislocation of patella

● S83.091   Other subluxation of right patella
● S83.092   Other subluxation of left patella
● S83.093   Other subluxation of unspecified patella
● S83.094   Other dislocation of right patella
● S83.095   Other dislocation of left patella
● S83.096   Other dislocation of unspecified patella

● S83.1   Subluxation and dislocation of knee

Excludes2   instability of knee prosthesis (T84.022, T84.023)

● S83.10   Unspecified subluxation and dislocation of knee

● S83.101   Unspecified subluxation of right knee
● S83.102   Unspecified subluxation of left knee
● S83.103   Unspecified subluxation of unspecified knee
● S83.104   Unspecified dislocation of right knee
● S83.105   Unspecified dislocation of left knee
● S83.106   Unspecified dislocation of unspecified knee

CHAPTER 19 (S00-T88)

● S83.11   **Anterior subluxation and dislocation of proximal end of tibia**
Posterior subluxation and dislocation of distal end of femur

  ● S83.111   Anterior subluxation of proximal end of tibia, right knee

  ● S83.112   Anterior subluxation of proximal end of tibia, left knee

  ● S83.113   Anterior subluxation of proximal end of tibia, unspecified knee

  ● S83.114   Anterior dislocation of proximal end of tibia, right knee

  ● S83.115   Anterior dislocation of proximal end of tibia, left knee

  ● S83.116   Anterior dislocation of proximal end of tibia, unspecified knee

● S83.12   **Posterior subluxation and dislocation of proximal end of tibia**
Anterior dislocation of distal end of femur

  ● S83.121   Posterior subluxation of proximal end of tibia, right knee

  ● S83.122   Posterior subluxation of proximal end of tibia, left knee

  ● S83.123   Posterior subluxation of proximal end of tibia, unspecified knee

  ● S83.124   Posterior dislocation of proximal end of tibia, right knee

  ● S83.125   Posterior dislocation of proximal end of tibia, left knee

  ● S83.126   Posterior dislocation of proximal end of tibia, unspecified knee

● S83.13   **Medial subluxation and dislocation of proximal end of tibia**

  ● S83.131   Medial subluxation of proximal end of tibia, right knee

  ● S83.132   Medial subluxation of proximal end of tibia, left knee

  ● S83.133   Medial subluxation of proximal end of tibia, unspecified knee

  ● S83.134   Medial dislocation of proximal end of tibia, right knee

  ● S83.135   Medial dislocation of proximal end of tibia, left knee

  ● S83.136   Medial dislocation of proximal end of tibia, unspecified knee

● S83.14   **Lateral subluxation and dislocation of proximal end of tibia**

  ● S83.141   Lateral subluxation of proximal end of tibia, right knee

  ● S83.142   Lateral subluxation of proximal end of tibia, left knee

  ● S83.143   Lateral subluxation of proximal end of tibia, unspecified knee

  ● S83.144   Lateral dislocation of proximal end of tibia, right knee

  ● S83.145   Lateral dislocation of proximal end of tibia, left knee

  ● S83.146   Lateral dislocation of proximal end of tibia, unspecified knee

● S83.19   **Other subluxation and dislocation of knee**

  ● S83.191   Other subluxation of right knee

  ● S83.192   Other subluxation of left knee

  ● S83.193   Other subluxation of unspecified knee

  ● S83.194   Other dislocation of right knee

  ● S83.195   Other dislocation of left knee

  ● S83.196   Other dislocation of unspecified knee

● S83.2   **Tear of meniscus, current injury**

Excludes1   old bucket-handle tear (M23.2)

● S83.20   **Tear of unspecified meniscus, current injury**
Tear of meniscus of knee NOS

  ● S83.200   Bucket-handle tear of unspecified meniscus, current injury, right knee

  ● S83.201   Bucket-handle tear of unspecified meniscus, current injury, left knee

  ● S83.202   Bucket-handle tear of unspecified meniscus, current injury, unspecified knee

  ● S83.203   Other tear of unspecified meniscus, current injury, right knee

  ● S83.204   Other tear of unspecified meniscus, current injury, left knee

  ● S83.205   Other tear of unspecified meniscus, current injury, unspecified knee

  ● S83.206   Unspecified tear of unspecified meniscus, current injury, right knee

  ● S83.207   Unspecified tear of unspecified meniscus, current injury, left knee

  ● S83.209   Unspecified tear of unspecified meniscus, current injury, unspecified knee

● S83.21   **Bucket-handle tear of medial meniscus, current injury**

  ● S83.211   Bucket-handle tear of medial meniscus, current injury, right knee

  ● S83.212   Bucket-handle tear of medial meniscus, current injury, left knee

  ● S83.219   Bucket-handle tear of medial meniscus, current injury, unspecified knee

● S83.22   **Peripheral tear of medial meniscus, current injury**

  ● S83.221   Peripheral tear of medial meniscus, current injury, right knee

  ● S83.222   Peripheral tear of medial meniscus, current injury, left knee

  ● S83.229   Peripheral tear of medial meniscus, current injury, unspecified knee

● S83.23   **Complex tear of medial meniscus, current injury**

  ● S83.231   Complex tear of medial meniscus, current injury, right knee

  ● S83.232   Complex tear of medial meniscus, current injury, left knee
Coding Clinic: 2019, Q2, P26

  ● S83.239   Complex tear of medial meniscus, current injury, unspecified knee

● S83.24   **Other tear of medial meniscus, current injury**

  ● S83.241   Other tear of medial meniscus, current injury, right knee

  ● S83.242   Other tear of medial meniscus, current injury, left knee

  ● S83.249   Other tear of medial meniscus, current injury, unspecified knee

● S83.25   **Bucket-handle tear of lateral meniscus, current injury**

  ● S83.251   Bucket-handle tear of lateral meniscus, current injury, right knee

  ● S83.252   Bucket-handle tear of lateral meniscus, current injury, left knee

  ● S83.259   Bucket-handle tear of lateral meniscus, current injury, unspecified knee

● S83.26   **Peripheral tear of lateral meniscus, current injury**

  ● S83.261   Peripheral tear of lateral meniscus, current injury, right knee

- S83.262   Peripheral tear of lateral meniscus, current injury, left knee
  - S83.269   Peripheral tear of lateral meniscus, current injury, unspecified knee
- S83.27   Complex tear of lateral meniscus, current injury
  - S83.271   Complex tear of lateral meniscus, current injury, right knee
  - S83.272   Complex tear of lateral meniscus, current injury, left knee
  - S83.279   Complex tear of lateral meniscus, current injury, unspecified knee
- S83.28   Other tear of lateral meniscus, current injury
  - S83.281   Other tear of lateral meniscus, current injury, right knee
  - S83.282   Other tear of lateral meniscus, current injury, left knee
  - S83.289   Other tear of lateral meniscus, current injury, unspecified knee
- S83.3   Tear of articular cartilage of knee, current
  - X S83.30   Tear of articular cartilage of unspecified knee, current
  - X S83.31   Tear of articular cartilage of right knee, current
  - X S83.32   Tear of articular cartilage of left knee, current
- S83.4   Sprain of collateral ligament of knee
  - S83.40   Sprain of unspecified collateral ligament of knee
    - S83.401   Sprain of unspecified collateral ligament of right knee
    - S83.402   Sprain of unspecified collateral ligament of left knee
    - S83.409   Sprain of unspecified collateral ligament of unspecified knee
  - S83.41   Sprain of medial collateral ligament of knee
    Sprain of tibial collateral ligament
    - S83.411   Sprain of medial collateral ligament of right knee
    - S83.412   Sprain of medial collateral ligament of left knee
    - S83.419   Sprain of medial collateral ligament of unspecified knee
  - S83.42   Sprain of lateral collateral ligament of knee
    Sprain of fibular collateral ligament
    - S83.421   Sprain of lateral collateral ligament of right knee
    - S83.422   Sprain of lateral collateral ligament of left knee
    - S83.429   Sprain of lateral collateral ligament of unspecified knee
- S83.5   Sprain of cruciate ligament of knee
  - S83.50   Sprain of unspecified cruciate ligament of knee
    - S83.501   Sprain of unspecified cruciate ligament of right knee
    - S83.502   Sprain of unspecified cruciate ligament of left knee
    - S83.509   Sprain of unspecified cruciate ligament of unspecified knee
  - S83.51   Sprain of anterior cruciate ligament of knee
    - S83.511   Sprain of anterior cruciate ligament of right knee
      Coding Clinic: 2016, Q2, P4
    - S83.512   Sprain of anterior cruciate ligament of left knee
    - S83.519   Sprain of anterior cruciate ligament of unspecified knee
  - S83.52   Sprain of posterior cruciate ligament of knee
    - S83.521   Sprain of posterior cruciate ligament of right knee

- S83.522   Sprain of posterior cruciate ligament of left knee
  - S83.529   Sprain of posterior cruciate ligament of unspecified knee
- S83.6   Sprain of the superior tibiofibular joint and ligament
  - X S83.60   Sprain of the superior tibiofibular joint and ligament, unspecified knee
  - X S83.61   Sprain of the superior tibiofibular joint and ligament, right knee
  - X S83.62   Sprain of the superior tibiofibular joint and ligament, left knee
- S83.8   Sprain of other specified parts of knee
  - S83.8X   Sprain of other specified parts of knee
    - S83.8X1   Sprain of other specified parts of right knee
    - S83.8X2   Sprain of other specified parts of left knee
    - S83.8X9   Sprain of other specified parts of unspecified knee
- S83.9   Sprain of unspecified site of knee
  - X S83.90   Sprain of unspecified site of unspecified knee
  - X S83.91   Sprain of unspecified site of right knee
  - X S83.92   Sprain of unspecified site of left knee

- S84   Injury of nerves at lower leg level
  Code also any associated open wound (S81.-)
  Excludes2   injury of nerves at ankle and foot level (S94.-)
  The appropriate 7th character is to be added to each code from category S84

A	initial encounter
D	subsequent encounter
S	sequela

  - S84.0   Injury of tibial nerve at lower leg level
    - X S84.00   Injury of tibial nerve at lower leg level, unspecified leg
    - X S84.01   Injury of tibial nerve at lower leg level, right leg
    - X S84.02   Injury of tibial nerve at lower leg level, left leg
  - S84.1   Injury of peroneal nerve at lower leg level
    - X S84.10   Injury of peroneal nerve at lower leg level, unspecified leg
    - X S84.11   Injury of peroneal nerve at lower leg level, right leg
    - X S84.12   Injury of peroneal nerve at lower leg level, left leg
  - S84.2   Injury of cutaneous sensory nerve at lower leg level
    - X S84.20   Injury of cutaneous sensory nerve at lower leg level, unspecified leg
    - X S84.21   Injury of cutaneous sensory nerve at lower leg level, right leg
    - X S84.22   Injury of cutaneous sensory nerve at lower leg level, left leg
  - S84.8   Injury of other nerves at lower leg level
    - S84.80   Injury of other nerves at lower leg level
      - S84.801   Injury of other nerves at lower leg level, right leg
      - S84.802   Injury of other nerves at lower leg level, left leg
      - S84.809   Injury of other nerves at lower leg level, unspecified leg
  - S84.9   Injury of unspecified nerve at lower leg level
    - X S84.90   Injury of unspecified nerve at lower leg level, unspecified leg
    - X S84.91   Injury of unspecified nerve at lower leg level, right leg
    - X S84.92   Injury of unspecified nerve at lower leg level, left leg

CHAPTER 19 (S00-T88)

S85 **Injury of blood vessels at lower leg level**

Code also any associated open wound (S81.-)

Excludes2   injury of blood vessels at ankle and foot level (S95.-)

The appropriate 7th character is to be added to each code from category S85

A	initial encounter
D	subsequent encounter
S	sequela

S85.0   **Injury of popliteal artery**

S85.00   Unspecified injury of popliteal artery

S85.001   Unspecified injury of popliteal artery, right leg

S85.002   Unspecified injury of popliteal artery, left leg

S85.009   Unspecified injury of popliteal artery, unspecified leg

S85.01   Laceration of popliteal artery

S85.011   Laceration of popliteal artery, right leg

S85.012   Laceration of popliteal artery, left leg

S85.019   Laceration of popliteal artery, unspecified leg

S85.09   Other specified injury of popliteal artery

S85.091   Other specified injury of popliteal artery, right leg

S85.092   Other specified injury of popliteal artery, left leg

S85.099   Other specified injury of popliteal artery, unspecified leg

S85.1   **Injury of tibial artery**

S85.10   Unspecified injury of unspecified tibial artery
Injury of tibial artery NOS

S85.101   Unspecified injury of unspecified tibial artery, right leg

S85.102   Unspecified injury of unspecified tibial artery, left leg

S85.109   Unspecified injury of unspecified tibial artery, unspecified leg

S85.11   Laceration of unspecified tibial artery

S85.111   Laceration of unspecified tibial artery, right leg

S85.112   Laceration of unspecified tibial artery, left leg

S85.119   Laceration of unspecified tibial artery, unspecified leg

S85.12   Other specified injury of unspecified tibial artery

S85.121   Other specified injury of unspecified tibial artery, right leg

S85.122   Other specified injury of unspecified tibial artery, left leg

S85.129   Other specified injury of unspecified tibial artery, unspecified leg

S85.13   Unspecified injury of anterior tibial artery

S85.131   Unspecified injury of anterior tibial artery, right leg

S85.132   Unspecified injury of anterior tibial artery, left leg

S85.139   Unspecified injury of anterior tibial artery, unspecified leg

S85.14   Laceration of anterior tibial artery

S85.141   Laceration of anterior tibial artery, right leg

S85.142   Laceration of anterior tibial artery, left leg

S85.149   Laceration of anterior tibial artery, unspecified leg

S85.15   Other specified injury of anterior tibial artery

S85.151   Other specified injury of anterior tibial artery, right leg

S85.152   Other specified injury of anterior tibial artery, left leg

S85.159   Other specified injury of anterior tibial artery, unspecified leg

S85.16   Unspecified injury of posterior tibial artery

S85.161   Unspecified injury of posterior tibial artery, right leg

S85.162   Unspecified injury of posterior tibial artery, left leg

S85.169   Unspecified injury of posterior tibial artery, unspecified leg

S85.17   Laceration of posterior tibial artery

S85.171   Laceration of posterior tibial artery, right leg

S85.172   Laceration of posterior tibial artery, left leg

S85.179   Laceration of posterior tibial artery, unspecified leg

S85.18   Other specified injury of posterior tibial artery

S85.181   Other specified injury of posterior tibial artery, right leg

S85.182   Other specified injury of posterior tibial artery, left leg

S85.189   Other specified injury of posterior tibial artery, unspecified leg

S85.2   **Injury of peroneal artery**

S85.20   Unspecified injury of peroneal artery

S85.201   Unspecified injury of peroneal artery, right leg

S85.202   Unspecified injury of peroneal artery, left leg

S85.209   Unspecified injury of peroneal artery, unspecified leg

S85.21   Laceration of peroneal artery

S85.211   Laceration of peroneal artery, right leg

S85.212   Laceration of peroneal artery, left leg

S85.219   Laceration of peroneal artery, unspecified leg

S85.29   Other specified injury of peroneal artery

S85.291   Other specified injury of peroneal artery, right leg

S85.292   Other specified injury of peroneal artery, left leg

S85.299   Other specified injury of peroneal artery, unspecified leg

S85.3   **Injury of greater saphenous vein at lower leg level**
Injury of greater saphenous vein NOS
Injury of saphenous vein NOS

S85.30   Unspecified injury of greater saphenous vein at lower leg level

S85.301   Unspecified injury of greater saphenous vein at lower leg level, right leg

S85.302   Unspecified injury of greater saphenous vein at lower leg level, left leg

S85.309   Unspecified injury of greater saphenous vein at lower leg level, unspecified leg

S85.31   Laceration of greater saphenous vein at lower leg level

S85.311   Laceration of greater saphenous vein at lower leg level, right leg

S85.312   Laceration of greater saphenous vein at lower leg level, left leg

S85.319   Laceration of greater saphenous vein at lower leg level, unspecified leg

CHAPTER 19 (S00-T88)

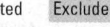

▶ New   ⇒ Revised   ~~deleted~~ Deleted   Excludes 1   Excludes 2   Includes   Use additional   Code first   Code also   Key words

OGCR Official Guidelines   X Assign placeholder X   ● Use Additional Character(s)   ▶ Manifestation Code   Hierarchical Condition Category   Coding Clinic

- ● S85.39   Other specified injury of greater saphenous vein at lower leg level
  - ● S85.391   Other specified injury of greater saphenous vein at lower leg level, right leg
  - ● S85.392   Other specified injury of greater saphenous vein at lower leg level, left leg
  - ● S85.399   Other specified injury of greater saphenous vein at lower leg level, unspecified leg
- ● S85.4   Injury of lesser saphenous vein at lower leg level
  - ● S85.40   Unspecified injury of lesser saphenous vein at lower leg level
    - ● S85.401   Unspecified injury of lesser saphenous vein at lower leg level, right leg
    - ● S85.402   Unspecified injury of lesser saphenous vein at lower leg level, left leg
    - ● S85.409   Unspecified injury of lesser saphenous vein at lower leg level, unspecified leg
  - ● S85.41   Laceration of lesser saphenous vein at lower leg level
    - ● S85.411   Laceration of lesser saphenous vein at lower leg level, right leg
    - ● S85.412   Laceration of lesser saphenous vein at lower leg level, left leg
    - ● S85.419   Laceration of lesser saphenous vein at lower leg level, unspecified leg
  - ● S85.49   Other specified injury of lesser saphenous vein at lower leg level
    - ● S85.491   Other specified injury of lesser saphenous vein at lower leg level, right leg
    - ● S85.492   Other specified injury of lesser saphenous vein at lower leg level, left leg
    - ● S85.499   Other specified injury of lesser saphenous vein at lower leg level, unspecified leg
- ● S85.5   Injury of popliteal vein
  - ● S85.50   Unspecified injury of popliteal vein
    - ● S85.501   Unspecified injury of popliteal vein, right leg
    - ● S85.502   Unspecified injury of popliteal vein, left leg
    - ● S85.509   Unspecified injury of popliteal vein, unspecified leg
  - ● S85.51   Laceration of popliteal vein
    - ● S85.511   Laceration of popliteal vein, right leg
    - ● S85.512   Laceration of popliteal vein, left leg
    - ● S85.519   Laceration of popliteal vein, unspecified leg
  - ● S85.59   Other specified injury of popliteal vein
    - ● S85.591   Other specified injury of popliteal vein, right leg
    - ● S85.592   Other specified injury of popliteal vein, left leg
    - ● S85.599   Other specified injury of popliteal vein, unspecified leg
- ● S85.8   Injury of other blood vessels at lower leg level
  - ● S85.80   Unspecified injury of other blood vessels at lower leg level
    - ● S85.801   Unspecified injury of other blood vessels at lower leg level, right leg
    - ● S85.802   Unspecified injury of other blood vessels at lower leg level, left leg

---

-     ● S85.809   Unspecified injury of other blood vessels at lower leg level, unspecified leg
- ● S85.81   Laceration of other blood vessels at lower leg level
  - ● S85.811   Laceration of other blood vessels at lower leg level, right leg
  - ● S85.812   Laceration of other blood vessels at lower leg level, left leg
  - ● S85.819   Laceration of other blood vessels at lower leg level, unspecified leg
- ● S85.89   Other specified injury of other blood vessels at lower leg level
  - ● S85.891   Other specified injury of other blood vessels at lower leg level, right leg
  - ● S85.892   Other specified injury of other blood vessels at lower leg level, left leg
  - ● S85.899   Other specified injury of other blood vessels at lower leg level, unspecified leg
- ● S85.9   Injury of unspecified blood vessel at lower leg level
  - ● S85.90   Unspecified injury of unspecified blood vessel at lower leg level
    - ● S85.901   Unspecified injury of unspecified blood vessel at lower leg level, right leg
    - ● S85.902   Unspecified injury of unspecified blood vessel at lower leg level, left leg
    - ● S85.909   Unspecified injury of unspecified blood vessel at lower leg level, unspecified leg
  - ● S85.91   Laceration of unspecified blood vessel at lower leg level
    - ● S85.911   Laceration of unspecified blood vessel at lower leg level, right leg
    - ● S85.912   Laceration of unspecified blood vessel at lower leg level, left leg
    - ● S85.919   Laceration of unspecified blood vessel at lower leg level, unspecified leg
  - ● S85.99   Other specified injury of unspecified blood vessel at lower leg level
    - ● S85.991   Other specified injury of unspecified blood vessel at lower leg level, right leg
    - ● S85.992   Other specified injury of unspecified blood vessel at lower leg level, left leg
    - ● S85.999   Other specified injury of unspecified blood vessel at lower leg level, unspecified leg

- ● S86   Injury of muscle, fascia and tendon at lower leg level

  Code also any associated open wound (S81.-)

  Excludes2   injury of muscle, fascia and tendon at ankle (S96.-)
  injury of patellar ligament (tendon) (S76.1-)
  sprain of joints and ligaments of knee (S83.-)

  The appropriate 7th character is to be added to each code from category S86

A	initial encounter
D	subsequent encounter
S	sequela

  - ● S86.0   Injury of Achilles tendon
    - ● S86.00   Unspecified injury of Achilles tendon
      - ● S86.001   Unspecified injury of right Achilles tendon
      - ● S86.002   Unspecified injury of left Achilles tendon
      - ● S86.009   Unspecified injury of unspecified Achilles tendon

● **S86.01** Strain of Achilles tendon
   ● S86.011 Strain of right Achilles tendon
   ● S86.012 Strain of left Achilles tendon
   ● S86.019 Strain of unspecified Achilles tendon
● **S86.02** Laceration of Achilles tendon
   ● S86.021 Laceration of right Achilles tendon
   ● S86.022 Laceration of left Achilles tendon
   ● S86.029 Laceration of unspecified Achilles tendon
● **S86.09** Other specified injury of Achilles tendon
   ● S86.091 Other specified injury of right Achilles tendon
   ● S86.092 Other specified injury of left Achilles tendon
   ● S86.099 Other specified injury of unspecified Achilles tendon
● **S86.1** Injury of other muscle(s) and tendon(s) of posterior muscle group at lower leg level
   ● **S86.10** Unspecified injury of other muscle(s) and tendon(s) of posterior muscle group at lower leg level
     ● S86.101 Unspecified injury of other muscle(s) and tendon(s) of posterior muscle group at lower leg level, right leg
     ● S86.102 Unspecified injury of other muscle(s) and tendon(s) of posterior muscle group at lower leg level, left leg
     ● S86.109 Unspecified injury of other muscle(s) and tendon(s) of posterior muscle group at lower leg level, unspecified leg
   ● **S86.11** Strain of other muscle(s) and tendon(s) of posterior muscle group at lower leg level
     ● S86.111 Strain of other muscle(s) and tendon(s) of posterior muscle group at lower leg level, right leg
     ● S86.112 Strain of other muscle(s) and tendon(s) of posterior muscle group at lower leg level, left leg
     ● S86.119 Strain of other muscle(s) and tendon(s) of posterior muscle group at lower leg level, unspecified leg
   ● **S86.12** Laceration of other muscle(s) and tendon(s) of posterior muscle group at lower leg level
     ● S86.121 Laceration of other muscle(s) and tendon(s) of posterior muscle group at lower leg level, right leg
     ● S86.122 Laceration of other muscle(s) and tendon(s) of posterior muscle group at lower leg level, left leg
     ● S86.129 Laceration of other muscle(s) and tendon(s) of posterior muscle group at lower leg level, unspecified leg
   ● **S86.19** Other injury of other muscle(s) and tendon(s) of posterior muscle group at lower leg level
     ● S86.191 Other injury of other muscle(s) and tendon(s) of posterior muscle group at lower leg level, right leg
     ● S86.192 Other injury of other muscle(s) and tendon(s) of posterior muscle group at lower leg level, left leg
     ● S86.199 Other injury of other muscle(s) and tendon(s) of posterior muscle group at lower leg level, unspecified leg
● **S86.2** Injury of muscle(s) and tendon(s) of anterior muscle group at lower leg level
   ● **S86.20** Unspecified injury of muscle(s) and tendon(s) of anterior muscle group at lower leg level
     ● S86.201 Unspecified injury of muscle(s) and tendon(s) of anterior muscle group at lower leg level, right leg

● S86.202 Unspecified injury of muscle(s) and tendon(s) of anterior muscle group at lower leg level, left leg
● S86.209 Unspecified injury of muscle(s) and tendon(s) of anterior muscle group at lower leg level, unspecified leg
● **S86.21** Strain of muscle(s) and tendon(s) of anterior muscle group at lower leg level
   ● S86.211 Strain of muscle(s) and tendon(s) of anterior muscle group at lower leg level, right leg
   ● S86.212 Strain of muscle(s) and tendon(s) of anterior muscle group at lower leg level, left leg
   ● S86.219 Strain of muscle(s) and tendon(s) of anterior muscle group at lower leg level, unspecified leg
● **S86.22** Laceration of muscle(s) and tendon(s) of anterior muscle group at lower leg level
   ● S86.221 Laceration of muscle(s) and tendon(s) of anterior muscle group at lower leg level, right leg
   ● S86.222 Laceration of muscle(s) and tendon(s) of anterior muscle group at lower leg level, left leg
   ● S86.229 Laceration of muscle(s) and tendon(s) of anterior muscle group at lower leg level, unspecified leg
● **S86.29** Other injury of muscle(s) and tendon(s) of anterior muscle group at lower leg level
   ● S86.291 Other injury of muscle(s) and tendon(s) of anterior muscle group at lower leg level, right leg
   ● S86.292 Other injury of muscle(s) and tendon(s) of anterior muscle group at lower leg level, left leg
   ● S86.299 Other injury of muscle(s) and tendon(s) of anterior muscle group at lower leg level, unspecified leg
● **S86.3** Injury of muscle(s) and tendon(s) of peroneal muscle group at lower leg level
   ● **S86.30** Unspecified injury of muscle(s) and tendon(s) of peroneal muscle group at lower leg level
     ● S86.301 Unspecified injury of muscle(s) and tendon(s) of peroneal muscle group at lower leg level, right leg
     ● S86.302 Unspecified injury of muscle(s) and tendon(s) of peroneal muscle group at lower leg level, left leg
     ● S86.309 Unspecified injury of muscle(s) and tendon(s) of peroneal muscle group at lower leg level, unspecified leg
   ● **S86.31** Strain of muscle(s) and tendon(s) of peroneal muscle group at lower leg level
     ● S86.311 Strain of muscle(s) and tendon(s) of peroneal muscle group at lower leg level, right leg
     ● S86.312 Strain of muscle(s) and tendon(s) of peroneal muscle group at lower leg level, left leg
     ● S86.319 Strain of muscle(s) and tendon(s) of peroneal muscle group at lower leg level, unspecified leg
   ● **S86.32** Laceration of muscle(s) and tendon(s) of peroneal muscle group at lower leg level
     ● S86.321 Laceration of muscle(s) and tendon(s) of peroneal muscle group at lower leg level, right leg
     ● S86.322 Laceration of muscle(s) and tendon(s) of peroneal muscle group at lower leg level, left leg

▶ New   ⇒ Revised   ~~deleted~~ Deleted   Excludes 1   Excludes 2   Includes   Use additional   Code first   Code also   Key words
OGCR Official Guidelines   X Assign placeholder X   ● Use Additional Character(s)   ▶ Manifestation Code   Hierarchical Condition Category   Coding Clinic

● S86.329   Laceration of muscle(s) and tendon(s) of peroneal muscle group at lower leg level, unspecified leg

● S86.39   Other injury of muscle(s) and tendon(s) of peroneal muscle group at lower leg level

   ● S86.391   Other injury of muscle(s) and tendon(s) of peroneal muscle group at lower leg level, right leg

   ● S86.392   Other injury of muscle(s) and tendon(s) of peroneal muscle group at lower leg level, left leg

   ● S86.399   Other injury of muscle(s) and tendon(s) of peroneal muscle group at lower leg level, unspecified leg

● S86.8   Injury of other muscles and tendons at lower leg level

 ● S86.80   Unspecified injury of other muscles and tendons at lower leg level

   ● S86.801   Unspecified injury of other muscle(s) and tendon(s) at lower leg level, right leg

   ● S86.802   Unspecified injury of other muscle(s) and tendon(s) at lower leg level, left leg

   ● S86.809   Unspecified injury of other muscle(s) and tendon(s) at lower leg level, unspecified leg

 ● S86.81   Strain of other muscles and tendons at lower leg level

   ● S86.811   Strain of other muscle(s) and tendon(s) at lower leg level, right leg

   ● S86.812   Strain of other muscle(s) and tendon(s) at lower leg level, left leg

   ● S86.819   Strain of other muscle(s) and tendon(s) at lower leg level, unspecified leg

 ● S86.82   Laceration of other muscles and tendons at lower leg level

   ● S86.821   Laceration of other muscle(s) and tendon(s) at lower leg level, right leg

   ● S86.822   Laceration of other muscle(s) and tendon(s) at lower leg level, left leg

   ● S86.829   Laceration of other muscle(s) and tendon(s) at lower leg level, unspecified leg

 ● S86.89   Other injury of other muscles and tendons at lower leg level

   ● S86.891   Other injury of other muscle(s) and tendon(s) at lower leg level, right leg

   ● S86.892   Other injury of other muscle(s) and tendon(s) at lower leg level, left leg

   ● S86.899   Other injury of other muscle(s) and tendon(s) at lower leg level, unspecified leg

● S86.9   Injury of unspecified muscle and tendon at lower leg level

 ● S86.90   Unspecified injury of unspecified muscle and tendon at lower leg level

   ● S86.901   Unspecified injury of unspecified muscle(s) and tendon(s) at lower leg level, right leg

   ● S86.902   Unspecified injury of unspecified muscle(s) and tendon(s) at lower leg level, left leg

   ● S86.909   Unspecified injury of unspecified muscle(s) and tendon(s) at lower leg level, unspecified leg

 ● S86.91   Strain of unspecified muscle and tendon at lower leg level

   ● S86.911   Strain of unspecified muscle(s) and tendon(s) at lower leg level, right leg

● S86.912   Strain of unspecified muscle(s) and tendon(s) at lower leg level, left leg

● S86.919   Strain of unspecified muscle(s) and tendon(s) at lower leg level, unspecified leg

● S86.92   Laceration of unspecified muscle and tendon at lower leg level

   ● S86.921   Laceration of unspecified muscle(s) and tendon(s) at lower leg level, right leg

   ● S86.922   Laceration of unspecified muscle(s) and tendon(s) at lower leg level, left leg

   ● S86.929   Laceration of unspecified muscle(s) and tendon(s) at lower leg level, unspecified leg

● S86.99   Other injury of unspecified muscle and tendon at lower leg level

   ● S86.991   Other injury of unspecified muscle(s) and tendon(s) at lower leg level, right leg

   ● S86.992   Other injury of unspecified muscle(s) and tendon(s) at lower leg level, left leg

   ● S86.999   Other injury of unspecified muscle(s) and tendon(s) at lower leg level, unspecified leg

● S87   Crushing injury of lower leg

Use additional code(s) for all associated injuries

Excludes2   crushing injury of ankle and foot (S97.-)

The appropriate 7th character is to be added to each code from category S87

A	initial encounter
D	subsequent encounter
S	sequela

 ● S87.0   Crushing injury of knee

   X● S87.00   Crushing injury of unspecified knee

   X● S87.01   Crushing injury of right knee

   X● S87.02   Crushing injury of left knee

 ● S87.8   Crushing injury of lower leg

   X● S87.80   Crushing injury of unspecified lower leg

   X● S87.81   Crushing injury of right lower leg

   X● S87.82   Crushing injury of left lower leg

● S88   Traumatic amputation of lower leg

An amputation not identified as partial or complete should be coded to complete

Excludes1   traumatic amputation of ankle and foot (S98.-)

The appropriate 7th character is to be added to each code from category S88

A	initial encounter
D	subsequent encounter
S	sequela

 ● S88.0   Traumatic amputation at knee level

   ● S88.01   Complete traumatic amputation at knee level

    ● S88.011   Complete traumatic amputation at knee level, right lower leg A, D, S 🔖
      Coding Clinic: 2023, Q1, P28-29

    ● S88.012   Complete traumatic amputation at knee level, left lower leg A, D, S 🔖
      Coding Clinic: 2023, Q1, P28-29

    ● S88.019   Complete traumatic amputation at knee level, unspecified lower leg A, D, S 🔖

   ● S88.02   Partial traumatic amputation at knee level

    ● S88.021   Partial traumatic amputation at knee level, right lower leg A, D, S 🔖

● S88.022   Partial traumatic amputation at knee
             level, left lower leg A, D, S 🐾

● S88.029   Partial traumatic amputation at knee
             level, unspecified lower leg A, D, S 🐾

● S88.1   Traumatic amputation at level between knee and ankle

   ● S88.11   Complete traumatic amputation at level
              between knee and ankle

      ● S88.111   Complete traumatic amputation at
                  level between knee and ankle, right
                  lower leg A, D, S 🐾

      ● S88.112   Complete traumatic amputation at
                  level between knee and ankle, left
                  lower leg A, D, S 🐾

      ● S88.119   Complete traumatic amputation at
                  level between knee and ankle,
                  unspecified lower leg A, D, S 🐾

   ● S88.12   Partial traumatic amputation at level between
              knee and ankle

      ● S88.121   Partial traumatic amputation at level
                  between knee and ankle, right lower
                  leg A, D, S 🐾

      ● S88.122   Partial traumatic amputation at level
                  between knee and ankle, left lower
                  leg A, D, S 🐾

      ● S88.129   Partial traumatic amputation at level
                  between knee and ankle, unspecified
                  lower leg A, D, S 🐾

● S88.9   Traumatic amputation of lower leg, level unspecified

   ● S88.91   Complete traumatic amputation of lower leg,
              level unspecified

      ● S88.911   Complete traumatic amputation of
                  right lower leg, level unspecified
                  A, D, S 🐾

      ● S88.912   Complete traumatic amputation of
                  left lower leg, level unspecified
                  A, D, S 🐾

      ● S88.919   Complete traumatic amputation of
                  unspecified lower leg, level
                  unspecified A, D, S 🐾

   ● S88.92   Partial traumatic amputation of lower leg, level
              unspecified

      ● S88.921   Partial traumatic amputation of right
                  lower leg, level unspecified A, D, S 🐾

      ● S88.922   Partial traumatic amputation of left
                  lower leg, level unspecified A, D, S 🐾

      ● S88.929   Partial traumatic amputation of
                  unspecified lower leg, level
                  unspecified A, D, S 🐾

● S89   Other and unspecified injuries of lower leg

   Note: A fracture not indicated as open or closed should be
   coded to closed

   Excludes2   other and unspecified injuries of ankle and foot
                   (S99.-)

   The appropriate 7th character is to be added to each code from
   subcategories S89.0, S89.1, S89.2, and S89.3

A	initial encounter for closed fracture
D	subsequent encounter for fracture with routine healing
G	subsequent encounter for fracture with delayed healing
K	subsequent encounter for fracture with nonunion
P	subsequent encounter for fracture with malunion
S	sequela

● S89.0   Physeal fracture of upper end of tibia

   ● S89.00   Unspecified physeal fracture of upper end of
              tibia

      ● S89.001   Unspecified physeal fracture of
                  upper end of right tibia

      ● S89.002   Unspecified physeal fracture of
                  upper end of left tibia

      ● S89.009   Unspecified physeal fracture of upper
                  end of unspecified tibia

   ● S89.01   Salter-Harris Type I physeal fracture of upper
              end of tibia

      ● S89.011   Salter-Harris Type I physeal fracture
                  of upper end of right tibia

      ● S89.012   Salter-Harris Type I physeal fracture
                  of upper end of left tibia

      ● S89.019   Salter-Harris Type I physeal fracture
                  of upper end of unspecified tibia

   ● S89.02   Salter-Harris Type II physeal fracture of upper
              end of tibia

      ● S89.021   Salter-Harris Type II physeal fracture
                  of upper end of right tibia

      ● S89.022   Salter-Harris Type II physeal fracture
                  of upper end of left tibia

      ● S89.029   Salter-Harris Type II physeal fracture
                  of upper end of unspecified tibia

   ● S89.03   Salter-Harris Type III physeal fracture of upper
              end of tibia

      ● S89.031   Salter-Harris Type III physeal fracture
                  of upper end of right tibia

      ● S89.032   Salter-Harris Type III physeal fracture
                  of upper end of left tibia

      ● S89.039   Salter-Harris Type III physeal fracture
                  of upper end of unspecified tibia

   ● S89.04   Salter-Harris Type IV physeal fracture of upper
              end of tibia

      ● S89.041   Salter-Harris Type IV physeal fracture
                  of upper end of right tibia

      ● S89.042   Salter-Harris Type IV physeal fracture
                  of upper end of left tibia

      ● S89.049   Salter-Harris Type IV physeal fracture
                  of upper end of unspecified tibia

   ● S89.09   Other physeal fracture of upper end of tibia

      ● S89.091   Other physeal fracture of upper
                  end of right tibia

      ● S89.092   Other physeal fracture of upper end
                  of left tibia

      ● S89.099   Other physeal fracture of upper
                  end of unspecified tibia

● S89.1   Physeal fracture of lower end of tibia

   ● S89.10   Unspecified physeal fracture of lower end of
              tibia

      ● S89.101   Unspecified physeal fracture of lower
                  end of right tibia

      ● S89.102   Unspecified physeal fracture of lower
                  end of left tibia

      ● S89.109   Unspecified physeal fracture of lower
                  end of unspecified tibia

   ● S89.11   Salter-Harris Type I physeal fracture of lower
              end of tibia

      ● S89.111   Salter-Harris Type I physeal fracture
                  of lower end of right tibia

      ● S89.112   Salter-Harris Type I physeal fracture
                  of lower end of left tibia

      ● S89.119   Salter-Harris Type I physeal fracture
                  of lower end of unspecified tibia

   ● S89.12   Salter-Harris Type II physeal fracture of lower
              end of tibia

      ● S89.121   Salter-Harris Type II physeal fracture
                  of lower end of right tibia

      ● S89.122   Salter-Harris Type II physeal fracture
                  of lower end of left tibia

      ● S89.129   Salter-Harris Type II physeal fracture
                  of lower end of unspecified tibia

   ● S89.13   Salter-Harris Type III physeal fracture of lower
              end of tibia

         Excludes1   fracture of medial malleolus
                         (adult) (S82.5-)

▶ New   ⇒ Revised   d̶e̶l̶e̶t̶e̶d̶ Deleted   Excludes 1   Excludes 2   Includes   Use additional   Code first   Code also   Key words

OGCR Official Guidelines   X Assign placeholder X   ● Use Additional Character(s)   ▶ Manifestation Code   🐾 Hierarchical Condition Category   Coding Clinic

● S89.131 Salter-Harris Type III physeal fracture of lower end of **right** tibia

● S89.132 Salter-Harris Type III physeal fracture of lower end of **left** tibia

● S89.139 Salter-Harris Type III physeal fracture of lower end of **unspecified** tibia

● S89.14 Salter-Harris Type IV physeal fracture of lower end of tibia

Excludes1 fracture of medial malleolus (adult) (S82.5-)

● S89.141 Salter-Harris Type IV physeal fracture of lower end of **right** tibia

● S89.142 Salter-Harris Type IV physeal fracture of lower end of **left** tibia

● S89.149 Salter-Harris Type IV physeal fracture of lower end of **unspecified** tibia

● S89.19 Other physeal fracture of lower end of tibia

● S89.191 Other physeal fracture of lower end of **right** tibia

● S89.192 Other physeal fracture of lower end of **left** tibia

● S89.199 Other physeal fracture of lower end of **unspecified** tibia

● S89.2 Physeal fracture of **upper** end of fibula

● S89.20 **Unspecified** physeal fracture of upper end of fibula

● S89.201 Unspecified physeal fracture of upper end of **right** fibula

● S89.202 Unspecified physeal fracture of upper end of **left** fibula

● S89.209 Unspecified physeal fracture of upper end of **unspecified** fibula

● S89.21 Salter-Harris Type I physeal fracture of upper end of fibula

● S89.211 Salter-Harris Type I physeal fracture of upper end of **right** fibula

● S89.212 Salter-Harris Type I physeal fracture of upper end of **left** fibula

● S89.219 Salter-Harris Type I physeal fracture of upper end of **unspecified** fibula

● S89.22 Salter-Harris Type II physeal fracture of upper end of fibula

● S89.221 Salter-Harris Type II physeal fracture of upper end of **right** fibula

● S89.222 Salter-Harris Type II physeal fracture of upper end of **left** fibula

● S89.229 Salter-Harris Type II physeal fracture of upper end of **unspecified** fibula

● S89.29 Other physeal fracture of upper end of fibula

● S89.291 Other physeal fracture of upper end of **right** fibula

● S89.292 Other physeal fracture of upper end of **left** fibula

● S89.299 Other physeal fracture of upper end of **unspecified** fibula

● S89.3 Physeal fracture of **lower** end of fibula

● S89.30 **Unspecified** physeal fracture of lower end of fibula

● S89.301 Unspecified physeal fracture of lower end of **right** fibula

● S89.302 Unspecified physeal fracture of lower end of **left** fibula

● S89.309 Unspecified physeal fracture of lower end of **unspecified** fibula

● S89.31 Salter-Harris Type I physeal fracture of lower end of fibula

● S89.311 Salter-Harris Type I physeal fracture of lower end of **right** fibula

● S89.312 Salter-Harris Type I physeal fracture of lower end of **left** fibula

● S89.319 Salter-Harris Type I physeal fracture of lower end of **unspecified** fibula

● S89.32 Salter-Harris Type II physeal fracture of lower end of fibula

● S89.321 Salter-Harris Type II physeal fracture of lower end of **right** fibula

● S89.322 Salter-Harris Type II physeal fracture of lower end of **left** fibula

● S89.329 Salter-Harris Type II physeal fracture of lower end of **unspecified** fibula

● S89.39 Other physeal fracture of lower end of fibula

● S89.391 Other physeal fracture of lower end of **right** fibula

● S89.392 Other physeal fracture of lower end of **left** fibula

● S89.399 Other physeal fracture of lower end of **unspecified** fibula

● S89.8 Other specified injuries of lower leg

The appropriate 7th character is to be added to each code in subcategory S89.8

A	initial encounter
D	subsequent encounter
S	sequela

X ● S89.80 Other specified injuries of **unspecified** lower leg

X ● S89.81 Other specified injuries of **right** lower leg

X ● S89.82 Other specified injuries of **left** lower leg

● S89.9 Unspecified injury of lower leg

The appropriate 7th character is to be added to each code in subcategory S89.9

A	initial encounter
D	subsequent encounter
S	sequela

X ● S89.90 Unspecified injury of **unspecified** lower leg

X ● S89.91 Unspecified injury of **right** lower leg

X ● S89.92 Unspecified injury of **left** lower leg

INJURIES TO THE ANKLE AND FOOT (S90-S99)

Excludes2 burns and corrosions (T20-T32)
fracture of ankle and malleolus (S82.-)
frostbite (T33-T34)
insect bite or sting, venomous (T63.4)

● S90 Superficial injury of ankle, foot and toes

The appropriate 7th character is to be added to each code from category S90

A	initial encounter
D	subsequent encounter
S	sequela

● S90.0 Contusion of ankle

X ● S90.00 Contusion of **unspecified** ankle

X ● S90.01 Contusion of **right** ankle

X ● S90.02 Contusion of **left** ankle

● S90.1 Contusion of **toe** without damage to nail

● S90.11 Contusion of **great** toe without damage to nail

● S90.111 Contusion of **right** great toe without damage to nail

● S90.112 Contusion of **left** great toe without damage to nail

● S90.119 Contusion of **unspecified** great toe without damage to nail

● S90.12 Contusion of **lesser** toe without damage to nail

● S90.121 Contusion of **right** lesser toe(s) without damage to nail

● S90.122 Contusion of **left** lesser toe(s) without damage to nail

● S90.129   Contusion of unspecified lesser toe(s) without damage to nail
     Contusion of toe NOS

● S90.2   Contusion of toe with damage to nail

   ● S90.21   Contusion of great toe with damage to nail

     ● S90.211   Contusion of right great toe with damage to nail

     ● S90.212   Contusion of left great toe with damage to nail

     ● S90.219   Contusion of unspecified great toe with damage to nail

   ● S90.22   Contusion of lesser toe with damage to nail

     ● S90.221   Contusion of right lesser toe(s) with damage to nail

     ● S90.222   Contusion of left lesser toe(s) with damage to nail

     ● S90.229   Contusion of unspecified lesser toe(s) with damage to nail

● S90.3   Contusion of foot

     Excludes2   contusion of toes (S90.1-, S90.2-)

X ● S90.30   Contusion of unspecified foot
     Contusion of foot NOS

X ● S90.31   Contusion of right foot

X ● S90.32   Contusion of left foot

● S90.4   Other superficial injuries of toe

   ● S90.41   Abrasion of toe

     ● S90.411   Abrasion, right great toe

     ● S90.412   Abrasion, left great toe

     ● S90.413   Abrasion, unspecified great toe

     ● S90.414   Abrasion, right lesser toe(s)

     ● S90.415   Abrasion, left lesser toe(s)

     ● S90.416   Abrasion, unspecified lesser toe(s)

   ● S90.42   Blister (nonthermal) of toe

     ● S90.421   Blister (nonthermal), right great toe

     ● S90.422   Blister (nonthermal), left great toe

     ● S90.423   Blister (nonthermal), unspecified great toe

     ● S90.424   Blister (nonthermal), right lesser toe(s)

     ● S90.425   Blister (nonthermal), left lesser toe(s)

     ● S90.426   Blister (nonthermal), unspecified lesser toe(s)

   ● S90.44   External constriction of toe
     Hair tourniquet syndrome of toe

     ● S90.441   External constriction, right great toe

     ● S90.442   External constriction, left great toe

     ● S90.443   External constriction, unspecified great toe

     ● S90.444   External constriction, right lesser toe(s)

     ● S90.445   External constriction, left lesser toe(s)

     ● S90.446   External constriction, unspecified lesser toe(s)

   ● S90.45   Superficial foreign body of toe
     Splinter in the toe

     ● S90.451   Superficial foreign body, right great toe

     ● S90.452   Superficial foreign body, left great toe

     ● S90.453   Superficial foreign body, unspecified great toe

     ● S90.454   Superficial foreign body, right lesser toe(s)

     ● S90.455   Superficial foreign body, left lesser toe(s)

     ● S90.456   Superficial foreign body, unspecified lesser toe(s)

   ● S90.46   Insect bite (nonvenomous) of toe

     ● S90.461   Insect bite (nonvenomous), right great toe

● S90.462   Insect bite (nonvenomous), left great toe

● S90.463   Insect bite (nonvenomous), unspecified great toe

● S90.464   Insect bite (nonvenomous), right lesser toe(s)

● S90.465   Insect bite (nonvenomous), left lesser toe(s)

● S90.466   Insect bite (nonvenomous), unspecified lesser toe(s)

● S90.47   Other superficial bite of toe

     Excludes1   open bite of toe (S91.15-, S91.25-)

● S90.471   Other superficial bite of right great toe

● S90.472   Other superficial bite of left great toe

● S90.473   Other superficial bite of unspecified great toe

● S90.474   Other superficial bite of right lesser toe(s)

● S90.475   Other superficial bite of left lesser toe(s)

● S90.476   Other superficial bite of unspecified lesser toe(s)

● S90.5   Other superficial injuries of ankle

   ● S90.51   Abrasion of ankle

     ● S90.511   Abrasion, right ankle

     ● S90.512   Abrasion, left ankle

     ● S90.519   Abrasion, unspecified ankle

   ● S90.52   Blister (nonthermal) of ankle

     ● S90.521   Blister (nonthermal), right ankle

     ● S90.522   Blister (nonthermal), left ankle

     ● S90.529   Blister (nonthermal), unspecified ankle

   ● S90.54   External constriction of ankle

     ● S90.541   External constriction, right ankle

     ● S90.542   External constriction, left ankle

     ● S90.549   External constriction, unspecified ankle

   ● S90.55   Superficial foreign body of ankle
     Splinter in the ankle

     ● S90.551   Superficial foreign body, right ankle

     ● S90.552   Superficial foreign body, left ankle

     ● S90.559   Superficial foreign body, unspecified ankle

   ● S90.56   Insect bite (nonvenomous) of ankle

     ● S90.561   Insect bite (nonvenomous), right ankle

     ● S90.562   Insect bite (nonvenomous), left ankle

     ● S90.569   Insect bite (nonvenomous), unspecified ankle

   ● S90.57   Other superficial bite of ankle

     Excludes1   open bite of ankle (S91.05-)

     ● S90.571   Other superficial bite of ankle, right ankle

     ● S90.572   Other superficial bite of ankle, left ankle

     ● S90.579   Other superficial bite of ankle, unspecified ankle

● S90.8   Other superficial injuries of foot

   ● S90.81   Abrasion of foot

     ● S90.811   Abrasion, right foot

     ● S90.812   Abrasion, left foot

     ● S90.819   Abrasion, unspecified foot

   ● S90.82   Blister (nonthermal) of foot

     ● S90.821   Blister (nonthermal), right foot

     ● S90.822   Blister (nonthermal), left foot

     ● S90.829   Blister (nonthermal), unspecified foot

▶ New   ⇛ Revised   ~~deleted~~ Deleted   Excludes 1   Excludes 2   Includes   Use additional   Code first   Code also   Key words

OGCR Official Guidelines   X Assign placeholder X   ● Use Additional Character(s)   ▶ Manifestation Code   🔁 Hierarchical Condition Category   **Coding Clinic**

- S90.84   **External constriction** of foot
  - S90.841   External constriction, right foot
  - S90.842   External constriction, left foot
  - S90.849   External constriction, unspecified foot
- S90.85   **Superficial foreign body** of foot
  - Splinter in the foot
  - S90.851   Superficial foreign body, right foot
  - S90.852   Superficial foreign body, left foot
  - S90.859   Superficial foreign body, unspecified foot
- S90.86   **Insect bite (nonvenomous)** of foot
  - S90.861   Insect bite (nonvenomous), right foot
  - S90.862   Insect bite (nonvenomous), left foot
  - S90.869   Insect bite (nonvenomous), unspecified foot
- S90.87   **Other superficial bite** of foot
  - **Excludes1**   open bite of foot (S91.35-)
  - S90.871   Other superficial bite of right foot
  - S90.872   Other superficial bite of left foot
  - S90.879   Other superficial bite of unspecified foot
- S90.9   **Unspecified superficial injury of ankle, foot and toe**
  - S90.91   Unspecified superficial injury of ankle
    - S90.911   Unspecified superficial injury of right ankle
    - S90.912   Unspecified superficial injury of left ankle
    - S90.919   Unspecified superficial injury of unspecified ankle
  - S90.92   Unspecified superficial injury of foot
    - S90.921   Unspecified superficial injury of right foot
    - S90.922   Unspecified superficial injury of left foot
    - S90.929   Unspecified superficial injury of unspecified foot
  - S90.93   Unspecified superficial injury of toes
    - S90.931   Unspecified superficial injury of right great toe
    - S90.932   Unspecified superficial injury of left great toe
    - S90.933   Unspecified superficial injury of unspecified great toe
    - S90.934   Unspecified superficial injury of right lesser toe(s)
    - S90.935   Unspecified superficial injury of left lesser toe(s)
    - S90.936   Unspecified superficial injury of unspecified lesser toe(s)

- S91   **Open wound of ankle, foot and toes**
  - Code also any associated wound infection
  - **Excludes1**   open fracture of ankle, foot and toes (S92.-with 7th character B)
    - traumatic amputation of ankle and foot (S98.-)
  - The appropriate 7th character is to be added to each code from category S91

A	initial encounter
D	subsequent encounter
S	sequela

  - S91.0   **Open wound of ankle**
    - S91.00   **Unspecified open wound** of ankle
      - S91.001   Unspecified open wound, right ankle
      - S91.002   Unspecified open wound, left ankle
      - S91.009   Unspecified open wound, unspecified ankle

- S91.01   **Laceration without foreign body** of ankle
  - S91.011   Laceration without foreign body, right ankle
  - S91.012   Laceration without foreign body, left ankle
    - **Coding Clinic: 2021, Q1, P8**
  - S91.019   Laceration without foreign body, unspecified ankle
- S91.02   **Laceration with foreign body** of ankle
  - S91.021   Laceration with foreign body, right ankle
  - S91.022   Laceration with foreign body, left ankle
  - S91.029   Laceration with foreign body, unspecified ankle
- S91.03   **Puncture wound without foreign body** of ankle
  - S91.031   Puncture wound without foreign body, right ankle
  - S91.032   Puncture wound without foreign body, left ankle
  - S91.039   Puncture wound without foreign body, unspecified ankle
- S91.04   **Puncture wound with foreign body** of ankle
  - S91.041   Puncture wound with foreign body, right ankle
  - S91.042   Puncture wound with foreign body, left ankle
  - S91.049   Puncture wound with foreign body, unspecified ankle
- S91.05   **Open bite** of ankle
  - **Excludes1**   superficial bite of ankle (S90.56-, S90.57-)
  - S91.051   Open bite, right ankle
  - S91.052   Open bite, left ankle
  - S91.059   Open bite, unspecified ankle
- S91.1   **Open wound of toe without damage to nail**
  - S91.10   **Unspecified open wound** of toe without damage to nail
    - S91.101   Unspecified open wound of right great toe without damage to nail
    - S91.102   Unspecified open wound of left great toe without damage to nail
    - S91.103   Unspecified open wound of unspecified great toe without damage to nail
    - S91.104   Unspecified open wound of right lesser toe(s) without damage to nail
    - S91.105   Unspecified open wound of left lesser toe(s) without damage to nail
    - S91.106   Unspecified open wound of unspecified lesser toe(s) without damage to nail
    - S91.109   Unspecified open wound of unspecified toe(s) without damage to nail
  - S91.11   **Laceration without foreign body** of toe without damage to nail
    - S91.111   Laceration without foreign body of right great toe without damage to nail
    - S91.112   Laceration without foreign body of left great toe without damage to nail
    - S91.113   Laceration without foreign body of unspecified great toe without damage to nail
    - S91.114   Laceration without foreign body of right lesser toe(s) without damage to nail
    - S91.115   Laceration without foreign body of left lesser toe(s) without damage to nail

CHAPTER 19 (S00-T88)

● S91.116   Laceration without foreign body of unspecified lesser toe(s) without damage to nail

● S91.119   Laceration without foreign body of unspecified toe without damage to nail

● S91.12   Laceration with foreign body of toe without damage to nail

● S91.121   Laceration with foreign body of right great toe without damage to nail

● S91.122   Laceration with foreign body of left great toe without damage to nail

● S91.123   Laceration with foreign body of unspecified great toe without damage to nail

● S91.124   Laceration with foreign body of right lesser toe(s) without damage to nail

● S91.125   Laceration with foreign body of left lesser toe(s) without damage to nail

● S91.126   Laceration with foreign body of unspecified lesser toe(s) without damage to nail

● S91.129   Laceration with foreign body of unspecified toe(s) without damage to nail

● S91.13   Puncture wound without foreign body of toe without damage to nail

● S91.131   Puncture wound without foreign body of right great toe without damage to nail

● S91.132   Puncture wound without foreign body of left great toe without damage to nail

● S91.133   Puncture wound without foreign body of unspecified great toe without damage to nail

● S91.134   Puncture wound without foreign body of right lesser toe(s) without damage to nail

● S91.135   Puncture wound without foreign body of left lesser toe(s) without damage to nail

● S91.136   Puncture wound without foreign body of unspecified lesser toe(s) without damage to nail

● S91.139   Puncture wound without foreign body of unspecified toe(s) without damage to nail

● S91.14   Puncture wound with foreign body of toe without damage to nail

● S91.141   Puncture wound with foreign body of right great toe without damage to nail

● S91.142   Puncture wound with foreign body of left great toe without damage to nail

● S91.143   Puncture wound with foreign body of unspecified great toe without damage to nail

● S91.144   Puncture wound with foreign body of right lesser toe(s) without damage to nail

● S91.145   Puncture wound with foreign body of left lesser toe(s) without damage to nail

● S91.146   Puncture wound with foreign body of unspecified lesser toe(s) without damage to nail

● S91.149   Puncture wound with foreign body of unspecified toe(s) without damage to nail

● S91.15   Open bite of toe without damage to nail
       Bite of toe NOS

     Excludes1   superficial bite of toe (S9Ø.46-, S9Ø.47-)

● S91.151   Open bite of right great toe without damage to nail

● S91.152   Open bite of left great toe without damage to nail

● S91.153   Open bite of unspecified great toe without damage to nail

● S91.154   Open bite of right lesser toe(s) without damage to nail

● S91.155   Open bite of left lesser toe(s) without damage to nail

● S91.156   Open bite of unspecified lesser toe(s) without damage to nail

● S91.159   Open bite of unspecified toe(s) without damage to nail

● S91.2   Open wound of toe with damage to nail

● S91.2Ø   Unspecified open wound of toe with damage to nail

● S91.2Ø1   Unspecified open wound of right great toe with damage to nail

● S91.2Ø2   Unspecified open wound of left great toe with damage to nail

● S91.2Ø3   Unspecified open wound of unspecified great toe with damage to nail

● S91.2Ø4   Unspecified open wound of right lesser toe(s) with damage to nail

● S91.2Ø5   Unspecified open wound of left lesser toe(s) with damage to nail

● S91.2Ø6   Unspecified open wound of unspecified lesser toe(s) with damage to nail

● S91.2Ø9   Unspecified open wound of unspecified toe(s) with damage to nail

● S91.21   Laceration without foreign body of toe with damage to nail

● S91.211   Laceration without foreign body of right great toe with damage to nail

● S91.212   Laceration without foreign body of left great toe with damage to nail

● S91.213   Laceration without foreign body of unspecified great toe with damage to nail

● S91.214   Laceration without foreign body of right lesser toe(s) with damage to nail

● S91.215   Laceration without foreign body of left lesser toe(s) with damage to nail

● S91.216   Laceration without foreign body of unspecified lesser toe(s) with damage to nail

● S91.219   Laceration without foreign body of unspecified toe(s) with damage to nail

● S91.22   Laceration with foreign body of toe with damage to nail

● S91.221   Laceration with foreign body of right great toe with damage to nail

● S91.222   Laceration with foreign body of left great toe with damage to nail

● S91.223   Laceration with foreign body of unspecified great toe with damage to nail

● S91.224   Laceration with foreign body of right lesser toe(s) with damage to nail

● S91.225   Laceration with foreign body of left lesser toe(s) with damage to nail

● S91.226   Laceration with foreign body of unspecified lesser toe(s) with damage to nail

● S91.229   Laceration with foreign body of unspecified toe(s) with damage to nail

▶ New   ⇒ Revised   ~~deleted~~ Deleted   Excludes 1   Excludes 2   Includes   Use additional   Code first   Code also   Key words

OGCR Official Guidelines   X Assign placeholder X   ● Use Additional Character(s)   ▶ Manifestation Code   ⬛ Hierarchical Condition Category   **Coding Clinic**

● S91.23   Puncture wound without foreign body of toe with damage to nail

    ● S91.231   Puncture wound without foreign body of right great toe with damage to nail

    ● S91.232   Puncture wound without foreign body of left great toe with damage to nail

    ● S91.233   Puncture wound without foreign body of unspecified great toe with damage to nail

    ● S91.234   Puncture wound without foreign body of right lesser toe(s) with damage to nail

    ● S91.235   Puncture wound without foreign body of left lesser toe(s) with damage to nail

    ● S91.236   Puncture wound without foreign body of unspecified lesser toe(s) with damage to nail

    ● S91.239   Puncture wound without foreign body of unspecified toe(s) with damage to nail

● S91.24   Puncture wound with foreign body of toe with damage to nail

    ● S91.241   Puncture wound with foreign body of right great toe with damage to nail

    ● S91.242   Puncture wound with foreign body of left great toe with damage to nail

    ● S91.243   Puncture wound with foreign body of unspecified great toe with damage to nail

    ● S91.244   Puncture wound with foreign body of right lesser toe(s) with damage to nail

    ● S91.245   Puncture wound with foreign body of left lesser toe(s) with damage to nail

    ● S91.246   Puncture wound with foreign body of unspecified lesser toe(s) with damage to nail

    ● S91.249   Puncture wound with foreign body of unspecified toe(s) with damage to nail

● S91.25   Open bite of toe with damage to nail

    Bite of toe with damage to nail NOS

    Excludes1   superficial bite of toe (S90.46-, S90.47-)

    ● S91.251   Open bite of right great toe with damage to nail

    ● S91.252   Open bite of left great toe with damage to nail

    ● S91.253   Open bite of unspecified great toe with damage to nail

    ● S91.254   Open bite of right lesser toe(s) with damage to nail

    ● S91.255   Open bite of left lesser toe(s) with damage to nail

    ● S91.256   Open bite of unspecified lesser toe(s) with damage to nail

    ● S91.259   Open bite of unspecified toe(s) with damage to nail

● S91.3   Open wound of foot

    ● S91.30   Unspecified open wound of foot

      ● S91.301   Unspecified open wound, right foot

      ● S91.302   Unspecified open wound, left foot

      ● S91.309   Unspecified open wound, unspecified foot

    ● S91.31   Laceration without foreign body of foot

      ● S91.311   Laceration without foreign body, right foot

      ● S91.312   Laceration without foreign body, left foot

      ● S91.319   Laceration without foreign body, unspecified foot

    ● S91.32   Laceration with foreign body of foot

      ● S91.321   Laceration with foreign body, right foot

      ● S91.322   Laceration with foreign body, left foot

      ● S91.329   Laceration with foreign body, unspecified foot

    ● S91.33   Puncture wound without foreign body of foot

      ● S91.331   Puncture wound without foreign body, right foot

      ● S91.332   Puncture wound without foreign body, left foot

      ● S91.339   Puncture wound without foreign body, unspecified foot

    ● S91.34   Puncture wound with foreign body of foot

      ● S91.341   Puncture wound with foreign body, right foot

      ● S91.342   Puncture wound with foreign body, left foot

      ● S91.349   Puncture wound with foreign body, unspecified foot

    ● S91.35   Open bite of foot

      Excludes1   superficial bite of foot (S90.86-, S90.87-)

      ● S91.351   Open bite, right foot

      ● S91.352   Open bite, left foot

      ● S91.359   Open bite, unspecified foot

● S92   Fracture of foot and toe, except ankle

    Note: A fracture not indicated as displaced or nondisplaced should be coded to displaced

    A fracture not indicated as open or closed should be coded to closed

    Excludes2   fracture of ankle (S82.-)

        fracture of malleolus (S82.-)

        traumatic amputation of ankle and foot (S98.-)

    The appropriate 7th character is to be added to each code from category S92

A	initial encounter for closed fracture
B	initial encounter for open fracture
D	subsequent encounter for fracture with routine healing
G	subsequent encounter for fracture with delayed healing
K	subsequent encounter for fracture with nonunion
P	subsequent encounter for fracture with malunion
S	sequela

● S92.0   Fracture of calcaneus

    Heel bone   Os calcis

    Excludes2   Physeal fracture of calcaneus (S99.0-)

    ● S92.00   Unspecified fracture of calcaneus

      ● S92.001   Unspecified fracture of right calcaneus

      ● S92.002   Unspecified fracture of left calcaneus

      ● S92.009   Unspecified fracture of unspecified calcaneus

    ● S92.01   Fracture of body of calcaneus

      ● S92.011   Displaced fracture of body of right calcaneus

      ● S92.012   Displaced fracture of body of left calcaneus

      ● S92.013   Displaced fracture of body of unspecified calcaneus

      ● S92.014   Nondisplaced fracture of body of right calcaneus

      ● S92.015   Nondisplaced fracture of body of left calcaneus

      ● S92.016   Nondisplaced fracture of body of unspecified calcaneus

● S92.02   Fracture of anterior process of calcaneus
   ● S92.021   Displaced fracture of anterior process of right calcaneus
   ● S92.022   Displaced fracture of anterior process of left calcaneus
   ● S92.023   Displaced fracture of anterior process of unspecified calcaneus
   ● S92.024   Nondisplaced fracture of anterior process of right calcaneus
   ● S92.025   Nondisplaced fracture of anterior process of left calcaneus
   ● S92.026   Nondisplaced fracture of anterior process of unspecified calcaneus

● S92.03   Avulsion fracture of tuberosity of calcaneus
   ● S92.031   Displaced avulsion fracture of tuberosity of right calcaneus
   ● S92.032   Displaced avulsion fracture of tuberosity of left calcaneus
   ● S92.033   Displaced avulsion fracture of tuberosity of unspecified calcaneus
   ● S92.034   Nondisplaced avulsion fracture of tuberosity of right calcaneus
   ● S92.035   Nondisplaced avulsion fracture of tuberosity of left calcaneus
   ● S92.036   Nondisplaced avulsion fracture of tuberosity of unspecified calcaneus

● S92.04   Other fracture of tuberosity of calcaneus
   ● S92.041   Displaced other fracture of tuberosity of right calcaneus
   ● S92.042   Displaced other fracture of tuberosity of left calcaneus
   ● S92.043   Displaced other fracture of tuberosity of unspecified calcaneus
   ● S92.044   Nondisplaced other fracture of tuberosity of right calcaneus
   ● S92.045   Nondisplaced other fracture of tuberosity of left calcaneus
   ● S92.046   Nondisplaced other fracture of tuberosity of unspecified calcaneus

● S92.05   Other extraarticular fracture of calcaneus
   ● S92.051   Displaced other extraarticular fracture of right calcaneus
   ● S92.052   Displaced other extraarticular fracture of left calcaneus
   ● S92.053   Displaced other extraarticular fracture of unspecified calcaneus
   ● S92.054   Nondisplaced other extraarticular fracture of right calcaneus
   ● S92.055   Nondisplaced other extraarticular fracture of left calcaneus
   ● S92.056   Nondisplaced other extraarticular fracture of unspecified calcaneus

● S92.06   Intraarticular fracture of calcaneus
   ● S92.061   Displaced intraarticular fracture of right calcaneus
   ● S92.062   Displaced intraarticular fracture of left calcaneus
   ● S92.063   Displaced intraarticular fracture of unspecified calcaneus
   ● S92.064   Nondisplaced intraarticular fracture of right calcaneus
   ● S92.065   Nondisplaced intraarticular fracture of left calcaneus
   ● S92.066   Nondisplaced intraarticular fracture of unspecified calcaneus

● S92.1   Fracture of talus
   Astragalus
  ● S92.10   Unspecified fracture of talus
   ● S92.101   Unspecified fracture of right talus

● S92.102   Unspecified fracture of left talus
● S92.109   Unspecified fracture of unspecified talus

● S92.11   Fracture of neck of talus
   ● S92.111   Displaced fracture of neck of right talus
   ● S92.112   Displaced fracture of neck of left talus
   ● S92.113   Displaced fracture of neck of unspecified talus
   ● S92.114   Nondisplaced fracture of neck of right talus
   ● S92.115   Nondisplaced fracture of neck of left talus
   ● S92.116   Nondisplaced fracture of neck of unspecified talus

● S92.12   Fracture of body of talus
   ● S92.121   Displaced fracture of body of right talus
   ● S92.122   Displaced fracture of body of left talus
   ● S92.123   Displaced fracture of body of unspecified talus
   ● S92.124   Nondisplaced fracture of body of right talus
   ● S92.125   Nondisplaced fracture of body of left talus
   ● S92.126   Nondisplaced fracture of body of unspecified talus

● S92.13   Fracture of posterior process of talus
   ● S92.131   Displaced fracture of posterior process of right talus
   ● S92.132   Displaced fracture of posterior process of left talus
   ● S92.133   Displaced fracture of posterior process of unspecified talus
   ● S92.134   Nondisplaced fracture of posterior process of right talus
   ● S92.135   Nondisplaced fracture of posterior process of left talus
   ● S92.136   Nondisplaced fracture of posterior process of unspecified talus

● S92.14   Dome fracture of talus
   Excludes1   osteochondritis dissecans (M93.2)
   ● S92.141   Displaced dome fracture of right talus
   ● S92.142   Displaced dome fracture of left talus
   ● S92.143   Displaced dome fracture of unspecified talus
   ● S92.144   Nondisplaced dome fracture of right talus
   ● S92.145   Nondisplaced dome fracture of left talus
   ● S92.146   Nondisplaced dome fracture of unspecified talus

● S92.15   Avulsion fracture (chip fracture) of talus
   ● S92.151   Displaced avulsion fracture (chip fracture) of right talus
   ● S92.152   Displaced avulsion fracture (chip fracture) of left talus
   ● S92.153   Displaced avulsion fracture (chip fracture) of unspecified talus
   ● S92.154   Nondisplaced avulsion fracture (chip fracture) of right talus
   ● S92.155   Nondisplaced avulsion fracture (chip fracture) of left talus
   ● S92.156   Nondisplaced avulsion fracture (chip fracture) of unspecified talus

▶ New   ⇒ Revised   ~~deleted~~ Deleted   Excludes 1   Excludes 2   Includes   Use additional   Code first   Code also   Key words
OGCR Official Guidelines   X Assign placeholder X   ● Use Additional Character(s)   ▷ Manifestation Code   Hierarchical Condition Category   Coding Clinic

- S92.19   Other fracture of talus
  - S92.191   Other fracture of right talus
  - S92.192   Other fracture of left talus
  - S92.199   Other fracture of unspecified talus
- S92.2   Fracture of other and unspecified tarsal bone(s)
  - S92.20   Fracture of unspecified tarsal bone(s)
    - S92.201   Fracture of unspecified tarsal bone(s) of right foot
    - S92.202   Fracture of unspecified tarsal bone(s) of left foot
    - S92.209   Fracture of unspecified tarsal bone(s) of unspecified foot
  - S92.21   Fracture of cuboid bone
    - S92.211   Displaced fracture of cuboid bone of right foot
    - S92.212   Displaced fracture of cuboid bone of left foot
    - S92.213   Displaced fracture of cuboid bone of unspecified foot
    - S92.214   Nondisplaced fracture of cuboid bone of right foot
    - S92.215   Nondisplaced fracture of cuboid bone of left foot
    - S92.216   Nondisplaced fracture of cuboid bone of unspecified foot
  - S92.22   Fracture of lateral cuneiform
    - S92.221   Displaced fracture of lateral cuneiform of right foot
    - S92.222   Displaced fracture of lateral cuneiform of left foot
    - S92.223   Displaced fracture of lateral cuneiform of unspecified foot
    - S92.224   Nondisplaced fracture of lateral cuneiform of right foot
    - S92.225   Nondisplaced fracture of lateral cuneiform of left foot
    - S92.226   Nondisplaced fracture of lateral cuneiform of unspecified foot
  - S92.23   Fracture of intermediate cuneiform
    - S92.231   Displaced fracture of intermediate cuneiform of right foot
    - S92.232   Displaced fracture of intermediate cuneiform of left foot
    - S92.233   Displaced fracture of intermediate cuneiform of unspecified foot
    - S92.234   Nondisplaced fracture of intermediate cuneiform of right foot
    - S92.235   Nondisplaced fracture of intermediate cuneiform of left foot
    - S92.236   Nondisplaced fracture of intermediate cuneiform of unspecified foot
  - S92.24   Fracture of medial cuneiform
    - S92.241   Displaced fracture of medial cuneiform of right foot
    - S92.242   Displaced fracture of medial cuneiform of left foot
    - S92.243   Displaced fracture of medial cuneiform of unspecified foot
    - S92.244   Nondisplaced fracture of medial cuneiform of right foot
    - S92.245   Nondisplaced fracture of medial cuneiform of left foot
    - S92.246   Nondisplaced fracture of medial cuneiform of unspecified foot
  - S92.25   Fracture of navicular [scaphoid] of foot
    - S92.251   Displaced fracture of navicular [scaphoid] of right foot
    - S92.252   Displaced fracture of navicular [scaphoid] of left foot
    - S92.253   Displaced fracture of navicular [scaphoid] of unspecified foot
    - S92.254   Nondisplaced fracture of navicular [scaphoid] of right foot
    - S92.255   Nondisplaced fracture of navicular [scaphoid] of left foot
    - S92.256   Nondisplaced fracture of navicular [scaphoid] of unspecified foot
- S92.3   Fracture of metatarsal bone(s)

  Excludes2   Physeal fracture of metatarsal (S99.1-)

  - S92.30   Fracture of unspecified metatarsal bone(s)
    - S92.301   Fracture of unspecified metatarsal bone(s), right foot
    - S92.302   Fracture of unspecified metatarsal bone(s), left foot
    - S92.309   Fracture of unspecified metatarsal bone(s), unspecified foot
  - S92.31   Fracture of first metatarsal bone
    - S92.311   Displaced fracture of first metatarsal bone, right foot
    - S92.312   Displaced fracture of first metatarsal bone, left foot
    - S92.313   Displaced fracture of first metatarsal bone, unspecified foot
    - S92.314   Nondisplaced fracture of first metatarsal bone, right foot
    - S92.315   Nondisplaced fracture of first metatarsal bone, left foot
    - S92.316   Nondisplaced fracture of first metatarsal bone, unspecified foot
  - S92.32   Fracture of second metatarsal bone
    - S92.321   Displaced fracture of second metatarsal bone, right foot
    - S92.322   Displaced fracture of second metatarsal bone, left foot
    - S92.323   Displaced fracture of second metatarsal bone, unspecified foot
    - S92.324   Nondisplaced fracture of second metatarsal bone, right foot
    - S92.325   Nondisplaced fracture of second metatarsal bone, left foot
    - S92.326   Nondisplaced fracture of second metatarsal bone, unspecified foot
  - S92.33   Fracture of third metatarsal bone
    Coding Clinic: 2018, Q1, P3
    - S92.331   Displaced fracture of third metatarsal bone, right foot
    - S92.332   Displaced fracture of third metatarsal bone, left foot
    - S92.333   Displaced fracture of third metatarsal bone, unspecified foot
    - S92.334   Nondisplaced fracture of third metatarsal bone, right foot
    - S92.335   Nondisplaced fracture of third metatarsal bone, left foot
    - S92.336   Nondisplaced fracture of third metatarsal bone, unspecified foot
  - S92.34   Fracture of fourth metatarsal bone
    - S92.341   Displaced fracture of fourth metatarsal bone, right foot
    - S92.342   Displaced fracture of fourth metatarsal bone, left foot
    - S92.343   Displaced fracture of fourth metatarsal bone, unspecified foot
    - S92.344   Nondisplaced fracture of fourth metatarsal bone, right foot
    - S92.345   Nondisplaced fracture of fourth metatarsal bone, left foot
    - S92.346   Nondisplaced fracture of fourth metatarsal bone, unspecified foot

CHAPTER 19 (S00-T88)

CHAPTER 19 (S00-T88)

- ● S92.35   Fracture of fifth metatarsal bone
  - ● S92.351   Displaced fracture of fifth metatarsal bone, right foot
  - ● S92.352   Displaced fracture of fifth metatarsal bone, left foot
  - ● S92.353   Displaced fracture of fifth metatarsal bone, unspecified foot
  - ● S92.354   Nondisplaced fracture of fifth metatarsal bone, right foot
  - ● S92.355   Nondisplaced fracture of fifth metatarsal bone, left foot
  - ● S92.356   Nondisplaced fracture of fifth metatarsal bone, unspecified foot
- ● S92.4   Fracture of great toe
  - **Excludes2**   Physeal fracture of phalanx of toe (S99.2-)
  - ● S92.40   Unspecified fracture of great toe
    - ● S92.401   Displaced unspecified fracture of right great toe
    - ● S92.402   Displaced unspecified fracture of left great toe
    - ● S92.403   Displaced unspecified fracture of unspecified great toe
    - ● S92.404   Nondisplaced unspecified fracture of right great toe
    - ● S92.405   Nondisplaced unspecified fracture of left great toe
    - ● S92.406   Nondisplaced unspecified fracture of unspecified great toe
  - ● S92.41   Fracture of proximal phalanx of great toe
    - ● S92.411   Displaced fracture of proximal phalanx of right great toe
    - ● S92.412   Displaced fracture of proximal phalanx of left great toe
    - ● S92.413   Displaced fracture of proximal phalanx of unspecified great toe
    - ● S92.414   Nondisplaced fracture of proximal phalanx of right great toe
    - ● S92.415   Nondisplaced fracture of proximal phalanx of left great toe
    - ● S92.416   Nondisplaced fracture of proximal phalanx of unspecified great toe
  - ● S92.42   Fracture of distal phalanx of great toe
    - ● S92.421   Displaced fracture of distal phalanx of right great toe
    - ● S92.422   Displaced fracture of distal phalanx of left great toe
    - ● S92.423   Displaced fracture of distal phalanx of unspecified great toe
    - ● S92.424   Nondisplaced fracture of distal phalanx of right great toe
    - ● S92.425   Nondisplaced fracture of distal phalanx of left great toe
    - ● S92.426   Nondisplaced fracture of distal phalanx of unspecified great toe
  - ● S92.49   Other fracture of great toe
    - ● S92.491   Other fracture of right great toe
    - ● S92.492   Other fracture of left great toe
    - ● S92.499   Other fracture of unspecified great toe
- ● S92.5   Fracture of lesser toe(s)
  - **Excludes2**   Physeal fracture of phalanx of toe (S99.2-)
  - ● S92.50   Unspecified fracture of lesser toe(s)
    - ● S92.501   Displaced unspecified fracture of right lesser toe(s)
    - ● S92.502   Displaced unspecified fracture of left lesser toe(s)
    - ● S92.503   Displaced unspecified fracture of unspecified lesser toe(s)

- ● S92.504   Nondisplaced unspecified fracture of right lesser toe(s)
- ● S92.505   Nondisplaced unspecified fracture of left lesser toe(s)
- ● S92.506   Nondisplaced unspecified fracture of unspecified lesser toe(s)
- ● S92.51   Fracture of proximal phalanx of lesser toe(s)
  - ● S92.511   Displaced fracture of proximal phalanx of right lesser toe(s)
  - ● S92.512   Displaced fracture of proximal phalanx of left lesser toe(s)
  - ● S92.513   Displaced fracture of proximal phalanx of unspecified lesser toe(s)
  - ● S92.514   Nondisplaced fracture of proximal phalanx of right lesser toe(s)
  - ● S92.515   Nondisplaced fracture of proximal phalanx of left lesser toe(s)
  - ● S92.516   Nondisplaced fracture of proximal phalanx of unspecified lesser toe(s)
- ● S92.52   Fracture of middle phalanx of lesser toe(s)
  - ● S92.521   Displaced fracture of middle phalanx of right lesser toe(s)
  - ● S92.522   Displaced fracture of middle phalanx of left lesser toe(s)
  - ● S92.523   Displaced fracture of middle phalanx of unspecified lesser toe(s)
  - ● S92.524   Nondisplaced fracture of middle phalanx of right lesser toe(s)
  - ● S92.525   Nondisplaced fracture of middle phalanx of left lesser toe(s)
  - ● S92.526   Nondisplaced fracture of middle phalanx of unspecified lesser toe(s)
- ● S92.53   Fracture of distal phalanx of lesser toe(s)
  - ● S92.531   Displaced fracture of distal phalanx of right lesser toe(s)
  - ● S92.532   Displaced fracture of distal phalanx of left lesser toe(s)
  - ● S92.533   Displaced fracture of distal phalanx of unspecified lesser toe(s)
  - ● S92.534   Nondisplaced fracture of distal phalanx of right lesser toe(s)
  - ● S92.535   Nondisplaced fracture of distal phalanx of left lesser toe(s)
  - ● S92.536   Nondisplaced fracture of distal phalanx of unspecified lesser toe(s)
- ● S92.59   Other fracture of lesser toe(s)
  - ● S92.591   Other fracture of right lesser toe(s)
  - ● S92.592   Other fracture of left lesser toe(s)
  - ● S92.599   Other fracture of unspecified lesser toe(s)
- ● S92.8   Other fracture of foot, except ankle
  - ● S92.81   Other fracture of foot
    - Sesamoid fracture of foot
    - **Coding Clinic: 2016, Q4, P68**
    - ● S92.811   Other fracture of right foot
    - ● S92.812   Other fracture of left foot
    - ● S92.819   Other fracture of unspecified foot
- ● S92.9   Unspecified fracture of foot and toe
  - ● S92.90   Unspecified fracture of foot
    - ● S92.901   Unspecified fracture of right foot
    - ● S92.902   Unspecified fracture of left foot
    - ● S92.909   Unspecified fracture of unspecified foot
  - ● S92.91   Unspecified fracture of toe
    - ● S92.911   Unspecified fracture of right toe(s)
    - ● S92.912   Unspecified fracture of left toe(s)
    - ● S92.919   Unspecified fracture of unspecified toe(s)

▶ New   ⇒ Revised   ~~deleted~~ Deleted | Excludes 1 | | Excludes 2 | | Includes | | Use additional | | Code first | | Code also | | Key words |

1324   **OGCR** Official Guidelines   **X** Assign placeholder X   ● Use Additional Character(s)   ▌ Manifestation Code   🔖 Hierarchical Condition Category   **Coding Clinic**

● S93   **Dislocation and sprain of joints and ligaments at ankle, foot and toe level**

     Includes   avulsion of joint or ligament of ankle, foot and toe
                 laceration of cartilage, joint or ligament of ankle, foot and toe
                 sprain of cartilage, joint or ligament of ankle, foot and toe
                 traumatic hemarthrosis of joint or ligament of ankle, foot and toe
                 traumatic rupture of joint or ligament of ankle, foot and toe
                 traumatic subluxation of joint or ligament of ankle, foot and toe
                 traumatic tear of joint or ligament of ankle, foot and toe

     Code also any associated open wound

     Excludes2   strain of muscle and tendon of ankle and foot (S96.-)

     The appropriate 7th character is to be added to each code from category S93

A	initial encounter
D	subsequent encounter
S	sequela

● S93.0   **Subluxation and dislocation of ankle joint**
     Subluxation and dislocation of astragalus
     Subluxation and dislocation of fibula, lower end
     Subluxation and dislocation of talus
     Subluxation and dislocation of tibia, lower end

   X ● S93.01   **Subluxation of right ankle joint**
   X ● S93.02   **Subluxation of left ankle joint**
   X ● S93.03   **Subluxation of unspecified ankle joint**
   X ● S93.04   **Dislocation of right ankle joint**
   X ● S93.05   **Dislocation of left ankle joint**
   X ● S93.06   **Dislocation of unspecified ankle joint**

● S93.1   **Subluxation and dislocation of toe**

   ● S93.10   **Unspecified subluxation and dislocation of toe**
       Dislocation of toe NOS
       Subluxation of toe NOS

     ● S93.101   Unspecified subluxation of right toe(s)
     ● S93.102   Unspecified subluxation of left toe(s)
     ● S93.103   Unspecified subluxation of unspecified toe(s)
     ● S93.104   Unspecified dislocation of right toe(s)
     ● S93.105   Unspecified dislocation of left toe(s)
     ● S93.106   Unspecified dislocation of unspecified toe(s)

   ● S93.11   **Dislocation of interphalangeal joint**
     ● S93.111   Dislocation of interphalangeal joint of right great toe
     ● S93.112   Dislocation of interphalangeal joint of left great toe
     ● S93.113   Dislocation of interphalangeal joint of unspecified great toe
     ● S93.114   Dislocation of interphalangeal joint of right lesser toe(s)
     ● S93.115   Dislocation of interphalangeal joint of left lesser toe(s)
     ● S93.116   Dislocation of interphalangeal joint of unspecified lesser toe(s)
     ● S93.119   Dislocation of interphalangeal joint of unspecified toe(s)

   ● S93.12   **Dislocation of metatarsophalangeal joint**
     ● S93.121   Dislocation of metatarsophalangeal joint of right great toe
     ● S93.122   Dislocation of metatarsophalangeal joint of left great toe
     ● S93.123   Dislocation of metatarsophalangeal joint of unspecified great toe

     ● S93.124   Dislocation of metatarsophalangeal joint of right lesser toe(s)
     ● S93.125   Dislocation of metatarsophalangeal joint of left lesser toe(s)
     ● S93.126   Dislocation of metatarsophalangeal joint of unspecified lesser toe(s)
     ● S93.129   Dislocation of metatarsophalangeal joint of unspecified toe(s)

   ● S93.13   **Subluxation of interphalangeal joint**
     ● S93.131   Subluxation of interphalangeal joint of right great toe
     ● S93.132   Subluxation of interphalangeal joint of left great toe
     ● S93.133   Subluxation of interphalangeal joint of unspecified great toe
     ● S93.134   Subluxation of interphalangeal joint of right lesser toe(s)
     ● S93.135   Subluxation of interphalangeal joint of left lesser toe(s)
     ● S93.136   Subluxation of interphalangeal joint of unspecified lesser toe(s)
     ● S93.139   Subluxation of interphalangeal joint of unspecified toe(s)

   ● S93.14   **Subluxation of metatarsophalangeal joint**
     ● S93.141   Subluxation of metatarsophalangeal joint of right great toe
     ● S93.142   Subluxation of metatarsophalangeal joint of left great toe
     ● S93.143   Subluxation of metatarsophalangeal joint of unspecified great toe
     ● S93.144   Subluxation of metatarsophalangeal joint of right lesser toe(s)
     ● S93.145   Subluxation of metatarsophalangeal joint of left lesser toe(s)
     ● S93.146   Subluxation of metatarsophalangeal joint of unspecified lesser toe(s)
     ● S93.149   Subluxation of metatarsophalangeal joint of unspecified toe(s)

● S93.3   **Subluxation and dislocation of foot**
     Excludes2   dislocation of toe (S93.1-)

   ● S93.30   **Unspecified subluxation and dislocation of foot**
       Dislocation of foot NOS
       Subluxation of foot NOS

     ● S93.301   Unspecified subluxation of right foot
     ● S93.302   Unspecified subluxation of left foot
     ● S93.303   Unspecified subluxation of unspecified foot
     ● S93.304   Unspecified dislocation of right foot
     ● S93.305   Unspecified dislocation of left foot
     ● S93.306   Unspecified dislocation of unspecified foot

   ● S93.31   **Subluxation and dislocation of tarsal joint**
     ● S93.311   Subluxation of tarsal joint of right foot
     ● S93.312   Subluxation of tarsal joint of left foot
     ● S93.313   Subluxation of tarsal joint of unspecified foot
     ● S93.314   Dislocation of tarsal joint of right foot
     ● S93.315   Dislocation of tarsal joint of left foot
     ● S93.316   Dislocation of tarsal joint of unspecified foot

   ● S93.32   **Subluxation and dislocation of tarsometatarsal joint**
     ● S93.321   Subluxation of tarsometatarsal joint of right foot
     ● S93.322   Subluxation of tarsometatarsal joint of left foot
     ● S93.323   Subluxation of tarsometatarsal joint of unspecified foot

CHAPTER 19 (S00-T88)

● S93.324   Dislocation of tarsometatarsal joint of right foot

● S93.325   Dislocation of tarsometatarsal joint of left foot

● S93.326   Dislocation of tarsometatarsal joint of unspecified foot

● S93.33   Other subluxation and dislocation of foot

  ● S93.331   Other subluxation of right foot

  ● S93.332   Other subluxation of left foot

  ● S93.333   Other subluxation of unspecified foot

  ● S93.334   Other dislocation of right foot

  ● S93.335   Other dislocation of left foot

  ● S93.336   Other dislocation of unspecified foot

● S93.4   Sprain of ankle

Injury to ligaments when one or more is stretched/torn

Excludes2   injury of Achilles tendon (S86.0-)

● S93.40   Sprain of unspecified ligament of ankle

     Sprain of ankle NOS

     Sprained ankle NOS

  ● S93.401   Sprain of unspecified ligament of right ankle

  ● S93.402   Sprain of unspecified ligament of left ankle

  ● S93.409   Sprain of unspecified ligament of unspecified ankle

● S93.41   Sprain of calcaneofibular ligament

  ● S93.411   Sprain of calcaneofibular ligament of right ankle

  ● S93.412   Sprain of calcaneofibular ligament of left ankle

  ● S93.419   Sprain of calcaneofibular ligament of unspecified ankle

● S93.42   Sprain of deltoid ligament

  ● S93.421   Sprain of deltoid ligament of right ankle

  ● S93.422   Sprain of deltoid ligament of left ankle

  ● S93.429   Sprain of deltoid ligament of unspecified ankle

● S93.43   Sprain of tibiofibular ligament

  ● S93.431   Sprain of tibiofibular ligament of right ankle

  ● S93.432   Sprain of tibiofibular ligament of left ankle

  ● S93.439   Sprain of tibiofibular ligament of unspecified ankle

● S93.49   Sprain of other ligament of ankle

     Sprain of internal collateral ligament

     Sprain of talofibular ligament

  ● S93.491   Sprain of other ligament of right ankle

  ● S93.492   Sprain of other ligament of left ankle

  ● S93.499   Sprain of other ligament of unspecified ankle

● S93.5   Sprain of toe

● S93.50   Unspecified sprain of toe

  ● S93.501   Unspecified sprain of right great toe

  ● S93.502   Unspecified sprain of left great toe

  ● S93.503   Unspecified sprain of unspecified great toe

  ● S93.504   Unspecified sprain of right lesser toe(s)

  ● S93.505   Unspecified sprain of left lesser toe(s)

  ● S93.506   Unspecified sprain of unspecified lesser toe(s)

  ● S93.509   Unspecified sprain of unspecified toe(s)

● S93.51   Sprain of interphalangeal joint of toe

  ● S93.511   Sprain of interphalangeal joint of right great toe

  ● S93.512   Sprain of interphalangeal joint of left great toe

  ● S93.513   Sprain of interphalangeal joint of unspecified great toe

  ● S93.514   Sprain of interphalangeal joint of right lesser toe(s)

  ● S93.515   Sprain of interphalangeal joint of left lesser toe(s)

  ● S93.516   Sprain of interphalangeal joint of unspecified lesser toe(s)

  ● S93.519   Sprain of interphalangeal joint of unspecified toe(s)

● S93.52   Sprain of metatarsophalangeal joint of toe

  ● S93.521   Sprain of metatarsophalangeal joint of right great toe

  ● S93.522   Sprain of metatarsophalangeal joint of left great toe

  ● S93.523   Sprain of metatarsophalangeal joint of unspecified great toe

  ● S93.524   Sprain of metatarsophalangeal joint of right lesser toe(s)

  ● S93.525   Sprain of metatarsophalangeal joint of left lesser toe(s)

  ● S93.526   Sprain of metatarsophalangeal joint of unspecified lesser toe(s)

  ● S93.529   Sprain of metatarsophalangeal joint of unspecified toe(s)

● S93.6   Sprain of foot

Excludes2   sprain of metatarsophalangeal joint of toe (S93.52-)

              sprain of toe (S93.5-)

● S93.60   Unspecified sprain of foot

  ● S93.601   Unspecified sprain of right foot

  ● S93.602   Unspecified sprain of left foot

  ● S93.609   Unspecified sprain of unspecified foot

● S93.61   Sprain of tarsal ligament of foot

  ● S93.611   Sprain of tarsal ligament of right foot

  ● S93.612   Sprain of tarsal ligament of left foot

  ● S93.619   Sprain of tarsal ligament of unspecified foot

● S93.62   Sprain of tarsometatarsal ligament of foot

  ● S93.621   Sprain of tarsometatarsal ligament of right foot

  ● S93.622   Sprain of tarsometatarsal ligament of left foot

  ● S93.629   Sprain of tarsometatarsal ligament of unspecified foot

● S93.69   Other sprain of foot

  ● S93.691   Other sprain of right foot

  ● S93.692   Other sprain of left foot

  ● S93.699   Other sprain of unspecified foot

● S94   Injury of nerves at ankle and foot level

The appropriate 7th character is to be added to each code from category S94

A	initial encounter
D	subsequent encounter
S	sequela

Code also any associated open wound (S91.-)

● S94.0   Injury of lateral plantar nerve

  X ● S94.00   Injury of lateral plantar nerve, unspecified leg

  X ● S94.01   Injury of lateral plantar nerve, right leg

  X ● S94.02   Injury of lateral plantar nerve, left leg

● S94.1   Injury of medial plantar nerve

  X ● S94.10   Injury of medial plantar nerve, unspecified leg

  X ● S94.11   Injury of medial plantar nerve, right leg

  X ● S94.12   Injury of medial plantar nerve, left leg

▶ New   ⇒ Revised   ~~deleted~~ Deleted   Excludes 1   Excludes 2   Includes   Use additional   Code first   Code also   Key words

OGCR Official Guidelines   X Assign placeholder X   ● Use Additional Character(s)   ▶ Manifestation Code   🝰 Hierarchical Condition Category   **Coding Clinic**

● **S94.2**   Injury of deep peroneal nerve at ankle and foot level
     Injury of terminal, lateral branch of deep peroneal nerve
X● **S94.20**   Injury of deep peroneal nerve at ankle and foot level, unspecified leg
X● **S94.21**   Injury of deep peroneal nerve at ankle and foot level, right leg
X● **S94.22**   Injury of deep peroneal nerve at ankle and foot level, left leg
● **S94.3**   Injury of cutaneous sensory nerve at ankle and foot level
X● **S94.30**   Injury of cutaneous sensory nerve at ankle and foot level, unspecified leg
X● **S94.31**   Injury of cutaneous sensory nerve at ankle and foot level, right leg
X● **S94.32**   Injury of cutaneous sensory nerve at ankle and foot level, left leg
● **S94.8**   Injury of other nerves at ankle and foot level
   ● **S94.8X**   Injury of other nerves at ankle and foot level
     ● **S94.8X1**   Injury of other nerves at ankle and foot level, right leg
     ● **S94.8X2**   Injury of other nerves at ankle and foot level, left leg
     ● **S94.8X9**   Injury of other nerves at ankle and foot level, unspecified leg
● **S94.9**   Injury of unspecified nerve at ankle and foot level
X● **S94.90**   Injury of unspecified nerve at ankle and foot level, unspecified leg
X● **S94.91**   Injury of unspecified nerve at ankle and foot level, right leg
X● **S94.92**   Injury of unspecified nerve at ankle and foot level, left leg

● **S95**   **Injury of blood vessels at ankle and foot level**
     Code also any associated open wound (S91.-)
     Excludes2   injury of posterior tibial artery and vein (S85.1-, S85.8-)
     The appropriate 7th character is to be added to each code from category S95

A	initial encounter
D	subsequent encounter
S	sequela

● **S95.0**   Injury of dorsal artery of foot
   ● **S95.00**   Unspecified injury of dorsal artery of foot
     ● **S95.001**   Unspecified injury of dorsal artery of right foot
     ● **S95.002**   Unspecified injury of dorsal artery of left foot
     ● **S95.009**   Unspecified injury of dorsal artery of unspecified foot
   ● **S95.01**   Laceration of dorsal artery of foot
     ● **S95.011**   Laceration of dorsal artery of right foot
     ● **S95.012**   Laceration of dorsal artery of left foot
     ● **S95.019**   Laceration of dorsal artery of unspecified foot
   ● **S95.09**   Other specified injury of dorsal artery of foot
     ● **S95.091**   Other specified injury of dorsal artery of right foot
     ● **S95.092**   Other specified injury of dorsal artery of left foot
     ● **S95.099**   Other specified injury of dorsal artery of unspecified foot
● **S95.1**   Injury of plantar artery of foot
   ● **S95.10**   Unspecified injury of plantar artery of foot
     ● **S95.101**   Unspecified injury of plantar artery of right foot
     ● **S95.102**   Unspecified injury of plantar artery of left foot
     ● **S95.109**   Unspecified injury of plantar artery of unspecified foot

   ● **S95.11**   Laceration of plantar artery of foot
     ● **S95.111**   Laceration of plantar artery of right foot
     ● **S95.112**   Laceration of plantar artery of left foot
     ● **S95.119**   Laceration of plantar artery of unspecified foot
   ● **S95.19**   Other specified injury of plantar artery of foot
     ● **S95.191**   Other specified injury of plantar artery of right foot
     ● **S95.192**   Other specified injury of plantar artery of left foot
     ● **S95.199**   Other specified injury of plantar artery of unspecified foot
● **S95.2**   Injury of dorsal vein of foot
   ● **S95.20**   Unspecified injury of dorsal vein of foot
     ● **S95.201**   Unspecified injury of dorsal vein of right foot
     ● **S95.202**   Unspecified injury of dorsal vein of left foot
     ● **S95.209**   Unspecified injury of dorsal vein of unspecified foot
   ● **S95.21**   Laceration of dorsal vein of foot
     ● **S95.211**   Laceration of dorsal vein of right foot
     ● **S95.212**   Laceration of dorsal vein of left foot
     ● **S95.219**   Laceration of dorsal vein of unspecified foot
   ● **S95.29**   Other specified injury of dorsal vein of foot
     ● **S95.291**   Other specified injury of dorsal vein of right foot
     ● **S95.292**   Other specified injury of dorsal vein of left foot
     ● **S95.299**   Other specified injury of dorsal vein of unspecified foot
● **S95.8**   Injury of other blood vessels at ankle and foot level
   ● **S95.80**   Unspecified injury of other blood vessels at ankle and foot level
     ● **S95.801**   Unspecified injury of other blood vessels at ankle and foot level, right leg
     ● **S95.802**   Unspecified injury of other blood vessels at ankle and foot level, left leg
     ● **S95.809**   Unspecified injury of other blood vessels at ankle and foot level, unspecified leg
   ● **S95.81**   Laceration of other blood vessels at ankle and foot level
     ● **S95.811**   Laceration of other blood vessels at ankle and foot level, right leg
     ● **S95.812**   Laceration of other blood vessels at ankle and foot level, left leg
     ● **S95.819**   Laceration of other blood vessels at ankle and foot level, unspecified leg
   ● **S95.89**   Other specified injury of other blood vessels at ankle and foot level
     ● **S95.891**   Other specified injury of other blood vessels at ankle and foot level, right leg
     ● **S95.892**   Other specified injury of other blood vessels at ankle and foot level, left leg
     ● **S95.899**   Other specified injury of other blood vessels at ankle and foot level, unspecified leg
● **S95.9**   Injury of unspecified blood vessel at ankle and foot level
   ● **S95.90**   Unspecified injury of unspecified blood vessel at ankle and foot level
     ● **S95.901**   Unspecified injury of unspecified blood vessel at ankle and foot level, right leg

● S95.902   Unspecified injury of unspecified blood vessel at ankle and foot level, left leg

● S95.909   Unspecified injury of unspecified blood vessel at ankle and foot level, unspecified leg

● S95.91   Laceration of unspecified blood vessel at ankle and foot level

● S95.911   Laceration of unspecified blood vessel at ankle and foot level, right leg

● S95.912   Laceration of unspecified blood vessel at ankle and foot level, left leg

● S95.919   Laceration of unspecified blood vessel at ankle and foot level, unspecified leg

● S95.99   Other specified injury of unspecified blood vessel at ankle and foot level

● S95.991   Other specified injury of unspecified blood vessel at ankle and foot level, right leg

● S95.992   Other specified injury of unspecified blood vessel at ankle and foot level, left leg

● S95.999   Other specified injury of unspecified blood vessel at ankle and foot level, unspecified leg

● S96   Injury of muscle and tendon at ankle and foot level

Code also any associated open wound (S91.-)

Excludes2   injury of Achilles tendon (S86.0-)
sprain of joints and ligaments of ankle and foot (S93.-)

The appropriate 7th character is to be added to each code from category S96

A	initial encounter
D	subsequent encounter
S	sequela

● S96.0   Injury of muscle and tendon of long flexor muscle of toe at ankle and foot level

● S96.00   Unspecified injury of muscle and tendon of long flexor muscle of toe at ankle and foot level

● S96.001   Unspecified injury of muscle and tendon of long flexor muscle of toe at ankle and foot level, right foot

● S96.002   Unspecified injury of muscle and tendon of long flexor muscle of toe at ankle and foot level, left foot

● S96.009   Unspecified injury of muscle and tendon of long flexor muscle of toe at ankle and foot level, unspecified foot

● S96.01   Strain of muscle and tendon of long flexor muscle of toe at ankle and foot level

● S96.011   Strain of muscle and tendon of long flexor muscle of toe at ankle and foot level, right foot

● S96.012   Strain of muscle and tendon of long flexor muscle of toe at ankle and foot level, left foot

● S96.019   Strain of muscle and tendon of long flexor muscle of toe at ankle and foot level, unspecified foot

● S96.02   Laceration of muscle and tendon of long flexor muscle of toe at ankle and foot level

● S96.021   Laceration of muscle and tendon of long flexor muscle of toe at ankle and foot level, right foot

● S96.022   Laceration of muscle and tendon of long flexor muscle of toe at ankle and foot level, left foot

● S96.029   Laceration of muscle and tendon of long flexor muscle of toe at ankle and foot level, unspecified foot

● S96.09   Other injury of muscle and tendon of long flexor muscle of toe at ankle and foot level

● S96.091   Other injury of muscle and tendon of long flexor muscle of toe at ankle and foot level, right foot

● S96.092   Other injury of muscle and tendon of long flexor muscle of toe at ankle and foot level, left foot

● S96.099   Other injury of muscle and tendon of long flexor muscle of toe at ankle and foot level, unspecified foot

● S96.1   Injury of muscle and tendon of long extensor muscle of toe at ankle and foot level

● S96.10   Unspecified injury of muscle and tendon of long extensor muscle of toe at ankle and foot level

● S96.101   Unspecified injury of muscle and tendon of long extensor muscle of toe at ankle and foot level, right foot

● S96.102   Unspecified injury of muscle and tendon of long extensor muscle of toe at ankle and foot level, left foot

● S96.109   Unspecified injury of muscle and tendon of long extensor muscle of toe at ankle and foot level, unspecified foot

● S96.11   Strain of muscle and tendon of long extensor muscle of toe at ankle and foot level

● S96.111   Strain of muscle and tendon of long extensor muscle of toe at ankle and foot level, right foot

● S96.112   Strain of muscle and tendon of long extensor muscle of toe at ankle and foot level, left foot

● S96.119   Strain of muscle and tendon of long extensor muscle of toe at ankle and foot level, unspecified foot

● S96.12   Laceration of muscle and tendon of long extensor muscle of toe at ankle and foot level

● S96.121   Laceration of muscle and tendon of long extensor muscle of toe at ankle and foot level, right foot

● S96.122   Laceration of muscle and tendon of long extensor muscle of toe at ankle and foot level, left foot

● S96.129   Laceration of muscle and tendon of long extensor muscle of toe at ankle and foot level, unspecified foot

● S96.19   Other specified injury of muscle and tendon of long extensor muscle of toe at ankle and foot level

● S96.191   Other specified injury of muscle and tendon of long extensor muscle of toe at ankle and foot level, right foot

● S96.192   Other specified injury of muscle and tendon of long extensor muscle of toe at ankle and foot level, left foot

● S96.199   Other specified injury of muscle and tendon of long extensor muscle of toe at ankle and foot level, unspecified foot

● S96.2   Injury of intrinsic muscle and tendon at ankle and foot level

● S96.20   Unspecified injury of intrinsic muscle and tendon at ankle and foot level

● S96.201   Unspecified injury of intrinsic muscle and tendon at ankle and foot level, right foot

● S96.202   Unspecified injury of intrinsic muscle and tendon at ankle and foot level, left foot

● S96.209   Unspecified injury of intrinsic muscle and tendon at ankle and foot level, unspecified foot

● S96.21   Strain of intrinsic muscle and tendon at ankle and foot level

● S96.211   Strain of intrinsic muscle and tendon at ankle and foot level, right foot

● S96.212   Strain of intrinsic muscle and tendon at ankle and foot level, left foot

● S96.219   Strain of intrinsic muscle and tendon at ankle and foot level, unspecified foot

● S96.22   Laceration of intrinsic muscle and tendon at ankle and foot level

● S96.221   Laceration of intrinsic muscle and tendon at ankle and foot level, right foot

● S96.222   Laceration of intrinsic muscle and tendon at left ankle and foot level, left foot

● S96.229   Laceration of intrinsic muscle and tendon at ankle and foot level, unspecified foot

● S96.29   Other specified injury of intrinsic muscle and tendon at ankle and foot level

● S96.291   Other specified injury of intrinsic muscle and tendon at ankle and foot level, right foot

● S96.292   Other specified injury of intrinsic muscle and tendon at ankle and foot level, left foot

● S96.299   Other specified injury of intrinsic muscle and tendon at ankle and foot level, unspecified foot

● S96.8   Injury of other specified muscles and tendons at ankle and foot level

● S96.80   Unspecified injury of other specified muscles and tendons at ankle and foot level

● S96.801   Unspecified injury of other specified muscles and tendons at ankle and foot level, right foot

● S96.802   Unspecified injury of other specified muscles and tendons at ankle and foot level, left foot

● S96.809   Unspecified injury of other specified muscles and tendons at ankle and foot level, unspecified foot

● S96.81   Strain of other specified muscles and tendons at ankle and foot level

● S96.811   Strain of other specified muscles and tendons at ankle and foot level, right foot

● S96.812   Strain of other specified muscles and tendons at ankle and foot level, left foot

● S96.819   Strain of other specified muscles and tendons at ankle and foot level, unspecified foot

● S96.82   Laceration of other specified muscles and tendons at ankle and foot level

● S96.821   Laceration of other specified muscles and tendons at ankle and foot level, right foot

● S96.822   Laceration of other specified muscles and tendons at ankle and foot level, left foot

● S96.829   Laceration of other specified muscles and tendons at ankle and foot level, unspecified foot

● S96.89   Other specified injury of other specified muscles and tendons at ankle and foot level

● S96.891   Other specified injury of other specified muscles and tendons at ankle and foot level, right foot

● S96.892   Other specified injury of other specified muscles and tendons at ankle and foot level, left foot

● S96.899   Other specified injury of other specified muscles and tendons at ankle and foot level, unspecified foot

● S96.9   Injury of unspecified muscle and tendon at ankle and foot level

● S96.90   Unspecified injury of unspecified muscle and tendon at ankle and foot level

● S96.901   Unspecified injury of unspecified muscle and tendon at ankle and foot level, right foot

● S96.902   Unspecified injury of unspecified muscle and tendon at ankle and foot level, left foot

● S96.909   Unspecified injury of unspecified muscle and tendon at ankle and foot level, unspecified foot

● S96.91   Strain of unspecified muscle and tendon at ankle and foot level

● S96.911   Strain of unspecified muscle and tendon at ankle and foot level, right foot

● S96.912   Strain of unspecified muscle and tendon at ankle and foot level, left foot

● S96.919   Strain of unspecified muscle and tendon at ankle and foot level, unspecified foot

● S96.92   Laceration of unspecified muscle and tendon at ankle and foot level

● S96.921   Laceration of unspecified muscle and tendon at ankle and foot level, right foot

● S96.922   Laceration of unspecified muscle and tendon at ankle and foot level, left foot

● S96.929   Laceration of unspecified muscle and tendon at ankle and foot level, unspecified foot

● S96.99   Other specified injury of unspecified muscle and tendon at ankle and foot level

● S96.991   Other specified injury of unspecified muscle and tendon at ankle and foot level, right foot

● S96.992   Other specified injury of unspecified muscle and tendon at ankle and foot level, left foot

● S96.999   Other specified injury of unspecified muscle and tendon at ankle and foot level, unspecified foot

● S97   Crushing injury of ankle and foot

Use additional code(s) for all associated injuries

The appropriate 7th character is to be added to each code from category S97

A	initial encounter
D	subsequent encounter
S	sequela

● S97.0   Crushing injury of ankle

X ● S97.00   Crushing injury of unspecified ankle

X ● S97.01   Crushing injury of right ankle

X ● S97.02   Crushing injury of left ankle

- S97.1   Crushing injury of toe
  - S97.10   Crushing injury of unspecified toe(s)
    - S97.101   Crushing injury of unspecified right toe(s)
    - S97.102   Crushing injury of unspecified left toe(s)
    - S97.109   Crushing injury of unspecified toe(s)
      Crushing injury of toe NOS
  - S97.11   Crushing injury of great toe
    - S97.111   Crushing injury of right great toe
    - S97.112   Crushing injury of left great toe
    - S97.119   Crushing injury of unspecified great toe
  - S97.12   Crushing injury of lesser toe(s)
    - S97.121   Crushing injury of right lesser toe(s)
    - S97.122   Crushing injury of left lesser toe(s)
    - S97.129   Crushing injury of lesser toe(s), unspecified toe(s)
- S97.8   Crushing injury of foot
  - X ● S97.80   Crushing injury of foot, unspecified side
    Crushing injury of foot NOS
  - X ● S97.81   Crushing injury of right foot
  - X ● S97.82   Crushing injury of left foot
- S98   Traumatic amputation of ankle and foot
  An amputation not identified as partial or complete should be coded to complete
  The appropriate 7th character is to be added to each code from category S98

A	initial encounter
D	subsequent encounter
S	sequela

  - S98.0   Traumatic amputation of foot at ankle level
    - S98.01   Complete traumatic amputation of foot at ankle level
      - S98.011   Complete traumatic amputation of right foot at ankle level A, D, S 🐾
      - S98.012   Complete traumatic amputation of left foot at ankle level A, D, S 🐾
      - S98.019   Complete traumatic amputation of unspecified foot at ankle level A, D, S 🐾
    - S98.02   Partial traumatic amputation of foot at ankle level
      - S98.021   Partial traumatic amputation of right foot at ankle level A, D, S 🐾
      - S98.022   Partial traumatic amputation of left foot at ankle level A, D, S 🐾
      - S98.029   Partial traumatic amputation of unspecified foot at ankle level A, D, S 🐾
  - S98.1   Traumatic amputation of one toe
    - S98.11   Complete traumatic amputation of great toe
      - S98.111   Complete traumatic amputation of right great toe A, D, S 🐾
      - S98.112   Complete traumatic amputation of left great toe A, D, S 🐾
      - S98.119   Complete traumatic amputation of unspecified great toe A, D, S 🐾
    - S98.12   Partial traumatic amputation of great toe
      - S98.121   Partial traumatic amputation of right great toe A, D, S 🐾
      - S98.122   Partial traumatic amputation of left great toe A, D, S 🐾
      - S98.129   Partial traumatic amputation of unspecified great toe A, D, S 🐾
    - S98.13   Complete traumatic amputation of one lesser toe
      Traumatic amputation of toe NOS
      - S98.131   Complete traumatic amputation of one right lesser toe A, D, S 🐾
      - S98.132   Complete traumatic amputation of one left lesser toe A, D, S 🐾
      - S98.139   Complete traumatic amputation of one unspecified lesser toe A, D, S 🐾
    - S98.14   Partial traumatic amputation of one lesser toe
      - S98.141   Partial traumatic amputation of one right lesser toe A, D, S 🐾
      - S98.142   Partial traumatic amputation of one left lesser toe A, D, S 🐾
      - S98.149   Partial traumatic amputation of one unspecified lesser toe A, D, S 🐾
  - S98.2   Traumatic amputation of two or more lesser toes
    - S98.21   Complete traumatic amputation of two or more lesser toes
      - S98.211   Complete traumatic amputation of two or more right lesser toes A, D, S 🐾
      - S98.212   Complete traumatic amputation of two or more left lesser toes A, D, S 🐾
      - S98.219   Complete traumatic amputation of two or more unspecified lesser toes A, D, S 🐾
    - S98.22   Partial traumatic amputation of two or more lesser toes
      - S98.221   Partial traumatic amputation of two or more right lesser toes A, D, S 🐾
      - S98.222   Partial traumatic amputation of two or more left lesser toes A, D, S 🐾
      - S98.229   Partial traumatic amputation of two or more unspecified lesser toes A, D, S 🐾
  - S98.3   Traumatic amputation of midfoot
    - S98.31   Complete traumatic amputation of midfoot
      - S98.311   Complete traumatic amputation of right midfoot A, D, S 🐾
      - S98.312   Complete traumatic amputation of left midfoot A, D, S 🐾
      - S98.319   Complete traumatic amputation of unspecified midfoot A, D, S 🐾
    - S98.32   Partial traumatic amputation of midfoot
      - S98.321   Partial traumatic amputation of right midfoot A, D, S 🐾
      - S98.322   Partial traumatic amputation of left midfoot A, D, S 🐾
      - S98.329   Partial traumatic amputation of unspecified midfoot A, D, S 🐾
  - S98.9   Traumatic amputation of foot, level unspecified
    - S98.91   Complete traumatic amputation of foot, level unspecified
      - S98.911   Complete traumatic amputation of right foot, level unspecified A, D, S 🐾
      - S98.912   Complete traumatic amputation of left foot, level unspecified A, D, S 🐾
      - S98.919   Complete traumatic amputation of unspecified foot, level unspecified A, D, S 🐾
    - S98.92   Partial traumatic amputation of foot, level unspecified
      - S98.921   Partial traumatic amputation of right foot, level unspecified A, D, S 🐾
      - S98.922   Partial traumatic amputation of left foot, level unspecified A, D, S 🐾
      - S98.929   Partial traumatic amputation of unspecified foot, level unspecified A, D, S 🐾

▶ New   ⇒ Revised   ~~deleted~~ Deleted   Excludes 1   Excludes 2   Includes   Use additional   Code first   Code also   Key words

OGCR Official Guidelines   X Assign placeholder X   ● Use Additional Character(s)   ▷ Manifestation Code   🐾 Hierarchical Condition Category   Coding Clinic

● S99 Other and unspecified injuries of ankle and foot
Coding Clinic: 2016, Q4, P68

● S99.0 Physeal fracture of calcaneus

The appropriate 7th character is to be added to each
code from subcategories S99.0

A	initial encounter for closed fracture
B	initial encounter for open fracture
D	subsequent encounter for fracture with routine healing
G	subsequent encounter for fracture with delayed healing
K	subsequent encounter for fracture with nonunion
P	subsequent encounter for fracture with malunion
S	sequela

● S99.00 Unspecified physeal fracture of calcaneus

● S99.001 Unspecified physeal fracture of right calcaneus

● S99.002 Unspecified physeal fracture of left calcaneus

● S99.009 Unspecified physeal fracture of unspecified calcaneus

● S99.01 Salter-Harris Type I physeal fracture of calcaneus
Coding Clinic: 2016, Q4, P69

● S99.011 Salter-Harris Type I physeal fracture of right calcaneus

● S99.012 Salter-Harris Type I physeal fracture of left calcaneus

● S99.019 Salter-Harris Type I physeal fracture of unspecified calcaneus

● S99.02 Salter-Harris Type II physeal fracture of calcaneus
Coding Clinic: 2016, Q4, P69

● S99.021 Salter-Harris Type II physeal fracture of right calcaneus

● S99.022 Salter-Harris Type II physeal fracture of left calcaneus

● S99.029 Salter-Harris Type II physeal fracture of unspecified calcaneus

● S99.03 Salter-Harris Type III physeal fracture of calcaneus
Coding Clinic: 2016, Q4, P69

● S99.031 Salter-Harris Type III physeal fracture of right calcaneus

● S99.032 Salter-Harris Type III physeal fracture of left calcaneus

● S99.039 Salter-Harris Type III physeal fracture of unspecified calcaneus

● S99.04 Salter-Harris Type IV physeal fracture of calcaneus
Coding Clinic: 2016, Q4, P69

● S99.041 Salter-Harris Type IV physeal fracture of right calcaneus

● S99.042 Salter-Harris Type IV physeal fracture of left calcaneus

● S99.049 Salter-Harris Type IV physeal fracture of unspecified calcaneus

● S99.09 Other physeal fracture of calcaneus
Coding Clinic: 2016, Q4, P69

● S99.091 Other physeal fracture of right calcaneus

● S99.092 Other physeal fracture of left calcaneus

● S99.099 Other physeal fracture of unspecified calcaneus

● S99.1 Physeal fracture of metatarsal

The appropriate 7th character is to be added to each
code from subcategories S99.1

A	initial encounter for closed fracture
B	initial encounter for open fracture
D	subsequent encounter for fracture with routine healing
G	subsequent encounter for fracture with delayed healing
K	subsequent encounter for fracture with nonunion
P	subsequent encounter for fracture with malunion
S	sequela

● S99.10 Unspecified physeal fracture of metatarsal

● S99.101 Unspecified physeal fracture of right metatarsal

● S99.102 Unspecified physeal fracture of left metatarsal

● S99.109 Unspecified physeal fracture of unspecified metatarsal

● S99.11 Salter-Harris Type I physeal fracture of metatarsal
Coding Clinic: 2016, Q4, P69

● S99.111 Salter-Harris Type I physeal fracture of right metatarsal

● S99.112 Salter-Harris Type I physeal fracture of left metatarsal
Coding Clinic: 2018, Q1, P3

● S99.119 Salter-Harris Type I physeal fracture of unspecified metatarsal

● S99.12 Salter-Harris Type II physeal fracture of metatarsal
Coding Clinic: 2016, Q4, P69

● S99.121 Salter-Harris Type II physeal fracture of right metatarsal

● S99.122 Salter-Harris Type II physeal fracture of left metatarsal

● S99.129 Salter-Harris Type II physeal fracture of unspecified metatarsal

● S99.13 Salter-Harris Type III physeal fracture of metatarsal
Coding Clinic: 2016, Q4, P69

● S99.131 Salter-Harris Type III physeal fracture of right metatarsal

● S99.132 Salter-Harris Type III physeal fracture of left metatarsal

● S99.139 Salter-Harris Type III physeal fracture of unspecified metatarsal

● S99.14 Salter-Harris Type IV physeal fracture of metatarsal
Coding Clinic: 2016, Q4, P69

● S99.141 Salter-Harris Type IV physeal fracture of right metatarsal

● S99.142 Salter-Harris Type IV physeal fracture of left metatarsal

● S99.149 Salter-Harris Type IV physeal fracture of unspecified metatarsal

● S99.19 Other physeal fracture of metatarsal
Coding Clinic: 2016, Q4, P69

● S99.191 Other physeal fracture of right metatarsal

● S99.192 Other physeal fracture of left metatarsal

● S99.199 Other physeal fracture of unspecified metatarsal

CHAPTER 19 (S00-T88)

● **S99.2**   Physeal fracture of phalanx of toe

The appropriate 7th character is to be added to each code from subcategories S99.2

A	initial encounter for closed fracture
B	initial encounter for open fracture
D	subsequent encounter for fracture with routine healing
G	subsequent encounter for fracture with delayed healing
K	subsequent encounter for fracture with nonunion
P	subsequent encounter for fracture with malunion
S	sequela

● **S99.20**   Unspecified physeal fracture of phalanx of toe

     ● **S99.201**   Unspecified physeal fracture of phalanx of right toe

     ● **S99.202**   Unspecified physeal fracture of phalanx of right toe

     ● **S99.209**   Unspecified physeal fracture of phalanx of unspecified toe

● **S99.21**   Salter-Harris Type I physeal fracture of phalanx of toe
     Coding Clinic: 2016, Q4, P69

     ● **S99.211**   Salter-Harris Type I physeal fracture of phalanx of right toe

     ● **S99.212**   Salter-Harris Type I physeal fracture of phalanx of left toe

     ● **S99.219**   Salter-Harris Type I physeal fracture of phalanx of unspecified toe

● **S99.22**   Salter-Harris Type II physeal fracture of phalanx of toe
     Coding Clinic: 2016, Q4, P69

     ● **S99.221**   Salter-Harris Type II physeal fracture of phalanx of right toe

     ● **S99.222**   Salter-Harris Type II physeal fracture of phalanx of left toe

     ● **S99.229**   Salter-Harris Type II physeal fracture of phalanx of unspecified toe

● **S99.23**   Salter-Harris Type III physeal fracture of phalanx of toe
     Coding Clinic: 2016, Q4, P69

     ● **S99.231**   Salter-Harris Type III physeal fracture of phalanx of right toe

     ● **S99.232**   Salter-Harris Type III physeal fracture of phalanx of left toe

     ● **S99.239**   Salter-Harris Type III physeal fracture of phalanx of unspecified toe

● **S99.24**   Salter-Harris Type IV physeal fracture of phalanx of toe
     Coding Clinic: 2016, Q4, P69

     ● **S99.241**   Salter-Harris Type IV physeal fracture of phalanx of right toe

     ● **S99.242**   Salter-Harris Type IV physeal fracture of phalanx of left toe

     ● **S99.249**   Salter-Harris Type IV physeal fracture of phalanx of unspecified toe

● **S99.29**   Other physeal fracture of phalanx of toe
     Coding Clinic: 2016, Q4, P69

     ● **S99.291**   Other physeal fracture of phalanx of right toe

     ● **S99.292**   Other physeal fracture of phalanx of left toe

     ● **S99.299**   Other physeal fracture of phalanx of unspecified toe

● **S99.8**   Other specified injuries of ankle and foot

The appropriate 7th character is to be added to each code from subcategory S99.8

A	initial encounter
D	subsequent encounter
S	sequela

● **S99.81**   Other specified injuries of ankle

     ● **S99.811**   Other specified injuries of right ankle

     ● **S99.812**   Other specified injuries of left ankle

     ● **S99.819**   Other specified injuries of unspecified ankle

● **S99.82**   Other specified injuries of foot

     ● **S99.821**   Other specified injuries of right foot

     ● **S99.822**   Other specified injuries of left foot

     ● **S99.829**   Other specified injuries of unspecified foot

● **S99.9**   Unspecified injury of ankle and foot

The appropriate 7th character is to be added to each code from subcategory S99.9

A	initial encounter
D	subsequent encounter
S	sequela

● **S99.91**   Unspecified injury of ankle

     ● **S99.911**   Unspecified injury of right ankle

     ● **S99.912**   Unspecified injury of left ankle

     ● **S99.919**   Unspecified injury of unspecified ankle

● **S99.92**   Unspecified injury of foot

     ● **S99.921**   Unspecified injury of right foot

     ● **S99.922**   Unspecified injury of left foot

     ● **S99.929**   Unspecified injury of unspecified foot

INJURY, POISONING AND CERTAIN OTHER CONSEQUENCES OF EXTERNAL CAUSES (T07-T88)

INJURIES INVOLVING MULTIPLE BODY REGIONS (T07)

Excludes1   burns and corrosions (T20-T32)
                     frostbite (T33-T34)
                     insect bite or sting, venomous (T63.4)
                     sunburn (L55.-)

X ● **T07**   Unspecified multiple injuries

The appropriate 7th character is to be added to code T07

A	initial encounter
D	subsequent encounter
S	sequela

Excludes1   injury NOS (T14.90)

INJURY OF UNSPECIFIED BODY REGION (T14)

● **T14**   Injury of unspecified body region

The appropriate 7th character is to be added to each code from category T14

A	initial encounter
D	subsequent encounter
S	sequela

Excludes1   multiple unspecified injuries (T07)

X ● **T14.8**   Other injury of unspecified body region
     Abrasion NOS   Skin injury NOS
     Contusion NOS   Vascular injury NOS
     Crush injury NOS   Wound NOS
     Fracture NOS

● **T14.9**   Unspecified injury

     X ● **T14.90**   Injury, unspecified
                Injury NOS

     X ● **T14.91**   Suicide attempt A, D, S 🏥
                Attempted suicide NOS

▶ New   ⇒ Revised   ~~deleted~~ Deleted   Excludes 1   Excludes 2   Includes   Use additional   Code first   Code also   Key words

OGCR Official Guidelines   X Assign placeholder X   ● Use Additional Character(s)   ▶ Manifestation Code   🏥 Hierarchical Condition Category   Coding Clinic

EFFECTS OF FOREIGN BODY ENTERING THROUGH NATURAL ORIFICE (T15–T19)

Use additional code, if known, for foreign body entering into or through a natural orifice (W44.-)

Excludes2   foreign body accidentally left in operation wound (T81.5-)
foreign body in penetrating wound - see open wound by body region
residual foreign body in soft tissue (M79.5)
splinter, without open wound - see superficial injury by body region

● T15   Foreign body on external eye

Excludes2   foreign body in penetrating wound of orbit and eye ball (S05.4-, S05.5-)
open wound of eyelid and periocular area (S01.1-)
retained foreign body in eyelid (H02.8-)
retained (old) foreign body in penetrating wound of orbit and eye ball (H05.5-, H44.6-, H44.7-)
superficial foreign body of eyelid and periocular area (S00.25-)

The appropriate 7th character is to be added to each code from category T15

A	initial encounter
D	subsequent encounter
S	sequela

● T15.0   Foreign body in cornea
X● T15.00   Foreign body in cornea, unspecified eye
X● T15.01   Foreign body in cornea, right eye
X● T15.02   Foreign body in cornea, left eye
● T15.1   Foreign body in conjunctival sac
X● T15.10   Foreign body in conjunctival sac, unspecified eye
X● T15.11   Foreign body in conjunctival sac, right eye
X● T15.12   Foreign body in conjunctival sac, left eye
● T15.8   Foreign body in other and multiple parts of external eye
Foreign body in lacrimal punctum
X● T15.80   Foreign body in other and multiple parts of external eye, unspecified eye
X● T15.81   Foreign body in other and multiple parts of external eye, right eye
X● T15.82   Foreign body in other and multiple parts of external eye, left eye
● T15.9   Foreign body on external eye, part unspecified
X● T15.90   Foreign body on external eye, part unspecified, unspecified eye
X● T15.91   Foreign body on external eye, part unspecified, right eye
X● T15.92   Foreign body on external eye, part unspecified, left eye

● T16   Foreign body in ear

Includes   foreign body in auditory canal

The appropriate 7th character is to be added to each code from category T16

A	initial encounter
D	subsequent encounter
S	sequela

X● T16.1   Foreign body in right ear
X● T16.2   Foreign body in left ear
X● T16.9   Foreign body in ear, unspecified ear

● T17   Foreign body in respiratory tract

The appropriate 7th character is to be added to each code from category T17

A	initial encounter
D	subsequent encounter
S	sequela

X● T17.0   Foreign body in nasal sinus
X● T17.1   Foreign body in nostril
Foreign body in nose NOS
● T17.2   Foreign body in pharynx
Foreign body in nasopharynx
Foreign body in throat NOS
● T17.20   Unspecified foreign body in pharynx
● T17.200   Unspecified foreign body in pharynx causing asphyxiation
● T17.208   Unspecified foreign body in pharynx causing other injury
● T17.21   Gastric contents in pharynx
Aspiration of gastric contents into pharynx
Vomitus in pharynx
● T17.210   Gastric contents in pharynx causing asphyxiation
● T17.218   Gastric contents in pharynx causing other injury
● T17.22   Food in pharynx
Bones in pharynx
Seeds in pharynx
● T17.220   Food in pharynx causing asphyxiation
● T17.228   Food in pharynx causing other injury
● T17.29   Other foreign object in pharynx
● T17.290   Other foreign object in pharynx causing asphyxiation
● T17.298   Other foreign object in pharynx causing other injury
● T17.3   Foreign body in larynx
● T17.30   Unspecified foreign body in larynx
● T17.300   Unspecified foreign body in larynx causing asphyxiation
● T17.308   Unspecified foreign body in larynx causing other injury
● T17.31   Gastric contents in larynx
Aspiration of gastric contents into larynx
Vomitus in larynx
● T17.310   Gastric contents in larynx causing asphyxiation
● T17.318   Gastric contents in larynx causing other injury
● T17.32   Food in larynx
Bones in larynx
Seeds in larynx
● T17.320   Food in larynx causing asphyxiation
● T17.328   Food in larynx causing other injury
● T17.39   Other foreign object in larynx
● T17.390   Other foreign object in larynx causing asphyxiation
● T17.398   Other foreign object in larynx causing other injury
● T17.4   Foreign body in trachea
● T17.40   Unspecified foreign body in trachea
● T17.400   Unspecified foreign body in trachea causing asphyxiation
● T17.408   Unspecified foreign body in trachea causing other injury
● T17.41   Gastric contents in trachea
Aspiration of gastric contents into trachea
Vomitus in trachea
● T17.410   Gastric contents in trachea causing asphyxiation

CHAPTER 19 (S00–T88)

● T17.418   Gastric contents in trachea causing other injury
● T17.42   Food in trachea
   Bones in trachea
   Seeds in trachea
   ● T17.420   Food in trachea causing asphyxiation
   ● T17.428   Food in trachea causing other injury
● T17.49   Other foreign object in trachea
   ● T17.490   Other foreign object in trachea causing asphyxiation
   ● T17.498   Other foreign object in trachea causing other injury
● T17.5   Foreign body in bronchus
   ● T17.50   Unspecified foreign body in bronchus
     ● T17.500   Unspecified foreign body in bronchus causing asphyxiation
     ● T17.508   Unspecified foreign body in bronchus causing other injury
   ● T17.51   Gastric contents in bronchus
     Aspiration of gastric contents into bronchus
     Vomitus in bronchus
     ● T17.510   Gastric contents in bronchus causing asphyxiation
     ● T17.518   Gastric contents in bronchus causing other injury
   ● T17.52   Food in bronchus
     Bones in bronchus
     Seeds in bronchus
     ● T17.520   Food in bronchus causing asphyxiation
     ● T17.528   Food in bronchus causing other injury
   ● T17.59   Other foreign object in bronchus
     ● T17.590   Other foreign object in bronchus causing asphyxiation
     ● T17.598   Other foreign object in bronchus causing other injury
● T17.8   Foreign body in other parts of respiratory tract
   Foreign body in bronchioles
   Foreign body in lung
   ● T17.80   Unspecified foreign body in other parts of respiratory tract
     ● T17.800   Unspecified foreign body in other parts of respiratory tract causing asphyxiation
     ● T17.808   Unspecified foreign body in other parts of respiratory tract causing other injury
   ● T17.81   Gastric contents in other parts of respiratory tract
     Aspiration of gastric contents into other parts of respiratory tract
     Vomitus in other parts of respiratory tract
     ● T17.810   Gastric contents in other parts of respiratory tract causing asphyxiation
     ● T17.818   Gastric contents in other parts of respiratory tract causing other injury
   ● T17.82   Food in other parts of respiratory tract
     Bones in other parts of respiratory tract
     Seeds in other parts of respiratory tract
     ● T17.820   Food in other parts of respiratory tract causing asphyxiation
     ● T17.828   Food in other parts of respiratory tract causing other injury
   ● T17.89   Other foreign object in other parts of respiratory tract
     ● T17.890   Other foreign object in other parts of respiratory tract causing asphyxiation
     ● T17.898   Other foreign object in other parts of respiratory tract causing other injury

● T17.9   Foreign body in respiratory tract, part unspecified
   ● T17.90   Unspecified foreign body in respiratory tract, part unspecified
     ● T17.900   Unspecified foreign body in respiratory tract, part unspecified causing asphyxiation
     ● T17.908   Unspecified foreign body in respiratory tract, part unspecified causing other injury
   ● T17.91   Gastric contents in respiratory tract, part unspecified
     Aspiration of gastric contents into respiratory tract, part unspecified
     Vomitus in trachea respiratory tract, part unspecified
     ● T17.910   Gastric contents in respiratory tract, part unspecified causing asphyxiation
     ● T17.918   Gastric contents in respiratory tract, part unspecified causing other injury
   ● T17.92   Food in respiratory tract, part unspecified
     Bones in respiratory tract, part unspecified
     Seeds in respiratory tract, part unspecified
     ● T17.920   Food in respiratory tract, part unspecified causing asphyxiation
     ● T17.928   Food in respiratory tract, part unspecified causing other injury
   ● T17.99   Other foreign object in respiratory tract, part unspecified
     ● T17.990   Other foreign object in respiratory tract, part unspecified in causing asphyxiation
      Coding Clinic: 2019, Q3, P15
     ● T17.998   Other foreign object in respiratory tract, part unspecified causing other injury

● T18   Foreign body in alimentary tract
   Excludes2   foreign body in pharynx (T17.2-)
   The appropriate 7th character is to be added to each code from category T18
   A   initial encounter
   D   subsequent encounter
   S   sequela

X ● T18.0   Foreign body in mouth
X ● T18.1   Foreign body in esophagus
   Excludes2   foreign body in respiratory tract (T17.-)
   ● T18.10   Unspecified foreign body in esophagus
     ● T18.100   Unspecified foreign body in esophagus causing compression of trachea
      Unspecified foreign body in esophagus causing obstruction of respiration
     ● T18.108   Unspecified foreign body in esophagus causing other injury
   ● T18.11   Gastric contents in esophagus
     Vomitus in esophagus
     ● T18.110   Gastric contents in esophagus causing compression of trachea
      Gastric contents in esophagus causing obstruction of respiration
     ● T18.118   Gastric contents in esophagus causing other injury
   ● T18.12   Food in esophagus
     Bones in esophagus
     Seeds in esophagus

▶ New   ⇒ Revised   ~~deleted~~ Deleted   Excludes 1   Excludes 2   Includes   Use additional   Code first   Code also   Key words
OGCR Official Guidelines   X Assign placeholder X   ● Use Additional Character(s)   ▶ Manifestation Code   Hierarchical Condition Category   Coding Clinic

- ● T18.120 **Food in esophagus causing compression of trachea**
  Food in esophagus causing obstruction of respiration
  - ● T18.128 **Food in esophagus causing other injury**
- ● T18.19 **Other foreign object in esophagus**
  - ● T18.190 **Other foreign object in esophagus causing compression of trachea**
    Other foreign body in esophagus causing obstruction of respiration
    Coding Clinic: 2015, Q1, P24
  - ● T18.198 **Other foreign object in esophagus causing other injury**
    Coding Clinic: 2015, Q1, P24
- X ● T18.2 **Foreign body in stomach**
- X ● T18.3 **Foreign body in small intestine**
- X ● T18.4 **Foreign body in colon**
- X ● T18.5 **Foreign body in anus and rectum**
  Foreign body in rectosigmoid (junction)
- X ● T18.8 **Foreign body in other parts of alimentary tract**
- X ● T18.9 **Foreign body of alimentary tract, part unspecified**
  Foreign body in digestive system NOS
  Swallowed foreign body NOS

- ● T19 **Foreign body in genitourinary tract**
  - Excludes2 complications due to implanted mesh (T83.7-)
    mechanical complications of contraceptive device (intrauterine) (vaginal) (T83.3-)
    presence of contraceptive device (intrauterine) (vaginal) (Z97.5)

  The appropriate 7th character is to be added to each code from category T19

A	initial encounter
D	subsequent encounter
S	sequela

- X ● T19.0 **Foreign body in urethra**
- X ● T19.1 **Foreign body in bladder**
- X ● T19.2 **Foreign body in vulva and vagina**
- X ● T19.3 **Foreign body in uterus**
- X ● T19.4 **Foreign body in penis**
- X ● T19.8 **Foreign body in other parts of genitourinary tract**
- X ● T19.9 **Foreign body in genitourinary tract, part unspecified**

BURNS AND CORROSIONS (T20-T32)

Includes burns (thermal) from electrical heating appliances
burns (thermal) from electricity
burns (thermal) from flame
burns (thermal) from friction
burns (thermal) from hot air and hot gases
burns (thermal) from hot objects
burns (thermal) from lightning
burns (thermal) from radiation chemical
burn [corrosion] (external) (internal) scalds

Excludes2 erythema [dermatitis] ab igne (L59.0)
radiation-related disorders of the skin and subcutaneous tissue (L55-L59)
sunburn (L55.-)

OGCR Section I.C.19.d.

Burns and Corrosions
The ICD-10-CM makes a distinction between burn and corrosions. The burn codes are for thermal burns, except sunburns, that come from a heat source, such as a fire or hot appliance. The burn codes are also for burns resulting from electricity and radiation. Corrosions are burns due to chemicals. The guidelines for burns and corrosions are the same.

Current burns (T20-T25) are classified by depth, extent and by agent (X code). Burns are classified by depth as first degree (erythema), second degree (blistering), and third degree (full-thickness involvement). Burns of the eye and internal organs (T26-T28) are classified by site, but not by degree.

1) Sequencing of burn and related condition codes
Sequence first the code that reflects the highest degree of burn when more than one burn is present.

a. When the reason for the admission or encounter is for treatment of external multiple burns, sequence first the code that reflects the burn of the highest degree.

b. When a patient has both internal and external burns, the circumstances of admission govern the selection of the principal diagnosis or first-listed diagnosis.

c. When a patient is admitted for burn injuries and other related conditions such as smoke inhalation and/or respiratory failure, the circumstances of admission govern the selection of the principal or first-listed diagnosis.

2) Burns of the same local site
Classify burns of the same local site (three-character category level, T20-T28) but of different degrees to the subcategory identifying the highest degree recorded in the diagnosis.

BURNS AND CORROSIONS OF EXTERNAL BODY SURFACE, SPECIFIED BY SITE (T20-T25)

Includes burns and corrosions of first degree [erythema]
burns and corrosions of second degree [blisters] [epidermal loss]
burns and corrosions of third degree [deep necrosis of underlying tissue] [full-thickness skin loss]

Use additional code from category T31 or T32 to identify extent of body surface involved

- ● T20 **Burn and corrosion of head, face, and neck**
  - Excludes2 burn and corrosion of ear drum (T28.41, T28.91)
    burn and corrosion of eye and adnexa (T26.-)
    burn and corrosion of mouth and pharynx (T28.0)

  The appropriate 7th character is to be added to each code from category T20

A	initial encounter
D	subsequent encounter
S	sequela

  - ● T20.0 **Burn of unspecified degree of head, face, and neck**
    Use additional external cause code to identify the source, place and intent of the burn (X00-X19, X75-X77, X96-X98, Y92)
    - X ● T20.00 **Burn of unspecified degree of head, face, and neck, unspecified site**
    - ● T20.01 **Burn of unspecified degree of ear [any part, except ear drum]**
      - Excludes2 burn of ear drum (T28.41-)
      - ● T20.011 **Burn of unspecified degree of right ear [any part, except ear drum]**
      - ● T20.012 **Burn of unspecified degree of left ear [any part, except ear drum]**
      - ● T20.019 **Burn of unspecified degree of unspecified ear [any part, except ear drum]**

Figure 19-15 **A.** Second-degree burn. **B.** Third-degree burn. (A. From Black J, Hawks J: Medical-Surgical Nursing: Clinical Management for Positive Outcomes, 8e, Saunders, 2008. B. From Marx J, Hockberger R, Walls R: Rosen's Emergency Medicine - Concepts and Clinical Practice, 7e, Mosby, 2009)

X● T20.02   Burn of unspecified degree of lip(s)
X● T20.03   Burn of unspecified degree of chin
X● T20.04   Burn of unspecified degree of nose (septum)
X● T20.05   Burn of unspecified degree of scalp [any part]
X● T20.06   Burn of unspecified degree of forehead and cheek
X● T20.07   Burn of unspecified degree of neck
X● T20.09   Burn of unspecified degree of multiple sites of head, face, and neck

● T20.1   Burn of first degree of head, face, and neck

Use additional external cause code to identify the source, place and intent of the burn (X00-X19, X75-X77, X96-X98, Y92)

X● T20.10   Burn of first degree of head, face, and neck, unspecified site
● T20.11   Burn of first degree of ear [any part, except ear drum]

    Excludes2   burn of ear drum (T28.41-)

● T20.111   Burn of first degree of right ear [any part, except ear drum]
● T20.112   Burn of first degree of left ear [any part, except ear drum]
● T20.119   Burn of first degree of unspecified ear [any part, except ear drum]

X● T20.12   Burn of first degree of lip(s)
X● T20.13   Burn of first degree of chin
X● T20.14   Burn of first degree of nose (septum)
X● T20.15   Burn of first degree of scalp [any part]
X● T20.16   Burn of first degree of forehead and cheek
X● T20.17   Burn of first degree of neck
X● T20.19   Burn of first degree of multiple sites of head, face, and neck

● T20.2   Burn of second degree of head, face, and neck

Use additional external cause code to identify the source, place and intent of the burn (X00-X19, X75-X77, X96-X98, Y92)

X● T20.20   Burn of second degree of head, face, and neck, unspecified site
● T20.21   Burn of second degree of ear [any part, except ear drum]

    Excludes2   burn of ear drum (T28.41-)

● T20.211   Burn of second degree of right ear [any part, except ear drum]
● T20.212   Burn of second degree of left ear [any part, except ear drum]
● T20.219   Burn of second degree of unspecified ear [any part, except ear drum]

X● T20.22   Burn of second degree of lip(s)
X● T20.23   Burn of second degree of chin
X● T20.24   Burn of second degree of nose (septum)
X● T20.25   Burn of second degree of scalp [any part]

    Coding Clinic: 2015, Q1, P19

X● T20.26   Burn of second degree of forehead and cheek
X● T20.27   Burn of second degree of neck
X● T20.29   Burn of second degree of multiple sites of head, face, and neck

● T20.3   Burn of third degree of head, face, and neck

Use additional external cause code to identify the source, place and intent of the burn (X00-X19, X75-X77, X96-X98, Y92)

X● T20.30   Burn of third degree of head, face, and neck, unspecified site
● T20.31   Burn of third degree of ear [any part, except ear drum]

    Excludes2   burn of ear drum (T28.41-)

● T20.311   Burn of third degree of right ear [any part, except ear drum]
● T20.312   Burn of third degree of left ear [any part, except ear drum]
    Coding Clinic: 2015, Q1, P18
● T20.319   Burn of third degree of unspecified ear [any part, except ear drum]

X● T20.32   Burn of third degree of lip(s)
X● T20.33   Burn of third degree of chin
X● T20.34   Burn of third degree of nose (septum)
X● T20.35   Burn of third degree of scalp [any part]
X● T20.36   Burn of third degree of forehead and cheek
X● T20.37   Burn of third degree of neck
X● T20.39   Burn of third degree of multiple sites of head, face, and neck

● T20.4   Corrosion of unspecified degree of head, face, and neck

Code first (T51-T65) to identify chemical and intent

Use additional external cause code to identify place (Y92)

X● T20.40   Corrosion of unspecified degree of head, face, and neck, unspecified site
● T20.41   Corrosion of unspecified degree of ear [any part, except ear drum]

    Excludes2   corrosion of ear drum (T28.91-)

● T20.411   Corrosion of unspecified degree of right ear [any part, except ear drum]
● T20.412   Corrosion of unspecified degree of left ear [any part, except ear drum]
● T20.419   Corrosion of unspecified degree of unspecified ear [any part, except ear drum]

X● T20.42   Corrosion of unspecified degree of lip(s)
X● T20.43   Corrosion of unspecified degree of chin
X● T20.44   Corrosion of unspecified degree of nose (septum)
X● T20.45   Corrosion of unspecified degree of scalp [any part]
X● T20.46   Corrosion of unspecified degree of forehead and cheek
X● T20.47   Corrosion of unspecified degree of neck
X● T20.49   Corrosion of unspecified degree of multiple sites of head, face, and neck

● T20.5   Corrosion of first degree of head, face, and neck

Code first (T51-T65) to identify chemical and intent

Use additional external cause code to identify place (Y92)

X● T20.50   Corrosion of first degree of head, face, and neck, unspecified site
● T20.51   Corrosion of first degree of ear [any part, except ear drum]

    Excludes2   corrosion of ear drum (T28.91-)

● T20.511   Corrosion of first degree of right ear [any part, except ear drum]
● T20.512   Corrosion of first degree of left ear [any part, except ear drum]
● T20.519   Corrosion of first degree of unspecified ear [any part, except ear drum]

X● T20.52   Corrosion of first degree of lip(s)
X● T20.53   Corrosion of first degree of chin

▶ New   ⇒ Revised   ~~deleted~~ Deleted   Excludes 1   Excludes 2   Includes   Use additional   Code first   Code also   Key words

OGCR Official Guidelines   X Assign placeholder X   ● Use Additional Character(s)   ▶ Manifestation Code   🅗 Hierarchical Condition Category   **Coding Clinic**

X● **T20.54**   Corrosion of first degree of nose (septum)

X● **T20.55**   Corrosion of first degree of scalp [any part]

X● **T20.56**   Corrosion of first degree of forehead and cheek

X● **T20.57**   Corrosion of first degree of neck

X● **T20.59**   Corrosion of first degree of multiple sites of head, face, and neck

● **T20.6**   Corrosion of second degree of head, face, and neck

Code first (T51-T65) *to identify chemical and intent*

Use additional external cause code to identify place (Y92)

X● **T20.60**   Corrosion of second degree of head, face, and neck, unspecified site

● **T20.61**   Corrosion of second degree of ear [any part, except ear drum]

Excludes2   corrosion of ear drum (T28.91-)

● **T20.611**   Corrosion of second degree of right ear [any part, except ear drum]

● **T20.612**   Corrosion of second degree of left ear [any part, except ear drum]

● **T20.619**   Corrosion of second degree of unspecified ear [any part, except ear drum]

X● **T20.62**   Corrosion of second degree of lip(s)

X● **T20.63**   Corrosion of second degree of chin

X● **T20.64**   Corrosion of second degree of nose (septum)

X● **T20.65**   Corrosion of second degree of scalp [any part]

X● **T20.66**   Corrosion of second degree of forehead and cheek

X● **T20.67**   Corrosion of second degree of neck

X● **T20.69**   Corrosion of second degree of multiple sites of head, face, and neck

● **T20.7**   Corrosion of third degree of head, face, and neck

Code first (T51-T65) *to identify chemical and intent*

Use additional external cause code to identify place (Y92)

X● **T20.70**   Corrosion of third degree of head, face, and neck, unspecified site

● **T20.71**   Corrosion of third degree of ear [any part, except ear drum]

Excludes2   corrosion of ear drum (T28.91-)

● **T20.711**   Corrosion of third degree of right ear [any part, except ear drum]

● **T20.712**   Corrosion of third degree of left ear [any part, except ear drum]

● **T20.719**   Corrosion of third degree of unspecified ear [any part, except ear drum]

X● **T20.72**   Corrosion of third degree of lip(s)

X● **T20.73**   Corrosion of third degree of chin

X● **T20.74**   Corrosion of third degree of nose (septum)

X● **T20.75**   Corrosion of third degree of scalp [any part]

X● **T20.76**   Corrosion of third degree of forehead and cheek

X● **T20.77**   Corrosion of third degree of neck

X● **T20.79**   Corrosion of third degree of multiple sites of head, face, and neck

● **T21**   **Burn and corrosion of trunk**

Includes   burns and corrosion of hip region

Excludes2   burns and corrosion of axilla (T22.- with fifth character 4)

burns and corrosion of scapular region (T22.- with fifth character 6)

burns and corrosion of shoulder (T22.- with fifth character 5)

The appropriate 7th character is to be added to each code from category T21

A	initial encounter
D	subsequent encounter
S	sequela

● **T21.0**   Burn of unspecified degree of trunk

Use additional external cause code to identify the source, place and intent of the burn (X00-X19, X75-X77, X96-X98, Y92)

X● **T21.00**   Burn of unspecified degree of trunk, unspecified site

X● **T21.01**   Burn of unspecified degree of chest wall
Burn of unspecified degree of breast

X● **T21.02**   Burn of unspecified degree of abdominal wall
Burn of unspecified degree of flank
Burn of unspecified degree of groin

X● **T21.03**   Burn of unspecified degree of upper back
Burn of unspecified degree of interscapular region

X● **T21.04**   Burn of unspecified degree of lower back

X● **T21.05**   Burn of unspecified degree of buttock
Burn of unspecified degree of anus

X● **T21.06**   Burn of unspecified degree of male genital region
Burn of unspecified degree of penis
Burn of unspecified degree of scrotum
Burn of unspecified degree of testis

X● **T21.07**   Burn of unspecified degree of female genital region
Burn of unspecified degree of labium (majus) (minus)
Burn of unspecified degree of perineum
Burn of unspecified degree of vulva

Excludes2   burn of vagina (T28.3)

X● **T21.09**   Burn of unspecified degree of other site of trunk

● **T21.1**   Burn of first degree of trunk

Use additional external cause code to identify the source, place and intent of the burn (X00-X19, X75-X77, X96-X98, Y92)

X● **T21.10**   Burn of first degree of trunk, unspecified site

X● **T21.11**   Burn of first degree of chest wall
Burn of first degree of breast

X● **T21.12**   Burn of first degree of abdominal wall
Burn of first degree of flank
Burn of first degree of groin

X● **T21.13**   Burn of first degree of upper back
Burn of first degree of interscapular region

X● **T21.14**   Burn of first degree of lower back

X● **T21.15**   Burn of first degree of buttock
Burn of first degree of anus

X● **T21.16**   Burn of first degree of male genital region
Burn of first degree of penis
Burn of first degree of scrotum
Burn of first degree of testis

X● **T21.17**   Burn of first degree of female genital region
Burn of first degree of labium (majus) (minus)
Burn of first degree of perineum
Burn of first degree of vulva

Excludes2   burn of vagina (T28.3)

X● **T21.19**   Burn of first degree of other site of trunk

● **T21.2**   Burn of second degree of trunk

Use additional external cause code to identify the source, place and intent of the burn (X00-X19, X75-X77, X96-X98, Y92)

X● **T21.20**   Burn of second degree of trunk, unspecified site

X● **T21.21**   Burn of second degree of chest wall
Burn of second degree of breast

X● **T21.22**   Burn of second degree of abdominal wall
Burn of second degree of flank
Burn of second degree of groin

X● **T21.23 Burn of second degree of upper back**
Burn of second degree of interscapular region

X● **T21.24 Burn of second degree of lower back**

X● **T21.25 Burn of second degree of buttock**
Burn of second degree of anus

X● **T21.26 Burn of second degree of male genital region**
Burn of second degree of penis
Burn of second degree of scrotum
Burn of second degree of testis

X● **T21.27 Burn of second degree of female genital region**
Burn of second degree of labium (majus) (minus)
Burn of second degree of perineum
Burn of second degree of vulva

     Excludes2   burn of vagina (T28.3)

X● **T21.29 Burn of second degree of other site of trunk**

● **T21.3 Burn of third degree of trunk**
Use additional external cause code to identify the source, place and intent of the burn (X00-X19, X75-X77, X96-X98, Y92)

X● **T21.30 Burn of third degree of trunk, unspecified site**

X● **T21.31 Burn of third degree of chest wall**
Burn of third degree of breast
Coding Clinic: 2016, Q2, P6

X● **T21.32 Burn of third degree of abdominal wall**
Burn of third degree of flank
Burn of third degree of groin

X● **T21.33 Burn of third degree of upper back**
Burn of third degree of interscapular region

X● **T21.34 Burn of third degree of lower back**

X● **T21.35 Burn of third degree of buttock**
Burn of third degree of anus

X● **T21.36 Burn of third degree of male genital region**
Burn of third degree of penis
Burn of third degree of scrotum
Burn of third degree of testis

X● **T21.37 Burn of third degree of female genital region**
Burn of third degree of labium (majus) (minus)
Burn of third degree of perineum
Burn of third degree of vulva

     Excludes2   burn of vagina (T28.3)

X● **T21.39 Burn of third degree of other site of trunk**

● **T21.4 Corrosion of unspecified degree of trunk**
Code first (T51-T65) to identify chemical and intent
Use additional external cause code to identify place (Y92)

X● **T21.40 Corrosion of unspecified degree of trunk, unspecified site**

X● **T21.41 Corrosion of unspecified degree of chest wall**
Corrosion of unspecified degree of breast

X● **T21.42 Corrosion of unspecified degree of abdominal wall**
Corrosion of unspecified degree of flank
Corrosion of unspecified degree of groin

X● **T21.43 Corrosion of unspecified degree of upper back**
Corrosion of unspecified degree of interscapular region

X● **T21.44 Corrosion of unspecified degree of lower back**

X● **T21.45 Corrosion of unspecified degree of buttock**
Corrosion of unspecified degree of anus

X● **T21.46 Corrosion of unspecified degree of male genital region**
Corrosion of unspecified degree of penis
Corrosion of unspecified degree of scrotum
Corrosion of unspecified degree of testis

X● **T21.47 Corrosion of unspecified degree of female genital region**
Corrosion of unspecified degree of labium (majus) (minus)
Corrosion of unspecified degree of perineum
Corrosion of unspecified degree of vulva

     Excludes2   corrosion of vagina (T28.8)

X● **T21.49 Corrosion of unspecified degree of other site of trunk**

● **T21.5 Corrosion of first degree of trunk**
Code first (T51-T65) to identify chemical and intent
Use additional external cause code to identify place (Y92)

X● **T21.50 Corrosion of first degree of trunk, unspecified site**

X● **T21.51 Corrosion of first degree of chest wall**
Corrosion of first degree of breast

X● **T21.52 Corrosion of first degree of abdominal wall**
Corrosion of first degree of flank
Corrosion of first degree of groin

X● **T21.53 Corrosion of first degree of upper back**
Corrosion of first degree of interscapular region

X● **T21.54 Corrosion of first degree of lower back**

X● **T21.55 Corrosion of first degree of buttock**
Corrosion of first degree of anus

X● **T21.56 Corrosion of first degree of male genital region**
Corrosion of first degree of penis
Corrosion of first degree of scrotum
Corrosion of first degree of testis

X● **T21.57 Corrosion of first degree of female genital region**
Corrosion of first degree of labium (majus) (minus)
Corrosion of first degree of perineum
Corrosion of first degree of vulva

     Excludes2   corrosion of vagina (T28.8)

X● **T21.59 Corrosion of first degree of other site of trunk**

● **T21.6 Corrosion of second degree of trunk**
Code first (T51-T65) to identify chemical and intent
Use additional external cause code to identify place (Y92)

X● **T21.60 Corrosion of second degree of trunk, unspecified site**

X● **T21.61 Corrosion of second degree of chest wall**
Corrosion of second degree of breast

X● **T21.62 Corrosion of second degree of abdominal wall**
Corrosion of second degree of flank
Corrosion of second degree of groin

X● **T21.63 Corrosion of second degree of upper back**
Corrosion of second degree of interscapular region

X● **T21.64 Corrosion of second degree of lower back**

X● **T21.65 Corrosion of second degree of buttock**
Corrosion of second degree of anus

X● **T21.66 Corrosion of second degree of male genital region**
Corrosion of second degree of penis
Corrosion of second degree of scrotum
Corrosion of second degree of testis

X● **T21.67 Corrosion of second degree of female genital region**
Corrosion of second degree of labium (majus) (minus)
Corrosion of second degree of perineum
Corrosion of second degree of vulva

     Excludes2   corrosion of vagina (T28.8)

X● **T21.69 Corrosion of second degree of other site of trunk**

● **T21.7**   **Corrosion of third degree of trunk**
Code first (T51-T65) to identify chemical and intent
Use additional external cause code to identify place (Y92)

X ● **T21.70**   Corrosion of third degree of trunk, **unspecified site**

X ● **T21.71**   Corrosion of third degree of **chest wall**
Corrosion of third degree of breast

X ● **T21.72**   Corrosion of third degree of **abdominal wall**
Corrosion of third degree of flank
Corrosion of third degree of groin

X ● **T21.73**   Corrosion of third degree of **upper back**
Corrosion of third degree of interscapular region

X ● **T21.74**   Corrosion of third degree of **lower back**

X ● **T21.75**   Corrosion of third degree of **buttock**
Corrosion of third degree of anus

X ● **T21.76**   Corrosion of third degree of **male genital region**
Corrosion of third degree of penis
Corrosion of third degree of scrotum
Corrosion of third degree of testis

X ● **T21.77**   Corrosion of third degree of **female genital region**
Corrosion of third degree of labium (majus) (minus)
Corrosion of third degree of perineum
Corrosion of third degree of vulva
Excludes2   corrosion of vagina (T28.8)

X ● **T21.79**   Corrosion of third degree of **other site** of trunk

● **T22**   **Burn and corrosion of shoulder and upper limb, except wrist and hand**
Excludes2   burn and corrosion of interscapular region (T21.-)
burn and corrosion of wrist and hand (T23.-)

The appropriate 7th character is to be added to each code from category T22

A	initial encounter
D	subsequent encounter
S	sequela

● **T22.0**   **Burn of unspecified degree of shoulder and upper limb, except wrist and hand**
Use additional external cause code to identify the source, place and intent of the burn (X00-X19, X75-X77, X96-X98, Y92)

X ● **T22.00**   Burn of unspecified degree of shoulder and upper limb, except wrist and hand, **unspecified site**

● **T22.01**   Burn of unspecified degree of **forearm**
● **T22.011**   Burn of unspecified degree of **right** forearm
● **T22.012**   Burn of unspecified degree of **left** forearm
● **T22.019**   Burn of unspecified degree of **unspecified** forearm

● **T22.02**   Burn of unspecified degree of **elbow**
● **T22.021**   Burn of unspecified degree of **right** elbow
● **T22.022**   Burn of unspecified degree of **left** elbow
● **T22.029**   Burn of unspecified degree of **unspecified** elbow

● **T22.03**   Burn of unspecified degree of **upper arm**
● **T22.031**   Burn of unspecified degree of **right** upper arm
● **T22.032**   Burn of unspecified degree of **left** upper arm
● **T22.039**   Burn of unspecified degree of **unspecified** upper arm

● **T22.04**   Burn of unspecified degree of **axilla**
● **T22.041**   Burn of unspecified degree of **right** axilla
● **T22.042**   Burn of unspecified degree of **left** axilla
● **T22.049**   Burn of unspecified degree of **unspecified** axilla

● **T22.05**   Burn of unspecified degree of **shoulder**
● **T22.051**   Burn of unspecified degree of **right** shoulder
● **T22.052**   Burn of unspecified degree of **left** shoulder
● **T22.059**   Burn of unspecified degree of **unspecified** shoulder

● **T22.06**   Burn of unspecified degree of **scapular region**
● **T22.061**   Burn of unspecified degree of **right** scapular region
● **T22.062**   Burn of unspecified degree of **left** scapular region
● **T22.069**   Burn of unspecified degree of **unspecified** scapular region

● **T22.09**   Burn of unspecified degree of **multiple sites** of shoulder and upper limb, except wrist and hand
● **T22.091**   Burn of unspecified degree of multiple sites of **right** shoulder and upper limb, except wrist and hand
● **T22.092**   Burn of unspecified degree of multiple sites of **left** shoulder and upper limb, except wrist and hand
● **T22.099**   Burn of unspecified degree of multiple sites of **unspecified** shoulder and upper limb, except wrist and hand

● **T22.1**   **Burn of first degree of shoulder and upper limb, except wrist and hand**
Use additional external cause code to identify the source, place and intent of the burn (X00-X19, X75-X77, X96-X98, Y92)

X ● **T22.10**   Burn of first degree of shoulder and upper limb, except wrist and hand, **unspecified site**

● **T22.11**   Burn of first degree of **forearm**
● **T22.111**   Burn of first degree of **right** forearm
● **T22.112**   Burn of first degree of **left** forearm
● **T22.119**   Burn of first degree of **unspecified** forearm

● **T22.12**   Burn of first degree of **elbow**
● **T22.121**   Burn of first degree of **right** elbow
● **T22.122**   Burn of first degree of **left** elbow
● **T22.129**   Burn of first degree of **unspecified** elbow

● **T22.13**   Burn of first degree of **upper arm**
● **T22.131**   Burn of first degree of **right** upper arm
● **T22.132**   Burn of first degree of **left** upper arm
● **T22.139**   Burn of first degree of **unspecified** upper arm

● **T22.14**   Burn of first degree of **axilla**
● **T22.141**   Burn of first degree of **right** axilla
● **T22.142**   Burn of first degree of **left** axilla
● **T22.149**   Burn of first degree of **unspecified** axilla

● **T22.15**   Burn of first degree of **shoulder**
● **T22.151**   Burn of first degree of **right** shoulder
● **T22.152**   Burn of first degree of **left** shoulder
● **T22.159**   Burn of first degree of **unspecified** shoulder

CHAPTER 19 (S00-T88)

CHAPTER 19 (S00-T88)

- ● T22.16   Burn of first degree of scapular region
  - ● T22.161   Burn of first degree of right scapular region
  - ● T22.162   Burn of first degree of left scapular region
  - ● T22.169   Burn of first degree of unspecified scapular region
- ● T22.19   Burn of first degree of multiple sites of shoulder and upper limb, except wrist and hand
  - ● T22.191   Burn of first degree of multiple sites of right shoulder and upper limb, except wrist and hand
  - ● T22.192   Burn of first degree of multiple sites of left shoulder and upper limb, except wrist and hand
  - ● T22.199   Burn of first degree of multiple sites of unspecified shoulder and upper limb, except wrist and hand
- ● T22.2   Burn of second degree of shoulder and upper limb, except wrist and hand

  Use additional external cause code to identify the source, place and intent of the burn (X00-X19, X75-X77, X96-X98, Y92)
  - X ● T22.20   Burn of second degree of shoulder and upper limb, except wrist and hand, unspecified site
  - ● T22.21   Burn of second degree of forearm
    - ● T22.211   Burn of second degree of right forearm
    - ● T22.212   Burn of second degree of left forearm
    - ● T22.219   Burn of second degree of unspecified forearm
  - ● T22.22   Burn of second degree of elbow
    - ● T22.221   Burn of second degree of right elbow
    - ● T22.222   Burn of second degree of left elbow
    - ● T22.229   Burn of second degree of unspecified elbow
  - ● T22.23   Burn of second degree of upper arm
    - ● T22.231   Burn of second degree of right upper arm
    - ● T22.232   Burn of second degree of left upper arm
    - ● T22.239   Burn of second degree of unspecified upper arm
  - ● T22.24   Burn of second degree of axilla
    - ● T22.241   Burn of second degree of right axilla
    - ● T22.242   Burn of second degree of left axilla
    - ● T22.249   Burn of second degree of unspecified axilla
  - ● T22.25   Burn of second degree of shoulder
    - ● T22.251   Burn of second degree of right shoulder
    - ● T22.252   Burn of second degree of left shoulder
    - ● T22.259   Burn of second degree of unspecified shoulder
  - ● T22.26   Burn of second degree of scapular region
    - ● T22.261   Burn of second degree of right scapular region
    - ● T22.262   Burn of second degree of left scapular region
    - ● T22.269   Burn of second degree of unspecified scapular region
  - ● T22.29   Burn of second degree of multiple sites of shoulder and upper limb, except wrist and hand
    - ● T22.291   Burn of second degree of multiple sites of right shoulder and upper limb, except wrist and hand

- ● T22.292   Burn of second degree of multiple sites of left shoulder and upper limb, except wrist and hand
- ● T22.299   Burn of second degree of multiple sites of unspecified shoulder and upper limb, except wrist and hand
- ● T22.3   Burn of third degree of shoulder and upper limb, except wrist and hand

  Use additional external cause code to identify the source, place and intent of the burn (X00-X19, X75-X77, X96-X98, Y92)
  - X ● T22.30   Burn of third degree of shoulder and upper limb, except wrist and hand, unspecified site
  - ● T22.31   Burn of third degree of forearm
    - ● T22.311   Burn of third degree of right forearm
    - ● T22.312   Burn of third degree of left forearm
    - ● T22.319   Burn of third degree of unspecified forearm
  - ● T22.32   Burn of third degree of elbow
    - ● T22.321   Burn of third degree of right elbow
    - ● T22.322   Burn of third degree of left elbow
    - ● T22.329   Burn of third degree of unspecified elbow
  - ● T22.33   Burn of third degree of upper arm
    - ● T22.331   Burn of third degree of right upper arm
    - ● T22.332   Burn of third degree of left upper arm
    - ● T22.339   Burn of third degree of unspecified upper arm
  - ● T22.34   Burn of third degree of axilla
    - ● T22.341   Burn of third degree of right axilla
    - ● T22.342   Burn of third degree of left axilla
    - ● T22.349   Burn of third degree of unspecified axilla
  - ● T22.35   Burn of third degree of shoulder
    - ● T22.351   Burn of third degree of right shoulder
    - ● T22.352   Burn of third degree of left shoulder
    - ● T22.359   Burn of third degree of unspecified shoulder
  - ● T22.36   Burn of third degree of scapular region
    - ● T22.361   Burn of third degree of right scapular region
    - ● T22.362   Burn of third degree of left scapular region
    - ● T22.369   Burn of third degree of unspecified scapular region
  - ● T22.39   Burn of third degree of multiple sites of shoulder and upper limb, except wrist and hand
    - ● T22.391   Burn of third degree of multiple sites of right shoulder and upper limb, except wrist and hand
    - ● T22.392   Burn of third degree of multiple sites of left shoulder and upper limb, except wrist and hand
    - ● T22.399   Burn of third degree of multiple sites of unspecified shoulder and upper limb, except wrist and hand
- ● T22.4   Corrosion of unspecified degree of shoulder and upper limb, except wrist and hand

  Code first (T51-T65) to identify chemical and intent

  Use additional external cause code to identify place (Y92)
  - X ● T22.40   Corrosion of unspecified degree of shoulder and upper limb, except wrist and hand, unspecified site
  - ● T22.41   Corrosion of unspecified degree of forearm
    - ● T22.411   Corrosion of unspecified degree of right forearm

▶ New   ⇒ Revised   ~~deleted~~ Deleted   Excludes 1   Excludes 2   Includes   Use additional   Code first   Code also   Key words

OGCR Official Guidelines   X Assign placeholder X   ● Use Additional Character(s)   ▶ Manifestation Code   ℗ Hierarchical Condition Category   Coding Clinic

● T22.412   Corrosion of unspecified degree of left forearm

● T22.419   Corrosion of unspecified degree of unspecified forearm

● T22.42   Corrosion of unspecified degree of elbow

   ● T22.421   Corrosion of unspecified degree of right elbow

   ● T22.422   Corrosion of unspecified degree of left elbow

   ● T22.429   Corrosion of unspecified degree of unspecified elbow

● T22.43   Corrosion of unspecified degree of upper arm

   ● T22.431   Corrosion of unspecified degree of right upper arm

   ● T22.432   Corrosion of unspecified degree of left upper arm

   ● T22.439   Corrosion of unspecified degree of unspecified upper arm

● T22.44   Corrosion of unspecified degree of axilla

   ● T22.441   Corrosion of unspecified degree of right axilla

   ● T22.442   Corrosion of unspecified degree of left axilla

   ● T22.449   Corrosion of unspecified degree of unspecified axilla

● T22.45   Corrosion of unspecified degree of shoulder

   ● T22.451   Corrosion of unspecified degree of right shoulder

   ● T22.452   Corrosion of unspecified degree of left shoulder

   ● T22.459   Corrosion of unspecified degree of unspecified shoulder

● T22.46   Corrosion of unspecified degree of scapular region

   ● T22.461   Corrosion of unspecified degree of right scapular region

   ● T22.462   Corrosion of unspecified degree of left scapular region

   ● T22.469   Corrosion of unspecified degree of unspecified scapular region

● T22.49   Corrosion of unspecified degree of multiple sites of shoulder and upper limb, except wrist and hand

   ● T22.491   Corrosion of unspecified degree of multiple sites of right shoulder and upper limb, except wrist and hand

   ● T22.492   Corrosion of unspecified degree of multiple sites of left shoulder and upper limb, except wrist and hand

   ● T22.499   Corrosion of unspecified degree of multiple sites of unspecified shoulder and upper limb, except wrist and hand

● T22.5   Corrosion of first degree of shoulder and upper limb, except wrist and hand

   Code first (T51-T65) *to identify chemical and intent*

   Use additional external cause code to identify place (Y92)

X ● T22.50   Corrosion of first degree of shoulder and upper limb, except wrist and hand unspecified site

● T22.51   Corrosion of first degree of forearm

   ● T22.511   Corrosion of first degree of right forearm

   ● T22.512   Corrosion of first degree of left forearm

   ● T22.519   Corrosion of first degree of unspecified forearm

● T22.52   Corrosion of first degree of elbow

   ● T22.521   Corrosion of first degree of right elbow

   ● T22.522   Corrosion of first degree of left elbow

   ● T22.529   Corrosion of first degree of unspecified elbow

● T22.53   Corrosion of first degree of upper arm

   ● T22.531   Corrosion of first degree of right upper arm

   ● T22.532   Corrosion of first degree of left upper arm

   ● T22.539   Corrosion of first degree of unspecified upper arm

● T22.54   Corrosion of first degree of axilla

   ● T22.541   Corrosion of first degree of right axilla

   ● T22.542   Corrosion of first degree of left axilla

   ● T22.549   Corrosion of first degree of unspecified axilla

● T22.55   Corrosion of first degree of shoulder

   ● T22.551   Corrosion of first degree of right shoulder

   ● T22.552   Corrosion of first degree of left shoulder

   ● T22.559   Corrosion of first degree of unspecified shoulder

● T22.56   Corrosion of first degree of scapular region

   ● T22.561   Corrosion of first degree of right scapular region

   ● T22.562   Corrosion of first degree of left scapular region

   ● T22.569   Corrosion of first degree of unspecified scapular region

● T22.59   Corrosion of first degree of multiple sites of shoulder and upper limb, except wrist and hand

   ● T22.591   Corrosion of first degree of multiple sites of right shoulder and upper limb, except wrist and hand

   ● T22.592   Corrosion of first degree of multiple sites of left shoulder and upper limb, except wrist and hand

   ● T22.599   Corrosion of first degree of multiple sites of unspecified shoulder and upper limb, except wrist and hand

● T22.6   Corrosion of second degree of shoulder and upper limb, except wrist and hand

   Code first (T51-T65) *to identify chemical and intent*

   Use additional external cause code to identify place (Y92)

X ● T22.60   Corrosion of second degree of shoulder and upper limb, except wrist and hand, unspecified site

● T22.61   Corrosion of second degree of forearm

   ● T22.611   Corrosion of second degree of right forearm

   ● T22.612   Corrosion of second degree of left forearm

   ● T22.619   Corrosion of second degree of unspecified forearm

● T22.62   Corrosion of second degree of elbow

   ● T22.621   Corrosion of second degree of right elbow

   ● T22.622   Corrosion of second degree of left elbow

   ● T22.629   Corrosion of second degree of unspecified elbow

● T22.63   Corrosion of second degree of upper arm

   ● T22.631   Corrosion of second degree of right upper arm

● T22.632   Corrosion of second degree of left upper arm

● T22.639   Corrosion of second degree of unspecified upper arm

● T22.64   Corrosion of second degree of axilla

  ● T22.641   Corrosion of second degree of right axilla

  ● T22.642   Corrosion of second degree of left axilla

  ● T22.649   Corrosion of second degree of unspecified axilla

● T22.65   Corrosion of second degree of shoulder

  ● T22.651   Corrosion of second degree of right shoulder

  ● T22.652   Corrosion of second degree of left shoulder

  ● T22.659   Corrosion of second degree of unspecified shoulder

● T22.66   Corrosion of second degree of scapular region

  ● T22.661   Corrosion of second degree of right scapular region

  ● T22.662   Corrosion of second degree of left scapular region

  ● T22.669   Corrosion of second degree of unspecified scapular region

● T22.69   Corrosion of second degree of multiple sites of shoulder and upper limb, except wrist and hand

  ● T22.691   Corrosion of second degree of multiple sites of right shoulder and upper limb, except wrist and hand

  ● T22.692   Corrosion of second degree of multiple sites of left shoulder and upper limb, except wrist and hand

  ● T22.699   Corrosion of second degree of multiple sites of unspecified shoulder and upper limb, except wrist and hand

● T22.7   Corrosion of third degree of shoulder and upper limb, except wrist and hand

  Code first (T51-T65) to identify chemical and intent

  Use additional external cause code to identify place (Y92)

X ● T22.70   Corrosion of third degree of shoulder and upper limb, except wrist and hand, unspecified site

● T22.71   Corrosion of third degree of forearm

  ● T22.711   Corrosion of third degree of right forearm

  ● T22.712   Corrosion of third degree of left forearm

  ● T22.719   Corrosion of third degree of unspecified forearm

● T22.72   Corrosion of third degree of elbow

  ● T22.721   Corrosion of third degree of right elbow

  ● T22.722   Corrosion of third degree of left elbow

  ● T22.729   Corrosion of third degree of unspecified elbow

● T22.73   Corrosion of third degree of upper arm

  ● T22.731   Corrosion of third degree of right upper arm

  ● T22.732   Corrosion of third degree of left upper arm

  ● T22.739   Corrosion of third degree of unspecified upper arm

● T22.74   Corrosion of third degree of axilla

  ● T22.741   Corrosion of third degree of right axilla

  ● T22.742   Corrosion of third degree of left axilla

  ● T22.749   Corrosion of third degree of unspecified axilla

● T22.75   Corrosion of third degree of shoulder

  ● T22.751   Corrosion of third degree of right shoulder

  ● T22.752   Corrosion of third degree of left shoulder

  ● T22.759   Corrosion of third degree of unspecified shoulder

● T22.76   Corrosion of third degree of scapular region

  ● T22.761   Corrosion of third degree of right scapular region

  ● T22.762   Corrosion of third degree of left scapular region

  ● T22.769   Corrosion of third degree of unspecified scapular region

● T22.79   Corrosion of third degree of multiple sites of shoulder and upper limb, except wrist and hand

  ● T22.791   Corrosion of third degree of multiple sites of right shoulder and upper limb, except wrist and hand

  ● T22.792   Corrosion of third degree of multiple sites of left shoulder and upper limb, except wrist and hand

  ● T22.799   Corrosion of third degree of multiple sites of unspecified shoulder and upper limb, except wrist and hand

● T23   Burn and corrosion of wrist and hand

  The appropriate 7th character is to be added to each code from category T23

A	initial encounter
D	subsequent encounter
S	sequela

● T23.0   Burn of unspecified degree of wrist and hand

  Use additional external cause code to identify the source, place and intent of the burn (X00-X19, X75-X77, X96-X98, Y92)

● T23.00   Burn of unspecified degree of hand, unspecified site

  ● T23.001   Burn of unspecified degree of right hand, unspecified site

  ● T23.002   Burn of unspecified degree of left hand, unspecified site

  ● T23.009   Burn of unspecified degree of unspecified hand, unspecified site

● T23.01   Burn of unspecified degree of thumb (nail)

  ● T23.011   Burn of unspecified degree of right thumb (nail)

  ● T23.012   Burn of unspecified degree of left thumb (nail)

  ● T23.019   Burn of unspecified degree of unspecified thumb (nail)

● T23.02   Burn of unspecified degree of single finger (nail) except thumb

  ● T23.021   Burn of unspecified degree of single right finger (nail) except thumb

  ● T23.022   Burn of unspecified degree of single left finger (nail) except thumb

  ● T23.029   Burn of unspecified degree of unspecified single finger (nail) except thumb

● T23.03   Burn of unspecified degree of multiple fingers (nail), not including thumb

  ● T23.031   Burn of unspecified degree of multiple right fingers (nail), not including thumb

▶ New   ⇒ Revised   ~~deleted~~ Deleted   Excludes 1   Excludes 2   Includes   Use additional   Code first   Code also   Key words

OGCR Official Guidelines   X Assign placeholder X   ● Use Additional Character(s)   ▶ Manifestation Code   Hierarchical Condition Category   Coding Clinic

● T23.032   Burn of unspecified degree of multiple left fingers (nail), not including thumb

● T23.039   Burn of unspecified degree of unspecified multiple fingers (nail), not including thumb

● T23.04   Burn of unspecified degree of multiple fingers (nail), including thumb

    ● T23.041   Burn of unspecified degree of multiple right fingers (nail), including thumb

    ● T23.042   Burn of unspecified degree of multiple left fingers (nail), including thumb

    ● T23.049   Burn of unspecified degree of unspecified multiple fingers (nail), including thumb

● T23.05   Burn of unspecified degree of palm

    ● T23.051   Burn of unspecified degree of right palm

    ● T23.052   Burn of unspecified degree of left palm

    ● T23.059   Burn of unspecified degree of unspecified palm

● T23.06   Burn of unspecified degree of back of hand

    ● T23.061   Burn of unspecified degree of back of right hand

    ● T23.062   Burn of unspecified degree of back of left hand

    ● T23.069   Burn of unspecified degree of back of unspecified hand

● T23.07   Burn of unspecified degree of wrist

    ● T23.071   Burn of unspecified degree of right wrist

    ● T23.072   Burn of unspecified degree of left wrist

    ● T23.079   Burn of unspecified degree of unspecified wrist

● T23.09   Burn of unspecified degree of multiple sites of wrist and hand

    ● T23.091   Burn of unspecified degree of multiple sites of right wrist and hand

    ● T23.092   Burn of unspecified degree of multiple sites of left wrist and hand

    ● T23.099   Burn of unspecified degree of multiple sites of unspecified wrist and hand

● T23.1   Burn of first degree of wrist and hand

    Use additional external cause code to identify the source, place and intent of the burn (X00-X19, X75-X77, X96-X98, Y92)

    ● T23.10   Burn of first degree of hand, unspecified site

      ● T23.101   Burn of first degree of right hand, unspecified site

      ● T23.102   Burn of first degree of left hand, unspecified site

      ● T23.109   Burn of first degree of unspecified hand, unspecified site

    ● T23.11   Burn of first degree of thumb (nail)

      ● T23.111   Burn of first degree of right thumb (nail)

      ● T23.112   Burn of first degree of left thumb (nail)

      ● T23.119   Burn of first degree of unspecified thumb (nail)

    ● T23.12   Burn of first degree of single finger (nail) except thumb

      ● T23.121   Burn of first degree of single right finger (nail) except thumb

      ● T23.122   Burn of first degree of single left finger (nail) except thumb

      ● T23.129   Burn of first degree of unspecified single finger (nail) except thumb

    ● T23.13   Burn of first degree of multiple fingers (nail), not including thumb

      ● T23.131   Burn of first degree of multiple right fingers (nail), not including thumb

      ● T23.132   Burn of first degree of multiple left fingers (nail), not including thumb

      ● T23.139   Burn of first degree of unspecified multiple fingers (nail), not including thumb

    ● T23.14   Burn of first degree of multiple fingers (nail), including thumb

      ● T23.141   Burn of first degree of multiple right fingers (nail), including thumb

      ● T23.142   Burn of first degree of multiple left fingers (nail), including thumb

      ● T23.149   Burn of first degree of unspecified multiple fingers (nail), including thumb

    ● T23.15   Burn of first degree of palm

      ● T23.151   Burn of first degree of right palm

      ● T23.152   Burn of first degree of left palm

      ● T23.159   Burn of first degree of unspecified palm

    ● T23.16   Burn of first degree of back of hand

      ● T23.161   Burn of first degree of back of right hand

      ● T23.162   Burn of first degree of back of left hand

      ● T23.169   Burn of first degree of back of unspecified hand

    ● T23.17   Burn of first degree of wrist

      ● T23.171   Burn of first degree of right wrist

      ● T23.172   Burn of first degree of left wrist

      ● T23.179   Burn of first degree of unspecified wrist

    ● T23.19   Burn of first degree of multiple sites of wrist and hand

      ● T23.191   Burn of first degree of multiple sites of right wrist and hand

      ● T23.192   Burn of first degree of multiple sites of left wrist and hand

      ● T23.199   Burn of first degree of multiple sites of unspecified wrist and hand

● T23.2   Burn of second degree of wrist and hand

    Use additional external cause code to identify the source, place and intent of the burn (X00-X19, X75-X77, X96-X98, Y92)

    ● T23.20   Burn of second degree of hand, unspecified site

      ● T23.201   Burn of second degree of right hand, unspecified site

      ● T23.202   Burn of second degree of left hand, unspecified site

      ● T23.209   Burn of second degree of unspecified hand, unspecified site

    ● T23.21   Burn of second degree of thumb (nail)

      ● T23.211   Burn of second degree of right thumb (nail)

      ● T23.212   Burn of second degree of left thumb (nail)

      ● T23.219   Burn of second degree of unspecified thumb (nail)

    ● T23.22   Burn of second degree of single finger (nail) except thumb

      ● T23.221   Burn of second degree of single right finger (nail) except thumb

CHAPTER 19 (S00-T88)

- T23.222   Burn of second degree of single left finger (nail) except thumb
  - T23.229   Burn of second degree of unspecified single finger (nail) except thumb
- T23.23   Burn of second degree of multiple fingers (nail), not including thumb
  - T23.231   Burn of second degree of multiple right fingers (nail), not including thumb
  - T23.232   Burn of second degree of multiple left fingers (nail), not including thumb
  - T23.239   Burn of second degree of unspecified multiple fingers (nail), not including thumb
- T23.24   Burn of second degree of multiple fingers (nail), including thumb
  - T23.241   Burn of second degree of multiple right fingers (nail), including thumb
  - T23.242   Burn of second degree of multiple left fingers (nail), including thumb
  - T23.249   Burn of second degree of unspecified multiple fingers (nail), including thumb
- T23.25   Burn of second degree of palm
  - T23.251   Burn of second degree of right palm
  - T23.252   Burn of second degree of left palm
  - T23.259   Burn of second degree of unspecified palm
- T23.26   Burn of second degree of back of hand
  - T23.261   Burn of second degree of back of right hand
  - T23.262   Burn of second degree of back of left hand
  - T23.269   Burn of second degree of back of unspecified hand
- T23.27   Burn of second degree of wrist
  - T23.271   Burn of second degree of right wrist
  - T23.272   Burn of second degree of left wrist
  - T23.279   Burn of second degree of unspecified wrist
- T23.29   Burn of second degree of multiple sites of wrist and hand
  - T23.291   Burn of second degree of multiple sites of right wrist and hand
  - T23.292   Burn of second degree of multiple sites of left wrist and hand
  - T23.299   Burn of second degree of multiple sites of unspecified wrist and hand
- T23.3   Burn of third degree of wrist and hand

  Use additional external cause code to identify the source, place and intent of the burn (X00-X19, X75-X77, X96-X98, Y92)

  - T23.30   Burn of third degree of hand, unspecified site
    - T23.301   Burn of third degree of right hand, unspecified site

      Coding Clinic: 2015, Q1, P19
    - T23.302   Burn of third degree of left hand, unspecified site

      Coding Clinic: 2016, Q2, P5
    - T23.309   Burn of third degree of unspecified hand, unspecified site
  - T23.31   Burn of third degree of thumb (nail)
    - T23.311   Burn of third degree of right thumb (nail)
    - T23.312   Burn of third degree of left thumb (nail)
    - T23.319   Burn of third degree of unspecified thumb (nail)

- T23.32   Burn of third degree of single finger (nail) except thumb
  - T23.321   Burn of third degree of single right finger (nail) except thumb
  - T23.322   Burn of third degree of single left finger (nail) except thumb
  - T23.329   Burn of third degree of unspecified single finger (nail) except thumb
- T23.33   Burn of third degree of multiple fingers (nail), not including thumb
  - T23.331   Burn of third degree of multiple right fingers (nail), not including thumb
  - T23.332   Burn of third degree of multiple left fingers (nail), not including thumb
  - T23.339   Burn of third degree of unspecified multiple fingers (nail), not including thumb
- T23.34   Burn of third degree of multiple fingers (nail), including thumb
  - T23.341   Burn of third degree of multiple right fingers (nail), including thumb
  - T23.342   Burn of third degree of multiple left fingers (nail), including thumb
  - T23.349   Burn of third degree of unspecified multiple fingers (nail), including thumb
- T23.35   Burn of third degree of palm
  - T23.351   Burn of third degree of right palm
  - T23.352   Burn of third degree of left palm
  - T23.359   Burn of third degree of unspecified palm
- T23.36   Burn of third degree of back of hand
  - T23.361   Burn of third degree of back of right hand
  - T23.362   Burn of third degree of back of left hand
  - T23.369   Burn of third degree of back of unspecified hand
- T23.37   Burn of third degree of wrist
  - T23.371   Burn of third degree of right wrist
  - T23.372   Burn of third degree of left wrist
  - T23.379   Burn of third degree of unspecified wrist
- T23.39   Burn of third degree of multiple sites of wrist and hand
  - T23.391   Burn of third degree of multiple sites of right wrist and hand
  - T23.392   Burn of third degree of multiple sites of left wrist and hand
  - T23.399   Burn of third degree of multiple sites of unspecified wrist and hand
- T23.4   Corrosion of unspecified degree of wrist and hand

  Code first (T51-T65) to identify chemical and intent

  Use additional external cause code to identify place (Y92)

  - T23.40   Corrosion of unspecified degree of hand, unspecified site
    - T23.401   Corrosion of unspecified degree of right hand, unspecified site
    - T23.402   Corrosion of unspecified degree of left hand, unspecified site
    - T23.409   Corrosion of unspecified degree of unspecified hand, unspecified site
  - T23.41   Corrosion of unspecified degree of thumb (nail)
    - T23.411   Corrosion of unspecified degree of right thumb (nail)
    - T23.412   Corrosion of unspecified degree of left thumb (nail)
    - T23.419   Corrosion of unspecified degree of unspecified thumb (nail)

▶ New   ⇒ Revised   ~~deleted~~ Deleted   Excludes 1   Excludes 2   Includes   Use additional   Code first   Code also   Key words

OGCR Official Guidelines   X Assign placeholder X   ● Use Additional Character(s)   ▶ Manifestation Code   🔖 Hierarchical Condition Category   Coding Clinic

● **T23.42**   Corrosion of unspecified degree of single finger (nail) except thumb
  ● **T23.421**   Corrosion of unspecified degree of single right finger (nail) except thumb
  ● **T23.422**   Corrosion of unspecified degree of single left finger (nail) except thumb
  ● **T23.429**   Corrosion of unspecified degree of unspecified single finger (nail) except thumb

● **T23.43**   Corrosion of unspecified degree of multiple fingers (nail), not including thumb
  ● **T23.431**   Corrosion of unspecified degree of multiple right fingers (nail), not including thumb
  ● **T23.432**   Corrosion of unspecified degree of multiple left fingers (nail), not including thumb
  ● **T23.439**   Corrosion of unspecified degree of unspecified multiple fingers (nail), not including thumb

● **T23.44**   Corrosion of unspecified degree of multiple fingers (nail), including thumb
  ● **T23.441**   Corrosion of unspecified degree of multiple right fingers (nail), including thumb
  ● **T23.442**   Corrosion of unspecified degree of multiple left fingers (nail), including thumb
  ● **T23.449**   Corrosion of unspecified degree of unspecified multiple fingers (nail), including thumb

● **T23.45**   Corrosion of unspecified degree of palm
  ● **T23.451**   Corrosion of unspecified degree of right palm
  ● **T23.452**   Corrosion of unspecified degree of left palm
  ● **T23.459**   Corrosion of unspecified degree of unspecified palm

● **T23.46**   Corrosion of unspecified degree of back of hand
  ● **T23.461**   Corrosion of unspecified degree of back of right hand
  ● **T23.462**   Corrosion of unspecified degree of back of left hand
  ● **T23.469**   Corrosion of unspecified degree of back of unspecified hand

● **T23.47**   Corrosion of unspecified degree of wrist
  ● **T23.471**   Corrosion of unspecified degree of right wrist
  ● **T23.472**   Corrosion of unspecified degree of left wrist
  ● **T23.479**   Corrosion of unspecified degree of unspecified wrist

● **T23.49**   Corrosion of unspecified degree of multiple sites of wrist and hand
  ● **T23.491**   Corrosion of unspecified degree of multiple sites of right wrist and hand
  ● **T23.492**   Corrosion of unspecified degree of multiple sites of left wrist and hand
  ● **T23.499**   Corrosion of unspecified degree of multiple sites of unspecified wrist and hand

● **T23.5**   Corrosion of first degree of wrist and hand
  Code first (T51-T65) to identify chemical and intent
  Use additional external cause code to identify place (Y92)
  ● **T23.50**   Corrosion of first degree of hand, unspecified site
    ● **T23.501**   Corrosion of first degree of right hand, unspecified site
    ● **T23.502**   Corrosion of first degree of left hand, unspecified site

● **T23.509**   Corrosion of first degree of unspecified hand, unspecified site
● **T23.51**   Corrosion of first degree of thumb (nail)
  ● **T23.511**   Corrosion of first degree of right thumb (nail)
  ● **T23.512**   Corrosion of first degree of left thumb (nail)
  ● **T23.519**   Corrosion of first degree of unspecified thumb (nail)

● **T23.52**   Corrosion of first degree of single finger (nail) except thumb
  ● **T23.521**   Corrosion of first degree of single right finger (nail) except thumb
  ● **T23.522**   Corrosion of first degree of single left finger (nail) except thumb
  ● **T23.529**   Corrosion of first degree of unspecified single finger (nail) except thumb

● **T23.53**   Corrosion of first degree of multiple fingers (nail), not including thumb
  ● **T23.531**   Corrosion of first degree of multiple right fingers (nail), not including thumb
  ● **T23.532**   Corrosion of first degree of multiple left fingers (nail), not including thumb
  ● **T23.539**   Corrosion of first degree of unspecified multiple fingers (nail), not including thumb

● **T23.54**   Corrosion of first degree of multiple fingers (nail), including thumb
  ● **T23.541**   Corrosion of first degree of multiple right fingers (nail), including thumb
  ● **T23.542**   Corrosion of first degree of multiple left fingers (nail), including thumb
  ● **T23.549**   Corrosion of first degree of unspecified multiple fingers (nail), including thumb

● **T23.55**   Corrosion of first degree of palm
  ● **T23.551**   Corrosion of first degree of right palm
  ● **T23.552**   Corrosion of first degree of left palm
  ● **T23.559**   Corrosion of first degree of unspecified palm

● **T23.56**   Corrosion of first degree of back of hand
  ● **T23.561**   Corrosion of first degree of back of right hand
  ● **T23.562**   Corrosion of first degree of back of left hand
  ● **T23.569**   Corrosion of first degree of back of unspecified hand

● **T23.57**   Corrosion of first degree of wrist
  ● **T23.571**   Corrosion of first degree of right wrist
  ● **T23.572**   Corrosion of first degree of left wrist
  ● **T23.579**   Corrosion of first degree of unspecified wrist

● **T23.59**   Corrosion of first degree of multiple sites of wrist and hand
  ● **T23.591**   Corrosion of first degree of multiple sites of right wrist and hand
  ● **T23.592**   Corrosion of first degree of multiple sites of left wrist and hand
  ● **T23.599**   Corrosion of first degree of multiple sites of unspecified wrist and hand

● **T23.6**   Corrosion of second degree of wrist and hand
  Code first (T51-T65) to identify chemical and intent
  Use additional external cause code to identify place (Y92)
  ● **T23.60**   Corrosion of second degree of hand, unspecified site
    ● **T23.601**   Corrosion of second degree of right hand, unspecified site

● T23.602   Corrosion of second degree of left hand, unspecified site

● T23.609   Corrosion of second degree of unspecified hand, unspecified site

● T23.61   Corrosion of second degree of thumb (nail)

● T23.611   Corrosion of second degree of right thumb (nail)

● T23.612   Corrosion of second degree of left thumb (nail)

● T23.619   Corrosion of second degree of unspecified thumb (nail)

● T23.62   Corrosion of second degree of single finger (nail) except thumb

● T23.621   Corrosion of second degree of single right finger (nail) except thumb

● T23.622   Corrosion of second degree of single left finger (nail) except thumb

● T23.629   Corrosion of second degree of unspecified single finger (nail) except thumb

● T23.63   Corrosion of second degree of multiple fingers (nail), not including thumb

● T23.631   Corrosion of second degree of multiple right fingers (nail), not including thumb

● T23.632   Corrosion of second degree of multiple left fingers (nail), not including thumb

● T23.639   Corrosion of second degree of unspecified multiple fingers (nail), not including thumb

● T23.64   Corrosion of second degree of multiple fingers (nail), including thumb

● T23.641   Corrosion of second degree of multiple right fingers (nail), including thumb

● T23.642   Corrosion of second degree of multiple left fingers (nail), including thumb

● T23.649   Corrosion of second degree of unspecified multiple fingers (nail), including thumb

● T23.65   Corrosion of second degree of palm

● T23.651   Corrosion of second degree of right palm

● T23.652   Corrosion of second degree of left palm

● T23.659   Corrosion of second degree of unspecified palm

● T23.66   Corrosion of second degree of back of hand

● T23.661   Corrosion of second degree back of right hand

● T23.662   Corrosion of second degree back of left hand

● T23.669   Corrosion of second degree back of unspecified hand

● T23.67   Corrosion of second degree of wrist

● T23.671   Corrosion of second degree of right wrist

● T23.672   Corrosion of second degree of left wrist

● T23.679   Corrosion of second degree of unspecified wrist

● T23.69   Corrosion of second degree of multiple sites of wrist and hand

● T23.691   Corrosion of second degree of multiple sites of right wrist and hand

● T23.692   Corrosion of second degree of multiple sites of left wrist and hand

● T23.699   Corrosion of second degree of multiple sites of unspecified wrist and hand

● T23.7   Corrosion of third degree of wrist and hand

Code first (T51-T65) to identify chemical and intent

Use additional external cause code to identify place (Y92)

● T23.70   Corrosion of third degree of hand, unspecified site

● T23.701   Corrosion of third degree of right hand, unspecified site

● T23.702   Corrosion of third degree of left hand, unspecified site

● T23.709   Corrosion of third degree of unspecified hand, unspecified site

● T23.71   Corrosion of third degree of thumb (nail)

● T23.711   Corrosion of third degree of right thumb (nail)

● T23.712   Corrosion of third degree of left thumb (nail)

● T23.719   Corrosion of third degree of unspecified thumb (nail)

● T23.72   Corrosion of third degree of single finger (nail) except thumb

● T23.721   Corrosion of third degree of single right finger (nail) except thumb

● T23.722   Corrosion of third degree of single left finger (nail) except thumb

● T23.729   Corrosion of third degree of unspecified single finger (nail) except thumb

● T23.73   Corrosion of third degree of multiple fingers (nail), not including thumb

● T23.731   Corrosion of third degree of multiple right fingers (nail), not including thumb

● T23.732   Corrosion of third degree of multiple left fingers (nail), not including thumb

● T23.739   Corrosion of third degree of unspecified multiple fingers (nail), not including thumb

● T23.74   Corrosion of third degree of multiple fingers (nail), including thumb

● T23.741   Corrosion of third degree of multiple right fingers (nail), including thumb

● T23.742   Corrosion of third degree of multiple left fingers (nail), including thumb

● T23.749   Corrosion of third degree of unspecified multiple fingers (nail), including thumb

● T23.75   Corrosion of third degree of palm

● T23.751   Corrosion of third degree of right palm

● T23.752   Corrosion of third degree of left palm

● T23.759   Corrosion of third degree of unspecified palm

● T23.76   Corrosion of third degree of back of hand

● T23.761   Corrosion of third degree of back of right hand

● T23.762   Corrosion of third degree of back of left hand

● T23.769   Corrosion of third degree of back of unspecified hand

● T23.77   Corrosion of third degree of wrist

● T23.771   Corrosion of third degree of right wrist

● T23.772   Corrosion of third degree of left wrist

● T23.779   Corrosion of third degree of unspecified wrist

● **T23.79**   Corrosion of third degree of multiple sites of wrist and hand

    ● **T23.791**   Corrosion of third degree of multiple sites of right wrist and hand

    ● **T23.792**   Corrosion of third degree of multiple sites of left wrist and hand

    ● **T23.799**   Corrosion of third degree of multiple sites of unspecified wrist and hand

● **T24**   Burn and corrosion of lower limb, except ankle and foot

    Excludes2   burn and corrosion of ankle and foot (T25.-)
                burn and corrosion of hip region (T21.-)

    The appropriate 7th character is to be added to each code from category T24

A	initial encounter
D	subsequent encounter
S	sequela

● **T24.0**   Burn of unspecified degree of lower limb, except ankle and foot

    Use additional external cause code to identify the source, place and intent of the burn (X00-X19, X75-X77, X96-X98, Y92)

    ● **T24.00**   Burn of unspecified degree of unspecified site of lower limb, except ankle and foot

       ● **T24.001**   Burn of unspecified degree of unspecified site of right lower limb, except ankle and foot

       ● **T24.002**   Burn of unspecified degree of unspecified site of left lower limb, except ankle and foot

       ● **T24.009**   Burn of unspecified degree of unspecified site of unspecified lower limb, except ankle and foot

    ● **T24.01**   Burn of unspecified degree of thigh

       ● **T24.011**   Burn of unspecified degree of right thigh

       ● **T24.012**   Burn of unspecified degree of left thigh

       ● **T24.019**   Burn of unspecified degree of unspecified thigh

    ● **T24.02**   Burn of unspecified degree of knee

       ● **T24.021**   Burn of unspecified degree of right knee

       ● **T24.022**   Burn of unspecified degree of left knee

       ● **T24.029**   Burn of unspecified degree of unspecified knee

    ● **T24.03**   Burn of unspecified degree of lower leg

       ● **T24.031**   Burn of unspecified degree of right lower leg

       ● **T24.032**   Burn of unspecified degree of left lower leg

       ● **T24.039**   Burn of unspecified degree of unspecified lower leg

    ● **T24.09**   Burn of unspecified degree of multiple sites of lower limb, except ankle and foot

       ● **T24.091**   Burn of unspecified degree of multiple sites of right lower limb, except ankle and foot

       ● **T24.092**   Burn of unspecified degree of multiple sites of left lower limb, except ankle and foot

       ● **T24.099**   Burn of unspecified degree of multiple sites of unspecified lower limb, except ankle and foot

● **T24.1**   Burn of first degree of lower limb, except ankle and foot

    Use additional external cause code to identify the source, place and intent of the burn (X00-X19, X75-X77, X96-X98, Y92)

    ● **T24.10**   Burn of first degree of unspecified site of lower limb, except ankle and foot

       ● **T24.101**   Burn of first degree of unspecified site of right lower limb, except ankle and foot

       ● **T24.102**   Burn of first degree of unspecified site of left lower limb, except ankle and foot

       ● **T24.109**   Burn of first degree of unspecified site of unspecified lower limb, except ankle and foot

    ● **T24.11**   Burn of first degree of thigh

       ● **T24.111**   Burn of first degree of right thigh

       ● **T24.112**   Burn of first degree of left thigh

       ● **T24.119**   Burn of first degree of unspecified thigh

    ● **T24.12**   Burn of first degree of knee

       ● **T24.121**   Burn of first degree of right knee

       ● **T24.122**   Burn of first degree of left knee

       ● **T24.129**   Burn of first degree of unspecified knee

    ● **T24.13**   Burn of first degree of lower leg

       ● **T24.131**   Burn of first degree of right lower leg

       ● **T24.132**   Burn of first degree of left lower leg

       ● **T24.139**   Burn of first degree of unspecified lower leg

    ● **T24.19**   Burn of first degree of multiple sites of lower limb, except ankle and foot

       ● **T24.191**   Burn of first degree of multiple sites of right lower limb, except ankle and foot

       ● **T24.192**   Burn of first degree of multiple sites of left lower limb, except ankle and foot

       ● **T24.199**   Burn of first degree of multiple sites of unspecified lower limb, except ankle and foot

● **T24.2**   Burn of second degree of lower limb, except ankle and foot

    Use additional external cause code to identify the source, place and intent of the burn (X00-X19, X75-X77, X96-X98, Y92)

    ● **T24.20**   Burn of second degree of unspecified site of lower limb, except ankle and foot

       ● **T24.201**   Burn of second degree of unspecified site of right lower limb, except ankle and foot

       ● **T24.202**   Burn of second degree of unspecified site of left lower limb, except ankle and foot

       ● **T24.209**   Burn of second degree of unspecified site of unspecified lower limb, except ankle and foot

    ● **T24.21**   Burn of second degree of thigh

       ● **T24.211**   Burn of second degree of right thigh

       ● **T24.212**   Burn of second degree of left thigh

       ● **T24.219**   Burn of second degree of unspecified thigh

    ● **T24.22**   Burn of second degree of knee

       ● **T24.221**   Burn of second degree of right knee

       ● **T24.222**   Burn of second degree of left knee

       ● **T24.229**   Burn of second degree of unspecified knee

    ● **T24.23**   Burn of second degree of lower leg

       ● **T24.231**   Burn of second degree of right lower leg

       ● **T24.232**   Burn of second degree of left lower leg

       ● **T24.239**   Burn of second degree of unspecified lower leg

    ● **T24.29**   Burn of second degree of multiple sites of lower limb, except ankle and foot

CHAPTER 19 (S00-T88)

● **T24.291** Burn of second degree of multiple sites of right lower limb, except ankle and foot
● **T24.292** Burn of second degree of multiple sites of left lower limb, except ankle and foot
● **T24.299** Burn of second degree of multiple sites of unspecified lower limb, except ankle and foot
● **T24.3** Burn of third degree of lower limb, except ankle and foot

Use additional external cause code to identify the source, place and intent of the burn (X00-X19, X75-X77, X96-X98, Y92)

● **T24.30** Burn of third degree of unspecified site of lower limb, except ankle and foot
● **T24.301** Burn of third degree of unspecified site of right lower limb, except ankle and foot
● **T24.302** Burn of third degree of unspecified site of left lower limb, except ankle and foot
● **T24.309** Burn of third degree of unspecified site of unspecified lower limb, except ankle and foot
● **T24.31** Burn of third degree of thigh
● **T24.311** Burn of third degree of right thigh
● **T24.312** Burn of third degree of left thigh
● **T24.319** Burn of third degree of unspecified thigh
● **T24.32** Burn of third degree of knee
● **T24.321** Burn of third degree of right knee
● **T24.322** Burn of third degree of left knee
● **T24.329** Burn of third degree of unspecified knee
● **T24.33** Burn of third degree of lower leg
● **T24.331** Burn of third degree of right lower leg
● **T24.332** Burn of third degree of left lower leg
● **T24.339** Burn of third degree of unspecified lower leg
● **T24.39** Burn of third degree of multiple sites of lower limb, except ankle and foot
● **T24.391** Burn of third degree of multiple sites of right lower limb, except ankle and foot
   Coding Clinic: 2016, Q2, P5
● **T24.392** Burn of third degree of multiple sites of left lower limb, except ankle and foot
● **T24.399** Burn of third degree of multiple sites of unspecified lower limb, except ankle and foot
● **T24.4** Corrosion of unspecified degree of lower limb, except ankle and foot

Code first (T51-T65) to identify chemical and intent
Use additional external cause code to identify place (Y92)

● **T24.40** Corrosion of unspecified degree of unspecified site of lower limb, except ankle and foot
● **T24.401** Corrosion of unspecified degree of unspecified site of right lower limb, except ankle and foot
● **T24.402** Corrosion of unspecified degree of unspecified site of left lower limb, except ankle and foot
● **T24.409** Corrosion of unspecified degree of unspecified site of unspecified lower limb, except ankle and foot

● **T24.41** Corrosion of unspecified degree of thigh
● **T24.411** Corrosion of unspecified degree of right thigh
● **T24.412** Corrosion of unspecified degree of left thigh
● **T24.419** Corrosion of unspecified degree of unspecified thigh
● **T24.42** Corrosion of unspecified degree of knee
● **T24.421** Corrosion of unspecified degree of right knee
● **T24.422** Corrosion of unspecified degree of left knee
● **T24.429** Corrosion of unspecified degree of unspecified knee
● **T24.43** Corrosion of unspecified degree of lower leg
● **T24.431** Corrosion of unspecified degree of right lower leg
● **T24.432** Corrosion of unspecified degree of left lower leg
● **T24.439** Corrosion of unspecified degree of unspecified lower leg
● **T24.49** Corrosion of unspecified degree of multiple sites of lower limb, except ankle and foot
● **T24.491** Corrosion of unspecified degree of multiple sites of right lower limb, except ankle and foot
● **T24.492** Corrosion of unspecified degree of multiple sites of left lower limb, except ankle and foot
● **T24.499** Corrosion of unspecified degree of multiple sites of unspecified lower limb, except ankle and foot
● **T24.5** Corrosion of first degree of lower limb, except ankle and foot

Code first (T51-T65) to identify chemical and intent
Use additional external cause code to identify place (Y92)

● **T24.50** Corrosion of first degree of unspecified site of lower limb, except ankle and foot
● **T24.501** Corrosion of first degree of unspecified site of right lower limb, except ankle and foot
● **T24.502** Corrosion of first degree of unspecified site of left lower limb, except ankle and foot
● **T24.509** Corrosion of first degree of unspecified site of unspecified lower limb, except ankle and foot
● **T24.51** Corrosion of first degree of thigh
● **T24.511** Corrosion of first degree of right thigh
● **T24.512** Corrosion of first degree of left thigh
● **T24.519** Corrosion of first degree of unspecified thigh
● **T24.52** Corrosion of first degree of knee
● **T24.521** Corrosion of first degree of right knee
● **T24.522** Corrosion of first degree of left knee
● **T24.529** Corrosion of first degree of unspecified knee
● **T24.53** Corrosion of first degree of lower leg
● **T24.531** Corrosion of first degree of right lower leg
● **T24.532** Corrosion of first degree of left lower leg
● **T24.539** Corrosion of first degree of unspecified lower leg
● **T24.59** Corrosion of first degree of multiple sites of lower limb, except ankle and foot
● **T24.591** Corrosion of first degree of multiple sites of right lower limb, except ankle and foot

● T24.592   Corrosion of first degree of multiple sites of left lower limb, except ankle and foot

● T24.599   Corrosion of first degree of multiple sites of unspecified lower limb, except ankle and foot

● T24.6   Corrosion of second degree of lower limb, except ankle and foot

Code first (T51-T65) to identify chemical and intent

Use additional external cause code to identify place (Y92)

● T24.60   Corrosion of second degree of unspecified site of lower limb, except ankle and foot

● T24.601   Corrosion of second degree of unspecified site of right lower limb, except ankle and foot

● T24.602   Corrosion of second degree of unspecified site of left lower limb, except ankle and foot

● T24.609   Corrosion of second degree of unspecified site of unspecified lower limb, except ankle and foot

● T24.61   Corrosion of second degree of thigh

● T24.611   Corrosion of second degree of right thigh

● T24.612   Corrosion of second degree of left thigh

● T24.619   Corrosion of second degree of unspecified thigh

● T24.62   Corrosion of second degree of knee

● T24.621   Corrosion of second degree of right knee

● T24.622   Corrosion of second degree of left knee

● T24.629   Corrosion of second degree of unspecified knee

● T24.63   Corrosion of second degree of lower leg

● T24.631   Corrosion of second degree of right lower leg

● T24.632   Corrosion of second degree of left lower leg

● T24.639   Corrosion of second degree of unspecified lower leg

● T24.69   Corrosion of second degree of multiple sites of lower limb, except ankle and foot

● T24.691   Corrosion of second degree of multiple sites of right lower limb, except ankle and foot

● T24.692   Corrosion of second degree of multiple sites of left lower limb, except ankle and foot

● T24.699   Corrosion of second degree of multiple sites of unspecified lower limb, except ankle and foot

● T24.7   Corrosion of third degree of lower limb, except ankle and foot

Code first (T51-T65) to identify chemical and intent

Use additional external cause code to identify place (Y92)

● T24.70   Corrosion of third degree of unspecified site of lower limb, except ankle and foot

● T24.701   Corrosion of third degree of unspecified site of right lower limb, except ankle and foot

● T24.702   Corrosion of third degree of unspecified site of left lower limb, except ankle and foot

● T24.709   Corrosion of third degree of unspecified site of unspecified lower limb, except ankle and foot

● T24.71   Corrosion of third degree of thigh

● T24.711   Corrosion of third degree of right thigh

● T24.712   Corrosion of third degree of left thigh

● T24.719   Corrosion of third degree of unspecified thigh

● T24.72   Corrosion of third degree of knee

● T24.721   Corrosion of third degree of right knee

● T24.722   Corrosion of third degree of left knee

● T24.729   Corrosion of third degree of unspecified knee

● T24.73   Corrosion of third degree of lower leg

● T24.731   Corrosion of third degree of right lower leg

● T24.732   Corrosion of third degree of left lower leg

● T24.739   Corrosion of third degree of unspecified lower leg

● T24.79   Corrosion of third degree of multiple sites of lower limb, except ankle and foot

● T24.791   Corrosion of third degree of multiple sites of right lower limb, except ankle and foot

● T24.792   Corrosion of third degree of multiple sites of left lower limb, except ankle and foot

● T24.799   Corrosion of third degree of multiple sites of unspecified lower limb, except ankle and foot

● T25   Burn and corrosion of ankle and foot

The appropriate 7th character is to be added to each code from category T25

A	initial encounter
D	subsequent encounter
S	sequela

● T25.0   Burn of unspecified degree of ankle and foot

Use additional external cause code to identify the source, place and intent of the burn (X00-X19, X75-X77, X96-X98, Y92)

● T25.01   Burn of unspecified degree of ankle

● T25.011   Burn of unspecified degree of right ankle

● T25.012   Burn of unspecified degree of left ankle

● T25.019   Burn of unspecified degree of unspecified ankle

● T25.02   Burn of unspecified degree of foot

Excludes2   burn of unspecified degree of toe(s) (nail) (T25.03-)

● T25.021   Burn of unspecified degree of right foot

● T25.022   Burn of unspecified degree of left foot

● T25.029   Burn of unspecified degree of unspecified foot

● T25.03   Burn of unspecified degree of toe(s) (nail)

● T25.031   Burn of unspecified degree of right toe(s) (nail)

● T25.032   Burn of unspecified degree of left toe(s) (nail)

● T25.039   Burn of unspecified degree of unspecified toe(s) (nail)

● T25.09   Burn of unspecified degree of multiple sites of ankle and foot

● T25.091   Burn of unspecified degree of multiple sites of right ankle and foot

● T25.092   Burn of unspecified degree of multiple sites of left ankle and foot

CHAPTER 19 (S00-T88)

● T25.Ø99   Burn of unspecified degree of multiple sites of unspecified ankle and foot

● T25.1   Burn of first degree of ankle and foot

Use additional external cause code to identify the source, place and intent of the burn (XØØ-X19, X75-X77, X96-X98, Y92)

   ● T25.11   Burn of first degree of ankle

     ● T25.111   Burn of first degree of right ankle

     ● T25.112   Burn of first degree of left ankle

     ● T25.119   Burn of first degree of unspecified ankle

   ● T25.12   Burn of first degree of foot

     Excludes2   burn of first degree of toe(s) (nail) (T25.13-)

     ● T25.121   Burn of first degree of right foot

     ● T25.122   Burn of first degree of left foot

     ● T25.129   Burn of first degree of unspecified foot

   ● T25.13   Burn of first degree of toe(s) (nail)

     ● T25.131   Burn of first degree of right toe(s) (nail)

     ● T25.132   Burn of first degree of left toe(s) (nail)

     ● T25.139   Burn of first degree of unspecified toe(s) (nail)

   ● T25.19   Burn of first degree of multiple sites of ankle and foot

     ● T25.191   Burn of first degree of multiple sites of right ankle and foot

     ● T25.192   Burn of first degree of multiple sites of left ankle and foot

     ● T25.199   Burn of first degree of multiple sites of unspecified ankle and foot

● T25.2   Burn of second degree of ankle and foot

Use additional external cause code to identify the source, place and intent of the burn (XØØ-X19, X75-X77, X96-X98, Y92)

   ● T25.21   Burn of second degree of ankle

     ● T25.211   Burn of second degree of right ankle

     ● T25.212   Burn of second degree of left ankle

     ● T25.219   Burn of second degree of unspecified ankle

   ● T25.22   Burn of second degree of foot

     Excludes2   burn of second degree of toe(s) (nail) (T25.23-)

     ● T25.221   Burn of second degree of right foot

     ● T25.222   Burn of second degree of left foot

     ● T25.229   Burn of second degree of unspecified foot

   ● T25.23   Burn of second degree of toe(s) (nail)

     ● T25.231   Burn of second degree of right toe(s) (nail)

     ● T25.232   Burn of second degree of left toe(s) (nail)

     ● T25.239   Burn of second degree of unspecified toe(s) (nail)

   ● T25.29   Burn of second degree of multiple sites of ankle and foot

     ● T25.291   Burn of second degree of multiple sites of right ankle and foot

     ● T25.292   Burn of second degree of multiple sites of left ankle and foot

     ● T25.299   Burn of second degree of multiple sites of unspecified ankle and foot

● T25.3   Burn of third degree of ankle and foot

Use additional external cause code to identify the source, place and intent of the burn (XØØ-X19, X75-X77, X96-X98, Y92)

● T25.31   Burn of third degree of ankle

   ● T25.311   Burn of third degree of right ankle

   ● T25.312   Burn of third degree of left ankle

   ● T25.319   Burn of third degree of unspecified ankle

● T25.32   Burn of third degree of foot

   Excludes2   burn of third degree of toe(s) (nail) (T25.33-)

   ● T25.321   Burn of third degree of right foot

   ● T25.322   Burn of third degree of left foot

   ● T25.329   Burn of third degree of unspecified foot

● T25.33   Burn of third degree of toe(s) (nail)

   ● T25.331   Burn of third degree of right toe(s) (nail)

   ● T25.332   Burn of third degree of left toe(s) (nail)

   ● T25.339   Burn of third degree of unspecified toe(s) (nail)

● T25.39   Burn of third degree of multiple sites of ankle and foot

   ● T25.391   Burn of third degree of multiple sites of right ankle and foot

   ● T25.392   Burn of third degree of multiple sites of left ankle and foot

   ● T25.399   Burn of third degree of multiple sites of unspecified ankle and foot

● T25.4   Corrosion of unspecified degree of ankle and foot

Code first (T51-T65) to identify chemical and intent

Use additional external cause code to identify place (Y92)

● T25.41   Corrosion of unspecified degree of ankle

   ● T25.411   Corrosion of unspecified degree of right ankle

   ● T25.412   Corrosion of unspecified degree of left ankle

   ● T25.419   Corrosion of unspecified degree of unspecified ankle

● T25.42   Corrosion of unspecified degree of foot

   Excludes2   corrosion of unspecified degree of toe(s) (nail) (T25.43-)

   ● T25.421   Corrosion of unspecified degree of right foot

   ● T25.422   Corrosion of unspecified degree of left foot

   ● T25.429   Corrosion of unspecified degree of unspecified foot

● T25.43   Corrosion of unspecified degree of toe(s) (nail)

   ● T25.431   Corrosion of unspecified degree of right toe(s) (nail)

   ● T25.432   Corrosion of unspecified degree of left toe(s) (nail)

   ● T25.439   Corrosion of unspecified degree of unspecified toe(s) (nail)

● T25.49   Corrosion of unspecified degree of multiple sites of ankle and foot

   ● T25.491   Corrosion of unspecified degree of multiple sites of right ankle and foot

   ● T25.492   Corrosion of unspecified degree of multiple sites of left ankle and foot

   ● T25.499   Corrosion of unspecified degree of multiple sites of unspecified ankle and foot

● T25.5   Corrosion of first degree of ankle and foot

Code first (T51-T65) to identify chemical and intent

Use additional external cause code to identify place (Y92)

● T25.51   Corrosion of first degree of ankle

● T25.511   Corrosion of first degree of right ankle

● T25.512   Corrosion of first degree of left ankle

● T25.519   Corrosion of first degree of unspecified ankle

● T25.52   Corrosion of first degree of foot

     Excludes2   corrosion of first degree of toe(s) (nail) (T25.53-)

● T25.521   Corrosion of first degree of right foot

● T25.522   Corrosion of first degree of left foot

● T25.529   Corrosion of first degree of unspecified foot

● T25.53   Corrosion of first degree of toe(s) (nail)

● T25.531   Corrosion of first degree of right toe(s) (nail)

● T25.532   Corrosion of first degree of left toe(s) (nail)

● T25.539   Corrosion of first degree of unspecified toe(s) (nail)

● T25.59   Corrosion of first degree of multiple sites of ankle and foot

● T25.591   Corrosion of first degree of multiple sites of right ankle and foot

● T25.592   Corrosion of first degree of multiple sites of left ankle and foot

● T25.599   Corrosion of first degree of multiple sites of unspecified ankle and foot

● T25.6   Corrosion of second degree of ankle and foot

     Code first (T51-T65) to identify chemical and intent

     Use additional external cause code to identify place (Y92)

● T25.61   Corrosion of second degree of ankle

● T25.611   Corrosion of second degree of right ankle

● T25.612   Corrosion of second degree of left ankle

● T25.619   Corrosion of second degree of unspecified ankle

● T25.62   Corrosion of second degree of foot

     Excludes2   corrosion of second degree of toe(s) (nail) (T25.63-)

● T25.621   Corrosion of second degree of right foot

● T25.622   Corrosion of second degree of left foot

● T25.629   Corrosion of second degree of unspecified foot

● T25.63   Corrosion of second degree of toe(s) (nail)

● T25.631   Corrosion of second degree of right toe(s) (nail)

● T25.632   Corrosion of second degree of left toe(s) (nail)

● T25.639   Corrosion of second degree of unspecified toe(s) (nail)

● T25.69   Corrosion of second degree of multiple sites of ankle and foot

● T25.691   Corrosion of second degree of right ankle and foot

● T25.692   Corrosion of second degree of left ankle and foot

● T25.699   Corrosion of second degree of unspecified ankle and foot

● T25.7   Corrosion of third degree of ankle and foot

     Code first (T51-T65) to identify chemical and intent

     Use additional external cause code to identify place (Y92)

● T25.71   Corrosion of third degree of ankle

● T25.711   Corrosion of third degree of right ankle

● T25.712   Corrosion of third degree of left ankle

● T25.719   Corrosion of third degree of unspecified ankle

● T25.72   Corrosion of third degree of foot

     Excludes2   corrosion of third degree of toe(s) (nail) (T25.73-)

● T25.721   Corrosion of third degree of right foot

● T25.722   Corrosion of third degree of left foot

● T25.729   Corrosion of third degree of unspecified foot

● T25.73   Corrosion of third degree of toe(s) (nail)

● T25.731   Corrosion of third degree of right toe(s) (nail)

● T25.732   Corrosion of third degree of left toe(s) (nail)

● T25.739   Corrosion of third degree of unspecified toe(s) (nail)

● T25.79   Corrosion of third degree of multiple sites of ankle and foot

● T25.791   Corrosion of third degree of multiple sites of right ankle and foot

● T25.792   Corrosion of third degree of multiple sites of left ankle and foot

● T25.799   Corrosion of third degree of multiple sites of unspecified ankle and foot

BURNS AND CORROSIONS CONFINED TO EYE AND INTERNAL ORGANS (T26-T28)

● T26   Burn and corrosion confined to eye and adnexa

     The appropriate 7th character is to be added to each code from category T26

A	initial encounter
D	subsequent encounter
S	sequela

● T26.0   Burn of eyelid and periocular area

     Use additional external cause code to identify the source, place and intent of the burn (X00-X19, X75-X77, X96-X98, Y92)

X ● T26.00   Burn of unspecified eyelid and periocular area

X ● T26.01   Burn of right eyelid and periocular area

X ● T26.02   Burn of left eyelid and periocular area

● T26.1   Burn of cornea and conjunctival sac

     Use additional external cause code to identify the source, place and intent of the burn (X00-X19, X75-X77, X96-X98, Y92)

X ● T26.10   Burn of cornea and conjunctival sac, unspecified eye

X ● T26.11   Burn of cornea and conjunctival sac, right eye

X ● T26.12   Burn of cornea and conjunctival sac, left eye

● T26.2   Burn with resulting rupture and destruction of eyeball

     Use additional external cause code to identify the source, place and intent of the burn (X00-X19, X75-X77, X96-X98, Y92)

X ● T26.20   Burn with resulting rupture and destruction of unspecified eyeball

X ● T26.21   Burn with resulting rupture and destruction of right eyeball

X ● T26.22   Burn with resulting rupture and destruction of left eyeball

● T26.3   Burns of other specified parts of eye and adnexa

     Use additional external cause code to identify the source, place and intent of the burn (X00-X19, X75-X77, X96-X98, Y92)

X ● T26.30   Burns of other specified parts of unspecified eye and adnexa

X ● T26.31   Burns of other specified parts of right eye and adnexa

X ● T26.32   Burns of other specified parts of left eye and adnexa

CHAPTER 19 (S00-T88)

● **T26.4 Burn of eye and adnexa, part unspecified**

> Use additional external cause code to identify the source, place and intent of the burn (X00-X19, X75-X77, X96-X98, Y92)

   X● **T26.40** Burn of **unspecified** eye and adnexa, part unspecified

   X● **T26.41** Burn of **right** eye and adnexa, part unspecified

   X● **T26.42** Burn of **left** eye and adnexa, part unspecified

● **T26.5 Corrosion of eyelid and periocular area**

> *Code first (T51-T65) to identify chemical and intent*
> Use additional external cause code to identify place (Y92)

   X● **T26.50** Corrosion of **unspecified** eyelid and periocular area

   X● **T26.51** Corrosion of **right** eyelid and periocular area

   X● **T26.52** Corrosion of **left** eyelid and periocular area

● **T26.6 Corrosion of cornea and conjunctival sac**

> *Code first (T51-T65) to identify chemical and intent*
> Use additional external cause code to identify place (Y92)

   X● **T26.60** Corrosion of cornea and conjunctival sac, **unspecified** eye

   X● **T26.61** Corrosion of cornea and conjunctival sac, **right** eye

   X● **T26.62** Corrosion of cornea and conjunctival sac, **left** eye

● **T26.7 Corrosion with resulting rupture and destruction of eyeball**

> *Code first (T51-T65) to identify chemical and intent*
> Use additional external cause code to identify place (Y92)

   X● **T26.70** Corrosion with resulting rupture and destruction of **unspecified** eyeball

   X● **T26.71** Corrosion with resulting rupture and destruction of **right** eyeball

   X● **T26.72** Corrosion with resulting rupture and destruction of **left** eyeball

● **T26.8 Corrosions of other specified parts of eye and adnexa**

> *Code first (T51-T65) to identify chemical and intent*
> Use additional external cause code to identify place (Y92)

   X● **T26.80** Corrosions of other specified parts of **unspecified** eye and adnexa

   X● **T26.81** Corrosions of other specified parts of **right** eye and adnexa

   X● **T26.82** Corrosions of other specified parts of **left** eye and adnexa

● **T26.9 Corrosion of eye and adnexa, part unspecified**

> *Code first (T51-T65) to identify chemical and intent*
> Use additional external cause code to identify place (Y92)

   X● **T26.90** Corrosion of **unspecified** eye and adnexa, part unspecified

   X● **T26.91** Corrosion of **right** eye and adnexa, part unspecified

   X● **T26.92** Corrosion of **left** eye and adnexa, part unspecified

● **T27 Burn and corrosion of respiratory tract**

> Use additional external cause code to identify the source and intent of the burn (X00-X19, X75-X77, X96-X98)
> Use additional external cause code to identify place (Y92)
> The appropriate 7th character is to be added to each code from category T27

A	initial encounter
D	subsequent encounter
S	sequela

   X● **T27.0 Burn of larynx and trachea**

   X● **T27.1 Burn involving larynx and trachea with lung**

   X● **T27.2 Burn of other parts of respiratory tract**
        Burn of thoracic cavity

   X● **T27.3 Burn of respiratory tract, part unspecified**

   X● **T27.4 Corrosion of larynx and trachea**
> *Code first (T51-T65) to identify chemical and intent*

   X● **T27.5 Corrosion involving larynx and trachea with lung**
> *Code first (T51-T65) to identify chemical and intent*

   X● **T27.6 Corrosion of other parts of respiratory tract**
> *Code first (T51-T65) to identify chemical and intent*

   X● **T27.7 Corrosion of respiratory tract, part unspecified**
> *Code first (T51-T65) to identify chemical and intent*

● **T28 Burn and corrosion of other internal organs**

> Use additional external cause code to identify the source and intent of the burn (X00-X19, X75-X77, X96-X98)
> Use additional external cause code to identify place (Y92)
> The appropriate 7th character is to be added to each code from category T28

A	initial encounter
D	subsequent encounter
S	sequela

   X● **T28.0 Burn of mouth and pharynx**

   X● **T28.1 Burn of esophagus**

   X● **T28.2 Burn of other parts of alimentary tract**

   X● **T28.3 Burn of internal genitourinary organs**

   X● **T28.4 Burns of other and unspecified internal organs**

      X● **T28.40** Burn of **unspecified** internal organ

      ● **T28.41** Burn of **ear drum**

         ● **T28.411** Burn of **right** ear drum

         ● **T28.412** Burn of **left** ear drum

         ● **T28.419** Burn of **unspecified** ear drum

      X● **T28.49** Burn of **other** internal organ

   X● **T28.5 Corrosion of mouth and pharynx**
> *Code first (T51-T65) to identify chemical and intent*

   X● **T28.6 Corrosion of esophagus**
> *Code first (T51-T65) to identify chemical and intent*

   X● **T28.7 Corrosion of other parts of alimentary tract**

> *Code first (T51-T65) to identify chemical and intent*

   X● **T28.8 Corrosion of internal genitourinary organs**
> *Code first (T51-T65) to identify chemical and intent*

   ● **T28.9 Corrosions of other and unspecified internal organs**
> *Code first (T51-T65) to identify chemical and intent*

      X● **T28.90** Corrosions of **unspecified** internal organs

      ● **T28.91** Corrosions of **ear drum**

         ● **T28.911** Corrosions of **right** ear drum

         ● **T28.912** Corrosions of **left** ear drum

         ● **T28.919** Corrosions of **unspecified** ear drum

      X● **T28.99** Corrosions of **other** internal organs

OGCR Section I.C.19.d.5.

Assign separate code for each burn site

When coding burns, assign separate codes for each burn site. Category T30, Burn and corrosion, body region unspecified is extremely vague and should rarely be used.

BURNS AND CORROSIONS OF MULTIPLE AND UNSPECIFIED BODY REGIONS (T30-T32)

● **T30 Burn and corrosion, body region unspecified**

   T30.0 Burn of unspecified body region, unspecified degree
> This code is not for inpatient use. Code to specified site and degree of burns
> Burn NOS
> Multiple burns NOS

▶ New   ⇒ Revised   ~~deleted~~ Deleted   Excludes 1   Excludes 2   Includes   Use additional   Code first   Code also   Key words

OGCR Official Guidelines   X Assign placeholder X   ● Use Additional Character(s)   ▶ Manifestation Code   🞢 Hierarchical Condition Category   **Coding Clinic**

CHAPTER 19 (S00-T88)

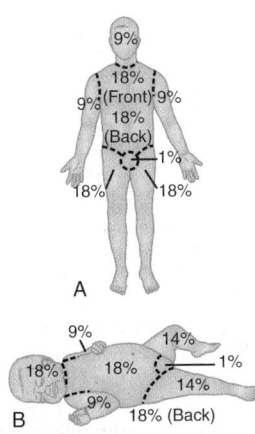

Figure 19-16 Rule of nines: percentages of total body area. (From Marx: Rosen's Emergency Medicine: Concepts and Clinical Practice, ed 6, Mosby, 2006)

T30.4 **Corrosion of unspecified body region, unspecified degree**
This code is not for inpatient use. Code to specified site and degree of corrosion
Corrosion NOS
Multiple corrosion NOS

● **T31** **Burns classified according to extent of body surface involved**

Note: This category is to be used as the primary code only when the site of the burn is unspecified. It should be used as a supplementary code with categories T20-T25 when the site is specified.

T31.0 Burns involving less than 10% of body surface

● **T31.1** Burns involving 10-19% of body surface

    T31.10 Burns involving 10-19% of body surface with 0% to 9% third degree burns
        Burns involving 10-19% of body surface NOS

    T31.11 Burns involving 10-19% of body surface with 10-19% third degree burns 🔏

● **T31.2** Burns involving 20-29% of body surface

    T31.20 Burns involving 20-29% of body surface with 0% to 9% third degree burns
        Burns involving 20-29% of body surface NOS

    T31.21 Burns involving 20-29% of body surface with 10-19% third degree burns 🔏

    T31.22 Burns involving 20-29% of body surface with 20-29% third degree burns 🔏

● **T31.3** Burns involving 30-39% of body surface

    T31.30 Burns involving 30-39% of body surface with 0% to 9% third degree burns
        Burns involving 30-39% of body surface NOS

    T31.31 Burns involving 30-39% of body surface with 10-19% third degree burns 🔏

    T31.32 Burns involving 30-39% of body surface with 20-29% third degree burns 🔏

    T31.33 Burns involving 30-39% of body surface with 30-39% third degree burns 🔏

● **T31.4** Burns involving 40-49% of body surface

    T31.40 Burns involving 40-49% of body surface with 0% to 9% third degree burns
        Burns involving 40-49% of body surface NOS

    T31.41 Burns involving 40-49% of body surface with 10-19% third degree burns 🔏

    T31.42 Burns involving 40-49% of body surface with 20-29% third degree burns 🔏

    T31.43 Burns involving 40-49% of body surface with 30-39% third degree burns 🔏

    T31.44 Burns involving 40-49% of body surface with 40-49% third degree burns 🔏

● **T31.5** Burns involving 50-59% of body surface

    T31.50 Burns involving 50-59% of body surface with 0% to 9% third degree burns
        Burns involving 50-59% of body surface NOS

    T31.51 Burns involving 50-59% of body surface with 10-19% third degree burns 🔏

    T31.52 Burns involving 50-59% of body surface with 20-29% third degree burns 🔏

    T31.53 Burns involving 50-59% of body surface with 30-39% third degree burns 🔏

    T31.54 Burns involving 50-59% of body surface with 40-49% third degree burns 🔏

    T31.55 Burns involving 50-59% of body surface with 50-59% third degree burns 🔏

● **T31.6** Burns involving 60-69% of body surface

    T31.60 Burns involving 60-69% of body surface with 0% to 9% third degree burns
        Burns involving 60-69% of body surface NOS

    T31.61 Burns involving 60-69% of body surface with 10-19% third degree burns 🔏

    T31.62 Burns involving 60-69% of body surface with 20-29% third degree burns 🔏

    T31.63 Burns involving 60-69% of body surface with 30-39% third degree burns 🔏

    T31.64 Burns involving 60-69% of body surface with 40-49% third degree burns 🔏

    T31.65 Burns involving 60-69% of body surface with 50-59% third degree burns 🔏

    T31.66 Burns involving 60-69% of body surface with 60-69% third degree burns 🔏

● **T31.7** Burns involving 70-79% of body surface

    T31.70 Burns involving 70-79% of body surface with 0% to 9% third degree burns
        Burns involving 70-79% of body surface NOS

    T31.71 Burns involving 70-79% of body surface with 10-19% third degree burns 🔏

    T31.72 Burns involving 70-79% of body surface with 20-29% third degree burns 🔏

    T31.73 Burns involving 70-79% of body surface with 30-39% third degree burns 🔏

    T31.74 Burns involving 70-79% of body surface with 40-49% third degree burns 🔏

    T31.75 Burns involving 70-79% of body surface with 50-59% third degree burns 🔏

    T31.76 Burns involving 70-79% of body surface with 60-69% third degree burns 🔏

    T31.77 Burns involving 70-79% of body surface with 70-79% third degree burns 🔏

● **T31.8** Burns involving 80-89% of body surface

    T31.80 Burns involving 80-89% of body surface with 0% to 9% third degree burns
        Burns involving 80-89% of body surface NOS

    T31.81 Burns involving 80-89% of body surface with 10-19% third degree burns 🔏

    T31.82 Burns involving 80-89% of body surface with 20-29% third degree burns 🔏

    T31.83 Burns involving 80-89% of body surface with 30-39% third degree burns 🔏

    T31.84 Burns involving 80-89% of body surface with 40-49% third degree burns 🔏

    T31.85 Burns involving 80-89% of body surface with 50-59% third degree burns 🔏

    T31.86 Burns involving 80-89% of body surface with 60-69% third degree burns 🔏

    T31.87 Burns involving 80-89% of body surface with 70-79% third degree burns 🔏

    T31.88 Burns involving 80-89% of body surface with 80-89% third degree burns 🔏

CHAPTER 19 (S00-T88)

● T31.9   **Burns involving 90% or more of body surface**

 T31.90   Burns involving 90% or more of body surface with 0% to 9% third degree burns
          Burns involving 90% or more of body surface NOS

 T31.91   Burns involving 90% or more of body surface with 10-19% third degree burns 🐾

 T31.92   Burns involving 90% or more of body surface with 20-29% third degree burns 🐾

 T31.93   Burns involving 90% or more of body surface with 30-39% third degree burns 🐾

 T31.94   Burns involving 90% or more of body surface with 40-49% third degree burns 🐾

 T31.95   Burns involving 90% or more of body surface with 50-59% third degree burns 🐾

 T31.96   Burns involving 90% or more of body surface with 60-69% third degree burns 🐾

 T31.97   Burns involving 90% or more of body surface with 70-79% third degree burns 🐾

 T31.98   Burns involving 90% or more of body surface with 80-89% third degree burns 🐾

 T31.99   Burns involving 90% or more of body surface with 90% or more third degree burns 🐾

● T32   **Corrosions classified according to extent of body surface involved**

 Note: This category is to be used as the primary code only when the site of the corrosion is unspecified. It may be used as a supplementary code with categories T20-T25 when the site is specified.

 T32.0   **Corrosions involving less than 10% of body surface**

● T32.1   **Corrosions involving 10-19% of body surface**

 T32.10   Corrosions involving 10-19% of body surface with 0% to 9% third degree corrosion
          Corrosions involving 10-19% of body surface NOS

 T32.11   Corrosions involving 10-19% of body surface with 10-19% third degree corrosion 🐾

● T32.2   **Corrosions involving 20-29% of body surface**

 T32.20   Corrosions involving 20-29% of body surface with 0% to 9% third degree corrosion

 T32.21   Corrosions involving 20-29% of body surface with 10-19% third degree corrosion 🐾

 T32.22   Corrosions involving 20-29% of body surface with 20-29% third degree corrosion 🐾

● T32.3   **Corrosions involving 30-39% of body surface**

 T32.30   Corrosions involving 30-39% of body surface with 0% to 9% third degree corrosion

 T32.31   Corrosions involving 30-39% of body surface with 10-19% third degree corrosion 🐾

 T32.32   Corrosions involving 30-39% of body surface with 20-29% third degree corrosion 🐾

 T32.33   Corrosions involving 30-39% of body surface with 30-39% third degree corrosion 🐾

● T32.4   **Corrosions involving 40-49% of body surface**

 T32.40   Corrosions involving 40-49% of body surface with 0% to 9% third degree corrosion

 T32.41   Corrosions involving 40-49% of body surface with 10-19% third degree corrosion 🐾

 T32.42   Corrosions involving 40-49% of body surface with 20-29% third degree corrosion 🐾

 T32.43   Corrosions involving 40-49% of body surface with 30-39% third degree corrosion 🐾

 T32.44   Corrosions involving 40-49% of body surface with 40-49% third degree corrosion 🐾

● T32.5   **Corrosions involving 50-59% of body surface**

 T32.50   Corrosions involving 50-59% of body surface with 0% to 9% third degree corrosion

 T32.51   Corrosions involving 50-59% of body surface with 10-19% third degree corrosion 🐾

 T32.52   Corrosions involving 50-59% of body surface with 20-29% third degree corrosion 🐾

 T32.53   Corrosions involving 50-59% of body surface with 30-39% third degree corrosion 🐾

 T32.54   Corrosions involving 50-59% of body surface with 40-49% third degree corrosion 🐾

 T32.55   Corrosions involving 50-59% of body surface with 50-59% third degree corrosion 🐾

● T32.6   **Corrosions involving 60-69% of body surface**

 T32.60   Corrosions involving 60-69% of body surface with 0% to 9% third degree corrosion

 T32.61   Corrosions involving 60-69% of body surface with 10-19% third degree corrosion 🐾

 T32.62   Corrosions involving 60-69% of body surface with 20-29% third degree corrosion 🐾

 T32.63   Corrosions involving 60-69% of body surface with 30-39% third degree corrosion 🐾

 T32.64   Corrosions involving 60-69% of body surface with 40-49% third degree corrosion 🐾

 T32.65   Corrosions involving 60-69% of body surface with 50-59% third degree corrosion 🐾

 T32.66   Corrosions involving 60-69% of body surface with 60-69% third degree corrosion 🐾

● T32.7   **Corrosions involving 70-79% of body surface**

 T32.70   Corrosions involving 70-79% of body surface with 0% to 9% third degree corrosion

 T32.71   Corrosions involving 70-79% of body surface with 10-19% third degree corrosion 🐾

 T32.72   Corrosions involving 70-79% of body surface with 20-29% third degree corrosion 🐾

 T32.73   Corrosions involving 70-79% of body surface with 30-39% third degree corrosion 🐾

 T32.74   Corrosions involving 70-79% of body surface with 40-49% third degree corrosion 🐾

 T32.75   Corrosions involving 70-79% of body surface with 50-59% third degree corrosion 🐾

 T32.76   Corrosions involving 70-79% of body surface with 60-69% third degree corrosion 🐾

 T32.77   Corrosions involving 70-79% of body surface with 70-79% third degree corrosion 🐾

● T32.8   **Corrosions involving 80-89% of body surface**

 T32.80   Corrosions involving 80-89% of body surface with 0% to 9% third degree corrosion

 T32.81   Corrosions involving 80-89% of body surface with 10-19% third degree corrosion 🐾

 T32.82   Corrosions involving 80-89% of body surface with 20-29% third degree corrosion 🐾

 T32.83   Corrosions involving 80-89% of body surface with 30-39% third degree corrosion 🐾

 T32.84   Corrosions involving 80-89% of body surface with 40-49% third degree corrosion 🐾

 T32.85   Corrosions involving 80-89% of body surface with 50-59% third degree corrosion 🐾

 T32.86   Corrosions involving 80-89% of body surface with 60-69% third degree corrosion 🐾

 T32.87   Corrosions involving 80-89% of body surface with 70-79% third degree corrosion 🐾

 T32.88   Corrosions involving 80-89% of body surface with 80-89% third degree corrosion 🐾

● T32.9   **Corrosions involving 90% or more of body surface**

 T32.90   Corrosions involving 90% or more of body surface with 0% to 9% third degree corrosion

 T32.91   Corrosions involving 90% or more of body surface with 10-19% third degree corrosion 🐾

 T32.92   Corrosions involving 90% or more of body surface with 20-29% third degree corrosion 🐾

 T32.93   Corrosions involving 90% or more of body surface with 30-39% third degree corrosion 🐾

 T32.94   Corrosions involving 90% or more of body surface with 40-49% third degree corrosion 🐾

▶ New   ⇒ Revised   ~~deleted~~ Deleted   Excludes 1   Excludes 2   Includes   Use additional   Code first   Code also   Key words
OGCR Official Guidelines   X Assign placeholder X   ● Use Additional Character(s)   ▶ Manifestation Code   🐾 Hierarchical Condition Category   **Coding Clinic**

T32.95   Corrosions involving 90% or more of body surface with 50-59% third degree corrosion 🔖

T32.96   Corrosions involving 90% or more of body surface with 60-69% third degree corrosion 🔖

T32.97   Corrosions involving 90% or more of body surface with 70-79% third degree corrosion 🔖

T32.98   Corrosions involving 90% or more of body surface with 80-89% third degree corrosion 🔖

T32.99   Corrosions involving 90% or more of body surface with 90% or more third degree corrosion 🔖

FROSTBITE (T33-T34)

Excludes2   hypothermia and other effects of reduced temperature (T68, T69.-)

● T33   **Superficial frostbite**

Includes   frostbite with partial thickness skin loss

The appropriate 7th character is to be added to each code from category T33

A	initial encounter
D	subsequent encounter
S	sequela

● T33.0   **Superficial frostbite of head**

   ● T33.01   Superficial frostbite of ear

     ● T33.011   Superficial frostbite of right ear

     ● T33.012   Superficial frostbite of left ear

     ● T33.019   Superficial frostbite of unspecified ear

   X● T33.02   Superficial frostbite of nose

   X● T33.09   Superficial frostbite of other part of head

X● T33.1   **Superficial frostbite of neck**

X● T33.2   **Superficial frostbite of thorax**

X● T33.3   **Superficial frostbite of abdominal wall, lower back and pelvis**

● T33.4   **Superficial frostbite of arm**

   Excludes2   superficial frostbite of wrist and hand (T33.5-)

   X● T33.40   Superficial frostbite of unspecified arm

   X● T33.41   Superficial frostbite of right arm

   X● T33.42   Superficial frostbite of left arm

● T33.5   **Superficial frostbite of wrist, hand, and fingers**

   ● T33.51   Superficial frostbite of wrist

     ● T33.511   Superficial frostbite of right wrist

     ● T33.512   Superficial frostbite of left wrist

     ● T33.519   Superficial frostbite of unspecified wrist

   ● T33.52   Superficial frostbite of hand

     Excludes2   superficial frostbite of fingers (T33.53-)

     ● T33.521   Superficial frostbite of right hand

     ● T33.522   Superficial frostbite of left hand

     ● T33.529   Superficial frostbite of unspecified hand

   ● T33.53   Superficial frostbite of finger(s)

     ● T33.531   Superficial frostbite of right finger(s)

     ● T33.532   Superficial frostbite of left finger(s)

     ● T33.539   Superficial frostbite of unspecified finger(s)

● T33.6   **Superficial frostbite of hip and thigh**

   X● T33.60   Superficial frostbite of unspecified hip and thigh

   X● T33.61   Superficial frostbite of right hip and thigh

   X● T33.62   Superficial frostbite of left hip and thigh

● T33.7   **Superficial frostbite of knee and lower leg**

   Excludes2   superficial frostbite of ankle and foot (T33.8-)

   X● T33.70   Superficial frostbite of unspecified knee and lower leg

   X● T33.71   Superficial frostbite of right knee and lower leg

   X● T33.72   Superficial frostbite of left knee and lower leg

● T33.8   **Superficial frostbite of ankle, foot, and toe(s)**

   ● T33.81   Superficial frostbite of ankle

     ● T33.811   Superficial frostbite of right ankle

     ● T33.812   Superficial frostbite of left ankle

     ● T33.819   Superficial frostbite of unspecified ankle

   ● T33.82   Superficial frostbite of foot

     ● T33.821   Superficial frostbite of right foot

     ● T33.822   Superficial frostbite of left foot

     ● T33.829   Superficial frostbite of unspecified foot

   ● T33.83   Superficial frostbite of toe(s)

     ● T33.831   Superficial frostbite of right toe(s)

     ● T33.832   Superficial frostbite of left toe(s)

     ● T33.839   Superficial frostbite of unspecified toe(s)

● T33.9   **Superficial frostbite of other and unspecified sites**

   X● T33.90   Superficial frostbite of unspecified sites

     Superficial frostbite NOS

   X● T33.99   Superficial frostbite of other sites

     Superficial frostbite of leg NOS

     Superficial frostbite of trunk NOS

● T34   **Frostbite with tissue necrosis**

The appropriate 7th character is to be added to each code from category T34

A	initial encounter
D	subsequent encounter
S	sequela

● T34.0   **Frostbite with tissue necrosis of head**

   ● T34.01   Frostbite with tissue necrosis of ear

     ● T34.011   Frostbite with tissue necrosis of right ear

     ● T34.012   Frostbite with tissue necrosis of left ear

     ● T34.019   Frostbite with tissue necrosis of unspecified ear

   X● T34.02   Frostbite with tissue necrosis of nose

   X● T34.09   Frostbite with tissue necrosis of other part of head

X● T34.1   **Frostbite with tissue necrosis of neck**

X● T34.2   **Frostbite with tissue necrosis of thorax**

X● T34.3   **Frostbite with tissue necrosis of abdominal wall, lower back and pelvis**

● T34.4   **Frostbite with tissue necrosis of arm**

   Excludes2   frostbite with tissue necrosis of wrist and hand (T34.5-)

   X● T34.40   Frostbite with tissue necrosis of unspecified arm

   X● T34.41   Frostbite with tissue necrosis of right arm

   X● T34.42   Frostbite with tissue necrosis of left arm

● T34.5   **Frostbite with tissue necrosis of wrist, hand, and finger(s)**

   ● T34.51   Frostbite with tissue necrosis of wrist

     ● T34.511   Frostbite with tissue necrosis of right wrist

     ● T34.512   Frostbite with tissue necrosis of left wrist

     ● T34.519   Frostbite with tissue necrosis of unspecified wrist

   ● T34.52   Frostbite with tissue necrosis of hand

     Excludes2   frostbite with tissue necrosis of finger(s) (T34.53-)

● T34.521   Frostbite with tissue necrosis of right hand

● T34.522   Frostbite with tissue necrosis of left hand

● T34.529   Frostbite with tissue necrosis of unspecified hand

● T34.53   Frostbite with tissue necrosis of finger(s)

   ● T34.531   Frostbite with tissue necrosis of right finger(s)

   ● T34.532   Frostbite with tissue necrosis of left finger(s)

   ● T34.539   Frostbite with tissue necrosis of unspecified finger(s)

● T34.6   Frostbite with tissue necrosis of hip and thigh

  X ● T34.60   Frostbite with tissue necrosis of unspecified hip and thigh

  X ● T34.61   Frostbite with tissue necrosis of right hip and thigh

  X ● T34.62   Frostbite with tissue necrosis of left hip and thigh

● T34.7   Frostbite with tissue necrosis of knee and lower leg

    Excludes2   frostbite with tissue necrosis of ankle and foot (T34.8-)

  X ● T34.70   Frostbite with tissue necrosis of unspecified knee and lower leg

  X ● T34.71   Frostbite with tissue necrosis of right knee and lower leg

  X ● T34.72   Frostbite with tissue necrosis of left knee and lower leg

● T34.8   Frostbite with tissue necrosis of ankle, foot, and toe(s)

  ● T34.81   Frostbite with tissue necrosis of ankle

    ● T34.811   Frostbite with tissue necrosis of right ankle

    ● T34.812   Frostbite with tissue necrosis of left ankle

    ● T34.819   Frostbite with tissue necrosis of unspecified ankle

  ● T34.82   Frostbite with tissue necrosis of foot

    ● T34.821   Frostbite with tissue necrosis of right foot

    ● T34.822   Frostbite with tissue necrosis of left foot

    ● T34.829   Frostbite with tissue necrosis of unspecified foot

  ● T34.83   Frostbite with tissue necrosis of toe(s)

    ● T34.831   Frostbite with tissue necrosis of right toe(s)

    ● T34.832   Frostbite with tissue necrosis of left toe(s)

    ● T34.839   Frostbite with tissue necrosis of unspecified toe(s)

● T34.9   Frostbite with tissue necrosis of other and unspecified sites

  X ● T34.90   Frostbite with tissue necrosis of unspecified sites
         Frostbite with tissue necrosis NOS

  X ● T34.99   Frostbite with tissue necrosis of other sites
         Frostbite with tissue necrosis of leg NOS
         Frostbite with tissue necrosis of trunk NOS

OGCR See Section I.C.19.e.

Adverse Effects, Poisoning, Underdosing and Toxic Effects

Codes in categories T36-T65 are combination codes that include the substance that was taken as well as the intent. No additional external cause code is required for poisonings, toxic effects, adverse effects and underdosing codes.

POISONING BY, ADVERSE EFFECTS OF AND UNDERDOSING OF DRUGS MEDICAMENTS AND BIOLOGICAL SUBSTANCES (T36-T50)

Includes   adverse effect of correct substance properly administered
     poisoning by overdose of substance
     poisoning by wrong substance given or taken in error
     underdosing by (inadvertently) (deliberately) taking less substance than prescribed or instructed

Code first, for adverse effects, the nature of the adverse effect, such as:
   adverse effect NOS (T88.7)
   aspirin gastritis (K29.-)
   blood disorders (D56-D76)
   contact dermatitis (L23-L25)
   dermatitis due to substances taken internally (L27.-)
   nephropathy (N14.0-N14.2)

Note: The drug giving rise to the adverse effect should be identified by use of codes from categories T36-T50 with fifth or sixth character 5.

Use additional code(s) to specify:
   manifestations of poisoning
   underdosing or failure in dosage during medical and surgical care (Y63.6, Y63.8-Y63.9)
   underdosing of medication regimen (Z91.12-, Z91.13-)

Excludes1   toxic reaction to local anesthesia in pregnancy (O29.3-)

Excludes2   abuse and dependence of psychoactive substances (F10-F19)
     abuse of non-dependence-producing substances (F55.-)
     drug reaction and poisoning affecting newborn (P00-P96)
     immunodeficiency due to drugs (D84.821)
     pathological drug intoxication (inebriation) (F10-F19)

● T36   Poisoning by, adverse effect of and underdosing of systemic antibiotics

  Excludes1   antineoplastic antibiotics (T45.1-)
     locally applied antibiotic NEC (T49.0)
     topically used antibiotic for ear, nose and throat (T49.6)
     topically used antibiotic for eye (T49.5)

  The appropriate 7th character is to be added to each code from category T36

A	initial encounter
D	subsequent encounter
S	sequela

● T36.0   Poisoning by, adverse effect of and underdosing of penicillins

  ● T36.0X   Poisoning by, adverse effect of and underdosing of penicillins

    ● T36.0X1   Poisoning by penicillins, accidental (unintentional)
         Poisoning by penicillins NOS

    ● T36.0X2   Poisoning by penicillins, intentional self-harm A, S 🅗🅒

    ● T36.0X3   Poisoning by penicillins, assault

    ● T36.0X4   Poisoning by penicillins, undetermined

    ● T36.0X5   Adverse effect of penicillins

    ● T36.0X6   Underdosing of penicillins

● T36.1   Poisoning by, adverse effect of and underdosing of cephalosporins and other betalactam antibiotics

  ● T36.1X   Poisoning by, adverse effect of and underdosing of cephalosporins and other beta-lactam antibiotics

---

▶ New   ⇒ Revised   ~~deleted~~ Deleted   Excludes 1   Excludes 2   Includes   Use additional   Code first   Code also   Key words

OGCR Official Guidelines   X Assign placeholder X   ● Use Additional Character(s)   ▶ Manifestation Code   🅗🅒 Hierarchical Condition Category   **Coding Clinic**

- T36.1X1 Poisoning by cephalosporins and other beta-lactam antibiotics, accidental (unintentional)
    - Poisoning by cephalosporins and other beta-lactam antibiotics NOS
- T36.1X2 Poisoning by cephalosporins and other beta-lactam antibiotics, intentional self-harm A, S 🐷
- T36.1X3 Poisoning by cephalosporins and other beta-lactam antibiotics, assault
- T36.1X4 Poisoning by cephalosporins and other beta-lactam antibiotics, undetermined
- T36.1X5 Adverse effect of cephalosporins and other beta-lactam antibiotics
- T36.1X6 Underdosing of cephalosporins and other beta-lactam antibiotics

- T36.2 Poisoning by, adverse effect of and underdosing of chloramphenicol group
    - T36.2X Poisoning by, adverse effect of and underdosing of chloramphenicol group
        - T36.2X1 Poisoning by chloramphenicol group, accidental (unintentional)
            - Poisoning by chloramphenicol group NOS
        - T36.2X2 Poisoning by chloramphenicol group, intentional self-harm A, S 🐷
        - T36.2X3 Poisoning by chloramphenicol group, assault
        - T36.2X4 Poisoning by chloramphenicol group, undetermined
        - T36.2X5 Adverse effect of chloramphenicol group
        - T36.2X6 Underdosing of chloramphenicol group

- T36.3 Poisoning by, adverse effect of and underdosing of macrolides
    - T36.3X Poisoning by, adverse effect of and underdosing of macrolides
        - T36.3X1 Poisoning by macrolides, accidental (unintentional)
            - Poisoning by macrolides NOS
        - T36.3X2 Poisoning by macrolides, intentional self-harm A, S 🐷
        - T36.3X3 Poisoning by macrolides, assault
        - T36.3X4 Poisoning by macrolides, undetermined
        - T36.3X5 Adverse effect of macrolides
        - T36.3X6 Underdosing of macrolides

- T36.4 Poisoning by, adverse effect of and underdosing of tetracyclines
    - T36.4X Poisoning by, adverse effect of and underdosing of tetracyclines
        - T36.4X1 Poisoning by tetracyclines, accidental (unintentional)
            - Poisoning by tetracyclines NOS
        - T36.4X2 Poisoning by tetracyclines, intentional self-harm A, S 🐷
        - T36.4X3 Poisoning by tetracyclines, assault
        - T36.4X4 Poisoning by tetracyclines, undetermined
        - T36.4X5 Adverse effect of tetracyclines
        - T36.4X6 Underdosing of tetracyclines

- T36.5 Poisoning by, adverse effect of and underdosing of aminoglycosides
    - Poisoning by, adverse effect of and underdosing of streptomycin
    - T36.5X Poisoning by, adverse effect of and underdosing of aminoglycosides

- T36.5X1 Poisoning by aminoglycosides, accidental (unintentional)
    - Poisoning by aminoglycosides NOS
- T36.5X2 Poisoning by aminoglycosides, intentional self-harm A, S 🐷
- T36.5X3 Poisoning by aminoglycosides, assault
- T36.5X4 Poisoning by aminoglycosides, undetermined
- T36.5X5 Adverse effect of aminoglycosides
- T36.5X6 Underdosing of aminoglycosides

- T36.6 Poisoning by, adverse effect of and underdosing of rifampicins
    - T36.6X Poisoning by, adverse effect of and underdosing of rifampicins
        - T36.6X1 Poisoning by rifampicins, accidental (unintentional)
            - Poisoning by rifampicins NOS
        - T36.6X2 Poisoning by rifampicins, intentional self-harm A, S 🐷
        - T36.6X3 Poisoning by rifampicins, assault
        - T36.6X4 Poisoning by rifampicins, undetermined
        - T36.6X5 Adverse effect of rifampicins
        - T36.6X6 Underdosing of rifampicins

- T36.7 Poisoning by, adverse effect of and underdosing of antifungal antibiotics, systemically used
    - T36.7X Poisoning by, adverse effect of and underdosing of antifungal antibiotics, systemically used
        - T36.7X1 Poisoning by antifungal antibiotics, systemically used, accidental (unintentional)
            - Poisoning by antifungal antibiotics, systemically used NOS
        - T36.7X2 Poisoning by antifungal antibiotics, systemically used, intentional self-harm A, S 🐷
        - T36.7X3 Poisoning by antifungal antibiotics, systemically used, assault
        - T36.7X4 Poisoning by antifungal antibiotics, systemically used, undetermined
        - T36.7X5 Adverse effect of antifungal antibiotics, systemically used
        - T36.7X6 Underdosing of antifungal antibiotics, systemically used

- T36.8 Poisoning by, adverse effect of and underdosing of other systemic antibiotics
    - T36.8X Poisoning by, adverse effect of and underdosing of other systemic antibiotics
        - T36.8X1 Poisoning by other systemic antibiotics, accidental (unintentional)
            - Poisoning by other systemic antibiotics NOS
        - T36.8X2 Poisoning by other systemic antibiotics, intentional self-harm A, S 🐷
        - T36.8X3 Poisoning by other systemic antibiotics, assault
        - T36.8X4 Poisoning by other systemic antibiotics, undetermined
        - T36.8X5 Adverse effect of other systemic antibiotics
            - **Coding Clinic: 2017, Q1, P39**
        - T36.8X6 Underdosing of other systemic antibiotics

- T36.9 Poisoning by, adverse effect of and underdosing of unspecified systemic antibiotic
    - X● T36.91 Poisoning by unspecified systemic antibiotic, accidental (unintentional)
        - Poisoning by systemic antibiotic NOS

CHAPTER 19 (S00-T88)

X● T36.92   Poisoning by unspecified systemic antibiotic, intentional self-harm A, S 🦠

X● T36.93   Poisoning by unspecified systemic antibiotic, assault

X● T36.94   Poisoning by unspecified systemic antibiotic, undetermined

X● T36.95   Adverse effect of unspecified systemic antibiotic

X● T36.96   Underdosing of unspecified systemic antibiotic

● T37   Poisoning by, adverse effect of and underdosing of other systemic anti-infectives and antiparasitics

Excludes1   anti-infectives topically used for ear, nose and throat (T49.6-)
anti-infectives topically used for eye (T49.5-)
locally applied anti-infectives NEC (T49.0-)

The appropriate 7th character is to be added to each code from category T37

A   initial encounter
D   subsequent encounter
S   sequela

● T37.0   Poisoning by, adverse effect of and underdosing of sulfonamides

● T37.0X   Poisoning by, adverse effect of and underdosing of sulfonamides

● T37.0X1   Poisoning by sulfonamides, accidental (unintentional)
Poisoning by sulfonamides NOS

● T37.0X2   Poisoning by sulfonamides, intentional self-harm A, S 🦠

● T37.0X3   Poisoning by sulfonamides, assault

● T37.0X4   Poisoning by sulfonamides, undetermined

● T37.0X5   Adverse effect of sulfonamides

● T37.0X6   Underdosing of sulfonamides

● T37.1   Poisoning by, adverse effect of and underdosing of antimycobacterial drugs

Excludes1   rifampicins (T36.6-) streptomycin (T36.5-)

● T37.1X   Poisoning by, adverse effect of and underdosing of antimycobacterial drugs

● T37.1X1   Poisoning by antimycobacterial drugs, accidental (unintentional)
Poisoning by antimycobacterial drugs NOS

● T37.1X2   Poisoning by antimycobacterial drugs, intentional self-harm A, S 🦠

● T37.1X3   Poisoning by antimycobacterial drugs, assault

● T37.1X4   Poisoning by antimycobacterial drugs, undetermined

● T37.1X5   Adverse effect of antimycobacterial drugs

● T37.1X6   Underdosing of antimycobacterial drugs

● T37.2   Poisoning by, adverse effect of and underdosing of antimalarials and drugs acting on other blood protozoa

Excludes1   hydroxyquinoline derivatives (T37.8-)

● T37.2X   Poisoning by, adverse effect of and underdosing of antimalarials and drugs acting on other blood protozoa

● T37.2X1   Poisoning by antimalarials and drugs acting on other blood protozoa, accidental (unintentional)
Poisoning by antimalarials and drugs acting on other blood protozoa NOS

● T37.2X2   Poisoning by antimalarials and drugs acting on other blood protozoa, intentional self-harm A, S 🦠

● T37.2X3   Poisoning by antimalarials and drugs acting on other blood protozoa, assault

● T37.2X4   Poisoning by antimalarials and drugs acting on other blood protozoa, undetermined

● T37.2X5   Adverse effect of antimalarials and drugs acting on other blood protozoa

● T37.2X6   Underdosing of antimalarials and drugs acting on other blood protozoa

● T37.3   Poisoning by, adverse effect of and underdosing of other antiprotozoal drugs

● T37.3X   Poisoning by, adverse effect of and underdosing of other antiprotozoal drugs

● T37.3X1   Poisoning by other antiprotozoal drugs, accidental (unintentional)
Poisoning by other antiprotozoal drugs NOS

● T37.3X2   Poisoning by other antiprotozoal drugs, intentional self-harm A, S 🦠

● T37.3X3   Poisoning by other antiprotozoal drugs, assault

● T37.3X4   Poisoning by other antiprotozoal drugs, undetermined

● T37.3X5   Adverse effect of other antiprotozoal drugs

● T37.3X6   Underdosing of other antiprotozoal drugs

● T37.4   Poisoning by, adverse effect of and underdosing of anthelminthics

● T37.4X   Poisoning by, adverse effect of and underdosing of anthelminthics

● T37.4X1   Poisoning by anthelminthics, accidental (unintentional)
Poisoning by anthelminthics NOS

● T37.4X2   Poisoning by anthelminthics, intentional self-harm A, S 🦠

● T37.4X3   Poisoning by anthelminthics, assault

● T37.4X4   Poisoning by anthelminthics, undetermined

● T37.4X5   Adverse effect of anthelminthics

● T37.4X6   Underdosing of anthelminthics

● T37.5   Poisoning by, adverse effect of and underdosing of antiviral drugs

Excludes1   amantadine (T42.8-)
cytarabine (T45.1-)

● T37.5X   Poisoning by, adverse effect of and underdosing of antiviral drugs

● T37.5X1   Poisoning by antiviral drugs, accidental (unintentional)
Poisoning by antiviral drugs NOS

● T37.5X2   Poisoning by antiviral drugs, intentional self-harm A, S 🦠

● T37.5X3   Poisoning by antiviral drugs, assault

● T37.5X4   Poisoning by antiviral drugs, undetermined

● T37.5X5   Adverse effect of antiviral drugs

● T37.5X6   Underdosing of antiviral drugs

● T37.8   Poisoning by, adverse effect of and underdosing of other specified systemic anti-infectives and antiparasitics
Poisoning by, adverse effect of and underdosing of hydroxyquinoline derivatives

Excludes1   antimalarial drugs (T37.2-)

● T37.8X   Poisoning by, adverse effect of and underdosing of other specified systemic anti-infectives and antiparasitics

▶ New   ➡ Revised   deleted Deleted   Excludes 1   Excludes 2   Includes   Use additional   Code first   Code also   Key words
OGCR Official Guidelines   X Assign placeholder X   ● Use Additional Character(s)   ▌ Manifestation Code   🦠 Hierarchical Condition Category   Coding Clinic

● T37.8X1   Poisoning by other specified systemic anti-infectives and antiparasitics, accidental (unintentional)
　　　　Poisoning by other specified systemic anti-infectives and antiparasitics NOS

● T37.8X2   Poisoning by other specified systemic anti-infectives and antiparasitics, intentional self-harm A, S 🔒

● T37.8X3   Poisoning by other specified systemic anti-infectives and antiparasitics, assault

● T37.8X4   Poisoning by other specified systemic anti-infectives and antiparasitics, undetermined

● T37.8X5   Adverse effect of other specified systemic anti-infectives and antiparasitics

● T37.8X6   Underdosing of other specified systemic anti-infectives and antiparasitics

● T37.9   Poisoning by, adverse effect of and underdosing of unspecified systemic anti-infective and antiparasitics

X● T37.91   Poisoning by unspecified systemic anti-infective and antiparasitics, accidental (unintentional)
　　　　Poisoning by, adverse effect of and underdosing of systemic anti-infective and antiparasitics NOS

X● T37.92   Poisoning by unspecified systemic anti-infective and antiparasitics, intentional self-harm A, S 🔒

X● T37.93   Poisoning by unspecified systemic anti-infective and antiparasitics, assault

X● T37.94   Poisoning by unspecified systemic anti-infective and antiparasitics, undetermined

X● T37.95   Adverse effect of unspecified systemic anti-infective and antiparasitic

X● T37.96   Underdosing of unspecified systemic anti-infectives and antiparasitics

● T38   Poisoning by, adverse effect of and underdosing of hormones and their synthetic substitutes and antagonists, not elsewhere classified

> **Excludes1**   mineralocorticoids and their antagonists (T50.0-)
> oxytocic hormones (T48.0-)
> parathyroid hormones and derivatives (T50.9-)

The appropriate 7th character is to be added to each code from category T38

A	initial encounter
D	subsequent encounter
S	sequela

● T38.0   Poisoning by, adverse effect of and underdosing of glucocorticoids and synthetic analogues

> **Excludes1**   glucocorticoids, topically used (T49.-)

● T38.0X   Poisoning by, adverse effect of and underdosing of glucocorticoids and synthetic analogues

● T38.0X1   Poisoning by glucocorticoids and synthetic analogues, accidental (unintentional)
　　　　Poisoning by glucocorticoids and synthetic analogues NOS

● T38.0X2   Poisoning by glucocorticoids and synthetic analogues, intentional self-harm A, S 🔒

● T38.0X3   Poisoning by glucocorticoids and synthetic analogues, assault

● T38.0X4   Poisoning by glucocorticoids and synthetic analogues, undetermined

● T38.0X5   Adverse effect of glucocorticoids and synthetic analogues

● T38.0X6   Underdosing of glucocorticoids and synthetic analogues

● T38.1   Poisoning by, adverse effect of and underdosing of thyroid hormones and substitutes

● T38.1X   Poisoning by, adverse effect of and underdosing of thyroid hormones and substitutes

● T38.1X1   Poisoning by thyroid hormones and substitutes, accidental (unintentional)
　　　　Poisoning by thyroid hormones and substitutes NOS

● T38.1X2   Poisoning by thyroid hormones and substitutes, intentional self-harm A, S 🔒

● T38.1X3   Poisoning by thyroid hormones and substitutes, assault

● T38.1X4   Poisoning by thyroid hormones and substitutes, undetermined

● T38.1X5   Adverse effect of thyroid hormones and substitutes

● T38.1X6   Underdosing of thyroid hormones and substitutes

● T38.2   Poisoning by, adverse effect of and underdosing of antithyroid drugs

● T38.2X   Poisoning by, adverse effect of and underdosing of antithyroid drugs

● T38.2X1   Poisoning by antithyroid drugs, accidental (unintentional)
　　　　Poisoning by antithyroid drugs NOS

● T38.2X2   Poisoning by antithyroid drugs, intentional self-harm A, S 🔒

● T38.2X3   Poisoning by antithyroid drugs, assault

● T38.2X4   Poisoning by antithyroid drugs, undetermined

● T38.2X5   Adverse effect of antithyroid drugs

● T38.2X6   Underdosing of antithyroid drugs

● T38.3   Poisoning by, adverse effect of and underdosing of insulin and oral hypoglycemic [antidiabetic] drugs

● T38.3X   Poisoning by, adverse effect of and underdosing of insulin and oral hypoglycemic [antidiabetic] drugs

● T38.3X1   Poisoning by insulin and oral hypoglycemic [antidiabetic] drugs, accidental (unintentional)
　　　　Poisoning by insulin and oral hypoglycemic [antidiabetic] drugs NOS

● T38.3X2   Poisoning by insulin and oral hypoglycemic [antidiabetic] drugs, intentional self-harm

● T38.3X3   Poisoning by insulin and oral hypoglycemic [antidiabetic] drugs, assault A, S 🔒

● T38.3X4   Poisoning by insulin and oral hypoglycemic [antidiabetic] drugs, undetermined

● T38.3X5   Adverse effect of insulin and oral hypoglycemic [antidiabetic] drugs

● T38.3X6   Underdosing of insulin and oral hypoglycemic [antidiabetic] drugs

● T38.4   Poisoning by, adverse effect of and underdosing of oral contraceptives
　　　Poisoning by, adverse effect of and underdosing of multiple- and single-ingredient oral contraceptive preparations

● T38.4X   Poisoning by, adverse effect of and underdosing of oral contraceptives

● T38.4X1   Poisoning by oral contraceptives, accidental (unintentional)
　　　　Poisoning by oral contraceptives NOS

● T38.4X2   Poisoning by oral contraceptives, intentional self-harm A, S 🦠

● T38.4X3   Poisoning by oral contraceptives, assault

● T38.4X4   Poisoning by oral contraceptives, undetermined

● T38.4X5   Adverse effect of oral contraceptives

● T38.4X6   Underdosing of oral contraceptives

● T38.5   Poisoning by, adverse effect of and underdosing of other estrogens and progestogens

Poisoning by, adverse effect of and underdosing of estrogens and progestogens mixtures and substitutes

● T38.5X   Poisoning by, adverse effect of and underdosing of other estrogens and progestogens

● T38.5X1   Poisoning by other estrogens and progestogens, accidental (unintentional)

Poisoning by other estrogens and progestogens NOS

● T38.5X2   Poisoning by other estrogens and progestogens, intentional self-harm A, S 🦠

● T38.5X3   Poisoning by other estrogens and progestogens, assault

● T38.5X4   Poisoning by other estrogens and progestogens, undetermined

● T38.5X5   Adverse effect of other estrogens and progestogens

● T38.5X6   Underdosing of other estrogens and progestogens

● T38.6   Poisoning by, adverse effect of and underdosing of antigonadotrophins, antiestrogens, antiandrogens, not elsewhere classified

Poisoning by, adverse effect of and underdosing of tamoxifen

● T38.6X   Poisoning by, adverse effect of and underdosing of antigonadotrophins, antiestrogens, antiandrogens, not elsewhere classified

● T38.6X1   Poisoning by antigonadotrophins, antiestrogens, antiandrogens, not elsewhere classified, accidental (unintentional)

Poisoning by antigonadotrophins, antiestrogens, antiandrogens, not elsewhere classified NOS

● T38.6X2   Poisoning by antigonadotrophins, antiestrogens, antiandrogens, not elsewhere classified, intentional self-harm A, S 🦠

● T38.6X3   Poisoning by antigonadotrophins, antiestrogens, antiandrogens, not elsewhere classified, assault

● T38.6X4   Poisoning by antigonadotrophins, antiestrogens, antiandrogens, not elsewhere classified, undetermined

● T38.6X5   Adverse effect of antigonadotrophins, antiestrogens, antiandrogens, not elsewhere classified

● T38.6X6   Underdosing of antigonadotrophins, antiestrogens, antiandrogens, not elsewhere classified

● T38.7   Poisoning by, adverse effect of and underdosing of androgens and anabolic congeners

● T38.7X   Poisoning by, adverse effect of and underdosing of androgens and anabolic congeners

● T38.7X1   Poisoning by androgens and anabolic congeners, accidental (unintentional)

Poisoning by androgens and anabolic congeners NOS

● T38.7X2   Poisoning by androgens and anabolic congeners, intentional self-harm A, S 🦠

● T38.7X3   Poisoning by androgens and anabolic congeners, assault

● T38.7X4   Poisoning by androgens and anabolic congeners, undetermined

● T38.7X5   Adverse effect of androgens and anabolic congeners

● T38.7X6   Underdosing of androgens and anabolic congeners

● T38.8   Poisoning by, adverse effect of and underdosing of other and unspecified hormones and synthetic substitutes

● T38.80   Poisoning by, adverse effect of and underdosing of unspecified hormones and synthetic substitutes

● T38.801   Poisoning by unspecified hormones and synthetic substitutes, accidental (unintentional)

Poisoning by unspecified hormones and synthetic substitutes NOS

● T38.802   Poisoning by unspecified hormones and synthetic substitutes, intentional self-harm A, S 🦠

● T38.803   Poisoning by unspecified hormones and synthetic substitutes, assault

● T38.804   Poisoning by unspecified hormones and synthetic substitutes, undetermined

● T38.805   Adverse effect of unspecified hormones and synthetic substitutes

● T38.806   Underdosing of unspecified hormones and synthetic substitutes

● T38.81   Poisoning by, adverse effect of and underdosing of anterior pituitary [adenohypophyseal] hormones

● T38.811   Poisoning by anterior pituitary [adenohypophyseal] hormones, accidental (unintentional)

Poisoning by anterior pituitary [adenohypophyseal] hormones NOS

● T38.812   Poisoning by anterior pituitary [adenohypophyseal] hormones, intentional self-harm A, S 🦠

● T38.813   Poisoning by anterior pituitary [adenohypophyseal] hormones, assault

● T38.814   Poisoning by anterior pituitary [adenohypophyseal] hormones, undetermined

● T38.815   Adverse effect of anterior pituitary [adenohypophyseal] hormones

● T38.816   Underdosing of anterior pituitary [adenohypophyseal] hormones

● T38.89   Poisoning by, adverse effect of and underdosing of other hormones and synthetic substitutes

● T38.891   Poisoning by other hormones and synthetic substitutes, accidental (unintentional)

Poisoning by other hormones and synthetic substitutes NOS

● T38.892   Poisoning by other hormones and synthetic substitutes, intentional self-harm A, S 🦠

● T38.893   Poisoning by other hormones and synthetic substitutes, assault

● T38.894   Poisoning by other hormones and synthetic substitutes, undetermined

▶ New   ⇒ Revised   ~~deleted~~ Deleted   Excludes 1   Excludes 2   Includes   Use additional   Code first   Code also   Key words

OGCR Official Guidelines   X Assign placeholder X   ● Use Additional Character(s)   ▶ Manifestation Code   🦠 Hierarchical Condition Category   **Coding Clinic**

● T38.895 Adverse effect of other hormones and synthetic substitutes

● T38.896 Underdosing of other hormones and synthetic substitutes

● T38.9 Poisoning by, adverse effect of and underdosing of other and unspecified hormone antagonists

● T38.90 Poisoning by, adverse effect of and underdosing of unspecified hormone antagonists

● T38.901 Poisoning by unspecified hormone antagonists, accidental (unintentional)
Poisoning by unspecified hormone antagonists NOS

● T38.902 Poisoning by unspecified hormone antagonists, intentional self-harm A, S 🔖

● T38.903 Poisoning by unspecified hormone antagonists, assault

● T38.904 Poisoning by unspecified hormone antagonists, undetermined

● T38.905 Adverse effect of unspecified hormone antagonists

● T38.906 Underdosing of unspecified hormone antagonists

● T38.99 Poisoning by, adverse effect of and underdosing of other hormone antagonists

● T38.991 Poisoning by other hormone antagonists, accidental (unintentional)
Poisoning by other hormone antagonists NOS

● T38.992 Poisoning by other hormone antagonists, intentional self-harm A, S 🔖

● T38.993 Poisoning by other hormone antagonists, assault

● T38.994 Poisoning by other hormone antagonists, undetermined

● T38.995 Adverse effect of other hormone antagonists

● T38.996 Underdosing of other hormone antagonists

● T39 Poisoning by, adverse effect of and underdosing of nonopioid analgesics, antipyretics and antirheumatics

The appropriate 7th character is to be added to each code from category T39

A	initial encounter
D	subsequent encounter
S	sequela

● T39.0 Poisoning by, adverse effect of and underdosing of salicylates

● T39.01 Poisoning by, adverse effect of and underdosing of aspirin
Poisoning by, adverse effect of and underdosing of acetylsalicylic acid

● T39.011 Poisoning by aspirin, accidental (unintentional)

● T39.012 Poisoning by aspirin, intentional self-harm A, S 🔖

● T39.013 Poisoning by aspirin, assault

● T39.014 Poisoning by aspirin, undetermined

● T39.015 Adverse effect of aspirin
Coding Clinic: 2016, Q1, P15

● T39.016 Underdosing of aspirin

● T39.09 Poisoning by, adverse effect of and underdosing of other salicylates

● T39.091 Poisoning by salicylates, accidental (unintentional)
Poisoning by salicylates NOS

● T39.092 Poisoning by salicylates, intentional self-harm A, S 🔖

● T39.093 Poisoning by salicylates, assault

● T39.094 Poisoning by salicylates, undetermined

● T39.095 Adverse effect of salicylates

● T39.096 Underdosing of salicylates

● T39.1 Poisoning by, adverse effect of and underdosing of 4-Aminophenol derivatives

● T39.1X Poisoning by, adverse effect of and underdosing of 4-Aminophenol derivatives

● T39.1X1 Poisoning by 4-Aminophenol derivatives, accidental (unintentional)
Poisoning by 4-Aminophenol derivatives NOS

● T39.1X2 Poisoning by 4-Aminophenol derivatives, intentional self-harm A, S 🔖

● T39.1X3 Poisoning by 4-Aminophenol derivatives, assault

● T39.1X4 Poisoning by 4-Aminophenol derivatives, undetermined

● T39.1X5 Adverse effect of 4-Aminophenol derivatives

● T39.1X6 Underdosing of 4-Aminophenol derivatives

● T39.2 Poisoning by, adverse effect of and underdosing of pyrazolone derivatives

● T39.2X Poisoning by, adverse effect of and underdosing of pyrazolone derivatives

● T39.2X1 Poisoning by pyrazolone derivatives, accidental (unintentional)
Poisoning by pyrazolone derivatives NOS

● T39.2X2 Poisoning by pyrazolone derivatives, intentional self-harm A, S 🔖

● T39.2X3 Poisoning by pyrazolone derivatives, assault

● T39.2X4 Poisoning by pyrazolone derivatives, undetermined

● T39.2X5 Adverse effect of pyrazolone derivatives

● T39.2X6 Underdosing of pyrazolone derivatives

● T39.3 Poisoning by, adverse effect of and underdosing of other nonsteroidal anti-inflammatory drugs [NSAID]

● T39.31 Poisoning by, adverse effect of and underdosing of propionic acid derivatives
Poisoning by, adverse effect of and underdosing of fenoprofen
Poisoning by, adverse effect of and underdosing of flurbiprofen
Poisoning by, adverse effect of and underdosing of ibuprofen
Poisoning by, adverse effect of and underdosing of ketoprofen
Poisoning by, adverse effect of and underdosing of naproxen
Poisoning by, adverse effect of and underdosing of oxaprozin

● T39.311 Poisoning by propionic acid derivatives, accidental (unintentional)

● T39.312 Poisoning by propionic acid derivatives, intentional self-harm A, S 🔖

● T39.313 Poisoning by propionic acid derivatives, assault

● T39.314 Poisoning by propionic acid derivatives, undetermined

● T39.315 Adverse effect of propionic acid derivatives

● T39.316 Underdosing of propionic acid derivatives

CHAPTER 19 (S00-T88)

● **T39.39**   Poisoning by, adverse effect of and underdosing of other nonsteroidal anti-inflammatory drugs [NSAID]

  ● **T39.391**   Poisoning by other nonsteroidal anti-inflammatory drugs [NSAID], accidental (unintentional)
      Poisoning by other nonsteroidal anti-inflammatory drugs NOS

  ● **T39.392**   Poisoning by other nonsteroidal anti-inflammatory drugs [NSAID], intentional self-harm A, S 🐾

  ● **T39.393**   Poisoning by other nonsteroidal anti-inflammatory drugs [NSAID], assault

  ● **T39.394**   Poisoning by other nonsteroidal anti-inflammatory drugs [NSAID], undetermined

  ● **T39.395**   Adverse effect of other nonsteroidal anti-inflammatory drugs [NSAID]

  ● **T39.396**   Underdosing of other nonsteroidal anti-inflammatory drugs [NSAID]

● **T39.4**   Poisoning by, adverse effect of and underdosing of antirheumatics, not elsewhere classified

  Excludes1   poisoning by, adverse effect of and underdosing of glucocorticoids (T38.0-)
      poisoning by, adverse effect of and underdosing of salicylates (T39.0-)

  ● **T39.4X**   Poisoning by, adverse effect of and underdosing of antirheumatics, not elsewhere classified

    ● **T39.4X1**   Poisoning by antirheumatics, not elsewhere classified, accidental (unintentional)
       Poisoning by antirheumatics, not elsewhere classified NOS

    ● **T39.4X2**   Poisoning by antirheumatics, not elsewhere classified, intentional self-harm A, S 🐾

    ● **T39.4X3**   Poisoning by antirheumatics, not elsewhere classified, assault

    ● **T39.4X4**   Poisoning by antirheumatics, not elsewhere classified, undetermined

    ● **T39.4X5**   Adverse effect of antirheumatics, not elsewhere classified

    ● **T39.4X6**   Underdosing of antirheumatics, not elsewhere classified

● **T39.8**   Poisoning by, adverse effect of and underdosing of other nonopioid analgesics and antipyretics, not elsewhere classified

  ● **T39.8X**   Poisoning by, adverse effect of and underdosing of other nonopioid analgesics and antipyretics, not elsewhere classified

    ● **T39.8X1**   Poisoning by other nonopioid analgesics and antipyretics, not elsewhere classified, accidental (unintentional)
       Poisoning by other nonopioid analgesics and antipyretics, not elsewhere classified NOS

    ● **T39.8X2**   Poisoning by other nonopioid analgesics and antipyretics, not elsewhere classified, intentional self-harm A, S 🐾

    ● **T39.8X3**   Poisoning by other nonopioid analgesics and antipyretics, not elsewhere classified, assault

    ● **T39.8X4**   Poisoning by other nonopioid analgesics and antipyretics, not elsewhere classified, undetermined

    ● **T39.8X5**   Adverse effect of other nonopioid analgesics and antipyretics, not elsewhere classified

    ● **T39.8X6**   Underdosing of other nonopioid analgesics and antipyretics, not elsewhere classified

● **T39.9**   Poisoning by, adverse effect of and underdosing of unspecified nonopioid analgesic, antipyretic and antirheumatic

  X ● **T39.91**   Poisoning by unspecified nonopioid analgesic, antipyretic and antirheumatic, accidental (unintentional)
      Poisoning by nonopioid analgesic, antipyretic and antirheumatic NOS

  X ● **T39.92**   Poisoning by unspecified nonopioid analgesic, antipyretic and antirheumatic, intentional self-harm A, S 🐾

  X ● **T39.93**   Poisoning by unspecified nonopioid analgesic, antipyretic and antirheumatic, assault

  X ● **T39.94**   Poisoning by unspecified nonopioid analgesic, antipyretic and antirheumatic, undetermined

  X ● **T39.95**   Adverse effect of unspecified nonopioid analgesic, antipyretic and antirheumatic

  X ● **T39.96**   Underdosing of unspecified nonopioid analgesic, antipyretic and antirheumatic

● **T40**   Poisoning by, adverse effect of and underdosing of narcotics and psychodysleptics [hallucinogens]

  Excludes2   drug dependence and related mental and behavioral disorders due to psychoactive substance use (F10.-F19.-)

  The appropriate 7th character is to be added to each code from category T40

A	initial encounter
D	subsequent encounter
S	sequela

● **T40.0**   Poisoning by, adverse effect of and underdosing of opium

  ● **T40.0X**   Poisoning by, adverse effect of and underdosing of opium

    ● **T40.0X1**   Poisoning by opium, accidental (unintentional)
       Poisoning by opium NOS

    ● **T40.0X2**   Poisoning by opium, intentional self-harm A, S 🐾

    ● **T40.0X3**   Poisoning by opium, assault

    ● **T40.0X4**   Poisoning by opium, undetermined

    ● **T40.0X5**   Adverse effect of opium

    ● **T40.0X6**   Underdosing of opium

● **T40.1**   Poisoning by and adverse effect of heroin

  ● **T40.1X**   Poisoning by and adverse effect of heroin

    ● **T40.1X1**   Poisoning by heroin, accidental (unintentional)
       Poisoning by heroin NOS

    ● **T40.1X2**   Poisoning by heroin, intentional self-harm A, S 🐾

    ● **T40.1X3**   Poisoning by heroin, assault

    ● **T40.1X4**   Poisoning by heroin, undetermined

● **T40.2**   Poisoning by, adverse effect of and underdosing of other opioids

  ● **T40.2X**   Poisoning by, adverse effect of and underdosing of other opioids

    ● **T40.2X1**   Poisoning by other opioids, accidental (unintentional)
       Poisoning by other opioids NOS

    ● **T40.2X2**   Poisoning by other opioids, intentional self-harm A, S 🐾

    ● **T40.2X3**   Poisoning by other opioids, assault

    ● **T40.2X4**   Poisoning by other opioids, undetermined

    ● **T40.2X5**   Adverse effect of other opioids

    ● **T40.2X6**   Underdosing of other opioids

▶ New   ⟾ Revised   ~~deleted~~ Deleted   Excludes 1   Excludes 2   Includes   Use additional   Code first   Code also   Key words
OGCR Official Guidelines   X Assign placeholder X   ● Use Additional Character(s)   ▷ Manifestation Code   🐾 Hierarchical Condition Category   **Coding Clinic**

● T40.3   Poisoning by, adverse effect of and underdosing of methadone
   ● T40.3X   Poisoning by, adverse effect of and underdosing of methadone
     ● T40.3X1   Poisoning by methadone, accidental (unintentional)
         Poisoning by methadone NOS
     ● T40.3X2   Poisoning by methadone, intentional self-harm A, S 🐾
     ● T40.3X3   Poisoning by methadone, assault
     ● T40.3X4   Poisoning by methadone, undetermined
     ● T40.3X5   Adverse effect of methadone
     ● T40.3X6   Underdosing of methadone

● T40.4   Poisoning by, adverse effect of and underdosing of other synthetic narcotics
   ● T40.41   Poisoning by, adverse effect of and underdosing of fentanyl or fentanyl analogs
     T40.411   Poisoning by fentanyl or fentanyl analogs, accidental (unintentional)
     T40.412   Poisoning by fentanyl or fentanyl analogs, intentional self-harm
     T40.413   Poisoning by fentanyl or fentanyl analogs, assault
     T40.414   Poisoning by fentanyl or fentanyl analogs, undetermined
     T40.415   Adverse effect of fentanyl or fentanyl analogs
     T40.416   Underdosing of fentanyl or fentanyl analogs
   ● T40.42   Poisoning by, adverse effect of and underdosing of tramadol
     T40.421   Poisoning by tramadol, accidental (unintentional)
     T40.422   Poisoning by tramadol, intentional self-harm
     T40.423   Poisoning by tramadol, assault
     T40.424   Poisoning by tramadol, undetermined
     T40.425   Adverse effect of tramadol
     T40.426   Underdosing of tramadol
   ● T40.49   Poisoning by, adverse effect of and underdosing of other synthetic narcotics
     T40.491   Poisoning by other synthetic narcotics, accidental (unintentional)
     T40.492   Poisoning by other synthetic narcotics, intentional self-harm
     T40.493   Poisoning by other synthetic narcotics, assault
     T40.494   Poisoning by other synthetic narcotics, undetermined
     T40.495   Adverse effect of other synthetic narcotics
     T40.496   Underdosing of other synthetic narcotics

● T40.5   Poisoning by, adverse effect of and underdosing of cocaine
   ● T40.5X   Poisoning by, adverse effect of and underdosing of cocaine
     ● T40.5X1   Poisoning by cocaine, accidental (unintentional)
         Poisoning by cocaine NOS
         Coding Clinic: 2016, Q2, P9
     ● T40.5X2   Poisoning by cocaine, intentional self-harm A, S 🐾
     ● T40.5X3   Poisoning by cocaine, assault
     ● T40.5X4   Poisoning by cocaine, undetermined
     ● T40.5X5   Adverse effect of cocaine
     ● T40.5X6   Underdosing of cocaine

● T40.6   Poisoning by, adverse effect of and underdosing of other and unspecified narcotics
   ● T40.60   Poisoning by, adverse effect of and underdosing of unspecified narcotics
     ● T40.601   Poisoning by unspecified narcotics, accidental (unintentional)
         Poisoning by narcotics NOS
     ● T40.602   Poisoning by unspecified narcotics, intentional self-harm A, S 🐾
     ● T40.603   Poisoning by unspecified narcotics, assault
     ● T40.604   Poisoning by unspecified narcotics, undetermined
     ● T40.605   Adverse effect of unspecified narcotics
     ● T40.606   Underdosing of unspecified narcotics
   ● T40.69   Poisoning by, adverse effect of and underdosing of other narcotics
     ● T40.691   Poisoning by other narcotics, accidental (unintentional)
         Poisoning by other narcotics NOS
     ● T40.692   Poisoning by other narcotics, intentional self-harm A, S 🐾
     ● T40.693   Poisoning by other narcotics, assault
     ● T40.694   Poisoning by other narcotics, undetermined
     ● T40.695   Adverse effect of other narcotics
     ● T40.696   Underdosing of other narcotics

● T40.7   Poisoning by, adverse effect of and underdosing of cannabis (derivatives)
   ● T40.71   Poisoning by, adverse effect of and underdosing of cannabis (derivatives)
     T40.711   Poisoning by cannabis, accidental (unintentional)
     T40.712   Poisoning by cannabis, intentional self-harm
     T40.713   Poisoning by cannabis, assault
     T40.714   Poisoning by cannabis, undetermined
     T40.715   Adverse effect of cannabis
     T40.716   Underdosing of cannabis
   ● T40.72   Poisoning by, adverse effect of and underdosing of synthetic cannabinoids
     T40.721   Poisoning by synthetic cannabinoids, accidental (unintentional)
     T40.722   Poisoning by synthetic cannabinoids, intentional self-harm
     T40.723   Poisoning by synthetic cannabinoids, assault
     T40.724   Poisoning by synthetic cannabinoids, undetermined
     T40.725   Adverse effect of synthetic cannabinoids
     T40.726   Underdosing of synthetic cannabinoids

● T40.8   Poisoning by and adverse effect of lysergide [LSD]
   ● T40.8X   Poisoning by and adverse effect of lysergide [LSD]
     ● T40.8X1   Poisoning by lysergide [LSD], accidental (unintentional)
         Poisoning by lysergide [LSD] NOS
     ● T40.8X2   Poisoning by lysergide [LSD], intentional self-harm A, S 🐾
     ● T40.8X3   Poisoning by lysergide [LSD], assault
     ● T40.8X4   Poisoning by lysergide [LSD], undetermined

● T40.9   Poisoning by, adverse effect of and underdosing of other and unspecified psychodysleptics [hallucinogens]
   ● T40.90   Poisoning by, adverse effect of and underdosing of unspecified psychodysleptics [hallucinogens]

CHAPTER 19 (S00-T88)

- T40.901 Poisoning by unspecified psychodysleptics [hallucinogens], **accidental (unintentional)**
- T40.902 Poisoning by unspecified psychodysleptics [hallucinogens], **intentional self-harm** A, S 🦠
- T40.903 Poisoning by unspecified psychodysleptics [hallucinogens], assault
- T40.904 Poisoning by unspecified psychodysleptics [hallucinogens], **undetermined**
- T40.905 **Adverse effect** of unspecified psychodysleptics [hallucinogens]
- T40.906 **Underdosing** of unspecified psychodysleptics [hallucinogens]
- T40.99 Poisoning by, adverse effect of and underdosing of **other psychodysleptics** [hallucinogens]
  - T40.991 Poisoning by other psychodysleptics [hallucinogens], **accidental (unintentional)**
    Poisoning by other psychodysleptics [hallucinogens] NOS
  - T40.992 Poisoning by other psychodysleptics [hallucinogens], **intentional self-harm** A, S 🦠
  - T40.993 Poisoning by other psychodysleptics [hallucinogens], **assault**
  - T40.994 Poisoning by other psychodysleptics [hallucinogens], **undetermined**
  - T40.995 **Adverse effect** of other psychodysleptics [hallucinogens]
  - T40.996 **Underdosing** of other psychodysleptics [hallucinogens]

- T41 Poisoning by, adverse effect of and underdosing of anesthetics and therapeutic gases

  Excludes1 benzodiazepines (T42.4-)
  cocaine (T40.5-)
  complications of anesthesia during pregnancy (O29.-)
  complications of anesthesia during labor and delivery (O74.-)
  complications of anesthesia during the puerperium (O89.-) opioids (T40.0-T40.2-)

  The appropriate 7th character is to be added to each code from category T41

A	initial encounter
D	subsequent encounter
S	sequela

  - T41.0 Poisoning by, adverse effect of and underdosing of inhaled anesthetics

    Excludes1 oxygen (T41.5-)

    - T41.0X Poisoning by, adverse effect of and underdosing of **inhaled anesthetics**
      - T41.0X1 Poisoning by inhaled anesthetics, **accidental (unintentional)**
        Poisoning by inhaled anesthetics NOS
      - T41.0X2 Poisoning by inhaled anesthetics, **intentional self-harm** A, S 🦠
      - T41.0X3 Poisoning by inhaled anesthetics, **assault**
      - T41.0X4 Poisoning by inhaled anesthetics, undetermined
      - T41.0X5 **Adverse effect** of inhaled anesthetics
      - T41.0X6 **Underdosing** of inhaled anesthetics
  - T41.1 Poisoning by, adverse effect of and underdosing of intravenous anesthetics
    Poisoning by, adverse effect of and underdosing of thiobarbiturates
    - T41.1X Poisoning by, adverse effect of and underdosing of **intravenous anesthetics**

- T41.1X1 Poisoning by intravenous anesthetics, **accidental (unintentional)**
  Poisoning by intravenous anesthetics NOS
- T41.1X2 Poisoning by intravenous anesthetics, **intentional self-harm** A, S 🦠
- T41.1X3 Poisoning by intravenous anesthetics, **assault**
- T41.1X4 Poisoning by intravenous anesthetics, **undetermined**
- T41.1X5 **Adverse effect** of intravenous anesthetics
- T41.1X6 **Underdosing** of intravenous anesthetics
- T41.2 Poisoning by, adverse effect of and underdosing of other and unspecified general anesthetics
  - T41.20 Poisoning by, adverse effect of and underdosing of **unspecified general anesthetics**
    - T41.201 Poisoning by unspecified general anesthetics, **accidental (unintentional)**
      Poisoning by general anesthetics NOS
    - T41.202 Poisoning by unspecified general anesthetics, **intentional self-harm** A, S 🦠
    - T41.203 Poisoning by unspecified general anesthetics, **assault**
    - T41.204 Poisoning by unspecified general anesthetics, **undetermined**
    - T41.205 **Adverse effect** of unspecified general anesthetics
      Coding Clinic: 2016, Q4, P73
    - T41.206 **Underdosing** of unspecified general anesthetics
  - T41.29 Poisoning by, adverse effect of and underdosing of **other general anesthetics**
    - T41.291 Poisoning by other general anesthetics, **accidental (unintentional)**
      Poisoning by other general anesthetics NOS
    - T41.292 Poisoning by other general anesthetics, **intentional self-harm** A, S 🦠
    - T41.293 Poisoning by other general anesthetics, **assault**
    - T41.294 Poisoning by other general anesthetics, **undetermined**
    - T41.295 **Adverse effect** of other general anesthetics
    - T41.296 **Underdosing** of other general anesthetics
- T41.3 Poisoning by, adverse effect of and underdosing of **local anesthetics**
  Cocaine (topical)

  Excludes2 poisoning by cocaine used as a central nervous system stimulant (T40.5X1-T40.5X4)

  - T41.3X Poisoning by, adverse effect of and underdosing of **local anesthetics**
    - T41.3X1 Poisoning by local anesthetics, **accidental (unintentional)**
      Poisoning by local anesthetics NOS
    - T41.3X2 Poisoning by local anesthetics, **intentional self-harm** A, S 🦠
    - T41.3X3 Poisoning by local anesthetics, **assault**
    - T41.3X4 Poisoning by local anesthetics, **undetermined**
    - T41.3X5 **Adverse effect** of local anesthetics
    - T41.3X6 **Underdosing** of local anesthetics
- T41.4 Poisoning by, adverse effect of and underdosing of unspecified anesthetic
  - X ● T41.41 Poisoning by unspecified anesthetic, **accidental (unintentional)**
    Poisoning by anesthetic NOS
  - X ● T41.42 Poisoning by unspecified anesthetic, **intentional** self-harm A, S 🦠

▶ New   ⟹ Revised   ~~deleted~~ Deleted   Excludes 1   Excludes 2   Includes   Use additional   Code first   Code also   Key words

OGCR Official Guidelines   X Assign placeholder X   ● Use Additional Character(s)   ▶ Manifestation Code   🦠 Hierarchical Condition Category   Coding Clinic

X● **T41.43** Poisoning by unspecified anesthetic, assault
X● **T41.44** Poisoning by unspecified anesthetic, undetermined
X● **T41.45** Adverse effect of unspecified anesthetic
X● **T41.46** Underdosing of unspecified anesthetics
● **T41.5** Poisoning by, adverse effect of and underdosing of therapeutic gases
　● **T41.5X** Poisoning by, adverse effect of and underdosing of therapeutic gases
　　● **T41.5X1** Poisoning by therapeutic gases, accidental (unintentional)
　　　Poisoning by therapeutic gases NOS
　　● **T41.5X2** Poisoning by therapeutic gases, intentional self-harm A, S 🔖
　　● **T41.5X3** Poisoning by therapeutic gases, assault
　　● **T41.5X4** Poisoning by therapeutic gases, undetermined
　　● **T41.5X5** Adverse effect of therapeutic gases
　　● **T41.5X6** Underdosing of therapeutic gases

● **T42** Poisoning by, adverse effect of and underdosing of antiepileptic, sedative-hypnotic and antiparkinsonism drugs
　Excludes2 drug dependence and related mental and behavioral disorders due to psychoactive substance use (F10.--F19.-)
　The appropriate 7th character is to be added to each code from category T42
　　A initial encounter
　　D subsequent encounter
　　S sequela

● **T42.0** Poisoning by, adverse effect of and underdosing of hydantoin derivatives
　● **T42.0X** Poisoning by, adverse effect of and underdosing of hydantoin derivatives
　　● **T42.0X1** Poisoning by hydantoin derivatives, accidental (unintentional)
　　　Poisoning by hydantoin derivatives NOS
　　● **T42.0X2** Poisoning by hydantoin derivatives, intentional self-harm A, S 🔖
　　● **T42.0X3** Poisoning by hydantoin derivatives, assault
　　● **T42.0X4** Poisoning by hydantoin derivatives, undetermined
　　● **T42.0X5** Adverse effect of hydantoin derivatives
　　● **T42.0X6** Underdosing of hydantoin derivatives
● **T42.1** Poisoning by, adverse effect of and underdosing of iminostilbenes
　Poisoning by, adverse effect of and underdosing of carbamazepine
　● **T42.1X** Poisoning by, adverse effect of and underdosing of iminostilbenes
　　● **T42.1X1** Poisoning by iminostilbenes, accidental (unintentional)
　　　Poisoning by iminostilbenes NOS
　　● **T42.1X2** Poisoning by iminostilbenes, intentional self-harm A, S 🔖
　　● **T42.1X3** Poisoning by iminostilbenes, assault
　　● **T42.1X4** Poisoning by iminostilbenes, undetermined
　　● **T42.1X5** Adverse effect of iminostilbenes
　　● **T42.1X6** Underdosing of iminostilbenes

● **T42.2** Poisoning by, adverse effect of and underdosing of succinimides and oxazolidinediones
　● **T42.2X** Poisoning by, adverse effect of and underdosing of succinimides and oxazolidinediones
　　● **T42.2X1** Poisoning by succinimides and oxazolidinediones, accidental (unintentional)
　　　Poisoning by succinimides and oxazolidinediones NOS
　　● **T42.2X2** Poisoning by succinimides and oxazolidinediones, intentional self-harm A, S 🔖
　　● **T42.2X3** Poisoning by succinimides and oxazolidinediones, assault
　　● **T42.2X4** Poisoning by succinimides and oxazolidinediones, undetermined
　　● **T42.2X5** Adverse effect of succinimides and oxazolidinediones
　　● **T42.2X6** Underdosing of succinimides and oxazolidinediones
● **T42.3** Poisoning by, adverse effect of and underdosing of barbiturates
　Excludes1 poisoning by, adverse effect of and underdosing of thiobarbiturates (T41.1-)
　● **T42.3X** Poisoning by, adverse effect of and underdosing of barbiturates
　　● **T42.3X1** Poisoning by barbiturates, accidental (unintentional)
　　　Poisoning by barbiturates NOS
　　● **T42.3X2** Poisoning by barbiturates, intentional self-harm A, S 🔖
　　● **T42.3X3** Poisoning by barbiturates, assault
　　● **T42.3X4** Poisoning by barbiturates, undetermined
　　● **T42.3X5** Adverse effect of barbiturates
　　● **T42.3X6** Underdosing of barbiturates
● **T42.4** Poisoning by, adverse effect of and underdosing of benzodiazepines
　● **T42.4X** Poisoning by, adverse effect of and underdosing of benzodiazepines
　　● **T42.4X1** Poisoning by benzodiazepines, accidental (unintentional)
　　　Poisoning by benzodiazepines NOS
　　● **T42.4X2** Poisoning by benzodiazepines, intentional self-harm A, S 🔖
　　● **T42.4X3** Poisoning by benzodiazepines, assault
　　● **T42.4X4** Poisoning by benzodiazepines, undetermined
　　● **T42.4X5** Adverse effect of benzodiazepines
　　● **T42.4X6** Underdosing of benzodiazepines
● **T42.5** Poisoning by, adverse effect of and underdosing of mixed antiepileptics
　● **T42.5X** Poisoning by, adverse effect of and underdosing of antiepileptics
　　● **T42.5X1** Poisoning by mixed antiepileptics, accidental (unintentional)
　　　Poisoning by mixed antiepileptics NOS
　　● **T42.5X2** Poisoning by mixed antiepileptics, intentional self-harm A, S 🔖
　　● **T42.5X3** Poisoning by mixed antiepileptics, assault
　　● **T42.5X4** Poisoning by mixed antiepileptics, undetermined
　　● **T42.5X5** Adverse effect of mixed antiepileptics
　　● **T42.5X6** Underdosing of mixed antiepileptics

CHAPTER 19 (S00-T88)

CHAPTER 19 (S00-T88)

- T42.6 **Poisoning by, adverse effect of and underdosing of other antiepileptic and sedative-hypnotic drugs**
  Poisoning by, adverse effect of and underdosing of methaqualone
  Poisoning by, adverse effect of and underdosing of valproic acid
  Excludes1   poisoning by, adverse effect of and underdosing of carbamazepine (T42.1-)
  - T42.6X **Poisoning by, adverse effect of and underdosing of other antiepileptic and sedative-hypnotic drugs**
    - T42.6X1 **Poisoning by other antiepileptic and sedative-hypnotic drugs, accidental (unintentional)**
      Poisoning by other antiepileptic and sedative-hypnotic drugs NOS
    - T42.6X2 **Poisoning by other antiepileptic and sedative-hypnotic drugs, intentional self-harm A, S** 🔒
    - T42.6X3 **Poisoning by other antiepileptic and sedative-hypnotic drugs, assault**
    - T42.6X4 **Poisoning by other antiepileptic and sedative-hypnotic drugs, undetermined**
    - T42.6X5 **Adverse effect of other antiepileptic and sedative-hypnotic drugs**
    - T42.6X6 **Underdosing of other antiepileptic and sedative-hypnotic drugs**
- T42.7 **Poisoning by, adverse effect of and underdosing of unspecified antiepileptic and sedative-hypnotic drugs**
  - X● T42.71 **Poisoning by unspecified antiepileptic and sedative-hypnotic drugs, accidental (unintentional)**
    Poisoning by antiepileptic and sedative-hypnotic drugs NOS
  - X● T42.72 **Poisoning by unspecified antiepileptic and sedative-hypnotic drugs, intentional self-harm A, S** 🔒
  - X● T42.73 **Poisoning by unspecified antiepileptic and sedative-hypnotic drugs, assault**
  - X● T42.74 **Poisoning by unspecified antiepileptic and sedative-hypnotic drugs, undetermined**
  - X● T42.75 **Adverse effect of unspecified antiepileptic and sedative-hypnotic drugs**
  - X● T42.76 **Underdosing of unspecified antiepileptic and sedative-hypnotic drugs**
- T42.8 **Poisoning by, adverse effect of and underdosing of antiparkinsonism drugs and other central muscle-tone depressants**
  Poisoning by, adverse effect of and underdosing of amantadine
  - T42.8X **Poisoning by, adverse effect of and underdosing of antiparkinsonism drugs and other central muscle-tone depressants**
    - T42.8X1 **Poisoning by antiparkinsonism drugs and other central muscle-tone depressants, accidental (unintentional)**
      Poisoning by antiparkinsonism drugs and other central muscle-tone depressants NOS
    - T42.8X2 **Poisoning by antiparkinsonism drugs and other central muscle-tone depressants, intentional self-harm A, S** 🔒
    - T42.8X3 **Poisoning by antiparkinsonism drugs and other central muscle-tone depressants, assault**
    - T42.8X4 **Poisoning by antiparkinsonism drugs and other central muscle-tone depressants, undetermined**

- T42.8X5 **Adverse effect of antiparkinsonism drugs and other central muscle-tone depressants**
- T42.8X6 **Underdosing of antiparkinsonism drugs and other central muscle-tone depressants**

- T43 **Poisoning by, adverse effect of and underdosing of psychotropic drugs, not elsewhere classified**
  Excludes1   appetite depressants (T50.5-)
  barbiturates (T42.3-)
  benzodiazepines (T42.4-)
  methaqualone (T42.6-)
  psychodysleptics [hallucinogens] (T40.7-T40.9-)
  Excludes2   drug dependence and related mental and behavioral disorders due to psychoactive substance use (F10.--F19.-)

  The appropriate 7th character is to be added to each code from category T43

A	initial encounter
D	subsequent encounter
S	sequela

  - T43.0 **Poisoning by, adverse effect of and underdosing of tricyclic and tetracyclic antidepressants**
    - T43.01 **Poisoning by, adverse effect of and underdosing of tricyclic antidepressants**
      - T43.011 **Poisoning by tricyclic antidepressants, accidental (unintentional)**
        Poisoning by tricyclic antidepressants NOS
      - T43.012 **Poisoning by tricyclic antidepressants, intentional self-harm A, S** 🔒
      - T43.013 **Poisoning by tricyclic antidepressants, assault**
      - T43.014 **Poisoning by tricyclic antidepressants, undetermined**
      - T43.015 **Adverse effect of tricyclic antidepressants**
      - T43.016 **Underdosing of tricyclic antidepressants**
    - T43.02 **Poisoning by, adverse effect of and underdosing of tetracyclic antidepressants**
      - T43.021 **Poisoning by tetracyclic antidepressants, accidental (unintentional)**
        Poisoning by tetracyclic antidepressants NOS
      - T43.022 **Poisoning by tetracyclic antidepressants, intentional self-harm A, S** 🔒
      - T43.023 **Poisoning by tetracyclic antidepressants, assault**
      - T43.024 **Poisoning by tetracyclic antidepressants, undetermined**
      - T43.025 **Adverse effect of tetracyclic antidepressants**
      - T43.026 **Underdosing of tetracyclic antidepressants**
  - T43.1 **Poisoning by, adverse effect of and underdosing of monoamine-oxidase-inhibitor antidepressants**
    - T43.1X **Poisoning by, adverse effect of and underdosing of monoamine-oxidase-inhibitor antidepressants**
      - T43.1X1 **Poisoning by monoamine-oxidase-inhibitor antidepressants, accidental (unintentional)**
        Poisoning by monoamine-oxidase-inhibitor antidepressants NOS
      - T43.1X2 **Poisoning by monoamine-oxidase-inhibitor antidepressants, intentional self-harm A, S** 🔒

▶ New   ⟹ Revised   ~~deleted~~ Deleted   Excludes 1   Excludes 2   Includes   Use additional   Code first   Code also   Key words
OGCR Official Guidelines   X Assign placeholder X   ● Use Additional Character(s)   ▶ Manifestation Code   🔒 Hierarchical Condition Category   Coding Clinic

● T43.1X3   Poisoning by monoamine-oxidase-inhibitor antidepressants, assault

● T43.1X4   Poisoning by monoamine-oxidase-inhibitor antidepressants, undetermined

● T43.1X5   Adverse effect of monoamine-oxidase-inhibitor antidepressants

● T43.1X6   Underdosing of monoamine-oxidase-inhibitor antidepressants

● T43.2   Poisoning by, adverse effect of and underdosing of other and unspecified antidepressants

  ● T43.20   Poisoning by, adverse effect of and underdosing of unspecified antidepressants

    ● T43.201   Poisoning by unspecified antidepressants, accidental (unintentional)
       Poisoning by antidepressants NOS

    ● T43.202   Poisoning by unspecified antidepressants, intentional self-harm A, S 🐾

    ● T43.203   Poisoning by unspecified antidepressants, assault

    ● T43.204   Poisoning by unspecified antidepressants, undetermined

    ● T43.205   Adverse effect of unspecified antidepressants
       Antidepressant discontinuation syndrome

    ● T43.206   Underdosing of unspecified antidepressants

  ● T43.21   Poisoning by, adverse effect of and underdosing of selective serotonin and norepinephrine reuptake inhibitors
     Poisoning by, adverse effect of and underdosing of SSNRI antidepressants

    ● T43.211   Poisoning by selective serotonin and norepinephrine reuptake inhibitors, accidental (unintentional)

    ● T43.212   Poisoning by selective serotonin and norepinephrine reuptake inhibitors, intentional self-harm A, S 🐾

    ● T43.213   Poisoning by selective serotonin and norepinephrine reuptake inhibitors, assault

    ● T43.214   Poisoning by selective serotonin and norepinephrine reuptake inhibitors, undetermined

    ● T43.215   Adverse effect of selective serotonin and norepinephrine reuptake inhibitors

    ● T43.216   Underdosing of selective serotonin and norepinephrine reuptake inhibitors

  ● T43.22   Poisoning by, adverse effect of and underdosing of selective serotonin reuptake inhibitors
     Poisoning by, adverse effect of and underdosing of SSRI antidepressants

    ● T43.221   Poisoning by selective serotonin reuptake inhibitors, accidental (unintentional)

    ● T43.222   Poisoning by selective serotonin reuptake inhibitors, intentional self-harm A, S 🐾

    ● T43.223   Poisoning by selective serotonin reuptake inhibitors, assault

    ● T43.224   Poisoning by selective serotonin reuptake inhibitors, undetermined

    ● T43.225   Adverse effect of selective serotonin reuptake inhibitors
       Coding Clinic: 2022, Q2, P11

    ● T43.226   Underdosing of selective serotonin reuptake inhibitors

● T43.29   Poisoning by, adverse effect of and underdosing of other antidepressants

    ● T43.291   Poisoning by other antidepressants, accidental (unintentional)
       Poisoning by other antidepressants NOS

    ● T43.292   Poisoning by other antidepressants, intentional self-harm A, S 🐾

    ● T43.293   Poisoning by other antidepressants, assault

    ● T43.294   Poisoning by other antidepressants, undetermined

    ● T43.295   Adverse effect of other antidepressants

    ● T43.296   Underdosing of other antidepressants

● T43.3   Poisoning by, adverse effect of and underdosing of phenothiazine antipsychotics and neuroleptics

  ● T43.3X   Poisoning by, adverse effect of and underdosing of phenothiazine antipsychotics and neuroleptics

    ● T43.3X1   Poisoning by phenothiazine antipsychotics and neuroleptics, accidental (unintentional)
       Poisoning by phenothiazine antipsychotics and neuroleptics NOS

    ● T43.3X2   Poisoning by phenothiazine antipsychotics and neuroleptics, intentional self-harm A, S 🐾

    ● T43.3X3   Poisoning by phenothiazine antipsychotics and neuroleptics, assault

    ● T43.3X4   Poisoning by phenothiazine antipsychotics and neuroleptics, undetermined

    ● T43.3X5   Adverse effect of phenothiazine antipsychotics and neuroleptics

    ● T43.3X6   Underdosing of phenothiazine antipsychotics and neuroleptics

● T43.4   Poisoning by, adverse effect of and underdosing of butyrophenone and thiothixene neuroleptics

  ● T43.4X   Poisoning by, adverse effect of and underdosing of butyrophenone and thiothixene neuroleptics

    ● T43.4X1   Poisoning by butyrophenone and thiothixene neuroleptics, accidental (unintentional)
       Poisoning by butyrophenone and thiothixene neuroleptics NOS

    ● T43.4X2   Poisoning by butyrophenone and thiothixene neuroleptics, intentional self-harm A, S 🐾

    ● T43.4X3   Poisoning by butyrophenone and thiothixene neuroleptics, assault

    ● T43.4X4   Poisoning by butyrophenone and thiothixene neuroleptics, undetermined

    ● T43.4X5   Adverse effect of butyrophenone and thiothixene neuroleptics

    ● T43.4X6   Underdosing of butyrophenone and thiothixene neuroleptics

● T43.5   Poisoning by, adverse effect of and underdosing of other and unspecified antipsychotics and neuroleptics

   Excludes 1   poisoning by, adverse effect of and underdosing of rauwolfia (T46.5-)

  ● T43.50   Poisoning by, adverse effect of and underdosing of unspecified antipsychotics and neuroleptics

    ● T43.501   Poisoning by unspecified antipsychotics and neuroleptics, accidental (unintentional)
       Poisoning by antipsychotics and neuroleptics NOS

CHAPTER 19 (S00-T88)

● T43.502 **Poisoning by unspecified antipsychotics and neuroleptics, intentional self-harm** A, S 🐾

● T43.503 **Poisoning by unspecified antipsychotics and neuroleptics, assault**

● T43.504 **Poisoning by unspecified antipsychotics and neuroleptics, undetermined**

● T43.505 **Adverse effect of unspecified antipsychotics and neuroleptics**
Coding Clinic: 2022, Q4, P24

● T43.506 **Underdosing of unspecified antipsychotics and neuroleptics**

● T43.59 Poisoning by, adverse effect of and underdosing of **other antipsychotics and neuroleptics**

● T43.591 **Poisoning by other antipsychotics and neuroleptics, accidental (unintentional)**
Poisoning by other antipsychotics and neuroleptics NOS

● T43.592 **Poisoning by other antipsychotics and neuroleptics, intentional self-harm** A, S 🐾
Coding Clinic: 2017, Q1, P40

● T43.593 **Poisoning by other antipsychotics and neuroleptics, assault**

● T43.594 **Poisoning by other antipsychotics and neuroleptics, undetermined**

● T43.595 **Adverse effect of other antipsychotics and neuroleptics**
Coding Clinic: 2022, Q2, P11

● T43.596 **Underdosing of other antipsychotics and neuroleptics**

● T43.6 Poisoning by, adverse effect of and underdosing of psychostimulants

Excludes1 poisoning by, adverse effect of and underdosing of cocaine (T40.5-)

● T43.60 Poisoning by, adverse effect of and underdosing of **unspecified psychostimulant**

● T43.601 **Poisoning by unspecified psychostimulants, accidental (unintentional)**
Poisoning by psychostimulants NOS

● T43.602 **Poisoning by unspecified psychostimulants, intentional self-harm** A, S 🐾

● T43.603 **Poisoning by unspecified psychostimulants, assault**

● T43.604 **Poisoning by unspecified psychostimulants, undetermined**

● T43.605 **Adverse effect of unspecified psychostimulants**

● T43.606 **Underdosing of unspecified psychostimulants**

● T43.61 Poisoning by, adverse effect of and underdosing of **caffeine**

● T43.611 **Poisoning by caffeine, accidental (unintentional)**
Poisoning by caffeine NOS

● T43.612 **Poisoning by caffeine, intentional self-harm** A, S 🐾

● T43.613 **Poisoning by caffeine, assault**

● T43.614 **Poisoning by caffeine, undetermined**

● T43.615 **Adverse effect of caffeine**

● T43.616 **Underdosing of caffeine**

● T43.62 Poisoning by, adverse effect of and underdosing of **amphetamines**

● T43.621 **Poisoning by amphetamines, accidental (unintentional)**
Poisoning by amphetamines NOS
Coding Clinic: 2021, Q3, P8

● T43.622 **Poisoning by amphetamines, intentional self-harm** A, S 🐾

● T43.623 **Poisoning by amphetamines, assault**

● T43.624 **Poisoning by amphetamines, undetermined**

● T43.625 **Adverse effect of amphetamines**

● T43.626 **Underdosing of amphetamines**

● T43.63 Poisoning by, adverse effect of and underdosing of **methylphenidate**

● T43.631 **Poisoning by methylphenidate, accidental (unintentional)**
Poisoning by methylphenidate NOS

● T43.632 **Poisoning by methylphenidate, intentional self-harm** A, S 🐾

● T43.633 **Poisoning by methylphenidate, assault**

● T43.634 **Poisoning by methylphenidate, undetermined**

● T43.635 **Adverse effect of methylphenidate**

● T43.636 **Underdosing of methylphenidate**

● T43.64 Poisoning by ecstasy
Poisoning by MDMA
Poisoning by 3,4-methylenedioxymethamphetamine

● T43.641 **Poisoning by ecstasy, accidental (unintentional)**
Poisoning by ecstasy NOS
Coding Clinic: 2018, Q4, P31

● T43.642 **Poisoning by ecstasy, intentional self-harm** A, S 🐾

● T43.643 **Poisoning by ecstasy, assault**

● T43.644 **Poisoning by ecstasy, undetermined**

● T43.65 Poisoning by, adverse effect of and underdosing of **methamphetamines**

● T43.651 **Poisoning by methamphetamines accidental (unintentional)**
Poisoning by methamphetamines NOS
Coding Clinic: 2022, Q4, P46

● T43.652 **Poisoning by methamphetamines intentional self-harm**

● T43.653 **Poisoning by methamphetamines, assault**

● T43.654 **Poisoning by methamphetamines, undetermined**

● T43.655 **Adverse effect of methamphetamines**
Coding Clinic: 2022, Q4, P47

● T43.656 **Underdosing of methamphetamines**

● T43.69 Poisoning by, adverse effect of and underdosing of **other psychostimulants**

● T43.691 **Poisoning by other psychostimulants, accidental (unintentional)**
Poisoning by other psychostimulants NOS

● T43.692 **Poisoning by other psychostimulants, intentional self-harm** A, S 🐾

● T43.693 **Poisoning by other psychostimulants, assault**

● T43.694 **Poisoning by other psychostimulants, undetermined**

● T43.695 **Adverse effect of other psychostimulants**

● T43.696 **Underdosing of other psychostimulants**

CHAPTER 19 (S00-T88)

▶ New   ⇒ Revised   ~~deleted~~ Deleted   Excludes 1   Excludes 2   Includes   Use additional   Code first   Code also   Key words
OGCR Official Guidelines   X Assign placeholder X   ● Use Additional Character(s)   ▷ Manifestation Code   🐾 Hierarchical Condition Category   Coding Clinic

● **T43.8** Poisoning by, adverse effect of and underdosing of other psychotropic drugs

  ● **T43.8X** Poisoning by, adverse effect of and underdosing of other psychotropic drugs

    ● **T43.8X1** Poisoning by other psychotropic drugs, accidental (unintentional)
Poisoning by other psychotropic drugs NOS

    ● **T43.8X2** Poisoning by other psychotropic drugs, intentional self-harm A, S 🔇

    ● **T43.8X3** Poisoning by other psychotropic drugs, assault

    ● **T43.8X4** Poisoning by other psychotropic drugs, undetermined

    ● **T43.8X5** Adverse effect of other psychotropic drugs

    ● **T43.8X6** Underdosing of other psychotropic drugs

● **T43.9** Poisoning by, adverse effect of and underdosing of unspecified psychotropic drug

  X ● **T43.91** Poisoning by unspecified psychotropic drug, accidental (unintentional)
Poisoning by psychotropic drug NOS

  X ● **T43.92** Poisoning by unspecified psychotropic drug, intentional self-harm A, S 🔇

  X ● **T43.93** Poisoning by unspecified psychotropic drug, assault

  X ● **T43.94** Poisoning by unspecified psychotropic drug, undetermined

  X ● **T43.95** Adverse effect of unspecified psychotropic drug

  X ● **T43.96** Underdosing of unspecified psychotropic drug

● **T44** Poisoning by, adverse effect of and underdosing of drugs primarily affecting the autonomic nervous system

  The appropriate 7th character is to be added to each code from category T44

A	initial encounter
D	subsequent encounter
S	sequela

● **T44.0** Poisoning by, adverse effect of and underdosing of anticholinesterase agents

  ● **T44.0X** Poisoning by, adverse effect of and underdosing of anticholinesterase agents

    ● **T44.0X1** Poisoning by anticholinesterase agents, accidental (unintentional)
Poisoning by anticholinesterase agents NOS

    ● **T44.0X2** Poisoning by anticholinesterase agents, intentional self-harm A, S 🔇

    ● **T44.0X3** Poisoning by anticholinesterase agents, assault

    ● **T44.0X4** Poisoning by anticholinesterase agents, undetermined

    ● **T44.0X5** Adverse effect of anticholinesterase agents

    ● **T44.0X6** Underdosing of anticholinesterase agents

● **T44.1** Poisoning by, adverse effect of and underdosing of other parasympathomimetics [cholinergics]

  ● **T44.1X** Poisoning by, adverse effect of and underdosing of other parasympathomimetics [cholinergics]

    ● **T44.1X1** Poisoning by other parasympathomimetics [cholinergics], accidental (unintentional)
Poisoning by other parasympathomimetics [cholinergics] NOS

    ● **T44.1X2** Poisoning by other parasympathomimetics [cholinergics], intentional self-harm A, S 🔇

    ● **T44.1X3** Poisoning by other parasympathomimetics [cholinergics], assault

    ● **T44.1X4** Poisoning by other parasympathomimetics [cholinergics], undetermined

    ● **T44.1X5** Adverse effect of other parasympathomimetics [cholinergics]

    ● **T44.1X6** Underdosing of other parasympathomimetics [cholinergics]

● **T44.2** Poisoning by, adverse effect of and underdosing of ganglionic blocking drugs

  ● **T44.2X** Poisoning by, adverse effect of and underdosing of ganglionic blocking drugs

    ● **T44.2X1** Poisoning by ganglionic blocking drugs, accidental (unintentional)
Poisoning by ganglionic blocking drugs NOS

    ● **T44.2X2** Poisoning by ganglionic blocking drugs, intentional self-harm A, S 🔇

    ● **T44.2X3** Poisoning by ganglionic blocking drugs, assault

    ● **T44.2X4** Poisoning by ganglionic blocking drugs, undetermined

    ● **T44.2X5** Adverse effect of ganglionic blocking drugs

    ● **T44.2X6** Underdosing of ganglionic blocking drugs

● **T44.3** Poisoning by, adverse effect of and underdosing of other parasympatholytics [anticholinergics and antimuscarinics] and spasmolytics
Poisoning by, adverse effect of and underdosing of papaverine

  ● **T44.3X** Poisoning by, adverse effect of and underdosing of other parasympatholytics [anticholinergics and antimuscarinics] and spasmolytics

    ● **T44.3X1** Poisoning by other parasympatholytics [anticholinergics and antimuscarinics] and spasmolytics, accidental (unintentional)
Poisoning by other parasympatholytics [anticholinergics and antimuscarinics] and spasmolytics NOS

    ● **T44.3X2** Poisoning by other parasympatholytics [anticholinergics and antimuscarinics] and spasmolytics, intentional self-harm A, S 🔇

    ● **T44.3X3** Poisoning by other parasympatholytics [anticholinergics and antimuscarinics] and spasmolytics, assault

    ● **T44.3X4** Poisoning by other parasympatholytics [anticholinergics and antimuscarinics] and spasmolytics, undetermined

    ● **T44.3X5** Adverse effect of other parasympatholytics [anticholinergics and antimuscarinics] and spasmolytics

    ● **T44.3X6** Underdosing of other parasympatholytics [anticholinergics and antimuscarinics] and spasmolytics

● **T44.4** Poisoning by, adverse effect of and underdosing of predominantly alpha-adrenoreceptor agonists
Poisoning by, adverse effect of and underdosing of metaraminol

- T44.4X Poisoning by, adverse effect of and underdosing of predominantly alpha-adrenoreceptor agonists
  - T44.4X1 Poisoning by predominantly alpha-adrenoreceptor agonists, accidental (unintentional)
    Poisoning by predominantly alpha-adrenoreceptor agonists NOS
  - T44.4X2 Poisoning by predominantly alpha-adrenoreceptor agonists, intentional self-harm A, S 🗞
  - T44.4X3 Poisoning by predominantly alpha-adrenoreceptor agonists, assault
  - T44.4X4 Poisoning by predominantly alpha-adrenoreceptor agonists, undetermined
  - T44.4X5 Adverse effect of predominantly alpha-adrenoreceptor agonists
  - T44.4X6 Underdosing of predominantly alpha-adrenoreceptor agonists
- T44.5 Poisoning by, adverse effect of and underdosing of predominantly beta-adrenoreceptor agonists
  - Excludes1 poisoning by, adverse effect of and underdosing of beta-adrenoreceptor agonists used in asthma therapy (T48.6-)
  - T44.5X Poisoning by, adverse effect of and underdosing of predominantly beta-adrenoreceptor agonists
    - T44.5X1 Poisoning by predominantly beta-adrenoreceptor agonists, accidental (unintentional)
      Poisoning by predominantly beta-adrenoreceptor agonists NOS
    - T44.5X2 Poisoning by predominantly beta-adrenoreceptor agonists, intentional self-harm A, S 🗞
    - T44.5X3 Poisoning by predominantly beta-adrenoreceptor agonists, assault
    - T44.5X4 Poisoning by predominantly beta-adrenoreceptor agonists, undetermined
    - T44.5X5 Adverse effect of predominantly beta-adrenoreceptor agonists
    - T44.5X6 Underdosing of predominantly beta-adrenoreceptor agonists
- T44.6 Poisoning by, adverse effect of and underdosing of alpha-adrenoreceptor antagonists
  - Excludes1 poisoning by, adverse effect of and underdosing of ergot alkaloids (T48.0)
  - T44.6X Poisoning by, adverse effect of and underdosing of alpha-adrenoreceptor antagonists
    - T44.6X1 Poisoning by alpha-adrenoreceptor antagonists, accidental (unintentional)
      Poisoning by alpha-adrenoreceptor antagonists NOS
    - T44.6X2 Poisoning by alpha-adrenoreceptor antagonists, intentional self-harm A, S 🗞
    - T44.6X3 Poisoning by alpha-adrenoreceptor antagonists, assault
    - T44.6X4 Poisoning by alpha-adrenoreceptor antagonists, undetermined
    - T44.6X5 Adverse effect of alpha-adrenoreceptor antagonists
    - T44.6X6 Underdosing of alpha-adrenoreceptor antagonists
- T44.7 Poisoning by, adverse effect of and underdosing of beta-adrenoreceptor antagonists
  - T44.7X Poisoning by, adverse effect of and underdosing of beta-adrenoreceptor antagonists

- T44.7X1 Poisoning by beta-adrenoreceptor antagonists, accidental (unintentional)
  Poisoning by beta-adrenoreceptor antagonists NOS
- T44.7X2 Poisoning by beta-adrenoreceptor antagonists, intentional self-harm A, S 🗞
- T44.7X3 Poisoning by beta-adrenoreceptor antagonists, assault
- T44.7X4 Poisoning by beta-adrenoreceptor antagonists, undetermined
- T44.7X5 Adverse effect of beta-adrenoreceptor antagonists
- T44.7X6 Underdosing of beta-adrenoreceptor antagonists
- T44.8 Poisoning by, adverse effect of and underdosing of centrally-acting and adrenergic-neuron-blocking agents
  - Excludes2 poisoning by, adverse effect of and underdosing of clonidine (T46.5)
    poisoning by, adverse effect of and underdosing of guanethidine (T46.5)
  - T44.8X Poisoning by, adverse effect of and underdosing of centrally-acting and adrenergic-neuron-blocking agents
    - T44.8X1 Poisoning by centrally-acting and adrenergic-neuron-blocking agents, accidental (unintentional)
      Poisoning by centrally-acting and adrenergic-neuron-blocking agents NOS
    - T44.8X2 Poisoning by centrally-acting and adrenergic-neuron-blocking agents, intentional self-harm A, S 🗞
    - T44.8X3 Poisoning by centrally-acting and adrenergic-neuron-blocking agents, assault
    - T44.8X4 Poisoning by centrally-acting and adrenergic-neuron-blocking agents, undetermined
    - T44.8X5 Adverse effect of centrally-acting and adrenergic-neuron-blocking agents
    - T44.8X6 Underdosing of centrally-acting and adrenergic-neuron-blocking agents
- T44.9 Poisoning by, adverse effect of and underdosing of other and unspecified drugs primarily affecting the autonomic nervous system
  Poisoning by, adverse effect of and underdosing of drug stimulating both alpha and beta-adrenoreceptors
  - T44.90 Poisoning by, adverse effect of and underdosing of unspecified drugs primarily affecting the autonomic nervous system
    - T44.901 Poisoning by unspecified drugs primarily affecting the autonomic nervous system, accidental (unintentional)
      Poisoning by unspecified drugs primarily affecting the autonomic nervous system NOS
    - T44.902 Poisoning by unspecified drugs primarily affecting the autonomic nervous system, intentional self-harm A, S 🗞
    - T44.903 Poisoning by unspecified drugs primarily affecting the autonomic nervous system, assault
    - T44.904 Poisoning by unspecified drugs primarily affecting the autonomic nervous system, undetermined
    - T44.905 Adverse effect of unspecified drugs primarily affecting the autonomic nervous system

CHAPTER 19 (S00-T88)

▶ New   ⇒ Revised   ~~deleted~~ Deleted   Excludes 1   Excludes 2   Includes   Use additional   Code first   Code also   Key words

OGCR Official Guidelines   X Assign placeholder X   ● Use Additional Character(s)   ▸ Manifestation Code   🗞 Hierarchical Condition Category   Coding Clinic

● **T44.906**   Underdosing of unspecified drugs primarily affecting the autonomic nervous system

● **T44.99**   Poisoning by, adverse effect of and underdosing of other drugs primarily affecting the autonomic nervous system

    ● **T44.991**   Poisoning by other drug primarily affecting the autonomic nervous system, accidental (unintentional)
          Poisoning by other drugs primarily affecting the autonomic nervous system NOS

    ● **T44.992**   Poisoning by other drug primarily affecting the autonomic nervous system, intentional self-harm A, S 🔖

    ● **T44.993**   Poisoning by other drug primarily affecting the autonomic nervous system, assault

    ● **T44.994**   Poisoning by other drug primarily affecting the autonomic nervous system, undetermined

    ● **T44.995**   Adverse effect of other drug primarily affecting the autonomic nervous system

    ● **T44.996**   Underdosing of other drug primarily affecting the autonomic nervous system

● **T45**   Poisoning by, adverse effect of and underdosing of primarily systemic and hematological agents, not elsewhere classified

    The appropriate 7th character is to be added to each code from category T45

A	initial encounter
D	subsequent encounter
S	sequela

● **T45.0**   Poisoning by, adverse effect of and underdosing of antiallergic and antiemetic drugs

    Excludes1   poisoning by, adverse effect of and underdosing of phenothiazine-based neuroleptics (T43.3)

    ● **T45.0X**   Poisoning by, adverse effect of and underdosing of antiallergic and antiemetic drugs

       ● **T45.0X1**   Poisoning by antiallergic and antiemetic drugs, accidental (unintentional)
            Poisoning by antiallergic and antiemetic drugs NOS

       ● **T45.0X2**   Poisoning by antiallergic and antiemetic drugs, intentional self-harm A, S 🔖

       ● **T45.0X3**   Poisoning by antiallergic and antiemetic drugs, assault

       ● **T45.0X4**   Poisoning by antiallergic and antiemetic drugs, undetermined

       ● **T45.0X5**   Adverse effect of antiallergic and antiemetic drugs

       ● **T45.0X6**   Underdosing of antiallergic and antiemetic drugs

● **T45.1**   Poisoning by, adverse effect of and underdosing of antineoplastic and immunosuppressive drugs

    ▶ **Excludes1**   poisoning by, adverse effect of and underdosing of immune checkpoint inhibitors and immunostimulant drugs (T45.A)
        Coding Clinic: 2023, Q2, P10

    ● **T45.1X**   Poisoning by, adverse effect of and underdosing of antineoplastic and immunosuppressive drugs

       ● **T45.1X1**   Poisoning by antineoplastic and immunosuppressive drugs, accidental (unintentional)
            Poisoning by antineoplastic and immunosuppressive drugs NOS

       ● **T45.1X2**   Poisoning by antineoplastic and immunosuppressive drugs, intentional self-harm A, S 🔖

       ● **T45.1X3**   Poisoning by antineoplastic and immunosuppressive drugs, assault

       ● **T45.1X4**   Poisoning by antineoplastic and immunosuppressive drugs, undetermined

       ● **T45.1X5**   Adverse effect of antineoplastic and immunosuppressive drugs
         Coding Clinic: 2024, Q1, P25; 2021, Q3, P4; 2019, Q2, P25, 28; Q1, P17, 21

       ● **T45.1X6**   Underdosing of antineoplastic and immunosuppressive drugs

● **T45.2**   Poisoning by, adverse effect of and underdosing of vitamins

    Excludes2   poisoning by, adverse effect of and underdosing of nicotinic acid (derivatives) (T46.7)
           poisoning by, adverse effect of and underdosing of iron (T45.4)
           poisoning by, adverse effect of and underdosing of vitamin K (T45.7)

    ● **T45.2X**   Poisoning by, adverse effect of and underdosing of vitamins

       ● **T45.2X1**   Poisoning by vitamins, accidental (unintentional)
            Poisoning by vitamins NOS

       ● **T45.2X2**   Poisoning by vitamins, intentional self-harm A, S 🔖

       ● **T45.2X3**   Poisoning by vitamins, assault

       ● **T45.2X4**   Poisoning by vitamins, undetermined

       ● **T45.2X5**   Adverse effect of vitamins

       ● **T45.2X6**   Underdosing of vitamins
         Excludes1   vitamin deficiencies (E50-E56)

● **T45.3**   Poisoning by, adverse effect of and underdosing of enzymes

    ● **T45.3X**   Poisoning by, adverse effect of and underdosing of enzymes

       ● **T45.3X1**   Poisoning by enzymes, accidental (unintentional)
            Poisoning by enzymes NOS

       ● **T45.3X2**   Poisoning by enzymes, intentional self-harm A, S 🔖

       ● **T45.3X3**   Poisoning by enzymes, assault

       ● **T45.3X4**   Poisoning by enzymes, undetermined

       ● **T45.3X5**   Adverse effect of enzymes

       ● **T45.3X6**   Underdosing of enzymes

● **T45.4**   Poisoning by, adverse effect of and underdosing of iron and its compounds

    ● **T45.4X**   Poisoning by, adverse effect of and underdosing of iron and its compounds

       ● **T45.4X1**   Poisoning by iron and its compounds, accidental (unintentional)
            Poisoning by iron and its compounds NOS

       ● **T45.4X2**   Poisoning by iron and its compounds, intentional self-harm A, S 🔖

       ● **T45.4X3**   Poisoning by iron and its compounds, assault

       ● **T45.4X4**   Poisoning by iron and its compounds, undetermined

       ● **T45.4X5**   Adverse effect of iron and its compounds

       ● **T45.4X6**   Underdosing of iron and its compounds
         Excludes1   iron deficiency (E61.1)

● **T45.5** Poisoning by, adverse effect of and underdosing of anticoagulants and antithrombotic drugs

  ● **T45.51** Poisoning by, adverse effect of and underdosing of anticoagulants

    ● **T45.511** Poisoning by anticoagulants, accidental (unintentional)
       Poisoning by anticoagulants NOS

    ● **T45.512** Poisoning by anticoagulants, intentional self-harm A, S 🏥

    ● **T45.513** Poisoning by anticoagulants, assault

    ● **T45.514** Poisoning by anticoagulants, undetermined

    ● **T45.515** Adverse effect of anticoagulants
       Coding Clinic: 2021, Q1, P5; 2016, Q1, P14; 2013, Q2, P35

    ● **T45.516** Underdosing of anticoagulants

  ● **T45.52** Poisoning by, adverse effect of and underdosing of antithrombotic drugs
     Poisoning by, adverse effect of and underdosing of antiplatelet drugs

     Excludes2 poisoning by, adverse effect of and underdosing of aspirin (T39.01-)
       poisoning by, adverse effect of and underdosing of acetylsalicylic acid (T39.01-)

    ● **T45.521** Poisoning by antithrombotic drugs, accidental (unintentional)
       Poisoning by antithrombotic drug NOS

    ● **T45.522** Poisoning by antithrombotic drugs, intentional self-harm A, S 🏥

    ● **T45.523** Poisoning by antithrombotic drugs, assault

    ● **T45.524** Poisoning by antithrombotic drugs, undetermined

    ● **T45.525** Adverse effect of antithrombotic drugs
       Coding Clinic: 2016, Q1, P15

    ● **T45.526** Underdosing of antithrombotic drugs

● **T45.6** Poisoning by, adverse effect of and underdosing of fibrinolysis-affecting drugs

  ● **T45.60** Poisoning by, adverse effect of and underdosing of unspecified fibrinolysis-affecting drugs

    ● **T45.601** Poisoning by unspecified fibrinolysis-affecting drugs, accidental (unintentional)
       Poisoning by fibrinolysis-affecting drug NOS

    ● **T45.602** Poisoning by unspecified fibrinolysis-affecting drugs, intentional self-harm A, S 🏥

    ● **T45.603** Poisoning by unspecified fibrinolysis-affecting drugs, assault

    ● **T45.604** Poisoning by unspecified fibrinolysis-affecting drugs, undetermined

    ● **T45.605** Adverse effect of unspecified fibrinolysis-affecting drugs

    ● **T45.606** Underdosing of unspecified fibrinolysis-affecting drugs

  ● **T45.61** Poisoning by, adverse effect of and underdosing of thrombolytic drugs

    ● **T45.611** Poisoning by thrombolytic drug, accidental (unintentional)
       Poisoning by thrombolytic drug NOS

    ● **T45.612** Poisoning by thrombolytic drug, intentional self-harm A, S 🏥

    ● **T45.613** Poisoning by thrombolytic drug, assault

    ● **T45.614** Poisoning by thrombolytic drug, undetermined

    ● **T45.615** Adverse effect of thrombolytic drugs
       Coding Clinic: 2017, Q2, P10

    ● **T45.616** Underdosing of thrombolytic drugs

  ● **T45.62** Poisoning by, adverse effect of and underdosing of hemostatic drugs

    ● **T45.621** Poisoning by hemostatic drug, accidental (unintentional)
       Poisoning by hemostatic drug NOS

    ● **T45.622** Poisoning by hemostatic drug, intentional self-harm A, S 🏥

    ● **T45.623** Poisoning by hemostatic drug, assault

    ● **T45.624** Poisoning by hemostatic drug, undetermined

    ● **T45.625** Adverse effect of hemostatic drug

    ● **T45.626** Underdosing of hemostatic drugs

  ● **T45.69** Poisoning by, adverse effect of and underdosing of other fibrinolysis-affecting drugs

    ● **T45.691** Poisoning by other fibrinolysis-affecting drugs, accidental (unintentional)
       Poisoning by other fibrinolysis-affecting drug NOS

    ● **T45.692** Poisoning by other fibrinolysis-affecting drugs, intentional self-harm A, S 🏥

    ● **T45.693** Poisoning by other fibrinolysis-affecting drugs, assault

    ● **T45.694** Poisoning by other fibrinolysis-affecting drugs, undetermined

    ● **T45.695** Adverse effect of other fibrinolysis-affecting drugs

    ● **T45.696** Underdosing of other fibrinolysis-affecting drugs

● **T45.7** Poisoning by, adverse effect of and underdosing of anticoagulant antagonists, vitamin K and other coagulants

  ● **T45.7X** Poisoning by, adverse effect of and underdosing of anticoagulant antagonists, vitamin K and other coagulants

    ● **T45.7X1** Poisoning by anticoagulant antagonists, vitamin K and other coagulants, accidental (unintentional)
       Poisoning by anticoagulant antagonists, vitamin K and other coagulants NOS

    ● **T45.7X2** Poisoning by anticoagulant antagonists, vitamin K and other coagulants, intentional self-harm A, S 🏥

    ● **T45.7X3** Poisoning by anticoagulant antagonists, vitamin K and other coagulants, assault

    ● **T45.7X4** Poisoning by anticoagulant antagonists, vitamin K and other coagulants, undetermined

    ● **T45.7X5** Adverse effect of anticoagulant antagonists, vitamin K and other coagulants

    ● **T45.7X6** Underdosing of anticoagulant antagonist, vitamin K and other coagulants

       Excludes1 vitamin K deficiency (E56.1)

● **T45.8**   **Poisoning by, adverse effect of and underdosing of other primarily systemic and hematological agents**
> Poisoning by, adverse effect of and underdosing of liver preparations and other antianemic agents
> Poisoning by, adverse effect of and underdosing of natural blood and blood products
> Poisoning by, adverse effect of and underdosing of plasma substitute
>> **Excludes2**   poisoning by, adverse effect of and underdosing of immunoglobulin (T50.Z1)
>> poisoning by, adverse effect of and underdosing of iron (T45.4)
>> transfusion reactions (T80.-)

● **T45.8X**   **Poisoning by, adverse effect of and underdosing of other primarily systemic and hematological agents**
>> ● **T45.8X1**   **Poisoning by other primarily systemic and hematological agents, accidental (unintentional)**
>>> Poisoning by other primarily systemic and hematological agents NOS
>> ● **T45.8X2**   **Poisoning by other primarily systemic and hematological agents, intentional self-harm A, S** 🔄
>> ● **T45.8X3**   **Poisoning by other primarily systemic and hematological agents, assault**
>> ● **T45.8X4**   **Poisoning by other primarily systemic and hematological agents, undetermined**
>> ● **T45.8X5**   **Adverse effect of other primarily systemic and hematological agents**
>>> **Coding Clinic: 2016, Q4, P42**
>> ● **T45.8X6**   **Underdosing of other primarily systemic and hematological agents**

● **T45.9**   **Poisoning by, adverse effect of and underdosing of unspecified primarily systemic and hematological agent**
> X ● **T45.91**   **Poisoning by unspecified primarily systemic and hematological agent, accidental (unintentional)**
>> Poisoning by primarily systemic and hematological agent NOS
> X ● **T45.92**   **Poisoning by unspecified primarily systemic and hematological agent, intentional self-harm A, S** 🔄
> X ● **T45.93**   **Poisoning by unspecified primarily systemic and hematological agent, assault**
> X ● **T45.94**   **Poisoning by unspecified primarily systemic and hematological agent, undetermined**
> X ● **T45.95**   **Adverse effect of unspecified primarily systemic and hematological agent**
> X ● **T45.96**   **Underdosing of unspecified primarily systemic and hematological agent**

▶● **T45.A**   **Poisoning by, adverse effect of and underdosing of immune checkpoint inhibitors andimmunostimulant drugs**
>> ▶ **Excludes1**   poisoning by, adverse effect of and underdosing of antineoplastic andimmunosuppressive drug (T45.1)

▶● **T45.AX**   **Poisoning by, adverse effect of and underdosing of immune checkpoint inhibitorsand immunostimulant drugs**
>> ▶ **T45.AX1**   **Poisoning by immune checkpoint inhibitors and immunostimulant drugs,accidental (unintentional)**
>>> ▶ Poisoning by immune checkpoint inhibitors and immunosuppressive drugs NOS
>> ▶ **T45.AX2**   **Poisoning by immune checkpoint inhibitors and immunostimulant drugs, intentional self-harm**

▶ **T45.AX3**   **Poisoning by immune checkpoint inhibitors and immunostimulant drugs, assault**
▶ **T45.AX4**   **Poisoning by immune checkpoint inhibitors and immunostimulant drugs, undetermined**
▶ **T45.AX5**   **Adverse effect of immune checkpoint inhibitors and immunostimulant drugs**
▶ **T45.AX6**   **Underdosing of immune checkpoint inhibitors and immunostimulant drugs**

● **T46**   **Poisoning by, adverse effect of and underdosing of agents primarily affecting the cardiovascular system**
>> **Excludes1**   poisoning by, adverse effect of and underdosing of metaraminol (T44.4)

> The appropriate 7th character is to be added to each code from category T46

> | | |
> |---|---|
> | A | initial encounter |
> | D | subsequent encounter |
> | S | sequela |

● **T46.0**   **Poisoning by, adverse effect of and underdosing of cardiac-stimulant glycosides and drugs of similar action**
> ● **T46.0X**   **Poisoning by, adverse effect of and underdosing of cardiac-stimulant glycosides and drugs of similar action**
>> ● **T46.0X1**   **Poisoning by cardiac-stimulant glycosides and drugs of similar action, accidental (unintentional)**
>>> Poisoning by cardiac-stimulant glycosides and drugs of similar action NOS
>> ● **T46.0X2**   **Poisoning by cardiac-stimulant glycosides and drugs of similar action, intentional self-harm A, S** 🔄
>> ● **T46.0X3**   **Poisoning by cardiac-stimulant glycosides and drugs of similar action, assault**
>> ● **T46.0X4**   **Poisoning by cardiac-stimulant glycosides and drugs of similar action, undetermined**
>> ● **T46.0X5**   **Adverse effect of cardiac-stimulant glycosides and drugs of similar action**
>> ● **T46.0X6**   **Underdosing of cardiac-stimulant glycosides and drugs of similar action**

● **T46.1**   **Poisoning by, adverse effect of and underdosing of calcium-channel blockers**
> ● **T46.1X**   **Poisoning by, adverse effect of and underdosing of calcium-channel blockers**
>> ● **T46.1X1**   **Poisoning by calcium-channel blockers, accidental (unintentional)**
>>> Poisoning by calcium-channel blockers NOS
>> ● **T46.1X2**   **Poisoning by calcium-channel blockers, intentional self-harm A, S** 🔄
>> ● **T46.1X3**   **Poisoning by calcium-channel blockers, assault**
>> ● **T46.1X4**   **Poisoning by calcium-channel blockers, undetermined**
>> ● **T46.1X5**   **Adverse effect of calcium-channel blockers**
>> ● **T46.1X6**   **Underdosing of calcium-channel blockers**

● **T46.2**   **Poisoning by, adverse effect of and underdosing of other antidysrhythmic drugs, not elsewhere classified**
>> **Excludes1**   poisoning by, adverse effect of and underdosing of beta-adrenoreceptor antagonists (T44.7-)
> ● **T46.2X**   **Poisoning by, adverse effect of and underdosing of other antidysrhythmic drugs**

CHAPTER 19 (S00-T88)

- ● T46.2X1   Poisoning by other antidysrhythmic drugs, accidental (unintentional)
  Poisoning by other antidysrhythmic drugs NOS
- ● T46.2X2   Poisoning by other antidysrhythmic drugs, intentional self-harm A, S 🦠
- ● T46.2X3   Poisoning by other antidysrhythmic drugs, assault
- ● T46.2X4   Poisoning by other antidysrhythmic drugs, undetermined
- ● T46.2X5   Adverse effect of other antidysrhythmic drugs
- ● T46.2X6   Underdosing of other antidysrhythmic drugs
- ● T46.3   Poisoning by, adverse effect of and underdosing of coronary vasodilators
  Poisoning by, adverse effect of and underdosing of dipyridamole

  Excludes1   poisoning by, adverse effect of and underdosing of calcium-channel blockers (T46.1)

  - ● T46.3X   Poisoning by, adverse effect of and underdosing of coronary vasodilators
    - ● T46.3X1   Poisoning by coronary vasodilators, accidental (unintentional)
      Poisoning by coronary vasodilators NOS
    - ● T46.3X2   Poisoning by coronary vasodilators, intentional self-harm A, S 🦠
    - ● T46.3X3   Poisoning by coronary vasodilators, assault
    - ● T46.3X4   Poisoning by coronary vasodilators, undetermined
    - ● T46.3X5   Adverse effect of coronary vasodilators
    - ● T46.3X6   Underdosing of coronary vasodilators
- ● T46.4   Poisoning by, adverse effect of and underdosing of angiotensin-converting-enzyme inhibitors
  - ● T46.4X   Poisoning by, adverse effect of and underdosing of angiotensin-converting-enzyme inhibitors
    - ● T46.4X1   Poisoning by angiotensin-converting-enzyme inhibitors, accidental (unintentional)
      Poisoning by angiotensin-converting-enzyme inhibitors NOS
    - ● T46.4X2   Poisoning by angiotensin-converting-enzyme inhibitors, intentional self-harm A, S 🦠
    - ● T46.4X3   Poisoning by angiotensin-converting-enzyme inhibitors, assault
    - ● T46.4X4   Poisoning by angiotensin-converting-enzyme inhibitors, undetermined
    - ● T46.4X5   Adverse effect of angiotensin-converting-enzyme inhibitors
    - ● T46.4X6   Underdosing of angiotensin-converting-enzyme inhibitors
- ● T46.5   Poisoning by, adverse effect of and underdosing of other antihypertensive drugs

  Excludes2   poisoning by, adverse effect of and underdosing of beta-adrenoreceptor antagonists (T44.7)
  poisoning by, adverse effect of and underdosing of calcium-channel blockers (T46.1)
  poisoning by, adverse effect of and underdosing of diuretics (T50.0-T50.2)

  - ● T46.5X   Poisoning by, adverse effect of and underdosing of other antihypertensive drugs

- ● T46.5X1   Poisoning by other antihypertensive drugs, accidental (unintentional)
  Poisoning by other antihypertensive drugs NOS
- ● T46.5X2   Poisoning by other antihypertensive drugs, intentional self-harm A, S 🦠
- ● T46.5X3   Poisoning by other antihypertensive drugs, assault
- ● T46.5X4   Poisoning by other antihypertensive drugs, undetermined
- ● T46.5X5   Adverse effect of other antihypertensive drugs
- ● T46.5X6   Underdosing of other antihypertensive drugs
  Coding Clinic: 2022, Q1, P36
- ● T46.6   Poisoning by, adverse effect of and underdosing of antihyperlipidemic and antiarteriosclerotic drugs
  - ● T46.6X   Poisoning by, adverse effect of and underdosing of antihyperlipidemic and antiarteriosclerotic drugs
    - ● T46.6X1   Poisoning by antihyperlipidemic and antiarteriosclerotic drugs, accidental (unintentional)
      Poisoning by antihyperlipidemic and antiarteriosclerotic drugs NOS
    - ● T46.6X2   Poisoning by antihyperlipidemic and antiarteriosclerotic drugs, intentional self-harm A, S 🦠
    - ● T46.6X3   Poisoning by antihyperlipidemic and antiarteriosclerotic drugs, assault
    - ● T46.6X4   Poisoning by antihyperlipidemic and antiarteriosclerotic drugs, undetermined
    - ● T46.6X5   Adverse effect of antihyperlipidemic and antiarteriosclerotic drugs
    - ● T46.6X6   Underdosing of antihyperlipidemic and antiarteriosclerotic drugs
- ● T46.7   Poisoning by, adverse effect of and underdosing of peripheral vasodilators
  Poisoning by, adverse effect of and underdosing of nicotinic acid (derivatives)

  Excludes1   poisoning by, adverse effect of and underdosing of papaverine (T44.3)

  - ● T46.7X   Poisoning by, adverse effect of and underdosing of peripheral vasodilators
    - ● T46.7X1   Poisoning by peripheral vasodilators, accidental (unintentional)
      Poisoning by peripheral vasodilators NOS
    - ● T46.7X2   Poisoning by peripheral vasodilators, intentional self-harm A, S 🦠
    - ● T46.7X3   Poisoning by peripheral vasodilators, assault
    - ● T46.7X4   Poisoning by peripheral vasodilators, undetermined
    - ● T46.7X5   Adverse effect of peripheral vasodilators
    - ● T46.7X6   Underdosing of peripheral vasodilators
- ● T46.8   Poisoning by, adverse effect of and underdosing of antivaricose drugs, including sclerosing agents
  - ● T46.8X   Poisoning by, adverse effect of and underdosing of antivaricose drugs, including sclerosing agents
    - ● T46.8X1   Poisoning by antivaricose drugs, including sclerosing agents, accidental (unintentional)
      Poisoning by antivaricose drugs, including sclerosing agents NOS
    - ● T46.8X2   Poisoning by antivaricose drugs, including sclerosing agents, intentional self-harm A, S 🦠

▶ New   ⇒ Revised   ~~deleted~~ Deleted   Excludes 1   Excludes 2   Includes   Use additional   Code first   Code also   Key words

OGCR Official Guidelines   X Assign placeholder X   ● Use Additional Character(s)   ▶ Manifestation Code   🦠 Hierarchical Condition Category   **Coding Clinic**

● T46.8X3　Poisoning by antivaricose drugs, including sclerosing agents, assault

● T46.8X4　Poisoning by antivaricose drugs, including sclerosing agents, undetermined

● T46.8X5　Adverse effect of antivaricose drugs, including sclerosing agents

● T46.8X6　Underdosing of antivaricose drugs, including sclerosing agents

● T46.9　Poisoning by, adverse effect of and underdosing of other and unspecified agents primarily affecting the cardiovascular system

　● T46.90　Poisoning by, adverse effect of and underdosing of unspecified agents primarily affecting the cardiovascular system

　　● T46.901　Poisoning by unspecified agents primarily affecting the cardiovascular system, accidental (unintentional)

　　● T46.902　Poisoning by unspecified agents primarily affecting the cardiovascular system, intentional self-harm A, S 🔖

　　● T46.903　Poisoning by unspecified agents primarily affecting the cardiovascular system, assault

　　● T46.904　Poisoning by unspecified agents primarily affecting the cardiovascular system, undetermined

　　● T46.905　Adverse effect of unspecified agents primarily affecting the cardiovascular system

　　● T46.906　Underdosing of unspecified agents primarily affecting the cardiovascular system

　● T46.99　Poisoning by, adverse effect of and underdosing of other agents primarily affecting the cardiovascular system

　　● T46.991　Poisoning by other agents primarily affecting the cardiovascular system, accidental (unintentional)

　　● T46.992　Poisoning by other agents primarily affecting the cardiovascular system, intentional self-harm A, S 🔖

　　● T46.993　Poisoning by other agents primarily affecting the cardiovascular system, assault

　　● T46.994　Poisoning by other agents primarily affecting the cardiovascular system, undetermined

　　● T46.995　Adverse effect of other agents primarily affecting the cardiovascular system

　　● T46.996　Underdosing of other agents primarily affecting the cardiovascular system

● T47　Poisoning by, adverse effect of and underdosing of agents primarily affecting the gastrointestinal system

　The appropriate 7th character is to be added to each code from category T47

A	initial encounter
D	subsequent encounter
S	sequela

● T47.0　Poisoning by, adverse effect of and underdosing of histamine H2-receptor blockers

　● T47.0X　Poisoning by, adverse effect of and underdosing of histamine H2-receptor blockers

　　● T47.0X1　Poisoning by histamine H2-receptor blockers, accidental (unintentional)
　　　　Poisoning by histamine H2-receptor blockers NOS

　　● T47.0X2　Poisoning by histamine H2-receptor blockers, intentional self-harm A, S 🔖

● T47.0X3　Poisoning by histamine H2-receptor blockers, assault

● T47.0X4　Poisoning by histamine H2-receptor blockers, undetermined

● T47.0X5　Adverse effect of histamine H2-receptor blockers

● T47.0X6　Underdosing of histamine H2-receptor blockers

● T47.1　Poisoning by, adverse effect of and underdosing of other antacids and anti-gastric-secretion drugs

　● T47.1X　Poisoning by, adverse effect of and underdosing of other antacids and anti-gastric-secretion drugs

　　● T47.1X1　Poisoning by other antacids and anti-gastric-secretion drugs, accidental (unintentional)
　　　　Poisoning by other antacids and anti-gastric-secretion drugs NOS

　　● T47.1X2　Poisoning by other antacids and anti-gastric-secretion drugs, intentional self-harm A, S 🔖

　　● T47.1X3　Poisoning by other antacids and anti-gastric-secretion drugs, assault

　　● T47.1X4　Poisoning by other antacids and anti-gastric-secretion drugs, undetermined

　　● T47.1X5　Adverse effect of other antacids and anti-gastric-secretion drugs

　　● T47.1X6　Underdosing of other antacids and anti-gastric-secretion drugs

● T47.2　Poisoning by, adverse effect of and underdosing of stimulant laxatives

　● T47.2X　Poisoning by, adverse effect of and underdosing of stimulant laxatives

　　● T47.2X1　Poisoning by stimulant laxatives, accidental (unintentional)
　　　　Poisoning by stimulant laxatives NOS

　　● T47.2X2　Poisoning by stimulant laxatives, intentional self-harm A, S 🔖

　　● T47.2X3　Poisoning by stimulant laxatives, assault

　　● T47.2X4　Poisoning by stimulant laxatives, undetermined

　　● T47.2X5　Adverse effect of stimulant laxatives

　　● T47.2X6　Underdosing of stimulant laxatives

● T47.3　Poisoning by, adverse effect of and underdosing of saline and osmotic laxatives

　● T47.3X　Poisoning by and adverse effect of saline and osmotic laxatives

　　● T47.3X1　Poisoning by saline and osmotic laxatives, accidental (unintentional)
　　　　Poisoning by saline and osmotic laxatives NOS

　　● T47.3X2　Poisoning by saline and osmotic laxatives, intentional self-harm

　　● T47.3X3　Poisoning by saline and osmotic laxatives, assault A, S 🔖

　　● T47.3X4　Poisoning by saline and osmotic laxatives, undetermined

　　● T47.3X5　Adverse effect of saline and osmotic laxatives

　　● T47.3X6　Underdosing of saline and osmotic laxatives

● T47.4　Poisoning by, adverse effect of and underdosing of other laxatives

　● T47.4X　Poisoning by, adverse effect of and underdosing of other laxatives

　　● T47.4X1　Poisoning by other laxatives, accidental (unintentional)
　　　　Poisoning by other laxatives NOS

　　● T47.4X2　Poisoning by other laxatives, intentional self-harm A, S 🔖

● T47.4X3　Poisoning by other laxatives, assault
● T47.4X4　Poisoning by other laxatives, undetermined
● T47.4X5　Adverse effect of other laxatives
● T47.4X6　Underdosing of other laxatives

● T47.5　Poisoning by, adverse effect of and underdosing of digestants
　● T47.5X　Poisoning by, adverse effect of and underdosing of digestants
　　● T47.5X1　Poisoning by digestants, accidental (unintentional)
　　　　　　Poisoning by digestants NOS
　　● T47.5X2　Poisoning by digestants, intentional self-harm A, S 🐾
　　● T47.5X3　Poisoning by digestants, assault
　　● T47.5X4　Poisoning by digestants, undetermined
　　● T47.5X5　Adverse effect of digestants
　　● T47.5X6　Underdosing of digestants

● T47.6　Poisoning by, adverse effect of and underdosing of antidiarrheal drugs
　　Excludes2　poisoning by, adverse effect of and underdosing of systemic antibiotics and other anti-infectives (T36-T37)
　● T47.6X　Poisoning by, adverse effect of and underdosing of antidiarrheal drugs
　　● T47.6X1　Poisoning by antidiarrheal drugs, accidental (unintentional)
　　　　　　Poisoning by antidiarrheal drugs NOS
　　● T47.6X2　Poisoning by antidiarrheal drugs, intentional self-harm A, S 🐾
　　● T47.6X3　Poisoning by antidiarrheal drugs, assault
　　● T47.6X4　Poisoning by antidiarrheal drugs, undetermined
　　● T47.6X5　Adverse effect of antidiarrheal drugs
　　● T47.6X6　Underdosing of antidiarrheal drugs

● T47.7　Poisoning by, adverse effect of and underdosing of emetics
　● T47.7X　Poisoning by, adverse effect of and underdosing of emetics
　　● T47.7X1　Poisoning by emetics, accidental (unintentional)
　　　　　　Poisoning by emetics NOS
　　● T47.7X2　Poisoning by emetics, intentional self-harm A, S 🐾
　　● T47.7X3　Poisoning by emetics, assault
　　● T47.7X4　Poisoning by emetics, undetermined
　　● T47.7X5　Adverse effect of emetics
　　● T47.7X6　Underdosing of emetics

● T47.8　Poisoning by, adverse effect of and underdosing of other agents primarily affecting gastrointestinal system
　● T47.8X　Poisoning by, adverse effect of and underdosing of other agents primarily affecting gastrointestinal system
　　● T47.8X1　Poisoning by other agents primarily affecting gastrointestinal system, accidental (unintentional)
　　　　　　Poisoning by other agents primarily affecting gastrointestinal system NOS
　　● T47.8X2　Poisoning by other agents primarily affecting gastrointestinal system, intentional self-harm A, S 🐾
　　● T47.8X3　Poisoning by other agents primarily affecting gastrointestinal system, assault
　　● T47.8X4　Poisoning by other agents primarily affecting gastrointestinal system, undetermined

● T47.8X5　Adverse effect of other agents primarily affecting gastrointestinal system
● T47.8X6　Underdosing of other agents primarily affecting gastrointestinal system

● T47.9　Poisoning by, adverse effect of and underdosing of unspecified agents primarily affecting the gastrointestinal system
　X● T47.91　Poisoning by unspecified agents primarily affecting the gastrointestinal system, accidental (unintentional)
　　　　Poisoning by agents primarily affecting the gastrointestinal system NOS
　X● T47.92　Poisoning by unspecified agents primarily affecting the gastrointestinal system, intentional self-harm A, S 🐾
　X● T47.93　Poisoning by unspecified agents primarily affecting the gastrointestinal system, assault
　X● T47.94　Poisoning by unspecified agents primarily affecting the gastrointestinal system, undetermined
　X● T47.95　Adverse effect of unspecified agents primarily affecting the gastrointestinal system
　X● T47.96　Underdosing of unspecified agents primarily affecting the gastrointestinal system

● T48　Poisoning by, adverse effect of and underdosing of agents primarily acting on smooth and skeletal muscles and the respiratory system

　The appropriate 7th character is to be added to each code from category T48

A	initial encounter
D	subsequent encounter
S	sequela

● T48.0　Poisoning by, adverse effect of and underdosing of oxytocic drugs
　　Excludes1　poisoning by, adverse effect of and underdosing of estrogens, progestogens and antagonists (T38.4-T38.6)
　● T48.0X　Poisoning by, adverse effect of and underdosing of oxytocic drugs
　　● T48.0X1　Poisoning by oxytocic drugs, accidental (unintentional)
　　　　　　Poisoning by oxytocic drugs NOS
　　● T48.0X2　Poisoning by oxytocic drugs, intentional self-harm A, S 🐾
　　● T48.0X3　Poisoning by oxytocic drugs, assault
　　● T48.0X4　Poisoning by oxytocic drugs, undetermined
　　● T48.0X5　Adverse effect of oxytocic drugs
　　● T48.0X6　Underdosing of oxytocic drugs

● T48.1　Poisoning by, adverse effect of and underdosing of skeletal muscle relaxants [neuromuscular blocking agents]
　● T48.1X　Poisoning by, adverse effect of and underdosing of skeletal muscle relaxants [neuromuscular blocking agents]
　　● T48.1X1　Poisoning by skeletal muscle relaxants [neuromuscular blocking agents], accidental (unintentional)
　　　　　　Poisoning by skeletal muscle relaxants [neuromuscular blocking agents] NOS
　　● T48.1X2　Poisoning by skeletal muscle relaxants [neuromuscular blocking agents], intentional self-harm A, S 🐾
　　● T48.1X3　Poisoning by skeletal muscle relaxants [neuromuscular blocking agents], assault

▶ New　⇒ Revised　~~deleted~~ Deleted　Excludes 1　Excludes 2　Includes　Use additional　Code first　Code also　Key words
OGCR Official Guidelines　X Assign placeholder X　● Use Additional Character(s)　▶ Manifestation Code　🐾 Hierarchical Condition Category　Coding Clinic

● T48.1X4   Poisoning by skeletal muscle relaxants [neuromuscular blocking agents], undetermined

● T48.1X5   Adverse effect of skeletal muscle relaxants [neuromuscular blocking agents]

● T48.1X6   Underdosing of skeletal muscle relaxants [neuromuscular blocking agents]

● T48.2   Poisoning by, adverse effect of and underdosing of other and unspecified drugs acting on muscles

   ● T48.20   Poisoning by, adverse effect of and underdosing of unspecified drugs acting on muscles

     ● T48.201   Poisoning by unspecified drugs acting on muscles, accidental (unintentional)
            Poisoning by unspecified drugs acting on muscles NOS

     ● T48.202   Poisoning by unspecified drugs acting on muscles, intentional self-harm A, S 📖

     ● T48.203   Poisoning by unspecified drugs acting on muscles, assault

     ● T48.204   Poisoning by unspecified drugs acting on muscles, undetermined

     ● T48.205   Adverse effect of unspecified drugs acting on muscles

     ● T48.206   Underdosing of unspecified drugs acting on muscles

   ● T48.29   Poisoning by, adverse effect of and underdosing of other drugs acting on muscles

     ● T48.291   Poisoning by other drugs acting on muscles, accidental (unintentional)
            Poisoning by other drugs acting on muscles NOS

     ● T48.292   Poisoning by other drugs acting on muscles, intentional self-harm A, S 📖

     ● T48.293   Poisoning by other drugs acting on muscles, assault

     ● T48.294   Poisoning by other drugs acting on muscles, undetermined

     ● T48.295   Adverse effect of other drugs acting on muscles

     ● T48.296   Underdosing of other drugs acting on muscles

● T48.3   Poisoning by, adverse effect of and underdosing of antitussives

   ● T48.3X   Poisoning by, adverse effect of and underdosing of antitussives

     ● T48.3X1   Poisoning by antitussives, accidental (unintentional)
            Poisoning by antitussives NOS

     ● T48.3X2   Poisoning by antitussives, intentional self-harm A, S 📖

     ● T48.3X3   Poisoning by antitussives, assault

     ● T48.3X4   Poisoning by antitussives, undetermined

     ● T48.3X5   Adverse effect of antitussives

     ● T48.3X6   Underdosing of antitussives

● T48.4   Poisoning by, adverse effect of and underdosing of expectorants

   ● T48.4X   Poisoning by, adverse effect of and underdosing of expectorants

     ● T48.4X1   Poisoning by expectorants, accidental (unintentional)
            Poisoning by expectorants NOS

     ● T48.4X2   Poisoning by expectorants, intentional self-harm A, S 📖

     ● T48.4X3   Poisoning by expectorants, assault

     ● T48.4X4   Poisoning by expectorants, undetermined

● T48.4X5   Adverse effect of expectorants

● T48.4X6   Underdosing of expectorants

● T48.5   Poisoning by, adverse effect of and underdosing of other anti-common-cold drugs
     Poisoning by, adverse effect of and underdosing of decongestants

     Excludes2   poisoning by, adverse effect of and underdosing of antipyretics, NEC (T39.9-)
              poisoning by, adverse effect of and underdosing of non-steroidal antiinflammatory drugs (T39.3-)
              poisoning by, adverse effect of and underdosing of salicylates (T39.0-)

   ● T48.5X   Poisoning by, adverse effect of and underdosing of other anti-common-cold drugs

     ● T48.5X1   Poisoning by other anti-common-cold drugs, accidental (unintentional)
            Poisoning by other anti-common-cold drugs NOS

     ● T48.5X2   Poisoning by other anti-common-cold drugs, intentional self-harm A, S 📖

     ● T48.5X3   Poisoning by other anti-common-cold drugs, assault

     ● T48.5X4   Poisoning by other anti-common-cold drugs, undetermined

     ● T48.5X5   Adverse effect of other anti-common-cold drugs

     ● T48.5X6   Underdosing of other anti-common-cold drugs

● T48.6   Poisoning by, adverse effect of and underdosing of antiasthmatics, not elsewhere classified
     Poisoning by, adverse effect of and underdosing of beta-adrenoreceptor agonists used in asthma therapy

     Excludes1   poisoning by, adverse effect of and underdosing of beta-adrenoreceptor agonists not used in asthma therapy (T44.5)
              poisoning by, adverse effect of and underdosing of anterior pituitary [adenohypophyseal] hormones (T38.8)

   ● T48.6X   Poisoning by, adverse effect of and underdosing of antiasthmatics

     ● T48.6X1   Poisoning by antiasthmatics, accidental (unintentional)
            Poisoning by antiasthmatics NOS

     ● T48.6X2   Poisoning by antiasthmatics, intentional self-harm A, S 📖

     ● T48.6X3   Poisoning by antiasthmatics, assault

     ● T48.6X4   Poisoning by antiasthmatics, undetermined

     ● T48.6X5   Adverse effect of antiasthmatics

     ● T48.6X6   Underdosing of antiasthmatics

● T48.9   Poisoning by, adverse effect of and underdosing of other and unspecified agents primarily acting on the respiratory system

   ● T48.90   Poisoning by, adverse effect of and underdosing of unspecified agents primarily acting on the respiratory system

     ● T48.901   Poisoning by unspecified agents primarily acting on the respiratory system, accidental (unintentional)

     ● T48.902   Poisoning by unspecified agents primarily acting on the respiratory system, intentional self-harm A, S 📖

     ● T48.903   Poisoning by unspecified agents primarily acting on the respiratory system, assault

     ● T48.904   Poisoning by unspecified agents primarily acting on the respiratory system, undetermined

● T48.905   Adverse effect of unspecified agents primarily acting on the respiratory system
● T48.906   Underdosing of unspecified agents primarily acting on the respiratory system
● T48.99   Poisoning by, adverse effect of and underdosing of other agents primarily acting on the respiratory system
  ● T48.991   Poisoning by other agents primarily acting on the respiratory system, accidental (unintentional)
  ● T48.992   Poisoning by other agents primarily acting on the respiratory system, intentional self-harm A, S 🐵
  ● T48.993   Poisoning by other agents primarily acting on the respiratory system, assault
  ● T48.994   Poisoning by other agents primarily acting on the respiratory system, undetermined
  ● T48.995   Adverse effect of other agents primarily acting on the respiratory system
  ● T48.996   Underdosing of other agents primarily acting on the respiratory system

● T49   Poisoning by, adverse effect of and underdosing of topical agents primarily affecting skin and mucous membrane and by ophthalmological, otorhinolaryngological and dental drugs

Includes   poisoning by, adverse effect of and underdosing of glucocorticoids, topically used

The appropriate 7th character is to be added to each code from category T49

A	initial encounter
D	subsequent encounter
S	sequela

● T49.0   Poisoning by, adverse effect of and underdosing of local antifungal, anti-infective and anti-inflammatory drugs
  ● T49.0X   Poisoning by, adverse effect of and underdosing of local antifungal, anti-infective and anti-inflammatory drugs
    ● T49.0X1   Poisoning by local antifungal, anti-infective and anti-inflammatory drugs, accidental (unintentional)
                Poisoning by local antifungal, anti-infective and anti-inflammatory drugs NOS
    ● T49.0X2   Poisoning by local antifungal, anti-infective and anti-inflammatory drugs, intentional self-harm A, S 🐵
    ● T49.0X3   Poisoning by local antifungal, anti-infective and anti-inflammatory drugs, assault
    ● T49.0X4   Poisoning by local antifungal, anti-infective and anti-inflammatory drugs, undetermined
    ● T49.0X5   Adverse effect of local antifungal, anti-infective and anti-inflammatory drugs
    ● T49.0X6   Underdosing of local antifungal, anti-infective and anti-inflammatory drugs
● T49.1   Poisoning by, adverse effect of and underdosing of antipruritics
  ● T49.1X   Poisoning by, adverse effect of and underdosing of antipruritics
    ● T49.1X1   Poisoning by antipruritics, accidental (unintentional)
                Poisoning by antipruritics NOS
    ● T49.1X2   Poisoning by antipruritics, intentional self-harm A, S 🐵
    ● T49.1X3   Poisoning by antipruritics, assault

● T49.1X4   Poisoning by antipruritics, undetermined
● T49.1X5   Adverse effect of antipruritics
● T49.1X6   Underdosing of antipruritics
● T49.2   Poisoning by, adverse effect of and underdosing of local astringents and local detergents
  ● T49.2X   Poisoning by, adverse effect of and underdosing of local astringents and local detergents
    ● T49.2X1   Poisoning by local astringents and local detergents, accidental (unintentional)
                Poisoning by local astringents and local detergents NOS
    ● T49.2X2   Poisoning by local astringents and local detergents, intentional self-harm A, S 🐵
    ● T49.2X3   Poisoning by local astringents and local detergents, assault
    ● T49.2X4   Poisoning by local astringents and local detergents, undetermined
    ● T49.2X5   Adverse effect of local astringents and local detergents
    ● T49.2X6   Underdosing of local astringents and local detergents
● T49.3   Poisoning by, adverse effect of and underdosing of emollients, demulcents and protectants
  ● T49.3X   Poisoning by, adverse effect of and underdosing of emollients, demulcents and protectants
    ● T49.3X1   Poisoning by emollients, demulcents and protectants, accidental (unintentional)
                Poisoning by emollients, demulcents and protectants NOS
    ● T49.3X2   Poisoning by emollients, demulcents and protectants, intentional self-harm A, S 🐵
    ● T49.3X3   Poisoning by emollients, demulcents and protectants, assault
    ● T49.3X4   Poisoning by emollients, demulcents and protectants, undetermined
    ● T49.3X5   Adverse effect of emollients, demulcents and protectants
    ● T49.3X6   Underdosing of emollients, demulcents and protectants
● T49.4   Poisoning by, adverse effect of and underdosing of keratolytics, keratoplastics, and other hair treatment drugs and preparations
  ● T49.4X   Poisoning by, adverse effect of and underdosing of keratolytics, keratoplastics, and other hair treatment drugs and preparations
    ● T49.4X1   Poisoning by keratolytics, keratoplastics, and other hair treatment drugs and preparations, accidental (unintentional)
                Poisoning by keratolytics, keratoplastics, and other hair treatment drugs and preparations NOS
    ● T49.4X2   Poisoning by keratolytics, keratoplastics, and other hair treatment drugs and preparations, intentional self-harm A, S 🐵
    ● T49.4X3   Poisoning by keratolytics, keratoplastics, and other hair treatment drugs and preparations, assault
    ● T49.4X4   Poisoning by keratolytics, keratoplastics, and other hair treatment drugs and preparations, undetermined
    ● T49.4X5   Adverse effect of keratolytics, keratoplastics, and other hair treatment drugs and preparations

▶ New   ⇒ Revised   d̶e̶l̶e̶t̶e̶d̶ Deleted   Excludes 1   Excludes 2   Includes   Use additional   Code first   Code also   Key words

1378   OGCR Official Guidelines   X Assign placeholder X   ● Use Additional Character(s)   ▶ Manifestation Code   🐵 Hierarchical Condition Category   Coding Clinic

● T49.4X6   Underdosing of keratolytics, keratoplastics, and other hair treatment drugs and preparations

● T49.5   Poisoning by, adverse effect of and underdosing of ophthalmological drugs and preparations

  ● T49.5X   Poisoning by, adverse effect of and underdosing of ophthalmological drugs and preparations

    ● T49.5X1   Poisoning by ophthalmological drugs and preparations, accidental (unintentional)
        Poisoning by ophthalmological drugs and preparations NOS

    ● T49.5X2   Poisoning by ophthalmological drugs and preparations, intentional self-harm A, S 🔍

    ● T49.5X3   Poisoning by ophthalmological drugs and preparations, assault

    ● T49.5X4   Poisoning by ophthalmological drugs and preparations, undetermined

    ● T49.5X5   Adverse effect of ophthalmological drugs and preparations

    ● T49.5X6   Underdosing of ophthalmological drugs and preparations

● T49.6   Poisoning by, adverse effect of and underdosing of otorhinolaryngological drugs and preparations

  ● T49.6X   Poisoning by, adverse effect of and underdosing of otorhinolaryngological drugs and preparations

    ● T49.6X1   Poisoning by otorhinolaryngological drugs and preparations, accidental (unintentional)
        Poisoning by otorhinolaryngological drugs and preparations NOS

    ● T49.6X2   Poisoning by otorhinolaryngological drugs and preparations, intentional self-harm A, S 🔍

    ● T49.6X3   Poisoning by otorhinolaryngological drugs and preparations, assault

    ● T49.6X4   Poisoning by otorhinolaryngological drugs and preparations, undetermined

    ● T49.6X5   Adverse effect of otorhinolaryngological drugs and preparations

    ● T49.6X6   Underdosing of otorhinolaryngological drugs and preparations

● T49.7   Poisoning by, adverse effect of and underdosing of dental drugs, topically applied

  ● T49.7X   Poisoning by, adverse effect of and underdosing of dental drugs, topically applied

    ● T49.7X1   Poisoning by dental drugs, topically applied, accidental (unintentional)
        Poisoning by dental drugs, topically applied NOS

    ● T49.7X2   Poisoning by dental drugs, topically applied, intentional self-harm A, S 🔍

    ● T49.7X3   Poisoning by dental drugs, topically applied, assault

    ● T49.7X4   Poisoning by dental drugs, topically applied, undetermined

    ● T49.7X5   Adverse effect of dental drugs, topically applied

    ● T49.7X6   Underdosing of dental drugs, topically applied

● T49.8   Poisoning by, adverse effect of and underdosing of other topical agents
    Poisoning by, adverse effect of and underdosing of spermicides

  ● T49.8X   Poisoning by, adverse effect of and underdosing of other topical agents

    ● T49.8X1   Poisoning by other topical agents, accidental (unintentional)
        Poisoning by other topical agents NOS

    ● T49.8X2   Poisoning by other topical agents, intentional self-harm A, S 🔍

    ● T49.8X3   Poisoning by other topical agents, assault

    ● T49.8X4   Poisoning by other topical agents, undetermined

    ● T49.8X5   Adverse effect of other topical agents

    ● T49.8X6   Underdosing of other topical agents

● T49.9   Poisoning by, adverse effect of and underdosing of unspecified topical agent

  X ● T49.91   Poisoning by unspecified topical agent, accidental (unintentional)

  X ● T49.92   Poisoning by unspecified topical agent, intentional self-harm A, S 🔍

  X ● T49.93   Poisoning by unspecified topical agent, assault

  X ● T49.94   Poisoning by unspecified topical agent, undetermined

  X ● T49.95   Adverse effect of unspecified topical agent

  X ● T49.96   Underdosing of unspecified topical agent

● T50   Poisoning by, adverse effect of and underdosing of diuretics and other and unspecified drugs, medicaments and biological substances

    The appropriate 7th character is to be added to each code from category T50

A	initial encounter
D	subsequent encounter
S	sequela

● T50.0   Poisoning by, adverse effect of and underdosing of mineralocorticoids and their antagonists

  ● T50.0X   Poisoning by, adverse effect of and underdosing of mineralocorticoids and their antagonists

    ● T50.0X1   Poisoning by mineralocorticoids and their antagonists, accidental (unintentional)
        Poisoning by mineralocorticoids and their antagonists NOS

    ● T50.0X2   Poisoning by mineralocorticoids and their antagonists, intentional self-harm A, S 🔍

    ● T50.0X3   Poisoning by mineralocorticoids and their antagonists, assault

    ● T50.0X4   Poisoning by mineralocorticoids and their antagonists, undetermined

    ● T50.0X5   Adverse effect of mineralocorticoids and their antagonists

    ● T50.0X6   Underdosing of mineralocorticoids and their antagonists

● T50.1   Poisoning by, adverse effect of and underdosing of loop [high-ceiling] diuretics

  ● T50.1X   Poisoning by, adverse effect of and underdosing of loop [high-ceiling] diuretics

    ● T50.1X1   Poisoning by loop [high-ceiling] diuretics, accidental (unintentional)
        Poisoning by loop [high-ceiling] diuretics NOS

    ● T50.1X2   Poisoning by loop [high-ceiling] diuretics, intentional self-harm A, S 🔍

    ● T50.1X3   Poisoning by loop [high-ceiling] diuretics, assault

    ● T50.1X4   Poisoning by loop [high-ceiling] diuretics, undetermined

    ● T50.1X5   Adverse effect of loop [high-ceiling] diuretics

    ● T50.1X6   Underdosing of loop [high-ceiling] diuretics

CHAPTER 19 (S00-T88)

● **T50.2**   **Poisoning by, adverse effect of and underdosing of carbonic-anhydrase inhibitors, benzothiadiazides and other diuretics**
     Poisoning by, adverse effect of and underdosing of acetazolamide

   ● **T50.2X**   **Poisoning by, adverse effect of and underdosing of carbonic-anhydrase inhibitors, benzothiadiazides and other diuretics**

     ● **T50.2X1**   **Poisoning by carbonic-anhydrase inhibitors, benzothiadiazides and other diuretics, accidental (unintentional)**
         Poisoning by carbonic-anhydrase inhibitors, benzothiadiazides and other diuretics NOS

     ● **T50.2X2**   **Poisoning by carbonic-anhydrase inhibitors, benzothiadiazides and other diuretics, intentional self-harm A, S** 🐾

     ● **T50.2X3**   **Poisoning by carbonic-anhydrase inhibitors, benzothiadiazides and other diuretics, assault**

     ● **T50.2X4**   **Poisoning by carbonic-anhydrase inhibitors, benzothiadiazides and other diuretics, undetermined**

     ● **T50.2X5**   **Adverse effect of carbonic-anhydrase inhibitors, benzothiadiazides and other diuretics**

     ● **T50.2X6**   **Underdosing of carbonic-anhydrase inhibitors, benzothiadiazides and other diuretics**

● **T50.3**   **Poisoning by, adverse effect of and underdosing of electrolytic, caloric and water-balance agents**
     Poisoning by, adverse effect of and underdosing of oral rehydration salts

   ● **T50.3X**   **Poisoning by, adverse effect of and underdosing of electrolytic, caloric and water-balance agents**

     ● **T50.3X1**   **Poisoning by electrolytic, caloric and water-balance agents, accidental (unintentional)**
         Poisoning by electrolytic, caloric and water-balance agents NOS

     ● **T50.3X2**   **Poisoning by electrolytic, caloric and water-balance agents, intentional self-harm A, S** 🐾

     ● **T50.3X3**   **Poisoning by electrolytic, caloric and water-balance agents, assault**

     ● **T50.3X4**   **Poisoning by electrolytic, caloric and water-balance agents, undetermined**

     ● **T50.3X5**   **Adverse effect of electrolytic, caloric and water-balance agents**
         Coding Clinic: 2022, Q2, P11

     ● **T50.3X6**   **Underdosing of electrolytic, caloric and water-balance agents**

● **T50.4**   **Poisoning by, adverse effect of and underdosing of drugs affecting uric acid metabolism**

   ● **T50.4X**   **Poisoning by, adverse effect of and underdosing of drugs affecting uric acid metabolism**

     ● **T50.4X1**   **Poisoning by drugs affecting uric acid metabolism, accidental (unintentional)**
         Poisoning by drugs affecting uric acid metabolism NOS

     ● **T50.4X2**   **Poisoning by drugs affecting uric acid metabolism, intentional self-harm A, S** 🐾

     ● **T50.4X3**   **Poisoning by drugs affecting uric acid metabolism, assault**

     ● **T50.4X4**   **Poisoning by drugs affecting uric acid metabolism, undetermined**

     ● **T50.4X5**   **Adverse effect of drugs affecting uric acid metabolism**

     ● **T50.4X6**   **Underdosing of drugs affecting uric acid metabolism**

● **T50.5**   **Poisoning by, adverse effect of and underdosing of appetite depressants**

   ● **T50.5X**   **Poisoning by, adverse effect of and underdosing of appetite depressants**

     ● **T50.5X1**   **Poisoning by appetite depressants, accidental (unintentional)**
         Poisoning by appetite depressants NOS

     ● **T50.5X2**   **Poisoning by appetite depressants, intentional self-harm A, S** 🐾

     ● **T50.5X3**   **Poisoning by appetite depressants, assault**

     ● **T50.5X4**   **Poisoning by appetite depressants, undetermined**

     ● **T50.5X5**   **Adverse effect of appetite depressants**

     ● **T50.5X6**   **Underdosing of appetite depressants**

● **T50.6**   **Poisoning by, adverse effect of and underdosing of antidotes and chelating agents**
     Poisoning by, adverse effect of and underdosing of alcohol deterrents

   ● **T50.6X**   **Poisoning by, adverse effect of and underdosing of antidotes and chelating agents**

     ● **T50.6X1**   **Poisoning by antidotes and chelating agents, accidental (unintentional)**
         Poisoning by antidotes and chelating agents NOS

     ● **T50.6X2**   **Poisoning by antidotes and chelating agents, intentional self-harm A, S** 🐾

     ● **T50.6X3**   **Poisoning by antidotes and chelating agents, assault**

     ● **T50.6X4**   **Poisoning by antidotes and chelating agents, undetermined**

     ● **T50.6X5**   **Adverse effect of antidotes and chelating agents**

     ● **T50.6X6**   **Underdosing of antidotes and chelating agents**

● **T50.7**   **Poisoning by, adverse effect of and underdosing of analeptics and opioid receptor antagonists**

   ● **T50.7X**   **Poisoning by, adverse effect of and underdosing of analeptics and opioid receptor antagonists**

     ● **T50.7X1**   **Poisoning by analeptics and opioid receptor antagonists, accidental (unintentional)**
         Poisoning by analeptics and opioid receptor antagonists NOS

     ● **T50.7X2**   **Poisoning by analeptics and opioid receptor antagonists, intentional self-harm A, S** 🐾

     ● **T50.7X3**   **Poisoning by analeptics and opioid receptor antagonists, assault**

     ● **T50.7X4**   **Poisoning by analeptics and opioid receptor antagonists, undetermined**

     ● **T50.7X5**   **Adverse effect of analeptics and opioid receptor antagonists**

     ● **T50.7X6**   **Underdosing of analeptics and opioid receptor antagonists**

● **T50.8**   **Poisoning by, adverse effect of and underdosing of diagnostic agents**

   ● **T50.8X**   **Poisoning by, adverse effect of and underdosing of diagnostic agents**

     ● **T50.8X1**   **Poisoning by diagnostic agents, accidental (unintentional)**
         Poisoning by diagnostic agents NOS

     ● **T50.8X2**   **Poisoning by diagnostic agents, intentional self-harm A, S** 🐾

     ● **T50.8X3**   **Poisoning by diagnostic agents, assault**

     ● **T50.8X4**   **Poisoning by diagnostic agents, undetermined**

▶ New   ▥ Revised   ~~deleted~~ Deleted   Excludes 1   Excludes 2   Includes   Use additional   Code first   Code also   Key words

OGCR Official Guidelines   X Assign placeholder X   ● Use Additional Character(s)   ▪ Manifestation Code   🐾 Hierarchical Condition Category   **Coding Clinic**

● T50.8X5   Adverse effect of diagnostic agents
        Coding Clinic: 2023, Q3, P4-5; 2022, Q4, P33; 2021, Q3, P9-10

● T50.8X6   Underdosing of diagnostic agents

● T50.A   Poisoning by, adverse effect of and underdosing of bacterial vaccines

   ● T50.A1   Poisoning by, adverse effect of and underdosing of pertussis vaccine, including combinations with a pertussis component

     ● T50.A11   Poisoning by pertussis vaccine, including combinations with a pertussis component, accidental (unintentional)

     ● T50.A12   Poisoning by pertussis vaccine, including combinations with a pertussis component, intentional self-harm A, S ✎

     ● T50.A13   Poisoning by pertussis vaccine, including combinations with a pertussis component, assault

     ● T50.A14   Poisoning by pertussis vaccine, including combinations with a pertussis component, undetermined

     ● T50.A15   Adverse effect of pertussis vaccine, including combinations with a pertussis component

     ● T50.A16   Underdosing of pertussis vaccine, including combinations with a pertussis component

   ● T50.A2   Poisoning by, adverse effect of and underdosing of mixed bacterial vaccines without a pertussis component

     ● T50.A21   Poisoning by mixed bacterial vaccines without a pertussis component, accidental (unintentional)

     ● T50.A22   Poisoning by mixed bacterial vaccines without a pertussis component, intentional self-harm A, S ✎

     ● T50.A23   Poisoning by mixed bacterial vaccines without a pertussis component, assault

     ● T50.A24   Poisoning by mixed bacterial vaccines without a pertussis component, undetermined

     ● T50.A25   Adverse effect of mixed bacterial vaccines without a pertussis component

     ● T50.A26   Underdosing of mixed bacterial vaccines without a pertussis component

   ● T50.A9   Poisoning by, adverse effect of and underdosing of other bacterial vaccines

     ● T50.A91   Poisoning by other bacterial vaccines, accidental (unintentional)

     ● T50.A92   Poisoning by other bacterial vaccines, intentional self-harm A, S ✎

     ● T50.A93   Poisoning by other bacterial vaccines, assault

     ● T50.A94   Poisoning by other bacterial vaccines, undetermined

     ● T50.A95   Adverse effect of other bacterial vaccines

     ● T50.A96   Underdosing of other bacterial vaccines

● T50.B   Poisoning by, adverse effect of and underdosing of viral vaccines

   ● T50.B1   Poisoning by, adverse effect of and underdosing of smallpox vaccines

     ● T50.B11   Poisoning by smallpox vaccines, accidental (unintentional)

     ● T50.B12   Poisoning by smallpox vaccines, intentional self-harm A, S ✎

     ● T50.B13   Poisoning by smallpox vaccines, assault

     ● T50.B14   Poisoning by smallpox vaccines, undetermined

     ● T50.B15   Adverse effect of smallpox vaccines

     ● T50.B16   Underdosing of smallpox vaccines

   ● T50.B9   Poisoning by, adverse effect of and underdosing of other viral vaccines

     ● T50.B91   Poisoning by other viral vaccines, accidental (unintentional)

     ● T50.B92   Poisoning by other viral vaccines, intentional self-harm A, S ✎

     ● T50.B93   Poisoning by other viral vaccines, assault

     ● T50.B94   Poisoning by other viral vaccines, undetermined

     ● T50.B95   Adverse effect of other viral vaccines
        Coding Clinic: 2021, Q1, P43-44

     ● T50.B96   Underdosing of other viral vaccines

● T50.Z   Poisoning by, adverse effect of and underdosing of other vaccines and biological substances

   ● T50.Z1   Poisoning by, adverse effect of and underdosing of immunoglobulin

     ● T50.Z11   Poisoning by immunoglobulin, accidental (unintentional)

     ● T50.Z12   Poisoning by immunoglobulin, intentional self-harm A, S ✎

     ● T50.Z13   Poisoning by immunoglobulin, assault

     ● T50.Z14   Poisoning by immunoglobulin, undetermined

     ● T50.Z15   Adverse effect of immunoglobulin

     ● T50.Z16   Underdosing of immunoglobulin

   ● T50.Z9   Poisoning by, adverse effect of and underdosing of other vaccines and biological substances

     ● T50.Z91   Poisoning by other vaccines and biological substances, accidental (unintentional)

     ● T50.Z92   Poisoning by other vaccines and biological substances, intentional self-harm A, S ✎

     ● T50.Z93   Poisoning by other vaccines and biological substances, assault

     ● T50.Z94   Poisoning by other vaccines and biological substances, undetermined

     ● T50.Z95   Adverse effect of other vaccines and biological substances
        Coding Clinic: 2020, Q1, P19

     ● T50.Z96   Underdosing of other vaccines and biological substances

● T50.9   Poisoning by, adverse effect of and underdosing of other and unspecified drugs, medicaments and biological substances

   ● T50.90   Poisoning by, adverse effect of and underdosing of unspecified drugs, medicaments and biological substances

     ● T50.901   Poisoning by unspecified drugs, medicaments and biological substances, accidental (unintentional)
        Coding Clinic: 2015, Q1, P21

     ● T50.902   Poisoning by unspecified drugs, medicaments and biological substances, intentional self-harm A, S ✎

     ● T50.903   Poisoning by unspecified drugs, medicaments and biological substances, assault

     ● T50.904   Poisoning by unspecified drugs, medicaments and biological substances, undetermined

● **T50.905** Adverse effect of unspecified drugs, medicaments and biological substances

● **T50.906** Underdosing of unspecified drugs, medicaments and biological substances

● **T50.91** Poisoning by, adverse effect of and underdosing of multiple unspecified drugs, medicaments and biological substances

Multiple drug ingestion NOS

Code also any specific drugs, medicaments and biological substances

● **T50.911** Poisoning by multiple unspecified drugs, medicaments and biological substances, accidental (unintentional)

● **T50.912** Poisoning by multiple unspecified drugs, medicaments and biological substances, intentional self-harm

● **T50.913** Poisoning by multiple unspecified drugs, medicaments and biological substances, assault

● **T50.914** Poisoning by multiple unspecified drugs, medicaments and biological substances, undetermined

● **T50.915** Adverse effect of multiple unspecified drugs, medicaments and biological substances

● **T50.916** Underdosing of multiple unspecified drugs, medicaments and biological substances

● **T50.99** Poisoning by, adverse effect of and underdosing of other drugs, medicaments and biological substances

● **T50.991** Poisoning by other drugs, medicaments and biological substances, accidental (unintentional)

● **T50.992** Poisoning by other drugs, medicaments and biological substances, intentional self-harm A, S 🦠

● **T50.993** Poisoning by other drugs, medicaments and biological substances, assault

● **T50.994** Poisoning by other drugs, medicaments and biological substances, undetermined

● **T50.995** Adverse effect of other drugs, medicaments and biological substances

Coding Clinic: 2023, Q3, P4-5

● **T50.996** Underdosing of other drugs, medicaments and biological substances

---

TOXIC EFFECTS OF SUBSTANCES CHIEFLY NONMEDICINAL AS TO SOURCE (T51-T65)

Note: When no intent is indicated code to accidental. Undetermined intent is only for use when there is specific documentation in the record that the intent of the toxic effect cannot be determined.

Use additional code(s): for all associated manifestations of toxic effect, such as:
respiratory conditions due to external agents (J60-J70)
personal history of foreign body fully removed (Z87.821)
to identify any retained foreign body, if applicable (Z18.-)

Excludes1 contact with and (suspected) exposure to toxic substances (Z77.-)

● **T51** Toxic effect of alcohol

The appropriate 7th character is to be added to each code from category T51

A	initial encounter
D	subsequent encounter
S	sequela

● **T51.0** Toxic effect of ethanol
Toxic effect of ethyl alcohol

Excludes2 acute alcohol intoxication or 'hangover' effects (F10.129, F10.229, F10.929)
drunkenness (F10.129, F10.229, F10.929)
pathological alcohol intoxication (F10.129, F10.229, F10.929)

● **T51.0X** Toxic effect of ethanol

● **T51.0X1** Toxic effect of ethanol, accidental (unintentional)
Toxic effect of ethanol NOS

● **T51.0X2** Toxic effect of ethanol, intentional self-harm A, S 🦠

● **T51.0X3** Toxic effect of ethanol, assault

● **T51.0X4** Toxic effect of ethanol, undetermined

● **T51.1** Toxic effect of methanol
Toxic effect of methyl alcohol

● **T51.1X** Toxic effect of methanol

● **T51.1X1** Toxic effect of methanol, accidental (unintentional)
Toxic effect of methanol NOS

● **T51.1X2** Toxic effect of methanol, intentional self-harm A, S 🦠

● **T51.1X3** Toxic effect of methanol, assault

● **T51.1X4** Toxic effect of methanol, undetermined

● **T51.2** Toxic effect of 2-Propanol
Toxic effect of isopropyl alcohol

● **T51.2X** Toxic effect of 2-Propanol

● **T51.2X1** Toxic effect of 2-Propanol, accidental (unintentional)
Toxic effect of 2-Propanol NOS

● **T51.2X2** Toxic effect of 2-Propanol, intentional self-harm A, S 🦠

● **T51.2X3** Toxic effect of 2-Propanol, assault

● **T51.2X4** Toxic effect of 2-Propanol, undetermined

● **T51.3** Toxic effect of fusel oil
Toxic effect of amyl alcohol
Toxic effect of butyl [1-butanol] alcohol
Toxic effect of propyl [1-propanol] alcohol

● **T51.3X** Toxic effect of fusel oil

● **T51.3X1** Toxic effect of fusel oil, accidental (unintentional)
Toxic effect of fusel oil NOS

● **T51.3X2** Toxic effect of fusel oil, intentional self-harm A, S 🦠

● **T51.3X3** Toxic effect of fusel oil, assault

● **T51.3X4** Toxic effect of fusel oil, undetermined

● **T51.8** Toxic effect of other alcohols

● **T51.8X** Toxic effect of other alcohols

● **T51.8X1** Toxic effect of other alcohols, accidental (unintentional)
Toxic effect of other alcohols NOS

● **T51.8X2** Toxic effect of other alcohols, intentional self-harm A, S 🦠

● **T51.8X3** Toxic effect of other alcohols, assault

● **T51.8X4** Toxic effect of other alcohols, undetermined

● **T51.9** Toxic effect of unspecified alcohol

X ● **T51.91** Toxic effect of unspecified alcohol, accidental (unintentional)

X ● **T51.92** Toxic effect of unspecified alcohol, intentional self-harm A, S 🦠

X ● **T51.93** Toxic effect of unspecified alcohol, assault

X ● **T51.94** Toxic effect of unspecified alcohol, undetermined

---

▶ New   ⇒ Revised   ~~deleted~~ Deleted   Excludes 1   Excludes 2   Includes   Use additional   Code first   Code also   Key words

OGCR Official Guidelines   X Assign placeholder X   ● Use Additional Character(s)   ▶ Manifestation Code   🦠 Hierarchical Condition Category   Coding Clinic

● **T52**   **Toxic effect of organic solvents**

> **Excludes1**   halogen derivatives of aliphatic and aromatic hydrocarbons (T53.-)

> The appropriate 7th character is to be added to each code from category T52

> | | |
> |---|---|
> | A | initial encounter |
> | D | subsequent encounter |
> | S | sequela |

● **T52.0**   **Toxic effects of petroleum products**
> Toxic effects of gasoline [petrol]
> Toxic effects of kerosene [paraffin oil]
> Toxic effects of paraffin wax
> Toxic effects of ether petroleum
> Toxic effects of naphtha petroleum
> Toxic effects of spirit petroleum

>> ● **T52.0X**   **Toxic effects of petroleum products**

>>> ● **T52.0X1**   Toxic effect of petroleum products, **accidental (unintentional)**
>>>> Toxic effects of petroleum products NOS

>>> ● **T52.0X2**   Toxic effect of petroleum products, **intentional self-harm** A, S 🐾

>>> ● **T52.0X3**   Toxic effect of petroleum products, **assault**

>>> ● **T52.0X4**   Toxic effect of petroleum products, **undetermined**

● **T52.1**   **Toxic effects of benzene**
> **Excludes1**   homologues of benzene (T52.2)
> nitroderivatives and aminoderivatives of benzene and its homologues (T65.3)

>> ● **T52.1X**   **Toxic effects of benzene**

>>> ● **T52.1X1**   Toxic effect of benzene, **accidental (unintentional)**
>>>> Toxic effects of benzene NOS

>>> ● **T52.1X2**   Toxic effect of benzene, **intentional self-harm** A, S 🐾

>>> ● **T52.1X3**   Toxic effect of benzene, **assault**

>>> ● **T52.1X4**   Toxic effect of benzene, **undetermined**

● **T52.2**   **Toxic effects of homologues of benzene**
> Toxic effects of toluene [methylbenzene]
> Toxic effects of xylene [dimethylbenzene]

>> ● **T52.2X**   **Toxic effects of homologues of benzene**

>>> ● **T52.2X1**   Toxic effect of homologues of benzene, **accidental (unintentional)**
>>>> Toxic effects of homologues of benzene NOS

>>> ● **T52.2X2**   Toxic effect of homologues of benzene, **intentional self-harm** A, S 🐾

>>> ● **T52.2X3**   Toxic effect of homologues of benzene, **assault**

>>> ● **T52.2X4**   Toxic effect of homologues of benzene, **undetermined**

● **T52.3**   **Toxic effects of glycols**

>> ● **T52.3X**   **Toxic effects of glycols**

>>> ● **T52.3X1**   Toxic effect of glycols, **accidental (unintentional)**
>>>> Toxic effects of glycols NOS

>>> ● **T52.3X2**   Toxic effect of glycols, **intentional self-harm** A, S 🐾

>>> ● **T52.3X3**   Toxic effect of glycols, **assault**

>>> ● **T52.3X4**   Toxic effect of glycols, **undetermined**

● **T52.4**   **Toxic effects of ketones**

>> ● **T52.4X**   **Toxic effects of ketones**

>>> ● **T52.4X1**   Toxic effect of ketones, **accidental (unintentional)**
>>>> Toxic effects of ketones NOS

>>> ● **T52.4X2**   Toxic effect of ketones, **intentional self-harm** A, S 🐾

>>> ● **T52.4X3**   Toxic effect of ketones, **assault**

>>> ● **T52.4X4**   Toxic effect of ketones, **undetermined**

● **T52.8**   **Toxic effects of other organic solvents**

>> ● **T52.8X**   **Toxic effects of other organic solvents**

>>> ● **T52.8X1**   Toxic effect of other organic solvents, **accidental (unintentional)**
>>>> Toxic effects of other organic solvents NOS

>>> ● **T52.8X2**   Toxic effect of other organic solvents, **intentional self-harm** A, S 🐾

>>> ● **T52.8X3**   Toxic effect of other organic solvents, **assault**

>>> ● **T52.8X4**   Toxic effect of other organic solvents, **undetermined**

● **T52.9**   **Toxic effects of unspecified organic solvent**

> X ● **T52.91**   Toxic effect of unspecified organic solvent, **accidental (unintentional)**

> X ● **T52.92**   Toxic effect of unspecified organic solvent, **intentional self-harm** A, S 🐾

> X ● **T52.93**   Toxic effect of unspecified organic solvent, **assault**

> X ● **T52.94**   Toxic effect of unspecified organic solvent, **undetermined**

● **T53**   **Toxic effect of halogen derivatives of aliphatic and aromatic hydrocarbons**

> The appropriate 7th character is to be added to each code from category T53

> | | |
> |---|---|
> | A | initial encounter |
> | D | subsequent encounter |
> | S | sequela |

● **T53.0**   **Toxic effects of carbon tetrachloride**
> Toxic effects of tetrachloromethane

>> ● **T53.0X**   **Toxic effects of carbon tetrachloride**

>>> ● **T53.0X1**   Toxic effect of carbon tetrachloride, **accidental (unintentional)**
>>>> Toxic effects of carbon tetrachloride NOS

>>> ● **T53.0X2**   Toxic effect of carbon tetrachloride, **intentional self-harm** A, S 🐾

>>> ● **T53.0X3**   Toxic effect of carbon tetrachloride, **assault**

>>> ● **T53.0X4**   Toxic effect of carbon tetrachloride, **undetermined**

● **T53.1**   **Toxic effects of chloroform**
> Toxic effects of trichloromethane

>> ● **T53.1X**   **Toxic effects of chloroform**

>>> ● **T53.1X1**   Toxic effect of chloroform, **accidental (unintentional)**
>>>> Toxic effects of chloroform NOS

>>> ● **T53.1X2**   Toxic effect of chloroform, **intentional self-harm** A, S 🐾

>>> ● **T53.1X3**   Toxic effect of chloroform, **assault**

>>> ● **T53.1X4**   Toxic effect of chloroform, **undetermined**

● **T53.2**   **Toxic effects of trichloroethylene**
> Toxic effects of trichloroethene

>> ● **T53.2X**   **Toxic effects of trichloroethylene**

>>> ● **T53.2X1**   Toxic effect of trichloroethylene, **accidental (unintentional)**
>>>> Toxic effects of trichloroethylene NOS

>>> ● **T53.2X2**   Toxic effect of trichloroethylene, **intentional self-harm** A, S 🐾

>>> ● **T53.2X3**   Toxic effect of trichloroethylene, **assault**

>>> ● **T53.2X4**   Toxic effect of trichloroethylene, **undetermined**

● **T53.3**   **Toxic effects of tetrachloroethylene**
> Toxic effects of perchloroethylene
> Toxic effect of tetrachloroethene

>> ● **T53.3X**   **Toxic effects of tetrachloroethylene**

CHAPTER 19 (S00-T88)

● **T53.3X1** **Toxic effect of tetrachloroethylene, accidental (unintentional)**
Toxic effects of tetrachloroethylene NOS

● **T53.3X2** **Toxic effect of tetrachloroethylene, intentional self-harm A, S** 🐾

● **T53.3X3** **Toxic effect of tetrachloroethylene, assault**

● **T53.3X4** **Toxic effect of tetrachloroethylene, undetermined**

● **T53.4** Toxic effects of dichloromethane
Toxic effects of methylene chloride

● **T53.4X** Toxic effects of **dichloromethane**

● **T53.4X1** **Toxic effect of dichloromethane, accidental (unintentional)**
Toxic effects of dichloromethane NOS

● **T53.4X2** **Toxic effect of dichloromethane, intentional self-harm A, S** 🐾

● **T53.4X3** **Toxic effect of dichloromethane, assault**

● **T53.4X4** **Toxic effect of dichloromethane, undetermined**

● **T53.5** Toxic effects of chlorofluorocarbons

● **T53.5X** Toxic effects of **chlorofluorocarbons**

● **T53.5X1** **Toxic effect of chlorofluorocarbons, accidental (unintentional)**
Toxic effects of chlorofluorocarbons NOS

● **T53.5X2** **Toxic effect of chlorofluorocarbons, intentional self-harm A, S** 🐾

● **T53.5X3** **Toxic effect of chlorofluorocarbons, assault**

● **T53.5X4** **Toxic effect of chlorofluorocarbons, undetermined**

● **T53.6** Toxic effects of other halogen derivatives of aliphatic hydrocarbons

● **T53.6X** Toxic effects of **other halogen derivatives of aliphatic hydrocarbons**

● **T53.6X1** **Toxic effect of other halogen derivatives of aliphatic hydrocarbons, accidental (unintentional)**
Toxic effects of other halogen derivatives of aliphatic hydrocarbons NOS

● **T53.6X2** **Toxic effect of other halogen derivatives of aliphatic hydrocarbons, intentional self-harm A, S** 🐾

● **T53.6X3** **Toxic effect of other halogen derivatives of aliphatic hydrocarbons, assault**

● **T53.6X4** **Toxic effect of other halogen derivatives of aliphatic hydrocarbons, undetermined**

● **T53.7** Toxic effects of other halogen derivatives of aromatic hydrocarbons

● **T53.7X** Toxic effects of **other halogen derivatives of aromatic hydrocarbons**

● **T53.7X1** **Toxic effect of other halogen derivatives of aromatic hydrocarbons, accidental (unintentional)**
Toxic effects of other halogen derivatives of aromatic hydrocarbons NOS

● **T53.7X2** **Toxic effect of other halogen derivatives of aromatic hydrocarbons, intentional self-harm A, S** 🐾

● **T53.7X3** **Toxic effect of other halogen derivatives of aromatic hydrocarbons, assault**

● **T53.7X4** **Toxic effect of other halogen derivatives of aromatic hydrocarbons, undetermined**

● **T53.9** Toxic effects of **unspecified halogen derivatives of aliphatic and aromatic hydrocarbons**

X ● **T53.91** **Toxic effect of unspecified halogen derivatives of aliphatic and aromatic hydrocarbons, accidental (unintentional)**

X ● **T53.92** **Toxic effect of unspecified halogen derivatives of aliphatic and aromatic hydrocarbons, intentional self-harm A, S** 🐾

X ● **T53.93** **Toxic effect of unspecified halogen derivatives of aliphatic and aromatic hydrocarbons, assault**

X ● **T53.94** **Toxic effect of unspecified halogen derivatives of aliphatic and aromatic hydrocarbons, undetermined**

● **T54** Toxic effect of corrosive substances
The appropriate 7th character is to be added to each code from category T54

A	initial encounter
D	subsequent encounter
S	sequela

● **T54.0** Toxic effects of phenol and phenol homologues

● **T54.0X** Toxic effects of **phenol and phenol homologues**

● **T54.0X1** **Toxic effect of phenol and phenol homologues, accidental (unintentional)**
Toxic effects of phenol and phenol homologues NOS

● **T54.0X2** **Toxic effect of phenol and phenol homologues, intentional self-harm A, S** 🐾

● **T54.0X3** **Toxic effect of phenol and phenol homologues, assault**

● **T54.0X4** **Toxic effect of phenol and phenol homologues, undetermined**

● **T54.1** Toxic effects of other corrosive organic compounds

● **T54.1X** Toxic effects of other **corrosive organic compounds**

● **T54.1X1** **Toxic effect of other corrosive organic compounds, accidental (unintentional)**
Toxic effects of other corrosive organic compounds NOS

● **T54.1X2** **Toxic effect of other corrosive organic compounds, intentional self-harm A, S** 🐾

● **T54.1X3** **Toxic effect of other corrosive organic compounds, assault**

● **T54.1X4** **Toxic effect of other corrosive organic compounds, undetermined**

● **T54.2** Toxic effects of corrosive acids and acid-like substances
Toxic effects of hydrochloric acid
Toxic effects of sulfuric acid

● **T54.2X** Toxic effects of **corrosive acids and acid-like substances**

● **T54.2X1** **Toxic effect of corrosive acids and acid-like substances, accidental (unintentional)**
Toxic effects of corrosive acids and acid-like substances NOS

● **T54.2X2** **Toxic effect of corrosive acids and acid-like substances, intentional self-harm A, S** 🐾

● **T54.2X3** **Toxic effect of corrosive acids and acid-like substances, assault**

● **T54.2X4** **Toxic effect of corrosive acids and acid-like substances, undetermined**

● **T54.3** Toxic effects of corrosive alkalis and alkali-like substances
Toxic effects of potassium hydroxide
Toxic effects of sodium hydroxide

● T54.3X Toxic effects of corrosive alkalis and alkali-like substances
   ● T54.3X1 Toxic effect of corrosive alkalis and alkali-like substances, accidental (unintentional)
       Toxic effects of corrosive alkalis and alkali-like substances NOS
   ● T54.3X2 Toxic effect of corrosive alkalis and alkali-like substances, intentional self-harm A, S 🐾
   ● T54.3X3 Toxic effect of corrosive alkalis and alkali-like substances, assault
   ● T54.3X4 Toxic effect of corrosive alkalis and alkali-like substances, undetermined

● T54.9 Toxic effects of unspecified corrosive substance
  X ● T54.91 Toxic effect of unspecified corrosive substance, accidental (unintentional)
  X ● T54.92 Toxic effect of unspecified corrosive substance, intentional self-harm A, S 🐾
  X ● T54.93 Toxic effect of unspecified corrosive substance, assault
  X ● T54.94 Toxic effect of unspecified corrosive substance, undetermined

● T55 Toxic effect of soaps and detergents
   The appropriate 7th character is to be added to each code from category T55

A	initial encounter
D	subsequent encounter
S	sequela

● T55.0 Toxic effect of soaps
  ● T55.0X Toxic effect of soaps
   ● T55.0X1 Toxic effect of soaps, accidental (unintentional)
       Toxic effect of soaps NOS
   ● T55.0X2 Toxic effect of soaps, intentional self-harm A, S 🐾
   ● T55.0X3 Toxic effect of soaps, assault
   ● T55.0X4 Toxic effect of soaps, undetermined

● T55.1 Toxic effect of detergents
  ● T55.1X Toxic effect of detergents
   ● T55.1X1 Toxic effect of detergents, accidental (unintentional)
       Toxic effect of detergents NOS
   ● T55.1X2 Toxic effect of detergents, intentional self-harm A, S 🐾
   ● T55.1X3 Toxic effect of detergents, assault
   ● T55.1X4 Toxic effect of detergents, undetermined

● T56 Toxic effect of metals
  Includes toxic effects of fumes and vapors of metals
       toxic effects of metals from all sources, except medicinal substances
  Use additional code to identify any retained metal foreign body, if applicable (Z18.0-, T18.1-)
  Excludes1 arsenic and its compounds (T57.0)
       manganese and its compounds (T57.2)
  The appropriate 7th character is to be added to each code from category T56

A	initial encounter
D	subsequent encounter
S	sequela

● T56.0 Toxic effects of lead and its compounds
  ● T56.0X Toxic effects of lead and its compounds
   ● T56.0X1 Toxic effect of lead and its compounds, accidental (unintentional)
       Toxic effects of lead and its compounds NOS

● T56.0X2 Toxic effect of lead and its compounds, intentional self-harm A, S 🐾
● T56.0X3 Toxic effect of lead and its compounds, assault
● T56.0X4 Toxic effect of lead and its compounds, undetermined

● T56.1 Toxic effects of mercury and its compounds
  ● T56.1X Toxic effects of mercury and its compounds
   ● T56.1X1 Toxic effect of mercury and its compounds, accidental (unintentional)
       Toxic effects of mercury and its compounds NOS
   ● T56.1X2 Toxic effect of mercury and its compounds, intentional self-harm A, S 🐾
   ● T56.1X3 Toxic effect of mercury and its compounds, assault
   ● T56.1X4 Toxic effect of mercury and its compounds, undetermined

● T56.2 Toxic effects of chromium and its compounds
  ● T56.2X Toxic effects of chromium and its compounds
   ● T56.2X1 Toxic effect of chromium and its compounds, accidental (unintentional)
       Toxic effects of chromium and its compounds NOS
   ● T56.2X2 Toxic effect of chromium and its compounds, intentional self-harm A, S 🐾
   ● T56.2X3 Toxic effect of chromium and its compounds, assault
   ● T56.2X4 Toxic effect of chromium and its compounds, undetermined

● T56.3 Toxic effects of cadmium and its compounds
  ● T56.3X Toxic effects of cadmium and its compounds
   ● T56.3X1 Toxic effect of cadmium and its compounds, accidental (unintentional)
       Toxic effects of cadmium and its compounds NOS
   ● T56.3X2 Toxic effect of cadmium and its compounds, intentional self-harm A, S 🐾
   ● T56.3X3 Toxic effect of cadmium and its compounds, assault
   ● T56.3X4 Toxic effect of cadmium and its compounds, undetermined

● T56.4 Toxic effects of copper and its compounds
  ● T56.4X Toxic effects of copper and its compounds
   ● T56.4X1 Toxic effect of copper and its compounds, accidental (unintentional)
       Toxic effects of copper and its compounds NOS
   ● T56.4X2 Toxic effect of copper and its compounds, intentional self-harm A, S 🐾
   ● T56.4X3 Toxic effect of copper and its compounds, assault
   ● T56.4X4 Toxic effect of copper and its compounds, undetermined

● T56.5 Toxic effects of zinc and its compounds
  ● T56.5X Toxic effects of zinc and its compounds
   ● T56.5X1 Toxic effect of zinc and its compounds, accidental (unintentional)
       Toxic effects of zinc and its compounds NOS
   ● T56.5X2 Toxic effect of zinc and its compounds, intentional self-harm A, S 🐾

CHAPTER 19 (S00–T88)

CHAPTER 19 (S00–T88)

● T56.5X3   Toxic effect of zinc and its compounds, assault
● T56.5X4   Toxic effect of zinc and its compounds, undetermined
● T56.6   Toxic effects of tin and its compounds
   ● T56.6X   Toxic effects of tin and its compounds
     ● T56.6X1   Toxic effect of tin and its compounds, accidental (unintentional)
       Toxic effects of tin and its compounds NOS
     ● T56.6X2   Toxic effect of tin and its compounds, intentional self-harm A, S 🦠
     ● T56.6X3   Toxic effect of tin and its compounds, assault
     ● T56.6X4   Toxic effect of tin and its compounds, undetermined
● T56.7   Toxic effects of beryllium and its compounds
   ● T56.7X   Toxic effects of beryllium and its compounds
     ● T56.7X1   Toxic effect of beryllium and its compounds, accidental (unintentional)
       Toxic effects of beryllium and its compounds NOS
     ● T56.7X2   Toxic effect of beryllium and its compounds, intentional self-harm A, S 🦠
     ● T56.7X3   Toxic effect of beryllium and its compounds, assault
     ● T56.7X4   Toxic effect of beryllium and its compounds, undetermined
● T56.8   Toxic effects of other metals
   ● T56.81   Toxic effect of thallium
     ● T56.811   Toxic effect of thallium, accidental (unintentional)
       Toxic effect of thallium NOS
     ● T56.812   Toxic effect of thallium, intentional self-harm A, S 🦠
     ● T56.813   Toxic effect of thallium, assault
     ● T56.814   Toxic effect of thallium, undetermined
   ● T56.82   Toxic effect of gadolinium
     Excludes1   adverse effect of diagnostic agents (T50.8X5-)
     T56.821   Toxic effect of gadolinium, accidental (unintentional)
       Toxic effect of gadolinium NOS
     T56.822   Toxic effect of gadolinium, intentional self-harm
     T56.823   Toxic effect of gadolinium, assault
     T56.824   Toxic effect of gadolinium, undetermined
   ● T56.89   Toxic effects of other metals
     ● T56.891   Toxic effect of other metals, accidental (unintentional)
       Toxic effects of other metals NOS
     ● T56.892   Toxic effect of other metals, intentional self-harm A, S 🦠
     ● T56.893   Toxic effect of other metals, assault
     ● T56.894   Toxic effect of other metals, undetermined
● T56.9   Toxic effects of unspecified metal
   X ● T56.91   Toxic effect of unspecified metal, accidental (unintentional)
   X ● T56.92   Toxic effect of unspecified metal, intentional self-harm A, S 🦠
   X ● T56.93   Toxic effect of unspecified metal, assault
   X ● T56.94   Toxic effect of unspecified metal, undetermined

● T57   Toxic effect of other inorganic substances
   The appropriate 7th character is to be added to each code from category T57

A	initial encounter
D	subsequent encounter
S	sequela

● T57.0   Toxic effect of arsenic and its compounds
   ● T57.0X   Toxic effect of arsenic and its compounds
     ● T57.0X1   Toxic effect of arsenic and its compounds, accidental (unintentional)
       Toxic effect of arsenic and its compounds NOS
     ● T57.0X2   Toxic effect of arsenic and its compounds, intentional self-harm A, S 🦠
     ● T57.0X3   Toxic effect of arsenic and its compounds, assault
     ● T57.0X4   Toxic effect of arsenic and its compounds, undetermined
● T57.1   Toxic effect of phosphorus and its compounds
   Excludes1   organophosphate insecticides (T60.0)
   ● T57.1X   Toxic effect of phosphorus and its compounds
     ● T57.1X1   Toxic effect of phosphorus and its compounds, accidental (unintentional)
       Toxic effect of phosphorus and its compounds NOS
     ● T57.1X2   Toxic effect of phosphorus and its compounds, intentional self-harm A, S 🦠
     ● T57.1X3   Toxic effect of phosphorus and its compounds, assault
     ● T57.1X4   Toxic effect of phosphorus and its compounds, undetermined
● T57.2   Toxic effect of manganese and its compounds
   ● T57.2X   Toxic effect of manganese and its compounds
     ● T57.2X1   Toxic effect of manganese and its compounds, accidental (unintentional)
       Toxic effect of manganese and its compounds NOS
     ● T57.2X2   Toxic effect of manganese and its compounds, intentional self-harm A, S 🦠
     ● T57.2X3   Toxic effect of manganese and its compounds, assault
     ● T57.2X4   Toxic effect of manganese and its compounds, undetermined
● T57.3   Toxic effect of hydrogen cyanide
   ● T57.3X   Toxic effect of hydrogen cyanide
     ● T57.3X1   Toxic effect of hydrogen cyanide, accidental (unintentional)
       Toxic effect of hydrogen cyanide NOS
     ● T57.3X2   Toxic effect of hydrogen cyanide, intentional self-harm A, S 🦠
     ● T57.3X3   Toxic effect of hydrogen cyanide, assault
     ● T57.3X4   Toxic effect of hydrogen cyanide, undetermined
● T57.8   Toxic effect of other specified inorganic substances
   ● T57.8X   Toxic effect of other specified inorganic substances
     ● T57.8X1   Toxic effect of other specified inorganic substances, accidental (unintentional)
       Toxic effect of other specified inorganic substances NOS
     ● T57.8X2   Toxic effect of other specified inorganic substances, intentional self-harm A, S 🦠

▶ New   ⟹ Revised   ~~deleted~~ Deleted   Excludes 1   Excludes 2   Includes   Use additional   Code first   Code also   Key words
OGCR Official Guidelines   X Assign placeholder X   ● Use Additional Character(s)   ▷ Manifestation Code   🦠 Hierarchical Condition Category   **Coding Clinic**

● T57.8X3   Toxic effect of other specified inorganic substances, assault

● T57.8X4   Toxic effect of other specified inorganic substances, undetermined

● T57.9   Toxic effect of unspecified inorganic substance

X ● T57.91   Toxic effect of unspecified inorganic substance, accidental (unintentional)

X ● T57.92   Toxic effect of unspecified inorganic substance, intentional self-harm A, S 🔒

X ● T57.93   Toxic effect of unspecified inorganic substance, assault

X ● T57.94   Toxic effect of unspecified inorganic substance, undetermined

● T58   Toxic effect of carbon monoxide

Includes	asphyxiation from carbon monoxide
	toxic effect of carbon monoxide from all sources

The appropriate 7th character is to be added to each code from category T58

A	initial encounter
D	subsequent encounter
S	sequela

● T58.0   Toxic effect of carbon monoxide from motor vehicle exhaust
Toxic effect of exhaust gas from gas engine
Toxic effect of exhaust gas from motor pump

X ● T58.01   Toxic effect of carbon monoxide from motor vehicle exhaust, accidental (unintentional)

X ● T58.02   Toxic effect of carbon monoxide from motor vehicle exhaust, intentional self-harm A, S 🔒

X ● T58.03   Toxic effect of carbon monoxide from motor vehicle exhaust, assault

X ● T58.04   Toxic effect of carbon monoxide from motor vehicle exhaust, undetermined

● T58.1   Toxic effect of carbon monoxide from utility gas
Toxic effect of acetylene
Toxic effect of gas NOS used for lighting, heating, cooking
Toxic effect of water gas

X ● T58.11   Toxic effect of carbon monoxide from utility gas, accidental (unintentional)

X ● T58.12   Toxic effect of carbon monoxide from utility gas, intentional self-harm A, S 🔒

X ● T58.13   Toxic effect of carbon monoxide from utility gas, assault

X ● T58.14   Toxic effect of carbon monoxide from utility gas, undetermined

● T58.2   Toxic effect of carbon monoxide from incomplete combustion of other domestic fuels
Toxic effect of carbon monoxide from incomplete combustion of coal, coke, kerosene, wood

● T58.2X   Toxic effect of carbon monoxide from incomplete combustion of other domestic fuels

● T58.2X1   Toxic effect of carbon monoxide from incomplete combustion of other domestic fuels, accidental (unintentional)

● T58.2X2   Toxic effect of carbon monoxide from incomplete combustion of other domestic fuels, intentional self-harm A, S 🔒

● T58.2X3   Toxic effect of carbon monoxide from incomplete combustion of other domestic fuels, assault

● T58.2X4   Toxic effect of carbon monoxide from incomplete combustion of other domestic fuels, undetermined

● T58.8   Toxic effect of carbon monoxide from other source
Toxic effect of carbon monoxide from blast furnace gas
Toxic effect of carbon monoxide from fuels in industrial use
Toxic effect of carbon monoxide from kiln vapor

● T58.8X   Toxic effect of carbon monoxide from other source

● T58.8X1   Toxic effect of carbon monoxide from other source, accidental (unintentional)

● T58.8X2   Toxic effect of carbon monoxide from other source, intentional self-harm A, S 🔒

● T58.8X3   Toxic effect of carbon monoxide from other source, assault

● T58.8X4   Toxic effect of carbon monoxide from other source, undetermined

● T58.9   Toxic effect of carbon monoxide from unspecified source

X ● T58.91   Toxic effect of carbon monoxide from unspecified source, accidental (unintentional)

X ● T58.92   Toxic effect of carbon monoxide from unspecified source, intentional self-harm A, S 🔒

X ● T58.93   Toxic effect of carbon monoxide from unspecified source, assault

X ● T58.94   Toxic effect of carbon monoxide from unspecified source, undetermined

● T59   Toxic effect of other gases, fumes and vapors

Includes	aerosol propellants
Excludes1	chlorofluorocarbons (T53.5)

The appropriate 7th character is to be added to each code from category T59

A	initial encounter
D	subsequent encounter
S	sequela

● T59.0   Toxic effect of nitrogen oxides

● T59.0X   Toxic effect of nitrogen oxides

● T59.0X1   Toxic effect of nitrogen oxides, accidental (unintentional)
Toxic effect of nitrogen oxides NOS

● T59.0X2   Toxic effect of nitrogen oxides, intentional self-harm A, S 🔒

● T59.0X3   Toxic effect of nitrogen oxides, assault

● T59.0X4   Toxic effect of nitrogen oxides, undetermined

● T59.1   Toxic effect of sulfur dioxide

● T59.1X   Toxic effect of sulfur dioxide

● T59.1X1   Toxic effect of sulfur dioxide, accidental (unintentional)
Toxic effect of sulfur dioxide NOS

● T59.1X2   Toxic effect of sulfur dioxide, intentional self-harm A, S 🔒

● T59.1X3   Toxic effect of sulfur dioxide, assault

● T59.1X4   Toxic effect of sulfur dioxide, undetermined

● T59.2   Toxic effect of formaldehyde

● T59.2X   Toxic effect of formaldehyde

● T59.2X1   Toxic effect of formaldehyde, accidental (unintentional)
Toxic effect of formaldehyde NOS

● T59.2X2   Toxic effect of formaldehyde, intentional self-harm A, S 🔒

● T59.2X3   Toxic effect of formaldehyde, assault

● T59.2X4   Toxic effect of formaldehyde, undetermined

● T59.3   Toxic effect of lacrimogenic gas
Toxic effect of tear gas

● T59.3X   Toxic effect of lacrimogenic gas

● T59.3X1   Toxic effect of lacrimogenic gas, accidental (unintentional)
Toxic effect of lacrimogenic gas NOS

● T59.3X2   Toxic effect of lacrimogenic gas, intentional self-harm A, S 🔒

● T59.3X3   Toxic effect of lacrimogenic gas, assault

● T59.3X4   Toxic effect of lacrimogenic gas, undetermined

CHAPTER 19 (S00–T88)

● **T59.4**   **Toxic effect of chlorine gas**
  ● **T59.4X**   Toxic effect of chlorine gas
    ● **T59.4X1**   Toxic effect of chlorine gas, accidental (unintentional)
        Toxic effect of chlorine gas NOS
    ● **T59.4X2**   Toxic effect of chlorine gas, intentional self-harm A, S 🦠
    ● **T59.4X3**   Toxic effect of chlorine gas, assault
    ● **T59.4X4**   Toxic effect of chlorine gas, undetermined
● **T59.5**   **Toxic effect of fluorine gas and hydrogen fluoride**
  ● **T59.5X**   Toxic effect of fluorine gas and hydrogen fluoride
    ● **T59.5X1**   Toxic effect of fluorine gas and hydrogen fluoride, accidental (unintentional)
        Toxic effect of fluorine gas and hydrogen fluoride NOS
    ● **T59.5X2**   Toxic effect of fluorine gas and hydrogen fluoride, intentional self-harm A, S 🦠
    ● **T59.5X3**   Toxic effect of fluorine gas and hydrogen fluoride, assault
    ● **T59.5X4**   Toxic effect of fluorine gas and hydrogen fluoride, undetermined
● **T59.6**   **Toxic effect of hydrogen sulfide**
  ● **T59.6X**   Toxic effect of hydrogen sulfide
    ● **T59.6X1**   Toxic effect of hydrogen sulfide, accidental (unintentional)
        Toxic effect of hydrogen sulfide NOS
    ● **T59.6X2**   Toxic effect of hydrogen sulfide, intentional self-harm A, S 🦠
    ● **T59.6X3**   Toxic effect of hydrogen sulfide, assault
    ● **T59.6X4**   Toxic effect of hydrogen sulfide, undetermined
● **T59.7**   **Toxic effect of carbon dioxide**
  ● **T59.7X**   Toxic effect of carbon dioxide
    ● **T59.7X1**   Toxic effect of carbon dioxide, accidental (unintentional)
        Toxic effect of carbon dioxide NOS
    ● **T59.7X2**   Toxic effect of carbon dioxide, intentional self-harm A, S 🦠
    ● **T59.7X3**   Toxic effect of carbon dioxide, assault
    ● **T59.7X4**   Toxic effect of carbon dioxide, undetermined
● **T59.8**   **Toxic effect of other specified gases, fumes and vapors**
  ● **T59.81**   Toxic effect of smoke
        Smoke inhalation
        Excludes2   toxic effect of cigarette (tobacco) smoke (T65.22-)
    ● **T59.811**   Toxic effect of smoke, accidental (unintentional)
        Toxic effect of smoke NOS
    ● **T59.812**   Toxic effect of smoke, intentional self-harm A, S 🦠
    ● **T59.813**   Toxic effect of smoke, assault
    ● **T59.814**   Toxic effect of smoke, undetermined
  ● **T59.89**   Toxic effect of other specified gases, fumes and vapors
    ● **T59.891**   Toxic effect of other specified gases, fumes and vapors, accidental (unintentional)
    ● **T59.892**   Toxic effect of other specified gases, fumes and vapors, intentional self-harm A, S 🦠
    ● **T59.893**   Toxic effect of other specified gases, fumes and vapors, assault
    ● **T59.894**   Toxic effect of other specified gases, fumes and vapors, undetermined

● **T59.9**   **Toxic effect of unspecified gases, fumes and vapors**
  X ● **T59.91**   Toxic effect of unspecified gases, fumes and vapors, accidental (unintentional)
  X ● **T59.92**   Toxic effect of unspecified gases, fumes and vapors, intentional self-harm A, S 🦠
  X ● **T59.93**   Toxic effect of unspecified gases, fumes and vapors, assault
  X ● **T59.94**   Toxic effect of unspecified gases, fumes and vapors, undetermined
● **T60**   **Toxic effect of pesticides**
  Includes   toxic effect of wood preservatives
  The appropriate 7th character is to be added to each code from category T60

A	initial encounter
D	subsequent encounter
S	sequela

● **T60.0**   **Toxic effect of organophosphate and carbamate insecticides**
  ● **T60.0X**   Toxic effect of organophosphate and carbamate insecticides
    ● **T60.0X1**   Toxic effect of organophosphate and carbamate insecticides, accidental (unintentional)
        Toxic effect of organophosphate and carbamate insecticides NOS
    ● **T60.0X2**   Toxic effect of organophosphate and carbamate insecticides, intentional self-harm A, S 🦠
    ● **T60.0X3**   Toxic effect of organophosphate and carbamate insecticides, assault
    ● **T60.0X4**   Toxic effect of organophosphate and carbamate insecticides, undetermined
● **T60.1**   **Toxic effect of halogenated insecticides**
  Excludes1   chlorinated hydrocarbon (T53.-)
  ● **T60.1X**   Toxic effect of halogenated insecticides
    ● **T60.1X1**   Toxic effect of halogenated insecticides, accidental (unintentional)
        Toxic effect of halogenated insecticides NOS
    ● **T60.1X2**   Toxic effect of halogenated insecticides, intentional self-harm A, S 🦠
    ● **T60.1X3**   Toxic effect of halogenated insecticides, assault
    ● **T60.1X4**   Toxic effect of halogenated insecticides, undetermined
● **T60.2**   **Toxic effect of other insecticides**
  ● **T60.2X**   Toxic effect of other insecticides
    ● **T60.2X1**   Toxic effect of other insecticides, accidental (unintentional)
        Toxic effect of other insecticides NOS
    ● **T60.2X2**   Toxic effect of other insecticides, intentional self-harm A, S 🦠
    ● **T60.2X3**   Toxic effect of other insecticides, assault
    ● **T60.2X4**   Toxic effect of other insecticides, undetermined
● **T60.3**   **Toxic effect of herbicides and fungicides**
  ● **T60.3X**   Toxic effect of herbicides and fungicides
    ● **T60.3X1**   Toxic effect of herbicides and fungicides, accidental (unintentional)
        Toxic effect of herbicides and fungicides NOS
    ● **T60.3X2**   Toxic effect of herbicides and fungicides, intentional self-harm A, S 🦠
    ● **T60.3X3**   Toxic effect of herbicides and fungicides, assault
    ● **T60.3X4**   Toxic effect of herbicides and fungicides, undetermined

▶ New   ⇒ Revised   ~~deleted~~ Deleted   Excludes 1   Excludes 2   Includes   Use additional   Code first   Code also   Key words
OGCR Official Guidelines   X Assign placeholder X   ● Use Additional Character(s)   ▶ Manifestation Code   🦠 Hierarchical Condition Category   Coding Clinic

● **T60.4**   Toxic effect of rodenticides
    Excludes1   strychnine and its salts (T65.1)
                thallium (T56.81-)
    ● **T60.4X**   Toxic effect of rodenticides
       ● **T60.4X1**   Toxic effect of rodenticides, accidental (unintentional)
             Toxic effect of rodenticides NOS
       ● **T60.4X2**   Toxic effect of rodenticides, intentional self-harm A, S 🐾
       ● **T60.4X3**   Toxic effect of rodenticides, assault
       ● **T60.4X4**   Toxic effect of rodenticides, undetermined

● **T60.8**   Toxic effect of other pesticides
    ● **T60.8X**   Toxic effect of other pesticides
       ● **T60.8X1**   Toxic effect of other pesticides, accidental (unintentional)
             Toxic effect of other pesticides NOS
       ● **T60.8X2**   Toxic effect of other pesticides, intentional self-harm A, S 🐾
       ● **T60.8X3**   Toxic effect of other pesticides, assault
       ● **T60.8X4**   Toxic effect of other pesticides, undetermined

● **T60.9**   Toxic effect of unspecified pesticide
    X● **T60.91**   Toxic effect of unspecified pesticide, accidental (unintentional)
    X● **T60.92**   Toxic effect of unspecified pesticide, intentional self-harm A, S 🐾
    X● **T60.93**   Toxic effect of unspecified pesticide, assault
    X● **T60.94**   Toxic effect of unspecified pesticide, undetermined

● **T61**   Toxic effect of noxious substances eaten as seafood
    Excludes1   allergic reaction to food, such as:
              anaphylactic reaction or shock due to adverse food reaction (T78.0-)
              bacterial foodborne intoxications (A05.-)
              dermatitis (L23.6, L25.4, L27.2)
              food protein-induced enterocolitis syndrome (K52.21)
              food protein-induced enteropathy (K52.22)
              gastroenteritis (noninfective) (K52.29)
              toxic effect of aflatoxin and other mycotoxins (T64)
              toxic effect of cyanides (T65.0-)
              toxic effect of harmful algae bloom (T65.82-)
              toxic effect of hydrogen cyanide (T57.3-)
              toxic effect of mercury (T56.1-)
              toxic effect of red tide (T65.82-)
    The appropriate 7th character is to be added to each code from category T61

      | | |
      A   initial encounter
      D   subsequent encounter
      S   sequela

● **T61.0**   Ciguatera fish poisoning
    X● **T61.01**   Ciguatera fish poisoning, accidental (unintentional)
    X● **T61.02**   Ciguatera fish poisoning, intentional self-harm A, S 🐾
    X● **T61.03**   Ciguatera fish poisoning, assault
    X● **T61.04**   Ciguatera fish poisoning, undetermined

● **T61.1**   Scombroid fish poisoning
    Histamine-like syndrome
    X● **T61.11**   Scombroid fish poisoning, accidental (unintentional)
    X● **T61.12**   Scombroid fish poisoning, intentional self-harm A, S 🐾
    X● **T61.13**   Scombroid fish poisoning, assault
    X● **T61.14**   Scombroid fish poisoning, undetermined

● **T61.7**   Other fish and shellfish poisoning
    ● **T61.77**   Other fish poisoning
       ● **T61.771**   Other fish poisoning, accidental (unintentional)

● **T61.772**   Other fish poisoning, intentional self-harm A, S 🐾
● **T61.773**   Other fish poisoning, assault
● **T61.774**   Other fish poisoning, undetermined
    ● **T61.78**   Other shellfish poisoning
       ● **T61.781**   Other shellfish poisoning, accidental (unintentional)
       ● **T61.782**   Other shellfish poisoning, intentional self-harm A, S 🐾
       ● **T61.783**   Other shellfish poisoning, assault
       ● **T61.784**   Other shellfish poisoning, undetermined

● **T61.8**   Toxic effect of other seafood
    ● **T61.8X**   Toxic effect of other seafood
       ● **T61.8X1**   Toxic effect of other seafood, accidental (unintentional)
       ● **T61.8X2**   Toxic effect of other seafood, intentional self-harm A, S 🐾
       ● **T61.8X3**   Toxic effect of other seafood, assault
       ● **T61.8X4**   Toxic effect of other seafood, undetermined

● **T61.9**   Toxic effect of unspecified seafood
    X● **T61.91**   Toxic effect of unspecified seafood, accidental (unintentional)
    X● **T61.92**   Toxic effect of unspecified seafood, intentional self-harm A, S 🐾
    X● **T61.93**   Toxic effect of unspecified seafood, assault
    X● **T61.94**   Toxic effect of unspecified seafood, undetermined

● **T62**   Toxic effect of other noxious substances eaten as food
    Excludes1   allergic reaction to food, such as:
              anaphylactic shock (reaction) due to adverse food reaction (T78.0-)
              dermatitis (L23.6, L25.4, L27.2)
              food protein-induced enterocolitis syndrome (K52.21)
              food protein-induced enteropathy (K52.22)
              gastroenteritis (noninfective) (K52.29)
              bacterial food borne intoxications (A05.-)
         toxic effect of aflatoxin and other mycotoxins (T64)
         toxic effect of cyanides (T65.0-)
         toxic effect of hydrogen cyanide (T57.3-)
         toxic effect of mercury (T56.1-)
    The appropriate 7th character is to be added to each code from category T62

      A   initial encounter
      D   subsequent encounter
      S   sequela

● **T62.0**   Toxic effect of ingested mushrooms
    ● **T62.0X**   Toxic effect of ingested mushrooms
       ● **T62.0X1**   Toxic effect of ingested mushrooms, accidental (unintentional)
             Toxic effect of ingested mushrooms NOS
       ● **T62.0X2**   Toxic effect of ingested mushrooms, intentional self-harm A, S 🐾
       ● **T62.0X3**   Toxic effect of ingested mushrooms, assault
       ● **T62.0X4**   Toxic effect of ingested mushrooms, undetermined

● **T62.1**   Toxic effect of ingested berries
    ● **T62.1X**   Toxic effect of ingested berries
       ● **T62.1X1**   Toxic effect of ingested berries, accidental (unintentional)
             Toxic effect of ingested berries NOS
       ● **T62.1X2**   Toxic effect of ingested berries, intentional self-harm A, S 🐾

● **T62.1X3** Toxic effect of ingested berries, assault
● **T62.1X4** Toxic effect of ingested berries, undetermined
● **T62.2** Toxic effect of other ingested (parts of) plant(s)
   ● **T62.2X** Toxic effect of other ingested (parts of) plant(s)
      ● **T62.2X1** Toxic effect of other ingested (parts of) plant(s), accidental (unintentional)
         Toxic effect of other ingested (parts of) plant(s) NOS
      ● **T62.2X2** Toxic effect of other ingested (parts of) plant(s), intentional self-harm A, S 🐾
      ● **T62.2X3** Toxic effect of other ingested (parts of) plant(s), assault
      ● **T62.2X4** Toxic effect of other ingested (parts of) plant(s), undetermined
● **T62.8** Toxic effect of other specified noxious substances eaten as food
   ● **T62.8X** Toxic effect of other specified noxious substances eaten as food
      ● **T62.8X1** Toxic effect of other specified noxious substances eaten as food, accidental (unintentional)
         Toxic effect of other specified noxious substances eaten as food NOS
      ● **T62.8X2** Toxic effect of other specified noxious substances eaten as food, intentional self-harm A, S 🐾
      ● **T62.8X3** Toxic effect of other specified noxious substances eaten as food, assault
      ● **T62.8X4** Toxic effect of other specified noxious substances eaten as food, undetermined
● **T62.9** Toxic effect of unspecified noxious substance eaten as food
   X ● **T62.91** Toxic effect of unspecified noxious substance eaten as food, accidental (unintentional)
      Toxic effect of unspecified noxious substance eaten as food NOS
   X ● **T62.92** Toxic effect of unspecified noxious substance eaten as food, intentional self-harm A, S 🐾
   X ● **T62.93** Toxic effect of unspecified noxious substance eaten as food, assault
   X ● **T62.94** Toxic effect of unspecified noxious substance eaten as food, undetermined

● **T63** Toxic effect of contact with venomous animals and plants
   Includes   bite or touch of venomous animal
                  pricked or stuck by thorn or leaf
   Excludes2 ingestion of toxic animal or plant (T61.-, T62.-)

   The appropriate 7th character is to be added to each code from category T63

A	initial encounter
D	subsequent encounter
S	sequela

● **T63.0** Toxic effect of snake venom
   ● **T63.00** Toxic effect of unspecified snake venom
      ● **T63.001** Toxic effect of unspecified snake venom, accidental (unintentional)
         Toxic effect of unspecified snake venom NOS
      ● **T63.002** Toxic effect of unspecified snake venom, intentional self-harm A, S 🐾
      ● **T63.003** Toxic effect of unspecified snake venom, assault
      ● **T63.004** Toxic effect of unspecified snake venom, undetermined

● **T63.01** Toxic effect of rattlesnake venom
   ● **T63.011** Toxic effect of rattlesnake venom, accidental (unintentional)
      Toxic effect of rattlesnake venom NOS
   ● **T63.012** Toxic effect of rattlesnake venom, intentional self-harm A, S 🐾
   ● **T63.013** Toxic effect of rattlesnake venom, assault
   ● **T63.014** Toxic effect of rattlesnake venom, undetermined
● **T63.02** Toxic effect of coral snake venom
   ● **T63.021** Toxic effect of coral snake venom, accidental (unintentional)
      Toxic effect of coral snake venom NOS
   ● **T63.022** Toxic effect of coral snake venom, intentional self-harm A, S 🐾
   ● **T63.023** Toxic effect of coral snake venom, assault
   ● **T63.024** Toxic effect of coral snake venom, undetermined
● **T63.03** Toxic effect of taipan venom
   ● **T63.031** Toxic effect of taipan venom, accidental (unintentional)
      Toxic effect of taipan venom NOS
   ● **T63.032** Toxic effect of taipan venom, intentional self-harm A, S 🐾
   ● **T63.033** Toxic effect of taipan venom, assault
   ● **T63.034** Toxic effect of taipan venom, undetermined
● **T63.04** Toxic effect of cobra venom
   ● **T63.041** Toxic effect of cobra venom, accidental (unintentional)
      Toxic effect of cobra venom NOS
   ● **T63.042** Toxic effect of cobra venom, intentional self-harm A, S 🐾
   ● **T63.043** Toxic effect of cobra venom, assault
   ● **T63.044** Toxic effect of cobra venom, undetermined
● **T63.06** Toxic effect of venom of other North and South American snake
   ● **T63.061** Toxic effect of venom of other North and South American snake, accidental (unintentional)
      Toxic effect of venom of other North and South American snake NOS
   ● **T63.062** Toxic effect of venom of other North and South American snake, intentional self-harm A, S 🐾
   ● **T63.063** Toxic effect of venom of other North and South American snake, assault
   ● **T63.064** Toxic effect of venom of other North and South American snake, undetermined
● **T63.07** Toxic effect of venom of other Australian snake
   ● **T63.071** Toxic effect of venom of other Australian snake, accidental (unintentional)
      Toxic effect of venom of other Australian snake NOS
   ● **T63.072** Toxic effect of venom of other Australian snake, intentional self-harm A, S 🐾
   ● **T63.073** Toxic effect of venom of other Australian snake, assault
   ● **T63.074** Toxic effect of venom of other Australian snake, undetermined

CHAPTER 19 (S00-T88)

▶ New   ➡ Revised   ~~deleted~~ Deleted   Excludes 1   Excludes 2   Includes   Use additional   Code first   Code also   Key words
OGCR Official Guidelines   X Assign placeholder X   ● Use Additional Character(s)   ▶ Manifestation Code   🐾 Hierarchical Condition Category   Coding Clinic

- **T63.08**   Toxic effect of venom of other African and Asian snake
  - **T63.081**   Toxic effect of venom of other African and Asian snake, accidental (unintentional)
    Toxic effect of venom of other African and Asian snake NOS
  - **T63.082**   Toxic effect of venom of other African and Asian snake, intentional self-harm A, S 🜲
  - **T63.083**   Toxic effect of venom of other African and Asian snake, assault
  - **T63.084**   Toxic effect of venom of other African and Asian snake, undetermined
- **T63.09**   Toxic effect of venom of other snake
  - **T63.091**   Toxic effect of venom of other snake, accidental (unintentional)
    Toxic effect of venom of other snake NOS
  - **T63.092**   Toxic effect of venom of other snake, intentional self-harm A, S 🜲
  - **T63.093**   Toxic effect of venom of other snake, assault
  - **T63.094**   Toxic effect of venom of other snake, undetermined
- **T63.1**   Toxic effect of venom of other reptiles
  - **T63.11**   Toxic effect of venom of gila monster
    - **T63.111**   Toxic effect of venom of gila monster, accidental (unintentional)
      Toxic effect of venom of gila monster NOS
    - **T63.112**   Toxic effect of venom of gila monster, intentional self-harm A, S 🜲
    - **T63.113**   Toxic effect of venom of gila monster, assault
    - **T63.114**   Toxic effect of venom of gila monster, undetermined
  - **T63.12**   Toxic effect of venom of other venomous lizard
    - **T63.121**   Toxic effect of venom of other venomous lizard, accidental (unintentional)
      Toxic effect of venom of other venomous lizard NOS
    - **T63.122**   Toxic effect of venom of other venomous lizard, intentional self-harm A, S 🜲
    - **T63.123**   Toxic effect of venom of other venomous lizard, assault
    - **T63.124**   Toxic effect of venom of other venomous lizard, undetermined
  - **T63.19**   Toxic effect of venom of other reptiles
    - **T63.191**   Toxic effect of venom of other reptiles, accidental (unintentional)
      Toxic effect of venom of other reptiles NOS
    - **T63.192**   Toxic effect of venom of other reptiles, intentional self-harm A, S 🜲
    - **T63.193**   Toxic effect of venom of other reptiles, assault
    - **T63.194**   Toxic effect of venom of other reptiles, undetermined
- **T63.2**   Toxic effect of venom of scorpion
  - **T63.2X**   Toxic effect of venom of scorpion
    - **T63.2X1**   Toxic effect of venom of scorpion, accidental (unintentional)
      Toxic effect of venom of scorpion NOS
    - **T63.2X2**   Toxic effect of venom of scorpion, intentional self-harm A, S 🜲
    - **T63.2X3**   Toxic effect of venom of scorpion, assault
    - **T63.2X4**   Toxic effect of venom of scorpion, undetermined

- **T63.3**   Toxic effect of venom of spider
  - **T63.30**   Toxic effect of unspecified spider venom
    - **T63.301**   Toxic effect of unspecified spider venom, accidental (unintentional)
    - **T63.302**   Toxic effect of unspecified spider venom, intentional self-harm A, S 🜲
    - **T63.303**   Toxic effect of unspecified spider venom, assault
    - **T63.304**   Toxic effect of unspecified spider venom, undetermined
  - **T63.31**   Toxic effect of venom of black widow spider
    - **T63.311**   Toxic effect of venom of black widow spider, accidental (unintentional)
    - **T63.312**   Toxic effect of venom of black widow spider, intentional self-harm A, S 🜲
    - **T63.313**   Toxic effect of venom of black widow spider, assault
    - **T63.314**   Toxic effect of venom of black widow spider, undetermined
  - **T63.32**   Toxic effect of venom of tarantula
    - **T63.321**   Toxic effect of venom of tarantula, accidental (unintentional)
    - **T63.322**   Toxic effect of venom of tarantula, intentional self-harm A, S 🜲
    - **T63.323**   Toxic effect of venom of tarantula, assault
    - **T63.324**   Toxic effect of venom of tarantula, undetermined
  - **T63.33**   Toxic effect of venom of brown recluse spider
    - **T63.331**   Toxic effect of venom of brown recluse spider, accidental (unintentional)
    - **T63.332**   Toxic effect of venom of brown recluse spider, intentional self-harm A, S 🜲
    - **T63.333**   Toxic effect of venom of brown recluse spider, assault
    - **T63.334**   Toxic effect of venom of brown recluse spider, undetermined
  - **T63.39**   Toxic effect of venom of other spider
    - **T63.391**   Toxic effect of venom of other spider, accidental (unintentional)
    - **T63.392**   Toxic effect of venom of other spider, intentional self-harm A, S 🜲
    - **T63.393**   Toxic effect of venom of other spider, assault
    - **T63.394**   Toxic effect of venom of other spider, undetermined
- **T63.4**   Toxic effect of venom of other arthropods
  > Use additional code, if applicable, for anaphylactic shock (T78.2)
  - **T63.41**   Toxic effect of venom of centipedes and venomous millipedes
    - **T63.411**   Toxic effect of venom of centipedes and venomous millipedes, accidental (unintentional)
    - **T63.412**   Toxic effect of venom of centipedes and venomous millipedes, intentional self-harm A, S 🜲
    - **T63.413**   Toxic effect of venom of centipedes and venomous millipedes, assault
    - **T63.414**   Toxic effect of venom of centipedes and venomous millipedes, undetermined
  - **T63.42**   Toxic effect of venom of ants
    - **T63.421**   Toxic effect of venom of ants, accidental (unintentional)
    - **T63.422**   Toxic effect of venom of ants, intentional self-harm A, S 🜲

● T63.423 Toxic effect of venom of ants, assault
● T63.424 Toxic effect of venom of ants, undetermined
● T63.43 Toxic effect of venom of caterpillars
  ● T63.431 Toxic effect of venom of caterpillars, accidental (unintentional)
  ● T63.432 Toxic effect of venom of caterpillars, intentional self-harm A, S 🐾
  ● T63.433 Toxic effect of venom of caterpillars, assault
  ● T63.434 Toxic effect of venom of caterpillars, undetermined
● T63.44 Toxic effect of venom of bees
  ● T63.441 Toxic effect of venom of bees, accidental (unintentional)
  ● T63.442 Toxic effect of venom of bees, intentional self-harm A, S 🐾
  ● T63.443 Toxic effect of venom of bees, assault
  ● T63.444 Toxic effect of venom of bees, undetermined
● T63.45 Toxic effect of venom of hornets
  ● T63.451 Toxic effect of venom of hornets, accidental (unintentional)
  ● T63.452 Toxic effect of venom of hornets, intentional self-harm A, S 🐾
  ● T63.453 Toxic effect of venom of hornets, assault
  ● T63.454 Toxic effect of venom of hornets, undetermined
● T63.46 Toxic effect of venom of wasps
  Toxic effect of yellow jacket
  ● T63.461 Toxic effect of venom of wasps, accidental (unintentional)
  ● T63.462 Toxic effect of venom of wasps, intentional self-harm A, S 🐾
  ● T63.463 Toxic effect of venom of wasps, assault
  ● T63.464 Toxic effect of venom of wasps, undetermined
● T63.48 Toxic effect of venom of other arthropod
  ● T63.481 Toxic effect of venom of other arthropod, accidental (unintentional)
  ● T63.482 Toxic effect of venom of other arthropod, intentional self-harm A, S 🐾
  ● T63.483 Toxic effect of venom of other arthropod, assault
  ● T63.484 Toxic effect of venom of other arthropod, undetermined
● T63.5 Toxic effect of contact with venomous fish
  Excludes2 poisoning by ingestion of fish (T61.-)
● T63.51 Toxic effect of contact with stingray
  ● T63.511 Toxic effect of contact with stingray, accidental (unintentional)
  ● T63.512 Toxic effect of contact with stingray, intentional self-harm A, S 🐾
  ● T63.513 Toxic effect of contact with stingray, assault
  ● T63.514 Toxic effect of contact with stingray, undetermined
● T63.59 Toxic effect of contact with other venomous fish
  ● T63.591 Toxic effect of contact with other venomous fish, accidental (unintentional)
  ● T63.592 Toxic effect of contact with other venomous fish, intentional self-harm A, S 🐾
  ● T63.593 Toxic effect of contact with other venomous fish, assault
  ● T63.594 Toxic effect of contact with other venomous fish, undetermined

● T63.6 Toxic effect of contact with other venomous marine animals
  Excludes1 sea-snake venom (T63.09)
  Excludes2 poisoning by ingestion of shellfish (T61.78-)
● T63.61 Toxic effect of contact with Portuguese Man-o-war
  Toxic effect of contact with bluebottle
  ● T63.611 Toxic effect of contact with Portuguese Man-o-war, accidental (unintentional)
  ● T63.612 Toxic effect of contact with Portuguese Man-o-war, intentional self-harm A, S 🐾
  ● T63.613 Toxic effect of contact with Portuguese Man-o-war, assault
  ● T63.614 Toxic effect of contact with Portuguese Man-o-war, undetermined
● T63.62 Toxic effect of contact with other jellyfish
  ● T63.621 Toxic effect of contact with other jellyfish, accidental (unintentional)
  ● T63.622 Toxic effect of contact with other jellyfish, intentional self-harm A, S 🐾
  ● T63.623 Toxic effect of contact with other jellyfish, assault
  ● T63.624 Toxic effect of contact with other jellyfish, undetermined
● T63.63 Toxic effect of contact with sea anemone
  ● T63.631 Toxic effect of contact with sea anemone, accidental (unintentional)
  ● T63.632 Toxic effect of contact with sea anemone, intentional self-harm A, S 🐾
  ● T63.633 Toxic effect of contact with sea anemone, assault
  ● T63.634 Toxic effect of contact with sea anemone, undetermined
● T63.69 Toxic effect of contact with other venomous marine animals
  ● T63.691 Toxic effect of contact with other venomous marine animals, accidental (unintentional)
  ● T63.692 Toxic effect of contact with other venomous marine animals, intentional self-harm A, S 🐾
  ● T63.693 Toxic effect of contact with other venomous marine animals, assault
  ● T63.694 Toxic effect of contact with other venomous marine animals, undetermined
● T63.7 Toxic effect of contact with venomous plant
● T63.71 Toxic effect of contact with venomous marine plant
  ● T63.711 Toxic effect of contact with venomous marine plant, accidental (unintentional)
  ● T63.712 Toxic effect of contact with venomous marine plant, intentional self-harm A, S 🐾
  ● T63.713 Toxic effect of contact with venomous marine plant, assault
  ● T63.714 Toxic effect of contact with venomous marine plant, undetermined
● T63.79 Toxic effect of contact with other venomous plant
  ● T63.791 Toxic effect of contact with other venomous plant, accidental (unintentional)
  ● T63.792 Toxic effect of contact with other venomous plant, intentional self-harm A, S 🐾
  ● T63.793 Toxic effect of contact with other venomous plant, assault
  ● T63.794 Toxic effect of contact with other venomous plant, undetermined

▶ New   ➡ Revised   ~~deleted~~ Deleted   Excludes 1   Excludes 2   Includes   Use additional   Code first   Code also   Key words
OGCR Official Guidelines   X Assign placeholder X   ● Use Additional Character(s)   ▶ Manifestation Code   🐾 Hierarchical Condition Category   Coding Clinic

● **T63.8**   **Toxic effect of contact with other venomous animals**

  ● **T63.81**   Toxic effect of contact with venomous frog

     Excludes1   contact with nonvenomous frog (W62.0)

    ● **T63.811**   Toxic effect of contact with venomous frog, accidental (unintentional)

    ● **T63.812**   Toxic effect of contact with venomous frog, intentional self-harm A, S 🔖

    ● **T63.813**   Toxic effect of contact with venomous frog, assault

    ● **T63.814**   Toxic effect of contact with venomous frog, undetermined

  ● **T63.82**   Toxic effect of contact with venomous toad

     Excludes1   contact with nonvenomous toad (W62.1)

    ● **T63.821**   Toxic effect of contact with venomous toad, accidental (unintentional)

    ● **T63.822**   Toxic effect of contact with venomous toad, intentional self-harm A, S 🔖

    ● **T63.823**   Toxic effect of contact with venomous toad, assault

    ● **T63.824**   Toxic effect of contact with venomous toad, undetermined

  ● **T63.83**   Toxic effect of contact with other venomous amphibian

     Excludes1   contact with nonvenomous amphibian (W62.9)

    ● **T63.831**   Toxic effect of contact with other venomous amphibian, accidental (unintentional)

    ● **T63.832**   Toxic effect of contact with other venomous amphibian, intentional self-harm A, S 🔖

    ● **T63.833**   Toxic effect of contact with other venomous amphibian, assault

    ● **T63.834**   Toxic effect of contact with other venomous amphibian, undetermined

  ● **T63.89**   Toxic effect of contact with other venomous animals

    ● **T63.891**   Toxic effect of contact with other venomous animals, accidental (unintentional)

    ● **T63.892**   Toxic effect of contact with other venomous animals, intentional self-harm A, S 🔖

    ● **T63.893**   Toxic effect of contact with other venomous animals, assault

    ● **T63.894**   Toxic effect of contact with other venomous animals, undetermined

● **T63.9**   **Toxic effect of contact with unspecified venomous animal**

  X ● **T63.91**   Toxic effect of contact with unspecified venomous animal, accidental (unintentional)

  X ● **T63.92**   Toxic effect of contact with unspecified venomous animal, intentional self-harm A, S 🔖

  X ● **T63.93**   Toxic effect of contact with unspecified venomous animal, assault

  X ● **T63.94**   Toxic effect of contact with unspecified venomous animal, undetermined

● **T64**   **Toxic effect of aflatoxin and other mycotoxin food contaminants**

   The appropriate 7th character is to be added to each code from category T64

A	initial encounter
D	subsequent encounter
S	sequela

● **T64.0**   **Toxic effect of aflatoxin**

  X ● **T64.01**   Toxic effect of aflatoxin, accidental (unintentional)

  X ● **T64.02**   Toxic effect of aflatoxin, intentional self-harm A, S 🔖

  X ● **T64.03**   Toxic effect of aflatoxin, assault

  X ● **T64.04**   Toxic effect of aflatoxin, undetermined

● **T64.8**   **Toxic effect of other mycotoxin food contaminants**

  X ● **T64.81**   Toxic effect of other mycotoxin food contaminants, accidental (unintentional)

  X ● **T64.82**   Toxic effect of other mycotoxin food contaminants, intentional self-harm A, S 🔖

  X ● **T64.83**   Toxic effect of other mycotoxin food contaminants, assault

  X ● **T64.84**   Toxic effect of other mycotoxin food contaminants, undetermined

● **T65**   **Toxic effect of other and unspecified substances**

   The appropriate 7th character is to be added to each code from category T65

A	initial encounter
D	subsequent encounter
S	sequela

● **T65.0**   **Toxic effect of cyanides**

     Excludes1   hydrogen cyanide (T57.3-)

  ● **T65.0X**   Toxic effect of cyanides

    ● **T65.0X1**   Toxic effect of cyanides, accidental (unintentional)

       Toxic effect of cyanides NOS

    ● **T65.0X2**   Toxic effect of cyanides, intentional self-harm A, S 🔖

    ● **T65.0X3**   Toxic effect of cyanides, assault

    ● **T65.0X4**   Toxic effect of cyanides, undetermined

● **T65.1**   **Toxic effect of strychnine and its salts**

  ● **T65.1X**   Toxic effect of strychnine and its salts

    ● **T65.1X1**   Toxic effect of strychnine and its salts, accidental (unintentional)

       Toxic effect of strychnine and its salts NOS

    ● **T65.1X2**   Toxic effect of strychnine and its salts, intentional self-harm A, S 🔖

    ● **T65.1X3**   Toxic effect of strychnine and its salts, assault

    ● **T65.1X4**   Toxic effect of strychnine and its salts, undetermined

● **T65.2**   **Toxic effect of tobacco and nicotine**

     Excludes2   nicotine dependence (F17.-)

  ● **T65.21**   Toxic effect of chewing tobacco

    ● **T65.211**   Toxic effect of chewing tobacco, accidental (unintentional)

       Toxic effect of chewing tobacco NOS

    ● **T65.212**   Toxic effect of chewing tobacco, intentional self-harm A, S 🔖

    ● **T65.213**   Toxic effect of chewing tobacco, assault

    ● **T65.214**   Toxic effect of chewing tobacco, undetermined

  ● **T65.22**   Toxic effect of tobacco cigarettes

     Toxic effect of tobacco smoke

     Use additional code for exposure to second hand tobacco smoke (Z57.31, Z77.22)

    ● **T65.221**   Toxic effect of tobacco cigarettes, accidental (unintentional)

       Toxic effect of tobacco cigarettes NOS

    ● **T65.222**   Toxic effect of tobacco cigarettes, intentional self-harm A, S 🔖

    ● **T65.223**   Toxic effect of tobacco cigarettes, assault

    ● **T65.224**   Toxic effect of tobacco cigarettes, undetermined

CHAPTER 19 (S00-T88)

CHAPTER 19 (S00-T88)

- ● T65.29   Toxic effect of other tobacco and nicotine
  - ● T65.291   Toxic effect of other tobacco and nicotine, accidental (unintentional)
    Toxic effect of other tobacco and nicotine NOS
  - ● T65.292   Toxic effect of other tobacco and nicotine, intentional self-harm A, S 🦠
  - ● T65.293   Toxic effect of other tobacco and nicotine, assault
  - ● T65.294   Toxic effect of other tobacco and nicotine, undetermined
- ● T65.3   Toxic effect of nitroderivatives and aminoderivatives of benzene and its homologues
  - ⇛ Toxic effect of aniline [benzenamine]
    Toxic effect of nitrobenzene
    Toxic effect of trinitrotoluene
  - ● T65.3X   Toxic effect of nitroderivatives and aminoderivatives of benzene and its homologues
    - ● T65.3X1   Toxic effect of nitroderivatives and aminoderivatives of benzene and its homologues, accidental (unintentional)
      Toxic effect of nitroderivatives and aminoderivatives of benzene and its homologues NOS
    - ● T65.3X2   Toxic effect of nitroderivatives and aminoderivatives of benzene and its homologues, intentional self-harm A, S 🦠
    - ● T65.3X3   Toxic effect of nitroderivatives and aminoderivatives of benzene and its homologues, assault
    - ● T65.3X4   Toxic effect of nitroderivatives and aminoderivatives of benzene and its homologues, undetermined
- ● T65.4   Toxic effect of carbon disulfide
  - ● T65.4X   Toxic effect of carbon disulfide
    - ● T65.4X1   Toxic effect of carbon disulfide, accidental (unintentional)
      Toxic effect of carbon disulfide NOS
    - ● T65.4X2   Toxic effect of carbon disulfide, intentional self-harm A, S 🦠
    - ● T65.4X3   Toxic effect of carbon disulfide, assault
    - ● T65.4X4   Toxic effect of carbon disulfide, undetermined
- ● T65.5   Toxic effect of nitroglycerin and other nitric acids and esters
  Toxic effect of 1,2,3-Propanetriol trinitrate
  - ● T65.5X   Toxic effect of nitroglycerin and other nitric acids and esters
    - ● T65.5X1   Toxic effect of nitroglycerin and other nitric acids and esters, accidental (unintentional)
      Toxic effect of nitroglycerin and other nitric acids and esters NOS
    - ● T65.5X2   Toxic effect of nitroglycerin and other nitric acids and esters, intentional self-harm A, S 🦠
    - ● T65.5X3   Toxic effect of nitroglycerin and other nitric acids and esters, assault
    - ● T65.5X4   Toxic effect of nitroglycerin and other nitric acids and esters, undetermined
- ● T65.6   Toxic effect of paints and dyes, not elsewhere classified
  - ● T65.6X   Toxic effect of paints and dyes, not elsewhere classified
    - ● T65.6X1   Toxic effect of paints and dyes, not elsewhere classified, accidental (unintentional)
      Toxic effect of paints and dyes NOS

- ● T65.6X2   Toxic effect of paints and dyes, not elsewhere classified, intentional self-harm A, S 🦠
- ● T65.6X3   Toxic effect of paints and dyes, not elsewhere classified, assault
- ● T65.6X4   Toxic effect of paints and dyes, not elsewhere classified, undetermined
- ● T65.8   Toxic effect of other specified substances
  - ● T65.81   Toxic effect of latex
    - ● T65.811   Toxic effect of latex, accidental (unintentional)
      Toxic effect of latex NOS
    - ● T65.812   Toxic effect of latex, intentional self-harm A, S 🦠
    - ● T65.813   Toxic effect of latex, assault
    - ● T65.814   Toxic effect of latex, undetermined
  - ● T65.82   Toxic effect of harmful algae and algae toxins
    Toxic effect of (harmful) algae bloom NOS
    Toxic effect of blue-green algae bloom
    Toxic effect of brown tide
    Toxic effect of cyanobacteria bloom
    Toxic effect of Florida red tide
    Toxic effect of pfiesteria piscicida
    Toxic effect of red tide
    - ● T65.821   Toxic effect of harmful algae and algae toxins, accidental (unintentional)
      Toxic effect of harmful algae and algae toxins NOS
    - ● T65.822   Toxic effect of harmful algae and algae toxins, intentional self-harm A, S 🦠
    - ● T65.823   Toxic effect of harmful algae and algae toxins, assault
    - ● T65.824   Toxic effect of harmful algae and algae toxins, undetermined
  - ● T65.83   Toxic effect of fiberglass
    - ● T65.831   Toxic effect of fiberglass, accidental (unintentional)
      Toxic effect of fiberglass NOS
    - ● T65.832   Toxic effect of fiberglass, intentional self-harm A, S 🦠
    - ● T65.833   Toxic effect of fiberglass, assault
    - ● T65.834   Toxic effect of fiberglass, undetermined
  - ● T65.89   Toxic effect of other specified substances
    - ● T65.891   Toxic effect of other specified substances, accidental (unintentional)
      Toxic effect of other specified substances NOS
      Coding Clinic: 2018, Q1, P5
    - ● T65.892   Toxic effect of other specified substances, intentional self-harm A, S 🦠
    - ● T65.893   Toxic effect of other specified substances, assault
    - ● T65.894   Toxic effect of other specified substances, undetermined
- ● T65.9   Toxic effect of unspecified substance
  - X ● T65.91   Toxic effect of unspecified substance, accidental (unintentional)
    Poisoning NOS
  - X ● T65.92   Toxic effect of unspecified substance, intentional self-harm A, S 🦠
  - X ● T65.93   Toxic effect of unspecified substance, assault
  - X ● T65.94   Toxic effect of unspecified substance, undetermined

▶ New   ⇛ Revised   ~~deleted~~ Deleted   Excludes 1   Excludes 2   Includes   Use additional   Code first   Code also   Key words
OGCR Official Guidelines   X Assign placeholder X   ● Use Additional Character(s)   ▌ Manifestation Code   🦠 Hierarchical Condition Category   Coding Clinic

---

OTHER AND UNSPECIFIED EFFECTS OF EXTERNAL CAUSES (T66-T78)

● **T66**   **Radiation sickness, unspecified**
    Excludes1   specified adverse effects of radiation, such as:
              burns (T20-T31)
              leukemia (C91-C95)
              radiation gastroenteritis and colitis (K52.0)
              radiation pneumonitis (J70.0)
              radiation related disorders of the skin and
                 subcutaneous tissue (L55-L59)
              sunburn (L55.-)

    The appropriate 7th character is to be added to code T66

A	initial encounter
D	subsequent encounter
S	sequela

● **T67**   **Effects of heat and light**
    Excludes1   erythema [dermatitis] ab igne (L59.0)
              malignant hyperpyrexia due to anesthesia (T88.3)
              radiation-related disorders of the skin and
                 subcutaneous tissue (L55-L59)
    Excludes2   burns (T20-T31)
              sunburn (L55.-)
              sweat disorder due to heat (L74-L75)

    The appropriate 7th character is to be added to each code from
        category T67

A	initial encounter
D	subsequent encounter
S	sequela

X ● **T67.0**   **Heatstroke and sunstroke**
         Use additional code(s) to identify any associated
            complications of heatstroke, such as:
            coma and stupor (R40.-)
            rhabdomyolysis (M62.82)
            systemic inflammatory response syndrome (R65.1-)
         Coding Clinic: 2019, Q4, P18

   X ● **T67.01**   **Heatstroke and sunstroke**
              Heat apoplexy
              Heat pyrexia
              Siriasis
              Thermoplegia

   X ● **T67.02**   **Exertional heatstroke**
              Coding Clinic: 2019, Q4, P18

   X ● **T67.09**   **Other heatstroke and sunstroke**

X ● **T67.1**   **Heat syncope**
     Heat collapse

X ● **T67.2**   **Heat cramp**

X ● **T67.3**   **Heat exhaustion, anhydrotic**
     Heat prostration due to water depletion
     Excludes1   heat exhaustion due to salt depletion
                (T67.4)

X ● **T67.4**   **Heat exhaustion due to salt depletion**
     Heat prostration due to salt (and water) depletion

X ● **T67.5**   **Heat exhaustion, unspecified**
     Heat prostration NOS

X ● **T67.6**   **Heat fatigue, transient**

X ● **T67.7**   **Heat edema**

X ● **T67.8**   **Other effects of heat and light**

X ● **T67.9**   **Effect of heat and light, unspecified**

X ● **T68**   **Hypothermia**
     Accidental hypothermia
     Hypothermia NOS
     Use additional code to identify source of exposure:
         Exposure to excessive cold of man-made origin (W93)
         Exposure to excessive cold of natural origin (X31)
    Excludes1   hypothermia following anesthesia (T88.51)
              hypothermia not associated with low
                 environmental temperature (R68.0)
              hypothermia of newborn (P80.-)
    Excludes2   frostbite (T33-T34)

    The appropriate 7th character is to be added to code T68

A	initial encounter
D	subsequent encounter
S	sequela

● **T69**   **Other effects of reduced temperature**
    Use additional code to identify source of exposure:
         Exposure to excessive cold of man-made origin (W93)
         Exposure to excessive cold of natural origin (X31)
    Excludes2   frostbite (T33-T34)

    The appropriate 7th character is to be added to each code from
        category T69

A	initial encounter
D	subsequent encounter
S	sequela

   ● **T69.0**   **Immersion hand and foot**
     ● **T69.01**   **Immersion hand**
       ● **T69.011**   **Immersion hand, right hand**
       ● **T69.012**   **Immersion hand, left hand**
       ● **T69.019**   **Immersion hand, unspecified hand**
     ● **T69.02**   **Immersion foot**
         Trench foot
       ● **T69.021**   **Immersion foot, right foot**
       ● **T69.022**   **Immersion foot, left foot**
       ● **T69.029**   **Immersion foot, unspecified foot**

X ● **T69.1**   **Chilblains**

X ● **T69.8**   **Other specified effects of reduced temperature**

X ● **T69.9**   **Effect of reduced temperature, unspecified**

● **T70**   **Effects of air pressure and water pressure**
    The appropriate 7th character is to be added to each code from
        category T70

A	initial encounter
D	subsequent encounter
S	sequela

X ● **T70.0**   **Otitic barotrauma**
     Aero-otitis media
     Effects of change in ambient atmospheric pressure or
        water pressure on ears

X ● **T70.1**   **Sinus barotrauma**
     Aerosinusitis
     Effects of change in ambient atmospheric pressure on
        sinuses

   ● **T70.2**   **Other and unspecified effects of high altitude**
     Excludes2   polycythemia due to high altitude (D75.1)
     X ● **T70.20**   **Unspecified effects of high altitude**
     X ● **T70.29**   **Other effects of high altitude**
         Alpine sickness
         Anoxia due to high altitude
         Barotrauma NOS
         Hypobaropathy
         Mountain sickness

CHAPTER 19 (S00-T88)

CHAPTER 19 (S00-T88)

X● **T70.3**   **Caisson disease [decompression sickness]**
     Compressed-air disease
     Diver's palsy or paralysis

X● **T70.4**   **Effects of high-pressure fluids**
     Hydraulic jet injection (industrial)
     Pneumatic jet injection (industrial)
     Traumatic jet injection (industrial)

X● **T70.8**   **Other effects of air pressure and water pressure**

X● **T70.9**   **Effect of air pressure and water pressure, unspecified**

● **T71**   **Asphyxiation**
     Mechanical suffocation
     Traumatic suffocation

     Excludes1   acute respiratory distress (syndrome) (J80)
                 anoxia due to high altitude (T70.2)
                 asphyxia NOS (R09.01)
                 asphyxia from carbon monoxide (T58.-)
                 asphyxia from inhalation of food or foreign body
                     (T17.-)
                 asphyxia from other gases, fumes and vapors
                     (T59.-)
                 respiratory distress (syndrome) in newborn
                     (P22.-)

     The appropriate 7th character is to be added to each code from
     category T71

        A   initial encounter
        D   subsequent encounter
        S   sequela

● **T71.1**   **Asphyxiation due to mechanical threat to breathing**
     Suffocation due to mechanical threat to breathing

     ● **T71.11**   **Asphyxiation due to smothering under pillow**

         ● **T71.111**   **Asphyxiation due to smothering
                  under pillow, accidental**
                     Asphyxiation due to smothering
                       under pillow NOS

         ● **T71.112**   **Asphyxiation due to smothering
                  under pillow, intentional self-harm**
                  A, S ⬧

         ● **T71.113**   **Asphyxiation due to smothering
                  under pillow, assault**

         ● **T71.114**   **Asphyxiation due to smothering
                  under pillow, undetermined**

     ● **T71.12**   **Asphyxiation due to plastic bag**

         ● **T71.121**   **Asphyxiation due to plastic bag,
                  accidental**
                     Asphyxiation due to plastic bag
                       NOS

         ● **T71.122**   **Asphyxiation due to plastic bag,
                  intentional self-harm** A, S ⬧

         ● **T71.123**   **Asphyxiation due to plastic bag,
                  assault**

         ● **T71.124**   **Asphyxiation due to plastic bag,
                  undetermined**

     ● **T71.13**   **Asphyxiation due to being trapped in bed
              linens**

         ● **T71.131**   **Asphyxiation due to being trapped in
                  bed linens, accidental**
                     Asphyxiation due to being trapped
                       in bed linens NOS

         ● **T71.132**   **Asphyxiation due to being trapped in
                  bed linens, intentional self-harm**
                  A, S ⬧

         ● **T71.133**   **Asphyxiation due to being trapped in
                  bed linens, assault**

         ● **T71.134**   **Asphyxiation due to being trapped in
                  bed linens, undetermined**

● **T71.14**   **Asphyxiation due to smothering under another
         person's body (in bed)**

     ● **T71.141**   **Asphyxiation due to smothering
               under another person's body (in bed),
               accidental**
                 Asphyxiation due to smothering
                   under another person's body
                   (in bed) NOS

     ● **T71.143**   **Asphyxiation due to smothering
               under another person's body (in bed),
               assault**

     ● **T71.144**   **Asphyxiation due to smothering
               under another person's body (in bed),
               undetermined**

● **T71.15**   **Asphyxiation due to smothering in furniture**

     ● **T71.151**   **Asphyxiation due to smothering in
               furniture, accidental**
                 Asphyxiation due to smothering in
                   furniture NOS

     ● **T71.152**   **Asphyxiation due to smothering in
               furniture, intentional self-harm
               A, S** ⬧

     ● **T71.153**   **Asphyxiation due to smothering in
               furniture, assault**

     ● **T71.154**   **Asphyxiation due to smothering in
               furniture, undetermined**

● **T71.16**   **Asphyxiation due to hanging**
     Hanging by window shade cord
     Use additional code for any associated injuries,
        such as:
     crushing injury of neck (S17.-)
     fracture of cervical vertebrae (S12.0-S12.2-)
     open wound of neck (S11.-)

     ● **T71.161**   **Asphyxiation due to hanging,
               accidental**
                 Asphyxiation due to hanging NOS
                 Hanging NOS

     ● **T71.162**   **Asphyxiation due to hanging,
               intentional self-harm A, S** ⬧

     ● **T71.163**   **Asphyxiation due to hanging, assault**

     ● **T71.164**   **Asphyxiation due to hanging,
               undetermined**

● **T71.19**   **Asphyxiation due to mechanical**
     Threat to breathing due to other causes

     ● **T71.191**   **Asphyxiation due to mechanical
               threat to breathing due to other
               causes, accidental**
                 Asphyxiation due to other causes
                 NOS
                 Coding Clinic: 2016, Q4, P76

     ● **T71.192**   **Asphyxiation due to mechanical
               threat to breathing due to other
               causes, intentional self-harm A, S** ⬧

     ● **T71.193**   **Asphyxiation due to mechanical
               threat to breathing due to other
               causes, assault**

     ● **T71.194**   **Asphyxiation due to mechanical
               threat to breathing due to other
               causes, undetermined**

● **T71.2**   **Asphyxiation due to systemic oxygen deficiency due to
         low oxygen content in ambient air**
     Suffocation due to systemic oxygen deficiency due to
        low oxygen content in ambient air

X● **T71.20**   **Asphyxiation due to systemic oxygen deficiency
              due to low oxygen content in ambient air due to
              unspecified cause**

X● **T71.21**   **Asphyxiation due to cave-in or falling earth**
              Use additional code for any associated
                 cataclysm (X34-X38)

▶ New   ⟹ Revised   ~~deleted~~ Deleted   Excludes 1   Excludes 2   Includes   Use additional   Code first   Code also   Key words

OGCR Official Guidelines   X Assign placeholder X   ● Use Additional Character(s)   ▶ Manifestation Code   ⬧ Hierarchical Condition Category   Coding Clinic

● T71.22 Asphyxiation due to being trapped in a car trunk
    ● T71.221 Asphyxiation due to being trapped in a car trunk, accidental
    ● T71.222 Asphyxiation due to being trapped in a car trunk, intentional self-harm A, S 🚳
    ● T71.223 Asphyxiation due to being trapped in a car trunk, assault
    ● T71.224 Asphyxiation due to being trapped in a car trunk, undetermined

● T71.23 Asphyxiation due to being trapped in a (discarded) refrigerator
    ● T71.231 Asphyxiation due to being trapped in a (discarded) refrigerator, accidental
    ● T71.232 Asphyxiation due to being trapped in a (discarded) refrigerator, intentional self-harm A, S 🚳
    ● T71.233 Asphyxiation due to being trapped in a (discarded) refrigerator, assault
    ● T71.234 Asphyxiation due to being trapped in a (discarded) refrigerator, undetermined

X ● T71.29 Asphyxiation due to being trapped in other low oxygen environment

X ● T71.9 Asphyxiation due to unspecified cause
Suffocation (by strangulation) due to unspecified cause
Suffocation NOS
Systemic oxygen deficiency due to low oxygen content in ambient air due to unspecified cause
Systemic oxygen deficiency due to mechanical threat to breathing due to unspecified cause
Traumatic asphyxia NOS

● T73 Effects of other deprivation
The appropriate 7th character is to be added to each code from category T73

A	initial encounter
D	subsequent encounter
S	sequela

X ● T73.0 Starvation
Deprivation of food
X ● T73.1 Deprivation of water
X ● T73.2 Exhaustion due to exposure
X ● T73.3 Exhaustion due to excessive exertion
Exhaustion due to overexertion
X ● T73.8 Other effects of deprivation
X ● T73.9 Effect of deprivation, unspecified

● T74 Adult and child abuse, neglect and other maltreatment, confirmed
Use additional code, if applicable, to identify any associated current injury
Use additional external cause code to identify perpetrator, if known (Y07.-)
Excludes1 abuse and maltreatment in pregnancy (O9A.3-, O9A.4-, O9A.5-)
adult and child maltreatment, suspected (T76.-)
The appropriate 7th character is to be added to each code from category T74

A	initial encounter
D	subsequent encounter
S	sequela

● T74.0 Neglect or abandonment, confirmed
  X ● T74.01 Adult neglect or abandonment, confirmed A
  X ● T74.02 Child neglect or abandonment, confirmed P

● T74.1 Physical abuse, confirmed
Excludes2 sexual abuse (T74.2-)
  X ● T74.11 Adult physical abuse, confirmed A
  X ● T74.12 Child physical abuse, confirmed P
    Excludes2 shaken infant syndrome (T74.4)

● T74.2 Sexual abuse, confirmed
Rape, confirmed
Sexual assault, confirmed
  X ● T74.21 Adult sexual abuse, confirmed A
  X ● T74.22 Child sexual abuse, confirmed P

● T74.3 Psychological abuse, confirmed
Bullying and intimidation, confirmed
Intimidation through social media, confirmed
Target of threatened harm, confirmed
Target of threatened physical violence, confirmed
Target of threatened sexual abuse, confirmed
  X ● T74.31 Adult psychological abuse, confirmed A
  X ● T74.32 Child psychological abuse, confirmed P

X ● T74.4 Shaken infant syndrome P

● T74.5 Forced sexual exploitation, confirmed
  X ● T74.51 Adult forced sexual exploitation, confirmed P
  X ● T74.52 Child sexual exploitation, confirmed P

● T74.6 Forced labor exploitation, confirmed
  X ● T74.61 Adult forced labor exploitation, confirmed P
  X ● T74.62 Child forced labor exploitation, confirmed P

● T74.9 Unspecified maltreatment, confirmed
  X ● T74.91 Unspecified adult maltreatment, confirmed A
  X ● T74.92 Unspecified child maltreatment, confirmed P

● T74.A Financial abuse, confirmed
  T74.A1 Adult financial abuse, confirmed
  T74.A2 Child financial abuse, confirmed

● T75 Other and unspecified effects of other external causes
Excludes1 adverse effects NEC (T78.-)
Excludes2 burns (electric) (T20-T31)
The appropriate 7th character is to be added to each code from category T75

A	initial encounter
D	subsequent encounter
S	sequela

● T75.0 Effects of lightning
Struck by lightning
  X ● T75.00 Unspecified effects of lightning
Struck by lightning NOS
  X ● T75.01 Shock due to being struck by lightning
  X ● T75.09 Other effects of lightning
Use additional code for other effects of lightning

X ● T75.1 Unspecified effects of drowning and nonfatal submersion
Immersion
  Excludes1 specified effects of drowning code to effects
  Coding Clinic: 2023, Q1, P26

● T75.2 Effects of vibration
  X ● T75.20 Unspecified effects of vibration
  X ● T75.21 Pneumatic hammer syndrome
  X ● T75.22 Traumatic vasospastic syndrome
  X ● T75.23 Vertigo from infrasound
    Excludes1 vertigo NOS (R42)
  X ● T75.29 Other effects of vibration

X● **T75.3** **Motion sickness**
    Airsickness   Travel sickness
    Seasickness
    Use additional external cause code to identify vehicle or type of motion (Y92.81-)

X● **T75.4** **Electrocution**
    Shock from electric current
    Shock from electroshock gun (taser)

● **T75.8** **Other specified effects of external causes**

    X● **T75.81** **Effects of abnormal gravitation [G] forces**

    X● **T75.82** **Effects of weightlessness**

    X● **T75.89** **Other specified effects of external causes**

● **T76** **Adult and child abuse, neglect and other maltreatment, suspected**
    Use additional code, if applicable, to identify any associated current injury

    Excludes1   adult and child maltreatment, confirmed (T74.-)
        suspected abuse and maltreatment in pregnancy (O9A.3-, O9A.4-, O9A.5-)
        suspected adult physical abuse, ruled out (Z04.71)
        suspected adult sexual abuse, ruled out (Z04.41)
        suspected child physical abuse, ruled out (Z04.72)
        suspected child sexual abuse, ruled out (Z04.42)

    The appropriate 7th character is to be added to each code from category T76

> A   initial encounter
> D   subsequent encounter
> S   sequela

    Coding Clinic: 2016, Q4, P129

● **T76.0** **Neglect or abandonment, suspected**

    X● **T76.01** **Adult** neglect or abandonment, suspected   A

    X● **T76.02** **Child** neglect or abandonment, suspected   P

● **T76.1** **Physical abuse, suspected**

    X● **T76.11** **Adult** physical abuse, suspected   A

    X● **T76.12** **Child** physical abuse, suspected   P
        Coding Clinic: 2019, Q2, P12

● **T76.2** **Sexual abuse, suspected**
    Rape, suspected

    Excludes1   alleged abuse, ruled out (Z04.7)

    X● **T76.21** **Adult** sexual abuse, suspected   A

    X● **T76.22** **Child** sexual abuse, suspected   P

● **T76.3** **Psychological abuse, suspected**
    Bullying and intimidation, suspected
    Intimidation through social media, suspected
    Target of threatened harm, suspected
    Target of threatened physical violence, suspected
    Target of threatened sexual abuse, suspected

    X● **T76.31** **Adult** psychological abuse, suspected   A

    X● **T76.32** **Child** psychological abuse, suspected   P

● **T76.5** **Forced sexual exploitation, suspected**

    X● **T76.51** **Adult forced sexual exploitation, suspected**   P

    X● **T76.52** **Child sexual exploitation, suspected**   P

● **T76.6** **Forced labor exploitation, suspected**

    X● **T76.61** **Adult forced labor exploitation, suspected**   P

    X● **T76.62** **Child forced labor exploitation, suspected**   P

● **T76.9** **Unspecified maltreatment, suspected**

    X● **T76.91** Unspecified **adult** maltreatment, suspected   A

    X● **T76.92** Unspecified **child** maltreatment, suspected   P

● **T76.A** **Financial abuse, suspected**

    X● **T76.A1** **Adult financial abuse, suspected**

    X● **T76.A2** **Child financial abuse, suspected**

● **T78** **Adverse effects, not elsewhere classified**

    Excludes2   complications of surgical and medical care NEC (T80-T88)

    The appropriate 7th character is to be added to each code from category T78

> A   initial encounter
> D   subsequent encounter
> S   sequela

● **T78.0** **Anaphylactic reaction due to food**
    Anaphylactic reaction due to adverse food reaction
    Anaphylactic shock or reaction due to nonpoisonous foods
    Anaphylactoid reaction due to food

    X● **T78.00** **Anaphylactic reaction due to unspecified food**

    X● **T78.01** **Anaphylactic reaction due to peanuts**

    X● **T78.02** **Anaphylactic reaction due to shellfish (crustaceans)**

    X● **T78.03** **Anaphylactic reaction due to other fish**

    X● **T78.04** **Anaphylactic reaction due to fruits and vegetables**

    X● **T78.05** **Anaphylactic reaction due to tree nuts and seeds**

        Excludes2   anaphylactic reaction due to peanuts (T78.01)

    X● **T78.06** **Anaphylactic reaction due to food additives**

    X● **T78.07** **Anaphylactic reaction due to milk and dairy products**

    X● **T78.08** **Anaphylactic reaction due to eggs**

    X● **T78.09** **Anaphylactic reaction due to other food products**

X● **T78.1** **Other adverse food reactions, not elsewhere classified**
    Use additional code to identify the type of reaction, if applicable

    Excludes1   anaphylactic reaction or shock due to adverse food reaction (T78.0-)
        anaphylactic reaction due to food (T78.0-)
        bacterial food borne intoxications (A05.-)

    Excludes2   allergic and dietetic gastroenteritis and colitis (K52.29)
        allergic rhinitis due to food (J30.5)
        dermatitis due to food in contact with skin (L23.6, L24.6, L25.4)
        dermatitis due to ingested food (L27.2)
        food protein-induced enterocolitis syndrome (K52.21)
        food protein-induced enteropathy (K52.22)

X● **T78.2** **Anaphylactic shock, unspecified**
    Occurs when allergic response triggers large quantities of histamines, prostaglandins, leukotrienes resulting in systemic vasodilation
    Allergic shock
    Anaphylactic reaction
    Anaphylaxis

    Excludes1   anaphylactic reaction or shock due to adverse effect of correct medicinal substance properly administered (T88.6)
        anaphylactic reaction or shock due to adverse food reaction (T78.0-)
        anaphylactic reaction or shock due to serum (T80.5-)

X● **T78.3** **Angioneurotic edema**
    Allergic angioedema
    Giant urticaria
    Vascular disorder resulting from abnormalities of autonomic nervous system fibers supplying blood vessels
    Quincke's edema

    Excludes1   serum urticaria (T80.6-)
        urticaria (L50.-)

▶ New   ⇒ Revised   ~~deleted~~ Deleted   Excludes 1   Excludes 2   Includes   Use additional   Code first   Code also   Key words

OGCR Official Guidelines   X Assign placeholder X   ● Use Additional Character(s)   ▶ Manifestation Code   🔾 Hierarchical Condition Category   **Coding Clinic**

● **T78.4**   **Other and unspecified allergy**

     Excludes1   specified types of allergic reaction
                   such as:
                   allergic diarrhea (K52.29)
                   allergic gastroenteritis and colitis
                      (K52.29)
                   dermatitis (L23-L25, L27.-)
                   food protein-induced enterocolitis
                      syndrome (K52.21)
                   food protein-induced enteropathy
                      (K52.22)
                   hay fever (J30.1)

   X● **T78.40**   **Allergy, unspecified**
               Allergic reaction NOS
               Hypersensitivity NOS

   X● **T78.41**   **Arthus phenomenon**
               Arthus reaction

   X● **T78.49**   **Other allergy**
               Coding Clinic: 2021, Q1, P42

X● **T78.8**   **Other adverse effects, not elsewhere classified**

CERTAIN EARLY COMPLICATIONS OF TRAUMA (T79)

● **T79**   **Certain early complications of trauma, not elsewhere classified**

     Excludes2   acute respiratory distress syndrome (J80)
                   complications occurring during or following
                      medical procedures (T80-T88)
                   complications of surgical and medical care NEC
                      (T80-T88)
                   newborn respiratory distress syndrome (P22.0)

     The appropriate 7th character is to be added to each code from
     category T79

     | | |
     A   initial encounter
     D   subsequent encounter
     S   sequela

X● **T79.0**   **Air embolism (traumatic) A**

     Excludes1   air embolism complicating abortion
                   or ectopic or molar pregnancy
                      (O00-O07, O08.2)
                   air embolism complicating pregnancy,
                      childbirth and the puerperium (O88.0)
                   air embolism following infusion,
                      transfusion, and therapeutic injection
                      (T80.0)
                   air embolism following procedure NEC
                      (T81.7-)
                   Coding Clinic: 2024, Q2, P16

X● **T79.1**   **Fat embolism (traumatic) A**

     Excludes1   fat embolism complicating:
                   abortion or ectopic or molar pregnancy
                      (O00-O07, O08.2)
                   pregnancy, childbirth and the
                      puerperium (O88.8)

X● **T79.2**   **Traumatic secondary and recurrent hemorrhage and seroma A**

X● **T79.4**   **Traumatic shock A**
      Shock (immediate) (delayed) following injury

     Excludes1   anaphylactic shock due to adverse food
                      reaction (T78.0-)
                   anaphylactic shock due to correct
                      medicinal substance properly
                      administered (T88.6)
                   anaphylactic shock due to serum (T80.5-)
                   anaphylactic shock NOS (T78.2)
                   electric shock (T75.4)
                   nontraumatic shock NEC (R57.-)
                   obstetric shock (O75.1)
                   postprocedural shock (T81.1-)
                   septic shock (R65.21)
                   shock complicating abortion or ectopic or
                      molar pregnancy (O00-O07, O08.3)
                   shock due to anesthesia (T88.2)
                   shock due to lightning (T75.01)
                   shock NOS (R57.9)

X● **T79.5**   **Traumatic anuria A**
      Crush syndrome
      Renal failure following crushing

X● **T79.6**   **Traumatic ischemia of muscle A**
      Traumatic rhabdomyolysis
      Volkmann's ischemic contracture

     Excludes2   anterior tibial syndrome (M76.8)
                   compartment syndrome (traumatic)
                      (T79.A-)
                   nontraumatic ischemia of muscle (M62.2-)

X● **T79.7**   **Traumatic subcutaneous emphysema A**

     Excludes2   emphysema NOS (J43)
                   emphysema (subcutaneous) resulting
                      from a procedure (T81.82)

X● **T79.8**   **Other early complications of trauma A**
      Coding Clinic: 2024, Q2, P16

X● **T79.9**   **Unspecified early complication of trauma A**

● **T79.A**   **Traumatic compartment syndrome**

     Excludes1   fibromyalgia (M79.7)
                   nontraumatic compartment syndrome
                      (M79.A-)

     Excludes2   traumatic ischemic infarction of muscle
                      (T79.6)

   X● **T79.A0**   **Compartment syndrome, unspecified**
               Compartment syndrome NOS

   ● **T79.A1**   **Traumatic compartment syndrome of upper extremity**
               Traumatic compartment syndrome of shoulder,
                   arm, forearm, wrist, hand, and fingers

     ● **T79.A11**   **Traumatic compartment syndrome of right upper extremity A**

     ● **T79.A12**   **Traumatic compartment syndrome of left upper extremity A**

     ● **T79.A19**   **Traumatic compartment syndrome of unspecified upper extremity A**

   ● **T79.A2**   **Traumatic compartment syndrome of lower extremity**
               Traumatic compartment syndrome of hip,
                   buttock, thigh, leg, foot, and toes

     ● **T79.A21**   **Traumatic compartment syndrome of right lower extremity A**

     ● **T79.A22**   **Traumatic compartment syndrome of left lower extremity A**

     ● **T79.A29**   **Traumatic compartment syndrome of unspecified lower extremity**

   X● **T79.A3**   **Traumatic compartment syndrome of abdomen A**

   X● **T79.A9**   **Traumatic compartment syndrome of other sites A**

CHAPTER 19 (S00-T88)

COMPLICATIONS OF SURGICAL AND MEDICAL CARE NOT ELSEWHERE CLASSIFIED (T80-T88)

Use additional code for adverse effect, if applicable, to identify drug (T36-T50 with fifth or sixth character 5)

Use additional code(s) to identify the specified condition resulting from the complication.

Use additional code to identify devices involved and details of circumstances (Y62-Y82)

Excludes2   any encounters with medical care for postprocedural conditions in which no complications are present, such as:
artificial opening status (Z93.-)
closure of external stoma (Z43.-)
fitting and adjustment of external prosthetic device (Z44.-)
burns and corrosions from local applications and irradiation (T20-T32)
complications of surgical procedures during pregnancy, childbirth and the puerperium (O00-O9A)
mechanical complication of respirator [ventilator] (J95.850)
poisoning and toxic effects of drugs and chemicals (T36-T65 with fifth or sixth character 1-4 or 6)
postprocedural fever (R50.82)
specified complications classified elsewhere, such as:
cerebrospinal fluid leak from spinal puncture (G97.0)
colostomy malfunction (K94.0-)
disorders of fluid and electrolyte imbalance (E86-E87)
functional disturbances following cardiac surgery (I97.0-I97.1)
intraoperative and postprocedural complications of specified body systems (D78.-, E36.-, E89.-, G97.3-, G97.4, H59.3-, H59.-, H95.2-, H95.3, I97.4-, I97.5, J95.6-, J95.7, K91.6-, L76.-, M96.-, N99.-)
ostomy complications (J95.0-, K94.-, N99.5-)
postgastric surgery syndromes (K91.1)
postlaminectomy syndrome NEC (M96.1)
postmastectomy lymphedema syndrome (I97.2)
postsurgical blind-loop syndrome (K91.2)
ventilator associated pneumonia (J95.851)

● **T80**   **Complications following infusion, transfusion and therapeutic injection**

Includes   complications following perfusion

Excludes2   bone marrow transplant rejection (T86.01)
febrile nonhemolytic transfusion reaction (R50.84)
fluid overload due to transfusion (E87.71)
posttransfusion purpura (D69.51)
transfusion associated circulatory overload (TACO) (E87.71)
transfusion (red blood cell) associated hemochromatosis (E83.111)
transfusion related acute lung injury (TRALI) (J95.84)

The appropriate 7th character is to be added to each code from category T80

> A   initial encounter
> D   subsequent encounter
> S   sequela

X ● **T80.0**   **Air embolism** following infusion, transfusion and therapeutic injection

X ● **T80.1**   **Vascular complications following infusion, transfusion and therapeutic injection**

Use additional code to identify the vascular complication

Excludes2   extravasation of vesicant agent (T80.81-)
infiltration of vesicant agent (T80.81-)
vascular complications specified as due to prosthetic devices, implants and grafts (T82.8- T83.8-, T84.8-, T85.8-)
postprocedural vascular complications (T81.7-)

● **T80.2**   **Infections following infusion, transfusion and therapeutic injection**

Use additional code to identify the specific infection, such as:
sepsis (A41.9)

Use additional code (R65.2-) to identify severe sepsis, if applicable

Excludes2   infections specified as due to prosthetic devices, implants and grafts (T82.6-T82.7, T83.5-T83.6, T84.5-T84.7, T85.7)
postprocedural infections (T81.44)

Coding Clinic: 2018, Q4, P89

● **T80.21**   **Infection due to central venous catheter**

Infection due to pulmonary artery catheter (Swan-Ganz catheter)

Coding Clinic: 2019, Q1, P13-14; 2018, Q4, P89

● **T80.211**   **Bloodstream infection due to central venous catheter**

Catheter-related bloodstream infection (CRBSI) NOS
Central line-associated bloodstream infection (CLABSI)
Bloodstream infection due to Hickman catheter
Bloodstream infection due to peripherally inserted central catheter (PICC)
Bloodstream infection due to portacath (port-a-cath)
Bloodstream infection due to pulmonary artery catheter
Bloodstream infection due to triple lumen catheter
Bloodstream infection due to umbilical venous catheter

Coding Clinic: 2018, Q4, P89

● **T80.212**   **Local infection due to central venous catheter**

Exit or insertion site infection
Local infection due to Hickman catheter
Local infection due to peripherally inserted central catheter (PICC)
Local infection due to portacath (port-a-cath)
Local infection due to pulmonary artery catheter
Local infection due to triple lumen catheter
Local infection due to umbilical venous catheter
Port or reservoir infection
Tunnel infection

● **T80.218**   **Other infection due to central venous catheter**
     Other central line-associated infection
     Other infection due to Hickman catheter
     Other infection due to peripherally inserted central catheter (PICC)
     Other infection due to portacath (port-a-cath)
     Other infection due to pulmonary artery catheter
     Other infection due to triple lumen catheter
     Other infection due to umbilical venous catheter

● **T80.219**   **Unspecified infection due to central venous catheter**
     Central line-associated infection NOS
     Unspecified infection due to Hickman catheter
     Unspecified infection due to peripherally inserted central catheter (PICC)
     Unspecified infection due to portacath (port-a-cath)
     Unspecified infection due to pulmonary artery catheter
     Unspecified infection due to triple lumen catheter
     Unspecified infection due to umbilical venous catheter

X ● **T80.22**   **Acute infection following transfusion, infusion, or injection of blood and blood products**

X ● **T80.29**   **Infection following other infusion, transfusion and therapeutic injection**

● **T80.3**   **ABO incompatibility reaction due to transfusion of blood or blood products**
     Excludes1   minor blood group antigens reactions (Duffy) (E) (K) (Kell) (Kidd) (Lewis) (M) (N) (P) (S) (T80.A-)

X ● **T80.30**   **ABO incompatibility reaction due to transfusion of blood or blood products, unspecified**
     ABO incompatibility blood transfusion NOS
     Reaction to ABO incompatibility from transfusion NOS

● **T80.31**   **ABO incompatibility with hemolytic transfusion reaction**

   ● **T80.310**   **ABO incompatibility with acute hemolytic transfusion reaction**
     ABO incompatibility with hemolytic transfusion reaction less than 24 hours after transfusion
     Acute hemolytic transfusion reaction (AHTR) due to ABO incompatibility

   ● **T80.311**   **ABO incompatibility with delayed hemolytic transfusion reaction**
     ABO incompatibility with hemolytic transfusion reaction 24 hours or more after transfusion
     Delayed hemolytic transfusion reaction (DHTR) due to ABO incompatibility

   ● **T80.319**   **ABO incompatibility with hemolytic transfusion reaction, unspecified**
     ABO incompatibility with hemolytic transfusion reaction at unspecified time after transfusion
     Hemolytic transfusion reaction (HTR) due to ABO incompatibility NOS

X ● **T80.39**   **Other ABO incompatibility reaction due to transfusion of blood or blood products**
     Delayed serologic transfusion reaction (DSTR) from ABO incompatibility
     Other ABO incompatible blood transfusion
     Other reaction to ABO incompatible blood transfusion

● **T80.4**   **Rh incompatibility reaction due to transfusion of blood or blood products**
     Reaction due to incompatibility of Rh antigens (C) (c) (D) (E) (e)

X ● **T80.40**   **Rh incompatibility reaction due to transfusion of blood or blood products, unspecified**
     Reaction due to Rh factor in transfusion NOS
     Rh incompatible blood transfusion NOS

● **T80.41**   **Rh incompatibility with hemolytic transfusion reaction**

   ● **T80.410**   **Rh incompatibility with acute hemolytic transfusion reaction**
     Acute hemolytic transfusion reaction (AHTR) due to Rh incompatibility
     Rh incompatibility with hemolytic transfusion reaction less than 24 hours after transfusion

   ● **T80.411**   **Rh incompatibility with delayed hemolytic transfusion reaction**
     Delayed hemolytic transfusion reaction (DHTR) due to Rh incompatibility
     Rh incompatibility with hemolytic transfusion reaction 24 hours or more after transfusion

   ● **T80.419**   **Rh incompatibility with hemolytic transfusion reaction, unspecified**
     Rh incompatibility with hemolytic transfusion reaction at unspecified time after transfusion
     Hemolytic transfusion reaction (HTR) due to Rh incompatibility NOS

X ● **T80.49**   **Other Rh incompatibility reaction due to transfusion of blood or blood products**
     Delayed serologic transfusion reaction (DSTR) from Rh incompatibility
     Other reaction to Rh incompatible blood transfusion

● **T80.5**   **Anaphylactic reaction due to serum**
     Allergic reaction due to serum
     Anaphylactic shock due to serum
     Anaphylactoid reaction due to serum
     Anaphylaxis due to serum
     Excludes1   ABO incompatibility reaction due to transfusion of blood or blood products (T80.3-)
         allergic reaction or shock NOS (T78.2)
         anaphylactic reaction or shock NOS (T78.2)
         anaphylactic reaction or shock due to adverse effect of correct medicinal substance properly administered (T88.6)
         other serum reaction (T80.6-)

X ● **T80.51**   **Anaphylactic reaction due to administration of blood and blood products**

X ● **T80.52**   **Anaphylactic reaction due to vaccination**
     Coding Clinic: 2021, Q1, P43

X ● **T80.59**   **Anaphylactic reaction due to other serum**

● **T80.6**   **Other serum reactions**
     Intoxication by serum   Serum sickness
     Protein sickness   Serum urticaria
     Serum rash
     Excludes2   serum hepatitis (B16-B19)

X ● **T80.61**   **Other serum reaction due to administration of blood and blood products**

CHAPTER 19 (S00-T88)

X ● **T80.62**   **Other serum reaction due to vaccination**
       Coding Clinic: 2021, Q1, P42

X ● **T80.69**   **Other serum reaction due to other serum**
       Code also, if applicable, arthropathy in hypersensitivity reactions classified elsewhere (M36.4)

● **T80.8**   **Other complications following infusion, transfusion and therapeutic injection**

   ● **T80.81**   **Extravasation of vesicant agent**
       Infiltration of vesicant agent

     ● **T80.810**   **Extravasation of vesicant antineoplastic chemotherapy**
       Infiltration of vesicant antineoplastic chemotherapy

     ● **T80.818**   **Extravasation of other vesicant agent**
       Infiltration of other vesicant agent

   T80.82 Complication of immune effector cellular therapy
       Complication of chimeric antigen receptor (CAR-T) cell therapy
       Complication of IEC therapy

     ▶ **Excludes2**   adverse effect of immune checkpoint inhibitors and immunostimulant drugs (T45.AX5)
         complication of bone marrow transplant (T86.0)
         complication of stem cell transplant (T86.5)

     Use additional code to identify the specific complication, such as:
         cytokine release syndrome (D89.83-)
         immune effector cell-associated neurotoxicity syndrome (G92.0-)

   X ● **T80.89**   **Other complications following infusion, transfusion and therapeutic injection**
       Delayed serologic transfusion reaction (DSTR), unspecified incompatibility
       Use additional code to identify graft-versus-host reaction, if applicable, (D89.81-)

● **T80.9**   **Unspecified complication following infusion, transfusion and therapeutic injection**

   X ● **T80.90**   **Unspecified complication following infusion and therapeutic injection**

   ● **T80.91**   **Hemolytic transfusion reaction, unspecified incompatibility**

     Excludes1   ABO incompatibility with hemolytic transfusion reaction (T80.31-)
       Non-ABO incompatibility with hemolytic transfusion reaction (T80.A1-)
       Rh incompatibility with hemolytic transfusion reaction (T80.41-)

     ● **T80.910**   **Acute hemolytic transfusion reaction, unspecified incompatibility**

     ● **T80.911**   **Delayed hemolytic transfusion reaction, unspecified incompatibility**

     ● **T80.919**   **Hemolytic transfusion reaction, unspecified incompatibility, unspecified as acute or delayed**
       Hemolytic transfusion reaction NOS

   X ● **T80.92**   **Unspecified transfusion reaction**
       Transfusion reaction NOS

● **T80.A**   **Non-ABO incompatibility reaction due to transfusion of blood or blood products**
     Reaction due to incompatibility of minor antigens (Duffy) (Kell) (Kidd) (Lewis) (M) (N) (P) (S)

   X ● **T80.A0**   **Non-ABO incompatibility reaction due to transfusion of blood or blood products, unspecified**
       Non-ABO antigen incompatibility reaction from transfusion NOS

● **T80.A1**   **Non-ABO incompatibility with hemolytic transfusion reaction**

   ● **T80.A10**   **Non-ABO incompatibility with acute hemolytic transfusion reaction**
       Acute hemolytic transfusion reaction (AHTR) due to non-ABO incompatibility
       Non-ABO incompatibility with hemolytic transfusion reaction less than 24 hours after transfusion

   ● **T80.A11**   **Non-ABO incompatibility with delayed hemolytic transfusion reaction**
       Delayed hemolytic transfusion reaction (DHTR) due to non-ABO incompatibility
       Non-ABO incompatibility with hemolytic transfusion reaction 24 or more hours after transfusion

   ● **T80.A19**   **Non-ABO incompatibility with hemolytic transfusion reaction, unspecified**
       Hemolytic transfusion reaction (HTR) due to non-ABO incompatibility NOS
       Non-ABO incompatibility with hemolytic transfusion reaction at unspecified time after transfusion

   X ● **T80.A9**   **Other non-ABO incompatibility reaction due to transfusion of blood or blood products**
       Delayed serologic transfusion reaction (DSTR) from non-ABO incompatibility
       Other reaction to non-ABO incompatible blood transfusion

● **T81**   **Complications of procedures, not elsewhere classified**
     Use additional code for adverse effect, if applicable, to identify drug (T36-T50 with fifth or sixth character 5)

   Excludes2   complications following immunization (T88.0-T88.1)
       complications following infusion, transfusion and therapeutic injection (T80.-)
       complications of transplanted organs and tissue (T86.-)
       poisoning and toxic effects of drugs and chemicals (T36-T65 with fifth or sixth character 1-4)
       specified complications classified elsewhere, such as:
         complication of prosthetic devices, implants and grafts (T82-T85)
         dermatitis due to drugs and medicaments (L23.3, L24.4, L25.1, L27.0-L27.1)
         endosseous dental implant failure (M27.6-)
         floppy iris syndrome (IFIS) (intraoperative) H21.81
         intraoperative and postprocedural complications of specific body system (D78.-, E36.-, E89.-, G97.3-, G97.4, H59.3-, H59.-, H95.2-, H95.3, I97.4-, I97.5, J95, K91.-, L76.-, M96.-, N99.-)
         ostomy complications (J95.0-, K94.-, N99.5-)
         plateau iris syndrome (post-iridectomy) (postprocedural) H21.82

   Coding Clinic: 2019, Q2, P21-22; 2016, Q4, P29

   The appropriate 7th character is to be added to each code from category T81

A	initial encounter
D	subsequent encounter
S	sequela

▶ New   ⇒ Revised   ~~deleted~~ Deleted   Excludes 1   Excludes 2   Includes   Use additional   Code first   Code also   Key words

OGCR Official Guidelines   X Assign placeholder X   ● Use Additional Character(s)   ▶ Manifestation Code   🐾 Hierarchical Condition Category   Coding Clinic

● **T81.1 Postprocedural shock**
Shock during or resulting from a procedure, not elsewhere classified

> **Excludes1**   anaphylactic shock NOS (T78.2)
> anaphylactic shock due to correct substance properly administered (T88.6)
> anaphylactic shock due to serum (T80.5-)
> electric shock (T75.4)
> obstetric shock (O75.1)
> septic shock (R65.21)
> shock due to anesthesia (T88.2)
> shock following abortion or ectopic or molar pregnancy (O00-O07, O08.3)
> traumatic shock (T79.4)

X ● **T81.10 Postprocedural shock unspecified**
Collapse NOS during or resulting from a procedure, not elsewhere classified
Postprocedural failure of peripheral circulation
Postprocedural shock NOS

X ● **T81.11 Postprocedural cardiogenic shock A** 🔖

X ● **T81.12 Postprocedural septic shock A** 🔖
Postprocedural endotoxic shock resulting from a procedure, not elsewhere classified
Postprocedural gram-negative shock resulting from a procedure, not elsewhere classified
Code first underlying infection
Use additional code, to identify any associated acute organ dysfunction, if applicable

X ● **T81.19 Other postprocedural shock**
Postprocedural hypovolemic shock
Coding Clinic: 2021, Q1, P14

● **T81.3 Disruption of wound, not elsewhere classified**
Disruption of any suture materials or other closure methods

> **Excludes1**   breakdown (mechanical) of permanent sutures (T85.612)
> displacement of permanent sutures (T85.622)
> disruption of cesarean delivery wound (O90.0)
> disruption of perineal obstetric wound (O90.1)
> mechanical complication of permanent sutures NEC (T85.692)

X ● **T81.30 Disruption of wound, unspecified**
Disruption of wound NOS

X ● **T81.31 Disruption of external operation (surgical) wound, not elsewhere classified**

> **Excludes1**   dehiscence of amputation stump (T87.81)

Dehiscence of operation wound NOS
Disruption of operation wound NOS
Disruption or dehiscence of closure of cornea
Disruption or dehiscence of closure of mucosa
Disruption or dehiscence of closure of skin and subcutaneous tissue
Full-thickness skin disruption or dehiscence
Superficial disruption or dehiscence of operation wound
Coding Clinic: 2015, Q1, P20

X ● **T81.32 Disruption of internal operation (surgical) wound, not elsewhere classified**
~~Deep disruption or dehiscence of operation wound NOS~~
~~Disruption or dehiscence of closure of internal organ or other internal tissue~~
~~Disruption or dehiscence of closure of muscle or muscle flap~~
~~Disruption or dehiscence of closure of ribs or rib cage~~
~~Disruption or dehiscence of closure of skull or craniotomy~~
~~Disruption or dehiscence of closure of sternum or sternotomy~~
~~Disruption or dehiscence of closure of tendon or ligament~~
~~Disruption or dehiscence of closure of superficial or muscular fasci~~a
Coding Clinic: 2017, Q3, P4

▶ ● **T81.320 Disruption or dehiscence of gastrointestinal tract anastomosis, repair, or closure**

▶ ● **T81.321 Disruption or dehiscence of closure of internal operation (surgical) wound ofabdominal wall muscle or fascia**

▶ ● **T81.328 Disruption or dehiscence of closure of other specified internal operation(surgical) wound**
▷ Disruption or dehiscence of closure of muscle or muscle flap (other than abdominal wall muscle)
▷ Disruption or dehiscence of closure of ribs or rib cage
▷ Disruption or dehiscence of closure of skull or craniotomy
▷ Disruption or dehiscence of closure of sternum or sternotomy
▷ Disruption or dehiscence of closure of tendon or ligament
▷ Disruption or dehiscence of closure of superficial or muscular fascia (other than abdominal wall fascia)

▶ ● **T81.329 Deep disruption or dehiscence of operation wound, unspecified**
▷ Deep disruption or dehiscence of operation wound NOS

X ● **T81.33 Disruption of traumatic injury wound repair**
Disruption or dehiscence of closure of traumatic laceration (external) (internal)

● **T81.4 Infection following a procedure**
▶ Code also, if applicable, disruption of internal operation (surgical) wound (T81.32-)
Use additional code to identify infection
Use additional code (R65.2-) to identify severe sepsis, if applicable

> **Excludes2**   bleb associated endophthalmitis (H59.4-)
> infection due to infusion, transfusion and therapeutic injection (T80.2-)
> infection due to prosthetic devices, implants and grafts (T82.6-T82.7, T83.5-T83.6, T84.5-T84.7, T85.7)
> obstetric surgical wound infection (O86.0-)
> postprocedural fever NOS (R50.82)
> postprocedural retroperitoneal abscess (K68.11)

X ● **T81.40 Infection following a procedure, unspecified**
Coding Clinic: 2024, Q1, P19

X ● **T81.41 Infection following a procedure, superficial incisional surgical site**
Subcutaneous abscess following a procedure
Stitch abscess following a procedure
Coding Clinic: 2024, Q1, P19; 2018, Q4, P34

X ● **T81.42 Infection following a procedure, deep incisional surgical site**
Intra-muscular abscess following a procedure
Coding Clinic: 2024, Q1, P19

X ● **T81.43 Infection following a procedure, organ and space surgical site**
Intra-abdominal abscess following a procedure
Subphrenic abscess following a procedure
Coding Clinic: 2024, Q1, P19,20

X ● **T81.44 Sepsis following a procedure A** 🔖
Use additional code to identify the sepsis
Coding Clinic: 2024, Q1, P19

X ● **T81.49 Infection following a procedure, other surgical site**
Coding Clinic: 2024, Q1, P19; 2015, Q4, P37

CHAPTER 19 (S00-T88)

- ● **T81.5** Complications of foreign body accidentally left in body following procedure
  - ● **T81.50** Unspecified complication of foreign body accidentally left in body following procedure
    - ● **T81.500** Unspecified complication of foreign body accidentally left in body following surgical operation
    - ● **T81.501** Unspecified complication of foreign body accidentally left in body following infusion or transfusion
    - ● **T81.502** Unspecified complication of foreign body accidentally left in body following kidney dialysis A, D, S ✎
    - ● **T81.503** Unspecified complication of foreign body accidentally left in body following injection or immunization
    - ● **T81.504** Unspecified complication of foreign body accidentally left in body following endoscopic examination
    - ● **T81.505** Unspecified complication of foreign body accidentally left in body following heart catheterization
    - ● **T81.506** Unspecified complication of foreign body accidentally left in body following aspiration, puncture or other catheterization
    - ● **T81.507** Unspecified complication of foreign body accidentally left in body following removal of catheter or packing
    - ● **T81.508** Unspecified complication of foreign body accidentally left in body following other procedure
    - ● **T81.509** Unspecified complication of foreign body accidentally left in body following unspecified procedure
  - ● **T81.51** Adhesions due to foreign body accidentally left in body following procedure
    - ● **T81.510** Adhesions due to foreign body accidentally left in body following surgical operation
    - ● **T81.511** Adhesions due to foreign body accidentally left in body following infusion or transfusion
    - ● **T81.512** Adhesions due to foreign body accidentally left in body following kidney dialysis A, D, S ✎
    - ● **T81.513** Adhesions due to foreign body accidentally left in body following injection or immunization
    - ● **T81.514** Adhesions due to foreign body accidentally left in body following endoscopic examination
    - ● **T81.515** Adhesions due to foreign body accidentally left in body following heart catheterization
    - ● **T81.516** Adhesions due to foreign body accidentally left in body following aspiration, puncture or other catheterization
    - ● **T81.517** Adhesions due to foreign body accidentally left in body following removal of catheter or packing
    - ● **T81.518** Adhesions due to foreign body accidentally left in body following other procedure
    - ● **T81.519** Adhesions due to foreign body accidentally left in body following unspecified procedure
  - ● **T81.52** Obstruction due to foreign body accidentally left in body following procedure
    - ● **T81.520** Obstruction due to foreign body accidentally left in body following surgical operation

- ● **T81.521** Obstruction due to foreign body accidentally left in body following infusion or transfusion
- ● **T81.522** Obstruction due to foreign body accidentally left in body following kidney dialysis A, D, S ✎
- ● **T81.523** Obstruction due to foreign body accidentally left in body following injection or immunization
- ● **T81.524** Obstruction due to foreign body accidentally left in body following endoscopic examination
- ● **T81.525** Obstruction due to foreign body accidentally left in body following heart catheterization
- ● **T81.526** Obstruction due to foreign body accidentally left in body following aspiration, puncture or other catheterization
- ● **T81.527** Obstruction due to foreign body accidentally left in body following removal of catheter or packing
- ● **T81.528** Obstruction due to foreign body accidentally left in body following other procedure
- ● **T81.529** Obstruction due to foreign body accidentally left in body following unspecified procedure
- ● **T81.53** Perforation due to foreign body accidentally left in body following procedure
  - ● **T81.530** Perforation due to foreign body accidentally left in body following surgical operation
  - ● **T81.531** Perforation due to foreign body accidentally left in body following infusion or transfusion
  - ● **T81.532** Perforation due to foreign body accidentally left in body following kidney dialysis A, D, S ✎
  - ● **T81.533** Perforation due to foreign body accidentally left in body following injection or immunization
  - ● **T81.534** Perforation due to foreign body accidentally left in body following endoscopic examination
  - ● **T81.535** Perforation due to foreign body accidentally left in body following heart catheterization
  - ● **T81.536** Perforation due to foreign body accidentally left in body following aspiration, puncture or other catheterization
  - ● **T81.537** Perforation due to foreign body accidentally left in body following removal of catheter or packing
  - ● **T81.538** Perforation due to foreign body accidentally left in body following other procedure
  - ● **T81.539** Perforation due to foreign body accidentally left in body following unspecified procedure
- ● **T81.59** Other complications of foreign body accidentally left in body following procedure
  - **Excludes2** obstruction or perforation due to prosthetic devices and implants intentionally left in body (T82.0-T82.5, T83.0-T83.4, T83.7, T84.0-T84.4, T85.0-T85.6)
  - ● **T81.590** Other complications of foreign body accidentally left in body following surgical operation

● **T81.591**   Other complications of foreign body accidentally left in body following **infusion or transfusion**

● **T81.592**   Other complications of foreign body accidentally left in body following **kidney dialysis** A, D, S 🔖

● **T81.593**   Other complications of foreign body accidentally left in body following **injection or immunization**

● **T81.594**   Other complications of foreign body accidentally left in body following **endoscopic examination**

● **T81.595**   Other complications of foreign body accidentally left in body following **heart catheterization**

● **T81.596**   Other complications of foreign body accidentally left in body following **aspiration, puncture or other catheterization**

● **T81.597**   Other complications of foreign body accidentally left in body following **removal of catheter or packing**

● **T81.598**   Other complications of foreign body accidentally left in body following **other procedure**

● **T81.599**   Other complications of foreign body accidentally left in body following **unspecified** procedure

● **T81.6**   **Acute reaction to foreign substance accidentally left during a procedure**

     Excludes2   complications of foreign body accidentally left in body cavity or operation wound following procedure (T81.5-)

X ● **T81.60**   **Unspecified** acute reaction to foreign substance accidentally left during a procedure

X ● **T81.61**   **Aseptic peritonitis due to foreign substance accidentally left during a procedure**
       Chemical peritonitis

X ● **T81.69**   **Other** acute reaction to foreign substance accidentally left during a procedure

● **T81.7**   **Vascular complications following a procedure, not elsewhere classified**
     Air embolism following procedure NEC
     Phlebitis or thrombophlebitis resulting from a procedure

     Excludes1   embolism complicating abortion or ectopic or molar pregnancy (O00-O07, O08.2)
                embolism complicating pregnancy, childbirth and the puerperium (O88.-)
                traumatic embolism (T79.0)

     Excludes2   embolism due to prosthetic devices, implants and grafts (T82.8, T83.81, T84.8-, T85.1-)
                embolism following infusion, transfusion and therapeutic injection (T80.0)
     Coding Clinic: 2019, Q2, P23

● **T81.71**   **Complication of artery following a procedure, not elsewhere classified**
     Coding Clinic: 2019, Q2, P22

     ● **T81.710**   Complication of **mesenteric artery** following a procedure, not elsewhere classified

     ● **T81.711**   Complication of **renal artery** following a procedure, not elsewhere classified

     ● **T81.718**   Complication of **other artery** following a procedure, not elsewhere classified
            Coding Clinic: 2019, Q2, P22-23

     ● **T81.719**   Complication of **unspecified** artery following a procedure, not elsewhere classified

X ● **T81.72**   **Complication of vein following a procedure, not elsewhere classified**
     Coding Clinic: 2019, Q2, P22

● **T81.8**   **Other complications of procedures, not elsewhere classified**

     Excludes2   hypothermia following anesthesia (T88.51)
                malignant hyperpyrexia due to anesthesia (T88.3)

X ● **T81.81**   **Complication of inhalation therapy**

X ● **T81.82**   **Emphysema (subcutaneous) resulting from a procedure**

X ● **T81.83**   **Persistent postprocedural fistula**

     ▶ Code also, if applicable, disruption of internal operation (surgical) wound (T81.32-)

     Use additional code, if known, for site of fistula such as:
       ⟩ anal fistula (K60.3-)
       ⟩ anorectal fistula (K60.5-)
         bladder fistula (N32.2)
         other female intestinal-genital tract fistulae (N82.4)
     Coding Clinic: 2023, Q1, P30; 2017, Q3, P3-5

X ● **T81.89**   **Other complications of procedures, not elsewhere classified**

     Use additional code to specify complication, such as:
       postprocedural delirium (F05)

X ● **T81.9**   **Unspecified complication of procedure**

● **T82**   **Complications of cardiac and vascular prosthetic devices, implants and grafts**

     Excludes2   failure and rejection of transplanted organs and tissue (T86.-)

     The appropriate 7th character is to be added to each code from category T82

A	initial encounter
D	subsequent encounter
S	sequela

● **T82.0**   **Mechanical complication of heart valve prosthesis**
     Mechanical complication of artificial heart valve

     Excludes1   mechanical complication of biological heart valve graft (T82.22-)

X ● **T82.01**   **Breakdown (mechanical) of heart valve prosthesis**

X ● **T82.02**   **Displacement of heart valve prosthesis**
     Malposition of heart valve prosthesis

X ● **T82.03**   **Leakage of heart valve prosthesis**

X ● **T82.09**   **Other mechanical complication of heart valve prosthesis**
     Obstruction (mechanical) of heart valve prosthesis
     Perforation of heart valve prosthesis
     Protrusion of heart valve prosthesis

● **T82.1**   **Mechanical complication of cardiac electronic device**

     ● **T82.11**   **Breakdown (mechanical) of cardiac electronic device**

       ● **T82.110**   Breakdown (mechanical) of cardiac **electrode**

       ● **T82.111**   Breakdown (mechanical) of cardiac **pulse generator (battery)**

       ● **T82.118**   Breakdown (mechanical) of **other cardiac electronic device**

       ● **T82.119**   Breakdown (mechanical) of **unspecified cardiac electronic device**

     ● **T82.12**   **Displacement of cardiac electronic device**
       Malposition of cardiac electronic device

       ● **T82.120**   Displacement of cardiac **electrode**

CHAPTER 19 (S00–T88)

- ● T82.121   Displacement of cardiac pulse generator (battery)
- ● T82.128   Displacement of other cardiac electronic device
- ● T82.129   Displacement of unspecified cardiac electronic device
- ● T82.19   Other mechanical complication of cardiac electronic device
  - Leakage of cardiac electronic device
  - Obstruction of cardiac electronic device
  - Perforation of cardiac electronic device
  - Protrusion of cardiac electronic device
  - ● T82.190   Other mechanical complication of cardiac electrode
  - ● T82.191   Other mechanical complication of cardiac pulse generator (battery)
  - ● T82.198   Other mechanical complication of other cardiac electronic device
  - ● T82.199   Other mechanical complication of unspecified cardiac device
- ● T82.2   Mechanical complication of coronary artery bypass graft and biological heart valve graft
  - **Excludes1** mechanical complication of artificial heart valve prosthesis (T82.0-)
  - ● T82.21   Mechanical complication of coronary artery bypass graft
    - ● T82.211   Breakdown (mechanical) of coronary artery bypass graft
    - ● T82.212   Displacement of coronary artery bypass graft
      - Malposition of coronary artery bypass graft
    - ● T82.213   Leakage of coronary artery bypass graft
    - ● T82.218   Other mechanical complication of coronary artery bypass graft
      - Obstruction, mechanical of coronary artery bypass graft
      - Perforation of coronary artery bypass graft
      - Protrusion of coronary artery bypass graft
  - ● T82.22   Mechanical complication of biological heart valve graft
    - ● T82.221   Breakdown (mechanical) of biological heart valve graft
    - ● T82.222   Displacement of biological heart valve graft
      - Malposition of biological heart valve graft
    - ● T82.223   Leakage of biological heart valve graft
    - ● T82.228   Other mechanical complication of biological heart valve graft
      - Obstruction of biological heart valve graft
      - Perforation of biological heart valve graft
      - Protrusion of biological heart valve graft
- ● T82.3   Mechanical complication of other vascular grafts
  - ● T82.31   Breakdown (mechanical) of other vascular grafts
    - ● T82.310   Breakdown (mechanical) of aortic (bifurcation) graft (replacement) A 🦠
    - ● T82.311   Breakdown (mechanical) of carotid arterial graft (bypass) A 🦠
    - ● T82.312   Breakdown (mechanical) of femoral arterial graft (bypass) A 🦠

- ● T82.318   Breakdown (mechanical) of other vascular grafts A 🦠
- ● T82.319   Breakdown (mechanical) of unspecified vascular grafts A 🦠
- ● T82.32   Displacement of other vascular grafts
  - Malposition of other vascular grafts
  - ● T82.320   Displacement of aortic (bifurcation) graft (replacement) A 🦠
  - ● T82.321   Displacement of carotid arterial graft (bypass) A 🦠
  - ● T82.322   Displacement of femoral arterial graft (bypass) A 🦠
  - ● T82.328   Displacement of other vascular grafts A 🦠
  - ● T82.329   Displacement of unspecified vascular grafts A 🦠
- ● T82.33   Leakage of other vascular grafts
  - ● T82.330   Leakage of aortic (bifurcation) graft (replacement) A 🦠
  - ● T82.331   Leakage of carotid arterial graft (bypass) A 🦠
  - ● T82.332   Leakage of femoral arterial graft (bypass) A 🦠
  - ● T82.338   Leakage of other vascular grafts A 🦠
  - ● T82.339   Leakage of unspecified vascular graft A 🦠
- ● T82.39   Other mechanical complication of other vascular grafts
  - Obstruction (mechanical) of other vascular grafts
  - Perforation of other vascular grafts
  - Protrusion of other vascular grafts
  - ● T82.390   Other mechanical complication of aortic (bifurcation) graft (replacement) A 🦠
  - ● T82.391   Other mechanical complication of carotid arterial graft (bypass) A 🦠
  - ● T82.392   Other mechanical complication of femoral arterial graft (bypass) A 🦠
  - ● T82.398   Other mechanical complication of other vascular grafts A 🦠
  - ● T82.399   Other mechanical complication of unspecified vascular grafts A 🦠
- ● T82.4   Mechanical complication of vascular dialysis catheter
  - Mechanical complication of hemodialysis catheter
  - **Excludes1** mechanical complication of intraperitoneal dialysis catheter (T85.62)
  - X ● T82.41   Breakdown (mechanical) of vascular dialysis catheter A, D, S 🦠
  - X ● T82.42   Displacement of vascular dialysis catheter A, D, S 🦠
    - Malposition of vascular dialysis catheter
  - X ● T82.43   Leakage of vascular dialysis catheter A, D, S 🦠
  - X ● T82.49   Other complication of vascular dialysis catheter A, D, S 🦠
    - Obstruction (mechanical) of vascular dialysis catheter
    - Perforation of vascular dialysis catheter
    - Protrusion of vascular dialysis catheter
- ● T82.5   Mechanical complication of other cardiac and vascular devices and implants
  - **Excludes2** mechanical complication of epidural and subdural infusion catheter (T85.61)
  - ● T82.51   Breakdown (mechanical) of other cardiac and vascular devices and implants
    - ● T82.510   Breakdown (mechanical) of surgically created arteriovenous fistula A 🦠
    - ● T82.511   Breakdown (mechanical) of surgically created arteriovenous shunt A 🦠

● T82.512   Breakdown (mechanical) of artificial heart

● T82.513   Breakdown (mechanical) of balloon (counterpulsation) device A 🖠

● T82.514   Breakdown (mechanical) of infusion catheter A 🖠

● T82.515   Breakdown (mechanical) of umbrella device A 🖠

● T82.518   Breakdown (mechanical) of other cardiac and vascular devices and implants A 🖠

● T82.519   Breakdown (mechanical) of unspecified cardiac and vascular devices and implants

● T82.52   Displacement of other cardiac and vascular devices and implants

     Malposition of other cardiac and vascular devices and implants

   ● T82.520   Displacement of surgically created arteriovenous fistula A 🖠

   ● T82.521   Displacement of surgically created arteriovenous shunt A 🖠

   ● T82.522   Displacement of artificial heart

   ● T82.523   Displacement of balloon (counterpulsation) device A 🖠

   ● T82.524   Displacement of infusion catheter A 🖠

      Coding Clinic: 2019, Q3, P15

   ● T82.525   Displacement of umbrella device A 🖠

   ● T82.528   Displacement of other cardiac and vascular devices and implants A 🖠

   ● T82.529   Displacement of unspecified cardiac and vascular devices and implants

● T82.53   Leakage of other cardiac and vascular devices and implants

   ● T82.530   Leakage of surgically created arteriovenous fistula A 🖠

   ● T82.531   Leakage of surgically created arteriovenous shunt A 🖠

   ● T82.532   Leakage of artificial heart

   ● T82.533   Leakage of balloon (counterpulsation) device A 🖠

   ● T82.534   Leakage of infusion catheter A 🖠

   ● T82.535   Leakage of umbrella device A 🖠

   ● T82.538   Leakage of other cardiac and vascular devices and implants A 🖠

   ● T82.539   Leakage of unspecified cardiac and vascular devices and implants

● T82.59   Other mechanical complication of other cardiac and vascular devices and implants

     Obstruction (mechanical) of other cardiac and vascular devices and implants

     Perforation of other cardiac and vascular devices and implants

     Protrusion of other cardiac and vascular devices and implants

   ● T82.590   Other mechanical complication of surgically created arteriovenous fistula A 🖠

   ● T82.591   Other mechanical complication of surgically created arteriovenous shunt A 🖠

   ● T82.592   Other mechanical complication of artificial heart

   ● T82.593   Other mechanical complication of balloon (counterpulsation) device A 🖠

   ● T82.594   Other mechanical complication of infusion catheter A 🖠

   ● T82.595   Other mechanical complication of umbrella device A 🖠

   ● T82.598   Other mechanical complication of other cardiac and vascular devices and implants A 🖠

   ● T82.599   Other mechanical complication of unspecified cardiac and vascular devices and implants

X ● T82.6   Infection and inflammatory reaction due to cardiac valve prosthesis A 🖠

     Use additional code to identify infection

X ● T82.7   Infection and inflammatory reaction due to other cardiac and vascular devices, implants and grafts A 🖠

     Use additional code to identify infection

     Coding Clinic: 2019, Q1, P13-14; 2018, Q4, P89

● T82.8   Other specified complications of cardiac and vascular prosthetic devices, implants and grafts

● T82.81   Embolism due to cardiac and vascular prosthetic devices, implants and grafts

     Coding Clinic: 2016, Q4, P70

   ● T82.817   Embolism due to cardiac prosthetic devices, implants and grafts

      Coding Clinic: 2016, Q4, P70; 2015, Q1, P20

   ● T82.818   Embolism due to vascular prosthetic devices, implants and grafts A 🖠

● T82.82   Fibrosis due to cardiac and vascular prosthetic devices, implants and grafts

     Coding Clinic: 2016, Q4, P70

   ● T82.827   Fibrosis due to cardiac prosthetic devices, implants and grafts

   ● T82.828   Fibrosis due to vascular prosthetic devices, implants and grafts A 🖠

● T82.83   Hemorrhage due to cardiac and vascular prosthetic devices, implants and grafts

     Coding Clinic: 2016, Q4, P70

   ● T82.837   Hemorrhage due to cardiac prosthetic devices, implants and grafts

   ● T82.838   Hemorrhage due to vascular prosthetic devices, implants and grafts A 🖠

● T82.84   Pain due to cardiac and vascular prosthetic devices, implants and grafts

     Coding Clinic: 2016, Q4, P70

   ● T82.847   Pain due to cardiac prosthetic devices, implants and grafts

   ● T82.848   Pain due to vascular prosthetic devices, implants and grafts A 🖠

● T82.85   Stenosis due to cardiac and vascular prosthetic devices, implants and grafts

   ● T82.855   Stenosis of coronary artery stent

     In-stent stenosis (restenosis) of coronary artery stent

     Restenosis of coronary artery stent

     Coding Clinic: 2021, Q3, P6-7; 2016, Q4, P70

   ● T82.856   Stenosis of peripheral vascular stent A 🖠

     In-stent stenosis (restenosis) of peripheral vascular stent

     Restenosis of peripheral vascular stent

     Coding Clinic: 2016, Q4, P70

   ● T82.857   Stenosis of other cardiac prosthetic devices, implants and grafts

     Coding Clinic: 2016, Q4, P70

   ● T82.858   Stenosis of other vascular prosthetic devices, implants and grafts A 🖠

     Coding Clinic: 2016, Q4, P70

● T82.86   Thrombosis of cardiac and vascular prosthetic devices, implants and grafts

   ● T82.867   Thrombosis due to cardiac prosthetic devices, implants and grafts

   ● T82.868   Thrombosis due to vascular prosthetic devices, implants and grafts A 🖠

     Coding Clinic: 2023, Q2, P7

● T82.89   Other specified complication of cardiac and vascular prosthetic devices, implants and grafts

    ● T82.897   Other specified complication of cardiac prosthetic devices, implants and grafts
         Coding Clinic: 2019, Q2, P32-33

    ● T82.898   Other specified complication of vascular prosthetic devices, implants and grafts A 🦠

X ● T82.9   Unspecified complication of cardiac and vascular prosthetic device, implant and graft

● T83   Complications of genitourinary prosthetic devices, implants and grafts

     Excludes2   failure and rejection of transplanted organs and tissue (T86.-)

     The appropriate 7th character is to be added to each code from category T83

A	initial encounter
D	subsequent encounter
S	sequela

     Coding Clinic: 2016, Q4, P70-71

● T83.0   Mechanical complication of urinary catheter

     Excludes2   complications of stoma of urinary tract (N99.5-)
         Coding Clinic: 2016, Q4, P70

  ● T83.01   Breakdown (mechanical) of urinary catheter

    ● T83.010   Breakdown (mechanical) of cystostomy catheter A 🦠

    ● T83.011   Breakdown (mechanical) of indwelling urethral catheter A 🦠

    ● T83.012   Breakdown (mechanical) of nephrostomy catheter A 🦠

    ● T83.018   Breakdown (mechanical) of other urinary catheter A 🦠
         Breakdown (mechanical) of Hopkins catheter
         Breakdown (mechanical) of ileostomy catheter
         Breakdown (mechanical) urostomy catheter

  ● T83.02   Displacement of urinary catheter
     Malposition of urinary catheter

    ● T83.020   Displacement of cystostomy catheter A 🦠

    ● T83.021   Displacement of indwelling urethral catheter A 🦠

    ● T83.022   Displacement of nephrostomy catheter A 🦠

    ● T83.028   Displacement of other urinary catheter A 🦠
         Displacement of Hopkins catheter
         Displacement of ileostomy catheter
         Displacement of urostomy catheter

  ● T83.03   Leakage of urinary catheter

    ● T83.030   Leakage of cystostomy catheter A 🦠
         Coding Clinic: 2021, Q4, P19

    ● T83.031   Leakage of indwelling urethral catheter A 🦠

    ● T83.032   Leakage of nephrostomy catheter A 🦠

    ● T83.038   Leakage of other urinary catheter A 🦠
         Leakage of Hopkins catheter
         Leakage of ileostomy catheter
         Leakage of urostomy catheter

  ● T83.09   Other mechanical complication of urinary catheter
     Obstruction (mechanical) of urinary catheter
     Perforation of urinary catheter
     Protrusion of urinary catheter

    ● T83.090   Other mechanical complication of cystostomy catheter A 🦠

    ● T83.091   Other mechanical complication of indwelling urethral catheter A 🦠

    ● T83.092   Other mechanical complication of nephrostomy catheter A 🦠

    ● T83.098   Other mechanical complication of other urinary catheter A 🦠
         Other mechanical complication of Hopkins catheter
         Other mechanical complication of ileostomy catheter
         Other mechanical complication of urostomy catheter

● T83.1   Mechanical complication of other urinary devices and implants
     Coding Clinic: 2016, Q4, P70

  ● T83.11   Breakdown (mechanical) of other urinary devices and implants

    ● T83.110   Breakdown (mechanical) of urinary electronic stimulator device A 🦠
         Excludes2   Breakdown (mechanical) of electrode (lead) for sacral nerve neurostimulator (T85.111)
             Breakdown (mechanical) of implanted electronic sacral neurostimulator, pulse generator or receiver (T85.113)

    ● T83.111   Breakdown (mechanical) of implanted urinary sphincter A 🦠

    ● T83.112   Breakdown (mechanical) of indwelling ureteral stent A 🦠

    ● T83.113   Breakdown (mechanical) of other urinary stents A 🦠
         Breakdown (mechanical) of ileal conduit stent
         Breakdown (mechanical) of nephroureteral stent

    ● T83.118   Breakdown (mechanical) of other urinary devices and implants A 🦠

  ● T83.12   Displacement of other urinary devices and implants
     Malposition of other urinary devices and implants

    ● T83.120   Displacement of urinary electronic stimulator device A 🦠
         Excludes2   Displacement of electrode (lead) for sacral nerve neurostimulator (T85.121)
             Displacement of implanted electronic sacral neurostimulator, pulse generator or receiver (T85.123)

    ● T83.121   Displacement of implanted urinary sphincter A 🦠

    ● T83.122   Displacement of indwelling ureteral stent A 🦠

    ● T83.123   Displacement of other urinary stents A 🦠
         Displacement of ileal conduit stent
         Displacement of nephroureteral stent

    ● T83.128   Displacement of other urinary devices and implants A 🦠

▶ New   ⇒ Revised   ~~deleted~~ Deleted   Excludes 1   Excludes 2   Includes   Use additional   Code first   Code also   Key words

OGCR Official Guidelines   X Assign placeholder X   ● Use Additional Character(s)   ▶ Manifestation Code   🦠 Hierarchical Condition Category   Coding Clinic

● **T83.19** **Other mechanical complication** of other urinary devices and implants
Leakage of other urinary devices and implants
Obstruction (mechanical) of other urinary devices and implants
Perforation of other urinary devices and implants
Protrusion of other urinary devices and implants

● **T83.190** **Other mechanical complication of urinary electronic stimulator device** A 🐾

Excludes2 Other mechanical complication of electrode (lead) for sacral nerve neurostimulator (T85.191)
Other mechanical complication of implanted electronic sacral neurostimulator, pulse generator or receiver (T85.193)

● **T83.191** **Other mechanical complication of** implanted **urinary sphincter** A 🐾

● **T83.192** **Other mechanical complication of** indwelling **ureteral stent** A 🐾

● **T83.193** **Other mechanical complication of** other **urinary stent** A 🐾
Other mechanical complication of ileal conduit stent
Other mechanical complication of nephroureteral stent

● **T83.198** **Other mechanical complication of other urinary devices and implants** A 🐾

● **T83.2** **Mechanical complication of** graft of urinary organ
Coding Clinic: 2016, Q4, P70

X ● **T83.21** **Breakdown (mechanical) of graft of urinary organ** A 🐾

X ● **T83.22** **Displacement of graft of urinary organ** A 🐾
Malposition of graft of urinary organ

X ● **T83.23** **Leakage of graft of urinary organ** A 🐾

X ● **T83.24** **Erosion of graft of urinary organ** A 🐾
Coding Clinic: 2016, Q4, P70

X ● **T83.25** **Exposure of graft of urinary organ** A 🐾
Coding Clinic: 2016, Q4, P70

X ● **T83.29** **Other mechanical complication of graft of urinary organ** A 🐾
Obstruction (mechanical) of graft of urinary organ
Perforation of graft of urinary organ
Protrusion of graft of urinary organ

● **T83.3** **Mechanical complication of** intrauterine contraceptive device

X ● **T83.31** **Breakdown (mechanical) of intrauterine** contraceptive device

X ● **T83.32** **Displacement of intrauterine contraceptive** device
Malposition of intrauterine contraceptive device
Missing string of intrauterine contraceptive device

X ● **T83.39** **Other mechanical complication of intrauterine** contraceptive device
Leakage of intrauterine contraceptive device
Obstruction (mechanical) of intrauterine contraceptive device
Perforation of intrauterine contraceptive device
Protrusion of intrauterine contraceptive device

● **T83.4** **Mechanical complication of** other prosthetic devices, implants and grafts of genital tract
Coding Clinic: 2016, Q4, P71

● **T83.41** **Breakdown (mechanical) of other prosthetic** devices, implants and grafts of genital tract

● **T83.410** **Breakdown (mechanical) of implanted penile prosthesis** A 🐾
Breakdown (mechanical) of penile prosthesis cylinder
Breakdown (mechanical) of penile prosthesis pump
Breakdown (mechanical) of penile prosthesis reservoir

● **T83.411** **Breakdown (mechanical) of implanted testicular prosthesis** A 🐾

● **T83.418** **Breakdown (mechanical) of other prosthetic devices, implants and grafts of genital tract** A 🐾

● **T83.42** **Displacement of other prosthetic devices, implants and grafts of genital tract**
Malposition of other prosthetic devices, implants and grafts of genital tract

● **T83.420** **Displacement of implanted penile prosthesis** A 🐾
Displacement of penile prosthesis cylinder
Displacement of penile prosthesis pump
Displacement of penile prosthesis reservoir

● **T83.421** **Displacement of implanted testicular prosthesis** A 🐾

● **T83.428** **Displacement of other prosthetic devices, implants and grafts of genital tract** A 🐾
Coding Clinic: 2018, Q1, P6

● **T83.49** **Other mechanical complication of other prosthetic devices, implants and grafts of genital tract**
Leakage of other prosthetic devices, implants and grafts of genital tract
Obstruction, mechanical of other prosthetic devices, implants and grafts of genital tract
Perforation of other prosthetic devices, implants and grafts of genital tract
Protrusion of other prosthetic devices, implants and grafts of genital tract

● **T83.490** **Other mechanical complication of implanted penile prosthesis** A 🐾
Other mechanical complication of penile prosthesis cylinder
Other mechanical complication of penile prosthesis pump
Other mechanical complication of penile prosthesis reservoir

● **T83.491** **Other mechanical complication of implanted testicular prosthesis** A 🐾

● **T83.498** **Other mechanical complication of other prosthetic devices, implants and grafts of genital tract** A 🐾

● **T83.5** **Infection and inflammatory reaction due to prosthetic device, implant and graft in** urinary system
Use additional code to identify infection
Coding Clinic: 2016, Q4, P71

● **T83.51** **Infection and inflammatory reaction due to urinary catheter**

Excludes2 complications of stoma of urinary tract (N99.5-)

● **T83.510** **Infection and inflammatory reaction due to cystostomy catheter** A 🐾

● **T83.511** **Infection and inflammatory reaction due to** indwelling **urethral catheter** A 🐾
Coding Clinic: 2022, Q2, P7

CHAPTER 19 (S00–T88)

● T83.512　Infection and inflammatory reaction due to nephrostomy catheter A 🐾

● T83.518　Infection and inflammatory reaction due to other urinary catheter A 🐾
　　　　　Infection and inflammatory reaction due to Hopkins catheter
　　　　　Infection and inflammatory reaction due to ileostomy catheter
　　　　　Infection and inflammatory reaction due to urostomy catheter

● T83.59　Infection and inflammatory reaction due to prosthetic device, implant and graft in urinary system

● T83.590　Infection and inflammatory reaction due to implanted urinary neurostimulation device A 🐾
　　　　　Excludes2　Infection and inflammatory reaction due to electrode lead of sacral nerve neurostimulator (T85.732)
　　　　　　　　　Infection and inflammatory reaction due to pulse generator or receiver of sacral nerve neurostimulator (T85.734)

● T83.591　Infection and inflammatory reaction due to implanted urinary sphincter A 🐾

● T83.592　Infection and inflammatory reaction due to indwelling ureteral stent A 🐾

● T83.593　Infection and inflammatory reaction due to other urinary stents A 🐾
　　　　　Infection and inflammatory reaction due to ileal conduit stents
　　　　　Infection and inflammatory reaction due to nephroureteral stent

● T83.598　Infection and inflammatory reaction due to other prosthetic device, implant and graft in urinary system A 🐾

● T83.6　Infection and inflammatory reaction due to prosthetic device, implant and graft in genital tract
　　　　Use additional code to identify infection
　　　　Coding Clinic: 2016, Q4, P71

● T83.61　Infection and inflammatory reaction due to implanted penile prosthesis A 🐾
　　　　　Infection and inflammatory reaction due to penile prosthesis cylinder
　　　　　Infection and inflammatory reaction due to penile prosthesis pump
　　　　　Infection and inflammatory reaction due to penile prosthesis reservoir

● T83.62　Infection and inflammatory reaction due to implanted testicular prosthesis A 🐾

● T83.69　Infection and inflammatory reaction due to other prosthetic device, implant and graft in genital tract A 🐾

● T83.7　Complications due to implanted mesh and other prosthetic materials
　　　　Coding Clinic: 2016, Q4, P71

● T83.71　Erosion of implanted mesh and other prosthetic materials to surrounding organ or tissue
　　　　Coding Clinic: 2016, Q4, P71

● T83.711　Erosion of implanted vaginal mesh to surrounding organ or tissue A 🐾
　　　　　Erosion of implanted vaginal mesh into pelvic floor muscles
　　　　　Coding Clinic: 2016, Q4, P71

● T83.712　Erosion of implanted urethral mesh to surrounding organ or tissue A 🐾
　　　　　Erosion of implanted female urethral sling
　　　　　Erosion of implanted male urethral sling
　　　　　Erosion of implanted urethral mesh into pelvic floor muscles

● T83.713　Erosion of implanted urethral bulking agent to surrounding organ or tissue A 🐾

● T83.714　Erosion of implanted ureteral bulking agent to surrounding organ or tissue A 🐾

● T83.718　Erosion of other implanted mesh to organ or tissue A 🐾
　　　　　Coding Clinic: 2016, Q4, P71

● T83.719　Erosion of other prosthetic materials to surrounding organ or tissue A 🐾
　　　　　Coding Clinic: 2016, Q4, P71

● T83.72　Exposure of implanted mesh and other prosthetic materials into surrounding organ or tissue
　　　　Extrusion of implanted mesh
　　　　Coding Clinic: 2016, Q4, P71

● T83.721　Exposure of implanted vaginal mesh into vagina A 🐾
　　　　　Exposure of implanted vaginal mesh through vaginal wall

● T83.722　Exposure of implanted urethral mesh into urethra A 🐾
　　　　　Exposure of implanted female urethral sling
　　　　　Exposure of implanted male urethral sling
　　　　　Exposure of implanted urethral mesh through urethral wall

● T83.723　Exposure of implanted urethral bulking agent into urethra A 🐾

● T83.724　Exposure of implanted ureteral bulking agent into ureter A 🐾

● T83.728　Exposure of other implanted mesh into organ or tissue A 🐾
　　　　　Coding Clinic: 2016, Q4, P71

● T83.729　Exposure of other prosthetic materials into organ or tissue A 🐾
　　　　　Coding Clinic: 2016, Q4, P71

X ● T83.79　Other specified complications due to other genitourinary prosthetic materials A 🐾

● T83.8　Other specified complications of genitourinary prosthetic devices, implants and grafts

X ● T83.81　Embolism due to genitourinary prosthetic devices, implants and grafts A 🐾

X ● T83.82　Fibrosis due to genitourinary prosthetic devices, implants and grafts A 🐾

X ● T83.83　Hemorrhage due to genitourinary prosthetic devices, implants and grafts A 🐾

X ● T83.84　Pain due to genitourinary prosthetic devices, implants and grafts A 🐾

X ● T83.85　Stenosis due to genitourinary prosthetic devices, implants and grafts A 🐾

X ● T83.86　Thrombosis due to genitourinary prosthetic devices, implants and grafts A 🐾

X ● T83.89　Other specified complication of genitourinary prosthetic devices, implants and grafts A 🐾
　　　　　Coding Clinic: 2022, Q3, P13

X ● T83.9　Unspecified complication of genitourinary prosthetic device, implant and graft A 🐾

▶ New　⇒ Revised　d̶e̶l̶e̶t̶e̶d̶ Deleted　Excludes 1　Excludes 2　Includes　Use additional　Code first　Code also　Key words
OGCR Official Guidelines　X Assign placeholder X　● Use Additional Character(s)　▶ Manifestation Code　🐾 Hierarchical Condition Category　Coding Clinic

● **T84**   **Complications of internal orthopedic prosthetic devices, implants and grafts**

     Excludes2   failure and rejection of transplanted organs and tissues (T86.-)

                 fracture of bone following insertion of orthopedic implant, joint prosthesis or bone plate (M96.6)

     The appropriate 7th character is to be added to each code from category T84

> A   initial encounter
> D   subsequent encounter
> S   sequela

● **T84.0**   **Mechanical complication of internal joint prosthesis**

   ● **T84.01**   **Broken internal joint prosthesis**

           Breakage (fracture) of prosthetic joint

           Broken prosthetic joint implant

           Excludes1   periprosthetic joint implant fracture (M97.-)

           Coding Clinic: 2016, Q4, P42

     ● **T84.010**   Broken internal right hip prosthesis A ⚙

     ● **T84.011**   Broken internal left hip prosthesis A ⚙

     ● **T84.012**   Broken internal right knee prosthesis A ⚙

     ● **T84.013**   Broken internal left knee prosthesis A ⚙

     ● **T84.018**   Broken internal joint prosthesis, other site A ⚙

           Use additional code to identify the joint (Z96.6-)

     ● **T84.019**   Broken internal joint prosthesis, unspecified site A ⚙

   ● **T84.02**   **Dislocation of internal joint prosthesis**

           Instability of internal joint prosthesis

           Subluxation of internal joint prosthesis

     ● **T84.020**   Dislocation of internal right hip prosthesis A ⚙

     ● **T84.021**   Dislocation of internal left hip prosthesis A ⚙

           Coding Clinic: 2019, Q2, P27

     ● **T84.022**   Instability of internal right knee prosthesis A ⚙

     ● **T84.023**   Instability of internal left knee prosthesis A ⚙

     ● **T84.028**   Dislocation of other internal joint prosthesis A ⚙

           Use additional code to identify the joint (Z96.6-)

     ● **T84.029**   Dislocation of unspecified internal joint prosthesis A ⚙

   ● **T84.03**   **Mechanical loosening of internal prosthetic joint**

           Aseptic loosening of prosthetic joint

     ● **T84.030**   Mechanical loosening of internal right hip prosthetic joint A ⚙

     ● **T84.031**   Mechanical loosening of internal left hip prosthetic joint A ⚙

     ● **T84.032**   Mechanical loosening of internal right knee prosthetic joint A ⚙

     ● **T84.033**   Mechanical loosening of internal left knee prosthetic joint A ⚙

     ● **T84.038**   Mechanical loosening of other internal prosthetic joint A ⚙

           Use additional code to identify the joint (Z96.6-)

     ● **T84.039**   Mechanical loosening of unspecified internal prosthetic joint A ⚙

● **T84.05**   **Periprosthetic osteolysis of internal prosthetic joint**

           Use additional code to identify major osseous defect, if applicable (M89.7-)

     ● **T84.050**   Periprosthetic osteolysis of internal prosthetic right hip joint A ⚙

     ● **T84.051**   Periprosthetic osteolysis of internal prosthetic left hip joint A ⚙

     ● **T84.052**   Periprosthetic osteolysis of internal prosthetic right knee joint A ⚙

     ● **T84.053**   Periprosthetic osteolysis of internal prosthetic left knee joint A ⚙

     ● **T84.058**   Periprosthetic osteolysis of other internal prosthetic joint A ⚙

           Use additional code to identify the joint (Z96.6-)

     ● **T84.059**   Periprosthetic osteolysis of unspecified internal prosthetic joint A ⚙

● **T84.06**   **Wear of articular bearing surface of internal prosthetic joint**

     ● **T84.060**   Wear of articular bearing surface of internal prosthetic right hip joint A ⚙

     ● **T84.061**   Wear of articular bearing surface of internal prosthetic left hip joint A ⚙

     ● **T84.062**   Wear of articular bearing surface of internal prosthetic right knee joint A ⚙

     ● **T84.063**   Wear of articular bearing surface of internal prosthetic left knee joint A ⚙

     ● **T84.068**   Wear of articular bearing surface of other internal prosthetic joint A ⚙

           Use additional code to identify the joint (Z96.6-)

     ● **T84.069**   Wear of articular bearing surface of unspecified internal prosthetic joint A ⚙

● **T84.09**   **Other mechanical complication of internal joint prosthesis**

           Prosthetic joint implant failure NOS

     ● **T84.090**   Other mechanical complication of internal right hip prosthesis A ⚙

           Coding Clinic: 2019, Q1, P20

     ● **T84.091**   Other mechanical complication of internal left hip prosthesis A ⚙

     ● **T84.092**   Other mechanical complication of internal right knee prosthesis A ⚙

     ● **T84.093**   Other mechanical complication of internal left knee prosthesis A ⚙

     ● **T84.098**   Other mechanical complication of other internal joint prosthesis A ⚙

           Use additional code to identify the joint (Z96.6-)

     ● **T84.099**   Other mechanical complication of unspecified internal joint prosthesis A ⚙

● **T84.1**   **Mechanical complication of internal fixation device of bones of limb**

     Excludes2   mechanical complication of internal fixation device of bones of feet (T84.2-)

                 mechanical complication of internal fixation device of bones of fingers (T84.2-)

                 mechanical complication of internal fixation device of bones of hands (T84.2-)

                 mechanical complication of internal fixation device of bones of toes (T84.2-)

- **T84.11** Breakdown (mechanical) of internal fixation device of bones of limb
  - **T84.110** Breakdown (mechanical) of internal fixation device of right humerus A 🐾
  - **T84.111** Breakdown (mechanical) of internal fixation device of left humerus A 🐾
  - **T84.112** Breakdown (mechanical) of internal fixation device of bone of right forearm A 🐾
  - **T84.113** Breakdown (mechanical) of internal fixation device of bone of left forearm A 🐾
  - **T84.114** Breakdown (mechanical) of internal fixation device of right femur A 🐾
  - **T84.115** Breakdown (mechanical) of internal fixation device of left femur A 🐾
  - **T84.116** Breakdown (mechanical) of internal fixation device of bone of right lower leg A 🐾
  - **T84.117** Breakdown (mechanical) of internal fixation device of bone of left lower leg A 🐾
  - **T84.119** Breakdown (mechanical) of internal fixation device of unspecified bone of limb A 🐾
- **T84.12** Displacement of internal fixation device of bones of limb

  Malposition of internal fixation device of bones of limb
  - **T84.120** Displacement of internal fixation device of right humerus A 🐾
  - **T84.121** Displacement of internal fixation device of left humerus A 🐾
  - **T84.122** Displacement of internal fixation device of bone of right forearm A 🐾
  - **T84.123** Displacement of internal fixation device of bone of left forearm A 🐾
  - **T84.124** Displacement of internal fixation device of right femur A 🐾
  - **T84.125** Displacement of internal fixation device of left femur A 🐾
  - **T84.126** Displacement of internal fixation device of bone of right lower leg A 🐾
  - **T84.127** Displacement of internal fixation device of bone of left lower leg A 🐾
  - **T84.129** Displacement of internal fixation device of unspecified bone of limb A 🐾
- **T84.19** Other mechanical complication of internal fixation device of bones of limb

  Obstruction (mechanical) of internal fixation device of bones of limb

  Perforation of internal fixation device of bones of limb

  Protrusion of internal fixation device of bones of limb
  - **T84.190** Other mechanical complication of internal fixation device of right humerus A 🐾
  - **T84.191** Other mechanical complication of internal fixation device of left humerus A 🐾
  - **T84.192** Other mechanical complication of internal fixation device of bone of right forearm A 🐾
  - **T84.193** Other mechanical complication of internal fixation device of bone of left forearm A 🐾
  - **T84.194** Other mechanical complication of internal fixation device of right femur A 🐾

- **T84.195** Other mechanical complication of internal fixation device of left femur A 🐾
- **T84.196** Other mechanical complication of internal fixation device of bone of right lower leg A 🐾
- **T84.197** Other mechanical complication of internal fixation device of bone of left lower leg A 🐾
- **T84.199** Other mechanical complication of internal fixation device of unspecified bone of limb A 🐾
- **T84.2** Mechanical complication of internal fixation device of other bones
  - **T84.21** Breakdown (mechanical) of internal fixation device of other bones
    - **T84.210** Breakdown (mechanical) of internal fixation device of bones of hand and fingers A 🐾
    - **T84.213** Breakdown (mechanical) of internal fixation device of bones of foot and toes A 🐾
    - **T84.216** Breakdown (mechanical) of internal fixation device of vertebrae A 🐾
    - **T84.218** Breakdown (mechanical) of internal fixation device of other bones A 🐾
  - **T84.22** Displacement of internal fixation device of other bones

    Malposition of internal fixation device of other bones
    - **T84.220** Displacement of internal fixation device of bones of hand and fingers A 🐾
    - **T84.223** Displacement of internal fixation device of bones of foot and toes A 🐾
    - **T84.226** Displacement of internal fixation device of vertebrae A 🐾
    - **T84.228** Displacement of internal fixation device of other bones A 🐾
  - **T84.29** Other mechanical complication of internal fixation device of other bones

    Obstruction (mechanical) of internal fixation device of other bones

    Perforation of internal fixation device of other bones

    Protrusion of internal fixation device of other bones
    - **T84.290** Other mechanical complication of internal fixation device of bones of hand and fingers A 🐾
    - **T84.293** Other mechanical complication of internal fixation device of bones of foot and toes A 🐾
    - **T84.296** Other mechanical complication of internal fixation device of vertebrae A 🐾

      Coding Clinic: 2024, Q2, P12
    - **T84.298** Other mechanical complication of internal fixation device of other bones A 🐾
- **T84.3** Mechanical complication of other bone devices, implants and grafts

  Excludes2 other complications of bone graft (T86.83-)
  - **T84.31** Breakdown (mechanical) of other bone devices, implants and grafts
    - **T84.310** Breakdown (mechanical) of electronic bone stimulator A 🐾
    - **T84.318** Breakdown (mechanical) of other bone devices, implants and grafts A 🐾
  - **T84.32** Displacement of other bone devices, implants and grafts

    Malposition of other bone devices, implants and grafts

● T84.320   Displacement of electronic bone stimulator A 🦟

● T84.328   Displacement of other bone devices, implants and grafts A 🦟

● T84.39   Other mechanical complication of other bone devices, implants and grafts
  Obstruction (mechanical) of other bone devices, implants and grafts
  Perforation of other bone devices, implants and grafts
  Protrusion of other bone devices, implants and grafts

● T84.390   Other mechanical complication of electronic bone stimulator A 🦟

● T84.398   Other mechanical complication of other bone devices, implants and grafts A 🦟

● T84.4   Mechanical complication of other internal orthopedic devices, implants and grafts

● T84.41   Breakdown (mechanical) of other internal orthopedic devices, implants and grafts

● T84.410   Breakdown (mechanical) of muscle and tendon graft A 🦟

● T84.418   Breakdown (mechanical) of other internal orthopedic devices, implants and grafts A 🦟

● T84.42   Displacement of other internal orthopedic devices, implants and grafts
  Malposition of other internal orthopedic devices, implants and grafts

● T84.420   Displacement of muscle and tendon graft A 🦟

● T84.428   Displacement of other internal orthopedic devices, implants and grafts A 🦟

● T84.49   Other mechanical complication of other internal orthopedic devices, implants and grafts
  Mechanical complication of other internal orthopedic devices, implants and grafts NOS
  Obstruction (mechanical) of other internal orthopedic devices, implants and grafts
  Perforation of other internal orthopedic devices, implants and grafts
  Protrusion of other internal orthopedic devices, implants and grafts

● T84.490   Other mechanical complication of muscle and tendon graft A 🦟

● T84.498   Other mechanical complication of other internal orthopedic devices, implants and grafts A 🦟

● T84.5   Infection and inflammatory reaction due to internal joint prosthesis
  Use additional code to identify infection
  Coding Clinic: 2015, Q1, P16

X ● T84.50   Infection and inflammatory reaction due to unspecified internal joint prosthesis A 🦟
  Coding Clinic: 2015, Q1, P3

X ● T84.51   Infection and inflammatory reaction due to internal right hip prosthesis A 🦟
  Coding Clinic: 2015, Q4, P36

X ● T84.52   Infection and inflammatory reaction due to internal left hip prosthesis A 🦟
  Coding Clinic: 2015, Q1, P16-17

X ● T84.53   Infection and inflammatory reaction due to internal right knee prosthesis A 🦟

X ● T84.54   Infection and inflammatory reaction due to internal left knee prosthesis A 🦟
  Coding Clinic: 2019, Q3, P16

X ● T84.59   Infection and inflammatory reaction due to other internal joint prosthesis A 🦟

● T84.6   Infection and inflammatory reaction due to internal fixation device
  Use additional code to identify infection

X ● T84.60   Infection and inflammatory reaction due to internal fixation device of unspecified site A 🦟

● T84.61   Infection and inflammatory reaction due to internal fixation device of arm

● T84.610   Infection and inflammatory reaction due to internal fixation device of right humerus A 🦟

● T84.611   Infection and inflammatory reaction due to internal fixation device of left humerus A 🦟

● T84.612   Infection and inflammatory reaction due to internal fixation device of right radius A 🦟

● T84.613   Infection and inflammatory reaction due to internal fixation device of left radius A 🦟

● T84.614   Infection and inflammatory reaction due to internal fixation device of right ulna A 🦟

● T84.615   Infection and inflammatory reaction due to internal fixation device of left ulna A 🦟

● T84.619   Infection and inflammatory reaction due to internal fixation device of unspecified bone of arm A 🦟

● T84.62   Infection and inflammatory reaction due to internal fixation device of leg

● T84.620   Infection and inflammatory reaction due to internal fixation device of right femur A 🦟

● T84.621   Infection and inflammatory reaction due to internal fixation device of left femur A 🦟

● T84.622   Infection and inflammatory reaction due to internal fixation device of right tibia A 🦟

● T84.623   Infection and inflammatory reaction due to internal fixation device of left tibia A 🦟

● T84.624   Infection and inflammatory reaction due to internal fixation device of right fibula A 🦟

● T84.625   Infection and inflammatory reaction due to internal fixation device of left fibula A 🦟

● T84.629   Infection and inflammatory reaction due to internal fixation device of unspecified bone of leg A 🦟

X ● T84.63   Infection and inflammatory reaction due to internal fixation device of spine A 🦟

X ● T84.69   Infection and inflammatory reaction due to internal fixation device of other site A 🦟

● T84.7   Infection and inflammatory reaction due to other internal orthopedic prosthetic devices, implants and grafts A 🦟
  Use additional code to identify infection

● T84.8   Other specified complications of internal orthopedic prosthetic devices, implants and grafts

X ● T84.81   Embolism due to internal orthopedic prosthetic devices, implants and grafts A 🦟

X ● T84.82   Fibrosis due to internal orthopedic prosthetic devices, implants and grafts A 🦟

X ● T84.83   Hemorrhage due to internal orthopedic prosthetic devices, implants and grafts A 🦟

X ● T84.84   Pain due to internal orthopedic prosthetic devices, implants and grafts A 🦟
  Coding Clinic: 2024, Q2, P13

X ● T84.85   Stenosis due to internal orthopedic prosthetic devices, implants and grafts A 🦟

X● **T84.86** Thrombosis due to internal orthopedic prosthetic devices, implants and grafts A 🐾

X● **T84.89** Other specified complication of internal orthopedic prosthetic devices, implants and grafts A 🐾

X● **T84.9** Unspecified complication of internal orthopedic prosthetic device, implant and graft A 🐾

● **T85** Complications of other internal prosthetic devices, implants and grafts

Excludes2 failure and rejection of transplanted organs and tissue (T86.-)

The appropriate 7th character is to be added to each code from category T85

> A initial encounter
> D subsequent encounter
> S sequela

Coding Clinic: 2016, Q4, P71

● **T85.0** Mechanical complication of ventricular intracranial (communicating) shunt

X● **T85.01** Breakdown (mechanical) of ventricular intracranial (communicating) shunt A 🐾

X● **T85.02** Displacement of ventricular intracranial (communicating) shunt A 🐾
Malposition of ventricular intracranial (communicating) shunt

X● **T85.03** Leakage of ventricular intracranial (communicating) shunt A 🐾

X● **T85.09** Other mechanical complication of ventricular intracranial (communicating) shunt A 🐾
Obstruction (mechanical) of ventricular intracranial (communicating) shunt
Perforation of ventricular intracranial (communicating) shunt
Protrusion of ventricular intracranial (communicating) shunt

● **T85.1** Mechanical complication of implanted electronic stimulator of nervous system
Coding Clinic: 2016, Q4, P71

● **T85.11** Breakdown (mechanical) of implanted electronic stimulator of nervous system

● **T85.110** Breakdown (mechanical) of implanted electronic neurostimulator of brain electrode (lead) A 🐾

● **T85.111** Breakdown (mechanical) of implanted electronic neurostimulator of peripheral nerve electrode (lead) A 🐾
Breakdown of electrode (lead) for cranial nerve neurostimulators
Breakdown of electrode (lead) for gastric neurostimulator
Breakdown of electrode (lead) for sacral nerve neurostimulator
Breakdown of electrode (lead) for vagal nerve neurostimulators

● **T85.112** Breakdown (mechanical) of implanted electronic neurostimulator of spinal cord electrode (lead) A 🐾

● **T85.113** Breakdown (mechanical) of implanted electronic neurostimulator, generator A 🐾
Breakdown (mechanical) of implanted electronic neurostimulator generator, brain, peripheral, gastric, spinal
Breakdown (mechanical) of implanted electronic sacral neurostimulator, pulse generator or receiver

● **T85.118** Breakdown (mechanical) of other implanted electronic stimulator of nervous system A 🐾

● **T85.12** Displacement of implanted electronic stimulator of nervous system
Malposition of implanted electronic stimulator of nervous system

● **T85.120** Displacement of implanted electronic neurostimulator of brain electrode (lead) A 🐾

● **T85.121** Displacement of implanted electronic neurostimulator of peripheral nerve electrode (lead) A 🐾
Displacement of electrode (lead) for cranial nerve neurostimulators
Displacement of electrode (lead) for gastric neurostimulator
Displacement of electrode (lead) for sacral nerve neurostimulator
Displacement of electrode (lead) for vagal nerve neurostimulators

● **T85.122** Displacement of implanted electronic neurostimulator of spinal cord electrode (lead) A 🐾

● **T85.123** Displacement of implanted electronic neurostimulator, generator A 🐾
Displacement of implanted electronic neurostimulator generator, brain, peripheral, gastric, spinal
Displacement of implanted electronic sacral neurostimulator, pulse generator or receiver

● **T85.128** Displacement of other implanted electronic stimulator of nervous system A 🐾

● **T85.19** Other mechanical complication of implanted electronic stimulator of nervous system
Leakage of implanted electronic stimulator of nervous system
Obstruction (mechanical) of implanted electronic stimulator of nervous system
Perforation of implanted electronic stimulator of nervous system
Protrusion of implanted electronic stimulator of nervous system

● **T85.190** Other mechanical complication of implanted electronic neurostimulator of brain electrode (lead) A 🐾

● **T85.191** Other mechanical complication of implanted electronic neurostimulator of peripheral nerve electrode (lead) A 🐾
Other mechanical complication of electrode (lead) for cranial nerve neurostimulators
Other mechanical complication of electrode (lead) for gastric neurostimulator
Other mechanical complication of electrode (lead) for sacral nerve neurostimulator
Other mechanical complication of electrode (lead) for vagal nerve neurostimulators

● **T85.192** Other mechanical complication of implanted electronic neurostimulator of spinal cord electrode (lead) A 🐾

▶ New   ⟹ Revised   ~~deleted~~ Deleted   Excludes 1   Excludes 2   Includes   Use additional   Code first   Code also   Key words
OGCR Official Guidelines   X Assign placeholder X   ● Use Additional Character(s)   ▸ Manifestation Code   🐾 Hierarchical Condition Category   Coding Clinic

CHAPTER 19 (S00-T88)

● T85.193   Other mechanical complication of implanted electronic neurostimulator, generator A 🔐
        Other mechanical complication of implanted electronic neurostimulator generator, brain, peripheral, gastric, spinal
        Other mechanical complication of implanted electronic sacral neurostimulator, pulse generator or receiver

● T85.199   Other mechanical complication of other implanted electronic stimulator of nervous system A 🔐

● T85.2   Mechanical complication of intraocular lens
X ● T85.21   Breakdown (mechanical) of intraocular lens
X ● T85.22   Displacement of intraocular lens
        Malposition of intraocular lens

X ● T85.29   Other mechanical complication of intraocular lens
        Obstruction (mechanical) of intraocular lens
        Perforation of intraocular lens
        Protrusion of intraocular lens

● T85.3   Mechanical complication of other ocular prosthetic devices, implants and grafts
        Excludes2   other complications of corneal graft (T86.84-)

● T85.31   Breakdown (mechanical) of other ocular prosthetic devices, implants and grafts
  ● T85.310   Breakdown (mechanical) of prosthetic orbit of right eye
  ● T85.311   Breakdown (mechanical) of prosthetic orbit of left eye
  ● T85.318   Breakdown (mechanical) of other ocular prosthetic devices, implants and grafts

● T85.32   Displacement of other ocular prosthetic devices, implants and grafts
        Malposition of other ocular prosthetic devices, implants and grafts
  ● T85.320   Displacement of prosthetic orbit of right eye
  ● T85.321   Displacement of prosthetic orbit of left eye
  ● T85.328   Displacement of other ocular prosthetic devices, implants and grafts

● T85.39   Other mechanical complication of other ocular prosthetic devices, implants and grafts
        Obstruction (mechanical) of other ocular prosthetic devices, implants and grafts
        Perforation of other ocular prosthetic devices, implants and grafts
        Protrusion of other ocular prosthetic devices, implants and grafts
  ● T85.390   Other mechanical complication of prosthetic orbit of right eye
  ● T85.391   Other mechanical complication of prosthetic orbit of left eye
  ● T85.398   Other mechanical complication of other ocular prosthetic devices, implants and grafts

● T85.4   Mechanical complication of breast prosthesis and implant
X ● T85.41   Breakdown (mechanical) of breast prosthesis and implant
X ● T85.42   Displacement of breast prosthesis and implant
        Malposition of breast prosthesis and implant
X ● T85.43   Leakage of breast prosthesis and implant
X ● T85.44   Capsular contracture of breast implant

X ● T85.49   Other mechanical complication of breast prosthesis and implant
        Obstruction (mechanical) of breast prosthesis and implant
        Perforation of breast prosthesis and implant
        Protrusion of breast prosthesis and implant

● T85.5   Mechanical complication of gastrointestinal prosthetic devices, implants and grafts
● T85.51   Breakdown (mechanical) of gastrointestinal prosthetic devices, implants and grafts
  ● T85.510   Breakdown (mechanical) of bile duct prosthesis
  ● T85.511   Breakdown (mechanical) of esophageal anti-reflux device
  ● T85.518   Breakdown (mechanical) of other gastrointestinal prosthetic devices, implants and grafts

● T85.52   Displacement of gastrointestinal prosthetic devices, implants and grafts
        Malposition of gastrointestinal prosthetic devices, implants and grafts
  ● T85.520   Displacement of bile duct prosthesis
  ● T85.521   Displacement of esophageal anti-reflux device
  ● T85.528   Displacement of other gastrointestinal prosthetic devices, implants and grafts

● T85.59   Other mechanical complication of gastrointestinal prosthetic devices, implants and
        Obstruction, mechanical of gastrointestinal prosthetic devices, implants and grafts
        Perforation of gastrointestinal prosthetic devices, implants and grafts
        Protrusion of gastrointestinal prosthetic devices, implants and grafts
  ● T85.590   Other mechanical complication of bile duct prosthesis
  ● T85.591   Other mechanical complication of esophageal anti-reflux device
  ● T85.598   Other mechanical complication of other gastrointestinal prosthetic devices, implants and grafts

● T85.6   Mechanical complication of other specified internal and external prosthetic devices, implants and grafts
        Coding Clinic: 2016, Q4, P71

● T85.61   Breakdown (mechanical) of other specified internal prosthetic devices, implants and grafts
  ● T85.610   Breakdown (mechanical) of cranial or spinal infusion catheter
        Breakdown (mechanical) of epidural infusion catheter
        Breakdown (mechanical) of intrathecal infusion catheter
        Breakdown (mechanical) of subarachnoid infusion catheter
        Breakdown (mechanical) of subdural infusion catheter
  ● T85.611   Breakdown (mechanical) of intraperitoneal dialysis catheter A, D, S 🔐
        Excludes1   mechanical complication of vascular dialysis catheter (T82.4-)
  ● T85.612   Breakdown (mechanical) of permanent sutures
        Excludes1   mechanical complication of permanent (wire) suture used in bone repair (T84.1-T84.2)

CHAPTER 19 (S00-T88)

● T85.613   **Breakdown (mechanical) of artificial skin graft and decellularized allodermis**
Failure of artificial skin graft and decellularized allodermis
Non-adherence of artificial skin graft and decellularized allodermis
Poor incorporation of artificial skin graft and decellularized allodermis
Shearing of artificial skin graft and decellularized allodermis

● T85.614   **Breakdown (mechanical) of insulin pump**

● T85.615   **Breakdown (mechanical) of other nervous system device, implant or graft A** 🐾
Breakdown (mechanical) of intrathecal infusion pump

● T85.618   **Breakdown (mechanical) of other specified internal prosthetic devices, implants and grafts**

● T85.62   **Displacement of other specified internal prosthetic devices, implants and grafts**
Malposition of other specified internal prosthetic devices, implants and grafts

● T85.620   **Displacement of cranial or spinal infusion catheter**
Displacement of epidural infusion catheter
Displacement of intrathecal infusion catheter
Displacement of subarachnoid infusion catheter
Displacement of subdural infusion catheter

● T85.621   **Displacement of intraperitoneal dialysis catheter A, D, S** 🐾
Excludes1   mechanical complication of vascular dialysis catheter (T82.4-)

● T85.622   **Displacement of permanent sutures**
Excludes1   mechanical complication of permanent (wire) suture used in bone repair (T84.1-T84.2)

● T85.623   **Displacement of artificial skin graft and decellularized allodermis**
Dislodgement of artificial skin graft and decellularized allodermis

● T85.624   **Displacement of insulin pump**

● T85.625   **Displacement of other nervous system device, implant or graft A** 🐾
Displacement of intrathecal infusion pump

● T85.628   **Displacement of other specified internal prosthetic devices, implants and grafts**
Coding Clinic: 2015, Q1, P15

● T85.63   **Leakage of other specified internal prosthetic devices, implants and grafts**

● T85.630   **Leakage of cranial or spinal infusion catheter**
Leakage of epidural infusion catheter
Leakage of intrathecal infusion catheter
Leakage of subdural infusion catheter
Leakage of subarachnoid infusion catheter
Coding Clinic: 2022, Q3, P24

● T85.631   **Leakage of intraperitoneal dialysis catheter A, D, S** 🐾
Excludes1   mechanical complication of vascular dialysis catheter (T82.4)

● T85.633   **Leakage of insulin pump**

● T85.635   **Leakage of other nervous system device, implant or graft A** 🐾
Leakage of intrathecal infusion pump

● T85.638   **Leakage of other specified internal prosthetic devices, implants and grafts**

● T85.69   **Other mechanical complication of other specified internal prosthetic devices, implants and grafts**
Obstruction, mechanical of other specified internal prosthetic devices, implants and grafts
Perforation of other specified internal prosthetic devices, implants and grafts
Protrusion of other specified internal prosthetic devices, implants and grafts

● T85.690   **Other mechanical complication of cranial or spinal infusion catheter**
Other mechanical complication of epidural infusion catheter
Other mechanical complication of intrathecal infusion catheter
Other mechanical complication of subarachnoid infusion catheter
Other mechanical complication of subdural infusion catheter

● T85.691   **Other mechanical complication of intraperitoneal dialysis catheter A, D, S** 🐾
Excludes1   mechanical complication of vascular dialysis catheter (T82.4)

● T85.692   **Other mechanical complication of permanent sutures**
Excludes1   mechanical complication of permanent (wire) suture used in bone repair (T84.1-T84.2)

● T85.693   **Other mechanical complication of artificial skin graft and decellularized allodermis**

● T85.694   **Other mechanical complication of insulin pump**

● T85.695   **Other mechanical complication of other nervous system device, implant or graft A** 🐾
Other mechanical complication of intrathecal infusion pump

● T85.698   **Other mechanical complication of other specified internal prosthetic devices, implants and grafts**
Mechanical complication of nonabsorbable surgical material NOS

● T85.7   **Infection and inflammatory reaction due to other internal prosthetic devices, implants and grafts**
Use additional code to identify infection
Coding Clinic: 2016, Q4, P72

X ● T85.71   **Infection and inflammatory reaction due to peritoneal dialysis catheter A, D, S** 🐾

X ● T85.72   **Infection and inflammatory reaction due to insulin pump A** 🐾

● **T85.73**   **Infection and inflammatory reaction due to nervous system devices, implants and graft**

  ● **T85.730**   **Infection and inflammatory reaction due to ventricular intracranial (communicating) shunt** A 🐾

  ● **T85.731**   **Infection and inflammatory reaction due to implanted electronic neurostimulator of brain, electrode (lead)** A 🐾

  ● **T85.732**   **Infection and inflammatory reaction due to implanted electronic neurostimulator of peripheral nerve, electrode (lead)** A 🐾
      Infection and inflammatory reaction due to electrode (lead) for cranial nerve neurostimulators
      Infection and inflammatory reaction due to electrode (lead) for gastric neurostimulator
      Infection and inflammatory reaction due to electrode (lead) for sacral nerve neurostimulator
      Infection and inflammatory reaction due to electrode (lead) for vagal nerve neurostimulators

  ● **T85.733**   **Infection and inflammatory reaction due to implanted electronic neurostimulator of spinal cord, electrode (lead)** A 🐾

  ● **T85.734**   **Infection and inflammatory reaction due to implanted electronic neurostimulator, generator** A 🐾
      Generator pocket infection

  ● **T85.735**   **Infection and inflammatory reaction due to cranial or spinal infusion catheter** A 🐾
      Infection and inflammatory reaction due to epidural catheter
      Infection and inflammatory reaction due to intrathecal infusion catheter
      Infection and inflammatory reaction due to subarachnoid catheter
      Infection and inflammatory reaction due to subdural catheter

  ● **T85.738**   **Infection and inflammatory reaction due to other nervous system device, implant or graft** A 🐾
      Infection and inflammatory reaction due to intrathecal infusion pump

X ● **T85.79**   **Infection and inflammatory reaction due to other internal prosthetic devices, implants and grafts** A 🐾
      Coding Clinic: 2023, Q2, P28; 2022, Q2, P8; 2016, Q4, P72

● **T85.8**   **Other specified complications of internal prosthetic devices, implants and grafts, not elsewhere classified**
      Coding Clinic: 2016, Q4, P72

  ● **T85.81**   **Embolism due to internal prosthetic devices, implants and grafts, not elsewhere classified**

    ● **T85.810**   **Embolism due to nervous system prosthetic devices, implants and grafts** A 🐾

    ● **T85.818**   **Embolism due to other internal prosthetic devices, implants and grafts**

  ● **T85.82**   **Fibrosis due to internal prosthetic devices, implants and grafts, not elsewhere classified**

    ● **T85.820**   **Fibrosis due to nervous system prosthetic devices, implants and grafts** A 🐾

    ● **T85.828**   **Fibrosis due to other internal prosthetic devices, implants and grafts**

● **T85.83**   **Hemorrhage due to internal prosthetic devices, implants and grafts, not elsewhere classified**

  ● **T85.830**   **Hemorrhage due to nervous system prosthetic devices, implants and grafts** A 🐾

  ● **T85.838**   **Hemorrhage due to other internal prosthetic devices, implants and grafts**

● **T85.84**   **Pain due to internal prosthetic devices, implants and grafts, not elsewhere classified**

  ● **T85.840**   **Pain due to nervous system prosthetic devices, implants and grafts** A 🐾

  ● **T85.848**   **Pain due to other internal prosthetic devices, implants and grafts**

● **T85.85**   **Stenosis due to internal prosthetic devices, implants and grafts, not elsewhere classified**

  ● **T85.850**   **Stenosis due to nervous system prosthetic devices, implants and grafts** A 🐾

  ● **T85.858**   **Stenosis due to other internal prosthetic devices, implants and grafts**

● **T85.86**   **Thrombosis due to internal prosthetic devices, implants and grafts, not elsewhere classified**

  ● **T85.860**   **Thrombosis due to nervous system prosthetic devices, implants and grafts** A 🐾

  ● **T85.868**   **Thrombosis due to other internal prosthetic devices, implants and grafts**
      Coding Clinic: 2024, Q2, P7

● **T85.89**   **Other specified complication of internal prosthetic devices, implants and grafts, not elsewhere classified**
      Coding Clinic: 2024, Q2, P8; 2016, Q4, P72

  ● **T85.890**   **Other specified complication of nervous system prosthetic devices, implants and grafts** A 🐾

  ● **T85.898**   **Other specified complication of other internal prosthetic devices, implants and grafts**
      Coding Clinic: 2024, Q2, P8

X ● **T85.9**   **Unspecified complication of internal prosthetic device, implant and graft**
      Complication of internal prosthetic device, implant and graft NOS

OGCR Section I.C.19.g.3.

Organ Transplant Complications

Transplant Complications

(a) Transplant complications other than kidney

Codes under category T86, Complications of transplanted organs and tissues, are for use for both complications and rejection of transplanted organs. A transplant complication code is only assigned if the complication affects the function of the transplanted organ. Two codes are required to fully describe a transplant complication: the appropriate code from category T86 and a secondary code that identifies the complication.

Pre-existing conditions or conditions that develop after the transplant are not coded as complications unless they affect the function of the transplanted organs.

See I.C.21 for transplant organ removal status.

See I.C.2 for malignant neoplasm associated with transplanted organ.

● **T86**   **Complications of transplanted organs and tissue**
      Use additional code to identify other transplant complications, such as:
      graft-versus-host disease (D89.81-)
      malignancy associated with organ transplant (C80.2)
      post-transplant lymphoproliferative disorders (PTLD) (D47.Z1)

  ● **T86.0**   **Complications of bone marrow transplant**

     T86.00   **Unspecified complication of bone marrow transplant** 🐾

T86.01 Bone marrow transplant rejection 🅗
T86.02 Bone marrow transplant failure 🅗
T86.03 Bone marrow transplant infection 🅗
T86.09 Other complications of bone marrow transplant 🅗
    Coding Clinic: 2023, Q3, P20
T86.1 Complications of kidney transplant
  T86.10 Unspecified complication of kidney transplant
  T86.11 Kidney transplant rejection
  T86.12 Kidney transplant failure
    Coding Clinic: 2013, Q1, P24
  T86.13 Kidney transplant infection
    Use additional code to specify infection
  T86.19 Other complication of kidney transplant
    Coding Clinic: 2019, Q2, P7
T86.2 Complications of heart transplant
  Excludes1 complication of:
    artificial heart device (T82.5-)
    heart-lung transplant (T86.3-)
  T86.20 Unspecified complication of heart transplant 🅗
  T86.21 Heart transplant rejection 🅗
  T86.22 Heart transplant failure 🅗
  T86.23 Heart transplant infection 🅗
    Use additional code to specify infection
  T86.29 Other complications of heart transplant
    T86.290 Cardiac allograft vasculopathy 🅗
      Excludes1 atherosclerosis of coronary arteries (I25.75-, I25.76-, I25.81-)
    T86.298 Other complications of heart transplant 🅗
T86.3 Complications of heart-lung transplant
  T86.30 Unspecified complication of heart-lung transplant 🅗
  T86.31 Heart-lung transplant rejection 🅗
  T86.32 Heart-lung transplant failure 🅗
  T86.33 Heart-lung transplant infection 🅗
    Use additional code to specify infection
  T86.39 Other complications of heart-lung transplant 🅗
T86.4 Complications of liver transplant
  T86.40 Unspecified complication of liver transplant 🅗
  T86.41 Liver transplant rejection 🅗
  T86.42 Liver transplant failure 🅗
  T86.43 Liver transplant infection 🅗
    Use additional code to identify infection, such as:
    Cytomegalovirus (CMV) infection (B25.-)
  T86.49 Other complications of liver transplant 🅗
T86.5 Complications of stem cell transplant 🅗
  Complications from stem cells from peripheral blood
  Complications from stem cells from umbilical cord
T86.8 Complications of other transplanted organs and tissues
  T86.81 Complications of lung transplant
    Excludes1 complication of heart-lung transplant (T86.3-)
    T86.810 Lung transplant rejection 🅗
    T86.811 Lung transplant failure 🅗
    T86.812 Lung transplant infection 🅗
      Use additional code to specify infection
    T86.818 Other complications of lung transplant 🅗
      Coding Clinic: 2019, Q2, P7
    T86.819 Unspecified complication of lung transplant 🅗

T86.82 Complications of skin graft (allograft) (autograft)
  Excludes2 complication of artificial skin graft (T85.693)
  T86.820 Skin graft (allograft) rejection
  T86.821 Skin graft (allograft) (autograft) failure
  T86.822 Skin graft (allograft) (autograft) infection
    Use additional code to specify infection
  T86.828 Other complications of skin graft (allograft) (autograft)
  T86.829 Unspecified complication of skin graft (allograft) (autograft)
T86.83 Complications of bone graft
  Excludes2 mechanical complications of bone graft (T84.3-)
  T86.830 Bone graft rejection
  T86.831 Bone graft failure
  T86.832 Bone graft infection
    Use additional code to specify infection
  T86.838 Other complications of bone graft
    Coding Clinic: 2023, Q1, P31
  T86.839 Unspecified complication of bone graft
T86.84 Complications of corneal transplant
  Excludes2 mechanical complications of corneal graft (T85.3-)
  T86.840 Corneal transplant rejection
    T86.8401 Corneal transplant rejection, right eye
    T86.8402 Corneal transplant rejection, left eye
    T86.8403 Corneal transplant rejection, bilateral
    T86.8409 Corneal transplant rejection, unspecified eye
  T86.841 Corneal transplant failure
    T86.8411 Corneal transplant failure, right eye
    T86.8412 Corneal transplant failure, left eye
    T86.8413 Corneal transplant failure, bilateral
    T86.8419 Corneal transplant failure, unspecified eye
  T86.842 Corneal transplant infection 🅗
    Use additional code to specify infection
    T86.8421 Corneal transplant infection, right eye
    T86.8422 Corneal transplant infection, left eye
    T86.8423 Corneal transplant infection, bilateral
    T86.8429 Corneal transplant infection, unspecified eye
  T86.848 Other complications of corneal transplant
    T86.8481 Other complications of corneal transplant, right eye
    T86.8482 Other complications of corneal transplant, left eye
    T86.8483 Other complications of corneal transplant, bilateral

T86.8489   Other complications of corneal transplant, unspecified eye

● T86.849   Unspecified complication of corneal transplant

T86.8491   Unspecified complication of corneal transplant, right eye

T86.8492   Unspecified complication of corneal transplant, left eye

T86.8493   Unspecified complication of corneal transplant, bilateral

T86.8499   Unspecified complication of corneal transplant, unspecified eye

● T86.85   Complication of intestine transplant

T86.850   Intestine transplant rejection 🦠

T86.851   Intestine transplant failure 🦠

T86.852   Intestine transplant infection 🦠
     Use additional code to specify infection

T86.858   Other complications of intestine transplant 🦠

T86.859   Unspecified complication of intestine transplant 🦠

● T86.89   Complications of other transplanted tissue
     Transplant failure or rejection of pancreas

T86.890   Other transplanted tissue rejection

T86.891   Other transplanted tissue failure

T86.892   Other transplanted tissue infection
     Use additional code to specify infection

T86.898   Other complications of other transplanted tissue

T86.899   Unspecified complication of other transplanted tissue

● T86.9   Complication of unspecified transplanted organ and tissue

T86.90   Unspecified complication of unspecified transplanted organ and tissue

T86.91   Unspecified transplanted organ and tissue rejection

T86.92   Unspecified transplanted organ and tissue failure

T86.93   Unspecified transplanted organ and tissue infection
     Use additional code to specify infection

T86.99   Other complications of unspecified transplanted organ and tissue

● T87   Complications peculiar to reattachment and amputation

● T87.0   Complications of reattached (part of) upper extremity

● T87.0X   Complications of reattached (part of) upper extremity

T87.0X1   Complications of reattached (part of) right upper extremity 🦠

T87.0X2   Complications of reattached (part of) left upper extremity 🦠

T87.0X9   Complications of reattached (part of) unspecified upper extremity 🦠

● T87.1   Complications of reattached (part of) lower extremity

● T87.1X   Complications of reattached (part of) lower extremity

T87.1X1   Complications of reattached (part of) right lower extremity 🦠

T87.1X2   Complications of reattached (part of) left lower extremity 🦠

T87.1X9   Complications of reattached (part of) unspecified lower extremity 🦠

T87.2   Complications of other reattached body part 🦠

● T87.3   Neuroma of amputation stump

T87.30   Neuroma of amputation stump, unspecified extremity 🦠

T87.31   Neuroma of amputation stump, right upper extremity 🦠

T87.32   Neuroma of amputation stump, left upper extremity 🦠

T87.33   Neuroma of amputation stump, right lower extremity 🦠

T87.34   Neuroma of amputation stump, left lower extremity 🦠

● T87.4   Infection of amputation stump

T87.40   Infection of amputation stump, unspecified extremity 🦠

T87.41   Infection of amputation stump, right upper extremity 🦠

T87.42   Infection of amputation stump, left upper extremity 🦠

T87.43   Infection of amputation stump, right lower extremity 🦠

T87.44   Infection of amputation stump, left lower extremity 🦠

● T87.5   Necrosis of amputation stump

T87.50   Necrosis of amputation stump, unspecified extremity 🦠

T87.51   Necrosis of amputation stump, right upper extremity 🦠

T87.52   Necrosis of amputation stump, left upper extremity 🦠

T87.53   Necrosis of amputation stump, right lower extremity 🦠

T87.54   Necrosis of amputation stump, left lower extremity 🦠

● T87.8   Other complications of amputation stump

T87.81   Dehiscence of amputation stump 🦠

T87.89   Other complications of amputation stump 🦠
     Amputation stump contracture
     Amputation stump contracture of next proximal joint
     Amputation stump flexion
     Amputation stump edema
     Amputation stump hematoma
     Excludes2   phantom limb syndrome (G54.6-G54.7)
     Coding Clinic: 2022, Q3, P11

T87.9   Unspecified complications of amputation stump 🦠

● T88   Other complications of surgical and medical care, not elsewhere classified

     Excludes2   complication following infusion, transfusion and therapeutic injection (T80.-)
     complication following procedure NEC (T81.-)
     complications of anesthesia in labor and delivery (O74.-)
     complications of anesthesia in pregnancy (O29.-)
     complications of anesthesia in puerperium (O89.-)
     complications of devices, implants and grafts (T82-T85)
     complications of obstetric surgery and procedure (O75.4)
     dermatitis due to drugs and medicaments (L23.3, L24.4, L25.1, L27.0-L27.1)
     poisoning and toxic effects of drugs and chemicals (T36-T65 with fifth or sixth character 1-4)
     specified complications classified elsewhere

The appropriate 7th character is to be added to each code from category T88

A	initial encounter
D	subsequent encounter
S	sequela

CHAPTER 19 (S00-T88)

CHAPTER 19 (S00-T88)

X● **T88.0** **Infection following immunization**
Sepsis following immunization
Coding Clinic: 2019, Q1, P14;2018, Q4, P90

X● **T88.1** **Other complications following immunization, not elsewhere classified**
Generalized vaccinia
Rash following immunization

> **Excludes1**   vaccinia not from vaccine (B08.011)
> **Excludes2**   anaphylactic shock due to serum (T80.5-)
> other serum reactions (T80.6-)
> postimmunization arthropathy (M02.2)
> postimmunization encephalitis (G04 02)
> postimmunization fever (R50.83)

X● **T88.2** **Shock due to anesthesia**
Use additional code for adverse effect, if applicable, to identify drug (T41.- with fifth or sixth character 5)

> **Excludes1**   complications of anesthesia (in):
> labor and delivery (O74.-)
> pregnancy (O29.-)
> puerperium (O89.-)
> postprocedural shock NOS (T81.1-)

X● **T88.3** **Malignant hyperthermia due to anesthesia**
Use additional code for adverse effect, if applicable, to identify drug (T41.- with fifth or sixth character 5)

X● **T88.4** **Failed or difficult intubation**

● **T88.5** **Other complications of anesthesia**
Use additional code for adverse effect, if applicable, to identify drug (T41.- with fifth or sixth character 5)
Coding Clinic: 2016, Q4, P72

X● **T88.51** **Hypothermia following anesthesia**

X● **T88.52** **Failed moderate sedation during procedure**
Failed conscious sedation during procedure

> **Excludes2**   personal history of failed moderate sedation (Z92.83)

X● **T88.53** **Unintended awareness under general anesthesia during procedure**

> **Excludes2**   personal history of unintended awareness under general anesthesia (Z92.84)

Coding Clinic: 2016, Q4, P72-73

X● **T88.59** **Other complications of anesthesia**

X● **T88.6** **Anaphylactic reaction due to adverse effect of correct drug or medicament properly administered**
Anaphylactic shock due to adverse effect of correct drug or medicament properly administered
Anaphylactoid reaction NOS
Use additional code for adverse effect, if applicable, to identify drug (T36-T50 with fifth or sixth character 5)

> **Excludes1**   anaphylactic reaction due to serum (T80.5-)
> anaphylactic shock or reaction due to adverse food reaction (T78.0-)

Coding Clinic: 2020, Q1, P18

X● **T88.7** **Unspecified adverse effect of drug or medicament**
Drug hypersensitivity NOS
Drug reaction NOS
Use additional code for adverse effect, if applicable, to identify drug (T36-T50 with fifth or sixth character 5)

> **Excludes1**   specified adverse effects of drugs and medicaments (A00-R94 and T80-T88.6, T88.8)

X● **T88.8** **Other specified complications of surgical and medical care, not elsewhere classified**
Use additional code to identify the complication
Coding Clinic: 2022, Q2, P8

X● **T88.9** **Complication of surgical and medical care, unspecified**

▶ New   ⇒ Revised   ~~deleted~~ Deleted   Excludes 1   Excludes 2   Includes   Use additional   Code first   Code also   Key words
OGCR Official Guidelines   X Assign placeholder X   ● Use Additional Character(s)   ▌ Manifestation Code   🐄 Hierarchical Condition Category   Coding Clinic

CHAPTER 20

EXTERNAL CAUSES OF MORBIDITY
(V00-Y99)

OGCR Chapter-Specific Coding Guidelines

20. **Chapter 20: External Causes of Morbidity (V00-Y99)**
The external causes of morbidity codes should never be sequenced as the first-listed or principal diagnosis.

External cause codes are intended to provide data for injury research and evaluation of injury prevention strategies. These codes capture how the injury or health condition happened (cause), the intent (unintentional or accidental; or intentional, such as suicide or assault), the place where the event occurred the activity of the patient at the time of the event, and the person's status (e.g., civilian, military).

There is no national requirement for mandatory ICD-10-CM external cause code reporting. Unless a provider is subject to a state-based external cause code reporting mandate or these codes are required by a particular payer, reporting of ICD-10-CM codes in Chapter 20, External Causes of Morbidity, is not required. In the absence of a mandatory reporting requirement, providers are encouraged to voluntarily report external cause codes, as they provide valuable data for injury research and evaluation of injury prevention strategies.

a. **General External Cause Coding Guidelines**

1) **Used with any code in the range of A00.0-T88.9, Z00-Z99**
An external cause code may be used with any code in the range of A00.0-T88.9, Z00-Z99, classification that represents a health condition due to an external cause. Though they are most applicable to injuries, they are also valid for use with such things as infections or diseases due to an external source, and other health conditions, such as a heart attack that occurs during strenuous physical activity.

2) **External cause code used for length of treatment**
Assign the external cause code, with the appropriate 7th character (initial encounter, subsequent encounter or sequela) for each encounter for which the injury or condition is being treated.

Most categories in Chapter 20 have a 7th character requirement for each applicable code. Most categories in this chapter have three 7th character values: A, initial encounter, D, subsequent encounter and S, sequela. While the patient may be seen by a new or different provider over the course of treatment for an injury or condition, assignment of the 7th character for external cause should match the 7th character of the code assigned for the associated injury or condition for the encounter.

3) **Use the full range of external cause codes**
Use the full range of external cause codes to completely describe the cause, the intent, the place of occurrence and if applicable, the activity of the patient at the time of the event, and the patient's status, for all injuries, and other health conditions due to an external cause.

4) **Assign as many external cause codes as necessary**
Assign as many external cause codes as necessary to fully explain each cause. If only one external code can be recorded, assign the code most related to the principal diagnosis.

5) **The selection of the appropriate external cause code**
The selection of the appropriate external cause code is guided by the Alphabetic Index of External Causes and by Inclusion and Exclusion notes in the Tabular List.

6) **External cause code can never be a principal diagnosis**
An external cause code can never be a principal (first-listed) diagnosis.

7) **Combination external cause codes**
Certain of the external cause codes are combination codes that identify sequential events that result in an injury, such as a fall which results in striking against an object. The injury may be due to either event or both. The combination external cause code used should correspond to the sequence of events regardless of which caused the most serious injury.

8) **No external cause code needed in certain circumstances**
No external cause code from Chapter 20 is needed if the external cause and intent are included in a code from another chapter (e.g., T36.0X1- Poisoning by penicillins, accidental (unintentional)).

b. **Place of Occurrence Guideline**
Codes from category Y92, Place of occurrence of the external cause, are secondary codes for use after other external cause codes to identify the location of the patient at the time of injury or other condition.

Generally, a place of occurrence code is assigned only once, at the initial encounter for treatment. However, in the rare instance that a new injury occurs during hospitalization, an additional place of occurrence code may be assigned. No 7th characters are used for Y92. Only one code from Y92 should be recorded on a medical record.

Do not use place of occurrence code Y92.9 if the place is not stated or is not applicable.

c. **Activity Code**
Assign a code from category Y93, Activity code, to describe the activity of the patient at the time the injury or other health condition occurred.

An activity code is used only once, at the initial encounter for treatment. Only one code from Y93 should be recorded on a medical record.

The activity codes are not applicable to poisonings, adverse effects, misadventures or sequela.

Do not assign Y93.9, Unspecified activity, if the activity is not stated.

A code from category Y93 is appropriate for use with external cause and intent codes if identifying the activity provides additional information about the event.

d. **Place of Occurrence, Activity, and Status Codes Used with Other External Cause Code**
When applicable, place of occurrence, activity, and external cause status codes are sequenced after the main external cause code(s). Regardless of the number of external cause codes assigned, there should be only one place of occurrence code, one activity code, and one external cause status code assigned to an encounter.

e. If the Reporting Format Limits the Number of External Cause Codes

If the reporting format limits the number of external cause codes that can be used in reporting clinical data, report the code for the cause/intent most related to the principal diagnosis. If the format permits capture of additional external cause codes, the cause/intent, including medical misadventures, of the additional events should be reported rather than the codes for place, activity, or external status.

f. Multiple External Cause Coding Guidelines

More than one external cause code is required to fully describe the external cause of an illness or injury. The assignment of external cause codes should be sequenced in the following priority:

If two or more events cause separate injuries, an external cause code should be assigned for each cause. The first-listed external cause code will be selected in the following order:

External codes for child and adult abuse take priority over all other external cause codes.

See Section I.C.19., Child and Adult abuse guidelines.

External codes for terrorism events take priority over all other external cause codes except child and adult abuse.

External cause codes for cataclysmic events take priority over all other external cause codes except child and adult abuse and terrorism.

External cause codes for transport accidents take priority over all other external cause codes except cataclysmic events, child and adult abuse and terrorism.

Activity and external cause status codes are assigned following all causal (intent) external cause codes.

The first-listed external cause code should correspond to the cause of the most serious diagnosis due to an assault, accident, or self-harm, following the order of hierarchy listed above.

g. Child and Adult Abuse Guideline

Adult and child abuse, neglect and maltreatment are classified as assault. Any of the assault codes may be used to indicate the external cause of any injury resulting from the confirmed abuse.

For confirmed cases of abuse, neglect and maltreatment, when the perpetrator is known, a code from Y07, Perpetrator of maltreatment and neglect, should accompany any other assault codes.

See Section I.C.19. Adult and child abuse, neglect and other maltreatment

h. Unknown or Undetermined Intent Guideline

If the intent (accident, self-harm, assault) of the cause of an injury or other condition is unknown or unspecified, code the intent as accidental intent. All transport accident categories assume accidental intent.

1) Use of undetermined intent

External cause codes for events of undetermined intent are only for use if the documentation in the record specifies that the intent cannot be determined.

i. Sequelae (Late Effects) of External Cause Guidelines

1) Sequelae external cause codes

Sequela are reported using the external cause code with the 7th character "S" for sequela. These codes should be used with any report of a late effect or sequela resulting from a previous injury.

See Section I.B.10. Sequela, (Late Effects).

2) Sequela external cause code with a related current injury

A sequela external cause code should never be used with a related current nature of injury code.

3) Use of sequela external cause codes for subsequent visits

Use a late effect external cause code for subsequent visits when a late effect of the initial injury is being treated. Do not use a late effect external cause code for subsequent visits for follow-up care (e.g., to assess healing, to receive rehabilitative therapy) of the injury when no late effect of the injury has been documented.

j. Terrorism Guidelines

1) Cause of injury identified by the Federal Government (FBI) as terrorism

When the cause of an injury is identified by the Federal Government (FBI) as terrorism, the first-listed external cause code should be a code from category Y38, Terrorism. The definition of terrorism employed by the FBI is found at the inclusion note at the beginning of category Y38. Use additional code for place of occurrence (Y92.-). More than one Y38 code may be assigned if the injury is the result of more than one mechanism of terrorism.

2) Cause of an injury is suspected to be the result of terrorism

When the cause of an injury is suspected to be the result of terrorism a code from category Y38 should not be assigned. Suspected cases should be classified as assault.

3) Code Y38.9, Terrorism, secondary effects

Assign code Y38.9, Terrorism, secondary effects, for conditions occurring subsequent to the terrorist event. This code should not be assigned for conditions that are due to the initial terrorist act.

It is acceptable to assign code Y38.9 with another code from Y38 if there is an injury due to the initial terrorist event and an injury that is a subsequent result of the terrorist event.

k. External cause status

A code from category Y99, External cause status, should be assigned whenever any other external cause code is assigned for an encounter, including an Activity code, except for the events noted below. Assign a code from category Y99, External cause status, to indicate the work status of the person at the time the event occurred. The status code indicates whether the event occurred during military activity, whether a non-military person was at work, whether an individual including a student or volunteer was involved in a non-work activity at the time of the causal event.

A code from Y99, External cause status, should be assigned, when applicable, with other external cause codes, such as transport accidents and falls. The external cause status codes are not applicable to poisonings, adverse effects, misadventures or late effects.

Do not assign a code from category Y99 if no other external cause codes (cause, activity) are applicable for the encounter.

An external cause status code is used only once, at the initial encounter for treatment. Only one code from Y99 should be recorded on a medical record.

Do not assign code Y99.9, Unspecified external cause status, if the status is not stated.

CHAPTER 20

EXTERNAL CAUSES OF MORBIDITY (V00-Y99)

Note: This chapter permits the classification of environmental events and circumstances as the cause of injury, and other adverse effects. Where a code from this section is applicable, it is intended that it shall be used secondary to a code from another chapter of the Classification indicating the nature of the condition. Most often, the condition will be classifiable to Chapter 19, Injury, poisoning and certain other consequences of external causes (S00-T88). Other conditions that may be stated to be due to external causes are classified in Chapters 1 to 18. For these conditions, codes from Chapter 20 should be used to provide additional information as to the cause of the condition.

This chapter contains the following blocks:

V00-X58	Accidents
V00-V99	Transport accidents
V00-V09	Pedestrian injured in transport accident
V10-V19	Pedal cycle rider injured in transport accident
V20-V29	Motorcycle rider injured in transport accident
V30-V39	Occupant of three-wheeled motor vehicle injured in transport accident
V40-V49	Car occupant injured in transport accident
V50-V59	Occupant of pick-up truck or van injured in transport accident
V60-V69	Occupant of heavy transport vehicle injured in transport accident
V70-V79	Bus occupant injured in transport accident
V80-V89	Other land transport accidents
V90-V94	Water transport accidents
V95-V97	Air and space transport accidents
V98-V99	Other and unspecified transport accidents
W00-X58	Other external causes of accidental injury
W00-W19	Slipping, tripping, stumbling and falls
W20-W49	Exposure to inanimate mechanical forces
W50-W64	Exposure to animate mechanical forces
W65-W74	Accidental non-transport drowning and submersion
W85-W99	Exposure to electric current, radiation and extreme ambient air temperature and pressure
X00-X08	Exposure to smoke, fire and flames
X10-X19	Contact with heat and hot substances
X30-X39	Exposure to forces of nature
X50	Overexertion and strenuous or repetitive movements
X52, X58	Accidental exposure to other specified factors
X71-X83	Intentional self-harm
X92-Y09	Assault
Y21-Y33	Event of undetermined intent
Y35-Y38	Legal intervention, operations of war, military operations, and terrorism
Y62-Y84	Complications of medical and surgical care
Y62-Y69	Misadventures to patients during surgical and medical care
Y70-Y82	Medical devices associated with adverse incidents in diagnostic and therapeutic use
Y83-Y84	Surgical and other medical procedures as the cause of abnormal reaction of the patient, or of later complication, without mention of misadventure at the time of the procedure
Y90-Y99	Supplementary factors related to causes of morbidity classified elsewhere

ACCIDENTS (V00-X58)

TRANSPORT ACCIDENTS (V00-V99)

Note: This section is structured in 12 groups. Those relating to land transport accidents (V00-V89) reflect the victim's mode of transport and are subdivided to identify the victim's 'counterpart' or the type of event. The vehicle of which the injured person is an occupant is identified in the first two characters since it is seen as the most important factor to identify for prevention purposes. A transport accident is one in which the vehicle involved must be moving or running or in use for transport purposes at the time of the accident.

Use additional code to identify:
Airbag injury (W22.1)
Type of street or road (Y92.4-)
Use of cellular telephone and other electronic equipment at the time of the transport accident (Y93.C-)

Excludes1 agricultural vehicles in stationary use or maintenance (W31.-)
assault by crashing of motor vehicle (Y03.-)
automobile or motor cycle in stationary use or maintenance - code to type of accident
crashing of motor vehicle, undetermined intent (Y32)
intentional self-harm by crashing of motor vehicle (X82)

Excludes2 transport accidents due to cataclysm (X34-X38)

Note: Definitions related to transport accidents:

(a) A transport accident (V00-V99) is any accident involving a device designed primarily for, or used at the time primarily for, conveying persons or good from one place to another.

(b) A public highway [trafficway] or street is the entire width between property lines (or other boundary lines) of land open to the public as a matter of right or custom for purposes of moving persons or property from one place to another. A roadway is that part of the public highway designed, improved and customarily used for vehicular traffic.

(c) A traffic accident is any vehicle accident occurring on the public highway [i.e., originating on, terminating on, or involving a vehicle partially on the highway]. A vehicle accident is assumed to have occurred on the public highway unless another place is specified, except in the case of accidents involving only off-road motor vehicles, which are classified as nontraffic accidents unless the contrary is stated.

(d) A nontraffic accident is any vehicle accident that occurs entirely in any place other than a public highway.

(e) A pedestrian is any person involved in an accident who was not at the time of the accident riding in or on a motor vehicle, railway train, streetcar or animal-drawn or other vehicle, or on a pedal cycle or animal. This includes, a person changing a tire, working on a parked car, or a person on foot. It also includes the user of a pedestrian conveyance such as a baby stroller, ice-skates, skis, sled, roller skates, a skateboard, nonmotorized or motorized wheelchair, motorized mobility scooter, or nonmotorized scooter.

(f) A driver is an occupant of a transport vehicle who is operating or intending to operate it.

(g) A passenger is any occupant of a transport vehicle other than the driver, except a person traveling on the outside of the vehicle.

(h) A person on the outside of a vehicle is any person being transported by a vehicle but not occupying the space normally reserved for the driver or passengers, or the space intended for the transport of property. This includes a person travelling on the bodywork, bumper, fender, roof, running board or step of a vehicle, as well as, hanging on the outside of the vehicle.

(i) A pedal cycle is any land transport vehicle operated solely by nonmotorized pedals including a bicycle or tricycle.

(j) A pedal cyclist is any person riding a pedal cycle or in a sidecar or trailer attached to a pedal cycle.

(k) A motorcycle is a two-wheeled motor vehicle with one or two riding saddles and sometimes with a third wheel for the support of a sidecar. The sidecar is considered part of the motorcycle. This includes a moped, motor scooter, or motorized bicycle.

(l) A motorcycle rider is any person riding a motorcycle or in a sidecar or trailer attached to the motorcycle.

(m) A three-wheeled motor vehicle is a motorized tricycle designed primarily for on-road use. This includes a motor-driven tricycle, a motorized rickshaw, or a three-wheeled motor car.

(n) A car [automobile] is a four-wheeled motor vehicle designed primarily for carrying up to 7 persons. A trailer being towed by the car is considered part of the car. It does not include a van or minivan—see definition (o)

(o) A pick-up truck or van is a four or six-wheeled motor vehicle designed for carrying passengers as well as property or cargo weighing less than the local limit for classification as a heavy goods vehicle, and not requiring a special driver's license. This includes a minivan and a sport-utility vehicle (SUV).

(p) A heavy transport vehicle is a motor vehicle designed primarily for carrying property, meeting local criteria for classification as a heavy goods vehicle in terms of weight and requiring a special driver's license.

(q) A bus (coach) is a motor vehicle designed or adapted primarily for carrying more than 10 passengers, and requiring a special driver's license.

(r) A railway train or railway vehicle is any device, with or without freight or passenger cars coupled to it, designed for traffic on a railway track. This includes subterranean (subways) or elevated trains.

(s) A streetcar is a device designed and used primarily for transporting passengers within a municipality, running on rails, usually subject to normal traffic control signals, and operated principally on a right-of-way that forms part of the roadway. This includes a tram or trolley that runs on rails. A trailer being towed by a streetcar is considered part of the streetcar.

(t) A special vehicle mainly used on industrial premises is a motor vehicle designed primarily for use within the buildings and premises of industrial or commercial establishments. This includes battery-powered airport passenger vehicles or baggage/mail trucks, forklifts, coal-cars in a coal mine, logging cars and trucks used in mines or quarries.

(u) A special vehicle mainly used in agriculture is a motor vehicle designed specifically for use in farming and agriculture (horticulture), to work the land, tend and harvest crops and transport materials on the farm. This includes harvesters, farm machinery and tractor and trailers.

(v) A special construction vehicle is a motor vehicle designed specifically for use on construction and demolition sites. This includes bulldozers, diggers, earth levellers, dump trucks, backhoes, front-end loaders, pavers, and mechanical shovels.

(w) A special all-terrain vehicle is a motor vehicle of special design to enable it to negotiate over rough or soft terrain, snow or sand. Examples of special design are high construction, special wheels and tires, tracks, and support on a cushion of air. This includes snow mobiles, all-terrain vehicles (ATV), and dune buggies. It does not include passenger vehicle designated as sport utility vehicles (SUV).

(x) A watercraft is any device designed for transporting passengers or goods on water. This includes motor or sail boats, ships, and hovercraft.

(y) An aircraft is any device for transporting passengers or goods in the air. This includes hot-air balloons, gliders, helicopters and airplanes.

(z) A military vehicle is any motorized vehicle operating on a public roadway owned by the military and being operated by a member of the military.

PEDESTRIAN INJURED IN TRANSPORT ACCIDENT (V00-V09)

Includes   person changing tire on transport vehicle
person examining engine of vehicle broken down in (on side of) road

Excludes1   fall due to non-transport collision with other person (W03)
pedestrian on foot falling (slipping) on ice and snow (W00.-)
struck or bumped by another person (W51)

● **V00** **Pedestrian conveyance accident**

Use additional place of occurrence and activity external cause codes, if known (Y92.-, Y93.-)

Excludes1   collision with another person without fall (W51)
fall due to person on foot colliding with another person on foot (W03)
fall from non-moving wheelchair, nonmotorized scooter and motorized mobility scooter without collision (W05.-)
pedestrian (conveyance) collision with other land transport vehicle (V01-V09)
pedestrian on foot falling (slipping) on ice and snow (W00.-)

The appropriate 7th character is to be added to each code from category V00

A	initial encounter
D	subsequent encounter
S	sequela

● **V00.0** **Pedestrian on foot injured in collision with pedestrian conveyance**

X ● **V00.01** **Pedestrian on foot injured in collision with roller-skater**

X ● **V00.02** **Pedestrian on foot injured in collision with skateboarder**

● **V00.03** **Pedestrian on foot injured in collision with standing micro-mobility pedestrian conveyance**

    V00.031 **Pedestrian on foot injured in collision with rider of standing electric scooter**

    V00.038 **Pedestrian on foot injured in collision with rider of other standing micro-mobility pedestrian conveyance**
Pedestrian on foot injured in collision with rider of hoverboard
Pedestrian on foot injured in collision with rider of segway

X ● **V00.09** **Pedestrian on foot injured in collision with other pedestrian conveyance**

● **V00.1** **Rolling-type pedestrian conveyance accident**

Excludes1   accident with baby stroller (V00.82-)
accident with wheelchair (powered) (V00.81-)
accident with motorized mobility scooter (V00.83-)

● **V00.11** **In-line roller-skate accident**

● **V00.111** **Fall from in-line roller-skates**

● **V00.112** **In-line roller-skater colliding with stationary object**

● **V00.118** **Other in-line roller-skate accident**

Excludes1   roller-skater collision with other land transport vehicle (V01-V09 with 5th character 1)

● **V00.12** **Non-in-line roller-skate accident**

● V00.121   **Fall from non-in-line roller-skates**
● V00.122   **Non-in-line roller-skater colliding with stationary object**
● V00.128   **Other non-in-line roller-skating accident**
> **Excludes1**   roller-skater collision with other land transport vehicle (V01-V09 with 5th character 1)

● V00.13   **Skateboard accident**
● V00.131   **Fall from skateboard**
● V00.132   **Skateboarder colliding with stationary object**
● V00.138   **Other skateboard accident**
> **Excludes1**   skateboarder collision with other land transport vehicle (V01-V09 with 5th character 2)

● V00.14   **Scooter (nonmotorized) accident**
> **Excludes1**   motor scooter accident (V20-V29)

● V00.141   **Fall from scooter (nonmotorized)**
● V00.142   **Scooter (nonmotorized) colliding with stationary object**
● V00.148   **Other scooter (nonmotorized) accident**
> **Excludes1**   scooter (non-motorized) collision with other land transport vehicle (V01-V09 with fifth character 9)

● V00.15   **Heelies accident**
Rolling shoe
Wheeled shoe
Wheelies accident
● V00.151   **Fall from heelies**
● V00.152   **Heelies colliding with stationary object**
● V00.158   **Other heelies accident**
● V00.18   **Accident on other rolling-type pedestrian conveyance**
● V00.181   **Fall from other rolling-type pedestrian conveyance**
● V00.182   **Pedestrian on other rolling-type pedestrian conveyance colliding with stationary object**
● V00.188   **Other accident on other rolling-type pedestrian conveyance**
● V00.2   **Gliding-type pedestrian conveyance accident**
● V00.21   **Ice-skates accident**
● V00.211   **Fall from ice-skates**
● V00.212   **Ice-skater colliding with stationary object**
● V00.218   **Other ice-skates accident**
> **Excludes1**   ice-skater collision with other land transport vehicle (V01-V09 with 5th character 9)

● V00.22   **Sled accident**
● V00.221   **Fall from sled**
● V00.222   **Sledder colliding with stationary object**
● V00.228   **Other sled accident**
> **Excludes1**   sled collision with other land transport vehicle (V01-V09 with 5th character 9)

● V00.28   **Other gliding-type pedestrian conveyance accident**
● V00.281   **Fall from other gliding-type pedestrian conveyance**
● V00.282   **Pedestrian on other gliding-type pedestrian conveyance colliding with stationary object**
● V00.288   **Other accident on other gliding-type pedestrian conveyance**
> **Excludes1**   gliding-type pedestrian conveyance collision with other land transport vehicle (V01-V09 with 5th character 9)

● V00.3   **Flat-bottomed pedestrian conveyance accident**
● V00.31   **Snowboard accident**
● V00.311   **Fall from snowboard**
● V00.312   **Snowboarder colliding with stationary object**
● V00.318   **Other snowboard accident**
> **Excludes1**   snowboarder collision with other land transport vehicle (V01-V09 with 5th character 9)

● V00.32   **Snow-ski accident**
● V00.321   **Fall from snow-skis**
Coding Clinic: 2015, Q1, P12
● V00.322   **Snow-skier colliding with stationary object**
● V00.328   **Other snow-ski accident**
> **Excludes1**   snow-skier collision with other land transport vehicle (V01-V09 with 5th character 9)

● V00.38   **Other flat-bottomed pedestrian conveyance accident**
● V00.381   **Fall from other flat-bottomed pedestrian conveyance**
● V00.382   **Pedestrian on other flat-bottomed pedestrian conveyance colliding with stationary object**
● V00.388   **Other accident on other flat-bottomed pedestrian conveyance**
● V00.8   **Accident on other pedestrian conveyance**
● V00.81   **Accident with wheelchair (powered)**
● V00.811   **Fall from moving wheelchair (powered)**
> **Excludes1**   fall from non-moving wheelchair (W05.0)

● V00.812   **Wheelchair (powered) colliding with stationary object**
● V00.818   **Other accident with wheelchair (powered)**
● V00.82   **Accident with baby stroller**
● V00.821   **Fall from baby stroller**
● V00.822   **Baby stroller colliding with stationary object**
● V00.828   **Other accident with baby stroller**

● **V00.83   Accident with motorized mobility scooter**
   ● **V00.831   Fall from motorized mobility scooter**
     Excludes1   fall from non-moving motorized mobility scooter (W05.2)
   ● **V00.832   Motorized mobility scooter colliding with stationary object**
   ● **V00.838   Other accident with motorized mobility scooter**
● **V00.84   Accident with standing micro-mobility pedestrian conveyance**
   V00.841   Fall from standing electric scooter
   V00.842   Pedestrian on standing electric scooter colliding with stationary object
   V00.848   Other accident with standing micro-mobility pedestrian conveyance
     Accident with hoverboard
     Accident with segway
● **V00.89   Accident on other pedestrian conveyance**
   ● **V00.891   Fall from other pedestrian conveyance**
   ● **V00.892   Pedestrian on other pedestrian conveyance colliding with stationary object**
   ● **V00.898   Other accident on other pedestrian conveyance**
     Excludes1   other pedestrian (conveyance) collision with other land transport vehicle (V01-V09 with 5th character 9)

● **V01   Pedestrian injured in collision with pedal cycle**

The appropriate 7th character is to be added to each code from category V01

A   initial encounter
D   subsequent encounter
S   sequela

● **V01.0   Pedestrian injured in collision with pedal cycle in nontraffic accident**
  X ● **V01.00   Pedestrian on foot injured in collision with pedal cycle in nontraffic accident**
     Pedestrian NOS injured in collision with pedal cycle in nontraffic accident
  X ● **V01.01   Pedestrian on roller-skates injured in collision with pedal cycle in nontraffic accident**
  X ● **V01.02   Pedestrian on skateboard injured in collision with pedal cycle in nontraffic accident**
  ● **V01.03   Pedestrian on standing micro-mobility pedestrian conveyance injured in collision with pedal cycle in nontraffic accident**
   V01.031   Pedestrian on standing electric scooter injured in collision with pedal cycle in nontraffic accident
   V01.038   Pedestrian on other standing micro-mobility pedestrian conveyance injured in collision with pedal cycle in nontraffic accident
     Pedestrian on hoverboard injured in collision with pedal cycle in nontraffic accident
     Pedestrian on segway injured in collision with pedal cycle in nontraffic accident

X ● **V01.09   Pedestrian with other conveyance injured in collision with pedal cycle in nontraffic accident**
   Pedestrian with baby stroller injured in collision with pedal cycle in nontraffic accident
   Pedestrian in wheelchair (powered) injured in collision with pedal cycle in nontraffic accident
   Pedestrian in motorized mobility scooter injured in collision with pedal cycle in nontraffic accident
   Pedestrian on ice-skates injured in collision with pedal cycle in nontraffic accident
   Pedestrian on nonmotorized scooter injured in collision with pedal cycle in nontraffic accident
   Pedestrian on sled injured in collision with pedal cycle in nontraffic accident
   Pedestrian on snowboard injured in collision with pedal cycle in nontraffic accident
   Pedestrian on snow-skis injured in collision with pedal cycle in nontraffic accident
● **V01.1   Pedestrian injured in collision with pedal cycle in traffic accident**
  X ● **V01.10   Pedestrian on foot injured in collision with pedal cycle in traffic accident**
     Pedestrian NOS injured in collision with pedal cycle in traffic accident
  X ● **V01.11   Pedestrian on roller-skates injured in collision with pedal cycle in traffic accident**
  X ● **V01.12   Pedestrian on skateboard injured in collision with pedal cycle in traffic accident**
  ● **V01.13   Pedestrian on standing micro-mobility pedestrian conveyance injured in collision with pedal cycle in traffic accident**
   V01.131   Pedestrian on standing electric scooter injured in collision with pedal cycle in traffic accident
   V01.138   Pedestrian on other standing micro-mobility pedestrian conveyance injured in collision with pedal cycle in traffic accident
     Pedestrian on hoverboard injured in collision with pedal cycle in traffic accident
     Pedestrian on segway injured in collision with pedal cycle in traffic accident
  X ● **V01.19   Pedestrian with other conveyance injured in collision with pedal cycle in traffic accident**
   Pedestrian with baby stroller injured in collision with pedal cycle in traffic accident
   Pedestrian in wheelchair (powered) injured in collision with pedal cycle in traffic accident
   Pedestrian in motorized mobility scooter injured in collision with pedal cycle in traffic accident
   Pedestrian on ice-skates injured in collision with pedal cycle in traffic accident
   Pedestrian on nonmotorized scooter injured in collision with pedal cycle in traffic accident
   Pedestrian on sled injured in collision with pedal cycle in traffic accident
   Pedestrian on snowboard injured in collision with pedal cycle in traffic accident
   Pedestrian on snow-skis injured in collision with pedal cycle in traffic accident

CHAPTER 20 (V00-Y99)

▶ New   ⇒ Revised   ~~deleted~~ Deleted   Excludes 1   Excludes 2   Includes   Use additional   Code first   Code also   Key words
OGCR Official Guidelines   X Assign placeholder X   ● Use Additional Character(s)   ▶ Manifestation Code   Hierarchical Condition Category   Coding Clinic

● **V01.9**   **Pedestrian injured in collision with pedal cycle, unspecified whether traffic or nontraffic accident**

    X ● **V01.90**   **Pedestrian on foot injured in collision with pedal cycle, unspecified whether traffic or nontraffic accident**

       Pedestrian NOS injured in collision with pedal cycle, unspecified whether traffic or nontraffic accident

    X ● **V01.91**   **Pedestrian on roller-skates injured in collision with pedal cycle, unspecified whether traffic or nontraffic accident**

    X ● **V01.92**   **Pedestrian on skateboard injured in collision with pedal cycle, unspecified whether traffic or nontraffic accident**

    ● **V01.93**   **Pedestrian on standing micro-mobility pedestrian conveyance injured in collision with pedal cycle, unspecified whether traffic or nontraffic accident**

       V01.931   **Pedestrian on standing electric scooter injured in collision with pedal cycle, unspecified whether traffic or nontraffic accident**

       V01.938   **Pedestrian on other standing micro-mobility pedestrian conveyance injured in collision with pedal cycle, unspecified whether traffic or nontraffic accident**

          Pedestrian on hoverboard injured in collision with pedal cycle, unspecified whether traffic or nontraffic accident

          Pedestrian on segway injured in collision with pedal cycle, unspecified whether traffic or nontraffic accident

    X ● **V01.99**   **Pedestrian with other conveyance injured in collision with pedal cycle, unspecified whether traffic or nontraffic accident**

       Pedestrian with baby stroller injured in collision with pedal cycle, unspecified whether traffic or nontraffic accident

       Pedestrian in wheelchair (powered) injured in collision with pedal cycle, unspecified whether traffic or nontraffic accident

       Pedestrian in motorized mobility scooter injured in collision with pedal cycle, unspecified whether traffic or nontraffic accident

       Pedestrian on ice-skates injured in collision with pedal cycle unspecified, whether traffic or nontraffic accident

       Pedestrian on nonmotorized scooter injured in collision with pedal cycle, unspecified whether traffic or nontraffic accident

       Pedestrian on sled injured in collision with pedal cycle unspecified, whether traffic or nontraffic accident

       Pedestrian on snowboard injured in collision with pedal cycle, unspecified whether traffic or nontraffic accident

       Pedestrian on snow-skis injured in collision with pedal cycle, unspecified whether traffic or nontraffic accident

● **V02**   **Pedestrian injured in collision with two- or three-wheeled motor vehicle**

    The appropriate 7th character is to be added to each code from category V02

> A   initial encounter
> D   subsequent encounter
> S   sequela

    ● **V02.0**   **Pedestrian injured in collision with two- or three-wheeled motor vehicle in nontraffic accident**

    X ● **V02.00**   **Pedestrian on foot injured in collision with two- or three-wheeled motor vehicle in nontraffic accident**

       Pedestrian NOS injured in collision with two- or three-wheeled motor vehicle in nontraffic accident

    X ● **V02.01**   **Pedestrian on roller-skates injured in collision with two- or three-wheeled motor vehicle in nontraffic accident**

    X ● **V02.02**   **Pedestrian on skateboard injured in collision with two- or three-wheeled motor vehicle in nontraffic accident**

    ● **V02.03**   **Pedestrian on standing micro-mobility pedestrian conveyance injured in collision with two- or three-wheeled motor vehicle in nontraffic accident**

       V02.031   **Pedestrian on standing electric scooter injured in collision with two- or three-wheeled motor vehicle in nontraffic accident**

       V02.038   **Pedestrian on other standing micro-mobility pedestrian conveyance injured in collision with two- or three-wheeled motor vehicle in nontraffic accident**

          Pedestrian on hoverboard injured in collision with two-or three wheeled motor vehicle in nontraffic accident

          Pedestrian on segway injured in collision with two- or three-wheeled motor vehicle in nontraffic accident

    X ● **V02.09**   **Pedestrian with other conveyance injured in collision with two- or three-wheeled motor vehicle in nontraffic accident**

       Pedestrian with baby stroller injured in collision with two- or three-wheeled motor vehicle in nontraffic accident

       Pedestrian on ice-skates injured in collision with two- or three-wheeled motor vehicle in nontraffic accident

       Pedestrian in wheelchair (powered) injured in collision with two- or three-wheeled motor vehicle in nontraffic accident

       Pedestrian in motorized mobility scooter injured in collision with two- or three-wheeled motor vehicle in nontraffic accident

       Pedestrian on nonmotorized scooter injured in collision with two- or three-wheeled motor vehicle in nontraffic accident

       Pedestrian on sled injured in collision with two- or three-wheeled motor vehicle in nontraffic accident

       Pedestrian on snowboard injured in collision with two- or three-wheeled motor vehicle in nontraffic accident

       Pedestrian on snow-skis injured in collision with two- or three-wheeled motor vehicle in nontraffic accident

CHAPTER 20 (V00-Y99)

● **V02.1** **Pedestrian injured in collision with two- or three- wheeled motor vehicle in traffic accident**

X● **V02.10** **Pedestrian on foot injured in collision with two- or three-wheeled motor vehicle in traffic accident**

Pedestrian NOS injured in collision with two- or three-wheeled motor vehicle in traffic accident

X● **V02.11** **Pedestrian on roller-skates injured in collision with two- or three-wheeled motor vehicle in traffic accident**

X● **V02.12** **Pedestrian on skateboard injured in collision with two- or three-wheeled motor vehicle in traffic accident**

● **V02.13** **Pedestrian on standing micro-mobility pedestrian conveyance injured in collision with two- or three-wheeled motor vehicle in traffic accident**

V02.131 **Pedestrian on standing electric scooter injured in collision with two- or three-wheeled motor vehicle in traffic accident**

V02.138 **Pedestrian on other standing micro-mobility pedestrian conveyance injured in collision with two- or three-wheeled motor vehicle in traffic accident**

Pedestrian on hoverboard injured in collision with two-or three wheeled motor vehicle in traffic accident

Pedestrian on segway injured in collision with two- or three-wheeled motor vehicle in traffic accident

X● **V02.19** **Pedestrian with other conveyance injured in collision with two- or three-wheeled motor vehicle in traffic accident**

Pedestrian with baby stroller injured in collision with two- or three-wheeled motor vehicle in traffic accident

Pedestrian in wheelchair (powered) injured in collision with two- or three-wheeled motor vehicle in traffic accident

Pedestrian in motorized mobility scooter injured in collision with two- or three-wheeled motor vehicle in traffic accident

Pedestrian on ice-skates injured in collision with two- or three-wheeled motor vehicle in traffic accident

Pedestrian on nonmotorized scooter injured in collision with two- or three-wheeled motor vehicle in traffic accident

Pedestrian on sled injured in collision with two- or three-wheeled motor vehicle in traffic accident

Pedestrian on snowboard injured in collision with two- or three-wheeled motor vehicle in traffic accident

Pedestrian on snow-skis injured in collision with two- or three-wheeled motor vehicle in traffic accident

● **V02.9** **Pedestrian injured in collision with two- or three- wheeled motor vehicle, unspecified whether traffic or nontraffic accident**

X● **V02.90** **Pedestrian on foot injured in collision with two- or three-wheeled motor vehicle, unspecified whether traffic or nontraffic accident**

Pedestrian NOS injured in collision with two- or three-wheeled motor vehicle, unspecified whether traffic or nontraffic accident

X● **V02.91** **Pedestrian on roller-skates injured in collision with two- or three-wheeled motor vehicle, unspecified whether traffic or nontraffic accident**

X● **V02.92** **Pedestrian on skateboard injured in collision with two- or three-wheeled motor vehicle, unspecified whether traffic or nontraffic accident**

● **V02.93** **Pedestrian on standing micro-mobility pedestrian conveyance injured in collision with two-or three-wheeled motor vehicle, unspecified whether traffic or nontraffic accident**

V02.931 **Pedestrian on standing electric scooter injured in collision with two- or three wheeled motor vehicle, unspecified whether traffic or nontraffic accident**

V02.938 **Pedestrian on other standing micro-mobility pedestrian conveyance injured in collision with two- or three wheeled motor vehicle, unspecified whether traffic or nontraffic accident**

Pedestrian on hoverboard injured in collision with two-three-wheeled motor vehicle, unspecified whether traffic or nontraffic accident

Pedestrian on segway injured in collision with two- or three wheeled motor vehicle, unspecified whether traffic or nontraffic accident

X● **V02.99** **Pedestrian with other conveyance injured in collision with two- or three-wheeled motor vehicle, unspecified whether traffic or nontraffic accident**

Pedestrian with baby stroller injured in collision with two- or three-wheeled motor vehicle, unspecified whether traffic or nontraffic accident

Pedestrian in wheelchair (powered) injured in collision with two- or three-wheeled motor vehicle, unspecified whether traffic or nontraffic accident

Pedestrian in motorized mobility scooter injured in collision with two- or three-wheeled motor vehicle, unspecified whether traffic or nontraffic accident

Pedestrian on ice-skates injured in collision with two- or three-wheeled motor vehicle, unspecified whether traffic or nontraffic accident

Pedestrian on nonmotorized scooter injured in collision with two- or three-wheeled motor vehicle, unspecified whether traffic or nontraffic accident

Pedestrian on sled injured in collision with two- or three-wheeled motor vehicle, unspecified whether traffic or nontraffic accident

Pedestrian on snowboard injured in collision with two- or three-wheeled motor vehicle, unspecified whether traffic or nontraffic accident

Pedestrian on snow-skis injured in collision with two- or three-wheeled motor vehicle, unspecified whether traffic or nontraffic accident

▶ New   ⇒ Revised   ~~deleted~~ Deleted   Excludes 1   Excludes 2   Includes   Use additional   Code first   Code also   Key words

OGCR Official Guidelines   X Assign placeholder X   ● Use Additional Character(s)   ▷ Manifestation Code   🅡 Hierarchical Condition Category   Coding Clinic

● **V03   Pedestrian injured in collision with car, pick-up truck or van**

The appropriate 7th character is to be added to each code from category V03

> A   initial encounter
> D   subsequent encounter
> S   sequela

● **V03.0   Pedestrian injured in collision with car, pick-up truck or van in nontraffic accident**

X● **V03.00   Pedestrian on foot injured in collision with car, pick-up truck or van in nontraffic accident**
> Pedestrian NOS injured in collision with car, pick-up truck or van in nontraffic accident

X● **V03.01   Pedestrian on roller-skates injured in collision with car, pick-up truck or van in nontraffic accident**

X● **V03.02   Pedestrian on skateboard injured in collision with car, pick-up truck or van in nontraffic accident**

● **V03.03   Pedestrian on standing micro-mobility pedestrian conveyance injured in collision with car, pick-up or van in nontraffic accident**

V03.031   Pedestrian on standing electric scooter injured in collision with car, pick-up or van in nontraffic accident

V03.038   Pedestrian on other standing micro-mobility pedestrian conveyance injured in collision with car, pick-up or van in nontraffic accident
> Pedestrian on hoverboard injured in collision with car, pick-up or van in nontraffic accident
> Pedestrian on segway injured in collision with car, pick-up or van in nontraffic accident

X● **V03.09   Pedestrian with other conveyance injured in collision with car, pick-up truck or van in nontraffic accident**
> Pedestrian with baby stroller injured in collision with car, pick-up truck or van in nontraffic accident
> Pedestrian in wheelchair (powered) injured in collision with car, pick-up truck or van in nontraffic accident
> Pedestrian in motorized mobility scooter injured in collision with car, pick-up truck or van in nontraffic accident
> Pedestrian on ice-skates injured in collision with car, pick-up truck or van in nontraffic accident
> Pedestrian on nonmotorized scooter injured in collision with car, pick-up truck or van in nontraffic accident
> Pedestrian on sled injured in collision with car, pick-up truck or van in nontraffic accident
> Pedestrian on snowboard injured in collision with car, pick-up truck or van in nontraffic accident
> Pedestrian on snow-skis injured in collision with car, pick-up truck or van in nontraffic accident

● **V03.1   Pedestrian injured in collision with car, pick-up truck or van in traffic accident**

X● **V03.10   Pedestrian on foot injured in collision with car, pick-up truck or van in traffic accident**
> Pedestrian NOS injured in collision with car, pick-up truck or van in traffic accident

X● **V03.11   Pedestrian on roller-skates injured in collision with car, pick-up truck or van in traffic accident**

X● **V03.12   Pedestrian on skateboard injured in collision with car, pick-up truck or van in traffic accident**

● **V03.13   Pedestrian on standing micro-mobility pedestrian conveyance injured in collision with car, pick-up or van in traffic accident**

V03.131   Pedestrian on standing electric scooter injured in collision with car, pick-up or van in traffic accident

V03.138   Pedestrian on other standing micro-mobility pedestrian conveyance injured in collision with car, pick-up or van in traffic accident
> Pedestrian on hoverboard injured in collision with car, pick-up or van in traffic accident
> Pedestrian on segway injured in collision with car, pick-up or van in traffic accident

X● **V03.19   Pedestrian with other conveyance injured in collision with car, pick-up truck or van in traffic accident**
> Pedestrian with baby stroller injured in collision with car, pick-up truck or van in traffic accident
> Pedestrian in wheelchair (powered) injured in collision with car, pick-up truck or van in traffic accident
> Pedestrian in motorized mobility scooter injured in collision with car, pick-up truck or van in traffic accident
> Pedestrian on ice-skates injured in collision with car, pick-up truck or van in traffic accident
> Pedestrian on nonmotorized scooter injured in collision with car, pick-up truck or van in traffic accident
> Pedestrian on sled injured in collision with car, pick-up truck or van in traffic accident
> Pedestrian on snowboard injured in collision with car, pick-up truck or van in traffic accident
> Pedestrian on snow-skis injured in collision with car, pick-up truck or van in traffic accident

● **V03.9   Pedestrian injured in collision with car, pick-up truck or van, unspecified whether traffic or nontraffic accident**

X● **V03.90   Pedestrian on foot injured in collision with car, pick-up truck or van, unspecified whether traffic or nontraffic accident**
> Pedestrian NOS injured in collision with car, pick-up truck or van, unspecified whether traffic or nontraffic accident

X● **V03.91   Pedestrian on roller-skates injured in collision with car, pick-up truck or van, unspecified whether traffic or nontraffic accident**

X● **V03.92   Pedestrian on skateboard injured in collision with car, pick-up truck or van, unspecified whether traffic or nontraffic accident**

CHAPTER 20 (V00-Y99)

● **V03.93** **Pedestrian on standing micro-mobility pedestrian conveyance injured in collision with car, pick-up or van, unspecified whether traffic or nontraffic accident**

  V03.931 **Pedestrian on standing electric scooter injured in collision with car, pick-up or van, unspecified whether traffic or nontraffic accident**

  V03.938 **Pedestrian on other standing micro-mobility pedestrian conveyance injured in collision with car, pick-up or van, unspecified whether traffic or nontraffic accident**

    Pedestrian on hoverboard injured in collision with car, pick-up or van, unspecified whether traffic or nontraffic accident

    Pedestrian on segway injured in collision with car, pick-up or van, unspecified whether traffic or nontraffic accident

X● **V03.99** **Pedestrian with other conveyance injured in collision with car, pick-up truck or van, unspecified whether traffic or nontraffic accident**

  Pedestrian with baby stroller injured in collision with car, pick-up truck or van, unspecified whether traffic or nontraffic accident

  Pedestrian in wheelchair (powered) injured in collision with car, pick-up truck or van, unspecified whether traffic or nontraffic accident

  Pedestrian in motorized mobility scooter injured in collision with car, pick-up truck or van, unspecified whether traffic or nontraffic accident

  Pedestrian on ice-skates injured in collision with car, pick-up truck or van, unspecified whether traffic or nontraffic accident

  Pedestrian on nonmotorized scooter injured in collision with car, pick-up truck or van, unspecified whether traffic or nontraffic accident

  Pedestrian on sled injured in collision with car, pick-up truck or van in nontraffic accident

  Pedestrian on snowboard injured in collision with car, pick-up truck or van, unspecified whether traffic or nontraffic accident

  Pedestrian on snow-skis injured in collision with car, pick-up truck or van, unspecified whether traffic or nontraffic accident

● **V04** **Pedestrian injured in collision with heavy transport vehicle or bus**

  Excludes1 pedestrian injured in collision with military vehicle (V09.01, V09.21)

The appropriate 7th character is to be added to each code from category V04

A	initial encounter
D	subsequent encounter
S	sequela

● **V04.0** **Pedestrian injured in collision with heavy transport vehicle or bus in nontraffic accident**

X● **V04.00** **Pedestrian on foot injured in collision with heavy transport vehicle or bus in nontraffic accident**

  Pedestrian NOS injured in collision with heavy transport vehicle or bus in nontraffic accident

X● **V04.01** **Pedestrian on roller-skates injured in collision with heavy transport vehicle or bus in nontraffic accident**

X● **V04.02** **Pedestrian on skateboard injured in collision with heavy transport vehicle or bus in nontraffic accident**

● **V04.03** **Pedestrian on standing micro-mobility pedestrian conveyance injured in collision with heavy transport vehicle or bus in nontraffic accident**

  V04.031 **Pedestrian on standing electric scooter injured in collision with heavy transport vehicle or bus in nontraffic accident**

  V04.038 **Pedestrian on other standing micro-mobility pedestrian conveyance injured in collision with heavy transport vehicle or bus in nontraffic accident**

    Pedestrian on hoverboard injured in collision with heavy transport vehicle or bus in nontraffic accident

    Pedestrian on segway injured in collision with heavy transport vehicle or bus in nontraffic accident

X● **V04.09** **Pedestrian with other conveyance injured in collision with heavy transport vehicle or bus in nontraffic accident**

  Pedestrian with baby stroller injured in collision with heavy transport vehicle or bus in nontraffic accident

  Pedestrian in wheelchair (powered) injured in collision with heavy transport vehicle or bus in nontraffic accident

  Pedestrian in motorized mobility scooter injured in collision with heavy transport vehicle or bus in nontraffic accident

  Pedestrian on ice-skates injured in collision with heavy transport vehicle or bus in nontraffic accident

  Pedestrian on nonmotorized scooter injured in collision with heavy transport vehicle or bus in nontraffic accident

  Pedestrian on sled injured in collision with heavy transport vehicle or bus in nontraffic accident

  Pedestrian on snowboard injured in collision with heavy transport vehicle or bus in nontraffic accident

  Pedestrian on snow-skis injured in collision with heavy transport vehicle or bus in nontraffic accident

● **V04.1** **Pedestrian injured in collision with heavy transport vehicle or bus in traffic accident**

X● **V04.10** **Pedestrian on foot injured in collision with heavy transport vehicle or bus in traffic accident**

  Pedestrian NOS injured in collision with heavy transport vehicle or bus in traffic accident

X● **V04.11** **Pedestrian on roller-skates injured in collision with heavy transport vehicle or bus in traffic accident**

X● **V04.12** **Pedestrian on skateboard injured in collision with heavy transport vehicle or bus in traffic accident**

● **V04.13** **Pedestrian on standing micro-mobility pedestrian conveyance injured in collision with heavy transport vehicle or bus in traffic accident**

  V04.131 **Pedestrian on standing electric scooter injured in collision with heavy transport vehicle or bus in traffic accident**

V04.138 Pedestrian on other standing micro-mobility pedestrian conveyance injured in collision with heavy transport vehicle or bus in traffic accident
　　　Pedestrian on hoverboard injured in collision with heavy transport vehicle or bus in traffic accident
　　　Pedestrian on segway injured in collision with heavy transport vehicle or bus in traffic accident

X⬤ V04.19 Pedestrian with other conveyance injured in collision with heavy transport vehicle or bus in traffic accident
　　　Pedestrian with baby stroller injured in collision with heavy transport vehicle or bus in traffic accident
　　　Pedestrian in wheelchair (powered) injured in collision with heavy transport vehicle or bus in traffic accident
　　　Pedestrian in motorized mobility scooter injured in collision with heavy transport vehicle or bus in traffic accident
　　　Pedestrian on ice-skates injured in collision with heavy transport vehicle or bus in traffic accident
　　　Pedestrian on nonmotorized scooter injured in collision with heavy transport vehicle or bus in traffic accident
　　　Pedestrian on sled injured in collision with heavy transport vehicle or bus in traffic accident
　　　Pedestrian on snowboard injured in collision with heavy transport vehicle or bus in traffic accident
　　　Pedestrian on snow-skis injured in collision with heavy transport vehicle or bus in traffic accident

⬤ V04.9 Pedestrian injured in collision with heavy transport vehicle or bus, unspecified whether traffic or nontraffic accident

X⬤ V04.90 Pedestrian on foot injured in collision with heavy transport vehicle or bus, unspecified whether traffic or nontraffic accident
　　　Pedestrian NOS injured in collision with heavy transport vehicle or bus, unspecified whether traffic or nontraffic accident

X⬤ V04.91 Pedestrian on roller-skates injured in collision with heavy transport vehicle or bus, unspecified whether traffic or nontraffic accident

X⬤ V04.92 Pedestrian on skateboard injured in collision with heavy transport vehicle or bus, unspecified whether traffic or nontraffic accident

⬤ V04.93 Pedestrian on standing micro-mobility pedestrian conveyance injured in collision with heavy transport vehicle or bus, unspecified whether traffic or nontraffic accident

V04.931 Pedestrian on standing electric scooter injured in collision with heavy transport vehicle or bus, unspecified whether traffic or nontraffic accident

V04.938 Pedestrian on other standing micro-mobility pedestrian conveyance injured in collision with heavy transport vehicle or bus, unspecified whether traffic or nontraffic accident
　　　Pedestrian on hoverboard injured in collision with heavy transport vehicle or bus, unspecified whether traffic or nontraffic accident
　　　Pedestrian on segway injured in collision with heavy transport vehicle or bus, unspecified whether traffic or nontraffic accident

X⬤ V04.99 Pedestrian with other conveyance injured in collision with heavy transport vehicle or bus, unspecified whether traffic or nontraffic accident
　　　Pedestrian with baby stroller injured in collision with heavy transport vehicle or bus, unspecified whether traffic or nontraffic accident
　　　Pedestrian in wheelchair (powered) injured in collision with heavy transport vehicle or bus, unspecified whether traffic or nontraffic accident
　　　Pedestrian in motorized mobility scooter injured in collision with heavy transport vehicle or bus, unspecified whether traffic or nontraffic accident
　　　Pedestrian on ice-skates injured in collision with heavy transport vehicle or bus, unspecified whether traffic or nontraffic accident
　　　Pedestrian on nonmotorized scooter injured in collision with heavy transport vehicle or bus, unspecified whether traffic or nontraffic accident
　　　Pedestrian on sled injured in collision with heavy transport vehicle or bus, unspecified whether traffic or nontraffic accident
　　　Pedestrian on snowboard injured in collision with heavy transport vehicle or bus, unspecified whether traffic or nontraffic accident
　　　Pedestrian on snow-skis injured in collision with heavy transport vehicle or bus, unspecified whether traffic or nontraffic accident

⬤ V05 Pedestrian injured in collision with railway train or railway vehicle

The appropriate 7th character is to be added to each code from category V05

A	initial encounter
D	subsequent encounter
S	sequela

⬤ V05.0 Pedestrian injured in collision with railway train or railway vehicle in nontraffic accident

X⬤ V05.00 Pedestrian on foot injured in collision with railway train or railway vehicle in nontraffic accident
　　　Pedestrian NOS injured in collision with railway train or railway vehicle in nontraffic accident

X⬤ V05.01 Pedestrian on roller-skates injured in collision with railway train or railway vehicle in nontraffic accident

X⬤ V05.02 Pedestrian on skateboard injured in collision with railway train or railway vehicle in nontraffic accident

⬤ V05.03 Pedestrian on standing micro-mobility pedestrian conveyance injured in collision with railway train or railway vehicle in nontraffic accident

V05.031 Pedestrian on standing electric scooter injured in collision with railway train or railway vehicle in nontraffic accident

V05.038 Pedestrian on other standing micro-mobility pedestrian conveyance injured in collision with railway train or railway vehicle in nontraffic accident
　　　Pedestrian on hoverboard injured in collision with railway train or railway vehicle in nontraffic accident
　　　Pedestrian on segway injured in collision with railway train or railway vehicle in nontraffic accident

CHAPTER 20 (V00-Y99)

CHAPTER 20 (V00-Y99)

X ● **V05.09** **Pedestrian with other conveyance injured in collision with railway train or railway vehicle in nontraffic accident**
Pedestrian with baby stroller injured in collision with railway train or railway vehicle in nontraffic accident
Pedestrian in wheelchair (powered) injured in collision with railway train or railway vehicle in nontraffic accident
Pedestrian in motorized mobility scooter injured in collision with railway train or railway vehicle in nontraffic accident
Pedestrian on ice-skates injured in collision with railway train or railway vehicle in nontraffic accident
Pedestrian on nonmotorized scooter injured in collision with railway train or railway vehicle in nontraffic accident
Pedestrian on sled injured in collision with railway train or railway vehicle in nontraffic accident
Pedestrian on snowboard injured in collision with railway train or railway vehicle in nontraffic accident
Pedestrian on snow-skis injured in collision with railway train or railway vehicle in nontraffic accident

● **V05.1** **Pedestrian injured in collision with railway train or railway vehicle in traffic accident**

X ● **V05.10** **Pedestrian on foot injured in collision with railway train or railway vehicle in traffic accident**
Pedestrian NOS injured in collision with railway train or railway vehicle in traffic accident

X ● **V05.11** **Pedestrian on roller-skates injured in collision with railway train or railway vehicle in traffic accident**

X ● **V05.12** **Pedestrian on skateboard injured in collision with railway train or railway vehicle in traffic accident**

● **V05.13** **Pedestrian on standing micro-mobility pedestrian conveyance injured in collision with railway train or railway vehicle in traffic accident**

V05.131 **Pedestrian on standing electric scooter injured in collision with railway train or railway vehicle in traffic accident**

V05.138 **Pedestrian on other standing micro-mobility pedestrian conveyance injured in collision with railway train or railway vehicle in traffic accident**
Pedestrian on hoverboard injured in collision with railway train or railway vehicle in traffic accident
Pedestrian on segway injured in collision with railway train or railway vehicle in traffic accident

X ● **V05.19** **Pedestrian with other conveyance injured in collision with railway train or railway vehicle in traffic accident**
Pedestrian with baby stroller injured in collision with railway train or railway vehicle in traffic accident
Pedestrian in wheelchair (powered) injured in collision with railway train or railway vehicle in traffic accident
Pedestrian in motorized mobility scooter injured in collision with railway train or railway vehicle in traffic accident
Pedestrian on ice-skates injured in collision with railway train or railway vehicle in traffic accident
Pedestrian on nonmotorized scooter injured in collision with railway train or railway vehicle in traffic accident
Pedestrian on sled injured in collision with railway train or railway vehicle in traffic accident
Pedestrian on snowboard injured in collision with railway train or railway vehicle in traffic accident
Pedestrian on snow-skis injured in collision with railway train or railway vehicle in traffic accident

● **V05.9** **Pedestrian injured in collision with railway train or railway vehicle, unspecified whether traffic or nontraffic accident**

X ● **V05.90** **Pedestrian on foot injured in collision with railway train or railway vehicle, unspecified whether traffic or nontraffic accident**
Pedestrian NOS injured in collision with railway train or railway vehicle, unspecified whether traffic or nontraffic accident

X ● **V05.91** **Pedestrian on roller-skates injured in collision with railway train or railway vehicle, unspecified whether traffic or nontraffic accident**

X ● **V05.92** **Pedestrian on skateboard injured in collision with railway train or railway vehicle, unspecified whether traffic or nontraffic accident**

● **V05.93** **Pedestrian on standing micro-mobility pedestrian conveyance injured in collision with railway train or railway vehicle, unspecified whether traffic or nontraffic accident**

V05.931 **Pedestrian on standing electric scooter injured in collision with railway train or railway vehicle, unspecified whether traffic or nontraffic accident**

V05.938 **Pedestrian on other standing micro-mobility pedestrian conveyance injured in collision with railway train or railway vehicle, unspecified whether traffic or nontraffic accident**
Pedestrian on hoverboard injured in collision with railway train or railway vehicle, unspecified whether traffic or nontraffic accident
Pedestrian on segway injured in collision with railway train or railway vehicle, unspecified whether traffic or nontraffic accident

▶ New   ⇒ Revised   ~~deleted~~ Deleted   Excludes 1   Excludes 2   Includes   Use additional   Code first   Code also   Key words
OGCR Official Guidelines   X Assign placeholder X   ● Use Additional Character(s)   ▶ Manifestation Code   🏷 Hierarchical Condition Category   **Coding Clinic**

X ● **V05.99** **Pedestrian with other conveyance injured in collision with railway train or railway vehicle, unspecified whether traffic or nontraffic accident**
Pedestrian with baby stroller injured in collision with railway train or railway vehicle, unspecified whether traffic or nontraffic
Pedestrian in wheelchair (powered) injured in collision with railway train or railway vehicle, unspecified whether traffic or nontraffic
Pedestrian in motorized mobility scooter injured in collision with railway train or railway vehicle, unspecified whether traffic or nontraffic
Pedestrian on ice-skates injured in collision with railway train or railway vehicle, unspecified whether traffic or nontraffic
Pedestrian on nonmotorized scooter injured in collision with railway train or railway vehicle, unspecified whether traffic or nontraffic
Pedestrian on sled injured in collision with railway train or railway vehicle, unspecified whether traffic or nontraffic
Pedestrian on snowboard injured in collision with railway train or railway vehicle, unspecified whether traffic or nontraffic
Pedestrian on snow-skis injured in collision with railway train or railway vehicle, unspecified whether traffic or nontraffic

● **V06**   **Pedestrian injured in collision with other nonmotor vehicle**
Includes   collision with animal-drawn vehicle, animal being ridden, nonpowered streetcar
Excludes1   pedestrian injured in collision with pedestrian conveyance (V00.0-)

The appropriate 7th character is to be added to each code from category V06

A   initial encounter
D   subsequent encounter
S   sequela

● **V06.0**   **Pedestrian injured in collision with other nonmotor vehicle in nontraffic accident**
X ● **V06.00** **Pedestrian on foot injured in collision with other nonmotor vehicle in nontraffic accident**
Pedestrian NOS injured in collision with other nonmotor vehicle in nontraffic accident
X ● **V06.01** **Pedestrian on roller-skates injured in collision with other nonmotor vehicle in nontraffic accident**
X ● **V06.02** **Pedestrian on skateboard injured in collision with other nonmotor vehicle in nontraffic accident**
● **V06.03** **Pedestrian on standing micro-mobility pedestrian conveyance injured in collision with other nonmotor vehicle in nontraffic accident**
V06.031 **Pedestrian on standing electric scooter injured in collision with other nonmotor vehicle in nontraffic accident**
V06.038 **Pedestrian on other standing micro-mobility pedestrian conveyance injured in collision with other nonmotor vehicle in nontraffic accident**
Pedestrian on hoverboard injured in collision with other nonmotor vehicle in nontraffic accident
Pedestrian on segway injured in collision with other nonmotor vehicle in nontraffic accident

X ● **V06.09** **Pedestrian with other conveyance injured in collision with other nonmotor vehicle in nontraffic accident**
Pedestrian with baby stroller injured in collision with other nonmotor vehicle in nontraffic accident
Pedestrian in wheelchair (powered) injured in collision with other nonmotor vehicle in nontraffic accident
Pedestrian in motorized mobility scooter injured in collision with other nonmotor vehicle in nontraffic accident
Pedestrian on ice-skates injured in collision with other nonmotor vehicle in nontraffic accident
Pedestrian on nonmotorized scooter injured in collision with other nonmotor vehicle in nontraffic accident
Pedestrian on sled injured in collision with other nonmotor vehicle in nontraffic accident
Pedestrian on snowboard injured in collision with other nonmotor vehicle in nontraffic accident
Pedestrian on snow-skis injured in collision with other nonmotor vehicle in nontraffic accident

● **V06.1**   **Pedestrian injured in collision with other nonmotor vehicle in traffic accident**
X ● **V06.10** **Pedestrian on foot injured in collision with other nonmotor vehicle in traffic accident**
Pedestrian NOS injured in collision with other nonmotor vehicle in traffic accident
X ● **V06.11** **Pedestrian on roller-skates injured in collision with other nonmotor vehicle in traffic accident**
X ● **V06.12** **Pedestrian on skateboard injured in collision with other nonmotor vehicle in traffic accident**
● **V06.13** **Pedestrian on standing micro-mobility pedestrian conveyance injured in collision with other nonmotor vehicle in traffic accident**
V06.131 **Pedestrian on standing electric scooter injured in collision with other nonmotor vehicle in traffic accident**
V06.138 **Pedestrian on other standing micro-mobility pedestrian conveyance injured in collision with other nonmotor vehicle in traffic accident**
Pedestrian on hoverboard injured in collision with other nonmotor vehicle in traffic accident
Pedestrian on segway injured in collision with other nonmotor vehicle in traffic accident
X ● **V06.19** **Pedestrian with other conveyance injured in collision with other nonmotor vehicle in traffic accident**
Pedestrian with baby stroller injured in collision with other nonmotor vehicle in nontraffic accident
Pedestrian in wheelchair (powered) injured in collision with other nonmotor vehicle in traffic accident
Pedestrian in motorized mobility scooter injured in collision with other nonmotor vehicle in traffic accident
Pedestrian on ice-skates injured in collision with other nonmotor vehicle in traffic accident
Pedestrian on nonmotorized scooter injured in collision with other nonmotor vehicle in traffic accident
Pedestrian on sled injured in collision with other nonmotor vehicle in traffic accident
Pedestrian on snowboard injured in collision with other nonmotor vehicle in traffic accident
Pedestrian on snow-skis injured in collision with other nonmotor vehicle in traffic accident

● **V06.9** Pedestrian injured in collision with other nonmotor vehicle, unspecified whether traffic or nontraffic accident

X● **V06.90** Pedestrian on foot injured in collision with other nonmotor vehicle, unspecified whether traffic or nontraffic accident

Pedestrian NOS injured in collision with other nonmotor vehicle, unspecified whether traffic or nontraffic accident

X● **V06.91** Pedestrian on roller-skates injured in collision with other nonmotor vehicle, unspecified whether traffic or nontraffic accident

X● **V06.92** Pedestrian on skateboard injured in collision with other nonmotor vehicle, unspecified whether traffic or nontraffic accident

● **V06.93** Pedestrian on standing micro-mobility pedestrian conveyance injured in collision with other nonmotor vehicle, unspecified whether traffic or nontraffic accident

V06.931 Pedestrian on standing electric scooter injured in collision with other nonmotor vehicle, unspecified whether traffic or nontraffic accident

V06.938 Pedestrian on other standing micro-mobility pedestrian conveyance injured in collision with other nonmotor vehicle, unspecified whether traffic or nontraffic accident

Pedestrian on hoverboard injured in collision with other nonmotor, unspecified whether traffic or nontraffic accident

Pedestrian on segway injured in collision with other nonmotor vehicle, unspecified whether traffic or nontraffic accident

X● **V06.99** Pedestrian with other conveyance injured in collision with other nonmotor vehicle, unspecified whether traffic or nontraffic accident

Pedestrian with baby stroller injured in collision with other nonmotor vehicle, unspecified whether traffic or nontraffic accident

Pedestrian in wheelchair (powered) injured in collision with other nonmotor vehicle, unspecified whether traffic or nontraffic accident

Pedestrian in motorized mobility scooter injured in collision with other nonmotor vehicle, unspecified whether traffic or nontraffic accident

Pedestrian on ice-skates injured in collision with other nonmotor vehicle, unspecified whether traffic or nontraffic accident

Pedestrian on nonmotorized scooter injured in collision with other nonmotor vehicle, unspecified whether traffic or nontraffic accident

Pedestrian on sled injured in collision with other nonmotor vehicle, unspecified whether traffic or nontraffic accident

Pedestrian on snowboard injured in collision with other nonmotor vehicle, unspecified whether traffic or nontraffic accident

Pedestrian on snow-skis injured in collision with other nonmotor vehicle, unspecified whether traffic or nontraffic accident

● **V09** Pedestrian injured in other and unspecified transport accidents

The appropriate 7th character is to be added to each code from category V09

A	initial encounter
D	subsequent encounter
S	sequela

● **V09.0** Pedestrian injured in nontraffic accident involving other and unspecified motor vehicles

X● **V09.00** Pedestrian injured in nontraffic accident involving unspecified motor vehicles

X● **V09.01** Pedestrian injured in nontraffic accident involving military vehicle

X● **V09.09** Pedestrian injured in nontraffic accident involving other motor vehicles

Pedestrian injured in nontraffic accident by special vehicle

X● **V09.1** Pedestrian injured in unspecified nontraffic accident

● **V09.2** Pedestrian injured in traffic accident involving other and unspecified motor vehicles

X● **V09.20** Pedestrian injured in traffic accident involving unspecified motor vehicles

X● **V09.21** Pedestrian injured in traffic accident involving military vehicle

X● **V09.29** Pedestrian injured in traffic accident involving other motor vehicles

X● **V09.3** Pedestrian injured in unspecified traffic accident

X● **V09.9** Pedestrian injured in unspecified transport accident

PEDAL CYCLE RIDER INJURED IN TRANSPORT ACCIDENT (V10-V19)

Includes any non-motorized vehicle, excluding an animal-drawn vehicle, or a sidecar or trailer attached to the pedal cycle

Excludes2 rupture of pedal cycle tire (W37.0)

● **V10** Pedal cycle rider injured in collision with pedestrian or animal

Excludes1 pedal cycle rider collision with animal-drawn vehicle or animal being ridden (V16.-)

The appropriate 7th character is to be added to each code from category V10

A	initial encounter
D	subsequent encounter
S	sequela

X● **V10.0** Pedal cycle driver injured in collision with pedestrian or animal in nontraffic accident

X● **V10.1** Pedal cycle passenger injured in collision with pedestrian or animal in nontraffic accident

X● **V10.2** Unspecified pedal cyclist injured in collision with pedestrian or animal in nontraffic accident

X● **V10.3** Person boarding or alighting a pedal cycle injured in collision with pedestrian or animal

X● **V10.4** Pedal cycle driver injured in collision with pedestrian or animal in traffic accident

X● **V10.5** Pedal cycle passenger injured in collision with pedestrian or animal in traffic accident

X● **V10.9** Unspecified pedal cyclist injured in collision with pedestrian or animal in traffic accident

▶ New   ⇒ Revised   ~~deleted~~ Deleted   Excludes 1   Excludes 2   Includes   Use additional   Code first   Code also   Key words

OGCR Official Guidelines   X Assign placeholder X   ● Use Additional Character(s)   ▶ Manifestation Code   🕭 Hierarchical Condition Category   Coding Clinic

● **V11**   **Pedal cycle rider injured in collision with other pedal cycle**

The appropriate 7th character is to be added to each code from category V11

> A   initial encounter
> D   subsequent encounter
> S   sequela

X● **V11.0**   Pedal cycle driver injured in collision with other pedal cycle in nontraffic accident

X● **V11.1**   Pedal cycle passenger injured in collision with other pedal cycle in nontraffic accident

X● **V11.2**   Unspecified pedal cyclist injured in collision with other pedal cycle in nontraffic accident

X● **V11.3**   Person boarding or alighting a pedal cycle injured in collision with other pedal cycle

X● **V11.4**   Pedal cycle driver injured in collision with other pedal cycle in traffic accident

X● **V11.5**   Pedal cycle passenger injured in collision with other pedal cycle in traffic accident

X● **V11.9**   Unspecified pedal cyclist injured in collision with other pedal cycle in traffic accident

● **V12**   **Pedal cycle rider injured in collision with two- or three-wheeled motor vehicle**

The appropriate 7th character is to be added to each code from category V12

> A   initial encounter
> D   subsequent encounter
> S   sequela

X● **V12.0**   Pedal cycle driver injured in collision with two- or three-wheeled motor vehicle in nontraffic accident

X● **V12.1**   Pedal cycle passenger injured in collision with two- or three-wheeled motor vehicle in nontraffic accident

X● **V12.2**   Unspecified pedal cyclist injured in collision with two- or three-wheeled motor vehicle in nontraffic accident

X● **V12.3**   Person boarding or alighting a pedal cycle injured in collision with two- or three-wheeled motor vehicle

X● **V12.4**   Pedal cycle driver injured in collision with two- or three-wheeled motor vehicle in traffic accident

X● **V12.5**   Pedal cycle passenger injured in collision with two- or three-wheeled motor vehicle in traffic accident

X● **V12.9**   Unspecified pedal cyclist injured in collision with two- or three-wheeled motor vehicle in traffic accident

● **V13**   **Pedal cycle rider injured in collision with car, pick-up truck or van**

The appropriate 7th character is to be added to each code from category V13

> A   initial encounter
> D   subsequent encounter
> S   sequela

X● **V13.0**   Pedal cycle driver injured in collision with car, pick-up truck or van in nontraffic accident

X● **V13.1**   Pedal cycle passenger injured in collision with car, pick-up truck or van in nontraffic accident

X● **V13.2**   Unspecified pedal cyclist injured in collision with car, pick-up truck or van in nontraffic accident

X● **V13.3**   Person boarding or alighting a pedal cycle injured in collision with car, pick-up truck or van

X● **V13.4**   Pedal cycle driver injured in collision with car, pick-up truck or van in traffic accident

X● **V13.5**   Pedal cycle passenger injured in collision with car, pick-up truck or van in traffic accident

X● **V13.9**   Unspecified pedal cyclist injured in collision with car, pick-up truck or van in traffic accident

● **V14**   **Pedal cycle rider injured in collision with heavy transport vehicle or bus**

> **Excludes1**   pedal cycle rider injured in collision with military vehicle (V19.81)

The appropriate 7th character is to be added to each code from category V14

> A   initial encounter
> D   subsequent encounter
> S   sequela

X● **V14.0**   Pedal cycle driver injured in collision with heavy transport vehicle or bus in nontraffic accident

X● **V14.1**   Pedal cycle passenger injured in collision with heavy transport vehicle or bus in nontraffic accident

X● **V14.2**   Unspecified pedal cyclist injured in collision with heavy transport vehicle or bus in nontraffic accident

X● **V14.3**   Person boarding or alighting a pedal cycle injured in collision with heavy transport vehicle or bus

X● **V14.4**   Pedal cycle driver injured in collision with heavy transport vehicle or bus in traffic accident

X● **V14.5**   Pedal cycle passenger injured in collision with heavy transport vehicle or bus in traffic accident

X● **V14.9**   Unspecified pedal cyclist injured in collision with heavy transport vehicle or bus in traffic accident

● **V15**   **Pedal cycle rider injured in collision with railway train or railway vehicle**

The appropriate 7th character is to be added to each code from category V15

> A   initial encounter
> D   subsequent encounter
> S   sequela

X● **V15.0**   Pedal cycle driver injured in collision with railway train or railway vehicle in nontraffic accident

X● **V15.1**   Pedal cycle passenger injured in collision with railway train or railway vehicle in nontraffic accident

X● **V15.2**   Unspecified pedal cyclist injured in collision with railway train or railway vehicle in nontraffic accident

X● **V15.3**   Person boarding or alighting a pedal cycle injured in collision with railway train or railway vehicle

X● **V15.4**   Pedal cycle driver injured in collision with railway train or railway vehicle in traffic accident

X● **V15.5**   Pedal cycle passenger injured in collision with railway train or railway vehicle in traffic accident

X● **V15.9**   Unspecified pedal cyclist injured in collision with railway train or railway vehicle in traffic accident

● **V16**   **Pedal cycle rider injured in collision with other nonmotor vehicle**

> **Includes**   collision with animal-drawn vehicle, animal being ridden, streetcar

The appropriate 7th character is to be added to each code from category V16

> A   initial encounter
> D   subsequent encounter
> S   sequela

X● **V16.0**   Pedal cycle driver injured in collision with other nonmotor vehicle in nontraffic accident

X● **V16.1**   Pedal cycle passenger injured in collision with other nonmotor vehicle in nontraffic accident

X● **V16.2**   Unspecified pedal cyclist injured in collision with other nonmotor vehicle in nontraffic accident

X● **V16.3**   Person boarding or alighting a pedal cycle injured in collision with other nonmotor vehicle in nontraffic accident

X● **V16.4**   Pedal cycle driver injured in collision with other nonmotor vehicle in traffic accident

CHAPTER 20 (V00-Y99)

X ● **V16.5** Pedal cycle passenger injured in collision with other nonmotor vehicle in traffic accident

X ● **V16.9** Unspecified pedal cyclist injured in collision with other nonmotor vehicle in traffic accident

● **V17** Pedal cycle rider injured in collision with fixed or stationary object

The appropriate 7th character is to be added to each code from category V17

A	initial encounter
D	subsequent encounter
S	sequela

X ● **V17.0** Pedal cycle driver injured in collision with fixed or stationary object in nontraffic accident

X ● **V17.1** Pedal cycle passenger injured in collision with fixed or stationary object in nontraffic accident

X ● **V17.2** Unspecified pedal cyclist injured in collision with fixed or stationary object in nontraffic accident

X ● **V17.3** Person boarding or alighting a pedal cycle injured in collision with fixed or stationary object

X ● **V17.4** Pedal cycle driver injured in collision with fixed or stationary object in traffic accident

X ● **V17.5** Pedal cycle passenger injured in collision with fixed or stationary object in traffic accident

X ● **V17.9** Unspecified pedal cyclist injured in collision with fixed or stationary object in traffic accident

● **V18** Pedal cycle rider injured in noncollision transport accident

Includes fall or thrown from pedal cycle (without antecedent collision)
overturning pedal cycle NOS
overturning pedal cycle without collision

The appropriate 7th character is to be added to each code from category V18

A	initial encounter
D	subsequent encounter
S	sequela

X ● **V18.0** Pedal cycle driver injured in noncollision transport accident in nontraffic accident

X ● **V18.1** Pedal cycle passenger injured in noncollision transport accident in nontraffic accident

X ● **V18.2** Unspecified pedal cyclist injured in noncollision transport accident in nontraffic accident

X ● **V18.3** Person boarding or alighting a pedal cycle injured in noncollision transport accident

X ● **V18.4** Pedal cycle driver injured in noncollision transport accident in traffic accident

X ● **V18.5** Pedal cycle passenger injured in noncollision transport accident in traffic accident

X ● **V18.9** Unspecified pedal cyclist injured in noncollision transport accident in traffic accident

● **V19** Pedal cycle rider injured in other and unspecified transport accidents

The appropriate 7th character is to be added to each code from category V19

A	initial encounter
D	subsequent encounter
S	sequela

● **V19.0** Pedal cycle driver injured in collision with other and unspecified motor vehicles in nontraffic accident

X ● **V19.00** Pedal cycle driver injured in collision with unspecified motor vehicles in nontraffic accident

X ● **V19.09** Pedal cycle driver injured in collision with other motor vehicles in nontraffic accident

● **V19.1** Pedal cycle passenger injured in collision with other and unspecified motor vehicles in nontraffic accident

X ● **V19.10** Pedal cycle passenger injured in collision with unspecified motor vehicles in nontraffic accident

X ● **V19.19** Pedal cycle passenger injured in collision with other motor vehicles in nontraffic accident

● **V19.2** Unspecified pedal cyclist injured in collision with other and unspecified motor vehicles in nontraffic accident

X ● **V19.20** Unspecified pedal cyclist injured in collision with unspecified motor vehicles in nontraffic accident
Pedal cycle collision NOS, nontraffic

X ● **V19.29** Unspecified pedal cyclist injured in collision with other motor vehicles in nontraffic accident

X ● **V19.3** Pedal cyclist (driver) (passenger) injured in unspecified nontraffic accident
Pedal cycle accident NOS, nontraffic
Pedal cyclist injured in nontraffic accident NOS

● **V19.4** Pedal cycle driver injured in collision with other and unspecified motor vehicles in traffic accident

X ● **V19.40** Pedal cycle driver injured in collision with unspecified motor vehicles in traffic accident

X ● **V19.49** Pedal cycle driver injured in collision with other motor vehicles in traffic accident

● **V19.5** Pedal cycle passenger injured in collision with other and unspecified motor vehicles in traffic accident

X ● **V19.50** Pedal cycle passenger injured in collision with unspecified motor vehicles in traffic accident

X ● **V19.59** Pedal cycle passenger injured in collision with other motor vehicles in traffic accident

● **V19.6** Unspecified pedal cyclist injured in collision with other and unspecified motor vehicles in traffic accident

X ● **V19.60** Unspecified pedal cyclist injured in collision with unspecified motor vehicles in traffic accident
Pedal cycle collision NOS (traffic)

X ● **V19.69** Unspecified pedal cyclist injured in collision with other motor vehicles in traffic accident

● **V19.8** Pedal cyclist (driver) (passenger) injured in other specified transport accidents

X ● **V19.81** Pedal cyclist (driver) (passenger) injured in transport accident with military vehicle

X ● **V19.88** Pedal cyclist (driver) (passenger) injured in other specified transport accidents

X ● **V19.9** Pedal cyclist (driver) (passenger) injured in unspecified traffic accident
Pedal cycle accident NOS

MOTORCYCLE RIDER INJURED IN TRANSPORT ACCIDENT (V20-V29)

Includes electric bicycle
e-bike
e-bicycle
moped motorcycle with sidecar motorized bicycle
motor scooter

Excludes1 three-wheeled motor vehicle (V30-V39)

● **V20** Motorcycle rider injured in collision with pedestrian or animal

Excludes1 motorcycle rider collision with animal-drawn vehicle or animal being ridden (V26.-)

The appropriate 7th character is to be added to each code from category V20

A	initial encounter
D	subsequent encounter
S	sequela

X ● **V20.0** Motorcycle driver injured in collision with pedestrian or animal in nontraffic accident

X ● **V20.01** Electric (assisted) bicycle driver injured in collision with pedestrian or animal in nontraffic accident

X ● **V20.09** Other motorcycle driver injured in collision with pedestrian or animal in nontraffic accident

X● **V20.1** Motorcycle passenger injured in collision with pedestrian or animal in nontraffic accident

     X● **V20.11** Electric (assisted) bicycle passenger injured in collision with pedestrian or animal in nontraffic accident

     X● **V20.19** Other motorcycle passenger injured in collision with pedestrian or animal in nontraffic accident

X● **V20.2** Unspecified motorcycle rider injured in collision with pedestrian or animal in nontraffic accident

     X● **V20.21** Unspecified electric (assisted) bicycle rider injured in collision with pedestrian or animal in nontraffic accident

     X● **V20.29** Unspecified rider of other motorcycle injured in collision with pedestrian or animal in nontraffic accident

X● **V20.3** Person boarding or alighting a motorcycle injured in collision with pedestrian or animal

     X● **V20.31** Person boarding or alighting an electric (assisted) bicycle injured in collision with pedestrian or animal

     X● **V20.39** Person boarding or alighting other motorcycle injured in collision with pedestrian or animal

X● **V20.4** Motorcycle driver injured in collision with pedestrian or animal in traffic accident

     X● **V20.41** Electric (assisted) bicycle driver injured in collision with pedestrian or animal in traffic accident

     X● **V20.49** Other motorcycle driver injured in collision with pedestrian or animal in traffic accident

X● **V20.5** Motorcycle passenger injured in collision with pedestrian or animal in traffic accident

     X● **V20.51** Electric (assisted) bicycle passenger injured in collision with pedestrian or animal in traffic accident

     X● **V20.59** Other motorcycle passenger injured in collision with pedestrian or animal in traffic accident

X● **V20.9** Unspecified motorcycle rider injured in collision with pedestrian or animal in traffic accident

     X● **V20.91** Unspecified electric (assisted) bicycle rider injured in collision with pedestrian or animal in traffic accident

     X● **V20.99** Unspecified rider of other motorcycle injured in collision with pedestrian or animal in traffic accident

● **V21** Motorcycle rider injured in collision with pedal cycle

     The appropriate 7th character is to be added to each code from category V21

A	initial encounter
D	subsequent encounter
S	sequela

X● **V21.0** Motorcycle driver injured in collision with pedal cycle in nontraffic accident

     X● **V21.01** Electric (assisted) bicycle driver injured in collision with pedal cycle in nontraffic accident

     X● **V21.09** Other motorcycle driver injured in collision with pedal cycle in nontraffic accident

X● **V21.1** Motorcycle passenger injured in collision with pedal cycle in nontraffic accident

     X● **V21.11** Electric (assisted) bicycle passenger injured in collision with pedal cycle in nontraffic accident

     X● **V21.19** Other motorcycle passenger injured in collision with pedal cycle in nontraffic accident

X● **V21.2** Unspecified motorcycle rider injured in collision with pedal cycle in nontraffic accident

     X● **V21.21** Unspecified electric (assisted) bicycle rider injured in collision with pedal cycle in nontraffic accident

     X● **V21.29** Unspecified rider of other motorcycle injured in collision with pedal cycle in nontraffic accident

X● **V21.3** Person boarding or alighting a motorcycle injured in collision with pedal cycle

     X● **V21.31** Person boarding or alighting an electric (assisted) bicycle injured in collision with pedal cycle

     X● **V21.39** Person boarding or alighting other motorcycle injured in collision with pedal cycle

X● **V21.4** Motorcycle driver injured in collision with pedal cycle in traffic accident

     X● **V21.41** Electric (assisted) bicycle driver injured in collision with pedal cycle in traffic accident

     X● **V21.49** Other motorcycle driver injured in collision with pedal cycle in traffic accident

X● **V21.5** Motorcycle passenger injured in collision with pedal cycle in traffic accident

     X● **V21.51** Electric (assisted) bicycle passenger injured in collision with pedal cycle in traffic accident

     X● **V21.59** Other motorcycle passenger injured in collision with pedal cycle in traffic accident

X● **V21.9** Unspecified motorcycle rider injured in collision with pedal cycle in traffic accident

     X● **V21.91** Unspecified electric (assisted) bicycle rider injured in collision with pedal cycle in traffic accident

     X● **V21.99** Unspecified rider of other motorcycle injured in collision with pedal cycle in traffic accident

● **V22** Motorcycle rider injured in collision with two- or three-wheeled motor vehicle

     The appropriate 7th character is to be added to each code from category V22

A	initial encounter
D	subsequent encounter
S	sequela

X● **V22.0** Motorcycle driver injured in collision with two- or three-wheeled motor vehicle in nontraffic accident

     X● **V22.01** Electric (assisted) bicycle driver injured in collision with two- or three-wheeled motor vehicle in nontraffic accident

     X● **V22.09** Other motorcycle driver injured in collision with two- or three-wheeled motor vehicle in nontraffic accident

X● **V22.1** Motorcycle passenger injured in collision with two- or three-wheeled motor vehicle in nontraffic accident

     X● **V22.11** Electric (assisted) bicycle passenger injured in collision with two- or three-wheeled motor vehicle in nontraffic accident

     X● **V22.19** Other motorcycle passenger injured in collision with two- or three-wheeled motor vehicle in nontraffic accident

X● **V22.2** Unspecified motorcycle rider injured in collision with two- or three-wheeled motor vehicle in nontraffic accident

     X● **V22.21** Unspecified electric (assisted) bicycle rider injured in collision with two- or three-wheeled motor vehicle in nontraffic accident

     X● **V22.29** Unspecified rider of other motorcycle injured in collision with two- or three-wheeled motor vehicle in nontraffic accident

X● **V22.3** Person boarding or alighting a motorcycle injured in collision with two- or three-wheeled motor vehicle

     X● **V22.31** Person boarding or alighting an electric (assisted) bicycle injured in collision with two- or three-wheeled motor vehicle

     X● **V22.39** Person boarding or alighting other motorcycle injured in collision with two- or three-wheeled motor vehicle

CHAPTER 20 (V00-Y99)

X● V22.4   Motorcycle driver injured in collision with two- or three-wheeled motor vehicle in traffic accident
   X● V22.41   Electric (assisted) bicycle driver injured in collision with two- or three-wheeled motor vehicle in traffic accident
   X● V22.49   Other motorcycle driver injured in collision with two- or three-wheeled motor vehicle in traffic accident
X● V22.5   Motorcycle passenger injured in collision with two- or three-wheeled motor vehicle in traffic accident
   X● V22.51   Electric (assisted) bicycle passenger injured in collision with two- or three-wheeled motor vehicle in traffic accident
   X● V22.59   Other motorcycle passenger injured in collision with two- or three-wheeled motor vehicle in traffic accident
X● V22.9   Unspecified motorcycle rider injured in collision with two- or three-wheeled motor vehicle in traffic accident
   X● V22.91   Unspecified electric (assisted) bicycle rider injured in collision with two- or three-wheeled motor vehicle in traffic accident
   X● V22.99   Unspecified rider of other motorcycle injured in collision with two- or three-wheeled motor vehicle in traffic accident

● V23   Motorcycle rider injured in collision with car, pick-up truck or van
   The appropriate 7th character is to be added to each code from category V23

> A   initial encounter
> D   subsequent encounter
> S   sequela

X● V23.0   Motorcycle driver injured in collision with car, pick-up truck or van in nontraffic accident
   X● V23.01   Electric (assisted) bicycle driver injured in collision with car, pick-up truck or van in nontraffic accident
   X● V23.09   Other motorcycle driver injured in collision with car, pick-up truck or van in nontraffic accident
X● V23.1   Motorcycle passenger injured in collision with car, pick-up truck or van in nontraffic accident
   X● V23.11   Electric (assisted) bicycle passenger injured in collision with car, pick-up truck or van in nontraffic accident
   X● V23.19   Other motorcycle passenger injured in collision with car, pick-up truck or van in nontraffic accident
X● V23.2   Unspecified motorcycle rider injured in collision with car, pick-up truck or van in nontraffic accident
   X● V23.21   Unspecified electric (assisted) bicycle rider injured in collision with car, pick-up truck or van in nontraffic accident
   X● V23.29   Unspecified rider of other motorcycle injured in collision with car, pick-up truck or van in nontraffic accident
X● V23.3   Person boarding or alighting a motorcycle injured in collision with car, pick-up truck or van
   X● V23.31   Person boarding or alighting an electric (assisted) bicycle injured in collision with car, pick-up truck or van
   X● V23.39   Person boarding or alighting other motorcycle injured in collision with car, pick-up truck or van
X● V23.4   Motorcycle driver injured in collision with car, pick-up truck or van in traffic accident
   X● V23.41   Electric (assisted) bicycle driver injured in collision with car, pick-up truck or van in traffic accident
   X● V23.49   Other motorcycle driver injured in collision with car, pick-up truck or van in traffic accident

X● V23.5   Motorcycle passenger injured in collision with car, pick-up truck or van in traffic accident
   X● V23.51   Electric (assisted) bicycle passenger injured in collision with car, pick-up truck or van in traffic accident
   X● V23.59   Other motorcycle passenger injured in collision with car, pick-up truck or van in traffic accident
X● V23.9   Unspecified motorcycle rider injured in collision with car, pick-up truck or van in traffic accident
   X● V23.91   Unspecified electric (assisted) bicycle rider injured in collision with car, pick-up truck or van in traffic accident
   X● V23.99   Unspecified rider of other motorcycle injured in collision with car, pick-up truck or van in traffic accident

● V24   Motorcycle rider injured in collision with heavy transport vehicle or bus
   Excludes1   motorcycle rider injured in collision with military vehicle (V29.818)
   The appropriate 7th character is to be added to each code from category V24

> A   initial encounter
> D   subsequent encounter
> S   sequela

X● V24.0   Motorcycle driver injured in collision with heavy transport vehicle or bus in nontraffic accident
   X● V24.01   Electric (assisted) bicycle driver injured in collision with heavy transport vehicle or bus in nontraffic accident
   X● V24.09   Other motorcycle driver injured in collision with heavy transport vehicle or bus in nontraffic accident
X● V24.1   Motorcycle passenger injured in collision with heavy transport vehicle or bus in nontraffic accident
   X● V24.11   Electric (assisted) bicycle passenger injured in collision with heavy transport vehicle or bus in nontraffic accident
   X● V24.19   Other motorcycle passenger injured in collision with heavy transport vehicle or bus in nontraffic accident
X● V24.2   Unspecified motorcycle rider injured in collision with heavy transport vehicle or bus in nontraffic accident
   X● V24.21   Unspecified electric (assisted) bicycle rider injured in collision with heavy transport vehicle or bus in nontraffic accident
   X● V24.29   Unspecified rider of other motorcycle injured in collision with heavy transport vehicle or bus in nontraffic accident
X● V24.3   Person boarding or alighting a motorcycle injured in collision with heavy transport vehicle or bus
   X● V24.31   Person boarding or alighting an electric (assisted) bicycle injured in collision with heavy transport vehicle or bus
   X● V24.39   Person boarding or alighting other motorcycle injured in collision with heavy transport vehicle or bus
X● V24.4   Motorcycle driver injured in collision with heavy transport vehicle or bus in traffic accident
   X● V24.41   Electric (assisted) bicycle driver injured in collision with heavy transport vehicle or bus in traffic accident
   X● V24.49   Other motorcycle driver injured in collision with heavy transport vehicle or bus in traffic accident
X● V24.5   Motorcycle passenger injured in collision with heavy transport vehicle or bus in traffic accident
   X● V24.51   Electric (assisted) bicycle passenger injured in collision with heavy transport vehicle or bus in traffic accident
   X● V24.59   Other motorcycle passenger injured in collision with heavy transport vehicle or bus in traffic accident

▶ New   ⇢ Revised   ~~deleted~~ Deleted   Excludes 1   Excludes 2   Includes   Use additional   Code first   Code also   Key words
OGCR Official Guidelines   X Assign placeholder X   ● Use Additional Character(s)   ▷ Manifestation Code   🔖 Hierarchical Condition Category   Coding Clinic

X ● **V24.9**   Unspecified motorcycle rider injured in collision with heavy transport vehicle or bus in traffic accident

    X ● **V24.91**   Unspecified electric (assisted) bicycle rider injured in collision with heavy transport vehicle or bus in traffic accident

    X ● **V24.99**   Unspecified rider of other motorcycle injured in collision with heavy transport vehicle or bus in traffic accident

● **V25**   Motorcycle rider injured in collision with railway train or railway vehicle

    The appropriate 7th character is to be added to each code from category V25

A	initial encounter
D	subsequent encounter
S	sequela

X ● **V25.0**   Motorcycle driver injured in collision with railway train or railway vehicle in nontraffic accident

    X ● **V25.01**   Electric (assisted) bicycle driver injured in collision with railway train or railway vehicle in nontraffic accident

    X ● **V25.09**   Other motorcycle driver injured in collision with railway train or railway vehicle in nontraffic accident

X ● **V25.1**   Motorcycle passenger injured in collision with railway train or railway vehicle in nontraffic accident

    X ● **V25.11**   Electric (assisted) bicycle passenger injured in collision with railway train or railway vehicle in nontraffic accident

    X ● **V25.19**   Other motorcycle passenger injured in collision with railway train or railway vehicle in nontraffic accident

X ● **V25.2**   Unspecified motorcycle rider injured in collision with railway train or railway vehicle in nontraffic accident

    X ● **V25.21**   Unspecified electric (assisted) bicycle rider injured in collision with railway train or railway vehicle in nontraffic accident

    X ● **V25.29**   Unspecified rider of other motorcycle injured in collision with railway train or railway vehicle in nontraffic accident

X ● **V25.3**   Person boarding or alighting a motorcycle injured in collision with railway train or railway vehicle

    X ● **V25.31**   Person boarding or alighting an electric (assisted) bicycle injured in collision with railway train or railway vehicle

    X ● **V25.39**   Person boarding or alighting other motorcycle injured in collision with railway train or railway vehicle

X ● **V25.4**   Motorcycle driver injured in collision with railway train or railway vehicle in traffic accident

    X ● **V25.41**   Electric (assisted) bicycle driver injured in collision with railway train or railway vehicle in traffic accident

    X ● **V25.49**   Other motorcycle driver injured in collision with railway train or railway vehicle in traffic accident

X ● **V25.5**   Motorcycle passenger injured in collision with railway train or railway vehicle in traffic accident

    X ● **V25.51**   Electric (assisted) bicycle passenger injured in collision with railway train or railway vehicle in traffic accident

    X ● **V25.59**   Other motorcycle passenger injured in collision with railway train or railway vehicle in traffic accident

X ● **V25.9**   Unspecified motorcycle rider injured in collision with railway train or railway vehicle in traffic accident

    X ● **V25.91**   Unspecified electric (assisted) bicycle rider injured in collision with railway train or railway vehicle in traffic accident

    X ● **V25.99**   Unspecified rider of other motorcycle injured in collision with railway train or railway vehicle in traffic accident

● **V26**   Motorcycle rider injured in collision with other nonmotor vehicle

    Includes   collision with animal-drawn vehicle, animal being ridden, streetcar

    The appropriate 7th character is to be added to each code from category V26

A	initial encounter
D	subsequent encounter
S	sequela

X ● **V26.0**   Motorcycle driver injured in collision with other nonmotor vehicle in nontraffic accident

    X ● **V26.01**   Electric (assisted) bicycle driver injured in collision with other nonmotor vehicle in nontraffic accident

    X ● **V26.09**   Other motorcycle driver injured in collision with other nonmotor vehicle in nontraffic accident

X ● **V26.1**   Motorcycle passenger injured in collision with other nonmotor vehicle in nontraffic accident

    X ● **V26.11**   Electric (assisted) bicycle passenger injured in collision with other nonmotor vehicle in nontraffic accident

    X ● **V26.19**   Other motorcycle passenger injured in collision with other nonmotor vehicle in nontraffic accident

X ● **V26.2**   Unspecified motorcycle rider injured in collision with other nonmotor vehicle in nontraffic accident

    X ● **V26.21**   Unspecified electric (assisted) bicycle rider injured in collision with other nonmotor vehicle in nontraffic accident

    X ● **V26.29**   Unspecified rider of other motorcycle injured in collision with other nonmotor vehicle in nontraffic accident

X ● **V26.3**   Person boarding or alighting a motorcycle injured in collision with other nonmotor vehicle

    X ● **V26.31**   Person boarding or alighting an electric (assisted) bicycle injured in collision with other nonmotor vehicle

    X ● **V26.39**   Person boarding or alighting other motorcycle injured in collision with other nonmotor vehicle

X ● **V26.4**   Motorcycle driver injured in collision with other nonmotor vehicle in traffic accident

    X ● **V26.41**   Electric (assisted) bicycle driver injured in collision with other nonmotor vehicle in traffic accident

    X ● **V26.49**   Other motorcycle driver injured in collision with other nonmotor vehicle in traffic accident

X ● **V26.5**   Motorcycle passenger injured in collision with other nonmotor vehicle in traffic accident

    X ● **V26.51**   Electric (assisted) bicycle passenger injured in collision with other nonmotor vehicle in traffic accident

    X ● **V26.59**   Other motorcycle passenger injured in collision with other nonmotor vehicle in traffic accident

X ● **V26.9**   Unspecified motorcycle rider injured in collision with other nonmotor vehicle in traffic accident

    X ● **V26.91**   Unspecified electric (assisted) bicycle rider injured in collision with other nonmotor vehicle in traffic accident

    X ● **V26.99**   Unspecified rider of other motorcycle injured in collision with other nonmotor vehicle in traffic accident

CHAPTER 20 (V00-Y99)

● V27 **Motorcycle rider injured in collision with fixed or stationary object**

The appropriate 7th character is to be added to each code from category V27

> A initial encounter
> D subsequent encounter
> S sequela

X● **V27.0** Motorcycle driver injured in collision with fixed or stationary object in nontraffic accident

 X● **V27.01** Electric (assisted) bicycle driver injured in collision with fixed or stationary object in nontraffic accident

 X● **V27.09** Other motorcycle driver injured in collision with fixed or stationary object in nontraffic accident

X● **V27.1** Motorcycle passenger injured in collision with fixed or stationary object in nontraffic accident

 X● **V27.11** Electric (assisted) bicycle passenger injured in collision with fixed or stationary object in nontraffic accident

 X● **V27.19** Other motorcycle passenger injured in collision with fixed or stationary object in nontraffic accident

X● **V27.2** Unspecified motorcycle rider injured in collision with fixed or stationary object in nontraffic accident

 X● **V27.21** Unspecified electric (assisted) bicycle rider injured in collision with fixed or stationary object in nontraffic accident

 X● **V27.29** Unspecified rider of other motorcycle injured in collision with fixed or stationary object in nontraffic accident

X● **V27.3** Person boarding or alighting a motorcycle injured in collision with fixed or stationary object

 X● **V27.31** Person boarding or alighting an electric (assisted) bicycle injured in collision with fixed or stationary object

 X● **V27.39** Person boarding or alighting other motorcycle injured in collision with fixed or stationary object

X● **V27.4** Motorcycle driver injured in collision with fixed or stationary object in traffic accident

 X● **V27.41** Electric (assisted) bicycle driver injured in collision with fixed or stationary object in traffic accident

 X● **V27.49** Other motorcycle driver injured in collision with fixed or stationary object in traffic accident

X● **V27.5** Motorcycle passenger injured in collision with fixed or stationary object in traffic accident

 X● **V27.51** Electric (assisted) bicycle passenger injured in collision with fixed or stationary object in traffic accident

 X● **V27.59** Other motorcycle passenger injured in collision with fixed or stationary object in traffic accident

X● **V27.9** Unspecified motorcycle rider injured in collision with fixed or stationary object in traffic accident

 X● **V27.91** Unspecified electric (assisted) bicycle rider injured in collision with fixed or stationary object in traffic accident

 X● **V27.99** Unspecified rider of other motorcycle injured in collision with fixed or stationary object in traffic accident

● V28 **Motorcycle rider injured in noncollision transport accident**

> **Includes** fall or thrown from motorcycle (without antecedent collision)
> overturning motorcycle NOS
> overturning motorcycle without collision

The appropriate 7th character is to be added to each code from category V28

> A initial encounter
> D subsequent encounter
> S sequela

X● **V28.0** Motorcycle driver injured in noncollision transport accident in nontraffic accident

 X● **V28.01** Electric (assisted) bicycle driver injured in noncollision transport accident in nontraffic accident

 X● **V28.09** Other motorcycle driver injured in noncollision transport accident in nontraffic accident

X● **V28.1** Motorcycle passenger injured in noncollision transport accident in nontraffic accident

 X● **V28.11** Electric (assisted) bicycle passenger injured in noncollision transport accident in nontraffic accident

 X● **V28.19** Other motorcycle passenger injured in noncollision transport accident in nontraffic accident

X● **V28.2** Unspecified motorcycle rider injured in noncollision transport accident in nontraffic accident

 X● **V28.21** Unspecified electric (assisted) bicycle rider injured in noncollision transport accident in nontraffic accident

 X● **V28.29** Unspecified rider of other motorcycle injured in noncollision transport accident in nontraffic accident

X● **V28.3** Person boarding or alighting a motorcycle injured in noncollision transport accident

 X● **V28.31** Person boarding or alighting an electric (assisted) bicycle injured in noncollision transport accident

 X● **V28.39** Person boarding or alighting other motorcycle injured in noncollision transport accident

X● **V28.4** Motorcycle driver injured in noncollision transport accident in traffic accident

 X● **V28.41** Electric (assisted) bicycle driver injured in noncollision transport accident in traffic accident

 X● **V28.49** Other motorcycle driver injured in noncollision transport accident in traffic accident

X● **V28.5** Motorcycle passenger injured in noncollision transport accident in traffic accident

 X● **V28.51** Electric (assisted) bicycle passenger injured in noncollision transport accident in traffic accident

 X● **V28.59** Other motorcycle passenger injured in noncollision transport accident in traffic accident

X● **V28.9** Unspecified motorcycle rider injured in noncollision transport accident in traffic accident

 X● **V28.91** Unspecified electric (assisted) bicycle rider injured in noncollision transport accident in traffic accident

 X● **V28.99** Unspecified rider of other motorcycle injured in noncollision transport accident in traffic accident

● **V29 Motorcycle rider injured in other and unspecified transport accidents**

The appropriate 7th character is to be added to each code from category V29

> A   initial encounter
> D   subsequent encounter
> S   sequela

Coding Clinic: 2015, Q3, P20

● **V29.0 Motorcycle driver injured in collision with other and unspecified motor vehicles in nontraffic accident**

● **V29.00 Motorcycle driver injured in collision with unspecified motor vehicles in nontraffic accident**

● V29.001 Electric (assisted) bicycle driver injured in collision with unspecified motor vehicles in nontraffic accident

● V29.008 Other motorcycle driver injured in collision with unspecified motor vehicles in nontraffic accident

● **V29.09 Motorcycle driver injured in collision with other motor vehicles in nontraffic accident**

● V29.091 Electric (assisted) bicycle driver injured in collision with other motor vehicles in nontraffic accident

● V29.098 Other motorcycle driver injured in collision with other motor vehicles in nontraffic accident

● **V29.1 Motorcycle passenger injured in collision with other and unspecified motor vehicles in nontraffic accident**

● **V29.10 Motorcycle passenger injured in collision with unspecified motor vehicles in nontraffic accident**

● V29.101 Electric (assisted) bicycle passenger injured in collision with unspecified motor vehicles in nontraffic accident

● V29.108 Other motorcycle passenger injured in collision with unspecified motor vehicles in nontraffic accident

● **V29.19 Motorcycle passenger injured in collision with other motor vehicles in nontraffic accident**

● V29.191 Electric (assisted) bicycle passenger injured in collision with other motor vehicles in nontraffic accident

● V29.198 Other motorcycle passenger injured in collision with other motor vehicles in nontraffic accident

● **V29.2 Unspecified motorcycle rider injured in collision with other and unspecified motor vehicles in nontraffic accident**

● **V29.20 Unspecified motorcycle rider injured in collision with unspecified motor vehicles in nontraffic accident**
Motorcycle collision NOS, nontraffic

● V29.201 Unspecified electric (assisted) bicycle rider injured in collision with unspecified motor vehicles in nontraffic accident

● V29.208 Unspecified rider of other motorcycle injured in collision with unspecified motor vehicles in nontraffic accident
Motorcycle collision NOS, nontraffic

● **V29.29 Unspecified motorcycle rider injured in collision with other motor vehicles in nontraffic accident**

● V29.291 Unspecified electric (assisted) bicycle rider injured in collision with other motor vehicles in nontraffic accident

● V29.298 Unspecified rider of other motorcycle injured in collision with other motor vehicles in nontraffic accident

X ● **V29.3 Motorcycle rider (driver) (passenger) injured in unspecified nontraffic accident**
Motorcycle accident NOS, nontraffic
Motorcycle rider injured in nontraffic accident NOS

X ● **V29.31 Electric (assisted) bicycle (driver) (passenger) injured in unspecified nontraffic accident**

X ● **V29.39 Other motorcycle (driver) (passenger) injured in unspecified nontraffic accident**
Motorcycle accident NOS, nontraffic
Motorcycle rider injured in nontraffic accident NOS

● **V29.4 Motorcycle driver injured in collision with other and unspecified motor vehicles in traffic accident**

● **V29.40 Motorcycle driver injured in collision with unspecified motor vehicles in traffic accident**

● V29.401 Electric (assisted) bicycle driver injured in collision with unspecified motor vehicles in traffic accident

● V29.408 Other motorcycle driver injured in collision with unspecified motor vehicles in traffic accident

● **V29.49 Motorcycle driver injured in collision with other motor vehicles in traffic accident**

● V29.491 Electric (assisted) bicycle driver injured in collision with other motor vehicles in traffic accident

● V29.498 Other motorcycle driver injured in collision with other motor vehicles in traffic accident

● **V29.5 Motorcycle passenger injured in collision with other and unspecified motor vehicles in traffic accident**

● **V29.50 Motorcycle passenger injured in collision with unspecified motor vehicles in traffic accident**

● V29.501 Electric (assisted) bicycle passenger injured in collision with unspecified motor vehicles in traffic accident

● V29.508 Other motorcycle passenger injured in collision with unspecified motor vehicles in traffic accident

● **V29.59 Motorcycle passenger injured in collision with other motor vehicles in traffic accident**

● V29.591 Electric (assisted) bicycle passenger injured in collision with other motor vehicles in traffic accident

● V29.598 Other motorcycle passenger injured in collision with other motor vehicles in traffic accident

● **V29.6 Unspecified motorcycle rider injured in collision with other and unspecified motor vehicles in traffic accident**

● **V29.60 Unspecified motorcycle rider injured in collision with unspecified motor vehicles in traffic accident**
Motorcycle collision NOS (traffic)

● V29.601 Unspecified electric (assisted) bicycle rider injured in collision with unspecified motor vehicles in traffic accident

● V29.608 Unspecified rider of other motorcycle injured in collision with unspecified motor vehicles in traffic accident
Motorcycle collision NOS (traffic)

● **V29.69 Unspecified motorcycle rider injured in collision with other motor vehicles in traffic accident**

● V29.691 Unspecified electric (assisted) bicycle rider injured in collision with other motor vehicles in traffic accident

● V29.698 Unspecified rider of other motorcycle injured in collision with other motor vehicles in traffic accident

● **V29.8 Motorcycle rider (driver) (passenger) injured in other specified transport accidents**

CHAPTER 20 (V00-Y99)

- V29.81 Motorcycle rider (driver) (passenger) injured in transport accident with military vehicle
  - V29.811 Electric (assisted) bicycle rider (driver) (passenger) injured in transport accident with military vehicle
  - V29.818 Rider (driver) (passenger) of other motorcycle injured in transport accident with military vehicle
- V29.88 Motorcycle rider (driver) (passenger) injured in other specified transport accidents
  - V29.881 Electric (assisted) bicycle rider (driver) (passenger) injured in other specified transport accidents
  - V29.888 Rider (driver) (passenger) of other motorcycle injured in other specified transport accidents
- X● V29.9 Motorcycle rider (driver) (passenger) injured in unspecified traffic accident
  Motorcycle accident NOS
  - X● V29.91 Electric (assisted) bicycle rider (driver) (passenger) injured in unspecified traffic accident
  - X● V29.99 Rider (driver) (passenger) of other motorcycle injured in unspecified traffic accident
  Motorcycle accident NOS

OCCUPANT OF THREE-WHEELED MOTOR VEHICLE INJURED IN TRANSPORT ACCIDENT (V30-V39)

Includes	motorized tricycle
	motorized rickshaw
	three-wheeled motor car

Excludes 1	all-terrain vehicles (V86.-)
	motorcycle with sidecar (V20-V29)
	vehicle designed primarily for off-road use (V86.-)

- V30 Occupant of three-wheeled motor vehicle injured in collision with pedestrian or animal

  | Excludes 1 | three-wheeled motor vehicle collision with animal-drawn vehicle or animal being ridden (V36.-) |

  The appropriate 7th character is to be added to each code from category V30

A	initial encounter
D	subsequent encounter
S	sequela

  - X● V30.0 Driver of three-wheeled motor vehicle injured in collision with pedestrian or animal in nontraffic accident
  - X● V30.1 Passenger in three-wheeled motor vehicle injured in collision with pedestrian or animal in nontraffic accident
  - X● V30.2 Person on outside of three-wheeled motor vehicle injured in collision with pedestrian or animal in nontraffic accident
  - X● V30.3 Unspecified occupant of three-wheeled motor vehicle injured in collision with pedestrian or animal in nontraffic accident
  - X● V30.4 Person boarding or alighting a three-wheeled motor vehicle injured in collision with pedestrian or animal
  - X● V30.5 Driver of three-wheeled motor vehicle injured in collision with pedestrian or animal in traffic accident
  - X● V30.6 Passenger in three-wheeled motor vehicle injured in collision with pedestrian or animal in traffic accident
  - X● V30.7 Person on outside of three-wheeled motor vehicle injured in collision with pedestrian or animal in traffic accident
  - X● V30.9 Unspecified occupant of three-wheeled motor vehicle injured in collision with pedestrian or animal in traffic accident

- V31 Occupant of three-wheeled motor vehicle injured in collision with pedal cycle

  The appropriate 7th character is to be added to each code from category V31

A	initial encounter
D	subsequent encounter
S	sequela

  - X● V31.0 Driver of three-wheeled motor vehicle injured in collision with pedal cycle in nontraffic accident
  - X● V31.1 Passenger in three-wheeled motor vehicle injured in collision with pedal cycle in nontraffic accident
  - X● V31.2 Person on outside of three-wheeled motor vehicle injured in collision with pedal cycle in nontraffic accident
  - X● V31.3 Unspecified occupant of three-wheeled motor vehicle injured in collision with pedal cycle in nontraffic accident
  - X● V31.4 Person boarding or alighting a three-wheeled motor vehicle injured in collision with pedal cycle
  - X● V31.5 Driver of three-wheeled motor vehicle injured in collision with pedal cycle in traffic accident
  - X● V31.6 Passenger in three-wheeled motor vehicle injured in collision with pedal cycle in traffic accident
  - X● V31.7 Person on outside of three-wheeled motor vehicle injured in collision with pedal cycle in traffic accident
  - X● V31.9 Unspecified occupant of three-wheeled motor vehicle injured in collision with pedal cycle in traffic accident

- V32 Occupant of three-wheeled motor vehicle injured in collision with two- or three-wheeled motor vehicle

  The appropriate 7th character is to be added to each code from category V32

A	initial encounter
D	subsequent encounter
S	sequela

  - X● V32.0 Driver of three-wheeled motor vehicle injured in collision with two- or three-wheeled motor vehicle in nontraffic accident
  - X● V32.1 Passenger in three-wheeled motor vehicle injured in collision with two- or three-wheeled motor vehicle in nontraffic accident
  - X● V32.2 Person on outside of three-wheeled motor vehicle injured in collision with two- or three-wheeled motor vehicle in nontraffic accident
  - X● V32.3 Unspecified occupant of three-wheeled motor vehicle injured in collision with two- or three-wheeled motor vehicle in nontraffic accident
  - X● V32.4 Person boarding or alighting a three-wheeled motor vehicle injured in collision with two- or three-wheeled motor vehicle
  - X● V32.5 Driver of three-wheeled motor vehicle injured in collision with two- or three-wheeled motor vehicle in traffic accident
  - X● V32.6 Passenger in three-wheeled motor vehicle injured in collision with two- or three-wheeled motor vehicle in traffic accident
  - X● V32.7 Person on outside of three-wheeled motor vehicle injured in collision with two- or three-wheeled motor vehicle in traffic accident
  - X● V32.9 Unspecified occupant of three-wheeled motor vehicle injured in collision with two- or three-wheeled motor vehicle in traffic accident

▶ New   ▮▶ Revised   ~~deleted~~ Deleted   Excludes 1   Excludes 2   Includes   Use additional   Code first   Code also   Key words
OGCR Official Guidelines   X Assign placeholder X   ● Use Additional Character(s)   ▮ Manifestation Code   🄷 Hierarchical Condition Category   Coding Clinic

● **V33**   Occupant of three-wheeled motor vehicle injured in collision with car, pick-up truck or van

> The appropriate 7th character is to be added to each code from category V33

> | | |
> |---|---|
> | A | initial encounter |
> | D | subsequent encounter |
> | S | sequela |

X ● **V33.0**   Driver of three-wheeled motor vehicle injured in collision with car, pick-up truck or van in nontraffic accident

X ● **V33.1**   Passenger in three-wheeled motor vehicle injured in collision with car, pick-up truck or van in nontraffic accident

X ● **V33.2**   Person on outside of three-wheeled motor vehicle injured in collision with car, pick-up truck or van in nontraffic accident

X ● **V33.3**   Unspecified occupant of three-wheeled motor vehicle injured in collision with car, pick-up truck or van in nontraffic accident

X ● **V33.4**   Person boarding or alighting a three-wheeled motor vehicle injured in collision with car, pick-up truck or van

X ● **V33.5**   Driver of three-wheeled motor vehicle injured in collision with car, pick-up truck or van in traffic accident

X ● **V33.6**   Passenger in three-wheeled motor vehicle injured in collision with car, pick-up truck or van in traffic accident

X ● **V33.7**   Person on outside of three-wheeled motor vehicle injured in collision with car, pick-up truck or van in traffic accident

X ● **V33.9**   Unspecified occupant of three-wheeled motor vehicle injured in collision with car, pick-up truck or van in traffic accident

● **V34**   Occupant of three-wheeled motor vehicle injured in collision with heavy transport vehicle or bus

> **Excludes1**   occupant of three-wheeled motor vehicle injured in collision with military vehicle (V39.81)

> The appropriate 7th character is to be added to each code from category V34

> | | |
> |---|---|
> | A | initial encounter |
> | D | subsequent encounter |
> | S | sequela |

X ● **V34.0**   Driver of three-wheeled motor vehicle injured in collision with heavy transport vehicle or bus in nontraffic accident

X ● **V34.1**   Passenger in three-wheeled motor vehicle injured in collision with heavy transport vehicle or bus in nontraffic accident

X ● **V34.2**   Person on outside of three-wheeled motor vehicle injured in collision with heavy transport vehicle or bus in nontraffic accident

X ● **V34.3**   Unspecified occupant of three-wheeled motor vehicle injured in collision with heavy transport vehicle or bus in nontraffic accident

X ● **V34.4**   Person boarding or alighting a three-wheeled motor vehicle injured in collision with heavy transport vehicle or bus

X ● **V34.5**   Driver of three-wheeled motor vehicle injured in collision with heavy transport vehicle or bus in traffic accident

X ● **V34.6**   Passenger in three-wheeled motor vehicle injured in collision with heavy transport vehicle or bus in traffic accident

X ● **V34.7**   Person on outside of three-wheeled motor vehicle injured in collision with heavy transport vehicle or bus in traffic accident

X ● **V34.9**   Unspecified occupant of three-wheeled motor vehicle injured in collision with heavy transport vehicle or bus in traffic accident

● **V35**   Occupant of three-wheeled motor vehicle injured in collision with railway train or railway vehicle

> The appropriate 7th character is to be added to each code from category V35

> | | |
> |---|---|
> | A | initial encounter |
> | D | subsequent encounter |
> | S | sequela |

X ● **V35.0**   Driver of three-wheeled motor vehicle injured in collision with railway train or railway vehicle in nontraffic accident

X ● **V35.1**   Passenger in three-wheeled motor vehicle injured in collision with railway train or railway vehicle in nontraffic accident

X ● **V35.2**   Person on outside of three-wheeled motor vehicle injured in collision with railway train or railway vehicle in nontraffic accident

X ● **V35.3**   Unspecified occupant of three-wheeled motor vehicle injured in collision with railway train or railway vehicle in nontraffic accident

X ● **V35.4**   Person boarding or alighting a three-wheeled motor vehicle injured in collision with railway train or railway vehicle

X ● **V35.5**   Driver of three-wheeled motor vehicle injured in collision with railway train or railway vehicle in traffic accident

X ● **V35.6**   Passenger in three-wheeled motor vehicle injured in collision with railway train or railway vehicle in traffic accident

X ● **V35.7**   Person on outside of three-wheeled motor vehicle injured in collision with railway train or railway vehicle in traffic accident

X ● **V35.9**   Unspecified occupant of three-wheeled motor vehicle injured in collision with railway train or railway vehicle in traffic accident

● **V36**   Occupant of three-wheeled motor vehicle injured in collision with other nonmotor vehicle

> **Includes**   collision with animal-drawn vehicle, animal being ridden, streetcar

> The appropriate 7th character is to be added to each code from category V36

> | | |
> |---|---|
> | A | initial encounter |
> | D | subsequent encounter |
> | S | sequela |

X ● **V36.0**   Driver of three-wheeled motor vehicle injured in collision with other nonmotor vehicle in nontraffic accident

X ● **V36.1**   Passenger in three-wheeled motor vehicle injured in collision with other nonmotor vehicle in nontraffic accident

X ● **V36.2**   Person on outside of three-wheeled motor vehicle injured in collision with other nonmotor vehicle in nontraffic accident

X ● **V36.3**   Unspecified occupant of three-wheeled motor vehicle injured in collision with other nonmotor vehicle in nontraffic accident

X ● **V36.4**   Person boarding or alighting a three-wheeled motor vehicle injured in collision with other nonmotor vehicle

X ● **V36.5**   Driver of three-wheeled motor vehicle injured in collision with other nonmotor vehicle in traffic accident

X ● **V36.6**   Passenger in three-wheeled motor vehicle injured in collision with other nonmotor vehicle in traffic accident

X ● **V36.7**   Person on outside of three-wheeled motor vehicle injured in collision with other nonmotor vehicle in traffic accident

X ● **V36.9**   Unspecified occupant of three-wheeled motor vehicle injured in collision with other nonmotor vehicle in traffic accident

● V37 Occupant of three-wheeled motor vehicle injured in collision with fixed or stationary object

The appropriate 7th character is to be added to each code from category V37

> A   initial encounter
> D   subsequent encounter
> S   sequela

X ● **V37.0** Driver of three-wheeled motor vehicle injured in collision with fixed or stationary object in nontraffic accident

X ● **V37.1** Passenger in three-wheeled motor vehicle injured in collision with fixed or stationary object in nontraffic accident

X ● **V37.2** Person on outside of three-wheeled motor vehicle injured in collision with fixed or stationary object in nontraffic accident

X ● **V37.3** Unspecified occupant of three-wheeled motor vehicle injured in collision with fixed or stationary object in nontraffic accident

X ● **V37.4** Person boarding or alighting a three-wheeled motor vehicle injured in collision with fixed or stationary object

X ● **V37.5** Driver of three-wheeled motor vehicle injured in collision with fixed or stationary object in traffic accident

X ● **V37.6** Passenger in three-wheeled motor vehicle injured in collision with fixed or stationary object in traffic accident

X ● **V37.7** Person on outside of three-wheeled motor vehicle injured in collision with fixed or stationary object in traffic accident

X ● **V37.9** Unspecified occupant of three-wheeled motor vehicle injured in collision with fixed or stationary object in traffic accident

● V38 Occupant of three-wheeled motor vehicle injured in noncollision transport accident

> **Includes**   fall or thrown from three-wheeled motor vehicle
> overturning of three-wheeled motor vehicle NOS
> overturning of three-wheeled motor vehicle without collision

The appropriate 7th character is to be added to each code from category V38

> A   initial encounter
> D   subsequent encounter
> S   sequela

X ● **V38.0** Driver of three-wheeled motor vehicle injured in noncollision transport accident in nontraffic accident

X ● **V38.1** Passenger in three-wheeled motor vehicle injured in noncollision transport accident in nontraffic accident

X ● **V38.2** Person on outside of three-wheeled motor vehicle injured in noncollision transport accident in nontraffic accident

X ● **V38.3** Unspecified occupant of three-wheeled motor vehicle injured in noncollision transport accident in nontraffic accident

X ● **V38.4** Person boarding or alighting a three-wheeled motor vehicle injured in noncollision transport accident

X ● **V38.5** Driver of three-wheeled motor vehicle injured in noncollision transport accident in traffic accident

X ● **V38.6** Passenger in three-wheeled motor vehicle injured in noncollision transport accident in traffic accident

X ● **V38.7** Person on outside of three-wheeled motor vehicle injured in noncollision transport accident in traffic accident

X ● **V38.9** Unspecified occupant of three-wheeled motor vehicle injured in noncollision transport accident in traffic accident

● V39 Occupant of three-wheeled motor vehicle injured in other and unspecified transport accidents

The appropriate 7th character is to be added to each code from category V39

> A   initial encounter
> D   subsequent encounter
> S   sequela

● **V39.0** Driver of three-wheeled motor vehicle injured in collision with other and unspecified motor vehicles in nontraffic accident

X ● **V39.00** Driver of three-wheeled motor vehicle injured in collision with unspecified motor vehicles in nontraffic accident

X ● **V39.09** Driver of three-wheeled motor vehicle injured in collision with other motor vehicles in nontraffic accident

● **V39.1** Passenger in three-wheeled motor vehicle injured in collision with other and unspecified motor vehicles in nontraffic accident

X ● **V39.10** Passenger in three-wheeled motor vehicle injured in collision with unspecified motor vehicles in nontraffic accident

X ● **V39.19** Passenger in three-wheeled motor vehicle injured in collision with other motor vehicles in nontraffic accident

● **V39.2** Unspecified occupant of three-wheeled motor vehicle injured in collision with other and unspecified motor vehicles in nontraffic accident

X ● **V39.20** Unspecified occupant of three-wheeled motor vehicle injured in collision with unspecified motor vehicles in nontraffic accident

> Collision NOS involving three-wheeled motor vehicle, nontraffic

X ● **V39.29** Unspecified occupant of three-wheeled motor vehicle injured in collision with other motor vehicles in nontraffic accident

X ● **V39.3** Occupant (driver) (passenger) of three-wheeled motor vehicle injured in unspecified nontraffic accident

> Accident NOS involving three-wheeled motor vehicle, nontraffic
> Occupant of three-wheeled motor vehicle injured in nontraffic accident NOS

● **V39.4** Driver of three-wheeled motor vehicle injured in collision with other and unspecified motor vehicles in traffic accident

X ● **V39.40** Driver of three-wheeled motor vehicle injured in collision with unspecified motor vehicles in traffic accident

X ● **V39.49** Driver of three-wheeled motor vehicle injured in collision with other motor vehicles in traffic accident

● **V39.5** Passenger in three-wheeled motor vehicle injured in collision with other and unspecified motor vehicles in traffic accident

X ● **V39.50** Passenger in three-wheeled motor vehicle injured in collision with unspecified motor vehicles in traffic accident

X ● **V39.59** Passenger in three-wheeled motor vehicle injured in collision with other motor vehicles in traffic accident

● **V39.6** Unspecified occupant of three-wheeled motor vehicle injured in collision with other and unspecified motor vehicles in traffic accident

X ● **V39.60** Unspecified occupant of three-wheeled motor vehicle injured in collision with unspecified motor vehicles in traffic accident

> Collision NOS involving three-wheeled motor vehicle (traffic)

X ● **V39.69** Unspecified occupant of three-wheeled motor vehicle injured in collision with other motor vehicles in traffic accident

▶ New   ⇒ Revised   ~~deleted~~ Deleted   Excludes 1   Excludes 2   Includes   Use additional   Code first   Code also   Key words
OGCR Official Guidelines   X Assign placeholder X   ● Use Additional Character(s)   ❱ Manifestation Code   🔖 Hierarchical Condition Category   Coding Clinic

● V39.8   Occupant (driver) (passenger) of three-wheeled motor vehicle injured in other specified transport accidents

    X ● V39.81   Occupant (driver) (passenger) of three-wheeled motor vehicle injured in transport accident with military vehicle

    X ● V39.89   Occupant (driver) (passenger) of three-wheeled motor vehicle injured in other specified transport accidents

X ● V39.9   Occupant (driver) (passenger) of three-wheeled motor vehicle injured in unspecified traffic accident

      Accident NOS involving three-wheeled motor vehicle

CAR OCCUPANT INJURED IN TRANSPORT ACCIDENT (V40-V49)

Includes   a four-wheeled motor vehicle designed primarily for carrying passengers
                automobile (pulling a trailer or camper)

Excludes1   bus (V50-V59)
                minibus (V50-V59)
                minivan (V50-V59)
                motorcoach (V70-V79)
                pick-up truck (V50-V59)
                sport utility vehicle (SUV) (V50-V59)

● V40   Car occupant injured in collision with pedestrian or animal

    Excludes1   car collision with animal-drawn vehicle or animal being ridden (V46.-)

    The appropriate 7th character is to be added to each code from category V40

A	initial encounter
D	subsequent encounter
S	sequela

X ● V40.0   Car driver injured in collision with pedestrian or animal in nontraffic accident

X ● V40.1   Car passenger injured in collision with pedestrian or animal in nontraffic accident

X ● V40.2   Person on outside of car injured in collision with pedestrian or animal in nontraffic accident

X ● V40.3   Unspecified car occupant injured in collision with pedestrian or animal in nontraffic accident

X ● V40.4   Person boarding or alighting a car injured in collision with pedestrian or animal

X ● V40.5   Car driver injured in collision with pedestrian or animal in traffic accident

X ● V40.6   Car passenger injured in collision with pedestrian or animal in traffic accident

X ● V40.7   Person on outside of car injured in collision with pedestrian or animal in traffic accident

X ● V40.9   Unspecified car occupant injured in collision with pedestrian or animal in traffic accident

● V41   Car occupant injured in collision with pedal cycle

    The appropriate 7th character is to be added to each code from category V41

A	initial encounter
D	subsequent encounter
S	sequela

X ● V41.0   Car driver injured in collision with pedal cycle in nontraffic accident

X ● V41.1   Car passenger injured in collision with pedal cycle in nontraffic accident

X ● V41.2   Person on outside of car injured in collision with pedal cycle in nontraffic accident

X ● V41.3   Unspecified car occupant injured in collision with pedal cycle in nontraffic accident

X ● V41.4   Person boarding or alighting a car injured in collision with pedal cycle

X ● V41.5   Car driver injured in collision with pedal cycle in traffic accident

X ● V41.6   Car passenger injured in collision with pedal cycle in traffic accident

X ● V41.7   Person on outside of car injured in collision with pedal cycle in traffic accident

X ● V41.9   Unspecified car occupant injured in collision with pedal cycle in traffic accident

● V42   Car occupant injured in collision with two- or three-wheeled motor vehicle

    The appropriate 7th character is to be added to each code from category V42

A	initial encounter
D	subsequent encounter
S	sequela

X ● V42.0   Car driver injured in collision with two- or three-wheeled motor vehicle in nontraffic accident

X ● V42.1   Car passenger injured in collision with two- or three-wheeled motor vehicle in nontraffic accident

X ● V42.2   Person on outside of car injured in collision with two- or three-wheeled motor vehicle in nontraffic accident

X ● V42.3   Unspecified car occupant injured in collision with two- or three-wheeled motor vehicle in nontraffic accident

X ● V42.4   Person boarding or alighting a car injured in collision with two- or three-wheeled motor vehicle

X ● V42.5   Car driver injured in collision with two- or three-wheeled motor vehicle in traffic accident

X ● V42.6   Car passenger injured in collision with two- or three-wheeled motor vehicle in traffic accident

X ● V42.7   Person on outside of car injured in collision with two- or three-wheeled motor vehicle in traffic accident

X ● V42.9   Unspecified car occupant injured in collision with two- or three-wheeled motor vehicle in traffic accident

● V43   Car occupant injured in collision with car, pick-up truck or van

    The appropriate 7th character is to be added to each code from category V43

A	initial encounter
D	subsequent encounter
S	sequela

● V43.0   Car driver injured in collision with car, pick-up truck or van in nontraffic accident

    X ● V43.01   Car driver injured in collision with sport utility vehicle in nontraffic accident

    X ● V43.02   Car driver injured in collision with other type car in nontraffic accident

    X ● V43.03   Car driver injured in collision with pick-up truck in nontraffic accident

    X ● V43.04   Car driver injured in collision with van in nontraffic accident

● V43.1   Car passenger injured in collision with car, pick-up truck or van in nontraffic accident

    X ● V43.11   Car passenger injured in collision with sport utility vehicle in nontraffic accident

    X ● V43.12   Car passenger injured in collision with other type car in nontraffic accident

    X ● V43.13   Car passenger injured in collision with pick-up truck in nontraffic accident

    X ● V43.14   Car passenger injured in collision with van in nontraffic accident

● V43.2   Person on outside of car injured in collision with car, pick-up truck or van in nontraffic accident

    X ● V43.21   Person on outside of car injured in collision with sport utility vehicle in nontraffic accident

    X ● V43.22   Person on outside of car injured in collision with other type car in nontraffic accident

    X ● V43.23   Person on outside of car injured in collision with pick-up truck in nontraffic accident

    X ● V43.24   Person on outside of car injured in collision with van in nontraffic accident

CHAPTER 20 (V00-Y99)

CHAPTER 20 (V00-Y99)

- ● V43.3   Unspecified car occupant injured in collision with car, pick-up truck or van in nontraffic accident
    - X ● V43.31   Unspecified car occupant injured in collision with sport utility vehicle in nontraffic accident
    - X ● V43.32   Unspecified car occupant injured in collision with other type car in nontraffic accident
    - X ● V43.33   Unspecified car occupant injured in collision with pick-up truck in nontraffic accident
    - X ● V43.34   Unspecified car occupant injured in collision with van in nontraffic accident
- ● V43.4   Person boarding or alighting a car injured in collision with car, pick-up truck or van
    - X ● V43.41   Person boarding or alighting a car injured in collision with sport utility vehicle
    - X ● V43.42   Person boarding or alighting a car injured in collision with other type car
    - X ● V43.43   Person boarding or alighting a car injured in collision with pick-up truck
    - X ● V43.44   Person boarding or alighting a car injured in collision with van
- ● V43.5   Car driver injured in collision with car, pick-up truck or van in traffic accident
    - X ● V43.51   Car driver injured in collision with sport utility vehicle in traffic accident
    - X ● V43.52   Car driver injured in collision with other type car in traffic accident
    - X ● V43.53   Car driver injured in collision with pick-up truck in traffic accident
    - X ● V43.54   Car driver injured in collision with van in traffic accident
- ● V43.6   Car passenger injured in collision with car, pick-up truck or van in traffic accident
    - X ● V43.61   Car passenger injured in collision with sport utility vehicle in traffic accident
      Coding Clinic: 2015, Q1, P5-7
    - X ● V43.62   Car passenger injured in collision with other type car in traffic accident
    - X ● V43.63   Car passenger injured in collision with pick-up truck in traffic accident
    - X ● V43.64   Car passenger injured in collision with van in traffic accident
- ● V43.7   Person on outside of car injured in collision with car, pick-up truck or van in traffic accident
    - X ● V43.71   Person on outside of car injured in collision with sport utility vehicle in traffic accident
    - X ● V43.72   Person on outside of car injured in collision with other type car in traffic accident
    - X ● V43.73   Person on outside of car injured in collision with pick-up truck in traffic accident
    - X ● V43.74   Person on outside of car injured in collision with van in traffic accident
- ● V43.9   Unspecified car occupant injured in collision with car, pick-up truck or van in traffic accident
    - X ● V43.91   Unspecified car occupant injured in collision with sport utility vehicle in traffic accident
    - X ● V43.92   Unspecified car occupant injured in collision with other type car in traffic accident
    - X ● V43.93   Unspecified car occupant injured in collision with pick-up truck in traffic accident
    - X ● V43.94   Unspecified car occupant injured in collision with van in traffic accident

- ● V44   Car occupant injured in collision with heavy transport vehicle or bus
    - **Excludes 1**   car occupant injured in collision with military vehicle (V49.81)

    The appropriate 7th character is to be added to each code from category V44

A	initial encounter
D	subsequent encounter
S	sequela

    - X ● V44.0   Car driver injured in collision with heavy transport vehicle or bus in nontraffic accident
    - X ● V44.1   Car passenger injured in collision with heavy transport vehicle or bus in nontraffic accident
    - X ● V44.2   Person on outside of car injured in collision with heavy transport vehicle or bus in nontraffic accident
    - X ● V44.3   Unspecified car occupant injured in collision with heavy transport vehicle or bus in nontraffic accident
    - X ● V44.4   Person boarding or alighting a car injured in collision with heavy transport vehicle or bus
    - X ● V44.5   Car driver injured in collision with heavy transport vehicle or bus in traffic accident
    - X ● V44.6   Car passenger injured in collision with heavy transport vehicle or bus in traffic accident
    - X ● V44.7   Person on outside of car injured in collision with heavy transport vehicle or bus in traffic accident
    - X ● V44.9   Unspecified car occupant injured in collision with heavy transport vehicle or bus in traffic accident
- ● V45   Car occupant injured in collision with railway train or railway vehicle

    The appropriate 7th character is to be added to each code from category V45

A	initial encounter
D	subsequent encounter
S	sequela

    - X ● V45.0   Car driver injured in collision with railway train or railway vehicle in nontraffic accident
    - X ● V45.1   Car passenger injured in collision with railway train or railway vehicle in nontraffic accident
    - X ● V45.2   Person on outside of car injured in collision with railway train or railway vehicle in nontraffic accident
    - X ● V45.3   Unspecified car occupant injured in collision with railway train or railway vehicle in nontraffic accident
    - X ● V45.4   Person boarding or alighting a car injured in collision with railway train or railway vehicle
    - X ● V45.5   Car driver injured in collision with railway train or railway vehicle in traffic accident
    - X ● V45.6   Car passenger injured in collision with railway train or railway vehicle in traffic accident
    - X ● V45.7   Person on outside of car injured in collision with railway train or railway vehicle in traffic accident
    - X ● V45.9   Unspecified car occupant injured in collision with railway train or railway vehicle in traffic accident
- ● V46   Car occupant injured in collision with other nonmotor vehicle
    - **Includes**   collision with animal-drawn vehicle, animal being ridden, streetcar

    The appropriate 7th character is to be added to each code from category V46

A	initial encounter
D	subsequent encounter
S	sequela

    - X ● V46.0   Car driver injured in collision with other nonmotor vehicle in nontraffic accident
    - X ● V46.1   Car passenger injured in collision with other nonmotor vehicle in nontraffic accident

▶ New   ⇒ Revised   ~~deleted~~ Deleted   Excludes 1   Excludes 2   Includes   Use additional   Code first   Code also   Key words

OGCR Official Guidelines   X Assign placeholder X   ● Use Additional Character(s)   ▶ Manifestation Code   🏥 Hierarchical Condition Category   Coding Clinic

X ● **V46.2** Person on outside of car injured in collision with other nonmotor vehicle in nontraffic accident

X ● **V46.3** Unspecified car occupant injured in collision with other nonmotor vehicle in nontraffic accident

X ● **V46.4** Person boarding or alighting a car injured in collision with other nonmotor vehicle

X ● **V46.5** Car driver injured in collision with other nonmotor vehicle in traffic accident

X ● **V46.6** Car passenger injured in collision with other nonmotor vehicle in traffic accident

X ● **V46.7** Person on outside of car injured in collision with other nonmotor vehicle in traffic accident

X ● **V46.9** Unspecified car occupant injured in collision with other nonmotor vehicle in traffic accident

● **V47** Car occupant injured in collision with fixed or stationary object

The appropriate 7th character is to be added to each code from category V47

A	initial encounter
D	subsequent encounter
S	sequela

Coding Clinic: 2016, Q4, P73

X ● **V47.0** Car driver injured in collision with fixed or stationary object in nontraffic accident

X ● **V47.1** Car passenger injured in collision with fixed or stationary object in nontraffic accident

X ● **V47.2** Person on outside of car injured in collision with fixed or stationary object in nontraffic accident

X ● **V47.3** Unspecified car occupant injured in collision with fixed or stationary object in nontraffic accident

X ● **V47.4** Person boarding or alighting a car injured in collision with fixed or stationary object

X ● **V47.5** Car driver injured in collision with fixed or stationary object in traffic accident

X ● **V47.6** Car passenger injured in collision with fixed or stationary object in traffic accident

X ● **V47.7** Person on outside of car injured in collision with fixed or stationary object in traffic accident

X ● **V47.9** Unspecified car occupant injured in collision with fixed or stationary object in traffic accident

● **V48** Car occupant injured in noncollision transport accident

Includes overturning car NOS
overturning car without collision

The appropriate 7th character is to be added to each code from category V48

A	initial encounter
D	subsequent encounter
S	sequela

X ● **V48.0** Car driver injured in noncollision transport accident in nontraffic accident

X ● **V48.1** Car passenger injured in noncollision transport accident in nontraffic accident

X ● **V48.2** Person on outside of car injured in noncollision transport accident in nontraffic accident

X ● **V48.3** Unspecified car occupant injured in noncollision transport accident in nontraffic accident

X ● **V48.4** Person boarding or alighting a car injured in noncollision transport accident

X ● **V48.5** Car driver injured in noncollision transport accident in traffic accident

X ● **V48.6** Car passenger injured in noncollision transport accident in traffic accident

X ● **V48.7** Person on outside of car injured in noncollision transport accident in traffic accident

X ● **V48.9** Unspecified car occupant injured in noncollision transport accident in traffic accident

● **V49** Car occupant injured in other and unspecified transport accidents

The appropriate 7th character is to be added to each code from category V49

A	initial encounter
D	subsequent encounter
S	sequela

● **V49.0** Driver injured in collision with other and unspecified motor vehicles in nontraffic accident

X ● **V49.00** Driver injured in collision with unspecified motor vehicles in nontraffic accident

X ● **V49.09** Driver injured in collision with other motor vehicles in nontraffic accident

● **V49.1** Passenger injured in collision with other and unspecified motor vehicles in nontraffic accident

X ● **V49.10** Passenger injured in collision with unspecified motor vehicles in nontraffic accident

X ● **V49.19** Passenger injured in collision with other motor vehicles in nontraffic accident

● **V49.2** Unspecified car occupant injured in collision with other and unspecified motor vehicles in nontraffic accident

X ● **V49.20** Unspecified car occupant injured in collision with unspecified motor vehicles in nontraffic accident

Car collision NOS, nontraffic

X ● **V49.29** Unspecified car occupant injured in collision with other motor vehicles in nontraffic accident

X ● **V49.3** Car occupant (driver) (passenger) injured in unspecified nontraffic accident

Car accident NOS, nontraffic
Car occupant injured in nontraffic accident NOS

● **V49.4** Driver injured in collision with other and unspecified motor vehicles in traffic accident

X ● **V49.40** Driver injured in collision with unspecified motor vehicles in traffic accident

X ● **V49.49** Driver injured in collision with other motor vehicles in traffic accident

● **V49.5** Passenger injured in collision with other and unspecified motor vehicles in traffic accident

X ● **V49.50** Passenger injured in collision with unspecified motor vehicles in traffic accident

X ● **V49.59** Passenger injured in collision with other motor vehicles in traffic accident

● **V49.6** Unspecified car occupant injured in collision with other and unspecified motor vehicles in traffic accident

X ● **V49.60** Unspecified car occupant injured in collision with unspecified motor vehicles in traffic accident

Car collision NOS (traffic)

X ● **V49.69** Unspecified car occupant injured in collision with other motor vehicles in traffic accident

● **V49.8** Car occupant (driver) (passenger) injured in other specified transport accidents

X ● **V49.81** Car occupant (driver) (passenger) injured in transport accident with military vehicle

X ● **V49.88** Car occupant (driver) (passenger) injured in other specified transport accidents

X ● **V49.9** Car occupant (driver) (passenger) injured in unspecified traffic accident

Car accident NOS
Coding Clinic: 2015, Q1, P11

OCCUPANT OF PICK-UP TRUCK OR VAN INJURED IN TRANSPORT ACCIDENT (V50-V59)

Includes a four- or six-wheel motor vehicle designed primarily for carrying passengers and property but weighing less than the local limit for classification as a heavy goods vehicle
minibus
minivan
sport utility vehicle (SUV)
truck
van

Excludes1 heavy transport vehicle (V60-V69)

● **V50** Occupant of pick-up truck or van injured in collision with pedestrian or animal

Excludes1 pick-up truck or van collision with animal-drawn vehicle or animal being ridden (V56.-)

The appropriate 7th character is to be added to each code from category V50

A initial encounter
D subsequent encounter
S sequela

X ● **V50.0** Driver of pick-up truck or van injured in collision with pedestrian or animal in nontraffic accident

X ● **V50.1** Passenger in pick-up truck or van injured in collision with pedestrian or animal in nontraffic accident

X ● **V50.2** Person on outside of pick-up truck or van injured in collision with pedestrian or animal in nontraffic accident

X ● **V50.3** Unspecified occupant of pick-up truck or van injured in collision with pedestrian or animal in nontraffic accident

X ● **V50.4** Person boarding or alighting a pick-up truck or van injured in collision with pedestrian or animal

X ● **V50.5** Driver of pick-up truck or van injured in collision with pedestrian or animal in traffic accident

X ● **V50.6** Passenger in pick-up truck or van injured in collision with pedestrian or animal in traffic accident

X ● **V50.7** Person on outside of pick-up truck or van injured in collision with pedestrian or animal in traffic accident

X ● **V50.9** Unspecified occupant of pick-up truck or van injured in collision with pedestrian or animal in traffic accident

● **V51** Occupant of pick-up truck or van injured in collision with pedal cycle

The appropriate 7th character is to be added to each code from category V51

A initial encounter
D subsequent encounter
S sequela

X ● **V51.0** Driver of pick-up truck or van injured in collision with pedal cycle in nontraffic accident

X ● **V51.1** Passenger in pick-up truck or van injured in collision with pedal cycle in nontraffic accident

X ● **V51.2** Person on outside of pick-up truck or van injured in collision with pedal cycle in nontraffic accident

X ● **V51.3** Unspecified occupant of pick-up truck or van injured in collision with pedal cycle in nontraffic accident

X ● **V51.4** Person boarding or alighting a pick-up truck or van injured in collision with pedal cycle

X ● **V51.5** Driver of pick-up truck or van injured in collision with pedal cycle in traffic accident

X ● **V51.6** Passenger in pick-up truck or van injured in collision with pedal cycle in traffic accident

X ● **V51.7** Person on outside of pick-up truck or van injured in collision with pedal cycle in traffic accident

X ● **V51.9** Unspecified occupant of pick-up truck or van injured in collision with pedal cycle in traffic accident

● **V52** Occupant of pick-up truck or van injured in collision with two- or three-wheeled motor vehicle

The appropriate 7th character is to be added to each code from category V52

A initial encounter
D subsequent encounter
S sequela

X ● **V52.0** Driver of pick-up truck or van injured in collision with two- or three-wheeled motor vehicle in nontraffic accident

X ● **V52.1** Passenger in pick-up truck or van injured in collision with two- or three-wheeled motor vehicle in nontraffic accident

X ● **V52.2** Person on outside of pick-up truck or van injured in collision with two- or three-wheeled motor vehicle in nontraffic accident

X ● **V52.3** Unspecified occupant of pick-up truck or van injured in collision with two- or three-wheeled motor vehicle in nontraffic accident

X ● **V52.4** Person boarding or alighting a pick-up truck or van injured in collision with two- or three-wheeled motor vehicle

X ● **V52.5** Driver of pick-up truck or van injured in collision with two- or three-wheeled motor vehicle in traffic accident

X ● **V52.6** Passenger in pick-up truck or van injured in collision with two- or three-wheeled motor vehicle in traffic accident

X ● **V52.7** Person on outside of pick-up truck or van injured in collision with two- or three-wheeled motor vehicle in traffic accident

X ● **V52.9** Unspecified occupant of pick-up truck or van injured in collision with two- or three-wheeled motor vehicle in traffic accident

● **V53** Occupant of pick-up truck or van injured in collision with car, pick-up truck or van

The appropriate 7th character is to be added to each code from category V53

A initial encounter
D subsequent encounter
S sequela

X ● **V53.0** Driver of pick-up truck or van injured in collision with car, pick-up truck or van in nontraffic accident

X ● **V53.1** Passenger in pick-up truck or van injured in collision with car, pick-up truck or van in nontraffic accident

X ● **V53.2** Person on outside of pick-up truck or van injured in collision with car, pick-up truck or van in nontraffic accident

X ● **V53.3** Unspecified occupant of pick-up truck or van injured in collision with car, pick-up truck or van in nontraffic accident

X ● **V53.4** Person boarding or alighting a pick-up truck or van injured in collision with car, pick-up truck or van

X ● **V53.5** Driver of pick-up truck or van injured in collision with car, pick-up truck or van in traffic accident

X ● **V53.6** Passenger in pick-up truck or van injured in collision with car, pick-up truck or van in traffic accident

X ● **V53.7** Person on outside of pick-up truck or van injured in collision with car, pick-up truck or van in traffic accident

X ● **V53.9** Unspecified occupant of pick-up truck or van injured in collision with car, pick-up truck or van in traffic accident

● V54　Occupant of pick-up truck or van injured in collision with heavy transport vehicle or bus

　　Excludes1　occupant of pick-up truck or van injured in collision with military vehicle (V59.81)

　　The appropriate 7th character is to be added to each code from category V54

A	initial encounter
D	subsequent encounter
S	sequela

X ● V54.0　Driver of pick-up truck or van injured in collision with heavy transport vehicle or bus in nontraffic accident

X ● V54.1　Passenger in pick-up truck or van injured in collision with heavy transport vehicle or bus in nontraffic accident

X ● V54.2　Person on outside of pick-up truck or van injured in collision with heavy transport vehicle or bus in nontraffic accident

X ● V54.3　Unspecified occupant of pick-up truck or van injured in collision with heavy transport vehicle or bus in nontraffic accident

X ● V54.4　Person boarding or alighting a pick-up truck or van injured in collision with heavy transport vehicle or bus

X ● V54.5　Driver of pick-up truck or van injured in collision with heavy transport vehicle or bus in traffic accident

X ● V54.6　Passenger in pick-up truck or van injured in collision with heavy transport vehicle or bus in traffic accident

X ● V54.7　Person on outside of pick-up truck or van injured in collision with heavy transport vehicle or bus in traffic accident

X ● V54.9　Unspecified occupant of pick-up truck or van injured in collision with heavy transport vehicle or bus in traffic accident

● V55　Occupant of pick-up truck or van injured in collision with railway train or railway vehicle

　　The appropriate 7th character is to be added to each code from category V55

A	initial encounter
D	subsequent encounter
S	sequela

X ● V55.0　Driver of pick-up truck or van injured in collision with railway train or railway vehicle in nontraffic accident

X ● V55.1　Passenger in pick-up truck or van injured in collision with railway train or railway vehicle in nontraffic accident

X ● V55.2　Person on outside of pick-up truck or van injured in collision with railway train or railway vehicle in nontraffic accident

X ● V55.3　Unspecified occupant of pick-up truck or van injured in collision with railway train or railway vehicle in nontraffic accident

X ● V55.4　Person boarding or alighting a pick-up truck or van injured in collision with railway train or railway vehicle

X ● V55.5　Driver of pick-up truck or van injured in collision with railway train or railway vehicle in traffic accident

X ● V55.6　Passenger in pick-up truck or van injured in collision with railway train or railway vehicle in traffic accident

X ● V55.7　Person on outside of pick-up truck or van injured in collision with railway train or railway vehicle in traffic accident

X ● V55.9　Unspecified occupant of pick-up truck or van injured in collision with railway train or railway vehicle in traffic accident

● V56　Occupant of pick-up truck or van injured in collision with other nonmotor vehicle

　　Includes　collision with animal-drawn vehicle, animal being ridden, streetcar

　　The appropriate 7th character is to be added to each code from category V56

A	initial encounter
D	subsequent encounter
S	sequela

X ● V56.0　Driver of pick-up truck or van injured in collision with other nonmotor vehicle in nontraffic accident

X ● V56.1　Passenger in pick-up truck or van injured in collision with other nonmotor vehicle in nontraffic accident

X ● V56.2　Person on outside of pick-up truck or van injured in collision with other nonmotor vehicle in nontraffic accident

X ● V56.3　Unspecified occupant of pick-up truck or van injured in collision with other nonmotor vehicle in nontraffic accident

X ● V56.4　Person boarding or alighting a pick-up truck or van injured in collision with other nonmotor vehicle

X ● V56.5　Driver of pick-up truck or van injured in collision with other nonmotor vehicle in traffic accident

X ● V56.6　Passenger in pick-up truck or van injured in collision with other nonmotor vehicle in traffic accident

X ● V56.7　Person on outside of pick-up truck or van injured in collision with other nonmotor vehicle in traffic accident

X ● V56.9　Unspecified occupant of pick-up truck or van injured in collision with other nonmotor vehicle in traffic accident

● V57　Occupant of pick-up truck or van injured in collision with fixed or stationary object

　　The appropriate 7th character is to be added to each code from category V57

A	initial encounter
D	subsequent encounter
S	sequela

X ● V57.0　Driver of pick-up truck or van injured in collision with fixed or stationary object in nontraffic accident

X ● V57.1　Passenger in pick-up truck or van injured in collision with fixed or stationary object in nontraffic accident

X ● V57.2　Person on outside of pick-up truck or van injured in collision with fixed or stationary object in nontraffic accident

X ● V57.3　Unspecified occupant of pick-up truck or van injured in collision with fixed or stationary object in nontraffic accident

X ● V57.4　Person boarding or alighting a pick-up truck or van injured in collision with fixed or stationary object

X ● V57.5　Driver of pick-up truck or van injured in collision with fixed or stationary object in traffic accident

X ● V57.6　Passenger in pick-up truck or van injured in collision with fixed or stationary object in traffic accident

X ● V57.7　Person on outside of pick-up truck or van injured in collision with fixed or stationary object in traffic accident

X ● V57.9　Unspecified occupant of pick-up truck or van injured in collision with fixed or stationary object in traffic accident

CHAPTER 20 (V00-Y99)

● **V58**   **Occupant of pick-up truck or van injured in noncollision transport accident**

> **Includes**   overturning pick-up truck or van NOS
> overturning pick-up truck or van without collision

The appropriate 7th character is to be added to each code from category V58

> A   initial encounter
> D   subsequent encounter
> S   sequela

X● **V58.0**   **Driver of pick-up truck or van injured in noncollision transport accident in nontraffic accident**

X● **V58.1**   **Passenger in pick-up truck or van injured in noncollision transport accident in nontraffic accident**

X● **V58.2**   **Person on outside of pick-up truck or van injured in noncollision transport accident in nontraffic accident**

X● **V58.3**   **Unspecified occupant of pick-up truck or van injured in noncollision transport accident in nontraffic accident**

X● **V58.4**   **Person boarding or alighting a pick-up truck or van injured in noncollision transport accident**

X● **V58.5**   **Driver of pick-up truck or van injured in noncollision transport accident in traffic accident**

X● **V58.6**   **Passenger in pick-up truck or van injured in noncollision transport accident in traffic accident**

X● **V58.7**   **Person on outside of pick-up truck or van injured in noncollision transport accident in traffic accident**

X● **V58.9**   **Unspecified occupant of pick-up truck or van injured in noncollision transport accident in traffic accident**

● **V59**   **Occupant of pick-up truck or van injured in other and unspecified transport accidents**

The appropriate 7th character is to be added to each code from category V59

> A   initial encounter
> D   subsequent encounter
> S   sequela

● **V59.0**   **Driver of pick-up truck or van injured in collision with other and unspecified motor vehicles in nontraffic accident**

X● **V59.00**   **Driver of pick-up truck or van injured in collision with unspecified motor vehicles in nontraffic accident**

X● **V59.09**   **Driver of pick-up truck or van injured in collision with other motor vehicles in nontraffic accident**

● **V59.1**   **Passenger in pick-up truck or van injured in collision with other and unspecified motor vehicles in nontraffic accident**

X● **V59.10**   **Passenger in pick-up truck or van injured in collision with unspecified motor vehicles in nontraffic accident**

X● **V59.19**   **Passenger in pick-up truck or van injured in collision with other motor vehicles in nontraffic accident**

● **V59.2**   **Unspecified occupant of pick-up truck or van injured in collision with other and unspecified motor vehicles in nontraffic accident**

X● **V59.20**   **Unspecified occupant of pick-up truck or van injured in collision with unspecified motor vehicles in nontraffic accident**
> Collision NOS involving pick-up truck or van, nontraffic

X● **V59.29**   **Unspecified occupant of pick-up truck or van injured in collision with other motor vehicles in nontraffic accident**

X● **V59.3**   **Occupant (driver) (passenger) of pick-up truck or van injured in unspecified nontraffic accident**
> Accident NOS involving pick-up truck or van, nontraffic
> Occupant of pick-up truck or van injured in nontraffic accident NOS

● **V59.4**   **Driver of pick-up truck or van injured in collision with other and unspecified motor vehicles in traffic accident**

X● **V59.40**   **Driver of pick-up truck or van injured in collision with unspecified motor vehicles in traffic accident**

X● **V59.49**   **Driver of pick-up truck or van injured in collision with other motor vehicles in traffic accident**

● **V59.5**   **Passenger in pick-up truck or van injured in collision with other and unspecified motor vehicles in traffic accident**

X● **V59.50**   **Passenger in pick-up truck or van injured in collision with unspecified motor vehicles in traffic accident**

X● **V59.59**   **Passenger in pick-up truck or van injured in collision with other motor vehicles in traffic accident**

● **V59.6**   **Unspecified occupant of pick-up truck or van injured in collision with other and unspecified motor vehicles in traffic accident**

X● **V59.60**   **Unspecified occupant of pick-up truck or van injured in collision with unspecified motor vehicles in traffic accident**
> Collision NOS involving pick-up truck or van (traffic)

X● **V59.69**   **Unspecified occupant of pick-up truck or van injured in collision with other motor vehicles in traffic accident**

● **V59.8**   **Occupant (driver) (passenger) of pick-up truck or van injured in other specified transport accidents**

X● **V59.81**   **Occupant (driver) (passenger) of pick-up truck or van injured in transport accident with military vehicle**

X● **V59.88**   **Occupant (driver) (passenger) of pick-up truck or van injured in other specified transport accidents**

X● **V59.9**   **Occupant (driver) (passenger) of pick-up truck or van injured in unspecified traffic accident**
> Accident NOS involving pick-up truck or van

OCCUPANT OF HEAVY TRANSPORT VEHICLE INJURED IN TRANSPORT ACCIDENT (V60-V69)

> **Includes**   18 wheeler
> armored car
> panel truck

> **Excludes1**   bus
> motorcoach

● **V60**   **Occupant of heavy transport vehicle injured in collision with pedestrian or animal**

> **Excludes1**   heavy transport vehicle collision with animal-drawn vehicle or animal being ridden (V66.-)

The appropriate 7th character is to be added to each code from category V60

> A   initial encounter
> D   subsequent encounter
> S   sequela

X● **V60.0**   **Driver of heavy transport vehicle injured in collision with pedestrian or animal in nontraffic accident**

X● **V60.1**   **Passenger in heavy transport vehicle injured in collision with pedestrian or animal in nontraffic accident**

X● **V60.2**   **Person on outside of heavy transport vehicle injured in collision with pedestrian or animal in nontraffic accident**

X● **V60.3**   **Unspecified occupant of heavy transport vehicle injured in collision with pedestrian or animal in nontraffic accident**

X● **V60.4**   **Person boarding or alighting a heavy transport vehicle injured in collision with pedestrian or animal**

X● **V60.5**   **Driver of heavy transport vehicle injured in collision with pedestrian or animal in traffic accident**

▶ New   ⯈ Revised   ~~deleted~~ Deleted   Excludes 1   Excludes 2   Includes   Use additional   Code first   Code also   Key words

OGCR Official Guidelines   X Assign placeholder X   ● Use Additional Character(s)   ⯈ Manifestation Code   🅗 Hierarchical Condition Category   **Coding Clinic**

X ● **V60.6**   Passenger in heavy transport vehicle injured in collision with pedestrian or animal in traffic accident

X ● **V60.7**   Person on outside of heavy transport vehicle injured in collision with pedestrian or animal in traffic accident

X ● **V60.9**   Unspecified occupant of heavy transport vehicle injured in collision with pedestrian or animal in traffic accident

● **V61**   Occupant of heavy transport vehicle injured in collision with pedal cycle

> The appropriate 7th character is to be added to each code from category V61

> | A | initial encounter |
> |---|---|
> | D | subsequent encounter |
> | S | sequela |

X ● **V61.0**   Driver of heavy transport vehicle injured in collision with pedal cycle in nontraffic accident

X ● **V61.1**   Passenger in heavy transport vehicle injured in collision with pedal cycle in nontraffic accident

X ● **V61.2**   Person on outside of heavy transport vehicle injured in collision with pedal cycle in nontraffic accident

X ● **V61.3**   Unspecified occupant of heavy transport vehicle injured in collision with pedal cycle in nontraffic accident

X ● **V61.4**   Person boarding or alighting a heavy transport vehicle injured in collision with pedal cycle while boarding or alighting

X ● **V61.5**   Driver of heavy transport vehicle injured in collision with pedal cycle in traffic accident

X ● **V61.6**   Passenger in heavy transport vehicle injured in collision with pedal cycle in traffic accident

X ● **V61.7**   Person on outside of heavy transport vehicle injured in collision with pedal cycle in traffic accident

X ● **V61.9**   Unspecified occupant of heavy transport vehicle injured in collision with pedal cycle in traffic accident

● **V62**   Occupant of heavy transport vehicle injured in collision with two- or three-wheeled motor vehicle

> The appropriate 7th character is to be added to each code from category V62

> | A | initial encounter |
> |---|---|
> | D | subsequent encounter |
> | S | sequela |

X ● **V62.0**   Driver of heavy transport vehicle injured in collision with two- or three-wheeled motor vehicle in nontraffic accident

X ● **V62.1**   Passenger in heavy transport vehicle injured in collision with two- or three-wheeled motor vehicle in nontraffic accident

X ● **V62.2**   Person on outside of heavy transport vehicle injured in collision with two- or three-wheeled motor vehicle in nontraffic accident

X ● **V62.3**   Unspecified occupant of heavy transport vehicle injured in collision with two- or three-wheeled motor vehicle in nontraffic accident

X ● **V62.4**   Person boarding or alighting a heavy transport vehicle injured in collision with two- or three-wheeled motor vehicle

X ● **V62.5**   Driver of heavy transport vehicle injured in collision with two- or three-wheeled motor vehicle in traffic accident

X ● **V62.6**   Passenger in heavy transport vehicle injured in collision with two- or three-wheeled motor vehicle in traffic accident

X ● **V62.7**   Person on outside of heavy transport vehicle injured in collision with two- or three-wheeled motor vehicle in traffic accident

X ● **V62.9**   Unspecified occupant of heavy transport vehicle injured in collision with two- or three-wheeled motor vehicle in traffic accident

● **V63**   Occupant of heavy transport vehicle injured in collision with car, pick-up truck or van

> The appropriate 7th character is to be added to each code from category V63

> | A | initial encounter |
> |---|---|
> | D | subsequent encounter |
> | S | sequela |

X ● **V63.0**   Driver of heavy transport vehicle injured in collision with car, pick-up truck or van in nontraffic accident

X ● **V63.1**   Passenger in heavy transport vehicle injured in collision with car, pick-up truck or van in nontraffic accident

X ● **V63.2**   Person on outside of heavy transport vehicle injured in collision with car, pick-up truck or van in nontraffic accident

X ● **V63.3**   Unspecified occupant of heavy transport vehicle injured in collision with car, pick-up truck or van in nontraffic accident

X ● **V63.4**   Person boarding or alighting a heavy transport vehicle injured in collision with car, pick-up truck or van

X ● **V63.5**   Driver of heavy transport vehicle injured in collision with car, pick-up truck or van in traffic accident

X ● **V63.6**   Passenger in heavy transport vehicle injured in collision with car, pick-up truck or van in traffic accident

X ● **V63.7**   Person on outside of heavy transport vehicle injured in collision with car, pick-up truck or van in traffic accident

X ● **V63.9**   Unspecified occupant of heavy transport vehicle injured in collision with car, pick-up truck or van in traffic accident

● **V64**   Occupant of heavy transport vehicle injured in collision with heavy transport vehicle or bus

> **Excludes1**   occupant of heavy transport vehicle injured in collision with military vehicle (V69.81)

> The appropriate 7th character is to be added to each code from category V64

> | A | initial encounter |
> |---|---|
> | D | subsequent encounter |
> | S | sequela |

X ● **V64.0**   Driver of heavy transport vehicle injured in collision with heavy transport vehicle or bus in nontraffic accident

X ● **V64.1**   Passenger in heavy transport vehicle injured in collision with heavy transport vehicle or bus in nontraffic accident

X ● **V64.2**   Person on outside of heavy transport vehicle injured in collision with heavy transport vehicle or bus in nontraffic accident

X ● **V64.3**   Unspecified occupant of heavy transport vehicle injured in collision with heavy transport vehicle or bus in nontraffic accident

X ● **V64.4**   Person boarding or alighting a heavy transport vehicle injured in collision with heavy transport vehicle or bus while boarding or alighting

X ● **V64.5**   Driver of heavy transport vehicle injured in collision with heavy transport vehicle or bus in traffic accident

X ● **V64.6**   Passenger in heavy transport vehicle injured in collision with heavy transport vehicle or bus in traffic accident

X ● **V64.7**   Person on outside of heavy transport vehicle injured in collision with heavy transport vehicle or bus in traffic accident

X ● **V64.9**   Unspecified occupant of heavy transport vehicle injured in collision with heavy transport vehicle or bus in traffic accident

CHAPTER 20 (V00–Y99)

● V65   Occupant of heavy transport vehicle injured in collision with railway train or railway vehicle

The appropriate 7th character is to be added to each code from category V65

> A   initial encounter
> D   subsequent encounter
> S   sequela

X ● V65.0   Driver of heavy transport vehicle injured in collision with railway train or railway vehicle in nontraffic accident

X ● V65.1   Passenger in heavy transport vehicle injured in collision with railway train or railway vehicle in nontraffic accident

X ● V65.2   Person on outside of heavy transport vehicle injured in collision with railway train or railway vehicle in nontraffic accident

X ● V65.3   Unspecified occupant of heavy transport vehicle injured in collision with railway train or railway vehicle in nontraffic accident

X ● V65.4   Person boarding or alighting a heavy transport vehicle injured in collision with railway train or railway vehicle

X ● V65.5   Driver of heavy transport vehicle injured in collision with railway train or railway vehicle in traffic accident

X ● V65.6   Passenger in heavy transport vehicle injured in collision with railway train or railway vehicle in traffic accident

X ● V65.7   Person on outside of heavy transport vehicle injured in collision with railway train or railway vehicle in traffic accident

X ● V65.9   Unspecified occupant of heavy transport vehicle injured in collision with railway train or railway vehicle in traffic accident

● V66   Occupant of heavy transport vehicle injured in collision with other nonmotor vehicle

> **Includes**   collision with animal-drawn vehicle, animal being ridden, streetcar

The appropriate 7th character is to be added to each code from category V66

> A   initial encounter
> D   subsequent encounter
> S   sequela

X ● V66.0   Driver of heavy transport vehicle injured in collision with other nonmotor vehicle in nontraffic accident

X ● V66.1   Passenger in heavy transport vehicle injured in collision with other nonmotor vehicle in nontraffic accident

X ● V66.2   Person on outside of heavy transport vehicle injured in collision with other nonmotor vehicle in nontraffic accident

X ● V66.3   Unspecified occupant of heavy transport vehicle injured in collision with other nonmotor vehicle in nontraffic accident

X ● V66.4   Person boarding or alighting a heavy transport vehicle injured in collision with other nonmotor vehicle

X ● V66.5   Driver of heavy transport vehicle injured in collision with other nonmotor vehicle in traffic accident

X ● V66.6   Passenger in heavy transport vehicle injured in collision with other nonmotor vehicle in traffic accident

X ● V66.7   Person on outside of heavy transport vehicle injured in collision with other nonmotor vehicle in traffic accident

X ● V66.9   Unspecified occupant of heavy transport vehicle injured in collision with other nonmotor vehicle in traffic accident

● V67   Occupant of heavy transport vehicle injured in collision with fixed or stationary object

The appropriate 7th character is to be added to each code from category V67

> A   initial encounter
> D   subsequent encounter
> S   sequela

X ● V67.0   Driver of heavy transport vehicle injured in collision with fixed or stationary object in nontraffic accident

X ● V67.1   Passenger in heavy transport vehicle injured in collision with fixed or stationary object in nontraffic accident

X ● V67.2   Person on outside of heavy transport vehicle injured in collision with fixed or stationary object in nontraffic accident

X ● V67.3   Unspecified occupant of heavy transport vehicle injured in collision with fixed or stationary object in nontraffic accident

X ● V67.4   Person boarding or alighting a heavy transport vehicle injured in collision with fixed or stationary object

X ● V67.5   Driver of heavy transport vehicle injured in collision with fixed or stationary object in traffic accident

X ● V67.6   Passenger in heavy transport vehicle injured in collision with fixed or stationary object in traffic accident

X ● V67.7   Person on outside of heavy transport vehicle injured in collision with fixed or stationary object in traffic accident

X ● V67.9   Unspecified occupant of heavy transport vehicle injured in collision with fixed or stationary object in traffic accident

● V68   Occupant of heavy transport vehicle injured in noncollision transport accident

> **Includes**   overturning heavy transport vehicle NOS
> overturning heavy transport vehicle without collision

The appropriate 7th character is to be added to each code from category V68

> A   initial encounter
> D   subsequent encounter
> S   sequela

X ● V68.0   Driver of heavy transport vehicle injured in noncollision transport accident in nontraffic accident

X ● V68.1   Passenger in heavy transport vehicle injured in noncollision transport accident in nontraffic accident

X ● V68.2   Person on outside of heavy transport vehicle injured in noncollision transport accident in nontraffic accident

X ● V68.3   Unspecified occupant of heavy transport vehicle injured in noncollision transport accident in nontraffic accident

X ● V68.4   Person boarding or alighting a heavy transport vehicle injured in noncollision transport accident

X ● V68.5   Driver of heavy transport vehicle injured in noncollision transport accident in traffic accident

X ● V68.6   Passenger in heavy transport vehicle injured in noncollision transport accident in traffic accident

X ● V68.7   Person on outside of heavy transport vehicle injured in noncollision transport accident in traffic accident

X ● V68.9   Unspecified occupant of heavy transport vehicle injured in noncollision transport accident in traffic accident

▶ New   ⇒ Revised   ~~deleted~~ Deleted   Excludes 1   Excludes 2   Includes   Use additional   Code first   Code also   Key words

OGCR Official Guidelines   X Assign placeholder X   ● Use Additional Character(s)   ▶ Manifestation Code   ⦿ Hierarchical Condition Category   **Coding Clinic**

● **V69**   Occupant of heavy transport vehicle injured in other and unspecified transport accidents

> The appropriate 7th character is to be added to each code from category V69

> | A | initial encounter |
> |---|---|
> | D | subsequent encounter |
> | S | sequela |

● **V69.0**   Driver of heavy transport vehicle injured in collision with other and unspecified motor vehicles in nontraffic accident

    X● **V69.00**   Driver of heavy transport vehicle injured in collision with unspecified motor vehicles in nontraffic accident

    X● **V69.09**   Driver of heavy transport vehicle injured in collision with other motor vehicles in nontraffic accident

● **V69.1**   Passenger in heavy transport vehicle injured in collision with other and unspecified motor vehicles in nontraffic accident

    X● **V69.10**   Passenger in heavy transport vehicle injured in collision with unspecified motor vehicles in nontraffic accident

    X● **V69.19**   Passenger in heavy transport vehicle injured in collision with other motor vehicles in nontraffic accident

● **V69.2**   Unspecified occupant of heavy transport vehicle injured in collision with other and unspecified motor vehicles in nontraffic accident

    X● **V69.20**   Unspecified occupant of heavy transport vehicle injured in collision with unspecified motor vehicles in nontraffic accident

> Collision NOS involving heavy transport vehicle, nontraffic

    X● **V69.29**   Unspecified occupant of heavy transport vehicle injured in collision with other motor vehicles in nontraffic accident

X● **V69.3**   Occupant (driver) (passenger) of heavy transport vehicle injured in unspecified nontraffic accident

> Accident NOS involving heavy transport vehicle, nontraffic
> Occupant of heavy transport vehicle injured in nontraffic accident NOS

● **V69.4**   Driver of heavy transport vehicle injured in collision with other and unspecified motor vehicles in traffic accident

    X● **V69.40**   Driver of heavy transport vehicle injured in collision with unspecified motor vehicles in traffic accident

    X● **V69.49**   Driver of heavy transport vehicle injured in collision with other motor vehicles in traffic accident

● **V69.5**   Passenger in heavy transport vehicle injured in collision with other and unspecified motor vehicles in traffic accident

    X● **V69.50**   Passenger in heavy transport vehicle injured in collision with unspecified motor vehicles in traffic accident

    X● **V69.59**   Passenger in heavy transport vehicle injured in collision with other motor vehicles in traffic accident

● **V69.6**   Unspecified occupant of heavy transport vehicle injured in collision with other and unspecified motor vehicles in traffic accident

    X● **V69.60**   Unspecified occupant of heavy transport vehicle injured in collision with unspecified motor vehicles in traffic accident

> Collision NOS involving heavy transport vehicle (traffic)

    X● **V69.69**   Unspecified occupant of heavy transport vehicle injured in collision with other motor vehicles in traffic accident

● **V69.8**   Occupant (driver) (passenger) of heavy transport vehicle injured in other specified transport accidents

    X● **V69.81**   Occupant (driver) (passenger) of heavy transport vehicle injured in transport accidents with military vehicle

    X● **V69.88**   Occupant (driver) (passenger) of heavy transport vehicle injured in other specified transport accidents

X● **V69.9**   Occupant (driver) (passenger) of heavy transport vehicle injured in unspecified traffic accident

> Accident NOS involving heavy transport vehicle

BUS OCCUPANT INJURED IN TRANSPORT ACCIDENT (V70-V79)

> | **Includes** | motorcoach |
> |---|---|
> | **Excludes1** | minibus (V50-V59) |

● **V70**   Bus occupant injured in collision with pedestrian or animal

> | **Excludes1** | bus collision with animal-drawn vehicle or animal being ridden (V76.-) |
> |---|---|

> The appropriate 7th character is to be added to each code from category V70

> | A | initial encounter |
> |---|---|
> | D | subsequent encounter |
> | S | sequela |

    X● **V70.0**   Driver of bus injured in collision with pedestrian or animal in nontraffic accident

    X● **V70.1**   Passenger on bus injured in collision with pedestrian or animal in nontraffic accident

    X● **V70.2**   Person on outside of bus injured in collision with pedestrian or animal in nontraffic accident

    X● **V70.3**   Unspecified occupant of bus injured in collision with pedestrian or animal in nontraffic accident

    X● **V70.4**   Person boarding or alighting from bus injured in collision with pedestrian or animal

    X● **V70.5**   Driver of bus injured in collision with pedestrian or animal in traffic accident

    X● **V70.6**   Passenger on bus injured in collision with pedestrian or animal in traffic accident

    X● **V70.7**   Person on outside of bus injured in collision with pedestrian or animal in traffic accident

    X● **V70.9**   Unspecified occupant of bus injured in collision with pedestrian or animal in traffic accident

● **V71**   Bus occupant injured in collision with pedal cycle

> The appropriate 7th character is to be added to each code from category V71

> | A | initial encounter |
> |---|---|
> | D | subsequent encounter |
> | S | sequela |

    X● **V71.0**   Driver of bus injured in collision with pedal cycle in nontraffic accident

    X● **V71.1**   Passenger on bus injured in collision with pedal cycle in nontraffic accident

    X● **V71.2**   Person on outside of bus injured in collision with pedal cycle in nontraffic accident

    X● **V71.3**   Unspecified occupant of bus injured in collision with pedal cycle in nontraffic accident

    X● **V71.4**   Person boarding or alighting from bus injured in collision with pedal cycle

    X● **V71.5**   Driver of bus injured in collision with pedal cycle in traffic accident

    X● **V71.6**   Passenger on bus injured in collision with pedal cycle in traffic accident

    X● **V71.7**   Person on outside of bus injured in collision with pedal cycle in traffic accident

    X● **V71.9**   Unspecified occupant of bus injured in collision with pedal cycle in traffic accident

---

● **V72** **Bus occupant injured in collision with two- or three-wheeled motor vehicle**

The appropriate 7th character is to be added to each code from category V72

A	initial encounter
D	subsequent encounter
S	sequela

X● **V72.0** Driver of bus injured in collision with two- or three-wheeled motor vehicle in nontraffic accident

X● **V72.1** Passenger on bus injured in collision with two- or three-wheeled motor vehicle in nontraffic accident

X● **V72.2** Person on outside of bus injured in collision with two- or three-wheeled motor vehicle in nontraffic accident

X● **V72.3** Unspecified occupant of bus injured in collision with two- or three-wheeled motor vehicle in nontraffic accident

X● **V72.4** Person boarding or alighting from bus injured in collision with two- or three-wheeled motor vehicle

X● **V72.5** Driver of bus injured in collision with two- or three-wheeled motor vehicle in traffic accident

X● **V72.6** Passenger on bus injured in collision with two- or three-wheeled motor vehicle in traffic accident

X● **V72.7** Person on outside of bus injured in collision with two- or three-wheeled motor vehicle in traffic accident

X● **V72.9** Unspecified occupant of bus injured in collision with two- or three-wheeled motor vehicle in traffic accident

● **V73** **Bus occupant injured in collision with car, pick-up truck or van**

The appropriate 7th character is to be added to each code from category V73

A	initial encounter
D	subsequent encounter
S	sequela

X● **V73.0** Driver of bus injured in collision with car, pick-up truck or van in nontraffic accident

X● **V73.1** Passenger on bus injured in collision with car, pick-up truck or van in nontraffic accident

X● **V73.2** Person on outside of bus injured in collision with car, pick-up truck or van in nontraffic accident

X● **V73.3** Unspecified occupant of bus injured in collision with car, pick-up truck or van in nontraffic accident

X● **V73.4** Person boarding or alighting from bus injured in collision with car, pick-up truck or van

X● **V73.5** Driver of bus injured in collision with car, pick-up truck or van in traffic accident

X● **V73.6** Passenger on bus injured in collision with car, pick-up truck or van in traffic accident

X● **V73.7** Person on outside of bus injured in collision with car, pick-up truck or van in traffic accident

X● **V73.9** Unspecified occupant of bus injured in collision with car, pick-up truck or van in traffic accident

● **V74** **Bus occupant injured in collision with heavy transport vehicle or bus**

Excludes1 bus occupant injured in collision with military vehicle (V79.81)

The appropriate 7th character is to be added to each code from category V74

A	initial encounter
D	subsequent encounter
S	sequela

X● **V74.0** Driver of bus injured in collision with heavy transport vehicle or bus in nontraffic accident

X● **V74.1** Passenger on bus injured in collision with heavy transport vehicle or bus in nontraffic accident

X● **V74.2** Person on outside of bus injured in collision with heavy transport vehicle or bus in nontraffic accident

X● **V74.3** Unspecified occupant of bus injured in collision with heavy transport vehicle or bus in nontraffic accident

X● **V74.4** Person boarding or alighting from bus injured in collision with heavy transport vehicle or bus

X● **V74.5** Driver of bus injured in collision with heavy transport vehicle or bus in traffic accident

X● **V74.6** Passenger on bus injured in collision with heavy transport vehicle or bus in traffic accident

X● **V74.7** Person on outside of bus injured in collision with heavy transport vehicle or bus in traffic accident

X● **V74.9** Unspecified occupant of bus injured in collision with heavy transport vehicle or bus in traffic accident

● **V75** **Bus occupant injured in collision with railway train or railway vehicle**

The appropriate 7th character is to be added to each code from category V75

A	initial encounter
D	subsequent encounter
S	sequela

X● **V75.0** Driver of bus injured in collision with railway train or railway vehicle in nontraffic accident

X● **V75.1** Passenger on bus injured in collision with railway train or railway vehicle in nontraffic accident

X● **V75.2** Person on outside of bus injured in collision with railway train or railway vehicle in nontraffic accident

X● **V75.3** Unspecified occupant of bus injured in collision with railway train or railway vehicle in nontraffic accident

X● **V75.4** Person boarding or alighting from bus injured in collision with railway train or railway vehicle

X● **V75.5** Driver of bus injured in collision with railway train or railway vehicle in traffic accident

X● **V75.6** Passenger on bus injured in collision with railway train or railway vehicle in traffic accident

X● **V75.7** Person on outside of bus injured in collision with railway train or railway vehicle in traffic accident

X● **V75.9** Unspecified occupant of bus injured in collision with railway train or railway vehicle in traffic accident

● **V76** **Bus occupant injured in collision with other nonmotor vehicle**

Includes collision with animal-drawn vehicle, animal being ridden, streetcar

The appropriate 7th character is to be added to each code from category V76

A	initial encounter
D	subsequent encounter
S	sequela

X● **V76.0** Driver of bus injured in collision with other nonmotor vehicle in nontraffic accident

X● **V76.1** Passenger on bus injured in collision with other nonmotor vehicle in nontraffic accident

X● **V76.2** Person on outside of bus injured in collision with other nonmotor vehicle in nontraffic accident

X● **V76.3** Unspecified occupant of bus injured in collision with other nonmotor vehicle in nontraffic accident

X● **V76.4** Person boarding or alighting from bus injured in collision with other nonmotor vehicle

X● **V76.5** Driver of bus injured in collision with other nonmotor vehicle in traffic accident

X● **V76.6** Passenger on bus injured in collision with other nonmotor vehicle in traffic accident

X● **V76.7** Person on outside of bus injured in collision with other nonmotor vehicle in traffic accident

X● **V76.9** Unspecified occupant of bus injured in collision with other nonmotor vehicle in traffic accident

CHAPTER 20 (V00-Y99)

● **V77**   **Bus occupant injured in collision with fixed or stationary object**

The appropriate 7th character is to be added to each code from category V77

A	initial encounter
D	subsequent encounter
S	sequela

X● **V77.0**   **Driver of bus injured in collision with fixed or stationary object in nontraffic accident**

X● **V77.1**   **Passenger on bus injured in collision with fixed or stationary object in nontraffic accident**

X● **V77.2**   **Person on outside of bus injured in collision with fixed or stationary object in nontraffic accident**

X● **V77.3**   **Unspecified occupant of bus injured in collision with fixed or stationary object in nontraffic accident**

X● **V77.4**   **Person boarding or alighting from bus injured in collision with fixed or stationary object**

X● **V77.5**   **Driver of bus injured in collision with fixed or stationary object in traffic accident**

X● **V77.6**   **Passenger on bus injured in collision with fixed or stationary object in traffic accident**

X● **V77.7**   **Person on outside of bus injured in collision with fixed or stationary object in traffic accident**

X● **V77.9**   **Unspecified occupant of bus injured in collision with fixed or stationary object in traffic accident**

● **V78**   **Bus occupant injured in noncollision transport accident**

     Includes   overturning bus NOS
                      overturning bus without collision

The appropriate 7th character is to be added to each code from category V78

A	initial encounter
D	subsequent encounter
S	sequela

X● **V78.0**   **Driver of bus injured in noncollision transport accident in nontraffic accident**

X● **V78.1**   **Passenger on bus injured in noncollision transport accident in nontraffic accident**

X● **V78.2**   **Person on outside of bus injured in noncollision transport accident in nontraffic accident**

X● **V78.3**   **Unspecified occupant of bus injured in noncollision transport accident in nontraffic accident**

X● **V78.4**   **Person boarding or alighting from bus injured in noncollision transport accident**

X● **V78.5**   **Driver of bus injured in noncollision transport accident in traffic accident**

X● **V78.6**   **Passenger on bus injured in noncollision transport accident in traffic accident**

X● **V78.7**   **Person on outside of bus injured in noncollision transport accident in traffic accident**

X● **V78.9**   **Unspecified occupant of bus injured in noncollision transport accident in traffic accident**

● **V79**   **Bus occupant injured in other and unspecified transport accidents**

The appropriate 7th character is to be added to each code from category V79

A	initial encounter
D	subsequent encounter
S	sequela

● **V79.0**   **Driver of bus injured in collision with other and unspecified motor vehicles in nontraffic accident**

X● **V79.00**   Driver of bus injured in collision with unspecified motor vehicles in nontraffic accident

X● **V79.09**   Driver of bus injured in collision with other motor vehicles in nontraffic accident

● **V79.1**   **Passenger on bus injured in collision with other and unspecified motor vehicles in nontraffic accident**

X● **V79.10**   Passenger on bus injured in collision with unspecified motor vehicles in nontraffic accident

X● **V79.19**   Passenger on bus injured in collision with other motor vehicles in nontraffic accident

● **V79.2**   **Unspecified bus occupant injured in collision with other and unspecified motor vehicles in nontraffic accident**

X● **V79.20**   Unspecified bus occupant injured in collision with unspecified motor vehicles in nontraffic accident

         Bus collision NOS, nontraffic

X● **V79.29**   Unspecified bus occupant injured in collision with other motor vehicles in nontraffic accident

X● **V79.3**   **Bus occupant (driver) (passenger) injured in unspecified nontraffic accident**

         Bus accident NOS, nontraffic
         Bus occupant injured in nontraffic accident NOS

● **V79.4**   **Driver of bus injured in collision with other and unspecified motor vehicles in traffic accident**

X● **V79.40**   Driver of bus injured in collision with unspecified motor vehicles in traffic accident

X● **V79.49**   Driver of bus injured in collision with other motor vehicles in traffic accident

● **V79.5**   **Passenger on bus injured in collision with other and unspecified motor vehicles in traffic accident**

X● **V79.50**   Passenger on bus injured in collision with unspecified motor vehicles in traffic accident

X● **V79.59**   Passenger on bus injured in collision with other motor vehicles in traffic accident

● **V79.6**   **Unspecified bus occupant injured in collision with other and unspecified motor vehicles in traffic accident**

X● **V79.60**   Unspecified bus occupant injured in collision with unspecified motor vehicles in traffic accident

         Bus collision NOS (traffic)

X● **V79.69**   Unspecified bus occupant injured in collision with other motor vehicles in traffic accident

● **V79.8**   **Bus occupant (driver) (passenger) injured in other specified transport accidents**

X● **V79.81**   Bus occupant (driver) (passenger) injured in transport accidents with military vehicle

X● **V79.88**   Bus occupant (driver) (passenger) injured in other specified transport accidents

X● **V79.9**   **Bus occupant (driver) (passenger) injured in unspecified traffic accident**

         Bus accident NOS

OTHER LAND TRANSPORT ACCIDENTS (V80-V89)

● **V80**   **Animal-rider or occupant of animal-drawn vehicle injured in transport accident**

The appropriate 7th character is to be added to each code from category V80

A	initial encounter
D	subsequent encounter
S	sequela

● **V80.0**   **Animal-rider or occupant of animal drawn vehicle injured by fall from or being thrown from animal or animal-drawn vehicle in noncollision accident**

● **V80.01**   **Animal-rider injured by fall from or being thrown from animal in noncollision accident**

● **V80.010**   Animal-rider injured by fall from or being thrown from horse in noncollision accident

● **V80.018**   Animal-rider injured by fall from or being thrown from other animal in noncollision accident

X ● **V80.02** Occupant of animal-drawn vehicle injured by fall from or being thrown from animal-drawn vehicle in noncollision accident
    Overturning animal-drawn vehicle NOS
    Overturning animal-drawn vehicle without collision

● **V80.1** Animal-rider or occupant of animal-drawn vehicle injured in collision with pedestrian or animal
    Excludes1 animal-rider or animal-drawn vehicle collision with animal-drawn vehicle or animal being ridden (V80.7)

X ● **V80.11** Animal-rider injured in collision with pedestrian or animal

X ● **V80.12** Occupant of animal-drawn vehicle injured in collision with pedestrian or animal

● **V80.2** Animal-rider or occupant of animal-drawn vehicle injured in collision with pedal cycle

X ● **V80.21** Animal-rider injured in collision with pedal cycle

X ● **V80.22** Occupant of animal-drawn vehicle injured in collision with pedal cycle

● **V80.3** Animal-rider or occupant of animal-drawn vehicle injured in collision with two- or three-wheeled motor vehicle

X ● **V80.31** Animal-rider injured in collision with two- or three-wheeled motor vehicle

X ● **V80.32** Occupant of animal-drawn vehicle injured in collision with two- or three-wheeled motor vehicle

● **V80.4** Animal-rider or occupant of animal-drawn vehicle injured in collision with car, pick-up truck, van, heavy transport vehicle or bus
    Excludes1 animal-rider injured in collision with military vehicle (V80.910)
    occupant of animal-drawn vehicle injured in collision with military vehicle (V80.920)

X ● **V80.41** Animal-rider injured in collision with car, pick-up truck, van, heavy transport vehicle or bus

X ● **V80.42** Occupant of animal-drawn vehicle injured in collision with car, pick-up truck, van, heavy transport vehicle or bus

● **V80.5** Animal-rider or occupant of animal-drawn vehicle injured in collision with other specified motor vehicle

X ● **V80.51** Animal-rider injured in collision with other specified motor vehicle

X ● **V80.52** Occupant of animal-drawn vehicle injured in collision with other specified motor vehicle

● **V80.6** Animal-rider or occupant of animal-drawn vehicle injured in collision with railway train or railway vehicle

X ● **V80.61** Animal-rider injured in collision with railway train or railway vehicle

X ● **V80.62** Occupant of animal-drawn vehicle injured in collision with railway train or railway vehicle

● **V80.7** Animal-rider or occupant of animal-drawn vehicle injured in collision with other nonmotor vehicles

● **V80.71** Animal-rider or occupant of animal-drawn vehicle injured in collision with animal being ridden

● **V80.710** Animal-rider injured in collision with other animal being ridden

● **V80.711** Occupant of animal-drawn vehicle injured in collision with animal being ridden

● **V80.72** Animal-rider or occupant of animal-drawn vehicle injured in collision with other animal-drawn vehicle

● **V80.720** Animal-rider injured in collision with animal-drawn vehicle

● **V80.721** Occupant of animal-drawn vehicle injured in collision with other animal-drawn vehicle

● **V80.73** Animal-rider or occupant of animal-drawn vehicle injured in collision with streetcar

● **V80.730** Animal-rider injured in collision with streetcar

● **V80.731** Occupant of animal-drawn vehicle injured in collision with streetcar

● **V80.79** Animal-rider or occupant of animal-drawn vehicle injured in collision with other nonmotor vehicles

● **V80.790** Animal-rider injured in collision with other nonmotor vehicles

● **V80.791** Occupant of animal-drawn vehicle injured in collision with other nonmotor vehicles

● **V80.8** Animal-rider or occupant of animal-drawn vehicle injured in collision with fixed or stationary object

X ● **V80.81** Animal-rider injured in collision with fixed or stationary object

X ● **V80.82** Occupant of animal-drawn vehicle injured in collision with fixed or stationary object

● **V80.9** Animal-rider or occupant of animal-drawn vehicle injured in other and unspecified transport accidents

● **V80.91** Animal-rider injured in other and unspecified transport accidents

● **V80.910** Animal-rider injured in transport accident with military vehicle

● **V80.918** Animal-rider injured in other transport accident

● **V80.919** Animal-rider injured in unspecified transport accident
    Animal rider accident NOS

● **V80.92** Occupant of animal-drawn vehicle injured in other and unspecified transport accidents

● **V80.920** Occupant of animal-drawn vehicle injured in transport accident with military vehicle

● **V80.928** Occupant of animal-drawn vehicle injured in other transport accident

● **V80.929** Occupant of animal-drawn vehicle injured in unspecified transport accident
    Animal-drawn vehicle accident NOS

● **V81** Occupant of railway train or railway vehicle injured in transport accident
    Includes derailment of railway train or railway vehicle
    person on outside of train
    Excludes1 streetcar (V82.-)
    The appropriate 7th character is to be added to each code from category V81

> A   initial encounter
> D   subsequent encounter
> S   sequela

X ● **V81.0** Occupant of railway train or railway vehicle injured in collision with motor vehicle in nontraffic accident
    Excludes1 occupant of railway train or railway vehicle injured due to collision with military vehicle (V81.83)

X ● **V81.1** Occupant of railway train or railway vehicle injured in collision with motor vehicle in traffic accident
    Excludes1 occupant of railway train or railway vehicle injured due to collision with military vehicle (V81.83)

X ● **V81.2** Occupant of railway train or railway vehicle injured in collision with or hit by rolling stock

X ● **V81.3** Occupant of railway train or railway vehicle injured in collision with other object
    Railway collision NOS

X ● **V81.4** Person injured while boarding or alighting from railway train or railway vehicle

▶ New   ⇒ Revised   ~~deleted~~ Deleted   Excludes 1   Excludes 2   Includes   Use additional   Code first   Code also   Key words

OGCR Official Guidelines   X Assign placeholder X   ● Use Additional Character(s)   ▷ Manifestation Code   🏷 Hierarchical Condition Category   **Coding Clinic**

X● **V81.5** Occupant of railway train or railway vehicle injured by fall in railway train or railway vehicle

X● **V81.6** Occupant of railway train or railway vehicle injured by fall from railway train or railway vehicle

X● **V81.7** Occupant of railway train or railway vehicle injured in derailment without antecedent collision

● **V81.8** Occupant of railway train or railway vehicle injured in other specified railway accidents

     X● **V81.81** Occupant of railway train or railway vehicle injured due to explosion or fire on train

     X● **V81.82** Occupant of railway train or railway vehicle injured due to object falling onto train
         Occupant of railway train or railway vehicle injured due to falling earth onto train
         Occupant of railway train or railway vehicle injured due to falling rocks onto train
         Occupant of railway train or railway vehicle injured due to falling snow onto train
         Occupant of railway train or railway vehicle injured due to falling trees onto train

     X● **V81.83** Occupant of railway train or railway vehicle injured due to collision with military vehicle

     X● **V81.89** Occupant of railway train or railway vehicle injured due to other specified railway accident

X● **V81.9** Occupant of railway train or railway vehicle injured in unspecified railway accident
     Railway accident NOS

● **V82** Occupant of powered streetcar injured in transport accident

     Includes   interurban electric car
           person on outside of streetcar
           tram (car)
           trolley (car)

     Excludes1   bus (V70-V79)
           motorcoach (V70-V79)
           nonpowered streetcar (V76.-)
           train (V81.-)

The appropriate 7th character is to be added to each code from category V82

> A   initial encounter
> D   subsequent encounter
> S   sequela

X● **V82.0** Occupant of streetcar injured in collision with motor vehicle in nontraffic accident

X● **V82.1** Occupant of streetcar injured in collision with motor vehicle in traffic accident

X● **V82.2** Occupant of streetcar injured in collision with or hit by rolling stock

X● **V82.3** Occupant of streetcar injured in collision with other object

     Excludes1   collision with animal-drawn vehicle or animal being ridden (V82.8)

X● **V82.4** Person injured while boarding or alighting from streetcar

X● **V82.5** Occupant of streetcar injured by fall in streetcar

     Excludes1   fall in streetcar:
           while boarding or alighting (V82.4)
           with antecedent collision (V82.0-V82.3)

X● **V82.6** Occupant of streetcar injured by fall from streetcar

     Excludes1   fall from streetcar:
           while boarding or alighting (V82.4)
           with antecedent collision (V82.0-V82.3)

X● **V82.7** Occupant of streetcar injured in derailment without antecedent collision

     Excludes1   occupant of streetcar injured in derailment with antecedent collision (V82.0-V82.3)

X● **V82.8** Occupant of streetcar injured in other specified transport accidents
     Streetcar collision with military vehicle
     Streetcar collision with train or nonmotor vehicles

X● **V82.9** Occupant of streetcar injured in unspecified traffic accident
     Streetcar accident NOS

● **V83** Occupant of special vehicle mainly used on industrial premises injured in transport accident

     Includes   battery-powered airport passenger vehicle
           battery-powered truck (baggage) (mail)
           coal-car in mine
           forklift (truck)
           logging car
           self-propelled industrial truck
           station baggage truck (powered)
           tram, truck, or tub (powered) in mine or quarry

     Excludes1   special construction vehicles (V85.-)
           special industrial vehicle in stationary use or maintenance (W31.-)

The appropriate 7th character is to be added to each code from category V83

> A   initial encounter
> D   subsequent encounter
> S   sequela

X● **V83.0** Driver of special industrial vehicle injured in traffic accident

X● **V83.1** Passenger of special industrial vehicle injured in traffic accident

X● **V83.2** Person on outside of special industrial vehicle injured in traffic accident

X● **V83.3** Unspecified occupant of special industrial vehicle injured in traffic accident

X● **V83.4** Person injured while boarding or alighting from special industrial vehicle

X● **V83.5** Driver of special industrial vehicle injured in nontraffic accident

X● **V83.6** Passenger of special industrial vehicle injured in nontraffic accident

X● **V83.7** Person on outside of special industrial vehicle injured in nontraffic accident

X● **V83.9** Unspecified occupant of special industrial vehicle injured in nontraffic accident
     Special-industrial-vehicle accident NOS

● **V84** Occupant of special vehicle mainly used in agriculture injured in transport accident

     Includes   self-propelled farm machinery
           tractor (and trailer)

     Excludes1   animal-powered farm machinery accident (W30.8-)
           contact with combine harvester (W30.0)
           special agricultural vehicle in stationary use or maintenance (W30.-)

The appropriate 7th character is to be added to each code from category V84

> A   initial encounter
> D   subsequent encounter
> S   sequela

X● **V84.0** Driver of special agricultural vehicle injured in traffic accident

X● **V84.1** Passenger of special agricultural vehicle injured in traffic accident

X● **V84.2** Person on outside of special agricultural vehicle injured in traffic accident

X● **V84.3** Unspecified occupant of special agricultural vehicle injured in traffic accident

X● **V84.4** Person injured while boarding or alighting from special agricultural vehicle

X● **V84.5** Driver of special agricultural vehicle injured in nontraffic accident

X● **V84.6** Passenger of special agricultural vehicle injured in nontraffic accident

CHAPTER 20 (V00-Y99)

X ● **V84.7** **Person on outside of special agricultural vehicle injured in nontraffic accident**

X ● **V84.9** **Unspecified occupant of special agricultural vehicle injured in nontraffic accident**
Special-agricultural vehicle accident NOS

● **V85** **Occupant of special construction vehicle injured in transport accident**

Includes   bulldozer
digger
dump truck
earth-leveller
mechanical shovel
road-roller

Excludes1   special industrial vehicle (V83.-)
special construction vehicle in stationary use or maintenance (W31.-)

The appropriate 7th character is to be added to each code from category V85

A   initial encounter
D   subsequent encounter
S   sequela

X ● **V85.0** **Driver of special construction vehicle injured in traffic accident**

X ● **V85.1** **Passenger of special construction vehicle injured in traffic accident**

X ● **V85.2** **Person on outside of special construction vehicle injured in traffic accident**

X ● **V85.3** **Unspecified occupant of special construction vehicle injured in traffic accident**

X ● **V85.4** **Person injured while boarding or alighting from special construction vehicle**

X ● **V85.5** **Driver of special construction vehicle injured in nontraffic accident**

X ● **V85.6** **Passenger of special construction vehicle injured in nontraffic accident**

X ● **V85.7** **Person on outside of special construction vehicle injured in nontraffic accident**

X ● **V85.9** **Unspecified occupant of special construction vehicle injured in nontraffic accident**
Special-construction-vehicle accident NOS

● **V86** **Occupant of special all-terrain or other off-road motor vehicle, injured in transport accident**

Excludes1   special all-terrain vehicle in stationary use or maintenance (W31.-)
sport-utility vehicle (V50-V59)
three-wheeled motor vehicle designed for on-road use (V30-V39)

The appropriate 7th character is to be added to each code from category V86

A   initial encounter
D   subsequent encounter
S   sequela

● **V86.0** **Driver of special all-terrain or other off-road motor vehicle injured in traffic accident**

X ● **V86.01** **Driver of ambulance or fire engine injured in traffic accident**

X ● **V86.02** **Driver of snowmobile injured in traffic accident**

X ● **V86.03** **Driver of dune buggy injured in traffic accident**

X ● **V86.04** **Driver of military vehicle injured in traffic accident**

X ● **V86.05** **Driver of 3- or 4-wheeled all-terrain vehicle (ATV) injured in traffic accident**

X ● **V86.06** **Driver of dirt bike or motor/cross bike injured in traffic accident**

X ● **V86.09** **Driver of other off-road special all-terrain or other off-road vehicle injured in traffic accident**
Driver of go cart injured in traffic accident
Driver of golf cart injured in traffic accident

● **V86.1** **Passenger of special all-terrain or other off-road motor vehicle injured in traffic accident**

X ● **V86.11** **Passenger of ambulance or fire engine injured in traffic accident**

X ● **V86.12** **Passenger of snowmobile injured in traffic accident**

X ● **V86.13** **Passenger of dune buggy injured in traffic accident**

X ● **V86.14** **Passenger of military vehicle injured in traffic accident**

X ● **V86.15** **Passenger of 3- or 4-wheeled all-terrain vehicle (ATV) injured in traffic accident**

X ● **V86.16** **Passenger of dirt bike or motor/cross bike injured in traffic accident**

X ● **V86.19** **Passenger of other off-road special all-terrain or other off-road off-road motor vehicle injured in traffic accident**
Passenger of go cart injured in traffic accident
Passenger of golf cart injured in traffic accident

● **V86.2** **Person on outside of special all-terrain or other off-road motor vehicle injured in traffic accident**

X ● **V86.21** **Person on outside of ambulance or fire engine injured in traffic accident**

X ● **V86.22** **Person on outside of snowmobile injured in traffic accident**

X ● **V86.23** **Person on outside of dune buggy injured in traffic accident**

X ● **V86.24** **Person on outside of military vehicle injured in traffic accident**

X ● **V86.25** **Person on outside of 3- or 4-wheeled all-terrain vehicle (ATV) injured in traffic accident**

X ● **V86.26** **Person on outside of dirt bike or motor/cross bike injured in traffic accident**

X ● **V86.29** **Person on outside of other special all-terrain or other off-road motor vehicle injured in traffic accident**
Person on outside of go cart in traffic accident
Person on outside of golf cart injured in traffic accident

● **V86.3** **Unspecified occupant of special all-terrain or other off-road motor vehicle injured in traffic accident**

X ● **V86.31** **Unspecified occupant of ambulance or fire engine injured in traffic accident**

X ● **V86.32** **Unspecified occupant of snowmobile injured in traffic accident**

X ● **V86.33** **Unspecified occupant of dune buggy injured in traffic accident**

X ● **V86.34** **Unspecified occupant of military vehicle injured in traffic accident**

X ● **V86.35** **Unspecified occupant of 3- or 4-wheeled all-terrain vehicle (ATV) injured in traffic accident**

X ● **V86.36** **Unspecified occupant of dirt bike or motor/cross bike injured in traffic accident**

X ● **V86.39** **Unspecified occupant of other special all-terrain or other off-road motor vehicle injured in traffic accident**
Unspecified occupant of go cart injured in traffic accident
Unspecified occupant of golf cart injured in traffic accident

● **V86.4** **Person injured while boarding or alighting from special all-terrain or other off-road motor vehicle**

X ● **V86.41** **Person injured while boarding or alighting from ambulance or fire engine**

X ● **V86.42** **Person injured while boarding or alighting from snowmobile**

X ● **V86.43** **Person injured while boarding or alighting from dune buggy**

X ● **V86.44** **Person injured while boarding or alighting from military vehicle**

X ● **V86.45** **Person injured while boarding or alighting from a 3- or 4-wheeled all-terrain vehicle (ATV)**

▶ New   ⇥ Revised   ~~deleted~~ Deleted   Excludes 1   Excludes 2   Includes   Use additional   Code first   Code also   Key words
OGCR Official Guidelines   X Assign placeholder X   ● Use Additional Character(s)   ▶ Manifestation Code   ✿ Hierarchical Condition Category   Coding Clinic

X● **V86.46**   Person injured while boarding or alighting from a dirt bike or motor/cross bike

X● **V86.49**   Person injured while boarding or alighting from other special all-terrain or other off-road motor vehicle

     Person injured while boarding or alighting from go cart

     Person injured while boarding or alighting from golf cart

● **V86.5**   Driver of special all-terrain or other off-road motor vehicle injured in nontraffic accident

X● **V86.51**   Driver of ambulance or fire engine injured in nontraffic accident

X● **V86.52**   Driver of snowmobile injured in nontraffic accident

X● **V86.53**   Driver of dune buggy injured in nontraffic accident

X● **V86.54**   Driver of military vehicle injured in nontraffic accident

X● **V86.55**   Driver of 3- or 4-wheeled all-terrain vehicle (ATV) injured in nontraffic accident

X● **V86.56**   Driver of dirt bike or motor/cross bike injured in nontraffic accident

X● **V86.59**   Driver of other off-road special all-terrain or other off-road motor vehicle injured in nontraffic accident

     Driver of go cart injured in nontraffic accident

     Driver of golf cart injured in nontraffic accident

● **V86.6**   Passenger of special all-terrain or other off-road motor vehicle injured in nontraffic accident

X● **V86.61**   Passenger of ambulance or fire engine injured in nontraffic accident

X● **V86.62**   Passenger of snowmobile injured in nontraffic accident

X● **V86.63**   Passenger of dune buggy injured in nontraffic accident

X● **V86.64**   Passenger of military vehicle injured in nontraffic accident

X● **V86.65**   Passenger of 3- or 4-wheeled all-terrain vehicle (ATV) injured in nontraffic accident

X● **V86.66**   Passenger of dirt bike or motor/cross bike injured in nontraffic accident

X● **V86.69**   Passenger of other special all-terrain or other off-road vehicle injured in nontraffic accident

     Passenger of go cart injured in nontraffic accident

     Passenger of golf cart injured in nontraffic accident

● **V86.7**   Person on outside of special all-terrain or other off-road motor vehicle injured in nontraffic accident

X● **V86.71**   Person on outside of ambulance or fire engine injured in nontraffic accident

X● **V86.72**   Person on outside of snowmobile injured in nontraffic accident

X● **V86.73**   Person on outside of dune buggy injured in nontraffic accident

X● **V86.74**   Person on outside of military vehicle injured in nontraffic accident

X● **V86.75**   Person on outside of 3- or 4-wheeled all-terrain vehicle (ATV) injured in nontraffic accident

X● **V86.76**   Person on outside of dirt bike or motor/cross bike injured in nontraffic accident

X● **V86.79**   Person on outside of other special all-terrain or other off-road motor vehicles injured in nontraffic accident

     Person on outside of go cart injured in nontraffic accident

     Person on outside of golf cart injured in nontraffic accident

● **V86.9**   Unspecified occupant of special all-terrain or other off-road motor vehicle injured in nontraffic accident

X● **V86.91**   Unspecified occupant of ambulance or fire engine injured in nontraffic accident

X● **V86.92**   Unspecified occupant of snowmobile injured in nontraffic accident

X● **V86.93**   Unspecified occupant of dune buggy injured in nontraffic accident

X● **V86.94**   Unspecified occupant of military vehicle injured in nontraffic accident

X● **V86.95**   Unspecified occupant of 3- or 4-wheeled all-terrain vehicle (ATV) injured in nontraffic accident

X● **V86.96**   Unspecified occupant of dirt bike or motor/cross bike injured in nontraffic accident

X● **V86.99**   Unspecified occupant of other special all-terrain or other off-road motor vehicle injured in nontraffic accident

     Off-road motor-vehicle accident NOS

     Other motor-vehicle accident NOS

     Unspecified occupant of go cart injured in nontraffic accident

     Unspecified occupant of golf cart injured in nontraffic accident

     Unspecified occupant of race car injured in nontraffic accident

● **V87**   **Traffic accident of specified type but victim's mode of transport unknown**

     Excludes1   collision involving:

         pedal cycle (V10-V19)

         pedestrian (V01-V09)

     The appropriate 7th character is to be added to each code from category V87

A	initial encounter
D	subsequent encounter
S	sequela

X● **V87.0**   Person injured in collision between car and two- or three-wheeled powered vehicle (traffic)

X● **V87.1**   Person injured in collision between other motor vehicle and two- or three-wheeled motor vehicle (traffic)

X● **V87.2**   Person injured in collision between car and pick-up truck or van (traffic)

X● **V87.3**   Person injured in collision between car and bus (traffic)

X● **V87.4**   Person injured in collision between car and heavy transport vehicle (traffic)

X● **V87.5**   Person injured in collision between heavy transport vehicle and bus (traffic)

X● **V87.6**   Person injured in collision between railway train or railway vehicle and car (traffic)

X● **V87.7**   Person injured in collision between other specified motor vehicles (traffic)

X● **V87.8**   Person injured in other specified noncollision transport accidents involving motor vehicle (traffic)

X● **V87.9**   Person injured in other specified (collision) (noncollision) transport accidents involving nonmotor vehicle (traffic)

● **V88**   **Nontraffic accident of specified type but victim's mode of transport unknown**

     Excludes1   collision involving:

         pedal cycle (V10-V19)

         pedestrian (V01-V09)

     The appropriate 7th character is to be added to each code from category V88

A	initial encounter
D	subsequent encounter
S	sequela

X● **V88.0**   Person injured in collision between car and two- or three-wheeled motor vehicle, nontraffic

X● **V88.1**   Person injured in collision between other motor vehicle and two- or three-wheeled motor vehicle, nontraffic

X● **V88.2**   Person injured in collision between car and pick-up truck or van, nontraffic

X ● **V88.3** **Person injured in collision between car and bus, nontraffic**

X ● **V88.4** **Person injured in collision between car and heavy transport vehicle, nontraffic**

X ● **V88.5** **Person injured in collision between heavy transport vehicle and bus, nontraffic**

X ● **V88.6** **Person injured in collision between railway train or railway vehicle and car, nontraffic**

X ● **V88.7** **Person injured in collision between other specified motor vehicle, nontraffic**

X ● **V88.8** **Person injured in other specified noncollision transport accidents involving motor vehicle, nontraffic**

X ● **V88.9** **Person injured in other specified (collision) (noncollision) transport accidents involving nonmotor vehicle, nontraffic**

● **V89** **Motor- or nonmotor-vehicle accident, type of vehicle unspecified**

> The appropriate 7th character is to be added to each code from category V89

> | | |
> |---|---|
> | A | initial encounter |
> | D | subsequent encounter |
> | S | sequela |

X ● **V89.0** **Person injured in unspecified motor-vehicle accident, nontraffic**
> Motor-vehicle accident NOS, nontraffic

X ● **V89.1** **Person injured in unspecified nonmotor-vehicle accident, nontraffic**
> Nonmotor-vehicle accident NOS (nontraffic)

X ● **V89.2** **Person injured in unspecified motor-vehicle accident, traffic**
> Motor-vehicle accident [MVA] NOS
> Road (traffic) accident [RTA] NOS

X ● **V89.3** **Person injured in unspecified nonmotor-vehicle accident, traffic**
> Nonmotor-vehicle traffic accident NOS

X ● **V89.9** **Person injured in unspecified vehicle accident**
> Collision NOS

WATER TRANSPORT ACCIDENTS (V90-V94)

● **V90** **Drowning and submersion due to accident to watercraft**
> **Excludes 1** civilian water transport accident involving military watercraft (V94.81-)
> fall into water not from watercraft (W16.-)
> military watercraft accident in military or war operations (Y36.0-, Y37.0-)
> water-transport–related drowning or submersion without accident to watercraft (V92.-)

> The appropriate 7th character is to be added to each code from category V90

> | | |
> |---|---|
> | A | initial encounter |
> | D | subsequent encounter |
> | S | sequela |

● **V90.0** **Drowning and submersion due to watercraft overturning**

X ● **V90.00** **Drowning and submersion due to merchant ship overturning**

X ● **V90.01** **Drowning and submersion due to passenger ship overturning**
> Drowning and submersion due to ferry-boat overturning
> Drowning and submersion due to liner overturning

X ● **V90.02** **Drowning and submersion due to fishing boat overturning**

X ● **V90.03** **Drowning and submersion due to other powered watercraft overturning**
> Drowning and submersion due to hovercraft (on open water) overturning
> Drowning and submersion due to jet ski overturning

X ● **V90.04** **Drowning and submersion due to sailboat overturning**

X ● **V90.05** **Drowning and submersion due to canoe or kayak overturning**

X ● **V90.06** **Drowning and submersion due to (nonpowered) inflatable craft overturning**

X ● **V90.08** **Drowning and submersion due to other unpowered watercraft overturning**
> Drowning and submersion due to windsurfer overturning

X ● **V90.09** **Drowning and submersion due to unspecified watercraft overturning**
> Drowning and submersion due to boat NOS overturning
> Drowning and submersion due to ship NOS overturning
> Drowning and submersion due to watercraft NOS overturning

● **V90.1** **Drowning and submersion due to watercraft sinking**

X ● **V90.10** **Drowning and submersion due to merchant ship sinking**

X ● **V90.11** **Drowning and submersion due to passenger ship sinking**
> Drowning and submersion due to ferry-boat sinking
> Drowning and submersion due to liner sinking

X ● **V90.12** **Drowning and submersion due to fishing boat sinking**

X ● **V90.13** **Drowning and submersion due to other powered watercraft sinking**
> Drowning and submersion due to hovercraft (on open water) sinking
> Drowning and submersion due to jet ski sinking

X ● **V90.14** **Drowning and submersion due to sailboat sinking**

X ● **V90.15** **Drowning and submersion due to canoe or kayak sinking**

X ● **V90.16** **Drowning and submersion due to (nonpowered) inflatable craft sinking**

X ● **V90.18** **Drowning and submersion due to other unpowered watercraft sinking**

X ● **V90.19** **Drowning and submersion due to unspecified watercraft sinking**
> Drowning and submersion due to boat NOS sinking
> Drowning and submersion due to ship NOS sinking
> Drowning and submersion due to watercraft NOS sinking

● **V90.2** **Drowning and submersion due to falling or jumping from burning watercraft**

X ● **V90.20** **Drowning and submersion due to falling or jumping from burning merchant ship**

X ● **V90.21** **Drowning and submersion due to falling or jumping from burning passenger ship**
> Drowning and submersion due to falling or jumping from burning ferry-boat
> Drowning and submersion due to falling or jumping from burning liner

X ● **V90.22** **Drowning and submersion due to falling or jumping from burning fishing boat**

X ● **V90.23** **Drowning and submersion due to falling or jumping from other burning powered watercraft**
> Drowning and submersion due to falling and jumping from burning hovercraft (on open water)
> Drowning and submersion due to falling and jumping from burning jet ski

X ● **V90.24** **Drowning and submersion due to falling or jumping from burning sailboat**

X ● **V90.25** **Drowning and submersion due to falling or jumping from burning canoe or kayak**

▶ New   ⇒ Revised   ~~deleted~~ Deleted   Excludes 1   Excludes 2   Includes   Use additional   Code first   Code also   Key words

OGCR Official Guidelines   X Assign placeholder X   ● Use Additional Character(s)   ▶ Manifestation Code   ✿ Hierarchical Condition Category   Coding Clinic

X⬤ **V90.26**   Drowning and submersion due to falling or jumping from burning (nonpowered) inflatable craft

X⬤ **V90.27**   Drowning and submersion due to falling or jumping from burning water-skis

X⬤ **V90.28**   Drowning and submersion due to falling or jumping from other burning unpowered watercraft
       Drowning and submersion due to falling and jumping from burning surf-board
       Drowning and submersion due to falling and jumping from burning windsurfer

X⬤ **V90.29**   Drowning and submersion due to falling or jumping from unspecified burning watercraft
       Drowning and submersion due to falling or jumping from burning boat NOS
       Drowning and submersion due to falling or jumping from burning ship NOS
       Drowning and submersion due to falling or jumping from burning watercraft NOS

⬤ **V90.3**   Drowning and submersion due to falling or jumping from crushed watercraft

X⬤ **V90.30**   Drowning and submersion due to falling or jumping from crushed merchant ship

X⬤ **V90.31**   Drowning and submersion due to falling or jumping from crushed passenger ship
       Drowning and submersion due to falling and jumping from crushed ferry-boat
       Drowning and submersion due to falling and jumping from crushed liner

X⬤ **V90.32**   Drowning and submersion due to falling or jumping from crushed fishing boat

X⬤ **V90.33**   Drowning and submersion due to falling or jumping from other crushed powered watercraft
       Drowning and submersion due to falling and jumping from crushed hovercraft
       Drowning and submersion due to falling and jumping from crushed jet ski

X⬤ **V90.34**   Drowning and submersion due to falling or jumping from crushed sailboat

X⬤ **V90.35**   Drowning and submersion due to falling or jumping from crushed canoe or kayak

X⬤ **V90.36**   Drowning and submersion due to falling or jumping from crushed (nonpowered) inflatable craft

X⬤ **V90.37**   Drowning and submersion due to falling or jumping from crushed water-skis

X⬤ **V90.38**   Drowning and submersion due to falling or jumping from other crushed unpowered watercraft
       Drowning and submersion due to falling and jumping from crushed surf-board
       Drowning and submersion due to falling and jumping from crushed windsurfer

X⬤ **V90.39**   Drowning and submersion due to falling or jumping from crushed unspecified watercraft
       Drowning and submersion due to falling and jumping from crushed boat NOS
       Drowning and submersion due to falling and jumping from crushed ship NOS
       Drowning and submersion due to falling and jumping from crushed watercraft NOS

⬤ **V90.8**   Drowning and submersion due to other accident to watercraft

X⬤ **V90.80**   Drowning and submersion due to other accident to merchant ship

X⬤ **V90.81**   Drowning and submersion due to other accident to passenger ship
       Drowning and submersion due to other accident to ferry-boat
       Drowning and submersion due to other accident to liner

X⬤ **V90.82**   Drowning and submersion due to other accident to fishing boat

X⬤ **V90.83**   Drowning and submersion due to other accident to other powered watercraft
       Drowning and submersion due to other accident to hovercraft (on open water)
       Drowning and submersion due to other accident to jet ski

X⬤ **V90.84**   Drowning and submersion due to other accident to sailboat

X⬤ **V90.85**   Drowning and submersion due to other accident to canoe or kayak

X⬤ **V90.86**   Drowning and submersion due to other accident to (nonpowered) inflatable craft

X⬤ **V90.87**   Drowning and submersion due to other accident to water-skis

X⬤ **V90.88**   Drowning and submersion due to other accident to other unpowered watercraft
       Drowning and submersion due to other accident to surf-board
       Drowning and submersion due to other accident to windsurfer

X⬤ **V90.89**   Drowning and submersion due to other accident to unspecified watercraft
       Drowning and submersion due to other accident to boat NOS
       Drowning and submersion due to other accident to ship NOS
       Drowning and submersion due to other accident to watercraft NOS

⬤ **V91**   Other injury due to accident to watercraft

   Includes   any injury except drowning and submersion as a result of an accident to watercraft

   Excludes1   civilian water transport accident involving military watercraft (V94.81-)
       military watercraft accident in military or war operations (Y36, Y37.-)

   Excludes2   drowning and submersion due to accident to watercraft (V90.-)

   The appropriate 7th character is to be added to each code from category V91

A	initial encounter
D	subsequent encounter
S	sequela

⬤ **V91.0**   Burn due to watercraft on fire

   Excludes1   burn from localized fire or explosion on board ship without accident to watercraft (V93.-)

X⬤ **V91.00**   Burn due to merchant ship on fire

X⬤ **V91.01**   Burn due to passenger ship on fire
       Burn due to ferry-boat on fire
       Burn due to liner on fire

X⬤ **V91.02**   Burn due to fishing boat on fire

X⬤ **V91.03**   Burn due to other powered watercraft on fire
       Burn due to hovercraft (on open water) on fire
       Burn due to jet ski on fire

X⬤ **V91.04**   Burn due to sailboat on fire

X⬤ **V91.05**   Burn due to canoe or kayak on fire

X⬤ **V91.06**   Burn due to (nonpowered) inflatable craft on fire

X⬤ **V91.07**   Burn due to water-skis on fire

X⬤ **V91.08**   Burn due to other unpowered watercraft on fire

X⬤ **V91.09**   Burn due to unspecified watercraft on fire
       Burn due to boat NOS on fire
       Burn due to ship NOS on fire
       Burn due to watercraft NOS on fire

CHAPTER 20 (V00-Y99)

● **V91.1 Crushed between watercraft and other watercraft or other object due to collision**
> Crushed by lifeboat after abandoning ship in a collision
>
> **Note:** Select the specified type of watercraft that the victim was on at the time of the collision.

X● **V91.10 Crushed between merchant ship and other watercraft or other object due to collision**

X● **V91.11 Crushed between passenger ship and other watercraft or other object due to collision**
> Crushed between ferry-boat and other watercraft or other object due to collision
> Crushed between liner and other watercraft or other object due to collision

X● **V91.12 Crushed between fishing boat and other watercraft or other object due to collision**

X● **V91.13 Crushed between other powered watercraft and other watercraft or other object due to collision**
> Crushed between hovercraft (on open water) and other watercraft or other object due to collision
> Crushed between jet ski and other watercraft or other object due to collision

X● **V91.14 Crushed between sailboat and other watercraft or other object due to collision**

X● **V91.15 Crushed between canoe or kayak and other watercraft or other object due to collision**

X● **V91.16 Crushed between (nonpowered) inflatable craft and other watercraft or other object due to collision**

X● **V91.18 Crushed between other unpowered watercraft and other watercraft or other object due to collision**
> Crushed between surfboard and other watercraft or other object due to collision
> Crushed between windsurfer and other watercraft or other object due to collision

X● **V91.19 Crushed between unspecified watercraft and other watercraft or other object due to collision**
> Crushed between boat NOS and other watercraft or other object due to collision
> Crushed between ship NOS and other watercraft or other object due to collision
> Crushed between watercraft NOS and other watercraft or other object due to collision

● **V91.2 Fall due to collision between watercraft and other watercraft or other object**
> Fall while remaining on watercraft after collision
>
> **Note:** Select the specified type of watercraft that the victim was on at the time of the collision.
>
> **Excludes1** crushed between watercraft and other watercraft and other object due to collision (V91.1-)
> drowning and submersion due to falling from crushed watercraft (V90.3-)

X● **V91.20 Fall due to collision between merchant ship and other watercraft or other object**

X● **V91.21 Fall due to collision between passenger ship and other watercraft or other object**
> Fall due to collision between ferry-boat and other watercraft or other object
> Fall due to collision between liner and other watercraft or other object

X● **V91.22 Fall due to collision between fishing boat and other watercraft or other object**

X● **V91.23 Fall due to collision between other powered watercraft and other watercraft or other object**
> Fall due to collision between hovercraft (on open water) and other watercraft or other object
> Fall due to collision between jet ski and other watercraft or other object

X● **V91.24 Fall due to collision between sailboat and other watercraft or other object**

X● **V91.25 Fall due to collision between canoe or kayak and other watercraft or other object**

X● **V91.26 Fall due to collision between (nonpowered) inflatable craft and other watercraft or other object**

X● **V91.29 Fall due to collision between unspecified watercraft and other watercraft or other object**
> Fall due to collision between boat NOS and other watercraft or other object
> Fall due to collision between ship NOS and other watercraft or other object
> Fall due to collision between watercraft NOS and other watercraft or other object

● **V91.3 Hit or struck by falling object due to accident to watercraft**
> Hit or struck by falling object (part of damaged watercraft or other object) after falling or jumping from damaged watercraft
>
> **Excludes2** drowning or submersion due to fall or jumping from damaged watercraft (V90.2-, V90.3-)

X● **V91.30 Hit or struck by falling object due to accident to merchant ship**

X● **V91.31 Hit or struck by falling object due to accident to passenger ship**
> Hit or struck by falling object due to accident to ferry-boat
> Hit or struck by falling object due to accident to liner

X● **V91.32 Hit or struck by falling object due to accident to fishing boat**

X● **V91.33 Hit or struck by falling object due to accident to other powered watercraft**
> Hit or struck by falling object due to accident to hovercraft (on open water)
> Hit or struck by falling object due to accident to jet ski

X● **V91.34 Hit or struck by falling object due to accident to sailboat**

X● **V91.35 Hit or struck by falling object due to accident to canoe or kayak**

X● **V91.36 Hit or struck by falling object due to accident to (nonpowered) inflatable craft**

X● **V91.37 Hit or struck by falling object due to accident to water-skis**
> Hit by water-skis after jumping off of waterskis

X● **V91.38 Hit or struck by falling object due to accident to other unpowered watercraft**
> Hit or struck by surf-board after falling off damaged surf-board
> Hit or struck by object after falling off damaged windsurfer

X● **V91.39 Hit or struck by falling object due to accident to unspecified watercraft**
> Hit or struck by falling object due to accident to boat NOS
> Hit or struck by falling object due to accident to ship NOS
> Hit or struck by falling object due to accident to watercraft NOS

● **V91.8 Other injury due to other accident to watercraft**

X● **V91.80 Other injury due to other accident to merchant ship**

X● **V91.81 Other injury due to other accident to passenger ship**
> Other injury due to other accident to ferry-boat
> Other injury due to other accident to liner

X● **V91.82 Other injury due to other accident to fishing boat**

X● **V91.83 Other injury due to other accident to other powered watercraft**
> Other injury due to other accident to hovercraft (on open water)
> Other injury due to other accident to jet ski

CHAPTER 20 (V00-Y99)

X● **V91.84** Other injury due to other accident to <mark>sailboat</mark>

X● **V91.85** Other injury due to other accident to <mark>canoe or kayak</mark>

X● **V91.86** Other injury due to other accident to (nonpowered) <mark>inflatable craft</mark>

X● **V91.87** Other injury due to other accident to <mark>water-skis</mark>

X● **V91.88** Other injury due to other accident to <mark>other unpowered watercraft</mark>
> Other injury due to other accident to surf-board
> Other injury due to other accident to windsurfer

X● **V91.89** Other injury due to other accident to <mark>unspecified watercraft</mark>
> Other injury due to other accident to boat NOS
> Other injury due to other accident to ship NOS
> Other injury due to other accident to watercraft NOS

● **V92** Drowning and submersion due to accident on board watercraft, without accident to watercraft

> **Excludes1**   civilian water transport accident involving military watercraft (V94.81-)
> drowning or submersion due to accident to watercraft (V90-V91)
> drowning or submersion of diver who voluntarily jumps from boat not involved in an accident (W16.711, W16.721)
> fall into water without watercraft (W16.-)
> military watercraft accident in military or war operations (Y36, Y37)

The appropriate 7th character is to be added to each code from category V92

A	initial encounter
D	subsequent encounter
S	sequela

● **V92.0** Drowning and submersion due to <mark>fall off</mark> watercraft
> Drowning and submersion due to fall from gangplank of watercraft
> Drowning and submersion due to fall overboard watercraft

> **Excludes2**   hitting head on object or bottom of body of water due to fall from watercraft (V94.0-)

X● **V92.00** Drowning and submersion due to fall off <mark>merchant ship</mark>

X● **V92.01** Drowning and submersion due to fall off <mark>passenger ship</mark>
> Drowning and submersion due to fall off ferry-boat
> Drowning and submersion due to fall off liner

X● **V92.02** Drowning and submersion due to fall off <mark>fishing boat</mark>

X● **V92.03** Drowning and submersion due to fall off <mark>other powered watercraft</mark>
> Drowning and submersion due to fall off hovercraft (on open water)
> Drowning and submersion due to fall off jet ski

X● **V92.04** Drowning and submersion due to fall off <mark>sailboat</mark>

X● **V92.05** Drowning and submersion due to fall off <mark>canoe or kayak</mark>

X● **V92.06** Drowning and submersion due to fall off (nonpowered) <mark>inflatable craft</mark>

X● **V92.07** Drowning and submersion due to fall off <mark>water-skis</mark>

> **Excludes1**   drowning and submersion due to falling off burning water-skis (V90.27)
> drowning and submersion due to falling off crushed water-skis (V90.37)
> hit by boat while water-skiing NOS (V94.-)

X● **V92.08** Drowning and submersion due to fall off <mark>other unpowered watercraft</mark>
> Drowning and submersion due to fall off surf-board
> Drowning and submersion due to fall off windsurfer

> **Excludes1**   drowning and submersion due to fall off burning unpowered watercraft (V90.28)
> drowning and submersion due to fall off crushed unpowered watercraft (V90.38)
> drowning and submersion due to fall off damaged unpowered watercraft (V90.88)
> drowning and submersion due to rider of nonpowered watercraft being hit by other watercraft (V94.-)
> other injury due to rider of nonpowered watercraft being hit by other watercraft (V94.-)

X● **V92.09** Drowning and submersion due to fall off <mark>unspecified</mark> watercraft
> Drowning and submersion due to fall off boat NOS
> Drowning and submersion due to fall off ship
> Drowning and submersion due to fall off watercraft NOS

● **V92.1** Drowning and submersion due to being <mark>thrown overboard by motion of watercraft</mark>

> **Excludes1**   drowning and submersion due to fall off surf-board (V92.08)
> drowning and submersion due to fall off water-skis (V92.07)
> drowning and submersion due to fall off windsurfer (V92.08)

X● **V92.10** Drowning and submersion due to being thrown overboard by motion of <mark>merchant ship</mark>

X● **V92.11** Drowning and submersion due to being thrown overboard by motion of <mark>passenger ship</mark>
> Drowning and submersion due to being thrown overboard by motion of ferry-boat
> Drowning and submersion due to being thrown overboard by motion of liner

X● **V92.12** Drowning and submersion due to being thrown overboard by motion of <mark>fishing boat</mark>

X● **V92.13** Drowning and submersion due to being thrown overboard by motion of <mark>other powered watercraft</mark>
> Drowning and submersion due to being thrown overboard by motion of hovercraft

X● **V92.14** Drowning and submersion due to being thrown overboard by motion of <mark>sailboat</mark>

X● **V92.15** Drowning and submersion due to being thrown overboard by motion of <mark>canoe or kayak</mark>

X● **V92.16** Drowning and submersion due to being thrown overboard by motion of (nonpowered) <mark>inflatable craft</mark>

X● **V92.19** Drowning and submersion due to being thrown overboard by motion of <mark>unspecified</mark> watercraft
> Drowning and submersion due to being thrown overboard by motion of boat NOS
> Drowning and submersion due to being thrown overboard by motion of ship NOS
> Drowning and submersion due to being thrown overboard by motion of watercraft NOS

● **V92.2** **Drowning and submersion due to being washed overboard from watercraft**

Code first any associated cataclysm (X37.0-)

X● **V92.20** **Drowning and submersion due to being washed overboard from merchant ship**

X● **V92.21** **Drowning and submersion due to being washed overboard from passenger ship**
Drowning and submersion due to being washed overboard from ferry-boat
Drowning and submersion due to being washed overboard from liner

X● **V92.22** **Drowning and submersion due to being washed overboard from fishing boat**

X● **V92.23** **Drowning and submersion due to being washed overboard from other powered watercraft**
Drowning and submersion due to being washed overboard from hovercraft (on open water)
Drowning and submersion due to being washed overboard from jet ski

X● **V92.24** **Drowning and submersion due to being washed overboard from sailboat**

X● **V92.25** **Drowning and submersion due to being washed overboard from canoe or kayak**

X● **V92.26** **Drowning and submersion due to being washed overboard from (nonpowered) inflatable craft**

X● **V92.27** **Drowning and submersion due to being washed overboard from water-skis**

> **Excludes1**   drowning and submersion due to fall off water-skis (V92.07)

X● **V92.28** **Drowning and submersion due to being washed overboard from other unpowered watercraft**
Drowning and submersion due to being washed overboard from surf-board
Drowning and submersion due to being washed overboard from windsurfer

X● **V92.29** **Drowning and submersion due to being washed overboard from unspecified watercraft**
Drowning and submersion due to being washed overboard from boat NOS
Drowning and submersion due to being washed overboard from ship NOS
Drowning and submersion due to being washed overboard from watercraft NOS

● **V93** **Other injury due to accident on board watercraft, without accident to watercraft**

> **Excludes1**   civilian water transport accident involving military watercraft (V94.81-)
> other injury due to accident to watercraft (V91.-)
> military watercraft accident in military or war operations (Y36, Y37.-)

> **Excludes2**   drowning and submersion due to accident on board watercraft, without accident to watercraft (V92.-)

The appropriate 7th character is to be added to each code from category V93

> A   initial encounter
> D   subsequent encounter
> S   sequela

● **V93.0** **Burn due to localized fire on board watercraft**

> **Excludes1**   burn due to watercraft on fire (V91.0-)

X● **V93.00** **Burn due to localized fire on board merchant vessel**

X● **V93.01** **Burn due to localized fire on board passenger vessel**
Burn due to localized fire on board ferry-boat
Burn due to localized fire on board liner

X● **V93.02** **Burn due to localized fire on board fishing boat**

X● **V93.03** **Burn due to localized fire on board other powered watercraft**
Burn due to localized fire on board hovercraft
Burn due to localized fire on board jet ski

X● **V93.04** **Burn due to localized fire on board sailboat**

X● **V93.09** **Burn due to localized fire on board unspecified watercraft**
Burn due to localized fire on board boat NOS
Burn due to localized fire on board ship NOS
Burn due to localized fire on board watercraft NOS

● **V93.1** **Other burn on board watercraft**
Burn due to source other than fire on board watercraft

> **Excludes1**   burn due to watercraft on fire (V91.0-)

X● **V93.10** **Other burn on board merchant vessel**

X● **V93.11** **Other burn on board passenger vessel**
Other burn on board ferry-boat
Other burn on board liner

X● **V93.12** **Other burn on board fishing boat**

X● **V93.13** **Other burn on board other powered watercraft**
Other burn on board hovercraft
Other burn on board jet ski

X● **V93.14** **Other burn on board sailboat**

X● **V93.19** **Other burn on board unspecified watercraft**
Other burn on board boat NOS
Other burn on board ship NOS
Other burn on board watercraft NOS

● **V93.2** **Heat exposure on board watercraft**

> **Excludes1**   exposure to man-made heat not aboard watercraft (W92)
> exposure to natural heat while on board watercraft (X30)
> exposure to sunlight while on board watercraft (X32)

> **Excludes2**   burn due to fire on board watercraft (V93.0-)

X● **V93.20** **Heat exposure on board merchant ship**

X● **V93.21** **Heat exposure on board passenger ship**
Heat exposure on board ferry-boat
Heat exposure on board liner

X● **V93.22** **Heat exposure on board fishing boat**

X● **V93.23** **Heat exposure on board other powered watercraft**
Heat exposure on board hovercraft

X● **V93.24** **Heat exposure on board sailboat**

X● **V93.29** **Heat exposure on board unspecified watercraft**
Heat exposure on board boat NOS
Heat exposure on board ship NOS
Heat exposure on board watercraft NOS

● **V93.3** **Fall on board watercraft**

> **Excludes1**   fall due to collision of watercraft (V91.2-)

X● **V93.30** **Fall on board merchant ship**

X● **V93.31** **Fall on board passenger ship**
Fall on board ferry-boat
Fall on board liner

X● **V93.32** **Fall on board fishing boat**

X● **V93.33** **Fall on board other powered watercraft**
Fall on board hovercraft (on open water)
Fall on board jet ski

X● **V93.34** **Fall on board sailboat**

X● **V93.35** **Fall on board canoe or kayak**

X● **V93.36** **Fall on board (nonpowered) inflatable craft**

X● **V93.38** **Fall on board other unpowered watercraft**

X● **V93.39** **Fall on board unspecified watercraft**
Fall on board boat NOS
Fall on board ship NOS
Fall on board watercraft NOS

▶ New   ⇒ Revised   ~~deleted~~ Deleted   Excludes 1   Excludes 2   Includes   Use additional   Code first   Code also   Key words

OGCR Official Guidelines   X Assign placeholder X   ● Use Additional Character(s)   ▶ Manifestation Code   🝮 Hierarchical Condition Category   **Coding Clinic**

● **V93.4 Struck by falling object on board watercraft**
Hit by falling object on board watercraft

> **Excludes1** struck by falling object due to accident to
> watercraft (V91.3)

X● **V93.40 Struck by falling object on** merchant ship

X● **V93.41 Struck by falling object on** passenger ship
Struck by falling object on ferry-boat
Struck by falling object on liner

X● **V93.42 Struck by falling object on** fishing boat

X● **V93.43 Struck by falling object on** other powered watercraft
Struck by falling object on hovercraft

X● **V93.44 Struck by falling object on** sailboat

X● **V93.48 Struck by falling object on** other unpowered watercraft

X● **V93.49 Struck by falling object on** unspecified watercraft

● **V93.5 Explosion on board watercraft**
Boiler explosion on steamship

> **Excludes2** fire on board watercraft (V93.0-)

X● **V93.50 Explosion on board** merchant ship

X● **V93.51 Explosion on board** passenger ship
Explosion on board ferry-boat
Explosion on board liner

X● **V93.52 Explosion on board** fishing boat

X● **V93.53 Explosion on board** other powered watercraft
Explosion on board hovercraft
Explosion on board jet ski

X● **V93.54 Explosion on board** sailboat

X● **V93.59 Explosion on board** unspecified watercraft
Explosion on board boat NOS
Explosion on board ship NOS
Explosion on board watercraft NOS

● **V93.6 Machinery accident on board watercraft**

> **Excludes1** machinery explosion on board watercraft
> (V93.4-)
> machinery fire on board watercraft
> (V93.0-)

X● **V93.60 Machinery accident on board** merchant ship

X● **V93.61 Machinery accident on board** passenger ship
Machinery accident on board ferry-boat
Machinery accident on board liner

X● **V93.62 Machinery accident on board** fishing boat

X● **V93.63 Machinery accident on board** other powered watercraft
Machinery accident on board hovercraft

X● **V93.64 Machinery accident on board** sailboat

X● **V93.69 Machinery accident on board** unspecified watercraft
Machinery accident on board boat NOS
Machinery accident on board ship NOS
Machinery accident on board watercraft NOS

● **V93.8 Other injury due to other accident on board watercraft**
Accidental poisoning by gases or fumes on watercraft

X● **V93.80 Other injury due to other accident on board** merchant ship

X● **V93.81 Other injury due to other accident on board** passenger ship
Other injury due to other accident on board ferry-boat
Other injury due to other accident on board liner

X● **V93.82 Other injury due to other accident on board** fishing boat

X● **V93.83 Other injury due to other accident on board** other powered watercraft
Other injury due to other accident on board hovercraft
Other injury due to other accident on board jet ski

X● **V93.84 Other injury due to other accident on board** sailboat

X● **V93.85 Other injury due to other accident on board** canoe or kayak

X● **V93.86 Other injury due to other accident on board** (nonpowered) inflatable craft

X● **V93.87 Other injury due to other accident on board** water-skis
Hit or struck by object while waterskiing

X● **V93.88 Other injury due to other accident on board** other unpowered watercraft
Hit or struck by object while surfing
Hit or struck by object while on board windsurfer

X● **V93.89 Other injury due to other accident on board** unspecified watercraft
Other injury due to other accident on board boat NOS
Other injury due to other accident on board ship NOS
Other injury due to other accident on board watercraft NOS

● **V94 Other and unspecified water transport accidents**

> **Excludes1** military watercraft accidents in military or war
> operations (Y36, Y37)

The appropriate 7th character is to be added to each code from category V94

> A   initial encounter
> D   subsequent encounter
> S   sequela

X● **V94.0 Hitting object or bottom of body of water due to fall from watercraft**

> **Excludes2** drowning and submersion due to fall
> from watercraft (V92.0-)

● **V94.1 Bather struck by watercraft**
Swimmer hit by watercraft

X● **V94.11 Bather struck by** powered **watercraft**

X● **V94.12 Bather struck by** nonpowered **watercraft**

● **V94.2 Rider of nonpowered watercraft struck by other watercraft**

X● **V94.21 Rider of nonpowered watercraft struck by other** nonpowered **watercraft**
Canoer hit by other nonpowered watercraft
Surfer hit by other nonpowered watercraft
Windsurfer hit by other nonpowered watercraft

X● **V94.22 Rider of nonpowered watercraft struck by** powered **watercraft**
Canoer hit by motorboat
Surfer hit by motorboat
Windsurfer hit by motorboat

● **V94.3 Injury to rider of (inflatable) watercraft being pulled behind other watercraft**

X● **V94.31 Injury to rider of (inflatable)** recreational **watercraft being pulled behind other watercraft**
Injury to rider of inner-tube pulled behind motor boat

X● **V94.32 Injury to rider of** non-recreational **watercraft being pulled behind other watercraft**
Injury to occupant of dingy being pulled behind boat or ship
Injury to occupant of life-raft being pulled behind boat or ship

X● **V94.4 Injury to barefoot water-skier**
Injury to person being pulled behind boat or ship

● **V94.8 Other water transport accident**

● **V94.81 Water transport accident involving military watercraft**

● **V94.810 Civilian watercraft involved in water transport accident with military watercraft**
Passenger on civilian watercraft injured due to accident with military watercraft

● V94.811 Civilian in water injured by military watercraft
● V94.818 Other water transport accident involving military watercraft
X● V94.89 Other water transport accident
X● V94.9 Unspecified water transport accident
Water transport accident NOS

AIR AND SPACE TRANSPORT ACCIDENTS (V95-V97)

Excludes1 military aircraft accidents in military or war operations (Y36, Y37)

● V95 Accident to powered aircraft causing injury to occupant
The appropriate 7th character is to be added to each code from category V95

A	initial encounter
D	subsequent encounter
S	sequela

● V95.0 Helicopter accident injuring occupant
X● V95.00 Unspecified helicopter accident injuring occupant
X● V95.01 Helicopter crash injuring occupant
X● V95.02 Forced landing of helicopter injuring occupant
X● V95.03 Helicopter collision injuring occupant
Helicopter collision with any object, fixed, movable or moving
X● V95.04 Helicopter fire injuring occupant
X● V95.05 Helicopter explosion injuring occupant
X● V95.09 Other helicopter accident injuring occupant
● V95.1 Ultralight, microlight or powered-glider accident injuring occupant
X● V95.10 Unspecified ultralight, microlight or powered-glider accident injuring occupant
X● V95.11 Ultralight, microlight or powered-glider crash injuring occupant
X● V95.12 Forced landing of ultralight, microlight or powered-glider injuring occupant
X● V95.13 Ultralight, microlight or powered-glider collision injuring occupant
Ultralight, microlight or powered-glider collision with any object, fixed, movable or moving
X● V95.14 Ultralight, microlight or powered-glider fire injuring occupant
X● V95.15 Ultralight, microlight or powered-glider explosion injuring occupant
X● V95.19 Other ultralight, microlight or powered-glider accident injuring occupant
● V95.2 Other private fixed-wing aircraft accident injuring occupant
X● V95.20 Unspecified accident to other private fixed-wing aircraft, injuring occupant
X● V95.21 Other private fixed-wing aircraft crash injuring occupant
X● V95.22 Forced landing of other private fixed-wing aircraft injuring occupant
X● V95.23 Other private fixed-wing aircraft collision injuring occupant
Other private fixed-wing aircraft collision with any object, fixed, movable or moving
X● V95.24 Other private fixed-wing aircraft fire injuring occupant
X● V95.25 Other private fixed-wing aircraft explosion injuring occupant
X● V95.29 Other accident to other private fixed-wing aircraft injuring occupant

● V95.3 Commercial fixed-wing aircraft accident injuring occupant
X● V95.30 Unspecified accident to commercial fixed-wing aircraft injuring occupant
X● V95.31 Commercial fixed-wing aircraft crash injuring occupant
X● V95.32 Forced landing of commercial fixed-wing aircraft injuring occupant
X● V95.33 Commercial fixed-wing aircraft collision injuring occupant
Commercial fixed-wing aircraft collision with any object, fixed, movable or moving
X● V95.34 Commercial fixed-wing aircraft fire injuring occupant
X● V95.35 Commercial fixed-wing aircraft explosion injuring occupant
X● V95.39 Other accident to commercial fixed-wing aircraft injuring occupant
● V95.4 Spacecraft accident injuring occupant
X● V95.40 Unspecified spacecraft accident injuring occupant
X● V95.41 Spacecraft crash injuring occupant
X● V95.42 Forced landing of spacecraft injuring occupant
X● V95.43 Spacecraft collision injuring occupant
Spacecraft collision with any object, fixed, moveable or moving
X● V95.44 Spacecraft fire injuring occupant
X● V95.45 Spacecraft explosion injuring occupant
X● V95.49 Other spacecraft accident injuring occupant
X● V95.8 Other powered aircraft accidents injuring occupant
X● V95.9 Unspecified aircraft accident injuring occupant
Aircraft accident NOS
Air transport accident NOS

● V96 Accident to nonpowered aircraft causing injury to occupant
The appropriate 7th character is to be added to each code from category V96

A	initial encounter
D	subsequent encounter
S	sequela

● V96.0 Balloon accident injuring occupant
X● V96.00 Unspecified balloon accident injuring occupant
X● V96.01 Balloon crash injuring occupant
X● V96.02 Forced landing of balloon injuring occupant
X● V96.03 Balloon collision injuring occupant
Balloon collision with any object, fixed, moveable or moving
X● V96.04 Balloon fire injuring occupant
X● V96.05 Balloon explosion injuring occupant
X● V96.09 Other balloon accident injuring occupant
● V96.1 Hang-glider accident injuring occupant
X● V96.10 Unspecified hang-glider accident injuring occupant
X● V96.11 Hang-glider crash injuring occupant
X● V96.12 Forced landing of hang-glider injuring occupant
X● V96.13 Hang-glider collision injuring occupant
Hang-glider collision with any object, fixed, moveable or moving
X● V96.14 Hang-glider fire injuring occupant
X● V96.15 Hang-glider explosion injuring occupant
X● V96.19 Other hang-glider accident injuring occupant
● V96.2 Glider (nonpowered) accident injuring occupant
X● V96.20 Unspecified glider (nonpowered) accident injuring occupant
X● V96.21 Glider (nonpowered) crash injuring occupant
X● V96.22 Forced landing of glider (nonpowered) injuring occupant

X● **V96.23 Glider (nonpowered) collision injuring occupant**
> Glider (nonpowered) collision with any object, fixed, moveable or moving

X● **V96.24 Glider (nonpowered) fire injuring occupant**

X● **V96.25 Glider (nonpowered) explosion injuring occupant**

X● **V96.29 Other glider (nonpowered) accident injuring occupant**

X● **V96.8 Other nonpowered-aircraft accidents injuring occupant**
> Kite carrying a person accident injuring occupant

X● **V96.9 Unspecified nonpowered-aircraft accident injuring occupant**
> Nonpowered-aircraft accident NOS

● **V97 Other specified air transport accidents**
> The appropriate 7th character is to be added to each code from category V97

A	initial encounter
D	subsequent encounter
S	sequela

X● **V97.0 Occupant of aircraft injured in other specified air transport accidents**
> Fall in, on or from aircraft in air transport accident
> **Excludes1**   accident while boarding or alighting aircraft (V97.1)

X● **V97.1 Person injured while boarding or alighting from aircraft**

● **V97.2 Parachutist accident**

X● **V97.21 Parachutist entangled in object**
> Parachutist landing in tree

X● **V97.22 Parachutist injured on landing**

X● **V97.29 Other parachutist accident**

● **V97.3 Person on ground injured in air transport accident**

X● **V97.31 Hit by object falling from aircraft**
> Hit by crashing aircraft
> Injured by aircraft hitting house
> Injured by aircraft hitting car

X● **V97.32 Injured by rotating propeller**

X● **V97.33 Sucked into jet engine**

X● **V97.39 Other injury to person on ground due to air transport accident**

● **V97.8 Other air transport accidents, not elsewhere classified**
> **Excludes1**   aircraft accident NOS (V95.9)
> exposure to changes in air pressure during ascent or descent (W94.-)

● **V97.81 Air transport accident involving military aircraft**

● **V97.810 Civilian aircraft involved in air transport accident with military aircraft**
> Passenger in civilian aircraft injured due to accident with military aircraft

● **V97.811 Civilian injured by military aircraft**

● **V97.818 Other air transport accident involving military aircraft**

X● **V97.89 Other air transport accidents, not elsewhere classified**
> Injury from machinery on aircraft

OTHER AND UNSPECIFIED TRANSPORT ACCIDENTS (V98-V99)
> **Excludes1**   vehicle accident, type of vehicle unspecified (V89.-)

● **V98 Other specified transport accidents**
> The appropriate 7th character is to be added to each code from category V98

A	initial encounter
D	subsequent encounter
S	sequela

X● **V98.0 Accident to, on or involving cable-car, not on rails**
> Caught or dragged by cable-car, not on rails
> Fall or jump from cable-car, not on rails
> Object thrown from or in cable-car, not on rails

X● **V98.1 Accident to, on or involving land-yacht**

X● **V98.2 Accident to, on or involving ice yacht**

X● **V98.3 Accident to, on or involving ski lift**
> Accident to, on or involving ski chair-lift
> Accident to, on or involving ski-lift with gondola

X● **V98.8 Other specified transport accidents**

X● **V99 Unspecified transport accident**
> The appropriate 7th character is to be added to code V99

A	initial encounter
D	subsequent encounter
S	sequela

OTHER EXTERNAL CAUSES OF ACCIDENTAL INJURY (W00-X58)

SLIPPING, TRIPPING, STUMBLING AND FALLS (W00-W19)
> **Excludes1**   assault involving a fall (Y01-Y02)
> fall from animal (V80.-)
> fall (in) (from) machinery (in operation) (W28-W31)
> fall (in) (from) transport vehicle (V01-V99)
> intentional self-harm involving a fall (X80-X81)
>
> **Excludes2**   at risk for fall (history of fall) Z91.81
> fall (in) (from) burning building (X00.-)
> fall into fire (X00-X04, X08)

● **W00 Fall due to ice and snow**
> **Includes**   pedestrian on foot falling (slipping) on ice and snow
>
> **Excludes1**   fall on (from) ice and snow involving pedestrian conveyance (V00.-)
> fall from stairs and steps not due to ice and snow (W10.-)
>
> The appropriate 7th character is to be added to each code from category W00

A	initial encounter
D	subsequent encounter
S	sequela

X● **W00.0 Fall on same level due to ice and snow**
> Coding Clinic: 2016, Q2, P5

X● **W00.1 Fall from stairs and steps due to ice and snow**

X● **W00.2 Other fall from one level to another due to ice and snow**

X● **W00.9 Unspecified fall due to ice and snow**

● **W01 Fall on same level from slipping, tripping and stumbling**
> **Includes**   fall on moving sidewalk
>
> **Excludes1**   fall due to bumping (striking) against object (W18.0-)
> fall in shower or bathtub (W18.2-)
> fall on same level NOS (W18.30)
> fall on same level from slipping, tripping and stumbling due to ice or snow (W00.0)
> fall off or from toilet (W18.1-)
> slipping, tripping and stumbling NOS (W18.40)
> slipping, tripping and stumbling without falling (W18.4-)
>
> The appropriate 7th character is to be added to each code from category W01

A	initial encounter
D	subsequent encounter
S	sequela

X● **W01.0 Fall on same level from slipping, tripping and stumbling without subsequent striking against object**
> Falling over animal

● **W01.1 Fall on same level from slipping, tripping and stumbling with subsequent striking against object**

X ● **W01.10 Fall on same level from slipping, tripping and stumbling with subsequent striking against unspecified object**

● **W01.11 Fall on same level from slipping, tripping and stumbling with subsequent striking against sharp object**

● **W01.110 Fall on same level from slipping, tripping and stumbling with subsequent striking against sharp glass**

● **W01.111 Fall on same level from slipping, tripping and stumbling with subsequent striking against power tool or machine**

● **W01.118 Fall on same level from slipping, tripping and stumbling with subsequent striking against other sharp object**

● **W01.119 Fall on same level from slipping, tripping and stumbling with subsequent striking against unspecified sharp object**

● **W01.19 Fall on same level from slipping, tripping and stumbling with subsequent striking against other object**

● **W01.190 Fall on same level from slipping, tripping and stumbling with subsequent striking against furniture**
Coding Clinic: 2021, Q1, P5

● **W01.198 Fall on same level from slipping, tripping and stumbling with subsequent striking against other object**

X ● **W03 Other fall on same level due to collision with another person**
Fall due to non-transport collision with other person

Excludes1   collision with another person without fall (W51)
crushed or pushed by a crowd or human stampede (W52)
fall involving pedestrian conveyance (V00-V09)
fall due to ice or snow (W00)
fall on same level NOS (W18.30)

The appropriate 7th character is to be added to code W03

A   initial encounter
D   subsequent encounter
S   sequela

Coding Clinic: 2015, Q1, P9-10; 2012, Q4, P108

X ● **W04 Fall while being carried or supported by other persons**
Accidentally dropped while being carried
The appropriate 7th character is to be added to code W04

A   initial encounter
D   subsequent encounter
S   sequel

● **W05 Fall from non-moving wheelchair, nonmotorized scooter and motorized mobility scooter**

Excludes1   fall from moving wheelchair (powered) (V00.811)
fall from moving motorized mobility scooter (V00.831)
fall from nonmotorized scooter (V00.141)

The appropriate 7th character is to be added to each code from category W05

A   initial encounter
D   subsequent encounter
S   sequela

X ● **W05.0 Fall from non-moving wheelchair**
Coding Clinic: 2019, Q2, P27
X ● **W05.1 Fall from non-moving nonmotorized scooter**
X ● **W05.2 Fall from non-moving motorized mobility scooter**

X ● **W06 Fall from bed**
The appropriate 7th character is to be added to code W06

A   initial encounter
D   subsequent encounter
S   sequela

X ● **W07 Fall from chair**
The appropriate 7th character is to be added to code W07

A   initial encounter
D   subsequent encounter
S   sequela

X ● **W08 Fall from other furniture**
The appropriate 7th character is to be added to code W08

A   initial encounter
D   subsequent encounter
S   sequela

● **W09 Fall on and from playground equipment**
Excludes1   fall involving recreational machinery (W31)
The appropriate 7th character is to be added to each code from category W09

A   initial encounter
D   subsequent encounter
S   sequela

X ● **W09.0 Fall on or from playground slide**
X ● **W09.1 Fall from playground swing**
X ● **W09.2 Fall on or from jungle gym**
X ● **W09.8 Fall on or from other playground equipment**

● **W10 Fall on and from stairs and steps**
Excludes1   fall from stairs and steps due to ice and snow (W00.1)
The appropriate 7th character is to be added to each code from category W10

A   initial encounter
D   subsequent encounter
S   sequela

X ● **W10.0 Fall (on) (from) escalator**
X ● **W10.1 Fall (on) (from) sidewalk curb**
X ● **W10.2 Fall (on) (from) incline**
Fall (on) (from) ramp
X ● **W10.8 Fall (on) (from) other stairs and steps**
X ● **W10.9 Fall (on) (from) unspecified stairs and steps**

X ● **W11 Fall on and from ladder**
The appropriate 7th character is to be added to code W11

A   initial encounter
D   subsequent encounter
S   sequela

X ● **W12 Fall on and from scaffolding**
The appropriate 7th character is to be added to code W12

A   initial encounter
D   subsequent encounter
S   sequela

● **W13 Fall from, out of or through building or structure**
The appropriate 7th character is to be added to each code from category W13

A   initial encounter
D   subsequent encounter
S   sequela

▶ New   ⇒ Revised   ~~deleted~~ Deleted   Excludes 1   Excludes 2   Includes   Use additional   Code first   Code also   Key words
OGCR Official Guidelines   X Assign placeholder X   ● Use Additional Character(s)   ▸ Manifestation Code   🐾 Hierarchical Condition Category   Coding Clinic

CHAPTER 20 (V00-Y99)

X● **W13.0**   **Fall from, out of or through balcony**
Fall from, out of or through railing

X● **W13.1**   **Fall from, out of or through bridge**

X● **W13.2**   **Fall from, out of or through roof**

X● **W13.3**   **Fall through floor**

X● **W13.4**   **Fall from, out of or through window**
> **Excludes2**   fall with subsequent striking against sharp glass (W01.110-)

X● **W13.8**   **Fall from, out of or through other building or structure**
Fall from, out of or through viaduct
Fall from, out of or through wall
Fall from, out of or through flag-pole

X● **W13.9**   **Fall from, out of or through building, not otherwise specified**
> **Excludes1**   collapse of a building or structure (W20.-)
> fall or jump from burning building or structure (X00.-)

X● **W14**   **Fall from tree**
The appropriate 7th character is to be added to code W14

A	initial encounter
D	subsequent encounter
S	sequela

X● **W15**   **Fall from cliff**
The appropriate 7th character is to be added to code W15

A	initial encounter
D	subsequent encounter
S	sequela

● **W16**   **Fall, jump or diving into water**
> **Excludes1**   accidental non-watercraft drowning and submersion not involving fall (W65-W74)
> effects of air pressure from diving (W94.-)
> fall into water from watercraft (V90-V94)
> hitting an object or against bottom when falling from watercraft (V94.0)

> **Excludes2**   striking or hitting diving board (W21.4)

The appropriate 7th character is to be added to each code from category W16

A	initial encounter
D	subsequent encounter
S	sequela

● **W16.0**   **Fall into swimming pool**
Fall into swimming pool NOS
> **Excludes1**   fall into empty swimming pool (W17.3)

   ● **W16.01**   **Fall into swimming pool striking water surface**

     ● **W16.011**   **Fall into swimming pool striking water surface causing drowning and submersion**
> **Excludes1**   drowning and submersion while in swimming pool without fall (W67)

     ● **W16.012**   **Fall into swimming pool striking water surface causing other injury**

   ● **W16.02**   **Fall into swimming pool striking bottom**

     ● **W16.021**   **Fall into swimming pool striking bottom causing drowning and submersion**
> **Excludes1**   drowning and submersion while in swimming pool without fall (W67)

     ● **W16.022**   **Fall into swimming pool striking bottom causing other injury**

● **W16.03**   **Fall into swimming pool striking wall**

   ● **W16.031**   **Fall into swimming pool striking wall causing drowning and submersion**
> **Excludes1**   drowning and submersion while in swimming pool without fall (W67)

   ● **W16.032**   **Fall into swimming pool striking wall causing other injury**

● **W16.1**   **Fall into natural body of water**
Fall into lake
Fall into open sea
Fall into river
Fall into stream

● **W16.11**   **Fall into natural body of water striking water surface**

   ● **W16.111**   **Fall into natural body of water striking water surface causing drowning and submersion**
> **Excludes1**   drowning and submersion while in natural body of water without fall (W69)

   ● **W16.112**   **Fall into natural body of water striking water surface causing other injury**

● **W16.12**   **Fall into natural body of water striking bottom**

   ● **W16.121**   **Fall into natural body of water striking bottom causing drowning and submersion**
> **Excludes1**   drowning and submersion while in natural body of water without fall (W69)

   ● **W16.122**   **Fall into natural body of water striking bottom causing other injury**

● **W16.13**   **Fall into natural body of water striking side**

   ● **W16.131**   **Fall into natural body of water striking side causing drowning and submersion**
> **Excludes1**   drowning and submersion while in natural body of water without fall (W69)

   ● **W16.132**   **Fall into natural body of water striking side causing other injury**

● **W16.2**   **Fall in (into) filled bathtub or bucket of water**

● **W16.21**   **Fall in (into) filled bathtub**
> **Excludes1**   fall into empty bathtub (W18.2)

   ● **W16.211**   **Fall in (into) filled bathtub causing drowning and submersion**
> **Excludes1**   drowning and submersion while in filled bathtub without fall (W65)

   ● **W16.212**   **Fall in (into) filled bathtub causing other injury**

● **W16.22**   **Fall in (into) bucket of water**

   ● **W16.221**   **Fall in (into) bucket of water causing drowning and submersion**

   ● **W16.222**   **Fall in (into) bucket of water causing other injury**

● W16.3 **Fall into other water**
Fall into fountain
Fall into reservoir
  ● W16.31 **Fall into other water striking water surface**
    ● W16.311 **Fall into other water striking water surface causing drowning and submersion**
      Excludes1 drowning and submersion while in other water without fall (W73)
    ● W16.312 **Fall into other water striking water surface causing other injury**
  ● W16.32 **Fall into other water striking bottom**
    ● W16.321 **Fall into other water striking bottom causing drowning and submersion**
      Excludes1 drowning and submersion while in other water without fall (W73)
    ● W16.322 **Fall into other water striking bottom causing other injury**
  ● W16.33 **Fall into other water striking wall**
    ● W16.331 **Fall into other water striking wall causing drowning and submersion**
      Excludes1 drowning and submersion while in other water without fall (W73)
    ● W16.332 **Fall into other water striking wall causing other injury**
● W16.4 **Fall into unspecified water**
  X ● W16.41 **Fall into unspecified water causing drowning and submersion**
  X ● W16.42 **Fall into unspecified water causing other injury**
● W16.5 **Jumping or diving into swimming pool**
  ● W16.51 **Jumping or diving into swimming pool striking water surface**
    ● W16.511 **Jumping or diving into swimming pool striking water surface causing drowning and submersion**
      Excludes1 drowning and submersion while in swimming pool without jumping or diving (W67)
    ● W16.512 **Jumping or diving into swimming pool striking water surface causing other injury**
  ● W16.52 **Jumping or diving into swimming pool striking bottom**
    ● W16.521 **Jumping or diving into swimming pool striking bottom causing drowning and submersion**
      Excludes1 drowning and submersion while in swimming pool without jumping or diving (W67)
    ● W16.522 **Jumping or diving into swimming pool striking bottom causing other injury**

● W16.53 **Jumping or diving into swimming pool striking wall**
  ● W16.531 **Jumping or diving into swimming pool striking wall causing drowning and submersion**
    Excludes1 drowning and submersion while in swimming pool without jumping or diving (W67)
  ● W16.532 **Jumping or diving into swimming pool striking wall causing other injury**
● W16.6 **Jumping or diving into natural body of water**
Jumping or diving into lake
Jumping or diving into open sea
Jumping or diving into river
Jumping or diving into stream
  ● W16.61 **Jumping or diving into natural body of water striking water surface**
    ● W16.611 **Jumping or diving into natural body of water striking water surface causing drowning and submersion**
      Excludes1 drowning and submersion while in natural body of water without jumping or diving (W69)
    ● W16.612 **Jumping or diving into natural body of water striking water surface causing other injury**
  ● W16.62 **Jumping or diving into natural body of water striking bottom**
    ● W16.621 **Jumping or diving into natural body of water striking bottom causing drowning and submersion**
      Excludes1 drowning and submersion while in natural body of water without jumping or diving (W69)
    ● W16.622 **Jumping or diving into natural body of water striking bottom causing other injury**
● W16.7 **Jumping or diving from boat**
  Excludes1 fall from boat into water - see watercraft accident (V90-V94)
  ● W16.71 **Jumping or diving from boat striking water surface**
    ● W16.711 **Jumping or diving from boat striking water surface causing drowning and submersion**
    ● W16.712 **Jumping or diving from boat striking water surface causing other injury**
  ● W16.72 **Jumping or diving from boat striking bottom**
    ● W16.721 **Jumping or diving from boat striking bottom causing drowning and submersion**
    ● W16.722 **Jumping or diving from boat striking bottom causing other injury**

▶ New ⇒ Revised ~~deleted~~ Deleted Excludes 1 Excludes 2 Includes Use additional Code first Code also Key words
OGCR Official Guidelines X Assign placeholder X ● Use Additional Character(s) ▷ Manifestation Code Hierarchical Condition Category Coding Clinic

● **W16.8**   **Jumping or diving into other water**
Jumping or diving into fountain
Jumping or diving into reservoir

   ● **W16.81**   **Jumping or diving into other water striking water surface**

      ● **W16.811**   Jumping or diving into other water striking water surface causing drowning and submersion

        Excludes1   drowning and submersion while in other water without jumping or diving (W73)

      ● **W16.812**   Jumping or diving into other water striking water surface causing other injury

   ● **W16.82**   **Jumping or diving into other water striking bottom**

      ● **W16.821**   Jumping or diving into other water striking bottom causing drowning and submersion

        Excludes1   drowning and submersion while in other water without jumping or diving (W73)

      ● **W16.822**   Jumping or diving into other water striking bottom causing other injury

   ● **W16.83**   **Jumping or diving into other water striking wall**

      ● **W16.831**   Jumping or diving into other water striking wall causing drowning and submersion

        Excludes1   drowning and submersion while in other water without jumping or diving (W73)

      ● **W16.832**   Jumping or diving into other water striking wall causing other injury

   ● **W16.9**   **Jumping or diving into unspecified water**

     X ● **W16.91**   Jumping or diving into unspecified water causing drowning and submersion

     X ● **W16.92**   Jumping or diving into unspecified water causing other injury

● **W17**   **Other fall from one level to another**

The appropriate 7th character is to be added to each code from category W17

A	initial encounter
D	subsequent encounter
S	sequela

X ● **W17.0**   **Fall into well**

X ● **W17.1**   **Fall into storm drain or manhole**

X ● **W17.2**   **Fall into hole**
Fall into pit

X ● **W17.3**   **Fall into empty swimming pool**
Excludes1   fall into filled swimming pool (W16.0-)

X ● **W17.4**   **Fall from dock**

● **W17.8**   **Other fall from one level to another**

   X ● **W17.81**   **Fall down embankment (hill)**

   X ● **W17.82**   **Fall from (out of) grocery cart**
Fall due to grocery cart tipping over

   X ● **W17.89**   **Other fall from one level to another**
Fall from cherry picker
Fall from lifting device
Fall from mobile elevated work platform [MEWP]
Fall from sky lift
Coding Clinic: 2015, Q2, P6

● **W18**   **Other slipping, tripping and stumbling and falls**

The appropriate 7th character is to be added to each code from category W18

A	initial encounter
D	subsequent encounter
S	sequela

● **W18.0**   **Fall due to bumping against object**
Striking against object with subsequent fall
Excludes1   fall on same level due to slipping, tripping, or stumbling with subsequent striking against object (W01.1-)

   X ● **W18.00**   Striking against unspecified object with subsequent fall

   X ● **W18.01**   Striking against sports equipment with subsequent fall

   X ● **W18.02**   Striking against glass with subsequent fall

   X ● **W18.09**   Striking against other object with subsequent fall

● **W18.1**   **Fall from or off toilet**

   X ● **W18.11**   **Fall from or off toilet without subsequent striking against object**
Fall from (off) toilet NOS

   X ● **W18.12**   **Fall from or off toilet with subsequent striking against object**

X ● **W18.2**   **Fall in (into) shower or empty bathtub**
Excludes1   fall in full bathtub causing drowning or submersion (W16.21-)

● **W18.3**   **Other and unspecified fall on same level**

   X ● **W18.30**   **Fall on same level, unspecified**

   X ● **W18.31**   **Fall on same level due to stepping on an object**
Fall on same level due to stepping on an animal
Excludes1   slipping, tripping and stumbling without fall due to stepping on animal (W18.41)

   X ● **W18.39**   **Other fall on same level**

● **W18.4**   **Slipping, tripping and stumbling without falling**
Excludes1   collision with another person without fall (W51)

   X ● **W18.40**   **Slipping, tripping and stumbling without falling, unspecified**

   X ● **W18.41**   **Slipping, tripping and stumbling without falling due to stepping on object**
Slipping, tripping and stumbling without falling due to stepping on animal
Excludes1   slipping, tripping and stumbling with fall due to stepping on animal (W18.31)

   X ● **W18.42**   **Slipping, tripping and stumbling without falling due to stepping into hole or opening**

   X ● **W18.43**   **Slipping, tripping and stumbling without falling due to stepping from one level to another**

   X ● **W18.49**   **Other slipping, tripping and stumbling without falling**

X ● **W19**   **Unspecified fall**
Accidental fall NOS

The appropriate 7th character is to be added to code W19

A	initial encounter
D	subsequent encounter
S	sequela

CHAPTER 20 (V00-Y99)

EXPOSURE TO INANIMATE MECHANICAL FORCES (W20-W49)

Excludes1 assault (X92-Y09)
contact or collision with animals or persons
(W50-W64)
exposure to inanimate mechanical forces
involving military or war operations (Y36.-,
Y37.-)
intentional self-harm (X71-X83)

Coding Clinic: 2022, Q4, P45; 2021, Q2, P5; 2016, Q4, P129; 2012, Q4, P95

● W20 Struck by thrown, projected or falling object

Code first any associated:
cataclysm (X34-X39)
lightning strike (T75.00)

Excludes1 falling object in machinery accident (W24,
W28-W31)
falling object in transport accident (V01-V99)
object set in motion by explosion (W35-W40)
object set in motion by firearm (W32-W34)
struck by thrown sports equipment (W21.-)

The appropriate 7th character is to be added to each code from
category W20

A	initial encounter
D	subsequent encounter
S	sequela

X● W20.0 Struck by falling object in cave-in
Excludes2 asphyxiation due to cave-in (T71.21)

X● W20.1 Struck by object due to collapse of building
Excludes1 struck by object due to collapse of
burning building (X00.2, X02.2)

X● W20.8 Other cause of strike by thrown, projected or falling
object
Excludes1 struck by thrown sports equipment
(W21.-)

● W21 Striking against or struck by sports equipment
Excludes1 assault with sports equipment (Y08.0-)
striking against or struck by sports equipment
with subsequent fall (W18.01)

The appropriate 7th character is to be added to each code from
category W21

A	initial encounter
D	subsequent encounter
S	sequela

● W21.0 Struck by hit or thrown ball
X● W21.00 Struck by hit or thrown ball, unspecified type
X● W21.01 Struck by football
X● W21.02 Struck by soccer ball
X● W21.03 Struck by baseball
X● W21.04 Struck by golf ball
X● W21.05 Struck by basketball
X● W21.06 Struck by volleyball
X● W21.07 Struck by softball
X● W21.09 Struck by other hit or thrown ball
● W21.1 Struck by bat, racquet or club
X● W21.11 Struck by baseball bat
X● W21.12 Struck by tennis racquet
X● W21.13 Struck by golf club
X● W21.19 Struck by other bat, racquet or club
● W21.2 Struck by hockey stick or puck
● W21.21 Struck by hockey stick
● W21.210 Struck by ice hockey stick
● W21.211 Struck by field hockey stick

● W21.22 Struck by hockey puck
● W21.220 Struck by ice hockey puck
● W21.221 Struck by field hockey puck
● W21.3 Struck by sports foot wear
X● W21.31 Struck by shoe cleats
Stepped on by shoe cleats
X● W21.32 Struck by skate blades
Skated over by skate blades
X● W21.39 Struck by other sports foot wear
X● W21.4 Striking against diving board
Use additional code for subsequent falling into water, if
applicable (W16.-)
● W21.8 Striking against or struck by other sports equipment
X● W21.81 Striking against or struck by football helmet
X● W21.89 Striking against or struck by other sports
equipment
X● W21.9 Striking against or struck by unspecified sports
equipment

● W22 Striking against or struck by other objects
Excludes1 striking against or struck by object with
subsequent fall (W18.09)

The appropriate 7th character is to be added to each code from
category W22

A	initial encounter
D	subsequent encounter
S	sequela

● W22.0 Striking against stationary object
Excludes1 striking against stationary sports
equipment (W21.8)
X● W22.01 Walked into wall
X● W22.02 Walked into lamppost
X● W22.03 Walked into furniture
● W22.04 Striking against wall of swimming pool
● W22.041 Striking against wall of swimming
pool causing drowning and
submersion
Excludes1 drowning and
submersion
while swimming
without striking
against wall
(W67)

● W22.042 Striking against wall of swimming
pool causing other injury
X● W22.09 Striking against other stationary object
● W22.1 Striking against or struck by automobile airbag
X● W22.10 Striking against or struck by unspecified
automobile airbag
X● W22.11 Striking against or struck by driver side
automobile airbag
X● W22.12 Striking against or struck by front passenger
side automobile airbag
X● W22.19 Striking against or struck by other automobile
airbag
X● W22.8 Striking against or struck by other objects
Striking against or struck by object NOS
Excludes1 struck by thrown, projected or falling
object (W20.-)

▶ New   ⟹ Revised   ~~deleted~~ Deleted   Excludes 1   Excludes 2   Includes   Use additional   Code first   Code also   Key words
OGCR Official Guidelines   X Assign placeholder X   ● Use Additional Character(s)   ◗ Manifestation Code   🔍 Hierarchical Condition Category   Coding Clinic

● W23   **Caught, crushed, jammed or pinched in or between objects**

     Excludes1   injury caused by cutting or piercing instruments (W25-W27)
             injury caused by firearms malfunction (W32.1, W33.1-, W34.1-)
             injury caused by lifting and transmission devices (W24.-)
             injury caused by machinery (W28-W31)
             injury caused by nonpowered hand tools (W27.-)
             injury caused by transport vehicle being used as a means of transportation (V01-V99)
             injury caused by struck by thrown, projected or falling object (W20.-)

     The appropriate 7th character is to be added to each code from category W23

A	initial encounter
D	subsequent encounter
S	sequela

X● **W23.0**   Caught, crushed, jammed, or pinched between **moving** objects

X● **W23.1**   Caught, crushed, jammed, or pinched between **stationary** objects

X● **W23.2**   Caught, crushed, jammed or pinched between a moving and stationary object

● W24   **Contact with lifting and transmission devices, not elsewhere classified**

     Excludes1   transport accidents (V01-V99)

     The appropriate 7th character is to be added to each code from category W24

A	initial encounter
D	subsequent encounter
S	sequela

X● **W24.0**   Contact with **lifting** devices, not elsewhere classified
         Contact with chain hoist
         Contact with drive belt
         Contact with pulley (block)

X● **W24.1**   Contact with **transmission** devices, not elsewhere classified
         Contact with transmission belt or cable

X● W25   **Contact with sharp glass**

     Code first any associated:
         injury due to flying glass from explosion or firearm discharge (W32-W40)
         transport accident (V00-V99)

     Excludes1   fall on same level due to slipping, tripping and stumbling with subsequent striking against sharp glass (W01.110-)
               striking against sharp glass with subsequent fall (W18.02-)

     Excludes2   glass embedded in skin (W45.-)

     The appropriate 7th character is to be added to code W25

A	initial encounter
D	subsequent encounter
S	sequela

● W26   **Contact with other sharp objects**

     Excludes2   sharp object(s) embedded in skin (W45.-)

     The appropriate 7th character is to be added to each code from category W26

A	initial encounter
D	subsequent encounter
S	sequela

     Coding Clinic: 2016, Q4, P73

X● **W26.0**   Contact with **knife**

         Excludes1   contact with electric knife (W29.1)

X● **W26.1**   Contact with **sword or dagger**

X● **W26.2**   Contact with edge of **stiff paper**
         Paper cut
         Coding Clinic: 2016, Q4, P73

X● **W26.8**   Contact with **other** sharp object(s), not elsewhere classified
         Contact with tin can lid
         Coding Clinic: 2016, Q4, P73

X● **W26.9**   Contact with **unspecified** sharp object(s)
         Coding Clinic: 2016, Q4, P73

● W27   **Contact with nonpowered hand tool**

     The appropriate 7th character is to be added to each code from category W27

A	initial encounter
D	subsequent encounter
S	sequela

X● **W27.0**   Contact with **workbench tool**
         Contact with auger
         Contact with axe
         Contact with chisel
         Contact with handsaw
         Contact with screwdriver

X● **W27.1**   Contact with **garden tool**
         Contact with hoe
         Contact with nonpowered lawn mower
         Contact with pitchfork
         Contact with rake

X● **W27.2**   Contact with **scissors**

X● **W27.3**   Contact with **needle** (sewing)
         Excludes1   contact with hypodermic needle (W46.-)

X● **W27.4**   Contact with **kitchen utensil**
         Contact with fork
         Contact with ice-pick
         Contact with can-opener NOS

X● **W27.5**   Contact with **paper-cutter**

X● **W27.8**   Contact with **other** nonpowered hand tool
         Contact with nonpowered sewing machine
         Contact with shovel

X● W28   **Contact with powered lawn mower**

     Powered lawn mower (commercial) (residential)

     Excludes1   contact with nonpowered lawn mower (W27.1)

     Excludes2   exposure to electric current (W86.-)

     The appropriate 7th character is to be added to code W28

A	initial encounter
D	subsequent encounter
S	sequela

● W29   **Contact with other powered hand tools and household machinery**

     Excludes1   contact with commercial machinery (W31.82)
               contact with hot household appliance (X15)
               contact with nonpowered hand tool (W27.-)
               exposure to electric current (W86)

     The appropriate 7th character is to be added to each code from category W29

A	initial encounter
D	subsequent encounter
S	sequela

X● **W29.0**   Contact with powered **kitchen appliance**
         Contact with blender
         Contact with can-opener
         Contact with garbage disposal
         Contact with mixer

X● **W29.1**   Contact with **electric knife**

X● **W29.2**   Contact with other powered household machinery
         Contact with electric fan
         Contact with powered dryer (clothes) (powered) (spin)
         Contact with washing-machine
         Contact with sewing machine

CHAPTER 20 (V00-Y99)

X● **W29.3 Contact with powered garden and outdoor hand tools and machinery**
Contact with chainsaw
Contact with edger
Contact with garden cultivator (tiller)
Contact with hedge trimmer
Contact with other powered garden tool
> **Excludes1**   contact with powered lawn mower (W28)

X● **W29.4 Contact with nail gun**

X● **W29.8 Contact with other powered hand tools and household machinery**
Contact with do-it-yourself tool NOS

● **W30 Contact with agricultural machinery**
> **Includes**   animal-powered farm machine
> **Excludes1**   agricultural transport vehicle accident (V01-V99)
> explosion of grain store (W40.8)
> exposure to electric current (W86.-)

The appropriate 7th character is to be added to each code from category W30

A	initial encounter
D	subsequent encounter
S	sequela

X● **W30.0 Contact with combine harvester**
Contact with reaper
Contact with thresher

X● **W30.1 Contact with power take-off devices (PTO)**

X● **W30.2 Contact with hay derrick**

X● **W30.3 Contact with grain storage elevator**
> **Excludes1**   explosion of grain store (W40.8)

● **W30.8 Contact with other specified agricultural machinery**

X● **W30.81 Contact with agricultural transport vehicle in stationary use**
Contact with agricultural transport vehicle under repair, not on public roadway
> **Excludes1**   agricultural transport vehicle accident (V01-V99)

X● **W30.89 Contact with other specified agricultural machinery**

X● **W30.9 Contact with unspecified agricultural machinery**
Contact with farm machinery NOS

● **W31 Contact with other and unspecified machinery**
> **Excludes1**   contact with agricultural machinery (W30.-)
> contact with machinery in transport under own power or being towed by a vehicle (V01-V99)
> exposure to electric current (W86)

The appropriate 7th character is to be added to each code from category W31

A	initial encounter
D	subsequent encounter
S	sequela

X● **W31.0 Contact with mining and earth-drilling machinery**
Contact with bore or drill (land) (seabed)
Contact with shaft hoist
Contact with shaft lift
Contact with undercutter

X● **W31.1 Contact with metalworking machines**
Contact with abrasive wheel
Contact with forging machine
Contact with lathe
Contact with mechanical shears
Contact with metal drilling machine
Contact with milling machine
Contact with power press
Contact with rolling-mill
Contact with metal sawing machine

X● **W31.2 Contact with powered woodworking and forming machines**
Contact with band saw
Contact with bench saw
Contact with circular saw
Contact with molding machine
Contact with overhead plane
Contact with powered saw
Contact with radial saw
Contact with sander
> **Excludes1**   nonpowered woodworking tools (W27.0)

X● **W31.3 Contact with prime movers**
Contact with gas turbine
Contact with internal combustion engine
Contact with steam engine
Contact with water driven turbine

● **W31.8 Contact with other specified machinery**

X● **W31.81 Contact with recreational machinery**
Contact with roller-coaster

X● **W31.82 Contact with other commercial machinery**
Contact with commercial electric fan
Contact with commercial kitchen appliances
Contact with commercial powered dryer (clothes) (powered) (spin)
Contact with commercial washing-machine
Contact with commercial sewing machine
> **Excludes1**   contact with household machinery (W29.-)
> contact with powered lawn mower (W28)

X● **W31.83 Contact with special construction vehicle in stationary use**
Contact with special construction vehicle under repair, not on public roadway
> **Excludes1**   special construction vehicle accident (V01-V99)

X● **W31.89 Contact with other specified machinery**

X● **W31.9 Contact with unspecified machinery**
Contact with machinery NOS

● **W32 Accidental handgun discharge and malfunction**
> **Includes**   accidental discharge and malfunction of gun for single hand use
> accidental discharge and malfunction of pistol
> accidental discharge and malfunction of revolver
> handgun discharge and malfunction NOS
> **Excludes1**   accidental airgun discharge and malfunction (W34.010, W34.110)
> accidental BB gun discharge and malfunction (W34.010, W34.110)
> accidental pellet gun discharge and malfunction (W34.010, W34.110)
> accidental shotgun discharge and malfunction (W33.01, W33.11)
> assault by handgun discharge (X93)
> handgun discharge involving legal intervention (Y35.0-)
> handgun discharge involving military or war operations (Y36.4-)
> intentional self-harm by handgun discharge (X72)
> Very pistol discharge and malfunction (W34.09, W34.19)

The appropriate 7th character is to be added to each code from category W32

A	initial encounter
D	subsequent encounter
S	sequela

X● **W32.0 Accidental handgun discharge**

X● **W32.1 Accidental handgun malfunction**
Injury due to explosion of handgun (parts)
Injury due to malfunction of mechanism or component of handgun
Injury due to recoil of handgun
Powder burn from handgun

▶ New   ⇒ Revised   ~~deleted~~ Deleted   Excludes 1   Excludes 2   Includes   Use additional   Code first   Code also   Key words

OGCR Official Guidelines   X Assign placeholder X   ● Use Additional Character(s)   ▶ Manifestation Code   Hierarchical Condition Category   Coding Clinic

● W33   **Accidental rifle, shotgun and larger firearm discharge and malfunction**

     Includes   rifle, shotgun and larger firearm discharge and malfunction NOS

     Excludes1   accidental airgun discharge and malfunction (W34.010, W34.110)
                 accidental BB gun discharge and malfunction (W34.010, W34.110)
                 accidental handgun discharge and malfunction (W32.-)
                 accidental pellet gun discharge and malfunction (W34.010, W34.110)
                 assault by rifle, shotgun and larger firearm discharge (X94)
                 firearm discharge involving legal intervention (Y35.0-)
                 firearm discharge involving military or war operations (Y36.4-)
                 intentional self-harm by rifle, shotgun and larger firearm discharge (X73)

     The appropriate 7th character is to be added to each code from category W33

A	initial encounter
D	subsequent encounter
S	sequela

  ● W33.0   **Accidental rifle, shotgun and larger firearm discharge**

    X ● W33.00   **Accidental discharge of unspecified larger firearm**
                 Discharge of unspecified larger firearm NOS

    X ● W33.01   **Accidental discharge of shotgun**
                 Discharge of shotgun NOS

    X ● W33.02   **Accidental discharge of hunting rifle**
                 Discharge of hunting rifle NOS

    X ● W33.03   **Accidental discharge of machine gun**
                 Discharge of machine gun NOS

    X ● W33.09   **Accidental discharge of other larger firearm**
                 Discharge of other larger firearm NOS

  ● W33.1   **Accidental rifle, shotgun and larger firearm malfunction**
          Injury due to explosion of rifle, shotgun and larger firearm (parts)
          Injury due to malfunction of mechanism or component of rifle, shotgun and larger firearm
          Injury due to piercing, cutting, crushing or pinching due to (by) slide trigger mechanism, scope or other gun part
          Injury due to recoil of rifle, shotgun and larger firearm
          Powder burn from rifle, shotgun and larger firearm

    X ● W33.10   **Accidental malfunction of unspecified larger firearm**
                 Malfunction of unspecified larger firearm NOS

    X ● W33.11   **Accidental malfunction of shotgun**
                 Malfunction of shotgun NOS

    X ● W33.12   **Accidental malfunction of hunting rifle**
                 Malfunction of hunting rifle NOS

    X ● W33.13   **Accidental malfunction of machine gun**
                 Malfunction of machine gun NOS

    X ● W33.19   **Accidental malfunction of other larger firearm**
                 Malfunction of other larger firearm NOS

● W34   **Accidental discharge and malfunction from other and unspecified firearms and guns**

     The appropriate 7th character is to be added to each code from category W34

A	initial encounter
D	subsequent encounter
S	sequela

  ● W34.0   **Accidental discharge from other and unspecified firearms and guns**

    X ● W34.00   **Accidental discharge from unspecified firearms or gun**
                 Discharge from firearm NOS
                 Gunshot wound NOS
                 Shot NOS
                 Coding Clinic: 2015, Q1, P17

    ● W34.01   **Accidental discharge of gas, air or spring-operated guns**

       ● W34.010   **Accidental discharge of airgun**
                 Accidental discharge of BB gun
                 Accidental discharge of pellet gun

       ● W34.011   **Accidental discharge of paintball gun**
                 Accidental injury due to paintball discharge

       ● W34.018   **Accidental discharge of other gas, air or spring-operated gun**

    X ● W34.09   **Accidental discharge from other specified firearms**
                 Accidental discharge from Very pistol [flare]

  ● W34.1   **Accidental malfunction from other and unspecified firearms and guns**

    X ● W34.10   **Accidental malfunction from unspecified firearms or gun**
                 Firearm malfunction NOS

    ● W34.11   **Accidental malfunction of gas, air or spring-operated guns**

       ● W34.110   **Accidental malfunction of airgun**
                 Accidental malfunction of BB gun
                 Accidental malfunction of pellet gun

       ● W34.111   **Accidental malfunction of paintball gun**
                 Accidental injury due to paintball gun malfunction

       ● W34.118   **Accidental malfunction of other gas, air or spring-operated gun**

    X ● W34.19   **Accidental malfunction from other specified firearms**
                 Accidental malfunction from Very pistol [flare]

X ● W35   **Explosion and rupture of boiler**

     Excludes1   explosion and rupture of boiler on watercraft (V93.4)

     The appropriate 7th character is to be added to code W35

A	initial encounter
D	subsequent encounter
S	sequela

● W36   **Explosion and rupture of gas cylinder**

     The appropriate 7th character is to be added to each code from category W36

A	initial encounter
D	subsequent encounter
S	sequela

    X ● W36.1   **Explosion and rupture of aerosol can**

    X ● W36.2   **Explosion and rupture of air tank**

    X ● W36.3   **Explosion and rupture of pressurized-gas tank**

    X ● W36.8   **Explosion and rupture of other gas cylinder**

    X ● W36.9   **Explosion and rupture of unspecified gas cylinder**

● W37   **Explosion and rupture of pressurized tire, pipe or hose**

     The appropriate 7th character is to be added to each code from category W37

A	initial encounter
D	subsequent encounter
S	sequela

    X ● W37.0   **Explosion of bicycle tire**

    X ● W37.8   **Explosion and rupture of other pressurized tire, pipe or hose**

CHAPTER 20 (V00-Y99)

X⬤W38 **Explosion and rupture of other specified pressurized devices**
The appropriate 7th character is to be added to code W38

> A   initial encounter
> D   subsequent encounter
> S   sequela

X⬤W39 **Discharge of firework**
The appropriate 7th character is to be added to code W39

> A   initial encounter
> D   subsequent encounter
> S   sequela

⬤W40 **Explosion of other materials**
    Excludes1   assault by explosive material (X96)
                 explosion involving legal intervention (Y35.1-)
                 explosion involving military or war operations
                    (Y36.0-, Y36.2-)
                 intentional self-harm by explosive material (X75)
The appropriate 7th character is to be added to each code from
    category W40

> A   initial encounter
> D   subsequent encounter
> S   sequela

X⬤ W40.0 **Explosion of blasting material**
Explosion of blasting cap
Explosion of detonator
Explosion of dynamite
Explosion of explosive (any) used in blasting operations

X⬤ W40.1 **Explosion of explosive gases**
Explosion of acetylene
Explosion of butane
Explosion of coal gas
Explosion in mine NOS
Explosion of explosive gas
Explosion of fire damp
Explosion of gasoline fumes
Explosion of methane
Explosion of propane

X⬤ W40.8 **Explosion of other specified explosive materials**
Explosion in dump NOS
Explosion in factory NOS
Explosion in grain store
Explosion in munitions
    Excludes1   explosion involving legal intervention
                 (Y35.1-)
                 explosion involving military or war
                    operations (Y36.0-, Y36.2-)

X⬤ W40.9 **Explosion of unspecified explosive materials**
Explosion NOS

⬤W42 **Exposure to noise**
The appropriate 7th character is to be added to each code from
    category W42

> A   initial encounter
> D   subsequent encounter
> S   sequela

X⬤ W42.0 **Exposure to supersonic waves**
X⬤ W42.9 **Exposure to other noise**
Exposure to sound waves NOS

⬤W44 **Foreign body entering into or through a natural orifice**
    Excludes2   contact with other sharp objects (W26)
                 contact with sharp glass (W25)
                 foreign body or object entering through skin
                    (W45)
The appropriate 7th character is to be added to each code from
    category W44

> A   initial encounter
> D   subsequent encounter
> S   sequela

X⬤ W44.A **Battery entering into or through a natural orifice**
    W44.A0 **Battery unspecified, entering into or through a natural orifice**
    W44.A1 **Button battery entering into or through a natural orifice**
    W44.A9 **Other batteries entering into or through a natural orifice**
          Cylindrical battery

X⬤ W44.B **Plastic entering into or through a natural orifice**
    W44.B0 **Plastic object unspecified, entering into or through a natural orifice**
    W44.B1 **Plastic bead entering into or through a natural orifice**
        Excludes2   Plastic jewelry entering into or through a
                      natural orifice (W44.B4)
    W44.B2 **Plastic coin entering into or through a natural orifice**
    W44.B3 **Plastic toy and toy part entering into or through a natural orifice**
    W44.B4 **Plastic jewelry entering into or through a natural orifice**
        Excludes2   Plastic bead entering into or through a
                      natural orifice (W44.B1)
    W44.B5 **Plastic bottle entering into or through a natural orifice**
    W44.B9 **Other plastic object entering into or through a natural orifice**

X⬤ W44.C **Glass entering into or through a natural orifice**
    W44.C0 **Glass unspecified, entering into or through a natural orifice**
    W44.C1 **Sharp glass entering into or through a natural orifice**
          Glass shard entering into or through a natural
             orifice
    W44.C2 **Intact glass entering into or through a natural orifice**
          Intact glass bottle entering into or through a
             natural orifice

X⬤ W44.D **Magnetic metal entering into or through a natural orifice**
    W44.D0 **Magnetic metal object unspecified, entering into or through a natural orifice**
    W44.D1 **Magnetic metal bead entering into or through a natural orifice**
    W44.D2 **Magnetic metal coin entering into or through a natural orifice**
    W44.D3 **Magnetic metal toy entering into or through a natural orifice**
    W44.D4 **Magnetic metal jewelry entering into or through a natural orifice**
    W44.D9 **Other magnetic metal objects entering into or through a natural orifice**

X⬤ W44.E **Non-magnetic metal entering into or through a natural orifice**
    W44.E0 **Non-magnetic metal object unspecified, entering into or through a natural orifice**
    W44.E1 **Non-magnetic metal bead entering into or through a natural orifice**
    W44.E2 **Non-magnetic metal coin entering into or through a natural orifice**

▶ New   ⇒ Revised   ~~deleted~~ Deleted   Excludes 1   Excludes 2   Includes   Use additional   Code first   Code also   Key words
OGCR Official Guidelines   X Assign placeholder X   ⬤ Use Additional Character(s)   ▷ Manifestation Code   ❦ Hierarchical Condition Category   Coding Clinic

W44.E3   Non-magnetic metal toy entering into or through a natural orifice

W44.E4   Non-magnetic metal jewelry entering into or through a natural orifice

W44.E9   Other non-magnetic metal objects entering into or through a natural orifice

> Bottle cap entering into or through a natural orifice
> Can lid entering into or through a natural orifice
> Pull tab entering into or through a natural orifice

X● W44.F   Objects of natural or organic material entering into or through a natural orifice

W44.F0   Objects of natural or organic material unspecified, entering into or through a natural orifice

W44.F1   Bezoar entering into or through a natural orifice

W44.F2   Rubber band entering into or through a natural orifice

W44.F3   Food entering into or through a natural orifice

W44.F4   Insect entering into or through a natural orifice

W44.F9   Other object of natural or organic material, entering into or through a natural orifice

X● W44.G   Other non-organic objects entering into or through a natural orifice

W44.G0   Other non-organic objects unspecified, entering into or through a natural orifice

W44.G1   Audio device entering into or through a natural orifice

> Ear buds
> Hearing aids

W44.G2   Combination metal and plastic toy and toy part entering into or through natural orifice

W44.G3   Combination metal and plastic jewelry entering into or through a natural orifice

W44.G9   Other non-organic objects entering into or through a natural orifice

X● W44.H   Other sharp object entering into or through a natural orifice

W44.H0   Other sharp object unspecified, entering into or through a natural orifice

W44.H1   Needle entering into or through a natural orifice

> Dart entering into or through a natural orifice
> Hypodermic needle entering into or through a natural orifice
> Safety pin entering into or through a natural orifice
> Sewing needle entering into or through a natural orifice

W44.H2   Knife, sword or dagger entering into or through a natural orifice

W44.8   Other foreign body entering into or through a natural orifice

W44.9   Unspecified foreign body entering into or through a natural orifice

> Foreign body NOS entering into or through a natural orifice

● W45   Foreign body or object entering through skin

> **Includes**   foreign body or object embedded in skin
> nail embedded in skin

> **Excludes2**   contact with hand tools (nonpowered) (powered) (W27-W29)
> contact with other sharp object(s) (W26.-)
> contact with sharp glass (W25.-)
> struck by objects (W20-W22)

The appropriate 7th character is to be added to each code from category W45

> A   initial encounter
> D   subsequent encounter
> S   sequela

X● W45.0   Nail entering through skin

X● W45.8   Other foreign body or object entering through skin

> Splinter in skin NOS

● W46   Contact with hypodermic needle

The appropriate 7th character is to be added to each code from category W46

> A   initial encounter
> D   subsequent encounter
> S   sequela

X● W46.0   Contact with hypodermic needle

> Hypodermic needle stick NOS

X● W46.1   Contact with contaminated hypodermic needle

● W49   Exposure to other inanimate mechanical forces

> **Includes**   exposure to abnormal gravitational [G] forces
> exposure to inanimate mechanical forces NEC

> **Excludes1**   exposure to inanimate mechanical forces involving military or war operations (Y36.-, Y37.-)

The appropriate 7th character is to be added to each code from category W49

> A   initial encounter
> D   subsequent encounter
> S   sequela

● W49.0   Item causing external constriction

X● W49.01   Hair causing external constriction

X● W49.02   String or thread causing external constriction

X● W49.03   Rubber band causing external constriction

X● W49.04   Ring or other jewelry causing external constriction

X● W49.09   Other item causing external constriction

X● W49.9   Exposure to other inanimate mechanical forces

EXPOSURE TO ANIMATE MECHANICAL FORCES (W50-W64)

> **Excludes1**   toxic effect of contact with venomous animals and plants (T63.-)

● W50   Accidental hit, strike, kick, twist, bite or scratch by another person

> **Includes**   hit, strike, kick, twist, bite, or scratch by another person NOS

> **Excludes1**   assault by bodily force (Y04)
> struck by objects (W20-W22)

The appropriate 7th character is to be added to each code from category W50

> A   initial encounter
> D   subsequent encounter
> S   sequela

X● W50.0   Accidental hit or strike by another person

> Hit or strike by another person NOS

X● W50.1   Accidental kick by another person

> Kick by another person NOS

X● W50.2   Accidental twist by another person

> Twist by another person NOS
> **Coding Clinic: 2015, Q1, P8**

X● W50.3   Accidental bite by another person

> Human bite
> Bite by another person NOS

X● W50.4   Accidental scratch by another person

> Scratch by another person NOS

CHAPTER 20 (V00-Y99)

X● **W51 Accidental striking against or bumped into by another person**

> **Excludes1**   assault by striking against or bumping into by another person (Y04.2)
> fall due to collision with another person (W03)

The appropriate 7th character is to be added to code W51

A	initial encounter
D	subsequent encounter
S	sequela

X● **W52 Crushed, pushed or stepped on by crowd or human stampede**
> Crushed, pushed or stepped on by crowd or human stampede with or without fall

The appropriate 7th character is to be added to code W52

A	initial encounter
D	subsequent encounter
S	sequela

● **W53 Contact with rodent**

> **Includes**   contact with saliva, feces or urine of rodent

The appropriate 7th character is to be added to each code from category W53

A	initial encounter
D	subsequent encounter
S	sequela

● **W53.0 Contact with mouse**
    X● **W53.01   Bitten by mouse**
    X● **W53.09   Other contact with mouse**
● **W53.1 Contact with rat**
    X● **W53.11   Bitten by rat**
    X● **W53.19   Other contact with rat**
● **W53.2 Contact with squirrel**
    X● **W53.21   Bitten by squirrel**
    X● **W53.29   Other contact with squirrel**
● **W53.8 Contact with other rodent**
    X● **W53.81   Bitten by other rodent**
    X● **W53.89   Other contact with other rodent**

● **W54 Contact with dog**

> **Includes**   contact with saliva, feces or urine of dog

The appropriate 7th character is to be added to each code from category W54

A	initial encounter
D	subsequent encounter
S	sequela

X● **W54.0   Bitten by dog**
X● **W54.1   Struck by dog**
> Knocked over by dog
X● **W54.8   Other contact with dog**

● **W55 Contact with other mammals**

> **Includes**   contact with saliva, feces or urine of mammal
> **Excludes1**   animal being ridden - see transport accidents
> bitten or struck by dog (W54)
> bitten or struck by rodent (W53.-)
> contact with marine mammals (W56.X-)

The appropriate 7th character is to be added to each code from category W55

A	initial encounter
D	subsequent encounter
S	sequela

● **W55.0   Contact with cat**
    X● **W55.01   Bitten by cat**
    X● **W55.03   Scratched by cat**
    X● **W55.09   Other contact with cat**

● **W55.1   Contact with horse**
    X● **W55.11   Bitten by horse**
    X● **W55.12   Struck by horse**
    X● **W55.19   Other contact with horse**
● **W55.2   Contact with cow**
> Contact with bull
    X● **W55.21   Bitten by cow**
    X● **W55.22   Struck by cow**
> Gored by bull
    X● **W55.29   Other contact with cow**
● **W55.3   Contact with other hoof stock**
> Contact with goats
> Contact with sheep
    X● **W55.31   Bitten by other hoof stock**
    X● **W55.32   Struck by other hoof stock**
> Gored by goat
> Gored by ram
    X● **W55.39   Other contact with other hoof stock**
● **W55.4   Contact with pig**
    X● **W55.41   Bitten by pig**
    X● **W55.42   Struck by pig**
    X● **W55.49   Other contact with pig**
● **W55.5   Contact with raccoon**
    X● **W55.51   Bitten by raccoon**
    X● **W55.52   Struck by raccoon**
    X● **W55.59   Other contact with raccoon**
● **W55.8   Contact with other mammals**
    X● **W55.81   Bitten by other mammals**
    X● **W55.82   Struck by other mammals**
    X● **W55.89   Other contact with other mammals**

● **W56 Contact with nonvenomous marine animal**

> **Excludes1**   contact with venomous marine animal (T63.-)

The appropriate 7th character is to be added to each code from category W56

A	initial encounter
D	subsequent encounter
S	sequela

● **W56.0   Contact with dolphin**
    X● **W56.01   Bitten by dolphin**
    X● **W56.02   Struck by dolphin**
    X● **W56.09   Other contact with dolphin**
● **W56.1   Contact with sea lion**
    X● **W56.11   Bitten by sea lion**
    X● **W56.12   Struck by sea lion**
    X● **W56.19   Other contact with sea lion**
● **W56.2   Contact with orca**
> Contact with killer whale
    X● **W56.21   Bitten by orca**
    X● **W56.22   Struck by orca**
    X● **W56.29   Other contact with orca**
● **W56.3   Contact with other marine mammals**
    X● **W56.31   Bitten by other marine mammals**
    X● **W56.32   Struck by other marine mammals**
    X● **W56.39   Other contact with other marine mammals**
● **W56.4   Contact with shark**
    X● **W56.41   Bitten by shark**
    X● **W56.42   Struck by shark**
    X● **W56.49   Other contact with shark**
● **W56.5   Contact with other fish**
    X● **W56.51   Bitten by other fish**
    X● **W56.52   Struck by other fish**
    X● **W56.59   Other contact with other fish**

▶ New   ⟹ Revised   ~~deleted~~ Deleted   Excludes 1   Excludes 2   Includes   Use additional   Code first   Code also   Key words

OGCR Official Guidelines   X Assign placeholder X   ● Use Additional Character(s)   ▶ Manifestation Code   ⬧ Hierarchical Condition Category   Coding Clinic

● W56.8   Contact with other nonvenomous marine animals

   X● W56.81   Bitten by other nonvenomous marine animals

   X● W56.82   Struck by other nonvenomous marine animals

   X● W56.89   Other contact with other nonvenomous marine animals

X● W57   Bitten or stung by nonvenomous insect and other nonvenomous arthropods

   Excludes1   contact with venomous insects and arthropods (T63.2-, T63.3-, T63.4-)

   The appropriate 7th character is to be added to code W57

A	initial encounter
D	subsequent encounter
S	sequela

● W58   Contact with crocodile or alligator

   The appropriate 7th character is to be added to each code from category W58

A	initial encounter
D	subsequent encounter
S	sequela

 ● W58.0   Contact with alligator

   X● W58.01   Bitten by alligator

   X● W58.02   Struck by alligator

   X● W58.03   Crushed by alligator

   X● W58.09   Other contact with alligator

 ● W58.1   Contact with crocodile

   X● W58.11   Bitten by crocodile

   X● W58.12   Struck by crocodile

   X● W58.13   Crushed by crocodile

   X● W58.19   Other contact with crocodile

● W59   Contact with other nonvenomous reptiles

   Excludes1   contact with venomous reptile (T63.0-, T63.1-)

   The appropriate 7th character is to be added to each code from category W59

A	initial encounter
D	subsequent encounter
S	sequela

 ● W59.0   Contact with nonvenomous lizards

   X● W59.01   Bitten by nonvenomous lizards

   X● W59.02   Struck by nonvenomous lizards

   X● W59.09   Other contact with nonvenomous lizards
      Exposure to nonvenomous lizards

 ● W59.1   Contact with nonvenomous snakes

   X● W59.11   Bitten by nonvenomous snake

   X● W59.12   Struck by nonvenomous snake

   X● W59.13   Crushed by nonvenomous snake

   X● W59.19   Other contact with nonvenomous snake

 ● W59.2   Contact with turtles

   Excludes1   contact with tortoises (W59.8-)

   X● W59.21   Bitten by turtle

   X● W59.22   Struck by turtle

   X● W59.29   Other contact with turtle
      Exposure to turtles

 ● W59.8   Contact with other nonvenomous reptiles

   X● W59.81   Bitten by other nonvenomous reptiles

   X● W59.82   Struck by other nonvenomous reptiles

   X● W59.83   Crushed by other nonvenomous reptiles

   X● W59.89   Other contact with other nonvenomous reptiles

X● W60   Contact with nonvenomous plant thorns and spines and sharp leaves

   Excludes1   contact with venomous plants (T63.X7-)

   The appropriate 7th character is to be added to code W60

A	initial encounter
D	subsequent encounter
S	sequela

● W61   Contact with birds (domestic) (wild)

   Includes   contact with excreta of birds

   The appropriate 7th character is to be added to each code from category W61

A	initial encounter
D	subsequent encounter
S	sequela

 ● W61.0   Contact with parrot

   X● W61.01   Bitten by parrot

   X● W61.02   Struck by parrot

   X● W61.09   Other contact with parrot
      Exposure to parrots

 ● W61.1   Contact with macaw

   X● W61.11   Bitten by macaw

   X● W61.12   Struck by macaw

   X● W61.19   Other contact with macaw
      Exposure to macaws

 ● W61.2   Contact with other psittacines

   X● W61.21   Bitten by other psittacines

   X● W61.22   Struck by other psittacines

   X● W61.29   Other contact with other psittacines
      Exposure to other psittacines

 ● W61.3   Contact with chicken

   X● W61.32   Struck by chicken

   X● W61.33   Pecked by chicken

   X● W61.39   Other contact with chicken
      Exposure to chickens

 ● W61.4   Contact with turkey

   X● W61.42   Struck by turkey

   X● W61.43   Pecked by turkey

   X● W61.49   Other contact with turkey

 ● W61.5   Contact with goose

   X● W61.51   Bitten by goose

   X● W61.52   Struck by goose

   X● W61.59   Other contact with goose

 ● W61.6   Contact with duck

   X● W61.61   Bitten by duck

   X● W61.62   Struck by duck

   X● W61.69   Other contact with duck

 ● W61.9   Contact with other birds

   X● W61.91   Bitten by other birds

   X● W61.92   Struck by other birds

   X● W61.99   Other contact with other birds
      Contact with bird NOS

● W62   Contact with nonvenomous amphibians

   Excludes1   contact with venomous amphibians (T63.81-T63.83)

   The appropriate 7th character is to be added to each code from category W62

A	initial encounter
D	subsequent encounter
S	sequela

   X● W62.0   Contact with nonvenomous frogs

   X● W62.1   Contact with nonvenomous toads

   X● W62.9   Contact with other nonvenomous amphibians

X●W64 **Exposure to other animate mechanical forces**

> **Includes**   exposure to nonvenomous animal NOS
> **Excludes1**   contact with venomous animal (T63.-)

The appropriate 7th character is to be added to code W64

> A   initial encounter
> D   subsequent encounter
> S   sequela

ACCIDENTAL NON-TRANSPORT DROWNING AND SUBMERSION (W65-W74)

> **Excludes1**   accidental drowning and submersion due to fall into water (W16.-)
> accidental drowning and submersion due to water transport accident (V90.-, V92.-)
> **Excludes2**   accidental drowning and submersion due to cataclysm (X34-X39)

X●W65 **Accidental drowning and submersion while in bathtub**

> **Excludes1**   accidental drowning and submersion due to fall in (into) bathtub (W16.211)

The appropriate 7th character is to be added to code W65

> A   initial encounter
> D   subsequent encounter
> S   sequela

X●W67 **Accidental drowning and submersion while in swimming pool**

> **Excludes1**   accidental drowning and submersion due to fall into swimming pool (W16.011, W16.021, W16.031)
> accidental drowning and submersion due to striking into wall of swimming pool (W22.041)

Coding Clinic: 2023, Q1, P26

The appropriate 7th character is to be added to code W67

> A   initial encounter
> D   subsequent encounter
> S   sequela

X●W69 **Accidental drowning and submersion while in natural water**
Accidental drowning and submersion while in lake
Accidental drowning and submersion while in open sea
Accidental drowning and submersion while in river
Accidental drowning and submersion while in stream

> **Excludes1**   accidental drowning and submersion due to fall into natural body of water (W16.111, W16.121, W16.131)

The appropriate 7th character is to be added to code W69

> A   initial encounter
> D   subsequent encounter
> S   sequela

X●W73 **Other specified cause of accidental non-transport drowning and submersion**
Accidental drowning and submersion while in quenching tank
Accidental drowning and submersion while in reservoir

> **Excludes1**   accidental drowning and submersion due to fall into other water (W16.311, W16.321, W16.331)

The appropriate 7th character is to be added to code W73

> A   initial encounter
> D   subsequent encounter
> S   sequela

X●W74 **Unspecified cause of accidental drowning and submersion**
Drowning NOS

The appropriate 7th character is to be added to code W74

> A   initial encounter
> D   subsequent encounter
> S   sequela

EXPOSURE TO ELECTRIC CURRENT, RADIATION AND EXTREME AMBIENT AIR TEMPERATURE AND PRESSURE (W85-W99)

> **Excludes1**   exposure to:
> failure in dosage of radiation or temperature during surgical and medical care (Y63.2-Y63.5)
> lightning (T75.0-)
> natural cold (X31)
> natural heat (X30)
> natural radiation NOS (X39)
> radiological procedure and radiotherapy (Y84.2)
> sunlight (X32)

X●W85 **Exposure to electric transmission lines**
Broken power line

The appropriate 7th character is to be added to code W85

> A   initial encounter
> D   subsequent encounter
> S   sequela

●W86 **Exposure to other specified electric current**

The appropriate 7th character is to be added to each code from category W86

> A   initial encounter
> D   subsequent encounter
> S   sequela

X●W86.0 **Exposure to domestic wiring and appliances**
X●W86.1 **Exposure to industrial wiring, appliances and electrical machinery**
Exposure to conductors
Exposure to control apparatus
Exposure to electrical equipment and machinery
Exposure to transformers
X●W86.8 **Exposure to other electric current**
Exposure to wiring and appliances in or on farm (not farmhouse)
Exposure to wiring and appliances outdoors
Exposure to wiring and appliances in or on public building
Exposure to wiring and appliances in or on residential institutions
Exposure to wiring and appliances in or on schools

●W88 **Exposure to ionizing radiation**

> **Excludes1**   exposure to sunlight (X32)

The appropriate 7th character is to be added to each code from category W88

> A   initial encounter
> D   subsequent encounter
> S   sequela

X●W88.0 **Exposure to X-rays**
X●W88.1 **Exposure to radioactive isotopes**
X●W88.8 **Exposure to other ionizing radiation**

●W89 **Exposure to man-made visible and ultraviolet light**

> **Includes**   exposure to welding light (arc)
> **Excludes2**   exposure to sunlight (X32)

The appropriate 7th character is to be added to each code from category W89

> A   initial encounter
> D   subsequent encounter
> S   sequela

X●W89.0 **Exposure to welding light (arc)**
X●W89.1 **Exposure to tanning bed**
X●W89.8 **Exposure to other man-made visible and ultraviolet light**
X●W89.9 **Exposure to unspecified man-made visible and ultraviolet light**

▶ New   ⇒ Revised   ~~deleted~~ Deleted   Excludes 1   Excludes 2   Includes   Use additional   Code first   Code also   Key words
OGCR Official Guidelines   X Assign placeholder X   ● Use Additional Character(s)   ▶ Manifestation Code   🔖 Hierarchical Condition Category   Coding Clinic

● W90   **Exposure to other nonionizing radiation**

> **Excludes2**   exposure to sunlight (X32)
>
> The appropriate 7th character is to be added to each code from category W90

A	initial encounter
D	subsequent encounter
S	sequela

X ● W90.0   **Exposure to radiofrequency**
X ● W90.1   **Exposure to infrared radiation**
X ● W90.2   **Exposure to laser radiation**
X ● W90.8   **Exposure to other nonionizing radiation**

X ● W92   **Exposure to excessive heat of man-made origin**

> The appropriate 7th character is to be added to code W92

A	initial encounter
D	subsequent encounter
S	sequela

● W93   **Exposure to excessive cold of man-made origin**

> The appropriate 7th character is to be added to each code from category W93

A	initial encounter
D	subsequent encounter
S	sequela

   ● W93.0   **Contact with or inhalation of dry ice**
     X ● W93.01   **Contact with dry ice**
     X ● W93.02   **Inhalation of dry ice**
   ● W93.1   **Contact with or inhalation of liquid air**
     X ● W93.11   **Contact with liquid air**
         Contact with liquid hydrogen
         Contact with liquid nitrogen
     X ● W93.12   **Inhalation of liquid air**
         Inhalation of liquid hydrogen
         Inhalation of liquid nitrogen
   X ● W93.2   **Prolonged exposure in deep freeze unit or refrigerator**
   X ● W93.8   **Exposure to other excessive cold of man-made origin**

● W94   **Exposure to high and low air pressure and changes in air pressure**

> The appropriate 7th character is to be added to each code from category W94

A	initial encounter
D	subsequent encounter
S	sequela

X ● W94.0   **Exposure to prolonged high air pressure**
● W94.1   **Exposure to prolonged low air pressure**
   X ● W94.11   **Exposure to residence or prolonged visit at high altitude**
   X ● W94.12   **Exposure to other prolonged low air pressure**
● W94.2   **Exposure to rapid changes in air pressure during ascent**
   X ● W94.21   **Exposure to reduction in atmospheric pressure while surfacing from deep-water diving**
   X ● W94.22   **Exposure to reduction in atmospheric pressure while surfacing from underground**
   X ● W94.23   **Exposure to sudden change in air pressure in aircraft during ascent**
   X ● W94.29   **Exposure to other rapid changes in air pressure during ascent**
● W94.3   **Exposure to rapid changes in air pressure during descent**
   X ● W94.31   **Exposure to sudden change in air pressure in aircraft during descent**
   X ● W94.32   **Exposure to high air pressure from rapid descent in water**
   X ● W94.39   **Exposure to other rapid changes in air pressure during descent**

X ● W99   **Exposure to other man-made environmental factors**

> The appropriate 7th character is to be added to code W99

A	initial encounter
D	subsequent encounter
S	sequela

EXPOSURE TO SMOKE, FIRE AND FLAMES (X00-X08)

> **Excludes1**   arson (X97)
>
> **Excludes2**   explosions (W35-W40)
>   lightning (T75.0-)
>   transport accident (V01-V99)

● X00   **Exposure to uncontrolled fire in building or structure**

> **Includes**   conflagration in building or structure
>
> *Code first any associated cataclysm*
>
> **Excludes2**   exposure to ignition or melting of nightwear (X05)
>   exposure to ignition or melting of other clothing and apparel (X06.-)
>   exposure to other specified smoke, fire and flames (X08.-)
>
> The appropriate 7th character is to be added to each code from category X00

A	initial encounter
D	subsequent encounter
S	sequela

X ● X00.0   **Exposure to flames in uncontrolled fire in building or structure**
         Coding Clinic: 2016, Q2, P5-6; 2015, Q1, P19
X ● X00.1   **Exposure to smoke in uncontrolled fire in building or structure**
X ● X00.2   **Injury due to collapse of burning building or structure in uncontrolled fire**
> **Excludes1**   injury due to collapse of building not on fire (W20.1)
X ● X00.3   **Fall from burning building or structure in uncontrolled fire**
X ● X00.4   **Hit by object from burning building or structure in uncontrolled fire**
X ● X00.5   **Jump from burning building or structure in uncontrolled fire**
X ● X00.8   **Other exposure to uncontrolled fire in building or structure**

● X01   **Exposure to uncontrolled fire, not in building or structure**

> **Includes**   exposure to forest fire
>
> The appropriate 7th character is to be added to each code from category X01

A	initial encounter
D	subsequent encounter
S	sequela

X ● X01.0   **Exposure to flames in uncontrolled fire, not in building or structure**
X ● X01.1   **Exposure to smoke in uncontrolled fire, not in building or structure**
X ● X01.3   **Fall due to uncontrolled fire, not in building or structure**
X ● X01.4   **Hit by object due to uncontrolled fire, not in building or structure**
X ● X01.8   **Other exposure to uncontrolled fire, not in building or structure**

● X02   Exposure to controlled fire in building or structure

| **Includes** | exposure to fire in fireplace exposure to fire in stove |

The appropriate 7th character is to be added to each code from category X02

A	initial encounter
D	subsequent encounter
S	sequela

X● X02.0   Exposure to flames in controlled fire in building or structure

X● X02.1   Exposure to smoke in controlled fire in building or structure

X● X02.2   Injury due to collapse of burning building or structure in controlled fire

| **Excludes1** | injury due to collapse of building not on fire (W20.1) |

X● X02.3   Fall from burning building or structure in controlled fire

X● X02.4   Hit by object from burning building or structure in controlled fire

X● X02.5   Jump from burning building or structure in controlled fire

X● X02.8   Other exposure to controlled fire in building or structure

● X03   Exposure to controlled fire, not in building or structure

| **Includes** | exposure to bon fire exposure to camp fire exposure to trash fire |

The appropriate 7th character is to be added to each code from category X03

A	initial encounter
D	subsequent encounter
S	sequela

X● X03.0   Exposure to flames in controlled fire, not in building or structure
    Coding Clinic: 2015, Q1, P19

X● X03.1   Exposure to smoke in controlled fire, not in building or structure

X● X03.3   Fall due to controlled fire, not in building or structure

X● X03.4   Hit by object due to controlled fire, not in building or structure

X● X03.8   Other exposure to controlled fire, not in building or structure

X● X04   Exposure to ignition of highly flammable material
    Exposure to ignition of gasoline
    Exposure to ignition of kerosene
    Exposure to ignition of petrol

| **Excludes2** | exposure to ignition or melting of nightwear (X05) |
| | exposure to ignition or melting of other clothing and apparel (X06) |

The appropriate 7th character is to be added to code X04

A	initial encounter
D	subsequent encounter
S	sequela

Coding Clinic: 2016, Q2, P4

X● X05   Exposure to ignition or melting of nightwear

Excludes2	exposure to uncontrolled fire in building or structure (X00.-)
	exposure to uncontrolled fire, not in building or structure (X01.-)
	exposure to controlled fire in building or structure (X02.-)
	exposure to controlled fire, not in building or structure (X03.-)
	exposure to ignition of highly flammable materials (X04.-)

The appropriate 7th character is to be added to code X05

A	initial encounter
D	subsequent encounter
S	sequela

● X06   Exposure to ignition or melting of other clothing and apparel

Excludes2	exposure to uncontrolled fire in building or structure (X00.-)
	exposure to uncontrolled fire, not in building or structure (X01.-)
	exposure to controlled fire in building or structure (X02.-)
	exposure to controlled fire, not in building or structure (X03.-)
	exposure to ignition of highly flammable materials (X04.-)

The appropriate 7th character is to be added to each code from category X06

A	initial encounter
D	subsequent encounter
S	sequela

X● X06.0   Exposure to ignition of plastic jewelry

X● X06.1   Exposure to melting of plastic jewelry

X● X06.2   Exposure to ignition of other clothing and apparel

X● X06.3   Exposure to melting of other clothing and apparel

● X08   Exposure to other specified smoke, fire and flames

The appropriate 7th character is to be added to each code from category X08

A	initial encounter
D	subsequent encounter
S	sequela

● X08.0   Exposure to bed fire
    Exposure to mattress fire

X● X08.00   Exposure to bed fire due to unspecified burning material

X● X08.01   Exposure to bed fire due to burning cigarette
    Coding Clinic: 2015, Q1, P19

X● X08.09   Exposure to bed fire due to other burning material

● X08.1   Exposure to sofa fire

X● X08.10   Exposure to sofa fire due to unspecified burning material

X● X08.11   Exposure to sofa fire due to burning cigarette

X● X08.19   Exposure to sofa fire due to other burning material

● X08.2   Exposure to other furniture fire

X● X08.20   Exposure to other furniture fire due to unspecified burning material

X● X08.21   Exposure to other furniture fire due to burning cigarette

X● X08.29   Exposure to other furniture fire due to other burning material

X● X08.8   Exposure to other specified smoke, fire and flames

CHAPTER 20 (V00-Y99)

▶ New   ⇒ Revised   ~~deleted~~ Deleted   Excludes 1   Excludes 2   Includes   Use additional   Code first   Code also   Key words

OGCR Official Guidelines   X Assign placeholder X   ● Use Additional Character(s)   ▶ Manifestation Code   ❀ Hierarchical Condition Category   Coding Clinic

CONTACT WITH HEAT AND HOT SUBSTANCES (X10-X19)

Excludes1   exposure to excessive natural heat (X30)
exposure to fire and flames (X00-X08)

● **X10**   **Contact with hot drinks, food, fats and cooking oils**

The appropriate 7th character is to be added to each code from category X10

> A   initial encounter
> D   subsequent encounter
> S   sequela

X ● **X10.0**   **Contact with hot drinks**
X ● **X10.1**   **Contact with hot food**
X ● **X10.2**   **Contact with fats and cooking oils**

● **X11**   **Contact with hot tap-water**

Includes   contact with boiling tap-water
contact with boiling water NOS

Excludes1   contact with water heated on stove (X12)

The appropriate 7th character is to be added to each code from category X11

> A   initial encounter
> D   subsequent encounter
> S   sequela

X ● **X11.0**   **Contact with hot water in bath or tub**

Excludes1   contact with running hot water in bath or tub (X11.1)

X ● **X11.1**   **Contact with running hot water**
Contact with hot water running out of hose
Contact with hot water running out of tap

X ● **X11.8**   **Contact with other hot tap-water**
Contact with hot water in bucket
Contact with hot tap-water NOS

X ● **X12**   **Contact with other hot fluids**
Contact with water heated on stove

Excludes1   hot (liquid) metals (X18)

The appropriate 7th character is to be added to code X12

> A   initial encounter
> D   subsequent encounter
> S   sequela

● **X13**   **Contact with steam and other hot vapors**

The appropriate 7th character is to be added to each code from category X13

> A   initial encounter
> D   subsequent encounter
> S   sequela

X ● **X13.0**   **Inhalation of steam and other hot vapors**
X ● **X13.1**   **Other contact with steam and other hot vapors**

● **X14**   **Contact with hot air and other hot gases**

The appropriate 7th character is to be added to each code from category X14

> A   initial encounter
> D   subsequent encounter
> S   sequela

X ● **X14.0**   **Inhalation of hot air and gases**
X ● **X14.1**   **Other contact with hot air and other hot gases**

● **X15**   **Contact with hot household appliances**

Excludes1   contact with heating appliances (X16)
contact with powered household appliances (W29.-)
exposure to controlled fire in building or structure due to household appliance (X02.8)
exposure to household appliances electrical current (W86.0)

The appropriate 7th character is to be added to each code from category X15

> A   initial encounter
> D   subsequent encounter
> S   sequela

X ● **X15.0**   **Contact with hot stove (kitchen)**
X ● **X15.1**   **Contact with hot toaster**
X ● **X15.2**   **Contact with hotplate**
X ● **X15.3**   **Contact with hot saucepan or skillet**
Contact with hot cooking pan
Contact with hot cooking pot

X ● **X15.8**   **Contact with other hot household appliances**
Contact with cooker
Contact with kettle
Contact with light bulbs

X ● **X16**   **Contact with hot heating appliances, radiators and pipes**

Excludes1   contact with powered appliances (W29.-)
exposure to controlled fire in building or structure due to appliance (X02.8)
exposure to industrial appliances electrical current (W86.1)

The appropriate 7th character is to be added to code X16

> A   initial encounter
> D   subsequent encounter
> S   sequela

X ● **X17**   **Contact with hot engines, machinery and tools**

Excludes1   contact with hot heating appliances, radiators and pipes (X16)
contact with hot household appliances (X15)

The appropriate 7th character is to be added to code X17

> A   initial encounter
> D   subsequent encounter
> S   sequela

X ● **X18**   **Contact with other hot metals**
Contact with liquid metal

The appropriate 7th character is to be added to code X18

> A   initial encounter
> D   subsequent encounter
> S   sequela

X ● **X19**   **Contact with other heat and hot substances**

Excludes1   objects that are not normally hot, e.g., an object made hot by a house fire (X00-X08)

The appropriate 7th character is to be added to code X19

> A   initial encounter
> D   subsequent encounter
> S   sequela

EXPOSURE TO FORCES OF NATURE (X30-X39)

X ● **X30** **Exposure to excessive natural heat**
Exposure to excessive heat as the cause of sunstroke
Exposure to heat NOS

Excludes1 excessive heat of man-made origin (W92)
exposure to man-made radiation (W89)
exposure to sunlight (X32)
exposure to tanning bed (W89)

The appropriate 7th character is to be added to code X30

A	initial encounter
D	subsequent encounter
S	sequela

X ● **X31** **Exposure to excessive natural cold**
Excessive cold as the cause of chilblains NOS
Excessive cold as the cause of immersion foot or hand
Exposure to cold NOS
Exposure to weather conditions

Excludes1 cold of man-made origin (W93.-)
contact with or inhalation of dry ice (W93.-)
contact with or inhalation of liquefied gas (W93.-)

The appropriate 7th character is to be added to code X31

A	initial encounter
D	subsequent encounter
S	sequela

X ● **X32** **Exposure to sunlight**

Excludes1 man-made radiation (tanning bed) (W89)

Excludes2 radiation-related disorders of the skin and
subcutaneous tissue (L55-L59)

The appropriate 7th character is to be added to code X32

A	initial encounter
D	subsequent encounter
S	sequela

X ● **X34** **Earthquake**

Excludes2 tidal wave (tsunami) due to earthquake (X37.41)

The appropriate 7th character is to be added to code X34

A	initial encounter
D	subsequent encounter
S	sequela

X ● **X35** **Volcanic eruption**

Excludes2 tidal wave (tsunami) due to volcanic eruption
(X37.41)

The appropriate 7th character is to be added to code X35

A	initial encounter
D	subsequent encounter
S	sequela

● **X36** **Avalanche, landslide and other earth movements**

Includes victim of mudslide of cataclysmic nature

Excludes1 earthquake (X34)

Excludes2 transport accident involving collision with
avalanche or landslide not in motion
(V01-V99)

The appropriate 7th character is to be added to each code from
category X36

A	initial encounter
D	subsequent encounter
S	sequela

X ● **X36.0** **Collapse of dam or man-made structure causing earth
movement**

X ● **X36.1** **Avalanche, landslide, or mudslide**

● **X37** **Cataclysmic storm**
The appropriate 7th character is to be added to each code from
category X37

A	initial encounter
D	subsequent encounter
S	sequela

X ● **X37.0** **Hurricane**
Storm surge Typhoon

X ● **X37.1** **Tornado**
Cyclone Twister

X ● **X37.2** **Blizzard (snow) (ice)**

X ● **X37.3** **Dust storm**

● **X37.4** **Tidalwave**

X ● **X37.41** **Tidal wave due to earthquake or volcanic
eruption**
Tidal wave NOS
Tsunami

X ● **X37.42** **Tidal wave due to storm**

X ● **X37.43** **Tidal wave due to landslide**

X ● **X37.8** **Other cataclysmic storms**
Cloudburst
Torrential rain

Excludes2 flood (X38)

X ● **X37.9** **Unspecified cataclysmic storm**
Storm NOS

Excludes1 collapse of dam or man-made structure
causing earth movement (X36.0)

X ● **X38** **Flood**
Flood arising from remote storm
Flood of cataclysmic nature arising from melting snow
Flood resulting directly from storm

Excludes1 collapse of dam or man-made structure causing
earth movement (X36.0)
tidal wave NOS (X37.41)
tidal wave caused by storm (X37.42)

The appropriate 7th character is to be added to code X38

A	initial encounter
D	subsequent encounter
S	sequela

● **X39** **Exposure to other forces of nature**
The appropriate 7th character is to be added to each code from
category X39

A	initial encounter
D	subsequent encounter
S	sequela

● **X39.0** **Exposure to natural radiation**

Excludes1 contact with and (suspected) exposure to
radon and other naturally occurring
radiation (Z77.123)
exposure to man-made radiation
(W88-W90)
exposure to sunlight (X32)

X ● **X39.01** **Exposure to radon**

X ● **X39.08** **Exposure to other natural radiation**

X ● **X39.8** **Other exposure to forces of nature**

▶ New ⇒ Revised ~~deleted~~ Deleted Excludes 1 Excludes 2 Includes Use additional Code first Code also Key words

OGCR Official Guidelines X Assign placeholder X ● Use Additional Character(s) ▶ Manifestation Code 🗝 Hierarchical Condition Category **Coding Clinic**

OVEREXERTION AND STRENUOUS OR REPETITIVE MOVEMENTS (X50)

● **X50**   **Overexertion and strenuous or repetitive movements**

The appropriate 7th character is to be added to each code from category X50

> A   initial encounter
> D   subsequent encounter
> S   sequela

Coding Clinic: 2016, Q4, P73-74

X● **X50.0**   **Overexertion from strenuous movement or load**
Lifting heavy objects
Lifting weights
Coding Clinic: 2016, Q4, P74

X● **X50.1**   **Overexertion from prolonged static or awkward postures**
Prolonged bending
Prolonged kneeling
Prolonged reaching
Prolonged sitting
Prolonged standing
Prolonged twisting
Static bending
Static kneeling
Static reaching
Static sitting
Static standing
Static twisting

X● **X50.3**   **Overexertion from repetitive movements**
Use of hand as hammer

> **Excludes2**   Overuse from prolonged static or awkward postures (X50.1)

Coding Clinic: 2016, Q4, P74

X● **X50.9**   **Other and unspecified overexertion or strenuous movements or postures**
Contact pressure
Contact stress

ACCIDENTAL EXPOSURE TO OTHER SPECIFIED FACTORS (X52, X58)

X● **X52**   **Prolonged stay in weightless environment**
Weightlessness in spacecraft (simulator)

The appropriate 7th character is to be added to code X52

> A   initial encounter
> D   subsequent encounter
> S   sequela

X● **X58**   **Exposure to other specified factors**
Accident NOS
Exposure NOS

The appropriate 7th character is to be added to code X58

> A   initial encounter
> D   subsequent encounter
> S   sequela

INTENTIONAL SELF-HARM (X71-X83)

Purposely self-inflicted injury
Suicide (attempted)

● **X71**   **Intentional self-harm by drowning and submersion**

The appropriate 7th character is to be added to each code from category X71

> A   initial encounter
> D   subsequent encounter
> S   sequela

X● **X71.0**   **Intentional self-harm by drowning and submersion while in bathtub** A, D, S 🔾

X● **X71.1**   **Intentional self-harm by drowning and submersion while in swimming pool** A, D, S 🔾

X● **X71.2**   **Intentional self-harm by drowning and submersion after jump into swimming pool** A, D, S 🔾

X● **X71.3**   **Intentional self-harm by drowning and submersion in natural water** A, D, S 🔾

X● **X71.8**   **Other intentional self-harm by drowning and submersion** A, D, S 🔾

X● **X71.9**   **Intentional self-harm by drowning and submersion, unspecified** A, D, S 🔾

X●**X72**   **Intentional self-harm by handgun discharge** A, D, S 🔾
Intentional self-harm by gun for single hand use
Intentional self-harm by pistol
Intentional self-harm by revolver

> **Excludes1**   Very pistol (X74.8)

The appropriate 7th character is to be added to code X72

> A   initial encounter
> D   subsequent encounter
> S   sequela

● **X73**   **Intentional self-harm by rifle, shotgun and larger firearm discharge**

> **Excludes1**   airgun (X74.01)

The appropriate 7th character is to be added to each code from category X73

> A   initial encounter
> D   subsequent encounter
> S   sequela

X● **X73.0**   **Intentional self-harm by shotgun discharge** A, D, S 🔾

X● **X73.1**   **Intentional self-harm by hunting rifle discharge** A, D, S 🔾

X● **X73.2**   **Intentional self-harm by machine gun discharge** A, D, S 🔾

X● **X73.8**   **Intentional self-harm by other larger firearm discharge** A, D, S 🔾

X● **X73.9**   **Intentional self-harm by unspecified larger firearm discharge** A, D, S 🔾

● **X74**   **Intentional self-harm by other and unspecified firearm and gun discharge**

The appropriate 7th character is to be added to each code from category X74

> A   initial encounter
> D   subsequent encounter
> S   sequela

● **X74.0**   **Intentional self-harm by gas, air or spring-operated guns**

X● **X74.01**   **Intentional self-harm by airgun** A, D, S 🔾
Intentional self-harm by BB gun discharge
Intentional self-harm by pellet gun discharge

X● **X74.02**   **Intentional self-harm by paintball gun** A, D, S 🔾

X● **X74.09**   **Intentional self-harm by other gas, air or spring-operated gun** A, D, S 🔾

X● **X74.8**   **Intentional self-harm by other firearm discharge** A, D, S 🔾
Intentional self-harm by Very pistol [flare] discharge

X● **X74.9**   **Intentional self-harm by unspecified firearm discharge** A, D, S 🔾

X●**X75**   **Intentional self-harm by explosive material** A, D, S 🔾

The appropriate 7th character is to be added to code X75

> A   initial encounter
> D   subsequent encounter
> S   sequela

X●**X76**   **Intentional self-harm by smoke, fire and flames** A, D, S 🔾

The appropriate 7th character is to be added to code X76

> A   initial encounter
> D   subsequent encounter
> S   sequela

CHAPTER 20 (V00-Y99)

● X77   **Intentional self-harm by steam, hot vapors and hot objects**

The appropriate 7th character is to be added to each code from category X77

A	initial encounter
D	subsequent encounter
S	sequela

X ● X77.0   **Intentional self-harm by steam or hot vapors** A, D, S 🐾

X ● X77.1   **Intentional self-harm by hot tap water** A, D, S 🐾

X ● X77.2   **Intentional self-harm by other hot fluids** A, D, S 🐾

X ● X77.3   **Intentional self-harm by hot household appliances** A, D, S 🐾

X ● X77.8   **Intentional self-harm by other hot objects** A, D, S 🐾

X ● X77.9   **Intentional self-harm by unspecified hot objects** A, D, S 🐾

● X78   **Intentional self-harm by sharp object**

The appropriate 7th character is to be added to each code from category X78

A	initial encounter
D	subsequent encounter
S	sequela

X ● X78.0   **Intentional self-harm by sharp glass** A, D, S 🐾

X ● X78.1   **Intentional self-harm by knife** A, D, S 🐾

X ● X78.2   **Intentional self-harm by sword or dagger** A, D, S 🐾

X ● X78.8   **Intentional self-harm by other sharp object** A, D, S 🐾
     Coding Clinic: 2022, Q1, P27

X ● X78.9   **Intentional self-harm by unspecified sharp object** A, D, S 🐾

X ● X79   **Intentional self-harm by blunt object** A, D, S 🐾

The appropriate 7th character is to be added to code X79

A	initial encounter
D	subsequent encounter
S	sequela

X ● X80   **Intentional self-harm by jumping from a high place** A, D, S 🐾
Intentional fall from one level to another

The appropriate 7th character is to be added to code X80

A	initial encounter
D	subsequent encounter
S	sequela

● X81   **Intentional self-harm by jumping or lying in front of moving object**

The appropriate 7th character is to be added to each code from category X81

A	initial encounter
D	subsequent encounter
S	sequela

X ● X81.0   **Intentional self-harm by jumping or lying in front of motor vehicle** A, D, S 🐾

X ● X81.1   **Intentional self-harm by jumping or lying in front of (subway) train** A, D, S 🐾

X ● X81.8   **Intentional self-harm by jumping or lying in front of other moving object** A, D, S 🐾

● X82   **Intentional self-harm by crashing of motor vehicle**

The appropriate 7th character is to be added to each code from category X82

A	initial encounter
D	subsequent encounter
S	sequela

X ● X82.0   **Intentional collision of motor vehicle with other motor vehicle** A, D, S 🐾

X ● X82.1   **Intentional collision of motor vehicle with train** A, D, S 🐾

X ● X82.2   **Intentional collision of motor vehicle with tree** A, D, S 🐾

X ● X82.8   **Other intentional self-harm by crashing of motor vehicle** A, D, S 🐾

● X83   **Intentional self-harm by other specified means**

> **Excludes1**   intentional self-harm by poisoning or contact with toxic substance - see Table of Drugs and Chemicals

The appropriate 7th character is to be added to each code from category X83

A	initial encounter
D	subsequent encounter
S	sequela

X ● X83.0   **Intentional self-harm by crashing of aircraft** A, D, S 🐾

X ● X83.1   **Intentional self-harm by electrocution** A, D, S 🐾

X ● X83.2   **Intentional self-harm by exposure to extremes of cold** A, D, S 🐾

X ● X83.8   **Intentional self-harm by other specified means** A, D, S 🐾

ASSAULT (X92-Y09)

> **Includes**   homicide injuries inflicted by another person with intent to injure or kill, by any means

> **Excludes1**   injuries due to legal intervention (Y35.-)
> injuries due to operations of war (Y36.-)
> injuries due to terrorism (Y38.-)

● X92   **Assault by drowning and submersion**

The appropriate 7th character is to be added to each code from category X92

A	initial encounter
D	subsequent encounter
S	sequela

X ● X92.0   **Assault by drowning and submersion while in bathtub**

X ● X92.1   **Assault by drowning and submersion while in swimming pool**

X ● X92.2   **Assault by drowning and submersion after push into swimming pool**

X ● X92.3   **Assault by drowning and submersion in natural water**

X ● X92.8   **Other assault by drowning and submersion**

X ● X92.9   **Assault by drowning and submersion, unspecified**

X ● X93   **Assault by handgun discharge**
Assault by discharge of gun for single hand use
Assault by discharge of pistol
Assault by discharge of revolver

> **Excludes1**   Very pistol (X95.8)

The appropriate 7th character is to be added to code X93

A	initial encounter
D	subsequent encounter
S	sequela

● X94   **Assault by rifle, shotgun and larger firearm discharge**

> **Excludes1**   airgun (X95.01)

The appropriate 7th character is to be added to each code from category X94

A	initial encounter
D	subsequent encounter
S	sequela

X ● X94.0   **Assault by shotgun**

X ● X94.1   **Assault by hunting rifle**

X ● X94.2   **Assault by machine gun**

X ● X94.8   **Assault by other larger firearm discharge**

X ● X94.9   **Assault by unspecified larger firearm discharge**

▶ New   ⇒ Revised   ~~deleted~~ Deleted   Excludes 1   Excludes 2   Includes   Use additional   Code first   Code also   Key words

1486   OGCR Official Guidelines   X Assign placeholder X   ● Use Additional Character(s)   ⟩ Manifestation Code   🐾 Hierarchical Condition Category   Coding Clinic

● **X95**   **Assault by other and unspecified firearm and gun discharge**

> The appropriate 7th character is to be added to each code from category X95

A	initial encounter
D	subsequent encounter
S	sequela

     ● **X95.0**   **Assault by gas, air or spring-operated guns**

       X ● **X95.01**   **Assault by airgun discharge**
         Assault by BB gun discharge
         Assault by pellet gun discharge

       X ● **X95.02**   **Assault by paintball gun discharge**

       X ● **X95.09**   **Assault by other gas, air or spring-operated gun**

     X ● **X95.8**   **Assault by other firearm discharge**
       Assault by very pistol [flare] discharge

     X ● **X95.9**   **Assault by unspecified firearm discharge**
       Coding Clinic: 2023, Q3, P8,12; 2016, Q3, P24

● **X96**   **Assault by explosive material**

> **Excludes1**   incendiary device (X97)
>   terrorism involving explosive material (Y38.2-)

> The appropriate 7th character is to be added to each code from category X96

A	initial encounter
D	subsequent encounter
S	sequela

     X ● **X96.0**   **Assault by antipersonnel bomb**

> **Excludes1**   antipersonnel bomb use in military or war (Y36.2-)

     X ● **X96.1**   **Assault by gasoline bomb**
     X ● **X96.2**   **Assault by letter bomb**
     X ● **X96.3**   **Assault by fertilizer bomb**
     X ● **X96.4**   **Assault by pipe bomb**
     X ● **X96.8**   **Assault by other specified explosive**
     X ● **X96.9**   **Assault by unspecified explosive**

X ● **X97**   **Assault by smoke, fire and flames**
     Assault by arson
     Assault by cigarettes
     Assault by incendiary device

> The appropriate 7th character is to be added to code X97

A	initial encounter
D	subsequent encounter
S	sequela

● **X98**   **Assault by steam, hot vapors and hot objects**

> The appropriate 7th character is to be added to each code from category X98

A	initial encounter
D	subsequent encounter
S	sequela

     X ● **X98.0**   **Assault by steam or hot vapors**
     X ● **X98.1**   **Assault by hot tap water**
     X ● **X98.2**   **Assault by hot fluids**
     X ● **X98.3**   **Assault by hot household appliances**
     X ● **X98.8**   **Assault by other hot objects**
     X ● **X98.9**   **Assault by unspecified hot objects**

● **X99**   **Assault by sharp object**

> **Excludes1**   assault by strike by sports equipment (Y08.0-)

> The appropriate 7th character is to be added to each code from category X99

A	initial encounter
D	subsequent encounter
S	sequela

     X ● **X99.0**   **Assault by sharp glass**
     X ● **X99.1**   **Assault by knife**
     X ● **X99.2**   **Assault by sword or dagger**
     X ● **X99.8**   **Assault by other sharp object**
     X ● **X99.9**   **Assault by unspecified sharp object**
       Assault by stabbing NOS

X ● **Y00**   **Assault by blunt object**

> **Excludes1**   assault by strike by sports equipment (Y08.0)

> The appropriate 7th character is to be added to code Y00

A	initial encounter
D	subsequent encounter
S	sequela

X ● **Y01**   **Assault by pushing from high place**

> The appropriate 7th character is to be added to code Y01

A	initial encounter
D	subsequent encounter
S	sequela

● **Y02**   **Assault by pushing or placing victim in front of moving object**

> The appropriate 7th character is to be added to each code from category Y02

A	initial encounter
D	subsequent encounter
S	sequela

     X ● **Y02.0**   **Assault by pushing or placing victim in front of motor vehicle**
     X ● **Y02.1**   **Assault by pushing or placing victim in front of (subway) train**
     X ● **Y02.8**   **Assault by pushing or placing victim in front of other moving object**

● **Y03**   **Assault by crashing of motor vehicle**

> The appropriate 7th character is to be added to each code from category Y03

A	initial encounter
D	subsequent encounter
S	sequela

     X ● **Y03.0**   **Assault by being hit or run over by motor vehicle**
     X ● **Y03.8**   **Other assault by crashing of motor vehicle**

● **Y04**   **Assault by bodily force**

> **Excludes1**   assault by:
>   submersion (X92.-)
>   use of weapon (X93-X95, X99, Y00)

> The appropriate 7th character is to be added to each code from category Y04

A	initial encounter
D	subsequent encounter
S	sequela

     X ● **Y04.0**   **Assault by unarmed brawl or fight**
     X ● **Y04.1**   **Assault by human bite**
     X ● **Y04.2**   **Assault by strike against or bumped into by another person**
     X ● **Y04.8**   **Assault by other bodily force**
       Assault by bodily force NOS

CHAPTER 20 (V00-Y99)

OGCR Section I.C.19.f.

Adult and child abuse, neglect and other maltreatment

Sequence first the appropriate code from categories T74 or T76 for abuse, neglect and other maltreatment, followed by any accompanying mental health or injury code(s).

If the documentation in the medical record states abuse or neglect it is coded as confirmed (T74.-). It is coded as suspected if it is documented as suspected (T76.-).

For cases of confirmed abuse or neglect an external cause code from the assault section (X92-Y09) should be added to identify the cause of any physical injuries. A perpetrator code (Y07) should be added when the perpetrator of the abuse is known. For suspected cases of abuse or neglect, do not report external cause or perpetrator code.

If a suspected case of abuse, neglect or mistreatment is ruled out during an encounter code Z04.71, Encounter for examination and observation following alleged physical adult abuse, ruled out, or code Z04.72, Encounter for examination and observation following alleged adult rape, should be used, not a code from T76.

If a suspected case of alleged rape or sexual abuse is ruled out during an encounter code Z04.41, Encounter for examination and observation following alleged adult rape or code Z04.42, Encounter for examination and observation following alleged child rape should be used, not a code from T76.

CHAPTER 20 (V00-Y99)

● **Y07 Perpetrator of assault, maltreatment and neglect**

Note: Codes from this category are for use only in cases of confirmed abuse (T74.-)

Selection of the correct perpetrator code is based on the relationship between the perpetrator and the victim

Includes perpetrator of abandonment
perpetrator of emotional neglect
perpetrator of mental cruelty
perpetrator of physical abuse
perpetrator of physical neglect
perpetrator of sexual abuse
perpetrator of torture

Coding Clinic: 2016, Q4, P129

● **Y07.0 Spouse or partner, perpetrator of maltreatment and neglect**
Spouse or partner, perpetrator of maltreatment and neglect against spouse or partner

● **Y07.01 Husband, perpetrator of maltreatment and neglect**

Y07.010 Husband, current, perpetrator of maltreatment and neglect

Y07.011 Husband, former, perpetrator of maltreatment and neglect

● **Y07.02 Wife, perpetrator of maltreatment and neglect**

Y07.020 Wife, current, perpetrator of maltreatment and neglect

Y07.021 Wife, former, perpetrator of maltreatment and neglect

● **Y07.03 Male partner, perpetrator of maltreatment and neglect**
Male intimate or dating partner, perpetrator of maltreatment and neglect

Y07.030 Male partner, current, perpetrator of maltreatment and neglect

Y07.031 Male partner, former, perpetrator of maltreatment and neglect

● **Y07.04 Female partner, perpetrator of maltreatment and neglect**
Female intimate or dating partner, perpetrator of maltreatment and neglect

Y07.040 Female partner, current, perpetrator of maltreatment and neglect

Y07.041 Female partner, former, perpetrator of maltreatment and neglect

● **Y07.05 Non-binary partner, perpetrator of maltreatment and neglect**
Gender non-conforming partner, perpetrator of maltreatment and neglect

Y07.050 Non-binary partner, current, perpetrator of maltreatment and neglect

Y07.051 Non-binary partner, former, perpetrator of maltreatment and neglect

● **Y07.1 Parent (adoptive) (biological), perpetrator of maltreatment and neglect**

Y07.11 Biological father, perpetrator of maltreatment and neglect

Y07.12 Biological mother, perpetrator of maltreatment and neglect

Y07.13 Adoptive father, perpetrator of maltreatment and neglect

Y07.14 Adoptive mother, perpetrator of maltreatment and neglect

● **Y07.4 Other family member, perpetrator of maltreatment and neglect**

● **Y07.41 Sibling, perpetrator of maltreatment and neglect**

Excludes1 stepsibling, perpetrator of maltreatment and neglect (Y07.435, Y07.436)

Y07.410 Brother, perpetrator of maltreatment and neglect

Y07.411 Sister, perpetrator of maltreatment and neglect

● **Y07.42 Foster parent, perpetrator of maltreatment and neglect**

Y07.420 Foster father, perpetrator of maltreatment and neglect

Y07.421 Foster mother, perpetrator of maltreatment and neglect

● **Y07.43 Stepparent or stepsibling, perpetrator of maltreatment and neglect**

Y07.430 Stepfather, perpetrator of maltreatment and neglect

Y07.432 Male friend of parent (co-residing in household), perpetrator of maltreatment and neglect

Y07.433 Stepmother, perpetrator of maltreatment and neglect

Y07.434 Female friend of parent (co-residing in household), perpetrator of maltreatment and neglect

Y07.435 Stepbrother, perpetrator or maltreatment and neglect

Y07.436 Stepsister, perpetrator of maltreatment and neglect

● **Y07.44 Child, perpetrator of maltreatment and neglect**
Adopted child, perpetrator of maltreatment and neglect
Biological child, perpetrator of maltreatment and neglect
Daughter, perpetrator of maltreatment and neglect
Foster child, perpetrator of maltreatment and neglect
In-law child, perpetrator of maltreatment and neglect
Non-binary child, perpetrator of maltreatment and neglect
Son, perpetrator of maltreatment and neglect
Stepchild, perpetrator of maltreatment and neglect

● **Y07.45**   **Grandchild,** perpetrator of maltreatment and neglect
   Adopted grandchild, perpetrator of maltreatment and neglect
   Biological grandchild, perpetrator of maltreatment and neglect
   Foster grandchild, perpetrator of maltreatment and neglect
   Granddaughter, perpetrator of maltreatment and neglect
   Grandson, perpetrator of maltreatment and neglect
   In-law grandchild, perpetrator of maltreatment and neglect
   Non-binary grandchild, perpetrator of maltreatment and neglect
   Step grandchild, perpetrator of maltreatment and neglect

● **Y07.46**   **Grandparent,** perpetrator of maltreatment and neglect
   Grandfather, perpetrator of maltreatment and neglect
   Grandmother, perpetrator of maltreatment and neglect
   Non-binary grandparent, perpetrator of maltreatment and neglect

● **Y07.47**   **Parental sibling,** perpetrator of maltreatment and neglect
   Aunt, perpetrator of maltreatment and neglect
   Non-binary parental sibling, perpetrator of maltreatment and neglect
   Uncle, perpetrator of maltreatment and neglect

● **Y07.49**   **Other family member,** perpetrator of maltreatment and neglect

   Y07.490   **Male cousin,** perpetrator of maltreatment and neglect

   Y07.491   **Female cousin,** perpetrator of maltreatment and neglect

   Y07.499   **Other family member,** perpetrator of maltreatment and neglect

● **Y07.5**   **Non-family member,** perpetrator of maltreatment and neglect

   Y07.50   **Unspecified** non-family member, perpetrator of maltreatment and neglect

● **Y07.51**   **Daycare provider,** perpetrator of maltreatment and neglect

   Y07.510   **At-home childcare provider,** perpetrator of maltreatment and neglect

   Y07.511   **Daycare center childcare provider,** perpetrator of maltreatment and neglect

   Y07.512   **At-home adultcare provider,** perpetrator of maltreatment and neglect

   Y07.513   **Adultcare center provider,** perpetrator of maltreatment and neglect

   Y07.519   **Unspecified daycare provider,** perpetrator of maltreatment and neglect

● **Y07.52**   **Healthcare provider,** perpetrator of maltreatment and neglect

   Y07.521   **Mental** health provider, perpetrator of maltreatment and neglect

   Y07.528   **Other therapist or healthcare provider,** perpetrator of maltreatment and neglect
     Nurse perpetrator of maltreatment and neglect
     Occupational therapist perpetrator of maltreatment and neglect
     Physical therapist perpetrator of maltreatment and neglect
     Speech therapist perpetrator of maltreatment and neglect

   Y07.529   **Unspecified** healthcare provider, perpetrator of maltreatment and neglect

   Y07.53   **Teacher or instructor,** perpetrator of maltreatment and neglect
     Coach, perpetrator of maltreatment and neglect

   Y07.54   **Acquaintance or friend,** perpetrator of maltreatment and neglect

   Y07.59   **Other non-family member,** perpetrator of maltreatment and neglect

   Y07.6   Multiple perpetrators of maltreatment and neglect

   Y07.9   **Unspecified** perpetrator of maltreatment and neglect

● **Y08**   **Assault by other specified means**
   The appropriate 7th character is to be added to each code from category Y08

A	initial encounter
D	subsequent encounter
S	sequela

● **Y08.0**   **Assault by strike by sport equipment**
   X● **Y08.01**   Assault by strike by **hockey stick**
   X● **Y08.02**   Assault by strike by **baseball bat**
   X● **Y08.09**   Assault by strike by **other specified type of sport equipment**

● **Y08.8**   **Assault by other specified means**
   X● **Y08.81**   Assault by **crashing of aircraft**
   X● **Y08.89**   Assault by **other specified means**

● **Y09**   **Assault by unspecified means**
   Assassination (attempted) NOS
   Homicide (attempted) NOS
   Manslaughter (attempted) NOS
   Murder (attempted) NOS

EVENT OF UNDETERMINED INTENT (Y21-Y33)

Undetermined intent is only for use when there is specific documentation in the record that the intent of the injury cannot be determined. If no such documentation is present, code to accidental (unintentional)

● **Y21**   **Drowning and submersion, undetermined intent**
   The appropriate 7th character is to be added to each code from category Y21

A	initial encounter
D	subsequent encounter
S	sequela

   X● **Y21.0**   Drowning and submersion while **in bathtub,** undetermined intent
   X● **Y21.1**   Drowning and submersion after **fall into bathtub,** undetermined intent
   X● **Y21.2**   Drowning and submersion while **in swimming pool,** undetermined intent
   X● **Y21.3**   Drowning and submersion after **fall into swimming pool,** undetermined intent
   X● **Y21.4**   Drowning and submersion in **natural water,** undetermined intent
   X● **Y21.8**   **Other** drowning and submersion, undetermined intent
   X● **Y21.9**   **Unspecified** drowning and submersion, undetermined intent

X● **Y22**   **Handgun** discharge, undetermined intent
   Discharge of gun for single hand use, undetermined intent
   Discharge of pistol, undetermined intent
   Discharge of revolver, undetermined intent
   Excludes2   very pistol (Y24.8)
   The appropriate 7th character is to be added to code Y22

A	initial encounter
D	subsequent encounter
S	sequela

● Y23　Rifle, shotgun and larger firearm discharge, undetermined intent

Excludes2　airgun (Y24.0)

The appropriate 7th character is to be added to each code from category Y23

> A　initial encounter
> D　subsequent encounter
> S　sequela

X● Y23.0　Shotgun discharge, undetermined intent
X● Y23.1　Hunting rifle discharge, undetermined intent
X● Y23.2　Military firearm discharge, undetermined intent
X● Y23.3　Machine gun discharge, undetermined intent
X● Y23.8　Other larger firearm discharge, undetermined intent
X● Y23.9　Unspecified larger firearm discharge, undetermined intent

● Y24　Other and unspecified firearm discharge, undetermined intent

The appropriate 7th character is to be added to each code from category Y24

> A　initial encounter
> D　subsequent encounter
> S　sequela

X● Y24.0　Airgun discharge, undetermined intent
　　　　　BB gun discharge, undetermined intent
　　　　　Pellet gun discharge, undetermined intent
X● Y24.8　Other firearm discharge, undetermined intent
　　　　　Paintball gun discharge, undetermined intent
　　　　　Very pistol [flare] discharge, undetermined intent
X● Y24.9　Unspecified firearm discharge, undetermined intent

X● Y25　Contact with explosive material, undetermined intent

The appropriate 7th character is to be added to code Y25

> A　initial encounter
> D　subsequent encounter
> S　sequela

X● Y26　Exposure to smoke, fire and flames, undetermined intent

The appropriate 7th character is to be added to code Y26

> A　initial encounter
> D　subsequent encounter
> S　sequela

● Y27　Contact with steam, hot vapors and hot objects, undetermined intent

The appropriate 7th character is to be added to each code from category Y27

> A　initial encounter
> D　subsequent encounter
> S　sequela

X● Y27.0　Contact with steam and hot vapors, undetermined intent
X● Y27.1　Contact with hot tap water, undetermined intent
X● Y27.2　Contact with hot fluids, undetermined intent
X● Y27.3　Contact with hot household appliance, undetermined intent
X● Y27.8　Contact with other hot objects, undetermined intent
X● Y27.9　Contact with unspecified hot objects, undetermined intent

● Y28　Contact with sharp object, undetermined intent

The appropriate 7th character is to be added to each code from category Y28

> A　initial encounter
> D　subsequent encounter
> S　sequela

X● Y28.0　Contact with sharp glass, undetermined intent
X● Y28.1　Contact with knife, undetermined intent
X● Y28.2　Contact with sword or dagger, undetermined intent
X● Y28.8　Contact with other sharp object, undetermined intent
X● Y28.9　Contact with unspecified sharp object, undetermined intent

X● Y29　Contact with blunt object, undetermined intent

The appropriate 7th character is to be added to code Y29

> A　initial encounter
> D　subsequent encounter
> S　sequela

X● Y30　Falling, jumping or pushed from a high place, undetermined intent

Victim falling from one level to another, undetermined intent

The appropriate 7th character is to be added to code Y30

> A　initial encounter
> D　subsequent encounter
> S　sequela

X● Y31　Falling, lying or running before or into moving object, undetermined intent

The appropriate 7th character is to be added to code Y31

> A　initial encounter
> D　subsequent encounter
> S　sequela

X● Y32　Crashing of motor vehicle, undetermined intent

The appropriate 7th character is to be added to code Y32

> A　initial encounter
> D　subsequent encounter
> S　sequela

X● Y33　Other specified events, undetermined intent

The appropriate 7th character is to be added to code Y33

> A　initial encounter
> D　subsequent encounter
> S　sequela

LEGAL INTERVENTION, OPERATIONS OF WAR, MILITARY OPERATIONS, AND TERRORISM (Y35-Y38)

● Y35　Legal intervention

Includes　any injury sustained as a result of an encounter with any law enforcement official, serving in any capacity at the time of the encounter, whether on-duty or off-duty. Includes: injury to law enforcement official, suspect and bystander

The appropriate 7th character is to be added to each code from category Y35

> A　initial encounter
> D　subsequent encounter
> S　sequela

● Y35.0　Legal intervention involving firearm discharge

● Y35.00　Legal intervention involving unspecified firearm discharge
　　　　　Legal intervention involving gunshot wound
　　　　　Legal intervention involving shot NOS

● Y35.001　Legal intervention involving unspecified firearm discharge, law enforcement official injured
● Y35.002　Legal intervention involving unspecified firearm discharge, bystander injured
● Y35.003　Legal intervention involving unspecified firearm discharge, suspect injured

▶ New　⇨ Revised　~~deleted~~ Deleted　Excludes 1　Excludes 2　Includes　Use additional　Code first　Code also　Key words

OGCR Official Guidelines　X Assign placeholder X　● Use Additional Character(s)　▶ Manifestation Code　🅗 Hierarchical Condition Category　Coding Clinic

●Y35.009   Legal intervention involving unspecified firearm discharge, unspecified person injured

●Y35.01   Legal intervention involving injury by machine gun

  ●Y35.011   Legal intervention involving injury by machine gun, law enforcement official injured

  ●Y35.012   Legal intervention involving injury by machine gun, bystander injured

  ●Y35.013   Legal intervention involving injury by machine gun, suspect injured

  ●Y35.019   Legal intervention involving injury by machine gun, unspecified person injured

●Y35.02   Legal intervention involving injury by handgun

  ●Y35.021   Legal intervention involving injury by handgun, law enforcement official injured

  ●Y35.022   Legal intervention involving injury by handgun, bystander injured

  ●Y35.023   Legal intervention involving injury by handgun, suspect injured

  ●Y35.029   Legal intervention involving injury by handgun, unspecified person injured

●Y35.03   Legal intervention involving injury by rifle pellet

  ●Y35.031   Legal intervention involving injury by rifle pellet, law enforcement official injured

  ●Y35.032   Legal intervention involving injury by rifle pellet, bystander injured

  ●Y35.033   Legal intervention involving injury by rifle pellet, suspect injured

  ●Y35.039   Legal intervention involving injury by rifle pellet, unspecified person injured

●Y35.04   Legal intervention involving injury by rubber bullet

  ●Y35.041   Legal intervention involving injury by rubber bullet, law enforcement official injured

  ●Y35.042   Legal intervention involving injury by rubber bullet, bystander injured

  ●Y35.043   Legal intervention involving injury by rubber bullet, suspect injured

  ●Y35.049   Legal intervention involving injury by rubber bullet, unspecified person injured

●Y35.09   Legal intervention involving other firearm discharge

  ●Y35.091   Legal intervention involving other firearm discharge, law enforcement official injured

  ●Y35.092   Legal intervention involving other firearm discharge, bystander injured

  ●Y35.093   Legal intervention involving other firearm discharge, suspect injured

  ●Y35.099   Legal intervention involving other firearm discharge, unspecified person injured

●Y35.1   Legal intervention involving explosives

  ●Y35.10   Legal intervention involving unspecified explosives

    ●Y35.101   Legal intervention involving unspecified explosives, law enforcement official injured

    ●Y35.102   Legal intervention involving unspecified explosives, bystander injured

    ●Y35.103   Legal intervention involving unspecified explosives, suspect injured

    ●Y35.109   Legal intervention involving unspecified explosives, unspecified person injured

  ●Y35.11   Legal intervention involving injury by dynamite

    ●Y35.111   Legal intervention involving injury by dynamite, law enforcement official injured

    ●Y35.112   Legal intervention involving injury by dynamite, bystander injured

    ●Y35.113   Legal intervention involving injury by dynamite, suspect injured

    ●Y35.119   Legal intervention involving injury by dynamite, unspecified person injured

  ●Y35.12   Legal intervention involving injury by explosive shell

    ●Y35.121   Legal intervention involving injury by explosive shell, law enforcement official injured

    ●Y35.122   Legal intervention involving injury by explosive shell, bystander injured

    ●Y35.123   Legal intervention involving injury by explosive shell, suspect injured

    ●Y35.129   Legal intervention involving other explosives, unspecified person injured

  ●Y35.19   Legal intervention involving other explosives
    Legal intervention involving injury by grenade
    Legal intervention involving injury by mortar bomb

    ●Y35.191   Legal intervention involving other explosives, law enforcement official injured

    ●Y35.192   Legal intervention involving other explosives, bystander injured

    ●Y35.193   Legal intervention involving other explosives, suspect injured

    ●Y35.199   Legal intervention involving other explosives, unspecified person injured

●Y35.2   Legal intervention involving gas
  Legal intervention involving asphyxiation by gas
  Legal intervention involving poisoning by gas

  ●Y35.20   Legal intervention involving unspecified gas

    ●Y35.201   Legal intervention involving unspecified gas, law enforcement official injured

    ●Y35.202   Legal intervention involving unspecified gas, bystander injured

    ●Y35.203   Legal intervention involving unspecified gas, suspect injured

    ●Y35.209   Legal intervention involving unspecified gas, unspecified person injured

  ●Y35.21   Legal intervention involving injury by tear gas

    ●Y35.211   Legal intervention involving injury by tear gas, law enforcement official injured

    ●Y35.212   Legal intervention involving injury by tear gas, bystander injured

    ●Y35.213   Legal intervention involving injury by tear gas, suspect injured

    ●Y35.219   Legal intervention involving injury by tear gas, unspecified person injured

  ●Y35.29   Legal intervention involving other gas

    ●Y35.291   Legal intervention involving other gas, law enforcement official injured

● Y35.292 Legal intervention involving other gas, bystander injured

● Y35.293 Legal intervention involving other gas, suspect injured

● Y35.299 Legal intervention involving other gas, unspecified person injured

● Y35.3 Legal intervention involving blunt objects
Legal intervention involving being hit or struck by blunt object

● Y35.30 Legal intervention involving unspecified blunt objects

● Y35.301 Legal intervention involving unspecified blunt objects, law enforcement official injured

● Y35.302 Legal intervention involving unspecified blunt objects, bystander injured

● Y35.303 Legal intervention involving unspecified blunt objects, suspect injured

● Y35.309 Legal intervention involving unspecified blunt objects, unspecified person injured

● Y35.31 Legal intervention involving baton

● Y35.311 Legal intervention involving baton, law enforcement official injured

● Y35.312 Legal intervention involving baton, bystander injured

● Y35.313 Legal intervention involving baton, suspect injured

● Y35.319 Legal intervention involving baton, unspecified person injured

● Y35.39 Legal intervention involving other blunt objects

● Y35.391 Legal intervention involving other blunt objects, law enforcement official injured

● Y35.392 Legal intervention involving other blunt objects, bystander injured

● Y35.393 Legal intervention involving other blunt objects, suspect injured

● Y35.399 Legal intervention involving other blunt objects, unspecified person injured

● Y35.4 Legal intervention involving sharp objects
Legal intervention involving being cut by sharp objects
Legal intervention involving being stabbed by sharp objects

● Y35.40 Legal intervention involving unspecified sharp objects

● Y35.401 Legal intervention involving unspecified sharp objects, law enforcement official injured

● Y35.402 Legal intervention involving unspecified sharp objects, bystander injured

● Y35.403 Legal intervention involving unspecified sharp objects, suspect injured

● Y35.409 Legal intervention involving unspecified sharp objects, unspecified person injured

● Y35.41 Legal intervention involving bayonet

● Y35.411 Legal intervention involving bayonet, law enforcement official injured

● Y35.412 Legal intervention involving bayonet, bystander injured

● Y35.413 Legal intervention involving bayonet, suspect injured

● Y35.419 Legal intervention involving bayonet, unspecified person injured

● Y35.49 Legal intervention involving other sharp objects

● Y35.491 Legal intervention involving other sharp objects, law enforcement official injured

● Y35.492 Legal intervention involving other sharp objects, bystander injured

● Y35.493 Legal intervention involving other sharp objects, suspect injured

● Y35.499 Legal intervention involving other sharp objects, unspecified person injured

● Y35.8 Legal intervention involving other specified means

● Y35.81 Legal intervention involving manhandling

● Y35.811 Legal intervention involving manhandling, law enforcement official injured

● Y35.812 Legal intervention involving manhandling, bystander injured

● Y35.813 Legal intervention involving manhandling, suspect injured

● Y35.819 Legal intervention involving manhandling, unspecified person injured

● Y35.83 Legal intervention involving a conducted energy device
Electroshock device (taser)
Stun gun

● Y35.831 Legal intervention involving a conducted energy device, law enforcement official injured

● Y35.832 Legal intervention involving a conducted energy device, bystander injured

● Y35.833 Legal intervention involving a conducted energy device, suspect injured

● Y35.839 Legal intervention involving a conducted energy device, unspecified person injured

● Y35.89 Legal intervention involving other specified means

● Y35.891 Legal intervention involving other specified means, law enforcement official injured

● Y35.892 Legal intervention involving other specified means, bystander injured

● Y35.893 Legal intervention involving other specified means, suspect injured
Coding Clinic: 2018, Q1, P5

● Y35.899 Legal intervention involving other specified means, unspecified person injured

● Y35.9 Legal intervention, means unspecified

X ● Y35.91 Legal intervention, means unspecified, law enforcement official injured

X ● Y35.92 Legal intervention, means unspecified, bystander injured

X ● Y35.93 Legal intervention, means unspecified, suspect injured

X ● Y35.99 Legal intervention, means unspecified, unspecified person injured

● Y36   Operations of war

Includes   injuries to military personnel and civilians caused by war, civil insurrection, and peacekeeping missions

Excludes1   injury to military personnel occurring during peacetime military operations (Y37.-)
military vehicles involved in transport accidents with non-military vehicle during peacetime (V09.01, V09.21, V19.81, V29.818, V39.81, V49.81, V59.81, V69.81, V79.81)

The appropriate 7th character is to be added to each code from category Y36

A	initial encounter
D	subsequent encounter
S	sequela

● Y36.0   War operations involving explosion of marine weapons
Weapons and military watercraft

● Y36.00   War operations involving explosion of unspecified marine weapon
War operations involving underwater blast NOS

● Y36.000   War operations involving explosion of unspecified marine weapon, military personnel

● Y36.001   War operations involving explosion of unspecified marine weapon, civilian

● Y36.01   War operations involving explosion of depth-charge

● Y36.010   War operations involving explosion of depth-charge, military personnel

● Y36.011   War operations involving explosion of depth-charge, civilian

● Y36.02   War operations involving explosion of marine mine
War operations involving explosion of marine mine, at sea or in harbor

● Y36.020   War operations involving explosion of marine mine, military personnel

● Y36.021   War operations involving explosion of marine mine, civilian

● Y36.03   War operations involving explosion of sea-based artillery shell

● Y36.030   War operations involving explosion of sea-based artillery shell, military personnel

● Y36.031   War operations involving explosion of sea-based artillery shell, civilian

● Y36.04   War operations involving explosion of torpedo

● Y36.040   War operations involving explosion of torpedo, military personnel

● Y36.041   War operations involving explosion of torpedo, civilian

● Y36.05   War operations involving accidental detonation of onboard marine weapons

● Y36.050   War operations involving accidental detonation of onboard marine weapons, military personnel

● Y36.051   War operations involving accidental detonation of onboard marine weapons, civilian

● Y36.09   War operations involving explosion of other marine weapons

● Y36.090   War operations involving explosion of other marine weapons, military personnel

● Y36.091   War operations involving explosion of other marine weapons, civilian

● Y36.1   War operations involving destruction of aircraft

● Y36.10   War operations involving unspecified destruction of aircraft

● Y36.100   War operations involving unspecified destruction of aircraft, military personnel

● Y36.101   War operations involving unspecified destruction of aircraft, civilian

● Y36.11   War operations involving destruction of aircraft due to enemy fire or explosives
War operations involving destruction of aircraft due to air to air missile
War operations involving destruction of aircraft due to explosive placed on aircraft
War operations involving destruction of aircraft due to rocket propelled grenade [RPG]
War operations involving destruction of aircraft due to small arms fire
War operations involving destruction of aircraft due to surface to air missile

● Y36.110   War operations involving destruction of aircraft due to enemy fire or explosives, military personnel

● Y36.111   War operations involving destruction of aircraft due to enemy fire or explosives, civilian

● Y36.12   War operations involving destruction of aircraft due to collision with other aircraft

● Y36.120   War operations involving destruction of aircraft due to collision with other aircraft, military personnel

● Y36.121   War operations involving destruction of aircraft due to collision with other aircraft, civilian

● Y36.13   War operations involving destruction of aircraft due to onboard fire

● Y36.130   War operations involving destruction of aircraft due to onboard fire, military personnel

● Y36.131   War operations involving destruction of aircraft due to onboard fire, civilian

● Y36.14   War operations involving destruction of aircraft due to accidental detonation of onboard munitions and explosives

● Y36.140   War operations involving destruction of aircraft due to accidental detonation of onboard munitions and explosives, military personnel

● Y36.141   War operations involving destruction of aircraft due to accidental detonation of onboard munitions and explosives, civilian

● Y36.19   War operations involving other destruction of aircraft

● Y36.190   War operations involving other destruction of aircraft, military personnel

● Y36.191   War operations involving other destruction of aircraft, civilian

● Y36.2   War operations involving other explosions and fragments

Excludes1   war operations involving explosion of aircraft (Y36.1-)
war operations involving explosion of marine weapons (Y36.0-)
war operations involving explosion of nuclear weapons (Y36.5-)
war operations involving explosion occurring after cessation of hostilities (Y36.8-)

● **Y36.20** **War operations involving unspecified explosion and fragments**
War operations involving air blast NOS
War operations involving blast NOS
War operations involving blast fragments NOS
War operations involving blast wave NOS
War operations involving blast wind NOS
War operations involving explosion NOS
War operations involving explosion of bomb NOS

● **Y36.200** **War operations involving unspecified explosion and fragments, military personnel**

● **Y36.201** **War operations involving unspecified explosion and fragments, civilian**

● **Y36.21** **War operations involving explosion of aerial bomb**

● **Y36.210** **War operations involving explosion of aerial bomb, military personnel**

● **Y36.211** **War operations involving explosion of aerial bomb, civilian**

● **Y36.22** **War operations involving explosion of guided missile**

● **Y36.220** **War operations involving explosion of guided missile, military personnel**

● **Y36.221** **War operations involving explosion of guided missile, civilian**

● **Y36.23** **War operations involving explosion of improvised explosive device [IED]**
War operations involving explosion of person-borne improvised explosive device [IED]
War operations involving explosion of vehicle-borne improvised explosive device [IED]
War operations involving explosion of roadside improvised explosive device [IED]

● **Y36.230** **War operations involving explosion of improvised explosive device [IED], military personnel**

● **Y36.231** **War operations involving explosion of improvised explosive device [IED], civilian**

● **Y36.24** **War operations involving explosion due to accidental detonation and discharge of own munitions or munitions launch device**

● **Y36.240** **War operations involving explosion due to accidental detonation and discharge of own munitions or munitions launch device, military personnel**

● **Y36.241** **War operations involving explosion due to accidental detonation and discharge of own munitions or munitions launch device, civilian**

● **Y36.25** **War operations involving fragments from munitions**

● **Y36.250** **War operations involving fragments from munitions, military personnel**

● **Y36.251** **War operations involving fragments from munitions, civilian**

● **Y36.26** **War operations involving fragments of improvised explosive device [IED]**
War operations involving fragments of person-borne improvised explosive device [IED]
War operations involving fragments of vehicle-borne improvised explosive device [IED]
War operations involving fragments of roadside improvised explosive device [IED]

● **Y36.260** **War operations involving fragments of improvised explosive device [IED], military personnel**

● **Y36.261** **War operations involving fragments of improvised explosive device [IED], civilian**

● **Y36.27** **War operations involving fragments from weapons**

● **Y36.270** **War operations involving fragments from weapons, military personnel**

● **Y36.271** **War operations involving fragments from weapons, civilian**

● **Y36.29** **War operations involving other explosions and fragments**
War operations involving explosion of grenade
War operations involving explosions of land mine
War operations involving shrapnel NOS

● **Y36.290** **War operations involving other explosions and fragments, military personnel**

● **Y36.291** **War operations involving other explosions and fragments, civilian**

● **Y36.3** **War operations involving fires, conflagrations and hot substances**
War operations involving smoke, fumes, and heat from fires, conflagrations and hot substances

> **Excludes1** war operations involving fires and conflagrations aboard military aircraft (Y36.1-)
war operations involving fires and conflagrations aboard military watercraft (Y36.0-)
war operations involving fires and conflagrations caused indirectly by conventional weapons (Y36.2-)
war operations involving fires and thermal effects of nuclear weapons (Y36.53-)

● **Y36.30** **War operations involving unspecified fire, conflagration and hot substance**

● **Y36.300** **War operations involving unspecified fire, conflagration and hot substance, military personnel**

● **Y36.301** **War operations involving unspecified fire, conflagration and hot substance, civilian**

● **Y36.31** **War operations involving gasoline bomb**
War operations involving incendiary bomb
War operations involving petrol bomb

● **Y36.310** **War operations involving gasoline bomb, military personnel**

● **Y36.311** **War operations involving gasoline bomb, civilian**

● **Y36.32** **War operations involving incendiary bullet**

● **Y36.320** **War operations involving incendiary bullet, military personnel**

● **Y36.321** **War operations involving incendiary bullet, civilian**

● **Y36.33** **War operations involving flamethrower**

● **Y36.330** **War operations involving flamethrower, military personnel**

● **Y36.331** **War operations involving flamethrower, civilian**

● **Y36.39** **War operations involving other fires, conflagrations and hot substances**

● **Y36.390** **War operations involving other fires, conflagrations and hot substances, military personnel**

● **Y36.391** **War operations involving other fires, conflagrations and hot substances, civilian**

● **Y36.4** **War operations involving firearm discharge and other forms of conventional warfare**

● **Y36.41** **War operations involving rubber bullets**

● **Y36.410** **War operations involving rubber bullets, military personnel**

● **Y36.411** **War operations involving rubber bullets, civilian**

▶ New ⇒ Revised ~~deleted~~ Deleted Excludes 1 Excludes 2 Includes Use additional Code first Code also Key words
OGCR Official Guidelines X Assign placeholder X ● Use Additional Character(s) ▷ Manifestation Code 🔖 Hierarchical Condition Category Coding Clinic

● Y36.42   War operations involving firearms pellets
    ● Y36.420   War operations involving firearms pellets, military personnel
    ● Y36.421   War operations involving firearms pellets, civilian
● Y36.43   War operations involving other firearms discharge
      War operations involving bullets NOS
      Excludes1   war operations involving munitions fragments (Y36.25-)
              war operations involving incendiary bullets (Y36.32-)
    ● Y36.430   War operations involving other firearms discharge, military personnel
    ● Y36.431   War operations involving other firearms discharge, civilian
● Y36.44   War operations involving unarmed hand to hand combat
      Excludes1   war operations involving combat using blunt or piercing object (Y36.45-)
              war operations involving intentional restriction of air and airway (Y36.46-)
              war operations involving unintentional restriction of air and airway (Y36.47-)
    ● Y36.440   War operations involving unarmed hand to hand combat, military personnel
    ● Y36.441   War operations involving unarmed hand to hand combat, civilian
● Y36.45   War operations involving combat using blunt or piercing object
    ● Y36.450   War operations involving combat using blunt or piercing object, military personnel
    ● Y36.451   War operations involving combat using blunt or piercing object, civilian
● Y36.46   War operations involving intentional restriction of air and airway
    ● Y36.460   War operations involving intentional restriction of air and airway, military personnel
    ● Y36.461   War operations involving intentional restriction of air and airway, civilian
● Y36.47   War operations involving unintentional restriction of air and airway
    ● Y36.470   War operations involving unintentional restriction of air and airway, military personnel
    ● Y36.471   War operations involving unintentional restriction of air and airway, civilian
● Y36.49   War operations involving other forms of conventional warfare
    ● Y36.490   War operations involving other forms of conventional warfare, military personnel
    ● Y36.491   War operations involving other forms of conventional warfare, civilian
● Y36.5   War operations involving nuclear weapons
      War operations involving dirty bomb NOS
    ● Y36.50   War operations involving unspecified effect of nuclear weapon
       ● Y36.500   War operations involving unspecified effect of nuclear weapon, military personnel
       ● Y36.501   War operations involving unspecified effect of nuclear weapon, civilian

● Y36.51   War operations involving direct blast effect of nuclear weapon
      War operations involving blast pressure of nuclear weapon
    ● Y36.510   War operations involving direct blast effect of nuclear weapon, military personnel
    ● Y36.511   War operations involving direct blast effect of nuclear weapon, civilian
● Y36.52   War operations involving indirect blast effect of nuclear weapon
      War operations involving being thrown by blast of nuclear weapon
      War operations involving being struck or crushed by blast debris of nuclear weapon
    ● Y36.520   War operations involving indirect blast effect of nuclear weapon, military personnel
    ● Y36.521   War operations involving indirect blast effect of nuclear weapon, civilian
● Y36.53   War operations involving thermal radiation effect of nuclear weapon
      War operations involving direct heat from nuclear weapon
      War operation involving fireball effects from nuclear weapon
    ● Y36.530   War operations involving thermal radiation effect of nuclear weapon, military personnel
    ● Y36.531   War operations involving thermal radiation effect of nuclear weapon, civilian
● Y36.54   War operation involving nuclear radiation effects of nuclear weapon
      War operation involving acute radiation exposure from nuclear weapon
      War operation involving exposure to immediate ionizing radiation from nuclear weapon
      War operation involving fallout exposure from nuclear weapon
      War operation involving secondary effects of nuclear weapons
    ● Y36.540   War operation involving nuclear radiation effects of nuclear weapon, military personnel
    ● Y36.541   War operation involving nuclear radiation effects of nuclear weapon, civilian
● Y36.59   War operation involving other effects of nuclear weapons
    ● Y36.590   War operation involving other effects of nuclear weapons, military personnel
    ● Y36.591   War operation involving other effects of nuclear weapons, civilian
● Y36.6   War operations involving biological weapons
    ● Y36.6X   War operations involving biological weapons
       ● Y36.6XØ   War operations involving biological weapons, military personnel
       ● Y36.6X1   War operations involving biological weapons, civilian
● Y36.7   War operations involving chemical weapons and other forms of unconventional warfare
      Excludes1   war operations involving incendiary devices (Y36.3-, Y36.5-)
    ● Y36.7X   War operations involving chemical weapons and other forms of unconventional warfare
       ● Y36.7XØ   War operations involving chemical weapons and other forms of unconventional warfare, military personnel

● Y36.7X1 War operations involving chemical weapons and other forms of unconventional warfare, civilian

● Y36.8 War operations occurring after cessation of hostilities
War operations classifiable to categories Y36.0-Y36.8 but occurring after cessation of hostilities

● Y36.81 Explosion of mine placed during war operations but exploding after cessation of hostilities
● Y36.810 Explosion of mine placed during war operations but exploding after cessation of hostilities, military personnel
● Y36.811 Explosion of mine placed during war operations but exploding after cessation of hostilities, civilian

● Y36.82 Explosion of bomb placed during war operations but exploding after cessation of hostilities
● Y36.820 Explosion of bomb placed during war operations but exploding after cessation of hostilities, military personnel
● Y36.821 Explosion of bomb placed during war operations but exploding after cessation of hostilities, civilian

● Y36.88 Other war operations occurring after cessation of hostilities
● Y36.880 Other war operations occurring after cessation of hostilities, military personnel
● Y36.881 Other war operations occurring after cessation of hostilities, civilian

● Y36.89 Unspecified war operations occurring after cessation of hostilities
● Y36.890 Unspecified war operations occurring after cessation of hostilities, military personnel
● Y36.891 Unspecified war operations occurring after cessation of hostilities, civilian

● Y36.9 Other and unspecified war operations
X● Y36.90 War operations, unspecified
X● Y36.91 War operations involving unspecified weapon of mass destruction [WMD]
X● Y36.92 War operations involving friendly fire

● Y37 Military operations
Includes Injuries to military personnel and civilians occurring during peacetime on military property and during routine military exercises and operations
Excludes1 military aircraft involved in aircraft accident with civilian aircraft (V97.81-)
military vehicles involved in transport accident with civilian vehicle (V09.01, V09.21, V19.81, V29.818, V39.81, V49.81, V59.81, V69.81, V79.81)
military watercraft involved in water transport accident with civilian watercraft (V94.81-)
war operations (Y36.-)

The appropriate 7th character is to be added to each code from category Y37

A initial encounter
D subsequent encounter
S sequela

● Y37.0 Military operations involving explosion of marine weapons
● Y37.00 Military operations involving explosion of unspecified marine weapon
Military operations involving underwater blast NOS
● Y37.000 Military operations involving explosion of unspecified marine weapon, military personnel

● Y37.001 Military operations involving explosion of unspecified marine weapon, civilian

● Y37.01 Military operations involving explosion of depth-charge
● Y37.010 Military operations involving explosion of depth-charge, military personnel
● Y37.011 Military operations involving explosion of depth-charge, civilian

● Y37.02 Military operations involving explosion of marine mine
Military operations involving explosion of marine mine, at sea or in harbor
● Y37.020 Military operations involving explosion of marine mine, military personnel
● Y37.021 Military operations involving explosion of marine mine, civilian

● Y37.03 Military operations involving explosion of sea-based artillery shell
● Y37.030 Military operations involving explosion of sea-based artillery shell, military personnel
● Y37.031 Military operations involving explosion of sea-based artillery shell, civilian

● Y37.04 Military operations involving explosion of torpedo
● Y37.040 Military operations involving explosion of torpedo, military personnel
● Y37.041 Military operations involving explosion of torpedo, civilian

● Y37.05 Military operations involving accidental detonation of onboard marine weapons
● Y37.050 Military operations involving accidental detonation of onboard marine weapons, military personnel
● Y37.051 Military operations involving accidental detonation of onboard marine weapons, civilian

● Y37.09 Military operations involving explosion of other marine weapons
● Y37.090 Military operations involving explosion of other marine weapons, military personnel
● Y37.091 Military operations involving explosion of other marine weapons, civilian

● Y37.1 Military operations involving destruction of aircraft
● Y37.10 Military operations involving unspecified destruction of aircraft
● Y37.100 Military operations involving unspecified destruction of aircraft, military personnel
● Y37.101 Military operations involving unspecified destruction of aircraft, civilian

● Y37.11 Military operations involving destruction of aircraft due to enemy fire or explosives
Military operations involving destruction of aircraft due to air to air missile
Military operations involving destruction of aircraft due to explosive placed on aircraft
Military operations involving destruction of aircraft due to rocket propelled grenade [RPG]
Military operations involving destruction of aircraft due to small arms fire
Military operations involving destruction of aircraft due to surface to air missile

▶ New ⇒ Revised ~~deleted~~ Deleted | Excludes 1 | Excludes 2 | Includes | Use additional | Code first | Code also | Key words
OGCR Official Guidelines X Assign placeholder X ● Use Additional Character(s) ▷ Manifestation Code 🏷 Hierarchical Condition Category | Coding Clinic

● Y37.110   Military operations involving
             destruction of aircraft due to enemy
             fire or explosives, military personnel
● Y37.111   Military operations involving
             destruction of aircraft due to enemy
             fire or explosives, civilian
● Y37.12   Military operations involving destruction of
            aircraft due to collision with other aircraft
    ● Y37.120   Military operations involving
                 destruction of aircraft due to collision
                 with other aircraft, military personnel
    ● Y37.121   Military operations involving
                 destruction of aircraft due to collision
                 with other aircraft, civilian
● Y37.13   Military operations involving destruction of
            aircraft due to onboard fire
    ● Y37.130   Military operations involving
                 destruction of aircraft due to onboard
                 fire, military personnel
    ● Y37.131   Military operations involving
                 destruction of aircraft due to onboard
                 fire, civilian
● Y37.14   Military operations involving destruction of
            aircraft due to accidental detonation of onboard
            munitions and explosives
    ● Y37.140   Military operations involving
                 destruction of aircraft due to
                 accidental detonation of onboard
                 munitions and explosives, military
                 personnel
    ● Y37.141   Military operations involving
                 destruction of aircraft due to
                 accidental detonation of onboard
                 munitions and explosives, civilian
● Y37.19   Military operations involving other destruction
            of aircraft
    ● Y37.190   Military operations involving other
                 destruction of aircraft, military
                 personnel
    ● Y37.191   Military operations involving other
                 destruction of aircraft, civilian
● Y37.2   Military operations involving other explosions and
           fragments
    Excludes1   military operations involving explosion
                     of aircraft (Y37.1-)
                     military operations involving explosion
                     of marine weapons (Y37.0-)
                     military operations involving explosion
                     of nuclear weapons (Y37.5-)
    ● Y37.20   Military operations involving unspecified
                explosion and fragments
                Military operations involving air blast NOS
                Military operations involving blast NOS
                Military operations involving blast fragments
                   NOS
                Military operations involving blast wave NOS
                Military operations involving blast wind NOS
                Military operations involving explosion NOS
                Military operations involving explosion of
                   bomb NOS
        ● Y37.200   Military operations involving
                     unspecified explosion and fragments,
                     military personnel
        ● Y37.201   Military operations involving
                     unspecified explosion and fragments,
                     civilian
    ● Y37.21   Military operations involving explosion of
                aerial bomb
        ● Y37.210   Military operations involving
                     explosion of aerial bomb, military
                     personnel
        ● Y37.211   Military operations involving
                     explosion of aerial bomb, civilian

● Y37.22   Military operations involving explosion of
            guided missile
    ● Y37.220   Military operations involving
                 explosion of guided missile, military
                 personnel
    ● Y37.221   Military operations involving
                 explosion of guided missile, civilian
● Y37.23   Military operations involving explosion of
            improvised explosive device [IED]
            Military operations involving explosion of
               person-borne improvised explosive device
               [IED]
            Military operations involving explosion of
               vehicle-borne improvised explosive
               device [IED]
            Military operations involving explosion of
               roadside improvised explosive device [IED]
    ● Y37.230   Military operations involving
                 explosion of improvised explosive
                 device [IED], military personnel
    ● Y37.231   Military operations involving
                 explosion of improvised explosive
                 device [IED], civilian
● Y37.24   Military operations involving explosion due
            to accidental detonation and discharge of own
            munitions or munitions launch device
    ● Y37.240   Military operations involving
                 explosion due to accidental
                 detonation and discharge of own
                 munitions or munitions launch
                 device, military personnel
    ● Y37.241   Military operations involving
                 explosion due to accidental detonation
                 and discharge of own munitions or
                 munitions launch device, civilian
● Y37.25   Military operations involving fragments from
            munitions
    ● Y37.250   Military operations involving
                 fragments from munitions, military
                 personnel
    ● Y37.251   Military operations involving
                 fragments from munitions, civilian
● Y37.26   Military operations involving fragments of
            improvised explosive device [IED]
            Military operations involving fragments of
               person-borne improvised explosive device
               [IED]
            Military operations involving fragments of
               vehicle-borne improvised explosive
               device [IED]
            Military operations involving fragments of
               roadside improvised explosive device [IED]
    ● Y37.260   Military operations involving
                 fragments of improvised explosive
                 device [IED], military personnel
    ● Y37.261   Military operations involving
                 fragments of improvised explosive
                 device [IED], civilian
● Y37.27   Military operations involving fragments from
            weapons
    ● Y37.270   Military operations involving
                 fragments from weapons, military
                 personnel
    ● Y37.271   Military operations involving
                 fragments from weapons, civilian
● Y37.29   Military operations involving other explosions
            and fragments
            Military operations involving explosion of
               grenade
            Military operations involving explosions of
               land mine
            Military operations involving shrapnel NOS
    ● Y37.290   Military operations involving other
                 explosions and fragments, military
                 personnel

CHAPTER 20 (V00–Y99)

CHAPTER 20 (V00-Y99)

● Y37.291 Military operations involving other explosions and fragments, civilian
● Y37.3 Military operations involving fires, conflagrations and hot substances
Military operations involving smoke, fumes, and heat from fires, conflagrations and hot substances

Excludes1 military operations involving fires and conflagrations aboard military aircraft (Y37.1-)
military operations involving fires and conflagrations aboard military watercraft (Y37.0-)
military operations involving fires and conflagrations caused indirectly by conventional weapons (Y37.2-)
military operations involving fires and thermal effects of nuclear weapons (Y36.53-)

● Y37.30 Military operations involving unspecified fire, conflagration and hot substance
● Y37.300 Military operations involving unspecified fire, conflagration and hot substance, military personnel
● Y37.301 Military operations involving unspecified fire, conflagration and hot substance, civilian

● Y37.31 Military operations involving gasoline bomb
Military operations involving incendiary bomb
Military operations involving petrol bomb
● Y37.310 Military operations involving gasoline bomb, military personnel
● Y37.311 Military operations involving gasoline bomb, civilian

● Y37.32 Military operations involving incendiary bullet
● Y37.320 Military operations involving incendiary bullet, military personnel
● Y37.321 Military operations involving incendiary bullet, civilian

● Y37.33 Military operations involving flamethrower
● Y37.330 Military operations involving flamethrower, military personnel
● Y37.331 Military operations involving flamethrower, civilian

● Y37.39 Military operations involving other fires, conflagrations and hot substances
● Y37.390 Military operations involving other fires, conflagrations and hot substances, military personnel
● Y37.391 Military operations involving other fires, conflagrations and hot substances, civilian

● Y37.4 Military operations involving firearm discharge and other forms of conventional warfare
● Y37.41 Military operations involving rubber bullets
● Y37.410 Military operations involving rubber bullets, military personnel
● Y37.411 Military operations involving rubber bullets, civilian

● Y37.42 Military operations involving firearms pellets
● Y37.420 Military operations involving firearms pellets, military personnel
● Y37.421 Military operations involving firearms pellets, civilian

● Y37.43 Military operations involving other firearms discharge
Military operations involving bullets NOS
Excludes1 military operations involving munitions fragments (Y37.25-)
military operations involving incendiary bullets (Y37.32-)
● Y37.430 Military operations involving other firearms discharge, military personnel

● Y37.431 Military operations involving other firearms discharge, civilian
● Y37.44 Military operations involving unarmed hand to hand combat
Excludes1 military operations involving combat using blunt or piercing object (Y37.45-)
military operations involving intentional restriction of air and airway (Y37.46-)
military operations involving unintentional restriction of air and airway (Y37.47-)
● Y37.440 Military operations involving unarmed hand to hand combat, military personnel
● Y37.441 Military operations involving unarmed hand to hand combat, civilian

● Y37.45 Military operations involving combat using blunt or piercing object
● Y37.450 Military operations involving combat using blunt or piercing object, military personnel
● Y37.451 Military operations involving combat using blunt or piercing object, civilian

● Y37.46 Military operations involving intentional restriction of air and airway
● Y37.460 Military operations involving intentional restriction of air and airway, military personnel
● Y37.461 Military operations involving intentional restriction of air and airway, civilian

● Y37.47 Military operations involving unintentional restriction of air and airway
● Y37.470 Military operations involving unintentional restriction of air and airway, military personnel
● Y37.471 Military operations involving unintentional restriction of air and airway, civilian

● Y37.49 Military operations involving other forms of conventional warfare
● Y37.490 Military operations involving other forms of conventional warfare, military personnel
● Y37.491 Military operations involving other forms of conventional warfare, civilian

● Y37.5 Military operations involving nuclear weapons
Military operation involving dirty bomb NOS
● Y37.50 Military operations involving unspecified effect of nuclear weapon
● Y37.500 Military operations involving unspecified effect of nuclear weapon, military personnel
● Y37.501 Military operations involving unspecified effect of nuclear weapon, civilian

● Y37.51 Military operations involving direct blast effect of nuclear weapon
Military operations involving blast pressure of nuclear weapon
● Y37.510 Military operations involving direct blast effect of nuclear weapon, military personnel
● Y37.511 Military operations involving direct blast effect of nuclear weapon, civilian

● Y37.52 Military operations involving indirect blast effect of nuclear weapon
Military operations involving being thrown by blast of nuclear weapon
Military operations involving being struck or crushed by blast debris of nuclear weapon

● Y37.520   Military operations involving indirect blast effect of nuclear weapon, military personnel

● Y37.521   Military operations involving indirect blast effect of nuclear weapon, civilian

● Y37.53   Military operations involving thermal radiation effect of nuclear weapon

     Military operations involving direct heat from nuclear weapon

     Military operation involving fireball effects from nuclear weapon

  ● Y37.530   Military operations involving thermal radiation effect of nuclear weapon, military personnel

  ● Y37.531   Military operations involving thermal radiation effect of nuclear weapon, civilian

● Y37.54   Military operation involving nuclear radiation effects of nuclear weapon

     Military operation involving acute radiation exposure from nuclear weapon

     Military operation involving exposure to immediate ionizing radiation from nuclear weapon

     Military operation involving fallout exposure from nuclear weapon

     Military operation involving secondary effects of nuclear weapons

  ● Y37.540   Military operation involving nuclear radiation effects of nuclear weapon, military personnel

  ● Y37.541   Military operation involving nuclear radiation effects of nuclear weapon, civilian

● Y37.59   Military operation involving other effects of nuclear weapons

  ● Y37.590   Military operation involving other effects of nuclear weapons, military personnel

  ● Y37.591   Military operation involving other effects of nuclear weapons, civilian

● Y37.6   Military operations involving biological weapons

  ● Y37.6X   Military operations involving biological weapons

    ● Y37.6X0   Military operations involving biological weapons, military personnel

    ● Y37.6X1   Military operations involving biological weapons, civilian

● Y37.7   Military operations involving chemical weapons and other forms of unconventional warfare

     Excludes1   military operations involving incendiary devices (Y36.3-, Y36.5-)

  ● Y37.7X   Military operations involving chemical weapons and other forms of unconventional warfare

    ● Y37.7X0   Military operations involving chemical weapons and other forms of unconventional warfare, military personnel

    ● Y37.7X1   Military operations involving chemical weapons and other forms of unconventional warfare, civilian

● Y37.9   Other and unspecified military operations

  X● Y37.90   Military operations, unspecified

  X● Y37.91   Military operations involving unspecified weapon of mass destruction [WMD]

  X● Y37.92   Military operations involving friendly fire

● Y38   Terrorism

     These codes are for use to identify injuries resulting from the unlawful use of force or violence against persons or property to intimidate or coerce a government, the civilian population, or any segment thereof, in furtherance of political or social objective

     Use additional code for place of occurrence (Y92.-)

     The appropriate 7th character is to be added to each code from category Y38

A	initial encounter
D	subsequent encounter
S	sequela

● Y38.0   Terrorism involving explosion of marine weapons

     Terrorism involving depth-charge

     Terrorism involving marine mine

     Terrorism involving mine NOS, at sea or in harbor

     Terrorism involving sea-based artillery shell

     Terrorism involving torpedo

     Terrorism involving underwater blast

  ● Y38.0X   Terrorism involving explosion of marine weapons

    ● Y38.0X1   Terrorism involving explosion of marine weapons, public safety official injured

    ● Y38.0X2   Terrorism involving explosion of marine weapons, civilian injured

    ● Y38.0X3   Terrorism involving explosion of marine weapons, terrorist injured

● Y38.1   Terrorism involving destruction of aircraft

     Terrorism involving aircraft burned

     Terrorism involving aircraft exploded

     Terrorism involving aircraft being shot down

     Terrorism involving aircraft used as a weapon

  ● Y38.1X   Terrorism involving destruction of aircraft

    ● Y38.1X1   Terrorism involving destruction of aircraft, public safety official injured

    ● Y38.1X2   Terrorism involving destruction of aircraft, civilian injured

    ● Y38.1X3   Terrorism involving destruction of aircraft, terrorist injured

● Y38.2   Terrorism involving other explosions and fragments

     Terrorism involving antipersonnel (fragments) bomb

     Terrorism involving blast NOS

     Terrorism involving explosion NOS

     Terrorism involving explosion of breech block

     Terrorism involving explosion of cannon block

     Terrorism involving explosion (fragments) of artillery shell

     Terrorism involving explosion (fragments) of bomb

     Terrorism involving explosion (fragments) of grenade

     Terrorism involving explosion (fragments) of guided missile

     Terrorism involving explosion (fragments) of land mine

     Terrorism involving explosion of mortar bomb

     Terrorism involving explosion of munitions

     Terrorism involving explosion (fragments) of rocket

     Terrorism involving explosion (fragments) of shell

     Terrorism involving shrapnel

     Terrorism involving mine NOS, on land

     Excludes1   terrorism involving explosion of nuclear weapon (Y38.5)

                  terrorism involving suicide bomber (Y38.81)

  ● Y38.2X   Terrorism involving other explosions and fragments

    ● Y38.2X1   Terrorism involving other explosions and fragments, public safety official injured

    ● Y38.2X2   Terrorism involving other explosions and fragments, civilian injured

    ● Y38.2X3   Terrorism involving other explosions and fragments, terrorist injured

● **Y38.3 Terrorism involving fires, conflagration and hot substances**
Terrorism involving conflagration NOS
Terrorism involving fire NOS
Terrorism involving petrol bomb

    Excludes1 terrorism involving fire or heat of nuclear weapon (Y38.5)

  ● **Y38.3X Terrorism involving fires, conflagration and hot substances**

    ● **Y38.3X1 Terrorism involving fires, conflagration and hot substances, public safety official injured**

    ● **Y38.3X2 Terrorism involving fires, conflagration and hot substances, civilian injured**

    ● **Y38.3X3 Terrorism involving fires, conflagration and hot substances, terrorist injured**

● **Y38.4 Terrorism involving firearms**
Terrorism involving carbine bullet
Terrorism involving machine gun bullet
Terrorism involving pellets (shotgun)
Terrorism involving pistol bullet
Terrorism involving rifle bullet
Terrorism involving rubber (rifle) bullet

  ● **Y38.4X Terrorism involving firearms**

    ● **Y38.4X1 Terrorism involving firearms, public safety official injured**

    ● **Y38.4X2 Terrorism involving firearms, civilian injured**

    ● **Y38.4X3 Terrorism involving firearms, terrorist injured**

● **Y38.5 Terrorism involving nuclear weapons**
Terrorism involving blast effects of nuclear weapon
Terrorism involving exposure to ionizing radiation from nuclear weapon
Terrorism involving fireball effect of nuclear weapon
Terrorism involving heat from nuclear weapon

  ● **Y38.5X Terrorism involving nuclear weapons**

    ● **Y38.5X1 Terrorism involving nuclear weapons, public safety official injured**

    ● **Y38.5X2 Terrorism involving nuclear weapons, civilian injured**

    ● **Y38.5X3 Terrorism involving nuclear weapons, terrorist injured**

● **Y38.6 Terrorism involving biological weapons**
Terrorism involving anthrax
Terrorism involving cholera
    A serious, often deadly, infectious disease of the small intestine
Terrorism involving smallpox

  ● **Y38.6X Terrorism involving biological weapons**

    ● **Y38.6X1 Terrorism involving biological weapons, public safety official injured**

    ● **Y38.6X2 Terrorism involving biological weapons, civilian injured**

    ● **Y38.6X3 Terrorism involving biological weapons, terrorist injured**

● **Y38.7 Terrorism involving chemical weapons**
Terrorism involving gases, fumes, chemicals
Terrorism involving hydrogen cyanide
Terrorism involving phosgene
Terrorism involving sarin

  ● **Y38.7X Terrorism involving chemical weapons**

    ● **Y38.7X1 Terrorism involving chemical weapons, public safety official injured**

    ● **Y38.7X2 Terrorism involving chemical weapons, civilian injured**

    ● **Y38.7X3 Terrorism involving chemical weapons, terrorist injured**

● **Y38.8 Terrorism involving other and unspecified means**

  ● **Y38.80 Terrorism involving unspecified means**
Terrorism NOS

  ● **Y38.81 Terrorism involving suicide bomber**

    ● **Y38.811 Terrorism involving suicide bomber, public safety official injured**

    ● **Y38.812 Terrorism involving suicide bomber, civilian injured**

  ● **Y38.89 Terrorism involving other means**
Terrorism involving drowning and submersion
Terrorism involving lasers
Terrorism involving piercing or stabbing instruments

    ● **Y38.891 Terrorism involving other means, public safety official injured**

    ● **Y38.892 Terrorism involving other means, civilian injured**

    ● **Y38.893 Terrorism involving other means, terrorist injured**

● **Y38.9 Terrorism, secondary effects**
    Note: This code is for use to identify conditions occurring subsequent to a terrorist attack not those that are due to the initial terrorist attack.

  ● **Y38.9X Terrorism, secondary effects**

    ● **Y38.9X1 Terrorism, secondary effects, public safety official injured**

    ● **Y38.9X2 Terrorism, secondary effects, civilian injured categories**

COMPLICATIONS OF MEDICAL AND SURGICAL CARE (Y62-Y84)

    Includes complications of medical devices surgical and medical procedures as the cause of abnormal reaction of the patient, or of later complication, without mention of misadventure at the time of the procedure

---

MISADVENTURES TO PATIENTS DURING SURGICAL AND MEDICAL CARE (Y62-Y69)

    Excludes1 surgical and medical procedures as the cause of abnormal reaction of the patient, without mention of misadventure at the time of the procedure (Y83-Y84)

● **Y62 Failure of sterile precautions during surgical and medical care**

  Y62.0 Failure of sterile precautions during surgical operation

  Y62.1 Failure of sterile precautions during infusion or transfusion

  Y62.2 Failure of sterile precautions during kidney dialysis and other perfusion 🅚

  Y62.3 Failure of sterile precautions during injection or immunization

  Y62.4 Failure of sterile precautions during endoscopic examination

  Y62.5 Failure of sterile precautions during heart catheterization

  Y62.6 Failure of sterile precautions during aspiration, puncture and other catheterization

  Y62.8 Failure of sterile precautions during other surgical and medical care

  Y62.9 Failure of sterile precautions during unspecified surgical and medical care

● **Y63 Failure in dosage during surgical and medical care**

    Excludes2 accidental overdose of drug or wrong drug given in error (T36-T50)

  Y63.0 Excessive amount of blood or other fluid given during transfusion or infusion

  Y63.1 Incorrect dilution of fluid used during infusion

  Y63.2 Overdose of radiation given during therapy

  Y63.3 Inadvertent exposure of patient to radiation during medical care

  Y63.4 Failure in dosage in electroshock or insulin-shock therapy

---

▶ New ⇒ Revised ~~deleted~~ Deleted Excludes 1 Excludes 2 Includes Use additional Code first Code also Key words

OGCR Official Guidelines X Assign placeholder X ● Use Additional Character(s) ▶ Manifestation Code 🅚 Hierarchical Condition Category **Coding Clinic**

Y63.5   Inappropriate temperature in local application and packing

Y63.6   Underdosing and nonadministration of necessary drug, medicament or biological substance

Y63.8   Failure in dosage during other surgical and medical care

Y63.9   Failure in dosage during unspecified surgical and medical care

● Y64   Contaminated medical or biological substances

Y64.0   Contaminated medical or biological substance, transfused or infused

Y64.1   Contaminated medical or biological substance, injected or used for immunization

Y64.8   Contaminated medical or biological substance administered by other means

Y64.9   Contaminated medical or biological substance administered by unspecified means
Administered contaminated medical or biological substance NOS

● Y65   Other misadventures during surgical and medical care

Y65.0   Mismatched blood in transfusion

Y65.1   Wrong fluid used in infusion

Y65.2   Failure in suture or ligature during surgical operation

Y65.3   Endotracheal tube wrongly placed during anesthetic procedure

Y65.4   Failure to introduce or to remove other tube or instrument

● Y65.5   Performance of wrong procedure (operation)

● Y65.51   Performance of wrong procedure (operation) on correct patient
Wrong device implanted into correct surgical site
Excludes1   performance of correct procedure (operation) on wrong side or body part (Y65.53)

● Y65.52   Performance of procedure (operation) on patient not scheduled for surgery
Performance of procedure (operation) intended for another patient
Performance of procedure (operation) on wrong patient

● Y65.53   Performance of correct procedure (operation) on wrong side or body part
Performance of correct procedure (operation) on wrong side
Performance of correct procedure (operation) on wrong site

Y65.8   Other specified misadventures during surgical and medical care
Coding Clinic: 2019, Q2, P24

Y66   Nonadministration of surgical and medical care
Premature cessation of surgical and medical care
Excludes1   DNR status (Z66)
palliative care (Z51.5)

Y69   Unspecified misadventure during surgical and medical care

---

MEDICAL DEVICES ASSOCIATED WITH ADVERSE INCIDENTS IN DIAGNOSTIC AND THERAPEUTIC USE (Y70-Y82)

Includes   breakdown or malfunction of medical devices (during use) (after implantation) (ongoing use)

Excludes2   later complications following use of medical devices without breakdown or malfunctioning of device (Y83-Y84)
misadventure to patients during surgical and medical care, classifiable to (Y62-Y69)
surgical and other medical procedures as the cause of abnormal reaction of the patient, or of later complication, without mention of misadventure at the time of the procedure (Y83-Y84)

● Y70   Anesthesiology devices associated with adverse incidents

Y70.0   Diagnostic and monitoring anesthesiology devices associated with adverse incidents

Y70.1   Therapeutic (nonsurgical) and rehabilitative anesthesiology devices associated with adverse incidents

Y70.2   Prosthetic and other implants, materials and accessory anesthesiology devices associated with adverse incidents

Y70.3   Surgical instruments, materials and anesthesiology devices (including sutures) associated with adverse incidents

Y70.8   Miscellaneous anesthesiology devices associated with adverse incidents, not elsewhere classified

● Y71   Cardiovascular devices associated with adverse incidents

Y71.0   Diagnostic and monitoring cardiovascular devices associated with adverse incidents

Y71.1   Therapeutic (nonsurgical) and rehabilitative cardiovascular devices associated with adverse incidents

Y71.2   Prosthetic and other implants, materials and accessory cardiovascular devices associated with adverse incidents

Y71.3   Surgical instruments, materials and cardiovascular devices (including sutures) associated with adverse incidents

Y71.8   Miscellaneous cardiovascular devices associated with adverse incidents, not elsewhere classified

● Y72   Otorhinolaryngological devices associated with adverse incidents

Y72.0   Diagnostic and monitoring otorhinolaryngological devices associated with adverse incidents

Y72.1   Therapeutic (nonsurgical) and rehabilitative otorhinolaryngological devices associated with adverse incidents

Y72.2   Prosthetic and other implants, materials and accessory otorhinolaryngological devices associated with adverse incidents

Y72.3   Surgical instruments, materials and otorhinolaryngological devices (including sutures) associated with adverse incidents

Y72.8   Miscellaneous otorhinolaryngological devices associated with adverse incidents, not elsewhere classified

● Y73   Gastroenterology and urology devices associated with adverse incidents

Y73.0   Diagnostic and monitoring gastroenterology and urology devices associated with adverse incidents

Y73.1   Therapeutic (nonsurgical) and rehabilitative gastroenterology and urology devices associated with adverse incidents

Y73.2   Prosthetic and other implants, materials and accessory gastroenterology and urology devices associated with adverse incidents

Y73.3   Surgical instruments, materials and gastroenterology and urology devices (including sutures) associated with adverse incidents

Y73.8   Miscellaneous gastroenterology and urology devices associated with adverse incidents, not elsewhere classified

CHAPTER 20 (V00-Y99)

●Y74　**General hospital and personal-use** devices associated with adverse incidents

Y74.0　Diagnostic and monitoring general hospital and personal-use devices associated with adverse incidents

Y74.1　Therapeutic (nonsurgical) and rehabilitative general hospital and personal-use devices associated with adverse incidents

Y74.2　Prosthetic and other implants, materials and accessory general hospital and personal-use devices associated with adverse incidents

Y74.3　Surgical instruments, materials and general hospital and personal-use devices (including sutures) associated with adverse incidents

Y74.8　Miscellaneous general hospital and personal-use devices associated with adverse incidents, not elsewhere classified

●Y75　**Neurological** devices associated with adverse incidents

Y75.0　Diagnostic and monitoring neurological devices associated with adverse incidents

Y75.1　Therapeutic (nonsurgical) and rehabilitative neurological devices associated with adverse incidents

Y75.2　Prosthetic and other implants, materials and neurological devices associated with adverse incidents

Y75.3　Surgical instruments, materials and neurological devices (including sutures) associated with adverse incidents

Y75.8　Miscellaneous neurological devices associated with adverse incidents, not elsewhere classified

●Y76　**Obstetric and gynecological** devices associated with adverse incidents

Y76.0　Diagnostic and monitoring obstetric and gynecological devices associated with adverse incidents

Y76.1　Therapeutic (nonsurgical) and rehabilitative obstetric and gynecological devices associated with adverse incidents

Y76.2　Prosthetic and other implants, materials and accessory obstetric and gynecological devices associated with adverse incidents

Y76.3　Surgical instruments, materials and obstetric and gynecological devices (including sutures) associated with adverse incidents

Y76.8　Miscellaneous obstetric and gynecological devices associated with adverse incidents, not elsewhere classified

●Y77　**Ophthalmic** devices associated with adverse incidents

Y77.0　Diagnostic and monitoring ophthalmic devices associated with adverse incidents

●Y77.1　Therapeutic (nonsurgical) and rehabilitative ophthalmic devices associated with adverse incidents

Y77.11　Contact lens associated with adverse incidents
　Rigid gas permeable contact lens associated with adverse incidents
　Soft (hydrophilic) contact lens associated with adverse incidents

Y77.19　Other therapeutic (nonsurgical) and rehabilitative ophthalmic devices associated with adverse incidents

Y77.2　Prosthetic and other implants, materials and accessory ophthalmic devices associated with adverse incidents

Y77.3　Surgical instruments, materials and ophthalmic devices (including sutures) associated with adverse incidents

Y77.8　Miscellaneous ophthalmic devices associated with adverse incidents, not elsewhere classified

●Y78　**Radiological** devices associated with adverse incidents

Y78.0　Diagnostic and monitoring radiological devices associated with adverse incidents

Y78.1　Therapeutic (nonsurgical) and rehabilitative radiological devices associated with adverse incidents

Y78.2　Prosthetic and other implants, materials and accessory radiological devices associated with adverse incidents

Y78.3　Surgical instruments, materials and radiological devices (including sutures) associated with adverse incidents

Y78.8　Miscellaneous radiological devices associated with adverse incidents, not elsewhere classified

●Y79　**Orthopedic** devices associated with adverse incidents

Y79.0　Diagnostic and monitoring orthopedic devices associated with adverse incidents

Y79.1　Therapeutic (nonsurgical) and rehabilitative orthopedic devices associated with adverse incidents

Y79.2　Prosthetic and other implants, materials and accessory orthopedic devices associated with adverse incidents

Y79.3　Surgical instruments, materials and orthopedic devices (including sutures) associated with adverse incidents

Y79.8　Miscellaneous orthopedic devices associated with adverse incidents, not elsewhere classified

●Y80　**Physical medicine** devices associated with adverse incidents

Y80.0　Diagnostic and monitoring physical medicine devices associated with adverse incidents

Y80.1　Therapeutic (nonsurgical) and rehabilitative physical medicine devices associated with adverse incidents

Y80.2　Prosthetic and other implants, materials and accessory physical medicine devices associated with adverse incidents

Y80.3　Surgical instruments, materials and physical medicine devices (including sutures) associated with adverse incidents

Y80.8　Miscellaneous physical medicine devices associated with adverse incidents, not elsewhere classified

●Y81　**General- and plastic-surgery** devices associated with adverse incidents

Y81.0　Diagnostic and monitoring general- and plastic-surgery devices associated with adverse incidents

Y81.1　Therapeutic (nonsurgical) and rehabilitative general- and plastic-surgery devices associated with adverse incidents

Y81.2　Prosthetic and other implants, materials and accessory general- and plastic-surgery devices associated with adverse incidents

Y81.3　Surgical instruments, materials and general- and plastic-surgery devices (including sutures) associated with adverse incidents

Y81.8　Miscellaneous general- and plastic-surgery devices associated with adverse incidents, not elsewhere classified

●Y82　Other and unspecified medical devices associated with adverse incidents

Y82.8　Other medical devices associated with adverse incidents

Y82.9　Unspecified medical devices associated with adverse incidents

SURGICAL AND OTHER MEDICAL PROCEDURES AS THE CAUSE OF ABNORMAL REACTION OF THE PATIENT, OR OF LATER COMPLICATION, WITHOUT MENTION OF MISADVENTURE AT THE TIME OF THE PROCEDURE (Y83-Y84)

Excludes1　misadventures to patients during surgical and medical care, classifiable to (Y62-Y69)

Excludes2　breakdown or malfunctioning of medical device (after implantation) (during procedure) (ongoing use) (Y70-Y82)

●Y83　Surgical operation and other surgical procedures as the cause of abnormal reaction of the patient, or of later complication, without mention of misadventure at the time of the procedure

Y83.0　Surgical operation with transplant of whole organ as the cause of abnormal reaction of the patient, or of later complication, without mention of misadventure at the time of the procedure

Y83.1　Surgical operation with implant of artificial internal device as the cause of abnormal reaction of the patient, or of later complication, without mention of misadventure at the time of the procedure

▶ New　⇒ Revised　~~deleted~~ Deleted　Excludes 1　Excludes 2　Includes　Use additional　Code first　Code also　Key words

OGCR Official Guidelines　X Assign placeholder X　● Use Additional Character(s)　▶ Manifestation Code　Hierarchical Condition Category　**Coding Clinic**

Y83.2 Surgical operation with anastomosis, bypass or graft as the cause of abnormal reaction of the patient, or of later complication, without mention of misadventure at the time of the procedure

Y83.3 Surgical operation with formation of external stoma as the cause of abnormal reaction of the patient, or of later complication, without mention of misadventure at the time of the procedure

Y83.4 Other reconstructive surgery as the cause of abnormal reaction of the patient, or of later complication, without mention of misadventure at the time of the procedure

Y83.5 Amputation of limb(s) as the cause of abnormal reaction of the patient, or of later complication, without mention of misadventure at the time of the procedure

Y83.6 Removal of other organ (partial) (total) as the cause of abnormal reaction of the patient, or of later complication, without mention of misadventure at the time of the procedure

Y83.8 Other surgical procedures as the cause of abnormal reaction of the patient, or of later complication, without mention of misadventure at the time of the procedure
> Coding Clinic: 2023, Q2, P14

Y83.9 Surgical procedure, unspecified as the cause of abnormal reaction of the patient, or of later complication, without mention of misadventure at the time of the procedure

● **Y84** Other medical procedures as the cause of abnormal reaction of the patient, or of later complication, without mention of misadventure at the time of the procedure

Y84.0 Cardiac catheterization as the cause of abnormal reaction of the patient, or of later complication, without mention of misadventure at the time of the procedure

Y84.1 Kidney dialysis as the cause of abnormal reaction of the patient, or of later complication, without mention of misadventure at the time of the procedure

Y84.2 Radiological procedure and radiotherapy as the cause of abnormal reaction of the patient, or of later complication, without mention of misadventure at the time of the procedure
> Coding Clinic: 2019, Q1, P21; 2017, Q1, P34

Y84.3 Shock therapy as the cause of abnormal reaction of the patient, or of later complication, without mention of misadventure at the time of the procedure

Y84.4 Aspiration of fluid as the cause of abnormal reaction of the patient, or of later complication, without mention of misadventure at the time of the procedure

Y84.5 Insertion of gastric or duodenal sound as the cause of abnormal reaction of the patient, or of later complication, without mention of misadventure at the time of the procedure

Y84.6 Urinary catheterization as the cause of abnormal reaction of the patient, or of later complication, without mention of misadventure at the time of the procedure

Y84.7 Blood-sampling as the cause of abnormal reaction of the patient, or of later complication, without mention of misadventure at the time of the procedure

Y84.8 Other medical procedures as the cause of abnormal reaction of the patient, or of later complication, without mention of misadventure at the time of the procedure
> Coding Clinic: 2024, Q1, P26; 2023, Q2, P28; 2021, Q1, P5

Y84.9 Medical procedure, unspecified as the cause of abnormal reaction of the patient, or of later complication, without mention of misadventure at the time of the procedure

SUPPLEMENTARY FACTORS RELATED TO CAUSES OF MORBIDITY CLASSIFIED ELSEWHERE (Y90-Y99)

Note: These categories may be used to provide supplementary information concerning causes of morbidity. They are not to be used for single-condition coding.

● **Y90** Evidence of alcohol involvement determined by blood alcohol level
Code first any associated alcohol related disorders (F10)
> Coding Clinic: 2024, Q2, P10

Y90.0 Blood alcohol level of less than 20 mg/100 ml

Y90.1 Blood alcohol level of 20-39 mg/100 ml

Y90.2 Blood alcohol level of 40-59 mg/100 ml

Y90.3 Blood alcohol level of 60-79 mg/100 ml

Y90.4 Blood alcohol level of 80-99 mg/100 ml

Y90.5 Blood alcohol level of 100-119 mg/100 ml

Y90.6 Blood alcohol level of 120-199 mg/100 ml

Y90.7 Blood alcohol level of 200-239 mg/100 ml

Y90.8 Blood alcohol level of 240 mg/100 ml or more

Y90.9 Presence of alcohol in blood, level not specified

OGCR Section I.C.20.b.

Place of Occurrence Guideline

Codes from category Y92, Place of occurrence of the external cause, are secondary codes for use after other external cause codes to identify the location of the patient at the time of injury or other condition.

Generally, a place of occurrence code is assigned only once, at the initial encounter for treatment. However, in the rare instance that a new injury occurs during hospitalization, an additional place of occurrence code may be assigned. No 7th characters are used for Y92. Only one code from Y92 should be recorded on a medical record.

Do not use place of occurrence code Y92.9 if the place is not stated or is not applicable.

● **Y92** Place of occurrence of the external cause
The following category is for use, when relevant, to identify the place of occurrence of the external cause. Use in conjunction with an activity code.
Place of occurrence should be recorded only at the initial encounter for treatment

● **Y92.0** Non-institutional (private) residence as the place of occurrence of the external cause
> **Excludes1**   abandoned or derelict house (Y92.89)
> home under construction but not yet occupied (Y92.6-)
> institutional place of residence (Y92.1-)

● **Y92.00** Unspecified non-institutional (private) residence as the place of occurrence of the external cause

Y92.000 Kitchen of unspecified non-institutional (private) residence as the place of occurrence of the external cause

Y92.001 Dining room of unspecified non-institutional (private) residence as the place of occurrence of the external cause

Y92.002 Bathroom of unspecified non-institutional (private) residence as the place of occurrence of the external cause

Y92.003 Bedroom of unspecified non-institutional (private) residence as the place of occurrence of the external cause

Y92.007 Garden or yard of unspecified non-institutional (private) residence as the place of occurrence of the external cause

Y92.008 Other place in unspecified non-institutional (private) residence as the place of occurrence of the external cause

Y92.009 Unspecified place in unspecified non-institutional (private) residence as the place of occurrence of the external cause
Home (NOS) as the place of occurrence of the external cause
> Coding Clinic: 2021, Q2, P5

CHAPTER 20 (V00-Y99)

CHAPTER 20 (V00-Y99)

- **Y92.01 Single-family non-institutional (private) house as the place of occurrence of the external cause**
  Farmhouse as the place of occurrence of the external cause

  Excludes1   barn (Y92.71)
  chicken coop or hen house (Y92.72)
  farm field (Y92.73)
  orchard (Y92.74)
  single family mobile home or trailer (Y92.02-)
  slaughter house (Y92.86)

  - Y92.010 **Kitchen** of single-family (private) house as the place of occurrence of the external cause
  - Y92.011 **Dining room** of single-family (private) house as the place of occurrence of the external cause
  - Y92.012 **Bathroom** of single-family (private) house as the place of occurrence of the external cause
  - Y92.013 **Bedroom** of single-family (private) house as the place of occurrence of the external cause
  - Y92.014 **Private driveway** to single-family (private) house as the place of occurrence of the external cause
  - Y92.015 **Private garage** of single-family (private) house as the place of occurrence of the external cause
  - Y92.016 **Swimming pool** in single-family (private) house or garden as the place of occurrence of the external cause
  - Y92.017 **Garden or yard** in single-family (private) house as the place of occurrence of the external cause
  - Y92.018 **Other place** in single-family (private) house as the place of occurrence of the external cause
  - Y92.019 **Unspecified** place in single-family (private) house as the place of occurrence of the external cause

- **Y92.02 Mobile home as the place of occurrence of the external cause**
  - Y92.020 **Kitchen** in mobile home as the place of occurrence of the external cause
  - Y92.021 **Dining room** in mobile home as the place of occurrence of the external cause
  - Y92.022 **Bathroom** in mobile home as the place of occurrence of the external cause
  - Y92.023 **Bedroom** in mobile home as the place of occurrence of the external cause
  - Y92.024 **Driveway** of mobile home as the place of occurrence of the external cause
  - Y92.025 **Garage** of mobile home as the place of occurrence of the external cause
  - Y92.026 **Swimming pool** of mobile home as the place of occurrence of the external cause
  - Y92.027 **Garden or yard** of mobile home as the place of occurrence of the external cause
  - Y92.028 **Other place** in mobile home as the place of occurrence of the external cause
  - Y92.029 **Unspecified** place in mobile home as the place of occurrence of the external cause

- **Y92.03 Apartment as the place of occurrence of the external cause**
  Condominium as the place of occurrence of the external cause
  Co-op apartment as the place of occurrence of the external cause

  - Y92.030 **Kitchen** in apartment as the place of occurrence of the external cause
  - Y92.031 **Bathroom** in apartment as the place of occurrence of the external cause
  - Y92.032 **Bedroom** in apartment as the place of occurrence of the external cause
  - Y92.038 **Other place** in apartment as the place of occurrence of the external cause
  - Y92.039 **Unspecified** place in apartment as the place of occurrence of the external cause

- **Y92.04 Boarding-house as the place of occurrence of the external cause**
  - Y92.040 **Kitchen** in boarding-house as the place of occurrence of the external cause
  - Y92.041 **Bathroom** in boarding-house as the place of occurrence of the external cause
  - Y92.042 **Bedroom** in boarding-house as the place of occurrence of the external cause
  - Y92.043 **Driveway** of boarding-house as the place of occurrence of the external cause
  - Y92.044 **Garage** of boarding-house as the place of occurrence of the external cause
  - Y92.045 **Swimming pool** of boarding-house as the place of occurrence of the external cause
  - Y92.046 **Garden or yard** of boarding-house as the place of occurrence of the external cause
  - Y92.048 **Other place** in boarding-house as the place of occurrence of the external cause
  - Y92.049 **Unspecified** place in boarding-house as the place of occurrence of the external cause

- **Y92.09 Other non-institutional residence as the place of occurrence of the external cause**
  - Y92.090 **Kitchen** in other non-institutional residence as the place of occurrence of the external cause
  - Y92.091 **Bathroom** in other non-institutional residence as the place of occurrence of the external cause
  - Y92.092 **Bedroom** in other non-institutional residence as the place of occurrence of the external cause
  - Y92.093 **Driveway** of other non-institutional residence as the place of occurrence of the external cause
  - Y92.094 **Garage** of other non-institutional residence as the place of occurrence of the external cause
  - Y92.095 **Swimming pool** of other non-institutional residence as the place of occurrence of the external cause
  - Y92.096 **Garden or yard** of other non-institutional residence as the place of occurrence of the external cause
  - Y92.098 **Other place** in other non-institutional residence as the place of occurrence of the external cause
  - Y92.099 **Unspecified** place in other non-institutional residence as the place of occurrence of the external cause

  Coding Clinic: 2017, Q2, P10

▶ New   ⇒ Revised   ~~deleted~~ Deleted   Excludes 1   Excludes 2   Includes   Use additional   Code first   Code also   Key words
OGCR Official Guidelines   X Assign placeholder X   ● Use Additional Character(s)   ▶ Manifestation Code   ⬢ Hierarchical Condition Category   **Coding Clinic**

- **Y92.1** Institutional (nonprivate) residence as the place of occurrence of the external cause

  Y92.10 Unspecified residential institution as the place of occurrence of the external cause

- **Y92.11** Children's home and orphanage as the place of occurrence of the external cause

  Y92.110 Kitchen in children's home and orphanage as the place of occurrence of the external cause

  Y92.111 Bathroom in children's home and orphanage as the place of occurrence of the external cause

  Y92.112 Bedroom in children's home and orphanage as the place of occurrence of the external cause

  Y92.113 Driveway of children's home and orphanage as the place of occurrence of the external cause

  Y92.114 Garage of children's home and orphanage as the place of occurrence of the external cause

  Y92.115 Swimming pool of children's home and orphanage as the place of occurrence of the external cause

  Y92.116 Garden or yard of children's home and orphanage as the place of occurrence of the external cause

  Y92.118 Other place in children's home and orphanage as the place of occurrence of the external cause

  Y92.119 Unspecified place in children's home and orphanage as the place of occurrence of the external cause

- **Y92.12** Nursing home as the place of occurrence of the external cause

  Home for the sick as the place of occurrence of the external cause

  Hospice as the place of occurrence of the external cause

  Y92.120 Kitchen in nursing home as the place of occurrence of the external cause

  Y92.121 Bathroom in nursing home as the place of occurrence of the external cause

  Y92.122 Bedroom in nursing home as the place of occurrence of the external cause

  Y92.123 Driveway of nursing home as the place of occurrence of the external cause

  Y92.124 Garage of nursing home as the place of occurrence of the external cause

  Y92.125 Swimming pool of nursing home as the place of occurrence of the external cause

  Y92.126 Garden or yard of nursing home as the place of occurrence of the external cause

  Y92.128 Other place in nursing home as the place of occurrence of the external cause

  Y92.129 Unspecified place in nursing home as the place of occurrence of the external cause

  Coding Clinic: 2017, Q2, P10

- **Y92.13** Military base as the place of occurrence of the external cause

  Excludes1 military training grounds (Y92.83)

  Y92.130 Kitchen on military base as the place of occurrence of the external cause

  Y92.131 Mess hall on military base as the place of occurrence of the external cause

  Y92.133 Barracks on military base as the place of occurrence of the external cause

  Y92.135 Garage on military base as the place of occurrence of the external cause

  Y92.136 Swimming pool on military base as the place of occurrence of the external cause

  Y92.137 Garden or yard on military base as the place of occurrence of the external cause

  Y92.138 Other place on military base as the place of occurrence of the external cause

  Y92.139 Unspecified place military base as the place of occurrence of the external cause

- **Y92.14** Prison as the place of occurrence of the external cause

  Y92.140 Kitchen in prison as the place of occurrence of the external cause

  Y92.141 Dining room in prison as the place of occurrence of the external cause

  Y92.142 Bathroom in prison as the place of occurrence of the external cause

  Y92.143 Cell of prison as the place of occurrence of the external cause

  Y92.146 Swimming pool of prison as the place of occurrence of the external cause

  Y92.147 Courtyard of prison as the place of occurrence of the external cause

  Y92.148 Other place in prison as the place of occurrence of the external cause

  Y92.149 Unspecified place in prison as the place of occurrence of the external cause

- **Y92.15** Reform school as the place of occurrence of the external cause

  Y92.150 Kitchen in reform school as the place of occurrence of the external cause

  Y92.151 Dining room in reform school as the place of occurrence of the external cause

  Y92.152 Bathroom in reform school as the place of occurrence of the external cause

  Y92.153 Bedroom in reform school as the place of occurrence of the external cause

  Y92.154 Driveway of reform school as the place of occurrence of the external cause

  Y92.155 Garage of reform school as the place of occurrence of the external cause

  Y92.156 Swimming pool of reform school as the place of occurrence of the external cause

  Y92.157 Garden or yard of reform school as the place of occurrence of the external cause

  Y92.158 Other place in reform school as the place of occurrence of the external cause

  Y92.159 Unspecified place in reform school as the place of occurrence of the external cause

- **Y92.16** School dormitory as the place of occurrence of the external cause

  Excludes1 reform school as the place of occurrence of the external cause (Y92.15-)
  school buildings and grounds as the place of occurrence of the external cause (Y92.2-)
  school sports and athletic areas as the place of occurrence of the external cause (Y92.3-)

  Y92.160 Kitchen in school dormitory as the place of occurrence of the external cause

CHAPTER 20 (V00-Y99)

Y92.161   **Dining room** in school dormitory as the place of occurrence of the external cause

Y92.162   **Bathroom** in school dormitory as the place of occurrence of the external cause

Y92.163   **Bedroom** in school dormitory as the place of occurrence of the external cause

Y92.168   **Other place** in school dormitory as the place of occurrence of the external cause

Y92.169   **Unspecified** place in school dormitory as the place of occurrence of the external cause

● Y92.19   **Other specified residential institution** as the place of occurrence of the external cause

Y92.190   **Kitchen** in other specified residential institution as the place of occurrence of the external cause

Y92.191   **Dining room** in other specified residential institution as the place of occurrence of the external cause

Y92.192   **Bathroom** in other specified residential institution as the place of occurrence of the external cause

Y92.193   **Bedroom** in other specified residential institution as the place of occurrence of the external cause

Y92.194   **Driveway** of other specified residential institution as the place of occurrence of the external cause

Y92.195   **Garage** of other specified residential institution as the place of occurrence of the external cause

Y92.196   **Pool** of other specified residential institution as the place of occurrence of the external cause

Y92.197   **Garden or yard** of other specified residential institution as the place of occurrence of the external cause

Y92.198   **Other place** in other specified residential institution as the place of occurrence of the external cause
Coding Clinic: 2017, Q2, P11

Y92.199   **Unspecified** place in other specified residential institution as the place of occurrence of the external cause
Coding Clinic: 2017, Q2, P10

● Y92.2   **School, other institution and public administrative area** as the place of occurrence of the external cause
Building and adjacent grounds used by the general public or by a particular group of the public

Excludes1   building under construction as the place of occurrence of the external cause (Y92.6)
residential institution as the place of occurrence of the external cause (Y92.1)
school dormitory as the place of occurrence of the external cause (Y92.16-)
sports and athletics area of schools as the place of occurrence of the external cause (Y92.3-)

● Y92.21   **School (private) (public) (state)** as the place of occurrence of the external cause

Y92.210   **Daycare center** as the place of occurrence of the external cause

Y92.211   **Elementary school** as the place of occurrence of the external cause
Kindergarten as the place of occurrence of the external cause

Y92.212   **Middle school** as the place of occurrence of the external cause

Y92.213   **High school** as the place of occurrence of the external cause
Coding Clinic: 2012, Q4, P108

Y92.214   **College** as the place of occurrence of the external cause
University as the place of occurrence of the external cause

Y92.215   **Trade school** as the place of occurrence of the external cause

Y92.218   **Other school** as the place of occurrence of the external cause

Y92.219   **Unspecified** school as the place of occurrence of the external cause

Y92.22   **Religious institution** as the place of occurrence of the external cause
Church as the place of occurrence of the external cause
Mosque as the place of occurrence of the external cause
Synagogue as the place of occurrence of the external cause

● Y92.23   **Hospital** as the place of occurrence of the external cause

Excludes1   ambulatory (outpatient) health services establishments (Y92.53-)
home for the sick as the place of occurrence of the external cause (Y92.12-)
hospice as the place of occurrence of the external cause (Y92.12-)
nursing home as the place of occurrence of the external cause (Y92.12-)

Y92.230   **Patient room** in hospital as the place of occurrence of the external cause

Y92.231   **Patient bathroom** in hospital as the place of occurrence of the external cause

Y92.232   **Corridor** of hospital as the place of occurrence of the external cause

Y92.233   **Cafeteria** of hospital as the place of occurrence of the external cause

Y92.234   **Operating room** of hospital as the place of occurrence of the external cause

Y92.238   **Other place** in hospital as the place of occurrence of the external cause

Y92.239   **Unspecified** place in hospital as the place of occurrence of the external cause

● Y92.24   **Public administrative building** as the place of occurrence of the external cause

Y92.240   **Courthouse** as the place of occurrence of the external cause

Y92.241   **Library** as the place of occurrence of the external cause

Y92.242   **Post office** as the place of occurrence of the external cause

Y92.243   **City hall** as the place of occurrence of the external cause

Y92.248   **Other** public administrative building as the place of occurrence of the external cause

● Y92.25   **Cultural building** as the place of occurrence of the external cause

Y92.250   **Art gallery** as the place of occurrence of the external cause

Y92.251   **Museum** as the place of occurrence of the external cause

Y92.252   **Music hall** as the place of occurrence of the external cause

▶ New   ⇒ Revised   ~~deleted~~ Deleted   Excludes 1   Excludes 2   Includes   Use additional   Code first   Code also   Key words
OGCR Official Guidelines   X Assign placeholder X   ● Use Additional Character(s)   ▶ Manifestation Code   ⚒ Hierarchical Condition Category   Coding Clinic

Y92.253   **Opera house** as the place of occurrence of the external cause

Y92.254   **Theater (live)** as the place of occurrence of the external cause

Y92.258   **Other** cultural public building as the place of occurrence of the external cause

Y92.26   **Movie house or cinema** as the place of occurrence of the external cause

Y92.29   **Other specified public building** as the place of occurrence of the external cause
> Assembly hall as the place of occurrence of the external cause
> Clubhouse as the place of occurrence of the external cause

● Y92.3   **Sports and athletics area** as the place of occurrence of the external cause

  ● Y92.31   **Athletic court** as the place of occurrence of the external cause
> **Excludes1**   tennis court in private home or garden (Y92.09)

     Y92.310   **Basketball** court as the place of occurrence of the external cause

     Y92.311   **Squash** court as the place of occurrence of the external cause

     Y92.312   **Tennis** court as the place of occurrence of the external cause

     Y92.318   **Other** athletic court as the place of occurrence of the external cause

  ● Y92.32   **Athletic field** as the place of occurrence of the external cause

     Y92.320   **Baseball** field as the place of occurrence of the external cause

     Y92.321   **Football** field as the place of occurrence of the external cause

     Y92.322   **Soccer** field as the place of occurrence of the external cause

     Y92.328   **Other** athletic field as the place of occurrence of the external cause
> Cricket field as the place of occurrence of the external cause
> Hockey field as the place of occurrence of the external cause

  ● Y92.33   **Skating rink** as the place of occurrence of the external cause

     Y92.330   **Ice** skating rink (indoor) (outdoor) as the place of occurrence of the external cause

     Y92.331   **Roller** skating rink as the place of occurrence of the external cause

   Y92.34   **Swimming pool (public)** as the place of occurrence of the external cause
> **Excludes1**   swimming pool in private home or garden (Y92.016)

   Y92.39   **Other specified sports and athletic area** as the place of occurrence of the external cause
> Golf-course as the place of occurrence of the external cause
> Gymnasium as the place of occurrence of the external cause
> Riding-school as the place of occurrence of the external cause
> Stadium as the place of occurrence of the external cause

● Y92.4   **Street, highway and other paved roadways** as the place of occurrence of the external cause
> **Excludes1**   private driveway of residence (Y92.014, Y92.024, Y92.043, Y92.093, Y92.113, Y92.123, Y92.154, Y92.194)

  ● Y92.41   **Street and highway** as the place of occurrence of the external cause

Y92.410   **Unspecified** street and highway as the place of occurrence of the external cause
> Road NOS as the place of occurrence of the external cause

Y92.411   **Interstate** highway as the place of occurrence of the external cause
> Freeway as the place of occurrence of the external cause
> Motorway as the place of occurrence of the external cause

Y92.412   **Parkway** as the place of occurrence of the external cause

Y92.413   **State road** as the place of occurrence of the external cause

Y92.414   **Local residential or business street** as the place of occurrence of the external cause

Y92.415   **Exit ramp or entrance ramp** of street or highway as the place of occurrence of the external cause

● Y92.48   **Other paved roadways** as the place of occurrence of the external cause

     Y92.480   **Sidewalk** as the place of occurrence of the external cause

     Y92.481   **Parking lot** as the place of occurrence of the external cause

     Y92.482   **Bike path** as the place of occurrence of the external cause

     Y92.488   **Other** paved roadways as the place of occurrence of the external cause

● Y92.5   **Trade and service area** as the place of occurrence of the external cause
> **Excludes1**   garage in private home (Y92.015)
> schools and other public administration buildings (Y92.2-)

  ● Y92.51   **Private commercial establishments** as the place of occurrence of the external cause

     Y92.510   **Bank** as the place of occurrence of the external cause

     Y92.511   **Restaurant or café** as the place of occurrence of the external cause

     Y92.512   **Supermarket, store or market** as the place of occurrence of the external cause

     Y92.513   **Shop (commercial)** as the place of occurrence of the external cause

  ● Y92.52   **Service areas** as the place of occurrence of the external cause

     Y92.520   **Airport** as the place of occurrence of the external cause

     Y92.521   **Bus station** as the place of occurrence of the external cause

     Y92.522   **Railway station** as the place of occurrence of the external cause

     Y92.523   **Highway rest stop** as the place of occurrence of the external cause

     Y92.524   **Gas station** as the place of occurrence of the external cause
> Petroleum station as the place of occurrence of the external cause
> Service station as the place of occurrence of the external cause

CHAPTER 20 (V00-Y99)

● **Y92.53** **Ambulatory health services establishments** as the place of occurrence of the external cause

    Y92.530 **Ambulatory surgery center** as the place of occurrence of the external cause

        Outpatient surgery center, including that connected with a hospital as the place of occurrence of the external cause

        Same day surgery center, including that connected with a hospital as the place of occurrence of the external cause

    Y92.531 **Health care provider office** as the place of occurrence of the external cause

        Physician office as the place of occurrence of the external cause

    Y92.532 **Urgent care center** as the place of occurrence of the external cause

    Y92.538 **Other** ambulatory health services establishments as the place of occurrence of the external cause

        Coding Clinic: 2019, Q1, P21

  Y92.59 **Other** trade areas as the place of occurrence of the external cause

    Office building as the place of occurrence of the external cause

    Casino as the place of occurrence of the external cause

    Garage (commercial) as the place of occurrence of the external cause

    Hotel as the place of occurrence of the external cause

    Radio or television station as the place of occurrence of the external cause

    Shopping mall as the place of occurrence of the external cause

    Warehouse as the place of occurrence of the external cause

● **Y92.6** **Industrial and construction area** as the place of occurrence of the external cause

  Y92.61 **Building [any] under construction** as the place of occurrence of the external cause

  Y92.62 **Dock or shipyard** as the place of occurrence of the external cause

    Dockyard as the place of occurrence of the external cause

    Dry dock as the place of occurrence of the external cause

    Shipyard as the place of occurrence of the external cause

  Y92.63 **Factory** as the place of occurrence of the external cause

    Factory building as the place of occurrence of the external cause

    Factory premises as the place of occurrence of the external cause

    Industrial yard as the place of occurrence of the external cause

  Y92.64 **Mine or pit** as the place of occurrence of the external cause

    Mine as the place of occurrence of the external cause

  Y92.65 **Oil rig** as the place of occurrence of the external cause

    Pit (coal) (gravel) (sand) as the place of occurrence of the external cause

  Y92.69 **Other** specified industrial and construction area as the place of occurrence of the external cause

    Gasworks as the place of occurrence of the external cause

    Power-station (coal) (nuclear) (oil) as the place of occurrence of the external cause

    Tunnel under construction as the place of occurrence of the external cause

    Workshop as the place of occurrence of the external cause

● **Y92.7** **Farm** as the place of occurrence of the external cause

    Ranch as the place of occurrence of the external cause

    Excludes1   farmhouse and home premises of farm (Y92.01-)

  Y92.71 **Barn** as the place of occurrence of the external cause

  Y92.72 **Chicken coop** as the place of occurrence of the external cause

    Hen house as the place of occurrence of the external cause

  Y92.73 **Farm field** as the place of occurrence of the external cause

  Y92.74 **Orchard** as the place of occurrence of the external cause

  Y92.79 **Other farm location** as the place of occurrence of the external cause

● **Y92.8** **Other places** as the place of occurrence of the external cause

 ● **Y92.81** **Transport vehicle** as the place of occurrence of the external cause

    Excludes1   transport accidents (V00-V99)

    Y92.810 **Car** as the place of occurrence of the external cause

    Y92.811 **Bus** as the place of occurrence of the external cause

    Y92.812 **Truck** as the place of occurrence of the external cause

    Y92.813 **Airplane** as the place of occurrence of the external cause

    Y92.814 **Boat** as the place of occurrence of the external cause

    Y92.815 **Train** as the place of occurrence of the external cause

    Y92.816 **Subway** car as the place of occurrence of the external cause

    Y92.818 **Other** transport vehicle as the place of occurrence of the external cause

 ● **Y92.82** **Wilderness area**

    Y92.820 **Desert** as the place of occurrence of the external cause

    Y92.821 **Forest** as the place of occurrence of the external cause

    Y92.828 **Other wilderness area** as the place of occurrence of the external cause

        Swamp as the place of occurrence of the external cause

        Mountain as the place of occurrence of the external cause

        Marsh as the place of occurrence of the external cause

        Prairie as the place of occurrence of the external cause

 ● **Y92.83** **Recreation area** as the place of occurrence of the external cause

    Y92.830 **Public park** as the place of occurrence of the external cause

    Y92.831 **Amusement park** as the place of occurrence of the external cause

    Y92.832 **Beach** as the place of occurrence of the external cause

        Seashore as the place of occurrence of the external cause

    Y92.833 **Campsite** as the place of occurrence of the external cause

    Y92.834 **Zoological garden (zoo)** as the place of occurrence of the external cause

    Y92.838 **Other recreation area** as the place of occurrence of the external cause

  Y92.84 **Military training ground** as the place of occurrence of the external cause

  Y92.85 **Railroad track** as the place of occurrence of the external cause

▶ New   ⟹ Revised   ~~deleted~~ Deleted   Excludes 1   Excludes 2   Includes   Use additional   Code first   Code also   Key words

OGCR Official Guidelines   X Assign placeholder X   ● Use Additional Character(s)   ⟩ Manifestation Code   🌀 Hierarchical Condition Category   Coding Clinic

Y92.86   **Slaughter house** as the place of occurrence of the external cause

Y92.89   **Other specified places** as the place of occurrence of the external cause

     Derelict house as the place of occurrence of the external cause

OGCR Section I.C.20.b.

Do not use place of occurrence code Y92.9 if the place is not stated or is not applicable.

Y92.9   **Unspecified** place or not applicable

OGCR See Section I.C.20.c.

Activity Code

Assign a code from category Y93, Activity code, to describe the activity of the patient at the time the injury or other health condition occurred.

An activity code is used only once, at the initial encounter for treatment. Only one code from Y93 should be recorded on a medical record.

The activity codes are not applicable to poisonings, adverse effects, misadventures or sequela.

Do not assign Y93.9, Unspecified activity, if the activity is not stated.

A code from category Y93 is appropriate for use with external cause and intent codes if identifying the activity provides additional information about the event.

● **Y93**   **Activity codes**

     Note: Category Y93 is provided for use to indicate the activity of the person seeking healthcare for an injury or health condition, such as a heart attack while shoveling snow, which resulted from, or was contributed to, by the activity. These codes are appropriate for use for both acute injuries, such as those from Chapter 19, and conditions that are due to the long-term, cumulative effects of an activity, such as those from Chapter 13. They are also appropriate for use with external cause codes for cause and intent if identifying the activity provides additional information on the event. These codes should be used in conjunction with codes for external cause status (Y99) and place of occurrence (Y92).

     This section contains the following broad activity categories:

     Y93.0   Activities involving walking and running

     Y93.1   Activities involving water and water craft

     Y93.2   Activities involving ice and snow

     Y93.3   Activities involving climbing, rappelling, and jumping off

     Y93.4   Activities involving dancing and other rhythmic movement

     Y93.5   Activities involving other sports and athletics played individually

     Y93.6   Activities involving other sports and athletics played as a team or group

     Y93.7   Activities involving other specified sports and athletics

     Y93.A   Activities involving other cardiorespiratory exercise

     Y93.B   Activities involving other muscle strengthening exercises

     Y93.C   Activities involving computer technology and electronic devices

     Y93.D   Activities involving arts and handcrafts

     Y93.E   Activities involving personal hygiene and interior property and clothing maintenance

     Y93.F   Activities involving caregiving

     Y93.G   Activities involving food preparation, cooking and grilling

     Y93.H   Activities involving exterior property and land maintenance, building and construction

     Y93.I   Activities involving roller coasters and other types of external motion

     Y93.J   Activities involving playing musical instrument

     Y93.K   Activities involving animal care

     Y93.8   Activities, other specified

     Y93.9   Activity, unspecified

● **Y93.0**   **Activities involving walking and running**

     Excludes1   Activity, walking an animal (Y93.K1)
                   Activity, walking or running on a treadmill (Y93.A1)

Y93.01   **Activity, walking, marching and hiking**

     Activity, walking, marching and hiking on level or elevated terrain

     Excludes1   activity, mountain climbing (Y93.31)

Y93.02   **Activity, running**

● **Y93.1**   **Activities involving water and water craft**

     Excludes1   activities involving ice (Y93.2-)

Y93.11   **Activity, swimming**

Y93.12   **Activity, springboard and platform diving**

Y93.13   **Activity, water polo**

Y93.14   **Activity, water aerobics and water exercise**

Y93.15   **Activity, underwater diving and snorkeling**

     Activity, SCUBA diving

Y93.16   **Activity, rowing, canoeing, kayaking, rafting and tubing**

     Activity, canoeing, kayaking, rafting and tubing in calm and turbulent water

Y93.17   **Activity, water skiing and wake boarding**

Y93.18   **Activity, surfing, windsurfing and boogie boarding**

     Activity, water sliding

Y93.19   **Activity, other involving water and watercraft**

     Activity involving water NOS
     Activity, parasailing
     Activity, water survival training and testing

● **Y93.2**   **Activities involving ice and snow**

     Excludes1   activity, shoveling ice and snow (Y93.H1)

Y93.21   **Activity, ice skating**

     Activity, figure skating (singles) (pairs)
     Activity, ice dancing

     Excludes1   activity, ice hockey (Y93.22)

Y93.22   **Activity, ice hockey**

Y93.23   **Activity, snow (alpine) (downhill) skiing, snowboarding, sledding, tobogganing and snow tubing**

     Excludes1   activity, cross country skiing (Y93.24)

Y93.24   **Activity, cross country skiing**

     Activity, nordic skiing

Y93.29   **Activity, other activity involving ice and snow**

     Activity, activity involving ice and snow NOS

● **Y93.3**   **Activities involving climbing, rappelling and jumping off**

     Excludes1   activity, hiking on level or elevated terrain (Y93.01)
                   activity, jumping rope (Y93.56)
                   activity, trampoline jumping (Y93.44)

Y93.31   **Activity, mountain climbing, rock climbing and wall climbing**

Y93.32   **Activity, rappelling**

Y93.33   **Activity, BASE jumping**

     Activity, building, Antenna, Span, Earth jumping

Y93.34   **Activity, bungee jumping**

Y93.35   **Activity, hang gliding**

Y93.39   **Activity, other activity involving climbing, rappelling and jumping off**

● **Y93.4**   **Activities involving dancing and other rhythmic movement**

     Excludes1   activity, martial arts (Y93.75)

Y93.41   **Activity, dancing**

     Coding Clinic: 2012, Q4, P108

Y93.42   **Activity, yoga**

Y93.43　**Activity, gymnastics**
　　Activity, rhythmic gymnastics
　　Excludes1　activity, trampolining (Y93.44)

Y93.44　**Activity, trampolining**

Y93.45　**Activity, cheerleading**

Y93.49　**Activity, other involving dancing and other rhythmic movements**

●Y93.5　**Activities involving other sports and athletics played individually**
　　Excludes1　activity, dancing (Y93.41)
　　　　activity, gymnastic (Y93.43)
　　　　activity, trampolining (Y93.44)
　　　　activity, yoga (Y93.42)

Y93.51　**Activity, roller skating (inline) and skateboarding**

Y93.52　**Activity, horseback riding**

Y93.53　**Activity, golf**

Y93.54　**Activity, bowling**

Y93.55　**Activity, bike riding**

Y93.56　**Activity, jumping rope**

Y93.57　**Activity, non-running track and field events**
　　Excludes1　activity, running (any form) (Y93.02)

Y93.59　**Activity, other involving other sports and athletics played individually**
　　Excludes1　activities involving climbing, rappelling, and jumping (Y93.3-)
　　　　activities involving ice and snow (Y93.2-)
　　　　activities involving walking and running (Y93.0-)
　　　　activities involving water and watercraft (Y93.1-)

●Y93.6　**Activities involving other sports and athletics played as a team or group**
　　Excludes1　activity, ice hockey (Y93.22)
　　　　activity, water polo (Y93.13)

Y93.61　**Activity, American tackle football**
　　Activity, football NOS

Y93.62　**Activity, American flag or touch football**

Y93.63　**Activity, rugby**

Y93.64　**Activity, baseball**
　　Activity, softball

Y93.65　**Activity, lacrosse and field hockey**
　　Coding Clinic: 2015, Q1, P9

Y93.66　**Activity, soccer**

Y93.67　**Activity, basketball**
　　Coding Clinic: 2019, Q4, P18

Y93.68　**Activity, volleyball (beach) (court)**

Y93.6A　**Activity, physical games generally associated with school recess, summer camp and children**
　　Activity, capture the flag
　　Activity, dodge ball
　　Activity, four square
　　Activity, kickball

Y93.69　**Activity, other involving other sports and athletics played as a team or group**
　　Cricket

●Y93.7　**Activities involving other specified sports and athletics**

Y93.71　**Activity, boxing**

Y93.72　**Activity, wrestling**

Y93.73　**Activity, racquet and hand sports**
　　Activity, handball
　　Activity, racquetball
　　Activity, squash
　　Activity, tennis

Y93.74　**Activity, frisbee**
　　Activity, ultimate frisbee

Y93.75　**Activity, martial arts**
　　Activity, combatives

Y93.79　**Activity, other specified sports and athletics**
　　Excludes1　sports and athletics activities specified in categories Y93.0-Y93.6

●Y93.A　**Activities involving other cardiorespiratory exercise**
　　Activities involving physical training

Y93.A1　**Activity, exercise machines primarily for cardiorespiratory conditioning**
　　Activity, elliptical and stepper machines
　　Activity, stationary bike
　　Activity, treadmill

Y93.A2　**Activity, calisthenics**
　　Activity, jumping jacks
　　Activity, warm up and cool down

Y93.A3　**Activity, aerobic and step exercise**

Y93.A4　**Activity, circuit training**

Y93.A5　**Activity, obstacle course**
　　Activity, challenge course
　　Activity, confidence course

Y93.A6　**Activity, grass drills**
　　Activity, guerilla drills

Y93.A9　**Activity, other involving other cardiorespiratory exercise**
　　Excludes1　activities involving cardiorespiratory exercise specified in categories Y93.0-Y93.7

●Y93.B　**Activity involving other muscle strengthening exercises**

Y93.B1　**Activity, exercise machines primarily for muscle strengthening**

Y93.B2　**Activity, push-ups, pull-ups, sit-ups**

Y93.B3　**Activity, free weights**
　　Activity, barbells
　　Activity, dumbbells

Y93.B4　**Activity, pilates**

Y93.B9　**Activity, other involving other muscle strengthening exercises**
　　Excludes1　activities involving muscle strengthening specified in categories Y93.0-Y93.A

●Y93.C　**Activities involving computer technology and electronic devices**
　　Excludes1　activity, electronic musical keyboard or instruments (Y93.J-)

Y93.C1　**Activity, computer keyboarding**
　　Activity, electronic game playing using keyboard or other stationary device

Y93.C2　**Activity, hand held interactive electronic device**
　　Activity, cellular telephone and communication device
　　Activity, electronic game playing using interactive device
　　Excludes1　activity, electronic game playing using keyboard or other stationary device (Y93.C1)

Y93.C9　**Activity, other involving computer technology and electronic devices**

●Y93.D　**Activities involving arts and handcrafts**
　　Excludes1　activities involving playing musical instrument (Y93.J-)

Y93.D1　**Knitting and crocheting**

Y93.D2　**Sewing**

Y93.D3　**Furniture building and finishing**
　　Furniture repair

Y93.D9　**Activity, other involving arts and handcrafts**

● **Y93.E**   **Activities involving personal hygiene and interior property and clothing maintenance**

> **Excludes1**   activities involving cooking and grilling (Y93.G-)
> activities involving exterior property and land maintenance, building and construction (Y93.H-)
> activity involving caregiving (Y93.F-)
> activity, dishwashing (Y93.G1)
> activity, food preparation (Y93.G1)
> activity, gardening (Y93.H2)

Y93.E1   Activity, personal bathing and showering

Y93.E2   Activity, laundry

Y93.E3   Activity, vacuuming

Y93.E4   Activity, ironing

Y93.E5   Activity, floor mopping and cleaning

Y93.E6   Activity, residential relocation
> Activity, packing up and unpacking involved in moving to a new residence

Y93.E8   Activity, other personal hygiene activity

Y93.E9   Activity, other household maintenance

● **Y93.F**   **Activities involving person providing caregiving**
> Activity involving the provider of caregiving

Y93.F1   Activity, caregiving involving bathing

Y93.F2   Activity, caregiving involving lifting
> Coding Clinic: 2016, Q4, P74

Y93.F9   Activity, other caregiving

● **Y93.G**   **Activities involving food preparation, cooking and grilling**

Y93.G1   Activity, food preparation and clean up
> Activity, dishwashing

Y93.G2   Activity, grilling and smoking food

Y93.G3   Activity, cooking and baking
> Activity, use of stove, oven and microwave oven

Y93.G9   Activity, other activity involving cooking and grilling

● **Y93.H**   **Activities involving property and land maintenance, building and construction**

Y93.H1   Activity, digging, shoveling and raking
> Activity, dirt digging
> Activity, raking leaves
> Activity, snow shoveling

Y93.H2   Activity, gardening and landscaping
> Activity, pruning, trimming shrubs, weeding

Y93.H3   Activity, building and construction

Y93.H9   Activity, other activity involving property and land maintenance, building and construction

● **Y93.I**   **Activities involving roller coasters and other types of external motion**

Y93.I1   Activity, rollercoaster riding

Y93.I9   Activity, other involving external motion

● **Y93.J**   **Activities involving playing musical instrument**
> Activity involving playing electric musical instrument

Y93.J1   Activity, piano playing
> Activity, musical keyboard (electronic) playing

Y93.J2   Activity, drum and other percussion instrument playing

Y93.J3   Activity, string instrument playing

Y93.J4   Activity, winds and brass instrument playing

● **Y93.K**   **Activities involving animal care**

> **Excludes1**   activity, horseback riding (Y93.52)

Y93.K1   Activity, walking an animal

Y93.K2   Activity, milking an animal

Y93.K3   Activity, grooming and shearing an animal

Y93.K9   Activity, other activity involving animal care

● **Y93.8**   **Other activity**
> Coding Clinic: 2016, Q4, P74

Y93.81   Activity, refereeing a sports activity

Y93.82   Activity, spectator at an event

Y93.83   Activity, rough housing and horseplay
> Coding Clinic: 2015, Q1, P8

Y93.84   Activity, sleeping

Y93.85   Activity, choking game
> Activity, blackout game
> Activity, fainting game
> Activity, pass out game
> Coding Clinic: 2016, Q4, P74-76

Y93.89   Activity, other specified

OGCR   See Section I.C.20.c.

Do not assign Y93.9, Unspecified activity, if the activity is not stated.

● **Y93.9**   **Activity, unspecified**

Y95   **Nosocomial condition**

● **Y99**   **External cause status**

> **Note:** A single code from category Y99 should be used in conjunction with the external cause code(s) assigned to a record to indicate the status of the person at the time the event occurred.
> Coding Clinic: 2016, Q4, P74

Y99.0   Civilian activity done for income or pay
> Civilian activity done for financial or other compensation

> **Excludes1**   military activity (Y99.1)
> volunteer activity (Y99.2)

Y99.1   Military activity

> **Excludes1**   activity of off duty military personnel (Y99.8)

Y99.2   Volunteer activity

> **Excludes1**   activity of child or other family member assisting in compensated work of other family member (Y99.8)

Y99.8   Other external cause status
> Activity NEC
> Activity of child or other family member assisting in compensated work of other family member
> Hobby not done for income
> Leisure activity
> Off-duty activity of military personnel
> Recreation or sport not for income or while a student
> Student activity

> **Excludes1**   civilian activity done for income or compensation (Y99.0)
> military activity (Y99.1)
> Coding Clinic: 2012, Q4, P108

Y99.9   Unspecified external cause status

CHAPTER 21

FACTORS INFLUENCING HEALTH STATUS AND CONTACT WITH HEALTH SERVICES (Z00-Z99)

OGCR Chapter-Specific Coding Guidelines

21. **Chapter 21: Factors influencing health status and contact with health services (Z00-Z99)**
Note: The chapter specific guidelines provide additional information about the use of Z codes for specified encounters.

a. **Use of Z codes in any healthcare setting**
Z codes are for use in any healthcare setting. Z codes may be used as either a first-listed (principal diagnosis code in the inpatient setting) or secondary code, depending on the circumstances of the encounter. Certain Z codes may only be used as first-listed or principal diagnosis.

b. **Z Codes indicate a reason for an encounter**
Z codes are not procedure codes. A corresponding procedure code must accompany a Z code to describe any procedure performed.

c. **Categories of Z Codes**
1) **Contact/Exposure**
Category Z20 indicates contact with, and suspected exposure to, communicable diseases. These codes are for patients who do not show any sign or symptom of a disease but are suspected to have been exposed to it by close personal contact with an infected individual or are in an area where a disease is epidemic.

Category Z77, Other contact with and (suspected) exposures hazardous to health, indicates contact with and suspected exposures hazardous to health.

Contact/exposure codes may be used as a first-listed code to explain an encounter for testing, or, more commonly, as a secondary code to identify a potential risk.

2) **Inoculations and vaccinations**
Code Z23 is for encounters for inoculations and vaccinations. It indicates that a patient is being seen to receive a prophylactic inoculation against a disease. Procedure codes are required to identify the actual administration of the injection and the type(s) of immunizations given. Code Z23 may be used as a secondary code if the inoculation is given as a routine part of preventive health care, such as a well-baby visit.

3) **Status**
Status codes indicate that a patient is either a carrier of a disease or has the sequelae or residual of a past disease or condition. This includes such things as the presence of prosthetic or mechanical devices resulting from past treatment. A status code is informative, because the status may affect the course of treatment and its outcome. A status code is distinct from a history code. The history code indicates that the patient no longer has the condition.

A status code should not be used with a diagnosis code from one of the body system chapters, if the diagnosis code includes the information provided by the status code. For example, code Z94.1, Heart transplant status, should not be used with a code from subcategory T86.2, Complications of heart transplant. The status code does not provide additional information. The complication code indicates that the patient is a heart transplant patient.

For encounters for weaning from a mechanical ventilator, assign a code from subcategory J96.1, Chronic respiratory failure, followed by code Z99.11, Dependence on respirator [ventilator] status.

The status Z codes/categories are:

Z14	Genetic carrier

Genetic carrier status indicates that a person carries a gene, associated with a particular disease, which may be passed to offspring who may develop that disease. The person does not have the disease and is not at risk of developing the disease.

Z15	Genetic susceptibility to disease Genetic

susceptibility indicates that a person has a gene that increases the risk of that person developing the disease.

Codes from category Z15 should not be used as principal or first-listed codes. If the patient has the condition to which he/she is susceptible, and that condition is the reason for the encounter, the code for the current condition should be sequenced first. If the patient is being seen for follow-up after completed treatment for this condition, and the condition no longer exists, a follow-up

code should be sequenced first, followed by the appropriate personal history and genetic susceptibility codes. If the purpose of the encounter is genetic counseling associated with procreative management, code Z31.5, Encounter for genetic counseling, should be assigned as the first-listed code, followed by a code from category Z15. Additional codes should be assigned for any applicable family or personal history.

Z16	Resistance to antimicrobial drugs

This code indicates that a patient has a condition that is resistant to antimicrobial drug treatment. Sequence the infection code first.

Z17	Estrogen receptor status
Z18	Retained foreign body fragments
Z19	Hormone sensitivity malignancy status
Z21	Asymptomatic HIV infection status This code indicates that a patient has tested positive for HIV but has manifested no signs or symptoms of the disease.
Z22	Carrier of infectious disease Carrier status indicates that a person harbors the specific organisms of a disease without manifest symptoms and is capable of transmitting the infection.
Z28.3	Underimmunization status
Z33.1	Pregnant state, incidental This code is a secondary code only for use when the pregnancy is in no way complicating the reason for visit. Otherwise, a code from the obstetric chapter is required.
Z66	Do not resuscitate

This code may be used when it is documented by the provider that a patient is on do not resuscitate status at any time during the stay.

Z67	Blood type
Z68	Body mass index (BMI)

BMI codes should only be assigned when the associated diagnosis (such as overweight or obesity) meets the definition of a reportable diagnosis (see Section III, Reporting Additional Diagnoses). Do not assign BMI codes during pregnancy. See Section I.B.14 for BMI documentation by clinicians other than the patient's provider.

Z74.01	Bed confinement status
Z76.82	Awaiting organ transplant status
Z78	Other specified health status

Code Z78.1, Physical restraint status, may be used when it is documented by the provider that a patient has been put in restraints during the current encounter. Please note that this code should not be reported when it is documented by the provider that a patient is temporarily restrained during a procedure.

Z79	Long-term (current) drug therapy

Codes from this category indicate a patient's continuous use of a prescribed drug (including such things as aspirin therapy) for the long-term treatment of a condition or for prophylactic use. It is not for use for patients who have addictions to drugs. This subcategory is not for use of medications for detoxification or maintenance programs to prevent withdrawal symptoms in patients with drug dependence (e.g., methadone maintenance for opiate dependence). Assign the appropriate code for the drug dependence instead.

Assign a code from Z79 if the patient is receiving a medication for an extended period as a prophylactic measure (such as for the prevention of deep vein thrombosis) or as treatment of a chronic condition (such as arthritis) or a disease requiring a lengthy course of treatment (such as cancer). Do not assign a code from category Z79 for medication being administered for a brief period of time to treat an acute illness or injury (such as a course of antibiotics to treat acute bronchitis).

Z88	Allergy status to drugs, medicaments and biological substances Except: Z88.9, Allergy status to unspecified drugs, medicaments and biological substances status
Z89	Acquired absence of limb
Z90	Acquired absence of organs, not elsewhere classified
Z91.0-	Allergy status, other than to drugs and biological substances
Z92.82	Status post administration of tPA (rtPA) in a different facility within the last 24 hours prior to admission to a current facility Assign code Z92.82, Status post administration of tPA (rtPA) in a different facility within the last 24 hours prior to admission to current

facility, as a secondary diagnosis when a patient is received by transfer into a facility and documentation indicates they were administered tissue plasminogen activator (tPA) within the last 24 hours prior to admission to the current facility. This guideline applies even if the patient is still receiving the tPA at the time they are received into the current facility. The appropriate code for the condition for which the tPA was administered (such as cerebrovascular disease or myocardial infarction) should be assigned first. Code Z92.82 is only applicable to the receiving facility record and not to the transferring facility record.

Z93	Artificial opening status
Z94	Transplanted organ and tissue status
Z95	Presence of cardiac and vascular implants and grafts
Z96	Presence of other functional implants
Z97	Presence of other devices
Z98	Other postprocedural states

Assign code Z98.85, Transplanted organ removal status, to indicate that a transplanted organ has been previously removed. This code should not be assigned for the encounter in which the transplanted organ is removed. The complication necessitating removal of the transplant organ should be assigned for that encounter.
See Section I.C.19. for information on the coding of organ transplant complications.

Z99	Dependence on enabling machines and devices, not elsewhere classified

Note: Categories Z89-Z90 and Z93-Z99 are for use only if there are no complications or malfunctions of the organ or tissue replaced, the amputation site or the equipment on which the patient is dependent.

4) History (of)
There are two types of history Z codes, personal and family. Personal history codes explain a patient's past medical condition that no longer exists and is not receiving any treatment, but that has the potential for recurrence, and therefore may require continued monitoring.

Family history codes are for use when a patient has a family member(s) who has had a particular disease that causes the patient to be at higher risk of also contracting the disease.

Personal history codes may be used in conjunction with follow-up codes and family history codes may be used in conjunction with screening codes to explain the need for a test or procedure. History codes are also acceptable on any medical record regardless of the reason for visit. A history of an illness, even if no longer present, is important information that may alter the type of treatment ordered.

The history Z code categories are:

Z80	Family history of primary malignant neoplasm
Z81	Family history of mental and behavioral disorders
Z82	Family history of certain disabilities and chronic diseases (leading to disablement)
Z83	Family history of other specific disorders
Z84	Family history of other conditions
Z85	Personal history of malignant neoplasm
Z86	Personal history of certain other diseases
Z87	Personal history of other diseases and conditions
Z91.4-	Personal history of psychological trauma, not elsewhere classified
Z91.5	Personal history of self-harm
Z91.81	History of falling
Z91.82	Personal history of military deployment
Z92	Personal history of medical treatment Except: Z92.0, Personal history of contraception Except: Z92.82, Status post administration of tPA (rtPA) in a different facility within the last 24 hours prior to admission to a current facility

5) Screening
Screening is the testing for disease or disease precursors in seemingly well individuals so that early detection and treatment can be provided for those who test positive for the disease (e.g., screening mammogram).

The testing of a person to rule out or confirm a suspected diagnosis because the patient has some sign or symptom is a diagnostic examination, not a screening. In these cases, the sign or symptom is used to explain the reason for the test.

A screening code may be a first-listed code if the reason for the visit is specifically the screening exam. It may also be used as an additional code if the screening is done during an office visit for other health problems. A screening code is not necessary if the screening is inherent to a routine examination, such as a pap smear done during a routine pelvic examination.

Should a condition be discovered during the screening then the code for the condition may be assigned as an additional diagnosis.

The Z code indicates that a screening exam is planned. A procedure code is required to confirm that the screening was performed.

The screening Z codes/categories:

Z11	Encounter for screening for infectious and parasitic diseases
Z12	Encounter for screening for malignant neoplasms
Z13	Encounter for screening for other diseases and disorders Except: Z13.9, Encounter for screening, unspecified
Z36	Encounter for antenatal screening for mother

6) Observation
There are three observation Z code categories. They are for use in very limited circumstances when a person is being observed for a suspected condition that is ruled out. The observation codes are not for use if an injury or illness or any signs or symptoms related to the suspected condition are present. In such cases the diagnosis/symptom code is used with the corresponding external cause code.

The observation codes are to be used as principal diagnosis only. The only exception to this is when the principal diagnosis is required to be a code from category Z38, Liveborn infants according to place of birth and type of delivery. Then a code from category Z05, Encounter for observation and evaluation of newborn for suspected diseases and conditions ruled out, is sequenced after the Z38 code. Additional codes may be used in addition to the observation code but only if they are unrelated to the suspected condition being observed.

Codes from subcategory Z03.7 Encounter for suspected maternal and fetal conditions ruled out, may either be used as a first-listed or as an additional code assignment depending on the case. They are for use in very limited circumstances on a maternal record when an encounter is for a suspected maternal or fetal condition that is ruled out during that encounter (for example, a maternal or fetal condition may be suspected due to an abnormal test result). These codes should not be used when the condition is confirmed. In those cases, the confirmed condition should be coded. In addition, these codes are not for use if an illness or any signs or symptoms related to the suspected condition or problem are present. In such cases the diagnosis/symptom code is used.

Additional codes may be used in addition to the code from subcategory Z03.7, but only if they are unrelated to the suspected condition being evaluated.

Codes from subcategory Z03.7 may not be used for encounters for antenatal screening of mother. *See Section I.C.21. Screening.*

For encounters for suspected fetal condition that are inconclusive following testing and evaluation, assign the appropriate code from category O35, O36, O40 or O41.

The observation Z code categories:

Z03	Encounter for medical observation for suspected diseases and conditions ruled out
Z04	Encounter for examination and observation for other reasons Except: Z04.9, Encounter for examination and observation for unspecified reason
Z05	Encounter for observation and evaluation of newborn for suspected diseases and conditions ruled out

7) Aftercare
Aftercare visit codes cover situations when the initial treatment of a disease has been performed and the patient requires continued care during the healing or recovery phase, or for the long-term consequences of the disease. The aftercare Z code should not be used if treatment is directed at a current, acute disease. The diagnosis code is to be used in these cases.

Exceptions to this rule are codes Z51.0, Encounter for antineoplastic radiation therapy, and codes from subcategory Z51.1, Encounter for antineoplastic chemotherapy and immunotherapy. These codes are to be first-listed, followed by the diagnosis code when a patient's encounter is solely to receive radiation therapy, chemotherapy, or immunotherapy for the treatment of a neoplasm. If the reason for the encounter is more than one type of antineoplastic therapy, code Z51.0 and a code from subcategory Z51.1 may be assigned together, in which case one of these codes would be reported as a secondary diagnosis.

The aftercare Z codes should also not be used for aftercare for injuries. For aftercare of an injury, assign the acute injury code with the appropriate 7th character (for subsequent encounter).

The aftercare codes are generally first-listed to explain the specific reason for the encounter. An aftercare code may be used as an additional code when some type of aftercare is provided in addition to the reason for admission and no diagnosis code is applicable. An example of this would be the closure of a colostomy during an encounter for treatment of another condition.

Aftercare codes should be used in conjunction with other aftercare codes or diagnosis codes to provide better detail on the specifics of an aftercare encounter visit, unless otherwise directed by the classification. Should a patient receive multiple types of antineoplastic therapy during the same encounter, code Z51.0, Encounter for antineoplastic radiation therapy, and codes from subcategory Z51.1, Encounter for antineoplastic chemotherapy and immunotherapy, may be used together on a record. The sequencing of multiple aftercare codes depends on the circumstances of the encounter.

Certain aftercare Z code categories need a secondary diagnosis code to describe the resolving condition or sequelae. For others, the condition is included in the code title.

Additional Z code aftercare category terms include fitting and adjustment, and attention to artificial openings.

Status Z codes may be used with aftercare Z codes to indicate the nature of the aftercare. For example code Z95.1, Presence of aortocoronary bypass graft, may be used with code Z48.812, Encounter for surgical aftercare following surgery on the circulatory system, to indicate the surgery for which the aftercare is being performed. A status code should not be used when the aftercare code indicates the type of status, such as using Z43.0, Encounter for attention to tracheostomy, with Z93.0, Tracheostomy status.

The aftercare Z category/codes:

Z42	Encounter for plastic and reconstructive surgery following medical procedure or healed injury
Z43	Encounter for attention to artificial openings
Z44	Encounter for fitting and adjustment of external prosthetic device
Z45	Encounter for adjustment and management of implanted device
Z46	Encounter for fitting and adjustment of other devices
Z47	Orthopedic aftercare
Z48	Encounter for other postprocedural aftercare
Z49	Encounter for care involving renal dialysis
Z51	Encounter for other aftercare and medical care

8) Follow-up

The follow-up codes are used to explain continuing surveillance following completed treatment of a disease, condition, or injury. They imply that the condition has been fully treated and no longer exists. They should not be confused with aftercare codes, or injury codes with a 7th character for subsequent encounter, that explain ongoing care of a healing condition or its sequelae. Follow-up codes may be used in conjunction with history codes to provide the full picture of the healed condition and its treatment. The follow-up code is sequenced first, followed by the history code.

A follow-up code may be used to explain multiple visits. Should a condition be found to have recurred on the follow-up visit, then the diagnosis code for the condition should be assigned in place of the follow-up code.

The follow-up Z code categories:

Z08	Encounter for follow-up examination after completed treatment for malignant neoplasm
Z09	Encounter for follow-up examination after completed treatment for conditions other than malignant neoplasm
Z39	Encounter for maternal postpartum care and examination

9) Donor

Codes in category Z52, Donors of organs and tissues, are used for living individuals who are donating blood or other body tissue.

These codes are only for individuals donating for others, not for self-donations. They are not used to identify cadaveric donations.

10) Counseling

Counseling Z codes are used when a patient or family member receives assistance in the aftermath of an illness or injury, or when support is required in coping with family or social problems.

The counseling Z codes/categories:

Z30.0-	Encounter for general counseling and advice on contraception
Z31.5	Encounter for procreative genetic counseling
Z31.6-	Encounter for general counseling and advice on procreation
Z32.2	Encounter for childbirth instruction
Z32.3	Encounter for childcare instruction
Z69	Encounter for mental health services for victim and perpetrator of abuse
Z70	Counseling related to sexual attitude, behavior and orientation
Z71	Persons encountering health services for other counseling and medical advice, not elsewhere classified
Z76.81	Expectant mother prebirth pediatrician visit

11) Encounters for Obstetrical and Reproductive Services

See Section I.C.15. Pregnancy, Childbirth, and the Puerperium, for further instruction on the use of these codes.

Z codes for pregnancy are for use in those circumstances when none of the problems or complications included in the codes from the Obstetrics chapter exist (a routine prenatal visit or postpartum care). Codes in category Z34, Encounter for supervision of normal pregnancy, are always first listed and are not to be used with any other code from the OB chapter.

Codes in category Z3A, Weeks of gestation, may be assigned to provide additional information about the pregnancy. Category Z3A codes should not be assigned for pregnancies with abortive outcomes (categories O00-O08), elective termination of pregnancy (code Z33.2), nor for postpartum conditions, as category Z3A is not applicable to these conditions. The date of the admission should be used to determine weeks of gestation for inpatient admissions that encompass more than one gestational week.

The outcome of delivery, category Z37, should be included on all maternal delivery records. It is always a secondary code. Codes in category Z37 should not be used on the newborn record.

Z codes for family planning (contraceptive) or procreative management and counseling should be included on an obstetric record either during the pregnancy or the postpartum stage, if applicable.

Z codes/categories for obstetrical and reproductive services:

Z30	Encounter for contraceptive management
Z31	Encounter for procreative management
Z32.2	Encounter for childbirth instruction
Z32.3	Encounter for childcare instruction
Z33	Pregnant state
Z34	Encounter for supervision of normal pregnancy
Z36	Encounter for antenatal screening of mother
Z3A	Weeks of gestation
Z37	Outcome of delivery
Z39	Encounter for maternal postpartum care and examination
Z76.81	Expectant mother prebirth pediatrician visit

12) Newborns and Infants

See Section I.C.16. Newborn (Perinatal) Guidelines, for further instruction on the use of these codes.

Newborn Z codes/categories:

Z76.1	Encounter for health supervision and care of foundling
Z00.1-	Encounter for routine child health examination
Z38	Liveborn infants according to place of birth and type of delivery

13) Routine and administrative examinations

The Z codes allow for the description of encounters for routine examinations, such as, a general check-up, or, examinations for administrative purposes, such as, a pre-employment physical. The codes are not to be used if the examination is for diagnosis of a suspected condition or for treatment purposes. In such cases the diagnosis code is used. During a routine exam, should a diagnosis or condition be discovered, it should be coded as an additional code. Pre-existing and chronic conditions and history codes may also be included as additional codes as long as the examination is for administrative purposes and not focused on any particular condition.

Some of the codes for routine health examinations distinguish between "with" and "without" abnormal findings. Code assignment depends on the information that is known at the time the encounter is being coded. For example, if no abnormal findings were found during the examination, but the encounter is being coded before test results are back, it is acceptable to assign the code for "without abnormal findings." When assigning a code for "with abnormal findings," additional code(s) should be assigned to identify the specific abnormal finding(s).

Pre-operative examination and pre-procedural laboratory examination Z codes are for use only in those situations when a patient is being cleared for a procedure or surgery and no treatment is given.

The Z codes/categories for routine and administrative examinations:

Z00 Encounter for general examination without complaint, suspected or reported diagnosis
Z01 Encounter for other special examination without complaint, suspected or reported diagnosis
Z02 Encounter for administrative examination Except: Z02.9, Encounter for administrative examinations, unspecified
Z32.0- Encounter for pregnancy test

14) Miscellaneous Z codes
The miscellaneous Z codes capture a number of other health care encounters that do not fall into one of the other categories. Certain of these codes identify the reason for the encounter; others are for use as additional codes that provide useful information on circumstances that may affect a patient's care and treatment.

Prophylactic Organ Removal
For encounters specifically for prophylactic removal of an organ (such as prophylactic removal of breasts due to a genetic susceptibility to cancer or a family history of cancer), the principal or first-listed code should be a code from category Z40, Encounter for prophylactic surgery, followed by the appropriate codes to identify the associated risk factor (such as genetic susceptibility or family history).

If the patient has a malignancy of one site and is having prophylactic removal at another site to prevent either a new primary malignancy or metastatic disease, a code for the malignancy should also be assigned in addition to a code from subcategory Z40.0, Encounter for prophylactic surgery for risk factors related to malignant neoplasms. A Z40.0 code should not be assigned if the patient is having organ removal for treatment of a malignancy, such as the removal of the testes for the treatment of prostate cancer.

Miscellaneous Z codes/categories:

Z28 Immunization not carried out Except: Z28.3, Underimmunization status
Z29 Encounter for other prophylactic measures
Z40 Encounter for prophylactic surgery
Z41 Encounter for procedures for purposes other than remedying health state Except: Z41.9, Encounter for procedure for purposes other than remedying health state, unspecified
Z53 Persons encountering health services for specific procedures and treatment, not carried out
Z55 Problems related to education and literacy
Z56 Problems related to employment and unemployment
Z57 Occupational exposure to risk factors
Z58 Problems related to physical environment
Z59 Problems related to housing and economic circumstances
Z60 Problems related to social environment
Z62 Problems related to upbringing
Z63 Other problems related to primary support group, including family circumstances
Z64 Problems related to certain psychosocial circumstances
Z65 Problems related to other psychosocial circumstances
Z72 Problems related to lifestyle Note: These codes should be assigned only when the documentation specifies that the patient has an associated problem
Z73 Problems related to life management difficulty

Z74 Problems related to care provider dependency Except: Z74.01, Bed confinement status
Z75 Problems related to medical facilities and other health care
Z76.0 Encounter for issue of repeat prescription
Z76.3 Healthy person accompanying sick person
Z76.4 Other boarder to healthcare facility
Z76.5 Malingerer [conscious simulation]
Z91.1- Patient's noncompliance with medical treatment and regimen
Z91.83 Wandering in diseases classified elsewhere
Z91.84- Oral health risk factors
Z91.89 Other specified personal risk factors, not elsewhere classified

See Section I.B.14 for Z55-Z65 Persons with potential health hazards related to socioeconomic and psychosocial circumstances, documentation by clinicians other than the patient's provider.

15) Nonspecific Z codes
Certain Z codes are so non-specific, or potentially redundant with other codes in the classification, that there can be little justification for their use in the inpatient setting. Their use in the outpatient setting should be limited to those instances when there is no further documentation to permit more precise coding. Otherwise, any sign or symptom or any other reason for visit that is captured in another code should be used.

Nonspecific Z codes/categories:

Z02.9 Encounter for administrative examinations, unspecified
Z04.9 Encounter for examination and observation for unspecified reason
Z13.9 Encounter for screening, unspecified
Z41.9 Encounter for procedure for purposes other than remedying health state, unspecified
Z52.9 Donor of unspecified organ or tissue
Z86.59 Personal history of other mental and behavioral disorders
Z88.9 Allergy status to unspecified drugs, medicaments and biological substances status
Z92.0 Personal history of contraception

16) Z Codes That May Only Be Principal/First-Listed Diagnosis
The following Z codes/categories may only be reported as the principal/first-listed diagnosis, except when there are multiple encounters on the same day and the medical records for the encounters are combined:

Z00 Encounter for general examination without complaint, suspected or reported diagnosis Except: Z00.6
Z01 Encounter for other special examination without complaint, suspected or reported diagnosis
Z02 Encounter for administrative examination
Z03 Encounter for medical observation for suspected diseases and conditions ruled out
Z04 Encounter for examination and observation for other reasons
Z33.2 Encounter for elective termination of pregnancy
Z31.81 Encounter for male factor infertility in female patient
Z31.83 Encounter for assisted reproductive fertility procedure cycle
Z31.84 Encounter for fertility preservation procedure
Z34 Encounter for supervision of normal pregnancy
Z39 Encounter for maternal postpartum care and examination
Z38 Liveborn infants according to place of birth and type of delivery
Z40 Encounter for prophylactic surgery
Z42 Encounter for plastic and reconstructive surgery following medical procedure or healed injury
Z51.0 Encounter for antineoplastic radiation therapy
Z51.1- Encounter for antineoplastic chemotherapy and immunotherapy
Z52 Donors of organs and tissues Except: Z52.9, Donor of unspecified organ or tissue
Z76.1 Encounter for health supervision and care of foundling
Z76.2 Encounter for health supervision and care of other healthy infant and child
Z99.12 Encounter for respirator [ventilator] dependence during power failure

CHAPTER 21

FACTORS INFLUENCING HEALTH STATUS AND CONTACT WITH HEALTH SERVICES (Z00-Z99)

Note: Z codes represent reasons for encounters. A corresponding procedure code must accompany a Z code if a procedure is performed. Categories Z00-Z99 are provided for occasions when circumstances other than a disease, injury or external cause classifiable to categories A00-Y89 are recorded as "diagnoses" or "problems." This can arise in two main ways.

(a) When a person who may or may not be sick encounters the health services for some specific purpose, such as to receive limited care or service for a current condition, to donate an organ or tissue, to receive prophylactic vaccination (immunization), or to discuss a problem which is in itself not a disease or injury.

(b) When some circumstance or problem is present which influences the person's health status but is not in itself a current illness or injury.

This chapter contains the following blocks:

Z00-Z13	Persons encountering health services for examination
Z14-Z15	Genetic carrier and genetic susceptibility to disease
Z16	Resistance to antimicrobial drugs
Z17	Estrogen, and other hormones and factors receptor status
Z18	Retained foreign body fragments
Z19	Hormone sensitivity malignancy status
Z20-Z29	Persons with potential health hazards related to communicable diseases
Z30-Z39	Persons encountering health services in circumstances related to reproduction
Z40-Z53	Encounters for other specific health care
Z55-Z65	Persons with potential health hazards related to socioeconomic and psychosocial circumstances
Z66	Do not resuscitate status
Z67	Blood type
Z68	Body mass index (BMI)
Z69-Z76	Persons encountering health services in other circumstances
Z77-Z99	Persons with potential health hazards related to family and personal history and certain conditions influencing health status

PERSONS ENCOUNTERING HEALTH SERVICES FOR EXAMINATIONS (Z00-Z13)

Note: Nonspecific abnormal findings disclosed at the time of these examinations are classified to categories R70-R94.

Excludes1 examinations related to pregnancy and reproduction (Z30-Z36, Z39.-)

● **Z00** **Encounter for general examination without complaint, suspected or reported diagnosis**

Excludes1 encounter for examination for administrative purposes (Z02.-)

Excludes2 encounter for pre-procedural examinations (Z01.81-)
special screening examinations (Z11-Z13)

● **Z00.0** **Encounter for general adult medical examination**
Encounter for adult periodic examination (annual) (physical) and any associated laboratory and radiologic examinations

Excludes1 encounter for examination of sign or symptom - code to sign or symptom
general health check-up of infant or child (Z00.12.-)
Coding Clinic: 2016, Q4, P131

Z00.00 **Encounter for general adult medical examination without abnormal findings** A
Encounter for adult health check-up NOS
Coding Clinic: 2017, Q4, P95; 2016, Q1, P37

Z00.01 **Encounter for general adult medical examination with abnormal findings** A
Use additional code to identify abnormal findings
Coding Clinic: 2016, Q1, P36

● **Z00.1** **Encounter for newborn, infant and child health examinations**

● **Z00.11** **Newborn health examination**
Health check for child under 29 days old
Use additional code to identify any abnormal findings

Excludes1 health check for child over 28 days old (Z00.12-)

Z00.110 **Health examination for newborn under 8 days old** N
Health check for newborn under 8 days old

Z00.111 **Health examination for newborn 8 to 28 days old** N
Health check for newborn 8 to 28 days old
Newborn weight check

● **Z00.12** **Encounter for routine child health examination**
Immunizations appropriate for age
Health check (routine) for child over 28 days old
Routine developmental screening of infant or child
Routine vision and hearing testing

Excludes1 health check for child under 29 days old (Z00.11-)
health supervision of foundling or other healthy infant or child (Z76.1-Z76.2)
newborn health examination (Z00.11-)

Z00.121 **Encounter for routine child health examination with abnormal findings** P
Use additional code to identify abnormal findings
Coding Clinic: 2017, Q4, P95; 2016, Q1, P34-35

Z00.129 **Encounter for routine child health examination without abnormal findings** P
Encounter for routine child health examination NOS
Coding Clinic: 2016, Q1, P34

Z00.2 **Encounter for examination for period of rapid growth in childhood** P

Z00.3 **Encounter for examination for adolescent development state** P
Encounter for puberty development state

Z00.5 **Encounter for examination of potential donor of organ and tissue**

Z00.6 **Encounter for examination for normal comparison and control in clinical research program**
Examination of participant or control in clinical research program

● **Z00.7** **Encounter for examination for period of delayed growth in childhood**

Z00.70 **Encounter for examination for period of delayed growth in childhood without abnormal findings** P

Z00.71 **Encounter for examination for period of delayed growth in childhood with abnormal findings** P
Use additional code to identify abnormal findings

Z00.8 **Encounter for other general examination**
Encounter for health examination in population surveys

● **Z01   Encounter for other special examination without complaint, suspected or reported diagnosis**

> **Includes**   routine examination of specific system
>
> **Note:** Codes from category Z01 represent the reason for the encounter. A separate procedure code is required to identify any examinations or procedures performed.
>
> **Excludes1**   encounter for examination for administrative purposes (Z02.-)
> encounter for examination for suspected conditions, proven not to exist (Z03.-)
> encounter for laboratory and radiologic examinations as a component of general medical examinations (Z00.0-)
> encounter for laboratory, radiologic and imaging examinations for sign(s) and symptom(s) - code to the sign(s) or symptom(s)
>
> **Excludes2**   screening examinations (Z11-Z13)

● **Z01.0   Encounter for examination of eyes and vision**

> **Excludes1**   examination for driving license (Z02.4)

Z01.00   Encounter for examination of eyes and vision without abnormal findings
> Encounter for examination of eyes and vision NOS

Z01.01   Encounter for examination of eyes and vision with abnormal findings
> Use additional code to identify abnormal findings
> Coding Clinic: 2016, Q4, P21

● **Z01.02   Encounter for examination of eyes and vision following failed vision screening**
> **Excludes1**   encounter for examination of eyes and vision with abnormal findings (Z01.01)
> encounter for examination of eyes and vision without abnormal findings (Z01.00)

● **Z01.020   Encounter for examination of eyes and vision following failed vision screening without abnormal findings**

● **Z01.021   Encounter for examination of eyes and vision following failed vision screening with abnormal findings**
> Use additional code to identify abnormal findings

● **Z01.1   Encounter for examination of ears and hearing**

Z01.10   Encounter for examination of ears and hearing without abnormal findings
> Encounter for examination of ears and hearing NOS
> Coding Clinic: 2016, Q4, P25

● **Z01.11   Encounter for examination of ears and hearing with abnormal findings**
> Coding Clinic: 2016, Q3, P18

Z01.110   Encounter for hearing examination following failed hearing screening
> Coding Clinic: 2016, Q3, P18-19

Z01.118   Encounter for examination of ears and hearing with other abnormal findings
> Use additional code to identify abnormal findings
> Coding Clinic: 2016, Q3, P17

Z01.12   Encounter for hearing conservation and treatment

● **Z01.2   Encounter for dental examination and cleaning**

Z01.20   Encounter for dental examination and cleaning without abnormal findings
> Encounter for dental examination and cleaning NOS

Z01.21   Encounter for dental examination and cleaning with abnormal findings
> Use additional code to identify abnormal findings

● **Z01.3   Encounter for examination of blood pressure**

Z01.30   Encounter for examination of blood pressure without abnormal findings
> Encounter for examination of blood pressure NOS

Z01.31   Encounter for examination of blood pressure with abnormal findings
> Use additional code to identify abnormal findings

● **Z01.4   Encounter for gynecological examination**

> **Excludes2**   pregnancy examination or test (Z32.0-)
> routine examination for contraceptive maintenance (Z30.4-)

● **Z01.41   Encounter for routine gynecological examination**
> Encounter for general gynecological examination with or without cervical smear
> Encounter for gynecological examination (general) (routine) NOS
> Encounter for pelvic examination (annual) (periodic)
> Use additional code:
> for screening for human papillomavirus, if applicable (Z11.51)
> for screening vaginal pap smear, if applicable (Z12.72)
> to identify acquired absence of uterus, if applicable (Z90.71-)
>
> > **Excludes1**   gynecologic examination status-post hysterectomy for malignant condition (Z08)
> > screening cervical pap smear not a part of a routine gynecological examination (Z12.4)

Z01.411   Encounter for gynecological examination (general) (routine) with abnormal findings
> Use additional code to identify any abnormal findings

Z01.419   Encounter for gynecological examination (general) (routine) without abnormal findings

Z01.42   Encounter for cervical smear to confirm findings of recent normal smear following initial abnormal smear

● **Z01.8   Encounter for other specified special examinations**

● **Z01.81   Encounter for preprocedural examinations**
> Encounter for preoperative examinations
> Encounter for radiological and imaging examinations as part of preprocedural examination

Z01.810   Encounter for preprocedural cardiovascular examination

Z01.811   Encounter for preprocedural respiratory examination

Z01.812   Encounter for preprocedural laboratory examination
> Blood and urine tests prior to treatment or procedure
> Coding Clinic: 2023, Q2, P4; 2021, Q1, P38

Z01.818   Encounter for other preprocedural examination
> Encounter for preprocedural examination NOS
> Encounter for examinations prior to antineoplastic chemotherapy

Z01.82   Encounter for allergy testing
> **Excludes1**   encounter for antibody response examination (Z01.84)

Z01.83   Encounter for blood typing
> Encounter for Rh typing

Z01.84   **Encounter for antibody response examination**
Encounter for immunity status testing

> **Excludes1**   encounter for allergy testing
> (Z01.82)

Z01.89   **Encounter for other specified special examinations**

● **Z02   Encounter for administrative examination**

Z02.0   **Encounter for examination for admission to educational institution**
Encounter for examination for admission to preschool (education)
Encounter for examination for re-admission to school following illness or medical treatment

Z02.1   **Encounter for pre-employment examination**

Z02.2   **Encounter for examination for admission to residential institution**

> **Excludes1**   examination for admission to prison
> (Z02.89)

Z02.3   **Encounter for examination for recruitment to armed forces**

Z02.4   **Encounter for examination for driving license**

Z02.5   **Encounter for examination for participation in sport**

> **Excludes1**   blood-alcohol and blood-drug test
> (Z02.83)

Z02.6   **Encounter for examination for insurance purposes**

● Z02.7   **Encounter for issue of medical certificate**

> **Excludes1**   encounter for general medical
> examination (Z00-Z01, Z02.0-Z02.6,
> Z02.8-Z02.9)

Z02.71   **Encounter for disability determination**
Encounter for issue of medical certificate of incapacity
Encounter for issue of medical certificate of invalidity

Z02.79   **Encounter for issue of other medical certificate**

● Z02.8   **Encounter for other administrative examinations**

Z02.81   **Encounter for paternity testing**

Z02.82   **Encounter for adoption services**

Z02.83   **Encounter for blood-alcohol and blood-drug test**
Use additional code for findings of alcohol or drugs in blood (R78.-)

Z02.84   **Encounter for child welfare exam**
Encounter for child welfare screening exam

> **Excludes2**   encounter for examination and
> observation for alleged
> child physical abuse(Z04.72)
> encounter for examination and
> observation for alleged
> child rape (Z04.42)

Z02.89   **Encounter for other administrative examinations**
Encounter for examination for admission to prison
Encounter for examination for admission to summer camp
Encounter for immigration examination
Encounter for naturalization examination
Encounter for premarital examination

> **Excludes1**   health supervision of foundling
> or other healthy infant or
> child (Z76.1-Z76.2)

Z02.9   **Encounter for administrative examinations, unspecified**

OGCR   Section II.C.21.c.6.

Observation

There are three observation Z code categories. They are for use in very limited circumstances when a person is being observed for a suspected condition that is ruled out. The observation codes are not for use if an injury or illnesses or any signs or symptoms related to the suspected condition are present. In such cases the diagnosis/symptom code is used with the corresponding external cause code.

The observation codes are to be used as principal diagnosis only. The only exception to this is when the principal diagnosis is required to be a code from category Z38, Liveborn infants according to place of birth and type of delivery. Then a code from category Z05, Encounter for observation and evaluation of newborn for suspected diseases and conditions ruled out, is sequenced after the Z38 code. Additional codes may be used in addition to the observation code but only if they are unrelated to the suspected condition being observed.

Codes from subcategory Z03.7 Encounter for suspected maternal and fetal conditions ruled out, may either be used as a first listed or as an additional code assignment depending on the case. They are for use in very limited circumstances on a maternal record when an encounter is for a suspected maternal or fetal condition that is ruled out during that encounter (for example, a maternal or fetal condition may be suspected due to an abnormal test result). These codes should not be used when the condition is confirmed. In those cases, the confirmed condition should be coded. In addition, these codes are not for use if an illness or any signs or symptoms related to the suspected condition or problem are present. In such cases the diagnosis/symptom code is used.

Additional codes may be used in addition to the code from subcategory Z03.7, but only if they are unrelated to the suspected condition being evaluated.

Codes from subcategory Z03.7 may not be used for encounters for antenatal screening of mother. See Section I.C.21. Screening.

For encounters for suspected fetal condition that are inconclusive following testing and evaluation, assign the appropriate code from category O35, O36, O40 or O41.

The observation Z code categories:

Z03   Encounter for medical observation for suspected diseases and conditions ruled out

Z04   Encounter for examination and observation for other reasons
Except: Z04.9, Encounter for examination and observation for unspecified reason

Z05   Encounter for observation and evaluation of newborn for suspected diseases and conditions ruled out

● **Z03   Encounter for medical observation for suspected diseases and conditions ruled out**
This category is to be used when a person without a diagnosis is suspected of having an abnormal condition, without signs or symptoms, which requires study, but after examination and observation, is ruled out. This category is also for use for administrative and legal observation status.

> **Excludes1**   contact with and (suspected) exposures
> hazardous to health (Z77.-)
> encounter for observation and evaluation
> of newborn for suspected diseases and
> conditions ruled out (Z05.-)
> person with feared complaint in whom no
> diagnosis is made (Z71.1)
> signs or symptoms under study - code to signs or
> symptoms

Z03.6   **Encounter for observation for suspected toxic effect from ingested substance ruled out**
Encounter for observation for suspected adverse effect from drug
Encounter for observation for suspected poisoning

▶ New   ⇒ Revised   ~~deleted~~ Deleted   Excludes 1   Excludes 2   Includes   Use additional   Code first   Code also   Key words
OGCR Official Guidelines   X Assign placeholder X   ● Use Additional Character(s)   ▶ Manifestation Code   ❧ Hierarchical Condition Category   **Coding Clinic**

● **Z03.7**   **Encounter for suspected maternal and fetal conditions ruled out**
Encounter for suspected maternal and fetal conditions not found

> **Excludes1**   known or suspected fetal anomalies affecting management of mother, not ruled out (O26.-, O35.-, O36.-, O40.-, O41.-)

Z03.71   **Encounter for suspected problem with amniotic cavity and membrane ruled out**   **M**
Encounter for suspected oligohydramnios ruled out
Encounter for suspected polyhydramnios ruled out

Z03.72   **Encounter for suspected placental problem ruled out**   **M**

Z03.73   **Encounter for suspected fetal anomaly ruled out**   **M**
Coding Clinic: 2016, Q4, P6

Z03.74   **Encounter for suspected problem with fetal growth ruled out**   **M**

Z03.75   **Encounter for suspected cervical shortening ruled out**   **M**

Z03.79   **Encounter for other suspected maternal and fetal conditions ruled out**   **M**
Coding Clinic: 2016, Q4, P7

● **Z03.8**   **Encounter for observation for other suspected diseases and conditions ruled out**

● **Z03.81**   **Encounter for observation for suspected exposure to biological agents ruled out**

Z03.810   **Encounter for observation for suspected exposure to anthrax ruled out**

Z03.818   **Encounter for observation for suspected exposure to other biological agents ruled out**

● **Z03.82**   **Encounter for observation for suspected foreign body ruled out**

> **Excludes1**   retained foreign body (Z18.-)
> retained foreign body in eyelid (H02.81)
> residual foreign body in soft tissue (M79.5)

> **Excludes2**   confirmed foreign body ingestion or aspiration including:
> foreign body in alimentary tract (T18)
> foreign body in ear (T16)
> foreign body on external eye (T15)
> foreign body in respiratory tract (T17)

Z03.821   **Encounter for observation for suspected ingested foreign body ruled out**

Z03.822   **Encounter for observation for suspected aspirated (inhaled) foreign body ruled out**

Z03.823   **Encounter for observation for suspected inserted (injected) foreign body ruled out**
Encounter for observation for suspected inserted (injected) foreign body in eye ruled out
Encounter for observation for suspected inserted (injected) foreign body in orifice ruled out
Encounter for observation for suspected inserted (injected) foreign body in skin ruled out

Z03.83   **Encounter for observation for suspected conditions related to home physiologic monitoring device ruled out**
Encounter for observation for apnea alarm without findings
Encounter for observation for bradycardia alarm without findings
Encounter for observation for malfunction of home cardiorespiratory monitor
Encounter for observation for non-specific findings home physiologic monitoring device
Encounter for observation for pulse oximeter alarm without findings

> **Excludes1**   apnea NOS (R06.81)
> neonatal bradycardia (P29.12)
> newborn apnea (P28.4-)
> primary sleep apnea of newborn (P28.3-)
> sleep apnea (G47.3-)

Z03.89   **Encounter for observation for other suspected diseases and conditions ruled out**

● **Z04**   **Encounter for examination and observation for other reasons**

> **Includes**   encounter for examination for medicolegal reasons
> This category is to be used when a person without a diagnosis is suspected of having an abnormal condition, without signs or symptoms, which requires study, but after examination and observation, is ruled-out. This category is also for use for administrative and legal observation status.

Z04.1   **Encounter for examination and observation following transport accident**

> **Excludes1**   encounter for examination and observation following work accident (Z04.2)
Coding Clinic: 2019, Q2, P11

Z04.2   **Encounter for examination and observation following work accident**

Z04.3   **Encounter for examination and observation following other accident**

● **Z04.4**   **Encounter for examination and observation following alleged rape**
Encounter for examination and observation of victim following alleged rape
Encounter for examination and observation of victim following alleged sexual abuse
Coding Clinic: 2016, Q4, P129

Z04.41   **Encounter for examination and observation following alleged adult rape**   **A**
Suspected adult rape, ruled out
Suspected adult sexual abuse, ruled out

Z04.42   **Encounter for examination and observation following alleged child rape**   **P**
Suspected child rape, ruled out
Suspected child sexual abuse, ruled out

Z04.6   **Encounter for general psychiatric examination, requested by authority**

● **Z04.7**   **Encounter for examination and observation following alleged physical abuse**

Z04.71   **Encounter for examination and observation following alleged adult physical abuse**   **A**
Suspected adult physical abuse, ruled out

> **Excludes1**   confirmed case of adult physical abuse (T74.-)
> encounter for examination and observation following alleged adult sexual abuse (Z04.41)
> suspected case of adult physical abuse, not ruled out (T76.-)

Z04.72   **Encounter for examination and observation following alleged child physical abuse**   P
Suspected child physical abuse, ruled out
> **Excludes1**   confirmed case of child physical abuse (T74.-)
> encounter for examination and observation following alleged child sexual abuse (Z04.42)
> suspected case of child physical abuse, not ruled out (T76.-)

● **Z04.8**   **Encounter for examination and observation for other specified reasons**
Encounter for examination and observation for request for expert evidence

Z04.81   **Encounter for examination and observation of victim following forced sexual exploitation**

Z04.82   **Encounter for examination and observation of victim following forced labor exploitation**

Z04.89   **Encounter for examination and observation for other specified reasons**

Z04.9   **Encounter for examination and observation for unspecified reason**
Encounter for observation NOS

● **Z05**   **Encounter for observation and evaluation of newborn for suspected diseases and conditions ruled out**
This category is to be used for newborns, within the neonatal period (the first 28 days of life), who are suspected of having an abnormal condition, but without signs or symptoms, and which, after examination and observation, is ruled out.
Coding Clinic: 2022, Q1, P17-18; 2019, Q2, P11; 2016, Q4, P54, 77, 126-127, 130

Z05.0   **Observation and evaluation of newborn for suspected cardiac condition ruled out**   N

Z05.1   **Observation and evaluation of newborn for suspected infectious condition ruled out**   N
Coding Clinic: 2019, Q2, P11

Z05.2   **Observation and evaluation of newborn for suspected neurological condition ruled out**   N

Z05.3   **Observation and evaluation of newborn for suspected respiratory condition ruled out**   N

● **Z05.4**   **Observation and evaluation of newborn for suspected genetic, metabolic or immunologic condition ruled out**

Z05.41   **Observation and evaluation of newborn for suspected genetic condition ruled out**   N
Coding Clinic: 2016, Q4, P55

Z05.42   **Observation and evaluation of newborn for suspected metabolic condition ruled out**   N

Z05.43   **Observation and evaluation of newborn for suspected immunologic condition ruled out**   N

Z05.5   **Observation and evaluation of newborn for suspected gastrointestinal condition ruled out**   N

Z05.6   **Observation and evaluation of newborn for suspected genitourinary condition ruled out**   N

● **Z05.7**   **Observation and evaluation of newborn for suspected skin, subcutaneous, musculoskeletal and connective tissue condition ruled out**

Z05.71   **Observation and evaluation of newborn for suspected skin and subcutaneous tissue condition ruled out**   N

Z05.72   **Observation and evaluation of newborn for suspected musculoskeletal condition ruled out**   N

Z05.73   **Observation and evaluation of newborn for suspected connective tissue condition ruled out**   N

● **Z05.8**   **Observation and evaluation of newborn for other specified suspected condition ruled out**   N
Coding Clinic: 2022, Q1, P17-18

Z05.81   **Observation and evaluation of newborn for suspected condition related to home physiologic monitoring device ruled out**
Encounter for observation of newborn for apnea alarm without findings
Encounter for observation of newborn for bradycardia alarm without findings
Encounter for observation of newborn for malfunction of home cardiorespiratory monitor
Encounter for observation of newborn for non-specific findings home physiologic monitoring device
Encounter for observation of newborn for pulse oximeter alarm without findings
> **Excludes1**   encounter for observation for suspected conditions related to home physiologic monitoring device ruled out (Z03.83)
> neonatal bradycardia (P29.12)
> other newborn apnea (P28.4-)
> primary sleep apnea of newborn (P28.3-)

Z05.89   **Observation and evaluation of newborn for other specified suspected condition ruled out**

Z05.9   **Observation and evaluation of newborn for unspecified suspected condition ruled out**   N
OGCR See Section II.C.21.c.8.

> The follow-up codes are used to explain continuing surveillance following completed treatment of a disease, condition, or injury. They imply that the condition has been fully treated and no longer exists. They should not be confused with aftercare codes, or injury codes with 7th character "D," that explain ongoing care of a healing condition or its sequelae. Follow-up codes may be used in conjunction with history codes to provide the full picture of the healed condition and its treatment. The follow-up code is sequenced first, followed by the history code.
>
> A follow-up code may be used to explain multiple visits. Should a condition be found to have recurred on the follow-up visit, then the diagnosis code for the condition should be assigned in place of the follow-up code.
>
> The follow-up Z code categories:
>
> Z08   Encounter for follow-up examination after completed treatment for malignant neoplasm
>
> Z09   Encounter for follow-up examination after completed treatment for conditions other than malignant neoplasm
>
> Z39   Encounter for maternal postpartum care and examination

Z08   **Encounter for follow-up examination after completed treatment for malignant neoplasm**
Medical surveillance following completed treatment
Use additional code to identify any acquired absence of organs (Z90.-)
Use additional code to identify the personal history of malignant neoplasm (Z85.-)
> **Excludes1**   aftercare following medical care (Z43-Z49, Z51)

Z09   **Encounter for follow-up examination after completed treatment for conditions other than malignant neoplasm**
Medical surveillance following completed treatment
Use additional code to identify any applicable history of disease code (Z86.-, Z87.-)
> **Excludes1**   aftercare following medical care (Z43-Z49, Z51)
> surveillance of contraception (Z30.4-)
> surveillance of prosthetic and other medical devices (Z44-Z46)
Coding Clinic: 2022, Q3, P4; 2021, Q1, P33; 2017, Q1, P9; 2015, Q1, P8

▶ New   ⇒ Revised   ~~deleted~~ Deleted   Excludes 1   Excludes 2   Includes   Use additional   Code first   Code also   Key words
OGCR Official Guidelines   X Assign placeholder X   ● Use Additional Character(s)   ▶ Manifestation Code   🔗 Hierarchical Condition Category   Coding Clinic

● **Z11** **Encounter for screening for infectious and parasitic diseases**
Screening is the testing for disease or disease precursors in asymptomatic individuals so that early detection and treatment can be provided for those who test positive for the disease.

Excludes1 encounter for diagnostic examination - code to sign or symptom

Z11.0 **Encounter for screening for intestinal infectious diseases**
Encounter for screening for active tuberculosis disease

Z11.1 **Encounter for screening for respiratory tuberculosis**

Z11.2 **Encounter for screening for other bacterial diseases**

Z11.3 **Encounter for screening for infections with a predominantly sexual mode of transmission**

Excludes2 encounter for screening for human immunodeficiency virus [HIV] (Z11.4)
encounter for screening for human papillomavirus (Z11.51)

Z11.4 **Encounter for screening for human immunodeficiency virus [HIV]**

● **Z11.5** **Encounter for screening for other viral diseases**

Excludes2 encounter for screening for viral intestinal disease (Z11.0)

Z11.51 **Encounter for screening for human papillomavirus (HPV)**
Coding Clinic: 2023, Q2, P3

Z11.52 **Encounter for screening for COVID-19**
Coding Clinic: 2023, Q2, P4; 2021, Q1, P37, 42

Z11.59 **Encounter for screening for other viral diseases**
Coding Clinic: 2021, Q1, P37

Z11.6 **Encounter for screening for other protozoal diseases and helminthiases**
Diseases or infestations caused by parasitic worms

Excludes2 encounter for screening for protozoal intestinal disease (Z11.0)

Z11.7 **Encounter for testing for latent tuberculosis infection**

Z11.8 **Encounter for screening for other infectious and parasitic diseases**
Encounter for screening for chlamydia
Encounter for screening for rickettsial
Encounter for screening for spirochetal
Encounter for screening for mycoses

Z11.9 **Encounter for screening for infectious and parasitic diseases, unspecified**

● **Z12** **Encounter for screening for malignant neoplasms**
Screening is the testing for disease or disease precursors in asymptomatic individuals so that early detection and treatment can be provided for those who test positive for the disease.

Use additional code to identify any family history of malignant neoplasm (Z80.-)

Excludes1 encounter for diagnostic examination - code to sign or symptom

Z12.0 **Encounter for screening for malignant neoplasm of stomach**

● **Z12.1** **Encounter for screening for malignant neoplasm of intestinal tract**

Z12.10 **Encounter for screening for malignant neoplasm of intestinal tract, unspecified**

Z12.11 **Encounter for screening for malignant neoplasm of colon**
Encounter for screening colonoscopy NOS
Coding Clinic: 2018, Q1, P7; 2017, Q1, P8-9

Z12.12 **Encounter for screening for malignant neoplasm of rectum**

Z12.13 **Encounter for screening for malignant neoplasm of small intestine**

Z12.2 **Encounter for screening for malignant neoplasm of respiratory organs**

● **Z12.3** **Encounter for screening for malignant neoplasm of breast**

Z12.31 **Encounter for screening mammogram for malignant neoplasm of breast**

Excludes1 inconclusive mammogram (R92.2)
Coding Clinic: 2023, Q4, P44; 2015, Q1, P24

Z12.39 **Encounter for other screening for malignant neoplasm of breast**

Z12.4 **Encounter for screening for malignant neoplasm of cervix**
Encounter for screening pap smear for malignant neoplasm of cervix

Excludes1 when screening is part of general gynecological examination (Z01.4-)

Excludes2 encounter for screening for human papillomavirus (Z11.51)

Z12.5 **Encounter for screening for malignant neoplasm of prostate**

Z12.6 **Encounter for screening for malignant neoplasm of bladder**

● **Z12.7** **Encounter for screening for malignant neoplasm of other genitourinary organs**

Z12.71 **Encounter for screening for malignant neoplasm of testis**

Z12.72 **Encounter for screening for malignant neoplasm of vagina**
Vaginal pap smear status - post hysterectomy for non-malignant condition
Use additional code to identify acquired absence of uterus (Z90.71-)

Excludes1 vaginal pap smear status - post hysterectomy for malignant conditions (Z08)

Z12.73 **Encounter for screening for malignant neoplasm of ovary**

Z12.79 **Encounter for screening for malignant neoplasm of other genitourinary organs**

● **Z12.8** **Encounter for screening for malignant neoplasm of other sites**

Z12.81 **Encounter for screening for malignant neoplasm of oral cavity**

Z12.82 **Encounter for screening for malignant neoplasm of nervous system**

Z12.83 **Encounter for screening for malignant neoplasm of skin**

CHAPTER 21 (Z00-Z99)

Z12.89   Encounter for screening for malignant neoplasm of other sites
Coding Clinic: 2021, Q1, P15

Z12.9   Encounter for screening for malignant neoplasm, site unspecified

● **Z13**   Encounter for screening for other diseases and disorders
Screening is the testing for disease or disease precursors in asymptomatic individuals so that early detection and treatment can be provided for those who test positive for the disease.
Excludes1   encounter for diagnostic examination - code to sign or symptom

Z13.0   Encounter for screening for diseases of the blood and blood-forming organs and certain disorders involving the immune mechanism

Z13.1   Encounter for screening for diabetes mellitus

● **Z13.2**   Encounter for screening for nutritional, metabolic and other endocrine disorders

Z13.21   Encounter for screening for nutritional disorder

● **Z13.22**   Encounter for screening for metabolic disorder

Z13.220   Encounter for screening for lipoid disorders
Encounter for screening for cholesterol level
Encounter for screening for hypercholesterolemia
Encounter for screening for hyperlipidemia

Z13.228   Encounter for screening for other metabolic disorders

Z13.29   Encounter for screening for other suspected endocrine disorder
Excludes2   encounter for screening for diabetes mellitus (Z13.1)

● **Z13.3**   Encounter for screening examination for mental health and behavioral disorders

Z13.30   Encounter for screening examination for mental health and behavioral disorders, unspecified

Z13.31   Encounter for screening for depression
Encounter for screening for depression, adult
Encounter for screening for depression for child or adolescent

Z13.32   Encounter for screening for maternal depression
Encounter for screening for perinatal depression

Z13.39   Encounter for screening examination for other mental health and behavioral disorders
Encounter for screening for alcoholism
Encounter for screening for intellectual disabilities

● **Z13.4**   Encounter for screening for certain developmental disorders in childhood   P
Encounter for development testing of infant or child
Encounter for screening for developmental handicaps in early childhood
Excludes2   encounter for routine child health examination (Z00.12-)

Z13.40   Encounter for screening for unspecified developmental delays

Z13.41   Encounter for autism screening

Z13.42   Encounter for screening for global developmental delays (milestones)
Encounter for screening for developmental handicaps in early childhood

Z13.49   Encounter for screening for other developmental delays

Z13.5   Encounter for screening for eye and ear disorders
Excludes2   encounter for general hearing examination (Z01.1-)
encounter for general vision examination (Z01.0-)
Coding Clinic: 2016, Q3, P17

Z13.6   Encounter for screening for cardiovascular disorders

● **Z13.7**   Encounter for screening for genetic and chromosomal anomalies
Excludes1   genetic testing for procreative management (Z31.4-)

Z13.71   Encounter for nonprocreative screening for genetic disease carrier status

Z13.79   Encounter for other screening for genetic and chromosomal anomalies

● **Z13.8**   Encounter for screening for other specified diseases and disorders
Excludes2   screening for malignant neoplasms (Z12.-)

● **Z13.81**   Encounter for screening for digestive system disorders

Z13.810   Encounter for screening for upper gastrointestinal disorder

Z13.811   Encounter for screening for lower gastrointestinal disorder
Excludes1   encounter for screening for intestinal infectious disease (Z11.0)

Z13.818   Encounter for screening for other digestive system disorders

● **Z13.82**   Encounter for screening for musculoskeletal disorder

Z13.820   Encounter for screening for osteoporosis

Z13.828   Encounter for screening for other musculoskeletal disorder

Z13.83   Encounter for screening for respiratory disorder NEC
Excludes1   encounter for screening for respiratory tuberculosis (Z11.1)

Z13.84   Encounter for screening for dental disorders

● **Z13.85**   Encounter for screening for nervous system disorders

Z13.850   Encounter for screening for traumatic brain injury

Z13.858   Encounter for screening for other nervous system disorders

Z13.88   Encounter for screening for disorder due to exposure to contaminants
Excludes1   those exposed to contaminants without suspected disorders (Z57-Z77.-)

Z13.89   Encounter for screening for other disorder
Encounter for screening for genitourinary disorders

Z13.9   Encounter for screening, unspecified

GENETIC CARRIER AND GENETIC SUSCEPTIBILITY TO DISEASE (Z14-Z15)

● **Z14**   Genetic carrier

● **Z14.0**   Hemophilia A carrier

Z14.01   Asymptomatic hemophilia A carrier

Z14.02   Symptomatic hemophilia A carrier

Z14.1   Cystic fibrosis carrier

Z14.8   Genetic carrier of other disease

● **Z15**   Genetic susceptibility to disease
Excludes1   chromosomal anomalies (Q90-Q99)
Includes   confirmed abnormal gene
Use additional code, if applicable, for any associated family history of the disease (Z80-Z84)

▶ New   ⇒ Revised   ~~deleted~~ Deleted   Excludes 1   Excludes 2   Includes   Use additional   Code first   Code also   Key words
OGCR Official Guidelines   X Assign placeholder X   ● Use Additional Character(s)   ▸ Manifestation Code   🝜 Hierarchical Condition Category   Coding Clinic

● **Z15.0** **Genetic susceptibility to malignant neoplasm**

Code first if applicable, any current malignant neoplasm (C00-C75, C81-C96)

Use additional code, if applicable, for any personal history of malignant neoplasm (Z85.-)

Z15.01 **Genetic susceptibility to malignant neoplasm of breast**

Z15.02 **Genetic susceptibility to malignant neoplasm of ovary**

Z15.03 **Genetic susceptibility to malignant neoplasm of prostate**

Z15.04 **Genetic susceptibility to malignant neoplasm of endometrium**

Z15.09 **Genetic susceptibility to other malignant neoplasm**

Coding Clinic: 2021, Q1, P15

▷ **Z15.1** **Genetic susceptibility to epilepsy and neurodevelopmental disorders**

▷ Code also, if applicable, related disorders such as:
▷ developmental and epileptic encephalopathy (G93.45)
▷ developmental disorder of speech and language (F80.-)
▷ developmental disorders of scholastic skills (F81.-)
▷ epilepsy, by specific type (G40.-)
▷ intellectual disabilities (F70-F79)
▷ other neurodevelopmental disorder (F88)
▷ pervasive developmental disorders (F84.-)

▷ **Z15.2** **Genetic susceptibility to obesity**

▷ Code also, if applicable, any associated manifestations, such as:
▷ other obesity (E66.8-)
▷ polyphagia (R63.2)
▷ Use Additional code to identify body mass index (BMI), if known (Z68.-)

● **Z15.8** **Genetic susceptibility to other disease**

Z15.81 **Genetic susceptibility to multiple endocrine neoplasia [MEN]**

Excludes1   multiple endocrine neoplasia [MEN] syndromes (E31.2-)

Z15.89 **Genetic susceptibility to other disease**

RESISTANCE TO ANTIMICROBIAL DRUGS (Z16)

● **Z16** **Resistance to antimicrobial drugs**

Note: The codes in this category are provided for use as additional codes to identify the resistance and non-responsiveness of a condition to antimicrobial drugs.

Code first the infection

Excludes1   Methicillin resistant Staphylococcus aureus infection (A49.02)
Methicillin resistant Staphylococcus aureus pneumonia (J15.212)
Sepsis due to Methicillin resistant Staphylococcus aureus (A41.02)

● **Z16.1** **Resistance to beta lactam antibiotics**

Z16.10 **Resistance to unspecified beta lactam antibiotics**

Z16.11 **Resistance to penicillins**
Resistance to amoxicillin
Resistance to ampicillin

Z16.12 **Extended spectrum beta lactamase (ESBL) resistance**

Excludes2   Methicillin resistant Staphylococcus aureus infection in diseases classified elsewhere (B95.62)

Z16.13 **Resistance to carbapenem**

Z16.19 **Resistance to other specified beta lactam antibiotics**
Resistance to cephalosporins

● **Z16.2** **Resistance to other antibiotics**

Z16.20 **Resistance to unspecified antibiotic**
Resistance to antibiotics NOS

Z16.21 **Resistance to vancomycin**

Z16.22 **Resistance to vancomycin related antibiotics**

Z16.23 **Resistance to quinolones and fluoroquinolones**

Z16.24 **Resistance to multiple antibiotics**

Z16.29 **Resistance to other single specified antibiotic**
Resistance to aminoglycosides
Resistance to macrolides
Resistance to sulfonamides
Resistance to tetracyclines

● **Z16.3** **Resistance to other antimicrobial drugs**

Excludes1   resistance to antibiotics (Z16.1-, Z16.2-)

Z16.30 **Resistance to unspecified antimicrobial drugs**
Drug resistance NOS

Z16.31 **Resistance to antiparasitic drug(s)**
Resistance to quinine and related compounds

Z16.32 **Resistance to antifungal drug(s)**

Z16.33 **Resistance to antiviral drug(s)**

● **Z16.34** **Resistance to antimycobacterial drug(s)**
Resistance to tuberculostatics

Z16.341 **Resistance to single antimycobacterial drug**
Resistance to antimycobacterial drug NOS

Z16.342 **Resistance to multiple antimycobacterial drugs**

Z16.35 **Resistance to multiple antimicrobial drugs**

Excludes1   Resistance to multiple antibiotics only (Z16.24)

Z16.39 **Resistance to other specified antimicrobial drug**

ESTROGEN, AND OTHER HORMONES AND FACTORS RECEPTOR STATUS (Z17)

➡● **Z17** **Estrogen, and other hormones and factors receptor status**

▷ **Note:** Use one code, as available, for each receptor: Z17.0, Z17.1, Z17.2-. Z17.3-

Code first malignant neoplasm of breast (C50.-)

▷ *Code first malignant neoplasm, such as:*
▷ *malignant neoplasm of ovary (C56.-)*

Z17.0 **Estrogen receptor positive status [ER+]**
Coding Clinic: 2022, Q3, P15

Z17.1 **Estrogen receptor negative status [ER-]**

▷● **Z17.2** **Progesterone receptor status**

▷ **Z17.21** **Progesterone receptor positive status**
▷ PR+

▷ **Z17.22** **Progesterone receptor negative status**
▷ PR-

▷● **Z17.3** **Human epidermal growth factor 2 receptor**

▷ **Z17.31** **Human epidermal growth factor receptor 2 positive status**
▷ HER2+

▷ **Z17.32** **Human epidermal growth factor receptor 2 negative status**
▷ HER2-

▷● **Z17.4** **Combined receptor status**

▷ **Note:** Assign a code from subcategory Z17.4- when only a combined receptor status is documented

▷● **Z17.41** **Hormone receptor positive**
▷ HR+

▷ **Z17.410** **Hormone receptor positive with human epidermal growth factor receptor 2 positive status**
▷ HR+ with HER2+

▷ **Z17.411** **Hormone receptor positive with human epidermal growth factor receptor 2 negative status**
▷ HR+ with HER2-

▶● Z17.42   **Hormone receptor negative**
     ▶HR-
     ▶ Z17.420   **Hormone receptor negative with human epidermal growth factor receptor 2 positive status**
       ▶HR- with HER2+
     ▶ Z17.421   **Hormone receptor negative with human epidermal growth factor receptor 2 negative status**
       ▶HR- with HER2-
       ▶TNBC
       ▶Triple negative breast cancer

RETAINED FOREIGN BODY FRAGMENTS (Z18)

● Z18   Retained foreign body fragments

Includes   embedded fragment (status)
         embedded splinter (status)
         retained foreign body status

Excludes1   artificial joint prosthesis status (Z96.6-)
         foreign body accidentally left during a procedure (T81.5-)
         foreign body entering through orifice (T15-T19)
         in situ cardiac device (Z95.-)
         organ or tissue replaced by means other than transplant (Z96.-, Z97.-)
         organ or tissue replaced by transplant (Z94.-)
         personal history of retained foreign body fully removed Z87.821
         superficial foreign body (non-embedded splinter) - code to superficial foreign body, by site

● Z18.0   Retained radioactive fragments
     Z18.01   Retained depleted uranium fragments
     Z18.09   Other retained radioactive fragments
         Other retained depleted isotope fragments
         Retained nontherapeutic radioactive fragments

● Z18.1   Retained metal fragments
     Excludes1   retained radioactive metal fragments (Z18.01-Z18.09)
     Z18.10   Retained metal fragments, unspecified
         Retained metal fragment NOS
     Z18.11   Retained magnetic metal fragments
     Z18.12   Retained nonmagnetic metal fragments

Z18.2   Retained plastic fragments
     Acrylics fragments
     Diethylhexylphthalates fragments
     Isocyanate fragments

● Z18.3   Retained organic fragments
     Z18.31   Retained animal quills or spines
     Z18.32   Retained tooth
     Z18.33   Retained wood fragments
     Z18.39   Other retained organic fragments

● Z18.8   Other specified retained foreign body
     Z18.81   Retained glass fragments
     Z18.83   Retained stone or crystalline fragments
         Retained concrete or cement fragments
     Z18.89   Other specified retained foreign body fragments
         Coding Clinic: 2016, Q3, P24

Z18.9   Retained foreign body fragments, unspecified material

HORMONE SENSITIVITY MALIGNANCY STATUS (Z19)

● Z19   Hormone sensitivity malignancy status
     Code first malignant neoplasm —*see* Table of Neoplasms, by site, malignant
     Coding Clinic: 2016, Q4, P129

Z19.1   Hormone sensitive malignancy status
     Coding Clinic: 2016, Q4, P76

Z19.2   Hormone resistant malignancy status
     Castrate resistant prostate malignancy status
     Coding Clinic: 2016, Q4, P76

PERSONS WITH POTENTIAL HEALTH HAZARDS RELATED TO COMMUNICABLE DISEASES (Z20-Z29)

● Z20   Contact with and (suspected) exposure to communicable diseases
     Excludes1   carrier of infectious disease (Z22.-)
         diagnosed current infectious or parasitic disease - see Alphabetic Index
     Excludes2   personal history of infectious and parasitic diseases (Z86.1-)
     Coding Clinic: 2021, Q1, P37

● Z20.0   Contact with and (suspected) exposure to intestinal infectious diseases
     Z20.01   Contact with and (suspected) exposure to intestinal infectious diseases due to Escherichia coli (E. coli)
     Z20.09   Contact with and (suspected) exposure to other intestinal infectious diseases

Z20.1   Contact with and (suspected) exposure to tuberculosis

Z20.2   Contact with and (suspected) exposure to infections with a predominantly sexual mode of transmission

Z20.3   Contact with and (suspected) exposure to rabies

Z20.4   Contact with and (suspected) exposure to rubella

Z20.5   Contact with and (suspected) exposure to viral hepatitis

Z20.6   Contact with and (suspected) exposure to human immunodeficiency virus [HIV]
     Excludes1   asymptomatic human immunodeficiency virus [HIV]
         HIV infection status (Z21)

Z20.7   Contact with and (suspected) exposure to pediculosis, acariasis and other infestations

● Z20.8   Contact with and (suspected) exposure to other communicable diseases
     ● Z20.81   Contact with and (suspected) exposure to other bacterial communicable diseases
         Z20.810   Contact with and (suspected) exposure to anthrax
         Z20.811   Contact with and (suspected) exposure to meningococcus
         Z20.818   Contact with and (suspected) exposure to other bacterial communicable diseases
     ● Z20.82   Contact with and (suspected) exposure to other viral communicable diseases
         Z20.820   Contact with and (suspected) exposure to varicella
         Z20.821   Contact with and (suspected) exposure to Zika virus
         Z20.822   Contact with and (suspected) exposure to COVID-19
           Contact with and (suspected) exposure to SARS-CoV-2
           Coding Clinic: 2023, Q2, P3-4; 2022, Q2, P28,29; 2021, Q4, P109; 2021, Q1, P37-39, 42
         Z20.828   Contact with and (suspected) exposure to other viral communicable diseases
           Coding Clinic: 2022, Q3, P4; 2021, Q1, P37-39; 2016, Q4, P6-7, 121
     Z20.89   Contact with and (suspected) exposure to other communicable diseases

Z20.9   Contact with and (suspected) exposure to unspecified communicable disease

Z21   Asymptomatic human immunodeficiency virus [HIV] infection status 🔖

HIV positive NOS

Code first Human immunodeficiency virus [HIV] disease complicating pregnancy, childbirth and the puerperium, if applicable (O98.7-)

Excludes1	acquired immunodeficiency syndrome (B20)
	contact with human immunodeficiency virus [HIV] (Z20.6)
	exposure to human immunodeficiency virus [HIV] (Z20.6)
	human immunodeficiency virus [HIV] disease (B20)
	inconclusive laboratory evidence of human immunodeficiency virus [HIV] (R75)

Coding Clinic: 2022, Q1, P37; 2019, Q1, P10-11

● **Z22   Carrier of infectious disease**

Includes	colonization status
	suspected carrier

Excludes2	carrier of viral hepatitis (B18.-)

Z22.0   **Carrier of typhoid**

Z22.1   **Carrier of other intestinal infectious diseases**

Z22.2   **Carrier of diphtheria**

● Z22.3   **Carrier of other specified bacterial diseases**

 Z22.31   **Carrier of bacterial disease due to meningococci**

 ● Z22.32   **Carrier of bacterial disease due to staphylococci**

  Z22.321   **Carrier or suspected carrier of Methicillin susceptible Staphylococcus aureus**
   MSSA colonization

  Z22.322   **Carrier or suspected carrier of Methicillin resistant Staphylococcus aureus**
   MRSA colonization

 ● Z22.33   **Carrier of bacterial disease due to streptococci**

  Z22.330   **Carrier of Group B streptococcus**

Excludes1	Carrier of streptococcus group B (GBS) complicating pregnancy, childbirth and the puerperium (O99.82-)

  Z22.338   **Carrier of other streptococcus**

 ● Z22.34   **Carrier of Acinetobacter baumannii**

  Z22.340   **Carrier of carbapenem-resistant Acinetobacter baumannii**

  Z22.341   **Carrier of carbapenem-sensitive Acinetobacter baumannii**

  Z22.349   **Carrier of Acinetobacter baumannii, unspecified**

 ● Z22.35   **Carrier of Enterobacterales**
  Carrier of E. coli
  Carrier of K. pneumoniae

  Z22.350   **Carrier of carbapenem-resistant Enterobacterales**

  Z22.358   **Carrier of other Enterobacterales**
   Carrier of carbapenem-sensitive Enterobacterales
   Carrier of ESBL-producing Enterobacterales
   Carrier of extended-spectrum beta-lactamase producing Enterobacterales

  Z22.359   **Carrier of Enterobacterales, unspecified**

 Z22.39   **Carrier of other specified bacterial diseases**

Z22.4   **Carrier of infections with a predominantly sexual mode of transmission**

Z22.6   **Carrier of human T-lymphotropic virus type-1 [HTLV-1] infection**

Z22.7   **Latent tuberculosis**
Latent tuberculosis infection (LTBI)

Excludes1	nonspecific reaction to cell mediated immunity measurement of gamma interferon antigen response without active tuberculosis (R76.12)
	nonspecific reaction to tuberculin skin test without active tuberculosis (R76.11)

Z22.8   **Carrier of other infectious diseases**

Z22.9   **Carrier of infectious disease, unspecified**

Z23   **Encounter for immunization**

Code first any routine childhood examination

Note: Procedure codes are required to identify the types of immunizations given.

Code also, if applicable, encounter for immunization safety counseling (Z71.85)

● **Z28   Immunization not carried out and underimmunization status**

Includes	vaccination not carried out

Code also, if applicable, encounter for immunization safety counseling (Z71.85)

● Z28.0   **Immunization not carried out because of contraindication**

 Z28.01   **Immunization not carried out because of acute illness of patient**

 Z28.02   **Immunization not carried out because of chronic illness or condition of patient**

 Z28.03   **Immunization not carried out because of immune compromised state of patient**

 Z28.04   **Immunization not carried out because of patient allergy to vaccine or component**

 Z28.09   **Immunization not carried out because of other contraindication**

Z28.1   **Immunization not carried out because of patient decision for reasons of belief or group pressure**
Immunization not carried out because of religious belief

● Z28.2   **Immunization not carried out because of patient decision for other and unspecified reason**

 Z28.20   **Immunization not carried out because of patient decision for unspecified reason**

 Z28.21   **Immunization not carried out because of patient refusal**

 Z28.29   **Immunization not carried out because of patient decision for other reason**

Z28.3   **Underimmunization status**
Coding Clinic: 2021, Q4, P110

Use additional code, if applicable, to identify:
immunization not carried out because of contraindication (Z28.0-)
immunization not carried out because of patient decision for other and unspecified reason (Z28.2-)
immunization not carried out because of patient decision for reasons of belief or group pressure (Z28.1)
immunization not carried out for other reason (Z28.8-)

 Z28.31   **Underimmunization for COVID-19 status**

  Note: These codes should not be used for individuals who are not eligible for the COVID-19 vaccines, as determined by the healthcare provider.

  Z28.310   **Unvaccinated for COVID-19**

  Z28.311   **Partially vaccinated for COVID-19**

 Z28.39   **Other underimmunization status**
  Delinquent immunization status
  Lapsed immunization schedule status

● Z28.8   **Immunization not carried out for other reason**

 Z28.81   **Immunization not carried out due to patient having had the disease**

CHAPTER 21 (Z00-Z99)

Z28.82   **Immunization not carried out because of caregiver refusal**
      Immunization not carried out because of guardian refusal
      Immunization not carried out because of parent refusal
      Excludes1   immunization not carried out because of caregiver refusal because of religious belief (Z28.1)

Z28.83   **Immunization not carried out due to unavailability of vaccine**
      Delay in delivery of vaccine
      Lack of availability of vaccine
      Manufacturer delay of vaccine

Z28.89   **Immunization not carried out for other reason**

Z28.9   **Immunization not carried out for unspecified reason**

● **Z29**   **Encounter for other prophylactic measures**
    Excludes1   desensitization to allergens (Z51.6)
                prophylactic surgery (Z40.-)
    Coding Clinic: 2016, Q4, P130

  ● **Z29.1**   **Encounter for prophylactic immunotherapy**
      Encounter for administration of immunoglobulin
      Coding Clinic: 2016, Q4, P78-79

    Z29.11   **Encounter for prophylactic immunotherapy for respiratory syncytial virus (RSV)**

    Z29.12   **Encounter for prophylactic antivenin**

    Z29.13   **Encounter for prophylactic Rho(D) immune globulin**
        Coding Clinic: 2019, Q3, P5

    Z29.14   **Encounter for prophylactic rabies immune globin**

  Z29.3   **Encounter for prophylactic fluoride administration**
    Coding Clinic: 2016, Q4, P79

  ● **Z29.8**   **Encounter for other specified prophylactic measures**
    Coding Clinic: 2022, Q2, P27; 2016, Q4, P79

    Z29.81   **Encounter for HIV pre-exposure prophylaxis**
      Code also, if applicable, risk factors for HIV, such as: contact with and (suspected) exposure to human immunodeficiency virus [HIV](Z20.6)
           high risk sexual behavior (Z72.5-)

    Z29.89   **Encounter for other specified prophylactic measures**

  Z29.9   **Encounter for prophylactic measures, unspecified**
    Coding Clinic: 2016, Q4, P79

PERSONS ENCOUNTERING HEALTH SERVICES IN CIRCUMSTANCES RELATED TO REPRODUCTION (Z30-Z39)

● **Z30**   **Encounter for contraceptive management**

  ● **Z30.0**   **Encounter for general counseling and advice on contraception**

    ● **Z30.01**   **Encounter for initial prescription of contraceptives**
      Excludes1   encounter for surveillance of contraceptives (Z30.4-)

      Z30.011   **Encounter for initial prescription of contraceptive pills**

      Z30.012   **Encounter for prescription of emergency contraception**
          Encounter for postcoital contraception

      Z30.013   **Encounter for initial prescription of injectable contraceptive**

      Z30.014   **Encounter for initial prescription of intrauterine contraceptive device**
        Excludes1   encounter for insertion of intrauterine contraceptive device (Z30.430, Z30.432)

      Z30.015   **Encounter for initial prescription of vaginal ring hormonal contraceptive**
        Coding Clinic: 2016, Q4, P78

      Z30.016   **Encounter for initial prescription of transdermal patch hormonal contraceptive device**
        Coding Clinic: 2016, Q4, P78

      Z30.017   **Encounter for initial prescription of implantable subdermal contraceptive**
        Coding Clinic: 2016, Q4, P78

      Z30.018   **Encounter for initial prescription of other contraceptives**
        Encounter for initial prescription of barrier contraception
        Encounter for initial prescription of diaphragm

      Z30.019   **Encounter for initial prescription of contraceptives, unspecified**

    Z30.02   **Counseling and instruction in natural family planning to avoid pregnancy**

    Z30.09   **Encounter for other general counseling and advice on contraception**
      Encounter for family planning advice NOS

  Z30.2   **Encounter for sterilization**
    Coding Clinic: 2021, Q3, P13

  ● **Z30.4**   **Encounter for surveillance of contraceptives**

    Z30.40   **Encounter for surveillance of contraceptives, unspecified**

    Z30.41   **Encounter for surveillance of contraceptive pills**
      Encounter for repeat prescription for contraceptive pill

    Z30.42   **Encounter for surveillance of injectable contraceptive**

    ● **Z30.43**   **Encounter for surveillance of intrauterine contraceptive device**

      Z30.430   **Encounter for insertion of intrauterine contraceptive device**

      Z30.431   **Encounter for routine checking of intrauterine contraceptive device**

      Z30.432   **Encounter for removal of intrauterine contraceptive device**

      Z30.433   **Encounter for removal and reinsertion of intrauterine contraceptive device**
        Encounter for replacement of intrauterine contraceptive device

    Z30.44   **Encounter for surveillance of vaginal ring hormonal contraceptive device**
      Coding Clinic: 2016, Q4, P78

    Z30.45   **Encounter for surveillance of transdermal patch hormonal contraceptive device**
      Coding Clinic: 2016, Q4, P78

    Z30.46   **Encounter for surveillance of implantable subdermal contraceptive**
      Encounter for checking, reinsertion or removal of implantable subdermal contraceptive
      Coding Clinic: 2016, Q4, P78

    Z30.49   **Encounter for surveillance of other contraceptives**
      Encounter for surveillance of barrier contraception
      Encounter for surveillance of diaphragm

  Z30.8   **Encounter for other contraceptive management**
    Encounter for postvasectomy sperm count
    Encounter for routine examination for contraceptive maintenance
    Excludes1   sperm count following sterilization reversal (Z31.42)
          sperm count for fertility testing (Z31.41)

  Z30.9   **Encounter for contraceptive management, unspecified**

● **Z31**   **Encounter for procreative management**
    Excludes2   complications associated with artificial fertilization (N98.-)
             female infertility (N97.-)
             male infertility (N46.-)

▶ New   ⇒ Revised   ~~deleted~~ Deleted   Excludes 1   Excludes 2   Includes   Use additional   Code first   Code also   Key words

OGCR Official Guidelines   X Assign placeholder X   ● Use Additional Character(s)   ▶ Manifestation Code   🄗 Hierarchical Condition Category   Coding Clinic

Z31.0   Encounter for reversal of previous sterilization

● Z31.4   Encounter for procreative investigation and testing

      Excludes1   postvasectomy sperm count (Z30.8)

    Z31.41   **Encounter for fertility testing**
          Encounter for fallopian tube patency testing
          Encounter for sperm count for fertility testing

    Z31.42   **Aftercare following sterilization reversal**
          Sperm count following sterilization reversal

●   Z31.43   **Encounter for genetic testing of female for procreative management**
          Use additional code for recurrent pregnancy loss, if applicable (N96, O26.2-)

          Excludes1   nonprocreative genetic testing (Z13.7-)

      Z31.430   **Encounter of female for testing for genetic disease carrier status for procreative management**

      Z31.438   **Encounter for other genetic testing of female for procreative management**

●   Z31.44   **Encounter for genetic testing of male for procreative management**

          Excludes1   nonprocreative genetic testing (Z13.7-)

      Z31.440   **Encounter of male for testing for genetic disease carrier status for procreative management**

      Z31.441   **Encounter for testing of male partner of patient with recurrent pregnancy loss**   **A**

      Z31.448   **Encounter for other genetic testing of male for procreative management**   **A**

    Z31.49   **Encounter for other procreative investigation and testing**

Z31.5   Encounter for procreative genetic counseling

● Z31.6   Encounter for general counseling and advice on procreation

    Z31.61   **Procreative counseling and advice using natural family planning**

    Z31.62   **Encounter for fertility preservation counseling**
          Encounter for fertility preservation counseling prior to cancer therapy
          Encounter for fertility preservation counseling prior to surgical removal of gonads

    Z31.69   **Encounter for other general counseling and advice on procreation**

Z31.7   Encounter for procreative management and counseling for gestational carrier

      Excludes1   pregnant state, gestational carrier (Z33.3)
      Coding Clinic: 2016, Q4, P78

● Z31.8   Encounter for other procreative management

    Z31.81   **Encounter for male factor infertility in female patient**

    Z31.82   **Encounter for Rh incompatibility status**
          Coding Clinic: 2015, Q3, P40

    Z31.83   **Encounter for assisted reproductive fertility procedure cycle**
          Patient undergoing in vitro fertilization cycle
          Use additional code to identify the type of infertility

          Excludes1   pre-cycle diagnosis and testing - code to reason for encounter
          Coding Clinic: 2022, Q2, P15,16

    Z31.84   **Encounter for fertility preservation procedure**
          Encounter for fertility preservation procedure prior to cancer therapy
          Encounter for fertility preservation procedure prior to surgical removal of gonads

    Z31.89   **Encounter for other procreative management**

Z31.9   Encounter for procreative management, unspecified

| First trimester (0 to 14 weeks) | Second trimester (14 to 28 weeks) | Third trimester (28 weeks to delivery) |

Figure 21-1   Trimesters. (From Shiland, Betsy J. Medical Terminology & Anatomy for ICD-10 Coding, ed 2, Mosby, 2015)

● Z32   Encounter for pregnancy test and childbirth and childcare instruction

●   Z32.0   Encounter for pregnancy test

    Z32.00   **Encounter for pregnancy test, result unknown**
          Encounter for pregnancy test NOS

    Z32.01   **Encounter for pregnancy test, result positive**   **M**

    Z32.02   **Encounter for pregnancy test, result negative**

  Z32.2   Encounter for childbirth instruction

  Z32.3   Encounter for childcare instruction
      Encounter for prenatal or postpartum childcare instruction

● Z33   Pregnant state

  Z33.1   Pregnant state, incidental   **M**
      Pregnancy NOS
      Pregnant state NOS

      Excludes1   complications of pregnancy (O00-O9A) pregnant state, gestational carrier (Z33.3)

  Z33.2   Encounter for elective termination of pregnancy   **M**

      Excludes1   early fetal death with retention of dead fetus (O02.1)
          late fetal death (O36.4)
          spontaneous abortion (O03)
      Coding Clinic: 2023, Q2, P15; 2016, Q4, P130

  Z33.3   Pregnant state, gestational carrier

      Excludes1   encounter for procreative management and counseling for gestational carrier (Z31.7)
      Coding Clinic: 2016, Q4, P78

● Z34   Encounter for supervision of normal pregnancy

    Excludes1   any complication of pregnancy (O00-O9A)
          encounter for pregnancy test (Z32.0-)
          encounter for supervision of high risk pregnancy (O09.-)
    Coding Clinic: 2016, Q4, P6

●   Z34.0   Encounter for supervision of normal first pregnancy

    Z34.00   **Encounter for supervision of normal first pregnancy, unspecified trimester**   **M**

    Z34.01   **Encounter for supervision of normal first pregnancy, first trimester**   **M**

    Z34.02   **Encounter for supervision of normal first pregnancy, second trimester**   **M**

    Z34.03   **Encounter for supervision of normal first pregnancy, third trimester**   **M**

●   Z34.8   Encounter for supervision of other normal pregnancy

    Z34.80   **Encounter for supervision of other normal pregnancy, unspecified trimester**   **M**

    Z34.81   **Encounter for supervision of other normal pregnancy, first trimester**   **M**

    Z34.82   **Encounter for supervision of other normal pregnancy, second trimester**   **M**

    Z34.83   **Encounter for supervision of other normal pregnancy, third trimester**   **M**

CHAPTER 21 (Z00-Z99)

● **Z34.9** **Encounter for supervision of normal pregnancy, unspecified**

　　　Z34.90　Encounter for supervision of normal pregnancy, unspecified, **unspecified trimester**　　M

　　　Z34.91　Encounter for supervision of normal pregnancy, unspecified, **first trimester**　　M

　　　Z34.92　Encounter for supervision of normal pregnancy, unspecified, **second trimester**　　M

　　　Z34.93　Encounter for supervision of normal pregnancy, unspecified, **third trimester**　　M

● **Z36** **Encounter for antenatal screening of mother**

　　　Includes　　Encounter for placental sample (taken vaginally)
　　　　　　　　Screening is the testing for disease or disease precursors in asymptomatic individuals so that early detection and treatment can be provided for those who test positive for the disease.

　　　Excludes1　diagnostic examination - code to sign or symptom
　　　　　　　　encounter for suspected maternal and fetal conditions ruled out (Z03.7-)
　　　　　　　　suspected fetal condition affecting management of pregnancy - code to condition in Chapter 15

　　　Excludes2　abnormal findings on antenatal screening of mother (O28.-)
　　　　　　　　genetic counseling and testing (Z31.43-, Z31.5)
　　　　　　　　routine prenatal care (Z34)

　　Z36.0 **Encounter for antenatal screening for chromosomal anomalies**　　M

　　Z36.1 **Encounter for antenatal screening for raised alphafetoprotein level**　　M
　　　　Encounter for antenatal screening for elevated maternal serum alphafetoprotein level

　　Z36.2 **Encounter for other antenatal screening follow-up**　　M
　　　　Non-visualized anatomy on a previous scan

　　Z36.3 **Encounter for antenatal screening for malformations**　　M
　　　　Screening for a suspected anomaly

　　Z36.4 **Encounter for antenatal screening for fetal growth retardation**　　M
　　　　Intrauterine growth restriction (IUGR)/small-for-dates

　　Z36.5 **Encounter for antenatal screening for isoimmunization**　　M

● **Z36.8** **Encounter for other antenatal screening**

　　　Z36.81　Encounter for antenatal screening for **hydrops fetalis**　　M

　　　Z36.82　Encounter for antenatal screening for **nuchal translucency**　　M

　　　Z36.83　Encounter for fetal screening for **congenital cardiac abnormalities**　　M

　　　Z36.84　Encounter for antenatal screening for **fetal lung maturity**　　M

　　　Z36.85　Encounter for antenatal screening for **Streptococcus B**　　M

　　　Z36.86　Encounter for antenatal screening for **cervical length**　　M
　　　　　　Screening for risk of pre-term labor

　　　Z36.87　Encounter for antenatal screening for **uncertain dates**　　M

　　　Z36.88　Encounter for antenatal screening for **fetal macrosomia**　　M
　　　　　　Screening for large-for-dates

　　　Z36.89　Encounter for **other specified** antenatal screening　　M

　　　Z36.8A　Encounter for antenatal screening for **other genetic defects**　　M

　　Z36.9 **Encounter for antenatal screening, unspecified**　　M

● **Z3A** **Weeks of gestation**

　　　Note: Codes from category Z3A are for use, only on the maternal record, to indicate the weeks of gestation of the pregnancy, if known.
　　　Code first obstetric condition or encounter for delivery (O09-O60, O80-O82)
　　　Coding Clinic: 2022, Q2, P3-4; 2016, Q4, P130; 2013, Q2, P33

● **Z3A.0** **Weeks of gestation of pregnancy, unspecified or less than 10 weeks**

　　　Z3A.00　Weeks of gestation of pregnancy **not specified**　　M

　　　Z3A.01　**Less than 8 weeks** gestation of pregnancy　　M

　　　Z3A.08　**8 weeks** gestation of pregnancy　　M

　　　Z3A.09　**9 weeks** gestation of pregnancy　　M

● **Z3A.1** **Weeks of gestation of pregnancy, weeks 10-19**

　　　Z3A.10　**10 weeks** gestation of pregnancy　　M

　　　Z3A.11　**11 weeks** gestation of pregnancy　　M

　　　Z3A.12　**12 weeks** gestation of pregnancy　　M

　　　Z3A.13　**13 weeks** gestation of pregnancy　　M

　　　Z3A.14　**14 weeks** gestation of pregnancy　　M

　　　Z3A.15　**15 weeks** gestation of pregnancy　　M

　　　Z3A.16　**16 weeks** gestation of pregnancy　　M
　　　　　　Coding Clinic: 2016, Q4, P5

　　　Z3A.17　**17 weeks** gestation of pregnancy　　M

　　　Z3A.18　**18 weeks** gestation of pregnancy　　M
　　　　　　Coding Clinic: 2019, Q2, P11

　　　Z3A.19　**19 weeks** gestation of pregnancy　　M

● **Z3A.2** **Weeks of gestation of pregnancy, weeks 20-29**

　　　Z3A.20　**20 weeks** gestation of pregnancy　　M
　　　　　　Coding Clinic: 2016, Q4, P6

　　　Z3A.21　**21 weeks** gestation of pregnancy　　M

　　　Z3A.22　**22 weeks** gestation of pregnancy　　M
　　　　　　Coding Clinic: 2016, Q4, P6

　　　Z3A.23　**23 weeks** gestation of pregnancy　　M

　　　Z3A.24　**24 weeks** gestation of pregnancy　　M

　　　Z3A.25　**25 weeks** gestation of pregnancy　　M

　　　Z3A.26　**26 weeks** gestation of pregnancy　　M

　　　Z3A.27　**27 weeks** gestation of pregnancy　　M

　　　Z3A.28　**28 weeks** gestation of pregnancy　　M

　　　Z3A.29　**29 weeks** gestation of pregnancy　　M

● **Z3A.3** **Weeks of gestation of pregnancy, weeks 30-39**

　　　Z3A.30　**30 weeks** gestation of pregnancy　　M

　　　Z3A.31　**31 weeks** gestation of pregnancy　　M

　　　Z3A.32　**32 weeks** gestation of pregnancy　　M
　　　　　　Coding Clinic: 2016, Q4, P6

　　　Z3A.33　**33 weeks** gestation of pregnancy　　M

　　　Z3A.34　**34 weeks** gestation of pregnancy　　M

　　　Z3A.35　**35 weeks** gestation of pregnancy　　M

　　　Z3A.36　**36 weeks** gestation of pregnancy　　M

　　　Z3A.37　**37 weeks** gestation of pregnancy　　M

　　　Z3A.38　**38 weeks** gestation of pregnancy　　M
　　　　　　Coding Clinic: 2016, Q2, P34

　　　Z3A.39　**39 weeks** gestation of pregnancy　　M

● **Z3A.4** **Weeks of gestation of pregnancy, weeks 40 or greater**

　　　Z3A.40　**40 weeks** gestation of pregnancy　　M

　　　Z3A.41　**41 weeks** gestation of pregnancy　　M

　　　Z3A.42　**42 weeks** gestation of pregnancy　　M

　　　Z3A.49　**Greater than 42 weeks** gestation of pregnancy　　M

● **Z37** **Outcome of delivery**

　　　This category is intended for use as an additional code to identify the outcome of delivery on the mother's record. It is not for use on the newborn record.

　　　Excludes1　stillbirth (P95)

　　Z37.0 **Single live birth**　　M
　　　　Coding Clinic: 2016, Q2, P34

　　Z37.1 **Single stillbirth**　　M

　　Z37.2 **Twins, both liveborn**　　M

　　Z37.3 **Twins, one liveborn and one stillbirth**　　M

▶ New　⟹ Revised　~~deleted~~ Deleted　Excludes 1　Excludes 2　Includes　Use additional　Code first　Code also　Key words

OGCR Official Guidelines　X Assign placeholder X　● Use Additional Character(s)　▌Manifestation Code　🅗 Hierarchical Condition Category　Coding Clinic

Z37.4   Twins, both stillborn   M

● Z37.5   Other multiple births, all liveborn

     Z37.50   Multiple births, unspecified, all liveborn   M

     Z37.51   Triplets, all liveborn   M

     Z37.52   Quadruplets, all liveborn   M

     Z37.53   Quintuplets, all liveborn   M

     Z37.54   Sextuplets, all liveborn   M

     Z37.59   Other multiple births, all liveborn   M

● Z37.6   Other multiple births, some liveborn

     Z37.60   Multiple births, unspecified, some liveborn   M

     Z37.61   Triplets, some liveborn   M

     Z37.62   Quadruplets, some liveborn   M

     Z37.63   Quintuplets, some liveborn   M

     Z37.64   Sextuplets, some liveborn   M

     Z37.69   Other multiple births, some liveborn   M

Z37.7   Other multiple births, all stillborn   M

Z37.9   Outcome of delivery, unspecified   M
     Multiple birth NOS
     Single birth NOS

● Z38   Liveborn infants according to place of birth and type of delivery
     This category is for use as the principal code on the initial record of a newborn baby. It is to be used for the initial birth record only. It is not to be used on the mother's record.
     Coding Clinic: 2017, Q2, P6-7; 2016, Q4, P126-127, 130; 2015, Q2, P15

● Z38.0   Single liveborn infant, born in hospital
     Single liveborn infant, born in birthing center or other health care facility
     Coding Clinic: 2017, Q2, P5-7

     Z38.00   Single liveborn infant, delivered vaginally   N
         Coding Clinic: 2021, Q4, P23; 2018, Q4, P26; 2016, Q4, P7, 55

     Z38.01   Single liveborn infant, delivered by cesarean   N
         Coding Clinic: 2017, Q2, P7; 2016, Q3, P18

Z38.1   Single liveborn infant, born outside hospital   N

Z38.2   Single liveborn infant, unspecified as to place of birth   N
     Single liveborn infant NOS

● Z38.3   Twin liveborn infant, born in hospital

     Z38.30   Twin liveborn infant, delivered vaginally   N

     Z38.31   Twin liveborn infant, delivered by cesarean   N

Z38.4   Twin liveborn infant, born outside hospital   N

Z38.5   Twin liveborn infant, unspecified as to place of birth   N

● Z38.6   Other multiple liveborn infant, born in hospital

     Z38.61   Triplet liveborn infant, delivered vaginally   N

     Z38.62   Triplet liveborn infant, delivered by cesarean   N

     Z38.63   Quadruplet liveborn infant, delivered vaginally   N

     Z38.64   Quadruplet liveborn infant, delivered by cesarean   N

     Z38.65   Quintuplet liveborn infant, delivered vaginally   N

     Z38.66   Quintuplet liveborn infant, delivered by cesarean   N

     Z38.68   Other multiple liveborn infant, delivered vaginally   N

     Z38.69   Other multiple liveborn infant, delivered by cesarean   N

Z38.7   Other multiple liveborn infant, born outside hospital   N

Z38.8   Other multiple liveborn infant, unspecified as to place of birth   N

● Z39   Encounter for maternal postpartum care and examination

Z39.0   Encounter for care and examination of mother immediately after delivery   M
     Care and observation in uncomplicated cases when the delivery occurs outside a healthcare facility

     Excludes1   care for postpartum complication - see Alphabetic index
     Coding Clinic: 2021, Q3, P13

Z39.1   Encounter for care and examination of lactating mother   M
     Encounter for supervision of lactation

     Excludes1   disorders of lactation (O92.-)

Z39.2   Encounter for routine postpartum follow-up   M

ENCOUNTERS FOR OTHER SPECIFIC HEALTH CARE (Z40-Z53)

Categories Z40-Z53 are intended for use to indicate a reason for care. They may be used for patients who have already been treated for a disease or injury, but who are receiving aftercare or prophylactic care, or care to consolidate the treatment, or to deal with a residual state

     Excludes2   follow-up examination for medical surveillance after treatment (Z08-Z09)

● Z40   Encounter for prophylactic surgery

     Excludes1   organ donations (Z52.-)
         therapeutic organ removal - code to condition
     Coding Clinic: 2016, Q4, P79

● Z40.0   Encounter for prophylactic surgery for risk factors related to malignant neoplasms
     Admission for prophylactic organ removal
     Use additional code to identify risk factor

     Z40.00   Encounter for prophylactic removal of unspecified organ

     Z40.01   Encounter for prophylactic removal of breast

     Z40.02   Encounter for prophylactic removal of ovary(s)
         Encounter for prophylactic removal of ovary(s) and fallopian tube(s)

     Z40.03   Encounter for prophylactic removal of fallopian tube(s)

     Z40.09   Encounter for prophylactic removal of other organ

Z40.8   Encounter for other prophylactic surgery

Z40.9   Encounter for prophylactic surgery, unspecified

● Z41   Encounter for procedures for purposes other than remedying health state

Z41.1   Encounter for cosmetic surgery
     Encounter for cosmetic breast implant
     Encounter for cosmetic procedure

     Excludes1   encounter for plastic and reconstructive surgery following medical procedure or healed injury (Z42.-)
         encounter for post-mastectomy breast implantation (Z42.1)

Z41.2   Encounter for routine and ritual male circumcision

Z41.3   Encounter for ear piercing

Z41.8   Encounter for other procedures for purposes other than remedying health state

Z41.9   Encounter for procedure for purposes other than remedying health state, unspecified

● Z42   Encounter for plastic and reconstructive surgery following medical procedure or healed injury

     Excludes1   encounter for cosmetic plastic surgery (Z41.1)
         encounter for plastic surgery for treatment of current injury - code to relevent injury

Z42.1   Encounter for breast reconstruction following mastectomy   A

     Excludes1   deformity and disproportion of reconstructed breast (N65.1-)

Z42.8   Encounter for other plastic and reconstructive surgery following medical procedure or healed injury
     Coding Clinic: 2017, Q1, P42

CHAPTER 21 (Z00-Z99)

● **Z43   Encounter for attention to artificial openings**

Includes   closure of artificial openings
passage of sounds or bougies through artificial openings
reforming artificial openings
removal of catheter from artificial openings
toilet or cleansing of artificial openings

Excludes1   complications of external stoma (J95.0-, K94.-, N99.5-)

Excludes2   fitting and adjustment of prosthetic and other devices (Z44-Z46)

Z43.0   **Encounter for attention to tracheostomy** 🐾

Z43.1   **Encounter for attention to gastrostomy** 🐾

      Excludes2   artificial opening status only, without need for care (Z93.-)

Z43.2   **Encounter for attention to ileostomy** 🐾
      Coding Clinic: 2016, Q3, P5

Z43.3   **Encounter for attention to colostomy** 🐾

Z43.4   **Encounter for attention to other artificial openings of digestive tract** 🐾

Z43.5   **Encounter for attention to cystostomy** 🐾

Z43.6   **Encounter for attention to other artificial openings of urinary tract** 🐾
Encounter for attention to nephrostomy
Encounter for attention to ureterostomy
Encounter for attention to urethrostomy

Z43.7   **Encounter for attention to artificial vagina**

Z43.8   **Encounter for attention to other artificial openings** 🐾

Z43.9   **Encounter for attention to unspecified artificial opening** 🐾

● **Z44   Encounter for fitting and adjustment of external prosthetic device**

Includes   removal or replacement of external prosthetic device

Excludes1   malfunction or other complications of device - see Alphabetical Index presence of prosthetic device (Z97.-)

● **Z44.0**   **Encounter for fitting and adjustment of artificial arm**

● **Z44.00**   Encounter for fitting and adjustment of unspecified artificial arm

     Z44.001   Encounter for fitting and adjustment of unspecified right artificial arm

     Z44.002   Encounter for fitting and adjustment of unspecified left artificial arm

     Z44.009   Encounter for fitting and adjustment of unspecified artificial arm, unspecified arm

● **Z44.01**   Encounter for fitting and adjustment of complete artificial arm

     Z44.011   Encounter for fitting and adjustment of complete right artificial arm

     Z44.012   Encounter for fitting and adjustment of complete left artificial arm

     Z44.019   Encounter for fitting and adjustment of complete artificial arm, unspecified arm

● **Z44.02**   Encounter for fitting and adjustment of partial artificial arm

     Z44.021   Encounter for fitting and adjustment of partial artificial right arm

     Z44.022   Encounter for fitting and adjustment of partial artificial left arm

     Z44.029   Encounter for fitting and adjustment of partial artificial arm, unspecified arm

● **Z44.1**   **Encounter for fitting and adjustment of artificial leg**

● **Z44.10**   Encounter for fitting and adjustment of unspecified artificial leg

     Z44.101   Encounter for fitting and adjustment of unspecified right artificial leg 🐾

     Z44.102   Encounter for fitting and adjustment of unspecified left artificial leg 🐾

     Z44.109   Encounter for fitting and adjustment of unspecified artificial leg, unspecified leg 🐾

● **Z44.11**   Encounter for fitting and adjustment of complete artificial leg

     Z44.111   Encounter for fitting and adjustment of complete right artificial leg 🐾

     Z44.112   Encounter for fitting and adjustment of complete left artificial leg 🐾

     Z44.119   Encounter for fitting and adjustment of complete artificial leg, unspecified leg 🐾

● **Z44.12**   Encounter for fitting and adjustment of partial artificial leg

     Z44.121   Encounter for fitting and adjustment of partial artificial right leg 🐾

     Z44.122   Encounter for fitting and adjustment of partial artificial left leg 🐾

     Z44.129   Encounter for fitting and adjustment of partial artificial leg, unspecified leg 🐾

● **Z44.2**   **Encounter for fitting and adjustment of artificial eye**

Excludes1   mechanical complication of ocular prosthesis (T85.3)

Z44.20   Encounter for fitting and adjustment of artificial eye, unspecified

Z44.21   Encounter for fitting and adjustment of artificial right eye

Z44.22   Encounter for fitting and adjustment of artificial left eye

● **Z44.3**   **Encounter for fitting and adjustment of external breast prosthesis**

Excludes1   complications of breast implant (T85.4-)
encounter for adjustment or removal of breast implant (Z45.81-)
encounter for initial breast implant insertion for cosmetic breast augmentation (Z41.1)
encounter for breast reconstruction following mastectomy (Z42.1)

Z44.30   Encounter for fitting and adjustment of external breast prosthesis, unspecified breast

Z44.31   Encounter for fitting and adjustment of external right breast prosthesis

Z44.32   Encounter for fitting and adjustment of external left breast prosthesis

Z44.8   **Encounter for fitting and adjustment of other external prosthetic devices**

Z44.9   **Encounter for fitting and adjustment of unspecified external prosthetic device**

● **Z45   Encounter for adjustment and management of implanted device**

Includes   removal or replacement of implanted device

Excludes1   malfunction or other complications of device - see Alphabetical Index

Excludes2   encounter for fitting and adjustment of non-implanted device (Z46.-)

● **Z45.0**   **Encounter for adjustment and management of cardiac device**

● **Z45.01**   Encounter for adjustment and management of cardiac pacemaker
Encounter for adjustment and management of cardiac resynchronization therapy pacemaker (CRT-P)

Excludes1   encounter for adjustment and management of automatic implantable cardiac defibrillator with synchronous cardiac pacemaker (Z45.02)

     Z45.010   Encounter for checking and testing of cardiac pacemaker pulse generator [battery]
Encounter for replacing cardiac pacemaker pulse generator [battery]

1530

▶ New   ⇒ Revised   ~~deleted~~ Deleted   Excludes 1   Excludes 2   Includes   Use additional   Code first   Code also   Key words

OGCR Official Guidelines   X Assign placeholder X   ● Use Additional Character(s)   ▸ Manifestation Code   🐾 Hierarchical Condition Category   Coding Clinic

Z45.018   Encounter for adjustment and management of other part of cardiac pacemaker

> **Excludes1**   presence of other part of cardiac pacemaker (Z95.0)
>
> **Excludes2**   presence of prosthetic and other devices (Z95.1-Z95.5, Z95.811-Z97)

Z45.02   **Encounter for adjustment and management of automatic implantable cardiac defibrillator**

Encounter for adjustment and management of automatic implantable cardiac defibrillator with synchronous cardiac pacemaker

Encounter for adjustment and management of cardiac resynchronization therapy defibrillator (CRT-D)

Coding Clinic: 2024, Q1, P22,23

Z45.09   **Encounter for adjustment and management of other cardiac device**

Z45.1   **Encounter for adjustment and management of infusion pump**

Z45.2   **Encounter for adjustment and management of vascular access device**

Encounter for adjustment and management of vascular catheters

> **Excludes1**   encounter for adjustment and management of renal dialysis catheter (Z49.01)

● Z45.3   **Encounter for adjustment and management of implanted devices of the special senses**

Z45.31   **Encounter for adjustment and management of implanted visual substitution device**

● Z45.32   **Encounter for adjustment and management of implanted hearing device**

> **Excludes1**   encounter for fitting and adjustment of hearing aid (Z46.1)

Z45.320   **Encounter for adjustment and management of bone conduction device**

Z45.321   **Encounter for adjustment and management of cochlear device**

Z45.328   **Encounter for adjustment and management of other implanted hearing device**

● Z45.4   **Encounter for adjustment and management of implanted nervous system device**

Z45.41   **Encounter for adjustment and management of cerebrospinal fluid drainage device**

Encounter for adjustment and management of cerebral ventricular (communicating) shunt

Z45.42   **Encounter for adjustment and management of neuropacemaker**

Encounter for adjustment and management of brain neurostimulator

Encounter for adjustment and management of gastric neurostimulator

Encounter for adjustment and management of peripheral nerve neurostimulator

Encounter for adjustment and management of sacral nerve neurostimulator

Encounter for adjustment and management of spinal cord neurostimulator

Encounter for adjustment and management of vagus nerve neurostimulator

Z45.49   **Encounter for adjustment and management of other implanted nervous system device**

● Z45.8   **Encounter for adjustment and management of other implanted devices**

● Z45.81   **Encounter for adjustment or removal of breast implant**

Encounter for elective implant exchange (different material) (different size)

Encounter for removal of tissue expander with or without synchronous insertion of permanent implant

> **Excludes1**   complications of breast implant (T85.4-)
> encounter for initial breast implant insertion for cosmetic breast augmentation (Z41.1)
> encounter for breast reconstruction following mastectomy (Z42.1)

Z45.811   **Encounter for adjustment or removal of right breast implant**

Z45.812   **Encounter for adjustment or removal of left breast implant**

Z45.819   **Encounter for adjustment or removal of unspecified breast implant**

Z45.82   **Encounter for adjustment or removal of myringotomy device (stent) (tube)**

Z45.89   **Encounter for adjustment and management of other implanted devices**

Z45.9   **Encounter for adjustment and management of unspecified implanted device**

● Z46   **Encounter for fitting and adjustment of other devices**

> **Includes**   removal or replacement of other device
>
> **Excludes1**   malfunction or other complications of device - see Alphabetical Index
>
> **Excludes2**   encounter for fitting and management of implanted devices (Z45.-)
> issue of repeat prescription only (Z76.0)
> presence of prosthetic and other devices (Z95-Z97)

Z46.0   **Encounter for fitting and adjustment of spectacles and contact lenses**

Z46.1   **Encounter for fitting and adjustment of hearing aid**

> **Excludes1**   encounter for adjustment and management of implanted hearing device (Z45.32-)

Z46.2   **Encounter for fitting and adjustment of other devices related to nervous system and special senses**

> **Excludes2**   encounter for adjustment and management of implanted nervous system device (Z45.4-)
> encounter for adjustment and management of implanted visual substitution device (Z45.31)

Z46.3   **Encounter for fitting and adjustment of dental prosthetic device**

Encounter for fitting and adjustment of dentures

Z46.4   **Encounter for fitting and adjustment of orthodontic device**

● Z46.5   **Encounter for fitting and adjustment of other gastrointestinal appliance and device**

> **Excludes1**   encounter for attention to artificial openings of digestive tract (Z43.1-Z43.4)

Z46.51   **Encounter for fitting and adjustment of gastric lap band**

Z46.59   **Encounter for fitting and adjustment of other gastrointestinal appliance and device**

Z46.6   **Encounter for fitting and adjustment of urinary device**

> **Excludes2**   attention to artificial openings of urinary tract (Z43.5, Z43.6)

● **Z46.8   Encounter for fitting and adjustment of other specified devices**

    Z46.81   Encounter for fitting and adjustment of insulin pump
         Encounter for insulin pump instruction and training
         Encounter for insulin pump titration

    Z46.82   Encounter for fitting and adjustment of non-vascular catheter

    Z46.89   Encounter for fitting and adjustment of other specified devices
         Encounter for fitting and adjustment of wheelchair

Z46.9   Encounter for fitting and adjustment of unspecified device

● **Z47   Orthopedic aftercare**
    Excludes1   aftercare for healing fracture - code to fracture with 7th character D

Z47.1   Aftercare following joint replacement surgery
     Use additional code to identify the joint (Z96.6-)
     Coding Clinic: 2020, Q1, P23-24

Z47.2   Encounter for removal of internal fixation device
    Excludes1   encounter for adjustment of internal fixation device for fracture treatment - code to fracture with appropriate 7th character
         encounter for removal of external fixation device - code to fracture with 7th character D
         infection or inflammatory reaction to internal fixation device (T84.6-)
         mechanical complication of internal fixation device (T84.1-)

● **Z47.3   Aftercare following explantation of joint prosthesis**
     Aftercare following explantation of joint prosthesis, staged procedure
     Encounter for joint prosthesis insertion following prior explantation of joint prosthesis
     Coding Clinic: 2020, Q1, P23; 2015, Q1, P17

    Z47.31   Aftercare following explantation of shoulder joint prosthesis
        Excludes1   acquired absence of shoulder joint following prior explantation of shoulder joint prosthesis (Z89.23-)
             shoulder joint prosthesis explantation status (Z89.23-)

    Z47.32   Aftercare following explantation of hip joint prosthesis
        Excludes1   acquired absence of hip joint following prior explantation of hip joint prosthesis (Z89.62-)
             hip joint prosthesis explantation status (Z89.62-)
         Coding Clinic: 2015, Q1, P17

    Z47.33   Aftercare following explantation of knee joint prosthesis
        Excludes1   acquired absence of knee joint following prior explantation of knee prosthesis (Z89.52-)
             knee joint prosthesis explantation status (Z89.52-)

● **Z47.8   Encounter for other orthopedic aftercare**

    Z47.81   Encounter for orthopedic aftercare following surgical amputation
         Use additional code to identify the limb amputated (Z89.-)

    Z47.82   Encounter for orthopedic aftercare following scoliosis surgery

    Z47.89   Encounter for other orthopedic aftercare
         Coding Clinic: 2015, Q1, P8

● **Z48   Encounter for other postprocedural aftercare**
    Excludes1   encounter for aftercare following injury - code to Injury, by site, with appropriate 7th character for subsequent encounter
         encounter for follow-up examination after completed treatment (Z08-Z09)
    Excludes2   encounter for attention to artificial openings (Z43.-)
         encounter for fitting and adjustment of prosthetic and other devices (Z44-Z46)

● **Z48.0   Encounter for attention to dressings, sutures and drains**
    Excludes1   encounter for planned postprocedural wound closure (Z48.1)

    Z48.00   Encounter for change or removal of nonsurgical wound dressing
         Encounter for change or removal of wound dressing NOS

    Z48.01   Encounter for change or removal of surgical wound dressing
         Coding Clinic: 2019, Q2, P33; 2015, Q4, P38

    Z48.02   Encounter for removal of sutures
         Encounter for removal of staples
         Coding Clinic: 2015, Q1, P6

    Z48.03   Encounter for change or removal of drains

Z48.1   Encounter for planned postprocedural wound closure
    Excludes1   encounter for attention to dressings and sutures (Z48.0-)

● **Z48.2   Encounter for aftercare following organ transplant**

    Z48.21   Encounter for aftercare following heart transplant 🦠

    Z48.22   Encounter for aftercare following kidney transplant

    Z48.23   Encounter for aftercare following liver transplant 🦠

    Z48.24   Encounter for aftercare following lung transplant 🦠

    ● **Z48.28   Encounter for aftercare following multiple organ transplant**

        Z48.280   Encounter for aftercare following heart-lung transplant 🦠

        Z48.288   Encounter for aftercare following multiple organ transplant

    ● **Z48.29   Encounter for aftercare following other organ transplant**

        Z48.290   Encounter for aftercare following bone marrow transplant 🦠

        Z48.298   Encounter for aftercare following other organ transplant

Z48.3   Aftercare following surgery for neoplasm
     Use additional code to identify the neoplasm

● **Z48.8   Encounter for other specified postprocedural aftercare**

    ● **Z48.81   Encounter for surgical aftercare following surgery on specified body systems**
         These codes identify the body system requiring aftercare. They are for use in conjunction with other aftercare codes to fully explain the aftercare encounter. The condition treated should also be coded if still present.
        Excludes1   aftercare for injury - code the injury with 7th character D
             aftercare following surgery for neoplasm (Z48.3)
        Excludes2   aftercare following organ transplant (Z48.2-)
             orthopedic aftercare (Z47.-)

        Z48.810   Encounter for surgical aftercare following surgery on the sense organs

Z48.811   Encounter for surgical aftercare following surgery on the nervous system

     Excludes2   encounter for surgical aftercare following surgery on the sense organs (Z48.810)

Z48.812   Encounter for surgical aftercare following surgery on the circulatory system
     Coding Clinic: 2012, Q4, P96

Z48.813   Encounter for surgical aftercare following surgery on the respiratory system
     Coding Clinic: 2019, Q2, P33

Z48.814   Encounter for surgical aftercare following surgery on the teeth or oral cavity

Z48.815   Encounter for surgical aftercare following surgery on the digestive system
     Coding Clinic: 2015, Q4, P38

Z48.816   Encounter for surgical aftercare following surgery on the genitourinary system

     Excludes1   encounter for aftercare following sterilization reversal (Z31.42)

Z48.817   Encounter for surgical aftercare following surgery on the skin and subcutaneous tissue
     Coding Clinic: 2015, Q1, P6

Z48.89   Encounter for other specified surgical aftercare

● **Z49**   Encounter for care involving renal dialysis
     Code also associated end stage renal disease (N18.6)

● **Z49.0**   Preparatory care for renal dialysis
     Encounter for dialysis instruction and training

Z49.01   Encounter for fitting and adjustment of extracorporeal dialysis catheter 🔗
     Removal or replacement of renal dialysis catheter
     Toilet or cleansing of renal dialysis catheter

Z49.02   Encounter for fitting and adjustment of peritoneal dialysis catheter 🔗

● **Z49.3**   Encounter for adequacy testing for dialysis

Z49.31   Encounter for adequacy testing for hemodialysis 🔗

Z49.32   Encounter for adequacy testing for peritoneal dialysis 🔗
     Encounter for peritoneal equilibration test

● **Z51**   Encounter for other aftercare and medical care
     Code also condition requiring care

     Excludes1   follow-up examination after treatment (Z08-Z09)
     Coding Clinic: 2017, Q1, P49; 2016, Q4, P130

Z51.0   Encounter for antineoplastic radiation therapy
     Coding Clinic: 2017, Q4, P103

● **Z51.1**   Encounter for antineoplastic chemotherapy and immunotherapy

     Excludes2   encounter for chemotherapy and immunotherapy for nonneoplastic condition-code to condition

Z51.11   Encounter for antineoplastic chemotherapy
     Coding Clinic: 2022, Q1, P16; 2015, Q3, P19

Z51.12   Encounter for antineoplastic immunotherapy
     Coding Clinic: 2024, Q1, P24

Z51.5   Encounter for palliative care
     Coding Clinic: 2022, Q1, P19; 2017, Q1, P48-49

Z51.6   Encounter for desensitization to allergens
     Coding Clinic: 2016, Q4, P77-79

● **Z51.8**   Encounter for other specified aftercare

     Excludes1   holiday relief care (Z75.5)

Z51.81   Encounter for therapeutic drug level monitoring
     Code also any long-term (current) drug therapy (Z79.-)

     Excludes1   encounter for blood-drug test for administrative or medicolegal reasons (Z02.83)

Z51.89   Encounter for other specified aftercare
     Coding Clinic: 2012, Q4, P96-97

▶ **Z51.A**   Encounter for sepsis aftercare

● **Z52**   Donors of organs and tissues

     Includes   autologous and other living donors
     Excludes1   cadaveric donor - omit code
         examination of potential donor (Z00.5)
     Coding Clinic: 2012, Q4, P100

● **Z52.0**   Blood donor

● **Z52.00**   Unspecified blood donor

     Z52.000   Unspecified donor, whole blood
     Z52.001   Unspecified donor, stem cells
     Z52.008   Unspecified donor, other blood

● **Z52.01**   Autologous blood donor

     Z52.010   Autologous donor, whole blood
     Z52.011   Autologous donor, stem cells
     Z52.018   Autologous donor, other blood

● **Z52.09**   Other blood donor
     Volunteer donor

     Z52.090   Other blood donor, whole blood
     Z52.091   Other blood donor, stem cells
     Z52.098   Other blood donor, other blood

● **Z52.1**   Skin donor

     Z52.10   Skin donor, unspecified
     Z52.11   Skin donor, autologous
     Z52.19   Skin donor, other

● **Z52.2**   Bone donor

     Z52.20   Bone donor, unspecified
     Z52.21   Bone donor, autologous
     Z52.29   Bone donor, other

Z52.3   Bone marrow donor

Z52.4   Kidney donor

Z52.5   Cornea donor

Z52.6   Liver donor
     Coding Clinic: 2012, Q4, P100

● **Z52.8**   Donor of other specified organs or tissues

● **Z52.81**   Egg (Oocyte) donor

     Z52.810   Egg (Oocyte) donor under age 35, anonymous recipient
         Egg donor under age 35 NOS

     Z52.811   Egg (Oocyte) donor under age 35, designated recipient

     Z52.812   Egg (Oocyte) donor age 35 and over, anonymous recipient
         Egg donor age 35 and over NOS

     Z52.813   Egg (Oocyte) donor age 35 and over, designated recipient

     Z52.819   Egg (Oocyte) donor, unspecified

Z52.89   Donor of other specified organs or tissues

Z52.9   Donor of unspecified organ or tissue
     Donor NOS

CHAPTER 21 (Z00-Z99)

● **Z53**   **Persons encountering health services for specific procedures and treatment, not carried out**

  ● **Z53.0**   **Procedure and treatment not carried out because of contraindication**

    Z53.01   Procedure and treatment not carried out due to patient smoking

    Z53.09   Procedure and treatment not carried out because of other contraindication

  Z53.1   **Procedure and treatment not carried out because of patient's decision for reasons of belief and group pressure**

  ● **Z53.2**   **Procedure and treatment not carried out because of patient's decision for other and unspecified reasons**

    Z53.20   Procedure and treatment not carried out because of patient's decision for unspecified reasons

    Z53.21   Procedure and treatment not carried out due to patient leaving prior to being seen by health care provider

    Z53.29   Procedure and treatment not carried out because of patient's decision for other reasons

  ● **Z53.3**   **Procedure converted to open procedure**
    Coding Clinic: 2016, Q4, P79

    Z53.31   Laparoscopic surgical procedure converted to open procedure
      Coding Clinic: 2016, Q4, P100

    Z53.32   Thoracoscopic surgical procedure converted to open procedure

    Z53.33   Arthroscopic surgical procedure converted to open procedure

    Z53.39   Other specified procedure converted to open procedure

  Z53.8   **Procedure and treatment not carried out for other reasons**

  Z53.9   **Procedure and treatment not carried out, unspecified reason**

PERSONS WITH POTENTIAL HEALTH HAZARDS RELATED TO SOCIOECONOMIC AND PSYCHOSOCIAL CIRCUMSTANCES (Z55-Z65)

● **Z55**   **Problems related to education and literacy**
  Excludes1   disorders of psychological development (F80-F89)

  Z55.0   **Illiteracy and low-level literacy**

  Z55.1   **Schooling unavailable and unattainable**

  Z55.2   **Failed school examinations**

  Z55.3   **Underachievement in school**

  Z55.4   **Educational maladjustment and discord with teachers and classmates**

  Z55.5   **Less than a high school diploma**
    No general equivalence degree (GED)

  Z55.6   **Problems related to health literacy**
    Difficulty understanding health related information
    Difficulty understanding medication instructions
    Problem completing medical forms

  Z55.8   **Other problems related to education and literacy**
    Problems related to inadequate teaching

  Z55.9   **Problems related to education and literacy, unspecified**
    Academic problems NOS

● **Z56**   **Problems related to employment and unemployment**
  Excludes2   occupational exposure to risk factors (Z57.-)
    problems related to housing and economic circumstances (Z59.-)

  Z56.0   **Unemployment, unspecified**

  Z56.1   **Change of job**   A

  Z56.2   **Threat of job loss**

  Z56.3   **Stressful work schedule**

  Z56.4   **Discord with boss and workmates**

  Z56.5   **Uncongenial work environment**
    Difficult conditions at work

  Z56.6   **Other physical and mental strain related to work**

  ● **Z56.8**   **Other problems related to employment**

    Z56.81   Sexual harassment on the job

    Z56.82   Military deployment status
      Individual (civilian or military) currently deployed in theater or in support of military war, peacekeeping and humanitarian operations

    Z56.89   Other problems related to employment

  Z56.9   **Unspecified problems related to employment**
    Occupational problems NOS

● **Z57**   **Occupational exposure to risk factors**

  Z57.0   **Occupational exposure to noise**

  Z57.1   **Occupational exposure to radiation**

  Z57.2   **Occupational exposure to dust**

  ● **Z57.3**   **Occupational exposure to other air contaminants**

    Z57.31   Occupational exposure to environmental tobacco smoke
      Excludes2   exposure to environmental tobacco smoke (Z77.22)

    Z57.39   Occupational exposure to other air contaminants

  Z57.4   **Occupational exposure to toxic agents in agriculture**
    Occupational exposure to solids, liquids, gases or vapors in agriculture

  Z57.5   **Occupational exposure to toxic agents in other industries**
    Occupational exposure to solids, liquids, gases or vapors in other industries

  Z57.6   **Occupational exposure to extreme temperature**

  Z57.7   **Occupational exposure to vibration**

  Z57.8   **Occupational exposure to other risk factors**

  Z57.9   **Occupational exposure to unspecified risk factor**

● **Z58**   **Problems related to physical environment**
  Excludes2   occupational exposure (Z57.-)

  Z58.6   **Inadequate drinking-water supply**
    Lack of safe drinking water
    Excludes2   deprivation of water (T73.1)

  ● **Z58.8**   **Other problems related to physical environment**

    Z58.81   Basic services unavailable in physical environment
      Unable to obtain internet service, due to unavailability in geographic area
      Unable to obtain telephone service, due to unavailability in geographic area
      Unable to obtain utilities, due to inadequate physical environment

    Z58.89   Other problems related to physical environment

● **Z59**   **Problems related to housing and economic circumstances**
  Excludes2   problems related to upbringing (Z62.-)

  ● **Z59.0**   **Homelessness**

    Z59.00   Homelessness unspecified

    Z59.01   Sheltered homelessness
      Doubled up
      Living in a shelter such as: motel, scattered site housing, temporary or transitional living situation

    Z59.02   Unsheltered homelessness
      Residing in place not meant for human habitation such as: abandoned buildings, cars, parks, sidewalk
      Residing on the street

  ● **Z59.1**   **Inadequate housing**
    ~~**Excludes1**   problems related to the natural and physical environment (Z77.1-)~~

    ▶ **Excludes1**   problems related to the natural and physical environment (Z77.1-)

    Z59.10   Inadequate housing, unspecified
      Inadequate housing NOS

▶ New   ⟹ Revised   ~~deleted~~ Deleted   Excludes 1   Excludes 2   Includes   Use additional   Code first   Code also   Key words

OGCR Official Guidelines   X Assign placeholder X   ● Use Additional Character(s)   ▶ Manifestation Code   🔗 Hierarchical Condition Category   **Coding Clinic**

Z59.11   **Inadequate housing environmental temperature**
Lack of air conditioning
Lack of heating

Z59.12   **Inadequate housing utilities**
Lack of electricity services
Lack of gas services
Lack of oil services
Lack of water services

> **Excludes2**   basic services unavailable in physical environment (Z58.81)
> lack of adequate food (Z59.4-)
> other problems related to housing and economic circumstances (Z59.8-)

Z59.19   **Other inadequate housing**
Pest infestation
Restriction of space
Technical defects in home preventing adequate care
Unsatisfactory surroundings

Z59.2   **Discord with neighbors, lodgers and landlord**

Z59.3   **Problems related to living in residential institution**
Boarding-school resident

> **Excludes1**   institutional upbringing (Z62.22)

● Z59.4   **Lack of adequate food**

> **Excludes2**   deprivation of food (T73.0)
> effects of hunger (T73.0)
> inappropriate diet or eating habits (Z72.4)
> malnutrition (E40-E46)

Z59.41   **Food insecurity**

Z59.48   **Other specified lack of adequate food**
Inadequate food
Lack of food

Z59.5   **Extreme poverty**

Z59.6   **Low income**

Z59.7   **Insufficient social insurance and welfare support**

Z59.71   **Insufficient health insurance coverage**
Inadequate social insurance
Insufficient social insurance
No health insurance coverage

Z59.72   **Insufficient welfare support**
Inadequate welfare support

● Z59.8   **Other problems related to housing and economic circumstances**

> ● Z59.81   **Housing instability, housed**
> Foreclosure on home loan
> Past due on rent or mortgage
> Unwanted multiple moves in the last 12 months

Z59.811   **Housing instability, housed, with risk of homelessness**
Imminent risk of homelessness

Z59.812   **Housing instability, housed, homelessness in past 12 months**

Z59.819   **Housing instability, housed unspecified**

> **Excludes2**   extreme poverty (Z59.5)
> financial insecurity (Z59.86)
> low income (Z59.6)
> material hardship due to limited financial resources, not elsewhere classified (Z59.87)

Z59.82   **Transportation insecurity**
Excessive transportation time
Inaccessible transportation
Inadequate transportation
Lack of transportation
Unaffordable transportation
Unreliable transportation
Unsafe transportation

> **Excludes2**   unavailability and inaccessibility of healthcare facilities (Z75.3)

Z59.86   **Financial insecurity**
Bankruptcy
Burdensome debt
Economic strain
Financial strain
Money problems
Running out of money
Unable to make ends meet

> **Excludes2**   extreme poverty (Z59.5)
> low income (Z59.6)
> material hardship, not elsewhere classified (Z59.87)

Z59.87   **Material hardship due to limited financial resources, not elsewhere classified**
Material deprivation due to limited financial resources
Unable to obtain adequate childcare due to limited financial resources
Unable to obtain adequate clothing due to limited financial resources
Unable to obtain adequate utilities due to limited financial resources
Unable to obtain basic needs due to limited financial resources

> **Excludes2**   extreme poverty (Z59.5)
> financial insecurity, not elsewhere classified (Z59.86)
> low income (Z59.6)

Z59.89   **Other problems related to housing and economic circumstances**
Foreclosure on loan
Isolated dwelling
Problems with creditors

Z59.9   **Problem related to housing and economic circumstances, unspecified**

● Z60   **Problems related to social environment**

Z60.0   **Problems of adjustment to life-cycle transitions**
Empty nest syndrome
Phase of life problem
Problem with adjustment to retirement [pension]

Z60.2   **Problems related to living alone**

Z60.3   **Acculturation difficulty**
Problem with migration
Problem with social transplantation

Z60.4   **Social exclusion and rejection**
Exclusion and rejection on the basis of personal characteristics, such as unusual physical appearance, illness or behavior.
Social isolation

> **Excludes1**   target of adverse discrimination such as for racial or religious reasons (Z60.5)

Z60.5   **Target of (perceived) adverse discrimination and persecution**

> **Excludes1**   social exclusion and rejection (Z60.4)

Z60.8   **Other problems related to social environment**
Inadequate social support
Lack of emotional support

Z60.9   **Problem related to social environment, unspecified**

● Z62   **Problems related to upbringing**

> **Includes**   current and past negative life events in childhood
> current and past problems of a child related to upbringing

> **Excludes2**   maltreatment syndrome (T74.-)
> problems related to housing and economic circumstances (Z59.-)

Z62.0   **Inadequate parental supervision and control**

Z62.1   **Parental overprotection**

● Z62.2   **Upbringing away from parents**

> **Excludes1**   problems with boarding school (Z59.3)

Z62.21   **Child in welfare custody**   P
Child in foster care
Child in welfare guardianship

Z62.22   Institutional upbringing
Child living in group home
Child living in orphanage
Code also, if applicable, child in welfare custody
(Z62.21)

Z62.23   Child in custody of non-parental relative
Child in care of non-parental family member
Child in custody of grandparent
Child in kinship care
Guardianship by non-parental relative
Code also, if applicable, child in welfare custody
(Z62.21)

Z62.24   Child in custody of non-relative guardian
Code also, if applicable, child in welfare custody
(Z62.21)

Z62.29   Other upbringing away from parents

Z62.3   **Hostility towards and scapegoating of child**   P

Z62.6   **Inappropriate (excessive) parental pressure**

● Z62.8   **Other specified problems related to upbringing**
Code also, if applicable:
absence of family member (Z63.3-)
disappearance and death of family member (Z63.4)
disruption of family by separation and divorce (Z63.5)
other specified problems related to primary support
group (Z63.8)
other stressful life events affecting family and
household (Z63.7-)

● **Z62.81   Personal history of abuse in childhood**
Personal history of abuse in adolescence

**Z62.810   Personal history of physical and
sexual abuse in childhood**
Excludes1   current child physical
abuse (T74.12,
T76.12)
current child sexual
abuse (T74.22,
T76.22)

**Z62.811   Personal history of psychological
abuse in childhood**
Excludes1   current child
psychological
abuse (T74.32,
T76.32)

**Z62.812   Personal history of neglect in
childhood**
Excludes1   current child neglect
(T74.02, T76.02)

**Z62.813   Personal history of forced labor or
sexual exploitation in childhood**

**Z62.814   Personal history of child financial
abuse**
Excludes1   current child financial
abuse (T74.A2)

**Z62.815   Personal history of intimate partner
abuse in childhood**
Excludes2   adult and child abuse,
neglect and other
maltreatment,
confirmed (T74.-)

**Z62.819   Personal history of unspecified abuse
in childhood**
Excludes1   current child abuse
NOS (T74.92,
T76.92)

● **Z62.82   Parent-child conflict**

Z62.820   Parent-biological child conflict
Parent-child problem NOS

Z62.821   Parent-adopted child conflict

Z62.822   Parent-foster child conflict

Z62.823   Parent-step child conflict

● **Z62.83   Non-parental relative or guardian-child conflict**

Z62.831   Non-parental relative-child conflict
Grandparent-child conflict
Kinship-care child conflict
Non-parental relative legal
guardian-child conflict
Other relative-child conflict
Excludes1   group home staff-child
conflict (Z62.833)

Z62.832   Non-relative guardian-child conflict
Excludes1   group home staff-child
conflict (Z62.833)

Z62.833   Group home staff-child conflict

● **Z62.89   Other specified problems related to upbringing**

Z62.890   Parent-child estrangement NEC

Z62.891   Sibling rivalry

**Z62.892   Runaway [from current living
environment]**
Child leaving living situation
without permission

**Z62.898   Other specified problems related to
upbringing**

Z62.9   **Problem related to upbringing, unspecified**

● Z63   **Other problems related to primary support group, including
family circumstances**
Excludes2   maltreatment syndrome (T74.-, T76)
parent-child problems (Z62.-)
problems related to negative life events in
childhood (Z62.-)
problems related to upbringing (Z62.-)

Z63.0   **Problems in relationship with spouse or partner**
Relationship distress with spouse or intimate partner
Excludes1   counseling for spousal or partner abuse
problems (Z69.1)
counseling related to sexual attitude,
behavior, and orientation (Z70.-)

Z63.1   **Problems in relationship with in-laws**

● Z63.3   **Absence of family member**
Excludes1   absence of family member due to
disappearance and death (Z63.4)
absence of family member due to
separation and divorce (Z63.5)

**Z63.31   Absence of family member due to military
deployment**
Individual or family affected by other family
member being on military deployment
Excludes1   family disruption due to return of
family member from military
deployment (Z63.71)

Z63.32   Other absence of family member

Z63.4   **Disappearance and death of family member**
Assumed death of family member
Bereavement

Z63.5   **Disruption of family by separation and divorce**
Marital estrangement

Z63.6   **Dependent relative needing care at home**

● Z63.7   **Other stressful life events affecting family and household**

**Z63.71   Stress on family due to return of family
member from military deployment**
Individual or family affected by family
member having returned from military
deployment (current or past conflict)

Z63.72   Alcoholism and drug addiction in family

**Z63.79   Other stressful life events affecting family and
household**
Anxiety (normal) about sick person in family
Health problems within family
Ill or disturbed family member
Isolated family

Z63.8   **Other specified problems related to primary support group**
Family discord NOS
Family estrangement NOS
High expressed emotional level within family
Inadequate family support NOS
Inadequate or distorted communication within family

Z63.9   **Problem related to primary support group, unspecified**
Relationship disorder NOS

● Z64   **Problems related to certain psychosocial circumstances**

Z64.0   **Problems related to unwanted pregnancy**

Z64.1   **Problems related to multiparity**

Z64.4   **Discord with counselors**
Discord with probation officer
Discord with social worker

● Z65   **Problems related to other psychosocial circumstances**

Z65.0   **Conviction in civil and criminal proceedings without imprisonment**

Z65.1   **Imprisonment and other incarceration**

Z65.2   **Problems related to release from prison**

Z65.3   **Problems related to other legal circumstances**
Arrest
Child custody or support proceedings
Litigation
Prosecution

Z65.4   **Victim of crime and terrorism**
Victim of torture

Z65.5   **Exposure to disaster, war and other hostilities**
Excludes1   target of perceived discrimination or persecution (Z60.5)

Z65.8   **Other specified problems related to psychosocial circumstances**
At risk for feeling loneliness
Religious or spiritual problem

Z65.9   **Problem related to unspecified psychosocial circumstances**

DO NOT RESUSCITATE STATUS (Z66)

Z66   **Do not resuscitate**
DNR status

BLOOD TYPE (Z67)

● Z67   **Blood type**
Coding Clinic: 2015, Q3, P40

● Z67.1   **Type A blood**
Z67.10   Type A blood, Rh positive
Z67.11   Type A blood, Rh negative

● Z67.2   **Type B blood**
Z67.20   Type B blood, Rh positive
Z67.21   Type B blood, Rh negative

● Z67.3   **Type AB blood**
Z67.30   Type AB blood, Rh positive
Z67.31   Type AB blood, Rh negative

● Z67.4   **Type O blood**
Z67.40   Type O blood, Rh positive
Z67.41   Type O blood, Rh negative

● Z67.9   **Unspecified blood type**
Z67.90   Unspecified blood type, Rh positive
Z67.91   Unspecified blood type, Rh negative
Coding Clinic: 2015, Q3, P40

▶ Z67.A   **Duffy phenotype**
▶ Z67.A1   **Duffy null**
▶ Duffy phenotype Fy(a-b-)
▶ Z67.A2   **Duffy a positive**
▶ Duffy phenotype Fy(a+b-)
▶ Z67.A3   **Duffy b positive**
▶ Duffy phenotype Fy(a-b+)
▶ Z67.A4   **Duffy a and b positive**
▶ Duffy phenotype Fy(a+b+)

BODY MASS INDEX [BMI] (Z68)

OGCR Section I.B.14.

General Coding Guidelines

14. Documentation for BMI, Depth of Non-pressure ulcers, Pressure Ulcer Stages, Coma Scale, and NIH Stroke Scale

For the Body Mass Index (BMI), depth of non-pressure chronic ulcers, pressure ulcer stage, coma scale, and NIH stroke scale (NIHSS) codes, code assignment may be based on medical record documentation from clinicians who are not the patient's provider (i.e., physician or other qualified healthcare practitioner legally accountable for establishing the patient's diagnosis), since this information is typically documented by other clinicians involved in the care of the patient (e.g., a dietitian often documents the BMI, a nurse often documents the pressure ulcer stages, and an emergency medical technician often documents the coma scale). However, the associated diagnosis (such as overweight, obesity, acute stroke, or pressure ulcer) must be documented by the patient's provider. If there is conflicting medical record documentation, either from the same clinician or different clinicians, the patient's attending provider should be queried for clarification.

The BMI, coma scale, and NIHSS codes should only be reported as secondary diagnoses.

● Z68   **Body mass index [BMI]**
Kilograms per meters squared
Note: BMI adult codes are for use for persons 20 years of age or older.
BMI pediatric codes are for use for persons 2-19 years of age.
These percentiles are based on the growth charts published by the Centers for Disease Control and Prevention (CDC)
Coding Clinic: 2018, Q4, P81; 2016, Q4, P129

Z68.1   **Body mass index [BMI] 19.9 or less, adult**   A
Coding Clinic: 2017, Q1, P39

● Z68.2   **Body mass index [BMI] 20-29, adult**
Z68.20   Body mass index [BMI] 20.0-20.9, adult   A
Z68.21   Body mass index [BMI] 21.0-21.9, adult   A
Z68.22   Body mass index [BMI] 22.0-22.9, adult   A
Z68.23   Body mass index [BMI] 23.0-23.9, adult   A
Z68.24   Body mass index [BMI] 24.0-24.9, adult   A
Z68.25   Body mass index [BMI] 25.0-25.9, adult   A
Z68.26   Body mass index [BMI] 26.0-26.9, adult   A
Z68.27   Body mass index [BMI] 27.0-27.9, adult   A
Z68.28   Body mass index [BMI] 28.0-28.9, adult   A
Z68.29   Body mass index [BMI] 29.0-29.9, adult   A

● Z68.3   **Body mass index [BMI] 30-39, adult**
Z68.30   Body mass index [BMI] 30.0-30.9, adult   A
Z68.31   Body mass index [BMI] 31.0-31.9, adult   A
Z68.32   Body mass index [BMI] 32.0-32.9, adult   A
Z68.33   Body mass index [BMI] 33.0-33.9, adult   A
Z68.34   Body mass index [BMI] 34.0-34.9, adult   A
Z68.35   Body mass index [BMI] 35.0-35.9, adult   A
Coding Clinic: 2022, Q3, P6
Z68.36   Body mass index [BMI] 36.0-36.9, adult   A
Z68.37   Body mass index [BMI] 37.0-37.9, adult   A
Z68.38   Body mass index [BMI] 38.0-38.9, adult   A
Z68.39   Body mass index [BMI] 39.0-39.9, adult   A

● Z68.4   **Body mass index [BMI] 40 or greater, adult**
Z68.41   Body mass index [BMI] 40.0-44.9, adult ✆   A
Z68.42   Body mass index [BMI] 45.0-49.9, adult ✆   A
Z68.43   Body mass index [BMI] 50.0-59.9, adult ✆   A
Z68.44   Body mass index [BMI] 60.0-69.9, adult ✆   A
Z68.45   Body mass index [BMI] 70 or greater, adult ✆   A

● Z68.5   **Body mass index [BMI] pediatric**
Coding Clinic: 2018, Q4, P81
Z68.51   Body mass index [BMI] pediatric, less than 5th percentile for age
Coding Clinic: 2018, Q4, P82
Z68.52   Body mass index [BMI] pediatric, 5th percentile to less than 85th percentile for age

CHAPTER 21 (Z00-Z99)

Z68.53   Body mass index [BMI] pediatric, 85th percentile to less than 95th percentile for age

➡ Z68.54   Body mass index [BMI] pediatric, 95th percentile for age to less than 120% of the 95th percentile for age

▶ Z68.55   Body mass index [BMI] pediatric, 120% of the 95th percentile for age to less than 140% of the 95th percentile for age

▶ Z68.56   Body mass index [BMI] pediatric, greater than or equal to 140% of the 95th percentile for age

PERSONS ENCOUNTERING HEALTH SERVICES IN OTHER CIRCUMSTANCES (Z69-Z76)

● Z69   Encounter for mental health services for victim and perpetrator of abuse

Includes   counseling for victims and perpetrators of abuse

● Z69.0   Encounter for mental health services for child abuse problems

● Z69.01   Encounter for mental health services for parental child abuse

Z69.010   Encounter for mental health services for victim of parental child abuse   P
Encounter for mental health services for victim of child abuse by parent
Encounter for mental health services for victim of child neglect by parent
Encounter for mental health services for victim of child psychological abuse by parent
Encounter for mental health services for victim of child sexual abuse by parent

Z69.011   Encounter for mental health services for perpetrator of parental child abuse
Encounter for mental health services for perpetrator of parental child neglect
Encounter for mental health services for perpetrator of parental child psychological abuse
Encounter for mental health services for perpetrator of parental child sexual abuse

Excludes1   encounter for mental health services for non-parental child abuse (Z69.02-)

● Z69.02   Encounter for mental health services for non-parental child abuse

Z69.020   Encounter for mental health services for victim of non-parental child abuse P
Encounter for mental health services for victim of non-parental child neglect
Encounter for mental health services for victim of non-parental child psychological abuse
Encounter for mental health services for victim of non-parental child sexual abuse

Z69.021   Encounter for mental health services for perpetrator of non- parental child abuse
Encounter for mental health services for perpetrator of non-parental child neglect
Encounter for mental health services for perpetrator of non-parental child psychological abuse
Encounter for mental health services for perpetrator of non-parental child sexual abuse

● Z69.1   Encounter for mental health services for spousal or partner abuse problems

Z69.11   Encounter for mental health services for victim of spousal or partner abuse
Encounter for mental health services for victim of spouse or partner neglect
Encounter for mental health services for victim of spouse or partner psychological abuse
Encounter for mental health services for victim of spouse or partner violence, physical

Z69.12   Encounter for mental health services for perpetrator of spousal or partner abuse
Encounter for mental health services for perpetrator of spouse or partner neglect
Encounter for mental health services for perpetrator of spouse or partner psychological abuse
Encounter for mental health services for perpetrator of spouse or partner violence, physical
Encounter for mental health services for perpetrator of spouse or partner violence, sexual

● Z69.8   Encounter for mental health services for victim or perpetrator of other abuse

Z69.81   Encounter for mental health services for victim of other abuse
Encounter for mental health services for victim of non-spousal adult abuse
Encounter for mental health services for victim of spouse or partner violence, sexual
Encounter for rape victim counseling

Z69.82   Encounter for mental health services for perpetrator of other abuse
Encounter for mental health services for perpetrator of non-spousal adult abuse

● Z70   Counseling related to sexual attitude, behavior and orientation

Includes   encounter for mental health services for sexual attitude, behavior and orientation

Excludes2   contraceptive or procreative counseling (Z30-Z31)

Z70.0   Counseling related to sexual attitude

Z70.1   Counseling related to patient's sexual behavior and orientation
Patient concerned regarding impotence
Patient concerned regarding non-responsiveness
Patient concerned regarding promiscuity
Patient concerned regarding sexual orientation

Z70.2   Counseling related to sexual behavior and orientation of third party
Advice sought regarding sexual behavior and orientation of child
Advice sought regarding sexual behavior and orientation of partner
Advice sought regarding sexual behavior and orientation of spouse

Z70.3   Counseling related to combined concerns regarding sexual attitude, behavior and orientation

Z70.8   Other sex counseling
Encounter for sex education

Z70.9   Sex counseling, unspecified

● Z71   Persons encountering health services for other counseling and medical advice, not elsewhere classified

Excludes2   contraceptive or procreation counseling (Z30-Z31)
sex counseling (Z70.-)

Z71.0   Person encountering health services to consult on behalf of another person
Person encountering health services to seek advice or treatment for non-attending third party

Excludes2   anxiety (normal) about sick person in family (Z63.7)
expectant (adoptive) parent(s) pre-birth pediatrician visit (Z76.81)

Z71.1   Person with feared health complaint in whom no diagnosis is made
Person encountering health services with feared condition which was not demonstrated
Person encountering health services in which problem was normal state
"Worried well"

> **Excludes1**   medical observation for suspected diseases and conditions proven not to exist (Z03.-)

Coding Clinic: 2016, Q4, P7

Z71.2   Person consulting for explanation of examination or test findings

Z71.3   Dietary counseling and surveillance
Use additional code for any associated underlying medical condition
Use additional code to identify body mass index (BMI), if known (Z68.-)

● **Z71.4   Alcohol abuse counseling and surveillance**
Use additional code for alcohol abuse or dependence (F10.-)

     Z71.41   Alcohol abuse counseling and surveillance of alcoholic

     Z71.42   Counseling for family member of alcoholic
Counseling for significant other, partner, or friend of alcoholic

● **Z71.5   Drug abuse counseling and surveillance**
Use additional code for drug abuse or dependence (F11-F16, F18-F19)

     Z71.51   Drug abuse counseling and surveillance of drug abuser

     Z71.52   Counseling for family member of drug abuser
Counseling for significant other, partner, or friend of drug abuser

Z71.6   Tobacco abuse counseling
Use additional code for nicotine dependence (F17.-)

Z71.7   Human immunodeficiency virus [HIV] counseling

● **Z71.8   Other specified counseling**

> **Excludes2**   counseling for contraception (Z30.0-)

     Z71.81   Spiritual or religious counseling

     Z71.82   Exercise counseling

     Z71.83   Encounter for nonprocreative genetic counseling

> > **Excludes1**   counseling for procreative genetics (Z31.5)
> > counseling for procreative management (Z31.6)

     Z71.84   Encounter for health counseling related to travel
Encounter for health risk and safety counseling for (international) travel
Code also, if applicable, encounter for immunization (Z23)

> > **Excludes2**   encounter for administrative examination (Z02.-)
> > encounter for other special examination without complaint, suspected or reported diagnosis (Z01.-)

     Z71.85 Encounter for immunization safety counseling
Encounter for vaccine product safety counseling
Code also, if applicable, encounter for immunization (Z23)
Code also, if applicable, immunization not carried out (Z28.-)

> > **Excludes1**   encounter for health counseling related to travel (Z71.84)

     Z71.87   Encounter for pediatric-to-adult transition counseling
Code also chronic condition, if applicable, such as:
autism spectrum disorder (F84.0)
congenital malformations of the circulatory system (Q20-Q28)
cystic fibrosis (E84-)
sickle-cell disorder (D57-)

     Z71.88   Encounter for counseling for socioeconomic factors

     Z71.89   Other specified counseling

Z71.9   Counseling, unspecified
Encounter for medical advice NOS

● **Z72   Problems related to lifestyle**

> **Excludes2**   problems related to life-management difficulty (Z73.-)
> problems related to socioeconomic and psychosocial circumstances (Z55-Z65)

Coding Clinic: 2016, Q4, P130

Z72.0   Tobacco use
Tobacco use NOS

> **Excludes1**   history of tobacco dependence (Z87.891)
> nicotine dependence (F17.2-)
> tobacco dependence (F17.2-)
> tobacco use during pregnancy (O99.33-)

Z72.3   Lack of physical exercise

Z72.4   Inappropriate diet and eating habits

> **Excludes1**   behavioral eating disorders of infancy or childhood (F98.2.-F98.3)
> eating disorders (F50.-)
> lack of adequate food (Z59.48)
> malnutrition and other nutritional deficiencies (E40-E64)

● **Z72.5   High risk sexual behavior**
Promiscuity

> **Excludes1**   paraphilias (F65)

     Z72.51   High risk heterosexual behavior

     Z72.52   High risk homosexual behavior

     Z72.53   High risk bisexual behavior

Z72.6   Gambling and betting

> **Excludes1**   compulsive or pathological gambling (F63.0)

● **Z72.8   Other problems related to lifestyle**

     ● **Z72.81   Antisocial behavior**

> > **Excludes1**   conduct disorders (F91.-)

         Z72.810   Child and adolescent antisocial behavior   P
Antisocial behavior (child) (adolescent) without manifest psychiatric disorder
Delinquency NOS
Group delinquency
Offenses in the context of gang membership
Stealing in company with others
Truancy from school

         Z72.811   Adult antisocial behavior   A
Adult antisocial behavior without manifest psychiatric disorder

     ● **Z72.82   Problems related to sleep**

         Z72.820   Sleep deprivation
Lack of adequate sleep

> > > **Excludes1**   insomnia (G47.0-)

         Z72.821   Inadequate sleep hygiene
Bad sleep habits
Irregular sleep habits
Unhealthy sleep wake schedule

> > > **Excludes1**   insomnia (F51.0-, G47.0-)

CHAPTER 21 (Z00-Z99)

Z72.823　Risk of suffocation (smothering) under another while sleeping
　Child-caregiver co-sleeping
　Infant bed-sharing
Z72.89　Other problems related to lifestyle
　Self-damaging behavior
Z72.9　Problem related to lifestyle, unspecified

Z73　Problems related to life management difficulty
　Excludes2　problems related to socioeconomic and psychosocial circumstances (Z55-Z65)
Z73.0　Burn-out
Z73.1　Type A behavior pattern
Z73.2　Lack of relaxation and leisure
Z73.3　Stress, not elsewhere classified
　Physical and mental strain NOS
　Excludes1　stress related to employment or unemployment (Z56.-)
Z73.4　Inadequate social skills, not elsewhere classified
Z73.5　Social role conflict, not elsewhere classified
Z73.6　Limitation of activities due to disability
　Excludes1　care-provider dependency (Z74.-)
Z73.8　Other problems related to life management difficulty
　Z73.81　Behavioral insomnia of childhood
　　Z73.810　Behavioral insomnia of childhood, sleep-onset association type　P
　　Z73.811　Behavioral insomnia of childhood, limit setting type　P
　　Z73.812　Behavioral insomnia of childhood, combined type　P
　　Z73.819　Behavioral insomnia of childhood, unspecified type　P
　Z73.82　Dual sensory impairment
　Z73.89　Other problems related to life management difficulty
Z73.9　Problem related to life management difficulty, unspecified

Z74　Problems related to care provider dependency
　Excludes2　dependence on enabling machines or devices NEC (Z99.-)
Z74.0　Reduced mobility
　Z74.01　Bed confinement status
　　Bedridden
　Z74.09　Other reduced mobility
　　Chairridden
　　Reduced mobility NOS
　　Excludes2　wheelchair dependence (Z99.3)
Z74.1　Need for assistance with personal care
Z74.2　Need for assistance at home and no other household member able to render care
Z74.3　Need for continuous supervision
Z74.8　Other problems related to care provider dependency
Z74.9　Problem related to care provider dependency, unspecified

Z75　Problems related to medical facilities and other health care
Z75.0　Medical services not available in home
　Excludes1　no other household member able to render care (Z74.2)
Z75.1　Person awaiting admission to adequate facility elsewhere
Z75.2　Other waiting period for investigation and treatment
Z75.3　Unavailability and inaccessibility of health care facilities
　Excludes1　bed unavailable (Z75.1)
Z75.4　Unavailability and inaccessibility of other helping agencies
Z75.5　Holiday relief care

Z75.8　Other problems related to medical facilities and other health care
Z75.9　Unspecified problem related to medical facilities and other health care

Z76　Persons encountering health services in other circumstances
Z76.0　Encounter for issue of repeat prescription
　Encounter for issue of repeat prescription for appliance
　Encounter for issue of repeat prescription for medicaments
　Encounter for issue of repeat prescription for spectacles
　Excludes2　issue of medical certificate (Z02.7)
　　repeat prescription for contraceptive (Z30.4-)
Z76.1　Encounter for health supervision and care of foundling
Z76.2　Encounter for health supervision and care of other healthy infant and child　P
　Encounter for medical or nursing care or supervision of healthy infant under circumstances such as adverse socioeconomic conditions at home
　Encounter for medical or nursing care or supervision of healthy infant under circumstances such as awaiting foster or adoptive placement
　Encounter for medical or nursing care or supervision of healthy infant under circumstances such as maternal illness
　Encounter for medical or nursing care or supervision of healthy infant under circumstances such as number of children at home preventing or interfering with normal care
Z76.3　Healthy person accompanying sick person
Z76.4　Other boarder to healthcare facility
　Excludes1　homelessness (Z59.0-)
Z76.5　Malingerer [conscious simulation]
　Person feigning illness (with obvious motivation)
　Excludes1　factitious disorder (F68.1-, F68.A)
　　peregrinating patient (F68.1-)
Z76.8　Persons encountering health services in other specified circumstances
　Z76.81　Expectant parent(s) prebirth pediatrician visit
　　Pre-adoption pediatrician visit for adoptive parent(s)
　Z76.82　Awaiting organ transplant status
　　Patient waiting for organ availability
　Z76.89　Persons encountering health services in other specified circumstances
　　Persons encountering health services NOS
　　Coding Clinic:2022, Q3, P7

PERSONS WITH POTENTIAL HEALTH HAZARDS RELATED TO FAMILY AND PERSONAL HISTORY AND CERTAIN CONDITIONS INFLUENCING HEALTH STATUS (Z77-Z99)

Code also any follow-up examination (Z08-Z09)

Z77　Other contact with and (suspected) exposures hazardous to health
　Includes　contact with and (suspected) exposures to potential hazards to health
　Excludes2　contact with and (suspected) exposure to communicable diseases (Z20.-)
　　exposure to (parental) (environmental) tobacco smoke in the perinatal period (P96.81)
　　newborn affected by noxious substances transmitted via placenta or breast milk (P04.-)
　　occupational exposure to risk factors (Z57.-)
　　retained foreign body (Z18.-)
　　retained foreign body fully removed (Z87.821)
　　toxic effects of substances chiefly nonmedicinal as to source (T51-T65)
Z77.0　Contact with and (suspected) exposure to hazardous, chiefly nonmedicinal, chemicals
　Z77.01　Contact with and (suspected) exposure to hazardous metals
　　Z77.010　Contact with and (suspected) exposure to arsenic

Z77.011   Contact with and (suspected) exposure to lead

Z77.012   Contact with and (suspected) exposure to uranium
      Excludes1   retained depleted uranium fragments (Z18.01)

Z77.018   Contact with and (suspected) exposure to other hazardous metals
    Contact with and (suspected) exposure to chromium compounds
    Contact with and (suspected) exposure to nickel dust

● Z77.02   Contact with and (suspected) exposure to hazardous aromatic compounds

Z77.020   Contact with and (suspected) exposure to aromatic amines

Z77.021   Contact with and (suspected) exposure to benzene

Z77.028   Contact with and (suspected) exposure to other hazardous aromatic compounds
    Aromatic dyes NOS
    Polycyclic aromatic hydrocarbons

● Z77.09   Contact with and (suspected) exposure to other hazardous, chiefly nonmedicinal, chemicals

Z77.090   Contact with and (suspected) exposure to asbestos

Z77.098   Contact with and (suspected) exposure to other hazardous, chiefly nonmedicinal, chemicals
    Dyes NOS

● Z77.1   Contact with and (suspected) exposure to environmental pollution and hazards in the physical environment

● Z77.11   Contact with and (suspected) exposure to environmental pollution

Z77.110   Contact with and (suspected) exposure to air pollution

Z77.111   Contact with and (suspected) exposure to water pollution

Z77.112   Contact with and (suspected) exposure to soil pollution

Z77.118   Contact with and (suspected) exposure to other environmental pollution

● Z77.12   Contact with and (suspected) exposure to hazards in the physical environment

Z77.120   Contact with and (suspected) exposure to mold (toxic)

Z77.121   Contact with and (suspected) exposure to harmful algae and algae toxins
    Contact with and (suspected) exposure to (harmful) algae bloom NOS
    Contact with and (suspected) exposure to blue-green algae bloom
    Contact with and (suspected) exposure to brown tide
    Contact with and (suspected) exposure to cyanobacteria bloom
    Contact with and (suspected) exposure to Florida red tide
    Contact with and (suspected) exposure to pfiesteria piscicida
    Contact with and (suspected) exposure to red tide

Z77.122   Contact with and (suspected) exposure to noise

Z77.123   Contact with and (suspected) exposure to radon and other naturally occurring radiation
      Excludes2   radiation exposure as the cause of a confirmed condition (W88-W90, X39.0-)
              radiation sickness NOS (T66)

Z77.128   Contact with and (suspected) exposure to other hazards in the physical environment

● Z77.2   Contact with and (suspected) exposure to other hazardous substances

Z77.21   Contact with and (suspected) exposure to potentially hazardous body fluids

Z77.22   Contact with and (suspected) exposure to environmental tobacco smoke (acute) (chronic)
    Exposure to second hand tobacco smoke (acute) (chronic)
    Passive smoking (acute) (chronic)
      Excludes1   nicotine dependence (F17.-)
              tobacco use (Z72.0)
      Excludes2   occupational exposure to environmental tobacco smoke (Z57.31)

Z77.29   Contact with and (suspected) exposure to other hazardous substances
    Coding Clinic: 2016, Q2, P34

Z77.9   Other contact with and (suspected) exposures hazardous to health

● Z78   Other specified health status
    Excludes2   asymptomatic human immunodeficiency virus [HIV] infection status (Z21)
             postprocedural status (Z93-Z99)
             sex reassignment status (Z87.890)

Z78.0   Asymptomatic menopausal state   A
    Menopausal state NOS
    Postmenopausal status NOS
      Excludes2   symptomatic menopausal state (N95.1)

Z78.1   Physical restraint status
      Excludes1   physical restraint due to a procedure - omit code

Z78.9   Other specified health status

● Z79   Long term (current) drug therapy
    Includes   long term (current) drug use for prophylactic purposes
    Code also any therapeutic drug level monitoring (Z51.81)
    Excludes2   drug abuse and dependence (F11-F19)
             drug use complicating pregnancy, childbirth, and the puerperium (O99.32-)
    Coding Clinic: 2024, Q2, P26

● Z79.0   Long term (current) use of anticoagulants and antithrombotics/antiplatelets
      Excludes2   long term (current) use of aspirin (Z79.82)
    Coding Clinic: 2021, Q1, P12-13

Z79.01   Long term (current) use of anticoagulants
    Coding Clinic: 2023, Q2, P28; 2022, Q2, P17; 2021, Q1, P5

Z79.02   Long term (current) use of antithrombotics/antiplatelets

Z79.1   Long term (current) use of non-steroidal anti-inflammatories (NSAID)
      Excludes2   long term (current) use of aspirin (Z79.82)

Z79.2   Long term (current) use of antibiotics

Z79.3   Long term (current) use of hormonal contraceptives
    Long term (current) use of birth control pill or patch

Z79.4   **Long term (current) use of insulin** 🅗

     Excludes2   long-term (current) use of injectable non-insulin antidiabetic drugs (Z79.85)

            long term (current) use of oral hypoglycemic drugs (Z79.84)

            long term (current) use of oral antidiabetic drugs (Z79.84)

● **Z79.5**   **Long term (current) use of steroids**

    Z79.51   **Long term (current) use of inhaled steroids**

    Z79.52   **Long term (current) use of systemic steroids**

● **Z79.6**   **Long term (current) use of immunomodulators and immunosuppressants**

     Excludes2   long term (current) use of steroids (Z79.5-)

            long term (current) use of agents affecting estrogen receptors and estrogen levels (Z79.81-)

    Z79.60   **Long term (current) use of unspecified immunomodulators and immunosuppressants**

    Z79.61   **Long term (current) use of immunomodulator**

        Long term (current) use of apremilast

        Long term (current) use of immunomodulatory imide drug

        Long term (current) use of lenalidomide

        Long term (current) use of pomalidomide

  ● **Z79.62**   **Long term (current) use of immunosuppressant**

        Z79.620   **Long term (current) use of immunosuppressive biologic**

            Long term (current) use of adalimumab

            Long term (current) use of etanercept

            Long term (current) use of infliximab

            Long term (current) use of monoclonal antibodies

        Z79.621   **Long term (current) use of calcineurin inhibitor**

            Long term (current) use of cyclosporine

            Long term (current) use of tacrolimus

        Z79.622   **Long term (current) use of Janus kinase inhibitor**

            Long term (current) use of tofacitinib

        Z79.623   **Long term (current) use of mammalian target of rapamycin (mTOR) inhibitor**

            Long term (current) use of sirolimus

        Z79.624   **Long term (current) use of inhibitors of nucleotide synthesis**

            Long term (current) use of azathioprine

            Long term (current) use ⇒mycophenolate

            Long term (current) use of purine synthesis (IMDH) inhibitors

  ● **Z79.63**   **Long term (current) use of chemotherapeutic agent**

        Z79.630   **Long term (current) use of alkylating agent**

            Long term (current) use of chlorambucil

            Long term (current) use of cisplatin

            Long term (current) use of cyclophosphamide

        Z79.631   **Long term (current) use of antimetabolite agent**

            Long term (current) use of 5-fluorouracil

            Long term (current) use of 6-mercaptopurine

            Long term (current) use of cytarabine

            Long term (current) use of methotrexate

        Z79.632   **Long term (current) use of antitumor antibiotic**

            Long term (current) use of bleomycin

            Long term (current) use of doxorubicin

            Long term (current) use of mitomycin C

        Z79.633   **Long term (current) use of mitotic inhibitor**

            Long term (current) use of paclitaxel

            Long term (current) use of plant alkaloids

            Long term (current) use of vinblastine

            Long term (current) use of vincristine

        Z79.634   **Long term (current) use of topoisomerase inhibitor**

            Long term (current) use of etoposide

            Long term (current) use of irinotecan

            Long term (current) use of topotecan

    Z79.64   **Long term (current) use of myelosuppressive agent**

        Long term (current) use of hydroxyurea

    Z79.69   **Long term (current) use of other immunomodulators and immunosuppressants**

● **Z79.8**   **Other long term (current) drug therapy**

  ● **Z79.81**   **Long term (current) use of agents affecting estrogen receptors and estrogen levels**

      Code first, if applicable:

        malignant neoplasm of breast (C50.-)

        malignant neoplasm of prostate (C61)

      Use additional code, if applicable, to identify:

        estrogen receptor positive status (Z17.0)

        family history of breast cancer (Z80.3)

        genetic susceptibility to malignant neoplasm (cancer) (Z15.0-)

        personal history of breast cancer (Z85.3)

        personal history of prostate cancer (Z85.46)

        postmenopausal status (Z78.0)

     Excludes1   hormone replacement therapy (Z79.890)

    Z79.810   **Long term (current) use of selective estrogen receptor modulators (SERMs)**

        Long term (current) use of raloxifene (Evista)

        Long term (current) use of tamoxifen (Nolvadex)

        Long term (current) use of toremifene (Fareston)

        Coding Clinic: 2022, Q3, P15

    Z79.811   **Long term (current) use of aromatase inhibitors**

        Long term (current) use of anastrozole (Arimidex)

        Long term (current) use of exemestane (Aromasin)

        Long term (current) use of letrozole (Femara)

    Z79.818   **Long term (current) use of other agents affecting estrogen receptors and estrogen levels**

        Long term (current) use of estrogen receptor downregulators

        Long term (current) use of fulvestrant (Faslodex)

        Long term (current) use of gonadotropin-releasing hormone (GnRH) agonist

        Long term (current) use of goserelin acetate (Zoladex)

        Long term (current) use of leuprolide acetate (leuprorelin) (Lupron)

        Long term (current) use of megestrol acetate (Megace)

Z79.82   Long term (current) use of aspirin

Z79.83   Long term (current) use of bisphosphonates
       Coding Clinic: 2016, Q4, P42

Z79.84   Long term (current) use of oral hypoglycemic drugs
       Long term (current) use of oral antidiabetic drugs

       Excludes2   long-term (current) use of injectable non-insulin antidiabetic drugs (Z79.85)
                   long term (current) use of insulin (Z79.4)
       Coding Clinic: 2016, Q4, P76, 121-122, 126

Z79.85   Long-term (current) use of injectable non-insulin antidiabetic drugs

       Excludes2   long term (current) use of insulin (Z79.4)
                   long term (current) use of oral hypoglycemic drugs (Z79.84)

● **Z79.89**   Other long term (current) drug therapy

       Z79.890   Hormone replacement therapy

       Z79.891   Long term (current) use of opiate analgesic
            Long term (current) use of methadone for pain management

            Excludes1   methadone use NOS (F11.9-)
                   use of methadone for treatment of heroin addiction (F11.2-)

       Z79.899   Other long term (current) drug therapy
            Coding Clinic: 2023, Q3, P17-18; 2015, Q4, P34, Q3, P21

● **Z80**   Family history of primary malignant neoplasm

Z80.0   Family history of malignant neoplasm of digestive organs
       Conditions classifiable to C15-C26
       Coding Clinic: 2018, Q1, P7

Z80.1   Family history of malignant neoplasm of trachea, bronchus and lung
       Conditions classifiable to C33-C34

Z80.2   Family history of malignant neoplasm of other respiratory and intrathoracic organs
       Conditions classifiable to C30-C32, C37-C39

Z80.3   Family history of malignant neoplasm of breast
       Conditions classifiable to C50.-

● **Z80.4**   Family history of malignant neoplasm of genital organs
       Conditions classifiable to C51-C63

       Z80.41   Family history of malignant neoplasm of ovary

       Z80.42   Family history of malignant neoplasm of prostate

       Z80.43   Family history of malignant neoplasm of testis

       Z80.49   Family history of malignant neoplasm of other genital organs

● **Z80.5**   Family history of malignant neoplasm of urinary tract
       Conditions classifiable to C64-C68

       Z80.51   Family history of malignant neoplasm of kidney

       Z80.52   Family history of malignant neoplasm of bladder

       Z80.59   Family history of malignant neoplasm of other urinary tract organ

Z80.6   Family history of leukemia
       Conditions classifiable to C91-C95

Z80.7   Family history of other malignant neoplasms of lymphoid, hematopoietic and related tissues
       Conditions classifiable to C81-C90, C96.-

Z80.8   Family history of malignant neoplasm of other organs or systems
       Conditions classifiable to C00-C14, C40-C49, C69-C79

Z80.9   Family history of malignant neoplasm, unspecified
       Conditions classifiable to C80.1

● **Z81**   Family history of mental and behavioral disorders

Z81.0   Family history of intellectual disabilities
       Conditions classifiable to F70-F79

Z81.1   Family history of alcohol abuse and dependence
       Conditions classifiable to F10.-

Z81.2   Family history of tobacco abuse and dependence
       Conditions classifiable to F17.-

Z81.3   Family history of other psychoactive substance abuse and dependence
       Conditions classifiable to F11-F16, F18-F19

Z81.4   Family history of other substance abuse and dependence
       Conditions classifiable to F55

Z81.8   Family history of other mental and behavioral disorders
       Conditions classifiable elsewhere in F01-F99

● **Z82**   Family history of certain disabilities and chronic diseases (leading to disablement)

Z82.0   Family history of epilepsy and other diseases of the nervous system
       Conditions classifiable to G00-G99

Z82.1   Family history of blindness and visual loss
       Conditions classifiable to H54.-

Z82.2   Family history of deafness and hearing loss
       Conditions classifiable to H90-H91

Z82.3   Family history of stroke
       Conditions classifiable to I60-I64

● **Z82.4**   Family history of ischemic heart disease and other diseases of the circulatory system
       Conditions classifiable to I00-I5A, I65-I99

       Z82.41   Family history of sudden cardiac death

       Z82.49   Family history of ischemic heart disease and other diseases of the circulatory system

Z82.5   Family history of asthma and other chronic lower respiratory diseases
       Conditions classifiable to J40-J47

       Excludes2   family history of other diseases of the respiratory system (Z83.6)

● **Z82.6**   Family history of arthritis and other diseases of the musculoskeletal system and connective tissue
       Conditions classifiable to M00-M99

       Z82.61   Family history of arthritis

       Z82.62   Family history of osteoporosis

       Z82.69   Family history of other diseases of the musculoskeletal system and connective tissue

● **Z82.7**   Family history of congenital malformations, deformations and chromosomal abnormalities
       Conditions classifiable to Q00-Q99

       Z82.71   Family history of polycystic kidney

       Z82.79   Family history of other congenital malformations, deformations and chromosomal abnormalities

Z82.8   Family history of other disabilities and chronic diseases leading to disablement, not elsewhere classified

● **Z83**   Family history of other specific disorders

       Excludes2   contact with and (suspected) exposure to communicable disease in the family (Z20.-)

Z83.0   Family history of human immunodeficiency virus [HIV] disease
       Conditions classifiable to B20

Z83.1   Family history of other infectious and parasitic diseases
       Conditions classifiable to A00-B19, B25-B94, B99

Z83.2   Family history of diseases of the blood and blood-forming organs and certain disorders involving the immune mechanism
       Conditions classifiable to D50-D89

Z83.3   Family history of diabetes mellitus
       Conditions classifiable to E08-E13

CHAPTER 21 (Z00-Z99)

● **Z83.4** **Family history of other endocrine, nutritional and metabolic diseases**
Conditions classifiable to E00-E07, E15-E88

   Z83.41 **Family history of multiple endocrine neoplasia [MEN] syndrome**

   Z83.42 **Family history of familial hypercholesterolemia**
     Coding Clinic: 2016, Q4, P77

●   **Z83.43** **Family history of other disorder of lipoprotein metabolism and other lipidemias**

     Z83.430 **Family history of elevated lipoprotein(a)**
       Family history of elevated Lp(a)

     Z83.438 **Family history of other disorder of lipoprotein metabolism and other lipidemia**
       Family history of familial combined hyperlipidemia

   Z83.49 **Family history of other endocrine, nutritional and metabolic diseases**

● **Z83.5** **Family history of eye and ear disorders**

●   **Z83.51** **Family history of eye disorders**
     Conditions classifiable to H00-H53, H55-H59

     Excludes2 family history of blindness and visual loss (Z82.1)

     Z83.511 **Family history of glaucoma**

     Z83.518 **Family history of other specified eye disorder**

   Z83.52 **Family history of ear disorders**
     Conditions classifiable to H60-H83, H92-H95

     Excludes2 family history of deafness and hearing loss (Z82.2)

Z83.6 **Family history of other diseases of the respiratory system**
Conditions classifiable to J00-J39, J60-J99

   Excludes2 family history of asthma and other chronic lower respiratory diseases (Z82.5)

● **Z83.7** **Family history of diseases of the digestive system**
Conditions classifiable to D12, K00-K93

●   **Z83.71** **Family history of colonic polyps**

     Excludes2 family history of malignant neoplasm of digestive organs (Z80.0)

     Coding Clinic: 2021, Q1, P15

     Z83.710 **Family history of adenomatous and serrated polyps**
       Conditions classifiable to D12.-
       Family history of tubular adenoma polyps
       Family history of tubulovillous adenoma polyps
       Family history of villous adenoma polyps

     Z83.711 **Family history of hyperplastic colon polyps**

     Z83.718 **Other family history of colon polyps**
       Family history of inflammatory colon polyps

     Z83.719 **Family history of colon polyps, unspecified**
       Family history of colon polyps NOS

▶ **Z83.72** **Family history of familial adenomatous polyposis**

   Z83.79 **Family history of other diseases of the digestive system**

● **Z84** **Family history of other conditions**

  Z84.0 **Family history of diseases of the skin and subcutaneous tissue**
     Conditions classifiable to L00-L99

  Z84.1 **Family history of disorders of kidney and ureter**
     Conditions classifiable to N00-N29

  Z84.2 **Family history of other diseases of the genitourinary system**
     Conditions classifiable to N30-N99
     Coding Clinic: 2016, Q4, P77

  Z84.3 **Family history of consanguinity**

● **Z84.8** **Family history of other specified conditions**

   Z84.81 **Family history of carrier of genetic disease**
     Coding Clinic: 2021, Q1, P15

   Z84.82 **Family history of sudden infant death syndrome**
     Family history of SIDS

   Z84.89 **Family history of other specified conditions**

● **Z85** **Personal history of malignant neoplasm**

Code first any follow-up examination after treatment of malignant neoplasm (Z08)

Use additional code to identify:
  alcohol use and dependence (F10.-)
  exposure to environmental tobacco smoke (Z77.22)
  history of tobacco dependence (Z87.891)
  occupational exposure to environmental tobacco smoke (Z57.31)
  tobacco dependence (F17.-)
  tobacco use (Z72.0)

  Excludes2 personal history of benign neoplasm (Z86.01-)
     personal history of carcinoma-in-situ (Z86.00-)

Coding Clinic: 2022, Q3, P28

● **Z85.0** **Personal history of malignant neoplasm of digestive organs**

   Z85.00 **Personal history of malignant neoplasm of unspecified digestive organ**

   Z85.01 **Personal history of malignant neoplasm of esophagus**
     Conditions classifiable to C15

●   **Z85.02** **Personal history of malignant neoplasm of stomach**

     Z85.020 **Personal history of malignant carcinoid tumor of stomach**
       Conditions classifiable to C7A.092

     Z85.028 **Personal history of other malignant neoplasm of stomach**
       Conditions classifiable to C16

●   **Z85.03** **Personal history of malignant neoplasm of large intestine**

     Z85.030 **Personal history of malignant carcinoid tumor of large intestine**
       Conditions classifiable to C7A.022-C7A.025, C7A.029

     Z85.038 **Personal history of other malignant neoplasm of large intestine**
       Conditions classifiable to C18

●   **Z85.04** **Personal history of malignant neoplasm of rectum, rectosigmoid junction, and anus**

     Z85.040 **Personal history of malignant carcinoid tumor of rectum**
       Conditions classifiable to C7A.026

     Z85.048 **Personal history of other malignant neoplasm of rectum, rectosigmoid junction, and anus**
       Conditions classifiable to C19-C21

   Z85.05 **Personal history of malignant neoplasm of liver**
     Conditions classifiable to C22

●   **Z85.06** **Personal history of malignant neoplasm of small intestine**

     Z85.060 **Personal history of malignant carcinoid tumor of small intestine**
       Conditions classifiable to C7A.01-

     Z85.068 **Personal history of other malignant neoplasm of small intestine**
       Conditions classifiable to C17

▶ New   ⇒ Revised   ~~deleted~~ Deleted   Excludes 1   Excludes 2   Includes   Use additional   Code first   Code also   Key words
OGCR Official Guidelines   X Assign placeholder X   ● Use Additional Character(s)   ▶ Manifestation Code   🅗 Hierarchical Condition Category   Coding Clinic

Z85.07   Personal history of malignant neoplasm of pancreas
> Conditions classifiable to C25

Z85.09   Personal history of malignant neoplasm of other digestive organs

● Z85.1   Personal history of malignant neoplasm of trachea, bronchus and lung

   ● Z85.11   Personal history of malignant neoplasm of bronchus and lung

     Z85.110   Personal history of malignant carcinoid tumor of bronchus and lung
> Conditions classifiable to C7A.090

     Z85.118   Personal history of other malignant neoplasm of bronchus and lung
> Conditions classifiable to C34

   Z85.12   Personal history of malignant neoplasm of trachea
> Conditions classifiable to C33

● Z85.2   Personal history of malignant neoplasm of other respiratory and intrathoracic organs

   Z85.20   Personal history of malignant neoplasm of unspecified respiratory organ

   Z85.21   Personal history of malignant neoplasm of larynx
> Conditions classifiable to C32

   Z85.22   Personal history of malignant neoplasm of nasal cavities, middle ear, and accessory sinuses
> Conditions classifiable to C30-C31

   ● Z85.23   Personal history of malignant neoplasm of thymus

     Z85.230   Personal history of malignant carcinoid tumor of thymus
> Conditions classifiable to C7A.091

     Z85.238   Personal history of other malignant neoplasm of thymus
> Conditions classifiable to C37

   Z85.29   Personal history of malignant neoplasm of other respiratory and intrathoracic organs

Z85.3   Personal history of malignant neoplasm of breast
> Conditions classifiable to C50.-

● Z85.4   Personal history of malignant neoplasm of genital organs
> Conditions classifiable to C51-C63

   Z85.40   Personal history of malignant neoplasm of unspecified female genital organ

   Z85.41   Personal history of malignant neoplasm of cervix uteri

   Z85.42   Personal history of malignant neoplasm of other parts of uterus

   Z85.43   Personal history of malignant neoplasm of ovary

   Z85.44   Personal history of malignant neoplasm of other female genital organs
> **Coding Clinic: 2024, Q2, P11,12**

   Z85.45   Personal history of malignant neoplasm of unspecified male genital organ

   Z85.46   Personal history of malignant neoplasm of prostate
> **Coding Clinic: 2023, Q2, P5**

   Z85.47   Personal history of malignant neoplasm of testis

   Z85.48   Personal history of malignant neoplasm of epididymis

   Z85.49   Personal history of malignant neoplasm of other male genital organs

● Z85.5   Personal history of malignant neoplasm of urinary tract
> Conditions classifiable to C64-C68

   Z85.50   Personal history of malignant neoplasm of unspecified urinary tract organ

   Z85.51   Personal history of malignant neoplasm of bladder

● Z85.52   Personal history of malignant neoplasm of kidney

> **Excludes1**   personal history of malignant neoplasm of renal pelvis (Z85.53)

   Z85.520   Personal history of malignant carcinoid tumor of kidney
> Conditions classifiable to C7A.093

   Z85.528   Personal history of other malignant neoplasm of kidney
> Conditions classifiable to C64

Z85.53   Personal history of malignant neoplasm of renal pelvis

Z85.54   Personal history of malignant neoplasm of ureter

Z85.59   Personal history of malignant neoplasm of other urinary tract organ

Z85.6   Personal history of leukemia
> Conditions classifiable to C91-C95

> **Excludes1**   leukemia in remission C91.0-C95.9 with 5th character 1

● Z85.7   Personal history of other malignant neoplasms of lymphoid, hematopoietic and related tissues

   Z85.71   Personal history of Hodgkin lymphoma
> Conditions classifiable to C81

   Z85.72   Personal history of non-Hodgkin lymphomas
> Conditions classifiable to C82-C85
> **Coding Clinic: 2022, Q3, P28**

   Z85.79   Personal history of other malignant neoplasms of lymphoid, hematopoietic and related tissues
> Conditions classifiable to C88-C90, C96

> **Excludes1**   multiple myeloma in remission (C90.01)
> plasma cell leukemia in remission (C90.11)
> plasmacytoma in remission (C90.21)

● Z85.8   Personal history of malignant neoplasms of other organs and systems
> Conditions classifiable to C00-C14, C40-C49, C69-C75, C7A.098, C76-C79

   ● Z85.81   Personal history of malignant neoplasm of lip, oral cavity, and pharynx
> Conditions classifiable to C00-C14

     Z85.810   Personal history of malignant neoplasm of tongue

     Z85.818   Personal history of malignant neoplasm of other sites of lip, oral cavity, and pharynx

     Z85.819   Personal history of malignant neoplasm of unspecified site of lip, oral cavity, and pharynx

   ● Z85.82   Personal history of malignant neoplasm of skin

     Z85.820   Personal history of malignant melanoma of skin
> Conditions classifiable to C43
> **Coding Clinic: 2022, Q3, P9**

     Z85.821   Personal history of Merkel cell carcinoma
> Conditions classifiable to C4A

     Z85.828   Personal history of other malignant neoplasm of skin
> Conditions classifiable to C44

   ● Z85.83   Personal history of malignant neoplasm of bone and soft tissue
> Conditions classifiable to C40-C41; C45-C49

     Z85.830   Personal history of malignant neoplasm of bone

Z85.831 **Personal history of malignant neoplasm of soft tissue**

> **Excludes2**   personal history of malignant neoplasm of skin (Z85.82-)

● Z85.84 **Personal history of malignant neoplasm of eye and nervous tissue**
Conditions classifiable to C69-C72

Z85.840 **Personal history of malignant neoplasm of eye**

Z85.841 **Personal history of malignant neoplasm of brain**

Z85.848 **Personal history of malignant neoplasm of other parts of nervous tissue**

● Z85.85 **Personal history of malignant neoplasm of endocrine glands**
Conditions classifiable to C73-C75

Z85.850 **Personal history of malignant neoplasm of thyroid**

Z85.858 **Personal history of malignant neoplasm of other endocrine glands**
Coding Clinic: 2024, Q2, P10

Z85.89 **Personal history of malignant neoplasm of other organs and systems**
Conditions classifiable to C7A.098, C76, C77-C79

Z85.9 **Personal history of malignant neoplasm, unspecified**
Conditions classifiable to C7A.00, C80.1

● Z86 **Personal history of certain other diseases**
Code first any follow-up examination after treatment (Z09)

● Z86.0 **Personal history of in-situ and benign neoplasms and neoplasms of uncertain behavior**

> **Excludes2**   personal history of malignant neoplasms (Z85.-)

● Z86.00 **Personal history of in-situ neoplasm**
Conditions classifiable to D00-D09

Z86.000 **Personal history of in-situ neoplasm of breast**
Conditions classifiable to D05

Z86.001 **Personal history of in-situ neoplasm of cervix uteri**
Conditions classifiable to D06
Personal history of cervical intraepithelial neoplasia III [CIN III]

Z86.002 **Personal history of in-situ neoplasm of other and unspecified genital organs**
Conditions classifiable to D07
Personal history of high-grade prostatic intraepithelial neoplasia III [HGPIN III]
Personal history of vaginal intraepithelial neoplasia III [VAIN III]
Personal history of vulvar intraepithelial neoplasia III [VIN III]

Z86.003 **Personal history of in-situ neoplasm of oral cavity, esophagus and stomach**
Conditions classifiable to D00

Z86.004 **Personal history of in-situ neoplasm of other and unspecified digestive organs**
Conditions classifiable to D01
Personal history of anal intraepithelial neoplasia (AIN III)

Z86.005 **Personal history of in-situ neoplasm of middle ear and respiratory system**
Conditions classifiable to D02

Z86.006 **Personal history of melanoma in-situ**
Conditions classifiable to D03

> **Excludes2**   sites other than skin - code to personal history of in-situ neoplasm of the site

Z86.007 **Personal history of in-situ neoplasm of skin**
Conditions classifiable to D04
Personal history of carcinoma in situ of skin

Z86.008 **Personal history of in-situ neoplasm of other site**
Conditions classifiable to D09

● Z86.01 **Personal history of benign neoplasm**
Coding Clinic: 2017, Q1, P14

▶ Z86.010 **Personal history of colon polyps**
▶ Personal history of colorectal polyps
▶ Personal history of rectal polyps
Coding Clinic: 2021, Q1, P15; 2017, Q1, P9, P14

▶ Z86.0100 **Personal history of colon polyps, unspecified**
▶ Personal history of colon polyps NOS

▶ Z86.0101 **Personal history of adenomatous and serrated colon polyps**
▶ Personal history of tubular adenoma polyps
▶ Personal history of sessile adenomatous colon polyp
▶ Personal history of sessile serrated colon polyp
▶ Personal history of tubulovillous adenoma polyps
▶ Personal history of villous adenoma polyps
▶ Personal history of traditional serrated adenoma polyps

▶ Z86.0102 **Personal history of hyperplastic colon polyps**

▶ Z86.0109 **Personal history of other colon polyps**

Z86.011 **Personal history of benign neoplasm of the brain**

Z86.012 **Personal history of benign carcinoid tumor**

Z86.018 **Personal history of other benign neoplasm**
Coding Clinic: 2017, Q1, P14

Z86.03 **Personal history of neoplasm of uncertain behavior**

● Z86.1 **Personal history of infectious and parasitic diseases**
Conditions classifiable to A00-B89, B99

> **Excludes1**   personal history of infectious diseases specific to a body system sequelae of infectious and parasitic diseases (B90-B94)

Coding Clinic: 2016, Q4, P5

Z86.11 **Personal history of tuberculosis**

Z86.12 **Personal history of poliomyelitis**

Z86.13 **Personal history of malaria**

Z86.14 **Personal history of Methicillin resistant Staphylococcus aureus infection**
Personal history of MRSA infection

Z86.15 **Personal history of latent tuberculosis infection**

▶ New   ⇒ Revised   ~~deleted~~ Deleted   Excludes 1   Excludes 2   Includes   Use additional   Code first   Code also   Key words
OGCR Official Guidelines   X Assign placeholder X   ● Use Additional Character(s)   ▶ Manifestation Code   🦙 Hierarchical Condition Category   Coding Clinic

Z86.16   **Personal history of COVID-19**
     Excludes1   post COVID-19 condition (U09.9)
       Coding Clinic: 2022, Q3, P4; 2021, Q4, P103-105, 107-108;
       2021, Q1, P34-35, 40-42, 44, 46

Z86.19   **Personal history of other infectious and parasitic diseases**
     Coding Clinic: 2021, Q1, P34-35, 40-41

Z86.2   **Personal history of diseases of the blood and blood-forming organs and certain disorders involving the immune mechanism**
     Conditions classifiable to D50-D89

● Z86.3   **Personal history of endocrine, nutritional and metabolic diseases**
     Conditions classifiable to E00-E88

Z86.31   **Personal history of diabetic foot ulcer**
     Excludes2   current diabetic foot ulcer
       (E08.621, E09.621, E10.621,
       E11.621, E13.621)

Z86.32   **Personal history of gestational diabetes**
     Personal history of conditions classifiable to O24.4-
     Excludes1   gestational diabetes mellitus in current pregnancy (O24.4-)

Z86.39   **Personal history of other endocrine, nutritional and metabolic disease**
     Coding Clinic: 2020, Q1, P13

● Z86.5   **Personal history of mental and behavioral disorders**
     Conditions classifiable to F40-F59

Z86.51   **Personal history of combat and operational stress reaction**   **A**

Z86.59   **Personal history of other mental and behavioral disorders**

● Z86.6   **Personal history of diseases of the nervous system and sense organs**
     Conditions classifiable to G00-G99, H00-H95

Z86.61   **Personal history of infections of the central nervous system**
     Personal history of encephalitis
     Personal history of meningitis

Z86.69   **Personal history of other diseases of the nervous system and sense organs**
     Coding Clinic: 2016, Q4, P25

● Z86.7   **Personal history of diseases of the circulatory system**
     Conditions classifiable to I00-I99
     Excludes2   old myocardial infarction (I25.2)
       personal history of anaphylactic shock (Z87.892)
       postmyocardial infarction syndrome (I24.1)

● Z86.71   **Personal history of venous thrombosis and embolism**

Z86.711   **Personal history of pulmonary embolism**

Z86.718   **Personal history of other venous thrombosis and embolism**

Z86.72   **Personal history of thrombophlebitis**

Z86.73   **Personal history of transient ischemic attack (TIA), and cerebral infarction without residual deficits**
     Personal history of prolonged reversible ischemic neurological deficit (PRIND)
     Personal history of stroke NOS without residual deficits
     Excludes1   personal history of traumatic brain injury (Z87.820)
       sequelae of cerebrovascular disease (I69.-)
     Coding Clinic: 2023, Q1, P37; 2012, Q4, P3

Z86.74   **Personal history of sudden cardiac arrest**
     Personal history of sudden cardiac death successfully resuscitated
     Coding Clinic: 2024, Q1, P27

Z86.79   **Personal history of other diseases of the circulatory system**
     Coding Clinic: 2022, Q2, P15; 2020, Q1, P13

● Z87   **Personal history of other diseases and conditions**
     Code first any follow-up examination after treatment (Z09)

● Z87.0   **Personal history of diseases of the respiratory system**
     Conditions classifiable to J00-J99

Z87.01   **Personal history of pneumonia (recurrent)**

Z87.09   **Personal history of other diseases of the respiratory system**

● Z87.1   **Personal history of diseases of the digestive system**
     Conditions classifiable to K00-K93

Z87.11   **Personal history of peptic ulcer disease**

Z87.19   **Personal history of other diseases of the digestive system**
     Coding Clinic: 2017, Q1, P14

Z87.2   **Personal history of diseases of the skin and subcutaneous tissue**
     Conditions classifiable to L00-L99
     Excludes2   personal history of diabetic foot ulcer (Z86.31)

● Z87.3   **Personal history of diseases of the musculoskeletal system and connective tissue**
     Conditions classifiable to M00-M99
     Excludes2   personal history of (healed) traumatic fracture (Z87.81)

● Z87.31   **Personal history of (healed) nontraumatic fracture**

Z87.310   **Personal history of (healed) osteoporosis fracture**
     Personal history of (healed) fragility fracture
     Personal history of (healed) collapsed vertebra due to osteoporosis

Z87.311   **Personal history of (healed) other pathological fracture**
     Personal history of (healed) collapsed vertebra NOS
     Excludes2   personal history of osteoporosis fracture (Z87.310)

Z87.312   **Personal history of (healed) stress fracture**
     Personal history of (healed) fatigue fracture

Z87.39   **Personal history of other diseases of the musculoskeletal system and connective tissue**

● Z87.4   **Personal history of diseases of genitourinary system**
     Conditions classifiable to N00-N99

● Z87.41   **Personal history of dysplasia of the female genital tract**
     Excludes1   personal history of intraepithelial neoplasia III of female genital tract (Z86.001, Z86.008)
       personal history of malignant neoplasm of female genital tract (Z85.40-Z85.44)

Z87.410   **Personal history of cervical dysplasia**

Z87.411   **Personal history of vaginal dysplasia**

Z87.412   **Personal history of vulvar dysplasia**

Z87.42   **Personal history of other diseases of the female genital tract**

● Z87.43   **Personal history of diseases of male genital organs**

Z87.430   **Personal history of prostatic dysplasia**
     Excludes1   personal history of malignant neoplasm of prostate (Z85.46)

Z87.438   **Personal history of other diseases of male genital organs**

CHAPTER 21 (Z00-Z99)

- **Z87.44** Personal history of diseases of urinary system
  - **Excludes1** personal history of malignant neoplasm of cervix uteri (Z85.41)
  - **Z87.440** Personal history of urinary (tract) infections
  - **Z87.441** Personal history of nephrotic syndrome
  - **Z87.442** Personal history of urinary calculi
    Personal history of kidney stones
  - **Z87.448** Personal history of other diseases of urinary system
- **Z87.5** Personal history of complications of pregnancy, childbirth and the puerperium
  Conditions classifiable to O00-O9A
  - **Excludes2** recurrent pregnancy loss (N96)
  - **Z87.51** Personal history of pre-term labor
    - **Excludes1** current pregnancy with history of pre-term labor (O09.21-)
  - **Z87.59** Personal history of other complications of pregnancy, childbirth and the puerperium
    Personal history of trophoblastic disease
- **Z87.6** Personal history of certain (corrected) conditions arising in the perinatal period
  Conditions classifiable to P00-P96
  - **Excludes1** personal history of (corrected) congenital malformations (Z87.7-)
  - **Z87.61** Personal history of (corrected) necrotizing enterocolitis of newborn
  - **Z87.68** Personal history of other (corrected) conditions arising in the perinatal period
- **Z87.7** Personal history of (corrected) congenital malformations
  Conditions classifiable to Q00-Q89 that have been repaired or corrected
  - **Excludes1** congenital malformations that have been partially corrected or repair but which still require medical treatment - code to condition
  - **Excludes2** other postprocedural states (Z98.-)
    personal history of medical treatment (Z92.-)
    presence of cardiac and vascular implants and grafts (Z95.-)
    presence of other devices (Z97.-)
    presence of other functional implants (Z96.-)
    transplanted organ and tissue status (Z94.-)
  - **Z87.71** Personal history of (corrected) congenital malformations of genitourinary system
    - **Z87.710** Personal history of (corrected) hypospadias
    - **Z87.718** Personal history of other specified (corrected) congenital malformations of genitourinary system
  - **Z87.72** Personal history of (corrected) congenital malformations of nervous system and sense organs
    - **Z87.720** Personal history of (corrected) congenital malformations of eye
    - **Z87.721** Personal history of (corrected) congenital malformations of ear
    - **Z87.728** Personal history of other specified (corrected) congenital malformations of nervous system and sense organs
  - **Z87.73** Personal history of (corrected) congenital malformations of digestive system
    - **Z87.730** Personal history of (corrected) cleft lip and palate
    - **Z87.731** Personal history of (corrected) tracheoesophageal fistula or atresia
    - **Z87.732** Personal history of (corrected) persistent cloaca or cloacal malformations

- **Z87.738** Personal history of other specified (corrected) congenital malformations of digestive system
- **Z87.74** Personal history of (corrected) congenital malformations of heart and circulatory system
- **Z87.75** Personal history of (corrected) congenital malformations of respiratory system
- **Z87.76** Personal history of (corrected) congenital malformations of integument, limbs and musculoskeletal system
  - **Z87.760** Personal history of (corrected) congenital diaphragmatic hernia or other congenital diaphragm malformations
  - **Z87.761** Personal history of (corrected) gastroschisis
  - **Z87.762** Personal history of (corrected) prune belly malformation
  - **Z87.763** Personal history of other (corrected) congenital abdominal wall malformations
  - **Z87.768** Personal history of other specified (corrected) congenital malformations of integument, limbs and musculoskeletal system
- **Z87.79** Personal history of other (corrected) congenital malformations
  - **Z87.790** Personal history of (corrected) congenital malformations of face and neck
  - **Z87.798** Personal history of other (corrected) congenital malformations
- **Z87.8** Personal history of other specified conditions
  - **Excludes2** personal history of self harm (Z91.5-)
  - **Z87.81** Personal history of (healed) traumatic fracture
    - **Excludes2** personal history of (healed) nontraumatic fracture (Z87.31-)
  - **Z87.82** Personal history of other (healed) physical injury and trauma
    Conditions classifiable to S00-T88, except traumatic fractures
    - **Z87.820** Personal history of traumatic brain injury
      - **Excludes1** personal history of transient ischemic attack (TIA), and cerebral infarction without residual deficits (Z86.73)
    - **Z87.821** Personal history of retained foreign body fully removed
    - **Z87.828** Personal history of other (healed) physical injury and trauma
  - **Z87.89** Personal history of other specified conditions
    - **Z87.890** Personal history of sex reassignment
    - **Z87.891** Personal history of nicotine dependence
      - **Excludes1** current nicotine dependence (F17.2-)
      - Coding Clinic: 2017, Q2, P27
    - **Z87.892** Personal history of anaphylaxis
      Code also allergy status such as:
      allergy status to drugs, medicaments and biological substances (Z88.-)
      allergy status, other than to drugs and biological substances (Z91.0-)
    - **Z87.898** Personal history of other specified conditions
      Coding Clinic: 2013, Q1, P21

▶ New　⇒ Revised　~~deleted~~ Deleted　Excludes 1　Excludes 2　Includes　Use additional　Code first　Code also　Key words
OGCR Official Guidelines　X Assign placeholder X　● Use Additional Character(s)　▶ Manifestation Code　🔖 Hierarchical Condition Category　Coding Clinic

● **Z88**   **Allergy status to drugs, medicaments and biological substances**

     Excludes2   allergy status, other than to drugs and biological substances (Z91.0-)

     Z88.0   Allergy status to **penicillin**

     Z88.1   Allergy status to **other antibiotic agents**

     Z88.2   Allergy status to **sulfonamides**

         Coding Clinic: 2015, Q3, P23

     Z88.3   Allergy status to **other anti-infective agents**

     Z88.4   Allergy status to **anesthetic agent**

     Z88.5   Allergy status to **narcotic agent**

     Z88.6   Allergy status to **analgesic agent**

     Z88.7   Allergy status to **serum and vaccine**

     Z88.8   Allergy status to **other drugs, medicaments and biological substances**

     Z88.9   Allergy status to **unspecified drugs, medicaments and biological substances**

● **Z89**   **Acquired absence of limb**

     Includes   amputation status
                 postprocedural loss of limb
                 post-traumatic loss of limb

     Excludes1   acquired deformities of limbs (M20-M21)
                   congenital absence of limbs (Q71-Q73)

  ● **Z89.0**   **Acquired absence of thumb and other finger(s)**

    ● **Z89.01**   Acquired absence of **thumb**

         Z89.011   Acquired absence of **right thumb**

         Z89.012   Acquired absence of **left thumb**

         Z89.019   Acquired absence of **unspecified thumb**

    ● **Z89.02**   Acquired absence of **other finger(s)**

         Excludes2   acquired absence of thumb (Z89.01-)

         Z89.021   Acquired absence of **right finger(s)**

         Z89.022   Acquired absence of **left finger(s)**

         Z89.029   Acquired absence of **unspecified finger(s)**

  ● **Z89.1**   **Acquired absence of hand and wrist**

    ● **Z89.11**   Acquired absence of **hand**

         Z89.111   Acquired absence of **right hand**

         Z89.112   Acquired absence of **left hand**

         Z89.119   Acquired absence of **unspecified hand**

    ● **Z89.12**   Acquired absence of **wrist**
         Disarticulation at wrist

         Z89.121   Acquired absence of **right wrist**

         Z89.122   Acquired absence of **left wrist**

         Z89.129   Acquired absence of **unspecified wrist**

  ● **Z89.2**   **Acquired absence of upper limb above wrist**

    ● **Z89.20**   Acquired absence of **upper limb, unspecified level**

         Z89.201   Acquired absence of **right upper limb, unspecified level**

         Z89.202   Acquired absence of **left upper limb, unspecified level**

         Z89.209   Acquired absence of **unspecified upper limb, unspecified level**
               Acquired absence of arm NOS

    ● **Z89.21**   Acquired absence of **upper limb below elbow**

         Z89.211   Acquired absence of **right upper limb below elbow**

         Z89.212   Acquired absence of **left upper limb below elbow**

         Z89.219   Acquired absence of **unspecified upper limb below elbow**

    ● **Z89.22**   Acquired absence of **upper limb above elbow**
         Disarticulation at elbow

         Z89.221   Acquired absence of **right upper limb above elbow**

         Z89.222   Acquired absence of **left upper limb above elbow**

         Z89.229   Acquired absence of **unspecified upper limb above elbow**

    ● **Z89.23**   Acquired absence of **shoulder**
         Acquired absence of shoulder joint following explantation of shoulder joint prosthesis, with or without presence of antibiotic-impregnated cement spacer

         Z89.231   Acquired absence of **right shoulder**

         Z89.232   Acquired absence of **left shoulder**

         Z89.239   Acquired absence of **unspecified shoulder**

  ● **Z89.4**   **Acquired absence of toe(s), foot, and ankle**

    ● **Z89.41**   Acquired absence of **great toe**

         Z89.411   Acquired absence of **right great toe** 🦵

         Z89.412   Acquired absence of **left great toe** 🦵

         Z89.419   Acquired absence of **unspecified great toe** 🦵

    ● **Z89.42**   Acquired absence of **other toe(s)**

         Excludes2   acquired absence of great toe (Z89.41-)

         Z89.421   Acquired absence of **other right toe(s)** 🦵

         Z89.422   Acquired absence of **other left toe(s)** 🦵

         Z89.429   Acquired absence of **other toe(s), unspecified side** 🦵

    ● **Z89.43**   Acquired absence of **foot**

         Z89.431   Acquired absence of **right foot** 🦵

         Z89.432   Acquired absence of **left foot** 🦵

         Z89.439   Acquired absence of **unspecified foot** 🦵

    ● **Z89.44**   Acquired absence of **ankle**
         Disarticulation of ankle

         Z89.441   Acquired absence of **right ankle** 🦵

         Z89.442   Acquired absence of **left ankle** 🦵

         Z89.449   Acquired absence of **unspecified ankle** 🦵

  ● **Z89.5**   **Acquired absence of leg below knee**

    ● **Z89.51**   Acquired absence of **leg below knee**

         Z89.511   Acquired absence of **right leg below knee** 🦵

         Z89.512   Acquired absence of **left leg below knee** 🦵

         Z89.519   Acquired absence of **unspecified leg below knee** 🦵

    ● **Z89.52**   Acquired absence of **knee**
         Acquired absence of knee joint following explantation of knee joint prosthesis, with or without presence of antibiotic-impregnated cement spacer

         Z89.521   Acquired absence of **right knee**

         Z89.522   Acquired absence of **left knee**

         Z89.529   Acquired absence of **unspecified knee**

  ● **Z89.6**   **Acquired absence of leg above knee**

    ● **Z89.61**   Acquired absence of **leg above knee**
         Acquired absence of leg NOS
         Disarticulation at knee

         Z89.611   Acquired absence of **right leg above knee** 🦵

         Z89.612   Acquired absence of **left leg above knee** 🦵

         Z89.619   Acquired absence of **unspecified leg above knee** 🦵

CHAPTER 21 (Z00-Z99)

● **Z89.62**   **Acquired absence of hip**
Acquired absence of hip joint following explantation of hip joint prosthesis, with or without presence of antibiotic-impregnated cement spacer
Disarticulation at hip

     Z89.621   Acquired absence of right hip joint

     Z89.622   Acquired absence of left hip joint

     Z89.629   Acquired absence of unspecified hip joint

Z89.9   Acquired absence of limb, unspecified

● **Z90**   **Acquired absence of organs, not elsewhere classified**

Includes   postprocedural or post-traumatic loss of body part NEC

Excludes1   congenital absence - see Alphabetical Index

Excludes2   postprocedural absence of endocrine glands (E89.-)

● **Z90.0**   **Acquired absence of part of head and neck**

     Z90.01   Acquired absence of eye

     Z90.02   Acquired absence of larynx

     Z90.09   Acquired absence of other part of head and neck
Acquired absence of nose

         Excludes2   teeth (K08.1)

● **Z90.1**   **Acquired absence of breast and nipple**

     Z90.10   Acquired absence of unspecified breast and nipple

     Z90.11   Acquired absence of right breast and nipple

     Z90.12   Acquired absence of left breast and nipple

     Z90.13   Acquired absence of bilateral breasts and nipples
Coding Clinic: 2022, Q3, P8

Z90.2   Acquired absence of lung [part of]

Z90.3   Acquired absence of stomach [part of]

● **Z90.4**   **Acquired absence of other specified parts of digestive tract**

   ● **Z90.41**   Acquired absence of pancreas

Code also exocrine pancreatic insufficiency (K86.81)

Use additional code to identify any associated: diabetes mellitus, postpancreatectomy (E13.-)
insulin use (Z79.4)

       Z90.410   Acquired total absence of pancreas
Acquired absence of pancreas NOS

       Z90.411   Acquired partial absence of pancreas
Coding Clinic: 2024, Q2, P10

     Z90.49   Acquired absence of other specified parts of digestive tract

Z90.5   Acquired absence of kidney

Z90.6   Acquired absence of other parts of urinary tract
Acquired absence of bladder

● **Z90.7**   **Acquired absence of genital organ(s)**

Excludes1   personal history of sex reassignment (Z87.890)

Excludes2   female genital mutilation status (N90.81-)

   ● **Z90.71**   Acquired absence of cervix and uterus

       Z90.710   Acquired absence of both cervix and uterus
Acquired absence of uterus NOS
Status post total hysterectomy

       Z90.711   Acquired absence of uterus with remaining cervical stump
Status post partial hysterectomy with remaining cervical stump

       Z90.712   Acquired absence of cervix with remaining uterus

   ● **Z90.72**   Acquired absence of ovaries

       Z90.721   Acquired absence of ovaries, unilateral

       Z90.722   Acquired absence of ovaries, bilateral

     Z90.79   Acquired absence of other genital organ(s)
Coding Clinic: 2023, Q2, P5

● **Z90.8**   **Acquired absence of other organs**

     Z90.81   Acquired absence of spleen

     Z90.89   Acquired absence of other organs
Coding Clinic: 2023, Q3, P13

● **Z91**   **Personal risk factors, not elsewhere classified**

Excludes2   contact with and (suspected) exposures hazardous to health (Z77.-)
exposure to pollution and other problems related to physical environment (Z77.1-)
female genital mutilation status (N90.81-)
occupational exposure to risk factors (Z57.-)
personal history of physical injury and trauma (Z87.81, Z87.82-)

● **Z91.0**   **Allergy status, other than to drugs and biological substances**

Excludes2   allergy status to drugs, medicaments, and biological substances (Z88.-)

   ● **Z91.01**   Food allergy status

       Excludes2   food additives allergy status (Z91.02)

       Z91.010   Allergy to peanuts

       Z91.011   Allergy to milk products

          Excludes1   lactose intolerance (E73.-)

       Z91.012   Allergy to eggs

       Z91.013   Allergy to seafood
Allergy to shellfish
Allergy to octopus or squid ink

       Z91.014   Allergy to mammalian meats
Allergy to beef
Allergy to lamb
Allergy to pork
Allergy to red meats

       Z91.018   Allergy to other foods
Allergy to nuts other than peanuts

     Z91.02   Food additives allergy status

   ● **Z91.03**   Insect allergy status

       Z91.030   Bee allergy status

       Z91.038   Other insect allergy status

   ● **Z91.04**   Nonmedicinal substance allergy status

       Z91.040   Latex allergy status
Latex sensitivity status

       Z91.041   Radiographic dye allergy status
Allergy status to contrast media used for diagnostic X-ray procedure

       Z91.048   Other nonmedicinal substance allergy status

     Z91.09   Other allergy status, other than to drugs and biological substances

● **Z91.1**   **Patient's noncompliance with medical treatment and regimen**

Code also, if applicable, to identify underdosing of specific drug (T36-T50 with final character 6)

Excludes2   caregiver noncompliance with patient's medical treatment and regimen (Z91.A-)

   ● **Z91.11**   Patient's noncompliance with dietary regimen
Code also, if applicable, food insecurity (Z59.4-)

       Z91.110   Patient's noncompliance with dietary regimen due to financial hardship

▶ New   ⇒ Revised   ~~deleted~~ Deleted   Excludes 1   Excludes 2   Includes   Use additional   Code first   Code also   Key words

OGCR Official Guidelines   X Assign placeholder X   ● Use Additional Character(s)   ▶ Manifestation Code   🅗 Hierarchical Condition Category   Coding Clinic

Z91.118   Patient's noncompliance with dietary regimen for other reason
    Inability to comply with dietary regimen

Z91.119   Patient's noncompliance with dietary regimen due to unspecified reason

● Z91.12   Patient's intentional underdosing of medication regimen
    Code first underdosing of medication (T36-T50) with fifth or sixth character 6

    Excludes1   adverse effect of prescribed drug taken as directed - code to adverse effect
        poisoning (overdose) - code to poisoning

Z91.120   Patient's intentional underdosing of medication regimen due to financial hardship

Z91.128   Patient's intentional underdosing of medication regimen for other reason

● Z91.13   Patient's unintentional underdosing of medication regimen
    Code first underdosing of medication (T36-T50) with fifth or sixth character 6

    Excludes1   adverse effect of prescribed drug taken as directed - code to adverse effect
        poisoning (overdose) - code to poisoning

Z91.130   Patient's unintentional underdosing of medication regimen due to age-related debility

Z91.138   Patient's unintentional underdosing of medication regimen for other reason

● Z91.14   Patient's other noncompliance with medication regimen
    ▶*Code first if applicable, adverse effect of underdosing (T36-T50)*
    Patient's underdosing of medication NOS
    Coding Clinic: 2022, Q1, P36

Z91.141   Patient's other noncompliance with medication regimen due to financial hardship

Z91.148   Patient's other noncompliance with medication regimen for other reason

● Z91.15   Patient's noncompliance with renal dialysis 🔗

Z91.151   Patient's noncompliance with renal dialysis due to financial hardship

Z91.158   Patient's noncompliance with renal dialysis for other reason

Z91.19   Patient's noncompliance with other medical treatment and regimen
    Patient's nonadherence to medical treatment

Z91.190   Patient's noncompliance with other medical treatment and regimen due to financial hardship

Z91.198   Patient's noncompliance with other medical treatment and regimen for other reason
    Coding Clinic: 2024, Q1, P24

Z91.199   Patient's noncompliance with other medical treatment and regimen due to unspecified reason

● Z91.4   Personal history of psychological trauma, not elsewhere classified

● Z91.41   Personal history of adult abuse
    Excludes2   personal history of abuse in childhood (Z62.81-)

Z91.410   Personal history of adult physical and sexual abuse   A
    Excludes1   current adult physical abuse (T74.11, T76.11)
        current adult sexual abuse (T74.21, T76.11)

Z91.411   Personal history of adult psychological abuse   A

Z91.412   Personal history of adult neglect   A
    Excludes1   current adult neglect (T74.01, T76.01)

Z91.413   Personal history of adult financial abuse

Z91.414   Personal history of adult intimate partner abuse

Z91.419   Personal history of unspecified adult abuse   A

Z91.42   Personal history of forced labor or sexual exploitation

Z91.49   Other personal history of psychological trauma, not elsewhere classified

● Z91.5   Personal history of self-harm
    Code also mental health disorder, if known

Z91.51   Personal history of suicidal behavior
    Personal history of parasuicide
    Personal history of self-poisoning
    Personal history of suicide attempt

Z91.52   Personal history of nonsuicidal self-harm
    Personal history of nonsuicidal self-injury
    Personal history of self-inflicted injury without suicidal intent
    Personal history of self-mutilation

● Z91.8   Other specified personal risk factors, not elsewhere classified

Z91.81   History of falling
    At risk for falling

Z91.82   Personal history of military deployment   A
    Individual (civilian or military) with past history of military war, peacekeeping and humanitarian deployment (current or past conflict)
    Returned from military deployment
    Excludes2   personal history of military service (Z91.85)

▷ Z91.83   *Wandering in diseases classified elsewhere*
    Code first underlying disorder such as:
    Alzheimer's disease (G30.-)
    autism or pervasive developmental disorder (F84.-)
    intellectual disabilities (F70-F79)
    unspecified dementia with behavioral disturbance (F03.9-, F03.A-, F03.B-, F03.C-)

● Z91.84   Oral health risk factors

Z91.841   Risk for dental caries, low

Z91.842   Risk for dental caries, moderate

Z91.843   Risk for dental caries, high

Z91.849   Unspecified risk for dental caries

Z91.85   Personal history of military service
    Excludes2   personal history of military deployment(Z91.82)
        personal history of serving in the armed forces
        personal history of veteran

Z91.89   Other specified personal risk factors, not elsewhere classified
    Increased risk for social isolation
    Coding Clinic: 2017, Q1, P46

CHAPTER 21 (Z00-Z99)

CHAPTER 21 (Z00–Z99)

● **Z91.A** **Caregiver's noncompliance with patient's medical treatment and regimen**

  ● **Z91.A1** **Caregiver's noncompliance with patient's dietary regimen**

    Caregiver's inability to comply with patient's dietary regimen

    Code also, if applicable, food insecurity (Z59.4-)

    Z91.A10 **Caregiver's noncompliance with patient's dietary regimen due to financial hardship**

    Z91.A18 **Caregiver's noncompliance with patient's dietary regimen for other reason**

  ● **Z91.A2** **Caregiver's intentional underdosing of patient's medication regimen**

    Code first underdosing of medication (T36-T50) with fifth or sixth character 6

    Z91.A20 **Caregiver's intentional underdosing of patient's medication regimen due to financial hardship**

    Z91.A28 **Caregiver's intentional underdosing of medication regimen for other reason**

  Z91.A3 **Caregiver's unintentional underdosing of patient's medication regimen**

    Code first underdosing of medication (T36-T50) with fifth or sixth character 6

  ● **Z91.A4** **Caregiver's other noncompliance with patient's medication regimen**

    Caregiver's underdosing of patient's medication NOS

    Z91.A41 **Caregiver's other noncompliance with patient's medication regimen due to financial hardship**

    Z91.A48 **Caregiver's other noncompliance with patient's medication regimen for other reason**

  ● **Z91.A5** **Caregiver's noncompliance with patient's renal dialysis**

    Z91.A51 **Caregiver's noncompliance with patient's renal dialysis due to financial hardship**

    Z91.A58 **Caregiver's noncompliance with patient's renal dialysis for other reason**

  ● **Z91.A9** **Caregiver's noncompliance with patient's other medical treatment and regimen**

    Caregiver's nonadherence to patient's medical treatment

    Z91.A91 **Caregiver's noncompliance with patient's other medical treatment and regimen due to financial hardship**

    Z91.A98 **Caregiver's noncompliance with patient's other medical treatment and regimen for other reason**

● **Z92** **Personal history of medical treatment**

  Excludes2 postprocedural states (Z98.-)

  Z92.0 **Personal history of contraception**

    Excludes1 counseling or management of current contraceptive practices (Z30.-)

    long term (current) use of contraception (Z79.3)

    presence of (intrauterine) contraceptive device (Z97.5)

  ● **Z92.2** **Personal history of drug therapy**

    Excludes2 long term (current) drug therapy (Z79.-)

    Z92.21 **Personal history of antineoplastic chemotherapy**

    Z92.22 **Personal history of monoclonal drug therapy**

      ▶ **Excludes2** personal history of immune checkpoint inhibitor therapy (Z92.26)

    Z92.23 **Personal history of estrogen therapy**

  ● **Z92.24** **Personal history of steroid therapy**

    Z92.240 **Personal history of inhaled steroid therapy**

    Z92.241 **Personal history of systemic steroid therapy**

      Personal history of steroid therapy NOS

    Z92.25 **Personal history of immunosuppression therapy**

      Excludes2 personal history of steroid therapy (Z92.24)

    Z92.26 ▶ **Personal history of immune checkpoint inhibitor therapy**

      ▶ Personal history of ICI drug therapy

    Z92.29 **Personal history of other drug therapy**

  Z92.3 **Personal history of irradiation**

    Personal history of exposure to therapeutic radiation

    Excludes1 exposure to radiation in the physical environment (Z77.12)

    occupational exposure to radiation (Z57.1)

  ● **Z92.8** **Personal history of other medical treatment**

    Coding Clinic: 2016, Q4, P72

    Z92.81 **Personal history of extracorporeal membrane oxygenation (ECMO)**

    Z92.82 **Status post administration of tPA (rtPA) in a different facility within the last 24 hours prior to admission to current facility**

      Code first condition requiring tPA administration, such as:

      acute cerebral infarction (I63.-)

      acute myocardial infarction (I21.-, I22.-)

    Z92.83 **Personal history of failed moderate sedation**

      Personal history of failed conscious sedation

      Excludes2 failed moderate sedation during procedure (T88.52)

    Z92.84 **Personal history of unintended awareness under general anesthesia**

      Excludes2 unintended awareness under general anesthesia during procedure (T88.53)

      Coding Clinic: 2016, Q4, P72, 77

  ● **Z92.85** **Personal history of cellular therapy**

      ▶ **Excludes2** personal history of immune checkpoint inhibitor therapy (Z92.26)

    Z92.850 **Personal history of Chimeric Antigen Receptor T-cell therapy**

      Personal history of CAR T-cell therapy

    Z92.858 **Personal history of other cellular therapy**

    Z92.859 **Personal history of cellular therapy, unspecified**

    Z92.86 **Personal history of gene therapy**

    Z92.89 **Personal history of other medical treatment**

    Coding Clinic: 2020, Q1, P18

● **Z93** **Artificial opening status**

  Excludes1 artificial openings requiring attention or management (Z43.-)

  complications of external stoma (J95.0-, K94.-, N99.5-)

  Z93.0 **Tracheostomy status** 🔵

  Z93.1 **Gastrostomy status** 🔵

▶ New   ⟹ Revised   ~~deleted~~ Deleted   Excludes 1   Excludes 2   Includes   Use additional   Code first   Code also   Key words

OGCR Official Guidelines   X Assign placeholder X   ● Use Additional Character(s)   ▶ Manifestation Code   🔵 Hierarchical Condition Category   Coding Clinic

Z93.2   Ileostomy status 🔒

Z93.3   Colostomy status 🔒
   ▶ Ileal pouch status
   ▶ Kock pouch status

Z93.4   Other artificial openings of gastrointestinal tract status 🔒

● Z93.5   Cystostomy status
         Z93.50   Unspecified cystostomy status 🔒
         Z93.51   Cutaneous-vesicostomy status 🔒
         Z93.52   Appendico-vesicostomy status 🔒
         Z93.59   Other cystostomy status 🔒

Z93.6   Other artificial openings of urinary tract status 🔒
         Nephrostomy status
         Ureterostomy status
         Urethrostomy status

Z93.8   Other artificial opening status 🔒

Z93.9   Artificial opening status, unspecified 🔒

● Z94   Transplanted organ and tissue status
   Includes   organ or tissue replaced by heterogenous or homogenous transplant
   Excludes1   complications of transplanted organ or tissue - see Alphabetical Index
   Excludes2   presence of vascular grafts (Z95.-)

Z94.0   Kidney transplant status

Z94.1   Heart transplant status 🔒
   Excludes1   artificial heart status (Z95.812)
                    heart-valve replacement status (Z95.2-Z95.4)

Z94.2   Lung transplant status 🔒

Z94.3   Heart and lungs transplant status 🔒

Z94.4   Liver transplant status 🔒

Z94.5   Skin transplant status
         Autogenous skin transplant status

Z94.6   Bone transplant status

Z94.7   Corneal transplant status

● Z94.8   Other transplanted organ and tissue status
         Z94.81   Bone marrow transplant status 🔒
         Z94.82   Intestine transplant status 🔒
         Z94.83   Pancreas transplant status 🔒
         Z94.84   Stem cells transplant status 🔒
         Z94.89   Other transplanted organ and tissue status

Z94.9   Transplanted organ and tissue status, unspecified

● Z95   Presence of cardiac and vascular implants and grafts
   Excludes2   complications of cardiac and vascular devices, implants and grafts (T82.-)

Z95.0   Presence of cardiac pacemaker
         Presence of cardiac resynchronization therapy (CRT-P) pacemaker
   Excludes1   adjustment or management of cardiac device (Z45.0-)
                    adjustment or management of cardiac pacemaker (Z45.0)
                    presence of automatic (implantable) cardiac defibrillator with synchronous cardiac pacemaker (Z95.810)
         Coding Clinic: 2019, Q1, P33

Z95.1   Presence of aortocoronary bypass graft
         Presence of coronary artery bypass graft

Z95.2   Presence of prosthetic heart valve
         Presence of heart valve NOS

Z95.3   Presence of xenogenic heart valve

Z95.4   Presence of other heart-valve replacement

Z95.5   Presence of coronary angioplasty implant and graft
   Excludes1   coronary angioplasty status without implant and graft (Z98.61)

● Z95.8   Presence of other cardiac and vascular implants and grafts
   ● Z95.81   Presence of other cardiac implants and grafts
         Z95.810   Presence of automatic (implantable) cardiac defibrillator
                    Presence of automatic (implantable) cardiac defibrillator with synchronous cardiac pacemaker
                    Presence of cardiac resynchronization therapy defibrillator (CRT-D)
                    Presence of cardioverter-defibrillator (ICD)
         Coding Clinic: 2022, Q2, P15

         Z95.811   Presence of heart assist device 🔒

         Z95.812   Presence of fully implantable artificial heart 🔒

         Z95.818   Presence of other cardiac implants and grafts

   ● Z95.82   Presence of other vascular implants and grafts
         Z95.820   Peripheral vascular angioplasty status with implants and grafts
            Excludes1   peripheral vascular angioplasty without implant and graft (Z98.62)

         Z95.828   Presence of other vascular implants and grafts
                    Presence of intravascular prosthesis NEC

Z95.9   Presence of cardiac and vascular implant and graft, unspecified

● Z96   Presence of other functional implants
   Excludes2   complications of internal prosthetic devices, implants and grafts (T82-T85)
                    fitting and adjustment of prosthetic and other devices (Z44-Z46)

Z96.0   Presence of urogenital implants

Z96.1   Presence of intraocular lens
         Presence of pseudophakia

● Z96.2   Presence of otological and audiological implants
         Z96.20   Presence of otological and audiological implant, unspecified
         Z96.21   Cochlear implant status
         Z96.22   Myringotomy tube(s) status
         Z96.29   Presence of other otological and audiological implants
                    Presence of bone-conduction hearing device
                    Presence of eustachian tube stent
                    Stapes replacement

Z96.3   Presence of artificial larynx

● Z96.4   Presence of endocrine implants
         Z96.41   Presence of insulin pump (external) (internal)
         Z96.49   Presence of other endocrine implants

Z96.5   Presence of tooth-root and mandibular implants

● Z96.6   Presence of orthopedic joint implants
         Z96.60   Presence of unspecified orthopedic joint implant

   ● Z96.61   Presence of artificial shoulder joint
         Z96.611   Presence of right artificial shoulder joint
         Z96.612   Presence of left artificial shoulder joint
         Z96.619   Presence of unspecified artificial shoulder joint

   ● Z96.62   Presence of artificial elbow joint
         Z96.621   Presence of right artificial elbow joint
         Z96.622   Presence of left artificial elbow joint
         Z96.629   Presence of unspecified artificial elbow joint

CHAPTER 21 (Z00-Z99)

CHAPTER 21 (Z00-Z99)

● **Z96.63**   Presence of artificial wrist joint

     Z96.631   Presence of right artificial wrist joint

     Z96.632   Presence of left artificial wrist joint

     Z96.639   Presence of unspecified artificial wrist joint

● **Z96.64**   Presence of artificial hip joint

     Hip-joint replacement (partial) (total)

     Z96.641   Presence of right artificial hip joint
                 Coding Clinic: 2016, Q3, P17

     Z96.642   Presence of left artificial hip joint
                 Coding Clinic: 2015, Q1, P16

     Z96.643   Presence of artificial hip joint, bilateral

     Z96.649   Presence of unspecified artificial hip joint

● **Z96.65**   Presence of artificial knee joint

     Z96.651   Presence of right artificial knee joint

     Z96.652   Presence of left artificial knee joint
                 Coding Clinic: 2019, Q3, P16

     Z96.653   Presence of artificial knee joint, bilateral

     Z96.659   Presence of unspecified artificial knee joint

● **Z96.66**   Presence of artificial ankle joint

     Z96.661   Presence of right artificial ankle joint

     Z96.662   Presence of left artificial ankle joint

     Z96.669   Presence of unspecified artificial ankle joint

● **Z96.69**   Presence of other orthopedic joint implants

     Z96.691   Finger-joint replacement of right hand

     Z96.692   Finger-joint replacement of left hand

     Z96.693   Finger-joint replacement, bilateral

     Z96.698   Presence of other orthopedic joint implants

Z96.7   Presence of other bone and tendon implants

     Presence of skull plate

● **Z96.8**   Presence of other specified functional implants

     Z96.81   Presence of artificial skin

     Z96.82   Presence of neurostimulator

          Presence of brain neurostimulator

          Presence of gastric neurostimulator

          Presence of peripheral nerve neurostimulator

          Presence of sacral nerve neurostimulator

          Presence of spinal cord neurostimulator

          Presence of vagus nerve neurostimulator

     Z96.89   Presence of other specified functional implants

Z96.9   Presence of functional implant, unspecified

● **Z97**   **Presence of other devices**

     Excludes2   fitting and adjustment of prosthetic and other devices (Z44-Z46)

               presence of cerebrospinal fluid drainage device (Z98.2)

Z97.0   Presence of artificial eye

● **Z97.1**   Presence of artificial limb (complete) (partial)

     Z97.10   Presence of artificial limb (complete) (partial), unspecified

     Z97.11   Presence of artificial right arm (complete) (partial)

     Z97.12   Presence of artificial left arm (complete) (partial)

     Z97.13   Presence of artificial right leg (complete) (partial)

     Z97.14   Presence of artificial left leg (complete) (partial)

     Z97.15   Presence of artificial arms, bilateral (complete) (partial)

     Z97.16   Presence of artificial legs, bilateral (complete) (partial)

Z97.2   Presence of dental prosthetic device (complete) (partial)

     Presence of dentures (complete) (partial)

Z97.3   Presence of spectacles and contact lenses

Z97.4   Presence of external hearing-aid

Z97.5   Presence of (intrauterine) contraceptive device

     Excludes1   checking, reinsertion or removal of implantable subdermal contraceptive (Z30.46)

               checking, reinsertion or removal of intrauterine contraceptive device (Z30.43-)

Z97.8   Presence of other specified devices

● **Z98**   **Other postprocedural states**

     Excludes2   aftercare (Z43-Z49, Z51)

               follow-up medical care (Z08-Z09)

               postprocedural complication - see Alphabetical Index

Z98.0   Intestinal bypass and anastomosis status

     Excludes2   bariatric surgery status (Z98.84)

               gastric bypass status (Z98.84)

               obesity surgery status (Z98.84)

Z98.1   Arthrodesis status

Z98.2   Presence of cerebrospinal fluid drainage device

     Presence of CSF shunt

Z98.3   Post therapeutic collapse of lung status

     Code first underlying disease

● **Z98.4**   Cataract extraction status

     Use additional code to identify intraocular lens implant status (Z96.1)

     Excludes1   aphakia (H27.0)

     Z98.41   Cataract extraction status, right eye

     Z98.42   Cataract extraction status, left eye

     Z98.49   Cataract extraction status, unspecified eye

● **Z98.5**   Sterilization status

     Excludes1   female infertility (N97.-)

               male infertility (N46.-)

     Z98.51   Tubal ligation status

     Z98.52   Vasectomy status   A

● **Z98.6**   Angioplasty status

     Z98.61   Coronary angioplasty status

          Excludes1   coronary angioplasty status with implant and graft (Z95.5)

          Coding Clinic: 2022, Q4, P23

     Z98.62   Peripheral vascular angioplasty status

          Excludes1   peripheral vascular angioplasty status with implant and graft (Z95.820)

● **Z98.8**   Other specified postprocedural states

     Coding Clinic: 2016, Q4, P76

     ● **Z98.81**   Dental procedure status

          Z98.810   Dental sealant status

          Z98.811   Dental restoration status

              Dental crown status

              Dental fillings status

          Z98.818   Other dental procedure status

     Z98.82   Breast implant status

          Excludes1   breast implant removal status (Z98.86)

          Coding Clinic: 2022, Q3, P8

▶ New   ⟹ Revised   ~~deleted~~ Deleted   Excludes 1   Excludes 2   Includes   Use additional   Code first   Code also   Key words

OGCR Official Guidelines   X Assign placeholder X   ● Use Additional Character(s)   ▶ Manifestation Code   🝁 Hierarchical Condition Category   Coding Clinic

Z98.83   **Filtering (vitreous) bleb after glaucoma surgery status**

    Excludes1   inflammation (infection) of postprocedural bleb (H59.4-)

Z98.84   **Bariatric surgery status**
Gastric banding status
Gastric bypass status for obesity
Obesity surgery status

    Excludes1   bariatric surgery status complicating pregnancy, childbirth, or the puerperium (O99.84)

    Excludes2   intestinal bypass and anastomosis status (Z98.0)

    Coding Clinic: 2020, Q1, P12

Z98.85   **Transplanted organ removal status**
Transplanted organ previously removed due to complication, failure, rejection or infection

    Excludes1   encounter for removal of transplanted organ - code to complication of transplanted organ (T86.-)

Z98.86   **Personal history of breast implant removal**

● Z98.87   **Personal history of in utero procedure**

Z98.870   **Personal history of in utero procedure during pregnancy**

    Excludes2   complications from in utero procedure for current pregnancy (O35.7)
supervision of current pregnancy with history of in utero procedure during previous pregnancy (O09.82-)

Z98.871   **Personal history of in utero procedure while a fetus**

● Z98.89   **Other specified postprocedural states**
    Coding Clinic: 2016, Q4, P76

Z98.890   **Other specified postprocedural states**
Personal history of surgery, not elsewhere classified
    Coding Clinic: 2023, Q3, P13

Z98.891   **History of uterine scar from previous surgery**

    Excludes1   Maternal care due to uterine scar from previous surgery (O34.2-)

    Coding Clinic: 2016, Q4, P52, P76

● Z99   **Dependence on enabling machines and devices, not elsewhere classified**
    Coding Clinic: 2020, Q1, P11

Z99.0   **Dependence on aspirator**

● Z99.1   **Dependence on respirator**
Dependence on ventilator

Z99.11   **Dependence on respirator [ventilator] status** 🔧
    Coding Clinic: 2018, Q1, P14; 2015, Q1, P21

Z99.12   **Encounter for respirator [ventilator] dependence during power failure** 🔧

    Excludes1   mechanical complication of respirator [ventilator] (J95.850)

Z99.2   **Dependence on renal dialysis** 🔧
Hemodialysis status
Peritoneal dialysis status
Presence of arteriovenous shunt for dialysis
Renal dialysis status NOS

    Excludes1   encounter for fitting and adjustment of dialysis catheter (Z49.0-)

    Excludes2   noncompliance with renal dialysis (Z91.15-)

    Coding Clinic: 2022, Q3, P16; 2016, Q1, P13

Z99.3   **Dependence on wheelchair**
Wheelchair confinement status
Code first cause of dependence, such as:
muscular dystrophy (G71.0-)
obesity (E66.-)

● Z99.8   **Dependence on other enabling machines and devices**

Z99.81   **Dependence on supplemental oxygen**
Dependence on long-term oxygen

Z99.89   **Dependence on other enabling machines and devices**
Dependence on machine or device NOS
    Coding Clinic: 2020, Q1, P11

CHAPTER 21 (Z00-Z99)

CHAPTER 22

CODES FOR SPECIAL PURPOSES (U00–U85)

Note: Codes from this chapter are for use on newborn records only, never on maternal records.

This chapter contains the following blocks:

U00–U49	Provisional assignment of new diseases of uncertain etiology or emergency use

PROVISIONAL ASSIGNMENT OF NEW DISEASES OF UNCERTAIN ETIOLOGY OR EMERGENCY USE (U00–U49)

U07   **Emergency use of U07**

     U07.0   **Vaping-related disorder**

         Dabbing related lung damage
         Dabbing related lung injury
         E-cigarette, or vaping, product use associated lung injury [EVALI]
         Electronic cigarette related lung damage
         Electronic cigarette related lung injury

         Use additional code to identify manifestations, such as:
           abdominal pain (R10.84)
           acute respiratory distress syndrome (J80)
           diarrhea (R19.7)
           drug-induced interstitial lung disorder (J70.4)
           lipoid pneumonia (J69.1)
           weight loss (R63.4)

     U07.1   **COVID-19**

         Use additional code to identify pneumonia or other manifestations

         Use Additional code, if applicable, for associated conditions such as:
           COVID-19 associated coagulopathy (D68.8)
           disseminated intravascular coagulation (D65)
           hypercoagulable states (D68.69)
           thrombophilia (D68.69)

         Excludes1   coronavirus as the cause of diseases classified elsewhere (B97.2-)
                         pneumonia due to SARS-associated coronavirus (J12.81)

         Coding Clinic: 2022, Q2, P29; 2021, Q4, P109; 2021, Q1, P31-33, 36, 39-40, 47, 49

● **U09 Post COVID-19 condition**

     U09.9 Post COVID-19 condition, unspecified

     Note: This code enables establishment of a link with COVID-19.

         This code is not to be used in cases that are still presenting with active COVID-19. However, an exception is made in cases of re-infection with COVID-19, occurring with a condition related to prior COVID-19.

         Post-acute sequela of COVID-19

         Code first the specific condition related to COVID-19 if known, such as:
           chronic respiratory failure (J96.1-)
           loss of smell (R43.8)
           loss of taste (R43.8)
           multisystem inflammatory syndrome (M35.81)
           pulmonary embolism (I26.-)
           pulmonary fibrosis (J84.10)

         Coding Clinic: 2021, Q4, P102-104,106

▶ New   ⮕ Revised   ~~deleted~~ Deleted   Excludes 1   Excludes 2   Includes   Use additional   Code first   Code also   Key words

OGCR Official Guidelines   X Assign placeholder X   ● Use Additional Character(s)   ▶ Manifestation Code   🗣 Hierarchical Condition Category   Coding Clinic

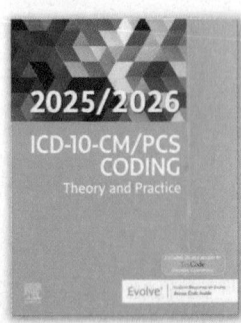